TIETZ TEXTBOOK OF

CLINICAL CHEMISTRY and MOLECULAR DIAGNOSTICS

SIXTH EDITION

NADER RIFAI, PhD
Professor of Pathology
Harvard Medical School
Louis Joseph Gay-Lussac Chair of Laboratory Medicine
Director of Clinical Chemistry
Boston Children's Hospital
Boston, Massachusetts

ANDREA RITA HORVATH, MD, PhD, FRCPath, FRCPA
Professor (Honorary), School of Public Health
University of Sydney
Professor (Conjoint), School of Medical Sciences
University of New South Wales
Clinical Director, SEALS Department of Clinical Chemistry and Endocrinology
New South Wales Health Pathology
Prince of Wales Hospital
Sydney, Australia

CARL T. WITTWER, MD, PhD
Professor of Pathology
University of Utah School of Medicine
Medical Director, Immunologic Flow Cytometry
ARUP Laboratories
Salt Lake City, Utah

ELSEVIER

ELSEVIER

3251 Riverport Lane
St. Louis, Missouri 63043

TIETZ TEXTBOOK OF CLINICAL CHEMISTRY AND MOLECULAR DIAGNOSTICS, SIXTH EDITION

ISBN: 978-0-323-35921-4

Library of Congress Cataloging-in-Publication Data

Names: Rifai, Nader, editor. | Horvath, Andrea R. (Andrea Rita), editor. | Wittwer, C. (Carl), 1955- editor.
Title: Tietz textbook of clinical chemistry and molecular diagnostics / [edited by] Nader Rifai ; senior editors, Andrea R. Horvath, Carl T. Wittwer.
Other titles: Textbook of clinical chemistry and molecular diagnostics | Clinical chemistry and molecular diagnostics
Description: Sixth edition. | St. Louis, Missouri : Elsevier, [2018] | Includes bibliographical references and index.
Identifiers: LCCN 2016038536 | ISBN 9780323359214 (hardcover : alk. paper)
Subjects: | MESH: Clinical Chemistry Tests | Chemistry, Clinical–methods | Molecular Diagnostic Techniques
Classification: LCC RB40 | NLM QY 90 | DDC 616.07/56–dc23 LC record available at https://lccn.loc.gov/2016038536

Executive Content Strategist: Kellie White
Senior Content Development Manager: Laurie Gower
Senior Content Development Specialist: Karen C. Turner
Publishing Services Manager: Patricia Tannian
Senior Project Manager: Amanda Mincher
Designer: Margaret Reid

Printed in the United States of America

Last digit is the print number: 9 8 7 6 5 4 3 2 1

To Ingibjörg, Tivadar, and Noriko, with our love and thanks.

ASSOCIATE EDITORS

Carey-Ann D. Burnham, PhD
Associate Professor of Pathology and Immunology
Washington University School of Medicine,
Director, Microbiology Laboratory
St. Louis, Missouri

Christopher M. Florkowski, MD, MRCP(UK), FRACP, FRCPA, FFSc
Clinical Associate Professor
University of Otago, Christchurch
Consultant in Chemical Pathology
Clinical Biochemistry Unit
Canterbury Health Laboratories
Christchurch, New Zealand

Andrew N. Hoofnagle, MD, PhD
Associate Professor
Head, Division of Clinical Chemistry
Department of Laboratory Medicine
University of Washington
Seattle, Washington

Gary Horowitz, MD
Associate Professor of Pathology
Harvard Medical School
Director, Clinical Chemistry
Beth Israel Deaconess Medical Center
Boston, Massachusetts

Graham R.D. Jones, MBBS, BSc(Med), D.Phil, FRCPA, FAACB
Conjoint Associate Professor
University of New South Wales
Faculty of Medicine, Department of Chemical Pathology, SydPath
St. Vincent's Hospital
New South Wales, Australia

Elaine Lyon, PhD
Professor of Pathology
University of Utah School of Medicine
Medical Director, Molecular Genetics
ARUP Laboratories
Salt Lake City, Utah

William J. Marshall, MA, PhD, MSc, MB, BS, FRCP, FRCPath, FRCPEdin, FRSC, FRSB
Emeritus Reader in Clinical Biochemistry
King's College London
London, United Kingdom

Jason Y. Park, MD, PhD
Associate Professor
Joint Appointment, Pathology and the Eugene McDermott Center for Human Growth and Development
University of Texas Southwestern Medical Center
Director, Advanced Diagnostics Laboratory
Department of Pathology
Children's Medical Center
Dallas, Texas

Kenneth Andrew Sikaris, BSc(Hons), MBBS, FRCPA, FAACB, FFSc, GAICD
Associate Professor of Pathology
Melbourne University
Director Clinical Support Systems, Sonic Healthcare
Chemical Pathology
Melbourne Pathology
Victoria, Australia

Jillian R. Tate, MSc, FFSc (RCPA)
Senior Scientist, Chemical Pathology
Royal Brisbane and Women's Hospital
Brisbane, Australia

Ian Young, MD, FRCP, FRCPath
Professor of Medicine
Centre for Public Health
Queen's University Belfast
Belfast, United Kingdom

REVIEWERS

Jude Abadie, PhD, DABCC(C&T), FACB
Chief, Core Laboratory
Tripler Army Medical Center
Honolulu, Hawaii

Ruth M. Ayling, PhD, FRCPath, FRCP
Consultant Chemical Pathologist
Clinical Biochemistry
Barts Health NHS Trust
London, United Kingdom

Linnea Baudhuin, PhD, DABMG
Associate Professor of Laboratory Medicine
Department of Laboratory Medicine and Pathology
Mayo Clinic
Rochester, Minnesota

David E. Bruns, MD
Professor of Pathology
University of Virginia
Director, Clinical Chemistry
Associate Director, Molecular Diagnostics
University of Virginia Health System
Charlottesville, Virginia

Susan Butler-Wu, PhD
Assistant Professor of Laboratory Medicine
University of Washington
Associate Director, Clinical Microbiology
Laboratory Medicine
University of Washington Medical Center
Seattle, Washington

Christa Cobbaert, PhD, EurSpLM
Professor of Clinical Chemistry and Laboratory Medicine
Director, Department of Clinical Chemistry and Laboratory Medicine
Leiden University Medical Centre
Leiden, The Netherlands

Marc Roger Couturier, PhD, D(ABMM)
Associate Professor of Pathology
University of Utah
Medical Director, Infectious Disease
ARUP Laboratories
Salt Lake City, Utah

Anne T. Daley, MS, CMQOE, CSSB, CLC, MT, DLM
President
Daley Consulting, LLC
Mesa, Arizona

Christina Ellervik, MD, PhD, DMSci
Associate Director of Clinical Chemistry
Department of Laboratory Medicine
Boston Children's Hospital
Boston, Massachusetts
Associate Professor of Clinical Chemistry
Department of Clinical Medicine
Faculty of Health and Medical Sciences
University of Copenhagen
Copenhagen, Denmark

John L. Frater, MD
Associate Professor
Department of Pathology and Immunology
Washington University School of Medicine
St. Louis, Missouri

Neil Selwyn Harris, MBChB, MD
Clinical Associate Professor
Medical Director, Core Laboratory
Department of Pathology, Immunology, and Laboratory Medicine
University of Florida College of Medicine
Gainesville, Florida

Mark D. Kellogg, PhD, MT(ASCP), DABCC
Assistant Professor of Pathology
Harvard Medical School
Associate Director, Clinical Chemistry
Boston Children's Hospital
Boston, Massachusetts

Stephen R. Master, MD, PhD
Associate Professor of Pathology and Laboratory Medicine
Director, Central Laboratory
Weill Cornell Medical College
New York, New York

Kerry L. O'Brien, MD
Assistant Professor of Pathology
Harvard Medical School
Associate Medical Director, Blood Bank
Department of Pathology
Beth Israel Deaconess Medical Center
Boston, Massachusetts

Ana-Maria Simundic, PhD
Professor, Specialist in Laboratory Medicine
Department of Medical Laboratory Diagnostics
Clinical Hospital Sveti Duh
Zagreb, Croatia

Vanessa Steenkamp, PhD
Professor
Department of Pharmacology
Faculty of Health Sciences
University of Pretoria
Pretoria, South Africa

Karen E. Weck, MD, FCAP
Professor of Pathology and Laboratory Medicine and Genetics
Director, Molecular Genetics
University of North Carolina
Chapel Hill, North Carolina

CONTRIBUTORS

Aasne K. Aarsand, MD, PhD
Consultant Medical Biochemist
Norwegian Porphyria Centre and Laboratory of Clinical Biochemistry
Haukeland University Hospital
Norwegian Quality Improvement of Primary Care Laboratories
Haraldsplass Deaconess Hospital
Bergen, Norway

April N. Abbott, PhD, D(ABMM)
Director, Microbiology Laboratory
Deaconess Health System
Evansville, Indiana

Khosrow Adeli, PhD, FCACB, DABCC
Professor of Clinical Biochemistry
The Hospital for Sick Children
University of Toronto
Toronto, Ontario, Canada

Neil W. Anderson, MD
Assistant Professor of Pathology and Immunology
Washington University School of Medicine
St. Louis, Missouri

Fred S. Apple, PhD
Professor of Laboratory Medicine and Pathology
University of Minnesota
Medical Director, Clinical Laboratories
Hennepin County Medical Center
Minneapolis, Minnesota

Ruth M. Ayling, PhD, FRCPath, FRCP
Consultant Chemical Pathologist
Clinical Biochemistry
Barts Health NHS Trust
London, United Kingdom

Esther Babady, PhD, D(ABMM)
Associate Attending Microbiologist
Director, Clinical Operations, Microbiology Laboratory Service
Director, Clinical Microbiology Fellowship Program
Department of Laboratory Medicine
Memorial Sloan Kettering Cancer Center
New York, New York

Michael N. Badminton, BSc, MBChB, PhD, FRCPath
Clinical Senior Lecturer
Centre for Medical Education
Cardiff University School of Medicine
Consultant Chemical Pathologist
Department of Medical Biochemistry and Immunology
University Hospital of Wales
Cardiff, Wales, United Kingdom

Tony Badrick, BAppSc, BSc, BA, MLitSt, MBA, PhD, FAACB, FAIMS, FRCPA(Hon), FACB, FFScRCPA
Chief Executive Officer
Royal College of Pathologists of Australasia Quality Assurance Programs
Sydney, Australia

Renze Bais, BSc(Hons), PhD, FFSc(RCPA), DipT
Director
RBaisconsulting.com
Sydney, Australia

Lindsay A.L. Bazydlo, PhD, DABCC
Assistant Professor of Pathology
University of Virginia School of Medicine
Director of Toxicology Laboratory
Associate Director of Clinical Chemistry Laboratory
Co-Director of Coagulation Laboratory
University of Virginia Health System
Charlottesville, Virginia

Laura K. Bechtel, PhD, DABCC
CLIA Laboratory Director
Colorado Antiviral Pharmacology Laboratory
University of Colorado Denver-Skaggs School of Pharmacy and Pharmaceutical Sciences
Laboratory Director
Cordant Health Solutions
Denver, Colorado

Roger L. Bertholf, PhD
Professor of Pathology and Laboratory Medicine
University of Florida Health Science Center Jacksonville
Director of Clinical Chemistry, Toxicology, and Point of Care Testing
UF Health Jacksonville
Jacksonville, Florida

D. Hunter Best, PhD
Associate Professor of Pathology
University of Utah School of Medicine
Medical Director, Molecular Genetics and Genomics
ARUP Laboratories
Salt Lake City, Utah

Ingvar Bjarnason, MD, MSc, FRCPath, FRCP, DSc
Professor of Digestive Disease
Consultant Physician and Gastroenterologist
King's College Hospital
London, United Kingdom

Darci R. Block, PhD, DABCC
Assistant Professor of Laboratory Medicine and Pathology
Mayo Clinic
Rochester, Minnesota

Lee M. Blum, PhD
Toxicologist
NMS Labs, Inc.
Willow Grove, Pennsylvania

Patrick M.M. Bossuyt, PhD
Professor of Clinical Epidemiology
Department of Clinical Epidemiology, Biostatistics, and Bioinformatics
University of Amsterdam
Amsterdam, The Netherlands

James C. Boyd, MD
Director of Clinical Pathology
Associate Professor of Pathology
University of Virginia Health System
Charlottesville, Virginia

Sarah M. Brown, PhD
Assistant Professor of Pediatrics
Washington University School of Medicine
Medical Director, Core Clinical Laboratory
Medical Director, Point of Care and Ancillary Services
Clinical Laboratories
St. Louis Children's Hospital
St. Louis, Missouri

Blake W. Buchan, PhD
Assistant Professor of Pathology
Medical College of Wisconsin
Associate Director
Microbiology and Molecular Diagnostics
Wisconsin Diagnostic Laboratories
Milwaukee, Wisconsin

David Burnett, OBE, PhD, FRCPath
Former Consultant Clinical Biochemist
St. Albans and Hemel Hempstead NHS Trust
St. Albans, Hertfordshire, United Kingdom

Leslie Burnett, MBBS, PhD, FRCPA
Kinghorn Centre for Clinical Genomics
Garvan Institute of Medical Research
St. Vincent's Clinical School
UNSW Australia
Darlinghurst, Australia
Sydney Medical School
University of Sydney
Sydney, Australia

Cory Bystrom, BS, MS, PhD
Vice President, Research and Development
Cleveland HeartLab
Cleveland, Ohio

Maria Domenica Cappellini, MD
Professor of Internal Medicine
Director of Community and Health Sciences Department
University of Milan
Director of Internal Medicine Department
Ca Granda Foundation IRCCS
Milan, Italy

Adam J. Caulfield, PhD
Director of Microbiology
Spectrum Health
Grand Rapids, Michigan

Ferruccio Ceriotti, MD
Laboratory Medicine Service
Ospedale San Raffaele
Milan, Italy

Devon Chabot-Richards, MD
Assistant Professor of Pathology
University of New Mexico School of Medicine
Department of Pathology
University of New Mexico Health Sciences Center
Albuquerque, New Mexico

Derrick J. Chen, MD
Assistant Professor of Pathology and Laboratory Medicine
University of Wisconsin–Madison
Madison, Wisconsin

Dong Chen, MD, PhD
Associate Professor of Laboratory Medicine and Pathology
Mayo Clinic
College of Medicine
Consultant
Special Coagulation Laboratory
Division of Hematopathology
Mayo Clinic
Rochester, Minnesota

Steven Cheng, MD
Associate Professor
Division of Nephrology
Washington University School of Medicine
Attending Physician
Internal Medicine–Division of Nephrology
Barnes-Jewish Hospital
St. Louis, Missouri

Nai-Kong V. Cheung, MD, PhD
Enid A. Haupt Chair in Pediatric Oncology
Department of Pediatrics
Memorial Sloan Kettering Cancer Center
New York, New York

Rossa W.K. Chiu, MBBS, PhD, FHKAM, FRCPA
Choh-Ming Li Professor of Chemical Pathology
Department of Chemical Pathology
The Chinese University of Hong Kong
Shatin, New Territories
Hong Kong, China

Nigel J. Clarke, BSc(Hons), PhD
Vice President, Advanced Technology
Quest Diagnostics Nichols Institute
San Juan Capistrano, California

Timothy J. Cole, PhD
Associate Professor of Biochemistry and Molecular Biology
Monash University
Clayton, Melbourne
Victoria, Australia

Mark Cooper, BMBCh, PhD, FRCP, FRACP
Professor of Medicine, Endocrinology
Concord Repatriation General Hospital
Professor of Medicine
University of Sydney
Sydney, Australia

Thomas D. Dayspring, MD, FACP, FNLA
Chief Academic Officer
True Health Diagnostics
Richmond, Virginia

Michael P. Delaney, BSc, MD, FRCP, LLM
Consultant Nephrologist
East Kent Hospitals University NHS Foundation Trust
Kent and Canterbury Hospital
Canterbury, Kent, United Kingdom

Dennis J. Dietzen, PhD
Professor of Pediatrics
Washington University School of Medicine
Medical Director, Core Laboratory and Metabolic Genetics Laboratory
St. Louis Children's Hospital
St. Louis, Missouri

Christopher D. Doern, PhD
Assistant Professor of Pathology
Associate Director of Microbiology
Virginia Commonwealth University Health System
Richmond, Virginia

Paul D'Orazio, PhD
Director, Critical Care Analytical
Instrumentation Laboratory
Bedford, Massachusetts

Graeme Eisenhofer, PhD
Professor and Chief, Division of Clinical Neurochemistry
Institute of Clinical Chemistry and Laboratory Medicine
Department of Medicine
Technische Universität Dresden
Dresden, Germany

Christina Ellervik, MD, PhD, DMSci
Associate Director of Clinical Chemistry
Department of Laboratory Medicine
Boston Children's Hospital
Boston, Massachusetts
Associate Professor of Clinical Chemistry
Department of Clinical Medicine
Faculty of Health and Medical Sciences
University of Copenhagen
Copenhagen, Denmark

Christopher M. Florkowski, MD, MRCP(UK), FRACP, FRCPA, FFSc
Clinical Associate Professor
University of Otago, Christchurch
Consultant in Chemical Pathology
Clinical Biochemistry Unit
Canterbury Health Laboratories
Christchurch, New Zealand

Betty A. Forbes, PhD
Professor of Pathology
Director of Clinical Microbiology Laboratory
Virginia Commonwealth University Medical Center
Richmond, Virginia

Callum G. Fraser, PhD
Professor
Centre for Research into Cancer Prevention and Screening
University of Dundee
Dundee, United Kingdom

William D. Fraser, BSc(Hons), MB ChB, MD (Hons), FRCP, FRCPath, EuSpLM
Professor of Medicine
Deputy Dean, Department of Medicine
University of East Anglia
Honorary Consultant in Metabolic Medicine/Chemical Pathology
Department of Endocrinology/Clinical Biochemistry
Norfolk and Norwich University Hospital Trust
Norwich, Norfolk, United Kingdom

Danielle B. Freedman, MBBS, FRCPath, EuSpLM
Consultant Chemical Pathologist
Associate Physician in Clinical Endocrinology
Clinical Biochemistry
Director of Pathology
Luton and Dunstable University Hospital NHS Foundation Trust
Luton, United Kingdom

Jonathan R. Genzen, MD, PhD
Assistant Professor of Pathology
University of Utah School of Medicine
Medical Director, Automated Core Laboratory
ARUP Laboratories
Salt Lake City, Utah

Tracy I. George, MD
Professor of Pathology
University of New Mexico School of Medicine
Vice Chair, Clinical Affairs and Hematopathology
Division Chief, Pathology
University of New Mexico Health Sciences Center
Albuquerque, New Mexico

Katherine B. Gettings, PhD
Research Biologist
Applied Genetics Group
National Institute of Standards and Technology
Gaithersburg, Maryland

Paul Glasziou, PhD
Professor of Evidence-Based Medicine
Centre for Research in Evidence-Based Practice
Faculty, Health Sciences and Medicine
Bond University
Gold Coast, Queensland, Australia

Jens Peter Goetze, MD, DMSc
Professor of Clinical Medicine
Aarhus University
Aarhaus, Denmark
Chief Physician, Department of Clinical Biochemistry
Rigshospitalet
Copenhagen, Denmark

Russell P. Grant, PhD
Vice President
Research and Development
Laboratory Corporation of America
Burlington, North Carolina

Stefan Grebe, MD, PhD
Professor of Laboratory Medicine and Pathology
Mayo Clinic
Rochester, Minnesota

Ralph Green, MD, PhD
Distinguished Professor of Pathology and Laboratory Medicine and Internal Medicine
University of California, Davis
Director, Medical Diagnostics
University of California, Davis Health Systems
Sacramento, California

Ann M. Gronowski, PhD
Professor of Pathology and Immunology and Obstetrics and Gynecology
Washington University School of Medicine
St. Louis, Missouri

Walter G. Guder, MD, PhD
Emeritus Head Physician, Clinical Chemistry
Community Hospitals
Emeritus Teacher of Clinical Biochemistry
Ludwig Maxmillian University
Munich, Germany

David S. Hage, PhD
Professor of Chemistry
University of Nebraska
Lincoln, Nebraska

David Halsall, PhD
Clinical Director, Blood Sciences
Addenbrooke's Hospital
Cambridge, United Kingdom

Doris M. Haverstick, PhD
Associate Professor of Pathology
University of Virginia
Charlottesville, Virginia

Charles D. Hawker, PhD, MBA, FACB, FACSc
Adjunct Professor of Pathology
University of Utah School of Medicine
Scientific Director, Automation and Special Projects
ARUP Laboratories
Salt Lake City, Utah

Phillip Heaton, MS, PhD
Technical Director of Microbiology and Molecular Diagnostics
Pathology and Laboratory Medicine
Children's Hospitals and Clinics of Minnesota
Minneapolis, Minnesota

Russell A. Higgins, MD
Associate Clinical Professor of Pathology
University of Texas Health Science Center San Antonio
Medical Director, Pathology Services
Section Chief, Hematology Laboratory
University Health System
San Antonio, Texas

Ingibjörg Hilmarsdóttir, MD
Assistant Professor of Medicine
University of Iceland
Consultant Microbiologist
Landspitali–The University Hospital of Iceland
Reykjavik, Iceland

Chris Holstege, MD
Professor of Emergency Medicine and Pediatrics
Chief, Division of Medical Toxicology
University of Virginia School of Medicine
Medical Director, Blue Ridge Poison Center
University of Virginia Health System
Charlottesville, Virginia

Andrew N. Hoofnagle, MD, PhD
Associate Professor
Head, Division of Clinical Chemistry
Department of Laboratory Medicine
University of Washington
Seattle, Washington

Dave Hoon, MSc, PhD
Professor of Translational Molecular Medicine
Division of Molecular Oncology
John Wayne Cancer Institute
Providence Health Systems
Santa Monica, California

Gary Horowitz, MD
Director, Clinical Chemistry
Beth Israel Deaconess Medical Center
Associate Professor of Pathology
Harvard Medical School
Boston, Massachusetts

Andrea Rita Horvath, MD, PhD, FRCPath, FRCPA
Professor (Honorary), School of Public Health
University of Sydney
Professor (Conjoint), School of Medical Sciences
University of New South Wales
Clinical Director, SEALS Department of Clinical Chemistry and Endocrinology
New South Wales Health Pathology
Prince of Wales Hospital
Sydney, Australia

John Greg Howe, PhD
Associate Professor of Laboratory Medicine
Yale University School of Medicine
New Haven, Connecticut

Romney M. Humphries, PhD
Assistant Professor of Pathology and Laboratory Medicine
University of California, Los Angeles
Los Angeles, California

Allan S. Jaffe, MD
Professor of Medicine/Cardiology and Laboratory Medicine and Pathology
Mayo Clinic
Rochester, Minnesota

Graham R.D. Jones, MBBS, BSc(Med), DPhil, FRCPA, FAACB
Conjoint Associate Professor
Department of Chemical Pathology, SydPath
St. Vincent's Hospital
Sydney, Australia
Faculty of Medicine
University of New South Wales
New South Wales, Australia

Patricia M. Jones, PhD
Professor of Pathology
University of Texas Southwestern Medical Center
Clinical Director, Chemistry
Department of Pathology
Children's Medical Center
Dallas, Texas

Emily Jungheim, MD, MSCI
Associate Professor of Department of Obstetrics and Gynecology
Washington University School of Medicine
St. Louis, Missouri

Todd W. Kelley, MD, MS
Associate Professor of Pathology
University of Utah
Medical Director, Molecular Hematopathology
ARUP Laboratories
Salt Lake City, Utah

Steve Kitchen, PhD
Clinical Scientist, Coagulation Department
Royal Hallamshire Hospital
Sheffield Teaching Hospitals
Sheffield, United Kingdom

Larry J. Kricka, DPhil, FACB, CChem, FRSC, FRCPath
Professor of Pathology and Laboratory Medicine
University of Pennsylvania Medical Center
Philadelphia, Pennsylvania

Mark M. Kushnir, PhD
Adjunct Assistant Professor of Pathology
University of Utah School of Medicine
Senior Scientist
ARUP Institute for Clinical and Experimental Pathology
Salt Lake City, Utah

Edmund J. Lamb, BSc, MSc, PhD, FRCPath
Consultant Clinical Scientist, Laboratory Medicine
East Kent Hospitals University NHS Foundation Trust
Kent and Canterbury Hospital
Canterbury, Kent, United Kingdom

James P. Landers, BS, PhD
Professor of Chemistry
University of Virginia
Charlottesville, Virginia

Loralie J. Langman, PhD
Professor of Laboratory Medicine and Pathology
Mayo Clinic College of Medicine
Director, Clinical and Forensic Toxicology Laboratory
Director, Clinical Mass Spectroscopy Laboratory
Department of Laboratory Medicine and Pathology
Mayo Clinic
Rochester, Minnesota

Omar Laterza, PhD
Executive Director
Translational Molecular Biomarkers
Merck & Co., Inc.
Rahway, New Jersey

Anna F. Lau, PhD, D(ABMM)
Co-Director Bacteriology, Parasitology, and Molecular Epidemiology
Department of Laboratory Medicine
Clinical Center, National Institutes of Health
Bethesda, Maryland

Evi Lianidou, PhD
Professor of Analytical Chemistry–Clinical Chemistry
National and Kapodistrian University of Athens
Athens, Greece

Rachael M. Liesman, PhD
Clinical Microbiology Fellow
Department of Laboratory Medicine and Pathology
Mayo Clinic
Rochester, Minnesota

Kristian Linnet, MD, PhD
Professor of Forensic Chemistry
University of Copenhagen
Copenhagen, Denmark

Stanley F. Lo, PhD
Associate Professor of Pathology
Medical College of Wisconsin
Milwaukee, Wisconsin

Y.M. Dennis Lo, DM, DPhil
Li Ka Shing Professor of Medicine
Department of Chemical Pathology
The Chinese University of Hong Kong
Shatin, New Territories, Hong Kong, China

Nicola Longo, MD, PhD, FACMG
Professor and Chief, Division of Medical Genetics
Department of Pediatrics
University of Utah School of Medicine
Medical Director, Biochemical Genetics and Newborn Screening
ARUP Laboratories
Salt Lake City, Utah

Mark Mackay, MSc(Hons)
Royal College of Pathologists of Australasia Quality Assurance Programs
Sydney, Australia

G. Mike Makrigiorgos, PhD
Professor and Director of Medical Physics and Biophysics
Radiation Oncology, Dana Farber Cancer Institute
Harvard Medical School
Boston, Massachusetts

John P. Manis, MD
Assistant Professor of Pathology
Department of Laboratory Medicine
Harvard Medical School
Associate Director, Transfusion Medicine Service
Boston Children's Hospital
Boston, Massachusetts

Elaine R. Mardis, PhD
Robert E. and Louise F. Dunn Distinguished Professor of Medicine
Washington University School of Medicine
Co-Director, McDonnell Genome Institute
St. Louis, Missouri

William J. Marshall, PhD, FRCP, FRCPath, FRCPEdin, FRSC, FLS
Emeritus Reader in Clinical Biochemistry
King's College London
London, United Kingdom

Ann McCormack, MBBS(Hons I), FRACP, PhD
Conjoint Lecturer of Medicine
University of New South Wales
Endocrinologist
St. Vincent's Hospital
Sydney, Australia

Gwendolyn A. McMillin, PhD
Professor of Pathology
University of Utah
Medical Director, Toxicology and Pharmacogenomics
ARUP Laboratories
Salt Lake City, Utah

Brenton M. Meier, BS, MD
Anesthesiology and Pain Medicine
Thedacare Health System
Appleton, Wisconsin

W. Greg Miller, PhD
Director, Clinical Chemistry and Pathology Information Systems
Professor of Pathology
Virginia Commonwealth University
Richmond, Virginia

Michael C. Milone, MD, PhD
Assistant Professor of Pathology and Laboratory Medicine
Perelman School of Medicine
University of Pennsylvania
Associate Director, Toxicology Laboratory
Hospital of the University of Pennsylvania
Philadelphia, Pennsylvania

Karel G.M. Moons, PhD
Professor
Jilius Centre
University Medical Center Utrecht
Utrecht, The Netherlands

Robert D. Nerenz, PhD
Assistant Professor of Pathology and Laboratory Medicine
Geisel School of Medicine at Dartmouth
Assistant Director of Clinical Chemistry
Dartmouth-Hitchcock Medical Center
Lebanon, New Hampshire

Michelle Nieuwesteeg, PhD
Pediatric Laboratory Medicine
The Hospital for Sick Children
Toronto, Ontario, Canada

Nora Nikolac, PhD
Specialist in Analytical Toxicology
University Department of Chemistry
Medical School University Hospital Sestre Milosrdnice
Zagreb, Croatia

Frederick S. Nolte, PhD, D(ABMM), F(AAM)
Professor and Vice-Chair for Laboratory Medicine
Department of Pathology and Laboratory Medicine
Director, Clinical Laboratories
Medical University of South Carolina
Charleston, South Carolina

Mauro Panteghini, MD
Full Professor of Clinical Biochemistry and Clinical Molecular Biology
Department of Biomedical and Clinical Biosciences
University of Milan Medical School
Director, Clinical Pathology Unit
Luigi Sacco University Hospital
Milan, Italy

Jason Y. Park, MD, PhD
Associate Professor
Joint Appointment, Pathology and the Eugene McDermott Center for Human Growth and Development
University of Texas Southwestern Medical Center
Director, Advanced Diagnostics Laboratory
Department of Pathology
Children's Medical Center Dallas
Dallas, Texas

Marzia Pasquali, PhD, FACMG
Professor of Pathology
University of Utah School of Medicine
Medical Director, Biochemical Genetics and Newborn Screening
ARUP Laboratories
Salt Lake City, Utah

Jay L. Patel, MD
Assistant Professor of Pathology
University of Utah School of Medicine
Salt Lake City, Utah

Robin Patel, MD, FRCP(C), D(ABMM), FIDSA, FACP, F(AAM)
Professor of Medicine and Microbiology
Chair, Division of Clinical Microbiology
Department of Laboratory Medicine and Pathology
Mayo Clinic
Rochester, Minnesota

Daniele S. Podini, PhD
Associate Professor of Forensic Sciences
George Washington University
Washington, D.C.

Victoria M. Pratt, PhD
Director, Pharmacogenomics Laboratory
Associate Professor of Medical and Molecular Genetics
Indiana University School of Medicine
Indianapolis, Indiana

Christopher P. Price, PhD, FRCPath, FRSC, FACB
Honorary Senior Fellow
Nuffield Department of Primary Care Health Sciences
University of Oxford
Oxford, United Kingdom

Bobbi S. Pritt, MD, MSc, DTM&H
Professor of Pathology and Laboratory Medicine
Director, Clinical Parasitology and Vector-borne Disease Laboratory Services
Department of Laboratory Medicine and Pathology
Division of Clinical Microbiology
Mayo Clinic
Rochester, Minnesota

Karen Quillen, MD, MPH
Professor of Pathology and Medicine
Boston University School of Medicine
Medical Director, Blood Bank
Boston Medical Center
Boston, Massachusetts

Brian A. Rappold, BS
Scientific Director
Essential Testing
Collinsville, Illinois

Hooman H. Rashidi, MD
Associate Professor of Pathology and Laboratory Medicine
University of California, Davis School of Medicine
Director, Flow Cytometry and Immunology
University of California, Davis Health Systems
Sacramento, California

Alan T. Remaley, MD, PhD
Senior Investigator
National Institutes of Health
National Heart, Lung and Blood Institute
Bethesda, Maryland

Nader Rifai, PhD
Professor of Pathology
Harvard Medical School
Louis Joseph Gay-Lussac Chair of Laboratory Medicine
Director of Clinical Chemistry
Boston Children's Hospital
Boston, Massachusetts

Norman B. Roberts, PhD, MSc, CChem
Clinical Biochemistry
The Royal Liverpool and Broadgreen University Hospitals
Liverpool, United Kingdom

Alan L. Rockwood, PhD, DABCC
Professor of Pathology
University of Utah School of Medicine
Scientific Director of Mass Spectrometry
ARUP Laboratories
Salt Lake City, Utah

William Rosenberg, **MA, MB, BS, DPhil, FRCP**
Peter Scheuer Chair of Liver Diseases
Institute for Liver and Digestive Health
Division of Medicine
University College London
London, United Kingdom

David B. Sacks, **MB, ChB, FRCPath**
Adjunct Professor of Medicine
Georgetown University
Clinical Professor of Pathology
George Washington University
Washington, D.C.
Honorary Professor of Clinical Laboratory Sciences
University of Cape Town
Cape Town, South Africa
Senior Investigator
Chief, Clinical Chemistry
National Institutes of Health
Bethesda, Maryland

Sverre Sandberg, **MD, PhD**
Professor, Medical Faculty
University of Bergen
Director, The Norwegian Quality
Improvement of Primary Care Laboratories
Haraldsplass Deaconess Hospital
Director, Norwegian Porphyria Centre
Laboratory of Clinical Biochemistry
Haukeland University Hospital
Bergen, Norway

Eliane Sardh, **MD, PhD, MSc**
Senior Registrar
Center of Inherited Metabolic Diseases
Department of Endocrinology, Metabolism, and Diabetes
Karolinska University Hospital
Stockholm, Sweden

Mark J. Sarno, **JD**
President
Vision Biotechnology Consulting
Escondido, California

Emily I. Schindler, **MD, PhD**
Fellow in Laboratory Medicine
Department of Pathology and Immunology
Washington University School of Medicine
St. Louis, Missouri

Audrey N. Schuetz, **MD, MPH, D(ABMM)**
Director, Initial Processing
Co-Director, Bacteriology
Division of Clinical Microbiology
Senior Associate Consultant
Department of Laboratory Medicine and Pathology
Mayo Clinic
Rochester, Minnesota

Mitchell G. Scott, **PhD**
Professor of Pathology and Immunology
Division of Laboratory and Genomic Medicine
Co-Medical Director, Clinical Chemistry
Washington University School of Medicine
St. Louis, Missouri

Amar A. Sethi, **MD, PhD**
President and Chief Scientific Officer
Pacific Biomarkers
Seattle, Washington

Howard M. Shapiro, **MD**
President
One World Cytometry, Inc.
West Newton, Massachusetts

Leslie M. Shaw, **BS, PhD**
Professor of Pathology and Laboratory Medicine
Director, Toxicology Laboratory
Director, Biomarker Research Laboratory
Perelman School of Medicine
University of Pennsylvania
Philadelphia, Pennsylvania

Roy A. Sherwood, **BSc, MSc, DPhil**
Professor of Clinical Biochemistry
King's College London
London, United Kingdom

Ana-Maria Simundic, **PhD**
Professor, Specialist in Laboratory Medicine
Department of Medical Laboratory Diagnostics
Clinical Hospital Sveti Duh
Zagreb, Croatia

Ravinder Sodi, **PhD, CSci, FRCPath**
Consultant Clinical Biochemist and Honorary Lecturer
Department of Biochemistry
Royal Lancaster Infirmary
University Hospitals of Morecambe Bay NHS Foundation Trust
Lancaster, Lancashire, United Kingdom

Andrew St John, **PhD**
Principal Consultant
ARC Consulting
Perth, Australia

Molly Stout, **MD**
Assistant Professor of Obstetrics and Gynecology
Washington University School of Medicine
St. Louis, Missouri

Frederick G. Strathmann, **PhD, DABCC (CC, TC)**
Assistant Professor
University of Utah
Medical Director of Toxicology
Associate Scientific Director of Mass Spectrometry
ARUP Laboratories
Salt Lake City, Utah

Catharine Sturgeon, **BSc, PhD, FRCPath**
Honorary Lecturer
University of Edinburgh
Consultant Clinical Scientist
Department of Laboratory Medicine
Royal Infirmary of Edinburgh
Edinburgh, United Kingdom

Dorine W. Swinkels, **MD, PhD**
Professor of Experimental Clinical Chemistry
Department of Laboratory Medicine
Translational Metabolic Laboratory
Radboudumc, Nijmegen, The Netherlands

Sudeep Tanwar, **MD, MRCP(UK)**
Consultant Gastroenterologist and Hepatologist
Barts Health NHS Trust
London, United Kingdom

Andrew Taylor, **BSc, MSc, PhD, FRSC, FRCPath**
Consultant Clinical Scientist
Clinical Biochemistry
Royal Surrey County Hospital
Surrey, Great Britain

Stephanie A. Thatcher, **MS**
Director of Systems Integration
BioFire Diagnostics
Salt Lake City, Utah

Wouter W. van Solinge, **PhD**
Professor of Laboratory Medicine
Chairman and Medical Director
Division Laboratories and Pharmacy
University Medical Centre Utrecht
Utrecht, The Netherlands

Richard van Wijk, **MD**
Associate Professor of Clinical Chemistry and Hematology
University Medical Center Utrecht
Utrecht, The Netherlands

Jim Vaught, **PhD**
Past President, International Society for Biological and Environmental Repositories
Editor-in-Chief, Biopreservation and Biobanking
Kensington, Maryland
Senior Research Fellow
International Prevention Research Institute
Lyon, France

Cindy L. Vnencak-Jones, **PhD**
Professor of Pathology, Microbiology, and Immunology
Vanderbilt University School of Medicine
Medical Director, Molecular Diagnostics Laboratory
Vanderbilt University Medical Center
Nashville, Tennessee

Mia Wadelius, **MD, PhD**
Associate Professor of Medical Sciences
Clinical Pharmacology
Uppsala University
Uppsala, Sweden

Natalie E. Walsham, **MBiochem, MSc, DipRCPath**
Lead Clinical Scientist
Department of Clinical Biochemistry
University Hospital Lewisham
London, United Kingdom

G. Russell Warnick, **MS, MBA**
Chief Science Officer
Prism Health Diagnostic Laboratory
Austin, Texas

Victor W. Weedn, **MD, JD**
Professor and Chair of Forensic Sciences
George Washington University
Washington, D.C.

David A. Wells, **PhD**
Founder and Principal Consultant
Wells Medical Research Services
Laguna Beach, California

Nancy L. Wengenack, **PhD**
Professor of Microbiology and Laboratory Medicine and Pathology
Division of Clinical Microbiology
Mayo Clinic
Rochester, Minnesota

Sharon D. Whatley, **MSc, PhD, FRCPath**
Clinical Scientist
Department of Medical Biochemistry and Immunology
Institute of Medical Genetics
University Hospital of Wales
Cardiff, Wales, United Kingdom

William E. Winter, **MD, DABCC, FACB, FCAP**
Professor of Pathology, Immunology, and Laboratory Medicine, Pediatrics, and Molecular Genetics and Microbiology
University of Florida
Gainesville, Florida

Carl T. Wittwer, **MD, PhD**
Professor of Pathology
University of Utah School of Medicine
Medical Director, Immunologic Flow Cytometry
ARUP Laboratories
Salt Lake City, Utah

Melanie L. Yarbrough, **PhD**
Clinical Chemistry Fellow
Department of Pathology and Immunology
Washington University School of Medicine
St. Louis, Missouri

Qian-Yun Zhang, **MD, PhD**
Professor of Pathology
University of New Mexico School of Medicine
Department of Pathology
University of New Mexico Health Sciences Center
Albuquerque, New Mexico

CONTRIBUTORS TO EXPERT CONSULT

Associate Editor
Roy W.A. Peake, PhD, FRCPath D(ABCC) D(ABMGG)
Associate Director of Clinical Chemistry
Boston Children's Hospital
Instructor
Harvard Medical School
Boston, Massachusetts
Tietz Atlas of Biochemical Genetics

John Coakley, MD, FRACP, FRCPA, MAACB
Head of Biochemistry Department (Retired)
The Children's Hospital at Westmead
Sydney, New South Wales, Australia
Tietz Clinical Vignettes: The Coakley Collection and Other Short Cases

Allan Deacon, PhD, FRCPath
Consultant Clinical Biochemist (Retired)
Kings College Hospital
London, United Kingdom
Tietz Biochemical Calculations: Deacon's Challenge

Julio C. Delgado, MD, MS
Associate Professor
Department of Pathology
University of Utah School of Medicine
Section Chief, Immunology Division
ARUP Laboratories
Salt Lake City, Utah
Tietz Atlas of Electrophoretic Patterns

Jonathan R. Genzen, MD, PhD
Assistant Professor of Pathology
University of Utah School of Medicine
Medical Director, Automated Core Laboratory
ARUP Laboratories
Salt Lake City, Utah
Tietz Atlas of Electrophoretic Patterns

Stephen Miller, BSc
Senior Medical Scientist
Pathology, Queensland
Core Haematology Central Laboratory
Royal Brisbane and Women's Hospitals
Herston, Queensland, Australia
Tietz Atlas of Electrophoretic Patterns

Bobbi S. Pritt, MD, MSc, DTM&H
Professor of Pathology and Laboratory Medicine
Director, Clinical Parasitology and Vector-borne Disease Laboratory Services
Department of Laboratory Medicine and Pathology
Division of Clinical Microbiology
Mayo Clinic
Rochester, Minnesota
Tietz Atlas of Parasitology: The Bobbi Pritt Collection
Tietz Teasers in Parasitology: The Bobbi Pritt Collection

Robert Rej, PhD
Associate Professor, School of Public Health
State University of New York at Albany
Rensselaer, New York
Director, Clinical Chemistry and Hematology
Wadsworth Center for Laboratories and Research
New York State Department of Health
Albany, New York
Podcasts

Melissa R. Snyder, PhD
Assistant Professor of Laboratory Medicine
College of Medicine
Mayo Clinic
Rochester, Minnesota
Tietz Atlas of Electrophoretic Patterns

Jillian R. Tate, MSc, FFSc (RCPA)
Senior Scientist, Chemical Pathology
Royal Brisbane and Women's Hospital
Brisbane, Australia
Tietz Atlas of Electrophoretic Patterns

FOREWORD

When I asked Michael Somogyi to write the foreword to the first edition of *Fundamentals of Clinical Chemistry* in 1969, little did I know that nearly 50 years later I would be asked by Nader Rifai, the editor of this edition, to do the same. As immigrants from war-torn countries, we both recognize the freedoms and opportunities afforded by life in America. It is that same sense of freedom and opportunity that this Web edition of the *Tietz Textbook of Clinical Chemistry and Molecular Diagnostics* brings to what originally was a rather classic textbook of defined but limited scope.

As both a veteran of World War II and a former prisoner of war, little did I know of the exciting and rewarding life that awaited me at Rockford Memorial Hospital. It was there that I had the good fortune to work under the guidance of Dr. Samuel Natelson. Dr. Natelson was an early pioneer in development of clinical laboratory methods, following in the footsteps of Otto Folin, Donald Van Slyke, and Michael Somogyi. It was the mid-1950s when instrumental methods of analysis were just becoming available. The first commercial flame photometers provided accurate measurements of sodium and potassium, and the first practical methods for clinically significant enzymes by UV spectrophotometry were developed. It was during this time that Wallace Coulter introduced the electronic cell counter and Technicon the Auto Analyzer, which signaled the beginning of automated chemical analysis. The experience with Dr. Natelson gave me both roots and wings as I learned of the medical needs and laboratory techniques that have become what we know as laboratory medicine today.

In 1959 I was offered a position as head of the clinical laboratory at Mount Sinai Hospital Medical Center in Chicago, which included an appointment at the Chicago Medical School. That gave me the inspiration to install and experience some of the early clinical chemistry automation and laboratory information systems. As important, however, was to understand the increasing dependence of medical staff on laboratory results. I began to realize the need for a textbook that documented contemporary and expanding knowledge in the field to guide laboratorians, teachers, and students.

The first edition was a grand success and in time with later editions became a bestseller. It was translated into Spanish, Italian, and Russian. But with each edition, it has become increasingly evident that a bridge was needed to fill the gap between the clinical laboratory and medical management by relating pathophysiology to analytical results in health and disease. It is this gap that Nader Rifai and his editorial team intend to fill with the Web edition. I will be in my 91st year as this edition becomes available. With it, my fondest dream of an authoritative, interactive source bridging the continuum between laboratory medicine and medical practice will finally be realized. My thanks to all who have contributed over the years to the textbook's success and to those who made this monumental task a reality.

Norbert W. Tietz
La Jolla, California

PREFACE

We are pleased to introduce the sixth edition of *Tietz Textbook of Clinical Chemistry and Molecular Diagnostics*. We built on the excellent work of our predecessors and used electronic tools to produce a unique and state-of-the-art product for students, trainees, and practicing professionals in laboratory medicine. Thus we introduce the concept of a *Platform*, of which the textbook is only a component (see Figure).

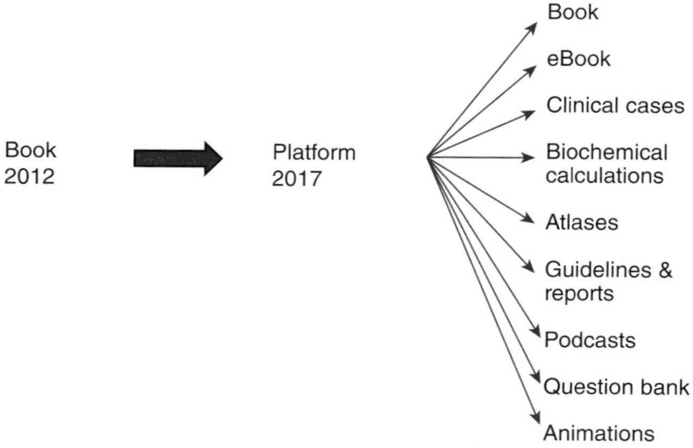

Although the textbook is available in print for most chapters with a selected list of references, the comprehensive product is only available electronically on the Platform. Using Elsevier's Expert Consult electronic system, we have created:

- User-friendly reading with great search capability and a built-in dictionary.
- Additional resources for an enhanced learning experience. These include hundreds of clinical case studies, biochemical calculations, morphology images, electrophoretic patterns, chromatograms and mass spectra, educational articles and documents, multiple choice questions, animations, and podcasts. These resources were either previously created by prominent laboratory medicine professionals (eg, Allan Deacon, Bobbi Pritt, and John Coakley) and scientific societies (ie, the United Kingdom Association for Clinical Biochemistry and Laboratory Medicine, Royal Society of Chemistry-London, and AACC) or produced de novo by accomplished scientists and physicians using materials from their own institutions (ie, Mayo Clinic, ARUP, Hôpitaux Universitaire La Pitié Salpêtrière-Paris, Pathology Queensland-Australia, and Boston Children's Hospital).
- A broadened scope that comprises the fundamentals of hematology, cytometry, microbiology, and transfusion medicine to provide trainees in laboratory medicine and clinical pathology with up-to-date information across an expanded range of topics. The growth of certain areas in laboratory medicine, such as clinical mass spectrometry and biomarker utility in the pharmaceutical industry, is reflected by the addition of several chapters. Compared with the previous edition, the number of chapters has increased from 59 to 82.
- A *living product* to which materials are periodically added and information is updated as necessary.

Our hope for this Platform is to serve as a resource center where important materials in laboratory medicine are deposited for use by and to the benefit of the community at large. Therefore, we encourage those who have similar materials and wish to have them considered for the Platform to contact one of the editors. The Platform can only be enhanced by the efforts of the community.

Unlike most textbooks, all chapters in this edition were reviewed by three individuals: a reviewer, an associate editor, and a senior editor. We believe that these efforts have led to a better product. In addition we have made a concerted effort to create an *International* rather than an *American* Platform; more than one-third of the authors, reviewers, and editors live outside of the United States. We have strongly encouraged authors to include European, Australasian, and other international guidelines in addition to the American ones in order to present different practices and points of view. Furthermore, all measurements are presented in both traditional and SI units.

We have aimed to harmonize the presentation of information among chapters while retaining the personality and unique style of each author, hoping for a readable, educational text with enough variety to amuse and occasionally delight.

This ambitious project has been a true group effort and represents the collective intellect, knowledge, and experience of over 200 leaders in laboratory medicine from 16 countries. We are in debt not only to the authors, reviewers, and editors of the chapters, but also to the contributors of the supplementary materials that greatly enrich the Platform. We are grateful to Elsevier, and particularly to Kellie White, Karen Turner, Melanie Cole, Kayci Wyatt, Alex Marden, Laurie Gower, and Amanda Mincher, for supporting us throughout this project to realize our vision and create this Platform.

We sincerely hope that this product will be a valuable educational and reference resource for the laboratory medicine community worldwide.

Nader Rifai
Andrea Rita Horvath
Carl T. Wittwer

CONTENTS

*Full versions of these chapters are available exclusively on ExpertConsult.com.

SECTION I

Basics of Laboratory Medicine

Exam questions, case studies, and additional resources are available on ExpertConsult.com.
*Full versions of these chapters are available electronically on ExpertConsult.com.

1

Clinical Chemistry and Molecular Diagnostics

*Nader Rifai, Andrea Rita Horvath, and Carl T. Wittwer**

ABSTRACT

Background

Clinical chemistry and molecular diagnostics are both disciplines of laboratory medicine that study molecules to aid clinical diagnoses. Both disciplines are greatly influenced by technology as methods, instrumentation, and automation continue to improve. Clinical chemistry was once a historical curiosity of questionable medical value but is now central to diagnostics with millions of tests performed daily to guide patient therapy. Molecular diagnostics focuses on DNA and RNA molecules, enabling the sequencing of entire genomes, as well as rapid near-to-the-patient identification of microbes responsible for infectious syndromes. Molecular approaches are necessary to achieve our hopes for companion diagnostics and for personalized and precision medicine. Although clinical chemistry and molecular diagnostic professionals are diverse in terms of their education, training, and career paths, their practice of laboratory medicine and their adherence to its guiding principles are the same. The goal is to generate relevant chemical and molecular data that can be integrated in professional knowledge to supplement the wisdom of physicians in clinical decision making.

Content

This chapter describes the evolution of both clinical chemistry and molecular diagnostics and discusses their similarities under the umbrella of laboratory medicine. The chapter examines the international practice of the profession, subdisciplines it may encompass, academic and postgraduate training, certification, career opportunities, and the skills and roles of the clinical chemist in the clinical laboratory and industry settings. Last, the chapter discusses the guiding principles of practicing the profession, which include maintaining confidentiality of genetic and medical information, using available resources appropriately, abiding by codes of conduct, avoiding conflict of interest, and following ethical publishing rules.

INTRODUCTION

The disciplines of "clinical chemistry" and "molecular diagnostics" elicit different images today. For clinical chemistry, one thinks of pH measurements or large chemistry analyzers, while molecular diagnostics conjures up the human genome project, companion diagnostics, and personalized and precision medicine. Whereas clinical chemistry is at the core of laboratory medicine, molecular diagnostics is a more recent but explosive upstart. Clinical chemistry excels in random access testing, but molecular diagnostics has evolved massively parallel methods. On the surface, these disciplines appear clearly different.

Consider, however, the meaning behind the words that compose "clinical chemistry" and "molecular diagnostics." Chemistry by its very nature is molecular, and the study of molecules is chemistry. There is no difference here. Perhaps the "molecular" in "molecular diagnostics" suggests complex polymers with meaningful sequence, excluding simpler chemicals. DNA and RNA sequence largely define life, and powerful technologies for nucleic acids now eclipse those for other complex polymers such as proteins and carbohydrates. In common parlance, molecular diagnostics is dominated by nucleic acids. The words "clinical" and "diagnostics" are also similar, connecting both fields to human disease. "Clinical" is more generic than "diagnostics," but again in common use, "molecular diagnostics" includes not only diagnostics but prognosis and genetic predisposition as well. In each two-word combination, the sum is greater than its parts, with combined meanings evolving to fit needs and interest. We believe that molecular diagnostics is best viewed as a subset of clinical chemistry.

According to the definition of the International Federation of Clinical Chemistry and Laboratory Medicine (IFCC), "Clinical Chemistry is the largest subdiscipline of Laboratory Medicine which is a multidisciplinary medical and scientific specialty with several interacting subdisciplines, such as hematology, immunology, clinical biochemistry, and others. Through these activities clinical chemists influence the practice of medicine for the benefit of the public."[1]

Hospital-based laboratory medicine departments as well as commercial clinical laboratories provide in vitro testing of chemical, biochemical, and genetic markers in various fluids or tissues of the human body to screen for a disease, confirm or exclude a diagnosis, help to select or monitor a treatment, or assess prognosis. The popular claim that 60% to 70% of clinical decisions are based on laboratory

*The authors gratefully acknowledge the contributions by David E. Bruns, Edward R. Ashwood, and Carl A. Burtis on which portions of this chapter are based.

tests is not backed by objectively measured data.[2,3] Nevertheless, laboratory testing impacts health care delivery to virtually every patient.

LOOKING BACK

The examination of body fluids for the diagnosis of disease is certainly not a modern concept. The Greeks noticed before 400 BC that ants are attracted to "sweet urine." Laboratory testing, however, was not always appreciated by clinicians; the famous Dublin physician Robert James Graves (1796–1853) once remarked, "Few and scanty, indeed, are the rays of light which chemistry has flung on the vital mysteries," and the pioneer Max Josef von Pettenkofer (1818–1901) stated that clinicians use their chemistry laboratory services only when needed for "luxurious embellishment for a clinical lecture."[4] Such views have changed throughout the years, and laboratory testing has proven to be a useful tool to clinicians who have grown to depend and rely on laboratory testing in the routine management of their patients.

Although it may be difficult to pinpoint the exact date at which the concept of the clinical laboratory was born, all indications point to the mid-19th century. One such indication is an article titled "Hospital Construction" by Francis H. Brown that was published in the *Boston Medical and Surgical Journal*, the precursor of the *New England Journal of Medicine*, in 1861. Dr. Brown stated: "[Every hospital should have] a small room at the end of the ward to serve as a general laboratory … necessary small cooking might be accomplished here; dishes and other articles washed etc.; and it would serve as a general store-room for brooms, pails, and other articles." Although Baron Justus von Liebig (1803–1873) boasted that his clinical laboratory performed more than 400 tests per annum, the average mid- to large-sized laboratory today performs several million tests yearly. The term *clinical chemistry* was purportedly coined by Charles Henry Ralfe (1842–1896) of London Hospital when he used it as the title of his 1883 treatise. The first laboratory attached to a hospital was established in 1886 in Munich, Germany, by Hugo Wilhelm von Ziemssen.[5] In the United States, the first clinical laboratory was reported to be The William Pepper Laboratory of Clinical Medicine, established in 1895 at the University of Pennsylvania in Philadelphia.[6]

Molecular diagnostics has more recent origins. "Molecular diagnosis" was first mentioned in 1968 as the title of a *New England Journal of Medicine* editorial, commenting on a new inborn error of metabolism that overproduced oxalic acid, resulting in kidney stones.[7] "Molecular" referred to an enzymatic pathway and the substrates, not nucleic acid variants. Twenty years later, additional articles describing "molecular diagnostics" began to appear. In 1986, molecular diagnostics was defined as, "… the detection and quantification of specific genes by nucleic acid hybridization procedures," exemplified by speciation of plant nematodes.[8] In 1987, molecular diagnostics was used to describe mapping of antigenic substances by affinity chromatography using immobilized antibodies.[9] In 1988, the term was used to describe methods for detecting gene amplification and rearrangement using Southern blotting.[10] With the advent of polymerase chain reaction (PCR), the term "molecular diagnostics" became more common, its use doubling in the medical literature every 6 to 7 years.[11] By 1997, commercial real-time PCR instruments solidified "molecular diagnostics" as a branch of clinical chemistry and laboratory medicine.

TRAINING IN CLINICAL CHEMISTRY

Clinical chemists are laboratory professionals with a medical or a doctorate degree (pharmacy, chemistry, biology, biochemistry) who are focused on clinical service. In North America, Australia, and Europe, a minimum of 9 years of academic education (a medical or a doctoral degree) and postgraduate professional training (residency and postdoctoral) is required before an individual becomes an independently practicing specialist (Fig. 1.1).[12] In some countries such as Austria, Lithuania, and Sweden, only physicians can practice the profession and direct a clinical laboratory. In most other European and North American countries, scientists, pharmacists, and physicians can be clinical chemists, yet those with a pharmacy degree are not allowed to be clinical laboratory directors in some of these countries, such as Italy. A pharmacy degree is a "professional" degree (but not equivalent to a PhD) in France.

Depending on the region, clinical chemistry may include components of microbiology, hematology, coagulation, and immunology, as well as molecular diagnostics. This diversity of subspecialties is reflected in the heterogeneity of postgraduate training across countries. Currently, in the United Kingdom and Ireland, chemical pathology training is restricted to the traditional subdiscipline of clinical chemistry. In all other European countries, trainees get exposed to not only clinical chemistry (45% of the curriculum) but also hematology (30%), microbiology (15%), and genetics (10%).[1,12] In the United States, PhD trainees primarily focus on clinical chemistry, but physician clinical pathologists are trained in all aspects of laboratory medicine.

Postgraduate professional training and certification examinations at the end of the training are not mandated in all countries (see Fig. 1.1). The European Communities Confederation of Clinical Chemistry and Laboratory Medicine (EC4) Register of the European Federation of Clinical Chemistry and Laboratory Medicine (http://www.ec-4.org) is attempting to standardize the minimum requirements for education and training for clinical chemists to facilitate the comparability of their professional training within the European Union.[1,12] These issues add to the complexity of defining the qualifications of clinical chemists and clinical laboratory directors.

EXPANDING BOUNDARIES DEFINED BY TECHNOLOGY

The diversity of background, training, and subspecialization has led to heterogeneity in what the profession is called throughout the world. Name designations include clinical chemistry, clinical biochemistry, chemical pathology, clinical pathology, laboratory diagnostics, clinical or medical biology, clinical laboratory, laboratory medicine, clinical analysis, and so on. The EC4 Register adopted the name "specialist in laboratory medicine" to represent clinical chemists in Europe.

Everyone, including laypeople, knows what a cardiologist is and does; the same is true for an infectious disease specialist and a surgeon. Within laboratory medicine, the function of certain specialists, such as clinical microbiologists or blood

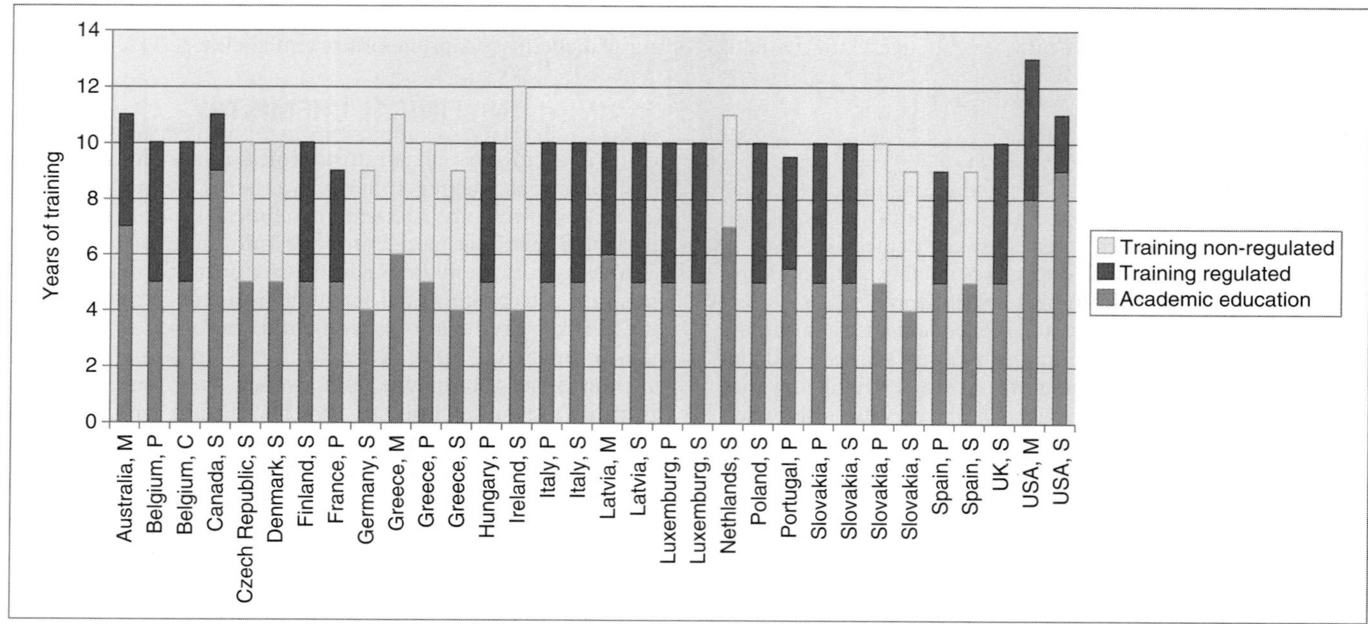

FIGURE 1.1 The number of years of education and training required to practice clinical chemistry in different countries varies from 9 to 13 years. Different training routes include medical (M), pharmacy (P), chemistry (C), and scientific (S). Both academic education *(light red bars)* and postgraduate training are required. Postgraduate training may be regulated *(dark red bars)* or nonregulated *(pink bars)* in different countries and even within the same country. (Modified from EU Directive 2013/55/EU. The recognition of professional qualifications. Proposing a common training framework for specialists in laboratory medicine across the European Union 2013. http://www.ukipg.org.uk/meetings/international_and_european_forum/ctf_e4_bid.)

bankers, is also clear. It is more difficult, however, to characterize a clinical chemist. Perhaps, unlike other specialties in laboratory medicine, clinical chemistry is very much influenced and shaped by technology. No discipline in laboratory medicine uses more technologies than clinical chemistry. Technologies that evolved over time not only changed practice but remodeled the boundaries of the traditional clinical chemistry laboratory. For example, with the emergence of immunochemical techniques in the 1970s, the U.S. Food and Drug Administration approved many tests for the measurement of proteins, small molecule hormones, and drugs, a development that profoundly changed clinical chemistry and its armamentarium of testing at the time. Integrated automated platforms later enabled the measurement of hormones and therapeutic drugs by immunoassays simultaneously with electrolytes, glucose, and other general chemistry tests, thus subsuming the "endocrine lab" and the "drug lab."

Serologic tests for hepatitis and HIV and tests for autoimmune diseases also moved from their traditional home in microbiology and immunology to chemistry analyzers.

Immunoglobulin analysis followed a similar path. In certain countries, coagulation is considered part of clinical chemistry because the measurement of coagulation proteins uses similar instruments to those used in the clinical chemistry laboratory. As a result, the typical clinical chemistry laboratory includes testing for general chemistries, specific proteins and immunoglobulins, therapeutic and abused drugs, blood gases, hormones, biogenic amines, porphyrins, vitamins, and trace elements. Testing for inborn errors of metabolism (such as the measurements of amino acids and organic acids), measurements of coagulation factors, general hematologic testing, and serologic assays can belong either to the clinical chemistry laboratory or to another subspecialty, depending on the institution and country. If amino acids and organic acids are measured in the clinical chemistry laboratory, that does not preclude a biochemical geneticist from providing the clinical interpretation. Similar arguments can be made for coagulation, hematology, and serology testing.

Clinical chemists have embraced technology over the years and used it effectively to derive answers to clinical questions. In modern clinical chemistry laboratories, technologies include spectrophotometry, atomic absorption, flame emission photometry, nephelometry, electrochemical and optical sensor technologies, electrophoresis, and chromatography. The influence of automation, information technology, and miniaturization is evident in today's clinical chemistry laboratory. Mass spectrometry, once thought of as a research tool, is playing an ever-growing role in clinical chemistry for the measurement of both small molecules and peptides and more recently proteins. In fact, matrix-assisted laser desorption ionization time-of-flight (MALDI-TOF) mass spectrometry is now routinely used in the identification of pathogens, so it is likely that the evolution in this technology will also bring the clinical chemistry and microbiology laboratories closer. Molecular diagnostics has forever changed virology and microbiology, introducing faster and more sensitive methods based on nucleic acid amplification rather than microbial replication. Nanotechnology, microfluidics, electrical impedance, reflectance spectroscopy, and time-resolved fluorescence are only a few of the technologies used in point-of-care testing for proteins, drugs, DNA, and analysis of metabolites in small samples of whole blood. Point-of-care testing is a disruptive innovation that decentralizes laboratory testing and presents the clinical chemist with many challenges and opportunities. Molecular diagnostics in particular impacts diverse specialties, including infectious disease, genetics, and oncology, providing new tools for study at a molecular detail never before considered. In summary, the boundaries of clinical chemistry expand with technology, making the profession vibrant, interesting, and ever evolving.

The scope of the profession is constantly changing for the very same reasons. Scientific and technological developments, medical needs, patient demands, and economic pressures bring various disciplines of medicine closer together, and further integration of diagnostic and therapeutic disciplines is envisaged in the pursuit of more integrated and effective health care delivery. For example, companion diagnostics, which help predict therapeutic responses and individualize patient treatment options, bring together pharmacy and medical laboratories. Point-of-care testing and use of biomarker measurements in real time with medical interventions break the walls of laboratories and bring the profession closer to clinicians and patients. Integrated diagnostics (a term coined by the medical device industry), whereby in vitro laboratory technology is combined with in vivo imaging technology, intends to provide fully coordinated, interpreted, action-oriented results for managing patient conditions, *and* it places laboratory testing into an integrated patient care pathway (see an example at http://www.healthcare.siemens.com.au/clinical-specialities/reproductive-endocrinology/integrated-diagnostics). New disruptive technologies (eg, "lab on a chip," nanotechnology, home monitoring) as well as movement toward patient empowerment and direct-to-consumer testing bring laboratory testing closer to patients. All of these developments present special challenges to the future generations of clinical chemists both in terms of how they should be trained and how they will have to practice.

Technology alone is not the answer to more effective clinical practice. There must be meaningful results behind the data obtained. The generation of more data does not necessarily lead to better patient management. Many technology platforms are great discovery tools, but these high-throughput platforms seldom provide cost-effective diagnostic or prognostic information that changes patient care. In the 1960s and 1970s, with the advent of automated clinical analyzers, pathologists reported (and charged for) chemistry panels of 10 to 20 results. Many were later sued for excessive production of data that increased their income without commensurate value to patient care. More recently, dense data from expression arrays, genome-wide association studies, epigenomics, and microRNA analyses excel in discovery research, but translation to clinical practice has been slower than anticipated. The promise of greater clinical significance with larger data sets seems intuitive, but history suggests caution. We strive for closure, and what could be more complete than the entire sequence of the genome? Unfortunately, disease has a way of winning in the end, and the best we can do is hope to delay the inevitable with clinical wisdom to increase the quality of remaining life.

Clinical chemists in this world of "big data" translate high-quality measurement *data* into clinically relevant *information*. This information—when integrated with clinical history and presentation, clinical signs, and an understanding of pathophysiology—becomes *knowledge*. Knowledge, in the context of the experience and judgment of the clinician, is converted to *wisdom* that translates to clinical action for improved patient outcomes. For example, a 2-week-old boy with a suspected inborn error of metabolism had a suppressed thyroid stimulating hormone and increased free T_4 concentrations. Acting on the basis of the data alone would have suggested treatment with methimazole for thyrotoxicosis. However, the patient was receiving biotin as part of his treatment for a metabolic disorder, and the biotin interfered with the immunoassays used in the thyroid function tests. Repeat measurement of these parameters with non–biotin-based immunoassays revealed a normal thyroid profile. Another example: A patient presented with Cushingoid appearance and a markedly decreased serum cortisol concentration. A further examination of his clinical history revealed that he was using topical corticosteroids for a skin condition, a treatment that caused adrenal suppression and thus a low cortisol level. Yet another example: A 55-year-old woman complained to her primary care physician about long-standing bony aches and pains. All results to exclude musculoskeletal problems came back normal except for a low alkaline phosphatase (ALP) enzyme activity. After excluding potential preanalytical errors (eg, contamination of sample by K-EDTA [potassium ethylenediaminetetraacetic acid] anticoagulant), the laboratory proposed the diagnosis of hypophosphatasia, and testing for mutations of the tissue nonspecific ALP gene confirmed the diagnosis both in the patient and in her daughter. The world of clinical chemistry is full of such examples that demonstrate the value of acting on information beyond the generated numbers. Knowledge is what we must provide to clinicians to support informed clinical decision making and for achieving improved patient outcomes.

HOW IS CLINICAL CHEMISTRY PRACTICED?

Both the training of clinical chemists and their career paths are heterogeneous. Although the majority of our colleagues choose a career in a clinical laboratory environment, many work in the in vitro diagnostics (IVD) and pharmaceutical industries. Clinical chemists, by virtue of their training, are translational researchers who are equipped for and capable of developing, evaluating, and validating biochemical and genetic assays for clinical use; they develop skills that are essential for new biomarker assays, reagent kits, and companion diagnostics. Clinical chemists also provide interfaces between researchers, clinicians, the clinical laboratory, and the IVD industry and help to translate biomarker research into clinically meaningful decisions and actions.

The functions of a clinical chemist and the molecular diagnostics specialist include:

- Develop and validate de novo laboratory tests to meet clinical needs.
- Evaluate and characterize the analytical and clinical performance of laboratory tests.
- Present laboratory results to clinicians in an effective manner.
- Provide education and advice on the selection and interpretation of laboratory tests as part of the clinical team.
- Determine the cost-effectiveness and intrinsic value of laboratory tests.

- Participate in the development of clinical testing algorithms and clinical practice guidelines.
- Assure compliance with regulatory requirements.
- Participate in quality assurance and improvement of the laboratory service.
- Teach and train future generations of laboratory specialists.
- Participate in basic or clinical research.

Clinical chemists practicing in the IVD or the pharmaceutical industry may not need to routinely interact with clinicians or interpret laboratory results, but they understand and appreciate the clinical utility and relevance of the assays and companion diagnostics they are developing and thus contribute more effectively to the development of diagnostics that improve health. The daily practice of the profession has changed over time. In the 1960s and 1970s, clinical chemists developed laboratory tests. However, as the profession matured and the instrumentation changed from open systems to "black boxes" that relied on manufacturers for assays, the traditional analytical focus of the profession has significantly diminished. At present, de novo assay development is still active only in certain areas such as chromatography, mass spectrometry, and molecular diagnostics.

Clinical chemists are now more active in the preanalytical and postanalytical phases of testing and in establishing processes such as how best to select the right test for the right patient and to communicate test results to clinicians in a medically meaningful way, how to build laboratory processes that reduce error, and how to continuously improve the quality of laboratory practices. In today's health care environment, there is increasing emphasis on clinical impact and cost-effectiveness. Laboratories are expected to demonstrate evidence of improved measurable clinical outcomes and the usefulness and added value of tests to clinical decision making. Proving the fact that laboratory testing contributes to improved patient outcomes is challenging because the relationship between testing and clinical outcomes is mostly indirect. Nevertheless, clinical chemists should move away from being just providers of high-quality data. Transforming laboratory data to information and knowledge requires more skills in information and information management technology, evidence-based medicine, epidemiology, data mining, and translational research. It also requires a shift of thinking from essentialism to consequentialism and from technology-driven to customer-focused and patient-centered laboratory medicine.[13,14]

To summarize, today's clinical chemists are laboratory professionals who are trained in pathophysiology and technology. The execution of their daily duties, which are more clinically or technology oriented, is influenced by their training (such as MD vs. PhD), interests, institutional needs, and the country where they practice. Clearly the practice of our profession has evolved over the past half a century, and there are even more challenges on the horizon that will expand and change its scope and role and enhance its diversity.

GUIDING PRINCIPLES OF PRACTICING THE PROFESSION

As in other branches of medicine, practitioners in the clinical laboratory are faced with ethical issues, often on a daily basis; examples are listed in Box 1.1.

BOX 1.1 Ethical Issues in Clinical Chemistry and Molecular Diagnostics

- Confidentiality of genetic information
- Confidentiality of patient medical information
- Allocation of resources
- Codes of conduct
- Publishing issues
- Conflicts of interest

Confidentiality of Genetic Information

Prominent in the news in the first and second decades of this millennium has been the issue of confidentiality of genetic information. Legislation was considered necessary to prevent denial of health insurance or employment to people found by DNA testing to be at risk of disease. Less appreciated is the fact that the issue of confidentiality of clinical laboratory data predated DNA testing. In fact, many non-DNA tests, old and new, also carry information about risks of illness and death. Clinical laboratory professionals have long been responsible for maintaining the confidentiality of all laboratory results, a situation made even more critical with the advent of increasingly powerful genetic testing.

Confidentiality of Patient Medical Information

New test development requires the use of patient samples and may involve the use of patient medical information.[15] Ethical judgments are required regarding the type of informed consent that is needed from patients for use of their samples and clinical information. Clinical laboratory physicians and scientists often serve on institutional review boards that examine proposed research on human subjects. In these discussions, ethical concepts such as clinical equipoise, which refers to the genuine uncertainty in the expert medical community over whether a particular treatment will be beneficial, and confidentiality, are central to decisions.

Allocation of Resources

Because resources are finite, clinical chemists must make ethically responsible decisions about allocation of resources. There is often a trade-off between cost and quality. What is best for patients generally? How can the most good be done with the available resources? For laboratorians in business, creative accounting may tarnish the profession if patient care is not kept paramount.

Codes of Conduct

Most professional organizations publish a code of conduct that requires adherence by their members. For example, the American Association for Clinical Chemistry (AACC) has published ethical guidelines that require AACC members to endorse principles of ethical conduct in their professional activities, including (1) selection and performance of clinical procedures, (2) research and development, (3) teaching, (4) management, (5) administration, and (6) other forms of professional service. A similar code of conduct has been developed and approved by the EC4 Register Commission and the European Federation of Clinical Chemistry and Laboratory Medicine.[16]

Publishing Issues

Publication of documents having high scientific integrity depends on editors, authors, and reviewers all working in concert in an environment governed by high ethical standards.[17]

Editors are responsible for the overall process, including identifying reviewers, evaluating the reviews and the authors' response to them, and making the final decision of whether to accept or reject a manuscript. Editors are also responsible for establishing policies and procedures to assure consistency in the editorial process. Finally, the editor-in-chief is responsible for developing a conflict of interest policy and monitoring it among his or her editors. Publishers, being commercial or scientific societies, should monitor any conflicts of interest of the editor-in-chief.

Authors are responsible for honest and complete reporting of original data produced in ethically conducted research studies. Practices such as fraud, plagiarism (verbatim, mosaic), and falsification or fabrication of data are unacceptable. The International Committee of Medical Journal Editors (ICMJE)[18] and the Committee on Publication Ethics (COPE)[19] have published policies that address such behavior. Other practices to be avoided include duplicate publication, redundant publication, and inappropriate authorship credit. In addition, ethical policies require that factors that might influence the interpretation of study findings must be revealed, such as (1) the role of the commercial sponsor in the design and conduct of the study, (2) interpretation of results, and (3) preparation of the manuscript. Additional undesirable and harmful practices are publication bias and selective reporting in which only studies with positive findings are reported and authors use "data dredging" and meaningless subanalyses to find a positive association rather than reporting the original hypothesis that was negative.[17] These practices inflate the actual value of observations or utility of markers and diminish the quality of meta-analyses. As a result, a comprehensive registry of diagnostic and prognostic studies, similar to the registry of clinical trials, has been advocated.[17,20,21]

To avoid publication of biased study results, reporting guidelines have been published for the main study types on the website of the EQUATOR Network (http://www.equator-network.org). For the laboratory profession, the STARD and TRIPOD statements for diagnostic and prognostic studies are probably the most important,[22,23] but reporting guidelines for randomized controlled trials (CONSORT), observational studies (STROBE), systematic reviews (PRISMA), quality improvement studies (SQUIRE), and economic evaluations (CHEERS) could also be relevant for the work of laboratory scientists active in research and publications.

Reviewers must provide a timely, fair, and impartial assessment of manuscripts. They must maintain confidentiality and never contact the authors until after the publication of the report. Finally, reviewers must excuse themselves from the review process if they perceive a conflict of interest.

Most journals now require authors to complete Conflict of Interest forms and delineate each author's contribution. Some journals, including *Clinical Chemistry,* publish this information along with the article for enhanced transparency. Some of the leading journals in clinical chemistry and molecular diagnostics are listed in Table 1.1.

TABLE 1.1 Major Journals in Clinical Chemistry and Molecular Diagnostics

Journal Name	URL
American Journal of Clinical Pathology	http://ajcp.ascpjournals.org
American Journal of Pathology	http://ajp.amjpathol.org
Annals of Clinical Biochemistry	http://acb.sagepub.com
Analytical Biochemistry	http://www.sciencedirect.com/science/journal/00032697
Analytical Chemistry	http://pubs.acs.org/journal/ancham
Archives of Pathology and Laboratory Medicine	http://www.archivesofpathology.org
Biochemical and Molecular Medicine	http://www.sciencedirect.com/science/journal/10773150
BioTechniques	http://www.biotechniques.com
Clinica Chimica Acta	http://www.journals.elsevier.com/clinica-chimica-acta
Clinical Chemistry	http://www.clinchem.org
Clinical Chemistry and Laboratory Medicine	http://www.degruyter.com/view/j/cclm
Clinical Biochemistry	http://www.journals.elsevier.com/clinical-biochemistry
Experimental and Molecular Pathology	http://www.journals.elsevier.com/experimental-and-molecular-pathology
Genetic Testing and Molecular Biomarkers	http://www.liebertpub.com/overview/genetic-testing-and-molecular-biomarkers/18
Genetics in Medicine	http://www.nature.com/gim/index.html
Human Mutation	http://onlinelibrary.wiley.com/journal/10.1002/(ISSN)1098-1004
Journal of Clinical Investigation	http://www.jci.org
Journal of Molecular Diagnostics	http://amp.org/JMD/index.cfm
Laboratory Investigation	http://www.nature.com/labinvest/index.html
Methods	http://www.journals.elsevier.com/methods
Nature Methods	http://www.nature.com/nmeth/index.html
Nucleic Acids Research	http://nar.oxfordjournals.org
Scandinavian Journal of Clinical and Laboratory Investigation	http://informahealthcare.com/loi/clb

Conflicts of Interest

The interrelationships between practitioners in the medical field and commercial suppliers of drugs, devices, and equipment can be positive or negative.[24] Concerns led the National Institutes of Health in 1995 to require official institutional review of financial disclosure by researchers and management in situations when disclosure indicates potential or actual conflicts of interest. In 2009, the Institute of Medicine issued a report[25] that questioned inappropriate relationships between pharmaceutical device companies and physicians and other health care professionals.[24] Similarly, the relationship between clinical laboratory professionals and manufacturers and providers of diagnostic equipment and supplies has been scrutinized.

As a consequence of these concerns and as a result of the enactment of various laws designed to prevent fraud, abuse, and waste in Medicare, Medicaid, and other federal programs, professional organizations that represent manufacturers of IVD and other device and health care companies have published codes of ethics. For example, the Advanced Medical Technology Association (AdvaMed) has published a revised code of ethics that became effective on July 1, 2009.[26] Topics discussed in this revised code include gifts and entertainment, consulting arrangements and royalties, reimbursement for testing, and education. Similarly, the European Diagnostic Manufacturers Association (EDMA) has published a code of ethics.[27] In Part A of the EDMA document, topics include member-sponsored product training and education, support for third-party educational conferences, sales and promotional meetings, arrangements and consultants, gifts, provision of reimbursements and other economic information, and donations for charitable and philanthropic purposes. Both documents address demands from regulators while nurturing the unique role that clinical chemists and other health care professionals play in developing and refining new technology.[24]

WHAT IS IN THIS TEXTBOOK?

In this textbook, we have assembled what is essential to effectively practice clinical chemistry and molecular diagnostics. We begin with introductory chapters that describe the basics of laboratory medicine, including statistics, sample handling, preanalytical processes, reference intervals, quality management, evidence-based laboratory medicine, biobanking, and biomarker and laboratory support for the pharmaceutical and IVD industries. This is followed by a section on analytical techniques and applications, detailing all of the methods used in clinical chemistry, including mass spectrometry, and the specialized topics of microfabrication and microfluidics, flow cytometry, and point-of-care testing. Next, all the major analytes are detailed, including enzymes, tumor markers, therapeutic drugs, and toxicology, among many others. This is followed by a section dedicated to molecular diagnostics, perhaps the fastest growing field in clinical chemistry. Finally, our last section on pathophysiology covers disease states and malfunction of different organ systems that correlate with abnormal laboratory findings. An appendix tabulates reference intervals for the clinical laboratory. The online version includes all of the above topics, while the print version is more selective to keep the tome manageable.

We have taken into account, to the best of our ability, the way clinical chemistry is currently practiced around the world and added chapters on basic hematology, microbiology, and transfusion medicine. Our aim is to provide current scientific and practical knowledge to support laboratory professionals as knowledge resources and an interface between science and technology on the one hand and the clinician and the patient on the other.

POINTS TO REMEMBER

- Clinical chemistry is the largest subdiscipline of laboratory medicine and molecular diagnostics is a subset of clinical chemistry.
- Clinical chemistry is a profession that has been shaped and defined by technology.
- Training of clinical chemists is heterogeneous and includes physicians and doctoral scientists in chemistry, pharmacy, biology, and biochemistry.
- The role of clinical chemists evolved over time from analytically and technology focused to customer and patient centered.
- Clinical chemists are translational researchers who convert laboratory data to clinical knowledge.
- Career paths of clinical chemists are heterogeneous and include work in clinical laboratories and IVD and pharmaceutical industries.
- Clinical chemists must adhere to guiding principles of practicing the profession, which include maintaining confidentiality of genetic and medical information, using resources appropriately, abiding by codes of conduct, following ethical publishing rules, and managing and disclosing conflict of interest.

REFERENCES

1. McMurray J, Zerah S, Hallworth M, et al. The European Register of Specialists in Clinical Chemistry and Laboratory Medicine: guide to the Register, version 3-2010. *Clin Chem Lab Med* 2010;**48**:999–1008.
2. Forsman RW. Why is the laboratory an afterthought for managed care organizations? *Clin Chem* 1996;**42**:813–16.
3. Hallworth MJ. The "70% claim": what is the evidence base? *Ann Clin Biochem* 2011;**48**:487–8.
4. Rifai N, Annesley T, Boyd J. International year of chemistry 2011: *Clinical Chemistry* celebrates. *Clin Chem* 2010;**56**: 1783–5.
5. Bruns DE, Ashwood ER, Burtis CA. Clinical chemistry, molecular diagnostics, and laboratory medicine. In: Bruns DE, Ashwood ER, Burtis CA, editors. *Tietz textbook of clinical chemistry and molecular diagnostics*. 5th ed. St Louis: Elsevier; 2012. p. 3–7.
6. Young DS, Berwick MC, Jarett L. Evolution of the William Pepper Laboratory. *Clin Chem* 1997;**43**:174–9.
7. Molecular diagnosis. *N Engl J Med* 1968;**278**:276–7.
8. Powers TO, Platzer EG, Hyman BC. Species-specific restriction site polymorphism in root-knot nematode mitochondrial DNA. *J Nematol* 1986;**18**:288–93.
9. Caliceti P, Fassina G, Chaiken IM. Molecular diagnostics using analytical immuno high performance liquid affinity chromatography. *Appl Biochem Biotechnol* 1987;**16**:119–28.

10. Fourney RM, Dietrich KD, Paterson MC. Rapid DNA extraction and sensitive alkaline blotting protocol: application for detection of gene rearrangement and amplification for clinical molecular diagnosis. *Dis Markers* 1989;**7**:15–26.
11. Chiu RW, Lo YM, Wittwer CT. Molecular diagnostics: a revolution in progress. *Clin Chem* 2015;**61**:1–3.
12. EU Directive 2013/55/EU. The recognition of professional qualifications. Proposing a common training framework for specialists in laboratory medicine across the European Union 2013. <http://www.ukipg.org.uk/meetings/international_and_european_forum/ctf_e4_bid>; 2013.
13. Hallworth MJ, Epner PL, Ebert C, et al. Current evidence and future perspectives on the effective practice of patient-centered laboratory medicine. *Clin Chem* 2015;**61**(4):589–99.
14. Hofmann BM. Too much technology. *BMJ* 2015;**350**:h705.
15. Council of Europe. Additional protocol to the convention for the protection of human rights and dignity of the human being with regard to the application of biology and medicine on biomedical research. *Law Hum Genome Rev* 2004;**21**:201–14.
16. McMurray J, Zerah S, Hallworth M, et al. The European Register of Specialists in Clinical Chemistry and Laboratory Medicine: code of conduct, version 2—2008. *Clin Chem* 2009;**47**:372–5.
17. Annesley TM, Boyd JC, Rifai N, et al. Publication ethics: clinical chemistry editorial standards. *Clin Chem* 2009;**55**:1–4.
18. International Committee of Medical Journal Editors. Uniform requirements for manuscripts submitted to biomedical journals: writing and editing for biomedical publication. <http://www.icmje.org/recommendations/browse/manuscript-preparation/>.
19. Graf CWE, Bowman A, Fiack S, et al. Best practice guidelines on publication ethics: a publisher's perspective. *Int J Clin Pract Suppl* 2007;**61**:1–26.
20. Rifai N, Bossuyt PM, Ioannidis JP, et al. Registering diagnostic and prognostic trials of tests: is it the right thing to do? *Clin Chem* 2014;**60**:1146–52.
21. Altman DG. The time has come to register diagnostic and prognostic research. *Clin Chem* 2014;**60**:580–2.
22. Bossuyt PM, Reitsma JB, Bruns DE, et al. The STARD statement for reporting studies of diagnostic accuracy: explanation and elaboration. *Clin Chem* 2003;**49**:7–18.
23. Moons KG, Altman DG, Reitsma JB, et al. Transparent reporting of a multivariable prediction model for individual prognosis or diagnosis (TRIPOD): explanation and elaboration. *Ann Intern Med* 2015;**162**:W1–73.
24. Malone B. Ethics code changes for diagnostics manufacturers. *Clin Lab News* 2009;**35**.
25. Institute of Medicine. Conflict of interest in medical research, education and practice. <http://www.nationalacademies.org/hmd/Reports/2009/Conflict-of-Interest-in-Medical-Research-Education-and-Practice.aspx>.
26. Advanced Medical Technology Association. Code of Eethics on interactions with health care professionals. <http://wwwadvamed.org/NR/rdonlyres/FA43745F-4C75-43B2-A900-C9470BA8DFA7/0/coe_with_faqs_41505.pdf>; 2009.
27. European Diagnostics Manufacturers Association. Part A: interaction with health care professionals. <http://www.edma-ivd.be/uploads/AboutUs/110519_global_compliance_statement2011.pdf>; 2011.

2

Statistical Methodologies in Laboratory Medicine: Analytical and Clinical Evaluation of Laboratory Tests

Kristian Linnet, Karel G.M. Moons, and James C. Boyd

ABSTRACT

Background

The careful selection and evaluation of laboratory tests are key steps in the process of implementing new measurement procedures in the laboratory for clinical use. Method evaluation in the clinical laboratory is complex and in most countries is a regulated process guided by various professional recommendations and quality standards on best laboratory practice.

Content

This chapter deals with the statistical aspects of both analytical and clinical evaluations of laboratory assays, tests, or markers. After a short overview on basic statistics, aspects such as accuracy, precision, trueness, limit of detection, and selectivity are considered in the first part. After dealing with comparison of assays in detail, including using difference plots and regression analysis, the focus is on quantification of the (added) diagnostic value of laboratory assays or tests. First, the evaluation of tests in isolation is outlined, which corresponds to simple diagnostic scenarios, when only a single test result is decisive (eg, in the screening context). Subsequently, the chapter addresses the more common clinical situation in which a laboratory assay or test is considered as part of a diagnostic workup and thus a test's added value is at issue. This involves use of receiver operating characteristic (ROC) areas, reclassification measures, predictiveness curves, and decision curve analysis. Finally, principles for considering the clinical impact of diagnostic tests on actual decision making and patient outcomes are discussed.

ASSAY SELECTION OVERVIEW

The introduction of new or revised laboratory tests, markers, or assays is a common occurrence in the clinical laboratory. Test selection and evaluation are key steps in the process of implementing new measurement procedures (Fig. 2.1). A new or revised test must be selected carefully and its analytical and clinical performance evaluated thoroughly before it is adopted for routine use in patient care (see later in this chapter and Chapter 9). Establishment of a new or revised laboratory test may also involve evaluation of the features of the automated analyzer on which the test will be implemented. When a new test is to be introduced to the routine clinical laboratory, a series of technical or analytical evaluations is commonly conducted. Assay imprecision is estimated, and comparison of the new assay versus an existing one is commonly undertaken. The allowable measurement range is assessed with estimation of the lower and upper limits of quantification. Interferences and carryover are evaluated when relevant. Depending on the situation, a limited verification of manufacturer claims may be all that is necessary, or, in the case of a newly developed test or assay, a full validation may be carried out. Subsequent subsections provide details for all these test evaluations. With regard to evaluation of reference intervals or medical decision limits, readers are referred to Chapter 8.

Evaluation of tests, markers, or assays in the clinical laboratory is influenced strongly by guidelines and accreditation or other regulatory standards.[1-3] The Clinical and Laboratory Standards Institute (CLSI, formerly the National Committee for Clinical Laboratory Standards [NCCLS]) has published a series of consensus protocols (CLIAs) for clinical chemistry laboratories and manufacturers to follow when evaluating methods (see the CLSI website at http://www.clsi.org). The International Organization for Standardization (ISO) has also developed several documents related to method evaluation (ISOs). In addition, meeting laboratory accreditation requirements has become an important aspect in the evaluation process with accrediting agencies placing increased focus on the importance of total quality management and assessment of trueness and precision of laboratory measurements. An accompanying trend has been the emergence of an international nomenclature to standardize the terminology used for characterizing laboratory test or assay performance.

This chapter presents an overview of considerations in and methods for the evaluation of laboratory tests. This includes explanation of graphical and statistical methods that are used to aid in the test evaluation process; examples of the application of these methods are provided, and current terminology within the area is summarized. Key terms and abbreviations are listed in Box 2.1.

Medical Need and Quality Goals

The selection of the appropriate clinical laboratory assays is a vital part of rendering optimal patient care. Advances in patient care are frequently based on the use of new or improved laboratory tests or measurements. Ascertainment

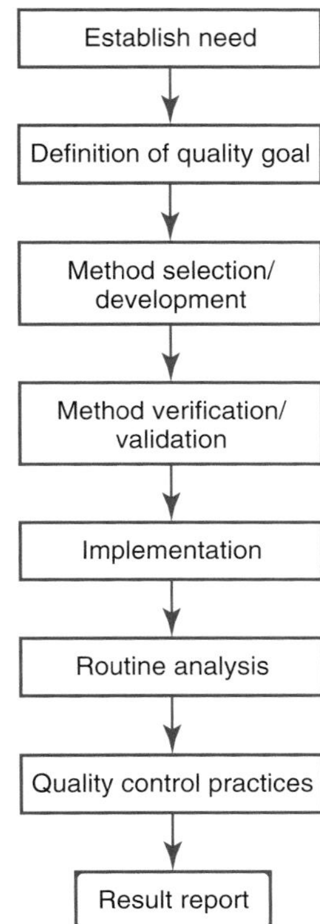

FIGURE 2.1 A flow diagram that illustrates the process of introducing a new assay into routine use.

of what is necessary clinically from a new or revised laboratory test is the first step in selecting the appropriate candidate test. Key parameters, such as desired turnaround time and necessary clinical utility for an assay, are often derived by discussions between laboratorians and clinicians. When new diagnostic assays are introduced, for example, reliable estimates of its diagnostic performance (eg, predictive values, sensitivity and specificity) must be considered. With established analytes, a common scenario is the replacement of an older, labor-intensive test with a new, automated assay that is more economical in daily use. In these situations, consideration must be given to whether the candidate assay has sufficient precision, accuracy, analytical measurement range, and freedom from interference to provide clinically useful results (see Fig. 2.1).

Analytical Performance Criteria

In evaluation of a laboratory test, (1) trueness (formerly termed accuracy), (2) precision, (3) analytical range, (4) detection limit, and (5) analytical specificity are of prime importance. The sections in this chapter on laboratory test evaluation and comparison contain detailed outlines of these concepts. Estimated test performance parameters should be related to analytical performance specifications that ensure acceptable clinical use of the test and its results. For more details related to the recommended models for setting analytical performance specifications, readers are referred to Chapters 6 and 7. From a practical point of view, the "ruggedness" of the test in routine use is of importance and reliable performance, when used by different operators and with different batches of reagents over long time periods, is essential.

When a new laboratory analyzer is at issue, various instrumental parameters require evaluation, including (1) pipetting, (2) specimen-to-specimen carryover, (3) reagent lot-to-lot variation, (4) detector imprecision, (5) time to first reportable result, (6) onboard reagent stability, (7) overall throughput, (8) mean time between instrument failures, and (9) mean time to repair. Information on most of these parameters should be available from the instrument manufacturer; the manufacturer should also be able to furnish information on what studies should be conducted in estimating these parameters for an individual analyzer. Assessment of reagent lot-to-lot variation is especially difficult for a user, and the manufacturer should provide this information.

Other Criteria

Various categories of laboratory tests may be considered. New tests may require "in-house" development. (Note: Such a test is also referred to as a laboratory-developed test [LDT].) Commercial kit assays, on the other hand, are ready for implementation in the laboratory, often in a "closed" analytical system on a dedicated instrument. When prospective assays are reviewed, attention should be given to the following:

1. Principle of the test or assay, with original references
2. Detailed protocol for performing the test
3. Composition of reagents and reference materials, the quantities provided, and their storage requirements (eg, space, temperature, light, humidity restrictions) applicable both before and after the original containers are opened
4. Stability of reagents and reference materials (eg, their shelf lives)
5. Technologist time and required skills
6. Possible hazards and appropriate safety precautions according to relevant guidelines and legislation
7. Type, quantity, and disposal of waste generated
8. Specimen requirements (eg, conditions for collection and transportation, specimen volume requirements, the necessity for anticoagulants and preservatives, necessary storage conditions)
9. Reference interval of the test and its results, including information on how such interval was derived, typical values obtained in both healthy and diseased individuals, and the necessity of determining a reference interval for one's own institution (See Chapter 8 for details on how to generate a reference interval of a laboratory test.)
10. Instrumental requirements and limitations
11. Cost-effectiveness
12. Computer platforms and interfacing with the laboratory information system
13. Availability of technical support, supplies, and service

Other questions concerning placement of the new or revised test in the laboratory should be taken into account. They include:

1. Does the laboratory possess the necessary measuring equipment? If not, is there sufficient space for a new instrument?
2. Does the projected workload match the capacity of a new instrument?
3. Is the test repertoire of a new instrument sufficient?
4. What is the method and frequency of (re)calibration?

BOX 2.1 Abbreviations and Vocabulary Concerning Technical Validation of Assays

Abbreviations

CI	Confidence interval
CV	Coefficient of variation (= SD/*x*, where *x* is the concentration)
CV%	= CV × 100%
CV_A	Analytical coefficient of variation
CV_G	Between-subject biological variation
CV_I	Within-subject biological variation
CV_{RB}	Sample-related random bias coefficient of variation
DoD	Distribution of differences (plot)
ISO	International Organization for Standardization
IUPAC	International Union of Pure and Applied Chemistry
OLR	Ordinary least-squares regression analysis
SD	Standard deviation
SEM	Standard error of the mean (= $SD/\sqrt{N}$)
SD_A	Analytical standard deviation
SD_{RB}	Sample-related random bias standard deviation
x_m	Mean
x_{mv}	Weighted mean
WLR	Weighted least-squares regression analysis

Vocabulary*

Analyte Compound that is measured.

Bias Difference between the average (strictly the expectation) of the test results and an accepted reference value (ISO 3534-1). Bias is a measure of trueness.[11]

Certified reference material (CRM) is a reference material, one or more of whose property values are certified by a technically valid procedure, accompanied by or traceable to a certificate or other documentation that is issued by a certifying body.

Commutability Ability of a material to yield the same results of measurement by a given set of measurement procedures.

Limit of detection The lowest amount of analyte in a sample that can be detected but not quantified as an exact value. Also called lower limit of detection or minimum detectable concentration (or dose or value).[23]

Lower limit of quantification (LLOQ) The lowest concentration at which the measurement procedure fulfills specifications for imprecision and bias (corresponds to the *lower limit of determination* mentioned under *Measuring interval*).

Matrix All components of a material system except the analyte.

Measurand The "quantity" that is actually measured (eg, the concentration of the analyte). For example, if the analyte is glucose, the measurand is the concentration of glucose. For an enzyme, the measurand may be the enzyme *activity* or the *mass concentration* of enzyme.

Measuring interval Closed interval of possible values allowed by a measurement procedure and delimited by the *lower limit of determination* and the *higher limit of determination*. For this interval, the total error of the measurements is within specified limits for the method. Also called the *analytical measurement range*.

Primary measurement standard Standard that is designated or widely acknowledged as having the highest metrologic qualities and whose value is accepted without reference to other standards of the same quantity.[73]

Quantity The amount of substance (eg, the concentration of substance).

Reference material (RM) A material or substance, one or more properties of which are sufficiently well established to be used for the calibration of a method or for assigning values to materials.

Random error Arises from unpredictable variations in influence quantities. These random effects give rise to variations in repeated observations of the measurand.

Reference measurement procedure Thoroughly investigated measurement procedure shown to yield values having an uncertainty of measurement commensurate with its intended use, especially in assessing the trueness of other measurement procedures for the same quantity and in characterizing reference materials.

Selectivity or specificity Degree to which a method responds uniquely to the required analyte.

Systematic error A component of error that, in the course of a number of analyses of the same measurand, remains constant or varies in a predictable way.

Traceability "The property of the result of a measurement or the value of a standard whereby it can be related to stated references, usually national or international standards, through an unbroken chain of comparisons all having stated uncertainties."[43] This is achieved by establishing a chain of calibrations leading to primary national or international standards, ideally (for long-term consistency) the Système Internationale (SI) units of measurement.

Uncertainty A parameter associated with the result of a measurement that characterizes the dispersion of values that could reasonably be attributed to the measurand. More briefly, *uncertainty* is a parameter characterizing the range of values within which the value of the quantity being measured is expected to lie.

Upper limit of quantification (ULOQ) The highest concentration at which the measurement procedure fulfills specifications for imprecision and bias (corresponds to the *upper limit of determination* mentioned under *Measuring interval*).

*A listing of terms of relevance in relation to analytical methods is displayed. Many of the definitions originate from Dybkær[12] with statement of original source where relevant (eg, International Organization for Standardization document number). Others are derived from the Eurachem/Citac guideline on uncertainty.[79] In some cases, slight modifications have been performed for the sake of simplicity.

5. Is staffing of the laboratory sufficient for the new technology?
6. If training the entire staff in a new technique is required, is such training worth the possible benefits?
7. How frequently will quality control (QC) samples be run?
8. What materials will be used to ensure QC?
9. What approach will be used for proficiency testing?
10. What is the estimated cost of performing an assay using the proposed method, including the costs of calibrators, QC specimens, and technologists' time? Questions applicable to implementation of new instrumentation in a particular laboratory may also be relevant. Does the instrument satisfy local electrical safety guidelines? What

are the power, water, drainage, and air conditioning requirements of the instrument? If the instrument is large, does the floor have sufficient load-bearing capacity?

A qualitative assessment of all these factors is often completed, but it is possible to use a value scale to assign points to the various features weighted according to their relative importance; the latter approach allows a more quantitative test evaluation process. Decisions are then made regarding the assays that best fit the laboratory's requirements and that have the potential for achieving the necessary analytical quality for clinical use.

BASIC STATISTICS

In this section, fundamental statistical concepts and techniques are introduced in the context of typical analytical investigations. The basic concepts of (1) populations, (2) samples, (3) parameters, (4) statistics, and (5) probability distributions are defined and illustrated. Two important probability distributions—Gaussian and Student *t*—are introduced and discussed.

Frequency Distribution

A graphical device for displaying a large set of laboratory test results is the *frequency distribution,* also called a *histogram.* Fig. 2.2 shows a frequency distribution displaying the results of serum gamma-glutamyltransferase (GGT) measurements of 100 apparently healthy 20- to 29-year-old men. The frequency distribution is constructed by dividing the measurement scale into cells of equal width; counting the number, n_i, of values that fall within each cell; and drawing a rectangle above each cell whose area (and height because the cell widths are all equal) is proportional to n_i. In this example, the selected cells were 5 to 9, 10 to 14, 15 to 19, 20 to 24, 25 to 29, and so on, with 60 to 64 being the last cell (range of values, 5–64 U/L). The ordinate axis of the frequency distribution gives the number of values falling within each cell. When this number is divided by the total number of values in the data set, the relative frequency in each cell is obtained.

Often, the position of the value for an individual within a distribution of values is useful medically. The *nonparametric* approach can be used to determine directly the *percentile* of a given subject. Having ranked *N* subjects according to their values, the *n*-percentile, Perc_n, may be estimated as the value of the $[N(n/100) + 0.5]$ ordered observation.[4] In the case of

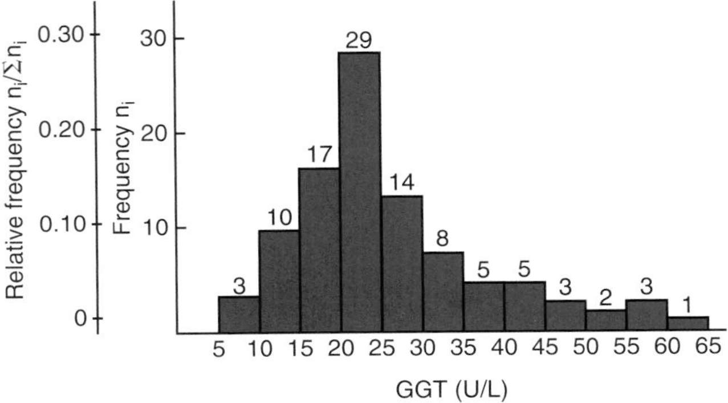

FIGURE 2.2 Frequency distribution of 100 gamma-glutamyltransferase (GGT) values.

a noninteger value, interpolation is carried out between neighbor values. The 50th percentile is the median of the distribution.

Population and Sample

It is useful to obtain information and draw conclusions about the characteristics of the test results for one or more target populations. In the GGT example, interest is focused on the location and spread of the population of GGT values for 20- to 29-year-old healthy men. Thus, a working definition of a *population* is the complete set of all observations that might occur as a result of performing a particular procedure according to specified conditions.

Most target populations of interest in clinical chemistry are in principle very large (millions of individuals) and so are impossible to study in their entirety. Usually a subgroup of observations is taken from the population as a basis for forming conclusions about population characteristics. The group of observations that has actually been selected from the population is called a *sample.* For example, the 100 GGT values make up a sample from a respective target population. However, a sample is used to study the characteristics of a population only if it has been properly selected. For instance, if the analyst is interested in the population of GGT values over various lots of materials and some time period, the sample must be selected to be representative of these factors, as well as of age, sex, and health factors of the individuals in the targeted population. Consequently, exact specification of the target population(s) is necessary before a plan for obtaining the sample(s) can be designed. In this chapter, a sample is also used as a specimen, depending on the context.

Probability and Probability Distributions

Consider again the frequency distribution in Fig. 2.2. In addition to the general location and spread of the GGT determinations, other useful information can be easily extracted from this frequency distribution. For instance, 96% (96 of 100) of the determinations are less than 55 U/L, and 91% (91 of 100) are greater than or equal to 10 but less than 50 U/L. Because the cell interval is 5 U/L in this example, statements such as these can be made only to the nearest 5 U/L. A larger sample would allow a smaller cell interval and more refined statements. For a sufficiently large sample, the cell interval can be made so small that the frequency distribution can be approximated by a continuous, smooth curve, similar to that shown in Fig. 2.3. In fact, if the sample is large enough, we can consider this a close representation of the "true" target *population frequency distribution.* In general, the functional form of the population frequency distribution curve of a variable *x* is denoted by $f(x)$.

The population frequency distribution allows us to make probability statements about the GGT of a randomly selected member of the population of healthy 20- to 29-year-old men. For example, the probability $\Pr(x > x_a)$ that the GGT value *x* of a randomly selected 20- to 29-year-old healthy man is greater than some particular value x_a is equal to the area under the population frequency distribution to the right of x_a. If $x_a = 58$, then from Fig. 2.3, $\Pr(x > 58) = 0.05$. Similarly, the probability $\Pr(x_a < x < x_b)$ that *x* is greater than x_a but less than x_b is equal to the area under the population frequency distribution between x_a and x_b. For example, if $x_a = 9$ and $x_b = 58$, then from Fig. 2.3, $\Pr(9 < x < 58) = 0.90$. Because the

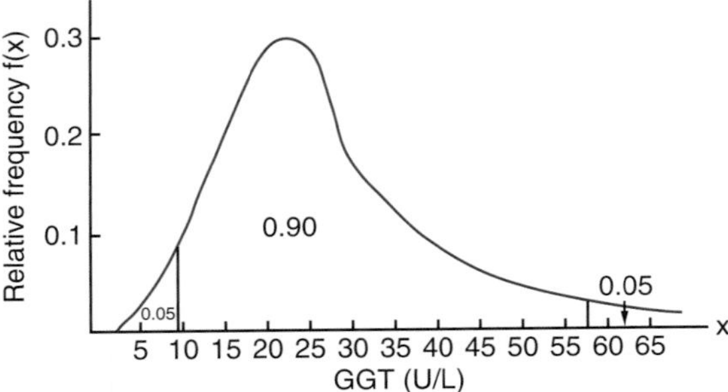

FIGURE 2.3 Population frequency distribution of gamma-glutamyltransferase (GGT) values.

population frequency distribution provides all information related to probabilities of a randomly selected member of the population, it is called the probability distribution of the population. Although the true probability distribution is never exactly known in practice, it can be approximated with a large sample of observations, that is, test results.

Parameters: Descriptive Measures of a Population

Any population of values can be described by measures of its characteristics. A *parameter* is a constant that describes some particular characteristic of a population. Although most populations of interest in analytical work are infinite in size, for the following definitions, we shall consider the population to be of finite size N, where N is very large.

One important characteristic of a population is its *central location*. The parameter most commonly used to describe the central location of a population of N values is the *population mean* (μ):

$$\mu = \frac{\sum x_i}{N}$$

An alternative parameter that indicates the central tendency of a population is the *median*, which is defined as the 50th percentile, Perc_{50}.

Another important characteristic is the *dispersion* of values about the population mean. A parameter very useful in describing this dispersion of a population of N values is the *population variance* σ^2 (sigma squared):

$$\sigma^2 = \frac{\sum (x_i - \mu)^2}{N}$$

The *population standard deviation (SD)* σ, the positive square root of the population variance, is a parameter frequently used to describe the population dispersion in the same units (eg, mg/dL) as the population values. For a Gaussian distribution, 95% of the population of values are located within the mean $\pm 1.96\ \sigma$. If a distribution is non-Gaussian (eg, asymmetric), an alternative measure of dispersion based on the percentiles may be more appropriate, such as the distance between the 25th and 75th percentiles (the interquartile interval).

Statistics: Descriptive Measures of the Sample

As noted earlier, clinical chemists usually have at hand only a sample of observations (ie, test results) from the overarching targeted population. A *statistic* is a value calculated from the observations in a sample to estimate a particular characteristic of the target population. As introduced earlier, the sample mean x_m is the arithmetical average of a sample, which is an estimate of μ. Likewise, the sample SD is an estimate of σ, and the coefficient of variation (CV) is the ratio of the SD to the mean multiplied by 100%. The equations used to calculate x_m, SD, and CV, respectively, are as follows:

$$x_m = \frac{\sum x_i}{N}$$

$$SD = \sqrt{\frac{\sum (x_i - x_m)^2}{N-1}} = \sqrt{\frac{\sum x_i^2 - \frac{\left(\sum x_i\right)^2}{N}}{N-1}}$$

$$CV = \frac{SD}{x_m} \times 100\%$$

where x_i is an individual measurement and N is the number of sample measurements.

The SD is an estimate of the dispersion of the distribution. Additionally, from the SD, we can derive an estimate of the uncertainty of X_m as an estimate of μ (see later discussion).

Random Sampling

A random sample of individuals from a target population is one in which each member of the population has an equal chance of being selected. A *random sample* is one in which each member of the sample can be considered to be a random selection from the target population. Although much of statistical analysis and interpretation depends on the assumption of a random sample from some population, actual data collection often does not satisfy this assumption. In particular, for sequentially generated data, it is often true that observations adjacent to each other tend to be more alike than observations separated in time.

The Gaussian Probability Distribution

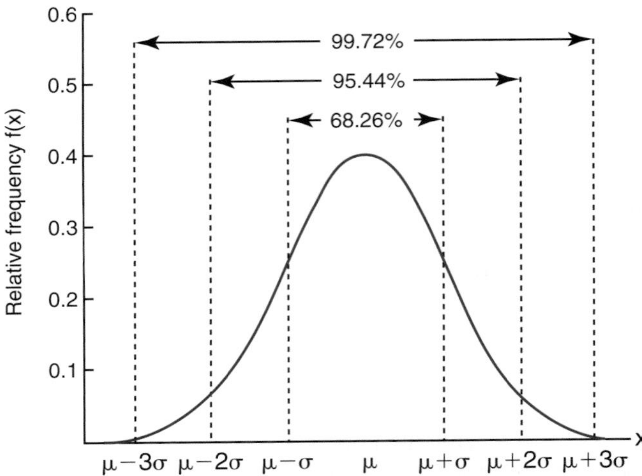

FIGURE 2.4 The Gaussian probability distribution.

The *Gaussian* probability distribution, illustrated in Fig. 2.4, is of fundamental importance in statistics for several reasons. As mentioned earlier, a particular test result x will not usually be equal to the true value μ of the specimen being measured. Rather, associated with this particular test result x will be a particular measurement error $\varepsilon = x - \mu$, which is the result of many contributing sources of error. Pure measurement errors tend to follow a probability distribution similar to that shown in Fig. 2.4, where the errors are symmetrically distributed, with smaller errors occurring more frequently than larger ones, and with an expected value of 0. This important fact is known as the central limit effect for distribution of errors: if a measurement error ε is the sum of many independent sources of error, such as $\varepsilon_1, \varepsilon_2, \ldots, \varepsilon_k$, several of which are major contributors, the probability distribution of the measurement error ε will tend to be Gaussian as the number of sources of error becomes large.

Another reason for the importance of the Gaussian probability distribution is that many statistical procedures are based on the assumption of a Gaussian distribution of values; this approach is commonly referred to as *parametric.* Furthermore, these procedures usually are not seriously invalidated by departures from this assumption. Finally, the magnitude of the uncertainty associated with sample statistics can be ascertained based on the fact that many sample statistics computed from large samples have a Gaussian probability distribution.

The Gaussian probability distribution is completely characterized by its mean μ and its variance σ^2. The notation $N(\mu, \sigma^2)$ is often used for the distribution of a variable that is Gaussian with mean μ and variance σ^2. Probability statements about a variable x that follows an $N(\mu, \sigma^2)$ distribution are usually made by considering the variable z,

$$z = \frac{x - \mu}{\sigma}$$

which is called the *standard Gaussian variable*. The variable z has a Gaussian probability distribution with $\mu = 0$ and $\sigma^2 = 1$, that is, z is $N(0, 1)$. The probably that x is within 2 σ of μ [ie, $\Pr(|x - \mu|<2\sigma) =$] is 0.9544. Most computer spreadsheet programs can calculate probabilities for all values of z.

Student *t* Probability Distribution

To determine probabilities associated with a Gaussian distribution, it is necessary to know the population SD σ. In actual practice, σ is often unknown, so we cannot calculate z. However, if a random sample can be taken from the Gaussian population, we can calculate the sample SD, substitute SD for σ, and compute the value t:

$$t = \frac{x - \mu}{SD}$$

Under these conditions, the variable t has a probability distribution called the *Student* t *distribution*. The t distribution is really a family of distributions depending on the degrees of freedom ν ($= N - 1$) for the sample SD. Several t distributions from this family are shown in Fig. 2.5. When the size of the sample and the degrees of freedom for SD are infinite, there is no uncertainty in SD, so the t distribution is identical to the standard Gaussian distribution. However, when the sample size is small, the uncertainty in SD causes the t distribution to have greater dispersion and heavier tails than the standard Gaussian distribution, as illustrated in Fig. 2.5. At sample sizes above 30, the difference between the t-distribution and the Gaussian distribution becomes relatively small and can usually be neglected. Most computer spreadsheet programs can calculate probabilities for all values of t, given the degrees of freedom for SD.

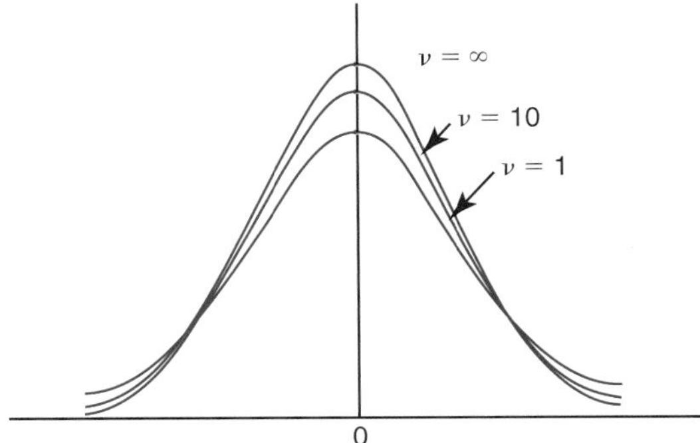

FIGURE 2.5 The t distribution for $\nu = 1$, 10, and ∞.

The Student t distribution is commonly used in significance tests, such as comparison of sample means, or in testing conducted if a regression slope differs significantly from 1. Descriptions of these tests can be found in statistics textbooks.[5] Another important application is the estimation of confidence intervals (CIs). CIs are intervals that indicate the uncertainty of a given sample estimate. For example, it can be proved that $X_m \pm t_{alpha}$ $(SD/N^{0.5})$ provides an approximate 2*alpha*-CI for the mean. A common value for *alpha* is 0.025 or 2.5%, which thus results in a 0.95% or 95% CI. Given sample sizes of 30 or higher, t_{alpha} is ca. 2. $(SD/N^{0.5})$ is called the standard error (SE) of the mean. A CI should be interpreted as follows. Suppose a sampling experiment of drawing 30 observations from a Gaussian population of values is repeated 100 times, and in each case, the 95% CI of the mean is calculated as described. Then, in 95% of the drawings, the true mean μ is included in the 95% CI. The popular interpretation is that for an estimated 95% CI, there is 95% chance that the true mean is within the interval. According to the central limit theorem, distributions of mean values converge toward the Gaussian distribution irrespective of the primary type of distribution of x. This means that the 95% CI is a robust estimate only minimally influenced by deviations from the Gaussian distribution. In the same way, the t-test is robust toward deviations from normality.

Nonparametric Statistics

Distribution-free statistics, often called nonparametric statistics, provides an alternative to parametric statistical procedures that assume data to have Gaussian distributions. For example, distributions of reference values are often skewed and so do not conform to the Gaussian distribution (see Chapter 8 on reference intervals). Formally, one can carry out a goodness of fit test to judge whether a distribution is Gaussian or not.[5] A commonly used test is the Kolmogorov-Smirnov test, in which the shape of the sample distribution is compared with the shape presumed for a Gaussian distribution. If the difference exceeds a given critical value, the hypothesis of a Gaussian distribution is rejected, and it is then appropriate to apply nonparametric statistics. A special problem is the occurrence of outlier, (ie, single measurements highly deviating from the remaining measurements). Outliers may rely on biological factors and so be of real significance (eg, in the context of estimating reference intervals or be related to clerical errors). Special tests exist for handling outliers.[5]

Given that a distribution is non-Gaussian, it is appropriate to apply nonparametric descriptive statistics based on the percentile or quantile concept. As stated under the earlier section Frequency Distribution, the n-percentile, Perc_n, of a sample of N values may be estimated as the value of the $[N(n/100) + 0.5]$ ordered observation.[4] In the case of a non-integer value, interpolation is carried out between neighbor values. The median is the 50th percentile, which is used as a measure of the center of the distribution. For the GGT example mentioned previously, we would order the $N = 100$ values according to size. The median or 50th percentile is then the value of the $[100(50/100) + 0.5 = 50.5]$ ordered observation (the interpolated value between the 50th and 51th ordered values. The 2.5th and 97.5th percentiles are values of the $[100(2.5/100) + 0.5 = 3]$ and $[100(97.5/100) + 0.5 = 98]$ ordered observations, respectively. When a 95% reference interval is estimated, a nonparametric approach is often preferable because many distributions of reference values are asymmetric. Generally, distributions based on the many biological sources of variation are often non-Gaussian compared with distributions of pure measurement errors that usually are Gaussian.

The nonparametric counterpart to the t-test is the Mann-Whitney test, which provides a significance test for the difference between median values of the two groups to be compared.[5] When there are more than two groups, the Kruskall-Wallis test can be applied.[5]

Categorical Variables

Hitherto focus has been on quantitative variables. When dealing with qualitative tests and in the context of evaluating diagnostic testing, categorical variables that only take the value positive or negative come into play. The performance is here given as proportions or percentages, which are proportions multiplied by 100. For example, the diagnostic sensitivity of a test is the proportion of diseased subjects who have a positive result. Having tested, for example, 100 patients, 80 might have had a positive test result. The sensitivity then is 0.8% or 80%. We are then interested in judging how precise this estimate is. Exact estimates of the uncertainty can be derived from the so-called binomial distribution, but for practical purposes, an approximate expression for the 95% CI is usually applied as the estimated proportion $P \pm 2\text{SE}$, where the SE in this context is derived as:

$$\text{SE} = [P(1-P)/N]^{0.5}$$

where P is here a proportion and not a percentage.[5] In the example, the SE equals 0.0016 and so the 95% CI is 0.77 to 0.83 or 77% to 83%. The applied approximate formula for the SE is regarded as reasonably valid when NP and $N(1 - P)$ both are equal to or higher than 5.

TECHNICAL VALIDITY OF ANALYTICAL ASSAYS

This section defines the basic concepts used in this chapter: (1) calibration, (2) trueness and accuracy, (3) precision, (4) linearity, (5) limit of detection, (6) limit of quantification, (7) specificity, and (8) others (see Box 2.1 for definitions).

POINTS TO REMEMBER

- Statistics as means, SDs, percentiles, proportions, and so on are computed from a sample of values drawn from a population and provide *estimates* of the unknown population characteristics.
- Whereas parametric statistics rely on the assumption of a Gaussian population of values, which typically applies for measurement errors, nonparametric statistics is a distribution-free approach that apply to, for example, asymmetric distributions often observed for biologic variables.
- The Gaussian distribution is characterized by the mean and the SD, and other types of distributions are described by the median and the percentile (quantile) values.
- Distributions of categorical variables are characterized by proportions or percentages and their SEs.

Calibration

The calibration function is the relation between instrument signal (y) and concentration of analyte (x), that is,

$$y = f(x)$$

The inverse of this function, also called the measuring function, yields the concentration from response:

$$x = f^{-1}(y)$$

This relationship is established by measurement of samples with known quantities of analyte[6] (calibrators). One may distinguish between solutions of pure chemical standards and samples with known quantities of analyte present in the typical matrix that is to be measured (eg, human serum). The first situation applies typically to a reference measurement procedure that is not influenced by matrix effects; the second case corresponds typically to a routine method that often is influenced by matrix components and so preferably is calibrated using the relevant matrix.[7] Calibration functions may be linear or curved and, in the case of immunoassays, may often take a special form (eg, modeled by the four-parameter logistic curve).[8] This model (logistic in log x) has been used for immunoassay techniques and is written in several forms (Table 2.1). An alternative, model-free approach is to estimate a smoothed spline curve, which often is

TABLE 2.1 The Four-Parameter Logistic Model Expressed in Three Different Forms

Algebraic Form	Variables*	Parameters†
$y = (a - d)/[1 + (x/c)^b] + d$	(x, y)	a, b, c, d
$R = R_0 + K_c/[1 + \exp(-\{a + b \log[C]\})]$	(C, R)	R_0, K_c, a, b
$y = y_0 + (y_¥ - y_0)(x^d)/(b + x^d)$	(x, y)	y_0, $y_¥$, b, d

*Concentration and instrument response variables shown in parentheses.

†Equivalent letters do not necessarily denote equivalent parameters.

performed for immunoassays; however, a disadvantage of the spline curve approach is that it is insensitive to aberrant calibration values, fitting these just as well as the correct values. If the assumed calibration function does not correctly reflect the true relationship between instrument response and analyte concentration, a systematic error or bias is likely to be associated with the analytical method. A common problem with some immunoassays is the "hook effect," which is a deviation from the expected calibration algorithm in the high-concentration range. (The hook effect is discussed in more detail in Chapter 23.)

The precision of the analytical method depends on the stability of the instrument response for a given quantity of analyte. In principle, a random dispersion of instrument signal (vertical direction) at a given true concentration transforms into dispersion on the measurement scale (horizontal direction), as is shown schematically (Fig. 2.6). The detailed statistical aspects of calibration are complex,[5,9] but in the following sections, some approximate relations are outlined. If the calibration function is linear and the imprecision of the signal response is the same over the analytical measurement range, the analytical SD (SD_A) of the method tends to be constant over the analytical measurement range (see Fig. 2.6). If the imprecision increases proportionally to the signal response, the analytical SD of the method tends to increase proportionally to the concentration *(x)*, which means that the *relative* imprecision ($CV = SD/x$) may be constant over the analytical measurement range if it is assumed that the intercept of the calibration line is zero.

With modern, automated clinical chemistry instruments, the relation between analyte concentration and signal can in some cases be very stable, and where this is the case, calibration is necessary relatively infrequently[10] (eg, at intervals of several months). Built-in process control mechanisms may help ensure that the relationship remains stable and may indicate when recalibration is necessary. In traditional chromatographic analysis (eg, high-performance liquid chromatography [HPLC]), on the other hand, it is customary to calibrate each analytical series (run), which means that calibration is carried out daily.

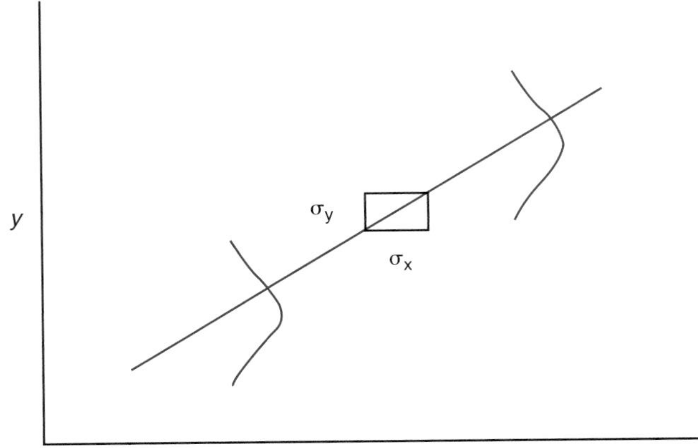

FIGURE 2.6 Relation between concentration *(x)* and signal response *(y)* for a linear calibration function. The dispersion in signal response (σ_y) is projected onto the *x*-axis and is called assay imprecision [σ_x (=σ_A)].

Trueness and Accuracy

Trueness of measurements is defined as closeness of agreement between the average value obtained from a large series of results of measurements and the true value.[11]

The difference between the average value (strictly, the mathematical expectation) and the true value is the *bias*, which is expressed numerically and so is inversely related to the trueness. *Trueness* in itself is a qualitative term that can be expressed, for example, as low, medium, or high. From a theoretical point of view, the exact true value for a clinical sample is not available; instead, an "accepted reference value" is used, which is the "true" value that can be determined in practice.[12] Trueness can be evaluated by comparison of measurements by the new test and by some preselected reference measurement procedure, both on the same sample or individuals.

The ISO has introduced the trueness expression as a replacement for the term *accuracy*, which now has gained a slightly different meaning. *Accuracy* is the closeness of agreement between the result of a measurement and a true concentration of the analyte.[11] Accuracy thus is influenced by both bias and imprecision and in this way reflects the total error. Accuracy, which in itself is a qualitative term, is inversely related to the "uncertainty" of measurement, which can be quantified as described later (Table 2.2).

In relation to trueness, the concepts *recovery*, *drift*, and *carryover* may also be considered. *Recovery* is the fraction or percentage increase in concentration that is measured in relation to the amount added. Recovery experiments are typically carried out in the field of drug analysis. One may distinguish between *extraction recovery*, which often is interpreted as the fraction of compound that is carried through an extraction process, and the recovery measured by the entire analytical procedure, in which the addition of an internal standard compensates for losses in the extraction procedure. A recovery close to 100% is a prerequisite for a high degree of trueness, but it does not ensure unbiased results because possible nonspecificity against matrix components (eg, an interfering substance) is not detected in a recovery experiment. *Drift* is caused by instrument or reagent instability over time, so that calibration becomes gradually biased. Assay *carryover* also must be close to zero to ensure unbiased results. Carryover can be assessed by placing a sample with a known, low value

TABLE 2.2 An Overview of Qualitative Terms and Quantitative Measures Related to Method Performance

Qualitative Concept	Quantitative Measure
Trueness	Bias
Closeness of agreement of mean value with "true value"	A measure of the systematic error
Precision	Imprecision (SD)
Repeatability (within run) Intermediate precision (long term) Reproducibility (inter-laboratory)	A measure of the dispersion of random errors
Accuracy	*Error of measurement*
Closeness of agreement of a single measurement with "true value"	Comprises both random and systematic influences

after a pathological sample with a high value, and an observed increase can be stated as a percentage of the high value.[13] Drift or carryover or both may be conveniently estimated by multifactorial evaluation protocols.[14,15]

Precision

Precision has been defined as the closeness of agreement between independent results of measurements obtained under stipulated conditions.[12] The degree of precision is usually expressed on the basis of statistical measures of imprecision, such as SD or CV (CV = SD/x, where x is the measurement concentration), which is inversely related to precision. Imprecision of measurements is solely related to the random error of measurements and has no relation to the trueness of measurements.

Precision is specified as follows:[11,12]

Repeatability: closeness of agreement between results of successive measurements carried out under the same conditions (ie, corresponding to within-run precision)

Reproducibility: closeness of agreement between results of measurements performed under changed conditions of measurements (eg, time, operators, calibrators, reagent lots). Two specifications of reproducibility are often used: total or between-run precision in the laboratory, often termed *intermediate precision,* and interlaboratory precision (eg, as observed in external quality assessment schemes [EQAS]) (see Table 2.2).

The total SD (σ_T) may be divided into within-run and between-run components using the principle of analysis of variance of components[5] (variance is the squared SD):

$$\sigma^2_T = \sigma^2_{\text{Within-run}} + \sigma^2_{\text{Between-run}}$$

It is not always clear in clinical chemistry publications what is meant by "between-run" variation. Some authors use the term to refer to the total variation of an assay, but others apply the term *between-run variance component* as defined earlier. The distinction between these definitions is important but is not always explicitly stated.

In laboratory studies of analytical variation, estimates of imprecision are obtained. The more observations, the more certain are the estimates. It is important to have an adequate number so that that analytical variation is not underestimated. Commonly, the number 20 is given as a reasonable number of observations (eg, suggested in the CLSI guideline for manufacturers).[16] To verify method precision by users, it has been recommended to run internal QC samples for 5 consecutive days in 5 replicates.[17] If too few replications are applied, it is likely that the analytical variation will be underestimated.

To estimate both the within-run imprecision and the total imprecision, a common approach is to measure duplicate control samples in a series of runs. Suppose, for example, that a control is measured in duplicate for 20 runs, in which case 20 observations are present with respect to both components. The dispersion of the means (x_m) of the duplicates is given as follows:

$$\sigma^2_{xm} = \sigma^2_{\text{Within-run}} / 2 + \sigma^2_{\text{Between-run}}$$

From the 20 sets of duplicates, we may derive the within-run SD using the following formula:

$$\text{SD}_{\text{Within-run}} = [\Sigma d_i^2 / (2 \times 20)]^{0.5}$$

where d_i refers to the difference between the ith set of duplicates. When SDs are estimated, the concept degrees of freedom (df) is used. In a simple situation, the number of degrees of freedom equals $N - 1$. For N duplicates, the number of degrees of freedom is $N(2 - 1) = N$. Thus, both variance components are derived in this way. The advantage of this approach is that the within-run estimate is based on several runs, so that an average estimate is obtained rather than only an estimate for one particular run if all 20 observations had been obtained in the same run. The described approach is a simple example of a *variance component analysis.* The principle can be extended to more components of variation. For example, in the CLSI EP05-A3 guideline,[16] a procedure is outlined that is based on the assumption of two analytical runs per day, in which case within-run, between-run, and between-day components of variance are estimated by a *nested* component of variance analysis approach.

Nothing definitive can be stated about the selected number of 20. Generally, the estimate of the imprecision improves as more observations become available. Exact confidence limits for the SD can be derived from the χ^2 distribution. Estimates of the variance, SD^2, are distributed according to the χ^2 distribution (tabulated in most statistics textbooks) as follows: $(N - 1)\ \text{SD}^2/\sigma^2 \approx \chi^2_{(N-1)}$, where $(N - 1)$ is the degrees of freedom.[5] Then the two-sided 95% CI is derived from the following relation:

$$\Pr[\chi^2_{97.5\%(N-1)} < (N-1)\ \text{SD}^2 / \sigma^2 < \chi^2_{2.5\%(N-1)}] = 0.95$$

which yields this 95% CI expression:

$$\text{SD} \times [(N-1)/\chi^2_{2.5\%(N-1)}]^{0.5} < \sigma < \text{SD} \times [(N-1)/\chi^2_{97.5\%(N-1)}]^{0.5}$$

Example

Suppose we have estimated the imprecision as an SD of 5.0 on the basis of $N = 20$ observations. From a table of the χ^2 distribution, we obtain the following 2.5 and 97.5 percentiles:

$$\chi^2_{2.5\%(19)} = 32.9 \text{ and } \chi^2_{97.5\%(19)} = 8.91$$

where 19 within the parentheses refers to the number of degrees of freedom. Substituting in the equation, we get

$$5.0 \times (19/32.9)^{0.5} < \sigma < 5.0 \times (19/8.91)^{0.5}$$

or

$$3.8 < \sigma < 7.3$$

A graphical display of 95% CIs at various sample sizes is shown in Fig. 2.7. For individual variance components, the relations are more complicated.

Precision Profile

Precision often depends on the concentration of analyte being considered. A presentation of precision as a function of analyte concentration is the precision profile, which usually

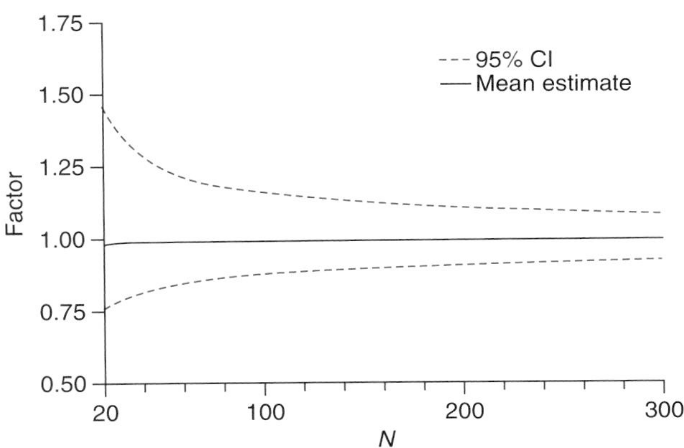

FIGURE 2.7 Relation between factors indicating the 95% confidence intervals (Cis) of standard deviations (SDs) and the sample size. The true SD is 1, and the solid line indicates the mean estimate, which is slightly downward biased at small sample sizes.

is plotted in terms of the SD or the CV as a function of analyte concentration (Fig. 2.8). Some typical examples may be considered. First, the SD may be constant (ie, independent of the concentration), as it often is for analytes with a limited range of values (eg, electrolytes). When the SD is constant, the CV varies inversely with the concentration (ie, it is high in the lower part of the range and low in the high range). For analytes with extended ranges (eg, hormones), the SD frequently increases as the analyte concentration increases. If a proportional relationship exists, the CV is constant. This may often apply approximately over a large part of the analytical measurement range. Actually, this relationship is anticipated for measurement error that arises because of imprecise volume dispensing. Often a more complex relationship exists. Not infrequently, the SD is relatively constant in the low range, so that the CV increases in the area approaching the lower limit of quantification. At intermediate concentrations, the CV may be relatively constant and perhaps may decline somewhat at increasing concentrations. A square root relationship can be used to model the relationship in some situations as an intermediate form of relation between the constant and the proportional case. The relationship between the SD and the concentration is of importance (1) when method specifications over the analytical measurement range are considered, (2) when limits of quantification are determined, and (3) in the context of selecting appropriate statistical methods for method comparison (eg, whether a difference or a relative difference plot should be applied, whether a simple or a weighted regression analysis procedure should be used) (see the "Relative Distribution of Differences Plot" and "Regression Analysis" sections later).

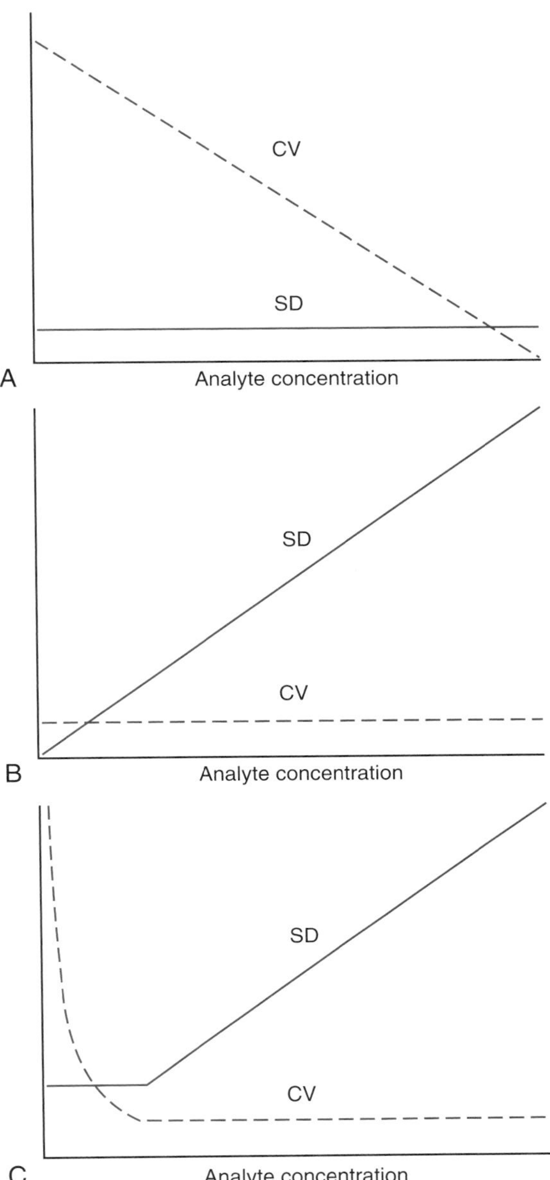

FIGURE 2.8 Relations between analyte concentration and standard deviation (SD)/coefficient of variation (CV). **A,** The SD is constant, so that the CV varies inversely with the analyte concentration. **B,** The CV is constant because of a proportional relationship between concentration and SD. **C,** A mixed situation with constant SD in the low range and a proportional relationship in the rest of the analytical measurement range.

Linearity

Linearity refers to the relationship between measured and expected values over the analytical measurement range. Linearity may be considered in relation to actual or relative analyte concentrations. In the latter case, a dilution series of a sample may be examined. This dilution series examines whether the measured concentration changes as expected according to the proportional relationship between samples introduced by the dilution factor. Dilution is usually carried out with an appropriate sample matrix (eg, human serum [individual or pooled serum] or a verified sample diluent).

Evaluation of linearity may be conducted in various ways. A simple, but subjective, approach is to visually assess whether the relationship between measured and expected concentrations is linear. A more formal evaluation may be carried out on the basis of statistical tests. Various principles may be applied here. When repeated measurements are available at each concentration, the random variation between measurements and the variation around an estimated regression line may be evaluated statistically[18] (by an *F*-test). This approach has been criticized because it relates only the magnitudes of random and systematic error without taking the absolute deviations from linearity into account. For example, if the random variation among measurements is large, a given deviation from linearity may not be declared statistically significant. On the other hand, if the random measurement variation is small, even a very small deviation from linearity that may be clinically unimportant is declared significant. When significant nonlinearity is found, it may be useful to explore nonlinear alternatives to the linear regression line (ie, polynomials of higher degrees).[19]

Another commonly applied approach for detecting nonlinearity is to assess the residuals of an estimated regression line and test whether positive and negative deviations are randomly distributed. This can be carried out by a runs test[20] (see "Regression Analysis" section). An additional consideration for evaluating proportional concentration relationships is whether an estimated regression line passes through zero or not. The presence of linearity is a prerequisite for a high degree of trueness. A CLSI guideline suggests procedure(s) for assessment of linearity.[21]

Analytical Measurement Range and Limits of Quantification

The analytical measurement range (measuring interval, reportable range) is the analyte concentration range over which measurements are within the declared tolerances for imprecision and bias of the method.[12] Taking drug assays as an example, there exist (arbitrary) requirements of a CV% of less than 15% and a bias of less than 15%.[22] The measurement range then extends from the lowest concentration (lower limit of quantification [LLOQ]) to the highest concentration (upper limit of quantification [ULOQ]) for which these performance specifications are fulfilled.

The LLOQ is medically important for many analytes. Thyroid-stimulating hormone (TSH) is a good example. As assay methods improved, lowering the LLOQ, low TSH results could be increasingly distinguished from the lower limit of the reference interval, making the test increasingly useful for the diagnosis of hyperthyroidism.

The limit of detection (LOD) is another characteristic of an assay. The LOD may be defined as the lowest value that significantly exceeds the measurements of a blank sample. Thus, the limit has been estimated on the basis of repeated measurements of a blank sample and has been *reported* as the mean plus 2 or 3 SDs of the blank measurements. In the interval from LOD up to LLOQ, one should report a result as "detected" but not provide a quantitative result. More complicated approaches for estimation of the LOD have been suggested.[23]

Analytical Sensitivity

The LLOQ of an assay should not be confused with analytical sensitivity. That is defined as ability of an analytical method to assess small differences in the concentration of analyte.[6] The smaller the random variation of the instrument response and the steeper the slope of the calibration function at a given point, the better is the ability to distinguish small differences in analyte concentrations. In reality, analytical sensitivity depends on the precision of the method. The smallest difference that will be statistically significant equals $2\sqrt{2}\ SD_A$ at a 5% significance level. Historically, the meaning of the term *analytical sensitivity* has been the subject of much discussion.

Analytical Specificity and Interference

Analytical specificity is the ability of an assay procedure to determine the concentration of the target analyte without influence from potentially interfering substances or factors in the sample matrix (eg, hyperlipemia, hemolysis, bilirubin, antibodies, other metabolic molecules, degradation products of the analyte, exogenous substances, anticoagulants). Interferences from hyperlipemia, hemolysis, and bilirubin are generally concentration dependent and can be quantified as a function of the concentration of the interfering compound.[24] In the context of a drug assay, specificity in relation to drug metabolites is relevant, and in some cases, it is desirable to measure the parent drug, as well as metabolites. A detailed protocol for evaluation of interference has been published by the CLSI.[25]

POINTS TO REMEMBER

- Technical validation of analytical methods focuses on (1) calibration, (2) trueness and accuracy, (3) precision, (4) linearity, (5) limit of detection, (6) limit of quantification, (7) specificity, and (8) others.
- The difference between the average measured value and the true value is the *bias*, which can be evaluated by comparison of measurements by the new test and by some preselected reference measurement procedure, both on the same sample or individuals.
- The degree of precision is usually expressed on the basis of statistical measures of imprecision, such as SD or CV ($CV = SD/x$, where x is the measurement concentration).
- The measurement range extends from the lowest concentration (LLOQ) to the highest concentration (ULOQ) for which the analytical performance specifications are fulfilled (imprecision, bias).
- Analytical specificity is the ability of an assay procedure to determine the concentration of the target analyte without influence from potentially interfering substances or factors in the sample matrix.

QUALITATIVE METHODS

Qualitative methods, which currently are gaining increased use in the form of point-of-care testing (POCT), are designed to distinguish between results below and above a predefined cutoff value. Note that the cutoff point should not be confused with the detection limit. These tests are assessed primarily on the basis of their ability to correctly classify results in relation to the cutoff value.

Diagnostic Accuracy Measures

The probability of classifying a result as positive (exceeding the cutoff) when the true value indeed exceeds the cutoff is called *sensitivity*. The probability of classifying a result as negative (below the cutoff) when the true value indeed is below the cutoff is termed *specificity*. Determination of sensitivity and specificity is based on comparison of test results with a gold standard. The gold standard may be an independent test that measures the same analyte, but it may also be a clinical diagnosis determined by definitive clinical methods

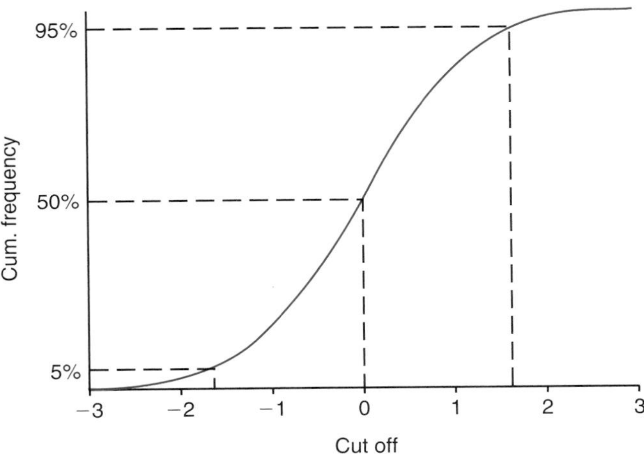

FIGURE 2.9 Cumulative frequency distribution of positive results. The *x*-axis indicates concentrations standardized to zero at the cutoff point (50% positive results) with unit standard deviation.

(eg, radiographic testing, follow-up, outcomes analysis). Determination of these performance measures is covered later on in the diagnostic testing part. Sensitivity and specificity may be given as a fraction or as a percentage after multiplication by 100. Standard errors of estimates are derived as described for categorical variables. The performance of two qualitative tests applied in the same groups of nondiseased and diseased subjects can be compared using the McNemar's test, which is based on a comparison of paired values of true and false-positive (FP) or false-negative (FN) results.[26]

One approach for determining the recorded performance of a test in terms of sensitivity and specificity is to determine the true concentration of analyte using an independent reference method. The closer the concentration is to the cutoff point, the larger the error frequencies are expected to be. Actually, the cutoff point is defined in such a way that for samples having a true concentration exactly equal to the cutoff point, 50% of results will be positive, and 50% will be negative.[27] Concentrations above and below the cutoff point at which repeated results are 95% positive or 95% negative, respectively, have been called the "95% interval" for the cutoff point for that method, which indicates a grey zone where the test does not provide reliable results[27,28] (Fig. 2.9).

Agreement Between Qualitative Tests

As outlined previously, if the outcome of a qualitative test can be related to a true analyte concentration or a definitive clinical diagnosis, it is relatively straightforward to express the performance in terms of clinical specificity and sensitivity. In the absence of a definitive reference or "gold standard," one should be cautious with regard to judgments on performance. In this situation, it is primarily *agreement* with another test that can be assessed. When replacement of an old or expensive routine assay with a new or less expensive assay is considered, it is of interest to know whether similar test results are likely to be obtained. If both assays are imperfect, however, it is not possible to judge which test has the better performance unless additional testing by a reference procedure is carried out.

In a comparison study, the same individuals are tested by both methods to prevent bias associated with selection of patients. Basically, the outcome of the comparison study should be presented in the form of a 2 × 2 table, from which various measures of agreement may be derived (Table 2.3). An obvious measure of agreement is the overall fraction or percentage of subjects tested who have the same test result (ie, both results negative or positive):

TABLE 2.3 2 × 2 Table for Assessing Agreement Between Two Qualitative Tests

		TEST 1	
		+	−
Test 2	+	a	b
	−	c	d
Total		a + c	b + d

$$\text{Overall percent agreement} = (a+d)/(a+b+c+d) \times 100\%$$

If agreement differs with respect to diseased and healthy individuals, the overall percent agreement measure becomes dependent on disease prevalence in the studied group of subjects. This is a common situation; accordingly, it may be desirable to separate this overall agreement measure into agreement concerning negative and positive results:

$$\text{Percent agreement given test 1 positive: } a/(a+c)$$

$$\text{Percent agreement given test 1 negative: } b/(b+d)$$

For example, if there is a close agreement with regard to positive results, overall agreement will be high when the fraction of diseased subjects is high; however, in a screening situation with very low disease prevalence, overall agreement will mainly depend on agreement with regard to negative results.

A problem with the simple agreement measures is that they do not take agreement by chance into account. Given independence, expected proportions observed in fields of the 2 × 2 table are obtained by multiplication of the fraction's negative and positive results for each test. Concerning agreement, it is excess agreement beyond chance that is of interest. More sophisticated measures have been introduced to account for this aspect. The most well-known measure is kappa, which is defined generally as the ratio of observed excess agreement beyond chance to maximum possible excess agreement beyond chance.[29] We have the following:

$$\text{Kappa} = (I_o - I_e)/(1 - I_e)$$

where I_o is the observed index of agreement and I_e is the expected agreement from chance. Given complete agreement, kappa equals +1. If observed agreement is greater than or equal to chance agreement, kappa is larger than or equal to zero. Observed agreement less than chance yields a negative kappa value.

Example

Table 2.4 shows a hypothetical example of observed numbers in a 2 × 2 table. The proportion of positive results for test 1

TABLE 2.4 2 × 2 Table With Example of Agreement of Data for Two Qualitative Tests

		TEST 1		
		+	–	Total
Test 2	+	60	20	80
	–	15	40	55
Total		75	60	135

is 75/(75 + 60) = 0.555, and for test 2, it is 80/(80 + 55) = 0.593. Thus, by chance, we expect the ++ pattern in 0.555 × 0.593 × 135 = 44.44 cases. Analogously, the — pattern is expected in (1 – 0.555) × (1 – 0.593) × 135 = 24.45 cases. The expected overall agreement percent by chance I_e is (44.44 + 24.45)/135 = 0.51. The observed overall percent agreement is I_o = (60 + 40)/135 = 0.74. Thus, we have

$$\text{Kappa} = (0.74 - 0.51)/(1 - 0.51) = 0.47$$

Generally, kappa values greater than 0.75 are taken to indicate excellent agreement beyond chance, values from 0.40 to 0.75 are regarded as showing fair to good agreement beyond chance, and values below 0.40 indicate poor agreement beyond chance. An SE for the kappa estimate can be computed.[29] Kappa is related to the intraclass correlation coefficient, which is a widely used measure of interrater reliability for quantitative measurements.[29] The considered agreement measures, percent agreement, and kappa can also be applied to assess the reproducibility of a qualitative test when the test is applied twice in a given context.

Various methodological problems are encountered in studies on qualitative tests. An obvious mistake is to let the result of the test being evaluated contribute to the diagnostic classification of subjects being tested (circular argument). This is also termed *incorporation bias*.[30,31] Another problem is partial as opposed to complete verification. When a new test is compared with an existing, imperfect test, a partial verification is sometimes undertaken, in which only discrepant results are subjected to further testing by a perfect test procedure. On this basis, sensitivity and specificity are reported for the new test. This procedure (called *discrepant resolution*) leads to biased estimates and should not be accepted.[30-33] The problem is that for cases with agreement, both the existing (imperfect) test and the new test may be wrong. Thus, only a measure of agreement should be reported, not specificity and sensitivity values. In the biostatistical literature, various procedures have been suggested to correct for bias caused by imperfect reference tests, but unrealistic assumptions concerning the independence of test results are usually put forward.

ASSAY COMPARISON

Comparison of measurements by two assays is a frequent task in the laboratory. Preferably, parallel measurements of a set of patient samples should be undertaken. To prevent artificial matrix-induced differences, fresh patient samples are the optimal material. A nearly even distribution of values over the analytical measurement range is also preferable. In an ordinary laboratory, comparison of two routine assays is the most frequently occurring situation. Less commonly, comparison of a routine assay with a reference measurement procedure is undertaken. When two routine assays are compared, the focus is on observed differences. In this situation, it is not possible to establish that one set of measurements is the correct one and thereby know by how much measurements deviate from the presumed correct concentrations. Rather, the question is whether the new assay can replace the existing one without a systematic change in result values. To address this question, the dispersion of observed differences between paired measurements may be evaluated by these assays. To carry out a formal, objective analysis of the data, a statistical procedure with graphics display should be applied. Various approaches may be used: (1) a frequency plot or histogram of the distribution of differences with measures of central tendency and dispersion (distribution of differences [DoD] plot), (2) a difference (bias) plot, which shows differences as a function of the average concentration of measurements (Bland-Altman plot), or (3) a regression analysis. In the following, a general error model is presented, and some typical measurement relationships are considered. Each of the statistical approaches mentioned is presented in detail along with a discussion of their advantages and disadvantages.

Basic Error Model

The occurrence of measurement errors is related to the performance characteristics of the assay. It is important to distinguish between pure, random measurement errors, which are present in all measurement procedures, and errors related to incorrect calibration and nonspecificity of the assay. Whereas a reference measurement procedure is associated only with pure, random error, a routine method, additionally, is likely to have some bias related to errors in calibration and limitations with regard to specificity. Whereas an erroneous calibration function gives rise to a systematic error, nonspecificity gives an error that typically varies from sample to sample. The error related to nonspecificity thus has a random character, but in contrast to the pure measurement error, it cannot be reduced by repeated measurements of a sample. Although errors related to nonspecificity for a group of samples look like random errors, for the individual sample, this type of error is a bias. Because this bias varies from sample to sample, it has been called a *sample-related random bias*.[34-36] In the following section, the various error components are incorporated into a formal error model.

Measured Value, Target Value, Modified Target Value, and True Value

Upon taking into account that an analytical method measures analyte concentrations with some random measurement error, one has to distinguish between the actual, measured value and the average result we would obtain if the given sample was measured an infinite number of times. If the assay is a reference assay without bias and nonspecificity, we have the following, simple relationship:

$$x_i = X_{\text{True}i} + \varepsilon_i$$

where x_i represents the measured value, $X_{\text{True}i}$ is the average value for an infinite number of measurements, and ε_i is the deviation of the measured value from the average value. If we were to undertake repeated measurements, the average of ε_i would be zero and the SD would equal the analytical SD (σ_A) of the reference measurement procedure. Pure, random, measurement error will usually be Gaussian distributed.

In the case of a routine assay, the relationship between the measured value for a sample and the true value becomes more complicated:

$$x_i = X_{Truei} + \text{Cal-Bias} + \text{Random-Bias}_i + \varepsilon_i$$

The *cal-bias* term (calibration bias) is a systematic error related to the calibration of the method. This systematic error may be a constant for all measurements corresponding to an offset error, or it may be a function of the analyte concentration (eg, corresponding to a slope deviation in the case of a linear calibration function). The *random-bias*$_i$ term is a bias that is specific for a given sample related to nonspecificity of the method. It may arise because of codetermination of substances that vary in concentration from sample to sample. For example, a chromogenic creatinine method codetermines some other components with creatinine in serum.[37] Finally, we have the random measurement error term ε_i.

If we performed an infinite number of measurements of a specific sample by the routine method, the random measurement error term ε_i would be zero. The cal-bias and the random-bias$_i$, however, would be unchanged. Thus, the average value of an infinite number of measurements would equal the sum of the true value and these bias terms. This average value may be regarded as the target value ($X_{Targeti}$) of the given sample for the routine method. We have:

$$X_{Targeti} = X_{Truei} + \text{Cal-Bias} + \text{Random-Bias}_i$$

As mentioned, the calibration bias represents a systematic error component in relation to the true values measured by a reference measurement procedure. In the context of regression analysis, this systematic error corresponds to the intercept and the slope deviation from unity when a routine method is compared with a reference measurement procedure (outlined in detail later). It is convenient to introduce a modified target value expression ($X'_{Targeti}$) for the routine method to delineate this systematic calibration bias, so that:

$$X'_{Targeti} = X_{Truei} + \text{Cal-Bias}$$

Thus, for a set of samples measured by a routine method, the $X_{Targeti}$ values are distributed around the respective $X'_{Targeti}$ values with an SD, which is called σ_{RB}.

If the assay is a reference method without bias and nonspecificity, the target value and the modified target value equal the true value, that is,

$$X_{Targeti} = X'_{Targeti} = X_{Truei}$$

The error model is outlined in Fig. 2.10.

Calibration Bias and Random Bias

For an individual measurement, the total error is the deviation of x_i from the true value, that is,

$$\text{Total error of } x_i = \text{Cal-Bias} + \text{Random-Bias}_i + \varepsilon_i$$

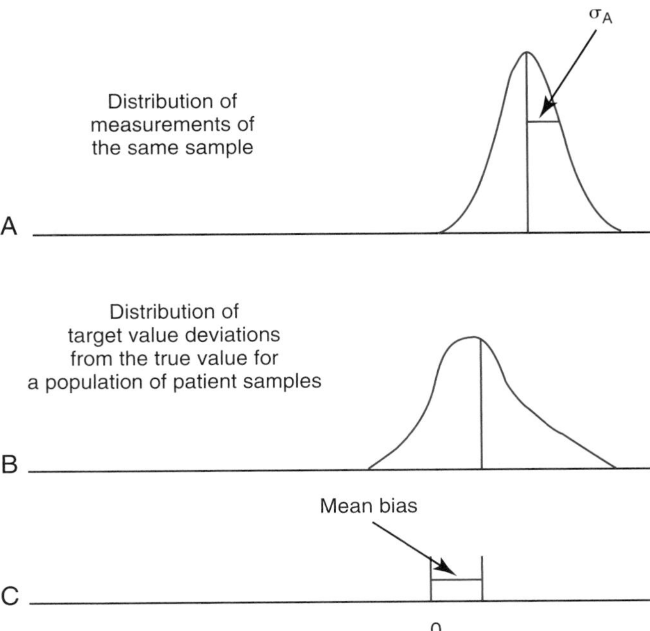

FIGURE 2.10 Outline of basic error model for measurements by a routine assay. **A,** The distribution of repeated measurements of the *same* sample, representing a normal distribution around the target value ($X_{Targeti}$) *(vertical line)* of the sample with a dispersion corresponding to the analytical standard deviation, σ_A. **B,** Schematic outline of the dispersion of target value deviations from the respective true values for a population of patient samples. A distribution of an arbitrary form is displayed. The standard deviation equals σ_{RB}. The vertical line indicates the mean of the distribution. **C,** The distance from zero to the mean of the target value deviations from the true values represents the calibration bias (mean bias = cal-bias) of the assay.

Estimation of the bias terms requires parallel measurements between the method in question and a reference method as outlined in detail later. With regard to calibration bias, one should be aware of the possibility of lot-to-lot variation in analytical kit sets. The manufacturer should provide documentation on this lot-to-lot variation because often it is not possible for the individual laboratory to investigate a sufficient number of lots to assess this variation. Lot-to-lot variation shows up as a calibration bias that changes from lot to lot.

The previous exposition defines the total error in somewhat broader terms than is often seen. A traditional total error expression is[38]:

$$\text{Total error} = \text{Bias} + 2\ \text{SD}_A$$

which often is interpreted as the calibration bias plus 2 SD_A. If a one-sided statistical perspective is taken, the expression is modified to Bias + 1.65 SD_A, indicating that 5% of results are located outside the limit. If a lower percentage is desired, the multiplication factor is increased accordingly, supposing a normal distribution. Interpreting the bias as identical with the calibration bias may lead to an underestimation of the total error.

Random bias related to sample-specific interferences may take several forms. It may be a regularly occurring additional random error component, perhaps of the same order of magnitude as the analytical error. In this context, it is natural to quantify the error in the form of an SD or CV. The most straightforward procedure is to carry out a method comparison study based on a set of patient samples in which one of the methods is a reference method, as outlined later. Krouwer[34] formally quantified sample-related random interferences in a comparison experiment of two cholesterol methods and found that the CV of the sample-related random interference component exceeded the analytical CV. Another form of sample-related random interference is more rarely occurring gross errors, which typically are seen in the context of immunoassays and are related to unexpected antibody interactions. Such an error usually shows up as an outlier in method comparison studies. A well-known source is the occurrence of heterophilic antibodies. Outliers should not just be discarded from the data analysis procedure. Rather, outliers must be investigated to identify their cause, which may be an important limitation in using a given assay. Supplementary studies may help clarify such random sample-related interferences and may provide specifications for the assay that limit its application in certain contexts (eg, with regard to samples from certain patient categories).

Assay Comparison Data Model

Here we consider the error model described earlier in relation to the method comparison situation. For a given sample measured by two analytical methods, 1 and 2, we have

$$x1_i = X1_{\mathrm{Target}i} + \varepsilon 1_i = X_{\mathrm{True}i} + \text{Cal-Bias1} + \text{Random-Bias1}_i + \varepsilon 1_i$$

$$\begin{aligned} x2_i &= X2_{\mathrm{Target}i} + \varepsilon 2_i \\ &= X_{\mathrm{True}i} + \text{Cal-Bias2} + \text{Random-Bias2}_i + \varepsilon 2_i \end{aligned}$$

From this general model, we may study some typical situations. First, comparison of a routine assay with a reference measurement procedure will be treated. Second, comparison of two routine assays is considered.

Comparison of a Routine Assay With a Reference Measurement Procedure

Assuming that method 1 is a reference method, the bias components disappear by definition, and we have the following situation:

$$x1_i = X1_{\mathrm{Target}i} + \varepsilon 1_i = X_{\mathrm{True}i} + \varepsilon 1_i$$

$$\begin{aligned} x2_i &= X2_{\mathrm{Target}i} + \varepsilon 2_i \\ &= X_{\mathrm{True}i} + \text{Cal-Bias2} + \text{Random-Bias2}_i + \varepsilon 2_i \end{aligned}$$

The paired differences become

$$(x2_i - x1_i) = \text{Cal-Bias2} + \text{Random-Bias2}_i + (\varepsilon 2_i - \varepsilon 1_i)$$

We thus have an expression consisting of a systematic error term (calibration bias of method 2) and two random terms. The random-bias2 term is distributed around cal-bias2 according to an undefined distribution. $(\varepsilon 2_i - \varepsilon 1_i)$ is a difference between two random measurement errors that are independent and, commonly, Gaussian distributed. However, we remind readers that the SD for analytical methods often depends on the concentration, as mentioned earlier. For analytes with a wide analytical measurement range (eg, some hormones), both sample-related random interferences and analytical SDs are likely to depend on the measurement concentration, often in a roughly proportional manner. It may then be more useful to evaluate the *relative* differences—$(x2_i - x1_i)/[(x2_i + x1_i)/2]$—and accordingly express mean and random bias and analytical error as proportions. An alternative is to partition the total analytical measurement range into segments (eg, three parts) and consider calibration bias, random bias, and analytical error separately for each of these segments. The segments may be divided preferably in relation to important decision concentrations (eg, in relation to reference interval limits, treatment decision concentrations, or both).

Comparison of Two Routine Assays

In the comparison of two routine methods, the paired differences become

$$\begin{aligned} (x2_i - x1_i) = {} & (\text{Cal-Bias2} - \text{Cal-Bias1}) + \\ & (\text{Random-Bias2}_i - \text{Random-Bias1}_i) + (\varepsilon 2_i - \varepsilon 1_i) \end{aligned}$$

The expression again consists of a constant term, the difference between the two calibration biases, and two random terms. The first random term is a difference between two random-bias components that may or may not be independent. If the two field methods are based on the same measurement principle, the random bias terms are likely to be correlated. For example, two chromogenic methods for creatinine are likely to be subject to interference from the same chromogenic compounds present in a given serum sample. On the other hand, a chromogenic method and an enzymatic creatinine method are subject to different types of interfering compounds, and the random bias terms may be relatively independent. In the $\varepsilon 2_i - \varepsilon 1_i$ term, the same relationships as described previously are likely to apply. One may note that the general form of the expressed differences is the same in the two situations. Thus, the same general statistical principles actually apply. In the following sections, we will consider the distribution of differences under various circumstances, as well as the measurement relations between methods 1 and 2 on the basis of regression analysis.

Preliminary Practical Work in Relation to a Method Comparison Study

When a method comparison study is to be conducted, the analytical methods to be examined first should be established in the laboratory according to written protocols and should be stable in routine performance. Reagents are commonly supplied as ready-made analytical kits, perhaps implemented on a dedicated analytical instrument (open or closed system). Technologists performing the study should be trained in the procedures and associated instrumentation. Furthermore, it is important that a QC system is in place to ensure that the methods being compared are running in an in-control state.

Planning a Method Comparison Study

In the planning phase of a method comparison study, several points require attention, including the (1) number of samples necessary, (2) distribution of analyte concentrations (preferably uniform over the analytical measurement range), and (3) representativeness of the samples. To address the latter point, samples from relevant patient categories should be included, so that possible interference phenomena can be discovered. For example, it may in a given context be relevant to include samples from patients with diabetes to exclude the possibility that aberrations in glucose metabolism may influence test results. Practical aspects related to storage and treatment of samples (eg, container) and possible artifacts induced by storage (eg, freezing of samples) and addition of anticoagulants should be considered. Comparison of measurements should preferably be undertaken over several days (eg, at least 5 days) so that the comparison of methods does not become dependent on the performance of the methods in one particular analytical run. Finally, ethical aspects (eg, informed consent from patients whose samples will be used) should be considered in relation to existing legislation.

When the comparison protocol is considered, various guidelines may be consulted. The CLSI Evaluation Protocol (EP) guidelines give advice on various aspects. For example, the CLSI guideline EP-09-A3, "Method Comparison and Bias Estimation Using Patient Samples," suggests measurement of 40 samples in duplicate by each method when a new method is introduced in the laboratory as a substitute for an established one.[39] Additionally, it is proposed that a vendor of an analytical test system should have made a comparison study based on at least 100 samples measured in duplicate by each method. The principle of a more demanding requirement for vendors appears reasonable. This initial validation should be comprehensive to disclose the performance of the assay system in detail. Then the requirement for the ordinary user may be more modest. The EP15 guideline "User Verification of Manufacturer's Claims" suggests a more condensed approach based on a bias or difference plot, which does not involve regression analysis and can be carried out using 20 samples.[17] Although these general guidelines on sample size are useful, additional aspects are important. The probability of detecting rarely occurring interferences showing up as outliers should be taken into account when the necessary sample size is considered. Finally, in relation to evaluation of automated methods, special consideration should be given to the sample sequence to evaluate drift, carryover, and nonlinearity (eg, by a multifactorial design).[14]

Distribution of Differences Plot (DoD Plot)

From the end-user viewpoint, it is the differences per se that matter. Thus, with regard to the outcome of replacing an established routine method with a new one that perhaps is less expensive or more practical, it is important to focus on the distribution of differences between paired measurements by the old and the new method. A graphic display with assessment of the central tendency and dispersion of differences in the form of an ordinary histogram or frequency polygon plot is useful. The differences may or may not be Gaussian distributed. Because both analytical error components and sample-related random interferences may contribute to the differences, the distribution may be irregular, and outliers may occur. Furthermore, the random dispersion elements may be dependent on analyte concentration. This is also termed the *heteroscedasticity* of the measurement. Therefore, a nonparametric approach for interpreting the distribution of differences may generally be preferable as a starting point.

Nonparametric Approach

Both the central tendency (median) and extreme percentiles are of interest when the nonparametric approach to the distribution of differences is used. With a traditional 95% level, the 2.5 and 97.5 percentiles are considered. A 99% or higher extreme level may be selected, and the related percentiles (0.5 and 99.5 percentiles, or more extreme ones) may then be applied for a description of method differences. Nonparametric estimation of the 2.5 and 97.5 percentiles requires 2.5 times as many observations as the parametric approach to obtain the same uncertainty, which implies that sample sizes cannot be too small.[40] Estimating confidence limits of the percentiles can give an indication of their imprecision. The CIs can be estimated from the ordered observations as described in Chapter 8 in the section on nonparametric estimation of the 95% reference interval. Alternatively, a bootstrap procedure can be applied as described.[40] The advantage of the bootstrap procedure is that SEs can be derived using smaller sample sizes than are used with the simple nonparametric approach.[41]

A method comparison example from the laboratory of one of the authors (K.L.) is considered. Two drug assays developed in house for serum concentrations of the antipsychotic drug clozapine are compared. The established assay (method 1) is an HPLC method based on manual liquid–liquid extraction. The new method (method 2) is an HPLC method with an automated on-column extraction step. An initial impression of the relation between $x1$ and $x2$ measurements can be obtained from a scatter plot of the 65 measurement sets ($x1$, $x2$) with the identity line outlined (Fig. 2.11). The $x1$ measurements range from 177 to 2650 nmol/L, and the range of $x2$ values is from 200 to 3004 nmol/L (ie, we have a relatively wide analytical measurement range in the present example). A histogram of the difference ($x2 - x1$) is shown in Fig. 2.12. Applying a nonparametric data description, we order the observed differences according to size and derive the median difference as the value of the $(0.5N + 0.5)^{th}$ ordered observation, here 26 nmol/L. In case the order is a noninteger, interpolation between neighbor-ordered values is carried out. A paired nonparametric test, the Wilcoxon test,[5] shows that the median difference was significantly different from zero (P <0.02). The 2.5 and 97.5 percentiles correspond

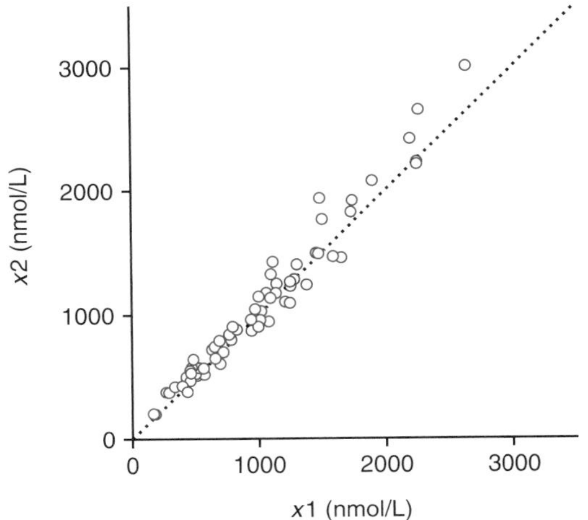

FIGURE 2.11 A scatter plot of $n = 65$ ($x1$, $x2$) data points for comparison of two drug assays. The *dashed line* is the line of identity.

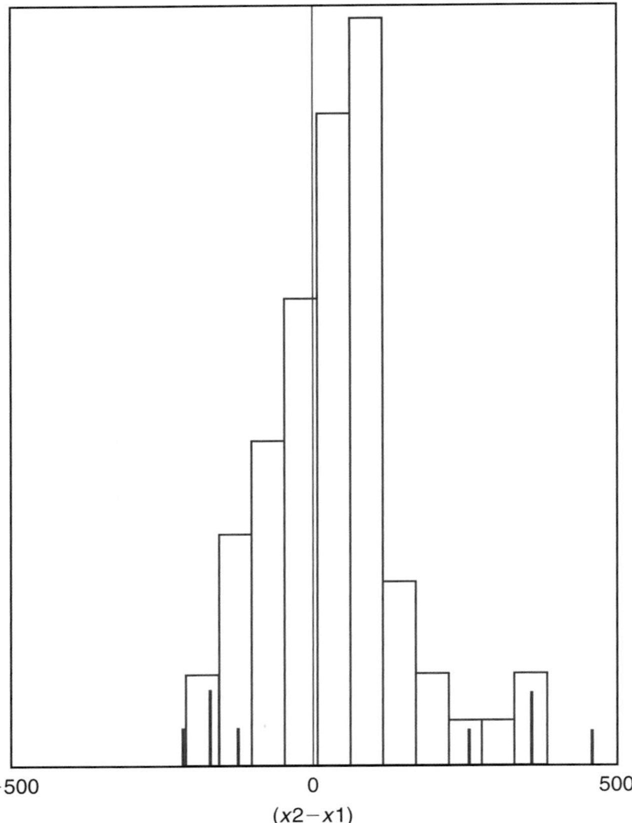

FIGURE 2.12 Distribution of differences (DoD) plot for comparison of two drug assays: nonparametric analysis. A histogram shows the relative frequency of $n = 65$ differences with demarcated 2.5 and 97.5 percentiles determined nonparametrically. The 90% confidence intervals (CIs) of the percentiles are shown. These were derived by the bootstrap technique.

to the values of the $(0.025N + 0.5)^{th}$ and $(0.975N + 0.5)^{th}$ ordered observations, respectively, as displayed in Table 2.5.[4,40] For a sample size smaller than 120, it is not possible to derive CIs for the percentiles by the simple nonparametric procedure. Therefore, we also applied the bootstrap procedure to estimate nonparametric percentiles with 90% CIs[40,42] (see Table 2.5). The bootstrap procedure, which is based on computerized random resampling of the observations, provides slightly different percentile estimates, as shown in Table 2.5. In this way, we obtain an estimation of the size of negative and positive differences with uncertainties. The present example shows a considerable range of differences, with the 2.5th percentile being −169 nmol/L (90%-CI: −214 to −123) and the 97.5 percentile being 356 nmol/L (90% CI: 255 to 457). These relatively large differences should be related to the considerable analytical measurement range for the analyte, and an evaluation of *relative* differences may be more relevant for the present example (see later in this chapter).

In the presented examples, no evident outliers were present. However, outliers deserve special attention.[4] Unless they are related to obvious method or apparatus malfunction, discarding of outliers should be considered with caution. Outliers may indicate the presence of large sample-related random interferences, which may be of major clinical importance (eg, interference by antibodies or degradation products that occur only rarely). Thus, a special investigation of outlying results with reanalysis and exploration of the reasons for the outlying observations should be considered.

Parametric Approach

If application of a goodness-of-fit test does not disprove that the distribution of differences is Gaussian distributed, a parametric statistical approach may be undertaken. In the example presented, a significant deviation from normality was present, as assessed by the Anderson-Darling test[43] (P <0.01); therefore, a parametric analysis in principle should not be carried out. However, to demonstrate the procedure, the parametric

TABLE 2.5 Analysis of Distribution of Differences for the Comparison of Drug Assays Example*

Total range of *x*1 measurements	177 to 2650		
Total range of *x*2 measurements	200 to 3004		
Total range of differences (*x*2 – *x*1)	–210.00 to 437.00		
Test for normality of differences (Anderson-Darling test)	*P* <0.01		
Statistical Analysis of Differences	**Simple Nonparametric**	**Bootstrap**	**Parametric**
Median	26.00 (*P* <0.02)		
Mean			42.00 (*P* <0.01)
SD			124.42
Coefficient of skewness			+0.83
Coefficient of kurtosis			+1.27
Outlier test (4 SD)			NS
2.5-percentile	–166.00	–169.11	–201.86
97.5 percentile	372.38	355.90	285.86
90% CI for 2.5 percentile		–214.73 to –123.50	–245.24 to –158.47
90% CI for 97.5 percentile		255.03 to 456.77	242.47 to 329.24

*$n = 65$ single (*x*1, *x*2 measurements). The units are nmol/L.
CI, Confidence interval; *NS*, not significant; *SD*, standard deviation.

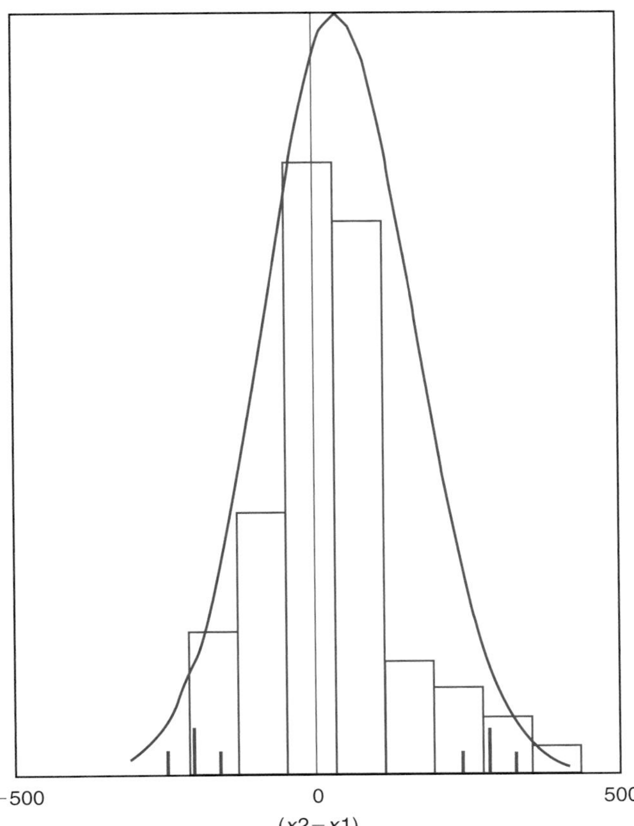

FIGURE 2.13 Distribution of differences (DoD) plot for comparison of two drug assays: parametric analysis. A histogram shows the relative frequency of $n = 65$ differences with the estimated Gaussian density distribution. Parametrically estimated 2.5 and 97.5 percentiles are shown with 90% confidence intervals (CIs).

approach is also carried out (Fig. 2.13 and Table 2.5). The mean and SD (SD_{Dif}) of the paired differences ($x2 - x1$) are estimated according to standard procedures. A paired t-test is used to determine whether the mean difference is significantly different from zero (P <0.01 in this case). The 2.5th and 97.5th percentiles for the differences are estimated as the mean $\pm t_{0.025(N-1)}$ SD_{Dif}. An SE for the percentiles (SE_{perc}) may be computed, and the 90% CI limits are then derived as ± 1.65 SE_{perc} around the percentiles (see Fig. 2.13 and Table 2.5). The parametrically derived 2.5 and 97.5 percentiles (−202 and 286 nmol/L) differ somewhat from the nonparametrically derived percentiles, which in the present context with proven non-normality may be regarded as the most reliable estimates.

Relative Distribution of Differences Plot (Rel DoD Plot)

In some cases in which a wide analytical measurement range (ie, corresponding to 1 or several decades) is used, the random error components depend on the concentration, as previously mentioned. Analytical SDs may be approximately proportional to the concentration over the major part of the analytical measurement range. In the present example, the initial scatter plot of ($x1$, $x2$) values suggests that the random error of the differences increases with the concentration (see Fig. 2.11). A formal test for this possible relation is to compute the correlation coefficient between the average concentration

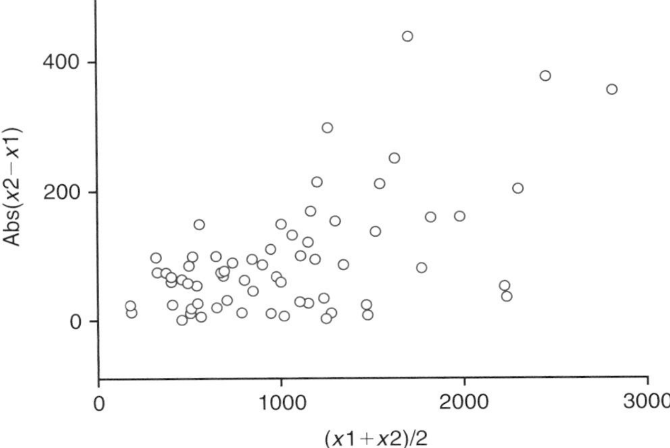

FIGURE 2.14 Plot of absolute differences (ordinate) against average concentration (abscissa) for the comparison of drug assays example. The scatter increases with the average concentration (r = +0.57).

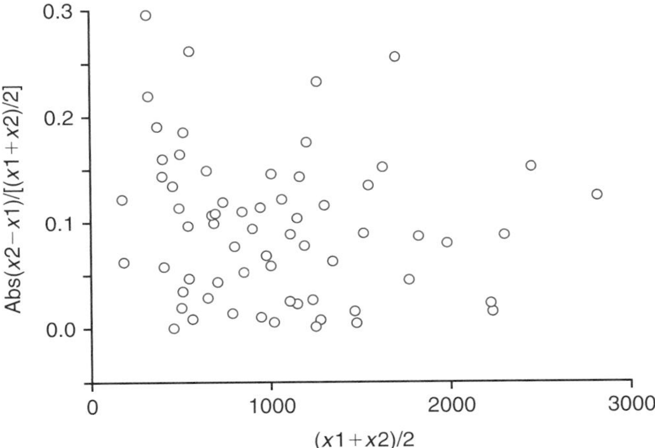

FIGURE 2.15 Plot of absolute *relative* differences (ordinate) against average concentration (abscissa) for the comparison of drug assays example. The scatter is not significantly correlated with the average concentration (r = −0.15, not significant).

and the *absolute* value of the differences. This correlation coefficient, r, is +0.57, which is significantly different from zero (P <0.001), and it confirms the relationship of scatter increasing with concentration, which also can be visualized in a scatter plot of the absolute differences against the average concentration (Fig. 2.14). A natural next step is to assess the *relative* differences in relation to the average concentration. The correlation coefficient between the absolute values of the relative differences [$|x2 - x1|/(\{x1 + x2\}/2)$] and the average concentration [$(x1 + x2)/2$] was not significantly different (P >0.05) from zero (r = −0.15); a scatter plot also suggests a more homogeneous dispersion (Fig. 2.15). In this situation, it is more reasonable to deal with *relative* differences or percentage differences [$(\{x2 - x1\}/\{x1 + x2\}/2) \times 100\%$]. The same nonparametric descriptive measures as used earlier may be applied for the central tendency and the dispersion (Fig. 2.16). The median relative difference amounts to 0.042, or 4.2%, which is significantly higher than zero (P <0.01) (Wilcoxon test) (Table 2.6). The 2.5 and 97.5 percentiles are −0.15 and 0.26, respectively. The 90% CIs derived by the

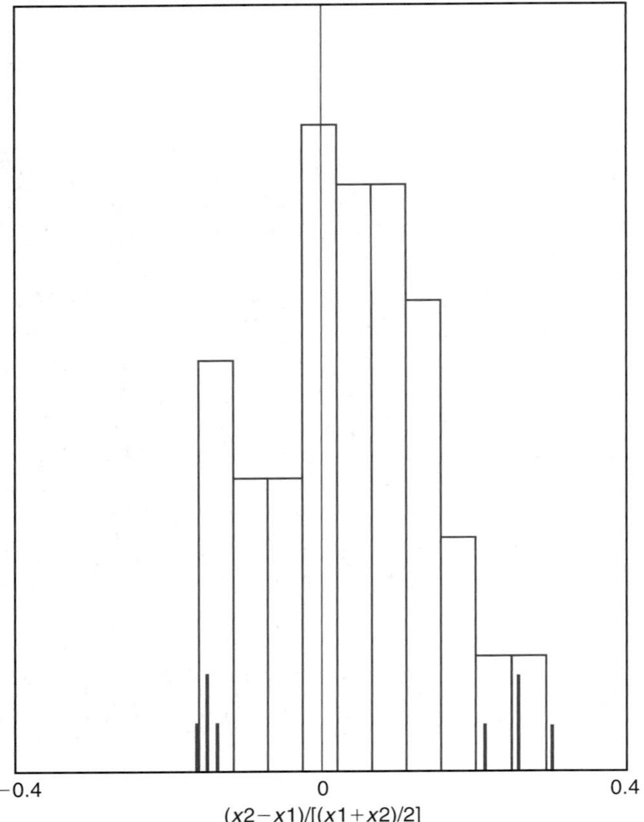

FIGURE 2.16 Relative distribution of differences (Rel DoD) plot for comparison of two drug assays: nonparametric analysis. A histogram shows the relative frequency of relative differences with demarcated 2.5 and 97.5 percentiles determined nonparametrically. The 90% confidence intervals (bootstrap) of the percentiles are shown.

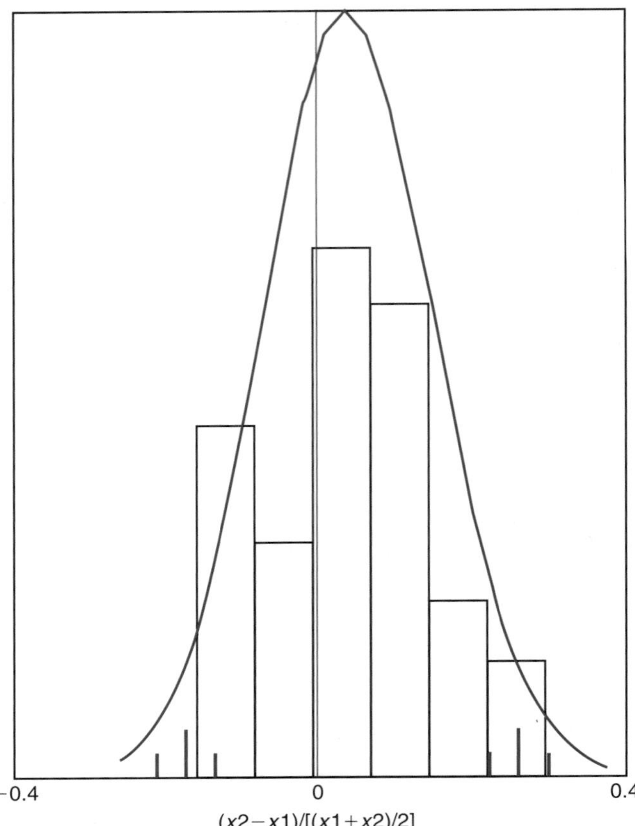

FIGURE 2.17 Distribution of *relative* differences plot for comparison of two drug assays: parametric analysis. A histogram shows the relative frequency of relative differences with the estimated Gaussian density distribution. Parametrically estimated 2.5 and 97.5 percentiles are shown with 90% confidence intervals.

TABLE 2.6 Analysis of Distribution of *Relative* Differences for the Comparison of Drug Assays Example; $n = 65$

Total range of relative differences	−0.1598 to 0.2953		
Test for normality (Anderson-Darling test)	NS		
Statistical Analysis	**Simple Nonparametric**	**Bootstrap**	**Parametric**
Median	0.0467 (P <0.01)		
Mean			0.0418 (P <0.01)
SD			0.1109
Coefficient of skewness			+0.05
Coefficient of kurtosis			−0.60
Outlier test			NS
2.5 percentile	−0.1487	−0.1492	−0.1754
97.5 percentile	0.2607	0.2570	0.2591
90% CI for 2.5 percentile		−0.1627 to −0.1357	−0.2141 to −0.1368
90% CI for 97.5 percentile		0.2135 to 0.3005	0.2204 to 0.2978

CI, Confidence interval; *NS*, not significant; *SD*, standard deviation.

bootstrap procedure were −0.16 to −0.14 and 0.21 to 0.30, respectively. Thus, from this analysis, we may conclude that the 95% interval for percentage differences ranges from about −15 to +26%.

Finally, we may consider a parametric analysis of the relative differences (Fig. 2.17 and Table 2.6). A goodness-of-fit test (Anderson-Darling test; P >0.05) showed that the relative differences did not depart significantly from a normal distribution, which in this case supports the parametric approach (Fig. 2.18). The parametric 2.5 and 97.5 percentiles were −0.18 and 0.26, respectively. The mean was 0.042, and the SD of the relative differences was 0.11. Thus, we may conclude

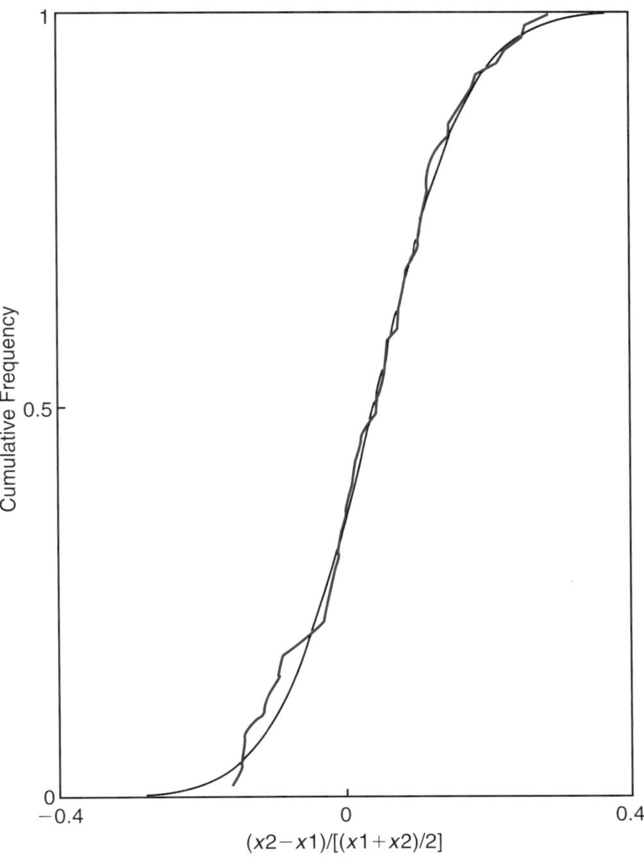

FIGURE 2.18 Cumulative frequency distribution of relative differences for the comparison of drug assays example. The black curve indicates the Gaussian cumulative frequency distribution curve. In accordance with the test for normality, good agreement is observed.

that there is an average bias of about 4%, which might rely on a calibration difference (an estimate of [cal-bias2 − cal-bias1]), and a random error corresponding to a CV of 11%. The random error CV of 11% is an estimate of the combined dispersion of [(Random-Bias2$_i$ − Random-Bias1$_i$) + ($\varepsilon 2_i - \varepsilon 1_i$)]. If we ascribe the random variation equally to the two assays, it corresponds to a random error level of $11\%/\sqrt{2} = 7.8\%$ for each assay. In the present example, the average bias of 4% and the estimated random variation of differences between the two assays were considered acceptable in relation to the clinical use of the assay, and it was decided to replace the manual assay with the new, automated assay.

Verification of Distribution of Differences in Relation to Specified Limits

In situations in which a field method is being considered for implementation, it may be desired primarily to *verify* whether the differences in relation to the existing method are located within given specified limits rather than *estimating* the distribution of differences. For example, one may set limits corresponding to ±15% as clinically acceptable and may desire that a majority (eg, 95% of differences) are located within this interval.

By counting, it may be determined whether the expected proportion of results is within the limits (ie, 95%). One may accept percentages that do not deviate significantly from the supposed percentage at the given sample size derived from the binomial distribution (Table 2.7). For example, if 50 paired measurements have been performed in a method comparison study, and if it is observed that 46 of these results (92%) are within specified limits (eg, ±15%), the study supports that the achieved goal has been reached because the lower boundary for acceptance is 90%. It is clear that a reasonable number of observations should be obtained for the assessment to have acceptable power. If very few observations are available, the risk is high of falsely concluding that at least 95% of the observations are within specified limits in case it is not true (ie, committing a type II error).

TABLE 2.7 Lower Bounds (One-Sided 95% Confidence Interval) of Observed Proportions (%) of Results Being Located Within Specified Limits for Paired Differences That Are in Accordance With the Hypothesis of at Least 95% of Differences Being Within the Limits

n	Observed Proportions
20	85
30	87
40	90
50	90
60	90
70	90
80	91
90	91
100	91
150	92
200	93
250	93
300	93
400	93
500	93
1000	94

Difference (Bland-Altman) Plot

The difference plot suggested by Bland and Altman is widely used for evaluating method comparison data.[44,45] The procedure was originally introduced for comparison of measurements in clinical medicine, but it has also been adopted in clinical chemistry.[46-48] The Bland-Altman plot is usually understood as a plot of the differences against the average results of the methods. Thus, the difference plot in this version provides information on the relation between differences and concentration, which is useful in evaluating whether problems exist at certain ranges (eg, in the high range) caused by nonlinearity of one of the methods. It may also be of interest to observe whether differences tend to increase proportionally with the concentration or whether they are independent of concentration. In some situations, particular interest may be directed toward the low-concentration region. Information on the relation between differences and concentration is useful in the context of how to adjust for an irregularity

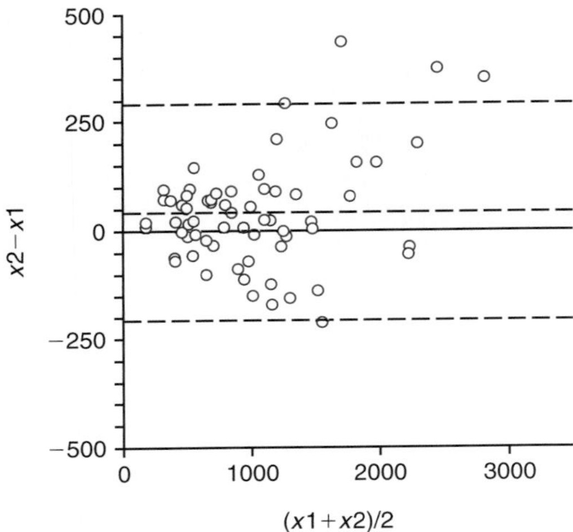

FIGURE 2.19 Bland-Altman plot of differences for the drug comparison example. The differences are plotted against the average concentration. The mean difference (42 nmol/L) with ±2 standard deviation of differences is shown *(dashed lines)*.

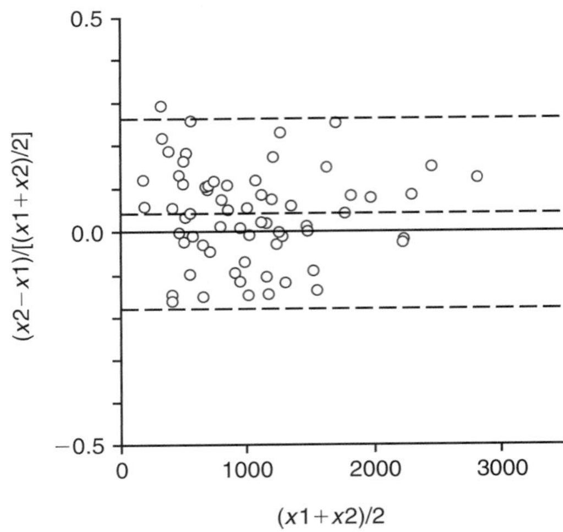

FIGURE 2.20 Bland-Altman plot of *relative* differences for the drug comparison example. The differences are plotted against the average concentration. The mean relative difference (0.042) with ±2 standard deviation of relative differences is shown *(dashed lines)*.

(eg, by changing the method to correct for nonlinearity, by restricting the analytical measurement range).

The basic version of the difference plot requires plotting of the differences against the average of the measurements. Fig. 2.19 shows the plot for the drug assay comparison data. The interval ±2 SD of the differences is often delineated around the mean difference (ie, corresponding to the mean and the 2.5 and 97.5 percentiles considered in the parametric DoD plot[45]). To assess whether the bias is significantly different from zero, the SE of the mean difference is estimated as the SD divided by the square root of the number of paired measurements ($SE = SD/N^{0.5}$) and tested against zero by a *t*-test ($t = [Mean - 0]/SE$).

Nonparametric limits may also be considered. The distribution of the differences as measured on the *y*-axis of the coordinate system corresponds to the relations outlined for the DoD plot, which represents a projection of the differences on the *y*-axis. A constant bias over the analytical measurement range changes the average concentration away from zero. The presence of sample-related random interferences increases the width of the distribution. If the calibration bias depends on the concentration, if the dispersion varies with the concentration, or if both occur, the relations become more complex, and the interval mean ±2 SD of the differences may not fit very well as a 95% interval throughout the analytical measurement range.

The displayed Bland-Altman plot for the drug assay comparison data (see Fig. 2.19) shows a tendency toward increasing scatter with increasing concentration, which is a reflection of increasing random error with concentration, as considered in detail in previous paragraphs. Thus, a plot of the relative differences against the average concentration is of relevance (Fig. 2.20). This plot has a more homogeneous dispersion of values, agreeing with the estimated limits for the dispersion, that is, the relative mean difference $\pm\, t_{0.025(N-1)}\ SD_{RelDif}$ equal to $0.042 \pm 1.998 \times 0.11$ corresponding to −0.18 and 0.26, analogous to the situation with the relative DoD plot considered earlier.

Use of *relative* differences in situations with a proportional random error relationship prevents very large differences in the high-concentration range from dominating the analysis and making a balanced interpretation difficult. In the low range, the proportional relationship may not necessarily hold true, and sometimes the relative difference plot overcompensates for lack of proportionality in this region. It is then possible to truncate the proportional relationship at some lower limit and assume a constant SD for differences below this limit[49] (ie, corresponding to the relationship in Fig. 2.3, *C*). In the actual drug example (see Fig. 2.20) with a slightly negative correlation coefficient between relative differences and average concentration, a tendency toward this pattern is seen. An alternative to the relative difference plot is to plot the logarithm of the differences against the average concentration, but this type of plot is more difficult to interpret, because the scale is changed.

Although it is customary to display the *estimated* limits for the differences (often, mean $\pm\, 2\ SD_{dif}$), one may, as an alternative, display specification limits considered reasonable, as mentioned for the DoD plot.[47] It may then be assessed whether the observed differences conform to these limits, as discussed earlier (see Table 2.7). Application of the difference plot in various specific contexts has been considered.[50,51] It has also been suggested to estimate a regression line for the differences as a function of the average measurement concentration.[52]

A Caution Against Incorrect Interpretation of Paired *t*-Tests in Method Comparison Studies

In association with the difference plot, the paired *t*-test is usually applied as described earlier,[44] but one should be careful with regard to the interpretation. For example, consider the case shown below, in which method 2 (*x*2) measurements tend to exceed method 1 (*x*1) measurements in the low range and vice versa at high concentrations (Fig. 2.21, *A*). This corresponds to a positive calibration bias in the low range, changing to a negative calibration bias in the high range. In this situation, the overall averages of both sets of measurements are nearly equal, and the paired *t*-test yields a nonsignificant result because the average paired difference

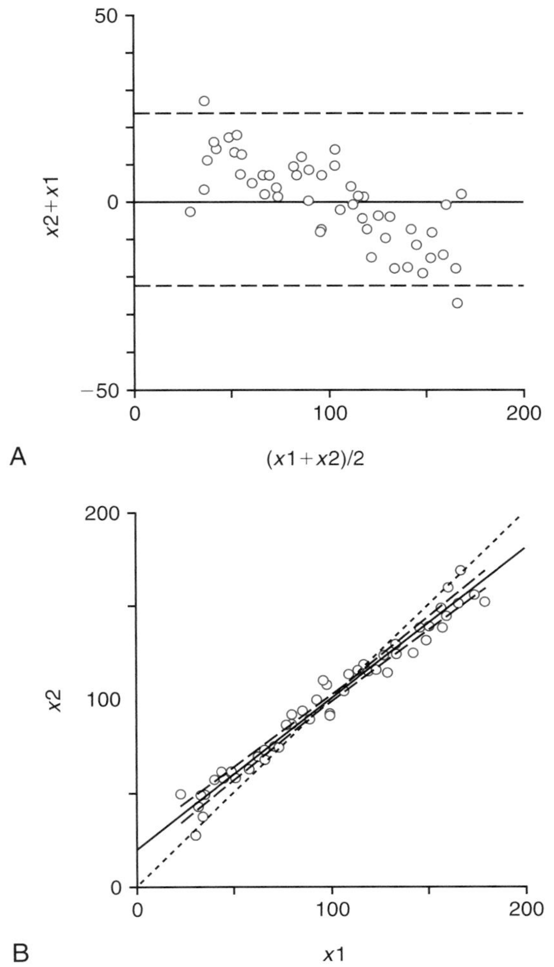

FIGURE 2.21 Simulated example with positive and negative differences in the low and high ranges, respectively. **A,** Bland-Altman plot. **B,** *x-y* Plot with diagonal *(dotted straight line)* and estimated Deming regression line *(solid line)* with 95% confidence curves *(dashed lines).*

(ie, the overall bias) is close to zero (Table 2.8). This does not mean that the measurements are equivalent. Subjecting the data to Deming regression analysis (see the next section) clearly discloses the relation[53] (Fig. 2.21, *B*). Results of the regression analysis confirm the existence of both a systematic constant error (intercept different from zero) and a systematic proportional error (slope different from 1). Therefore, as pointed out previously, the statistical significance revealed by the paired *t*-test cannot be used to indicate whether measurements are equivalent. The paired *t*-test is just a test for the average bias; it does not say anything about the equivalency of measurements throughout the analytical measurement range.

Regression Analysis

Regression analysis is commonly applied in comparing the results of analytical method comparisons. Typically, an experiment is carried out in which a series of paired values is collected when a new method is compared with an established method. This series of paired observations ($x1_i$, $x2_i$) is then used to establish the nature and strength of the relationship between the tests. This discussion outlines various regression models that may be used, gives criteria for when each should be used, and provides guidelines for interpreting the results.

Regression analysis has the advantage that it allows the relation between the target values for the two compared methods to be studied over the full analytical measurement range. If the systematic difference between target values (ie, the calibration bias between the two methods, or the systematic error) is related to the analyte concentration, such a relationship may not be clearly shown when the previously mentioned types of difference plots are used. Although nonlinear regression analysis may be applied, the focus is usually on linear regression analysis. In linear regression analysis, it is assumed that the systematic difference between target values can be modeled as a constant systematic difference (intercept deviation from zero) combined with a proportional systematic difference (slope deviation from unity), usually related to a discrepancy with regard to calibration of the methods. In situations when random errors have a constant SD, unweighted regression procedures are used (eg, Deming regression analysis). For cases with SDs that are proportional to the concentration, the weighted Deming regression procedure is preferred.

TABLE 2.8 Comparison of Paired *t*-Test Results and Deming Regression Results for a Simulated Method Comparison Example With Positive Intercept (a_0 = 20) and Slope Below Unity (*b* = 0.80), *n* = 50 (*x*1, *x*2) Measurements

	Paired *t*-Test	Regression Analysis (Deming)
Mean difference (SEM)	0.78 (1.63)	
t = mean difference/ SEM	0.78/1.63 = 0.48 (NS)	
Slope *(b)* [SE*(b)*]		0.80 (0.027)
t = (b − 1)/SE(b)		−7.4 (*P* <0.001)
Intercept (a0) [SE(a0)]		20.3 (2.82)
t = (a0 − 0)/SE(a0)		7.2 (*P* <0.001)

NS, Not significant; *SEM,* standard error of the mean.

Error Models in Regression Analysis

As outlined previously, we distinguish between the measured value (x_i) and the target value ($X_{\text{Target}i}$) of a sample subjected to analysis by a given method. In linear regression analysis, we assume a linear relationship between values devoid of random error of any kind.[54,55] Thus, to operate with a linear relationship between values without random measurement error and sample-related random bias, we have to introduce modified target values:

$$X1_{\text{Target}i} = X1'_{\text{Target}i} + \text{Random-Bias1}_i$$

$$X2_{\text{Target}i} = X2'_{\text{Target}i} + \text{Random-Bias2}_i$$

where we now assume a linear relationship between these modified target values:

$$X2'_{\text{Target}i} = \alpha_0 + \beta X1'_{\text{Target}i}$$

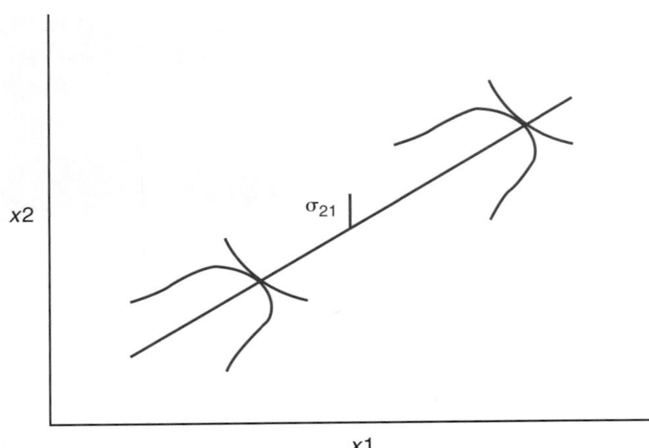

FIGURE 2.22 Outline of the relation between $x1$ and $x2$ values measured by two assays subject to random errors with constant standard deviations over the analytical measurement range. A linear relationship between the modified target values ($X1'_{\text{Target}i}$, $X2'_{\text{Target}i}$) is presumed. The $x1_i$ and $x2_i$ values are Gaussian distributed around $X1'_{\text{Target}i}$ and $X2'_{\text{Target}i}$, respectively, as schematically shown. σ_{21} (σ_{yx}) is demarcated.

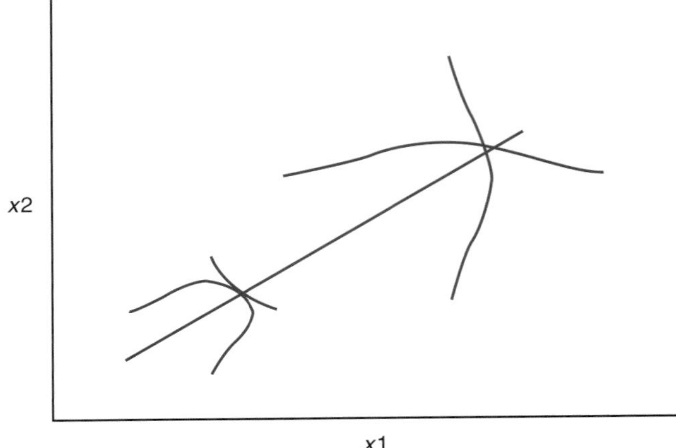

FIGURE 2.23 Outline of the relation between $x1$ and $x2$ values measured by two assays subject to proportional random errors. A linear relationship between the modified target values is assumed. The $x1_i$ and $x2_i$ values are Gaussian distributed around $X1'_{\text{Target}i}$ and $X2'_{\text{Target}i}$, respectively, with increasing scatter at higher concentrations, as is shown schematically.

In this model, α_0 corresponds to a constant difference with regard to calibration, and ($\beta - 1$) is a proportional deviation. Thus, the systematic error or calibration difference between the measurements corresponds to

$$X2'_{\text{Target}i} - X1'_{\text{Target}i} = \alpha_0 + (\beta - 1)X1'_{\text{Target}i}$$

Because of sample-related random interferences and measurement imprecision (of the type that can be described by a Gaussian distribution, eg, caused by pipetting variability, signal variability), individually measured pairs of values ($x1_i$, $x2_i$) will be scattered around the line expressing the relationship between $X1'_{\text{Target}i}$ and $X2'_{\text{Target}i}$. Fig. 2.22 outlines schematically how the random distribution of $x1$ and $x2$ values occurs around the regression line. We have

$$x1_i = X1_{\text{Target}i} + \varepsilon 1_i = X1'_{\text{Target}i} + \text{Random-Bias}1_i + \varepsilon 1_i$$

$$x2_i = X2_{\text{Target}i} + \varepsilon 2_i = X2'_{\text{Target}i} + \text{Random-Bias}2_i + \varepsilon 2_i$$

The random error components may be expressed as SDs, and generally we can assume that sample-related random bias (SD σ_{RB}) and analytical imprecision (SD σ_A) are independent for each analyte, yielding the relations

$$\sigma^2_{\text{ex}1} = \sigma^2_{\text{RB}1} + \sigma^2_{\text{A}1}$$

$$\sigma^2_{\text{ex}2} = \sigma^2_{\text{RB}2} + \sigma^2_{\text{A}2}$$

$\sigma_{\text{ex}1}$ and $\sigma_{\text{ex}2}$ are the total SDs of the distributions of $x1_i$ and $x2_i$ around their respective modified target values, $X1'_{\text{Target}i}$ and $X2'_{\text{Target}i}$. The sample-related random bias components for methods 1 and 2 may not necessarily be independent. They also may not be Gaussian distributed, contrary to the analytical components. Thus, when a regression procedure is applied, the explicit assumptions to take into account should be considered. In situations without random bias components of any significance, the relationships simplify to

$$\sigma^2_{\text{ex}1} = \sigma^2_{\text{A}1}$$

$$\sigma^2_{\text{ex}2} = \sigma^2_{\text{A}2}$$

In this situation, it usually can be assumed that the error distributions are Gaussian, and estimates of the analytical SDs may be available from QC data.

Another methodologic problem concerns the question of whether the dispersion of sample-related random bias and the analytical imprecision are constant or change with the analyte concentration, as considered previously in the difference plot sections. In cases with a considerable range (ie, a decade or longer), this phenomenon should also be taken into account when a regression analysis is applied. Fig. 2.23 schematically shows how dispersions may increase proportionally with concentration.

Deming Regression Analysis and Ordinary Least-Squares Regression Analysis (Constant Standard Deviations)

To reliably estimate the relationship between modified target values (ie, a_0 for α_0 and b for β), a regression procedure taking into account errors in both $x1$ and $x2$ is preferable[6] (ie, Deming approach) (see Fig. 2.22). Although the ordinary least-squares (OLR) procedure is commonly used in method comparison studies, it does not take errors in $x1$ into account but is based on the assumption that only the $x2$ measurements are subject to random errors (Fig. 2.24). In the Deming procedure, the sum of squared distances from measured sets of values ($x1_i$, $x2_i$) to the regression line is minimized at an angle determined by the ratio between SDs for the random variations of $x1$ and $x2$. It can be proven theoretically that, given Gaussian *error* distributions, this estimation procedure is optimal. It should here be noted that it is the *error* distributions that should be Gaussian, not the dispersion of values over the measurement range. This is often misunderstood. In Fig. 2.25, the symmetric case is illustrated with a regression slope of 1 and equal SDs for the random variations of $x1$ and

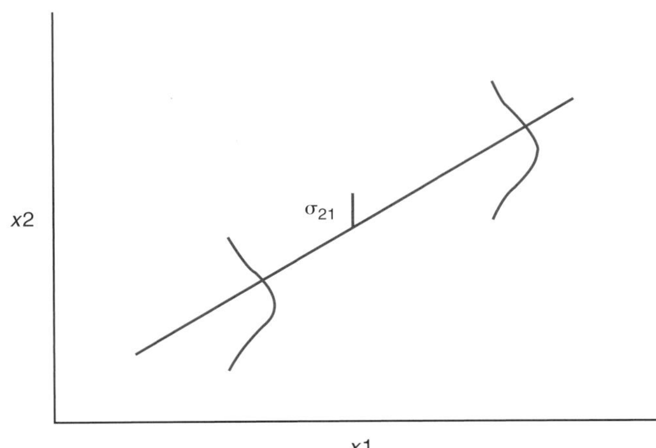

FIGURE 2.24 The model assumed in ordinary least-squares regression. The *x2* values are Gaussian distributed around the line with constant standard deviation over the analytical measurement range. The *x1* values are assumed to be without random error. σ_{21} (σ_{yx}) is shown.

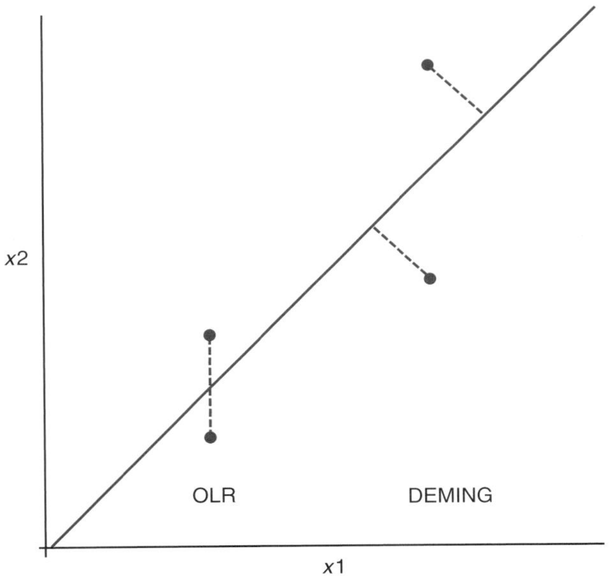

FIGURE 2.25 In ordinary least-squares regression (OLR), the sum of squared deviations from the line is minimized in the vertical direction. In Deming regression analysis, the sum of squared deviations is minimized at an angle to the line, depending on the random error ratio. Here the symmetric case is displayed with orthogonal deviations. (From Linnet K. The performance of Deming regression analysis in case of a misspecified analytical error ratio. *Clin Chem* 1998;44:1024–1031.)

$x2$, in which case the sum of squared distances is minimized orthogonally in relation to the line.

Ordinary least-squares regression is not recommended except in special situations. In OLR, the sum of squared distances is minimized in the vertical direction to the line (see Fig. 2.25). It can be proven theoretically that neglect of the random error in $x1$ induces a downward biased slope estimate

$$\beta' = \beta[\sigma^2_{X1'\text{target}} / (\sigma^2_{X1'\text{target}} + \sigma^2_{\text{ex}1})] = \beta / [1 + (\sigma_{\text{ex}1} / \sigma_{X1'\text{target}})^2]$$

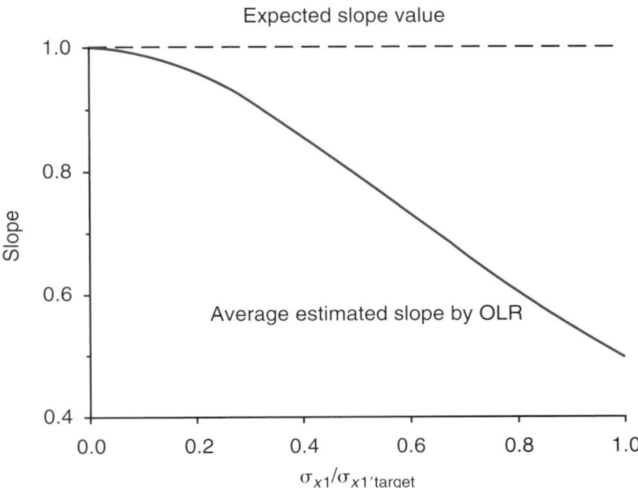

FIGURE 2.26 Relations between the true (expected) slope value and the average estimated slope by ordinary least-squares regression (OLR). The bias of the OLR slope estimate increases negatively for increasing ratios of the standard deviation (SD) random error in *x1* to the SD of the *X1* target value distribution.

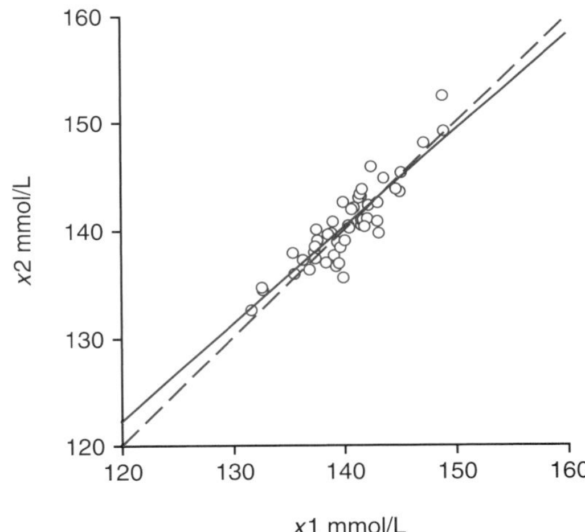

FIGURE 2.27 Simulated comparison of two sodium methods. The *solid line* indicates the average estimated ordinary least-squares regression (OLR) line, and the *dotted line* is the identity line. Even though no systematic difference is evident between the two methods, the average OLR line deviates from the identity line corresponding to a downward slope bias of about 10%.

where $\sigma_{X1'\text{target}}$ is the SD of $X1'$ target values.[5] The magnitude of the bias depends on the ratio between the SD for the random error in $x1$ and the SD of the $X1'$ target values. Fig. 2.26 shows the bias as a function of the ratio of the random error SD to the SD of the $X1'$ target value dispersion. For a ratio up to 0.1, the bias is less than 1%. At a ratio of 0.33, the bias amounts to 10%; it increases further for increasing ratios. In a given case, one can take the analytical SD (eg, from QC data) and divide by the SD of the measured $x1$ values, which approximately equals the SD of $X1'$ target values. As an example, a typical comparison study for two serum sodium methods may be associated with a downward directed slope bias of about 10% (Fig. 2.27).

In the example presented previously, the ratio of the analytical SD to the SD of the target value distribution is large because of the tight physiologic regulation of electrolyte concentrations, which means that the biological variation is limited. Most other types of analytes exhibit wider distributions, and the ratio of error to target value distribution is smaller. For example, for analytes with a distribution of longer than 1 decade and an analytical error corresponding to a CV of 5% at the middle of the analytical measurement range, the OLR slope bias amounts to about −1%.

Computation Procedures for Ordinary Least-Squares Regression and Deming Regression

Assuming no errors in $x1$ and a Gaussian error distribution of $x2$ with constant SD throughout the analytical measurement range, OLR is the optimal estimation procedure, as proved by Gauss in the 18th century. Given errors in both $x1$ and $x2$, the Deming approach is the method of choice.[56] It should be noted for these parametric procedures that only the *error* distributions must be Gaussian or normal. The least-squares principle does not require normality to be applied, but it is optimal under normality conditions, and the nominal type I errors for associated statistical tests for slope and intercept hold true under this assumption. The procedures are generally robust toward deviations from normality, but they are sensitive to outliers because of the squaring principle. Finally, the distribution of the $x1$ and $x2$ values over the measurement range does not have to be normal. A uniform distribution over the analytical measurement range is generally of advantage, but the distribution in principle may take any form. For both procedures, we may evaluate the SD of the dispersion in the *vertical* direction around the line (commonly denoted $SD_{y \cdot x}$ and here given as SD_{21}). We have

$$SD_{21} = [\Sigma(x2_i - X2'_{\text{Targetest}i})^2 / (N-2)]^{0.5}$$

Further discussion regarding the interpretation of SD_{21} will be given later.

To compute the slope in Deming regression analysis, the ratio between the SDs of the random errors of $x1$ and $x2$ is necessary, that is,

$$\lambda = (\sigma^2_{RB1} + \sigma^2_{A1}) / (\sigma^2_{RB2} + \sigma^2_{A2})$$

SD_As can be estimated from duplicate sets of measurements as

$$SD^2_{A1} = (1/2N)[\Sigma(x1_{2i} - x1_{1i})^2]$$

$$SD^2_{A2} = (1/2N)[\Sigma(x2_{2i} - x2_{1i})^2]$$

or they may be available from QC data. The latter is a practical approach that avoids the need for duplicate measurements by each measurement procedure.

If a specific value for λ is not available and the two routine methods that are compared are likely to be associated with random errors of the same order of magnitude, λ can be set to 1. The Deming procedure is generally relatively insensitive to a misspecification of the λ value.[57]

Formulas for computing slope (β), intercept (α_0), and their SEs are available from other sources[5,49,56] and are not provided here.

Evaluation of the Random Error Around an Estimated Regression Line

The estimated slope and intercept provide an estimate of the systematic difference or calibration bias between two methods over the analytical measurement range. Additionally, an estimate of the random error is important. It is common to consider the dispersion around the line in the vertical direction, which is quantified as $SD_{y.x}$ (here denoted SD_{21}). SD_{21} was originally introduced in the context of OLR, but it also can be considered in relation to Deming regression analysis.

Interpreting $SD_{y \cdot x}$ (SD_{21}) With Random Errors in Both *x1* and *x2*

With regard to σ_{21}, we have here without sample-related random interferences

$$\sigma^2_{21} = \beta^2\sigma^2_{A1} + \sigma^2_{A2}$$

Thus, σ_{21} reflects the random error both in $x1$ (with a rescaling) and in $x2$. Often β is close to unity, and in this case, σ^2_{21} becomes approximately the sum of the individual squared SDs. This relation holds true for both Deming and OLR analyses. Frequently, OLR is applied in situations associated with random measurement error in both $x1$ and $x2$, and in these situations, σ_{21} reflects the errors in both.

The presence of sample-related random interferences in both $x1$ and $x2$ gives the following expression:

$$\sigma^2_{21} = (\beta^2\sigma^2_{A1} + \sigma^2_{A2}) + (\beta^2\sigma^2_{RB1} + \sigma^2_{RB2})$$

Thus, the σ_{21} value is influenced by the slope value and the analytical error components σ_{A1} and σ_{A2} (grouped in the first bracket) and σ_{RB1} and σ_{RB2} (grouped in the second bracket). In many cases, the slope is close to unity, in which case we have simple addition of the components. As mentioned earlier, the sample-related random interferences may not be independent. In this case, simple addition of the components is not correct because a covariance term should be included. However, in a real case, we can estimate the combined effect corresponding to the bracket term. Information on the analytical components is usually available from duplicate sets of measurements or from QC data. On this basis, the combined random bias term in the second bracket can be derived by subtracting the analytical components from σ_{21}. Overall, it can be judged whether the total random error is acceptable or not. The systematic difference can be adjusted for relatively easily by rescaling one of the sets of measurements. However, if the random error term is very large, such a rescaling does not ensure equivalency of measurements with regard to individual samples. Thus, it is important to assess both the systematic difference and the random error when deciding whether a new routine method can replace an existing one.

Assessment of Outliers

The principle of minimizing the sum of squared distances from the line makes the described regression procedures sensitive to outliers, and an assessment of the occurrence of outliers should be carried out routinely. The distance from a suspected outlier to the line is recorded in SD units, and the outlier is rejected if the distance exceeds a predetermined limit (eg, 3 or 4 SD units). In the case of OLR, the SD unit

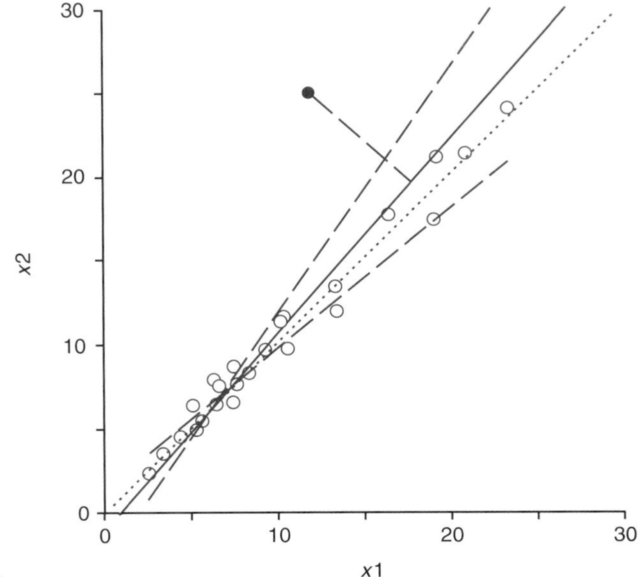

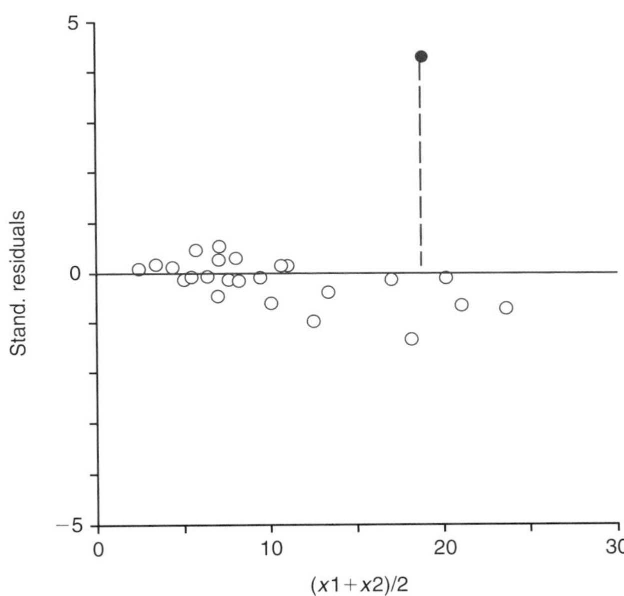

FIGURE 2.28 A, A scatter plot with the Deming regression line *(solid line)* with an outlier *(filled point)*. The *dotted straight line* is the diagonal, and the *curved dashed lines* demarcate the 95% confidence region. **B,** Standardized residuals plot with indication of the outlier.

equals SD_{21}, and the vertical distance is considered. For Deming regression analysis, the unit is the SD of the deviation of the points from the line at an angle determined by the error variance ratio λ. A plot of these deviations, a so-called residuals plot, conveniently illustrates the occurrence of outliers.[54] Fig. 2.28, *A*, illustrates an example of Deming regression analysis with occurrence of an outlier and the associated residuals plot *(B)*, which clearly shows the outlier pattern. In this example, the residuals plot was standardized to unit SD. Use of an outlier limit of 4 SD units in this example led to rejection of the outlier, and a reanalysis was undertaken. In this example, rejection of the outlier changed the slope from 1.14 to 1.03. With regard to outliers, these measurements should not be rejected automatically; the reason for their presence should be investigated as a method limitation (eg, possibly a nonspecificity for the analyte).

The Correlation Coefficient

Now that the random error components related to regression analysis have been outlined, some comments on the correlation coefficient may be appropriate. The ordinary correlation coefficient, ρ, also called the Pearson product moment correlation coefficient, is estimated as *r* from sums of squared deviations for $x1$ and $x2$ values as follows:

$$r = p/(uq)^{0.5}$$

where

$$p = \Sigma(x1_i - x1_m)(x2_i - x2_m)$$

$$u = \Sigma(x1_i - x1_m)^2 \text{ and } q = \Sigma(x2_i - x2_m)^2$$

and

$$x1_m = \Sigma x1_i / N \text{ and } x2_m = \Sigma x2_i / N$$

A look at the theoretical model reveals that ρ is related to the ratio between the SDs of the distributions of target values ($\sigma_{X1'\text{target}}$ and $\sigma_{X2'\text{target}}$) and the associated independent total random error components[58] (σ_{ex1} and σ_{ex2}):

$$\rho = \sigma_{X1'\text{target}}\sigma_{X2'\text{target}} / [(\sigma^2_{X1'\text{target}} + \sigma^2_{ex1})(\sigma^2_{X2'\text{target}} + \sigma^2_{ex2})]^{0.5}$$

The total random error components comprise both imprecision error and sample-related random interferences (ie, $\sigma^2_{ex1} = \sigma^2_{A1} + \sigma^2_{RB1}$ and $\sigma^2_{ex2} = \sigma^2_{A2} + \sigma^2_{RB2}$). Thus, ρ is a *relative* indicator of the amount of dispersion around the regression line. If the numeric interval of values is short, ρ tends to be low and vice versa for a long range of values. For example, consider simulated examples, where the random errors of $x1$ and $x2$ are the same but the width of the distributions of measured values differs (Fig. 2.29, *A* and *B*). In *A*, the target values are uniformly distributed over the range 1 to 3, and in *B*, the range is 1 to 6. The random error SD is presumed constant, and it is set to 0.15 for both $x1$ and $x2$, corresponding to a CV of 5% at the value 3. Given sets of 50 paired measurements, the correlation coefficient is 0.93 in case *A* and 0.99 in case *B*. Furthermore, a single point located outside the range of the rest of the observations exerts a strong influence (Fig. 2.29, *C*). In *C*, 49 of the observations are distributed within the range 1 to 3, with a single point located apart from the others around the value 6, other factors being equal. The correlation coefficient here takes an intermediate value, 0.97. Thus, a single point located away from the rest has a strong influence (a so-called influential point). Note that it is not an outlying point, just an aberrant point with regard to the range.

Although σ_{21} is the relevant measure for random error in method comparison studies, ρ is still incorrectly used as a supposed measure of agreement between two methods. It should be noted that a systematic difference due to a difference with regard to calibration is not expressed through ρ but solely in the form of an intercept (α_0) deviation from zero or a slope (β) deviation from unity. Thus, even though the

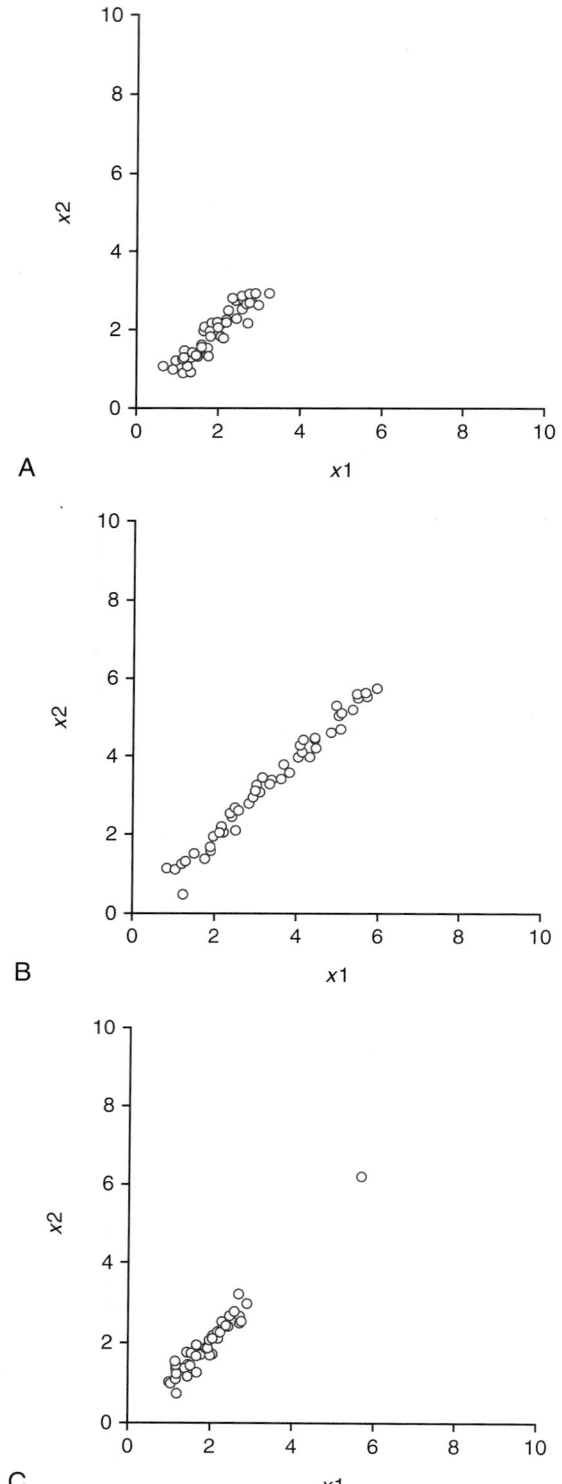

FIGURE 2.29 Scatter plots illustrating the effect of the range on the value of the correlation coefficient ρ. **A,** Target values are uniformly distributed over the range 1 to 3 with random errors of both *x*1 and *x*2 corresponding to a standard deviation (SD) of 5% of the target value at 3 (constant error SDs). **B,** The range is extended to 1 to 6 with the same random error levels. The correlation coefficient equals 0.93 in A and 0.99 in B. **C,** The effect of a single aberrant point is shown. Forty-nine of the target values are distributed over the range 1 to 3, with a single point at 6. The correlation coefficient is 0.97.

correlation coefficient is very high, a considerable calibration bias may be noted between the measurements of two methods.

Regression Analysis in Cases of Proportional Random Error

As discussed in relation to the precision profile, for analytes with extended ranges (eg, 1 or several decades), the SD_A is seldom constant. Rather, a proportional relationship may apply. This may also be true for the random bias components. In this situation, the regression procedures described previously may still be used, but they are not optimal because the SEs of slope and intercept become larger than is the case when a weighted form of regression analysis is applied. The optimal approaches are weighted forms of regression analysis that take into account the relationship between random error and analyte concentration.[49,54] Given a proportional relationship, a weighted procedure assigns larger weights to observations in the low range; low-range observations are more precise than measurements at higher concentrations that are subject to larger random errors. More specifically, weights are applied in the computations that are inversely proportional to the squared SDs (variances) that express the random error. In the weighted modification of the Deming procedure, distances from ($x1_i$, $x2_i$) to the line are inversely weighted according to the squared SDs at a given concentration (Fig. 2.30). The regression procedures are most conveniently performed using dedicated software.

Testing for Linearity

Splitting of the systematic error into a constant and a proportional component depends on the assumption of linearity, which should be tested. A convenient test is a runs test, which in principle assesses whether negative and positive deviations from the points to the line are randomly distributed over the

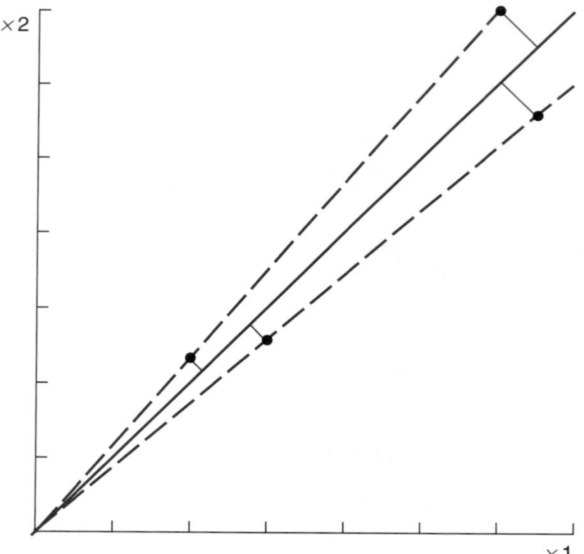

FIGURE 2.30 Distances from data points to the line in weighted Deming regression assuming proportional random errors in *x*1 and *x*2. The symmetric case is illustrated with equal random errors and a slope of unity yielding orthogonal projections onto the line. (Modified from Linnet K. Necessary sample size for method comparison studies based on regression analysis. *Clin Chem* 1999;45:882–894. Used with permission.)

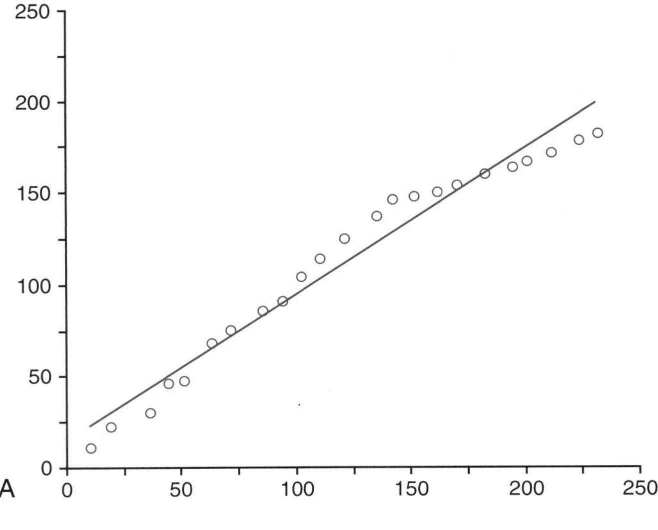

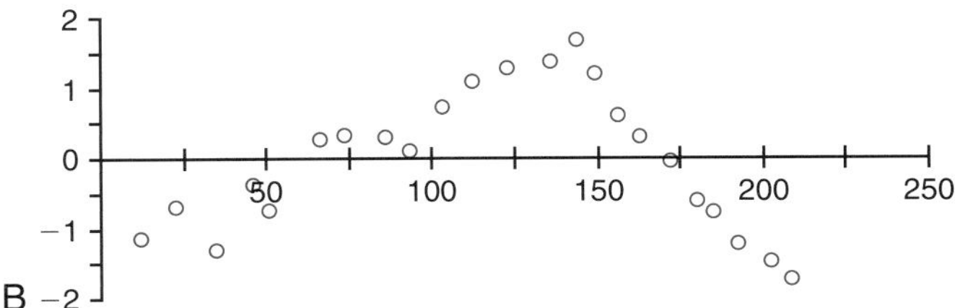

FIGURE 2.31 **A,** Scatter plot showing an example of nonlinearity in the form of downward-deviating x2 values at the upper part of the range. **B,** Plot of residuals showing the effects of nonlinearity. At the upper end of the analytical measurement range, a sequence (run) of negative residuals is present.

analytical measurement range. The term *run* here relates to a sequence of deviations with the same sign. Consider, for example, the situation with a downward trend of $x2$ values at the upper end of the analytical measurement range (Fig. 2.31, *A*). The SDs from the line (ie, the residuals) will tend to be negative in this area instead of being randomly distributed above and below the line[20] (Fig. 2.31, *B*). Given a sufficient number of points, such a sequence will turn out to be statistically significant in a runs test.

Nonparametric Regression Analysis (Passing-Bablok Procedure)

The slope and the intercept may be estimated by a nonparametric procedure, which is robust to outliers and requires no assumptions of Gaussian error distributions.[59,60] The method takes measurement errors for both $x1$ and $x2$ into account, but it presumes that the ratio between random errors is related to the slope in a fixed manner:

$$\lambda = (SD^2_{RB1} + SD^2_{A1}) / (SD^2_{RB2} + SD^2_{A2}) = 1/\beta^2$$

Otherwise, a biased slope estimate is obtained.[49,60] The procedure may be applied both in situations with random errors with constant SDs and in cases with proportional SDs. The method is not as efficient as the corresponding parametric procedures[49] (ie, Deming and weighted Deming procedures). Slope and intercept with CIs are provided, together with Spearman's rank correlation coefficient. A software program is required for the procedure.

Interpretation of Systematic Differences Between Methods Obtained on the Basis of Regression Analysis

A systematic difference between two methods is identified if the estimated intercept differs significantly from zero or if the slope deviates significantly from 1. This is decided on the basis of *t*-tests:

$$t = (a_0 - 0) / \mathrm{SE}(a_0)$$

$$t = (b - 1) / \mathrm{SE}(b)$$

The *t*-tests can be supplemented with 95% CIs.

SE(a_0) and SE*(b)* are the SEs of the estimated intercept a_0 and the slope *b,* respectively. Standard errors can be derived by a computerized resampling principle called *the jackknife procedure,* which in practice can be carried out using appropriate software.[61] Having estimated a_0 and *b,* we have the estimate of the systematic difference between the methods, D_c, at a selected concentration, $X1'_{\mathrm{Targetc}}$:

$$D_c = X2'_{\mathrm{Targetestc}} - X1'_{\mathrm{Targetc}} = a_0 + (b-1)X1'_{\mathrm{Targetc}}$$

$X2'_{\mathrm{Targetestc}}$ is the estimated $X2'$ target value at $X1'_c$. Note that D_c refers to the *systematic* difference (ie, the difference between modified target values corresponding to a calibration difference). The SE of D_c can be derived by the jackknife procedure using a software program. By evaluating the SE throughout the analytical measurement range, a confidence region for the estimated line can be displayed. If method comparison is performed to assess the calibration to a reference measurement procedure, correction of a significant systematic difference $Delta_c$ will often be performed by recalibration [$x2_{rec} = (x1 - a_0)/b$]. The associated standard uncertainty is the SE of $Delta_c$. Even though the intercept and the slope are not significantly different from zero and 1, respectively, the combined expression $Delta_c$ may be significantly different from zero.

Example of Application of Regression Analysis (Weighted Deming Analysis)

Application of weighted Deming regression analysis may be illustrated by the comparison of drug assays example [$N = 65$ ($x1$, $x2$) single measurements]. As outlined in the section on the Bland-Altman plot (see Fig. 2.15), in this example the random error of the differences increases with the concentration, suggesting that the weighted form of Deming regression analysis is appropriate. Fig. 2.32 shows *(A)* the estimated regression line with 95% confidence bands and *(B)* a plot of normalized residuals. The nearly homogeneous scatter in the residuals plot supports the assumed proportional random error model and the assumption of linearity. The slope estimate (1.014) is not significantly different from 1 (95% CI: 0.97–1.06), and the intercept is not significantly different from zero (95% CI: −6.7–47.4) (Table 2.9). A runs test for linearity does not contradict the assumption of linearity. The amount of random error is quantified in the form of the SD_{21} proportionality factor equal to 0.11, or 11%. In the present example, with a slope close to unity and two routine methods with assumed random errors of about the same magnitude, we divide the random error by the square root of 2 and get $CV_{x1} = CV_{x2} = 7.8\%$. QC data in the laboratory have provided CV_As of 6.1% and 7.2% for methods 1 and 2, respectively. Thus in this example, the random error may be attributed

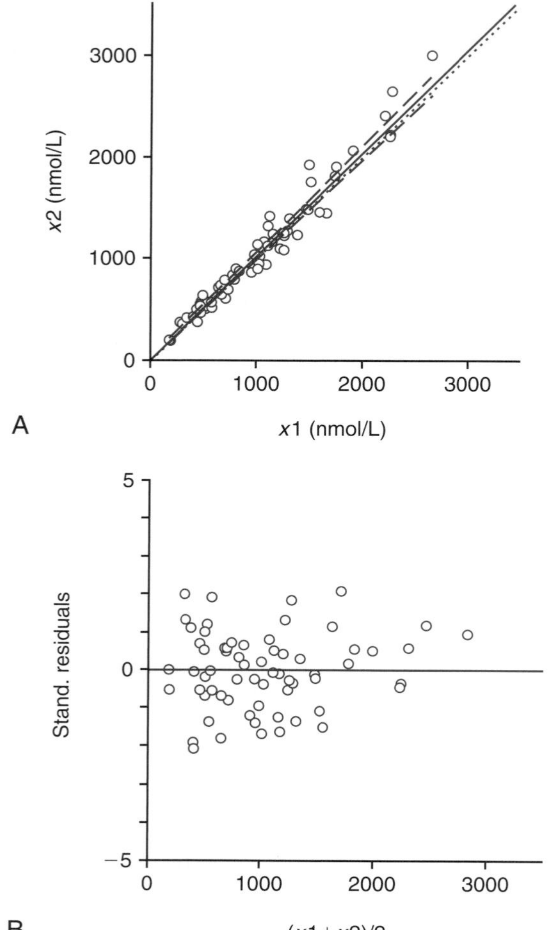

FIGURE 2.32 An example of weighted Deming regression analysis for the comparison of drug assays. **A,** The *solid line* is the estimated weighted Deming regression line, the *dashed curves* indicate the 95%-confidence region, and the *dotted line* is the line of identity. **B,** A plot of residuals standardized to unit standard deviation. The homogeneous scatter supports the assumed proportional error model and the assumption of linearity.

largely to analytical error. The assay principle for both methods is HPLC, which generally is a rather specific measurement principle; considerable random bias effects are not expected in this case.

In Table 2.9, estimated systematic differences at the limits of the therapeutic interval (300 and 2000 nmol/L) are displayed (24.6 and 48.9 nmol/L, respectively). This corresponds to percentage values of 8.2% and 2.4%, respectively. Estimated SEs by the jackknife procedure yield the 95% Cis, as shown in the table. At the low concentration, the difference is significant (95% CI: 5.7 to 44 nmol/L; does not include zero), which is not the case at the high level (95% CI: −19 to 117 nmol/L). Even though the intercept and slope estimates separately are not significantly different from the null hypothesis values of 0 and 1, respectively, the combined difference $Delta_c$ is significant at low concentrations in this example. If the difference is considered of medical importance and both methods are to be used simultaneously in the laboratory, recalibration of one of the methods might be considered.

TABLE 2.9 Results of Weighted Deming Regression Analysis for the Comparison of Drug Assays Example, $n = 65$ Single ($x1$, $x2$) Measurements

	Estimate	SE	95% CI
Slope *(b)*	1.014	0.022	0.97 to 1.06
Intercept (a_0)	20.3	13.5	−6.7 to 47.4
Weighted correlation coefficient	0.98		
SD_{21} proportionality factor	0.11		
Runs test for linearity	NS		
$Delta_c = X_2 - X_1$ at $X_c = 300$	24.6	9.5	5.72 to 43.6
$Delta_c = X_2 - X_1$ at $X_c = 2000$	48.9	34.2	−19.3 to 117

CI, Confidence interval; *NS,* not significant; *SD,* standard deviation; *SE,* standard error.

Discussion of Application of Regression Analysis

Generally, it is recommended that Deming or weighted Deming regression analysis should be used to operate with a type of regression analysis that is based on a correct error model. Most published method evaluations are based on unweighted regression analysis; here the use of unweighted analysis is considered in the setting of proportional random errors.

Basically, the Deming procedure provides unbiased estimates of slope and intercept when the SDs vary, provided that their ratio is constant throughout the analytical measurement range. This aspect is important and means that generally the estimates of slope and intercept are reliable in this frequently encountered situation. However, application of the unweighted Deming analysis in cases of proportional SD_As is less efficient than applying the weighted approach. For uniform distributions of values with range ratios from 2 to 100, 1.2 to 3.7 times as many samples are necessary to obtain the same uncertainty of the slope estimated by the unweighted compared with the weighted approach.[61] Thus, the larger the range ratio, the more inefficient is the unweighted method.

POINTS TO REMEMBER

- Comparison of two analytical methods is usually based on parallel measurement of a suitable number of patient samples (eg, 40 in a laboratory and 100 for a vendor of analytical kit methods).
- Data analysis can be based on either a difference plot or regression analysis, the latter providing more details.
- Differences between measurement results may rely on calibration differences, random measurement errors, and biologically based bias sources.
- The optimal regression technique takes measurement errors by both methods into account (eg, the parametric Deming approach or the nonparametric Passing-Bablok procedure).

MONITORING SERIAL RESULTS

An important aspect of clinical chemistry is monitoring of disease or treatment (eg, tumor markers in cases of cancer, drug concentrations in cases of therapeutic drug monitoring). To assess changes in a rational way, various imprecision components have to be taken into account. Biologic within-subject variation (SD_I) and preanalytical (SD_{PA}) and analytical variation (SD_A) all have to be recognized.[62] We assume in the following discussion that preanalytical variation is already included in the estimated within-subject variation SD, which often is the case. On this basis, using the principle of adding squared SDs (variances), a total SD (SD_T) can be estimated as follows:

$$SD_T^2 = SD_{Within\ B}^2 + SD_A^2$$

The limit for statistically significant changes then is $k\sqrt{2}\ SD_T$, where k depends on the desired probability level. Considering a two-sided 5% level, k is 1.96. The corresponding one-sided factor is 1.65. If a higher probability level is desired, k should be increased.

Limits for statistically significant changes ($Delta_{stat}$) may be related to changes that are considered of medical importance by clinicians[63] (ie, action limits [$Delta_{med}$]). Here we will consider a one-sided situation in which an increase is of importance and a 5% significance level is selected (ie, $Delta_{stat} = 1.65\sqrt{2}\ SD_T = 1.65\ SD_{delta}$). Suppose as a starting point that the true change ($Delta_{true}$) for a patient is zero (Fig. 2.33, *A*). If $Delta_{stat}$ is less than $Delta_{med}$, the frequency of FP alarms will be less than 5%. If, on the other hand, $Delta_{stat}$ exceeds $Delta_{med}$, the frequency of FP alarms will exceed 5% (ie, medical action will be taken too frequently). Fig. 2.33, *A*, illustrates the situation with $Delta_{stat}$ equal to $Delta_{med}$. We now consider the situation with a true change equal to the medically important change (ie, $Delta_{true} = Delta_{med}$) (Fig. 2.33, *B*), where exactly 50% of observed changes exceed the medically important limit. If $Delta_{stat}$ is less than or equal to $Delta_{med}$, fewer than 5% of patients will exhibit an observed delta value in the opposite direction of the true change (an obviously misleading trend). If the condition is not met, more than 5% will have a misleading change. Finally, when the true change equals the sum of $Delta_{med}$ and $Delta_{stat}$ (Fig. 2.33, *C*), more than 95% of observed changes exceed the medically important change, and appropriate action will be taken for most patients.

The outline presented previously illustrates that in the monitoring situation, not only the requirement for statistical significance (ie, the type I error problem concerning false alarms) but also the type II error problem or the risk of overlooking changes, should be addressed; the latter is an aspect that often is overlooked.[64] Provided that $Delta_{stat}$ is small relative to $Delta_{med}$, both type I and type II errors can be kept small. On the other hand, if $Delta_{stat}$ equals or exceeds $Delta_{med}$, the relative importance of type I and type II errors may be weighed against each other. If the consequences of

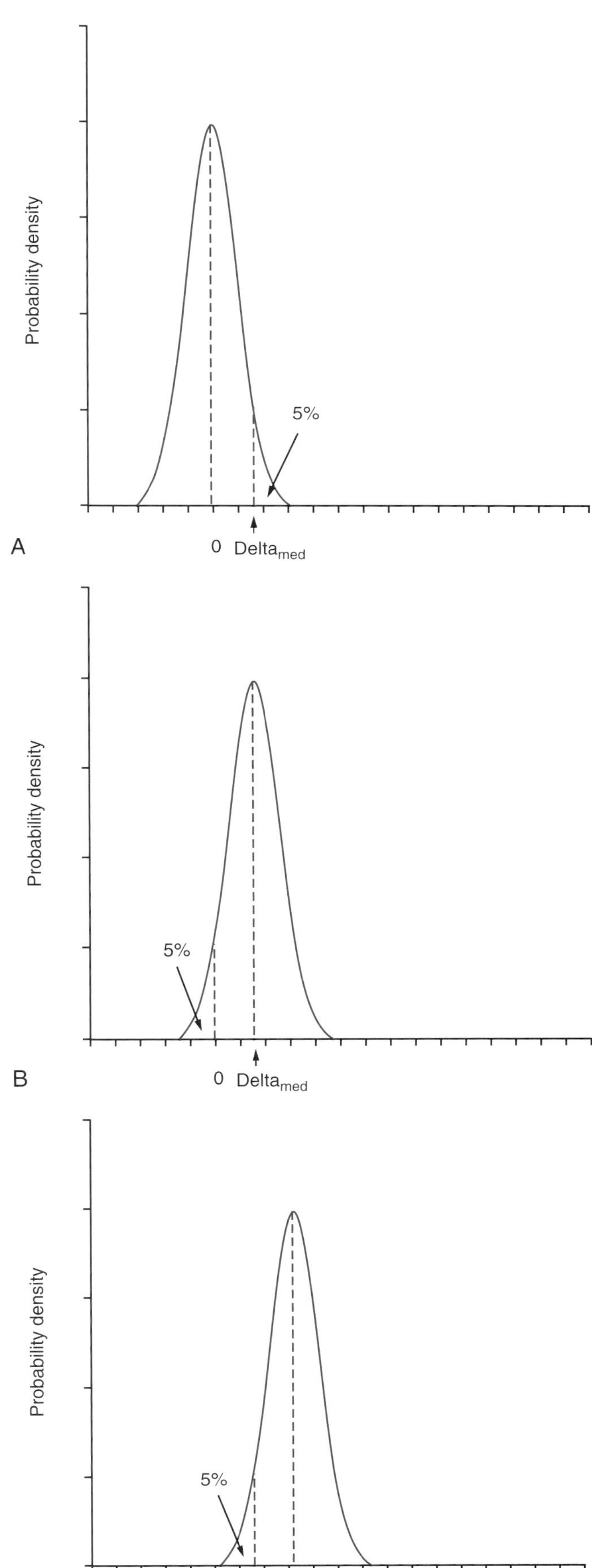

FIGURE 2.33 The monitoring situation. **A,** Distribution of observed changes given a true change of zero. **B,** A true change equal to $Delta_{med}$. **C,** A true change of ($Delta_{med}$ + 1.65 SD_{delta}). $Delta_{stat}$ (=1.65 SD_{delta}) equals $Delta_{med}$ in these examples.

overlooking a medically important change are serious, one should keep the type II error small and accept a relatively large type I error (ie, accept the occurrence of false alarms). On the contrary, if overlooking changes only gives rise to minor or transient problems, the priority may be to keep the type I error small. In addition to simple evaluation of a shift between two measurements, as considered here, sequential results may be analyzed using more refined time-series models.[65]

TRACEABILITY AND MEASUREMENT UNCERTAINTY

As outlined previously in the error model sections, laboratory results are likely to be influenced by systematic and random errors of various types. Obtaining agreement of measurements between laboratories or agreement over time in a given laboratory often can be problematic.

Traceability

To ensure reasonable agreement between measurements of routine methods, the concept of traceability comes into focus. (See also the "Calibration Traceability to a Reference System and Commutability Considerations" section in Chapter 6.) Traceability is based on an unbroken chain of comparisons of measurements leading to a known reference value (Fig. 2.34). A hierarchical approach for tracing the values of routine clinical chemistry measurements to reference measurement procedures was proposed by Tietz[66] and has been adapted by the ISO. For well-established analytes, a hierarchy of methods exists with *a reference measurement procedure* at the top, *selected measurement procedures* at an intermediate level, and finally *routine measurement procedures* at the bottom.[66-68] A reference measurement procedure is a fully understood procedure of highest analytical quality containing a complete uncertainty budget given in Système Internationale (SI) units.[12,69] Reference procedures are used to measure the analyte concentration in *secondary reference materials,* which typically have the same matrix as samples that are to be measured by routine procedures (eg, human serum). Secondary reference materials are usually of high analytical quality, and certified secondary reference materials must be validated for commutability with clinical samples if they are intended for use as trueness controls for routine methods.[70,71] Otherwise, their use is restricted to selected measurement procedures for which they are intended. The certificate of analysis should state the methods for which the secondary reference materials have been validated to be commutable with clinical samples. When no information is given for commutability, it must be assumed that the reference material is not commutable with clinical samples, and the user has the responsibility to validate commutability for the methods of interest.[72] Uncertainty of the measurement procedure results in increases from the top level to the bottom. ISO guidelines (15193 and 15194) address requirements for reference methods and reference materials.[69,73]

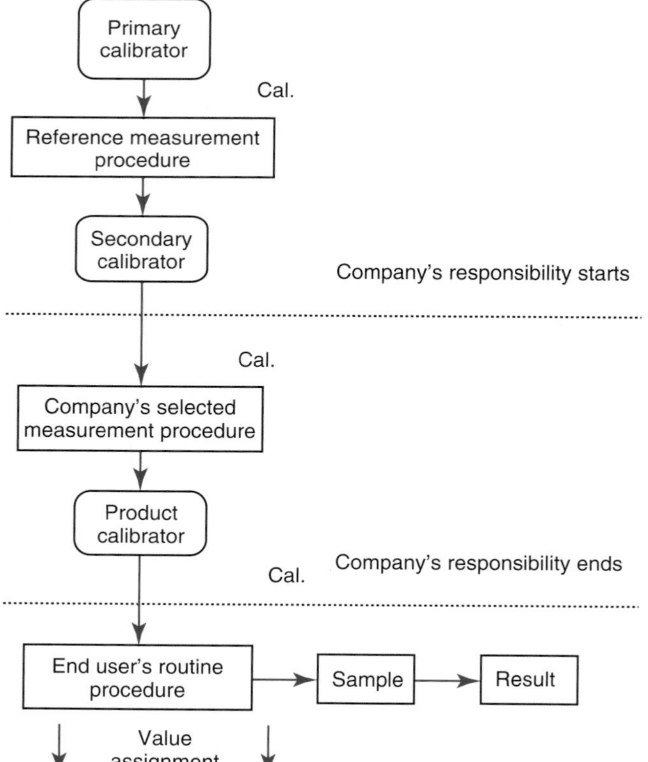

FIGURE 2.34 The calibration hierarchy from a reference measurement procedure to a routine assay. The uncertainty increases from top to bottom. *Cal., Calibration.*

The measurement uncertainty down the traceability chain can end up being too high. By repetition of independent measurements at each step, it may be possible to reduce the overall uncertainty so that it becomes acceptable in relation to analytical performance specification (eg, those based on biological variation).[74] For more detailed information on analytical performance specifications see "Performance of a Measurement Procedure for Its Intended Medical Use" section of Chapter 6 and the "Analytical Performance Specifications Based on Biological Variation" section of Chapter 7.

Using cortisol as an example, the primary reference material is crystalline cortisol with a chemical analysis for impurities[71] (National Institute of Standards and Technology [NIST] standard reference material 921, cortisol [hydrocortisone]). A primary calibrator is then a cortisol preparation with a stated mass fraction (purity) (eg, 0.998 and a 95% CI of ±0.001). The reference measurement procedure is an isotope-dilution gas chromatography–mass spectrometry method that is calibrated with the primary calibrator. A panel of individual frozen serum samples that have values assigned by the primary reference measurement procedure is available from the Institute for Reference Materials and Measurements (IRMM) as secondary reference materials (European Reference Material [ERM]-DA451/International Federation of Clinical Chemistry and Laboratory Medicine [IFCC]). A manufacturer's *selected measurement* procedure is calibrated with the secondary reference materials and is used for measurement of the quantity in the manufacturer's *product calibrator,* which is the calibrator used for the routine method in clinical laboratories.

At the time of writing, the Joint Committee for Traceability in Laboratory Medicine (JCTLM) Database (http://www.bipm.org/jctlm) lists reference materials, either pure or matrix matched, for more than 95 measurands, of which over 50 are traceable to the SI (list I). SI traceable measurands include electrolytes, some metabolites (eg, glucose, creatinine, urea, uric acid), drugs, metals, steroids, and thyroid and other hormones. Analytes listed in the database that are not traceable to the SI (list II) include 13 plasma proteins (eg, albumin, α1 acid glycoprotein, α1 antitrypsin, transferrin, transerythretin), using the ERM-DA470k/IFCC. The database also lists reference measurement procedures that define the top of the traceability chain for eight serum enzymes. There are also analytes traceable to higher-order international reference preparations not listed in the JCTLM database, which have been produced by National Measurement Institutes (eg, pH, pCO_2, pO_2, and ammonia) or by the World Health Organization (http://www.who.int/bloodproducts/catalogue/en) (eg, for allergens, various proteins and antigens, coagulation factors, and various hormones); however, these are not traceable to the SI. With protein hormones, the existence of heterogeneity or microheterogeneity complicates the problem of traceability.[75,76]

In case a reference measurement procedure exists for an analyte (measurand), comparable results among measurement procedures can be achieved as described earlier, so-called standardization. When reference measurement procedures are not available, so-called harmonization refers to the process of establishing comparable results among measurement procedures for the given analyte.[77] Harmonization is typically based on distribution among laboratories of commutable secondary reference materials with arbitrarily set target values. For more information on harmonization, readers are referred to the "Calibration Traceability to a Reference System and Commutability Considerations" section of Chapter 6.

Harmonization and standardization are especially important when disease is defined by clinical biochemistry results. This pertains to, for example, the diagnosis of diabetes based on plasma glucose determinations. The analytical quality in this instance becomes very critical for a correct evaluation. An analytical bias results in misclassification of subjects into diseased and nondiseased groups. With regard to imprecision, repeat testing may partly circumvent classification errors.[78]

The Uncertainty Concept

To assess in a systematic way errors associated with laboratory results, the *uncertainty* concept has been introduced into laboratory medicine.[79,80] According to the ISO's "Guide to the Expression of Uncertainty in Measurement" (GUM), *uncertainty* is formally defined as "a parameter associated with the result of a measurement that characterizes the dispersion of the values that could reasonably be attributed to the measurand." In practice, this means that the uncertainty is given as an interval around a reported laboratory result that specifies the location of the true value with a given probability (eg, 95%). In general, the uncertainty of a result, which is traceable to a particular reference, is the uncertainty of that reference together with the overall uncertainty of the traceability chain.[79] Updated information on traceability aspects is available on the website of the Joint Committee on Traceability in Laboratory Medicine (www.bipm.org/jctlm/).

The Standard Uncertainty (u_{st})

The uncertainty concept is directed toward the end user (clinician) of the result, who is concerned about the total error possible and who is not particularly interested in the question of whether the errors are systematic or random. In the outline of the uncertainty concept, it is assumed that any known systematic error components of a measurement method have been corrected, and the specified uncertainty includes uncertainty associated with correction of the systematic error(s).[80] Although this appears logical, one problem may be that some routine methods have systematic errors dependent on the patient category from which the sample originates. For example, kinetic Jaffe methods for creatinine are subject to positive interference by 2-OXO compounds and to negative interference by bilirubin and its metabolites, which means that the direction of systematic error will be patient dependent and not generally predictable.

In the theory on uncertainty, a distinction between type A and B uncertainties is made. Type A uncertainties are frequency-based estimates of SDs (eg, an SD of the imprecision). Type B uncertainties are uncertainty components for which frequency-based SDs are not available. Instead, uncertainty is estimated by other approaches or by the opinion of experts. Finally, the total uncertainty is derived from a combination of all sources of uncertainty. In this context, it is practical to operate with *standard uncertainties* (u_{st}), which are equivalent to SDs. By multiplication of a standard uncertainty with a *coverage factor (k),* the uncertainty corresponding to a specified probability level is derived. For example, multiplication with a coverage factor of 2 yields a probability level of ≈95%, given a Gaussian distribution. When the total uncertainty of an analytical result obtained by a routine method is considered (u_{st}), preanalytical variation (u_{PAst}), method imprecision (u_{Ast}), sample-related random interferences (u_{RBst}), and uncertainty related to calibration and bias corrections (traceability) (u_{Tracst}) should be taken into account. In expressing the uncertainty components as standard uncertainties, we have the following general relation:

$$u_{st} = [u_{PAst}^2 + u_{Ast}^2 + u_{RBst}^2 + u_{Tracst}^2]^{0.5}$$

Uncertainty can be assessed in various ways; often a combination of procedures is necessary. In principle, uncertainty can be judged *directly* from measurement comparisons ("top down")[81,82] or *indirectly* from an analysis of individual error sources according to the law of error propagation ("error budget," bottom up").[80] Measurement comparison may consist of a method comparison study with a reference method based on patient samples according to the principles outlined previously or by measurement of commutable certified matrix reference materials (CRMs). This approach demonstrates the actual uncertainty, which is an advantage. The indirect procedure, on the other hand, builds on an assumed error model, which may or may not be correct and so the uncertainty estimate. It may depend on the circumstances which procedure is feasible. Below, examples of the two types of approaches are outlined.

Example of Direct Assessment of Uncertainty on the Basis of Measurements of a Commutable Certified Reference Material

Suppose a CRM is available that was validated to be *commutable* with patient samples for a given routine method with a specified value 10.0 mmol/L and a standard uncertainty of 0.2 mmol/L. Ten repeated measurements in independent runs give a mean value of 10.3 mmol/L with SD 0.5 mmol/L. The SE of the mean is then $0.5/\sqrt{10} = 0.16$ mmol/L. The mean is not significantly different from the assigned value

[$t = (10.3 - 10.0)/(0.2^2 + 0.16^2)^{0.5} = 1.17$]. The total standard uncertainty with regard to traceability is then $u_{\text{Trac st}} = (0.16^2 + 0.2^2)^{0.5} = 0.26$ mmol/L. If the bias had been significant, one might have considered making a correction to the method, and the standard uncertainty would then be the same at the given concentration. Thus, measurements of the CRM provide an estimate of the uncertainty related to traceability, *given the assumption of commutability with patient samples.* The other components have to be estimated separately. Concerning method imprecision, long-term imprecision (eg, observed from QC measurements) should be used rather than the short-term SD observed for CRM material. Here we suppose that the long-term SD_A is 0.8 mmol/L. Data on preanalytical variation can be obtained by sampling in duplicates from a series of patients or can be a matter of judgment (type B uncertainty) based on literature data or data on similar analytes. We here suppose that SD_{PA} equals half the analytical SD (ie, 0.4 mmol/L). Finally, we lack data on a possible sample-related random bias component, which we may choose to ignore in the present example. The standard uncertainty of the results then becomes

$$\begin{aligned} u_{st} &= [u_{PAst}^2 + u_{Ast}^2 + u_{RBst}^2 + u_{Tracst}^2]^{0.5} \\ &= (0.4^2 + 0.8^2 + 0.26^2)^{0.5} \\ &= 0.93\,(\text{mmol/L}) \end{aligned}$$

In this case, the major uncertainty component is the long-term imprecision in the laboratory. To attain a reasonably precise uncertainty estimate, estimated SDs should be based on an appropriate number of repetitions. In the subsection on method precision, it can be seen that $N = 30$ repetitions provides SD estimates with 95% CIs extending from about 20% below to 35% above an estimated value (see Fig. 2.7), which may be regarded as reasonable.

Example of Direct Assessment of Uncertainty on the Basis of a Method Comparison Study With a Reference Measurement Procedure Using Patient Samples

Suppose a set of patient samples has been measured by a routine method ($X2$) in parallel with a reference measurement procedure ($X1$) and that a linear relationship exists between measurements. We want to assess a possible calibration bias and evaluate the standard uncertainty of results of the routine method on the basis of regression analysis results and information on standard uncertainty related to the traceability of reference method results. The imprecision of the reference method is 2.5% or, as a fraction (used in the following), 0.025 (= CV_{A1}), and the component related to the uncertainty of the traceability chain for the reference method is 0.020 (= $u_{\text{trac st}}$). Proportional measurement errors are assumed for both methods, and a weighted form of Deming regression analysis is applied. The error variance ratio λ is not known exactly, but the reference method is devoid of sample-related random bias, so it is assumed that the random error is about half that of the routine method (ie, λ is set to $1/2^2 = 1/4$). At a decision point ($X1'_{\text{Targetc}}$) (eg, corresponding to the upper limit of the 95% reference interval), the systematic difference between methods ($D_c = a_0 + [b - 1]\, X1'_{\text{Targetc}}$) is estimated with SE (see section on regression):

$$D_c = X2'_{\text{Targetc}} - X1'_{\text{Targetc}} = 20\text{ mg/L with SE}(D_c) = 1.0\text{ mg/L}$$

corresponding to a relative SE(D_c) of 0.050 (= [1.0 mg/L]/[20 mg/L]). For the Deming procedures, the SE can be conveniently computed by the jackknife procedure. We observe that the difference is highly significant and decide to recalibrate the routine method in relation to the reference method using the estimated slope and intercept (ie, the recalibrated $x2$ values equals [$x2 - a_0$]/b). Having done this, the routine method is assumed to have no systematic error in relation to the reference method, but when the uncertainty of the results is considered, we have to add the standard uncertainty of the bias correction. The uncertainty related to traceability for the routine method is now obtained as the uncertainty inherent to the reference method and the comparison step, that is:

$$u_{\text{Tracst}} = (0.020^2 + 0.050^2)^{0.5} = 0.054$$

We are now further interested in deriving estimates of random error components for the routine method from regression analysis results. Both analytical error (eg, estimated from QC data) and sample-related random bias should be assessed, and it should be recognized that the observed total random error is the result of contributions from both measurement methods. Suppose that CV_{21} of the regression analysis has been calculated to be 0.10 (CV_{21} is analogous to SD_{21} or SD_{yx}), given constant measurement errors over the analytical measurement range (ie, an expression for the random error in the vertical direction in the x-y plot). From the regression section, we have

$$CV_{21}^2 = [CV_{A1}^2 + CV_{A2}^2] + [CV_{RB1}^2 + CV_{RB2}^2]$$

By substituting $CV_{A1} = 0.025$, $CV_{RB1} = 0$, and $CV_{21} = 0.10$, we derive

$$CV_{RB2}^2 + CV_{A2}^2 = 0.009375$$

and get

$$[CV_{RB2}^2 + CV_{A2}^2]^{0.5} = 0.0968$$

Thus, the total random error of the routine method corresponds to a CV of 0.097. If we had measured samples in duplicate in the method comparison experiment or had available QC data, we could split the total random error into its components. CV_{A2} was here determined to be 0.035 from QC data, which gives 0.090 corresponding to CV_{RB2}. We may here note that the assumed error ratio λ of $(1/2)^2$ is not quite correct. According to our results, λ should be $(0.025/0.0968)^2$. Although the Deming regression principle is rather robust toward misspecified λ values, we could choose to carry out a reanalysis with the more correct λ value—a process that could be iterated. Finally, assuming a value of 0.03 for the preanalytical CV, we derive a total standard uncertainty estimate of

$$\begin{aligned} u_{st} &= [u_{PAst}^2 + u_{Ast}^2 + u_{RBst}^2 + u_{Tracst}^2]^{0.5} \\ &(0.03^2 + 0.0968^2 + 0.054^2)^{0.5} = 0.115 \end{aligned}$$

At the given decision level of 20 mg/L and with a coverage factor of 2, we obtain the 95% uncertainty interval of a single routine measurement as

$$20\text{ mg/L} \pm (2 \times 0.115 \times 20)\text{ mg/L} = 15.4 - 24.6\text{ mg/L}$$

Having estimated the uncertainty as outlined, additional uncertainty sources should be considered. If the comparison was undertaken within a short time period, one might consider adding an additional long-term imprecision component as a variance component to the standard uncertainty expression.

When the two approaches briefly outlined are compared, the latter is the more informative. Using a series of patient samples instead of a pooled sample, individual random bias components are included in the uncertainty estimation, assuming that the patient samples are representative. Also, natural patient samples are preferable to a stabilized pool that perhaps is distributed in freeze-dried form, which may introduce artefactual errors into some analytical systems. Using a commutable CRM, on the other hand, is more practical and in many situations is the only realistic alternative.

Care is necessary in estimating the uncertainty when it is derived from a comparison study of patient samples. First, it is important to estimate correctly the SE of the difference at selected decision points or at points covering the analytical measurement range (ie, at the lower limit, in the middle part, and at the upper limit). From the expression of the estimated difference $[D_c = a_0 + (b - 1)\ X1'_{\mathrm{Targetc}}]$, initially, one might estimate the SE (standard uncertainty) by adding (squared) the SEs of the intercept and the slope. However, simple squared addition of SEs is correct only when the independence of estimates is given (see later). Estimates of intercept and slope in regression analysis are negatively correlated, which implies that simple squared addition of standard errors leads to an overestimation of the total standard uncertainty.[83] Rather, a direct estimation procedure for the SE should be applied, as mentioned earlier.

As mentioned earlier a method comparison study based on genuine patient samples represents a real assessment of traceability. In Fig. 2.34, the focus is on the calibration aspect intended to *mediate* traceability. One should recognize that the matrix of product calibrators for practical reasons often is artificial (eg, the matrix of a calibrator may be bovine albumin instead of human serum). Many routine methods are matrix sensitive, which implies that calibrators and patient samples are not commutable. To ensure traceability in this situation, the assigned concentration of a calibrator has to be different from the real concentration.

Indirect Evaluation of Uncertainty by Quantification of Individual Error Source Components

On the basis of a detailed quantitative model of the analytical procedure, the standard approach is to assess the standard uncertainties associated with individual input parameters and combine them according to the law of propagation of uncertainties.[79,84] The relationship between the combined standard uncertainty $u_c(y)$ of a value y and the uncertainty of the *independent* parameters x_1, x_2, ... x_n, on which it depends, is

$$u_c[y(x_1,x_2,\ldots)] = [\Sigma c_i^2 u(x_1)^2]^{0.5}$$

where c_i is a sensitivity coefficient (the partial differential of y with respect to x_i). These sensitivity coefficients indicate how the value of y varies with changes in the input parameter x_i. If the variables are not independent, the relationship becomes

$$u_c[y(x_1,x_2,\ldots)] = [\Sigma c_i^2 u(x_1)^2 + \Sigma c_i c_k u(x_i,x_k)^2]^{0.5}$$

where $u(x_i, x_k)$ is the covariance between x_i and x_k, and c_i and c_k are the sensitivity coefficients. The covariance is related to the correlation coefficient ρ_{ik} by

$$u(x_i,x_k) = u(x_i)u(x_k)\rho_{ik}$$

This is a complex relationship that usually will be difficult to evaluate in practice. In many situations, however, the contributing factors are independent, thus simplifying the picture. Below, some simple examples of combined expressions are shown.[84] The rules are presented in the form of combining SDs or CVs given *independent* input components.

$$q = x + y \qquad \mathrm{SD}(q) = [SD(x)^2 + SD(y)^2]^{0.5}$$

$$q = x - y \qquad \mathrm{SD}(q) = [\mathrm{SD}(x)^2 + \mathrm{SD}(y)^2]^{0.5}$$

$$q = ax \qquad \mathrm{SD}(q) = a\mathrm{SD}(x) \text{ and } \mathrm{CV}(q) = \mathrm{CV}(x)$$

$$q = x^p \qquad \mathrm{CV}(q) = p\ \mathrm{CV}(x)$$

$$q = xy \qquad \mathrm{CV}(q) = [\mathrm{CV}(x)^2 + \mathrm{CV}(y)^2]^{0.5}$$

$$q = x/y \qquad \mathrm{CV}(q) = [\mathrm{CV}(x)^2 + \mathrm{CV}(y)^2]^{0.5}$$

The formulas shown may be used, for example, to calculate the combined uncertainty of a calibrator solution from the uncertainties of the reference compound, the weighting, and dilution steps) (see later).

The SD for certain non-Gaussian distributions may also be of relevance for uncertainty calculations (type B uncertainties) (Table 2.10). For example, if the uncertainty of a CRM value is given with some percentage, it may be understood as referring to a rectangular probability distribution. In relation to calibration of flasks, the triangular distribution is often assumed.

It has been suggested to apply the standard uncertainty estimate as the smallest analyte reporting interval.[85] Using a coverage factor of two, the uncertainty of a result becomes twice the smallest reporting interval, and the reference change value (RCV) becomes approximately three times (2sqrt(2)) the smallest reporting interval.

TABLE 2.10 Relations Between Standard Deviation and Range for Various Types of Distributions

Normal Distribution	Rectangular Distribution	Triangular Distribution
SD = Half width of 95% interval/$t_{0.975}(v)$ ≈Half width of 95% interval/2	SD = Half width/$\sqrt{3}$	SD = Half width/$\sqrt{6}$

SD, Standard deviation.

Example. Briefly, computation of the standard uncertainty of a calibrator solution will be outlined. The concentration C equals the mass M divided by the volume $V(C = M/V)$. We will here express the standard uncertainties as relative values and will derive the approximate total standard uncertainty by squared addition of the individual contributions. Starting with the mass, the purity is stated on the certificate as 99.4 ± 0.4%. Assuming a rectangular distribution, the relative SD becomes $0.004/\sqrt{3} = 0.0023$. The uncertainty of the weighing process is known in the laboratory to have a CV of 0.1%, or 0.0010. Thus, the relative standard uncertainty of the mass becomes

$$u_{M\,st} = (0.0023^2 + 0.0010^2)^{0.5} = 0.0025$$

The certificate of the flask (50 mL at 20°C) indicates ±0.1 mL as uncertainty. Assuming here a triangular distribution, we derive the standard uncertainty as $0.10\ \text{mL}/\sqrt{6} = 0.0408\ \text{mL}$, which is converted to a relative value of 0.000816. The temperature expansion coefficient is given as 0.020 mL per degree change of temperature. Assuming a variability of 20 ± 4 °C, this contribution amounts to ±0.080 mL. Assuming here a rectangular distribution, we get an SD of $0.080/\sqrt{3}$ mL, or 0.00092 as a relative SD. The repeatability of the volume dispensing process in the laboratory has been assessed to 0.020 mL expressed as an SD, which corresponds to a relative value of 0.00040. The total standard uncertainty of the volume dispensing process becomes

$$u_{V\,st} = (0.000816^2 + 0.00092^2 + 0.00040^2)^{0.5} = 0.0013$$

The total standard uncertainty of the calibrator solution is

$$\begin{aligned} u_{Cal\,st} &= (u_{M\,st}^2 + u_{v\,st}^2)^{0.5} \\ &= (0.0025^2 + 0.0013^2)^{0.5} \\ &= 0.0028, \text{ or } 0.28\% \end{aligned}$$

Generally, when squared CVs are added, minor contributions in practice can be ignored (eg, CVs less than a third or a quarter of the other components).[79]

The indirect procedure is mainly of relevance for relatively simple procedures. For closed, automated clinical chemistry procedures, it is often not possible to discern the individual error elements. Furthermore, the correlation aspect is difficult to take into account in practice. In these cases, the direct procedure of measurement comparison is preferable. However, the indirect procedure has been applied in clinical chemistry.[86,87]

In some situations, a simulation model of a complex analytical method may be established to estimate the combined uncertainty of the method on the basis of input uncertainties.[88,89] Farrance and Frenkel[89] investigated Monte Carlo simulations using Microsoft Excel for the calculation of uncertainties building on functional relationships and taking into account uncertainties in empirically derived constants. In this way, complex relationships can be evaluated relatively easily and a resulting standard uncertainty estimate of an analytical result estimated. This procedure is useful for generating standard uncertainties of derived expressions, such as the estimated glomerular filtration rate or the expression for the anion gap.

Uncertainty in Relation to Traditional Systematic and Random Error Classifications

As mentioned previously, systematic errors are not included in the uncertainty expression because it is assumed that they have been corrected. Therefore, the uncertainty of the correction procedure should be taken into account. Otherwise, systematic errors have been added linearly or squared in error propagation models.[90,91] One may further consider that the distinction between systematic effects and random effects may be a matter of the reference frame. For example, a systematic error over time may turn into a random error because a bias may change over time. Lot-to-lot reagent effects may be interpreted as systematic or random errors. When a laboratory changes from an old to a new lot, a shift in measurement values may occur. Initially, this will be considered a systematic change. However, over a long time period involving several lots of reagents, the recorded shifts typically will be up and down and will be regarded as a long-term random error component. Additionally, a bias in a particular laboratory may be viewed as a random error component when dealing with a whole group of laboratories because individual laboratory biases appear randomly distributed and are quantified as the interlaboratory SD. Thus, there are arguments for using the uncertainty concept as outlined earlier to end up with one overall uncertainty expression directed toward the end user of the laboratory result. Still, as mentioned previously, systematic errors linked to samples from specific patient subcategories may constitute a problem because a general correction is not possible. A way to quantify this error contribution is to include samples from all patient subgroups in a balanced way in a method comparison study so that this error type is incorporated into the uncertainty component related to traceability. Another problem with systematic errors is that they often depend on the analyte concentration. Thus, if a commutable CRM is measured at a particular concentration, one should consider whether a bias correction is valid only at the given concentration or generally over the analytical measurement range. Furthermore, the occurrence of outliers caused by rarely occurring interference (eg, heterophilic antibodies in relation to immunoassays) constitutes a problem.[92] If the uncertainty estimation is based on parametric statistics (standard uncertainty expanded by a coverage factor), inclusion of gross outliers may increase the standard uncertainty considerably and make the uncertainty specification useless. A solution might here be to omit the outliers in the first hand, compute the 95% uncertainty interval, and then finally add a special note with regard to the probability of occurrence of outliers in the uncertainty specification.

Although it may appear complicated to specify the uncertainty in a detailed manner, a rough estimate may be obtained by adding the squares of CVs corresponding to essential uncertainty elements (eg, grouped as factors outside the laboratory) (derived from the traceability chain), the analytical factors inside the laboratory (intermediate precision), and the preanalytical elements.[93] In estimating uncertainty, it is important to include relevant elements, but one must be careful to avoid counting the same elements twice. Application of the uncertainty concept and the pros and cons of "top-down" versus "bottom-up" approaches in the field of clinical chemistry are subject to some discussion.[81,92,94] Further reading and case studies with worked example calculations can be found in freely downloadable resources.[81,82]

POINTS TO REMEMBER

- For well-established analytes, a hierarchy of methods exists with *a reference measurement procedure* at the top, *selected measurement procedures* at an intermediate level, and finally *routine measurement procedures* at the bottom.
- The uncertainty is given as an interval around a reported laboratory result that specifies the location of the true value with a given probability (eg, 95%).
- The uncertainty of a result, which is traceable to a particular reference, is the uncertainty of that reference together with the overall uncertainty of the traceability chain.
- The uncertainty can be judged *directly* from measurement comparisons ("top down") or *indirectly* from an analysis of individual error sources according to the law of error propagation ("error budget," bottom up").

DIAGNOSTIC ACCURACY OF LABORATORY TESTS[a]

Application of diagnostic assays or tests represents a form of medical intervention and therefore requires systematic evaluation before the tests are put into clinical use. We here consider the basic steps for evaluation of the clinical accuracy of laboratory tests, although it applies to any type of diagnostic test, including imaging or electrophysiologic tests. In diagnostic accuracy studies, the measurements or results of one (or more) laboratory test under evaluation (ie, the so-called index test) are compared with the results of a reference standard or method. This reference is the best prevailing test or strategy that is used to establish the presence or absence of the disease of interest (ie, the so-called target disease that is to be detected or excluded by the index tests). This reference standard is conducted and its results interpreted as blindly for and independently from the index test(s) results as possible. Test accuracy studies show the concordance in results of the index test(s) with the presence or absence of disease as defined by the reference standard results.[98-100] These studies provide information regarding the frequency of types of errors (ie, FP and FN test results) by the index test in relation to the reference standard.

Diagnostic Accuracy of a Test in Isolation

Diagnostic Accuracy, Sensitivity, and Specificity

A systematic and unbiased evaluation and comparison of tests is important.[101-103] The basic approach for any diagnostic accuracy study is one in which the results of the index test are compared with those of a reference test in the same individuals, all of whom are suspected to have the target disease. The simplest situation is a comparison of a single index test, with only two result categories (ie, a dichotomous or binary index test) to a reference standard (ie, a single-test accuracy study). The ideal dichotomous index test correctly identifies all individuals as diseased or nondiseased with an error rate of zero. A zero error rate is only possible when there is no overlap between index test results in the diseased and nondiseased individuals. However, when there is overlap in index test results, some individuals are classified wrongly as shown below in an example concerning the diagnosis of deep venous thrombosis (DVT) using a D-dimer index test. When using a quantitative (continuous) index test to classify individuals as diseased or nondiseased, a cutoff value needs to be chosen to estimate these error rates. This results in a so-called dichotomized index test.

[a]This section relies on three published papers.[95-97]

	Disease status	
Test result	**Diseased**	**Nondiseased**
Positive	TP	FP
Negative	FN	TN

FIGURE 2.35 The basic 2-by-2 table for estimating the diagnostic accuracy of a dichotomized quantitative test result. Positive test results are divided into true positives (TPs) and false positives (FPs) and negative results into true negatives (TNs) and false negatives (FNs). (From Linnet K, Bossuyt PM, Moons KG, Reitsma JB. Quantifying the accuracy of a diagnostic test or marker. *Clin Chem* 2012;58:1292–1301.)

Values of the dichotomous or dichotomized index test that exceed the cutoff in individuals having the target disease are classified as true positives (TP) (Fig. 2.35). Similarly, index test results lower than the cutoff in nondiseased individuals are true negatives (TN). Accordingly, index test results below the cutoff in truly diseased subjects are FN, and correspondingly, index test results exceeding the cutoff in truly nondiseased subjects are FP. Based on the frequencies of FN and FP results, an overall error rate or non-error rate can be derived. The overall diagnostic accuracy of an index test is then defined as the fraction of true classifications out of all classifications:

$$\text{Diagnostic accuracy} = (TN + TP)/(TN + TP + FP + FN)$$

This is an overall non-error rate that can be subdivided into the non-error rate of the nondiseased individuals, which is the specificity of the test and the non-error rate of diseased individuals which is the sensitivity of the test

$$\text{Specificity} = TN/(TN + FP)$$

$$\text{Sensitivity} = TP/(TP + FN)$$

Whereas a very specific test provides negative results for all or almost all subjects who are free of the target disease, a very sensitive test detects all or almost all diseased subjects.

Confidence Intervals of Diagnostic Accuracy, Sensitivity, and Specificity

To assess the (im)precision of these estimates, CIs for either the estimates or the SEs should be specified. If the cutoff value of a quantitative index test is fixed and has not been estimated from the results obtained in the study, the binomial distribution can be applied. Given random sampling, the 95% CI of a proportion can be derived from tables or by applying simple computer programs. An approximation of the binomial to the normal distribution is often used for estimation of the 95% CI of proportions such as a sensitivity and specificity, ie,

TABLE 2.11 Relationship Between Sample Size and 95% Confidence Intervals of a Proportion (eg, a Sensitivity or Specificity): Selected Examples of Proportions of 0.05 and 0.8

Sample Size	95% CI of a Proportion of 0.05	95% CI of a Proportion of 0.80
20	0.00–0.25	0.56–0.94
60	0.01–0.14	0.68–0.90
100	0.02–0.11	0.71–0.87
500	0.03–0.07	0.76–0.83
1000	0.04–0.07	0.77–0.82

CI, Confidence interval.

±2 SE(P), where SE(P) = $[P(1 - P)/N]^{0.5}$ (P, proportion; N, sample size).

The normal approximation does not work well with small sample sizes or proportions close to 0 or 1. Both situations occur frequently in diagnostic accuracy research. The method of Wilson is an alternative.[104] Table 2.11 displays the widths of the 95% CIs at various sample sizes of 20 to 1000 for two selected proportions, corresponding to either a sensitivity or a specificity (for that threshold) of an index test. For example, at a sample size of 20, the 95% CI extends from 0.56 to 0.94 for a proportion of 0.80. Thus, rather wide estimates of specificity or sensitivity are obtained for small samples. Bachmann et al.[105] reported that for 43 nonscreening studies on diagnostic accuracy of tests, the median sample size was 118 (interquartile range, 71–350). For the diseased group, the median sample size was only 49 (interquartile range, 28–91), but for the nondiseased group, it was 76 (interquartile range, 27–209). The specificity and sensitivity of two tests applied in the same study subjects can be statistically compared using the McNemar's test, which is based on a comparison of paired values of true and FP or FN results.[26]

Clinical Example: Accuracy of D-Dimer Test in Diagnosis of Deep Venous Thrombosis

We illustrate the concepts using some of the empirical data of a previously published study in primary care patients suspected of having DVT, the target disease[106,107] (Fig. 2.36). The data given here are used for illustration purposes only and not to quantify the true diagnostic accuracy of the index test for this clinical situation.

The study consisted of 2086 patients suspected of DVT, where DVT was defined as present in patients manifesting at least one of the following symptoms or signs: presence of swelling, redness, or pain in the leg. All patients were given a standardized diagnostic workup, including medical history; clinical examination; and testing for D-dimer, the (quantitative) index test. The reference procedure consisted of repeated compression ultrasonography tests and was performed in all patients, blinded to and independent of the index test results. A total of 416 (20%) of the 2086 included patients had DVT. It should be noted that although the reference test is applied currently, it may not be infallible. The potential consequences of applying imperfect reference tests and how to cope with this problem are very important, but these aspects are beyond the scope of this chapter, and for this, we refer to the literature.[108-113]

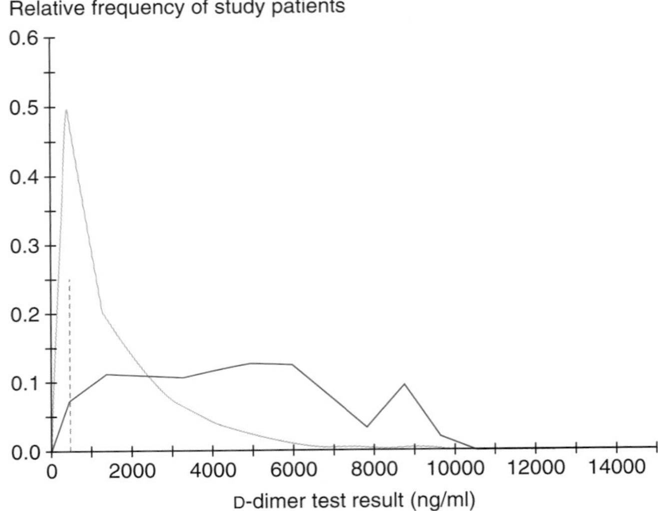

FIGURE 2.36 Distribution of the quantitative D-dimer values for deep venous thrombosis (DVT) and non-DVT subjects in the example study. *Light red line,* non-DVT; *red line,* DVT. The *dashed line* indicates the commonly used cutoff value of 500 µg/L. (From Linnet K, Bossuyt PM, Moons KG, Reitsma JB. Quantifying the accuracy of a diagnostic test or marker. *Clin Chem* 2012;58:1292–1301.)

Applying a commonly used cutoff of 500 µg/L or greater for the (originally) quantitative D-dimer assay (dashed line in Fig. 2.36), the sensitivity was 0.97 (ie, 3% of the subjects with DVT had a value <500 µg/L). The specificity was only 0.37. The resulting overall diagnostic accuracy was 0.50. Whereas the test displayed good sensitivity at this threshold, detecting all but 3% of those having DVT, its specificity at this test threshold was relatively low, resulting in many FP results. The sample size was high enough to provide precise estimates of specificity and sensitivity. The SEs were 0.012 for the specificity and 0.008 for the sensitivity, resulting in CIs of 0.356 to 0.402 and 0.955 to 0.987, respectively.

Receiver Operating Characteristic Curves

As said, for a quantitative index test, the specificity and sensitivity depend on the selected cutoff point. A plot of the sensitivity and specificity pairs for all possible cutoff values over the measurement range provides the so-called ROC curve, which is shown in Fig. 2.37 for the D-dimer example.[114-117] Usually, sensitivity (y) is plotted against (1 − specificity) (x) at each possible cutoff value. The better the performance of the test, the higher the ROC curve is located in the left, upper region of the plot. With use of the ROC curve, an appropriate combination of specificity and sensitivity, or rather for an acceptable FN and FP proportion, may be chosen, and the corresponding cutoff then selected. For the D-dimer test, in the example given, the commonly used cutoff of 500 µg/L corresponds to a sensitivity of 0.97 and (1 − specificity) of 0.63.

An area under the ROC curve (ie, the ROC area or so-called concordance or c-index) can be assessed statistically. The approach used for assessment should emulate the approach used to estimate the ROC curve, either parametric or

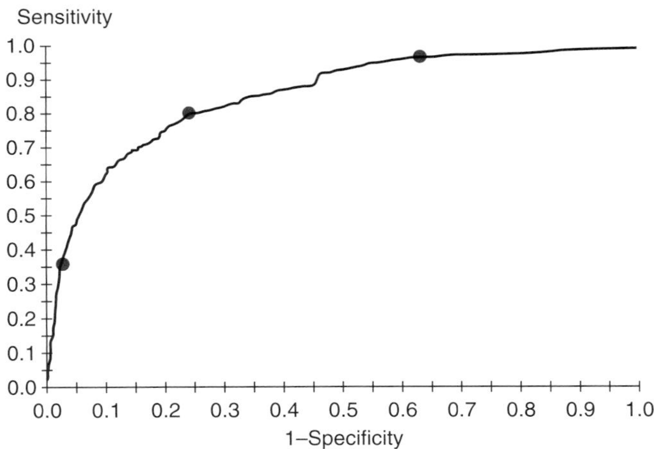

FIGURE 2.37 Receiver operating characteristic (ROC) curve of the D-dimer assay result for diagnosis of deep venous thrombosis (DVT) in our example study. The *red markers* correspond to various cutoff choices (from left to right, 5435 µg/L, 2133 µg/L, and 500 µg/L). (From Linnet K, Bossuyt PM, Moons KG, Reitsma JB. Quantifying the accuracy of a diagnostic test or marker. *Clin Chem* 2012;58:1292–1301.)

nonparametric, of which the latter approach generally is preferable. Standard computer programs to perform these calculations are widely available. Given an SE of the ROC area or c-index, it is possible to test whether the area significantly exceeds 0.5, which would demonstrate that the index test performs better than chance. A worthless test has an area of 0.5. Furthermore, using the SE also a 95% CI can be derived for the ROC area or c-index. For the D-dimer test in the earlier example, the area under the ROC curve was 0.86 (SE, 0.011), with a 95% CI of 0.84 to 0.88.

The ROC area provides an overall measure of an index test's diagnostic ability. It can be shown that the area under the ROC curve indicates, for all possible pairings of individuals, one with and one without the target disease, the proportion of pairs in which diseased individuals have a higher (more severe) index test result than individuals without the disease.[114-117] Although ROC curve evaluation has various advantages, it also has some drawbacks.[117-119] The ROC curve does not reflect directly the index test performance for a given cutoff value but can be used for this purpose depending on the desired sensitivity and specificity, or rather the acceptable FN and FP proportions; Fig. 2.37 also displays the sensitivity and specificity at various D-dimer cutoff points (including 500 µg/L, as well as the cutoff values used in Fig. 2.38 below).

Selection of Cutoff Value in Case of Quantitative Index Tests

The specificity and sensitivity determined for an index test almost always vary inversely over the range of possible cutoffs. One may select the cutoff point that provides the maximum of the sum of the specificity and sensitivity. In the D-dimer example, this cutoff would be close to 2000 µg/L, yielding a specificity of 0.76 and a sensitivity of 0.80 (Fig. 2.38, *A*). However, this method of cutoff selection is commonly not recommended. The selection should rather be based on the intended purpose of the index test. If an index test is applied primarily to rule out the presence of disease (eg, in the case of the D-dimer assay for exclusion of DVT), the cutoff point should be at the lower end of the distribution of values of diseased individuals (see Fig. 2.36) (eg, a cutoff of 500 µg/L). At this cutoff, the sensitivity approaches 1.0. But attaining such a high sensitivity is at the cost of a loss of specificity. How low the specificity becomes depends on the extent of overlap of test values in the diseased and nondiseased individuals. Conversely, when FP results are judged unacceptable, the cutoff should be toward the upper limit of the distribution of values for the nondiseased group. For the D-dimer test example, a cutoff value corresponding to the 97.5 percentile of the distribution of values for those not having DVT (5435 µg/L) resulted in a specificity of 0.975, but now the sensitivity was only 0.36 (ie, nearly the opposite of the situation with a cutoff of 500 µg/L) (see Fig. 2.38, *B*).

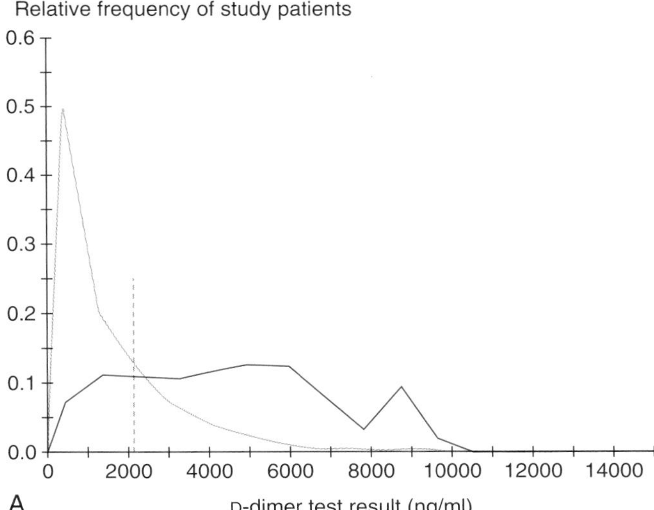

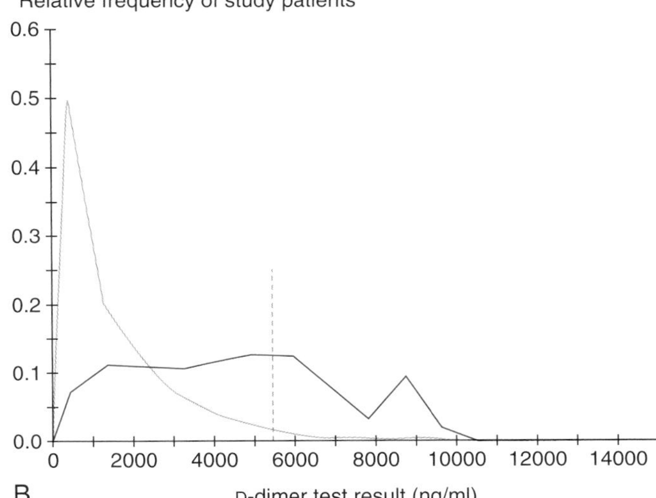

FIGURE 2.38 Alternative cutoffs to 500 µg/L in the D-dimer example. **A,** Cutoff (2133 µg/L) giving maximum value of the sum of the specificity and sensitivity. **B,** Cutoff (5435 µg/L) providing a high specificity (0.975). *Light red line,* non–deep venous thrombosis (DVT); *red line,* DVT. The *dashed line* indicates the cutoff value. (From Linnet K, Bossuyt PM, Moons KG, Reitsma JB. Quantifying the accuracy of a diagnostic test or marker. *Clin Chem* 2012;58:1292–1301.)

The estimation of an optimal cutoff point can be biased when the cutoff value is selected in the same study in which sensitivity and specificity of the index test have been estimated.[26,120] A good rule is to use independent samples for estimation of the optimal diagnostic cutoff value of the index test and for estimating the diagnostic accuracy measures. Evaluation of the index test in an independent sample also gives an indication of the robustness of the index test.

Posterior Probabilities (Predictive Values)

A straightforward question arising after the application of a diagnostic index test is what is the probability that the target disease is present given the index test value ($P[\mathrm{D}|\mathrm{Tpos}]$)? The sensitivity and specificity of a test do not directly relate to this question. The probability of presence of target disease given the index test result is an example of a so-called posterior disease probability, where the prior probability corresponds to the prevalence of the disease in the given situation. The prevalence of disease (P[D]) in the study sample is the a priori (pretest) probability of disease.

Given a positive test result (Tpos), the posterior disease probability is estimated as the fraction of TP out of all test result positives:

$$P(D|\mathrm{Tpos}) = \mathrm{TP}/(\mathrm{TP} + \mathrm{FP})$$

Analogously for a negative result (Tneg), the probability that the given disease is absent is

$$P(\text{Non-D}|\mathrm{Tneg}) = \mathrm{TN}/(\mathrm{TN} + \mathrm{FN})$$

Just as with sensitivity and specificity values, these posterior disease probabilities depend on the selected cutoff point for a quantitative test. In case of a dichotomous or dichotomized index test, these posterior probabilities are also called predictive values.[121] They are highly dependent on the disease prevalence.

From the Bayes rule, the following relations exist:

$$P(D|\mathrm{Tpos}) = [\text{Sensitivity} \times P(D)]/[\text{Sensitivity} \times P(D) + (1 - \text{Specificity})(1 - P(D))]$$

$$P(\text{Non-D}|\mathrm{Tneg}) = [\text{Sensitivity} \times (1 - P(D))]/[\text{Specificity} \times (1 - P(D)) + P(D) \times (1 - \text{Specificity})]$$

Likelihood Ratios and Odds Ratios

Besides the above parameters, one may also estimate the so-called diagnostic likelihood ratio (LR) for index test results. From relative frequency distributions for results of the index test in the nondiseased and diseased groups, one may calculate the LR of an index test result (X) as the ratio between the heights of the relative frequency (f) distributions at that specific test value.[122] We get:

$$\mathrm{LR}\ (X) = f_{\mathrm{D}}\ (X)/f_{\text{Non-D}}\ (X)$$

In case the relative frequency of the distribution of diseased individuals is higher than that of the nondiseased individuals, the ratio exceeds 1. This indicates that disease is more likely than nondisease given this particular index test result. More formally, the ratio can be used to calculate posterior disease probabilities given specific values of the index test (X) and the disease prevalence (D):

$$P(D|X) = P(D) \times \mathrm{LR}\ (X)/[P(D) \times \mathrm{LR}\ (X) + (1 - P(D)]$$

or a more simple calculation can be carried out using odds instead of probabilities:

$$\text{Odds}\ (D|X) = \text{Odds}\ (D) \times \mathrm{LR}\ (X)$$

based on the relation:

$$\text{Odds} = P/(1 - P)$$

Odds is an alternative way of expressing probabilities commonly used in betting games in Anglo-Saxon countries. For example, a probability of 0.80, or 80%, corresponds to an odds value of 4 according to the formula above. The higher the odds, the closer a probability is to one. From the equation, the posterior odds are equal to the prior odds multiplied by the diagnostic LR for the result X.

For a dichotomous or dichotomized index test, the following relationships apply:

$$\mathrm{LR}\ (\text{pos}) = \text{Sensitivity}/(1 - \text{Specificity})$$

$$\mathrm{LR}\ (\text{neg}) = (1 - \text{Sensitivity})/\text{Specificity}$$

Although the LR approach has been tried in various situations, generally the application of diagnostic LRs has been limited in clinical chemistry. Specific conditions are required for the concept to be applied in a practical and reliable way. A simple way of achieving the posttest probability of disease from the prevalence (pretest probability of disease) and the diagnostic LR is to use the Fagan nomogram.[123] A recent example is the estimation of the probability of DVT from testing for D-dimer.[124] Finally, it can be noted that the diagnostic LR of a result X equals the slope of the ROC curve at that index test value.

Comparison of Diagnostic Accuracy of Two Tests in Isolation

The diagnostic accuracy—that is, the ability to detect or exclude the target disease as determined by the reference method—of a new diagnostic index test is usually compared with another, established, index test. We here focus on the pure performances of the tests without consideration of other tests (ie, we consider each test in isolation). When comparing the accuracy of two or more diagnostic index tests, a paired design is generally preferable for reasons of both validity and efficiency. In the target disease-suspected patients, the two index tests under comparison and the reference standard are performed on all subjects, again independently and blinded with regard to each other's test results. Because both index tests are applied to the same nondiseased and diseased individuals (as classified by the same reference standard), any bias effects caused by differences in disease spectrum or comorbidity are automatically balanced.

A paired comparison of for example the sensitivities or specificities for two dichotomous or dichotomized index tests can be evaluated using the McNemar's test.[26,125] The principle of this statistical procedure is that the number of preferences for index test A (cases detected by index test A but not by index test B) is compared with the number of preferences for index test B, and if the difference exceeds some critical value, one index test is found to be superior to the other.

Receiving operating characteristic curve areas may also be compared. Here, a paired comparison should also be undertaken when the index tests have been applied in the same groups of individuals. An example of a paired comparison is displayed in Fig. 2.39. Parametric and nonparametric statistical procedures exist that usually are performed by computer programs.[116,126] Overall, the index test having the largest area under the ROC curve represents the best test, although this assessment becomes more difficult if the ROC curves of tests cross each other.[119] Preferably, CIs of areas and differences of areas should be provided.

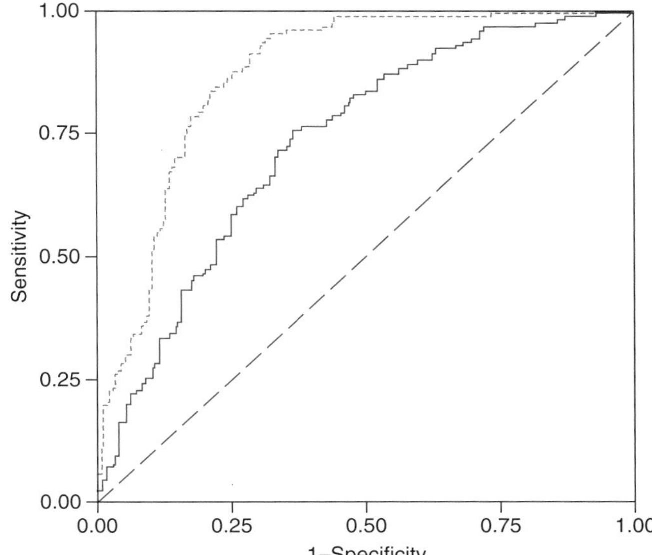

FIGURE 2.39 Comparison of the receiver operating characteristic (ROC) curves of two hypothetical index tests for the same target disease undertaken in the same individuals. The *dotted, red curve* represents a superior diagnostic test, both with regard to sensitivity and specificity over all possible cutoff points. The *dashed diagonal* represents a worthless test, with equal probability of a false-positive (1–Specificity) and false-negative (1–Sensitivity) result across all cutoff values (ie, flipping a coin test). (From Linnet K, Bossuyt PM, Moons KG, Reitsma JB. Quantifying the accuracy of a diagnostic test or marker. *Clin Chem* 2012;58:1292–1301.)

Shortcomings of Diagnostic Accuracy Studies of Tests in Isolation

The accuracy of a diagnostic test highly depends on the context. The estimated diagnostic accuracy measures of an index test (posterior probabilities, sensitivity, specificity, LR, or ROC area) preferably obtained from data of a cohort of target disease–suspected patients are not constant; they vary across other index test results, patient characteristics, disease prevalence, or disease severities.[127-129] We illustrate this for our D-dimer example in Table 2.12. The overall sensitivity and specificity for the 500 μg/L threshold were 0.97 and 0.37, respectively (upper row). However, when estimating these measures for patient subgroups within the study sample defined by other test results from patient history and physical examination, substantial differences appear with regard to specificity, especially for the malignancy, recent surgery, and pitting-edema subgroups. At a higher threshold (1000 μg/L)

TABLE 2.12 Variations in the Sensitivity and Specificity (at Cutoff Values 500 ng/mL and 1000 ng/mL) and the Receiver Operating Characteristic Area of the D-Dimer Test According to Various Other Test Results or Patient Characteristics.

	D-DIMER >500 ng/mL		D-DIMER >1000 ng/mL		D-DIMER (CONTINUOUS)
	Sensitivity	Specificity	Sensitivity	Specificity	AUC (CI)
Overall	0.97	0.37	0.89	0.55	0.86 (0.84;0.88)
Previous lung embolism					
Yes (n = 173)	1.00	0.37	0.84	0.53	0.82 (0.75;0.90)
No (n = 1913)	0.97	0.37	0.89	0.55	0.86 (0.84;0.88)
Malignancy					
Yes (n = 115)	0.95	0.25	0.95	0.44	0.86 (0.79;0.93)
No (n = 1971)	0.97	0.38	0.89	0.55	0.84 (0.83;0.87)
Recent surgery					
Yes (n = 278)	0.96	0.22	0.90	0.38	0.84 (0.78;0.90)
No (n = 1808)	0.97	0.39	0.89	0.57	0.86 (0.84;0.88)
Leg trauma					
Yes (n = 344)	0.96	0.32	0.85	0.48	0.79 (0.72;0.87)
No (n =1742)	0.97	0.38	0.89	0.56	0.86 (0.84;0.89)
Pitting edema					
Yes (n = 1301)	0.97	0.32	0.88	0.50	0.84 (0.82;0.87)
No (n = 785)	0.97	0.46	0.90	0.62	0.87 (0.84;0.91)
Pregnancy					
Yes (n = 45)	1.00	0.28	1.00	0.55	0.98 (0.00;1.00)
No (n = 2041)	0.97	0.37	0.89	0.55	0.85 (0.83;0.88)

AUC, Area under the Receiver Operating Characteristic curve; *CI*, 95% confidence interval.

variations in sensitivity also occur, for example, in the pregnancy and previous embolism subgroups. The last column of Table 2.12 reveals that this variation in single-test accuracy measures also holds true for non–threshold-dependent measures such as the ROC area. The ROC area was from 0.79 to 0.98, with 0.86 for the total study group. Although all these differences should not be overinterpreted, one must always be careful when judging a single test's diagnostic accuracy measures. A diagnostic laboratory test should always be considered in relation to a specific clinical situation and its results judged within the diagnostic pathway (ie, in view of the results of other usually applied tests) in which the test under study is to be applied.[128-130] How to do so is covered in the next section.

The STARD (Standards for Reporting of Diagnostic Accuracy Studies) initiative, originally launched in 2003[101] and updated in 2015,[102] aims to improve the quality and reporting of diagnostic accuracy studies. A checklist guides investigators regarding what information to report on patient selection, the order of test application, and the number of individuals undergoing the test under evaluation, the reference test, or both, and other characteristics important for unbiased study design[102] (Box 2.2). Similarly, the so-called QUADAS-2 (Quality Assessment Tool for Diagnostic Accuracy Studies) tool to critically appraise and assess risk of bias in primary diagnostic accuracy studies has been developed to assist systematic reviews of diagnostic accuracy studies[131] (http://www.quadas.org). For more information on STARD and QUADAS and the Diagnostic Test Accuracy Review Group of the Cochrane Collaboration, see Chapter 9 on evidence-based laboratory medicine.

POINTS TO REMEMBER

- The diagnostic accuracy of a test indicates the frequency and type of errors that a test will produce when differentiating between patients with and without the target disease.
- The cohort design based on patients suspected of the diseases targeted by the index test is generally preferable for evaluating diagnostic accuracy.
- It is not meaningful to regard estimates of diagnostic performance as properties of the test itself but rather to interpret them as depending on the setting in which the index test was applied and dependent on other tests that are commonly used in that setting.

Diagnostic Accuracy of a Test in the Clinical Context

The diagnostic process in practice begins with a patient having particular symptoms or signs. These symptoms and signs may direct the suspicion toward several possible diseases (the differential diagnosis). The diagnostic workup is often primarily targeted to include or exclude a particular disease or disorder, the so-called target disease, among several possible differential diagnoses.[99,101,132-135] For example, a woman showing up with a red, swollen leg may be suspected of having DVT; a man with blood in his stool may be suspected of having colon carcinoma; and a child with convulsions may be suspected of having bacterial meningitis. The target disorder in question can be the most severe disorder of the differential diagnoses ("the one not to miss") but also the most probable one.

The diagnostic process commonly consists of a series of sequential steps in which much diagnostic information (ie, diagnostic test results) is acquired. After each step, the physician intuitively judges the probability of the target disease being present. The initial step always consists of patient history and physical signs. If uncertainty about the presence and type of disease remains, subsequent tests are performed, often in another stepwise fashion. These supplementary tests may consist of simple blood or urine tests or be imaging, electrophysiology, or genetic tests or even later in the process more invasive testing such as biopsy, angiography, or arthroscopy. The supplementary information of each subsequent test is implicitly added to the yet collected diagnostic information, and the target disease probability is constantly updated. This process continues until the target disease can be included or excluded with sufficient certainty and some therapeutic management can be started, including the decision to refrain from treatment.

Hardly any diagnosis is based on a single test; for example, information from the history and the physical examination are almost always collected before any laboratory test is applied. Rather, the diagnostic context involves a multivariable (multiple-test) and phased process in which physicians decide whether the next test will add information to what is already established.[129,136,137]

Investigations of diagnostic laboratory tests should incorporate this multivariable clinical context in their studies. Laboratory tests should not be evaluated in isolation; rather, their studies should reflect the steps in the diagnostic process so that the added value of such tests in excess of the information that is already present can be assessed. Depending on the situation, studies may reveal that the diagnostic information of any subsequent test is already supplied by the simpler previous test results. When regarded in isolation such subsequent test or marker may indeed show diagnostic accuracy or value, but when assessed in the overall diagnostic workup, it does not. Such a case can arise because different tests may gauge the same underlying pathologic processes to varying degrees and thus provide related diagnostic information. From a statistical point of view, the various test values, whether obtained from patient history, physical signs, or subsequent testing, are to varying degrees mutually correlated.[127,128,130] The main point in diagnostic accuracy assessment, therefore, is not what the diagnostic accuracy of a particular (laboratory) test is, as covered in the previous section, but rather whether it is going to improve the diagnostic accuracy of the existing setup beyond what is present from the already acquired diagnostic information.

In the following, we focus on the extent to which a certain laboratory test adds information to test results that have already been obtained. How much the new test adds in terms of improved discrimination between the presence or absence of the target disease in relation to a reference standard is of interest in this section.

Clinical Example: Added Value of D-Dimer Testing in the Diagnosis of Suspected Deep Venous Thrombosis

The concept of assessing the added value of a subsequent diagnostic test will be illustrated by the same DVT case study described earlier.[106,107] In short, 2086 patients were suspected of DVT, having at least one of the following symptoms: swelling, redness, or pain in the leg. All patients had a standardized

BOX 2.2 STARD 2015: An Updated List of Essential Items for Reporting Diagnostic Accuracy Studies[102]

Title or Abstract

1. Identification as a study of diagnostic accuracy using at least one measure of accuracy (eg, sensitivity, specificity, predictive values, AUC)

Abstract

2. Structured summary of study design, methods, results, and conclusions (for specific guidance, see STARD for Abstracts)

Introduction

3. Scientific and clinical background, including the intended use and clinical role of the index test
4. Study objectives and hypotheses

Methods

Study Design

5. Whether data collection was planned before the index test and reference standard were performed (prospective study) or after (retrospective study)

Participants

6. Eligibility criteria
7. On what basis potentially eligible participants were identified (eg, symptoms, results from previous tests, inclusion in registry)
8. Where and when potentially eligible participants were identified (setting, location, and dates)
9. Whether participants formed a consecutive, random, or convenience series

Test Methods

10a. Index test, in sufficient detail to allow replication

10b. Reference standard, in sufficient detail to allow replication

11. Rationale for choosing the reference standard (if alternatives exist)

12a. Definition of and rationale for test positivity cutoffs or result categories of the index test, distinguishing pre-specified from exploratory

12b. Definition of and rationale for test positivity cutoffs or result categories of the reference standard, distinguishing prespecified from exploratory

13a. Whether clinical information and reference standard results were available to the performers or readers of the index test

13b. Whether clinical information and index test results were available to the assessors of the reference standard

Analysis

14. Methods for estimating or comparing measures of diagnostic accuracy
15. How indeterminate index test or reference standard results were handled
16. How missing data on the index test and reference standard were handled
17. Any analyses of variability in diagnostic accuracy, distinguishing pre-specified from exploratory
18. Intended sample size and how it was determined

Results

Participants

19. Flow of participants, using a diagram
20. Baseline demographic and clinical characteristics of participants

21a. Distribution of severity of disease in those with the target condition

21b. Distribution of alternative diagnoses in those without the target condition

22. Time interval and any clinical interventions between index test and reference standard

Test Results

23. Cross-tabulation of the index test results (or their distribution) by the results of the reference standard
24. Estimates of diagnostic accuracy and their precision (eg, 95% CIs)
25. Any adverse events from performing the index test or the reference standard

Discussion

26. Study limitations, including sources of potential bias, statistical uncertainty, and generalizability
27. Implications for practice, including the intended use and clinical role of the index test

Other Information

28. Registration number and name of registry
29. Where the full study protocol can be accessed
30. Sources of funding and other support; role of funders

AUC, Area under the curve; *CI,* confidence interval; *STARD,* Standards for Reporting of Diagnostic Accuracy Studies.
From Bossuyt PM, Reitsma JB, Bruns DE, et al; STARD Group. STARD 2015: an updated list of essential items for reporting diagnostic accuracy studies. *Clin Chem* 2015;61(12):1446–1452.

diagnostic workup consisting of index tests from medical history taking, physical examination, and quantitative D-dimer testing. The reference standard was repeated compression ultrasonography, according to current clinical practice. This reference test was carried out in all patients independent of the results of the index tests and blinded with regard to all preceding collected index test results. In total, 416 of the 2068 included patients (20%) had DVT confirmed by ultrasonography. In this section, we focus on estimating the added value of D-dimer testing to the information provided by history taking and physical examination (Table 2.13).

Table 2.13 displays the relationship between each diagnostic test result and the presence or absence of DVT. The values in fact correspond to single-test accuracy values, as discussed in the preceding section. It would be difficult, if not impossible, to select the most promising index tests from these

TABLE 2.13 Distribution and Accuracy of Each Diagnostic Variable Compared With the Reference Standard Outcome (Deep Venous Thrombosis Present or Absent Based on Repeated Compression Ultrasonography)

	DEEP VENOUS THROMBOSIS						
	YES (n = 416)			NO (n = 1670)			
	n	Sens (%) (95% CI)	PPV (%) (95% CI)	n	Spec (%) (95% CI)	NPV(%) (95% CI)	ROC Area* (95% CI)
Male gender	194	47 (42–51)	25 (22–29)	569	66 (64–68)	83 (81–85)	—
Mean age in years (SD)	62 (17)	—	—	59 (18)	—	—	0.53 (0.50–0.56)
Presence of malignancy	40	10 (7–13)	35 (27–44)	75	96 (94–96)	81 (79–83)	—
Recent surgery	76	18 (15–22)	27 (22–33)	202	88 (86–89)	81 (79–83)	—
Absence of recent leg trauma	47	89 (85–91)	21 (19–23)	297	18 (16–20)	86 (82–90)	—
Vein distension	115	28 (24–32)	28 (24–32)	302	82 (80–84)	82 (80–84)	—
Pain on walking	344	83 (79–86)	21 (19–23)	1325	21 (19–23)	83 (79–86)	—
Swelling whole leg	247	59 (55–64)	26 (23–29)	699	58 (56–60)	85 (83–87)	—
Mean difference in calf circumference in cm (SD)	3 (2)	—	—	2 (2)	—	—	0.69 (0.67–0.72)
Mean D-dimer in ng/mL (SD)	4549 (2665)	—	—	1424 (1791)	—	—	0.86 (0.84–0.88)

*A receiving operator characteristic (ROC) area lower than 0.5 means that overall this test result was better for excluding than including deep venous thrombosis (DVT) presence.

NPV, Negative predictive value, the proportion of subjects labeled no DVT by the diagnostic test with true absence of DVT; *PPV,* positive predictive value, the proportion of subjects labeled DVT by the diagnostic test with true DVT; *Sens,* sensitivity, the proportion of subjects with true DVT who are labeled as DVT by the diagnostic test; *Spec,* specificity, the proportion of subjects with true absence of DVT who are labeled as no DVT by the diagnostic test.

single-test accuracy values. None of the history and physical examination tests was pathognomonic for DVT. Some tests or investigations had a high sensitivity but a low specificity (eg, absence of leg trauma and pain on walking), but other tests exhibited a high specificity and low sensitivity (eg, presence of malignancy or recent surgery). Some tests would serve better for exclusion, others for inclusion. The ROC areas for the continuous tests, age and difference in calf circumference (but also for the D-dimer test), were all below 1 and above 0.5. One questions whether combinations of history and physical examination test results have better accuracy compared with their individual accuracy values and whether the D-dimer biomarker has incremental accuracy.

A multivariable statistical approach is needed to assess the diagnostic accuracy of combined index test results. Given a dichotomous outcome (DVT present or not), multivariable logistic regression modelling is the most appropriate approach. Logistic regression models express the probability of DVT (on the logit scale) as a linear function of the included index test results. Note that index test results may be included as binary, categorical, or even continuous results. The latter two do by no means need to be dichotomized first. Indeed, this is even contraindicated because it may often lose diagnostic value to the index test. Table 2.14 (model 1) shows the results from history and physical examination test results that were significantly related to DVT in the multivariable analysis, here defined as a multivariable odds ratio significantly (P <0.05) different from 1 (no association).

To quantify whether the quantitative D-dimer assay value has added diagnostic value beyond the history and physical examination results combined, the basic model 1 was simply extended by including the index test D-dimer value, resulting in model 2 (see Table 2.14). After the inclusion of the D-dimer assay result, the regression coefficients of most history and physical tests in model 2 are found to be different from those in model 1: They now express the contribution of the corresponding test results, given a specific D-dimer result. This change reveals that the history and physical and the D-dimer results are indeed correlated and partly provide the same diagnostic information regarding whether DVT is present or not. The trend of lower regression coefficients of most findings can be interpreted as follows: A portion of the information supplied by the history and physical items is now replaced by the D-dimer assay result. Notice that the influence of the variable, recent surgery, has completely disappeared after the addition of the D-dimer biomarker.

TABLE 2.14 The Basic and Extended Multivariable Diagnostic Model to Discriminate Between Deep Venous Thrombosis Presence versus Absence*

	MODEL 1 (BASIC MODEL)			MODEL 2 (BASIC MODEL + D-DIMER)		
	Regression Coefficient (SE)	OR (95% CI)	*P* Value	Regression Coefficient (SE)	OR (95% CI)	*P* Value
(Intercept)	−3.70 (0.26)	—	<0.01	−4.94 (0.32)	—	<0.01
Presence of malignancy	0.62 (0.22)	1.9 (1.2-2.9)	<0.01	0.22 (0.26)	1.2 (0.7-2.1)	0.41
Recent surgery	0.44 (0.16)	1.6 (1.1-2.1)	<0.01	0.003 (0.19)	1.0 (0.7-1.5)	0.99
Absence of leg trauma	0.75 (0.18)	2.1 (1.5-3.0)	<0.01	0.67 (0.20)	2.0 (1.3-2.9)	<0.01
Vein distension	0.48 (0.13)	1.6 (1.1-2.1)	<0.01	0.25 (0.16)	1.3 (0.9-1.8)	0.12
Pain on walking	0.41 (0.15)	1.5 (1.1-2.0)	<0.01	0.46 (0.18)	1.6 (1.1-2.3)	0.01
Swelling whole leg	0.36 (0.12)	1.4 (1.1-1.8)	<0.01	0.47 (0.14)	1.6 (1.2-2.1)	<0.01
Difference in calf circumference (per cm)	0.36 (0.04)	1.4 (1.3-1.5)	<0.01	0.29 (0.04)	1.3 (1.2-1.4)	<0.01
D-Dimer (per 500 ng/mL)	NA	NA	NA	0.29 (0.02)	1.3 (1.3-1.4)	<0.01

*Exp(regression coefficient) is the odds ratio (OR) of a diagnostic test result. For example, an odds ratio of 2 for absence leg trauma (model 2) means that a suspected patient without a recent leg trauma has a two times higher chance of having deep venous thrombosis (DVT) than a patient with a recent leg trauma (because in the latter the leg trauma would more likely be the cause of the presenting symptoms and signs). Similarly, an odds ratio of 1.3 for calf difference in cm (model 2) means that for every centimeter increase in calf circumference difference, a patient has a 1.3 times (or 30%) higher chance of having DVT.

A diagnostic model can be considered as a single overall or combined test consisting of different test results, with the probability of DVT presence as its test result. For example, for a male subject without malignancy, recent surgery, or leg trauma but with vein distension and a painful not swollen leg when walking with a calf difference of 6 cm the formula is (model1):

$Z = -3.70 + 0.62*0 + 0.44*0 + 0.75*0 + 0.48*1 + 0.41*1 + 0.36*0 + 0.36*6 = -0.65$

The probability for this patient of the presence of DVT based on the basic model then is $\exp(-0.65)/(1 + \exp(-0.65)) = 34\%$.

Diagnostic Accuracy of Combinations of Diagnostic Tests: Receiver Operating Characteristic Area

The multivariable diagnostic model, which is based on a combination of diagnostic index tests, as exemplified in models 1 and 2 in Table 2.14, can actually be considered as a single (overall or combined) quantitative index test, consisting of a composite of individual index tests. The test result of this "combined index test model" for each study patient is simply the calculated posterior probability of DVT presence given the observed pattern of the individual index test results in that patient. (See the footnote to Table 2.14 on how to calculate this probability of disease presence.) Note that this posterior probability is now the probability of DVT based on combination of multiple index test results rather than of a single index test result.

As for single continuous index tests described earlier, also for "test combinations" combined into a single multivariable model, one can calculate the ROC area (*c*-statistic) to indicate the ability of this "test combination" to discriminate between the presence versus absence of the target disease (here DVT).[115,138] Here the ROC area expresses the proportion out of all possible pairs of patients with and without DVT for which the patient with DVT has a higher estimated probability by the model than the patient without DVT. Fig. 2.40 shows the ROC curves and areas for models 1 and 2, which is not much different from the comparison of two continuous index tests in isolation described earlier except that in this section, all tests are not considered in isolation but in combination or within the diagnostic pathway.

Fig. 2.40 displays how adding the quantitative D-dimer assay to model 1 mediated an increase in the ROC area from 0.72 to 0.87, a considerable and statistically significant gain ($P<0.01$),[115,116] which can be estimated using the same method described earlier for comparing two quantitative index tests in isolation. This implies that the overall diagnostic accuracy of the information from patient history and physical examination can be improved substantially by addition of the D-dimer test.

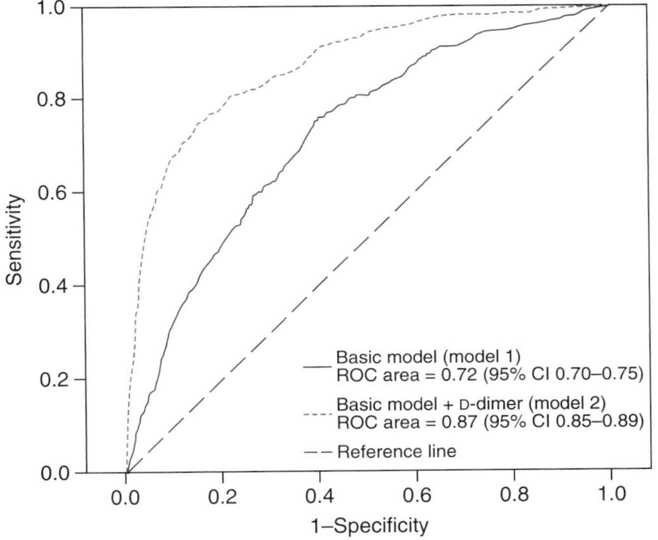

FIGURE 2.40 Receiver operating characteristic (ROC) curves for the combination of history and physical examination tests before and after addition of the D-dimer assay result. (From Moons KG, de Groot JA, Linnet K, et al. Quantifying the added value of a diagnostic test or marker. *Clin Chem* 2012;58: 1408–1417.)

The use of the difference in ROC area to express the added value of a new test or biomarker has been subject to criticism.[139-141] First, the AUC is a summary measure of discrimination and has no direct clinical implication in terms of correct or incorrect diagnostic classifications or absolute

TABLE 2.15 Reclassification Table From The Basic and Extended (With D-Dimer) Model at an Arbitrary DVT Probability Threshold of 25%*

DVT YES (n = 416)

		Model 2 with D-Dimer		
DVT probability threshold		≤25%	>25%	Total
Model 1 without D-dimer	≤25%	92	123	215
	>25%	26	175	201
	Total	118	298	416

DVT NO (n = 1670)

		Model 2 with D-Dimer		
DVT probability threshold		≤25%	>25%	Total
Model 1 without D-dimer	≤25%	1223	116	1339
	>25%	227	104	331
	Total	1450	220	1670

*A patient with a model's probability of greater than 25% is considered high probability of having deep venous thrombosis (DVT) and is further worked up or managed for DVT.

patient numbers. Various investigators have noticed that the increase in AUC commonly may be relatively small by adding new but still relevant biomarkers, particularly when the AUC of the baseline model already is large.[140-143] Several alternative measures have been suggested to quantify the added value of a novel test or biomarker to circumvent these limitations.

Reclassification Measures

To handle the problems associated with the difference in ROC areas, reclassification analysis has been proposed.[144] The reclassification table displays how many patients actually are regrouped by adding a new test to (a combination of) existing tests after defining a threshold for a given posterior probability for presence of disease. The reclassification table with a threshold at 25% is shown in Table 2.15. This means, in this theoretical example, that patients with a calculated posterior probability of 25% or higher are considered to be at high risk of having DVT and need to be referred for reference testing, but those of less than 25% receive no reference testing.

Table 2.15 displays the reclassification of patients according to model 2 instead of model 1 at a DVT probability threshold of 25%. For example, in patients with DVT, 36% (123/416 + 26/416) were reclassified by model 2 compared with model 1. For patients without DVT, this percentage was 21% (227/1670 + 116/1670).

The simple change in classification of individuals to different posterior probability categories of DVT presence, however, is not satisfactory for assessing improvement in diagnostic accuracy by a new test or biomarker; the changes should also be in the right direction. Otherwise, an increase in posterior probability categories for subjects with DVT implies improved diagnostic classification, and any movement in the other direction implies worse diagnostic categorization. The picture is opposite for individuals without DVT present.[145]

The overall improvement in diagnostic reclassification can be expressed in various ways depending on the selected denominators, but commonly it is quantified as the difference between two differences. This is done by first calculating the difference between the proportions of individuals moving up and the proportion of subjects moving down for those with DVT, computing the corresponding difference in proportions for those without DVT, and then taking the difference of these two differences. This measure has been proposed as the net reclassification improvement (NRI).[146] The NRI is thus estimated as follows:

$$\text{NRI} = [P(\text{up}|D=1) - P(\text{down}|D=1)] - [P(\text{up}|D=0) - P(\text{down}|D=0)]$$

where P is the proportion of patients, upward movement (up) is defined as a change into a higher probability of disease presence category based on model 2, and downward movement (down) is defined as a change in the opposite direction. D denotes the disease classification (in this case, DVT), present (1) or absent (0).

The NRI results for addition of D-dimer assay to the combination of history and physical examination using the numbers displayed in Table 2.15 were (0.30 − 0.06) − (0.07 − 0.14) = 0.31 (95% CI, 0.24–0.36). For 123 of 416 (ie, 0.30) of patients who experienced DVT events, classification improved with the model with D-dimer, and for 26 of 416 (0.06) people, it became worse, resulting in a net gain in reclassification proportion of 0.24. In subjects who did not have DVT, 116 of 1670 (0.07) individuals were reclassified worse by the model with the D-dimer, and 227 of 1670 (0.14) were reclassified better, resulting in a net gain in reclassification proportion of 0.07. The overall net gain in reclassification proportion therefore was 0.24 + 0.07 = 0.31. This estimate was significantly different from 0 (P <0.001). The 95% CI around the NRI estimate was computed as suggested by Pencina et al.[146]

Most investigators use three or four categories. But the NRI is clearly highly dependent on what probability threshold(s) are selected. Different thresholds may result in very different NRIs for the same added test result. To circumvent this problem of arbitrary cutoff choices, another possibility is to compute the so-called integrated discrimination improvement (IDI), which determines the magnitude of the reclassification probability improvements or deteriorations by a new test or biomarker over all possible categorizations or probability thresholds.[145-147]

The IDI is calculated as follows:

$$\text{IDI} = [(P_{\text{extended}}|D=1) - (P_{\text{basic}}|D=1)] - [(P_{\text{extended}}|D=0) - (P_{\text{basic}}|D=0)].$$

In this equation, $P_{\text{extended}}|D = 1$ and $P_{\text{extended}}|D = 0$ are the means of the predicted DVT probability by the extended model 2 (see Table 2.14) for, respectively, the patients with DVT and the patients without DVT, and $P_{\text{basic}}|D = 1$ and $P_{\text{basic}}|D = 0$ are the means of the predicted DVT probability by model 1 see (Table 2.14) for, respectively, the patients with DVT and the patients without DVT. The 95% CI around the NRI estimate again was calculated as outlined by Pencina et al.[146]

The IDI for the DVT example was (0.49 − 0.13) − (0.28 − 0.18) = 0.26 (95% CI, 0.23–0.28).

This implies that adding D-dimer to history and physical examination increased the difference in mean predicted probability between patients with DVT and patients without DVT by 0.26. This can also be interpreted as corresponding to the increase in mean sensitivity given an unchanged specificity.[146]

Although very popular and increasingly requested in reports on added value estimations, the NRI and IDI are only measures of discrimination between disease and nondiseased, as is also the case for ROC area. They give no information about whether the diagnostic probabilities calculated with a diagnostic model are in agreement with the observed disease prevalence (ie, whether the models' DVT probabilities are over- or underestimated compared with the observed DVT prevalence), nor do they account in any way for the consequences of diagnostic misclassifications when a diagnostic biomarker or test is added.[148,149] The following methods better address these issues.

Predictiveness Curve

The predictiveness curve[147,150] is a graphic outline of the distribution of the predictive disease probabilities. Accordingly, the predictive probabilities of model 1 (without D-dimer) are ordered from lowest to highest and then plotted (Fig. 2.41).

The x-axis delineates the cumulative percentage over all individuals in the study; the y-axis shows the probabilities according to model 1. Looking first at the results only for model 1, we observe for the DVT example that if individuals who have a posterior risk (after history and physical examination) of more than 25% are selected for further investigation (regarded as positive), then 74% of patients will actually be negative and 26% will be positive (vertical dividing line in Fig. 2.41).

The four areas defined by the vertical dividing line represent, respectively, the TNs (64%), FPs (16%), FNs (10%), and TPs (10%).

In this example (threshold of >25%), the sensitivity becomes TP/Prevalence × 100 = 0.10/0.2 × 100 = 50%.

The specificity becomes

$$\text{TN}/(1-\text{Prevalence})\times 100 = 0.64/0.8\times 100 = 80\%$$

The graph thus displays the estimated probabilities associated with the history and physical examination mode when applied to the source population from which the study patients theoretically originated.[151]

The graph may also be used to assess the two different diagnostic models and, accordingly, the added value of the D-dimer test for correct estimation of the probability of DVT presence. The predictiveness curve for model 1 is substantially inferior to that of the more comprehensive model including the D-dimer results (Fig. 2.42). For example, if we set less than 0.1 as a cutoff for low risk and greater than 0.4 as a threshold for high risk (on the y-axis), we observe that 90 − 20 = 70% of the predictions of model 1 are in the equivocal zone between these thresholds, but only 85 − 50 = 35% fall between these thresholds for the predictions of model 2. Thus, model 2 performs much better with regard to classifying patients into low (<0.1) versus high (>0.4) risk, as can be directly seen from the difference in steepness or slope of the predictiveness curve of the model with D-dimer (steeper) as opposed to the model without.[151]

Decision Curve Analysis

Decision curve analysis, according to Vickers and Elkin,[152] is a procedure that focuses on the explicit quantification of the clinical usefulness of a new index test when added to established ones in the intended clinical context. As opposed to the NRI, which is based on a single predefined probability threshold, this approach allows each professional (or even patient)

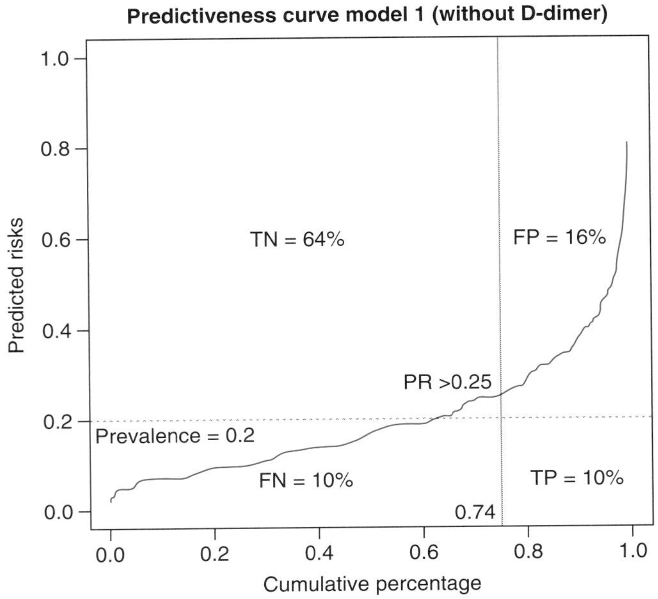

FIGURE 2.41 Predictiveness curve for model 1 (without D-dimer) showing the distribution of positive and negative patients at a posterior risk (PR) cutoff of 0.25. (From Moons KG, de Groot JA, Linnet K, et al. Quantifying the added value of a diagnostic test or marker. *Clin Chem* 2012;58:1408–1417.)

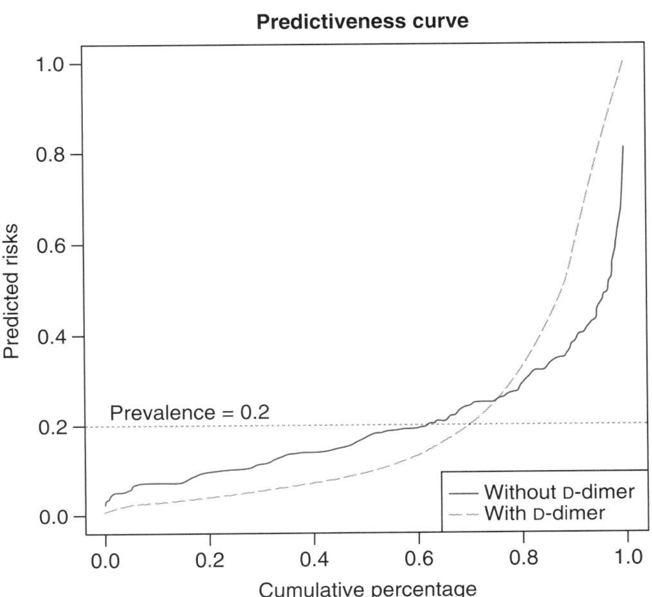

FIGURE 2.42 Comparison of predictiveness curves for the 2 models of Table 2.16 with and without D-dimer. (From Moons KG, de Groot JA, Linnet K, et al. Quantifying the added value of a diagnostic test or marker. *Clin Chem* 2012;58:1408–1417.)

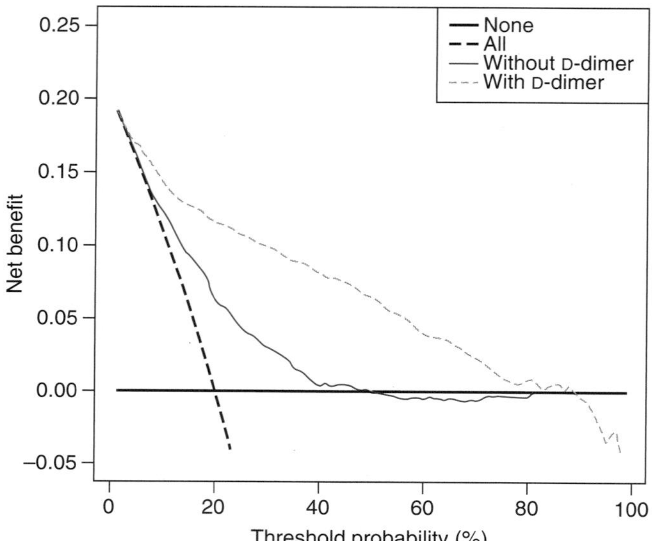

FIGURE 2.43 Decision curve analysis showing the net benefit of referring none of the patients for reference testing, referring all patients for reference testing, the basic prediction model, and the extended prediction model, in relation to the selected probability threshold for referral. (From Moons KG, de Groot JA, Linnet K, et al. Quantifying the added value of a diagnostic test or marker. *Clin Chem* 2012;58:1408–1417.)

to select his or her individual threshold to determine whether to take further steps such as referral for supplemental diagnostic investigations or for treatment initiation in the context of the intended use of the index test or index model. Accordingly, the corresponding net benefits can be considered without explicitly assigning weights or utilities to the wrong diagnostic classifications.

As displayed in Fig. 2.43, a posterior probability threshold of 50% would indicate that an incorrect referral (FP) is equivalent in consequences to a missed thrombosis (FN). To reduce the risk, the physician or patient might prefer reference testing or further management at a lower posterior probability threshold. This would be of particular relevance if the further testing were simple, noninvasive, or inexpensive or if the given treatment had relatively low risk of adverse reactions. In such a situation, the risk of DVT could be, for example, 20%. Such a lower cutoff for referral would lead to acceptance of a larger percentage of incorrect referrals (FPs) rather than missing a diseased DVT subject (FN) (ie, implicitly a higher weight is assigned to FN cases than to FP cases). On the contrary, another one might pay more attention to the costs or burden of further testing or initiation of treatment. This might be the case if the subsequent test was very invasive or complicated or therapy implied a heavy risk of adverse reactions. In this situation, a higher probability threshold of, for example, 70% might be relevant, implying a higher weight to incorrect referral of patients without the disease (FPs) and less weight to missed cases (FNs) with disease (DVT).

The graph displays the whole range of probability thresholds for further management on the x-axis and the net benefit of the diagnostic strategies or models on the y-axis.[153] To compute the net benefit, the proportion of all patients who are FP is subtracted from the proportion of all patients who are TP, weighting by the relative cost of an FP and an FN classification.[152] A numerical example shows the relations.

TABLE 2.16 The Relationship Between True Deep Venous Thrombosis Status and the Result of the Basic and Extended Prediction Model With Thresholds of 20% and 70% Predicted Probability

		DVT (n = 2086)	
		Present	**Absent**
Basic model (model 1):	Yes	263	528
probability of DVT ≥20%	No	153	1142
Extended model (model 2):	Yes	319	301
probability of DVT ≥20%	No	97	1369
Basic model (model 1):	Yes	3	6
probability of DVT ≥70%	No	413	1664
Extended model (model 2):	Yes	123	31
probability of DVT ≥70%	No	293	1639

Table 2.16, presenting results for this empirical study on DVT, shows for the above-mentioned threshold of 20% that the TP count for model 1 was 263, and the FP count was 528. The total number of patients (n) was 2086. The net benefit for model 1 at the threshold of 20% was $(263/2086) - (528/2086) \times (0.2/0.8) = 0.06$. The net benefit ratio 0.2/0.8 explicitly reveals that less weight is now assigned to the FPs compared with the FNs, as considered earlier. For model 2, the net benefit at the cutoff of 20% was $(319/2086) - (301/2086) \times (0.2/0.8) = 0.12$, two times larger. Although model 2 outperforms model 1, it should be noted that when the extended model is used at this threshold, 97 of 416 known cases would be missed and thus not treated or referred for additional testing. This implies that the overall diagnostic performance of our shown model 2 is relatively poor for this theoretically selected threshold.

At the threshold of 70%, the net benefit of model 1 was $(3/2086) - (6/2086) \times (0.7/0.3) = -0.01$, and for model 2, it was $(123/2086) - (31/2086) \times (0.7/0.3) = 0.02$.

The net benefit of model 1 of 0.06 for a threshold of 20% can be expressed as: "Compared with the case of no referrals, referral by model 1 is the equivalent of a strategy that correctly refers 6 patients with DVT of 100 suspected patients without having any unnecessary (ie, FP) referrals."

The important point of the decision curve (see Fig. 2.43) is to observe which diagnostic strategy provides the best net benefit given the doctor's or patient's individual choice for a probability cutoff. The horizontal black line along the x-axis in Fig. 2.43 presupposes that no patients will be referred to reference testing. Because this strategy refers 0 patients, the net benefit of this strategy becomes 0 (ie, corresponding to incorrect handling of all patients with DVT). The grey steep declining line in Fig. 2.43 shows the net benefit of the strategy of simply subjecting all individuals to reference testing. This line intersects the x-axis at the threshold probability of 20% (ie, the prevalence in the study). Accordingly, model 2 has the greatest net benefit (ie, it is the highest line) for all threshold probabilities. Thus, we can conclude that, irrespective of the applied probability thresholds, the extended model with D-dimer added is better than the basic model.

POINTS TO REMEMBER

- Focus has been on approaches and measures for quantification of the diagnostic accuracy of combinations of index tests and of the added value of a new diagnostic test beyond existing diagnostic tests.
- Reporting on the increase in discrimination and in (re)classification is important to gain insight into the full clinical value of a biomarker.
- Decision-curve analysis implicitly accounts for the consequences of the FP and FN classifications, complementing the information from the other measures.

Test Evaluation Beyond Diagnostic Accuracy

Despite the methods we have presented in this chapter for the evaluation of the analytical performance and diagnostic accuracy of laboratory tests, increasingly more information is demanded about the actual impact laboratory tests and test results have on medical decision making and indeed on patient outcomes.[97,137,154-161] For instance, government health policymakers and private insurers in the United States now want to see empirical evidence that testing quantifiably improves actual patient outcomes in relevant patient populations or that it enhances healthcare quality, efficiency, and cost-effectiveness before recommending diagnostic tests and markers for clinical use and before deciding on their reimbursement.[162] In Europe, a visionary document was recently issued stressing the importance of evaluating medical technology, including diagnostic devices, on their ability to actually improve medical care and patient outcomes.[163] When making decisions and considering recommendations about diagnostic tests, clinicians and other decision makers have to consider the (cost-) effectiveness of the test use.

Restricting ourselves to the above explained traditional diagnostic accuracy study designs and statistical measures (eg, sensitivity, specificity, predictive values, ROC curves), we cannot easily infer on a test's actual impact on patient health or healthcare. Addressing these challenges ideally requires comparative studies, wherein the use of a certain (new) test is examined in the clinical context compared with the current best alternatives of care, such as other form(s) of testing or no testing at all. Downstream effects of testing on clinical decision making and patient care and patients' health outcomes can be compared between both strategies. Furthermore, such studies allow for in-depth examination whether the diagnostic test improves patient outcomes and healthcare quality, efficiency and cost-effectiveness at large.[97,137,154-159,161] The terms *clinical utility* or *clinical effectiveness* and *impact* of a diagnostic test are often used to express the extent to which diagnostic testing or diagnostic test results improve decision making, patient outcomes, or (cost-)effectiveness of healthcare. A more detailed discussion of clinical effectiveness and the overall impact of diagnostic tests is provided in Chapter 9 on evidence-based laboratory medicine.

How Does Testing Yield Health(care) Benefits?

Tests, including laboratory tests that are diagnostic, prognostic, monitoring, or screening tests, do not by themselves alleviate diseases, symptoms, or signs directly but rather *indirectly*.[99,154,155,158,159,163] A test provides information to a user (eg, healthcare professional or patient), which in turn indicates subsequent actions or interventions, such as therapies or lifestyle changes. For example, a test provides information (test results) that can be used to better identify patients who will and who will not benefit from helpful downstream management actions, such as administration of effective interventions or actions in individuals with certain (positive) test results and alternative or no treatment for those with other (negative) results. These interventions or actions, if beneficial, yield benefits in terms of improved health outcomes of individuals or patients. Diagnostic tests may affect patient outcomes and healthcare cost-effectiveness by improving the selection of the most effective treatment modalities or methods; examples include companion diagnostics, molecular imaging devices, and imaging devices to guide surgery. Moreover, a certain (new) diagnostic test may be beneficial because it allows for less invasive or less costly detection of disorders. A new screening or monitoring test that leads to early detection makes it possible to administer the appropriate treatment at an early stage. Also, knowing certain diagnostic test results may affect the cognition, behavior, and lifestyle of individuals, which in turn may affect their health outcomes. Finally, besides intended effects (benefits) of testing, some tests may also lead to unintended (side) effects.

The Working Pathway

When thinking about approaches to evaluate the impact of diagnostic tests on medical decision making, patient outcomes, and healthcare at large, it is useful to describe the pathways through which benefits (and risks) of using the test are likely to occur. This so-called *working pathway* provides a framework (Fig. 2.44) to explain how a given test leads to benefits or risks for patients' health or healthcare. Such working pathways include:

1. The anticipated technical or analytical capabilities of the test
2. The unintended and intended results and effects of the test when applied in the targeted context
3. In whom these effects are likely to occur (eg, in the targeted patients or in the care providers)
4. The anticipated mechanisms through which these potential effect will occur
5. Existing care in the targeted context and individuals
6. The expected time frame in which potential risks and benefits might occur

A clear description of the working pathway of a new test can determine the current benefits (and risks) of prevailing care in the intended medical context. It also helps determine what added value or benefits the new test must provide to improve existing care and what evidence is necessary to quantify whether these (added) benefits are indeed achieved at what risks or costs.

Having a detailed description of the working pathway at an early stage is particularly useful for invasive and costly (new) tests. A detailed description of the working pathway can also be used when evidence is interpreted from different studies (eg, technical, safety, and clinical studies). For instance, if analytical performance studies fail to provide evidence for the intended technical capabilities of a test, further studies are unnecessary. If safety and analytical performance studies of a new version (modification) of an existing test show that its safety and analytical performance is similar to the preceding

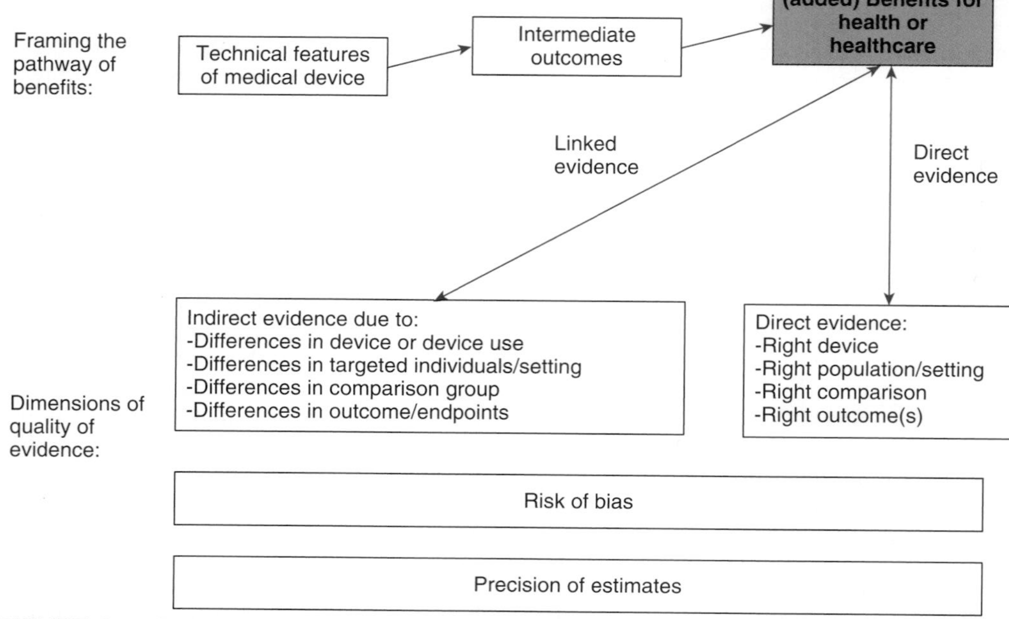

FIGURE 2.44 Relationship between the pathway through which devices may lead to benefits or added benefits for health or healthcare and the three dimensions of quality for evidence (indirectness of evidence, risk of bias, precision of estimates). (From KNAW. *Evaluation of new technology in health care. In need of guidance for relevant evidence.* Amsterdam, 2014, KNAW.)

version but that it is less burdensome or cheaper to use, then subsequent studies may not be needed.

Comparative Tests: Treatment Studies to Quantify the Impact of Tests

One could design a longitudinal study to validly quantify whether a certain (new) test has impact on patient's health or healthcare beyond what is achieved by current practice.[156,157,161,163-168] This is in fact a similar approach used to evaluate the *effectiveness* (not the efficacy) of medical drugs: so-called comparative or pragmatic randomized trial. The study should:

- Investigate the (new) test in the same targeted individuals (eg, professionals and patients) as it is intended to be used in practice.
- Investigate the test in the clinical pathway in which it is intended to be used in practice.
- Study the use of the test in combination with any subsequent management (eg, therapeutic) actions indicated by the test or its results.
- Compare the test and subsequent management actions to the best prevailing care. Ideally, this would be a randomized comparison: Individuals are allocated randomly to either the new test use or to the comparative strategy.
- Measure all outcomes or endpoints relevant for the targeted individuals, professionals, and ideally for society at large, including unintended outcomes, intended health outcomes (for patient and users), burden and ease of test use, speed of administering subsequent management, and even costs of test use.
- Be sufficiently long to investigate the long-term health care effects.
- Be sufficiently large to obtain precise estimates of the safety and health benefits of the test use.

The two comparison groups are thus created randomly. In the index group, the new test is used in combination with subsequent management or therapeutic actions, with the prevailing tests and management being applied in the comparison (control) group. Provided the two groups are large enough, any observed differences between the two groups in terms of benefits (and risks) can then be ascribed to the difference in tests plus subsequent management. Such randomized studies compare the use of the index test or tests combined with subsequent actions, directly with the best alternative strategy in the right population, measuring all relevant outcomes (for patients, users, and healthcare) in the short and long terms. Such studies thus generate the most *direct* and *valid evidence* as to whether the test use will indeed produce the intended relevant benefits at an acceptable level of risks and costs compared with prevailing care.

This randomized comparative study approach is not always feasible or possible.[156,157,161,168] Numerous alternative comparative study approaches may also produce (direct) evidence of the (added) benefits of test use for the relevant health outcomes in the intended medical context. These approaches may include alternative randomized designs as described.[169,170] Furthermore, there are also many nonrandomized comparative study approaches, ranging from quasi-randomized studies to controlled before-and-after studies and comparative cohort or even case-control studies.[133,171,172] These nonrandomized comparative studies are more prone to bias because of differences in demographic and clinical characteristics between the two groups being compared. Fortunately, there are various approaches to controlling or adjusting for such biases, for which we refer to the literature.[133,171,172]

Linked-Evidence Approaches to Quantify the Impact of Tests

Besides technical performance and cross-sectional diagnostic test accuracy studies described earlier, many clinical studies of (new) laboratory tests focus on measuring intermediate effects or outcomes along the working pathway for a given test. Each of these studies by themselves often do not allow for inferring on the desired longer-term (added) benefits and risks of the test use. However, it is possible to use the so-called quantitative linked-evidence approach in which the evidence of these different types of diagnostic test studies are quantitatively combined to estimate a test's effect on relevant health or healthcare outcomes.[158,159,173-177]

An example is the assessment of the analytical performance requirements for glucose monitoring devices to achieve clinically useful glucose control. Rather than conducting large-scale longitudinal comparative, expensive randomized studies using many different measuring devices as comparators, computers using a variety of underlying modeling schemes have been used to generate simulated glucose results from glucose measurement devices having varying amounts of bias and imprecision. The patient data used in these studies were derived from physiologic models of glucose metabolism or hospitalized patients.[178] The results of such linked-evidence modeling approaches can be used to evaluate the effects of measurement bias and imprecision on quantifiable intermediate results such as the percentage of the time glucose falls within the desired therapeutic range, the frequency and duration of hypoglycemic episodes, and the within-patient variability of glucose. Such intermediate results are known to have direct relationships with the rates of clinical complications in individuals with poor glucose control. For the evaluation of the impact or utility of (new) laboratory tests on patient and healthcare outcomes in the intended medical context, linked-evidence approaches offer an attractive alternative when direct evaluation of a test's benefits on long-term, patient-relevant outcomes is difficult or impossible. For the glucose example, it would be difficult to gain ethical approval for a randomized trial in which yet imprecise glucose analyzers were evaluated for their effects when used for patient glucose monitoring. The validity of a linked-evidence approach is dependent on how predictive the existing study results and evidence are and the relation of these intermediate outcomes with the long-term, relevant health or healthcare outcomes.

Linked-evidence studies can be particularly useful for laboratory test studies when there is evidence from cross-sectional studies on the diagnostic accuracy of a test and results of therapeutic studies provide a link to health outcomes. Simple modeling approaches might be used to link both types of evidence and to actually quantify the benefits (and risks) of the test use on these health outcomes. Such linked-evidence models might include various sensitivity analyses, for example, to account for the risks of using various types of evidence taken from different sources.[158,159,173-176] For example, a so-called Markov model was used to combine evidence from analytical performance studies, cross-sectional diagnostic accuracy studies, and long-term management studies to quantify the long-term cost-effectiveness of point-of-care D-dimer tests compared with the use of central laboratory D-dimer tests to rule out DVT in primary care.[179]

POINTS TO REMEMBER

- It is important to assess information concerning the actual impact or utility of the use of a diagnostic test on patient outcomes or health care at large.
- The impact of diagnostic tests on medical decision making and patient outcomes can be considered by describing the pathways through which benefits (and risks) of using the test are likely to occur (the so-called *working pathway*).
- *Direct and valid evidence* as to whether the new test will indeed produce the intended relevant benefits can be assessed by randomized studies comparing the outcome of use of the new test with that of the index test.
- A supplementary approach is the so-called quantitative linked-evidence procedure in which the evidence of different types of diagnostic test studies are quantitatively combined to estimate a test's effect on relevant health or health care outcomes.

SELECTED REFERENCES

For a full list of references for this chapter, please refer to ExpertConsult.com.

5. Snedecor GW, Cochran WG. *Statistical methods*. 8th ed. Ames, Iowa: Iowa State University Press; 1989. p. 75, 121, 140–2, 170–4, 177, 237–8, 279.
12. Dybkær R. Vocabulary for use in measurement procedures and description of reference materials in laboratory medicine. *Eur J Clin Chem Clin Biochem* 1997;**35**:141–73.
35. Krouwer JS. Setting performance goals and evaluating total analytical error for diagnostic assays. *Clin Chem* 2002;**48**: 919–27.
40. Linnet K. Nonparametric estimation of reference intervals by simple and bootstrap-based procedures. *Clin Chem* 2000;**46**:867–9.
44. Bland JM, Altman DG. Statistical methods for assessing agreement between two methods of clinical measurement. *Lancet* 1986;**i**:307–10.
49. Linnet K. Evaluation of regression procedures for methods comparison studies. *Clin Chem* 1993;**39**:424–32.
53. Linnet K. Limitations of the paired t-test for evaluation of method comparison data. *Clin Chem* 1999;**45**:314–15.
54. Linnet K. Estimation of the linear relationship between the measurements of two methods with proportional errors. *Stat Med* 1990;**9**:1463–73.
60. Passing H, Bablok W. Comparison of several regression procedures for method comparison studies and determination of sample sizes. *J Clin Chem Clin Biochem* 1984;**22**:431–45.
71. Vesper HW, Thienpont LM. Traceability in laboratory medicine. *Clin Chem* 2009;**55**:1067–75.
95. Linnet K, Bossuyt PM, Moons KG, et al. Quantifying the accuracy of a diagnostic test or marker. *Clin Chem* 2012;**58**: 1292–301.
96. Moons KG, de Groot JA, Linnet K, et al. Quantifying the added value of a diagnostic test or marker. *Clin Chem* 2012;**58**:1408–17.
97. Bossuyt PMM, Reitsma JB, Linnet K, et al. Beyond diagnostic accuracy: the clinical utility of diagnostic tests. *Clin Chem* 2012;**58**:1636–43.

102. Bossuyt PM, Reitsma JB, Bruns DE, et al. An updated list of essential items for reporting diagnostic accuracy studies. *Clin Chem* 2015;in press.
106. Oudega R, Moons KG, Hoes AW. Ruling out deep venous thrombosis in primary care. A simple diagnostic algorithm including D-dimer testing. *Thromb Haemost* 2005;**94**:200–5.
118. Obuchowski NA, Lieber ML, Wians FH Jr. ROC curves in clinical chemistry: uses, misuses, and possible solutions. *Clin Chem* 2004;**50**:1118–25.
137. Moons KG. Criteria for scientific evaluation of novel markers: a perspective. *Clin Chem* 2010;**56**:537–41.
143. Pencina MJ, D'Agostino RB, Vasan RS. Statistical methods for assessment of added usefulness of new biomarkers. *Clin Chem Lab Med* 2010;**48**:1703–11.
177. Horvath AR, Lord SJ, StJohn A, et al. From biomarkers to medical tests: the changing landscape of test evaluation. *Clin Chim Acta* 2014;**427**:49–57.
179. Hendriksen JMT, Geersing GJ, van Voorthuizen SC, et al. The cost–effectiveness of point-of-care D-dimer tests compared with a laboratory test to rule out deep venous thrombosis in primary care. *Expert Rev Mol Diagn* 2015;**15**:125–36.

3

Quality Management in the Medical Laboratory

David Burnett, Leslie Burnett, and Mark Mackay

ABSTRACT

Background

Quality management (QM) is an organization-wide framework to coordinate management activities to ensure that the organization meets at all times the requirements of its customers or users. Quality management systems (QMS) are structured frameworks for ensuring this consistency in the quality of products and services to meet user or customer needs. QMS evolved from quality control (QC) and external quality assessment/proficiency testing (EQA/PT) activities, and these still play important roles within the overall QMS. The International Organization for Standardization (ISO) has developed ISO 15189 as an internationally accepted standard suitable for accreditation of medical laboratories. In some countries, alternative or additional standards or accreditation requirements may apply.

Content

The most significant and widely adopted QMS used internationally (ISO 15189) is described in some detail, and it is compared with alternative or supplementary frameworks (eg, Clinical and Laboratory Standards Institute [CLSI] QMS01-A4). The differences between accreditation and certification are explained as is the role of standards and guidelines in self-assessment and in the accreditation and regulation of medical laboratories. Finally, various approaches to QM are summarized. The philosophy and principles of QM are described, and within this, the rationale is explained for using a QMS as a means of maintaining and controlling existing operations, as well as systematically improving the quality of test results and organizational services. Various pathways taken by laboratories to implementing QMS are considered, and various structured quality improvement tools and management approaches are described.

4

Specimen Collection and Processing

Doris M. Haverstick and Patricia M. Jones

ABSTRACT

Background

Proper specimen collection and processing is critical to avoiding common preanalytical errors. The specific steps and recommendations are designed to protect both the patient and the individual collecting the specimen.

Content

This chapter explicitly addresses in detail issues related to specimen collection. The most common types of specimens collected are addressed with the collection method(s) outlined, and some caveats for special populations, such as pediatric patients, are included. Details on collection devices and preservatives that should be used appropriately for an individual test request are outlined with attention to how to recognize when an incorrect sample is submitted for testing. The chapter concludes with the equally important details on proper specimen processing, handling, and transport to the testing facility and various circumstances in which additional testing might be required. It is stressed that specimen collection and handling must be done in a manner that is validated for the tests that will be performed. The information provided is designed to assist all laboratorians to ensure that the tests requested by the physician will be for the right person and will result in the right results in all cases.

INTRODUCTION

Proper collection, processing, storage, and transport of common sample types associated with requests for diagnostic testing are critical to the provision of quality test results. Each of the steps involved, as well as factors associated with the patient from whom the sample is being collected, can be the source of errors that cause inaccurate results. Minimizing these errors through careful adherence to the concepts discussed here and to individual institutional policies will result in more reliable information for use by healthcare professionals in providing quality patient care.

This chapter provides a review of the most common specimen types and discusses how they are (1) collected, (2) identified, (3) processed, (4) stored, and (5) transported. Body fluids other than blood and urine are covered in detail elsewhere (see Chapter 43) as are additional preanalytical factors (see Chapter 5). Attention to the differences between adult and pediatric collection are also discussed.

PATIENT IDENTIFICATION

Before any specimen is collected, the phlebotomist must confirm the identity of the patient. Two or three items of identification should be used (eg, name, medical record number, date of birth, social security number, address if the patient is an outpatient). The Joint Commission, a US hospital accreditation body, requires at least two of these unique identifiers be used to properly identify the patient.[1] In specialized situations, such as paternity testing or other tests of medicolegal importance, establishment of a chain of custody for the specimen may require that additional patient identification, such as a photograph, be provided as part of the identification process or taken to confirm the identity of the patient.

Identification must be an active process. When possible, the patient should state his or her name, and the phlebotomist should verify information on the patient's wrist band if the patient is hospitalized. If the patient is an outpatient, the phlebotomist should ask the patient to state his or her name and should confirm the information on the test requisition form with identifying information provided by the patient. In the case of pediatric patients, the parent or guardian should be present and should provide active identification of the child such as: "Please tell me the name of your child." Parents with young children are often distracted or worried about the upcoming procedure and may answer without paying attention to the question, so the question should always be posed in a manner to prevent a yes or no answer. Strict adherence to institutional policies is required.

TYPES OF SPECIMENS

Types of biologic specimens that are analyzed in clinical laboratories include (1) whole blood; (2) serum; (3) plasma; (4) urine; (5) feces; (6) saliva; (7) other body fluids such as spinal, synovial, amniotic, pleural, pericardial, and ascitic fluids; and (8) cells and various types of solid tissue. The World Health Organization[2] and the Clinical and Laboratory Standards Institute (CLSI) have published several guidelines for collecting many of these specimens under standardized conditions (Table 4.1). In addition, the CLSI has published

TABLE 4.1 Clinical and Laboratory Standards Institute Documents Related to Specimen Collection, Processing, and Transport

Document Name	Document Number
Accuracy in patient and sample identification: proposed guideline	GP33-P
Blood collection on filter paper for newborn screening programs: approved standard	LA4-A5
Body fluid analysis for cellular composition: approved guideline	H56-A
Collection, transport, and processing of blood specimens for testing plasma-based coagulation assays and molecular hemostasis assay: approved guideline	H21-A5
Collection, transport, preparation, and storage of specimens for molecular methods: approved guideline	MM13-A
Ionized calcium determinations: precollection variables, specimen choice, collection, and handling: approved guideline	C31-A2
Procedures and devices for the collection of diagnostic capillary blood specimens: approved standard	H04-A6
Procedures for the collection of arterial blood specimens: approved standard	H11-A4
Procedures for the collection of diagnostic blood specimens by venipuncture: approved standard	H3-A6
Procedures for the handling and transport of diagnostic specimens and etiologic agents: approved standard	H5-A3
Protection of laboratory workers from occupationally acquired infections: approved standard	M29-A3
Selecting and evaluating a referral laboratory: approved standard	GP9-A
Sweat testing: sample collection and quantitative chloride analysis: approved guideline	C34-A3

documents related to sample collection and analysis for specialized tests such as sweat chloride collection and testing (CLSI C34-A3, Table 4.1).

Blood

Blood for analysis may be obtained from veins, arteries, or capillaries. Venous blood is usually the specimen of choice, and venipuncture is the method for obtaining this specimen. Arterial puncture is used mainly for blood gas analyses. In young children and for many point-of-care tests, skin puncture is frequently used to obtain what is mostly capillary blood. The process of collecting blood is known as phlebotomy (from *phleb,* which means vein, and *tome,* to cut or incise) and should always be performed by a trained phlebotomist.

Venipuncture

In the clinical laboratory, venipuncture is defined as all of the steps involved in obtaining an appropriate and identified blood specimen from a patient's vein (CLSI H3-A6, Table 4.1).

Preliminary Steps. In many institutions, at this point in the process, the patient should be asked about latex allergies. If latex allergy is present and if latex gloves or a latex tourniquet may be used, the phlebotomist should secure an alternative tourniquet and put on gloves that are latex free. Finally, for some specialized tests such as testing for genetic diseases, the performing laboratory may request a signed consent form from the patient or the use of a special requisition; these should be completed at the time of collection if not provided by the requesting physician.

Before collection of a specimen, the phlebotomist should dress in personal protective equipment (PPE), such as an impervious gown and gloves applied immediately before approaching the patient, and adhere to standard precautions against potentially infectious material; the goal is to limit the spread of infectious disease from one patient to another and to promote the safety of the phlebotomist. Because small children are often frightened of anyone in a white coat or gown, pediatric phlebotomists often dress in bright, cheerful colors, including colored PPE rather than standard white. Pediatric drawing stations are also often brightly colored with lots of distracters for the patient. If the phlebotomist must collect a specimen from a patient in isolation in a hospital, the phlebotomist must put on a clean gown and gloves and a face mask and goggles before entering the patient's room. The face mask limits the spread of potentially infectious droplets, and the goggles limit the possible entry of infectious material into the eye. The extent of the precautions required varies with the nature of the patient's illness and the institution's policies and bloodborne pathogen plan, to which a phlebotomist must adhere. For example, if airborne precautions are indicated, the phlebotomist must wear an N95 tuberculosis respirator in the United States.

If appropriate, the phlebotomist should verify that the patient has fasted, identify what medications are being taken or have been discontinued as required, and determine any other relevant information required. Chapter 5 describes in more detail the effects of diet and fluid intake and the recommended steps for patient preparation, including fasting, before phlebotomy. The patient should be comfortable, seated or supine (if sitting is not feasible), and should have been in this position for as long as possible before the specimen is drawn. The correct interpretation of certain tests (eg, aldosterone, renin, plasma metanephrines) requires that the patient is in a supine position for at least 30 minutes before venipuncture. (For details on the effects of position, refer to Chapters 5 and 63.) For an outpatient, it is generally recommended that patients be seated before completion of the identification process to maximize their relaxation. At no time should venipuncture be performed on a standing patient.

Infants and young children may need to be held in order to restrain them and prevent movement. Young children may be held sitting upright in a parent's lap with the parent helping to support and hold the patient and arm still[2] (Fig. 4.1). Infants' blood is often drawn with the infant in a supine position, and the infant may be swaddled in a blanket, or a papoose board may be used to restrain movement. Occasionally, the parents will be more anxious than the child,

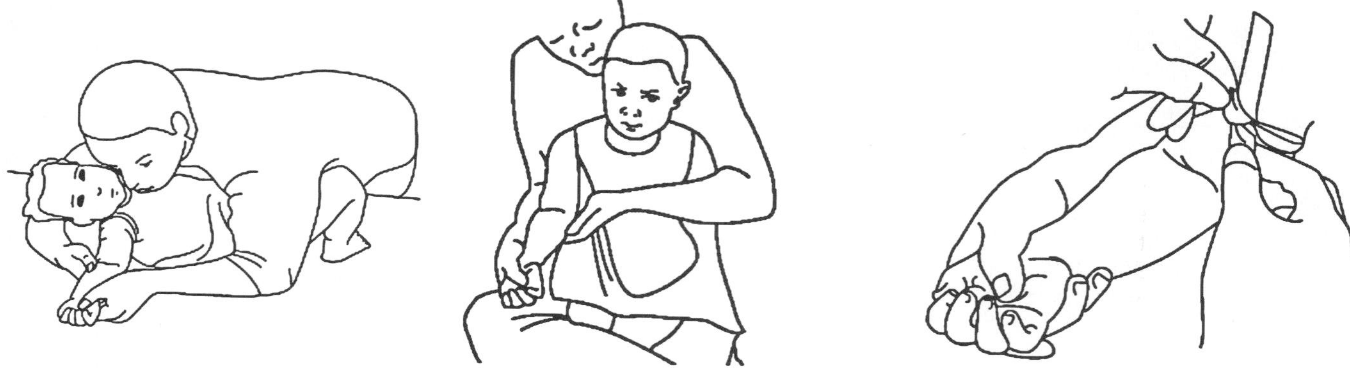

FIGURE 4.1 Holding a child for venipuncture. (Modified from World Health Organization. WHO guidelines on drawing blood: best practices in phlebotomy. *Pediatric and neonatal blood sampling.* Geneva: World Health Organization; 2010. http://www.ncbi.nlm.nih.gov/books/NBK138647.)

and the phlebotomist will need to make the decision to request help from a colleague phlebotomist to properly and safely perform the collection.[3,4]

Either of the patient's arms should be extended in a straight line from the shoulder to the wrist. An arm with an inserted intravenous (IV) line should be avoided, as should an arm with extensive scarring or a hematoma at the intended collection site. If a woman has had a mastectomy, arm veins on that side of the body should not be used because the surgery may have caused lymphostasis (blockade of normal lymph node drainage), affecting the blood composition. If a woman has had double mastectomies, blood should be drawn from the arm of the side on which the first procedure was performed. If the surgery was done within 6 months on both sides, a vein on the back of the hand or at the ankle should be used.

Before performing a venipuncture, the phlebotomist should estimate the volume of blood to be drawn and should select the appropriate number and types of tubes for the blood, plasma, or serum tests requested. In many settings, this is facilitated by computer-generated collection recommendations and should be designed to collect the minimum amount necessary for testing. Estimating volume of blood to be drawn is especially critical in a pediatric setting. An average-weight newborn infant has a total blood volume of approximately 350 mL. Collecting too much blood from an infant in a hospital setting will eventually result in the need to give the infant blood back in the form of a transfusion, risking exposure to bloodborne pathogens. Blood collection in the pediatric population should not exceed recommended volumes for the pediatric patient's weight.[5] The later sections on "Order of Draw for Multiple Collections" and "Collection with Evacuated Blood Tubes" discuss in greater detail the recommended order of draw for multiple specimens and types of tubes. Careful consideration should also be taken in the case of an adult patient as one study showed that on average, every 100 mL of phlebotomy was associated with a decrease in hemoglobin of 7.0 g/L and hematocrit of 1.9%.[6] Such iatrogenic blood loss can lead to the same possible unnecessary blood transfusion and an increased risk of exposure to bloodborne pathogens in adults as in children.

In addition to tubes, an appropriate needle must be selected. The most commonly used sizes for adults are 19 to 22 gauge. (The larger the gauge number, the smaller the bore.) The usual choice for an adult with normal veins is 20 gauge; if veins tend to collapse easily, a size 21 is preferred. For volumes of blood from 30 to 50 mL, an 18-gauge needle may be required to ensure adequate blood flow. In pediatric patients, 23- to 25-gauge needles are most commonly used, with 23-gauge being the preferred size. Venipuncture on infants and children younger than 2 years old is often performed on dorsal hand veins rather than arm veins, and the veins in either place are very small in this age group. Even for larger volumes of blood, rarely will a needle larger than a 21 gauge be used because it will not fit into the vein easily. A needle is typically 1.5 inches (3.7 cm) long, but 1-inch (2.5-cm) needles, usually attached to a winged or butterfly collection set, are also used and are common in pediatrics. All needles must be sterile and sharp and without barbs. If blood is drawn for trace element measurements, the needle should be stainless steel and should be known to be free from contamination.

Finally, the phlebotomist should ensure that all postdraw safety devices are in place. These include (for the person drawing) quick, convenient, and safe access to proper disposal devices for all (now) contaminated needles and associated devices and (for the patient) the appropriate post–blood draw supplies (gauze and bandage) are in place to ensure no adverse events might affect the patient.

Location. The median cubital vein in the antecubital fossa, or crook of the elbow, is the preferred site for collecting venous blood in adults because the vein is large and is close to the surface of the skin (CLSI H3-A6, Table 4.1). Veins on the back of the hand or at the ankle may be used, although these are less desirable and should be avoided in people with diabetes and other individuals with poor circulation. However, in infants and children younger than 2 years old, collection from superficial veins is recommended, and these sites may be preferred over the median cubital vein. In the inpatient setting, it is appropriate to collect blood through a cannula that is inserted for long-term fluid infusions at the time of first insertion to avoid the need for a second stick. This method of collection may increase the chances of a hemolyzed sample as well as contamination of the collected sample with fluids being infused. Careful adherence to withdrawal of a discard volume and discussions with the clinical team on alternative site for phlebotomy can greatly reduce these preanalytical variables. For severely ill individuals and those requiring many IV injections, an alternative blood-drawing site should be chosen. Selection of a vein for puncture is facilitated by palpation. An arm containing a cannula or an arteriovenous fistula should not be used without consent of the patient's physician. If fluid is being infused intravenously into a limb, the fluid should be shut off for 3 minutes (with clinician consent) before a specimen is obtained and a suitable note made in the patient's chart and on the result report form. Specimens obtained from the opposite arm are preferred. Specimens below the infusion site in the same arm may be satisfactory for most tests, except for analytes that are contained in the infused solution (eg, glucose, electrolytes).

Preparation of the Site. The area around the intended puncture site should be cleaned with whatever cleanser is approved for use by the institution. Three commonly used materials are a prepackaged alcohol swab, a gauze pad saturated with 70% isopropanol, and a benzalkonium chloride solution (eg, Zephiran chloride solution, 1:750). Cleaning of the puncture site should be done with a circular motion from the site outward. The skin should be allowed to dry in the air. No alcohol or cleanser should remain on the skin because traces may cause hemolysis and invalidate test results. After the skin has been cleaned, it should not be touched until after the venipuncture has been completed.

Timing. The time at which a specimen is obtained is important for blood constituents that undergo marked diurnal variation (eg, corticosteroids, iron), for those for which a fasting sample has been requested, and for those used to monitor drug therapy. In each case, the timing should match the conditions under which reference intervals or clinical decision points were determined (see Chapter 8). Furthermore, timing is important in relation to specimens for alcohol or drug measurements in association with medicolegal considerations. For most current molecular diagnostic tests, the time of day is unlikely to contribute to altered or invalid test results.

Venous Occlusion. After the skin is cleaned, a blood pressure cuff or a tourniquet is applied 4 to 6 inches (10–15 cm) above the intended puncture site (distance for adults). This obstructs the return of venous blood to the heart and distends the veins (venous occlusion). When a blood pressure cuff is used as a tourniquet, it is usually inflated to approximately 60 mm Hg (8.0 kPa). Tourniquets typically are made from precut soft rubber strips or from Velcro. If a dorsal hand vein is being accessed in infants and young children, no tourniquet is used. The phlebotomist applies enough pressure with the hand holding the patient's wrist and hand to occlude and distend the vein.

It is rarely necessary to leave a tourniquet in place for longer than 1 minute after venous access is secured and the tourniquet is removed, but even within this short time, the composition of blood changes, and adherence to institutional policies must be followed. Although the changes that occur in 1 minute are slight, marked changes have been observed after 3 minutes for some chemistry analytes, but there are no known changes that affect molecular diagnostic testing. The composition of blood drawn first—that is, the blood closest to the tourniquet—is most representative of the composition of circulating blood and the least affected by fluid shifts where protein bound components and other large molecules will be concentrated; water-soluble smaller molecules such as electrolytes may be less affected. The first-drawn specimen should therefore be used for analytes such as calcium and other analytes that are both protein bound and pertinent to critical medical decisions and may be affected by the collection process.[6,7] A uniform procedure for the order of draw for tests should therefore be established (see later discussion). If it is possible to collect only a small volume of blood, the priority of which tests to perform should be established.

Two special notes on the collection process: Pumping of the fist before venipuncture should be avoided because it causes an increase in plasma potassium, phosphate, and lactate concentrations. Lowering of blood pH by accumulation of lactate causes the plasma ionized calcium concentration to increase.[7] The ionized calcium concentration reverts to normal 10 minutes after the tourniquet is released.[8] Importantly, the stress associated with blood collection can have effects on patients at any age. As a consequence, plasma concentrations of analytes affected by stress, such as cortisol, thyroid-stimulating hormone, and growth hormone, may increase. Stress occurs particularly in young children who are frightened, struggling, and held in physical restraint. Collection under these conditions may cause adrenal stimulation, leading to an increased plasma glucose concentration, or may create increases in the serum activities of enzymes that originate in skeletal muscle.

Order of Draw for Multiple Blood Specimens. In a few patients, backflow from blood tubes into veins occurs owing to a decrease in venous pressure. The dangerous consequences of this occurrence may be prevented if only sterile tubes are used for collection of blood. Backflow is minimized if the arm is held downward and blood is kept from contact with the stopper during the collection procedure. When collecting multiple specimens with an evacuated tube system, one of the primary concerns is to prevent cross-contamination between tubes. For example, EDTA (ethylenediaminetetraacetic acid) contamination can cause an erroneously reported hyperkalemia or hypocalcemia when an inappropriate tube type is analyzed but should be recognized by the laboratorian releasing the results.[9] To minimize problems if backflow occurs and to optimize the quality of specimens by preventing cross-contamination with anticoagulants, blood should be collected into tubes in the order outlined in Table 4.2. This table also provides the recommended number of inversions for each tube type because it is critical that complete mixing of any additive with the blood collected be accomplished as quickly as possible. In addition, completing a blood collection within 2 minutes of starting, and getting the tubes mixed correctly as soon as possible, helps to prevent clotting in anticoagulated tubes. The order of collection when multiple tubes are drawn from a skin puncture is different than when an evacuated system is used (see the later section on skin puncture).

Collection With Evacuated Blood Tubes. Evacuated blood tubes are usually considered to be safer, less expensive, more convenient, and easier to use than syringes and thus are the collection device of choice in many institutions. Evacuated blood tubes may be made of soda-lime or borosilicate glass or plastic (polyethylene terephthalate). Because of the decreased likelihood of breakage and subsequent exposure to infectious materials, many, if not most, laboratories have converted from glass to plastic tubes. Several types of evacuated tubes may be used for venipuncture collection. They vary by the type of additive added and the volume of the tube. The

TABLE 4.2 Recommended Order of Draw for Multiple Specimen Collection

Stopper Color	Contents	Inversions
Yellow	Sterile media for blood culture	8
Royal blue	No additive	0
Clear	Nonadditive; discard tube if no royal blue used	0
Light blue	Sodium citrate	3–4
Gold/red	Serum separator tube	5
Red/red, orange/yellow, royal blue	Serum tube, with or without clot activator, with or without gel	5
Green	Heparin tube with or without gel	8
Tan (glass)	Sodium heparin	8
Royal blue	Sodium heparin, sodium EDTA (trace metal free)	8
Lavender, pearl white, pink/pink, tan (plastic)	EDTA tubes, with or without gel	8
Gray	Glycolytic inhibitor	8
Yellow (glass)	ACD for molecular studies and cell culture	8

ACD, Acid citrate dextrose; *EDTA,* ethylenediaminetetraacetic acid.
Modified from information in Clinical and Laboratory Standards Institute. *Tubes and additives for venous blood specimen collection: CLSI-approved standard H1-A5.* 5th ed. Wayne, PA: Clinical and Laboratory Standards Institute; 2003; and Kiechle FL, ed. *So you're going to collect a blood specimen: an introduction to phlebotomy.* 11th ed. Northfield, IL: College of American Pathologists, 2005.

different types of additives are identified by the color of the stopper used. Color coding of specimen collection tubes is not yet harmonized and may vary according to manufacturers. Table 4.3 presents the most common forms of color codes of various tube types. Serum or plasma separator tubes are available that contain an inert, polymer gel material with a specific gravity of approximately 1.04. Aspiration of blood into the tube and subsequent centrifugation displace the gel, which settles like a disk between cells and supernatant when the tube is centrifuged. A minimum relative centrifugal force (RCF) of 1100 ×g is required for gel release and barrier formation in most tubes. Release of intracellular components into the supernatant is prevented by the barrier for several hours or, in many cases, for 7 days or more, allowing for additional testing ("add-ons") from samples collected at a specific time in the patient's care. However, all laboratories need to review the specific manufacturers' recommendations of what may be allowed based on provided data or perform their own validation studies. Most important, these separator tubes may be used as primary containers from which serum or plasma can be directly aspirated by a number of analytical instruments, avoiding aspiration of red blood cells (RBCs) or possible errors of patient or sample identification during aliquoting. Additional tubes, not listed, are sold for special applications, such as RNA isolation. As with all specimen collection containers, these less common tubes must be validated by each laboratory before use if not approved by the manufacturer for the specific analysis to be conducted.

Stoppers may contain zinc, invalidating the use of evacuated blood tubes for zinc measurement, and TBEP (tris[2-butoxyethyl] phosphate), also a constituent of the stopper, which may interfere with the measurement of certain drugs. With time, the vacuum in evacuated tubes is lost and their effective draw diminishes. The silicone coating also decays with age. Therefore, the stock of these tubes should be rotated and careful attention paid to the expiration date. Blood collected into a tube containing one additive should never be transferred into other tubes because the first additive may interfere with tests for which a different additive is specified. Additionally, transfer of the additive from one tube to another should be minimized (or adverse effects reduced) through strict adherence to recommendations for order of tube use (see Table 4.2).

A typical system for collecting blood in evacuated tubes is shown in Fig. 4.2.[10] This is an example of a commonly used single-use device that incorporates a cover that is designed to be placed over the needle when collection of the blood is complete, thereby reducing the risk of puncture of the phlebotomist by the now contaminated needle. A needle or winged (butterfly) set is screwed into the collection tube holder, and the tube is then gently inserted into this holder. The tube should be gently tapped to dislodge any additive from the stopper before the needle is inserted into a vein; this prevents aspiration of the additive into the patient's vein.

After the skin has been cleaned, the needle should be guided gently into the patient's vein; when the needle is in place, the tube should be pressed forward into the holder to puncture the stopper and release the vacuum. As soon as blood begins to flow into the tube, the tourniquet should be released without moving the needle (see earlier discussion on venous occlusion). The tube is filled until the vacuum is exhausted. It is critically important that the evacuated tube be filled completely. Many additives, particularly for coagulation testing, are provided at concentrations in the tube based on a "full and proper" collection; both short and too-full draws can be a source of preanalytical error because they can significantly affect the established testing parameters that are based on a properly collected sample. Therefore, a vacuum tube should always be filled using the vacuum that is designed to fill it correctly. These tubes should never be opened and filled from a syringe or other source. After the tube is filled completely, it should be withdrawn from the holder, mixed gently by inversion, and replaced by another tube if necessary. Other tubes may be filled using the same technique with the holder in place.

Blood Collection With a Syringe. Syringes are customarily used for patients with difficult veins, including very small veins, and for blood gas analysis. If a syringe is used, the needle is placed firmly over the nozzle of the syringe, and the cover of the needle is removed. If the syringe has an eccentric nozzle, the needle should be arranged with the nozzle downward but the bevel of the needle upward. The syringe and the needle should be aligned with the vein to be entered and the needle pushed into the vein at an angle to the skin of approximately 15 degrees. When the initial resistance of the vein wall is overcome as it is pierced, forward pressure on the syringe is eased, and the blood is withdrawn by very gently pulling back the plunger of the syringe. If a second syringe is necessary, a gauze pad may be placed under the hub of the needle to absorb the spill; the first syringe is then quickly

TABLE 4.3 Coding of Stopper Color to Indicate Additive in Evacuated Blood Tube

Tube Type	Additive	Stopper Color	Alternative
Gel separation tubes	Polymer gel/silica activator	Red/black	Gold
	Polymer gel/silica activator/lithium heparin	Green/gray	Light gray
Serum tubes (nonadditive)	Silicone-coated interior	Red	None
	Uncoated interior	Red	Pink
Serum tubes (with additives)	Thrombin (dry additive)	Gray/yellow	Orange
	Particulate clot activator	Yellow/red	Red
	Thrombin (dry additive)	Light blue	Light blue
Whole blood/plasma tubes	K_2 EDTA (dry additive)	Lavender	Lavender
	K_3 EDTA (liquid additive)	Lavender	Lavender
	Na_2 EDTA (dry additive)	Lavender	Lavender
	Citrate, trisodium (coagulation)	Light blue	Light blue
	Citrate, trisodium (erythrocyte sedimentation rate)	Black	Black
	Sodium fluoride (antiglycolic agent)	Gray	Light/gray
	Heparin, lithium (dry or liquid additive)	Green	Green
	Potassium oxalate/sodium fluoride	Light gray	Light gray
	Lithium heparin/iodoacetate	Light gray	Light gray
Specialty Tubes (Microbiology)			
Blood culture	Sodium polyanethol sulfonate (SPS)	Light yellow	Light yellow
Specialty Tubes (Chemistry)			
Lead	Heparin, potassium (liquid additive)	Tan	Tan
	Heparin, sodium (dry additive)	Royal blue	Royal blue
Trace elements	Silicone-coated interior (serum tube)	Royal blue	Royal blue
Stat chemistry	Thrombin	Gray/yellow	Orange
Specialty Tubes (Molecular Diagnostics)			
Plasma	K_2 EDTA (dry additive)/polymer gel/silica activator	Opalescent white	Opalescent white
	ACD solution A (Na_3 citrate, 22.0 g/L; citric acid, 8.0 g/L; dextrose, 24.5 g/L)	Bright yellow	Bright yellow
	ACD solution B (Na_3 citrate, 13.2 g/L; citric acid, 4.8 g/L; dextrose, 14.7 g/L)	Bright yellow	Bright yellow
Mononuclear cell preparation tube	Sodium citrate with density gradient polymer fluid	Blue/black	Blue/black
	Sodium heparin with density gradient polymer fluid	Green/red	Green/red

ACD, Acid citrate dextrose; *EDTA,* ethylenediaminetetraacetic acid.
Modified from information in Clinical and Laboratory Standards Institute. *Tubes and additives for venous blood specimen collection: CLSI-approved standard H1-A5.* 5th ed. Wayne, PA: Clinical and Laboratory Standards Institute, 2003; and Becton Dickinson (http://www.bd.com).

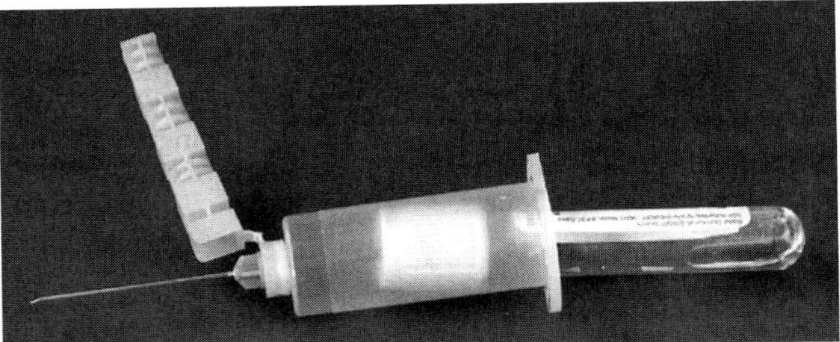

FIGURE 4.2 Assembled venipuncture set. (From Flynn JC. *Procedures in phlebotomy.* 3rd ed. St. Louis: Saunders, 2005.)

disconnected, and the second is put in place to continue the blood draw.

After filling the syringe and completing the collection, if the sample needs to be transferred to an evacuated tube, the same needle, a new needle, or a transfer device should be used to puncture the cap of the tube. The tube should be allowed to fill passively using its vacuum; uncapping the evacuated tube is not recommended for the reasons stated earlier. Vigorous withdrawal of blood into a syringe during collection or forceful transfer from the syringe to the receiving vessel may cause hemolysis of blood and will likely make the sample not valid for testing. Communication of this common preanalytical error to those not trained in routine sample collection is the responsibility of all laboratory directors and the experts, the phlebotomy team. Although safe use and disposal of sharps is important with any collection device, this is particularly important with the use of a needle and syringe. The phlebotomist must ensure an appropriate sharps disposal bin is available at the point of collection, that the location is free of interference or distractions that may increase the risk of a needle-stick injury, and that he or she has been trained in all procedures.

Completion of Collection. When blood collection is complete and the needle withdrawn, the patient should be instructed to hold a dry gauze pad tightly over the puncture site to stop residual bleeding and promote the clotting process with the arm raised. The pad should then be held in place firmly by a bandage or by a nonadhesive strap (which avoids pulling hairs on the arm when it is removed); these may be removed after 15 minutes. With a collection device, such as that shown in Fig. 4.2, the needle is covered, and the needle and the tube holder are immediately discarded into a sharps container that should be conveniently and safely positioned. In the event that a winged (butterfly) set is used, the wings are pushed forward to cover the needle, or with newer available equipment, a button is pressed, releasing a spring that retracts the needle. If a syringe was used, the needle should not be removed because of the danger of a needlestick on the part of the phlebotomist. All used supplies should be discarded in a hazardous waste receptacle.

All tubes should then be labeled per institutional policy. Most institutions have a written procedure prohibiting the advance labeling of tubes because this is seen as providing the potential for mislabeling, one of the most common sources of preanalytical error. Collectors should ensure that the correct labels are applied because this is a source of error for patient labels to be incorrectly filed in patient notes, files, or in the room of a hospitalized patient. Many US institutions recommend showing the labeled tube to the patient to further confirm correct identification. At the conclusion of this process, gloves should be discarded in a hazardous waste receptacle if visibly contaminated or in noncontaminated trash if not visibly contaminated. Before applying new gloves and proceeding to the next patient, and depending on institutional policy, all should use an alcohol-based cleanser or soap and water to wash their hands.

Venipuncture in Children. The techniques for venipuncture in children and adults are similar. However, children are likely to make unexpected movements, and assistance in holding them still is often desirable. Although a syringe or an evacuated blood tube system may be used to collect specimens, a syringe with a winged butterfly collection set is more commonly used in younger children. The pressure on a syringe can be more easily controlled by the phlebotomist than the vacuum pressure in an evacuated tube, thus preventing the pressure from pulling small veins closed instead of drawing blood from them. A syringe should be the tuberculin type or should have a 3-mL capacity, except when a large volume of blood is required for analysis. A 21- to 23-gauge needle or a 20- to 23-gauge butterfly needle with attached tubing is appropriate to collect specimens. In the pediatric population, alternative collection through skin puncture is often used.

Skin Puncture

Skin puncture is an open collection technique in which the skin is punctured by a lancet and a small volume of blood is collected into a microdevice. In practice, skin puncture is used in situations in which (1) sample volume is limited (eg, pediatric applications), (2) repeated venipunctures have resulted in severe vein damage, or (3) patients have been burned or bandaged and veins therefore are unavailable for venipuncture. This technique is also commonly used when the sample is to be applied directly to a testing device in a point-of-care testing situation or to filter paper. It is most often performed on the tip of the finger or the heels of infants. For example, in an infant younger than 6 months, the lateral or medial plantar surface of the foot should be used for skin puncture; suitable areas are illustrated in Fig. 4.3.[11] These areas are the fleshiest part of the foot in an infant, with the most distance between the skin surface and the underlying bone. Risk of inadvertently hitting bone and causing a bone infection is the lowest when these areas are used for a heel stick. For this reason, the back of the heel and the toes should not be used.[3] Blood collection from anywhere on the foot should be avoided on ambulatory patients; thus, when an infant starts walking, a heel stick should no longer be performed. In addition, devices are made specifically for a heel stick or a finger stick, and they should not be used interchangeably. These devices have different tip lengths and thus make a shallower or a deeper puncture (Table 4.4). The finger-stick procedure should not be performed on infants younger than 6 months old because no commercially available device punctures shallow enough to avoid bones. The complete procedure for collecting blood from infants using skin puncture is described in a CLSI document (CLSI H04-A6, Table 4.1).

To collect a blood specimen by skin puncture, the phlebotomist first thoroughly cleans the skin with a gauze pad saturated with an approved cleaning solution, as outlined earlier for venipuncture. If an alcohol swab is used, the alcohol must be allowed to evaporate from the skin so that hemolysis does not occur. When the skin is dry, it is quickly punctured by a sharp stab with a lancet. The depth of the incision should be less than 2.0 mm to prevent contact with bone. To minimize the possibility of infection, a different site should be selected for each puncture. The finger should be held in such a way that gravity assists collection of blood at the fingertip and the lancet held to make the incision as close

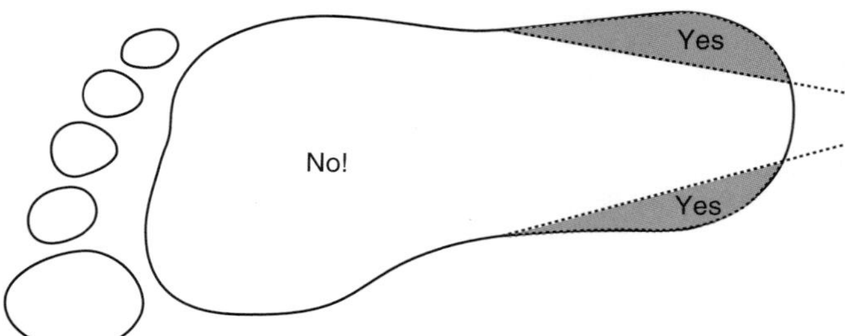

FIGURE 4.3 Acceptable sites for skin puncture to collect blood from an infant's foot. (Modified from Blumenfeld TA, Turi GK, Blanc WA. Recommended site and depth of newborn heel punctures based on anatomical measurements and histopathology. *Lancet* 1979;1:230–233. Reprinted with permission from Elsevier.)

TABLE 4.4 Tip Lengths in Finger- and Heel-Stick Devices

Collection Type and Age of Use	Tip Length (mm)
Heel stick: premature infants	0.85
Heel stick: term infants to 6 months old	1.25
Heel stick: 6 months to 1 year	1.25
Finger stick: walking to 8 years	1.5
Finger stick: >8 years	1.75–2.2

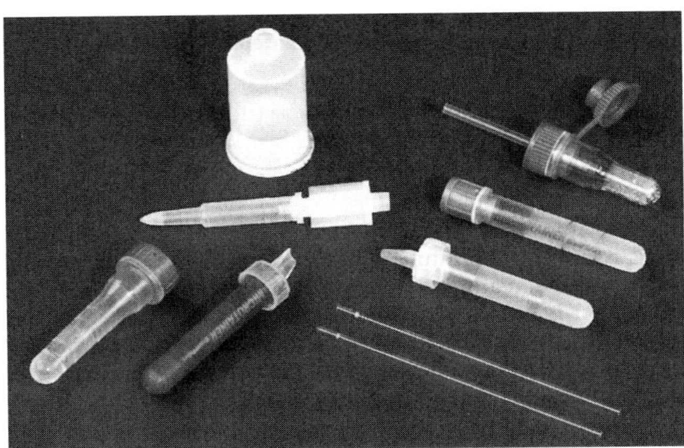

FIGURE 4.4 Microcollection tubes. (From Flynn JC. *Procedures in phlebotomy*. 3rd ed. St. Louis: Saunders, 2005.)

to perpendicular to the fingernail as possible.[11] Massage of the finger to stimulate blood flow should be avoided because it causes the outflow of debris and tissue fluid, which does not have the same composition as plasma. To improve circulation of the blood, the finger (or the heel in the case of a heel stick) may be warmed by application of a warm, wet washcloth or a specialized device, such as a heel warmer, for 3 minutes before the lancet is applied. Warming the heel or finger properly will not only cause the capillary blood to be free flowing and improve the ability to collect the sample, but the analytes in the sample will also approach arterial blood values in a properly warmed heel stick. In a cold heel, the values more approximate venous blood. Warming thus may be especially important for capillary blood gas collections. The first drop of blood is wiped off, and subsequent drops are transferred to the appropriate collection tube by gentle contact. Filling should be done rapidly to prevent clotting, and introduction of air bubbles should be prevented.

As the name suggests, blood is collected into capillary blood tubes by capillary action. A variety of collection tubes are commercially available (Fig. 4.4). Containers are available that contain different anticoagulants, such as sodium and lithium heparin, and some are available in brown glass for collection of light-sensitive analytes, such as bilirubin (see later section on anticoagulants). As with evacuated blood tubes and to prevent the possibility of breakage and the spread of infection, capillary devices frequently are plastic or coated with plastic. A disadvantage of some of the collection devices shown in Fig. 4.4 is that blood tends to pool in the mouth of the tube and must be flicked down the tube, creating a risk of hemolysis. Drop-by-drop collection and scooping along the skin with the edge of the tube to collect the blood should be avoided because both practices increase hemolysis. The correct order of filling of these devices is different than evacuated blood tubes because the concerns are different.[12] These samples are collected by dripping or capillary action from the puncture site into the small tubes that hold less than 1 mL each. There is less chance of cross-contamination with anticoagulant between tubes; however, the flow of blood also clots quickly in a heel or finger stick, and platelet levels drop quickly as the clots form. Thus, the anticoagulant tubes, especially the EDTA tube for the complete blood count (CBC), are drawn first rather than last. The serum tubes are drawn last (Table 4.5) because it does not matter if clots are formed in the sample.[13,14]

TABLE 4.5 Order of Draw for Skin Puncture: Capillary Blood

Usage or Additive	Tube Top Color
Blood gases (heparin)	Microhematocrit tubes
EDTA	Lavender
Heparin	Green
Other additives	Light blue, gray
Nonadditives	Red, tiger, yellow

EDTA, Ethylenediaminetetraacetic acid.

For collection of blood specimens on filter paper for molecular genetic testing and neonatal screening, the skin is cleaned and punctured as described previously. The first drop of blood should be wiped away. Then the filter paper is gently touched against a large drop of blood that is allowed to soak into the paper to fill the marked circle. Only a single application per circle should be made to prevent non-uniform analyte concentration. The paper is examined to verify that there has been complete penetration of the paper. The procedure is repeated to fill all the circles. As with all skin puncture collections, avoid milking or squeezing the finger or foot because this procedure contributes tissue fluids to the sample. The filter papers should be air dried (generally for 2 to 3 hours and horizontally placed to prevent mold or bacterial overgrowth and possible separation of blood components, respectively) before storage in a properly labeled paper envelope. Blood should never be transferred onto filter paper after it has been collected in nonanticoagulated capillary tubes because partial clotting may have occurred, compromising the quality of the specimen. However, blood collected into any type of tube containing an anticoagulant may be applied directly to the filter paper. This is a convenient way to store a sample for possible future molecular testing (with patient consent). These blood spots are handled in the same manner as neonatal screening specimens, with air drying and storage in a dry protected environment.

Arterial Puncture

Arterial puncture requires considerable skill and is usually performed only by physicians or specially trained technicians or nurses. Preferred sites of arterial puncture are, in order, the (1) radial artery at the wrist, (2) brachial artery in the elbow, and (3) femoral artery in the groin. Because leakage of blood from the femoral artery tends to be greater, especially in older adults, sites in the arm are used most often. The proper technique for arterial puncture is described in a CLSI document (CLSI H11-A4, Table 4.1).

In neonates, an indwelling catheter in the umbilical artery is best to obtain specimens for blood gas analysis. In older children and adults in whom it is impossible to perform an arterial puncture, a capillary puncture may be performed to obtain arterialized capillary blood. Such a specimen yields acceptable values for pH and PCO_2 but not always for PO_2 unless the site is properly warmed. In children and adults, the preferred puncture site is the finger; in infants, it is the heel. Capillary blood specimens are particularly inappropriate when blood circulation is poor and thus should be avoided when a patient has reduced cardiac output, hypotension, or vasoconstriction or has a condition of fluid overload. For each capillary puncture, the skin should be warmed first with a hot, moist towel to improve the circulation. The puncture itself should be performed as described previously; a free flow of blood is essential. Heparinized capillary tubes containing a small metal bar can be used to collect the blood. Tubes should be sealed quickly and the contents mixed well by using a magnet to move the metal bar up and down in the tube so that a uniform specimen is available for analysis.

Anticoagulants and Preservatives for Blood

Serum is defined as that portion of blood that remains after coagulation has occurred and the cells have been removed and is the specimen of choice for many analyses, including viral and antibody screening and protein electrophoresis. Samples are collected into tubes with no additive or with a clot activator and must be allowed to complete the coagulation process before further processing. Plasma is defined as the noncellular component of anticoagulated whole blood after the cellular components have been removed. There are multiple ways to produce a plasma sample detailed later. Heparin plasma is increasingly being used for routine chemistry testing to decrease turnaround time because it is not necessary to wait for the blood to clot. Sometimes considerable differences may be observed between the concentrations of analytes in serum and in plasma, as shown in Table 4.6. For molecular diagnostics, anticoagulated whole blood or plasma is more likely to be the specimen of choice for either genomic DNA isolation from the white blood cells (WBCs) still intact from a whole blood collection or from plasma that will yield viral identification and quantification. A number of anticoagulants are available, including heparin, EDTA, sodium fluoride, citrate, acid citrate dextrose, oxalate, and iodoacetate, which are covered in detail later.

For any assay provided for clinical use, manufacturers specify the appropriate sample type(s) for which they have validated the assay. Use of different sample types is acceptable only if the laboratory has validated the alternate type(s). For example, care should be taken with gel tubes because they may vary among tube manufacturers. Acceptability of a wide range of sample types can be advantageous because it can reduce the need for recollections if the preferred tube is not provided.

Heparin. Heparin is the most widely used anticoagulant for chemistry testing. It is a mucoitin polysulfuric acid and is available as sodium, potassium, lithium, and ammonium salts, all of which can adequately prevent coagulation. This anticoagulant accelerates the action of antithrombin III, which neutralizes thrombin and thus prevents the formation of fibrin from fibrinogen. Most blood tubes are prepared with approximately 0.2 mg of heparin for each milliliter of blood (1000 units/mL) to be collected. The heparin is usually present as a dry powder that is hygroscopic and dissolves rapidly assuming that the tube of blood is correctly mixed (see Table 4.2). Heparin is a naturally occurring anticoagulant and has the disadvantages of high cost and a more temporary action of anticoagulation than is attained by the chemicals discussed later. It produces a blue background in blood smears that are stained with Wright's stain. In addition, heparin can interfere with the binding of calcium to EDTA in analytical methods for calcium involving complexing with EDTA. Heparin, which is negatively charged, binds calcium and can reduce results for ionized calcium measurements. Thus, either serum tubes are required or blood gas syringes with either low heparin concentrations or so-called "balanced heparin" with added calcium to block the binding of further calcium are used. Of course, the use of lithium or ammonium heparin is unacceptable for lithium and ammonia measurements, respectively, because the tube contains an amount similar to that found in treated patients (lithium) or can elevate the clinically actionable value (ammonia).

It should be noted that heparin is unacceptable for most tests performed using polymerase chain reaction (PCR) because of inhibition of the polymerase enzyme by this large molecule. In some special circumstances, a heparin tube can be shared with a molecular diagnostic laboratory if a non-heparinized tube is not available. DNA can be extracted from heparinized samples, but amplification may be reduced, and the effect of heparin on any molecular diagnostic assay should be assessed as part of a method validation study.

Ethylenediaminetetraacetic Acid. Ethylenediaminetetraacetic acid is a chelating agent of divalent cations such as Ca^{2+} and Mg^{2+} that is particularly useful for (1) hematologic examinations including transfusion medicine applications, (2) measurement of intracellular drugs such as cyclosporine or tacrolimus, (3) HbA_{1c} analysis (4) isolation of genomic DNA, and (5) qualitative and quantitative virus determinations by molecular techniques because it preserves the cellular components of blood. It is used as the disodium, dipotassium, or tripotassium salt, the last two being more soluble with the tripotassium salt commonly provided as a liquid in the collection tube. It is effective at a final concentration of 1 to 2 g/L of blood. Higher concentrations hypertonically

TABLE 4.6 Differences in Composition Between Heparin Plasma and Serum*†

Plasma Value > Serum Value (%)		No Difference Between Serum and Plasma Values	Plasma Value <Serum Value (%)	
Lactate dehydrogenase	2.7	Bilirubin	Glucose	5.1
Total protein	4.0	Cholesterol	Phosphorus	7.0
		Creatinine	Potassium	8.4

*To estimate the probable effect of a factor on results, relate the percent increase or decrease shown in the table to analytical variation (±% coefficient of variation) routinely found for analytes.

†This list includes only differences that are of clinical significance and may need to be annotated with a comment on patient results that general (plasma) reference intervals may not apply.

Modified from Ladenson JH, Tsai L-MB, Michael JM, et al. Serum versus heparinized plasma for eighteen common chemistry tests. *Am J Clin Pathol* 1974;62:545–552. Copyright 1974 by the American Society of Clinical Pathologists. Reprinted with permission.

shrink the RBCs. EDTA prevents coagulation by binding calcium, which is essential for the clotting mechanism. Newer advances using EDTA include the inclusion of a gel barrier to separate plasma from cells when EDTA plasma is required (white tubes; see Table 4.3). In blue/black tubes, incorporation of a density gradient allows recovery of nucleated cells after centrifugation, thus increasing the yield of DNA.

Because it chelates calcium, magnesium, and iron, EDTA is unsuitable for specimens for these analyses using the most common photometric or titrimetric techniques. For many laboratories, an undetectable calcium value or a critical potassium value in an otherwise stable patient is often used as a flag that an inappropriate specimen type has been submitted for just this reason. Additionally, EDTA, probably by chelation of required metallic cofactors, inhibits alkaline phosphatase and creatine kinase activities. As an anticoagulant, it has little effect on other clinical tests, although the concentration of cholesterol has been reported to be decreased by 3% to 5%.

Sodium Fluoride. Sodium fluoride (NaF) is a weak anticoagulant that is often added as a preservative for blood glucose and lactate.[15] As a preservative, together with another anticoagulant such as potassium oxalate, it is effective at a concentration of approximately 2 g/L blood. It exerts its preservative action by inhibiting the enzyme systems involved in glycolysis, although such inhibition is not immediate,[14] and a certain amount of degradation occurs during the first hour after collection. Most specimens are then stable at 25°C for at least 24 hours or at 4°C for 48 hours. Without an antiglycolytic agent, the blood glucose concentration decreases approximately 100 mg/L (0.56 mmol/L) per hour at 25°C. The rate of decrease is faster in newborns because of the increased metabolic activity of their erythrocytes and in leukemic patients because of the high metabolic activity of the WBCs. Sodium fluoride is poorly soluble, and blood must be well mixed before effective antiglycolysis occurs (see Table 4.2). Because of the delay in onset of action, recent protocols recommend placing the tube on ice until the sample can be separated to ensure accurate glucose measurements. Newer NaF combination tubes include tubes containing NaF–citrate buffer–Na_2EDTA, NaF–Na-heparin, NaF–K_2oxalate, NaF–citrate, and NaF–Na_2EDTA. Acidification of specimens by citrate and addition of EDTA to a fluoride tube immediately inhibit glycolysis and preserve glucose in the specimen for at least 24 hours. These various tubes have all been found to be suitable for glucose preservation,[16] but care must be taken to ensure use according to manufacturers' guidelines when using different tube types.[17]

If sodium fluoride is used alone for anticoagulation, three to five times greater concentrations than the usual 2 g/L are required. This high concentration and inhibition of the glycolytic cycle are likely to cause fluid shifts and a change in the concentration of some analytes. Fluoride is also a potent inhibitor of many serum enzymes and in high concentrations also affects urease, which is used to measure urea nitrogen in many analytical systems.

Citrate. Sodium citrate solution, at a concentration of 34 to 38 g/L in a ratio of 1 part to 9 parts of blood, is widely used for coagulation studies. The correct ratio of blood to anticoagulant is critical (refer to the earlier discussion concerning proper filling of vacuum blood tubes) to achieve proper coagulation measurements because the anticoagulant effect is reversed by addition of standard amounts of Ca^{2+} that are based on a proper collection volume. Because citrate chelates calcium, it is unsuitable as an anticoagulant for specimens for measurement of this element. It also inhibits aminotransferases and alkaline phosphatase but stimulates acid phosphatase when phenylphosphate is used as a substrate. Because citrate complexes molybdate, it decreases the color yield in phosphate measurements that involve molybdate ions and produces low results.

Acid Citrate Dextrose. As indicated previously, the collection of specimens into EDTA is often used for isolation of genomic DNA from the patient. However, additional and complementary diagnostic tests, such as cytogenetic testing, may be requested at the same time. For this reason, samples for molecular diagnostics with an accompanying cytogenetic request are often collected into acid citrate dextrose (ACD) anticoagulant so as to preserve both the form and the function of the cellular components. There are two ACD tube designations: ACD A and ACD B. These differ only by the concentrations of the additives (see Table 4.3). Both enhance the vitality and recovery of WBCs for several days after collection of the specimen; thus, they are suitable for both molecular diagnostic testing and cytogenetic testing.

Whereas solution A is used for an 8.5-mL blood draw (10 mL total volume), solution B is used for a 3- or a 6-mL blood draw (7 mL total volume). The specific test(s) requested will determine the size of tube necessary for specimen collection.

Oxalates. Sodium, potassium, ammonium, and lithium oxalates inhibit blood coagulation by forming rather insoluble complexes with calcium ions. Potassium oxalate ($K_2C_2O_4 \cdot H_2O$), at a concentration of approximately 1 to 2 g/L of blood, is the most widely used oxalate. At concentrations of greater than 3 g oxalate per liter, hemolysis is likely to occur.

Combined ammonium and/or potassium oxalate does not cause shrinkage of erythrocytes. However, other oxalates have been known to cause shrinkage by drawing water into the plasma. Reduction in hematocrit may be as much as 10%, causing a reduction in the concentration of plasma constituents of 5%. As fluid is lost from the cells, an exchange of electrolytes and other constituents across the cell membrane occurs. Oxalate inhibits several enzymes, including acid and alkaline phosphatases, amylase, and lactate dehydrogenase (LDH), and may cause precipitation of calcium as the oxalate salt.

Iodoacetate. Sodium iodoacetate at a concentration of 2 g/L is an effective antiglycolytic agent (with the caveats mentioned earlier) and a substitute for sodium fluoride. Because it has no effect on urease, it can be used when glucose and urea tests are performed on a single specimen. It inhibits creatine kinase but appears to have no notable effects on other clinical tests.

Influence of Site of Collection on Blood Composition

Blood obtained from different sites differs in composition. In general, skin puncture blood is more similar to arterial blood than venous blood, depending on the collection condition as described earlier. Thus, there are no clinically significant differences between freely flowing capillary blood and arterial blood in pH, PCO_2, PO_2, and oxygen saturation. The PCO_2 of venous blood is up to 6 to 7 mm Hg (0.8 to

TABLE 4.7 Difference in Composition of Capillary and Venous Serum*

Capillary Value >Venous Value (%)		No Difference Between Capillary and Venous Values	Capillary Value <Venous Value (%)	
Glucose	1.4	Phosphate	Bilirubin	5.0
Potassium	0.9	Urea	Calcium	4.6
			Chloride	1.8
			Sodium	2.3
			Total protein	3.3

*To estimate the probable effect of a factor on results, relate the percent increase or decrease shown in the table to analytical variation (±% coefficient of variation) routinely found for analytes. From Kupke IR, Kather B, Zeugner S. On the composition of capillary and venous blood serum. *Clin Chim Acta* 1981;112:177–185.

0.9 kPa) higher. Venous blood glucose is as much as 70 mg/L (0.39 mmol/L) less than capillary blood glucose.

Blood obtained by skin puncture is contaminated to some extent with interstitial and intracellular fluids. The major differences between venous serum and capillary serum are illustrated in Table 4.7.

Collection of Blood From Intravenous or Arterial Lines

When blood is collected from a central venous catheter or arterial line, it is necessary to ensure that the composition of the specimen is not affected by the fluid that is infused into the patient. With clinical approval, fluid may be shut off using the stopcock on the catheter, and 10 mL of blood is aspirated through the stopcock and discarded before the specimen for analysis is withdrawn. In pediatric patients, 10 mL of blood going to waste is often not feasible, so lesser volumes are aspirated, although the goal is still to aspirate roughly three times the dead space of the line before collecting the sample for testing. Any infused fluid contamination may affect basic biochemical tests such as electrolytes, lactate, or glucose. Aspirating this blood and clearing the lines is equally important for molecular diagnostics and coagulation testing because the stopcock is often heavily saturated with heparin to prevent clotting. Collection of samples for therapeutic drug monitoring should not be done from the line used for the infusion irrespective of the time since infusion or amount of blood aspirated because the drug may adhere to the line and leak into the collected sample, causing false elevations. Blood properly collected from a central venous catheter and compared with blood drawn from a peripheral vein at the same time shows notable differences in composition.[18]

In theory, blood may be collected from the veins of an arm below an IV line without interference from the fluid being infused because retrograde blood flow does not occur in the veins and the fluid that is infused must first circulate through the heart and return to the tissue before it reaches the sampling site. However, as stated previously, collection from the arm without the IV line is strongly recommended.

Hemolysis

Hemolysis is defined as the disruption of the RBC membrane, resulting in the release of hemoglobin, and may be the consequence of intravascular events (in vivo hemolysis) or may occur subsequent to or during blood collection (in vitro hemolysis). Serum and plasma show visual evidence of hemolysis when the hemoglobin concentration exceeds 50 mg/dL (7.7 μmol/L). When the level exceeds 150 to 200 mg/dL (23–31 μmol/L), the plasma will appear bright red to most observers. Slight hemolysis has little effect on most but not all test values. A clinically significant interpretation of results at this lower concentration may be observed on those constituents that are present at a higher concentration in erythrocytes than in plasma. Thus, plasma activities or concentrations of LDH, aspartate transaminase (AST), potassium, magnesium, and phosphate are particularly increased by even a slight degree of hemolysis and may need to be explained to the clinician who insists that a value be reported despite noted sample problems to determine whether or not the result(s) represent in vivo or in vitro hemolysis and determine the implication(s) of the test result. Most manufacturers provide data on the effects of hemolysis on the analytical performance of individual tests, and this should be evaluated in the selection of individual methods. Each laboratory must define at what level of hemolysis results should be held and not reported to prevent poor clinical action on such unreliable test results.

Although the amount of free hemoglobin could be measured and a calculation made to correct test values affected by hemoglobin, this practice is undesirable because factors other than hemoglobin could contribute to the altered test values, and it would be impossible to assess their impact. Hemolysis may affect many unblanked or inadequately blanked analytical methods.[19] Currently, most large chemistry analyzers have the capability of measuring the amount of hemolysis, icterus, and lipemia (the HIL indices) in samples placed on the instrument. These are the three main interferents present in patient samples, and the instrument can be programmed to prevent release of results affected by a specific level of each of these. For some analytes, the effect of hemolysis is time dependent (eg, the degradation of insulin by released intracellular enzymes), and any hemolysis may give falsely low results. For more details about HIL indices and their assessment and management in the laboratory, refer to Chapter 5.

In molecular diagnostic testing, hemoglobin may interfere with the amplification reaction, particularly when reverse transcriptase (RT)-PCR is the first step in the analysis of RNA. In some situations, the isolation of nucleic acid is sufficiently selective that free hemoglobin from the ruptured cells is removed and will not cause a problem. However, with hemolyzed blood, alternative or additional extraction methods are usually needed to ensure that RNA is fully and accurately transcribed and that the greatest amplification of DNA is achieved.

Urine

The type of urine specimen to be collected is dictated by the tests to be performed. Untimed or random specimens are suitable for only a few chemical tests; usually, urine specimens must be collected over a predetermined interval of time, such as 4, 12, or 24 hours. A clean, early morning, fasting specimen is usually the most concentrated specimen and thus is preferred for microscopic examinations and for the detection of abnormal amounts of constituents, such as proteins, or of unusual compounds, such as chorionic gonadotropin. The clean timed specimen is one obtained at specific times of the day or during certain phases of the act of micturition. Whereas bacterial examination of the first 10 mL of urine voided is most appropriate to detect urethritis, the midstream specimen is best for investigating bladder disorders. The double-voided specimen is the urine excreted during a timed period after complete emptying of the bladder; it is used, for example, to assess glucose excretion during a glucose tolerance test. Its collection must be timed in relation to the ingestion of glucose. Similarly, in some metabolic disorders, urine must be collected during or immediately after symptoms of the disease appear (see Chapter 39 on porphyrins).

When they are to be tested for their alcohol and drugs of abuse content, urine specimens are collected under rigorous conditions. Such collections may begin with a requirement for formal identification such as a driver's license or other picture identification as discussed earlier. Patients are asked to leave all personal belongings outside of the restroom facility to prevent substitution of the patient's urine with urine brought from outside. Many locations that routinely perform these collections have the capacity to turn running water off to prevent dilution or put a coloring agent in the toilet water so such dilution attempts are easily identified; the temperature of the urine is often recorded as well to detect such attempts. Finally, patients are often asked to put their initials on the urine cup and sign the paperwork, accepting the sample as theirs. This chain of custody documentation is then sealed in a transport bag with the sample (also sealed) and transported to the testing laboratory directly, where the chain of custody documentation will be continued throughout the testing process. It is necessary for laboratories to be aware of the relevant legal requirements for this type of testing and plan in advance how these samples and the supporting paperwork will be collected and handled. Institutional policies should be in place and adhered to in all cases.

Catheter specimens are used for microbiologic examination in critically ill patients and in those with urinary tract obstruction but should not normally be obtained just for examination of chemical constituents. The suprapubic tap specimen is a useful alternative because the tap is unlikely to cause infection. After appropriate cleaning of the skin over the full bladder, a 22-gauge spinal needle is passed through a small wheal made by a local anesthetic. The bladder is penetrated and the urine withdrawn into the syringe.

Even though tests in the clinical laboratory are not usually affected by lack of sterile collection procedures, the patient's genitalia should be cleaned before each voiding to minimize the transfer of surface bacteria to the urine. Cleansing is essential if the true concentration of WBCs is to be obtained.

Currently, urine is an uncommon specimen type in the molecular diagnostic laboratory for genomic testing, although some laboratories use urine samples for bladder cancer screening and monitoring of therapy for bladder cancer. However, urine is frequently used for molecular testing for infectious agents, such as *Chlamydia*, a common sexually transmitted organism, or BK virus, associated with potential rejection or failure of transplanted kidneys. Because most requests involve a specific organism, an untimed or random urine specimen collected into a sterile container with no preservative is usually acceptable.

Timed Urine Specimens

The collection period for timed specimens should be long enough to minimize the influence of short-term biologic variations. When specimens are to be collected over a specified period of time, the patient's close adherence to instructions is critically important, and a common source of a preanalytical variable. The bladder must be emptied at the time the collection is to begin and this urine discarded. Thereafter, all urine must be collected until the end of the scheduled time, including emptying of the bladder at the end of the collection period. If a patient has a bowel movement during the collection period, precautions should be taken to prevent fecal contamination of the urine. If the collection has to be made over several hours, urine should be passed into a separate container at each voiding and then emptied into a larger container for the complete specimen. This two-step procedure prevents the danger of patients splashing themselves with a preservative, such as acid that may be included in the timed collection device. The large container generally should be stored at 4°C during the entire collection period.

Before beginning a timed collection, a patient should be given written instructions with regard to diet or drug ingestion, if appropriate, to avoid interference of ingested compounds with analytical procedures. Thus instructions for collection of specimens for 5-hydroxyindoleacetic acid measurements should specify avoidance of avocados, bananas, plums, walnuts, pineapples, eggplant, acetaminophen, and cough syrups containing glyceryl guaiacolate (guaifenesin). These dietary components are sources of 5-hydroxytryptamine and should be avoided for this reason; the other compounds interfere with certain analytical procedures but may not interfere with highly specific analytical methods. Each laboratory should determine its own requirements. See also specimen information for specific analytes in the respective chapters.

For 2-hour specimens, a prelabeled 1-L bottle is generally adequate. For a 12-hour collection, a 2-L bottle usually suffices; for a 24-hour collection, a 3- or 4-L bottle is appropriate for most patients. A single bottle allows adequate mixing of the specimen and prevents possible loss of some of the specimen if a second container does not reach the laboratory. Urine should not be collected at the same time for two or more tests requiring different preservatives. Aliquots for an analysis such as a microscopic examination should not be removed while a 24-hour collection is in process. Removal of aliquots is not permissible even when the volume removed is measured and corrected because excretion of most compounds varies throughout the day, and test results will be affected. Appropriate information regarding the collection, including warnings with respect to handling of the specimen, should appear on the bottle label.

When a timed collection is complete, the specimen should be delivered without delay to the clinical laboratory, where the volume should be measured. This may be done by using graduated cylinders or by weighing the container and the urine when preweighed or uniform containers are used. The mass in grams may be reported as if it were the volume in milliliters. There is rarely a need to measure the specific gravity of a weighed specimen because errors in analysis usually exceed the error arising from failure to correct the volume of urine for its mass.

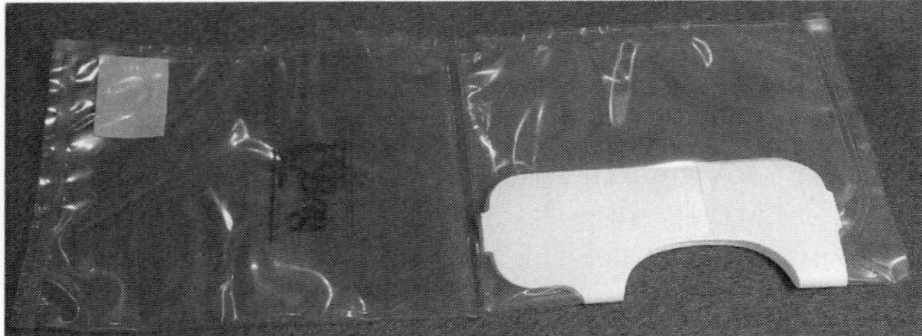

FIGURE 4.5 Urine collection device used in children.

Before a specimen is transferred into small containers for each of the ordered tests, it must be thoroughly mixed to ensure homogeneity because the specific gravity, volume, and composition of the urine all may vary throughout the collection period. The small container into which an aliquot is transferred should not be a plastic bottle if toluene or another organic compound has been used as a preservative; metal-free containers must be used for trace metal analyses. See the later discussion on appropriate labeling of such secondary containers.

Collection of Urine From Children

Collection of any type of urine specimen from an infant is difficult, with timed collections being the most problematic. Fortunately, timed collections are rarely required. The approved method for collecting a random urine specimen from an infant involves a process known as bagging. The scrotal or perineal area is cleaned and dried first, and any natural or applied skin oils are removed. Then a plastic bag (eg, U-Bag, Hollister, Chicago, or Tink-Col, C.R. Bard, Murray Hill, N.J.) is placed around the infant's genitalia and then is held in place by a mild adhesive (Fig. 4.5). The baby's diaper is reapplied to help hold the bag in place. As soon as voiding has occurred, the bag containing the urine sample is removed and emptied into a regular urine collection cup. The mild adhesive on the bag will often fail when it becomes wet with urine, so the infant should be monitored and the bag removed as soon as the urine sample is collected. Even a random or spot urine collection for something as simple as a urinalysis may require either catheterization or a suprapubic tap collection in an infant, especially if there is difficulty getting the infant to urinate or in collecting the sample when the infant does urinate. In infants and very young children requiring a rare 24-hour urine collection, hospitalization and catheterization are often required to obtain a complete collection.

Urine Preservatives

The most common preservatives and the tests for which preservatives are required are listed in Table 4.8. Preservatives have different roles but usually are added to reduce bacterial action or chemical decomposition or to solubilize constituents that otherwise might precipitate out of solution. Another application is to decrease atmospheric oxidation of unstable compounds. Some specimens should not have *any* preservatives added because of the possibility of interference with analytical methods.

One of the most acceptable forms of preservation of urine specimens is refrigeration immediately after collection; it is even more successful when combined with chemical preservation. Urinary preservative tablets that contain a mixture of chemicals, such as potassium acid phosphate, sodium benzoate, benzoic acid, hexamethylene tetramine, sodium bicarbonate, and mercuric oxide (Starplex Scientific, http://www.starplexscientific.com), have been used for chemical and microscopic examination. Because these tablets contain sodium and potassium salts, among others, they should not be used for analysis of these analytes. The preservative tablets act mainly by lowering the pH of the urine and by releasing formaldehyde. Formalin has also been used for preserving specimens, but in large amounts it precipitates urea and inhibits certain reactions (eg, the dipstick esterase test for leukocytes). Acidification to below a pH of 3 is widely used to preserve 24-hour specimens and is particularly useful for specimens for determination of calcium, steroids, adrenaline, noradrenaline, and vanillylmandelic acid. However, precipitation of urates will occur, thereby rendering a specimen unsuitable for measurement of uric acid.

TABLE 4.8 Commonly Used Urine Preservatives

Preservative	Concentrations or Volumes
HCl	6 mol/L; 30 mL per 24-hr collection
Acetic acid	50%; 25 mL per 24-hr collection
Na_2CO_3	5 g per 24-hr collection
HNO_3	6 mol/L; 15 mL 24-hr hour collection
Boric acid	10 g per 24-hr collection
Toluene	30 mL per 24-hr collection
Thymol	10% in isopropanol; 10 mL per 24-hr collection

Modified from information provided in Clinical and Laboratory Standards Institute. *Routine urinalysis and collection, transportation, and preservation of urine specimens: CLSI-approved guideline GP16-A3.* Wayne, PA: Clinical and Laboratory Standards Institute; 2009.

Sulfamic acid (10 g/L urine) has also been used to reduce pH. Boric acid (5 mg/30 mL) has been used, but it also causes precipitation of urates. Although thymol and chloroform were widely used in the past to preserve specimens for chemical and microscopic urinalysis, it is now recognized that specimens for these tests should be analyzed immediately and that the addition of preservatives is both largely ineffective and a source of interference with several analytical methods. Toluene is the only organic solvent that is still used as a preservative. When present in a large enough amount, it acts as a barrier between the air and the surface of the specimen. Toluene, however, does not prevent the growth of anaerobic microorganisms and, because of its flammable nature, is a safety hazard. A mild base, such as sodium bicarbonate or a small amount of sodium hydroxide, is used to preserve porphyrins, urobilinogen, and uric acid. A sufficient quantity should be added to adjust the pH to between 8 and 9.

Feces

Small aliquots of feces are frequently analyzed to detect the presence of "hidden" blood, so-called occult blood. Occult blood screening is included as part of many periodic health examinations. Guaiac-based occult blood tests are subject to many interferences (aspirin, vitamin C, steroids, various drugs, red meat, alcohol), causing both false-positive and false-negative results, and should be interpreted cautiously unless the intent is to identify current bleeding in any portion of the gastrointestinal (GI) tract in an emergent patient. Newer immunochemical-based tests, so called iFOB tests, have decreased the effects of food intake greatly for the purpose of identifying a lower GI tract bleed that may indicate the presence or possibility of malignant growth. In either case, tests for occult blood should be done on aliquots of excreted stools rather than on material obtained on the glove of a physician doing a rectal examination because this procedure may cause enough bleeding to produce a positive result. Conversely, the small amount of stool present on the glove may not be representative of the whole, so bleeding may not be recognized.

In newborns, the first specimen from the bowel (meconium) may be used for detection of maternal drug use during the gestational period, which requires specific attention to the details of collection and identification similar to the chain of custody procedure for urine collection discussed earlier. Feces from infants and children may be screened for tryptic activity or for increased fecal fat concentrations, both of which can be indicators of cystic fibrosis. Fecal material is also commonly collected in childhood for the detection of parasites (ova and parasites [O & P]), enteric disease organisms such as *Salmonella* and *Shigella*, and viruses, all of which are useful in sorting out the differential diagnosis of diarrhea. Fecal testing is also used for helping to determine causes of malabsorption. In infants, fecal material for these tests is usually recovered from the diaper.

In adults and children, measurement of fecal nitrogen and fat in 72-hour specimens is used to assess the severity of malabsorption; measurement of fecal porphyrins is occasionally required to characterize the type of porphyria. Usually, no preservative is added to the feces, but the container should be kept refrigerated throughout the collection period, and care should be taken to prevent contamination from urine. When the collection is complete, the container and feces are weighed, and the mass of excreted feces is calculated. The specimen is homogenized and aliquoted so that the amount of fat or nitrogen excreted per day and the proportion of dietary intake excreted can be calculated.

For metabolic balance studies, collections of stool are usually made over a 72-hour period. Many balance studies are carried out in conjunction with research on the metabolism of such elements as calcium. It is important for such studies that a patient be on a controlled diet for a sufficiently long time before commencement of the study, so that a steady state has been attained.

Testing of patient DNA in stool is uncommon, but DNA isolated from fecal samples is representative of the genetic composition of the colonic mucosa at the time of stool collection. The differential and quantitative analysis of stool DNA integrity has been proposed as a sensitive and specific biomarker useful for the detection of colorectal cancer.[20]

Other Body Fluids

Specimens may be collected for analysis from a range of different body fluids. These include cerebrospinal fluid (CSF), pleural fluid, ascitic fluid, pericardial fluid, amniotic fluid, synovial fluid, and others.[21,22] Readers are referred to Chapter 43 for a complete discussion of collection, analysis, and interpretation for these specimens.

Bronchoalveolar Lavage

Bronchoalveolar lavage (BAL) samples are another type of fluid sample that may be received in a laboratory. BAL is performed by a skilled clinician and involves passing a bronchoscope into a part of the lung, squirting a small amount of saline into that section, and then aspirating it back for examination. BAL is the most common method of sampling the internal lung milieu in the lower respiratory tract and is especially useful in patients with cystic fibrosis; immunocompromised patients; patients with pneumonia on ventilators; and patients with lung diseases, including cancers. Tests that are commonly ordered on BAL samples include cell count and WBC differential; cytospin and various histology slides for staining; and aerobic and anaerobic bacterial, mycobacterial, fungal, and viral cultures. Respiratory viral panels by PCR are also commonly ordered on BAL samples, as are acid-fast bacilli culture and stain and *Mycobacterium tuberculosis*–specific PCR testing.

Chorionic Villus Sampling

Chorionic villus sampling (CVS) allows for earlier diagnosis of inherited genetic disorders than is possible with amniotic fluid analysis. With CVS, testing can be performed at a gestation period of 10 to 12 weeks, but with amniotic fluid, testing generally is not performed until week 15 to 20 of gestation. CVS is the technique of inserting a catheter or needle into the placenta and removing some of the chorionic villi, or vascular projections, from the chorion. This tissue has the same chromosomal and genetic makeup as the fetus and can be used to test for disorders that may be present in the fetus. When chorionic villus is sampled, ultrasonography is performed to assess the placenta and determine its position. The sample of the placenta is obtained through the vagina or through the abdomen, depending on the location of the placenta. The specimen is examined under a microscope by a physician at the time of collection to determine the quality, quantity, and integrity of the chorionic villi. After it is received by the laboratory, the quality of the specimen is further assessed by examination for branching, budding, and veining. The specimen is then placed in culture medium and is allowed to grow for up to 3 weeks. When the cells are fully confluent, they are treated in the way that cells from amniotic fluid (earlier) are treated for DNA extraction. Better collection methods for cell-free nucleic acids are expected to become the collection method of choice in the future.

Maternal cell contamination testing is used to definitively identify the source of isolated cells in an amniotic fluid sample and in CVS. Such confirmation of the source of the sample is strongly recommended for any prenatal diagnostic testing and may be required as a quality monitor in some laboratories.

Buccal Cells

Collection of buccal cells (cells of the oral cavity of epithelial origin) has been identified as providing an excellent source of genomic DNA. Collection of buccal cells is often viewed as less invasive than collection of blood. It is particularly useful for collecting cells with the patient's genomic DNA when the patient has had blood transfusions and thus has blood with another person's (or persons') DNA. Similarly, it is useful after bone marrow transplantation when the circulating blood cells are derived wholly or partially from the donor of the bone marrow. Two methods are used commonly to collect buccal cells: rinsing with mouthwash and using swabs or cytobrushes.

Rinsing of the oral cavity generally provides a higher yield of cells than can be obtained by using swabs. For these collections, the patient is provided with a small amount of mouthwash and is instructed to rinse well for a minimum of 60 seconds; then the patient returns the mouthwash to a collection tube. There is no harm in doing this longer than 60 seconds, but shortening the time may decrease the yield of buccal cells. Mouthwash solutions high in phenol and ethanol are destructive to recovered cells and should be avoided. It is necessary for each laboratory to validate a list of acceptable solutions.

Swabs or cytobrushes have also been used to collect buccal cells for molecular genetics testing. For swabs, a sterile Dacron or rayon swab with a plastic shaft is preferred because calcium alginate swabs or swabs with wooden sticks may contain substances that inhibit PCR-based testing. After collection, the swab or cytobrush should be stored in an air-tight plastic container or immersed in liquid, such as phosphate-buffered saline or viral transport medium. In general, the yield of cells and nucleic acid is lower with physical scraping using swabs or cytobrushes than with rinsing.

Although collection of buccal cells from children is rare except in the situation of identification of paternity or maternity, the same process is followed.

Solid Tissue

Traditionally, the solid tissue most often analyzed in the clinical laboratory was malignant tissue from the breast for estrogen and progesterone receptors. During surgery, at least 0.5 to 1 g of tissue is removed and trimmed of fat and nontumor material. This tissue is quickly frozen, within 20 minutes, preferably snap frozen in liquid nitrogen or in a mixture of dry ice and alcohol. A histologic section should always be examined at the time of analysis of the specimen to confirm that the specimen is indeed malignant tissue. Another traditional use is measurement of liver iron or copper to assist with the diagnosis of hemochromatosis or Wilson's disease, respectively.

The same procedure may be used to obtain and prepare solid tissue for elemental or toxicologic analysis; however, when trace element determinations are to be made, all materials used in the collection or handling of the tissue should be made of plastic or materials known to be free of contaminating trace elements.

Somatic gene analysis such at T and B cell clonality and the identification of possible clinically actionable mutations in malignant tissue (*KRAS* mutations, *MGMT/MLH* methylation status) are now proving to be of increasing importance for clinicians in both diagnosis and direction of appropriate therapeutic options for the patient. For these studies, the molecular diagnostic laboratory often receives tissue that has been formalin-fixed and paraffin-embedded (FFPE) rather than fresh tissue because the request for further testing is generally made after the pathologist's diagnosis of the particular malignancy. In general, neutral buffered formalin, containing no heavy metals, will not interfere with amplification reactions. However, recovery of nucleic acids is greatly decreased if the tissue has been overfixed or if a decalcification process has been applied to, for example, bone marrow samples. DNA can still be extracted from tissue embedded in paraffin, but the DNA will be degraded to low-molecular-weight fragments. In most cases, segments of DNA will amplify in a PCR reaction, but Southern blot methods are problematic because most require high-molecular-weight DNA.

Tissue structure and better recovery of DNA can be retained without permanent fixation by freezing specimens in an optimal cutting temperature compound (OCT). OCT is a mixture of polyvinyl alcohol and polyethylene glycol that surrounds but does not infiltrate the tissue. The sample is then frozen at about −80°C, and sections are prepared for review by a pathologist. OCT is fully water soluble and should be completely removed from a tissue specimen before it is used as a source of DNA. In general, DNA of higher molecular weight can be extracted from OCT-fixed tissues compared with that extracted from FFPE samples.

Hair and Nails

Currently, the use of hair or nails in molecular diagnostics is limited to forensic analysis (genomic DNA identification). Hair and fingernails or toenails have been used for trace metal and drug analyses with the potential advantage of timing of exposure if separate segments of longer hair are analyzed, although no current standards for such testing currently exist. For the latter examinations, clear labeling of the follicular end of the sample is required. However, collection procedures have been poorly standardized, and quantitative measurements are better obtained from blood or urine. Use of such samples requires each laboratory to validate the processes because, again, there are no published standards for this unusual specimen type.

HANDLING OF SPECIMENS FOR ANALYSIS

Steps that are important for obtaining a valid specimen for analysis include (1) identification, (2) preservation, (3) separation and storage, and (4) transport.

Maintenance of Specimen Identification

Although the collection of an acceptable specimen is a key aspect of excellent testing, proper identification of the specimen must be maintained at each step of the testing process to ensure that the correct result is reported for the correct patient at all times. The minimum information on any label associated with a specific specimen should include the patient's name, location, and identifying number, as well as the date and time of collection. Many institutions also require the collecting person's initials or some means of identifying the person who collected the sample be included on the label of the primary collection device. All labels should conform to the laboratory's stated requirements to facilitate proper processing of specimens. In the United States, no specific labeling should be attached to specimens from patients with infectious diseases that are submitted to the routine laboratory to suggest that these specimens should be handled with special care. Universal precautions should always be used, meaning that all specimens should be treated as if they are potentially infectious with the following caveat. The exception will be samples from patients suspected to have known, high-risk pathogens (eg, hemorrhagic viruses such as Ebola) that must have separate, pre-prepared sample handling protocols that may or may not involve the routine laboratory. Proactive procedures must be in place including by whom and where such samples might be analyzed unless the sample can be rendered safe (eg, by heat treatment), in which case again standard universal precautions should be used.

In practice, every specimen container must be adequately labeled even if the specimen must be placed in ice or if the container is so small that a label cannot be placed along the tube, as might happen with a capillary blood tube. Direct labeling of a capillary blood tube by folding the label like a flag around the tube is preferred or recommended by most laboratories. For small volumes of urine submitted in screw-cap urine cups and any specimen submitted in a screw-cap test tube or cup, the label should be placed on the cup or tube directly, not just on the cap.

It is critical that samples be positively identified through all steps of processing and analysis, and this is especially important in pediatrics because the samples are often collected in small tubes that cannot be sampled from directly by an automated instrument. Aliquoting a sample from the primary collection container to one or more other containers configured for the instrumentation requires close attention to proper labeling and tracking of the sample identifiers to ensure samples are not switched. Good work practice includes "piece work" in which only a single patient's samples are in the work area at one time, the area is clean with no old labels present, and the worker is not disturbed. Although this may not be possible in a large laboratory facility, training that emphasizes the criticality of this function to achieve best patient care and adherence to all policies can be equally effective. Because the majority of samples received from pediatric patients are in microtubes, many samples need to be aliquoted; poured into a microsampling device; or hand entered into instruments that use whole blood, such as hematology instruments, because these systems are not made to deal with such small tubes. Additionally, many times bar codes do not fit these tubes. Bar code readers in instruments cannot be used unless the sample is aliquoted into a larger tube. This extra handling of the specimens offers more opportunities for error and thus requires more strict attention to detail and analysis of the possible risks during design of the process. Special attention should be placed on molecular diagnostics, forensic specimens, and transfusion medicine specimens as applicable.

Preservation of Specimens

The practitioner must ensure that specimens are collected into the correct container and are properly labeled; in addition, specimens must be properly treated both during transport to the laboratory and from the time the serum, plasma, or cells have been separated until analysis. For some tests, specimens must be kept at 4°C from the time the blood is drawn until the specimens are analyzed or until the serum or plasma is separated from the cells to minimize metabolism and degradation of sample components. Examples are specimens for ammonia and blood gas determinations, such as PCO_2, PO_2, and blood pH. Transfer of these specimens to the laboratory must be done by placing the specimen container on ice; a bag of ice is used to surround the sample to keep it cool while the sample and label are not subjected to possible water contamination. Specimens for lactate, pyruvate, and certain hormone tests (eg, adrenocorticotropic hormone [ACTH], gastrin and renin activity) should be treated the same way. A notable decrease in pyruvate and increase in lactate concentration occurs within a few minutes at ambient temperature.

For all test constituents that are thermally labile, serum and plasma should be separated from cells in a refrigerated centrifuge. Specimens for bilirubin or carotene and for some drugs, such as methotrexate, may need to be protected from both daylight and fluorescent light to prevent photodegradation, although the use of plastic, rather than glass, tubes has decreased this preanalytical variable.

For molecular diagnostic laboratories, the largest challenge is the recovery of RNA from transported specimens. Depending on the tissue source, RNA yields vary, primarily because of the amount of RNA present at the time of collection. Specimens from the liver, spleen, and heart have larger amounts of RNA than specimens from skin, muscle, and bone. Increasingly, creative solutions to this issue continue to be produced (eg, see http://www.dnagenoteck.com) with collection kits that contain stabilizers and even the first reagents required for extraction, all of which have the effect of maximizing the recoverable nucleic acid. Tissue samples should be frozen immediately. Alternatively, a blood specimen should never be frozen before separation of the cellular elements because of hemolysis and released hemoglobin that may interfere with subsequent amplification processes. For tissue samples, it is critical to choose the disruption method best suited for the specific type of tissue. Thorough cellular disruption is critical for high RNA quality and yield. RNA that is trapped in intact cells is often removed with cellular debris by centrifugation.[23]

For specimens that are collected in a remote facility with infrequent transportation by courier to a central laboratory, proper specimen processing must be done in the remote facility so that appropriately separated and preserved plasma or serum is delivered to the laboratory. This necessitates that the remote facility has ready access to appropriately calibrated centrifuges, all commonly used preservatives, and wet ice.

Add-on Requests

In the interest of preventing additional phlebotomies and to assess a clinical situation from a specimen collected at a specific time, many physicians request an "add-on" test, that is, for the laboratory to perform a test on a sample already in the laboratory and processed. This is especially true in specimens collected from pediatric patients, in whom more blood may not be able to be collected promptly, and for patients from an emergency department, where additional testing from the time of presentation with specific symptoms may be needed after a clinical diagnosis has been made or narrowed by the clinician. Each laboratory must establish its own guidelines for what will be allowed in what time frame. For example, evaporation of small or even routine samples with requests for volatile compounds such as ethanol or methanol can make them unsuitable for additional testing, so storage conditions and time in the laboratory are important considerations. Also, most samples are stored at refrigerated temperatures after initial analysis; this makes them unacceptable for LDH analysis later but does not affect, for example, alkaline phosphatase or electrolyte analysis, provided that evaporation and air exposure has been kept to a minimum.

Separation and Storage of Specimens

Plasma or serum should be separated from cells as soon as possible and certainly within 2 hours[24] for some but not all analytes. Premature separation of serum, however, may permit continued formation of fibrin, which can clog sampling devices in testing equipment. If it is impossible to centrifuge a blood specimen within 2 hours, the specimen should be held at room temperature rather than at 4°C to decrease any effect on potassium measurement caused by leakage from the RBCs by inhibition of the Na/K ATPase pump. For most plasma samples used for molecular diagnostics, the plasma should be removed from the primary tube promptly after centrifugation and held at −20°C in a freezer capable of maintaining this temperature. In all instances of freezing a sample, frost-free freezers should be avoided because they have a wide temperature swing during the freeze–thaw cycle. Although changes in concentration of test constituents have been observed when serum or plasma is stored in a gel separator tube in a refrigerator for 24 hours, these changes do not appear to be large enough to be of clinical significance.

Primary specimen tubes should always be centrifuged with the original cap in place. Such containment reduces evaporation, which occurs rapidly in a warm centrifuge with the air currents set up by centrifugation. Caps on the original tube also prevent aerosolization of infectious particles and thus provide a further safeguard for laboratorians. Specimen tubes with requested test for volatiles, such as ethanol, *must* have the initial cap in place while they are spun to prevent release of the volatile compound and result in an artificially reduced measurement of ethanol, methanol, or such compounds. Centrifuging specimens with the cap in place also maintains anaerobic conditions, which are important in the measurement of carbon dioxide and ionized calcium. Removal of the stopper before centrifugation allows loss of carbon dioxide and an increase in blood pH. Control of pH is especially important for the accurate measurement of ionized calcium.

Cryopreservation of WBC and DNA is one method to store and maintain samples for extended periods of time. Whole blood specimens can be centrifuged and WBCs removed and cryopreserved at −20°C in a temperature-controlled freezer until these cells are required for DNA extraction. For even longer periods of storage, isolated DNA can be stored at −70°C, although 4°C may be adequate for most purposes. The extracted DNA should not be exposed to repetitive cycles of freezing and thawing because this can lead to shearing of the DNA. After these extracted DNA samples have completely thawed, it is important to fully mix the sample to ensure a homogeneous specimen.

Transport of Specimens

Hemolysis may occur in pneumatic tube systems unless the tubes are completely filled and movement of the blood tubes inside the specimen carrier is prevented.[25] The pneumatic tube system should be designed to eliminate sharp curves and sudden stops of specimen carriers because these factors are responsible for much of any in vitro hemolysis that may occur. With many systems, however, the plasma hemoglobin concentration may be increased, and the serum activity of RBC enzymes, such as LDH and AST, may also be increased (see the earlier discussion on the effect of hemolysis). Nonetheless, the amount of hemolysis from transport issues is usually so small that it can be ignored. In special cases, such as a patient undergoing chemotherapy whose cells are fragile or leukemia patients with fragile leukocytes, samples should be centrifuged before they are placed in the pneumatic tube system or identified as "messenger delivery only" and delivered rapidly to the laboratory. There are also occasional tests that cannot be transported to the laboratory via a pneumatic tube system because of the effect the transport has on the test results. For example, sending blood gas samples through the tube system has been shown to adversely affect PO_2 results,[26] and samples for thromboelastography and rotational thromboelastometry or platelet function testing may also require hand delivery to the laboratory.

Although the remaining discussion uses the specific example of referral laboratory testing by another laboratory, many of the issues discussed, such as regulations related to shipping, are also relevant to a laboratory that receives specimens from outlying clinics via a courier service, which may be laboratory owned or operated. This may involve validating specific transport or storage conditions that are in conflict with existing CLSI recommendations.[27] For example, a laboratory may have a clinic that provides sweat chloride collection and sends the sweat samples to the main laboratory for chloride analysis. The appropriate transport parameters for these samples must be validated. This is a very specific example, but all parameters for any samples should be similarly examined and approved by the laboratory director.

Before a referral laboratory is used for any tests, the quality of its work should be verified by the referring laboratory. Guidelines for selection and evaluation of a referral laboratory have been published (GP 9-A, Table 4.1). For laboratories accredited by the College of American Pathologists (CAP), it is a requirement that the referring laboratory validate that the referral laboratory is CLIA'88 certified by obtaining a copy of the CLIA (Clinical Laboratory Improvement Act) certificate before specimens are shipped. For molecular diagnostic testing, this is of particular importance because often the latest genetic test being requested by a physician has not yet been moved from research interest status to patient care status and may not be available in a CLIA-certified laboratory.

Specimen type and quantity and specimen handling requirements of the referral laboratory must be observed, and in laboratories operating under CLIA'88 regulations, test results reported by a referral laboratory must be identified as such when they are filed in a patient's medical record. The director of a referring laboratory has the responsibility to ensure that specimens will be adequately transported to the referral laboratory. Also, the director should determine the benefits of different services and should keep in mind that the fastest service may be the most expensive. The director should also know that specimens should not be sent to a referral laboratory at the end of the week or in a holiday period because more delays in transit occur during these times than during the working week, and deterioration of specimens is more likely.

It should be assumed that transport from a referring laboratory to a referral laboratory may take as long as 72 hours. Under optimal conditions, a referring laboratory should retain enough of the original specimen for retesting in case an unanticipated problem arises during shipment, although this essentially never happens in pediatrics, in which sample volume is at a minimum. Most reference laboratories have lower minimum volume requirements for pediatric specimens than for adult specimens, but these lower minimums generally preclude being able to retest the sample if there is a problem with the initial analysis. The tube and transport condition for the specimen should be constructed such that the contents do not escape if the container is exposed to extremes of heat, cold, or sunlight. Reduced pressure of 0.50 atmosphere (50 kPa) may be encountered during air transport, together with vibration, and specimens should be protected from these adverse conditions by a suitable container. Variability in temperature is a significant factor causing instability of test constituents.

Polypropylene and polyethylene containers are usually suitable for specimen transport. Glass should be avoided. Polystyrene is unsuitable because it may crack when frozen. Containers must be leak-proof and should have a Teflon-lined screw cap that does not loosen under the variety of temperatures to which the container may be exposed. The materials of both stopper and container must be inert and must not have any effect on the concentration of the analyte.

In situations in which sample delivery for molecular analysis will be delayed, extracted nucleic acid, usually DNA only, can be transported in a buffer solution or water, or it can be dried down and shipped as a loose powder. With either method, DNA should be transported at ambient temperatures and should not be exposed to extremely high temperatures for an extended period of time because it will begin to degrade and testing may be compromised. Because dried blood spot samples are so easy to store and transport, and with an increasing number of DNA tests being developed using dried blood spots (eg, PCR testing for cystic fibrosis and severe combined immunodeficiency), such samples may become one of the best ways to collect, store, and ship samples for DNA testing.

The shipping or secondary container used to hold one or more specimen tubes or bottles must be constructed to prevent the tubes from contact with another specimen. Corrugated, fiberboard, or Styrofoam boxes designed to fit around a single specimen tube are commonly used. A padded shipping envelope provides adequate protection for shipping single specimens. When specimens are shipped as drops of blood on filter paper (eg, for neonatal screening), the paper should be enclosed in a paper envelope to ensure that the sample remains dry. The initial paper envelope can be placed in a shipping envelope and transported to the testing facility; rapid shipping is rarely required for dried blood on paper.

For transport of frozen or refrigerated specimens, a Styrofoam container should be used. The container walls should be 1 inch (2.5 cm) thick to provide effective insulation. The container should be vented to prevent buildup of carbon dioxide under pressure and a possible explosion. Solid carbon dioxide (dry ice) is the most convenient refrigerant material for keeping specimens frozen, and temperatures as low as −70°C can be achieved. The amount of dry ice required in a container depends on the size of the container, the efficiency of its insulation, and the length of time for which the specimens must be kept frozen. One piece of solid dry ice (about 3 inches × 4 inches × 1 inch) in a container with 1-inch Styrofoam walls and a volume of 125 cubic inches (2000 cm^3) will maintain a single specimen frozen for 48 hours. More commonly, smaller pieces of the solid will be used and it is critical that that the specimen be buried rather than sitting on top of this refrigerant.

Various laws and regulations apply to the shipment of biologic specimens. Although such regulations theoretically apply only to etiologic agents (known infectious agents), all specimens should be transported as if the same regulations apply. In many countries, airlines have rigid regulations covering the transport of specimens. Airlines deem dry ice a hazardous material; therefore, the transport of most clinical laboratory specimens is affected by the regulations and those who package the specimens should be trained in the appropriate regulations, such as those put forth by the US International Air Transport Association.

The various modes of transport of specimens influence the shipping time and cost, and each laboratory needs to make its own assessment as to adequate service. The objective is to ensure that the properly collected, processed, and identified specimen arrives at the testing facility in time and under the correct storage conditions so that the analytical phase can then proceed.

CONCLUSION

Accurate test results (ie, the right result for the right patient) begin and end with the integrity of the sample being tested. Integrity can only be assured by proper preparation of the patient; choice of sample container; collection of the sample; and finally transport, processing, and storage of the collected sample with each step maintaining proper identification. Every step of the process affects the quality of the end result. For these reasons, best laboratory practice demands attention to detail and following appropriate protocols. It is incumbent on laboratories and laboratory professionals to fully delineate their processes in complete policies and procedures that not only cover the routine and correct procedures but also cover the unusual. These should include how to handle the process when the system breaks down and steps are not properly performed and may need to be addressed case-by-case by the laboratory director. Finally, laboratories should fully validate protocols that may not be covered under normal procedures or that may deviate from local regulatory guidelines (eg, the US Food and Drug Administration or CLIA). Preanalytical variables can be lessened or even avoided if these steps are followed.

POINTS TO REMEMBER

- Proper identification of the patient is essential, and the sample should be properly labeled at all steps if separated from the primary collection container.
- Policies designed to ensure the safety of both the patient and the person collecting any sample should always be followed.
- Collection of all samples must be in the correct primary container with proper identification, and those collecting a specimen, most commonly blood and urine, should understand the biochemical or chemical actions of any additive and possible implications on the test result.
- Attention to the details related to processing of the collected sample (time, temperature, special handling) should always follow validated local policies.
- The accurate result for any patient's sample (that will be acted on by the clinician) depends on adherence to all policies and procedures, and those collecting specimens bear a tremendous responsibility to ensure that they do not contribute to errors that may impact patient care.

REFERENCES

1. The Joint Commission. National Patient Safety Goals. <http://www.jointcommission.org/assets/1/6/2015_HAP_NPSG_ER.pdf>; [accessed 27.07.15].
2. *WHO Guidelines on Drawing Blood: Best practices in phlebotomy*. Pediatric and neonatal blood sampling. World Health Organization; 2010 [Chapter 6] <http://www.ncbi.nlm.nih.gov/books/NBK138647/>; [accessed 27.07.15].
3. Garza D, Becan-McBride K. Pediatric procedures. In: Garza D, Becan-McBride K, editors. *Phlebotomy handbook: blood collection essentials*. 7th ed. Upper Saddle River, N.J.: Pearson Prentice Hall; 2005. p. 327–3594.
4. Hoeltke LB. Caring for the pediatric patient. In: Hoeltke LB, editor. *The complete textbook of phlebotomy*. 3rd ed. Clifton Park, NY: Thomas Delmar Learning; 2006. p. 249–2645.
5. Jones PM. Pediatric clinical biochemistry: why is it different? In: Dietzen DJ, Bennett MJ, Wong ECC, editors. *Biochemical and molecular basis of pediatric disease*. 4th ed. Washington DC: AACC Press; 2010. p. 1–9.
6. Thavendiranathan P, Bagai A, Ebidia A, et al. Do blood tests cause anemia in hospitalized patients? *J Gen Intern Med* 2005;**20**:520–4.
7. Renoe BW, McDonald JM, Ladenson JH. The effects of stasis with and without exercise on free calcium, various cations, and related parameters. *Clin Chim Acta* 1980;**103**:91–100.
8. McNair P, Nielsen SL, Christiansen C, et al. Gross errors made by routine blood sampling from two sites using a tourniquet applied at different positions. *Clin Chim Acta* 1979;**98**:113–18.
9. Cornes MP, Ford C, Gama R. Spurious hyperkalemia due to EDTA contamination: common and not always easy to identify. *Ann Clin Biochem* 2008;**45**:601–3.
10. Flynn JC. *Procedures in phlebotomy*. 3rd ed. St Louis: Saunders; 2005.
11. Blumenfeld TA, Turi GK, Blanc WA. Recommended site and depth of newborn heel skin punctures based on anatomic measurements and histopathology. *Lancet* 1979;**1**:230–3.
12. Kiechle FL, editor. *So you're going to collect a blood specimen: an introduction to phlebotomy*. 11th ed. Northfield, Ill: College of American Pathologists; 2005.
13. Green AMI, Gray J. *Neonatology & laboratory medicine*. London, UK: ACB Venture Publications; 2003.
14. Hoeltke LB. The challenge of phlebotomy. In: Hoeltke LB, editor. *The complete textbook of phlebotomy*. 3rd ed. Clifton Park, NJ: Thomas Delmar Learning; 2006. p. 227–48.
15. Mikesh LM, Bruns DE. Stabilization of glucose in blood specimens: mechanism of delay in fluoride inhibition of glycolysis. *Clin Chem* 2008;**54**:930–2.
16. Fokker M. Stability of glucose in plasma with different anticoagulants. *Clin Chem Lab Med* 2014;**52**:1057–60.
17. Ridefelt P, Akerfeldt T, Helmersson-Karlqvist J. Increased plasma glucose levels after change of recommendation from NaF to citrate blood collection tubes. *Clin Biochem* 2014;**47**:625–8.
18. Rommel K, Koch C-D, Spilker D. Einfluss der Materialgewinnung auf klinisch-chemische Parameter in Blut, Plasma und Serum bei Patienten mit stabilem und zentralisiertem Kreislauf. *J Clin Chem Clin Biochem* 1978;**16**:373–80.
19. Young DS. *Effects of preanalytical variable on clinical laboratory tests*. 3rd ed. Washington, DC: AACC Press; 2007.
20. Boynton KA, Summerhayes IC, Ahlquist DA, et al. DNA integrity as a potential marker for stool-based detection of colorectal cancer. *Clin Chem* 2003;**49**:2112–13.
21. Natsugoe S, Tokuda K, Matsumoto M. Molecular detection of free cancer cells in pleural lavage fluid from esophageal cancer patients. *Int J Mol Med* 2003;**12**:771–5.
22. Carroll T, Raff H, Findling JW. Late-night salivary cortisol for the diagnosis of Cushing's syndrome: a meta-analysis. *Endocr Pract* 2009;**6**:1–17.
23. Groszbach A. Nucleic acid preparation. Presented at: 4th Annual University of Connecticut Molecular Review Symposium, 26th Annual Meeting of the Association of Genetic Technologists, May 30, 2001, Minneapolis, Minn.
24. Laessig RH, Indriksons AA, Hassemer DJ, et al. Changes in serum chemical values as a result of prolonged contact with the clot. *Am J Clin Pathol* 1976;**66**:598–604.
25. Steige H, Jone JD. Evaluation of pneumatic tube system for delivery of blood specimens. *Clin Chem* 1971;**17**:1160–4.
26. Victor PJ, Patole S, Fleming JJ, et al. Agreement between paired blood gas values in samples transported either by a pneumatic tube system or by human courier. *Clin Chem Lab Med* 2011;**49**:1303–9.
27. Haverstick DM, Brill LB, Scott MG, et al. Preanalytical variables in measurement of free (ionized) calcium in lithium heparin-containing blood collection tubes. *Clin Chim Acta* 2009;**403**:102–4.

Preanalytical Variation and Preexamination Processes

Ana-Maria Simundic, Nora Nikolac, and Walter G. Guder

ABSTRACT

Background

The preanalytical phase has long been recognized as a source of substantial variability in laboratory medicine. Laboratory errors, mostly due to some defect in the preanalytical phase, may lead to diagnostic errors. Understanding preanalytical variation and reducing errors in the preexamination phase of the testing process are therefore important for improved safety and quality of laboratory services delivered to patients.

Content

There are numerous preanalytical factors that may affect the concentration of the analyte, the measurement procedure, or the test result. These factors may be divided into two major groups: influencing and interference factors. Influencing factors are effects on laboratory results of biological origin that most commonly occur in vivo but can also be derived from the sample in vitro during transport and storage. Biological influence factors lead to changes in the quantity of the analyte in a method-independent way. Interference factors (interferences) are defined as mechanisms and factors that lead to falsely increased or decreased results of laboratory tests of a defined analyte. Interference factors and their mechanisms differ with respect to the intended analyte and analytical method. Interference factors do not affect the concentration of the analyte. On the contrary, they alter the test result for a specific analyte after the sample has been collected. They are different from the measured analyte and interfere with the analytical procedure. Therefore their effect is method dependent and may thus be reduced or eliminated by selecting a more specific method. This chapter describes the most common preanalytical sources of variability (influences and interferences) and provides recommendations on how to deal with them in everyday practice.

INTRODUCTION

The annual incidence of premature patient deaths associated with some kind of preventable medical error has been estimated to be 98,000 per year.[1] More recent data indicate that the actual mortality caused by preventable medical errors is fourfold higher.[2] According to the European Commission (EC) and World Health Organization (WHO), 1 in 10 patients is being harmed while receiving hospital care in developed countries.[3,4] Errors in laboratory medicine can lead to increased health care expenditure, cause patient harm to various degrees, and lead to different diagnostic errors (ie, missed diagnosis, misdiagnosis, and delayed diagnosis).[5]

It has been estimated that laboratory test results affect approximately 70% of medical decisions, and this clearly explains why laboratory errors have a large contribution to the overall error frequency in health care.[6,7] Almost 40% of diagnostic errors are attributed to some error that has occurred within the area of radiology or laboratory medicine, and the majority of those laboratory errors are due to some defect in the preanalytical phase of the total testing process.[8]

Historical Perspective

The preanalytical or, according to ISO15189 terminology, *preexamination* phase of the laboratory testing process has been recognized since the early 1970s as an important source of variability, and it still represents one of the greatest challenges for specialists in laboratory medicine.[9,10]

In the second half of the 20th century, when quality assurance programs were introduced for the analytical processes, laboratories became aware that some factors outside the analytical phase also significantly impacted laboratory results.[11] Results that did not correspond with the patient's clinical condition have often been called "laboratory errors." It also became clear that these variables could not be standardized or controlled by analytical quality assurance programs. In the late 1970s, Statland and Winkel defined the phase prior to analysis as the "preinstrumental phase,"[12] which was later changed to the "preanalytical phase."[13]

Even before the preanalytical phase was recognized as an important issue in laboratory medicine, some experts from different areas of laboratory medicine defined these variables as *influencing* and *interference* factors,[14,15] which were not immediately recognized as important sources of "laboratory errors." It took some time for laboratory medicine professionals to gather knowledge about their causes and mechanisms and acknowledge their importance.

After years of discussion within several national and international expert groups in the 1960s and 1970s,[12,13,14,15,16] the term *biological influence factor* was introduced and distinguished from interference factors. This led to the definitions established in the 1980s,[17,18,19] which are still valid today.[20]

The Preanalytical Phase Today

The preanalytical phase is recognized as the most vulnerable part of the total testing process, and it accounts for two-thirds of all laboratory errors.[21] Preanalytical errors can occur at any step of the preanalytical phase—for example, during test requesting, patient preparation, sample collection, sample transport, handling, and storage.[22] This high frequency of preanalytical errors may be attributed to various reasons. Many preanalytical steps are performed outside the laboratory and are not under the direct supervision of laboratory staff. Furthermore, many individuals are involved in various preanalytical steps, and those individuals have different levels of education and professional background. Finally, safe practice standards for many activities and procedures are either not available, or are available but not evidence-based, or the level of compliance with those standards is low.

The ISO 15189 accreditation standard clearly defines that medical laboratories are responsible for the management and quality of the preexamination phase.[22] It is the role of the laboratorian that the right sample be taken from the right patient, at the right time, and that correct test results are provided to the requesting physician in a timely manner. If the quality of the specimen is compromised to a degree where the expected effect is larger than the allowable error, thus causing clinically significant bias, the sample should be rejected for analysis. Our guiding principle should be "No result is always better than a wrong result." Patient benefit should always be the top priority.

Influencing and Interference Factors

Influencing Factors

Influencing factors are the effects on laboratory results of biological origin that most commonly occur in vivo but can also be derived from the sample in vitro during transport and storage. Biological influence factors lead to changes in the quantity of the analyte to be measured in a defined matrix. They modify the concentration of the measured (affected) analyte in a method-independent way.

These factors are either present in the healthy individual, like circadian rhythms,[18] or they appear as side effects of a disease and its treatment. Influencing factors may be modifiable, such as diet, time of the day, or time of the year (season), or unmodifiable, such as gender, ethnicity, genetic background, and so on. Some modifiable biological influence factors can be controlled by patient action—for example, diet—whereas others—for example, age—are not controllable. Particular care should be taken with the influencing factors whose effects may be reduced through standardization of preanalytical conditions.

As already mentioned, modification of the concentration of certain analytes can also occur in vitro. For example, concentration glucose will decrease during prolonged storage of unseparated blood due to cell metabolism, whereas potassium concentration will increase if blood is kept at lower temperatures or refrigerated (+4°C). Such increase in potassium will occur even without visible hemolysis.

Interference Factors

Interferences are defined as mechanisms and factors that lead to falsely increased or decreased laboratory test results for a defined analyte. Interference factors and their mechanisms differ with respect to the intended analyte and analytical method, and they alter the result of a sample constituent after the specimen has been collected. They are different from the measured analyte and interfere with the analytical procedure. Therefore their effect is method dependent and may thus be reduced or eliminated by selecting a more specific method.[14]

Possible interferents include the following:

1. Biological constituents of the sample (one example is acetoacetate, which interferes with creatinine measurement by the Jaffe method)
2. Exogenous molecules present in the sample (drug interferences fall into this category)
3. Exogenous molecules added to the sample during sampling or after the sampling procedure (examples are anticoagulants, tube additives, intravenous infusions, etc.)

Because interference factors are analyte and method specific, they may be eliminated or at least reduced by changing the measurement method. This chapter provides an overview of the most common preanalytical sources of variability (influences and interferences) and provides recommendations on how to deal with them in practice.

POINTS TO REMEMBER

Influencing and Interference Factors

- Influencing factors lead to changes in the quantity of the analyte in a method-independent way.
- Influencing factors may be changeable (eg, diet, time of the day) or unchangeable (eg, gender, ethnicity, genetic background).
- The effect of influencing factors may be reduced through standardization of preanalytical conditions.
- Interferences are mechanisms and factors that lead to falsely increased or decreased results of laboratory tests.
- Interference factors and their mechanisms differ with respect to the intended analyte and analytical method and may be reduced or eliminated by selecting a more specific method.

INFLUENCING FACTORS

International recommendations for patient preparation that cover all aspects and all available sample types are limited and often not evidence based. Local and international guidelines cover certain aspects of patient preparation and blood and urine sampling.[23,24] These documents provide guidance on timing of sampling, diet and activities before sampling, body position and disinfection during sampling, and regulations regarding documentation of these variables for diagnostic and/or therapeutic purposes.

Decision About Sample Type

Before diagnostic samples are obtained, it has to be decided which analytes are going to be measured. The medical needs and clinical questions usually determine the source of the sample and time of sampling. Besides medical knowledge about the physiology of the analytes intended to be measured, criteria such as practicability of sampling and risk of patient harm may influence the decision. Average concentrations of different analytes commonly observed in different kinds of body fluids may guide the choice of the specimen. Venous blood is the most commonly used sample type, followed by capillary blood, which, because of the lower amount of sample needed, became the preferred sample in newborns and young children. Arterial blood, on the other hand, is mainly used for analyzing blood gases and acid base state. Other sample types, such as urine and saliva, are primarily used when a parameter of interest is predominantly present in that particular sample type.

Controllable Variables

Time of Sampling

Changes occurring in specimens due to the time factor should be taken into account in the preanalytical phase. Due to these changes, results sometimes cannot be compared longitudinally if they have not been taken at the same time of day, month, or year. Changes can be linear (in a chronological order) and cyclic (of a repetitive nature, such as seasonal changes, or changes due to the menstrual cycle). Both of these may affect the results of laboratory tests.

Therefore several key elements need to be considered when thinking about the best time for sampling: the best time of the day, time after the last meal, time after the last sample, time after the last dose of the drug, and so on.

Influence of Circadian Rhythm

Several analytes tend to fluctuate in terms of their plasma concentration over the course of a day.[25] Thus the concentration of potassium is lower in the afternoon than in the morning, whereas that of cortisol decreases during the day and increases at night (Fig. 5.1).[39]

The cortisol circadian rhythm may well be responsible for the poor results obtained from oral glucose tolerance testing in the afternoon. For this reason, reference intervals are preferentially defined for sampling between 7 and 9 AM. The circadian rhythm can also be influenced by individual responses to meals, exercise, and sleep. These influences should not be confused with real circadian changes. In some cases, seasonal influences also have to be considered. Thus total triiodothyronine (T3) is 20% lower in the summer than in the winter,[26] whereas 25 OH-cholecalciferol exhibits higher serum concentrations in the summer.[27]

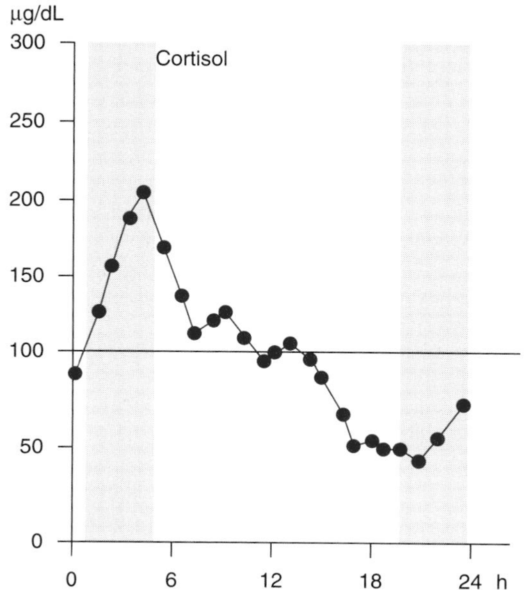

FIGURE 5.1 Daily variation of plasma concentrations of cortisol (shaded area = sleep period).[39]

Menstrual Cycle

Analytes can exhibit significant changes due to the biological changes that occur in hormone patterns during menstruation.[25] For example, aldosterone concentration in plasma is twice as high before ovulation than in the follicular phase. Likewise, renin can show a preovulatory increase. Even cholesterol exhibits a significant decrease during ovulation, and phosphate and iron decrease during menstruation.[25]

Influence of Diagnostic and Therapeutic Procedures

To ensure maximum quality of the samples, the exact time of sampling should always be documented in the medical charts and test requests. To prevent confounding preanalytical influences, samples should be taken before any diagnostic procedures with potential interfering effects. Likewise, interfering drugs should be administered after collecting a blood sample. On the other hand, in therapeutic drug monitoring (see Chapter 40), the exact timing of sampling is essential for correct interpretation of the drug level. The following diagnostic and therapeutic measures can result in both in vivo (frequent) and in vitro (less common) effects on laboratory tests:[28,29]

- Operations
- Infusions and transfusions
- Punctures, injections, biopsies, palpations, whole-body massage
- Endoscopy
- Dialysis
- Physical stress (eg, ergometry, exercise, ECG)
- Function tests (eg, oral glucose tolerance test)
- Immunoscintigraphy
- Contrast media, drugs
- Mental stress
- Ionizing radiation

When considering the appropriate time for the blood sampling, this simple rule should always be kept in mind: "A sample taken at the wrong time is worse than taking no sample."

Diet

Diet substantially affects the composition of plasma. Differences in serum composition may occur respective to the source of nutrients, number of meals, and proportion of nutrients in a diet. Moreover, malnutrition or obesity, prolonged fasting, starvation, and vegetarianism may also influence plasma composition. The effects from diet can be divided into long-term and acute effects.

Long-Term Effects of Diet. It is well known that changes in protein intake that occur over a couple of days may affect the composition of nitrogenous components of plasma and the excretion of end products of protein metabolism. Creatinine is an important example of the effect of diet on the composition of plasma. It has been shown that an increase of up to 20% of plasma creatinine concentration (measured by kinetic Jaffe method) is observed after ingesting a cooked meat.[30] Protein-rich foods affect not only the concentration of serum creatinine but also the concentration of urea and urate in serum.

A diet rich in fat leads to increased serum triglyceride concentration, reduced serum urate, and a depletion of the body's nitrogen pool. The nitrogen pool is affected because excretion of ammonium ions is required to maintain acid-base homeostasis.[31,32,33] The relative ratio in which various dietary fats are consumed closely relates to serum lipid concentrations. A diet rich in monounsaturated and polyunsaturated fats causes a reduction of LDL and HDL cholesterol concentrations,[34] although in some situations HDL cholesterol may be elevated.

A diet rich in carbohydrates decreases serum protein and lipid concentrations (triglycerides, and total and LDL cholesterol).[35] It should be emphasized that not only the proportion but also the source of nutrients in the diet affect the composition of serum. For example, some early studies have shown that serum ALP and LD activities are higher, whereas AST and ALT activities are lower in individuals who consume carbohydrates rich in sucrose or starch rather than other sugar types.[36] Moreover, total LDL and HDL cholesterol concentrations tend to be much lower in those who consume the same amount of food in many small meals throughout the day than in individuals who eat three meals per day.[31]

Compared to omnivorous subjects, vegetarians tend to have lower concentrations of plasma cholesterol, triglycerides, and creatinine, with reduced urinary excretion of creatinine and a higher urinary pH as a result of reduced intake of precursors of acid metabolites.[31] In malnourished individuals, the activity of most of the commonly measured proteins and enzymes is reduced.[37,38] Most of the above described changes are corrected following the restoration of good nutrition.

Acute Effects of Diet and Other Influencing Factors. Prior to blood sampling, the confounding influences of foods and fluid intake should be excluded. Diet and fluid intake are major factors influencing a number of analytes. From a practical point of view, one should distinguish acute effects from those observed over a longer period. Fig. 5.2 shows the percent of change in different analyte concentrations as a function of food intake.[39] Changes of 5% or less may be neglected (below 1.05 in Fig. 5.2) for being clinically insignificant. Therefore samples for these analytes do not require strict fasting.

The effect of food is dependent on the composition of diet and on the elapsed time between food intake and sampling. The activity of some enzymes (eg, ALP, AST, ALT) increases up to 20% following a meal. Triglyceride and glucose concentrations in serum increase during the absorptive phase. The turbidity of the plasma/serum sample, caused by chylomicrons following absorption of lipids, can also interfere with various measurement procedures and cause apparent changes in analyte concentrations.

The serum concentrations of cholesterol and triglycerides are influenced by various factors, such as food composition,[40] physical activity, smoking, and consumption of alcohol and coffee.[41] To avoid any misinterpretation, it is therefore recommended that blood sampling be done after 12 hours of fasting and reduced activity (bed rest).

In response to a meal, hydrochloric acid secretion in the parietal cells of the stomach is coupled with extraction of chloride from and release of bicarbonate into the plasma in order to maintain electrical neutrality. Thus venous blood leaving the stomach is enriched with bicarbonates, and this phenomenon is responsible for a mild postprandial metabolic alkalosis (ie, the alkaline tide) with concomitant increase of pCO_2 and a subsequent reduction of ionized calcium by 0.2 mg/dL (0.05 mmol/L).[31]

Effects of Fluid Intake Before Sampling

Whereas drinking coffee or small amounts of alcohol is largely seen as part of normal life and therefore not worth reporting to the physician, one should be aware of the influence of the intake of various fluids on the concentration of different analytes. Intake of various fluids may also exert acute and chronic effects.

Caffeine. Many beverages, such as tea, coffee, and cola drinks, contain caffeine. Caffeine stimulates the adrenal cortex and medulla, leading to the subsequent increase of the concentration of catecholamines and their metabolites, as

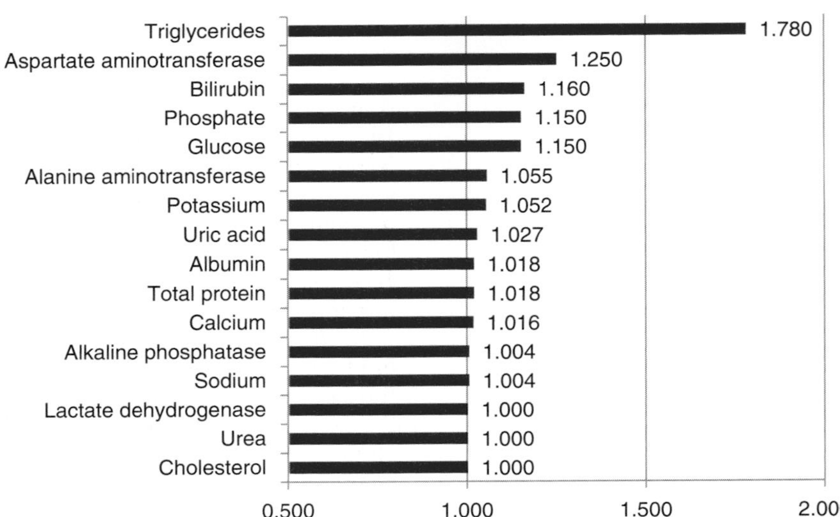

FIGURE 5.2 Change in serum concentration of different analytes 2 hours after a standard meal. (Reproduced from Guder WG, Narayanan S, Wisser H, Zawta B. *Diagnostic Samples: From the Patient to the Laboratory.* 4th updated ed. Weinheim: Wiley-Blackwell; 2009, with permission by Wiley-VCH-Verlag, Weinheim, Germany.)

well as free cortisol, 11-hydroxycorticoids, and 5-HIAA in serum. These hormonal changes are followed by the increase in plasma glucose concentration. Plasma renin activity may also be increased following caffeine ingestion.[28,31,42] Caffeine induces diuresis and inhibits the reabsorption of electrolytes, thus leading to a transient increase in their excretion. Total urine output of water and electrolytes (calcium, magnesium, sodium, chloride, potassium) increases within 2 hours following caffeine ingestion, and caffeine-induced urinary loss of calcium and magnesium is therefore largely attributable to a reduction of the renal reabsorption of calcium and magnesium.[43] Caffeine also has a marked effect on lipid metabolism. Ingestion of coffee increases the rate of lipid catabolism, thus leading to the increase of plasma lipids, free fatty acids, glycerol, and lipoproteins.[44,45] Finally, caffeine is a strong stimulant of gastrin release and gastric acid secretion and also induces the secretion of pepsin.[46]

Alcohol. Alcohol consumption, depending on its duration and extent, may affect a number of analytes. Among alcohol-related changes, acute and chronic effects should be considered separately. The decrease of plasma glucose and increase of lactate are the acute effects that occur within 2 to 4 hours of ethanol consumption. Ethanol is metabolized to acetaldehyde and then to acetate. This increases hepatic formation of uric acid[47] and inhibits renal urea excretion, thus causing an increase of uric acid in plasma.[48] Together with lactate, acetate decreases plasma bicarbonate, resulting in mild to severe metabolic acidosis, depending on the amount of ingested alcohol.

Acute alcohol ingestion increases the activity of serum GGT and some other enzymes (eg, isocitrate dehydrogenase, ornithine carbamoyltransferase).[49] Chronic effects of ethanol ingestion include the increase in serum triglyceride concentration due to decreased plasma triglyceride breakdown and an increase in the serum activity of many enzymes (GGT, AST, ALT),

Moreover, chronic alcohol consumption affects pituitary and adrenal function and is associated with numerous biochemical abnormalities. It affects lipid metabolism[25] and inhibits the salinization of transferrin that leads to the increase of serum concentration of carbohydrate-deficient forms of transferrins (CDT).[50] Increased mean corpuscular volume (MCV) is related to the direct toxic effect of alcohol on erythropoietic cells or a deficiency of folate.[51] Increased urine ethanol excretion leads to a decreased formation of vasopressin with increasing diuresis. Enhanced diuresis is followed by increased secretion of renin and aldosterone.[52]

To assess the effect of alcoholic drinks on test results and to avoid misinterpretations of laboratory results, it is recommended that the history of alcohol intake (ie, the ingested amount and frequency/time of ingestion) be documented in clinical records.

Smoking Tobacco

Smoking tobacco leads to a number of acute and chronic changes in analyte concentrations, with the chronic changes being rather modest. Smoking increases the serum concentrations of fatty acids, epinephrine, free glycerol, aldosterone, and cortisol.[25] These changes occur within 1 hour of smoking a cigarette. Through adrenal gland stimulation, nicotine causes the increase of the concentration of epinephrine in the plasma and the urinary excretion of catecholamines and their

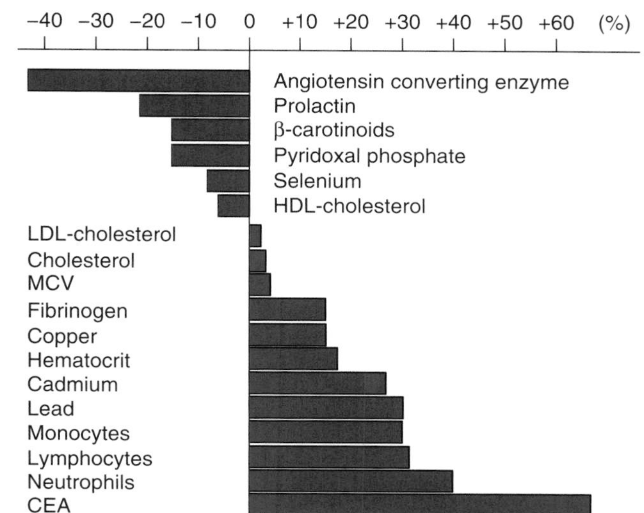

FIGURE 5.3 Chronic effects of smoking. Deviation (%) of blood analyte concentrations between current smokers and nonsmokers. (Reproduced from Guder WG, Narayanan S, Wisser H, Zawta B. *Diagnostic Samples: From the Patient to the Laboratory.* 4th updated ed. Weinheim: Wiley-Blackwell; 2009, with permission by Wiley-VCH-Verlag, Weinheim, Germany.)

metabolites.[53] Smoking leads to the acute increase in serum triglyceride, LDL, and total cholesterol concentrations.[54] Glucose metabolism is also dramatically affected by nicotine. Within only 10 minutes of smoking a single cigarette, glucose concentration increases by up to 10 mg/dL (0.56 mmol/L). This increase may persist for 1 hour.

Alterations in analytes induced by chronic smoking affect numerous blood components such as blood cell count, some enzymes, lipoproteins, carboxyhemoglobin, hormones, vitamins, tumor markers, and heavy metals (Fig. 5.3). These changes are induced by nicotine and its metabolites and reflect pathophysiological responses to toxic effects. To avoid a risk of misinterpretation of laboratory test results, smoking habits should be documented in clinical records.

In heavy smokers blood leukocyte count may be increased by as much as 30%, with a proportional increase of the lymphocyte count.[31] For CEA, different reference limits should be applied for smokers and nonsmokers due to the large differences between the two groups. The higher concentration found in smokers is caused by an increased synthesis and secretion of CEA in the colon. Tobacco smokers have higher carboxyhemoglobin concentration. To compensate for the impaired capacity for oxygen transport in heavy smokers, there is also an increase in red blood cell count. Partial pressure of oxygen (pO_2) is lower in tobacco smokers than in nonsmoking individuals by about 5 mm Hg (0.7 kPa).[31] Similar to caffeine, nicotine is also a very potent stimulant of the secretion of gastric juice and an inhibitor of duodenal bicarbonate secretion.[55] These effects may be observed within 1 hour of smoking several cigarettes. Smoking also affects the body's immune response and male fertility by affecting the sperm count, morphology, and motility.[31,56] The effect of smoking may persist even after smoking cessation. It usually takes 5 years, or even longer, for most parameters to normalize (eg, C-reactive protein and fibrinogen concentrations, hematocrit). Interestingly, for some parameters (eg, white blood cell count), it may take up to 20 years to return to baseline value.[57]

Body Position and Tourniquet

Body posture influences blood constituent concentrations. This is caused by the net capillary filtration (ie, the net result of the differences in the membrane permeability, hydrostatic pressure, colloid osmotic pressure of plasma, and interstitial fluid). Capillary filtration is increased in the lower extremities when changing from the supine to the upright position. The change in body posture from the supine to the upright position increases the concentration of all constituents that usually do not pass the capillary filtration barrier, including small molecular weight molecules bound to proteins. Thus free calcium does not change, whereas total calcium increases by 5% to 10%,[58] when changing from the supine to the upright position. Although this effect is observed in healthy and diseased individuals, the degree of the change is usually greater in some disease states—for example, in cardiac insufficiency. Therefore reference intervals should ideally be obtained under identical conditions with regard to body posture. Blood sampling should be performed after at least 15 minutes of rest in a supine or sitting position.

A similar mechanism occurs when a tourniquet is applied to facilitate finding appropriate veins for venipuncture. The higher pressure obtained in veins leads to the loss of water and low molecular weight substances, increasing the concentration of proteins, cells, and analytes bound to them. This becomes clinically significant after 1 to 2 minutes.[39] Therefore the tourniquet should be released 1 minute after it has been applied.

Muscular Activity

Physical activity of varying duration and intensity may lead to substantial changes in the plasma composition, and the extent of this change depends on several factors, such as training status, intake of fluid, electrolytes and carbohydrates, and even the ambient temperature.[59,60,61] For example, even a mild physical effort, like clenching the fist during venous blood sampling, can increase the concentration of potassium and should therefore be avoided.[62] This occurs due to the release of potassium from skeletal muscles and even without a tourniquet. Intensive exercise is associated with transient elevations of cardiac biomarkers, markers of muscle damage, enhanced platelet aggregation, leukocytosis, elevation of tissue-plasminogen activator levels, activation of the fibrinolytic system, and a decreased ability of the blood to clot and generate thrombin.[63,64,65,66] Concentrations of creatine kinase (CK), creatine kinase MB (CK-MB), alanine aminotransferase (ALT), and lactate dehydrogenase (LD) are increased in individuals where physical activity is greater than 12 hours per week.[67] Cardiac troponin (cTn) rises after maximal bicycle stress test.[68] Due to the substantial changes in plasma composition, in professional sportsmen (eg, marathon runners), a large proportion of laboratory results may fall outside the usual reference intervals.

Intensive physical activity (within 12 hours before blood sampling) may also affect homeostasis for numerous hormones: catecholamines and their derivatives, epinephrine, norepinephrine, dopamine, corticotropin (ACTH) and vasopressin, gastrin, thyroid-stimulating hormone (TSH), prolactin, growth hormone, aldosterone, cortisol, testosterone, human chorionic gonadotropin (hCG), insulin, glucagon, and β-endorphin.[69,70,71,72]

Preparing for Blood Sampling

Because food, fasting time, circadian rhythm, muscular activity, smoking, drugs, and ethanol consumption can affect the concentration of numerous analytes, standardization of all those controllable variables is highly recommended. Proper standardization of controllable variables leads to significant reduction of preanalytical variability. Until very recently, there has been a great heterogeneity in the definition of *fasting state* currently being used for different analytes by different health care facilities and in original reports throughout the literature. Obviously, agreement on the definition of *fasting state* and uniform and consistent compliance would greatly help to reduce the heterogeneity arising from such differences. The European Federation for Clinical Chemistry and Laboratory Medicine (EFLM) Working Group for Preanalytical Phase WG-PRE has therefore recently published a recommendation for the definition of fasting requirements as a guiding framework for harmonization of this important preanalytical aspect.[73]

According to these recommendations, the following general requirements should be applied to all blood tests:

1. Blood should be drawn preferably in the morning between 7 a.m. and 9 a.m.
2. Fasting should last for 12 hours, during which only water consumption is permitted.
3. Alcohol should be avoided for 24 hours before blood sampling.
4. In the morning before blood sampling, patients should refrain from cigarette smoking and caffeine-containing drinks (tea, coffee, etc.).

Professional associations and laboratories worldwide are encouraged to adopt, implement, and disseminate the EFLM WG-PRE recommendation for the definition of *fasting*. Moreover, laboratories worldwide should have policies for sample acceptance criteria related to fasting samples. Blood samples for routine testing should not be taken if a patient has not been appropriately prepared for sample collection.

Noncontrollable Variables

Various unavoidable biological factors can lead to changes in analyte concentration and can therefore only be considered during interpretation with the respective knowledge. Table 5.1 summarizes some of these influences and their respective effects. These factors should be considered when interpreting laboratory results because their influence cannot be prevented by preanalytical standardization.

Age and Gender

Due to dramatic physiological changes associated with growth and development, the reference intervals for many analytes differ substantially with respect to an individual's age and gender. In newborn subjects, the body fluids reflect the trauma of birth and early postnatal events related to the adaptation of the baby to new extrauterine life. Immediately after birth, infants usually experience a mild metabolic acidosis of transient nature, due to the accumulation of lactates. This acid-base disturbance is usually normalized within the first day after birth.[31] The Canadian CALIPER study is an excellent source of reference intervals in childhood.[78] In the

TABLE 5.1 Unavoidable Influences on Laboratory Results

Influence	Examples of Analyte Concentrations Changed	Remarks
Age[74,75]	Alkaline phosphatase, LDL-cholesterol, hormones, creatinine.	Provide age-dependent reference intervals
Race[75,76]	Creatine kinase higher in black than in white males. Granulocytes higher in white than in black males. Creatinine higher in black than in white males.	Provide race-specific reference intervals
Gender[74,77]	Alanine aminotransferase, γ-GT, creatinine	Provide gender-specific reference intervals
Pregnancy[25,39]	Triglycerides ↑, homocysteine ↓ during pregnancy	Document months of pregnancy with laboratory results
Altitude[39]	CRP, hemoglobin ↑, transferrin↓	Consider weeks of adaptation, when coming from or going to high altitude

early hours of extrauterine life, the concentration of some biochemical markers (AST, direct bilirubin, total bilirubin, creatinine, C-reactive protein, GGT, IgG, LDH, magnesium, phosphate, rheumatoid factor, uric acid) is increased, thus reflecting the maternal levels, but it then declines within the first 2 weeks of life.[79] Levels of other markers (eg, amylase, transferrin, antistreptolysin O, cholesterol, IgA, IgM) are very low in the neonatal period and gradually increase within the first 2 weeks of extrauterine life. This upward trend in analyte concentrations continues over time from birth to 18 years. Most of the biochemistry parameters (albumin, ALP, AST, total bilirubin, creatinine, IgM, iron, lipase, transferrin, HDL cholesterol, and uric acid) exert differences between genders during the early childhood years. However, these changes are most significant during puberty (age 14–18 years), due to the strong influence of sexual development and growth.[79]

Hemoglobin concentration, hematocrit, and the other red blood cell indices follow a similar pattern, showing the gradual increase during the first 10 years of life. First gender differences are observed at the age of 10 years, when levels in boys show a sharp increase during puberty and adolescence. Levels in females are much lower, but they also slowly increase throughout puberty. Such gender differences are related to the lower metabolic demand, decreased muscle mass, and lower iron stores in females.[80]

Concentration of thrombopoietin peaks shortly after birth and then slowly decreases. Subsequent to the change of thrombopoietin concentration, immediately after birth, there is a peak in platelet count, followed by a decline during childhood and into adulthood. The white blood cell count is also higher in the early extrauterine days, and throughout the first couple of years of childhood, values decline in older children. Females have slightly higher platelet count than men during adolescence and adulthood.[80]

INTERFERENCE FACTORS

As mentioned earlier, interference factors have the ability to interfere with the analytical procedure and alter the test results. The effect of interference factors depends on the method—that is, the same interferent may not necessarily affect two different methods used to measure the same analyte. Common interference factors are hemolysis, lipemia, icterus, drugs, paraproteins, and various sample contaminants such as gels, tube additives, and fibrin clots.

POINTS TO REMEMBER

Influencing Factors

- Samples should be taken before any therapeutic and diagnostic procedures that have a potential influencing effect.
- Tobacco smoking leads to several acute and chronic changes in the concentrations of numerous analytes.
- Even within only 1 hour of smoking 1 to 5 cigarettes, there is an increase in serum concentration of fatty acids, epinephrine, free glycerol, aldosterone, and cortisol.
- Diet substantially affects the composition of plasma. The effects of diet can be long term and acute.
- Physical activity of varying duration and intensity leads to changes in the plasma composition of many analytes. The extent of this change depends on training status, intake of liquid, electrolytes and carbohydrates, and even the ambient temperature.
- Most of the reference interval data for children are obtained from the Canadian CALIPER study.

Interfering factors are considered clinically relevant when the bias caused by their interference is greater than the maximum allowable deviation of a measurement procedure. How this "maximum allowable deviation" should be established is still debated. The Clinical Laboratory Standards Institute (CLSI) EP7-A2 guideline, for example, sets this criterion at ±10% as a rule of thumb. Others would argue that the degree of allowable deviation caused by interfering factors should be derived (1) from data on the biological variation of the analyte, (2) by simulation modeling based on the effect of preanalytical and analytical performance on clinical decisions or patient outcomes, or (3) from information on the state-of-the-art.[95] The choice of the method for determining the maximum allowable deviation for a certain analyte not only depends on the medical use of the test but also on the national and international regulations in use.

Interferences can be endogenous and exogenous. Endogenous interferences originate from the substances present in the patient sample, whereas exogenous interferences relate to the effect of various substances added to the patient sample, such as separator gels, anticoagulants, surfactants, and so on, all of which may cause significant interference.[96,97]

Hemolysis

Definition and Background

Hemolysis is defined as a process of membrane disruption of erythrocytes and other blood cells, accompanied by the subsequent release of cell components into the plasma and red coloration of the serum (or plasma) to various degrees after centrifugation.[81] Though hemoglobin is the most abundant protein in red blood cells, hemolysis is not necessarily always associated with the release of hemoglobin into the surrounding extracellular fluid. For example, if the blood sample is stored at a low temperature, low molecular intracellular components like electrolytes diffuse from the cells, but hemoglobin will not. Furthermore, efflux of cell components due to cell lysis affects all blood cells (ie, platelets and white blood cells) and not only erythrocytes. Therefore it is important to remember that red coloration of the serum or plasma can never accurately predict the concentration of blood cell components.

Hemolysis is the most common preanalytical error and the most common cause of sample rejection. It occurs with a frequency of up to 30%[82,83,84,85] and accounts for almost 60% of unsuitable specimens.[86] The frequency of hemolysis largely depends on the collection facility, characteristics of the patient population, and the type of professional who is doing the phlebotomy. The highest frequency of hemolysis has been observed in samples from emergency departments, pediatric departments, and intensive care units, whereas hemolysis has proven to be the least frequent in outpatient phlebotomy centers, where blood sampling is done by specialized laboratory staff.[87,88] These differences are due to the level of knowledge and skills of the staff who perform the blood collection.[23] One large study in Australia of five hospitals from October 2009 to September 2013 found that the hemolysis rate is much higher in emergency departments than in other inpatient settings. Interestingly, the hemolysis rate was highest in patients who were triaged in the most urgent category. Also, the hemolysis rate was higher if the phlebotomy was done by the clinical staff than by laboratory phlebotomists.[89]

The two major sources of hemolysis are in vivo hemolysis and in vitro hemolysis. In vivo hemolysis is a result of a pathological condition and occurs within the body before the blood has been drawn. It may occur as a result of numerous biochemical (enzyme deficiencies, erythrocyte membrane defects, hemoglobinopathies), physical (prolonged marching, drumming, prosthetic heart valves), chemical (ethanol, drug overdose, toxins, snake venom), immunological (autoantibodies) mechanisms, and infections (babesiosis, malaria). In vivo hemolysis can further be categorized as intravascular and extravascular, depending on the site of the destruction of red blood cells. Intravascular hemolysis occurs as a direct and immediate disruption of red blood cells due to the cell injury within the vasculature, whereas in extravascular hemolysis, red blood cell membranes are damaged by the reticuloendothelial system, primarily in the spleen.[90] The most common causes of in vivo hemolysis are reaction to incompatible transfusion and autoimmune hemolytic anemia.

In vivo hemolysis is not very common and accounts for only 3% of all hemolyzed samples.[91] Nevertheless, in vivo hemolysis is of great clinical importance because it reflects an underlying pathological process in a patient. Laboratories should therefore have a procedure in place for distinguishing in vivo and in vitro hemolysis. In vivo hemolysis should always be suspected when patient blood is hemolyzed over a longer period of time after different types of samples (eg, citrate, serum, and heparinated tube) are hemolized or repeated blood sampling, even after special care has been taken to avoid hemolysis. Decreased concentrations of haptoglobin in serum and free hemoglobin in urine are the most pronounced and specific laboratory signs of in vivo hemolysis. Haptoglobin is a protein that binds free hemoglobin in the circulation to prevent oxidative damage induced by hemoglobin.[92] Once released from the erythrocyte into the plasma, hemoglobin forms complexes with haptoglobin, and those complexes are removed from the circulation by macrophages. In more pronounced cases of in vivo hemolysis, haptoglobin in serum can be undetectable (ie, below the detection range), whereas its concentration in cases of in vitro hemolysis remains unchanged.[93,94] When in vivo hemolysis is confirmed, the laboratory should not reject hemolyzed samples for analysis, because parameters in hemolyzed samples reflect the actual patient condition and are extremely relevant for adequate patient care (diagnosis, therapy management, monitoring).

In vitro hemolysis occurs outside the patient at many steps of the preanalytical phase: blood sampling, sample handling and delivery to the laboratory, and sample storage. Causes of in vitro hemolysis are described in Chapter 4.

Mechanisms of Hemolysis Interference

Hemolysis is an endogenous interference that causes clinically relevant bias of patient results through the several distinct mechanisms described in the following.

Spectrophotometric Interference. Spectrophotometric interference of hemolysis occurs due to the ability of hemoglobin to absorb light at 415-, 540-, and 570-nm wavelengths.[98] This characteristic of hemoglobin causes optical interference that can lead to either falsely increased or decreased concentrations of the measured parameters. The direction and degree of the interference largely depend on the analyte and the method.

Release of the Cell Components Into the Sample. Some components are present in blood cells in concentrations that are several times higher than those in the extracellular space (ie, plasma or serum). Table 5.2 shows some of the most pronounced differences between intracellular and extracellular concentration in red cells.[99,100,101,102]

From this it follows that there is a dramatic increase in the concentration of the listed analytes measured in hemolyzed plasma (or serum) due to the efflux of those substances from erythrocytes into the sample. The most pronounced effect of hemolysis is seen for LDH. LDH activity may be increased by over 20% in mildly hemolyzed samples (at a concentration of only 0.27 g/L of free hemoglobin), by over 60% at 0.75 g/L free hemoglobin, and up to over 350% in grossly hemolyzed samples with 3.34 g/L free hemoglobin.[103]

Because intracellular components may also escape from platelets during clotting, there is a marked difference in the potassium concentration between serum and plasma. The mean estimated difference in the concentration of potassium in serum and plasma is 0.36 ± 0.18 mmol/L, and this difference is positively associated with the platelet count.[104] Plasma

TABLE 5.2 Ratio Between Intracellular and Extracellular Concentration of Various Parameters in Red Cells

Analyte	Intracellular Concentration (Compared to Extracellular)
Lactate dehydrogenase	↑ 160 ×
Inorganic phosphate	↑ 100 ×
Potassium	↑ 40 ×
Aaspartate aminotransferase	↑ 40 ×
Folic acid	↑ 30 ×
Aalanine aminotransferase	↑ 7 ×
Magnesium	↑ 3 ×

is therefore the recommended sample type for the accurate measurement of potassium.

Sample Dilution. Some analytes are present in much higher concentrations in plasma than in blood cells like albumin, bilirubin, glucose, sodium, and a few others.[100] For those parameters hemolysis will cause a dilution effect, and their concentrations will be lower in hemolyzed samples. The effect of sample dilution causes clinically significant bias only at higher degree of hemolysis. For example, glucose is negatively affected by severe hemolysis (−8.3%) only at the concentration of 3.34 g/L of free Hb if measured by the Beckman Coulter chemistry analyzer and reagents (Olympus AU2700, Beckman Coulter, O'Callaghan's Mills, County Clare, Ireland).[103]

Chemical Interference. Various blood cell components may affect the analyte measurement procedure by directly or indirectly competing for molecules in the reagents, inhibiting indicator reactions or modifying the analyte by complexation, proteolysis, or precipitation. One such effect is caused by the enzyme adenylate kinase, which is present in both erythrocytes and platelets.[105] Adenylate kinase (EC 2.7.4.3) is an enzyme that catalyzes the reversible conversion of ATP and AMP to two ADP molecules and maintains the adenine nucleotide cell content.[106] When released from the cells during hemolysis, adenylate kinase may compete for ADP with creatine kinase in a creatine kinase assay if inhibitors are not supplied in the reaction mixture.[107]

Hemoglobin released from erythrocytes during hemolysis may interfere with various assays through its pseudoperoxidase activity. Pseudo-peroxidase activity of free hemoglobin released from erythrocytes interferes in the assay for measurement of bilirubin concentration through the inhibition of the formation of diazonium salt.[108]

Hemolysis may cause a clinically significant interference on a wide range of analytes in immunochemistry assays. This interference is caused by modifying the reaction analytes (antigens and antibodies) by the proteolytic action of cathepsin E, the major proteolytic enzyme in mature erythrocytes. Proteolytic enzymes released from erythrocytes may mask or potentially enhance epitope recognition in various immunoassays. Interference caused by proteolytic activity may cause measurement bias of various degrees and various directions, depending on the assay. For example, current troponin assays have variable susceptibilitiy to hemolysis interference.

Hemolysis has been shown to cause negative interference with concentrations of cTnT, insulin, cortisol, testosterone, and vitamin B12, and false-positive increases for PSA and cTnI in a concentration-dependent manner.[109,110,111] However, the degree and direction of bias are analyte and method dependent. For example, hemolysis causes falsely decreased concentrations of cTnT assayed with the Roche hs cTnT assay on the Elecsys E170 immunochemistry analyzer, whereas concentrations of cTnI measured using the Ortho Clinical Diagnostics TnI ES assay on the Vitros 5600 Integrated System (Ortho Clinical Diagnostics, Rochester, N.Y.) are falsely elevated in hemolyzed samples.[112] Abbott Architect TnI assay appears to be more robust against interference from hemolysis.[113] The microparticle enzyme immunoassay for troponin I (Abbott Laboratories, Abbott Park, Ill.) is not affected by moderate hemolysis and exerts clinically relevant bias only for grossly hemolyzed samples.[114]

Lipemia

Lipemia is defined as a turbidity of the sample visible to the naked eye. Turbidity of the sample is caused by the light scattering due to the presence of large lipoprotein particles. The increase in concentration of lipoproteins in blood most commonly occurs due to postprandial triglyceride increase, parenteral lipid infusions, or some lipid disorders. Not all lipoproteins have equal contribution to the sample turbidity. The effect of lipoprotein particles on the sample turbidity depends on the size of the particles. Chylomicrons and VLDL lipoproteins, the largest lipoprotein particles in the circulation, have the greatest contribution to the sample turbidity. To avoid postprandial lipemia, patients are therefore requested to fast for 12 hours before the blood sampling.[73]

Mechanisms of Interference Caused by Lipemia

Lipemia is an important endogenous interference that may cause clinically relevant bias of patient results through the several mechanisms described in the following.

Spectrophotometric Interference. Lipemia causes interference by light absorbance and light scattering. The lipemic sample absorbs light, causing a decrease in the intensity of the light passing through the sample. The ability of lipoprotein particles to absorb light is manifested in the range of wavelengths (300–700 nm). Sample absorbance rises with the decreasing wavelengths and is maximal in the ultraviolet range. That is why many enzymatic methods in which the end product is measured at 340 nm (NAD[P] or NADP[H]) are strongly affected by lipemia.

Lipemic samples also cause light scattering. Light scattering occurs in all directions, and its intensity depends on the number and size of lipoprotein particles and the wavelength of measurement.[115] For this reason, light scattering of lipoprotein particles causes significant interference with turbidimetry and nephelometry. In methods where the transmittance of light is inversely proportional to the concentration of the analyte, in the absence of the sample blank, sample turbidity causes positive bias. However, in some competitive assays where the transmittance of light is directly proportional to the concentration of the analyte, sample turbidity will cause negative bias.

Interference Caused by the Volume Depletion Effect. Plasma in healthy individuals in the fasting state consists of only minor portion of lipids (<10% of the total plasma volume). The rest of the plasma is water. The increase in the concentration of lipoprotein particles leads to an increase in the plasma

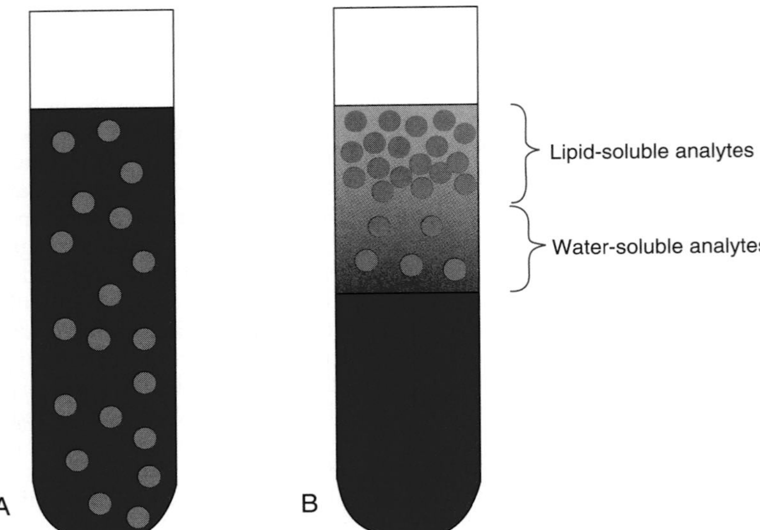

FIGURE 5.4 **A,** Lipids are distributed evenly in whole blood prior to centrifugation. **B,** Lipid gradient in centrifuged sample. Top lipid-rich layer contains lipid-soluble analytes. Lower plasma layer contains water-soluble analytes.

volume occupied by lipids. Particles that are not lipid soluble are displaced by the lipids to the water part of the plasma. Therefore lipemia leads to a false decrease in the concentration of the measured analyte in all methods in which the concentration of respective analyte is measured in the total plasma volume.

One example of interference caused by the volume depletion effect is the bias in electrolyte measurement, leading to so-called pseudo-hyponatremia. This type of interference affects electrolytes only if measured by flame photometry and by indirect measurement using ion-selective electrodes but not in direct potentiometry (for more details, see Chapters 14 and 35). However, it must be noted that the volume displacement effect of the lipemic sample will affect the electrolyte measurement only in grossly lipemic samples with concentrations of triglycerides greater than 17 mmol/L (1504 mg/dL).[116]

Interference Caused by Partitioning of the Sample. Upon centrifugation of a lipemic sample, lipoproteins are not homogeneously distributed in the serum or plasma due to the lipid gradient (Fig. 5.4). Water-soluble analytes are more concentrated in the lower layer of the plasma or serum, whereas lipids and lipid-soluble analytes, such as drugs and some lipid-soluble hormones, are more concentrated in the top lipid-rich layer. This is especially important in automated chemistry analyzers with fixed path lengths of the sample probe. Test results may differ for those analytes that are not evenly distributed between the lipid and water portion of the sample, depending on the part of the sample from which the sample probe is taking the sample for analysis.

Interference Caused by Physicochemical Mechanisms. An excess of lipoproteins in the blood may interfere in electrophoretic and chromatographic methods by causing abnormal peaks. Elevated levels of triglycerides and lipoprotein particles may disturb the electrophoretic pattern and morphology, as well as falsely increase the relative percentage of the prealbumin, albumin, and α1- and α2-globulin regions.[117,118] Moreover, lipemia may even affect some immunochemistry assays by masking the binding sites on antigens and antibodies and thus physically interfering with antigen–antibody binding.[119]

One additional complication of excessive lipemia is the increased sample susceptibility to hemolysis leading to the specific turbid and reddish appearance of the sample (the so-called "strawberry milk" appearance). This effect is most probably caused by the increased fragility of the erythrocyte membranes due to the alterations in the content of the phospholipid membrane layer and is more pronounced with the increase in lipid (particularly triglyceride) concentrations.[120]

Removal of Lipids From the Sample

In the hospital environment, lipemic samples are not infrequent. They most often originate from emergency departments, intensive care units, and endocrinology and gastrointestinal clinics from patients suffering from conditions that include acute pancreatitis, acute or chronic kidney failure, thyroid disorders, and diabetes mellitus. Lipemic samples quite commonly require immediate results. Unlike hemolysis, the interference caused by lipemia can be fully eliminated, or at least reduced, by removing the excess of lipids from the sample. Still, even if lipids have been successfully removed from the sample, any visible turbidity of a sample should be documented and reported with the test results because it offers clinically useful information about the patient.[121] Moreover, lipid testing and testing for lipid-soluble drugs (eg, benzodiazepines) and hormones (eg, thyroid hormones) should always be done on the native sample, before delipidation. Methods for lipid removal include ultracentrifugation, high-speed centrifugation, and some lipid-clearing agents.

Lipid Removal by Ultracentrifugation and High-Speed Centrifugation. According to the CLSI C56-A standard for Hemolysis, Icterus, and Lipemia/Turbidity Indices as Indicators of Interference in Clinical Laboratory Analysis, ultracentrifugation is the recommended method for the removal of the excess of lipids in the sample.[122] Ultracentrifuges use the centrifugation force of almost 200,000 *g* and are

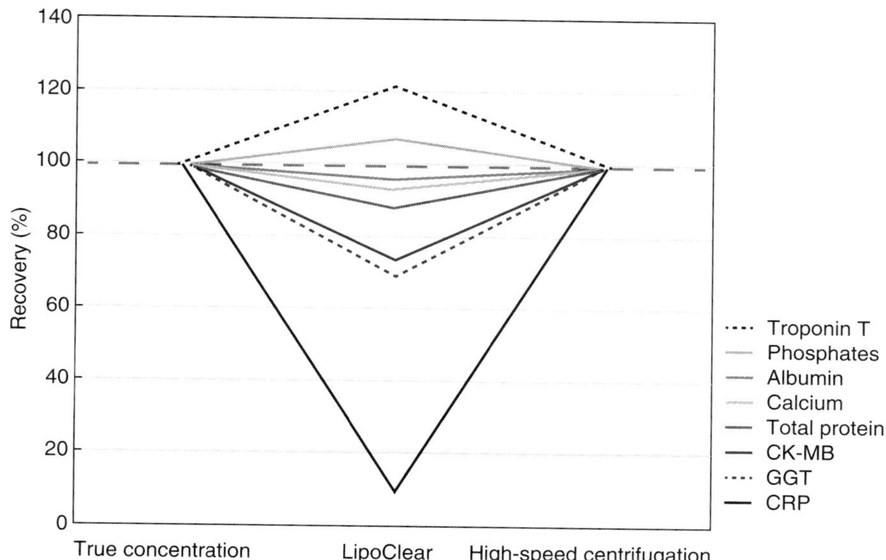

FIGURE 5.5 Recoveries for several chemistry assays after lipid removal from a lipemic sample with a lipid clearing agent (LipoClear, Iris International Inc., Westwood, Massachusetts) and high-speed centrifugation in Eppendorf Mini Spin centrifuge (Eppendorf, Hamburg, Germany) at 12,100 g for 5 minutes. *CK-MB,* Creatine kinase MB; *CRP,* C-reactive protein; *GGT,* gamma-glutamyl transferase. (Data from Saracevic A, Nikolac N, Simundic AM. The evaluation and comparison of consecutive high-speed centrifugation and LipoClear reagent for lipemia removal. *Clin Biochem* 2014;47:309–14.)

very effective in clearing lipemic sera by separating lipids, especially chylomicrons (top layer) from the aqueous part (lower layer) of the sample. After centrifugation, the infranatant (lower part of the sample) can be transferred into the clean tube and analyzed. It should be kept in mind that by removing the upper lipid layer, one also removes lipid-soluble analytes like drugs and hormones. Results reported from ultracentrifuged samples or samples from which lipids have been removed in any other way should be appropriately annotated to ensure clinicians are aware that the sample has been manipulated to obtain the reported results.

Though considered a gold standard, ultracentrifugation is not widely available in many laboratories. High-speed centrifugation using the microcentrifuge with a maximum centrifugation speed of up to 20,000 *g* may therefore serve as an acceptable alternative and is the method of choice for most laboratories.[123] The effectiveness of high-speed centrifugation depends on the concentration of lipids in the lipemic sample. However, it must be emphasized that ultracentrifugation is superior to high-speed centrifugation for grossly lipemic samples. By using the ultracentrifuge, triglyceride concentration may be reduced 7-fold (from 59.2 to 8.1 mmol/L; or 5239 to 717 mg/dL), whereas the high-speed centrifuge may achieve only 3.4-fold reduction.[124]

Lipid Removal by Lipid-Clearing Agents. Lipid-clearing agents are widely used in many laboratories due to their low cost, convenience, and ease of use. Those agents (cyclodextrin, polyethylene glycol, dextran sulphate, hexane, and others) may vary in their ability to extract lipids from a lipemic sample and may also lead to reduction of a significant amount of protein from the sample.[125] It is therefore extremely important for laboratories to verify the performance of such reagents before their routine use because they may not be appropriate for a wide range of analytes due to their low recovery. For example, LipoClear spin columns (Iris International Inc., Westwood, Mass.) may lead to serious underestimation of CRP (−92%), CK-MB (−25%), and GGT (−30%) and overestimation of Troponin T (+20%) and phosphates (+7%) (Fig. 5.5).[126]

Lipid removal takes time and may cause delays in reporting the results. It is up to each individual laboratory to establish its own procedure for managing lipemic samples, bearing in mind to ensure the highest possible accuracy of results and speed. To minimize the prolongation of the turnaround time and subsequent delays in reporting the results for grossly lipemic samples, laboratories may consider analyzing electrolytes using the blood gas analyzers (direct ISE methodology) while manipulating the rest of the sample to remove the lipids.

Intravenous Lipid Emulsion Therapy as an Antidote to Drug Overdose

Lipid emulsions were introduced in 2006 as a remedy for systemic toxic effects caused by local anesthetic and are used increasingly today in emergency settings to treat patients who have overdosed on antiepileptic, cardiovascular. or psychotropic drugs.[127,128] Their use is recommended in patients suffering from severe systemic cardiovascular toxic effects who have not otherwise responded to conventional resuscitation protocol and antidotal therapies.[127] The American College of Medical Toxicology recommends it as a reasonable therapeutic option in circumstances where there is serious hemodynamic or other instability from a lipid-soluble drug, even if the patient is not in cardiac arrest.[129] The exact mechanism of action of lipid emulsions is not known. In patients treated with large doses of lipid emulsions, possible side effects include severe hypertriglyceridemia, pancreatitis, lipemia, and numerous interferences in laboratory assays.[130] To avoid compromising patient outcome caused by reporting of incorrect results and delays in reporting of critical results, it is important that blood samples in such cases are collected prior to initiating the intravenous lipid emulsion therapy whenever possible.[131] If intravenous lipid emulsion therapy has already been initiated before the blood sampling, the laboratory should make an effort to remove the lipids and ensure acceptable accuracy of results as well as turnaround time. Good communication between the laboratory and the clinical staff in such cases of life-threatening toxicity from lipophilic drugs is of paramount importance.

Icterus

The normal concentration of bilirubin in human plasma (or serum) is up to 20 μmol/L. Change in the color of the serum (or plasma) becomes detectable when bilirubin concentration exceeds 34 μmol/L. Bilirubin concentrations above 100 μmol/L are clinically defined as *icterus*. Icteric plasma is commonly seen in patients from intensive care units, gastroenterology centers, and pediatric clinics. Bilirubin interferes with numerous chemistry tests such as enzymes (ALT, alkaline phosphatase, creatine kinase, lipase), electrolytes, metabolites (urea, creatinine, glucose), lipids (cholesterol, triglycerides), proteins (albumin, total proteins, IgG), hormones (estradiol, beta-HCG, free T3), and even some drugs (gentamicin, phenobarbital, theophylline, tobramycin).[132,133,134]

Just as with hemolysis and lipemia, interference caused by bilirubin differs among instruments and assays. For example, bilirubin exerts interference of different magnitudes (strong, moderate, or negligible) and directions (positive and negative interferences), both with Jaffe and enzymatic methods for the measurement of serum creatinine from different manufacturers. While some methods are not affected by bilirubin at all, others may exhibit strong interference by bilirubin, causing clinically significant bias for creatinine measurement and compromising the adequate management of patients with kidney disease.[135,136] It has been demonstrated that even if two methods have identical reagents, differences in their susceptibility to interference by bilirubin may still occur. These differences may be due to the different incubation times and temperatures and some other parameters related to the assay setup.[137] Interestingly, although enzymatic methods are often considered the method of choice due to being less susceptible to various interferences, bilirubin has been reported to cause greater interference in some enzymatic creatinine assays than in Jaffe methods.[138]

Bilirubin is present in the blood in several distinct forms: as unconjugated and conjugated (mono- and diglucuronide conjugates). Unconjugated bilirubin is not soluble in water and is therefore transported in blood bound to albumin. Bilirubin conjugates are soluble in water. Additionally, bilirubin photoisomers may be found in the blood of neonates.[139] All these different molecular forms of bilirubin have different physical and chemical properties and behave differently in different chemistry assays. The total amount of measured bilirubin in the patient is a mixture of these different forms. Different forms of bilirubin cause interference to various degrees with different laboratory methods, and the same forms of bilirubin can act differently with the same assays on different instruments.

Most interference studies performed by manufacturers and most original studies published by different authors were done on commercially available forms of unconjugated bilirubin that may not correspond to what is found in the blood. This is why sometimes data obtained by interference studies does not mimic real scenarios in human blood and cannot be extrapolated to define rules for adequate detection and management of icteric samples.

Unfortunately, laboratories cannot do much about removing or minimizing the effect of icteric interference. Bilirubin oxidase and blanking procedures have been recommended.[20] Possible options are dilution of the sample (possible only for analytes present at high enough concentrations in the blood) and testing the requested analytes with a different method or on a different instrument for which icterus does not cause clinically significant interference. For maximal patient benefit, laboratories may consider having special protocols (dilutions or different methods) for some critical analytes in icteric samples to avoid unnecessary sample rejections.

Mechanisms of Interference Caused by Icterus

Icterus interferes through two mechanisms: spectrophotometric interference and by interfering with chemical reaction. It is important to recognize that both mechanisms may occur simultaneously in one sample.

Spectrophotometric Interference of Bilirubin. Bilirubin causes spectrophotometric interference due to its ability to absorb light in the wide range of wavelengths between 400 and 540 nm.

Chemical Interference of Bilirubin. Bilirubin produces negative bias on assays that involve H_2O_2 as an intermediate reaction (eg, cholesterol, glucose, uric acid, triglycerides).

Detection of Hemolytic, Icteric, and Lipemic Samples

Hemolysis becomes visible at the concentration of 0.3 to 0.5 g/L of free hemoglobin, and the intensity of the red color of the serum or plasma further increases with the increase in concentration of free serum hemoglobin (Fig. 5.6A). Lipemia causes sample turbidity, which approximately corresponds to the concentration of serum triglycerides (Fig. 5.6B). Increased concentrations of serum bilirubin lead to yellow to orange coloration of the serum, and the change of the color correlates to the increasing concentration of the bilirubin in the serum (Fig. 5.6C).

Free hemoglobin, triglycerides, and bilirubin have characteristic absorption peaks in a wide wavelength range of 300 to 600 nm. This is also the range where sample absorbance is measured in spectrophotometric methods, and that is why hemolysis, icterus, and lipemia cause spectral interferences. Fig. 5.7 presents the characteristic absorption curves of oxyhemoglobin, triglycerides, and bilirubin. Serum indices may be detected by visual inspection and by the use of automated detection systems.

Visual Detection of Serum Indices

Although detection of the degree of hemolysis, icterus, or lipemia has historically been done by visual inspection, such an approach is highly unreliable.[140] Laboratory personnel are not able to accurately assess the degree of hemolysis, icterus, or lipemia in serum, even if well trained and when using a color standard for comparison.[141] Moreover, there is a poor interrater agreement (reproducibility) in estimating the degree of serum indices between different members of laboratory staff, reflecting the substantial interindividual differences in visual sensitivity to different colors.[142] For example, it has been demonstrated that visual inspection of the degree of hemolysis is influenced by the sample type (serum or plasma) and the test requested, thus leading to either over- or

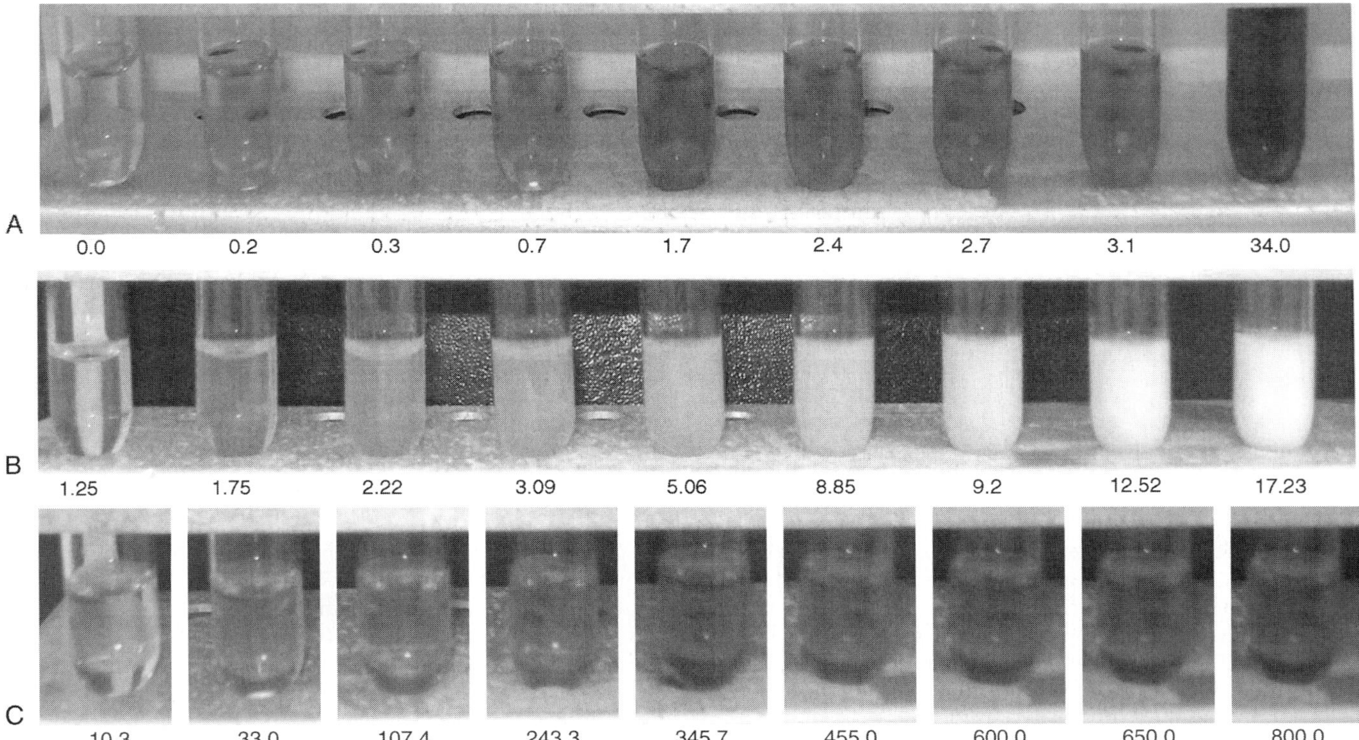

FIGURE 5.6 A, Hemolysis: the intensity of the red color of the serum and corresponding concentrations of free serum hemoglobin (in g/L). B, Lipemia: the degree of turbidity and corresponding concentrations (in mmol/L) of tryglicerides. C, Icterus: the intensity of the yellow color of the serum and corresponding concentrations of bilirubin (in μmol/L). (Color standard scales provided by Clinical Institute of Chemistry, University Hospital Center "Sestre milosrdnice," Zagreb, Croatia. Please see the online version of this figure for full color.)

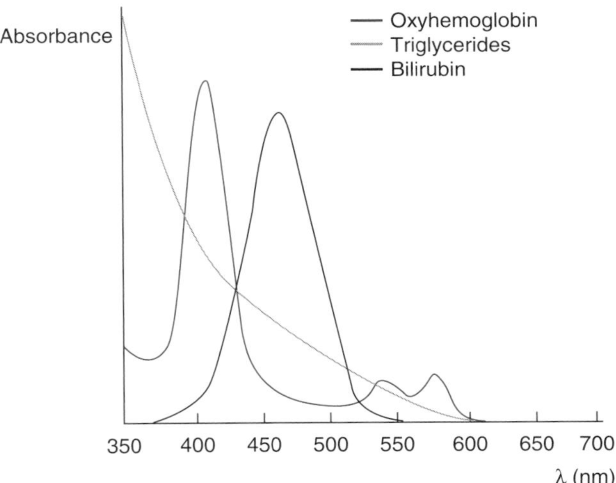

FIGURE 5.7 Absorption curves of oxyhemoglobin in serum with characteristic peaks at 415, 540, and 570 nm *(red line)*; triglycerides absorption curve cover wide range of wavelengths, with a maximum in the lower part of the spectrum *(dotted gray line)*; bilirubin has one distinct peak at 460 nm *(black line)*.

underestimation of the actual degree of hemolysis, depending on the expected effect of hemolysis on the measured analyte.[143] The ability to detect hemolysis by visual inspection is further impaired in samples that are both hemolyzed and icteric.[144] This is especially important in neonatal samples, where elevated bilirubin concentrations are quite common.

Other substances, such as medical contrast media, may also influence the human ability to detect not only hemolysis but also icterus and lipemia.[145] One such example is Patent Blue dye, which is commonly used for sentinel lymph node biopsy in breast cancer patients. The presence of this dye in serum negatively affects the ability of laboratory personnel to reliably detect hemolysis, as well as icterus and lipemia. For the above-mentioned reasons, visual detection of the degrees of hemolysis, lipemia, and icterus is not recommended and should be replaced with automated detection systems whenever and wherever possible.

Automated Serum Indices

Today, most mainstream chemistry analyzers can detect serum indices by the use of semiquantitative, spectrophotometric measurement and grading the interfering substances into categories. The serum index is automatically reported for every sample and can be used to determine the degree of interference and its effect on the requested parameters. Where an automated detection system for serum indices is not available, grading of interference factors by visual inspection is still a practical alternative used by many laboratories.[146,147,148]

Automated serum index detection systems have numerous advantages. Such systems are highly reproducible and provide an objective and standardized way to screen for common interferences and manage specimen rejection via built-in rules. Moreover, their implementation improves laboratory turnaround time, leads to an increase in laboratory efficiency, and minimizes waste by reducing the number of rejected samples.[149] However, there are still some problems and challenges associated with the automated detection of serum indices on various analytical platforms, which are detailed below.

Variability Between Different Analytical Platforms. There is a large variability across different chemistry analyzers in analytical characteristics of their serum index measurement. Different analyzers have different sensitivities, measurement ranges of, and decision thresholds for hemolysis, icterus, and lipemia. Moreover, they differ in the sample volume necessary for the estimation of serum indices and the type of solution used (saline, sample diluent, etc.). Different analyzers measure sample absorbance at different wavelengths and use different algorithms for determining the degree of serum indices. Finally, different manufacturers have employed different reporting systems to report the results of serum indices. Some are reporting qualitative results using the ordinal scale, whereas others are reporting semiquantitative results using actual concentrations of the interferent.[150,151]

Necessity to Verify Manufacturers' Claims. It is the responsibility of the manufacturers of in vitro diagnostic systems and reagents to validate the analytical performance characteristics of their reagents and provide this information to the customer. The instructions for use must particularly contain the information about the effect of all known relevant interferences (eg, serum indices) on laboratory assays. The Clinical Laboratory Standards Institute (CLSI) EP7-A2 standard for interference testing in clinical chemistry[152] recommends that validation of the effect of an interferent on clinical chemistry assay be done at two concentrations of an analyte and at five concentrations of an interferent. The maximum concentration of an interferent must reflect the maximum expected concentration of that interferent in the clinical laboratory on patient samples. Moreover, the acceptance limits for allowable interference should be derived whenever possible from biological variability or clinically established thresholds. Due to financial constraints and the lack of time and staff, laboratories often rely on the information provided by the manufacturers, and only a minority of laboratories verify manufacturer declarations.[146] However, manufacturers do not always comply with the recommended procedure for testing interferences, and their claims are often not accurate, reproducible, and reliable.[153,154] It is therefore good practice for a laboratory to perform its own verification of serum indices. Alternatively, laboratories may rely on the evidence from the literature if such exists and only if the evidence is of adequate quality.

Necessity to Implement a Systematic Approach to Internal and External Quality Control of Serum Indices. Like all other laboratory methods, analytical quality of the method for detection of serum indices should be continuously monitored by using appropriate internal quality control (IQC) and through participation in an external quality assessment program (EQA). The ISO 15189:2012 International Standard for medical laboratories states, "EQA programs should, as far as possible, provide clinically relevant challenges that mimic patient samples and have the effect of checking the entire examination process, including pre- and postexamination procedures."[22] EQA for serum indices may be run by sending out samples with varying degrees of lipemia, hemolysis, and icterus, and participants are then asked to provide their serum indices value and to report results as they would for a patient sample.[155,156] Unfortunately, IQC and EQA are not widely available for serum indices. EQA for serum indices is currently available from only one provider (WEQAS), and IQC material for serum indices has been recently made available on the market by only one manufacturer.[157]

Potential Sources of Interferences Affecting Serum Indices. Some medical contrast media are known to interfere with serum indices and impair the accurate determination of hemoglobin, bilirubin, and sample turbidity. It is important that laboratory staff be aware of this issue and that each sample be visually checked whenever serum index measurements raise suspicion or do not match the sample appearance or clinical condition of the patient. Patent Blue dye, which negatively affects the ability to detect changes in the sample's color, has also been found to interfere with serum indices measurement on the Roche Modular Pre-Analytics system and the Abbott Architect chemistry analyzer.[158,159] Patent Blue exerts positive interference on the lipemia index and a negative interference on hemolytic and icteric indices in a linear, dose-responsive fashion.

Rose Bengal has a peak absorbance at 562 nm and is a component of a drug that is used for intralesional therapy in patients with refractory cutaneous or subcutaneous metastatic melanoma.[160] Used in a treatment trial for severe melanoma lesions, it was found to cause false-positive interference on the hemolysis index on Roche Modular D in a sample with a red/pink tinge collected 20 minutes after the injection of a drug.[161]

Monoclonal proteins may also give an abnormal reading of serum lipemic index in apparently clear serum.[162] Markedly elevated serum lipemia indices in clear sera were also quite frequently observed in patients with high concentrations of polyclonal immunoglobulins.[163] Nevertheless, unusually high lipemia indices in otherwise clear sera do not occur in all patients with monoclonal or biclonal peaks.

One serum index may also adversely affect the other when two or three HIL indices are abnormal in the same sample (eg, serum hemolyzed and icteric, hemolyzed and lipemic). In these cases the magnitude and direction of the bias of one index on the measurement of the other will vary greatly among different instruments and will depend on the respective wavelengths used.[122]

Management of Hemolytic, Icteric, and Lipemic Samples

Laboratories should be aware of the effect of preanalytical interferences on their assays. When there is a significant deviation from the true value of the analyte caused by the presence of cell compounds released by sample hemolysis, bilirubin, or increased concentration of serum lipids, such a result is a threat to patient safety. Biased and inaccurate results may cause diagnostic errors and affect patient management. To ensure the accuracy of their results, laboratories should have procedures in place to systematically detect the presence of potential interferences and how to address them. Unfortunately, there is a large discrepancy among the ways results are reported from samples with interferences, among different countries, institutions, and even individuals (eg, analyze and report all components, reject the sample and not analyze anything, or analyze only selected components that are not affected by the interferent).[89,122,147,148] There is room for improvement and harmonization in this respect.

When interferences from hemolysis, icterus, and lipemia are causing unacceptable bias and results are clinically inaccurate, such results should not be reported and sample redraw should be requested.[121,164,165] Such a test report should always be accompanied with comments informing the clinical staff about the reasons for not reporting the originally requested test results. It is also important that a laboratory notify the staff when sample appearance (color, turbidity) deviates from a normal state by including a comment on a test report (eg, sample hemolyzed, icteric, lipemic, or turbid), even if the tests are not affected by this change in appearance. Such comments provide useful information to the clinicians. Comments should also indicate if the sample has been treated in any way to minimize the effect of interfering substances (eg, delipidation).

Unfortunately, each time a redraw is requested, there is a delay in providing the requested test results, and this leads to delays in patient management. In a previously mentioned study by Vecellio and colleagues, the length of stay in emergency departments of five large Australian hospitals was on average 18 minutes longer if one or more samples for a particular patient was hemolyzed.[89] To avoid such delays, a laboratory should make a thorough investigation of the causes of the unsuitable specimens and be actively engaged in process improvement to reduce the frequency of errors that affect the quality of the sample.

POINTS TO REMEMBER

Hemolysis, Lipemia, and Icterus

- Visual assessment of the degree of hemolysis, lipemia, and icterus is not reliable and leads to errors.
- Hemolysis is the most common preanalytical error and most common cause of sample rejection.
- Hemolysis may cause clinically relevant bias through spectrophotometric and chemical interference, sample dilution, and release of the cell components into the sample.
- Lipemia causes interference by spectrophotometric interference (light absorbtion and light scattering), the volume depletion effect, partitioning of the sample, and physicochemical mechanisms (eg, disturbance of the electrophoretic pattern).
- Laboratories should verify the performance of lipid removal reagents before their routine use because they may not be appropriate for a wide range of analytes due to their low recovery.
- Different forms of bilirubin cause varying degrees of interference with different laboratory methods, and the same forms of bilirubin act differently with the same assays on different instruments.

Drug Influences (Drug effects) and Interferences

Exogenous interferences are quite complex and difficult to identify and deal with.[124,152] In the case of exogenous interferences, interfering substance is not normally present in the patient blood and can be introduced into the sample via several different sources:

- Interferences from the prescribed medication used for patient treatment
- Interferences from supportive medical therapy, including parenteral emulsions, contrast media agents, and infusion solutions
- Interferences from natural preparations (herbal and animal remedies) and dietary supplements
- Interferences occurring in the cases of accidental exposures and poisonings
- Interferences introduced by contamination during sample handling (from rubber tube stoppers, lubricants, anticoagulants, or surfactants) or sample analysis (antibiotics used for reagent and buffer stability)

Mechanisms of Interference

According to the mechanism of action, drug interferences on laboratory tests can be categorized as either biological or chemical. Biological influences are the result of an in vivo action of a drug or metabolite. Drugs can alter levels of a large number of tests by several mechanisms:

- Induction of hepatic microsomal enzymes (phenytoin raises levels of gamma-glutamyl transferase through this mechanism)[166]
- Enzyme inhibition (finasteride and dutasteride cause a decrease in prostate-specific antigen concentration by inhibition of 5α-reductase)[167]
- Displacement of the drug from the protein-binding site (tizoxanide alters free warfarin fraction by its displacement from the protein-binding site; this effect can be monitored by alterations in coagulation parameters)[168]

All of these drug actions occur in vivo, and changes in parameters reflect a true state in the human body. Therefore alteration in concentration of the measured parameter is not an analytical error.

Analytical (chemical) interference is caused when the presence of the drug directly or indirectly leads to falsely elevated or decreased concentration/result of a measured analyte. The parent drug or its metabolite can have structural similarity to the tested analyte and therefore interfere in immunochemical or photometric methods. Reaction interference can occur when the compound or its metabolites catalyze or inhibit some steps of the chemical or immunochemical reaction. Some drugs can interfere with the integrity of the sample by changing sample density (viscosity) and cause obstruction problems on analytical systems (eg, iodine-based contrast media). Chemical mechanisms of interference are discussed in more detail in the following.

Manufacturer Claims Regarding Drug Interferences

Manufacturers of laboratory reagents are responsible for identifying potential errors that can occur as a result of interfering substances. Therefore they conduct extensive testing and provide information about interference susceptibility to their users. Laboratory professionals are responsible for verifying interference claims, investigating any discrepant result that might be caused by an interfering substance, and providing feedback to the manufacturers.[152]

Besides interferences of endogenous components that are listed in manufacturers' claims (lipids, hemoglobin, bilirubin, proteins), manufacturers usually include the results of interference testing for drugs that could potentially affect the measurement. The drug list is adjusted for any specific analyte. Drugs and metabolites that are likely to interfere based on their chemical and physical properties and also drugs most often prescribed in the patient population for which the test is ordered should be tested.[152] Tested drug concentrations should be chosen in order to cover expected

TABLE 5.3 List of Interfering Drugs Tested for Potential Interference With HbA1c Enzymatic Assay

	HIGH TEST LEVEL		% INTERFERENCE*	
Interfering Substance	**Conventional Units**	**SI Units**	**6.0 to 7.0% HbA1c**	**≥8.0% HbA1c**
Acarbose	50 mg/dL	0.77 mmol/L	0.0	0.0
Acetaminophen	200 µg/mL	1324 µmol/L	−1.5	−1.1
Acetylsalicylate	50.8 mg/dL	2.82 mmol/L	0.0	0.0
Atorvastatin	600 µg Eq/L	600 µg Eq/L	0.0	0.0
Captopril	0.5 mg/dL	23 µmol/L	−1.5	−1.1
Chloropropamide	74.7 mg/dL	2.7 mmol/L	0.0	0.0
Cyanate	50 mg/dL	6.16 mmol/L	0.0	1.1
Furosemide	6.0 mg/dL	181 µmol/L	0.0	0.0
Gemfibrozil	7.5 mg/dL	300 µmol/L	0.0	0.0
Ibuprofen	0.5 mg/mL	2524 µmol/L	0.0	0.0
Insulin	450 µU/mL	450 µU/mL	0.0	0.0
Losartan	5 mg/dL	0.11 mmol/L	0.0	0.0
Metformin	5.1 mg/dL	310 µmol/L	0.0	0.0
Nicotinic acid	61 mg/dL	4.95 mmol/L	0.0	0.0
Propranolol	0.2 mg/dL	7.71 µmol/L	0.0	0.0
Repaglinide	60 ng/mL	132.57 nmol/L	0.0	0.0

Interference effects were assayed by comparing test samples containing potential drug interferents to the reference samples. According to the CLSI EP7-A2 protocol for interference testing in clinical chemistry,[152] two clinically relevant analyte concentrations were used (6.0% to 7.0% and ≥8.0% HbA1c). Various potential interfering drugs are added into the samples (listed in column 1). Concentrations of the analyte (HbA1c) were measured in the sample with added interferent (test result) and in the reference sample without interferent (control result). Interference effect was calculated as bias according to the formula: Interference = (Test result − Control result)/Control result × 100%. However, calculated bias values are representative of potential drug interferences only up to the tested concentrations listed in columns 2 and 3. Some of these drugs might have a stronger impact on HbA1c concentration measurements when they are present in higher concentrations.

From reagent insert sheet provided with the Abbott HbA1c reagent (REF 4P52-21). From Abbott Laboratories, Lake Bluff, Illinois.

blood concentrations. To minimize the risk of unrecognized drug effect due to the low tested concentration, the highest expected concentration should be tested at least three times. A list of proposed tested drug concentrations is provided in Clinical Laboratory Standards Institute document EP7-A2, *Interference Testing in Clinical Chemistry.*[152] Table 5.3 presents an example of drug interferences listed in the reagent insert sheet provided with the Abbott Hemoglobin A1c enzymatic assay (Abbott Laboratories, Lake Bluff, Ill.).

Unfortunately, information about patient medication is often not available to laboratory staff. Hospital electronic medical records can help identify whether any potentially interfering drug is prescribed to the patient. However, for most of the drugs there is no way of knowing if the drug concentration in patient blood exceeds the allowable threshold. For most of the drugs listed in Table 5.3, concentration can be measured only in specialized laboratories. Therefore many drug interferences remain undetected. Only a clear discrepancy between the test result and clinical information prompts the laboratory staff to suspect drug interference and proceed to further investigation.[169]

Prescribed Medication

Prescribed medication can often interfere with the measurement and cause erroneous laboratory results. Although all laboratory methods can be affected by drug interferences, specific enzymatic chemistry methods are usually not as sensitive as colorimetric tests. Creatinine is one of the most commonly measured parameters in a clinical chemistry laboratory. Laboratories worldwide use either the Jaffé colorimetric assay with alkaline picrate or an enzymatic assay for creatinine measurement (Fig. 5.8).

Some commonly prescribed antibiotics and analgesic drugs can interfere with creatinine measurement. For example, cephalosporin antibiotics cause falsely increased creatinine levels (measured by the Jaffe method) in sera drawn shortly after intravenous administration of cefpirome.[170,171] Falsely elevated creatinine concentration measured by the Jaffe method has also been observed after adding subtherapeutic, therapeutic, and toxic concentrations of acetaminophen, acetylsalicylic acid, and metamizole to the serum. Although the Jaffe method has always been considered to be more susceptible to interference compared to the enzymatic assay, it is now known that even the enzymatic assay is not free from the interfering effects of various drugs. While the enzymatic dry chemistry creatinine method is not affected by the addition of any tested amounts of acetylsalicylic acid and acetaminophen, the addition of toxic levels of metamizole causes falsely decreased creatinine concentrations (Fig. 5.9).[172]

Ethamsylate is a hemostatic drug indicated in cases of capillary bleeding.[173] This drug causes a significant decrease in creatinine concentration (approximately by 50%) measured by enzymatic assay. Interestingly, the Jaffe method is not influenced by ethamsylate. The interference is probably caused by the presence of a hydrochinone structure in the ethamsylate molecule. Hydrochinone interferes in the last reaction of creatinine quantification (see Fig. 5.8A). Therefore the other methods that are using the same indicator reaction are also

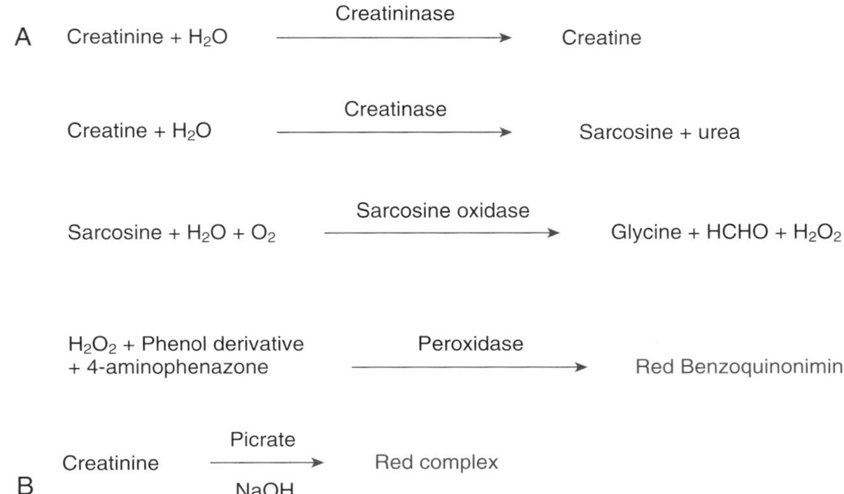

FIGURE 5.8 Methods for the measurement of creatinine. **A,** Enzymatic assay: the absorption at 546 nm of the red-colored product of the indicator reaction is proportional to creatinine concentration. **B,** Jaffe colorimetric assay: creatinine reacts with picrate in alkaline media and forms a red complex. Change in absorption at 509 nm is proportional to creatinine concentration.

affected by the administration of this drug. There is evidence that ethamsylate also causes significant false declines in the concentrations of cholesterol (9.2%), triglycerides (15.6%), and uric acid (15.4%).[174,175] A similar problem with the enzymatic creatinine assay was found in the presence of high concentrations of therapeutically administered catecholamines. Dopamine, dobutamine, epinephrine, and norepinephrine cause strong negative interference with the Creatinine Plus enzymatic (Roche Diagnostics GmbH, Penzberg, Germany) assay. The Vitros (Ortho Clinical Diagnostics) enzymatic creatinine assay demonstrates slight negative interference, while the i-STAT enzymatic (Abbott) and Jaffe methods (Roche Diagnostics and Siemens [Siemens Healthcare Diagnostics, Munich, Germany]) are unaffected by the presence of catecholamines.[176]

The active metabolite of leflunomide (teriflunomide), a synthetic isoxazole-derivative drug with immunosuppressive and antiviral properties, exerts interference with ionized calcium. Ionized calcium is a best indicator of calcium homeostasis in patients with suspected or known derangements of calcium metabolism.[177] In kidney transplant patients, low ionized calcium concentrations are sometimes observed without any clinical signs of hypocalcemia. These patients are treated with leflunomide. After oral administration, leflunomide is rapidly converted into its active metabolite teriflunomide, which causes falsely decreased ionized calcium concentrations. The interference is dependent on the type of the blood gas analyzer and was found to affect the Rapidlab-1265 (Siemens Diagnostics) and i-Stat point-of-care analyzer (Abbott), but not the ABL800-FLEX blood gas analyzer (Radiometer, Copenhagen, Denmark).[178] Because this drug is widely used not only in kidney transplant patients but also in patients with rheumatoid arthritis, every hypocalcemia in laboratories using Rapidlab or i-Stat point-of-care analyzers should be interpreted with caution and compared with the patient's clinical condition. Unfortunately, this is not the only reported interference for ionized calcium measurement. Sodium perchlorate is used as an oral drug to treat hyperthyroidism. There is a significant false decrease in calcium results in the presence of perchlorate when using Radiometer and Siemens Rapidlab POCT instruments for measuring ionized calcium.[179]

Thiopental is a barbiturate used for the treatment of elevated intracranial pressure. The central laboratory analyzer Dimension Vista (Siemens), which uses the V-LYTE Integrated Multisensor Technology system for electrolyte measurement, produces falsely elevated sodium concentrations in the presence of thiopental. However, when the sodium is measured on a point-of-care analyzer using direct potentiometry (Rapidlab 1200, Siemens), there is no evidence of thiopental interference.[180]

Drug interferences are also observed in coagulation testing. Dabigatran etexilate, a new oral direct thrombin inhibitor, is used as an anticoagulant drug. Application of this drug causes significant bias in many coagulation tests. Dabigatran causes dose-dependent prolongation of prothrombin time (PT) and activated partial thromboplastin time (aPTT), and thus significantly changes the results of various other coagulation tests, including antithrombin III and coagulation factors II, V, VII, VIII, IX, X, XI, XII, and XIII. Falsely decreased factor activities and falsely positive misdiagnosis of lupus anticoagulant are observed in the presence of dabigatran.[181]

Carbohydrate-deficient transferrin (CDT) is a biomarker for long-term alcohol consumption. There is evidence that the sensitivity of the test can be affected by the use of several dugs like amlodipine (calcium channel blocker), perindopril (ACE inhibitor), atorvastatin (statin), isosorbide mononitrate (nitrate), carvedilol (beta blocker), ticlopidine (inhibitor of platelet aggregation), and pantoprazole (gastric acid pump inhibitor).[182] It is still not clear if the false-negative measurement is a result of polytherapy where unexpected metabolic pathways can be activated. Even if some or all of the drugs are listed as potential interfering substances, manufacturers usually do not declare what effects can occur in vivo when multiple drugs are combined.

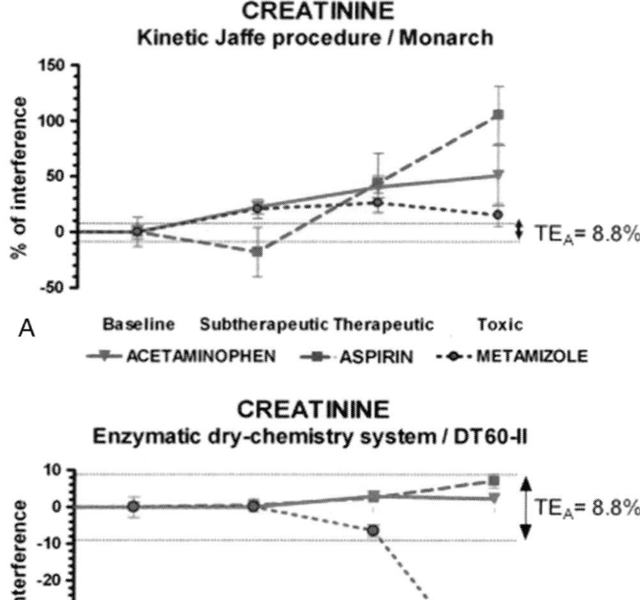

FIGURE 5.9 Analgesic drug interference with creatinine measurement. **A,** Interference of acetaminophen, acetylsalicylic acid (aspirin), and metamizole on creatinine measurement by Jaffe method. All tested drugs cause interference error over acceptance criteria based on biological variations (dashed line; total error = 8.8%). **B,** Interference of acetaminophen, acetylsalicylic acid (aspirin), and metamizole on creatinine measurement by enzymatic method. Only toxic concentrations of metamizole cause a falsely decreased concentration of creatinine. (Reproduced from Luna-Záizar H, Virgen-Montelongo M, Cortez-Álvarez CR, et al. In vitro interference by acetaminophen, aspirin, and metamizole in serum measurements of glucose, urea, and creatinine. *Clin Biochem* 2015;48:538–44, with permission by Elsevier.)

Supportive Medical Therapy

Medical contrast media are used during medical imaging procedures to enhance the contrast of organs and fluids. Iodine-based compounds (iohexol, iodixanol, and ioversol) are mostly used for the x-ray methods, while gadolinium contrast agents (ionic, neutral, albumin-bound, or polymeric) are typically used in magnetic resonance imaging.[145] Iodine-based compounds can interfere with chemical reactions in several ways. Any measurement can be obstructed because of the interference with the sample integrity. Iodine molecules have high density and can prevent proper formation of the barrier in the serum gel separator tubes.[183,184] Also, some specific interferences with chemistry parameters are observed. Iopromide is used as a contrast media agent in coronary angiography. A false increase in troponin I concentration measured by Opus Magnum reagent (Opus cTnI immunoassay system; Behring Diagnostics, Siemens) is detected if the sample is taken immediately after the procedure. This interference was found to be reagent specific because no similar finding was observed when using troponin assay by a different manufacturer (ACCESS cTnI immunoassay; Beckman Coulter, Tokyo, Japan).[185]

Gadolinium contrast agents act as chelators, and that seems to be the main interference mechanism. Therefore calcium measurement is mostly affected by the presence of these compounds. Colorimetric calcium assays (o-cresolphthalein complexone or methylthymol blue) are affected by the presence of gadodiamide, while ion selective electrode and inductively coupled plasma-atomic emission spectroscopy can reliably determine calcium concentration.[186,187,188]

Inductively coupled mass spectrometry (ICP-MS) is often used for the measurement of trace elements. There is ample evidence that gadolinium (Gd) interferes with ICP-MS measurement of selenium and causes false elevations of selenium concentrations in patients undergoing magnetic resonance imaging. Ryan and colleagues published a case report of a 30-year-old man with no history of Se exposure or toxicity symptoms who had lethal concentrations of plasma selenium (Se) measured by ICP-MS.[189] This patient had undergone magnetic resonance imaging with a gadolinium contrast agent prior to measurement of selenium concentration. It was postulated that the $^{156}Gd^{2+}$ isotope was causing interference on $^{78}Se^{+}$, the isotope used for the selenium measurement, by having an identical mass-to-charge ratio. If this interference is not recognized, potential selenium exposure can be suspected for these patients, and the patient could be misdiagnosed and mistreated. To avoid this interference, another Se isotope (^{82}Se) that has a different mass-to-charge ratio, and thus is not affected by Gd, should be measured, or pure hydrogen should be used in the collision cell.[190,191]

Other clinical chemistry assays are also influenced by several different gadolinium contrast agents: angiotensin-converting enzyme, total iron-binding capacity, zinc, magnesium, and creatinine.[192,193] All of these interferences were found to be assay specific, and different contrast media agents displayed different degrees of interferences.

Natural Preparations

Today, it is becoming more common to use natural preparations for self-medication or supportive therapy. Patients consume herbal and other dietary products, but they fail to report the usage to their doctors or to laboratory staff when they come in for blood sampling.[194] The influence of these products on laboratory tests is not fully known. Herbal medicines can cause direct interference with immunoassays due to cross-reactivity. Due to their structural similarity to the tested analyte, active compounds that are present in herbal products can react with the antibody in the assay and, based on the structure and design of the immunoassay, result in both falsely elevated and decreased analyte concentrations. The concept of cross-reactivity in immunoassays is described in more detail in Chapter 23.

Another potential problem is unexpected reactions, because the exact content of these preparations is not always known.[195] Preparations used in Chinese medicine, like Chan Su, can contain some physiologically highly active molecules, like bufadienolides (bufalin, cinobufagin, and resibufogenin) that are extracted from the glands of Chinese toads. This preparation is used for the treatment of a variety of conditions, such as tonsillitis, sore throat, furuncle, and heart palpitations.[196] The structural similarity of bufadienolides and digoxin is responsible for both cardiotoxicity and interference in the immunochemistry method. Ingestion of this medicine can cause both false-positive and false-negative results for the digoxin measurement, depending on the assay format. The most affected assays are those that are using polyclonal antibodies, like fluorescence polarization immunoassay or microparticle enzyme immunoassay, but the assays using monoclonal antibodies are also susceptible to interference by bufadienolides.[197,198] Herbal supplements that are used widely throughout the world, like ginseng, can also interfere with digoxin measurement, even though some more recently introduced chemiluminescent microparticle assays seem to be free of such interference.[199,200] Labeling of herbal products may not accurately reflect their content, and adverse events or interactions attributed to a specific herb may be due to misidentification of plants, contamination of plants with pharmaceuticals or heavy metals, or quality control problems.[195] For example, it has been recognized that some Chinese herbal remedies may contain steroids, with the potential to interfere with some assays and to cause suppression of the hypothalamic-pituitary-adrenal axis. Similarly, it is also well documented that some Ayurvedic herbal medicine products may be contaminated with lead, with the potential to cause toxicity.[201,202]

Accidental Exposures and Poisonings

In the case of accidental poisonings with herbs, household cleaning products, or any other exogenous compounds, interferences on laboratory test results can potentially prolong the diagnostic procedures in acute patient care and cause harm to the patient. Due to their structural similarity to the digoxin molecule, cardiotonic glycosides can interfere with the digoxin measurement. Numerous cases of poisonings by cardiac glycoside–containing plants like lily of the valley *(Convallaria majalis)* or oleander *(Nerium oleander)* are reported. Ingestion of oleander is potentially fatal due to cardiotoxicity of its active component, oleandrin. Positive and negative interferences of oleandrin and oleander extract on a Loci digoxin assay using the Vista 1500 analyzer have been reported.[203] Convallatoxin is a glycoside extracted from *Convallaria majalis*. Due to the significant cross-reactivity between convallatoxin and digoxin, the digoxin assay is proposed to be used as a screening tool for detection of convallatoxin ingestion.[204]

Accidental intoxications often occur as a result of children ingesting cleaning products commonly found in the home. Miniature racing cars run on nitromethane, which has been shown to interfere with creatinine measurement, producing a falsely elevated concentration.[205,206,207] Nitromethane is also used in racing cars to enhance combustion. Extreme creatinine concentration (8270 µmol/L) without evident renal failure has been observed in a suicide attempt in which Blue Thunder fuel containing nitromethane was ingested.[208] In a Jaffe method, nitromethane also reacts with alkaline picrate and forms a red chromophore with absorbance similar to the creatinine picrate chromophore. This reaction causes falsely elevated creatinine concentration. When an enzymatic assay is used, creatinine can be accurately measured in the presence of nitromethane.[209,210]

Potential drug interferences are numerous, and not all of them can be recognized or predicted. The largest available online source for analytical interferences is the *Effects on Clinical Laboratory Tests* series, edited by Young and colleagues.[211] This database has compiled the large body of evidence from the published literature and is the most extensive source of analytical interferences. For example, the database lists 307 results of potential drug interferences for creatinine. Laboratory professionals should be alerted by any unexpected result and discuss it with the clinical staff. If the source of suspected interference cannot be determined, laboratories should try to involve manufacturers of the reagents to identify the potential interfering substance and quantify its effect.

Sample Contaminants

Blood samples can be contaminated by several different exogenous substances during phlebotomy, sample handling, or even test measurement. Several components of the blood collection tubes can interfere with the measurement and influence laboratory results, including lubricants, anticoagulants, separator gels, clot activators, and surfactants.[96] Lubricants like silicone oils and glycerol facilitate insertion and removal of the stoppers. Glycerol should not be used for the lubrication of stoppers in tubes that will be used for triglyceride measurement because glycerol interferes with most triglyceride assays.[212] Silicone-based lubricants are less likely to interfere with assays, although silicone can falsely elevate ionized magnesium and triiodothyronine levels.[213] Additional peaks in mass spectrometry in the presence of silicone-based lubricants can interfere with interpretation of results.[214] Plastic tubes require clot activators to ensure rapid clot formation. Some clot activators based on silica particles affect the measurement of some analytes like lithium[215] and testosterone.[216] Silicone surfactants used to decrease nonspecific adsorption of components on tube walls may interfere with measurement of vitamin B12 and cancer antigen 15-3.[213]

Antibiotics are commonly added into reagents and buffer solutions to prevent microbial growth. Carryover from reagents containing gentamicin may cause spuriously high gentamicin results. Gentamicin is present in some diagnostic reagents (glucose, urate, direct bilirubin, CK, ALT, AST, beta-hydroxybutyrate) as an antibacterial additive and is known to cause spuriously high gentamicin results on the Beckman Coulter AU480 analyzer (Beckman Coulter, Inc., Brea, Calif.) due to reagent carryover.[217,218] Therefore gentamicin measurement should be processed in a separate batch (ie, before or after the measurement of any of the listed parameters) to prevent carryover.

Interferences in Immunoassays

Interferences in immunoassays may occur due to numerous endogenous and exogenous causes.[219] Endogenous sources of interferences in immunoassays are discussed in Chapter 23, but exogenous sources of preanalytical variability in immunoassays are briefly addressed here.

Exogenous interferences occur in the preanalytical phase due to the action of some external factors or conditions that are not normally present in properly collected, transported, handled, and stored specimens.[220] Although exogenous preanalytical interferences are not rare, they are often neglected and overlooked in everyday routine work. If they go undetected, preanalytical interferences in immunoassays may cause unnecessary harm to the patient and increase health care–related costs. Some examples of harmful results due to erroneous immunoassay findings are listed in Table 5.4.

TABLE 5.4 **Effects of Laboratory Errors on Patient Outcome**[221]

Wrong Result	Consequence
Elevated Result	
Raised human chorionic gonadotrophin (hCG) indicating gonadal tumor	Unnecessary surgery, chemotherapy
Raised calcitonin indicating medullary thyroid cancer	Unnecessary fine-needle aspiration
Raised prolactin level	Misdiagnosis of prolactinoma
Increase in urine free cortisol	Unnecessary diagnostic follow-up
Elevated testosterone in women	Unnecessary diagnostic follow-up
Elevated LH and FSH levels	Unnecessary diagnostic follow-up
Low Result	
Low 25-hydroxyvitamin D result despite replacement therapy	Incorrect diagnosis of hypovitaminosis D
Negative hCG level	Missed diagnosis of choriocarcinoma
False low digoxin results	Wrong treatment (overdosing with digoxin, risk of digoxin toxicity)
Low insulin level	Missed diagnosis of insulinoma
False negative troponin results	Missed diagnosis of myocardial infarction

Modified from Jones AM, Honour JW. Unusual results from immunoassays and the role of the clinical endocrinologist. *Clin Endocrinol (Oxf)* 2006;64:234–44.

Potential exogenous sources of preanalytical interferences in immunochemistry assays include the following[119,219,220]:

- Sample type (type of additive)
- Underfilling the tube
- Sample stability during transport and storage
- Hemolysis
- Lipemia or sample turbidity
- Icterus (hyperbilirubinemia)
- Fibrin clots
- Carryover
- Administration of radioactive or fluorescent compounds
- Drugs
- Herbal medicines
- Nutritional supplements

Mechanisms of preanalytical interferences in immunoassays are numerous, and not all assays are equally susceptible to every interfering factor. This is why it is important that laboratory staff have a thorough knowledge and understanding of their own assays and instruments and potential sources of interference. Some major preanalytical issues related to immunochemistry assays are discussed below.

Tube Additives as Potential Interfering Factors in Immunoassays

Many laboratories prefer plasma over serum because of the shorter turnaround time and greater plasma yield and the ability to eliminate the problem of the formation of fibrin clots in serum. For particularly urgent analytes, such as cardiac markers, plasma was formerly the preferred specimen.[222] Nevertheless, due to the interfering effect of some plasma additives (EDTA, heparin, sodium citrate), serum is an acceptable alternative.

Heparin interferes with numerous immunoassays by affecting the binding of antibody and antigen and thus affecting the rate of reaction.[96] Heparin plasma has been documented to cause significant negative bias (up to 30%) in cardiac troponin measurement with different earlier-generation troponin assays by several major manufacturers.[223,224] The observed bias did not correlate with the

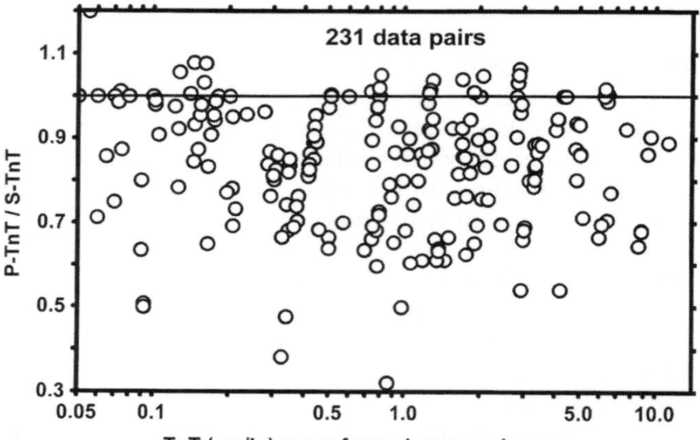

FIGURE 5.10 Differences (ratio) in the concentration of cardiac troponin T (cTnT) in plasma versus serum (P-TnT/S-TnT) relative to the average troponin concentrations in plasma and serum (log transformed and presented as natural logarithm). (From Gerhardt W, Nordin G, Herbert AK, Burzell BL, Isaksson A, Gustavsson E, et al. Troponin T and I assays show decreased concentrations in heparin plasma compared with serum: Lower recoveries in early than in late phase of myocardial injury. *Clin Chem* 2000;46:817–21, with permission by American Association for Clinical Chemistry.)

concentration of cardiac troponin (Fig. 5.10). Heparin interference occurs due to its negative charge and its binding to positively charged troponin. Binding of heparin and troponin leads to the conformational change of troponin and affects the antibody-antigen interaction. This interference was neutralized in the fourth-generation troponin T assay by adding cationic heparin blocking agent to the assay's mixture, although in certain cases there is still poor comparability between serum and plasma values.[225] For this reason, it is essential that the sample type for troponin testing remain consistent for a given patient.[226]

Ethylenediamine tetraacetic acid (EDTA) is a commonly used additive, especially in hematology and endocrinology, because it offers increased stability of cells and analytes.[227] Most hormones (except ACTH) are stable for up to 5 days in EDTA plasma if they are kept refrigerated at 4°C.[228] The main action of EDTA is chelation of cations (eg, calcium, magnesium, and zinc). If EDTA is present in higher concentrations in the sample (when tubes are underfilled), its chelating activity is enhanced. This may lead to interferences in some chemiluminescence immunoassays that use conjugated alkaline phosphatase as a secondary enzyme in their reactions. For example, it has been shown that underfilling the EDTA tubes by half or more causes clinically significant bias (the reported concentration was <75% of the true value) in the measurement of intact parathyroid hormone with the DPC IMMULITE assay.[229]

Potassium oxalate also acts as calcium chelating anticoagulant and is often combined with antiglycolytic agents (sodium fluoride and sodium iodoacetate). As with EDTA, oxalate can also inhibit some enzymes (eg, amylase, lactate dehydrogenase, alkaline phosphatase) by chelating bivalent cations that are necessary for their activity.[97]

Interferences in Immunoassays Caused by Hemolysis, Lipemia, and Icterus

As previously described, hemolysis interferes with a wide range of immunochemistry assays through the proteolytic action of cathepsin E, a major proteolytic enzyme in mature erythrocytes. Increased lipid concentration and consequent sample turbidity may affect some immunochemistry assays by affecting the light scatter pattern or by masking the binding sites on antigens and antibodies and thus physically interfering with antigen–antibody binding.

Formation of Fibrin Clots

Under optimal clotting conditions, serum is considered to be free of fibrin, fibrinogen, and cells, and it is a preferred matrix for the most immunoassays. To allow complete clot formation, serum tubes should be allowed to clot for a minimum of 30 minutes. This delay due to clotting time is a major shortcoming of the serum, especially in emergency settings. However, with new tube types containing clot activators (thrombin-based clotting agent), serum clotting time is substantially reduced (on average <2.5 minutes) without compromising the sample quality and stability for most chemistry analytes.[230,231]

Blood from patients who are receiving heparin therapy may require a longer time to completely clot, and there is a greater likelihood for latent postcentrifugation clot formation. Insoluble fibrin has been found in both serum and plasma.[232,233,234,235] Insoluble fibrin, fibrin strands, and microclots as a result of delayed and latent clotting may affect instrument performance and cause interferences. Some analyzers have the ability to detect clots and flag such samples for rerun, but if this feature is not available on the instrument being used, clots may interfere with assay measurements and cause erroneous results and unnecessary delays.

If fibrin is aspirated for analysis and goes undetected, there is a high likelihood of getting false-positive results for that sample.[232] This is manifested by duplicate measurement errors (ie, unacceptable deviations in two measurements on the same sample). The false-positive result is caused by the nonspecific binding by insoluble fibrin strands present in the sample. Duplicate errors due to latent clotting or incomplete fibrin removal during centrifugation have been repeatedly reported for cardiac troponin measurements (Fig. 5.11), and laboratories have been implementing different strategies to minimize the risk of reporting erroneous troponin results due to fibrin clots.[236] A possible approach is to recentrifuge all positive troponin samples (eg, cTnI concentration >0.1 mg/L, measured on DxI 800 analyzer, Beckman Coulter) at a high speed (6700 g for 5 min) and then repeat the analysis.[236,237] This approach, however, has been questioned by some authors and is not widely implemented.[238] Another approach employs a reflex rule to analyze samples in duplicate whenever the result is below or above some predefined value (eg, cTnI concentration <0.04 or >5.00 μg/L). If a reflex measurement exceeds the limits of acceptance (>20%), an aliquot is recentrifuged and the sample is reanalyzed.[232]

Obviously, neither serum nor plasma has sufficient quality for certain sensitive analyses, such as cardiac troponins. Also, many instruments cannot consistently detect and appropriately respond to samples of questionable quality due to residual and latent fibrin strands. Until the quality of blood collection systems and instrument performance is improved, laboratory professionals must stringently monitor reported results and implement corrective strategies to minimize the risk of such preanalytical errors.

Interference Caused by Separator Gels

Separator gels are used to ensure rapid and prolonged separation of serum/plasma from clotted blood and cells, respectively. Separation of the sample is enabled due to the specific gravity of the gel (1.03–1.06), its ability to undergo a temporary change in viscosity during centrifugation, and its ability to lodge between the packed cells and the top serum/plasma layer.[97]

Hydrophobic compounds may bind to the gel, which is why tubes containing separator gels are not appropriate for some hydrophobic drugs and hormones such as the following:[240,241,242,243]

1. Drugs: phenytoin, phenobarbitol, carbamazepine, tricyclic antidepressants, quinidine, lidocaine
2. Hormones: testosterone, estradiol, cortisol, free thyroxine, total triiodothyronine

Due to differences in the gel composition among different manufacturers, it is quite possible that one manufacturer's gel tube may be used for a particular analyte but another manufacturer's may not.

Moreover, if kept under improper storage conditions (time and temperature), the gel may degrade and release small particles or globules into the supernatant. These particles may affect instrument performance by interfering with the sample probe, coating the inner surface of the reaction cuvettes, and causing interference in immunoassays.[96] It is therefore important to strictly follow recommendations provided by the tube manufacturers on the appropriate storage and handling of gel tubes.

Interference Caused by Sample Carryover

Sample carryover in automated analyzers occurs due to the inefficient probe and cuvette washing and subsequent inability of an instrument to successfully remove any remnants of the sample or reagent. Due to improper washing, a certain amount of reagent or analyte can be transferred (carried) by the measuring system from one assay reaction

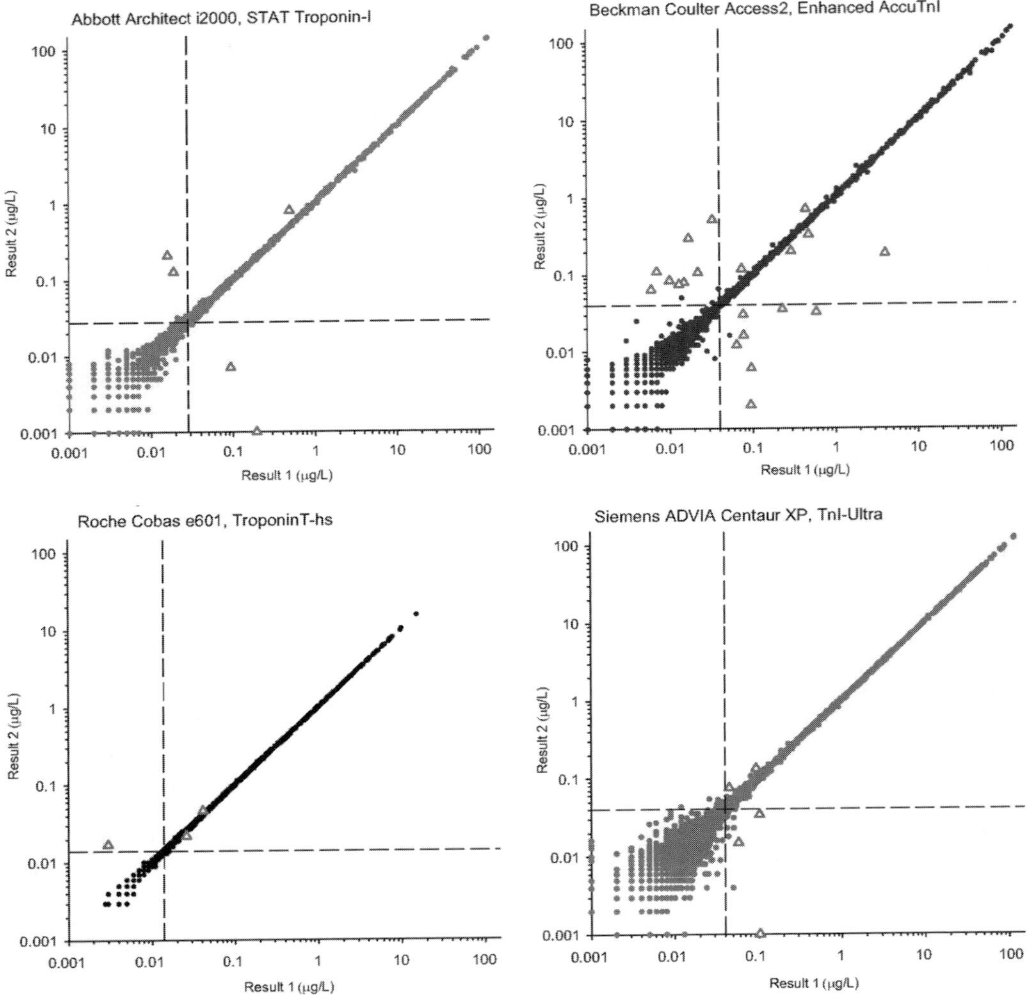

FIGURE 5.11 Distribution of duplicate results for cardiac troponin measurement on four analyzers for a series of duplicate measurements in 2391 patient sera. Samples were analyzed with (1) Abbott Architect i2000SR analytical system with STAT Troponin-I reagent (Abbott Diagnostics); (2) Beckman Coulter Access2 analyzer with Enhanced AccuTnI reagent; (3) Roche Cobas e601 with TroponinT hs reagent (Roche Diagnostics); and (4) Siemens ADVIA Centaur XP with TnI-Ultra reagent (Siemens Healthcare Diagnostics). Dashed line marks the 99th percentile, as declared by the manufacturer. Red triangles represent outliers. (From[239] Pretorius CJ, Dimeski G, O'Rourke PK, Marquart L, Tyack SA, Wilgen U, Ungerer JP. Outliers as a cause of false cardiac troponin results: Investigating the robustness of four contemporary assays. *Clin Chem* 2011;57:710–8, with permission by American Association for Clinical Chemistry.)

to a subsequent reaction, thereby erroneously affecting test results. Those instruments that do not use disposable probes are more susceptible to carryover problems with some highly sensitive assays. Carryover is, of course, not unique to immunoassays and may occur in all assay types. Nevertheless, the effect of carryover is more pronounced in sensitive assays, such as highly sensitive immunoassays.

Sample carryover has been reported for the Enzymun-Test carcinoembryonic antigen (CEA) assay on the ES-300 automated immunochemistry instrument (Boehringer-Mannheim, Germany).[244] Carryover was observed in samples being tested subsequent to the sample with extremely high CEA concentrations.

Though not confirmed by all authors,[245] sample carryover as a cause of faulty results was also reported for cTnI on Beckman Access 2, UniCel DxI600, and UniCel DxI800 immunochemistry analyzers (Beckman Coulter, Inc., Brea, Calif.). Specimens with extremely high troponin concentrations have been causing false elevations that resulted in clinically significant changes in subsequent patients tested for cTnI.[246,247] To mitigate this problem, a reflex rule may be implemented to reanalyze cTnI in two subsequent specimens. Also, additional probe and cuvette washing may be performed after the extremely elevated results with an increased risk for carryover.

Finally, it is highly recommended that laboratories perform testing for interferences due to sample carryover where evidence for the absence of an analyte is of clinical importance (ie, at the limit of quantification), such as cardiac markers, tumor markers, and infectious disease (eg, hepatitis) markers.

According to International Union of Pure and Applied Chemistry (IUPAC), sample carryover testing is performed

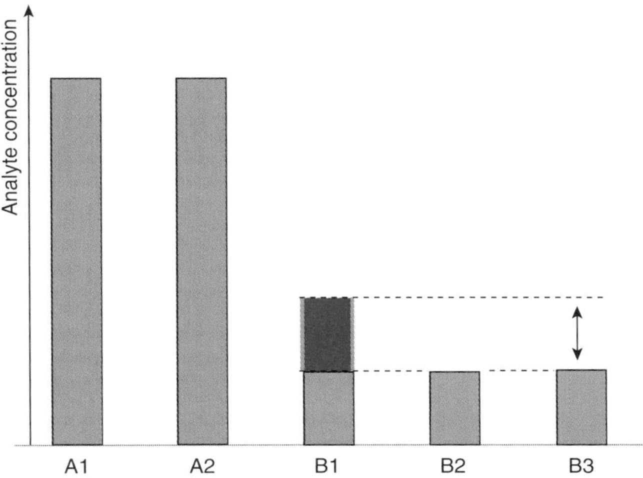

FIGURE 5.12 Carryover analysis. Samples A1 and A2 Have a high concentration of an analyte. Samples B1, B2, and B3 have a low concentration of the same analyte. The red rectangle depicts the amount of an analyte transferred from sample A2 to sample B1.

by running one sample with high concentration of an analyte at least two times, followed by at least three runs of a sample with low concentration of that analyte.[248] If the instrument probe washing procedure is not done correctly, the results in the sample with low analyte concentration will be higher, and subsequent results will show a gradually decreasing pattern. The performance of the cuvette washing procedure is somewhat more difficult to assess because it may require multiple runs of a sample with high and low analyte concentrations (the exact number of runs depends on the number of cuvettes).[124]

According to CLSI, carryover testing for immunoassays is done by running four consecutive analyses of two samples at different levels (samples with extremely high analyte concentrations (A), followed by samples with very low (B) concentrations for the same analyte).[249] The order of samples may be as follows:

A1, A2, A3, A4, B1, B2, B3, B4

According to the IUPAC protocol, carryover is expressed as the amount of analyte transferred from sample A2 to sample B1 (Fig. 5.12), and it may be calculated as follows:[248]

$$\text{Carryover, \%} = 100 \times (\text{B1} - \text{B3})/(\text{A2} - \text{B3})$$

Interferences Caused by Paraproteins

Paraprotein interferences are not uncommon. The frequency of paraprotein interference has been estimated to be as high as 3% or 4% in hospitals,[250] and it has been reported to affect numerous laboratory assays (Table 5.5). Laboratory staff should carefully review every case in which a measured concentration of an analyte does not correlate with the clinical condition of the patient after all potential sources of errors have been investigated.

Paraprotein interferences have been observed on different analytical instruments, and they appear to be methodology and concentration dependent. They affect not only turbidimetry and nephelometry but also some common chemistry assays with spectrophotometric detection. The likelihood of paraprotein-caused interferences increases with an increasing paraprotein concentration.[263]

TABLE 5.5. Paraprotein Interference With Different Assays

Group of Analytes	Molecule
Enzymes	Alkaline phosphatase[251]
	Gamma-glutamyl transferase[252]
	Lactate dehydrogenase[251]
Electrolytes, minerals, and microelements	Calcium[253]
	Inorganic phosphorus[254,255,256,257,258]
	Iron[259]
Metabolites	Bilirubin[260,261,262,263]
	Cholesterol[260,264,265]
	Creatinine[264]
	Glucose[252]
	Urea[266]
	Uric acid[251]
Proteins	C-reactive protein[264,267,268]
	IgA, IgG[269]
Hormones	Thyroid-stimulating hormone[270,271]
	Human chorionic gonadotropin[270]
Drugs	Gentamicin[272]
	Vancomycin[272,273,274,275]
	Valproic acid[272]
	Phenytoin[276]
Cardiac markers	Troponin I[270]
Tumor markers	α-fetoprotein[270]
	CA-125[270]

Mechanisms of Paraprotein Interference. Paraprotein interference may affect chemistry assays through several distinct mechanisms, including precipitation, volume displacement, and change of sample viscosity.

Precipitation of the Paraprotein. Paraprotein interference has been reported in a 93-year-old female with severe dementia who presented with cellulitis on the leg and sepsis. Gentamicin was not measurable due to the paraprotein interference caused by the IgM monoclonal protein.[272] The IgM concentration was 18.9 g/L (reference interval: 0.4–2.3 g/L). Paraprotein interference was observed on a Beckman DxC600 general chemistry analyzer with a particle-enhanced turbidimetric inhibition immunoassay method (Beckman Coulter, Brea, Calif.), and it was a result of the persistent high blank absorbance readings. Gentamicin concentration for that patient was successfully measured (3.3 mg/L) on a Roche Cobas system (Roche Diagnostics, Mannheim, Germany) where interference was not present.

Paraprotein interference can be detected by reviewing the reaction curve on the instrument for that specific patient. The reaction curve for the sample without interference shows that precipitation of the gentamicin occurs when precipitating reagent is added to the reaction mixture. The reaction curve for the sample affected by the paraprotein interference showed that IgM precipitation occurs in the blanking phase even before precipitating reagent is added to the reaction mixture. This phenomenon was also observed in a sample that was diluted with a normal saline with a ratio of 1:20

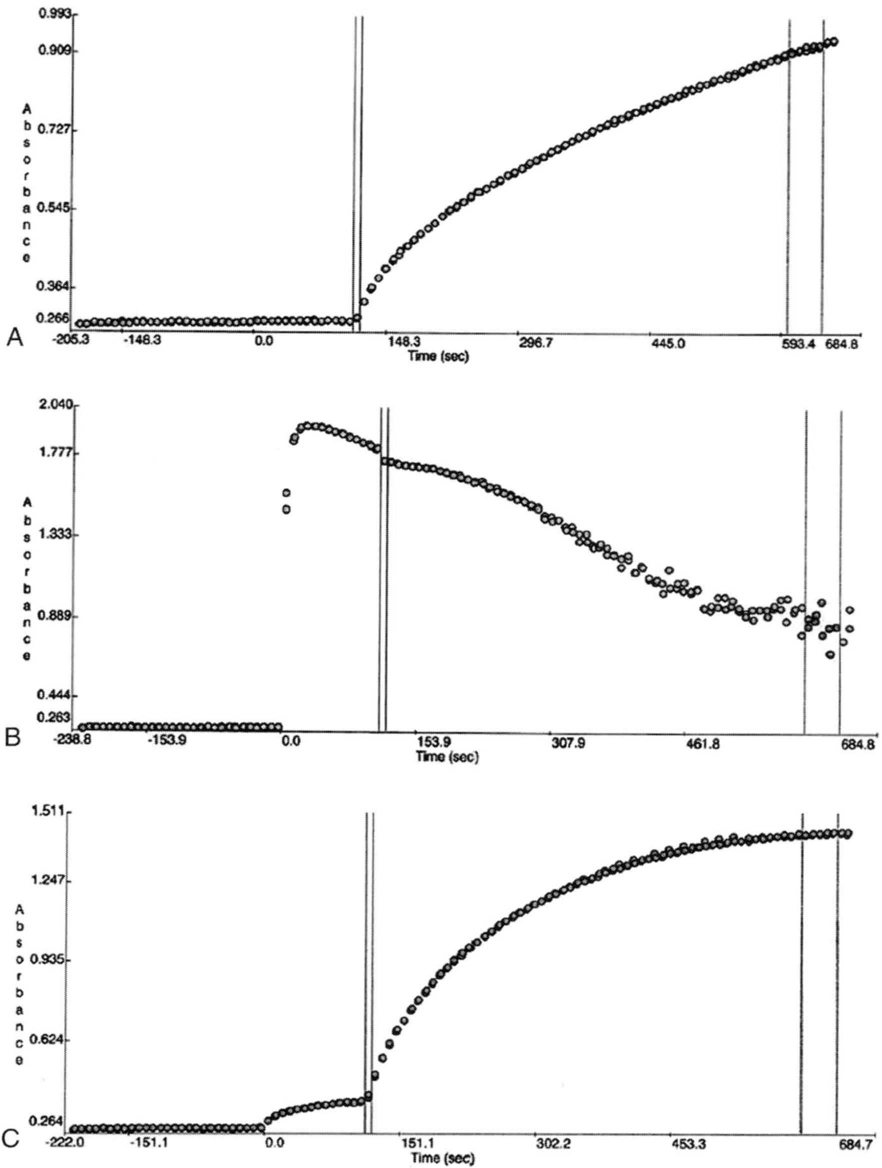

FIGURE 5.13 Reaction curve for the gentamicin particle–enhanced turbidimetric inhibition immunoassay method on the Beckman DxC600 general chemistry analyzer in a patient in whom gentamicin was not measurable due to the paraprotein interference caused by the IgM monoclonal protein. **A,** Precipitation of the analyte occurs when precipitating reagent is added to the reaction mixture. The reaction curve for the sample is affected by the paraprotein interference (IgM). **B,** Precipitation of the analyte occurs in the blanking phase (unexpectedly high blank absorbance readings), even before the precipitating reagent is added to the reaction mixture. **C,** The change in the reaction curve is visible even in a sample that has been diluted with a normal saline in a ratio of 1 : 20. (From Dimeski G, Bassett K, Brown N. Paraprotein interference with turbidimetric gentamicin assay. *Biochem Med* 2015;25:117–24, with permission by the Croatian Society of Medical Biochemistry and Laboratory Medicine.)

(Fig. 5.13A–C). The manufacturer's instructions for the gentamicin assay states that there is no interference by IgM up to 5 g/L. However, IgM concentration in this patient was fourfold higher.

Precipitation depends on various assay parameters, such as reaction components, presence of assay additives such as preservatives and surfactants, ionic strength, pH (protein precipitation can occur at both very low and very high pH), and the physicochemical characteristics of the paraprotein. This explains why some assays are affected and others are not by the same paraprotein on the same instrument.

Monoclonal proteins have been reported to appear in serum with a concentration of up to 104.1 g/L.[262] Manufacturers should improve the way they test and report data from interference studies. Paraprotein interference should be studied in the whole range of expected concentrations of paraproteins.

Laboratories must carefully read the declarations provided by manufacturers and perform their own interference studies to verify the absence or presence of paraprotein interference.

Paraprotein interference may vary according to the type of specimen or the choice of anticoagulant in specimen tubes. For example, IgM interfered with a hexokinase method for glucose and a Szasz method for gamma-glutamyltransferase (GGT) using reagents on Hitachi Modular D and P systems (Roche Diagnostics GmbH).[252] Glucose in lithium heparin plasma was extremely low in that patient, but the interference was not present in serum tubes. Moreover, the interference was absent when glucose and GGT were tested with dry-chemistry on a Vitros 950 analyzer (Ortho Clinical Diagnostics). Precipitation of a paraprotein has occurred due to fibrinogen precipitation resulting from the action of heparin. In this case, the best solution is to request a serum sample for that patient or run the tests affected by the interference using a different method.

Precipitation of paraprotein may occur due to the reaction of paraprotein and the solubilizing agent in the reagent for the measurement of the concentration for total bilirubin. This mechanism of paraprotein interference has been reported to affect bilirubin measurement by Hitachi Modular P random access autoanalyzer using Roche test kits (Roche Diagnostics GmbH). Such interference leads to a false increase of bilirubin concentration in serum with otherwise normal (anicteric) appearance and in the absence of hemolysis or lipemia and while direct bilirubin measurement is normal.[262,277]

Binding of Paraprotein to Assay Components. Paraproteins may bind to the analyte or any other component of the reaction mixture. The effect of such interference depends on the component to which the paraprotein is bound. Binding of an IgM paraprotein to latex particles resulted in high CRP and antistreptolysin O (ASO) values in a young Japanese female myeloma patient.[268] The IgM concentration was grossly elevated at 70.0 g/L (reference interval: 1.31–2.83 g/L). Concentrations of CRP, ASO, IgG, IgA, and IgM were measured by a Behring nephelometer II automated analyzer (Behringwerke AG, Marburg, Germany) that used latex particles coated with anti-CRP rabbit antibody, streptolysin-O antigen, and anti-human IgG, IgA, and IgM rabbit antibody (Behringwerke AG), respectively. When measured with another method, CRP and ASO concentrations were within the reference interval.

This kind of interference does not cause sample turbidity. Reaction kinetics for the unaffected sample and a sample with an interferring paraprotein are very similar, and therefore this type of interference cannot be detected by reviewing the reaction curve on the instrument (Fig. 5.14).[278]

Paraprotein Interference Due to Volume Displacement. Paraproteins affect chemistry assays by the same mechanism as lipemia—that is, due to the volume displacement effect. Most pronounced are changes in serum electrolytes and especially in serum sodium measurement by indirect ion-selective technology (ISE). A high concentration of paraproteins leads to false hyponatremia if sodium is measured by indirect ISE. As a general rule, in samples with total protein concentration greater than 100 g/L or less than 40 g/L, electrolytes (and especially sodium) should be measured by direct ISE technology.[279,280] Otherwise, clinically significant bias is possible that may lead to adverse patient outcomes.

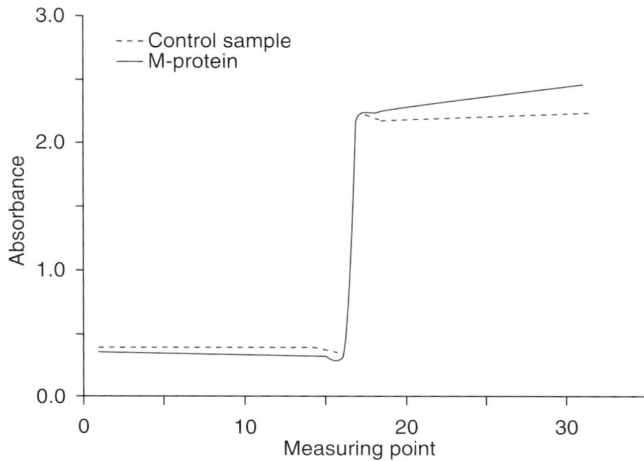

FIGURE 5.14 An example of IgM (7.45 g/L) paraprotein interference with measurement of ferritin concentration on the Roche/Hitachi 911 analyzer, caused by binding of the paraprotein to the components of the reaction mixture. The ferritin concentration was 492 mg/L on the Roche/Hitachi 911 analyzer and six times lower (80 mg/L) when measured with a different assay on another instrument. (From Bakker AJ, Mücke M. Gammopathy interference in clinical chemistry assays: Mechanisms, detection and prevention. *Clin Chem Lab Med* 2007;45:1240–43, with permission by Walter de Gruyter.)

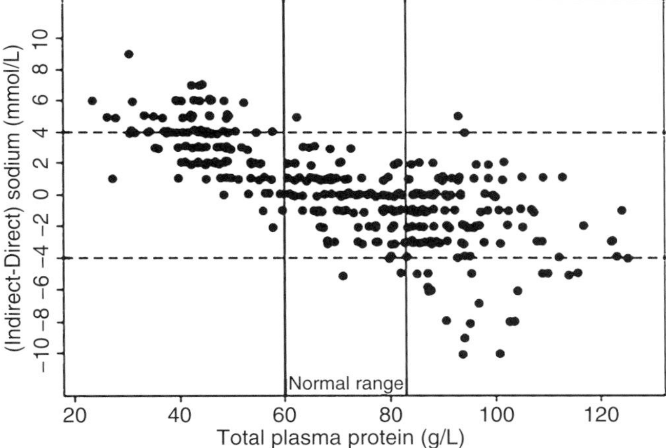

FIGURE 5.15 The association of the difference between direct and indirect ISE measurement of plasma sodium relative to plasma protein concentration. Vertical lines demonstrate the reference interval for total plasma protein. Dashed line shows disagreement of 4 mmol/L or greater in sodium measurements. (From Dimeski G, Morgan TJ, Presneill JJ, Venkatesh B. Disagreement between ion selective electrode direct and indirect sodium measurements: Estimation of the problem in a tertiary referral hospital. *J Crit Care* 2012;27:326.e9–16, with permission from Elsevier.)

The concentration of plasma sodium, measured by indirect ISE methods, is inversely proportional to the concentration of plasma proteins. The greater the concentration of plasma proteins, the lower the concentration of plasma sodium (Fig. 5.15).

Paraprotein Interference Due to Change in Sample Viscosity. Paraproteins may exert their interference simply by affecting the viscosity of the sample. Viscosity is much higher in samples with very high paraprotein concentration or in refrigerated samples in which a gel has been formed (eg, in the case of cryoglobulinemia).[278] Sample viscosity affects the volume of the sample pipetted in the reaction mixture. Many instruments are able to detect such changes in sample viscosity and trigger an alarm if viscosity is not within predefined limits. In such cases, a rerun in a dilution mode is the recommended corrective action, provided the analyte can be accurately measured in the diluted specimen. In instruments where this feature is not available, increased sample viscosity may lead to incorrect sample volume and cause falsely elevated or decreased results, depending on the assay format.

Paraprotein Interference. Laboratories can put safeguards in place to automatically detect interference caused by paraproteins:

- Have the instrument sound an alarm if the difference in absorbance between selected points is unexpectedly greater than some predetermined value.[260]
- In cases of interference of paraproteins on bilirubin concentration, have the instrument flag the results for confirmation when the bilirubin concentration in a sample is higher than some predetermined value and the icterus index is normal.[250]
- Have the instrument flag and block all test results that are preceded by a minus sign.[263]
- Have the instrument block all test results for patients who have erroneous results, such as higher direct bilirubin than total bilirubin or higher albumin than total proteins.

Hopefully, future chemistry analyzers will be able to monitor analytical reactions in real time and automatically screen for potential interferences similarly to the detection of serum indices.

Laboratories may also apply various approaches to eliminate paraprotein interference:[124]

- Samples can be analyzed on an alternative instrument with a different method.
- Proteins in the sample can be precipitated by a blocking agent, ethanol, ammonium sulphate, or polyethyleneglycol, while the analyte of interest remains in the supernatant.
- Serial dilutions of the sample may be performed.
- The sample can be filtered to remove the proteins.

SPECIFIC CONSIDERATIONS

Besides the general features of preanalytical quality (ie, patient and sample identification, controllable and noncontrollable variables), some specific aspects related to urine, saliva, and blood gas testing are of particular relevance to laboratory medicine. The following sections examine the preanalytical aspects sample types other than serum and plasma, and other types of testing that deserve special preanalytical considerations.

Influences and Interferences in Urine Testing

Urine composition is usually more variable and exhibits a broader reference interval compared to plasma.[281] Fluid intake, eating, starvation, and muscular activity all influence the excreted amounts of urine constituents. Immobilization has also been shown to affect calcium excretion.[282] Calcium excretion increased 2.5-fold over 6 weeks of immobilization, reflecting bone degradation, and returned to normal when the patient was remobilized.[39] Some of the most important preanalytical issues in the analysis of urine are patient preparation, choice of urine type, type of collection vessel, sample stability during transport and storage, sample homogeneity, and sample contamination.[283,284] These aspects are covered below.

TABLE 5.6 Urine Specimens and Their Diagnostic Use

Urine Type	Use
First morning urine	Urine sediment, test strip
Second morning urine	Proteins, urinalysis
Timed urine (6–24 h)	Hormones, drugs
First void urine	Chlamydia
Midstream urine	Urinalysis, microbiological examination
Urine obtained through a catheter or sterile suprapubic aspiration	Exclusion and confirmation of urinary tract infection

Types of Urine

Not every urine sample is suitable for every type of laboratory testing. Whereas some samples are well suited for hormone or drug testing, other types are appropriate for microbiological examinations. The possible types of urine samples and their intended uses are described in Table 5.6.

When collecting urine specimens, to prevent contamination with bacteria that normally reside on the skin, hygiene of the hands and genitalia is essential. Hands should be washed with soap, thoroughly rinsed with water, and dried. The positive predictive value of urinalysis for urinary tract infection is significantly higher and the contamination rate is much lower in urine specimens collected after proper hand and genital hygiene.[285] Thorough rinsing is also extremely important because baby soaps, for example, are known to cause significant interference with tetrahydrocannabinol (THC) immunoassays.[286] To prevent sample contamination by skin microorganisms, it is very important not to touch the inner surface of the cap and the container during collection. Urine should be collected while holding the skin folds (labia) apart (females) or retracting the foreskin (uncircumcised men) during voiding.

First morning urine (also called "overnight" or "early morning" specimen) is collected immediately after arising from bed. In the cases of patients who suffer from insomnia or work the night shift, another 8-hour period can be used for first morning urine collection. It is important that the patient's bladder is emptied immediately before going to sleep and that any amount of urine voided during the night is also collected and added to the first morning voided specimen.[287]

Timed urine specimens are collected at a specified time or in relation to some activity (before a meal, after a meal, before therapy, after exercise, etc.) during the 24-hour period. The exact time of the collection should always be reported with a test report.

First void urine comprises the first portion of the urine (usually the first 15–50 mL) voided at any time of the day. It

TABLE 5.7 Stability of Urine Particles at Different Storage Conditions (Temperatures)

Particle	−20°C	4–8°C	20–25°C
Red blood cell	NA	1 to 4 h	1 to 24 h (>300 mOsmol/kg)
White blood cell	NA	1 to 4 h	1 h (ph >7.5) to 24 h (ph <6.5)
Acanthocytes	NA	2 days	1 day (>300 mOsmol/kg)
Casts	Not allowed	NA	2 days
Bacteria	NA	24 h	1 to 2 h
Epithelial cells	NA	NA	3 h

NA, Data not available.
From Delanghe J, Speeckaert M. Preanalytical requirements of urinalysis. *Biochemia Medica* 2014;24:89–104, with permission by Croatian Society of Medical Biochemistry and Laboratory Medicine.

is collected after a patient has not urinated for at least 1 to 2 hours. The exact time depends on the sensitivity of the actual test method and is usually designated on the method insert sheet.

Midstream urine (also called a "clean catch specimen") is a urine specimen collected during the middle of a urine flow after the urinary opening has been carefully cleaned. The first few drops of urine should go into the toilet. This prevents contamination with skin, vaginal, or urethral cells and bacteria. The midstream of the urine is collected, and once the container is filled, the rest of urine is voided into the toilet until the bladder is empty.

Suprapubic aspiration and catheterization are procedures that are usually applied for bacteriologic studies to obtain uncontaminated bladder urine. A catheter specimen is collected after inserting a catheter into the bladder through the urethra. A suprapubic specimen is collected by aspirating urine from the distended bladder through the abdominal wall. Both collection methods use sterile techniques and serve as an alternative to traditional methods of obtaining urine due to their high sensitivity and low risk of contamination.

Patient Preparation and Sampling

European Urinalysis Guidelines provide recommendations on the proper patient preparation and sampling techniques to ensure the most accurate and reliable test results.[288] It is the responsibility of the laboratory to explain to a patient why a urine specimen needs to be collected and provide correct information regarding optimal preparation and sampling procedure. Proper interpretation of laboratory reports is possible only if these conditions are fulfilled. Patients should be informed of all practical aspects of urine sampling and the possible effects of diet and fluid intake, diuresis, exercise, and other interferents.

The ideal container for any urine specimen is a wide-mouthed bottle of appropriate size. Containers should be clean, leakproof, particle-free, and preferably made of a clear, disposable material that is inert with regard to urinary constituents.[287] If the urine is to be transported, the container should have a secure lid that will not leak during transport. If the urine is to be analyzed bacteriologically, the container must be sterile.

Nonspecific adsorption of various compounds (hormones, drugs, and proteins) to container surfaces in which the samples are collected, stored, or processed can cause analyte losses and affect the accuracy of quantification methods.[289,290] This is especially significant for protein

TABLE 5.8 The Effect of Urine Storage Temperature on Chemical Constituents Examined by Urine Test Strips

Analyte	4–8°C	20–25°C
Red blood cells	1 to 3 h	4 to 8 h
White blood cells	1 day	1 day
Proteins	NA	>2 h (unstable at ph >7.5)
Glucose	2 h	<2 h
Nitrites	8 h	4 days

NA, Data not available.
From Delanghe J, Speeckaert M. Preanalytical requirements of urinalysis. *Biochemia Medica* 2014;24:89–104, with permission by Croatian Society of Medical Biochemistry and Laboratory Medicine.

analytes present in urine in low concentrations. For example, at low albumin concentrations, the adsorption of albumin to the surface of the urine container can cause a significant relative loss.[291] Analyte absorption to the vessel wall is avoided, or at least minimized, by the addition of some agents that either increase analyte solubility or minimize the interaction of analytes with the surface of a urine container.[292]

For pediatric and newborn patients, urine specimen collection bags with hypoallergenic skin adhesive should be used. First, the pubic and perineal areas should be cleaned with soap and water. Then the adhesive strip should be pressed all around the vagina or the bag fixed over the penis and the flaps pressed to the perineum.

Transport and Storage of the Sample

Because some urine parameters have limited stability in unpreserved urine, temperature and time conditions during transport and storage of urine are of utmost importance for adequate sample quality. The stability of different particles in urine (Table 5.7) and test strip parameters (Table 5.8) is limited and decreases during prolonged storage and at higher temperatures. Urine samples may be stored for up to 1 hour at room temperature and up to 4 hours if refrigerated without significant variation in the results of the physical, chemical, and morphological analyses of particles.[281,293] With prolonged storage, urine particles lyse and bacteria grow. Bacterial growth causes the increase of urine pH. The stability of urine particles is lower in urine with alkaline pH (vegetarian diet), low relative density, and low osmolality (polyuria). Also, some preservatives (eg, ethanol, polyethylene glycol, sodium fluoride, mercuric chloride, boric acid, formaldehyde- and formate-based solutions, etc.) may enhance the stability of urine particles.

As a general rule, if test strip analysis is performed within 2 to 4 hours from urine collection and urine has been kept at room temperature, preservatives for chemical constituents examined with test strips are not necessary. In unrefrigerated urine, bacterial growth may occur, leading to false-positive test strip results.

The addition of stabilizers inhibits the bacterial growth, metabolic processes, and degradation of urine analytes and particles. While the addition of some preservatives and the use of commercially available preservative tubes may be beneficial if sample transport time is more than 2 hours, it must be kept in mind that these preservatives can affect some chemical properties of the urine and particle integrity.[294] It is therefore important to select appropriate preservatives, taking into account potential effects on the analyte of interest. Table 5.9 provides data on the influence of the most common preservatives on the stability of urine particles. Data about the influence of preservatives on the stability of some chemical constituents examined by urine test strips are provided in Table 5.10.

TABLE 5.9 Stability of Urine Particles in the Most Commonly Used Urinary Preservatives

Particle	Borate + Formiate + Sorbitol	10 mL/L Formaline 0.15 mol/L NaCl	80 mL/L Ethanol + 20 g/L PEG
Red blood cell	Good	Not good	Not good
White blood cell	Very good	Very good	Very good
Casts	Good	Not good	Not good
Epithelial cells	Very good	Good	Not good
Bacteria	Very good	Very good	Good

From Delanghe J, Speeckaert M. Preanalytical requirements of urinalysis. *Biochemia Medica* 2014;24:89–104, with permission by Croatian Society of Medical Biochemistry and Laboratory Medicine.

POINTS TO REMEMBER

Urine

- The contamination rate is much lower in urine specimens collected after proper hand and genital hygiene.
- Laboratories should provide instructions to patients about reasons for urine collection, how to prepare for urine sampling (eg, effects of diet and fluid intake, diuresis, exercise, and other interferents), and how to properly collect urine.
- The stability of different analytes in urine is limited and decreases during prolonged storage and at higher temperatures.
- Preservatives like ethanol, polyethylene glycol, sodium fluoride, mercuric chloride, boric acid, and formaldehyde- and formate-based solutions may enhance the stability of urine particles.
- The addition of urine stabilizers inhibits the bacterial growth, metabolic processes, and degradation of urine analytes and particles.

Saliva

Saliva is produced by the major salivary glands (parotid, submandibular, and sublingual glands) and by oral secretion of the mucus by hundreds of minor salivary glands. The major function of saliva is to provide oral protection by lubrication, digestion, and immune response.[295] Saliva is an attractive alternative to blood because it is collected noninvasively. As a diagnostic sample, saliva offers many advantages as well as some challenges (Box 5.1). Today, saliva is increasingly used for assessing the genetic susceptibility to various conditions and for testing numerous analytes, as shown in Table 5.11.[296,297]

Types of Saliva Samples

The easiest way to collect saliva is to collect whole oral fluid (whole saliva). Whole saliva is representative of the oral milieu. However, depending on the intended aim of the sample collection and analyte to be tested, some other sample types are also possible. Various sampling techniques and devices are available. Whereas collection of whole oral fluid is an easy procedure, other sampling methods are more complicated, they require trained staff, and they are not commonly used.[298]

Whole saliva may be collected as both unstimulated and stimulated samples. Stimulation of saliva is obtained by oral

TABLE 5.10 The Influence of Preservatives on the Stability of Some Chemical Constituents Examined by Urine Test Strips

Analyte	Boric Acid	Formaldehyde	Hg Salts	Chloral Hexidine
Red blood cells	Stabilization	No stabilization	Stabilization	Limited stabilization
White blood cells	No stabilization	No stabilization	Limited stabilization	Limited stabilization
Proteins	No stabilization	Stabilization	Stabilization	Stabilization
Glucose	No stabilization	No stabilization	No stabilization	No stabilization
pH	No stabilization	No stabilization	No stabilization	No stabilization
Bacteria	Stabilization	Stabilization	Stabilization	Stabilization

From Delanghe J, Speeckaert M. Preanalytical requirements of urinalysis. *Biochemia Medica* 2014;24:89–104 with permission by Croatian Society of Medical Biochemistry and Laboratory Medicine.

movements (yawning, chewing gum) or by the use of a cotton ball soaked with citric acid. It must be noted that stimulated and unstimulated saliva are of different origins (produced by different salivary glands) and compositions (concentration of some analytes may vary) and are thus not equally suitable for all assays.[299] Unstimulated saliva is mostly produced by the submandibular glands, while stimulated saliva predominantly originates from the parotid glands.[300] Moreover, saliva stimulated by citric acid has a much lower pH (~3.0), and this may affect antigen antibody binding and interfere with immunoassays.[301]

BOX 5.1 Advantages and Challenges of Using Saliva as a Diagnostic Specimen

Advantages

- Rapid and easy collection by minimally trained individuals
- Sampling can be done by patients, at home, or outside hospital
- Multiple sample collection is possible
- Procedure is safe and painless for the patient
- Convenient in children, psychiatric patients, and stress research
- Availability
- Low cost associated with sampling (skilled staff not required)
- Convenient method for population screening programs
- Low risk of infections associated with sampling

Challenges

- Low analyte concentration
- Some analytes may be affected by circadian cycle
- Questionable recovery for some analytes
- Risk of contamination during collection
- Difficult sampling and low patient compliance (in small children)

Several commercially available devices may be used for the collection of saliva. Unstimulated whole saliva can be collected by passive drooling into a plastic vial or spitting into a collector vial. Passive drooling is considered by many to be the gold standard collection method for many analytes because it enables collection of a representative portion of saliva in the oral cavity.[302] Moreover, passive drooling is preferred over spitting because saliva collected by spitting is more likely to be contaminated with bacteria.[303]

Stimulated saliva can be obtained by adsorbing saliva with cotton balls, cotton swabs, or filter paper. Cotton is not an ideal collection material because of its unpleasant texture and because it may induce some variations in salivary immunoassays (some analytes are difficult to elute from cotton). To address this problem, some synthetic materials were made available, like inert polymers, polystyrene, rayon, and polyester.[298] Saliva is collected by placing the cotton ball in the patient's mouth. Placement of the ball or swab may vary depending on the analyte of interest. The ball is gently chewed for a couple of minutes and then placed in the vial. Saliva is obtained from the ball by centrifugation or expressed by a syringe. It must be emphasised that the composition of saliva collected by the use of various adsorbent devices may differ from the whole saliva because adsorbent devices mostly collect localized saliva. It is therefore very important to be well aware of the collection method, its characteristics, and its performance.

Saliva collection in the elderly may be challenging, mostly due to xerostomia (dry mouth), which is quite common in the geriatric population, and low compliance. Challenges characteristic to infants and small children include the following:[301]

- Irregular cycles of sleep and periods of being awake
- Frequent napping (small babies often fall asleep, even during collection),
- Residue from liquids (eg, milk in babies, juices in children) in the patient's mouth

TABLE 5.11 Suitability of Different Specimens for Downstream Analyses

	Whole Blood	Plasma	Serum	Buffy	ACP	DBS	Urine	Saliva
Chemistry		✓	✓			✓	✓	✓
Hematology	✓					✓	✓	
Coagulation		✓						
Glucose	✓	✓				✓	✓	✓
Hemoglobin A_{1c}	✓					✓		
Hormones		✓	✓			✓	✓	✓
Inflammation		✓	✓			✓	✓	✓
Cytokines			✓			✓	✓	✓
Vitamins			✓			✓		
Live cells				✓				
Proteomics		✓	✓			✓	✓	✓
Metabolomics		✓	✓			✓	✓	✓
Genomics/germline DNA	✓			✓	✓	✓	✓	✓
ccfDNA		✓					✓	✓
Transcriptomics/mRNA	✓			✓		✓	✓	✓
miRNA (circulating)		✓	✓				✓	✓

ACP, All-cell pellet; *DBS,* dried blood spot; *ccfDNA,* circulating cell-free DNA; *miRNA,* microRNA.

From Ellervik C, Vaught J. Preanalytical variables affecting the integrity of human biospecimens in biobanking. *Clin Chem* 2015;61:914–34, with permission by American Association for Clinical Chemistry.

- Food residue in an infant's mouth
- Anxiety about strangers (in children)
- Low compliance

Patient Preparation for Saliva Sampling

The laboratory is responsible for providing information to the patient about the purpose of saliva collection, as well as how to prepare for collection and how to collect saliva. Gloves should be worn during saliva collection to avoid sample contamination. Here are some important measures to minimize errors and ensure a high-quality saliva sample:

- If not otherwise decided by the requesting physician, saliva should be collected in the morning, preferably in the fasting state (the exact time of collection is important because some analytes may have diurnal variations).
- The patient should wash his or her face with water and soap and rinse it thoroughly to avoid contamination with facial creams and lotions.
- The patient should not consume alcohol 12 hours before the collection.
- The patient should not brush or floss his or her teeth at least 30 minutes before the collection.
- The patient should not have any dental work done 2 days before the collection (dental bleeding may affect test results).
- The patient should not ingest any food or drink (except water) within 30 minutes before the collection.
- The patient should not chew gum for at least 30 minutes before collection.
- Before the collection, the patient should rinse his or her mouth with water to remove any food particles. To avoid sample dilution with water, the sample should be collected 10 to 15 minutes after rinsing the mouth.

Any sample that is visibly contaminated with blood or food remnants should be rejected for analysis, and sample recollection should be requested.

Storage of Saliva

After taking the sample, the saliva should be properly stored to prevent bacterial growth and protein degradation and to maintain sample integrity. Storage recommendation depends on the intended use of the saliva and duration of storage (Table 5.12). Some additives may also be used to inhibit the protease activity and retard bacterial growth (sodium azide).[296]

TABLE 5.12 Recommendations for Different Storage Conditions for Saliva Specimens

Storage Condition	Storage Time
Room temperature	30–90 minutes
+4°C	3–6 hours
–80°C	Several months

From reference 298.

Preanalytical Aspects of Arterial Blood Gas Testing

Arterial blood gas testing requires attention for several reasons[304]:

POINTS TO REMEMBER

Saliva

- Saliva is increasingly used for assessing the genetic susceptibility to various conditions and for testing numerous analytes.
- The advantages of saliva as a diagnostic specimen are that it is inexpensive, convenient, rapid, easy, safe, and painless.
- The easiest way to collect saliva is to collect whole oral fluid (whole saliva), which is representative of the oral milieu.
- Whole saliva may be collected as either an unstimulated or a stimulated sample.
- Stimulation of saliva is obtained by oral movements (yawning, chewing gum) or by using a cotton ball soaked with citric acid.
- Stimulated and unstimulated saliva are of different origin and composition.

- Blood gas testing is commonly requested in patients with a critical, life-threatening condition or who are experiencing some unexpected deterioration. Such patients may have a serious metabolic (acute complications of diabetes mellitus, drug intoxication) or respiratory disorder (respiratory failure, sepsis, or multiorgan failure) and need immediate medical intervention.
- Arterial blood sampling is an invasive procedure associated with a risk of complications such as bruising, bleeding, infections, and arterial thrombosis.
- Arterial blood samples have very limited stability. Due to the low biological variability of many blood gas parameters, allowable total error is quite low, and even small differences in serial measurements can be clinically meaningful.

International standards are available and may serve as a good resource for standardization of preanalytical steps respective to laboratory testing for blood gases, pH analysis, and ionized calcium.[305,306,307]

Patient Condition

To ensure that test results reflect the actual condition of the patient, blood sampling should be done when a patient is in a stable, resting state. Furthermore, the exact time of the blood collection should always be recorded and reported with a test result. Any deviation from the steady state should be noted as a comment and accompany the test result in order to allow proper interpretation of the results and patient management.

Relevant patient condition determinants (at the time of blood collection) include the following:

- Patient status (resting, exercising, crying (children), anxious)
- Ventilatory setting (spontaneous breathing or assisted mechanical ventilation)
- Mode of oxygen delivery (fraction of inspired oxygen (FiO2) through nasal cannula or Ventouri mask)
- Respiratory rate (hyperventilation, hypoventilation)
- Body temperature

If the patient's condition is changing, a sufficient time should be allowed for the patient to stabilize.[308,309] For example, crying leads to a rapid decrease of oxygen saturation.[310] It has been shown that even a short walk or mild exercise may lead to a significant decrease in oxygen saturation in patients who are suffering from chronic obstructive pulmonary disease.[311] Hypoventilation and increasing body temperature are associated with an increase in ionized calcium and pCO_2 and a decrease in pH.[312] Thus if patient temperature deviates from normal body temperature, information about that should accompany the test report to allow proper interpretation of results. Although blood gas instruments offer temperature corrected values, their use is not recommended because currently data are not available to quantify the balance between oxygen delivery and oxygen demand at temperatures other than 37°C.[313] If the temperature-adjusted results are reported anyway, it is absolutely mandatory that the report be clearly labeled as such and that the uncorrected values (at 37°C) are also made available on the test report.[314]

If there has been any change in the ventilatory setting or mode of oxygen delivery, the patient should be left in a resting state to stabilize. For patients without pulmonary disease, a period of 3 to 5 minutes is usually enough to stabilize. However, in patients with pulmonary disease, this period is significantly longer. According to the CLSI C46-A2 standard for blood gas and pH analysis and related measurements, adequate time for most patients to reach a stable state following ventilatory changes is 20 to 30 minutes.[306]

Sample Type

In healthy individuals, oxygen content in arterial blood is higher than in venous blood. The composition of arterial blood is constant throughout the body, whereas the composition of venous blood largely depends on the time of blood sampling, local and global circulatory conditions, and metabolic activity of the organ or tissue from which it carries blood to the heart. The major difference between arterial and venous blood is in their oxygen content. However, other parameters (pCO_2, pH) may also vary. The differences are more pronounced in conditions associated with compromised local or global circulation. Although venous blood is the specimen of choice for most routine laboratory tests, it is not the appropriate sample choice for the assessment of oxygen content in the blood. Arterial blood collected under anaerobic conditions is therefore the only acceptable sample type for an accurate evaluation of the gas exchange function of the lungs (pO_2 and pCO_2).[314]

If arterial blood is not available (eg, neonates, small children, patients with burns) and during medical transport and prehospital critical care, a capillary sample is an acceptable alternative. Capillary blood is obtained by puncturing the dermis layer of the skin and collecting it from the capillary beds running through the subcutaneous layer of the skin. Capillary blood is therefore a mixture of unknown proportions of the blood from the smallest veins (venules) and arteries (arterioles), the capillaries, and surrounding interstitial and intracellular fluids. Due to large differences in oxygen content between arterial and capillary blood, the results obtained from a capillary sample should be interpreted with extra caution.

Whereas capillary blood, if sampled properly, may accurately reflect arterial pCO_2 and pH over a wide range of values, it unfortunately may never serve as an adequate substitute for arterial blood for accurate pO_2 measurement.[315,316] The difference in oxygen content between arterial and capillary blood is even more pronounced in hypotensive patients and in patients with an increase of arterial pO_2.[317,318] Moreover, capillary blood sampling is not recommended in patients with circulatory shock or with poorly perfused (cyanotic), infected, inflamed, swollen, or edematous tissues. Capillary blood should be collected using an arterialization technique by warming the skin to 40 to 45°C with a warm towel or by using a vasodilating cream containing, for example, methyl nicotinate or capsaicin. Arterialization increases the blood flow through the capillary beds and thus the proportion of arterial blood relative to venous blood in the capillary sample. An earlobe is better sampling site than a fingertip because the blood sampled from an arterialized earlobe better reflects arterial blood values. Arterialized earlobe capillary blood gas sampling is widely used across primary and secondary health care settings, especially in patients requiring frequent monitoring of blood gas parameters.[319] To circumvent difficulties in capillary blood collection from an earlobe and minimize room air contamination, some special devices have been designed and are currently being evaluated.[320] These devices have been primarily designed to improve medical emergency management of patients in some extreme environments (eg, space, high altitudes), but they could also become routinely used in the near future.

Anticoagulants

The recommended anticoagulant for arterial blood gas and ionized calcium testing is lyophilized balanced Li-heparin. According to the CLSI C46-A2 standard on blood gas and pH analysis and related measurements, the final heparin concentration in the sample should be 20 IU/mL blood. Because the pH of heparin is 7.0 (slightly acidic) and its pO_2 and pCO_2 values are near room air values, the excess of heparin in the sample can alter sample pH, pO_2, and pCO_2.[321]

Why Use Balanced Heparin? Heparin is traditionally used to prevent blood sample coagulation. However, heparin is negatively charged and binds various cations (eg, Ca++, Na+, K+) in a dose-dependent manner. This may cause underestimation of electrolyte concentration. To prevent such direct binding of heparin and cations from the sample, balanced heparin was introduced. The binding sites of balanced heparin are presaturated with calcium.

Why Use Lyophilized Heparin? Most commercially available dedicated syringes for arterial blood sampling contain spray-dried balanced heparin as an anticoagulant. Syringes with liquid heparin are also available. Whereas liquid heparin enables better sample mixing, it may introduce sample dilution in cases of incomplete draw. Using ordinary syringes (without heparin) and flushing them before use are strongly discouraged. Flushing the syringe with liquid heparin causes sample contamination with heparin and sample dilution, resulting in significant differences among blood gas parameters (Fig. 5.16).[322]

Sample Contamination

Sample contamination may substantially affect blood sample quality and cause significant bias. Arterial blood gas samples are most commonly contaminated with liquid heparin (discussed above), venous blood, or air bubbles. Contamination of an arterial sample with venous blood occurs if a vein is

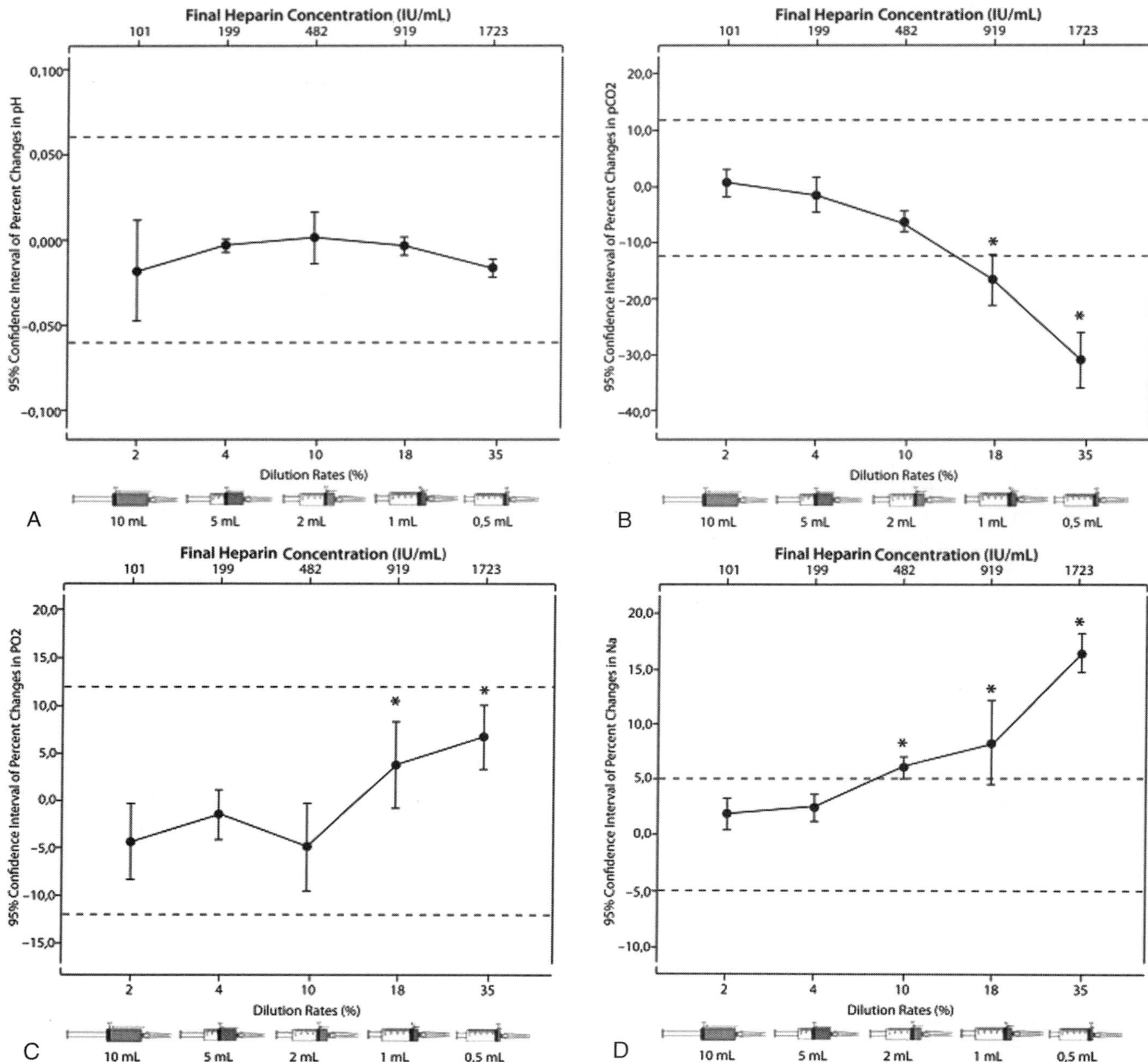

FIGURE 5.16 The changes in pH (A) and the percent changes in pCO_2 (B), pO_2 (C), Na+ (D), K+ (E), iCa+2 (F), and iMg+2 (G) at different dilutions and final heparin concentrations. The horizontal dotted line indicates the acceptable total analytical error (TEa) limits according to RiliBAK. *$P < 0.05$ for differences from the true values (full sampling done to the full volume without dilution). (From Küme T, Şişman AR, Solak A, Tuğlu B, Çinkooğlu B, Çoker C. The effects of different syringe volume, needle size and sample volume on blood gas analysis in syringes washed with heparin. *Biochem Med* 2012;22:189–201, with permission from Croatian Society of Medical Biochemistry and Laboratory Medicine.)

accidentally punctured. This may happen if the needle is not correctly positioned during arterial blood sampling. In an arterial blood sample contaminated with venous blood, pO_2 and sO_2 may be falsely decreased, while pCO_2 may be falsely elevated.

When making an arterial puncture, the needle should be inserted at a 30 to 45 degree angle. Moreover, it is also recommended that short-beveled needles be used because they are much easier to position inside the artery. Self-filling dedicated syringes are also highly recommended. These syringes fill more quickly and much easier when a needle is puncturing an artery instead of a vein as a result of the difference in blood pressure between the vein and the artery.[323]

The aspiration of air during arterial blood sampling or bubble formation can result in significant changes in the concentration of some blood gas parameters (↑pH, ↑pO_2, ↑sO_2, ↓pCO_2). The exchange between the air bubble and the arterial blood sample is rapid. It starts immediately and

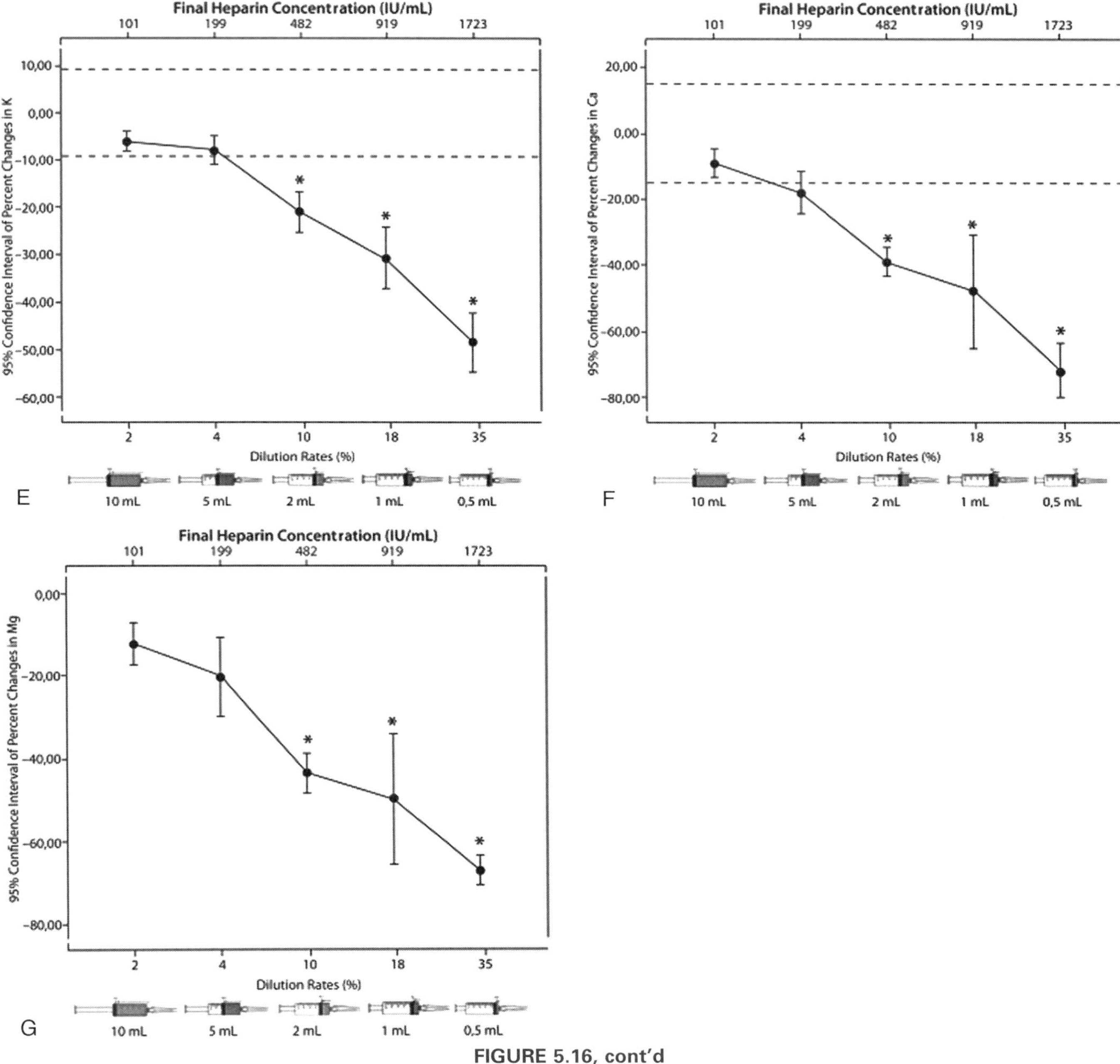

FIGURE 5.16, cont'd

becomes significant after only 1 to 2 minutes. The exchange rate does not depend on the size of the bubble.[324] The longer the delay between blood sampling and sample analysis, the greater the effect of the contamination with atmospheric air and deviation from the true patient values. It should be noted that even a bubble as small as 1% of the total sample volume may cause significant changes in the oxygen content of the specimen.

Contamination with air bubbles can be prevented by visual inspection of the specimen immediately after blood sampling. If air bubbles are present in the sample, they should be expelled as soon as possible and certainly prior to the sample mixing. If there is a visible froth in the sample, such samples should not be analyzed because froth may contain a significant amount of atmospheric air.

The degree of contamination also depends on sample agitation during transport. The increment in pO_2 in the presence of air bubbles in the sample is even more pronounced if the samples are transported by pneumatic tubes due to the exaggerated oxygen movement between the blood sample and ambient air caused by sample turbulences in the pneumatic tube.[325,326,327] Pneumatic tubes are thus not recommended for the transport of arterial blood samples.

The use of blood gas syringes with a vented mechanism is also recommended to avoid sample contamination with air. Once such a syringe has been filled up to the dedicated volume, the vent allows the air to be pushed out from the syringe. After the air has been pushed out, the vent is closed, preventing the subsequent contamination of the sample with atmospheric air.

Without milking		Milking applied	
ELECTROLYTES		ELECTROLYTES	
Na^+	140.1	Na^+	137.1
K^+	3.76	K^+	4.12
Ca^{++}	0.97 ↓	Ca^{++}	0.70 ↓
Ca^{++} (7.4)	0.99	Ca^{++} (7.4)	0.71
Cl^-	104	Cl^-	101

FIGURE 5.17 Example of the effect of excessive repetitive pressure (the so-called sample "milking") on sample hemolysis and sample contamination with tissue fluid. These two samples were obtained from the same patient in the resting state within 2 minutes. Sample without milking was obtained after an arterialization with a warm towel, while the other sample was obtained by the use of excessive finger pressure. (Laboratory data from the Clinical Institute of Chemistry, Clinical Hospital Center "Sestre milosrdcnice," Zagreb, Croatia. Data used with patient consent.)

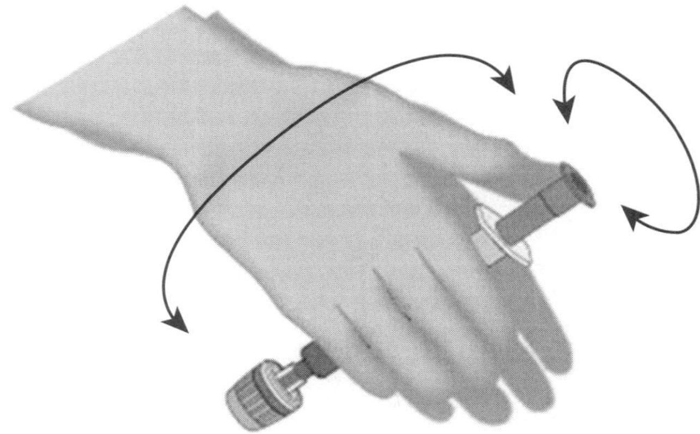

FIGURE 5.18 Manual sample mixing is done by gently inverting the syringe several times and rolling it between the palms. If manual sample mixing is not done properly, the sample is unsuitable for analysis.

Hemolysis

Sample hemolysis is another big concern related to blood gas testing. Although sample hemolysis is difficult (or almost impossible) to assess in arterial blood samples, it has been demonstrated that a significant proportion (up to 4%) of arterial blood samples are hemolyzed.[328,329] Hemolysis leads to a significant decrease in pO_2 and an increase in pCO_2.[330] Electrolyte concentrations (potassium, calcium) are also dramatically affected by hemolysis. Hemolysis can occur during sampling and due to the inadequate transport and storage conditions.

Because sample hemolysis cannot be detected in arterial blood gas samples, all necessary precautions should be taken to minimize the risk of sample hemolysis. The following conditions should be avoided to minimize the risk of hemolysis:

- Vigorous mixing. Sample mixing should be done gently.
- Any source of sample turbulence
- Pneumatic tube systems
- High force during sample aspiration
- Cooling the sample directly on ice cubes. If the sample needs to be cooled, an ice slurry should be used instead.

If capillary blood is collected, excessive pressure ("milking") should be avoided. Sample milking leads to significant hemolysis and contamination of the sample with surrounding tissue fluid. If milking is applied, many parameters in the sample will substantially deviate from the true values (Fig. 5.17). Possible difficulties during capillary blood sampling should always be recorded and reported with the test results to enable proper interpretation of test results by the clinician.

Sample Mixing

Blood samples must be properly mixed to prevent clot formation, promote heparin dissolution, and ensure that blood cells are uniformly suspended in the sample. Blood samples should be mixed immediately after the sampling but only after visible air bubbles have been expelled. Mixing should be done gently to avoid hemolysis. Samples can be mixed manually and automatically. Manual sample mixing is done by gently inverting the syringe several times and rolling it between the palms (Fig. 5.18). If manual mixing is not performed properly, the sample is unsuitable for analysis. The automatic arterial sample mixing is done with the use of a small metal ball located in the syringe barrel. The ball in the sample is moved through the sample by the force of the external magnet.

A clotted sample will cause analyzer malfunction. Moreover, if a clotted sample is analyzed, potassium concentration will be increased due to the efflux of the potassium from the platelets during blood clotting.

If the analysis is not done immediately and the sample needs to be transported to another location, the sample must be mixed again immediately prior to analysis. This is necessary to obtain a homogeneous sample and to ensure accurate test results. Mixing time depends on the time span between the sample collection and analysis. A shorter mixing time (<1 minute) is acceptable if the time span from sampling to analysis is no longer than a couple of minutes. If longer delays occur between sampling and analysis, longer mixing intervals are required. The longer the time span, the longer the mixing time required. In samples that have been left to stand for 20 to 30 minutes, the homogeneity of the samples can be achieved by continuous mixing for at least 2 minutes.[331]

Sample Transport

Arterial blood samples should be transported by hand and at room temperature. As already mentioned, vigorous movement during sample transport should be avoided. Time is a critical variable in blood gas testing. It is important to avoid delays and to analyze the sample as soon as possible. Prolonged storage prior to analysis introduces significant bias due to cell metabolism and oxygen exchange between the sample and the atmosphere. Moreover, prolonged storage may also cause spurious results due to blood sedimentation. To avoid that, samples should be visually inspected and properly mixed to homogenize the blood inside the syringe.

As a general rule, samples drawn in plastic syringes should be analyzed immediately. If analysis is delayed, the samples should be stored in glass syringes.[332] Plastic syringes should not be cooled because plastic molecules contract when cooled to 0 to 4°C. Contraction of plastic molecules creates pores in the syringe wall through which oxygen easily diffuses. Because carbon dioxide is a much larger molecule

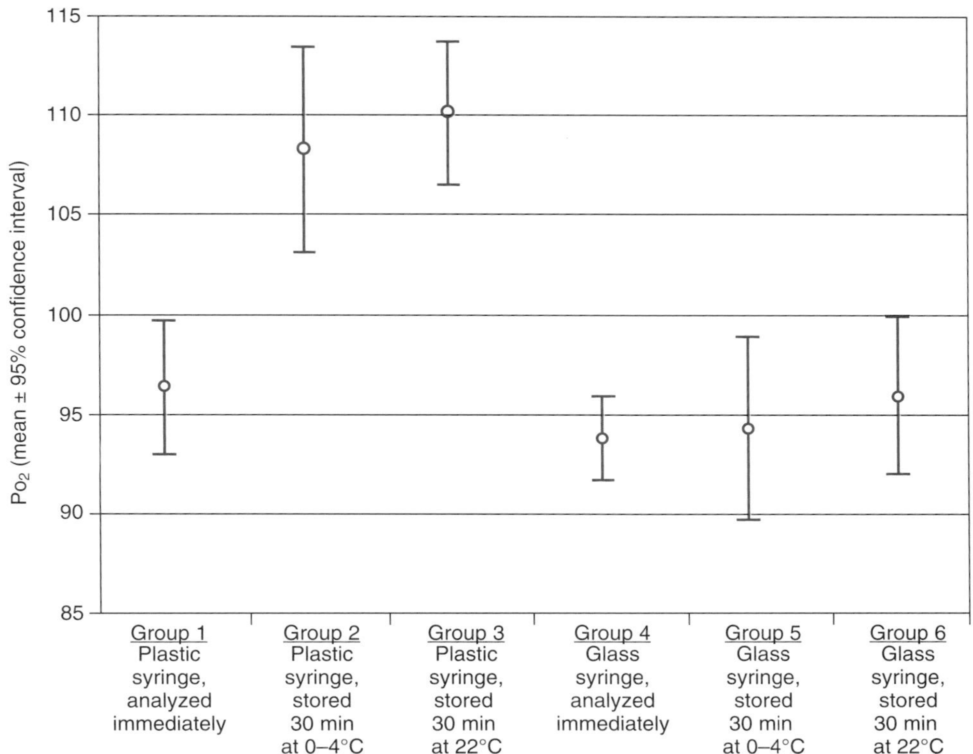

FIGURE 5.19 Plastic syringes should not be cooled because plastic molecules contract when cooled to 0 to 4°C. Contraction of plastic molecules creates pores in the syringe wall, through which oxygen easily diffuses. If samples must be cooled, glass syringes should be used to avoid the exchange of oxygen through the syringe wall. This graph shows the differences in pO_2 values in arterial blood samples stored at different temperatures for different periods of time. (From Knowles TP, Mullin RA, Hunter JA, Douce FH. Effects of syringe material, sample storage time, and temperature on blood gases and oxygen saturation in arterialized human blood samples. *Respir Care* 2006;51:732–36, with permission by Dallas, Texas: Daedalus Enterprises for the American Association for Respiratory Therapy.)

than oxygen, it cannot diffuse through the syringe wall (Fig. 5.19). The deviation in an inappropriately cooled plastic syringe is therefore greatest for oxygen and oxygen-related parameters.

According to the CLSI C46-A2 standard (blood gas and pH analysis and related measurements), samples should be transported by hand in a plastic syringe at room temperature and analyzed within 30 minutes of collection. In cases when expected delivery time is longer than 30 minutes, glass syringes should be used and the sample should be transported on ice to reduce the rate of metabolism and exchange of gases between the sample and the ambient air.[306] For more information on blood gas measurement and interpretation of results, refer to Chapter 35.

Hemostasis Testing

Some specific considerations related to hemostasis testing are associated with the type of anticoagulant, sampling technique (fasting state, length of the venous stasis, order of draw, sampling from a catether), sample handling (centrifugation), transport, and storage prior to analysis.[333,334,335] Samples for hemostasis testing should be anticoagulated with 3.2% sodium citrate, although 3.8% may also be acceptable. It is important that the same concentration of sodium citrate be used within the laboratory because clotting times may be longer in 3.8% than in 3.2% sodium citrate. Also, it has been reported that PT and APTT may be overestimated in 3.8% sodium citrate, whereas fibrinogen is underestimated compared to values obtained in 3.2% citrated samples.[336]

Mixing of samples is extremely important for adequate sample coagulation. Samples must be promptly mixed to avoid in vitro clot formation. Tubes should be mixed by gently inverting the tubes (at 180 degrees) several times. For proper mixing, instructions from the tube manufacturer should be followed. Vigorous mixing and shaking the tubes are discouraged because that may lead to sample hemolysis; the activation of platelets and coagulation factors, resulting in false shortening of clotting times; and even possibly a false increase in clotting factor activity. Transport of samples by pneumatic tubes is still under debate. While some claim that pneumatic tube transport is acceptable for the transport of coagulation samples for routine hematology and coagulation parameters,[334,337] others argue that samples transported by pneumatic tube are not suitable for platelet aggregation assays.[338] It is therefore recommended that each institution should verify the acceptability of its tube transport systems by comparing paired samples for differences.

Samples for hemostasis testing that contain visible clots should not be accepted for analysis and must be rejected. To prevent clot formation, some precautionary measures should be taken during blood sampling, handling, and transport, and the following errors should be avoided:

- Blood flow (during blood sampling) too slow
- Collection of the sample into a syringe and then transfer into a citrated tube
- Tubes underfilled
- Prolonged use of a tourniquet
- Considerable manipulation of the vein by the needle
- Incomplete mixing

Clot formation induces the activation of platelets and clotting factors, allows the release of granules from the platelets, and may cause false results in coagulation assays. It is very important to keep in mind that even small clots that are invisible to the human eye may significantly impact coagulation assays.

The required blood to anticoagulant ratio is 9 : 1, and it is therefore very important that tubes for coagulation assays be filled to the mark noted on the tube. Acceptable deviation is maximum 10% of the total volume; filling the tube over 10% (overfilling) or less than 10% (underfilling) of the designated volume is strictly discouraged because this can introduce bias into test results. Laboratories should have preanalytical procedures in place for the rejection of over- or underfilled tubes. Other anticoagulants (eg, EDTA or heparin) are not acceptable for hemostasis testing because they can lead to erroneous results and can cause clinically significant errors. For some analyses, especially platelet function assays, buffered citrate solution or other anticoagulants, such as lepirudin or synthetic inhibitors of thrombin and factor Xa are used.[339,340,341]

Longer venous stasis should be avoided because it results in hemoconcentration, activation of fibrinolysis, and other changes, such as an increase in fibrinogen and factors VII, VIII, and XII.[342] A standardized order of draw has been recommended, with the coagulation tube as the first tube and a tube drawn and discarded before the citrate tube.[343] However, more recent evidence suggests that a "discard" tube may not be necessary.[344] If intravenous catheter systems are used for blood sampling, five to six times the dead space volume of the catheter should be discarded prior to blood sampling, or the first tube should be used for other analyses. If the catheter might be contaminated with heparin due to heparin infusion or flushing with heparin-containing fluid, only laboratory tests insensitive to heparin may be undertaken.[345]

Following collection, citrated samples should ideally be transported to the laboratory immediately and at room temperature but no later than within 1 hour of blood draw.[335] Blood samples for coagulation testing must be kept at room temperature (20 to 25°C) until analysis. Storage at lower temperatures or on ice is discouraged because cold activates some coagulation factors. For example, in citrated whole blood stored in an ice bath or refrigerated (2 to 8°C), the activation of platelets, activation of factor VII, and significant time-dependent loss of both FVIII and von Willebrand factor (VWF) will occur.[335] Prothrombin time (PT) and aPTT should generally be performed using fresh plasma within 4 hours after blood sampling and stored at room temperature.[346] If the centrifuged plasma is left to sit on the blood cells, this may result in shortening of PT and prolongation of aPTT.[347] Stability data for all coagulation factors can be found in the literature.[348]

Whole blood coagulation assays should be performed within 4 hours after blood sampling. For platelet function assays, samples should rest (at room temperature) for 30 minutes before analysis. Centrifugation is normally performed at 1500 g at room temperature for 10 to 15 minutes to obtain platelet-poor plasma. Higher speeds with shorter centrifugation times are not recommended because this may induce hemolysis and activation of platelets. Moreover, centrifuge breaks should also be avoided to prevent remixing of samples.[349]

The preparation of platelet-rich plasma (PRP) for platelet function assays requires special care, and centrifugation speeds and duration need to be carefully optimized to ensure optimal results. Generally, centrifugation is performed at 200 to 250 *g* for 10 minutes without application of a rotor brake.[350,351]

If possible, all coagulation analyses should be performed using fresh material; freezing of samples should be an exception. PT and aPTT should not be performed in samples that were stored frozen because freezing results in changes, especially aPTT, and also PT. Freezing leads to a marked decrease, especially in factor VIII activity, and to an apparent increase in fibrinogen levels.[352] For more information on coagulation and platelet function tests and interpretation of results, refer to Chapter 71.

Hematology

Being of supreme efficacy for preserving cellular morphology, EDTA (ethylenediaminetetraacetic acid) is the anticoagulant of choice for hematology testing. Anticoagulant function of EDTA is exerted through its potential to chelate calcium. Because EDTA as a free acid is not water soluble, it comes as disodium, dipotassium, and tripotassium salt. Potassium EDTA salts are more soluble than sodium salts. EDTA salts cause osmotically induced cell shrinkage and swelling to a different degree. Also, pH of EDTA increases with the number of ions bound to EDTA. Whereas the pH of EDTA in a free acid form is 2.5, tripotassium EDTA has a pH of 7.5. In dipotassium and disodium EDTA, cell swelling is counteracted by cell shrinkage (due to the lower pH in dipotassium salts). Because cell shrinkage is less apparent, dipotassium EDTA salts are superior to tripotassium EDTA. Also, mean cell corpuscular volume (MCV) based on the minihematocrit values in disodium and dipotassium EDTA samples provide acceptable results, as opposed to tripotassium EDTA samples.[353] For these reasons, due to its higher solubility, lower osmotic effect, and best overall performance, the International Council for Standardization in Haematology (ICSH) recommends dipotassium EDTA salt as the anticoagulant of choice for hematology testing.[354]

Tube mixing is essential for the quality of hematology samples. Tubes need to be mixed immediately after the blood is drawn to allow proper mixing of additive with blood and to prevent sample clotting. Adequate mixing is achieved by gently inverting the tube at 180 degrees and back to the upright position. The number of turns depends on the tube type, and for optimal results, manufacturer instructions should be followed.

Blood tubes should be filled to ±10% of the stated draw volume. In underfilled EDTA tubes, cell count and hematocrit might be falsely decreased due to the excess EDTA. In overfilled tubes, clot formation and platelet clumping are likely to occur due to the difficulty of appropriate mixing.[355]

EDTA may in some individuals cause pseudothrombocytopenia—that is, platelet clumping or platelet satellitism (platelets adhering to neutrophils) and subsequently inaccurate platelet results.[356,357] Because most cell counters are not able to identify this preanalytical problem, platelets are thus counted as white blood cells, resulting in spurious leukocytosis and false thrombocytopenia. EDTA-induced pseudothrombocytopenia has so far been observed in healthy and diseased individuals and is not related to gender and age. The hypothesized mechanism in pseudothrombocytopenia involves IgM autoantibodies directed against platelet IIb/IIIa fibrinogen receptors. This is further supported by the fact that platelets from patients with Glanzmann thrombasthenia (in which platelets have either defective or low levels of glycoprotein IIb/IIIa) do not react to autoantibodies from pseudothrombocytopenic patients.[355,358]

Stability during transport and storage has been studied for a number of analytes.[359] As a general rule, the EDTA anticoagulated blood should be stored at room temperature and analyzed within 3 hours of collection. It should be noted that analyte stability may differ depending on the parameters that are being measured, instrument type, and transport and storage conditions.[360] Therefore on some occasions, a shorter time is necessary to ensure accurate and reliable results, whereas some parameters show excellent stability even over much longer time intervals. Some parameters are very stable (hemoglobin and red blood cells), while others are not (reticulocytes, mean cell volume, and hematocrit). The stability of hematological parameters is improved if samples are kept at 4°C. Here are the International Council for Standardization in Haematology data on the stability of some hematology parameters:[361]

- Hemoglobin concentration and red blood cell count are stable up to 72 hours if blood is kept at 4°C.
- Platelet and reticulocyte counts are stable for 24 to 72 hours if blood is stored at 4°C.
- WBC count with automated differential count is stable for at least 24 hours if blood is kept at 4°C and up to 6 hours at room temperature.[362]
- Peripheral blood smear should be made from blood stored not more than 3 hours at room temperature (18 to 25°C).

As already emphasized above, the stability may vary depending on the instrument. It is therefore the responsibility of the individual laboratory to verify the stability of hematological parameters on their instruments.

Antibodies may affect the cell count of erythrocytes, leukocytes, and platelets. The following antibodies are known to interfere with hematological analytes:

- Cold agglutinins (erythrocyte specific)
- Cryoglobulins
- EDTA-dependent antibodies with thrombocyte and leukocyte specificity

Cold Agglutinins

Cold agglutinins are antibodies that are specific for erythrocyte surface carbohydrate antigens, which bind to the erythrocyte surface at temperatures of 0 to 4°C. Binding of agglutinins causes agglutination of erythrocytes, induces complement activation and hemolysis, and impairs peripheral circulation.[363] Cold agglutinins may be monoclonal or polyclonal. Monoclonal agglutinins are found in patients with idiopathic forms of cold agglutinin disease or lymphoproliferative disorders, whereas polyclonal antibodies are often found in patients recovering from some infectious diseases.[364] Some rare cases of cold agglutinins toward platelets have also been described, causing pseudothrombocytopenia independent of EDTA.[365]

Cold agglutinins, if undetected, may cause diagnostic confusion and lead to subsequent extensive diagnostic workup as well as incorrect and unnecessary therapy, risking patient safety and increasing health care costs. It is therefore very important to recognize cold agglutinins promptly. Cold agglutinins should be suspected if the following anomalies are observed[365a]:

- Red blood cell count too low even at normal hemoglobin concentration
- Grossly enhanced MCV values
- Excessively low values of calculated hematocrit in samples with too high MCH and MCHC values without any obvious explanation
- Falsely elevated white blood cell count and platelet count

White blood cell and platelet counts may be falsely elevated because agglutinates, depending on their size, are counted in either the leucocyte or platelet channel. The blood smear may also show agglutination of erythrocytes. For adequate analysis of samples in which cold agglutinins are suspected, it is essential to warm up the EDTA blood sample at 37°C and analyze immediately afterward. This anomaly will appear again if a sample is kept at 4°C and analyzed while it is cold.

Cryoglobulins

Cryoglobulins are immunoglobulins with temperature-dependent solubility that precipitate at temperatures below 37°C. Cryoglobulins are often associated with infections, autoimmune disorders, and malignancies, and they can cause organ damage through immune-mediated mechanisms and vascular damage due to increased viscosity of the blood.[366] The precipitation of cryoglobulins depends on the immunoglobulin class to which they belong. Also, precipitation is absent at pH less than 5.0 or greater than 8.0.[355]

In samples kept at room temperature, cryoglobulins tend to form globular or cylindric precipitates that are then counted by automated hematological analyzers as cells, thus affecting hematological laboratory tests and leading to false leucocytosis (pseudoleucocytosis) or false thrombocytosis (pseudothrombocytosis). The degree of pseudoleucocytosis and pseudothrombocytosis depends on the time of exposure, temperature, cryoglobulin concentration, and the interaction of cryoglobulins with other plasma proteins.[367] The following indices may point to the presence of cryoglobulins:

- Very different cell counts in different investigations
- Blue sediments in differential count samples
- In a sample warmed up to 37°C, significantly lower cell counts

As in the case of cold agglutinins, for adequate analysis of samples in which cryoglobulins are suspected, blood samples should be kept warm at 37°C and analyzed immediately afterward.

MANAGEMENT OF THE QUALITY OF THE PREANALYTICAL PHASE

The ultimate goal of preanalytical quality management is not to improve the quality of the sample per se but to improve patient outcome.[156] Preanalytical quality management achieves its primary goal only if (1) the importance of preanalytical processes in the total testing process (TTP) is fully understood; (2) all sources of preanalytical variability and their effects are known; (3) patient-centered and evidence-based guidelines are available; (4) compliance with guidelines can be ensured; and (5) quality is continuously monitored and improved.[156]

Unfortunately, the preanalytical part of the TTP is not fully understood by all involved (laboratory staff, nurses, clinicians, and patients). Patients are usually not aware of the importance of proper preanalytical procedures and how improper sample collection could affect the results of requested tests.[368,369] Education is the key to the improvement of the level of understanding of the importance of the preanalytical phase.[370,371,372] However, the effects of educational interventions are usually short-lived, and education should therefore be a continuous quality improvement activity.

Outcome-Based Preanalytical Studies

Although many potential sources of variability and how they affect the quality of samples and test results are well recognized, there is little evidence demonstrating the effect of preanalytical variation on patient outcomes and how particular errors may affect health care organization and expenditure. Most studies so far have been descriptive and reported failures of processes without linking those to patient harm. Quality improvement should focus on reducing patient harm rather than just eliminating process defects and waste.[373] Original studies need to focus more on patient-relevant outcomes—for example, how some preanalytical errors, such as improper sampling, delayed transport, or hemolyzed or

TABLE 5.13 Proposed Preanalytical (Priority 1) QIs Based on a Harmonized Consensus Model

Quality Indicator	Reporting Systems
Misidentification errors	Samples suspected to be from wrong patients
	Percentage of "Number of misidentified requests/Total number of requests"
	Percentage of "Number of misidentified samples/Total number of samples"
	Percentage of "Number of samples with fewer than two identifiers initially supplied/Total number of samples"
	Percentage of "Number of unlabeled samples/Total number of samples"
Test transcription errors	Percentage of "Number of outpatient requests with erroneous data entry (test name)/Total number of outpatient requests"
	Percentage of "Number of outpatient requests with erroneous data entry (missed test)/Total number of outpatient requests"
	Percentage of "Number of outpatient requests with erroneous data entry (added test)/Total number of outpatient requests"
	Percentage of "Number of inpatient requests with erroneous data entry (test name)/Total number of inpatient requests"
	Percentage of "Number of inpatient requests with erroneous data entry (missed test)/Total number of inpatient requests"
	Percentage of "Number of inpatient requests with erroneous data entry (added test)/Total number of inpatient requests"
Incorrect sample type	Percentage of "Number of samples with wrong or inappropriate type (ie, whole blood instead of plasma)/Total number of samples"
	Percentage of "Number of samples collected in wrong containers/Total number of samples"
Incorrect fill level	Percentage of "Number of samples with insufficient sample volume/Total number of samples"
	Percentage of "Number of samples with inappropriate sample-anticoagulant volume ration/Total number of samples with anticoagulant"
Unsuitable samples for transportation and storage problems	Percentage of "Number of samples not received/Total number of samples"
	Percentage of "Number of samples not properly stored before analysis/Total number of samples"
	Percentage of "Number of samples damaged during transportation/Total number of samples"
	Percentage of "Number of samples transported at inappropriate temperature/Total number of samples"
	Percentage of "Number of samples with excessive transportation time/Total number of samples"
Contaminated samples	Percentage of "Number of contaminated samples rejected/Total number of samples"
Samples hemolyzed	Percentage of "Number of samples with free Hb >0.5 g/L/Total number of samples (clinical chemistry)"*
Samples clotted	Percentage of "Number of samples clotted/Total number of samples with an anticoagulant"

*Clinical chemistry: all samples that are analyzed on the chemistry analyzer that is used for detection of HIL indices. If laboratories are detecting hemolysis visually, they count all samples with visible hemolysis (clinical chemistry). A color chart should be provided for this purpose.

From Plebani M, Astion ML, Barth JH, Chen W, de Oliveira Galoro CA, Escuer MI, et al. Harmonization of quality indicators in laboratory medicine: a preliminary consensus. *Clin Chem Lab Med* 2014;52:951–8, with permission by Walter de Gruyter.

clotted samples, may lead to patient discomfort, additional diagnostic workup, increased length of stay (LOS) in the hospital, increased costs, disease prevalence, and so on.[374,375,376,377] Error reduction strategies should focus on those most critical errors that have the greatest potential to impact patient outcomes.

Quality Indicators

Preanalytical quality should continuously be monitored and improved. To measure the degree of improvement, quality indicators (QI) should be used. Quality indicators are measurable, objective, quantitative measures of key system elements that show to what extent a laboratory meets the needs and expectations of the customers.[378] To allow consistent and comparable use across settings over time, a unique definition is needed for QIs.[379,380,381] While different professional groups have proposed some interesting programs on the use of QI in the TTP, until very recently there was no consensus on the definition, measurement methodology, and reporting practices for QI. Recently, a harmonized model of QI has been established by an expert panel during a consensus conference in Padua in October 2013.[382] The proposed QI model is based on a patient-centered approach, and the essential prerequisites taken into account were the following:

1. Importance and applicability to a wide range of clinical laboratories worldwide
2. Scientific soundness (focused on some most important areas in laboratory medicine)
3. Definition of evidence-based thresholds for acceptable performance
4. Timeliness and possible utilization as a measure of laboratory improvement

The model proposes 22 high-priority and 6 lower-priority preanalytical QIs (Table 5.13).

QIs enable the measurement of the quality of care and services, with the aim of assisting in quality improvement efforts. Collecting data on QI per se does not automatically mean quality improvement. Laboratories should strive for a system of continuous preanalytical quality improvement based on the "plan-do-check-act" cycle and using corrective and preventive actions with subsequent system redesign. Only then can patient outcomes be improved, preanalytical errors be reduced, and waste be eliminated.

POINTS TO REMEMBER

Management of the Quality of the Preanalytical Phase

- Quality improvement should focus on how to improve patient outcomes and reduce patient harm rather than to eliminate process defects and waste.
- Original studies need to focus more on outcomes and provide evidence for the effect of preanalytical errors (eg, improper sampling, delayed transport, hemolyzed or clotted sample) on patient discomfort or harm, additional diagnostic workup, increased length of stay, increased costs, disease prevalence, and so on.
- Knowing the errors with the greatest potential to impact patient outcomes helps to prioritize error-reduction strategies and focus on the most critical errors.

SELECTED REFERENCES

For a full list of references for this chapter, please refer to ExpertConsult.com.

20. Guder WG, Narayanan S. *Pre-examination procedures in laboratory diagnostics*. Berlin: Walter de Gruyter; 2015.
73. Simundic AM, Cornes M, Grankvist K, et al. Standardization of collection requirements for fasting samples: For the Working Group on Preanalytical Phase (WG-PA) of the European Federation of Clinical Chemistry and Laboratory Medicine (EFLM). *Clin Chim Acta* 2014;**432**:33–7.
80. Adeli K, Raizman JE, Chen Y, et al. Complex biological profile of hematologic markers across pediatric, adult, and geriatric ages: Establishment of robust pediatric and adult reference intervals on the basis of the Canadian Health Measures Survey. *Clin Chem* 2015;**61**:1075–86.
89. Vecellio E, Li L, Mackay M, et al. A benchmark study of the frequency and variability of haemolysis reporting across pathology laboratories—The implications for quality use of pathology and safe and effective patient care. Report to Royal College of Pathologists Australasia. Australian Institute of Health Innovation, Macquarie University, Sydney. July 2015.
96. Bowen RA, Remaley AT. Interferences from blood collection tube components on clinical chemistry assays. *Biochem Med* 2014;**24**:31–44.
97. Bowen RA, Hortin GL, Csako G, et al. Impact of blood collection devices on clinical chemistry assays. *Clin Biochem* 2010;**43**:4–25.
104. Nijsten MWN, Dofferhoff ASM. Pseudohyperkalemia and platelet counts. *N Engl J Med* 1991;**325**:1107.
116. Nikolac N. Lipemia: Causes, interference mechanisms, detection and management. *Biochem Med* 2014;**24**:57–67.
123. Dimeski G, Jones BW. Lipaemic samples: Effective process for lipid reduction using high-speed centrifugation compared with ultracentrifugation. *Biochem Med* 2011;**21**:86–94.
124. Dimeski G. Interference testing. *Clin Biochem Rev* 2008;**29**(Suppl. 1):S43–8.
126. Saracevic A, Nikolac N, Simundic AM. The evaluation and comparison of consecutive high-speed centrifugation and LipoClear reagent for lipemia removal. *Clin Biochem* 2014;**47**:309–14.
145. Lippi G, Daves M, Mattiuzzi C. Interference of medical contrast media on laboratory testing. *Biochem Med* 2014;**24**:80–8.
150. Dolci A, Panteghini M. Harmonization of automated hemolysis index assessment and use: Is it possible? *Clin Chim Acta* 2014;**432**:38–43.
154. Nikolac N, Simundic AM, Miksa M, et al. Heterogeneity of manufacturers' declarations for lipemia interference—An urgent call for standardization. *Clin Chim Acta* 2013;**426**:33–40.
217. Dimeski G, Johnston J, Bassett K, et al. Cuvette carryover with the gentamicin assay on the Beckman AU480 analyser. *Clin Chem Lab Med* 2015;**53**:e293–95.
218. Lima-Oliveira G, Salvagno GL, Danese E, et al. Contamination of lithium heparin blood by K2-ethylenediaminetetraacetic acid (EDTA): An experimental evaluation. *Biochem Med* 2014;**24**:359–67.
219. Dodig S. Interferences in quantitative immunochemical methods. *Biochem Med* 2009;**19**:50–62.
283. Delanghe J, Speeckaert M. Preanalytical requirements of urinalysis. *Biochem Med (Zagreb)* 2014;1:89–104.

296. Nunes LA, Mussavira S, Bindhu OS. Clinical and diagnostic utility of saliva as a non-invasive diagnostic fluid: a systematic review. *Biochem Med (Zagreb)* 2015;**25**:177–92.
298. Chiappin S, Antonelli G, Gatti R, et al. Saliva specimen: a new laboratory tool for diagnostic and basic investigation. *Clin Chim Acta* 2007;**383**:30–40.
304. Baird G. Preanalytical considerations in blood gas analysis. *Biochem Med* 2013;**23**:19–27. <http://dx.doi.org/10.11613/BM.2013.005>.
314. Davis MD, Walsh BK, Sittig SE, et al. AARC clinical practice guideline: Blood gas analysis and hemoximetry: 2013. *Respir Care* 2013;**58**:1694–703.
322. Küme T, Şişman AR, Solak A, et al. The effects of different syringe volume, needle size and sample volume on blood gas analysis in syringes washed with heparin. *Biochem Med* 2012;**22**:189–201. <http://dx.doi.org/10.11613/BM.2012.022>.

6

Quality Control of the Analytical Examination Process

*W. Greg Miller and Sverre Sandberg**

ABSTRACT

Background

The purpose of a clinical laboratory test is to provide information on the pathophysiologic condition of an individual patient to assist with diagnosis, to guide or monitor therapy, or to assess risk for developing a disease or for progression of a disease. Quality control (QC) of the analytical examination process monitors a measurement procedure to verify that it meets performance specifications appropriate for patient care or that an error condition exists that must be corrected.

Content

Internal QC ensures that measurement procedures meet specifications at the time patient testing occurs. QC samples are measured at intervals along with patient samples. Recovery of the expected target values for the QC samples allows the laboratory to verify that a measurement procedure is working correctly and the results for patient samples can be released. The QC plan specifies the number of controls, the frequency they are to be measured, and the rules to determine if the QC results are consistent with expected measurement procedure performance. External QC, also called *external quality assessment (EQA)* or *proficiency testing (PT)*, is a monitoring process in which control samples are received from an independent external organization and the expected values are not known by the laboratory. The results for the EQA/PT samples are compared with results from other laboratories to verify that a laboratory's measurement procedures conform to expected performance. In addition to internal and external QC, the results from patient sample testing can be used to assess and monitor the performance of measurement procedures.

INTRODUCTION

The purpose of a clinical laboratory test is to provide information on the pathophysiologic condition of an individual patient to assist with diagnosis, to guide or monitor therapy, or to assess risk for developing a disease or for progression of a disease. Quality control (QC) of the analytical examination process monitors a measurement procedure to verify that it meets performance specifications appropriate for patient care or that an error condition exists that must be corrected. QC includes both internal and external components. Internal QC includes control procedures performed within a laboratory using surrogate samples that are intended to simulate clinical samples from patients. The QC samples are measured at intervals along with patient samples. Recovery of the expected target values for the QC samples allows the laboratory to verify that a measurement procedure is working correctly and the results for patient samples are reliable enough to be released. Note the term internal QC is more comprehensive than control processes and fluids that are "built-in" to a measurement technology or to the reagent cartridges or strips used by a measurement procedure. External QC, also called external quality assessment (EQA) or proficiency testing (PT), is a monitoring process in which surrogate samples are received from an independent external organization and the expected values are not known by the laboratory. The results for the EQA/PT samples are compared with results from other laboratories to verify that a laboratory's measurement procedures conform to expected performance. Another component of QC uses the results from patient samples as part of the QC monitoring process.

Fig. 6.1 illustrates that QC is part of a laboratory quality management system described in Chapter 3. The quality management system integrates good laboratory practices to ensure that results are suitable for use in patient care decisions. The items in red font are addressed in this chapter. Internal QC is in the process management category of the quality management system because its primary function is to ensure that measurement procedures meet specifications at the time patient testing occurs. EQA/PT is in the evaluation and audits category because its primary function is external assessment that measurement procedures conform to specifications for agreement of results among laboratories. Quality indicators are also part of the evaluation and audits category and are used to assess the performance of the QC plan and to identify opportunities for continuous quality improvement. This chapter includes recommendations for quality indicators that are useful for the QC function. Other quality management system components also influence the implementation of QC and EQA/PT but are not addressed in this chapter. In particular, written standard operating procedures

*Some of this material was previously published in McPherson RA and Pincus MR, editors. *Henry's clinical diagnosis and management by laboratory methods.* 23rd ed. St. Louis: Elsevier; 2016.

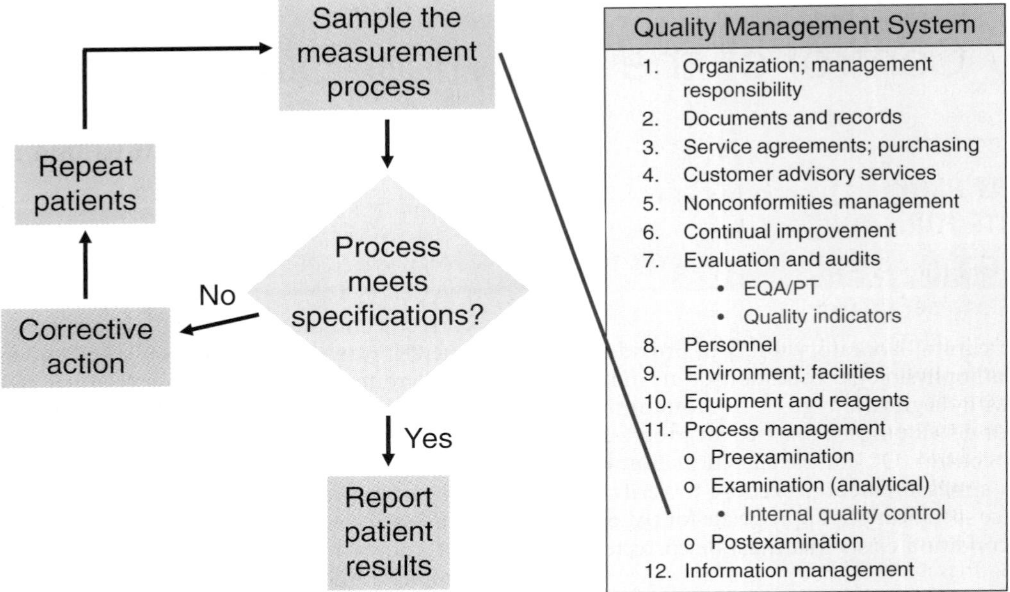

FIGURE 6.1 Overview of internal statistical quality control and its integration into a quality management system. The topics in *red font* are addressed in this chapter. *EQA,* External quality assessment; *PT,* proficiency testing.

(SOPs) are required for the QC plan and should include instructions for all aspects of the QC program as described in this chapter, as well as who is responsible for the various QC activities and who is authorized to approve and to make changes to the QC program.

As illustrated in Fig. 6.1, internal QC evaluates a measurement procedure by periodically measuring a QC sample for which the expected result is known in advance. If the result for a QC material is within acceptable limits of the known value, the measurement procedure is verified to be stable, which means that it is performing as expected, and results for patient samples can be reported with high probability that they are suitable for clinical use. If a QC result is not within acceptable limits, the measurement procedure is not performing correctly, there is a high probability that results for patient samples are not suitable for clinical use, and corrective action is necessary. Note that QC acceptance criteria may be designed to provide a warning of gradual changes in, for example, calibration drift that can be corrected before the error becomes large enough to adversely affect patient results. If corrective action is indicated, patient sample measurements will need to be repeated when the measurement procedure has been restored to its stable performance condition. If erroneous results have already been reported before an error condition is identified, a corrected report must be issued.

Measurement procedures fall into one of two general categories from a QC plan perspective. One type of procedure is a "batch" measurement process in which the results for patient samples and QC samples are completed before the results are reported. For batch measurement procedures, results are not reported if an error condition is identified by the QC sample measurements. The other type of procedure is a "continuous" measurement process in which patient sample results are reported during the interval between QC sample measurements and continue to be reported after a QC measurement event with no intervention made to the measuring system. For continuous measurement procedures, there is a possibility that erroneous results have already been reported if an error condition is identified by the next QC sample measurement(s). In either category, a measurement error that affects only one or a few patient results, called a nonpersistent (random) error, may not be identified by the results for the QC samples. QC procedures only identify persistent error conditions at the point in time when a QC sample is actually measured. Consequently, the choice of criteria to evaluate QC results and the frequency that QC results are measured become important QC plan design considerations.

The design of a QC plan must consider the analytical performance capability of a measurement procedure and the risk of harm to a patient that might occur if an erroneous laboratory test result is used for a clinical care decision. An erroneous laboratory test result is a hazardous condition that may or may not cause harm to a patient depending on what action or inaction is taken by a clinical care provider based on the erroneous result. The following sections in this chapter explain how to use information about a measurement procedure's analytical performance, the analytical performance required to meet medical care requirements, and the risk of harm from an erroneous result to establish a QC plan for monitoring a measurement procedure. However, it must be emphasized that establishing the analytical performance specifications to meet medical requirements and evaluating the probability of harm from an erroneous result are challenging because the link between analytical performance and the outcome for the patient can be difficult to establish.[1]

POINTS TO REMEMBER

Quality Control

- The primary role of internal QC is to ensure release of correct patient results.
- The primary role of EQA/PT is to compare performance between laboratories and, if possible, with a true value to determine that a laboratory's measurement procedures conform to expected performance.

MEASUREMENT PROCEDURE PERFORMANCE AS A PREREQUISITE FOR A QUALITY CONTROL PLAN

Calibration Traceability to a Reference System and Commutability Considerations

Whenever possible, calibration of clinical laboratory measurement procedures should be traceable to a higher order reference measurement procedure or certified reference material.[2-4] Ensuring that calibrations of clinical laboratory measurement procedures are traceable to the highest order reference system components available ensures that results for patient samples are equivalent within medically acceptable limits irrespective of the measurement procedure or laboratory making the measurements.

Calibration traceability is described in International Organization for Standardization (ISO) standard 17511:2003, "In vitro diagnostic medical devices-measurement of quantities in biological samples-metrological traceability of values assigned to calibrators and control materials"[2] and is illustrated in Fig. 6.2. A complete reference system provides traceability of the results from a routine clinical laboratory measurement procedure to the Système Internationale (SI) unit based on a series of calibrations that link the routine measurement procedure calibrator to a higher order reference material or reference measurement procedure. The highest order primary calibrator in the traceability chain is prepared from a well-characterized pure substance primary reference material that realizes the SI unit for the measurand in a well-defined solution that is suitable for use as a calibrator for a secondary reference measurement procedure such as isotope dilution mass spectrometry. Note that a measurand is the substance intended to be measured and includes the analyte name with the sample type and specification of the molecular substance intended to be measured.[5] Gravimetry is commonly used as a primary reference measurement procedure to determine the quantity of the measurand in the primary calibrator.

A secondary reference measurement procedure is then used to assign quantity values of a measurand to a secondary

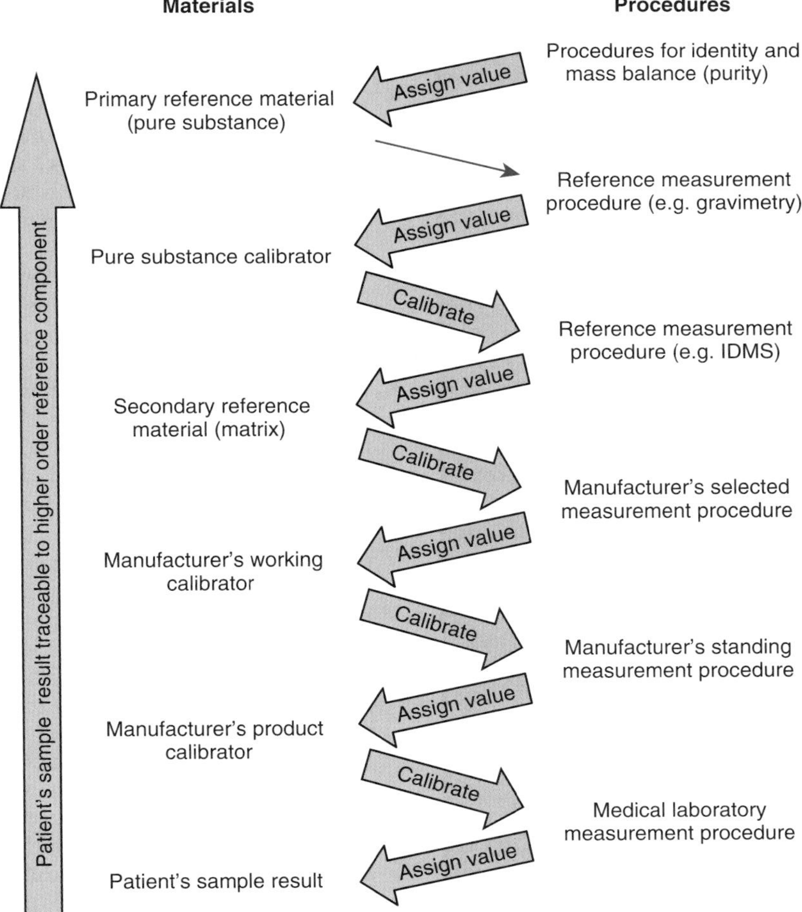

FIGURE 6.2 Traceability of calibration of measurement procedures based on International Organization for Standardization standard 17511.[2] *IDMS,* Isotope dilution mass spectrometry. (Modified with permission from Miller WG, Tate JR, Barth JH, Jones GR. Harmonization: the sample, the measurement and the report. *Ann Lab Med* 2014;34:187–197.)

reference material that typically has a matrix similar or identical to that of a clinical specimen or may be a panel of clinical patient specimens. A secondary reference measurement procedure is one with high selectivity for the measurand, very small imprecision, and minimal influence by sample matrix components. Secondary reference materials are typically provided by a national metrology institute, such as the National Institute for Standards and Technology in the United States or the Institute for Reference Materials and Measurements in the European Union, or other national or international organizations.

The secondary reference material is then used as a calibrator for a manufacturer's internal selected measurement procedure that is used to assign values to a working calibrator, frequently called a *master lot of calibrator,* that is used in the manufacturing process to assign values to the product calibrators that are used to calibrate routine measurement procedures used by clinical laboratories. Note that the manufacturer's selected and standing measurement procedures may be the same but used to fulfill two purposes in the calibration traceability scheme. A master lot of working calibrator is typically used for many years to transfer traceable calibration to many lots of product calibrator. The same traceability chain is applicable when laboratories develop measurement procedures in which case the steps assigned to manufacturers are the responsibility of the laboratory that develops a measurement procedure.

The Joint Committee for Traceability in Laboratory Medicine (JCTLM) lists certified reference materials, reference measurement procedures, and reference laboratories that conform to the ISO standards for such reference system components.[6-9] When there is no primary reference material or secondary reference measurement procedure for a measurand, then the calibration traceability chain stops at an intermediate position. For example, there may be a certified secondary reference material that is characterized by its producer as suitable for its intended use as a calibrator and a value for the measurand may be assigned by an agreed consensus process. Such a secondary reference material is called a *conventional reference material* and may be listed by JCTLM if it conforms to the requirements in the ISO standard 15194:2009.[8]

A category of traceability that is not well described in the current ISO 17511 standard but is under discussion for the revised standard has calibration traceable to a harmonization protocol (personal communication). A harmonization protocol is an internationally agreed approach to achieve equivalent results among a group of clinical laboratory measurement procedures when neither a reference measurement procedure nor a certified reference material is available. Examples of harmonization protocols have been described in which equivalent results can be achieved by aligning calibration of clinical laboratory measurement procedures so that results for a panel of individual patient samples agree among the different measurement procedures.[4,10-12]

In laboratory medicine, there are a large number of measurands for which there are no higher order reference materials. In these situations, the calibration traceability ends with the manufacturer's or laboratory's internal working calibrator. In this situation, results for patient samples frequently differ depending on the routine measurement procedure used or the laboratory performing the measurements.

The terms *standardized* and *harmonized* are frequently used interchangeably to refer to clinical laboratory measurement procedures that are calibrated such that results for patient samples are equivalent among different measurement procedures. The term *standardized* has traditionally been used when a calibration is traceable to a higher order reference measurement procedure or certified reference material. However, *standardized* is more appropriately used when calibration is traceable to any category of traceability described in ISO standard 17511 that is of higher order than to a manufacturer's or laboratory's internal working calibrator. The term *harmonized* has been used to refer to conformance to a harmonization protocol, but this usage is expected to be modified in the revision of ISO standard 17511. *Harmonized* remains a term that can be used whenever results measured by any clinical laboratory procedure are equivalent irrespective of the process used to achieve that condition.

Reference materials intended for use as calibrators or to establish calibration traceability for routine clinical laboratory measurement procedures must have the property called *commutability*.[4,13,14] As illustrated in Fig. 6.3, *A*, a commutable reference material has a numeric relationship between (or among) two (or more) measurement procedures that closely agrees with the relationship observed for a panel of clinical patient samples. Consequently, a commutable reference material (that may be used as a calibrator) reacts in a measurement procedure to give a numeric result that would be in close agreement to that observed for a patient sample with the same amount of analyte. Commutability is a challenge for secondary reference materials because their matrix may be modified from that of a clinical patient specimen during preparation. Differences in matrix-related bias between a reference material (or calibrator) and clinical patient samples cause a noncommutable relationship between the reference material (or calibrator) and the patient samples as illustrated in Fig. 6.3, *B*. Commutability is also a desirable property of QC materials. However, most QC materials are noncommutable, and this limitation influences how they are used as described in later sections.

Calibrators provided by in vitro device (IVD) manufacturers typically have matrix characteristics and target values that are intended only for use with that specific measurement procedure and cannot be used with any other manufacturer's measurement procedures. An IVD manufacturer can assign a target value to a measurement procedure–specific calibrator that corrects for any matrix-related bias (noncommutability) that may be present so that results for clinical samples are correctly traceable to the reference system for a measurand. However, if such a measurement procedure–specific calibrator is used with a different measurement procedure, it will cause miscalibration because it does not compensate for a different matrix-related bias with that different measurement procedure (ie, the calibrator is not commutable with clinical samples when used with a different measurement procedure).

A clinical laboratory may wish to verify that a measurement procedure's calibration conforms to an IVD manufacturer's claim for traceability to the reference system used for a given measurand. Some measurement procedure manufacturers provide materials specifically intended for this purpose. Such materials may be provided as measurement procedure-specific QC materials. As for measurement procedure–specific calibrators, such measurement procedure–specific

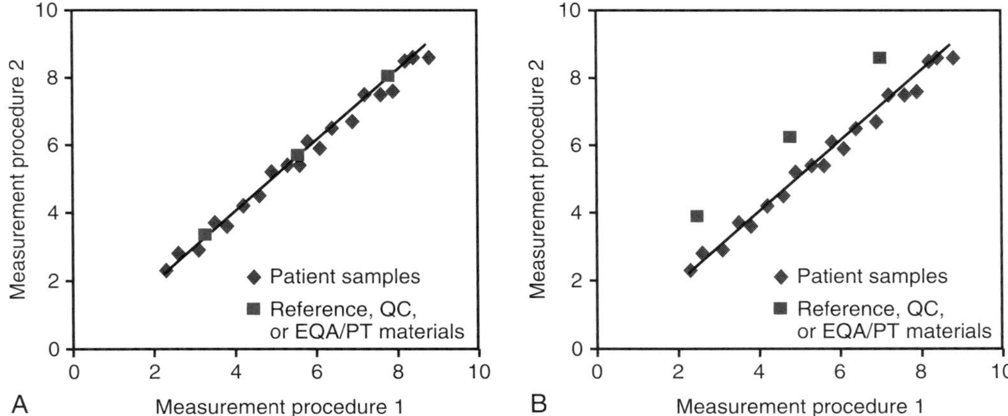

FIGURE 6.3 Illustration of commutable and noncommutable materials. **A,** Commutable materials *(red squares)* have the same relationship between two measurement procedures as observed for patient samples *(gray diamonds)*. **B,** Noncommutable materials have a different relationship than observed for patient samples. The materials to be examined for commutability represent preparations at different concentrations irrespective of how they are prepared. *EQA,* External quality assessment; *PT,* proficiency testing; *QC,* quality control.

QC materials typically have matrix characteristics and target values that are intended only for use with the specific measurement procedures claimed in the instructions for use and cannot be used with any other manufacturer's measurement procedure. Such measurement procedure–specific materials to verify calibration traceability may have target values that are specific for stated reagent lots, or they may have values certified by the IVD manufacturer to be suitable for all reagent lots.

A clinical laboratory has limited resources to verify the calibration traceability of a commercially available or laboratory developed routine measurement procedure. National and international certified reference materials are available for some measurands. Not all reference materials listed by JCTLM have been validated for commutability, and some are not intended for use with routine clinical laboratory measurement procedures. Rather, they are only intended for higher order reference measurement procedures that have better selectivity for the measurand. A reference material's certificate of analysis should be reviewed for commutability documentation. If a reference material is commutable with patient samples for a given measurement procedure, it can be used for calibration or to verify the traceability of calibration to the reference system. Using a noncommutable reference material as a calibrator will cause the routine measurement procedure to be miscalibrated and produce erroneous patient results.[4,13,15,16] Similarly, use of a noncommutable reference material to verify calibration traceability will give incorrect information regarding the traceability of a measurement procedure. Many higher order reference materials listed by JCTLM or provided by the World Health Organization have not been evaluated for commutability with patient samples measured using clinical laboratory measurement procedures. If a reference material's commutability status is unknown, it must be assumed not to be commutable with patient samples, and validation of suitability for use should be conducted.

Third-party QC materials intended for statistical process control (ie, those provided by a manufacturer other than the routine measurement procedure's manufacturer) are not suitable to verify calibration traceability. These materials are not validated for commutability with clinical samples for different routine measurement procedures, and they do not have target values that are traceable to higher-order reference measurement procedures. Such QC materials are designed to be used as QC samples, with target values and standard deviation (SD) values assigned as described later in this chapter. When third-party QC materials are used in an interlaboratory comparison program with measurement procedure-specific peer group mean values, these values can be used to confirm that a laboratory is using a specific measurement procedure in conformance with other users of the same measurement procedure (see External Quality Assessment or Proficiency Testing section).

Calibration of a Measurement Procedure and Verification of Calibration Stability

Calibration of an analytical measurement procedure is an essential step for achieving quality results. Fig. 6.4, *A*, shows that calibration of a measurement procedure establishes the relationship between the signal measured and the quantitative value of a measurand in the calibrator materials. This relationship is used to convert the measurement signal from a patient sample into a reportable concentration for the measurand. Specific techniques for calibration are unique to individual measurement procedures and are not covered here. However, some general principles for implementing calibration procedures can contribute to the stability and clinical reliability of laboratory results.

In principle, a measurement procedure should be calibrated only when evidence indicates that the current calibration is no longer valid. A recalibration event may introduce a small change in the relationship between analytical system response and sample concentration that contributes to overall long-term variability in measurement procedure performance. Evidence that a recalibration is needed could come from QC sample results that demonstrate a shift or trend in bias over a time period. However, QC results have random variability that may make it difficult to identify when recalibration is needed. Consequently, it is common practice to recalibrate measurement procedures on a time schedule that

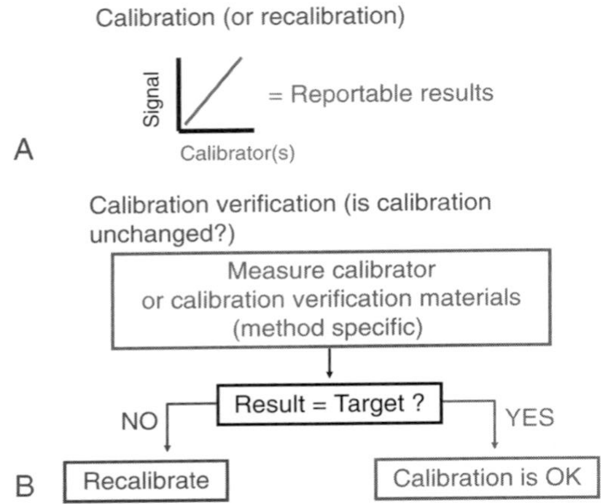

FIGURE 6.4 Calibration (**A**) and calibration verification (**B**) using measurement procedure–specific calibrators (or other measurement procedure–specific calibration verification materials). (From Miller WG. Quality control. In: *Henry's Clinical Diagnosis and Management by Laboratory Methods.* 23rd ed. Philadelphia: Elsevier; 2016.)

is established based on experience with stable QC results used as a metric for the suitability of the recalibration frequency. The IVD manufacturers frequently specify calibration intervals.

When no change in performance parameters has occurred, it is acceptable to verify that the current calibration has not changed (referred to as calibration verification) rather than perform a recalibration. Fig. 6.4, *B*, illustrates that a measurement procedure's current calibration can be verified not to have changed rather than performing a recalibration. Not performing a recalibration can avoid introducing small changes in the calibration relationship and thus minimize one potential source of long term variability. A common procedure to verify calibration is to assay the calibrator materials as "unknowns." Recovery of target values for the calibrators indicates that the measurement procedure's calibration has not changed (ie, the current calibration is verified to be correct), and there is no reason to perform a recalibration to reestablish the same relationship between measurement signal and calibrator concentration that is already in use. The laboratory must establish criteria for agreement with the calibrator target value for calibration verification. Conservative criteria for agreement, such as ±1 SD from the target value, should be considered to avoid misinterpretation of calibration status.

Analytical Bias and Imprecision

Fig. 6.5 illustrates the meaning of bias and imprecision for a measurement procedure that must be known to develop a QC plan. The horizontal axis represents the numeric value for an individual result, and the vertical axis represents the number of repeated measurements with the same value made on aliquots of a QC material. The *red line* shows the dispersion of results for repeated measurements of aliquots of the same QC material, which is the random imprecision of the measurement. Assuming that the dispersion follows a Gaussian (normal) distribution, it is described by the SD. The SD is a measure of expected imprecision in a measurement procedure when it is performing within specifications. Note that results near the mean (average value) occur more frequently than results farther away from the mean. An interval of ±1 SD includes 68% of the measured values, and an interval of ±2 SDs includes 95% of the values. A result that is more than 2 SDs from the mean is expected to occur 5% of the time (100% − 95%) in a positive or a negative direction from the mean value. Correct calibration of a measurement procedure eliminates systematic bias (within uncertainty limits), so the mean of repeated measurements of a QC sample becomes the expected value for that QC sample when the measurement procedure is performing within specifications.

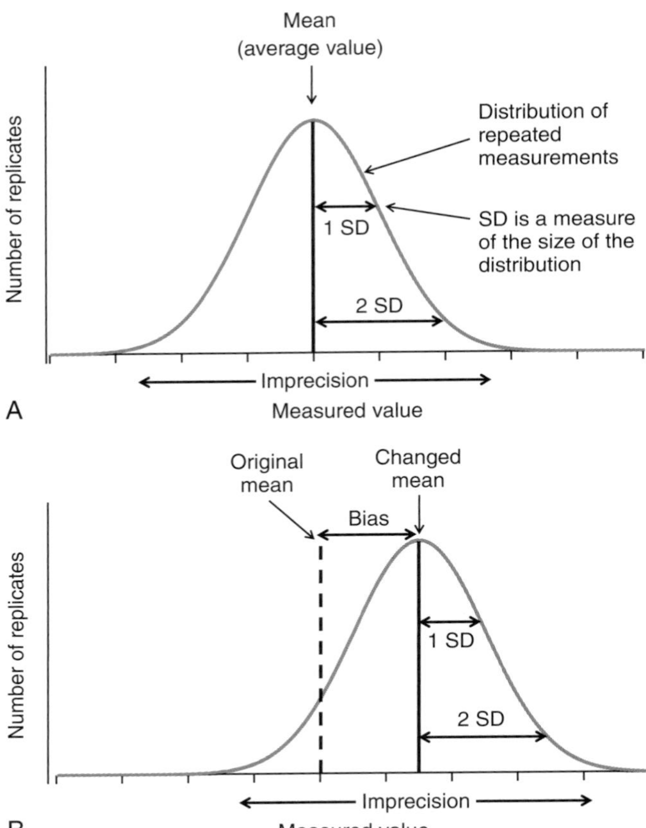

FIGURE 6.5 **A,** Distribution of results showing the mean value and expected imprecision for repeated measurements of a quality control sample. **B,** Bias when a change in calibration has occurred. *SD,* Standard deviation. (From Miller WG. Quality control. In: *Henry's Clinical Diagnosis and Management by Laboratory Methods.* 23rd ed. Philadelphia: Elsevier; 2016.)

Fig. 6.5, *B*, illustrates that if the calibration changes for any reason, a systematic bias is introduced into the results. The bias is the difference between the observed mean and the expected value for a QC material (for more discussion on bias, refer to Chapter 2). Note that the imprecision is the same as before the bias occurred because it is unlikely, although not impossible, that a change in imprecision would occur at the same time as a bias shift. The primary purpose of measuring QC samples is to statistically evaluate the measurement procedure to verify that it continues to perform within the specifications consistent with its acceptable expected stable condition or to identify that a change in performance occurred that needs to be corrected. QC result acceptance criteria, discussed in a later section, are based on the probability for an individual QC result to be different from the variability in results expected when the measurement procedure is performing within specifications.

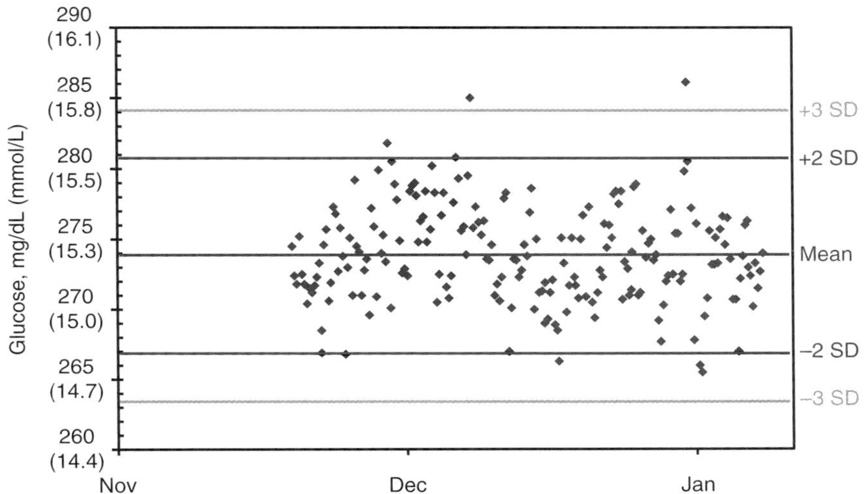

FIGURE 6.6 Levey-Jennings plot of quality control (QC) results ($n = 199$) for a single lot of QC material used for a 49-day period. *SD*, Standard deviation. (From Miller WG. Quality control. In: *Henry's Clinical Diagnosis and Management by Laboratory Methods*. 23rd ed. Philadelphia: Elsevier; 2016.)

The term *accuracy* is used for an individual result and is the combination of bias and imprecision that occurred for that specific measurement (for more discussion on accuracy, refer to Chapter 2). The result for an individual patient sample may also be influenced by interfering substances that could be present in that sample. Total error for a patient sample measurement is the combination of measurement procedure bias, imprecision, and sample specific bias caused by any interfering substances that may be present. An individual QC sample is only influenced by systematic bias and imprecision of the measurement procedure. Statistical QC does not evaluate possible interfering substances that may affect results for an individual patient sample. The influence of interfering substances needs to be examined during the evaluation that a measurement procedure is suitable for use[17] (for additional discussion on interference, please refer to Chapter 5). However, the imprecision observed for QC results provides a measure of the variability expected for an individual patient result caused by the inherent imprecision of a measurement procedure and is usually independent of interfering substances that typically affect the bias.

The term *trueness* is inversely related to a bias that may be present in a measurement procedure. Trueness is an attribute of a measurement procedure that reflects how correctly its calibration is traceable to a reference system.

Fig. 6.6 shows a Levey-Jennings[18] plot that was an adaptation for clinical laboratory measurements of the Shewhart[19] plot developed for statistical control in manufacturing. The Levey-Jennings plot is the most common presentation for evaluating QC results. This format shows each QC result sequentially over time and allows a quick visual assessment of performance. Assuming the measurement procedure is performing in a stable condition consistent with its specifications, the mean value represents the target (or expected) value for the QC result, and the SD lines represent the expected imprecision. Assuming a Gaussian (normal) distribution of imprecision, the results should be distributed uniformly around the mean with results observed more frequently closer to the mean than near the extremes of the distribution. Note that a few results in Fig. 6.6 are greater than 2 SDs, and two results slightly exceed 3 SDs, which is expected for a Gaussian distribution of imprecision. For a large number of repeated measurements, the number of results expected within the SD intervals is:

- ±1 SD = 68.3% of observations
- ±2 SD = 95.4% of observations
- ±3 SD = 99.7% of observations

Interpretation of an individual QC result is based on its probability to be part of the expected distribution of results for the measurement procedure when the procedure is performing correctly. A later section provides details regarding interpretive rules for evaluation of QC results. Note that evaluation of individual QC results may be performed by computer algorithms without visual examination of a Levey-Jennings chart. However, the underlying logic of such algorithms is illustrated by the Levey-Jennings chart example.

Performance of a Measurement Procedure for Its Intended Medical Use

It is necessary to determine how the performance of a measurement procedure relates to the medical requirements for interpreting results in order to determine the frequency to measure QC samples and the criteria to use to evaluate the QC results. The sigma metric is commonly used to assess how well a measurement procedure performs relative to the medical requirement. Sigma is the Greek letter used to denote SD. The sigma scale expresses the variability of a measurement process in SDs to the variability that is acceptable because it will not cause an error in diagnosis or treatment of a patient.

For laboratory measurements, the sigma metric is calculated as:

$$\text{Sigma} = (\text{TE}_a - \text{bias})/\text{SD}$$

where TE_a is the total error allowed based on medical requirements, and bias and SD refer to performance characteristics of the measurement procedure. The SD is estimated from the QC data as previously described. It is critically important that the estimate of SD be made using QC data that represent all or most components of variability that occur over an extended time period (see the section called Establishing the Quality

Control Target Value and Standard Deviation That Represent a Stable Measurement Operating Condition). The bias is difficult for a laboratory to estimate because it is difficult to evaluate if a particular measurement procedure has a bias compared with a reliable estimate of a true value such as based on a reference measurement procedure. For internal QC, a laboratory is usually interested to determine if a bias has occurred compared with the condition established by calibration of a measurement procedure. Such a bias represents a QC result that is sufficiently different from its target value that corrective action is needed. Consequently, the bias is usually assumed to be zero for calculating sigma.

However, a bias term may be needed in situations when there are two or more different measurement procedures used for the same measurand and those different measurement procedures have a bias between them that cannot be removed or when changes in lots of reagents or calibrators introduce shifts in bias that cannot otherwise be corrected. Note that it is preferable to adjust the calibration of different measurement procedures or different lots of reagents or calibrators to provide equivalent results but this solution may not be applicable for some technologies. In such cases, this relative bias can be estimated based on comparison of results for patient samples following a procedure such as described in Clinical and Laboratory Standards Institute (CLSI) document EP9[20] and that bias should be considered in determining the sigma metric and in establishing a QC plan for such measurement procedures.

TE_a represents the measurement procedure performance required to enable suitable medical decisions based on a test result. TE_a can be estimated using three models.[21] The preferred model (model 1) to set a performance specification is to base it on an outcome study (ie, investigating the impact of analytical performance of the measurement procedure on the clinical outcome). Outcome studies can be direct assessment of clinical outcome for a group of patients or "indirect" outcome when the consequences of analytical performance on, for example, clinical classifications or decisions and thereby on the probability of patient outcomes can be investigated. These probabilities can be discussed with clinical experts who then can recommend a performance specification.[21]

Indirect outcome studies are often used to set TE_a in laboratory practice guidelines. For example, the National Cholesterol Education Program recommends that total cholesterol be measured with a TE_a of 9% or less,[22] and the National Kidney Disease Education Program recommends that creatinine be measured with a TE_a of less than 7% to 10% in the concentration interval 1 to 1.5 mg/dL (76.3–114.4 mmol/L).[23] The disadvantage with this model is that it is only useful when the links between the measurand, clinical decision-making, and clinical outcomes are strong, which is only the case for a minority of measurands.

Model 2 bases the TE_a on a fraction of the within and between individual biologic variations of the measurand.[24,25] This model is not related to the clinical effect or medical requirement of the analytical quality. Instead, this model tries to minimize the ratio of the "analytical" noise to the "biologic signal" with an assumption that a small ratio will identify measurement procedure performance that relates to the medical requirements. Tables of optimal, desirable, and minimal TE_a based on biologic variation are available and may provide useful information when other information is not available.[26] However, biologic variation based estimates of TE_a should be used with caution because the estimates of biologic variation in many cases are based on minimal data, and the experimental designs of the estimates and the process to select the estimates to list in the tables have been challenged.[27,28] The estimates of biologic variation typically vary among different investigations, making it challenging to have confidence in a given value. For example, reports of biologic variation for aspartate aminotransferase, alanine aminotransferase, and gamma glutamyl transferase varied between 11% and 58%, 3% and 32%, and 4% and 14%, respectively, among different studies.[29] In addition, the way the TE_a is calculated is flawed because the calculation combines maximum allowable imprecision with maximum allowable bias (both based on a fraction of biologic variation) that has no theoretical basis and leads to overestimation of the TE_a.[30] There are now initiatives to improve the data on biologic variation and to address how TE_a can be estimated from biologic variation.[31] Another limitation is that the biologic variability has typically been derived from data for nondiseased individuals and may be different for pathological conditions. Additional examples and discussion of biologic variation are provided in Chapter 7.

Model 3 bases the performance specifications on the "state of the art." The advantage of this model is that data are readily available. The disadvantage is that there may be no relationship between what is technically achievable and what is needed to make a medical decision for diagnosis or treatment of a patient. It is generally agreed that preference should be given to model 1 whenever such information is available or to model 2 as a starting point to estimate TE_a.[21] A laboratory director could consult with clinical care providers to agree on an appropriate TE_a for the patient population served.

Because sigma assumes a Gaussian or normal distribution for repeated measurements, the probability of a defect (ie, an erroneous laboratory result) can be predicted as shown in Table 6-1. The sigma metric represents the probability that a given number of erroneous results, that could cause risk of harm to a patient, are expected to occur when the test measurement procedure is performing to its specifications. The phrase "six sigma" refers to a condition when the variability in the measurement process is sufficiently smaller than the medical requirement that erroneous results are very uncommon. A "four-sigma" measurement procedure would be less

TABLE 6.1 Probability of Acceptable or Erroneous Results Based on the Sigma Scale

Sigma Value	Percent of Results Within Specification	Percent of Results With an Error (Defect)	Errors (Defects) per Million Opportunities
1	68	32	317,311
2	95.5	4.5	45,500
3	99.7	0.3	2,700
4	99.994	0.006	63
5	99.99994	0.00006	0.6
6	99.9999998	0.0000002	0.002

(From Miller WG. Quality control. In: *Henry's Clinical Diagnosis and Management by Laboratory Methods.* 23rd ed. Philadelphia: Elsevier; 2016.)

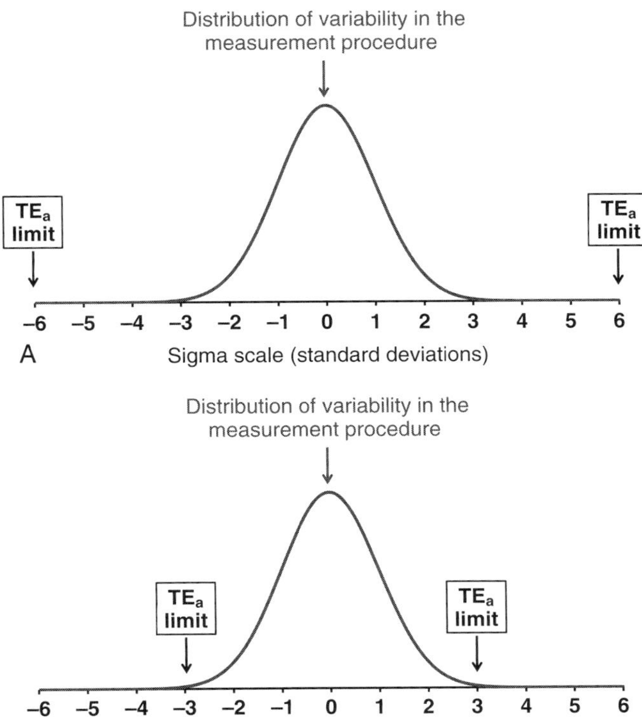

FIGURE 6.7 Test performance relative to the sigma scale to describe how well performance meets medical requirements expressed as the allowable total error (TE_a). **A,** A "six-sigma" measurement procedure. **B,** A "three-sigma" measurement procedure. (From Miller WG. Quality control. In: *Henry's Clinical Diagnosis and Management by Laboratory Methods.* 23rd ed. Philadelphia: Elsevier; 2016.)

robust and have a higher probability that erroneous results could be produced but still at a fairly low frequency. A "two-sigma" measurement procedure would produce enough erroneous results even though it met its performance specifications that it would not be very reliable for patient care.

Fig. 6.7 shows how the sigma metric describes the performance of a laboratory test relative to the TE_a. Parts *A* and *B* show that a measurement procedure with the same analytical performance characteristics can have different sigma metrics depending on how the imprecision relates to the TE_a. Fig. 6.7, *A*, shows a "six-sigma" test that has the TE_a limits 6 SDs away from the center point of the distribution of variability in measurements when the measurement procedure is performing to its analytical specifications. In the "six-sigma" situation, a small amount of bias or increased imprecision will have little influence on the number of erroneous results produced, and less stringent QC will be appropriate because the risk of producing an erroneous result even with some loss of performance is very low.

Fig. 6.7, *B*, shows a "three-sigma" measurement procedure that has the TE_a limits 3 SDs away from the center point of the expected distribution of variability in measurements when the measurement procedure is performing to its analytical specifications. In the "three-sigma" situation, a small amount of bias or increased imprecision will cause the number of erroneous results to increase substantially, and more stringent QC is needed to identify when such an error condition occurs. Note that no amount of QC will improve the performance of a marginal measurement procedure. However, more frequent QC and more stringent acceptance criteria will allow the laboratory to identify when small changes in performance occur so they can be corrected to minimize the risk of harm to a patient from erroneous results being acted on to make clinical care decisions. It is important to emphasize that the sigma calculations are dependent on what TE_a is chosen. As discussed earlier, an "objective" TE_a is often difficult to establish, and good data to set a TE_a are often lacking.

POINTS TO REMEMBER

Measurement Procedure Performance as a Prerequisite for a Quality Control Plan

- The performance characteristics of a measurement procedure when it is performing in a stable in-control condition must be understood.
- The allowable total error for a measurement procedure must be established based on clinical requirements for using a laboratory result in patient care decisions.
- The sigma metric represents the probability that a given number of erroneous results that could cause risk of harm to a patient are expected to occur when the test measurement procedure is performing to its specifications.

DEVELOPING A QUALITY CONTROL PLAN AND IMPLEMENTING QUALITY CONTROL PROCEDURES

Selection of Quality Control Materials

Generally, two different concentrations are necessary for adequate statistical QC. For quantitative measurement procedures, QC materials should be selected to provide measurand concentrations that monitor the analytical measuring interval of the measurement procedure. In practice, laboratories are frequently limited by concentrations available in commercial QC products. When possible, it is important to confirm that measurement procedure performance is stable near the limits of its analytical measuring interval because defects may affect these concentrations before others. Many quantitative measurement procedures have a linear response over the analytical measuring interval, and it is reasonable to assume that their performance over the interval is acceptable if the results near the interval limits are acceptable. In the case of nonlinear analytical response, it may be necessary to use additional controls at intermediate concentrations. Critical concentrations for clinical decisions (eg, glucose, therapeutic drugs, thyroid-stimulating hormone, prostate-specific antigen, hemoglobin A_{1c} [HbA_{1c}], troponin) may also be appropriate for QC monitoring. In many cases, the imprecision near the limit of quantitation may be relatively large, in which case the concentration should be chosen to provide adequate SD for practical evaluation of QC results. For procedures with extraction or other pretreatment steps, controls must be used to include any pretreatment steps.

This chapter primarily focuses on QC procedures for quantitative measurement procedures. However, the principles can be adapted to most qualitative procedures with allowances for the lack of numeric results. For measurement procedures based on qualitative interpretation of quantitative measurements (eg, drugs of abuse, human chorionic gonadotropin, hepatitis markers), the same principles of QC assessment can be applied to the numeric results even if they are only expressed as instrument signal values. For qualitative results, the negative and positive controls should be selected to have concentrations relatively near the threshold to adequately control for discrimination between negative and positive. For qualitative procedures with graded responses (eg, dipstick urinalysis), negative, positive, and graded response controls are required. For qualitative tests based on other properties (eg, electrophoretic procedures, stain adequacy, immunofluorescence, organism identification), it is necessary to ensure that the QC procedure will appropriately evaluate that the measurement procedure correctly discriminates normal from pathologic conditions.

The QC materials selected must be manufactured to provide a stable product that can be used for an extended time period, preferably 1 or more years for stable measurands. Use of a single lot for an extended period allows reliable interpretive criteria to be established that will permit efficient identification of a measurement problem, avoid false alerts caused by poorly defined expected ranges for the QC results, and minimize limitations in interpreting values after reagent and calibrator lot changes.

Limitations of Quality Control Materials

Limitations are inherent in currently available QC materials. One limitation is that the QC material is frequently noncommutable with clinical patient samples. A commutable QC material is one that reacts in a measurement procedure to give a result that would closely agree with that expected for an authentic patient sample with the same amount of measurand. QC as well as EQA/PT materials are typically noncommutable with clinical patient samples because the serum or other biologic fluid matrix is usually altered from that of a patient sample.[15,32-35] The matrix alteration is due to processing of the biologic fluid during product manufacturing; use of partially purified human and nonhuman additives to achieve desired concentrations of the measurands; and various stabilization processes that alter proteins, cells, and other components. The impact of the matrix alteration on the recovery of a measurand is not predictable and is frequently different for different lots of QC material, for different lots of reagent within a given measurement procedure, and for different measurement procedures.[36,37] Because of the noncommutability limitation, special procedures are required (discussed in later sections) when changing lots of reagent or comparing QC results among two or more measurement procedures.

A second limitation of QC materials is deterioration of the measurand during storage. Measurand stability during unopened storage is generally excellent, but slow deterioration eventually limits the shelf life of a product and can introduce a gradual drift into QC data that may require correction over the life of a lot of QC material. Measurand stability after reconstitution, thawing, or vial opening can be an important source of variability in QC results and can vary substantially among measurands in the same vial. Variables to be controlled are the time spent at room temperature and the time spent uncapped with the potential for evaporation. An expiration time after opening is provided by the QC manufacturer but may need to be established by a laboratory for each QC material under the conditions of use in that laboratory and may be different for different measurands in the same QC product. For QC materials reconstituted by adding a diluent, vial-to-vial variability can be minimized by standardizing the pipetting procedure (eg, using the same pipet or filling device, preferably an automated device, and having the same person prepare the controls) whenever practical.

Another limitation is that measurand concentrations in multiconstituent control materials may not be at levels optimal for all measurement procedures. This limitation may be caused by solubility considerations or potential interactions between different constituents, particularly at higher concentrations. It may be necessary to use supplementary QC materials to adequately monitor the measuring interval.

Frequency to Measure Quality Control Samples

The frequency to measure QC samples is a function of several parameters:

- Analytical stability of the measurement procedure
- Risk of harm to a patient from clinical action being taken before a significant error is detected at the next scheduled QC event
- Number of patient results produced in a period of time when an error condition could exist but was not yet detected
- Events such as recalibration or maintenance that may alter the current performance condition of the measurement procedure
- Training and competency of the test operator, particularly for manual or semiautomated measurement procedures

Analytical Stability of the Measurement Procedure

The stability of the measurement procedure is a fundamental determinant of how frequently a QC sample needs to be measured. The more stable the measurement procedure, the less frequently a QC evaluation needs to be performed. Note, however, that all of the considerations in the preceding list must be evaluated together to determine a suitable frequency to perform QC. Some measurement procedures have been designed with sophisticated built-in control procedures to mitigate the risk that an erroneous result may be produced. Built-in control procedures may include calibrators and QC materials integrated with reagent packaging and sensors that monitor electronic components and the measurement process with algorithms that prevent a result from being produced if any monitored conditions fail to meet criteria. Examples of built-in controls are frequently found in point-of-care (POC) instruments. These measurement systems may be sufficiently stable and self-monitored to justify reduced frequency of traditional surrogate QC sample testing. However, there is little information in the literature that has examined the optimal frequency or control rules to be used in these cases.

Risk of Harm to a Patient and Number of Patients Who May Be at Risk

The risk of clinical action being taken before a significant measurement error is detected is an important consideration for more frequent QC sampling than one based strictly on analytical stability of the measurement procedure or on regulatory minimum requirements. More frequent QC sampling is appropriate to avoid the situation of discovering a measurement procedure defect many hours after a physician has made a clinical treatment or nontreatment decision based on an erroneous result. For example, QC sampling performed on a

24-hour cycle might be performed at 9 AM. If QC results indicate a measurement procedure problem, the erroneous condition could have started at any time during the previous 24 hours. If the problem had occurred at 3 PM the previous day, erroneous results could have been reported for 18 hours, likely putting a large number of patients at risk of an inappropriate care decision. Parvin[38] reported an assessment of the frequency of QC testing and the number of potentially incorrect patient results that could be reported before errors of different magnitudes were detected.

The medical risk of harm to a patient from erroneous results must be considered and the frequency of QC testing established to minimize risk. From a practical perspective, the cost of a medical error, or simply the cost of repeating questionable patient samples since the last acceptable QC results, could be more expensive than a more frequent QC sampling schedule that would detect an error condition in a timelier manner.

The CLSI has published the guideline EP23 addressing risk-based QC procedures.[39] The document provides guidance to clinical laboratories on how to develop a QC plan based on evaluation of risk of harm to a patient and assessment of the effectiveness of risk mitigation procedures using information from the manufacturer and from other sources combined with the clinical requirements of the local health care setting and conditions in the laboratory. In general terms, the laboratory director is responsible to ensure that a result has a high probability to be correct at the time it is reported for clinical use. To make this judgment, the laboratory director needs to understand the risks that can cause a measurement technology to perform incorrectly, needs to evaluate the effectiveness of built-in control processes to mitigate those risks, and needs to ensure that adequate control procedures are in place to confirm that a result is correct at the time it is reported. A combination of built-in and external monitoring procedures using surrogate QC samples can be used to ensure that all risks have been appropriately mitigated or monitored at a frequency commensurate with the risk of malfunction and the risk of harm to a patient if an incorrect result was reported.

Event Based Quality Control Sample Measurement

It is necessary when using a continuous measurement system to measure QC samples before and after scheduled events such as recalibration or maintenance that may alter the current performance condition. It is necessary to measure QC samples before these operations alter the condition of the measurement system to verify that no significant errors in results have occurred since the last time QC samples were measured. Each of these operations is intended to restore the measurement conditions to optimal specifications and to correct for any calibration drift or component deterioration that may have occurred. If QC samples are not measured before such scheduled events, a laboratory will not know if an error condition may have occurred that could have caused erroneous results for patient testing to have been reported. It is also necessary to measure QC samples after these events to verify that the operations were performed correctly and that measurement procedure performance meets specifications before restarting to measure patient samples.

Establishing the Quality Control Target Value and Standard Deviation That Represent a Stable Measurement Operating Condition

QC target values and acceptable performance limits are established to optimize the probability to detect a measurement defect that is large enough to have an impact on clinical care while minimizing the frequency of "false alerts" caused by statistical limitations of the criteria used to evaluate QC results. The measurement system must be correctly calibrated and operating within acceptable performance specifications before the statistical parameters to establish QC interpretive rules can be established. Some sources of measurement variability that are expected to occur during typical operation of a measurement procedure are listed in Table 6-2. Measurement

TABLE 6.2 Common Sources of Measurement Variability

Source	Time Interval for Fluctuation	Likely Statistical Distribution
Pipet volume	Short	Gaussian
Pipet seal deterioration	Long	Drift
Instrument temperature control	Short or long	Gaussian or other
Electronic noise in the measuring system	Short	Gaussian
Calibration cycles	Short to long	Gaussian or periodic shift
Reagent deterioration in storage	Long	Drift
Reagent deterioration after opening	Intermediate	Cyclic, periodic drift or shift
Calibrator deterioration in storage	Long	Drift
Calibrator deterioration after opening	Intermediate	Cyclic, periodic drift or shift
Control material deterioration in storage	Long	Drift
Control material deterioration after opening	Intermediate	Cyclic, periodic drift or shift
Environmental temperature and humidity	Variable	Variable
Reagent lot changes*	Long	Periodic shift
Calibrator lot changes	Long	Periodic shift
Instrument maintenance	Variable	Cyclic or periodic shift
Deterioration of instrument components	Variable	Cyclic, periodic drift or shift

*Note that reagent lot changes can have an artifactual influence on quality control values and require special handling as discussed in the section Verifying Quality Control Evaluation Parameters After a Reagent Lot Change.

From Miller WG. Quality control. In: *Henry's Clinical Diagnosis and Management by Laboratory Methods.* 23rd ed. Philadelphia: Elsevier; 2016.

variability includes sources with short time interval frequencies, many of which can be described by Gaussian error distributions, and intermittent and longer time interval sources, which can cause cyclic fluctuations over several days or weeks, gradual drift over weeks or months, and intermittent abrupt small shifts in results. The SD used in QC interpretive rules needs to adequately represent all sources of variability in results that are expected to occur over time when the measurement procedure is performing to specifications (see Table 6-2).

Quality Control Material Target Value

A QC material must have a reliable target value that represents the condition when systematic bias is as small as possible. This condition requires the measurement procedure to be calibrated correctly and adequate replicate measurements to be obtained over a sufficient time interval to include the typical sources of measurement variability that will ensure that a representative mean value is calculated from the data. For practical reasons, this objective is rarely met for the longer term variability components in Table 6-2; consequently, the target value has some uncertainty and may need to be refined if measurement conditions fluctuate but remain within performance specifications.

The generally accepted minimum protocol for target value assignment is to use the mean value from a minimum of 10 measurements of the QC material on 10 different days.[40] When applicable, more than one calibration should be represented in the 10 measured values to include this source of variability in the target value. The 10 or more measurements can be performed over a longer time interval to include other important sources of variability in the estimate of target value. If a QC material will be used for longer than 1 day, a single vial should be stored correctly and assayed on as many days as the material is planned to be used to allow variability caused by opened storage to be represented in the target value. If a 10-day protocol is not possible (eg, if an emergency replacement of a lot of QC material is necessary), a provisional target value can be established with fewer data but should be updated when additional replicate results are available.

Because all sources of variability cannot be captured in 10 measurements, it is recommended to update the target value after more data have been acquired during use of the QC material. Target values may also need to be updated after reagent lot changes or other alterations in measurement conditions as described in a later section called Verifying Quality Control Evaluation Parameters After a Reagent Lot Change.

Quality Control Material Standard Deviation

SD is the conventional way to express measurement procedure variability and assumes the QC data can be described by a Gaussian (normal) distribution even though non-Gaussian components of variability influence the QC results. The statistical QC packages in instrument and laboratory computer systems are designed with the assumption that the SD for a Gaussian distribution is used for the QC rules criteria. Because there are non-Gaussian components to measurement variability over time, it is very important that they be represented in the data used to estimate an SD. We use an estimate of SD to make conclusions regarding the acceptability of an individual QC value, so the SD must be as realistic as possible to represent the variability expected for a measurement procedure when its performance meets its specifications.

When a measurement procedure has been established in a laboratory and a new lot of QC material is being introduced, the target value for the new lot of QC material is used along with the well-established SD from the previous lot. This practice is appropriate because in most cases, measurement imprecision is a property of the measurement procedure and equipment used and is unlikely to change with a different lot of QC material.[40] When a new QC material from a different manufacturer is introduced, it is possible for the observed SD to be different than the historic value because of matrix differences, and the SD should be monitored and adjusted as experience with the new material is accumulated. If target values for the old and new lots are substantially different, a different SD may be needed. Assuming the coefficient of variation (CV) is approximately constant over the difference in concentration between target values for the old and new QC lots, the SD can be calculated by applying the existing CV to the new target value and then converting to the corresponding SD value. Because it is possible for the SD to be influenced by a lot of QC material, adjustment to the SD may be necessary as additional experience with the new lot is accumulated.

If a new measurement procedure is introduced for which no historical performance information is available, the SD for stable performance can be established using QC data obtained during the measurement procedure validation. An SD that represents the typical imprecision of the measurement procedure when it is performing according to its design specifications is needed but may not be possible to determine because not all of the sources of variability in Table 6.2 can be included in the initial estimate of SD. A minimum of 20 observations on different days is recommended for the initial estimation of the SD.[40] It is desirable to have some of the events that contribute to measurement variability, in particular calibration and maintenance, included during the time interval over which the SD is estimated. Note that reagent lot changes should not be included in the estimate of SD because QC results are frequently artifactually influenced by different reagent lots (see the section Verifying Quality Control Evaluation Parameters After a Reagent Lot Change). The CLSI document EP05 provides guidance on establishing the SD for a measurement procedure.[41] Note that EP05 does not include longer term sources of variability, so the SD is underestimated by this protocol.

When a new measurement procedure replaces an existing procedure, the SD for the existing procedure can in many cases be used to inform the initial estimate of the SD for the new measurement procedure. With the assumption that the SD for the existing measurement procedure was appropriate to ensure the results were suitable for use in medical decisions, that SD can be used as the basis for QC decisions for the new measurement procedure. This approach is suitable when the initial estimates of SD for the new procedure are smaller than the SD in use for the old procedure. This approach may allow an initial estimate of SD that is consistent with medical use requirements until sufficient QC results have been obtained for the new measurement procedure to estimate a new SD that includes sources of variability that are not possible to include in the initial estimate of SD determined during validation of the new measurement procedure.

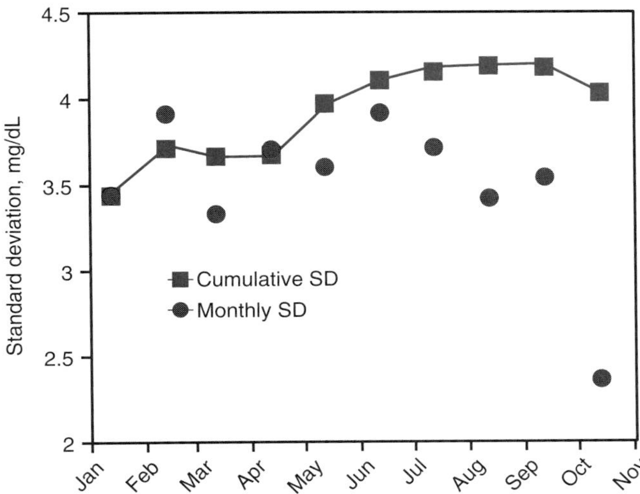

FIGURE 6.8 Cumulative standard deviation (SD) versus single monthly values calculated from the data in Fig. 6.11. (From Miller WG. Quality control. In: *Henry's Clinical Diagnosis and Management by Laboratory Methods*. 23rd ed. Philadelphia: Elsevier; 2016.)

The initial estimate of SD will likely not include contributions from all expected sources of variability and will need to be updated when additional QC data are available. An SD that represents stable measurement performance can usually be estimated from the cumulative SD over a 6- to 12-month period for a single lot of QC material. This approach is likely to include most expected sources of variation. Fig. 6.8 illustrates using data for a glucose measurement procedure the fluctuation in SD that occurred when calculated for monthly intervals compared with the relatively stable value observed for the cumulative SD after a period of 6 months. Note that the cumulative SD is not the average of the monthly values but is the SD determined from all individual results obtained over a time interval since the lot of QC material was first used. Different sources of long-term variability occur at different times during the use of a measurement procedure. The monthly SD does not adequately reflect the longer term components of variability. Consequently, the cumulative SD is typically larger than the monthly values because it includes more sources of variability (see Table 6-2) and better represents the actual variability of the measurement procedure. If the imprecision expected during normal stable operation is underestimated, the acceptable range for QC results will be too small, and the false-alert rate will be unacceptably high. If imprecision for the stable condition is overestimated, the acceptable range will be too large, and a significant measurement error might go undetected.

It may be useful to combine data from more than one lot of QC material or for more than one lot of reagent to obtain a long-term estimate of SD that represents most sources of variability in a measurement procedure. For example, this approach may be needed when the stability of a QC product is limited and a single lot is not available for an extended time interval or when reagent stability is limited and a new lot must be used frequently. See the later section called Verifying Quality Control Evaluation Parameters After a Reagent Lot Change that explains why QC results can be artifactually influenced by reagent lot changes. Pooling of data to obtain an SD requires the SD for each stable interval of use to be determined separately; then the SD for each stable interval can be combined using the following formula where n is the number of QC results in a given time interval from 1 to i.

$$SD_{pooled} = \sqrt{\frac{(n_1 - 1)\times SD_1^2 + (n_2 - 1)\times SD_2^2 + \cdots + (n_i - 1)\times SD_i^2}{n_1 + n_2 + \cdots + n_i - i}}$$

It is important to include all valid QC results in the calculation of SD to ensure that the SD correctly represents expected measurement procedure variability. A valid QC result is one that was, or would have been in the case of preliminary value assignment, used to verify acceptable assay performance and supported reporting patient results. Only QC results that were, or would have been, responsible for not releasing patient results should be excluded from summary calculations.

Quality Control Materials With Preassigned Values

Some QC materials are provided by the measurement procedure manufacturer with preassigned target values and acceptable ranges intended to confirm that the measurement procedure meets the manufacturer's specifications. Such assigned values may be used to verify the manufacturer's specifications. However, it is recommended that both the target value and the SD should be reevaluated and assigned by the laboratory after adequate replicate results have been obtained because the QC interpretive rules used in a single laboratory should reflect performance for the measurement procedure in that laboratory. The acceptability limits (product insert ranges) suggested by a manufacturer typically account for sources of variability, such as among instruments, among reagent lots, and among calibrator lots, that will be greater than the variability expected in an individual laboratory. Use of product insert ranges that are too large will reduce a laboratory's ability to detect an erroneous measurement condition. It is often a problem for POC devices that the manufacturer's preset limits must be used which can reduce the possibilities to detect errors. A laboratory can institute additional QC testing, but such options may be limited for some technologies.

QC materials with assigned target values and SDs are also available from third-party manufacturers (ie, manufacturers not affiliated with the measurement procedure manufacturer) and typically have values that are applicable to specifically stated measurement procedures to accommodate the influence of noncommutability. Caution should be used with target values and SDs assigned by third-party QC material providers because the target values may have been assigned by a small number of measurements and using reagent and calibrator lots that are no longer available. The SD values will not be suitable for use in QC acceptance rules because they do not reflect the measurement conditions in an individual laboratory. Of particular concern is, for example, if a manufacturer assigned SD is larger than that observed in an individual laboratory, the acceptable limits for QC results will be too large, and an erroneous measurement condition may not be identified appropriately. Some QC material providers offer an interlaboratory comparison program to which participants send QC results for aggregation with those of other laboratories. Such interlaboratory summary data are similar to those from EQA/PT programs and can be useful to laboratories to compare their target values to those from a group

TABLE 6.3 Abbreviation Nomenclature for Quality Control Evaluation Rules

Rule	Meaning	Detects
1_{2S}	One observation exceeds 2 SDs from the target value. The 1_{2S} rule is not recommended except for low sigma measurement procedures because it has a high false-alert rate.	Bias or imprecision
1_{3S}	One observation exceeds 3 SDs from the target value.	Bias or large imprecision
2_{2S} ($2_{2.5S}$)	Two sequential observations, or observations for two QC samples measured at approximately the same time, exceed 2 SDs (or 2.5 SDs) from the target value in the same direction.	Bias
$2of3_{2S}$	Two observations for three QC samples measured at approximately the same time exceed 2 SDs from the target value in the same direction. Note that this type of rule is used when three QC materials are used for a measurement procedure.	Bias
R_{4S}	Range between observations for two QC samples measured at approximately the same time, or for two sequential observations of the same QC sample, exceeds 4 SDs.	Imprecision
10_x or 10_m	Ten sequential observations for the same QC sample are on the same side of the target value (x or mean). The 10_x rule is not recommended because it has an excessive false-alert rate.	Not recommended
8_{1S} ($8_{1.5S}$)	Eight sequential observations for the same QC sample exceed 1 SD (or 1.5 SD) in the same direction from the target value.	Bias trend
CUSUM	CUSUM of SDI for the current and previous results.	Bias trend
EWMA	EWMA for the current and previous results with newer results having more influence (weight).	Bias trend

CUSUM, Cumulative sum; *EWMA*, exponentially weighted moving averages; *QC*, quality control; *SD*, standard deviation; *SDI*, standard deviation interval.
From Miller WG. Quality control. In: *Henry's Clinical Diagnosis and Management by Laboratory Methods*. 23rd ed. Philadelphia: Elsevier; 2016.

of laboratories using the same measurement procedure and lot of QC material (see the section called External Quality Assessment or Proficiency Testing).

Establishing Rules to Evaluate Quality Control Results

The acceptable range and rules for interpretation of QC results are based on the probability of detecting a significant analytical error condition with an acceptably small false-alert rate. The desired process control performance characteristics must be established for each measurand before the appropriate QC rules can be selected.

The conventional way to express QC interpretive rules is by using an abbreviation nomenclature popularized among clinical laboratories by Westgard[42] and summarized in Table 6.3. Note that fractional standard deviation intervals (SDIs) can be used as in the $2_{2.5S}$ and $8_{1.5S}$ examples and that combinations of numbers of controls and limits can be used as appropriate for QC interpretive rules. Statistical procedures, such as cumulative sum (CUSUM) or exponentially weighted moving averages (EWMA), are preferred to monitor for bias trends.[43] It is recommended to use one of these more advanced trend detection procedures if supported by an available computer system because they are more powerful for detecting trends than approaches based on a number of sequential observations exceeding a specified SD interval from the target value.

CUSUM expresses the difference between a QC result and its target value as an SDI, or *z*-score, that is the fraction of SD represented by the difference. For example, if the target value is 25.3 and the SD is 1.4, a QC result of 27.5 would have an SDI of (27.5 − 25.3)/1.4 = 1.6. Fig. 6.9 illustrates the CUSUM of SDI values for the most recent QC result and previous results for the same QC material since the last

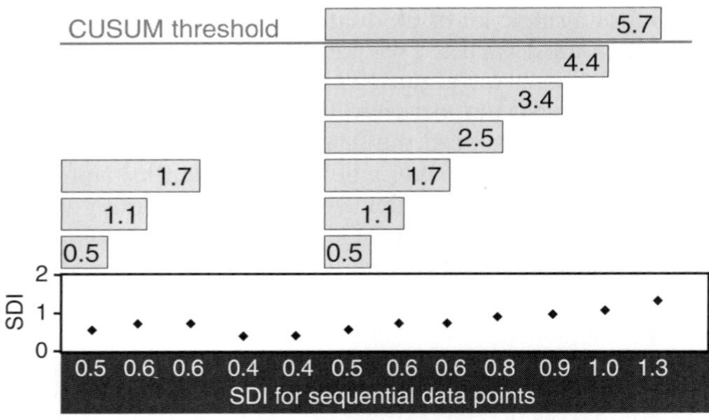

FIGURE 6.9 Cumulative sum (CUSUM) process to identify trends in sequential results. The SDI (standard deviation interval for a result vs. its target value) to initiate a CUSUM is 0.45, and the threshold for an alert is 5.0.

CUSUM reset. A minimum value for the SDI is required to initiate the cumulative summation to prevent relatively small increments from giving false alerts. If a QC value does not exceed the minimum SDI, the CUSUM is reset to zero. When the CUSUM exceeds a threshold value, an alert is given. The CUSUM alert may occur before a trend in bias causes the result for an individual QC value to be recognized as exceeding its QC evaluation rules. The threshold value for the CUSUM and the minimum value for the SDI to initiate the summation are set to provide a high probability to identify a trend in bias that may represent a defect in the measurement procedure that needs to be investigated. The threshold can be set to provide a warning that may not require immediate corrective action but rather an alert to a potential problem.

EWMA operates similarly to CUSUM by taking the average of the most recent QC result and previous results. A function in the calculation gives more "weight" or influence to the more recent values in determining the "average" of all the results. The function decreases the weights in an exponential manner such that recent results contribute a greater proportion, and older results contribute very little to the current EWMA value. Consequently, the EWMA value represents a bias trend in the QC results, and a threshold is set that may represent a defect in the measurement procedure that needs to be investigated. As for CUSUM, the threshold can be set to provide a warning that may not require immediate corrective action but rather an alert to a potential problem.

Power function graphs have been used to express the probability that a QC interpretive rule will detect an analytical error of a given magnitude.[44] Software to calculate power function graphs assumes Gaussian (normal) error distributions. Consequently, because there are influences on QC results that are non-Gaussian, the conclusions about QC rule performance from power function graphs are most useful as general guidance for selecting rules to interpret QC data. Other literature reports have addressed rule selection criteria using various statistical models and assumptions regarding distribution of errors.[45-47]

Power function graphs have been useful to indicate relationships and relative effectiveness among different QC rules. Fig. 6.10 shows an example power function graph that plots the probability to detect a measurement error (*y*-axis), which is the probability that a result will exceed a particular interpretive rule, versus a systematic bias of known magnitude in a result (*x*-axis) with a fixed random imprecision of 1 SD when there are two QC samples being measured along with the group of patient samples. The three lines in Fig. 6.10 represent the probabilities of different interpretive rules to detect biases of various magnitudes. For example, for the 1_{2S} rule, a result with a bias of 1 SD (*x*-axis) has a 0.35 (35%) probability (*y*-axis) of violating the rule (ie, of having a result >2 SDs from the target value). Note that this figure shows

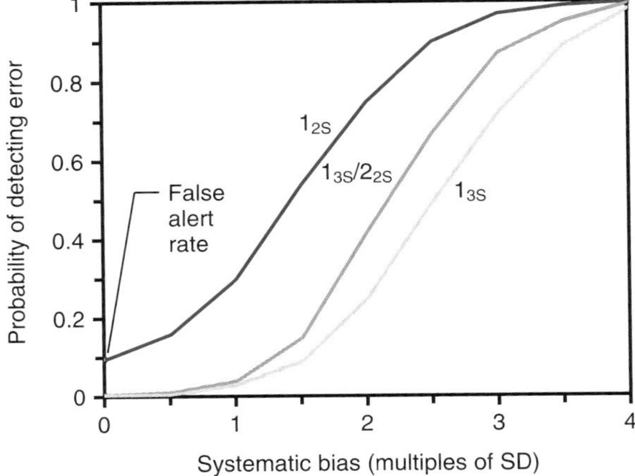

FIGURE 6.10 Power function graphs for the ability of different quality control interpretive rules to detect systematic error using two controls. Systematic error is expressed as number of standard deviations (SDs) from the target value. (Modified with permission from Westgard JO, Groth T. Power functions for statistical control rules. *Clin Chem* 1979;25:863–869.)

only bias as SD on the *x*-axis, and a result with 1 SD bias will also have an imprecision component that may cause the 1_{2S} rule to be exceeded. Thus, a 1_{2S} interpretive rule has a 35% probability to detect a systematic error that is 1 SD in magnitude. Similar graphs can be created for other interpretive rules for both bias and imprecision error conditions.

Note in Fig. 6.10 that none of these interpretive rules has a 100% probability to detect a systematic bias until the error becomes relatively large. The 1_{2S} rule has a good probability of detecting errors (eg, almost 90% probability of detecting a 2.5-SD bias) but has a high false-alert rate as indicated by the *y*-intercept that indicates that because of imprecision, the probability of indicating an error condition for zero bias is approximately 10%. Because of this high false-alert rate, it is generally not recommended to use a 1_{2S} rule unless the measurement procedure has marginal performance (ie, is a "low sigma" measurement procedure) and the laboratory desires to identify small biases that could cause inappropriate risk for a patient care decision. The 1_{3S} rule has a low false-alert rate but a lower probability to detect an error (eg, a 50% probability to detect a 2.5-SD bias).

It is recommended to improve the efficiency of QC interpretive rules by combining two or more rules and applying them simultaneously as multi-rule criteria. For example, the $1_{3S}/2_{2S}$ multi-rule identifies an error condition if one control exceeds ±3 SD from the target value or if two controls exceed ±2 SDs in the same direction from the target value. The $1_{3S}/2_{2S}$ multi-rule has a low false-alert rate similar to the 1_{3S} rule but improved probability to detect an error (eg, a 65% probability to detect a 2.5-SD bias and a 90% probability to detect a 3.2-SD bias). In this multi-rule example, whereas the 1_{3S} component is sensitive to imprecision or large bias, the 2_{2S} component is sensitive to bias.

A challenge in selecting interpretive rules for evaluating QC results is that the different longer term sources of variation listed in Table 6-2 occur at different times when using a measurement procedure. These types of variability are not adequately described by Gaussian models for rules selection. At certain periods of time, the short-term SD will be noticeably smaller than the long-term cumulative value (see Fig. 6.8). One must avoid concluding, based on a short-term estimate of SD, that the SD used for evaluation is too large because, over time, the cumulative value will be more consistent with measurement procedure performance as periodic sources of variability are encountered. Using an estimate of SD that is inappropriately small will lead to increased frequency of false alerts.

Fig. 6.11 shows how non-Gaussian error sources influenced results for a single lot of QC material used over a 10-month period for an automated glucose measurement procedure. The stability and performance over the 10 months were considered acceptable for clinical use. Data for the first 49 days are the same as in Fig. 6.6 and represent the initial experience with this lot of QC material. Examination of these data shows several fluctuations that cannot be described by a Gaussian statistical model. The first reagent lot change caused a step shift to higher values that was too small to initiate a change in target value. The second reagent lot change had no effect on QC results. Between March and April, a transition to lower values occurred that did not correspond to any maintenance, reagent lot change, or calibration events. Throughout the 10-month period, intervals of several weeks'

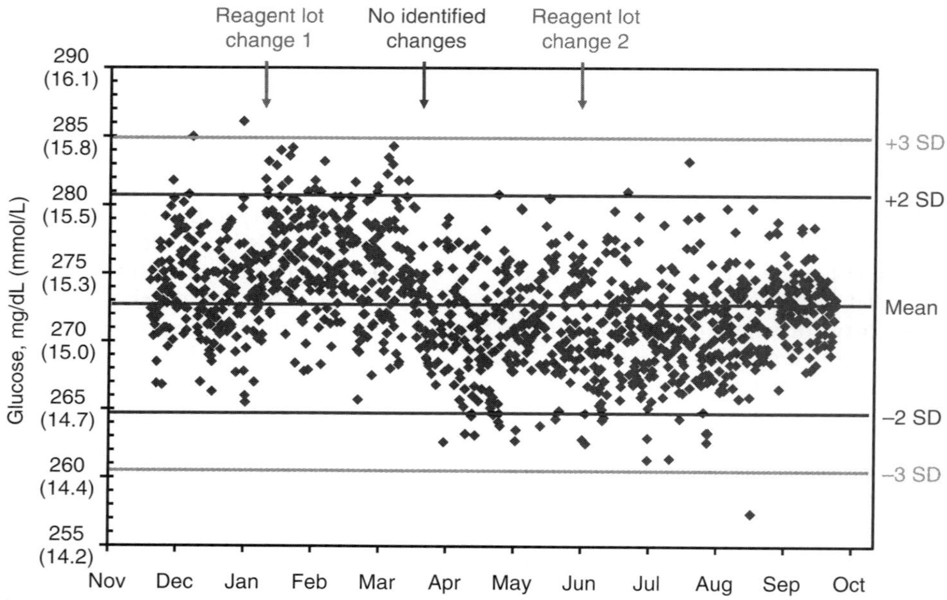

FIGURE 6.11 Levey-Jennings plot of quality control (QC) results (n = 1232) for a single lot of QC material used over a 10-month period. *SD,* Standard deviation. (Reprinted with permission from Miller WG, Nichols JH. Quality control. In: Clarke WA, editor. *Contemporary practice in clinical chemistry.* 2nd ed. Washington, DC: AACC Press; 2010.)

TABLE 6.4 Empirical Multi-Rule for the Quality Control Data Presented in Fig. 6.11

Multi-Rule Components	Type of Variability Detected
1_{3S}	Imprecision or bias
$2_{2.5S}$	Bias
R_{4S}	Imprecision
$8_{1.5S}$	Bias trend

QC, Quality control.
From Miller WG. Quality control. In: *Henry's Clinical Diagnosis and Management by Laboratory Methods.* 23rd ed. Philadelphia: Elsevier; 2016.

duration occurred when the imprecision was better or worse than at other time periods (also see Fig. 6.8 calculated from the same data).

In practice, empirical judgment is frequently used to establish acceptance criteria (rules) to evaluate QC results based on data acquired over a long enough time to adequately estimate the expected variability when a measurement procedure is working correctly. It is recommended not to select QC rules based only on Gaussian models of imprecision because the rules will not correctly accommodate all the types of variability observed for many analytical systems.

Table 6.4 gives an example of an empirically developed multi-rule based on the data in Fig. 6.11. An empirical approach can be used by obtaining a set of QC data that represents a time interval expected to include most sources of variability. Using those data, the false-alert rate for a rule can be determined, and bias errors of different magnitudes can be added to estimate the ability of a rule, or a combination of rules, to identify that error. This multi-rule had 0.6% false alerts when applied to the data in Fig. 6.11 using the mean from the November to January (see Fig. 6.6) period as the target value and the cumulative SD for the 10-month period to represent overall imprecision. If a 2_{2S} rule was used instead of a $2_{2.5S}$ rule, the false-alert rate would increase by 1.2%, but the rule would detect slightly smaller biases. An $8_{1.5S}$ rule was used to provide detection of bias trends because it had a 0% false-alert rate (compared with 0.5% for an 8_{1S} rule) and was adequate to detect a developing trend before it became clinically important because the CV was small, 1.5%, at the concentration of the QC material. If a 10% TE_a is considered acceptable for glucose at this concentration, then the sigma metric for this measurement procedure is 6.7, suggesting that it has a very low error rate, and these QC rules with a low false-alert rate will be suitable to alert the laboratory to an error condition that might affect patient care decisions. Such control rules should allow the laboratory to detect errors before they are of a magnitude that will affect clinical actions. At other clinical concentration ranges or for other analytes, a different set of QC evaluations rules may be more appropriate. A 10_x rule was not used because it would have increased the false-alert rate by 10.6%. A 10_x rule or other rule that counts the number of sequential QC results on one side of the target value is not recommended because this condition does not indicate a problem with clinical interpretation of patient results when the magnitude of the difference from the target value is small. Counting the number of sequential results that exceed a larger SD from the target value, such as $8_{1.5S}$ in this example, is more likely to represent a measurement condition that might need investigation.

The balance between false alerts and the probability of detecting an error is improved when multiple rules are used in combination. When establishing rules to interpret QC results, it is important to remember that statistical process control can only verify at a point in time that a measurement procedure is producing results that conform to the expected variability when the procedure is performing in a stable operating condition. It is important to remember that periodic measurement of QC samples does not identify random events (eg, a temporary clot in a sample pipet, a random reagent pipet error) that do not persist until the next QC sample is measured. QC rules are chosen to detect changes in calibration and changes in imprecision that persist until the next QC measurement and are significant enough to require correction before patient results are reported.

In the process of reviewing statistical parameters for QC data, a measurement procedure's performance may be identified as marginal or inadequate to meet medical requirements. Determining the sigma metric is helpful to make this assessment because the sigma value gives a prediction of the number of erroneous results expected. If the measurement procedure performance cannot be improved and a better measurement procedure is not available, the laboratory can either discontinue the test if the performance is inadequate or apply more stringent QC practices to identify small deviations from the expected performance. More stringent QC practices include selecting rules that will give an alert at smaller error conditions, using additional rules in a multirule set, measuring QC more frequently, using more than two QC samples, and not releasing patient results until QC assessment is complete for the time interval during which patient samples were measured. It is usually necessary to measure QC samples more frequently for lower sigma measurement procedures. It is important to recognize that more stringent QC rules will not improve measurement procedure performance but will identify smaller changes in measurement procedure performance that could affect patient care decisions based on the results. More stringent QC rules will have more false alerts, but this is an unavoidable cost when lower sigma measurement procedures are used. Because the analytical requirements are not easy to establish and are themselves somewhat uncertain, one should regularly readdress the requirements to see if they remain appropriate or should be updated and should reconsider that the QC rules are appropriate to identify an error condition. In addition, the measurement procedure limitations should be communicated to patient care providers.

Specifying the Quality Control Plan

The preceding subsections describe the considerations for each component in a QC plan. The laboratory director is responsible for considering the components, making judgments regarding the considerations, and approving the final plan for each analyte measured in a laboratory. A plan for internal QC using surrogate samples specifies the following components:

- The number of controls to be measured and the approximate concentrations of analytes in those controls
- The target values for each control
- The SD to be used in the QC rules
- The rules for evaluating the QC results
- The frequency to test the QC samples

Overall, the choice of the parameters in the QC plan depends on the performance characteristics of the measurement procedure, the number of potentially erroneous patient results that could occur before the error condition is identified, and the risk of harm to a patient if potentially erroneous results were used in clinical care decisions. Yundt-Pacheco and Parvin described a methodology to compute the expected number of unreliable patient results produced based on an out-of-control condition and the performance characteristics of a measurement procedure.[48]

Considerations for Point-of-Care Testing

Internal QC of POC instruments offer extra challenges compared with those addressed at the central laboratory. The main reasons for this are that POC instruments are often operated by persons without laboratory training; they often use methodologic principles that are different from those in the central laboratory; they often have "built-in" controls; and the number of measurements is rather small, making the use of QC samples in the traditional way expensive. Because the instruments are used by nonlaboratory personnel who also should run the QC program, these people have to be convinced that measuring QC samples is useful and will detect errors important for patient safety. Unfortunately, the evidence for measuring QC samples is scarce, probably because there is little agreement on how to implement QC for POC instruments and how to handle the QC alerts. In the ISO 22870 document[49] it is stated that if an institution wants to be accredited to this standard, internal and external QC of POC instruments should be done, but it is not stated how this should be done. Recommendations from different countries generally state that it is "mandatory" to measure QC samples, but they are usually vague concerning how it should be done, from analyzing two levels of QC materials a day to one level of QC material every sixth month or as "recommended by the manufacturer" or "recommended to use control material independent from the manufacturer" and use specifications as defined by the local laboratory.[50]

It is not surprising that there are no uniform or concrete recommendations because POC instruments use different methodologies and technologies, and they are used at different locations, from wards at a hospital to remote areas. Before establishing an internal QC program for POC instruments, at least three issues should be taken into consideration: (1) the type of POC instrument and what "built-in" control processes it has, (2) the location of the instrument, and (3) the operator of the instrument. Broadly, the current instruments have been divided into three categories: (1) instruments that are similar to the wet chemistry instruments used in the central laboratory, (2) cartridge-based instruments, and (3) strip-based instruments,[51] although there is a significant "overlap" between the two last categories. The instruments using wet chemistry and similar technologies to those used in the central laboratory should follow the principles for internal QC as outlined in this chapter albeit taking into consideration the number of measurements per day. In cartridge-based and some strip-based instruments, the manufacturer often has placed the technology in the cartridge or strip together with QCs, and in some cases, QC rules are built in so that patient results cannot be reported unless the QC is "satisfactory." The instrument is then merely an electronic reader that often has incorporated an "electronic quality control" where the electronics of the measurement procedure are verified. The electronic instrument checks do not verify the reagents in the cartridges or strips, and unless each cartridge has internal QC materials, the reagent cartridges or strips should be checked at delivery and then at intervals (eg, with the arrival of a new shipment or lot or at a suitable interval such as monthly).

Not all POC instruments include enhanced QC features. In these cases, one must rely on daily liquid surrogate QC performed by the operator.[52] The limitation of using the liquid QC sample in this situation is that it only checks if one disposable cartridge or strip meets the performance specifications. Inevitably, this limitation requires an assumption that all devices in a lot were manufactured uniformly and will perform equivalently. Some tests, such as dipstick urinalysis, require liquid QC because there are no built-in control mechanisms. Others, such as urine pregnancy tests, have a built-in positive control band to ensure that the device is functioning properly, but this may not be an adequate substitute for a traditional QC sample that can assess suitable recovery of concentrations. Some POC protocols run patients' samples on a POC instrument and send the same samples to a central laboratory as a form of internal QC. It has been shown for international normalized ratio that this periodic split patients' samples procedure cannot be recommended because it had a lower probability of error detection and a higher rate of false alarms compared with using commercial lyophilized QC material.[53] The operator of the instrument is also important. In patient self-testing, it is difficult to implement internal QC procedures other than what is built into the instruments or strips or cartridges.

How internal QC should be performed and supervised also depend on the location of the POC instruments. In a hospital, it is now possible with real-time bidirectional connectivity between the POC devices and the central laboratory to transfer both patient and QC results and to set lock out parameters for conformance to a QC protocol. As technology advances, the general trend is for more sophisticated POC devices with built-in control systems to be incorporated to minimize or prevent the possibility for an incorrect result.[54]

Corrective Action When a Quality Control Result Indicates a Measurement Problem

A QC alert occurs when a QC result fails an evaluation rule, which indicates that an analytical problem may exist. A QC alert means there is a high probability that the measurement procedure is producing results that have the potential to be unreliable for patient care. When this condition occurs, it is necessary to take corrective action to investigate the cause of the QC alert. Fig. 6.12 presents a generalized troubleshooting sequence. Remeasuring the same QC sample is not recommended because, with properly designed control rules, it is more likely that a measurement procedure problem exists than the QC result was a statistical outlier or gave a false alert. However, QC materials can deteriorate after opening because of improper handling and storage or because of unstable measurands. Thus, repeating the measurement on a new vial of the QC material is a useful step to determine if the alert was caused by deteriorated QC material rather than by a measurement procedure problem. In this situation, if the result for the new QC sample is acceptable, testing of patient samples can resume. One caution when the repeat QC result is near acceptability limits, is to consider whether the repeat and original results are essentially the same. In this situation, the probability is fairly high that a measurement problem exists, and this possibility should be investigated. In addition, current and preceding QC results should be examined for a trend in bias that indicates a measurement issue that needs to be corrected. These precautions in evaluating repeat results for a new QC sample can be challenging or impossible for automated evaluation by computer systems, thus requiring the laboratory technologist to be vigilant in reviewing results.

When repeat testing of a new QC sample does not resolve the alert situation, the instrument and reagents should be inspected for component deterioration, empty reagent containers, mechanical problems, and so on. In many cases, it will be necessary to recalibrate (or verify calibration).

When the problem is identified and corrected, QC samples should be measured to verify the correction, and all patient samples since the time of the last acceptable QC results, or the time when the error condition occurred, should be measured again. It may be difficult to establish the time when an error condition occurred, but repeating selected patient results may be considered. For example, every few samples can be repeated back to the time of the last acceptable QC results. The repeated results are then compared with acceptable criteria for repeated results agreement (see later discussion) to identify a point in time when the error condition occurred. When selecting the samples to repeat, it is important to ensure that a substantial representation of the potentially erroneous samples is repeated and that samples at a concentration consistent with that of the unacceptable QC are represented. Alternatively, groups of 10 patient samples can be repeated, again ensuring that samples at a concentration consistent with that of the unacceptable QC are represented, until all repeat results in at least two sequential groups are within acceptable criteria for repeated results. When the point at which the error condition was likely to have occurred is identified, all patient samples must be repeated from that point until the unacceptable QC result was obtained. Any assessment of the point at which an error condition occurred by repeating selected patient samples has a risk to incorrectly identify that point and laboratories are encouraged to repeat enough patient samples to have confidence in the assessment.

The laboratory director must establish acceptable criteria to determine if the repeat results agree adequately to permit reporting of original results without issuing a corrected report. Otherwise, corrected results must be reported. As an example, Table 6-5 lists empirical criteria used in one author's laboratory for this purpose. The criteria for acceptability of repeated tests are based on measurement procedure performance characteristics and clinical requirements of the medical services. The considerations for determining the TE_a described in the section Performance of a Measurement Procedure for its Intended Medical Use and in Chapter 7 related to the reference change value may be helpful to set acceptance criteria for repeated patient sample results.

In some cases, residual sample volume may not be adequate for repeat testing (quantity not sufficient [QNS]). In these situations, no results can be reported unless it is documented that the impact of the measurement procedure defect on the original results was small enough to have minimal effect on clinical interpretation. A protocol to evaluate the clinical impact of the measurement defect involves repeating those samples that have adequate volume. The repeated samples must represent the concentration range of the QNS samples and the time span since the previous acceptable

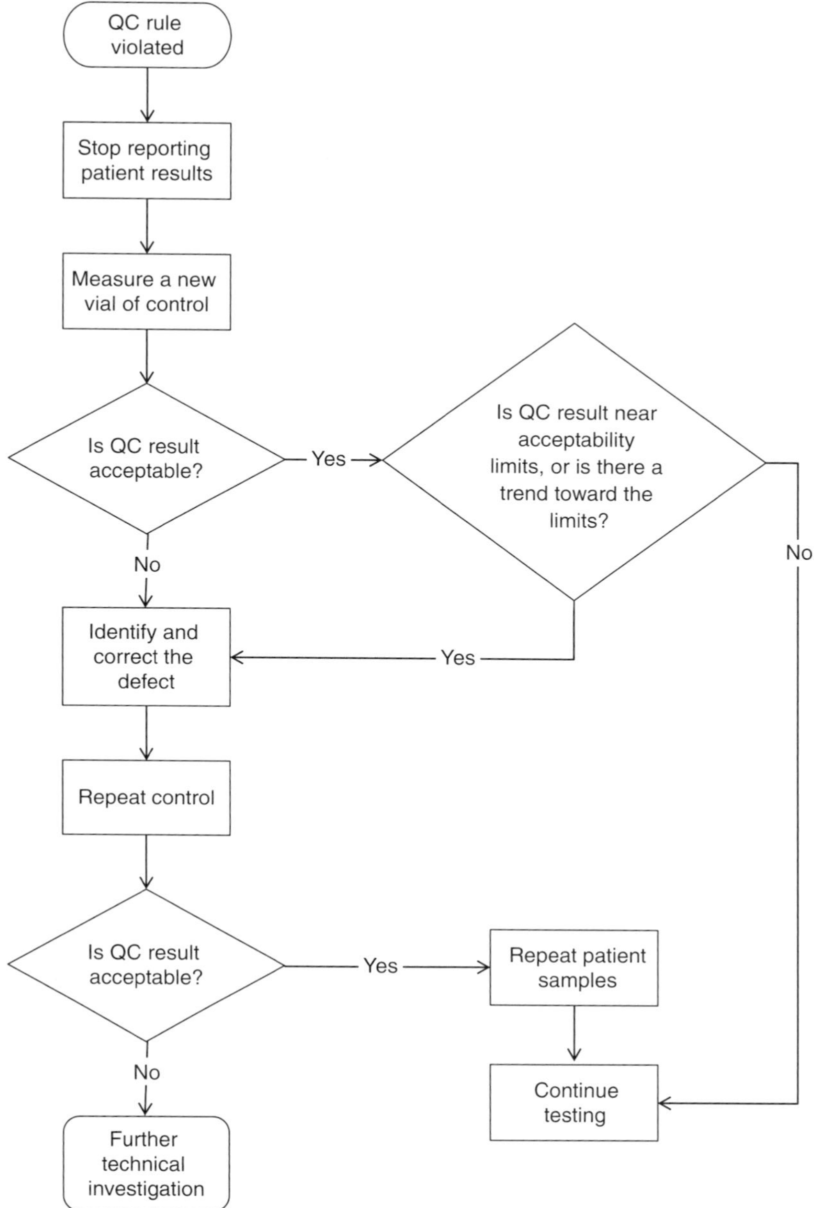

FIGURE 6.12 Generalized troubleshooting sequence showing the initial steps after an unacceptable quality control (QC) result. The details of troubleshooting the defect may be different for different rules violations or if more than one unacceptable QC result was obtained.

QC results and should include a substantial proportion of the total samples originally assayed while the measurement procedure was in the unacceptable condition. If the repeat results for this sample group are within established "acceptable" criteria for repeat testing of patient samples, the original results for the QNS samples can be reported. Otherwise, the original results for the QNS samples are considered erroneous; no results can be reported, and any original results already reported need to be corrected to a "no result" condition.

Alternatively, for QNS samples, when there was not an outright malfunction but rather a drift or shift in calibration, it may be possible to estimate the magnitude of a bias error from the results for other patient samples that were repeated, apply that bias as a correction to the QNS samples, and report the corrected result with a comment regarding the increased uncertainty in the values. When there are inadequate data to estimate a correction factor from repeated results for other patients, the laboratory may consider reporting the original result for a QNS sample with a comment regarding its uncertainty. This approach can be useful especially in cases when it might be difficult or take a long time to obtain a new sample or in cases when the clinical question can be answered by whether the result is very high or very low (eg, hypo- or hyperthyroidism). The laboratory director should be consulted for guidance in reporting results for QNS samples that may have greater uncertainty than the usual quality performance for a laboratory.

TABLE 6.5 Example for Selected Chemistry Analytes of Empirical Criteria for Patient Test Result Agreement Between Repeated Assays and for Agreement Among Results for a Single Patient Sample Measured on Multiple Instruments

Analyte	Acceptance Criteria (Difference Between Results)
Albumin	0.4 g/dL (4.0 g/L)
ALP	10 U/L or 10%*
ALT	10 U/L or 10%*
Amylase	15 U/L or 10%*
AST	10 U/L or 10%*
Bilirubin, total	0.3 mg/dL (5 μmol/L) or 10%*
Calcium, total	0.5 mg/dL (0.125 mmol/L)
Chloride	4 mmol/L
Cholesterol	5%
CK	10 U/L or 10%*
CO_2	4 mmol/L
Creatinine	0.2 mg/dL (0.018 mmol/L) or 10%*
GGT	10 U/L or 10%*
Glucose	6 mg/dL (0.33 mmol/L) or 5%*
Iron	10 μg/dL (1.8 μmol/L) or 10%*
Lactate	0.32 mmol/L
LDH	10 U/L or 10%*
Lipase	10 U/L or 10%*
Magnesium	0.3 mg/dL (0.1 mmol/L)
Phosphorus	0.4 mg/dL (0.13 mmol/L)
Potassium	0.3 mmol/L
Protein, total	0.4 g/dL (4.0 g/L)
Sodium	4 mmol/L
Triglycerides	10%
Urea nitrogen (BUN)	3 mg/dL (1.1 mmol/L urea) or 10%*
Uric acid	0.4 mg/dL (24 μmol/L)

*Whichever is greater.

ALP, Alkaline phosphatase; *ALT*, alanine aminotransferase; *AST*, aspartate aminotransferase; *BUN*, blood urea nitrogen; *CK*, creatine kinase; *CO_2*, carbon dioxide; *GGT*, γ-glutamyl transferase; *LDH*, lactate dehydrogenase.

From Miller WG. Quality control. In: *Henry's Clinical Diagnosis and Management by Laboratory Methods*. 23rd ed. Philadelphia: Elsevier; 2016.

Verifying Quality Control Evaluation Parameters After a Reagent Lot Change

Changing reagent lots can have an unexpected impact on QC results. Careful reagent lot crossover evaluation of QC target values is necessary. Because the matrix-related interaction between a QC material and a reagent can change with a different reagent lot, QC results may not be a reliable indicator of a measurement procedure's performance for patient samples after a reagent lot change. In a large study of 661 reagent lot changes for eight QC materials assayed for 82 analytes using seven different instrument platforms, 41% of 1483 QC material–reagent lot combinations had significant differences in QC values between the reagent lots that were not observed for patient samples.[36] In the example in Fig. 6.13, QC values for the high-concentration control shifted after the change to a new lot of reagents, but there was no change in results for the low control. A comparison of results

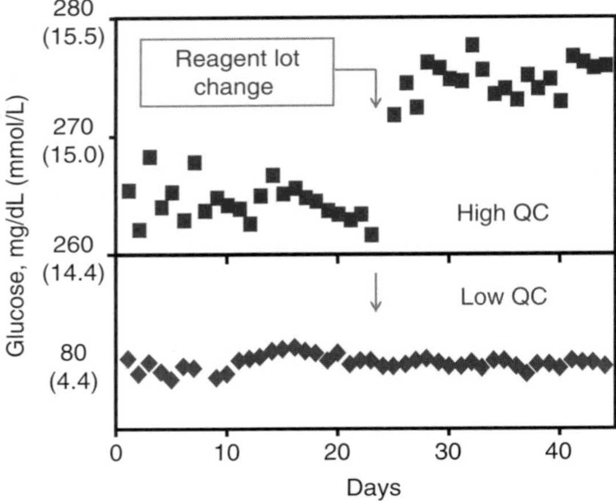

FIGURE 6.13 Levey-Jennings plot showing impact of a reagent lot change on matrix bias with quality control (QC) samples. (Modified with permission from Miller WG, Nichols JH. Quality control. In: Clarke WA, editor. *Contemporary practice in clinical chemistry*. 2nd ed. Washington DC: AACC Press; 2010.)

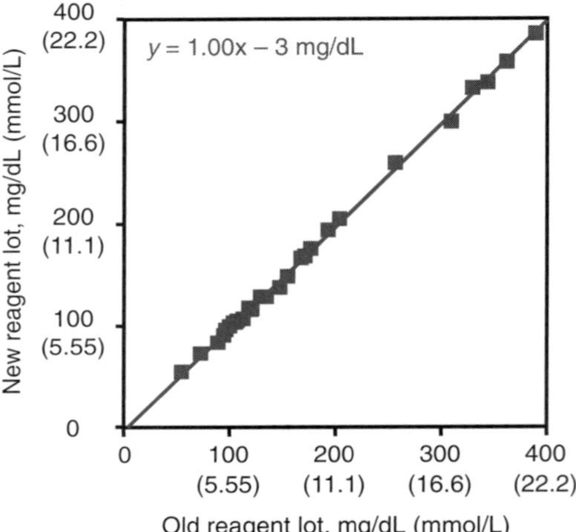

FIGURE 6.14 Deming regression analysis of results from a patient sample comparison between the same old and new lots of reagent shown in Fig. 6.13 for quality control samples. (From Miller WG. Quality control. In: *Henry's Clinical Diagnosis and Management by Laboratory Methods*. 23rd ed. Philadelphia: Elsevier; 2016.)

for a panel of patient samples assayed using the new and old reagent lots, as shown in Fig. 6.14, verified that patient results were the same when either lot of reagents was used. Patient results spanning the measuring interval had nearly identical values, as indicated by the slope of 1.00 and the small intercept of −3 mg/dL (0.17 mmol/L). Consequently, the change in QC values for the high-concentration material was due to a difference in matrix-related bias between the QC material and each of the reagent lots.

It is necessary to use clinical patient samples to verify the consistency of results between old and new lots of reagents because of the unpredictability of a matrix-related bias being present for QC materials. Fig. 6.15 presents a protocol to verify or adjust QC material target values after a reagent lot change. A group of patient samples and the QC samples are measured using both the current (old) and new reagent lots. The first step is to verify that results for a group of patient samples measured with the new reagent lot are consistent

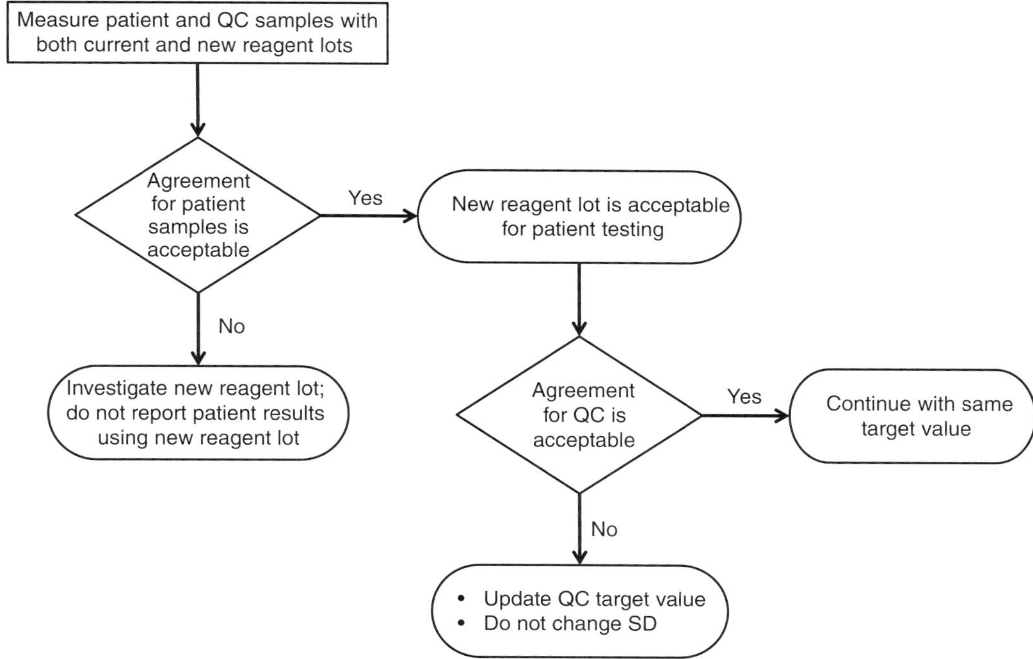

FIGURE 6.15 Process for assessment of potential matrix impact on quality control (QC) samples after a reagent lot change. *SD*, Standard deviation. (From Miller WG. Quality control. In: *Henry's Clinical Diagnosis and Management by Laboratory Methods*. 23rd ed. Philadelphia: Elsevier; 2016.)

with results from the current (old) lot. The patient sample results, not the QC results, provide the basis for verifying that the new reagent lot is acceptable for use. If a problem is identified, the calibration of the new reagent lot must be investigated and corrected, or the new reagent lot may be defective and should not be used. When evaluating the patient results, keep in mind that the calibration of the old reagent lot may have drifted and should be verified before concluding that the new reagent lot is not giving acceptable results for the patient samples.

The number of patient samples to use for verifying the performance of a new reagent lot will depend on the measuring interval, the imprecision of a measurement procedure, and the concentrations at which clinical decisions are made. CLSI document EP26[55] recommends a minimum of three patient samples and more patient samples depending on the number of important clinical decision concentrations and the imprecision of a measurement procedure. This CLSI guideline includes a statistical analysis to determine if a difference in patient results is less than a critical difference that would represent risk for an inappropriate patient care decision based on a particular laboratory test result. An alternate approach is to select 10 or more patient samples that span the measuring interval and use orthogonal regression analysis or a difference plot to evaluate average performance over the interval of concentrations represented by the patient samples.

There are no well-established clinical acceptance criteria for agreement between results; consequently, the laboratory must establish acceptance criteria consistent with the relatively small number of samples used, the analytical performance characteristics of a measurement procedure, and the clinical requirements for interpreting results. As an example, empirical acceptance criteria used in one author's laboratory for assessment of individual results are provided in Table 6-5.

When the results for patients are acceptable, the second step in Fig. 6.15 evaluates results for each QC material to determine if its target value is correct for use with the new lot of reagent(s). If the target value has changed, it must be adjusted to correct for the change in matrix-related bias between old and new lots of reagent(s). This adjustment keeps the expected variability centered around the QC target value so that QC interpretive rules will remain valid. Failure to make a target value adjustment will introduce an artifactual bias in subsequent QC results, causing both an increased false-alert rate and a decreased ability to detect some error conditions. These effects are illustrated in Fig. 6.16 where the shift in target value would cause some of the results shown by *squares* to exceed the old upper QC rule limit when in reality there is no defect in patient results because the QC results are artifactually increased because of the matrix-related bias with the new reagent lot. Similarly, the increased magnitude of the gap to the old lower QC rule limit will permit a low bias condition, as shown by the square red points at sequence number 29 and 30, to be undetected until the low bias becomes larger than the QC rule is intended to detect.

The SD used to evaluate QC results will not typically change when a new lot of reagent(s) is put into use. The SD represents expected variability when the measurement procedure is stable and is performing according to specifications. In most cases, the variability of a measurement procedure will be the same with any lot of reagent(s). However, occasional exceptions may occur; for example, if the new reagent lot is a reformulation, it may be necessary to adjust the SD after additional numbers of QC results are accumulated with the new reagent lot. A reagent lot verification is typically performed on a single day and will likely provide only a few QC results from which to evaluate if the target value has changed. Consequently, it is necessary to carefully monitor QC results

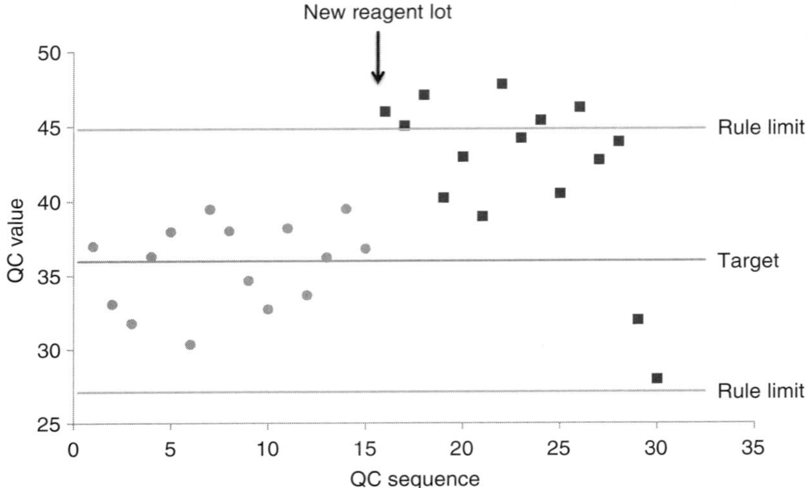

FIGURE 6.16 Illustration of the influence on the failure rate for a quality control (QC) rule when failing to adjust the target value for a matrix-related shift. QC results before a new reagent lot are shown as *gray circles* and after the new reagent lot as *red squares*. *SD,* Standard deviation. (From Miller WG. Quality control. In: *Henry's Clinical Diagnosis and Management by Laboratory Methods.* 23rd ed. Philadelphia: Elsevier; 2016.)

as more data are acquired using the new reagent lot and, if needed, to further refine the new target value.

Note that a reagent lot induced matrix-related change in the numeric values for the QC results will cause an artifactual increase in the cumulative SD, thus making it larger than the inherent measurement variability and not suitable for use in QC rules. For this reason, it is recommended to use the cumulative SD from a single reagent lot or the pooled SD from more than one reagent lot (see subsection called Quality Control Material Standard Deviation) when determining the SD to use for interpreting QC rules.

Experience in clinical laboratories has shown that there are changes, other than reagent lot changes, in measurement procedures that can also affect the QC values but not the results for patient samples. Such changes could be caused by instrument component replacement or other causes. In theory, there should be an assignable cause for such effects, but such a cause is not always identifiable. In practice, any condition that affects QC results but does not affect patient results is treated in the same manner as described for reagent lot changes. The important QC principle is that if the results for patient samples are consistent between the two conditions, then the target value for the QC sample should be adjusted, if necessary, to reflect its value under the new condition. Failure to adjust the QC target value will cause inappropriate acceptability criteria to be used for evaluating the QC results.

Verifying Measurement Procedure Performance After Use of a New Lot of Calibrator

When a new lot of calibrator is used, with no change in reagents, there is no change in matrix interaction between the QC material and the reagents. In this situation, QC results provide a reliable indication of calibration status with the new lot of calibrator. If the QC results indicate a bias after use of a new lot of calibrator, the calibration has changed and needs to be corrected to ensure consistent results for patient samples.

Some measurement procedures are packaged as kits that include reagents, calibrators, and QC materials. In this case, QC results could fail to identify a calibration shift when a new kit lot is used, and it is necessary to measure patient samples with the old and new kit lots to verify consistency of patient results. When possible, it is recommended to use QC materials that are independent of the kit lot and to avoid changing lots of QC material at the same time as changing lots of reagent or calibrators. Measuring patient samples always provides a reliable approach to verify the consistency of results after changes in lots of reagents or calibrators as well as changes in other measurement conditions.

Review of Quality Control Data and the Effectiveness of the Quality Control Plan

The immediate use of QC data is to determine if the results for patient samples can be reported for use in clinical care decisions as described in the preceding sections. In addition, QC data must be reviewed by laboratory management on a regular schedule. Typical review schedules are weekly by senior technologists or supervisors and at least monthly by the laboratory director. However, the laboratory director should promptly review items such as reagent or calibrator lot change validations, changes in QC target values associated with reagent lot or other changes, EQA/PT results review, and other occurrences that may affect quality of the laboratory results.

The weekly review process should determine that correct follow up of any QC alerts was conducted, that all patient samples that may have had erroneous results were repeated, that any corrected reports were issued, and that the process was properly documented in QC records. The monthly review should include any issues identified by the weekly review process as well as examination of the Levey-Jennings chart or other tool to identify trends or changes in assay performance that may need to be addressed before they have effects on clinical care decisions. Note that automated systems to assist in the review of QC data are acceptable, and individual

TABLE 6.6 **Examples of Quality Indicators for the Examination Process**

Quality Indicator	Interpretation
Frequency of QC alerts	Compare with the frequency expected for the measurement procedure sigma metric and QC rules used. A higher frequency may indicate an issue with the measurement procedure or inappropriate QC rules. A lower frequency may indicate inappropriate QC rules.
Frequency of recalibration based on QC alerts	May indicate that recalibration should be performed more frequently.
Number of reagent changes due to QC alerts	May indicate that reagents are not stable and smaller quantities should be used or perhaps more frequent recalibration should be performed to compensate for reagent changes.
Number of times controls were repeated without confirming a measurement error	May indicate that the QC rules allow too high frequency of false alerts or the QC material is not stable after opening, is stored incorrectly, or other QC handling issue.
Frequency of unscheduled maintenance due to QC alerts	May indicate that maintenance is needed on a more frequent schedule.
Number of patient samples repeated based on QC alerts	May indicate that QC should be performed more frequently to minimize the risk of an erroneous result causing harm to a patient.
Frequency that patient samples are repeated based on QC alerts	May indicate inadequate calibration or maintenance schedules, that QC rules are inappropriate, or the QC sample target value or SD is not a correct reflection of measurement procedure performance.
Number of patient results corrected	May indicate an unstable measurement procedure and that QC should be performed more frequently to minimize the risk of an erroneous result causing harm to a patient.
Number of EQA/PT unacceptable results	May indicate that a measurement procedure is not calibrated correctly or some part of the measurement is not being performed correctly.

EQA, External quality assessment; *PT,* proficiency testing; *QC,* quality control; *SD,* standard deviation.

Levey-Jennings charts do not need to be examined every month. A report that compares the mean and SD for QC results over a defined time interval, such as 1 month, to the expected values consistent with stable performance can be useful to focus the review on measurement procedures that may need attention. For example, the report might identify a QC mean value that is more than a specified amount, such as 1 SD, from its target value, an SD that exceeds its expected value, or the number of individual results that exceed 2 or 3 SDs from the target value. QC values that are identified as needing further examination can then be followed up with review of a Levey-Jennings chart or other records of measurement procedure performance such as maintenance, calibration, and reagent change. The monthly review should also include any patient data–based QC procedures described in the following sections, as well as notation of any adjustments made to QC parameters during the month.

The QC review process serves three major functions, which are to (1) verify that the measurement procedures are stable and meeting their performance specifications, (2) identify measurement procedures that may need intervention to address performance issues, and (3) make adjustments as needed to the QC plan based on review of relevant quality indicators. Quality indicators and implementation of the laboratory quality management program are described in Chapter 3. Table 6-6 lists some useful quality indicators related to the examination process and its QC plan. The quality indicators should be reviewed at regular intervals as part of the overall quality management program and can also be reviewed at suitable intervals during regularly scheduled QC review meetings to determine if changes in the QC plan may be needed.

POINTS TO REMEMBER

Internal Quality Control/Statistical Process Control

- QC material is measured along with patient samples.
- The target value and SD expected for a control material are established by the laboratory.
- Results from control samples are evaluated using interpretive rules that are established after considering the probability for false alerts and the probability for detecting errors that represent a risk of harm to a patient.
- The QC plan is designed to confirm acceptable performance of a measurement procedure and to identify error conditions that may cause risk of harm to a patient.

USING PATIENT DATA IN QUALITY CONTROL PROCEDURES

In addition to using patient samples to verify consistency of patient results when changing lots of reagent or calibrators for a measurement procedure discussed previously, patient data are used in other QC applications. A delta check process compares current with previous results for a patient to identify inconsistencies that may represent a preexamination or measurement error. Comparison of patient results among different measurement procedures used in a healthcare system for the same measurand is used to ensure that calibration of the different measurement procedures produces consistent results. Patient results can also be used to monitor the performance of a measurement procedure in a statistical QC process as a supplement to the surrogate QC sample approach.

Delta Check With a Previous Result for a Patient

Some types of laboratory errors can be identified by comparing a patient's current test result against a previous result for the same measurand. This comparison is called a "delta check." Delta check values can be developed in three ways.[56] The first approach is to set delta check values based empirically on experience and then adjust them with time so as not to generate too many delta check failures that are false alerts. The second involves collecting large numbers of consecutive pairs of patient data that are similar to the patient data to which the delta check values will be applied. Then the differences (the delta values) are calculated and plotted in a frequency distribution histogram. Delta check values are identified to flag a certain percentage, for example, 5% or 1% of the observed delta values. The third approach is to calculate the reference change value based on analytical and within-subject variation (see Chapter 7). Reference change values can then be used to flag reports to alert users to those serial results in an individual where, for example, there is less than 1% probability that the change can be explained by analytical and biologic variation.

Delta checks can be used for different purposes but are most useful to detect mislabeled samples and samples altered by dilution with intravenous fluid. Consequently, an effective delta check process can be established using a limited number of measurands. The difference between results that cause a delta check alert must be sufficiently large to avoid excessive numbers of false alerts yet adequate to allow identification of samples that may be compromised and require follow-up investigation. Table 6-7 shows, as an example, the delta check parameters for automated chemistry used in one author's laboratory designed to identify compromised patient samples. The delta criteria were based on assessment of the delta values for consecutive pairs of patient data that had differences likely to be greater than physiological variation and that had an alert rate less than 1%.

Delta checks can detect analytical measurement errors; however, the threshold values necessary to identify analytical errors is fairly small compared with physiologic changes and may cause a large number of false alerts that reduce the efficiency of laboratory workflow. A well-designed statistical QC plan is more effective to detect analytical errors. However, delta checks might be useful to identify an interfering substance (eg, from a drug) that may appear in a patient's sample. Kazmierczak[57] has reviewed and presented recommendations for using delta check and other patient data–based QC procedures. CLSI has published guideline EP33 for using delta checks in the clinical laboratory.[58]

TABLE 6.7 Example Delta Check Criteria Intended to Identify Samples That Are Potentially Mislabeled or Contaminated With Intravenous Fluids Because of Incorrect Collection

Test	Delta Criteria
Sodium	5% change within previous 48 hours
Urea nitrogen	60% change within previous 48 hours
Creatinine	50% change within previous 48 hours
Calcium	25% change within previous 48 hours
Osmolality	5% change within previous 48 hours

From Miller WG. Quality control. In: *Henry's Clinical Diagnosis and Management by Laboratory Methods*. 23rd ed. Philadelphia: Elsevier; 2016.

Verify Consistency of Results Between More Than One Instrument or Measurement Procedure

Another common use of patient results as part of the QC process is to verify the consistency of patient results when a measurand is measured using more than one instrument or measurement procedure within the same health delivery system. Verification of consistent results is necessary even when identical measurement procedures from the same manufacturer are used. Good laboratory practice requires that multiple instruments or measurement procedures for the same measurand be calibrated to produce the same results for patient samples whenever possible. It may be necessary to modify the calibration settings of one measurement procedure so that results for patient samples will be equivalent to those for another measurement procedure. This strategy allows a common reference interval to be used, provides continuity in results among different laboratory testing locations, and avoids clinical confusion regarding interpretation of laboratory results.

As illustrated in Fig. 6.17, consistency of patient results is verified by measuring clinical patient sample aliquots using each of two or more measurement procedures to evaluate and, if necessary, adjust the calibration or use a postmeasurement correction function as needed to achieve agreement in results for patient samples. Such an analysis design is called a "round robin." One procedure may be chosen to represent the primary measurement procedure (or designated comparison measurement procedure) to which others will be adjusted to achieve equivalent results. The primary measurement procedure should be chosen based on quality and reliability of results with consideration of its calibration traceability to a national or international reference system, its performance stability, its analytical selectivity for the analyte, and its susceptibility to interfering substances. An alternate approach is to evaluate each measurement procedure for agreement with the mean of all measurement procedures and to adjust the calibration of any measurement procedures as necessary to produce equivalent results among the group.

There are no well-established guidelines regarding the number of samples to use for a round robin exchange. The laboratory needs to establish the frequency of evaluation and the number of samples based on the stability of the measurement procedures, the frequency of reagent and calibrator lot changes, and the clinical requirements of the health delivery system. Common practices include a round robin exchange of one or more individual patient samples or a pool prepared from several samples on a weekly basis for high-volume measurement procedures or on a monthly or quarterly basis for lower volume or very stable measurement procedures. For frequent comparisons with one or two samples, concentrations should be chosen to evaluate the measuring interval over a period of several examinations. For less frequent comparisons, a larger number of patient samples is recommended to cover the measuring interval. When establishing interpretation criteria, the laboratory needs to consider the limited statistical power for the number of results available. CLSI document EP31 provides a statistical approach suitable for using one to five samples in a comparison.[59]

Table 6.5 provides, as an example, empirical criteria used in one author's laboratory for evaluation of agreement among

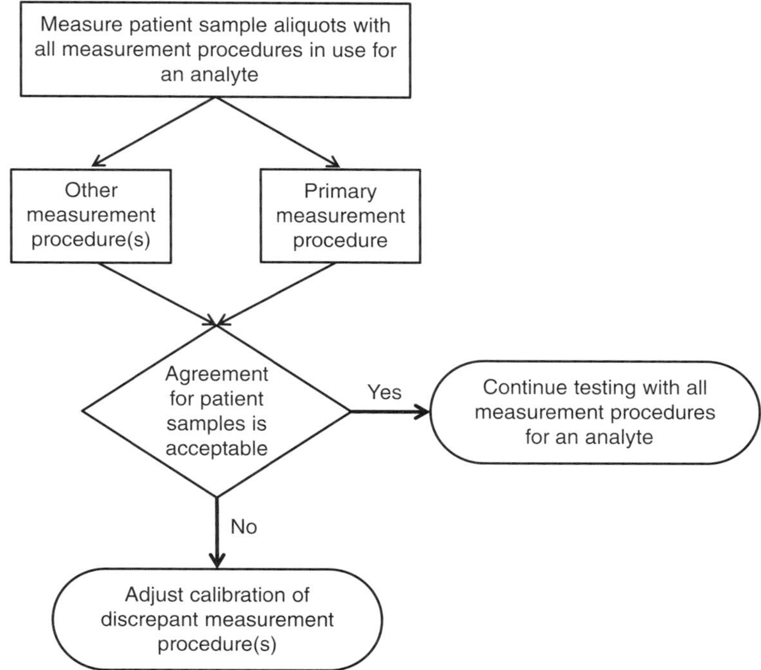

FIGURE 6.17 Process used to evaluate agreement between measurement procedures and to adjust calibration, if necessary, to achieve equivalent results from different measurement procedures. (From Miller WG. Quality control. In: *Henry's Clinical Diagnosis and Management by Laboratory Methods.* 23rd ed. Philadelphia: Elsevier; 2016.)

results for a single patient sample assayed weekly among multiple analyzers. These criteria were established based on the expected imprecision of the measurement procedures used and the clinical impact of discrepant results. To allow for the limitations of a single measurement of a single sample in a comparison, a result outside a criterion is typically not acted on unless the magnitude of a difference is much larger than the criterion or the situation persists for 2 or more weeks.

It is recommended to use patient samples to verify agreement between multiple measurement procedures or instruments of the same type even when from the same manufacturer. Results for QC materials should not be used for the purpose of verifying consistency of results for patient samples measured using different measurement procedures or instruments. As discussed in an earlier section, QC materials are not validated to be commutable with patient samples between different measurement procedures. Even when more than one measurement procedure from the same manufacturer is used, differences may be seen in the measured values for QC materials between different reagent lots and different instruments. In principle, if more than one of the same model of an instrument with the same reagent lots is used, all should have the same results for the same lot of QC material. In practice, differences in measurement details or maintenance condition between different instruments frequently cause small differences in QC results. The acceptance criteria for QC result can be set to allow for such differences. However, more reliable conclusions will be drawn when patient samples are used to evaluate agreement among different instruments.

Using Patient Data for Statistical Quality Control

Patient results can be used in a statistical QC process to monitor measurement procedure performance. For a sufficiently large number of results, the mean (or preferably, median) value may be sufficiently stable to be used as an indicator of measurement procedure consistency over time. This approach can be used on a periodic basis by extracting data for a specified time period (eg, 1 month), calculating the mean and SD for the distribution of results, and comparing one time period versus another to determine whether any changes have occurred. This type of periodic evaluation can identify changes in calibration stability or in overall imprecision for a measurement procedure. The mean and SD can also be compared for consistency among two or more measurement procedures for the same measurand.

An important limitation for using patient data to evaluate consistency within a single measurement procedure or between different measurement procedures for the same measurand is the physiologic homogeneity of results. Fig. 6.18 shows an example of the potential impact of a nonhomogeneous sample of patients on distribution of albumin results for hospital general medicine inpatients compared with a student health outpatient clinic. The histograms are very different because the two patient groups differ in severity of disease and in recumbent versus supine position for blood collection, which influences vascular water volume and the concentration of albumin.

Automated approaches to use the mean (or median) for groups of sequential patient results as a continuous process control parameter have been described. These approaches are called "average of normals" or "moving average" techniques and are suitable for use in higher volume measurement procedures in chemistry and hematology. In general, these approaches evaluate sequential patient results over time intervals such as several hours to 1 or more days. The time interval that can be confidently used depends on the number of results in the time interval and the relative homogeneity of the clinical conditions represented in the patients. For

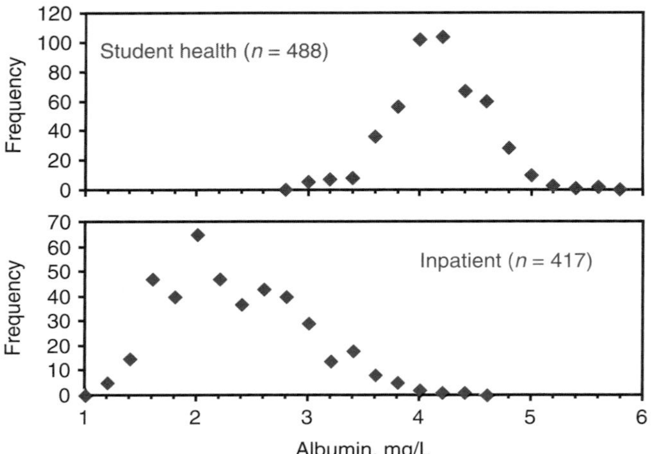

FIGURE 6.18 Histograms for distribution of sequential patient results for albumin from a student health outpatient clinic and a hospital general medicine inpatient unit. (From Miller WG. Quality control. In: *Henry's Clinical Diagnosis and Management by Laboratory Methods*. 23rd ed. Philadelphia: Elsevier; 2016.)

some measurands, patients may need to be partitioned to obtain subgroups whose results are expected to be homogeneous. Considerations for partitioning include age, gender, ethnicity, and disease conditions. Some approaches have arbitrarily ignored abnormal results in an attempt to restrict results to more normal health conditions. Removing abnormal results must be used with caution because excessive deletion will create an artificial subset of results that may not reflect a measurement procedure's calibration condition. The median of a group of patient results is sensitive to the overall distribution of results but is minimally influenced by extreme values and is recommended as the most robust estimate for tracking measurement procedure stability over time.

There is no consensus approach to determine the number of sequential patient results to include in a single group for which the mean or median is calculated. Estimates have differed widely, and the statistical models and assumptions used in investigations have been different and contributed to different conclusions.[57,60-63] An empirical approach based on extracting patient data from the laboratory computer system and simulating different group sizes in a spreadsheet can identify group sizes that have sufficiently small variation over time to provide useful information for tracking consistency of a measurement procedure. The same data can be used to assess the influence of partitioning considerations and to determine the group statistical parameters to use for interpreting the data described in the next paragraph.

The mean or median for groups of patient results is tracked over sequential time intervals to monitor measurement procedure performance. The mean or median for groups of patient results can be treated as a QC sample value. A target value for the average mean or median and an SD for the distribution of mean or median values is determined, and these parameters are used to establish acceptance rules similar to those used to interpret an individual surrogate QC sample result. Process control using patient data is primarily useful to identify bias and is less useful to identify changes in imprecision because of the inherent differences in measurand values among a group of patient results. It is recommended to use statistical procedures such as CUSUM or EWMA to monitor trends in calibration status based on patient data.

Patient data for statistical process control can be useful for supplementing traditional surrogate QC sample techniques to monitor a measurement procedure's calibration stability and to monitor calibration uniformity among multiple measurement procedures in higher volume settings. However, patient-based monitoring procedures have not been widely adopted because of lack of consensus guidelines for their use and lack of computer support from instrument and laboratory information system suppliers.

EXTERNAL QUALITY ASSESSMENT OR PROFICIENCY TESTING

EQA/PT is a program used to evaluate measurement procedure performance by comparing a laboratory's results with those of other laboratories for the same set of samples.[64] Ideally, an EQA/PT program should provide participants with results that inform them if their measurement procedure has a bias from a true value. In principle, the EQA/PT provider should circulate commutable materials that are measured in replicates by the participating laboratories. Unfortunately, commutable materials are often not used, and in some cases, circulation of unsuitable EQA/PT materials can cause harm by misclassifying measurement procedure performance.

EQA/PT providers circulate a set of samples among a group of laboratories. Each laboratory measures the EQA/PT samples as if they were patient samples and reports the results to the EQA/PT provider for evaluation. The EQA/PT provider assigns or obtains a target value for the EQA/PT samples and determines if the results for an individual laboratory are in close enough agreement with the target value to be consistent with acceptable measurement procedure performance. When commutable EQA/PT materials are used, a laboratory can verify that its results are consistent with a true value when a reference measurement procedure is available for target value assignment or with results from all other routine measurement procedures. When noncommutable materials are used, a laboratory is only able to verify that its results are consistent with other laboratories using the same measurement procedure.

EQA/PT is not available for some measurands because a particular measurement procedure may be new to the clinical laboratory or is not commonly performed or because measurand stability makes it difficult to include in an EQA/PT material. In these situations, the laboratory should use an alternate approach to periodically verify acceptable performance of the measurement procedure. CLSI guideline GP27 provides approaches for verifying measurement procedure performance when formal EQA/PT is not available.[65]

QC material manufacturers may provide a data analysis service that compares results from different laboratories using the same QC material by calculating group statistics for performance evaluation. As with EQA/PT evaluation, this type of interlaboratory QC data analysis allows a laboratory to verify that it is producing QC results that are consistent with those of other laboratories using the same measurement procedure. This information can be helpful for troubleshooting measurement procedure issues and for assessing performance of a new measurement procedure being introduced to a laboratory.

Before enrolling in an EQA/PT program, the laboratory should consider the quality of the program. The following questions have to be addressed: (1) How closely does the EQA/PT material match typical patient samples? (2) Is the EQA/PT material commutable? 3) How many replicates are measured? (4) How is the target value established? (5) What is the number of participants in the scheme and in a particular method group? And (6) How are the performance specifications set? This information is necessary to be able to interpret the feedback report from the organizer in a sensible way. Types of EQA/PT schemes are summarized in Table 6.8, with the most desirable type of program listed first and schemes that provide less information at the bottom.

External Quality Assessment or Proficiency Testing Programs That Use Commutable Samples

EQA/PT programs that use commutable samples are preferred whenever available.[64] Commutable samples are typically prepared by using an individual donor's specimen or by pooling clinical patient samples with minimal processing or additives to avoid any alteration of the sample matrix. To achieve samples with abnormal values for measurands, donors can be identified with known pathologic conditions, or blood, plasma, serum or urine units from a general donor population can be prescreened for a selected measurand. Supplementing donor samples or pools with purified analytes may be acceptable in some cases, but assessment of commutability should be performed to confirm that supplementation did not inappropriately alter the matrix. When commutable EQA/PT samples can be prepared, the results reflect what would be expected if individual patient samples were sent to each of the different laboratories. Thus, agreement among different laboratories and measurement procedures (harmonization) can be correctly evaluated. The agreement between an individual laboratory result measured in singlicate and a reference measurement result gives an assessment of accuracy, the agreement between an individual laboratory result measured in replicate and a reference measurement result gives an assessment of trueness, and the agreement between a measurement procedure group mean value and the reference measurement result gives an assessment of trueness and calibration traceability for the measurement procedure group. The latter information is of particular interest to the producers of measurement procedures and can be used as part of a surveillance program for the traceability scheme.[10]

For example, the College of American Pathologists, the Norwegian Quality Improvement of Primary Care Laboratories (Noklus), and the External Quality Assessment for Clinical Laboratory Investigations in Sweden (EQUALIS) EQA/PT programs for HbA_{1c} all use pooled, freshly collected whole blood from both normal and diabetic donors. The target values for the pooled blood are assigned by reference measurement procedures for HbA_{1c}. In these surveys, the accuracy of individual laboratory results and the trueness of measurement procedure group means versus the reference measurement procedure values can be evaluated because the EQA/PT samples are commutable with clinical patient samples. In these cases, the performance of different measurement procedures has been used to monitor and improve the calibration traceability processes used by the measurement procedure manufacturers for the benefit of improved patient care decisions regarding diabetes.[66,67]

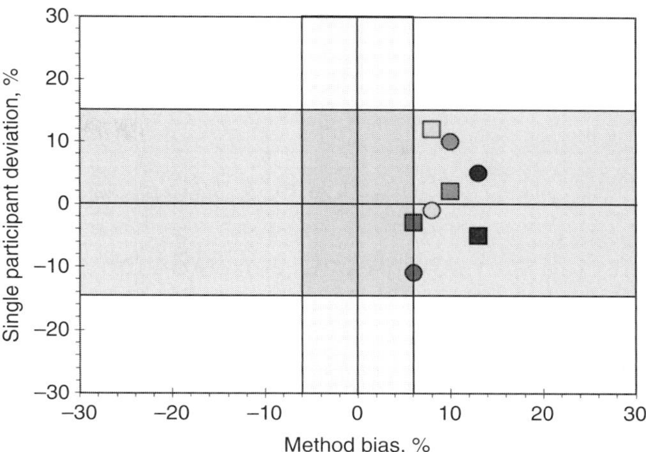

FIGURE 6.19 Example of part of an international normalized ratio external quality control report from the Norwegian Quality Improvement of Primary Care Laboratories (Noklus). The bias of each measurement procedure from the conventional true value was obtained using native patient samples for each measurement procedure (*x*-axis). A single participant was evaluated against the peer group target value for a given measurement procedure (*y*-axis). *Vertical lines* represent acceptable bias for measurement procedure performance, and *horizontal lines* represent acceptable deviation from a peer group target value. The *circle* and *square* represent two samples in one survey with each color representing a different survey (four surveys). The results show that whereas the measurement procedure had a bias of about 10%, the participant's deviation from the peer group target value was within the performance specifications. This graph indicates that the participant performs the measurement procedure correctly, but the measurement procedure has an unacceptable positive bias. (Modified with permission from Stavelin A, Petersen PH, Sølvik UØ, Sandberg S. External quality assessment of point-of-care methods: model for combined assessment of method bias and single-participant performance by the use of native patient samples and noncommutable control materials. *Clin Chem* 2013;59:363–371.)

It has been challenging to prepare commutable materials for use in large EQA/PT programs. An alternative is to combine commutable and noncommutable material in the same EQA/PT event. An example from such a survey is shown in Fig. 6.19. The measurement procedure bias was evaluated based on results from a smaller group of the participating laboratories that measured the commutable samples and individual participants' performance was evaluated based on agreement within a measurement procedure peer group using the noncommutable materials.[68] Use of commutable materials adds substantial value to the information obtained from EQA/PT survey results and should be encouraged.[64] Procedures have been developed to validate the commutability of QC, EQA/PT, and reference materials.[14,69]

External Quality Assessment or Proficiency Testing Programs That Use Noncommutable Samples

Table 6.8 includes EQA/PT programs that use noncommutable samples. The materials commonly used for

TABLE 6.8 **Evaluation Capabilities of External Quality Assessment or Proficiency Testing Related to Scheme Design**

				EVALUATION CAPABILITY						
				ACCURACY					STANDARDIZATION OR HARMONIZATION*	
				INDIVIDUAL LABORATORY						
	SAMPLE CHARACTERISTICS				RELATIVE TO PARTICIPANT RESULTS		REPRODUCIBILITY		MEASUREMENT PROCEDURE CALIBRATION TRACEABILITY	
Category	**Commutable**	**Value Assigned With RMP or CRM**	**Replicate Samples in Survey**	**Absolute vs. RMP or CRM**	**Overall**	**Peer Group**	**Individual Laboratory Intralaboratory CV**	**Measurement Procedure Interlaboratory CV**	**Absolute vs. RMP or CRM**	**Relative to Participant Results**
1	Yes	Yes	Yes	X	X	X	X	X	X	X
2	Yes	Yes	No	X	X	X		X	X	X
3	Yes	No	Yes		X	X	X	X		X
4	Yes	No	No		X	X		X		X
5	No	No	Yes			X	X	X		
6	No	No	No			X		X		

*Standardization when patient results are equivalent between measurement procedures and calibration is traceable to the Système Internationale using a reference measurement procedure, harmonization when patient results are equivalent between measurement procedures, and calibration traceability is not based on a reference measurement procedure.

CRM, Certified reference material; *CV,* coefficient of variation; *RMP,* reference measurement procedure.

Reproduced with permission from Miller WG, Jones GRD, Horowitz GL, Weykamp C. Proficiency testing/external quality assessment: current challenges and future directions. *Clin Chem* 2011;57:1670–1680.

EQA/PT samples are derived from blood, urine, or other body fluids but are altered in the process to manufacture EQA/PT samples such that the matrix is modified and the samples frequently do not have the same measurement characteristics as observed for unaltered clinical patient samples.[32-35,64,70] In addition, some EQA/PT samples (eg, cerebrospinal fluid or blood gas) are prepared as synthetic materials that are not derived from patient fluids. Consequently, many EQA/PT samples, as for QC samples, are noncommutable with authentic patient samples. The results for a noncommutable EQA/PT sample will have a different relationship in their numeric values between different measurement procedures and sometimes for different reagent lots within a measurement procedure than would be observed for patient samples.

Because EQA/PT samples are frequently noncommutable with patient samples, it is a common practice for EQA/PT providers to organize results into "peer groups" of measurement procedures that represent similar technology expected to have the same result for a noncommutable EQA/PT sample. The mean or median value of the peer group results is the target value. Because the peer group mean value may be influenced by a matrix-related bias, that value can only be used to evaluate laboratories using the same or very similar measurement procedures and cannot be used to evaluate laboratories using other measurement procedures or to evaluate if results from different measurement procedures agree with each other. Peer groups may be formed arbitrarily based on the apparent agreement among results for different measurement procedures, but there is no scientific basis for this practice, and unexpected changes may occur, such as when new reagent lots or formulations are introduced by a manufacturer.

However, even within a peer group using the same measurement procedure, differences can occur because of different reagent lots used by the measurement procedures in different laboratories because the matrix of the EQA/PT material can influence the results from different reagent lots even if the patient samples give similar results.[37] Therefore, in some cases, reagent lots should be registered, and even reagent lot–specific target values may need to be assigned.[71,72] When target values are set for noncommutable materials, it is important how the target values are calculated, how outlier results are treated, and what uncertainty is associated with the target value. When target values are assigned from relatively small numbers of results in a peer group, the target value should be given with an uncertainty and the criteria for acceptable performance should be "extended" to high and low values that include the uncertainty.

Fig. 6.20 illustrates the effects of noncommutable materials on interpretation of EQA/PT results and demonstrates why "peer group" evaluation is used. In this older but still valid example, pooled patient sera and EQA/PT samples were assayed by the duPont Dimension Analyzer and by the Abell-Kendall reference measurement procedure for cholesterol.[73] The Abell-Kendall measurement procedure was shown to be unaffected by matrix-induced changes in EQA/PT samples.[74] The patient samples showed excellent agreement between the two measurement procedures (average bias, 0.2%). However, the EQA/PT samples had a large negative bias (−9.5%) between measurement procedures, caused by a matrix-related bias with the duPont measurement procedure that was not present with the reference measurement procedure.[75]

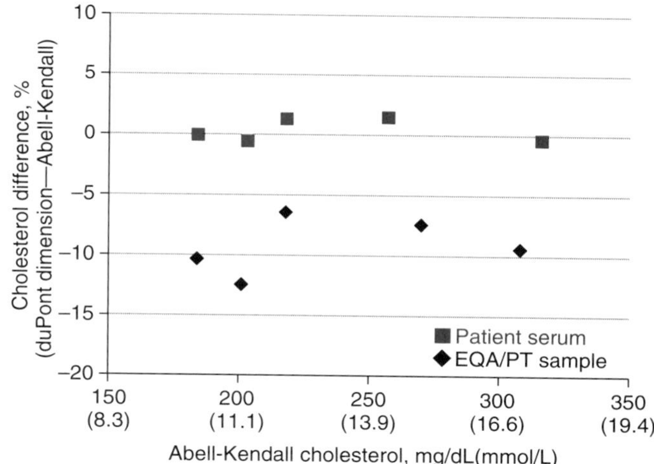

FIGURE 6.20 Example of noncommutable results between proficiency testing materials and pooled patient samples for a specific measurement procedure. *EQA,* External quality assessment; *PT,* proficiency testing. (Data from Naito HK, Kwak YS, Hartfiel JL, et al. Matrix effects on proficiency testing materials: impact on accuracy of cholesterol measurement in laboratories in the nation's largest hospital system. *Arch Pathol Lab Med* 1993;117:345–51.)

In this example, the routine measurement procedure was correctly calibrated and produced results for patient samples that were traceable to the reference measurement procedure. However, EQA/PT results gave an incorrect impression of the measurement procedure's calibration relationship to the reference measurement procedure. If the routine measurement procedure's calibration had been erroneously adjusted on the basis of EQA/PT results, the results for patient samples would then be incorrect. EQA/PT results were useful for evaluating the performance of all laboratories using the duPont measurement procedure because the matrix-related bias was uniform within this peer group. Consequently, if an individual laboratory's results agreed with those of the peer group, the individual laboratory could conclude that the measurement procedure was performing in conformance with the manufacturer's specifications. In general, an individual laboratory depends on the manufacturer to correctly calibrate a clinical laboratory routine measurement procedure to be traceable to the reference system for an analyte.

External Quality Assessment or Proficiency Testing Programs for Measurements on a Nominal or Ordinal Scale

Many constituents in laboratory medicine can be measured on a nominal scale (all types of classification of a quantity irrespective of magnitude, eg, type of virus, bacteria, or mutations) or an ordinal scale (all types of grading, eg, urine strips or pregnancy tests). Often, measurements performed on an ordinal scale are measurements that can also be performed on a ratio or interval scale. The quantities are often measured on an ordinal scale because a more rapid result can be obtained and because such tests can be performed by nonprofessional users (eg, in a physician's office or by lay people using a POC instrument). When setting up an EQA/PT program for such measurement procedures, it is important to notice that all aspects concerning QC material regarding commutability and thereby the establishment of target values will be the same as for measurement procedures on the interval or ratio scale.

EQA/PT programs addressing identifications of species or mutations often circulate multiple samples where different mutations of species should be identified and the participants are classified according to the percentage of correct identifications.[76,77]

Results from measurement procedures using the ordinal scale can be dichotomous or multinary with more steps (often called semiquantitative tests) in which each category can be considered as a dichotomous test. It is possible to evaluate the results from these tests using a rankit ordinal model.[78,79] The performance characteristics of the measurement procedure should be described from the manufacturer giving a detection limit for dichotomous tests and, for example, the concentrations below which 5% of the samples should be negative, the concentration at which 50% of the samples should be positive, and the concentration above which 95% of the samples should be positive (C_5, C_{50}, C_{95}, respectively) when related to a ratio scale. Performance specifications for such measurement procedures should use the same models as described earlier[21] and can, for example, relate to the percentage of results that should be positive or negative above or below a certain concentration.[79] These performance specifications are, however, easier to apply for method evaluation than for single participant evaluation in an EQA/PT scheme because numerous samples are necessary.

In an EQA/PT, it is useful to circulate samples with concentrations that are expected to give "positive" or "negative" results as well as samples with an intermediate concentration that can result in both positive and negative results. In the feedback report, participants will typically be evaluated with respect to the positive or negative samples because failure to obtain the expected results will be evaluated as "poor" performance. Samples with intermediate concentrations may be included to assess the robustness of threshold values by reporting to the participants how many obtained positive results and how many obtained negative results. However, intermediate concentrations are typically not graded because the results are expected to be mixed between "positive" and "negative." Such information is useful to assess and to monitor the performance of the measurement procedure. For example, a study using EQA/PT results showed that six of eight POC measurement procedures for human chorionic gonadotropin gave 3% to 11% false-positive results.[79] Using a commutable EQA/PT material, different measurement procedures can be compared and monitored over time, and it is possible to identify opportunities when the threshold discrimination needs to be improved among different measurement procedures.[80,81]

Some EQA/PT programs, often for rare diseases, are examining the whole testing procedure (eg, the correct measurands to request for a certain diagnostic problem, the appropriate sample collection and transportation, the performance of the analytical measurement procedures, the adequacy of the diagnosis, and the report provided to the clinicians).[77,82,83] These programs are often run on an international level.

Reporting External Quality Assessment or Proficiency Testing Results When One Measurement Procedure Is Adjusted to Agree With Another Measurement Procedure

It is good laboratory practice to adjust the calibration of different measurement procedures for the same measurand used within a large hospital system that can have several satellite laboratories or a collection of several hospitals with the same management structure so that the results for patient samples are consistent, irrespective of which measurement procedure is used. Such harmonization of results is important for uniform use of reference intervals and decision thresholds within a hospital or clinic system. In this situation, it is important to report EQA/PT results such that they can be properly evaluated against the peer group target value. The peer group target value will reflect the measurement procedure calibration established by the measurement procedure manufacturer. For an individual laboratory's EQA/PT result to be evaluated against the peer group mean, that individual result must be reported to the EQA/PT provider after removing any calibration adjustments so that the reported result is consistent with the manufacturer's nonadjusted calibration. The most convenient way to remove a calibration adjustment is to first measure the EQA/PT samples with the calibration adjustment applied to the measurement procedure, as would be the usual measurement process for patient samples. After the measurement, the EQA/PT results should be adjusted "in reverse" by mathematically removing the calibration adjustment factors, and the results should be reported to the EQA/PT provider with any adjustment factors removed. One should not recalibrate the instrument with a new set of calibrators for the purpose of measuring the EQA/PT samples because this practice would violate regulations requiring the EQA/PT material to be measured in the same manner as patient samples.

For example, a laboratory has performed a patient sample comparison between measurement procedure A used in the main laboratory and measurement procedure B used in a satellite laboratory. Measurement procedure B consistently gave 10% higher results (ie, a slope of 1.10 and a negligible intercept were observed for a regression analysis). Measurement procedure B was adjusted to agree with measurement procedure A by putting the adjustment factor 1/1.10 = 0.9091 in the measurement procedure B instrument to automatically multiply each measured result by 0.9091 to lower the reported result to be equivalent to a value that would have been reported by method A. When EQA/PT results from measurement procedure B are reported, it is necessary to remove the 0.9091 factor to allow the reported result to be compared with the peer group mean of results from all laboratories using measurement procedure B. Removing the 0.9091 factor is accomplished by multiplying the reported EQA/PT result from measurement procedure B by the factor 1/0.9091 = 1.100 to increase its numeric value by 10% to the nonadjusted value that was actually measured according to the manufacturer's defined calibration procedure for measurement procedure B. This process allows the EQA/PT result measured by measurement procedure B to be appropriately evaluated in comparison with its peer group mean, which will reflect the manufacturer's established calibration. This process permits the EQA/PT sample to be measured in the same manner as patient samples and the numeric result reported to the EQA/PT provider to reflect the actual measured result using the manufacturer's calibration settings.

Interpretation of External Quality Assessment or Proficiency Testing Results

Many countries have regulations requiring EQA/PT and specifying the evaluation criteria for acceptable performance. When criteria are set by regulations, an EQA/PT provider is required to use them. When criteria are not set by regulations, the EQA/PT provider sets evaluation criteria on the basis of clinically acceptable performance, biologic variation, or the analytical capability of the measurement procedures in use. EQA/PT evaluation criteria are usually designed to evaluate the total error of a single measurement. In some cases, measurements are made several times, and it is possible to separately assess the bias and the imprecision. The acceptability limits for EQA/PT include bias and imprecision components considered acceptable for a measurand plus other error components that are unique to EQA/PT samples such as between-laboratory variation in calibration; variable matrix-related bias with different lots of reagent within a peer group; uncertainty in the target value; stability variability in the EQA/PT material, both in storage and shipping, and after reconstitution or opening in the laboratory; and homogeneity of the EQA/PT material vials. Consequently, the acceptability limits for EQA/PT samples are frequently larger than what might be expected for clinically acceptable total error with patient samples.

The acceptability limits are partly dependent on the quality of the EQA/PT material (eg, its commutability, stability, homogeneity, and methods of reconstitution). A commutable EQA/PT material often has a target value assigned by a reference measurement procedure or by value transfer from suitable measurement procedures calibrated using commutable certified reference materials. A commutable EQA/PT material should in principle have the same results for all measurement procedures and lots of reagent and routine measurement procedure calibrator. In this case, the variation in the results will reflect the different measurement procedures, reagent lots, and calibrator lots in use from all of the manufacturers represented in the survey.

With a noncommutable EQA/PT material, the target value is set by the mean or median of the peer group that should include only very similar measurement procedures, and the acceptance criteria could be stricter because the variability only includes variation within the same measurement procedure. However, in some cases, a noncommutable EQA/PT material is not even commutable among reagent lots for the same measurement procedure, and in theory, each reagent lot could have its own target value with even stricter acceptability limits.[36,37]

Fig. 6.21 is an example of a typical evaluation report sent to a participating laboratory. Each reported result is compared with the mean result for the peer group using the same measurement procedure. The report also includes the SD for the distribution of results in the peer group, the number of laboratories in the peer group, and the SDI, which expresses the reported result as the number of SDs it is from the mean value (SDI = [Result − Mean]/SD). The limits of acceptability are shown. Acceptability criteria may be a number of SDs from the mean value, a fixed percent from the mean value, or a fixed concentration from the mean value. For example, in Fig. 6.21, calcium acceptability criteria are ±1 mg/dL (0.25 mmol/L) from the mean value, and iron criteria are ±20% from the mean value.

Peer group evaluation allows a laboratory to verify that its EQA/PT results are consistent with those of other laboratories using the same measurement procedure and by extension that its results for patient results are in agreement with those of other laboratories in the peer group. Consequently, the laboratory can conclude that it is using a commercially available measurement procedure according to the manufacturer's specifications.[64] In Fig. 6.21, the calcium results are in close agreement with the peer group mean (SDI ranges from

A External Quality Assessment (Proficiency Testing) Participant Report
Shipment date: 1 May 2015
Evaluation date: 12 June 2015

Analyte Units Method	Specimen	Reported Result	Mean	SD	Labs (*n*)	SDI	Limits of Acceptability Lower	Limits of Acceptability Upper
Calcium	1	9.6	9.92	0.23	587	−1.4	8.9	11.0
mg/dL	2	8.8	8.86	0.26	592	−0.2	7.8	9.9
Arsenazo dye	3	7.5	7.65	0.23	587	−0.7	6.6	8.7
Manufacturer A	4	8.2	8.43	0.23	590	−1.0	7.4	9.5
	5	10.8	10.87	0.25	589	−0.3	9.8	11.9
Iron	1	190	192.5	7.0	397	−0.4	154	232
μg/dL	2	65	65.0	3.4	394	0.0	51	78
Pyridylazo dye	3	74	69.2	3.2	395	+1.5	55	83
Manufacturer A	4	124	107.9	4.6	395	+3.5	86	130
	5	277	260.9	8.8	396	+1.8	208	314

FIGURE 6.21 Example of an external proficiency testing evaluation report sent to a participating laboratory. Part **A** uses conventional units and part **B** uses SI units. *SD,* Standard deviation; *SDI,* standard deviation interval. (From Miller WG. Quality control. In: *Henry's Clinical Diagnosis and Management by Laboratory Methods*. 23rd ed. Philadelphia: Elsevier; 2016.)

Continued

B External Quality Assessment (Proficiency Testing) Participant Report
Shipment date: 1 May 2015
Evaluation date: 12 June 2015

Analyte Units Method	Specimen	Reported Result	Mean	SD	Labs (*n*)	SDI	Limits of Acceptability Lower	Limits of Acceptability Upper
Calcium	1	2.40	2.48	0.06	587	−1.4	2.22	2.74
mmol/L	2	2.20	2.21	0.06	592	−0.2	1.95	2.47
Arsenazo dye	3	1.87	1.91	0.06	587	−0.7	1.65	2.17
Manufacturer A	4	2.05	2.10	0.06	590	−1.0	1.85	2.37
	5	2.69	2.71	0.06	589	−0.3	2.45	2.97
Iron	1	34.0	34.5	1.3	397	−0.4	27.6	41.5
µmol/L	2	11.6	11.6	0.6	394	0.0	9.1	14.0
Pyridylazo dye	3	13.3	12.4	0.6	395	+1.5	9.8	14.9
Manufacturer A	4	22.2	19.3	0.8	395	+3.5	15.4	23.3
	5	49.6	46.7	1.6	396	+1.8	37.2	56.2

FIGURE 6.21, cont'd

−0.2 to −1.4). However, the iron results show greater variability, with one result +3.5 SDI. Although this iron result is within the acceptability criteria, it is recommended to investigate the measurement procedure because a +3.5 SDI is more likely to be different from than to be in agreement with the peer group.

Fig. 6.22 shows a typical evaluation report sent to a primary care office for HbA_{1c} for one of two EQA/PT samples. In this situation the EQA/PT provider is communicating directly with the user of the measurement procedure, the clinician or the coworker in the general practice office, and the feedback must be easy to understand for nonlaboratory professionals. The EQA/PT result is evaluated as "good," "acceptable," or "poor." The lot numbers of the reagent are always registered so that the participant, in case of an aberrant result, can get information if the result was due to the measurement procedure used, the reagent lot used, or the performance of the user. When noncommutable material is used, comments to results for aberrant reagent lots will typically include a sentence that the EQA/PT result may not necessarily reflect results for patient samples. When commutable material is used, in addition to participants, manufacturers will be informed of aberrant reagent lots. In all cases, the participants are encouraged to contact the organizers to sort out problems.

Fig. 6.23 shows a similar report from the same HbA_{1c} survey provided to hospital laboratories. In addition to the figures about the distribution of results, information is provided on how different measurement procedures performed as well as a historical overview of performance on consecutive EQA/PT samples and performance related to the concentration of the sample. The EQA/PT material used for the HbA_{1c} is pooled fresh patient blood (commutable), and the target value is set by a reference measurement procedure and is therefore the same for all measurement procedures. Each sample was measured in duplicate (as requested by the EQA/PT provider), and the mean of the duplicate was used to estimate bias versus the reference measurement procedure. In the present example, the performance was within the acceptability limits but with a generally high bias during the

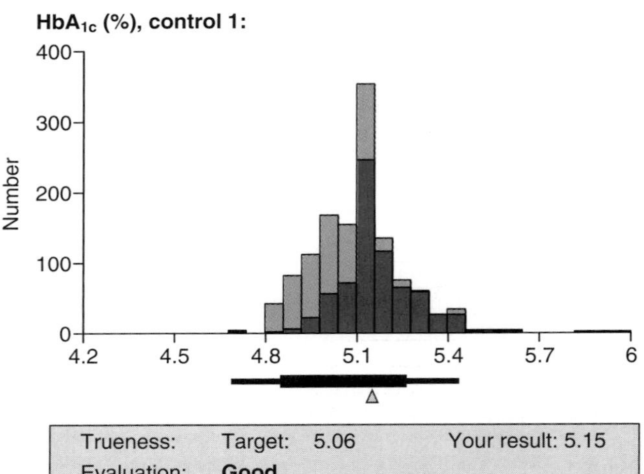

FIGURE 6.22 Example of part of a feedback report to hemoglobin A_{1c} (HbA_{1c}) point-of-care (POC) users in a survey for general practitioners' offices and nursing homes. Commutable EQA/PT material was circulated in two levels and measured in duplicate. The participant is informed about the bias (mean of the two results) compared with a reference measurement procedure target (*x*-axis) and "precision" as the difference between the two results. The histogram represents the distribution of results among all participants *(pink)* and for the participant's method group *(red)*. The *thick black line* represents the interval for "good" results, and the *thin black line* represents the interval for "acceptable" results. Results outside these limits are characterized as "poor." The *triangle* points to the result of the participant. (Modified with permission from the Norwegian Quality Improvement of Primary Care Laboratories, the external quality assessment provider in Norway.)

whole period. Because this observation was true for all the instruments using this measurement procedure, the EQA/PT organizer discussed the results with the manufacturer to solve the problem. Until the problem was solved (the manufacturer had to make a new calibrator), the participants were advised

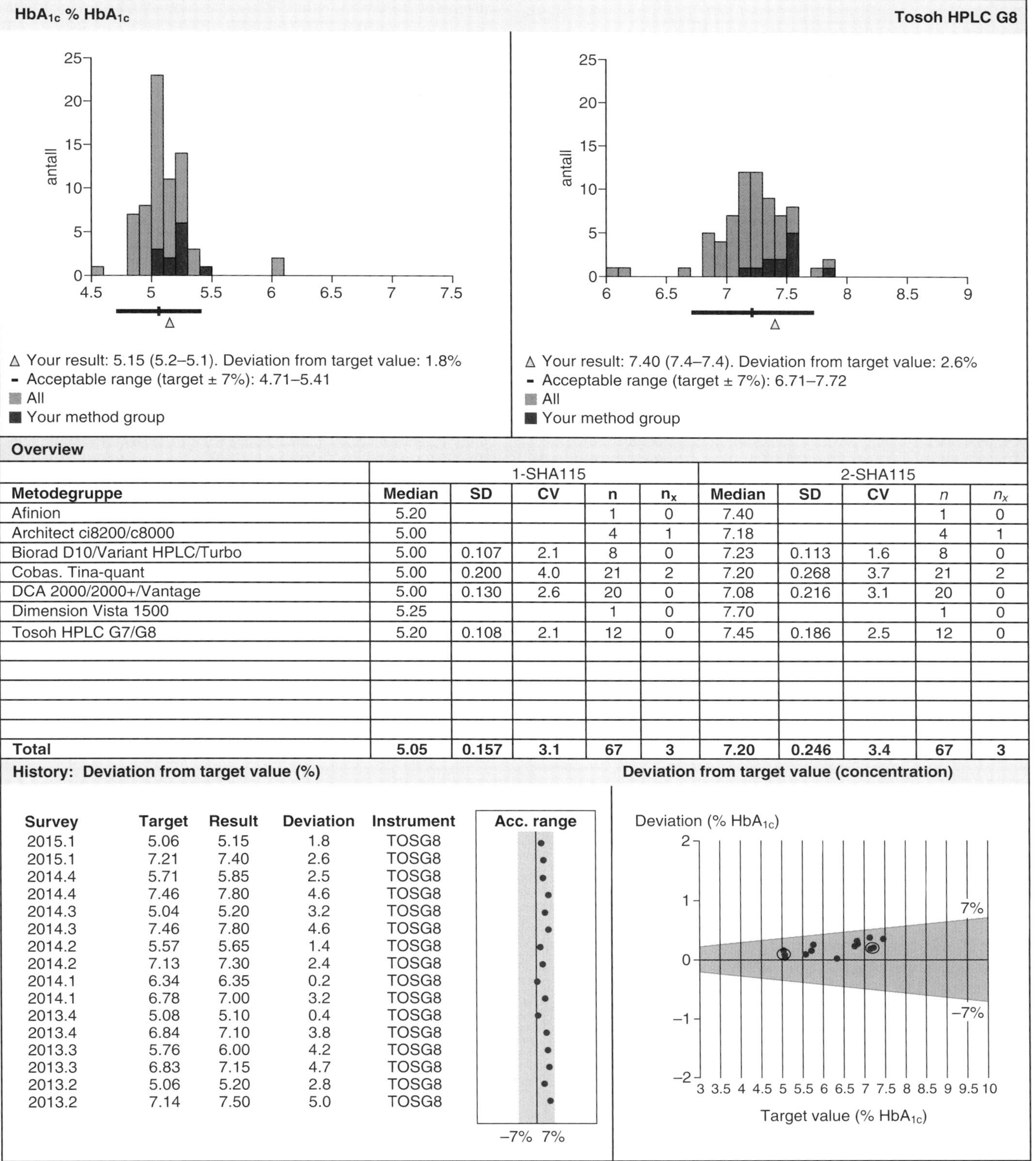

Metodegruppe	1-SHA115 Median	SD	CV	n	n_x	2-SHA115 Median	SD	CV	n	n_x
Afinion	5.20			1	0	7.40			1	0
Architect ci8200/c8000	5.00			4	1	7.18			4	1
Biorad D10/Variant HPLC/Turbo	5.00	0.107	2.1	8	0	7.23	0.113	1.6	8	0
Cobas. Tina-quant	5.00	0.200	4.0	21	2	7.20	0.268	3.7	21	2
DCA 2000/2000+/Vantage	5.00	0.130	2.6	20	0	7.08	0.216	3.1	20	0
Dimension Vista 1500	5.25			1	0	7.70			1	0
Tosoh HPLC G7/G8	5.20	0.108	2.1	12	0	7.45	0.186	2.5	12	0
Total	**5.05**	**0.157**	**3.1**	**67**	**3**	**7.20**	**0.246**	**3.4**	**67**	**3**

Survey	Target	Result	Deviation	Instrument
2015.1	5.06	5.15	1.8	TOSG8
2015.1	7.21	7.40	2.6	TOSG8
2014.4	5.71	5.85	2.5	TOSG8
2014.4	7.46	7.80	4.6	TOSG8
2014.3	5.04	5.20	3.2	TOSG8
2014.3	7.46	7.80	4.6	TOSG8
2014.2	5.57	5.65	1.4	TOSG8
2014.2	7.13	7.30	2.4	TOSG8
2014.1	6.34	6.35	0.2	TOSG8
2014.1	6.78	7.00	3.2	TOSG8
2013.4	5.08	5.10	0.4	TOSG8
2013.4	6.84	7.10	3.8	TOSG8
2013.3	5.76	6.00	4.2	TOSG8
2013.3	6.83	7.15	4.7	TOSG8
2013.2	5.06	5.20	2.8	TOSG8
2013.2	7.14	7.50	5.0	TOSG8

FIGURE 6.23 Example of a part of a feedback report to hemoglobin A_{1c} (HbA_{1c}) users in hospital laboratories. Same survey and same materials as presented in Fig. 6.22. The histogram represents the distribution of results among all participants *(pink)* and for the participant's method group *(red)*. Only limits for "acceptable" (Acc.) results are given (*thin black lines* in figures). Information about performance of measurement procedures is given in addition to a historical overview of percentage deviation from target values dependent on time and concentration of HbA_{1c}. *CV,* Coefficient of variation; *HPLC,* high pressure liquid chromatography; *SD,* standard deviation. (Modified with permission from the Norwegian Quality Improvement of Primary Care Laboratories, the external quality assessment provider in Norway.)

by the EQA/PT provider to use a correction factor when reporting their results for patient samples.[84]

If an unacceptable EQA/PT result is identified, the measurement procedure must be investigated for possible causes and the necessary corrective action taken. Even when an EQA/PT result is within acceptability criteria, it is a good laboratory practice to investigate results that are more than approximately 2.5 SDI from the peer group mean. When the SDI is 2.5, there is only a 0.6% probability that the result will be within the expected distribution for the peer group; consequently, the probability is reasonable that a measurement procedure problem may need to be corrected. In addition, EQA/PT results that have been near the failure limit for more than one EQA/PT event, even if the results have met the EQA/PT acceptance criteria, should initiate a review for systematic problems with the measurement procedure. These practices support identification of potential problems before they progress to more serious situations. When results are investigated, a limitation of SD-based grading criteria should be considered. A peer group with very precise measurement procedures may have a very small SD, and even if a result is outside an SD limit, the finding may be inconsequential regarding the use of results for medical decisions.

Common causes for EQA/PT failure are listed in Box 6.1. Incorrect handling and reporting are unique to EQA/PT events and may not reflect the process used in the laboratory for patient samples. Nonetheless, these situations reflect the attention to detail, which is a necessary attribute for quality laboratory testing. Occasionally, the EQA/PT material may have a defect that causes it to perform inappropriately for all or a subgroup of measurement procedures or reagent lots. In this case, the EQA/PT provider should recognize the problem and not grade participants for that sample. Because the influence of reagent lots on noncommutability related bias is well documented,[36,37] it would be appropriate for EQA/PT reports to register reagent lots as part of the reporting process so this limitation can be more appropriately addressed in the scoring schemes.[71,72]

EQA/PT results are usually received several weeks after the date of testing. Consequently, investigation of unacceptable results requiring review of QC, reagent lots, calibration frequency and lots, and maintenance records for the date of the test and the preceding several weeks or months is necessary. It is common practice to save any remaining EQA/PT samples for use to investigate an unacceptable result. Care must be taken to store the residual EQA/PT samples to preserve the stability of the measurands. In some cases, the measurand will not be stable during storage. In addition, when remeasuring stored samples, degradation may have occurred during or possibly before storage, while the materials were still being tested in the laboratory for the EQA/PT event, that could affect any remeasured value. It may be possible to obtain additional vials from the EQA/PT provider. If a review of records suggests a stable operating condition, and a review of

BOX 6.1 Classification of Potential Problems Identified When Investigating Unacceptable External Quality Assessment or Proficiency Testing Results*

1. Clerical errors
   - Incorrectly transcribed EQA/PT result from the instrument read-out to the report form
   - The EQA/PT sample was mislabeled in the laboratory
   - Incorrect instrument or measurement procedure was reported on the results submission form
   - Incorrect units were reported
   - Decimal point was misplaced
2. Measurement procedure problems
   - Inadequate standard operating procedure (SOP)
   - Problem with manufacture or preparation of reagents or calibrators (eg, unstable)
   - Lot-to-lot variation in reagents or calibrators
   - Incorrect value assignment of calibrators
   - Measurement procedure lacks adequate specificity for the measurand
   - Measurement procedure lacks adequate sensitivity to measure the concentration
   - Carry-over from a previous sample
   - Inadequate QC procedures used
3. Equipment problems
   - Obstruction of instrument tubing or orifice by clot
   - Misalignment of instrument probes
   - Incorrect instrument data processing functions
   - Incorrect instrument setting
   - Automatic pipetter not calibrated to acceptable precision and accuracy
   - Equipment component malfunction (eg, light source, membrane, fluidics, detector)
   - Incorrect instrument conditions (eg, water quality, surrounding temperature)
   - Instrument maintenance not performed appropriately
4. Technical problems caused by personnel errors
   - Did not operate equipment correctly or did not conform to measurement procedure SOP
   - Incorrect storage, preparation, or handling of reagents or calibrators
   - Delay causing evaporation or deterioration of the EQA/PT sample
   - Failure to follow recommended instrument function checks or maintenance
   - Pipetting or dilution error
   - Calculation error
   - Misinterpretation of test result
5. A problem with the EQA/PT material such as:
   - Incorrect storage, preparation, or handling of EQA/PT materials
   - Differences between EQA/PT samples and patient samples (eg, matrix, additives, stabilizers)
   - Sample deteriorated in transit or during laboratory storage
   - Sample had weak or borderline reaction
   - Sample contained interfering factors (which may be measurement procedure specific)
   - Sample was not homogeneous among vials

*This classification scheme assists in developing an appropriate corrective action plan.
EQA, External quality assessment; *PT,* proficiency testing; *QC,* quality control.
From Miller WG, Jones GRD, Horowitz GL, Weykamp C. Proficiency testing/external quality assessment: current challenges and future directions. *Clin Chem* 2011;57:1670–80.

the EQA/PT material handling and documentation does not identify a cause for the erroneous EQA/PT result, it can be concluded that the EQA/PT failure was a random event. Investigative steps, data reviews, conclusions, and all corrective actions must be documented in a written report to address the unacceptable EQA/PT results and reviewed by the laboratory director. Some EQA/PT programs provide the participants with flow charts to be used to identify the reason for the EQA/PT failure.

Interpreting External Quality Assessment or Proficiency Testing Summary Reports

EQA/PT providers typically provide a summary report, which includes the mean and SD for all peer groups represented by the participants' results (see Figs. 6.21 to 6.23). Similar reports are available from interlaboratory QC programs. When commutable materials were used in the surveys, the trueness compared with a reference measurement procedure or the harmonization among different measurement procedures can be assessed.

When summary reports are for surveys with noncommutable materials, assessment of mean results among different peer groups or to a reference measurement procedure is not possible. The EQA/PT results are not reliable to infer agreement or lack of agreement for patient results among different measurement procedures for the same measurand. In this case, the peer group mean and SD are useful for evaluating the uniformity of results among laboratories using the same measurement procedure and to evaluate the consistency of an individual measurement procedure's performance over time intervals from one EQA/PT event to the next (trend monitoring). A limitation using EQA/PT results for trend monitoring is that differences in matrix-related bias in different sample materials can be different within the same peer group over time.

Summary information also allows evaluation of the imprecision of various measurement procedure groups, within the limitations of EQA/PT material and reagent lot matrix-bias differences. The number of users in each measurement procedure group reveals which measurement procedures are commonly used.

Responsibility of the External Quality Assessment or Proficiency Testing Provider

The EQA/PT provider is responsible for producing programs that fulfill the goal of evaluating a measurement procedure performance of a single laboratory to that of other laboratories or to a true value when possible.[85] EQA/PT providers should strive to use commutable materials whenever possible.[64] The frequency to distribute EQA/PT samples must address the need of the laboratory and conform to applicable regulatory requirements.

The EQA/PT provider should have the knowledge to advise the participants when they have questions regarding their EQA/PT results. Some EQA/PT providers organize "user meetings" to address and evaluate the results of the different schemes, facilitate discussions on topics of common interest, provide a "national overview" of the performance of measurement procedures and laboratories, and develop national "expert" groups within different topics.[86,87]

The EQA/PT providers should communicate directly with manufacturers concerning findings related to their measurement procedures. Furthermore, they should, especially when commutable control materials are used, perform postmarketing surveillance and report any deficiency that could affect patient safety to the appropriate regulatory body.[88]

POINTS TO REMEMBER

External Quality Assessment or Proficiency Testing

- An independent external organization circulates control materials with unknown target values.
- The quality of the EQA/PT material is critical for interpretation of the results.
- When commutable, "patient-like," material is used, a laboratory can compare its own results with results from all other measurement procedures and often with a true value from a reference measurement procedure.
- When noncommutable material is used, a laboratory can only compare its own results with results from participants using a similar measurement procedure.

SELECTED REFERENCES

For a full list of references for this chapter, please refer to ExpertConsult.com.

1. Horvath AR, Bossuyt PMM, Sandberg S, et al. Setting analytical performance specifications based on outcome studies—is it possible? *Clin Chem Lab Med* 2015;**53**:841–8.
2. ISO 17511:2003. In vitro diagnostic medical devices—measurement of quantities in biological samples—metrological traceability of values assigned to calibrators and control materials. ISO, Geneva, Switzerland, 2003.
3. Vesper HW, Thienpont LM. Traceability in laboratory medicine. *Clin Chem* 2009;**55**:1067–75.
4. Miller WG, Tate JR, Barth JH, et al. Harmonization: the sample, the measurement and the report. *Ann Lab Med* 2014;**34**:187–97.
10. Miller WG, Myers GL, Gantzer ML, et al. Roadmap for harmonization of clinical laboratory measurement procedures. *Clin Chem* 2011;**57**:1108–17.
13. Miller WG, Myers GL. Commutability still matters. *Clin Chem* 2013;**59**:1291–3.
20. CLSI. Measurement procedure comparison and bias estimation using patient samples; approved guideline EP09-A3. Wayne, PA: Clinical and Laboratory Standards Institute; 2013.
21. Sandberg S, Fraser CG, Horvath AR, et al. Defining analytical performance specifications: consensus statement from the 1st Strategic Conference of the European Federation of Clinical Chemistry and Laboratory Medicine. *Clin Chem Lab Med* 2015;**53**:833–5.
27. Roraas T, Petersen PH, Sandberg S. Confidence intervals and power calculations for within-person biological variation: effect of analytical imprecision, number of replicates, number of samples, and number of individuals. *Clin Chem* 2012;**58**:1306–13.
28. Aarsand AK, Røraas T, Sandberg S. Biological variation—reliable data is essential. *Clin Chem Lab Med* 2015;**53**:153–4.

30. Oosterhuis WP. Gross overestimation of total allowable error based on biological variation. *Clin Chem* 2011;**57**:1334–6.
31. Panteghini M, Sandberg S. Defining analytical performance specifications 15 years after the Stockholm conference. *Clin Chem Lab Med* 2015;**53**:829–32.
36. Miller WG, Erek A, Cunningham TD, et al. Commutability limitations influence quality control results with different reagent lots. *Clin Chem* 2011;**57**:76–83.
38. Parvin CA. Assessing the impact of the frequency of quality control testing on the quality of reported patient results. *Clin Chem* 2008;**54**:2049–54.
39. CLSI. Laboratory quality control based on risk management; approved guideline EP23-A. Wayne, PA: Clinical and Laboratory Standards Institute; 2011.
40. CLSI. Statistical quality control for quantitative measurement procedures: principles and definitions; approved guideline C24-A4. Wayne, PA: Clinical and Laboratory Standards Institute; 2016.
55. CLSI. User evaluation of between-reagent lot variation; approved guideline EP26-A. Wayne, PA: Clinical and Laboratory Standards Institute; 2013.
59. CLSI. Verification of Comparability of Patient Results Within One Healthcare System; approved guideline EP31-A-IR. Wayne, PA: Clinical and Laboratory Standards Institute; 2012.
64. Miller WG, Jones GRD, Horowitz GL, et al. Proficiency testing/external quality assessment: current challenges and future directions. *Clin Chem* 2011;**57**:1670–80.
65. CLSI. Using proficiency testing to improve the clinical laboratory; approved guideline GP27-A3. Wayne, PA: Clinical and Laboratory Standards Institute; 2016.
68. Stavelin A, Petersen PH, Sølvik UØ, et al. External quality assessment of point-of-care methods: model for combined assessment of method bias and single-participant performance by the use of native patient samples and noncommutable control materials. *Clin Chem* 2013;**59**:363–71.

7

Biological Variation

Callum G. Fraser and Sverre Sandberg

ABSTRACT

Background
There are many sources of variation in numerical results generated by examinations performed in laboratory medicine. Although some measurands have biological variations over the span of life and others have predictable cyclical variation, most measurands have random variation around homeostatic setting points, which differ between individuals. Knowledge of the generation and application of data on within-subject and between-subject variation is essential for the correct interpretation of results.

Content
In this chapter, we explain that numerical estimates of analytical, within-subject, and between-subject biological variation are generated by examination of a series of specimens taken from a cohort of individuals, which is then followed by statistical analysis of the sources of variation. Databases of estimates are available that facilitate applications. The individuality of a measurand and the use of conventional population-based reference intervals are determined by comparison of the within-subject and between-subject biological variations. Within-subject biological variation and analytical imprecision can be used to create reference change values (RCVs) to assess the statistical significance of changes in serial results from an individual or the probability that any change seen is significant. Analytical performance specifications for imprecision, bias, total error allowable, measurement uncertainty, and other characteristics can be created using within-subject and between-subject variation. The data have many other uses. Currently, there are concerns regarding the robustness of some data and estimates for some measurands that show considerable heterogeneity. We support recent recommendations on the evaluation, generation, and application of biological variation data. If followed, more evidence-based data on biological variation will be published.

NATURE OF BIOLOGICAL VARIATION

There are many sources of variation that contribute to the uncertainty of any result generated in laboratory medicine. Biological variation is one of the most important and should be taken into account in any interpretation made. In the previous edition of this textbook, a footnote to the section on Biological Variability stated: the author has based much of the discussion on a monograph (and) this source should be consulted for further details.[1] This still holds true, although there has been considerable progress in this field, which will be particularly highlighted in this chapter.

There are various types of biological variation. The concentration or activity of some measurands changes over the span of life, some slowly and some more quickly, particularly at times of rapid physiologic development, such as the neonatal period, childhood, puberty, menopause, and old age. The concentration or activity of measurands can also differ between men and women. This variation is taken care of by the creation of age- and/or sex-stratified (partitioned) reference intervals when these are needed, although a disadvantage is that age-stratified reference intervals are based on chronological age rather than biological age. A number of measurands have predictable cyclical rhythms in their concentrations. These can be daily, monthly, or seasonal in nature. The major ramifications for interpretation are that reference intervals cannot be generated for every point during cycles, knowledge of the expected values throughout the cycle is vital for clinical interpretation, specimen collection must be at appropriate times, and absence of rhythm may indicate disease. These types of biological variations have been described in detail in Chapter 5, and the stratification (or partitioning) of reference intervals is explained in Chapter 8.

The most important type of biological variation is random biological variation. As an example, four specimens were taken from four individuals at daily intervals, and serum sodium activity was examined (reference interval: 135–147 mmol/L). The results are provided in Table 7.1. It is evident that the results for each individual vary from day to day; this is due to three sources of variation, namely, preanalytical, analytical, and within-subject biological variations. The mean value is termed the homeostatic setting point. In addition, each individual has a different average serum sodium activity; the variation among the homeostatic setting points of individuals is the between-subject variation that can translate into reference intervals, whereas the average variation within each individual is the within-subject variation.

TABLE 7.1 Serum Sodium Activity in Four Specimens Collected at Daily Intervals From Each of a Cohort of Four Individuals

Sodium	Day 1	Day 2	Day 3	Day 4
Individual 1	137	139	136	138
Individual 2	144	146	145	144
Individual 3	141	143	142	140
Individual 4	139	138	141	140

Values are measured in millimoles per liter.

Generation and subsequent application of numerical data on the components of biological variation are crucial facets of laboratory medicine, and both of these are described in detail in this chapter.

TERMINOLOGY

There is little doubt that global harmonization in laboratory medicine needs to go beyond the examination phase and must include all steps within the total process, including terminology, symbols, and units. Unfortunately, the range of terms and variety of symbols used to define the components of biological variation has grown with the increasing body of literature, which undoubtedly causes confusion. A recent study that investigated papers on biological variation in the 13 most highly cited journals of laboratory medicine found that, from 2009 to 2013, 62 papers contained terms and symbols for components of biological variation. There were 68 terms and 25 symbols for the components applicable to individuals and 47 terms and 18 symbols for the component applicable to groups of individuals.[2] It was proposed that the following terms and symbols should be used, because they were mostly applied and were also suggested by Fraser and Harris in their highly cited review of 1989[3]:

- CV_I: within-subject biological variation (variation within a single individual estimated as a pooled variation from a [homogenous] group of individuals)
- CV_G: between-subject biological variation (variation between the central tendencies of a group of individuals)
- CV_A: analytical variation (analytical imprecision).

These terms and symbols are used throughout this chapter, and the other recommendations in the publication by Fraser and Harris[3] are followed. This work has been supported by a prestigious, high-impact journal of laboratory medicine: the journal now recommends that both authors and referees comply with the use of these terms and symbols.[4]

GENERATION OF DATA ON COMPONENTS OF BIOLOGICAL VARIATION

Production of data on biological variation is very similar to derivation of population-based reference intervals (see Chapter 8) except that, instead of one specimen being taken from a large number of reference individuals, a number of specimens are taken from a smaller cohort of reference individuals. In general terms, the traditional approach recommends that numerical estimates of CV_A and both CV_I and CV_G components of biological variation should be generated using the following experimental approach: select a group of reference individuals (usually apparently healthy volunteers); take a set of specimens from each of the individuals at regular time intervals while minimizing all sources of pre-examination variation in preparation of the subjects for collection, and the collection and handling and transport of specimens; store the samples derived from the specimens until ready for examination; and undertake the examination in duplicate while minimizing examination sources of variation. Then, after removal of statistical outliers and confirmation that all results from the individuals are homogenous, dissect out the CV_A, CV_I, and CV_G components using nested analysis of variance. This approach is described in detail in the review by Fraser and Harris,[3] where it is stated that "the components of variation can be obtained from a relatively small number of specimens collected from a small group of subjects over a reasonably short period of time," although good evidence for this subjective statement was not provided and has been lacking until recently.[5]

Design of Studies

The preceding general design has been widely used and is very suitable for those measurands that have low CV_I and tight homeostatic control, but it is somewhat simplistic for a number of reasons. The measurand may be unstable, and examinations must be performed soon after the collection of specimens (eg, for some hematological measurands, such as mean cell volume, and numbers of erythrocytes and leukocytes per volume). In this case, to obtain the necessary statistically unconfounded estimate of CV_I, the CV_A can be estimated by analyzing all of the samples in duplicate, but this is a within-run CV. Thus, quality control materials have to be analyzed between each run during the examinations to ascertain that variance due to systematic deviations in the analytical procedure between each examination is not introduced. If the CV_A estimated from examination of the duplicates is less than the CV_A estimated from the between-run control material, the CV_I might be overestimated. Using this strategy, it must be assured that the concentrations or activities of the quality control materials are similar to those of the specimens from the subjects studied because CV_A often varies with concentration or activity. Moreover, it must be assured that the analytical variation of the examinations of specimens from the individuals and the quality control materials are not significantly different. This can be assessed by examining a number of the specimens from the individuals in duplicate, calculating the analytical SD, using the formula: SD = [(sum of differences between duplicates – $\Sigma d)^2/2 \times$ number of pairs – $n]^{1/2}$, $SD = (\Sigma d^2/2n)^{1/2}$, and then comparing this SD with that obtained with the quality control materials, using the F-test for comparison of variances.

There is a school of thought that most biological data are naturally logarithmically distributed, and if this is the case, the calculations must be performed on the natural logarithms of the observations to make the data distribution closer to normal.[6] Furthermore, it may be that the measurand is not present in matrices from apparently healthy subjects (such as unusual proteins found in myeloma) or that it would be unacceptable or unethical to collect specimens from the individuals in whom the measurand is most interesting, such as children. In such cases, specimens could be collected from patients with stable disease, as discussed later and described in recent reviews and editorials.[7-9]

Estimates in laboratory medicine are usually accompanied by confidence intervals (CIs); this is rarely done in reports that provide estimates of the components of biological variation. The determination of CIs for different balanced designs for a two-level nested variance analysis model with varying analytical imprecision has been examined in detail.[5] Data sets based on the model were created to calculate the power of different study designs for estimation of CV_I. It was found that the reliability of an estimate for CV_I and the power are greatly influenced by the study design and by the ratio between CV_A and CV_I. For a fixed number of measurements, it is preferable to have a high number of specimens from each individual. If the CV_A is high compared with the CV_I, the number of replicate examinations should be increased. The study provided tables that indicated the effects of increasing the number of individuals studied and the number of replicates at different levels of imprecision. This work is mandatory reading before studies generating data on the components of biological variation are performed. In addition, estimates of the components of biological variation should always be reported with CIs.

Methods for Data Analysis

The currently accepted best method for data analysis is that described by Fraser and Harris.[3] Duplicate examinations are performed on specimens from a cohort of individuals. However, before any estimation of components of variation are made, it is important to examine the data set for outliers, that is, values that do not belong to the set. This assessment of outliers is important because this process might detect either contamination of specimens or an error in the analysis (eg, insufficient sampling); such aberrant values will lead to erroneous inflated values. This assessment is done at three levels. First, the duplicate variances from the individuals are examined; each variance is calculated by squaring the difference between the duplicate results and dividing by two (as per the preceding formula for calculation of the SD of the set of duplicate results). To decide whether an extreme value is different from the remainder of the distribution, the ratio of the maximum variance to the sum of the variances is calculated, and the Cochrane test is applied. This assumes that each variance is based on an equal number of observations (two in this case), and that only one variance appears to be an outlier. Failure to examine for outliers of the duplicates can result in a falsely high CV_A and a falsely low CV_I, with wide CIs. Second, again using the Cochrane test, outliers in the variances of the specimen mean values are examined to assess whether any duplicate values are different from the remainder; this is vital—because if the difference between any duplicate results is not significantly different from the rest, it does not mean that both duplicates are not different from those from the other individuals. Although the Cochrane test of the variances of the mean values of the specimens is primarily an outlier test, it can also be used as a simple alternative for a homogeneity test, such as Bartlett's test (see later). Failure to examine for outliers in the mean results from each individual can result in a falsely increased CV_I. Finally, outliers among the mean values of the individuals are assessed; a simple strategy to perform this process is to use Reed's criterion—that the difference between any mean value and the next value in the series should be less than one-third of the overall range of all values. In the assessment of outliers, one of the most useful tools to use is a simple graphical approach in which the mean values and the range of all these values are plotted for each individual (on the *y*-axis) against concentration or activity (on the *x*-axis); an example is provided in Fig. 7.1[10] and discussed later in this chapter. Failure to exclude outliers of the mean values will result in a falsely large CV_G, and because the mean value will be different, it will also affect the CV_I. After exclusion of the outliers, a nested analysis of variance is used to derive the components of analytical and biological variations.

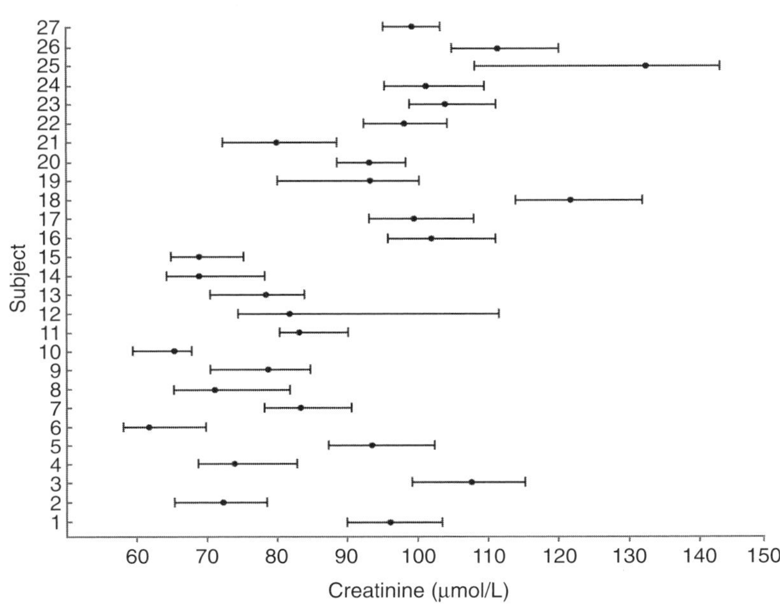

FIGURE 7.1 Means and extreme values for serum creatinine in 27 older adults.[33] Note: 100 μmol/L = 1.13 mg/dL.

Many have not used formal analysis of variance but instead have used simply subtracted variances. The thesis is that because pre-examination sources of variation have been minimized and can be considered negligible, the total CV (CV_T) of a set of results from each cohort of individuals includes CV_A, CV_I, and CV_G. Then, because

$$CV_T = [(CV_A)^2 + (CV_I)^2 + (CV_G)^2]^{1/2}$$

the components can be calculated. Outliers are often not looked for, and a normal distribution is assumed, but the detection of the former and the checking of the latter assumption (using Kolmogorov-Smirnov or Anderson-Darling or other techniques for assessment of normality) should now be considered mandatory. Usually what is done in practice is that, first, the results from each individual are taken and the mean, SD, and CV are calculated. This CV (CV_B) is comprised of CV_A and CV_I:

$$CV_B = [(CV_A)^2 + (CV_I)^2]^{1/2}$$

Overall, CV_A is then calculated from the duplicate or replicate assays, or from assessment using quality control materials (with the previously noted caveats). Then, by simple subtraction, an estimate of $CV_I = [(CV_B)^2 - (CV_A)^2]^{1/2}$ is generated for each individual. If replicates are used and the mean of the values calculated for subsequent examination, then the analytical imprecision is reduced by $n^{1/2}$, where n is the number of replicates and the correct formula is $CV_I = [(CV_B)^2 - (CV_A)^2/n]^{1/2}$. This is not required if only the first result is used, but this also appears to be a waste of half of the results generated. Then an overall estimate of the CV_I is calculated by taking the individual CV_I, squaring all of these, adding the squares (the variances), dividing by the number of subjects and taking the square root; thus, average $CV_I = (\Sigma CV_I^2/n)^{1/2}$. Following this, then CV_G can be generated using the formula:

$$CV_G = [(CV_T)^2 - \{(CV_A)^2 + (CV_I)^2\}]^{1/2}.$$

Many publications dealing with the generation of estimates of the components of biological variation do not dissect out CV_A and simply report the previously noted CV_B, which is $[(CV_A)^2 + (CV_I)^2]^{1/2}$, as the "within-subject biological variation"; this is clearly incorrect. Pure unconfounded estimates of the components of analytical and biological variation are required so that they can be applied correctly, as described in the following.

Homogeneity and Heterogeneity

The calculation of biological variation data assumes that the individuals examined are in a "steady state," that is, the measurand does not change during the time span of the study. Moreover, data on within-subject biological variation can be applied, particularly for estimation of RCVs, only if the estimates are homogeneous and do not show heteroscedasticity. If the data are not homogenous, the results are not representative of the population, and ubiquitous application of the estimates is fraught with difficulties. Although estimates of CV_I and RCVs can clearly be calculated, these cannot be generalized for the entire population. It is therefore important to know that the variances of samples drawn from one and the same population are "homogeneous" by definition, and consequently, the ranked cumulative distributions of these variances are distributed around the true variance of the population according to χ^2/df (χ^2 distribution for degrees of freedom [df] according to the individual sample sizes). In contrast, when a series of different variances have a dispersion around the pooled variance according to a χ^2/df distribution, they are considered to be heterogeneous. This can be illustrated by plotting the cumulated ranked fractions of within-subject variation values as a function of the within-subject variation estimates on a rankit scale. If homogeneous, this curve will fit to the theoretical of the square root of the pooled variance times χ^2/df. Variance homogeneity can be tested further by Bartlett's test.[6,10]

Alternatively, an index of heterogeneity (IH) has been proposed, and the simple mathematical estimation of this and its interpretation are given in the review of Fraser and Harris.[3] The IH provides a means of determining whether individuals within a population have similar within-subject variation for a given analyte. It is defined as the ratio of the overall CV of the $(SD_A^2 + SD_I^2)^{1/2}$ of the subjects to $[2/(n - 1)]1/2$, where SD_A and SD_I are the examination and within-subject biological variations as standard deviations, and n is the number of specimens per subject. The higher the index of heterogeneity is, the greater the heterogeneity of within-subject biological variation. It is important to test for homogeneity (eg, with the Bartlett or Cochrane test) and indicate how many individuals have had to be removed to obtain homogeneity of the estimate of CV_I. This again would provide an indication of the representative nature of the data and underscore its suitability for wide application.

Many data have been generated over the last 45 years on the components of biological variation in a broad range of measurands. Before considering the uses of the existing data, it is necessary to consider their reliability. A small number of the measurands that have been assessed have had a number of studies done, which has allowed a few reviews to be performed on the robustness of estimates; examples are blood glycated hemoglobin (HbA_{1c}),[11,12] serum C-reactive protein (CRP),[13] and three serum enzymes.[14] Published studies on the biological variation of HbA_{1c} were examined to check the consistency of the available data to accurately define analytical performance specifications; the authors found nine studies and considered that these were limited in a number of ways, including choice of analytical methodology, population selection, protocol application, and statistical analyses.[12] A similar evaluation of the 11 available studies on CRP again found deficiencies in all aspects of the generation of the estimates, and only 1 study fulfilled all major preexamination, examination, and postexamination requirements.[13] A search of the literature found 10 publications with data on the components of biological variation of alanine aminotransferase (ALT), 14 on aspartate aminotransferase (AST), and 9 on γ-glytamyl transferase (GGT).[14] The protocols used for the derivation of the components were varied. The ranges of CV_I reported were 11.1 to 58.1% for ALT, 3.0 to 32.3% for AST, and 3.9 to 14.5% for GGT. The range of values is shown in Fig. 7.2. Available CIs are shown: the dark diamond is the estimate in the current database. The median values (ALT: 18.0%, AST: 11.9%, and GGT: 13.8%) were, possibly as expected, similar to those listed in a database commonly used as a reference source. These three studies, and other similar studies, suggest that

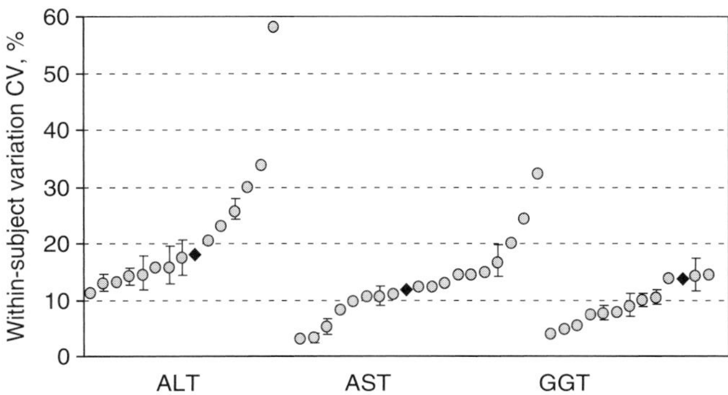

FIGURE 7.2 Estimates of within-subject biological variation for three enzyme activities as components of variations [CV] (%). *ALT,* Alanine aminotransferase; *AST,* aspartate aminotransferase; *GGT,* γ-glutamyl transferase. (From Carobene A, Braga F, Roraas T, et al. A systematic review of data on biological variation for alanine aminotransferase, aspartate aminotransferase and γ-glutamyl transferase. *Clin Chem Lab Med* 2013;51: 1997–2007.)

there are some concerns regarding the usefulness of the currently available data.

DATABASES

Current Databases and Their Merits and Disadvantages

As stated previously, derivation of the components of biological variation is not without difficulties and requires expenditure of considerable resources of various types, so the need for a database of published information found in the literature was perceived some years ago. In view of the concern over some of the data available on the components of biological variation, examination of these available databases is a necessary prerequisite to their use. Compilations of data were generated,[15-17] but these simply provided lists of published data. It was believed that publication of a database giving one value for each measurand for which data were available, based on the objective assessment of the reliability of the data in the literature and updated regularly, would be of major benefit. Generation of such a comprehensive database was initiated in 1997 by the Analytical Quality Commission of the Spanish Society of Clinical Chemistry (SEQC), and it was first published in 1999.[18] An update of this table is made available biannually on the Internet,[19] and the information documented contains a brief introduction concerning the aims of provision of the database, the changes that have been made compared with the previous edition, and three important appendices, namely, a list of the measurands studied with the within-subject and between-subject components of biological variation. These are expressed as CV (CV_I and CV_G, respectively), the derived examination quality specifications for imprecision, bias, and total allowable error at three different levels (desirable, minimum, and optimum), the number of publications examined for each measurand, a list of the publications examined by measurand, and documentation of the full citation for every publication. Full details of the structure and derivation of the database have been recently published,[20] including the criteria for inclusion of published estimates into the database. The criteria for acceptance state that the ratio $CV_A/0.5\ CV_I$, originally called the index of fiduciality,[21] must be less than 2.0, which ensures that the estimates of CV_I are not confounded by CV_A.

The database, which has been much cited and widely used, has a number of advantages. CV_I has been determined for 358 measurands in 247 articles, and this large resource has been developed and refined over nearly 20 years. Data are available on measurands in a number of matrices, namely, serum (n =185), plasma (n = 74), whole blood (n = 55), and urine (n = 47). In addition, as stated previously, data are systematically updated every 2 years and made available on the Internet.[19] Moreover, an introduction informs of changes made to existing estimates and information on included new measurands.

The disadvantages include lack of data for many measurands of interest in laboratory medicine. There is a paucity of new publications available each year for inclusion in the database, with only 25% published since 2000; few data are documented for some measurands because 202 were found in a single publication, 129 had data from 2 to 9 publications, and 27 had data from 10 or more publications. Further, as discussed previously, there appears to be heterogeneity for some measurands, including blood HbA_{1c},[12] serum CRP,[13] AST, ALT, and GGT,[14] prostate-specific antigen,[22] and urinary albumin.[23] However, it must be realized that these data are estimates, and as such, it should not be expected that they will be identical across studies in numerical terms, but they will have a distribution. Therefore, in future, CIs for the estimates should be provided to allow for comparison of these. In the current database, in which most of the published papers have no CIs given, the robustness of the data is difficult to assess objectively. However, this was examined in the current database by calculation of the ratio of the maximum CV_I to the minimum CV_I (CV_I max/CV_I min), and it was considered that a ratio below seven indicates robustness. This criterion was achieved or surpassed by 86% of the measurands included in the database.[20] It has been suggested, in an editorial about the database, that it is difficult to use the data for setting performance specifications or RCVs if the estimates can vary with a factor of seven, and that a ratio of no more than two is more than likely to indicate a significant difference between the estimates.[6]

It is generally assumed that the data on the components of biological variation are robust, and that the estimates are representative for the specific population and setting in which they will be applied. In view of the growing concerns about the apparent heterogeneity of the estimates, which is probably due in part to the less than ideal methods used in many of the studies, and therefore, their general applicability, an Expert Working Group on Biological Variation of the European Federation of Clinical Chemistry and Laboratory Medicine (EFLM) has produced a checklist to enable standardized assessment of existing and future publications of biological variation data.[24] The checklist identifies key elements to be reported in studies to enable safe, accurate, and effective transfer of biological variation data sets across healthcare systems. The checklist is mapped to the domains of a minimum data set required to enable this process. Following this work, a new EFLM Task and Finish Group has evolved the checklist into a practical tool that will enable existing studies to be classified according to how well the work fulfils all the required attributes. In addition, work is already in progress to examine the data in the existing database; a new database with high-quality estimates generated in studies that fulfill the criteria laid down will be generated and made available on the EFLM website.[25] Moreover, compliance with the checklist for new studies will enable authors, reviewers, and journal editors to ensure that studies are fit for purpose, appropriately powered, share common terminology, and deliver robust estimates of CV_I and CV_G, accompanied by the key metadata required to enable valid application of the data described.[26] It is anticipated that this ongoing work will define a standard for the reporting of studies on biological variation akin to the well-known standard for reporting of studies on diagnostic accuracy (STARD),[27] and will mean that only studies accompanied by a complete checklist will be considered acceptable by reviewers and editors. It is hoped that this standard will be included in the requirements documented in instructions for authors.

Biological Variation in Health and Disease

Some argue that many of the data on the components of biological variation are inappropriate for wide use in laboratory medicine because they have been derived, in general, from studies on healthy individuals, and not on patients with disease who are the source of most requests for examinations.[28] A database on the components of biological variation in disease has been published[29]; the group from the Analytical Quality Commission of the SEQC have continued to collect such data and have prepared an update that has recently been made available on the Internet.[30] The 2014 database has information on 97 measurands in subjects with 41 disease states. This work has led to further evidence that estimates of CV_I are generally independent of the state of health, except when the measurand is one that is pathologically changed, such as tumor markers in patients with cancers.

It is generally assumed that CV_I is independent of age, sex, time span of study (unless very frequent specimens are collected when serial correlation of data exist), geographical area, health, and disease, as well as the measurement procedure used. This is hardly surprising because CV_I are numerical estimates of the homeostatic mechanisms of the measurands.

As a consequence, it can be considered that estimates of the components of biological variation should be relatively easily available and can be used in a large number of applications fundamental to laboratory medicine. However, because the quality of published papers varies, it is strongly recommended that all users investigate the sources and quality of the data selected before application in their individual laboratories (eg, by using the proposed check list).[24]

Generation of Data From Patient Populations

Because estimates of CV_I, a measure of the homeostatic mechanisms in individuals, seem constant in general, this characteristic can be used to determine this component of biological variation in difficult settings. For example, estimation of CV_I of HbA_{1c} was done in specimens taken routinely from children with cystic fibrosis who had no evidence of diabetes mellitus or impaired glucose tolerance.[31] Similarly, it would be difficult to justify taking multiple samplings from apparently healthy individuals for examinations such as arterial pH, gas partial pressures, and electrolytes; derivation of CV_I from results of a number of examinations in diseased individuals performed regularly in the intensive care unit provided reliable estimates.[32] These interesting examples showed that, although it might be ideal to undertake the well-documented, previously noted experimental protocols and statistical analyses, further studies using novel approaches such as these might be required for examinations for which the generation and application of traditional estimates of CV_I are difficult.

INTERPRETATION AND USE OF DATA

Individuality

The results of most examinations in laboratory medicine are compared with conventional population-based reference intervals or sometimes fixed clinical decision-making limits. This is mandatory when previous results are unavailable, as is often the case in clinical settings of diagnosis, case finding, and screening. However, reference intervals represent the values found in a fractile (usually 0.95) of the reference population rather than the values found in a single individual. The ramification of biological variation on the use of reference intervals is determined by the individuality of the measurand; this has been explained in detail.[33] The example therein is reproduced in part here.

Fig. 7.1 shows a graph, which as stated earlier, should be prepared by all who are generating data on the components of biological variation to assess the presence of outlying observations visually. This shows the means and extreme values on a cohort of 27 older adults for serum creatinine concentration. Subjects 1 to 13 were women and subjects 14 to 27 were men. The conventional reference intervals for creatinine in individuals older than 55 years of age generated in the laboratory were 60 to 98 μmol/L (0.68–1.10 mg/dL) for women and 66 to 128 μmol/L (0.75–1.45 mg/dL) for men. As documented previously,[10] analysis of the data in Fig. 7.1 allows the following conclusions to be drawn:

- No individual has observed values that span the entire reference interval, and the range of values from each individual occupies only a small part of the dispersion of the reference interval.
- Most individuals have all observed values within the reference interval.
- The means of the observed values of most individuals lie within the reference interval, but they are different from each other.
- A few individuals have observed values that span the lower reference limit, and these individuals have values that change from usual to unusual over time.
- A few individuals have observed values that span the upper reference limit, and these individuals also have values that change from usual to unusual.

It is clear that the CV_I of creatinine (the variation around the homeostatic setting points) is smaller than the CV_G (the difference among homeostatic setting points). In numerical terms, CV_I was 4.3% and CV_G was 18.3%. Thus, CV_I is less than CV_G, and in such situations, the measurand is said to have marked individuality. This characteristic can be expressed mathematically as an index of individuality (II) and is best calculated as the ratio of examination plus within-subject biological variations to between-subject biological variation, mathematically: $II = (CV_A^2 + CV_I^2)^{1/2}/CV_G$. However, it is common now for II to be simply calculated as CV_I/CV_G. This is satisfactory if CV_A is less than $0.5CV_I$, as is often the case with modern analytical technology and methodology, because CV_A will then contribute little analytical noise to the numerator $(CV_A^2 + CV_I^2)^{1/2}$. Calculation of II from the most recent database shows that most commonly examined measurands have a low II, meaning that they have marked individuality.

This example provides a biological explanation for the fact that serum creatinine concentration, compared with conventional reference intervals, even if partitioned by age or sex, does not have high sensitivity for the detection of mild renal impairment, and provides the reason for the undoubted benefits of estimated glomerular filtration rate. The estimated glomerular filtration rate uses formulas that take age, sex, and ethnicity into account. This example also provides a sound rationale for the well-established fact that most measurands examined in laboratory medicine are not very useful in population screening or in case finding.

Consequences for Population-Based Reference Intervals

The consequences of individuality were first postulated by Harris[34,35] who showed that, when CV_I/CV_G is high (the criterion usually applied is $CV_I/CV_G > 1.4$), the distribution of values from any single individual will cover much of the entire dispersion of the reference interval derived from values found in reference individuals. In contrast, if CV_I/CV_G is low (especially when CV_I/CV_G is <0.6), the dispersion of values for any individual will span only a small part of the conventional population-based reference interval.

The ramifications of this individuality on the interpretation of the results of examinations are profound. When II is low, most individuals can have values that are unusual for them, but these will often lie within the reference interval. As a consequence, these results would not be flagged by laboratories as deserving of further attention because, although they are unusual for that individual, they are within the reference interval. Moreover, the users of the laboratory results would be highly unlikely to pay attention to such unusual values. Thus, taking one specimen from an individual and comparing the result of an examination with the population-based reference interval will not, as shown previously for creatinine, be an effective way of picking up the small changes often seen in early pathological processes. However, when only one sample is examined in an individual, the II will have no influence on the percentage of false positives and true positives detected, irrespective of whether the upper reference limit or a selected clinical decision-making value is used. However, if a "confirmatory" measurement is performed, the II is of importance. For quantities with a very low II, which is the usual situation in laboratory medicine, a new result of measurement will be close to the first and only provide limited new information. For quantities with a high II, a repeat measurement will decrease the number of true positives and false positives. In a low prevalence situation (eg, in screening and case finding), in which it is important to prevent healthy individuals being incorrectly labelled, a positive result will "confirm" the first. In a relatively high prevalence situation (eg, in diagnosis) in which the number of false positives is low, and it is important to discover most of the diseased patients, the measurement should not be repeated. Thus, the only clear reason for a "confirmation" measurement is in a low prevalence situation when the II is high; this is rare in laboratory medicine.[36,37]

TABLE 7.2 Within-Subject (CV_I) and Between-Subject (CV_G) Biological Variation of Urine Creatinine and Indices of Individuality (II)

Group	CV_I (%)	CV_G (%)	II
Men (n = 7)	11.0	6.0	1.83
Women (n = 8)	15.7	11.0	1.42
Total	13.0	28.2	0.46

If II is defined as CV_I/CV_G, this ratio must be made larger to make conventional population-based reference intervals of higher clinical usefulness, especially in diagnosis, case finding, and screening, when no previous results on an individual are available. This is actually sometimes easily achieved because CV_G can be made smaller by stratifying (or partitioning) the data.[36] An example is shown in Table 7.2.

Table 7.2 shows that, for the total cohort, II is 0.46, and therefore, the reference intervals will be of low usefulness, especially for monitoring individuals. However, for men and women taken separately, the II are 1.83 and 1.42,[†] respectively, and reference intervals will be very useful. Stratification according to gender has vastly increased the usefulness of conventional population-based reference intervals. Because most measurands have low II, stratification must be considered when reference intervals are being developed (see Chapter 8). Knowledge of individuality gives a sound scientific basis for stratification; II must be high for conventional, population-based reference intervals to be of high usefulness. Because CV_I is generally considered constant and rarely stratified, it must be CV_G that is made smaller, if possible.

REFERENCE CHANGE VALUES AND DIFFERENCES IN SERIAL RESULTS

The results of examinations in laboratory medicine are used for many purposes; most are used for monitoring, either of acute disease in the short term in secondary and tertiary care institutions, or for chronic disease, which is often done in primary care. Monitoring, by definition, means assessment of results over time. Because most measurands have marked individuality and low II, conventional population-based reference intervals have disadvantages as aids to interpretation of serial results in an individual.

Harris and Yasaka[38] introduced the concept of the RCV (as discussed earlier), which is also sometimes called the critical difference; the former term is much preferred to indicate an analogy with population-based reference intervals. The generation and application of RCVs have been recently reviewed in depth.[6-8]

The result of one examination will have: dispersion = $Z \times (CV_A^2 + CV_I^2)^{1/2}$, where Z is the Z-score equal to the number of standard deviations appropriate for the probability desired. The result of a second examination will have the same dispersion, and so the total dispersion of two results will be $2^{1/2} \times Z \times (CV_A^2 + CV_I^2)^{1/2}$. Thus, for two results on the same individual to be different, this inherent difference due to CV_A and CV_I must be exceeded, and this is the RCV. It is assumed that preexamination sources of variation are considered negligible, and in clinical and laboratory practice, this means having well-documented standard operating procedures for patient preparation and specimen collection, transport, and handling before examination, and also good training of healthcare staff performing these tasks. Moreover, it is important to realize that changes in the bias of the examination between the collections of the serial specimens can also add to the RCV; if these can be quantitated, as a difference due to bias in percentage terms, ΔB, the formula becomes $RCV = \Delta B + 2^{1/2} \times Z \times (CV_A^2 + CV_I^2)^{1/2}$. However, in a single laboratory in practice, the main source of ΔB over time is due to recalibration, and this random bias is usually an integral component of the longer term CV_A as estimated from replicate examinations of internal quality control materials. Thus, it can be assumed that the bias of the examination does not change during the period between the two examinations, and the simpler formula applies.

It is often assumed that a Z-score of 1.96 for $P < 0.05$ (and sometimes also 2.58 for $P < 0.01$) are appropriate. It is almost ubiquitously stated in studies on biological variation that the RCV is calculated as $2.77 \times (CV_A^2 + CV_I^2)^{1/2}$. This is incorrect for a number of reasons.

First, these Z-scores are termed bidirectional (or two-tailed or two-sided), and this infers that the difference between the two serial results can be either an increase or a decrease. However, in most clinical situations, the decision-making is the assessment of a significant fall (decline, decrease or reduction, for example, HbA_{1c} after treatment for diabetes mellitus or in blood glucose after adjustment of insulin dosage), or a significant rise (for example, an increase in serum creatinine to assess acute kidney injury or serum troponin after acute chest pain). Thus, unidirectional (one-tailed or one-sided) Z-scores must be used in most clinical situations to facilitate correct interpretation; these are 1.65 for $P < 0.05$ and 2.33 for $P < 0.01$. Correct definitions of the clinical decision-making context and the major differences between the terms "change" and "rise or fall," and their synonyms, are required for correct calculation of appropriate RCVs.

Second, clinical decision-making is not always done at $P < 0.05$, which is the most commonly used probability in analysis of research data. The semantics used are crucial to understanding the probability that is appropriate. An example was given in a recent study on RCVs for dehydration markers, which, in addition to graphs that showed probability against change for plasma osmolality, urine specific gravity, and body mass, integrated a series of semantic interpretative anchors, namely, change was likely at $P > 0.80$, more likely at $P > 0.90$, very likely at $P > 0.95$, and virtually certain at $P > 0.99$.[39] RCVs should be used in a spectrum of post-examination processes, including provision of graphs and tables of change versus probability, Δ-checking, and flagging of significant changes at different levels of probability on electronic and paper reports of results of examinations.[1]

In addition, because RCV is calculated as $RCV = 2^{1/2} \times Z \times (CV_A^2 + CV_I^2)^{1/2}$, the magnitude of what the RCV for each laboratory is will depend on the CV_A achieved. Furthermore, generation of data on CV_I is not easy, and it is important that the CV_I used is obtained from a population with a homogenous CV_I and that is similar to the population for whom the RCV is being created. In addition, the time interval used for obtaining the CV_I must be comparable to the one used in practice. An overview of the source publications on CV_I can be found in the available database,[19] and these should be examined for their usefulness[23] until the new EFLM database (which is being developed) is available. Thus, laboratories can calculate relevant RCVs by using CV_A derived from their own internal quality control programs, using data close to clinical decision-making concentrations or activities, along with the CV_I estimates from publications cited in the most up-to-date database to create a RCV to use for a variety of purposes. The RCV is commonly calculated assuming that CV_I for the both examinations is identical (ie, CV_I is constant). A formula has been developed, which specifies that, even if CV_A is constant, because the concentrations or activities will be different, the SD of the two examinations can also differ.[40] Using the proposed more complex formula, the RCV becomes larger for increases than for decreases. This interesting proposal does not seem to have been translated into routine practice.

Moreover, it is obvious that the RCV generated using the traditional formula will depend on the number of significant figures to which the results of examinations are reported; these should be determined by consideration of the CV_A achieved in practice.[41] However, it has been suggested that, for examinations in which small changes in results may be of clinical significance for monitoring purposes, the effect of the number of significant figures reported on the RCV should also be taken into consideration.[42]

Traditional RCVs are believed by some to be rather simplistic, especially because they only address how likely it is that a certain change can be explained by CV_A and CV_I, but not the probability that a change in the disease state has occurred. It has been suggested that a tool for better understanding and interpretation of measured differences in monitoring is needed; the concepts of sensitivity, specificity, likelihood ratios, and odds used for diagnostic test evaluations were applied to monitoring by substituting measured concentrations with measured differences.[43] It was suggested that this idea expanded the earlier concept of RCV by making it possible to have an estimate of the post-test odds for a certain difference to occur. Consequently, the likelihood ratio for change increases with a larger measured difference, and when used together with the pretest odds or pretest probability, the post-test odds and post-test probability, which are related to the clinical situation, can be calculated.

It has been proposed[6-8] that the probability of significance of any difference seen in clinical practice between two results can be readily calculated using a simple rearrangement of the RCV equation making the Z-score (and thus, the probability) the unknown, namely: $Z = \text{difference}/[2^{1/2} \times (CV_A^2 + CV_I^2)^{1/2}]$. This does not seem to have been applied in practice, but there is clearly scope for adoption of this technique to enhance interpretation of serial results. Exactly as for RCVs, this application would have important consequences for CV_A: the smaller the CV_A, the smaller the RCV will be for any probability, and the significance of any difference seen will be of higher probability.

Reference Change Values When the Distribution Is Not Normal

Some would argue that biological variables are not normally distributed but have a natural logarithm distribution. The traditional approach to generation of RCV does assume that CV_A is random and also assumes that CV_I is a random fluctuation around a homeostatic setting point, both distributed normally. However, recently, a number of examinations have been evaluated, making the assumption that the distributions of results in an individual were ln-normal rather than normal. The strategy proposed[44] has since been adopted by others who are investigating examinations such as serum troponin.[45,46] CV_I was calculated from the total imprecision (CV_T) for duplicate examinations by the often used formula: $CV_I = (CV_T^2 - CV_A^2)^{1/2}$. With the ln-normal approach, the median normal deviation of the n-normal distribution (σ) was calculated as $\sigma = [\ln(CV_T^2 + 1)]^{1/2}$. The asymmetrical limits for the upward (positive) value for the ln-normal RCV (RCV_{pos}) and for the downward (negative) value for the ln-normal RCV (RCV_{neg}), were calculated as: $RCV_{pos} = [\exp(1.96 \times 2^{1/2} \times \sigma) - 1] \times 100$ and $RCV_{neg} = [\exp(1.96 \times 2^{1/2}\ \sigma) - 1] \times 100$, respectively. This approach gives different RCVs for increases in concentration or activity to the RCV for decreases. This approach is likely to be used more often in the future when the measurand has a ln-normal rather than a normal distribution.[47] The CV_T term used in this calculation is equal to $(CV_A^2 + CV_I^2)^{1/2}$, and where it is difficult to dissect out numerical estimates of CV from the total variation of individuals, then calculation of RCV as $RCV = 2^{1/2} \times Z \times CV_T$ seems appropriate and does provide an estimate of RCV that can be used in clinical and laboratory practices, assuming the CV_A is similar between that derived in the assessment of $(CV_A^2 + CV_I^2)^{1/2}$ and in the practice in which it is going to be used.

Reference Change Values for More Than Two Serial Examinations

Frequently, in practice, more than two results of examinations are available for the individuals over time. Using the traditional RCVs described previously, it is only possible to calculate the significance of changes between each of the two consecutive examinations. Thus, a RCV method including all available serial results might be useful for interpretation of significant differences over time.

Mathematical methods have been developed to assess serial results from an individual, which is sometimes called methods for time series analysis.[34] One model is called the "homeostatic model." The model assumes that the measurand varies randomly around a homeostatic setting point. After collection of results from a small number of examinations, the mean and standard deviation are calculated. The next result should fall within the range calculated from the mean and the standard deviation. Then, new data from the same individual is used in an ongoing manner to refine the estimates of the mean and standard deviation for that individual to interpret whether the next new result has changed significantly from previous data. In contrast, the "random walk" model assumes that the measurand behaves randomly, and there is no homeostatic setting point. The dispersion of each result is calculated. However, instead of calculating a mean for the individual and recalculating this mean as further data are gathered, it is assumed that the most recent result is the starting point from which to assess whether change has occurred. These models have not been widely applied; they generate many false positive signals that change has occurred, when there is no obvious usual or pathological change. They also seem too complex and time consuming to be used in everyday practice.

Recently, studies on both unidirectional and bidirectional changes in serial results that used computer simulations have been performed.[48,49] Factors used to multiply the first result from an individual were calculated to create the limits for constant cumulated significant differences. The factors were shown to become a simple function of the number of results and the total CV. The first result is multiplied by the appropriate factor for an increase or a decrease, which gives the limits for a significant difference. It remains to be seen if such apparently simple techniques become used in practice.

ANALYTICAL PERFORMANCE SPECIFICATIONS BASED ON BIOLOGICAL VARIATION

Analytical performance specifications are the numerical standards of examination performance required to facilitate optimum patient care. There are many strategies available to set these specifications, and these have been described over time as this facet of laboratory medicine has evolved.[50,51] A concise historical perspective has been published recently.[52]

Following pioneering studies done in the United States[53] on the definition of the components of biological variation, a College of America Pathologists conference held in 1976 supported the concept that specifications should be best based on biology.[54] The consensus statement, restated in current terms and symbols, was: "For group screening, in which an individual is to be selected from a population, a specification for imprecision (CV_A) is defined as: $CV_A = 0.5 \times (CV_I^2 + CV_G^2)^{1/2}$" and "For individual single and multipoint testing, in which an individual is evaluated on the basis of discrimination values: $CV_A = 0.5 \times CV_I$."

Specifications for Examination Imprecision

This approach became of even greater interest as the quantity of data on the components of biological variation increased. In most cases, the examination performance specification for CV_A was simply taken as $CV_A = 0.5 \times CV_I$, with the rationale that the same technology and methodology were used to examine specimens in both of the previously described clinical settings (and other situations). In consequence, the most stringent situation would allow both specifications to be met.

Specifications for Examination Bias

Examination bias was not mentioned at that time, possibly because the thesis was that laboratories all had their own reference intervals to which the results of their examinations were compared. However, as interest in harmonization of data across time and geography developed, it was realized that harmonization of reference intervals was important, and it was proposed that the examination performance specification for bias (*B*), to allow use of harmonized reference intervals, was $B < 0.25 \times (CV_I^2 + CV_G^2)^{1/2}$.[55]

Specifications for Total Error Allowable

As the concepts of total laboratory quality management evolved, and the idea that random and systematic sources of variation (imprecision and bias) were both important, it became clear that total analytical error was the most important clinically.[56] It was proposed that the linear model of combining imprecision and bias could be used to set analytical performance specifications for total error allowable (TEa) as a simple linear addition; for $P < 0.05$: TEa $< 0.1.65 \times 0.5\ CV_A + 0.25\ (CV_I^2 + CV_G^2)^{1/2}$. It should be noted that this model for combining bias and imprecision is only one of the models available; the advantages and disadvantages of these have been discussed in detail,[57] and the disadvantages of this particular model have been recently restated.[58] EFLM has established a Task and Finish Group to address the difficulties with the total error concept and to try to evolve new models that are sounder. However, the present model is widely used in current practice in laboratory medicine, albeit sometimes with a different multiplier for the imprecision term, to deliver different levels of probability.

Application of this has become very widespread because the formula is simple, much data on biological variations exist, and they are directly related to the general use of results of examinations in laboratory medicine. However, concerns have been expressed. First, because the biological variation data currently used for some measurands vary,[6] and second, because the analytical performance standards derived using biological variation are unattainable for some measurands with current technology and methodology, including serum sodium, chloride, and calcium. However, some analytical performance standards were easy to obtain for others, including serum urea, triglycerides, and many enzyme activities. A three-tier model to cater for this was proposed, giving minimum, desirable, and maximum examination performance specifications based on biological variation using 0.25 CV_A, 0.5 CV_A, and 0.75 CV_A for imprecision and 0.125 $(CV_I^2 + CV_G^2)^{1/2}$, 0.25 $(CV_I^2 + CV_G^2)^{1/2}$, and 0.325 $(CV_I^2 + CV_G^2)^{1/2}$ for bias, respectively.[59] Numerical data on these three levels of analytical performance specifications are included for the 358 measurands in the eighth edition of the biological variation database on the Internet.[19] Furthermore, because analytical technology has evolved rapidly of late, and analytical performance has improved, it has been suggested that a fourth "ideal" level should be introduced with multipliers of 0.1 for both imprecision and bias.[60] Combinations of the three (or four) levels can be done to obtain relevant analytical performance specifications for TEa.

Specifications Derived From Opinions of Clinicians

Because it is the users of the results of examinations in laboratory medicine that make use of the data provided, it might be believed that they should be able to inform about the analytical quality required to facilitate decision-making. One way of attempting to do this is with clinical vignettes, whereby the clinician provides information about the change in serial results that is required to stimulate a clinical decision. Some early studies were carried out, but these were completely unsatisfactory, in that it was assumed that changes were all due to analytical imprecision, and within-subject biological variation was not considered. The probability used was bidirectional, and always at $P < 0.05$ despite the very large differences in probability attributable to words used in the statements.[61,62] The principle behind the studies should be that a difference in serial results is due to preexamination sources of variation (CV_P), CV_A, CV_I, and changes in bias (ΔB):

$$\text{difference} = 2^{1/2} \times Z \times [CV_P^2 + CV_I^2 + CV_A^2]^{1/2} + \Delta B$$

now, let CV_P and ΔB be zero and rearrange the equation:

$$CV_A = [\text{difference}/(2^{1/2} \times Z + CV_I^2)]^{1/2}.$$

Studies have been done using this model on a variety of measurands, and have included some studies that involved patients undertaking self-testing. An early example is provided by the studies on blood hemoglobin[63]; other studies performed since then have investigated HbA_{1c}, glucose, prothrombin time, erythrocyte sedimentation rate, and urinary albumin.[64] It was found that the derived analytical performance specification depends on the clinical setting, the semantics of the questions posed, how close the result was to a decision limit or reference limit, and probably on current examination performance. Moreover, there was large interclinician variation in responses. This approach is probably possible only for assessment of a single measurand in a specific clinical situation. In addition, it has been suggested that this strategy is possible only for analytes that have a major role in monitoring and/or diagnosis.

Specifications for Measurement Uncertainty

Because there is now a requirement for medical laboratories to document the measurement uncertainty to comply with ISO 15189, there should be consideration of the setting of analytical performance specifications for this characteristic. Because the fundamental principles are that bias should be eliminated (if possible) and all sources of variation should be added linearly as variances, then the only possible analytical performance specifications for measurement uncertainty are that $CV_A < f \times CV_I$, where $f = 0.10, 0.25, 0.50, 0.75$ for ideal, optimum, desirable, and minimum levels of performance, respectively,[60] but again this is dependent on reliable data being available for CV_I.

Specifications for Other Applications

Data on biological variation have been used to generate analytical performance specifications in other than general clinical settings, including an evaluation of systems,[65] reference methods,[66] and for the allowable difference in bias (ΔB) between two systems used to generate results on the same individuals, which is $\Delta B < 0.33\ CV_I$.[67]

Role of Biological Variation in Setting Analytical Performance Specifications

The setting of analytical performance specifications in laboratory medicine has been a topic of discussion and debate for more than 50 years; 15 years ago, as this topic matured and a profusion of recommendations appeared, a number of leading professionals in laboratory medicine realized that there was a need for a global consensus on the setting of such specifications. The Stockholm Conference held in 1999 on "Strategies to set global analytical quality specifications in laboratory medicine" achieved this and advocated the ubiquitous application of a hierarchical structure of approaches, based on a model proposed by Fraser and Petersen.[68] The hierarchy has five levels, namely: (1) evaluation of the effect of analytical performance on clinical outcomes in specific clinical settings; (2) evaluation of the effect of analytical performance on clinical decisions in general, using (a) data based on components of biological variation or (b) analysis of clinicians' opinions; (3) published professional recommendations from (a) national and international expert bodies or (b) expert local groups or individuals; (4) performance goals set by (a) regulatory bodies or (b) organizers of external quality assessment (EQA) schemes; and (5) goals based on the current state of the art as (a) demonstrated by data from EQA or proficiency testing scheme, or (b) found in current publications on methodology.[69] This approach has mostly been used, and there is considerable evidence that the specifications advocated in level 2, which are based on biological variation, are widely implemented. A number of EQA schemes, including those in Australia,[70] base their acceptable standards of examination performance on the Stockholm consensus conference recommendations, especially the use of biological variation data. Three convocations of experts in quality control in laboratory medicine discussed the generation and application of analytical performance specifications, and these strategies, based on biological variation, are used by many.[60,71,72] Furthermore, a recent survey with more than 450 responses from professionals in more than 80 countries demonstrated the wide use of specifications based on biological variation.[73] Since the Stockholm conference, there have been further proposals for setting performance specifications for examination performance characters,[74,75] but it is interesting that all of these include biological variation data in their considerations.[76]

Because laboratory medicine has evolved considerably over the last few years, the EFLM organized the 1st Strategic Conference on defining analytical goals 15 years after the Stockholm conference; the many insightful presentations are available on the Internet.[77] The consensus statement and formal papers emanating from the speakers are included in a Special Issue of *Clinical Chemistry and Laboratory Medicine*,[78] and represent an invaluable up-to-date resource on all aspects of setting analytical performance standards, and on generation and application of data on biological variation. The consensus was that the Stockholm hierarchical approach was supported, but could be simplified. In this revision, the hierarchy was simplified and represented by three different models to set analytical performance specifications. Model 1 is based on the effect of analytical performance on clinical outcomes using direct (1a) or indirect (1b) outcome studies, which basically investigate the impact of analytical performance of the test on clinical outcomes. Model 2 is based on components of biological variation of the measurand. Model 3 is based on state of the art. The three models use different principles, and some models will be better suited for certain measurands than for others. Application of model 1 is difficult and will probably be limited to a few measurands. It has been considered that generally applicable analytical performance specifications will be best based on biological variation data for some time to come. In view of the caveats regarding the reliability of certain data on the components of biological variation, it will be significant when the EFLM group on biological variation fulfills its remit and evaluates the current database, creates a database of high quality, and its recommendations on standards of generation and reporting of data are carried through into practice.

OTHER APPLICATIONS

Calculation of Reliability Coefficient

The individuality of tests and the consequences of the marked individuality (low II) of most measurands in laboratory medicine in diagnosis, case finding, screening, and monitoring has been discussed. Epidemiologists and others use similar information to the II, but in a slightly different way. The reliability coefficient is used, which is calculated as $CV_G^2/(CV_A^2 + CV_I^2 + CV_G^2)^{1/2}$, which is the between-subject variance divided by the total variance.[1] The reliability coefficient, usually called R, is numerically equal to the correlation coefficient of repeated measurements. It can be between 0 and 1. If R approached 0, II would be high, and if R approached 1, then II would be low. Most measurands have high values for R.

Number of Samples Needed

In usual clinical practice, only one sample is taken. Examination result variation can be reduced by multiple sampling (or multiple examinations), and the variation is made smaller by the square root of the number of replicates. To estimate the number of specimens needed to determine the homeostatic setting point within a certain percentage error with a stated probability, a simple rearrangement of the usual standard error of the mean formula is used, namely: $n = (Z \times [CV_A^2 + CV_I^2]^{1/2}/D)^2$, where Z is the Z-score appropriate for the probability, and D is the desired percentage closeness to the homeostatic setting point. It is important to note that taking multiple specimens and undertaking replicate analyses does affect the overall variability of the individual examination result; the dispersion (expressed as 1 CV) can be calculated as: dispersion $= Z \times [(CV_A^2/nA) + (CV_I^2/nS)]^{1/2}$, where Z is the number of standard deviations appropriate to the probability selected, nA is the number of replicate examinations, and nS is the number of specimens. The relative magnitudes of CV_A and CV_I are important in deciding if a lower dispersion is required, whether it is better to undertake replicate examinations on one specimen or singleton examinations on multiple specimens. Calculators for this can be found, along with a more detailed discussion of this topic, with real examples.[79] A review has documented further examples and detailed the reasons why knowledge of numerical data on the components of biological variation is of crucial importance.[80]

Reporting Results, Selecting the Best Specimen to Collect, and Choosing the Best Examination

It is sometimes possible to report the results of examinations in different ways. For example, measurands in urine such as creatinine can be reported as concentration or output per day, and many are reported as a ratio with creatinine concentration. Moreover, for some measurands, it is possible to collect different samples for the same clinical purpose (eg, early morning or random or timed urine specimens for low concentration albumin and protein examinations). In certain clinical situations, examinations that might be considered to have a somewhat similar purpose are available, such as serum creatinine and cystatin-C, or blood HbA_{1c} and serum fructosamine. Knowledge of the components of biological variation can assist in making decisions about reporting results, selecting the best specimen to collect, and choosing the best test.[1]

To undertake such comparisons, the influences of biological variation should be considered. The ideal measurand would have low CV_I so that a single examination will give a good measure of the true value for that individual. Moreover, this would allow easy monitoring over time and detection of significant differences, because the RCV would be low, provided that the CV_A was also low. In addition, the ideal measurand would have no heterogeneity of CV_I among individuals and across studies, and would not be dependent on age and gender and other possible confounding factors so that the simple general formulas given in this chapter would hold for all.

Method Development and Evaluation

Introduction of new examinations is an ongoing task for most medical laboratories. Some years ago, Zweig and Robertson suggested that the introduction of a new procedure should be similar to the structured evolution of a new drug through phase trials.[81] They suggested that the phases should be the following: analytical investigation and assessment of reliability and practicability characteristics; overlap investigation involving generation of reference intervals and assessment of values in disease; clinical investigation and evaluation of sensitivity, specificity, and predictive value; outcome investigation of whether individuals gain an advantage; and, finally, investigation of usefulness, which is a cost–benefit analysis with respect to individuals and the population. In contrast to the linear models, another approach has been proposed in which the essential components of analytical and clinical performance, clinical and cost-effectiveness, and the broader impact of testing are assembled in a dynamic cycle. This approach emphasizes the interaction of the different components, and that clinical effectiveness data should be fed back to refine analytical and clinical performances to achieve improved outcomes.[82]

One aspect that is not covered in any of these phases, however, is the need to generate and apply data on biological variation early in the evolution of any examination. Data can be generated on the components of biological variation through duplicate analysis of a small number of samples from a small cohort of healthy individuals. This allows the setting of analytical performance specifications, calculation of the significance of changes in an individual (otherwise unobtainable and not mentioned in any of the phases), and assessment of the use of the generated population-based reference intervals. Generation and application of data on biological variation are essential prerequisites for introducing new examinations.[83] Moreover, the data are also necessary for objective analysis of the often somewhat subjective guidelines from professional bodies that give recommendations on interpretation of the numerical results of examinations and on examination performance specifications; unfortunately, these recommendations are often flawed.[80]

OVERALL CONCLUSIONS

Numerical estimates of within-subject and between-subject biological variation are best generated by examination of a series of specimens taken from a cohort of individuals, followed by statistical analysis of the sources of variation. The proper design and performance of such studies is complex. However, databases of estimates are available that facilitate application in determining the individuality of a measurand and the usefulness of conventional population-based reference intervals, the statistical significance of changes in serial results from an individual, analytical performance specifications for imprecision, bias, total error allowable, measurement uncertainty, and other characteristics. The estimates have many other uses. There are current concerns regarding the robustness of certain of these data and estimates because some measurands show considerable heterogeneity. Recent recommendations should be followed in the generation and application of biological variation data.

POINTS TO REMEMBER

Biological variation may be daily, monthly or seasonal, but most measurands have random variation around homeostatic setting points.

It is challenging to generate data on within-subject and between-subject components of biological variation, but available databases facilitate application; users should ensure applicability of published data to their applications.

Data on biological variation are used, inter alia, to determine:

- the individuality of a measurand and the usefulness of conventional population-based reference intervals
- the statistical significance of changes in serial results from an individual and the probability that any change documented is significant
- examination performance specifications for imprecision, bias, TEa, measurement uncertainty, and other characteristics.

SELECTED REFERENCES

For a full list of references for this chapter, please refer to ExpertConsult.com.

1. Fraser CG. *Biological variation: from principles to practice.* Washington, DC: AACC Press; 2001.
3. Fraser CG1, Harris EK. Generation and application of data on biological variation in clinical chemistry. *Crit Rev Clin Lab Sci* 1989;**27**:409–37.
5. Røraas T, Petersen PH, Sandberg S. Confidence intervals and power calculations for within-person biological variation: effect of analytical imprecision, number of replicates, number of samples, and number of individuals. *Clin Chem* 2012;**58**: 1306–13.
8. Fraser CG. Reference change values. *Clin Chem Lab Med* 2011;**50**:807–12.
19. Minchinela J, Ricós C, Perich C, et al. Biological variation database and quality specifications for imprecision, bias and total error (desirable and minimum). The 2014 update. http://www.westgard.com/biodatabase-2014-update.htm>.
20. Perich C, Minchinela J, Ricós C, et al. Biological variation database: structure and criteria used for generation and update. *Clin Chem Lab Med* 2015;**53**:299–305.
24. Bartlett WA, Braga F, Carobene A, et al. A checklist for critical appraisal of studies of biological variation. *Clin Chem Lab Med* 2015;**53**:879–85.

29. Ricos C, Iglesias N, Garcia-Lario JV, et al. Within-subject biological variation in disease: collated data and clinical consequences. *Ann Clin Biochem* 2007;**44**:343–52.
33. Fraser CG. Inherent biological variation and reference values. *Clin Chem Lab Med* 2004;**42**:758–64.
37. Petersen PH, Sandberg S, Fraser CG, et al. Influence of index of individuality on false positives in repeated sampling from healthy individuals. *Clin Chem Lab Med* 2001;**39**:160–5.
43. Hyltoft Petersen P, Sandberg S, Iglesias N, et al. Likelihood-ratio and odds applied to monitoring of patients as a supplement to reference change value (RCV). *Clin Chem Lab Med* 2007;**46**:157–64.
59. Fraser CG, Hyltoft Petersen P, Libeer JC, et al. Proposals for setting generally applicable quality goals solely based on biology. *Ann Clin Biochem* 1997;**34**:8–12.
68. Fraser CG, Petersen PH. Analytical performance characteristics should be judged against objective quality specifications. *Clin Chem* 1999;**45**:321–3.
69. Hyltoft Petersen P, Fraser CG, Kallner A, et al., editors. Strategies to set global analytical quality specifications in laboratory medicine. *Scand J Clin Lab Invest* 1999;**59**: 475–585.
75. Klee GG. Establishment of outcome-related analytic performance goals. *Clin Chem* 2010;**56**:714–22.
78. Sandberg S, Fraser CG, Horvath AR, et al. Defining analytical performance specifications: Consensus Statement from the 1st Strategic Conference of the European Federation of Clinical Chemistry and Laboratory Medicine. *Clin Chem Lab Med* 2015;833–5.
80. Fraser CG. Test result variation and the quality of evidence-based clinical guidelines. *Clin Chim Acta* 2004;**346**: 19–24.
83. Fraser CG. Data on biological variation; essential prerequisites for introducing new procedures. *Clin Chem* 1994;**40**: 1671–3.

8

Establishment and Use of Reference Intervals

Gary Horowitz and Graham R.D. Jones

ABSTRACT

Background

One of the most important elements of a laboratory test is the reference interval, the values to which physicians compare their patients' test results, facilitating interpretation. It is extremely important, therefore, that laboratories devote sufficient resources to ensure that the reference limits they provide are well-founded. Most frequently, these reference limits represent values for healthy, adult patients, but other sets of values can be provided (such as values for pregnancy or for children). Sometimes, clinical decision limits are provided in place of conventional reference limits (such as for treating patients with diabetes or for diagnosing acute coronary syndromes).

Content

In this chapter, we describe the techniques for properly establishing reference intervals, including selection of appropriate reference individuals, implementation of preanalytical standardization, considerations for eliminating outliers and partitioning the reference group, and performance of statistical methods to calculate reference limits and their confidence intervals. In addition, since formal establishment of reference intervals may be beyond the capacity of many laboratories, we discuss alternative sources for reference limits (including manufacturers' package inserts, peer-reviewed literature, multicenter trials, historical laboratory data), along with techniques to verify the transferability of these data. Consideration will be given to issues related to enhancing the display of patient test results with the appropriate reference limits. Even though most of the chapter is devoted to single tests (univariate) and population-based reference limits, we will also briefly describe the concept of subject-based reference intervals. Lastly, we discuss techniques for ongoing verification of reference limits.

CONCEPT OF REFERENCE LIMITS

Interpretation by Comparison

Laboratory test results play a vital role in clinical medicine. Physicians use these results when screening for diseases in apparently healthy people, for confirming, excluding, or changing the probability of specific diseases in patients with certain symptoms and signs, and for monitoring changes in a patient over time. To achieve these goals, interpretation is made by comparison to population reference limits, clinical decision limits, or previous results or sets of results from the same patient. Population reference limits are derived from relevant patients with (or without) similar diseases, whereas clinical decision limits are generally based on clinical categories or outcomes of patients separated on the basis of laboratory results. To facilitate these comparisons it is critical that laboratories provide not only the patient's test result but appropriate *reference limits* to which the patient's results can be compared. Ideally, for comparison with population limits, such reference limits should be available not only from healthy individuals but also from patients with relevant diseases, though usually only health-associated reference limits are available. These limits have been described as the most common decision support tool in laboratory medicine, and their inclusion on a pathology report is endorsed by the international clinical laboratory standard ISO 15189[1] and required by the College of American Pathologists (CAP).[2] A detailed history and commentary on the development of reference intervals has recently been written.[3]

Normal Values/Normal Ranges: Obsolete Terms

Historically, the term ***normal values*** was used to describe the laboratory data provided for purposes of comparison, and *normal ranges* as the expression of these on pathology reports. However, use of these terms often leads to confusion because the word "normal" has several different connotations.[4] For example, three medically important but very different meanings of "normal" are:

1. *Statistical sense:* Values can be described as "normal" if their observed distribution seems to follow closely the theoretical *normal distribution* of statistics—the Gaussian probability distribution. This use of "normal" has sometimes misled people to believe that the distribution of biological data is always symmetric and bell shaped, like the Gaussian distribution. But on closer examination, this usually is not correct. To exorcize the "ghost of Gauss," Elveback and colleagues recommend not using the term *normal limits*.[5] For a similar reason, the term *normal distribution* should be avoided and replaced by the term *Gaussian distribution*.
2. *Epidemiologic sense:* Another meaning of "normal" is illustrated by the following statement: It is "normal"

to find that the activity of gamma-glutamyltransferase (GGT) in serum is between 7 and 47 IU/L, whereas it is considered "abnormal" to have a serum GGT value outside these limits. Here a more exact statement would read as follows: Approximately 95% of the values obtained, when the activity of GGT in sera collected from individuals considered to be healthy is measured, are included in the interval 7 to 47 IU/L. The obsolete concept of *normal values* in part carried this meaning. Alternative terms for "normal" in this sense are *common, frequent, habitual, usual,* and *typical.*

3. *Clinical sense:* The term "normal" also is often used to indicate that values show the absence of certain diseases or the absence of risks for the development of diseases. In this sense, a *normal value* is considered a sign of health. Better descriptive terms for such values are *healthy, nonpathologic,* and *harmless.* As a corollary, when results are discussed with patients, it may be unhelpful to describe results outside reference limits as "abnormal" because this may be taken to indicate the presence of disease or ill health and therefore create unnecessary anxiety or concern.

Because of confusion resulting from the different meanings of normal, the terms *normal values* and *normal ranges* are obsolete and should not be used.

To prevent the ambiguities inherent in the term *normal values,* the concept of *reference values* from which the terms *reference intervals* and *reference limits* are derived, was introduced and implemented in the 1980s.[6,7] The term *reference* is appropriate because these values provide something to refer to when interpreting a result. This was an important event in establishing a scientific basis for clinical interpretation of laboratory data.[8] The term *reference range* is sometimes used in place of the term *reference interval* recommended by the International Federation of Clinical Chemistry and Laboratory Medicine (IFCC). This use is incorrect because the statistical term *range* denotes the difference (a single value!) between maximum and minimum values in a distribution.[9]

Terminology

The IFCC recommends use of the term *reference values* and related terms, such as *reference individual, reference limit, reference interval,* and *observed values.*[7,10-15]* The definitions and the presentation in the following sections of this chapter are in accordance with IFCC recommendations,[10-15] which have been adopted by the Clinical Laboratory Standards Institute (CLSI).[16]

The definition of *reference values* is based on that of the reference individual.

Reference individual: An individual selected for comparison using defined criteria.

As mentioned previously, for the interpretation of values obtained from an individual under clinical investigation, appropriate comparison values are needed. To provide such values, suitable individuals must be selected. The characteristics of the individuals in each group chosen for comparison should be clearly defined. Their age and sex must be specified, along with the conditions for the specimen collection, and whether they should be healthy or have a certain disease. The definition of a reference individual also covers cases in which the individual under clinical investigation is his or her own reference, as discussed in a later section on subject-based reference values.

A reference value may then be defined as follows[10-15]:

Reference value: A value obtained by observation or measurement of a particular type of quantity on a reference individual.

If, for example, the activity of GGT is measured in sera collected from a group of reference individuals selected for comparison according to a sufficiently exact set of criteria, the GGT results are considered reference values.

The observed value is defined as follows[10-15]:

Observed value: A value of a particular type of quantity obtained by observation or measurement and produced to make a medical decision. Observed values can be compared with reference values, reference distributions, reference limits, or reference intervals.

Or, rephrased: An observed value is the result obtained by analysis of a specimen collected from *an individual under clinical investigation.* Some call such values "test values," but the word "test" in this term is ambiguous (a laboratory test? a statistical test?), and it should be avoided. The equivalent term used in the International Vocabulary of Metrology (VIM) is *measurement result.*[17]

The IFCC also defines other terms related to the concept of reference values: reference population, reference sample group, reference distribution, reference limit, and reference interval.[10-15] Some of these terms are introduced in later sections of this chapter.

Clinical Decision Limits

The terms ***reference limits*** and ***clinical decision limits*** should not be confused.[8,18] ***Reference limits*** are descriptive of the reference distribution; they tell us something about the variation of values in the selected subset of reference individuals. Comparison of new values with these limits conveys information about similarity to the given reference values. In contrast, ***clinical decision limits*** provide separation based on clinical categories or outcomes. The latter limits may be based on analysis of reference values from several groups of individuals (healthy persons and patients with relevant diseases) and are used for the purpose of differential diagnosis.[6,18,19] Alternatively, such values are established on the basis of outcome studies and are used as clinical guidelines for treatment. Examples of current decision limits include recommended concentrations for therapeutic drug levels (see Chapter 40), the National Cholesterol Education Program guidelines related to cholesterol,[20] the American Diabetes Association recommendations for diagnosis of diabetes with HbA1c or plasma glucose,[21] and the American Academy of Pediatrics guidelines on neonatal bilirubin.[22] A key factor with clinical decision limits is that each assumes that measurements of the involved analytes are accurate, with the accuracy base being the method used in the clinical studies on which the clinical decision points were established.

In this context, it is critical to point out another difference between reference limits and clinical decision limits. For most analytes, a laboratory should establish (or verify) its own

*A note on the literature: The Expert Panel on Theory of Reference Values of the IFCC produced a series of six documents with recommendations on the establishment and use of reference values.[10-15] In 1989, Solberg and Grasbeck published an in-depth review of this information.[7]

reference limits. The processes to do this are described later in this chapter. But for other analytes, in particular those with clinical decision limits, physicians tend to use national (or international) guidelines. In the 2010 CLSI guidelines,[16] this point is given much-deserved emphasis. Laboratory efforts that once would have been dedicated to establishing or verifying reference intervals should, for these analytes, be redirected toward establishing accuracy. It does little good to establish one's own reference limits if physicians will (and should) use national guidelines. Methods to establish the accuracy of one's method are discussed in Chapter 6. It is also important for laboratories to communicate to clinicians the nature of reference limits provided with results, specifying whether these are population reference intervals or clinical decision limits, as well as any additional information required for appropriate use. In particular, information on populations with and without specified diseases allows for determination of important characteristics of diagnostic tests, including their sensitivity, specificity, predictive values, and likelihood ratios, all of which are discussed in detail in Chapter 2.

Types of Reference Limits

In practice it is often necessary or convenient to give a short description associated with the term ***reference limits,*** such as ***health-associated reference limits*** (close to what was understood by the obsolete term ***normal values). With conditions, such as obesity, that are prevalent in many populations and associated with poorer health outcomes, the definition of health-associated reference limits becomes more difficult, both to define (this is discussed in subsequent text with exclusions from the reference population) and to communicate to the end-user.*** Other examples of such qualifying words could be *hospital inpatient*, *pregnancy*, and *patients with well-controlled diabetes*. These short descriptions prevent the common misunderstanding that reference values are associated only with health.

Subject-Based and Population-Based Reference Values

Subject-based reference values are previous values from the same individual, obtained when he or she was in a known state of health. *Population-based* reference limits are those obtained from a group of well-defined reference individuals and are usually the types of values referred to when the term *reference limits* is used with no qualifying words. This chapter deals primarily with population-based values. It should be noted, however, that for some tests, intraindividual variation may be small relative to interindividual differences. The relationship of within to between individual variation is known as the index of individuality (see Chapter 7), and in cases in which this is low (eg, creatinine,[23] immunoglobulins[24]), the use of population-based reference intervals may distract from clinically significant intra-individual changes, as noted later in this chapter.

It is also important to note that this chapter focuses on population-based *univariate reference limits* and quantities derived from them. For example, if separate reference limits for calcium and parathyroid hormone (PTH) in plasma are used, two sets of univariate reference limits are produced. The term *multivariate reference limits* denotes that results of two or more analytes obtained from the same set of reference individuals are treated in combination. Plasma calcium and PTH values may be used, for example, to define a bivariate reference region, which would reflect the fact that, as calcium concentrations decrease, even within healthy reference limits, PTH levels rise. Thus a PTH level that is within health-associated univariate reference limits might not be within the health-associated bivariate reference limits. This subject is addressed briefly in a later section.

Requirements

Certain conditions apply for a valid comparison between a patient's laboratory results and reference values[25]:

1. All groups of reference individuals should be clearly defined.
2. The patient examined should sufficiently resemble the reference individuals (in all groups selected for comparison) in all respects other than those under investigation.
3. The conditions under which the reference specimens were obtained and processed for analysis should be known and these conditions should be the same as for the patient specimen.
4. The measurand under examination in the patient and the reference individuals should be the same.
5. All laboratory results should be produced using adequately standardized methods under sufficient analytical quality control (see Chapter 6). The standardization should be sufficient that any bias or difference in precision or analytical specificity between the analytical system used for the patient sample and that used for the reference samples does not affect the interpretation.

To these general requirements one may add others that become necessary when more detailed and sophisticated approaches to decision making are applied.[8]

6. Stages in the pathogenesis of diseases that are the objectives for diagnosis should be demarcated beyond the separation between presence and absence of the disease. For example, although some overlap occurs, the clinical grades of congestive heart failure (CHF) are distinguished by progressive increases in levels of N-terminal pro-brain natriuretic peptide (NTproBNP).[26]
7. Clinical diagnostic sensitivity and specificity, prevalence, and clinical costs of misclassification should be known for all laboratory tests used. For example, in some instances, one might want to know whether a given NTproBNP value is "healthy," in which case one would want to use reference limits for age- and sex-matched individuals with no evidence of CHF. In contrast, when faced with a patient complaining of shortness of breath in the emergency room, one might want instead to know, not so much whether any degree of CHF is present, but whether the patient's CHF is sufficiently advanced to be the cause of the shortness of breath.[27,28]

SELECTION OF REFERENCE INDIVIDUALS

A set of *selection criteria* determines which individuals should be included in the group of reference individuals.[7,10-15] Such selection criteria include statements describing the source population and specifications of criteria for health or for the disease of interest.

Often, separate reference values for each sex and for different age groups,[29] as well as other criteria, are necessary. The overall group of reference individuals therefore may have to be divided into more homogeneous subgroups. For this purpose, specific rules for the division, called *stratification* or *partitioning criteria,* are needed.

It is important to distinguish between selection and partitioning criteria. First, selection criteria are applied to obtain a group of reference individuals. Thereafter, this group is divided into subgroups using partitioning criteria. Whether a specific criterion (eg, sex) is a selection or a partitioning criterion depends on the purpose of the actual project. For example, sex is a selection criterion if reference values only from female subjects are necessary. Sex can also be a selection criteria where the data will be partitioned using this criterion to ensure sufficient numbers of each sex are collected.

Concept of Health in Relation to Reference Values

There is an obvious requirement for health-associated reference values for quantities measured in the clinical laboratory. But the concept of health[30] is problematic; much confusion may arise if the selection criteria for health are not clearly stated for a specific project.

Gräsbeck suggested the following general definition of health, which summarizes the relative, privative, and goal-oriented aspects discussed previously[30]: "*Health is characterized by a minimum of subjective feelings and objective signs of disease, assessed in relation to the social situation of the subject and the purpose of the medical activity, and it is in the absolute sense an unattainable ideal state.*"

When reference values are produced, the following questions are asked: (1) Why are these values needed? (2) How are they going to be used? (3) To what extent does the intended purpose of the project determine how health is identified? For example when setting reference limits for cardiac-specific troponins, a "cardio-healthy" population is required that is in other ways similar to the patients who are likely to present with possible acute coronary syndrome (ie, they should be of similar age and gender, and they may have hypertension or hyperlipidemia).[31,32]

Strategies for Selection of Reference Individuals

Several methods have been suggested for the selection of reference individuals. Table 8.1 shows a variety of concepts that may be used to describe a sampling scheme. The concepts can be considered as pairs, each of which is mutually exclusive. For example, the sampling may be direct or indirect, and direct sampling may be a priori or a posteriori.

The merits and disadvantages of these strategies are described in the following sections. It is not possible to recommend one sampling scheme that is superior in all respects and applicable to all situations. One must choose the optimal approach for a given project and state clearly what has been done.

Direct or Indirect Sampling?

Selection of reference intervals by *direct* sampling involves collection of specimens from selected members of the reference population for the purpose of establishing reference limits. *Indirect* sampling involves deriving reference limits from using results of samples collected for other purposes. Direct selection of reference individuals (see Table 8.1) concurs with the concept of reference values as recommended by the IFCC,[10-15] and it is the basis for the presentation in this chapter. Its major disadvantages are the problems and costs of obtaining a representative group of reference individuals.

TABLE 8.1 Strategies for Selection of Reference Individuals

Direct vs. Indirect	
Direct	Individuals are selected from a parent population using defined criteria
Indirect	Individuals are not considered, but certain statistical methods are applied to analytical values in a laboratory database
A Priori vs. A Posteriori	
A Priori	Individuals are selected for specimen collection and analysis if they fulfil defined inclusion criteria
A Posteriori	Use of an already existing database containing both relevant clinical information and analytical results. Values of individuals meeting defined inclusion criteria are selected.
Random vs. Nonrandom	
Random	Process of selection giving each item (individual or test result) in the parent population an equal chance of being chosen
Nonrandom	Process of selection that does not ensure that each item in the parent population has an equal chance of being chosen

These practical problems have led to the search for simpler and less expensive approaches such as *indirect* methods.[6,33] This approach is based on the observation that most analysis results produced in the clinical laboratory seem to be "normal." Two main concepts have been used to extract information about reference distributions from this type of data. The first is the identification of a distribution within the database which is then taken to represent the reference population. Note that for this approach no attempt is made to classify individual results as representing the reference population. The alternate method is to use additional clinical information to classify individual results and derive reference intervals from these data.

An example of the former indirect method is shown in Fig. 8.1. As seen, the values of serum sodium concentrations from hospitalized patients have a distribution with a preponderant central peak and a shape similar to a Gaussian distribution. The underlying assumption of the indirect method is that this peak is composed mainly of *normal values* or, more specifically, are derived from patients without the condition of interest or diseases that may affect the analyte under consideration. Advocates of the method therefore claim that it is possible to estimate a *reference interval* if the distribution of unaffected values from this distribution is extracted. However, as shown in Fig. 8.1, reference limits determined by the indirect method on the basis of this distribution would be seriously biased compared with the health-associated reference limits. Note, for example, the substantial proportion of values below 135 mmol/L—the true, health-associated lower reference limit. This may be due to the presence of a significant proportion of the samples being derived from patients with a condition affecting the results, for example, in

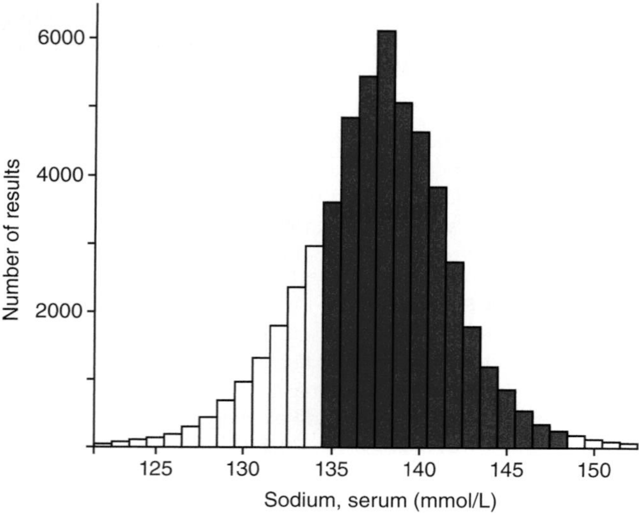

FIGURE 8.1 Distribution of sodium concentrations in serum obtained in a routine laboratory. The histogram shows the distribution of 53,128 serum sodium concentrations measured in consecutive clinical specimens during a 6-month period in 1982 at Rikshospitalet, Oslo, Norway. The *shaded area* is within health-associated reference limits (135 to 148 mmol/L), as determined by a direct method (193 healthy adults of both sexes).

the case of serum sodium, diuretic use, dehydration and other fluid imbalances. It may also be due to systematic preanalytical differences, such as recumbence in inpatients compared with ambulatory outpatients. Several mathematical methods have been used to extract a distribution for the derivation of reference limits from routine laboratory data.[6,33]

In short, the indirect method has at least two potential major deficiencies:

1. Estimates of the reference limits can depend heavily on the particular mathematical method used and on its underlying assumptions.
2. Estimates of the reference limits can be affected by the prevalence, nature, and severity of disease included in the laboratory database. This may be a particular problem with databases containing only hospital inpatients. The use of ambulatory outpatients and general practice patients can reduce this variability remarkably.

However, the alternate method of indirect sampling from pathology databases may be used for the establishment of reference values in a way that is fully concordant with IFCC recommendations.[34,35] The requirement for this approach is that laboratory data should be *combined with information stored in clinical databases* (ie, to combine an *a posteriori* strategy with the indirect method). Laboratory results are to be used as reference values only if stated clinical criteria are fulfilled. One may define criteria for selecting individuals who have a specified state of health or the disease for which reference data are necessary. Certain constraints are usually imposed on the use of their laboratory results, such as allowing only one result for each analyte under study from each selected individual.

Reference values produced by indirect sampling techniques have a number of significant potential advantages over those based on direct sampling. With any indirect method, the preanalytical and analytical factors are exactly the same for the patient sample and the reference setting process, and indeed the reference population matches that of the patient. This can provide a more appropriate comparison group, as the role of clinical decision-making is to separate patients with the same clinical presentation on the basis of disease, rather than separating sick from healthy. For example, the need is to distinguish chest pain patients having a myocardial infarction from chest pain patients who are not.

A Priori or a Posteriori Sampling?

When carefully performed, both *a priori* (before) and *a posteriori* (after) sampling (see Table 8.1) may result in reliable reference values. The choice is often a question of practicality. Both require the same set of successive steps, but the order of some of these operations differs depending on the mode of selection: a priori or a posteriori.[6]

The first step in the process of producing reference values for a laboratory test should always be the collection of quantitative information about sources of biological, preanalytical and analytical variation for the analyte studied. In this setting, biological variation includes expected variation with time of day, with meals, with seasons and with life stages. A search through relevant literature may yield the required information.[36,37] If relevant information cannot be found in the literature, pilot studies may be necessary before the selection of reference individuals is planned in detail. Serum sodium is an example of a biological analyte that is affected by only a few sources of biological variation. However, the list of factors may be rather long for other analytes, such as serum enzymes, proteins, and hormones.

It is important to distinguish between controllable and noncontrollable sources of biological variation. Some factors may be controlled by standardization of the procedure for preparation of reference individuals and specimen collection (see a later section of this chapter). Other factors, such as age and gender, may be relevant partitioning criteria. Remaining sources of variation should be considered when criteria for the selection of reference individuals are defined.

The *a priori* strategy is best suited for smaller studies and for analytes for which there are very specific confounding factors or for which the analytical process is very difficult or expensive. One such example is male sex hormone–related reference intervals.[38] Potential reference individuals from the parent population should be interviewed and examined clinically and by selected laboratory methods to decide whether they fulfill the defined inclusion criteria. If the decision is positive, specimens for analysis are collected by a standardized procedure (including the necessary preparation of individuals before the collection).

The *a posteriori* method is based on the availability of a large collection of data on medically examined individuals and measured quantities. Studies thoroughly planned by centers for health screening or preventive medicine may provide such data. It is important that data be collected by a strictly standardized and comprehensive protocol concerning (1) sampling from the parent population, (2) registration of demographic and clinical data on participating individuals, (3) preparation for and execution of specimen collection, and (4) handling and analysis of the specimens. If these requirements are met, values may be selected after application of the defined inclusion criteria to individuals found in the database. The selection of individuals from large pathology databases (see earlier discussion) is another example of the application of an *a posteriori* method. In this case, however, the quality of data may be lower than that in well-planned population studies.

A study performed in Kristianstad, Sweden,[39] highlights a practical problem often met when reference individuals are selected: the number of subjects fulfilling the inclusion criteria may be too small. In this study, only 17% of participants were accepted into the study, according to the criteria used, leaving an insufficient reference sample group. The frequency of exclusion was higher among women and in older age groups.

This problem has two possible solutions:

1. The exclusion criteria may be relaxed. As already discussed, the set of relevant sources of biological variation differs among different analytes. One may define a minimum set of exclusion criteria for a given laboratory test. In the Kristianstad study, the complete group of individuals could probably be used for establishment of reference values for serum sodium, and most of the individuals would be acceptable for the determination of reference values for several other analytes.[39]
2. Another design of the sampling procedure could reduce the practical problems and costs of obtaining a sufficiently large group of reference individuals. The Kristianstad study showed that 75% of excluded subjects could have been identified using only a simple questionnaire.[39] In the upper age group, this percentage was even higher. Therefore, preliminary screening of a large number of individuals from the parent population, using a carefully designed questionnaire (ie, of or related to the current or previous medical history of a patient), would result in a much smaller sample of individuals for examination clinically and by laboratory methods. If 3000 individuals had been prescreened in Kristianstad, and if only the individuals remaining in the reduced sample were subjected to a closer examination, a group of 240 reference individuals would have been obtained.

The two modifications of the protocol may also be combined.

Random or Nonrandom Sampling?

Ideally, the group of reference individuals should be a random sample of all individuals fulfilling the inclusion criteria defined in the parent population. Statistical estimation of distribution parameters (and their confidence intervals) and statistical hypothesis testing require this assumption.

For several reasons, most collections of reference values are, in fact, obtained by a nonrandom process.[40] This means that all possible reference individuals in the entire population under study do not have an equal chance of being chosen for inclusion in the usually much smaller sample of individuals studied. A strictly random sampling scheme in most cases is impossible for practical reasons. It would imply the examination of and application of inclusion criteria to the entire population (thousands or millions of persons), and then the random selection of a subset of individuals from among those accepted. This approach has been used by national organizations, such as the National Health and Nutrition Examination Survey (NHANES)[41] in the United States and the Australian Bureau of Statistics,[42] to select individuals at random to provide a cohort that is representative of the full population.

Usually the situation is less satisfactory. The sampling process is highly affected by convenience and cost. For example, samples of reference individuals are commonly obtained by selecting (1) from blood donors, (2) from persons working in a nearby factory, (3) from hospital staff, or (4) from hospital databases, none of which represent a random sampling of possible reference individuals in the general population.

The conclusions are obvious: (1) the best reference sample obtainable should be used with a balance between practical considerations and consideration of possible biases that may be introduced by the selection process, and (2) the data should be used and interpreted with due caution, with awareness of the possible bias introduced by the nonrandomness of the sample selection process. For example, lower iron stores may be expected in a sample of regular blood donors, and higher vitamin D concentrations may be expected in a sample drawn from outdoor workers.

Selection Criteria and Evaluation of Subjects

The selection of reference individuals consists essentially of applying defined criteria to a group of examined candidate persons.[10-15] The required characteristics of the reference values determine which criteria should be used in the selection process. Table 8.2 lists some important criteria to consider when production of health-associated reference values is the aim.

In practice, consideration of which *diseases* and *risk factors* to exclude is difficult (see the discussion on the concept of health earlier in this chapter). The answer lies in part in the intended purpose of establishing reference values; the project must be goal oriented.

Once a factor has been selected as an exclusion factor, a relevant and practical definition is required. For example,

TABLE 8.2 Examples of Exclusion and Partitioning Criteria

Exclusion	Partitioning
Age	Age
Alcohol intake	Blood group
Blood donation (recent)	Circadian variation
Drug abuse	Ethnicity
Exercise intensity (recent)	Exercise intensity (recent)
Fasting vs. nonfasting	Fasting vs. nonfasting
Sex	Sex
Hospitalization (recent)	Menstrual cycle (by stage)
Hypertension	
Illness (recent)	
Lactation	
Obesity	Obesity
Occupation	Posture (when sampled)
Oral contraceptives	
Pregnancy	Pregnancy (by stage)
Prescription drugs	Prescription drugs
Recent transfusion	

As indicated by the *shaded boxes,* some criteria may be considered as either exclusion criteria or partitioning criteria.

obesity is a common condition that is associated with a number of diseases; however, the definition of *obesity* is problematic. A definition might be based on a known assumed contribution to the risk of a development of specified disease. However, scientific data of this type are seldom available for the studied population. Another possibility for establishing obesity is to use upper limits based on weight measurements in different age, gender, and height groups of the general population (for example, more than 20% above the national age-, sex-, and height-specific mean weight). For obesity, a common approach is to use definitions based on the body mass index (BMI),[43] although limiting subjects to the healthy range will exclude over 50% of some populations. Tables of optimum or ideal weights have been published by life insurance companies; they may be more appropriate for delineation of obesity. Similar problems relate to the definition of hypertension. And what if a potential reference individual is no longer obese as a result of bariatric surgery or is currently normotensive on drug therapy?

In addition, is it permissible to use exclusion criteria based on *laboratory measurements*? It has been argued that a circular process might happen when laboratory tests are used to assess the health of subjects who are subsequently used as healthy control subjects for laboratory tests. But actually there is no difference, in this context, between measuring height, weight, and blood pressure and performing selected laboratory tests, provided that these laboratory tests are neither those for which reference values are produced nor tests that are significantly correlated with them.[30]

It is particularly difficult to define selection criteria when establishing reference values for a geriatric population.[44] In higher age groups, it is "normal" (ie, common) to have minor or major diseases and to take therapeutic drugs. One solution is to collect values at one time and to use the values of survivors after a defined number of years.[30,45]

Usually the clinical evaluation of candidate individuals is based on (1) a detailed interview or questionnaire (ie, the complete history recalled and recounted by a patient), (2) a physical examination, and (3) supplementary investigations. Questionnaires and examination forms tailored to the requirements of the actual project facilitate the evaluation and document the decisions made.

Partitioning of the Reference Group

It may also be necessary to define *partitioning criteria* for the subclassification of the set of selected reference individuals into more homogeneous groups (see Table 8.2).[10-15] (The question of determining when stratification of the reference sample group is necessary and justified is discussed in later sections.) In practice, the number of partitioning criteria should usually be kept as small as possible to ensure sufficient sample sizes to derive valid estimates.

Age and *sex* are the most frequently used criteria for subgrouping, because several analytes vary notably among different age and sex groups.[36,37,44] Age may be categorized by equal intervals (eg, by decades) or by intervals that are narrower in the periods of life when greater variation is observed. In some cases, more appropriate intervals can be obtained from qualitative age groups, such as (1) postnatal, (2) infancy, (3) childhood, (4) prepubertal, (5) pubertal, (6) adult, (7) premenopausal, (8) menopausal, and (9) geriatric. Further subdivision may also be needed based on Tanner stage of puberty or based on phase of the menstrual cycle. Height and weight also have been used as criteria for categorizing children. The use of age and sex for partitioning has the advantage that reference limits derived from subpopulations on these criteria can be easily applied on pathology reports where these factors are usually known about the patient. In contrast, the application of limits based on other criteria requires knowledge not usually available to the laboratory.[36,37]

SPECIMEN COLLECTION

Several preanalytical factors can influence the values of measured biological quantities, such as the concentrations of components in a blood sample or the amount excreted in feces, urine, or sweat.[46,47] This topic is covered elsewhere (see Chapters 4 and 5). In this discussion, only aspects of special relevance to the generation of reliable reference values are highlighted.[10-15,46]

Preanalytical standardization of the (1) preparation of individuals before specimen collection, (2) procedure of specimen collection itself, and (3) handling of the specimen before analysis may eliminate or minimize bias or variation from these factors. This reduces the "noise" that might otherwise conceal important biological "signals" of disease, risk, or treatment effect.

Preanalytical Standardization

Preanalytical procedures used before routine analysis of patient specimens and when reference values are established should be as similar as possible. In general, it is much easier to standardize routines for studies of reference values than those used in the daily clinical setting, especially when specimens are collected in emergency or other unplanned situations. Thus two general approaches have been suggested:

1. Only such factors that may be relatively easily controlled in the clinical setting should be part of the standardization when reference values are produced.
2. The rules for preanalytical standardization when reference values are produced should also be used for the clinical situation. Such rules include food and beverage restrictions, exercise restrictions, time sitting (or lying down) prior to phlebotomy, and tourniquet time. It has been shown that it is possible to apply these rules rather closely in the clinical setting for both hospitalized and ambulatory patients.[7] The same philosophy forms the basis for recommendations concerning sample preparation preceding analysis.

However, either philosophy is concordant with the concept of reference values, provided that the conditions under which reference values are produced are clearly stated.

Analyte-Specific Considerations

The types and magnitudes of preanalytical sources of variation clearly are not equal for different analytes (see Chapter 5). In fact, some believe that only those factors that cause unwanted variation in the biological quantities for which reference values are being generated should be considered. For example, body posture during specimen collection is highly relevant for the establishment of reference values for analytes that do not diffuse across blood vessel walls, such as albumin in serum or red cell count in blood, but posture is irrelevant for establishment of serum sodium values.[47]

Alternatively, several constituents are analyzed routinely in the same clinical specimen. Therefore, it would be impractical to devise special systems for every single type of quantity.[7] Consequently, three standardized procedures for blood specimen collection by venipuncture have been recommended[6,46]: (1) collection in the morning from hospitalized patients, (2) collection in the morning from ambulatory patients, and (3) collection in the afternoon from ambulatory patients. Such schemes have to be modified depending on local conditions and necessities and on the intended use of the reference values produced. Published checklists[7,10-15] may be helpful in the design of a scheme.

A special problem is caused by drugs taken by individuals before specimen collection,[48-50] and it may be necessary to distinguish between indispensable and dispensable medications. If possible, dispensable medication should be avoided for at least 48 hours. The use of indispensable drugs, such as contraceptive pills or essential medication, may be a criterion for exclusion or partitioning if these affect the analyte of interest.

In emergency or other unplanned clinical situations, even a partial application of the standardized procedure for collection has been shown to be of great value.[6] When collections have been made under conditions other than those specified for a specific analyte, interpretation of results against reference limits requires awareness of the type and magnitude of variation that may be expected under those circumstances. For example, a serum cortisol collected in the evening cannot usually be compared with reference limits established for morning collections, the exception being that a high result is still of great clinical relevance because the upper limit for evening values is typically much lower than the upper limit for morning values.

Necessity for Additional Information

The clinical situation is often different from a controlled research situation; for example, specimens have to be taken (1) during operations, (2) in emergency situations, and (3) when patients are unwilling or unable to follow instructions. Therefore the clinician may need additional information for interpretation of a patient's values in relation to reference values obtained under fairly standardized conditions.

An *empirical approach*[7] is to produce other sets of reference values, such as postprandial values, post-exercise values, or postpartum values.[6] Such a method, however, is very expensive and does not cover all situations that could possibly arise. This approach is also limited by the variability in these events (ie, for postprandial samples, the size of the meal, the types of food consumed, and the number of hours since the meal).

Another, more general solution to the problem is called the *predictive approach*.[7] Starting from a set of ordinary reference values and using quantitative information on the effects of various factors (eg, intake of food, alcohol, and drugs; exercise; stress; posture; or time of day), expected reference values that fit the actual clinical setting could be estimated.[36,37] An interesting example is provided by thyroid-stimulating hormone (TSH), where the effect of diurnal variation needs to be considered.[51]

More studies of such effects are needed, especially for the combined effect of two or more sources of variation. For example, is the combined effect of alcohol and contraceptive drugs on GGT activity in serum less than, equal to, or greater than the sum of their individual effects?

ANALYTICAL PROCEDURES AND QUALITY CONTROL

Essential components of the required definition of a set of reference values are specifications concerning (1) the analysis method (including information on traceability, equipment, reagents, calibrators, type of raw data, and calculation method; see Chapter 2), (2) quality control (see Chapter 6), and (3) reliability criteria.[6,10-15]

Specifications should be so carefully described that another investigator will be able to reproduce the study, and the user of reference values will then be able to evaluate their comparability with values obtained by methods used for producing the patients' values in a routine laboratory. To ensure comparability between reference values and observed values a method with the same performance characteristics of traceability, reproducibility, and analytical specificity should be used.

It is often claimed that analytical quality should be better when reference values rather than routine values are produced. This is certainly correct for trueness; all measures should be taken to select an appropriate reference standard (materials or methods) for traceability base and minimizing bias from that standard. The use of methods traceable to the Joint Committee for Traceability in Laboratory Medicine (JCTLM)-listed reference materials, methods, and services[52] (if available) increases the likelihood that reference limits are transferable among different laboratories. The question of imprecision is more difficult because it depends in part on the intended use of the reference values. Increases in analytical random variation result in widening of the reference interval.[6†] For some special uses of reference values, the narrower reference interval obtained by a more precise analytical method may be appropriate. However, this usually is not true for routine clinical use of reference values. Interpretation is simplest if a patient's values and reference values are comparable with regard to analytical imprecision. For the same reason, it is advisable to analyze specimens from reference individuals in several runs to include between-run components of variation. A safe way to obtain comparability is to include these specimens in routine runs together with real patient specimens.

STATISTICAL TREATMENT OF REFERENCE VALUES

This section deals with two main topics: the partitioning of reference values into more homogeneous classes, and the

†The width of a reference interval is a combination of the within-subject biological variation (coefficient of variation [CV_i]), the between-subject biological variation (CV_g), the preanalytical variation (CV_{pa}), and the analytical variation (CV_a). Assuming for demonstration that these factors are all distributed in a Gaussian manner, the CV of the results produced in a reference interval study (CV_{ri}) is $CVri = \sqrt{CVi^2 + CVg^2 + CVpa^2 + CVa^2}$. Thus a greater analytical imprecision leads to a wider reference interval.

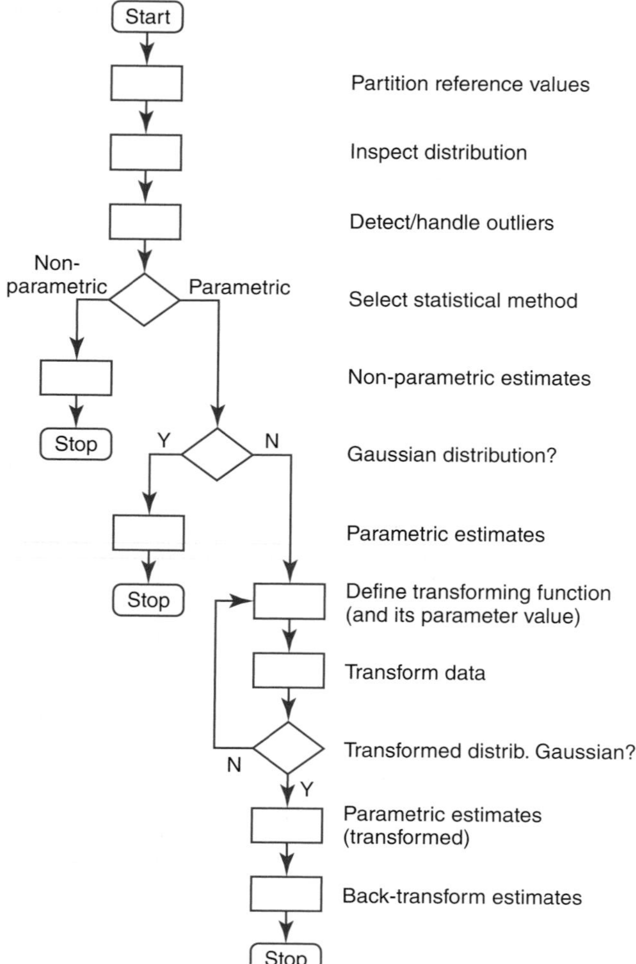

FIGURE 8.2 The statistical treatment of reference values. The *boxes* in the flow chart refer to sections in the text. The order of the three first actions (partitioning, inspection, and detection and/or handling of outliers) may vary, depending on the distribution and the statistical methods applied. *Y,* Yes; *N,* no.

determination of reference limits and intervals.[53] The subject matter is presented in the order in which data are often treated. Fig. 8.2 gives an outline and refers to corresponding sections in the text. Before the presentation of methods, some statistical concepts used are briefly discussed (see also Chapter 2). A textbook by Harris and Boyd gives an excellent summary of the statistical bases of reference values in laboratory medicine.[54]

Basic Statistical Concepts

Sample

The first step in the establishment of reference values is the selection of a group of reference individuals. In practice, it is not feasible to gather observations on all possible reference individuals of a certain category of the general population. Therefore, a smaller group (sometimes called the reference *sample* group) is examined. This *subset* is chosen so that it is expected to give the desired information about the characteristics of the complete *set* of individuals (the reference *population*).[10-15]

The reference *population* is often considered to be *hypothetical* because its characteristics are not observed directly; neither the number (the set size) nor the properties of all of its individuals are known. An obvious requirement is that individuals in the subset are typical of those in the complete set. Statistical theory usually assumes that items in the subset are selected at *random* from among those in the set; otherwise, the subset may be biased. If items are not randomly selected, statistical techniques are still used, but only with due caution and with awareness of the possible bias introduced.

Two main types of inferences may be made from values obtained from the subset (sample group) to the set (total reference population): estimating properties of the reference population (eg, reference limits) and testing hypotheses related to the reference population (eg, whether the distribution is Gaussian).

Estimating Properties

In practice, properties of the set are estimated. A *reference limit* (a percentile) of a biological quantity, such as the activity of serum GGT, based on subset reference values, is an example of a *point estimate* (a single value). It is considered representative of the property that might have been found if all possible values in the set had been observed. If many randomly selected subsets from the same set are examined, several estimates with some variation around the "true" value of the set are obtained. Also, it is possible to produce an *interval estimate* bounded by limits within which the "true" value is located with a specified confidence: the *confidence interval*. The parameter is expressed as a percentage between 0% and 100%, indicating the degree on the scale between "never" and "always" that the point estimate lies within the interval estimate. A reference limit for serum GGT can thus be associated with a confidence interval showing its region of uncertainty (eg, the 97.5th percentile for serum GGT is 47 IU/L, with 90% confidence limits of 39 to 50 IU/L).

Testing Hypotheses

Hypotheses about the population distribution can be also tested. For example, one can state the *null hypothesis* that the distribution of values for serum GGT activities is Gaussian. If true, this will enable determination of the reference limits with relatively few points. If deviations of subset values from the Gaussian distribution are small, they can be ascribed to variation caused by chance alone. In that case, it is reasonable to use statistical methods based on the Gaussian distribution. However, the hypothesis must be rejected if it is unlikely that observed deviations from the Gaussian distribution are caused by chance alone. *Statistical tests* provide quantitative approaches to these types of decisions; the null hypothesis is rejected if the statistical test shows that the probability of the hypothesis being true is less than a stated *significance level*. The *probability (P)* is a number in the interval of 0 to 1, with higher values indicating a greater certainty. If a significance level of 0.05 is stated, the Gaussian hypothesis is tested for the distribution of serum GGT activities; it should be rejected if the probability obtained by the test is below this value (eg, if $P = 0.01$, there is only a 1% chance that the distribution is Gaussian). Then the alternative hypothesis that the distribution is non-Gaussian is accepted. The *power* of a statistical test is the probability of rejection when the null hypothesis is false.

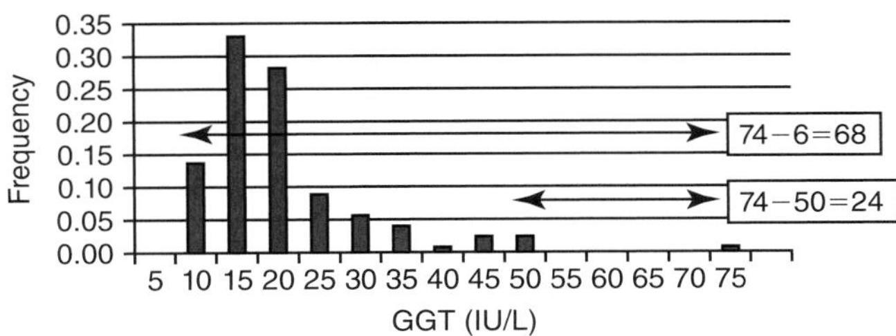

FIGURE 8.3 Observed distribution of 124 gamma-glutamyltransferase (GGT) values in serum (IU/L). The *upper arrow* indicates the range of the observed values (highest − lowest, or 74 − 6 = 68); the *lower arrow* indicates the difference between the highest value and the next highest value (74 − 50 = 24). Since the quotient (24/68 = 0.35) exceeds 0.33, Dixon's range test indicates that the highest value is an outlier and is therefore omitted from all further analyses.

Describing the Distribution

In the following sections, the term *reference distribution*[10-15] is used for the distribution of reference values *(x)*. For Gaussian distributions the two statistics *arithmetic mean* ($\overline{x}$) and *standard deviation* (s_x) are measures of the location (based on a measure of the center of the distribution) and the dispersion of values in it, respectively. They are defined as follows:

$$\overline{x} = \frac{\sum x}{n}$$

$$s_x = \sqrt{\frac{\sum (x-\overline{x})^2}{n-1}} = \sqrt{\frac{\sum x^2 - \frac{\left(\sum x\right)^2}{n}}{n-1}}$$

where ***x*** represents each of the *n* reference values in the subset (or a subclass of it). The equations can be described in words to facilitate understanding. The arithmetic mean is the sum of all the values divided by the number of values. The standard deviation is the square root of the result of the following calculation: the sum of the squares of all the differences of each value from the arithmetic mean divided by the number of samples minus one.

An observed distribution should be presented as a table or, preferably, as a graph (histogram) showing the number of observations in small intervals (Fig. 8.3). The number of observations in an interval divided by the total number of observations in the distribution (its size) is an estimator of the probability of finding a value in the corresponding interval of the hypothetical *probability distribution* of the population (assuming random sampling). By consecutive summing of all these ratios, starting with the leftmost interval of the observed distribution, an estimate is obtained of the hypothetical *cumulative probability distribution,* shown as a normal probability plot in Fig. 8.4B.

Reference Limits: Interpercentile Interval

As mentioned previously, reference values provide a basis for interpretation of laboratory data. In clinical practice, one usually compares a patient's result with the corresponding *reference interval,* which is bounded by a pair of *reference limits.*[10-15] This interval, which may be defined in different

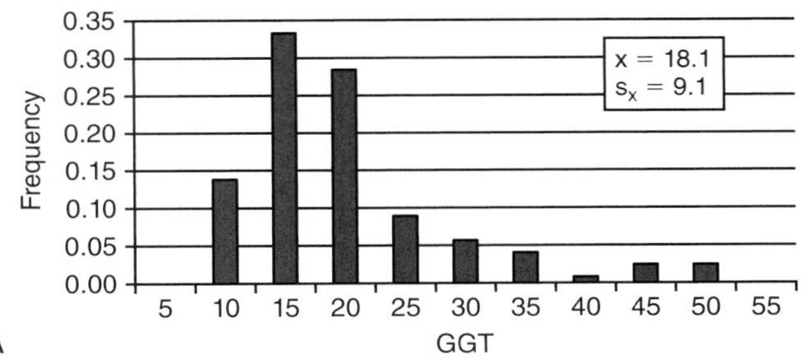

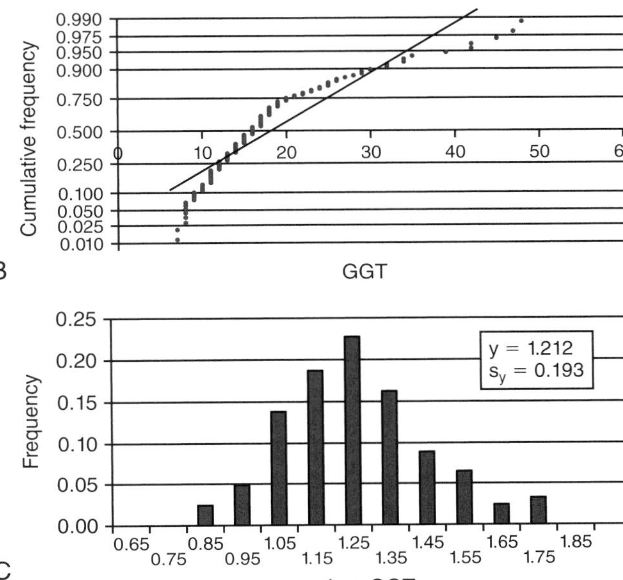

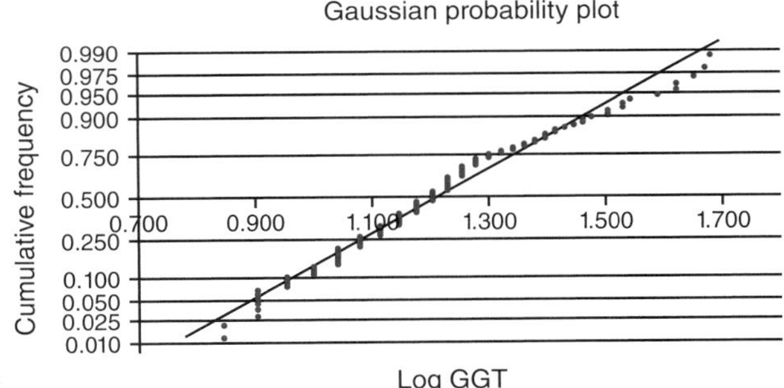

FIGURE 8.4 Distribution of 123 remaining gamma-glutamyltransferase (GGT) values from reference subjects. **A** is a histogram of the original, untransformed data. **B** shows the cumulative frequency of the data from **A** plotted on Gaussian probability paper. **C** is a histogram of the logarithmic transformed data. **D** shows the cumulative frequency of the data from **C** using a "normal probability plot."

ways, is a useful condensation of the information carried by the total set of reference values.

This discussion will be confined to the *interpercentile interval,* which is (1) simple to estimate, (2) commonly used, and (3) recommended by the IFCC[10-15] and CLSI.[16] It is defined as an interval bounded by two percentiles of the reference distribution. A *percentile* denotes a value that divides the reference distribution such that specified percentages of

TABLE 8.3 Notable Differences Between Analysis Methods

	Nonparametric	Parametric
Sample Size (minimum number of reference individuals per partition)	120	40
Reference Value Distribution	No requirements Any distribution is acceptable	Gaussian distribution required
Ease of Analysis	Straightforward No expertise required	Can be complicated Proof that distribution is Gaussian required Transformation of data may be required
Endorsements	IFCC, CLSI	

its values have magnitudes less than or equal to the limiting value. For example, if 47 IU/L is the 97.5th percentile of serum GGT values, then 97.5% of the values are equal to or below this value.

It is an arbitrary but common convention to define the reference interval as the *central 95%-interval* bounded by the 2.5th and 97.5th percentiles.[10-15] Another size or an asymmetric location of the reference interval may be more appropriate in particular cases. For example, the 99th percentile has been recommended for cardiac troponins,[55] and the 80th percentile for lipoprotein(a).[56] To prevent ambiguity, the definition of the interval should always be stated. The estimation of percentiles presented in the following sections is based on the conventional central 95% interval, but the techniques are easily adapted to other locations of the limits.

The percentiles are point estimates of population parameters. Accordingly, they are unbiased estimates only if the subset of values was selected randomly from the population. But, as was discussed earlier, random sampling is often difficult to achieve. An interpercentile interval may always be used, however, as a summary or description of the *subset* reference distribution.

The precision of a percentile as an estimate of a population value depends on the size of the subset and the scatter of results around the percentile; it is less precise when few observations are reported or when data points are more widely scattered. If the assumption of random sampling is fulfilled, the *confidence interval* of the percentile (ie, the limits within which the true percentile is located with a specified degree of confidence) can be determined. The 90% confidence interval of the 2.5th percentile (lower reference limit) for serum GGT values may, for example, be 6 to 8 IU/L, whereas the 90% confidence interval of the 97.5th percentile could be 39 to 50 IU/L. The upper limit confidence interval is wider because of a skewed distribution leading to more scattered data points.

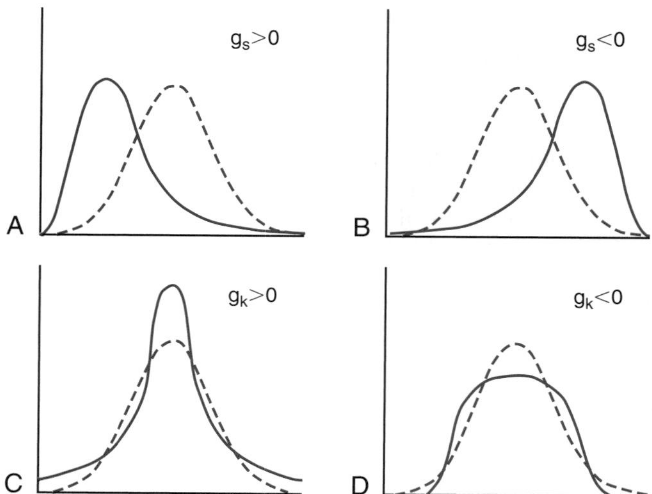

FIGURE 8.5 Skewness and kurtosis. The two *upper figures* show asymmetric distributions (**A,** positive skewness; **B,** negative skewness). The two *lower figures* show distributions with non-Gaussian peakedness (**C,** positive kurtosis; **D,** negative kurtosis). The Gaussian distribution *(dashed curve)* is shown in all graphs for comparison. The values of the coefficients of skewness *(g_s)* and kurtosis *(g_k)* are also shown.

Methods Used to Determine Interpercentile Intervals

The interpercentile interval is typically determined based on one of two major method principles: parametric or nonparametric (Table 8.3).[10-16]

The *parametric method* has as its major advantage the need for fewer reference values to determine percentiles and their confidence intervals. It can be applied when the distribution can be described completely by a small number of population parameters. For example, in a Gaussian distribution, determination of the mean and standard deviation allow for calculation of the 2.5th and 97.5th reference limits as the values located roughly two standard deviations below and above the mean. In fact, most of the parametric methods are based on the Gaussian distribution. If the reference distribution does not appear to be Gaussian, mathematical functions may be used to transform data to a distribution that approximates a Gaussian shape. Some positively skewed distributions (Fig. 8.5A) may, for example, be made symmetric by using logarithmic, Box-Cox or other transformations of the data values.

In contrast, the *nonparametric method* has as its major advantage that it makes no assumptions concerning the type of distribution and does not use estimates of distribution parameters. Percentiles are determined simply by eliminating the required percentage of values in each tail of the subset reference distribution (typically 2.5%).

The simple nonparametric method for determination of percentiles is recommended by IFCC[10-15] and CLSI.[16] The parametric method, which can be fairly complex, is seldom necessary, but it will be presented here because of its popularity and frequent misapplication.

Two other methods will be mentioned later in this chapter, but they are more complex and require the use of computer techniques (though these techniques are widely available in commercial software). It is worth emphasizing that, when results obtained using proper application of any of these methods are compared, it is usually found that estimates of the percentiles are very similar. Detailed descriptions of nonparametric and parametric methods are given later in this chapter.

Sample Size

For the parametric method, the theoretical lower limit of the sample size required for estimation of the $100p$ and $100(1 - p)$ percentiles is equal to $1/p$. Thus, estimation of the 2.5th percentile requires at least $1/0.025 = 40$ observations (per partition).

In contrast, for the nonparametric approach, a sample size of at least 120 reference values (per partition) has been recommended (the actual minimum is 119; however, this is commonly rounded up to 120); otherwise, one cannot determine confidence intervals for the reference limits.[10-16] It is important to note that 120 reference values allows for calculation of statistically valid 90% confidence limits; it does not necessarily provide the user with reference limits that would be considered clinically adequate.

It should be noted that for any method (parametric or nonparametric), the precision of the percentiles increases as the number of observations increases. For example, it requires 299 samples to determine the 90% confidence limit for the 99th percentile (vs. 120 for the 97.5th percentile). Also, the more highly skewed a distribution is, the larger is the number of reference values needed to obtain clinically reasonable confidence intervals at the tail end of the distribution.[57] The NORIP study[58] provides a particularly good example of this phenomenon. The value for the 97.5th percentile for serum alanine aminotransferase (ALT) in males was 68, with 90% confidence limits of 63.4 to 73.6. Even though the study was based on 1080 subjects, the confidence interval represented more than 15% of the reference interval.

Partitioning of Reference Values

The best order of the first three actions outlined in Fig. 8.2 (1—partitioning of reference values, 2—inspection of the distribution, and 3—detection/handling of outliers) may in some cases be different from that shown in the figure. For example, it might be more appropriate to detect outliers before testing for partitioning. No strict rules for the order of these actions can be given because it depends on data and the statistical methods applied. In addition, it can be argued that inspection of the data is important at each of the processes in the figure. With these cautions in mind, the presentation in this chapter follows Fig. 8.2.

The subset of reference individuals and corresponding reference values may be partitioned according to sex, age, and other characteristics (see Table 8.2). The process of partitioning is also referred to as stratification, categorization, or subgrouping, and its results have been called partitions, strata, categories, classes, or subgroups. In this chapter, the terms *partitioning* (for the process) and *(sub)classes* (for its result) are used.

The aim of partitioning is to create more homogeneous subsets of data so as to provide a better basis for comparison of clinical laboratory results: *class-specific* reference intervals (eg, age- and sex-specific reference intervals). An initial step is to graph the data against the relevant parameter. For example, plotting reference values against age will allow assessment as to whether partitioning is likely to be needed and, if so, which ages should be included in each class.

Various statistical criteria for partitioning have been suggested.[54,59] For example, an intuitive criterion states that partitioning is necessary if differences between classes are statistically significant (rejection of the "null" hypothesis of equal distributions). The distribution of reference values in the classes may show different locations (the mean values vary) or different intraclass variations (the standard deviations vary). These differences may be tested by statistical methods, which are not described here. The reader is referred to Chapter 2 and to standard textbooks of parametric[60,61] and nonparametric statistics.[62]

Differences in location or variation, however, may be statistically significant and still may be too small to justify replacing a single total reference interval with several class-specific intervals. In practice it is common to use a clinical assessment as to whether the proposed differences are likely to be important for patient care. For example, a difference within the analytical variation of the assay may be deemed sufficiently small to ignore. Alternatively, statistically nonsignificant differences can lead to situations in which the proportions of each subclass above the upper or below the lower reference limits (without partitioning) are much different from the desired 2.5% on each side. Harris and Boyd[54] therefore suggested criteria based on the ratio between subclass standard deviations, a normal deviate test of means, and calculation of critical decision values dependent on the sample size. Lahti and coworkers[59,63] suggested focusing directly on the proportions of each subgroup falling outside the combined population reference limits in order to determine whether partitioning is indicated. According to their approach, subgroup specific reference limits are needed when more than 4.1% or less than 0.9% of any subgroup falls outside the combined reference limits. Advantages of their method are that it can be used with non-Gaussian as well as Gaussian distributions and that it takes into account differences in subgroup prevalences.

Partitioning requires large samples of reference values. If these are not used, subclass sizes may be too small for reliable estimates of reference intervals and there may be limited statistical power to identify true differences between classes.

To solve the subclass size problem, it has been suggested to estimate regression-based reference intervals. Instead of dividing, for example, the total material into several age classes, one may construct continuous age-dependent reference limits and their confidence regions. Simulation studies have shown that this method produces reliable estimates with small sample sizes.[64,65] When the intended purpose of the reference interval is to detect individual changes in biochemical status, subject-based reference values may be more appropriate than class-specific reference intervals for interpretation.[54,66,67]

In the following sections, a homogeneous reference distribution and either the complete distribution (if partitioning has been shown to be unnecessary) or a subclass distribution (after partitioning) are assumed.

Inspection of the Distribution

It is always advisable to display the reference distribution graphically and to inspect it. A *histogram*, as shown in Fig. 8.3, is easily prepared and is the type of data display best suited for visual inspection. Examination of the histogram serves as a safeguard against misapplication or misinterpretation of statistical methods, and it may reveal valuable information about the data. Data should be evaluated for the following characteristics of the distribution:

1. Highly deviating values *(outliers)* may represent erroneous values.
2. *Bimodal* or *polymodal* distributions have more than one peak and may indicate that the distribution is nonhomogeneous because of mixing of two or more distributions. If so, the criteria used to select reference individuals should be reevaluated, or partitioning of the values according to age, sex, or other relevant factors should be attempted.
3. The shape of the distribution should be noticed. It may be asymmetrical, or it may be more or less peaked than the symmetrical and bell-shaped Gaussian distribution (see Fig. 8.5). The asymmetry most frequently observed with clinical chemistry data is positive *skewness* (see Fig. 8.5A). A symmetric distribution with positive *kurtosis* has a high and slim peak and a greater number of values in both tails than the Gaussian type of distribution (see Fig. 8.5C). Conversely, negative kurtosis indicates that the distribution has a broad and flat top with relatively few observations in the tails (see Fig. 8.5D). Asymmetry and non-Gaussian peakedness may be combined.

The visual inspection may also provide initial estimates of the location of reference limits that are useful as checks on the validity of computations. Assessment of the shape of the distribution can lead to a number of actions. It can guide the choice of approach (ie, parametric or nonparametric) or the necessity for transformation before using a parametric approach. As noted earlier, a skewed distribution may be a true reflection of the population, but it, or a secondary population, may also raise a question about possible causes: for example, the effect of a co-variate (eg, age affecting part of the population), an analytical problem (eg, bias during one analytical run), or a preanalytical problem (eg, samples from one site handled differently from other sites).

Identification and Handling of Erroneous Values

An *erroneous value* may occur due to a gross deviation from the prescribed procedure for establishment of reference values.[40] Such values may deviate significantly from proper reference values *(outliers)* or may be hidden in the reference distribution. Only a strict experimental protocol, with adequate controls at each step, can eliminate the latter type of erroneous values.

An outlier has been defined as "an observation whose discordancy from the majority of the sample is excessive in relation to the assumed distribution model for the sample, thereby leading to the suspicion that it is not generated by this model."[68] This definition has some particular utility because it focuses on the possible nature of the expected distribution as outlined in the subsequent text.

As stated previously, *visual inspection* of a histogram is a reliable method for identification of possible outliers. It is important to keep in mind, however, that values far out in the long tail of a skewed distribution may easily be misinterpreted as outliers. If the distribution is positively skewed, inspection of a histogram displaying logarithms or some other transformation of the values may aid in the visual identification of outliers. Indeed, the importance of visual inspection is supported in a number of CLSI documents (enter "outlier" as a search term at http://htd.clsi.org): "Statistical tests can be used to identify outliers, but the 'common-sense' judgment using visual inspection of the data is often more effective."

Some outliers may also be identified by statistical tests, but no single method is capable of detecting outliers in every situation that may occur. The number of techniques suggested or recommended is, for this reason, very large.[54,69,70] The two main problems encountered can be described as follows:

1. Many tests assume that the type of the true distribution is known before the test is used. Some of these specifically require that the distribution be Gaussian. However, biological distributions often are non-Gaussian, and their types are seldom known in advance. Furthermore, statistical tests of types of distribution are unreliable in the presence of outliers. This unreliability poses a difficult dilemma; some tests for outliers assume that the type of distribution is known, but tests for determining the type of distribution require that outliers be absent! As a consequence, it may be difficult to transform the distribution to Gaussian form before outliers are identified by statistical tests. Some tests are relatively insensitive to departures from a Gaussian distribution. This is the case with Dixon's *range test,* in which a value is identified as an extreme outlier if the difference between the two highest (or lowest) values in the distribution exceeds one third of the range of all values (see Fig. 8.3).[10-15,54,71]
2. Several tests for outliers assume that a data set contains only a single outlier. The limitation of these tests is obvious. Some tests may detect a specified number of outliers, or they may be run several times, discarding one outlier in each pass of data. The range test, however, usually fails in the presence of several outliers. It is possible to estimate the standard deviation using data remaining after *trimming* of both tails of the distribution by a specified percentage of observations.[54,72] Outliers could be identified by this method as the values lying 3 or 4 standard deviations from the arithmetic mean. This method assumes, however, that the true distribution is Gaussian.

Horn and coworkers[73] published a novel method in two stages for outlier detection that seems to provide a promising solution to both of the problems just mentioned. With this method, one executes the following:

1. Mathematically transform the data to approximate a Gaussian distribution. Horn used the Box-Cox transformation,[74] but other transformations that correct for skewness (see later) probably would also work. As mentioned earlier, it is impossible to achieve exact symmetry by transformation in the presence of outliers, but this does not seem to be critical with Horn's method.
2. Identify (or eliminate) outliers using a criterion based on the central 50% of the distribution, thus reducing the masking effect of several outliers. Compute the interquartile range (IQR) between the lower and upper quartiles of the distribution (Q_1 and Q_3, respectively): $IQR = Q_3 - Q_1$. Then identify as outliers data lying outside the two fences

$$Q_1 - 1.5 \times IQR \text{ and } Q_3 + 1.5 \times IQR.$$

Deviating values identified as possible outliers cannot always be discarded automatically. Values should be included or excluded on a rational basis. For example, records of the dubious values should be checked and errors corrected. In some cases, deviating values should be rejected because noncorrectable causes have been found, such as in previously unrecognized conditions that qualify individuals for exclusion from the group of reference individuals or analytical errors.

Methods for Determining Reference Limits

More details regarding four different approaches to determining reference limits are discussed in this section. In addition to the nonparametric and parametric methods described in general terms earlier, overviews of the bootstrap and robust methods are provided. In all four cases, it is important to remember that, at this stage, a homogeneous reference distribution, with outliers removed, is assumed.

Nonparametric Method

The nonparametric method is notable for at least three reasons: it is simple to perform, it does not require that the distribution is Gaussian, and it is recommended by both IFCC[10-15] and CLSI.[16] On the other hand, for estimates of the central 95 percentiles, it does require a minimum of 120 values (per partition). It consists essentially of eliminating a specified percentage of the values from each tail of the reference distribution. Very simple and reliable methods are based on *rank numbers.*[10-15,71,75] These methods also allow nonparametric estimation of the confidence intervals of the percentiles[71] and can easily be applied manually or with a spreadsheet program.

The rank-based method as recommended by the IFCC[10-15] and CLSI[16] requires the following steps:

1. First, the n reference values are sorted in ascending order of magnitude.
2. Next, the individual values are ranked. For example, the minimum value has rank number 1, the next value has rank number 2, and so on, until the maximum value, which has rank number n. Consecutive rank numbers should be given to two or more values that are equal ("ties").
3. The rank numbers of the $100p$ and $100(1 - p)$ percentiles are computed as $p(n + 1)$ and $(1 - p)(n + 1)$, respectively. Thus the limits of the conventional 95% reference interval have rank numbers equal to $0.025(n + 1)$ and $0.975(n + 1)$; in a data set of 120, these are the 3rd and 118th ranked results.
4. The percentiles are determined by finding the original reference values that correspond to the computed rank numbers, provided that the rank numbers are integers. Otherwise, one should interpolate between the two limiting values.
5. Finally, the confidence interval of each percentile is determined by using the binomial distribution.[71] Table 8.4 provides data for the 0.90 confidence interval of the 2.5th and 97.5th percentiles. For the relevant sample size n, rank numbers for the lower and upper limits should be found for the 2.5th percentile; those same values are subtracted from $(n + 1)$ to find the rank numbers for the 97.5th percentile.

Table 8.5 provides a detailed example of the nonparametric determination of 95% reference limits using the serum GGT reference values first shown in Fig. 8.3.

TABLE 8.4 Nonparametric Confidence Intervals of Reference Limits*

Sample Size	RANK NUMBERS Lower 0.90 CI Limit	2.5th Percentile	Upper 0.90 CI Limit
119–132	1	4	7
133–160	1	4	8
161–187	1	5	9
188–189	2	5	9
190–200	2	5	10
201–219	2	6	10
219–240	2	7	10
240–248	2	7	11
249–249	2	7	12
250–279	3	7	12
280–307	3	8	13
308–309	4	8	13
310–320	4	8	14
321–340	4	9	14
341–360	4	9	15
361–363	4	10	15
364–372	5	10	15
373–400	5	9	16
401–403	5	11	16
404–417	5	11	17
418–435	6	11	17
436–440	6	11	18
441–468	6	12	18
469–470	6	12	19
471–481	6	13	19
471–500	7	13	19

*The table shows the rank numbers of the 2.5th percentile together with the lower and upper limits of the 0.90 confidence interval for samples with 119 to 500 values. To obtain the corresponding rank numbers of the 97.5th percentile, subtract the rank numbers in the table from $(n + 1)$, where n is the sample size. Note that the 2.5th percentile values are the nearest number from the data set and may differ from results derived from statistical software packages that commonly derive the percentile values by interpolation between results from the data set when the rank value does not correspond to the exact percentile.

It is claimed that the nonparametric process is less affected by outliers than parametric methods, a statement that has some truth. For example, a single extreme outlier in a set of 120 results will affect the calculated mean and standard deviation, but it will not affect the 2.5th and 97.5th percentiles. It will, however, affect the 90% confidence interval of the nonparametric method, as the extreme result is the boundary of the confidence limit with these numbers. It can be easily seen, however, that a larger number of outliers will influence the percentile limits as well.

It should be emphasized that Table 8.4 is specific for the 2.5th and 97.5th percentiles and 90% confidence limits. It can be seen from the table that 0.90 CI are not available for fewer than 119 samples. For this reason, when fewer than 120 samples are included in reference interval studies provided by manufacturers, a narrower reference interval is sometimes provided (eg, the central 90% [5th through 95th percentiles]).

TABLE 8.5 Nonparametric Determination of Reference Interval*

Calculation of Rank Numbers of Percentiles

Lower:	0.025 (123 + 1) = 3.1 (i.e., Rank #3)
Upper:	0.975 (123 + 1) = 120.9 (i.e., Rank #121)

Original Values Corresponding to These Rank Numbers

Lower limit (2.5-percentile):	7 IU/L
Upper limit (97.5-percentile):	47 IU/L

Rank Numbers and Values of the 0.90-Confidence Limits

Lower Reference Limits

Rank numbers (see Table 8-4):	#1 and #7
Values:	6 and 8 IU/L

Upper Reference Limits

Rank numbers (see Table 8-4):	(123 + 1) − 7 = #117 and (123 + 1) − 1 = #123
Values:	39 and 50 IU/L

Summary

Lower reference limit:	7 (6 to 8) IU/L
Upper reference limit:	47 (39 to 50) IU/L

GGT Value	Frequency	Rank Order
6	1	1
7	2	2, 3
8	6	4-9
9	4	10-13
10	4	14-17
11	9	18-26
12	7	27-33
13	7	34-40
14	9	41-49
15	9	50-58
16	8	59-66
17	11	67-77
18	8	78-85
19	5	86-90
20	3	91-93
21	2	94, 95
22	2	96, 97
23	2	98, 99
24	2	100, 101
25	3	101-104
26	2	105, 106
27	1	107
28	1	108
29	2	109, 110
30	1	111
32	2	112, 113
34	2	114, 115
35	1	116
39	1	117
42	2	118, 119
45	1	120
47	1	121
48	1	122
50	1	123

*This table shows an example using the 123 serum gamma-glutamyltransferase (GGT) values displayed in Fig. 8.4A. See text for a description of the nonparametric method.

In general, a larger number of samples is required to generate 0.90 CI for wider reference intervals (eg, the central 98%, or 1st through 99th percentiles); a smaller number is required for narrower reference limits (eg, the central 90%, or 5th through 95th percentiles).

Parametric Method

Although it can be more complicated, usually involving relatively sophisticated statistical software, the parametric method is advantageous (in comparison to the nonparametric method) in requiring fewer reference values to determine reference limits. The method is presented here under separate headings for testing the type of distribution, for transforming the data, and for estimating percentiles and their confidence intervals.

It should be noted that commonly used statistical computer program packages aid in the estimation of reference limits, but these packages may lack some of the techniques described in this chapter. Several programs have been designed with clinical laboratories in mind and have specific functions to perform many of these processes, including CBstat,[76] MedCalc,[77] and Analyse-it.[78] The availability of these and other specialized programs will change over time, but it can be most useful to select a program that meets the needs of the laboratory, gain skills in its correct use, and maintain use of the same program over time. Basic statistical analysis can also be performed in common spreadsheet programs (eg, Microsoft Excel), but the more sophisticated features like confidence limits may require writing special functions into the spreadsheet.

Testing Fit to Gaussian Distribution. The parametric method for estimating percentiles assumes that the true distribution is Gaussian. This fact was frequently ignored in the past and caused Elveback[5] to warn against "the ghost of Gauss." Negligence often results in seriously biased estimates of reference limits.[79] After elimination of the outlier from the GGT reference values in Fig. 8.3, the mean and standard deviation of the remaining 123 serum GGT reference values are 18.1 and 9.1 (see Fig. 8.4A), from which the reference interval is calculated as $\bar{x} \pm 1.96 \times s_x$, or 0 to 36 IU/L (vs. the nonparametric values of 7 and 47 IU/L; Table 8.6). More highly positively skewed distributions may even result in negative values for the lower reference limit.

Therefore, a critical phase in the parametric method is testing the goodness-of-fit of the reference distribution to a hypothetical Gaussian distribution. If the Gaussian hypothesis must be rejected at a specified significance level, one is left with two alternatives (see Fig. 8.2): either the nonparametric method can be used, or a mathematical transformation of data can be applied to approximate the Gaussian distribution. Only when the Gaussian hypothesis is not rejected by the test can one pass directly to parametric estimation of percentiles and their confidence intervals (see Fig. 8.2). Simple signs that a distribution is highly unlikely to be Gaussian are skewed distribution on visual inspection of the distribution, a mean and median that are markedly different, and S_x above approximately 30% of the mean value. In any of these cases, formal assessment for Gaussian distribution is unnecessary.

Formal goodness-of-fit tests have been reviewed by Mardia.[80] These tests can be broadly classified as (1) graphical

TABLE 8.6 Summary of GGT Reference Interval Determination by Three Methods

Method	Lower Limit (CI)	Upper Limit (CI)	Values Below Lower Limit	Values Above Upper Limit
Nonparametric	7 (6 to 8)	47 (39 to 50)	1	2
Parametric—untransformed data	0 (−2 to 2)	36 (34 to 38)	0	7
Parametric—transformed data	7 (6 to 8)	40 (35 to 44)	1	6

The table summarizes the 95% reference intervals and associated 90% confidence limits generated by each of three methods for the same data set. The numbers of observed values deemed lower and higher than the corresponding interval for each method are given in the last two columns. Because the original data are positively skewed, note that the parametric techniques generate intervals that are biased low. Note, too, that the parametric technique on untransformed data has a lower confidence interval, which is actually less than 0.
CI, Confidence interval; *GGT*, gamma-glutamyltransferase.

procedures, (2) coefficient-based tests, and (3) tests that are based on shape differences between observed and theoretical distributions.

1. *The graphical procedure* consists of plotting the cumulative distribution on probability paper, which has a nonlinear vertical axis based on the Gaussian distribution (see Fig. 8.4B and D). The plot should be close to a straight line if the distribution is Gaussian.
2. *Coefficient-based tests* use statistical measures of skewness and kurtosis (see Fig. 8.5). Formulas for calculating these parameters are available elsewhere.[10-15] For Gaussian (and other symmetric distributions), the *coefficient of skewness* is zero; the sign of a nonzero coefficient indicates the type of skewness present in the data (see Fig. 8.5A and B). The *coefficient of kurtosis* is approximately zero for the Gaussian distribution. The sign of a nonzero coefficient indicates the type of kurtosis present in the data (see Fig. 8.5C and D). The statistical significance of these two coefficients may be found by referring to tables for testing skewness and kurtosis.[61]
3. Tests of *shape differences* that have been used to evaluate goodness-of-fit include the (1) Kolmogorov-Smirnov, (2) Cramer-von Mises, and (3) Anderson-Darling tests.[10-15,81] The Anderson-Darling test is recommended by the IFCC.[10-15]

Transformation of Data. In the previous section, it was shown that $\bar{x} \pm 1.96 \times s_x$ of the serum GGT data in Fig. 8.4A resulted in biased reference limits (too low values), as was to be expected with this positively skewed distribution. However, it is often possible to transform data mathematically to obtain a distribution of transformed values that approximates a Gaussian distribution. With these new values, the 2.5th and 97.5th percentiles are again localized at 1.96 standard deviations on both sides of the mean. The estimates may then be transformed back to the original measurement scale by using the inverse mathematical function.

It is frequently observed that *logarithmically transformed* values, $y = log(x)$, of a positively skewed distribution fit the Gaussian distribution rather closely. In other cases, *square roots* of the values, $y = \sqrt{x}$, result in a better approximation to the Gaussian distribution. In theory, any mathematical transformation of the data can be used. From a practical perspective, the family of Box-Cox transformations provides solutions in the vast majority of situations.[79]

The following example uses the logarithmic transformation for convenience, but any other transformation can be used in the same way. The procedure is as follows:

1. Test the fit of the distribution of original data to the Gaussian distribution. If the distribution has approximately a Gaussian shape, the 2.5th and 97.5th percentiles are calculated directly as $\bar{x} \pm 1.96 \times s_x$. Otherwise, continue with the following steps.
2. Transform data by the logarithmic function $y = log(x)$ (or by another selected function), then test the fit to the Gaussian distribution. If the transformed distribution is significantly different from Gaussian shape, try another transformation or estimate the percentiles by the nonparametric method (see earlier in this chapter). Continue with the next step if the transformation resulted in a Gaussian distribution.
3. Compute the mean $\bar{y}$ and the standard deviation s_y of transformed data. Then estimate the 2.5th and 97.5th percentiles in the transformed data scale as $\bar{y} \pm 1.96 \times s_y$.
4. The final step is reconversion of these percentiles to the original data scale. The inverse function for the logarithmic transformation $y = \log x$ is $x = 10^y$.
5. It is now possible to use the properties of the Gaussian distribution to estimate the reference limits and their confidence intervals. This method is presented in a later section.

Example: As noted earlier, the original GGT data reference distribution is not Gaussian but is, similar to many biological distributions, skewed to the right (see Fig. 8.4A). However, by using the logarithm of the serum GGT values, a distribution very close to Gaussian shape (see Fig. 8.4C) is obtained. This observation is confirmed in Fig. 8.4B and D where the cumulative probabilities are shown graphed on Gaussian probability paper; the original data are not linear, but the transformed data form a reasonably good line.

Parametric Estimates of Percentiles and Their Confidence Intervals. Once the distribution of reference data (original or transformed) is shown to be Gaussian, calculations of the $100p$ and $100(1 - p)$ percentiles and their 0.90 confidence intervals are straightforward:

As noted earlier, the $100p$ and $100(1 - p)$ *percentiles* are calculated as follows:

$$\text{mean} \pm c \times (\text{standard deviation})$$

where c is the $(1 - p)$ standard Gaussian deviate, as can be found in statistical tables. For the 2.5th and 97.5th percentiles, the $(1 - 0.025) = 0.975$ standard Gaussian deviate, c, has a value of 1.960.

The 0.9-*confidence intervals* of these percentiles are then determined as follows[7,10-15]:

$$percentile = \pm 2.81 \frac{S_y}{\sqrt{n}}$$

where s_y is the standard deviation of the reference values (original or transformed) and n is the number of values.[‡]

Example: The mean and standard deviation of the transformed data in Fig. 8.4 are $\bar{y} = 1.212$ and $s_y = 0.193$, respectively; that is, the mean value is 1.212 (corresponding to $10^{1.212}$, or 16 in the original scale). The transformed 2.5th percentile is then 1.212 − (1.960 × 0.193) = 0.835. On reconversion to the original data scale, a value of $10^{0.835}$ = 6.84 is obtained. The lower reference limit of serum GGT is thus 7 IU/L. Similarly, it is found that the upper reference limit is 39 IU/L. These values are in closer agreement with those found by the nonparametric method: 7 and 47 IU/L (see Tables 8.5 and 8.6).

The 0.90 confidence limits of the lower percentile are then

$$0.835 - 2.81 * \left(0.193/\sqrt{123}\right) = 0.786 \quad 10^{0.786} = 6.1$$

$$0.835 + 2.81 * \left(0.193/\sqrt{123}\right) = 0.884 \quad 10^{0.884} = 7.7$$

Thus the complete estimate of the 2.5th percentile (and its 0.90 confidence interval) is 7 (6 to 8) IU/L. The 97.5th percentile is, by the same method, found to be 39 (35 to 43) IU/L.

Table 8.6 summarizes data from the three methods used to determine reference intervals from GGT data. It can be seen that the application of parametric statistics to transformed data yields similar reference limits to those obtained by nonparametric methods. While nonparametric methods have the advantage of simpler mathematical processes and determining reference limits without assumptions on the underlying distribution, there can be some advantages to using parametric methods. If an underlying distribution can be defined, it can assist in assessing the likelihood of a result being a member of the reference population based on the parameters defining the population.

Other Methods for Calculating Reference Limits

As a brief introduction to the bootstrap and robust methods for determining reference limits, it is worth noting that they share two similarities. First, neither of these methods makes assumptions about the underlying distribution; it need not be Gaussian. Second, both require the use of computer software because they involve numerous iterations and somewhat complicated calculations.

Bootstrap Method. There are a number of variations on the "bootstrap" method, all of which can be used to generate reliable reference limits.[54,75,82] In principle, the technique is simple, but it involves many iterations (100 to 1000) and thus requires computers. As is the case with the nonparametric method, there is no requirement that the distribution be Gaussian. For reliable estimates of confidence intervals for the reference limits, it is recommended that there be a minimum of 100 reference values (per partition).[75] The following steps are involved in a typical bootstrap procedure:

1. First, random samples, each of size *m*, are selected, with replacement, from the original set of *n* reference values. One selects "with replacement" if each value randomly selected from the original set remains available, so that it may be selected again in the random selection of the next value. In other words, even if there is only one occurrence of a specific value in the original set of *n* values, it may appear more than once in one, or more, random samples of size *m*. The number of resamples should be high (500 is a reasonable number of iterations).
2. For each resample, the upper and lower reference limits (percentiles) are next estimated by the rank-based nonparametric procedure described previously. These estimates from each iteration are saved.
3. Upon completion of all iterations, the final lower reference limit is calculated as the mean of the estimates of the lower reference limit; similarly, the final upper reference limit is calculated as the mean of the estimates of the upper reference limit.
4. Finally, the 0.90 confidence interval of each reference limit is calculated from the distribution of the percentile estimates, that is, with 500 iterations, the 25th rank order value represents the 5th percentile, and the 475th rank order value represents the 95th percentile.

The reader should note that the bootstrap version described here uses rank-based nonparametric percentile estimates. However, the bootstrap principle may be employed with any kind of estimation, parametric or nonparametric.

Robust Method. The robust method has the form of the parametric method described earlier, but instead of using the mean and the standard deviation of the sample, it uses robust measures of location and spread. For example, instead of using the mean, it uses the median: in a series of 10 values, if the highest value is doubled, the mean changes appreciably, but the median does not change at all. The process involves weighting the data to place more value on results near the middle of the distribution and less weight on more distant results. The rationale is that the scattered data are more likely to reflect results that are not members of the desired distribution. This resistance to the effect of outliers is the basis for the term *Robust Method.* This method has particular value with small sample sizes.

Briefly, the steps involved are as follows:

1. Symmetry of the data is ensured, using transformations if necessary (eg, Box-Cox transformation[74]).
2. Initial robust measures of location (median) and spread (median absolute deviation) are found.
3. Using a *biweight estimation* technique, in which more weight is given to observations closer to the center and progressively less to values farther from the center, new estimates of location and spread are found until successive results are satisfactorily close.
4. With final robust values of location and spread, the upper and lower limits are calculated, in a manner analogous to that described for the parametric technique.

[‡]This formula is a special case of a general formula that can be used for confidence intervals of other sizes or for other percentiles derived from Gaussian distributions. CI for percentiles are calculated as follows: mean $\pm z_1 \times s_y \pm z_2 \times [s_y^2/n + (z_1^2 \times s_y^2)/(2 \times n)]^{0.5}$ where mean is the population mean, s_y is the population SD, n is the sample size, z_1 is the probit value related to the selected percentile (= 1.96 for 97.5th percentile) and z_2 is the covering factor for the CI (= 1.64 for 90%). (http://www.statsdirect.com/help/Default.htm#parametric_methods/reference_range.htm.)

5. Confidence intervals are then estimated using the bootstrapping technique described in the previous section.

Similar to the bootstrap method, this method does not require a Gaussian distribution. It is resistant to outliers and may be applied to very small numbers of observations. Details on the method are available.[83]

TRANSFERABILITY OF REFERENCE LIMITS FROM OTHER SOURCES

Determination of reliable reference values for each test in the laboratory's repertoire is a major task that is often far beyond the capabilities of the individual laboratory. This is especially important when ethical or practical considerations limit the number of available individuals (eg, when establishing pediatric or cerebrospinal fluid [CSF] reference values). But, even in the absence of such considerations, most of the methods discussed in the previous sections require qualification of, and analysis of samples from, relatively large numbers of reference individuals.

Two issues are critical in considering adopting reference intervals derived from the other sources discussed in the following sections. First, the populations under consideration must be comparable (ie, no major ethnic, social, or environmental differences should be noted between them that may be relevant to the analyte in question). If they are not, a separate reference interval study may well need to be done. Second, even if the populations are comparable, the analytical methods under consideration must be comparable. The optimal, but often unrealistic, situation assumes that analytical methods, including their calibration and quality assurance, are identical in the laboratories. The provision of methods from different manufacturers that are all traceable to equivalent higher-order reference materials and methods, such as are listed on the Joint Committee for Traceability in Laboratory Medicine (JCTLM) database, is facilitating the sharing of reference intervals.[84] In the absence of verified traceable methods, a pragmatic approach involves (1) standardization of analytical protocols, (2) common calibration, (3) design of a sufficiently efficient external quality control scheme, and (4) the use of mathematical transfer functions if results still are not directly comparable.[85] The parameters of transfer functions may be estimated from results obtained by analysis of a sufficient number of patient specimens spanning the relevant range of concentrations in all participating laboratories.[16] Provided both assays are linear, functions of the form $y = \alpha \times x + \beta$ are generally appropriate, where the constant term β compensates for systematic shifts among methods, whereas the coefficient term α adjusts for proportional differences. Care should be taken to ensure that errors do not occur due to the use of inappropriate statistical techniques. For example, simple linear regression can be affected by outlier values, variation in data dispersion at different analyte concentrations (heteroscedasticity), and a limited range of analyte concentrations. The use of Passing and Bablok[86] (or weighted linear regression) provides a more robust estimate of the linear function (see Chapter 2). It should be noted that the mentioned transfer functions account only for analytical bias; however, adjustments for differences in imprecision may also be designed.

Specific Examples of Other Sources for Reference Limits

One of the most common sources used for reference limits by clinical laboratories is manufacturers' package inserts. At the outset, it is important to note that, in some cases, manufacturers do not actually perform reference limit studies with their methods but instead cite other literature as the source for their reference limits (including earlier versions of this textbook). As stated earlier, some manufacturer's limits are central 90% rather than the usual central 95%. If, however, the manufacturer has indeed performed a good reference limit study using its method, and the laboratory uses the method exactly as prescribed by the manufacturer, it is reasonable to infer that the issue of method comparability has been addressed. Even after method comparability has been assured, though, it remains to be shown that the package insert data addresses the population comparability. Because supporting information is commonly not supplied in the manufacturers' Instructions for Use, it may be necessary to contact the manufacturer. The information required should include the age and sex distribution of the reference population, exclusion criteria, confidence intervals of the reference limits, and the statistical processes used. If relevant, additional information (eg, ethnicity; lifestyle factors; body composition data, such as body mass index or waist circumference) may be helpful. For example, in a recent study, the creatine kinase (CK) upper reference limits cited in a package insert based on a Caucasian population underestimated, by several-fold, the upper reference limits for blacks and Asians.[87]

A second source for reference limits is peer-reviewed publications. In this case, both method comparability and population comparability are at issue. Laboratories seeking to adopt these limits must proceed carefully, but it may well be considerably easier to address these issues than it would be to repeat the studies themselves. To return to the CK example just cited,[87] laboratories using the same method that was used in that publication, or other methods with demonstrated traceability to the same reference method (which is stated in the paper), could presumably adopt the reference limits determined in the study, whereas laboratories using other methods without this traceability would be aware of a potential problem but could not simply adopt those same reference limits for those ethnic groups. Another excellent example is the CALIPER initiative,[88] which established, using the methods described earlier, pediatric reference intervals, partitioned by age, sex, and ethnicity, for 40 different assays. As the authors emphasized, the published reference limits were specific to the methods they used. (In later publications[89] the authors provide reference limits for additional analytical methods based on transference studies alluded to in the previous section.) A third example, involving adult reference intervals, was structured along the same lines as the original CALIPER studies.[90]

A third source for reference limits is becoming increasingly popular—multicenter trials. In contrast to the CALIPER initiative, in which all the analyses were done in a single laboratory, these studies seek to pool data from many laboratories spread over large regions and potentially among different countries. Although this decreases the number of reference individuals needed to be recruited from each laboratory, it also typically increases the number of analytical methods involved for each assay. Despite global efforts at harmonization and standardization, these multicenter trials have repeatedly shown that current methods do not always produce interchangeable results, and therefore methods to ensure method comparability are still needed. Nonetheless, once these issues have been addressed, multicenter trials are proving to be an excellent way to generate data for establishing reference limits.[58,91]

Another potential source of data to generate reference limits is a laboratory's own historical data. A laboratory's database is attractive on several counts: it encompasses the laboratory's own populations; it is generated with the laboratory's own methods and own preanalytical conditions; and it may include large quantities of data. When the database consists strictly of relatively healthy outpatients (or techniques are used to limit the data to such patients), these techniques are capable of working reasonably well.[92] On the other hand, typical laboratory databases include data from unhealthy as well as healthy subjects, which is problematic because, in most cases, laboratories are trying to establish reference limits for healthy populations. There are methods (often referred to as "data mining" techniques) of extracting usable reference limit data from such databases (eg, Hoffmann[93] and Bhattacharya[94]), but they usually involve some assumptions and often involve relatively complicated data manipulation. Both the Hoffman and the Bhattacharya methods, for example, assume that the data include a genuine reference population and that this reference population follows a Gaussian distribution (either the original data or a transformed version). Simply analyzing data that has (or can be transformed into) a Gaussian distribution is not sufficient because population differences (eg, hospital inpatients vs. healthy outpatients) may produce misleading results.[95] With proper attention to the origins of the data (ie, that there are sufficient numbers of reference individuals, the populations are matched), the Hoffman and Bhattacharya techniques have been used to generate reliable reference limits.[96-98]

In summary, there are multiple different sources of information on reference intervals, including local formal reference interval studies, manufacturer's data, peer-reviewed publications, data mining techniques, and textbooks, including a compilation of reference interval data in various chapters and at the end of this textbook. Such information can be used as yet another source of data, with the same caveats noted at the beginning of this section and in the following section on verification. As is the case with any scientific process, it is good practice, when setting reference intervals, to access all available sources of information. This process allows for identification of discordant data sources and unexpected causes of variation, as well as for confirmation when different data sources provide the same information.

POINTS TO REMEMBER

Sources for Reference Limits (Other Than Establishing One's Own)

- Manufacturers' package inserts*
- Peer-reviewed literature*
- Multicenter trials*
- Analysis of laboratory's own historical data ("data mining")*

*Verification of the transferability of these values is ***required.***

Verification of Transferability

Whether a laboratory adopts reference values from (1) a manufacturer's package insert, (2) a peer-reviewed publication or textbooks, (3) a multicenter trial, or (4) a data mining exercise, it is important that the laboratory verifies the appropriateness of those values for its own use.[54] This verification is the final check that the laboratory has implemented the analytical method correctly, and that the laboratory's own population is comparable with that used for the original reference value study.

Comparison of a locally produced, small subset of values with the large set produced elsewhere using traditional statistical tests often is not appropriate because the underlying statistical assumptions are not fulfilled and the sample sizes are unbalanced. Relatively sophisticated methods using nonparametric tests[99] or Monte Carlo sampling[100] have been described. In addition to providing its own recommendations for relatively sophisticated tests for verification, CLSI suggests a reasonably practical alternative that most laboratories should be able to adopt: with a sample size of 20 reference values, one verifies the appropriateness of a proposed reference interval so long as no more than two values are outside the proposed limits.[16] One obvious deficiency of this test is that it does not detect the situation in which the reference interval of the local group is narrower than that of the study group. Nonetheless, it does provide reasonable assurance that a proposed reference interval can be used. The use of a larger number of local samples can give greater assurance that the intervals are satisfactory and more chance to detect inappropriate intervals. If the data exists, local data mining techniques can also be used to verify, or at least assess, transferred reference intervals. For example, the median or mode of an outpatient population should be close to the central point of the transferred reference interval, and the effect of the transferred interval on flagging rates, high and low, can be assessed.

PROCESS OF SELECTING REFERENCE INTERVALS

Laboratories are responsible for, and usually take the lead in, providing reference limits for their test results. However, as indicated in the previous sections of this chapter, there are a large number of potentially complicated decisions involved in the process, and the final selection of reference limits will influence the decisions of many physicians about their patients. As a result, it is important for organizations to include individuals from outside the laboratory in the process of selecting reference limits for use. A multidisciplinary group should be involved in making decisions, such as whether to perform a reference interval study or to transfer intervals from another source; if the decision is made to do a local study, whether partitioning will be necessary (which will affect the number of subjects) and which preanalytical variables are relevant; and if limits will be transferred from another source, whether the methods and populations from that source are comparable. Some issues are more subjective: whether to set exclusion criteria in an effort to change sensitivity (eg, exclude individuals who are obese or drink alcohol in order to increase sensitivity to detect the effects of these conditions); whether statistically significant differences in partitions are clinically significant; consideration of "rounding" the reference limits for ease of memory and to avoid an unwarranted impression of precision (eg, whether the GGT upper limit calculated earlier could be rounded from 47 to 50 IU/L). As suggested earlier, even if a local reference limit study is performed, it is appropriate to review all available data from the literature and from local data mining. When all data sources are concordant, there can be greater confidence in the limits. In contrast, when there is variability among the sources, it serves as a flag to assess possible reasons for the differences. There should be a written record of the people, decisions, and data used in selecting reference intervals, which will facilitate review and understanding in the future.

PRESENTATION OF AN OBSERVED VALUE IN RELATION TO REFERENCE VALUES

The purpose of reference limits is to allow a point of comparison for an observed value (patient's value). This comparison is similar to hypothesis testing, but it is seldom statistical testing in the strict sense. Ideally, the patient and the reference individuals should match (ie, the hypothesis is stated that they were all picked from the same set [population]) in all aspects other than the presence of the medical condition for which the test has been requested. Often, however, this is not the case. Thus it is advisable to consider the reference values as the yardstick for a less formal assessment than hypothesis testing. It is this less formal assessment that typically directs the attention of the interpreting doctor to those results most likely to represent pathology.

The clinician should always have access to as much information about the reference values as needed to use them appropriately. Reference values for all laboratory tests may be presented to clinicians in a booklet, web page or other medium, together with information about (1) analytical methods, (2) their imprecision, (3) descriptions of the reference values (eg, whether they represent the central 90% rather than 95% of values) and any relevant limitations necessary for basic interpretation (eg, diurnal variation). Graphical representations of the reference distributions can be informative (eg, the use of a histogram [see Fig. 8.4A and C]), or a plot of the cumulative distribution [see Fig. 8.4B and D]), particularly with skewed distributions and tests with which the clinician is less familiar. If a reference limit is a clinical decision limit, it is important to make this distinction and to provide supporting documentation. The goal is to provide sufficient information to clinicians for them to make rational clinical judgments.

In addition, a convenient presentation of an observed value in relation to reference values may be of great help for the busy clinician.[6,10-15,25,101] The most common presentation format for reference limits is the provision of the upper and lower reference limits on the same line of a report as the test name, test result (observed value), and units used for the result. Typically, when the result is outside the reference limits, the test result is accompanied by a "flag," which may be an asterisk, the letter H for "High" (ie, above the upper reference limit), the letter L for "Low" (ie, below the lower reference limit), or some other combinations of symbols. This format for reference limits has some significant strengths and weaknesses. The key strengths are the close proximity of the limits to the results, the ability to highlight values outside the reference limits, and the potential to tailor the displayed limits based on patient demographics typically available to the laboratory (such as age, sex, and fasting status). To the extent that additional factors about the patient are available (eg, time since last drug dose or stage of pregnancy), even more specific limits can be supplied with the result. Limitations to this process include situations in which relevant factors are not available (eg, stage of puberty or phase of the menstrual cycle). In these cases, a list of reference limits covering those factors can be included in the report, and the ordering clinician with knowledge of the patient can make the correct interpretation.

The preceding comments relate to reports in paper format and rendered electronic formats (eg, PDF), situations in which the laboratory controls the way the data are presented. Recognizing that ease of reading pathology reports is a patient safety issue (a misread report can lead to a wrong medical decision; a report that is difficult to read will waste important clinical time), an Australian group has recommended strict formatting requirements for reports, including the placement and formatting of reference limits and flagging.[102]

A more difficult, and often under-appreciated, issue is the need to transfer reference limits along with patient results when they are communicated in other ways. For example, when individual patient values are transferred into third-party systems or common pathology databases, it is important to ensure that the laboratory-specific reference limits be as easily accessible as the patient values themselves. This issue is one driver towards developing common reference intervals.[103]

In addition, a very informative presentation of the observed value involves showing its location graphically relative to the reference limits. In the era of information overload, and review of pathology reports by patients and other nonmedical personnel, a number of graphical tools are being developed to convey the information contained in a result and its relationship to reference limits.[104]

As stated earlier, results outside the reference limits may be flagged. A more detailed division of these results has been advocated to indicate how unusual the observed value is. For example, some laboratories highlight critical or extreme values with different flags. In such cases, it is important for laboratories to educate their clinicians about these flags because their use and meaning may vary considerably between laboratories and among tests. Similarly, subdivisions within the reference interval may also have clinical meaning and require communication to clinicians. For example, high-sensitivity C-reactive protein (hsCRP) results may be used not only for cardiovascular risk prediction but also as an indicator of acute inflammation.

Another method that can be used to express the observed value is by a *statistical distance measure.* All such distances are ratios of the following type:

$$\frac{\text{observed value} - \text{measure of location}}{\text{measure of dispersion}}$$

The *standard deviation (SD) unit,* or normal equivalent deviate, is such a measure. It is calculated as the difference between the observed value and the mean of the reference values divided by their standard deviation.[105] Several similar ratios under different names have been suggested and discussed.[44,106-108] This approach can be used to produce a graphical report for multiple analytes where the reference limits for different tests are aligned, and the observed values plotted as an SD unit against the reference limits. This allows a rapid assessment as to which results on a report are the "most abnormal." One issue with these protocols is the need to develop methods for non-Gaussian distributions. Such methods include using transformed data[109] or using split data with different SDs for the upper and lower half of the reference population.[110]

A related concept is the use of *multiples of the median* (MoM), where observed values are expressed as a multiple of the median reference value. This is most commonly used in antenatal testing. By maintaining a current database comprising a large number of subjects unaffected by disease, this process seeks to reduce the effect of analytical bias by normalizing current reported values against current assay performance; the extent to which this is achieved has been questioned.[111]

Reporting the observed value as a *percentile* of the reference distribution provides a very accurate measure of the relation for results within the interval.[25,112] An observed serum GGT value of 48 IU/L may, for example, be reported as 48 IU/L (99th percentile). Results outside the reference interval will have very high or low percentiles and the accuracy of the assignment is likely to be limited. Alternatively, the probability of finding a value closer to the mean than the observed value, the *index of atypicality,* can be estimated.[101,113]

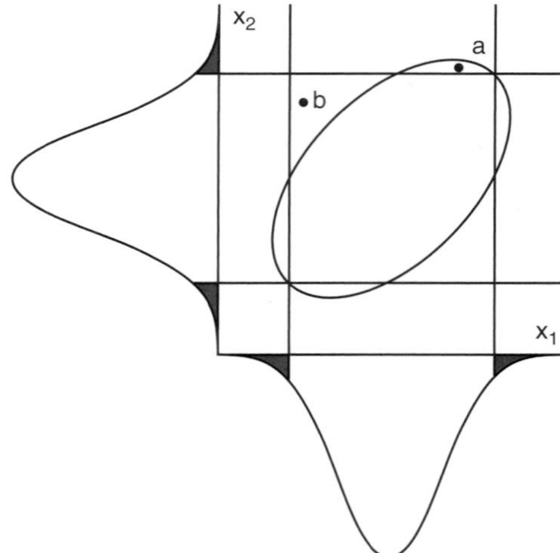

FIGURE 8.6 Bivariate reference region *(ellipse)* compared with the region defined by the two univariate reference intervals *(box).*

ADDITIONAL TOPICS

Multivariate, Population-Based Reference Regions

The topic of previous sections of this chapter has been univariate population-based reference values and quantities derived from them. However, such values do not fit the common clinical situation in which observed values of several different laboratory tests are available for interpretation and decision making. For example, the average number of individual clinical chemistry tests requested on each specimen received in the authors' laboratories is roughly 10; in many laboratories, this number is even larger. Two models are used for interpretation by comparison in this situation. Each observed value can be compared with the corresponding reference values or interval (ie, a *multiple, univariate comparison is performed*), or the set of observed values can be considered as a single multivariate observation and can be interpreted as such by a *multivariate comparison.* In this section, the relative merits of these two approaches are discussed, and methods for the latter type of comparison are presented.

Multivariate Concept

A univariate observation, such as a single laboratory result, may be represented graphically as a point on a line—the axis. Results obtained by two different laboratory tests performed on the same specimen (a bivariate observation) are then displayed as a point in a plane defined by two perpendicular axes. With three results, a trivariate observation and a point in a space are defined by three perpendicular axes, and so forth. The possibility of visualization of a multivariate observation is lost when there are more than three dimensions. Still, one can consider the multivariate observation as a point in a multidimensional hyperspace with as many mutually perpendicular axes as there are results of different tests. The prefix *hyper-* signifies, in this context, "more than three dimensions." Such multivariate observations are also called *patterns* or *profiles.* A multivariate distribution thus is represented by a cluster of points on a plane, in a space, or in a hyperspace, depending on the dimensionality of the observation.[69,109,114,115] Several statistical methods are based on multivariate methods, some of which are straightforward extensions of well-known univariate methods.[116]

Multiple, Univariate Reference Region

The univariate reference interval is bounded by two reference limits (lower and upper) on the result axis. Fig. 8.6 shows the univariate reference intervals for two laboratory tests: one depicted on the *x*-axis, and the other, on the *y*-axis. Together, they describe a square in the plane of the two axes. Similarly, three or more univariate reference intervals define boxes or hyperboxes in the (hyper)space. By multiple, univariate comparison, it can be decided whether a multivariate observation point lies inside or outside this square, box, or hyperbox. However, this method has two very serious deficiencies[117]: an observation may lie outside the limits of the region without being unusual (see Fig. 8.6, point *a*), or it may be found on the inside and still be an atypical observation (see Fig. 8.6, point *b*). If the central 95% interval is used, 5% of the values by definition are expected to be located in the two tails of the univariate reference distribution. However, more than 5% of the values would be located outside the square or (hyper)box created by several 95% intervals. To be exact, $100(1 - 0.95^m)$ percent of multivariate reference values would be excluded by the method of multiple, univariate comparison (*m* being the number of different tests, or the dimensionality). For example, provided the results are independent of each other, one would expect to find $100(1 - 0.95^{10}) = 40\%$ of healthy subjects (members of the reference population) to have at least one result flagged as "abnormal" (ie, 40% of healthy subjects will have false-positive results when 10 laboratory tests are performed). While this description is based on a multi-dimensional analysis, it is a model of standard laboratory practice. Additionally, an unusual combination (eg, a low serum urea and high serum creatinine, each within its reference interval) would not be detected as abnormal, reflecting a limited sensitivity for abnormal patterns of results. This discouraging result has been verified in several multiphasic screening programs. Therefore, a better method is needed.

Multivariate Reference Region

It is possible to define a common multivariate reference region[54,113-115,117,118] on the basis of joint distribution of reference values for two or more laboratory tests. This multivariate region is not a right-angled area, or hyperbox, but is more like an ellipse in the plane (see Fig. 8.6) or an ellipsoid hyperbody in hyperspace. This region may be a straightforward extension of the univariate 95% interval to the multivariate situation; it may be set to enclose 95% of central multivariate reference data points. In this case, one would expect to find only 5% false positives.

The use of multivariate reference regions usually requires the assistance of a computer program, which takes a set of results obtained by several laboratory tests on the same clinical specimen and calculates an index. Interpretation of a multivariate observation in relation to reference values is then the task of comparing the index with a threshold value estimated from the reference values. Obviously, this is much simpler than comparing each result with its proper reference interval.

This index is essentially a distance measure and is known as *Mahalanobis' squared distance* (D^2). It is analogous to the square of the standard deviation for single reference values. It expresses the multivariate distance between the observation point and the common mean of the reference values, taking into account the dispersion and the correlation of the variables.[54,113-115,117,118] More interpretational guidance may be obtained from this distance by expressing it as a percentile analogous to the percentile presentation of univariate observed values.[118] Also, the index of atypicality has a multivariate counterpart.[113,114]

Although the theory of multivariate reference regions has been known for a while, surprisingly few applications of it have been reported in the literature. An important report reviews the topic and presents the results of a very careful study on the multivariate 95% region for a 20-test chemistry profile.[118] Some of the most important findings can be summarized as follows:

1. Sixty-eight percent of subjects had at least one test result outside univariate reference intervals, which was close to what was theoretically expected: $100(1 - 0.95^{20}) = 64\%$.
2. By contrast, only 5% of patterns were outside the multivariate reference region (as expected).
3. Transformation to approximately Gaussian shape of the univariate distributions was necessary.
4. A test profile may be distinctly unusual in the multivariate sense even though each individual result is within its proper reference interval (eg, see point *b* in Fig. 8.6).
5. The multivariate reference region could detect minor deviations of multiple analytes.
6. Conversely, it could also be insensitive to highly deviating results for a single analyte.
7. Sensitivity could be increased by defining multivariate reference regions for subsets of physiologically related tests.

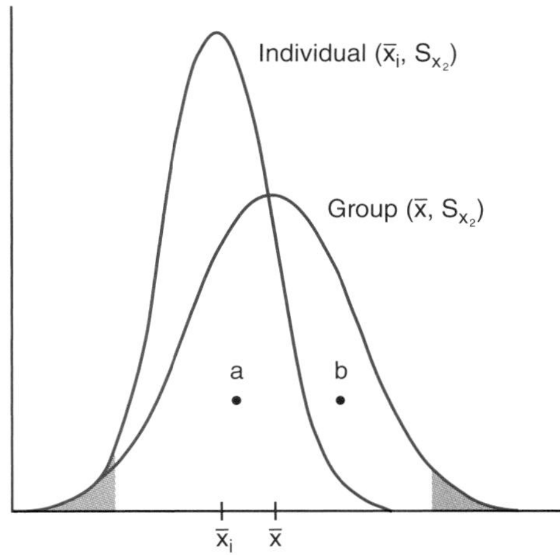

FIGURE 8.7 Relationship between population- and subject-based reference distributions and reference intervals. The example is hypothetical, and the two distributions are, for simplicity, Gaussian. Note that both points *a* and *b* are within the population-based reference interval, but only point *a* would be "normal" for this particular subject. (Modified from Harris EK: Effects of intraindividual and interindividual variation on the appropriate use of normal ranges. *Clin Chem* 1974;20:1536.)

Subject-Based Reference Values

Fig. 8.7 depicts the inherent problem associated with population-based reference values. It shows two hypothetical reference distributions. One represents the common reference distribution based on single specimens obtained from a group of different reference individuals. It has a true (hypothetical) mean $\bar{x}$ and a standard deviation s_x. The other distribution is based on several specimens collected over time in a single individual, the *i*th individual. Its hypothetical mean is $\bar{x}_i$ and its standard deviation s_{xi}.

If an observed value is located outside the subject's 2.5th and 97.5th percentiles, the personal or *subject-based reference interval,* the cause may be a change in biochemical status, suggesting the presence of disease. Fig. 8.7 shows that such an observed value may still be within the population-based reference interval. The sensitivity of the latter interval to changes in a subject's biochemical status depends accordingly on the location of the individual's mean x_i relative to the common mean x and to the relative magnitudes of the corresponding standard deviations s_{xi} and s_x. A mean s_{xi} close to s_x and a small s_{xi} relative to s_x may conceal the individual's changes entirely within the population-based reference interval.

Harris[66,67] analyzed this topic and found that the ratio *R* of intraindividual (personal) variation over interindividual (among subjects) variation provides a criterion for the usefulness of the population-based reference interval. This is also known as the Index of Individuality (II). The population-based reference interval has less than the desired sensitivity to changes in biochemical status if the ratio value is $R \leq 0.6$. This interval is a more trustworthy reference if $R > 1.4$, at least for the individual whose standard deviation σ_i is close to the average value. Published data[66,119] usually show that homeostatically tightly controlled quantities, such as serum electrolytes, have high ratio values. Population-based reference intervals of such analytes suffice for clinical use. In contrast, serum proteins and enzymes have very low ratios

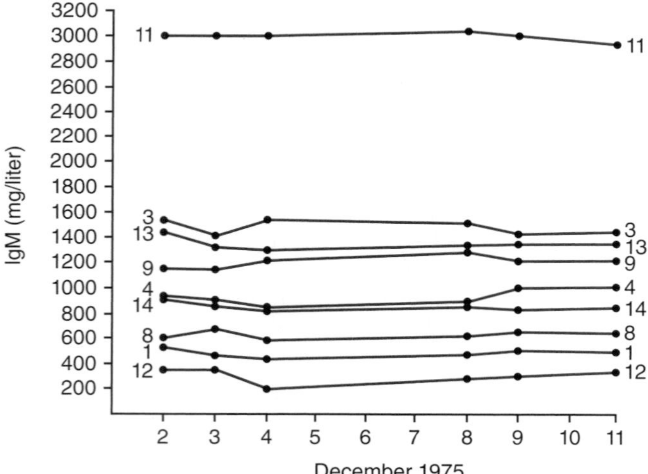

FIGURE 8.8 Serial immunoglobulin (Ig)M values over several days from reference individuals. Note that the intraindividual variability is very small compared to the interindividual variability. (From Statland BE, Winkel P, Killingsworth LM. Factors contributing to intra-individual variation of serum constituents: physiological day-to-day variation in concentrations of 10 specific proteins in sera. *Clin Chem* 1976;22:1635-163.)

because they are not under the same degree of metabolic control. Here, subject-based reference intervals seem more appropriate, although limitations to the meaning of a low value for the II have been raised.[120]

Two specific examples mentioned earlier may help to clarify this concept further. Fig. 8.8 depicts immunoglobulin (Ig)M values from several healthy individuals over the course of several days. As illustrated, the intraindividual differences are small compared with interindividual differences. Even though the population-based reference interval might extend from 200 to 1600 mg/dL, it would be most unusual (abnormal) for any patient's IgM value to change by more than 200 mg/dL, even if the value remained within the population-based reference interval. Similarly, it is well known that any given patient's serum creatinine value is reasonably constant,[23] which is related both to glomerular filtration rate (GFR) and to lean muscle mass. If the latter is constant, then changes in GFR are inversely proportional to the serum creatinine (see Chapter 32). That is, even though a typical (population-based) reference interval for serum creatinine might extend from 62 to 106 μmol/L (0.7 to 1.2 mg/dL), a change from 65 to 105 μmol/L in a given patient would be distinctly abnormal, representing the loss of almost half of the GFR, a finding of great clinical importance.

Two solutions can be proposed to the problem of the clinical insensitivity of population-based reference intervals:

1. One can try to reduce variation in reference values by *partitioning* into more homogeneous subclasses, as was discussed in a previous section. However, increasing the ratio, *R*, for example, from 0.6 to 1.4 by partitioning requires that one can obtain the rather dramatic reduction of 37% in standard deviation.[67] This is often difficult to attain in practice.
2. The other possibility is to use the patient's previous values, obtained when the patient was in a defined state of health, as the reference for any future value. Application of *subject-based reference values* becomes more feasible as health screening by laboratory tests and computer storage of results become available to large segments of the general population.

Two not completely separated classes of models may be used for construction of subject-based reference intervals: statistical and physiologic models.[54]

1. Harris has developed several models based on statistical *time series analysis*[40,54,66,67,121] At one extreme, a stationary or *homeostatic model* is suitable for analytes showing relatively fast, random fluctuations around a constant mean (set point). The set point is estimated from past values that are given equal weights. Another model, the nonstationary *random-walk model,* allows a changing set point over time in healthy subjects. Then, more recent values are given heavier weights during estimation of the current set point. Intermediate and more or less complex models exist. Some of these data-following methods are suitable for adaptive forecasting in situations in which the time intervals are short (eg, during hospitalization).[40] They might thus be implemented on a computer as part of a laboratory cumulative reporting system. The reader is referred to papers by Harris for details on statistical time series models.[40,54,66,67,121]
2. It is also possible to construct *physiologic models* that use known physiologic and biochemical time-dependent relationships. Winkel has developed a time series model for monitoring plasma progesterone in pregnancy using the assumption of a simple exponential growth curve for the size of the placenta.[119]

When "Normal" May Appear to Be "Abnormal," and Vice Versa

Some, if not many, clinical laboratory test results are related to other clinical laboratory test results. For example, consider the relatively common situation of a patient with a low serum albumin. Because of the relationship between total calcium and albumin in serum (see Chapter 64), a total serum calcium concentration in the healthy reference interval might actually be pathologically high in this patient, and a total serum calcium concentration below the lower reference limit might be healthy. (For this reason, clinicians may choose to calculate an "adjusted calcium concentration" or to measure the "free calcium" concentration in these patients). In these types of situations, it is important not to consider the normal (or abnormal) test results out of context. In most cases, laboratory reports do not take these situations into account.

As another example, consider a pregnant woman with typically high concentrations of serum binding proteins, including thyroxine binding globulin. She might well have what appears to be an "abnormally" high concentration of serum total thyroxine when compared with conventional reference limits (see Chapter 67), when in fact this is typical of a healthy pregnant state. Other such examples in clinical medicine abound. Consider the prostate specific antigen (PSA) level in a postprostatectomy patient or the thyroglobulin level in a postthyroidectomy patient. In these cases, it would be "healthy" to have abnormally low (undetectable) concentrations of these measurands, and it would be distinctly abnormal to have healthy (detectable) levels. In all of these cases, the problem is that the traditional reference population (nonpregnant, healthy individuals) is not appropriate.

Indeed, interpretations in the entire field of endocrinology are based not so much on "healthy" concentrations but rather on "appropriate" concentrations. For example, in a patient with a very high free T4 concentration, a TSH within the traditional reference limits is used for differential diagnosis rather than likelihood of health. It should be undetectable in primary hyperthyroidism; otherwise, it may well represent secondary or tertiary hyperthyroidism (see Chapter 67). Similarly, in a patient with hypercalcemia, a PTH within the traditional healthy reference limits is distinctly abnormal.

In other words, even when reference limit studies are done well, one needs to remember there are dependencies that can render those reference limits misleading.

Special Populations

As noted in the previous section, there are groups of patients for whom the typical populations used in establishing reference limits may not be appropriate. Such groups include, but are not limited to, children, pregnant women, and the elderly. Even within these groups there may be important subgroups (partitions): for example, children may need to be further divided by age, sex, ethnicity, and/or Tanner stage; pregnant women, by trimester; elderly, by age, sex, and ethnicity. Over the past decade a number of studies have been conducted to establish reference intervals for these populations.

As noted earlier, the CALIPER initiative, a multicenter trial, recruited several thousand healthy pediatric subjects from across Canada and established reference limits, partitioned by age, sex, and ethnicity, for 40 measurands using one analytical system.[88] Its database was later extended by transference to several additional analytical systems as well as to an additional 29 measurands.[89] A recent study from Denmark established reference limits for 36 measurands based on 801 normal pregnancies in Caucasian women.[122] These limits might be extended to other analytical systems by transference, but additional pregnancies in non-Caucasian women will be required to determine whether the limits can be extended to other ethnic groups. Another study from Denmark established reference limits for 27 measurands based on 1016 70-year old Caucasians.[123] Again, this involved a single set of analytical systems and a single ethnic group, so the authors were careful to point out that additional work will be required to determine to what extent their reference limits can be adopted by others.

In each of these cases, important differences from the traditional reference intervals were uncovered.

Special Cases of Laboratory Test Result Interpretation

In the search for improved diagnostic performance, several individual test results may be combined to form an index or score with the aim of combining the discriminating power of the individual results. Examples include the "triple" and "quad" screens used to calculate risk for Down syndrome and trisomy 18 in early pregnancy (see Chapter 69), a variety of proprietary "liver fibrosis" screens to estimate the likelihood of cirrhosis (see Chapter 61), and the prostate health index from Beckman Coulter.[124] Although a discussion of these methods is beyond the scope of this chapter, the basic concepts of reference populations, sampling, outlier exclusion, and so on, remain vital to the process. Typically, the reference limit is a clinical decision point rather than a population reference interval limit. In these cases, the goal is not so much to determine whether the patient is healthy but to determine whether the likelihood of abnormality is high enough that additional testing is warranted (triple and quad screens) or to determine whether certain therapies are likely to be helpful without resorting to an invasive liver[124] or prostate biopsy.[125]

Ongoing Verification of Reference Limits

Whether a laboratory establishes values with its own reference limit studies or adopts reference limits after verification from another source, it is rare for any laboratory to assess those reference limits on a regular basis. Typically, the reference limits are not reevaluated until the laboratory implements new instrumentation, at which point it may be necessary to make changes. Even with changes in methods, though, there is no guarantee that a reassessment will occur. In an interesting report from Australia,[84] studies showed that reference limits for common measurands differed significantly among laboratories, even when they used the same analytical systems; additional studies indicated that common reference intervals for these measurements could, and should, be implemented across all these laboratories.

Laboratories can, however, use "data mining" techniques discussed earlier to perform ongoing audits of reference limits and to investigate specific concerns when they arise. For example, with these techniques, a laboratory could determine the median of the distribution of bicarbonate values from its healthy outpatients, which should be extremely stable.[126,127] Similarly, it could determine what percentage of these values fall outside the reference limits. Assuming those limits were set to include the central 95% of healthy outpatient values, no more than 2.5% of the values should be below the lower limit or above the upper limit. If a change in median occurs, or if too many samples fall outside the limits, there may well be a problem. The laboratory could then investigate further by using the technique to see when the problem started, by reviewing whether any changes in methods were made, by investigating performance on proficiency testing, and even by repeating a short reference interval study with 20 individuals as described earlier. These data mining studies are relatively inexpensive, involving only retrieval and manipulation of data that already exists, but they provide great reassurance to the laboratory and its users of the accuracy of its test results and reference limits.

CONCLUSION

In this chapter, we have emphasized the importance of reference limits, which provide physicians with values to which they can compare their patients' results, thereby facilitating interpretation. In most, but not all, cases, reference limits reflect values seen in healthy individuals.

When generating, verifying, or reporting reference limits, it is critical that the populations be well-defined and that the patients for whom the limits are used be comparable in terms of gender, age, and ethnicity where relevant, and any other measurable characteristics determined to be of importance. We have described in detail ways to ensure collection of high-quality data, methods to eliminate outliers when appropriate, and techniques to analyze the data (including nonparametric [preferred], parametric, bootstrap, and robust).

Recognizing that many laboratories do not have the resources to generate their own reference limits, we have described alternative sources (including manufacturers' package inserts, peer-reviewed literature, multicenter trials, historical laboratory data) and techniques to verify the transferability of such data.

We have recommended a multidisciplinary approach to selecting and implementing reference limits, and we have discussed a number of considerations related to the display of reference limits along with patient results.

We have also included discussion of several special topics, including multivariate reference limits, subject-based reference limits, reference limits for special populations, and ongoing verification of reference limits.

It is quite clear that laboratories face many issues and a great deal of effort in ensuring that their reference limits are valid, but we would argue that, in the absence of this effort, much of the data we generate would not be interpretable. The validity of our reference limits is at least as important as the accuracy and precision of our analytical techniques and should therefore warrant at least as much attention.

SELECTED REFERENCES

For a full list of references for this chapter, please refer to ExpertConsult.com.

7. Solberg HE, Grasbeck R. Reference values. *Adv Clin Chem* 1989;**27**:1–79.
16. Clinical and Laboratory Standards Institute. *Defining, establishing, and verifying reference intervals in the clinical laboratory*. 3rd ed. Wayne, PA: Clinical and Laboratory Standards Institute; 2010.
35. Solberg HE. Using a hospitalized population to establish reference intervals: pros and cons. *Clin Chem* 1994;**40**:2205–6.
53. Ichihara K, Boyd JC. An appraisal of statistical procedures used in derivation of reference intervals. *Clin Chem Lab Med* 2010;**48**:1537–51.
54. Harris EK, Boyd JC. *Statistical bases of reference values in laboratory medicine*. New York: Marcel Dekker; 1995.
58. Rustad P, Felding P, Franzson L, et al. The Nordic Reference Interval Project 2000: recommended reference intervals for 25 common biochemical properties. *Scand J Clin Lab Invest* 2004;**64**:271–84.
68. Horn PS, Pesce AJ. Reference intervals: an update. *Clin Chim Acta* 2003;**334**:5–23.
79. Pavlov IY, Wilson AR, Delgado JC. Reference interval computation: which method (not) to choose? *Clin Chim Acta* 2012;**413**:1107–14.
83. Horn PS, Pesce AJ. *Reference intervals: a user's guide*. Washington, DC: AACC Press; 2005.
84. Tate JR, Sikaris KA, Jones GR, et al. Harmonising adult and paediatric reference intervals in Australia and New Zealand: an evidence-based approach for establishing a first panel of chemistry analytes. *Clin Biochem Rev* 2014;**35**:213–35.
88. Colantonio DA, Kyriakopoulou L, Chan MK, et al. Closing the gaps in pediatric laboratory reference intervals: a CALIPER database of 40 biochemical markers in a healthy and multiethnic population of children. *Clin Chem* 2012;**58**:854–68.
89. Karbasy K, Ariadne P, Gaglione S, et al. Advances in pediatric reference intervals for biochemical markers: establishment of the CALIPER database in healthy children and adolescents. *J Med Biochem* 2015;**34**:23–30.
91. Yamamoto Y, Hosogaya S, Osawa S, et al. Nationwide multicenter study aimed at the establishment of common reference intervals for standardized clinical laboratory tests in Japan. *Clin Chem Lab Med* 2013;**51**:1663–72.
92. Grossi E, Colombo R, Cavuto S, et al. The ReaLab project: a new method for the formulation of reference intervals based on current data. *Clin Chem* 2005;**51**:1232–40.
95. Shaw JL, Cohen A, Konforte D, et al. Validity of establishing pediatric reference intervals based on hospital patient data: a comparison of the modified Hoffmann approach to caliper reference intervals obtained in healthy children. *Clin Biochem* 2014;**47**:166–72.
97. Katayev A, Fleming JK, Luo D, et al. Reference intervals data mining: no longer a probability paper method. *Am J Clin Pathol* 2015;**143**:134–42.
102. Flatman R, Legg M, Jones GR, et al. Recommendations for reporting and flagging of reference limits on pathology reports. *Clin Biochem Rev* 2014;**35**:199–202.
104. O'Connor JD. Reducing post analytical error: perspectives on new formats for the blood sciences pathology report. *Clin Biochem Rev* 2015;**36**:7–20.

9

Evidence-Based Laboratory Medicine

Patrick M.M. Bossuyt, Paul Glasziou, and Andrea Rita Horvath

ABSTRACT

Background

Evidence-based laboratory medicine (EBLM) is an approach to medical practice that integrates the best available research evidence about laboratory investigations with the expertise of clinicians and with patient values to improve the health and healthcare outcomes of individual patients. Practicing EBLM enables laboratory professionals to translate test results to clinically relevant information that helps clinicians deliver effective and cost-effective patient care.

Content

This chapter provides an overview on how evidence about laboratory tests is generated, how it is synthesized, and how it can be applied to questions about diagnosis, screening, prognosis, or monitoring. The topics covered introduce the methodological and practical aspects of EBLM. They include (1) the process and methods of practicing EBLM; (2) the key components and types of evidence used in the evaluation of biomarkers; (3) tools for the assessment of the validity and applicability of the evidence; (4) key aspects of synthesizing the evidence in systematic reviews and meta-analyses; (5) basic principles of how EBLM is applied to other purposes of testing than diagnosis; (6) the challenges and tools of implementing the evidence for achieving best laboratory practice; and (7) the history and future challenges of EBLM.

Understanding the general principles and approaches of EBLM will help laboratory professionals to become resources for information and knowledge who are able to add value to laboratory testing.

10

Biobanking

Christina Ellervik and Jim Vaught

ABSTRACT

Background

Biobanks were originally primarily for treatment and diagnostic purposes, but during the past 40 years more extensive epidemiological and clinical trial collections have contributed to advances in biomedical research. Biobank planning is essential for biospecimen integrity in support of such research.

Content

This chapter focuses on best practices procedures for collection, processing, storage, and retrieval of biospecimens with regard to downstream analyses of blood, urine, and saliva. Security measures, disaster planning, quality management, accreditation and certification, staff education, chain-of-custody, annotation of data, cost, and sustainability issues are reviewed. Ethical, legal, and social issues, as well as administrative issues regarding governance, ownership, custodianship, and access criteria are discussed.

11

Laboratory Support of Pharmaceutical, In Vitro Diagnostics, and Epidemiologic Studies

*Mark J. Sarno, Amar A. Sethi, Omar Laterza, and Nader Rifai**

ABSTRACT

Background

Biomarkers are used in the clinical laboratory for routine patient care, in the pharmaceutical industry during drug development, and in establishing safety and efficacy of a candidate drug. Biomarkers are also used in clinical and epidemiologic research to gain a better insight into pathophysiology, to identify predictors of disease, and to refine treatment strategies. The in vitro diagnostic (IVD) industry develops most of the biomarker assays and makes them commercially available. The pharmaceutical and IVD industries, as well as epidemiological researchers, often seek the help of clinical laboratories in their biomarker studies, thus providing a mutually beneficial and rewarding relationship.

Content

This chapter describes, in detail, the various areas in which the pharmaceutical and IVD industries and epidemiological and clinical researchers use biomarkers, and illustrates the ways in which the clinical laboratory can be involved in providing such services, which can be both financially and intellectually rewarding. However, these opportunities have their own challenges, including the need for strict regulatory rules, extensive documentation requirements, and particular data access and storage specifications. The regulatory requirements for performing biomarker testing are described in this chapter; results may be used in premarket approval (PMA) submissions to governmental agencies, for both drugs and assay kits. The relevant documents for analytical and clinical evaluations of biomarkers are identified and discussed. Due to the daunting task of summarizing worldwide regulations, the regulatory requirements in the United States are primarily referred to as examples of typical requirements. The reader should refer to their local agencies when assessing the exact needs applicable to their situation. Overall, the goal of this chapter is to provide a general blueprint to those in the clinical laboratory who are interested in biomarker research collaborations.

*The authors acknowledge that a small portion of this chapter was based on Cole TG, Warnick GR, Rifai N. Providing laboratory support for clinical trials, epidemiological studies, and *in vitro* diagnostic evaluations. In: Rifai N, Warnick GR, Dominiczak MH, editors. *Handbook of Lipoprotein Testing*. AACC Press, with permission.

SECTION II

Analytical Techniques and Applications

Exam questions, case studies, and additional resources are available on ExpertConsult.com.
*Full versions of these chapters are available electronically on ExpertConsult.com.

12

Principles of Basic Techniques and Laboratory Safety

*Stanley F. Lo**

ABSTRACT

Background

In order to appropriately interpret clinical laboratory test results and adequately validate assays, the basic principles and techniques of analytical chemistry need to be understood. These techniques should be used by laboratory professionals in a safe testing environment.

Content

Factors that affect the analytical process and operation of the clinical laboratory are described in this chapter. The concepts of solute and solution, and the international system of units used to standardize their expression and reporting are described. These solutions are composed of various types of chemicals used in the development of clinical laboratory assays. The importance of water purity, appropriate reagent preparation, and the different types of reference materials are addressed. The principles of basic techniques in the clinical laboratory, including pipetting, centrifugation, radioactivity, gravimetry, and thermometry, are also discussed. These techniques are used in a variety of laboratory tasks such as making buffers, performing dilutions, evaporation, lyophilization, and filtration. Safety is a constant and crucial concern for laboratory personnel. Each laboratory must create a comprehensive safety program. Plans for the handling of chemicals, exposure to blood-borne pathogens, tuberculosis (TB), and other highly infectious agents, are necessary components of a safety plan. The training of laboratory personnel to identify various types of biological, chemical, and electrical hazards, and to react appropriately to fire, must be addressed in such a plan.

*The author gratefully acknowledges the original contributions of Drs. Edward W. Bermes, Stephen E. Kahn, Donald S. Young, Edward R. Powsner, and John C. Widman, on which portions of this chapter are based.

13

Optical Techniques

*Larry J. Kricka and Jason Y. Park**

ABSTRACT

Background

Measurement of radiant energy (light) is used throughout the clinical laboratory. Radiant energy is used to measure a vast array of analytes, including proteins, metals, enzymes, antigens, and antibodies.

Content

This chapter describes the range of optical techniques used in clinical laboratory analysis. The techniques and instrumentation used for these measurements range from simple visualization by the naked eye to complex analysis with semiconductor-based lasers matched to solid-state, charge-coupled detectors. With the naked eye, white light is the radiant energy that is used to observe the presence or absence of turbidity or a chromogen (eg, latex agglutination or lateral-flow point-of-care test). In sophisticated instrumentation, the radiant energy may take the form of white light (eg, halogen light bulb), but the radiant energy may also be selectively chosen for a specific wavelength or range of wavelengths (eg, laser excitation of a fluorophore). The radiant energy in an instrument may be used to energize or be scattered by molecules of interest. The basic components of all optical analytical systems include a source for radiant energy, a device for selecting wavelength(s) of light, and a detector.

Although the optical components of a test system may be hidden away in the deep recesses of high-throughput instrumentation, electromagnetic radiation is a critical component of modern clinical chemistry methods (eg, spectrophotometry, fluorometry, nephelometry, turbidimetry).

Many determinations made in the clinical laboratory are based on measurements of radiant energy emitted, transmitted, absorbed, scattered, or reflected under controlled conditions. The principles involved in such measurements are considered in this chapter.

NATURE OF LIGHT

Electromagnetic radiation includes radiant energy that extends from cosmic rays with wavelengths as short as 10 nm up to radio waves longer than 1000 km. However, in this chapter, the term *light* is used to describe radiant energy from the ultraviolet (UV) and visible portions of the spectrum (380 to 750 nm).

The wavelength of light is defined as the distance between two peaks as the light travels in a wavelike manner. This distance is expressed in nanometers (nm) for wavelengths commonly used in photometry. Other units include:

$$1\ \text{nm} = 1\ \text{millimicron}\ (\text{m}\mu) = 10\ \text{Angstroms}\ (\text{Å}) = 10^{-9}\ \text{m}$$

In addition to possessing wavelength characteristics, light has properties that indicate that it is composed of discrete energy packets called *photons*. The relationship between the energy of photons and their frequency is given by the equation:

$$E = h\nu \qquad \textbf{13.1}$$

where E = energy in ergs, ν = frequency of light in cycles per second, and h = Planck's constant (6.62×10^{27} erg seconds). The ν is related to the wavelength by an equation:

$$\nu = \frac{c}{\lambda} \qquad \textbf{13.2}$$

where c = speed of light in a vacuum (3×10^{10} cm/s), and λ = wavelength in centimeters. Combining Eqs. 13.1 and 13.2 results in:

$$E = \frac{hc}{\lambda} \qquad \textbf{13.3}$$

This equation shows that the energy of light is inversely proportional to the wavelength. For example, UV radiation at 200 nm possesses greater energy than infrared (IR) radiation at 750 nm.

The human eye is able to detect radiant energy with wavelengths between approximately 380 and 750 nm, but modern instrumentation permits measurements at both shorter wavelength (UV) and longer wavelength (IR) portions of the spectrum. Sunlight, or light emitted from a tungsten filament, is a mixture of wavelengths or a spectrum of

*The authors gratefully acknowledge the original contributions by Dr. Merle A. Evenson and Dr. Thomas O. Tiffany, upon which portions of this chapter are based.

TABLE 13.1 Ultraviolet, Visible, and Short Infrared Spectrum Characteristics

Wavelength (nm)	Region Name	Color Observed*
<380	UV†	Invisible
380–440	Visible	Violet
440–500	Visible	Blue
500–580	Visible	Green
580–600	Visible	Yellow
600–620	Visible	Orange
620–750	Visible	Red
800–2500	Near infrared	Not visible
2500–15,000	Mid infrared	Not visible
15,000–1,000,000	Far infrared	Not visible

*Because of the subjective nature of color, the wavelength intervals shown are only approximations.
†The ultraviolet (UV) portion of the spectrum is sometimes further divided into "near" UV (200–380 nm) and "far" UV (<220 nm). This arbitrary distinction has a practical basis, because silica used to make cuvets transmits light effectively at wavelengths ≥220 nm.

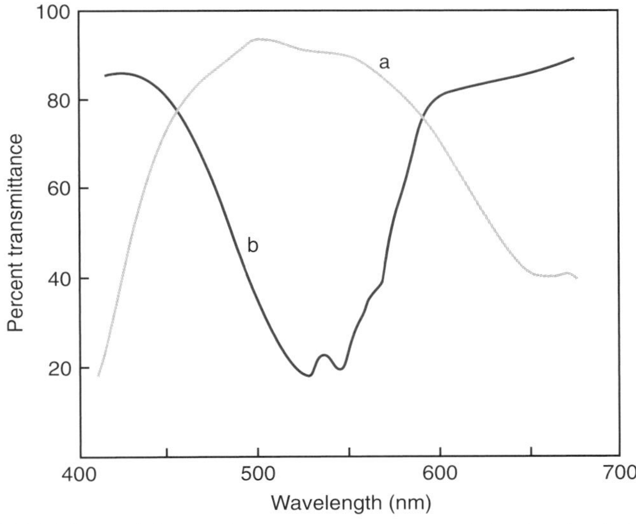

FIGURE 13.1 Spectral transmittance curves of *(a)* nickel sulfate and *(b)* potassium permanganate. Arbitrary concentrations read versus water as a blank (Beckman DB-G spectrophotometer).

radiant energy of different wavelengths that the eye recognizes as "white." Table 13.1 shows approximate relationships between wavelengths and color characteristics for the UV, visible, and short IR portions of the spectrum. Thus, a solution will appear green when viewed against white light if it transmits light maximally between 500 and 580 nm but absorbs light at other wavelengths. Similarly, a solid object appears green if it reflects light in this region (500 to 580 nm) but absorbs light at other portions of the spectrum. In general, if the intensity of light transmitted by a colored solution is compared with that of a reference solution over the entire spectrum, a typical spectral transmittance curve characteristic for that spectrum is obtained. Such curves are shown in Fig. 13.1 for solutions of (*a*) nickel sulfate and (*b*) potassium permanganate. Inspection of the curves should lead to the prediction that the color of the solution (*a*) is green because light is transmitted maximally near the green portion of the spectrum. In contrast, curve (*b*) illustrates the spectrum of a solution that transmits light maximally in the blue, violet, and red portions of the spectrum. The eye recognizes this mixture of colors as purple.

POINTS TO REMEMBER

Radiant Energy

- Wavelength size has a wide distribution, ranging from as small as 10 nm to greater than 1000 km.
- The visible portion of the spectrum ranges from approximately 380 to approximately 750 nm.
- The energy of light is inversely proportional to the wavelength; shorter wavelengths have greater energy.
- Light possesses both wavelength and energy packet characteristics; the packets are described as photons.

SPECTROPHOTOMETRY

Photometry is defined as the measurement of light; spectrophotometry is defined as the measurement of the intensity of light at selected wavelengths. Spectrophotometric analysis is a widely used method of quantitative and qualitative analysis in the chemical and biological sciences. The method depends on the light-absorbing properties of the substance or a derivative of the substance being analyzed. The intensity of transmitted light passing through a solution containing an absorbing substance (chromogen) is decreased by the absorbed fraction. This fraction is detected, measured, and used to relate the light transmitted or absorbed to the concentration of the analyte in question.

Basic Concepts

Consider an incident light beam with intensity I_0 passing through a square cell containing a solution of a compound that absorbs light of a certain wavelength, λ. Because the intensity of the transmitted light beam is I_S, then transmittance *(T)* of light is defined as:

$$T = \frac{I_S}{I_0} \qquad \textbf{13.4}$$

However, a portion of the incident light may be reflected by the surface of the cell or may be absorbed by the cell wall or solvent. To focus attention on the compound of interest, elimination of these factors is necessary. This is achieved using a reference cell identical to the sample cell, except that the compound of interest is omitted from the solvent in the reference cell. The transmittance *(T)* through this reference cell is I_R divided by I_O; the transmittance for the compound in solution is then defined as I_S divided by I_R. In practice, the light beam is blocked, the detector signal is set to zero transmittance, then a reference cell is inserted, and the detector signal is adjusted to an arbitrary scale reading of 100 (corresponding to 100% transmittance), followed by the cell containing the sample to be measured, and the percent transmittance reading is made on the sample. As the concentration of the compound in solution is increased, the transmittance varies inversely and logarithmically with the concentration (Fig. 13.2). Consequently, it is more convenient to define a new term, absorbance *(A)*, which will be directly proportional to the concentration. Thus, the amount of light

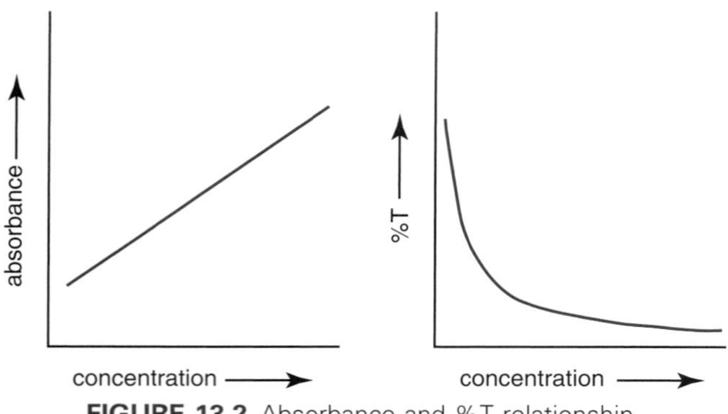

FIGURE 13.2 Absorbance and %T relationship.

absorbed *(A)* as the incident light passes through the sample is equivalent to:

$$A = -\log\frac{I_S}{I_R} = -\log T \qquad \textbf{13.5}$$

Analytically, the amount of light absorbed or transmitted is related mathematically to the concentration of the analyte in question by Beer's law.

Beer's Law: Relationship Among Transmittance, Absorbance, and Concentration

Beer's law (also known as the Beer-Lambert law) states that the concentration of a substance is directly proportional to the amount of light absorbed or inversely proportional to the logarithm of the transmitted light (see Fig. 13.2). Mathematically, Beer's law is expressed as:

$$A = abc \qquad \textbf{13.6}$$

where A = absorbance; a = proportionality constant defined as absorptivity; b = light path (in centimeters); and c = concentration of the absorbing compound (usually expressed in moles per liter).

This equation forms the basis of quantitative analysis by absorption photometry. When b is 1 cm and c is expressed in moles per liter, the constant a is called the molar absorptivity. The value for a is a constant for a given compound at a given wavelength under prescribed conditions of solvent, temperature, pH, and so forth. The nomenclature of spectrophotometry is summarized in Table 13.2. Values for a are useful for characterizing compounds, establishing their purity, and comparing the sensitivity of measurements obtained on derivatives. Pure bilirubin, for example, when dissolved in chloroform at 25°C, has a molar absorptivity of 60,700 ± 1600 $cm^{-1}M^{-1}$ at 453 nm. The molecular weight of bilirubin is 584. Hence, a solution containing 5 mg/L (0.005 g/L) should have a concentration c of 0.005 g/L × $(584\ g/mole)^{-1}$ which is 0.005/584 moles/L (M). This results in:

$$A = abc = \left(\frac{60{,}700}{cm^{-1}\cdot M^{-1}}\right)\times(1cm)\times\left(\frac{0.005}{584}M\right) = 0.520 \qquad \textbf{13.7}$$

The molar absorptivity of the complex between ferrous iron and *s*-tripyridyltriazine is 22,600, whereas that with 1,10-phenanthroline is 11,000. Thus, for a given concentration of iron, *s*-tripyridyltriazine produces a complex with an absorbance approximately twice that of the complex with 1,10-phenanthroline. Consequently, *s*-tripyridyltriazine is a more sensitive reagent to use in the measurement of iron.

TABLE 13.2 Spectrophotometry Nomenclature

Name	Symbol	Definition
Absorbance	A	$-\log T$ or $\log I_0/I$
Absorptivity	a	A/bc (c in g/L)
Molar absorptivity	ε	A/bc (c in mol/L)
Path length	b	Internal cell or sample length, in cm
Transmittance	T	I_S/I_0*
Wavelength unit	nm	10^{-9} m
Absorption maximum	λmax	Wavelength at which maximum absorption occurs

*I_S/I_0 is the ratio of the intensity of transmitted light to incident light.

Application of Beer's Law

In practice, a calibration relationship between absorbance and concentration is established experimentally for a given instrument under specified conditions using a series of reference solutions that contain increasing concentrations of analyte. Frequently, a linear relationship exists up to a certain concentration or absorbance. When this linear relationship exists, the solution is said to obey Beer's law up to this point. Within this limitation, a calibration constant may be derived and used to calculate the concentration of an unknown solution by comparison with a calibrating solution.

Certain precautions must be observed with the use of such calibration constants. For example, under no circumstances should the calibration constants be used when the calibrator or unknown readings exceed the linear portion of the calibration relationship. In other words, calibration constants are used only when the curve obeys Beer's law. At least two and preferably more calibrators should be included in each series of determinations to permit direct comparison of unknown readings with calibrators or to calculate the calibration constant. These multiple calibrators are necessary because variations in reagents, working conditions, and cell diameters, and deterioration or changes in instruments may result in day-to-day changes in the absorbance value for the calibrator. A nonlinear calibration curve may be used if a sufficient number of calibrators of varying concentrations are included to cover the entire range encountered for readings of unknowns.

In some cases, a pure reference material may not be readily available, and constants may be provided that were obtained on pure materials and reported in the literature. In general, published constants should only be used if the method is followed in detail and readings are made on a spectrophotometer capable of providing light of high spectral purity at a verified wavelength. Use of broader band light sources usually leads to some decrease in absorbance. For example, the absorbance of nicotinamide adenine dinucleotide at 340 nm is frequently used as a reference for determination of enzyme activity, based on a molar absorptivity of 6220 $cm^{-1}M^{-1}$ (see Chapter 22). This value is acceptable only under the carefully

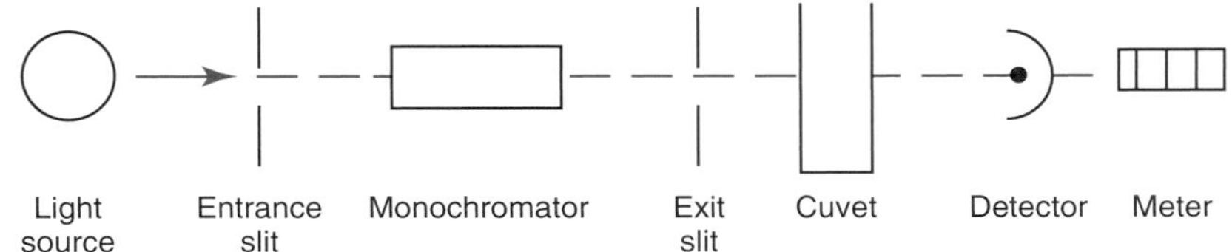

FIGURE 13.3 Major components of a single-beam spectrophotometer.

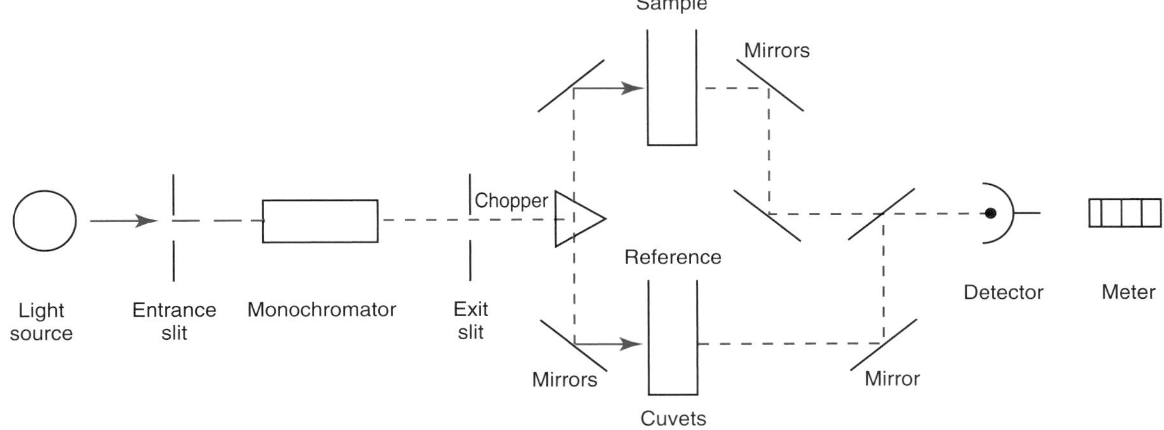

FIGURE 13.4 Major components of a double-beam spectrophotometer.

controlled conditions previously described and should not be used unless these conditions are met. Published values for molar absorptivities and absorption coefficients should be used only as guidelines until they are verified by readings on pure reference materials for a given instrument. In addition, Beer's law is followed only if the following conditions are met:

- Incident radiation on the substance of interest is monochromatic.
- The solvent absorption is insignificant compared with the solute absorbance.
- The solute concentration is within given limits.
- An optical interferent is not present.
- A chemical reaction does not occur between the molecule of interest and another solute or solvent molecule.

Instrumentation

Modern instruments isolate a narrow wavelength range of the spectrum for measurements. Those that use filters for this purpose are referred to as filter photometers; those that use prisms or gratings are called spectrophotometers. Spectrophotometers are classified as single or double beam.

The major components of a single-beam spectrophotometer are shown in Fig. 13.3. In such an instrument, a beam of light is passed through a monochromator that isolates the desired region of the spectrum to be used for measurements. The light next passes through an absorption cell (cuvet), where a portion of the radiant energy is absorbed, depending on the nature and concentration of the substance in the solution. Any light not absorbed is transmitted to a detector, which converts light energy to electrical energy that is registered on a meter or recorder, or digitally displayed.

In operation, an opaque block is substituted for the cuvet, so that no light reaches the photocell, and the meter is adjusted to read 0% *T*. Next, a cuvet containing a reagent blank is inserted, and the meter is adjusted to read 100% *T* (zero absorbance). The composition of the reagent blank should be identical to that of the calibrating or unknown solutions except for the substance to be measured. Calibrating solutions containing various known concentrations of the substance are inserted, and readings are recorded. Finally, a reading is made of the unknown solution, and its concentration is determined by comparison with readings obtained on the calibrators. In most spectrophotometers, digital hardware and software are integral components and perform these functions automatically.

Fig. 13.4 illustrates a typical double-beam instrument that uses a light-beam chopper (a rotating wheel with alternate silvered sections and cutout sections) inserted after the exit slit. A system of mirrors passes portions of the light reflected off the chopper alternately through the sample and a reference cuvet onto a common detector. The chopped-beam approach, using one detector, compensates for light source variation and for sensitivity changes in the detector.

Components

The basic components of a spectrophotometer include (1) a light source, (2) a device to isolate light of a desired wavelength, (3) a cuvet, (4) a photodetector, (5) a readout device, and (6) a data system.

Light Sources. Types of light sources used in spectrophotometers include incandescent lamps, xenon discharge lamps, laser, and light-emitting diodes (LEDs).

Incandescent, Arc, and Cathode Lamps. The light source for measurements in the visible portion of the spectrum is usually a tungsten light bulb. The lifetime of a tungsten filament is greatly increased by the presence of a low pressure of iodine or bromine vapor within the lamp. An example is the quartz-halogen lamp, which has a fused-silica envelope and provides high-intensity light over a wide spectrum for extended operating periods (2000 to 5000 hours) before replacement is necessary.

However, a tungsten light source does not supply sufficient radiant energy for measurements in the UV region (<320 nm). In the UV region of the spectrum, hydrogen and deuterium lamps, as well as high-pressure mercury and xenon arc lamps, are sources of continuous spectra in the UV region with sharp emission lines. These sources are more commonly used in UV absorption measurements. Low-pressure mercury vapor lamps also provide spectra in the UV region and are useful for calibration purposes, but because of their limited wavelengths, they are not practical for absorbance measurements.

Mercury arc lamps emit an intense 254 nm resonance line and are widely used as detectors in high-pressure liquid chromatography (HPLC) (see Chapter 16). Alternatively, some HPLCs use a miniature hollow cathode lamp as a very narrow wavelength intense source. For example, a zinc hollow cathode lamp emits a line at 214 nm that is close to the maximum wavelength of peptide bond absorption (206 nm); this emission property permits the usage of such lamps to measure peptides and proteins. Details on the hollow cathode lamp are found in the section on Atomic Absorption Spectrophotometry. The hollow cathode lamp also has a long, useful lifetime if a lower current, nonpulsed power supply is used.

Laser Sources. A laser (light amplification by stimulated emission of radiation) is a device that controls the way that energized atoms release photons; lasers are used as light sources in spectrophotometers because they provide intense light of a narrow wavelength. Through selection of different materials, different wavelength(s) of light are emitted by different types of lasers (Table 13.3).

TABLE 13.3 Various Types of Lasers and the Wavelengths at Which They Operate

Laser	Wavelengths (nm)
Argon fluoride	193
Argon fluoride	248
Helium-cadmium	325 or 442
Nitrogen	337
Argon (blue)	488
Argon (green)	514
Helium-neon (green)	543
Light-emitting diode (GaP)	550 or 700
Rhodamine 6G dye (tunable)	570–650
Laser diode (AlGaInP, GaAlAs)	633–1660
Helium-neon (red)	633
Ruby ($CrAlO_3$) (red)	694
Light-emitting diode (GaAs)	880
Light-emitting diode (Si)	1100
Neodymium-YAG (yttrium aluminum garnet)	1064
Carbon dioxide	9300, 9600, 10,300, or 10,600

AlGaInP, Aluminum gallium indium phosphide; *GaAlAs,* aluminum gallium arsenide; *GaAs,* gallium arsenide; *GaP,* gallium phosphide; *Si,* silicon.

Three properties of laser sources distinguish them from "conventional" sources: (1) spatial coherence is a property of lasers that allows beam diameters in the range of several micrometers; (2) lasers produce monochromatic light; and (3) lasers have pulse widths that vary from microseconds (flash lamp–pulsed lasers) to nanoseconds (nitrogen lasers) to picoseconds or less (mode-locked lasers) in duration. Air-cooled argon ion lasers produce approximately 25 mW of energy output at 488 nm and have plasma tube lifetimes of 6000 hours or longer. Continuous-wave dye lasers typically use an argon ion laser with an output of 1 W or less as an energy pump and use different fluorescent dyes to achieve excitation wavelength ranges of 400 to 800 nm. Helium-neon and helium-cadmium lasers are useful because of their low cost and ease of operation, and because they emit a number of excitation wavelengths; however, the power output of helium-neon lasers has been limited to approximately 2 mW at 594 nm.

Diode lasers are used in compact disc players and laser printers, and in bar code readers (see Chapter 26). They are solid-state devices, typically constructed of gallium arsenide, and energy is pumped into them at a low potential of −1.5 V. Depending on its construction, the wavelength output of the laser ranges from 350 to 29,000 nm. Development of inexpensive near-IR lasers has led to interest in using reflective techniques in the near-IR region of the spectrum (0.8- to 2.5-μm wavelength). Reflectance spectrophotometry is now used clinically for the transcutaneous measurement of bilirubin in neonates.[1] Another application of reflectance spectrophotometry is measurement of blood oxygen saturation in near-IR and IR regions.

Spectral Isolation. Radiant energy of a desired wavelength can be isolated and that of other wavelengths excluded in various ways, including the use of (1) filters (interference or dichroic filters), (2) prisms, and (3) diffraction gratings. Combinations of lenses and slits may be inserted before or after the monochromatic device to render light rays parallel or to isolate narrow portions of the light beam. Variable slits may be used to permit adjustments in total radiant energy to reach the photocell.

Filters. The simplest type of filter is a thin layer of colored glass. Certain metal complexes or salts, dissolved or suspended in glass, produce colors corresponding to the predominant wavelengths transmitted. The spectral purity of a filter or other monochromator is usually described in terms of its spectral bandwidth. This is defined as the width, in nanometers, of the spectral transmittance curve at a point equal to one half the peak transmittance. Glass filters have spectral bandwidths of approximately 50 nm, and are referred to as wide bandpass filters.

Other glass filters include narrow bandpass and sharp cutoff types. Operationally, a cutoff filter typically shows a sharp rise in transmittance over a narrow portion of the spectrum and is used to eliminate light below a given wavelength. Historically, narrow bandpass filters were constructed by combining two or more sharp cutoff filters or regular filters. Currently, however, the availability of high-intensity light sources now favors the use of narrow bandpass interference filters.

A narrow bandpass interference or dichroic filter uses a dielectric material of controlled thickness sandwiched between two thinly silvered pieces of glass. The thickness of the layer determines the wavelength of energy transmitted after constructive and destructive wavelength interference caused by reflections between the glass surfaces separated by the dielectric spacing. These filters have narrow spectral bandwidths, usually from 5 to 15 nm. Because they also transmit harmonics, or multiples, of the desired wavelength, accessory glass filters are required to eliminate undesired wavelengths. For example, an interference filter designed for 620 nm will also transmit some radiation at 310 and 1240 nm unless accessory cutoff filters are provided to absorb this undesired stray light.

Prisms and Gratings. Prisms and diffraction gratings are widely used as monochromators. A prism separates white light into a continuous spectrum because shorter wavelengths are bent, or refracted, more than longer wavelengths as they pass through the prism. A diffraction grating is prepared by depositing a thin layer of aluminum-copper alloy on the surface of a flat glass plate, and then fabricating many small parallel grooves into the metal coating. Better gratings contain 1000 to 2000 lines/mm and must be made with great care. These are then used as molds to prepare less expensive replicas for general use in instruments.

Modern holographic gratings are made using a laser in a "high-precision machining" mode. The focused beam of the laser is accurately scanned over a photosensitive material termed a photoresist. After multiple lines have been scribed on the photoresist, chemicals are used to dissolve and elute the exposed photoresist to create channels that become the lines of the grating. A layer of a highly reflective material is then deposited onto the surface of the laser-etched channels, and the grating is then ready for use. A flat photoresistive surface or a concave surface can be used to make this type of grating. These types of gratings are extremely accurate, have low light scatter, and are widely used in the spectrophotometers found in clinical chemistry instruments. For example, most UV-visible spectrophotometers and virtually all IR spectrophotometers use reflective gratings. In addition, HPLC detectors frequently use a concave holographic reflective grating in their optical system.

Each line ruled on the grating, when illuminated, reflects light and gives rise to a tiny spectrum. An array of parallel wavefronts is formed that reinforce those wavelengths in phase and cancel those wavelengths not in phase. The net result is a uniform linear spectrum. Some instruments contain diffraction gratings that produce spectral bandwidths of 20 nm or more; higher priced instruments may have a resolution of 0.5 nm or less.

The flat surface grating discussed previously is called a plane transmission grating. Lines are engraved on the surface of a mirror, which may be a polished metal slab or a glass plate on which a thin, metallic film has been deposited. A grating may also be ruled at a specified angle, so that a maximum fraction of the radiant energy is directed into wavelengths diffracted at a selected angle. This type of grating is called an echelette and is said to have been given a blaze at a particular angle or to have been blazed at a certain wavelength (eg, 250 nm).

Selection of a Wavelength Isolation Device. The type of monochromator chosen depends on the analytical purpose for which it is to be used. For example, narrow spectral bandwidths are required in spectrophotometers for resolving and identifying sharp absorption peaks that are closely adjacent. Lack of agreement with Beer's law will occur when a part of the spectral energy transmitted by the monochromator is not absorbed by the substance being measured. This is more commonly observed with wide bandpass instruments. In practice, an increase in absorbance and improved linearity with concentration are usually observed with instruments that operate at narrower bandwidths of light. This is especially true for substances that exhibit a sharp peak of absorption.

The natural bandwidth of an absorbing substance is defined as "the bandwidth of the spectral absorbance curve at a point equal to one half of the maximum absorbance." As a general rule, for peak absorbance readings to be within 99.5% of true values, the spectral bandwidth should not exceed 10% of the natural bandwidth. For example, many chemistry procedures used in the clinical laboratory produce an absorbing species for which the natural bandwidth ranges from 40 to more than 200 nm. The natural bandwidth of nicotinamide adenine dinucleotide is 58 nm (λmax = 339 nm). Therefore, for accurate measurements of this compound, a spectral bandwidth of 6 nm or less should be used.

In practice, the wavelength selected is usually at the peak of maximum absorbance to attain the maximum measurement; however, it may be desirable to choose another wavelength to minimize interfering substances. For example, turbidity readings on a spectrophotometer are greater in the blue region than in the red region of the spectrum, but the latter region is chosen for turbidity measurements to avoid absorption of light by bilirubin (460 nm) or hemoglobin (417 and 575 nm). The absorbing species developed in the alkaline picrate procedure for creatinine produces a relatively flat peak in the visible region of the spectrum at approximately 480 nm, but the reagent blank itself absorbs light strongly at less than 500 nm. A compromise is made by selecting a wavelength at 520 nm to minimize the contribution of the blank. Blank readings should be kept to a minimum. A small difference between two large numbers is subject to greater uncertainty; hence, minimizing absorbance of the blank improves precision and accuracy. The linear working range of a method can be expanded by not measuring at the peak absorbance. However, measurements should not be taken on the steep slope of an absorption curve, because a slight error in wavelength adjustment will introduce a significant error in absorbance readings.

Cuvets. A cuvet (also often termed a cuvette) is a small vessel used to hold a liquid sample to be analyzed in the light path of a spectrometer. Cuvets may be round, square, or rectangular, and are constructed from glass, silica (quartz), or plastic. Square or rectangular cuvets have plane-parallel optical surfaces and a constant light path. The most popular cuvets have a 1.0-cm light path, held to close tolerances. Ordinary borosilicate glass or plastic cuvets are suitable for measurements in the visible portion of the spectrum. However, quartz cells are usually required for readings at less than 340 nm. Some plastic cells have good clarity in both the visible and UV range, but they can present problems related to tolerances, cleaning, etching by solvents, and temperature deformations. Many plastic cuvets are designed for disposable, single-use applications. However, in many clinical analyzers, cuvets are cleaned and reused many times before optical degradation requires them to be replaced.

Cuvets must be clean and optically clear, because etching or deposits on the surface affect absorbance values. Cuvets used in the visible range are cleaned by copious rinsing with tap water and distilled water. Alkaline solutions should not be left standing in cuvets for prolonged periods, because alkali slowly dissolves glass and produces etching. Cuvets may be cleaned in mild detergent or soaked in a mixture of concentrated hydrogen chloride to water to ethanol (1:3:4). Cuvets should never be soaked in dichromate cleaning solution because the solution is hazardous and tends to adsorb onto and discolor the glass.

Cuvets used for measurements in the UV region should be handled with special care. Invisible scratches, fingerprints, or residual traces of previously measured substances may be present and may absorb significantly. A good practice is to fill all such cuvets with distilled water and measure the absorbance for each against a reference blank over the wavelengths to be used. This value should be essentially zero.

Photodetectors. A photodetector is a device that converts light into an electric signal that is proportional to the number of photons striking its photosensitive surface. The photomultiplier tube is a commonly used photodetector for measuring light intensity in the UV and visible regions of the spectrum. Alternatively, photodiodes are solid-state devices that are also used in modern instruments. In older instruments, barrier layer cells (also known as photovoltaic cells) were used as photodetectors, because they were rugged and less expensive.

Photomultiplier Tubes. A photomultiplier tube (PMT) contains (1) a cathode, (2) a light-sensitive metal, and (3) a series of dynodes, all of which are enclosed in an evacuated glass enclosure. As many as 10 to 15 stages or dynodes are present in common photomultipliers. Photons that strike the photoemissive cathode emit electrons that are accelerated toward the dynodes. Additional electrons are generated at each dynode. Depending on the number of dynodes and the accelerating voltage, the cascading effect creates 10^5 to 10^7 electrons for each photon hitting the first cathode. This amplified signal is finally collected at the anode, where it can be measured.

When such a tube is operated, voltage is applied between the photocathode and each successive stage. The normal incremental increase in voltage at each photomultiplier stage is from 50 to 100 V greater than that of the previous stage (Fig. 13.5). Typically, a conventional PMT tube has approximately 1500 V applied to it.

PMTs have (1) extremely rapid response times, (2) are very sensitive, and (3) are slow to fatigue. Because these tubes are very sensitive and have a rapid response, they must be carefully shielded from all stray light. A PMT with the voltage applied should never be exposed to room light because it will burn out. The rapid response times of PMTs are needed when a spectrophotometer is being used to determine an absorption spectrum of a compound. Also, PMTs are sensitive over a wide range of wavelengths.

When voltage is applied to a PMT in the absence of any incident light, some current is usually produced. This current is called dark current. It is desirable to have the dark current of a PMT at its lowest level because this current appears as background noise.

Photodiodes. Photodiodes are solid-state photodetectors that are fabricated from photosensitive semiconductor materials such as (1) silicon, (2) gallium arsenide, (3) indium antimonide, (4) indium arsenide, (5) lead selenide, and (6) lead sulfide. These materials absorb light over a characteristic wavelength range (eg, 250 to 1100 nm for silicon). Their development and use as detectors in spectrophotometers have resulted in instruments capable of measuring light at a multitude of wavelengths. When a photodetector consists of two-dimensional arrays of diodes, it is known as a photodiode array. Each photodetector within the array responds to a specific wavelength. For example, photodiode arrays have been designed to have a 2-nm resolution per diode from 200 to 340 nm, and a 1-nm resolution per diode from 340 to 800 nm.

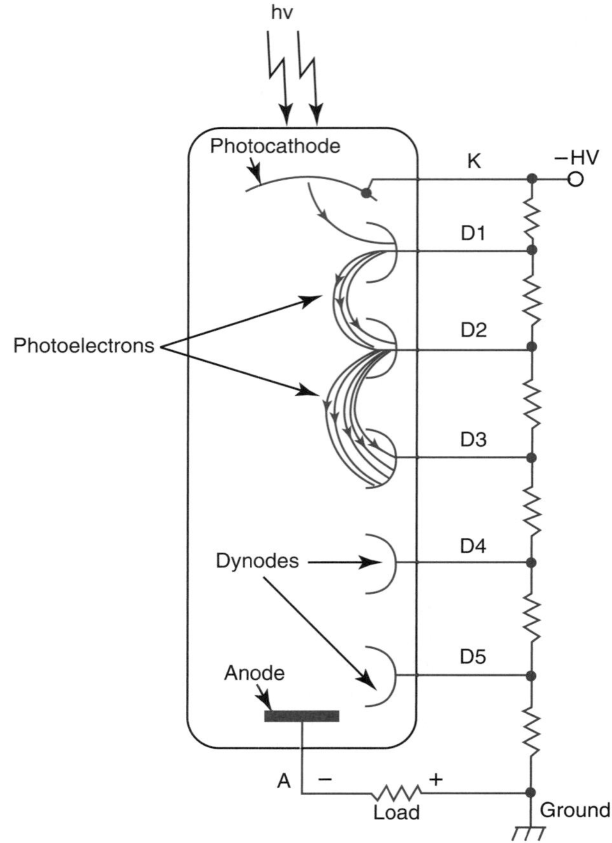

FIGURE 13.5 Schematic diagrams of a glass photomultiplier tube. Energy from photons of light (hv) are converted into electrons at the photocathode. Electrons from the photocathode travel to the chain of dynodes *(D1, D2, D3, D4, D5)* (HV, high voltage). At each dynode, additional electrons are generated, leading to a multiplying effect. The photoelectrons terminate at the anode.

In practice, all diodes are initially charged to 5 V, and they discharge when they are struck by light. Each diode then is sequentially scanned and recharged to 5 V. The amount of energy required for recharging is proportional to the quantity of light striking that diode. Because scan time for all diodes is in the millisecond range, many scans are typically taken. The resultant data are processed using a variety of algorithms, including signal averaging, background subtraction, and correction for scattered light. Consequently, an optical spectrum of an ongoing chemical reaction can be monitored as a function of time with a high degree of resolution and accuracy.

Readout Devices. Electrical energy from a detector is displayed on some type of meter or readout system. In the past, analog devices were widely used as readout devices in spectrophotometers. However, they have been replaced by digital readout devices that provide a visual numeric display of absorbance or converted values of concentrations. Spectrophotometers may be equipped with recorders in addition to or instead of a digital display. These are synchronized to provide line traces of transmittance or absorbance as a function of time or wavelength. When a continuous tracing of absorbance versus wavelength is recorded, the resultant display is called an absorption spectrum. If a substance absorbs light, distinct peaks of absorbance will be observed (see Fig. 13.1). Measuring the absorption spectra of an unknown sample and comparing them with spectra from known compounds is useful for qualitative purposes. For example, this type of procedure is especially useful for identification of drugs that absorb in the UV region.

Performance Parameters

In most spectrophotometric analytical procedures, the absorbance of an unknown is compared directly with that of a calibrator or a series of calibrators. Under these circumstances, minor errors in wavelength calibration, variation in spectral bandwidths, and the presence of stray light are compensated for and usually do not contribute serious errors. Use of a series of calibrators covering a wide range of concentrations also provides a measure of linearity (ie, agreement with Beer's law for a given procedure and instrument). However, when calculations are based on published or previously determined values for molar absorptivities or absorption coefficients, the spectrophotometer must be checked more rigorously. Performance verification of spectrophotometers on a periodic basis also improves reliability of routine comparative analyses.

To verify that a spectrophotometer is performing satisfactorily, the following parameters should be tested: (1) wavelength accuracy, (2) spectral bandwidth, (3) stray light, (4) linearity, and (5) photometric accuracy.

The National Institute of Standards and Technology (NIST) provides several standard reference materials (SRMs) for spectrophotometry that are useful in the calibration or verification of the performance of photometers or spectrophotometers (eg, SRM 930e is for the verification and calibration of the transmittance and absorbance scales of visible absorption spectrometers) (http://www.nist.gov/srm).

The Institute for Reference Materials and Measurements (IRMM) belongs to the European Commission and provides reference materials for verification of the performance of photometers or spectrophotometers. These materials are listed in the Joint Research Centre's Reference Materials Catalogue (https://ec.europa.eu/jrc/en/reference-materials).

Wavelength Calibration. With narrow spectral bandwidth instruments, a holmium oxide glass may be scanned over the range of 280 to 650 nm. This material shows sharp absorbance peaks at defined wavelengths, and the operator may compare the wavelength scale readings that produce maximum absorbance with established values. If compared values do not coincide, a calibration correction table can be constructed to relate scale readings to true wavelengths. A typical spectral transmittance curve for holmium oxide glass is shown in Fig. 13.6. Selected absorption peaks for this filter, which are suitable for calibration purposes, occur at the following wavelengths: 279.3, 418.5, 287.6, 536.4, 333.8, 637.5, and 360.8 nm. Solutions of holmium oxide in dilute perchloric acid have also been recommended and may be used with any spectrophotometer.

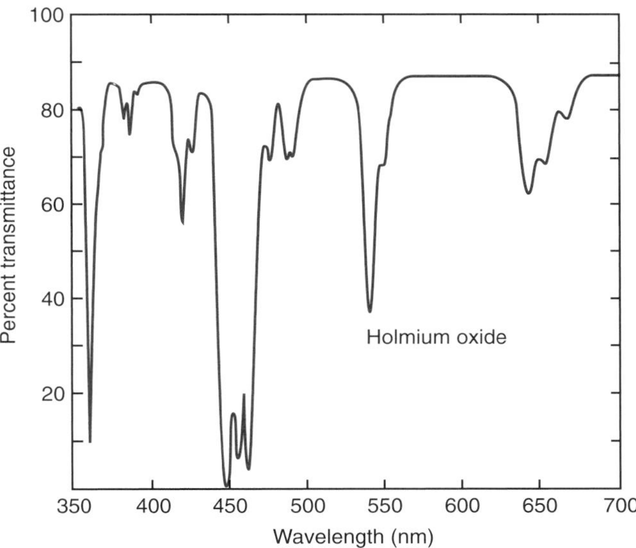

FIGURE 13.6 Spectral transmittance curve of holmium oxide filter.

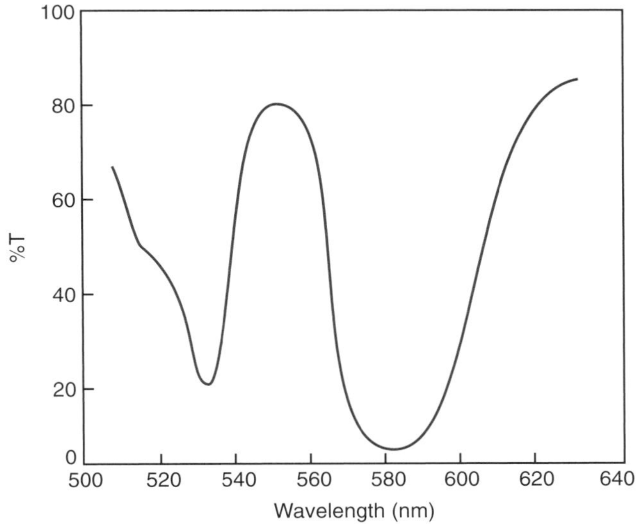

FIGURE 13.7 Spectral transmittance curve of a didymium filter (Perkin-Elmer Model 35 spectrophotometer, 8-nm nominal spectral bandwidth).

With broader bandpass instruments, a didymium filter may be used to verify wavelength settings. These filters should show a minimum percent transmittance at 530 nm against an air blank (Fig. 13.7). Because didymium has several absorption peaks, the setting should be verified grossly by visual examination of transmitted light. This light should appear green at 530 nm.

Spectral Bandwidth. The apparent width of an emission band at half-peak height is taken to be the spectral bandwidth of the instrument. The spectral bandwidth may also be calculated from the manufacturer's specifications. Interference filters with spectral bandwidths of 1 to 2 nm are available and may be used to check those instruments with a nominal spectral bandwidth of 8 nm or more.

Stray Light. Stray light, in general terms, is radiation of wavelengths outside the narrow band nominally transmitted by the monochromator that hits the detector. A perfect monochromator would transmit light only within its bandpass. In practice, scattering and diffraction inside the monochromator generate light of other wavelengths into the exit beam. This light is further modified by other components of the spectrophotometer and by the sample itself. Stray light is usually defined as a ratio or percent to the total detected light.

Other sources of unwanted light include light leaks and fluorescence of the sample. Light leaks should be excluded by covering the cell compartments. Light arising from fluorescence can increase the signal to the detector and cause an apparent decrease in absorbance. These sources of light are not included in the usual definition of stray light.

The major effect of stray light on the performance of a spectrophotometer is an absorbance error, especially in the upper end of the absorbance range of the instrument. Most spectrophotometers are equipped with one or more stray-light filters. Thus a blue filter is used with a tungsten lamp for wavelength settings below approximately 400 nm. For example, when the spectrophotometer is set to 350 nm, most of the stray light is of wavelengths in the visible range. The blue filter absorbs most of the visible light but transmits well in this UV portion of the spectrum. By analogy, a red filter is used for wavelengths in the range of 650 to 800 nm.

Cutoff filters are satisfactory for the detection of stray light. These may be of glass, similar to the stray-light filters discussed previously, and produce a sharp cut in the spectrum, with almost complete absorption on one side and high transmittance on the other. Liquid cutoff filters are satisfactory and convenient in the UV range, where stray light is usually more of a problem. A 50 g/L aqueous solution of sodium nitrite should show essentially 0% T when read against water over the range of 300 to 385 nm. Acetone, read against water, should show 0% T over the range of 250 to 320 nm.

Photometric Accuracy. Neutral density filters (eg, SRM 1930; NIST) are used to check an instrument's photometric accuracy. In addition, solutions of potassium dichromate ($K_2Cr_2O_7$) may be used for overall checks on photometric accuracy. In practice, analytical reagent grade $K_2Cr_2O_7$ is dried at 110°C for 1 hour, and then the following solutions in 0.005 mol/L sulfuric acid are prepared: (1) solution A: 0.0500 g/L for the absorbance range from 0.2 to 0.7; and (2) solution B: 0.1000 g/L for the absorbance range from 0.4 to 1.4.

Measurements are made in 10-mm cells with the temperature controlled in the range of 15°C to 25°C, using 0.005 mol/L sulfuric acid as the reference. Table 13.4 gives the expected values for the two absorbance maxima and minima of the solutions based on literature values. Because the natural bandwidth of solution A at 350 nm is approximately 63 nm, the values shown are applied strictly to spectrophotometers with a spectral bandwidth of 6 nm or less.

Multiple-Wavelength Readings. Background interference due to interfering chromogens can often be eliminated or minimized by inclusion of blanks or by reading absorbance at two or three wavelengths. In one approach, termed bichromatic, absorbance is measured at two wavelengths—one corresponding to peak absorbance and another at a point near the base of the peak that serves as a baseline. The difference in absorbance at the two wavelengths is related to concentration.

TABLE 13.4 Absorbance Values for Acidic Potassium Dichromate Solutions on a Calibrated Spectrophotometer

	ABSORBANCE	
Wavelength (nm)	**Solution A**	**Solution B**
235 (min)	0.626 ± 0.009	1.251 ± 0.019
257 (max)	0.727 ± 0.007	1.454 ± 0.015
313 (min)	0.244 ± 0.004	0.488 ± 0.007
350 (max)	0.536 ± 0.005	1.071 ± 0.011

Before the correction is used, knowledge of the shape of the absorption curve for the substance of interest and of the interference is required. The linearity of the baseline shift should be verified by measuring the absorption spectrum of commonly encountered interferences. Care should be exercised in the use of the correction because if it is not properly used, it may introduce larger errors than would be observed without correction. For example, such a situation may occur if the background reading is not linear over the region measured.

REFLECTANCE PHOTOMETRY

In reflectance photometry, diffuse reflected light is measured. The reaction mixture in a carrier is illuminated with diffused light, and the intensity of the reflected light from the chromogen is compared with the intensity of light reflected from a reference surface. Because the intensity of reflected light is nonlinear in relation to the concentration of the analyte, the Kubelka-Munk equation or the Clapper-Williams transformation is commonly used to convert the data into a linear format (see Chapter 26). The electro-optical components used in reflectance photometry are essentially the same as those required for absorbance photometry, except that the geometry of the system is modified so that the light source and the detector are located next to each other on one side of the sample, as opposed to on opposite sides of the sample cuvet, as in absorption photometry. Reflectance photometry is used as the measurement method with dry-film chemistry systems.

FLAME EMISSION AND INDUCTIVELY COUPLED PLASMA SPECTROPHOTOMETRY

Flame emission spectrophotometry is based on the characteristic emission of light by atoms of many metallic elements when given sufficient energy, such as that supplied by a hot flame. The wavelength to be used for the measurement of an element depends on the selection of a line of sufficient intensity to provide adequate sensitivity and freedom from other interfering lines at or near the selected wavelength. For example, lithium produces a red, sodium a yellow, potassium a violet, rubidium a red, and magnesium a blue color in a flame. These colors are characteristic of the metal atoms that are present as cations in solution. Under constant and controlled conditions, the light intensity of the characteristic

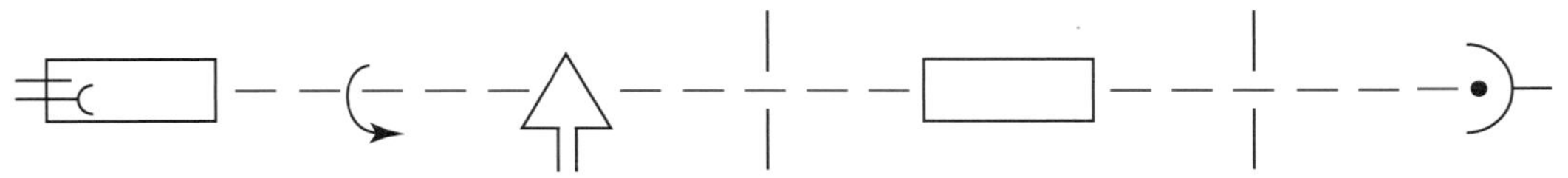

FIGURE 13.8 Basic components of an atomic absorption spectrophotometer.

wavelength produced by each of the atoms is directly proportional to the number of atoms that are emitting energy, which in turn is directly proportional to the concentration of the substance of interest in the sample. Although this technique once was used widely for analysis of sodium, potassium, and lithium in body fluids, it now has been replaced largely by electrochemical techniques.

Inductively coupled plasma (ICP) atomic emission spectroscopy is a technique for elemental analysis (eg, trace metals) that uses an ICP to produce excited species that emit light at wavelengths characteristic of a particular element present in the sample. An ICP spectrometer consists of an optical spectrometer and an ICP torch. The torch produces argon gas plasma (10,000 K) using a radiofrequency induction coil and an electric spark. A nebulized sample is injected into the argon gas plasma; elements in the sample become excited, and the electrons emit energy at a characteristic wavelength as they return to ground state. The emitted light is then measured by optical spectrometry.

ATOMIC ABSORPTION SPECTROPHOTOMETRY

Atomic absorption (AA) spectrophotometry is used widely in clinical laboratories to measure elements such as aluminum, calcium, copper, lead, lithium, magnesium, zinc, and other metals. A method for metal analysis that has begun to replace atomic absorption is inductively coupled plasma mass spectrometry (ICP-MS). AA retains advantages over ICP-MS in terms of overall cost and ease of use. However, a single ICP-MS instrument has greater flexibility in measuring multiple metals simultaneously and with greater sensitivity (see Chapters 37 and 42).

Basic Concepts

AA is an absorption spectrophotometric technique in which a metallic atom in the sample absorbs light of a specific wavelength. However, the element is not appreciably excited in the flame, but is merely dissociated from its chemical bonds (atomized) and placed in an unexcited or ground state (neutral atom). Thus, the ground state atom absorbs radiation at a very narrow bandwidth corresponding to its own line spectrum. A hollow cathode lamp with the cathode made of the material to be analyzed is used to produce a wavelength of light specific for the atom. Thus, if the cathode were made of sodium, sodium light at predominantly 589 nm would be emitted by the lamp. When the light from the hollow cathode lamp enters the flame, some of it is absorbed by the ground-state atoms in the flame, resulting in a net decrease in the intensity of the beam from the lamp. This process is referred to as atomic absorption.

A specific hollow cathode lamp serves as the light source, and the sample heated in the flame is the sample in the cuvet. The path length of the flame is the light path through the cuvet. Hence, most of the atoms are in the ground state and are able to absorb light emitted by the cathode lamp. In general, AA methods are approximately 100 times more sensitive than flame emission methods. In addition, because of the unique specificity of the wavelength from the hollow cathode lamp, these methods are highly specific for the element being measured.

Instrumentation

Fig. 13.8 shows the basic components of an AA spectrophotometer. The hollow cathode lamp is made of the metal of the substance to be analyzed and is different for each metal analysis. In some cases, an alloy is used to make the cathode, resulting in a multielement lamp. The hollow cathode lamp usually contains argon or neon gas at a pressure of a few millimeters of mercury. An argon-filled lamp produces a blue-to-purple glow during operation, and the neon produces a reddish-orange glow inside the hollow cathode lamp. Quartz, or a special glass that allows transmission of the proper wavelength, is used as a window. A current is applied between the two electrodes inside the hollow cathode lamp, and metal is deposited from the cathode into the gases inside the glass envelope. When the metal atoms collide with the neon or argon gases, they lose energy and emit their characteristic radiation. Calcium has a sharp, intense, analytical emission line at 422.7 nm, which is used most frequently for calcium analysis. In an ideal interference-free system, only calcium atoms absorb the calcium light from the hollow cathode as it passes through the flame.

A pulsed hollow cathode lamp and a tuned amplifier are incorporated into most AA instruments. Operationally, the power to the hollow cathode lamp is pulsed, so that light is emitted by the lamp at a certain number of pulses per second. In contrast, all of the light originating from the flame is continuous. When light leaves the flame, it is composed of pulsed, unabsorbed light from the lamp and a small amount of non-pulsed flame spectrum and sample emission light. The detector senses all light, but the amplifier is electrically tuned to the pulsed signals and can subtract the background light measured when the lamp is off and the total light that includes both the lamp and flame background light. In this way, the electronics, in conjunction with the monochromator, discriminates between the flame background emission and the sample atomic absorption.

Fig. 13.9 shows a laminar flow premix burner and illustrates how the sample is aspirated, volatilized, and burned to form atoms of the metal in the gas phase. Note that the gases are mixed and the sample is atomized before it is burned. An advantage of this system is that the larger droplets go to waste while the fine mist enters the flame, thus producing a less noisy signal.

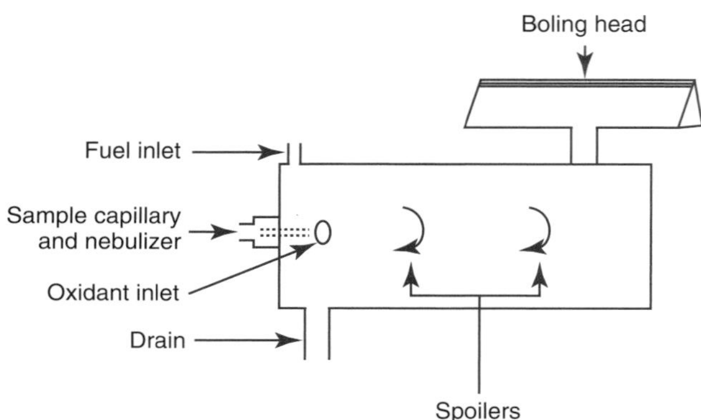

FIGURE 13.9 Laminar flow pre-mix burner.

In flameless AA techniques (carbon rod or "graphite furnace"), the sample is placed in a depression on a carbon rod in an enclosed chamber. Strips of tantalum or platinum metal may also be used as sample cups. In successive steps, the temperature of the rod is raised to dry, char, and, finally, atomize the sample into the gas phase in the chamber. The atomized element then absorbs energy from the corresponding hollow cathode lamp. This approach is more sensitive than conventional flame methods and permits determination of trace metals in small samples of blood or tissue.

With flameless AA, a novel approach used to correct for background absorption is called the Zeeman correction.[2] In Zeeman background correction, the light source or the atomizer is placed in a strong magnetic field. In practice, because Zeeman correction requires special lamps, the analyte is placed in the magnetic field. The intense magnetic field splits the degenerate (ie, of equal energy) atomic energy levels into two components that are polarized parallel and perpendicular to the magnetic field, respectively. The parallel component is at the resonance line of the source, whereas the two perpendicular components are shifted to different wavelengths. The two components interact differently with polarized light. A polarizer is placed between the source and the atomizer, and two absorption measurements are taken at different polarizer settings. One measures both analyte and background absorptions, A_t, the other only the background absorption, A_{bc}. The difference between the two absorption readings is the corrected absorbance.

The major advantage of the Zeeman correction method is that the same light source at the same wavelength is used to measure the total and the background absorption. The implementation is complex and expensive, and the strength of the magnetic field needs to be optimized for every element, but the method gives more accurate results at higher background levels than those attained with the other correction techniques.

Interferences in Atomic Absorption Spectrophotometry

Interferences in AA spectroscopy are divided into spectral and nonspectral interferences.

Spectral Interferences

Spectral interferences include absorption by other closely absorbing atomic species, absorption by molecular species, scattering by nonvolatile salt particles or oxides, and background emission (which can be electronically filtered). Absorption by other atomic species usually is not a problem because of the extremely narrow bandwidth (0.01 nm) used in the absorption measurements. Absorption and scattering by molecular species are particularly problematic in lower atomizing temperatures.

Nonspectral Interferences

Nonspectral interferences may be nonspecific or specific. Nonspecific interferences affect nebulization by altering the viscosity, surface tension, or density of the analyte solution, and consequently, the sample flow rate. Certain contaminants also decrease desolvation and atomization efficiency by lowering the atomizer temperature. Specific interferences are also called chemical interferences because they are more analyte-dependent. Solute volatilization interference refers to the situation in which the contaminant forms nonvolatile species with the analyte. An example is phosphate interference in the determination of calcium that is caused by the formation of calcium–phosphate complexes. The phosphate interference is overcome by adding a cation, usually lanthanum or strontium; the cation competes with the calcium for the phosphate. Enhancement effects are also observed, in which the addition of contaminants increases the volatilization efficiency. Such is the case with aluminum, which normally forms nonvolatile oxides, but in the presence of hydrofluoric acid forms more volatile aluminum fluoride. Dissociation interferences affect the degree of dissociation of the analyte. Analytes that form oxides or hydroxides are especially susceptible to dissociation interferences. Ionization interference occurs when the presence of an easily ionized element, such as potassium, affects the degree of ionization of the analyte, which leads to changes in the analyte signal. Ionization interference is controlled by adding a relatively high concentration of an element that is easily ionized to maintain a more consistent concentration of ions in the flame and to suppress ionization of the analyte. In the case of excitation interference, the analyte atoms are excited in the atomizer, with subsequent emission at the absorption wavelength. This type of interference is more pronounced at higher temperatures.

FLUOROMETRY

Fluorescence refers to the condition when a molecule absorbs light at one wavelength and reemits light at a longer wavelength. An atom or molecule that fluoresces is termed a fluorophore. Fluorometry is defined as the measurement of emitted fluorescent light. Fluorometric analysis is a widely used method of quantitative analysis in the chemical and biological sciences; it is a very accurate and sensitive technique.

Basic Concepts

Fig. 13.10 illustrates the relationship among absorption, fluorescence, and phosphorescence. As indicated, each molecule contains a series of closely spaced energy levels. Absorption of a quantum of light energy by a molecule causes the transition of an electron from the singlet ground state to one of a number of possible vibrational levels of its first singlet state. The actual number of molecules in the excited state under typical reaction conditions and excited with a typical 150-W light source is very small and is estimated to be approximately 10^{-13} mol/mol of fluorophore. Once the molecule is in an

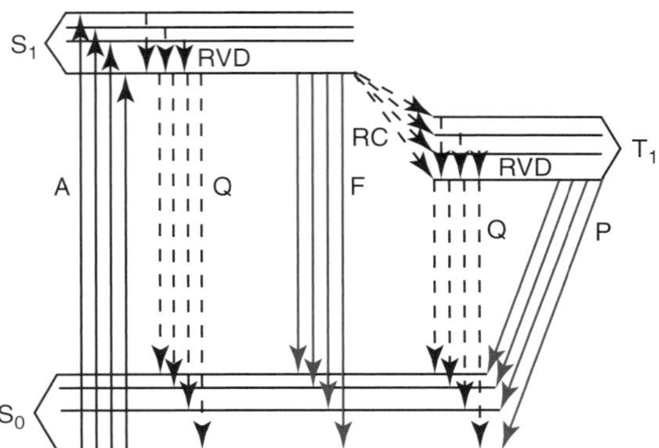

FIGURE 13.10 Luminescence Energy-Level Diagram of Typical Organic Molecule. *A*, Absorption process; *F*, fluorescence process from the first excited singlet state; *P*, phosphorescence process from the first excited triplet state; *Q*, quenching of the excited singlet or triplet state; *RC*, radiation-less crossover from the first excited singlet state to the first excited triplet state; *RVD*, radiation-less vibrational deactivation; S_0, ground-level singlet state; S_1, first excited singlet state; T_1, first excited triplet state.

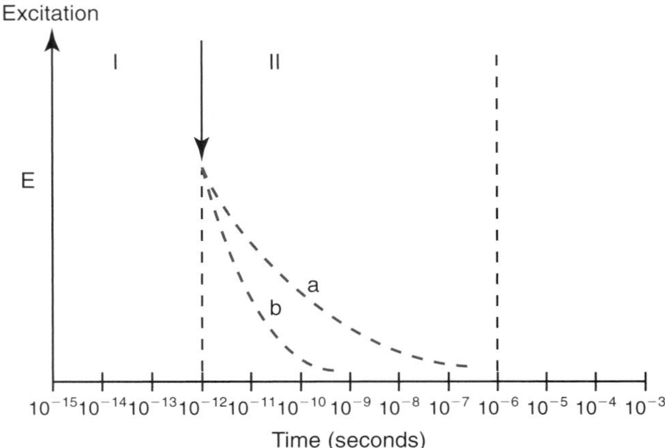

FIGURE 13.11 Fluorescence Decay Process. *a*, Long fluorescence decay time; *b*, short fluorescence decay time; *E*, absorption of energy; *I*, vibrational deactivation time phase; *II*, fluorescence emission time phase.

excited state, it returns to its original energy state in several ways. These include (1) radiation-less vibrational equilibration, (2) the fluorescence process from the excited singlet state, (3) quenching of the excited singlet state, (4) radiation-less crossover to a triplet state, (5) quenching of the first triplet state, and (6) the phosphorescence process of light emission from the triplet state.

As shown in Fig. 13.10, vibrational equilibration before fluorescence results in some loss of the excitation energy. The emitted fluorescence light is therefore of less energy or has a longer wavelength than the excitation light. The difference between the maximum wavelength of the excitation light and the maximum wavelength of the emitted fluorescence light is a constant referred to as the Stokes shift. This constant is a measure of energy lost during the lifetime of the excited state (radiation-less vibrational deactivation) before returning to the ground singlet level (fluorescence emission).

Time Relationships of Fluorescence Emission

The time required for a molecule to absorb radiant energy and to be promoted to an excited state is approximately 10^{-15} s. The length of time for vibrational equilibration to occur to the lowest excited state is 10^{-14} to 10^{-12} s. The length of time required for fluorescence emission to occur is 10^{-8} to 10^{-7} s. Relatively speaking, there is a considerable time delay among the (1) absorption of light energy, (2) return to the lowest excited state, and (3) emission of fluorescence light. This time relationship is shown in Fig. 13.11. In this figure, phase I represents the time period between the absorbance of light energy and the radiation-less loss of energy during vibrational rearrangement to the lowest excited energy state. This time period is represented by the up and down arrows in the diagram. Phase II shows the emission and decay of a (*b*) short- and (*a*) a long-lived fluorophore. If the fluorescence emission is measured over time following a pulse of light from an excitation source, such as a xenon lamp or laser, the intensity of the emitted light decays as a first-order process similar to radioactive decay (ie, phase II of Fig. 13.11). The time required for the emitted light to reach $1/e$ of its initial intensity, where e is the Naperian base 2.718, is called the average lifetime of the excited state of the molecule, or the fluorescence decay time.

The time delay between absorption of quanta of energy and fluorescence is used in fluorescence instrumentation called time-resolved fluorometers.[3] Advantages of a time-resolved fluorometer include the elimination of background light scattering due to Rayleigh and Raman signals and a short-lived fluorescence background with a consequent dramatic increase in signal-to-noise and detection sensitivity.

Time-resolved fluorometry[4] falls into one of two categories, depending on how the fluorescence emission response is measured: (1) pulse fluorometry, in which the sample is illuminated with an intense brief pulse of light and the intensity of the resulting fluorescence emission is measured as a function of time with a fast detector system; or (2) phase fluorometry, in which a continuous-wave laser illuminates the sample, and the fluorescence emission response is monitored for impulse and frequency response.[3]

Relationship of Concentration and Fluorescence Intensity

The relationship of concentration to the intensity of fluorescence emission is derived from the Beer-Lambert law. By expansion through a Taylor series, rearrangement, logarithm base conversion, and basic assumptions about dilute solutions, the following equation is obtained:

$$F = \varphi [I_0(2.3 - abc)] \qquad \textbf{13.8}$$

where F = relative fluorescence intensity; φ = fluorescence efficiency (ie, the ratio between quanta of light emitted and quanta of light absorbed); I_0 = initial excitation intensity; a = molar absorptivity; b = volume element defined by geometry of the excitation and emission slits; and c = the concentration in moles per liter.

Eq. 13.8 indicates that fluorescence intensity is directly proportional to the concentration of the fluorophore and the excitation intensity. This relationship holds only for dilute solutions, in which absorbance is less than 2% of the exciting radiation; the fluorescence intensity becomes nonlinear as the absorbance of the solution increases to greater than 2% of the exciting radiation. This phenomenon, called the inner filter effect, is discussed in more detail in a later section. Other factors influencing the measurement of fluorescence intensity include the sensitivity of the detector and the degree of background light scatter seen by the detector.

Fluorescence intensity measurements are more sensitive than absorbance measurements. The magnitude of absorbance of a chromophore in solution is determined by its concentration and the path length of the cuvet. The magnitude of fluorescence intensity of a fluorophore is determined by its concentration, the path length, and the intensity of the light source. The sensitivity of fluorescence measurements can be 100 to 1000 times greater than the sensitivity of absorbance measurements using more intense light sources, digital signal filtering techniques, and sensitive emission photometers. All of these are incorporated into conventional spectrofluorometric instrumentation, described later in this chapter.

Frequently, fluorescence measurements are expressed in units of relative intensity. The word *relative* is used because the intensity measured is not an absolute quantity. It is a small part of the total fluorescence emission, and its magnitude is defined by the instrument slit width, detector sensitivity, monochromator efficiency, and excitation intensity. Because these are instrument-related variables, establishing an absolute intensity unit for a given concentration of a fluorophore that is valid from instrument to instrument is difficult, if not impossible.

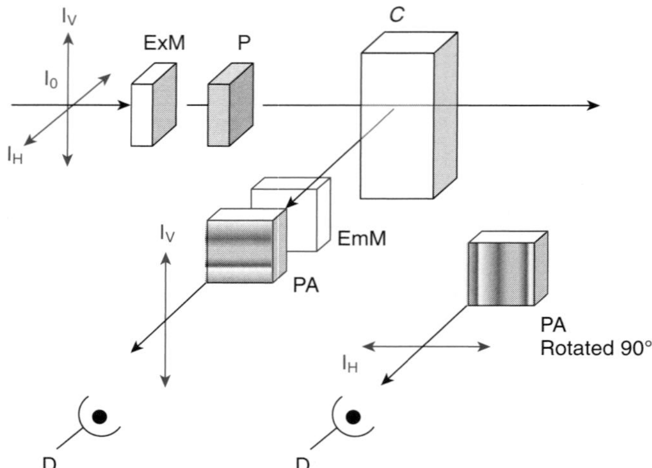

FIGURE 13.12 Schematic Diagram of a Fluorescence Polarization Analyzer. *Top panel,* the nonpolarized excitation light (I_0) has both vertical (I_V) and horizontal (I_H) components. The light travels through excitation monochromator and polarizer to energize the sample in the cuvet. The light from the sample travels through the emission monochromator and polarizer analyzer as light in the vertical plane I_V, which is measured by the detector. *Bottom panel,* the polarizer analyzer has been rotated 90 degrees and light in the horizontal plane I_H is measured by the detector. *C,* Reaction cell or cuvet; *D,* detector; *EmM,* emission monochromator; *ExM,* excitation monochromator; *P,* polarizer used to provide polarized excitation light; *PA,* polarizer analyzer, which is rotated to provide measurements of parallel and perpendicular polarized fluorescence emission intensity.

Fluorescence Polarization

Light is composed of electrical and magnetic waves at right angles to each other. Light waves produced by standard excitation sources have their electrical vectors oriented randomly. Light waves, passed through certain crystalline materials (polarizers), have their electrical vectors oriented in a single plane and are said to be plane-polarized. Fluorophores absorb light most efficiently in the plane of their electronic energy levels. If their rotational relaxation (Brownian movement) is slower than their fluorescence decay time, as is the case for large fluorescent-labeled molecules, the emitted fluorescence light will remain polarized. Because small molecules have rotational relaxation times that are much shorter than their fluorescence decay time, their emitted fluorescence light is depolarized. However, if the small fluorescent molecule is attached to a macromolecule, or if it is placed in a viscous solution, the small molecule will emit polarized light. Fluorescence polarization, *P,* is defined by the following equation:

$$P = \frac{(I_v - I_h)}{(I_v + I_h)} \quad \textbf{13.9}$$

where I_v = intensity of the emitted fluorescence light in the vertical plane; and I_h = intensity of the emitted fluorescence light in the horizontal plane.

As indicated, *P* is the difference between the two observed intensities divided by their sum. Fluorescence polarization is measured by placing a mechanically or electrically driven polarizer between the sample cuvet and the detector. A diagram of a fluorescence polarization measurement system is shown in Fig. 13.12. In the normal instrumentation mode, the sample is excited with polarized light to obtain maximum sensitivity. First, the polarization analyzer is positioned to measure the intensity of the emitted fluorescence light in the vertical plane (I_v); then the polarization analyzer is rotated 90° to measure the emitted fluorescence light intensity in the horizontal plane (I_h). *P* is then calculated manually or automatically by using Eq. 13.9.

Fluorescence polarization is used to quantitate analytes by using the change in fluorescence depolarization following immunologic reactions (see Chapter 23). Quantitation is accomplished by adding a known quantity of fluorescent-labeled analyte molecules to a reaction solution containing an antibody specific to the analyte. The labeled analyte binds to the antibody, and the slowed rotation and longer relaxation time results in an increased degree of fluorescence polarization. The addition of a nonlabeled analyte, such as an unknown quantity of a therapeutic drug in a serum specimen, will result in competition for binding to the antibody with the fluorescent-labeled analyte. This change in binding of the fluorophore-labeled analyte causes a change in fluorescence polarization that is inversely proportional to the amount of analyte contained in a given sample. Because the change in fluorescence polarization is a direct response to the reaction mixture, the bound fluorophore need not be separated from free fluorophore. Thus, fluorescence polarization is applicable to homogeneous assays of low-molecular-weight analytes, such as therapeutic drugs.[5]

Instrumentation

Fluorometers and spectrofluorometers are used to measure fluorescence. Operationally, a fluorometer uses interference filters, glass filters, gratings, or prisms to produce monochromatic light for sample excitation and for isolation of fluorescence emission.

Components

Basic components of fluorometers and spectrofluorometers include (1) an excitation source, (2) an excitation monochromator, (3) a cuvet, (4) an emission monochromator, and (5) a detector.

Excitation Source. The absorption spectra of most fluorescent compounds of interest are in the spectral region of 300 to 700 nm. The fluorescence emission intensity is proportional to the initial excitation intensity and to the concentration and size of the volume element being measured in the sample cell. Therefore, an intense lamp capable of emitting radiant energy over a large spectral region is desirable. Excitation sources used in fluorometers and spectrophotometers include xenon, quartz halogen, and mercury arc lamps and lasers. Some provide high-intensity spectra at one or more wavelengths; others provide a continuum over the spectral range of interest.

Xenon Lamp. The xenon lamp is a popular excitation source because it provides a continuum of relatively high-intensity radiant energy over the spectral region of 250 to 800 nm. It is widely used for certain fluorescence applications because of its high energy output, stability of lamp flashes, and higher UV and visible spectral output. These flash lamps can be pulsed at rates up to 2500 pulses/s. Light output is typically in the 0.01- to 0.1-J interval, with a spectral distribution ranging from 250 to 800 nm. The life of flash lamps varies from 10^6 to 10^9 flashes, with spectral stability maintained throughout the life of the flash lamp. A limitation of xenon lamps for analytical use is arc wandering or flicker. However, the use of current-stabilized power supplies has minimized this problem and improved the performance of fluorescence instrumentation using xenon lamps.

Lasers. Laser sources (discussed earlier in the Spectrophotometry section) are widely used in fluorescence applications in which highly intense, well-focused, and essentially monochromatic light is required. Examples of these applications include time-resolved fluorometry, flow cytometry, pulsed laser confocal microscopy, laser-induced fluorometry, and light scattering measurements for particle size and shape. Several different types of lasers are available as an excitation source for fluorescence measurements (see Table 13.3).

Light-Emitting Diode. LEDs are similar to laser diodes in that they are both solid-state devices. However, LEDs are fabricated from different semiconductor materials and produce incoherent light, compared with the coherent, narrow wavelength of light from laser diodes.[6] For spectrophotometry and typical fluorescence assays, laser diodes with coherent, narrow wavelength light are preferred; however, LED light sources can be used instead of conventional light sources (mercury vapor lamp) in fluorescence microscopy. In 2011, the World Health Organization issued a policy statement supporting the use of fluorescence LED microscopy for the diagnosis of tuberculosis.[7]

Excitation and Emission Monochromators. Monochromators used in fluorescence instrumentation include interference filters, colored glass filters, gratings, and prisms. Most modern analytical instruments using interference filters use the all-dielectric multicavity filter or a hybrid Fabry-Perot–coupled dielectric layer filter (a filter with metal reflective layers). Either type of filter is combined with appropriate sharp cutoff glass filters to form a single filter package, which removes undesired transmission of higher orders and provides narrow bandwidth, higher peak wavelength transmission, and increased band slope. The increased slope of the spectral band makes the transition from peak transmission to nontransmission more abrupt, which is very important for the spectral separation of excitation and emission bands with a small Stokes shift.

Colored glass filters selectively absorb certain wavelengths of light. These filters have been used for both excitation and emission wavelength selection, but they are more susceptible to transmitting stray light and unwanted fluorescence.

Grating monochromators are devices that isolate regions of the spectrum. The spectral resolution of the light at the slit is a function of slit width and resolution of the grating. Spectrofluorometers generally use larger slit widths than absorbance spectrophotometers to obtain higher excitation intensities. An advantage of the grating monochromator is that it provides selectivity of the excitation and emission wavelengths required when working with new fluorophores with absorbance and emission maxima for which specially fabricated interference filters may not exist. The rotation of the grating is digitally controlled when spectral scans of fluorescence excitation and emission are automated. In the conventional operation of a spectrofluorometer, the excitation wavelength or the emission wavelength is held constant, and the other is scanned. With more automated instrumentation, both excitation and emission monochromators are synchronized and scanned together at programmed rates. This provides a change in emission intensity as a function of change in excitation and emission wavelength, and gives an additional dimension of specificity to fluorescence measurements. Because of their high degree of monochromaticity, lasers are used as both the excitation light source and the monochromator. When a laser is used as a combination excitation source and monochromator, a narrowband interference filter is usually placed before the detector to eliminate additional orders of emission.

Cuvet. As with spectrophotometers, cuvets are used in fluorometers and spectrofluorometers to hold the liquid sample to be analyzed. For fluorescence instruments, the cuvets used are typically square or rectangular, and are constructed from a material that allows the excitation and the emitting light to pass (glass or plastic for visible light; quartz for UV light). However, some plastic cuvets contain UV absorbers that fluoresce, causing unwanted background signal and loss of sensitivity.

With fluorometers and spectrofluorometers, placement of the cuvet and excitation beam relative to the photodetector is critical in establishing the optical geometry for fluorescence measurements. Because fluorescence light is emitted in all directions from a molecule, several excitation and/or emission geometries are used to measure fluorescence (Fig. 13.13). Although the end-on approach allows the adaptation of a fluorescence detector to existing 180 degree absorption instruments, it is not widely used because its sensitivity is limited by the quality of the excitation and/or emission interference filter pair, the excitation and/or emission spectral band overlap, and the inner filter effect. In practice, most commercial spectrofluorometers and fluorometers use the

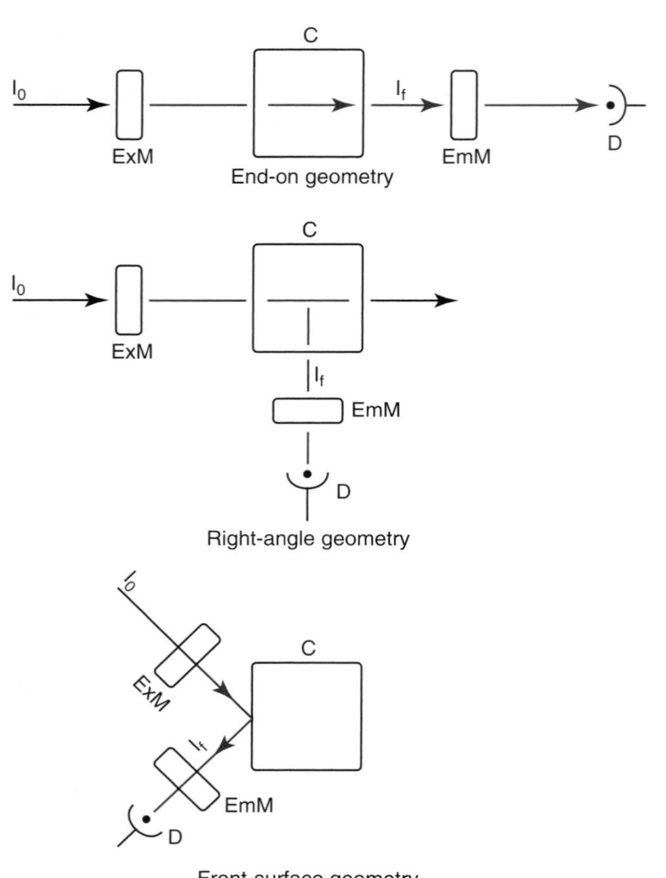

FIGURE 13.13 Fluorescence Excitation/Emission Geometries. *C*, Sample cuvet; *D*, detector; *EmM*, emission monochromator; *ExM*, excitation monochromator; I_0, initial excitation energy; I_f, fluorescence intensity.

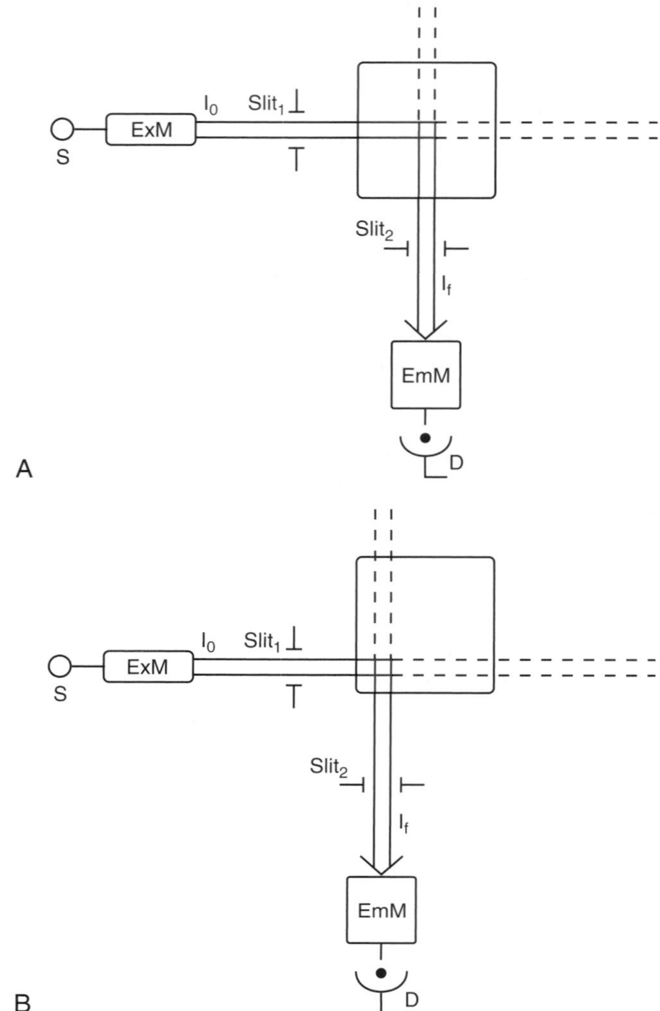

FIGURE 13.14 Two Right-Angle Fluorescence Sample Cuvet Positions. **A**, The standard 90 degree configuration. **B**, The offset positioning of the cuvet to minimize the inner filter effect. *D*, Detector; *ExM*, excitation monochromator; *EmM*, emission monochromator; I_0, Initial excitation energy; I_f, fluorescence intensity; *S*, excitation source; $Slit_1$, excitation slit; $Slit_2$, emission slit.

right angle–detector approach because it minimizes the background signal that limits analytical sensitivity. The front surface approach provides the greatest linearity over a broad range of concentration because it minimizes the inner filter effect. The front surface approach shows similar sensitivity to the right-angle detectors but is more susceptible to background light scatter (see section on Inner Filter Effects). Front surface fluorometry has been widely applied to heterogeneous solid-phase fluorescence immunoassay systems.

To accommodate these different geometries, the sample cell is oriented at different angles in relation to the excitation source and the detector. Major concerns related to the geometry of the sample cell include light scattering, the inner filter effect, and the sample volume element seen by the detector. Fig. 13.14A shows the sample cell and slit arrangement for a conventional fluorescence spectrophotometer, with the excitation and emission slits oriented at a right angle. $Slit_1$ and $Slit_2$ designate the excitation and emission slits, respectively. The position of the emission slit and the width of the slit are important. If the emission slit is located near the front edge of the sample cell, as shown in Fig. 13.14B, the inner filter effect is minimized. If the emission slit width is increased, sensitivity will increase, but specificity may decrease.

Photodetectors. As with spectrophotometric instruments, a number of devices are used as photodetectors in fluorometric instruments, including the PMT and the charge-coupled detector (CCD). In addition, visual observation is used for some applications.

Visual Observation. Because the human eye is a sensitive detector with a wide range of spectral recognition, qualitative fluorescent thin-layer chromatographic (TLC) methods in the clinical laboratory use short- and long-wavelength UV lamp sources coupled with visual observation. TLC is used as a routine screening method in analytical toxicology laboratories and in testing for counterfeit drugs in resource poor settings (Global Pharma Health Fund–Minilab).[8]

Photomultiplier Tube. For quantitative assays, the most commonly used detector in fluorometers and spectrofluorometers is the PMT. Important features of the PMT for fluorescence measurements consist of (1) a wide choice of spectral responses, (2) nanosecond photon response time, and (3) sensitivity. Sensitivity is due to the possible gain of 10^6

electrons at the anode of the PMT for each incident photon hitting the photo cathode.

Depending on the light level (photon flux) striking the PMT cathode and the desired sensitivity, measurement of electron flow at the PMT anode is accomplished in different ways. At high light intensities, analog techniques for measurement of PMT current are used. The analog signal is converted to a digital signal for computer use or for panel digital display. At low light levels, spikes or pulses generated at the cathode of the PMT are counted. The number of pulses that occur per unit of time is directly proportional to the intensity of emitted fluorescence light striking the PMT. This method is called photon counting. The use of photon counting increases the signal-to-noise ratio and decreases the lower limit of detection of the measurement of fluorophores at low concentrations.

Charge-Coupled Detector. CCDs are multichannel devices with a dynamic range and a signal-to-noise ratio that is superior to those of PMTs.[9,10] These solid-state devices are composed of a large number of photo-detecting shift registers that are read horizontally and vertically. CCDs were first used for astronomy applications and in ground-based optical telescopes, in which sensitive low-light measurements are required. Because of their ability to detect low levels of light, they have been used for molecular fluorescence measurement of low concentrations of fluorescent molecules and as quantitative electronic imagers for quantitative confocal microscopy.[11] A data-reading technique called *binning* has been developed that allows multielement devices to have functional elements linked together, much like rectangular slit widths. A related solid-state device, the avalanche photodiode, is also finding use for low-level light detection as a detector in confocal microscopy.[12]

Performance Verification

As with spectrophotometers, NIST provides a number of SRMs for use in calibration or verification of the performance of fluorometers or fluorospectrophotometers. These include SRM 936a (quinine sulfate dihydrate) for calibrating such instruments and SRM 1932 (fluorescein) for establishing a reference scale for fluorescence measurements (http://www.nist.gov/srm).

Types of Fluorometers and Spectrofluorometers

Fluorometers and fluorescence spectrophotometers that offer a variety of features are available. These features include ratio referencing, microprocessor-controlled excitation and emission monochromators, pulsed xenon light sources, photon counting, rhodamine cells for corrected spectra, polarizers, flow cells, front-surface viewing adapters, multiple cell holders, and microprocessor-based data reduction systems.

In addition to the basic spectrofluorometer discussed earlier, other types of fluorometric instruments include a ratio-referencing spectrofluorometer, a time-resolved fluorometer, a flow cytometer, and a hematofluorometer.

Ratio-Referencing Spectrofluorometer. The xenon lamp energy source in single-beam spectrofluorometers is unstable (ie, arc flicker and lamp decay). This is a source of laboratory error and requires frequent calibration. The unstable energy source in single-beam spectrofluorometry can be addressed by ratio-referencing spectrofluorometry. The ratio-referencing spectrofluorometer splits the energy from the light source to energize both a sample PMT and a reference PMT. Thus any instability of the energy source will affect both the reference and sample PMT and reduce the possibility of measurement error.

A typical ratio-referencing spectrofluorometer is illustrated in Fig. 13.15. Basically, this is a right-angle instrument that uses two monochromators (ExM and EmM), two PMT detectors (D1 and D2, the reference, and sample PMTs), and a xenon lamp source. The light from the exciter monochromator (ExM) is split, and a small portion (10%) is directed to the reference PMT (D1) for ratio-referencing purposes. The remaining excitation light is focused into the sample compartment. Emission optics are positioned at a right angle to the excitation optics. An emission monochromator (EmM) is used to select or scan the desired portion of the emission spectra, which is directed to the sample PMT (D2) for measurement of emission intensity. Output signals from the reference and sample PMTs are amplified (A1 and A2), and the ratio of the sample to the reference signal is provided by a digital display or a chart recorder. The operational mode of a ratio fluorometer is similar to that of a spectrofluorometer; however, only discrete excitation and emission wavelengths are available, and use of this type of instrument is precluded from scanning fluorophores to obtain emission and excitation spectra. The ratio filter fluorometer is most useful for obtaining concentration measurements at defined excitation and emission wavelengths.

The ratio-referencing spectrofluorometer is operated at fixed excitation and emission wavelength settings for concentration measurements; alternatively, it is used to measure the excitation or emission spectrum of a given compound. Measurement of the concentration of a specimen is accomplished in a similar manner as with a single-beam fluorometer. A blank and a calibrating solution are measured first; then the unknown specimens are measured (see Fig. 13.15).

Time-Resolved Fluorometer. The time-resolved fluorometer was introduced in the mid-1970s, when Weider developed a pulsed nitrogen laser fluorometer in conjunction with a lanthanide-based immunoassay system to measure the fluorescence decay of lanthanide chelates as a means of eliminating background interferences from light scatter and short decay time fluorescence compounds. The time-resolved fluorometer[4,13] is similar to the ratio-referencing fluorometer, with the exceptions that the light source is pulsed, and the detector monitors the exponential decay of the fluorescence signal after excitation in a fast photon-counting mode. Time-resolved fluorometry requires the use of long-lived fluorophores, such as the lanthanide (rare earth) metal ions europium (Eu^{3+}) and samarium (Sm^{3+}). Although most fluorescence compounds have decay times of 5 to 100 ns, Eu^{3+} chelates decay in 0.6 to 100 s. Thus, time-resolved fluorescence assays take advantage of the difference in lifetimes of fluorophore and background fluorescence by measuring the decaying fluorescence signal. This eliminates background interferences and at the same time averages the signal to improve the precision of measurement. Detection limits of approximately 10^{-13} mol/L can be achieved with time-resolved fluorometry; this is an improvement of approximately four orders of magnitude compared with conventional fluorometric measurements. For example, Eu^{3+}-labeled nanoparticles in combination with time-resolved fluorometry have been used to develop a highly sensitive immunoassay for free and

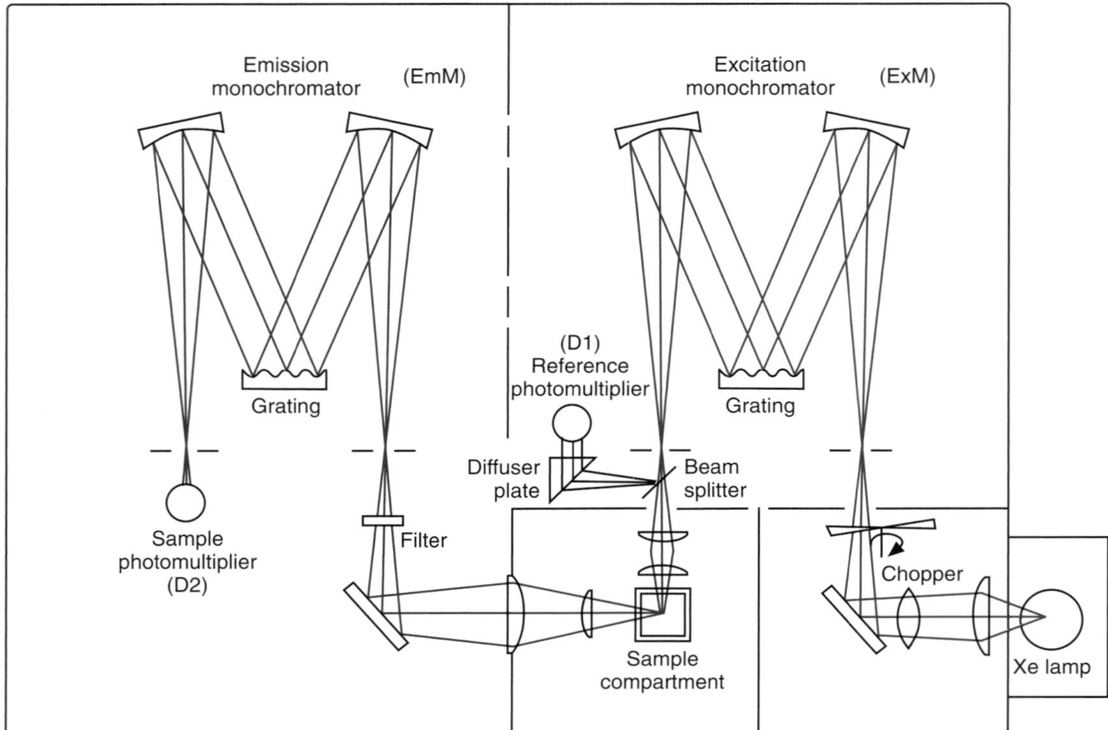

FIGURE 13.15 Diagram of a Typical Ratio-Referencing Spectrofluorometer. *Xe,* Xenon.

total prostate-specific antigen with a functional sensitivity of 0.5 ng/L.[14-16]

Flow Cytometer. Cytometry refers to the measurement of physical and/or chemical characteristics of cells, or by extension, of other biological particles. Flow cytometry is a process in which such measurements are made while cells or particles pass, preferably in single file, through the measuring apparatus in a fluid stream. Flow sorting extends flow cytometry by using electrical or mechanical means to divert and collect cells with one or more measured characteristics that fall within a range or ranges of values set by the user.[17,18]

Operationally, flow cytometry combines laser-induced fluorometry with particle light scattering analysis that allows different populations of molecules, cells, or particles to be differentiated by size and shape using low-light and right-angle light scattering. The use of a laser is ideally suited for low-angle light scattering. These cells, molecules, or particles are labeled with specific fluorescent labels, such as β-phycoerythrin, fluorescein isothiocyanate, rhodamine-6G, and other dye-labeled antibodies. As they move in a fluid stream through the flow cell, simultaneous fluorescence and light scattering measurements are automatically performed by the flow cytometer. Most flow cytometers incorporate two or more fluorescence emission detection systems, so that multiple fluorescent labels can be used. In this manner, molecules, cells, or particles can be classified by size, shape, and type according to their light scattering and fluorescent properties. A schematic diagram of a flow cytometer is shown in Fig. 13.16. An optical stop is placed in the 180° beam after the flow capillary to block the main laser beam and permit low-angle forward light scattering measurements. The 90° emission signal is split and directed to two PMTs to determine right-angle light scattering and detect at least two separate fluorescence emission signals. Two narrow bandpass interference filters (530 and 596 nm) are placed in front of the two 90° fluorescence emission PMTs. A computer with substantial resident software is used to reduce the acquired data to appropriate histograms for final result reporting. Cell-sorting electrodes are shown in the schematic drawing. Most commercial flow cytometers use one or more laser light sources. For example, the LSR II (BD Biosciences, Rockville, Maryland) can be equipped with 7 lasers (355 nm [UV], 405 nm [violet], 488 nm [blue], 532 nm [green], 594 nm [yellow], 638 nm [red], and 785 nm [IR]), which are used to simultaneously measure 18 emission spectra.

Flow cytometers are able to measure multiple parameters, including cell size (forward scatter), granularity (90° scatter), DNA content, RNA content, DNA (A + T)/(G + C) nucleotide ratios, chromatin structure, antigens, total protein content, cell receptors, membrane potential, and calcium ion concentration as a function of pH. These parameters are used in hematology, immunology (eg, in T-cell subsets, tissue typing, lymphocyte stimulation, and antigen antibody reactions), oncology (eg, in diagnosis, prognosis, and treatment monitoring), microbiology (eg, in bacterial identification and antibiotic sensitivity), virology (eg, viral particles), and genetics (eg, in karyotyping and carrier state detection) (for additional information on flow cytometry, refer to Chapter 25). Flow cytometry also has potential applications for the development of sensitive laser-induced fluoroimmunoassays. Phycoerythrin is a large phycobiliprotein molecule (molecular weight = 250,000 Da) with the fluorescence emission equivalent of 25 rhodamine-6G molecules, a quantum yield of 0.98, a broad emission spectrum of 530 to 630 nm, and low photodecomposition. It is an excellent label for cells and possibly for use in new fluoroimmunoassays.

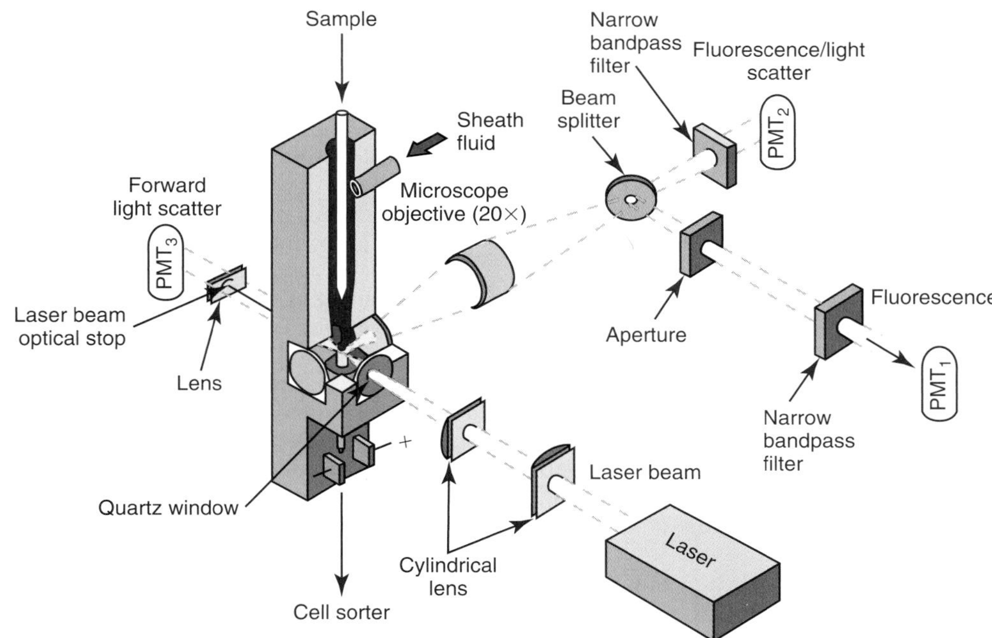

FIGURE 13.16 Schematic Diagram of a Flow Cytometer. *PMT*, Photomultiplier tube.

The development and use of particle-based flow cytometric assays should be noted. With this technology, a flow cytometer is combined with microspheres that are used as the solid support for conventional immunoassay, affinity assay, or DNA hybridization assay.[19] The microspheres are comprised of different proportions of two fluorescent dyes to generate 100 different signatures. Each of these signatures can be assigned to a specific analyte to multiplex 100 analytes in the same sample. The resultant system is flexible, and its use has led to the development of small volume assays that simultaneously assess a wide variety of analytes in the same sample.

Hematofluorometer. The hematofluorometer is a single-channel, front-surface photofluorometer dedicated to the analysis of zinc protoporphyrin in whole blood (see Chapter 39). A typical hematofluorometer uses a quartz-tungsten lamp, a narrow bandpass excitation filter (420 nm), front-surface optics, a narrow bandpass filter (594 nm), and a PMT. A drop of whole blood is placed on a small rectangular glass slide that serves as a cuvet. Zinc protoporphyrin analysis by a hematofluorometer is used for lead screening in adults and may have additional usefulness in screening for iron deficiency in pediatric populations.[20]

Limitations of Fluorescence Measurements

Factors that influence fluorescence measurements include concentration effects (eg, inner filter effects, concentration quenching), background effects (due to Rayleigh and Raman scattering), solvent effects (eg, interfering nonspecific fluorescence, quenching from the solvent), sample effects (eg, light scattering, interfering fluorescence, sample adsorption), temperature effects, and photodecomposition (bleaching) of the sample.

Inner Filter Effects

The linear relationship between concentration and fluorescence emission (Eq. 13.8) is valid when solutions that absorb less than 2% of the exciting light are used. As the absorbance of the solution increases above this amount, the relationship becomes nonlinear, a phenomenon known as the inner filter effect. It is caused by loss of excitation intensity across the cuvet path length as excitation light is absorbed by the fluorophore. Thus, as the fluorophore becomes more concentrated, absorbance of the excitation intensity increases, and loss of the excitation light as it travels through the cuvet increases. This effect is most often encountered with a right-angle fluorescence instrument, in which the emission slits are set to monitor the center of the sample cell, where absorbance of excitation light is greater than that at the front surface of the cuvet. Therefore, it is less problematic if a front-surface fluorescence instrument is used. However, most fluorescence measurements are made on dilute solutions, and therefore, the inner filter effect is not a problem.

Concentration Quenching

Another related phenomenon that results in a lower quantum yield than expected is called concentration quenching. This can occur when a macromolecule, such as an antibody, is heavily labeled with a fluorophore, such as fluorescein isothiocyanate. When this compound is excited, the fluorescence labels are in such close proximity that radiation-less energy transfer occurs. Thus, the resulting fluorescence is much lower than expected for the concentration of the label. This is a common problem in flow cytometry and laser-induced fluorescence when attempts are made to enhance detection sensitivity by increasing the density of the fluorescing label.

Light Scattering

Light scattering—Rayleigh and Raman—limits the use of fluorescence measurements. Rayleigh scattering occurs with no change in wavelength. For fluorophores with small Stokes shifts, the excitation and emission spectra overlap and are particularly susceptible to loss of sensitivity because of background light scatter. Rayleigh-type light scatter is controlled by using well-defined emission and excitation interference filters or by appropriate monochromator settings and the use of polarizers.

Raman scattering occurs with lengthening of a wavelength. This type of light scattering is independent of excitation wavelength and is a property of the solvent. Because Raman light scattering appears at longer wavelengths than the exciting radiation, it is a difficult interference to eliminate when working at very low fluorophore concentrations. As an example, the wavelength shift in water is approximately 50 nm at an excitation wavelength of 365 nm and approximately 75 nm at an excitation wavelength of 436 nm. This shift will represent a problem if the excitation maximum of a fluorophore is 365 nm, and the emission maximum is 415 nm. Raman light scattering is controlled by setting the excitation and emission wavelengths far enough apart to prevent the Raman scatter. It is also controlled by narrowing the slit width on the excitation monochromator. However, both options tend to decrease sensitivity.

Cuvet Material and Solvent Effects

Certain quartz glass and plastic materials that contain UV absorbers will fluoresce. Some solvents, such as ethanol, are also known to cause appreciable fluorescence. It is therefore important when developing a fluorescence assay to assess the background fluorescence of all components of the reaction mixture. Solvents and cuvets with minimal fluorescence emissions are commercially available; these reagents minimize background fluorescence problems.

Quenching by the solvent can be a problem and should be investigated when a new fluorometric method is established. Quenching is related to the interaction of the fluorophore with the solvent or with a solute dissolved in the solvent. Such interaction results in loss of fluorescence because of energy transfer or other mechanisms, but no effect on the absorbance spectrum of the fluorophore has been noted. Although unintended fluorescence quenching can be detrimental in fluorometric assays, fluorescence quenching has been used in assays for analytical measurements. In TaqMan DNA probes (Thermo Fisher Scientific Inc., Waltham, Massachusetts), a reporter fluorescent dye is linked to a nearby quencher fluorescent dye; in the presence of target DNA sequence, the quencher is separated from the reporter, which allows the reporter fluorescent dye to be detected (see Chapter 47). Quenching can be a useful tool for studying molecular structure, because fluorescence emission is sensitive to and specific for changes in atomic and molecular structure.

Sample Matrix Effects

A serum or urine sample contains many compounds that fluoresce. Thus, the sample matrix is a potential source of unwanted background fluorescence and must be examined when new methods are developed. The most serious contributors to unwanted fluorescence are proteins and bilirubin. However, because protein excitation maxima are in the spectral region of 260 to 290 nm, their contribution to overall background fluorescence is minor when excitation at more than 300 nm occurs.

Light scattering of proteins and other macromolecules in the sample matrix has been known to cause unwanted background signal. For example, lipemic samples are noted for their intense light scattering, and the relative contributions of lipids to the background signal of a fluorescence measurement should be investigated when setting up a new method.

In addition to background interferences, dilute solutions of some fluorophores in the concentration range of 10^{-9} mol/L or less will adsorb to the walls of glass cuvets and other reaction vessels. Also, dilute solutions of fluorophores, when excited over long periods of time, are susceptible to photodecomposition by intense excitation light. Operationally, these problems are avoided by selecting proper reaction vessels, adding wetting agents, and minimizing the length of time a sample is exposed to the excitation light.

Temperature Effects

The fluorescence quantum efficiency of many compounds is sensitive to temperature fluctuations. Therefore, the temperature of the reaction must be regulated to within ±0.1°C. In general, fluorescence intensity decreases with increasing temperature by approximately 1% to 5% per degree Celsius. Increased temperatures result in more frequent molecular collisions and quenching. Collisional quenching can be decreased by lowering the temperature or by increasing the viscosity.

Photodecomposition

In conventional fluorometry, excitation of weakly fluorescing or dilute solutions with intense light sources will cause photochemical decomposition of the analyte (photobleaching).

The following steps help to minimize photodecomposition effects:

1. Always use the longest feasible wavelength for excitation that does not introduce light scattering effects.
2. Decrease the duration of excitation of the sample by measuring the fluorescence intensity immediately after excitation.
3. Protect unstable solutions from ambient light by storing them in dark bottles.
4. Remove dissolved oxygen from the solution.

In addition, fluorescence-based assays for analytes at ultralow concentrations require optimization of laser intensity and use of a sensitive detector. Highly intense laser light sources with an energy output greater than 5 to 10 mW have higher sensitivity and are used in applications that have low concentrations of analyte, such as flow cytometry, fluorescence microscopy, and laser-induced fluorescence measurements. However, these intense light sources rapidly photodecompose some fluorescence analytes. This decomposition introduces nonlinear response curves and loss of most of the sample fluorescence. Thus, optimization of laser intensity balances higher sensitivity with increased photodecomposition.

PHOSPHORESCENCE

Phosphorescence is the luminescence produced by certain substances (eg, zinc sulfide) after radiant energy or other types of energy are absorbed. Phosphorescence is distinguished from fluorescence in that light emission results from the relaxation of molecules in an excited triplet electronic state, as opposed to an excited singlet electronic state in fluorescence emission. The decay time of emission of phosphorescence light is usually longer (10^{-4} to 10^{2} s) than the decay time of fluorescence emission because of the longer lifetime of molecules in an excited triplet state. Phosphorescence shows a larger shift in emitted light wavelength than that seen with fluorescence. There have been many proposed assay formats based on phosphorescence, but few of them are currently commercialized (see Chapter 14 and Chapter 23).

CHEMILUMINESCENCE, BIOLUMINESCENCE, AND ELECTROCHEMILUMINESCENCE

Chemiluminescence, bioluminescence, and electrochemiluminescence are types of luminescence in which the excitation event is caused by a chemical,[21] biochemical, or an electrochemical reaction, and not by photoillumination.

Basic Concepts

The physical event of light emission in chemiluminescence, bioluminescence, and electrochemiluminescence is similar to fluorescence in that it occurs from an excited singlet state, and light is emitted when the electron returns to the ground state.

Chemiluminescence and Bioluminescence

Chemiluminescence is the emission of light when an electron returns from an excited or higher energy level to a lower energy level. The excitation event is caused by a chemical reaction and involves the oxidation of an organic compound, such as luminol, isoluminol, acridinium esters, or luciferin, by an oxidant (eg, hydrogen peroxide, hypochlorite, oxygen); light is emitted from the excited product formed in the oxidation reaction. These reactions occur in the presence of catalysts, such as enzymes (eg, alkaline phosphatase, horseradish peroxidase), metal ions, or metal complexes (eg, hemin).[22,23]

Bioluminescence is a special form of chemiluminescence found in biological systems. In bioluminescence, an enzyme or a photoprotein increases the efficiency of the luminescence reaction. Luciferase and aequorin are two examples of these biological catalysts. The quantum yield (eg, total photons emitted per total molecules reacting) is approximately 0.1% to 10% for chemiluminescence, and typically, 10% to 30% for bioluminescence.

Chemiluminescence assays are ultrasensitive (attomole to zeptomole detection limits) and have wide dynamic ranges. They are now widely used in automated immunoassay and DNA probe assay systems (eg, acridinium ester and acridinium sulfonamide labels, 1,2-dioxetane substrates for alkaline phosphatase labels, enhanced luminol reaction for horseradish peroxidase labels [see Chapter 23]).

Electrochemiluminescence

Electrochemiluminescence differs from chemiluminescence in that the reactive species that produce the chemiluminescent reaction are electrochemically generated from stable precursors at the surface of an electrode.[24] A ruthenium, tris(bipyridyl) chelate is the most commonly used electrochemiluminescence label, and electrochemiluminescence is generated at an electrode via an oxidation reduction–type reaction with tripropylamine. This chelate is stable and relatively small, and has been used to label haptens or large molecules (eg, proteins, oligonucleotides). The electrochemiluminescence process has been used in both immunoassays and nucleic acid assays. Advantages of this process include (1) improved reagent stability, (2) simple reagent preparation, and (3) enhanced sensitivity. With its use, detection limits of 200 fmol/L and a dynamic range extending over six orders of magnitude can be obtained.

Instrumentation

Luminometers are instruments used to measure chemiluminescence and electrochemiluminescence.[22] Basic components are (1) the sample cell housed in a light-tight chamber, (2) the injection system used to add reagents to the sample cell, and (3) the detector. The detector is usually a PMT. However, CCD, x-ray film, or photographic film has been used to image chemiluminescence reactions on a membrane or in the wells of a microplate. For electrochemiluminescence, the reaction vessel incorporates an electrode, at which electrochemiluminescence is generated.

Limitations of Chemiluminescence and Electrochemiluminescence Measurements

Light leaks, light piping, and high background luminescence from assay reagents and reaction vessels (eg, plastic tubes exposed to light) are common factors that degrade analytical performance. The extreme sensitivity of chemiluminescence assays requires stringent controls on the purity of reagents and the solvents (eg, water) used to prepare reagent solutions. Efficient capture of light emission from reactions that produce a flash of light requires an efficient injector that provides adequate mixing when the triggering reagent is added to the reaction vessel. Chemiluminescent and electrochemiluminescent assays have a wide linear range that are usually several orders of magnitude, but high-intensity light emission can lead to pulse pile-up in PMTs, and this can lead to a serious underestimation of true light emission intensity.

POINTS TO REMEMBER

Radiant Energy in Analytical Measurements

- Fluorescence: light is absorbed by a molecule and subsequently emitted as light at a longer wavelength.
- Phosphorescence: light is absorbed by a molecule, but in contrast to fluorescence, the subsequently emitted light is from relaxation from an excited triplet state; compared with fluorescence, the emission time and wavelength of light are both much longer.
- Chemiluminescence: light is emitted as a result of chemical energy; no light is absorbed.
- Electrochemiluminescence: light is generated from precursor molecules at the surface of an electrode.

NEPHELOMETRY AND TURBIDIMETRY

Light scattering is a physical phenomenon that results from the interaction of light with particles in solution. Nephelometry and turbidimetry are analytical techniques used to measure scattered light. Light scattering measurements have been applied to immunoassays of specific proteins and haptens.

Basic Concepts

Light scattering occurs when radiant energy passing through a solution encounters a molecule in an elastic collision, which results in scattering of the light in all directions. Unlike fluorescence emission, the scattered light is of the same frequency as the incident light.

Factors that influence light scattering include effects of particle size, wavelength dependence, distance of observation, effects of polarization of incident light, concentration of the particles, and molecular weight of the particles.

Particle Size

The Rayleigh scattering equation (see next section) applies to the scattering of light from small particles with much smaller dimensions than the wavelength of incident light (eg, particle size less than $\lambda/10$). When the dimensions of the particles are much smaller than the wavelength of the incident light, each particle is subjected to the same electric field strength at the same time. Reradiated or scattered light waves from the small particle are in phase and reinforce each other. As the particles become larger than the incident light wave, radiated light waves are no longer all in phase. Reinforcement of radiation occurs in some directions, and destructive interference occurs in others. Scattering patterns from these large particles are characteristic of the size and shape of the particle.

Wavelength Dependence of Light Scattering

In 1871, Lord Rayleigh derived the following equation, which demonstrates the relationship of the intensity (I_S) of scattered light to the intensity (I_0) of incident light:

$$\frac{I_S}{I_0} = \frac{16\pi^2 a \sin^2\theta}{\lambda^4 r^2} \qquad \textbf{13.10}$$

where I_s = intensity of scattered light; I_0 = intensity of the excitation light; a = polarizability of the small particle; θ = angle of observation; λ = wavelength of incident light; *and* r = distance from light scattering to the detector.

As indicated, the intensity of light scattering is inversely proportional to the wavelength of the incident light. Another useful observation from Eq. 13.10 is the fact that scattered light intensity is also inversely proportional to the distance r from the light scattering particles to the detector. Thus, the detector should be located close to the analytical cell by the juxtaposition of the cell to the detector or by the use of good collection optics.

Concentration and Molecular Weight Factors in Light Scattering

The direct relationship of light scattering to the concentration of particles and to the molecular weight of particles is derived from Eq. 13.10, showing that

$$\frac{I_S}{I_0} = \frac{4\pi^2\left(\frac{dn}{dc}\right)^2 Mc\sin^2\theta}{N_a\lambda^4 r^2} \qquad \textbf{13.11}$$

where I_s = intensity of scattered light from small particles excited by polarized light; I_0 = incident intensity; dn/dc = change in refractive index of the solvent with respect to change in solute concentration; M = molecular weight (grams per mole); c = concentration (grams per milliliter) of the particles; θ = angle of observation; N_a = Avogadro's number; λ = wavelength of the incident light; and r = distance from light scattering to the detector.

The important observation to be made from Eq. 13.11 is the direct relationship of light scattering to the concentration and the molecular weight of particles.

Effects of Polarized Light on Light Scattering

Eqs. 13.10 and 13.11 are different forms of the Rayleigh expression for light scattering from small particles if excited by polarized light. Fig. 13.17A shows the effects of polarized and nonpolarized light on light scattering intensity from small particles as a function of the scattering angle. Polarized light generates scattering intensity diagrams shown by curves 1 and 2 as predicted by Eq. 13.10. Nonpolarized light results in the curve 3 intensity diagram and is the summation of curves 1 and 2. Curves 1 and 2 represent intensity diagrams from vertically and horizontally polarized light components that are considered to comprise nonpolarized light. The Rayleigh light scattering expression for small particles excited by nonpolarized light is given by Eq. 13.12:

$$\frac{I_S}{I_0} = \frac{2\pi^2\left(\frac{dn}{dc}\right)^2 Mc\,(1+\cos\theta)}{N_a\lambda^4 r^2} \qquad \textbf{13.12}$$

Two important observations can be made from Eq. 13.12 and Fig. 13.17A. First, the total light scattered by small particles is less when excited by polarized light than that by nonpolarized light, and reduction of background signal from

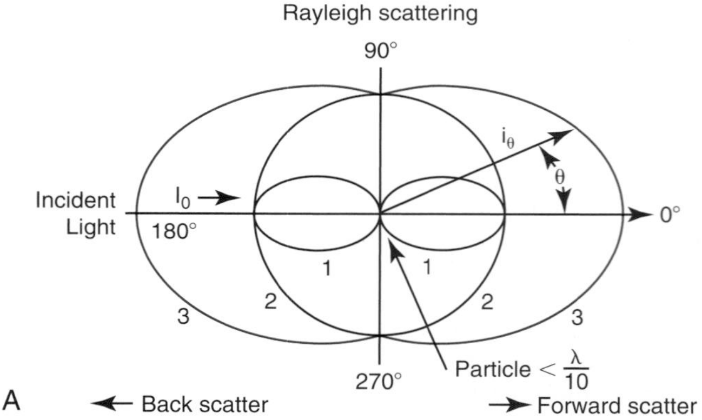

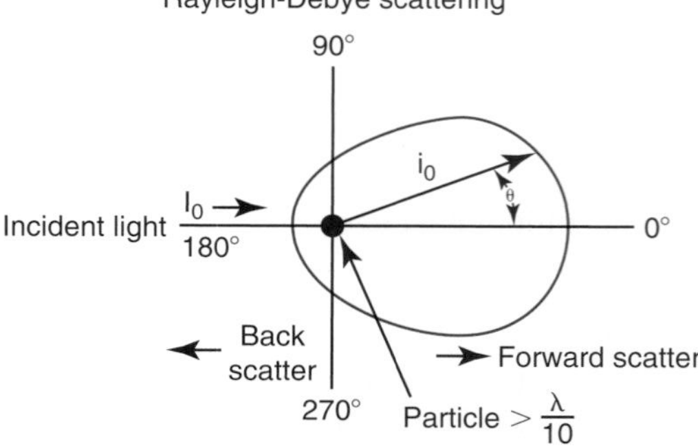

FIGURE 13.17 **Intensity of Scatter in Different Directions Under Different Particle Size Conditions Relative to the Wavelength of Light. A,** The angular dependence of light scattering intensity with nonpolarized and polarized incident light for small particles (*1, 2,* and *3*). **B,** The angular dependence of light scattering with nonpolarized light for larger particles.

light scattering in fluorescence measurements is achieved if an appropriately oriented polarizer is used in front of the emission detector. Second, light scattering intensity from small particles excited by nonpolarized light shows symmetric angular dependence of light scattering about the 90 degree axis (refer to Fig. 13.17A, curve 3).

Angular Dependence of Light Scattering

The angular dependence of light scattering from small particles (ie, less than λ/10), as indicated in the previous section, is represented by Fig. 13.17A. Examination of Fig. 13.17A (curve 3) shows that light scatter intensity values for forward scatter and back scatter (I_0 at 0 degree and 180 degrees) from small particles excited by nonpolarized light are equal. However, light scatter intensity at 90 degrees is much less. As particles become larger (eg, greater than λ/10), the angular dependence of light scatter takes on the dissymmetric relationship known as Rayleigh-Debye scattering (Fig. 13.17B). In this situation, light scattering intensities at forward and back angles are not equal; forward scatter intensity is much larger. Also, light scattering intensity at 90 degrees is much less than the intensity at the forward (0 degree) angle. As particles become even larger, this dissymmetry increases even further. This dissymmetry and the change in angular dependence of light scattering with change in the size of particles are very useful for characterization and differentiation of various classes of macromolecules and cells. As was previously mentioned, this property of light scattering is being used in the design of flow cytometers. These instruments measure near-forward light scattering and right-angle light scattering from cellular particles flowing through an optical cell and excited by a high-intensity laser. The ratio of near-forward light scattering intensity to right-angle light intensity is used in these instruments to distinguish among cell sizes.

Light Scattering and Plasma Proteins

The expression for light scattering given in Eq. 13.10 holds true in dilute solution for small particles if the largest dimension is less than one-tenth the wavelength of the incident light. Thus, the upper limit on the size of particles exhibiting Rayleigh scattering is approximately 40 nm when visible light is used at 400 nm. Many of the plasma proteins—such as immunoglobulins, β-lipoproteins, and albumin—are below this limit. For larger particles (approximately 40 to 400 nm), the angular dependence of the scattered light loses symmetry around the 90 degree axis, as seen in Fig. 13.17, and shows an increase in forward scattering. Some plasma proteins of the immunoglobulin-M class, chylomicrons, and aggregating immunoglobulin–antigen complexes fall into the size range described by Rayleigh-Debye scattering. Particles such as red blood cells and bacteria are larger yet (ie, 7000 to 40,000 nm). These particles show a complex angular dependence of light scattering, and this type of scattering from large particles is called Mie scattering. These large particles produce a predominance of scattered light in a narrow angular region in the forward direction.

Measurement of Scattered Light

Turbidimetry and nephelometry are methods used to measure scattered light. Such measurement has proven useful for the quantitation of serum proteins (see Chapter 28).

Turbidimetry

Because of the light scattering that occurs with turbidity, the intensity of light reaching the detector at 180 degrees is reduced. Measurement of this decrease in intensity is called turbidimetry. Analogous to absorption spectroscopy, turbidity is defined as follows:

$$I = I_0 e^{-bt} \quad \textbf{13.13}$$

or

$$t = \frac{1}{b} \ln \frac{I_0}{I} \quad \textbf{13.14}$$

where t = turbidity; b = path length of incident light through the solution of light scattering particles; I_S= intensity of transmitted light; and I_0 = intensity of incident light.

Turbidity is measured at 180 degrees from the incident beam, or more simply, in the same manner as absorbance measurements are made in a spectrophotometer. Turbidity can be measured on most spectrophotometers and automated clinical chemistry analyzers. The stability and resolution of modern microprocessor-driven spectrophotometers and photometers have greatly improved their ability to measure turbidity with accuracy and precision.

Nephelometry

Nephelometry is defined as the detection of light energy scattered or reflected toward a detector that is not in the direct path of the transmitted light.[25] Common nephelometers measure scattered light at right angles to the incident light. The ideal nephelometric instrument would be free of stray light, and neither light scatter nor any other signal would be seen by the detector when the solution in front of the detector is free from particles. However, because of stray light-generating components in the optical system and in the sample cuvet or the sample itself, a truly dark field situation is difficult to obtain when making nephelometric measurements. Some nephelometers are designed to measure scattered light at an angle other than 90 degrees to take advantage of the increased forward scatter intensity caused by light scattering from larger particles (eg, immune complexes).

Selection of Method

The choice between turbidimetry and nephelometry depends on the application and the available instrumentation. However, nephelometry still offers some advantage in terms of sensitivity when low-level antigen–antibody reactions are measured.

Instrumentation

Turbidimeters and nephelometers are used to measure the intensity of light scattering.

Turbidimeter

Turbidimetric measurements are easily performed on photometers or spectrophotometers and require little optimization. The principal concern of turbidimetric measurements is signal-to-noise ratio. Photometric systems with electro-optical noise in the range of ±0.0002 absorbance unit or less are useful for turbidity measurements.

Nephelometer

Although light scattering can be measured with standard analytical fluorometers or photometers, the angular dependence of light scattering intensity has resulted in the design of special nephelometers. These devices place the PMT detector at appropriate angles to the excitation light beam. The design principle of a nephelometer is similar to the design principle applied in fluorescence measurement. The major operational difference between the fluorometer and the nephelometer is that the excitation and detection wavelengths will be set to the same value when operating a nephelometer. The principal concerns of light scatter instrumentation include excitation intensity, wavelength, distance of the detector from the sample cuvet, and minimization of external stray light. As shown in Fig. 13.18, the basic components of a nephelometer include (1) a light source, (2) collimating optics, (3) a sample cell, and (4) collection optics, which include light scattering optics, a detector optical filter, and a detector. The schematic diagram also shows the different angles from the incident light beam where the detector, filter, and optics are placed to measure light scattering. Fig. 13.18 *a* shows the straight-through arrangement for turbidimetry, whereas Figs. 13.18 *b* and *c* show arrangements frequently found in nephelometers. The detector arrangement shown in Fig. 13.18 *b* is used for measurement of forward scatter at 30 degrees, which is the optical arrangement used with some commercial nephelometers.

Operationally, the optical components used in turbidimeters and nephelometers are similar to those used in fluorometers and photometers. For example, the light sources commonly used are quartz-halogen lamps, xenon lamps, and lasers. Helium-neon lasers, which operate at 633 nm, typically have been used for light scattering applications, such as nephelometric immunoassays, and particle size and shape determinations. The laser beam is used specifically in some nephelometers because of its high intensity; in addition, the coherent nature of laser light makes it ideally suited for nephelometric applications. In addition, ratio-referencing fluorometers are well suited for nephelometric measurements.

Limitations of Light Scattering Measurements

Antigen excess and matrix effects are limitations encountered in the use of turbidimeters and nephelometers for measurement of analytes of clinical interest.

Antigen Excess

Antigen–antibody reactions are complex and appear to result in a mixture of aggregate sizes. As turbidity increases during addition of antigen to antibodies, the signal increases to a maximum value and then decreases. The point at which the decrease begins marks the beginning of the phase of antigen excess; this phenomenon is explained in Chapter 23. Consequently, light scattering methods for quantitation of antigen–antibody reactions must provide a method for detecting antigen excess. The kinetics of immune complex formation measured by nephelometry or turbidimetry is sufficiently different in each of the three phases—antibody excess, equivalence, and antigen excess—that computer algorithms have been developed to flag antigen excess automatically.[25,26]

Matrix Effects

Particles, solvent, and all serum macromolecules scatter light. Lipoproteins and chylomicrons in lipemic serum provide the highest background turbidity or nephelometric intensity. With appropriate dilutions, the relative intensity of light scattering from a lipemic sample is less than that of the

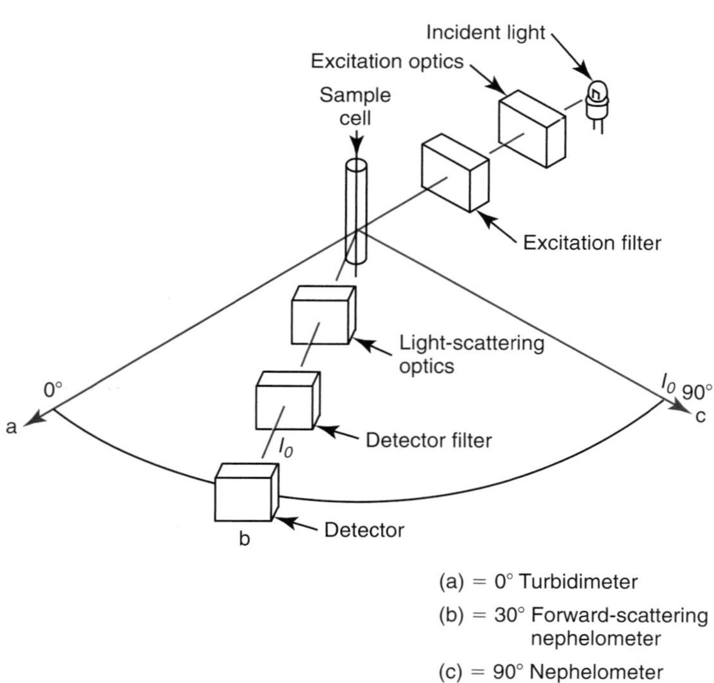

FIGURE 13.18 Schematic diagram of light scattering instrumentation showing *(a)* the optics position for a turbidimeter, *(b)* the optics position for a forward scattering nephelometer, and *(c)* the optics position for a right-angle nephelometer.

antiserum blank. However, as the concentration of the antigen in serum decreases and correspondingly less dilute samples are used, background interference from lipemic samples becomes greater. An effective method for minimizing this background interference is the use of rate measurements, in which the initial sample blank is eliminated. Large particles, such as suspended dust, also cause significant background interference. This background interference is controlled by filtering all buffers and diluted antisera before analysis is attempted.

POINTS TO REMEMBER

Light Scattering Assays

- Turbidity assays measure light scattering to determine the formation of antigen–antibody complexes.
- Interferences in light scattering include:
  - an excess of antigen decreases the turbidity
  - macromolecules, such as lipoproteins, chylomicrons, and dust in the sample matrix, which will increase the background turbidity
- Macromolecule interference in light scattering can be decreased by using rate measurements rather than directly assessing light scattering.

REFERENCES

1. Petersen JR, Okorodudu AO, Mohammad AA, et al. Association of transcutaneous bilirubin testing in hospital with decreased readmission rate for hyperbilirubinemia. *Clin Chem* 2005;**51**:540–4.
2. Slavin W. Atomic absorption spectroscopy: the present and future. *Anal Chem* 1982;**54**:685A–94A.
3. Heiftje GM, Vogelstein EE. A linear response theory approach to time-resolved fluorometry. In: Wehry EL, editor. *Modern fluorescence spectroscopy*, vol. 4. New York: Plenum Press; 1981. p. 25–50.
4. Diamandis E, Christopoulos TK. Europium chelate labels in time-resolved fluorescence immunoassays and DNA hybridization assays. *Anal Chem* 1990;**62**:1149A–57A.
5. Jolley ME, Stroupe SD, Schwenzer KS, et al. Fluorescence polarization immunoassay. III. An automated system for therapeutic drug determination. *Clin Chem* 1981;**27**:1575–9.
6. Bergh AA. Blue laser diode (LD) and light emitting diode (LED) applications. *Physica Status Solidi (a)* 2004;**201**: 2740–54.
7. World Health Organization. *Fluorescent light-emitting diode (LED) microscopy for diagnosis of tuberculosis*. Geneva, Switzerland: World Health Organization; 2011.
8. Visser BJ, Meerveld-Gerrits J, Kroo D, et al. Assessing the quality of anti-malarial drugs from Gabonese pharmacies using the MiniLab: a field study. *Malar J* 2015;**14**:273.
9. Epperson PM, Sweedler JV, Billhorn RB, et al. Applications of charge transfer devices in spectroscopy. *Anal Chem* 1988;**60**: 327A–35A.
10. Sweedler JV, Billhorn RB, Epperson PM, et al. High performance charge transfer devices. *Anal Chem* 1988;**60**: 282A–91A.
11. Masters BR, Kino GS. Charge coupled devices for quantitative Nipkow Disk real-time scanning confocal microscopy. In: Shotton D, editor. *Electron light microscopy: the principles and practice of video-enhanced contrast, digital intensified fluorescence, and confocal scanning light microscopy*. New York: Wiley-Liss; 1993.
12. Vukojevic V, Heidkamp M, Ming Y, et al. Quantitative single-molecule imaging by confocal laser scanning microscopy. *Proc Natl Acad Sci USA* 2008;**104**:18176–81.
13. Soini E, Kojola H. Time-resolved fluorometer for lanthanide chelates: a new generation of nonisotopic immunoassays. *Clin Chem* 1983;**29**:65–8.
14. Harma H, Soukka T, Lovgren T. Europium nanoparticles and time-resolved fluorescence for ultrasensitive detection of prostate-specific antigen. *Clin Chem* 2001;**47**:561–8.
15. Soukka T, Paukkunen J, Harma H, et al. Supersensitive time-resolved immunofluorometric assay of free prostate-specific antigen with nanoparticle label technology. *Clin Chem* 2001;**47**:1269–78.
16. Soukka T, Antonen K, Harma H, et al. Highly sensitive immunoassay of free prostate-specific antigen in serum using europium(III) nanoparticle label technology. *Clin Chim Acta* 2003;**328**:45–8.
17. Patrick CW. Clinical flow cytometry: milestones along the pathway of progress. *MLO Med Lab Obs* 2002;**34**:10–11, 14–16.
18. Shapiro HM. *Practical flow cytometry*. 4th ed. Hoboken, NJ: John Wiley & Sons; 2003.
19. Vignali DA. Multiplexed particle-based flow cytometric assays. *J Immunol Methods* 2000;**243**:243–55.
20. Magge H, Sprinz P, Adams WG, et al. Zinc protoporphyrin and iron deficiency screening. *JAMA Pediatr* 2013;**167**: 361–7.
21. Rodríguez-Orozco AR, Ruiz-Reyes H, Medina-Serriteño N. Recent applications of chemiluminescence assays in clinical immunology. *Mini Rev Med Chem* 2010;**10**:1393–400.
22. DeLuca M, McElroy WD. Bioluminescence and chemiluminescence, part B. In: *Methods in enzymology*, vol. 133. San Diego, CA: Academic Press; 1986.
23. Ziegler MM, Baldwin TO, editors. Bioluminescence and chemiluminescence, part C. In: *Methods in enzymology*, vol. 305. San Diego, CA: Academic Press; 2000.
24. Blackburn GF, Shah HP, Kenten JH, et al. Electrochemiluminescence detection for development of immunoassays and DNA probe assays for clinical diagnostics. *Clin Chem* 1991;**37**:1534–9.
25. Hills LP, Tiffany TO. Comparison of turbidimetric and light scattering measurements of immunoglobulins by use of a centrifugal analyzer with absorbance and fluorescence light scattering optics. *Clin Chem* 1980;**26**:1459–66.
26. Sternberg J. A rate nephelometer for measuring specific proteins by immunoprecipitin reactions. *Clin Chem* 1977;**25**: 1456–64.

14

Electrochemistry and Chemical Sensors

*Paul D'Orazio**

ABSTRACT

Background

Chemical sensors, which are primarily based on electrochemical and optical measurements, have been firmly established as analytical tools in clinical chemistry, especially for measurement of critical care analytes (blood gases, electrolytes, metabolites) directly in whole blood. Coupling transducers to biological recognition elements for construction of biosensors is expanding the role of chemical sensors for measurement of analytes without direct electrochemical or optical activity.

Content

This chapter reviews fundamental aspects of electrochemical and optical measurements and their application in practical systems for measurements of blood gases (pH, partial pressure of oxygen [PO_2], partial pressure of carbon dioxide [PCO_2]) and electrolytes (sodium [Na^+], potassium [K^+], calcium [Ca^{2+}], chloride [Cl^-], magnesium [Mg^{2+}], lithium [Li^+]) directly in whole blood. The same electrochemical and optical sensors are applied as building blocks for enzyme-based biosensors for measurement of important metabolites directly in whole blood (glucose, lactate, urea, creatinine), which are ideally suited as measurement technologies in systems for point-of-care testing. Affinity sensors are expanding the role of biological recognition elements in biosensors to include antibodies, nucleic acids, and aptamers. These molecules, when coupled to electrochemical, optical, and other transducers, produce biosensors for sensitive detection of biomarkers for cancer, cardiac disease, and DNA analysis. Although there are few practical embodiments for affinity sensors, key research points to future possibilities. This chapter discusses nanotechnology to further enhance sensitivity of biosensors. The same sensor technologies applied successfully for in vitro measurements of important critical care analytes (blood gases, glucose) are being adapted for in vivo and minimally invasive measurements, including solutions to problems such as biocompatibility and calibration stability.

INTRODUCTION

Electrochemical and optical sensors (and associated biosensors) are firmly established in clinical analysis systems. Sensors for measurement of blood gases, electrolytes, and metabolites are particularly well suited for incorporation into automated, point-of-care, and critical care analyzers (see Chapters 26, 27, and 35, respectively), because of their ease of use, low maintenance, and ability to measure clinically important analytes in undiluted blood.[1] When integrated into chromatographic systems (see Chapter 16), electrochemical detectors provide a highly sensitive and selective means of detecting a variety of other analytes, such as therapeutic drugs, neurotransmitters, glutathione, and homocysteine. Electrochemical detection has also been applied successfully for monitoring coagulation reactions, detecting toxic lead in blood samples, and developing novel ultrasensitive immunoassays. When bioelements are integrated with electrodes, the resultant biosensors further expand the analytical capabilities of such devices. In addition, the development and application of *optodes,* which are based on some of the same selective chemistries used in electrochemical devices, have resulted in another analytical tool for measuring blood gases and electrolytes.

In this chapter, the fundamental electrochemical principles of (1) potentiometry, (2) voltammetry and/or amperometry, (3) conductance, and (4) coulometry are summarized, and their clinical applications are presented. Optodes and biosensors are also discussed. The chapter concludes with a discussion of in vivo and minimally invasive sensors.

POTENTIOMETRY AND ION-SELECTIVE ELECTRODES

Potentiometry is widely used clinically for the measurement of pH, PCO_2, and electrolytes (Na^+, K^+, Cl^-, Ca^{2+}, Mg^{2+}, Li^+) in whole blood, serum, plasma, and urine, and as the basis for some biosensors for metabolites of clinical interest.

Basic Concepts

Potentiometry is the measurement of an electrical potential difference between two electrodes (half-cells) in an electrochemical cell (Fig. 14.1) when the cell current is zero (galvanic cell). Such a cell consists of two electrodes (electron and metallic conductors) that are connected by an electrolyte solution (ion conductor). An electrode, or half-cell, consists of a single metallic conductor that is in contact with an

*The author gratefully acknowledges the contributions of Drs. Richard A. Durst, Ole Siggard-Andersen, and Mark E. Meyerhoff to earlier versions of this chapter.

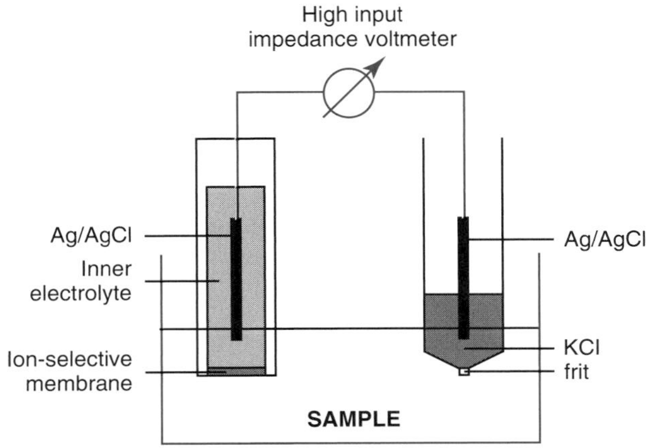

FIGURE 14.1 Schematic of Ion-Selective Membrane Electrode–Based Potentiometric Cell. *Ag/AgCl,* Silver-silver chloride; *KCl,* potassium chloride.

electrolyte solution. Ion conductors are composed of one or more phases that are either in direct contact with each other or separated by membranes permeable only to specific cations or anions (see Fig. 14.1). One of the electrolyte solutions is the unknown or test solution; this solution may be replaced by an appropriate reference solution for calibration purposes. By convention, the cell notation is shown so that the left electrode (M_L) is the reference electrode, and the right electrode (M_R) is the indicator (measuring) electrode (see Eq. 3).[2]

The electromotive force (*E* or EMF) is defined as the maximum difference in potential between the two electrodes (right minus left) obtained when the cell current is zero. The cell potential is measured using a potentiometer, of which the common pH meter is a special type. The direct-reading potentiometer is a voltmeter that measures the potential across the cell (between the two electrodes); however, to obtain an accurate potential measurement, it is necessary that no current flow through the cell. This is accomplished by incorporating high resistance within the voltmeter (input impedance greater than 10^{12} Ω). Modern direct-reading potentiometers are accurate and can be modified to provide direct digital displays or printouts.

Within any one conductive phase, the potential is constant as long as the current flow is zero. However, a potential difference arises between two different phases in contact with each other. The overall potential of an electrochemical cell is the sum of all potential gradients that exist between different phases of the cell. The potential of a single electrode with respect to the surrounding electrolyte and the absolute magnitude of the individual potential gradients between phases are unknown and cannot be measured. Only potential differences between two electrodes (half-cells) can be measured. Potential gradients can be classified as (1) redox potentials, (2) membrane potentials, or (3) diffusion potentials. Generally, it is possible to devise a cell in such a manner that all potential gradients except one are constant. This potential then can be related to the activity of a specific ion of interest (eg, hydrogen [H^+] or Na^+).

Types of Electrodes

Many different types of electrodes are used for potentiometric applications. They include redox, ion-selective membrane (glass and polymer), and PCO_2 electrodes.

Redox Electrodes

Redox potentials are the result of chemical equilibria involving electron transfer reactions:

$$\text{Oxidized form (Ox)} + ne^- \leftrightarrow \text{Reduced form (Red)} \quad \textbf{(1)}$$

where n = the number of electrons involved in the reaction. Any substance that accepts electrons is an oxidant (Ox), and any substance that donates electrons is a reductant (Red). The two forms, Ox and Red, represent a redox couple (conjugate redox pair). Usually, homogeneous redox processes take place only between two redox couples. In such cases, electrons are transferred from Red_1 to an Ox_2. In this process, Red_1 is oxidized to its conjugate Ox_1, whereas Ox_2 is reduced to Red_2:

$$\text{Red}_1 + \text{Ox}_2 \leftrightarrow \text{Ox}_1 + \text{Red}_2 \quad \textbf{(2)}$$

In an electrochemical cell, electrons may be accepted from or donated to an inert metallic conductor (eg, platinum [Pt]). A reduction process tends to charge the electrode positively (remove electrons), and an oxidation process tends to charge the electrode negatively (add electrons). By convention, a heterogeneous redox equilibrium (Eq. 2) is represented by the cell:

$$M_L|\text{Red}_1 - \text{Ox}_1 :: \text{Ox}_2 - \text{Red}_2|M_R \quad \textbf{(3)}$$

A positive potential ($E > 0$) for this cell signifies that the cell reaction proceeds spontaneously from left to right; $E < 0$ signifies that the reaction proceeds from right to left, and $E = 0$ indicates that the two redox couples are at mutual equilibrium.

The electrode potential (reduction potential) for a redox couple is defined as the couple's potential measured with respect to the standard H_2 electrode, which is set equal to zero (see later discussion of the H_2 electrode). This potential, by convention, is the electromotive force of a cell, where the standard H_2 electrode is the reference electrode (left electrode) and the given half-cell is the indicator electrode (right electrode). The reduction potential for a given redox couple is shown by the Nernst equation:

$$E = E^0 - \frac{N}{n} \times \log\frac{a\text{Red}}{a\text{Ox}} = E^0 - \frac{0.0592\text{V}}{n} \times \log\frac{a\text{Red}}{a\text{Ox}} \quad \textbf{(4)}$$

where E = electrode potential of the half-cell; E^0 = standard electrode potential when $a_{Red}/a_{Ox} = 1$; n = number of electrons involved in the reduction reaction; $N = (R \times T \times \ln 10)/F$ (the Nernst factor if $n = 1$); $N = 0.0592$ V if $T = 298.15$ K (25°C); $N = 0.0615$ V if $T = 310.15$ K (37°C); R = gas constant (= 8.31431 J × K^{-1} × mol^{-1}); T = absolute temperature (in kelvins); F = Faraday constant (= 96,487 Coulombs × mol^{-1}); ln 10 = natural logarithm of 10 = 2.303; a = activity; and aRed/aOx = product of mass action for the reduction reaction.

Redox electrodes currently in use include (1) inert metal electrodes immersed in solutions containing redox couples and (2) metal electrodes whose metal functions as a member of the redox couple.

Inert Metal Electrodes. Platinum and gold (Au) are examples of inert metals used to record the redox potential of a redox couple dissolved in an electrolyte solution. The H_2

electrode is a special redox electrode for pH measurement. It consists of a Pt or Au electrode that is electrolytically coated (platinized) with highly porous Pt (Pt black) to catalyze the electrode reaction:

$$H^+ + e^- \leftrightarrow \frac{1}{2}H_2 \quad (5)$$

The electrode potential is given by

$$E = E^0 - N \times \log\frac{(fH_2)^{1/2}}{aH^+} \quad (6)$$

or

$$E = E^0 - N \times [\log(fH_2)^{1/2} - \log aH^+] \quad (7)$$

where $E^0 = 0$ at all temperatures (by convention); fH_2 = fugacity of H_2 gas; aH^+ = activity of H^+ ions; and $-\log aH^+$ = negative log of H^+ activity (paH^+ or pH).

When the partial pressure of H_2 (PH_2) in the solution (and hence, fH_2) is maintained constant by bubbling H_2 through the solution, the potential is a linear function of log aH^+ (= −pH). In the standard H_2 electrode, the electrolyte consists of an aqueous solution of HCl with aHCl equal to 1.000 (or cHCl = 1.2 mol/L) in equilibrium with a gas phase, and with fH_2 equal to 1.000 (or PH_2 = 101.3 kPa = 1 atm). The standard H_2 electrode is also used as a reference electrode.

Metal Electrodes Participating in Redox Reactions. The silver-silver chloride (Ag/AgCl) electrode is an example of a metal electrode that participates as a member of a redox couple. The Ag/AgCl electrode consists of a Ag wire or rod coated with $AgCl_{(solid)}$ in contact with a Cl^- solution of constant activity; this sets the half-cell potential. The Ag/AgCl electrode is itself considered a potentiometric electrode because its phase boundary potential is governed by an oxidation-reduction electron transfer equilibrium reaction that occurs at the surface of Ag:

$$AgCl_{(solid)} + e^- \leftrightarrow Ag^{\circ}_{(solid)} + Cl^- \quad (8)$$

The Nernst equation for the reference half-cell potential of an Ag/AgCl reference electrode is written as follows:

$$E_{Ag/AgCl} = E^0_{Ag/AgCl} + \frac{RT}{nF} \times \ln\frac{a_{AgCl}}{a_{Ag}a_{Cl-}} \quad (9)$$

Because AgCl and Ag are both solids, their activities are equal to unity ($a_{AgCl} = a^0_{Ag} = 1$). Therefore, from Eq. 9, the half-cell potential is controlled by the activity of the Cl^- ion in solution (a_{Cl-}) contacting the electrode.

The Ag/AgCl electrode is used both as an internal reference element in potentiometric ion-selective electrodes (ISEs) and as an external reference electrode half-cell of constant potential, which is required to complete a potentiometric cell (see Fig. 14.1). In both cases, the Ag/AgCl electrode must be in equilibrium with a solution of constant Cl^- ion activity.

The Ag/AgCl element of the external reference electrode half-cell is in contact with a high-concentration solution of a soluble Cl^- salt. Saturated KCl is commonly used. A porous membrane or frit is frequently employed to separate the concentrated KCl from the sample solution. The frit serves both as a mechanical barrier to hold the concentrated electrolyte within the electrode and as a diffusional barrier to prevent proteins and other species in the sample from coming into contact with the internal Ag/AgCl element, which could poison and alter its potential. The interface between two dissimilar electrolytes (concentrated KCl/calibrator or sample) occurs within the frit and develops the liquid–liquid junction potential (E_j), a source of error in potentiometric measurements. The difference in E_j between the calibrator and sample (residual liquid junction potential) is responsible for this error and can be minimized and usually neglected in practice if the compositions of the calibrating solutions are matched as closely as possible to the sample with respect to ionic content and ionic strength. An equitransferant electrolyte at high concentration as the reference electrolyte further helps to minimize the residual liquid junction potential. KCl at a concentration 2 mol/L or more is preferred. Differences of approximately −2% in the measurement of sodium by ISEs have been demonstrated when the KCl concentration in the reference electrolyte is lowered from 3 to 0.5 mol/L.[3] The magnitude of the residual liquid junction potential may also be estimated by the Henderson equation[4] with sufficient knowledge of ionic activities, ionic charges, and ionic mobilities for each electrolyte on both sides of the junction and the temperature. Using this estimate, a correction to the overall cell potential may be applied.

The presence of erythrocytes in the sample may affect the magnitude of the residual liquid junction potential in a less predictable manner. For example, erythrocytes in blood of normal hematocrit are estimated to produce approximately 1.8 mmol/L positive error in the measurement of Na by ISEs when an open, unrestricted liquid–liquid junction is used.[5] This bias may be minimized if a restrictive membrane or frit is used to modify the liquid–liquid junction.

The saturated calomel electrode is another example of a metal electrode that participates as a member of a redox couple. The calomel electrode consists of mercury (Hg) covered by a layer of relatively insoluble calomel (Hg_2Cl_2) (or present as insoluble salt dispersed in the electrolyte), which is in contact with an electrolyte solution containing Cl^-. The oxidation-reduction equilibrium reaction is as shown:

$$Hg_2Cl_2 + 2e^- \leftrightarrow 2Hg^{\circ} + 2Cl^- \quad (10)$$

As with the Ag/AgCl electrode, the half-cell potential is controlled by the activity of Cl^- ion contacting the electrode. Calomel electrodes are frequently used as reference electrodes for pH measurements using glass pH electrodes, but are not commonly used in clinical instrumentation using electrochemical sensors.

Ion-Selective Electrodes

Membrane potentials are caused by the permeability of certain types of membranes to selected anions or cations. Such membranes are used to fabricate ISEs that selectively interact with a single ionic species. The potential produced at the membrane–sample solution interface is proportional to the logarithm of the ionic activity or concentration of the ion in question. Measurements with ISEs are simple, often rapid, nondestructive, and applicable to a wide range of concentrations.

The ion-selective membrane is the "heart" of an ISE because it controls the selectivity of the electrode. Ion-selective membranes are typically composed of glass, crystalline, or polymeric materials. The chemical composition of the membrane is designed to achieve an optimal permselectivity toward the ion of interest. In practice, other ions exhibit finite interaction with membrane sites and display some degree of interference for determination of an analyte ion. In clinical practice, if the interference exceeds an acceptable quantity, a correction is required.

The Nicolsky-Eisenman equation describes the selectivity of an ISE for the ion of interest over interfering ions:

$$E = E^0 + \left[\frac{2.303\,RT}{z_i F}\right]\log\left(a_i + \sum K_{i/j}\, a_j^{z_i/z_j}\right) \tag{11}$$

where a_i = activity of the ion of interest; a_j = activity of the interfering ion; and $K_{i/j}$ = selectivity coefficient for the primary ion over the interfering ion. Low values indicate good selectivity for the analyte i over the interfering ion j; z_i = charge of the primary ion; and z_j = charge of the interfering ion.

All other terms are identical to those in the Nernst equation (Eq. 4).

Various approaches may be used to determine the selectivity of an ISE for a primary ion over an interfering ion.[6,7] A straightforward approach is the separate solution method, in which the potential of an ISE is determined in solutions of the primary and interfering ions separately, but at equal ionic activities. The selectivity coefficient is then calculated as follows:

$$\log K_{ij} = \frac{E_j - E_i}{\dfrac{2.303\,RT}{nF}} + \left(1 - \frac{z_i}{z_j}\right)\log a_i \tag{12}$$

An alternate approach to determine selectivity coefficient is the fixed interference method, in which the potential response of an ISE to the primary ion is determined in solutions of constant activity of the interfering ion. The potential values obtained are plotted versus the logarithm of the activity of the primary ion a_i. The intersection of the extrapolation of the linear portions of this plot indicates the value of a_i to be used to calculate $K_{i/j}$:

$$K_{i/j} = a_i / a_j^{z_i/z_j} \tag{13}$$

where all terms have the same definition as in Eq. 12. Traditionally, the fixed interference method has been preferred because it more closely resembles a practical application of the sensor, in that primary and interfering ions are present simultaneously in solution and must compete for complexation sites in the ISE membrane.

Most ISEs used in clinical practice have sufficient selectivity and do not require correction for interfering ions. Oesch and colleagues[8] have published required ISE selectivity coefficients for ions commonly measured in clinical chemistry over other ions found in blood. Table 14.1 shows required selectivity coefficients for the measurement of cations of interest in clinical chemistry over potentially interfering cations, assuming an acceptable maximum interference of 1% for the ion of interest.

TABLE 14.1 Required Selectivities for Cation-Selective Ion-Selective Electrodes for Whole Blood, Plasma, and Serum Measurements

Primary Ion (i)	REQUIRED SELECTIVITY COEFFICIENT ($LOGK_{I/J}$) FOR INTERFERING CATION (J)					
	H^+	Li^+	Na^+	K^+	Mg^{2+}	Ca^{2+}
H^+	—	−6.5	−8.5	−7.0	−7.7	−7.7
Li^+*	2.1	—	−4.3	−2.8	−3.5	−3.6
Na^+	4.4	−0.1	—	−0.6	−1.2	−1.3
K^+	2.8	−1.7	−3.6	—	−2.8	−2.9
Mg^{2+}	8.9	0.1	−3.9	−0.9	—	−2.4
Ca^{2+}	9.3	0.4	−3.6	−0.6	−1.9	—

*Assumes a therapeutic range for Li^+ between 0.7 and 1.5 mmol/L.
Ca, Calcium; *H*, hydrogen; *K*, potassium; *Li*, lithium; *Mg*, magnesium; *Na*, sodium.

Glass membrane and polymer membrane electrodes are two types of ISEs that are commonly used in clinical chemistry applications.

The Glass Electrode. Glass membrane electrodes are used to measure pH and Na^+, and as an internal transducer for PCO_2 sensors. The H^+ response of thin glass membranes was first demonstrated in 1906 by Cremer.[9] In the 1930s, practical application of this phenomenon for measurement of acidity in lemon juice was made possible by the invention of the pH meter by Beckman.[2] Glass electrode membranes are formulated from melts of silicon and/or aluminum oxide (Al_2O_3) mixed with oxides of alkaline earth or alkali metal cations. By varying the glass composition, electrodes with selectivity for H^+, Na^+, K^+, Li^+, rubidium (Rb^+), cesium (Cs^+), Ag^+, thallium (Tl^+), and ammonium (NH_4^+) have been demonstrated.[10] However, glass electrodes for H^+ and Na^+ are currently the only types with sufficient selectivity over interfering ions to allow practical application in clinical chemistry. A typical formulation for H^+ selective glass is 72% silicon dioxide (SiO_2), 22% Na_2O, and 6% calcium oxide (CaO), which has a selectivity order of $H^+ \ggg Na^+ > K^+$. This glass membrane has sufficient selectivity for H^+ over Na^+ to allow error-free measurements of pH in the range of 7.0 to 8.0 ($[H^+] = 10^{-7}$ to 10^{-8} mol/L) in the presence of >0.1 mol/L Na^+. Glass pH electrodes with selectivity coefficients ($K_{H/Na}$) over Na^+ of 10^{-7} and better have been realized. By altering the formulation of the glass membrane slightly to 71% SiO_2, 11% Na_2O, and 18% Al_2O_3, its selectivity order becomes $H^+ > Na^+ > K^+$. Thus, the preference of the glass membrane for H^+ over Na^+ is greatly reduced, resulting in a practical sensor for Na^+ at pH values typically found in blood.[11]

Polymer Membrane Electrodes. Polymer membrane ISEs are used for monitoring pH and for measuring electrolytes, including K^+, Na^+, Cl^-, Ca^{2+}, Li^+, Mg^{2+}, and carbonate (CO_3^{2-}) (for total CO_2 measurements). They are the predominant class of potentiometric electrodes used in modern clinical analysis instruments.

Mechanisms of response of these ISEs fall into three categories: (1) charged, dissociated ion exchanger; (2) charged associated carrier; and (3) neutral ion carrier (ionophore).[12,13] An early charged-associated, ion-exchanger type ISE for Ca^{2+}

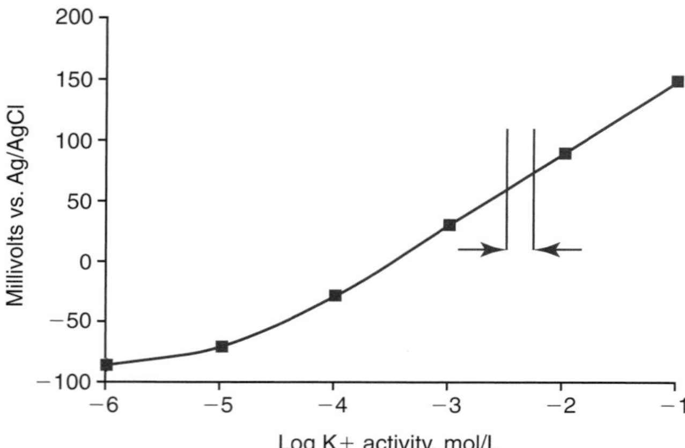

FIGURE 14.2 Typical Electromotive Force (EMF) Response of Potassium (K^+) Selective Membrane Electrode to Changes in Activity of K^+ in the Sample Solution. Bracketed interval represents the normal reference interval of K^+ concentration in blood. *Ag/AgCl,* Silver-silver chloride. (From D'Orazio P. In: Lewendrowski K, editor. Clinical chemistry: laboratory management and clinical correlations. Philadelphia: Lippincott, Williams and Wilkins, 2002:455.)

was developed and commercialized for clinical application in the 1960s based on the Ca^{2+}-selective, ion-exchange/complexation properties of 2-ethylhexyl phosphoric acid dissolved in dioctyl phenyl phosphonate.[14] A porous membrane was impregnated with this cocktail and mounted at the end of an electrode body. This type of sensor was referred to as the "liquid membrane" ISE. Later, a method was devised in which these ingredients could be cast into a plasticized poly(vinyl Cl) (PVC) membrane that was more rugged and convenient to use. This same approach is still used today to formulate PVC-based ISEs for clinical use.[15]

A major breakthrough in the development and routine application of PVC-type ISEs was the discovery by Simon and colleagues that the neutral antibiotic valinomycin could be incorporated into organic liquid membranes (and later plasticized PVC membranes), resulting in a sensor with high selectivity for K^+ over Na^+ ($K_{K/Na} = 2.5 \times 10^{-4}$).[16] The K^+ ISE based on valinomycin was the first example of a neutral carrier ISE and is used extensively today for the routine measurement of K^+ in blood. Fig. 14.2 shows the response of the valinomycin-based K^+ ISE in the presence of physiologic concentrations of Na^+, Ca^{2+}, and Mg^{2+}. The wide linear range and excellent selectivity of this ISE over three orders of magnitude makes it suitable for the measurement of K^+ in blood and urine. The K^+ range in blood is only a small portion of the electrode linear range and is spanned by a total ΔEMF of approximately 9 mV. Interference from other cations, which is seen as deviation from linearity, is not apparent at K^+ activities more than 10^{-4} mol/L. Other, less selective polymer-based ISEs (eg, for the measurement of Mg^{2+} and Li^+) are subject to interference from Ca^{2+} and Na^+ and Na^+, respectively, requiring simultaneous determination and correction for the presence of significant concentrations of these interfering ions.[17,18]

Studies regarding the relationship between molecular structure and ionic selectivity have resulted in the development of polymer-based ISEs using a number of naturally occurring and synthetic ionophores, with sufficient selectivity for application in clinical analysis. The chemical structures of several of these neutral ionophores are illustrated in Fig. 14.3.

Dissociated anion exchanger-based electrodes using lipophilic quaternary NH_4^+ salts as active membrane components are still used commercially for the determination of Cl^- in whole blood, serum, and plasma, despite some limitations.[19] Selectivity for this type of ISE is controlled by extraction of the ion into the organic membrane phase and is a function of the lipophilic character of the ion (because, unlike the carriers described earlier, no direct binding interaction occurs between the exchanger site and the anion in the membrane phase). Thus, the selectivity order for a Cl^- ISE based on an anion exchanger is fixed as lipophilic anion R^- > perchlorate (ClO_4^-) > iodide (I^-) > nitrate (NO_3^-) > bromide (Br^-) > Cl^- > fluoride (F^-), where R^- represents anions with greater lipophilic character than ClO_4^-. Application of the Cl^- ion-exchange electrode is therefore limited to samples without significant concentrations of anions more lipophilic than Cl^-. For example, blood samples containing salicylate or thiocyanate will produce positive interference for the measurement of Cl^-. Repeated exposure of the electrode to the anticoagulant heparin will lead to loss of electrode sensitivity toward Cl^- because of the extraction of negatively charged heparin into the membrane. This extraction process has been used successfully to devise a method to detect heparin concentrations in blood by potentiometry[20] and to develop a simple potentiometric technique to screen for the presence of toxic, high-charge density polyanion contaminants (eg, oversulfated chondroitin sulfate) in biomedical-grade heparin preparations.[21]

High selectivity for the CO_3^{2-} anion can be achieved using a neutral carrier ionophore that possesses trifluoroacetophenone groups doped within a polymeric membrane.[22,23] Such ionophores form negatively charged adducts with CO_3^{2-} anions, and the resulting electrodes have proven useful in commercial instruments for determination of total CO_2 in serum and/or plasma, after dilution of the blood to a pH value in the range of 8.5 to 9.0, where a significant fraction of total CO_2 will exist as CO_3^{2-} anions.

A typical formulation of a PVC membrane ISE used in clinical instrumentation consists of the following in % by weight (wt%):

1 to 3 wt% ionophore;
≈64 wt% plasticizer;
≈30 wt% PVC; and <1 wt% additives.

The plasticizer is crucial in controlling the polarity of the membrane, and thus, along with the ionophore, plays a pivotal role in determining the selectivity of the membrane toward the ion of interest. A large lipophilic anion (eg, tetraphenylborate derivative) is often included as an additive for preparation of cation-selective ISE membranes. This anion serves as a counter-anion for the cation of interest as it is extracted into the membrane phase, forming a positively charged complex with the neutral ionophore. However, it is the ratio of the bound-to-unbound ionophore sites at the membrane surface that determines the magnitude of the phase boundary potential generated by the ISE membrane.[24] Thus, the selective response to the activity of the ion of interest is an interfacial property of the given ISE membrane.

Studies have demonstrated that the ultimate detection limits of polymer membrane–type ISEs are controlled in part by the leakage of analyte ions from the internal solution to

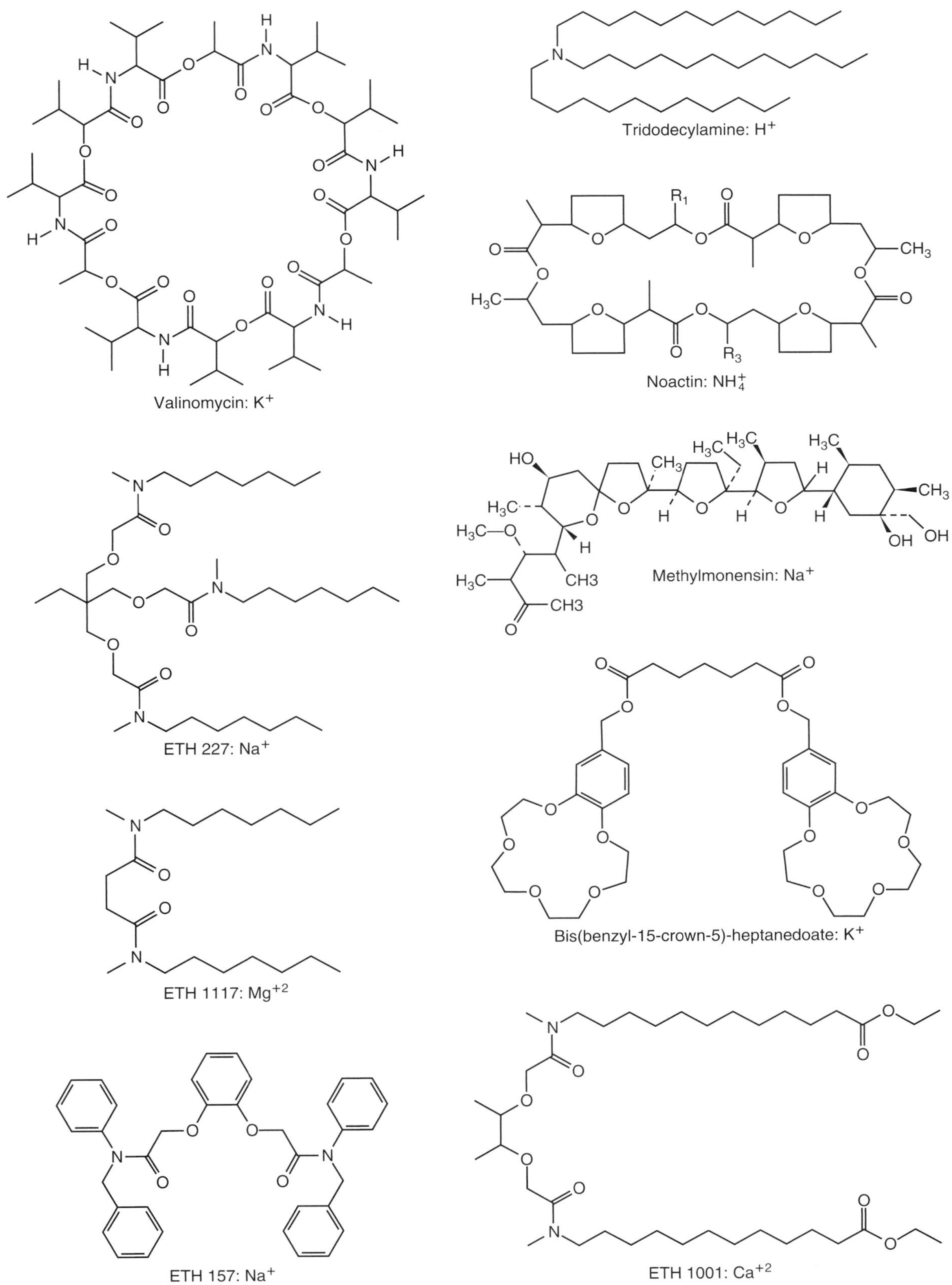

Valinomycin: K^+

Tridodecylamine: H^+

Noactin: NH_4^+

Methylmonensin: Na^+

ETH 227: Na^+

Bis(benzyl-15-crown-5)-heptanedoate: K^+

ETH 1117: Mg^{+2}

ETH 157: Na^+

ETH 1001: Ca^{+2}

FIGURE 14.3 Structures of Common Ionophores Used to Fabricate Polymer Membrane–Type Ion-Selective Electrodes for Clinical Analysis.

the outer surface of the membrane and into the sample phase in close contact with the membrane.[25] Hence, lower limits of detection can be achieved by decreasing the concentration of the primary analyte ion within the internal solution of the electrode. Furthermore, this leakage of analyte ions, coupled with an ion exchange process at the membrane sample interface when the selectivity of the membrane over other ions is assessed, can often yield a measured potentiometric selectivity coefficient that underestimates the true selectivity of the membrane. To determine "unbiased" selectivity coefficients by the separate solution method, the membrane should not be exposed to the analyte ion for extended periods of time, and the concentration of the analyte ion in the internal solution should be low.[26] To avoid leakage of primary ions from the inner solution of conventional polymer membrane ISEs, new, more stable designs for solid-state ion sensors have been suggested, in which the ionophore-doped, polymer ion–sensing membrane (based on a more water-repellent poly[methylmethacrylate]/poly[decylmethacrylate copolymer]) is coated onto a conductive poly(3-octylethiophene 2,5-diyl) (POT) polymer layer on the surface of an underlying Au electrode.[27]

An interesting application of Na^+ selective polymer (or glass) membrane electrodes is seen in the determination of whole blood hematrocrit.[28] Because intracellular Na^+ concentrations are much lower than those in the plasma phase, the change in Na^+ concentration (dilution) measured potentiometrically before and after erythrocyte lysis can be used to assess the hematocrit of the blood sample. This approach can be coupled with simultaneous measurement of changes in K^+ ion concentration as determined with a valinomycin-based polymer membrane ISE to quantify the concentration of K^+ ions within red blood cells.[29]

Recently, a reversible polymer membrane ISE for measurement of polyions was described.[30] The sensor consists of a highly lipophilic electrolyte (tetradodecylammonium-dinonylnaphthalenesulfonate), which is free of intrinsic ion-exchange properties, added to a plasticized PVC membrane at high concentration (approximately 10 wt%). Application of a cathodic current pulse across the membrane results in reversible extraction and potentiometric response to the polycation protamine. Protamine is a polypeptide administered to neutralize heparin activity. A response to heparin in whole blood was demonstrated via protamine titration. Later, it was found that by changing the lipophilic cation in the membrane to tridodecylmethylammonium, application of an anodic current pulse resulted in a direct potentiometric response to heparin.[31] Testing of other polyanions in addition to heparin led to the conclusion that the magnitude of the potentiometric response is a function of charge density of the polyanion.

Electrodes for Partial Pressure of Carbon Dioxide. Electrodes have been developed to measure PCO_2 in body fluids. The first PCO_2 electrode, developed in the 1950s by Stow and Severinghaus, used a glass pH electrode as the internal element in a potentiometric cell for measurement of the PCO_2.[32] This important development paved the way for commercial availability of the three-channel blood analyzer (pH, PCO_2, PO_2) which gives the complete picture of the oxygenation and acid-base status of blood.

Fig. 14.4 shows a diagram of a typical Severinghaus-style electrode for PCO_2. A thin membrane (approximately 20 μm), permeable only to gases and water vapor, is in contact with the sample. Membranes of silicone rubber, Teflon, and other polymeric materials are suitable for this purpose. On the opposite side of the membrane is a thin electrolyte layer consisting of a weak bicarbonate salt (approximately 5 mmol/L) and a Cl^- salt. A pH electrode and an Ag/AgCl reference electrode are in contact with this solution. The PCO_2 electrode is a self-contained potentiometric cell. CO_2 gas from the sample or calibration matrix diffuses through the membrane and dissolves in the internal electrolyte layer. Carbonic acid is formed and dissociates, shifting the pH of the bicarbonate solution in the internal layer as follows:

$$CO_2 + H_2O \rightleftarrows H_2CO_3 \leftrightarrow H^+ + HCO_3^- \quad \textbf{(14)}$$

and

$$\Delta \log PCO_{2(\text{sample})} \approx \Delta pH_{(\text{internal layer})} \quad \textbf{(15)}$$

The relationship between the sample PCO_2 and the signal generated by the internal pH electrode is logarithmic and is governed by the Nernst equation. The electrode may be calibrated using precision gas mixtures or using solutions with stable PCO_2 concentrations. Although Severinghaus-style electrodes for PCO_2 have gained widespread use in modern blood gas analyzers, the format in which such sensors may be constructed is limited by size, shape, and the ability to fabricate the internal pH sensitive element.

A slightly different potentiometric cell for PCO_2 is shown in Fig. 14.5. This cell arrangement uses two PVC-type, pH-selective electrodes in a differential mode. The electrode membranes contain a lipophilic amine-type neutral ionophore that exhibits high selectivity for H^+ (see Fig. 14.3). One electrode has an internal layer that is buffered, and the other is unbuffered, consisting of a low concentration of bicarbonate salt. CO_2 gas from the sample or calibration matrix diffuses across the outer H^+-selective PVC membranes of both sensors. On the unbuffered side, CO_2 diffusion produces a potential shift at the internal interface of the pH-responsive membrane proportional to the sample PCO_2 concentration. The signal at the electrode with the buffered internal layer is unaffected by the CO_2 that diffuses across the membrane. Consequently, one half of the sensor responds to pH alone, and the other half responds to both pH and PCO_2. The signal difference between the two electrodes cancels any contribution of sample pH to the overall measured cell potential. The differential signal is proportional only to PCO_2. Unlike the traditional Severinghaus-style electrode, this differential potentiometric cell PCO_2 sensor has been commercialized in a planar format and is more easily adaptable to mass production in sensor arrays.[33]

Direct Potentiometry by Ion-Selective Electrodes: Units of Measure and Reporting for Clinical Applications

Older analytical methods such as flame photometry for the measurement of electrolytes provide the total concentration *(c)* of a given ion in the sample, usually expressed in units of millimoles of ion per liter of sample. Molality *(m)* is a measure of the moles of ion per mass of water (millimoles per kilogram) in the sample. Using the Na^+ ion as an example,

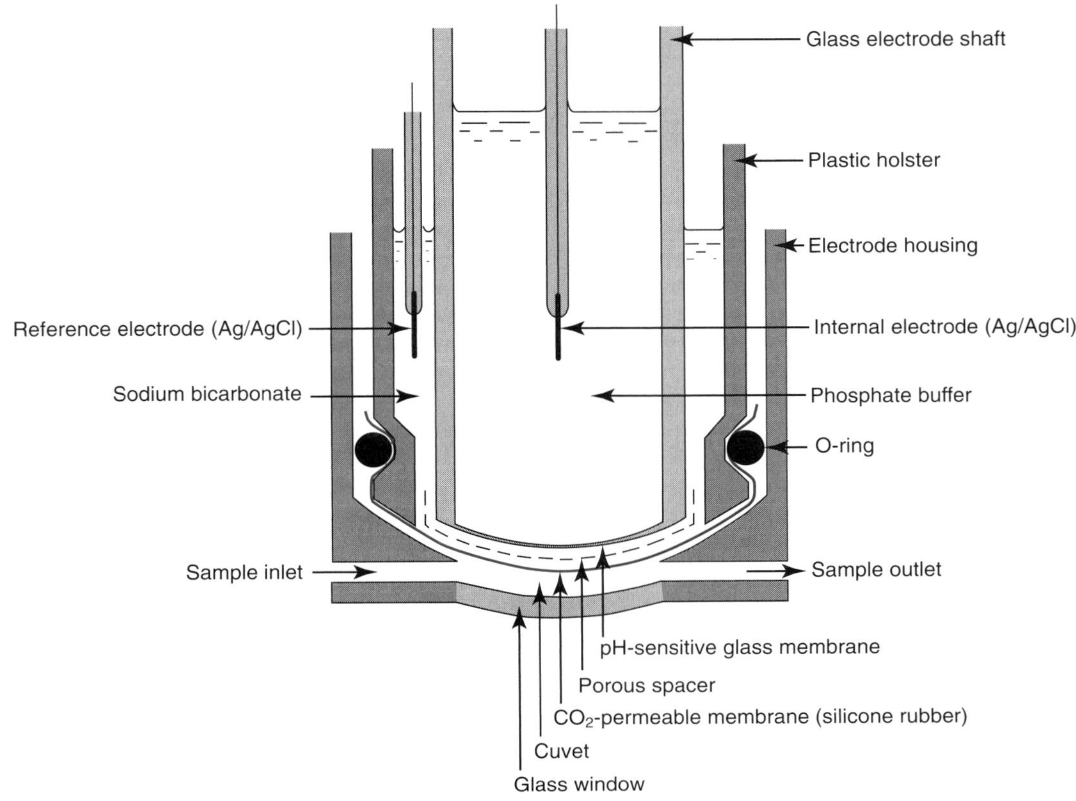

FIGURE 14.4 **Schematic of Severinghaus-Style Partial Pressure of Carbon Dioxide (PCO_2) Sensor Used to Monitor CO_2 Concentrations in Blood Samples.** *Ag/AgCl,* Silver-silver chloride. (From Siggard-Andersen O. The acid-base status of the blood. 4th ed. Baltimore, MD: Williams & Wilkins, 1974:172.)

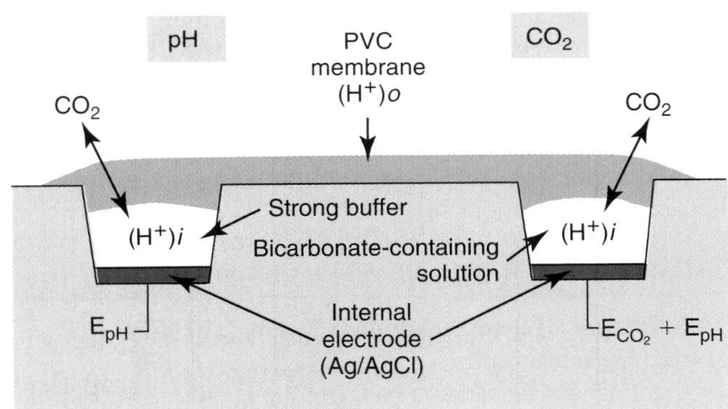

FIGURE 14.5 **Differential Planar Partial Pressure of Carbon Dioxide (PCO_2) Potentiometric Sensor Design, Based on Two Identical Polymeric Membrane pH Electrodes, but With Different Internal Reference Electrolyte Solutions.** Both pH sensing membranes are prepared with a hydrogen (H^+)-selective ionophore. *Ag/AgCl,* Silver-silver chloride; *PVC,* poly(vinyl chloride).

the relationship between concentration and molality is given by

$$c_{Na^+} = m_{Na^+} \times \rho H_2O \qquad \textbf{(16)}$$

where ρH_2O = mass concentration of water in kilograms per liter. For normal blood plasma, the mass concentration of water is approximately 0.93 kg/L, but in specimens with increased lipids or protein, the value may be as low as 0.8 kg/L. In these specimens, the difference between concentration and molality may be as great as 20%. A significant advantage of direct potentiometry by ISE for the measurement of electrolytes is that the technique is sensitive to molality, and therefore, is not affected by variations in the concentration of protein or lipids in the sample. Techniques such as flame photometry, ISE methods that require sample dilution (also called indirect potentiometry), and other photometric methods that require sample dilution are affected by the presence of protein and lipids. In these methods, only the water phase of the sample is diluted, which produces results lower than molality as a function of the concentration of protein and lipids in the sample. Thus, there is a risk for errors, such as a falsely low Na^+ concentration (pseudohyponatremia), in cases of extremely increased protein and lipid concentrations (see also Chapter 35).[34]

In addition to the difference between molality and concentration, measurement of ions by direct potentiometry provides yet another unit of measurement known as activity *(a)*, the concentration of free, unbound ion in solution. Unlike methods sensitive to ion concentration, ISEs do not sense the presence of complexed or electrostatically "hindered" ions in the sample. The relationship between activity and concentration, using Na^+ ion as an example, is expressed as

$$a_{Na^+} = \gamma_{Na^+} \times c_{Na^+} \qquad \textbf{(17)}$$

where γ = dimensionless quantity known as the activity coefficient. The activity coefficient is primarily dependent on ionic strength of the sample as described by the Debye-Huckel equation:

$$\log \gamma = -\frac{(A \times z^2 \times I^{0.5})}{1 + B \times a \times I^{0.5}} \quad \textbf{(18)}$$

where A and B = temperature-dependent constants (A = 0.5213 and B = 3.305 in water at 37°C); a = ion size parameter for a specific ion; and I = ionic strength ($I = 0.5\ \Sigma m \times z^2$, where z is the charge number of the ions). Eq. 18 shows that a decrease in the activity coefficient occurs with an increase in ionic strength. This effect is more pronounced when the charge *(z)* of the ion is higher. Activity coefficients for ions in biological fluids, such as blood and serum, are difficult to calculate with accuracy because of the uncertain contribution of macromolecular ions, such as proteins, to the overall ionic strength. However, assuming that the normal ionic strength of blood plasma is 0.160 mol/kg, estimates of activity coefficients at 37°C are as follows: Na^+ = 0.75, K^+ = 0.74, and Ca^{2+} = 0.31. Referring to Eq. 17, activity and concentration will differ greatly in samples of physiologic ionic strength, especially for divalent ions.

Physiologically, ionic activity is assumed to be more relevant than concentration when chemical equilibria or biological processes are considered. Practically, however, ionic concentration is the more familiar term in clinical practice, forming the basis of reference intervals and medical decision concentrations for electrolytes. Early in the evolution of ISEs as practical tools in clinical chemistry, it was decided that changing clinical reference intervals to a system based on activity instead of concentration was impractical and carried the risk for clinical misinterpretation. A pragmatic approach for using ISEs in modern analyzers without changing established concentration-based reference intervals is to formulate calibration solutions with ionic strengths and ionic compositions as close as possible to those of blood plasma. In this way, the activity coefficient of each ion in the calibrating solutions approximates that in the sample matrix, which allows calibration and measurement of electrolytes in units of concentration instead of activity.[35]

A typical set of solutions for multi-ISE calibration in an analyzer is shown in Table 14.2. Two points are used to calibrate each ISE. The difference in the cell potential generated by these two solutions (ΔE) is used to calculate the response slope of the cell (slope = $\Delta E/\Delta \log c$), where c is the concentration of ion in each calibrating solution, substituted for activity. The standard electrode potential, E^0, is calculated as the y-intercept. Determination of the ion concentration in an unknown sample is then a straightforward solution of the Nickolsky-Eisenman equation (Eq. 11), after the cell potential generated by the sample is measured. The measured slope is used in place of the $2.303RT/z_iF$ term of Eq. 11. In the absence of significant influence from interfering ions on measurement of the primary ion (eg., ≤1% interference on the measured value), contributions from a_j in Eq. 11 may be ignored.

Calibration of the cell is done in units of concentration; however, as mentioned earlier, direct potentiometry is sensitive to the molality of the ion, which is related to concentration by the water content of the sample (Eq. 16). The water

TABLE 14.2 Examples of Two-Value Calibrating Solutions for Measurement of pH and Electrolytes by Direct Potentiometry*

Analyte	Calibration Point (mmol/L)	Slope Point (mmol/L)	Expected Signal Δ, (mV)
Na^+	140	110	6.6
K^+	4.0	8.0	18
Ca^{2+}	1.25	2.50	9
Cl^-	100	80	6
pH	7.38 (pH units)	6.84 (pH units)	32.4

*Ionic strength adjusted to 160 mmol/kg with buffer salts and inert electrolytes. *Ca^{2+}*, Calcium; *Cl^-*, chloride; *K^+*, potassium; *Na^+*, sodium.

content of the aqueous calibrating solutions shown in Table 14.2 is approximately 0.99 kg/L. The water content of normal blood plasma is approximately 0.93 kg/L. Molality is 7% greater than the concentration in this normal plasma specimen. The direct potentiometric cell will report results approximately 6% greater than the concentration in normal specimens because of this difference in water content between the sample and the calibrator (0.99/0.93 = 1.06). Direct potentiometry presents an advantage in that the technique is not affected by the presence of protein and lipids in the sample; however, the application of clinical reference intervals based on concentration again poses a risk for confusion and clinical misinterpretation. Most manufacturers of electrolyte measurement systems have overcome this problem in a practical way by following Clinical and Laboratory Standards Institute (CLSI) guidelines that recommend the use of correlation factors to standardize ISE measurements to units of concentration. These factors may be obtained by standardizing the ISE measurement to certified reference materials based on human serum, with electrolyte values assigned in units of concentration.[36-38] Appropriate correlation factors are then applied to sample calculations using algorithms resident in the instrument software.

POINTS TO REMEMBER

Advantages of Electrochemical Sensors for Whole Blood Measurements

- Electrochemical sensors measure the most important critical care analytes (gases, electrolytes, glucose) directly in whole blood without need for sample pretreatment or dilution.
- Measurement is rapid and nondestructive.
- Measurement is not affected by sample turbidity (red cells, lipids); only the analyte present in the water phase of plasma is measured.
- Simultaneous measurement of multiple analytes in the same blood sample is possible.

VOLTAMMETRY AND/OR AMPEROMETRY

Voltammetric and amperometric techniques are among the most sensitive and widely applicable of all electroanalytical methods.

Basic Concepts

In contrast to potentiometry, voltammetric and amperometric methods are based on electrolytic electrochemical cells in which an external voltage is applied to a polarizable working electrode (measured vs. a suitable reference electrode: $E_{appl} = E_{work} - E_{ref}$), and the resulting cathodic (for analytical reductions) or anodic (for analytical oxidations) current of the cell is monitored and is proportional to the concentration of the analyte present in the test sample. Current flows only if E_{appl} is greater than a certain voltage (decomposition voltage) determined by the thermodynamics for a given redox reaction of interest ($Ox + ne^- \rightleftharpoons Red$, which is defined by the E^0 value for that reaction [standard reduction potential]) and the kinetics for heterogeneous electron transfer at the interface of the working electrode. Often, slow kinetics of electron transfer for the redox reaction on a given inert working electrode (Pt, carbon, Au, and so on) mandates use of a much more negative (for reductions) or positive (for oxidations) E_{appl} than that predicted based merely on the E^0 for a given redox reaction. This is called an overpotential (η). Regardless of whether an overpotential for electron transfer exists, a specific oxidation or reduction reaction occurs at the surface of the working electrode in voltammetry and/or amperometry, and it is the charge transfer at this interface (current flow) that provides the analytical information.

For electrolytic cells that form the basis of voltammetric and amperometric methods:

$$E_{appl} = E_{cell} + \eta - iR_{cell} \quad \mathbf{(19)}$$

where E_{cell} = thermodynamic potential between the working and reference electrodes in the absence of an applied external voltage. When the external voltage is greater or less than this equilibrium potential, plus or minus any overpotential (η), then current will flow because of an oxidation or reduction reaction at the working electrode. A voltammogram is simply the plot of observed current, i, versus E_{appl} (Fig. 14.6). In amperometry (see later), a fixed voltage is applied, and the resulting current is monitored. The amount of current is inversely related to the resistance of the electrolyte solution and to any "apparent" resistance that develops because of mass transfer of the analyte species to the surface of the working electrode. Because electrochemical reactions are heterogeneous, occurring only at the surface of the working electrode, the amount of current observed is also highly dependent on the surface area (A) of the working electrode.

When a potential is applied to a working electrode that will oxidize or reduce a species in the solution phase contacting the electrode, the electrochemical reaction causes the concentration of electroactive species to decrease at the surface of the electrode (Fig. 14.7), a process termed concentration polarization. This, in turn, causes a concentration gradient of analyte species between the bulk sample solution and the surface of the electrode.[39] When the bulk solution is stirred, the diffusion layer of the analyte grows out from the surface of the electrode quickly to a fixed distance, which is controlled by how vigorously the solution is stirred. This diffusion layer is termed the Nernst layer and has a finite thickness (δ) after a relatively short time period (see Fig. 14.7) when the solution is moving (convection). Voltammetry carried out in the presence of convection (by stirring the solution, rotating the electrode, flowing solution by electrode, and so on) is called steady-state voltammetry. When the solution is not moving, the diffusion layer grows further and further with time (ie, not constant), creating larger and larger δ values over time. This is termed non–steady-state voltammetry and often results in peak currents in i versus E_{appl} plots for electrolytic cells.

In steady-state voltammetry, when the potential of the working electrode is scanned past a value that will cause an electrochemical reaction, the current will rise rapidly and then will plateau, even as E_{appl} changes further. Fig. 14.6

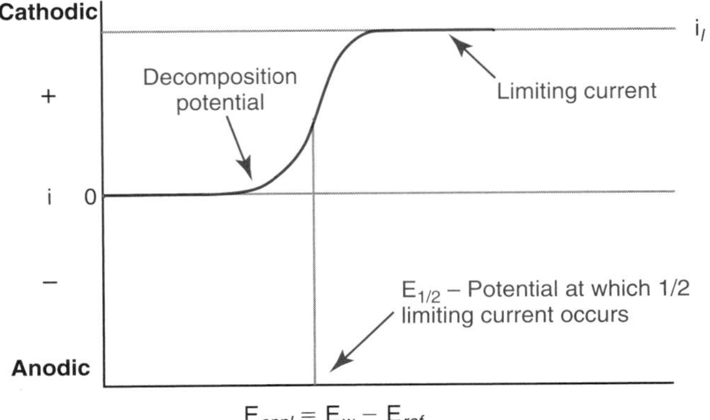

FIGURE 14.6 Current Versus Voltage Curve (Voltammogram) Obtained for Oxidized Species (Ox) Reduced (Red) at the Surface of the Working Electrode, as the Eappl Is Scanned More Negatively and the Solution Is Stirred to Yield a Steady-State Response.

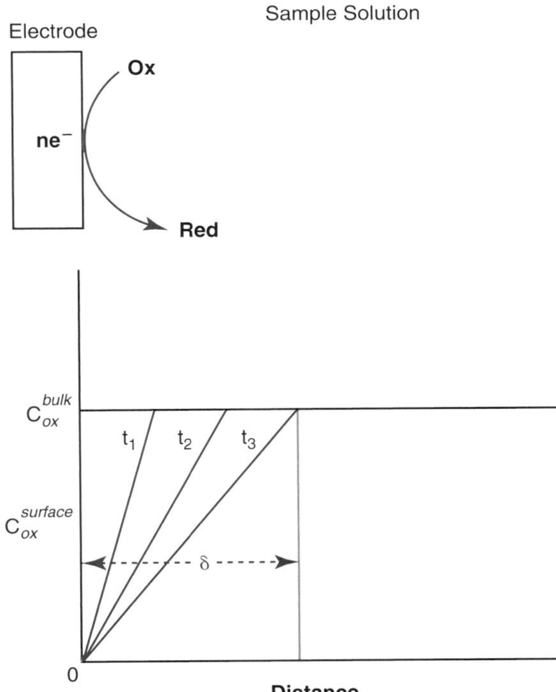

FIGURE 14.7 Concept of Electrochemical Reaction Increasing Diffusion Layer Thickness (Concentration Polarization) of Analytes via Reduction (Red) (or Oxidation [Ox]) at the Surface of the Working Electrode. As time *(t)* increases, the diffusion layer thickness grows quickly to a value determined by the degree of convection in the sample solution.

illustrates such a wave for a hypothetical reduction of an oxidized species (Ox) via an n electron reduction to a reduced species (Red). When the applied potential is much more negative than required, the current reaches a limiting value (termed the limiting current, i_l). This limiting current is proportional to the concentration of the electroactive species (Ox in this case) as expressed by the following equation:

$$i_l = nFA\left(\frac{D}{\delta}\right)C_{\text{ox}} \quad (20)$$

where i = measured current in amperes; n = the number of electrons in the electrochemical reaction (reduction in this case); F = Faraday's constant (96,487 coulombs/mol); A = electrochemical surface area of the working electrode (in square centimeters) (assuming a planar electrode geometry); D = diffusion coefficient (in square centimeters per second) of the electroactive species (Ox in this case); δ = diffusion layer thickness (in centimeters); and C = concentration of the analyte species (in moles per cubic meter). The D/δ term is often denoted as m_o, the mass transfer coefficient of the Ox species to the surface of the working electrode. Note that Eq. 20 indicates a linear relationship for limiting current and concentration. The exact same equation applies for detecting reduced species by an oxidation reaction at the working electrode. In this case, by convention, the resulting anodic current is considered a negative current. As shown in Fig. 14.6, the potential of the working electrode that corresponds to a current that is exactly one-half the limiting current is termed the $E_{1/2}$ value. This value is not dependent on analyte concentration. The $E_{1/2}$ is determined by the thermodynamics (E^0) of the given redox reaction, the solution conditions (eg, if protons are involved in reaction, then the pH will influence the $E_{1/2}$ value), and any overpotential caused by slow electron transfer, and so on, at a particular working electrode surface. The $E_{1/2}$ values are indicative of a given species undergoing an electrochemical reaction under specified conditions; hence, the $E_{1/2}$ values enable distinguishing one electroactive species from another in the same sample. If the $E_{1/2}$ values for various species differ significantly (eg, more than 120 mV), then measurements of several limiting currents in a given voltammogram can yield quantitative results for several different species simultaneously.

Electrochemical cells used to carry out voltammetric or amperometric measurements can involve a two- or three-electrode configuration. In the two-electrode mode, external voltage is applied between the working electrode and a reference electrode, and the current is monitored. Because the current must also pass through the reference electrode, such current flow can potentially alter the surface concentration of electroactive species that poise the actual half-cell potential of the reference electrode, changing its value by a concentration polarization process. For example, if an Ag/AgCl reference electrode were used in a cell in which a reduction reaction for the analyte occurs at the working electrode, then an oxidation reaction would take place at the surface of the reference electrode:

$$Ag^0 + Cl^- \rightarrow AgCl_{(s)} + 1\,e^- \quad (21)$$

Hence, the activity and/or concentration of Cl^- ions near the surface of the electrode would decrease, which would make the potential of the reference electrode more positive than its true equilibrium value based on the actual activity of the Cl^- ion in the reference half-cell, because the Nernst equation for this half-cell is:

$$E_{Ag/AgCl} = E^0_{Ag/AgCl} - 0.059\log(a^{\text{surface}}_{Cl^-}) \quad (22)$$

Such concentration polarization of the reference electrode is prevented by keeping the current density (amperes per square centimeter) low at the reference electrode. This is achieved in practice by making sure that the area of the working electrode in the electrochemical cell is much smaller than the surface area of the reference electrode; hence, the total current flow will be limited by this much smaller area, and current density values for the reference will be very small, as desired, to prevent concentration polarization.

A three-electrode potentiostat is often used to completely eliminate changes in reference electrode half-cell potentials. In simple terms, the potentiostat applies a voltage to the working electrode, which is measured versus a reference electrode via a zero current potentiometric-type measurement, but the current flow is between the working electrode and a third electrode, called the counter electrode. Thus, if reduction takes place at the working electrode, oxidation would occur at the counter electrode, but no net reaction would take place at the surface of the reference electrode because no current flows through this electrode. A potentiostat circuit is relatively simple to construct using modern operational amplifiers.

In voltammetric methods, the E_{appl} is varying via some waveform to alter the working electrode potential as a function of time and the resulting current measured. The current change occurs at the decomposition potential range, which is best when specific for a given analyte. However, the location of the current response as a function of E_{appl} provides information on the nature of the species present (eg, $E_{1/2}$), along with a concentration-dependent signal. This scan of E_{appl} can be linear (linear sweep voltammetry) or it can have more complex shapes that enable greatly enhanced sensitivity to be achieved for monitoring the concentration of a given electroactive species (eg, normal pulsed voltammetry, differential pulse voltammetry, square wave voltammetry).[40] When a dropping Hg electrode is used, such voltammetric methods are considered polarographic methods of analysis.

Amperometric methods differ from voltammetry, in that E_{appl} is fixed, generally at a potential value that occurs in the limiting current plateau region of the voltammogram, which simply monitors the resulting current and will be proportional to concentration. Amperometry can be more sensitive than common voltammetric methods because background charging currents, which arise from changing the E_{appl} as a function of time in voltammetry, do not exist. Hence, when selectivity can be assured at a given E_{appl} value, amperometry may be preferred to voltammetric methods for more sensitive quantitative measurements.

Applications

Molecular O_2 is capable of undergoing several reduction reactions, all with a significant overpotential at solid electrodes, such as Pt, Au, or Ag. For example, the following reaction:

$$\begin{gathered} O_2 + 2H_2O + 4e^- \rightarrow 4OH^- \\ (E^0 = +0.179 \quad \text{vs} \quad Ag/AgCl; 1\,M\ Cl^-) \end{gathered} \quad (23)$$

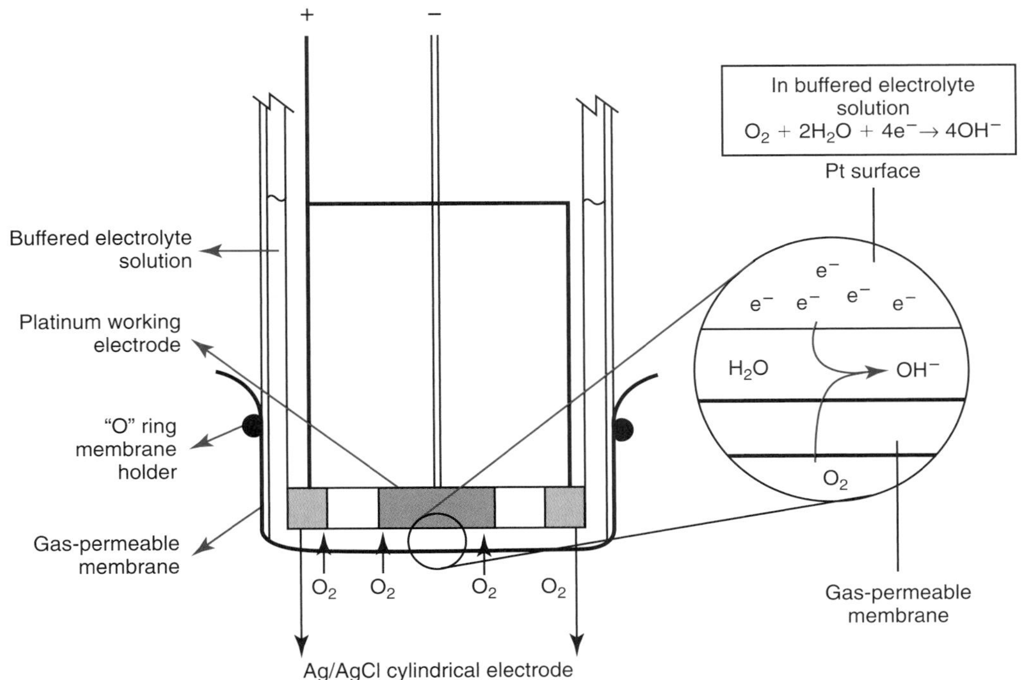

FIGURE 14.8 Design of Clark-Style Amperometric Oxygen Sensor Used to Monitor Partial Pressure of Oxygen (PO_2) in Blood. *H_2O*, Water; Pt, platinum.

exhibits an $E_{1/2}$ at approximately −0.500 V on a Pt electrode (vs. a Ag/AgCl reference electrode), with a limiting current plateau beginning at approximately −0.600 V. This reaction is used to monitor the PO_2 in blood, which is the basis of the widely used Clark-style amperometric O_2 sensor (Fig. 14.8). This device uses a small area planar Pt electrode as a working electrode (encased in insulating glass or other material) and an Ag/AgCl reference electrode, typically with a cylindrical design (see Fig. 14.8). This two-electrode electrolytic cell is placed within sensor housing, on which a gas-permeable membrane (eg, polypropylene, silicone rubber, Teflon) is held at the distal end. The inner working Pt electrode is pressed tightly against the gas-permeable membrane to create a thin film of internal electrolyte solution (usually buffer with KCl added). O_2 in the sample can permeate across the membrane and can be reduced in accordance with the preceding electrochemical reaction. An E_{appl} of −0.650 or −0.700 V versus Ag/AgCl (within the limiting current regime) to the Pt working electrode will result in an observed current that is proportional to the PO_2 present in the sample (including whole blood). In the absence of any O_2, the current at this applied voltage under amperometric conditions will be near zero.

The outer gas-permeable membrane enables the Clark electrode to detect O_2 with high selectivity over other easily reduced species that might be present in a given sample (eg, metal ions, cystine). Only other gas species or highly lipophilic organic species can partition into and pass through such gas-permeable membranes. One type of interference in clinical samples can be caused by certain anesthesia gases, such as nitrous oxide, halothane, and isoflurane. These species can also diffuse through the outer membrane of the sensor, can be electrochemically reduced at the Pt electrode, and can yield a false-positive value for the measurement of PO_2.[41] However, optimized gas-permeable membrane materials and appropriate control of the applied potential to the cathode of the sensor have greatly reduced this problem in modern instruments. The outer gas-permeable membranes also help restrict the diffusion of analyte to the inner working electrode; hence, the membrane can control the mass transport of analyte (D/δ term in Eq. 20), such that in the presence or absence of sample convection, mass transport of O_2 to the surface of the Pt working electrode is essentially the same.

The basic design of the Clark amperometric PO_2 sensor can be used to detect other gas species by altering the applied voltage to the working electrode. For example, it is possible to detect nitric oxide (NO) with high selectivity using a similar gas electrode design in which the Pt is polarized at +0.900 versus Ag/AgCl to oxidize diffusing NO to nitrate at the Pt anode.[42] Such NO sensors can be used for a variety of biomedically important studies to deduce the amount of NO locally at or near the surface of various NO-producing cells.

Beyond amperometric devices, one specialized method of detecting trace concentrations of toxic metal ions in clinical samples is anodic stripping voltammetry (ASV). In ASV, a carbon working electrode is used (sometimes further coated with an Hg film), and the E_{appl} is first fixed at a negative E_{appl} voltage so that all metal ions in the solution will be reduced to elemental metals (M^0) within the Hg film and/or on the surface of the carbon. Then, the E_{appl} is scanned more positively, and reduced metals deposited in and/or on the surface of the working electrode are reoxidized, giving a large anodic current peak proportional to the concentration of metal ions in the original sample. The potential at which these peaks are observed indicates which metal is present, and the height of the stripping peak current is directly proportional to the concentration of the metal ion in the original sample. Such ASV techniques can be used to detect the total concentration of lead in whole blood samples, providing a rapid screening method for lead exposure and poisoning.[43]

Another biomedical example of modern voltammetry is a rapid scan cyclic voltammetric technique that has been used to quantify dopamine in brain tissue of freely moving animals.[44] In this application, oxidation of dopamine to a quinone species at an implanted microcarbon electrode (at approximately +0.600 V vs. Ag/AgCl) yields peak currents proportional to dopamine concentrations. The electrode can be used to measure this neurotransmitter in different regions of the brain or in a fixed location. Often, pharmacologic or electrical stimulation can be used to measure the change in local dopamine concentrations due to such stimulation techniques.

Although voltammetric and/or amperometric techniques can be applied to detect a wide range of species, the selectivity offered for measurements in complex clinical samples—where many species can be electroactive—is rather limited. For example, as stated in the previous discussion relevant to the Clark O_2 sensor, in the absence of the gas-permeable membrane, other species that can be reduced at or near the same E_{appl} as O_2 would cause significant interference.

To expand the range of analytes that can be detected with voltammetric and/or amperometric methods, electrochemical techniques can be used as highly sensitive detectors for modern high-performance liquid chromatography systems (see Chapter 16). In liquid chromatography with electrochemical detection (LC-EC), eluting solutes are detected by flow-through electrodes (usually carbon or Hg) designed to have extremely low dead volumes (Fig. 14.9). The electrodes can be operated in amperometric or voltammetric modes (with high scan speeds), and several electrodes can be operated simultaneously in series or in parallel flow arrangements to gain additional selectivity.[45] For example, homocysteine can be measured with (1) the addition of reducing agents to a serum sample to generate free homocysteine, (2) precipitation of proteins in the sample (with trichloroacetic acid), and (3) separation of the serum components on a reversed-phase octadecylsilane high-performance liquid chromatography column. The eluting homocysteine is detected and measured with online electrochemical detection via homocysteine oxidation to the corresponding mercuric dithiolate complex:

$$2RSH + Hg \rightarrow Hg(RS)_2 + 2H^+ + 2e^- \quad \textbf{(24)}$$

using a thin-layer Hg/Au amalgam electrode poised at +0.150 V versus Ag/AgCl.[46] Integration of the eluting band for homocysteine provides quantitative results, with high selectivity. Similarly, catechols and catecholamines can be readily detected in serum by a similar LC-EC method, with eluted catechols oxidized to quinones at a flow-through carbon working electrode poised at potentials typically more than 0.200 V versus Ag/AgCl. Furthermore, a host of therapeutic drugs can also be quantitated in serum or urine via LC-EC methods.

POINTS TO REMEMBER

Predominant Types of Electrochemical Sensor Technologies Used in Whole Blood Analyzers

- Potentiometry: for measurement of pH, PCO_2, and electrolytes
- Amperometry: for measurement of PO_2 and as the basis for whole blood glucose and lactate biosensors
- Conductometry: for measurement of hematocrit

CONDUCTOMETRY

Conductometry is an electrochemical technique used to determine the quantity of an analyte present in a mixture by measurement of its effects on the electrical conductivity of the mixture. It is the measure of the ability of ions in solution to carry current under the influence of a potential difference. In a conductometric cell, potential is applied between two inert metal electrodes. An alternating potential with a frequency between 100 and 3000 Hz is used to prevent

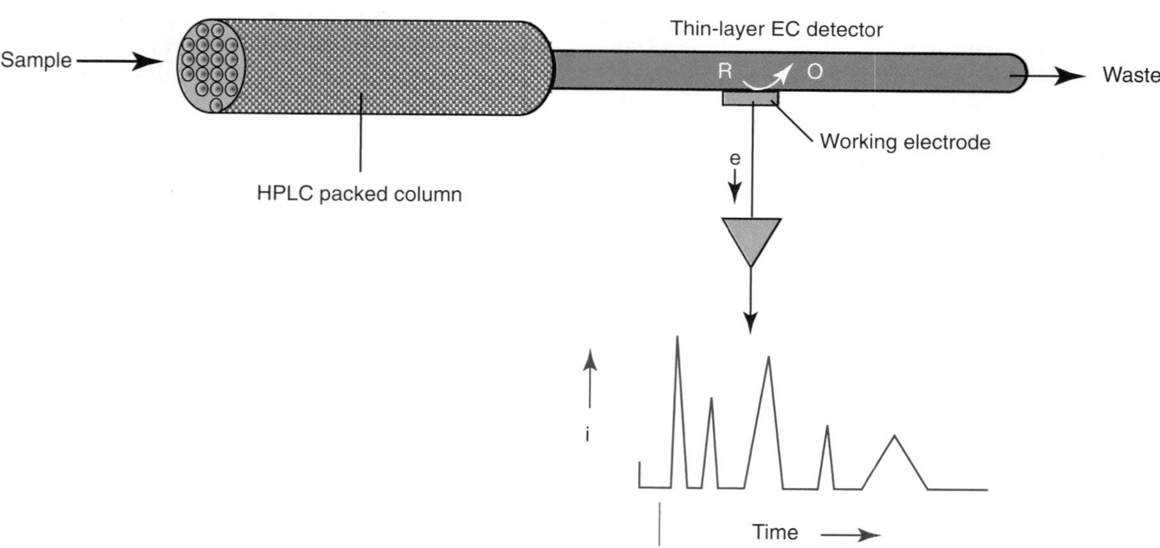

FIGURE 14.9 Schematic of liquid chromatography with electrochemical detection (LC-EC) system, with electrochemical detector monitoring elution of analytes from a high-performance liquid chromatography (HPLC) column by their oxidation or reduction (shown here as example) at a suitable thin-layer working electrode.

polarization of the electrodes. A decrease in solution resistance results in an increase in conductance, and more current is passed between the electrodes. The resulting current flow is also alternating. The current is directly proportional to solution conductance. Conductance is considered the inverse of resistance and may be expressed in units of ohm^{-1} (siemens). In clinical analysis, conductometry is frequently used for measurement of the volume fraction of erythrocytes in whole blood (hematocrit) and as the transduction mechanism for some biosensors (see the following).

Erythrocytes act as electrical insulators because of their lipid-based membrane composition. This phenomenon was used first in the 1940s to measure the volume fraction of erythrocytes in whole blood (hematocrit) by conductivity[47] and is used today to measure hematocrit on multianalyte instruments for clinical analysis. The conductivity of whole blood depends not only on the volume fraction and shape of the erythrocytes, but also on the conductivity of the surrounding plasma. An increase in the volume fraction of erythrocytes that are less conductive than the surrounding plasma leads to a decrease in conductivity shown by the following relationship[48]:

$$G_b = \frac{a}{1} + \frac{H}{100 - H} \times c \quad \textbf{(25)}$$

where G_b = conductivity of whole blood; a = plasma conductivity; H = percent of hematocrit; and c = factor for erythrocyte orientation. In practice, plasma conductivity also contains correction factors for Na^+ and K^+ concentrations. These cations are usually measured in conjunction with hematocrit on systems designed for clinical analysis.

Conductivity-based hematocrit measurements have limitations.[49] Abnormal protein concentrations will change plasma conductivity and interfere with measurement. Low protein concentrations resulting from dilution of blood with protein-free electrolyte solutions during cardiopulmonary bypass surgery will result in erroneously low hematocrit values by conductivity. Preanalytical variables, such as insufficient mixing of the sample, will also lead to errors.[50] Hemoglobin is the preferred analyte to monitor blood loss and the need for transfusion during trauma and surgery. However, electrochemical measurement of hematocrit in conjunction with blood gases and electrolytes remains in use mainly because of its simplicity and convenience, despite some limitations.

Another clinical application of conductance is for electronic counting of blood cells in suspension. Termed the Coulter principle, it relies on the fact that the conductivity of blood cells is lower than that of a salt solution used as a suspension medium.[51] The cell suspension is forced to flow through a tiny orifice. Two electrodes are placed on either side of the orifice, and a constant current is established between the electrodes. Each time a cell passes through the orifice, resistance increases; this causes a spike in the electrical potential difference between the electrodes. The pulses are then amplified and counted.

COULOMETRY

Coulometry measures the electrical charge passing between two electrodes in an electrochemical cell. The amount of charge passing between the electrodes is directly proportional to oxidation or reduction of an electroactive substance at one of the electrodes. The number of coulombs transferred in this process is related to the absolute amount of electroactive substance by Faraday's law:

$$Q = n \times N \times F \quad \textbf{(26)}$$

where Q = amount of charge passing through the cell (unit: C = coulomb = ampere × second); n = the number of electrons transferred in the oxidation or reduction reaction; N = the amount of substance reduced or oxidized in moles; and F = Faraday constant (96,487 coulombs/mol).

The measurement of current is related to the charge as the amount of charge passed per unit time (ampere = coulomb per second). Coulometry is used in clinical applications for the determination of Cl^- in serum or plasma and as the mode of transduction in certain types of biosensors.

Commercial coulometric titrators have been developed for determination of Cl^-. A constant current is applied between a Ag wire (anode) and a Pt wire (cathode). At the anode, Ag is oxidized to Ag^+. At the cathode, H^+ is reduced to H_2 gas. At a constant applied current, the number of coulombs passed between the anode and the cathode is directly proportional to time (coulombs = amperes × seconds). Therefore, the absolute number of Ag^+ ions produced at the anode may be calculated from the amount of time current passes through it. In the presence of Cl^-, Ag^+ ions formed are precipitated as $AgCl_{(s)}$, and the amount of free Ag^+ in solution is low. When all Cl^- ions have been complexed, a sudden increase in the concentration of Ag^+ in solution is noted. Excess Ag^+ is sensed amperometrically at a second Ag electrode, which is polarized at negative potential. The excess Ag^+ is reduced to Ag, producing a current. When this current exceeds a certain value, the titration is stopped. The absolute number of Cl^- ions present in the sample is calculated from the time during which titration with Ag^+ was in progress. Because of the volumetric amount of serum or plasma sample originally used, it is possible to calculate the concentration of Cl^- in the sample. Coulometric titration is one of the most accurate electrochemical techniques because the method measures the absolute quantity of electroactive substance in the sample. Coulometry is considered the gold standard for determination of Cl^- in serum or plasma. However, the method is subject to interference from anions in the sample that have affinity for Ag^+ more than Cl^- (eg, bromide)[52] and is not commonly used in today's clinical laboratories.

OPTICAL CHEMICAL SENSORS

An optode is an optical sensor used in analytical instruments to measure blood gases and electrolytes. Optodes have certain advantages over electrodes, including (1) ease of miniaturization, (2) less noise (no transduction wires), (3) potential long-term stability using ratiometric-type measurements at multiple wavelengths,[53] and (4) they do not require a separate reference electrode. These advantages initially promoted the development of optical sensor technology for the design of intravascular blood gas sensors (see the section on the In Vivo Sensor). However, the same basic sensing principles can be used in clinical chemistry instrumentation designed for more classic in vitro measurements on discrete samples. In such

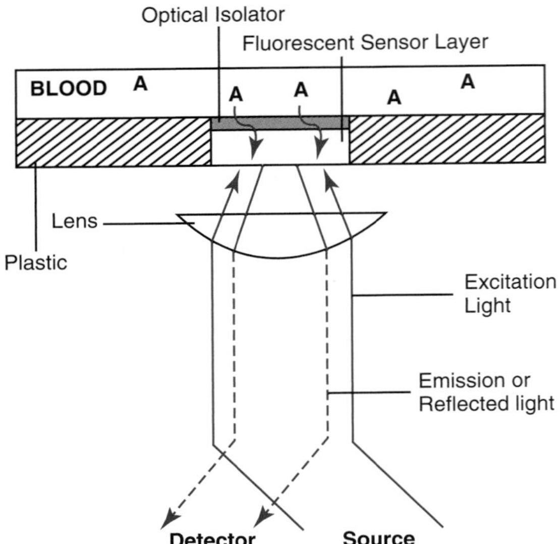

FIGURE 14.10 General Design for in Vitro Optical Sensor Designed to Detect Given Analyte in Blood Sample. Polymer film contains dye that changes spectral properties in proportion to the amount of analyte in the sample phase. Example shown is for sensing film that changes luminescence (fluorescence or phosphorescence).

systems, light can be brought to and from the sensing site by optical fibers or simply by appropriate positioning of light sources (light-emitting diodes), filters, and photodetectors to monitor absorbance (by reflectance), fluorescence, or phosphorescence (Fig. 14.10).

Basic Concepts

Optical sensors devised for PO_2 measurements are typically based on immobilization of certain organic dyes (eg, pyrene, diphenylphenanthrene, phenanthrene, fluoranthene) or metal ligand complexes (eg, ruthenium[II] tris[dipyridine], Pt and palladium metalloporphyrins) within hydrophobic polymer films (eg, silicone rubber) in which O_2 is soluble.[54] The fluorescence or phosphorescence of such species at a given wavelength is often quenched in the presence of paramagnetic species, including molecular O_2. In the case of embedded fluorescent dyes, the intensity of the emitted fluorescence of such films will decrease in proportion to the PO_2 in the sample in contact with the polymer film, in accordance with the Stern-Volmer equation for quenching:

$$\frac{I_0}{I_{PO_2}} = 1 + kPO_2 \quad \textbf{(27)}$$

where I_0 = fluorescence intensity in the absence of any O_2; I_{PO_2} = fluorescence intensity at a given PO_2; and k = quenching constant for the particular fluorophore used.

Hence, a linear relationship exists between the ratio I_0/I_{PO2} and the PO_2 in the sample phase. The larger the Stern-Volmer constant, the greater is the degree of quenching for the given fluorophore. However, it is important that the quenching constant is in a range that will yield linear Stern-Volmer behavior over the physiologically relevant range of PO_2 in blood. For example, if k is too large, then the maximum quenching possible will occur over a range of PO_2 that is less than physiologic.

Phosphorescence intensity or phosphorescence lifetime measurements of immobilized metal ligand complexes can also be used (ie, binding of O_2 decreases excited state lifetimes). Sensors based on changes in luminescent lifetime have the inherent advantage of being insensitive to perturbations in the optical path length and the amount of active dye present in the sensing layer.

Optical pH sensors require immobilization of appropriate pH indicators (eg, fluorescein, 8-hydroxy-1,2,6-pyrene trisulfonate, phenol red) within thin layers of hydrophilic polymers (eg, hydrogels) because equilibrium access of protons to the indicator is essential. The absorbance or fluorescence of the protonated or deprotonated form of the species can be used for sensing purposes.[53] One issue with respect to using immobilized indicators for accurate physiologic pH measurements is the effect of ionic strength on the acid dissociation constant (pKa) of the indicator. Because optical sensors measure the concentration of protonated or deprotonated dye as an indirect measure of H^+ ion activity, variations in ionic strength of the physiologic sample can influence the accuracy of the pH measurement.

Applications

Optical sensors suitable for the determination of PCO_2 use optical pH transducers (with immobilized indicators) as inner transducers in an arrangement similar to the classic Severinghaus-style electrochemical sensor design (see Fig. 14.4). The addition of bicarbonate salt within the pH sensing hydrogel layer creates the required electrolyte film layer, which varies in pH depending on the PCO_2 in equilibrium with the film. The optical pH sensor is covered by an outer gas-permeable hydrophobic film (eg, silicone rubber) to prevent proton access, yet it allows CO_2 equilibration with the pH sensing layer. As the PCO_2 in the sample increases, the pH of the bicarbonate layer decreases, and the corresponding decrease in the deprotonated form of the indicator (or increase in the protonated form) is sensed optically.

Two approaches have been used to sense electrolyte ions optically in physiologic samples. One method uses many of the same lipophilic ionophores developed for polymer membrane–type ISEs (see Fig. 14.3).[12,13] These species are doped into thin hydrophobic polymeric films along with a lipophilic pH indicator. In the case of cation ionophores (eg, valinomycin for sensing K^+), when cations from the sample are extracted by the ionophore into the thin film, the pH indicator (RH) loses a proton to the sample phase to maintain charge neutrality within the organic film (yielding R^-). This results in a change in the optical absorption or fluorescence spectrum of the polymer layer. If the thickness of the films is kept at less than 10 μm, equilibrium response times on the order of less than 1 minute have been achieved. The main limitation of this design is that the pH of the sample phase also influences the overall extraction equilibrium for ions into the film. Thus, simultaneous and independent measurement of sample pH is required, or buffered dilution and/or pH control of the sample phase is necessary to obtain accurate measurements of electrolytes.

A second technique used to sense electrolyte ions is immobilization of a cation and/or anion recognition agent within a hydrogel matrix, similar to the pH sensors described earlier. The recognition agent in this case is not usually lipophilic; therefore, it must be covalently anchored to the hydrogel, so

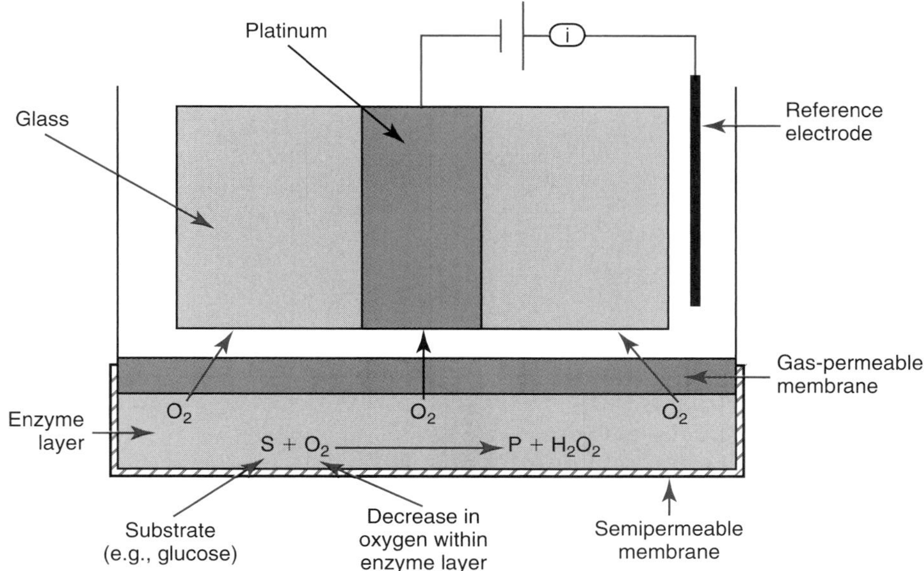

FIGURE 14.11 Illustration of Enzyme Electrode Prepared Using Oxidase Enzyme Immobilized at the Surface of an Amperometric Partial Pressure of Oxygen (PO_2) Sensor. Increase in substrate concentration *(S)* reduces the amount of oxygen present at the surface of the sensor. H_2O_2, Hydrogen peroxide.

that it does not leach into the sample phase. The agent is designed so that selective cation or anion binding alters the absorbance or fluorescence spectrum of the species within the hydrogel. Typically, this is achieved by linking ion recognition and chromophoric properties within a single organic molecule. Such ion sensors have been used successfully in at least one commercial blood gas-electrolyte analyzer using an array of sensors of the generic design similar to that in Fig. 14.10.

BIOSENSORS

A biosensor is a specific type of chemical sensor consisting of a biological recognition element and a physicochemical transducer, often an electrochemical[55,56] or an optical device. The biological element is capable of recognizing the presence and activity and/or concentration of a specific analyte in solution. The recognition may be a biocatalytic reaction (enzyme-based biosensor) or a binding process (affinity-based biosensor) when the recognition element is, for example, an antibody, DNA segment, or cell receptor. Interaction of the recognition element with a target analyte results in a measurable change in a solution property locally at the surface of the device, such as formation of a product or consumption of a reactant. The transducer converts the change in solution property into a quantifiable electrical signal. The mode of transduction may be one of several, including electrochemical or optical measurement and measurement of mass or heat. The present discussion is limited to biosensors based on electrochemical and optical modes of transduction because they constitute most biosensors used for clinical applications.

Enzyme-Based Biosensors With Amperometric Detection

Enzyme-based biosensors based on electrochemical transducers, specifically amperometric electrodes, are the most commonly used for clinical analyses and the most frequently cited in the literature.[57] Most of the current blood glucose meters are based on measurements using enzyme-based biosensors with amperometric detection, with glucose sensors produced in single-use formats. Clark and Lyons developed the first amperometric biosensor; it was used to measure glucose in blood and was based on immobilizing glucose oxidase on the surface of an amperometric PO_2 sensor.[58] A solution of glucose oxidase was physically entrapped between the gas-permeable membrane of the PO_2 electrode and an outer semipermeable membrane (Fig. 14.11; see general design). The outer membrane was of a low-molecular-weight cutoff to allow the substrate (glucose) and O_2 from the sample to pass, but not proteins and other macromolecules. In this way, enzymes could be concentrated at the

POINTS TO REMEMBER

Biosensors

- Biosensors measure substances lacking direct electroactive or optical properties.
- Biosensors consist of a biological recognition element and a physicochemical (eg, electrochemical or optical) transducer.
- Interaction of a biological recognition element and an analyte results in either a biocatalytical reaction or a binding process, producing a measurable signal.
- Biosensors are used in most commercial blood glucose meters.
- Sensors for whole blood measurements without a biological recognition element (eg., ISEs) are not considered biosensors.

sensor's surface. Oxidation of glucose, catalyzed by glucose oxidase as follows:

$$\text{Glucose} + O_2 \xrightarrow{\text{glucose oxidase}} \text{gluconic acid} + H_2O_2 \quad \textbf{(28)}$$

consumes O_2 near the surface of the sensor. The rate of decrease in PO_2 is a function of the glucose concentration and is monitored by the PO_2 electrode. A steady-state PO_2 can be achieved at the surface in a short period of time, yielding a steady-state current value that decreases as a function of glucose concentration in the sample.

If the polarizing voltage of the PO_2 electrode is reversed, making the Pt electrode positive (anode) relative to the Ag/AgCl reference electrode, and if the gas-permeable membrane is replaced with a hydrophilic membrane containing the immobilized enzyme, it is possible to oxidize the hydrogen peroxide (H_2O_2) produced by the glucose oxidase as follows:

$$H_2O_2 \rightarrow 2H^+ + O_2 + 2e^- \quad \textbf{(29)}$$

The steady-state current produced is now directly proportional to the concentration of glucose in the sample.

In practice, a sufficiently high voltage (overpotential) must be applied to the platinum anode to drive the oxidation of the H_2O_2. An applied voltage of +0.7 V or greater (relative to Ag/AgCl) is typically used. Fig. 14.12 illustrates this basic H_2O_2 detection design, which is suitable for use in devising clinically useful sensors for glucose, but also for a host of other substrates for which suitable oxidase enzymes generate H_2O_2.

Immobilization of enzymes in the early biosensors was a simple entrapment method behind a membrane of low-molecular-weight cutoff; this approach is still used in some commercial applications. Many other schemes for enzyme immobilization for biosensor development have been suggested.[59] The most common are cross-linking of the enzyme with an inert protein (eg, bovine serum albumin), using glutaraldehyde, simple adsorption of enzyme to electrode surfaces, and covalent binding of enzymes to insoluble carriers (eg, nylon or glass). Another immobilization technique involves bulk modification of an electrode material, mixing enzymes with carbon paste, which serves as both the enzyme immobilization matrix and the electroactive surface.[60]

One of the first biosensor-based systems for the measurement of glucose in blood was commercialized by Yellow Springs Instruments, Inc. in 1975, and used the amperometric detection of H_2O_2 as the measurement principle (see Fig. 14.12). Dependence of the measured glucose value on O_2 concentration in the sample was a problem because significantly less than the stoichiometric amount of dissolved O_2 is present in blood to support the glucose oxidase reaction and to produce a linear relationship of signal with glucose concentration. This is especially true at high concentrations of glucose found in samples from patients with diabetes (more than 500 mg/dL; 27.8 mmol/L). In the case of the Yellow Spring Instrument system, sample and calibration solutions are diluted at least 1:10 in buffer (depending on the model), which is in equilibrium with atmospheric PO_2 and fixes the O_2 concentration in the calibrator and sample at a constant value.

The problem of O_2 limitations of biosensors based on oxidase enzymes has been addressed by designing semipermeable membranes that restrict diffusion of the primary

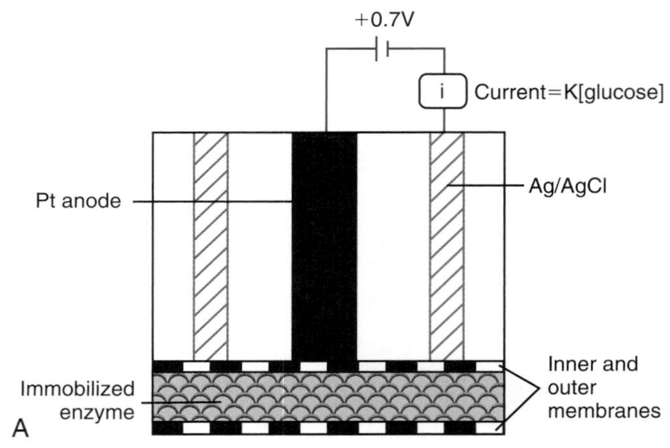

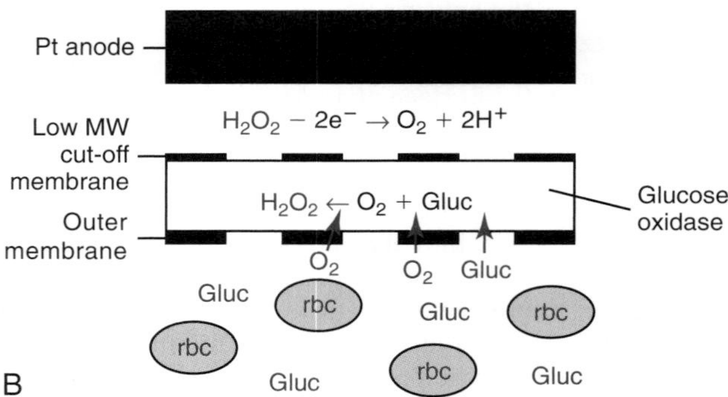

FIGURE 14.12 **A**, Design of amperometric enzyme electrode based on anodic detection of hydrogen peroxide (H_2O_2) generated from oxidase enzymatic reaction (eg, glucose oxidase). **B**, Expanded view of the sensing surface shows the different membranes and electrochemical processes that yield the anodic current proportional to the substrate concentration in the sample. *Ag/AgCl*, Silver-silver chloride; *K*, proportionality constant; *MW*, molecular weight; *Pt*, platinum; *rbc*, red blood cells. (From Meyerhoff M. New in vitro analytical approaches for clinical chemistry measurements in critical care. *Clin Chem* 1990;36:1570.)

analyte (substrate) to the enzyme layer, which avoids saturation of the enzyme and keeps the ratio of O_2 to analyte always in excess of 1. This extends the linearity of response to analyte concentrations substantially higher than the K_m of the enzyme and reduces the signal dependence on O_2. Outer track–etched polycarbonate membranes are commonly used,[61] as are membranes of poly(vinyl Cl), polyurethanes, and silicone emulsions.[62] Another approach has been to use an O_2-rich electrode material as a reservoir of O_2 to support the bioreaction. A fluorocarbon (Kel-F Oil) has been used to formulate a carbon paste electrode to act as a source of O_2 and as the working electrode.[63]

Electron acceptors other than O_2 can serve as mediators in the glucose oxidase reaction and completely eliminate any dependence of the amperometric response on the O_2 concentration of the sample. The mediator, which is usually co-immobilized with the enzyme, transports electrons to the anode surface, where it is reoxidized, resulting in a cyclic reaction mechanism (Fig. 14.13). Mediators with electron transfer kinetics (little or no overpotential) more favorable

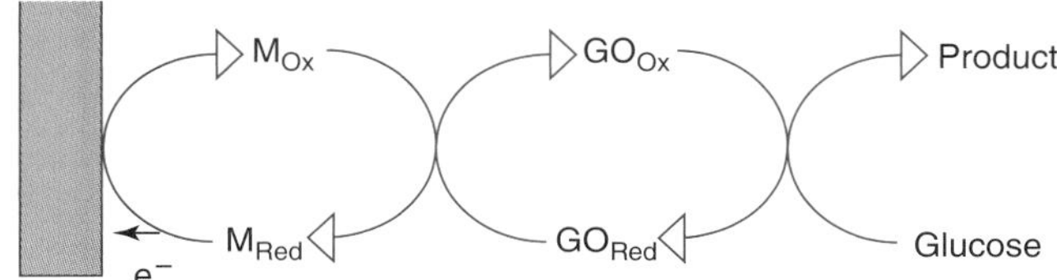

FIGURE 14.13 The Use of an Electroactive Mediator in the Design of an Amperometric Enzyme Electrode. The mediator accepts electrons directly from the enzyme and is oxidized at the surface of the working electrode, creating more oxidized mediator to continue this process. (From D'Orazio P. In: Lewendrowski K, editor. Clinical chemistry: laboratory management and clinical correlations. Philadelphia: Lippincott, Williams & Wilkins, 2002:464.)

than that of O_2 allow operation of the sensor at lower applied potentials (+0.2 V vs. Ag/AgCl or lower) than those that are typically used for the oxidation of H_2O_2. This approach not only eliminates dependency of the reaction rate on O_2, it also serves to reduce the contribution from oxidizable interfering substances (eg, uric acid, ascorbic acid, acetaminophen) to the sensor response. Examples of mediators that have been used include quinones and conductive organic salts, such as tetrathiafulvalene-tetracyanoquinodimethane.[64,65] Ferricyanide and ferrocene derivatives have also been used,[66] including commercial applications in a first-generation device for home blood glucose monitoring. Dimethylferrocene is impregnated into a graphite electrode to which glucose oxidase has been immobilized. Reduced glucose oxidase from the enzymatic reaction is reoxidized by the electrochemically generated ferricinium ion. Current produced during this cycling mechanism is proportional to the concentration of glucose in the blood sample.

Another technique used to decrease interferences from easily oxidized species in a blood sample when traditional H_2O_2 electrochemical detection is used is to employ selectively permeable membranes in proximity to the electrode surface that allow transport of H_2O_2 to the electrode surface, but reject the interfering substances based on size exclusion (see Fig. 14.12B). An example is as simple as a low-molecular-weight cutoff membrane, such as cellulose acetate, which is used in many commercial amperometric biosensors.[67] Electropolymerized films, such as poly(phenylenediamine) formed in situ, are also used, to reject interfering substances based on size.[68] Another approach used in a commercial application involves using a second correcting electrode, identical to the working electrode, but without an enzyme that is sensitive only to the presence of oxidizable interfering substances. The resulting differential signal is proportional to the concentration of analyte.

A novel approach used for elimination of electroactive interfering substances in a commercially available glucose sensor is to directly "wire" the redox center of the enzyme glucose oxidase to a metallic, amperometric electrode using an osmium (III/IV)-based redox hydrogel.[69] Osmium sites effectively serve as mediators and can accept electrons directly from the entrapped enzyme, without the need for O_2. This approach allows the operating potential of the electrode to be dramatically lowered to +0.2 V versus the saturated calomel reference electrode, where currents resulting from electro-oxidation of ascorbate, urate, acetaminophen, and L-cysteine are negligible.

Substitution of other oxoreductase enzymes for glucose oxidase allows amperometric biosensors for other substrates of clinical interest to be constructed. Practical sensors with commercial application in critical care analyzers for blood lactate have been realized.[70] By using the multiple enzyme cascade shown in the reactions discussed here, an amperometric biosensor for creatinine is also possible. Electrochemical oxidation of H_2O_2 is the detection mechanism:

$$\text{Creatinine} + H_2O \xrightarrow{\text{creatinine amidohydrolase}} \text{Creatine} \quad (30)$$

$$\text{Creatine} + H_2O \xrightarrow{\text{creatine amidinohydrolase}} \text{Sarcosine} + \text{Urea} \quad (31)$$

$$\text{Sarcosine} + H_2O + O_2 \xrightarrow{\text{sarcosine oxidase}} \text{Glycine} + \text{formaldehyde} + H_2O_2 \quad (32)$$

This three-enzyme scheme suffers interference from endogenous creatine in the sample, requiring correction. Low concentrations of creatinine found in blood (1.13 mg/dL or less; 100 µmol/L or less) must be measured in the presence of oxidizable interfering substances, which are sometimes present at higher concentrations than the analyte.[71] Special electroactive layers within the biosensor have been proposed to remove redox-active interfering substances.[72] Because the useful life of the creatinine biosensor based on these reactions requires three enzymes to retain activity, reusable commercial biosensors for creatinine based on this measurement principle typically have a short (few days) useful life, but improvements in enzyme immobilization methods and/or use of stabilizers and/or activators within calibrating reagents may yield creatinine sensor devices with much longer lifetimes. The importance of developing creatinine sensors and progress to date in this field have recently been summarized in detail by Lad and colleagues.[73]

Enzyme-Based Biosensors With Potentiometric and Conductometric Detection

ISEs can be used as transducers in potentiometric biosensors. An example is a biosensor for urea (blood urea nitrogen [BUN]) based on a polymer membrane ISE (poly[vinyl Cl]) for NH_4^+ ion (Fig. 14.14).[74] The enzyme urease is immobilized at the surface of the NH_4^+-selective ISE based on the antibiotic nonactin (see structure of ionophore in Fig. 14.3) and catalyzes the hydrolysis of urea to NH_3 and CO_2:

$$\text{Urea} \xrightarrow{\text{urease}} 2NH_3 + CO_2 \quad (33)$$

The ammonia (NH_3) produced forms NH_4^+, which is sensed by the ISE. The signal generated by the NH_4^+ produced is proportional to the logarithm of the concentration of urea in the sample. The response may be steady state or transient. Typically, correction for background K^+ is required, because the nonactin ionophore has limited selectivity for NH_4^+ over K^+ ($K_{NH4/K} = 0.1$). Potassium is measured simultaneously with urea and is used to correct the output of the urea sensor using the Nicolsky-Eisenman equation (Eq. 11).

The approach already described for measurement of urea using an enzyme-based potentiometric biosensor assumes

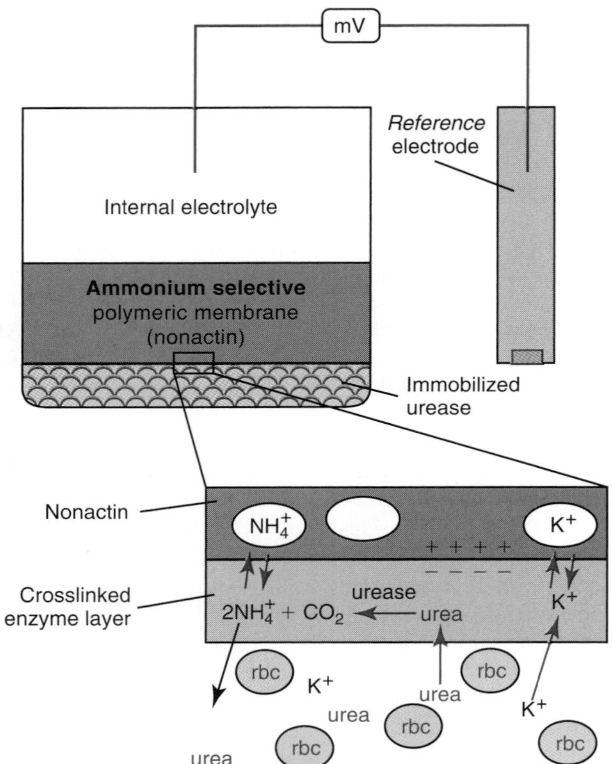

FIGURE 14.14 Potentiometric Enzyme Electrode for Determination of Blood Urea, Based on Urease Enzyme Immobilized on the Surface of an Ammonium Ion–Selective Polymeric Membrane Electrode. *CO_2*, Carbon Dioxide; K^+, Potassium; *NH_4^+*, ammonium; *rbc,* red blood cells.

that the turnover of urea to NH_4^+ at steady state provides a constant ratio of NH_4^+ ions to urea, independent of concentration. This is rarely the case, especially at higher substrate concentrations, which results in a nonlinear sensor response. The linearity of the sensor is also limited by the fact that hydrolysis of urea produces a local alkaline pH in the vicinity of the NH_4^+-sensing membrane, partially converting NH_4^+ to NH_3 (pKa = 9.3). Ammonia is not sensed by the ISE. The degree of nonlinearity may be reduced by the placement of a semipermeable membrane between the enzyme and the sample to restrict diffusion of urea to the immobilized enzyme layer.

A change in solution conductivity has also been used as a transduction mechanism in enzyme-based biosensors. Examples include the measurement of glucose, creatinine, and acetaminophen using interdigitated electrodes.[75] There are few practical applications of conductometric biosensors because of the variable ionic background of clinical samples and the requirement to measure small conductivity changes in media of high ionic strength. A commercial system for the measurement of urea in serum, plasma, and urine is a BUN analyzer (Beckman-Coulter, Brea, California) based on the enzyme urease.[76] Dissolution of products to NH_4^+ and HCO_3^- produces a change in sample conductivity. The initial rate of change in conductivity is measured to compensate for the background conductivity of the sample. This approach is limited to the measurement of analytes at relatively high concentrations because of small changes in conductivity produced by low concentrations of analyte.

Enzyme-Based Biosensors With Optical Detection

Optical sensors with immobilized enzymes and indicator dyes have been developed for the measurement of glucose and other substrates of clinical interest.[77] These biosensors are based on optical detection chemistries for pH and O_2, described earlier in this chapter, and rely on absorbance and/or reflectance, fluorescence, and luminescence as modes of detection. Enzyme immobilization methods resemble those used to construct electrochemical biosensors, including physical entrapment or encapsulation in a gel matrix, physical adsorption onto substrates, and covalent binding or absorption on an insoluble support. Using an example based on an optode for PO_2, a sensitive indicator is co-immobilized with an oxidase enzyme at the end of a fiber optic probe. The probe is used to monitor fluorescence of the indicator. Quenching of fluorescence of the indicator by O_2 is followed. A decrease in PO_2 resulting from a reaction catalyzed by the enzyme will result in less quenching of the indicator and a fluorescent signal directly proportional to the concentration of the substrate. In an example of an optical biosensor probe for glucose, an O_2-sensitive cationic dye, $Ru(phen)_3^{2+}$, is immobilized along with glucose oxidase on the surface of an optical fiber.[78] A decrease in PO_2 arising from the enzyme-catalyzed oxidation of glucose results in an increase in luminescence intensity of the ruthenium tris(phenanthrene).

Similar optical biosensors have been prepared for many other analytes. For example, a cholesterol optical biosensor has been devised based on fluorescence quenching of an O_2-sensitive dye that is coupled to the consumption of O_2 resulting from the enzyme-catalyzed oxidation of cholesterol by the enzyme cholesterol oxidase.[79] Serum bilirubin has been detected using bilirubin oxidase, co-immobilized with a ruthenium dye, on an optical fiber.[80] The bilirubin sensor was reported to exhibit a lower detection limit of 0.6 mg/dL (10 µmol/L), a linear range up to 1.8 mg/dL (30 mmol/L), and a typical reproducibility of 3% (coefficient of variation), which is adequate for clinical application.

The pH change resulting from enzyme-catalyzed reactions has also been measured optically. The indicator dye fluorescein is often used as a pH-sensitive indicator to construct such sensors. The protonated form of fluorescein does not fluoresce, but the conjugate base strongly fluoresces at 530 nm, when excited at 490 nm. Using glucose oxidase as the enzyme, a pH optode has been used to follow the formation of gluconic acid.[81] A disadvantage of optical sensors based on pH changes is that they are strongly dependent on the pH and buffer capacity of the sample. Moreover, the working range of the sensor is determined by the pKa of the indicator, 6.8 to 7.2 for fluorescein, depending on ionic strength of the sample matrix. A pH-sensitive indicator may also be used to follow enzymatic reactions that produce ammonia (eg, urease action on urea).

Affinity Sensors

Affinity sensors are a special class of biosensors in which the immobilized biological recognition element is a binding protein, antibody (immunosensors), or oligonucleotide (eg, DNA, aptamers, covered in more detail in the following) with high binding affinity and high specificity toward a clinically important analyte and/or partner. Such sensors are being developed as alternatives to conventional binding assays to enhance the speed and convenience of a wide range of assays that normally would be run on large, sophisticated instruments in a central laboratory. Affinity sensors may be more easily adapted than traditional assays to systems developed for point-of-care testing for infectious disease, cardiac markers, or other cases where speed and ease of use are required. Ideally, direct binding of the immobilized species with its target in a clinical sample should yield a sensor signal proportional to the concentration of the analyte. However, direct sensing (without use of exogenous labels and/or tracers) of the binding events at analyte concentrations that would cover the full range for clinical applications is very difficult to achieve. Furthermore, high affinity of such binding reactions, which are required to achieve optimal sensitivity, also limits the reversibility of such devices (slow reverse rate constant). Unlike ISEs, O_2 sensors, and many of the enzyme-based biosensors described previously, affinity sensors based on electrochemical, optical, or other transduction modes are typically single-use devices. For repeated multiuse applications, some type of regeneration step (pH change, temperature change, and so on) to dissociate the tight binding between the recognition element and the target is required. An example of a thermally reversible immunosensor, demonstrated to retain activity and specificity for up to 30 assays, has recently been described.[82] The sensor consists of an antibody conjugated to a polymer, which undergoes a reversible phase transition in response to temperature. Altering temperature produces a change in orientation of the conjugated polymer and affinity between the conjugate and a target antigen, resulting in a reversible antigen–antibody binding reaction.

Most affinity-type sensors appearing in the literature with a promise of clinical usefulness are based on labeled reagents, such as enzymes, fluorophores, and electrochemical tags, and hence, they function more like traditional binding and/or immunoassays, except that one recognition element is immobilized on the surface of a suitable electrode or another type of transducer.[83-85] For example, electrochemical O_2 sensors have been used to carry out heterogeneous enzyme immunoassays (sandwich or competitive type), using catalase as a labeling enzyme (catalyzes $H_2O_2 \rightarrow 2H^+$ and O_2) and immobilizing capture antibodies on the outer surface of the gas-permeable membrane. After binding equilibration and washing steps, the amount of bound enzyme is detected by adding the substrate and following the increase in current generation caused by local production of O_2 near the surface of the sensor.

The number of research reports related to affinity biosensors continues to increase, with potential application for detection of markers of cardiac disease, cancer, and autoimmune disease.[86] Affinity sensors for DNA analysis are covered in more detail in the following. Commercialization has lagged behind research output, and movement of affinity biosensors from the research laboratory to the clinical laboratory has been slow. Some commercial examples of immunosensors do exist, primarily in the unit-use, disposable format designed for point-of-care testing. One successful commercial example is a cartridge-based device for cardiac troponin I on the i-STAT handheld analyzer (Abbott Point of Care, Abbott Laboratories, Abbott Park, Illinois).[87] This sensor uses a sandwich immunoassay format with electrochemical detection. A capture antibody is immobilized on a Au electrode for recognition and capture of troponin in the blood sample. A second reporter antibody is labeled with alkaline phosphatase and binds with surface-captured troponin antigen. Following incubation and washing steps, the substrate p-aminophenyl phosphate is introduced, and the product of the enzymatic reaction (p-aminophenol) is detected amperometrically by oxidation. Magnitude of the oxidative current is proportional to concentration of troponin in the sample.

The basic advantage of immobilizing affinity reagents on the surfaces of electrodes and optical sensing devices is somewhat diminished when separate washing steps are required to remove unbound label species. As discussed previously, true affinity biosensors should yield analytically useful responses in the presence of undiluted physiologic samples, without the need for discrete incubation and washing steps. One example of an electrochemical-based immunosensor method that partially achieves this goal is a technique termed nonseparation electrochemical enzyme immunoassay.[88] The basic concept is illustrated in Fig. 14.15. As indicated, no separation or washing steps are required. This method was used to detect prostate-specific antigen (PSA) and human chorionic gonadotropin at nanogram per milliliters concentrations in undiluted plasma and whole blood. A number of other direct-reading affinity sensors have been proposed, based on electrochemical (including capacitance and impedance changes), optical, thermal, mass, and acoustic detection methods.[83-85,89,90] Direct affinity sensors eliminate the need for labeled reagents because the binding reaction

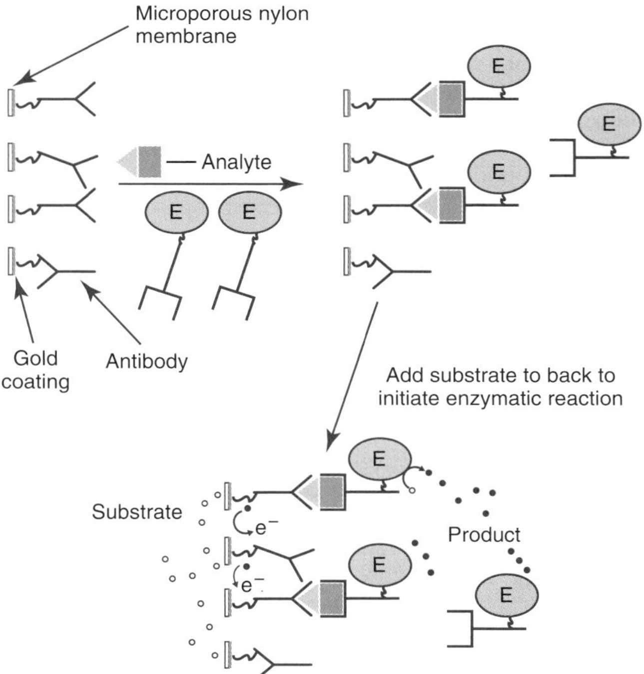

FIGURE 14.15 Principle of Nonseparation Electrochemical Enzyme Immunoassay Concept, Configured in Sandwich Immunoassay Mode to Detect a Given Protein Analyte. Enzyme label on reporter antibody generates an electroactive product that is detected at the surface of the porous gold electrode when the substrate for the enzyme is added to the back of the membrane.

results in a change in a property that may be monitored directly. Of these, few have adequate specificity to be used in complex clinical samples because of significant signals arising from nonspecific binding. However, one report has suggested that α-fetoprotein can be detected reliably in serum samples via a quartz crystal microbalance mass detector, which possesses immobilized anti–α-fetoprotein antibodies on the surface of the quartz crystal transducer.[91] Increasing concentrations of analyte in the sample yield increased binding to the surface, changing the mass loaded because of the immunologic reaction. Incubation times as low as 20 minutes are required to achieve results that compare favorably with those of a conventional radioimmunoassay method for serum samples. Direct immunosensors for sensitive assays of tumor markers have been reported. Examples include an electrochemical immunosensor for PSA with an enhanced lower limit of detection, based on an alternating current impedance measurement,[92] and an assay for carcinoma antigen-125 using a quartz crystal microbalance.[93] The former uses a control sensor with an immobilized immunoglobulin-G antibody instead of anti-PSA to subtract out effects from nonspecific binding to achieve a limit of detection of 1 pg/mL toward PSA.

Affinity Sensors for DNA Analysis Using Fluorescent Labels

Affinity-type sensors based on oligonucleotide binding represent perhaps the most promising application of affinity sensors to clinical chemistry. Fluorescent labels were the first to be used in an early commercial biosensor for DNA analysis, introduced in 1996 (GeneChip, Affymetrix, Santa Clara, California). High-density oligonucleotide arrays are formed on glass substrates. Target DNA is isolated and amplified using the polymerase chain reaction (PCR) while a fluorescent label is incorporated. The sample is incubated on the array, and detection of hybridization of labeled DNA to its complementary strands takes place by monitoring light emitted by the fluorescent labels. The primary application of the device has been for DNA sequencing, so the focus has been primarily on increasing the density of the DNA arrays. Applications of the device continue to expand with a variety of arrays developed for gene expression and whole genomic analysis related to (1) cancer, (2) inflammatory disease, (3) infectious disease, and (4) diabetes. Another commercial example of affinity sensors for DNA analysis using fluorescent labels is the BeadArray technology (Illumina, San Diego, California).[94,95] Silica microbeads with covalently attached, single-stranded DNA probes are randomly assembled on a fiberoptic bundle or planar silica surface. Each bead carries hundreds of thousands of copies of a gene-specific probe sequence. Due to the high-density packing of beads, with a possibility of approximately 50,000 beads on a 1.4-mm diameter array, a large number of probe sequences may be investigated in parallel, and multiple copies of each probe sequence are possible, which increases measurement precision. Fluorescently labeled target sequences in the sample to be analyzed hybridize with their complementary probe sequences. Arrays are scanned in a BeadArray reader for image analysis and data extraction. This versatile platform has been adapted for various genetic analyses, such as single nucleotide polymorphism genotyping, DNA methylation detection, and gene expression profiling.[96]

Affinity Sensors for DNA Analysis Using Electrochemical Labels

DNA sensors in which a segment of DNA complementary to a target strand is immobilized on a suitable electrochemical sensor have been demonstrated. These devices operate in direct (based on electrochemical oxidation of guanine in target DNA; Fig. 14.16A) or indirect (with exogenous electrochemical markers and/or labels, see later and Fig. 14.16B) transduction modes. Although most of the proposed electrochemical DNA biosensors require amplification methods, such as PCR, to multiply small amounts of DNA into measurable quantities, some are sensitive enough to eliminate the need for target amplification. Nanotechnology has been proposed, in the indirect format, for signal amplification. For example, a capture probe DNA is immobilized on a Au electrode. Reporter probes with electrostatically bound ruthenium complexes $(Ru[NH_3]_6)^{3+}$ are loaded onto Au nanoparticles (AuNP) and are capable of hybridizing with one of two sequences on target DNA. The other sequence on the target DNA is capable of hybridizing with the immobilized capture probe. Hybridization events on the electrode surface bring multiple reporter probes for each AuNP. Electroactive $(Ru[NH_3]_6)^{3+}$ is reduced at the electrode surface, and the coulometric signal is proportional to the concentration of target DNA.[97] A commercial example of electrochemical DNA sensing, along with AuNP probes without need for PCR amplification, is the Verigene system (Nanosphere, Chicago, Illinois), which is capable of detecting single-nucleotide polymorphisms related to common genetic disorders, such as (1) thrombophilia, (2) alterations of folate metabolism, (3) cystic fibrosis, and (4) hemochromatosis. Another commercially available, electrochemically based platform for nucleic acid detection without the need for sample purification or target amplification is from GeneFluidics (Irwindale, California). The system uses a sensor array chip consisting of 16 nanoscale Au electrodes, modified with thiol self-assembled monolayers, optimized for biomolecule immobilization.[98] Horseradish peroxidase is the preferred target label because of its fast electron transfer kinetics, when used with amperometric detection.

Another example of an electrochemical "gene" sensor array uses electrochemical probes that are selectively inserted into hybridized DNA duplexes. In one approach, after the immobilized capture of oligo anchored to the electrode surface is allowed to bind the target sequence, hybridization is detected by exposing the surface of the electrode to an exogenous electroactive species (Co[III]tris-phenanthroline, ruthenium complexes, and so on) that intercalates within the duplex, but not to single-stranded DNA. After unbound electroactive species are removed by washing, the presence of hybridization is readily detected by voltammetry, scanning the potential of the underlying electrode to oxidize or reduce any intercalated electroactive species, with the current detected being proportional to the number of duplex DNA species on the surface of the electrode.

Affinity Sensors Based on Aptamers (Aptasensors)

Apatmers have been explored as versatile recognition elements for a variety of biosensing applications, including small molecules, proteins, and cells.[99] Aptamers are synthetic single-stranded nucleic acids capable of folding into three-dimensional structures to selectively bind target molecules.

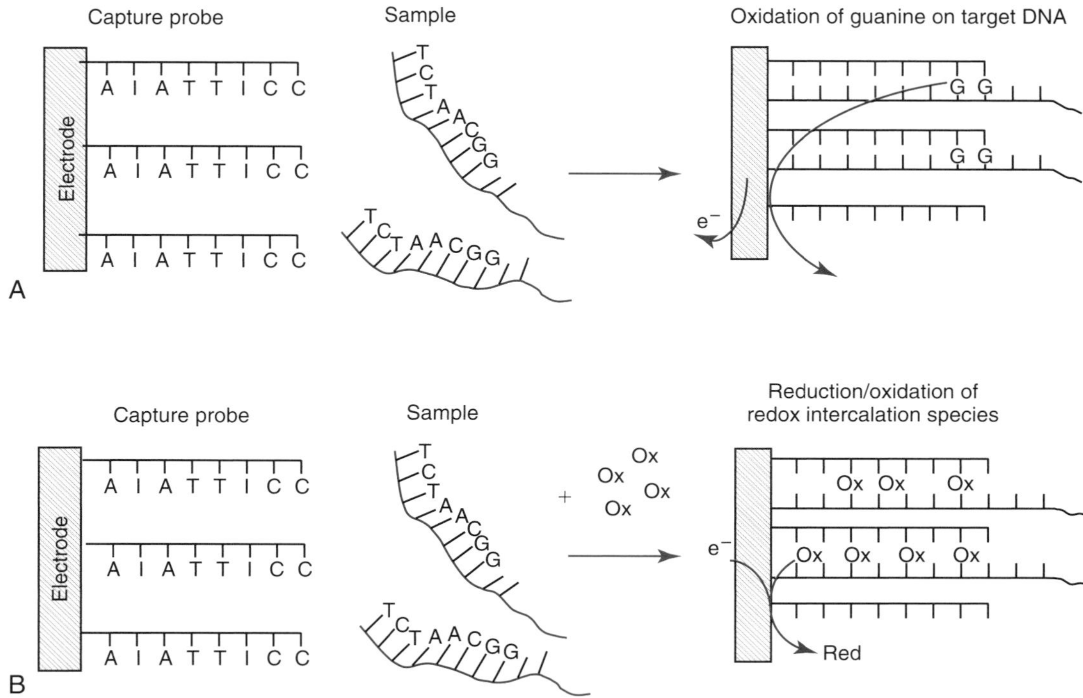

FIGURE 14.16 Examples of DNA Biosensor Configurations. A, Direct electro-oxidation (Ox) detection of guanosine bases in target DNA after hybridization with immobilized capture probe on electrode surface. **B,** Electrochemical detection of hybridization using exogenous redox (Red) species that intercalates into hybridized complex between the immobilized capture DNA probe and target DNA.

In practice, aptamers may be generated and selected in vitro to bind targets for which antibodies and other protein receptors are not easily obtained, using a process known as systematic evolution of ligands by exponential enrichment (SELEX).[99] During the SELEX process, a large, random DNA or RNA library goes through an iterative process of selective binding toward a target analyte. After separation of bound and unbound DNA, the binding DNA is amplified using PCR for a subsequent round of selection and isolation of the optimum binding segment. This method, by which aptamers are selected against their targets, makes them inherently suited to displacement assays because of greatly reduced affinity for the labeled form of a target. Another inherent advantage of aptamer-based affinity sensors is reduced nonspecific binding because of the conformational change of the aptamer during the binding event, making the aptamer less susceptible to recognition of many potential interfering substances in a complex sample matrix (eg, blood serum).[100] The same conformational change may optimize performance of a labeled target following a binding event; for example, by altering the local environment of a fluorescent label or changing the position of an electrochemical label with respect to a sensing electrode. Although few aptamer-based diagnostic products have been commercialized at present, reported practical applications for aptamer-based affinity sensors in clinical chemistry are increasing in the literature.

Aptamers have been demonstrated to function in biosensors using various transduction methods, including optical sensing (using fluorescently labeled aptamers),[101] and acoustic, mass (cantilever-based), and electrochemical sensing, which use, for example, aptamer probes labeled with a redox species (eg, Ferrocene).[102,103] Many transduction modes, such as fluorescence, have a background signal in a complex sample matrix (eg, blood serum), which limits the sensitivity of the method. One transduction mode, demonstrated using an aptasensor, to reduce background fluorescence in a complex sample matrix is time-resolved fluorescence, in which the fluorescence lifetime of the detection signal is differentiated from nonspecific fluorescence background in the sample matrix. Lanthanides, such as europium ions, are attractive candidates as fluorescent labels because of their long fluorescent lifetimes (up to 1 ms).[104] As is the case with most affinity-based biosensors, electrochemical sensing for aptasensors may still be the preferred transduction mode because redox labels may be chosen to operate at an applied potential away from potentially interfering electroactive species in the sample matrix. By taking advantage of the conformational change of the aptamer during a binding event, it changes the relative proximity of an electrochemical label to an electrode surface.[102,105] Using thrombin as a model analyte and methylene blue (MB) as an electroactive label, an aptasensor was constructed by immobilizing a MB-labeled, thrombin-binding aptamer to a thiol modified Au electrode.[106] In the absence of thrombin, the apatmer chain is flexible, and the MB label is close to the electrode surface for high electron transfer efficiency. Upon binding to the thrombin target, the folding of the aptamer moves the label away from the electrode surface, inhibiting electron transfer. A sensitivity down to 6.4-nmol thrombin was demonstrated. The opposite transduction approach (in which target binding by the aptamer brings an electroactive label closer to an electrode surface) was demonstrated as a sensor for platelet-derived growth factor (PDGF) in blood serum.[107] In this case, the MB label was attached at one end of the PDGF aptamer, and in the absence of a target, the label was relatively far from the electrode surface. Binding of the PDGF target brought the MB label close to the electrode surface in a stable configuration, enhancing an electron transfer. Detection of PDGF down to 50 pmol was shown.

POINTS TO REMEMBER

Affinity Biosensors

- Affinity biosensors are a specific type of biosensor in which an immobilized recognition element exhibits a high binding constant for the analyte of interest.
- Examples of recognition elements are antibodies and oligonucleotides (DNA segments).
- Affinity biosensor binding reactions are typically irreversible and best suited to single-use sensors.
- Most affinity biosensors for clinical application use indirect modes of transduction, based on reagent label such as enzymes, fluorescent, and electrochemical labels.

CHEMICAL SENSORS BASED ON NANOTECHNOLOGY

Nanotechnology is defined as the study of the synthesis, properties, and application of structures and materials having at least one critical dimension in the range of 1 to 100 nm.[108,109] Structures such as nanowires, nanoparticles, quantum dots, and carbon nanotubes offer unique electrical, optical, and magnetic properties that can be exploited for chemical sensing. The large surface area available on nanostructures for immobilization of labels and biological recognition elements offers the potential for high signal amplification by increasing the signal-to-noise ratio. Nanomaterials and their applications, particularly for the development of sensors for cancer biomarkers with improved lower limits of detection, have recently been reviewed.[109,110] Developments in the field of DNA nanodevices have resulted in complex molecular detection and amplification schemes, which may outperform PCR in terms of sensitivity and ease of use.[111]

The flexibility and the unique shape of carbon nanotubes and the presence of reactive groups on their surface has led to their being used as biocatalytic and affinity biosensors.[112,113] Direct electron transfer between immobilized glucose oxidase and carbon nanotubes allows construction of glucose biosensors without mediators. In addition, enhanced electron transfer between proteins and carbon nanotubes results in lower overpotentials and higher peak currents observed for the voltammetric response of several molecules at electrodes modified with carbon nanotubes.[112] For DNA sensors, using carbon nanotubes in a detector for the hybridization event provides an efficient way to amplify the label-free electrochemical detection of DNA hybridization and to enhance charge transfer between surface-anchored DNA sequences and carbon nanotubes.[90,114]

Nanomaterial labels, including Au, Ag, and semiconductor nanoparticles, have been shown to result in large signal enhancements and to lower limits of detection in electrochemical immunosensors for disease-related protein biomarkers, and for detection of DNA hybridization events.[115] Au nanoparticles have been used as both immobilization platforms and labels for electrochemical immunosensors.[116] Electrodes with layers of densely packed 5-nm AuNP were used as a matrix for immobilization of horseradish peroxidase in a sandwich immunoassay for PSA with a detection limit of 0.5 pg/mL.[117] In an optical assay, oligonucleotide targets labeled with AuNP instead of fluorophore probes have been shown to enhance sensitivity toward the oligonucleotide target by up to two orders of magnitude.[118] A commercial system using AuNP for electrochemical DNA sensing is the Verigene System, which was reviewed previously.

Other examples of nanotechnology applied to chemical sensing are emerging. For example, nanopores down to 1.4 nm in diameter have been created in lipid bilayers through the action of the protein α-hemolysin. A pore with nanometer-scale dimensions has a size comparable to that of a single large molecule (protein, single-stranded DNA). The molecule must be charged to be driven through the pore by an electric field. The contribution of the large molecule to the passage of electric (ionic) current through the pore is small compared with that of mobile small ions, allowing detection of the target analyte down to a single molecule.[119] Microfabricated cantilevers made of silicon or silicon nitride have been used as transducers in affinity biosensors for monitoring (1) DNA hybridization, (2) antigen–antibody interactions, or (3) absorption of bacteria. Mechanical bending of the cantilever on the order of nanometers, in response to affinity reactions, is monitored. Although the sensitivity of cantilever biosensors is limited by nonspecific binding, the technology is equivalent in sensitivity to that of other label-free methods, for example, in the picomolar range for detection of oligonucleotides, and in the nanogram per milliliter range for measurement of antigens.[120]

IN VIVO AND MINIMALLY INVASIVE SENSORS

Progress has been made in the development of miniaturized, implantable electrochemical and optical sensors that can be used for in vivo, real-time monitoring of clinically important species. Unfortunately, the biological response toward such sensors (eg, clotting) can have a dramatic impact on the analytical accuracy of such indwelling probes[121-124] and has prevented their widespread use in clinical practice. However, progress is being made toward improving the reliability of in vivo measurements, and some commercial products for subcutaneous glucose monitoring are already on the market (see later).

Analytical sensors that can be implanted within human blood vessels or subcutaneously mandate that such sensing devices have an outside diameter of less than 0.6 mm. Both electrochemical and optical sensor technologies have been used to create devices of the required size. These are basically miniaturized versions of the previously described in vitro electrochemical and optical sensor devices. However, in addition to their small size, such devices must exhibit stable output signals because reliable calibration of the probes with calibrating solutions is not possible once the probes are inserted. Although so-called in situ calibration is possible (periodically removing an in vitro blood sample to obtain current values of analytes and updating in vivo sensor output to this value), if the frequency of such in situ calibrations is high, the true advantage of having an in vivo probe is greatly diminished.

Continuous in vivo measurement of oxygen saturation (SaO_2) has been achieved by placing small optical fibers into the bloodstream via a catheter and then measuring the reflective absorbance of the blood at two or three appropriately selected wavelengths based on the absorbance spectra of oxy- and deoxy-Hb.[125] In addition, implantable analytical sensors that provide continuous readings of blood gases ($pH/PCO_2/PO_2$), when inserted within the radial artery, especially for critically ill patients already fitted with an arterial line, have been developed.[126] Such sensors are usually based on the classical Clark-style design, in which O_2 is reduced at a micro-Pt, -Ag, or -Au working electrode confined (along with Ag/AgCl reference) within a narrow-diameter gas-permeable catheter tube made of a given polymer (Fig.14.17A), with the resulting current being proportional to the PO_2 in the medium surrounding the catheter. Indwelling electrochemical pH and PCO_2 sensors are typically potentiometric devices, based on polymer membrane pH electrode technology or the use of solid-state metal oxide–based pH sensors. Incorporation of lipophilic proton ionophores (eg, tridodecylamine; see Fig.14.3) within the walls of plastic tubing provides a convenient means of preparing a novel dual-lumen pH/PCO_2 sensing design that has been demonstrated in animal experiments to provide accurate in vivo results.[127]

However, miniaturization of electrode designs that enable several sensors to be bundled into a single implantable device remains a significant engineering challenge. Consequently, many efforts aimed at developing commercially viable intravascular blood gas sensors for simultaneously monitoring pH, PCO_2, and PO_2 have used modern optical fiber–based technology alone or in combination with a single electrochemical device. Because the outer diameter of available fibers continues to decrease, it is now possible to bundle three or more separate chemically sensitive fibers within a single catheter with an outer diameter of less than 600 μm for implantation within human radial arteries, without dampening the pressure waveform detected by a microelectronic pressure transducer within the arterial line. Absorbance-,

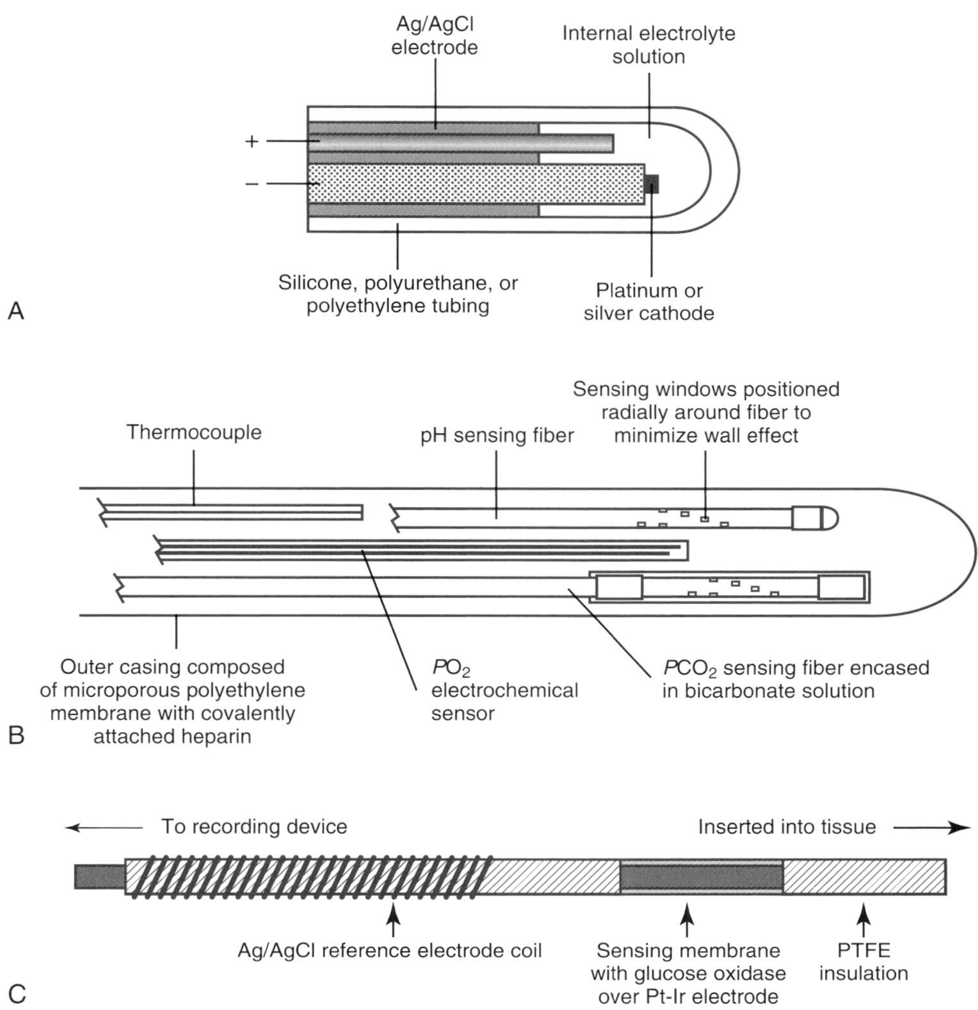

FIGURE 14.17 Schematics of Various Implantable Electrochemical and/or Optical Sensors Useful for Continuous in Vivo Monitoring. A, Catheter-style amperometric oxygen sensor. **B,** Design of Paratrend intravascular combined partial pressure of oxygen (PO_2), partial pressure of carbon dioxide (PCO_2), and pH sensor (hybrid electrochemical/optical design). **C,** Needle-type electrochemical glucose sensor useful for monitoring glucose subcutaneously to track blood glucose concentrations continuously. *Ag/AgCl,* Silver-silver chloride; *Pt-Ir,* platinum-iridium; *PTFE,* Teflon.

fluorescence-, and phosphorescence-based chemistries have been investigated in the design of sensors with suitable selectivity and calibration stability.[124] Appropriate indicators are usually immobilized on the distal ends of the fibers, although alternate configurations and/or locations have also been proposed. Most optical O_2 measurements are made with indicators whose luminescence is quenched in the presence of O_2, whereas pH sensors are prepared by immobilizing pH indicators (eg, phenol red) in hydrogel type films.[53] Optical sensors for PCO_2 can be easily prepared from the same pH sensors by incorporating bicarbonate salt in the hydrogel layer and then covering this layer with a gas-permeable polymeric film (usually silicone rubber material), as described previously in the section on Optical Sensors.

Despite significant efforts by a number of large biomedical companies in the 1980s and 1990s, only the Paratrend probe was commercially available for a period of time for the intravascular measurement of blood gases. As shown in Fig. 14.17B, this indwelling sensor consisted of a novel hybrid design, in which O_2 was sensed electrochemically (catheter form of Clark sensor), whereas pH and PCO_2 were determined via fiber-based optical fluorescence sensors.[128] Although acceptable clinical performance of the Paratrend was reported, frequent in situ recalibrations were suggested.[129] A later version of this product replaced the electrochemical O_2 sensor with an optical fiber design. However, continued problems with in vivo performance and concomitant costs of using the device prevented widespread use, and the product is no longer available.

Another class of in vivo chemical sensors consists of glucose sensors designed to help manage patients with diabetes by continuous monitoring of glucose in interstitial fluid (ISF) using glucose sensors implanted subcutaneously. Continuous monitors for measuring glucose in ISF first appeared commercially in the late 1990s. Currently, devices from at least two manufacturers continue to be offered. Sensor designs are similar to electrochemical sensors used for in vitro measurement of blood glucose, as described previously. Subcutaneously implanted glucose sensors require periodic calibration using results from fingerstick blood glucose and require replacement every 3 to 7 days, depending on the device. Despite limited commercial success, continuous glucose monitors, based on subcutaneously implanted sensors, have been shown to detect and predict hypoglycemic events and reduce time spent in the hypoglycemic range in adults and children with type 1 diabetes.[130] Several clinical trials have shown significant reduction in glycosylated hemoglobin concentration among users of continuous glucose monitors.[130,131]

Implantable glucose (and lactate) sensors have been based, almost exclusively, on electrochemical transducers. For example, one such sensor is based on using dual O_2 sensors in a single catheter design for indwelling blood glucose and lactate measurements.[132] One O_2 sensor with immobilized glucose or lactate oxidase provides response to substrate concentrations (decreasing surface O_2 in response to increased glucose or lactate), whereas the second matched O_2 sensor, without enzyme, is able to correct for unknown and varying amounts of endogenous PO_2. Others have focused on the design of probes with amperometric detection of H_2O_2 (via oxidation) at an underlying iridium/Pt anode, similar in operation to those used in vitro in commercial instruments.[133] With such designs, the use of outer polymer films to restrict glucose (or lactate) diffusion relative to O_2 is critical to achieve a linear electrochemical response to glucose from normal (90 mg/dL; 5 mmol/L) to increased concentrations found in patients with diabetes (greater than 500 mg/dL; 27.8 mmol/L). Fig. 14.17C illustrates a design in which the needle-type probe is constructed by multiple membrane coatings and electrodeposition of the glucose oxidase layer.[134] Designs similar to this are among the currently US Food and Drug Administration–cleared sensors available for subcutaneous monitoring of glucose.[135-137] In one instance, the sensor is actually fabricated on a narrow planar substrate, rather than on a cylindrical wire-based system. Relatively frequent calibration of all such sensors is still required via periodic in vitro blood tests, especially in the early stages after subcutaneous implantation.[135]

Instead of implanting glucose sensors intravascularly or subcutaneously, an alternative approach that is considered minimally invasive uses electrochemical glucose sensors to monitor glucose concentrations in ISF collected through the skin.[135] Techniques for drawing ISF include iontophoresis (a low electric current applied across the skin to cause charged and uncharged species to move through the skin pores), sonophoresis (application of low-frequency ultrasound to increase skin permeability of ISF), and micropore technology (laser ablation to create an array of microscopic holes in the skin and collection of ISF using a small vacuum).[138] In all cases, ISF is collected and assayed externally using a glucose sensor. One such commercial device is the Symphony continuous glucose monitor (CGM) (Echo Therapeutics, Philadelphia, Pennsylvania), which collects ISF transdermally and assays the glucose concentration using an electrochemical biosensor. The device was recently reported to show acceptable accuracy when used to monitor glucose in critically ill cardiac surgery patients, with 99.6% of results within Zones A and B of the Clarke error grid.[131] The device required a 1-hour warm-up period after attachment to the patient, after which glucose readings were collected every minute. To evaluate accuracy of the device, arterial blood samples were taken at 30- to 60-minute intervals and analyzed using an in vitro blood glucose reference instrument. The CGM sensor was recalibrated every 4 hours after sensor application using glucose results from the reference device. The CGM sensor requires replacement every 24 hours.

Current research and development efforts have focused on the use of more biocompatible coatings to reduce the biological response of intravascular and subcutaneous devices. These efforts are based on the expectation that such developments will be critical to the ultimate success in developing implanted sensors that yield continuous analytical results that closely match those attained by conventional in vitro test methods. One new approach in this direction uses novel NO release and/or generating polymers to coat the surface of intravascular sensors.[139-141] The potent antiplatelet activity of NO has been shown to greatly reduce the formation of thrombus on the surface of implantable electrochemical O_2 sensing catheters and to yield much more accurate continuous PO_2 values in animal experiments. Furthermore, NO has been shown to decrease the inflammatory response that occurs for glucose sensors implanted subcutaneously[142,143] and for glucose and lactate sensors implanted intravenously.[144]

SELECTED REFERENCES

For a full list of references for this chapter, please refer to ExpertConsult.com.

2. Bates RG. *Determination of pH: theory and practice*. New York: John Wiley & Sons; 1973.
7. Buck RP, Lindner E. Recommendations for nomenclature of ion-selective electrodes. *Pure Appl Chem* 1994;**66**:2527–36.
8. Oesch U, Ammann D, Simon W. Ion-selective membrane electrodes for clinical use. *Clin Chem* 1986;**32**:1448–59.
12. Bakker E, Bühlmann P, Pretsch E. Carrier-based ion-selective electrodes and bulk optodes. 1. General characteristics. *Chem Rev* 1997;**97**:3083–132.
16. Pioda LA, Simon W, Bosshard HR, et al. Determination of potassium ion concentration in serum using a highly selective liquid-membrane electrode. *Clin Chim Acta* 1970;**29**:289–93.
30. Shvarev A, Bakker E. Response characteristics of a reversible electrochemical sensor for the polyion protamine. *Anal Chem* 2005;**77**:5221–8.
32. Astrup P, Severinghaus JW. *The history of blood gases, acids and bases*. Copenhagen, Denmark: Munksgaard; 1986.
34. Apple FS, Koch DD, Graves S, et al. Relationship between direct potentiometric and flame photometric measurement of sodium in blood. *Clin Chem* 1982;**28**:1931–5.
35. Osswald HF, Wuhrmann HR. Calibration standards for multi ion analysis in whole blood samples. In: Lubbers DW, Acker H, Buck RP, et al., editors. *Progress in enzyme and ion-selective electrodes*. Berlin: Springer-Verlag; 1981. p. 74–8.
49. Stott RAW, Hortin GL, Wilhite TR, et al. Analytical artifacts in hematocrit measurements by whole blood chemistry analyzers. *Clin Chem* 1995;**41**:306–11.
53. Seitz WR. Chemical sensors based on fiber optics. *Anal Chem* 1984;**56**:16A–34A.
56. Thevenot DR, Toth K, Durst RA, et al. Electrochemical biosensors: recommended definitions and classifications. *Biosens Bioelectron* 2001;**16**:121–31.
57. Heller A. Amperometric biosensors. *Curr Opin Biotechnol* 1996;**7**:50–4.
58. Clark LC Jr, Lyons C. Electrode systems for continuous monitoring in cardiovascular surgery. *Ann N Y Acad Sci* 1962;**102**:29–45.
59. Guilbault GG. *Handbook of immobilized enzymes*. New York: Marcel-Dekker; 1984.
77. Leiner MJP. Luminescence chemical sensors for biomedical applications: scope and limitations. *Anal Chim Acta* 1991;**255**:209–22.
83. Luppa PB, Sokoll LJ, Chan DW. Immunosensors—principles and applications to clinical chemistry. *Clin Chim Acta* 2001;**314**:1–26.
86. D'Orazio P. Biosensors in clinical chemistry—2011 update. *Clin Chim Acta* 2011;**412**:1749–61.
99. Zhou W, Huang PJ, Ding J, et al. Aptamer-based biosensors for biomedical diagnostics. *Analyst* 2014;**139**: 2627–60.
109. Ronkainen NJ, Okon SL. Nanomaterial-based electrochemical immunosensors for clinically significant biomarkers. *Materials* 2014;**7**:4669–709.

15

Electrophoresis

*Lindsay A.L. Bazydlo and James P. Landers**

ABSTRACT

Background

Developments in DNA testing, improvements in ease of performance through automation, and advantages of speed and miniaturization afforded by the technique of *capillary electrophoresis (CE)* have led to a renaissance and growth of *electrophoresis* as an analytical tool that is widely used in clinical laboratories. These developments and improvements have enabled clinical laboratories to keep pace with higher volumes of testing and to introduce more sophisticated technology to meet the demands of modern clinical practice.

Content

This chapter will review the principles and practice of the technique and will separately discuss conventional, capillary, and microchip electrophoresis. Traditional electrophoresis has been performed in the slab gel format, and many laboratories today still use that approach. Based on the same inherent principles, CE has recently been gaining popularity in clinical laboratory use. Capillary zone electrophoresis (CZE) allows for higher voltages to be applied to facilitate the separation, which can translate to faster separation times. Taking faster separations one step further, electrophoresis also can be performed in the microfluidic format. This allows for even faster separations and in recent years has seen an increase in commercialization. Clinical applications are mentioned throughout the chapter to illustrate the utility of this technique and the analysis of relevant biological analytes.

POINTS TO REMEMBER

Electrophoresis

- Refers to the migration of ions in an electrical field
- Separation occurs based on the inherent electrophoretic mobility of an analyte
- Electrophoretic mobility is directly proportional to the net charge and inversely proportional to the size of the molecule and the viscosity of the electrophoresis medium

BASIC CONCEPTS AND DEFINITIONS

Electrophoresis is a comprehensive term that refers to the migration of charged solutes or particles of any size in a liquid medium under the influence of an electrical field. *Iontophoresis* and *isotachophoresis* (ITP) are similar terms but refer specifically to the migration of small ions. The first electrophoresis method used to study proteins was the free solution or moving boundary method devised by Tiselius in 1937. This technique was used in research to measure electrophoretic mobility and study protein-protein interaction. It was able to resolve the serum proteins into only four component mixtures, with the α_1 fraction incompletely separated from albumin.

Zone electrophoresis refers to the migration of charged molecules of proteins, usually in a porous supporting medium such as agarose gel film, so that each protein zone is sharply separated from neighboring zones by a protein-free area. Zones are visualized by staining with a protein-specific stain to produce an *electropherogram* that is then scanned and quantified using a densitometer. The support medium also can be handled after drying and kept as a permanent record. This is the most commonly applied technique in clinical chemistry and is used to separate proteins in serum, urine, cerebrospinal fluid (CSF), other physiologic fluids, erythrocytes and tissue, and nucleic acids in various tissue cells.

Although electrophoretic separation of biologically relevant macromolecules in gels (or paper) has been the workhorse of modern biomedical research, the advent of CE has revolutionized separations. Intense interest in carrying out electrophoretic separation in capillaries with inner diameters ranging from 20 to 75 μm has resulted from its unprecedented resolving power, separation speed, and small sample analysis capabilities. However, the true significance of CE to the separations community can be seen in its ability to apply these separation principles in a multimodal approach to a variety of analytes that obviously included proteins and polynucleic acids, but also peptides, small drug-like molecules, and even ions.

THEORY OF ELECTROPHORESIS

Depending on the charge they carry, ionized solutes move toward either the cathode (negative electrode) or the anode

*The authors gratefully acknowledge the original contributions of Drs. Emmanuel Epstein, Raymond Karcher, and Kern L. Nuttall, on which portions of this chapter are based.

BOX 15.1 Factors Affecting the Motility of Ions in an Electrophoretic System

- Net charge of the molecules
- Size and shape of the molecules
- Strength of the electrical field
- Support medium properties
- Ionic strength of the buffer
- Temperature

(positive electrode) in an electrophoresis system. For example, positive ions (cations) migrate to the cathode and negative ions (anions) to the anode. An ampholyte (a molecule that is either positively or negatively charged, formerly called a *zwitterion*) becomes positively charged in a solution that is more acidic than its isoelectric point (pI)[†] and migrates toward the cathode. In a more alkaline solution, the ampholyte becomes negatively charged and migrates toward the anode. Because proteins contain many ionizable amino (—NH_2) and carboxyl (—COOH) groups and because the bases in nucleic acids also may be positively or negatively charged, they both behave as ampholytes in solution.

The rate of migration of ions in an electrical field depends on the factors listed in Box 15.1. The equation expressing the driving force in such a system is given by the following:

$$F = (X)(Q) = \frac{(EMF)\ (Q)}{d}$$

where

F = the force exerted on an ion
X = the current field strength (V/cm) (ie, voltage drop per unit length of medium)
Q = the net charge on the ion
EMF = the electromotive force [voltage (V) applied]
d = the length of the electrophoretic medium (cm)

Steady acceleration of the migrating ion is counteracted by a resisting force characteristic of the solution in which migration occurs. This force, expressed by Stokes' law, is:

$$F' = 6\pi r \eta v$$

where

F' = the counter force
π = 3.1416
r = the ionic radius of the solute
η = the viscosity of the buffer solution in which migration is occurring
v = the rate of migration of the solute = velocity, length (l) traveled per unit of time (cm/s)

The force F' counteracts the acceleration that would be produced by F if no counter force were present, and the result of the two forces is a constant velocity. Therefore, when

$$F = F'$$

then

$$6\pi r \eta v = (X)(Q)$$

[†]The isoelectric point of a molecule is the pH at which it has no net charge and will not move in an electrical field.

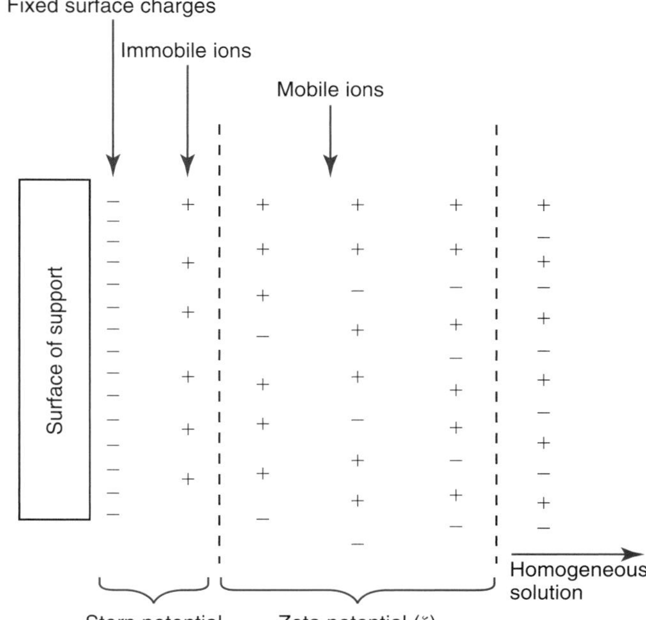

FIGURE 15.1 Distribution of + and – ions around the surface of an electrophoretic support. Fixed on the surface of the solid is a layer of – ions. (These may be + ions under suitable conditions). A second layer of + ions is attracted to the surface. These two layers compose the Stern potential. The large, diffuse layer containing mostly + ions is the electrokinetic or zeta potential. Extending farther from the surface of the solid is homogeneous solution. The Stern potential plus the zeta potential equals the electrochemical potential, or epsilon potential.

or

$$\frac{v}{X} = \frac{1 \times d}{t \times E} = \frac{Q}{6\pi r \eta} = \mu$$

where v/X is the rate of migration (cm/s) per unit field strength (E/cm), defined as the electrophoretic mobility and expressed by the symbol μ.

Electrophoretic mobility is directly proportional to the net charge and inversely proportional to the size of the molecule and the viscosity of the electrophoresis medium. Mobility may be positive or negative, depending on whether a protein migrates in the same or the opposite direction as the electrophoretic field (defined as extending from the anode to the cathode).

In addition to the factors listed in Box 15.1, other factors that affect electrophoretic mobility include electroendosmosis (endosmosis) and wick flow. Electroendosmosis affects mobility by causing uneven movement of water through the support medium. An electrophoretic support medium, such as a gel in contact with water, takes on a negative charge caused by adsorption of hydroxyl ions. These ions are fixed to the surface and are immobile. Positive ions in solution cluster about the fixed negative charge sites, forming an ionic cloud of mostly positive ions. The number of negative ions in the solution increases with increasing distance from the fixed negative charge sites until eventually positive and negative ions are present in equal concentrations (Fig. 15.1).

When current is applied to such a system, charges attached to the immobile support remain fixed but the cloud of ions in solution moves to the electrode of opposite polarity. Because ions in solution are highly hydrated, this results in movement of the solvent as well. Movement of solvent and its solutes relative to the fixed support is referred to as *endosmosis* and causes preferential movement of water in one direction. Macromolecules in solution that move in the direction opposite this flow may remain immobile or even may be swept back toward the opposite pole if they are insufficiently charged. In media in which endosmosis is strong, such as conventional cellulose acetate and unpurified agarose gel, γ-globulins are swept back from the application point. Because the inner surface of a glass capillary contains many such charged groups, endosmosis is very strong and is actually the primary driving force for migration in CE systems. The endosmosis in CE can be manipulated, however, to modify the magnitude of the endosmotic effect. In electrophoretic media in which surface charges are minimal (starch gel, purified agarose gel, or polyacrylamide gel), endosmosis is minimal.

Wick flow results from the movement of buffer into the support medium. During electrophoresis, heat that evolves because of the passage of current through a resistive medium can cause evaporation of solvent from the electrophoretic support. This drying effect draws buffer into the support, and, if significant, the flow of buffer can affect protein migration and hence the calculated mobility.

CLINICAL ELECTROPHORESIS

In this section, focus will be on the electrophoresis methodology that is frequently used in clinical laboratories. Refer to Chapter 28 for a thorough discussion on the various electrophoretic fractions present in clinical protein electrophoresis.

Slab Gel Electrophoresis

Traditional methods, using a rectangular gel regardless of thickness, are referred to collectively by the term *slab gel electrophoresis.* Its main advantage is its ability to simultaneously separate several samples in one run. Starch, agarose, and polyacrylamide media have been used in this format. It is the primary method used in clinical chemistry laboratories for separation of various classes of serum or CSF proteins and DNA and RNA fragments. Gels (usually agarose) may be cast on a sheet of plastic backing or completely encased within a plastic-walled cell, which allows horizontal or vertical electrophoresis and submersion for cooling, if necessary.

General Operations

General operations performed in conventional electrophoresis include separation, detection, and quantification, and "blotting" techniques.

Electrophoretic Separation. When electrophoresis is performed on precast microzone agarose gels, the following steps are typical: (1) excess buffer is removed from the support surface by blotting, taking care that bubbles are not present; (2) 5 to 7 μL of sample is applied using a comb or a plastic template and is allowed to diffuse into the gel; it is then blotted to remove the excess; (3) the gel is placed into the electrode chamber; (4) electrophoresis is performed at specified current, voltage, or power; (5) the gel is fixed, rinsed, and then dried; (6) the gel is stained and redried; and (7) the gel is scanned in a densitometer. If isoenzymes are to be determined, substrate dye solution is incubated on the gel to stain zones before fixing and drying. Alternative procedures would be required if the more sophisticated methods described later are used.

Detection and Quantification. Once separated, proteins may be detected by staining followed by quantification using a densitometer or by direct measurement using an optical detection system set at 210 nm.

Staining. If staining is used to visualize separated proteins, the proteins usually are fixed first by precipitating them in the gel with a chemical agent such as acetic acid or methanol. This prevents diffusion of proteins out of the gel when submersed in the stain solution. The amount of dye taken up by the sample is affected by many factors, such as the type of protein and the degree of denaturation of the proteins by fixing agents.

Table 15.1 lists dyes commonly used in electrophoresis, along with suggested wavelengths for quantification by densitometry. Most commercial methods for serum protein electrophoresis use Amido Black B or members of the Coomassie Brilliant Blue series of dyes for staining. Isoenzymes are typically visualized by incubating the gel in contact with a solution of substrate, which is linked structurally or chemically to a dye before fixing. Silver nitrate and silver diamine stain proteins and polypeptides with sensitivity 10- to 100-fold greater than that of conventional dyes.[1] Selective fixing and staining of protein subclasses also can be achieved by combining a stain molecule with an antiglobulin, as is done in immunofixation electrophoresis (IFE).

Improvements in conducting sensitive measurements have been achieved by linking an enzyme such as alkaline phosphatase or peroxidase to a single or double antibody specific for particular proteins such as oligoclonal immunoglobulin (Ig)[2] or by spraying separated proteins with luminal and peroxide to develop chemiluminescence, which, in turn, exposes x-ray film to form a permanent image.[3] Chemiluminescence

TABLE 15.1 Suggested Wavelengths for Quantitation of Protein Zones by Direct Densitometry

Separation Type	Stain	Nominal Wavelength (nm)
Serum proteins in general	Amido Black (Naphthol Blue Black)	640
	Coomassie Brilliant Blue G-250 (Brilliant Blue G)	595
	Coomassie Brilliant Blue R-250 (Brilliant Blue R)	560
	Ponceau S	520
Isoenzymes	Nitrotetrazolium Blue	570
Lipoprotein zones	Fat Red 7B (Sudan Red 7B)	540
	Oil Red O	520
	Sudan Black B	600
DNA fragments	Ethidium bromide (fluorescent)	254 (Ex) 590 (Em)
CSF proteins	Silver nitrate	—

CSF, Cerebrospinal fluid; *Em,* emission; *Ex,* excitation.

has been used in this way to quantify IgE (Lumi-Phos 530, Lumigen, Southfield, Mich),[4] and DNA fragments have been detected by linking with a fluorescent dye label.[5]

In practice, a typical stain solution may be used several times before it is replaced. A good rule of thumb is that a stain solution of 100 mL may be used for a combined total of 387 cm^2 (60 in^2) of agarose film. The stain solution may be considered faulty if leaching of stained protein zones occurs in the 5% acetic acid wash solution. Whenever protein zones appear too lightly stained, the stain or substrate reagent—in the case of isoenzymes—always should be suspected. Stain solution must be stored tightly covered to prevent evaporation.

Quantification. A *densitometer* is used to quantify stained zones. This instrument measures the absorbance of each fraction as the gel (or other medium) is moved past a photometric optical system and displays an *electropherogram* on a computer display. The software is able to automatically integrate the area under each peak and report each as a percent of total or as absolute concentration or activity computed from the total protein or activity of enzyme in the sample.

Reliable densitometric quantitation requires (1) light of an appropriate wavelength, (2) linear response from the instrument, and (3) a transparent background in the medium being scanned. Linearity may be tested with a neutral density filter designed with separated or adjacent areas of linearly increasing density. The densities are permanent and have expected absorbance values. The very small sample sizes used and the transparency of agarose gels satisfy the requirement for a clear background. Nevertheless, problems can occur with densitometry because of differences in the quantity of stain taken up by individual proteins and differences in protein zone sizes.

Essential features of a densitometer include (1) the ability to scan gels 25 to 100 mm in length; (2) electronic adjustment of the most intense peak to full scale; (3) automatic background zeroing (peaks are not lost or "cut off"); (4) variable wavelength control over the range of 400 to 700 nm; (5) variable slits to allow adjustment of the beam size; (6) an integrating device with both automatic and manual selection of cut points between peaks; and (7) automatic indexing, a feature that advances the electrophoresis strip from one sample channel to the next.

Desirable features of a densitometer include computerized integration and printout, built-in diagnostics for instrument troubleshooting, choice of one of several scanning speeds, and ability to measure in the reflectance mode. Models with a separate computer for data processing permit storage and reformatting of data, if desired, and reprinting or delayed transmission to a host computer.

DNA analysis requires the ability to scan larger gels, which may contain several dozen bands of DNA fragments of different length. Modern automated electrophoresis systems also use larger gels containing 30 or more samples, which are scanned on a new generation of densitometers referred to as *flatbed scanners* or *digital image analyzers.* These instruments are capable of scanning and storing digitized light intensity readings from large areas and use ultrasensitive charge-coupled device detectors having a resolution of up to 1200 dots per inch (21 μm). Sophisticated data processing software permits manipulation of stored image information to produce conventional scans and computations or more complex outputs, such as overlaying and subtraction of patterns from two different samples.

Blotting Techniques. In 1975, Edward Southern developed a technique that is widely used to detect fragments of DNA. This technique, known as *Southern blotting,*[6] first requires electrophoretic separation of DNA or DNA fragments by agarose gel electrophoresis (AGE). Next, a strip of nitrocellulose or a nylon membrane is laid over the agarose gel, and the DNA or DNA fragments are transferred or "blotted" onto it by capillary blotting, electro-blotting, or vacuum blotting. They are then detected and identified by hybridization with a labeled, complementary nucleic acid probe. This technique is widely used in molecular biology for identifying a particular DNA sequence; determining the presence, position, and number of copies of a gene in a genome; and typing DNA.

Northern and *Western* blotting techniques,[6] named by analogy to Southern blotting, were subsequently developed to separate and detect RNAs and proteins, respectively. Northern blotting is carried out identically to Southern blotting except that a labeled RNA probe is used for hybridization. Western blotting is used to separate, detect, and identify one or more proteins in a complex mixture. It involves first separating the individual proteins by polyacrylamide gel and then transferring or blotting onto an overlying strip of nitrocellulose or a nylon membrane by electro-blotting. The strip or membrane is then reacted with a reagent that contains an antibody raised against the protein of interest.

Instrumentation

Although modern electrophoresis equipment and systems vary considerably in form and degree of automation, the essential components common to all systems (Fig. 15.2) include two reservoirs (1), which contain the buffer used in the process, a means of delivering current from a power supply via platinum or carbon electrodes (2), which contact the buffer, and a support medium (3) in which separation takes place connecting the two reservoirs. In some systems, wicks (4) may connect the medium to the buffer solution or directly to the electrodes. The entire apparatus is enclosed (5) to minimize evaporation and protect both the system and the operator. The direct current power supply sets the polarity of the electrodes and delivers current to the medium.

Power Supplies. The power supply drives the movement of ionic species in the medium and allows adjustment and control of the current or the voltage. With more sophisticated units, the power may be controlled as well and conditions may be programmed to change during electrophoresis. Capillary systems use power supplies capable of providing voltages in the kilovolt range.

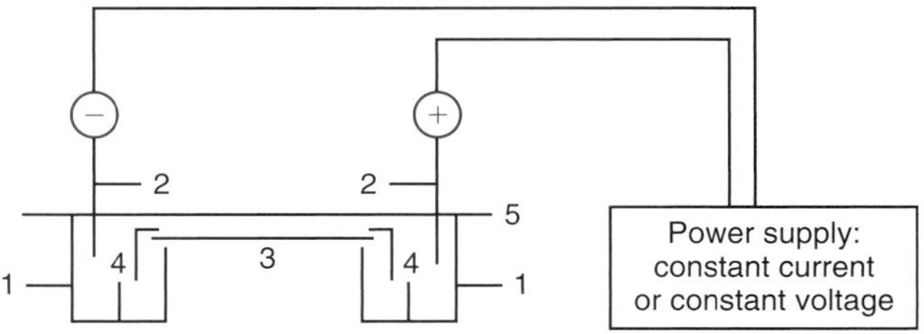

FIGURE 15.2 A schematic diagram of a typical electrophoresis apparatus showing two buffer boxes with baffle plates *(1)*, electrodes *(2)*, electrophoretic support *(3)*, wicks *(4)*, cover *(5)*, and power supply.

Current flowing through a medium that has resistance produces heat:

$$Heat = (E)(I)(t)$$

where

E = electromotive force (EMF) in volts (V)

I = current in amperes (A)

T = time in seconds (s)

This heat is released into the medium and increases the thermal agitation of all dissolved ions and therefore the conductance of the system (decreases resistance). With constant-voltage power supplies, the resultant rise in current increases both protein migration and evaporation of water from the medium. Any water loss increases the ion concentration and further decreases the resistance *(R)*. Under these circumstances, the current and therefore the migration rate will progressively increase. To minimize these effects, it is best to use a constant-current power supply. According to Ohm's law,

$$E = (I)(R)$$

Therefore if R decreases, the applied EMF also decreases, keeping the current constant. This in turn decreases the heat effect and stabilizes the migration rate.

Buffers. Buffer ions have a twofold purpose in electrophoresis: they carry the applied current, and they fix the pH at which electrophoresis is carried out. Thus they determine (1) the type of electrical charge on the solute; (2) the extent of ionization of the solute, and therefore (3) the electrode toward which the solute will migrate. The buffer's ionic strength determines the thickness of the ionic cloud (buffer and nonbuffer ions) surrounding a charged molecule, the rate of its migration, and the sharpness of the electrophoretic zones. With increasing concentration of ions, the ionic cloud increases in size and the molecule becomes more hindered in its movement.

According to Joule's law, power produced when current flows through a resistive medium is dissipated as heat. This heat increases in direct proportion to the resistance, but also in proportion to the square of the current. The reduction in resistance caused by a high ionic strength buffer therefore leads to increased current and excessive heat. These buffers yield sharper band separations, but the benefits of sharper resolution are diminished by the Joule (heat) effect that leads to denaturation of heat-labile proteins or degradation of other components.

Ionic strength (also denoted by the symbol μ) is computed according to the following:

$$\mu = 0.5\sum c_i z_i^2$$

where

c_i = ion concentration in mol/L

z_i = the charge on the ion

The ionic strength μ of an electrolyte (buffer) composed of monovalent ions is equal to its molarity (mol/L). The ionic strength of a 1-mol/L electrolyte solution with one monovalent and one divalent ion is 3 mol/L, and for a doubly divalent electrolyte it is 4 mol/L.

A buffer of relatively high ionic strength used in *high-resolution electrophoresis* improves the separation of serum proteins into as many as 13 bands, with 2 or more bands in the α_1-, α_2-, and β-globulin regions and one or more additional bands seen in various pathologic conditions. Because of higher conductivity and the associated heat produced, it is necessary to reduce the temperature of the system to 10° to 14°C. "Submarine" techniques, in which gels are submersed in circulating buffer cooled by an external cooling device or are supported on an electrophoresis chamber cooled by circulating water or an integral Peltier plate, provide exact temperature control. Effective cooling with less precise temperature control also may be achieved using chambers designed with a sealed compartment of cooled ethylene glycol, which is in contact with the gel during running.

Because buffers used in electrophoresis are good culture media for the growth of microorganisms, they should be refrigerated when not in use. Moreover, a cold buffer is preferred in an electrophoretic run, because it improves resolution and decreases evaporation from the electrophoretic support. Buffer used in a small-volume apparatus should be discarded after each run because of pH changes resulting from the electrolysis of water that accompany electrophoresis. If volumes used are larger than 100 mL, buffer from both reservoirs may be combined, mixed, and reused up to four times.

Support Media. The support medium provides the matrix in which protein separation takes place. Various types of support media have been used in electrophoresis and range from pure buffer solutions in a capillary to insoluble gels (eg, sheets, slabs, or columns of starch, agarose, or polyacrylamide) or membranes of cellulose acetate. Gels are cast in a solution of the same buffer to be used in the procedure and may be used in a horizontal or vertical direction. In either case, maximum resolution is achieved if the sample is applied in a very fine starting zone. Separation is based on differences in charge-to-mass ratio of the proteins and, depending on the pore size of the medium, possibly molecular size.

Cellulose Acetate. Cellulose acetate, a thermoplastic resin made by treating cellulose with acetic anhydride to acetylate the hydroxyl groups, also is primarily of historical interest. When dry, the membranes contain approximately 80% air space within the interlocking cellulose acetate fibers and are opaque, brittle films. As the film is soaked in buffer, the air spaces fill with liquid and it becomes pliable. Samples are applied with a twin-wire applicator or the edge of a glass slide. Because of their opacity, stained membranes need to be made transparent (cleared) for densitometry by soaking in 95:5 methanol to glacial acetic acid. Cleared membranes are strong and could be stored as a permanent record, but because of the necessity for presoaking and clearing, cellulose acetate has largely been replaced by agarose gel in most clinical applications.

Agarose. Agarose is a linear polymer containing alternating D-galactose and 3,6-anhydro-L-galactose monomers. It is the purified, essentially neutral fraction of agar obtained by separating agarose from agaropectin, a more highly charged fraction containing acidic sulfate and carboxylic side groups. Because the pore size in agarose gel is large enough for all proteins to pass through unimpeded, separation is based only on the charge-to-mass ratio of the protein. Advantages of agarose gel include its lower affinity for proteins and its native clarity after drying, which permits excellent densitometry. It

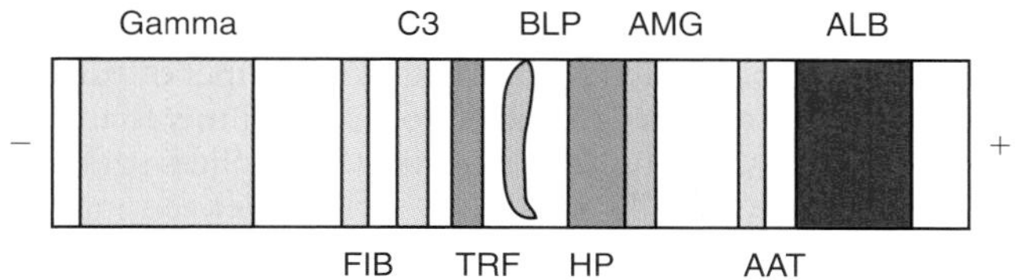

FIGURE 15.3 A simplified schematic drawing of a protein pattern from the serum of a subject with haptoglobin type 2-1 (separation by polyacrylamide gel electrophoresis [PAGE]). Some zones contain more than the one protein shown, as demonstrated by immunologic techniques. *AAT,* α_1-Antitrypsin; *ALB,* albumin; *AMG,* α_2-macroglobulin; *BLP,* β-lipoprotein; *C3,* complement 3; *FIB,* fibrinogen; *gamma,* γ-globulin; *HP,* haptoglobin; *TRF,* transferrin.

is essentially free of ionizable groups and so exhibits little endosmosis.

Most routine procedures for AGE are now performed using commercially produced, prepackaged microzone gels, and the sample is applied by means of a comb or a thin plastic template, with small slots corresponding to sample application points. The template is placed on the agarose surface, and 5- to 7-μL samples are placed on each slot. The serum sample is allowed to diffuse into the agarose for 5 minutes, excess sample is removed by blotting, and the template is removed. AGE separation for most routine serum applications requires an electrophoresis time of 20 to 30 minutes.

Polyacrylamide Gel. Polyacrylamide is a polymeric matrix consisting of linear chains of acrylamide cross-linked with bis-acrylamide. It is thermostable, transparent, strong, and relatively chemically inert, and—depending on concentration—can be made in a wide range of pore sizes. Its average pore size in a typical 7.5% gel is approximately 5 nm (50 Å)—large enough to allow most serum proteins to migrate unimpeded. However, proteins with a molecular radius and/or length that exceeds critical limits will be impeded in their migration. Some of these proteins are fibrinogen, β-lipoprotein, α_2-macroglobulin, and γ-globulins; a schematic representation of serum protein electrophoresis by polyacrylamide gel electrophoresis (PAGE) is shown in Fig. 15.3. The separation is based on both charge-to-mass ratio and molecular size (a phenomenon referred to as *molecular sieving*), and serum proteins can be resolved into more individual fractions than with agarose gel. Furthermore, these gels are uncharged, thus eliminating electroendosmosis. Precast minigels are available in a variety of concentrations and ratios of acrylamide to bis-acrylamide suitable for most protein or nucleic acid separations. Because of the known neurotoxicity of acrylamide, however, appropriate caution must be exercised when handling this material if gels are prepared by hand.

Attempts to improve the hydrophilic nature of polyacrylamide have led to the development of mono- and di-substituted monomers, one of which is *N*-acryloyl-tris(hydroxymethyl) aminomethane, or poly(NAT) (Elchrom Scientific, Cham, Switzerland).[7] This material is more hydrophilic than polyacrylamide and its matrix has larger pores, thereby presenting less resistance to the passage of large molecules. It is ideally suited to the separation of DNA fragments up to 20 kilobases (kb) using a homogeneous (nonpulsed) electric field. Fragments that differ in size by as little as 2% can be resolved. Gels are submersed in buffer during use, allowing temperatures to be tightly controlled at values between 50° and 60°C. Use of increased temperatures results in shorter run times and more reproducible band migration.

Automated Systems. Because of increased volume of testing, primarily for serum proteins, many laboratories are converting to automated systems for electrophoresis. Such a system is the Helena SPIFE 4000 (Helena Laboratories, Beaumont, Tex.), an automated electrophoresis system providing automated reagent application and a variety of gel sizes that permit analysis of 10 to 100 samples simultaneously. It also features in-line sample application, automated electrophoretic separation and staining of analytes, multiple stain ports, and positive sample identification. The Interlab Microgel system (Interlab Srl, Rome, Italy) also fully automates the process and integrates sample application, temperature-controlled electrophoresis, staining, and densitometry into a single unit with the capability of managing four gels simultaneously. Other systems that have partially automated the procedure or incorporated the ability to process sequentially multiple gels of different compositions include the Phast System (Pharmacia LKB, Gaithersburg, Md.), the HITE Fractoscan (Olympus, Invicon, München, Germany), the Hydragel-Hydrasys (Sebia, Durham, N.C.), and the High-Performance Gel Electrophoresis (HPGE)-1000 system (LabIntelligence, Belmont, Calif.). Most CE systems (see section on Capillary Electrophoresis) have autosampling capability for sequentially processing specimens, but the Sebia Capillarys permits simultaneous processing of seven samples by using multiple capillaries. Newer microchip-based analyzers such as the Agilent 2100 Bioanalyzer (Agilent Technologies, Santa Clara, Calif.) significantly miniaturize and increase the speed of the process for separating proteins, nucleic acids, or even entire cells. These advances substantially reduce the labor component associated with this technique.

Capillary Electrophoresis

With CE, the classic techniques of zone electrophoresis, ITP, isoelectric focusing (IEF), and gel electrophoresis are carried out in a small-bore (10- to 100-μm internal diameter) fused silica capillary tube, 20 to 200 cm in length.[8]

Two distinct advantages of the capillary format include the ability to apply much higher voltages than in traditional electrophoresis and the ease of automation. Applications are also more extensive and include separation of low molecular weight ions, in addition to proteins and other macromolecules. Even uncharged molecules can be separated using CE in the micellar electrokinetic chromatography (MEKC) mode, discussed later. CE has also proved useful for separation of inorganic ions, amino acids, organic acids, drugs, vitamins, porphyrins, carbohydrates, oligonucleotides, proteins, and DNA fragments.[9-12]

General Operations

A schematic diagram of a typical instrumental configuration for CE is shown in Fig. 15.4. As indicated, the capillary serves as an electrophoretic chamber, analogous to a lane on a gel, which is connected to buffer reservoirs at both ends, which, in turn, are connected to a high-voltage power supply. It is important to note that at some point along the length of the capillary (typically close to the end), a detector is interfaced for online detection. Improved heat dissipation from the cap-

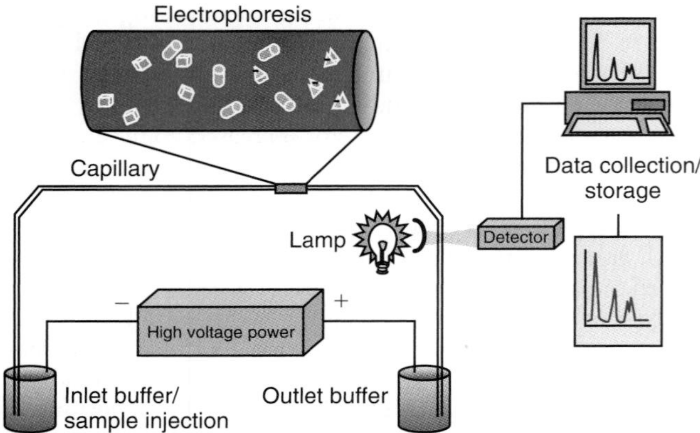

FIGURE 15.4 A schematic for capillary electrophoresis instrumentation.

illary (as opposed to a slab gel) permits the application of voltages in the range of 10 to 30 kV, which enhances separation efficiency and reduces separation time, in some cases to less than 1 minute. Only a few microliters of the sample are required, with injected volumes in the nanoliter range. The small sample plug volume minimizes distortions in the applied field caused by the presence of analytes or other sample species.

In contrast to the cumbersome and time-consuming tasks of conventional electrophoresis, CE is easily automated. Analogous to high-performance liquid chromatography (HPLC) technology, samples typically are stored in a temperature-controlled environment and are automatically injected into the capillary, with a variety of detector types available; the resulting electropherograms are analyzed and manipulated in much the same manner as chromatograms.

The capillaries used as separation columns in CE are most commonly made from fused silica (ie, pure glass) coated with a thin exterior covering of polyimide to provide strength and flexibility. Although capillaries can be made from other materials, such as polyethylene or Teflon, such capillaries have seen limited use. The polyimide coating is usually removed from a small portion of the capillary close to the terminal end, creating a window for online optical detection. The outer diameter of the capillary tubing typically varies from 180 to 375 μm, the inner diameter from 20 to 180 μm, and the total length from 20 cm up to several meters. Noncylindrical capillary tubing suitable for CE is now available from some commercial providers. For example, rectangular capillaries (Polymicro Technologies, Phoenix, Arizona) provide a flat surface that is more amenable to optical detection than their curved counterparts.

CE is distinguished from other forms of electrophoresis by the fact that extraordinarily high voltage (30,000 V) has been used to obtain rapid, high-efficiency separations. The problems encountered with noncapillary platforms (eg, slab gels) are avoided because of the effective dissipation of Joule heat by forced air convection or liquid cooling of the narrow-bore capillary.

Sample Injection. In CE, sample volumes of 1 to 50 nL are loaded into the capillary by *hydrodynamic injection* or *electrokinetic (EK) injection.* With hydrodynamic injection, an aliquot of a sample is introduced by applying positive pressure at the inlet vial or vacuum at the outlet vial. The volume of sample loaded is governed by a number of parameters, including (but not restricted to) (1) the inner diameter of the capillary, (2) buffer viscosity, (3) applied pressure, (4) temperature, and (5) time. With some earlier commercial or homemade systems, gravity was used as the source of pressure by raising the inlet vial (or lowering the outlet vial), thus allowing "siphoning" to occur for a timed interval. With EK injection, an aliquot of a sample is introduced by applying a voltage for a timed interval. The magnitude of the voltage depends on the analyte and buffer system used but typically involves field strength three to five times lower than that used for separation. It is important to note that although hydrodynamic methods introduce a sample representative of the bulk specimen, EK injection favors the preferential movement of more electrokinetically mobile analytes into the capillary.

In practice, to maintain high separation efficiency, the sample plug length is usually less than 2% of the total capillary length.

Direct Detection. With CE, separated analytes are detected and measured as they migrate past a point on the capillary that is optically interrogated. Optical detection is based on classic methods, such as photometric absorbance, refractive index, and fluorescence (see Chapter 13). As with HPLC, ultraviolet (UV)-visible photometers are widely used as detectors to monitor CE separations.[13] To interface such online detectors with the capillary, a *detection window* is created toward the outlet end of the capillary. This "window," which serves as an inline cuvet, typically is formed by burning off the polyimide with a small flame and cleaning the window with ethanol. Although this configuration allows high-efficiency separation, the inner diameter of the capillary tube defines the optical path length (OPL) of the inline cuvet. Because absorbance is directly proportional to the length of the cuvet used in an optical system, the 20- to 100-μm inner diameter of the capillary limits UV-visible absorbance detection limits to concentrations of 10^{-8} to 10^{-6} molar.

More sensitive optical techniques that have been used with CE include (1) fluorescence, (2) refractive index, (3) chemiluminescence, (4) Raman spectrophotometry, and (5) circular dichroism.[11] The most sensitive optical detection method used in CE is laser-induced fluorescence (LIF), which is capable of detection limits in the 10^{-9} to 10^{-12} molar (or better) range. This detection mode is easily accomplished with analytes that may be labeled with a fluorescent substrate (eg, intercalators for double-stranded [ds]DNA) or may be naturally fluorescent (eg, proteins or peptides containing tryptophan). CE systems also have been interfaced with mass spectrometers,[14] and electrochemical detection methods[15] have been developed, although such detectors must be isolated electrically from the electrophoretic voltages.

Indirect Detection. When strong chromophores are lacking in the analyte of interest, absorbance and fluorescence detection have been used in an indirect mode.[16-18] In this mode, a strongly absorbing ion is added to the running electrolyte and is monitored at a wavelength that gives a constant high background absorbance. As solute ions move into their discrete zones during the electrophoretic process, they displace the indirect detection agent through mutual repulsion, and this produces a decrease in background absorbance as the zone passes through the detector. Reagents with appropriate fluorescence properties have been employed in a similar manner. Indirect detection of amino acids by CE has been demonstrated, with the potential for use in diagnosis of aminoacidurias.[19] Investigators have demonstrated the direct extrapolation of this technique to microchip detection when UV detection is difficult, if not impossible.

Types of Electrophoresis

Capillary Zone Electrophoresis. CZE, also called *open-tube* or *free-solution* CE, is the simplest form of CE. It includes *capillary ion electrophoresis,* which refers to the analysis of inorganic ions by CZE, often using indirect detection. The power of the CZE mode is its ability to electrophoretically resolve charged species without a sieving matrix; this applies to a broad spectrum of analytes ranging from proteins, peptides, and amino acids to small molecules (eg, drugs) and ions.

Capillary Gel Electrophoresis. Capillary gel electrophoresis (CGE) is directly comparable with traditional slab or tube gel electrophoresis because the separation mechanisms are identical. Size separation is achieved with a suitable polymer, which acts as a molecular sieve or sizing mechanism. As charged analytes migrate through the polymer network, they become hindered to a degree that is governed by their size (larger molecules are hindered more than smaller ones). Macromolecules, such as DNA and sodium dodecyl sulfate (SDS)-saturated proteins, cannot be separated without a gel or some other separation mechanism, because they have a mass-to-charge ratio that is size independent. The term *gel* in CGE is a misnomer, primarily because cross-linked "gels," as we know them in slab format, are not routinely used in CE. A more suitable term is a *sieving matrix* or *soluble polymer network,* a linear polymeric structure that is soluble, has reasonably low viscosity, and is capable of self-entangling in a manner that forms pores through which sieving can occur. A variety of polymeric matrices have been defined for DNA (eg, polyacrylamide, cellulosic materials) and protein analysis (eg, dextran-base matrices), provided that pores can be formed inherently that have diameters in the range of tens to hundreds of nanometers. One of the requirements that often accompanies this type of analysis is reduction of electroosmotic flow (EOF). This is accomplished by covalently, adsorptively, or dynamically coating the surface. Cross-linked polyacrylamide was the main polymer of choice for this but recently has been supplanted by a host of polymeric matrices that not only provide effective molecular sieving but also adsorptively coat the capillary surface.[20,21]

POINTS TO REMEMBER

Capillary Electrophoresis

- CZE uses EOF to mobilize the sample plug pass the detector.
- CGE is best used with macromolecules such as DNA or large proteins and uses a sieving matrix for separation.
- Higher voltages can be applied because of more efficient dissipation of heat—this can translate to faster separations.

TECHNICAL CONSIDERATIONS

Gel

In performing electrophoretic separations, a number of technical and practical aspects need to be considered because they affect the process.

Sampling

To achieve a proper balance between sensitive measurements and resolution, the amount of serum protein applied to an electrophoretic support must be optimum. Albumin is approximately 10 times more concentrated in serum than the smallest fraction, the α_1-globulins. Therefore the amount of serum applied should prevent overloading with albumin but still should be adequate to quantify α_1-globulin. For separation of serum proteins using PAGE, 3 μL of serum containing approximately 210 μg of total protein is applied. For alkaline phosphatase isoenzymes, up to 25 μL of a normal serum may be applied (less may be used if activity is greatly increased). Urine specimens require 50- to 100-fold concentration or extended application time for adequate sensitivity, and CSF may or may not require concentration, depending on the staining approach used.

Discontinuities in Sample Application

Discontinuities in sample application may be caused by (1) dirty applicators, (2) uneven absorption by sample combs, or (3) inclusion of an air bubble if sample is pipetted onto the gel. The pipette tip should be checked for air bubbles before the sample is applied to the agarose gel template.

Unequal Migration Rates

Unequal migration of samples across the width of the gel may be caused by dirty electrodes, which may cause uneven application of the electric field, or by uneven wetting of the gel. If wicks are used to connect the gel to a power supply, uneven wetting of the wicks could cause unequal migration or bowing of sample lanes at the gel edges. Gels must be kept horizontal during storage to avoid sagging and uneven thickness. Finally, gels that may have been stored too close to heat sources (eg, in a cabinet over a light fixture) could have partially and unevenly dried areas, contributing to similar problems.

Distorted, Unusual, or Atypical Bands

Distorted protein zones may be caused by (1) bent applicators, (2) incorporation of an air bubble during sample application, (3) overapplication, or (4) inadequate blotting of the sample. Excessive drying of the electrophoretic support before or during electrophoresis may also cause distorted zones. Irregularities (other than broken zones) in the sample application probably are due to excessively wet agarose gels. Portions of applied samples may look washed out.

In most cases, unusual bands are artifacts that may be easily recognized. Hemolyzed samples are frequent causes of increased β-globulin (where free hemoglobin migrates) or an unusual band between the α_2- and β-globulins, the result of a hemoglobin-haptoglobin complex. A band occurring at the starting point of an electropherogram may be fibrinogen. The sample should be verified as being serum before this band is reported as an abnormal protein. The α- and β-lipoproteins may migrate ahead of their normal positions in some samples. Occasionally, a split albumin zone is observed in the rare, benign, genetically related condition of bis-albuminemia. However, a grossly widened albumin zone could be due to albumin-bound medication and not faulty practice of electrophoresis.

Capillary

Temperature and surface effects influence the separation capabilities of CE. Artifacts also have been known to arise with CE.

Temperature Effects

In most slab or tube platforms for electrophoresis, moderate electric fields (up to 1000 V) are used, because the Joule heating that accompanies the use of higher field strengths causes nonuniform temperature gradients, local changes in viscosity, and subsequent zone broadening. CE is distinguished from other forms of electrophoresis by the fact that extraordinarily high fields (30,000 V) are used to obtain rapid, high-efficiency separations. The problems encountered with noncapillary platforms are prevented by effective dissipation of Joule heat by forced air convection or liquid cooling of the capillary, both of which are possible because of the narrow bore of the capillary. The Joule heat produced is a function of (1) buffer type, (2) concentration, (3) voltage applied, (4) capillary inner diameter, and (5) length, and can be determined for any given system by generating an *Ohm's law plot,* which allows easy determination of the maximum voltage that can be used effectively.[22] Reducing the inner diameter of the capillary, the ionic strength of the running buffer, or the applied voltage will reduce the heat produced by the electrophoretic process. It should be noted that reducing the inner diameter will compromise the detection limit of UV measurements (smaller OPL); reducing the applied field is less desirable in that resolution is directly proportional to the applied field. Consequently, attempts should be made to alter other parameters before reducing inner diameter or the applied field.

Surface Effects

As in electrophoresis in general, the flow of fluid (electro-osmotic or EOF) in CE is a consequence of surface charge on the solid support. In CE, EOF has been known to play a significant role in the separation process. The charge on the inner surface of a fused silica capillary is determined by the ionization state of the silanol groups that populate it. Interaction of positively charged buffer species with bound surface anions generates a layer of mobile cations that move toward the cathode when voltage is applied. This induces a very strong EOF that mobilizes all analytes in the same direction, regardless of their charge. Separation is consequently achieved because of differences in the electrophoretic migration rates of analytes superimposed on this EOF.

Because the driving force of the flow is distributed along the wall of the capillary, the flow profile is nearly flat or plug-like, contrasting with the laminar or parabolic flow generated by a pressure-driven system caused by shear forces at the wall. A flat flow profile is beneficial because it does not contribute to the dispersion of solute zones. The magnitude and direction of the EOF are influenced by several parameters, including (1) type of electrolyte used, (2) pH, (3) ionic strength, (4) use of additives (eg, surfactants, organic solvents), and (5) polarity and magnitude of the applied electric field.

Although advantageous for dissipation of Joule heat, the large ratio of surface area to volume of the inner capillary space increases the likelihood of analyte adsorption onto the surface of its inner wall. This causes phenomena such as peak tailing and even total and irreversible adsorption of the analyte. Adsorption is typically noted between cationic solutes and the negatively charged inner wall of the capillary, primarily through ionic interactions (with deprotonated silanols), but also involves hydrophobic interactions (with siloxanes). Because of the numerous charges and hydrophobic regions, significant adsorptive effects have been noted, especially for highly cationic proteins. In practice, adsorption of substances, whether from the sample or from the buffer, to the inner surface of the capillary will alter migration times and other separation characteristics; unaddressed, the capillary eventually may become "fouled." Buffer components and/or additives such as surfactants often can render permanent changes to the inner surface of the capillary (through adsorption) and may warrant dedication of specific capillaries for use with particular surfactants.

To minimize these inner wall effects, capillaries are conditioned by chemical treatment, most commonly with base, to remove adsorbates and rejuvenate the surface. A typical wash method includes flushing the chamber with 10 to 20 capillary volumes of 0.1 to 1.0 mol/L NaOH, followed by flushing with "run" buffer. To prevent exposing the capillary surface to drastic fluctuations in pH, conditioning procedures for separations at low pH may be better served by using strong acids (eg, HNO_3), surfactants (eg, SDS), or organic solvents, such as acetonitrile or methanol.

Serum Protein Analysis

Compared with AGE and cellulose acetate electrophoresis (CAE), CZE is more advantageous for serum protein analysis.[8,23,24] Fig. 15.5 shows a comparison of the separation of serum proteins by CAE, AGE, and CE. The presence of the classic zones with CE is apparent, albeit in reversed order, as is the identification of serum protein abnormalities in gamma regions. Retrospective studies have shown CE to be effective for detecting monoclonal proteins, which could then be immunotyped by conventional techniques (IFE and IEF).[8] Moreover, one study demonstrated the utility of CE in doing both serum protein electrophoresis and immunotyping for more than 1500 serum samples.[23] These and other studies put forth the same conclusion—that CE is more sensitive than AGE in identifying abnormalities. More recent studies have shown the value of CZE in serum protein analysis. In 2005, Luraschi and associates[25] described the use of CZE coupled with immunosubtraction to detect and characterize low concentrations of free γ heavy chains in serum. In this study, they showed that γ heavy chain disease could be detected by serum protein analysis in CZE in tandem with immunosubtraction. However, although studies have proved the clear utility of CZE for serum protein analysis, Bossuyt and coworkers[26] point to the fact that CZE is not flawless, describing a case in which CZE failed to detect μ heavy chain disease in a 90-year-old woman. This is countered by Maisnar and colleagues,[27] who submit that the laboratory diagnosis of patients with μ heavy chain disease is typically challenging and that detection of the monoclonal protein by standard electrophoretic approaches may fail in up to 75% of cases of μ heavy chain disease. They describe a patient who had multiple

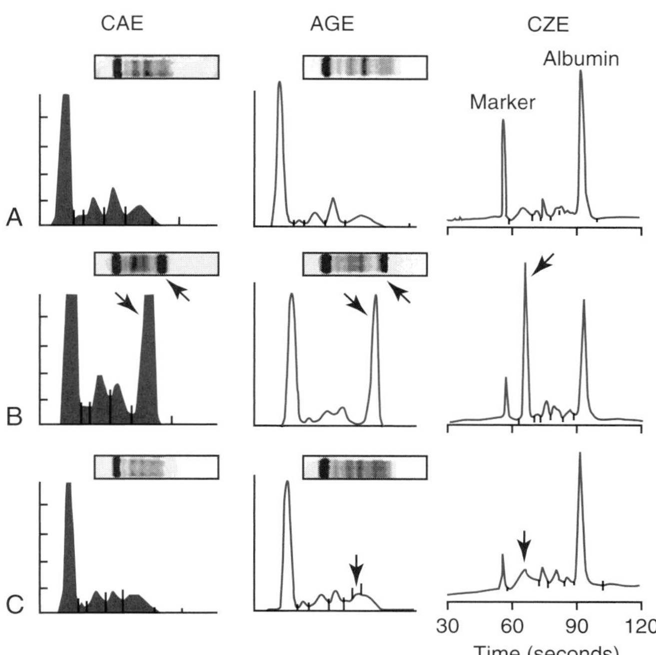

FIGURE 15.5 Rapid protein electrophoresis of serum protein; comparison with scanning densitometry profiles obtained from cellulose acetate *(CAE)* and agarose *(AGE)* electrophoresis. **A,** Normal serum. **B,** Patient serum containing a large M-protein. **C,** Patient serum containing a small monoclonal protein. *Arrows* indicate the position of the monoclonal proteins. *CZE,* Capillary zone electrophoresis.

malignancies, which included vulvar carcinoma and Hodgkin lymphoma, for whom CZE with immunotyping allowed the detection and characterization of monoclonal μ heavy chains.

Finally, CZE for serum protein analysis is evolving in a high-throughput format that has leveraged the success of multiplexed CE systems developed for DNA analysis. Two commercial systems have evolved: the Beckman Paragon 2000 (Beckman Analytical, Milan, Italy) and Sebia Capillarys. Although several studies have illustrated the potential of these systems for serum paraprotein characterization (essentially supplanting AGE and IFE),[28-30] studies have not yet settled the issue of paraprotein detection sensitivity and specificity for the clinical community.[28,31,32] For example, Yang and associates[33] compared the Capillarys 2 system versus standard serum protein AGE for the detection and identification of monoclonal proteins in patient serum samples. After defining sensitivity for both, they concluded that AGE and CZE had the same specificity for detection of monoclonal proteins, but that CZE/immunosubtraction was slightly less sensitive than standard immunofixation in the detection of IgM and free light chains.

Artifacts in Serum Protein Analysis

With CE using online optical detection, artifacts can occur in the form of "system peaks." These often originate from the sample or from the interfaces between the sample and the separation buffer, because any species that absorbs at the detection wavelength will generate a response. This differs from protein slab gel electrophoresis, wherein detection specificity is governed by a protein-specific stain. It is not uncommon, for example, for buffer species present in the sample but not in the separation buffer to generate system peaks.

One problem associated with conventional electrophoresis of serum proteins is its proclivity for point-of-application artifacts. These are bands that result from the fact that electrophoretic mobility (eg, with AGE) is bidirectional from the point of application. Consequently, the point of application remains part of the scanned area of interest. These bands must be immunotyped to distinguish real monoclonal proteins from artifacts—a process that is costly and time-consuming. CE prevents point-of-application artifacts in two ways. First, net mobility in CE results from the vectorial addition of both protein electrophoretic mobility and EOF. As a result of this unidirectional movement (toward the detector), the point of application remains removed from the detector. Second, unlike AGE, in which precipitates cannot exit the loading well and enter the gel (thus appearing as a band in the scanned region of the gel), no gel matrix is present in CZE to impede electrophoretic migration, because analysis occurs in free solution (ie, CZE). This was demonstrated by Clark and colleagues,[34] who evaluated a small subset of serum samples containing application artifacts resembling monoclonal proteins on agarose gels (and cellulose acetate) but were eliminated by CZE. These precipitates may be euglobulin or cryoprecipitates and may contain a monoclonal protein; only immunoelectrophoresis or IFE can identify the presence of monoclonal proteins.

Improving Limits of Detection

Several approaches have been devised to improve the limit of detection of online CE detectors. These include increasing the length of the OPL and online concentration of the sample.

Increased Optical Path Length. Capillary tubes modified at the detector window with a "bubble" cell (a glass-blown expansion of the internal diameter of the capillary tube) can expand the OPL by almost an order of magnitude, with concomitant lowering of the system's limit of detection. Alternatively, a "Z" geometry has been developed that increases the OPL via detection down the core of the capillary, with possible lengths up to 1 mm.

Online Sample Concentration. Another technique used in CE systems to increase their limit of detection is preconcentration of the sample. One of the simplest methods for sample preconcentration is to induce a "stacking" effect with the sample components, which is easily accomplished by exploiting the ionic strength differences between the sample matrix and the separation buffer.[35] This results from the fact that sample ions have decreased electrophoretic mobility in a higher conductivity environment. When voltage is applied to the system, sample ions in the sample plug instantaneously accelerate toward the adjacent separation buffer zone. On crossing the boundary, the higher conductivity environment induces a decrease in electrophoretic velocity and subsequent stacking of the sample components into a smaller buffer zone than the original sample plug. Within a short time, the ionic strength gradient dissipates and the charged analyte molecules begin to move from the stacked sample zone toward the cathode. Stacking has been used with hydrostatic or EK injection and typically yields a 10-fold enhancement in sample concentration, resulting in a lower limit of detection.

An alternative approach to stacking is "focusing" that is based on pH differences between the sample plug and the separation buffer. This has been shown to be very useful for analysis of peptides, mainly because of their relative stability over a wide pH range.[36] By increasing the pH of the sample to above that of the net isoelectric point (pI) of the analytes of interest and flanking the sample plug with low-pH separation buffer zones (ie, an equivalent volume of low-pH separation buffer after introduction of the sample plug), negatively charged peptides are electrophoretically driven toward the anode. On entering the lower pH separation buffer, a pH-induced change in their charge state causes a reversal in their electrophoretic mobility, resulting in "focusing" of the peptides at the interface of the sample (high pH) and low-pH buffer plugs (similar to those in IEF). After the pH gradient dissipates, the peptides, again positively charged, migrate toward the cathode as a sharp zone. This approach has been applied to a variety of analytes but is limited to those able to withstand inherent changes in pH without substantial denaturation and may yield as much as a fivefold enhancement of a system's limit of detection.[37]

Other types of sample concentration enhancement approaches applicable to CE include ITP[38] and those involving concentration of an online solid phase.[39] This latter method shows much promise for both small and large molecules and is discussed in detail in the review by Wettstein and Strausbauch.[40]

SPECIALTY ELECTROPHORESIS TECHNIQUES

With different media in different physical formats and a variety of instrumental configurations, several different types of electrophoretic techniques are used for the separation of a diverse range of analytes.

Starch Gel

Starch gel was the first gel medium to be used for electrophoresis and is only of historical interest. It separated proteins by both charge-to-mass ratio and molecular size, and, because proteins compacted on the surface of the gel before migrating into it, they formed narrow bands with improved resolution.

Disc Electrophoresis

Protein electrophoresis using agarose gel yields only five zones: (1) albumin and (2) α_1-, (3) α_2-, (4) β-, and (5) γ-globulins, although some subfractionation of the α_2- and β-globulins is possible with high-resolution gels. *Disc electrophoresis* was developed by Davis and Ornstein to improve this situation and derived its name from *discontinuities* in the electrophoretic matrix caused by layers of polyacrylamide or starch gel that differ in composition and pore size. These gels may yield 20 or more fractions and were widely used to study individual proteins in serum, especially genetic variants and isoenzymes.

With this technique, samples were separated in a three-gel system prepared in situ. A small-pore *separation gel,* followed by a thin segment of large-pore *spacer gel,* then a thin layer of large-pore monomer solution containing a small amount of serum—approximately 3 μL—was polymerized in open-ended glass tubes. When electrophoresis begins, all protein ions stack up on the separation gel in a very thin zone. This process improves resolution and concentrated protein components so that preconcentration of specimens with low protein content (eg, CSF) may not be necessary.

Isoelectric Focusing Electrophoresis

IEF separates amphoteric compounds, such as proteins, with increased resolution in a medium possessing a stable pH gradient. The protein becomes "focused" at a point on the gel as it migrates to a zone where the pH of the gel matches the protein's pI. At this point, the charge of the protein becomes zero and its migration ceases. Fig. 15.6 illustrates the procedure and shows the electrophoretic conditions before and after current is applied. The protein zones are very sharp, because the region associated with a given pH is very narrow. Ordinary diffusion is also counteracted by the acquisition of a charge, as a protein varies from its pI position and subsequently migrates back because of electrophoretic forces (Fig. 15.7). Proteins that differ in their pI values by only 0.02 pH unit have been separated by IEF.

The pH gradient is created with *carrier ampholytes,* a group of amphoteric polyaminocarboxylic acids that have slight differences in pKa value and molecular weights of 300 to 1000. Mixtures of 50 to 100 different compounds are added to the medium and create a "natural pH gradient" when individual ampholytes reach their pI values during electrophoresis. They establish narrow buffered zones, with stable but slightly different pH values, through which the slower moving proteins migrate and stop at their individual pIs.

As Fig. 15.4 illustrates, the anode is surrounded by a dilute acid solution, and the cathode by a dilute alkaline solution. After focusing, the most negatively charged carrier ampholytes and proteins will be found at the anodal end and the most positively charged near the cathodal end of the electrophoretic matrix. The other carrier ampholytes and proteins focus at intermediate points according to their pI values.

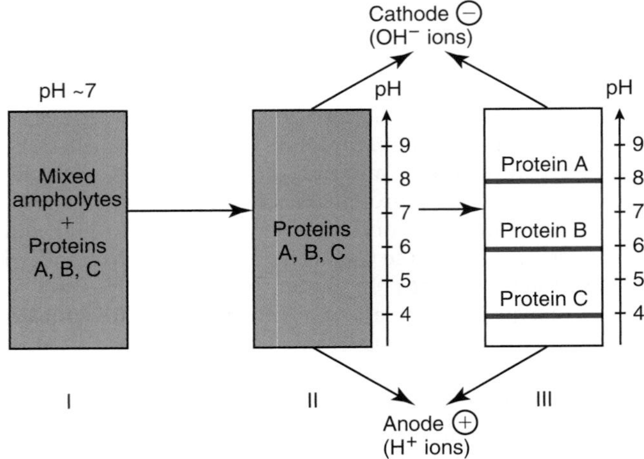

FIGURE 15.6 Schematic of an isoelectric focusing (IEF) procedure. *I,* A homogeneous mixture of carrier ampholytes, pH range 3 to 10, to which proteins A, B, and C, with isoelectric point (pI) of 8, 6, and 4, respectively, were added. *II,* Current is applied and carrier ampholytes rapidly migrate to pH zones where the net charge is zero (the pI value). *III,* Proteins A, B, and C migrate more slowly to their respective pI zones, where migration ceases. The high buffering capacity of the carrier ampholyte creates stable pH zones in which each protein may reach its pI.

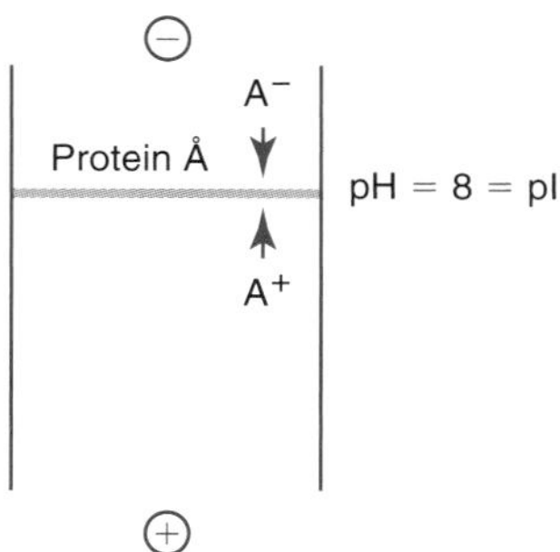

FIGURE 15.7 After the pH where protein A has a net charge of zero (Å) is attained, diffusion toward the cathode bestows a negative charge on A (A^-), and migration in the electric field forces A^- back to Å. Diffusion toward the anode causes A to take on the opposite charge A^+, and migration is toward the cathode and toward the point where Å exists. Isoelectric focusing processes of this type cause focusing of proteins and formation of sharp zones.

Because carrier ampholytes are generally used in relatively high concentrations, a high-voltage power source (up to 2000 V) is necessary (power is in the vicinity of 2 to 50 W, depending on experimental conditions). As a result, the electrophoretic matrix must be cooled. A modification of this technique (immobilized pH gradient [IPG]-IEF), in which an immobilized pH gradient is produced in the gel before the sample is applied, is reported to improve resolution and reproducibility.[41]

PAGE-IEF is widely used in analytical work, because it is essentially free of electroendosmosis. The polyacrylamide gel must have a sufficiently large pore size, however, that protein migration will not be impeded by molecular sieving effects. In actual practice, impeded migration of some proteins, such as IgM, cannot be prevented. AGE-IEF has the advantages that operating conditions are simple and large pore sizes make it unlikely that any proteins will be excluded on the basis of molecular size. IEF has been applied to the separation of alkaline phosphatase isoenzymes and is widely used in neonatal screening programs to test for variant hemoglobins (see Chapter 38). Off-gel techniques carry out the separation in free solution with sample containing ampholytes loaded into each of a linear series of wells separated by semipermeable membranes and in contact with a pH gradient strip. Electrophoresis separates sample proteins into different wells depending on their pI values. Separated fractions can be further resolved in a second similar focusing step or taken directly to further separation by two-dimensional (2D) electrophoresis (see later section) or liquid chromatography–mass spectrometry (LC-MS/MS).[42,43] This technique has been useful in the study of the human proteome.

For *IEF*, a power supply that provides constant power is advisable. During electrophoresis, current drops significantly because of lower conductivity as carrier ampholytes focus at their pI values and because of creation of zones of pure water. If a constant voltage supply is used, frequent voltage adjustments may be necessary. As a result, constant current power supplies are not customarily used in IEF. *Pulsed-power* or *pulsed-field* techniques (see later section) require a power supply that can periodically change the orientation of the applied field relative to the direction of migration.

Isotachophoresis

ITP completely separates smaller ionic substances into adjacent zones that contact one another with no overlap, and all migrate at the same rate. In this technique, background electrolyte (buffer) is not mixed with the sample, so current flow is carried entirely by charged sample ions. An aliquot of a sample is typically placed in a capillary between a leading electrolyte solution that contains faster migrating ions than any in the sample and a trailing solution containing slower migrating ions than any in the sample. Once a faster moving component separates completely from a slower moving one, any further separation creates a region of depleted charge and increases the resistance and therefore the local voltage in that region. Increased voltage causes the slower component to migrate faster and close the gap, thereby concentrating it and increasing the conductivity of its zone until it matches that of the faster ion. Ultimately, all ions migrate at the rate of the fastest ion in zones that differ in size depending on their original concentrations. Zone size is determined by measuring UV absorbance, temperature difference, or conductivity as the sample passes a detector. Applications include the separation of small anions and cations, organic and amino acids, and peptides, nucleotides, nucleosides, and proteins.

Pulsed-Field Electrophoresis

In pulsed-field electrophoresis, power is alternately applied to different pairs of electrodes or electrode arrays, so the electrophoretic field is cycled between two directions. The directions can differ spatially by 105 to 180 degrees, and molecules must reorient themselves to the new field direction during each cycle before migration can continue. Because reorientation time depends on molecular size, net migration becomes a function of the frequency of field alteration. This permits separation of very large molecules, such as DNA fragments greater than 50 kb, which cannot be resolved by the relatively small pores in agarose or polyacrylamide gels.[44] Fragments of 50 to 400 kb can be resolved using 10-s pulse times, whereas larger fragments up to 7 Mb in size or intact chromosomes require pulse times of several hours for complete resolution. This technique has been applied to typing various strains of bacterial DNA for research or epidemiologic studies.[45-48]

Two-Dimensional Electrophoresis

2D electrophoresis is extensively used in the field of proteomics to study families of proteins and search for genetic- or disease-based differences or to study the protein content of cells of various types.[49] It also has been applied to the study of human gene mutations[50] and the DNA of various bacteria and tumor cells as a means to earlier diagnosis.[51,52] By combining charge-dependent IEF in the first dimension with molecular weight–dependent electrophoresis in the second, the technique is able to resolve up to 1100 separate protein spots using autoradiographic detection, and up to 400 using Coomassie dyes. The first-dimension separation is carried out in a large-pore medium, such as agarose gel or large-pore polyacrylamide gel. The second dimension is often polyacrylamide in a linear or gradient format.

Conventional 2D electrophoresis uses PAGE-IEF in 130 × 2.5-mm (internal diameter) tubes for the first dimension and covers a pH range of 3 to 10 units. After electrophoresis is complete, the gel is extruded from the tube and placed in contact with a thin, polyacrylamide gradient gel slab that incorporates SDS. At the end of the process, the polypeptides are detected by one of several different methods. SDS is commonly used in the second dimension because it denatures proteins to polypeptides by reducing disulfide bonds and depolymerizing proteins. When native proteins, such as enzymes, are desired for further study, nondenaturing sample preparation and electrophoresis conditions must be used.

Separated proteins are detected with Coomassie dyes, silver staining, radiography (exposure of photographic film to emissions of isotopically labeled polypeptides or chemiluminescence), or fluorographic analysis (x-ray film exposed to tritium-labeled polypeptides in the presence of a scintillator). The latter two methods represent the most sensitive methods and are 100 to 1000 times more sensitive than Coomassie dyes. Difference gel electrophoresis permits two samples to be compared on the same 2D gel by labeling each with a different fluorophor. Although each separated spot contains protein from the two different samples, selective excitation and scanning software allow differences in expression to be qualitatively identified.[53,54]

Newer developments in this area combine analytical techniques to achieve 2D separation by linking, for example, liquid IEF with nonporous silica reverse-phase HPLC (for additional information on chromatography see Chapter 16) and detecting intact proteins by electrospray ionization, time of flight, and mass spectrometry[21,55] (see Chapter 17).

Micellar Electrokinetic Chromatography

MEKC is a hybrid of electrophoresis and chromatography. MEKC, a mode that is separate and distinct from capillary electrokinetic chromatography, is an effective electrophoretic technique, because it can be used for separation of neutral and charged solutes. The separation of neutral species is accomplished by exploiting micelles formed in the running buffer when the concentration of surfactant exceeds the critical micelle concentration (eg, 8 to 9 mmol/L for SDS). During electrophoresis, neutral micelles can interact with analytes in a chromatographic manner through hydrophobic interactions in which analytes are micellized based on their degree of hydrophobicity. Under these conditions, partitioning into the micelle is the driving force for separation. With charged micelles (eg, SDS), analytes also can interact through electrostatic interactions via the charge on the surface of the micelle.[56]

Capillary Isoelectric Focusing Electrophoresis

Capillary isoelectric focusing electrophoresis (cIEF) is comparable with tube IEF and is governed by the same principles and procedures. It differs from conventional IEF in that it can be carried out using a free solution of ampholytes or a precast gel. As expected with a CE mode, and unlike conventional IEF, the focused zones migrate past the online detector during the focusing process or following it. Fig. 15.8 shows an example of this in which separation by cIEF is completed in ≈15 minutes, circumventing conventional IEF protocols and/or the necessity for other electrophoretic methods (eg, CAE to detect hemoglobin variants), both of which are much less time efficient.[57]

Capillary Isotachophoresis

Capillary ITP has essentially the same features as ITP in other formats, except that conditions of pure ITP usually are not achieved. This is not commonly used as a bona fide CE mode, but instead is more typically used for online sample preconcentration (as described earlier). Most of the time, it functions as a preconcentrating step in a mixed mode with CZE, MEKC, or CGE. However, ITP may be undergoing a renaissance. Research being performed by the Santiago Group at Stanford is beginning to show that rigorous modeling of the process may begin to tease new capabilities and applications out of a technique that has been largely unheralded over the decades since Eaverarts first described it as a sample preparation technique for liquid chromatography.[58]

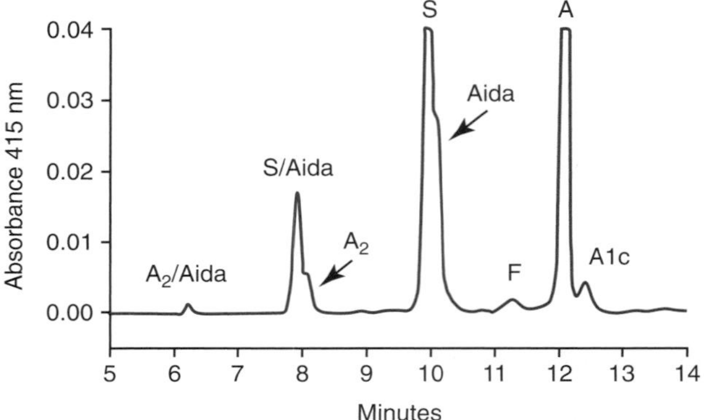

FIGURE 15.8 Capillary electrophoresis (CE)-based identification of uncommon hemoglobin (Hb) variants by capillary isoelectric focusing electrophoresis.[57] Analysis of blood from a patient with Hb S/Aida trait detected the presence of seven different normal and abnormal structural Hb variants, some of which are not detectable by conventional electrophoresis because of lack of sensitivity or inadequate resolution. The four abnormal variants include Hb S, Aida, S/Aida hybrid, and A_2/Aida. Glycated Hb A (HbA_{1c}) is also apparent in the electropherogram.

Microchip Electrophoresis

Over the past decade, microchip electrophoresis has undergone substantial development, including integrated microchip designs, advanced detection systems, and new applications.[59-62] In the arena of clinical diagnosis, the main analytes of interest for extrapolation to the microchip platform are proteins and DNA. This section provides a very brief overview; for a more comprehensive discussion see Chapter 24.

Among the attributes of microchip electrophoresis separation, the most notable is high speed—normally 4-fold to 10-fold faster than conventional CE, and at least an order of magnitude faster than the slab gel format. Other advantages of microchips include simplicity, capability for chip integration of multiple functions, and certainly the potential for automation.

Instrumentation

Although similar in principle, the microchip system differs from its CE counterpart. For example, with the microchip approach, separation channels, sample injection channels, reservoirs, and sample preparation and/or precolumn or postcolumn reactors can be fabricated onto the surface of a microchip, using photolithographic processes defined by the microelectronics industry. Thus, creation of a truly multifunctional, "integrated" analytical device embedded in a single monolithic substrate is possible. The classic "cross-T" design of a single-channel microchip involves a short (injection) channel that intersects a longer (separation) channel and includes a reservoir at the end of each of these, as shown in Fig. 15.9. The setup for LIF detection on a single-channel microchip is shown in Fig. 15.10.

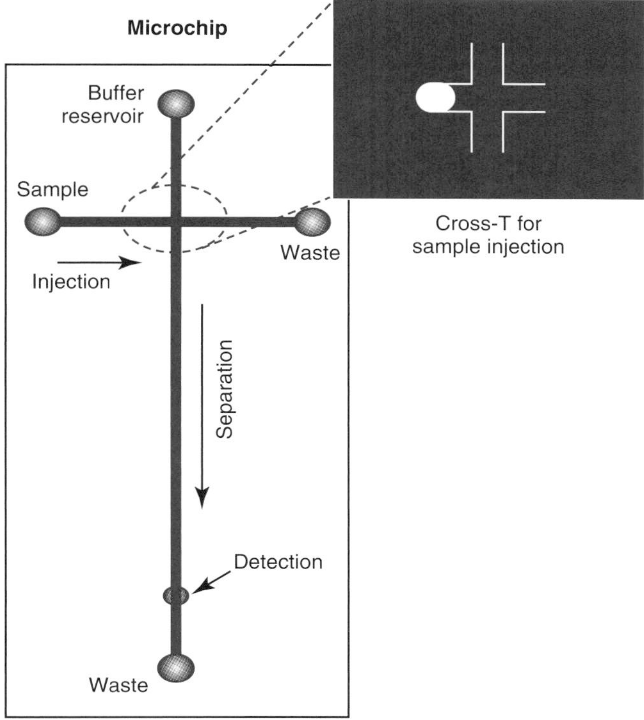

FIGURE 15.9 Simple cross-T microstructure design on chips used for electrophoretic separation.

When solution volumes required to fill the architecture are compared, it is seen that the volume of the separation channel on a microchip is roughly an order of magnitude smaller (low nanoliters) than conventional capillary systems. With their decreased volume requirements (nanoliter and even picoliter range), pressure injection is more challenging (but not impossible), and the EK sample injection mode is used primarily. In practice, an injection voltage of several hundred volts is applied across the sample and sample waste reservoirs to migrate the sample to the injection cross, which typically represents an injection volume of 50 to 100 pL. A separation voltage (1 to 4 kV) is then applied to the separation channel; this induces separation of the analyte zones before they reach the detection window downstream. It is important to note that, although the sample volume injected is ≈100 to 500 pL, the actual sample volume necessary (for handling) is still ≈2 to 4 μL, depending on the reservoir size.

Detection with a microchip occurs primarily through LIF, because this is easily implemented with the planar configuration of the microchip (see Fig. 15.10). Limits of detection for fluorescein have been easily demonstrated at 10^{-15} molar.[63] This allows for detection, for example, of polymerase chain reaction (PCR)-amplified DNA fragments at a level that competes with phosphorus-32 autoradiography from Southern blots.[64] Typical microchip separation times are around 50 to 200 seconds.

Fabrication of Microchips

Standard cross-T configuration microchips can be obtained commercially from several small vendors, but chips of more complex architecture tend to be fabricated in the laboratories that use them. They can be constructed from substrates such as glass (Pyrex-like or soda lime), silicon (as per microelectronic chips), or a variety of polymeric materials (plastics),

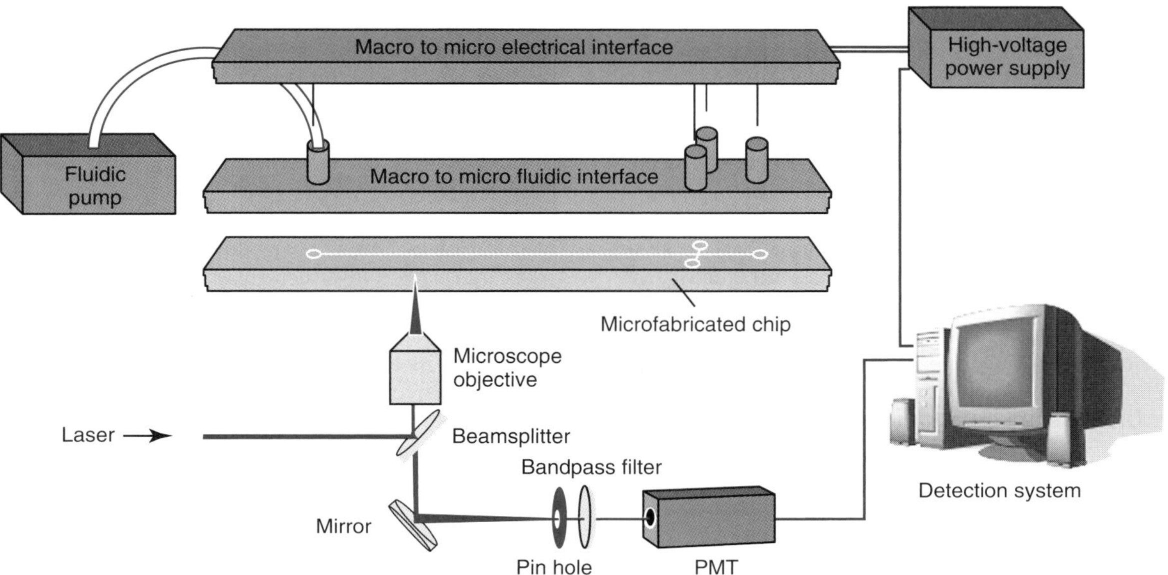

FIGURE 15.10 Detection system for laser-induced fluorescence detection on microchips. Fluidic and electrical interfaces are indirectly fundamental to the detection system. The fluidic interface drives the preparation and flushing of the chip before separation and after separation, and the electrical interface drives the electrophoretic separation and controls the flow of fluid through the chip architecture via electrokinetic valving. *PMT,* Photomultiplier tube.

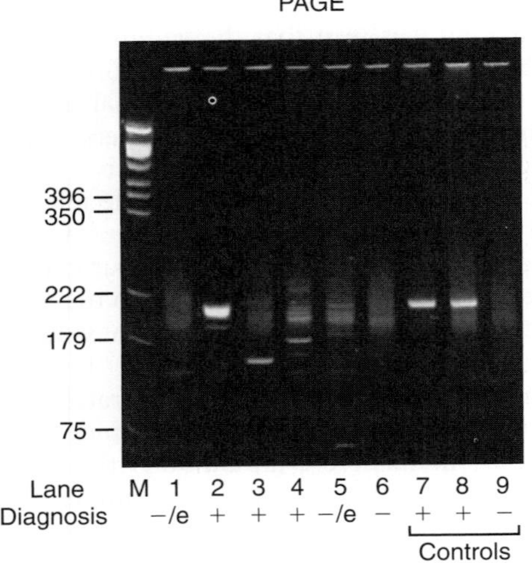

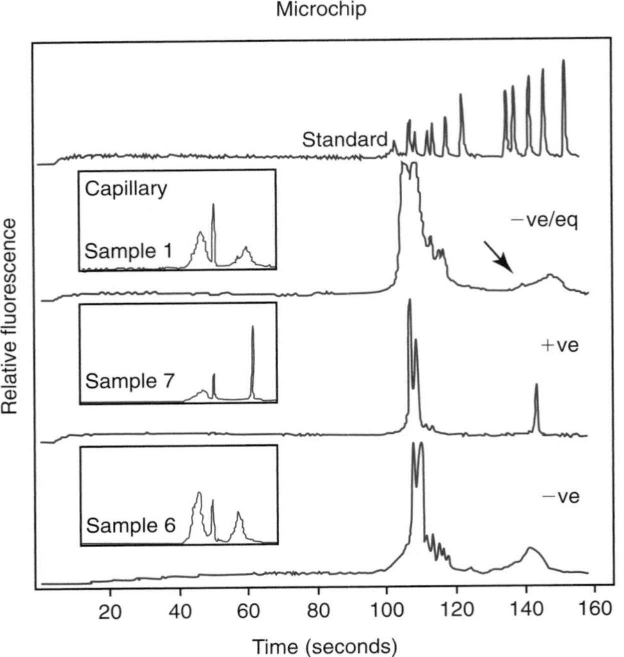

FIGURE 15.11 Electrophoretic detection of T cell receptor γ-gene rearrangement products. *Left,* Slab gel electrophoresis of amplified products resulting from polymerase chain reaction of nine patient samples. *Right,* Capillary *(inset)* and microchip separations of select samples analyzed by gel electrophoresis on the left. The top profile results from separation of a DNA sizing standard. *Sample 6* was consistent with a negative diagnosis for gene rearrangement; *sample 7* was positive, as indicated by the dominant peak signifying clonality (peak at 142 s); *sample 1* was deemed negative and/or equivocal based on the suspicious peak indicated by the *arrow.* Separation in both systems used hydroxyethylcellulose as a polymeric sieving matrix and applied fields of 300 V/cm and 275 V/cm, respectively, for the capillary and microchip systems.[70] *eq,* Equivocal; *+ve,* positive; *−ve,* negative.

or they may be cast from silicone-like materials (polydimethylsiloxane).[65] Historically, the first two of these types constituted the vast majority of electrophoretic devices described in the literature.

A buffered solution of hydrofluoric acid is used to etch the desired structures into a glass wafer, thereby producing a series of U-shaped troughs (typically 70 μm [w] × 20 μm [d]) that interconnect appropriately. Smooth walls are typically achieved, but channels are U-shaped because of downward and lateral etching by the etch solution. Consequently, features are often designed to be smaller than they have to be to allow for this type of spreading. After successful etching, the etched wafer is bonded to a second piece of glass, into which reservoirs have been drilled, to enclose chambers and channels of the device.

Molecular Diagnostics Using Microchips

As a result of the ease with which dsDNA can be made to fluoresce via high-affinity dsDNA fluorescent intercalators, and the excellent detection sensitivity that results from LIF, DNA separations on microchips have developed more rapidly than protein separations. Consequently, capillary and microchip types of electrophoresis have emerged as alternatives to traditional slab gel electrophoresis for DNA analysis; this is exemplified by sequencing of the human genome by Celera using primarily CE-based separation. A variety of polymers have been defined as *sieving matrices,* effective for molecular sieving and size-based microchip DNA separations, many of which had been used previously in CE.

As described in the CE section, the chemical nature of the microchannel surface is equally important in DNA separation, in which EOF has to be minimized or eliminated. For microchip-based electrophoretic DNA analysis, the chip surface must be passivated to reduce EOF. This can be accomplished through covalent modification with polymers such as polyacrylamide[66]; however, PCR samples must be desalted to achieve optimal resolution and acceptable longevity.[67,68] More attractive alternatives developed for CE involve polymers that have dual functionality, in that they both coat the microchannel surface and act as effective sieving polymers. Polydimethylacrylamide and the cellulosic polymers hydroxyethyl cellulose and hydroxypropyl cellulose have been shown to be very effective in this respect.[69]

An almost exponential growth of literature has occurred with respect to the application of microchip electrophoresis to the molecular diagnosis of disease based on PCR amplification of DNA.[20] Rudimentary microchip designs have been used to demonstrate the application of this platform in the most simplistic form, that is, detecting the presence of a PCR product of diagnostic significance. This has been demonstrated with multiple applications, including detection of herpes simplex viral DNA in CSF for diagnosis of encephalitis, detection of gene rearrangements correlative with lymphoproliferative disorders, detection of polymorphisms in the methylenetetrahydrofolate reductase gene, diagnosis of fragile X syndrome, detection of tetranucleotide repeats associated with hypercholesterolemia, and diagnosis of muscular dystrophy. More complicated DNA assays have been accomplished on electrophoretic microchips, including single-stranded conformation polymorphism and heteroduplex analysis for the detection of common mutations in the breast cancer susceptibility genes, *BRCA1* and *BRCA2*.[20]

An example of microchip DNA separation applied to the diagnosis of lymphoproliferative disorders is shown in Fig. 15.11.[70] The high-resolution (8%) acrylamide slab gel used for conventional analysis is given on the left for comparison. Because of the short separation length of the electrophoretic chamber (≈4 cm) and the use of applied electrical fields comparable with those used in CE, separation on the microchip is complete in 160 seconds (in comparison with 8 hours for the slab gel). More recent examples are seen in chip-based methods for DNA extraction from sample, PCR amplification of purified DNA, and a method to inject this material with a DNA ladder for electrophoretic interrogation, with all processes interfaced on a single chip. Using whole blood from a mouse infected with *Bacillus anthracis,* analysis of less than 1 μL of blood allowed the detection of an *anthracis*-specific PCR product in less than 30 minutes, demonstrating the power of integrated microchip-based analysis.

More complicated microchip systems have been developed to address the high-throughput requirements of molecular diagnostics laboratories. For example, high-throughput genetic typing has been performed on a 96-channel radial capillary array electrophoresis microplate with an unprecedented sample throughput of ≈0.6 samples/s.[62,68] This has been extrapolated to a variety of other applications, including genotyping of the marker gene for diagnosis of hereditary hemochromatosis.[71]

SELECTED REFERENCES

For a full list of references for this chapter, please refer to ExpertConsult.com.

2. Sadaba MC, Gonzalez Porque P, Masjuan J, et al. An ultrasensitive method for the detection of oligoclonal IgG bands. *J Immunol Methods* 2004;**284**:141–5.
4. Vesterberg O, Acevedo F, Bayard C. Sensitive quantification of proteins by electrophoresis in gels by use of chemiluminescence. *Electrophoresis* 1995;**16**:1390–3.
8. Oda RP, Clark R, Katzmann JA, et al. Capillary electrophoresis as a clinical tool for the analysis of protein in serum and other body fluids. *Electrophoresis* 1997;**18**:1715–23.
18. Nielen MWF. Quantitative aspects of indirect UV detection in capillary zone electrophoresis. *J Chromatogr* 1991;**588**:321–6.
24. Katzmann JA, Clark R, Wiegert E, et al. Identification of monoclonal proteins in serum: a quantitative comparison of acetate, agarose gel, and capillary electrophoresis. *Electrophoresis* 1997;**18**:1775–80.
25. Luraschi P, Infusino I, Zorzoli I, et al. Heavy chain disease can be detected by capillary zone electrophoresis. *Clin Chem* 2005;**51**:247–9.
29. Gay-Bellile C, Bengoufa D, Houze P, et al. Automated multicapillary electrophoresis for analysis of human serum proteins. *Clin Chem* 2003;**49**:1909–15.
33. Yang Z, Harrison K, Park YA, et al. Performance of the Sebia Capillarys 2 for detection and immunotyping of serum monoclonal paraproteins. *Am J Clin Pathol* 2007;**128**:293–9.
34. Clark R, Katzmann JA, Kyle RA, et al. Differential diagnosis of gammopathies by capillary electrophoresis and immunosubtraction: analysis of serum samples problematic by agarose gel electrophoresis. *Electrophoresis* 1998;**19**: 2479–84.
37. Shihabi Z. Effects of sample matrix on capillary electrophoretic analysis. In: Landers JP, editor. *Handbook of capillary electrophoresis*. 2nd ed. Boca Raton, FL: CRC Press; 1997. p. 457–77.
43. Xiao Z, Conrads TP, Lucas DA, et al. Direct ampholyte-free liquid-phase isoelectric peptide focusing: application to the human serum proteome. *Electrophoresis* 2004;**25**:128–33.
45. Drinka PJ, Stemper ME, Gauerke CD, et al. The identification of genetically related bacterial isolates using pulsed field gel electrophoresis on nursing home units: a clinical experience. *J Am Geriatr Soc* 2004;**52**:1373–7.
51. Gurtler V, Barrie HD, Mayall BC. Use of denaturing gradient gel electrophoresis to detect mutation in VS2 of the 16S-23S rDNA spacer amplified from *Staphylococcus aureus* isolates. *Electrophoresis* 2001;**22**:1920–4.
55. Wittmann-Liebold B, Graack HR, Pohl T. Two-dimensional gel electrophoresis as tool for proteomics studies in combination with protein identification by mass spectrometry. *Proteomics* 2006;**6**:4688–703.
57. Hempe J, Vargas A, Craver R. Clinical analysis of structural hemoglobin variants and Hb A1c by capillary isoelectric focusing. In: Petersen J, Mohammad A, editors. *Clinical and forensic applications of capillary electrophoresis*. Totowa, NJ: Humana Press; 2001. p. 145–63.
58. Schoots AC, Everaerts FM. Isotachophoresis as a preseparation technique for liquid chromatography. *J Chromatogr* 1983;**277**: 328–32.
59. Colyer CL, Mangru SD, Harrison DJ. Microchip-based capillary electrophoresis of human serum proteins. *J Chromatogr A* 1997;**781**:271–6.
60. Harrison DJ, Manz A, Fan ZH, et al. Capillary electrophoresis and sample injection systems integrated on a planar glass chip. *Anal Chem* 1992;**64**:1926–32.
62. Medintz I, Wong WW, Sensabaugh G, et al. High speed single nucleotide polymorphism typing of a hereditary haemochromatosis mutation with capillary array electrophoresis microplates. *Electrophoresis* 2000;**21**:2352–8.
67. Carrilho E. DNA sequencing by capillary array electrophoresis and microfabricated array systems. *Electrophoresis* 2000;**21**: 55–65.

16

Chromatography

*David S. Hage**

ABSTRACT

Background

Clinical tests often involve the use of one or more separation steps to isolate, enrich, or separate a target compound from other chemicals in the sample. Chromatography is one of the most common methods for achieving this type of separation. In this method, the components of a mixture are separated based on their differential interactions with two chemical or physical phases: a mobile phase and a stationary phase that is held in place by a supporting material. There are many forms of chromatography based on the different mobile phases, stationary phases, and supports that can be used in this method, which has led to a wide range of applications for this technique.

Content

This chapter describes the basic principles of chromatography and discusses various forms of this method that are used for chemical analysis or to prepare specimens for analysis by other techniques. The methods of gas chromatography and liquid chromatography are discussed, as well as the techniques of planar chromatography, supercritical fluid chromatography, and multidimensional separations. The mobile phases, stationary phases, and supports that are used in each of these methods are described. The instrumentation and detection schemes that are employed in these methods are also discussed.

Biological fluids are complex mixtures of chemicals. This means that clinical tests for specific components in these fluids often involve the use of one or more separation steps to isolate, enrich, or separate the target compound of interest from other chemicals in the sample. Chromatography is one of the most common methods for achieving this type of separation. This chapter describes the basic principles of chromatography and discusses various forms of this method that are used for chemical analysis or to prepare specimens for analysis by other techniques.

BASIC PRINCIPLES OF CHROMATOGRAPHY

General Terms and Components of Chromatography

Chromatography is a method in which the components of a mixture are separated based on their differential interactions with two chemical or physical phases: a mobile phase and a stationary phase.[1-4] The basic components and operation of a typical chromatographic system are illustrated in Fig. 16.1. The mobile phase travels through the system and carries sample components with it once the sample has been applied or injected. The stationary phase is held within the system by a support and does not move. As a sample's components pass through this system, the components that have the strongest interactions with the stationary phase will be more highly retained by this phase and move through the system more slowly than components that have weaker interactions with the stationary phase and spend more time in the mobile phase. This leads to a difference in the rate of travel for these components and their separation as they move through the chromatographic system.

*The author gratefully acknowledges the contributions of Drs. Glen L. Hortin, Bruce A. Goldberger, M. David Ullman, Carl A. Burtis, and Larry D. Bowers to this chapter in previous editions.

The type of chromatographic system that is shown in Fig. 16.1 uses a column (or a tube) to contain the stationary phase and support, while also allowing the mobile phase and sample to pass through the system. This approach was first described in 1903 by Mikhail Tswett, who used this method to separate plant pigments into colored bands by using a column that contained calcium carbonate as both the support and stationary phase.[5] Tswett gave the name *chromatography* to this method. This name is derived from Greek words *chroma* and *graphein,* which mean "color" and "to write." This term is still used to describe this technique, even though most modern chromatographic separations do not involve colored sample components.

The type of chromatography that was used by Tswett, in which the stationary phase and support are held within a column, is known as "column chromatography." In chromatography, the stationary phase may be the surface of the support, a coating on this support, or a chemical layer that is cross-linked or bonded to the support.[2,6,7] In column chromatography, the support may be the interior wall of the column or it may be a material that is placed or packed into the column. A column is the most common format for chromatography. However, it is also possible to use a support and stationary phase that are present on a plane or open surface.

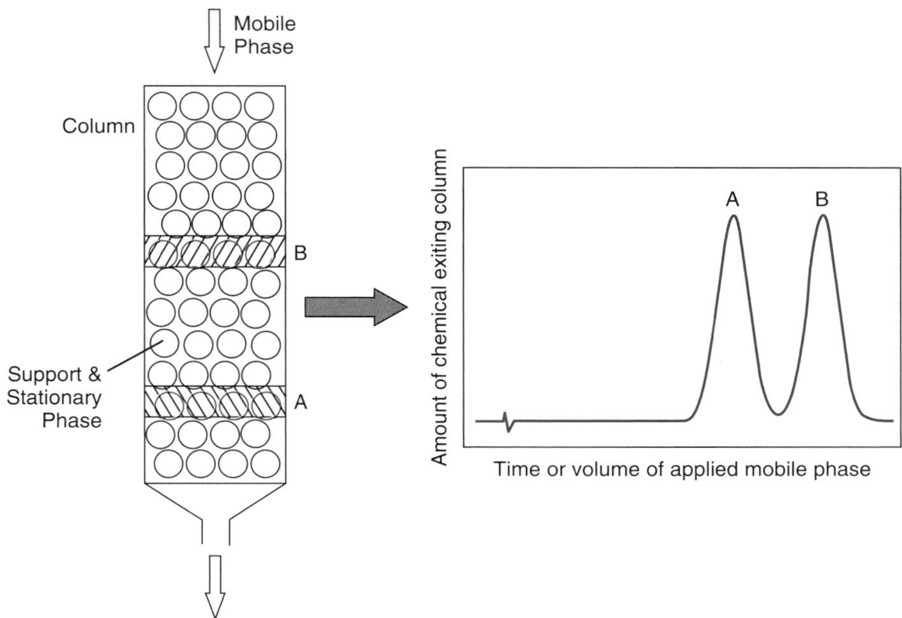

FIGURE 16.1 The general components of a chromatographic system, as illustrated here by using a column to separate two chemicals, *A* and *B*.

This second format is known as "planar chromatography," as will be discussed in more detail later in this chapter.[2,7]

One way of classifying chromatographic methods is based on the type of support that they employ; two examples are the techniques of column chromatography and planar chromatography. Chromatographic methods also can be classified based on the mobile phase that is present. For instance, a chromatographic method that uses a mobile phase that is a gas is called gas chromatography (GC),[8] and a chromatographic method that uses a liquid mobile phase is known as liquid chromatography (LC).[9] It is also possible to divide chromatographic methods according to the type of stationary phase that is present or the way in which this stationary phase is interacting with sample components. Examples of these classifications include the GC methods of gas-solid chromatography (GSC) or gas-liquid chromatography (GLC) and the LC methods of adsorption chromatography, partition chromatography, or ion-exchange chromatography (IEC). Each of these categories, as well as others, will also be discussed later in this chapter.

The instrument that is used to perform a separation in chromatography is known as a chromatograph.[7,10] For instance, in GC the instrument is a gas chromatograph, and in LC the instrument used to carry out this method is a liquid chromatograph. These instruments can provide a response that is related to the amount of a compound that is exiting (or eluting) from the column as a function of the elution time or the volume of mobile phase that has passed through the system. The resulting plot of the response versus time or volume is known as a chromatogram,[7,10] as is illustrated in Figs. 16.1 and 16.2.

The average time or volume that is required for a particular chemical to pass through the column is known as that chemical's retention time (t_R) or retention volume (V_R). These values both increase with the strength and degree to which the chemical is interacting with the stationary phase. The elution time or volume for a compound that is nonretained or that does not interact with the stationary phase is known as the void time (t_M) or void volume (V_M). If the retention time or retention volume is corrected for the void time or void volume, the resulting measure of retention is known as the adjusted retention time (t_R', where $t_R' = t_R - t_M$) or the adjusted retention volume (V_R', where $V_R' = V_R - V_M$). For two chemicals to be separated by chromatography, it is necessary for these chemicals to have different values for t_R and V_R (or t_R' and V_R').[2,7,10]

Most separations that are used for chemical analysis in column chromatography are carried out by injecting a relatively small volume or amount of sample onto the chromatographic system. This situation results in a chromatogram that consists of a series of peaks that represent the different compounds in the sample as they each elute from the column. The retention time or retention volume of each peak can be used to help identify the eluting compound, whereas the area or height of the peak can be used to measure the amount of the compound that is present.

The width of each peak is also of interest in a chromatogram. The peak width reflects the separating performance or efficiency of the chromatographic system. The width of a peak in a chromatogram is often represented by its baseline width (W_b) or its half-height width (W_h) (Fig. 16.3).[2,7,10] As the widths for the peaks in a chromatogram become sharper, it becomes easier for the chromatographic system to separate two peaks with similar interactions with the system and to separate more peaks in a given amount of time. Sharper peaks are also easier to measure than broader peaks and tend to produce better limits of detection.

Retention and Selectivity

For two chemicals to be separated by chromatography, these chemicals need to have some differences in how they are interacting with the stationary phase versus the mobile phase.

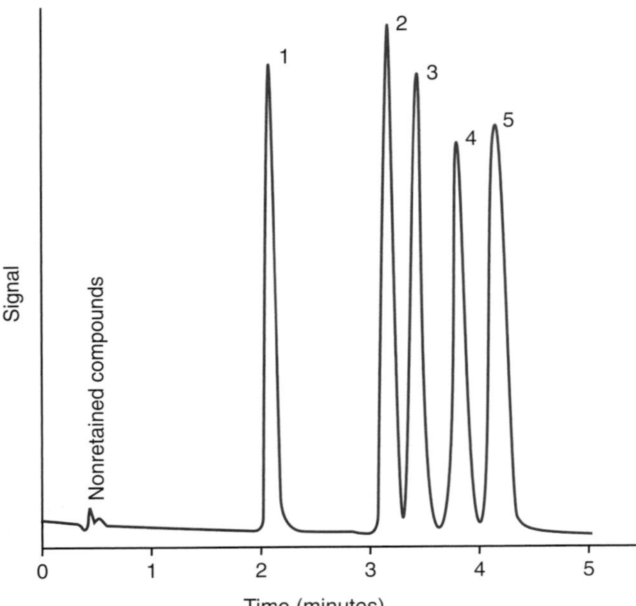

FIGURE 16.2 Chromatogram from a separation of tricyclic antidepressants based on reversed-phase chromatography and high-performance liquid chromatography. Detection was based on the use of an absorbance detector that monitored the column eluent at 215 nm. *Note:* the signal is displayed at 0.1 absorbance units-full scale *(AUFS)*. (Courtesy Vydac/Grace Materials Technologies, Columbia, Maryland.)

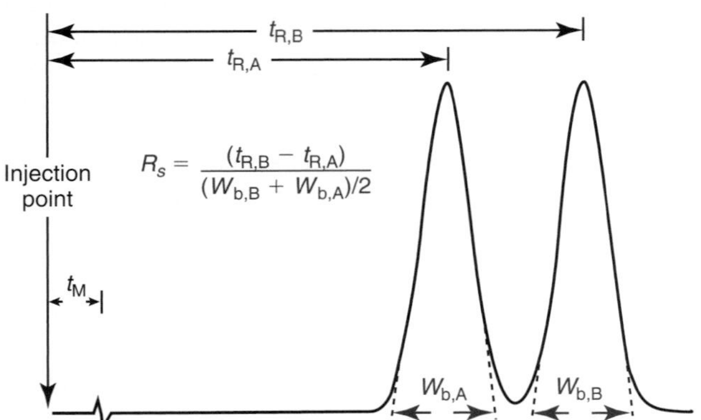

FIGURE 16.3 An example of a general chromatogram that may be obtained when using a column. In this example, compound B is eluted later than compound A. R_s, Resolution; t_M, void time; $t_{R,A}$ and $t_{R,B}$, retention times for solutes A and B; $W_{b,A}$ and $W_{b,B}$, baseline peak widths for compounds A and B.

Besides using the retention time and retention volume (or adjusted retention time and adjusted retention volume) to describe these differences, another way of representing retention in chromatography is by using the retention factor (k). This term is also sometimes represented as k' or called the capacity factor.[7,10] The retention factor is a measure of the average time a chemical resides in the stationary phase versus the time it spends in the mobile phase. This value can be calculated from experimental data by using any of the following equivalent relationships.[2,7,10]

$$k = (t_R - t_M)/t_M = (t_R')/t_M$$

or

$$k = (V_R - V_M)/V_M = (V_R')/V_M$$

As these equations suggest, the retention factor is a unitless number where a value of 0 indicates that no binding or interactions are occurring between a chemical and the stationary phase or that this compound is eluting from the system at the void time. As the chemical undergoes greater interactions with the stationary phase, this will result in longer retention times and an increased value of k. In practice, it is desirable to have a value for k that is between 1 and 10 to provide reasonable separations between compounds without the need for excessive lengths of time for their elution from the column.

The retention factor is useful in describing a compound's retention in chromatography for several reasons. First, the value of k should be independent of the flow rate and column size. Also, k can be directly related to the strength of the interactions that are occurring between a chemical and the stationary phase or mobile phase, as well as the relative amount of stationary phase versus mobile phase that is present in the column. This last feature is illustrated by the following equation for a chromatographic system in which a chemical is separated based on its ability to partition between the mobile phase and stationary phase. Similar relationships can be written for other types of separation mechanisms.[2]

$$k = K_D(V_S/V_M)$$

In this relationship, the value of k is directly related to (1) the distribution equilibrium constant (K_D) for partitioning of the analyte into the stationary phase versus the mobile phase and (2) the relative amount of stationary phase in the column (as represented here by V_S) versus the amount of mobile phase that is present (as represented by V_M, the void volume). The value of k in this situation will increase if there is either an increase in K_D, which reflects the tendency of the chemical to enter the stationary phase over the mobile phase, or the ratio (V_S/V_M), which is a term also known as the *phase ratio*.[2,7]

Any separation in chromatography requires that there be some difference in retention for the chemicals that are to be separated from each other. One way of describing this difference in retention is by using the separation factor or selectivity factor (α).[7,10] The separation factor for two compounds (A and B) is equal to the ratio of their retention factors (k_A and k_B),

$$\alpha = k_B/k_A$$

where the retention factor for the later eluting component is given in the numerator. If two chemicals have the same retention in a chromatographic system, the value of α will equal 1 and no separation will be possible. If the peaks for A and B do have different retention, the value of α will be greater than 1 and will increase as the degree of separation increases.

The values of both the retention factor and selectivity factor are determined by the chemicals that are being separated, as well as the stationary phase and mobile phases that are present in the chromatographic system. A large difference in retention and a large separation factor are desirable when the goal is to selectively isolate one chemical from others in a sample. However, smaller differences in retention and in separation factors are often used when the chromatographic system is used to separate several chemicals and peaks from the same sample. In this second situation, a value for α of 1.1 or greater represents an adequate separation in many common types of chromatography. However, chromatographic methods that result in broad peaks may need even larger values of α to produce a good separation between two chemicals.

Band-Broadening and Efficiency

Besides needing a difference in retention for a separation to occur, the peaks for two neighboring chemicals must be sufficiently narrow to allow this difference to be observed. The injection of even a sample with a small volume will experience some increase in width, or band-broadening, as this peak travels through the chromatographic system. This broadening of peaks is produced by various processes related to the rate of movement or diffusion of the applied chemicals as they pass around or within the support and within or between the mobile phase and stationary phase. These band-broadening processes, in turn, are affected by factors such as the diameter or type of support within the chromatographic system, the flow rate, the diffusion coefficient of the chemical in the mobile phase and stationary phases, and the degree of retention of the chemical in the column (Box 16.1). Together, these processes and factors determine the overall efficiency or extent of band-broadening obtained.

The efficiency and degree of band-broadening in a chromatographic system are related experimentally to the final observed width of a chemical's peak. This width can be described by measures such as the baseline width (W_b), the half-height width (W_h), or the standard deviation (σ) of the peak. These values, in turn, can be used to find another measure of chromatographic efficiency known as the number of theoretical plates, or plate number *(N)*. The value of N for any type of chromatographic peak can be calculated by using the following formula:

$$N = (t_R/\sigma)^2$$

where t_R is the retention time for the peak and σ is the standard deviation of the peak in the same units of time as t_R.[7,10] This equation takes on the following two equivalent forms for a Gaussian-shaped peak[2,7]:

$$N = 16(t_R/W_b)^2 \quad \text{or} \quad N = 5.545(t_R/W_h)^2$$

These last two equations make use of the fact that a Gaussian peak has a baseline width, as measured by the intersection of the baseline with tangents along either side of the peak, that is equal to 4 σ, and a half-width width that is equal to 2.355 σ.

The value of N can be thought of as representing the effective number of times that a chemical has been distributed between the mobile phase and stationary phase as this chemical has passed through the chromatographic system. A larger value for N represents many such steps, which makes it easier to distinguish between two chemicals that have only small differences in their retention. Experimentally, a large value of N results in a high chromatographic efficiency and sharp peaks, which are both desirable for either separating chemicals with similar retention or quickly separating many chemicals in the same sample.

There are several other ways in which the efficiency of a chromatographic system can be described. One way is by using the number of theoretical plates *(N)* per unit length of the chromatographic system (L), as given by the ratio (N/L). This ratio helps in comparing systems with different lengths, because the value of N increases in direct proportion to the length of the column or support bed that is used in a separation for chromatography. Although this means that a longer chromatographic system will always lead to a larger value for N and greater efficiency, the use of a longer system also results in longer separation times.

Another way of describing column efficiency is the height equivalent of a theoretical plate or plate height (HETP, or H).[7,10] The value of H is found by dividing the length of the chromatographic system by the number of theoretical plates for this system.

$$H = L/N$$

The value of H represents the length of the column or chromatographic system that makes up one theoretical plate or one distribution step for a chemical between the mobile phase and stationary phase. Although a large value of N (or N/L) represents a chromatographic system with high efficiency, the same system would be represented by a small value for H (or L/N).

A valuable feature of using H to describe chromatographic efficiency is that this term can be related directly to the parameters and processes that affect band-broadening. A common example of this is the *van Deemter equation*,[11] which shows how the overall value of H is affected by the linear

BOX 16.1 Factors That Can Affect Chromatographic Efficiency

- Column length (affecting the number of theoretical plates, N, but not the plate height, H)
- Particle size of support (packed bed column) or tube diameter (open tubular column)
- Uniformity in size, shape, and packing of the support
- Flow rate and linear velocity
- Temperature and rate of solute diffusion
- Mobile phase viscosity
- Degree of compound retention
- Initial injection volume
- Volume of connecting tubing, detector, and system components besides the column

velocity of the mobile phase (u), which is directly related to the flow rate (F) through the relationship $u = (F \times L)/V_M$.[10,12]

$$H = A + B/u + C\,u$$

The terms A, B, and C in this equation are constants that represent the contributions of several types of band-broadening processes. For instance, the A term represents the contributions of band-broadening processes that are independent of the linear velocity and flow rate, such as eddy diffusion and mobile phase mass transfer. The B term is the contribution to the plate height by longitudinal diffusion, which is a process that becomes more important as the flow rate and linear velocity are decreased. Finally, the C term represents the contributions from processes that lead to an increase in H as the flow rate or linear velocity is increased. The processes that make up the C term are stagnant mobile phase mass transfer and stationary phase mass transfer. The van Deemter equation predicts that the combined effect of these band-broadening processes will be an optimum range of flow rates and linear velocities over which the lowest plate heights, and best efficiencies, will be obtained.[11] In practice, the usual goal in varying the flow rate in chromatography is to identify those conditions that provide the most rapid separation times while still providing adequate resolution of all peaks that are of interest in the samples being separated.

Several factors that affect chromatographic efficiency are listed in Box 16.1. For instance, efficiency can be improved by using longer columns, which increases the value of N but does not alter H. It is also possible to change the flow rate to its optimum value, to use smaller diameter support particles, to use nonporous or pellicular particles instead of fully porous support particles, or to use a relatively narrow-diameter coated capillary instead of a packed bed column. All of these latter factors help to lower the value of H, which in turn increases the value of N for a given length of column or chromatographic bed. However, there are practical limits to how much some of these experimental parameters can be changed. As an example, a reduction in the diameter of the support particle will lead to greater efficiency, but it will also result in higher back pressures across the chromatographic system, require the use of lower flow rates, or both.

Resolution and Peak Capacity

The overall extent to which two peaks are separated in chromatography can be described by using a term known as the resolution (R_s), as is illustrated in Fig. 16.3. The resolution between two neighboring peaks can be found by using the following formula.[7,10]

$$R_s = \frac{(t_{R,B} - t_{R,A})}{(W_{b,B} + W_{b,A})/2}$$

In this equation, $t_{R,A}$ and $t_{R,B}$ are the average retention times for compounds A and B (where B elutes after A), while $W_{b,A}$ and $W_{b,B}$ are the baseline widths for the peaks of these compounds (in time units, in this case). An equivalent equation can be written in terms of the retention volumes of A and B and their baseline widths in volume units. The use of either approach will give a unit-less value for R_s that represents the average number of baseline widths that separate the centers of the two peaks.

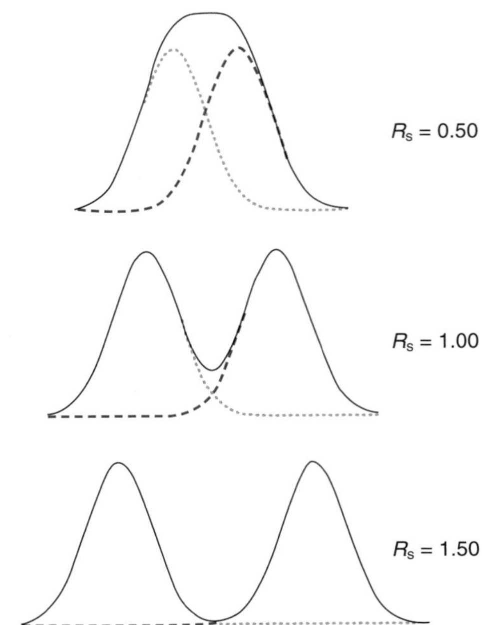

FIGURE 16.4 Degree of separation obtained for two chromatographic peaks that are present in a 1 : 1 area ratio as the resolution between these peaks (R_s) is varied.

Fig. 16.4 shows how the separation of two neighboring peaks changes as the value of R_s increases for these peaks. An R_s value of 0 is obtained when there is no separation between the peaks and they have exactly the same retention times or retention volumes. The degree of peak separation increases as the value of R_s increases. An R_s value of 1.5 or greater is often said to represent a complete separation between two equally sized peaks, or baseline resolution. However, for many separations, resolution values between 1.0 or 1.25 and 1.5 also may be adequate, especially if the peaks are about the same size and are to be measured using their peak heights rather than their peak areas.

Several approaches can be used to alter or improve the resolution between two peaks in chromatography (Fig. 16.5). These approaches are indicated by the following expression, which is sometimes known as the resolution equation of chromatography.[13]

$$R_s = [(N^{1/2})/4] \times [(\alpha - 1)/\alpha] \times [k/(1+k)]$$

In this equation, k is the retention factor for the second of two neighboring peaks, α is the separation factor between the first and second peaks, and N is the number of theoretical plates for the chromatographic system. This relationship indicates that resolution of two peaks in chromatography can be changed in three ways: (1) by altering the efficiency of the system, as represented by N; (2) by changing the overall degree of peak retention, as represented by k; or (3) by changing the selectivity of the column for one compound versus another, as represented by α. An increase in N, such as can be obtained through the use of a longer column, will lead to an increase in R_s that is proportional to $N^{1/2}$. An increase in the retention factor (k) or selectivity (α) will also lead to a nonlinear increase in resolution.

Another way of describing a chromatographic separation is in terms of the *peak capacity*. The peak capacity is the

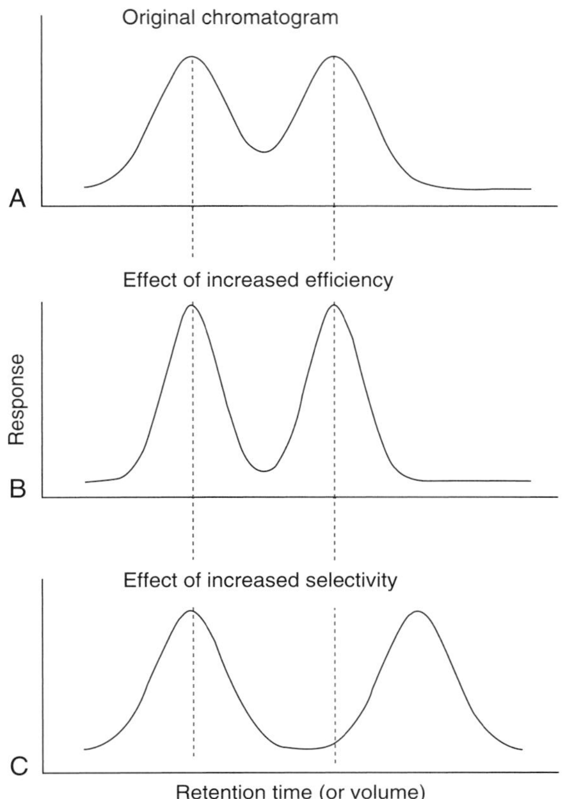

FIGURE 16.5 Effects of selectivity and efficiency on the resolution of peaks in chromatography. These three situations represent cases in which there is **(A)** poor or moderate resolution between two neighboring peaks, **(B)** good resolution between the peaks as a result of high column efficiency, or **(C)** good resolution between the peaks as a result of good column selectivity.

maximum number of peaks (or sample components) that can be separated, in theory, during a single chromatographic separation.[14-16] The value of the peak capacity can be found by assuming there is a continuous distribution of peaks that are separated by an average baseline width (or 4 standard deviations). In practice, the number of components that can be separated in a single run by a given system will be lower than the theoretical peak capacity because the retention times of their peaks will not be evenly distributed. The peak capacity of a system that is used for high-performance liquid chromatography (HPLC) is usually limited to several hundred peaks, whereas higher values can be obtained in methods such as capillary GC. Factors that can be used to increase the peak capacity include increasing the efficiency of the system (eg, by using a longer column) and using gradient elution or extended run times. Another approach for increasing the peak capacity is to use a multidimensional separation, as will be discussed later in this chapter.

Analyte Identification and Quantification

Chromatography is often used as an analytical tool to qualitatively identify analytes in a sample and to measure the concentrations of these analytes. For example, the retention time, retention volume, and retention factor for an analyte are all characteristic values that reflect how this chemical is interacting within a particular chromatographic system. These retention values can be compared to those for a known sample of the same compound to help confirm its identity. However, other confirmation also may be needed because other compounds may have similar retention characteristics.

One way additional confirmation can be obtained is if the unknown compound and reference compound have the same retention under several types of chromatographic conditions, such as on different columns or column/mobile phase combinations. In the case of capillary GC or LC columns, it is possible to simultaneously introduce samples onto two columns that contain different stationary phases and that are connected to separate detectors. If the unknown compound and a reference compound match in their retention properties on the two columns, this greatly enhances the chance for correctly identifying the unknown analyte. An alternative and even more reliable approach for identification is to use a detection method that provides structural information on the analyte, such as mass spectrometry (see Chapters 17 and 19 to 21).

The peak area or peak height can be used to produce quantitative information on an analyte that is separated from other sample components by chromatography. Peak areas tend to provide a more precise means for measuring an analyte, whereas peak heights are easier to use if there is not complete resolution between the analyte and its neighboring peaks. Both external and internal calibration techniques can be used in chromatography for such measurements.[2,17] In external calibration, standard solutions containing known quantities of the analytes are processed and separated in the same manner as samples that contain one or more of these analytes (Fig. 16.6). A calibration curve is then constructed by plotting the peak height or peak area (or the spot density, in the case of planar methods) versus the concentration or mass of analyte that was applied in the standard solutions. This curve can then be used with the peak area or peak height that is determined for the same analyte in the samples to find the concentration or amount of this analyte present.

In the method of internal calibration (also called internal standardization), standard solutions of the analyte are again prepared; however, a constant amount of a different compound known as the internal standard is also now added to each standard solution and sample (Fig. 16.7). The internal standard should be a chemical that was not originally present in either the sample or the standard, is similar in its chemical and physical properties to the analyte, and can be measured independently from the analyte. This internal standard is typically added to the samples and standards before they are processed by any pretreatment steps, such as extraction or derivatization. The addition of this agent can help normalize the results for any variations that may occur during the

POINTS TO REMEMBER

General Ways to Improve Peak Resolution in Chromatography

- Increase the efficiency of the system
- Increase the overall degree of peak retention
- Increase the selectivity of the column for the peak of one compound versus another

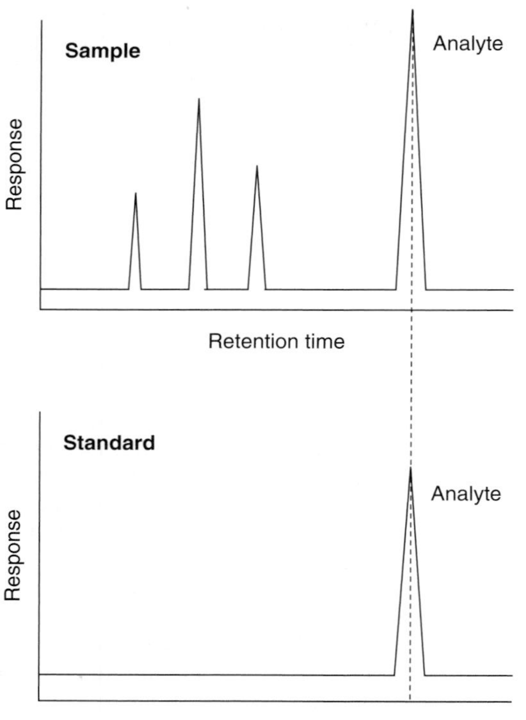

FIGURE 16.6 Use of external calibration and standards to quantify an analyte based on its peak height or area in a chromatogram for an injected sample.

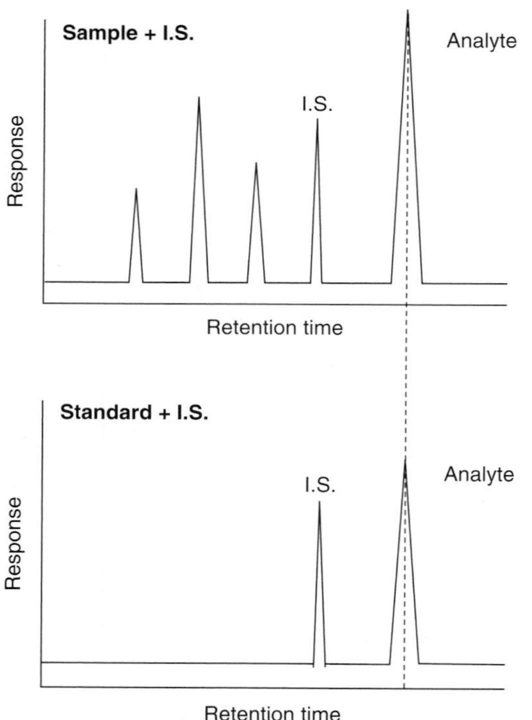

FIGURE 16.7 Use of internal calibration and samples or standards containing an internal standard (I.S.) to quantify an analyte based on its peak height or area in a chromatogram for an injected sample.

pretreatment steps or during sample/standard injection onto the chromatographic system. This normalization is made by constructing a calibration curve in which the *y*-axis is based on the ratio of the peak height or peak area for the analyte in a given standard or sample divided by the peak height or peak area for the internal standard in the same standard or sample. This ratio is plotted versus the concentration or amount of analyte in each standard. This calibration plot can then be used to find the concentration or amount of the analyte that was present in each sample.[2,17]

GAS CHROMATOGRAPHY

GC is a common type of chromatography often used in chemical separations and analysis. GC can be defined as a chromatographic method in which the mobile phase is a gas.[7] The first modern GC system was developed in the mid-1940s by Cremer[18,19] and became popular after work by James and Martin in 1952, who used this method to separate fatty acids.[20]

In GC, a gaseous mobile phase is used to pass a mixture of volatile solutes through a column containing the stationary phase.[7,8] The mobile phase is typically an inert gas such as nitrogen, helium, or argon or a low mass gas such as hydrogen. Because of the low densities of gases under typical GC operating conditions, the compounds injected onto a GC column do not have any appreciable interactions with the gaseous mobile phase. Instead, this gas acts to merely carry samples through the column. As a result, the term carrier gas is commonly used to refer to the mobile phase in GC.[7]

Solute separation in GC is based on differences in the vapor pressures of the injected compounds and in the different interactions of these compounds with the stationary phase. For instance, a more volatile chemical will spend more time in the gaseous mobile phase than a less volatile solute and will tend to elute more quickly from the column. In addition, a chemical that selectively interacts with the stationary phase more strongly than another chemical will tend to stay longer in the column. The overall result is a separation of these chemicals based on their volatility and interactions with the stationary phase.

Types of Gas Chromatography

There are several ways of classifying GC methods based on the type of stationary phase present. These categories include GSC, GLC, and bonded phase GC.

Gas-Solid Chromatography

GSC is a type of GC in which the same material acts as both the stationary phase and the support.[7] In this method, chemicals are retained by their adsorption to the surface of the support. This support is often an inorganic material such as silica or alumina. Other supports that can be used in this method are molecular sieves, which are porous materials that are made from a mixture of silica and alumina, or organic polymers such as porous polystyrene.[2,12,21]

The retention of an analyte on a GSC support will be affected by several factors. These factors include the surface area of the support, the size of the pores in the support, and the types of functional groups that are present on the surface of the support. Using a support with a high surface area will lead to higher retention than a support with a lower surface

TABLE 16.1 Stationary Phases Commonly Used in Gas-Liquid Chromatography and as Bonded Phases in Gas Chromatography

Composition	Polarity	Commercial Examples	Typical Applications
100% Methylpolysiloxane	Nonpolar	OV-1, SE-30	Drugs, amino acid derivatives
5% Phenyl–95% methylpolysiloxane	Nonpolar	OV-23, SE-54	Drugs
50% Phenyl–50% methylpolysiloxane	Intermediate polarity	OV-17	Drugs, steroids, glycols
50% Cyanopropylmethyl–50% phenylmethylpolysiloxane	Intermediate polarity	OV-225	Fatty acid methyl esters, carbohydrate derivatives
Polyethylene glycol	Polar	Carbowax 20M	Acids, alcohols, glycols, ketones

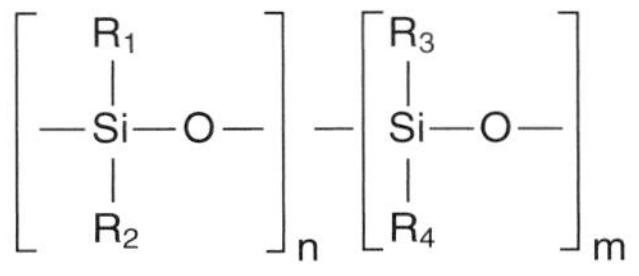

$$\left[-\underset{R_2}{\overset{R_1}{\mathrm{Si}}}-\mathrm{O}- \right]_n \left[-\underset{R_4}{\overset{R_3}{\mathrm{Si}}}-\mathrm{O}- \right]_m$$

FIGURE 16.8 General structure of a polysiloxane. The side groups are represented by R_1 through R_4, while *n* and *m* represent the relative lengths (or amounts) of each type of segment in the overall polymer.

area. The selection of an appropriate pore size may be important if the analytes are large enough to be able to access the surface within only some of these pores. The functional groups and polarity of the support and its surface will also determine which types of analytes will have the strongest adsorption to this surface. Polar materials such as silica, alumina, and molecular sieves will usually have strong binding to polar compounds and to those that can form hydrogen bonds. Polystyrene and other less polar supports will have weaker and less selective interactions with chemicals and tend to give separations that are based more on the volatility of the components in an applied sample.

Gas-Liquid Chromatography and Bonded Phases

In GLC, the stationary phase is a liquid that is placed as a coating or layer on the support.[7] This is the most common type of GC for chemical analysis. Various types of liquids can be used for this purpose (see examples in Table 16.1). All of these liquids must have a low volatility to allow them to stay within the column at the high temperatures that are often used in GC separations. Many GLC stationary phases are based on polysiloxanes, which have the basic structure shown in Fig. 16.8.[12] The molar mass of the -Si-O-Si- chain in a polysiloxane can range in size from a few thousand to over a million grams per mole. The side chains that are attached to the silicon atoms in this chain can have structures that range from nonpolar methyl groups to polar cyanopropyl groups. These side chains also can be present in various ratios as mixtures. The overall polarity and types of chemicals that will be retained the most by this type of stationary phase will be determined by the amounts and types of side chains that are present.

One issue in using a liquid as a stationary phase in GC is that some of this liquid will eventually leave the column over time. This loss of the stationary phase is known as column bleed.[12,22] This process is not desirable because it will result in a change in the amount of stationary phase present and a change in the ability of the GC system to retain chemicals. This process also may cause the signal of the GC detector to have a high background or to be noisy as the liquid stationary phase leaves the column and passes through the detector.

Column bleed can be minimized by using a bonded phase instead of a liquid as the stationary phase in the GC column. The resulting method is sometimes known as bonded phase GC. A bonded phase can be produced by reacting functional groups on a stationary phase such as a polysiloxane with silanol groups on the surface of silica. Alternatively, the stationary phase can be cross-linked to make it less volatile and more stable. Besides providing a stationary phase that is more stable, a bonded phase also can provide a stationary phase that has a thinner and more uniform coating than a stationary phase based on a liquid coating. Although bonded phases are more expensive than liquid stationary phases, bonded phases are often preferred for analytical work because of their better thermal stability and better efficiencies.[12,22]

POINTS TO REMEMBER

Types of Gas Chromatography Based on the Stationary Phase

- GSC
- GLC
- Bonded phase GC

Gas Chromatography Instrumentation

The typical components of a gas chromatograph are illustrated in Fig. 16.9.[21] The first major component is the source of the gaseous mobile phase, which is used to supply the carrier gas at a controlled pressure and flow rate. Next, there is the injection system, through which samples are placed into the gas chromatograph and converted into a volatile form. This is followed by the column, which contains the support and the stationary phase. This column is held in an oven for temperature control. The fourth part of the GC system is a detector that monitors sample components as they leave the column. Finally, there is a computer or control system that acquires data from the detector and allows control of the GC system.[21]

Carrier Gas Sources and Flow Control

The function of the carrier gas source is to provide the gas that will be used as the mobile phase for the GC separation. The carrier gas is usually supplied by a standard gas cylinder. However, the carrier gas is sometimes provided by using a gas

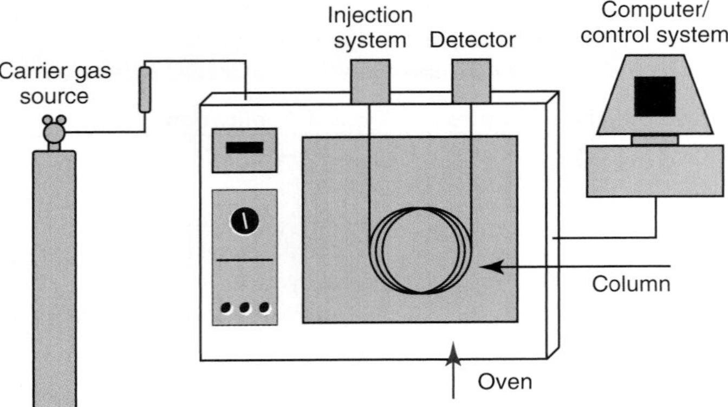

FIGURE 16.9 General design of a gas chromatograph. (Modified from a figure courtesy Restek Corporation, Bellefonte, Pennsylvania.)

generator that is connected to the GC system. Such a generator can be used to isolate nitrogen from air or produce hydrogen gas through the electrolysis of water.[2]

Good flow control is needed in GC to provide a constant or well-defined flow of the carrier gas. This control makes it possible to maintain good column efficiency and obtain reproducible elution times. Systems that are used to provide constant flow rates may use a simple mechanical device, such as a pressure regulator, or a more sophisticated electronic control device. Methods in GC such as temperature programming, as will be discussed later, require electronic pressure control to regulate the carrier gas flow rate and pressure during a chromatographic run. Such a controller may be operated in a constant-flow or constant-pressure mode. In the constant-flow mode, the pressure required to provide a flow rate that is independent of the carrier gas viscosity is determined and maintained by the system through the use of a pressure transducer and pressure regulator.

The magnitude of the carrier gas flow rate will depend on the type of column being used. For example, packed columns require typical flow rates that range from 10 to 60 mL/min. Capillary columns use much lower flow rates (eg, 1 to 2 mL/min). Because of the greater efficiencies of capillary columns versus packed columns, operating at a consistent flow rate is even more critical for the operation of the capillary columns.

Various gases can be used as the mobile phase in GC. The choice of carrier gas will depend on factors such as the type of column and detector used, as well as the expense, purity, and chemical or physical properties of the gas. Hydrogen and helium are the carrier gases of choice with capillary columns. Only high-purity hydrogen and helium should be used for this purpose. For packed columns, the most frequently used carrier gas is nitrogen.

Carrier gas impurities such as water, oxygen, and hydrocarbons can (1) harm or alter the column, (2) negatively influence the performance of some detectors, and (3) adversely affect the measurement of chemicals. The carrier gas should be as pure as possible to avoid such problems. The carrier gas should be dry, and the tubing used to connect the gas source to the GC system should be free from contamination. Molecular sieve beds and specialized inline traps are often used to remove water, hydrocarbons, oxygen, and particulate matter that may be present in the carrier gas.[23]

Many GC detectors work best with certain types of carrier gases. For instance, work with packed columns often involves the use of nitrogen as the carrier gas when working with a flame ionization detector (FID), electron capture detector (ECD), or thermal conductivity detector (TCD), which are each described in more detail later. Helium is often used with capillary columns and in work with a FID or TCD, whereas nitrogen/argon-methane mixtures are used with an ECD.

Injection Systems and Sample Derivatization

The injection of a sample into a GC system has to be done with minimal disruption of gas flow into the column. Most clinical GC methods make use of liquid-phase samples, for which the sample components are first extracted into or dissolved in a nonaqueous liquid or adsorbed onto a microextraction fiber (see Chapter 18). This liquid or microextraction fiber is then placed into the chromatographic system by using a precise and rapid online injector (eg, an autosampler or automated injection system). With packed columns, a glass microsyringe is used to inject a 1- to 10-μL portion of the sample through a septum, which serves as the interface between the injector and the chromatographic system. On the other side of the septum is located a heated injection port. Volatile chemicals in the sample and the solvent are flash-vaporized in this heated port and swept into the column by the carrier gas. To ensure rapid and complete volatilization, the temperature of the heated injection port is usually maintained at a temperature that is at least 30 to 50° C higher than the column temperature.

Common problems during injection include septum leaks and the adsorption of sample components onto the septum. In addition, because the injection port is heated, thermal decomposition products may be produced here from the sample and enter into the column. This process can result in spurious peaks, or "ghost" peaks, in the chromatogram. This type of contamination is most likely to occur at high injection temperatures. A Teflon-coated septum, or low-bleed septum, can be used to minimize this problem. In addition, the inner surface of the septum can be purged with the carrier gas and vented before the purge gas passes into the column. This approach is especially effective in reducing septum-related problems, and most commercial injectors are equipped with continuous-purge capabilities. The septum is a consumable component of the gas chromatograph and should be replaced at least once every 100 injections.

Because of the low sample capacities and slow carrier gas flow rates that are used with capillary columns, split and splitless injection techniques are used to introduce samples into such columns.[2,22] In the method of split injection, only a small portion of the vaporized sample enters the column, with the remainder being passed through a side vent. In splitless injection, most of the sample enters the column.[4] The split flow injection mode is used for samples that contain relatively high concentrations of the target analytes, whereas the splitless mode is used for samples that contain relatively low concentrations of the analytes.

Temperature-programmable injection ports are available and may be used in either the split or splitless injection mode. In this type of port, the sample is injected at a temperature slightly higher than the boiling point of the solvent that contains the sample. Under these conditions, most of the sample components will condense on a glass or fused silica wool insert that is present in the injector, while the solvent is vaporized and removed. The injector is then rapidly heated at rates of up to 100°C/min. The rapid heating vaporizes the analytes, which then move into the column. This rapid heating is advantageous because any thermally labile compounds that may be present in the sample are exposed to the high temperatures for only a short time. The ability of this approach to provide separate steps for solvent removal and analyte vaporization can allow the injection of sample volumes of up to hundreds of microliters. This ability can improve analyte detection when the amount of sample that is available is not a limiting factor.

Headspace analysis is a sample introduction technique that can be used with aqueous solutions or samples that contain some nonvolatile components.[22] In this method, a portion of the vapor phase (or "headspace") that is above a liquid or solid sample is used for the analysis. This vapor phase contains a portion of some of the more volatile components of the sample and can be directly injected onto a GC system for analysis. Headspace analysis can be carried out using either a static method or a dynamic method. In the static method, the sample is placed in an enclosed container and allowed to reach equilibrium for the distribution of its components between the sample and the vapor phase above the sample. A portion of the vapor phase is then injected onto the GC system for analysis. In the dynamic method, an inert gas is passed through the sample and used to sweep away the volatile components. These components are then captured by a solid adsorbent or a cold trap and later injected onto the GC system for analysis.

Although a fairly large number of low-mass chemicals can be injected directly onto a GC system, many more are not sufficiently volatile or thermally stable for their direct application to a GC system. A common way of making a chemical more volatile and thermally stable is to alter its structure through derivatization.[2,24] This usually involves replacing one or more polar groups on the analyte with less polar groups. This change tends to make the chemical more volatile by reducing dipole-related interactions or hydrogen bonding and also often makes the chemical more thermally stable. Various types of reactions can be used for this purpose in GC. A common example is the replacement of an active hydrogen on an alcohol, phenol, amine, or carboxylic acid group with a trimethylsilyl (TMS) group, producing a TMS derivative. Other examples include the use of alkylation (eg, the formation of a methyl ester through the esterification of a carboxylic acid) or acylation (eg, the production of an acetate derivative from an alcohol or amine).[24] Along with increasing the volatility and thermal stability of a compound, some of these derivatization reactions also can be used to change the response of the analyte to certain detectors, such as an ECD through the addition of halogen atoms to a compound's structure.

Columns and Supports

Both packed columns and capillary columns are used in GC.[2,7,21,25] Packed GC columns are filled with support particles that are based on either uncoated supports, as used in GSC, or that have liquid coatings or bonded stationary phases, as used in GLC and bonded phase GC. These packed columns vary from 1 to 4 mm in inner diameter and have typical lengths of 1 to 2 m, with the outside of the column being fabricated from tubes of glass or stainless steel. Packed GC columns are useful when it is necessary to apply a relatively large amount of a sample onto the GC system. However, packed columns also tend to have lower efficiencies than capillary columns. This last factor results in packed columns being mainly used for separations in which a relatively small number of compounds are to be separated.

Capillary columns, which are also known as open-tubular columns, consist of a column that has the stationary phase attached to or coated on its interior surface. Capillary columns have typical inner diameters of 0.1 to 0.75 mm and lengths that often range from 10 to 150 m. The capillary columns with narrow bores are more efficient, and the wider bore columns have greater sample capacities. Capillary GC columns are usually made from fused silica capillaries that have a polyimide or aluminum coating on the outside to give the capillary sufficient strength and flexibility for use in a GC system. Although capillary columns have lower sample capacities than packed columns, they also provide better peak resolution and higher efficiencies. These properties make capillary columns the most common type of support used in GC for analytical applications.

There are several types of capillary columns. Three common types are (1) porous-layer open tubular (PLOT) columns, (2) support-coated open tubular (SCOT) columns, and (3) wall-coated open tubular (WCOT) columns.[2,7,21,25] In PLOT columns, a porous layer is placed on the inner wall of the capillary columns. This porous layer is made by either chemical means (eg, etching) or by depositing a layer of porous particles on the wall from a suspension. The porous layer serves as a support and/or stationary phase for use in GSC. PLOT columns are primarily used for analysis of gases and separation of low-mass hydrocarbons.

SCOT columns have an inner wall with a thin layer of a support onto which a stationary phase is coated or attached. This type of column is used with liquid stationary phases or bonded phases. WCOT columns consist of a capillary tube whose inner wall is coated directly with a liquid stationary phase or a bonded phase. WCOT columns tend to be more efficient than SCOT columns but also have a smaller sample capacity.

In addition to traditional packed columns and capillary columns, research has been carried out in the development of GC columns on microchips.[26] These devices have great potential for use in high-speed GC and miniaturized GC systems.[27]

Temperature Control

All types of GC columns and systems require careful control of temperature. The accurate, precise control of the column and injector temperatures is required to obtain optimal performance and reliable results in a GC system. Control of the column temperature is achieved by using a column oven, in which the column is heated directly by resistive heating.[21,28] The temperatures of the injection system and detectors are also usually controlled by resistance heating. Temperature control of the column is especially important, particularly in applications in which the retention times or volumes of eluting peaks are compared with those of standards for compound identification. For instance, a change of only 1°C in column temperature can lead to a 5% change in retention time.

Depending on the type of GC separation being carried out and the complexity of the sample, the column may be maintained at a constant temperature during the separation (ie, a method known as isothermal elution) or the temperature may be varied as a function of time (ie, a technique known as temperature programming).[7] Temperature programming is used for most clinical applications. In temperature programming, the sample components with the lowest boiling points and weakest interactions with the GC column will elute first, followed by chemicals that have higher boiling points and/or stronger interactions with the column. As a result, it is possible with temperature programming to separate a complex mixture of chemicals with a wide range of boiling points and volatilities. Temperature programming also usually provides sharper and more distinct peaks in less time than can be obtained with isothermal elution. The main advantage of isothermal elution is that it can be faster for simple samples that do not contain a wide range of chemicals with different volatilities. Also, it is essential with temperature programming to use computer control to provide a reproducible and well-defined temperature gradient during the analysis.

The thermal stability of the stationary phase is important to consider during the development of a GC method. Because each stationary phase has a specific temperature range over which it is stable, it is necessary to keep the column temperature within this usable range. For nonpolar stationary phases in silica capillary columns, the upper temperature limit is often determined by the stability of the polyimide coating on the capillary. The introduction of aluminum clad columns has broadened this usable temperature range. Oxidation reactions that may occur at high temperatures tend to limit the operating temperature of stationary phases that have an intermediate polarity or that have a higher polarity.

Before any GC column is used for routine analysis, it must be "thermally conditioned" by heating the column at various temperatures and for different lengths of time. This process helps to remove volatile contaminants, including residual monomers from a polymeric stationary phase that may be initially present in the column. Furthermore, the thermal conditioning of used columns can remove nonvolatile contaminants that have accumulated on this column and that can lead to unstable baselines.

To thermally condition a column, the column should be disconnected from the detector and purged for at least 5 minutes with pure carrier gas. The column should then be heated to a temperature that is above 50°C. The column temperature is then passed through a normal temperature program for three or four cycles. Alternatively, the column can be maintained at the maximum operating temperature for 12 to 24 hours. Thermal conditioning at lower temperatures can prolong the life of the column, but longer conditioning times are required under these conditions to achieve good baseline stability. Preconditioned capillary columns are also available to minimize such problems.

Gas Chromatography Detectors

A variety of detectors can be used in GC systems (Table 16.2). These include universal detectors that can detect a broad range of analytes and more selective devices that may detect only specific groups of analytes. Examples that will be examined in this section include the (1) FID, (2) nitrogen-phosphorus detector, (3) ECD, (4) photoionization detector (PID), (5) TCD, and (6) mass spectrometric detectors.[12,21,22]

TABLE 16.2 Examples of Detectors Used in Gas Chromatography

Type of Detector	Principle of Operation	Selectivity	Approximate Limit of Detection
Flame ionization detector (FID)	Production of gas phase ions from combustion of organic compounds	General: Organic compounds	10^{-12} g carbon
Nitrogen-phosphorus detector (NPD; thermionic detector, TSD)	Heated alkali bead selectively ionizes nitrogen- or phosphorus-containing compounds	Nitrogen- or phosphorus-containing compounds	10^{-14}–10^{-13} g nitrogen or phosphorus
Electron capture detector (ECD)	Capture of electrons by chemicals with electronegative groups	Chemicals with electronegative groups	10^{-15}–10^{-13} g
Mass spectrometry (MS)	Production of gas phase ions, followed by separation/analysis of these ions based on their mass-to-charge ratios	Universal: Full-scan mode Selective: Selected ion monitoring mode (SIM)	10^{-10}–10^{-9} g Full-scan mode 10^{-12}–10^{-11} g SIM mode
Thermal conductivity detector (TCD)	Measurement of change in thermal conductivity of carrier gas as compounds elute from the column	Universal	10^{-9} g
Photoionization detector (PID)	Measurement of gas phase ions that are produced due to chemical ionization with light	General: Organic compounds	10^{-12}–10^{-11} g
Flame photometric detector (FPD)	Phosphorus- and sulfur-containing compounds emit light when burned in a flame; emitted light is detected	Phosphorus and sulfur-containing compounds	10^{-12} g phosphorus 10^{-11} g sulfur
Infrared (IR) spectroscopy	Absorption of IR light	IR-absorbing compounds	10^{-9} g

Portions of this table are based on data from Hage, DS, Carr, JD. *Analytical chemistry and quantitative analysis*. New York: Pearson; 2011, and references cited therein.

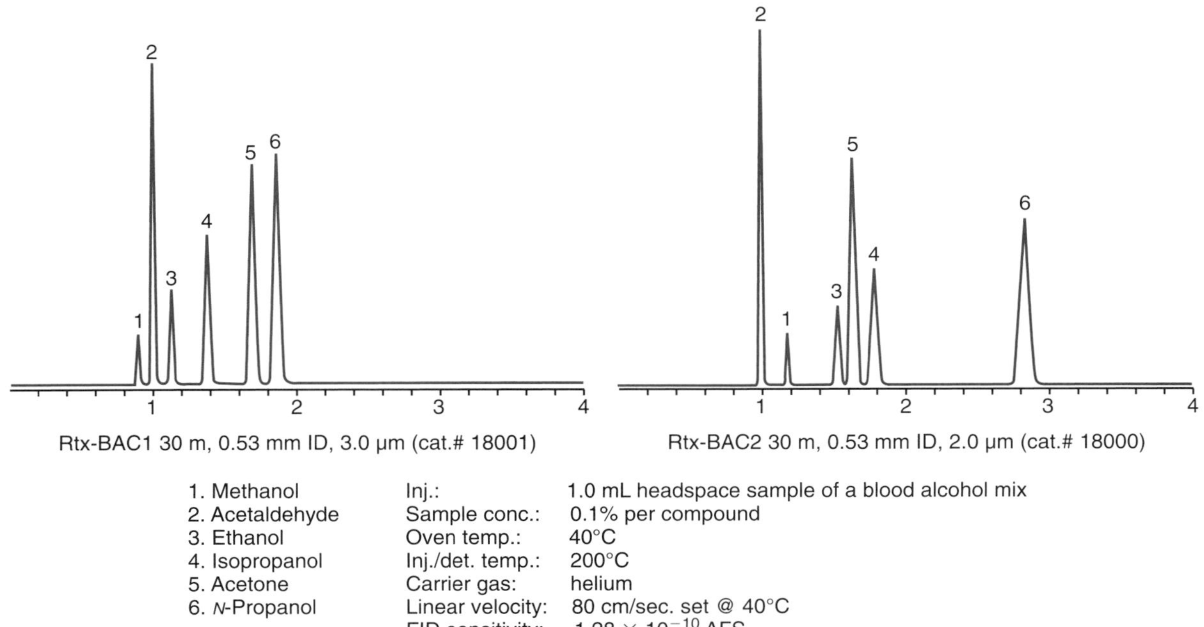

FIGURE 16.10 Chromatograms obtained during the analysis of volatile organic compounds when using headspace analysis and gas chromatography. (Courtesy Restek Corporation, Bellefonte, Pennsylvania.)

Many other types of detectors have been used in GC, and it has become common to place two or more detectors in series to enhance the specificity and sensitivity of GC systems.

Flame Ionization Detector. An FID is a common detector used for GC in clinical laboratories.[12,21,22] This type of detector is often used during GC analysis of ethanol and other volatiles in blood or other aqueous samples. Typical chromatograms are shown in Fig. 16.10 of volatile compounds that have been examined by using headspace analysis and a GC system equipped with an FID. During the operation of an FID, the carrier gas that is leaving the column is mixed with hydrogen, and the eluting compounds are burned by a flame that is surrounded by air and an oxygen-rich environment. Approximately one organic molecule in 10,000 results in the production of a gas-phase ion. These ions are detected by a collector electrode that is positioned above the flame. The magnitude of the current that is generated by these ions is related to the mass of carbon that was delivered to the detector. This signal can then be used for both the detection and quantification of organic compounds that are eluting from the column.

The advantages of an FID include its simplicity, reliability, versatility, and ease of operation. Another advantage of using an FID is that this detector gives little or no signal for common carrier gases (eg, He, Ar, or N_2) or typical contaminants in such gases (eg, O_2 and H_2O). An FID is easy to use with temperature programming and is a good general detector for the routine clinical analysis of organic compounds. One disadvantage of the FID is its destructive nature, so it cannot be connected directly to other GC detectors. However, an FID still can be used in combination with another detector if part of the carrier gas stream is split between the FID and the other detector.

Nitrogen-Phosphorus Detector. The nitrogen-phosphorus detector (NPD) is also known as a thermionic selective detector (TSD). This detector is similar to an FID but instead of a flame uses an electrically heated alkali bead, which is generally made of rubidium. This heated bead is placed directly above where the mixture of the carrier gas and hydrogen enter the detector.[12,21,22] Ions are generated at or above the surface of the heated alkali bead, which supplies electrons to electronegative compounds that surround the bead and leads to the formation of negatively charged ions. These ions are then collected at an electrode and generate a current that is used to detect and quantify the eluting compounds.

Nitrogen- or phosphorus-containing compounds are especially good at creating ions in an NPD. This feature makes the NPD particularly useful for monitoring low concentrations of analytes that have nitrogen or phosphorus in their structures. The NPD is frequently used in GC for detection of organic bases and acids. This type of detector does not respond to common GC carrier gases or their impurities, and several types of carrier gases can be used with this detector. However, it is necessary to have the alkali bead in this detector changed on a regular basis because this material will slowly degrade over time.

Electron Capture Detector. The ECD is another example of a selective GC detector. The operation of an ECD is based on the capture of secondary electrons by electronegative compounds that are eluting from the column.[12,21,22] High-energy electrons, or beta particles, are provided in an ECD by a radioactive source such as ^{63}Ni or ^{3}H that is housed in the detector. As the beta particles are produced, they collide with the carrier gas and lead to the release of a large number of secondary electrons. When only the carrier gas is passing through this detector, a consistent supply of the secondary electrons is created. These secondary electrons are collected at a positive electrode and measured. When a chemical with electronegative groups elutes from the column, some of these secondary electrons are captured and fewer reach the electrode. The resulting change in current is used to detect and measure the amount of analyte that was eluting from the column.

An ECD can provide both selective and sensitive detection for chemicals that contain electronegative groups. This includes chemicals that contain halogen atoms (I, Br, Cl, and F) or nitro groups ($-NO_2$). It also includes chemicals that are polynuclear aromatic hydrocarbons, anhydrides, or conjugated carbonyl compounds, along with many among others. Derivatization with reagents containing polychlorinated or polyfluorinated groups can be used with some chemicals to also allow them to be monitored with an ECD.

Argon and nitrogen are usually employed as the carrier gases for a GC system with an ECD because their relatively large size makes it easy for them to collide with beta particles and produce secondary electrons. Some methane is also usually combined with these carrier gases to produce a steady stream of secondary electrons and provide a stable detector response. It is important that these gases be pure and dry because the presence of oxygen and water can foul this type of detector. Because an ECD uses a radioactive source, this source needs to be replaced on a regular basis by a certified technician.

Mass Spectrometry. Mass spectrometers are also used as detectors for GC. This combination is known as gas chromatography/mass spectrometry (GC/MS).[12] GC/MS is a powerful method for identifying analytes and quantifying them as they elute from a GC column. Ionization methods that are often used in GC/MS include electron impact ionization and chemical ionization, which are both discussed in Chapter 17. Some mass analyzers that are commonly used in GC/MS are quadrupole mass analyzers and ion traps (see Chapter 17), although other types of mass analyzers can be used as well.

In the full-scan mode of GC/MS, information is acquired by the MS system on a wide range of ions. This mode is used when the goal is to detect many compounds in a single run or provide data that can be used to identity an unknown compound from its mass spectrum. In this mode, the mass spectrometer acts as a general detector for the GC system. GC/MS also can monitor specific analytes by using selected ion monitoring (SIM). This mode uses the mass spectrometer to monitor only a few ions that are representative of the analytes of interest. SIM is used when selective detection and low detection limits are desired, but does require that information be available in advance on the types of ions that will be generated from the analytes.

The response of a GC/MS system can be represented in several ways. For instance, in the full-scan mode a plot can be made of the number of ions measured at each elution time. This type of graph is known as a mass chromatogram, or total ion chromatogram, and can be used to show the overall response of the system to the eluting analytes. It is also possible in the full-scan mode to use all of the collected data to show the mass spectrum that is acquired at a given elution time. This plot can be used to help identify a compound that is eluting at that time from the GC/MS system. Finally, a plot can be made of the number of ions that are detected at only specific mass-to-charge ratios as a function of the elution time. This last plot is called a selected ion chromatogram and is used in the SIM mode or the full-scan mode when looking for specific compounds that may be eluting from the GC/MS system.

Other Gas Chromatography Detectors. A variety of other detectors can be part of a GC system. One example is the TCD. A TCD is a general detector that can monitor both inorganic and organic compounds. It detects and measures these compounds based on their ability to change how the carrier gas/analyte mixture will conduct heat away from a hot wire filament (ie, a property referred to as thermal conductivity).[12,21,22] The carrier gas used with a TCD is often helium or hydrogen, which have the greatest differences in their thermal conductivities from most organic or inorganic compounds. However, nitrogen or other carrier gases also can be used with a TCD.

The primary advantage of a TCD is its ability to detect many types of chemicals, as long as they are present at sufficient quantities to be detected. This detector is nondestructive and can be easily combined with a second detector. However, a TCD also can respond to contaminants in the carrier gas and can give a change in the background response during temperature programming. In addition, the TCD tends to have much higher detection limits than other common GC detectors.

Another group of GC detectors make use of the interactions of chemicals with light. One example is the PID.[12,21] The PID is similar in design and operation to an FID in that both use electrodes to detect and measure ions produced from chemicals eluting from the column. However, in the PID these ions are produced through interaction of the eluting chemicals with ultraviolet (UV) radiation rather than through the use of a flame. Another GC detector that makes use of light is a flame photometric detector (FPD).[12] An FPD is a selective detector for phosphorus- or sulfur-containing compounds. Like an FID, an FPD passes the eluting chemicals into a flame, but with the FPD measuring the release of light from excited-state phosphorus- or sulfur-containing species rather than the production of ions. It is also possible to combine GC with infrared (IR) spectroscopy, giving a method known as gas chromatography/infrared spectroscopy (GC/IR).[12] This combination can be used for both chemical measurement and identification by looking at the absorption of IR radiation by chemicals as they elute from a GC column.

Data Acquisition and System Control

As with most modern analytical instruments, computers are used to both control and automate GC systems, as well as collect and process data from these systems. With regard to system control, the computer can regulate parameters such as (1) the carrier gas composition and flow rate; (2) the column back pressure; (3) the column and detector temperatures, including temperature programming; (4) the sample injection process; (5) detector selection and operation; and (6) the timing steps that are used during system operation and a chemical analysis.

In terms of data acquisition and processing, the computer can monitor the signals generated by the GC system's detectors, including the acquisition and storage of data at specified time intervals. From this information, the area or height of each chromatographic peak can be measured, and this information can be used to determine the analyte concentration represented by each peak. Algorithms are available for this process in modern GC systems that allow for the generation of calibration curves or conversion factors based on either internal or external calibration methods. The computer system also can be used to search databases to aid in identification of analytes based on their retention times or response at the detector (eg, their mass spectra).[21,29] If desired, the data acquisition system can then be used to generate a report on the results for each chromatographic run. Alternatively, these data can be stored for later examination or reprocessing.

Laboratory Safety in Gas Chromatography

Standard safety precautions should be followed when placing and securing the gas cylinder or mobile phase source that is used for GC. If hydrogen is used as the carrier gas, extra precautions should be taken in training laboratory personnel in the handling and use of this flammable and potentially explosive gas. Proper ventilation facilities should be available in the work area to deal with carrier gas that has passed through the GC system. All samples, reagents, and solutions that are used during a GC analysis should also be handled and stored using appropriate laboratory procedures (see Chapter 12).

LIQUID CHROMATOGRAPHY

LC is a type of chromatography in which the mobile phase is a liquid. Separations in LC are based on the distribution of chemicals between a liquid mobile phase and a stationary phase.[9] This was the type of chromatography used by Tswett when he first began to practice column chromatography in 1903. Although LC was mainly a preparative tool until the 1960s, it is now the dominant type of chromatography used for chemical analysis in clinical or biomedical laboratories. A key advantage of this method over GC is the ability of LC to work directly with liquid samples, such as those encountered with clinical or biological specimens.

Before the mid-1960s, the supports used in LC columns were based on large and irregularly shaped particulate supports such as those used in packed columns for GC. These supports were useful in preparative work but were not suitable for many analytical applications because they tended to result in broad peaks and separations with low resolution. In addition, these supports generally had limited mechanical stability and could be used only at relatively low operating pressures.

Developments began to occur in the 1960s to produce smaller, more mechanically stable and more efficient supports for LC, along with the instrumentation that could be used with such materials.[30] This resulted in a method that is now known as HPLC.[10,30-32] The use of these more efficient supports made it possible to obtain narrower peaks, better separations, and lower limits of detection in LC. These reasons, along with the ability of HPLC to be used as an automated method, have made this technique the method of choice for most routine chemical separations and analysis methods in modern laboratories, including those in a clinical setting. Other advantages of HPLC and LC include the wide range of separation mechanisms, stationary phases, solvents, and detectors that can be employed in such methods.

In HPLC, particulate supports with relatively small diameters are often used to hold the stationary phase within the column. Because the pressure drop across a packed bed column is related to the square of a support particle's diameter, relatively high pressures can be required to pump liquids through HPLC columns with even moderate lengths. As a result, this technique has also been referred to as high-pressure liquid chromatography, although HPLC is the preferred name. Most modern HPLC systems can work at pressures up to 5000 to 6000 psi. Specialized systems that can operate at even higher pressures have recently been developed for a method known as ultra-high-performance liquid chromatography or ultra-high-pressure liquid chromatography."[33-36]

One important difference between LC and GC is that the retention of chemicals in LC can depend on the interactions of these chemicals with both the mobile phase and stationary phase. This means the composition and nature of the mobile phase are important to consider when adjusting the retention of a chemical in an LC system. The term strong mobile phase is used to describe a mobile phase that leads to weak retention for an analyte on a given type of stationary phase. The weakest retention for a chemical will occur when this substance favors staying in the mobile phase instead of the stationary phase. The term weak mobile phase refers to the opposite situation in which a chemical favors the stationary phase versus the mobile phase and has its highest retention within a given column.[2]

POINTS TO REMEMBER

Mobile Phase Strength in Liquid Chromatography

- The mobile phase is important in LC in determining chemical retention.
- A strong mobile phase is a mobile phase that leads to weak retention for an analyte on a given type of stationary phase and column.
- A weak mobile phase is a mobile phase in which a chemical favors the stationary phase and has its highest retention within a given column.

Types of Liquid Chromatography

Liquid chromatographic methods are classified according to the chemical or physical mechanisms by which they separate chemicals (Fig. 16.11). The five main types of LC based on the separation mechanism are (1) adsorption chromatography, (2) partition chromatography, (3) IEC, (4) size-exclusion chromatography (SEC), and (5) affinity chromatography.[2,7] Most clinical applications use LC separations that are based on partition chromatography or IEC; however, the other types of LC also have valuable clinical applications.

Adsorption Chromatography

Adsorption chromatography is a type of LC in which chemicals are retained based on their adsorption and desorption at the surface of the support, which also acts as the stationary phase (see Fig. 16.11). This method is also sometimes referred to as liquid-solid chromatography.[10] Retention in this method

Adsorption chromatography
Separation based on adsorption of chemicals to the surface of a support

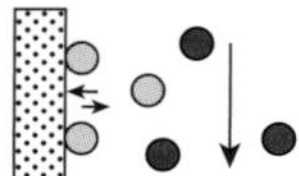

Partition chromatography
Separation based on partitioning of chemicals into a layer of the stationary phase

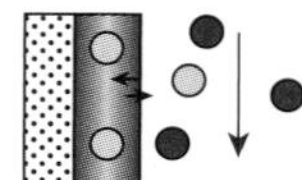

Ion-exchange chromatography
Separation of ions based on their binding to fixed charges on a support

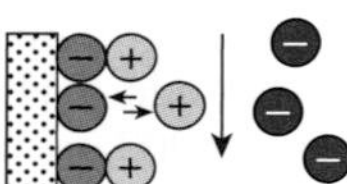

Size-exclusion chromatography
Separation of chemicals based on their size and ability to enter a porous support

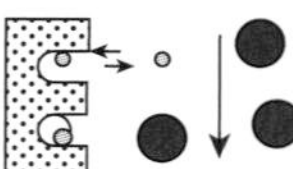

Affinity chromatography
Separation of chemicals based on their interactions with a biologically related binding agent

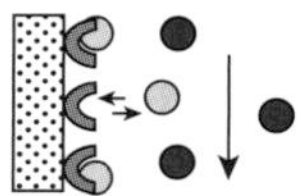

FIGURE 16.11 Main types of liquid chromatography based on their separation mechanisms.

is based on the competition of the analyte with molecules of the mobile phase as both bind to the surface of the support. The degree of a chemical's retention in adsorption chromatography will depend on (1) the binding strength of this chemical to the support, (2) the surface area of the support, (3) the amount of mobile phase displaced from the support by the chemical, and (4) the binding strength of the mobile phase to the support.[12] Electrostatic interactions, hydrogen bonding, dipole-dipole interactions, and dispersive interactions (ie, van der Waals forces) all may affect retention in this type of chromatography.[37,38]

The binding strength of the mobile phase with the support in adsorption chromatography is described by the mobile phase's elutropic strength.[10,12,39] A liquid or solution that has a large elutropic strength for a given support will act as a strong mobile phase for that material because this mobile phase will tend to bind tightly to the support and cause the analyte to elute more quickly as it spends more time in the mobile phase. As an example, a relatively polar solvent such as methanol will have a higher elutropic strength for a polar support such as silica than a nonpolar solvent such as carbon tetrachloride. In the same manner, a liquid or solution that has a low elutropic strength for a support would represent a weak mobile phase for that support in adsorption chromatography (eg, carbon tetrachloride on silica).

Three types of adsorbents are generally used in adsorption chromatography: (1) polar acidic supports, (2) polar basic supports, and (3) nonpolar supports. The most common polar and acidic support used in adsorption chromatography is silica. The surface silanol groups on this support tend to adsorb polar compounds and work particularly well for basic substances. Alumina is the main type of polar and basic adsorbent that is used in adsorption chromatography. Like silica, alumina retains polar compounds, but alumina works especially well for polar acidic substances. Florisil is an alternative polar and basic support that can be used in place of alumina, such as when catalytic decomposition of an analyte is observed with this latter material. Other types of supports that can be used in adsorption chromatography are nonpolar adsorbents such as charcoal and polystyrene.

Partition Chromatography

The second major type of LC based on the separation mechanism is partition chromatography. Partition chromatography is an LC method in which solutes are separated based on their partitioning between a liquid mobile phase and a stationary phase that is coated or bonded onto a solid support (see Fig. 16.11).[40-42] The support in most types of partition chromatography is silica, although other types of supports also can be employed. This method originally involved coatings of liquid stationary phases that were immiscible with the desired mobile phase. However, most current columns used in partition chromatography employ stationary phases that are bonded to the support. These bonded phases are more stable than the coated layers of stationary phases that were initially used in partition chromatography and provide better column efficiencies.

The two main types of partition chromatography based on the polarity of the stationary phase are normal-phase chromatography and reversed-phase chromatography.[7,10,12,39] Normal-phase chromatography is a type of partition chromatography in which a polar stationary phase is used.[7,10,43] This is the first type of partition chromatography that was developed, and it is also known as normal-phase liquid chromatography. The stationary phase in this method typically contains groups that can form hydrogen bonds or undergo dipole-related interactions. Examples of bonded stationary phases for normal-phase chromatography are those that contain aminopropyl groups, cyano groups, and diol groups. Because this method has a polar stationary phase, it will have its highest retention for polar compounds. A weak mobile phase in this method will be a nonpolar liquid. A strong mobile phase in normal-phase chromatography is a polar liquid, such as methanol or water.

Normal-phase chromatography can be used in many of the same applications as separations in adsorption chromatography that use silica or alumina supports. These applications usually involve the separation or analysis of chemicals that are present in organic solvents and of substances that contain one or more polar functional groups. Examples of chemicals that are of clinical interest and for which normal-phase chromatography has been used include steroids and sugars.[12,31,32,44]

The second major type of partition chromatography is reversed-phase chromatography, which is also known as reversed-phase liquid chromatography. Reversed-phase chromatography is a type of partition chromatography that uses a nonpolar stationary phase.[7,10] It is the most popular type of liquid chromatography and the most common type found in clinical laboratories.[12,31,32,45] One reason for this is that the weak mobile phase in reversed-phase chromatography is a polar solvent, such as water. This property makes this type of LC convenient for the analysis and separation of chemicals in aqueous-based systems, such as serum, urine, and blood.[12,31,32,39] A strong mobile phase in this method is a liquid that is less polar than water, such as acetonitrile or methanol. Because of the presence of a nonpolar stationary phase, nonpolar compounds will have the highest retention in reversed-phase chromatography.

Reversed-phase chromatography has many applications in the areas of clinical chemistry and biomedical research. Examples of chemicals that have been separated or analyzed by this method include drugs, drug metabolites, amino acids, peptides, proteins, carbohydrates, lipids, and bile acids. A separation of antidepressant drugs by reversed-phase chromatography was shown earlier in Fig. 16.2. Compounds representing the greatest challenge for reversed-phase separations are highly polar compounds such as sugars or amino acids, which tend to be weakly retained by reversed-phase columns, and basic compounds, which may exhibit peak tailing as the result of their interactions with silica. Derivatization of some compounds (eg, amino acids) has been employed to improve their retention on reversed-phase columns.[3] It is also important to consider both the type of analyte and support that are being used in these separations. For instance, large chemicals such as peptides or proteins will require reversed-phase supports with larger pore sizes than those routinely used for the separation of small molecules.[46-48]

A relatively wide range of stationary phases and supports are available for reversed-phase separations.[6,49-51] The most common stationary phases used in reversed-phase chromatography are those based on octadecyl (C_{18}), octyl (C_8), phenyl, or butyl (C_4) groups that are attached to a support such as silica. Similar materials are commonly used in solid-phase extraction (see Chapter 18). The retention characteristics of these silica-based columns will depend on (1) the nature of bonded phase, (2) the amount of the bonded phase (often expressed as the percent of carbon load), (3) the surface area of the support, (4) the pore size of the support, and (5) the quantity of accessible groups on the support (eg, silanol groups on silica) that can be used to prepare the bonded phase. Alternative reversed-phase materials such as porous graphite, fluorinated hydrocarbons, and hydrophobic stationary phases with embedded polar groups offer different selectivities than C_{18}- or C_8-silica. Silica tends to dissolve slowly at a pH greater than 8.0 or at a pH below 2.0, so separations that make use of silica supports are usually done in this pH range unless the silica has been stabilized by surface treatment.[49] Some of the other supports that are available for reversed-phase chromatography, such as polystyrene or porous graphite, are stable over a broader pH range (eg, pH 2.0 to 13.0).

During the bonding of a reversed-phase stationary phase to silica it usually is not possible to cover all of the available silanol groups. These remaining silanol groups may interact with some analytes and lead to mixed-mode interactions that produce broad peaks and result in a decrease in peak resolution. For instance, the peak tailing that may occur for some basic compounds on silica is caused by coulombic interactions of these compounds with the conjugate base form of silanol groups. These interactions can be minimized by reacting many of the silanol groups with a small organosilane such as trimethylchlorosilane in a method known as endcapping.[10] In addition, the pH of the mobile phase can be lowered to decrease the amount of silanol groups that are present in their charged form. Additives such as trifluoroacetic acid or triethylamine can be added to the mobile phase to minimize interactions of the silanol groups with analytes.[12,39,44]

The strength of a mobile phase in both normal-phase chromatography and reversed-phase chromatography can be described by using the solvent polarity index. A weak mobile phase for normal-phase chromatography will be a solvent or solvent mixture that has a low value for the solvent polarity index, whereas a strong mobile phase in this method would be one with a high solvent polarity index. The opposite trend occurs in reversed-phase chromatography, in which a weak mobile phase will have a high solvent polarity index, and a strong mobile phase will have a low solvent polarity index. Some large aliphatic stationary phases in reversed-phase chromatography, such as C_{18}-silica, may undergo phase collapse if they are used in only an aqueous mobile phase; this process probably represents the folding of the aliphatic groups down onto the surface to decrease their exposure to water. This effect can be minimized by including a small amount of organic modifier in the mobile phase or by using a bonded phase with a shorter chain length.

Samples are usually applied or injected onto a reversed-phase column in the presence of an aqueous solution or water that contains a low concentration of an organic solvent such as methanol or acetonitrile. The partitioning of chemicals that are weak acids or weak bases can be adjusted in reversed-phase chromatography by changing the pH to minimize the charge of these solutes. Because most acid-base reactions are fast, this situation will usually result in only one observed peak with a retention time that is the weighted average of what would be seen for the acid or base forms of the compound. The same type of effect and shifts in retention can occur for chemicals that undergo other rapid reactions, such as complex formation with mobile phase additives.[12] The mobile phase strength in normal-phase chromatography and reversed-phase chromatography is often changed by using mixtures of solvents or solutions and gradients in which the proportions of solvents or solutions are changed during an analysis (see Fig. 16.12).[52] It is also possible to modify the polarity of aqueous solutions in reversed-phase chromatography by changing the salt concentration of the mobile phase.

This last approach is employed in a variation of reversed-phase chromatography that is known as hydrophobic interaction chromatography (HIC).[12] This method is applied mainly in the separation of large biomolecules such as proteins. HIC

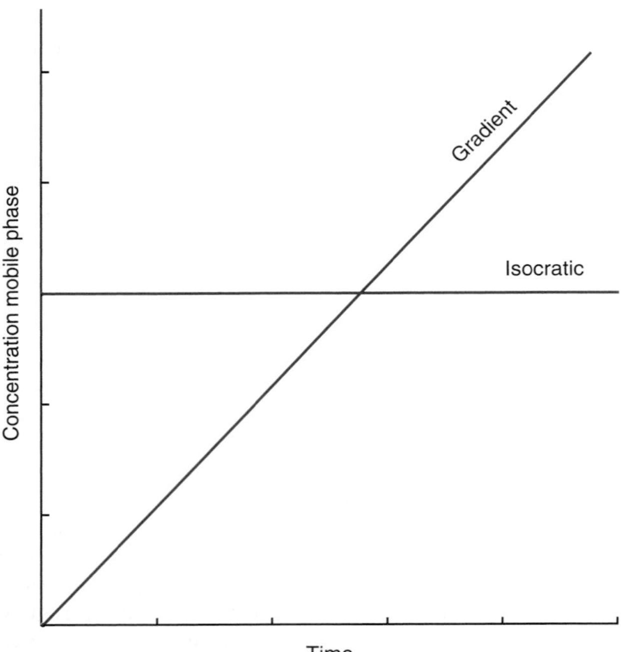

FIGURE 16.12 Examples of isocratic elution (ie, constant mobile phase composition) or gradient elution based on solvent programming (ie, varying mobile phase composition).

makes use of a weakly hydrophobic stationary phase that is made up of small nonpolar groups such as phenyl or butyl residues. The weak mobile phase that is used with this type of column, and which promotes the binding of proteins or related biomolecules to the stationary phase, is an aqueous solution that contains a high salt concentration. The retained biomolecules are eluted by using a strong mobile phase that is less polar, which in this case is an aqueous solution that has a lower salt concentration.

Ion-Exchange Chromatography

The third type of liquid chromatography is IEC. IEC is a type of liquid chromatography in which ions are separated by their adsorption onto a support that contains fixed charges on its surface.[7,10] This method relies on the interaction (or exchange) of ions in the sample or mobile phase with fixed ionic groups of the opposite charge that are bound to the support and act as the stationary phase (see Fig. 16.11). Depending on the charge of the groups that make up the stationary phase, the types of ions that bind to the column may be either cations (ie, positively charged ions) or anions (ie, negatively charged ions). These two methods are referred to as cation-exchange chromatography and anion-exchange chromatography, respectively.[12]

Supports for cation-exchange chromatography contain negatively charged functional groups. These groups may be the conjugate bases of strong acids, such as sulfonate ions that are formed by the deprotonation of sulfonic acid, or the conjugate bases of weak acids, such as those produced from carboxyl or carboxymethyl groups. The supports used in anion-exchange chromatography are usually the conjugate acids of strongly basic quaternary amines, such as triethylaminoethyl groups, or the conjugate acids of weak bases, such as aminoethyl or diethylaminoethyl groups. Supports that can be modified to contain these charged groups for use in IEC include silica and polystyrene, as well as carbohydrate-based materials such as agarose, dextran, or cellulose.[10,12,44] The carbohydrate-based supports are particularly useful in preparative work with biological agents, which can have strong binding to materials such as underivatized silica or polystyrene. The large pore size of supports such as agarose also makes these materials valuable in separations involving biological macromolecules such as proteins and nucleic acids.[10,12,44]

A strong mobile phase in IEC is usually a mobile phase that contains a high concentration of competing ions. The presence of these competing ions will make it more difficult for a charged analyte to bind to the fixed charges that act as the stationary phase. A weak mobile phase in IEC is one that contains few or no competing ions or that otherwise promotes binding by charged analytes to the column. Changing the competing ion concentration is the most common approach for adjusting the retention of analyte ions in IEC. The retention of ions in this method also may be affected by (1) pH, (2) the type of competing ion used, (3) the type of fixed charges used as the stationary phase, and (4) the density of these fixed charges on the support. Many stationary phases in IEC can exhibit mixed-mode retention through a combination of coulombic interactions and adsorption. As an example, ion-exchange resins that are used for amino acid analysis are able to separate amino acids with virtually the same charge because of differences in the adsorption of these amino acids onto the stationary phase.

IEC has a number of clinical applications. Common examples are the use of this method in the separation and analysis of amino acids and hemoglobin variants. IEC is also frequently used as a preparative tool in biomedical research for purifying proteins, peptides, and nucleotides. A modified form of IEC, known as ion chromatography, can be used with a conductivity detector to analyze small inorganic and organic ions.[12] The water purification systems that are used in many laboratories are another important application of IEC. In these purification systems, supports containing a mixture of cation- and anion-exchange groups are used to remove anions and cations from water, in which hydrogen ions are exchanged for other cations and hydroxide ions are exchanged for other anions. Most of these hydrogen ions and hydroxide ions then combine to form deionized water.[2]

Size-Exclusion Chromatography

SEC is an LC technique that separates molecules or other particles based on size (Figs. 16.11 and 16.13).[2,12,44] In this method, a porous support is used that has an inert surface and few or no interactions with the injected sample components. This support also should have a range of pore sizes that approach, or are similar to, the sizes of the compounds that are to be separated. As a sample travels through a column that contains this support, small components of the sample can enter all or most of the pores and larger components may enter only a few or none of the pores. The result is a separation based on size or molar mass, in which the larger components elute first from the column.

In SEC, all of the injected components will elute in a fairly narrow volume range. This range extends from the volume of mobile phase that is outside of all the pores of the support

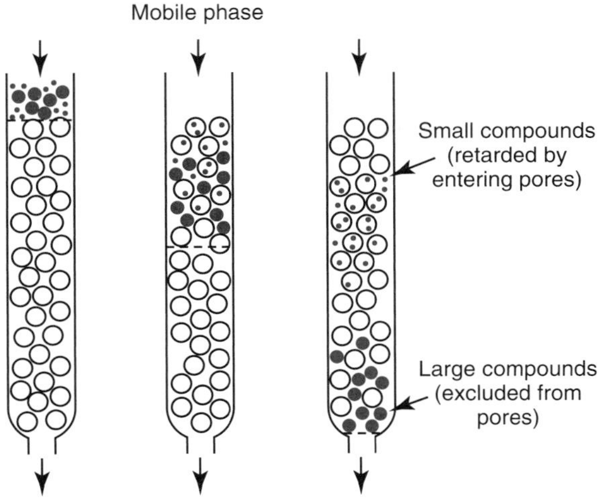

FIGURE 16.13 General principle of size-exclusion chromatography. This method separates compounds based on their size and by using a column that contains a porous support. (Modified from Bennett TP. *Graphic biochemistry, vol 1: chemistry of biological molecules.* New York: Macmillan; 1968.)

(also known as the excluded volume, V_E) to the total amount of mobile phase in the column, as represented by the void volume (V_M). The stationary phase in SEC can be thought of as the volume of the mobile phase in the pores of the support that can be entered by a given solute. The extent of retention in this method can be described by using the measured t_R or retention volume V_R for an injected component or by using the ratio K_o, which is calculated by using the following equation[44]:

$$K_o = \frac{(V_R - V_E)}{(V_M - V_E)}$$

The value of K_o represents the fraction of the volume between V_M and V_E in which a given sample component elutes. Small components will have a value for K_o that is equal to or approaches 1, whereas large components will have a K_o value that is equal to or approaches 0. Components with intermediate sizes will have values for K_o between 0 and 1.

Many types of porous supports have been used in SEC. Cross-linked carbohydrate-based supports such as dextran and agarose are often used in this method for work with aqueous-based samples and biological compounds such as proteins or nucleic acids. Polyacrylamide gel and silica or glass beads that have been modified into a diol-bonded form also can be used for aqueous samples and biological compounds. Polystyrene is usually employed as the support when SEC is to be used with synthetic polymers and samples that are present in organic solvents.[12,31,44] For each of these supports, the range of pore sizes that are present will determine the range of sizes for the injected compounds that can be separated. In the case of carbohydrate-based supports and polymeric supports, this range will become smaller as the degree of cross-linking of the support is increased.

The mobile phase in SEC can be a polar solvent, such as water, or a nonpolar solvent, which is usually tetrahydrofuran. Because the stationary phase is based on a physical difference in the accessible pore volume for the solutes, rather than on chemical interactions, there is no weak mobile phase or strong mobile phase in this method. The choice of the mobile phase is instead determined by the solubility of the desired analytes and the stability of the support and the column. If water or an aqueous mobile phase is used in SEC (which typically involves a carbohydrate-based support, polyacrylamide or diol-bonded silica or glass), the resulting method is often called gel filtration chromatography. If an organic mobile phase is used (which generally involves the use of polystyrene as the support), the size-exclusion method is referred to as gel permeation chromatography.[10] Other names that are sometimes used for SEC are steric exclusion, molecular exclusion, and molecular sieve chromatography.

SEC in the gel filtration mode allows the separation of molecules under physiologic salt conditions. This feature is useful for identifying intact complexes of agents such as lipoproteins, antibody-antigen complexes, and the binding of proteins with their target compounds. SEC is often used as a rapid preparative technique to exchange buffers or to remove salts from large sample components. In addition, this method can be used to remove small molecules from large biomolecules, such as in the isolation of drugs, fatty acids, and peptides from proteins.

SEC also can be used to estimate the molecular weight of a biomolecule, such as a protein or nucleic acid, or to characterize the distribution of molecular weights for a polymer. This is done by first calibrating the size-exclusion column with compounds that are similar to the desired analytes in structure but that have known molecular weights.[53] A calibration curve can be made by plotting the logarithm of the molecular weight versus the measured retention time, retention volume, or calculated value of K_o for each standard compound. This plot is then used to determine the molecular weight of the unknown compounds based on their measured retention on the same column. This approach can be used to provide a good estimate of the molecular weight; however, it is a relatively low-resolution technique that does require substantial differences in molecular weight to create significant shifts in retention. For example, the diameters of globular proteins change in proportion to the cube root of their molecular weights, so roughly an eightfold difference in molecular weight is required to yield a twofold change in diameter.[53] Linear polymers, such as DNA and proteins that have been denatured and treated with sodium dodecyl sulfate or guanidine hydrochloride, have a much larger diameter for the same molecular weight, and their diameter changes approximately in proportion to the square root of molecular weight. This latter effect allows for smaller differences in molecular weight to be observed by SEC for linear molecules compared to globular molecules (eg, nondenatured globular proteins).

Affinity Chromatography and Chiral Separations

The fifth main type of LC is affinity chromatography. Affinity chromatography is an LC method that makes use of biologically related interactions for the retention and separation of chemicals (see Figs. 16.11 and 16.14).[7,10,54-56] This method uses the selective, reversible interactions found in many biological

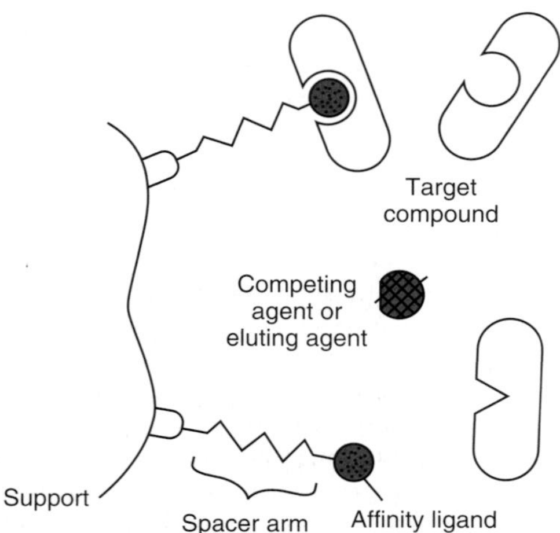

FIGURE 16.14 General mechanism of separation in affinity chromatography. The target analyte is first allowed to bind to the immobilized affinity ligand in the column. After the nonretained sample components have been washed from the column, the retained analyte is later released by using an elution buffer. This elution may be based on a nonspecific method (eg, the addition of a chaotropic agent or a change in pH), or it may be accomplished by adding a biospecific competing agent to the mobile phase to displace the analyte from the column.

systems, such as the binding of an antibody with an antigen, the interactions of an enzyme with a substrate or inhibitor, the binding of a hormone with a receptor, and the interactions of a lectin with a carbohydrate. These selective interactions are used in affinity chromatography by immobilizing one of a pair of interacting compounds onto a support for use as the stationary phase. This immobilized binding agent is called the affinity ligand,[55] and it is used to create a column that can selectively bind and capture the complementary compound from applied samples.

The stationary phase for affinity chromatography is usually prepared by covalently immobilizing the affinity ligand to the support.[55] This is often done through the reaction of amine, sulfhydryl, carboxyl, or carbonyl groups on the affinity ligand with activated sites on the support, although other types of groups can be employed. During this process, the orientation of the affinity ligand and its accessibility to its target compound are both important to consider in providing good activity for the binding agent. Use of a spacer between the surface of the support and the affinity ligand also may be needed with smaller binding agents. Besides covalent immobilization, it is also sometimes possible to adsorb the affinity ligand to the support. This can be done in a general manner, such as through polar or ionic interactions; it also can be done through biospecific adsorption to a secondary binding agent. Examples of this latter approach include the biospecific adsorption of antibodies to an immobilized immunoglobulin-binding protein such as protein A or protein G, and the biospecific adsorption of biotin-labeled agents to immobilized avidin or strepavidin.[55] Another alternative approach for preparing affinity ligands is to form a molecularly imprinted polymer in the presence of the desired target or a target analog.[55,57] In this case, the shape and structure of the binding pockets that remain in the polymer after release of the target template can be used to selectively bind to the same or similar targets from samples.

Affinity chromatography is usually carried out by applying a sample to the column under conditions that allow strong and specific binding of the affinity ligand to its target compound.[55] This is done in the presence of a mobile phase solution, known as the application buffer, which mimics the pH and natural or preferred conditions for binding between the affinity ligand and the target. As the target binds to the column under these conditions, most other sample components are washed away as a result of the selective nature of this interaction. The retained target is then later released from the column by using an elution buffer that either contains a competing agent that will displace the target from the affinity ligand (a method known as biospecific elution) or uses a change in conditions such as pH, ionic strength, or polarity of the mobile phase to decrease the strength of binding between the target and affinity ligand (a technique called nonspecific elution). After the target has been eluted for detection or further use, the application buffer can be passed again through the column and the system is allowed to regenerate before application of the next sample. For systems with weak to moderate binding strengths, it is also possible to use isocratic elution for both sample application and target elution. This second type of elution is usually employed in chiral separations and in a method known as weak affinity chromatography.[55,58]

Various supports can be used in affinity chromatography. For preparative work, it is most common to use carbohydrate-based materials such as cross-linked agarose and various modified forms of cellulose. Silica and glass also have been used as supports for both preparative and analytical applications of affinity chromatography. This first requires that these supports be modified to give them low nonspecific binding for biological molecules and to provide groups that can be used for the immobilization of affinity ligands. In addition, several polymeric materials have been used in this method, ranging from hydroxylated polystyrene to azlactone beads, agarose-acrylamide or dextran-acrylamide copolymers, and derivatives of polyacrylamide or polymethacrylate.[55,59]

The power of affinity chromatography lies in its selectivity and in the wide range of binding agents that can be used in this method. This has led to many applications for this type of LC in work with biological compounds. Bioaffinity chromatography (or biospecific adsorption) is the most common type of affinity chromatography and involves the use of a biological binding agent as the affinity ligand.[55,59] The purification of an enzyme by using an immobilized inhibitor, coenzyme, substrate, or cofactor is an example of this approach.[55,60,61] Another example is the use of affinity ligands that are lectins or nonimmune system proteins that can bind certain types of carbohydrate residues.[55] Lectins such as concanavalin A (Con A, which binds to α-D-mannose and α-D-glucose residues) and wheat germ agglutinin (which binds to D-*N*-acetylglucosamines) have been popular in recent years for the isolation of carbohydrate-containing compounds, such as glycopeptides, glycoproteins, and glycolipids. This method is sometimes referred to as lectin affinity chromatography.[55] Another set of binding agents that are used in bioaffinity chromatography are immunoglobulin-binding proteins, such as protein A (from *Staphylococcus aureus*) and protein G (from group G streptococci), which have been used for antibody purification and as secondary ligands for the biospecific adsorption of antibodies.[55]

Immunoaffinity chromatography (IAC) is a subset of bioaffinity chromatography that uses an antibody or antibody-related agent as the affinity ligand. The selectivity of this method has made it popular for the isolation of targets that have ranged from antibodies, hormones, and recombinant proteins to receptors, viruses, and cellular components. This method also can be used to detect specific target compounds directly or indirectly in a set of techniques known as chromatographic immunoassays (or flow-injection immunoanalysis).[55,62] Another important application of IAC is as a tool for target isolation and sample pretreatment before analysis by other methods. The use of IAC to isolate a specific target from a sample is known as immunoextraction, which can be combined either off-line or online with other analytical methods.[55,63] A related technique is immunodepletion, which is used to remove certain compounds from a sample before analysis of the remaining sample components. This last approach has been used in proteomics to remove high-abundance proteins from biological samples before the measurement and detection of lower abundance proteins in the same samples.[63]

Another group of methods in affinity chromatography are those that use nonbiological binding agents. Dye-ligand affinity chromatography uses an affinity ligand that is a synthetic dye such as Cibacron Blue 3GA, Procion Red HE-3B, or Procion Yellow H-A. This method is commonly used for the large- and small-scale purification of enzymes and proteins, including many protein-based biopharmaceuticals.[55,64] Dye-ligand affinity chromatography is a type of biomimetic affinity chromatography that uses an affinity ligand that is a mimic of a natural compound. Besides synthetic dyes, other binding agents that are used in this method are those generated by combinatorial chemistry and computer modeling or that are derived from peptide libraries, phage display libraries, aptamer libraries, and ribosome display libraries.[55]

Two other types of affinity chromatography that use nonbiological binding agents are immobilized metal-ion affinity chromatography (IMAC) and boronate affinity chromatography. In IMAC, the affinity ligand is a metal ion that is complexed with an immobilized chelating agent, such as Ni^{2+} complexed to a support containing iminodiacetic acid.[55] This technique is frequently used to isolate recombinant histidine-tagged proteins and has been used for the isolation or analysis of phosphorylated proteins in proteomics.[55] Boronate affinity chromatography uses an affinity ligand that is boronic acid or a related derivative. These affinity ligands are able to form covalent bonds with compounds that contain *cis*-diol groups; this feature makes these binding agents useful in the purification and analysis of polysaccharides, glycoproteins, ribonucleic acids, and catecholamines.[55,65] An important clinical application of boronate affinity chromatography is its use in the analysis and isolation of glycosylated hemoglobin in blood samples from diabetic patients.[66,67]

Many biological molecules occur as specific stereoisomers. Examples are amino acids, peptides, and proteins. As a result, it is not unusual for the different chiral forms of a drug to have some variations in their interactions with these biological agents. This, in turn, can lead to differences in the activity and toxicity of these drugs in the body.[68-70] In some cases only a particular stereoisomer of a drug may be active. In the absence of any chiral binding agent, the two mirror-image forms of a drug (or enantiomers) will have identical physical and chemical properties. These forms will not be separated in most types of chromatography, which generally use non-stereoselective (or achiral) stationary phases. However, it may be possible to separate the enantiomers and stereoisomers of a drug or target compound if the stationary phase is also chiral and can interact with these compounds in a stereospecific manner. This type of medium is known as a chiral stationary phase (CSP).[55,68,69]

The use of a CSP can be viewed as a subset of affinity chromatography, in that the resulting separation makes use of a biologically related binding agent or a mimic of such an agent.[55,71-73] For instance, carbohydrates, peptides, and proteins (including some enzymes and serum transport proteins) have all been used as CSPs because they are composed of chiral amino acids and sugars.[55,68] Cyclodextrins, which are cyclic polymers of glucose, are an important set of carbohydrates that have been used for separating many types of chiral compounds in both LC and GC.[68,69] CSPs also can be based on synthetic binding agents or molecularly imprinted polymers.[12,55,68-70] It is further possible in LC to carry out a chiral separation with an achiral column, such as a reversed-phase support, by placing a chiral binding agent such as a cyclodextrin in the mobile phase. In this last case, the separate forms of a chiral drug or compound may have different interactions with this mobile phase additive, which then leads to differences in their observed retention on the column.[68,69]

Hydrophilic Interaction Liquid Chromotography and Mixed-Mode Methods

Besides the traditional categories of LC, there are other methods that combine several separation modes. One example is hydrophilic interaction liquid chromatography (HILIC). HILIC is a type of partition chromatography that uses a polar stationary phase and in which chemicals partition between an organic-rich region in the mobile phase and a more polar water-enriched layer that is at or near the surface of a polar support. The surface of the support, which can often undergo hydrogen bonding or dipole-related interactions with the applied solutes, also may have charged groups that can take part in ionic interactions with these compounds while they are in the water-enriched layer.[74-76] These features make HILIC a variation of normal-phase chromatography that is combined with some of the retention characteristics of reversed-phase chromatography and IEC.

Several types of supports can be used in HILIC. The conventional form of HILIC uses a polar but noncharged surface, such as is present on unmodified silica. Other neutral groups that may be present on the supports for HILIC are amide, diol, or cyano groups. One variation of this method is the technique of electrostatic repulsion hydrophilic interaction liquid chromatography (ERLIC, or eHILIC), in which charged groups such as protonated amines or deprotonated carboxylic acids are present on the support and used to repel injected compounds with the same charge. Another form of HILIC is zwitterionic hydrophilic interaction liquid chromatography (ZIC-HILIC), in which zwitterionic groups are present on the support; these groups can interact with analytes that have a positive charge or negative charge or that are also zwitterions.[74-76]

HILIC and related methods have become popular in areas such as proteomics and glycomics. Advantages of these methods include (1) their ability to give better separations for polar compounds than can be obtained by reversed-phase chromatography, (2) the greater ease with which they can be used with aqueous samples and in solubilizing polar compounds compared to normal-phase chromatography, and (3) the ability to couple these methods with mass spectrometry. A possible limitation of HILIC for use in clinical laboratories is that biological fluids are highly polar and include a substantial quantity of salts that also can interact with polar stationary phases. Therefore, these specimens may need to be extracted or modified by the addition of a less polar solvent such as acetonitrile to promote compound interactions in HILIC.

Ion-pair chromatography (IPC) is another example of a mixed-mode LC method.[12] This technique combines columns that are used in reversed-phase chromatography with the ability to separate ionic compounds based on their charges, as is done in IEC. This method is carried out by adding an ion-pairing agent to the mobile phase for a reversed-phase column. The ion-pairing agent is usually a surfactant that has a charged group at one end and a nonpolar tail or group at the other end. Examples of ion-pairing agents are sodium dodecyl sulfate and perchlorate, for binding to positively charged ions, and *t*-butyl ammonium, for binding to negatively charged ions.

The purpose of the ion-pairing agent is to combine with ions of the opposite charge in the sample. This may involve the sample ions interacting with the charged end of the ion-pairing agent while the nonpolar tail of the same agent partitions into the nonpolar stationary phase of the reversed-phase column. Alternatively, the sample ion and ion-pairing agent may interact in the mobile phase and form a neutral complex that then interacts with the nonpolar stationary phase. The result in either case is the retention of charged analytes based on their ability to interact with the ion-pairing agent.

IPC is useful in the separation of charged compounds that are poorly resolved by IEC. This method not only combines the better efficiencies that are normally produced by reversed-phase columns, but it also has several parameters that can be varied to control and adjust its separations. These parameters include (1) the strength and type of solvent used in the mobile phase for the reversed-phase column, (2) the concentration and type of ion-pairing agent placed into this mobile phase, and (3) the ion content and pH of the mobile phase. Applications in which IPC has been employed include the separation and analysis of catecholamines, drugs, and nucleic acids.[12]

Restricted access media are a set of supports that combine SEC with another type of LC, which is usually reversed-phase chromatography.[12] This type of material is prepared in a manner so that the exterior of the support is inert or protected by a hydrophilic network with low nonspecific binding for proteins and biological compounds. The interior contains a stationary phase such as a nonpolar bonded phase. If the sizes of the pores or the size-exclusion properties are chosen properly, small solutes such as drugs can pass into the interior and be retained by the stationary phase that is located there. Larger compounds, such as proteins, will not be able to access this inner region and pass nonretained through the column. Columns that contain a restricted access support can be used for the direct injection of biological samples that may contain high concentrations of proteins (ie, which will elute nonretained) and are being used for measurement of small analytes. This approach can greatly simplify the process of sample preparation for such analytes.

Liquid Chromatography Instrumentation

The major components of an LC system used in HPLC are shown in Fig. 16.15.[21,77] First, there is a source for the mobile phase, or a solvent reservoir, which supplies a solvent or solution that goes into a pump for delivery to the rest of the LC system. This is followed by an injection valve or injection system, which allows samples to be placed into the mobile phase stream. Next, the mobile phase and sample enter and pass through the column, which contains the support and stationary phase. A control system also may be present to maintain a constant or well-defined temperature within the column. The column is followed by a detector to observe and measure the components of the sample as they exit the system. Modern systems also have a computer or control system to operate the liquid chromatograph and to gather data from the LC detector.

Mobile Phase Reservoirs and Delivery Systems

Solvents and solutions that are used as mobile phases in LC are contained in solvent reservoirs. In their simplest form, these reservoirs are glass bottles or flasks into which feed lines to the pump are inserted. Filters are often placed at the inlets of the feed lines to prevent any particles in the mobile phase from moving on to the rest of the LC system. Most mobile phase reservoirs also have a means of "sparging" the mobile phase by bubbling through a gas such as helium or nitrogen to remove dissolved air or oxygen that may interfere with the response of some detectors. The removal of air and oxygen, or degassing, also can be achieved by applying a vacuum to the reservoir by placing gas exchange devices or gas filters in the flow path leading from the mobile phase reservoir.[12]

The composition and strength of the mobile phase are factors that can be used to adjust and control a separation in LC. If the same mobile phase is used throughout the separation, this approach is known as isocratic elution.[7,10] If the composition of the mobile phase is varied over time, the method is called solvent programming.[7,12] Solvent programming begins with a weak mobile phase to allow chemicals with weak retention to have their strongest possible interactions with the column. A change is then made over time to a stronger mobile phase to also elute chemicals with moderate or high retention. This change in mobile phase composition can be made in one or more steps and may involve the use of a linear change or a nonlinear change over time.

A variety of techniques have been used to vary the composition of the mobile phase over time.[12,21] For instance, this might be done by using valves that alternate which solvents or solutions are being passed into the LC system at a given time. Solvent gradients may be generated by using the same type of valve linked to two or more solvent reservoirs and that passes these mobile phases into a mixing chamber and onto the inlet of a single pump. This method is known as low-pressure mixing. A second approach, known as high-pressure mixing, uses two or more pumps that are each linked to a different solvent or solution; the flow rates of the mobile phases that are being passed through these pumps are then varied to control the mixing ratio of these solvents or solutions. This combined solution is then passed through a mixing chamber and onto the column. These solvents and

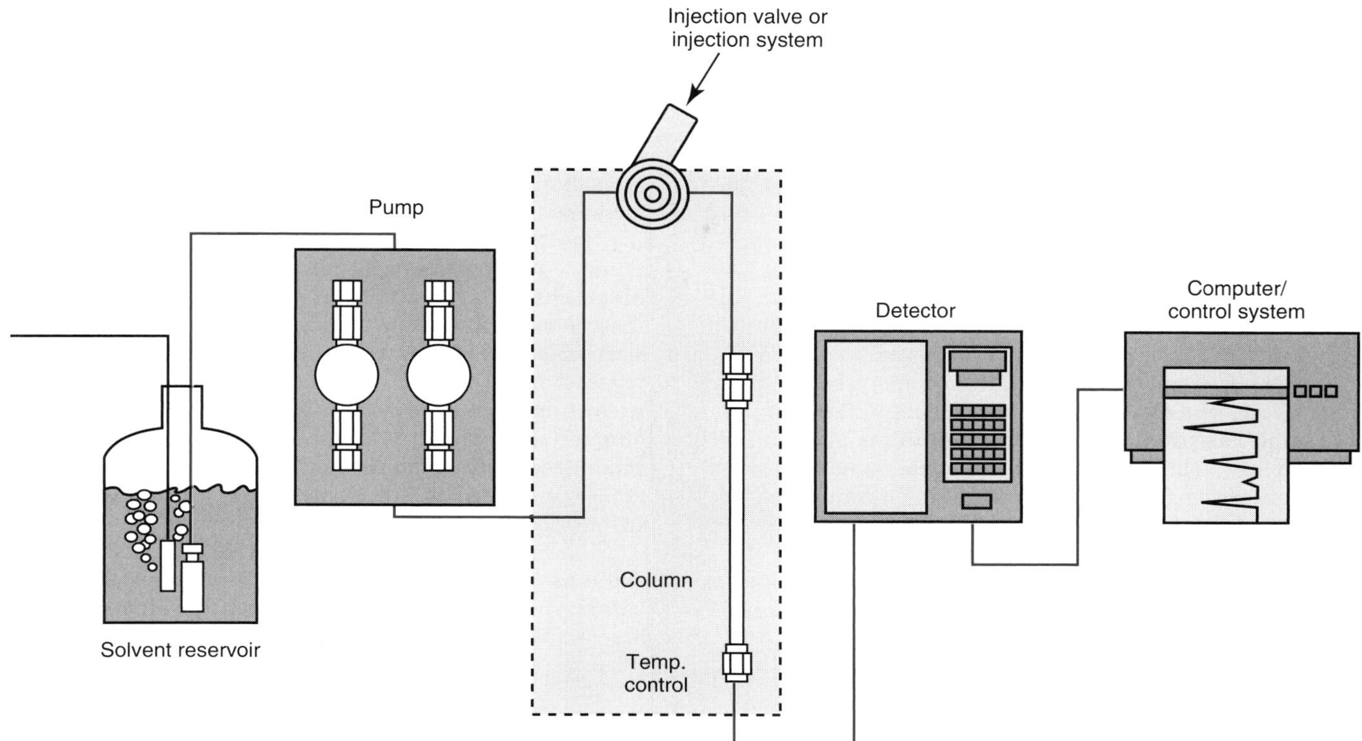

FIGURE 16.15 General design of a liquid chromatograph, as used in high-performance liquid chromatography. (Modified from a figure courtesy Restek Corporation, Bellefonte, Pennsylvania.)

solutions can be mixed by using static mixers, which rely on flow-generated turbulence, or dynamic mixers, which use magnetic stirrers. Solvent miscibility and viscosity are two factors to consider when choosing which solvents or solutions are to be used in a solvent program. Both of these factors can affect the mixing characteristics of the two liquids, where inadequate mixing may result in poor chromatographic performance and inadequate separations.[21]

Several types of pumps have been used in LC.[12,21] Peristaltic and diaphragm-type pumps can be used with columns that can be operated at low pressures, as are encountered in classic and low- to medium-performance LC; however, these pumps are not usually suitable for HPLC. Reciprocating pumps and syringe pumps are instead used to achieve the higher pressures needed to deliver the mobile phase through HPLC columns. Reciprocating pumps are commonly used in HPLC for work at flow rates in the milliliter-per-minute range. In these pumps, a piston moves in and out of the solvent chamber, with check valves being used to keep the flow of the mobile phase moving from the pump inlet to the outlet. The reciprocating action of the piston in this type of pump does generate some pulsation in the pressure and mobile phase flow, which can increase the baseline noise seen with many LC detectors. These pulsations can be minimized by electronic control of the pump and by placing pulse dampers in the flow path. Syringe pumps make use of the continuous application of a syringe to the solvent chamber to deliver the mobile phase to the rest of the system. These pumps can deliver essentially pulse-free flow and can be used at much lower flow rates than reciprocal pumps (eg, flow rates in the microliter-to-minute range). However, syringe pumps are not as convenient to use as reciprocating pumps when carrying out solvent programming or during the application of even modest volumes of the mobile phase to a column.[12,21]

Until recently, the upper pressure limit of most HPLC applications has been approximately 6000 psi (41 MPa or 414 bar). In recent years, commercial instrumentation for LC has been developed that can operate up to 15,000 psi (103 MPa or 1034 bar).[33,36,78-80] These higher pressures are needed for work with small-diameter supports, which offer the potential for more efficient separations but also produce higher column back pressures. The use of these smaller support particles and these higher pressures has resulted in a method that is often called ultra-high performance liquid chromatography (UPLC or UHPLC).[33-36] Work at these higher pressures not only requires special pumps that are designed to operate under these conditions, but also requires tubing, connections, and columns that can be used under the same conditions.

Systems for HPLC have pressure sensors to detect any obstruction to flow. These sensors can shut down the entire system once a defined pressure limit has been reached, which is done to prevent damage to the components of the LC system. At very high pressures, some solvents become slightly compressible and a compensation for this solvent compression needs to be made to achieve constant flow rates.[33]

Another extreme condition that may be encountered during the operation of an LC system is when work is to be carried out at quite low flow rates, as might be needed for small-bore microfluidic columns or capillary columns. Work at flow rates below 10 μL/min may require specially designed pumping systems or flow splitting of the output from a standard HPLC pump. The use of low rates in the nanoliter-per-minute range is sometimes called nanoflow chromatography and has been combined with mass spectrometry through the use of nanospray interfaces, which can provide high ionization efficiencies.

Injection Systems and Sample Derivatization

Various approaches can be used to introduce a sample into an LC system.[12,21] The most widely used approach in HPLC is a fixed-loop injector that is switched into or out of the flow path by manual control or through the use of an autoinjector. When this valve is in the inject mode, the sample loop is switched into the flow path and the sample is carried downstream and into the column. The loop continues to be part of this flow path until it is switched back into the load or fill position.

Some important characteristics to consider when selecting an injection system are its (1) reproducibility, (2) the amount of sample carryover from one injection to the next, and (3) the range of volumes that can be injected. Some automated injection systems have the capability of injecting multiple aliquots of the same sample or of mixing a sample and a reagent for derivatization before injection. Some of these systems also are able to control the temperature of the samples before their injection. For instance, the refrigeration of samples before injection may be important during the analysis of specimens or analytes that have limited stability or when large batches of samples are to be analyzed.

Derivatization is sometimes used in LC to improve the response of a given compound or group of compounds to a particular detector (eg, an absorbance, fluorescence, or electrochemical detector, as will be discussed later). It is also possible to use derivatization in LC to alter the separation of a compound from other chemicals by changing the structure and retention of this compound on the column. The two main ways of carrying out derivatization in LC are (1) precolumn derivatization and (2) postcolumn derivatization. Precolumn derivatization is done before the sample is injected and can be used to alter a compound's retention or to increase its response to a particular type of detector. Postcolumn derivatization is carried out online as compounds elute from a column and is used only to improve the response of one or more of these compounds on the LC detector.[44,81]

Columns and Supports

A wide selection of columns are available for LC. These columns can have various combinations of packing materials and diameters or lengths. Columns for LC, and especially those used in HPLC, often include an inlet filter to remove particulate matter. In the use of LC and HPLC for chemical analysis, a short guard column that contains the same packing material also may be placed before a longer analytical column to protect and extend the usable life of the more expensive analytical column.[12]

The size used for a column in LC will depend on the desired application for this column. The column size used for off-line sample pretreatment or the low-performance isolation of compounds is often determined by the sample capacity that is needed for the separation. Examples of these columns include those used for applications such as desalting, purification of compounds based on IEC, and many types of affinity-based separations for sample pretreatment. Size-exclusion columns, such as small centrifugation columns that are used for desalting, can accommodate specimens with sizes up to about 10% of the column volume. The size of ion-exchange or affinity columns that are used for sample pretreatment and compound isolation will depend on the amount of compound that needs to be separated and the binding capacity of the packing material. This principle also applies to the use of other types of LC for sample pretreatment or compound isolation.

Modern column technology for HPLC has produced columns having various dimensions, with a trend toward smaller internal volumes.[12] These small volume columns are useful in combining LC with other methods, such as mass spectrometry, to produce hyphenated techniques (see Chapter 17). In the clinical laboratory, most conventional packed HPLC columns consist of tubes that are made of 316 stainless steel; however, polymers that are suitable for work at high liquid pressures also can be employed. These columns have typical internal diameters that range from 4 to 5 mm and lengths ranging from 5 to 30 cm (Table 16.3). Column end fittings, which ideally have a zero dead volume and frits to hold the support particles in the column, are used to connect the column to the injector and to a detector or other postcolumn devices.

In general, better efficiencies and lower detection limits are achieved with HPLC columns that have longer lengths and smaller inner diameters. These smaller inner diameter columns include narrow-bore columns, with approximate inner diameters of 2 to 3 mm, and microbore columns, with approximate inner diameters of 1 to 2 mm. In addition to providing improved efficiencies, these columns with small inner diameters also can require lower flow rates and smaller volumes of the mobile phase for their operation than conventional packed columns.

Capillary columns are sometimes used in LC. For instance, packed capillary columns can be used that have inner diameters of 0.1 to 0.5 mm and lengths of 20 to 200 cm. Open tubular capillary columns for LC also can be constructed by placing a thin film or coating of the stationary

TABLE 16.3 Typical Column Sizes Used in Analytical High-Performance Liquid Chromatography

Type of Column	Typical Inner Diameter (ID) and Lengths	Typical Flow Rate Range
Conventional packed column	4–5 mm ID × 5–30 cm	1–3 mL/min
Narrow-bore column	2–3 mm ID × 5–15 cm	0.2–0.6 mL/min
Microbore column	1–2 mm ID × 10–100 cm	0.05–0.2 mL/min
Packed capillary	0.1–0.5 mm ID × 20–200 cm	0.1–20 µL/min
Open tubular column	0.01–0.075 mm ID × 1–100 cm	0.05–2 µL/min

Portions of the data in this table are based on Poole, CF, Poole, SK. *Chromatography today.* New York: Elsevier, 1991.

phase onto the inner wall of a fused silica tube. These open tubular columns have typical inner diameters of 0.01 to 0.075 mm and lengths of 1 to 100 cm. Both types of capillary columns are used with flow rates in the mid-to-low microliter-per-minute range.

Many types of particles and support formats have been developed for LC.[30,82] The most common type of support in LC is a packed bed of small particles.[82] The supports in modern HPLC columns may have particle diameters for porous supports that are in the range of 1.8 to 10 μm, with a typical value of 5 μm. The lower end of this diameter range is representative of the supports that are used in the UPLC.[36] A smaller diameter for these supports provides better efficiency for the chromatographic system, but it also leads to an increase in back pressure across the column. As mentioned previously, the back pressure generated by a packed bed that contains such a support will vary inversely with the square of the particle diameter. Thus a twofold reduction in the particle size will result in approximately a fourfold increase in back pressure. Low-to-medium performance separations, which have much lower operating pressures than HPLC, typically use packing materials such as cross-linked dextran or agarose that have support particles with diameters of 50 to 200 μm.

In the porous support particles that are usually employed in LC, the mobile phase flows around the support but not through the particle. However, this means compounds must travel within the particle by means of diffusion, which is a relatively slow process that can be a major source of band-broadening. The distance that these compounds must diffuse can be reduced by using a nonporous support or a pellicular support, in which the latter has a thin porous layer or porous shell.[10,30] The use of these supports results in a more efficient separation and less band-broadening because of diffusion-based processes. Another approach for minimizing this band-broadening is to use perfusion particles. This type of support has small pores that contain most of the stationary phase and larger pores that allow the mobile phase to pass both through and around the support particles. The presence of these large flow-through pores decreases the distance compounds must diffuse to reach the stationary phase and helps decrease band-broadening.[10,30]

Another alternative support that can be used to improve efficiency is a monolithic support.[83-85] This type of support consists of a continuous porous bed that is prepared from an inorganic or organic polymer. Monoliths may be made from silica or various polymers. Monolith columns have bimodal pore structures with large pores (approximately a few microns in diameter) that allow the mobile phase to flow through the support and smaller pores (with typical pore sizes of 10 to 20 nm) that provide a large internal surface area to contain the stationary phase. These supports can provide efficient and fast separations, while also providing lower back pressures than particle-based columns at high flow rates. The low back pressure of a monolithic column makes it possible to use this type of column with a flow gradient (eg, increasing the flow rate at the end of a separation) and allow several such columns to be coupled in series to improve the efficiency and resolution of an LC separation. These columns also can have reasonably high sample capacities. Commercial monolithic rods are encased in inert polytetrafluoroethylene tubing and housed in stainless steel tubes. The inert tubing eliminates voids that may occur at the interface between the stainless steel and the monolith, thus improving the resolution of the column. Capillary monolithic columns also are available. One area of clinical interest in which monolithic columns have been used is in reversed-phase separations of peptides and proteins.[46-48,86]

Temperature Control

The control of column temperature can be an important factor in determining the reproducibility and efficiency of an LC separation.[21] Unlike in GC, in which temperature gradients are often employed, in LC a constant column temperature is usually maintained. Temperature control of an LC column can be achieved by a variety of techniques. These techniques include the use of temperature-controlled (1) column chambers, (2) water jackets, (3) blankets, and (4) heating/cooling blocks. In addition, operation at high flow rates might require a heater/exchanger, which is usually a coil of tubing with good heat exchange properties that is placed before the column inlet.

During the operation of an LC separation, a stable column temperature is required to generate reproducible retention times. In addition, an increase in the column temperature will (1) lower the mobile phase viscosity, (2) increase the rates of mass transfer between mobile phase and stationary phase, and (3) allow the use of higher flow rates, which in turn will lead to a shorter analysis time. The degree to which the temperature can be increased is determined by the boiling point and vapor pressure of the mobile phase, as well as the thermal stability of the analytes in the injected samples. In some instances, the stability of the samples and analytes may require separations to be carried out at reduced temperatures. One common example of this occurs in the use of LC for the isolation and preparation of proteins, which is often performed in cold rooms or in refrigerated cabinets to decrease the rates of protein denaturation and proteolytic degradation. Some systems for temperature control have the ability to operate below room temperature through the action of Peltier coolers or other types of refrigeration. Features to consider in selecting a system for temperature control in LC include (1) the usable temperature range of the system, (2) the constancy of the temperatures it can provide, and (3) the number and sizes of columns that the system can accommodate.

Liquid Chromatography Detectors

Many types of detectors can be used in LC (Table 16.4).[12,21] Some common LC detectors are (1) absorbance detectors, (2) fluorescence detectors, (3) electrochemical detectors, (4) refractive index detectors, and (5) mass spectrometric detectors. A key component for most of these detectors is the flow cell through which the mobile phase and eluting compounds from the column must pass. As these components travel through the flow cell or into the detector, a signal is generated that can be used to monitor the eluting chemicals and measure the amount of these chemicals that are present. Many LC detectors are nondestructive and can be used individually or linked together in series. In addition, a postcolumn reactor may be present between the column and detector to derivatize some of the eluting compounds and generate products that have a stronger and more specific signal on the detector.

Absorbance Detectors. The absorption of UV or visible light is often used to detect compounds as they elute from a

TABLE 16.4 Examples of Detectors Used in Liquid Chromatography

Type of Detector	Principle of Operation	Range of Application	Detection Limit
Absorbance detector	Measures absorbance of light at a given wavelength or set of wavelengths	Compounds with chromophores that can absorb ultraviolet or visible light	10^{-10}–10^{-9} g
Fluorescence detector	Measures ability of chemicals to absorb and reemit light through fluorescence	Compounds with fluorophores	10^{-12}–10^{-9} g
Electrochemical detector	Measures current or charge as a result of chemical oxidation or reduction	Electrochemically active compounds	10^{-11}–10^{-9} g
Conductivity detector	Measures change in conductivity of the mobile phase as ions elute from the column	General for ionic solutes	10^{-9} g
Refractive index detector	Measures change in refractive index of the mobile phase as compounds elute the column	Universal	10^{-7}–10^{-6} g
Mass spectrometry	Production of gas phase ions, followed by separation/analysis of these ions based on their mass-to-charge ratios	Universal: Full-scan mode Selective: Selected ion monitoring mode	10^{-10}–10^{-9} g (full-scan mode) $\leq 10^{-12}$ g (SIM mode)
Evaporative light scattering detector	Light scattering by chemicals after solvent evaporation	Nonvolatile compounds	10^{-9} g
Charged aerosol detector	Measurement of ions produced from chemicals by using a corona discharge	Nonvolatile compounds	$<10^{-9}$ g

Portions of the data in this table are based on Poole, CF, Poole, SK. *Chromatography today.* New York: Elsevier, 1991.

liquid chromatographic column.[12,21] Many of the absorbance detectors (also referred to as photometers or spectrophotometers) used in LC can measure the absorption of UV light with wavelengths in the range 190 to 400 nm or of visible light with wavelengths in the range of 400 to 700 nm. Many organic compounds with aromatic groups or double or triple bonds absorb UV light between 250 and 300 nm. Many other organic compounds can absorb in the range of 190 to 220 nm, at which amide bonds, carboxylic acids, and many other groups can have substantial absorption of light. In addition, some ions, inorganic compounds and metal complexes can be detected by their absorption of light in the UV or visible range.

There are several types of absorbance detectors that can be used in LC.[2,12,21] Fixed-wavelength absorbance detectors have the simplest design and are used to monitor absorbance at a particular wavelength or wavelength band. For instance, detection is often done with a UV absorbance detector at 254 nm, which is a wavelength absorbed by many unsaturated organic compounds and corresponds to an intense emission line that is produced by a mercury arc lamp. A fixed-wavelength absorbance detector can be extremely sensitive and is capable of operating with detection at 0.005 absorbance unit full scale. Fixed-wavelength absorbance detectors that have greater flexibility in their design can be obtained by using other, less intense emission lines of a mercury arc lamp. In addition, a phosphor can be placed between the light source and the flow cell, with the light that is emitted by this agent then being passed through the flow cell. This approach is used in dual-wavelength detectors that operate at two fixed wavelengths (eg, 254 and 280 nm). The intense emission lines at 214 or 229 nm that are produced by a zinc or cadmium arc lamp, respectively, may be used for detection at lower wavelengths, where many organic compounds have strong absorption of light.

A second type of detector in this category is a variable-wavelength absorbance detector.[2,12,21] This detector operates at a wavelength that is selected from a given wavelength range. The ability to have a detector that operates at the absorption maximum for a given chemical or set of chemicals can greatly enhance the applicability and selectivity of such a device. Another advantage of this detector is its ability to operate at low-UV wavelengths (eg, 190 nm), at which a number of clinically important compounds absorb light (eg, cholesterol). However, at these lower wavelengths many solvents and mobile phases also absorb light. Important exceptions are water, acetonitrile, and methanol, which are frequently used in reversed-phase chromatography.

A photodiode array detector also can be used in LC.[2,12,21] This is an absorbance detector that uses an array of small detector cells to measure the change in absorbance at many wavelengths simultaneously. This array makes it possible to record an entire spectrum for a compound because it elutes from a column, which can be valuable in identifying overlapping peaks.[12,32,44] This type of detector can yield spectral data over a wide wavelength range (eg, 190 to 600 nm) in approximately 10 ms. During operation, the photodiode array detector passes polychromatic light through the flow cell. The transmitted light is then dispersed by a diffraction grating and directed to a photodiode array, at which the intensity of transmitted light is measured at multiple wavelengths across the spectrum. Such detectors have been helpful in the identification of drugs in samples such as urine and serum.[87]

During the use of an absorbance detector, it is necessary to use solvents, ion-pairing agents, and buffers that have little or no absorption of light at the wavelengths of interest; this is needed to maintain a low background signal. Water, acetonitrile, methanol, isopropanol, and hexane are solvents that allow UV detection down to wavelengths of 200 nm. Phosphate buffers also can be used under these detection conditions. Many other solvents and buffers have substantial absorbance in the UV, which may limit their use over this wavelength range.

There are a number of other factors to consider in the use of absorbance detectors. For instance, flow cells with small volumes should be used in absorbance detectors for HPLC to avoid the introduction of significant extracolumn band-broadening. Another issue with the operation of these detectors is the outgassing and bubble formation that can occur as the mobile phase exits the high-pressure region within the column and enters the lower pressure region in the flow cell. Because these detectors can be quite sensitive, these bubbles can lead to noise in their response and degrade their signal-to-noise ratio. Effective degassing of the mobile phase and the use of some back pressure across the detector can help minimize this bubble formation. However, care must also be taken in this last approach to avoid exceeding the usable pressure range of the detector.

Fluorescence Detectors. As discussed in Chapter 13, fluorescence occurs when a chemical absorbs light at one wavelength and reemits light at a different, longer wavelength.[12,21] Fluorescence detectors with flow cells are used in LC to detect fluorescent compounds as they elute from the column. These detectors are generally much more selective and have better limits of detection than absorbance detectors for chemicals that are naturally fluorescent or can be converted into a fluorescent derivative. Both precolumn and postcolumn derivatization have been used to modify chemicals for use with this type of detector.[81] For example, amino acids and other primary amines are often labeled with a dansyl or fluorescamine tag, followed by their HPLC separation and detection through fluorescence. Some fluorescence detectors for LC use fixed wavelengths for both the excitation and emission wavelengths that are employed for monitoring compounds. However, variable-wavelength fluorescence detectors are also available. Deuterium lamps, xenon arc lamps, and lasers have all been used as light sources in such detectors.

Electrochemical and Conductivity Detectors. Various types of electrochemical detectors can be used in LC. This combination is sometimes known as liquid chromatography/electrochemical detection (LC-EC).[2,12] In an amperometric electrochemical detector (see Chapter 14), an electroactive chemical enters the flow cell, where it may be oxidized or reduced at an electrode that is held at a constant potential; the current needed for or generated by this process is then detected.[88] The use of multiple electrodes and cyclic changes in the applied voltage can allow the detection of multiple components at different potentials and provides for regular cleaning of the electrode. Electroactive compounds that are of clinical interest and that can be readily examined by HPLC with electrochemical detection include urinary catecholamines (see Chapter 63), ascorbic acid, and thiol-containing compounds such as homocysteine. In addition, electrochemically active tags (eg, bromine) can be added to compounds such as unsaturated fatty acids or prostaglandins for use with this type of detector.

Coulometric detectors are also used in LC. This type of detector measures the amount of charge that is required for a given electrochemical reaction. When placed in series, such detectors can be used to detect and measure coeluting compounds that differ in their half-wave potentials (ie, the potential at half of the maximum signal) by 60 mV or more. These detectors are selective, sensitive, and have reasonably wide linear ranges. Coulometric detectors are used in clinical laboratories during the analysis of metanephrines, vanillylmandelic acid, homovanillic acid, and 5-hydroxyindole acetic acid in human urine (see Chapter 63).

A conductivity detector in LC measures the ability of the mobile phase and its contents to conduct a current when they are placed in an electrical field.[2,12] This type of detector is often used in combination with IEC. For instance, conductivity detectors with relatively low sensitivities have been used to monitor salt gradients during IEC. Conductivity detectors are also used to monitor the elution of charged analytes in ion chromatography.[2,89] The signal resulting from the conductivity of a specific ion will be related to its concentration, charge, and mobility. This means such a detector is best suited for work with small inorganic and organic ions, which have high mobilities. Conductivity detectors have been used to measure compounds such as sulfate in biological fluids.

Refractive Index Detectors. A refractive index detector in LC measures the change in the refraction of light as chemicals pass with the mobile phase through a flow cell.[12,21] An important advantage for this type of detector is that it can monitor substances such as alcohols, polyethylene glycol, salts, and sugars that do not give a usable response on absorbance or fluorescence detectors.[90] An RI detector also can be valuable in work in which the nature or spectroscopic properties of an analyte have not yet been determined. One disadvantage of this type of detector is it does not have limits of detection as low as absorbance or fluorescence detectors, and it has a response that can be sensitive to changes in the mobile phase composition and temperature.

Mass Spectrometry. LC can be combined with mass spectrometry, giving a combined technique known as LC-MS.[91-94] This is a sensitive and specific technique that has seen increasing applications in clinical and research laboratories and in fields such as proteomics, metabolomics, and small molecule analysis (see Chapters 17, 19, and 20).[60,95-99] This method is similar to GC-MS in that the combined use of LC with mass spectrometry makes it possible to both measure chemicals and identify them based on the masses of their molecular ions or fragment ions. When used in the full-scan mode to look at all or most ions, the mass spectrometer in LC-MS acts as a general detector. If the mass spectrometer is instead used for looking at particular ions, this device then acts as a selective detector.

Several types of ionization methods and mass analyzers can be employed in LC-MS (see Chapter 17). A common combination is the use of electrospray ionization with a quadrupole mass analyzer.[2] Other possible ionization methods that can be used in LC-MS are chemical ionization or photoionization (see Chapter 17). For many applications, the specificity of tandem mass spectrometers allows short HPLC separations to be used because most compounds do not need to be completely separated for them to be detected by the mass spectrometer.

A critical element in linking HPLC to a mass spectrometer is their interface. For example, the interface between an LC and a mass spectrometer has the challenging task of removing solvent from the mobile phase and placing the remaining sample components in a charged form and in the gas phase that can be analyzed by the mass spectrometer. This process requires that the buffers used in LC-MS be sufficiently volatile to avoid overloading and contaminating the interface. For the same reason, a switching valve is often used to divert salts and other nonretained components that elute early in the LC separation to a waste container. The same switching valve can then direct later eluting components to the mass spectrometer for analysis (see Chapter 17 for an extensive discussion of mass spectrometry).

Other Liquid Chromatography Detectors. Several detectors have been developed for LC to detect nonvolatile compounds.[90,100] An example is an evaporative light-scattering detector (ELSD). In an ELSD, the solvent is evaporated by nebulizing it with a stream of gas as the mobile phase and its contents exit the column. Nonvolatile chemicals that were present in the mobile phase will remain as particles in the gas phase, and these particles can be detected by measuring their ability to scatter light. The degree of this light scattering will be proportional to the mass of the nonvolatile substances. Potential applications for an ELSD include its use in the analysis of lipids, sugars, and other compounds that are difficult to monitor by absorbance or fluorescence detectors.

Another type of evaporative detector is a charged aerosol detector.[100] This detector ionizes chemicals by using a corona discharge and measures the ion current that is produced. This type of detector has a good response for many compounds. A disadvantage of both the ELSD and the charged aerosol detector is that they are destructive. This means sample components cannot be collected for further analysis after passing through these detectors and that these detectors cannot be followed directly online by another detector.

A number of other detectors have been used in LC, although many of these have been used primarily for research applications. Dynamic light-scattering detectors measure the scattering of light by chemicals that are eluting from a column, which provides a signal that is related to the size of these chemicals. This type of detector has been useful in characterizing the size of large molecules and complexes.[101] Nuclear magnetic resonance (NMR) spectroscopy has been combined with LC[12] for applications such as lipoprotein analysis, metabolomics, and the characterization of drug metabolites.

Data Acquisition and System Control

When using simple LC systems it is possible to perform injections and make pump adjustments manually, with the results being recorded by a computer or comparable data acquisition device. For automated or high-volume applications, there usually is a need to automate both the injection of samples and the chromatographic system. The system controller for an HPLC will often manage (1) sample injections, (2) solvent delivery, (3) system flow rate and temperature, (4) control the detectors, and (5) acquisition of data from these detectors. Modern control systems also usually provide an auditable record of the analyst, LC method, calibration conditions, control samples, and specimens that were analyzed.

Data acquisition systems can collect thousands of data points from an individual run. These data can then be used to identify and characterize a set of peaks based on parameters such as the retention times, areas, heights, and widths of these peaks. Comparison of these parameters with those that have been generated by reference materials and standards makes it possible to identify and measure the compounds in these peaks. The hardware and software that are used for data analysis in LC become more critical as the amount of collected data becomes large, as can often occur during the use of photodiode array detectors or LC-MS. Libraries of spectra or other databases can be searched as part of this process to aid in the identification of chemicals (eg, peptides and nucleic acid sequences) based on the chromatograms and signals that are generated during the separation.

Laboratory Safety in Liquid Chromatography

Standard laboratory procedures for the storage, handling, and disposal of chemicals and solvents should be followed when using LC and HPLC. For instance, many of the organic solvents that are used as mobile phases or solvents in LC are flammable and should be treated with appropriate precautions for such chemicals (see Chapter 12). The waste solvents, samples, and column effluent should be collected in a suitable container and stored appropriately before disposal. The release of pressure in a traditional LC system or HPLC system is not usually a major hazard, because liquids compress only slightly and therefore accumulate little energy; however, work at the higher pressures of UPLC may require some additional precautions.

OTHER CHROMATOGRAPHIC METHODS

In addition to LC and GC, and the use of columns or open tubular supports, there are a variety of other chromatographic methods that can be used for chemical separation and analysis. Some important examples are supercritical fluid chromatography (SFC) and planar chromatography. The use of multidimensional separations based on chromatography is another area of continued interest.

Supercritical Fluid Chromatography

SFC is a type of chromatography in which the mobile phase is a supercritical fluid.[12,102,103] A supercritical fluid is a state of matter that has properties between those of a gas and a liquid and that is formed when the temperature and pressure exceed a particular critical point in a chemical's phase diagram. Carbon dioxide is one chemical that can be easily converted into a supercritical fluid for use in SFC. The formation of supercritical fluid carbon dioxide occurs at or above a temperature of 31.1°C and at or above a pressure of 73.9 bar (72.9 atm). Under these conditions, carbon dioxide has a density that approaches that of a liquid, so it can interact with and solvate chemicals; this feature allows supercritical fluid carbon dioxide to be used in dissolving many hydrophobic compounds.[104,105] However, a supercritical fluid also has a lower viscosity and a higher diffusion coefficient than liquid, which allows it to provide efficiencies that are closer to those seen when using a gas as the mobile phase. As a result, SFC has performance characteristics that are between those of LC and GC.[102,103]

SFC can be used with many columns that are available for either LC or GC and can be carried out on systems that are modified versions of LC or GC instruments. It is necessary for these systems to have both pressure and temperature control to keep the mobile phase in the state of a supercritical fluid as it passes through the column. A variety of organic modifiers have been mixed with carbon dioxide to serve as the mobile phase, and solvent programming or temperature programming can be used for elution in this method. It is

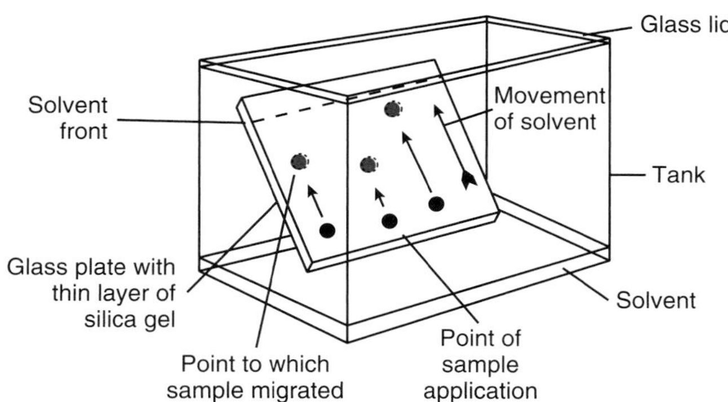

FIGURE 16.16 General operation and system components of thin-layer chromatography. In this example, the mobile phase moves up the glass plate and thin layer of adsorbent by means of capillary action. (Modified from Bennett TP. *Graphic biochemistry, vol 1: chemistry of biological molecules.* New York: Macmillan; 1968.)

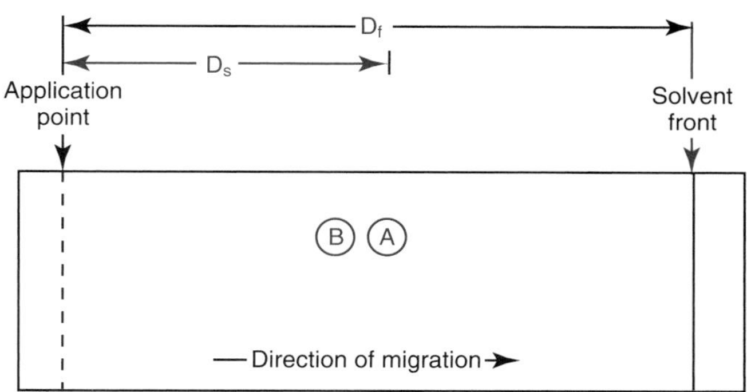

FIGURE 16.17 General example of a separation obtained by planar chromatography. In this example, compound *B* is more strongly retained and migrates a shorter distance than compound *A*. D_f, distance traveled by the mobile phase, or solvent front, from the point of sample application in the same amount of time as allowed for sample migration; D_s, distance traveled by an analyte (*A*, in this example) from the point of sample application.

also common for pressure programming (or density programming) to be used in SFC, as the mobile phase strength of a supercritical fluid will change with its density.[21,102] This technique has been used for the analysis of lipids and other hydrophobic compounds. In addition, SFC has been applied to pharmaceutical research and to the analysis of natural products. However, because of its need for specialized equipment, SFC has found limited use in clinical laboratories.

Planar Chromatography

Another alternative type of chromatographic method is planar chromatography. In planar chromatography, the stationary phase is coated or placed onto a flat surface, or plane.[12] The sample is added as a small spot or band on this surface. This support is then placed into an enclosed container with the bottom edge in contact with the mobile phase and the sample band located above this point of contact (Fig. 16.16). The mobile phase is usually allowed to travel across the plane by means of capillary action. After this movement has occurred for a given period, the support is removed from the mobile phase and dried before the analysis or measurement of the separated sample components.

The planar surface that is used in this method may be a sheet of paper, giving a method known as paper chromatography, or some other type of surface, resulting in a method known as thin-layer chromatography (TLC).[12,106] In paper chromatography, the stationary phase is a layer of water or a polar solvent that is coated onto paper. In TLC, a thin layer of particles (made from a material such as silica, microparticulate cellulose, or alumina) is usually spread uniformly on a glass plate, plastic sheet, or aluminum sheet. When this layer of particles is made up of a material with a small diameter (eg, silica with diameter of around 4.5 μm), the resulting technique is known as high-performance thin-layer chromatography.[12]

In planar chromatography, retention is described as a function of the distance that compounds have traveled in a given amount of time (Fig. 16.17). This differs from column chromatography or open tubular chromatography, in which retention is instead described by using the time or volume of mobile phase that is needed for compounds to travel a given distance (eg, the length of the column). The retention of chemicals in methods such as paper chromatography and TLC can be described either in terms of the migration distances that these chemicals have traveled from their point of application in a set amount of time, or by comparing these distances to the distance that has been traveled by the mobile phase in the same amount of time. This second approach can be used to calculate a measure of retention that is known as the retardation factor (R_f), which is defined as follows,

$$R_f = D_s/D_f$$

where D_s is the distance traveled by a chemical from its point of application, and D_f is the distance traveled by the mobile phase, or solvent front, in the same amount of time. The value for R_f will always be between 0 and 1. Chemicals that have high retention with the stationary phase will have low values R_f, and chemicals that have low retention will have R_f values that approach 1.[7,12]

Chemicals can be identified in planar chromatography based on the position of their bands and by comparing their retention to reference compounds that have been examined on the same plate or surface as the unknown samples. The detection characteristics of the reference compounds also can be compared with the chemicals in the unknown sample. If the R_f value for an unknown substance and the R_f value for a reference compound do not match within the allowed tolerance, the compounds can be said to be different. If the R_f values do match, then confirmation can be made by comparing the detection properties of these compounds (eg, the color of their bands or their response to a color-forming reagent). Software and databases are also available for compound identification in planar chromatography that allow for searching libraries of both absorption spectra and R_f values. Additional confirmation can be obtained by comparing the unknown compound and the reference compound under a different set of separation conditions.

The separated components in planar chromatography often can be detected by their natural color, by their response to UV light (eg, through their fluorescence), or through their visualization with chemical reagents that form colored products.[12] In some cases, these chemicals may be allowed to react with labeled antibodies for their detection or they may be detected by using radiolabels and autoradiography. Their bands also may be removed from the planar surface for analysis by a method such as mass spectrometry or NMR spectroscopy.

Paper chromatography and TLC tend to be used primarily for qualitative analysis. In addition, they can be used in multidimensional separations (see next section). One application of these techniques in clinical laboratories is their use in the analysis of amniotic fluid to determine lecithin-to-sphingomyelin ratios. Another application is their use in the screening of urine for drugs or metabolites such as amino acids that accumulate during hereditary disorders. Planar chromatography is relatively simple, inexpensive to conduct, and can be used for the simultaneous analysis of multiple samples. However, the application of these methods in clinical laboratories has been decreasing in recent years because of the lack of automation in traditional planar methods and their general lack of ability to perform precise quantitative measurements for chemicals.

Multidimensional Separations

Another area of growing interest in chromatography is in the area of multidimensional separations. These separations involve the use of two or more separation methods on a sample, in which each of these methods ideally uses a different mechanism for resolving components of the sample. A multidimensional separation can allow a large increase in peak capacity by combining chromatographic methods in which each separation step (or dimension) is performed sequentially.

Multidimensional separations can be carried out in various ways. For instance, this might be done by collecting fractions from one method and then analyzing these fractions by a second method. It is also possible in some cases to couple two chromatographic methods together. This can be done if the second method is faster than the first and if the mobile phase used for elution in the first method is compatible with the conditions needed for sample application in the second method.[14,107]

Planar chromatography is one approach that can be used for two-dimensional separations, but HPLC methods also can be employed. Peak capacities greater than 10,000 have been achieved for two-dimensional HPLC separations; however, this can require prolonged analysis times for the sample and usually means that multiple runs per sample must be conducted in the second dimension.

It is possible to link chromatographic methods with other analytical methods or detectors to create multidimensional methods. One common example is liquid chromatography-tandem mass spectrometry (LC-MS/MS), in which LC is used to separate chemicals based on their interactions with a given mobile phase and stationary phase, while a mass spectrometer is used to separate and analyze the gas phase ions that are generated at any given point in the chromatogram.[91] The addition of another dimension based on mass spectrometry, as occurs in LC-MS/MS to look at fragment ions that are produced from a given parent ion,[92,93,94,108] can further increase the ability to resolve or detect multiple components without extending the chromatographic component of the analysis time. This combined approach can enable the practical analysis of hundreds or thousands of components in a single specimen, as occurs during the analysis of samples in metabolomics[109] and proteomics.[110]

SELECTED REFERENCES

For a full list of references for this chapter, please refer to ExpertConsult.com.

2. Hage DS, Carr JD. *Analytical chemistry and quantitative analysis*. New York: Pearson; 2011.
3. Miller JM. *Chromatography: concepts and contrasts*. 2nd ed. Malden, Mass: Wiley-InterScience; 2009.
8. McNair HM, Miller JM. *Basic gas chromatography*. 2nd ed. Malden, Mass: Wiley-InterScience; 2009.
9. Snyder LR, Kirkland JJ, Dolan JW. *Introduction to modern liquid chromatography*. 3rd ed. New York: Wiley; 2009.
21. Ewing GW, editor. *Analytical instrumentation handbook*. 2nd ed. New York: Marcel Dekker; 1997.
24. Drozd J. *Chemical derivatization in gas chromatography*. Amsterdam: Elsevier; 1981.
30. Majors RE. A review of HPLC column packing technology. *Am Lab* 2003;**10**:46–54.
32. Lough WJ, Wainer IW. *High performance liquid chromatography: fundamentals principles and practice*. New York: Blackie Academic; 1995.
39. Karger BL, Snyder LR, Horvath C. *An introduction to separation science*. New York: Wiley; 1973.
44. Ravindranath B. *Principles and practice of chromatography*. New York: Wiley; 1989.
55. Hage DS, editor. *Handbook of affinity chromatography*. 2nd ed. Boca Raton: CRC Press; 2005.
64. Janson JC, editor. *Protein purification: principles, high resolution methods, and applications*. 3rd ed. Hoboken: Wiley; 2011.
68. Allenmark S. *Chromatographic enantioseparations: methods and applications*. 2nd ed. New York: Ellis Horwood; 1991.
79. Jorgenson JW. Capillary liquid chromatography at ultrahigh pressures. *Annu Rev Anal Chem (Palo Alto Calif)* 2010;**3**: 129–50.
81. Lunn G, Hellwig GC. *Handbook of derivatization reactions for HPLC*. New York: Wiley-InterScience; 1998.
85. Svec F, Huber CG. Monolithic materials: promises, challenges, achievements. *Anal Chem* 2006;**78**:2100–8.
91. Gross ML, Caprioli RM, Niessen W. *The encyclopedia of mass spectrometry*, vol. 8. hyphenated methods. Amsterdam: Elsevier; 2006.
92. Shushan B. A review of clinical diagnostic applications of liquid chromatography-tandem mass spectrometry. *Mass Spectrom Rev* 2010;**29**:930–44.
103. Taylor LT. Supercritical fluid chromatography. *Anal Chem* 2008;**80**:4285–94.
106. Sherma J, Fried B, editors. *Planar chromatography*. New York: Taylor & Francis; 2003.

17

Mass Spectrometry

*Alan L. Rockwood, Mark M. Kushnir, and Nigel J. Clarke**

ABSTRACT

Background
Mass spectrometry is a powerful analytical technique used to identify and quantify analytes using the mass-to-charge ratio *(m/z)* of ions generated from a sample. It is useful for the analysis of a wide range of clinically relevant analytes, including small molecules, proteins, and peptides. When mass spectrometry is coupled with either gas or liquid chromatographs, the resultant analyzers have expanded analytical capabilities with widespread clinical applications, including quantitation of analytes from myriad body tissues and fluids. In addition, because of its ability to identify and quantify proteins, mass spectrometry is widely used in the field of proteomics.

Content
This chapter describes the basic concepts and definitions of mass spectrometry. Techniques based on mass spectrometry require an ionization step wherein an ion is produced from neutral atoms or molecules. Electron impact and chemical ionization (CI) are often used in gas chromatography–mass spectrometry. In liquid chromatography–mass spectrometry, electrospray ionization (ESI) and atmospheric pressure CI are the most commonly used techniques. In microbiology, a desorption/ionization technique termed MALDI (matrix-assisted laser desorption ionization) is employed. Each of these ionization techniques is described in detail, and advantages of the techniques are highlighted. Once molecules are ionized, resultant ions are analyzed using either beam type analyzers (eg, quadrupole, or time-of-flight [TOF]) or trapping mass analyzers (eg, ion trap). Mass analyzers also can be combined to form tandem mass spectrometers, which allow further expending capabilities of the technique. Clinical applications of mass spectrometry are provided to illustrate the role of this technique in the analysis of clinically relevant analytes.

Mass spectrometry (MS) is a powerful qualitative and quantitative analytical technique that is used to identify and quantify a wide range of clinically relevant analytes. When coupled with gas or liquid chromatographs, mass spectrometers allow expansion of analytical capabilities to a variety of clinical applications. In addition, because of its ability to identify and quantify proteins, MS is a key analytical tool in the field of proteomics.

We begin this chapter with a discussion of the basic concepts and definitions of MS, followed by discussions of MS instrumentation and clinical applications, and we end the chapter with a discussion of logistic, operational, and quality issues. In this chapter it is impossible to cover all concepts in a field as vast as MS, even if focus is limited to clinical applications. The Clinical and Laboratory Standards Institute (CLSI) has published recommendations on clinical MS that can serve as a good next step to study this topic and another gateway into the extensive literature on this topic.[1,2]

BASIC CONCEPTS AND DEFINITIONS

MS is the branch of physical chemistry (often also considered a branch of analytical chemistry) that deals with all aspects of instrumentation and the applications of this technique. *Molecular mass* (sometimes referred to as *molecular weight*) is measured in *unified atomic mass units* (u), also known as the *dalton* (Da), equal to 1/12 of the atomic mass of the most abundant isotope of a carbon atom in its lowest energy state, defined as 12 Da. Although the term *atomic mass unit* (amu) has been regarded as equivalent to the Da, it is only approximately equal to the dalton and now is considered an obsolete unit; its use to refer to the dalton is strongly discouraged.

Most MS data are presented in units of mass-to-charge ratio, or *m/z,* where *m* is the molecular weight of the ion (in daltons) and *z* is the number of charges present on the measured molecule. For small molecules (<1000 Da) there is typically only a single charge and therefore the *m/z* value is the same as the mass of the molecular ion. However, when larger molecules such as proteins or peptides are measured, they typically carry multiple ionic charges and therefore the *z* value is an integer greater than 1. In these cases the *m/z* value will be a fraction of the mass of the ion.

*The authors gratefully acknowledge the original contributions by Thomas M. Annesley, Nicholas E. Sherman, and Larry D. Bowers on which portions of this chapter are based. We also wish to acknowledge technical assistance by Leita Rogers, Jacquelyn McCowen-Rose, and Martha Fowles and helpful suggestions from N. Leigh Anderson, Julianne C. Botelho, Pierre Chaurand, David K. Crockett, Ulrich Eigner, Steven A. Hofstadler, Andrew N. Hoofnagle, Gary H. Kruppa, Donald Mason, Michael Morris, Maria M. Ospina, and Hubert W. Vesper.

All MS techniques require an initial *ionization* step in which an ion is produced from a neutral atom or molecule. Ions are formed in the ion source of the mass spectrometer. The development of versatile ionization techniques has allowed MS to become the excellent broad-spectrum analytical technique it is today; this was highlighted when, in 2002, John Fenn and Koichi Tanaka shared the Nobel Prize for their development of electrospray[3,4] and laser desorption[5-7] ionization, respectively. In the ion sources most commonly used with MS instruments in clinical chemistry, ionization in positive ion mode results from the addition of one (or more) protons to the basic sites on the molecule. This is referred to as protonation and leads to formation of a positively charged ion. The mass of the ion is greater than the mass of the uncharged neutral molecule by the added mass of one proton, approximately 1 Da, or multiples of a single proton mass (in case of multiply charged ions). Negatively charged ions (negative ion mode of MS operation) can be generated by the loss of a proton or addition of a negatively charged moiety (such as a hydroxyl group).

Ions may also be produced by removal of one or more electrons from a molecule using electron ionization (EI). This ionization method is historically the dominant ionization method used in MS (most commonly in gas chromatography–mass spectrometry [GC-MS] instruments) and is still used in some applications, but other ionization methods are now more frequently used in clinical laboratories. The removal of one electron produces a positively charged ion and reduces the mass by approximately 5×10^{-4} Da relative to the neutral molecule from which the ion is produced. This relatively small mass shift is often considered to be negligible and therefore ignored. More rarely, ions may be produced by addition of one electron to a molecule, producing a negative ion with mass approximately 5×10^{-4} Da greater than the neutral molecule from which the ion is produced. This small mass increment is also often considered to be negligible relative to the neutral molecule.

Ions formed in the ion source are separated according to *m/z* values in a mass analyzer. The term *mass analyzer* is in common use, although more correctly it would be termed an *m/z analyzer* given the fact that mass spectrometers separate ions according to *m/z*, not mass. This chapter will use the terms *mass analyzer* and *m/z analyzer* interchangeably.

While in a mass analyzer, ions may undergo *fragmentation,* whereby energy is imparted into the ionized analyte, causing internal bonds to break and resulting in the production of multiple independent unconnected chemical species. *Fragmentation can occur within different regions of the mass spectrometer and can occur due to the deliberate action of the operator or excessive energy imparted into the parent molecule as it is being ionized or passes through the vacuum region of the* mass analyzer. An unfragmented ion of the intact molecule is referred to as the *molecular ion, whereas the species that occur on fragmentation of the molecular ion are called the fragment ions. There is a certain ambiguity in the term molecular ion because in many cases the structure of the ion is not identical to the structure of the original neutral molecule* (eg, differing by the addition or removal of one or more protons, so the term *molecular ion* must be thought of in terms of an unfragmented ion whose structure is closely related to, but not necessarily identical to, the original uncharged molecule.

If the ionization of the analyte in the source produces little fragmentation, it is referred to as being soft, and the most abundant peak in the mass spectrum (the *base* peak) is often the molecular ion. If the ion source produces extensive fragmentation it is referred to as hard ionization, and the base peak in the resulting spectra may be one of the fragment ions. By convention, the base peak in a mass spectrum is assigned a relative abundance value of 100%.

Fragment ions that are formed in a separate dissociation cell (also known as the collision cell) inside a *tandem mass spectrometer* are known as *product ions, and the technique is called tandem mass spectrometry (MS/MS).* Ions that give rise to product ions are known as precursor ions. A tandem mass spectrometer consists of two mass spectrometers operated in sequence (MS/MS in space) or a single mass spectrometer capable of sequential fragmentation and measurement of ions within a single region of space (MS/MS in time). Most commonly in the clinical diagnostic methods, precursor ions are dissociated into product ions between the two stages of *m/z* analysis (MS/MS in space).

A *mass spectrum* is represented by the relative abundance of each ion plotted as a function of *m/z* (Fig. 17.1). As

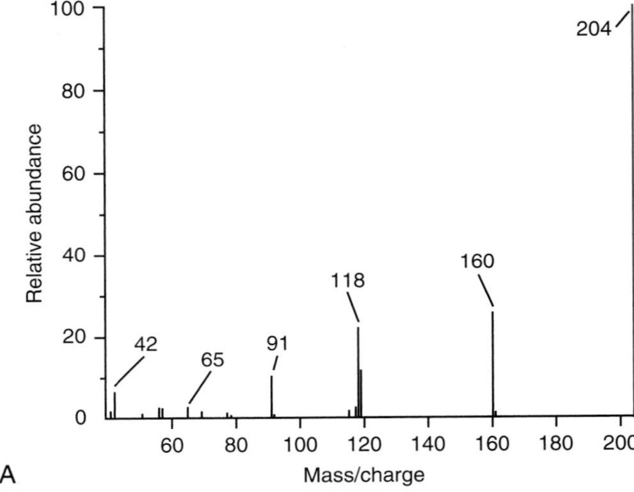

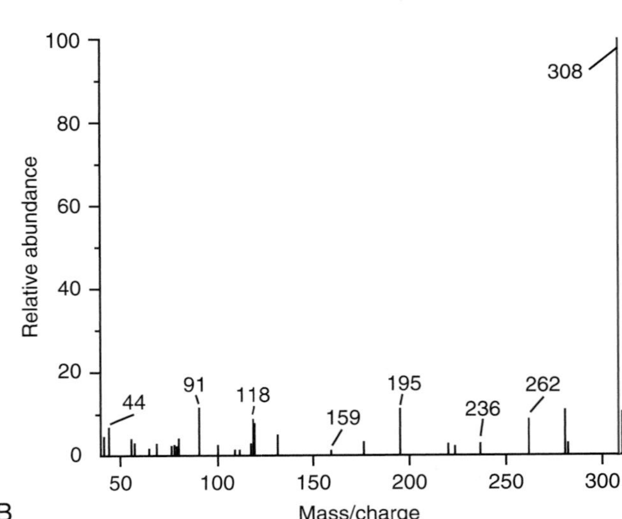

FIGURE 17.1 Mass spectrum of the pentafluoropropionyl **(A)** and carbethoxyhexafluorobutyryl **(B)** derivatives of D-methamphetamine.

mentioned earlier, for small molecules, usually each ion has a single charge ($z = 1$); thus the m/z ratio is equal to the mass of the ion and is approximately 1 Da greater than the neutral molecule from which the ion is formed. However, in some cases, the charge may be represented by an integer number greater than 1, in which case the m/z ratio is not equal to the mass of the ion, but rather is some fraction of the mass of the ion.

An ion may be positively charged, in which case the number of electrons in the ion is less than the sum of the number of protons in all nuclei of the ion, or negatively charged, in which case the number of electrons is greater than the number of protons. By convention, in MS z is taken as an absolute value. For example, $z = 1$ for both Na^+ and Cl^-.

Chemical interferences as well as higher background noise are more common for analytes with m/z 200 to 500 than for m/z less than 200 and m/z greater than 500. Monitoring ions with higher m/z often results in lower limits of detection because of the lower background noise and lower occurrence of isomers and isobars of the targeted molecules (ie, superior signal to noise).

A peak in a mass spectrum can be characterized by its *resolution* $[(m/z)/(\Delta m/z)]$, where $\Delta m/z$ is the width of the mass spectral peak. This parameter characterizes the ability of a mass spectrometer to separate nearby masses from each other. Typically the width of the peak is measured at 50% of the height of the peak and is referred to as the full width half height (FWHH) or full width half maximum (FWHM) resolution. A second frequently encountered definition for resolution is 10% valley. It defines *Δm/z as the distance between two peaks of equal intensity, spaced so that the valley between the peaks is 10% of the peak height* (Fig. 17.2). *This is a more conservative definition than FWHM because for a given quoted resolution (eg, 2000) the peaks are narrower under the 10% valley definition, hence better separated. High resolution is a desirable property in MS because it can help reduce interferences from nearby peaks in the mass spectrum, thereby allowing it to achieve a higher specificity.*

By setting the relative abundance of the base peak to 100% and therefore using the relative, rather than absolute, abundance of each ion fragment, instrument-dependent variability is minimized and the mass spectrum can be compared

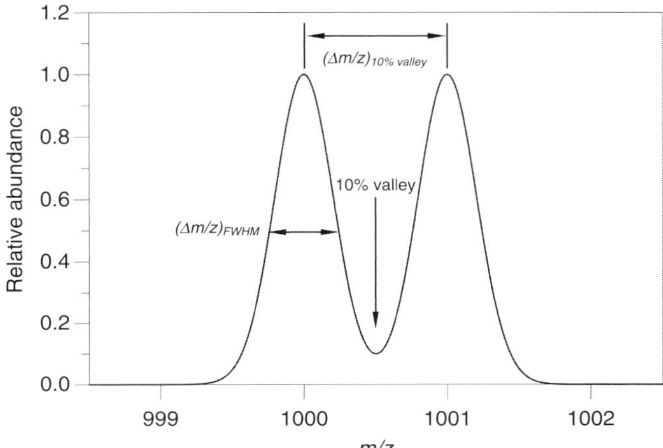

FIGURE 17.2 Parameters used to define resolution in mass spectrometry. *FWHM,* Full width half maximum.

with mass spectra obtained on other instruments. Because fragmentation at specific bonds depends on their chemical nature and strength of the bonds, the mass spectrum can be interpreted in terms of the molecular structure of the analyte. In some cases, the chemical structure of the analyte can be deduced or at least reconciled with features found in the mass spectrum. Computer-based libraries of mass spectra are also available to assist in identification of the analyte(s) based on fragmentation pattern. In some applications, the mass spectrum of an analyte may be matched against mass spectra in a database, thereby identifying the analyte by its mass spectral *fingerprint*. In general, an unknown is considered to be identified if the relative abundances of three or four ion fragments agree within ±20% of those from a reference compound and the relative abundances of the fragments, monoisotopic and isotopic ions of the molecular ion are in agreement with the relative abundances of the reference mass spectrum.

When interfaced to a liquid or gas chromatograph, the mass spectrometer functions as a powerful detector, providing structural information in real time on individual analytes as they elute from a chromatographic column. Depending on the operating characteristics of the mass spectrometer and the chromatographic peak width, multiple mass spectral scans can be acquired across the peak. The data also can be displayed as a function of time to yield a *total ion chromatogram in which at each time point in the chromatogram the abundances of all ions in a mass spectrum are summed to constitute a single point in the ion chromatogram, regardless of m/z.*

The mass spectrometer can be considered to be close to a universal detector because molecules of many identities may be ionized and then detected in a mass spectrometer. Furthermore there are different MS operation modes and different types of fragmentation that can be applied to provide different types of data, giving more information about the measured compound(s). Finally, the instrument data system can analyze and display the collected data in various manners, allowing the operator to selectively extract information from the acquired data.

For example, it is possible to display chromatograms of only preselected ions acquired during data acquisition—that is, representing data from only part of the mass spectrum. The resultant display of data is called an *extracted ion chromatogram,* displaying signal intensity plotted as a function of time; peak heights or peak areas can be integrated for use in quantitative analysis. Use of the extracted ion chromatogram allows selecting data corresponding to the analyte of interest, as identified by its m/z, while disregarding data corresponding to different m/z. With high-resolution instruments, specificity of analysis can be improved by use of narrow m/z windows for plotting extracted ion chromatograms. Such data processing results in a reduced number of overlapping chromatographic peaks from ions of nearby m/z thus improving the quantitative accuracy and the specificity (Fig. 17.3).

Sample preparation is critical to successful MS, particularly when dealing with complex matrices, such as are commonly encountered in clinical chemistry. This typically involves one or more of the following steps: (1) protein precipitation followed by centrifugation or filtration, (2) solid-phase extraction, (3) liquid-liquid extraction, (4) affinity enrichment, or (5) *derivatization* (see Chapter 18).

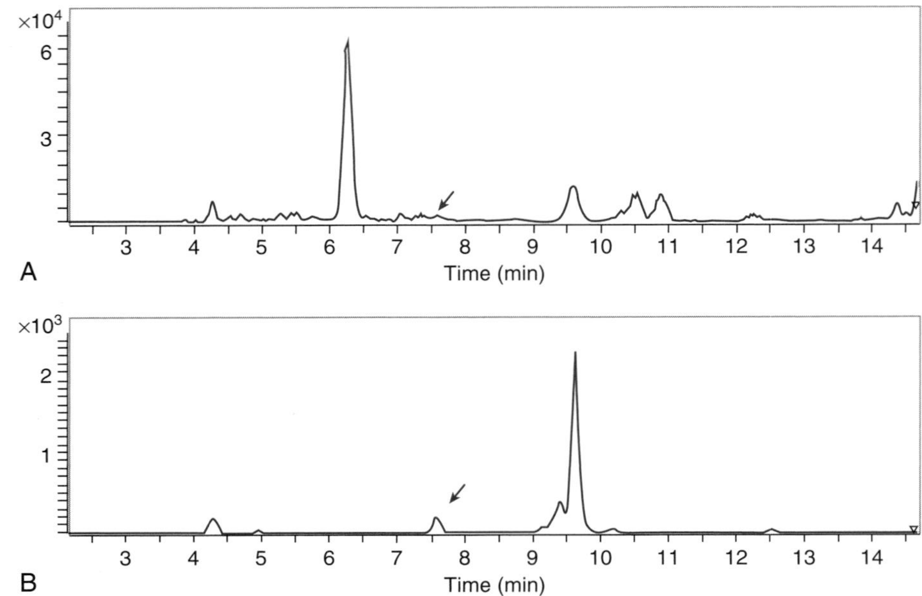

FIGURE 17.3 Extracted ion chromatograms for a peptide ion of *m/z* 761.3718 using a window of 1 Da **(A)** and 0.0076 Da **(B)**. *Arrows* point on peak that is completely hidden in the chemical background noise while resolved from the noise using mass extraction window of 0.0076 Da.

Derivatization is the process of chemically modifying the target compound(s) to be more favorably analyzed by MS. Derivatization usually involves the addition of some well-defined functional group. The goals of derivatization vary, depending on the application, but typically include (1) increased volatility, (2) greater thermal stability, (3) modified chromatographic properties, (4) greater ionization efficiency, (5) favorable fragmentation properties, or a combination of these.

Analysis by MS can be used to target specific known compounds (targeted analysis) or seek to identify one or more unknown compounds in a sample (screening). When only one or a few targeted analytes are of interest for quantitative analysis and their mass spectrum is known, the mass spectrometer is set to monitor only those ions of interest. This selective detection technique is known as *selected ion monitoring* (SIM). Because SIM focuses on a limited number of ions, more data points are collected for the selected *m/z, which results in better, more precise measurements.* The SIM data acquisition increases the signal-to-noise ratio for the analyte of interest, improves the lower limit of detection, and enables more accurate quantitation. One drawback of SIM is that it is based around measurement of a nominal analyte mass. Most biological samples are highly complex, and thus it is not unexpected to find multiple compounds with very close or identical masses in the matrix. In those cases, chromatography can aid in separation of these isobars; however, they still can affect a SIM result should the isobar not be separated completely from the analyte to be measured. By using a triple-quadrupole mass analyzer, a method known as selected reaction monitoring (SRM) (or generalized for the analysis of many ions at the same time, multiple reaction monitoring [MRM]) can be used to help alleviate such potential issues. This is where the first quadrupole instrument is set to transmit the *m/z* of the molecular ion, the analyte is caused to fragment in the second quadrupole and the third quadrupole is set to transmit the *m/z* of one or more known fragment ions from the analyte. In this manner data similar to those gathered by SIM can be produced but with added specificity from the structural information gathered by the use of the fragment ion as a gatekeeper. A more detailed description of MRM is given in the section of this chapter on tandem mass spectrometers.

Screening methods (used here in the analytical chemistry sense, not to be confused with screening in a clinical or medical sense) are less common in clinical chemistry than the analysis of target compounds; the main task for screening methods is qualitative identification of unknowns in a sample. In most cases this reduces to the problem of matching chromatographic retention time and fragment ion patterns, that is, mass and abundance patterns of either fragment ions generated in the source of a single-stage mass spectrometer or product ions from a collision cell in a tandem mass spectrometer.

A chemical element may be composed of a single or multiple isotopes. Each isotope of an element has the same number of protons in its nucleus but different numbers of neutrons. For example, naturally occurring carbon is composed primarily of two isotopes: ^{12}C, whose nuclei contain six protons and six neutrons, and ^{13}C, whose nuclei contain six protons and seven neutrons. (Here we ignore ^{14}C, which is generally of negligible abundance compared to the other two isotopes.) The natural abundance of ^{12}C is approximately 98.9%, and the natural abundance of ^{13}C is approximately 1.1%. Some elements, such as arsenic, have only a single isotope in the naturally occurring state, whereas other elements, such as tin, may have as many as 10 naturally occurring isotopes.

When a compound is made of multiple atoms the isotope pattern is a convolution of the isotope patterns of the individual atoms. To illustrate with a simple example, carbon monoxide (CO) has the following combinations of isotopes $^{12}C^{16}O$ (molecular weight 28), $^{13}C^{16}O$ (molecular weight 29),

$^{12}C^{17}O$ (molecular weight 29), $^{12}C^{18}O$ (molecular weight 30), and $^{13}C^{18}O$ (molecular weight 31).

Nitrogen (N_2) is isobaric with CO; that is, it has nearly the same mass. However, the accurate masses of the isotope peaks of isobars may differ. For example, the monoisotopic mass of $^{12}C^{16}O^+$ (the isotopic peak composed of the most abundant atomic isotopes) has an accurate mass of 27.9944 Da, whereas the isobaric mass 28 Da peak of N_2^+ has an accurate molecular mass of 28.0056 Da. The small difference in masses of isobars can be used to infer the chemical formula of a compound or to confirm the identity of a target compound. This technique requires a mass analyzer capable of mass accuracy of a few parts per million, is limited to compounds of a few hundred Da or less, and it is not capable of discriminating between isobars of the same chemical formula.

Compounds that have the same chemical formulas but different chemical structures are also isobars and might therefore be referred to as strict isobars because they have exactly the same mass. Succinic acid and methylmalonic acid provide an example of a pair of compounds that are strict isobars because they have the same chemical formula ($C_4H_6O_4$). Unlike isobars that have nearly the same masses but different accurate masses, strict isobars cannot be separated or distinguished by MS alone, although they often can be separated if MS is combined with a separation method or if tandem MS is applied.

Isotopic information also can be used to identify a compound in a different way. Using CO^+ and N_2^+ as examples, the first three isotopic peaks of CO^+ have a relative abundance pattern of 0.986, 0.011, and 0.002, whereas the first three isotope peaks of N_2^+ has a pattern of 0.993, 0.007, and 0.000. Differences in the isotopic pattern can be used to infer the chemical formula of an unknown or to confirm chemical identity of a target compound. This technique requires accurate measurement of relative isotopic peak abundances and is sometimes used in conjunction with accurate mass measurements, particularly when using TOF mass spectrometers.

A distinct advantage of the mass spectrometer is that it can distinguish between ions of the same chemical formula that have different masses because of the different isotopic composition. To illustrate with a trivial and simple example, $^{12}C^{16}O^+$ has a different mass than $^{12}C^{18}O^+$, and these two forms can be separated and detected in a mass spectrometer. One can take advantage of this fact by using artificially labeled forms of a target analyte. The labeling consists of substitution of a less common isotope for one or more of the atoms in the analyte, for example, substituting ^2H for ^1H, ^{13}C for ^{12}C, or ^{15}N for ^{14}N. The substituted molecule is prepared artificially and added to the sample as an internal standard, which behaves nearly identically to the native compounds during sample preparation and chromatographic separation. In this respect, ^{13}C or ^{15}N is generally preferred over ^2H labeling because ^2H-labeled compounds sometimes exhibit chromatographic shifts compared to unlabeled compounds, whereas ^{13}C- or ^{15}N-labeled compounds generally do not. A quantitative analysis can then be carried out by comparison of the signal from the native compound versus the artificially added labeled version of the compound spiked into the sample.

An internal standard should be selected to have a sufficient number of isotopic ions so that no naturally occurring isotopes (such as ^2H or ^{13}C) of the analyte of interest would significantly contribute to the signal of the internal standard. For the methamphetamine derivatives shown in Figure 17.4, *A*, an internal standard with at least three ^2H or ^{13}C atoms is preferred, because contribution of the natural abundance of these isotopes to the molecular ion [$(M + 3)^+$] would be ≈0.1%. The position of the stable isotope atoms within the molecule and the number of isotopic ions within the structure is also important for adequate performance of the methods.[8] For example, the *m/z* 204 ion for methamphetamine represents the aliphatic portion of the molecule (loss of the aromatic ring). If three deuterium atoms were located on the aromatic ring of the pentafluoropropionyl derivative of methamphetamine, the native and the isotope-labeled

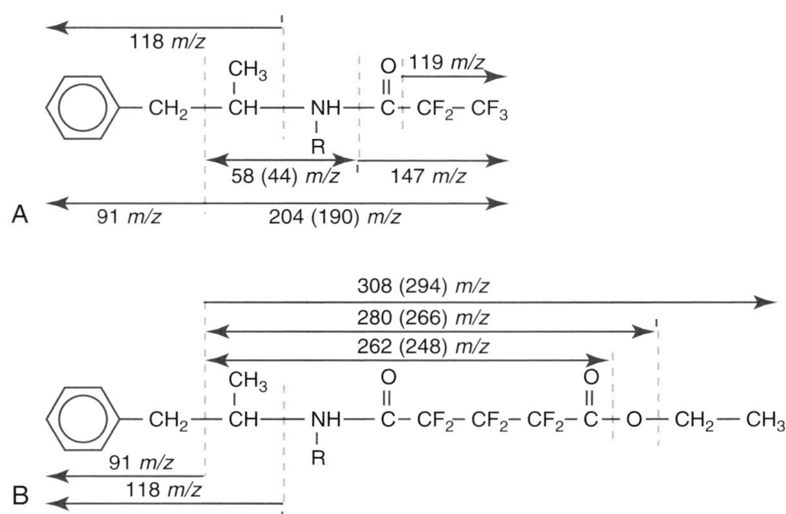

FIGURE 17.4 Fragmentation patterns for the pentafluoropropionyl **(A)** and carbethoxyhexafluorobutyryl **(B)** derivatives of methamphetamine (R = CH_3) and amphetamine (R = H; *masses in parentheses*). Compare the predicted masses with the spectrum shown in Figure 17.1. Note that for the pentafluoropropionyl derivative, only one ion [204 (190) *m/z*] is characteristic of the aliphatic portion of the molecule.

molecules would both yield the *m/z* 204 ion. This *m/z* 204 ion would therefore fail to distinguish the native compound from the isotope-labeled compound and would therefore not be useful as an internal standard. On the other hand, if ^2H labeling were to occur in the aliphatic portion of the molecule, the fragment ion analogous to the *m/z* 204 fragment ion would be labeled, producing a higher *m/z* than 204 (eg, 207), and the ion could be useful as an internal standard. The same comments apply to the compound illustrated in Figure 17.4, *B*.

These concepts of internal standard selection must be modified slightly when applied to tandem MS. For example, it is possible for a native compound and the internal standard to have product ions of the same *m/z*, because they can be distinguished by their differing precursor ion masses.

When using hydrogen (^2H) labeling the stable isotope must be located on atoms from which it will not be exchangeable with hydrogen atoms in solution or in gas phase (in the ion source). For example, deuterium labeling of an acidic hydrogen position would be useless because the ^2H would easily exchange with protons in the matrix, making the original labeling moot. Certain other labeling positions also must be avoided. The hydrogen atoms in the constituent groups of alcohols, amines, amides, and thiols all may readily exchange with hydrogen ions in an aqueous matrix.

A technique of quantitative analysis of compounds relative to their isotopic analogs added to the samples at known or fixed concentration is called *isotope dilution analysis* or isotope dilution mass spectrometry (IDMS). The IDMS technique has been used to develop definitive methods for a number of clinically relevant analytes, including drugs of abuse and disease markers.

MS is often referred to as a highly sensitive technique. *Sensitivity* is a somewhat problematic term because it is used in two different ways. In an official definition[9,10] it means the slope of a calibration curve (or more generally, a change in signal vs the change in concentration), but far more commonly it is used to signify the ability to detect or quantify an analyte at very low concentration; that is, a highly sensitive technique would be able to detect or quantify a very low concentration of the target analyte.

INSTRUMENTATION

A mass spectrometer consists of (1) an ion source, (2) a vacuum system, (3) a mass analyzer, (4) a detector, and (5) a computer (Fig. 17.5).

Ion Source

Many approaches have been used to form ions in both high-vacuum and near-atmospheric pressure conditions. EI and CI are ionization techniques used when gas-phase molecules are introduced directly into an ion source operated at very low pressure, often from a gas chromatograph. In other analyses, such as high-performance liquid chromatography–mass spectrometry (HPLC-MS), ESI, *atmospheric pressure chemical ionization* (APCI), and *atmospheric pressure photoionization* (APPI) ion sources are often used.[11-14] Ionization in these three ion sources takes place at atmospheric pressure. Other ionization techniques include (1) *inductively coupled plasma* (ICP), (2) MALDI (see Chapter 19), (3) *atmospheric pressure matrix-assisted laser desorption ionization*, and others. This chapter will limit its discussion primarily to ion sources of interest to clinical applications of MS. The CLSI documents C-50A and C-62A contain recommendations for matching the capabilities of different ion source technologies to various application classes.[1,2]

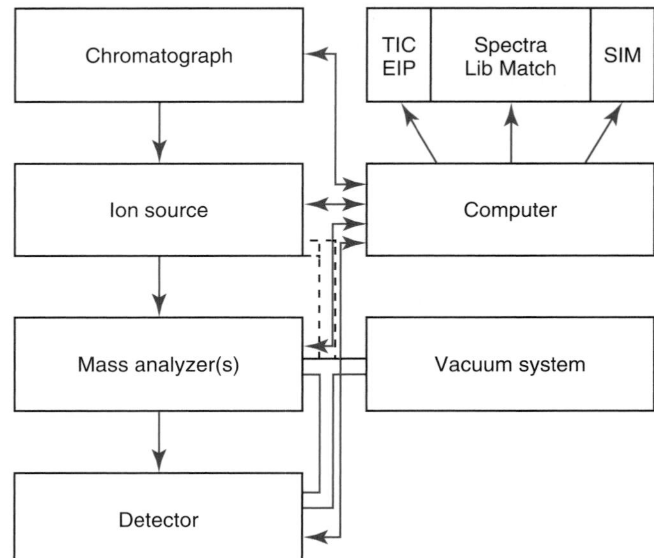

FIGURE 17.5 Block diagram of the components of a chromatograph–mass spectrometer system. The mass analyzer and the detector are always under vacuum. The ion source may be under vacuum or under near-atmospheric pressure conditions, depending on the ionization mode. The computer system is an integral part of data acquisition and output. *EIP*, Extracted ion profile; *SIM*, selected ion monitoring; *TIC*, total ion current.

Electron Ionization

In EI, gas-phase molecules are bombarded by electrons emitted from a heated filament and attracted to a collector electrode (Fig. 17.6). To prevent filament oxidation, as well as to minimize scattering of the electron beam, this process must occur in a vacuum. EI is typically performed using electrons with a kinetic energy of 70 eV; collision of electrons having such energy with most organic molecules results in formation of *radical* cations, that is, a structure that is both a positively charged ion and a radical.[15] A radical is a molecule or ion with an unpaired electron. The radical ion then often undergoes unimolecular rearrangement and dissociation to produce a cation and an uncharged radical:

$$AB^{+\cdot} \rightarrow A^{+} + B^{\cdot}$$

Positive ions are drawn out of the ionization chamber by an electrical field. The cations are then electrostatically focused and introduced into the mass analyzer. EI is primarily used as an ion source in GC-MS. Because the same ion energy (70 eV) is used in commercial instruments using EI, and because the fragmentation pattern is only weakly dependent on small deviations from 70 eV, fragmentation patterns observed using an EI source are reasonably reproducible among the GC-MS instruments. The fragmentation pattern is therefore often used as a fingerprint to identify compounds by matching mass spectra of unknowns to the entries in the mass spectral libraries.

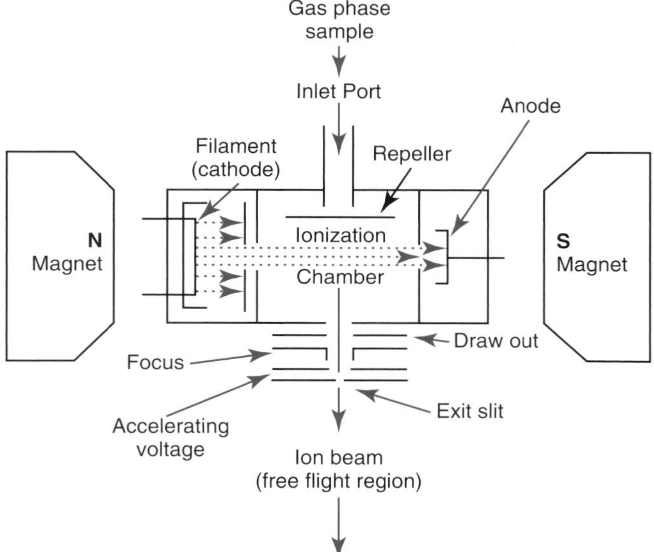

FIGURE 17.6 Electron impact ion source. The small magnets are used to collimate a dense electron beam, which is drawn from a heated filament placed at a negative potential. The electron beam is positioned in front of a repeller, which is at a slightly positive potential compared with the ion source. The repeller sends any positively charged fragment ions toward the opening at the front of the ion source. The accelerating plates strongly attract the positively charged fragment ions.

Chemical Ionization

CI is a soft ionization technique in which a proton is transferred to, or abstracted from, a gas-phase molecule by a reagent gas molecule such as methane, ammonia (NH_3), isobutane, or water. The reagent gas is supplied into a CI ion source at a pressure of about 0.1 torr. (*Note:* For virtually all practical purposes, torr is equivalent to millimeters of mercury and is the more customary term used in the field of MS). An electron beam produces reactive species through a series of ion-molecule reactions, intermediate species (such as methonium [CH_5^+] if methane is the CI reagent gas); further ion-molecule reactions can cause analyte ions to become charged, usually via attachment of a proton. In most cases, relatively little fragmentation occurs, and for the majority of the molecules, only molecular ions (in the form of a protonated version of the neutral molecule) are observed in the mass spectra; the lack of fragmentation enhances sensitivity of detection. Negative ion electron capture CI has become popular for quantification of drugs such as benzodiazepines. Negative ions are formed when thermalized electrons are captured by electronegative functional groups, such as chlorine or fluorine atoms within structure of the molecule. Negative ion CI often leads to very low limits of detection.

Electrospray Ionization

ESI is a soft ionization technique in which a sample is ionized at atmospheric pressure before introduction into the mass analyzer.[16,17] An effluent from a separation device, typically an HPLC, is passed through a narrow metal or fused silica capillary to which a 1- to 5-kV voltage has been applied (Fig. 17.7, *A*). The partial charge separation between the liquid and the capillary results in instability in the liquid that

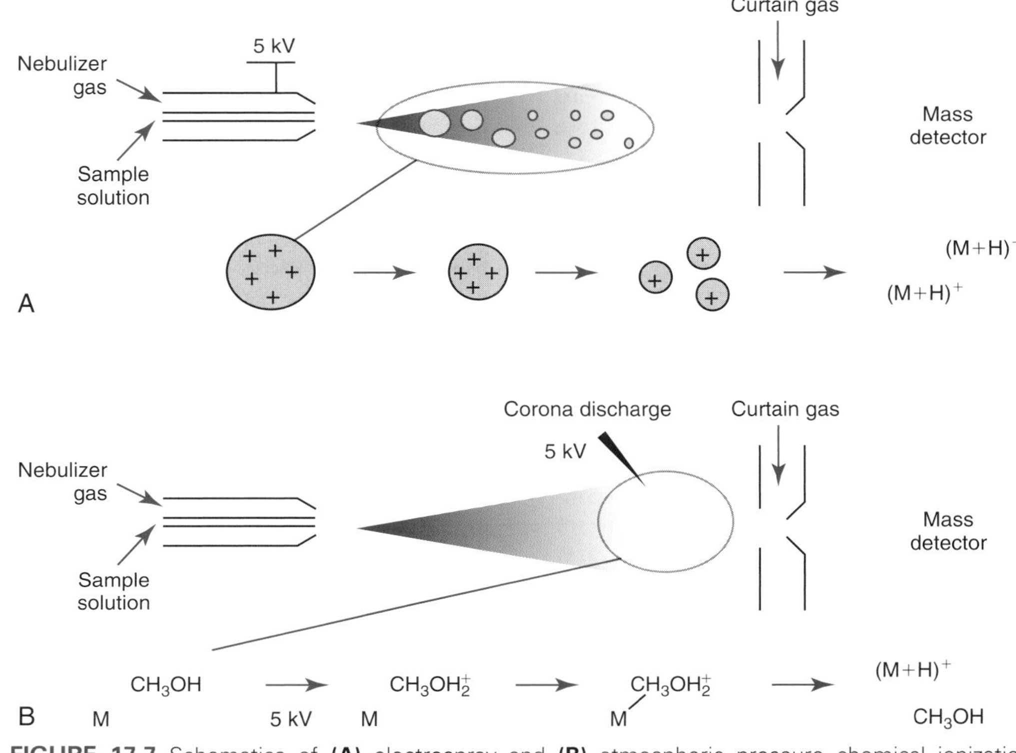

FIGURE 17.7 Schematics of **(A)** electrospray and **(B)** atmospheric pressure chemical ionization sources. Note the different points where ionization occurs, as described in the text.

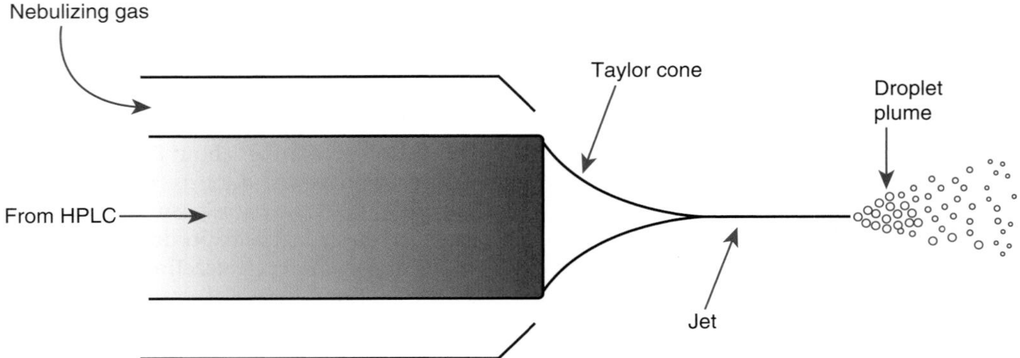

FIGURE 17.8 Simplified conceptual schematic of electrospray ion source showing Taylor cone. *HPLC,* High-performance liquid chromatography. (Published with permission from Eclipse Business Media Ltd. Reprinted from MS Solutions, Issue 7 [2010]. http://www.sepscience.com/Information/Archive/MS-Solutions/235-/MS-Solutions-7-Adjusting-Electrospray-Voltage-for-Optimum-Results.)

in turn results in expulsion of charged droplets from a Taylor cone, which forms at the tip of the capillary (Fig. 17.8). In many variations of ESI a coaxial nebulizing gas aids in nebulization and helps direct the charged droplets toward a counter-electrode as well as speeding up the evaporative process. As droplets evaporate while migrating through the atmospheric pressure region, they expel smaller droplets as the charge-to-volume ratio exceeds the Raleigh instability limit. The adducts of the molecules (with solvent molecules, NH_3, etc.) are desolvated to form bare ions that are typically formed in the ionization process. However, other ionization products are sometimes observed, such as metal ion adducts, or ions formed by redox processes. Ions then pass through a sampling cone and one or more extraction cones (skimmers) before entering the high-vacuum region of the mass analyzer.

One feature of ESI is the production of multiple charged ions, particularly from peptides and proteins. It is common to observe approximately one charge for every 10 to 15 amino acid residues in a protein. For example, for a molecule of mass 20,000, 20 charges supplied by the addition of 20 protons would be detected at m/z approximately 1000 [or more correctly, m/z 1001 = (20,000 + 20)/20]. This phenomenon greatly extends the accessible mass range of an instrument. It is frequently observed that a distribution of charges occurs; in cases of multiple charged molecules, one usually observes a series of peaks, with each peak corresponding to a different number of charges. Multiply charged ions are also observed for nucleic acid polymers, particularly when ESI mass spectra are acquired in negative ion mode.

It should be noted that Figure 17.7 is a simplified illustration of the probe being directed toward the sampling cone of the mass detector. To enhance performance and minimize contamination of the mass analyzer, modern hardware configurations have offset the probe and/or the mass detector relative to the sampling cone; in some instruments the spray is orthogonal to the sampling cone.

ESI tends to be an efficient ion source for polar compounds or for molecules that are present as ions in solution, which includes a majority of biomolecules. ESI, along with APCI, allows an effective interface between a liquid chromatograph and a mass spectrometer. ESI and APCI have become the most widely used ion sources in mass spectrometers used in clinical laboratories.

As already mentioned, electrospray is considered a soft ionization source. However, it is also possible to generate fragment ions before mass analysis using a technique known as nozzle-skimmer dissociation,[18] infrared multiphoton dissociation,[19] and thermally induced dissociation.[20] In these methods, ions are heated before entering the mass analyzer, and this causes ions to dissociate into fragment ions. In nozzle-skimmer dissociation, a higher than normal voltage gradient is applied in the first low-pressure region of the electrospray interface, resulting in collisional heating of the ions. In infrared multiphoton dissociation, ions are subjected to an intense bombardment of infrared photons, resulting in heating of the ions, followed by dissociation. In thermally induced dissociation, ions are activated and dissociated by excess heating of the gas used to transport ions from atmospheric pressure to the vacuum system of the mass spectrometer.

Atmospheric Pressure Chemical Ionization

APCI is similar to ESI in the sense that ionization takes place at atmospheric pressure, involves nebulization and desolvation, and uses the same design of the ion extraction cone as ESI. The major difference lies in the mode of ionization. In APCI, no high voltage is applied to the inlet capillary. Instead, the mobile phase from the separation device gets evaporated and the vapor passes by a needle with applied current.[21] This process generates a corona discharge. Somewhat analogously to the processes occurring in a CI source, ions generated by the corona discharge undergo variety of ion-molecule reactions such as the following:

$$CH_3OH + H^+ \rightarrow CH_3OH_2^+$$

$$A(\text{analyte}) + CH_3OH_2^+ \rightarrow AH^+ + CH_3OH$$

or

$$H_2O + H^+ \rightarrow H_3O^+$$

$$A(\text{analyte}) + H_3O^+ \rightarrow AH^+ + H_2O$$

Because solvent molecules from the evaporated mobile phase (eg, water, methanol, acetonitrile) are present in the vapor in excess relative to the sample constituents, they are predominantly ionized early in the ion molecule cascade of reactions and then act as a reagent gas that reacts secondarily to ionize analyte molecules (see Fig. 17.7, *B*). The products of these secondary reactions may contain clusters of solvent and analyte molecules, and thus a heated transfer tube or a countercurrent flow of a curtain gas, such as nitrogen, is used to decluster the ions. As with ESI, APCI is a soft ionization technique that produces relatively little fragmentation. However, unlike ESI, APCI uses much higher heat and this can cause pyrolysis of the compound leading to loss of metabolically induced modifications to targeted compounds (glucuronidation, glutathionylation, etc.) and therefore can cause issues with analyses (in the methods that do not chromatographically resolve peaks of unconjugated and conjugated targeted molecules). On the other hand, in methods using ESI at lower temperature, those modifications tend to remain intact. When compared with EI, the mass spectra produced by APCI, ESI, and other soft ionization techniques typically have fewer fragments and are less useful for analyte identification by mass spectral fingerprinting. However, because the ion current is concentrated into a single mass spectral peak (or relatively few mass spectral peaks), APCI and other soft ionization sources are well matched to the requirements of tandem MS (discussed later) and are well suited for quantitative analysis. APCI and ESI are the most commonly used ion sources in quantitative analysis. However, in the case of nonpolar compounds such as steroids and some drug molecules, APCI is often a more efficient ion source than ESI.

Atmospheric Pressure Photoionization

APPI is a relatively new and less frequently used ion source in clinical chemistry that provides a complementary ionization approach to ESI or APCI. The physical configuration of an APPI source is similar to that for APCI, but an ultraviolet photon flux (typically Krypton lamp that emits photons at 10 Ev) is used instead of a corona discharge needle to generate ions in the gas phase.[22-24] In APPI, an ionizable dopant, such as toluene or acetone, is often infused coaxially to the nebulizer to provide a source of ions that participate in charge or proton transfer to analyte molecules, thus increasing the efficiency of analyte ionization. APPI has a similar range of application to APCI and could be more useful than APCI for compounds of very low polarity, such as some steroids.

Inductively Coupled Plasma

ICP, as ESI, APCI, and APPI, is an atmospheric pressure ionization method. However, unlike most atmospheric pressure ionization methods, which are soft (ie, producing little fragmentation), ICP is the ultimate in hard ionization, typically leading to complete atomization of the sample during ionization. Consequently, its primary use is for elemental analysis. In the clinical laboratory, it is particularly useful for trace element analysis in tissues or body fluids. ICP is extremely sensitive (eg, parts per trillion limits of detection) and is capable of extremely wide dynamic ranges.

After sample preparation, which generally includes the addition of an internal standard such as yttrium and sometimes includes an acid digestion step, the sample is introduced into the ion source, usually via a nebulizer fed by a peristaltic pump. The nebulized sample is transmitted into hot plasma generated at atmospheric pressure by inductively coupling power into the plasma using a high-powered, radiofrequency (RF) generator (Fig. 17.9).[25] The temperature of the plasma is typically 6000 to 10,000 K (comparable to the temperature of the surface of the sun). Sample is introduced in the plasma, and ions are transmitted to the mass analyzer through a series of differential pumping stages. The atmospheric sampling apparatus is conceptually similar to that of other atmospheric pressure ion sources, such as electrospray, except that the device must withstand the extremely high temperatures generated by the plasma.

ICP-MS is comparatively free from most interference. However, some interfering species can be extremely troublesome. Most interfering species are small polyatomic ions formed in the torch via ion-molecule reactions. For example, argon oxide (ArO^+) interferes with iron at *m/z* 56. One solution to this problem is to use a reaction cell, which consists of a moderate-pressure gas region in front of the *m/z* analyzer,[26] with a reactant gas, such as NH_3, bled into the reaction cell. The reactant gas reacts with polyatomic interferences and removes them before introduction into the *m/z* analyzer. A

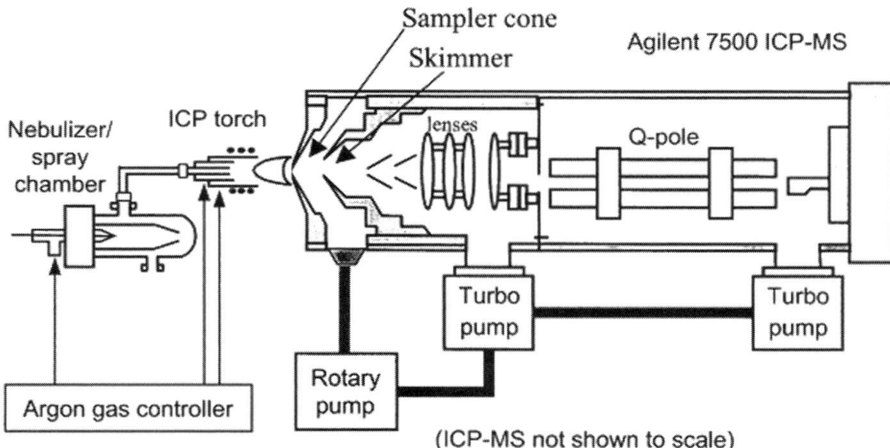

FIGURE 17.9 Simplified conceptual schematic of inductively coupled plasma–mass spectrometer *(ICP-MS). Q-pole,* Quadrupole. (From Kannamkumarath S, Wrobel K, Wrobel K, et al. Capillary electrophoresis–inductively coupled plasma-mass spectrometry: an attractive complementary technique for elemental speciation analysis. *J Chromatogr A* 2002;975:245–266.)

related technique uses a nonreactive collision gas, which removes interferences using collisions, relying on differences in collision cross-sections between polyatomic ions and atomic ions. Another approach to removing interferences of the same nominal mass is to use a high-resolution mass spectrometer, which is capable of resolving species with similar nominal mass.[26] For example, the masses of ArO^+ and $^{56}Fe^+$ differ by 0.022 Da—a difference that may be resolved using a high-resolution mass spectrometer.

Matrix-Assisted Laser Desorption Ionization

MALDI is another type of soft ionization method that typically produces singly charged ions. MALDI and related techniques rely on energy transfer processes from a pulsed laser beam to the sample for ion generation. In most cases, the analyte is dissolved in a solution containing a solid phase matrix, a small molecular weight UV-absorbing compound, and this solution is placed on a target and dried. A pulsed laser irradiates the dried spots, triggering ablation, and desorption of the sample and matrix material; ions produced in the process are accelerated and introduced into the mass analyzer (Fig. 17.10). In other cases a layer of the solid matrix is deposited on the target and allowed to crystalize, and then the sample applied on top. The sample causes the top portion of the matrix to solubilize and mix with the sample before recrystallizing. In this way the sample is maintained in the very outer layer of the matrix, and this can help with enhancing the sensitivity and reducing the background noise. A related technique includes atmospheric pressure matrix-assisted laser desorption/ionization, in which the MALDI process occurs at atmospheric pressure rather than reduced pressure (see Chapter 19).

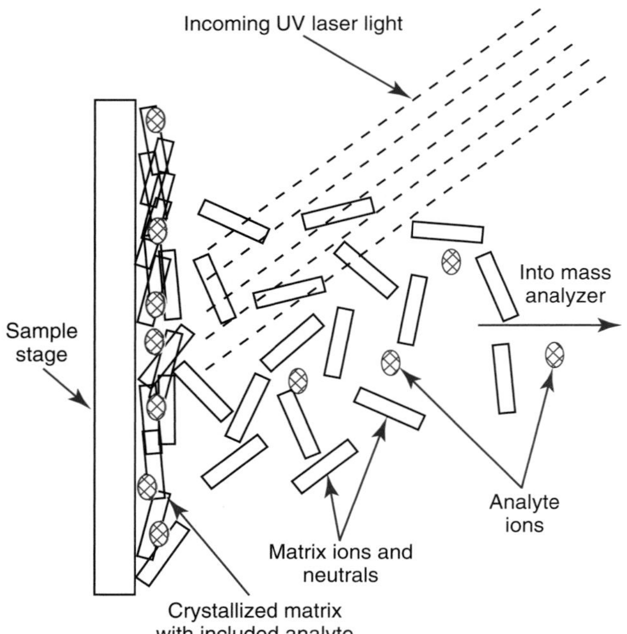

FIGURE 17.10 A generic view of the process of matrix-assisted laser desorption ionization. Co-crystallized matrix and analyte molecules are irradiated with an ultraviolet *(UV)* laser. The laser vaporizes the matrix, producing a plume of matrix ions, analyte ions, and neutrals. Gas-phase ions are directed into a mass analyzer.

Ionization Methods of Potential Interest

Desorption electrospray ionization (DESI)[27] and direct analysis in real time (DART)[28] are two relatively new ionization methods that generate ions from surfaces at atmospheric pressure. Most applications of DESI and DART to date have been directed toward minimal sample preparation. Paper spray MS is another emerging ionization method of potential interest. It is essentially a version of electrospray MS, but the spray is generated at the point of a triangular cut in a solvent-wetted piece of paper rather than from a capillary. It has the feature of easily integrating paper chromatography with MS.[29] It also has been used for rapid measurement of therapeutic drugs from dried blood spots without the need for complex sample preparation and separation.[30]

Ionization Methods of Historical Interest

The older literature includes several ionization methods or sample introduction methods that, although promising, or even widely used at one time, hold little interest for current practice in clinical chemistry. Nevertheless, it is useful to be aware of them because they may still be referred to in the literature from time to time. Some of these include (1) *fast atom bombardment*, (2) *thermospray*, (3) *direct liquid introduction*, (4) *plasma desorption*, (5) *field ionization*, (6) *field desorption*, (7) *secondary ion mass spectrometry*, and (8) *laser desorption*. ESI and APCI ion sources have largely rendered these techniques obsolete.

Vacuum System

With the exception of certain ion trap mass spectrometers, ion separation in any of the mass analyzers requires that the ions do not collide with other molecules during their interaction with magnetic or electric fields. This requires the use of a vacuum from 10^{-3} to 10^{-9} torr, depending on mass analyzer type. The length of the ion path in the analyzer must be less than the mean free path length, unless collisions play a role in mass analysis.

Fourier transform ion cyclotron resonance (FT-ICR) requires the lowest pressure (10^{-9} torr). The quadrupole ion trap (QIT) tolerates the highest pressure (10^{-3} to 10^{-5} torr), a pressure range in which some collisions occur between ions and background gas. Routine quality assurance checks for vacuum leaks should include evaluation of the presence of air and water in the mass spectra.

Efficient high-vacuum pumps generally do not operate well near atmospheric pressure. Thus the vacuum system must have a positive displacement (mechanical) vacuum pump to evacuate the system to a pressure at which the high-vacuum pumps are effective. Mechanical pumps require routine maintenance, such as ballasting and replacing the pump oil.

Although diffusion pumps are the least expensive and most reliable high-vacuum pump, they are rarely used outside of some very specialized mass spectrometers that typically are not used in the clinical laboratory. Cryopumps are another class of pumps that are sometimes used in specialized mass spectrometers but not in the clinical laboratory. In modern instruments, the most common high-vacuum pumps are turbomolecular (often referred to as "turbo") pumps; they have largely replaced diffusion pumps and cryopumps because they are more convenient to use. A key consideration in the design of the vacuum system is pumping speed. The ability of the pump to maintain the vacuum by removing any gas (or solvent vapor) that enters the system determines the maximum flow rate of gas introduced into the mass spectrometer. In general, higher pump capacities are associated with lower detection limits because noise arising from the gas background is reduced.

Mass Analyzers, Tandem Mass Spectrometers, and Ion Detectors

The term *mass spectrometry* is somewhat a misnomer because mass spectrometers do not measure molecular mass, but rather they measure the mass-to-charge ratio. This fact is fundamental to the physical operating principles of mass spectrometers and consequently affects all aspects of instrumentation design, instrument operation, and interpretation of results. The symbol *m/z* is used to denote mass-to-charge ratio and conventionally has been defined as a dimensionless quantity[31] (see also http://goldbook.iupac.org/M03752.html).

However, a "dimensionless" mass-to-charge ratio is not consistent with equations of ion motion in the presence of electric and magnetic fields, which require units of mass divided by charge. Furthermore, the *m/z* scale sometimes is loosely discussed in terms of daltons (also known as unified atomic mass units [u]), although strictly speaking, Da is a unit of mass, not mass-to-charge ratio. Despite these somewhat confusing nomenclature issues, the present chapter generally follows convention by discussing *m/z* in terms of mass and Da.

To help avoid some of the confusion surrounding the use of *m/z,* it has been proposed that it should be defined explicitly as quantity having units of mass-to-charge ratio, with mass specified in daltons and charge specified in elementary charges; this proposed unit would be called the *Thomson* (Th) in honor of one of the pioneers of MS.[32-34] This terminology is sometimes seen in the literature but has not been widely adopted.

General Classes of Mass Spectrometers

Mass spectrometers are broadly classified into two groups: beam-type instruments and trapping-type instruments. In a beam-type instrument, the ions make one pass through the instrument and then strike the detector, where they are destructively detected. The entire process, from the time an ion enters the analyzer until the time it is detected, generally takes microseconds to milliseconds.

In a trapping-type analyzer, ions are held in a spatially confined region of space through a combination of magnetic and/or electrostatic and/or RF electrical fields. The trapping fields or supplemental fields are applied and manipulated in ways that allow *m/z* measurements to be performed. Trapping times may range from a fraction of a second to minutes, although most clinical applications are at the low end of this range.

Examples of trapping-type instruments include QITs, linear ion traps (which, along with QITs, also depend on RF electric fields), ICR mass spectrometers, electrostatic ion traps, and orbitraps (which are a type of electrostatic ion traps).

Detection of the ions in a trapping-type instrument may be destructive or nondestructive, depending on the specific type of mass spectrometer used. In this context, *destructive* means that ions are destroyed in the detection process. Additional discussions of mass analyzers, tandem mass spectrometers, and ion detectors can be found in the literature,[33,35] and the CLSI documents C-50A and C-62A contain recommendations for matching the capabilities of different *m/z* analyzers to various application classes.[1,2]

Beam-Type Designs. The main beam-type mass spectrometer designs are (1) quadrupole, (2) magnetic sector, and (3) TOF. It is convenient to categorize beam-type instruments into two broad categories, those that produce a mass spectrum by scanning the *m/z* range over a period (quadrupole and magnetic sectors) and those that acquire instantaneous snapshots of the mass spectrum (TOF). This categorization is not hard and fast. Certain instrument designs have been adapted to scanning or nonscanning operations. Nevertheless, the categorization is a useful one because it covers the majority of instruments currently available and because scanning and nonscanning instruments are adapted for different optimal usages.

Quadrupole. Quadrupole mass spectrometers, sometimes known as quadrupole mass filters (QMFs), are currently the most widely used mass spectrometers, having displaced magnetic sector mass spectrometers as the standard instrument. Although these instruments lag behind magnetic sector instruments in terms of (1) sensitivity, (2) upper mass range, (3) resolution, and (4) mass accuracy, they offer an attractive and practical set of features that account for their popularity, including (1) ease of use, (2) flexibility, (3) adequate performance for most applications, (4) relatively low cost, (5) small size, (6) noncritical site requirements, and (7) highly developed data collection software systems.

A quadrupole mass spectrometer consists of four parallel electrically conductive rods arranged in a square array (Fig. 17.11). The four rods form a long channel through which the ion beam passes. The beam enters near the axis at one end of the array, passes through the array in a direction generally parallel to the axis, and exits at the far end of the array. The ion beam entering the quadrupole array may contain a

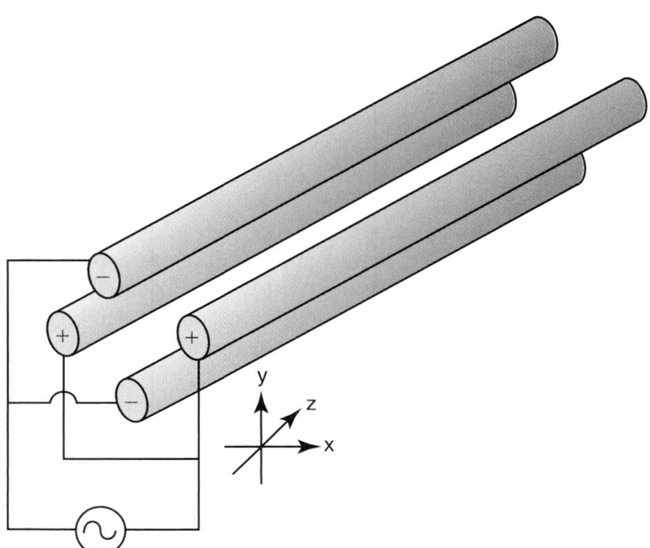

FIGURE 17.11 Diagram of quadrupole mass filter, including the radiofrequency part of voltages applied to the quadrupole rods.

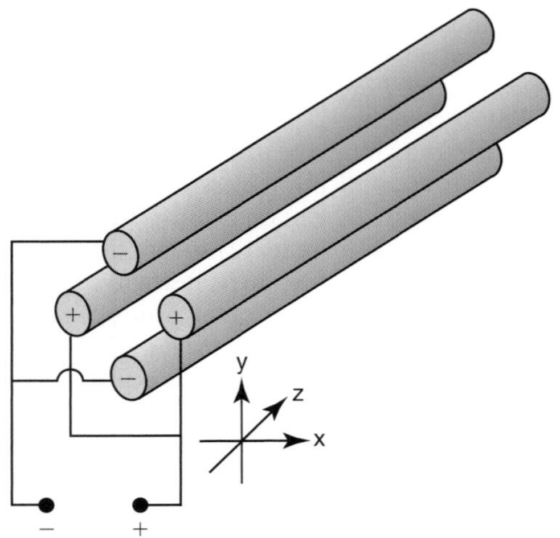

FIGURE 17.12 Direct current voltages applied to quadrupole rod assembly.

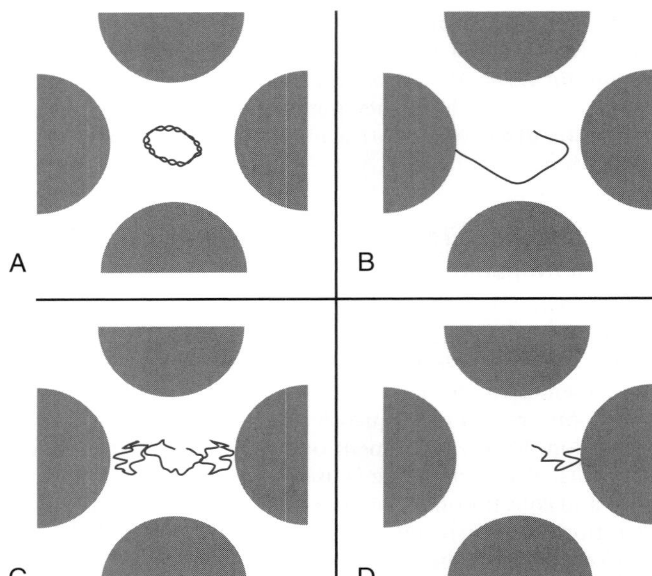

FIGURE 17.13 Ion trajectories showing confinement and ejection in quadrupole mass filters. **A,** Ion confinement by radiofrequency (RF)-only field. **B,** Ion ejection by RF-only field. **C,** Ion confinement with a combination of RF and direct current (DC) fields. **D,** Ion ejection with a combination of RF and DC fields. All trajectories were simulated using Simion software. (Courtesy Scientific Instrument Services, Ringoes, New Jersey.)

mixture of ions of various *m/z* values, and in different modes of operation, different mass ranges can be selected. If a very narrow *m/z* range is selected (eg, $\Delta m/z < 1$) only ions of the specified *m/z* will be transported through the device to reach the detector. Ions outside this narrow range are ejected radially. The $\Delta m/z$ range represents a pass band, analogous to the pass band of an interference filter in optics (see Chapter 13). This is why quadrupole mass spectrometers are often referred to as *mass filters* rather than *mass spectrometers*.

Separation of ions in QMS is based on a superposition of RF and constant direct current, or DC potentials applied to the quadrupole rods. DC voltages are applied to the electrodes in a quadrupolar pattern. For example, a positive DC potential is applied to electrodes 1 and 3, as indicated in Figure 17.12, and an equivalent negative DC potential is applied to electrodes 2 and 4. The DC potentials are relatively small, on the order of a few volts. Superimposed on the DC potentials are RF potentials, also applied in a quadrupolar fashion. RF potentials range up to the kilovolt range, and frequency is on the order of 1 MHz. In the most frequently used mode of operation the frequency is fixed and highly stable, derived from a crystal controlled oscillator.

The physical principles underlying the operation of a quadrupole mass spectrometer are rigorously described by solutions of a complicated differential equation, the Mathieu equation.[36] When an ion is subjected to a quadrupolar RF field, its trajectory is described qualitatively as a combination of fast and slow oscillatory motions. For descriptive purposes, the fast component will be ignored here. The slow component oscillates about the quadrupolar axis; this resembles the motion of a particle in a fictitious harmonic *pseudopotential.* The frequency of this oscillation is sometimes called the *secular frequency.*

Effective force associated with the pseudopotential is directed inward toward the quadrupolar axis and is proportional to the distance from the axis. It therefore acts as a confining force, preventing ions from being ejected radially from the quadrupolar assembly. Figure 17.13, *A,* shows an example of an ion confined by an RF-only quadrupole. Below a certain *m/z* cutoff frequency (which depends on the frequency and amplitude of the RF field), ions are ejected rather than confined. Figure 17.13, *B,* shows an example of an ion ejected by an RF-only quadrupolar field. This establishes the low mass cutoff for the *m/z* pass band. The effective confining force is strongest just above the low *m/z* cutoff and then decreases asymptotically toward zero at high *m/z.*

The DC part of the quadrupolar potential is independent of *m/z.* Positive ions are attracted toward the negative poles. Negative ions are attracted toward the positive poles. Attraction increases as the distance from the quadrupolar axis increases. Because a quadrupolar DC potential always has both negative and positive poles, the quadrupolar DC potential always contributes to ejection in at least one direction. Whether ejection of an ion of a particular *m/z* actually occurs depends on whether the ejecting force caused by the quadrupolar DC potential overcomes the effective confining force caused by the pseudopotential generated by the RF field. Above a certain *m/z* value, the DC part dominates and ions are ejected radially from the device. This establishes an upper *m/z* limit for ion transmission. Figures 17.13, *C* and *D,* show examples of ion trajectories under the influence of combined RF-DC fields, one being confined and the other being ejected. Trajectories in Figure 17.13 were calculated using the Simion ion optics computer program.[37]

A rigorous description of low- and high-mass cutoffs is found in so-called stability diagrams, which graphically describe the lower and upper *m/z* cutoffs of a quadrupole mass spectrometer in terms of parameters related to voltages, frequencies, and *m/z.* However, a full discussion of the stability diagram is outside of the scope of this chapter.

The combination of lower and upper *m/z* limits establishes a pass band ($\Delta m/z$) and ultimately a resolution [(*m/z*)/

($\Delta m/z$)]. With relatively few exceptions, quadrupole instruments are limited to a resolution of a few hundred to several thousand, which is sufficient to achieve isotopic resolution for singly charged ions of m/z as high as several thousand.

A quadrupole MS may be operated in SIM mode or scanning mode. In SIM mode, both DC and RF voltages are fixed. Consequently, both the center of the pass band and the width of the pass band are fixed. For example, the mass spectrometer may be set to pass ions of m/z 363 ± 0.5. Both the center m/z and the $\Delta m/z$ are adjusted by the appropriate choice of DC and RF.

In the scanning mode of operation, the RF and/or DC voltages are continuously varied to scan a range of the specified m/z values. As with the SIM mode, the $\Delta m/z$ is determined by the RF and DC voltages. Usually the scan function is designed to maintain a constant $\Delta m/z$ across the full m/z range. Thus the resolution increases as m/z increases. The value of $\Delta m/z$ is frequently chosen in the range 0.5 to 0.7 to resolve isotopic peaks of singly charged species across the full m/z range.

Magnetic Sector. Because magnetic sector mass spectrometers are rarely used in clinical laboratories, they will not be described in detail here. It should be noted, however, that these classic mass spectrometers are easy to understand (given a basic understanding of physics); are versatile, reliable, and highly sensitive; and in their "double focusing" design are capable of very high m/z resolution and mass accuracy. However, they are typically very large, expensive, and have the reputation of being difficult to use. Consequently, other instruments have largely displaced magnetic sector mass spectrometers.

Time-of-Flight. TOF mass spectrometry (TOF-MS) is a nonscanning technique whereby a full mass spectrum is acquired as a snapshot rather than by sweeping through a sequential series of m/z values while acquiring the data. It is described here as a snapshot because, although ions of different m/z arrive at the detector sequentially (low m/z first), the samples are loaded into the ion source with little or no m/z discrimination with regard to time, and the duration of the acquisition of a single mass spectrum is measured in microseconds. One implication of this is that if the composition of the sample stream being presented to the mass spectrometer changes with time, there is essentially no distortion of the mass spectrum resulting from this time dependence, whereas with scanning-type mass spectrometers the mass spectrum may be distorted because of the interaction between scan time of the mass spectrometer and the changing concentration of the sample stream. This is particularly significant when dealing with fast chromatography coupled to MS.

TOF mass spectrometers have several advantages, including (1) a nearly unlimited m/z range, (2) high acquisition speed, (3) high mass accuracy, (4) moderate to high resolution, (5) moderate to high sensitivity, (6) absence of spectral distortions when used in conjunction with fast separations and narrow chromatographic peaks, and (7) reasonable cost. TOF-MS is also well adapted to pulsed ionization sources, which is an advantage in some applications, particularly with MALDI and related techniques.[38]

A major advantage of modern TOF mass spectrometers is that they are capable of acquiring accurate mass measurements, sometimes loosely referred to as *exact mass,* which is typically accurate to a few parts per million (ppm). This allows TOF measurements to confirm the molecular formula of a compound and assist with identification of unknowns in the mass spectra. TOF mass spectrometers are conceptually simple to understand because they are based on the fact that in vacuum a lighter ion travels faster than a heavier ion, provided that both have the same kinetic energy.

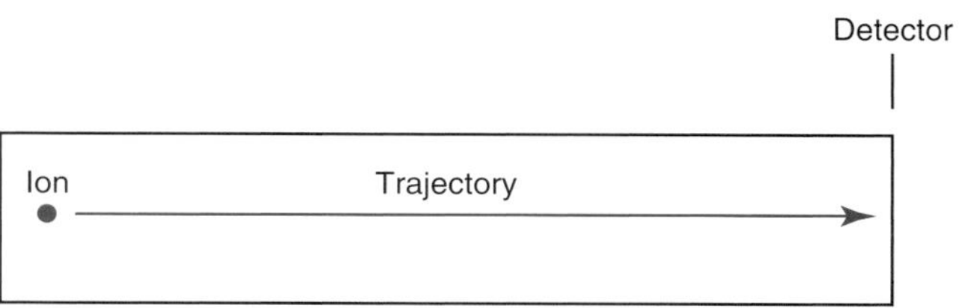

FIGURE 17.14 Diagram of simplified time-of-flight mass spectrometer.

Figure 17.14 presents a simplified conceptual diagram of a TOF mass spectrometer. It resembles a long pipe wherein ions are created or injected at the source end of the device and are then accelerated by the applied potential of several kilovolts. The ions travel down the flight tube and strike the detector at the far end. The time it takes to traverse the tube is known as the flight time; this is related to the mass-to-charge ratio of the ion.

The flight time for an ion of mass m and kinetic energy E to travel a distance L in a region free of electric fields is given by:

$$t = L\left(\frac{m}{2E}\right)^{1/2}$$

A sample calculation for an ion of molecular weight 200 Da (3.32×10^{-25} kg) with a kinetic energy of 10 keV (1.60×10^{-15} J), traveling through a distance of 1 m, yields a flight time of 10.18 μs, and an ion of molecular weight 201 takes just 25 ns longer. To accurately capture such fleeting signals, the data recording system must operate on an approximately 1 ns or shorter time-scale. Advances in signal processing electronics have made these mass analyzers possible at a modest cost, and this has been a major factor in the rise in popularity of TOF-MS.

TOF is inherently a pulsed technique; it couples readily to pulsed ionization methods, with MALDI being the most common example, although TOF is also coupled with continuous ion sources such as EI, ESI, and APCI. However, the continuous nature of these sources causes a mismatch between continuous introduction of ions from the ion source and a pulsed detection with TOF-MS. This mismatch is overcome by using a technique known as orthogonal acceleration TOF-MS (OA-TOF-MS), in which the ion beam is injected orthogonal to the axis of the TOF-MS.[39-41]

During the injection period, the acceleration voltage is turned off. Once the injection region is filled with the traversing beam, the acceleration voltage is quickly turned on and the TOF timing cycle starts. The process is cycled repeatedly. The overall duty cycle for this method can be more than 10%; this represents a vast improvement over the traditional method of gating the ion beam for TOF analysis. For full spectrum capability with continuous ion sources, orthogonal injection TOF mass spectrometers are generally considered to have the lowest detection limits of all mass spectrometers.

However, for the monitoring of a single *m/z* rather than a full mass spectrum, the use of SIM mode with a quadrupole MS provides superior sensitivity.

Improved resolution is an additional benefit conferred by OA-TOF-MS. Although a complete explanation is beyond the scope of this chapter, in brief, orthogonal acceleration reduces the resolution-degrading effects that would normally accompany the kinetic energy variations of individual ions in the ion beam.

Use of an ion mirror is another technique often employed in TOF-MS design to improve resolution by compensating for kinetic energy variations.[42,43] Such instruments are known as *reflectrons.* To date, TOF-MS has had a limited impact in clinical chemistry with only a few commercially offered TOF-MS assays, such as insulin-like growth factor I[44,45] and drug screening,[46] but it could potentially play a greater role in the future. For example, full-spectrum capability, high resolution (up to 40,000 in some current instruments), high speed (10 to 100 stored spectra per second), and high mass accuracy of TOF-MS seem ideally suited to applications such as high-speed drug screens in toxicology when combined with fast chromatographic sample introduction.

Another area in which TOF-MS provides an advantage is high-mass analysis, where its mass range is nearly unlimited. In MALDI-TOF, for example, it is not unusual to detect proteins with molecular weights exceeding 100,000 (see Chapter 19). The ability for high-mass analysis is expected to increase in importance as clinical laboratories embrace proteomic-based diagnostic methods.

Trapping Mass Spectrometers. In contrast to beam-type designs, these mass spectrometers are based on the trapping of ions to capture and hold ions for an extended length of time in a small region of space. Trapping times vary from a fraction of a second to minutes. Compared with beam-type instruments, the division between scanning and nonscanning instruments has less meaning for ion-trapping instruments. The main practical difference between scanning and nonscanning instruments is related to distortions in chromatographic peak shape (or peak skewing). These arise from the finite scan time of a mass spectrometer relative to the timescale of the width of a chromatographic peak. The result is that the abundances of the peaks in mass spectra collected during the rising or falling portions of a chromatographic peak are distorted relative to the true mass spectrum. In other words, as an instrument collects a mass spectrum, scanning from low *m/z* to high *m/z,* the peak intensities observed for low *m/z* will reflect the concentration of analyte that elutes earlier than the concentration of analyte that elutes when detecting high *m/z.* As a result, mass spectra collected at the beginning of a chromatographic peak may have different relative peak intensities compared with those of spectra collected at the end of a chromatographic peak. In terms of producing skewed spectra, trapping devices are more similar to nonscanning instruments, such as TOF (does not cause skewing), than to scanning instruments. This is because the sample is captured in an instant and then analyzed at leisure. Because the sample is captured in an instant, no skewing of the spectra occurs, regardless of whether the *mass* analysis is performed by a scanning or a nonscanning technique.

Traditionally, ion traps have been classified as (1) a QIT, which relies on RF fields to provide ion trapping; (2) a linear ion trap, which is closely related to the QIT in its operating principles; (3) an ion cyclotron resonance (ICR) mass spectrometer, which relies on a combination of magnetic fields and electrostatic fields for trapping, and (4) an orbitrap, a more recent introduction into the field of ion trap MS.[47]

Quadrupole Ion Trap. QITs are relatively compact, inexpensive, and versatile instruments that are excellent for (1) exploratory studies, (2) structural characterization, and (3) qualitative identification. They are also used for quantitative analysis, although precision of measurements is inferior when compared with quadrupole-based instruments.

Operation of the QIT is based on the same physical principle as the quadrupole mass spectrometer described earlier. Both devices make use of the ability of RF fields to confine ions. However, the RF field of an ion trap is designed to trap ions in three dimensions rather than to allow the ions to pass through as in a QMF, which confines ions in two dimensions. This difference has a large impact on the operation and limitations of the QIT.

The physical arrangement of a QIT is different from that of a QMF. If an imaginary axis is drawn through the *y*-axis of the quadrupole rods, and the rods are rotated around the axis, a solid ring with a hyperbolic inner surface results from the *x*-axis pair of rods. The two *y*-axis rods form two solid end caps. A diagram of an ion trap is given in Figure 17.15. The description of the fields within the electrodes must now include a radial component and an axial (between the end caps) component. These design features have an effect on the conditions required for ion confinement when compared with a QMF, although the qualitative description of ion confinement discussed previously is valid.

A discussion of the several types of scanning experiments in QIT is beyond the scope of this chapter, except to mention that ions may be ejected from the trap in an *m/z*-dependent fashion for detection using an external electron multiplier.

Some advantages of QITs are an ability to perform multiple stages of tandem MS (MS^n), high sensitivity, and decoupling of the mass analysis from scanning, so no mass spectral peak skewing is seen in GC-MS and HPLC-MS. However,

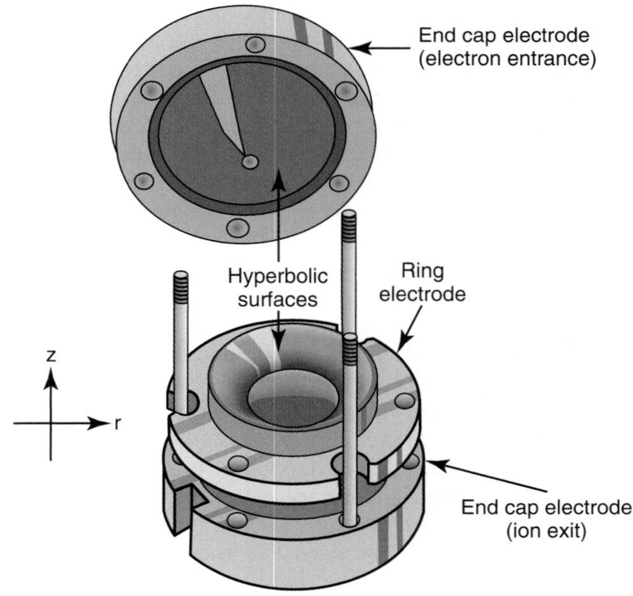

FIGURE 17.15 Diagram of quadrupole ion trap. *r,* Radial direction; *z,* axial direction.

ion-ion repulsion effects (caused by large numbers of similarly charged species in a small space within the trap) limit the number of ions that can be trapped, simultaneously reducing dynamic range and producing mass mis-assignments at high signal levels. The previously mentioned features make QITs not well suited for quantitative analyses, which are typically required for majority of applications in clinical laboratories.

Linear Ion Trap. The linear trap is an RF ion trap that is based on a modified linear QMF. Rather than being a pass-through device, as in a traditional linear QMF, electrostatic fields are applied to the ends to prevent ions from exiting out the ends of the device. When trapped in this manner, ions can be manipulated in many of the same ways as in a QIT. An advantage of the linear quadrupole ion trap is that the trapping field can be turned off at will and the device operated as a normal QMF. Furthermore the trapping volume available within the QMF is much greater than the traditional QIT, allowing greater capacity of the ions to be trapped before ion-ion repulsion becomes an issue. Thus a single device combines most of the features of a QIT and QMF and is extremely versatile. Commercial triple quadrupole mass spectrometers are being offered in which the third quadrupole is modified to function either as a linear trap or as a conventional third quadrupole mass spectrometer as selected by the user.

Ion Cyclotron Resonance. The ICR-MS excels in high-resolution and high mass accuracy measurements.[48] Measurements at resolution exceeding 1 million are not unusual. ICR is a trapping technique that shares many of the advantages of RF ion traps (QIT or linear ion traps). However, there are even more ways to manipulate ions in an ICR-MS than in RF ion traps, and MS^n (multiple stages of MS/MS) measurements are easily done with an ICR-MS. Sensitivity of an ICR-MS is generally high. Furthermore, sampling is decoupled from spectral acquisition, so no peak skewing is seen in chromatographic experiments—a feature that ICR shares with TOF and QIT, and the signal acquisition times are typically longer than for other types of mass analyzers.

Fourier transform ion cyclotron resonance–mass spectrometry (ICR-MS) is based on the principle that ions immersed in a magnetic field undergo circular motion (cyclotron motion). A typical ICR-MS uses a high-field (3 to 12 tesla) superconducting magnet. Within this field and within a high vacuum is mounted a cell typically composed of six metal electrodes, arranged as the faces of a cube. Ions are suspended inside the cell and undergo cyclotron motion, which keeps ions from being lost radially (the radial direction being defined as perpendicular to the magnetic field lines). A low (~1 V) potential is applied to the end caps to keep ions from leaving the trap axially. Thus the combination of electric and magnetic fields keeps ions confined within the cell.

Ions circulating in the ICR cell induce an electrical current in two parallel detection electrodes. The detection electrodes are on opposite sides of the ICR cell and are arranged parallel to the magnetic field. After certain mathematical operations are performed on the signal (principally a Fourier transform [FT]), a mass spectrum is recovered. Each *m/z* is associated with a specific cyclotron frequency, and each *m/z* value that is present in the sample produces a peak in the transformed signal. Because of the frequent use of FT in ICR, the technique is often referred to as FT-ICR or FTMS.

Although this technique has many advantages, including (1) high mass accuracy, (2) ultra-high resolution, and (3) the ability to perform MS^n, ICR-MS has several disadvantages, including (1) high instrument costs; (2) very demanding site requirements, in terms of both space and access restrictions; (3) requirement for a high-field superconducting magnet; (4) relatively long signal acquisition time, which limits the number of scans that can be acquired during the elution of a chromatographic peak; (5) safety concerns related to high magnetic fields; (6) demagnetization of credit cards and other magnetically encoded strips; (7) high costs of operation and maintenance because the instruments consume liquid helium and must never be allowed to run out of helium; and (8) necessity of a highly skilled individual to operate the instrument.

Orbitrap. The suitability of a new type of mass analyzer, the orbitrap, for clinical analysis has yet to be proved. However, the high resolution and mass accuracy of the orbitrap suggest that it has potential for use in clinical laboratories. The orbitrap mass analyzer has resolution and mass accuracy approaching that of an ICR mass spectrometer but does not require a magnetic field. This innovation minimizes many of the ICR disadvantages listed previously. The principles of mass analysis in an orbitrap are based on an early ion storage device—the Kingdon trap.[49] After many variations over the years, Makarov and associates[47,50-52] developed a modified version that was commercialized in 2006. The commercial instrument can easily achieve resolutions up to 100,000 and parts per million or even sub–parts per million mass accuracy, has four orders of magnitude dynamic range, and has sampling decoupled from spectral acquisition (as in the ICR). The resolution and mass accuracy are typically approximately 2 orders of magnitude greater than with a quadrupole mass spectrometer.

Orbitrap-MS is based on trapping within electrostatic fields.[53] The actual device is a spindle-like central electrode surrounded by a barrel-like outer electrode.[54] When ions are introduced perpendicular to the central electrode and a radial potential is applied between electrodes, the ions spiral (orbit) around the central electrode and are effectively trapped in a radial direction. Trapping in the axial direction is assisted by the shape of the electrodes, together with the potentials that are applied to the electrodes. Ion trapping therefore involves both orbital motion around the central electrode and axial oscillations.

The trapping potential in the axial direction is of the form of a harmonic oscillator, and because the frequency of a harmonic oscillator is independent of oscillation amplitude, this frequency is very stable and well behaved. The *m/z* can be calculated from the frequency of axial oscillation:

$$\omega = 2\pi f = (km/z)^{-1/2}$$

where ω is angular velocity, *f* is frequency, *m/z* is the mass-to-charge ratio, and *k* is a constant determined by the trap geometry, dimensions, and applied potential. (To be dimensionally correct, *m/z* in this equation must have units of mass divided by charge, which differs from the currently accepted definition of *m/z* as a unitless number[31] (see also http://goldbook.iupac.org/M03752.html).

The image current (current induced by a motion of ions passing near a conductor) made in the outer electrode induced by the ion motion is acquired in the time domain and can be Fourier-transformed to produce a frequency spectrum that is then converted to *m/z* using the previous equation.

With the ability to perform accurate mass measurements, especially when combined with a linear ion trap or quadrupole to form a hybrid tandem mass spectrometer, orbitrap mass analyzers have excellent capabilities for proteomics research. One recent publication noted anomalous isotope ratios observed under high-resolution operating conditions.[55] It is a curious point that the anomalies are compound-dependent, and generally increase with increasing resolution. A theoretical explanation for these anomalies has been given.[56]

Tandem Mass Spectrometers

Tandem MS, or MS/MS, has become the dominant MS-based technique used in clinical laboratories, where it has found extensive application in the quantitative analysis of routine samples.[57] However, it is also a useful technique for structural characterization and compound identification and therefore often used for exploratory work. The most important features of this technique are its very high selectivity, ability to measure very low concentrations of analyte(s), and ability to multiplex the measurement of multiple analytes in a single method. Susceptibility of MS/MS to interferences is typically very low, especially if MS/MS is combined with chromatographic separation. The reason is that a detected compound is separated and characterized by three physical properties: chromatographic retention time, precursor ion mass, and product ion mass. Because of its high specificity, low consumable cost, and a potentially high sample throughput, increasingly more clinical laboratories are using tandem mass spectrometers for the routine analysis of samples.

The physical principle of MS/MS is based on the use of two mass spectrometers (or mass filters) arranged sequentially in tandem, with a collision cell placed between the two mass filters. The first filter is used to select a *precursor ion* of a particular *m/z*. The precursor ion is directed into the collision cell, where ions collide with background gas molecules and are broken into smaller product ions. The second mass filter acquires the mass spectrum of the product ions.

A variety of scan functions are possible with MS/MS. A product ion scan involves setting the first mass spectrometer (also called mass filter 1, MF1, MF1, MS1, or Q1) to select a given *m/z*, and scanning through the full mass spectrum of product ions using the second mass spectrometer or mass filter, MF2. This scan function is often used for structural characterization.

A precursor ion scan reverses this relationship, with the second mass filter, MF2, set to select a specific product ion, and MF1 is scanned through the spectrum of precursor ions. The scan tells which precursor ions produce a specific product ion—a capability that is often used to analyze for specific classes of compounds. For example, acylcarnitines are often analyzed using precursor ion scan mode by acquiring signal from all the precursors of the *m/z* 85.

In a constant neutral loss scan, the two mass filters are scanned synchronously, with a constant *m/z* offset between precursor and product ion. This scan indicates which ions lose a particular neutral fragment. For example, an offset of 176 *m/z* units would select for ions losing a glucuronide moiety in the dissociation process.

The most commonly used scan function in MS/MS is MRM (also referred as SRM). In this type of acquisition a series of precursor/product ion pairs are monitored, with the mass spectrometer set to step through the table of parent/product ion pairs in a cyclic fashion. MRM acquisition is primarily used for quantitative analysis of target compounds and is an analog to the SIM type of acquisition used in GC-MS.

As with single-stage mass spectrometers, MS/MS are roughly categorized as beam-type instruments and trapping instruments. The most popular beam-type instrument is the triple quadrupole. In this instrument, the first quadrupole (Q1) functions as MF1 and the third quadrupole (Q3) functions as MF2. Between these two quadrupoles is another quadrupole, Q2, which functions as the collision cell. The pressure is raised in Q2 (eg, $>10^{-3}$ torr) by the addition of a nonreactive gas (nitrogen, helium, argon, etc.) to the point that ions traversing Q2 undergo multiple collisions, leading to deposition of energy onto the analyte and subsequent fragmentation of the precursor ion(s) into smaller fragments, followed by separation and detection of the product ions in a subsequent stage of mass analysis. The Q2 is operated as an RF-only quadrupole, ideally passing all ions regardless of *m/z*. The technique is typically used to fragment molecular or pseudomolecular ions in order to obtain analyte-specific fragments, which can be used for elucidating structure of the molecules of interest or in selective analysis of targeted molecules. In cases in which the collision-induced dissociation spectrum contains a large number of ions, the experienced investigator often can deduce the structure of a molecule from the mass spectrum of the product ion.

Two magnetic sector instruments also have been operated in tandem, with a collision cell placed between the two mass analyzers. These instruments permit high-resolution selection of both precursor and product ions. However, they are now rarely used because of the high cost and cumbersome operation. A single magnetic sector mass spectrometer (in the form of a double focusing mass spectrometer) has also been used as an MS/MS by a technique known as *linked scanning*. A product ion scan by linked scanning involves low resolution for the first *m/z* selection and high resolution for the second *m/z* selection.

Hybrid mass spectrometers include a combination of two different types of mass spectrometers in a tandem arrangement. The combination of a magnetic sector mass spectrometer with a quadrupole mass spectrometer was an early instrument of this type. More popular today is the combination of a quadrupole for the first stage of *m/z* selection and a TOF for the second *m/z* analyzer. Subsequently, linear ion trap and quadrupole mass analyzers have been combined with an orbitrap. Hybrid instruments are presently used mainly for proteomics research. These instruments cannot perform the true precursor ion scans or constant neutral loss scans, though it is possible to mimic these functions by post-processing data, provided the full precursor-product ion map was generated in the experiment.

QIT, linear ion trap, and ICR mass spectrometers also can be used as MS/MS. Unlike beam-type instruments, which are referred to as "tandem in space," trapping mass spectrometers are "tandem in time," meaning that ions are held in one region of space while the parent ion is selected and dissociated and the daughter ion is analyzed sequentially in time in the same region of space. The ability to perform MS/MS is inherent in the design of most trapping mass spectrometers. Generally, little or no additional hardware is required, and tandem capability is supplied via software. An exception is the orbitrap, which is not amenable to MS/MS when used alone. However, when incorporated into a hybrid instrument, with a different type of mass spectrometer supplying the first stage of MS (such as a linear ion trap or a quadrupole), and with the orbitrap providing the final stage of MS, MS/MS is possible in an orbitrap-based instrument.

Most trap-based instruments are capable of multiple stages of MS. Thus, product ions may be further dissociated to produce another generation of product ions (MS/MS/MS, or MS^3). In principle, any number of dissociation stages may be performed (MS^n). This capability finds its greatest use in structural characterization, such as in the sequencing of peptides, and is less useful for quantitative analysis. Although trapping designs are extremely versatile (such as allowing multiple stages of fragmentation), these instruments are unable to perform true precursor ion scans or constant neutral loss scans, as illustrated in Figure 17.16, *C* and *D*, respectively. However, it is possible to simulate the effect of precursor ion scans or constant neutral loss scans by taking a series of product ion scans, one for each possible parent ion

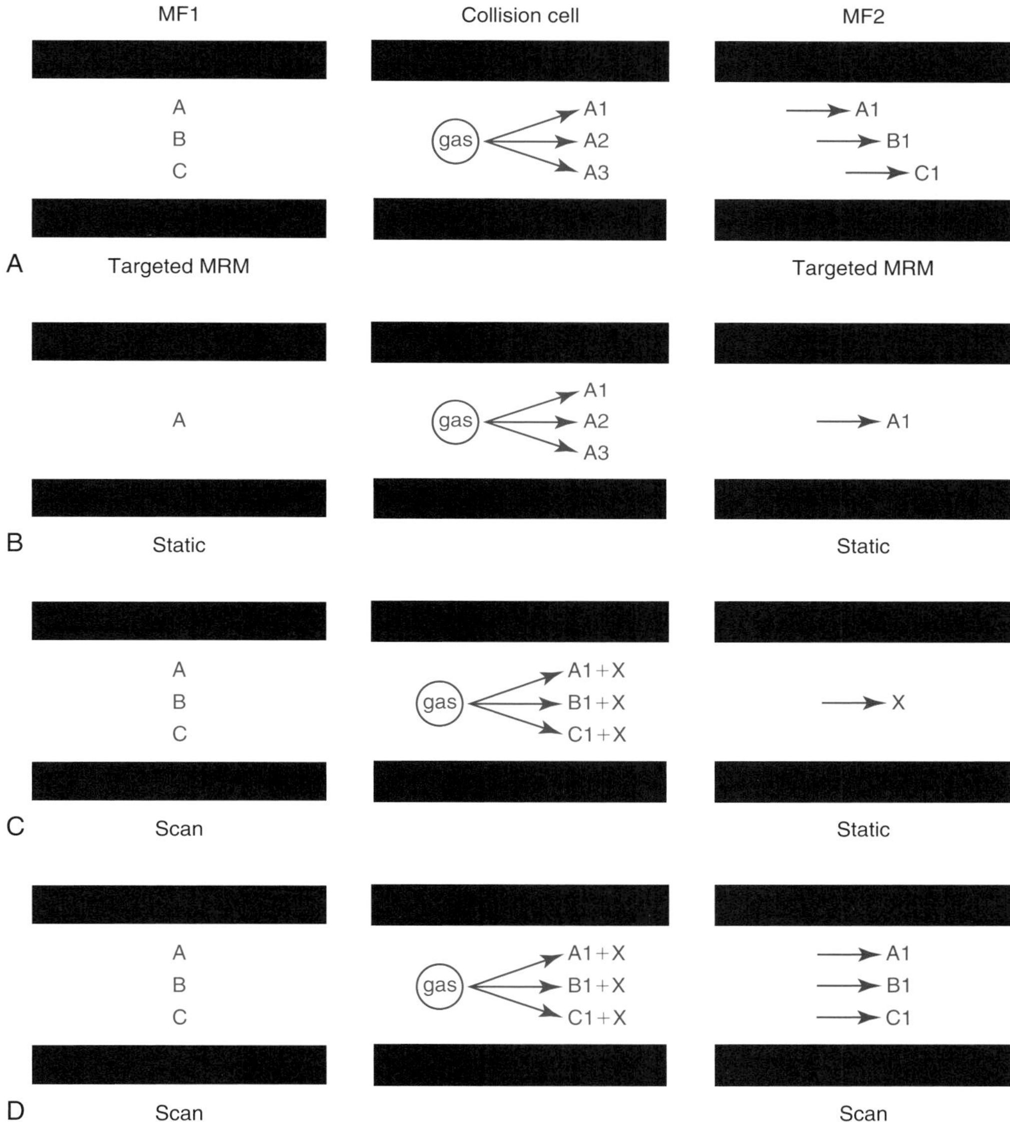

FIGURE 17.16 Scan modes in mass spectrometry/mass spectrometry (MS/MS). **A,** Multiple reaction monitoring (MRM), in which *A, B, C, A1, B1,* and *C1* are ions. Monitoring of MS/MS transitions *A* → *A1, B* → *B1,* and *B* → *C1* is multiplexed. For simplicity, only the dissociation of *A* is shown in a collision cell in the figure. **B,** MRM of a single compound, where only one MS/MS transition is monitored. **C,** Precursor ion scan, in which *A, B, C,* and *X* are all ions. The second mass filter (MF2) is fixed to monitor the mass-to-charge ratio *(m/z)* corresponding to ionic species *X,* and the first mass filter (MF1) is scanned through a range of *m/z* values. **D,** Constant neutral loss scan, in which *X* is uncharged and *A, B, C, A1, B1,* and *C1* are ions. The two mass filters are scanned with a constant *m/z* offset between the two corresponding to the mass of *X.*

m/z. This will generate a complete MS/MS map. From this complete map data can be selected to simulate these two scan modes because a precursor ion scan is just a subset of the complete MS/MS map, as is a constant neutral loss scan. However, this procedure can be quite time-consuming, which would make it impractical in some applications.

Ion Mobility

Although strictly speaking, ion mobility spectrometers (IMS) are not mass analyzers, they are nevertheless often included as part of the field of MS, either as part of a hyphenated technique (eg, IMS-MS) or as a substitute for an MS analyzer.[58-60] Ion mobility spectrometers are like mass spectrometers in the sense that they require the analyte to be ionized, but the separation mechanism is different. Rather than separating ions by their mass-to-charge ratio, ions are separated according to their mobility in an electric field. Thus ion mobility can be regarded in some respects as a form of gas phase electrophoresis.

The simplified schematic of a conventional ion mobility spectrometer strongly resembles a TOF-MS, but rather than following a collisionless trajectory, ions undergo many collisions as they drift under the influence of an electric field. Other configurations for measuring gas phase mobility are also possible,[58-60] but these will not be reviewed in detail here.

An IMS may operate at atmospheric pressure or at reduced pressure but not under a high vacuum because collisions are necessary for its operation. When used in conjunction with a mass spectrometer it is possible to place the mobility device before the first mass analyzer or following one or more stage of mass analysis.

A technique known as field asymmetric ion mobility spectrometry (FAIMS) is also based on ion mobility, but in this case ions are not separated strictly according to their mobility. FAIMS, sometimes known as differential mobility spectrometry (DMS), is based on the fact that the mobility of a gas phase ion is not strictly constant; that is, the drift velocity is not simply proportional to the electric field, but rather at high field there is a deviation from the proportional relationship. FAIMS uses a combination of an asymmetrical high-voltage RF field and a smaller DC field to separate ions according to a combination of low-field mobility and high-field mobility. FAIMS is beginning to find applications in clinical MS when used as a filtering device positioned between the ion source and the mass analyzer.[61]

IMS also has been used alone for clinical applications, without being combined with MS. Notably, it has been used to separate unmodified lipoproteins on the basis of size using a differential mobility analyzer (DMA, not to be confused with DMS). The instrument configuration differs from a conventional drift tube IMS, but like a drift tube IMS (and unlike FAIMS), the physical property being measured is gas phase ion mobility. After the separation, each lipoprotein particle is directly detected and counted as it exits the separation chamber, and the lipoprotein subfraction categorization is made based on the mobility of the particles.[62-64]

Detectors

With the exception of ICR-MS, orbitrap, and some ICP-MS instruments, most modern mass spectrometers use electron multipliers for ion detection. The main classes of electron multipliers used as MS detectors include the (1) discrete dynode multipliers; (2) continuous dynode electron multipliers (CDEMs), also known as channel electron multipliers; and (3) microchannel plate electron multipliers, also known as multichannel plate electron multipliers. Although different in design, all three work on the same physical principle. Additional types of detectors used in mass spectrometers are the Faraday cup, image current detection, and photomultipliers.

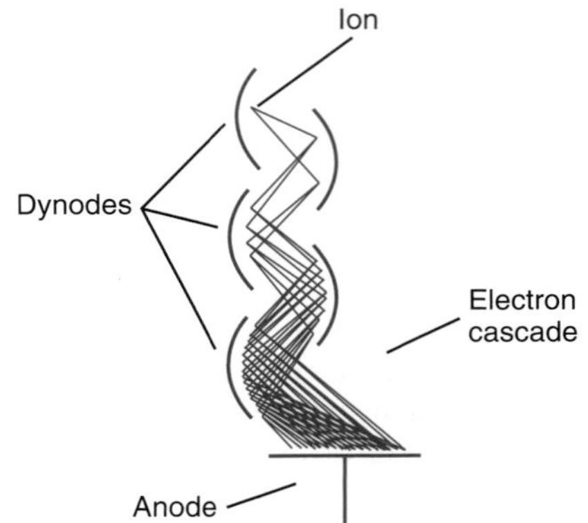

FIGURE 17.17 Discrete dynode electron multiplier showing dynode structure and generation of electron cascade.

Figure 17.17 presents a conceptual diagram of the operation of a discrete dynode electron multiplier. When an ion strikes the first dynode, it causes the ejection of one or more electrons (secondary electrons) from the dynode surface. The electron is accelerated toward the second dynode by a voltage difference of approximately 100 V. On striking the second dynode, this electron causes the ejection of additional electrons, typically 2 or 3. The second group of electrons is then accelerated toward the third dynode and, on striking the third dynode, causes the ejection of several more electrons. This process is repeated through a chain of dynodes, numbering between 12 and 24 for most designs. The cascade process typically produces a gain of 10^4 to 10^8, meaning that one ion striking the first electrode produces a pulse of 10^4 to 10^8 electrons at the end of the cascade. The duration of the pulse is very short, typically less than 10 ns.

A CDEM works on the same principle as a discrete dynode electron multiplier but differs in design. The set of dynodes of a discrete dynode electron multiplier is replaced by a single continuous resistive surface that acts both as a (continuous) voltage divider to establish the potential gradient and as the secondary electron-generating surface. A microchannel plate electron multiplier is essentially a monolithic array of miniaturized CDEMs fabricated in a single wafer or disk of glass. Sometimes these are stacked into a chevron configuration for added gain.

The Faraday cup is not an electron-multiplying device, but rather a simple electrode that intercepts the ion beam directly. This current is amplified using electronic amplifiers. Because the Faraday cup measures signal intensity directly, rather than indirectly (as in saturation-prone electron multipliers), it provides an absolute measure of ion current and is useful when the magnitude of the signal is too high for electron multiplier–based detection. Some instruments use both electron multiplier and Faraday cup–based detection to provide extended dynamic range—a capability that is especially useful for elemental analysis of trace and toxic elements by ICP-MS.

Detection in ICR occurs via image current detection. This is closely related to the Faraday detection cup in the sense that the ion current is detected directly. However, ions are not destroyed in the process of image current detection and are available for remeasurement. This feature is one of the keys to the versatility of ICR mass spectrometers. Image current detection is also used in the orbitrap.

Closely linked to the detection system is the electronic and signal processing system. In instruments that use electron multiplier detection (the vast majority of mass spectrometers), the raw signal from the detector is processed in one of two ways: (1) individual pulses (corresponding to individual ions) may be counted, as in ion counting systems, or (2) the signal may be converted to a digital representation of the analog signal using an analog-to-digital converter, as in analog detection.

Computer and Software

Because of their (1) mass resolution capabilities, (2) scanning functions, (3) ability to automatically switch between positive to negative ionization modes, and (4) speed with which multiple *m/z* signals are acquired, modern MS instruments generate enormous quantities of raw data. In addition, the use of MS in such areas as (1) proteomics, (2) biomarker discovery, (3) synthetic combinatorial chemistry, (4) high-throughput drug discovery, (5) pharmacogenomics, (6) toxicology, and (7) therapeutic drug monitoring requires that MS manufacturers provide powerful computers and software.

In toxicology laboratories, one important function of the data system is library searching to assist in compound identification. Several commercial libraries, including the Wiley Registry of Mass Spectral Data; the NIST Mass Spectral Database; and the Pfleger, Maurer, and Weber drug libraries, are available. In addition, many laboratories generate their own libraries. The quality and number of available spectra, the search algorithm, and whether condensed or full spectra are searched are all important factors in spectral matching.

In proteomics and biomarker discovery, complex mass spectra from single proteins, protein mixtures, or protein digests corresponding to complex samples are obtained. Data systems aid in characterization of spectral data to identify such properties as intact protein mass, amino acid subsequences, and posttranslational modifications. Fragmentation information also can be compared with peptide databases to identify structural mutations that may be present.

The most important function of software in MS systems is data collection and processing. Chromatographic peaks are integrated using data analysis software, and integrated peak intensities or peak areas serve as the basis for quantitative analysis. Calibration curves are generated during data processing, and quantitative results from individual samples are generated using the calibration curves; the data systems also contain report generation capabilities.

Deconvolution protocols have been developed that identify and characterize the mass spectra corresponding to the coeluting peaks. In addition to proprietary deconvolution protocols embedded in the data systems of mass spectrometers supplied by some vendors, there is a freely available deconvolution software program known as AMDIS.[65]

CLINICAL APPLICATIONS

Mass spectrometers coupled with gas or liquid chromatographs (GC-MS or LC-MS) serve as versatile analytical instruments that combine the resolving power of a chromatograph with the specificity of a mass spectrometer.[66] Such instruments are powerful analytical tools that are used by clinical laboratories to identify and quantify biomolecules. The instruments are capable of providing structural and quantitative information in real time on individual analytes as they elute from a chromatographic column. Specific applications of these coupled instruments can be found in Chapters 20, 21, 40, and 41.

Gas Chromatography–Mass Spectrometry

GC-MS has been used for the analysis of biological samples for several decades. This technique is used by the US National Institute of Standards and Technology and other agencies for the development of definitive methods to qualify standard reference materials and assign accurate concentration to reference materials of many clinically relevant analytes, including cholesterol, glucose, steroid hormones, creatinine, and urea nitrogen (see Chapter 12).

One of the most common applications of GC-MS is drug testing for clinical or forensic purposes (see Chapter 41). Many drugs have relatively low molecular weight and nonpolar and/or volatile properties, making these compounds particularly suitable for analysis by GC. Electron impact ionization with full scan mass detection is the most widely used approach for comprehensive drug screening. Unknown compounds can be identified by matching full mass spectrum of unknown peaks with a mass spectral library or a database. In addition, vendors have recently introduced GC tandem quadrupole (GC-MS/MS) mass spectrometers, which should expand the capability of GC-MS to perform improved targeted and untargeted analysis, thus enhancing existing screening and mass spectral identification capabilities of GC-MS.

GC-MS has many applications beyond drug testing. Numerous xenobiotic compounds are readily analyzed by GC-MS. Applications for anabolic steroids, pesticides, pollutants, and inborn errors of metabolism have been described.[67-69]

One important limitation to GC-MS is the requirement that compounds be sufficiently volatile to allow transfer from the liquid phase to the mobile carrier gas and thus to elute from the analytical column to the detector. Although many biologic compounds are amenable to chromatographic separation with GC, numerous other compounds are too polar or too large to be analyzed with this technique. In many cases, chemical derivatization is necessary to create sufficiently volatile forms of compounds. Knapp's classic work on derivatization[70] may be consulted for more information.

Despite its limitations, GC-MS has several positive attributes. High-efficiency separations have been achieved with numerous commercial capillary columns. This technique allows achieving high-efficiency chromatographic separation and excellent limits of quantification, and it allows use of commercial mass spectral libraries for identification of sample constituents. For some of the analytes, such as organic acids, GC-MS has advantages of higher specificity compared to soft ionization techniques used in LC-MS.

Liquid Chromatography–Mass Spectrometry

As discussed earlier, several interface techniques have been developed for coupling a liquid chromatograph to a mass spectrometer, notably ESI and APCI, which have allowed LC-MS and LC-MS/MS to be successfully applied to analysis of a wide range of compounds. In theory, as long as a compound can be dissolved in a liquid, it can be introduced into an LC-MS system. Thus, in addition to low molecular weight polar and nonpolar analytes, large molecular weight compounds, such as proteins, can be analyzed using this technique (see Chapter 21).

LC-MS/MS has gained momentum in the arena of toxicology screening and confirmation.[71-73] A majority of the currently used methods for targeted analysis use MRM acquisition using mass transitions corresponding to drugs of interest (see Fig. 17.16, *A*). For example, within the chromatographic time window of 1.0 to 2.0 minutes, the MRM transitions for selected sympathomimetic amines might be monitored. During the next defined time window, a new set of MRM transitions are monitored and so on for the rest of the chromatographic run. A related approach is the use of targeted MRM, in which recognition of a chromatographic peak containing a preselected MRM transition triggers a product ion scan in a process called *information-dependent acquisition,* also known as *data-dependent acquisition*. One benefit of this approach is the ability to provide confirmation of the identity of the peaks identified during the analysis.

Coupling of TOF-MS to GC or LC provides a new approach to the identification of unknowns.[46,74] Because TOF is capable of achieving high mass resolution and high sensitivity, the need for compound fragmentation may be minimized, allowing compound identification based on retention time and accurate mass.[75]

The number of quantitative LC-MS/MS assays introduced for the measurement of clinically important compounds has markedly increased. For example, a few compounds that have been of special interest include (1) immunosuppressant drugs,[76] (2) biogenic amines,[77] (3) 25(OH)-vitamin D,[78] (4) antiretroviral drugs,[79,80] (5) psychoactive drugs,[81-83] (6) methylmalonic acid,[84,85] (7) thyroid hormones,[86] and (8) steroids.[87,88] When quantification of a specific compound is desired, the most effective approach is MRM analysis (see Fig. 17.16, *B*). With MRM acquisition, both mass filters MF1 and MF2 are set in a static mode, whereby only precursor ions specific for the compound and the internal standard being measured are passed through MF1. This preselected precursor ion is then fragmented in the collision cell, and molecule-specific fragment ions derived from the compound of interest are passed by MF2 to the detector. Because only one ion is monitored in MF1 and typically two molecule-specific fragment ions monitored in MF2, as opposed to scanning for multiple ions, the MRM approach allows much greater specificity as well as lower limits of quantification.

Another area in which MS/MS is used clinically is screening and confirmation of genetic disorders and inborn errors of metabolism (see Chapter 70).[89,90] The ability to analyze multiple compounds in a single analytical run makes this technique an efficient tool for screening purposes. In this application, in some cases MS/MS is of sufficient selectivity to eliminate the need to incorporate LC separation, a simplification that allows high-throughput analysis.

Electrospray-MS/MS is also used for carnitine and acylcarnitine analysis to detect organic acidemias and fatty acid oxidation defects.[91,92] In the methods for acylcarnitine and amino acid analysis, these compounds vary widely in their polarity, which creates problems with consistency of response factors. To address this issue, most methods use a butyl ester derivatization of the carboxyl group to force cationic character on the amino acids and thus enhance the ionization efficiency.[93]

Acylcarnitines can be analyzed without derivatization,[94] but most often are analyzed as butyl esters using a *precursor ion scan* mode of acquisition (see Fig. 17.16, *C*).[95,96] This type of acquisition makes use of the fact that acylcarnitines have a common collision-induced *m/z* 85 product ion (represented by *X* in Fig. 17.16, *C*) that is selectively monitored in MF2. MF1 is set to scan for precursors with *m/z* 85, thus detecting and identifying acylcarnitines present in the sample (see Fig. 17.16, *C*). By incorporating in the method stable isotope-labeled analogs of the targeted acetylcarnitines, it is possible in addition to identification, to establish concentration of the acylcarnitines of interest.

Analysis of amino acids by LC-MS/MS is typically performed using traditional MRM monitoring but also can be performed using a data acquisition mode known as *constant neutral loss* (see Fig. 17.16, *D*).[88] Butyl derivatives of α-amino acids share a common neutral product, butylformate, which has a mass of 102 Da (represented by *X* in Fig. 17.16, *D*). By scanning for both product (MF2) and precursor (MF1) ions, and by keeping a constant offset between the two mass *m/z* analyzers (eg, a difference of 102 *m/z* units), any *m/z* differences that equal 102 Da can be used to detect and identify amino acids present in the samples.

One advantage of LC-MS/MS relative to GC-MS is that in many cases it allows avoidance of derivatization of the target compounds, but in some cases derivatization is useful for LC-MS/MS as well. An example of butyl ester derivatization was discussed previously. In this example, the derivative has more favorable fragmentation properties than the underivatized compounds. Similarly, the dibutyl ester of methylmalonic acid (MMA), when run in positive ion mode ESI, has more favorable MS/MS spectra than the underivatized compound run in negative ion mode ESI; in addition, the dibutyl esters of dicarboxylic acids are selectively ionized in positive ion mode ESI, whereas monocarboxylic organic acids are not efficiently ionized and are therefore not detected by the mass spectrometer.[84] By using MMA extraction at conditions specific for acidic compounds and detection specific for polycarboxylic acids, it is possible to perform the LC-MS/MS analysis using isocratic chromatographic separation without the need for reconditioning and reequilibration of the chromatographic column between injections.[84]

The most frequent reason for using derivatization in LC-MS and LC-MS/MS is to achieve improved ionization efficiency. Gao and colleagues[97] have emphasized this issue in an extensive discussion of derivatization in ESI and APCI MS.

Product ion scan is another mode of acquisition using MS/MS; in this scan mode, the first mass filter is fixed to pass a specific *m/z* and the second mass filter is scanned over a specified range of *m/z* values. Product ion scan mode is very useful for structural elucidation, such as in peptide sequencing, but is less useful for routine quantitative analysis.

Matrix-Assisted Laser Desorption Ionization Mass Spectrometry

MALDI (typically coupled with a TOF analyzer) has been used to analyze many different classes of compounds. Notably, it has been widely applied in discovery applications for the detection and identification of proteins and peptides (see Chapter 21). Primary limitations include high background noise and a higher coefficient of variation that seems inherent in the MALDI ionization process. In addition, MALDI is essentially a batch-type process that does not interface naturally with online separation processes using chromatographic techniques (eg, HPLC, capillary electrophoresis).

MALDI-TOF is often used to determine the identity of proteins through peptide mass fingerprinting. This technique has been used to identify a large number of two-dimensional (2D) gel spots for the bacterial pathogen *Pseudomonas aeruginosa*.[98] The procedure generally involves in-gel tryptic digestion followed by accurate mass measurement of the peptides produced during the digestion. The generated mass list is then compared with theoretical tryptic masses for proteins in a database (Fig. 17.18 and Table 17.1). This procedure, which works best for organisms with complete and annotated genomes, is very rapid because 100 or more samples may be deposited on a single MALDI target plate and automatically processed. In the previous example,[98] the group rapidly identified a large number of proteins that were expressed differently among the studied bacteria. In addition, it was found that some proteins were listed as "hypothetical," meaning they were previously undescribed or confirmed to be expressed, and that the theoretical molecular weight and/or isoelectric point (pI) in some cases were different from those measured in the gel, indicating possible loss of terminal amino acids and/or posttranslational modifications.

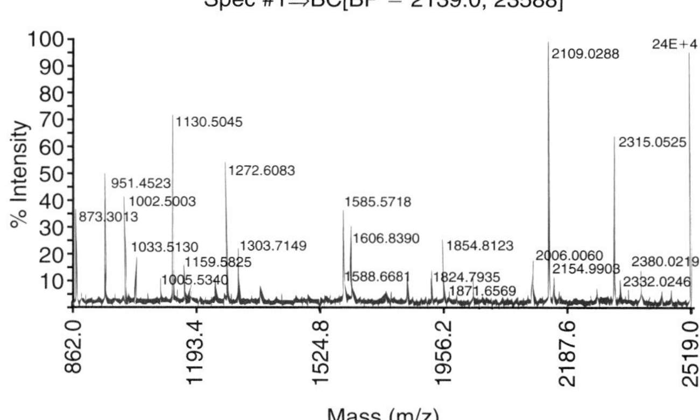

FIGURE 17.18 Example of a matrix-assisted laser desorption ionization–time-of-flight spectrum showing peptides generated in a tryptic digest of a spot cored from a two-dimensional sodium dodecyl sulfate polyacrylamide gel electrophoresis. The 16 most abundant *m/z* values were submitted to the MS-Fit database for searching against the nonredundant database. The results for this search are shown in Table 17.1.

TABLE 17.1 Example of Printout of Bacterial Identification Through Peptide Mass Fingerprinting Using Matrix-Assisted Laser Desorption Ionization MALDI-Time of Flight*

Rank	Mowse Score	# (%) Masses Matched	Protein Mw (Da)/pI	Species	NCBInr.81602 Accession #	Protein Name
1	1.07e+008	14/16 (87%)	101754.9/ 9.15	*Saccharomyces cerevisiae*	6321275	(Z72685) ORF YGL163c

1. 14/16 matches (87%). 101754.9 Da, pI = 9.15. Acc. #6321275. *Saccharomyces cerevisiae*. (Z72685) ORF YGL163c.

m/z Submitted	MH+ Matched	Delta ppm	Start	End	Peptide Sequence (Click for Fragment Ions)	Modifications
870.4746	870.4797	−5.8732	598	606	(K) GVGGSQPLR(A)	
873.3981	873.3929	5.9793	774	779	(K) DCFIYR(F)	$C^2H^2O^2$
951.4901	951.4900	0.1050	814	821	(R) LFSSDNLR(Q)	
1002.5385	1002.5373	1.2224	515	522	(K) NFENPILR(G)	
1033.5513	1033.5543	−2.8793	46	55	(K) NTHIPPAAGR(I)	
1130.6349	1130.6322	2.4037	120	128	(R) LSHIQYTLR(R)	
1130.6349	1130.6322	2.4037	514	522	(R) KNFENPILR(G)	
1159.6039	1159.6071	−2.7957	56	67	(R) IATGSDNIVGGR(S)	
1272.6508	1272.6483	1.9865	734	746	(K) AGGCGINLIGANR(L)	$C^2H^2O^2$
1303.7573	1303.7599	−1.9457	270	280	(K) ILRPHQVEGVR(F)	
1585.7190	1585.7215	−1.5602	446	459	(K) NCNVGLMLADEGHR(L)	$C^2H^2O^2$
1606.8861	1606.9029	−10.4650	22	35	(R) LVPRPINVQDSVNR(L)	
2138.0756	2138.0704	2.4250	747	765	(R) LILMDPDWNPAADQQALAR(V)	
2315.1093	2315.0951	6.1321	401	423	(K) SSMGGGNTTVSQAIHAWAQAQGR(N)	
2388.0671	2388.0731	−2.5004	293	313	(K) DYLEAEAFNTSSEDPLKSDEK(A)	

*A generated mass list is compared with theoretical tryptic masses for proteins in a database. Match quality is used for pathogen identification.

MH+, Ion formed by attachment of a proton to molecule M; *MOWSE*, MOlecular Weight SEarch method; *MW*, molecular weight; *m/z*, mass-to-charge ratio.

One clinical application of MALDI-TOF that has proved its clinical utility is identification of microorganisms (discussed in more depth in Chapter 19). Identification of the bacteria is performed by fingerprinting proteins and peptides extracted from cultures using gentle conditions.[99] The basis of this technique is that different bacteria express unique mixtures of proteins and peptides; when samples are analyzed using MALDI-TOF, the bacteria-specific mass spectra are observed in the 2- to 20-kDa mass range, allowing database searching and classification based on the protein mass fingerprint. One of the disadvantages[99] of the technique is the lack of actual protein information and the relative lack of specificity to different strains of the same bacteria. The protein mass fingerprints must be catalogued (entered in mass spectral library) for each bacterium and validated to be specific and reproducible for a given extraction method.

Some of these drawbacks were addressed in a MALDI technique that targets ribosomal proteins.[100] This technique was evaluated using 1116 isolates collected in a routine clinical microbiology laboratory and was described as being fast, reliable, and easy to use. More than 95% of clinical isolates were correctly identified, and most of the previously incorrectly identified isolates were assigned to the correct genus or a closely related genus. Bacterial identification by MALDI MS is rapidly becoming a routine method in microbiology laboratories.

MALDI MS has the reputation of being a nonquantitative technique. However, some progress has been made toward its use as a quantitative technique.[101] If this application becomes routine, it could have major benefits for clinical MS because the time to acquire a mass spectrum by MALDI is only a few seconds. This could dramatically improve throughput. However, it seems likely that this application will require offline separation (or sample fractionation) before loading on the MALDI target, to obtain sufficient selectivity necessary for clinical applications.

Inductively Coupled Plasma Mass Spectrometry

ICP-MS is used for the determination of trace and toxic elements in many types of samples (see Chapters 37 and 42 and references 10, 102, and 103). However, it is known that the toxicity of an element may depend on the organic or inorganic state in which the element is present. In these cases, it is more important to ascertain the concentrations of toxic species rather than the total concentration of the element. To extend the usefulness of this technique, GC and HPLC systems have been coupled to ICP-MS to separate different compounds containing the targeted element before ICP-MS analysis.[104]

Proteomics, Genomics, and Metabolomics

The past 20+ years have seen tremendous progress in genomics, with hundreds of genomes completed or near completion and many now parsed and annotated. This information is highly complex, mainly because of the myriad changes that occur to proteins produced from the genome throughout the life cycle of a cell, but potentially will provide a better understanding of the cellular functions and allow discovery of novel disease biomarkers.[105] In the mid-1990s, MS came to the forefront of analytical techniques used to study proteins, and the term *proteomics* was coined. Although the definition of proteomics is still debated, for the present discussion it is taken to encompass knowledge of the structure, function, and expression of all proteins in the biochemical or biological contexts of all organism.[106] In a more basic and practical sense, proteomics refers to the identification and quantification of proteins and their posttranslational modifications in a given system or systems. Proteome analysis is a powerful tool for investigating (1) biomarkers of disease, (2) antigens of pathogens, (3) drug target proteins, and (4) posttranslational modifications, as well as for other investigations. This is a challenging task in that a given gene may have many distinct chemical protein isoforms. In addition, many other molecules (metals, lipids, etc.) interact with proteins in a noncovalent fashion. Therefore in a genome, such as the human genome, a repertoire of more than a million proteins may require identification and quantification. Two foundations are necessary to begin this daunting challenge. The first is the basic sequence expected for each possible protein in a cell (ie, information from a completed genome). The second is instrumentation, which currently consists of advanced mass spectrometers that identify and quantify protein isoforms in an automated fashion at very low limits of detection. Both foundations are now essentially in place. However, the goals previously stated are far from being reached, and considerable advances will need to be made in the field of systems biology for better understanding of the biological systems.

Currently, MS is routinely used to accomplish many tasks in proteomics. The most basic task is protein identification. The typical approach is known as the *bottom-up* method, whereby proteins are separated—by gel electrophoresis or by solution-based methods—and then digested. The resulting enzymatic fragments are analyzed and used to identify the protein(s) present. This process is time-consuming and has many pitfalls. Increasingly, much research has been devoted to analysis of mixtures of proteins. These mixtures are derived from biological fluids, cellular compartments, tissue, or immunoprecipitation. Currently, both instrumentation and data analysis software are not sufficiently advanced to allow unambiguous identification of all the proteins in highly complex biological samples. As a result, much emphasis has been placed on separation methods and enrichment techniques for preparing samples for analysis of proteins and peptides.

Another approach that was shown to enable sequencing of intact proteins and posttranslational modifications is known as the top-down method. Top-down proteomics involves identification of proteins in complex mixtures without prior digestion of proteins into peptides. Approaches used for protein top-down characterization include extraction of the proteins from samples, fractionation and analysis of the samples using high-resolution accurate mass MS/MS with CID, higher energy collision dissociation, and electron-transfer dissociation fragmentation. Main benefits of the top-down analysis are in the ability to detect in the samples proteins containing posttranslational modifications and their sequence variants.

Many research groups have introduced methods allowing handling of highly complex biological samples. The most popular approaches include subcellular fractionation, multidimensional chromatography, affinity enrichment, and multiplexing. By combining these approaches, several thousand protein species can be identified routinely. Obviously these numbers are better than those obtained through bottom-up methods from gels, but they still fall far short of those necessary for complete understanding of biological systems.

The term *proteomics* is often used in the context of biomarker discovery. To date, very few markers have been discovered using proteomics methods that have migrated to the clinical laboratory. Some of the reasons for the dearth of new protein biomarkers have recently been discussed.[107] From a broader view, however, proteomics also may include the application of MS for the analysis of known protein and peptide biomarkers. For example, mass spectrometric methods for the analysis of carbohydrate-deficient transferrin have been developed, including a reference method[108] and a method for routine patient testing. Additional areas of application of MS include analysis of the proteome of the pathogenic mold *Aspergillus fumigatus* with the aim of identifying vaccine candidates and new allergens.[109]

Analysis of thyroglobulin, a widely used marker of the recurrence of thyroid cancer, has been described by several groups.[110-112] The initial digestion of the thyroglobulin by trypsin also digests and therefore removes autoantibodies which cause interference in immunoassays. Currently assays based on the above principle are offered in several commercial laboratories and represents substantial progress in the application of MS for routine analysis of proteins as well as providing important information to treating physicians.

Promising proof-of-principle research has been performed on the characterization of hemoglobinopathies by MS.[113,114] Most methods for hemoglobin analysis use MS to detect separate hemoglobin chains or peptide products from enzymatic digests of hemoglobin. However, as shown by Rockwood and coworkers,[115] and shortly thereafter by Ganem and associates,[116,117] the retention of higher order structure, such as noncovalent complexes, is possible when ions are transferred from solution to gas phase, and hemoglobin tetramers have been observed by MS.[118] Another hemoglobin application, a reference method for hemoglobin A_{1c} using MS, has been approved by the International Federation of Clinical Chemistry and Laboratory Medicine.[119] LC-MS methods for quantitative analysis of hepcidin, a peptide hormone believed to be a master regulator of iron status, have been published.[120-122]

Genetic applications for clinical MS are beginning to emerge. For example, MALDI-TOF has been used for mutation detection in myeloproliferative disorders,[123] DNA methylation analysis,[124,125] and gene expression analysis.[126]

A promising genomic approach for pathogen identification uses polymerase chain reaction amplification of selected regions of a pathogen genome, followed by accurate mass measurement using ESI-TOF-MS. From the accurate mass information, a DNA base composition is computed, and the results are matched to pathogen DNA base compositions in a database.[127,128]

A burgeoning area in which MS plays a role is the emerging field of *metabolomics*. This scientific area involves the investigation and characterization of small molecules, including intermediates and products of metabolism, present in biological fluids under different conditions that include (1) normal homeostasis, (2) disease states, (3) stress, (4) dietary modification, (5) treatment protocols, and (6) aging. In a fashion similar to a mass spectrum providing a fingerprint signature for a specific molecule, it has been speculated that compounds identified and evaluated in metabolomic studies may provide a fingerprint signature for different physiologic states.

In practice, metabolites are identified through comparison with (1) known reference materials, (2) commercial or in-house developed mass spectral libraries or metabolite databases, (3) interpretation of mass spectra, or (4) ancillary techniques such as nuclear magnetic resonance. As with other applications of MS, both GC-MS and LC-MS have a place in such studies. GC-MS has some potential advantages that were described earlier. To use GC-MS, however, the metabolites in the sample must be volatile, or derivatization needs to be used to enhance detectability of a larger number of compounds.

LC-MS has its own usefulness in metabolomics because it has potentially wider applicability to polar and nonpolar compounds and allows the observation of the molecular or pseudomolecular ions. However, because reference materials or isotope-labeled internal reference materials do not exist for validating ionization efficiencies or recoveries for some of the biologically relevant compounds, the effects of ion suppression (discussed later) remain a potential confounding factor. Compared with proteomic research, metabolomics faces the added difficulties in that the MS/MS spectra are more difficult to interpret, scarce information is available in the MS/MS libraries, and DNA and protein sequence databases are of no use in interpreting the results.

Mass spectral imaging of tissue sections is another emerging technology that has potential for clinical applications and holds a great promise. The most common approach is to apply MALDI MS to image tissue sections.[129,130] A mass spectrum is acquired at each spot on a regularly spaced array across the sample. From these data, an image is constructed for each *m/z*. The images provide a spatial map of chemical composition (peptides or small molecules) from the sample. Another approach uses laser ablation, followed by ICP-MS, to provide a spatial map of the inorganic elemental composition of the sample.[131] This technique can be extended to immunohistochemical imaging by using metal-labeled antibodies.[132] With this scheme, it is possible to use different labels on different antibodies to do multiplexed imaging of several different targets on the same sample. However, it should be noted that at the present time mass spectral imaging is an extremely time-consuming process because the beam has to be rastered across the tissue by the laser many thousands of times and very large amounts of data need to be processed and analyzed. At this time this is mainly a research technique that is not used in routine diagnostic laboratories.

Practical Aspects of Mass Spectrometry: Logistics, Operations, and Quality

In many respects, the logistics, operations, quality control, and quality assurance processes for clinical MS laboratories follow the well-established clinical laboratory standards and guidelines. However, mass spectrometers are complex instruments and most manufacturers of instrumentation are still learning how to best support their clients in clinical laboratories. Consequently, the adoption of MS, and especially the more complex technologies such as LC-MS/MS, places added demands on training, competency, and manufacturers' support beyond those of more familiar and well-established technologies used in clinical laboratories.

In contrast to techniques such as optical spectrophotometry, mass spectrometers tend to require more frequent troubleshooting, tuning, calibration, and optimization, and the laboratory inspection checklist of the College of American Pathologists specifies that mass spectrometer performance should be verified daily.[133] In addition, the frequency of calibrations and optimizations needed to maintain instruments in fit-for-purpose condition will vary, depending on the requirements of the assays being performed, the instrumentation used, and other factors.

The term *calibration* in relation to MS is used in at least two distinct ways. The first is calibration of the *m/z* scale of the instrument, usually referred to as *mass calibration.* The other is calibration for quantitative analysis.

Schedules for mass calibration vary among laboratories, types of instruments used, and types of assays being run. For example, if accurate mass measurements are an important part of a method, as with many assays that employ TOF-MS, then very frequent mass calibration is typically required. In some cases, internal mass reference materials are included within each run, or even within each sample. For applications that are less dependent on mass accuracy, such as most quantitative methods performed on quadruple mass analyzers, mass calibration may be performed less frequently. For example, mass calibration may be performed every few weeks, with verification of mass calibration performed more frequently—as often as daily in some laboratories.

Similarly, based on validation results obtained in individual laboratories, schedules for calibration for quantitative analysis may vary. For example, some laboratories calibrate an assay daily, whereas others calibrate with every run.

One advantage of MS is that most methods in the MS laboratories avoid the use of highly specialized reagents such as commercial kits of reagents and antibodies. Consumables are mostly generic items, such as solvents, chromatographic columns, and sample vials or 96-well plates. This tends to buffer the laboratory from supply disruptions of specialized reagents, and in some cases can decrease consumable costs as well. However, consumables must be carefully selected and monitored for quality, because contaminated reagents and supplies may negatively affect performance of the methods; this problem is far too common. Solvent quality is of particular concern. For example, one study documented wide variations in methanol quality from different suppliers, which can lead to large differences in ionization efficiency and cause interferences in the analysis.[134]

Whenever possible, a quantitative method should use isotopically labeled internal standards, which typically differ from the analyte of interest by substitution of monoisotopic ions with isotope labels (typically deuterium, ^{13}C, or ^{15}N). However, it is not always possible to obtain isotopically labeled versions of each target analyte, in which case a closely related chemical analog should be selected as an internal standard.

MS provides several opportunities for enhancing analytical quality and therefore improving patient care. The high degree of selectivity of MS, particularly when included as a part of hyphenated techniques (GC-MS, LC-MS, LC-MS/MS, etc.) reduces the likelihood of interference compared with immunoassays or separation-based techniques (GC or LC) using nonspecific detection, particularly for small molecule analysis, where cross-reactivity is a concern.[135] Perhaps as important as a high degree of selectivity, MS provides a means to detect the presence of interferences when they occur. With methods that produce fragmentation, in the ion source (as in EI) or in a collision cell (as in MS/MS), fragment ions are produced with reproducible relative intensity (compared to the base peak). By monitoring one or more ratios of the ion fragments, and by comparing these ratios to ratios obtained from authentic reference materials measured in the same run, it is possible to detect the presence of interfering compounds on a sample-by-sample basis.[136]

In addition, accurate mass measurements are useful for detecting interferences if one is using an instrument capable of such measurements, such as a TOF mass spectrometer. To illustrate, the accurate mass of protonated cortisol ($C_{21}H_{31}O_5^+$) is 363.2166 Da, whereas the accurate mass of one of the isotope peaks of protonated molecule of the drug fenofibrate ($C_{20}H_{22}ClO_4^+$) is 363.1180 Da—a difference of 271 ppm. Therefore an interference of even a few percent by fenofibrate (drug used for treating patients with high cholesterol and high triglycerides) in a cortisol analysis would be detectable as a shift in mass of the observed peak on an instrument capable of low single-digit parts per million mass accuracy.[137]

Obviously, detection of interferences by accurate mass measurement alone becomes more difficult as the mass of the interfering compound approaches that of the target compound, but given the ability to detect interferences at a $\approx 20\%$ level or better, and assuming a mass spectrometer of ≈ 3 ppm mass accuracy, a reasonable estimate is that interferences could be detected for all compounds with $|\Delta m/z|$ greater than 30 ppm relative to the target compound. Given the cortisol example discussed earlier, 22 chemical formulas for ions are within 30 ppm of the mass of protonated cortisol, provided we limit our list to the composition constraints listed earlier. Interferences from these would be difficult or impossible to detect by mass measurement alone. Thus accurate mass would likely detect the majority of possible interferences, but some of the potentially interfering compounds would be difficult or impossible to detect.

OPTIMIZATION OF INSTRUMENT CONDITIONS

When developing an MS-based method there are many parameters to optimize. This applies to both the mass spectrometer and the separation method.

Selection of Mass Transitions and Operating Conditions

MRM is the most commonly used type of acquisition in LC-MS/MS methods for targeted analysis. MRM-based methods allow sensitive and specific quantitation of analytes in samples with complex matrices. Typical MRM chromatograms contain one peak or a few peaks, which are easy to integrate, particularly if the sample preparation has been well designed.

When developing MRM methods, it is useful to start with identifying all analyte-specific mass transitions. The typical approach for selection and optimization of mass transitions is through infusion of solution of pure standard of the targeted compound using syringe pump. During the infusion, the signal can be optimized by adjusting the ion source conditions, declustering potential, the ion transmission conditions, and collisional fragmentation. When ions are transported from atmospheric pressure to the vacuum region, they typically exist in the form of clusters. Application of the declustering potential during the ion focusing causes low-energy collisions, which lead to declustering of the ions.

The MRM experiments are set by specifying *m/z* of the precursor ion (typically the molecular ion) of the targeted molecule and the *m/z* of the molecule-specific fragments, produced by fragmentation in the collision cell. While developing a method, it is important to carefully assess which mass transitions to be used in the method. The best sensitivity and specificity are typically achieved using high-intensity unique fragment ions, which have minimal background noise and no interfering peaks coeluting with the analyte of interest. Use of fragment ions corresponding to the loss of water, ammonia, carbonyl (CO), and CO_2 groups generally should be avoided because they result in nonspecific mass transitions.

The optimal values of the voltages needed for declustering the molecular ion and the ion transmission are established by scanning the voltages and finding the apex values that correspond to the maximum signal intensity. Optimization of the collision energy (CE) is accomplished by scanning the CE used for fragmentation of the molecular ion, and plotting the abundances as a function of CE produces a profile, called a breakdown curve (Fig. 17.19).

In the majority of cases, the voltage corresponding to the apex is selected for use in the method. At this value of the CE there is maximum signal intensity. A second advantage of operating at the apex is that slight fluctuations in the instrument conditions do not result in large changes in the signal intensity, so the acquired signal is more stable. However, on some occasions, when unresolved chromatographic peaks could interfere with the analysis, it is beneficial to select CE on the leading slope or the trailing slope of the breakdown curve (more commonly on the leading slope) to improve specificity of analysis by avoiding fragmentation of the substance that potentially interferes with target analyte. This can be useful in cases in which the breakdown curve of an MS/MS transition of a potentially interfering compound partially overlaps that of the target compound. In such cases, by operating on the slope of the breakdown curve of the selected MS/MS transition of the target compound it may be possible to more strongly discriminate from the interfering substances.

In addition to evaluating breakdown curves, CE should be selected with the following principles in mind. If the CE is too low, ion fragmentation will be inefficient, and the signal abundance will be low. If the CE is too high, fragmentation can become too extensive; the number of peaks in the product ion spectrum may increase intensity of the peaks that are selective to the product ion of interest may have insufficient intensity to be useful, and the possibility of interfering peaks from coeluting isobars may increase.

Depending on the type of ionization source used, ionizability of molecules is influenced by their volatility, pKa, proton affinity, electronegativity, hydrophilicity/hydrophobicity, surfactant properties, solution pH, ionization energy, electron collision cross-section, etc. Of the ionization methods most commonly used in the MS applications in clinical laboratories, ESI is typically used for analysis of polar and ionizable molecules and APCI and APPI are used for nonpolar molecules. When a new method is being developed, available ionization techniques and polarity modes should be evaluated to assess effect of the conditions on the signal response and specificity of the detection.

The electrospray voltage and ion source conditions have a great effect on the ionization efficiency; the optimal voltage depends on the molecular structure, mobile phase composition, and flow rate. At higher electrospray voltages, greater fluctuation in the ionization efficiency can be observed and a larger number of impurities present in the sample may get ionized, potentially causing the loss of specificity and poor reproducibility. Therefore the lowest voltage resulting in an adequate sensitivity for the analyte is typically preferred. In general terms, there tends to be a threshold voltage, below which ionization is very inefficient; if the ESI voltage is too high, corona discharge or other undesirable effects may occur.

Online Two-Dimensional Separations

Two-dimensional chromatographic separation is a technique in which separation is performed using two HPLC columns with phases having different selectivity. The chromatographic columns are connected to each other through a switching valve, the sample is injected in the first column, and effluent of the column is directed to waste. At the time when the targeted peak is eluted from the the first column, the effluent is redirected into the second column, then during the column reconditioning and equilibration the switching valve is turned

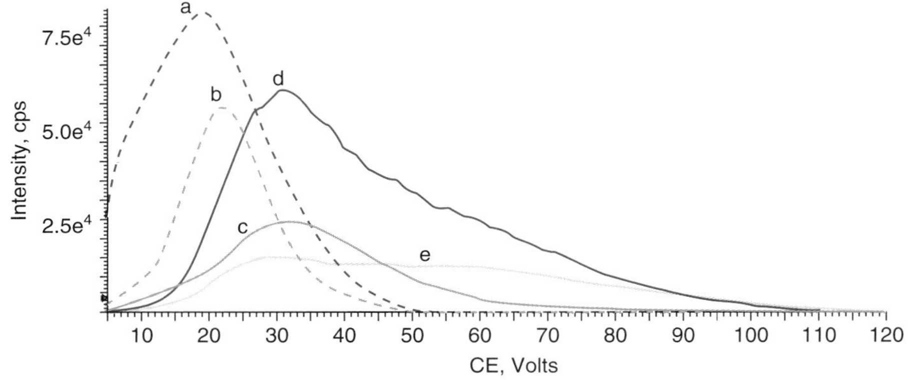

FIGURE 17.19 Breakdown curves for collision energy scans of cortisol. Curves correspond to mass transitions: *a*—*m/z* 363 → 345, *b*—*m/z* 363 → 327, *c*—*m/z* 363 → 171, *d*—*m/z* 363 → 121, *e*—*m/z* 363 → 97. *cps*, Counts per second; *CE*, collision energy.

back to the original position. Using this approach, chromatographic columns with complementary (orthogonal or partially orthogonal) selectivity are typically used, so that peaks that are poorly resolved or unresolved by the first column would get separated on the second column.

In addition to the use of different stationary phases with complementary retention mechanisms, the selectivity may be modified through selection of the optimum for each separation mobile phase and temperature. Some advantages of well-designed 2D separations may include greater resolving power, faster analysis time (while the separation takes place on one column, the other column could be conditioned and reequilibrated), reduced contamination of the mass analyzer (major fraction of the effluent from the first column is directed to waste and not transferred into the second column), and ability to use for the second separation a mobile phase that is favorable for the optimal ionization efficiency. Various coupling strategies have been developed for the switching valve configuration and the peak transfer from the first to the second column; the choice of the specific strategy is method-dependent and would affect the robustness of the assay. Two-dimensional separations are more difficult to develop and troubleshoot, but in many cases the benefits in the methods' performance overweigh the drawbacks.

Conventional Versus Microflow Separations

As more LC-MS methods are developed, greater sensitivity and reduced sample volume are often required. This is especially true for analysis of novel biomarkers. Other trends in modern analytical laboratories are aimed at reducing the volume of solvents used, the cost of the used mobile phase disposal, and the costs of labor. The benefits of microflow separations in LC-MS analysis have been widely reported[138]; they include a higher sensitivity, greater efficiency of ion sampling, reduced solvent consumption and waste, and reduced contamination of the ion source. Despite the advantages, there are relatively few micro-flow based LC-MS methods currently used in routine laboratories. The main reasons are related to the fact that these separations historically were insufficiently rugged, required greater technical expertise of the staff, and caused frequent interruptions in the workflow of a laboratory. However, recent publications on comparison of the microflow and high-flow-rate traditional LC-MS/MS methods demonstrated the rugged method's performance with up to 10-fold gain in the signal-to-noise ratios and up to 20-fold reduction in the use of the solvents.[138]

Ion Suppression

Ion suppression is another quality issue that should be evaluated during method development and validation.[139] First described in 1993,[140,141] ion suppression is a matrix effect that results from the presence of coeluting nonvolatile or less volatile compounds (or compounds with greater proton affinity) that change the efficiency of spray droplet formation, ionic properties, and evaporation. These interfering substances, which include salts, ion-pairing agents, endogenous compounds, surfactants, drugs and/or metabolites, compete with analyte ions for access to the droplet surface or transfer to the gas phase, which, in turn, affects the number of charged ions in the gas phase that ultimately reach the detector.[142] Anions, such as phosphate or borate in buffers, also can neutralize the effective ionization of an analyte. Phospholipids present in biological samples and impurities introduced during the sample preparation and analysis have been demonstrated to be major contributors to ion suppression.[134,143]

Ion suppression refers to the effect of the constituents of the sample that suppresses ionization of the analyte of interest. Factors contributing to ion suppression include greater ionizability of the substances coeluting with the peak of interest, and concentration of the coeluting substance causing ion suppression. Ion suppression can have an adverse effect on the accuracy, precision, and sensitivity of the assay, particularly if the internal standard does not perfectly coelute with the targeted analyte, in which case the internal standard and the analyte may undergo different extents of ion suppression and thus compromise quantitative measurements. This is most likely to happen if the internal standard is highly deuterated. Ion suppression also may reduce the signal of the target analyte to nearly undetectable levels, in which case it is essentially impossible to obtain an accurate quantitative result. Of the different types of ionization techniques used in LC-MS methods, ESI tends to be most susceptible to ion suppression; methods using APCI are typically less prone to the effects of ion suppression, but the possibility of ion suppression in APCI should not be dismissed without validation.

Considering that biological samples contain a large number of endogenous molecules with concentrations ranging over a very wide dynamic range, ion suppression should be expected and the effects of ion suppression should be evaluated for all new or modified methods. The presence of ion suppression or other deleterious matrix effects can be evaluated via several experimental protocols.[1] One involves comparison of (1) the instrument response for reference materials (including any internal standards) injected directly in the mobile phase, and (2) the same amount of compound spiked into preextracted samples.[144] Data for the standard in the mobile phase provide a relative 100% response value. Data for the same amount of compound spiked into preextracted samples show the effects of sample matrix on MS response (ion suppression).

A second, more commonly used and preferred protocol involves postcolumn continuous infusion of compound into the MS detector, while analyzing samples (type intended for the evaluated method, eg, serum, plasma, urine) prepared according to the protocol of the evaluated method.[145-147] The instrumental setup includes a syringe pump connected via a tee to the column effluent (Fig. 17.20). Because the compound being tested is introduced into the ion source at a constant rate, a constant instrument response should be observed if no ionization suppression or enhancement occurs while analyzing biological specimens (Fig. 17.21, *A*). Typically there is suppression of the signal at the portion of the analysis that corresponds to the void volume of the HPLC column (see Fig. 17.21, *B*). The void volume is that portion of a chromatogram corresponding to no retention other than the time it takes for the mobile phase to flow through the column. Thus it represents a chromatographic time region, despite the word *volume* in the terminology.

The degree of ion suppression and the recovery time to full response can vary from assay to assay[145] and among the samples and can be dependent on the sample preparation method, chromatographic column used, and LC separation conditions. Because endogenous compounds from the specimen matrix may elute at any time during the chromatographic

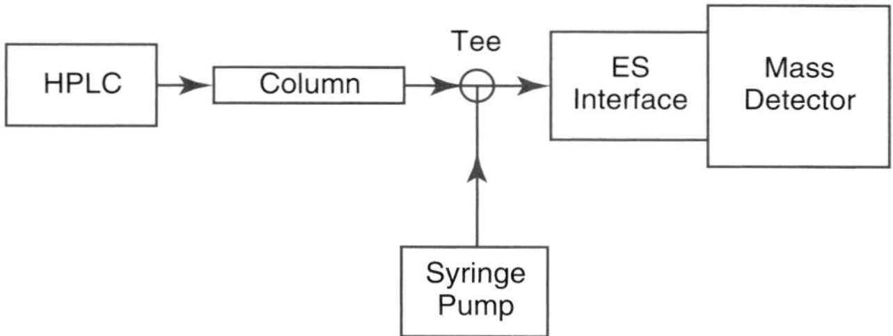

FIGURE 17.20 Postcolumn infusion system. Mobile phase or specimen extracts are injected into the high-performance liquid chromatography *(HPLC)* system. The analyte being evaluated is continuously infused, post column, and is mixed with the column effluent through a tee before entering the electrospray interface *(ES)*.

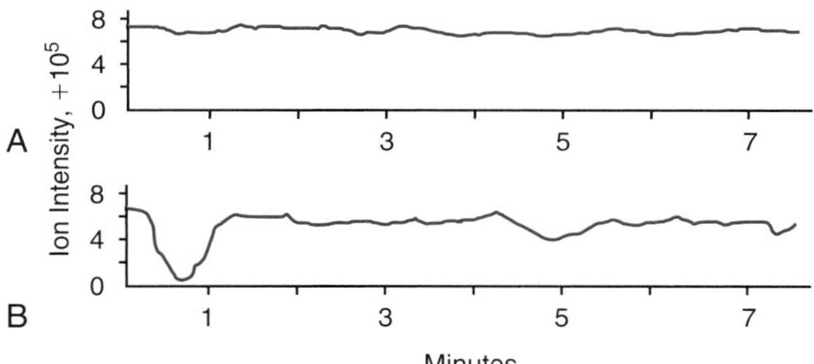

FIGURE 17.21 Infusion chromatograms for hypothetical analytes. **A,** Mobile-phase injection. **B,** Serum liquid-liquid extract injection. These profiles illustrate that ion suppression can be greater than 90%, that a recovery time may exist, and that suppression is not limited to the solvent front region. For a comprehensive presentation of these types of effects, the reader is referred to references 145 to 147.

run, ion suppression is not limited to the column void and not limited to the analysis time of the evaluated sample. In the case of strongly retained compounds, substances causing ion suppression may elute in subsequent injections. Considering this, the detector response should be monitored during analysis of multiple patient samples, to ensure that ion suppression will not affect subsequent injections. The observed degree of ion suppression also can be dependent on the sample volume aliquotted for the analysis, the injection volume, and the concentration of the analyte being monitored,[148] which is related to the matrix-to-analyte concentration ratio.[149] It should be noted that the degree of the matrix effect might differ among the samples of the same biological material, as has been ably shown by Matuszewski and colleagues.[150,151]

To control for ion suppression, it is highly desirable to use matrix-matched calibration standards and controls. It is important to evaluate ion suppression for all types of sample matrices intended for analysis by the method; in addition, considering the complexity of biological samples and the between-subject differences, there may be substantial fluctuations in the concentrations of the ion-suppressing species among samples. Because of this, a significant number of individual samples of all sample matrices intended for the method (serum, plasma, urine, etc.) should be used during the evaluation of the ion suppression.

In cases in which the isotope-labeled internal standards do not completely coelute with the analytes of interest, ion suppression cannot be completely compensated by the internal standard. This problem is particularly acute when using an internal standard that is highly deuterated, because these compounds are likely to not totally coelute with the native compound, and this can lead to significant quantitative errors in the analysis.[152] The ^{13}C- or ^{15}N-labeled compounds are chromatographically retained identically to the nonlabeled analogs and are not susceptible to the previously described problem.

Ion suppression is not limited to HPLC-MS or ESI/APCI ion sources. For MALDI analysis, arginine-containing peptides have been reported to dominate over the signal from other peptides in protein digests,[153] with the extent depending on the matrix used. The presence of ionic detergents, such as Triton X-100 and Tween 20, has also been shown to cause signal suppression in MALDI experiments, which can be countered by modifications to the matrix.[154]

Noise Reduction Techniques

In MS, background noise refers to the sum of electronic and chemical noise, which is independent of the data signal. Presence of the background noise interferes with the measurements and affects accuracy and specificity of analysis, especially at low concentrations. Reduction of chemical noise has been one of the aims for improvement since introduction of MS as an analytical technique. This is sometimes known as the "peak-at-every-mass" problem. The problem has long been known to mass spectrometrists, and it affects virtually all ionization methods to some degree.

Chemical noise is often dominant over electronic noise in MS. Background ions are inherent of atmospheric pressure ionization and related to the presence of impurities in the samples and in the mobile phases, residues accumulating on the surfaces of the ion source, and in part the high efficiency of atmospheric pressure ionization. Approaches used for noise reduction include optimizing the sample preparation, improving selectivity of ionization, optimization of the declustering conditions and ion transmission, maintaining cleanliness of the ion sources, and the flow path of the separation device.

One effective way for significant reduction of the effect of the background noise on the methods' performance is the use of MS/MS acquisition (MRM, neutral loss scan, product ion scan, and precursor ion scan), which allows substantial improvement of the detection specificity and reduction of the effects of chemical noise. Other approaches for reduction of the background noise include the use of mass analyzers with high resolving power (see Fig. 17.3); the use of multidimensional separations along with MS, such as ion mobility separations (IMS); high FAIMS; multidimensional chromatographic separations; and the incorporation of additional stages of fragmentation (MS/MS/MS). Software-based approaches (eg, dynamic background subtraction, active background noise reduction) also have been applied as noise reduction techniques. The previously mentioned techniques allow a reduction in the interference from the chemical background noise, but do not affect its cause. The best approach to the reduction of chemical background noise is the use of more extensive and efficient sample cleanup (as a way of minimizing introduction of contaminants into the ion source) and the use of high-purity solvents and additives for the mobile phases. This brings up the general issue of developing methods that are fit for purpose, but not so complex or expensive that their use will be impractical. Every laboratory needs to balance these factors in a way that is consistent with their goals, throughput, and constraints.

With regard to reducing background noise by using mass analyzers with high resolving power, it is important to understand the relationships among resolution, background noise (primarily chemical noise), electronic noise, and total signal level. A complete discussion is beyond the scope of the chapter, but a few general concepts can be useful to the clinical chemist without necessarily delving into all of the subtleties. For the sake of discussion, let us consider TOF detection. As mentioned earlier, this type of mass spectrometer acquires the full mass spectrum; that is, it is not possible to operate the instrument in SIM mode (or MRM mode in the case of a quadrupole TOF). However, it is possible to simulate SIM or MRM mode in postprocessing by integrating the mass spectrum over a limited *m/z* range and plotting the result as a function of spectrum number or chromatographic retention time.

If the *m/z* window is wide compared to the mass spectral peak width, the portion of the integrated signal arising from the targeted peak is independent of peak width. However, the signal arising from chemical noise generally increases with increasing width of the *m/z* window. This corresponds to the conditions in Figure 17.3, *A*—the FWHM of the TOF mass spectrometer was approximately 0.06 Da, whereas the window for generating the simulated SIM was 1 Da. Thus one would expect the chemical noise to decrease as the width of the integration window decreases.

The simulated SIM in Figure 17.3, *B* has the integration window set at 0.0072 Da, nearly an order of magnitude narrower than the peak width of the mass spectrometer. Under these conditions (ie, with the integration window much narrower than the peak width), narrowing the integration window still further affects chemical noise and target analyte signal nearly equally, so there is very little to be gained in terms of improving the signal-to-noise ratio by making the integration window narrower. Furthermore, in some cases there is a danger of increased statistical noise in the signal because ion numbers are quantized, which shows up as shot noise in the integrated signal. The signal-to-noise ratio in the shot noise-limit scales as 1 over the square root of the integration window width—that is, it gets worse as the window is made narrower. Discussion of the effect of the electronic noise on the noise budget is outside of the scope of this chapter, but it can be evaluated using methods analogous to those discussed previously.

Thus, in many cases, there is an optimum operating condition wherein the optimal integration window is often roughly equal to the peak width of the mass spectrometer. One additional comment is in order. Narrowing the integration window does nothing to reduce chemical noise if an interfering species is strictly isobaric with the targeted species. This implies that it is not at all useful if the goal is to reduce interferences from isomers. Furthermore, it is of very little usefulness if the mass offset of the interfering compound from the targeted compound is less than the peak width of the mass spectrometer. Nevertheless, as Figure 17.3 illustrates, a narrow window can be useful in improving the quality of chromatograms, and, as one can infer from the earlier discussion, this technique works best when using a high-resolution mass spectrometer.

POINTS TO REMEMBER

- MS is a highly sensitive and selective technique for analyzing a wide variety of clinically relevant analytes.
- MS relies on ionizing analytes in a sample, followed by separation of the ions according to their mass to charge ratios.
- When coupled with a separation technology such as gas chromatography or liquid chromatography, the hybrid technique is well suited for the quantitative analysis of clinically relevant molecules from bodily tissues and fluids.
- The use of MS for clinical applications has led to the development of highly specific assays that can overcome many of the issues faced when using immunoassays, such as cross-reactivity.
- Although highly selective, MS is not immune from interferences; molecules with same *m/z* (isomers and isobars) and similar fragmentation pattern may interfere with analysis

SELECTED REFERENCES

For a full list of references for this chapter, please refer to ExpertConsult.com.

1. Clinical Laboratory Standards Institute. *Mass spectrometry in the clinical laboratory. General principles and practice: approved guideline*, vol. C-50A. Wayne, Penn.: Clinical Laboratory Standards Institute; 2007.
2. Clinical Laboratory Standards Institute. *Liquid chromatography-mass spectrometry methods*, vol. C-62A. Wayne, Penn.: Clinical Laboratory Standards Institute; 2014.
3. Fenn JB. Electrospray wings for molecular elephants (Nobel lecture). *Angew Chem Int Ed Engl* 2003;**42**:3871–94.
10. Calvert J. Glossary of atmospheric chemistry terms 1990. *Pure Appl Chem* 1990;**62**:2167–219.
13. Glish GL, Vachet RW. The basics of mass spectrometry in the twenty-first century. *Nat Rev Drug Discov* 2003;**2**:140–50.
33. de Hoffman E, Stroobant V. *Mass spectrometry principles and applications*. 2nd ed. New York: John Wiley & Sons; 2001. p. 63–122, 132–155, 361.
36. Dawson PH. *Quadrupole mass spectometry and its applications*. New York: Elsevier; 1976. p. 65–78.
42. Mamyrin B, Karataev V, Shmikk D, et al. Mass reflectron: new non-magnetic time-of-flight high-resolution mass spectrometer. *Zh Eksp Teor Fiz.* 1973;**64**:82–9.
45. Bystrom C, Sheng S, Zhang K, et al. Clinical utility of insulin-like growth factor 1 and 2; determination by high resolution mass spectrometry. *PLoS ONE* 2012;**7**:e43457.
54. Hu Q, Noll RJ, Li H, et al. The orbitrap: a new mass spectrometer. *J Mass Spectrom* 2005;**40**:430–43.
75. Annesley T, Majzoub J, Hsing A, et al. Mass spectrometry in the clinical laboratory: how have we done, and where do we need to be? *Clin Chem* 2009;**55**:1236–9.
95. Chace DH. Mass spectrometry in newborn and metabolic screening: historical perspective and future directions. *J Mass Spectrom* 2009;**44**:163–70.
97. Gao S, Zhang ZP, Karnes HT. Sensitivity enhancement in liquid chromatography/atmospheric pressure ionization mass spectrometry using derivatization and mobile phase

additives. *J Chromatogr B Analyt Technol Biomed Life Sci* 2005;**825**:98–110.

111. Hoofnagle AN, Becker JO, Wener MH, et al. Quantification of thyroglobulin, a low-abundance serum protein, by immunoaffinity peptide enrichment and tandem mass spectrometry. *Clin Chem* 2008;**54**:1796–804.
119. Jeppsson JO, Kobold U, Barr J, et al. Approved IFCC reference method for the measurement of HbA1c in human blood. *Clin Chem Lab Med* 2002;**40**:78–89.
130. Cornett DS, Reyzer ML, Chaurand P, et al. MALDI imaging mass spectrometry: molecular snapshots of biochemical systems. *Nat Methods* 2007;**4**:828–33.
135. Hoofnagle AN, Wener MH. The fundamental flaws of immunoassays and potential solutions using tandem mass spectrometry. *J Immunol Methods* 2009;**347**:3–11.
136. Kushnir MM, Rockwood AL, Nelson GJ, et al. Assessing analytical specificity in quantitative analysis using tandem mass spectrometry. *Clin Biochem* 2005;**38**:319–27.
144. Matuszewski BK, Constanzer ML, Chavez-Eng CM. Matrix effect in quantitative LC/MS/MS analyses of biological fluids: a method for determination of finasteride in human plasma at picogram per milliliter concentrations. *Anal Chem* 1998;**70**:882–9.
145. Bonfiglio R, King RC, Olah TV, et al. The effects of sample preparation methods on the variability of the electrospray ionization response for model drug compounds. *Rapid Commun Mass Spectrom* 1999;**13**:1175–85.

18

Sample Preparation for Mass Spectrometry Applications

David A. Wells

ABSTRACT

Background
Biological samples require one or more pretreatment steps before analysis and detection by mass spectrometry. This chapter discusses the different sample preparation steps performed in laboratories analyzing drugs and proteins in the clinical and research setting and introduces high-throughput applications.

Content
The general techniques discussed are dilution, centrifugation, sonication, and homogenization. Separation techniques are filtration and ultrafiltration, dialysis and microdialysis, desalting, buffer exchange, enzymatic hydrolysis, and acid-base digestion. The precipitation technique discussed is protein precipitation. Enrichment techniques are evaporation, solvent exchange, and derivatization. Extraction techniques reviewed are liquid-liquid extraction, solid-supported liquid-liquid extraction, and solid-phase extraction (off-line and online sample processing). The chromatographic techniques discussed are column-switching (single and dual column modes) for turbulent flow chromatography, restricted access media, monolithic columns, and immunoaffinity extraction. The evolving techniques described are dried blood spots, capillary microsampling, and tissue imaging.

19

Mass Spectrometry Applications in Infectious Disease and Pathogens Identification

*Phillip Heaton and Robin Patel**

ABSTRACT

Background

Matrix-assisted laser desorption ionization time-of-flight mass spectrometry (MALDI-TOF-MS) is a powerful tool in the clinical microbiology laboratory enabling accurate identification of bacteria, fungi, and mycobacteria. First adopted in European microbiology laboratories, its ease of use, accuracy, rapid turnaround times, and low cost have led to its widespread adoption in microbiology laboratories worldwide. In contrast, polymerase chain reaction electrospray ionization–mass spectrometry (PCR-ESI-MS) is an emerging technology for clinical microbiology with the potential for direct-from-sample testing and actionable results in a few hours.

Content

This first half of this chapter briefly discusses the history of MALDI-TOF-MS leading to its commercialization and adoption in clinical microbiology laboratories. Identification of aerobic and anaerobic organisms as well as mycobacteria and fungi is discussed. Additional applications, such as direct identification from blood and urine cultures as well as antimicrobial susceptibility testing are also reviewed. Additionally, implementation of MALDI-TOF-MS into routine laboratory workflows is addressed. The second half of this chapter discusses PCR-ESI-MS and its potential applications in the clinical microbiology laboratory in its current state.

*This chapter expands upon the previous review: Patel R. *Clin Chem* 2015;61:100–111, with permission.

20

Development and Validation of Small Molecule Analytes by Liquid Chromatography-Tandem Mass Spectrometry

Russell P. Grant and Brian A. Rappold

ABSTRACT

Background

The application of liquid chromatography coupled to tandem mass spectrometry (LC-MS/MS) represents one of the most compelling opportunities for advancements in human health through the combination of reference measurement procedure capabilities, broad chemical coverage, and a rich history in support of drug development from the 1990s onward. Clinical application of these technologies has begun to gather pace in many laboratories, with diverse applications ranging from expanded newborn screening to identification of emerging toxicants. The promise of these technologies is vast and the need is palpable; however, the journey can be exacting. Perhaps somewhat unique among analytical techniques, LC-MS/MS assay development and validation requires significant knowledge of a number of specialties: a mastery of chemistry (sample preparation, chromatography, ionization), physics (ion manipulation), engineering principles (automation, order of experiments, programming), and mathematics (data reduction and interpretation) applied to questions of a biological origin (normal, disease, metabolism).

Content

This chapter provides a stepwise roadmap for systematically developing and validating an LC-MS/MS assay for small molecule analytes. Starting from first principles (salt correction in gravimetric weighing), each component of the LC-MS/MS assay (mass spectrometer tuning, ionization enhancements, chromatography, extraction) is detailed with best-practice experiments for development and data reduction techniques to fulfill performance goals. After refinement of each component of the assay, prevalidation experiments are described to enable efficient execution of validation. Finally, an array of validation guidance documents is reduced to a coherent process for burden of proof.

21

Proteomics

Andrew N. Hoofnagle and Cory Bystrom

ABSTRACT

Background
Clinical proteomics has traditionally referred to experiments that attempt to discover novel biomarkers for disease diagnosis, prognosis, or therapeutic management by using tools that measure the abundance of hundreds or thousands of proteins in a single sample. These discovery experiments began with protein electrophoresis, particularly two-dimensional (2D) gel electrophoresis, and have evolved into workflows that rely very heavily on mass spectrometry (MS). Using the workflows developed for discovery proteomics, clinical laboratories have developed quantitative assays for proteins in human samples that solve many of the issues associated with the measurement of proteins by immunoassay. The technology is changing clinical research and is poised to significantly transform protein measurements used in patient care.

Content
This chapter begins with the history of clinical proteomics, with a special emphasis on 2D gel electrophoresis of serum and plasma proteins. It then describes discovery techniques that use MS, including data-dependent acquisition and data-independent acquisition. It finishes with a discussion of targeted quantitative proteomic methods, both bottom-up and top-down, as replacement methodologies for immunoassays and Western blotting. Special attention is paid to peptide selection, denaturation and digestion, peptide and protein enrichment, internal standards, and calibration.

22

Enzyme and Rate Analysis

Renze Bais and Mauro Panteghini

ABSTRACT

Background

Enzymes are biological catalysts that can be used in the monitoring and diagnosis of disease, and their remarkable properties make them sensitive indicators of pathologic change.

Metabolism can be regarded as an integrated series of enzymatic reactions and some diseases as a derangement of the physiologic pattern of metabolism. Many enzymes exist in multiple forms, and differences in their properties help in differentiating them and understanding organ-specific pathophysiology. Genetically determined variations in enzyme structure among individuals are used to account for such characteristics as differences in sensitivity to drugs and differences in metabolism that manifest as hereditary metabolic diseases.

Content

The properties and mechanism of action of enzymes that influence the specificity and sensitivity of these proteins and enables them to be used in disease management are described. In addition, the existence of multiple forms of some enzymes provides opportunities to increase the diagnostic specificity and sensitivity of enzyme assays in body fluids. The principles of enzyme kinetics are described, as well as how these properties are affected by activators and inhibitors. Kinetic properties are used to develop optimal conditions for measuring enzymatic activity. It is shown how these properties also enable enzymes to be used as biological reagents in the measurement of metabolites and as indicator reactions in many immunoassays.

Enzymes are proteins with catalytic properties, and clinical enzymology is the application of the science of enzymes to the diagnosis and treatment of disease. The principles of clinical enzymology will be introduced and discussed in this chapter, as will information on how enzymes are measured and how they are used as analytical reagents in various types of rate analysis. Individual topics include basic principles, enzyme kinetics, analytical enzymology, and rate analyses.

BASIC PRINCIPLES

This section discusses enzyme nomenclature followed by a description of enzymes as proteins and biological catalysts.

Enzyme Nomenclature

Historically, individual enzymes were identified using the name of the substrate or group on which they act and then adding the suffix *-ase.* For example, the enzyme hydrolyzing urea was ure*ase.* Later, the type of reaction involved was identified, as in carbonic anhydrase, D-amino acid oxidase, and succinate dehydrogenase. In addition, some enzymes were given empirical names such as trypsin, diastase, ptyalin, pepsin, and emulsin.

Because this combination of trivial common names and semisystematic names was found to be inadequate, in 1955 the International Union of Biochemistry (IUB) appointed an Enzyme Commission (EC) to study the problem of enzyme nomenclature. Its subsequent recommendations, with periodic updating, provide a rational and practical basis for identifying all enzymes now known and enzymes that will be discovered in the future.[1]

With the IUB system, a systematic and trivial name is provided for each enzyme. The systematic name describes the nature of the reaction catalyzed and is associated with a unique numeric code. The trivial or practical name, which may be identical to the systematic name but is often a simplification of it, is suitable for everyday use. The unique numeric designation for each enzyme consists of four numbers, separated by periods (eg, 2.2.8.11), and is prefixed by the letters *EC,* denoting *Enzyme Commission.* The first number defines the class to which the enzyme belongs. All enzymes are assigned to one of six classes, characterized by the type of reaction they catalyze: (1) oxidoreductases, (2) transferases, (3) hydrolases, (4) lyases, (5) somerases, and (6) ligases. The next two numbers indicate the subclass and the sub-subclass to which the enzyme is assigned. For example, these may differentiate the amino-transferring subclass from the phosphate-transferring category, or the ethanol acceptor sub-subclass from that accepting acyl groups. The last number is the specific serial number given to each enzyme within its sub-subclass.

To illustrate how this system is used to name an enzyme, consider the enzyme creatine kinase, which catalyzes the following reaction:

$$\text{ATP} + \text{creatine} \rightleftharpoons \text{ADP} + \text{creatine phosphate}$$

TABLE 22.1 Enzyme Commission Numbers, Systematic and Trivial Names, and Frequently Adopted Abbreviations of Enzymes of Major Clinical Importance

EC Number	Systematic Name	Trivial Name	Abbreviation
1.1.1.27	L-Lactate: NAD$^+$ oxidoreductase	Lactate dehydrogenase	LD
1.4.1.3	L-Glutamate: NAD(P)$^+$ oxidoreductase (deaminating)	Glutamate dehydrogenase	GLD
2.3.2.2	(γ-Glutamyl)-peptide: amino acid γ-glutamyltransferase	γ-Glutamyltransferase	GGT
2.6.1.1	L-Aspartate: 2-oxoglutarate aminotransferase	Aspartate aminotransferase (transaminase)	AST
2.6.1.2	L-Alanine: 2-oxoglutarate aminotransferase	Alanine aminotransferase (transaminase)	ALT
2.7.3.2	ATP: creatine *N*-phosphotransferase	Creatine kinase	CK
3.1.1.3	Triacylglycerol acylhydrolase	Lipase	LPS
3.1.1.7	Acetylcholine acetylhydrolase	Acetylcholinesterase, true cholinesterase, choline esterase I	—
3.1.1.8	Acylcholine acylhydrolase	Pseudocholinesterase, butyryl cholinesterase, choline esterase II (serum cholinesterase)	CHE
3.1.3.1	Orthophosphoric-monoester phosphohydrolase (alkaline optimum)	Alkaline phosphatase	ALP
3.1.3.2	Orthophosphoric-monoester phosphohydrolase (acid optimum)	Acid phosphatase	ACP
3.1.3.5	5′-Ribonucleotide phosphohydrolase	5′-Nucleotidase	NTP
3.2.1.1	1,4-α-D-Glucan glucanohydrolase	Amylase	AMY
3.4.21.4		Trypsin	TRY
4.1.2.13	D-Fructose-1,6-bisphosphate D-glyceraldehyde-3-phosphate-lyase	Aldolase	ALD

EC, Enzyme Commission; *NAD*, nicotinamide adenine dinucleotide; *NAD(P)*, NAD phosphate.

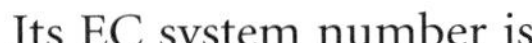
Its EC system number is

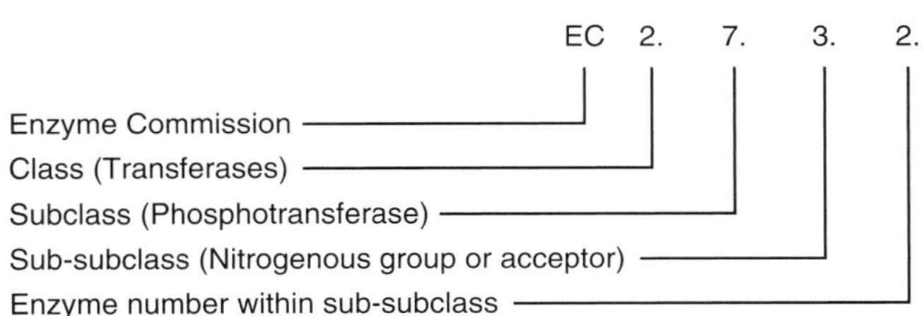

Table 22.1 lists selected enzymes of clinical interest, identified by trivial, abbreviated, and systematic names and by their code numbers.

Although not recommended by the EC, it is a common and convenient practice to use capital letter abbreviations for the names of certain enzymes, such as ALT for alanine aminotransferase, AST for aspartate aminotransferase, LD for lactate dehydrogenase, and CK for creatine kinase (see Table 22.1).

Enzymes as Proteins

Enzymes are proteins that possess the primary, secondary, and tertiary structural characteristics of proteins (see Chapter 28), and most also exhibit quaternary structure. The *primary* structure, the linear sequence of amino acids linked through their α-carboxyl and α-amino groups by peptide bonds, is specific for each type of enzyme molecule. Each polypeptide chain is coiled into three-dimensional (3D) secondary and tertiary structures. Secondary structure refers to the conformation of limited segments of the polypeptide chain, namely α-helices, β-pleated sheets, random coils, and β-turns. The arrangement of secondary structural elements and amino acid side chain interactions that define the 3D structure of the folded protein is referred to as its tertiary structure. In many cases, biological activity, such as the catalytic activity of enzymes, requires two or more folded polypeptide chains (subunits) to associate to form a functional molecule. The arrangement of these subunits defines the quaternary structure. The subunits may be copies of the same polypeptide chain (eg, the MM isoenzyme of CK, the H_4 isoenzyme of LD), or they may represent distinct polypeptides (eg, the MB isoenzyme of CK).

In general, no feature of primary structures is common to all enzyme molecules. However, considerable homologies of sequence are found between enzymes that appear to share a common evolutionary origin, such as the proteases trypsin and chymotrypsin, and similarities of sequence are even more marked among the members of a family of isoenzymes. The amino acid sequence in the immediate neighborhood of the active center of the enzyme (discussed later) is often similar in enzymes with related function (eg, the *serine proteases* are so called because they all have this amino acid in the active center).

Enzyme molecules differ in the proportion of secondary structures—such as α-helices—they contain, although no enzyme molecule studied thus far approaches the large proportion of α-helices found in myoglobin and hemoglobin. The tertiary structures of different types of enzyme molecules are as individually characteristic as their primary structures; nevertheless, some common features exist. Enzyme molecules are roughly globular in overall shape, with a preponderance of polar amino acid side chains on the outside of the molecule and nonpolar side chains in the interior. The ionizable residues in contact with the surrounding medium are responsible for many of the properties of the enzyme molecules in solution, such as their migration in an electric field and their solubility. Covalent disulfide bridges may link different parts of the polypeptide chains in some enzyme molecules, but the 3D structure is mainly stabilized by the large number of hydrophobic interactions formed between the nonpolar side chains in the interior of the molecule.

The application of physical methods, such as x-ray crystallography and multidimensional nuclear magnetic resonance, has provided structural insights on which enzyme mechanisms have been built. Furthermore, the tools of molecular biology, such as molecular cloning, have enabled the purification and characterization of enzymes that previously were available only in minute amounts. Molecular biology also enables the manipulation of the amino acid sequence of enzymes, and site-directed mutagenesis (substituting one amino acid residue for another) and deletion mutagenesis (eliminating sections of the primary structure) have enabled the identification of chemical groups that participate in ligand binding and specific chemical steps during catalysis. There are a number of free online databases describing various properties of enzymes, including structure[2] and reaction mechanisms.[3]

The biological activity of a protein molecule depends generally on the integrity of its structure, and any disruption of its structure is accompanied by a loss of activity, a process known as *denaturation.* If the process of denaturation is minimal, it may be reversed with the recovery of enzyme activity on removal of the denaturing agent. However, prolonged or severe denaturing conditions result in an irreversible loss of activity. Denaturing conditions include increased temperatures, extremes of pH, and chemical addition. Heat inactivation of most enzymes takes place at an appreciable rate at room temperature and in most cases becomes almost instantaneous above 60°C. The polymerases are an exception and retain activity at temperatures as high as 90°C—a property that has been made use of in the polymerase chain reaction (see Chapter 44). Low temperatures are used to preserve enzyme activity, especially in aqueous solutions, such as serum (see Chapter 29). Extremes of pH also cause unfolding of enzyme molecular structures and, except for a few exceptions, should be avoided when enzyme samples are preserved. Addition of chemicals, such as urea and detergents, disrupts hydrogen bonds and hydrophobic interactions so that exposure of enzymes to strong solutions of these reagents results in inactivation.

Specificity and the Active Center

With the exception of enzymes such as proteases, nucleases, and amylases, which act on macromolecular substrates, enzyme molecules are considerably larger than the molecules of their substrates. Consideration of the structure of an enzyme's active site and its relationship to the structures of the enzyme's substrate(s) in its ground and transition states is necessary to understand the rate enhancement and specificity of the chemical reactions performed by an enzyme. The active site of an enzyme will vary among enzymes but in general[4]:

1. The active site of an enzyme is relatively small compared with the total size of the enzyme molecule and may involve less than 5% of the total amino acids in the molecule.
2. The active sites of enzymes are 3D structures that are formed as a result of the overall tertiary structure of the protein. This results in the amino acids and cofactors in the active site of an enzyme being spatially structured in an exact, 3D relationship with respect to one another and reflects the structure of the substrate molecule.
3. Typically, the attraction between the molecules of the enzyme and its substrate molecules is noncovalent binding. Physical forces used in this type of binding include hydrogen bonding, electrostatic and hydrophobic interactions, and van der Waals interactions.
4. Active sites of enzymes typically occur in clefts and crevices in the protein.

The specificity of substrate binding is a function of the exact spatial arrangement of atoms in the enzyme active site that complements the structure of the substrate molecule.[5]

Isoenzymes and Other Multiple Forms of Enzymes

The IUB recommends that isoenzyme or isozyme should apply only to those multiple forms of enzymes arising from genetically determined differences in primary structure and not to those derived by modification of the same primary sequence.[5] The term *multiple forms of the enzyme* should be used as a broad term covering all proteins catalyzing the same reaction and occurring naturally in a single species, for example, to an enzyme that has undergone posttranslational modification.

Isoenzymes may occur within a single organ or even within a single type of cell. The forms can be distinguished on the basis of differences in various physical properties, such as electrophoretic mobility and resistance to chemical or thermal inactivation. They often have significant quantifiable differences in catalytic properties, but all forms of a particular enzyme retain the ability to catalyze its characteristic reaction.

The existence of multiple forms of enzymes in human tissue has important implications in the study of human disease. The presence in different organs of isoenzymes with distinctive properties helps in understanding organ-specific patterns of metabolism, but genetically determined variations in enzyme structure among individuals account for such characteristics as differences in sensitivity to drugs and differences in metabolism, which manifest themselves as hereditary metabolic diseases. For diagnostic enzymology, the existence of multiple forms of enzymes, whether the result of genetic or nongenetic causes, provides opportunities to increase the diagnostic specificity and sensitivity of enzyme assays in body fluid samples.

Similar to other proteins, enzymes usually elicit the production of antibodies when they are injected into animals of a species other than those in which they originate. Even small structural differences among closely similar molecules, such as the members of a family of isoenzymes, are often sufficient to render them antigenically distinct, allowing antibodies to be produced specific to a single type of molecule. The availability of enzyme-specific antisera opens up a wide range of methods in enzyme analysis, some of which—such as immunoassay—do not depend on the catalytic activity of the enzyme molecules. The availability of immunochemical methods has been particularly important in the analysis of isoenzyme mixtures. Many commercial immunoassays now use monoclonal antibodies to increase specificity.

Genetic Origins of Enzyme Variants

True isoenzymes result from the existence of more than one gene locus coding for the structure of the enzyme protein. Many human enzymes (more than one-third) are known to be determined by more than one structural gene locus. Genes at the different loci have undergone differential modifications during the course of evolution, so that the enzyme proteins coded by them no longer have identical structures, although they are recognizably similar; in other words, they are isoenzymes.

The multiple genes that determine a particular group of isoenzymes are not necessarily closely linked on one chromosome. For example, the structural genes that code for human salivary and pancreatic amylases both are located on chromosome 1, whereas the genes that code for cytoplasmic and mitochondrial malate dehydrogenase are carried on chromosomes 2 and 7, respectively. Among the enzymes of clinical importance that exist as isoenzymes because of the presence of multiple-gene loci are LD, CK, α-amylase, and some forms of alkaline phosphatase (ALP).

An enzyme can exist in molecular forms that differ from one individual to another because of the existence of alternative alleles that are inherited according to mendelian laws. These give rise to gene products with the same function and isoenzymes that result from the existence of allelic genes that are termed *allozymes*. The proportion of human gene loci subject to allelic variation is considerable, and the probability that individual human beings will differ to some degree in their isoenzyme patterns is correspondingly high.

The number of allelic variants and the frequency with which particular variants occur within the population vary considerably across enzymes. For example, mutations at either of the two principal loci that determine human LD are extremely rare, but a high incidence of mutant alleles occurs at the single locus that determines the structure of placental ALP. More than 400 mutations in the glucose-6-phosphate dehydrogenase gene have now been identified on the X chromosome (up-to-date genetic information on this and other enzymes can be obtained from the Online Mendelian Inheritance in Man [OMIM] database).[6] When isoenzymes, because of variation at a single locus, occur with appreciable frequency in a human population, the population is said to be *polymorphic* with respect to the isoenzymes in question.

Another category of multiple molecular forms can arise when enzymes are oligomeric, consisting of molecules made up of subunits. The association of different types of subunits in various combinations gives rise to a range of active enzyme molecules. When the subunits are derived from different structural genes—multiple loci or multiple alleles—the hybrid molecules so formed are called *hybrid isoenzymes*. The ability to form hybrid isoenzymes is evidence of considerable structural similarities among the different subunits. Hybrid isoenzymes can be formed in vitro, but they are also formed in vivo in cells in which different types of constituent subunits are present in the same subcellular compartment.

The number of different hybrid isoenzymes that can be formed from two nonidentical protomers depends on the number of subunits in the complete enzyme molecule. For a dimeric enzyme, one mixed dimer (hybrid isoenzyme) can be formed. If the enzyme is a tetramer, three heteropolymeric isoenzymes may be formed (Fig. 22.1). Examples of hybrid isoenzymes include the mixed MB dimer of CK and the three hybrid isoenzymes, LD-2, LD-3, and LD-4, of LD.

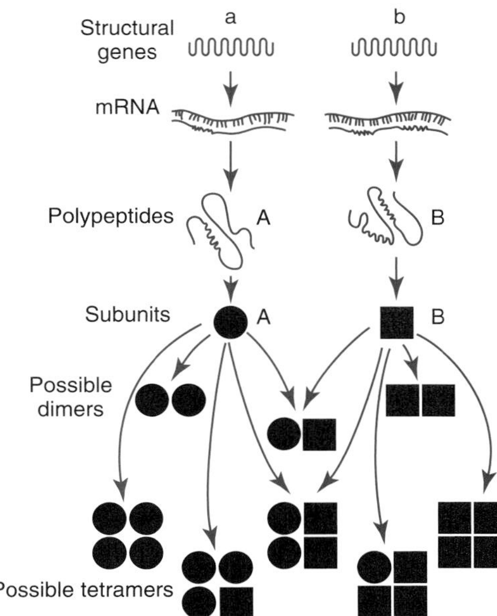

FIGURE 22.1 Diagram showing the origin of isoenzymes, assuming the existence of two distinct gene loci. When the active enzymes are polymers containing more than one subunit, hybrid isoenzymes consisting of mixtures of different subunits may be formed. One such isoenzyme can be formed in the case of a dimeric enzyme, such as creatine kinase and three if the enzyme is a tetramer (eg, lactate dehydrogenase). In both cases, two homopolymeric isoenzymes also can exist. (From Moss DW. Isoenzyme analysis. London: The Chemical Society, 1979. Reproduced by permission of The Royal Society of Chemistry.)

Nongenetic Causes of Multiple Forms of Enzymes

Posttranslational modifications of enzyme molecules give rise to multiple forms known as *isoforms* (Fig. 22.2).

Modifications of residues in the polypeptide chains of enzyme molecules take place in living cells to yield multiple forms. For example, removal of amide groups accounts for some of the heterogeneity of amylase and carbonic anhydrase (each of these enzymes also exists as a true isoenzyme). Modification also can take place as a result of extraction procedures. Many erythrocyte enzymes, including adenosine deaminase, acid phosphatase, and some forms of phosphoglucomutase, contain sulfhydryl groups that are susceptible to oxidation. In hemolysates, oxidation may be brought about by the action of oxidized glutathione, although in intact cells, this compound is present in its reduced form. Thus variant enzyme molecules with altered molecular charge may be generated.

Serum isoforms of CK are formed as part of the normal clearance process of the cell. Human myocardial and skeletal muscle tissues have the CK-MM and CK-MB isoenzymes, which are modified on release into the circulation. This modification is due to sequential removal of the C-terminal amino acid, lysine, by the action of carboxypeptidase.

Modifications affecting nonprotein components of enzyme molecules also may lead to molecular heterogeneity. Many enzymes are glycoproteins, and variations in

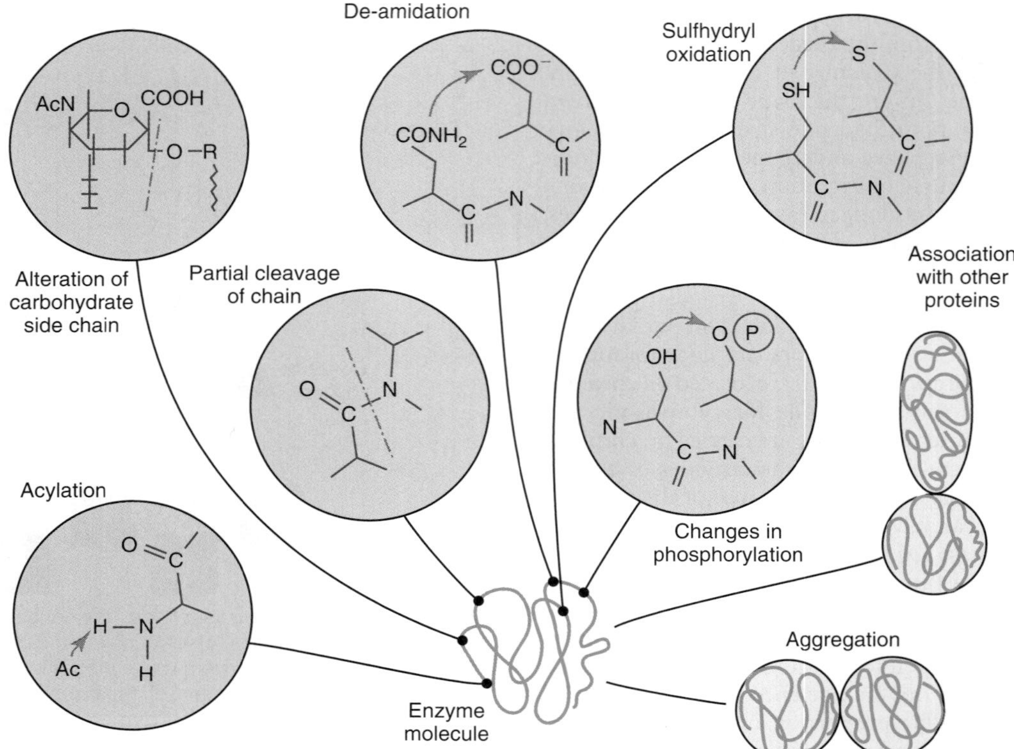

FIGURE 22.2 Nongenetic modifications that may give rise to multiple forms of enzymes. (From Moss DW. *Isoenzymes.* London: Chapman & Hall, 1982.)

carbohydrate side chains are a common cause of nonhomogeneity of preparations of these enzymes. Some carbohydrate moieties, notably *N*-acetylneuraminic acid (sialic acid), are strongly ionized and consequently have a profound effect on some properties of enzyme molecules.[7] For example, removal of terminal sialic acid groups from human liver and/or bone ALP with neuraminidase greatly reduces the electrophoretic heterogeneity of the enzyme.

Aggregation of enzyme molecules with each other or with nonenzymatic proteins may give rise to multiple forms that can be separated by techniques that depend on differences in molecular size. For example, four catalytically active cholinesterase components with molecular weights ranging from approximately 80,000 to 340,000 are found in most sera, with the heaviest component, carbon (C_4), contributing most of the enzyme activity. Other enzyme forms are also occasionally present, but it appears that the principal serum cholinesterase fractions can be attributed to different states of aggregation of a single monomer.

A specific form of interaction between enzymatic and nonenzymatic proteins, such as immunoglobulins, results in the formation of an enzyme-protein complex (macrocomplex). Since the identification of macroamylase, the first such enzyme–immunoglobulin complex to be identified, similar complexes have been observed involving LD, CK, ALP, and other enzymes.

A single polypeptide chain in theory exists in an infinite number of different conformations. However, one specific conformation generally appears to be the most stable for any given sequence of amino acids, and this conformation is assumed by the chain as it is synthesized within the cell. Thus the primary structure of the polypeptide chain also determines its 3D secondary and tertiary structures. It is conceivable that in some cases, several alternative conformations (conformers) of a single chain that are almost equally stable may be present, and therefore these alternative forms may coexist. However, no multiple-enzyme forms have been shown unequivocally to be due to conformational isomerism.

Changes in Isoenzyme Distribution During Development and Disease

The patterns of many isoenzymes change during physiologic development in tissues from many species. For example, during the embryonic development of skeletal muscle, the proportions of the electrophoretically more cathodal isoenzymes—both LD and CK—progressively increase in this tissue until approximately the sixth month of intrauterine life, when the pattern resembles that of differentiated muscle.

The liver also shows characteristic changes in the patterns of several isoenzymes during embryogenesis. In early fetal development, three aldolase isoenzymes—A, B, and C—together with various hybrid tetramers, can be detected in extracts of liver. However, at birth, as in the adult liver, aldolase B is the predominant isoenzyme. Striking changes in the distribution of isoenzymes of alcohol dehydrogenase also occur in human liver during prenatal development.

Changes in isoenzyme patterns during development result from changes in the relative activities of gene loci within developing cells of a particular type (eg, muscle cells). Other alterations in the balance of isoenzymes within the whole organism may derive from changes in the number or activity of cells that contain large amounts of a characteristic isoenzyme. An example of this is the increased number and activity of the osteoblasts, which are responsible for mineralization of the skeleton between the early postnatal period and the beginning of the third decade of life. An excess of ALP from active osteoblasts enters the circulation, where its presence can be recognized by its characteristic properties and where it increases the total serum ALP activity of young individuals to values higher than in skeletally mature adults. An ALP from the liver also contributes to the total activity of this enzyme in the plasma of healthy individuals, and the amount of this form in plasma shows a small, progressive increase with age. The reason for the latter age-dependent change is not known, but it may result from increased synthesis of the enzyme by hepatocytes in response to continuing exposure to inducing factors.

Certain diseases, such as the progressive muscular dystrophies, appear to involve failure of the affected tissues to mature normally or maintain a normal state. The distributions of isoenzymes of aldolase, LD, and CK in the muscles of patients with progressive muscular dystrophy have been found to be similar to those in the earlier stages of development of fetal muscle. Isoenzyme abnormalities in dystrophic muscle have been interpreted as failure to reach or maintain a normal degree of differentiation. Isoenzyme patterns seen in regenerating tissues also may show some tendency to approach fetal distributions. This tendency may result from relaxation or modification of control systems in rapidly dividing cells and may account for some of the isoenzyme changes noted (eg, in muscle in acute polymyositis).

Cancer cells show progressive loss of the structure and metabolism of the healthy cells from which they arise. Therefore the pattern of isoenzymes of mature, differentiated tissue may be lost or modified if normal differentiation is arrested or reversed, and many examples of isoenzyme changes accompanying such processes have been reported. Reemergence of fetal patterns of isoenzyme distribution is a feature of malignant transformation in many tissues. This phenomenon was first studied extensively in the case of LD isoenzymes. Malignant tumors in general show a significant shift in the balance of isoenzymes toward electrophoretically more cathodal forms such as LD-4 and LD-5. The decline in activity of the LD-1 and LD-2 isoenzymes results in patterns that are reminiscent of those occurring in embryonic tissues. Tumors of prostate, cervix, breast, brain, stomach, colon, rectum, bronchus, and lymph nodes are among those that show this transformation. In contrast, comparatively benign gliomas show a relative increase in anionic isoenzymes. A relative increase in the proportion of cathodal isoenzymes of LD has been observed in tissue adjacent to malignant tumors (eg, the colon), although the cells in these regions are morphologically normal.

Differences in Properties Among Multiple Forms of Enzymes

Structural differences among the multiple forms of an enzyme give rise to greater or lesser differences in physicochemical properties, such as electrophoretic mobility, resistance to inactivation, and solubility or in catalytic characteristics, such as the ratio of reaction with substrate analogs or response to inhibitors. Methods of isoenzyme analysis have therefore been designed to investigate a wide range of catalytic and structural properties of enzyme molecules.[8] However, it is usually possible to make only limited deductions about the nature of the underlying structural differences between isoenzymes that are responsible for the dissimilar properties. Equally, the changes in catalytic and other properties that may result from specific structural alterations in enzyme molecules are difficult to predict from current theoretical knowledge of the relationship between structure and function of proteins.[9]

Techniques of molecular biology, such as gene cloning and sequencing, have revolutionized investigation of the primary structures of isoenzymes. Differences in primary structures among isoenzymes, whether derived from multiple-gene loci or from different alleles, are now known to exist in a growing number of cases. Furthermore, many questions have been answered about whether multiple-enzyme forms represented true (genetically determined) isoenzymes or arose from posttranslational modification.

Isoenzymes caused by the existence of multiple-gene loci usually differ quantitatively in catalytic properties. These differences may be manifested in such characteristics as molecular activity, K_m values for substrate(s), sensitivity to various inhibitors, and relative rates of activity with substrate analogs (when the specificity of the isoenzymes allows the substrate to be varied), underscoring the biological importance of isoenzymatic variation. In contrast, multiple-enzyme forms that arise by such posttranslational modifications as aggregation usually have similar catalytic properties.

Multilocus isoenzymes also usually differ in terms of antigenic specificity, although these differences may be less pronounced among isoenzymes that have emerged relatively recently in evolutionary history and are closely related in structure. Immunologic cross-reaction is not uncommon among multilocus isoenzymes. Multiple-enzyme forms caused by posttranslational modification frequently have common antigenic determinants. Isoenzymes derived from allelic genes (allozymes) are also often antigenically similar, even to the extent that they may cross-react with antisera to the common isoenzyme despite a mutation having abolished enzyme activity altogether. The capacity for detecting differences among antigenically similar isoenzyme molecules depends on the extent of monoclonal antibody specificity.

Differences in resistance to denaturation (eg, by heat, concentrated urea solutions, detergents) are commonly found among true isoenzymes, whether these are the products of multiple loci or multiple alleles. Other multiple forms of enzymes often do not differ or differ only slightly in this respect. The most commonly exploited difference among isoenzymes is the difference in net molecular charge that results from the altered amino acid compositions of the molecules; this forms the basis of separation by zone electrophoresis, ion-exchange chromatography, or isoelectric focusing. Separation methods that depend on differences in molecular size, such as gel filtration, do not distinguish among the small size differences that often exist among true isoenzyme molecules but are important in the detection of multiple forms that involve aggregation or association of enzyme molecules with other proteins, such as immunoglobulins.

Enzymes as Catalysts

A catalyst is a substance that modifies and increases the rate of a particular chemical reaction without being consumed or permanently altered. Enzymes are protein catalysts of biological origin. Metabolism is a coordinated series of chemical reactions that occur within a living cell to provide energy and accomplish biosynthesis. The process can be regarded as an integrated series of enzymatic reactions and some diseases as a derangement of the normal pattern of metabolism. Apart from these fundamental considerations, it is the remarkable properties of enzymes that make them such sensitive indicators of pathologic change.

Because of their catalytic activity, a given number of enzyme molecules convert an enormous number of substrate molecules to products within a short time. This property is used to measure increased amounts of enzymes in the bloodstream, although the amount of enzyme protein released from damaged cells is small compared with the total quantity of nonenzymatic proteins in blood. Thus a change in the quantity of a particular enzyme is recognized by its characteristic effect on a given chemical reaction.

Units for Expressing Enzyme Activity

When enzymes are measured by their catalytic activities, the results of such determinations are expressed in terms of the concentration of the number of activity units present in a convenient volume or mass of specimen. The unit of activity is the measure of the rate at which the reaction proceeds (eg, the quantity of substrate consumed or product formed in a unit of time). In clinical enzymology, the activity of an enzyme is generally reported in terms of unit of volume, such as activity per 100 mL, per liter of serum, or per 1.0 mL of packed erythrocytes. Because the rate of the reaction depends on experimental parameters, such as pH, type of buffer, temperature, nature of substrate, ionic strength, concentration of activators, and other variables, these parameters must be specified in the definition of the unit.

To standardize how enzyme activities are expressed, the EC proposed that the unit of enzyme activity should be defined as the quantity of enzyme that catalyzes the reaction of 1 μmol of substrate per minute and that this unit should be termed the international unit (U). Catalytic concentration is to be expressed in terms of units per liter (U/L) or kilounits (kU/L), whichever gives the more convenient numeric value. In this chapter, the symbol U is used to denote the international unit. In those instances in which there is some uncertainty about the exact nature of the substrate, or when difficulty is encountered in calculating the number of micromoles reacting (as with macromolecules such as starch, protein, and complex lipids), the unit is to be expressed in terms of the chemical group or residue measured in the following reaction (eg, glucose units, amino acid units formed).

The International System of Units (SI)-derived unit for catalytic activity is the katal, defined as moles converted per second. The name *katal* had been used for this unit for decades but did not become an official SI-derived unit until 1999 with Resolution 12 of the 21st French Conférence Général des Poids et Mesures, on the recommendation of the International Federation of Clinical Chemistry and Laboratory Medicine. Both the International Union of Pure and Applied Chemistry and the IUB now recommend that enzyme activity be expressed in moles per second and that the enzyme concentration be expressed in terms of katals per liter (kat/L).[8] Thus 1 U = 10^{-6} mol/60 s = 16.7×10^{-9} mol/s, or 1.0 nkat/L = 0.06 U/L.

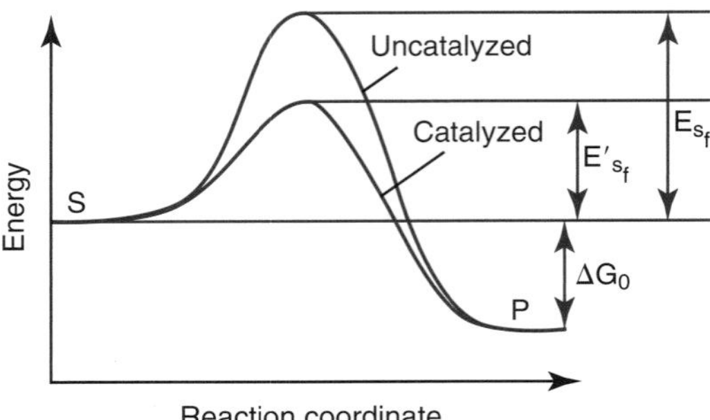

FIGURE 22.3 Activation energy barrier and reaction course, with and without enzyme catalysis. E_{Sf} is the activation energy for the forward reaction ($S \rightarrow P$) in the absence of a catalyst, and E'_{Sf} is the activation energy in the presence of a catalyst. ΔG_0 is the change in free energy for the reaction.

ENZYME KINETICS

The Enzyme-Substrate Complex

Enzymes act through the formation of an enzyme–substrate (ES) complex, in which a molecule of substrate is bound to the active center of the enzyme molecule. The binding process transforms the substrate molecule to its activated state. The energy required for this transformation is provided by the free energy of binding of S to E. Therefore activation takes place without the addition of external energy, so that the energy barrier to the reaction is lowered and the breakdown to products is accelerated (Fig. 22.3). The ES complex breaks down to give the reaction products (P) and free enzyme (E):

$$E + S \rightleftharpoons ES \longrightarrow P + E \quad (1)$$

All reactions catalyzed by enzymes are in theory reversible. However, in practice, the reaction is usually found to be more rapid in one direction than in the other, so that an equilibrium is reached in which the product of the forward or the backward reaction predominates, sometimes so markedly that the reaction is virtually irreversible.

If the product of the reaction in one direction is removed as it is formed (eg, because it is the substrate of a second enzyme present in the reaction mixture), the equilibrium of the first enzymatic process will be displaced so that the reaction will proceed to completion in that direction. Reaction sequences in which the product of one enzyme-catalyzed reaction becomes the substrate of the next enzyme and so on, often through many stages, are characteristic of biological processes. In the laboratory also, several enzymatic reactions may be linked together to provide a means of measuring the activity of the first enzyme or the concentration of the initial substrate in the chain. For example, the activity of CK is usually measured by a series of linked reactions, and the concentration of glucose is determined by consecutive reactions catalyzed by hexokinase and glucose-6-phosphate dehydrogenase.

When a secondary enzyme-catalyzed reaction, known as an indicator reaction, is used to determine the activity of a different enzyme, the primary reaction catalyzed by the enzyme to be determined must be the rate-limiting step. Reaction conditions must ensure that the rate of reaction catalyzed by the indicator enzyme is directly proportional to the rate of product formation in the first reaction.

Factors Governing the Rate of Enzyme-Catalyzed Reactions

Factors that affect the rate of enzyme-catalyzed reactions include enzyme and substrate concentration, pH, temperature, and the presence of inhibitors, activators, coenzymes, and prosthetic groups.

Enzyme Concentration

The simplest enzymatically catalyzed reaction for converting substrate S into product P with the intermediate formation of an ES complex is as follows:

$$E_f + S \underset{k_{-1}}{\overset{k_1}{\rightleftarrows}} ES \xrightarrow{k_2} E_f + P \quad \textbf{(2)}$$

where

E_f = free enzyme
k_1 = rate constant for the association of the complex
k_{-1} = rate constant for the dissociation of the complex
ES = enzyme–substrate complex
k_2 = rate constant for breakdown of ES to E_f and P
P = product

Michaelis and Menten assumed that equilibrium is attained rapidly among E, S, and ES, with the effect of product formation (ES → P) on the concentration of ES being negligible. In addition, the formation of product is written as an irreversible process because there is no product in the solution under initial conditions. Therefore the overall rate of the reaction under otherwise constant conditions is proportional to the concentration of the ES complex.

Provided that an excess of free substrate molecules is present, addition of more enzyme molecules to the reaction system increases the concentration of the ES complex and thus the overall rate of reaction. This accounts for the observation that the rate of reaction is generally proportional to the concentration of enzyme present in the system and is the basis for the quantitative determination of enzymes by measurement of reaction rates. Reaction conditions are selected to ensure that the observed reaction rate is proportional to enzyme concentration over as wide a range as possible.

Substrate Concentration

In addition to explaining the dependence of reaction rate on enzyme concentration under conditions in which excess substrate is present, the formation of an ES complex accounts for the hyperbolic relationship between reaction velocity and substrate concentration (Fig. 15.4). In the next sections, single-substrate, two-substrate, and consecutive enzyme reactions will be discussed.

Single-Substrate Reactions. If the enzyme concentration is fixed and the substrate concentration is varied, the rate of reaction is first order with respect to substrate concentration and proportional to substrate concentration at low values of the latter. Under these conditions, only a fraction of the enzyme is associated with substrate, and the rate observed reflects the low concentration of the ES complex. At high substrate concentrations, variation in substrate concentration has no effect on rate, and the reaction is zero order with respect to substrate concentration. Under these conditions, all the enzyme is bound to the substrate and a much higher rate of reaction is obtained. Moreover, because all the enzyme is now present in the form of the complex, no further increase in complex concentration and no further increment in reaction rate are possible. The maximum possible velocity for the reaction has been reached. The significance of substrate-rate curves was first emphasized by Michaelis and Menten, and such curves are referred to as Michaelis-Menten plots.

Referring again to Eq. 22.2, the overall rate of the reaction *(v)* is determined by the rate at which product is formed:

$$v = \frac{d[P]}{dt} = k_2[ES] \quad \textbf{(3)}$$

The formation of ES will depend on the rate constant k_1 and the availability of enzyme and substrate. If it is assumed that the system is in a steady state with the ES complex being formed and broken down at the same rate so that overall *(ES)* is constant, then the steady-state equation is

$$k_1[E][S] = k_{-1}[ES] + k_2[ES] \quad \textbf{(4)}$$

This equation can be rearranged to:

$$[ES] = \frac{k_1[E][S]}{k_{-1} + k_2} \quad \textbf{(5)}$$

when these rate constants are combined into a single term; writing the Michaelis constant (K_m) as

$$K_m = \frac{k_{-1} + k_2}{k_1} \quad \textbf{(6)}$$

and then substituting this into Eq. 22.5 gives

$$[ES] = \frac{[E][S]}{K_m} \quad \textbf{(7)}$$

Because the total amount of enzyme in the system does not change,

$$[E_t] = [ES] + [E] \quad \textbf{(8)}$$

and on substituting Eq. 22.3 into Eq. 22.7 and eliminating (ES) using Eq. 22.8,

$$v = k_2 \times \frac{[E_t] \times [S]}{K_m + [S]} \quad \textbf{(9)}$$

For a given amount of enzyme, the maximum reaction velocity (V_{max}) is reached when all of the enzyme is saturated with substrate (ie, $[ES]$ = $[Et]$), and therefore $V_{max} = k_2 \times [Et]$. Substituting this in Eq. 22.9 gives

$$v = \frac{V_{max}[S]}{K_m + [S]} \quad \textbf{(10)}$$

A plot of v against *[S]* gives a section of a rectangular hyperbola (see Fig. 22.4), and this is the shape of the curve that is found experimentally for most enzyme reactions. When

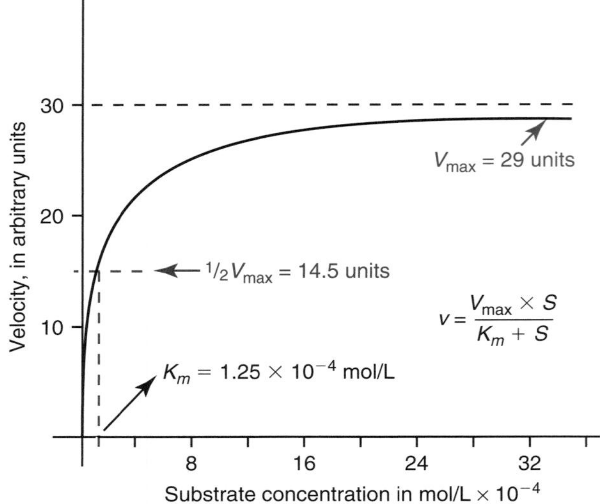

FIGURE 22.4 Michaelis-Menten curve relating velocity (rate) of an enzyme-catalyzed reaction to substrate concentration. The value of K_m is given by the substrate concentration at which half of the maximum velocity is obtained.

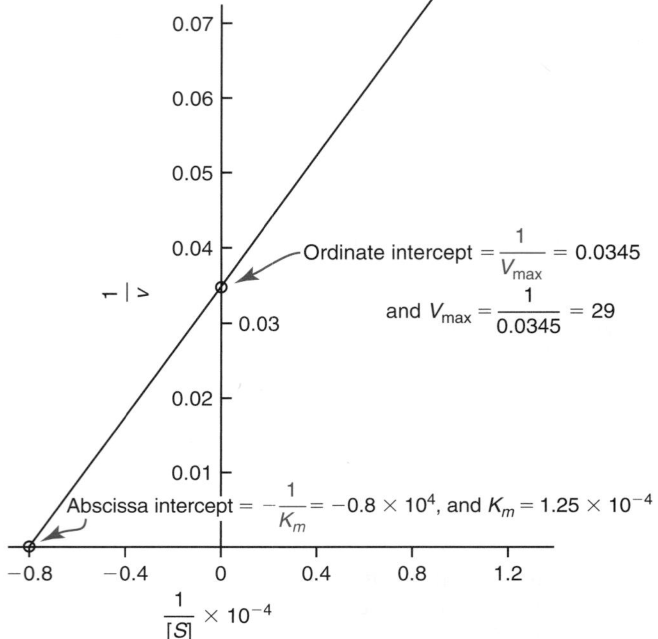

FIGURE 22.5 Lineweaver-Burk transformation of the curve in Fig. 22.4, with 1/*v* plotted on the ordinate (*y*-axis), and 1/[*S*] on the abscissa (*x*-axis). The indicated intercepts permit calculation of V_{max} and K_m. The units of *v* and [*S*] are those given in Fig. 22.4.

$[S] = K_m$, it can be shown with manipulation of Eq. 22.10 that K_m is the substrate concentration at which the reaction proceeds at half of its maximum velocity. In practice, it is now customary to restrict K_m to the experimentally determined substrate concentration at which $v = 0.5\ V_{max}$ and to use the symbol K_s to represent the true ES association constant, where this is known.

Although it is simple to set up an experiment to determine the variation of *v* with *[S]*, the exact value of V_{max} is not easily determined from hyperbolic curves. Furthermore, many enzymes deviate from ideal behavior at high substrate concentrations and may even be inhibited by the excess of substrate, so the calculated value of V_{max} cannot be achieved in practice. In the past, it was common practice to transform the Michaelis-Menten Eq. 22.10 into one of several reciprocal forms (Eqs. 22.11 and 12), and either $1/v$ was plotted against $1/[S]$ or $[S]/v$ was plotted against $[S]$.

$$\frac{1}{v} = \left(\frac{K_m}{V_{max}} \times \frac{1}{[S]}\right) + \frac{1}{V_{max}} \quad \textbf{(11)}$$

$$\frac{[S]}{v} = \left(\frac{1}{V_{max}} \times [S]\right) + \frac{K_m}{V_{max}} \quad \textbf{(12)}$$

Eq. 22.11, for example, when plotted, results in a Lineweaver-Burk plot that gives a straight line with intercepts at $1/V_{max}$ on the ordinate and $-1/K_m$ on the abscissa. For illustrative purposes, the data for Fig. 22.4 are replotted in Lineweaver-Burk form in Fig. 22.5.

It is now routine practice to determine kinetic constants such as K_m and V_{max} using a software package. A large number of such packages are available; these vary from specialized routines for kinetic simulations or for data fitting to general mathematical, statistical, or graphical packages.[10] These packages are free (public domain, shareware, or free license) or are commercially available. An example of the former is the ENCORA 1.2 freeware package available from RJW Slats and colleagues at the Delft University of Technology, which was developed for an enzymatic kinetic parameter fitting using progressive curve analysis.[11] DynaFit (BioKin, Watertown, Massachusetts) is an example of a commercially available product that performs nonlinear least-squares regression of chemical kinetic, enzyme kinetic, or ligand receptor binding data. The data can be initial reaction velocities for different concentrations of varied species (eg, inhibitor concentration vs. velocity) or reaction progress curves (eg, time vs. absorbance).[12] SigmaPlot 13 (Systat Software, San Jose, California) is another example of commercially available software that will compute and plot enzyme kinetic data.[13]

The value of K_m, has been used to compare the binding of homologous or related substrates to the same enzyme. Also, if measured against the same substrate under defined conditions, the K_m value can be used to compare the properties of similar enzymes from different sources. Isoenzymes determined by distinct genetic loci typically differ in their K_m (eg, for the isoenzymes of LD).

When setting up methods of enzyme assay, it is necessary to (1) explore the relationship between reaction velocity and substrate concentration over a wide range, (2) determine K_m, and (3) detect any inhibition at high substrate concentrations. Zero-order kinetics is maintained if the substrate is present in large excess (ie, concentrations at least 10 and preferably 100 times that of the value of K_m). When $[S] = 10 \times K_m$, *v* is approximately 91% of the theoretical V_{max}. The K_m values for the majority of enzymes are on the order of 10^{-5} to 10^{-3} mol/L; therefore substrate concentrations are usually chosen to be in the range of 0.001 to 0.10 mol/L. On occasion, the optimal concentrations of substrate cannot be used, for example, when the substrate has limited solubility or when the concentration of a given substrate inhibits the activity of another enzyme needed in a coupled reaction system.

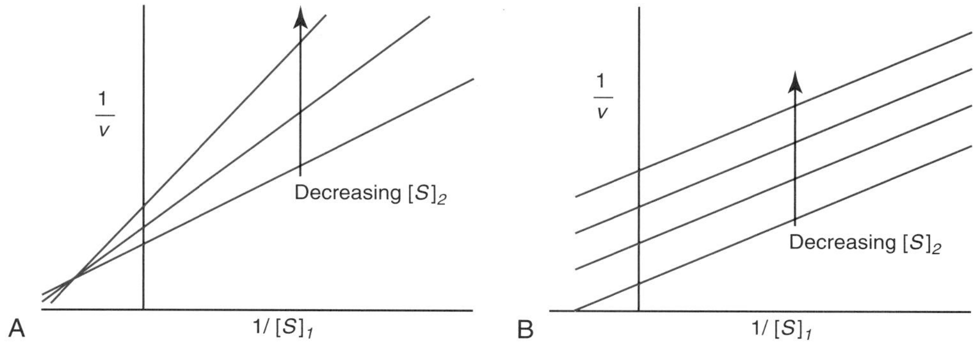

FIGURE 22.6 Double-reciprocal plots of $1/v$ against $1/[S_1]$ for two-substrate reactions, showing the effect of falling concentration of the second substrate, $[S_2]$. **A,** In a dehydrogenase reaction in which a ternary complex is formed. **B,** In a *ping-pong bi-bi* reaction mechanism (eg, aminotransferase) in which no ternary complex is formed. (From Moss DW. Measurement of enzymes. In: Hearse DJ, de Leiris J, editors. *Enzymes in cardiology: diagnosis and research.* New York: John Wiley & Sons, 1979. Reprinted by permission of John Wiley & Sons.)

Two-Substrate Reactions. Most enzymes catalyze reactions with two or more interacting substrates symbolized by the following equation:

$$\underset{S_1}{Substrate\,1} + \underset{S_2}{Substrate\,2} \overset{E}{\rightleftharpoons} \underset{P_1}{Product\,1} + \underset{P_2}{Product\,2} \quad (13)$$

When one of the substrates is water (ie, when the process is one of hydrolysis), with the reaction taking place in aqueous solution, only a fraction of the total number of water molecules present participates in the reaction. The small change in the concentration of water has no effect on the rate of reaction and these pseudo–one substrate reactions are described by one-substrate kinetics. More generally, the concentrations of both substrates may be variable and both may affect the rate of reaction. Among the bisubstrate reactions important in clinical enzymology are the reactions catalyzed by dehydrogenases, in which the second substrate is a specific coenzyme, such as the oxidized or reduced forms of nicotinamide adenine dinucleotide (NADH), or nicotinamide adenine dinucleotide phosphate (NADPH), and the amino-group transfers catalyzed by the aminotransferases.

If a bisubstrate reaction proceeds by way of intermediate ES complexes, so that

$$E + S_1 \rightleftharpoons ES_1 \quad (14)$$

followed by

$$ES_1 + S_2 \rightleftharpoons ES_1S_2 \longrightarrow P_1 + P_2 + E \quad (15)$$

and if S_1 and S_2 combine with separate sites on the enzyme molecule, the rate of reaction is given by

$$v = \frac{V_{max} \times [S_1][S_2]}{[S_1][S_2] + [S_2]K_m^1 + [S_1]K_m^2 + K_S^1 K_m^2} \quad (16)$$

K^1_m and K^2_m are the K_m values for the two substrates, and $[S_1]$ and $[S_2]$ are their concentrations. K^1_s is the equilibrium constant for the reversible reaction between the enzyme and S_1. If the equation is rearranged into the double reciprocal form,

$$\frac{1}{v} = \frac{1}{[S_1]}\left(\frac{K_m^1}{V_{max}} + \frac{K_m^2 K_S^1}{[S_2]V_{max}}\right) + \frac{1}{V_{max}}\left(1 + \frac{K_m^2}{[S_2]}\right) \quad (17)$$

a plot of $1/v$ against $1/[S_1]$ gives a straight line, but both the slope of the line and its intercept on the ordinate are dependent on $[S_2]$, the concentration of the second substrate (Fig. 22.6A). Similarly, a plot of $1/v$ against $1/[S_2]$ is rectilinear but with the slope and intercept dependent on $[S_1]$.

In some bisubstrate reactions, no ternary complex ES_1S_2 is formed, because the binding of the first substrate is followed by release of the first product before the second substrate is bound and the second product is released. This sequence is described as a *ping-pong bi-bi* type of reaction. It occurs in reactions catalyzed by aminotransferases.

The relationship between reaction velocity and the concentrations of the two substrates in *ping-pong bi-bi* reactions reduces to the form

$$v = \frac{V_{max} \times [S_1][S_2]}{[S_1][S_2] + [S_2]K_m^1 + [S_1]K_m^2} \quad (18)$$

The reciprocals of v and $[S_1]$ are related by the equation

$$\frac{1}{v} = \frac{1}{[S_1]} \times \frac{K_m^1}{V_{max}} + \frac{1}{V_{max}}\left(1 + \frac{K_m^2}{[S_2]}\right) \quad (19)$$

so that a plot of $1/v$ against $1/[S_1]$ is unchanged in slope by variation in $[S_2]$, but the intercept on the ordinate and therefore the value of V_{max} changes as $[S_2]$ is varied (see Fig. 22.6B). Similar equations describe the variation of V_{max} with $[S_1]$ when $1/v$ is plotted as a function of $1/[S_2]$.

Values of K_m and V_{max} for each substrate are derived from experiments in which the concentration of the first substrate is held constant at saturating quantities while the concentration of the second substrate is varied, and vice versa. There is no reason why the K_m values for the two substrates should be the same or even similar (eg, pyruvate and NADH, the two-substrate pair in the reaction catalyzed by LD of beef heart, have K_m values of 2×10^{-5} mol/L and 3×10^{-6} mol/L, respectively).

The selection of reaction conditions for the measurement of enzymatic activity involving two substrates is approached similarly by varying the concentration of the first substrate and keeping the concentration of the second substrate constant until maximum activity is reached. The process is then repeated with the concentration of the first substrate held at the value thus determined, whereas the concentration of the second substrate is varied.

In practice, the choice of substrate concentrations is limited by such considerations as the solubility of the substrates, the viscosity and initial absorbance of concentrated solutions, and the relative costs of the reagents. Furthermore, the selection of appropriate substrate concentrations is only one of the factors to be considered in formulating an optimal assay system for the measurement of a specific enzyme activity. Critical choices also must be made with respect to other, frequently interdependent, factors that affect reaction rate, such as the concentrations of activators and the nature and pH of the buffer system.

Consecutive Enzymatic Reactions. As discussed previously, an enzymatic reaction is usually found to be more rapid in one direction than the other, so that the reaction is essentially irreversible. If the product of the reaction in one direction is removed as it is formed (ie, because it is the substrate of a second enzyme present in the reaction mixture), the equilibrium of the first enzymatic process is displaced so that the reaction may continue to completion in that direction. Analytically, several enzymatic reactions also may be linked together to provide a means of measuring the activity of the first enzyme or the concentration of the initial substrate in the chain.

When a linked enzyme assay, known as an *indicator reaction,* is used to determine the activity of a different enzyme, it is essential that the primary reaction be the rate-limiting step. For example, in the determination of aspartate aminotransferase activity, the indicator reaction is the reduction of the 2-oxoglutarate formed in the aminotransferase reaction to malate by malate dehydrogenase and NADH. The activity of the indicator enzyme must be sufficient to ensure the virtually instantaneous removal of the product of the first reaction so as to prevent significant reversal of the first reaction. The measured enzyme typically is acting under conditions of saturation with respect to its substrate; however, the concentration of the substrate of the indicator enzyme (ie, the product of the first reaction) remains in the region of the Michaelis-Menten curve, in which v is directly proportional to $[S]$. Therefore the rate of reaction catalyzed by the indicator enzyme is directly proportional to the rate of product formation in the first reaction.

During a lag period that occurs after the start of the first reaction, the concentration of its product reaches a steady state. Because the rate of the second reaction depends on the activity of the indicator enzyme and on the concentration of its substrate (the product of the primary reaction), the duration of the lag period is reduced by increasing the concentration of the indicator enzyme, thus lowering the steady-state concentration of the product of the primary reaction.

The rate of the indicator reaction, v_i, is related to substrate concentration and therefore to the product concentration $[P]$ by the Michaelis-Menten equation

$$v_i = \frac{V^i_{\max} \times [P]}{[P] + K^i_m} \tag{20}$$

in which $V^i_{\max}$ and K^i_m are the maximum velocity and K_m of the indicator enzyme, respectively. For the rate of the indicator reaction not to be the rate limiting factor, v_i must at least equal the limiting velocity of the primary reaction, v_t, which the assay system is expected to measure. Therefore the minimum activity of indicator enzyme needed is given by

$$v_t = \frac{V^i_{\max} \times [P]}{[P] + K^i_m} \tag{21}$$

or is rearranged as

$$V^i_{\max} = v_t \left(1 + \frac{K^i_m}{[P]}\right) \tag{22}$$

The ratio of activities of the indicator and primary enzymes varies from one assay method to another, depending on (1) the range of activity measured, (2) the K_m of the indicator enzyme, and (3) the lag period that is considered acceptable. Nevertheless, the catalytic concentration of the indicator enzyme in the reaction mixture always must be much greater than that of the enzyme being determined.

Effect of pH

The rate of enzyme-catalyzed reactions typically shows a marked dependence on pH (Fig. 22.7). Many of the enzymes in blood plasma show maximum activity in vitro in the pH range from 7 to 8. However, activity has been observed at pH values as low as 1.5 (pepsin) and as high as 10.5 (ALP). The optimal pH for a given forward reaction may be different

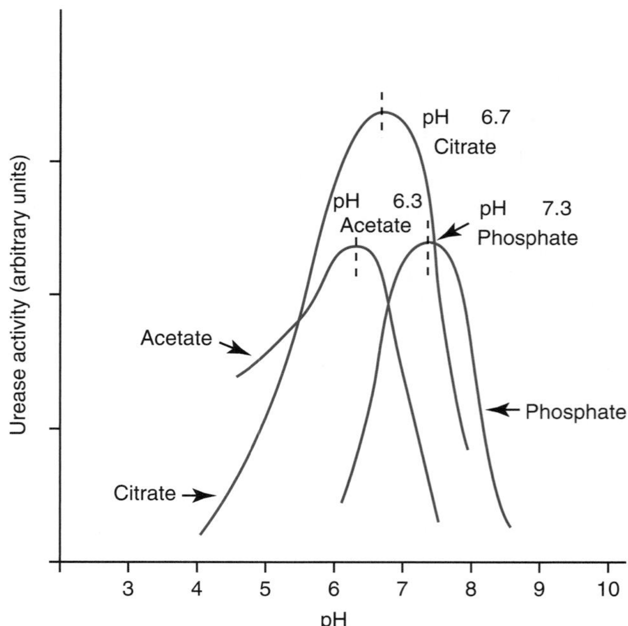

FIGURE 22.7 The pH activity curves for urease show the effects of buffer species on pH optimum. (Modified from Howell SF, Sumner JB. The specific effects of buffers upon urease activity. *J Biol Chem* 1934;104:619.)

from the optimal pH found for the corresponding reverse reaction. The form of the pH-dependence curve is the result of a number of separate effects, including ionization of the substrate and the extent of dissociation of certain key amino acid side chains in the protein molecule, both at the active center and elsewhere in the molecule. Both pH and ionic environment also will have an effect on the 3D conformation of the protein and therefore on enzyme activity to such an extent that enzymes may be irreversibly denatured at extreme values of pH.

The pronounced effects of pH on enzyme reactions emphasize the need to control this variable by means of adequate buffer solutions. Enzyme assays should be carried out at the pH of optimal activity, because the pH-activity curve has its minimum slope near this pH, and a small variation in pH will cause a minimal change in enzyme activity. The buffer system must be capable of counteracting the effect of adding the specimen (eg, serum itself is a powerful buffer) to the assay system, as well as the effects of acids or bases formed during the reaction (eg, formation of fatty acids by the action of lipase). Because buffers have their maximum buffering capacity close to their pK_a values, whenever possible a buffer system should be chosen with a pK_a value within 1 pH unit of the desired pH of the assay (see Chapter 12). Interaction between buffer ions and other components of the assay system (eg, activating metal ions) may eliminate certain buffers from consideration.

Temperature

The rate of an enzymatic reaction is proportional to its reaction temperature. For most enzymatic reactions, values of Q_{10} (the relative reaction rates at two temperatures differing by 10°C) vary from 1.7 to 2.5. However, an increase in the rate of the catalyzed reaction is not the only effect of increasing temperature on an enzymatic reaction. In theory, the initial rate of reaction measured instantaneously will increase with a rising temperature. In practice, however, a finite time is needed to allow the components of the reaction mixture, including the enzyme solution, to reach temperature equilibrium and permit the formation of a measurable amount of the product. During this period, the enzyme is undergoing thermal inactivation and denaturation, a process that has a very large temperature coefficient for most enzymes and thus becomes virtually instantaneous at temperatures of 60 to 70°C. The counteracting effects of the increased rate of the catalyzed reaction and more rapid enzyme inactivation as the temperature increases account for the existence of an apparent optimal temperature for enzyme activity (Fig. 22.8).

As stated earlier, at some critical temperature, an enzyme will undergo thermal inactivation influenced by a number of factors. These include the presence of substrate and its concentration, the pH, and the nature and ionic strength of the buffer. The presence of other proteins, as in serum samples, may help to stabilize enzymes. Storage of serum samples at low temperatures is necessary to minimize loss of enzyme activity while awaiting analysis, although repeated freezing and thawing should be avoided. However, individual enzymes vary in their stability characteristics, and appropriate storage conditions vary correspondingly. In serum, amylase, for example, is stable at room temperature (22 to 25°C) for 24 hours, whereas acid phosphatase is exceedingly unstable, even when refrigerated, unless kept at a pH below 6.0. ALP exhibits an unusual property; in sera stored at refrigerated temperatures, ALP increases slowly (2% per day), which is thought to be due to the reincorporation of cations required for full activity. Frozen specimens should be thawed and kept at room temperature for 18 to 24 hours before measurement to achieve full enzyme reactivation. This effect is shared by reconstituted, lyophilized preparations of the enzyme and affects their use for quality control purposes. A few enzymes are inactivated at refrigerator temperatures; a clinically important example is the liver-type isoenzyme of LD, LD-5, which appears to be less stable at lower temperatures. As a result, sera for LD determinations should be kept at room temperature and not refrigerated.

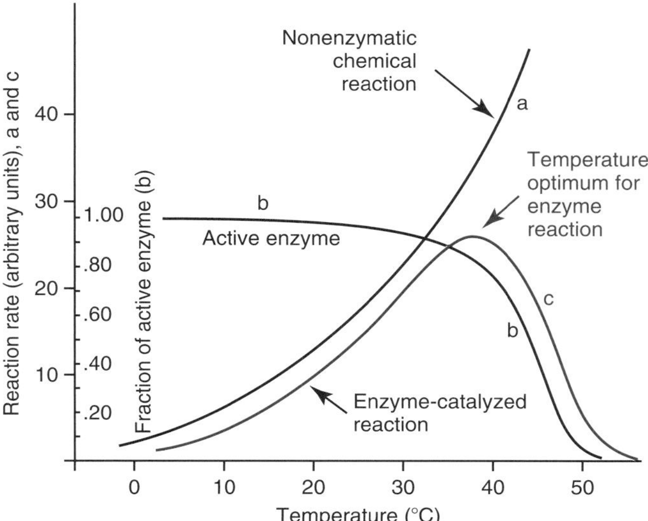

FIGURE 22.8 Schematic diagram showing effects of temperature on the rate of non–enzyme-catalyzed and enzyme-catalyzed reactions.

Historically, the choice of temperature for the assay of enzymes of clinical importance was the subject of extensive debate. The choice of reaction temperature has become a nonissue because most analytical systems operate at 37°C, and reference methods for several clinically relevant enzymes have now been developed at this temperature.[14-21] In practice, accurate temperature control to within ±0.1°C during the enzymatic reaction is essential.

Inhibitors and Activators

The rates of enzymatic reactions are often affected by substances other than the enzyme or substrate. These modifiers may be inhibitors because their presence reduces the reaction rate or activators because they increase the rate of reaction. Activators and inhibitors are usually small molecules (compared with the enzyme itself) or even ions. They vary in specificity from modifiers that exert similar effects on a wide range of different enzymatic reactions at one extreme, to substances that affect only a single reaction. Reagents, such as strong acids or multivalent anions and cations that denature or precipitate proteins, destroy enzyme activity and thus may be regarded as extreme examples of nonspecific enzyme inhibitors. These effects usually are not included in discussions of enzyme inhibition, although they have obvious practical implications in the treatment and storage of specimens in which enzyme activity is to be measured. The activity of some enzymes depends on the presence of particular chemical groups, such as reduced sulfhydryl (–SH) groups, in the active center. Reagents that alter these groups (eg, oxidants of SH groups) therefore act as general inhibitors of such enzymes.

Some phenomena of enzyme activation or inhibition are caused by interactions between the modifier and a nonenzymatic component of the reaction system, such as the substrate (eg, magnesium [Mg^{2+}] combining with ATP to form MgATP, the required substrate for the CK reaction). In most cases, however, the modifier combines with the enzyme itself in a manner analogous to the combination of enzyme and substrate.

Inhibition of Enzyme Activity. Inhibitors are classified as reversible or irreversible. *Reversible inhibition* implies that the activity of the enzyme is fully restored when the inhibitor is removed from the system in which the enzyme acts by some physical separative process, such as dialysis, gel filtration, or chromatography. An *irreversible inhibitor* combines covalently with the enzyme so that physical methods are ineffective in separating the two. For example, organophosphorus compounds are extremely potent irreversible inhibitors of esterases, including acetylcholinesterase. The enzyme breaks one of the bonds in the inhibitor, but part of the molecule is left bound to the active center of the enzyme, preventing further activity. In some cases, enzymes that have combined with irreversible inhibitors can be reactivated by a chemical reaction that removes the blocking group (eg, the phosphoryl enzymes formed with organophosphorus compounds sometimes can be reactivated by treatment with oximes or hydroxamic acids).

Reversible Inhibition. Reversible inhibition is characterized by the existence of equilibrium between enzyme, *E*, and inhibitor, *I*:

$$E + I \rightleftharpoons EI \quad \textbf{(23)}$$

The equilibrium constant of the reaction, K_i (the *inhibitor constant*), is a measure of the affinity of the inhibitor for the enzyme, just as K_m generally reflects the affinity of the enzyme for its substrate.

A *competitive* inhibitor is usually a structural analog of the substrate that can combine with the free enzyme in such a way that it competes with the normal substrate for binding at the active site. The rate of the reaction is strictly dependent on the relative concentrations of substrate and inhibitor. Two equilibriums are therefore possible:

$$E + S \rightleftharpoons ES \longrightarrow E + Products \quad \textbf{(24)}$$

and

$$E + I \rightleftharpoons EI \quad \textbf{(25)}$$

The equation that relates the observed reaction velocity to the concentrations of substrate, [*S*], and inhibitor, [*I*], is as follows:

$$v = \frac{V_{\max}[S]}{[S] + K_m\left(1 + \frac{[I]}{K_i}\right)} \quad \textbf{(26)}$$

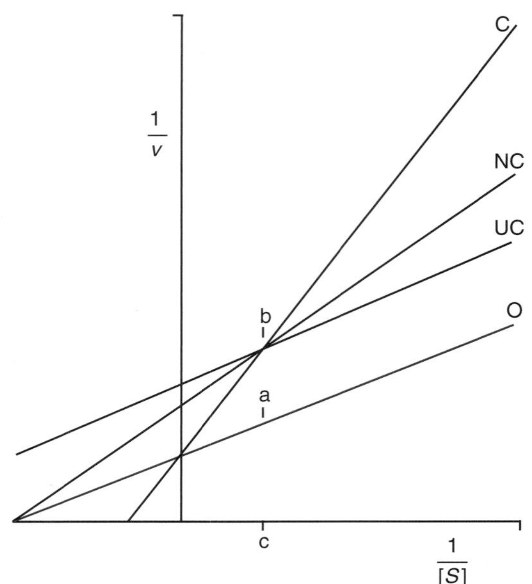

FIGURE 22.9 Effects of different types of inhibitors on the double-reciprocal plot of 1/*v* against 1/[*S*]. Each of the inhibitors has been assumed to reduce the activity of the enzyme by the same amount, represented by the change in 1/*v* from *a* to *b* at a substrate concentration of *c*. *Line O* is the plot for enzyme without inhibitor, *C* with a competitive inhibitor, *NC* with a noncompetitive inhibitor, and *UC* with an uncompetitive inhibitor. (From Moss DW. Measurement of enzymes. In: Hearse DJ, de Leiris J, editors. *Enzymes in cardiology: diagnosis and research.* New York: John Wiley & Sons, 1979. Reprinted by permission of John Wiley & Sons.)

This is the Michaelis-Menten equation, but with K_m modified by a term including the inhibitor concentration and the inhibitor constant while V_{max} remains unaltered. Therefore curves of *v* against [*S*] in the presence and absence of inhibitor reach the same limiting value at high substrate concentrations, but when the inhibitor is present, K_m is apparently greater. Plots of 1/*v* against 1/[*S*] with and without inhibitor intersect the ordinate at the same point but have different slopes and intercepts on the abscissa (Fig. 22.9).

Competitive inhibition is responsible for the inhibition of some enzymes by excess substrate because of competition between substrate molecules for a single binding site. In two-substrate reactions, high concentrations of the second substrate may compete with binding of the first substrate. For example, aspartate aminotransferase is inhibited by excess concentrations of the substrate 2-oxoglutarate, and this inhibition is competitive with respect to L-aspartate. Therefore to maintain a given velocity at high 2-oxoglutarate concentrations, the concentration of L-aspartate has to be increased above the value needed at lower concentrations of 2-oxoglutarate.

Competitive inhibition also contributes to the reduction in the rate of an enzymatic reaction over time. For example, rate reduction can occur because increasing concentrations of reaction products tend to drive the reaction backward, if it is freely reversible. A product may be an inhibitor of the forward reaction, so even if the reaction is not readily reversible, it proceeds against a rising concentration of inhibitor. A familiar example of product inhibition is the release of the competitive inhibitor inorganic phosphate by the action of

ALP on its substrates. In this case, both organic phosphates and inorganic phosphates bind to the active center of the enzyme with similar affinities (ie, K_m and K_i are of the same order of magnitude).

Product inhibition is a cause of nonlinearity of reaction progress curves during fixed-time methods of enzyme assay. For example, oxaloacetate produced by the action of AST inhibits the enzyme, particularly the mitochondrial isoenzyme. The inhibitory product may be removed as it is formed by a coupled enzymatic reaction; malate dehydrogenase converts the oxaloacetate to malate and at the same time oxidizes NADH to NAD^+.

Competitive inhibition by metal ions occurs when two metal ions compete for the same binding site on the enzyme. Sodium and lithium are potent inhibitors of pyruvate kinase, for which potassium is an obligatory activator.

A noncompetitive inhibitor is usually structurally different from the substrate. It is assumed to bind at a site on the enzyme molecule that is different from the substrate-binding site; thus there is no competition between inhibitor and substrate, and a ternary enzyme substrate–inhibitor (ESI) complex is formed. Attachment of the inhibitor to the enzyme does not alter the affinity of the enzyme for its substrate (ie, K_m is unaltered), but the ESI complex does not break down to give products. Because the substrate does not compete with the inhibitor for binding sites on the enzyme molecule, increasing the substrate concentration does not overcome the effect of a noncompetitive inhibitor. Thus V_{max} is reduced in the presence of such an inhibitor, whereas K_m is not altered, as the Lineweaver-Burk plot shows (see Fig. 22.9).

Uncompetitive inhibition is produced by a combination of the inhibitor with the ES complex. It is more common in two-substrate reactions, in which a ternary ESI complex forms after the first substrate has combined with the enzyme. In uncompetitive inhibition, parallel lines are obtained when plots of $1/v$ against $1/[S]$ with and without the inhibitor are compared (see Fig. 22.9); that is, both K_m and V_{max} are decreased.

Irreversible Inhibition. Irreversible inhibitors render the enzyme molecule inactive by covalently and permanently modifying a functional group required for catalysis. An irreversible inhibitor is not in equilibrium with the enzyme. Its effect is progressive with time, becoming complete if the amount of inhibitor present exceeds the total amount of enzyme. The rate of the reaction between enzyme and inhibitor is expressed as the fraction of the enzyme activity that is inhibited in a fixed time by a given concentration of inhibitor. The velocity constant of the reaction of the inhibitor with the enzyme is a measure of the effectiveness of the inhibitor.

When the inhibitor is added to the enzyme in the presence of its substrate, the reaction between the enzyme and the inhibitor may be delayed because some of the enzyme molecules are combined with the substrate and are therefore protected from reacting with the inhibitor. However, when the substrate molecules react chemically, the active centers become available, and inhibition eventually will become complete, even though an excess of substrate may have been present initially. Furthermore, the addition of more substrate is ineffective in reversing the inhibition in contrast to its effect on reversible competitive inhibition.

Irreversible inhibitors have been useful in mapping active sites by covalently modifying different types of functional groups in the enzyme molecule to establish whether such groups are necessary for catalytic activity.

A physiologically important category of irreversible enzyme inhibition is exemplified by various trypsin inhibitors. These are proteins that bind to trypsin irreversibly, nullifying its proteolytic activity. One such inhibitor is present in the α_1-globulin fraction of serum proteins; others are found in soybeans and lima beans. Similar proteolysis inhibitors present in plasma prevent the accumulation of excess thrombin and other coagulation enzymes, thus keeping the coagulation process under control.

Inhibition by Antibodies. The combination of enzyme molecules with specific antibodies often has no effect on catalytic activity, which is retained by the enzyme-antibody complex.[7] However, in some cases, the reaction of the enzyme and antibody reduces or even abolishes enzymatic activity. The most probable explanation for this type of inhibition is that the antibody molecule restricts access of the substrate molecules to the active center by steric hindrance or, in extreme cases, completely masks the substrate-binding site. However, it appears that some examples of enzyme inhibition by combination with antibodies are caused by a conformational change induced in the enzyme molecule.

Inhibition of the activity of an enzyme molecule labeled with a hapten (eg, morphine) as a result of combination with a specific antibody forms the basis for a homogeneous enzyme immunoassay (see Chapter 23).

Enzyme Activation. Activators increase the rates of enzyme-catalyzed reactions by promoting formation of the most active state of the enzyme or of other reactants, such as the substrate. This generalization covers a wide variety of mechanisms of activation.

Many enzymes contain metal ions as an integral part of their structures (eg, zinc in ALP and carboxypeptidase A). The function of the metal may be to stabilize tertiary and quaternary protein structures. Removal of divalent metal ions by treatment with an appropriate quantity of ethylenediaminetetraacetic acid (EDTA) solution is accompanied by conformational changes and inactivation of the enzyme. The enzyme often can be reactivated by dialysis against a solution of the appropriate metal ion or simply by addition of the ion to the reaction mixture. Reactivation may take some time, because rearrangement of polypeptide chains into the active conformation is not instantaneous.

When the activator ion is an essential part of the functional enzyme molecule, whether as a purely structural element or with an additional catalytic role, it is usually incorporated quite firmly into the enzyme molecule. Therefore it is not usually necessary to add the activator to reaction mixtures and an excess of the ion may even have an inhibitory effect. However, in some cases, the activating ion is attached only weakly or transiently to the enzyme (or its substrate) during catalysis. Enzyme samples therefore may be deficient in the ion, so that addition of the ion increases the reaction rate or indeed may be essential for the reaction to take place. For example, all phosphate transfer enzymes (kinases), such as CK, require the essential presence of Mg^{2+} ions. Other common activating cations are manganese (Mn^{2+}), iron (Fe^{2+}), calcium (Ca^{2+}), zinc (Zn^{2+}), and potassium (K^+). More rarely, anions may act as activators. Amylase functions at its maximal rate only if chlorine (Cl^-) or other monovalent anions, such as bromide (Br^-) or nitrate (NO_3^-), are present. Addition of

5 mmol/L of chloride increases amylase activity almost threefold, at the same time shifting the pH optimum from 6.5 to 7.0. The Cl^- ion may combine with a positively charged group in the enzyme, changing the ionization constant of a group important in catalysis. However, other anions—such as Br^-—are less effective activators of amylase, so some degree of specificity is involved in the process of activation. Some enzymes require the obligate presence of two activating ions. K^+ and Mg^{2+} are essential for the activity of pyruvate kinase, and both Mg^{2+} and Zn^{2+} are required for ALP activity.

The velocity of the reaction depends on the concentration of a reversible activator in a fashion similar to its dependence on substrate concentration, and an activator constant, K_a, analogous to K_m, can be determined from data relating enzyme activity to increasing activator concentration in the presence of excess substrate. The simplest interpretation of K_a is that it is the dissociation constant of the equilibrium between E and the activator, A. However, this is true only when the combination of enzyme and activator is independent of the reaction between E and S, and the same value for K_a is obtained at all concentrations of the substrate. If the free enzyme and the ES complex have different affinities for the activator, the value for K_a varies with $[S]$.

Apparent activation of an enzyme may be observed whenever a substance that can counteract the presence of some inhibiting agent is added.

Coenzymes and Prosthetic Groups

Coenzymes are usually more complex molecules than activators, although they are smaller molecules than the enzyme proteins. Some compounds, such as the dinucleotides NAD and NADP, are classified as coenzymes and are specific substrates in two-substrate reactions. Their effects on the rate of reaction follow the Michaelis-Menten pattern of dependence on substrate concentration. The structures of these two coenzymes are identical except for the presence of an additional phosphate group in NADP; nevertheless, individual dehydrogenases, for which these coenzymes are substrates, are predominantly or even absolutely specific for one or the other form.

Coenzymes such as NAD and NADP are bound only momentarily to the enzyme during the course of the reaction, as is the case for substrates in general. Therefore no reaction takes place unless the appropriate coenzyme is present in solution (eg, by adding it to the reaction mixture in the assay of dehydrogenase activity). In contrast to these entirely soluble coenzymes, some coenzymes are more or less permanently bound to the enzyme molecules, where they form part of the active center and undergo cycles of chemical change during the reaction. In this case, the coenzyme is known as a prosthetic group. Prosthetic groups, such as activators with a structural role, do not usually have to be added to elicit full catalytic activity of the enzyme unless previous treatment has caused the prosthetic group to be lost from some enzyme molecules.

The active *holoenzyme* results from the combination of the inactive *apoenzyme* with the prosthetic group. An example of a prosthetic group is pyridoxal-5′-phosphate (P-5′-P), a component of AST and ALT. The P-5′-P prosthetic group undergoes a cycle of conversion of the pyridoxal moiety to pyridoxamine and back again during the transfer of an amino group from an amino acid to an oxoacid. However, both normal and pathologic serum samples contain appreciable quantities of apoaminotransferases, which are converted to active holoenzymes through a suitable period of incubation with P-5′-P.

A study of the formulas of coenzyme and prosthetic groups shows that many contain structures derived from vitamins (see Chapter 37). Thus the nicotinamide portion of NAD and NADP derives from the vitamin niacin, whereas the P-5′-P prosthetic group of the aminotransferases is a derivative of pyridoxine, vitamin B_6.

ANALYTICAL ENZYMOLOGY

Analytically, the clinical laboratorian is concerned with measuring the activity or mass in serum or plasma of enzymes that are predominantly intracellular and that are physiologically present in the serum in low concentrations only. By measuring changes in the concentrations of these enzymes in disease, it is possible to infer the location and nature of pathologic changes in body tissues.

Measurement of Reaction Rates

The rate of an enzyme-catalyzed reaction is directly proportional to the amount of active enzyme present in the system. Consequently, determination of the rate of reaction under defined and controlled conditions provides a measurement of the amount of enzyme in a sample such as serum.

Determination of reaction rate involves the kinetic measurement of the amount of change produced within a defined time interval.[22,23] Both *fixed-time* and *continuous-monitoring* methods are used to measure reaction rates. In the fixed-time method, the amount of change produced by the enzyme is measured after the reaction is stopped at the end of a fixed-time interval. In the continuous-monitoring method, the progress of the reaction is monitored continuously. These two methods have different advantages and limitations. To appreciate them, it is necessary to consider the way in which the rate of an enzymatic reaction varies with time.

The progress of conversion of the substrate into products in the presence of an enzyme is monitored by measuring the decreasing concentration of the substrate or the increasing concentration of the products. Measurement of product formation is preferable because determination of the increase in concentration of a substance above an initially zero or low concentration is analytically more reliable than measurement of a decline from an initially high concentration.

At the moment when the enzyme and the substrate are mixed, the rate of the reaction is zero. The rate then typically rises rapidly to a maximum value, which remains constant for a period (Fig. 22.10). During the period of constant reaction rate, the rate depends only on enzyme concentration and is completely independent of substrate concentration. The reaction is said to follow zero-order kinetics, because its rate is proportional to the zero power of the substrate concentration. Ultimately, however, as more substrate is consumed, the reaction rate declines and enters a phase of first-order dependence on substrate concentration. Other factors that contribute to the decline in reaction rate include accumulation of products that may be inhibitory, the growing importance of the reverse reaction, and even enzyme denaturation. Although it is possible to compare the rates of reaction produced by different amounts of an enzyme under first-order conditions,

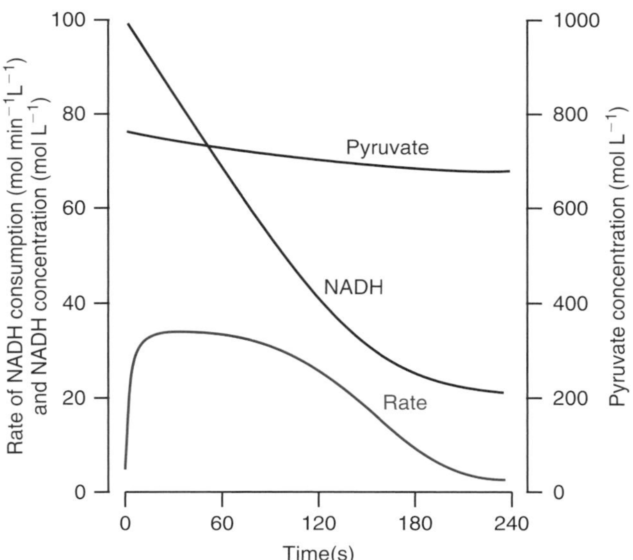

FIGURE 22.10 Changes in substrate concentrations and rates of reaction during an assay of lactate dehydrogenase activity at 37°C in phosphate buffer, with pyruvate and nicotinamide adenine dinucleotide (NADH) as substrates. The reaction is followed by observing the fall in absorbance at 340 nm as NADH is oxidized to NAD^+. The rate of reaction rises rapidly to a maximum value, from which it declines only slightly until about half the NADH has been used up. During this phase of the reaction, the rate is essentially zero order with respect to substrate concentration. At the point at which the rate falls below about 90% of its maximum value, NADH concentration is approximately $10 \times K_m$. The K_m for NADH is on the order of 5×10^{-6} mol/L, whereas for pyruvate it is 9×10^{-5} mol/L. Thus an initial pyruvate concentration approximately 10 times that of NADH is used. (Concentrations are per liter of reaction mixture.) (From Moss DW. Measurement of enzymes. In: Hearse DJ, de Leiris J, editors. *Enzymes in cardiology: diagnosis and research.* New York: John Wiley & Sons, 1979. Reprinted by permission of John Wiley & Sons.)

it is obviously easier to standardize such comparisons when the enzyme concentration is the only variable that influences the reaction rate. Therefore enzyme assays are usually made under conditions that are initially saturating with respect to substrate concentration. The rate of reaction during the zero-order phase is determined by measuring the product formed during a fixed period of incubation in which the rate remains constant. This is illustrated in Fig. 22.11. Measurement of reaction rates at any portion of *curve A* gives results that are identical to the true *initial rate.* However, *curve B* deviates from linearity over its entire course, and rates fall off with time. From *curve C,* correct results are obtained only if the rate is measured along segment II. Incorrect results are obtained if the rate is measured during the lag phase (I) or during phase III.

Careful selection of reaction conditions, such as the concentrations of substrates and cofactors, improves the reaction progress curves, eliminating lag phases and prolonging the period of linearity, so that fixed-time methods of analysis become feasible. Improvements in optical techniques, leading to more reliable and sensitive measurement of product formation, also have allowed the duration of incubation to be shortened compared with that of older assays. This has resulted in a corresponding increase in the interval over which enzyme activity is measured. Nevertheless, an upper limit of activity exists in all fixed-time methods, above which progress curves will no longer be linear. In this case, the amount of change measured over the fixed-time interval no longer represents true zero-order rate conditions.

The upper limit of activity acceptable in the unmodified method must be chosen so samples with activities below it are presumed with a high degree of certainty to give linear progress curves; alternatively, if the limit is set too low, many samples will be reanalyzed unnecessarily. Samples that are above the limit should ideally be reassayed by shortening the incubation period until a constant reaction rate is obtained. However, this is difficult or impossible in some automated

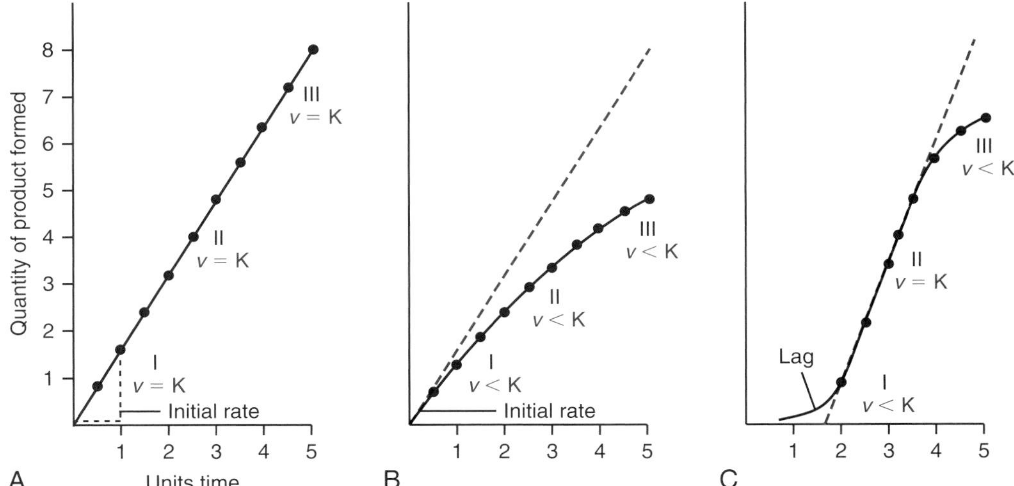

FIGURE 22.11 Forms of graphs showing change in enzyme reaction rate as a function of time. In **A,** the rate is constant during the entire run, and rates calculated as *I, II,* and *III* will be identical to the initial rate. In **B,** the rate falls off continuously; rates calculated at *I, II,* and *III* will be different and less than the true initial rate. In **C,** a measurement at *II* will be representative of the maximum rate, but at *I* (lag period) and *III* (substrate depletion), it will be less than at *II.*

methods, in which the duration of incubation is fixed by the configuration of the apparatus. It then becomes necessary to dilute the specimen; however, dilution may not always result in a proportional change in activity.

The initial rate of reaction theoretically increases without limit as enzyme concentration increases, as long as no other factor, such as substrate concentration, becomes limiting. In practice, the reaction rate becomes so rapid at high enzyme activities that it is impossible to measure the initial rate of reaction, even with continuous monitoring methods. Therefore an upper limit of activity that is measurable without modification of the assay procedure exists even in continuous monitoring methods, but this limit is usually much higher than that applicable in corresponding fixed-time methods. Therefore fewer samples require special treatment. Furthermore, continuous monitoring allows identification of the appropriate zero-order portion of the progress curve for each sample and identification of samples that require special treatment. Continuous-monitoring methods therefore provide a decisive advantage in enzyme assay and should be used whenever possible.

Measurement of Substrates

The amount of substrate transformed into products during an enzyme-catalyzed reaction can be measured with any appropriate analytical method, such as spectrophotometry, fluorometry, or chemiluminescence (see Chapter 13). For example, if an enzyme reaction is accompanied by a change in the absorbance characteristics of some component of the assay system, in the visible or ultraviolet spectrum, it can be photometrically observed while it is proceeding. *Self-indicating* reactions of this type are particularly valuable because they allow continuous monitoring. Important examples of self-indicating reactions are determination of dehydrogenase activity by monitoring the change in absorbance at 339 (340) nm of the coenzyme NADH or NADPH during oxidation or reduction and measurement of ALP activity by the generation of the yellow *p*-nitrophenolate ion from the substrate *p*-nitrophenyl phosphate in alkaline solution. These indicator reactions are so versatile that coupled reactions are frequently used to provide an observable optical change accompanying a primary reaction in which such a change is not present.

The introduction of prism or diffraction-grating spectrophotometers capable of isolating a narrow beam of monochromatic light in the ultraviolet or visible spectrum and with stable and sensitive photomultipliers as detectors has greatly improved the reproducibility of photometric measurements (see Chapter 13). Consequently, it is customary to make use of the known molar absorptivity of well-defined reaction products (such as NADH) when calculating changes in their concentrations based on measurements made with spectrophotometers.

Optimization and Standardization

To measure enzyme activity reliably, all factors that affect the reaction rate—other than the concentration of active enzyme—need to be optimized and rigidly controlled because when the reaction velocity is at or near its maximum under optimal conditions, a larger analytical signal is obtained that can be more accurately measured than the smaller signal obtained under suboptimal conditions. Much effort therefore has been devoted to determining optimal conditions for measuring the activities of enzymes of clinical importance.

Optimization

Optimization of reaction conditions for enzyme assays traditionally has been carried out by varying a single factor and studying its effect on the reaction rate, then repeating the experiment with a second factor and so on, until effects of all the variables have been tested. An optimal combination of variables is selected on the basis of these experiments, and the validity of the chosen conditions is verified. Not only is this approach labor intensive, it also is difficult to adapt in situations in which the effects of different variables are interdependent, as is frequently the case in enzyme analysis. This traditional empirical approach to optimization has been replaced by techniques of simplex cooptimization and response surface methodology.[24]

Standardization

Despite considerable effort, the goal of a single universally used procedure to measure the catalytic activity of a given enzyme has not been achieved. Consequently, current enzyme standardization efforts are focused on the development of a system that allows comparability of test results, independent of the measurement method. To achieve this, a reference measurement system based on the concepts of metrologic traceability and on the hierarchy of analytical methods has been proposed.[25-27] A reference procedure and certified reference materials form the basis of the metrological traceability chain

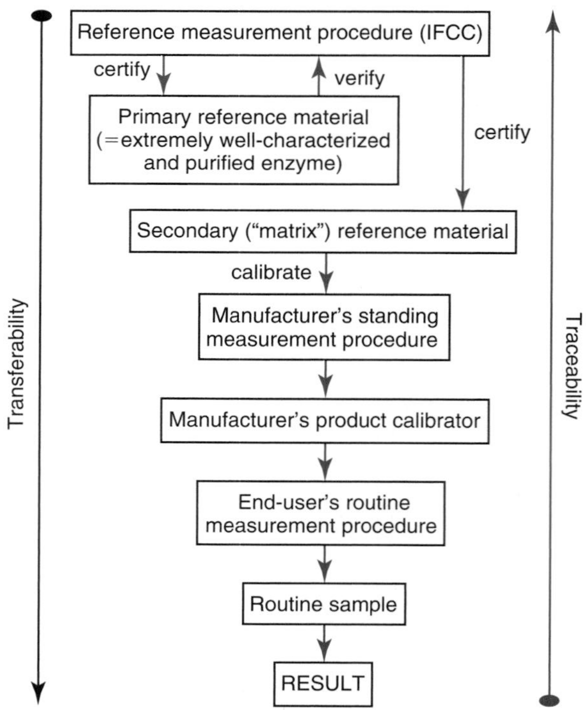

FIGURE 22.12 The proposed reference system for enzyme measurement showing the traceability of the laboratory result to the reference measurement procedure. (From Panteghini M, Ceriotti F, Schumann G, Siekmann L. Establishing a reference system in clinical enzymology. *Clin Chem Lab Med* 2001;39:795–800. Reprinted with permission of Walter de Gruyter.)

(Fig. 22.12).[26,28,29] As part of this hierarchy, reference procedures at 37°C for the most common enzymes have been developed,[25] and some reference laboratories use these reference procedures to perform enzyme measurements at an appropriately high metrologic level.[25]

Reference procedures set standards of precision and trueness against which the relative performance of methods intended for clinical use are judged. The reference procedure is used to assign a certified value to reference material, and this certified material is then used by the manufacturers to assign values to commercial calibrators, resulting in traceability of the value obtained in the laboratory.[25,30]

Several studies have demonstrated that enzyme preparations with reproducible properties and purity and having ensured stability can be made. These may be derived from animal sources in which the enzymes closely resemble their human counterparts, although new possibilities have been created by gene transfer and recombinant techniques.

For a reference system to be capable of standardizing the results of different assays of a given enzyme activity, some conditions must be satisfied.[31] First, the reference procedure used to assign the value of the reference material and the field method(s) to be calibrated must have similar, if not identical, specificities for the analyte enzyme isoenzyme or isoform under study. Second, the properties of the calibrator material must be the same as or closely similar to those of the analyte enzyme in its natural matrix and "commutable" and capable of being exchanged for another or for something else that is equivalent with human serum samples for that particular method.

Measurement of Enzyme Mass Concentration

Many immunoassays for human enzymes and isoenzymes measuring protein mass instead of catalytic activity have been described. To develop such assays, purified enzyme protein has to be prepared to (1) act as a calibrator, (2) be labeled, and (3) be used to raise the enzyme-specific antibody. These methods identify all molecules with the antigenic determinants necessary for recognition by the antibody, so that inactive enzyme molecules that are immunologically unaltered are measured along with active molecules. This has been found to be significant in the determination of some digestive enzymes, such as trypsin, when inactive precursors and inhibitors of catalytic activity are present in plasma. In the majority of cases, however, no degradation or changes in the active enzyme occur in blood so that the clinical equivalence of the different measurement approaches (ie, estimation of catalytic activity and mass concentration) is obtained.

Immunoassays typically are not used for determination of total activities for the more important diagnostic enzymes because these assays generally cannot compete in terms of speed, precision, and cost with automated measurements of catalytic activity. Furthermore, several enzyme activities in serum are due to mixtures of immunologically distinct forms, so an assay using a single type of antibody usually determines only one of the enzyme forms. However, this disadvantage in the determination of total enzyme activity becomes a marked advantage in the measurement of specific isoenzymes and isoforms, and immunologic methods have been used routinely in the isoenzyme analysis of CK amylase, and alkaline phosphatase.

Enzymes as Analytical Reagents

Enzymes are used as analytical reagents for measurement of several metabolites and substrates and in immunoassays to detect and quantify immunologic reactions.

Measurement of Metabolites

The use of enzymes as analytical reagents to measure metabolites frequently offers the advantage of great specificity for the substance being determined. This high specificity typically removes the need for preliminary separation or purification steps, so the analysis can be carried out directly on complex mixtures such as serum. Uricase (urate oxidase), urease, and glucose oxidase are examples of highly specific enzymes used in clinically important assays, such as the measurement of uric acid, urea, and glucose in biological fluids. However, high specificity cannot always be achieved in practice and knowledge of the substrate specificities of reagent enzymes is therefore essential to allow possible interferences with the assay to be anticipated and corrected. Coupled reactions are often necessary to construct an enzymatic analytical system for specifically determining a particular compound. For example, in the enzymatic determination of glucose, hexokinase converts a number of sugars to their 6-phosphate esters, but the indicator reaction used to monitor this change is catalyzed by glucose-6-phosphate dehydrogenase, which is highly specific for glucose; therefore the overall process is a highly specific glucose assay.

Equilibrium Methods. Most assays used to determine the amount of a substance enzymatically are allowed to continue to completion, so that all substrate has been converted into a measurable product. These methods are called *end point* or, more correctly, *equilibrium* methods, because the reaction ceases when equilibrium is reached. Reactions in which the equilibrium point corresponds virtually to complete conversion of the substrate are obviously preferable for this type of analysis. However, an unfavorable equilibrium often can be displaced in the desired direction by additional enzymatic or nonenzymatic reactions that convert or trap a product of the first reaction (eg, in measuring lactate with LD, the pyruvate formed can be trapped by the addition of hydrazine, with which it forms an irreversible hydrazone).

Theoretically, the time required to transform a fixed quantity, Q, of substrate into products is inversely proportional to the amount of enzyme, $[E]$, present:

$$Q = k_1 + [E] \times t \tag{27}$$

and

$$[E] = \frac{Q}{k_1} \times \frac{1}{t} \tag{28}$$

where k_l is the rate constant and t is the elapsed time. Equilibrium methods therefore may require the use of appreciable amounts of enzyme for each sample, to avoid inconveniently long incubation periods. As the substrate concentration falls to low quantities toward the end of the reaction, the K_m of the enzyme becomes important in determining the reaction rate. Enzymes with high affinities for their substrates (low K_m values) are most suitable for equilibrium analysis. Equilibrium methods are largely insensitive to minor changes in reaction conditions so it is not necessary to have exactly the same amount of enzyme in each reaction mixture or to maintain the pH or temperature absolutely constant, provided that the variations are not so great that the reaction is not completed within the fixed time allowed.

Kinetic Methods. First-order or pseudo–first-order reactions are the most important reactions for the kinetic determination of substrate concentration. For any first-order reaction, the substrate concentration $[S]$ at a given time t after the start of the reaction is given by

$$[S]=[S_0]\times e^{-kt} \quad \textbf{(29)}$$

where $[S_0]$ is the initial substrate concentration, e is the base of the natural log, and k is the rate constant.

The change in substrate concentration $\Delta[S]$ over a fixed time interval, t_1 to t_2, is related to $[S_0]$ by the equation

$$[S_0]=\frac{-\Delta[S]}{e^{-kt_1}-e^{kt_2}} \quad \textbf{(30)}$$

As this equation indicates, the change in substrate concentration over a fixed time interval is directly proportional to its initial concentration. This is a general property of first-order reactions.

For an enzymatic reaction, first-order kinetics is followed when $[S]$ is small compared with K_m. Thus

$$v=\frac{V_{max}}{K_m}\times[S] \quad \textbf{(31)}$$

or

$$v=k[S] \quad \textbf{(32)}$$

Therefore the first-order rate constant, k, is equal to $\frac{V_{max}}{K_m}$.

Methods in which some property related to substrate concentration (eg, absorbance, fluorescence, chemiluminescence) is measured at two fixed times during the course of the reaction are known as *two-point* kinetic methods. Theoretically, they are most accurate for the enzymatic determination of substrates. However, these methods are technically more demanding than equilibrium methods and all factors that affect reaction rate, such as pH, temperature, and amount of enzyme, must be kept constant from one assay to the next, as must the timing of the two measurements. These conditions can be readily achieved in automated analyzers. A reference solution of the analyte (substrate) is used for calibration. To ensure first-order reaction conditions, the substrate concentration must be low compared with the K_m (ie, in the order of less than $0.2 \times K_m$). Enzymes with high K_m values therefore are preferred for kinetic analysis to obtain a wider usable range of substrate concentrations.

Immunoassay

In enzyme immunoassay, enzyme-labeled antibodies or antigens first are allowed to react with ligand; then an enzyme substrate is added. Enzymes such as (1) ALP all have been used as enzyme labels. A modification of this methodology is the enzyme-linked immunosorbent assay (ELISA), in which one of the reaction components is bound to a solid-phase surface. In this technique, an aliquot of sample is allowed to interact with the solid-phase antibody. After washing, a second antibody labeled with enzyme is added to form an Ab–Ag–Ab–enzyme complex. Excess free enzyme-labeled antibody is then washed away, and the substrate is added; the conversion of substrate is proportional to the quantity of antigen. In immunoassays, it is not the specificity of labeled enzymes that is important, but rather their sensitivity.

Analytical Applications of Immobilized Enzymes

For some types of enzymatic analyses, enzyme consumption is reduced by the use of immobilized enzymes that are reused for several analyses. Immobilized enzymes have been chemically bonded to adsorbents, such as (1) microcrystalline cellulose, (2) diethylaminoethyl (DEAE) cellulose, (3) carboxymethyl cellulose, and (4) agarose. Diazo, triazine, and azide groups are used to join the enzyme protein to the insoluble matrix, forming particles in contact with the substrate solution or a surface in contact with substrate solution, such as a membrane or a coating on the inner surface of a vessel holding the substrate solution. Among enzymes available in such immobilized form are (1) urease, (2) hexokinase, (3) α-amylase, (4) glucose oxidase, (5) trypsin, and (6) leucine aminopeptidase. Temperature stability and other forms of inactivation are considerably increased compared with enzymes in solution. Immobilized proteolytic enzymes are not subject to autodigestion. However, some properties of the enzyme, such as its K_m or its pH optimum, may be altered.

Electrochemical techniques such as (1) potentiometry, (2) polarography, and (3) microcalorimetry have been chosen in exploiting the benefits of immobilized enzymes (see Chapters 13 and 14). Enzymes incorporated into membranes form part of enzyme electrodes such as on blood gas analyzers. The surface of an ion-sensitive electrode is coated with a layer of porous gel in which an enzyme has been polymerized. When the electrode is immersed in a solution of the appropriate substrate, the action of the enzyme produces ions to which the electrode is sensitive.

Measurement of Isoenzymes and Isoforms

A number of analytical techniques have been used to measure isoenzymes or isoforms. They include (1) electrophoresis (see Chapter 15), (2) chromatography (see Chapter 16), (3) chemical inactivation, and (4) differences in catalytic properties, but the most widely used methods are now based on immunochemical principles (Chapter 23).

Electrophoresis

Various forms of electrophoresis have been used to separate isoenzymes. The methods are time-consuming, difficult to quantify, and relatively expensive and thus tend to be restricted to larger, reference laboratories.

Chromatography

Ion-exchange chromatography makes use of differences in net molecular charge at a given pH to separate isoenzymes. A typical ion-exchange material is DEAE cellulose, in which ionizable DEAE groups are attached to an inert cellulose matrix. Ion-exchange chromatography is not in general as highly resolving of closely similar proteins as is zone electrophoresis, but relatively large quantities of proteins can be separated with good recovery of enzymatic activity, so the method is of great value in enzyme purification.

Other forms of chromatography that have been applied to fractionation of isoenzyme mixtures include high-performance liquid chromatography and affinity chromatography. The latter makes use of differences between isoenzymes in their affinities for a specific ligand that is attached to an inert insoluble support used as the stationary phase in a chromatography column or in a batch technique.

Chemical Inactivation and Differences in Catalytic Properties

Selective inactivation under controlled conditions has been used in isoenzyme characterization. The method is based on differences in stability that result from small changes in the structure of protein molecules. Increased temperatures or concentrated solutions of urea or other reagents are used to denature the enzyme. Rates of enzyme inactivation by these agents are critically dependent on the conditions of the experiment, which therefore must be strictly controlled if reliable comparisons between samples are to be made.

Differences in catalytic properties, such as (1) differences in K_m, relative rates of reaction with substrate analogs (when the specificity of the enzyme allows for variation in the structure of the substrate), (2) pH optima, and (3) response to inhibitors, typically exist between isoenzymes that are the products of multiple-gene loci. These differences can serve as the basis of methods of identification and measurement of particular isoenzymes.

These techniques are no longer used routinely because they have been largely superseded by other, more convenient methods such as immunoassay methods.

Immunochemical Assays

Immunochemical methods of isoenzyme analysis are particularly applicable to isoenzymes derived from multiple-gene loci because these are usually most clearly antigenically distinct. However, the greater discriminating power of monoclonal antibodies has potentially brought all multiple forms of an enzyme within the scope of immunochemical analysis. Some of these methods detect catalytic activity of the isoenzymes. For example, residual activity may be measured after reaction with antiserum. Radioimmunoassays in which isoenzyme labeled with a radioactive tracer competes with unlabeled isoenzyme for antibody-binding sites have been applied in the past to isoenzyme measurement. However, with the development of automated immunoassay systems, the preferred method for measuring isoenzymes in the clinical laboratory is a solid-phase sandwich ELISA assay because of its convenience and relative low cost. These methods do not depend on the catalytic activity of the isoenzyme being determined.

The choice and application of various methods of isoenzyme analysis in clinical enzymology in relation to specific isoenzyme systems are discussed in Chapter 29.

POINTS TO REMEMBER

- Enzymes are proteins with the ability to accelerate or catalyze chemical reactions.
- The characteristics of the reactions catalyzed by an enzyme depend on the structure of its active site and relationship to its substrates.
- Enzymes exist in multiple forms, isoenzymes, the properties and distribution of which are important in diagnosis.
- The catalytic properties of enzymes can be described by equations based on the formation of an ES complex.
- Enzyme reactions are affected by temperature, pH, enzyme concentration, substrate concentration, and the presence of any inhibitors or activators.
- Because of their specificity, enzymes can be used as analytical reagents to measure compounds such as metabolites in complex mediums.

23

Immunochemical Techniques

*Larry J. Kricka and Jason Y. Park**

ABSTRACT

Background

Immunoassay is a powerful qualitative and quantitative analytical technique used to detect and measure a wide range of clinically important analytes. The extreme sensitivity and specificity of immunoassay has allowed detection and quantitation of analytes present at very low concentrations not easily measured by other analytical techniques.

Content

This chapter describes the scope of immunologic assays, including the basics of antigen-antibody binding, antibody production, and nonantibody binding agents (eg, aptamers, molecularly imprinted polymers, boronates). Qualitative methods described include the precipitin reaction, the agglutination reaction, passive gel diffusion, immunoelectrophoresis (crossed and counterimmunoelectrophoresis), immunofixation, blotting (western and dot blotting), and cell- and tissue-based immunochemical techniques. Quantitative methods include radial immunodiffusion, electroimmunoassay, turbidimetric and nephelometric assays, surface plasmon resonance–based immunoassay, and labeled immunochemical assays. Important aspects of the latter assay category are considered, including methodologic principles (competitive vs. noncompetitive and heterogeneous vs. homogeneous immunochemical assays), and analytical and functional sensitivity. Important types of labeled immunoassays are outlined, including radioimmunoassay, enzyme immunoassay (eg, enzyme-linked immunosorbent assay, enzyme multiplied immunoassay technique, cloned enzyme donor immunoassay, fluoroimmunoassay [eg, fluorescence resonance energy transfer]), phosphor immunoassay, chemiluminescence and bioluminescence immunoassay, electrochemiluminescence immunoassay, magnetic particle immunoassay, immuno–polymerase chain reaction, bio-barcode immunoassay and digital immunoassay. Multiplexed immunoassays based on distinguishable labels and location of a solid support (eg, protein microarray) are illustrated, as well as simplified immunoassays designed for point-of-care applications.

Immunologic assays are prone to interferences, and the scope of these interferences is described and exemplified (eg, hook effect, false-negative or false-positive results resulting from anti–animal immunoglobulin antibodies).

Immunochemical reactions form the basis of a diverse range of sensitive and specific clinical assays. In a typical immunochemical analysis, an antibody is used as a reagent to detect an antigen of interest. The exquisite specificity and high affinity of antibodies for their antigens, coupled with the ability of antibodies to cross-link antigens, allow the identification and quantitation of specific substances by a variety of methods. The principles of the methods most commonly used in the clinical laboratory are discussed in this chapter. This introduction is intended to acquaint the reader with the structure and function of antibodies (immunoglobulins) in relation to their use as reagents in immunoanalyses.

BASIC CONCEPTS

The binding of antibodies and their complementary antigens forms the basis of all immunochemical techniques.

Antibodies

Antibodies are immunoglobulins capable of binding specifically to a wide array of natural and synthetic antigens, including proteins, carbohydrates, nucleic acids, lipids, and other molecules. Immunoglobulins consist of five general classes designated as immunoglobulin (Ig)G, IgA, IgM, IgD, and IgE. IgG is used most commonly in immunochemical reagents. A schematic diagram of the IgG molecule is shown in Fig. 23.1. IgG is a glycoprotein (molecular weight [MW], 158,000 Da) composed of two heavy (γ) and two light (κ or λ) chains joined by disulfide bonds. Each chain (H or L) is the product of three (L) or four (H) distinct gene segments. These are the constant (C), joining (J), diversity (D), and variable (V) genes that undergo combinatorial joining during B cell development. Several hundred germline V genes, 5 to 10 J genes, 15 D genes (H chain only), and a single C gene have been identified for each heavy or light chain class. During B cell development, the V, D, and J (H chain) or V and J (L chain) undergo random rearrangement and splicing, and this recombined product then is spliced to the constant region gene. This combinatorial diversity, along with somatic mutations

*The authors gratefully acknowledge the original contribution by Dr. Gregory Buffone, on which portions of this chapter are based.

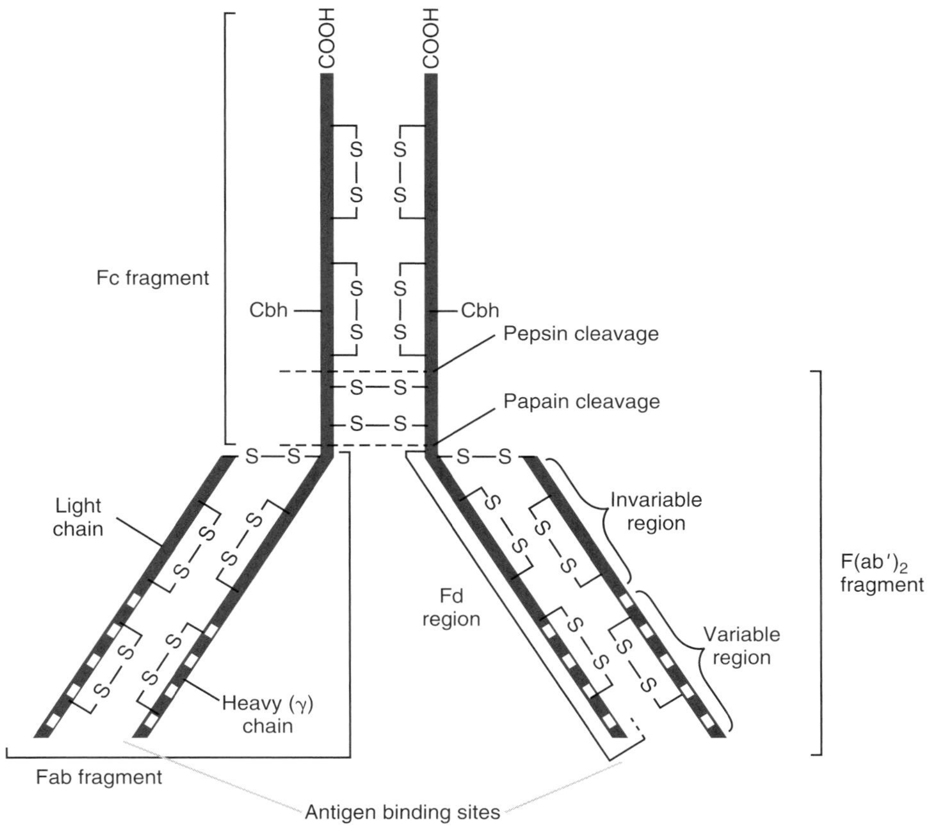

FIGURE 23.1 Schematic diagram of immunoglobulin (Ig)G antibody molecule showing carbohydrate (Cbh), disulfide bonds (—S—S—), and major fragments produced by proteolytic enzyme treatment ($F[ab']_2$, Fc, Fab, Fd).

that occur at the splicing sites, generates a tremendous diversity of antibody specificities. When a B cell clone expressing a particular antibody specificity on its surface is selected by an antigen, it expands and differentiates into a plasma cell that secretes the specific antibody.

The variable amino acid sequence at the amino terminal end (~105 amino acids) of each chain determines the antigenic specificity of the particular antibody. Each unique variable region is a product of a single plasma cell line or clone. A complex antigen is capable of eliciting a multiplicity of antibodies with different specificities that are derived from different cell lines. Antibodies derived in this manner are termed *polyclonal* and exhibit diverse specificities in their reactivity with the immunogen. Each unique region of the antigen molecule that will bind a complementary antibody is termed an *epitope* (antigenic determinant).

Immunogens

An immunogen is a protein or a substance coupled to a carrier that when introduced into a foreign host is capable of inducing the formation of an antibody in the host. The antibody produced may be circulating (humoral) or tissue bound (cellular).

A hapten is a small, chemically defined determinant that when conjugated to an immunogenic carrier stimulates the synthesis of antibody specific for the hapten. It is capable of binding an antibody but cannot by itself stimulate an immune response.

Continued stimulation by an immunogen results in increased production of immunoglobulins of different types and of high-affinity binding characteristics for antigens. After the first exposure to an immunogen, a latent period (induction) occurs during which no antibody is present in serum; this period may last from 5 to 10 days.

The strength or energy of interaction between the antibody and the antigen is described by two terms. Affinity refers to the thermodynamic quantity defining the energy of interaction of a single antibody-combining site and its corresponding epitope on the antigen. Avidity refers to the overall strength of binding of an antibody and its antigen and includes the sum of the binding affinities of all the individual combining sites on the antibody. For example, IgG has two antigen-binding sites, whereas IgM has 10 antigen-binding sites per antibody molecule. Thus affinity is a property of the substance bound (antigen), and avidity is a property of the binder (antibody). For polyclonal antibodies, avidity is difficult to determine primarily because of the diversity of the antibody population.

Polyclonal antiserum is raised in a normal animal host in response to immunogen administration. In contrast, monoclonal antibodies are produced in a very different manner and represent the product of a single clone or plasma cell line, rather than a heterogeneous mixture of antibodies produced by many plasma cell clones in response to immunization. Monoclonal antibodies are now widely used as reagents in immunoassay techniques.[1] The usual method of production of monoclonal antibodies involves fusing antibody-producing plasma cells from the spleens or lymph nodes of immunized mice with a murine myeloma cell line from tissue culture.

Because of the unique ability of a monoclonal antibody to react with a single epitope on a multivalent antigen, the majority of monoclonal antibodies will not cross-link and precipitate macromolecular antigens. Consequently, monoclonal antibodies have not found broad applicability in traditional precipitin methods. A practical advantage of using monoclonal antibodies is that two different antibody specificities can be used in a single incubation step. A solid-phase antibody specific for a unique epitope and another labeled antibody specific for a different epitope can react with an antigen in a single step. This eliminates the incubating and washing steps that usually would be required for polyclonal antibodies.

Phage display technology provides an in vitro approach for producing antibodies (single-chain Fv fragments, Fab fragments, and whole antibody molecules) that mimic the immune system but do not require B cell immortalization.[2] V genes coding for the heavy- and light-chain variable domains of immunoglobulin isolated from lymphocytes are amplified by the polymerase chain reaction (PCR) and ligated into a filamentous bacteriophage vector to form combinatorial libraries of V_H and V_L genes. Individual bacteriophages display copies of a specific antibody on their surface, and the phage library can be screened for the antibody of a defined specificity using immobilized antigen ("panning"). Large libraries displaying antibodies formed from more than 10^{12} different V_H and V_L combinations can be constructed; this provides a rich source of antibodies with binding constants of 10^8 to 10^9 L/mol.

ANTIGEN-ANTIBODY BINDING

Binding Forces

The strength of the binding of an antigen to an antibody depends on several forces acting cooperatively. These include van der Waals-London dipole-dipole interaction, hydrophobic interaction, and ionic coulombic bonding.[3]

Van der Waals-London Dipole-Dipole Interactions

Van der Waals-London binding is caused by the attraction between atoms when they are brought together in close proximity. These interactions are basically electrostatic and are applicable to polarizable, noncharged molecules whose structure allows the electron cloud around the molecule to be distorted by outside forces in such a way that a transient dipole is produced. These forces operate over short distances (4 to 6 nm) and are more significant for larger molecules. Because polarizability varies inversely with temperature, the attractive force is inversely proportional to the temperature.

Hydrophobic Interaction

Hydrophobic interactions result because the association of nonpolar groups is energetically favored in aqueous or other polar solutions. In proteins, hydrophobic interactions bend and fold a molecule in a way that brings nonpolar groups inside to the less polar interior; polar groups are oriented outside toward the more polar aqueous environment. Thus hydrophobic bonding forms an interior, hydrophobic protein core, in which most hydrophobic side chains can closely associate and weakly bind. Hydrophobic interaction enhances or stabilizes antigen-antibody binding but is not necessarily the major force in such binding.[4]

Coulombic Bonds

Coulombic bonding results from the attraction between charged groups on the antigen and the antibody, primarily carboxylate (COO^-) and ammonium (NH_4^+). The attraction between the charged groups is greatest in a medium with a low dielectric constant caused by reduced interaction of the solvent or other solute (salts) with the macromolecular ions. In a medium of high dielectric constant (aqueous solutions containing added salt), a diffuse double layer of charged particles will tend to shield the attraction of the charged species in the reactive sites of the antigen and antibody. This inhibition under certain circumstances can considerably reduce the binding constant for many antigen-antibody systems.

Given these forces, one would predict that changing pH, temperature, and ionic strength of the reaction medium should influence the binding of antigen and antibody. However, given a lower and upper limit of pH of 6.0 and 8.0 and an incubation temperature between 25° and 35°C, these variables have only minimal effect on the rate of association and immune complex formation.[5] Extremes in pH (<4.0 and >8.0), however, can cause inhibition of binding or dissociation of already formed antigen-antibody complexes. In addition, changes in ionic strength will produce a significant effect on the rate of binding of antigen and antibody. This concept is studied further in the following sections.

Reaction Mechanism

The binding of antigen to antibody is not static but is an equilibrium reaction that proceeds in three phases. The initial reaction (phase 1) of a multivalent antigen (Ag_n) and a bivalent antibody (Ab) occurs very rapidly in comparison with subsequent growth of the complexes (phase 2) and is depicted by the following equation:

$$Ag_n + Ab \underset{k_{-1}}{\overset{k_1}{\rightleftharpoons}} Ag_nAb \underset{k_{-2}}{\overset{k_2}{\rightleftharpoons}} Ag_aAb_b \qquad \textbf{(23.1)}$$

where $k_1 \gg> k_2$, n is the number of epitopes per molecule, and a and b are the numbers of antigen and antibody molecules per complex. Phase 3 of the reaction involves precipitation of the complex after a critical size is reached. The speed of these reactions depends on electrolyte concentration, pH, and temperature, and on antigen structure and antibody class and the binding affinity of the antibody. The concentration of sodium chloride (NaCl) is important, and in most cases saline (NaCl, 0.15 mol/L) is used. Higher concentrations of NaCl can lead to smaller amounts of precipitate; this is due not to increased solubility of the antigen-antibody complex, but to an equilibrium shift causing a given amount of antigen to combine with smaller amounts of antibody. Decreasing the NaCl concentration can lead to increased precipitation of other proteins.

It is best to use dilute Ab and Ag solutions for determining the influence of such factors as (1) ionic species, (2) ionic strength, and (3) pH. Use of dilute solutions slows the growth of antigen-antibody complexes; this results in more stable and homogeneous complexes.

Factors Influencing Binding

Factors that influence the strength of binding between an antigen and an antibody include ion species, ionic strength, and polymers used in the solution.

Ion Species and Ionic Strength Effects

Cationic salts produce an inhibition of the binding of antibody with a cationic hapten.[6] The order of inhibition by various cations is cesium (Cs^+) > rubidium (Rb^+) > ammonium (NH_4^+) > potassium (K^+) > sodium (Na^+) > lithium (Li^+). This order corresponds to the decreasing ionic radius and the increasing radius of hydration. Similar results are observed with anionic haptens and anionic salts. For example, the order of inhibition of binding for anionic salts is thiocyanate (CNS^-) > nitrate (NO_3^-) > iodide (I^-) > bromide (Br^-) > chloride (Cl^-) > fluoride (F^-), which again is in the order of decreasing ionic radius and increasing radius of hydration. If the competition theory as suggested by these experiments is correct, the degree of inhibition would be expected to be a concentration-dependent phenomenon, and indeed the rate of formation of immune complexes is slower in normal saline (NaCl, 0.15 mol/L) than the same reaction carried out in deionized water. Given the previous observation, F^- should be the anion of choice for immunochemical reaction buffers. In fact, F^- does provide a modest improvement over Cl^-, but the advantage is so small that laboratories rarely substitute toxic fluoride ion for innocuous chloride ion in buffer solutions.

Polymer Effect

In general, the solubility of a protein in the presence of different linear polymers is inversely proportional to the MW of the polymer (ie, the higher the MW of the polymer, the lower is the solubility of the protein). For example, in the presence of Dextran 500, the solubility of α-crystalline < fibrinogen < γ-globulin < albumin ⋘ tyrosine.[7] Laurent thus proposed a steric exclusion mechanism to explain the effects of polymers on protein solubility. Assuming a fixed total volume (V_T) of solvent being occupied by both polymer and protein and defining the volume occupied by polymer as V_E (excluded volume, ie, volume not accessible to proteins) and the volume occupied by protein as V′, then the relation

$$V_T = V' + V_E \qquad (23.2)$$

implies that any increase in V_E caused by an increase in number or size of polymer molecules forces a decrease in V′ and an effective increase in the concentration of protein molecules. Hence, as V_E is increased the effective protein concentration is increased, the probability of collision and self-association of protein molecules is increased, and large insoluble aggregates are formed.

Studies have provided support for the steric exclusion model[8] and have demonstrated that (1) the composition of the immune complex formed is not affected by the presence of a polymer; (2) no complex is formed between the polymer and the antigen, antibody, or immune complex; (3) the polymer effect depends on the MW of both antigen and polymer; and (4) the use of polymer in a reaction mixture can increase the precipitation of an immune complex with low-avidity antibody. Addition of polymer to a mixture of antigen and antibody causes a notable increase in the rate of immune complex growth, especially during the early phase of the reaction. Numerous polymer species have been tested (eg, polyethylene glycol, dextran) for applications in immunochemical methods. The most desirable characteristics of the polymer are high MW, a high degree of linearity (minimal branching), and high aqueous solubility. Most investigators have found the polymer polyethylene glycol (PEG) 6000, in concentrations of 3 to 5 g/dL to be most useful in promoting immune complex formation.

Types of Reactions

Types of antigen-antibody reactions that are of analytical importance include the precipitin reaction and those noted at a solid-liquid interface.

Precipitin Reaction

If the number of antibody-combining sites is notably greater than the antigen-epitope sites ([Ab] ⋙ [Ag]), then antigen-binding sites are quickly saturated by antibodies before cross-linking can occur, along with the formation of small insoluble antigen-antibody complexes (Fig. 23.2A). When an antibody is in moderate excess (ie, [Ab] > [Ag]), the probability of cross-linking of Ag by Ab is more likely and hence large insoluble complex formation is favored (see Fig. 23.2B). When [Ag] is in great excess, large complexes would be less probable (see Fig. 23.2C). This model describes the results observed when antigens and antibodies are mixed in various concentration ratios. The curve shown in Fig. 23.3 is a schematic diagram of the classic precipitin curve. Although the concentration of total antibody is constant, the concentration of free antibody $[Ab]_f$ (ie, not bound to antigen) and free antigen $[Ag]_f$ varies throughout the range for any given Ag/Ab ratio. A low Ag/Ab ratio exists in *A* of Fig. 23.3 (zone of antibody excess). Under these conditions, $[Ab]_f$ exists in solution but $[Ag]_f$ does not. As total antigen increases, the size of the immune complexes increases up to equivalence (see Fig. 23.3B), in which little or no $[Ab]_f$ or $[Ag]_f$ exists. This is the zone of maximum immune complex size. This equivalence zone does not represent a ratio of exact molar equivalence of reactants but is the optimal combining ratio for cross-linking in the particular system under evaluation. As Ag/Ab increases (see Fig. 23.3C), the immune complex size will decrease and $[Ag]_f$ will increase (zone of antigen excess). No $[Ab]_f$ should exist in this area of the curve. However, for a given Ag/Ab ratio, the population of immune complexes formed at equilibrium will be heterogeneous with respect to size and composition.

Reactions at a Solid-Liquid Interface

If the antigen or antibody of interest is bound to a solid phase such as a synthetic particle (polystyrene or cellulose), the protein will exist in a microenvironment that is different from that of a protein in free solution. Water surrounding the protein is more highly ordered near the surface of the solid phase, and the condition that results is more favorable for van der Waals-London dipole-dipole interaction and coulombic bonding. This situation favors the formation of both low- and high-avidity antigen-antibody complexes and hence can provide lower detection limits for analytical applications.

Because of the exquisite specificity and the high affinity of antibodies for specific antigens, thousands of immunoassays have been developed to detect and measure a wide variety of

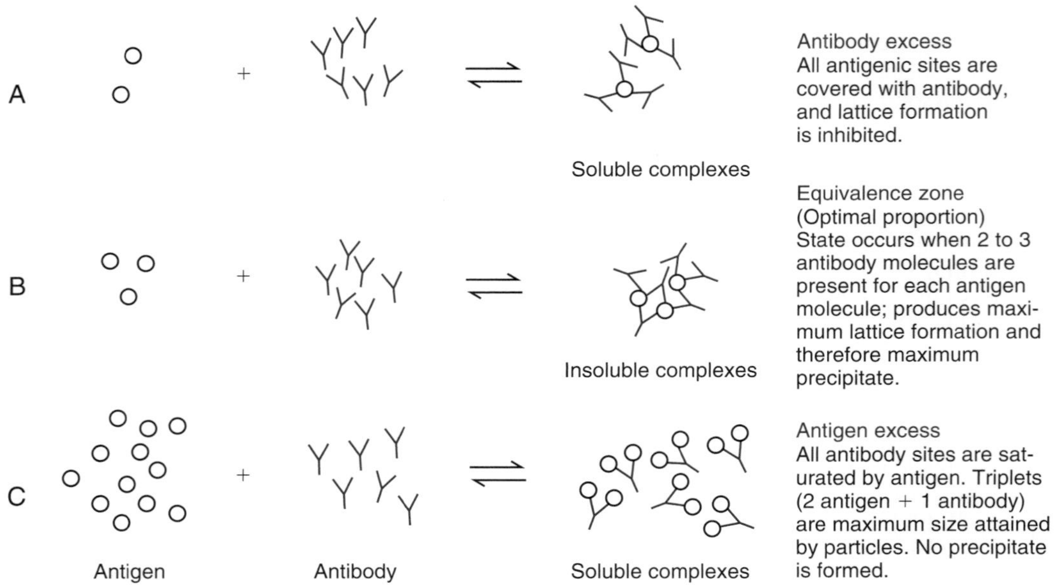

A

Soluble complexes

Antibody excess
All antigenic sites are covered with antibody, and lattice formation is inhibited.

B

Insoluble complexes

Equivalence zone
(Optimal proportion)
State occurs when 2 to 3 antibody molecules are present for each antigen molecule; produces maximum lattice formation and therefore maximum precipitate.

C

Antigen

Antibody

Soluble complexes

Antigen excess
All antibody sites are saturated by antigen. Triplets (2 antigen + 1 antibody) are maximum size attained by particles. No precipitate is formed.

FIGURE 23.2 Schematic diagram for precipitin reaction.

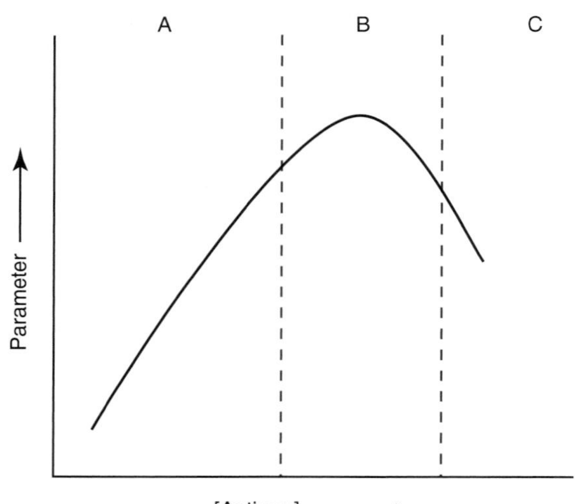

FIGURE 23.3 Schematic diagram of precipitin curve illustrating zones of antibody excess *(A)*, equivalence *(B)*, and antigen excess *(C)*. The parameter measured may be the quantity of protein precipitated, light scattering, or another measurable parameter. Antibody concentration is held constant in this example.

biological analytes. In the next two sections, qualitative and quantitative immunotechniques are discussed.

QUALITATIVE METHODS

Various types of immunotechniques have been used for qualitative purposes; these include passive gel diffusion, immunoelectrophoresis (IEP), and western and dot blotting.

Passive Gel Diffusion

Many qualitative and quantitative immunochemical methods are performed in a semisolid medium, such as agar or agarose. The primary advantage of using a gelatinous medium is that the diffusion process is stabilized with regard to mixing caused by vibration, and visualization of precipitin bands is allowed for qualitative and quantitative evaluation of the reaction. Antigen-to-antibody ratio, salt concentration, and polymer enhancement have the same influence on the antigen-antibody reaction in gels that they have on reactions in solution.

The initial concentration of antigen and antibody is critical. Each molecule in the system will achieve a unique concentration gradient with time. When the leading fronts of antigen and antibody diffusion overlap, the reaction will begin, but formation of a precipitin line will not occur until moderate antibody excess is achieved. A precipitin band may form and be dissolved many times by an incoming antigen before equilibrium is established and the position of the precipitin band becomes stable. Because heavier molecules diffuse more slowly, the position of the precipitin band is in part a function of the molecular masses of both antigen and antibody. The precipitin band acts as a specific barrier; neither specific antigen nor antibody can penetrate without being precipitated by the other, but unrelated molecules can cross the band of precipitation freely. Basic approaches to passive diffusion include simple diffusion and double diffusion. With simple diffusion, a concentration gradient is established for only a single reactant. Single immunodiffusion usually depends on diffusion of an antigen into agar impregnated with antibody. A quantitative technique based on this principle is radial immunodiffusion (RID), which is discussed later. The second approach is double diffusion, in which a concentration gradient is established for both reactants (antigen and antibody).

Double immunodiffusion in two dimensions is a historical immunotechnique known as the Ouchterlony method. It allows direct comparison of two or more test materials and provides a simple method for determining whether the antigens in the test specimens are identical, cross-reactive, or nonidentical.

The simplest method uses an agar dish or slide with holes cut as shown in Fig. 23.4. When the same antigen is in adjacent

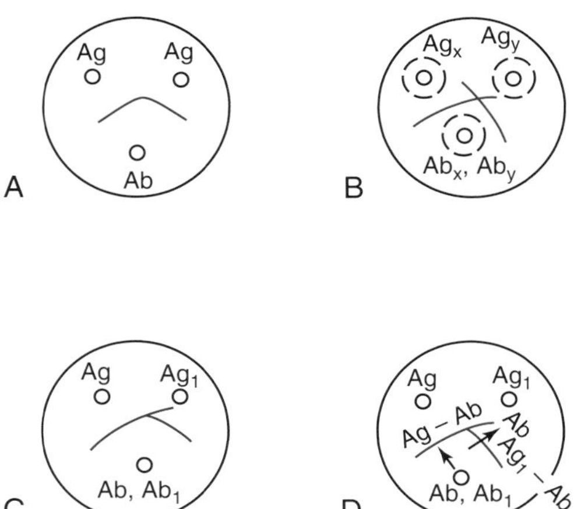

FIGURE 23.4 Double immunodiffusion in two dimensions by the Ouchterlony technique. **A,** Reaction of identity; **B,** reaction of nonidentity; **C,** reaction of partial identity; **D,** scheme for spur formation. *Ab,* Antibody; *Ag,* antigen.

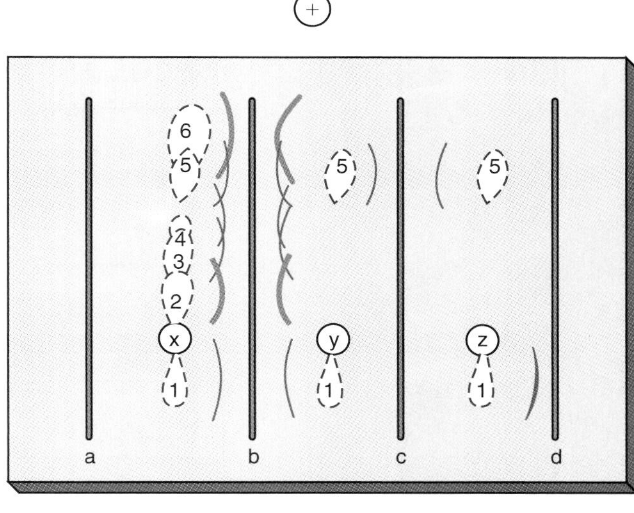

FIGURE 23.5 Configuration for immunoelectrophoresis. Sample wells are punched in the agar and/or agarose, sample is applied, and electrophoresis is carried out to separate the proteins in the sample. Antiserum is loaded into the troughs and the gel incubated in a moist chamber at 4°C for 24 to 72 hours. Track *x* represents the shape of the protein zones after electrophoresis; tracks *y* and *z* show the reactions of proteins 5 and 1 with their specific antisera in troughs *c* and *d.* Antiserum against protein *1* to *6* is present in trough *b.*

wells, the lines of precipitation fuse and are continuous—this is a reaction of identity (see Fig. 23.4A). When the precipitin bands cross each other, this is a reaction of nonidentity (see Fig. 23.4B); if the two antigens are related but are not identical, a reaction of partial identity is observed (see Fig. 23.4C). Here the cardinal point is that the precipitate serves as a barrier that does not block unrelated diffusing reactants. As shown in Fig. 23.4D, when the two related antigens Ag and Ag_1 are in separate wells and the respective antibodies, Ab and Ab_1, are in the third well, an AgAb precipitate forms on one side and blocks further diffusion of Ab from the antibody well. However, on the other side, the Ag_1Ab_1 precipitate does not stop Ab from migrating further and forming an AgAb spur.

Note that a negative reaction does not necessarily imply absence of antibody or antigen. A negative reaction can result from using amounts of material too small for the detection limit of the method, or the antibody may be nonprecipitating.

Immunoelectrophoresis

If several antigens of interest exist in a solution (eg, spinal fluid or serum), the various protein species can be separated and identified by IEP. This technique has been used extensively for the study of antigen mixtures and evaluation of the specificity of antiserum.[9]

The procedure is performed using an agarose gel medium poured onto a thin plastic sheet. The sample to be analyzed is placed in a reservoir in the gel, and an electrical field is applied across the gel surface. During electrophoresis, the proteins in the serum are separated according to their electrophoretic mobilities (Fig. 23.5). After electrophoresis, an antiserum against the protein of interest is placed in a trough parallel and adjacent to the electrophoresed sample. Simultaneous diffusion of the antigen from the separated sample and the antibody from the trough leads to the formation of precipitin arcs, whose shape and position are characteristic of individual separated proteins within the specimen. By comparison with a known control separated on the same plate, individual proteins can be tentatively identified.

Crossed Immunoelectrophoresis

This technique, also known as two-dimensional IEP, is a variation of IEP in which electrophoresis is also used in the second dimension to drive the antigen into a gel containing antibodies specific for the antigens of interest.[10] This technique is more sensitive and produces higher resolution than IEP.

Counterimmunoelectrophoresis

With counterimmunoelectrophoresis (CIE), two parallel lines of wells are punched in the agar. One row is filled with antigen solution, and the opposing row is filled with antibody solution (Fig. 23.6). If the solutions were allowed to passively diffuse, a precipitin line would form between the opposing wells in 18 to 24 hours. With CIE, this process is accelerated by applying a voltage across the gel so that the antigen and the antibody move toward each other. Qualitative information (ie, identification of antigen) is provided within 1 to 2 hours. Historically, this method has found application in the detection of bacterial antigens in blood, urine, and cerebrospinal fluid (CSF).

Immunofixation

This technique has gained widespread acceptance as an immunochemical method for identifying proteins.[11] As in IEP and crossed radioimmunoelectrophoresis (CRIE), a first-dimension electrophoresis is performed in agarose gel to separate proteins in the sample. Subsequently, antiserum spread directly on the gel causes the protein(s) of interest to precipitate. The immune precipitate is trapped within the gel matrix, and all other nonprecipitated proteins are removed by washing the gel. The gel may then be stained for

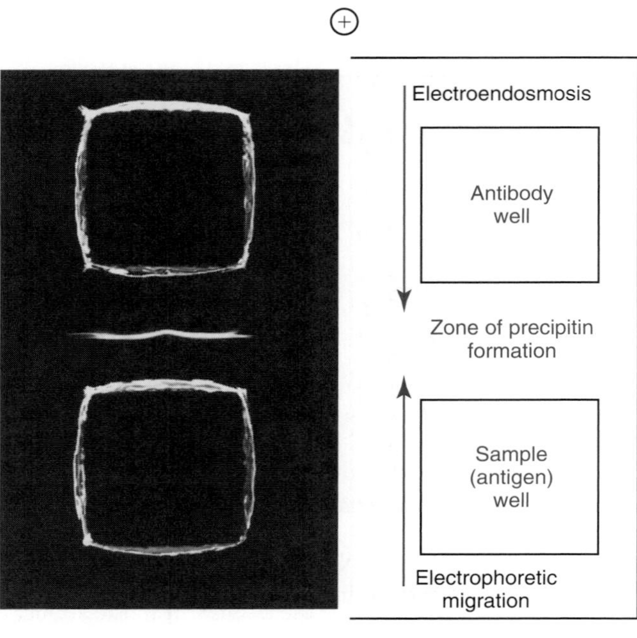

FIGURE 23.6 Counterimmunoelectrophoresis showing positive reaction between anti–*Haemophilus influenzae* B *(upper well)* and a cerebrospinal fluid sample containing *H. influenzae* B *(lower well).*

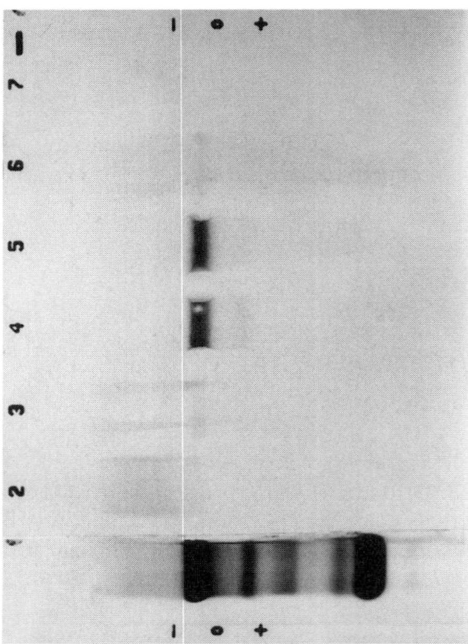

FIGURE 23.7 Immunofixation of a serum containing an immunoglobulin (Ig)M kappa paraprotein. *Lane 1,* Serum electrophoresis stained for protein; *lane 2,* anti-IgG, Fc piece specific; *lane 3,* anti-IgA, α-chain specific; *lane 4,* anti-IgM, μ-chain specific; *lane 5,* anti-κ light chain; *lane 6,* anti-λ light chain. (Courtesy Katherine Bayer, Protein Laboratory, Hospital of the University of Pennsylvania, Philadelphia, Pennsylvania.)

identification of the proteins. Immunofixation is technically more efficient than IEP or CRIE, and it produces patterns that are interpreted more easily. The usefulness of immunofluorescence, which is now widely used for the evaluation of monoclonal gammopathies (eg, multiple myeloma) is illustrated in Fig. 23.7.

Western Blotting

The techniques discussed previously use direct evaluation of the immunoprecipitation of the protein(s) in a gel. However, certain media, such as polyacrylamide, do not lend themselves to direct immunoprecipitation, nor is there always sufficient antigen concentration to produce an immunoprecipitate that will be retained in the gel during subsequent processing. Under these circumstances, western blotting can be used.[12] This technique involves an electrophoresis step followed by transfer of separated proteins onto an overlying strip of nitrocellulose or a nylon membrane by the process of electro-blotting. Once the proteins are in the membrane, they can be detected using antibodies labeled with probes, such as radioactive isotopes or enzymes. When such probes are used, the limits of detection can be 10 to 100 times lower than when direct immunoprecipitation and staining of proteins are conducted. This technique is analogous to Southern blotting (electrophoresed DNA blotted onto a membrane), and northern blotting (electrophoresed RNA blotted onto a membrane).

An example of this technique applied to the detection of human immunodeficiency virus type 1 (HIV-1) antibodies is shown in Fig. 23.8. HIV-1 antigens are separated according to MW by gel electrophoresis and then transferred to a nitrocellulose membrane by electro-blotting. A serum sample is then incubated with a strip of the membrane. HIV-1

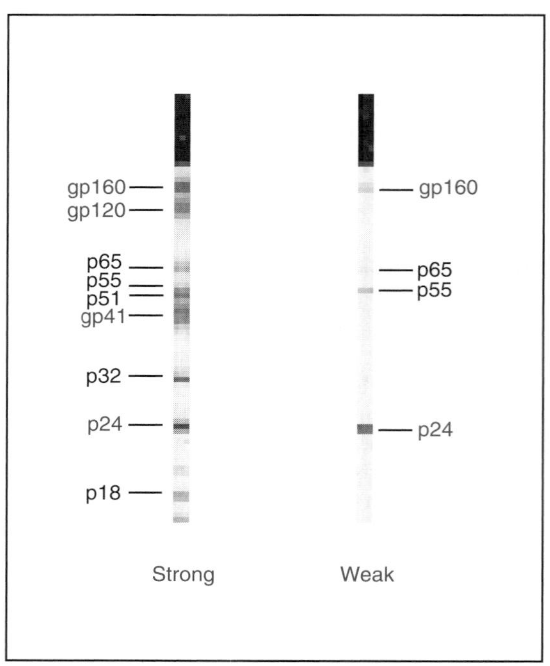

FIGURE 23.8 Western blot analysis of serum samples strongly positive and weakly positive for human immunodeficiency virus type 1 (HIV-1) antibody. Core proteins (GAG, group-specific antigens) p18, p24, and p55; polymerase (POL) p32, p51, and p65; envelope proteins (ENV) gp41, gp120, and gp160. (Courtesy Bio-Rad Laboratories Diagnostics Group, Irvine, California.)

antibodies in the sample bind to the viral antigens transferred to the strip as discrete bands. After washing, the strip is incubated with an alkaline phosphatase antihuman immunoglobulin conjugate. After a further washing step, the nitrocellulose strip is incubated with an alkaline phosphatase substrate solution (5-bromo-4-chloro-3-indolyl phosphate and nitroblue tetrazolium) to reveal where anti–HIV-1 antibody is bound to specific viral antigens fixed in the membrane.

Protein transfer and immobilization after separation by electrophoresis, isoelectric focusing, sodium dodecyl sulfate polyacrylamide electrophoresis, or other methods provide a powerful tool for analytical study of proteins present in low concentrations in cell culture or body fluids. When applied to antigen assays, concentrations of antigen as low as 500 ng/mL or 2.5 ng/band in the gel can be detected by this method. The detection limit of the technique can be lowered to approximately 100 pg by using chemiluminescence labels on the antibody.[13]

Dot Blotting

A technique similar to western blotting that bypasses the electrophoretic separation step is known as dot immunobinding (or dot blotting). A sample containing the protein to be analyzed (eg, a viral protein) is applied to a membrane surface as a small dot and dried. The membrane is then exposed to a labeled antibody specific for the test antigen contained in the dotted protein mixture. After washing, bound labeled antibody is detected with a photometric or chemiluminescent detection system.[14]

QUANTITATIVE METHODS

Several immunochemical techniques have been used to quantify analytes of clinical interest. They include RID and electroimmunoassays, turbidimetric and nephelometric assays, and labeled immunochemical antibody assays.

Radial Immunodiffusion and Electroimmunoassay

Historically, the two most commonly encountered gel-based methods for quantitative immunochemical studies were RID immunoassay and electroimmunoassay ("rocket" technique), but these methods have been mostly supplanted by other types of immunodetection techniques.

Radial Immunodiffusion Immunoassay

With this technique, a concentration gradient is established for a single reactant, usually the antigen. The antibody is uniformly dispersed in the gel matrix. Antigen is allowed to passively diffuse from a well into the gel, and immune precipitation occurs until antibody excess exists. The antigen-antibody interaction is manifested by a defined ring of precipitation around the antigen well, and ring diameter will increase with increased antigen concentration. Calibrators are run at the same time as the sample, and a calibration curve of ring diameter versus concentration is plotted. Under equilibrium conditions, a linear relationship exists between antigen concentration and the square of the precipitin ring diameter.[15] In addition, the precision of the measurement of the ring diameter is better when equilibrium is established. However, quantitative data also can be derived by reading the ring diameter before equilibrium is established.[16] This approach obviously is less precise. Antigen concentrations are calculated in both the preequilibrium and equilibrium methods by plotting the square of the precipitin ring diameter against calibrating antigen concentrations. RID can be made more sensitive by using PEG to enhance precipitin line formation or by using ^{125}I- or enzyme-labeled reagents.[17]

Electroimmunoassay

In electroimmunoassay, as in RID, a single concentration gradient is established for the antigen, but in this case, an applied voltage is used to drive the antigen from the application well into a homogeneous suspension of antibody in the gel (Fig. 23.9).[18] Unlike RID, this produces a unidirectional migration of antigen and results in a lower limit of detection for electroimmunoassay methods. The height of the resulting rocket-shaped precipitin line is proportional to the antigen concentration. Quantitation is affected by using calibrators on the same plate and estimating the concentrations of unknowns from the heights of the "rockets" obtained. The calibration curve is linear only over a narrow concentration range, so samples may have to be diluted or concentrated as necessary. Electroimmunoassay methods produce the best results, with antigens having a strong anodic mobility and intermediate to low MW. Proteins such as transferrin, C3, or IgG, with low anodal mobility or virtually no net charge at pH 8.6 (the most common pH used for the method), can be modified by carbamylation or can be run at a lower pH to make their measurements by electroimmunoassay feasible. Other modifications, such as use of an intermediate gel that causes precipitation of C3, allow measurement of C3d in human serum and illustrate the exceptional versatility of this method.[19]

Turbidimetric and Nephelometric Assays

Turbidimetry and nephelometry are convenient techniques for measuring the rate of formation of immune complexes in vitro. The reaction between antigen and antibody begins within milliseconds and continues for hours and both turbidimetric and nephelometric immunochemical methods

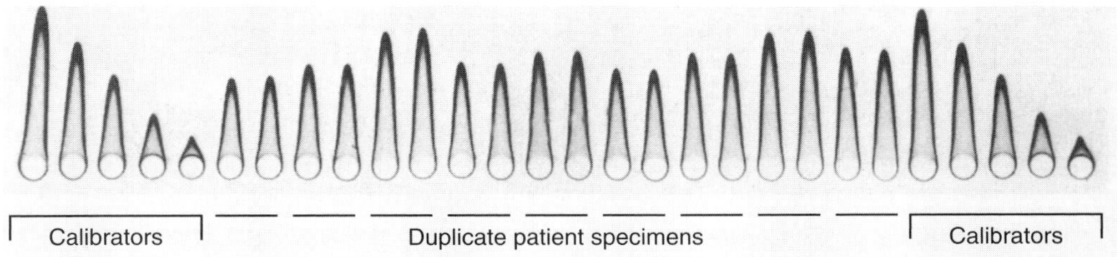

FIGURE 23.9 Rocket immunoelectrophoresis of human serum albumin. Patient samples were applied in duplicate. Standards were placed at opposite ends of the plate.

using rate and pseudoequilibrium protocols can be devised for proteins, antigens, and haptens. In rate assays, measurements are usually made within the first few minutes of the reaction, when the largest change *(dIs/dt)* in intensity of scattered light *(Is)* with respect to time occurs. For so-called equilibrium assays, it is necessary to wait 30 to 60 minutes. For the purpose of this discussion, such conditions are referred to as pseudoequilibrium because true equilibrium is not reached within the time allowed for these assays. Measurement of the rate of immune complex formation also can be used for quantitative immunochemical studies. Either *dIs/dt* or the time required to reach peak rate can be related to antigen concentration in a manner analogous to any other rate methodology. Rate nephelometric assays have the advantage that blank correction is not required and that several samples can be assayed in a few minutes instead of the 30 to 60 minutes required for pseudoequilibrium methods.[20] The analytical performance of nephelometric or turbidimetric assays can be significantly improved by increasing the reaction rate by adding water-soluble linear polymers. This allows the use of much lower reactant concentrations and results in more stable immune complexes.

Nephelometric methods in general are more sensitive than turbidimetric assays and have an average lower limit of detection of 0.1 to 10 mg/L for a serum protein. Lower detection limits are obtained in CSF and urine because of their lower lipid and protein concentrations, resulting in a better signal-to-noise ratio. In addition, for low-MW proteins (eg, myoglobin [MW, 17,800 Da]), assay detection limits can be lowered using a latex-enhanced procedure based on antibody-coated latex beads.[21]

Nephelometric and turbidimetric assays also have been applied to the measurement of drugs (haptens). An example of this type of assay is the particle-enhanced turbidimetric inhibition immunoassay (PETINIA), which measures decreasing agglutination in the presence of increasing concentrations of analyte (eg, digoxin).[22] The reagents comprise an antibody to the analyte of interest and a reagent containing the analyte of interest linked to a latex bead. In the absence of analyte in a specimen, reagent antibody binds to the reagent containing the analyte linked to the latex bead, resulting in increased turbidity. When a specimen with high analyte concentrations is added to the reagent mixture, the reagent antibody is bound by the analyte in the specimen and not to the reagent containing the analyte linked to the latex bead. Thus the presence of specimen analyte results in less turbidity.

POINTS TO REMEMBER

- Turbidimetric (turbidity) and nephelometric (light scattering) immunoassays provide simple, rapid nonseparation (homogeneous) format immunoassays that can be adapted to small molecules by attaching the antigen to a latex microparticle (eg, PETINIA).
- The major types of nonseparation (homogeneous) immunoassays based on modulation of signal from the label are as follows:
  - CEDIA: Cloned enzyme donor immunoassay
  - EMIT: Enzyme multiplied immunoassay technique
  - FPIA: Fluorescent polarization immunoassay
  - LOCI: Luminescent oxygen channeling immunoassay

Surface Plasmon Resonance–Based Immunoassay (Immunosensor)

An important type of label-free immunoassay is based on surface plasmon resonance (SPR), an optical phenomenon that enables detection of unlabeled reactants in real time based on changes in the index of refraction at the surface where the binding interaction occurs. The assay is conducted on an electrically conducting gold-coated glass slide mounted on a prism. The binding agent is immobilized on the gold surface, over which reactant is flowed. Polarized light is directed underneath the glass slide and interacts with the gold surface to produce electron charge density waves called plasmons at the sample and gold surface interface. This results in a reduction in the intensity of the reflected light. Slight changes in the refractive index at the interface lead to a change in the signal, thus facilitating real-time detection of surface molecular interactions (eg, association and dissociation of biomolecules with the binder immobilized on the gold surface). SPR assays (eg, Biacore, Marlborough, Massachusetts) are used to characterize binding reactions, such as antibody affinity, kinetics, cross-reactivity.[23]

Labeled Immunochemical Assays

The previously discussed methods rely on immune complex formation as an index of antigen-antibody reaction. As demonstrated previously in equation (1), the overall reaction occurs in sequential phases and only the final phase is the formation of the immune complex. However, the initial binding of the antibody and antigen has been demonstrated to be very useful analytically and has been used with labeled antigens and antibodies to develop many sensitive and specific immunochemical assays. The reaction describing this initial binding and the kinetic constant for the overall reaction are shown in equations (3a) and (3b), respectively:

$$\mathrm{Ab} + \mathrm{Ag} \underset{k_{-1}}{\overset{k_1}{\rightleftharpoons}} \mathrm{AbAg} \qquad \textbf{(23.3a)}$$

$$K = \frac{[\mathrm{AbAg}]}{[\mathrm{Ab}][\mathrm{Ag}]} \qquad \textbf{(23.3b)}$$

where

k_1 = the rate constant for the forward reaction
k_{-1} = the rate constant for the reverse reaction
K = the equilibrium constant for the overall reaction

As would be predicted from the law of mass action, the concentration of Ab, Ag, and AbAg will depend on the magnitude of k_1 and k_{-1}. For polyclonal antiserum, the average avidity of the antibody populations will determine *K* (typically 10^8 to 10^{10} L/mol) and the magnitude of k_1 compared with k_{-1} will determine the ultimate limit of detection attainable with a given antibody population.

The original immunochemical assays used radioactivity for labeling, but concerns about safe handling and disposal of radioactive reagents and waste have led to the development of alternative nonisotopic labels (Table 23.1).[24] In this section, the methodologic principles on which these assays are based and the factors that affect their analytical sensitivity are discussed. In addition, specific examples of these assays and the types of labels that are used in them are evaluated.

Competitive (limited reagent)

Simultaneous

$$\underset{\text{(free)}}{Ab + Ag + Ag - L} \rightleftharpoons \underset{\text{(bound)}}{Ab{:}Ag + Ab{:}Ag - L}$$

Sequential

$$\text{Step 1 } Ab + Ag \underset{k_{-1}}{\overset{k_1}{\rightleftharpoons}} Ab{:}Ag + Ab$$

$$\text{Step 2 } Ab{:}Ag + Ab + Ag - L \rightleftharpoons Ab{:}Ag + Ab{:}Ag - L + Ag - L$$

Noncompetitive (excess reagent, two-site, sandwich)

$$\blacksquare - Ab \xrightarrow{+\ Ag} \blacksquare - Ab{:}Ag \xrightarrow{+\ Ab\ -\ L} \blacksquare - Ab{:}Ag{:}Ab - L$$

FIGURE 23.10 Immunoassay designs. *L*, Label.

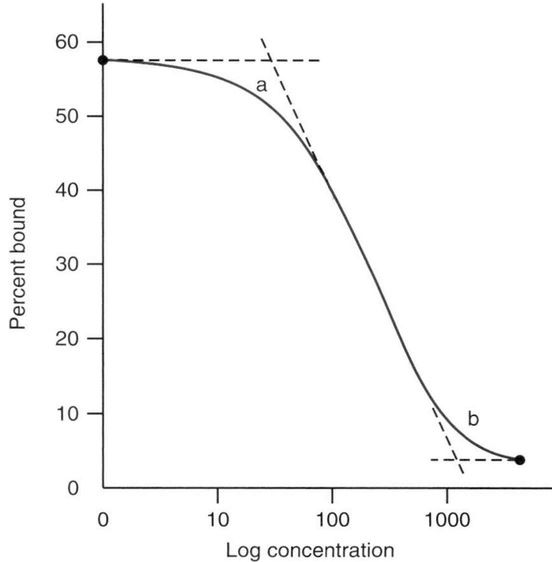

FIGURE 23.11 A schematic diagram of the dose-response curve for a typical competitive immunoassay. The analytically useful portion of the curve is bracketed by points *a* and *b*.

TABLE 23.1 Labels Used for Nonisotopic Immunoassay

Type of Label	Examples
Chemiluminescent	Acridinium ester, sulfonyl acridinium ester, isoluminol
Cofactor	Adenosine triphosphate, flavin adenine dinucleotide
Enzyme	Alkaline phosphatase, marine bacterial luciferase, β-galactosidase, firefly luciferase, glucose oxidase, glucose-6-phosphate dehydrogenase, horseradish peroxidase, lysozyme, malate dehydrogenase, microperoxidase, urease, xanthine oxidase
Fluorophore	Cyanine dye, fluorescein, lanthanide chelate (europium, terbium), phycoerythrin
Free radical	Nitroxide
Inhibitor	Methotrexate
Metal	Gold sol, selenium sol, silver sol
Particle	Bacteriophage, carbon, erythrocyte, latex bead, liposome, magnetic nanoparticle, nanorod, nanotube, quantum dot
Phosphor	Upconverting lanthanide-containing nanoparticle
Polynucleotide	DNA
Substrate	Galactosyl-umbelliferone

Methodologic Principles

To exploit the exquisite specificity and enhanced sensitivity that are possible with immunochemical assays, various methodologic principles have been applied in their development. These include competitive and noncompetitive reaction formats and different processing schemes for performing the assays.

Competitive Versus Noncompetitive Reaction Formats. The two major reaction formats that are used in immunochemical assays (Fig. 23.10) are termed *competitive* (limited reagent assays) and *noncompetitive* (excess reagent, two-site, or sandwich assays).

Competitive Immunoassays. In a competitive immunochemical assay, all reactants are mixed together simultaneously or sequentially. In the simultaneous approach, the labeled antigen (Ag*) and the unlabeled antigen (Ag) compete for binding to the antibody. Under these conditions, the probability of the antibody binding the labeled antigen is inversely proportional to the concentration of unlabeled antigen; hence, bound label is inversely proportional to unlabeled antigen concentration. Any differences in the avidity of the antibody for the labeled and unlabeled antigen is not an issue as long as the calibrators are comparable to the patient samples.

In a sequential competitive assay, unlabeled antigen is first mixed with excess antibody and binding is allowed to reach equilibrium (see Fig. 23.10, *step 1*). Labeled antigen is then sequentially added *(step 2)* and is allowed to equilibrate. After separation, the bound labeled antigen is determined and is used to calculate the unlabeled antigen concentration. Using this two-step method, a larger fraction of the unlabeled antigen is bound by the antibody than in the simultaneous assay, especially at low antigen concentrations. Consequently, this strategy provides a twofold to fourfold improvement in the detection limit of provided $k_1 \gg k_{-1}$. This improvement in detection limit results from an increase in AgAb binding (and thus a decrease in Ag* binding), which is favored by the sequential addition of Ag and Ag*. If $k_1 \ll k_{-1}$, dissociation of AgAb becomes more likely, resulting in increased competition between Ag* and Ag. A typical competitive immunochemical assay binding curve is shown in Fig. 23.11.

Noncompetitive Immunoassays. In a noncompetitive immunochemical assay, a capture antibody first is passively adsorbed or covalently bound to the surface of a solid phase. However, this can lead to some loss of antibody-binding capacity because of steric factors or attachment of the antibody via its Fab region. To protect the binding properties of the antibody, more complex sequences have been devised. For example, the solid support is coated with an antispecies antibody, and then the antispecies antibody used to immobilize the capture antibody via an antigen-antibody reaction.

In the first stage of the assay, the antigen from the sample is allowed to react with the solid phase, capture antibody; other proteins are washed away, and a labeled antibody (conjugate) is added that reacts with the bound antigen through a second and distinct epitope. After washing again, the bound label is determined and its concentration or activity is directly proportional to the concentration of the antigen.

In noncompetitive assays, the capture and labeled antibody can be polyclonal or monoclonal. If monoclonal antibodies having specificity for distinct epitopes are used, it is possible to incubate the sample and conjugate simultaneously with the capture antibody, thus simplifying the assay protocol.

Noncompetitive immunoassays are performed in a simultaneous (one-step) or sequential (two-step) mode. However, in the simultaneous mode, a situation can occur in which a high concentration of analyte can saturate both capture and labeled antibodies. When this occurs, the calibration curve of the assay exhibits a "hook effect," in which the assay response drops off at high analyte concentrations. Under these conditions, the analyte is present in such high concentrations that it reacts simultaneously with the capture antibody and the labeled antibody. This reduces the number of complexes formed and produces a falsely low result. Assays for analytes for which the normal pathologic concentration range is very wide (eg, tumor markers) are particularly prone to this problem. Dilutions of a sample are usually reanalyzed to check for this type of analytical interference. One way of minimizing or eliminating the hook effect is by ensuring that the concentrations of capture and labeled antibody are sufficiently high to cover analyte concentrations over the entire analytical range of the assay. Unfortunately, with modern automated immunoassays, hook-effects may occur silently and be undetectable. Immunoassays cleared by the US Food and Drug Administration typically define the upper limit of the assay, which is not affected by the hook-effect.

Noncompetitive immunoassays rely on different epitopes on a large analyte molecule so as to provide a binding site for both the capture antibody and for the labeled antibody. In the past, a small molecule could not be measured using the conventional sandwich format because a small molecule had too few epitopes. Various strategies have been developed to expand the scope of the sandwich assay to small molecules.[25] A strategy, exemplified by a 25-hydroxyvitamin D assay (25OH-D), has made small molecules amenable to a routine sandwich immunoassay format. In this commercial assay format, 25OH-D binds to an immobilized capture antibody and a second antibody (an antimetatype antibody) specifically recognizes the immunocomplex formed between the 25OH-D molecule and the capture antibody, hence facilitating a sandwich assay design.[26]

Heterogeneous Versus Homogeneous Immunochemical Assays. Immunochemical assays that require separation of free from bound labels are termed *heterogeneous;* those that do not are called *homogeneous.*

Heterogeneous Assays. Heterogeneous assays implicitly assume that $k_1 \gg k_{-1}$ and that a variety of physical separation techniques are used to separate the free-label (Ag*) from the bound-label antigen (Ag*Ab). The most widely used of these techniques are precipitation and solid-phase adsorption.

Precipitation of the bound labeled antigen (Ag*Ab) from the reaction mixture can be achieved chemically by the addition of a protein-precipitating chemical, such as $(NH_4)_2SO_4$, or immunologically by the addition of a second, precipitating antibody. In the latter approach, if the primary antibody was obtained from rabbit antiserum, the precipitating antibody would be contained in a goat or sheep antiserum raised against rabbit globulin. This approach has the advantage that it can be used for practically any assay; however, it has the disadvantage that it usually requires longer assay times and additional processing steps.

Solid-phase adsorption is the separation technique that currently is the most popular and widely used in both manual and automated heterogeneous immunoassays. In this technique, the binding and competition of labeled and unlabeled antigens for the binding sites of the antibody occur on the surface of a solid support onto which the capture antibody has been attached by physical adsorption or covalent bonding. Several different types of solid support have been used, including the inner surface of plastic tubes or wells of microtiter plates and the outer surface of insoluble materials, such as cellulose or magnetic latex beads or particles. With the tubes and microtiter plates, the solid surface containing the attached antibody and the bound antigen is washed in place and indicator reagents are subsequently added to complete the assay. When beads or particles are used, they are added directly to the reaction mixture and after incubation are removed by centrifugation or magnetic separation. After the supernatant has been removed by siphoning or decanting, the beads or particles are washed and indicator reagents subsequently added to complete the assay.

Homogeneous Assays. The development of homogeneous assays that do not require separation of bound and free labeled antibody or antigen was a major advance in the field of immunochemical analysis. In this type of assay, the activity of the label attached to the antigen is directly modulated by antibody binding, with the magnitude of the modulation being proportional to the concentration of the antigen or antibody being measured. Consequently, in practice it is necessary to incubate only the sample containing the analyte antigen with the labeled antigen and antibody and then to directly measure the activity of the label in place, thus making these assays technically easier and faster. The original homogeneous immunoassay was developed for drug analysis and used a nitroxide spin label; this was termed a *free radical immunoassay technique.*[27] The electron spin resonance spectrum of this label was modulated when the nitroxide-labeled drug was bound by a drug-specific antibody. This procedure was quickly superseded by homogeneous immunoassays that used enzyme labels and could be performed on spectrophotometric analyzers (see subsequent descriptions of EMIT[28] and CEDIA).[29]

A homogeneous sandwich format chemiluminescent immunoassay also has been developed that expands the scope of homogeneous assays to large molecules (see subsequent description of LOCI).[30] In addition, a diverse range of homogeneous fluoroimmunoassays based on fluorescence energy transfer (FRET) between fluorescent donor and acceptor dye-labeled assay components represent a further expansion of

TABLE 23.2 Detection Limits for Isotopic and Nonisotopic Immunoassay Labels Based on Commonly Used Detection Methods

Label	Detection Limit in Zeptomoles* (10^{-21} moles)	Method
Alkaline phosphatase	50,000	Photometry
	300	Time-resolved fluorescence
	100	Fluorescence
	10	Chemiluminescence
β-D-Galactosidase	5,000	Chemiluminescence
	1,000	Fluorescence
Europium chelate	10,000	Time-resolved fluorescence
Glucose-6-phosphate dehydrogenase	1,000	Chemiluminescence
Horseradish peroxidase	2,000,000	Photometry
	1	Chemiluminescence
Iodine-125	1,000	Scintillation
Ruthenium (II) tris(bipyridyl)	20	Electrochemiluminescence

*One zeptomole = 10^{-3} attomoles or 10^{-6} femtomoles.

the scope of homogeneous immunoassays (see subsequent descriptions of FRET).

Analytical and Functional Sensitivity

The analytical detection limits (sensitivity) of competitive and noncompetitive immunoassays are determined principally by the affinity of the antibody and the detection limit of the label used, respectively.[31,32] Calculations have indicated that a lower limit of detection of 10 fmol/L (ie, 600,000 molecules of analyte in a typical sample volume of 100 μL) is possible in a competitive assay using an antibody with an affinity of 10^{12} L/mol. Table 23.2 illustrates theoretical detection limits for isotopic and nonisotopic labels. A radioactive label, such as ^{125}I, has low specific activity (7.5 million labels necessary for detection of 1 disintegration/s) compared with enzyme labels and chemiluminescent and fluorescent labels. Enzyme labels provide an amplification (each enzyme label produces many detectable product molecules), and the detection limit for an enzyme can be improved by replacing the conventional photometric detection reaction by a chemiluminescent or bioluminescent reaction. The combination of amplification and an ultrasensitive detection reaction makes noncompetitive chemiluminescent immunoassays among the most sensitive types of immunoassay. Fluorescent labels also have high specific activity, and a single high-quantum yield fluorophor can produce 100 million photons/s. In practice, several factors degrade the detection limit of an immunoassay; these include background signal from the detector, assay reagents, and nonspecific binding of the labeled reagent.

Secondary labels, such as biotin, can be used to introduce amplification into an immunoassay. The binding constant of the biotin-avidin complex is extremely high (10^{15} L/mol); capitalizing on this system allows immunoassay systems to be devised that are even more sensitive than simple antibody systems. A biotin-avidin system uses a biotin-labeled soluble antibody. Biotin can be attached to the antibody in relatively high proportion without loss of immunoreactivity.[33,34] When an avidin-conjugated label is added, a complex of Ag:Ab-biotin:avidin label is formed. Further amplification can be achieved by a biotin:avidin:biotin linkage, because the binding ratio of biotin:avidin is 4:1. If the label is an enzyme, large numbers of enzyme molecules in the complete complex provide a large increase in enzymatic activity coupled with the small amount of antigen being determined, and the assay is correspondingly more sensitive.

Another type of sensitivity is termed functional sensitivity. This is defined as the lowest concentration of an assay that can be measured with an interassay coefficient of variation of 20%[35] (for further information on definitions of various measures of sensitivity including limit of detection and lowest limit of quantification, refer to Chapter 2). This is used to establish a more realistic and robust detection limit for an assay used in patient care. Functional sensitivity is associated with concept of assay generations, each successive generation representing a 1-log concentration improvement in sensitivity (eg, for a thyroid-stimulating hormone [TSH] immunoassay first generation 1 mIU/L, second generation 0.1 mIU/L, third generation 0.01 mIU/L, etc).

Examples of Labeled Immunoassays

In the decade after the pioneering developments of Yalow and Berson,[36] all competitive and noncompetitive immunoassays used a radioactive label in a competitive assay format. Since the introduction of enzyme immunochemical assays in the 1970s, a vast array of sophisticated immunochemical assays have evolved; some of the major types are discussed in the following sections.

Radioimmunoassay. Radioimmunoassays (RIAs) were developed in the 1960s and used radioactive isotopes of iodine (^{125}I, ^{131}I) and tritium (^{3}H) as labels.[36] Labeled antibody noncompetitive assays (immunoradiometric or sandwich assay) have the advantage of not requiring a quantity of purified antigen because the antigen does not have to be labeled. This also obviates potential problems that may be caused by iodination of labile antigens. Antibodies are relatively stable proteins that are less difficult to label without damaging the function of the protein. Combinations of labels (eg, cobalt [^{57}Co] and ^{125}I) have been used for simultaneous assays of lutropin and follitropin.[37]

Enzyme Immunoassay. Enzyme immunoassays (EIAs) use the catalytic properties of enzymes to detect and quantify immunologic reactions. In practice, enzyme-labeled

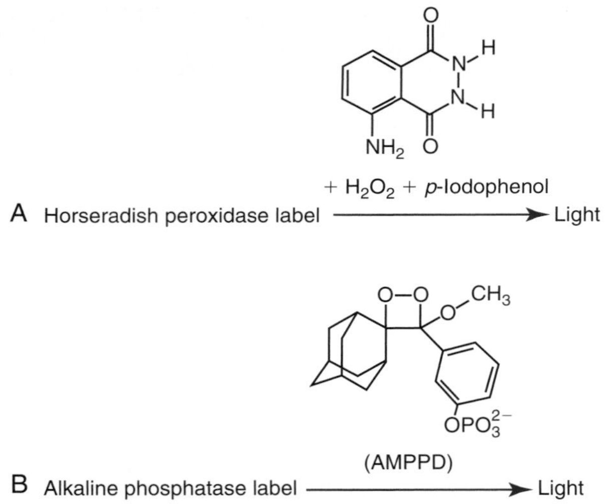

FIGURE 23.12 Ultrasensitive assays for horseradish peroxidase and alkaline phosphatase labels. **A,** Chemiluminescent assay for horseradish peroxidase label using luminol. **B,** Chemiluminescent assay for an alkaline phosphatase label using 3-(2′-spiroadamantyl)-4-methoxy-4-(3″-phosphoryloxy)-phenyl-1,2-dioxetane (AMPPD).

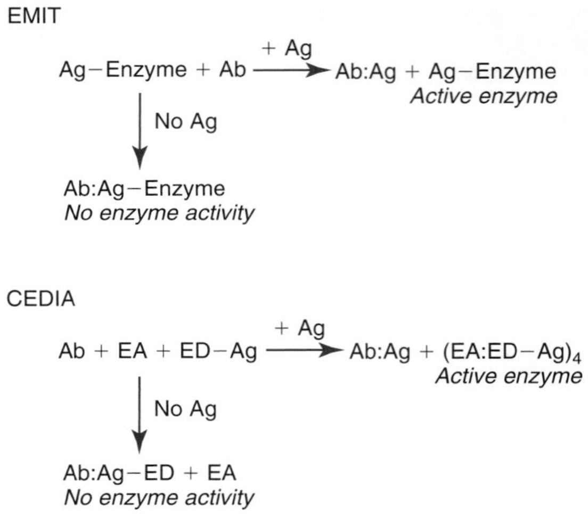

FIGURE 23.13 Enzyme multiplied immunoassay technique *(EMIT)* and cloned enzyme donor immunoassay *(CEDIA)* homogeneous immunoassays. *EA,* Enzyme acceptor; *ED,* enzyme donor.

antibodies or antigens (ie, conjugates) are first allowed to react with ligands. Bound label is then separated, and enzyme substrates are subsequently added. Measurement of the resultant increase in product concentration is used to detect or quantify the antigen-antibody reaction. Alkaline phosphatase, horseradish peroxidase, glucose-6-phosphate dehydrogenase, and β-galactosidase enzyme labels predominate in EIA.[38,39]

Various detection systems have been used to monitor and quantify EIAs. Assays that produce compounds that can be monitored photometrically are very popular, because compact, high-performance photometers are available. However, EIAs that use fluorescent- or chemiluminescent-labeled substrates or products are often preferred to photometry-based assays owing to the inherent sensitivity of fluorescent and chemiluminescent measurements (Table 23.2). Immunoassays that incorporate horseradish peroxidase as a label can be assayed by chemiluminescence using a mixture of luminol, peroxide, and an enhancer such as *p*-iodophenol (Fig. 23.12A)[40] or by using an acridan derivative.[41] A very sensitive assay for alkaline phosphatase labels uses a chemiluminescent adamantyl 1,2-dioxetane aryl phosphate substrate (see Fig. 23.12B).[42] The enzyme dephosphorylates the substrate, which decomposes with a concomitant long-lived glow of light (detection limit for alkaline phosphatase using this assay is 10 zeptomoles [10^{-20} moles]).[42]

Types of enzyme-linked immunoassay include enzyme-linked immunosorbent assay (ELISA), EMIT, and CEDIA.

Enzyme-Linked Immunosorbent Assay. ELISA is a heterogeneous EIA technique used in clinical analyses. In this type of assay, one of the reaction components is nonspecifically adsorbed or covalently bound to the surface of a solid phase, such as a microtiter well, a magnetic particle, or a plastic bead. This attachment facilitates separation of bound and free labeled reactants. In the most common approach to using the ELISA technique, an aliquot of sample or calibrator containing the antigen to be quantitated is added to and allowed to bind with a solid-phase antibody. After washing, enzyme-labeled antibody is added and forms a "sandwich complex" of solid-phase Ab-Ag-Ab enzyme. Unbound antibody is then washed away, and enzyme substrate is added. The amount of product generated is proportional to the quantity of antigen in the sample. Specific antibodies in a sample also can be quantified using an ELISA procedure in which antigen instead of antibody is bound to a solid phase and the second reagent is an enzyme-labeled antibody specific for the analyte antibody. Also, ELISA assays have been used extensively for detection of antibodies to viruses and autoantigens in serum or whole blood.[43] In addition, enzyme conjugates coupled with substrates that produce visible products have been used to develop ELISA-type assays with results that can be interpreted visually. Such assays have been found very useful in screening, point-of-care, and home testing applications.

Enzyme Multiplied Immunoassay Technique. EMIT is a homogeneous EIA that is very widely used in clinical analyses, an illustration of which is shown in Fig. 23.13. Because EMIT does not require a separation step, it is simple to perform and has been used to develop a wide variety of drug, hormone, and metabolite assays.[28] Because of their operational simplicity, EMIT-type assays are easily automated and are included in the repertoire of many automated clinical and immunoassay analyzers. In this technique, antibody against the analyte drug, hormone, or metabolite is added together with substrate to the patient's sample. Binding of the antibody and analyte occurs. An aliquot of the enzyme conjugate of the analyte is then added as a second reagent; the enzyme hapten (analyte) conjugate binds with the excess analyte antibody, forming an antigen-antibody complex. This binding of the analyte antibody with the enzyme analyte conjugate affects enzyme activity by physically blocking access of the substrate to the active site of the enzyme or by changing the conformation of the enzyme molecule and thus altering its activity. To complete the assay, the resultant enzyme activity is measured. The relative change in enzyme activity resulting from the formation of the antigen-antibody complex is proportional to the hapten concentration in the patient's sample. Concentration of the analyte is calculated from a calibration

TABLE 23.3 Properties of Fluorescent Labels

Fluorophore	Excitation (nm)	Emission (nm)	Fluorescence Quantum Yield*	Lifetime (ns)
Cy3 (cyanine dye)	550	570	0.15	—
Cy5 (cyanine dye)	650	670	0.28	—
Europium (β-naphthoyl trifluoroacetone)	340	590, 613	—	500,000
Fluorescein isothiocyanate	492	520	0.0–0.85	4.5
NN382	778	806	0.59	—
	550–620	580–660	0.5–0.98	—
Rhodamine B isothiocyanate	550	585	0.0–0.7	3.0
Umbelliferone	380	450	—	—

*Fluorescence quantum yield: fraction of molecules that emit a photon.

Ag−F + Ab —(Variable amount of Ag)→ [Ab:Ag−F, High polarization (slow rotation)] + Ab:Ag + [Ag−F, Low polarization (fast rotation)]

FIGURE 23.14 Homogeneous polarization fluoroimmunoassay. *F*, Fluorescein.

curve prepared by analyzing calibrators that contain known quantities of the analyte in question.

Cloned Enzyme Donor Immunoassay. As shown in Fig. 23.13, CEDIA is a homogeneous EIA; it was the first EIA designed and developed using genetic engineering techniques.[29] Inactive fragments (the enzyme donor and acceptor) of β-galactosidase are prepared by manipulation of the Z gene of the *lac* operon of *Escherichia coli.* These two fragments spontaneously reassemble to form active enzyme even if the enzyme donor is attached to an antigen. However, binding of antibody to the enzyme donor antigen conjugate inhibits reassembly and no active enzyme is formed. Thus competition between the antigen and the enzyme donor antigen conjugate for a fixed amount of antibody in the presence of the enzyme acceptor modulates the measured enzyme activity (high concentrations of the analyte antigen result in the least inhibition of enzyme activity; low concentrations result in the greatest inhibition).

Fluoroimmunoassay. Examples of fluorophores that are used as labels in fluoroimmunoassay and their properties are listed in Table 23.3. Initially, background fluorescence from drugs, drug metabolites, and protein-bound substances, such as bilirubin, limited the usefulness of this technique. However, this problem has largely been overcome by the use of rare earth (lanthanide) chelates and background rejection (time-resolved) procedures.[44,45] Fluorescent emissions from lanthanide chelates (eg, europium, terbium, samarium) are long lived (greater than 1 μs) compared with the typical background fluorescence encountered in biological specimens. In a time-resolved fluoroimmunoassay, a europium chelate label is excited by a pulse of excitation light (0.5 μs), and the long-lived fluorescence emission from the label is measured after a delay (400 to 800 μs). The measurement after the delay ensures that any short-lived background signal has decayed.

FPIA is a type of homogeneous fluoroimmunoassay that is widely used to measure drugs and other small molecules (Fig. 23.14).[46] The polarization of the fluorescence from a fluorescein-antigen conjugate is determined by its rate of rotation during the lifetime of the excited state in solution. When the fluorescein-antigen conjugate is bound to the large antibody molecule the fluorophore is constrained from rotating in the time between absorption of the incident radiation and emission of fluorescence; hence the fluorescence emission is still highly polarized. In contrast, when the fluorescein-antigen conjugate is free in solution it can rotate more rapidly and the emitted light is depolarized. Thus binding to antibody modulates polarization, and a homogeneous assay is possible.

Förster or fluorescence resonance energy transfer (FRET) is the distance-dependent transfer of energy from a fluorescent donor dye to a fluorescent acceptor dye. Distances at which there is 50% transfer efficiency are typically 1 to 20 nm, but up to approximately 20 nm is possible for some donor-acceptor pairs (eg, lanthanide chelate – quantum dot).[47,48] For example, in a sandwich FRET immunoassay format used in the time-resolved amplified cryptate emission (TRACE) assays, an antibody labeled with a europium chelate (donor) is matched with an antibody labeled with an allophycocyanin dye (XL665; acceptor). The two antibodies form a sandwich immunocomplex with the antigen and after irradiation with excitation light (337 nm) energy transfer occurs from the donor europium chelate to the XL665 acceptor. In the absence of immunocomplex formation, the XL665 fluorescence is short lived (nanoseconds). However, with immunocomplex formation, the europium chelate provides energy to prolong the normally short-lived fluorescence of the XL665 dye (microseconds). Intensity of the 665-nm emission is proportional to antigen concentration. Another strategy used in the Triage system (Alere, Waltham, Massachusetts) for cardiac markers uses an antibody-coated latex particle containing a donor dye (a silicon [intravenous] phthalocyanine bis[7-oct-1-enyldimethylsilyloxide]) and a second antibody-coated latex particle containing an acceptor dye (2^1, 2^6,12^1,12^6-tetraphenyldinaphtho [b,1]-7,17-dibenzo[g,q]-5,10,15,20-tetraazoporphyrinato] silicon bis(7-oct-1-enyldimethylsilyloxide). Analyte in the sample binds to create donor particle:analyte:acceptor particle complexes. Excitation at 670 nm excites the donor dye, and energy transfer to the acceptor dye occurs as a result of the proximity of the two different types of particle. The acceptor particle then emits light at 760 nm (long wavelength in the red portion of the spectrum). An advantage of this red emission is that scattering and fluorescence from blood plasma is minimized.[49] Other examples of donor-acceptor pairs include Cy3-Cy5, fluorescein-gold or Cy3-gold nanoparticles, Blue Fluorescent Protein–Green Fluorescent protein, lanthanide chelate–quantum dot, europium cryptate–allophycocyanin, and upconverting phosphor–B-phycoerythrin.

Multiplexed fluoroimmunoassays can be achieved using fluorophores with different fluorescent emissions, for example, lanthanide chelates. Multiplexing is also possible using quantum dot labels. A quantum dot is a nanometer-sized highly fluorescent nanocrystal composed of cadmium selenide (CdSe), cadmium sulfide (CdS), zinc selenide (ZnSe), indium phosphide (InP), or indium arsenide (InAs) or a layer of zinc sulfide (ZnS) or CdS on, for example, a CdSe core. Multiplexing is possible with these labels because their emission properties can be modulated by changing the size and composition of the nanocrystal (eg, CdS emits blue light, InP emits red light).[50]

Phosphor Immunoassay. A phosphor is a material that emits light (phosphorescence) over a relatively long time scale after exposure to excitation energy (see Chapter 13). A particular type of phosphor, an upconverting phosphor nanoparticle, can be used as a label for immunoassay.[51] In one application, the upconverting phosphor nanoparticle (200- to 400-nm diameter) was a crystalline lanthanide oxysulfide. This nanoparticle absorbs two or more photons of infrared light (980 nm) and produces light emission at a shorter wavelength (anti-Stokes shift). The phosphorescence is not influenced by reaction conditions (eg, temperature, buffer), and no upconverted signal is received from biological components in the sample (low background). Multiplexing is possible because different types of particles produce different wavelengths of phosphorescence (eg, yttrium/erbium oxysulfides are green [550 nm], yttrium/thulium oxysulfide particles are blue [475 nm]).

Chemiluminescence and Bioluminescence Immunoassay. Chemiluminescence is the name given to light emission produced during a chemical reaction. Isoluminol and acridinium esters are important examples of chemiluminescent labels used in chemiluminescent immunoassay. Oxidation of isoluminol by hydrogen peroxide in the presence of a catalyst, such as microperoxidase, produces a relatively long-lived light emission at 425 nm, and oxidation of an acridinium ester by alkaline hydrogen peroxide in the presence of a detergent (eg, Triton X-100) produces a rapid flash of light at 429 nm. Acridinium and sulfonyl acridinium esters are high-specific activity labels (detection limit for the label is 800 zeptomoles) that can be used to label both antibodies and haptens (Fig. 23.15A).[52,53]

LOCI is a particularly important type of chemiluminescent immunoassay. It is one of the few homogeneous immunoassays that operate in a noncompetitive (sandwich) format and can be used to assay large molecules. LOCI uses two reagent particles (sensitizer and chemiluminescer particles) that form a complex with the analyte of interest.[30]

The presence of analyte links the two reagent latex particles in close proximity. The first particle contains a photosensitizer (eg, phthalocyanine) and in the presence of light converts oxygen to singlet oxygen. The second chemiluminescer particle contains a chemiluminescent agent (eg, olefin) that reacts with singlet oxygen to form a dioxetane that decomposes and emits light. This reaction occurs only if the two particles are in close proximity and the singlet oxygen can diffuse efficiently from the sensitizer particle to the chemiluminescer particle. Singlet oxygen does not react with unbound chemiluminescer particles because of the short lifetime of this transient species in an aqueous environment. An example of a LOCI assay for TSH is illustrated in Fig. 23.16. TSH binds to a biotinylated anti-TSH antibody, and this complex links the streptavidin-coated sensitizer particle to the anti-TSH antibody–coated chemiluminescer particle. Exposure of light results in emission of singlet oxygen from the photosensitive particle. The singlet oxygen activates the chemiluminescent particle to emit light that is then measured.

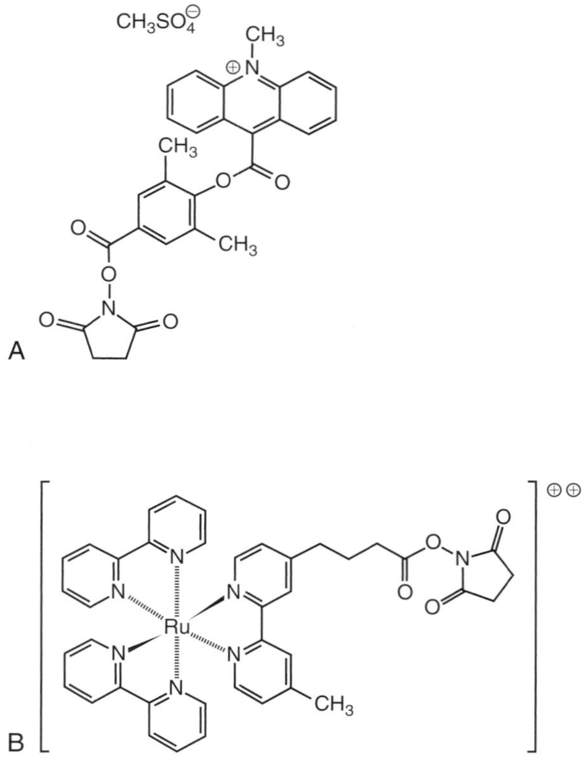

FIGURE 23.15 Luminescent labels. **A,** Chemiluminescent acridinium ester label. **B,** Electrochemiluminescent ruthenium (II) tris(bipyridyl) NHS ester label. (From Law S-J, Miller T, Piran U, Klukas C, Chang S, Unger J. Novel poly-substituted aryl acridinium esters and their use in immunoassay. *J Biolumin Chemilumin* 1989;4:88–98. Reprinted by permission of John Wiley & Sons.)

Components of bioluminescent reactions (light-emitting reactions that occur in living organisms) have also been exploited as labels. One example is the use of native or recombinant apoaequorin (from the bioluminescent jellyfish *Aequorea*) as a label. This protein is activated by reaction with coelenterazine, and light emission at 469 nm is triggered by reaction with calcium ions (calcium chloride).[54]

Electrochemiluminescence Immunoassay. Ruthenium (II) tris(bipyridyl) (see Fig. 23.15B) undergoes an electrochemiluminescent reaction (620 nm) with tripropylamine at an electrode surface, and this chelate is now used as a label in competitive and sandwich electrochemiluminescence immunoassays. Using this label, various assays have been developed using magnetic beads as the solid phase. Beads are captured by a magnet at an electrode surface in a flow cell, and unbound label is washed out of the cell by a wash buffer. Label bound to the bead undergoes an electrochemiluminescent reaction, and the light emission is measured by an adjacent photomultiplier.[55]

Magnetic Particle Immunoassay. A magnetic particle has found application as a label in immunoassay. In one immunoassay design, a superparamagnetic particle (300 nm diameter) is used as the label and is detected by its magnetic properties using a giant magneto-resistance sensor.[56] A magnetic particle also can be detected based on its reflective and light-scattering properties (optomagnetic immunoassay). The assay is performed in a flow-through cartridge having a localized region with surface-immobilized capture antibodies. Magnetic nanoparticles coated with detection antibody bind to captured antigens. The bound magnetic particle labels are detected using frustrated total internal reflection. In the absence of binding, light projected onto the capture region is reflected at full strength and detected using a camera. Binding of the magnetic particle labels causes reflection and scattering of the light and the intensity of the light arriving at the camera is reduced in proportion to the number of the magnetic particle bound. An advantage of this assay format is speed (external fields are used to manipulate the magnetic particles), and it has been applied to a fast-turnaround intraoperative parathyroid hormone assay.[57]

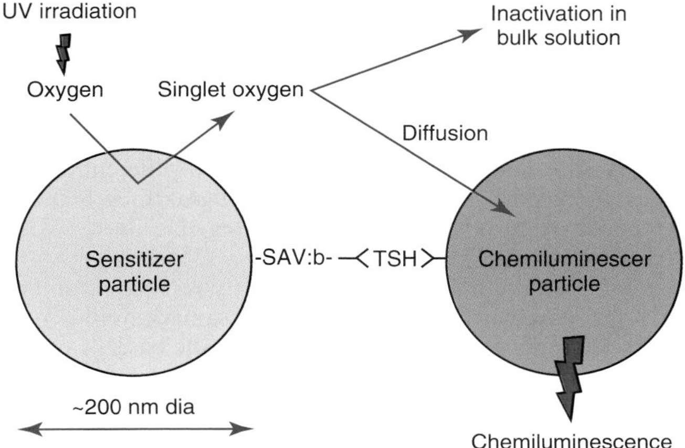

FIGURE 23.16 Example of luminescent oxygen channeling immunoassay (LOCI) for thyroid-stimulating hormone (TSH). In this assay, TSH links two latex microbeads—one containing a photosensitive reagent and the other a precursor of a chemiluminescent reagent. *UV,* Ultraviolet.

Nuclear magnetic resonance (NMR) detection of magnetic particle labels facilitates a homogeneous immunoassay design. The assay uses magnetic nanoparticles (~20 nm diameter) coated with antibody that binds to and clusters around analyte in solution. A consequence of the binding and clustering is that the microscopic environment of water in the reaction mixture is altered, and this can be detected by NMR as a change in the T2 relaxation signal[58] (Fig. 23.17). An advantage of this type of immunoassay is that the signal is unaffected by the sample matrix (eg, opacity), and this allows direct detection in various types of specimens, such as whole blood and sputum.

Immuno–Polymerase Chain Reaction and Bio-Barcode Immunoassay. DNA has been employed in a number of different immunoassay designs. Immuno-PCR (Innova Biosciences, Cambridge, United Kingdom) is a heterogeneous immunoassay in which a piece of single- or double-stranded DNA is used as a label for an antibody in a sandwich assay.[59] Bound DNA label is amplified using polymerase chain reaction (PCR). The amplified DNA product is separated by gel electrophoresis and quantitated by densitometric scanning of an ethidium-stained gel.

In the bio-barcode assay, capture antibody immobilized on a magnetic particle binds to the analyte (eg, a protein) and the bound analyte is reacted with a gold particle (30 nm diameter) decorated with detection antibody and barcode dsDNA (Fig. 23.18; refer to the figure legend for details). After complex formation and washing, one strand of the barcode, dsDNA is released from the gold particle. Next, the released barcode dsDNA is hybridized to an immobilized capture DNA probe and to a gold particle–labeled detection probe.

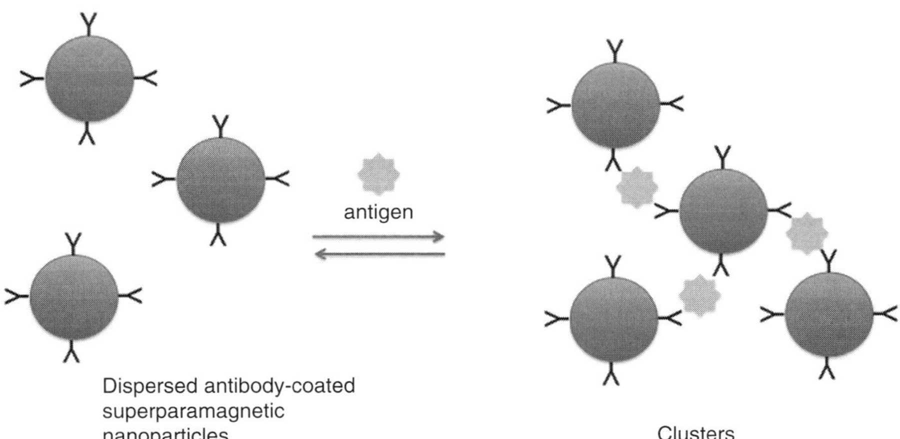

FIGURE 23.17 Magnetic particle immunoassay. Antigen binds to magnetic nanoparticles (~20 nm diameter) coated with antibody. The binding and resulting clustering of the particles alters the microscopic environment of water in the reaction mixture, and this can be detected by nuclear magnetic resonance (change in the T2 relaxation signal).

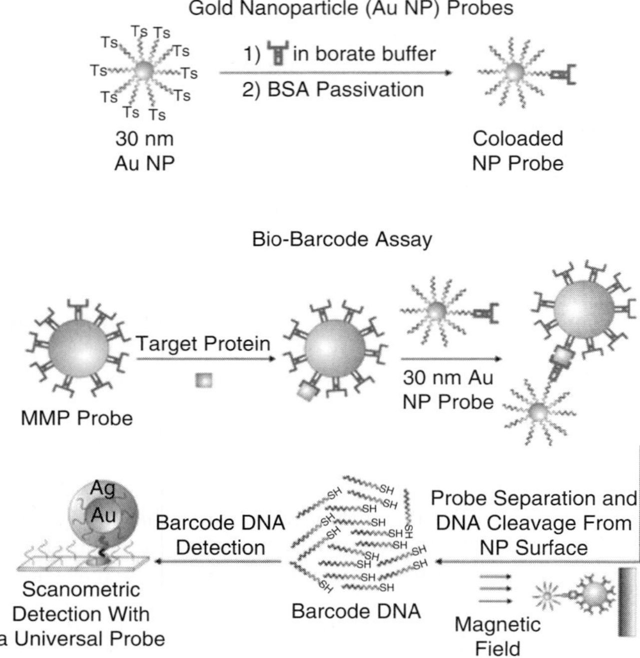

FIGURE 23.18 Bio-barcode assay for a protein target. Barcode DNA-functionalized gold nanoparticles *(Au-NP)* (30 nm diameter) are conjugated to target protein-specific antibodies (via tosyl [Ts] groups) to generate the coloaded target protein Au-NP probes that are then passivated with bovine serum albumin. The next steps in the sandwich immunoassay are reaction of the target protein with magnetic microparticle probes *(MMPs)* (1 μm diameter) coated with monoclonal antibodies to target protein, washing to remove excess serum components, and then reaction with the *Au-NP*. After magnetic separation and wash steps, the target protein-specific DNA barcodes are released into solution and detected using the scanometric assay (includes an Au-NP catalyzed silver enhancement step). Approximately half of the barcode DNA sequence is complementary to the universal scanometric Au-NP probe DNA, and the other half is complementary to a surface immobilized DNA sequence that is responsible for sorting and binding barcodes complementary to the target protein barcode sequence. (From Thaxton CS, Elghanian R, Thomas AD, Stoeva SI, Lee J-S, Smith ND, et al. Nanoparticle-based bio-barcode assay redefines "undetectable" PSA and biochemical recurrence after radical prostatectomy. *PNAS* 2009;106:18437-18442 [with permission]).

The bound gold particle–labeled detection probe is first decorated with silver and then detected scanometrically. This type of assay has achieved very low detection limits, for example, the picogram per milliliter range for serum prostate-specific antigen.[60]

Multiplexed Immunoassays and Protein Microarrays. Simultaneous multianalyte immunoassays in which two or more analytes are detected in a single assay (multiplex) improve the efficiency of detecting multiple analytes. Two different strategies have been developed based on discrete reaction zones or combinations of different labels.

In the Triage point-of-care device (Alere) for testing for drugs of abuse, simultaneous detection of up to nine drugs is achieved using discrete test zones on a small piece of nylon membrane.[61] Each test zone consists of antibodies for a specific drug immobilized on the membrane surface. This zone captures free gold-drug conjugate from the sample, antidrug antibody, and gold-drug conjugate reaction mixture and appears as a purple band.

Microarrays provide a further increase in the scale of testing. Arrays of hundreds or thousands of micrometer-sized dots of antigens or antibodies immobilized on the surface of a glass or plastic chip are emerging as an important tool in proteomic studies and in assessing protein-protein interactions. This format facilitates simultaneous multianalyte immunoassays using, for example, enzyme- or fluorophore-labeled conjugates. The arrays are made by printing or spotting 1-nL drops of protein solutions onto a flat surface, such as a glass microscope slide. In a typical sandwich assay, the array on the surface of the slide is incubated with sample and then with conjugate. Bound conjugate is detected with chemiluminescence or fluorescence using a scanning device. The pattern of the signal provides information on the presence and amount of individual analytes in the sample or the reactivity of a single analyte with the range of proteins arrayed on the surface of the slide.[62]

Another type of microarray is the so-called liquid array exemplified by the Luminex xMAP (Austin, Texas) type assay based on collections of microbeads optically coded with fluorescent dyes.[63] Each type of fluorescent bead is coated with a different antibody, and after the immunologic reaction with sample and labeled antibody the formation of an immunocomplex on each bead is assessed using flow cytometric or fluorescence imaging principles. Up to 500 different signatures can be created, allowing multiplexing of up to 500 different assays in a single assay vessel (eg, Luminex xMAP technology).

Combinations of distinguishable labels, such as europium (613 nm; emission lifetime, 730 μs) and samarium (643 nm; emission lifetime 50 μs) chelates, provide the basis of quantitative simultaneous immunoassays. These two chelates have different fluorescence emission maxima and different fluorescence decay times and thus can be easily distinguished by making measurements at 613 nm, delay time 0.4 ms (europium), and 643 nm, delay time 0.05 ms (samarium). Apart from fluorophores, many other label combinations have been developed, including different radioisotopes, and nano-sized objects such as quantum dots, and other particles of different shapes and sizes.[64]

Digital Immunoassay. A long-cherished goal in immunoassay has been single molecule sensitivity. A new digital immunoassay design (Simoa, Quanterix, Lexington, Massachusetts) led to dramatic improvements in sensitivity (Fig. 23.19). This ELISA type of assay is performed on small antibody-coated paramagnetic microbeads. At the end of the incubation of the capture antibody-coated beads with sample and β-galactosidase–labeled antibody, the beads, in the presence of a fluorogenic substrate, are distributed into an array of 216,000 wells (one bead per well), each with a volume of 40 fL. A single target molecule captured onto the bead in a femtoliter-sized well generates sufficient fluorescence signal for detection. The signal from the array of wells is imaged using a charge-coupled device camera and the number of fluorescent wells is counted (a digital read-out), thus counting the number of molecules in the sample. At the 10 : 1 bead-to-molecule ratio used in the assay the number of beads that carry a labeled immunocomplex follows a Poisson distribution, such that at low protein concentrations each bead will capture one labeled immunocomplex or none. The combination of the sensitive label detection method and the low

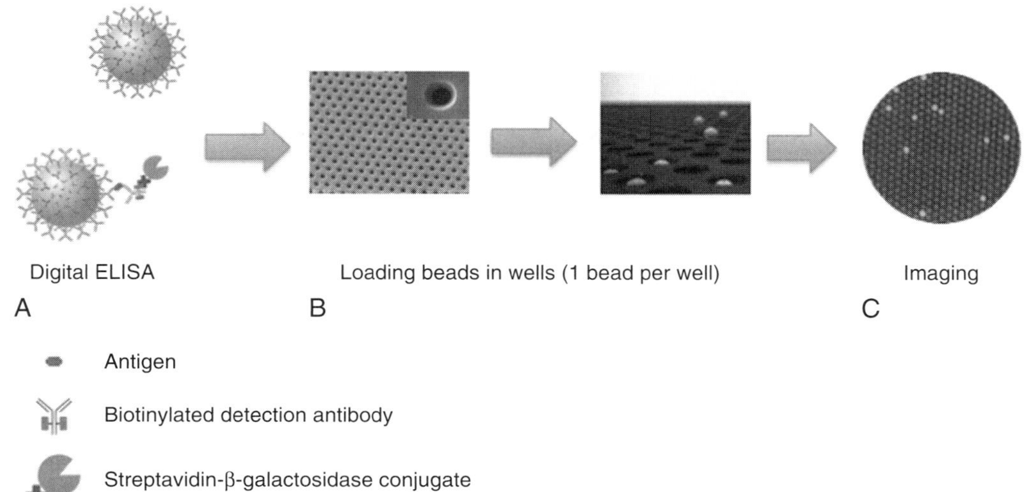

FIGURE 23.19 Design of a digital immunoassay (Simoa). **A,** Reaction of the antigen with capture antibody-coated magnetic beads and biotinylated detection antibody. This is then followed by reaction of the bound complex with streptavidin-β-galactosidase conjugate to form single immunocomplexes of the magnetic beads. **B,** The beads are loaded into wells, one bead per well and then treated with a fluorometric substrate for β-galactosidase and fluorescence from the beads in the array of wells imaged. *ELISA,* Enzyme-linked immunosorbent assay. (Images used with permission of Quanterix, Lexington, Massachusetts.)

background achieved by the signal counting leads to protein assays with femtogram per milliliter sensitivity.[65]

Fluoroimmunoassays also can be operated in a digital mode as exemplified by the Erenna Immunoassay System (Singulex, Alameda, California). This system combines a magnetic microparticle-based sandwich fluoroimmunoassay and single-molecule counting technology. It integrates capillary flow, laser-induced fluorescence, and a highly sensitive detection optics module for sample analysis. On completion of sandwich formation the fluorescent dye–labeled detection antibody is released from the captured antigen and eluted into a very small volume (20 μL) for counting. Fluorescence detection occurs in a flow system in a very small interrogation space (5 μm) that is illuminated by a laser. Signals above the background are counted as digital events, and the sum of the digital events is related to the original concentration of the analyte in the sample.[66]

Simplified Immunoassays. Integration of the technical advances made in molecular immunology with those made in the material and processing sciences has resulted in the development of simplified immunoassays for use in physicians' offices or the home (ie, the point-of-care market). Early efforts were directed toward pregnancy and fertility testing and were based on agglutination and inhibition of agglutination using labeled red blood cells or latex particles in a slide format. Subsequently, sandwich immunoassays have been adapted for similar applications.

These tests only require the addition of sample, thus simplifying the assay protocol and minimizing possible malfunction resulting from operator error. Numerous one-step pregnancy tests are now available.[67] For example, one popular test device uses an absorbent strip that contains blue beads attached to an anti–human chorionic gonadotropin (hCG) monoclonal antibody. As urine moves by capillary action through the strip, labeled antibodies are mobilized and move up the test strip, which contains regions of immobilized antibodies loaded with a blue dye. Each strip has separate windows for the positive, negative, and procedural controls. If hCG is present at a concentration of 25 mIU/mL or greater, a blue line becomes visible in the test region window. This region remains clear if the test is negative. A blue line appears in the reference region of the result window to show the test is complete and has worked correctly.

POINTS TO REMEMBER

The most commonly used nonisotopic labels in immunoassay are:

- Enzyme labels: Alkaline phosphatase, horseradish peroxidase, β-galactosidase
- Fluorophore labels: Fluorescein
- Chemiluminescent labels: Acridinium esters
- Electrochemiluminescent labels: Ruthenium chelates

Interferences in Immunoassays

Immunologic assays are prone to interferences, in spite of the use of highly specific antibodies for molecular recognition of the analyte. Falsely low results can occur because of the hook effect at high antigen concentrations (see earlier discussion). False-negative or false-positive results are encountered if the sample contains anti–animal immunoglobulin antibodies. For example, in a two-site sandwich assay for hCG based on mouse antibodies, any human antimouse antibodies (HAMAs) present in the specimen will recognize the immobilized mouse capture, and mouse conjugate antibodies and will form a complex that is indistinguishable from an immobilized capture antibody:hCG:conjugate complex. This leads to a false-positive result. A false-negative result will be obtained if the HAMAs react with the capture antibody or the conjugate to such an extent that specific antibody binding to hCG is prevented. Many different types of circulating anti–animal immunoglobulin antibodies have been detected (eg, human anti-goat, human anti-bovine antibodies) and shown to interfere in immunoassays. In practice, this type of interference is minimized by including additives in the immunoassay reagents such as nonimmune serum or IgG from the species used to raise the antibodies used in the assay. In practice this type of interference can sometimes be uncovered by performing dilution studies (nonlinear response) or from changes in values after incubation of the sample in a heterophile blocking tube.[68]

CELL-BASED AND TISSUE-BASED IMMUNOCHEMICAL TECHNIQUES

Other analytical methods of clinical interest that employ antibodies include immunohistochemistry and agglutination assays.

Immunohistochemistry

The use of labeled antibody reagents as specific probes for protein and peptide antigens allows the researcher and the pathologist to evaluate single cells or pieces of tissue for their synthetic capability and/or phenotypic identity. Immunohistochemistry has been rapidly expanded by immunoenzymatic methods, especially with regard to the use of horseradish peroxidase–labeled (immunoperoxidase) assays. Using enzyme labels provides several advantages over fluorescent labels. They permit the use of fixed tissue embedded in paraffin, which provides excellent preservation of cell morphology and eliminates the problem of autofluorescence from tissue. In addition, immunoperoxidase stains are permanent and only a standard light microscope is necessary to identify labeled features. The immunoperoxidase methods are also applicable to electron microscopy. Several approaches for immunoenzymatic assays have been used, including direct, indirect, peroxidase-antiperoxidase, and enzyme bridge methods.

Agglutination Assays

Agglutination assays have been used for many years for the qualitative and quantitative measurement of antigens and antibodies. In an agglutination method, the visible clumping of particulates, such as cells and latex particles, is used as an indicator of the primary reaction of antigen and antibody. Agglutination methods require stable and uniform particulates, pure antigen, and specific antibody. IgM antibodies are more likely to produce complete agglutination than are IgG antibodies because of the size and valence of the IgM molecule. Therefore, when only IgG antibodies are involved, it may be necessary to use chemical enhancement or an antiglobulin agglutination method. As with all immunochemical reactions in which aggregation is the measured end point, the ratio of antigen to antibody is critical. Extremes in antigen or antibody concentration will result in inhibition of aggregation.

An incomplete agglutination reaction is one in which the primary reaction occurs, but no or only minimal aggregation of the particles occurs. Many particles, such as erythrocytes and bacteria in solution, have a net negative charge (zeta potential), which causes mutual repulsion. For successful agglutination, the antigen-antibody reaction must overcome this normal resistance. In the case of a weak antigen-antibody reaction, or one in which only IgG is involved, this mutual repulsion may be sufficient to inhibit agglutination completely or partially. In systems in which incomplete agglutination results, enhancement may be achieved by lowering the ionic strength or by introducing polymeric molecules, such as polymerized albumin (5% to 30%), dextran, hexadimethrine bromide (Polybrene, Santa Cruz Biotechnology, Dallas, Texas), polyvinylpyrrolidone, or PEG.[69]

Hemagglutination refers to agglutination reactions in which the antigen is located on an erythrocyte. Erythrocytes not only are good passive carriers of antigen, they also are easily coated with foreign proteins and can be easily obtained and stored.

Direct testing of erythrocytes for blood group, Rh, and other antigenic types is used widely in blood banks; specific antisera, such as anti-A, anti-C, and anti-Kell, are used to detect such antigens on the erythrocyte surface.

In indirect or passive hemagglutination, the erythrocytes are used as a particulate carrier of foreign antigen (and in some tests of antibodies); this technique has wide applications. Other materials available in the form of fine particles, such as bentonite and latex, also have been used as antigen carriers, but they are more difficult to coat, standardize, and store. In a related variation of this technique, known as hemagglutination inhibition, the ability of antigens, haptens, or other substances to specifically inhibit hemagglutination of sensitized (coated) cells by antibody is determined.

In general, agglutination methods are sensitive but are not as quantitative as other immunochemical methods discussed thus far. Nonisotopic immunoassays, especially EIAs, are as convenient as agglutination reactions and therefore are replacing agglutination methods in many laboratories.

NONANTIBODY BINDING AGENTS

This chapter has focused on antibodies as binding agents in assays. However, a variety of nonantibody alternatives are emerging, notably aptamers,[70] molecularly imprinted polymers (MIPs),[71] and boronates[72] (compare the use of thyroxine-binding globulin in the thyroxine assay that was contemporaneous with the original RIA for insulin).[73]

Nucleic acid aptamers are single-stranded oligonucleotides (eg, DNA, RNA) that bind to a specific target molecule. Aptamers against a specific target are identified by a selection process (eg, systematic evolution of ligands by exponential enrichment [Selex]), in vitro selection). Binding properties of DNA aptamers can be improved by genetic alphabet expansion using unnatural bases (nucleotide triphosphates analogs). Aptamers with high affinity and specificity toward a wide range of target molecules have been developed and tested in various types of binding assays.

MIP is a polymer that has been synthesized in the presence of a template molecule. During the polymerization process, complementary cavities are formed in the polymer and hence the resulting polymer (a "plastic antibody") has affinity for the template molecule. These synthetic binding agents represent an emerging type of alternative to an antibody as a binding agent.

Boronic acids have the property of binding to carbohydrates (*cis*-diols) and thus can serve as a binding agent for glycoproteins. An example of the use of a pair of boronate affinity reagents is shown in Fig. 23.20.[72] The assay used a solid-phase boronate affinity MIP array as the capture component and a boronic acid–coated silver nanoparticle as the

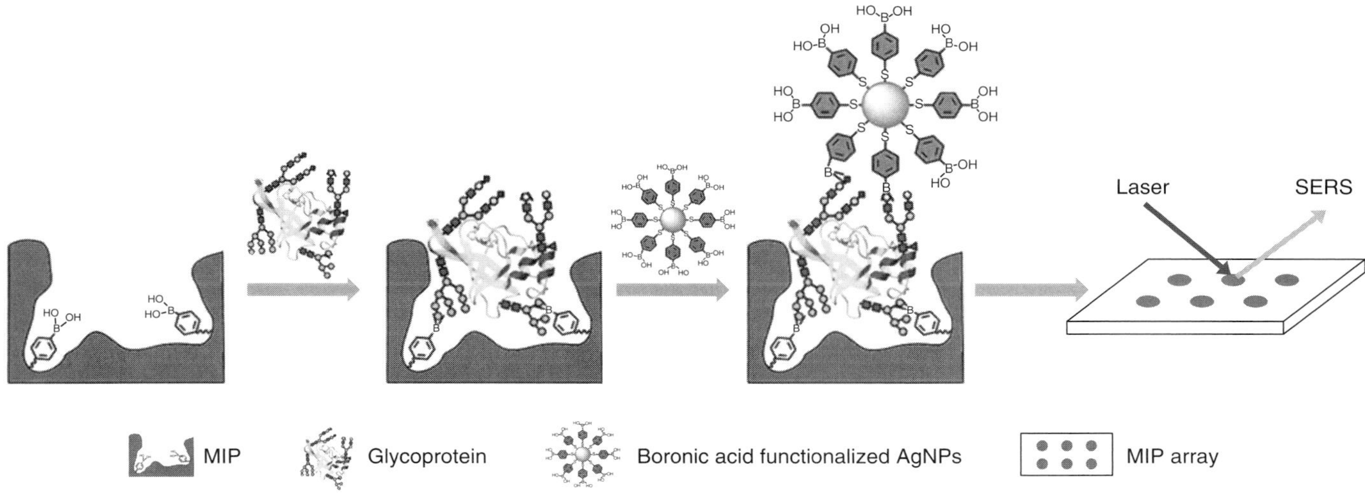

FIGURE 23.20 A boronate affinity sandwich assay for glycoproteins At the *left* of the figure is a molecularly imprinted polymer *(MIP)*, which is a three-dimensional cavity synthesized from a 4-vinylboronic acid monomer; this cavity complements the structure of a specific glycoprotein. Next in the reaction, the glycoprotein of interest is bound by the MIP. A detection reagent based on a boronic acid and silver nanoparticles *(AgNPs)* is bound to the glycoprotein of interest. Finally, the binding of the AgNP detection reagent is detected by surface-enhanced Raman scattering *(SERS)*. (Reproduced with permission of John Wiley & Sons from Ye J, Chen Y, Liu Z. A boronate affinity sandwich assay: an appealing alternative to immunoassays for determination of glycoproteins. *Angew Chem Int Ed* 2014;53:10386–10389.)

detection reagent. The glycoprotein (eg, α-fetoprotein) was sandwiched between these two reagents (a boronate affinity sandwich), and after washing away unbound material the bound complex was detected via the surface-enhanced Raman scattering signal originating from the bound silver nanoparticles.

SELECTED REFERENCES

For a full list of references for this chapter, please refer to ExpertConsult.com.

14. Stott DI. Immunoblotting and dot blotting. *J Immunol Methods* 1989;**119**:153–87.
21. Grange J, Roch AM, Quash GA. Nephelometric assay of antigens and antibodies with latex particles. *J Immunol Methods* 1977;**18**:365–75.
23. Safsten P, Klakamp SL, Drake AW, et al. Screening antibody-antigen interactions in parallel using Biacore A100. *Anal Biochem* 2006;**353**:181–90.
24. Price CP, Newman DJ, editors. *Principles and practice of immunoassay*. 2nd ed. New York: Stockton Press; 1996.
26. Omi K, Ando T, Sakyu S, et al. Noncompetitive immunoassay detection system for haptens on the basis of antimetatype antibodies. *Clin Chem* 2015;**61**:627–35.
28. Rubenstein KE, Schneider RS, Ullman EF. "Homogeneous" enzyme immunoassay: new immunochemical technique. *Biochem Biophys Res Commun* 1972;**47**:846–51.
29. Henderson DR, Friedman SB, Harris JB, et al. CEDIA, a new homogeneous immunoassay system. *Clin Chem* 1986;**32**: 1637–41.
30. Ullman EF, Kirakossian H, Switchenko AC, et al. Luminescent oxygen channeling assay (LOCI): sensitive, broadly applicable homogeneous immunoassay method. *Clin Chem* 1996;**42**: 1518–26.
34. Guesdon JL, Ternynck T, Avrameas S. The use of avidin-biotin interaction in immunoenzymatic techniques. *J Histochem Cytochem* 1979;**27**:1131–9.
36. Yalow RS, Berson SA. Assay of plasma insulin in human subjects by immunological methods. *Nature* 1959;**184**:1648–69.
38. Engvall E, Perlmann P. Enzyme-linked immunosorbent assay (ELISA): quantitative assay of immunoglobulin G. *Immunochemistry* 1971;**8**:871–4.
39. Van Weeman BK, Schuurs AH. Immunoassay using antigen-enzyme conjugates. *FEBS Letts* 1971;**15**:232–6.
40. Thorpe GHG, Kricka LJ. Enhanced chemiluminescent reactions catalyzed by horseradish peroxidase. *Methods Enzymol* 1986;**133**:331–53.
42. Bronstein I, Edwards B, Voyta JC. 1,2-Dioxetanes: novel chemiluminescent enzyme substrates: applications to immunoassays. *J Biolumin Chemilumin* 1989;**4**:99–111.
55. Blackburn GF, Shah HP, Kenten JH, et al. Electrochemiluminescence detection for development of immunoassays and DNA probe assays for clinical diagnostics. *Clin Chem* 1991;**37**:1534–9.
59. Sano T, Smith CL, Cantor CR. Immuno-PCR: very sensitive antigen detection by means of specific antibody-DNA conjugates. *Science* 1992;**258**:120–2.
65. Rissin DM, Fournier DR, Piech T, et al. Simultaneous detection of single molecules and singulated ensembles of molecules enables immunoassays with broad dynamic range. *Anal Chem* 2011;**83**:2279–85.
66. Todd J, Freese B, Lu A, et al. Ultrasensitive flow-based immunoassays using single-molecule counting. *Clin Chem* 2007;**53**:1990–5.
67. Braunstein GD. The long gestation of the modern home pregnancy test. *Clin Chem* 2014;**60**:18–21.
68. Park JY, Kricka LJ. Interferences in immunoassay. In: Wild D, editor. *The immunoassay handbook*. 4th ed. Amsterdam: Elsevier; 2013. p. 403–16.

24

Microfabrication and Microfluidics and Their Application in Clinical Diagnostics

Lindsay A.L. Bazydlo and James P. Landers

ABSTRACT

Background

Microfluidics is a burgeoning area of analytical chemistry that will impact many fields, including clinical diagnostics. The ability to miniaturize and expedite chemistry with smaller volumes presents the possibility for testing with expedited turnaround times at lower cost and possibly in a portable and handheld format.

Content

This chapter describes the basic concepts necessary to understand microfluidics at a fundamental level. This includes the methods and materials used for fabrication, both historically and currently, as well aspects of microfluidic architecture necessary to carry out reactions, chemistry, labeling, and detection. The chapter highlights some of the basic developments associated with the microfluidic manipulation or analysis of diagnostically relevant analytes such as cells, nucleic acid (NA), proteins, and small molecules. It also presents some exemplary applications (eg, circulating tumor cell capture and pathogen detection) that have paved the path for the development and adoption of microfluidics in clinical chemistry and molecular diagnostics.

25

Cytometry

Howard M. Shapiro

ABSTRACT

Background

Cytometry, or "cell measurement," can describe any process by which individual biologic cells are counted or characterized, whether or not a human observer is involved. An apparatus used in the process is called a cytometer. From the 1950s on, cytometers, nearly all automated to some degree, have replaced microscopy in an increasing number of applications in both clinical and research laboratories. Some chemical assays can also be done using cytometers or similar instruments.

Flow cytometers, in which individual cells are measured as they pass through a series of optical or electronic sensors (or both), represent the majority of instruments now in use, and at least a plurality of clinical cytometric analyses are performed on cells from the blood and immune system. Apparatus, reagents, and other tools for cytometry now represent a multibillion-dollar market.

Although the sophistication and cost of high-end cytometers continue to increase, advances in optics and electronics during the past two decades could make cytometric technology affordable and applicable for a broader range of tasks worldwide within the next few years, including point-of-care assays for diagnosis and management of infectious diseases in both affluent and resource-poor countries.

Content

This chapter provides a historical overview of how cytometry evolved from microscopy; explains how cytometers work, with examples of what is measured and why; and considers some likely directions for future developments.

26

Automation in the Clinical Laboratory

*Charles D. Hawker, Jonathan R. Genzen, and Carl T. Wittwer**

ABSTRACT

Background
Automation has dramatically changed both the analytical and nonanalytical aspects of clinical laboratory operations. Automation of test procedures began more than 50 years ago, but nonanalytical automation—including conveyor systems, interfaced analyzers, and automated specimen processing and storage—began in earnest in the 1990s. Today there is a wide selection of automation options designed to improve the quality, throughput, and efficiency of laboratory testing.

Content
This chapter covers automation from both nonanalytical and analytical perspectives. Historical contexts are provided. The discussion of preanalytical automation includes a review of labeling, barcoding, and portable wireless labeling systems along with the use of pneumatic tube systems and mobile robots for transport of specimens. Single-function robotic systems and multifunction systems for specimen processing are discussed. Some of these systems have pre- and postanalytical capabilities. Total laboratory automation (TLA) systems are discussed extensively. Several TLA systems include post-analytical functions; thus, the chapter also addresses storage and retrieval systems. The second half of the chapter discusses automation from the analytical perspective, including specimen and reagent handling on analytical instrumentation, as well as common measurement approaches used by automated analyzers. The chapter concludes with area-specific considerations of how analytical automation has impacted all subdisciplines of laboratory medicine.

*The authors would like to acknowledge the original contributions of Ernest Maclin, PE; Donald S. Young, MB, PhD; and James C. Boyd, MD, upon which portions of this chapter are based.

27

Point-of-Care Testing

Andrew St John and Christopher P. Price

ABSTRACT

Background

Point-of-care testing (POCT) is essentially any form of laboratory testing that takes place outside of the conventional or central laboratory and encompasses a wide variety of locations. Utilization of POCT has steadily increased over the 40 or so years since its introduction, principally driven by technology developments and changes in health care delivery that are aimed at delivering less costly and more effective care closer to the patient's home.

Content

This chapter describes the various POCT technologies, including those currently in use and those developed more than several decades ago such as glucose strips and lateral flow technologies. The succeeding years have seen these technologies refined and improved to deliver easier-to-use devices with incremental improvements in analytical performance. Other major technological developments include miniaturization and co-developments in consumer electronics. The developments have enabled what are essentially laboratory instruments to be reduced in both size and complexity so that they can be used in point-of-care locations. Thus the menu of tests that can be measured with POCT devices has grown to include most of the commonly requested analytes, and most recently, is being extended to infectious disease testing. Developments in information technology and informatics are described that make management of POCT devices easier and allow the generation of accurate and timely results. The importance of careful implementation of POCT is also discussed with various case histories to show the clinical and cost-effectiveness of POCT compared with central laboratory testing.

SECTION III

Analytes

Exam questions, case studies, and additional resources are available on ExpertConsult.com.
*Full versions of these chapters are available electronically on ExpertConsult.com.

28

Amino Acids, Peptides, and Proteins

*Dennis J. Dietzen**

ABSTRACT

Background

Amino acids are the building blocks of proteins, but they also play diverse roles in the provision of energy and the formation of a number of other important biomolecules, including hormones, neurotransmitters, and signaling molecules. The polymers of amino acids, peptides, and proteins orchestrate and control the vast array of human physiologic and biochemical processes. The catalog of amino acids, peptides, and proteins in various biological fluids is a target-rich environment for the detection of pathological states.

Content

This chapter first describes the chemistry, metabolism, transport, and analysis of amino acids. Polymers of amino acids may be relatively short (peptides) or long (proteins). The human genome contains the information to dictate formation of approximately 20,000 polypeptides, but the actual diversity of the human proteome and peptidome is manifold more expansive. Proteome diversity arises from linear amino acid sequence and an array of modifications that include acylation, phosphorylation, glycosylation, and isoprenylation. Systems of short peptides, larger protein monomers, and multimeric protein complexes are the tools that orchestrate and control human physiologic and biochemical processes. Proper synthesis, folding, subcellular targeting, and catabolism of proteins and peptides, therefore, are essential for human health. Analytic exploitation of biologic fluids including blood, urine, and cerebrospinal fluid using chemical, immunologic, and mass spectrometric methods enables informed diagnosis and therapy in a multitude of disease states.

INTRODUCTION

Amino acids, peptides, and proteins are crucial for virtually all biologic processes. Amino acids serve as structural subunits of peptides and proteins but also play diverse roles in metabolism, neurotransmission, and intercellular signaling. Peptides serve as autocrine and endocrine signaling molecules that control appetite, vascular tone, and electrolyte homeostasis, as well as carbohydrate and mineral metabolism. Proteins, longer peptide chains with molecular mass typically greater than approximately 6000 Daltons (Da) serve as (1) intracellular and extracellular structural components, (2) biologic catalysts, (3) mediators of contractility and motility, (4) agents of molecular assembly, (5) ion channels and pumps, (6) molecular transporters, (7) mediators of immunity, and (8) components of intracellular and intercellular signaling networks.

The human genome contains more than 20,000 open reading frames that encode proteins. The actual number of proteins is far greater, however, because of alternative splicing of messenger RNA (mRNA), somatic recombination, mutation, proteolytic processing, and posttranslational modification. The *proteome* represents the complete set of proteins in an organism or compartment of an organism such as the plasma space. Efforts to catalog the proteome include those by the Human Proteome Organization (hupo.org), the National Center for Biotechnology Information (ncbi.nlm.nih.gov), the Swiss Institute of Bioinformatics (expasy.org), and the Healthy Human Individual's Integrated Plasma Proteome Database (bio.informatics.iupui.edu/HIP2). Most databases were designed mainly to assist with peptide and protein identification, but efforts have shifted to characterizing the abundance of specific protein components in healthy and diseased populations, the usual basis for diagnostic applications.

This chapter begins with a discussion of the chemistry, metabolism, and analysis of amino acids. Inherited disorders of amino acid metabolism are discussed in Chapter 70. A description of the chemistry and biochemistry of the peptide bond is then followed by a description of several clinically relevant peptide systems and methods for in vitro assessment. The protein narrative begins with an account of protein structure and cellular compartmentalization followed by discussion of co- and posttranslational modifications. Constituents of the proteome in body fluids are also addressed, followed lastly by a description of methods for specific and global assessment of the proteome for clinical purposes. More in-depth treatment of other specific proteins and protein networks may be found in Chapters 29 (serum enzymes), 30 (enzymes of the red blood cell [RBC]), 31 (tumor markers),

*The author gratefully acknowledges the preceding foundation for this chapter laid by Glen L. Hortin and A. Myron Johnson, as well as generous assistance from Carl H. Smith on the topic of amino acid transport.

34 (lipoproteins), and 38 (hemoglobin), as well as other chapters dedicated to the specific pathophysiology of cardiac, liver, renal, bone, pituitary, thyroid, and adrenal disease. In-depth treatment of measurement modalities for amino acids, peptides, and proteins such as electrophoresis, chromatography, mass spectrometry (MS), and immunoassay may be found in Chapters 15, 16, 17, and 23, respectively.

AMINO ACIDS

Amino acids were likely among the first organic molecules to emerge from the mix of methane, hydrogen, ammonia, and water in earth's primordial atmosphere.[1] Only 20 of the hundreds of known amino acids account for the vast majority of residues in human polypeptide chains. Their structure and molecular properties are summarized in Table 28.1. These 20 along with dozens of non–protein-forming amino acids are critical to the form and function of the human body. Disrupted amino acid metabolism is not surprisingly associated with a multitude of pathologic processes.

Basic Biochemistry

Amino acids are organic compounds containing both an amino group ($-NH_2$) and a carboxyl group ($-COOH$) or another acidic group such as a sulfonate group ($-SO_3$). In a majority of biologically relevant amino acids, the amine moiety is primary ($-NH_2$), but some (eg, sarcosine) are secondary ($-NH-$) amines, and others containing tertiary amines (eg, proline) are referred to as imino ($=N-$) acids. With the exception of proline, the amino acids that occur in protein are α-amino acids (below).

$$H_2N-C(H)(R)-C(=O)OH$$

α-Carbon atom

The R group represents the unique side chains responsible for the chemical properties of individual amino acids. Not all biologic amino acids are α amino acids. β amino acids such as β-alanine and taurine as well as γ-amino acids such as γ-aminobutyric acid (GABA) also play key biochemical roles (Fig. 28.1).

With the exception of glycine, all α amino acids contain four distinct moieties asymmetrically arranged around the α carbon. As a consequence, amino acids may exist as mirror images (enantiomers) referred to as the *D* or *L* configuration. With few exceptions, the biologically relevant amino acids exist in the *L* configuration. Small quantities of *D* amino acids occur in physiological fluids but typically do not have specific functions. An exception is *D* serine, which represents 5% to

TABLE 28.1 Structure and Chemical Properties of the 20 Proteogenic Amino Acids

Amino Acid	MW (Da)	Structure (pH 7.0)	pK_1	pK_2	pK_3	pI	HI
Alanine (ALA, A)	89.09	$H_3C-CH(NH_3^+)-COO^-$	2.4	9.7		6.0	1.8
Arginine (ARG, R)	174.20	$(H_2N)(H_2N^+{=})C-NH-CH_2-CH_2-CH_2-CH(NH_3^+)-COO^-$	2.2	9.0	12.5	10.8	−4.5
Asparagine (ASN, N)	132.12	$H_2N-C(=O)-CH_2-CH(NH_3^+)-COO^-$	2.0	8.8		5.4	−3.5
Aspartate (ASP, D)	133.10	$^-OOC-CH_2-CH(NH_3^+)-COO^-$	2.1	9.8	3.9	2.9	−3.5
Cysteine (CYS, C)	121.16	$HS-CH_2-CH(NH_3^+)-COO^-$	1.7	10.8	8.3	5.1	2.5
Glycine (GLY, G)	75.07	$H-CH(NH_3^+)-COO^-$	2.3	9.6		6.0	−0.4
Glutamate (GLU, E)	147.13	$^-OOC-CH_2-CH_2-CH(NH_3^+)-COO^-$	2.2	9.7	4.3	3.2	−3.5

TABLE 28.1 Structure and Chemical Properties of the 20 Proteogenic Amino Acids—cont'd

Amino Acid	MW (Da)	Structure (pH 7.0)	pK_1	pK_2	pK_3	pI	HI
Glutamine (GLN, Q)	146.15	$H_2N-C(=O)-CH_2-CH_2-CH(NH_3^{\oplus})-C(=O)O^{\ominus}$	2.2	9.1		5.7	–3.5
Histidine (HIS, H)	155.16	$(HN^{\oplus}$ imidazole ring, N–H$)-CH_2-CH(NH_3^{\oplus})-C(=O)O^{\ominus}$	1.8	9.2	6.0	7.6	–3.2
Isoleucine (ILE, I)	131.17	$H_3C-CH_2-CH(CH_3)-CH(NH_3^{\oplus})-C(=O)O^{\ominus}$	2.4	9.7		6.0	4.5
Leucine(LEU, L)	131.17	$(H_3C)_2CH-CH_2-CH(NH_3^{\oplus})-C(=O)O^{\ominus}$	2.4	9.6		6.0	3.8
Lysine (LYS, K)	146.19	$H_3N^{\oplus}-CH_2-CH_2-CH_2-CH_2-CH(NH_3^{\oplus})-C(=O)O^{\ominus}$	2.2	9.0	10.5	9.7	–3.9
Methionine (MET, M)	149.21	$H_3C-S-CH_2-CH_2-CH(NH_3^{\oplus})-C(=O)O^{\ominus}$	2.3	9.2		5.8	1.9
Phenylalanine (PHE, F)	165.19	$C_6H_5-CH_2-CH(NH_3^{\oplus})-C(=O)O^{\ominus}$	1.8	9.1		5.5	2.8
Proline (PRO, P)	115.13	(pyrrolidine ring, $NH_2^{\oplus}$)$-C(=O)O^{\ominus}$	2.1	10.6		6.1	1.6
Serine (SER, S)	105.09	$HO-CH_2-CH(NH_3^{\oplus})-C(=O)O^{\ominus}$	2.2	9.2		5.7	–0.8
Threonine (THR, T)	119.12	$(HO)(H_3C)CH-CH(NH_3^{\oplus})-C(=O)O^{\ominus}$	2.6	10.4		6.5	–0.7
Tryptophan (TRP, W)	201.22	(indole ring, N)$-CH_2-CH(NH_3^{\oplus})-C(=O)O^{\ominus}$	2.5	9.4		5.9	–0.9
Tyrosine (TYR, Y)	181.19	$HO-C_6H_4-CH_2-CH(NH_3^{\oplus})-C(=O)O^{\ominus}$	2.2	9.2	10.5	5.7	–1.3
Valine (VAL, V)	117.17	$(H_3C)_2CH-CH(NH_3^{\oplus})-C(=O)O^{\ominus}$	2.3	9.6		6.0	4.2

HI, Hydropathy index; *MW*, molecular weight; *pk*, acid ionization constant; *pI*, isoelectric point.

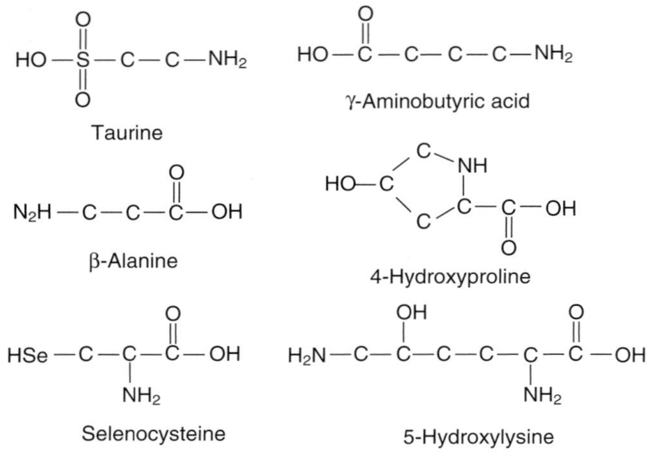

FIGURE 28.1 Planar structures of rare or unusual, naturally occurring amino acids.

20% of total serine in cerebrospinal fluid and may serve as a neurotransmitter. Amino acids with the *D* configuration occur in some bacterial products, foods, and pharmaceuticals. *D* amino acid oxidases in liver and kidney convert *D* amino acids to ketoacids, which can be further metabolized. *L* amino acids in proteins undergo slow racemization to a *DL* mixture over many years. Aspartic acid undergoes the most rapid racemization, and this rate can be used to estimate the time of synthesis of proteins with very slow turnover, such as ocular lens proteins or intervertebral collagen in which half-lives may exceed 50 years. Two amino acids, threonine and isoleucine, have a second asymmetric carbon, and their stereoisomers are referred to as *allothreonine* and *alloisoleucine.* The latter compound has utility in the diagnosis of maple syrup urine disease (MSUD; OMIM #248600).

In addition to the 20 well-known protein-forming amino acids, a number of rare amino acids are recovered from protein hydrolysates. For example, 4-hydroxyproline and 5-hydroxylysine are found in collagen lysates, and desmosine and isodesmosine are recovered in elastin hydrolysates. These amino acids are formed by posttranslational mechanisms because no codon is responsible for their incorporation into growing polypeptides. Selenocysteine is a special case of an amino acid synthesized on a specific transfer RNA and incorporated into a few sites in only about 25 proteins that include members of the thyroid hormone deiodinase and glutathione peroxidase families.[2] Some of these rare amino acids are shown in Fig. 28.1.

Acid–base properties of amino acids depend on the amino and carboxyl groups attached to the α carbon and on the basic or acidic groups occurring on some sidechains (R). At a physiologic pH near 7.4, the α-carboxyl group is ionized and carries a negative charge, and the α amino group is protonated and carries a positive charge. Molecules existing simultaneously as cations and anions are referred to as zwitterions (diagrammed below).

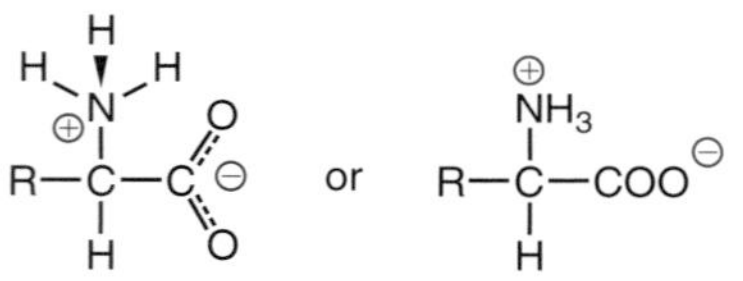

$$R-CH(NH_3^{\oplus})-COO^{\ominus} \quad \text{or} \quad R-CH(NH_3^{\oplus})-COO^{\ominus}$$

The pH at which ionizable groups exist equally as charged and uncharged forms is referred to as the pK. Amino acids thus have two or more pKs—one for the carboxyl, one for the amino group, and an additional one in the presence of an ionizable side chain. The isoelectric point (pI) is the pH at which an amino acid or other molecule has a net charge of 0. For a typical neutral amino acid such as glycine, the pI of 5.97 is midway between the pK of 2.34 for the carboxylic acid and the pK of 9.60 for the amino group. The pKs of amino acid side chains in proteins vary somewhat from those in free amino acids because of the influence of neighboring amino acids. The buffering capacity of ionizable groups is primarily in a pH range within ±1 unit of the pK for the respective groups. Amino acids and proteins therefore have a limited buffering capacity near physiologic pH. The imidazole side chain of histidine is an exception with a pK near 6.0. Glycine, for example, is used as a buffer near pH 2.5 or 9.5.

The structural diversity of side chains permits formation of proteins with a variety of structure and function. Sidechain diversity is dictated not only by pK but by size and hydrophobicity as well. Amino acids with longer aliphatic or aromatic side chains such as isoleucine, leucine, and phenylalanine have greater hydrophobicity than shorter side chains such as the methyl group found in alanine. Neutral amino acids with polar groups such as hydroxyl or amide groups in their side chains are more hydrophilic. Acidic amino acids have side chains with carboxylic acids, and basic amino acids have side chains with amino, guanidino, or imidazole groups. The thiol side chain (–SH) of cysteine oxidizes easily and may become linked to other molecules via disulfide. In plasma, cysteine occurs as cystine (cysteine homodimer linked via a disulfide) or as a mixed disulfide with albumin or other proteins.

With some exceptions, amino acids are water soluble and stable in plasma. The most soluble amino acids have small side chains with polar or ionizable moieties such as glycine, alanine, arginine, serine, and threonine. Less soluble amino acids such as phenylalanine, tyrosine, leucine, and tryptophan tend to have larger, nonpolar aliphatic or alicyclic side chains. Amino acid solubility is rarely limiting in vivo except in some metabolic disorders. Deposition of tyrosine crystals in the eye and skin is common in tyrosinemia (particularly type II; OMIM #276600). Likewise, cystine may crystallize in the renal parenchyma in patients with cystinuria (OMIM #220100). Structural and chemical details for the 20 protein-forming amino acids are displayed in Table 28.1.

Amino Acid Supply and Transport

Amino acids participate in many metabolic pathways in addition to serving as substrates for protein synthesis. In the healthy state, women require approximately 46 g/d and men approximately 56 g/d of dietary protein (0.8 g/kg body weight), and substantial increases in demand occur during growth and in many disease states.[3] Dietary protein is digested by proteases in the stomach (eg, pepsin) and small intestine (eg, trypsin, chymotrypsin) to yield amino acids. Endogenous protein turnover serves as another source of free amino acids. Eight amino acids used for protein synthesis (isoleucine, leucine, lysine, methionine, phenylalanine, threonine, tryptophan, and valine) are not synthesized by humans and therefore are considered "essential" constituents of the diet. Meat, milk, eggs, and fish contain a full range of essential amino acids. Gelatin is deficient in tryptophan, and some plant sources of protein may be additionally deficient in lysine or methionine. Therefore, diets based on a single source of plant protein may be deficient in some amino acids. When liver function is compromised, cysteine and tyrosine become essential because they are not converted from their usual precursors, methionine and phenylalanine.[4] Arginine may be conditionally essential as well because endogenous rates of synthesis may be insufficient to meet requirements in adults under metabolic stress or in growing children.[5]

Requirements for dietary protein to maintain nitrogen balance increase in infancy and childhood when there are increased demands for growth.[6,7] Daily requirements increase by up to 3.5 to 4 g protein/kg body weight for premature infants, for example.[8] Protein demand is also increased in pregnancy, lactation, and states of protein loss or catabolic states (eg, burn patients). Persistent negative nitrogen balance results in a number of undesirable phenotypic features. A diet severely deficient in protein and consisting primarily of high-starch foods can lead to kwashiorkor, a disorder characterized by decreased serum albumin, immune deficiency, edema, ascites, growth failure, apathy, and many other symptoms.[9] Marasmus results when protein and energy sources such as carbohydrates are deficient, causing wasting of muscles and subcutaneous tissues. Albumin or prealbumin concentrations are used to assess adequacy of the amino acid supply. The shorter biologic half-life of prealbumin compared with albumin (2 vs. 20 days) makes it a valuable marker for acute dietary assessment.[10,11]

Homeostasis of cellular amino acid concentrations is dependent on supply, catabolism, and excretion. Supply and excretion are regulated by a series of transport systems with overlapping substrate specificity, strategic tissue expression, and polarized cellular distribution.[12,13] Amino acids are derived from dietary protein precursors through the action of proteolytic enzymes in the stomach and small intestine that produce shorter oligopeptides and individual amino acids. Enteral absorption of di- and tripeptides is mediated by a single proton-coupled transport system termed PEPT1 (encoded by *SLC15A1*).[14] Transport of individual amino acids across the intestinal and renal epithelium as well as the blood–brain barrier is far more specialized.

Early biochemical characterization of amino acid transport was technologically limited to studies of the plasma membrane. These broad-specificity transport systems function as co-transporters, exchange transporters, or facilitative transporters. Nomenclature was based on substrate specificity, co-transport requirements, and sensitivity to inhibitors. By convention, capital letters indicate a requirement for Na^+, and lower case descriptors imply the lack of Na^+ dependence. Systems A and ASC are responsible for Na^+-mediated symport of neutral species with small side chains. System L facilitates exchange of amino acids with large, hydrophobic side chains. Cationic amino acid transport is mediated by a system termed y^+. System y^+L facilitates exchange of neutral amino acids with cationic species. System B^o catalyzes Na^+ mediated transport of branched-chain and aromatic amino acids, and system b^o enables exchange of bulky neutral and cationic side chains. Finally, system X^- mediates transport of anionic amino acids. These systems act in a coordinated way to achieve amino acid homeostasis.[15]

Distinct transport systems cooperate to achieve net amino acid transport across epithelial barriers. For example, transcellular transport of cationic amino acids across the renal brush border is achieved by a combination of two exchange systems, b^o and y^+L. On the apical surface, positively charged amino acids are imported in exchange for an uncharged amino acid via system b^o. System b^o uses the transmembrane electrical potential to drive transport. Efflux across the basolateral membrane is also achieved via exchange transport via system y^+L. System y^+L uses the driving force of the transmembrane sodium gradient. Lack of proper polarized expression in appropriate tissue types results in transport disorders such as cystinuria (OMIM #220100) and lysinuric protein intolerance (OMIM #222700).[16]

Intracellular amino acid compartments are maintained by a distinct set of transport systems. These systems are important for metabolizing, sequestering, and recycling various amino acids. Substrate concentrations in the urea cycle are regulated in part via the mitochondrial ornithine-citrulline antiporter. Defects in this transport system leads to HHH (hyperornithinemia, hyperammonemia, homocitrullinuria) syndrome (OMIM #238970). Reclamation of amino acids from lysosomal protein digestion also relies on transport systems. Defects in the *CTNS* gene, for example, inhibits lysosomal cystine transport and results in the clinical disorder known as cystinosis (OMIM #219750). Finally, neuronal vesicles must concentrate synaptic transmitters to achieve interneuronal communication. Two of these transmitters, glycine and glutamate, are actively transported across vesicle membranes.

The rather coarse biochemical definition of amino acid transport is being redefined as the genetic basis for these systems is clarified.[17] Table 28.2 summarizes selected connections between gene and functional transport systems. Genes of the SLC (solute carrier) family encode integral transmembrane spanning proteins that catalyze amino acid transport. The *SLC1* family, for example, encodes transporters primarily responsible for transport of anionic amino acids that are particularly important in brain and neural tissues.[18] Neutral amino acid transporters (eg, System A) are encoded by the *SLC38* family.[19] Mitochondrial transport systems are expressed by the *SLC25* gene family.[20] The *SLC3* and *SLC7* gene families encode a wide array of heterodimeric transporters, including the aforementioned b^o and y^+L transport systems.[21] Each of these transporters contains one of two *SLC3* genes that encode membrane-targeting subunits that are disulfide linked to one of at least a dozen *SLC7* gene products dictating transport specificity. Metabolic flux of amino acid carbon is critically dependent on the proper expression and regulation of transport as well as enzyme-catalyzed chemical transformation.

Amino Acid Metabolism

Amino acids serve as scaffolds for the synthesis of many hormones, nucleotides, lipids, signaling molecules, and metabolic intermediates that play a role in energy production. As portrayed in Fig. 28.2, the transformation of amino acid carbon to energetic intermediate typically begins with transamination. Excess nitrogen is excreted as urea. Resulting α-ketoacids may enter the Krebs cycle; undergo conversion to ketone bodies, fatty acids, or glucose; or be completely oxidized to CO_2 depending on cellular energy demands. A vast array of enzyme networks has evolved to orchestrate demand for amino acids. Information regarding the substrates, products,

TABLE 28.2 Genetic Basis of Selected Amino Acid Transport Systems

Gene Family	System	Expression	Substrates	Disease Link
SLC1	X^-, ASC	Brain, gut, kidney, liver	D,E, A, S, T, C, N, Q	
SLC3A1 (rBAT)	y^+, L, y^+L, b^0	Broad	R, K, H, M, L, A, C, L, I, V	Cystinuria
SLC3A2 (4F2hc)				Lysinuric protein intolerance
SLC7 (A1-A13)				
SLC6	B^0	Brain, kidney, gut, liver	F, Y, L, I, V, P, C, A, Q, S, H, G, M	Hartnup disorder Iminoglycinuria
SLC17		Neurons	E	
SLC25	ASP/GLU ORN/CIT	Broad, (mitochondria)	D, E, ornithine, citrulline	Type II citrullinemia HHH syndrome
SLC32		Neurons	G, γ-aminobutyrate	
SLC38	A, N	Broad	Q, A, N, C, H, S, T	
SLC43	L	Liver, kidney, gut, muscle	L, I, V	
CTS		Broad	Cystine	Cystinosis

HHH, Hyperornithinemia, hyperammonemia, homocitrullinuria.

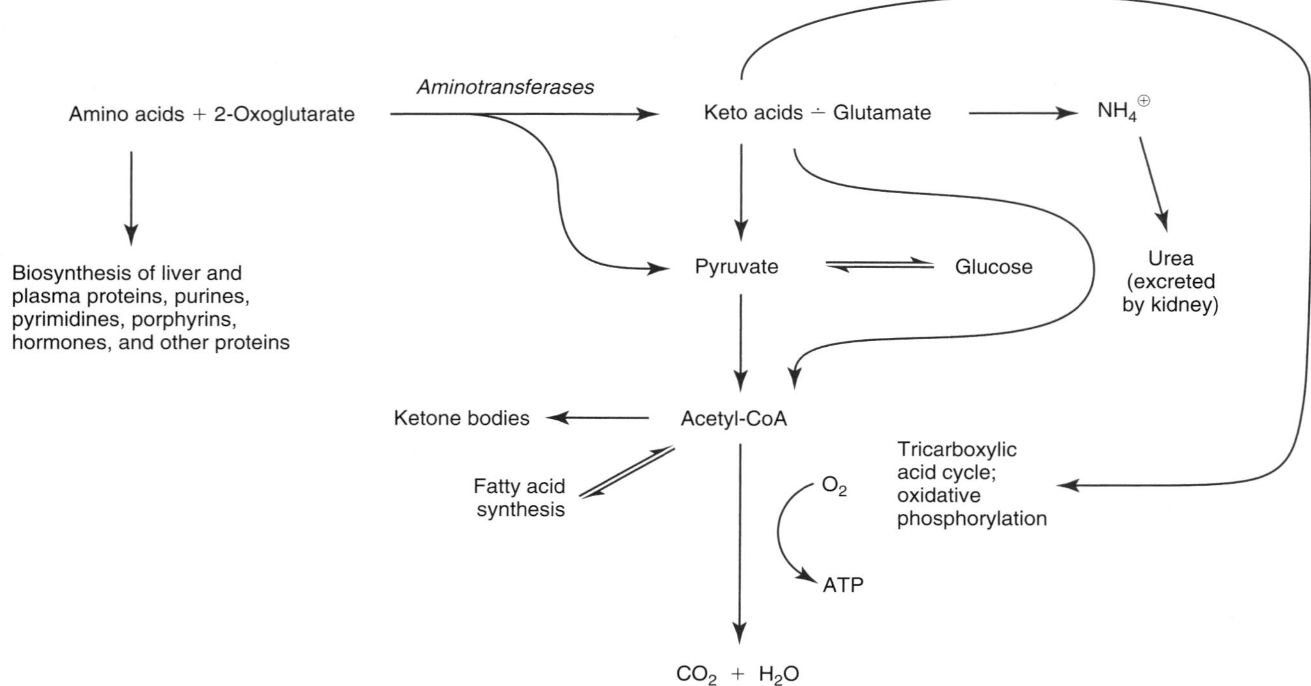

FIGURE 28.2 A generalized scheme of amino acid metabolism in the liver. After transamination, amino acid carbon may be used to in the Krebs cycle directly or transformed into other respiratory fuels such as glucose and ketones. Waste nitrogen is disposed of via the urea cycle. *ATP,* Adenosine triphosphate.

kinetics, and inhibitors of these enzymes may be found in multiple databases, including BRENDA (brenda-enzymes.org), ExPASy-enzyme, (enzyme.expasy.org), and ExplorEnz (enzyme-database.org). Pathway databases include KEGG (genome.jp/kegg), GenMAPP (genmapp.org), and BioCyc (biocyc.org).

Glucose, fatty acids, and ketones are primary respiratory substrates in humans. These substrates generate adenosine triphosphate (ATP) via the mitochondrial Krebs cycle. Amino acids play two key roles in energy provision. First, amino acids are converted to Krebs cycle intermediates to maintain the activity of the cycle in a process called anaplerosis. Glutamine and glutamate, for example, are converted to α-ketoglutarate via loss of the epsilon and alpha amino groups. Fumarate may be derived from asparagine and aspartate, and succinate is derived from methionine, threonine, and valine. Second, amino acids may be mobilized to generate fuels for a variety of organ systems. Five amino acids (LEU, ILE, LYS, PHE, and TYR) may be converted to ketones. All of the amino acids except for leucine may be used to produce glucose. In times of high energy demand and limiting fuel sources, therefore, flux of amino acid carbon through proper pathways becomes an important source of respiratory fuel.

Excess tissue nitrogen is disposed of as urea, which contains two moles of nitrogen per mole (see also Chapter 70). Urea production is limited to the liver, so selected amino acids, primarily glutamine and alanine, serve to shuttle excess nitrogen to the liver. Nitrogen in the form of ammonium ion is first converted to carbamoyl phosphate, which is transferred to ornithine to form citrulline. Aspartic acid and citrulline are condensed to form arginosuccinic acid, which, in turn, is cleaved to arginine and fumaric acid. Arginase hydrolyzes arginine to urea and ornithine to allow the cycle to repeat. Urea is usually viewed simply as waste, but it is also the primary contributor to the high osmolality in the renal medulla and enables maximal urinary concentrating ability.

Amino acids are precursors for many hormones and signaling molecules. Tyrosine provides a scaffold for thyroxine, dopamine, and adrenaline synthesis. Tryptophan is a precursor of serotonin and melatonin. The potent vasodilator nitric oxide (NO) is produced from arginine. Glycine, aspartate, glutamine, and serine contribute atoms to purine and pyrimidine synthesis. Glycine and arginine are precursors for creatine synthesis.

Creatine synthesis and many other biochemical processes rely on a series of single-carbon transfer reactions mediated by serine, glycine, histidine, and methionine. Transfer of fully oxidized carbonyl carbon (=C=O) to molecules such as propionyl CoA (to form methylmalonyl CoA) is mediated by biotin. Glycine, serine, and histidine contribute less oxidized carbon units such as methylidine (=CH–), and methylene ($-CH_2-$) groups that enable purine and pyrimidine synthesis via folate derivatives. Folate also mediates transfer of methyl ($-CH_3$) groups to homocysteine to form methionine. The resulting methionine is, in turn, activated to S-adenosylmethionine becoming a methyl donor to a vast array of substrates including DNA, RNA, histones, choline, and catecholamines. The importance of folate and single-carbon metabolism to cell growth and division cannot be overstated. Folate deficiency in a developing embryo can lead to death or severe neurologic birth defects. The use of folate antimetabolites such as methotrexate has been a mainstay in the treatment of cancer for many decades. These pathways are treated in more detail in Chapter 37.

Amino Acid Concentrations

Plasma amino acid concentrations collectively span a 4-order-of-magnitude dynamic range from very low micromolar quantities (eg, β-alanine, cystathionine) to near 1 mmol/L (eg, glutamine, glycine). With protein intake of 1 to 2 g/kg, daily variation of approximately 30% in healthy adults has been observed.[22] Concentrations of both essential and nonessential amino acids vary in a coordinated way, suggesting that mechanisms beyond diet and enteral extraction are responsible. Amino acid concentrations tend to peak between 12 and 8 PM with a nadir between midnight and 4 AM.[23,24] After an ingested protein bolus, dietary amino acids rise and tend to return to preprandial levels in 3 to 6 hours. Determination of "fasting" amino acid concentrations, therefore, requires extended periods of dietary abstinence.

Most amino acids in blood undergo glomerular filtration but are efficiently reabsorbed in proximal renal tubules by previously described saturable transport systems. Increased renal excretion of amino acids *(aminoaciduria)* results from filtration of excessive plasma concentrations, generalized tubular impairment, or heritable defects in amino acid transport systems. Glycine tends to be most abundant in normal urine followed by histidine, glutamine, and serine. Increased concentrations of proteogenic amino acids in plasma tend to precipitate only mildly elevated excretion because of efficient reabsorption. Other amino acids that accumulate in plasma secondary to metabolic errors (eg, argininosuccinate, homocitrulline) demonstrate pronounced excretion because of the absence of specific tubular mechanisms enabling reclamation from the filtrate.

With the exception of glutamine, CSF amino acid concentrations are typically less than 10% of those found in plasma. This high plasma to CSF gradient suggests active net brain to blood transport across the blood–brain barrier.[25,26] Glutamine concentrations in CSF are generally equal to those in plasma, suggesting a bidirectional facilitative transport process. Insofar as CSF concentrations reflect synaptic concentrations, regulation of neurotransmitter amino acid concentrations is critical for normal neural action potential propagation. Glutamate is the most abundant amino acid in the brain and is the primary excitatory transmitter. Glycine and GABA are the predominant inhibitory transmitters. Lumbar puncture to access the CSF amino acid pool must be done with great care to avoid overestimation of central amino acid concentrations secondary to contamination with peripheral blood.

Assessment of amino acid concentrations in blood, urine, and spinal fluid has been historically applied to the detection of inborn errors of metabolism. These are comprehensively covered in Chapter 70. Aside from the measurement of homocysteine as a marker of vitamin B_{12} and folate status, clinical applications of amino acid measurement are promising but presently limited. Future applications may include the assessment of immune status using tryptophan and its metabolites such as kynurenine.[27] Increased plasma concentrations of α-aminobutyric acid may be useful in detecting liver regeneration.[28] Branched-chain amino acid concentrations may be early indicators of diabetes,[29] while a combination of phenylalanine, glutamate, and alanine has some value to predict the onset of preeclampsia.[30] Finally, quantitation of arginine and its dimethylated derivatives (asymmetric and symmetric dimethylarginine) may have utility in assessing endothelial function.[31,32] These applications require further clinical validation.

Analysis of Amino Acids

For decades, the standard method of amino acid analysis was cation-exchange chromatography with postcolumn spectrophotometric or fluorescent detection of various primary amine derivatives. Derivatizing agents have included dansyl chloride, o-phthalaldehyde, and ninhydrin. The ninhydrin approach developed by Stein and Moore in the 1950s was initially applied to determination of amino acid content of protein hydrolysates and then adapted for profiling of free amino acids in deproteinized body fluids.[33] Other systems commercialized by Beckman (Brea, California) and Hitachi (Tokyo, Japan) were large floor models and required as long as 2 to 3 hours to quantitate 30 to 50 physiologic amino acids in a single patient specimen. These systems have given way to smaller bench-top systems using ninhydrin (Biochrom; Cambridge, United Kingdom) or fluorescent (quinolyl-*N*-hydroxysuccinimidyl) amine derivatives (Waters; Milford, Massachusetts) that still require 90 to 120 minutes for full sample analysis. In addition to long cycle times, these methods are subject to interference from co-eluting amines, leading to overestimation of some amino acid concentrations. Common co-eluting compounds include methionine with homocitrulline, phenylalanine with aminoglycosides, and histidine with gabapentin.

Mass spectrometry is increasingly being adopted as the method of choice for amino acid profiling. Newborn screening programs quantitate amino acid butyl esters derived from dried blood spots using flow-injection MS protocols. These methods do not use chromatographic separation and so cannot distinguish between isomeric or isobaric amino acids such as leucine, isoleucine, alloisoleucine, and hydroxyproline. Liquid chromatography–tandem mass spectrometry (LC-MS/MS) methods for detection of amino acids in plasma and other body fluids that use liquid chromatography have also been developed.[34-36] Some of these use amine-targeted derivatives, others target the carboxyl group, and some others use no chemical derivatization. Advantages of MS-based techniques include improved analytic specificity, a 3- to 4-order-of-magnitude dynamic range, and rapid (20-minute) throughput. MS methods may also be optimized for profiling multiple molecular species in addition to amino acids. Such approaches promise to improve the scope of metabolic disorders detectable with a single patient specimen in a single analytic run.

PEPTIDES

This section describes the basic biochemistry of peptides. In general, the term *peptide* applies to relatively short polymers of amino acids with molecular weights less than 6,000 Da (<~50 amino acid residues). The chemistry of the peptide bond and the physical characteristics of the peptide backbone are discussed in this section along with a number of clinically relevant peptide systems.

Peptide Bond

A peptide bond, also referred to as an amide bond, is formed between the α-nitrogen atom of one amino acid and the carbonyl carbon of a second (diagrammed below).

$$R_1-CH(NH_2)-COOH + HN(H)-CH(R_2)-COOH \xrightarrow{-H_2O} H_2N-CH(R_1)-C(=O)-NH-CH(R_2)-COOH$$

First amino acid — Second amino acid — Dipeptide

So-called isopeptide bonds refer to amide bonds between sidechain amines or carbonyl carbons on the side chain rather than α-amine or α-carbonyl. In glutathione, for example, the γ-carboxyl group of glutamic acid is linked to the α-amino group of cysteine. During translation, peptide bonds are formed from the amino (N) to the carboxyl (C) terminus by removal of water (also referred to as dehydration or condensation) and catalyzed by RNA (referred to as a ribozyme) that forms part of the ribosome.[37] Peptides are also synthesized in vitro for therapeutic and experimental purposes. Such chemical peptide synthesis proceeds from C to N terminus using N-protected amino acids and catalyzed by N,N'-dicylohexylcarbodiimide.[38,39] In this scheme, the nucleophilic amine group reacts with a carbodiimide:carbonyl intermediate, resulting in the formation of a new peptide bond and dicyclohexylurea. Dicyclohexylurea is insoluble in most solvents and can be easily removed from the maturing peptide. Cleavage of peptide bonds may be nonspecifically achieved by acid hydrolysis or accomplished specifically by a host of proteolytic enzymes with affinity for bonds between specific amino acid residues. These protease systems are described later in this chapter.

Electron sharing in the amide bond (also known as the ω bond) is delocalized effectively preventing rotation about this bond. This bond is fixed in one plane. Conformational flexibility of the peptide backbone results entirely from rotation about the axes of the two bonds to the α-carbon. Angles of rotation about these bonds are referred to as Ramachandran angles.[40] The nitrogen to α-carbon bond angle is referred to as the Φ angle, and the α-carbon to carbonyl bond is referred to as the Ψ angle (below).

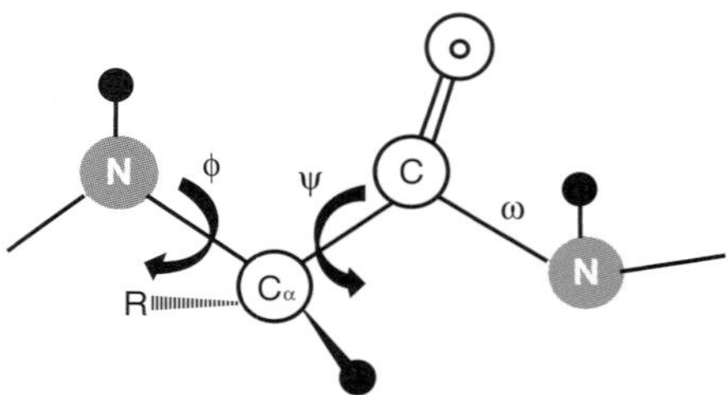

Theoretically, free rotation about these bonds allows angles ranging from -180 to 180 degrees. In reality, steric and energetic factors limit the possible combinations. These bond angles play a key role in dictating the secondary structure of proteins. For example, values of Φ and Ψ in α-helices are approximately −60 and −45 degrees, respectively. Secondary structure is addressed more extensively later in this chapter.

Peptide Heterogeneity and Analysis

Assessment of circulating peptide concentrations has a number of limitations. In the absence of enzymatic activity, peptide measurements have been historically limited to immunologic techniques (discussed in more detail in Chapter 23). Antibodies may recognize linear sequence epitopes or discontinuous, conformational epitopes. These epitopes typically involve 10 to 20 amino acids binding exposed areas of 600 to 1000 Å.[41] Measurement of short peptides (<20–30 amino acids) are therefore limited to single-site, competitive assays that lack the analytic specificity of two-site (sandwich) immunoassays. The molecular specificity issues may be addressed using MS as an alternative. Small peptides may be ionized via electrospray (ESI) or matrix-assisted laser desorption (MALDI) and interfaced to tandem quadrupole mass analyzers (see Chapter 17).

Absolute analytic specificity is not always ideal when applied to biologic peptide systems. Peptide populations may consist of species with a variable number of amino acid residues with sometimes unknown biologic potency. Hepcidin, for example, is an iron transport regulatory peptide that circulates principally as a 25–amino acid peptide but also as shorter peptides of 22 and 20 amino acids with diminished biologic activity. Likewise, dozens of truncated forms of the mature 32–amino acid B-type natriuretic peptide ranging from 24 to 31 amino acids are detectable in heart failure patients (see Chapter 58). Some of these truncated forms are present in vivo, and others likely develop in vitro. Thus, narrowly targeted MS assays may exclude active peptide species and run the risk of underestimating bioactive peptide. Cross-reactive immunoassays, on the other hand, may stoichiometrically detect both active and inactive peptide, thus running the risk of overestimating bioactive peptide concentrations. Examples of several important biologic peptide systems and their analytic considerations follow.

Clinically Relevant Peptide Systems

Pro-Opiomelanocortin System

The pro-opiomelanocortin *(POMC)* gene on chromosome 2 is expressed primarily in the pituitary gland, arcuate nucleus of the hypothalamus, and skin melanocytes. The gene produces a 241–amino acid prohormone that can yield as many as 10 distinct biologically active peptides depending on patterns of cleavage in specific tissue types. The POMC peptides have diverse effects on glucose and electrolyte homeostasis (via adrenocorticotropic hormone [ACTH]), body mass and appetite (via lipotropins and melanocortins), pigmentation (also via melanocortins), and pain (via endorphins).[42-44]

Clinical exploitation of this complex peptide system is currently limited to the impact of ACTH on the adrenal gland and subsequent feedback by cortisol. Measurement of circulating ACTH concentrations may be used to clarify the mechanism of adrenal disease. For example, Cushing's disease may result from autonomous adrenal function or may be fueled by ectopic ACTH production. Likewise, Addison's disease may result from adrenal or pituitary failure. The pathophysiology of this axis is treated more extensively in Chapters 65 and 66. Full-length ACTH consists of 39 amino acid residues and circulates with a half-life ranging from 10 to 15 minutes. The biologic activity of ACTH is contained in residues 1 to18, and the length of the C-terminus mediates circulating half-life. Two-site immunoassays typically target the extreme N and C termini to avoid detection of shorter, inactive circulating species. This approach, however, can lead to cross-reactivity with longer precursor forms of ACTH such as pro-ACTH and the full POMC gene product.[45] These precursors typically circulate at concentrations that are five times greater (5–50 pmol/L) than ACTH (1–10 pmol/L). ACTH assays are poorly standardized.

Natriuretic Peptides

This peptide family consists of atrial natriuretic peptide (ANP), B-type natriuretic peptide (BNP, formerly brain natriuretic peptide), and C-type natriuretic peptide (CNP).[46] ANP and BNP are highly expressed in cardiac tissue relative to CNP, which is expressed at low levels in a broad variety of tissue types. The mature forms of these peptides contain a 17–amino acid loop stabilized by an intramolecular disulfide bond. Each peptide acts via a specific guanylate cyclase-coupled receptor to promote sodium and water excretion, blunt activation of the renin–angiotensin system, and decrease vascular resistance. Circulating concentrations of ANP and BNP (but not CNP) increase rapidly in response to increased cardiac filling pressures that are characteristic of heart failure. Clinical measurement of BNP has become a widely used tool to detect heart failure and monitor its progression.

B-type natriuretic peptide is synthesized as a 108–amino acid precursor (pro-BNP) that is cleaved upon cellular release to the active 32–amino acid peptide and an N-terminal fragment (NT-proBNP), which lacks biologic activity.[47] The diagnostic and prognostic role of these peptides is treated extensively in Chapter 58. Two-site immunoassays for both BNP and NT-proBNP are commercially available and widely used. NT-proBNP circulates at higher concentration than BNP by virtue of its longer biologic half-life (~60 minutes vs. ~20 minutes). Recent evidence suggests that the BNP detected immunologically in heart failure is not the bioactive form of BNP. Using MS, almost no mature 32–amino acid peptide was detected in heart failure patients despite the significant presence of immunoreactive BNP.[48,49] Further studies suggest that the immunoreactive BNP in the plasma of heart failure patients may be attributed to higher molecular weight forms such as proBNP that exhibit a fraction of the bioactivity of the mature peptide.[50,51] This new analytic information may prompt a reevaluation of the role of BNP in the pathophysiology, diagnosis, and treatment of heart failure.

Hepcidin

Hepcidin was initially described as an antimicrobial peptide.[52] The role of hepcidin in iron metabolism was noted by Nicolas et al. in 2001.[53] The mature 25–amino acid molecule is derived from a 60–amino acid precursor expressed from 3 exons of the *HAMP* gene on chromosome 19. The tightly looped structure of hepcidin is stabilized by four intramolecular disulfide bonds. The biologic activity of hepcidin is mediated via its interaction with ferroportin, the transport protein that mediates iron transport from duodenal enterocytes and macrophages. Hepcidin binding promotes the internalization and degradation of ferroportin, thus inhibiting mobilization of iron stores.[54,55] Physiologic states such as chronic inflammation are characterized by microcytic anemia with paradoxically adequate iron stores known as anemia of chronic disease. Increased hepcidin expression is at the pathologic root of this condition. In addition to its diagnostic role in differentiating iron deficiency anemia from the anemia of chronic disease, hepcidin measurement may aid in the treatment of hemochromatosis, transfusion-associated iron overload, and anemia associated with chronic renal failure.[56]

Despite the important role of hepcidin in iron metabolism, its clinical use remains infrequent partly because of difficulties associated with its measurement. Antibodies toward hepcidin have been difficult to develop because of its small, compact size and because it is highly conserved across multiple species. Immunoassays have largely been limited to single-site, competitive formats that cross-react significantly with shorter versions of the molecule (22-, 20-mers).[57] This can lead to overestimation of circulating hepcidin compared with MS techniques[58] when applied to patients with renal failure in whom shorter hepcidin peptides tend to accumulate in the plasma.[59] Improvements in the molecular specificity and harmonization of hepcidin determination will further clarify the role of hepcidin in both normal and pathologic physiology and also promise to enhance its clinical utility. For additional discussion on hepcidin, see Chapter 38.

Angiotensins

Renin is secreted by the afferent arterioles of the kidney in response to decreased flow, pressure, and sodium delivery to the renal juxtaglomerular apparatus.[60] Renin acts on circulating angiotensinogen to initiate the formation of vasoactive peptides that act to reestablish glomerular flow. The N-terminal decapeptide cleaved from the 452–amino acid angiotensinogen molecule by renin is referred to as angiotensin I. Angiotensin-converting enzyme (ACE) cleaves 2 C-terminal residues from angiotensin I to form the octapeptide, angiotensin II, which promotes contraction of vascular smooth muscle and stimulates proximal tubular sodium reabsorption to increase blood pressure. ACE inhibitors (eg, captopril, enalapril, quinapril) are important pharmacologic tools used to treat hypertension.

Although the renin–angiotensin–aldosterone axis is an important therapeutic target, it is a far more infrequent target for diagnostic laboratory studies. Plasma renin activity is assessed to explore the possibility of renovascular hypertension. In this condition, unilateral restriction of renal blood flow results in inappropriate release of renin and severe hypertension. Renin activity in the plasma is normally very low (<10 ng/mL/h) and is typically measured by assessing the production of angiotensin I from endogenous angiotensinogen after a long (>12 hours) incubation period. Angiotensin I generation is most commonly monitored via a competitive immunoassay with the potential to crossreact with shorter peptides. MS approaches that address peptide specificity and stability may mitigate these analytic limitations.[61,62]

Endothelins

Endothelins (ETs) are peptides with 21 amino acids derived from the vascular endothelium (ET-1), intestinal and renal tissue (ET-2), and neural tissue (ET-3).[63] ET-1 is produced from a 203–amino acid precursor (preproendothelin) and smaller, 30– to 40–amino acid "big" ET molecules that are inactive. ET-1 is a potent vasoconstrictor and may mediate pathology associated with diabetic nephropathy and hypertension.[64] Increased circulating concentrations of ET after myocardial infarction suggest a negative survival prognosis.[65] The reliability of these observations using currently available immunoassays and other potential clinical applications for ET measurement remain unclear.

Vasopressin

Vasopressin (arginine vasopressin [AVP]), also known as antidiuretic hormone (ADH), is a nonapeptide stored in and secreted from the posterior pituitary gland. Its primary target organ is the distal convoluted tubule and collecting duct, where it acts to promote water reabsorption. ADH circulates at very low concentrations (<40 pmol/L) and has a very short half-life (15–20 minutes), making routine diagnostic measurement impractical. Diabetes insipidus (DI) may result from faulty secretion (central DI) or from end-organ resistance (nephrogenic DI). Head injury, tumors, and some medications may also induce pathologic secretion of ADH, resulting in fluid overload referred to as the syndrome of inappropriate antidiuretic hormone secretion (SIADH). A synthetic analog referred to as DDAVP (1-desamino, 8-D-arginine vasopressin) is used therapeutically to treat DI and some forms of coagulopathy. DDAVP stimulates release of von Willebrand factor from endothelial cells and extends the half-life of circulating factor VIII, thereby mediating improvements of circulating hemostatic factors associated with various forms of von Willebrand disease and hemophilia A.

Glutathione

Glutathione consists of a glutamate residue linked to cysteine via its γ-carboxyl rather than the α-carboxyl group and followed by a conventional peptide bond between cysteine and glycine.[66] This ubiquitous tripeptide is the most abundant intracellular thiol (1–10 mmol/L) and circulates in the blood at micromolar concentrations. The cellular ratio of reduced glutathione (GSH) to oxidized glutathione (GSSG) ranges from 10 to 100. Intracellular glutathione performs a variety of important functions. It plays an important role in maintaining the proper ratio of oxidized to reduced forms of metabolically important thiols such as coenzyme A. It also provides reducing equivalents that detoxify reactive oxygen species such as peroxides (catalyzed by glutathione peroxidase). Through the activity of glutathione-S-transferase, glutathione also serves to detoxify other xenobiotic compounds via formation of a thioether derivative, which can then be excreted. Amines and peptides are transported across the plasma membrane via the γ-glutamyl moiety of glutathione, a reaction catalyzed by γ-glutamyl-transpeptidase. The tripeptide is then regenerated through the concerted action enzymes in the so-called γ-glutamyl cycle (Fig. 28.3).

Determination of circulating GSH and GSSG is not routinely called for in clinical practice as the site of action is intracellular. Nonetheless, a variety of techniques to measure glutathione have been used.[67] Measurement of total glutathione requires prior reduction of the sample to release all oxidized forms. The simplest techniques employ the colorimetric detection of free thiol using 5,5′-dithio-bis-2-nitrobenzoic acid (DTNB). Reaction of DTNB with thiols results in the formation of 2-thio-5-thiobenzoate, which absorbs with high extinction (~14,000 L cm^{-1} mol^{-1}) at 410 nm. Other techniques use derivatization and stabilization of GSH followed by high-performance liquid chromatography or MS. Inborn errors of glutathione metabolism such as glutathione synthetase deficiency are detected via the accumulation of components of the γ-glutamyl cycle such as pyroglutamic acid (5-oxoproline).

PROTEINS

The structural diversity of proteins may be described using the following features:

1. Primary structure is the linear sequence of amino acids in a peptide or protein. Posttranslational modifications of amino acids contribute to increased diversity.
2. Secondary structure describes the nature of the peptide backbone dictated by the peptide bond angles described earlier and stabilized by hydrogen bonds. Examples of secondary structure include α-helix, β-sheet, and β-turn. An α-helix has about 3.6 residues per turn and is stabilized by hydrogen bonds between the N–H and C=O group of the fourth following amino acid. A β-sheet involves hydrogen bonds between the peptide bonds of adjacent peptide chains arranged in parallel or antiparallel configurations. Random coils refer to segments of peptide that lack defined secondary structure.
3. Tertiary structure refers to the folding of the polypeptide chain and elements of secondary structure into a compact three-dimensional (3D) shape. Folding is a complex process driven by energy minimization of intramolecular and solvent interactions. Hydrophobic groups tend to fold into the interior with less exposure to solvent, while charged and polar sidechains tend to be located on the surface. The 3D structure is stabilized by intramolecular hydrogen bonds, van der Waals forces, and hydrophobic interactions.

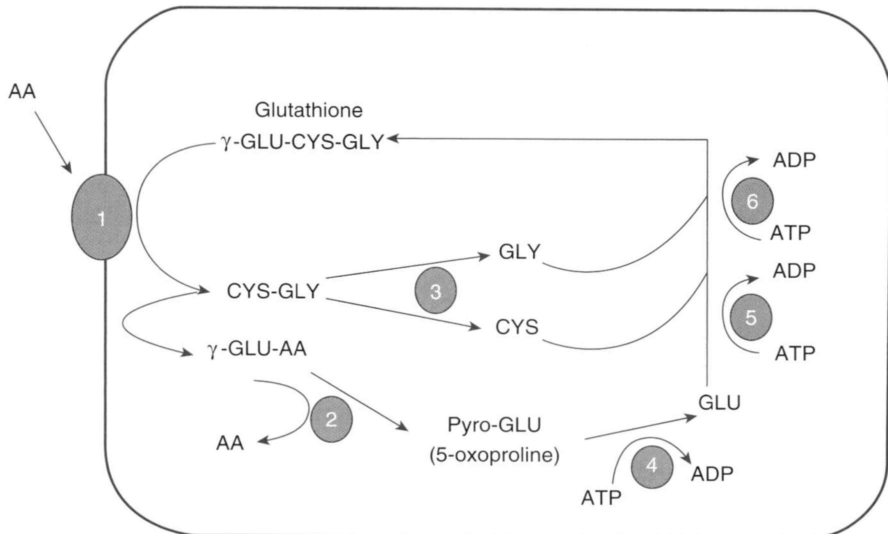

FIGURE 28.3 Transmembrane transport of amino acids (AAs) using the γ-glutamyl cycle. Three-letter AA abbreviations are used. Extracellular AA is transferred to glutathione via activity of membrane-bound γ-glutamyl transpeptidase *(1)*. AA is released in the cytoplasm via the activity of γ-glutamyl cyclotransferase *(2)*, which also results in the formation of pyroglutamate (5-oxoproline). Cysteine and glycine generated via dipeptidase activity *(3)* are recycled with pyroglutamate to reform glutathione via successive activities of 5-oxoprolinase *(4)*, γ-glutamyl-cysteine synthetase *(5)*, and glutathione synthetase *(6)*. *ADP*, Adenosine diphosphate; *ATP*, adenosine triphosphate; *CYS*, cysteine; *GLU*, glutamate; *GLY*, glycine.

Disulfide bonds between cysteine residues also stabilize 3D structure. Denaturation of protein refers to unfolding that occurs with temperature change or in the presence of organic solvents, detergents, or reagents that disrupt hydrogen bonds. Limited denaturation can be reversible, but extensive unfolding and denaturation of proteins often lead to irreversible aggregation and precipitation.

4. Quaternary structure refers to the incorporation of two or more polypeptide chains or subunits into a larger multimeric unit. Examples range from the relatively simple creatine kinase, a heterodimer of M and B subunits, to branched chain α-ketoacid dehydrogenase, which is a heteromeric complex of 12 E1, 24 E2, and 6 E3 subunits.
5. Ligands and prosthetic groups provide additional functional and structural elements, such as metals in metalloenzymes, heme in hemoglobin and cytochromes, and lipids in lipoproteins. Proteins without their associated ligands are often referred to as apoproteins (eg, apotransferrin without iron, apolipoproteins without lipid).

Physical Properties of Proteins

The diverse structural features of proteins result in unique physical properties that can be exploited for analysis. For example, tyrosine and tryptophan residues absorb light at 280 nm, and the abundance of these amino acids determines the extinction coefficient of a peptide or protein. A pure protein, therefore, may be quantitated using A_{280}. Some prosthetic groups such as heme also possess intrinsic absorbance that may be monitored to assess the presence of specific proteins. Automated clinical analyzers assess the presence of hemoglobin at 540–570 nm, for example, to detect hemolyzed plasma or serum specimens. Ionizable groups exert a strong effect on physical properties depending on the pH of the surrounding solution. Differing physical properties serve as the basis of methods to separate proteins (see also Chapter 12). Some important characteristics include the following:

1. *Differential solubility*. The solubility of proteins is affected by pH, ionic strength, temperature, and the characteristics of the solvent. Changing solvent pH affects the net charge of a protein. Changing ionic strength affects the hydration and solubility of proteins. "Salting-in" and "salting-out" procedures were early methods for separating and characterizing protein. Albumin, for example, stays in solution at high concentrations of ammonium sulfate that precipitate globulins. Addition of organic solvents and polyethylene glycol is also useful for differential precipitation. Fractional precipitation of plasma with ethanol, using protocols developed by Cohn and coworkers,[67a] enables isolation of plasma fractions that are enriched in immunoglobulins, α- and β-globulins, or albumin (fraction V). Polyethylene glycols induce precipitation by steric exclusion and therefore preferentially precipitate large proteins or complexes.
2. *Molecular size*. Separation of small and large molecules is commonly achieved by differential migration through molecular filters. Examples are size exclusion chromatography (also known as gel filtration), ultracentrifugation, and electrophoresis. These techniques may be used under conditions when proteins and peptides are in native globular states or under denaturing conditions. Addition of reducing agents allows separation of disulfide-linked components.
3. *Molecular mass*. Advances in MS allow the determination of masses of peptides and proteins with increasing accuracy. Peptides and proteins can be ionized by MALDI or by ESI (see Chapter 21).

4. *Electrical charge.* Ion-exchange chromatography, isoelectric focusing, and electrophoresis separate peptides and proteins based on charge (see Chapters 15 and 16).
5. *Surface adsorption.* The affinity of peptides and proteins for a variety of physical surfaces may also be used as the basis for separation. Reverse-phase chromatography, for example, exploits the interaction of hydrophobic molecular moieties with hydrophobic surfaces (C8 or C18 alkyl chains) when the ratio of water to organic solvent is high but not when organic content is increased.
6. *Affinity chromatography.* Specific ligands, antibodies, and other recognition molecules have been used to separate peptides or proteins selectively.

Protein Formation

Folding

Proteins are synthesized by ribosomes reading from the 5′-end of mRNA. Triplet codons in mRNA are matched with complementary sequence in transfer RNA carrying specific amino acids. Protein synthesis begins with an AUG codon encoding methionine, and the polypeptide chain is synthesized from the N-terminus. During translation, the initiator methionine is typically cleaved and the resulting N-terminal residue commonly acetylated. Although 80% to 90% of proteins carry an N-terminal acetyl group, the function of this modification is not entirely clear, but it may play a role in stabilizing the growing peptide chain.

Instructions for folding are largely contained in the primary amino acid sequence of the growing polypeptide chain. The rate of elongation (typically 5–10 amino acids per second in eukaryotes) may have a significant impact on folding. The use of rare codons, secondary structural elements of the mRNA, and polybasic stretches may dictate pauses in translation and enhance formation of secondary structural elements.[68,69] Folding begins as the chain is elongated and still associated with the ribosome, assisted by a family of proteins referred to as chaperones.[70] The function of chaperones was originally ascribed to a group of proteins called "heat shock proteins" that prevented protein denaturation and aggregation in response to heat and other extreme environmental conditions.

Many gene products that share common 3D features have arisen from common ancestral genes. The serpin (serine proteinase inhibitor) superfamily consists of more than 1000 related proteins in different organisms.[71] Humans have 36 serpins, 29 of which are protease inhibitors and 7 of which lack protease inhibitor function. Serpins that act as protease inhibitors in plasma include α_1-antitrypsin (AAT), α_1-antichymotrypsin, α_2-antiplasmin, antithrombin, C1 inhibitor, heparin cofactor II, protein C inhibitor, and plasminogen activator inhibitor-1 (PAI-1). Serpins without known protease inhibitor function are cortisol-binding globulin, thyroxine-binding globulin, angiotensinogen, intracellular proteins, heat shock protein 47, and the tumor suppressor maspin. Serpins illustrate how a common structure motif may be adapted to multiple functions. Other examples of plasma protein families are the albumin and lipocalin families. The albumin family includes albumin, α-fetoprotein, and afamin. The lipocalin family includes several plasma proteins such as α_1-acid glycoprotein, retinol-binding protein, apolipoprotein D, α_1-microglobulin, prostaglandin D synthase (β-trace), β-lactoglobulin, neutrophil gelatinase-associated lipocalin (NGAL), inter-α-trypsin inhibitor, and C8 γ-chain. Lipocalins generally have a barrel-shaped structure that is well suited to serve as a carrier for small molecules.

Protein folding is an error-prone process, and many molecular chaperones work to refold, prevent aggregation, or degrade misfolded proteins.[72] Several heat shock proteins that increase in response to a variety of stresses are molecular chaperones. Increased accumulation of misfolded proteins induces an adaptive mechanism—the unfolded protein response.[73] This response increases production of chaperones and slows general protein synthesis to allow more time to fold new proteins.

Despite these protective mechanisms, several families of age-related, genetic, and infectious diseases appear connected to disorders of protein folding and protein aggregation. Prion diseases are infectious diseases in which the transmissible protein agent may catalyze misfolding of endogenous proteins. In Alzheimer's disease, deposits of amyloid may contribute to pathogenesis. Polyglutamine diseases result from genetic expansion of repeat units encoding glutamine and are associated with Huntington's disease and other neurodegenerative disorders.[74] These expanded polyglutamine sequences tend to aggregate as β-sheets. TDP-43 proteinopathies include amyotrophic lateral sclerosis (Lou Gehrig's disease), resulting from aggregation of transactive DNA-binding proteins.[75] Several inherited disorders related to mutations in specific proteins probably result from problems in protein folding. In AAT deficiency, hepatic injury results from aggregation and accumulation of misfolded protein.[76,77] The most common cause of cystic fibrosis results from a single amino acid deletion (ΔF508), which results in rapid degradation of the cystic fibrosis transmembrane conductance regulator (CFTR). Accumulation of misfolded proteins has been suggested as a pathogenic mechanism contributing to vascular, cardiac, and β-cell failure in diabetes.[73] Small molecule therapeutics capable of modulating protein folding have shown some promise in mitigating disease caused by abnormal protein aggregation.[78]

Targeting

As originally outlined by Lingappa and Blobel,[79] proteins that are secreted, located in vesicular compartments, or oriented on the external surface of cell membranes usually contain a hydrophobic N-terminal signal peptide about 15 to 30 amino acids in length. Signal peptides interact with signal recognition particles (SRPs) and mediate interaction with the endoplasmic reticulum (ER). Nascent peptide chains are inserted through the membrane of the ER as the protein is synthesized. Signal peptides of most secretory proteins are removed even before synthesis of the entire protein chain is completed. Co-translational membrane retention may be achieved via an uncleaved signal sequence, by one or more hydrophobic transmembrane domains, or by lipid modifications such as N-myristoylation.[80]

Newly synthesized proteins ultimately reside in a number of membranous or soluble compartments, including the nucleus, lysosome, peroxisome, mitochondrion, or plasma membrane. Plasma membrane sorting is further complicated in polarized epithelial cells where proteins may be targeted to basolateral or apical environments. In the so-called "secretory" pathway, proteins are shuttled via membrane-bound vesicles bearing COP II (coat protein II) from ER through the

Golgi apparatus.[81,82] Intra-Golgi transport and retrograde Golgi to ER transport is mediated by COP I vesicles. Upon fusion of vesicle with specific membranes, soluble components are extruded, and lipid-associated components take up residence as stable membrane components. Sorting in polarized epithelia is mediated by association of proteins with unique membrane domains. For example, proteins anchored to the membrane via a glycosylphosphatidylinositol (GPI) anchor tend to cluster in cholesterol- and sphingolipid-rich domains called lipid rafts that are selectively sorted to apical surfaces.[83] Proteins destined for mitochondria contain a unique N-terminal targeting sequence that mediates their interaction and import into the proper submitochondrial location (eg, outer membrane, inner membrane, matrix, intermembrane space).[84]

Posttranslational Modifications

Fatty Acylation

The activity and localization of a variety of proteins may be modulated by covalent attachment of fatty acyl chains. Co-translational attachment of myristate via a glycine residue has been previously mentioned as a mechanism for membrane association. The most common acylation of eukaryotic proteins involves thioester linkage of palmitate to membrane proximal cysteine residues.[85] S-palmitoylation reversibly controls localization to membrane microdomains such as lipid rafts and thus regulates interaction of proteins with signaling and other effector molecules. Examples of palmitoylated proteins include caveolin-1, some members of the SRC protein kinase family, nitric oxide synthase (NOS), β-adrenergic receptor, and transferrin receptor. Ghrelin, a potent growth hormone secretagogue, is modified by covalent attachment of an octanoyl moiety at serine 3 of the polypeptide.[86,87] Only octanoylated ghrelin promotes growth hormone release.

Phosphorylation

Reversible phosphorylation may impact as many as one third of all human cellular proteins.[88] O-phosphorylation occurs at serine, threonine, and tyrosine residues. The human genome encodes approximately 1000 kinases, enzymes responsible for phosphorylation, and about 500 phosphatases responsible for removal of covalent phosphate groups. Detailed treatment of reversible phosphorylation is beyond the scope of this chapter but, in general, serine and threonine phosphorylation acutely modifies enzyme activity (eg, glycogen phosphorylase)[89] and subcellular localization (eg, cAMP-dependent protein kinase).[90] Tyrosine phosphorylation, on the other hand, regulates a plethora of signaling pathways (eg, mitogen activated protein kinase, Janus kinase pathways) in part by providing docking site proteins that propagate a transmembrane signal such as those of the SRC kinase family (lyn, lck, fyn).[91] Mitochondria contain members of a primitive kinase family that modulate flux through the pyruvate dehydrogenase and branched chain α-ketoacid dehydrogenase complex via a unique phosphohistidine intermediate.[92-94]

Prenylation

Isoprenoid compounds such as farnesyl pyrophosphate (15 carbons) and geranylgeranyl pyrophosphate (20 carbons) are hydrophobic moieties formed from 3-hydroxy-3-methylglutaryl CoA and mevalonate via HMG CoA reductase. These groups modify more than 300 members of the human proteome via enzymatic attachment to a cysteine residue in a so-called "CaaX" motif where C is cysteine, a is an aliphatic amino acid such as glycine or alanine, and X is typically serine, methionine, glutamine, alanine, or threonine.[95,96] Isoprenylation regulates membrane and molecular association of a number of proteins important for signal transduction (H-Ras, K-Ras), vesicular trafficking (Rab2, Rab3a), cyctoskeletal function (RhoA, RhoB), and the integrity of the nuclear membrane (lamin A).[97]

Glycosylphosphatidylinositol Anchor

The GPI anchor is a glycoglycero-phospholipid construct that mediates membrane attachment for a variety of proteins. The anchor is presynthesized in the ER and then transferred to the target protein via a C-terminal hydrophobic signal sequence. After modification, this hydrophobic sequence is removed, leaving a protein that is uniquely membrane anchored via interdigitation of two fatty acyl chains with a single membrane leaflet.[98,99] The purpose of the GPI anchor remains unclear, although it has been proposed that such lipid-anchored proteins diffuse in the lateral plane of biologic membranes more rapidly than transmembrane proteins.[100] GPI-anchored proteins also uniquely associate with cholesterol- and glycosphingolipid-rich plasma membrane domains referred to as lipid rafts and caveolae.[83] Notable examples of GPI-anchored proteins include decay accelerating factor (DAF, CD55), membrane inhibitor of reactive lysis (MIRL, CD59), alkaline phosphatase, 5′-nucleotidase, and glypican family members. Defects in the PIG-A gene product that mediates GPI synthesis are responsible for paroxysmal nocturnal hemoglobinuria (PNH). PNH is characterized by abnormal complement-mediated lysis of erythrocytes deficient in CD55 and CD59.

γ-Carboxylation

Glutamic acid is a five-carbon α-amino dicarboxylic acid. Vitamin K acts as a cofactor in the enzymatic addition of a second carboxyl group to the γ-carbon.[101] A cluster of γ-carboxylated glutamyl residues is referred to as a "gla" domain. This modification mediates calcium-dependent membrane association and is required for full functional activity. Many proteins of the coagulation cascade contain the gla domain, including thrombin, factors VII, IX, and X, and protein C, S, and Z. Warfarin exerts its anticoagulant effect by abrogating the activities of the vitamin K–dependent factors.

Glycosylation

Secreted proteins and the extracellular domains of transmembrane proteins are commonly modified with carbohydrate. Carbohydrate plays an important role in folding, secretion, and stability of the modified polypeptide. Sugar chains are added in the ER and Golgi apparatus via O-linkage to serine and threonine residues or N-linkage to the amide nitrogen of asparagine residues.[102] O-linked sugar modifications are typically simple and consist of one to four residues. The sugars are transferred to the nascent polypeptide via the energy of the phosphoester bonds of nucleotide sugars such as uridine diphosphate–galactose and guanosine diphosphate–mannose. N-linked sugars are far more complex. A core glycan consisting of 2 *N*-acetylglucosamine, 9 mannose, and 2 glucose moieties is pre-assembled on a membrane embedded isoprenoid molecule, dolichol, and then transferred en bloc to the newly synthesized peptide chain. The core glycan structure may then be lengthened and trimmed by a host of enzymatic processes. Approximately 200 human gene products are involved in glycosylation, and more than 100 genetic defects in this process have now been documented.[103]

Sulfation

Sulfation of proteins on tyrosine residues was originally described in 1954.[104,105] Nearly 50 secreted and transmembrane proteins carry this irreversible modification that occurs in the Golgi apparatus. Examples of sulfated proteins include coagulation factors V, VIII, and IX, fibrinogen, thyroglobulin, and α-fetoprotein. The sulfation reaction is catalyzed by two widely expressed isoforms of tyrosylprotein phosphotransferase (TPST) and uses 3′-phosphoadenosine-5′-phosphosulfate as the sulfonic acid donor.[106] The consensus peptide sulfation site is poorly understood aside from the fact that acidic residues surrounding the target tyrosine appear to promote this modification. The function of sulfation is likewise not well understood beyond its capacity to enhance the affinity of molecular recognition events. A naturally occurring Tyr → Phe at position 1680 of factor VIII, for example, prevents sulfation and weakens its interaction with von Willebrand factor, causing a mild form of hemophilia.[107]

Hydroxylation

Hydroxylation is the most prevalent posttranslational modification of human proteins. Hydroxylation most commonly occurs at the 4-position of the proline ring. Approximately 30% of proline residues in collagen are modified in this way. Hydroxyproline residues are, therefore, more common in proteins than many other common amino acid residues, including cysteine, histidine, methionine, phenylalanine, tryptophan, and tyrosine.[108] Hydroxylation of proline residues is thought to alter the flexibility ("pucker") of the pyrrolidine ring, thereby stabilizing the triple helical structure of collagen[109] and other connective tissue proteins (eg, elastin).

Proline hydroxylation also plays a unique role in mediating the cellular response to oxygen through hypoxia inducible factor-1 (HIF-1). Under hypoxic conditions, HIF-1α/HIF-1β heterodimers induce expression of genes that mediate angiogenesis, erythropoiesis, vascular tone, citric acid cycle activity, and iron metabolism.[110] During normoxia, proline residues at position 402 or 564 are targets for enzymatic hydroxylation, which mediates ubiquitination by a protein complex containing von Hippel-Lindau (VHL) protein.[111] Ubiquitination of HIF-1α mediates its degradation via the proteasome (see section on protein catabolism) and subsequent blunting of the genetic response to hypoxia.

Nitrosylation

Nitric oxide is a volatile free radical produced from arginine via three human NOS enzyme systems: neuronal (nNOS), endothelial (eNOS), and an inducible form (iNOS). NO exerts its primary biologic effects (eg, vasodilation) via guanylate cyclase–coupled receptors, but it also forms covalent nitrosothiol (S–N=O) derivatives with free cysteine thiol groups.[112,113] Thousands of proteins with a diverse array of functions are reversibly modified in this way.[114] Although no rigorous determinants of nitrosylation sites have been defined, solvent exposed cysteine residues in alpha helices within 6 Å of charged residues seem to be preferred targets.[112] Nitrosylation may occur directly with the possible aid of metal catalysis via transfer of SNO groups from low molecular weight thiols such as glutathione, or through exchange mediated by disulfide reducing enzymes such as thioredoxin.[115,116] Effects of nitrosylation are pleiotropic. Whereas nitrosylation of the *N*-methyl-D-aspartate receptor in neurons blunts its activity,[117] nitrosylation of matrix metalloprotease-9 (MMP-9) stimulates its activity.[118] The role of protein nitrosylation in health and disease remains to be fully clarified.

Protein Catabolism

The steady-state concentration of any specific intra- or extracellular protein reflects not only its rate of synthesis but also its rate of degradation. The degradative process is much more than a passive, nonspecific mechanism for disposing of unwanted cellular material. It is highly specific and tightly controlled. As supporting evidence, consider that the human genome contains more than 500 proteases. These proteases belong to one of four families based on the catalytic mechanism for hydrolyzing peptide bonds. Representative members of the four protease families are detailed in Table 28.3.

Protease Families

Serine Proteases. The serine proteases are the most abundant family in humans and are so named because serine serves as the nucleophilic residue at the active site of the enzyme.[119] Peptide bond hydrolysis is achieved via a conserved "catalytic triad" of spatially adjacent histidine, serine, and aspartate residues. These enzymes enable a vast array of physiologic processes, including protein digestion, complement activation, and blood coagulation. A family of endogenous serine protease inhibitors (serpins) inactivates a broad variety of protease enzymes via formation of a covalent complex with the active site serine. Members of the serpin superfamily with antiprotease activity include AAT, antithrombin, PAI-1, and protein C. Some members of the serpin family, including angiotensinogen and thyroxine-binding globulin, do not possess known activity against specific proteases. Serine protease activity in vitro can be mitigated with a number of inhibitors, including phenylmethanesulfonylfluoride (PMSF), [4-(2-aminoethyl)benzenesulfonyl fluoride] (AEBSF), aprotinin, and leupeptin.

Cysteinyl Proteases. This group of proteases uses a cysteine thiol in nucleophilic attack on the peptide bond.[120] A thioester intermediate with the carbonyl carbon of the peptide bond is formed before hydrolysis and formation of two peptides with new C and N termini. In humans, cysteine proteases mediate apoptosis via a series of enzymes referred to as caspases.[121] Other notable cysteine proteases include some in the cathepsin family and interleukin 1β converting enzyme (ICE). Cystatins are endogenous inhibitors of cysteine protease activities. Some chemical inhibitors of serine proteases such as PMSF and leupeptin also exhibit activity toward cysteine proteases. Unique in vitro inhibitors of cysteine proteases include L-trans-epoxysuccinyl-leucylamide-(4-guanido)-butane (E-64) and N-[N-(*N*-acetyl-L-leucyl)-L-leucyl]-L-norleucine (ALLN).

Aspartyl Proteases. In contrast to the serine and cysteinyl proteases, aspartyl proteases do not act via a covalent acyl enzyme intermediate. Instead, peptide bond lysis is achieved

TABLE 28.3 **Selected Members of the Four Protease Families**

Protease/Family	Gene Loci	Tissue Expression	Subcellular Localization	Substrate, Function, Pathology
Serine				
Corin	4p13	Broad	Plasma membrane	Natriuretic peptides (heart failure)
Trypsin	7q34	Pancreas	Secreted	Promiscuous (cleavage of LYS-X, ARG-X)
Chymotrypsin	16q23	Pancreas	Secreted	Promiscuous (cleavage of TRP-X, PHE-X, TYR-X)
Neutrophil elastase	19p13	Myeloid cells	Cytoplasm, secreted	Promiscuous (cleavage of VAL-X, ALA-X)
Factor IX	Xq27	Liver	Secreted, plasma membrane	Conversion of factor X to Xa (hemophilia B)
Activated protein C	2q14	Liver		Factor V_a, factor VIII_a (coagulopathy)
PSA (kallikrein)	19q13	Prostate	Secreted	Semen liquefaction; marker of prostate mass and cancer
C1s	12p13	Broad	Secreted	Complement C1r, C2, and C4 (angioedema)
Cysteinyl				
Caspase-3	4q34	Broad	Cytosol, nucleus, mitochondria	ASP-X-X-ASP (apoptosis)
Cathepsin C	8p23	Broad	Lysosome	Amyloid precursor (Alzheimer disease)
Aspartyl				
Renin	1q32	Ovary, broad	Secreted	Angiotensinogen (hypertension)
Pepsin	6p21	GI tract, lung	Secreted	Cleavage at adjacent hydrophobic residues (PHE-VAL, ALA-LEU, LEU-TYR)
Presenilin	14q24	Broad	Endoplasmic reticulum/ Golgi	Amyloid precursor (Alzheimer disease)
Metallo				
ADAMTS13	9q34	Liver, erythroid precursors, broad	Secreted	von Willebrand factor (thrombotic thrombocytopenic purpura)
MMP-1	11q22	Muscle	Secreted	Collagen (tissue remodeling, embryogenesis, metastasis)
Angiotensin I converting enzyme	17q23	Testes, broad	Secreted	Angiotensin I (hypertension)

in a single step through the coordination of a water molecule between two highly conserved aspartate residues. One aspartate residue abstracts a proton from water, which then becomes a nucleophile, attacking the carbonyl carbon of the peptide bond.[122] Human aspartyl protease enzymes include members of the pepsin, cathepsin, and renin families. The target for HIV protease inhibitors (eg, indinavir, ritonavir) is also an aspartyl protease. Pepstatin is a potent hexa-peptide inhibitor of aspartyl protease activity.

Metalloproteases. Members of this protease family, commonly referred to as MMPs, include approximately 25 Zn^{2+} dependent enzymes sub-classified by their reactivity to collagen, gelatin, and other extracellular matrix proteins.[123-125] MMPs contain a conserved motif in which a Zn atom is coordinated by three histidine residues and a glutamate residue. MMPs achieve peptide bond fission through nucleophilic activation of a water molecule bound between Zn and the γ-carboxyl of glutamate.[126] MMPs play a multitude of roles in wound healing and repair, pathogen defense, cancer metastasis, and rheumatoid arthritis. Endogenous control of MMP activity is achieved through an endogenous group of four proteins referred to as tissue inhibitors of matrix metalloproteases (TIMPs). TIMPs act via formation of an equimolar complex with target MMPs. Chemical inhibition of MMP activity may be achieved by metal chelation and hydroxamic acid derivatives.

The Ubiquitin-Proteasome System

Ubiquitin is a highly conserved 76–amino acid polypeptide containing seven lysine residues encoded by four human genes.[127] Intracellular polypeptide chains may be modified with ubiquitin through the concerted action of three ubiquitin ligase enzymes (E1–E3). In the presence of ATP, ubiquitin is first activated via formation of a thioester bond between E1–cysteine residue and the C-terminal carboxyl of ubiquitin. Activated ubiquitin is then trans-esterified to the E2 ligase, which cooperates with E3 to effect the formation of an isopeptide bond between the C-terminal glycine of ubiquitin and a lysine residue on the target protein.[128] The target protein may be modified by a single ubiquitin moiety, or multiple molecules may be added to the original ubiquitin at one or more of the seven ubiquitin lysine residues. Limited ubiquitination of target proteins generally modifies their subcellular location or intermolecular interactions, and

TABLE 28.4 High-Abundance Plasma Proteins

	RANKED BY MASS ABUNDANCE (mg/L)		RANKED BY MOLECULAR ABUNDANCE (μmol/L)	
Rank	Protein	Concentration	Protein	Concentration
1	Albumin	35,000–52,000	Albumin	500–800
2	Immunoglobulin G	7000–16,000	Immunoglobulin G	40–120
3	Transferrin	2000–3600	Apolipoprotein A-I	30–70
4	Immunoglobulin A	700–4000	Apolipoprotein A-II	30–60
5	α_2-Macroglobulin	1300–3000	Transferrin	25–45
6	Fibrinogen	2000–4000	α_1-Antitrypsin	18–40
7	α_1-Antitrypsin	900–2000	Haptoglobin	6–40
8	Apolipoprotein A-I	910–1940	α_1-Acid glycoprotein	15–30
9	C3	900–1800	α_2HS-glycoprotein	9–30
10	IgM	400–2300	Immunoglobulin A	5–30
11	Haptoglobin	300–2000	Hemopexin	9–20
12	Apolipoprotein B	600–1550	Apolipoprotein C-III	6–20
13	α_1-Acid glycoprotein	500–1200	Fibrinogen	5–18
14	α_2HS-glycoprotein	400–1300	Gc-globulin	8–14
15	Hemopexin	500–1150	Apolipoprotein C-I	6–12
16	Gc-globulin (vitamin D–BP)	400–700	C3	5–10
17	Factor H	240–740	α_1-Antichymotrypsin	4–9
18	α_1-Antichymotrypsin	300–600	Apolipoprotein D	2–10
19	Inter-α-trypsin inhibitor	200–700	Prealbumin	4–8
20	Apolipoprotein A-II	260–510	β_2-Glycoprotein I	3–6
21	C4b-binding protein	200–530	Apolipoprotein A-IV	3–6
22	Ceruloplasmin	200–500	Apolipoprotein C-II	2–7
23	Factor B	180–460	Serum amyloid A4	3–6
24	Prealbumin	200–400	Inter-α-trypsin inhibitor	3–5
25	Gelsolin	200–400	Antithrombin III	3–5
26	Fibronectin	300	α_1B-glycoprotein	3–5
27	C1 inhibitor	190–370	Gelsolin	3–5
28	C4	100–400	Ceruloplasmin	2–5
29	Plasminogen	150–350	Factor H	2–5
30	Antithrombin III	170–300	Factor B	2–5

Data from in Hortin GL, Sviridov D, Anderson L. High-abundance polypeptides of the human plasma proteome comprising the top 4 logs of polypeptide abundance. *Clin Chem* 2008;54:1608–1616.

polyubiquitination targets the protein for destruction. Proteolysis occurs in the 26S proteasome, consisting of a 20S catalytic and 19S regulatory subunit constructed from greater than 60 polypeptides.[129] After recognition of the protein target by the 19S subunit, the unfolded polypeptide is threaded into the 20S subunit, where peptide bond fission occurs via a threonine-mediated nucleophilic attack.

Proteins in Human Serum and Plasma

The circulating proteome is a complex mixture of thousands of gene products. The most abundant products are proteins secreted directly into the circulation primarily by the liver and immunoglobulins contributed by lymphatic tissue. Classical methods for protein fractionation and purification over several decades led to isolation and characterization of about 100 of the most abundant proteins.[130] The 12 most abundant proteins represent more than 95% of total protein mass. Albumin alone represents more than 50% of the total mass of protein and an even higher proportion of the number of molecules so that albumin is the main contributor to colloid osmotic pressure (oncotic pressure). The distinction between mass and molar concentrations of circulating proteins may be significant in considering oncotic pressure, protease inhibition, and the binding capacity for ions, drugs, or small molecules. Table 28.4 lists the 30 most abundant proteins by mass and molecular abundance. An exhaustive list of the contents of the circulating proteome would exceed 12,000 entries.[131]

The range of protein concentrations measured in clinical assays spans more than 10 orders of magnitude and thus poses a significant analytic challenge. In decreasing order of abundance, the source of circulating proteins include (1) proteins secreted directly into plasma, (2) proteins associated with the cell membrane and shed into the circulation, (3) secretory proteins in exocrine secretions, (4) high-abundance cytoplasmic proteins, (5) low-abundance cytoplasmic proteins, (6) transmembrane proteins, and (7) organellar proteins that must traverse more than one membrane to exit cells. Many of these serve as useful markers of physiology and disease.

Circulating concentrations of proteins depend not only on rates of production and efficiency of entry to the circulation but also on rates of clearance. Proteins and peptides substantially smaller than albumin are cleared from the circulation by glomerular filtration unless they are bound to larger carrier molecules. Peptides and small proteins not bound to carriers are cleared with half-lives of about 2 hours under conditions of normal kidney function and accumulate in kidney failure. Examples of proteins and peptides that increase dramatically in renal failure include β_2-microglobulin (BMG), cystatin C, immunoglobulin light chains, parathyroid hormone fragments, complement factor D, atrial natriuretic peptide, and interleukins.[132,133] Other proteins and bioactive peptides such as insulin, intact parathyroid hormone, and growth hormone have much shorter circulating half-lives of only a few minutes, indicating receptor-mediated uptake or degradation by exopeptidases or endopeptidases.[134]

For all circulating proteins, the choice of measurement using plasma or serum is not without consequence. Plasma refers to the fluid portion of blood in the presence of an anticoagulant after the cells are removed by centrifugation. Common anticoagulants include dry heparin or ethylenediaminetetraacetic acid (EDTA) or solutions containing citrate. Small molecular weight additives such as EDTA may introduce osmotic effects on plasma volume, and citrate solutions introduce some specimen dilution. Variation in platelet concentration is noted, depending on the time of centrifugation and the force applied. Preparation of platelet-poor plasma commonly requires spinning specimens twice to ensure platelet removal and remove their contribution to plasma proteins. Serum is the fluid component of blood after blood is allowed to clot. It differs from plasma in several respects. An approximate 4% decrease in total protein content is related mainly to removal of fibrinogen during coagulation. Because of the absence of fibrinogen, serum has a lower viscosity than plasma. Intact clotting factors are consumed during the clotting process and in their place proteolytic fragments and the contents of platelet granules produced by the clotting process may be recovered in serum.[135]

Abundant Components of the Circulating Proteome

Prealbumin (Transthyretin)

Prealbumin (molecular weight, 35 kDa) is composed of four identical noncovalently bound subunits with the capacity to bind and transport 10% of circulating triiodothyronine (T_3) and thyroxine (T_4). Prealbumin concentrations are often used as an indicator of adequacy of protein nutrition because of its relatively short half-life (~2 days), high proportion of essential amino acids, and small pool size.[6,10,11] Concentrations also fall in cirrhosis of the liver and protein-losing diseases of the gut or kidneys. Prealbumin migrates as a minor component anodal to albumin on routine serum electrophoresis and is not routinely observed by most methods. It is a proportionately greater component of CSF. Prealbumin is most commonly assessed using immunonephelometric or immunoturbidimetric methods.

Albumin

The name *albumin* (*L. albus,* meaning white) originated from the white precipitate formed during the boiling of acidic urine from patients with proteinuria. Normally, albumin is the most abundant plasma protein from the fetal period onward, accounting for about half of the plasma protein mass. It is a major component of most body fluids, including interstitial fluid, CSF, urine, and amniotic fluid. More than half of the total pool of albumin is in the extravascular space.

Albumin has a nonglycosylated polypeptide chain of 585 amino acids and a calculated molecular weight of 66,438 Da. It is synthesized in the liver and has a 3D structure stabilized by 17 intrachain S-S bonds.[136] It is both chemically and biologically stable because it resists denaturation at higher temperatures than most plasma proteins and circulates with a half-life of 15 to 19 days. Albumin has a high abundance of charged amino acids that contribute to high solubility, and it has a net negative charge of about −12 at neutral pH.[137] Albumin therefore contributes about 6 to 10 mmol/L to the anion gap at normal albumin concentrations of 0.5 to 0.8 mmol/L (3.5–5.2 g/dL) and lesser amounts at lower albumin concentrations. At a pH of 8.6 for alkaline electrophoresis, albumin has a net charge of about −25, resulting in high mobility toward the anode. One unpaired cysteine at position 34 occurs partially in reduced form and partially in exchangeable disulfide bonds with other free thiols.

Albumin has two critical biologic functions. First, it serves as the major component of colloid osmotic pressure. Patients with hypoalbuminemia caused by nephrotic syndrome, for example, develop edema. Second, it serves as a transporter for a diverse range of substances, including fatty acids and other lipids, bilirubin, foreign substances such as drugs, thiol-containing amino acids, tryptophan, calcium, and metals. Some of these substances, such as fatty acids and unconjugated bilirubin, have very low solubility in water in the absence of a carrier molecule.

Most clinical laboratories assay albumin in plasma or serum samples by dye-binding methods, which rely on a shift in the absorption spectrum of dyes such as bromcresol green (BCG) or purple (BCP) upon albumin binding. The affinity of these dyes is higher for albumin than for other proteins, providing some specificity for albumin. BCP generally is slightly more specific for albumin and yields lower values than BCG, particularly for patients with kidney failure.[138] Heparin in collection tubes is reported to affect some dye-binding methods.[139] Dye-binding assays also tend to be less accurate when the serum or plasma protein composition is abnormal. The many ligands of albumin do not typically affect dye-binding assays of serum or plasma significantly unless their concentrations are very high.

α_1-Antitrypsin

Schultze et al.[140] described the inhibition of trypsin in the 1950s. However, AAT inhibits a variety of serine proteinases, leading to the term *α_1-proteinase inhibitor. AAT* is the term commonly used by clinicians and clinical laboratorians, but phenotypes are commonly abbreviated as Pi (protease inhibitor). AAT is synthesized by hepatocytes as a single polypeptide chain with 394 amino acid residues and 3 *N*-linked oligosaccharides, yielding a total molecular weight of approximately 51 kDa. It belongs to the serpin superfamily, a group of suicide inhibitors of serine proteases, which abortively cleave the inhibitor at the reactive site residue but remain covalently linked to the reactive site. Serpins usually occur in a "stressed" conformation, and cleavage leads to a dramatic conformational shift to a "relaxed" form. AAT and other serpins serve as important models for conformational change in protein function and aggregation.[76]

More than 75 genetic variants of AAT have been noted. Clinical AAT deficiency is inherited in an autosomal codominant fashion with a prevalence of 1 in 3000 to 5000 in the United States. AAT alleles are designated B to Z in order of decreasing electrophoretic mobility.[141] The allele designated

M is the wild type. Clinically important variants are the S allele characterized by a Glu → Val substitution at position p264 and the Z allele characterized by a Lys → Glu missense mutation at position p340. Whereas individuals homozygous for the S allele have serum concentrations approximately 60% of normal, those homozygous for the Z allele possess about 15% of normal levels.[77] The lung disease of AAT deficiency is thought to be associated with unchecked elastase activity. Pulmonary disease is characterized by onset of emphysema in the third to fifth decades of life. The onset is particularly early in smokers. Liver manifestations include neonatal cholestasis or hepatitis, cirrhosis, and hepatocellular carcinoma.

Assessment of circulating AAT concentrations is usually performed by immunoturbidimetry or immunonephelometry. Normal concentrations range from 70 to 200 mg/dL (14–50 μmol/L). Concentrations are higher in patients with inflammatory disorders, malignancy, or trauma and in women who are pregnant, on estrogen therapy, or taking oral contraceptives. Neonates also have increased concentrations, possibly secondary to maternal estrogen. Individuals with decreased AAT may be phenotyped using electrophoresis or MS or alternatively, genotyped.

Ceruloplasmin

Ceruloplasmin (Cp) is an α_2-globulin that contains about 95% of serum copper. Each molecule of Cp contains 6 to 8 tightly bound copper atoms. A solution of Cp is blue (*L. caeruleus*, meaning blue), and increased concentrations of Cp may lend plasma a green tint. Cp is a polypeptide chain with 1046 amino acids and three asparagine-linked oligosaccharides yielding a molecular weight of approximately 132 kDa. Cp is synthesized primarily by hepatic parenchymal cells, with small amounts from macrophages and lymphocytes. The peptide chain is formed first and then copper is added via the activity of an intracellular ATPase (ATP7B). ATP7B is commonly mutated in Wilson disease.[142] Cp synthesized in the absence of copper or the ATPase is degraded intracellularly, but some apoCp reaches the circulation, where it has a shortened half-life of a few hours (normal, 4–5 days). Consequently, serum Cp is low in those with Wilson disease (see Chapter 61).[143]

Haptoglobin

Haptoglobin (Hp) is an α_2-glycoprotein that binds hemoglobin (*G. haptein*, meaning to bind). Hp is synthesized as a single peptide chain by hepatocytes and cleaved into α- and β-chains. Variable numbers of α- and β-chains combine and become covalently linked by disulfides to form Hp.[144] Hp scavenges hemoglobin in the vascular space. Hp–hemoglobin complexes are bound by CD163 receptors and rapidly cleared by the reticuloendothelial system, which degrades protein and recycles heme and iron. This process prevents renal clearance of hemoglobin until Hp-binding capacity is exceeded. Because Hp is degraded after complexing with hemoglobin, its concentration drops severely in the event of intravascular hemolysis. The normal plasma half-life of Hp is about 5.5 days. Hemolysis of specimens after blood collection does not decrease Hp. Hp has a capacity to bind only about 1% of the hemoglobin in RBCs at usual hematocrits, so minimal intravascular lysis completely depletes plasma Hp. When Hp capacity is exceeded, free hemoglobin in the circulation increases. Free hemoglobin can oxidize to methemoglobin (Fe^{3+}) followed by dissociation of metheme from globin. Metheme binds to hemopexin (high affinity) or albumin (low affinity), keeping it in solution. Hemopexin–heme complexes are removed by the reticuloendothelial system. Hp depletion is usually a sensitive biochemical indicator of intravascular hemolysis followed by hemopexin depletion and finally by the presence of methemalbuminemia, hemoglobinuria, or both. Hp measurement, typically by immunoturbidimetry or immunonephelometry, is therefore part of the assessment of possible transfusion reactions or other causes of hemolysis.

Transferrin

Transferrin (originally named *siderophilin*) is the principal plasma transport protein for iron (Fe^{3+}). Chapter 38 describes iron metabolism. Transferrin has a molecular weight of 79.6 kDa, including 5.5% carbohydrate. It is a single polypeptide chain, with two *N*-linked oligosaccharides and two homologous domains, each with an Fe^{3+}-binding site. It is synthesized mainly in the liver and circulates with a half-life of 8-10 days. Transferrin reversibly binds two ferric (Fe^{3+}) ions with high affinity at physiologic pH but lower affinity at decreased pH, which allows release of iron in intracellular compartments. After cellular delivery of iron via receptor-mediated endocytosis, apotransferrin is recycled back into the circulation. Clinical indications for direct measurement of transferrin are few. Indirect assessment of transferrin concentration may be inferred by total iron-binding capacity (TIBC).

Under normal circumstances, transferrin oligosaccharides terminate in four sialic acid residues, but this pattern is altered under both normal and pathologic conditions. Transferrin glycan structure is widely used to detect congenital disorders of glycosylation.[145] These forms are generically referred to as carbohydrate-deficient transferrin (CDT).[146] A desialated version of transferrin, termed tau-transferrin or β_2-transferrin, is a substantial component of CSF but not serum. It has been used as an indicator of CSF leakage in fluid from the ear or nasal passages (see later section on CSF proteins).[147,148] Increased CDT in plasma also has been used as an indicator of alcohol abuse.[149] The decreased amount of sialic acid and the reduced negative charge of CDT may be detected by electrophoresis, isoelectric focusing, ion-exchange chromatography, or MS.

β_2-Microglobulin

β_2-Microglobulin is a small, nonglycosylated 99 residue protein with a molecular weight of 11.8 kDa. It is the noncovalently bound light chain subunit of class I major histocompatibility complex molecules present on the surface of all nucleated cells. BMG is shed into the blood, particularly by B lymphocytes, and some tumor cells. Its small size allows efficient glomerular filtration, resulting in a plasma half-life of approximately 100 minutes. In addition to renal failure, therefore, high plasma concentrations occur in inflammation and neoplasms, especially those associated with B lymphocytes. In patients with chronic lymphocytic leukemia, high BMG concentrations are a negative prognostic marker for decreased survival. Plasma BMG concentrations are used as a staging criterion in multiple myeloma.[150] BMG concentrations are also increased in states of immune activation and have been applied as an indicator of transplant rejection.

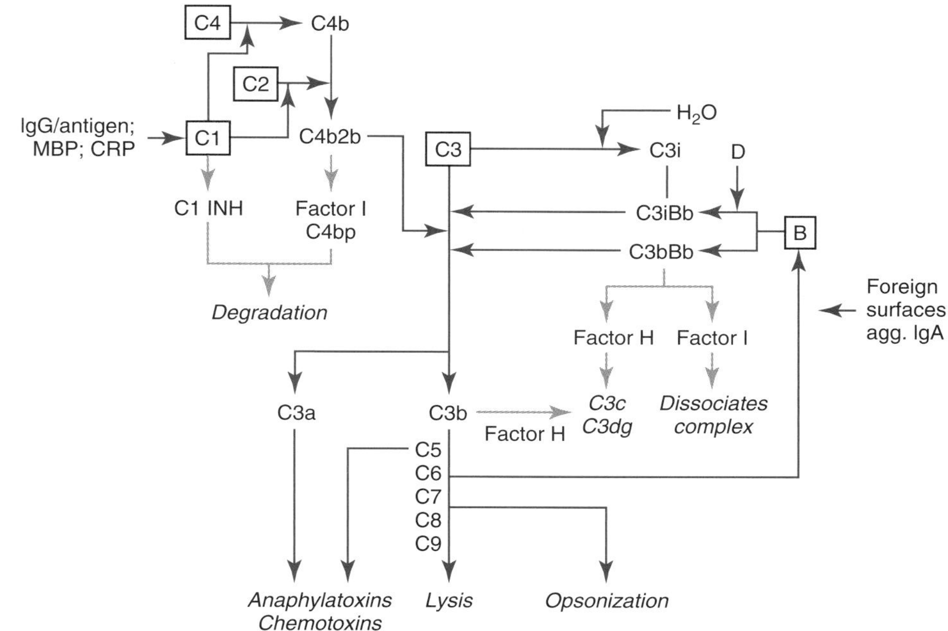

FIGURE 28.4 The complement cascade. Activation via the classical pathway is shown on the *left* and via the alternative pathway on the *right.* Both pathways converge at the level of C3 convertase. Direct activation of C3 by neutrophil and plasma proteases also may occur. *CRP,* C-reactive protein; *IgA,* immunoglobulin A; *MBP,* mannan-binding protein. (Courtesy J.W. Whicher, with modifications.)

C-Reactive Protein

In 1930, Tillet and Francis described a substance in the sera of acutely ill patients that bound cell wall C-polysaccharide of *Streptococcus pneumoniae* and agglutinated the organisms.[151] In 1941, the substance was shown to be a protein and named C-reactive protein (CRP).[152] CRP consists of five identical, nonglycosylated 23 kDa subunits noncovalently associated to form a disk-shaped structure with radial symmetry and total mass of approximately 115 kDa. CRP aids in nonspecific host defense against infectious organisms by activating the classical complement pathway.

C-reactive protein is one of the strongest acute-phase reactants, with plasma concentrations rising up to 1000-fold after myocardial infarction, stress, trauma, infection, inflammation, surgery, or neoplastic proliferation.[153] Concentrations greater than 5 to 10 mg/L suggest the presence of an infection or inflammatory process. Concentrations are generally higher in bacterial than viral infection, although concentrations greater than 100 mg/L (10 mg/dL) may be seen in uncomplicated influenza and infectious mononucleosis. The increase with inflammation occurs within 6 to 12 hours and peaks at about 48 hours and is generally proportional to the extent of tissue damage. Because the increase is nonspecific, however, it cannot be interpreted without other clinical information.

C-reactive protein is normally present in plasma at a concentration below 5 mg/L. High concentrations in inflammatory states are measured with direct immunoturbidimetric or immunonephelometric assays. Epidemiologic studies demonstrate that mildly increased CRP concentrations are associated with risk of cardiovascular disease (see Chapter 34).[154] Increased concentrations may reflect low-grade, chronic intimal inflammation. The use of CRP for these purposes requires assays with detection limits below 0.3 mg/L that generally are referred to as high-sensitivity CRP assays. High-sensitivity assays require particle-enhanced (also termed *latex-enhanced*) light scattering assays or sandwich-type immunoassay formats.

Complement

The complement system consists of more than 20 proteins, synthesized primarily by the liver. A basic schematic of the complement cascade is presented in Fig. 28.4. The basic functions of the complement cascade are to recruit effector phagocytes for opsonization and clearance of foreign pathogens as well as trigger direct destruction of the foreign organism. Activation of the cascade proceeds by three different stimuli. The classical pathway is activated primarily by IgM or IgG binding to antigens, which activates a complex consisting of C1q, C1r, and C1s. The alternative pathway is triggered by activation of C3, factor B, and factor D on a variety of pathogenic surfaces in the absence of antibodies. The lectin pathway is activated by binding of mannan-binding protein (MBP) to mannose-rich oligosaccharides that are present in the cell walls of many microorganisms.[155] This event triggers activation of MBP-associated serine proteases termed MASP-1 and MASP-2.

During activation, many complement components are enzymatically cleaved into two or more fragments. The larger fragments are designated by a lowercase *b* and the smaller ones by a lowercase *a.* The larger fragments usually contain a binding site for membranes, immune complexes, and protein association, or in some cases, yield new protease activities that activate subsequent component(s) of the cascade. Smaller fragments typically serve as anaphylatoxic or chemotactic peptides. Inactivated fragments are designated

TABLE 28.5 Inherited Deficiencies of Complement Components

Component	Frequency of Deficiency	Associated Disorders
Ficolins 1-3	Rare?	Recurrent infection
MBP	5%	Infection in infancy; less effect on adults
MASP	Rare?	Recurrent infection (eg, pneumococcal); inflammation
C1q*	Relatively rare	SLE; DLE; GN
C1r, C1s	Rare	SLE; DLE; infection
C2	≥0.0003% (homozygous)	Recurrent infection, vasculitis; SLE, DLE (no antinuclear antibody); half of affected individuals are asymptomatic
C3	Rare	Severe and recurrent bacterial infection, especially with encapsulated, pyogenic bacteria
C4a	13% (heterozygous)	SLE, DLE
C4b	13% (heterozygous)	IgA nephropathy; infection
Combined C4	35% one null; 8%–10% 2 nulls; ≈1% 3 nulls; <0.1% 4 null alleles	Total deficiency: SLE, GN, DLE (many are anti-dsDNA negative but anti-Ro/SSA positive)
C5-C9	Rare	Severe or recurrent infection with Neisseria species
Properdin	Rare	*X*-linked; neisserial infection
Factor D	Rare	Recurrent infection
Factor H or I	Rare	Hypercatabolism of C3; recurrent bacterial infection; HUS in factor H deficiency
C1 inhibitor	0.002%	Hereditary angioedema (autosomal dominant)
Decay accelerating factor (DAF, CD 55)	Rare	PNH related to decreased DAF and CD59 on cell surfaces

*Both quantitative and qualitative (functional) deficiencies reported.

DLE, Discoid lupus erythematosus; *GN,* glomerulonephritis; *HUS,* hemolytic-uremic syndrome; *MBP,* mannan-binding protein; *PNH,* paroxysmal nocturnal hematuria; *SLE,* systemic lupus erythematosus (or SLE-like disease).

Data from Colten HR, Rosen FS. Complement deficiencies. *Annu Rev Immunol* 1992;10:809–834; and Unsworth DJ. Complement deficiency and disease. *J Clin Pathol* 2008;61:1013–1017.

by the letter *i* (eg, C3bi). Activated complexes are indicated by a bar over the components (eg, $\overline{C567}$).

Via coordinated proteolysis, all three pathways converge at the C3 convertase. The classical and lectin pathway C3 convertase consists of C4b and C2b, and the alternative pathway C3 convertase consists of C3b and factor Bb. C3 convertase catalyzes formation of C3b and C3a. Surface-bound C3b serves as a docking site for phagocyte receptors. The C3 convertase also triggers the formation of the classical (C4b2a3b) and alternative (C3bBb3b) C5 convertase, which ultimately leads to the formation of a membrane attack complex (MAC) consisting of components C5 to C9. The MAC forms an ion channel in the membrane of the foreign pathogen triggering lysis and destruction of the target organism.

The constant slow ongoing activation of complement factors would have devastating circumstances were it not for a host of regulatory proteins designed to limit complement activity. A few of these factors include decay-accelerating factor (DAF or CD55), membrane inhibitor of reactive lysis (CD59), membrane cofactor protein (MCP), C1 esterase inhibitor, and factor H. Deficiency of DAF and CD59 can lead to abnormal lysis of RBCs.[156] Defects in C1 esterase inhibitor are linked to hereditary angioedema.[157] Factor H plays a role in age-related macular degeneration.[158] Proper function of complement regulatory factors prevents destruction of endogenous cells at the same time that foreign cells are destroyed by complement.

Despite its complexities, the function of the complement system in vivo is probed with relatively few tools. Total serum complement is a screening test that demonstrates an intact complement pathway from activation to formation of the MAC. The classic version of this assay tests the capacity of patient sera to lyse sheep RBCs coated with rabbit antisheep antibodies. Progress of the reaction is monitored using hemoglobin release from the RBCs. CH50 refers to the amount of serum required to lyse 50% of the added erythrocytes. Assessment of circulating C3 and C4 is also common. C3 and C4 are typically determined with immunoturbidimetry or immunonephelometry. Measurement of C3 may be complicated by in vitro conversion of C3 to C3c. Because of differences in antibody reactivity toward C3 and C3c, C3 concentrations measured on fresh samples may be lower than those determined after long-term storage. Measurement of C3 and C4 are used to assess activation of the alternative and classical pathways, respectively. Low concentrations are observed in complement deficiency, glomerulonephritis, lupus erythematosus, and sepsis. Clinical disorders of inherited complement deficiency are listed in Table 28.5.

Immunoglobulins

Immunoglobulins (antibodies) are generated against foreign immunogens and initiate clearance of the foreign molecule or organism. Human immunoglobulin molecules consist of one or more basic units built of two identical heavy (H) chains and two identical light (L) chains. Each of the four chains has one variable and one (L chain) or three to four (H chain) constant domains, with the variable region involved in antigen recognition and binding (see Chapter 23). Extensive diversity in the variable domains is generated by somatic recombination and mutation of the immunoglobulin genes. Individual plasma cells or clonally expanded cells are committed to synthesis of a single variable domain sequence for heavy and light chains. The amino acid sequences of the variable domains at the N-terminal ends of the four chains form two antigen-binding sites with a high degree of variation in binding specificity. The constant domains are the same for every immunoglobulin molecule of a given subclass and carry sites for binding to complement receptors and activation of complement.

The variable domains contain the antigen-binding regions and the constant domains of the heavy chains contain sites for complement activation and receptor binding. Cleavage of immunoglobulins with pepsin or papain can yield antigen-binding fragments (Fab) and constant region fragments (Fc). Variations in the constant domains of heavy chains (Fc region) result in the classes and subclasses into which immunoglobulins are grouped: IgM, IgG (four subclasses), IgA (two subclasses), IgD, and IgE, respectively. Light chains, which are produced independently and in slight excess of heavy chains, are of two types—kappa (κ) and lambda (λ). The heavy-chain genes are located on chromosome 14; whereas κ light chains are encoded by a gene on chromosome 2, the λ-chain gene is on chromosome 22.

Immunoglobulins are synthesized by plasma cells, the progeny of B-lymphocyte stem cells in bone marrow. More mature B lymphocytes, found mainly in lymph nodes and in blood, develop receptor immunoglobulins on their surface membranes. Upon binding a target antigen, these B lymphocytes proliferate and develop into a clone of plasma cells, producing antibody to the target antigen. Somatic mutation of immunoglobulins leads to further diversity of immunoglobulin variable region and antibody maturation, generally leading to antibodies with higher affinity. B lymphocytes at first have IgM surface receptors and secrete IgM as the first or "primary" response to an antigen. Membrane and secreted forms of the antibody arise from differential splicing of the messenger RNA for heavy chains, which adds a transmembrane segment to the membrane-bound form. Heavy chains of the IgM surface receptor molecules undergo class switching to produce immunoglobulins with γ- or α-heavy chains (IgG or IgA), but the variable regions remain unchanged; as the cells change into plasma cells, second exposure to the same antigen causes a larger secondary or anamnestic response of IgG secretion.

Individual Immunoglobulins and Light Chains

Immunoglobulin G. Immunoglobulin G (IgG) accounts for 70% to 75% of the total immunoglobulins in plasma. Only 35% is found in the plasma space, and 65% is extravascular. IgG consists of two γ-heavy and two light chains, linked by disulfides (see Chapter 23). The molecular weight of IgG is approximately 150 kDa, including one N-linked oligosaccharide on each heavy chain. The oligosaccharide structure may change in inflammatory states and affect interactions with receptors.[159] On agarose gel electrophoresis, IgG migrates broadly in the γ- and slow β-regions as a result of its heterogeneity of charge from sequence variation.

Immunoglobulin G has four subclasses: IgG_1, IgG_2, IgG_3, and IgG_4. The circulating half-life of IgG_1, IgG_2, and IgG_4 is about 22 days. IgG_3 has a half-life of 7 days. IgG_1 and IgG_3 strongly activate complement via the classical pathway, IgG_2 is weakly complement fixing, and IgG_4 does not activate complement. Clustering of multiple IgG molecules is required to activate complement. Both IgG_1 and IgG_3 bind Fc receptors on phagocytic cells, activate killer monocytes, and cross the placenta via receptor-mediated active transport. IgG_1 is the principal IgG to cross the placenta, and neonatal concentrations are similar to maternal concentrations. Neonates have low production of IgG as the result of immaturity of their immune systems, and IgG concentrations fall through infancy as maternally acquired antibody is cleared.

Immunoglobulin M. Immunoglobulin M (IgM) is produced at earlier stages of B-cell development. In the immature immune systems of neonates, IgM is the major immunoglobulin synthesized. In adult serum, it is the third most abundant immunoglobulin, usually accounting for 5% to 10% of total circulating immunoglobulins. IgM as a membrane receptor molecule is monomeric, but most of the serum IgM is a pentamer containing five monomers linked via disulfides to the small J (joining) chain. Plasma cell malignancies may secrete monomeric IgM in addition to, or instead of, pentamers. The high molecular weight of IgM (970 kDa; approximately 10% carbohydrate) prevents its ready passage into extravascular spaces. IgM is not transported across the placenta and therefore is not involved in hemolytic disease of neonates. It activates complement even more efficiently than IgG. Binding of one IgM molecule may be adequate to activate complement. In rare hyper-IgM syndromes, class switching to IgG and IgA is deficient. Affected patients have deficiency of IgG and IgA and increased susceptibility to infection.[160]

Immunoglobulin A. Immunoglobulin A (IgA) has a molecular weight of 160 kDa, including about 10% carbohydrate derived from both N- and O-linked oligosaccharide chains. IgA accounts for about 10% to 15% of serum immunoglobulin and has a half-life of 6 days. In its monomeric form, its structure is similar to that of IgG, but 10% to 15% of IgA in serum is dimeric, particularly IgA_2, which is more resistant to destruction by pathogenic bacteria than IgA_1. On electrophoresis, IgA migrates in the β-γ region, anodal to most IgG. IgA is an important component of mucosal immunity.[161] Secretory IgA is found in tears, sweat, saliva, milk, colostrum, and gastrointestinal (GI) and bronchial secretions. Secretory IgA has a molecular weight of 380 kDa and consists of two molecules of IgA: a secretory component (70 kDa) and a J chain (15.6 kDa). It is synthesized mainly by plasma cells in the mucous membranes of the gut and bronchi and in the ductules of the lactating breast. The secretory component assists with transport of secretory IgA across mucosal epithelium and into secretions. Secretory IgA in colostrum and milk is more abundant than IgG and may aid in protection of neonates from intestinal infection. IgA can activate complement by the alternative pathway, but the exact role of IgA in serum is not clear.

Immunoglobulin D. Immunoglobulin D (IgD) accounts for less than 1% of serum immunoglobulin. It is monomeric, contains about 12% carbohydrate, and has a molecular weight of 184 kDa. Its structure is similar to that of IgG. Similar to IgM, IgD is a surface receptor for antigen on B lymphocytes, but its primary function is unknown.

Immunoglobulin E. Immunoglobulin E (IgE) contains 15% carbohydrate and has a molecular weight of 188 kDa. IgE is so rapidly and firmly bound to specific IgE receptors on mast cells that only trace amounts of it are normally present in serum. IgE binds to mast cells via sites on its Fc region. When the antigen (allergen) cross-links two of the attached IgE molecules, the mast cell is stimulated to release histamine and other vasoactive amines that increase vascular

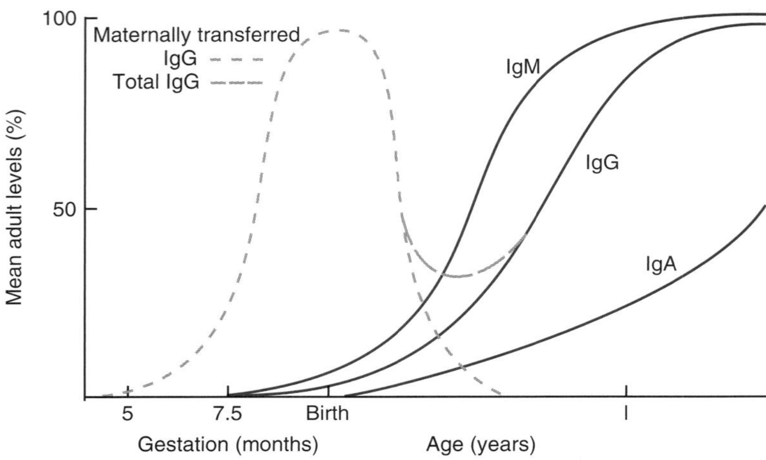

FIGURE 28.5 Serum immunoglobulin concentrations as percent of mean adult concentrations before birth and for the first year of life. *IgA,* Immunoglobulin A; *IgG,* immunoglobulin G; *IgM,* immunoglobulin M.

permeability and smooth muscle contraction, mediating type 1 hypersensitivity reactions such as hay fever, asthma, urticaria, and eczema. Rare regulatory disorders with hyperproduction of IgE lead to a primary immunodeficiency disorder, Job's syndrome, with eczema, recurrent infection, and markedly increased IgE.[162] IgE molecules specific for particular allergens are analyzed to identify the specificity of allergies. The total serum concentration of IgE may be increased in individuals with allergic disorders.

Free Immunoglobulin Light Chains. Light chains are usually synthesized in slight excess versus quantities required for intact immunoglobulins. Consequently, small amounts of free light chain, representing only about 0.1% of total immunoglobulin, are present in serum or plasma. Amounts in plasma are kept low by renal clearance. Free κ-light chains (23 kDa) are cleared about two to three times faster than free λ-light chains (a disulfide-linked dimer of 46 kDa), which have a half-life of 4 to 6 hours. Consequently, even though production of κ-light chains is about twice as great as that of λ-light chains, the plasma concentration of free λ-light chains is usually higher, except in renal failure.[163] Free light chains usually are not functional, but immunoassays specific for free light chains are applied to detect plasma cell disorders.[164]

Clinical Utility of Immunoglobulin Measurement. Serum normally contains a diverse, polyclonal mixture of antibodies with varying amino acid sequences, which represent multiple "idiotypes" (ie, the products of many different clones of plasma cells, each producing a specific immunoglobulin molecule). Benign or malignant proliferation of one such clone produces a high concentration of a single monoclonal antibody, which may appear as a sharp, narrow band on protein electrophoresis. Unbalanced production of free light chains might also lead to a second band representing free light chains. If a few clones proliferate, several sharp bands may be seen. Therefore, disease may be associated with a decrease or an increase in normal polyclonal immunoglobulins or an increase in one or more monoclonal immunoglobulins. These disease states are detailed below.

Immunoglobulin Deficiency. Immunodeficiency states may be the result of deficiency of a single factor or combinations affecting multiple systems of immune defense. The diagnosis of major deficiencies in immunoglobulin production is clinically important to avoid infection as their maternally acquired antibodies decline. Severe combined immune deficiency (SCID) is a disorder of B-cell development or activation affecting 1 in 100,000 newborns and resulting in broad-spectrum immunoglobulin deficiency. The more common primary deficiencies[165] involve only one or two immunoglobulin classes (IgA) or subclasses (IgA or IgG subclasses) or ability to generate antibodies against polysaccharide antigens. IgA deficiency occurs in about 1 in 500 whites but much less frequently in Asian populations. IgA deficiency usually is not associated with severe infection, but the risk of clinically mild infection with *Giardia* or other organisms may be increased. IgA deficiency may lead to false-negative assays for celiac disease detection, and some affected individuals are at risk for anaphylaxis if they receive blood products containing IgA.[166] Selective deficiency of IgG subclasses is not rare, but it is unclear whether it is an important risk for infection. Deficiency of IgG2 may be related to poorer responses to polysaccharide antigens and increased risk of infection with encapsulated organisms.[165]

Infants have transient physiologic deficiency of IgG, with a nadir at about 3 months of age (Fig. 28.5). Prolonged or severe physiologic deficiency may be associated with increased infection rates, especially with encapsulated bacteria. Concentrations of maternal IgG, transferred across the placenta, rise rapidly in the fetus during the last half of pregnancy but then drop over a few months after birth. Two groups of neonates are at risk for clinically significant IgG deficiency: premature infants who begin life with less maternal IgG and infants with delayed initiation of IgG synthesis. Monitoring of IgG concentrations can identify this problem. Rising IgM and normal salivary IgA concentrations at 6 weeks of age suggest a favorable prognosis. Contact of the neonate with environmental antigens normally causes B lymphocytes to begin to multiply and IgM concentrations to start to rise, followed weeks to months later by IgA and IgG.

Polyclonal Hyperimmunoglobulinemia. Polyclonal increases in plasma immunoglobulins are the normal response to infection. IgG predominates in autoimmune responses. IgA is increased in skin, gut, respiratory, and renal infections, and IgM is increased in primary viral infections and bloodstream infection with parasites such as malaria. Chronic

TABLE 28.6 Monoclonal Immunoglobulins (Paraproteins) in Multiple Myeloma

Plasma Paraprotein	Incidence* (%)	Mean Age of Occurrence* (yr)	Incidence of Free Light Chain in Urine (%)	Comments
IgG	50	65	60	Patients more susceptible to infection; paraproteins reach highest concentrations
IgA	25	65	70	Tend to have hypercalcemia and amyloidosis
Free light chain only	20	56	100	Often renal failure; bone lesions; amyloidosis; poor prognosis
IgD	2	57	100	90% λ type; often have extraosseous lesion, amyloidosis, renal failure; poor prognosis
IgM	1	—	100	May or may not have hyperviscosity syndrome
IgE	0.1	—	Most	—
Biclonal	1	—	—	—
None detected	<1	—	0	Usually reduction of normal immunoglobulins; increased plasma cells in bone marrow biopsy

*Approximate.
Ig, Immunoglobulin.

bacterial infection may cause increased concentrations of all immunoglobulins. Measurements of total IgE are used in the management of asthma and other allergic conditions, especially in children. Measurements of allergen-specific IgE assist in identifying the stimulus for hypersensitivity responses.

Monoclonal Immunoglobulins (Paraproteins). A single clone of plasma cells produces immunoglobulin molecules with a single defined amino acid sequence. If the clone expands greatly, it may produce a discrete band on electrophoresis, often referred to as an M-spike or M-protein. These monoclonal immunoglobulins, termed *paraproteins,* may be polymers, monomers, individual immunoglobulin chains such as free light chains or heavy chains, or fragments of immunoglobulins. Clinical, epidemiologic, and biochemical characteristics of monoclonal paraprotein diseases are summarized in Table 28.6. About 60% of paraproteins are associated with plasma cell malignancies (multiple myeloma or solitary plasmacytoma), and approximately 15% are caused by overproduction by B lymphocytes, mainly in lymph nodes (lymphomas, chronic lymphocytic leukemia, Waldenström's macroglobulinemia, or heavy-chain disease). Up to 25% of paraproteins are benign and have been termed *monoclonal gammopathy of undetermined significance (MGUS).* The incidence of MGUS increases with age, with 1% incidence for people 50 to 70 years of age and 3% incidence for people older than 70. The occurrence of MGUS is associated with increased risk of progression to multiple myeloma that should be monitored. Multiple myeloma appears to be preceded consistently by MGUS.[167]

The primary clinical interest in identifying paraproteins is to detect or monitor proliferative disorders of B cells. However, from the laboratory standpoint, paraproteins are also significant as a potentially unpredictable source of interference with many assays. Paraproteins may aggregate or precipitate, causing interference in a variety of photometric reactions and in light-scattering hematology analyzers.

Many patients with paraproteins have nonspecific presentations such as anemia or infection. Identification of paraproteins in serum usually is based on serum protein electrophoresis and immunofixation electrophoresis (IFE) (described in a later section). Urine protein electrophoresis and urine IFE are helpful mainly in identifying patients with free immunoglobulin light chains. Urinary free light chains, as described by Bence Jones in the 1850s, were the first tumor marker. Free light chains are often referred to as *Bence Jones proteins.*[168]

Acute Phase Response

Systemic inflammation in response to infection, tissue injury, or inflammatory disease triggers changes in hepatic production of multiple plasma proteins, as indicated in Box 28.1. This process, mediated by the action of interleukin-6 (IL-6) and other cytokines has been termed the *acute-phase response* (APR).[153] It is a nonspecific reaction to inflammation, analogous to the increase in temperature or leukocyte count. In the APR, synthesis of a few proteins, including albumin, transferrin, and prealbumin, is downregulated. These proteins are termed *negative acute-phase reactants.* Albumin concentrations fall because of acutely decreased synthesis and from redistribution to extracellular fluids. Production of a number of proteins, including AAT, α_1-acid glycoprotein (AAG), Hp, Cp, C4, C3, fibrinogen, and CRP, increases several-fold. Plasma concentrations of individual acute-phase proteins rise at different rates, and all reach maxima within 2 to 5 days after an acute insult. Qualitative changes in proteins, such as altered glycosylation, are also observed secondary to the APR. Changes to glycosylation of immunoglobulins may have an immunomodulatory effect.

Methods for Analyzing Proteins

Determination of Total Protein

Plasma normally contains about 6.5 to 8.5 g/dL protein and serum about 4% less. Determination of total protein in biologic fluids in some respects represents a greater challenge than analysis of a specific protein because variable protein composition of biologic fluids leads to variable carbohydrate composition, charge, and physical characteristics of proteins in the mixture. Many methods of protein analysis respond differentially to different proteins and present problems when applied to specimens of varying protein composition. Most methods other than the biuret method have not been thoroughly examined for interactions with small peptide components as well as intact proteins, and this may become a

BOX 28.1 The Acute Phase Response: Changes in Plasma Protein Concentrations

Positive Acute Phase Response
C-reactive protein (extreme)
Serum amyloid A (extreme)
α1-Acid glycoprotein
α1-Antitrypsin
α1-Antichymotrypsin
Antithrombin III
C3, C4, and C9
C1 inhibitor
C4b-binding protein
Ceruloplasmin
Factor B
Ferritin
Fibrinogen
Haptoglobin
Hemopexin
Lipopolysaccharide-binding protein
Mannan-binding protein (lectin)
Plasminogen
Procalcitonin

Negative Acute Phase Response
Albumin
Apolipoprotein A-I
Apolipoprotein B
α2-HS glycoprotein
Insulin-like growth factor I
Prealbumin
Retinol-binding protein
Thyroxine-binding globulin
Transferrin

Data from Craig WY, Ledue TB, Ritchie RF. *Plasma proteins: clinical utility and interpretation.* Scarborough, ME: Foundation for Blood Research, 2001; Gabay C, Kushner I. Acute-phase proteins and other systemic responses to inflammation. *N Engl J Med* 1999;340:448–454; and Vollmer T, Piper C, Kleesiek K, Dreier J. Lipopolysaccharide-binding protein: a new biomarker for infectious endocarditis? *Clin Chem* 2009;55:295–302.

significant issue in renal failure with increased accumulation of peptides and small proteins. Many methods have been developed to measure the total protein content of biologic fluids. Several are reviewed here.

Kjeldahl Method. This method is rarely used in clinical laboratories but is of historical importance and is sometimes used as a reference method. Protein nitrogen is converted to ammonium ion by heating with sulfuric acid in the presence of a catalyst. Ammonium ion is measured by alkalinization, distillation, and acid titration or by Nessler's reagent. Protein is estimated to contain 16% nitrogen. Errors in protein estimation occur if the amino acid composition is unusual and if nitrogen content differs from 16%. Nonprotein nitrogen, such as from urea and amino acids, also is measured, so a protein precipitation step may be required. The Kjeldahl method was one of the first methods used for reproducible total protein measurement, but it is time consuming and impractical for routine use. This method has been used to assign values to reference materials for the biuret method.

Biuret Method. Under strongly alkaline conditions, Cu^{2+} ions form multivalent complexes with peptide bonds in proteins. Binding shifts the absorption spectrum of Cu^{2+} ions to shorter wavelengths, leading to a color change from blue to violet that has been termed the *biuret reaction*. Absorbance attributable to protein is measured spectrophotometrically at 540 nm. Absorbance changes at 540 nm also result from binding of Cu^{2+} ions by many compounds that can form chelates with five- or six-member rings where amino, amide, or hydroxyl groups bind to Cu^{2+} ions. Such compounds include serine, asparagine, ethanolamine, and TRIS buffer, among others.[169] Small compounds lead to a smaller spectral shift than proteins. Historically, the biuret method was not considered to react with free amino acids and dipeptides, but absorbance changes occur with some amino acids, with amino acid amides, and with dipeptides. The biuret action also was considered to react equally with all proteins and peptides longer than two amino acids, but subsequently, peptides containing proline were noted to have reduced reactivity. As long as proteins are not extremely proline rich or do not have a very unusual composition, different proteins probably have similar reactivities as long as the biuret reaction is performed in the typical endpoint manner. Biuret rate assays are also available but should be considered as a separate category from endpoint assays. Cu^{2+} ions complex with small molecules and accessible sites in proteins almost instantaneously while additional absorbance change depends on the rate of unfolding of a protein and exposure of additional binding sites for Cu^{2+} ions under strongly alkaline conditions.

Direct Optical Methods. Absorbance of ultraviolet (UV) light between 200 to 225 nm and 270 to 290 nm has been used to measure protein concentrations and is commonly applied to monitor chromatographic separations of peptides and proteins. Absorbance at 280 nm depends primarily on the tryptophan and tyrosine content of a protein. This technique works best for purified proteins with known absorptivity. For complex mixtures, accuracy and specificity suffer from variable content of tryptophan and tyrosine and from absorbance of low molecular weight compounds such as free amino acids, uric acid, and bilirubin. From 200 to 225 nm, peptide bonds are chiefly responsible for UV absorbance. Absorptivity by proteins at these shorter wavelengths is 10 to 30 times greater than at 280 nm. Many low molecular weight compounds such as urea also have absorbance at wavelengths below 220 nm. Accurate measurement of proteins by this method may require removal of low molecular weight molecules before absorbance measurements are performed. Several other optical methods using infrared or Raman analysis of specimens offer methods for total protein determination based on complex spectral analysis.

Dye-Binding Methods. Dye-binding methods depend on shifts in the absorbance spectra of dyes when they bind to proteins. Variable binding of dyes to different proteins is a limitation. Calibration with a protein mixture is particularly difficult to define consistently. Calibration with a pure protein such as albumin may not simulate binding to the complex mixture of proteins in serum or plasma. Using Coomassie blue, for example, immunoglobulins often give only 60% of the response of an equivalent concentration of albumin or transferrin. This dye binds to polypeptide chains under acidic conditions, resulting in decreased absorbance at 465 nm and increased absorbance at 595 nm. Some dyes offer sensitivity at low protein concentrations. Pyrogallol red, for instance, has become one of the most commonly used dyes for analysis of fluids with lower protein concentrations such as urine and CSF.

Lowry (Folin-Ciocalteu) Method. The detection limit of the Lowry method is about 100 times lower than that of the biuret method.[170] In this technique, specimens are mixed with an alkaline copper solution followed by addition of the Folin-Ciocalteu reagent. Phosphotungstic acid and phosphomolybdic acid are reduced to tungsten blue and molybdenum blue by copper complexed with peptide and by tyrosine and tryptophan residues. Absorbance of products is measured between 650 and 750 nm. Reactivity of proteins varies with the content of tyrosine and tryptophan. Low molecular weight compounds, including tryptophan and tyrosine as well as drugs such as salicylates, chlorpromazine, tetracyclines, and some sulfa drugs, also interfere. Analysis of a fluid such as urine with high concentrations of phenolic compounds requires removal of low molecular weight substances before protein is measured.

Refractometry. Refractometry is a method used to rapidly estimate protein at high concentrations. Accuracy decreases at protein concentrations below 3.5 g/dL, where salts, glucose, and other low molecular weight compounds have a larger proportional effect on refractive index. Refractometry is used more often in clinical laboratories to assess the concentration of solutes in urine specimens than for determining total protein.

Light-Scattering Methods. Many different reagents have been used to aggregate protein for turbidimetric or nephelometric assays, including trichloroacetic acid, sulfosalicylic acid, benzethonium chloride, and benzalkonium salts under alkaline conditions. Precipitation methods for total protein assay depend on forming a suspension of uniform, insoluble protein particles, which scatter incident light. Albumin and globulins often give different reactivities in precipitation methods.

Variables Affecting Measured Protein Concentrations. Calibration of biuret methods commonly uses bovine or human albumin. Protein mixtures with specific albumin-to-globulin ratios often have been recommended for calibration of other methods. Using these calibration schemes, the total protein concentration of plasma obtained from healthy ambulatory adults is typically 6.5 to 8.5 g/dL. Serum usually contains a protein concentration about 0.3 g/dL less because of the content of fibrinogen and other proteins removed during clotting to form serum. Hemoconcentration and relative hyperproteinemia, with increased concentrations of all plasma proteins, occur with inadequate water intake or excessive water loss as in severe vomiting, diarrhea, Addison's disease, or diabetic ketoacidosis. Some hemoconcentration also occurs with standing (reduced intravascular volume) or prolonged tourniquet time during blood collection. Hemodilution and relative hypoproteinemia, with decreased concentrations of all plasma proteins, occur with water intoxication or salt retention syndromes, during massive intravenous infusions, and physiologically when a recumbent position is assumed. A recumbent position decreases total protein concentration by 0.3 to 0.5 g/dL and many individual proteins, including albumin, by up to 10%. This reflects the redistribution of extracellular fluid from the extravascular space to the intravascular space and therefore dilution of a constant amount of plasma protein in a larger volume.

Immunochemical Techniques for Specific Proteins

Nephelometric and turbidimetric methods are performed as equilibrium or rate methods for measuring the amount of light scattering by antigen–antibody complexes (see Chapter 13). Limits of detection of approximately 10 mg/L are attained with routine nephelometric and turbidimetric methods using antibodies in solution. Binding antibodies to particles of latex or other materials enhances light scattering and can lower limits of detection by 10- to 100-fold. Such assays may be described as latex-enhanced or as particle-enhanced assays. Nephelometric and turbidimetric assays commonly offer within-run coefficients of variation (CVs) of less than 5% except as limits of detection are approached. Turbidimetric methods can be applied on most automated chemistry analyzers capable of performing photometric methods. Nephelometry requires instrumentation capable of measuring light scattering at an angle to the incident light.

Electrophoresis

Electrophoresis is used to separate proteins by charge and thereby to assess protein variants or the concentrations of specific components in serum or other fluids. Electrophoretic techniques commonly performed in clinical laboratories include nondenaturing electrophoresis on cellulose acetate strips or agarose gels, capillary electrophoresis (CE), immunofixation, and "Western blotting." Protein separation in one or two dimensions with polyacrylamide gel is a powerful separation technique frequently used for research.

Serum Protein Electrophoresis. Generally, serum rather than plasma is used for electrophoresis of proteins on agarose gels to avoid the fibrinogen band at the β-γ interface. The principles of electrophoresis are described in Chapter 15. Fig. 28.6 illustrates examples of serum electrophoretic patterns for normal and pathologic specimens. Analysis usually is performed with low ionic strength buffers (0.05 mol/L) at slightly basic pH (~8.6). For agarose gels, the usual sample is 3 to 5 µL. Much smaller volumes are injected for CE. Separation and processing times are typically about 1 hour for agarose gels and a few minutes for CE. A variety of stains are used to visualize proteins in gels, including amido black, Ponceau S, acid violet, and Coomassie blue. Levels of detection and linearity of protein detection vary with different dyes. Only a few of the most abundant proteins are visualized, and intensities of bands with protein stains usually relate to the mass of peptide; oligosaccharides and lipids may reduce rather than contribute to band intensities. Therefore, glycoproteins with a high proportion of carbohydrate (eg, α_1 acid glycoprotein) have lower detection responses than a nonglycosylated protein such as albumin. Quantitative analysis relies on densitometry, which provides relative proportions of different components rather than absolute amounts. Quantitation of individual components relies on calculations derived from total protein concentration. Lipophilic stains such as Sudan black are needed to visualize lipoproteins such as high-density lipoprotein (α_1-lipoprotein), very-low-density lipoprotein (pre-β-region), low-density lipoprotein (LDL; β-lipoprotein), or chylomicrons (origin) (see also Chapter 34). CE detects proteins passing through a flow cell by their light absorbance at wavelengths below 220 nm. This offers a more unbiased

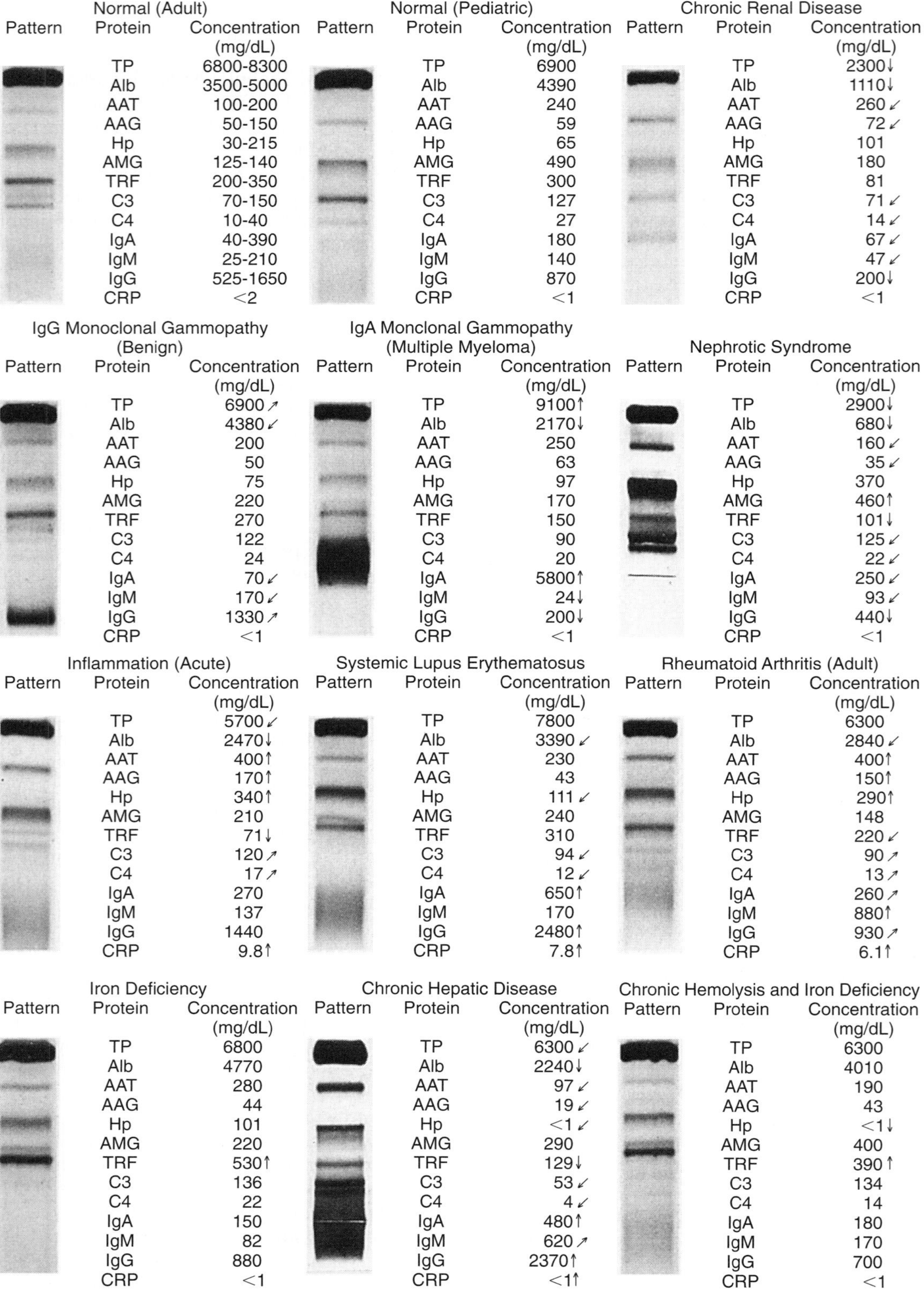

Protein	Normal (Adult) Concentration (mg/dL)	Normal (Pediatric) Concentration (mg/dL)	Chronic Renal Disease Concentration (mg/dL)	IgG Monoclonal Gammopathy (Benign) Concentration (mg/dL)	IgA Monclonal Gammopathy (Multiple Myeloma) Concentration (mg/dL)	Nephrotic Syndrome Concentration (mg/dL)	Inflammation (Acute) Concentration (mg/dL)	Systemic Lupus Erythematosus Concentration (mg/dL)	Rheumatoid Arthritis (Adult) Concentration (mg/dL)	Iron Deficiency Concentration (mg/dL)	Chronic Hepatic Disease Concentration (mg/dL)	Chronic Hemolysis and Iron Deficiency Concentration (mg/dL)
TP	6800-8300	6900	2300↓	6900↗	9100↑	2900↓	5700↙	7800	6300	6800	6300↙	6300
Alb	3500-5000	4390	1110↓	4380↙	2170↓	680↓	2470↓	3390↙	2840↙	4770	2240↓	4010
AAT	100-200	240	260↙	200	250	160↙	400↑	230	400↑	280	97↙	190
AAG	50-150	59	72↙	50	63	35↙	170↑	43	150↑	44	19↙	43
Hp	30-215	65	101	75	97	370	340↑	111↙	290↑	101	<1↙	<1↓
AMG	125-140	490	180	220	170	460↑	210	240	148	220	290	400
TRF	200-350	300	81	270	150	101↓	71↓	310	220↙	530↑	129↓	390↑
C3	70-150	127	71↙	122	90	125↙	120↗	94↙	90↗	136	53↙	134
C4	10-40	27	14↙	24	20	22↙	17↗	12↙	13↗	22	4↙	14
IgA	40-390	180	67↙	70↙	5800↑	250↙	270	650↑	260↗	150	480↑	180
IgM	25-210	140	47↙	170↙	24↓	93↙	137	170	880↑	82	620↗	170
IgG	525-1650	870	200↓	1330↗	200↓	440↓	1440	2480↑	930↗	880	2370↑	700
CRP	<2	<1	<1	<1	<1	<1	9.8↑	7.8↑	6.1↑	<1	<1↑	<1

FIGURE 28.6 Electrophoretic patterns typical of normal conditions and of some pathologic conditions (agarose gel). The *upward-* and *downward-pointing arrows* indicate increase and decrease from the reference interval, respectively. *Right-* and *left-slanting arrows* indicate variation from normal to an increase or from normal to a decrease from the reference interval, respectively. *AAG,* Alpha-1 acid glycoprotein; *AAT,* alpha-1 antitrypsin; *Alb,* albumin; *AMG,* alpha-2 macroglobulin; *C3,* complement component 3; *C4,* complement component 4; *CRP,* C-reactive protein; *Hp,* haptoglobin; *Ig,* immunoglobulin; *TP,* total protein concentration; *TRF,* transferrin.

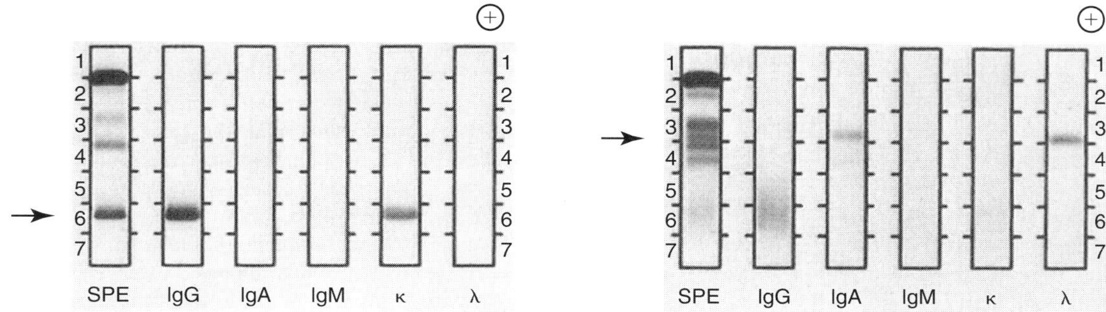

FIGURE 28.7 Immunofixation electrophoresis (IFE). *Left,* Patient specimen with an immunoglobulin G (IgG; κ) monoclonal protein. *Right,* Patient specimen with an immunoglobulin A (IgA; λ) monoclonal protein. The *arrow* indicates the position of monoclonal protein.

assessment of protein concentration than staining intensity because absorbance of proteins in the low ultraviolet region is more consistently related to mass. Small molecules at high concentrations, such as metabolites, radiocontrast dyes, or drugs, may also yield absorbance peaks, and this presents problems with analysis of urine specimens.

The major clinical application of serum protein electrophoresis is the detection of monoclonal immunoglobulins (paraproteins) to assist in the diagnosis and monitoring of multiple myeloma and related disorders. Most monoclonal immunoglobulins are observed in the β-region or γ-region. Quantitation of monoclonal components serves as a means of monitoring disease progression and response to therapy. Identification of paraproteins requires distinction from a variety of other sources of additional bands or pseudoparaproteins by means such as IFE as described later. Incompletely clotted specimens contain fibrinogen. Genetic or posttranslational variants of proteins such as transferrin, Hp, and C3 may migrate in different positions than usual. Large increases in CRP may yield a detectable band in the β- or γ-region. Increased lysozyme in monocytic leukemia may produce a band in the post-γ-region. Hemoglobin will yield a band in hemolyzed specimens.

Protein electrophoresis is capable of being informative in many other clinical circumstances. Changes in the α_1-region are typically related to AAT. Decreases are associated with AAT deficiency or protein-losing disorders. Increases are related to inflammation. Changes in the α_2-region usually relate to changes in Hp and α_2 macroglobulin (AMG). Migration of Hp varies with genotype. Hp decreases with in vivo hemolysis and increases with inflammation. AMG and high molecular weight forms of Hp increase in nephrotic syndrome, but most other protein components decrease. Bands in the β-region are related to transferrin, C3, and LDL. Migration of transferrin may change from the β_1-region to the β_2-region when significant carbohydrate deficient forms are present. An increase between β- and γ-bands, so-called bridging of β- and γ-bands, suggests an increase in IgA as seen with cirrhosis, respiratory tract or skin infection, and rheumatoid arthritis. Finally, increases or decreases in the γ-region suggest changes in immunoglobulins. Increases result from chronic infection or paraproteins. Decreases occur with many immunodeficiency states. Multiple myeloma may suppress global production of immunoglobulins other than from the expanded clone. A decrease in the γ-region may suggest the need for additional studies such as IFE to detect paraproteins.

Immunofixation Electrophoresis. Immunofixation electrophoresis is complementary to serum protein electrophoresis and employs antisera targeted to specific proteins rather than nonspecific dyes. Examples of IFE from two patients with monoclonal gammopathies are shown in Fig. 28.7. Specific lanes of the gel are overlaid with antisera against κ and λ light chains or γ, μ, and α-immunoglobulin heavy chains. Antibody dilutions are adjusted to provide approximate equivalence with immunoglobulins separated in the gel so as to form immune complexes precipitated in the gel. Proteins not precipitated are washed from the gel to lower background, and precipitated proteins are stained. Paraproteins characteristically yield sharper precipitin bands than the heterogeneous polyclonal immunoglobulins. IFE provides more sensitive detection of paraproteins because of the lower background and signal amplification from immune complex formation. Additionally, immunofixation helps identify the immunoglobulin type of the paraprotein. Sometimes more than one clone may be expanded, or free light chain may occur together with intact immunoglobulin. Uncommonly, paraproteins may be of the IgD or IgE class. These paraproteins should be detected by antisera versus light chains but require δ or ε heavy chain–specific antisera to distinguish them from free light chains. High concentrations of paraproteins may interfere with fixation (prozone effect) requiring specimen dilution for optimal studies. For paraproteins present in high concentrations, quantitative analysis of immunoglobulins can confirm the unbalanced production of a specific class of immunoglobulin and may assist in proper dilution of specimens for immunofixation.

Capillary Electrophoresis. Capillary electrophoresis of proteins relies on zone electrophoresis in small-bore (10–100 μm), fused silica capillary tubes 20 to 200 cm in length (see Chapter 15). Electrokinetic or hydrostatic injection introduces a small amount of protein that is resolved rapidly under high voltage. One of the challenges is to avoid adsorption of proteins to the surface of the capillary. CE is suitable for automation and offers rapid analysis with no need for gel handling or staining. Direct UV detection offers slightly different specificity than protein staining and offers better reproducibility of quantitation than densitometry. Immunofixation cannot be performed with CE. Immunosubtraction with specific antisera is used as an alternative procedure to identify paraproteins.[171]

Western Blotting. For Western blotting, proteins separated on a gel are transferred by diffusion or electroblotting onto a membrane made of nitrocellulose or polyvinylidene fluoride. Proteins bound on the membrane are identified with specific antibodies conjugated to enzymes such as peroxidase or alkaline phosphatase that act on photometric, fluorescent, or chemiluminescent signaling molecules.

Mass Spectrometry. Multiple types of MS instrumentation provide qualitative or quantitative information about proteins (see Chapter 21). An advantage of MS is the ability to analyze a large number of components in a single analysis, including rapid-sequence analysis of peptides. MS, therefore, has been an enabling technology in *proteomics,* defined as the effort to study the complete set of proteins in an organism or in subcompartments of an organism such as plasma. Ionization of peptides and proteins has been accomplished by electrospray or MALDI sources. Electrospray is better suited to analyzing small peptides than larger intact proteins. After ionization, proteins can be separated by quadrupoles, ion traps, time-of-flight, and other types of mass analyzers. Use of tandem MS with an intermediate fragmentation step between two stages of MS separation offers high sensitivity and specificity for the quantitative analysis of peptides, as it does for most small molecules.

Advantages of using MS for quantitative analysis include the ability to analyze components without developing specific antibodies and the ability to multiplex a large number of measurements. MS can provide information about posttranslational modifications that is difficult to assess by immunoassays and chromatographic or electrophoretic techniques. Examples of clinical applications include identification of genetic variants of prealbumin and CDT. The use of MS is likely to increase for accurate determination of protein concentrations as recently applied for standardization of hemoglobin A_{1c}, insulin, and C-peptide.[172,173] Likewise, MS is also able to distinguish peptides differing in length by one or two amino acids or by a posttranslational modification. For these reasons, MS is likely to find increased use for clinical laboratory analysis of bioactive peptides and other components of the peptidome.

Proteins in Other Body Fluids

Complex mixtures of proteins are present in all biologic fluids; analysis of a variety of other specimens is diagnostically useful, including analyses of urine (see Chapter 32), CSF, pleural and peritoneal fluids (see Chapter 43), amniotic fluid (see Chapter 69), saliva, and feces.

Saliva

Saliva has a very different protein composition compared with plasma.[174,175] Protein composition varies with the site and method of sampling of saliva. In addition to the well-known presence of amylase, proteomic approaches have detected sequence from hundreds of different proteins in saliva. Proteins involved in host defense against pathogens such as immunoglobulins, lysozyme, and lactoferrin are also particularly abundant. Efforts are under way to exploit the salivary proteome to detect and characterize susceptibility to dental caries, periodontal disease, head and neck cancers, diabetes, and cystic fibrosis. Patients with Sjögren syndrome exhibit increased concentrations of β_2 MG and other inflammatory proteins compared with normal patients. Interrogation of saliva for the presence of secretory IgA is common in the diagnostic workup of hypogammaglobulinemia.

Cerebrospinal Fluid

Cerebrospinal fluid is the extracellular fluid around the brain and spinal column. CSF usually has total protein concentrations about 100-fold lower than plasma and a different protein composition because most proteins have limited passage across the blood–brain barrier. CSF for testing is most frequently obtained by a spinal tap in the lumbar region. CSF is secreted by the choroid plexus, around the cerebral vessels, and along the walls of the ventricles of the brain. It fills the ventricles and cisternae, bathes the spinal cord, and is reabsorbed into the blood through the arachnoid villi. CSF turnover is rapid, exchanging totally about four times daily. More than 80% of CSF protein content originates from plasma by ultrafiltration and pinocytosis; the remainder is derived from intrathecal synthesis. The lowest protein concentration and the smallest proportion of larger protein molecules are in the ventricular fluid. As the CSF passes down to the lumbar spine (where specimens are usually collected), the protein concentration increases.

Low to intermediate molecular weight plasma proteins such as prealbumin, albumin, and transferrin normally predominate because CSF is mainly an ultrafiltrate of plasma. No protein with a molecular weight greater than that of IgG is present in sufficient concentration to be visible on electrophoresis. The normal plasma/CSF gradient is about 14 for prealbumin, 240 for albumin, 140 for transferrin, 800 for IgG, and more than 1000 for larger proteins such as IgA, AMG, fibrinogen, IgM, and β-lipoprotein.[176]

The electrophoretic pattern of normal CSF after concentration of the fluid has two striking features—a prealbumin band and two transferrin bands—one at β_2 in addition to the usual β_1 position. As mentioned previously, β_2-transferrin has decreased charge because its glyosyl chains lack terminal sialic acid residues. Both β_2-transferrin and another relatively abundant CSF protein, prostaglandin D synthase or β-trace, have been used to determine whether clear fluids from nasal or ear passages represent leakage of CSF, so-called CSF rhinorrhea and otorrhea.[147] The utility of β2-transferrin in this context is compromised in patients with congenital disorders of glycosylation. Prostaglandin D synthase is a protein of about 30 kDa that is relatively enriched in CSF relative to serum or plasma, where it normally is cleared rapidly by glomerular filtration. Apolipoprotein E (ApoE) is also abundant in CSF because it plays a primary role in lipid transport rather than apo AI– and apo B100–containing lipoproteins, which are relatively scarce in CSF.

The blood–brain or blood–CSF barrier limits exchange of many compounds, particularly large compounds such as proteins. Analyses of total protein and specific proteins in CSF are used primarily to detect increased permeability of the blood–CSF barrier, increased intrathecal synthesis, or increased release of proteins from neural and glial tissue. Conditions such as viral meningitis, encephalitis, increased intracranial pressure, trauma, and hemorrhage may all compromise the blood–brain barrier, resulting in increased CSF protein. Protein concentrations associated with these conditions are displayed in Table 28.7. Increased intrathecal synthesis of immunoglobulins, particularly IgG, occurs in demyelinating diseases of the CNS, especially multiple sclerosis. Methods used to assess potential abnormalities in CSF protein content are detailed next.

TABLE 28.7 Cerebrospinal Fluid Total Protein in Various Diseases

Clinical Condition	Appearance and Cells × 10^6/L	Total Protein, mg/dL
Normal	Clear, colorless; 0–5 lymphocytes	15–45*
INCREASED ADMIXTURE OF PROTEINS FROM BLOOD		
Increased capillary permeability		
• Bacterial meningitis	Turbid, opalescent, purulent, usually >500 polymorphs	80–500
• Cryptococcal meningitis	Clear or turbid; 50–150 polymorphs or lymphocytes	25–200
• Leptospiral meningitis	Clear to slight haze; polymorphs early, then 5–100 lymphocytes	50–100
• Viral meningitis	Clear or slight haze, colorless; usually ≤500 lymphocytes	30–100
• Encephalitis	Clear or slight haze, colorless; usually ≤500 lymphocytes	15–100
• Poliomyelitis	Clear, colorless; ≤500 lymphocytes	10–300
• Brain tumor	Usually clear; 0–80 lymphocytes	15–200 (usually normal)
Mechanical obstruction:		
• Spinal cord tumor†	Clear, colorless, or yellow	100–2000
Hemorrhage		
Cerebral hemorrhage	Colorless, yellow, or bloody; blood cells	30–150
Local immunoglobulin production		
• Neurosyphilis	Clear, colorless; 10–100 lymphocytes	50–150
• Multiple sclerosis‡	Clear, colorless; 0–10 lymphocytes	25–50
Both increased capillary permeability and local immunoglobulin production:		
• Tuberculous meningitis	Colorless, fibrin clot, or slightly turbid; 50–500 lymphocytes	50–300 (occasionally ≤1000)
• Brain abscess	Clear or slightly turbid	20–120
After myelography (inflammatory reaction)		Slight increase

*Premature infants: ≤400 mg/dL; children: 30–100 mg/dL; older adults: ≤60 mg/dL.
†Froin syndrome: Lumbar fluid values are much higher than cisternal fluid values.
‡Similar values may occur in certain other chronic inflammatory conditions of the nervous system.

Total Protein in Cerebrospinal Fluid. The total protein concentration in CSF is an indicator of blood–CSF permeability. The protein concentration of CSF usually is more than 100-fold lower than for plasma, and methods with greater sensitivity or increased specimen volume are required for measuring total serum or plasma protein. In practice, methods commonly used by clinical laboratories to measure total CSF protein include (1) pyrogallol red, (2) benzethonium chloride, (3) reverse-biuret, and (4) biuret. The reverse-biuret method measures free copper remaining after formation of biuret complexes by reduction and complexation with a chelating dye. Analyzers often use the same method, possibly with some adjustment of specimen volume, for CSF and urine protein. The usual reference interval for CSF total protein is 15 to 45 mg/dL. Total protein concentrations are considerably higher in neonates and in healthy elderly adults. In CSF from premature and full-term neonates, concentrations up to 400 mg/dL are observed. In term newborns, a progressive decline in the reference interval CSF protein is seen over the first few weeks of life, with values approaching adult concentrations after 4 months of age.[177]

Permeability of the Blood–Brain Barrier. A more specific measure of the permeability of the blood–CSF barrier involves determination of the ratio of albumin concentration in CSF versus plasma. This ratio, the *CSF/serum albumin index,* usually is calculated for CSF albumin in milligrams per deciliter and for serum protein in grams per liter, effectively multiplying values by 1000. A CSF–serum albumin index less than 9 indicates an intact blood–CSF barrier. Values of 9 to 14 represent slight impairment, 14 to 30 moderate impairment, and greater than 30 severe impairment. The index helps correct for variation in serum albumin concentration.

Intrathecal Protein Synthesis. Measurement of the CSF–serum immunoglobulin ratio and assessment of oligoclonal immunoglobulin bands on electrophoretic separations of CSF serve as assays for intrathecal immunoglobulin synthesis. At least 90% of cases of multiple sclerosis give positive findings, but increased immunoglobulins and oligoclonal immunoglobulins may be found in other inflammatory diseases of the CNS, such as infection caused by bacteria, viruses, fungi, or parasites; neurosyphilis; subacute sclerosing panencephalitis; and Guillain-Barré syndrome. Multiple sclerosis is less likely if CSF total protein exceeds 100 mg/dL or if the CSF leukocyte count is greater than 50/μL. The CSF albumin concentration in 70% of cases of multiple sclerosis is within the reference interval. Increases in CSF IgG concentration or in the CSF–serum IgG ratio may result from increased permeability of the blood–CSF barrier, increased local production of IgG, or both. To identify intrathecal production specifically, correction for increased permeability is necessary. Corrections use *CSF and serum* albumin and IgG concentrations in one of several ways:

1. Concentrations *in CSF* of IgG and albumin are measured, and the IgG–albumin ratio is calculated. A ratio greater than 0.27 is considered indicative of increased synthesis;

in about 70% of cases of multiple sclerosis, the ratio exceeds 0.27.

$$\text{Ratio} = \frac{\text{IgG}_{\text{CSF}}\,(\text{mg/dL})}{\text{Albumin}_{\text{CSF}}\,(\text{mg/dL})}$$

2. Concentrations in *CSF and serum* of IgG and albumin are measured, and the CSF immunoglobulin index is calculated.

$$\text{Index} = \frac{\text{IgG}_{\text{CSF}}\,(\text{mg/dL}) \times \text{Albumin}_{\text{serum}}\,(\text{g/dL})}{\text{Albumin}_{\text{CSF}}\,(\text{mg/dL}) \times \text{IgG}_{\text{serum}}\,(\text{g/dL})}$$

The reference interval for the index is 0.30 to 0.70. Values greater than 0.70 indicate increased IgG synthesis; in more than 80% of cases of multiple sclerosis, this index exceeds 0.70. This CSF immunoglobulin index is now frequently used.

3. The rate of intrathecal IgG synthesis is estimated by Tourtellotte's formula.[178] The rate of synthesis of IgG in milligrams per day is equal to:

$$5\ \text{dL/d}\left[\left\{\text{IgG}_{\text{CSF}} - \frac{\text{IgG}_{\text{serum}}}{369}\right\} - \left\{\left(\text{Albumin}_{\text{CSF}} - \frac{\text{Albumin}_{\text{serum}}}{230}\right) \times \frac{0.43\,(\text{IgG}_{\text{serum}})}{\text{Albumin}_{\text{serum}}}\right\}\right]$$

where protein concentrations are in mg/dL. The 5 dL/d term is daily CSF production. The first bracketed term represents the difference between IgG found in CSF and the IgG expected if the blood–brain barrier is intact. The second bracketed term represents the same for albumin but is corrected by a factor of 0.43, corresponding to the ratio of molecular weights of albumin to IgG, assuming that 1 mole of IgG accompanies every mole of albumin that passes the blood-brain barrier. The constants 369 and 230 originate from the normal serum–CSF ratios for IgG and albumin. The reference interval for the synthesis rate is 0 to 3.3 mg/d. Values exceeding 8 mg/d are found in most cases of multiple sclerosis. This estimator provides no more clinical information than the IgG index; the complex formula merely rearranges the results for serum and CSF IgG and albumin and then factors in several constants.

In addition to albumin and IgG, the concentrations of other CSF proteins may shed light on other disease processes. Myelin basic protein concentrations may be an indicator of myelin turnover in multiple sclerosis.[179] A number of other proteins such as S100B and neuron-specific enolase are potential markers of traumatic or ischemic brain injury.[180] In acute leukemia and lymphoma with central nervous system involvement, the concentration of β_2 MG is increased in CSF. Concentrations of tau and β-amyloid isoforms may be useful in the diagnosis and prognosis of Alzheimer disease.[181]

Peritoneal and Pleural Fluids

Pathologic accumulations of fluid in the peritoneal and pleural cavities or elsewhere vary greatly in protein content. These fluids may be ultrafiltrates with low-protein concentrations relative to plasma and scant amounts of large proteins (transudates). Alternatively, fluids may have protein concentrations approaching those of plasma and significant amounts of large proteins such as immunoglobulins and AMG (exudates) in response to local inflammation and increased vascular permeability. Distinction between transudates and exudates assists in diagnosing the cause of fluid accumulation. The major cause of pleural transudates is congestive heart failure. Exudates occur with infection, pleuritis, pulmonary embolism, and cancer. Criteria for identifying exudates in pleural fluid were proposed by Light.[182] According to these criteria ratios of (1) pleural fluid protein to serum protein greater than 0.5, (2) pleural lactate dehydrogenase (LDH) to serum LDH activity greater than 0.6, and (3)c) total pleural fluid LDH greater than 200 IU/L likely result from an exudative process.[183] Pleural fluid may be turbid from large numbers of white blood cells (WBCs), fibrin particles, or chylomicrons. Chylous effusions (containing chylomicrons) result from lymphatic obstruction related to cancer, surgery, trauma, sarcoidosis, or other causes.[184] Lymphatics, particularly the major trunk, the thoracic duct, serve as the major route for chylomicrons from the intestines to the blood circulation. Entry of chylomicrons into the pleural space, therefore, is related in part to dietary fat intake to generate chylomicrons, and fasting lowers the fat content of chylous effusions. Chylomicrons in fluids may be identified by separation of a cream layer upon standing or by triglycerides analysis. For peritoneal fluid, the serum to ascites albumin gradient (ie, the difference between serum and peritoneal fluid albumin) helps distinguish transudates (mainly in portal hypertension from cirrhosis) from infection and other causes of ascites. Usually, the serum to ascites albumin gradient is greater than 1.1 g/dL in portal hypertension and is lower than 1.1 g/dL for other causes that generate exudates.[185]

Fecal Material

The use of fecal material for protein analysis is relatively infrequent but indicated in some specific clinical circumstances. Assessment of protein content in feces is fraught with a number of limitations. Results of fecal protein content are often normalized to fecal weight. Thus, watery stool specimens generally provides decreased estimates of protein concentration. Extraction is likewise dependent on stool consistency and homogeneity, leading to considerable within-subject and between-subject variability.

Protein loss in the GI tract may be assessed using an assay of fecal AAT. The amount of fecal AAT excreted over time is determined as a function of the serum AAT concentration. Correction for serum AAT concentration is necessary because of variation in serum AAT from severe enteric losses or from acute-phase responses. AAT is relatively stable in the lower digestive tract but is digested in the stomach at acid pH. Therefore, suppression of acid secretion is necessary to use AAT excretion as a measure of gastric protein-losing enteropathy.[186] An alternative measure of increased GI loss of protein has been the assessment of stool radioactivity following the injection of radiolabeled albumin.

Inflammatory bowel disease (IBD) includes Crohn's disease and ulcerative colitis. Although GI histology remains the gold standard for diagnosis, a number of fecal protein markers have been employed as tools for screening and response to therapy. In the setting of IBD, it may be more useful to have indicators of inflammation rather than leakage of plasma proteins. Fecal products secreted by WBCs, such as lactoferrin and calprotectin, have been used as a measure of disease activity in IBD.[187] Lactoferrin has diagnostic sensitivity and specificity ranging from 47% to 92% and 60% to 100%, respectively, for the diagnosis of IBD. The sensitivity and specificity of calprotectin is similar and ranges from 61% to 100% and 72% to 100%, respectively.[188]

Exocrine pancreatic disease occurs in the setting of multiple pathologic states, including chronic alcoholism, diabetes, HIV, celiac disease, and cystic fibrosis. Determination of fecal proteins such as elastase that are derived from pancreatic secretions provides an alternative for the diagnosis of pancreatic insufficiency compared with gold standard duodenal sampling after secretin administration.[189,190] For example, fecal elastase concentrations of less than 100 µg/mg stool suggest severe functional deficiency with sensitivity ranging from 72% to 100% and specificity ranging from 29% to 96%.[188]

POINTS TO REMEMBER

- Amino acids are the building blocks of protein but also serve as substrates for energy generation and other important biomolecules.
- Amino acid homeostasis depends on enteral extraction, a host of broad-specificity transport systems, as well as metabolism.
- An array of small peptide systems derived from larger protein precursors dictate control of numerous physiologic processes, including glucose and electrolyte homeostasis (ACTH), fluid retention (natriuretic peptides, vasopressin), iron metabolism (hepcidin), and vascular tone (angiotensins, ETs).
- Protein diversity is derived from linear amino acid sequence and an array of cotranslational and posttranslational modifications, including acylation, prenylation, phosphorylation, and glycosylation.
- Current catalogs of the circulating human proteome contain more than 12,000 components.

SELECTED REFERENCES

For a full list of references for this chapter, please refer to ExpertConsult.com.

1. Miller SL. A production of amino acids under possible primitive earth conditions. *Science* 1953;**117**(3046):528–9.
3. Otten JJHJ, Meyers LD. *Dietary Reference Intakes: the essential guide to nutrient requirements*. Washington, DC: National Academy of Sciences Press; 2006.
12. Broer S. Amino acid transport across mammalian intestinal and renal epithelia. *Physiol Rev* 2008;**88**(1):249–86.
24. Feigin RD, Beisel WR, Wannemacher RW Jr. Rhythmicity of plasma amino acids and relation to dietary intake. *Am J Clin Nutr* 1971;**24**(3):329–41.
29. Wang TJ, Larson MG, Vasan RS, et al. Metabolite profiles and the risk of developing diabetes. *Nat Med* 2011;**17**(4):448–53.
34. Dietzen DJ, Weindel AL, Carayannopoulos MO, et al. Rapid comprehensive amino acid analysis by liquid chromatography/tandem mass spectrometry: comparison to cation exchange with post-column ninhydrin detection. *Rapid Commun Mass Spectrom* 2008;**22**(22):3481–8.
36. Nagy K, Takats Z, Pollreisz F, et al. Direct tandem mass spectrometric analysis of amino acids in dried blood spots without chemical derivatization for neonatal screening. *Rapid Commun Mass Spectrom* 2003;**17**(9):983–90.
46. Pandey KN. Biology of natriuretic peptides and their receptors. *Peptides* 2005;**26**(6):901–32.
54. Ganz T. Hepcidin, a key regulator of iron metabolism and mediator of anemia of inflammation. *Blood* 2003;**102**(3):783–8.
69. Kramer G, Boehringer D, Ban N, et al. The ribosome as a platform for co-translational processing, folding and targeting of newly synthesized proteins. *Nat Struct Mol Biol* 2009;**16**(6):589–97.
70. Saibil H. Chaperone machines for protein folding, unfolding and disaggregation. *Nat Rev Mol Cell Biol* 2013;**14**(10):630–42.
76. Carrell RW, Lomas DA. Alpha1-antitrypsin deficiency—a model for conformational diseases. *N Engl J Med* 2002;**346**(1):45–53.
79. Lingappa VR, Blobel G. Early events in the biosynthesis of secretory and membrane proteins: the signal hypothesis. *Recent Prog Horm Res* 1980;**36**:451–75.
88. Cohen P. The regulation of protein function by multisite phosphorylation—a 25 year update. *Trends Biochem Sci* 2000;**25**(12):596–601.
102. Fares F. The role of O-linked and N-linked oligosaccharides on the structure-function of glycoprotein hormones: development of agonists and antagonists. *Biochim Biophys Acta* 2006;**1760**(4):560–7.
128. Hochstrasser M. Origin and function of ubiquitin-like proteins. *Nature* 2009;**458**(7237):422–9.
153. Gabay C, Kushner I. Acute-phase proteins and other systemic responses to inflammation. *N Engl J Med* 1999;**340**(6):448–54.
170. Lowry OH, Rosebrough NJ, Farr AL, et al. Protein measurement with the Folin phenol reagent. *J Biol Chem* 1951;**193**(1):265–75.
173. Kaiser P, Akerboom T, Ohlendorf R, et al. Liquid chromatography-isotope dilution-mass spectrometry as a new basis for the reference measurement procedure for hemoglobin A1c determination. *Clin Chem* 2010;**56**(5):750–4.

29

Serum Enzymes

Mauro Panteghini and Renze Bais

ABSTRACT

Background

Serum enzymes are measured in medical diagnosis to detect injury to a tissue that makes up the measured enzyme. Clinical applications have concentrated mostly on enzymes such as creatine kinase, alanine transaminase, aspartate transaminase, alkaline phosphatase, γ-glutamyltransferase, lactate dehydrogenase, lipase, and (pancreatic) amylase.

Content

This chapter describes the use of the clinically most important enzymes as the preferred markers in various disease states such as skeletal muscle disease, hepatocellular damage and cholestasis, pancreatitis, bone disorders, and cancer. In many conditions, they may provide a unique insight into the disease process by diagnosis, prognosis, and assessment of response to therapy. As the literature on the use of enzymes in various clinical conditions has accumulated, the scope of this chapter is to provide a comprehensive and updated analysis of this relevant topic, exploiting the evidence supporting the clinical usefulness of these biomarkers and highlighting all testing aspects (including pre- and postanalytical) that may influence their correct application.

INTRODUCTION

Injury to tissue releases cellular substances that can be used as plasma markers of tissue damage. For a substance to serve as a biochemical marker of damage to a specific organ or tissue, it must arise predominantly from the organ or tissue of interest. Many of the clinically useful markers of cellular damage are enzymes.

Measurements of enzymes are used in medicine in two major ways. Enzymes are measured in serum and other body fluids to detect injury to a tissue that makes up the enzyme and are also measured, often within a tissue, to identify abnormalities or absence of the enzyme, which may cause disease. Some enzymes are found predominantly in specialized tissue (eg, lipase in the pancreas); others, more widely distributed, have tissue-specific isoenzymes or isoforms (eg, the pancreatic isoenzyme of α-amylase, the bone isoform of alkaline phosphatase) that can be evaluated to enhance tissue and organ specificity.

The timing of the enzyme's diagnostic window is another important aspect to be considered when these markers are used to evaluate acute injury. According to Noe,[1] the diagnostic window for an injury marker is the interval of time after an episode of injury during which plasma concentrations of the marker are increased, thereby demonstrating the occurrence of injury. Marker substances that rapidly enter the circulation (ie, early indicators) tend to have diagnostic windows that begin soon after onset of the injury. On the contrary, biomarkers that are slowly released into the circulation or are slowly cleared from the circulation (ie, late indicators) generally have diagnostic windows that begin later and last long after the time of injury.

DIAGNOSTIC ENZYMOLOGY

In general, clinical laboratorians use changes in activity in the serum or plasma of enzymes that are predominantly intracellular and physiologically present in the blood at low activity concentrations only. Increases in the serum activities of these enzymes are used to infer the location and nature of pathologic changes in tissues of the body. Therefore, an understanding of the factors that affect the rate of release of enzymes from their cells of origin and the rate at which they are cleared from the circulation is necessary to interpret correctly changes in activity that occur with disease.

Factors Affecting Enzyme Concentrations in Blood[2]

The measured activity of an enzyme in blood is the result not only of the total amount released from its cells of origin but also of the rate of enzyme catabolism in the circulation, the escape to the extracellular enzyme pool, and the rate at which it is inactivated or removed.

Leakage of Enzymes From Cells

Enzymes are retained within their cells of origin by the plasma membrane surrounding the cell. The plasma membrane is a metabolically active part of the cell, and its integrity depends on the cell's production of adenosine triphosphate (ATP). Any process that impairs ATP production by depriving the cell of oxidizable substrates or by reducing the efficiency of energy production by restricting the access of oxygen (ischemia or anoxia) promotes deterioration of the cell membrane. The earliest sign of impaired energy metabolism is the efflux of potassium with influx of sodium; water thus accumulates within the cell, causing it to swell. The next

TABLE 29.1 **Causes of Cell Injury or Death**

Category	Examples
Hypoxia (an extremely common accompaniment of clinical disease)	Loss of blood supply caused by narrowing (atheromatous plaques) or blocking (thrombosis) of artery or vein; ischemic-perfusion injury; inadequate oxygenation due to cardiorespiratory failure; loss of oxygen-carrying capacity, carbon monoxide poisoning, anemia
Chemicals and drugs	Environmental pollutants—lead, mercury; drugs—use and abuse (therapeutic and "recreational"); alcohol; tobacco
Physical agents	Trauma; extremes of heat and radiation; electrical energy; toxic chemicals
Infectious agents	Bacteria, viruses, fungi, protozoa, and helminths
Immune mechanisms	Immune disorders can cause tissue damage by a number of mechanisms: **1.** Anaphylaxis (causing release of vasoactive amines) **2.** Cytotoxicity (causing the target cell to be lysed) **3.** Immune complex disease (leading to release of lysosomal enzymes) **4.** Cell-mediated hypersensitivity (leading to cytotoxicity)
Genetic factors	Disorders with polygenic inheritance—diabetes mellitus, gout Mendelian disorders—X-linked disorders, autosomal dominant and recessive disorders, disorders with variable modes of transmission and inborn errors of metabolism
Nutritional imbalances	Protein-calorie malnutrition, vitamin deficiencies, mineral deficiencies; obesity and its consequences

Modified from Kumar V, Abbas AK, Aster JC, editors. In: *Basic pathology*. 9th ed. Philadelphia: Saunders; 2012.

and most serious stage is the entry of calcium, which stimulates intracellular enzymes, leading to both cell damage and disruption of the cell membrane. Finally, free radicals formed during these processes may cause further damage. The membrane becomes leaky; if cellular injury becomes irreversible, the cell will die, although enzyme loss may also occur without the occurrence of irreversible injury. Small molecules are the first to leak from damaged or dying cells followed by larger molecules, such as enzymes and other proteins. Cytosolic proteins appear early on in the plasma followed much later by mitochondrial and membrane-bound enzymes. It appears that ATP must decline to below a certain level before substantial enzyme release occurs. Ultimately, the complete content of the necrotic cells is discharged.[3]

Because of very high concentrations of enzymes within the cells—thousands or even tens of thousands times greater than concentrations in extracellular fluid—and because extremely small amounts of enzyme can be detected by their catalytic activity, increased enzyme activity in the extracellular fluid or plasma is an extremely sensitive indicator of even minor cellular damage, some causes of which are listed in Table 29.1.

A reduction in the supply of oxygenated blood perfusing any tissue will promote enzyme release, such as occurs in myocardial infarction (MI). Cells of the affected region rapidly begin to deteriorate and die, releasing their protein and enzyme contents to the systemic circulation, which accounts for the rapid rise in serum biomarkers that is characteristic of this condition. The liver is also very sensitive to hypoxia, which can result from diminished cardiac output (heart failure) or other causes. Direct attack on the cell membranes by such agents as viruses or organic chemicals also causes enzyme release, which is particularly important in the case of the liver. Skeletal muscles also contribute enzymes to blood. Again, the cause may be poor perfusion, hypothermia, or direct trauma to the muscles (crush injuries). Infection, inflammation (polymyositis), degenerative changes (dystrophies), drugs, and alcohol (alcoholic myopathy) cause enzyme leakage from myocytes.

Efflux of Enzymes From Damaged Cells

When conditions for leakage of enzymes from cells have occurred, the speed and extent to which the process is reflected in enzyme changes in the blood depend on several factors.

The driving force of enzyme release is the steep concentration gradient that exists between the interior and the exterior of the cells. The rate of escape of enzyme molecules is presumably controlled to some extent by diffusion; therefore, smaller enzyme molecules might be expected to appear in the extracellular fluid earlier than larger ones.

The way in which released enzyme molecules are transferred from the interstitial fluid to the blood varies from one tissue to another; they may pass directly through the capillary wall, or lymphatic transfer may occur. Direct transfer occurs to a large extent in the liver, which is a highly vascular tissue with many permeable capillaries, although evidence suggests that liver enzymes may also be subject to lymphatic transfer. On the other hand, the capillaries of skeletal muscle are relatively impermeable, and in this tissue it is probable that released enzymes mainly reach the circulatory system through drainage from the lymphatic system. Lymph drainage is also important in transporting enzymes released from damaged intestinal, pancreatic, and myocardial cells to the circulation, although after MI, a minor proportion of myocardial enzymes reaches the circulation also by direct capillary transfer.

The intracellular location of the leaking enzymes affects the rates at which they appear in the circulation. As would be expected, the most sensitive indicators of cell damage are the molecules that are present in the soluble fraction of the cell. Release of structurally bound membrane proteins requires both a leaky cell membrane and a dissociation or degradation, which is a slower process.[3] Enzymes associated with subcellular structures, such as mitochondria, are less readily released into the circulation and often indicate irreversible cellular injury. This fact has been used in attempts to distinguish reversible leakage, presumed to reflect damage only to the cell membrane, from necrotic lesions, in which intracellular structures are destroyed.

The relation between tissue injury and the appearance of enzymes in the circulation is most clearly seen in MI, in which a relatively short episode of damage is followed by a rapid transfer of enzymes to the circulatory system. About 24 hours after an MI, the pattern of relative activity of various enzymes in the circulatory system closely resembles that in myocardial tissue. These relationships are less clearly recognized in other conditions, such as chronic liver disease, in which enzyme release is a process that continues over a period of time. The pattern of relative enzyme activities in serum in chronic disease may also become distorted by differential rates of removal of enzymes from the circulation and possibly by differential changes in rates of enzyme synthesis in affected tissue.

Release of enzymes from damaged or dying cells and changes in the rate of enzyme production constitute the most important mechanisms by which changes in enzyme activity in the serum or plasma are produced. However, other possibilities exist and appear to account for some changes of diagnostic importance. For example, much of the γ-glutamyltransferase (GGT) activity of liver cells is located on their exterior surfaces. It is possible that ectoenzymes such as this may be eluted from the surfaces, especially where the detergent action of the blood is increased through accumulation of bile salts. This process does not involve cell damage in the sense of increased membrane permeability, as evidenced by lack of correlation between activities in the serum of GGT and the aminotransferases in liver disease of different types.

Altered Enzyme Production

Small amounts of intracellular enzymes physiologically present in the plasma can be assumed to result from wear and tear of cells or leakage of enzyme from healthy cells. This contribution of enzymes to the circulating blood may decrease as the result of a genetic deficiency of enzyme production (eg, as is the case for alkaline phosphatase in hypophosphatasia or in individuals homozygous for the "silent" gene for serum cholinesterase) or when enzyme production is depressed as a result of disease (eg, cholinesterase in liver disease). However, cases in which enzyme production is increased are generally of more interest in diagnostic enzymology. For example, an increase in the number and activity of alkaline phosphatase–producing osteoblasts of bone is responsible for the increased concentration of alkaline phosphatase in the serum of normally growing children. Increased osteoblastic activity also accounts for increased concentrations of this enzyme in the serum in various types of bone disease.

The process of enzyme induction also increases enzyme production. An example of such induction is the increased activity of GGT in serum, which results from administration of drugs such as barbiturates or phenytoin, and from intake of ethanol.

Clearance of Enzymes

Significant evidence is available about the way in which enzymes are cleared from the circulation. Few enzyme molecules are small enough to pass through the glomerulus of the kidney; therefore, urinary excretion is not a major route for elimination of enzymes from the circulation. An exception to this is α-amylase (molecular weight, 54–62 kDa), which is the only plasma enzyme physiologically found in urine; increased concentrations of this enzyme in the blood (eg, after acute pancreatitis) are accompanied by increased excretion in the urine.

Evidence now suggests that many enzymes are not inactivated in the plasma but are rapidly removed, probably by the reticuloendothelial system, such as the bone marrow, spleen, and liver (Kupffer cells), or, to a lesser extent, by nearly all cells in the body. The mechanism appears to consist of receptor-mediated endocytosis (the process of recognition, specific accumulation, and uptake of protein by specific cell surface receptors followed by fusion with lysosomes, digestion of ingested protein, and recycling of the receptor back to the cell membrane). For example, hepatic Kupffer cells have been shown to take up several tissue-derived enzymes—such as creatine kinase, adenylate kinase, cytoplasmic and mitochondrial aspartate aminotransferase, and malate and alcohol dehydrogenases—by receptor-mediated endocytosis, which may have affinity for lysine residues on these enzymes. The adult isoform of intestinal alkaline phosphatase is a galactosyl-terminal glycoprotein that reacts with a galactosyl-specific receptor on the hepatocyte membrane and undergoes subsequent endocytosis. This process is rapid, accounting for the extremely short plasma half-life of this isoform. However, in hepatic cirrhosis, in which considerable reduction in parenchymal cell mass often occurs, the plasma concentration and half-life of the isoform increase. Other alkaline phosphatase isoenzymes and isoforms are sialoglycoproteins that do not react with the galactosyl receptor and therefore are protected from rapid uptake from blood. Indeed, examples are known of excessive sialylation of alkaline phosphatases produced by malignant cells, prolonging their plasma half-lives and facilitating their detection. This example illustrates the importance of understanding the processes by which enzymes are cleared from plasma.

The half-lives of enzymes in plasma vary from a few hours to several days, but in most cases, the average half-life ($t_{1/2}$) is 6 to 48 hours. Rates of decay may also be expressed as k_d values with units of hour^{-1}—the fractional disappearance rate—and the relationship to $t_{1/2}$ values is as follows:

$$k_d = 2.303 \log \frac{2}{t_{1/2}} = \frac{0.693}{t_{1/2}}$$

Typical disappearance rates from human blood for several clinically relevant enzymes are shown in Fig. 29.1.

POINTS TO REMEMBER

The pattern of appearance of an enzyme in blood after an acute injury depends on:

- The intracellular location and whether molecules are bound or free
- Molecular weight (because heavier molecules diffuse at a slower rate)
- Local blood and lymphatic flow
- The rate of elimination from blood

Selection of Enzyme Tests

The selection of which enzyme to measure in serum for diagnostic or prognostic purposes depends on a number of factors. An important factor is the distribution of enzymes among the various tissues, shown, for example, for aspartate aminotransferase, alanine aminotransferase, and creatine

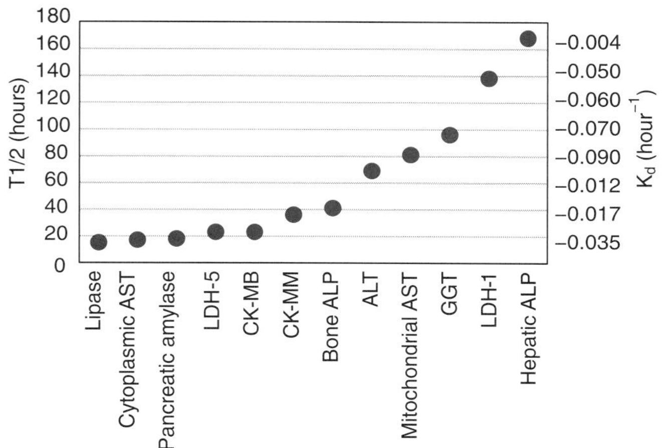

FIGURE 29.1 Fractional disappearance rates (k_d, in hour^{-1}) from human blood of the most important enzymes. *ALP,* Alkaline phosphatase; *ALT,* alanine aminotransferase; *AST,* aspartate aminotransferase; *CK-MB,* creatine kinase isoenzyme MB; *CK-MM,* creatine kinase isoenzyme MM; *GGT,* γ-glutamyltransferase; *LDH,* lactate dehydrogenase.

kinase in Fig. 29.2. The main enzymes of established clinical value, together with their tissues of origin and their major clinical applications, are listed in Table 29.2.

The mass of the damaged or malfunctioning organ, together with the enzyme cell/blood gradient, obviously has a profound influence on the resulting increase of enzyme activity in blood. As an example, the gradient of activity of prostatic acid phosphatase between prostate and blood is about 10^3 : 1, and the mass of that organ is 20 g. By contrast, the cell or blood gradient of alanine aminotransferase in the liver cell is 10^4 : 1, and the mass of the liver can exceed 1000 g. Obviously, fewer cells have to be damaged in the liver than in the prostate for the abnormality to be detected by an enzyme increase in blood. If, on the other hand, total organ involvement occurs, then clearly the vast number of affected liver cells will markedly elevate blood concentrations of any liver enzyme. It has been estimated that if only 1 liver cell in every 750 is damaged, the increase in the blood concentration of alanine aminotransferase would be detectable.

Knowledge of the intracellular location of enzymes can assist in determining the nature and severity of a pathologic

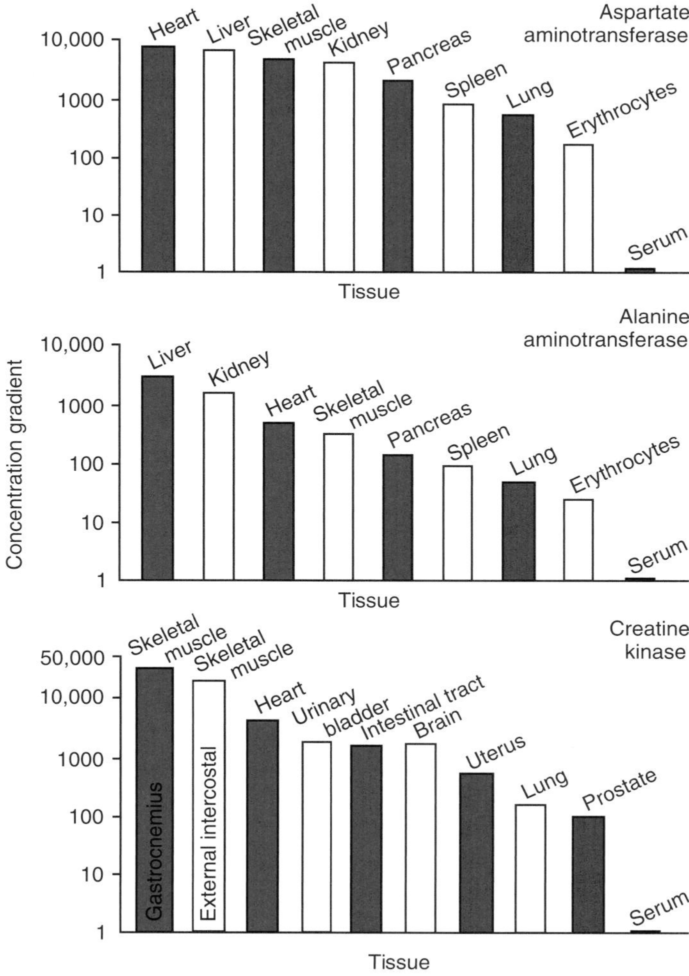

FIGURE 29.2 The concentration gradients between some human tissues and serum for aspartate aminotransferase, alanine aminotransferase, and creatine kinase. The concentration gradient axis is logarithmic.

TABLE 29.2 Distribution of Clinically Important Enzymes

Enzyme	Principal Sources of Enzyme in Blood	Principal Clinical Applications
Alanine aminotransferase	Liver	Hepatic parenchymal disease
Alkaline phosphatase	Liver, bone, intestinal mucosa, placenta	Hepatobiliary disease, bone disease
Amylase	Salivary glands, pancreas	Pancreatic disease
Aspartate aminotransferase	Heart, liver, skeletal muscle, erythrocytes	Hepatic parenchymal disease
Creatine kinase	Skeletal muscle, heart	Muscle disease, myocardial infarction
γ-Glutamyltransferase	Liver, pancreas, kidney	Hepatobiliary disease
Lactate dehydrogenase	Heart, erythrocytes, lymph nodes, skeletal muscle, liver	Hemolytic and megaloblastic anemias, leukemia and lymphomas, oncology
Lipase	Pancreas	Pancreatic disease
5′-Nucleotidase	Liver	Hepatobiliary disease

process if suitable enzymes are assayed in the blood. For instance, a mild, reversible viral inflammation of the liver, such as a mild attack of viral hepatitis, is likely to increase only the permeability of the cell membrane while allowing cytoplasmic enzymes to leak out into the blood, but a severe attack causing cell necrosis also disrupts the mitochondrial membrane, and both cytoplasmic and mitochondrial enzymes are detected in the blood. Finally, in selecting a suitable enzyme to assay in blood for diagnostic purposes, the clearance way and the rate at which its activity disappears from the blood are of significance. As previously indicated, the most commonly assayed enzymes are those with half-lives in the range of 12 hours or greater.

Several enzymes of diagnostic utility are discussed in this chapter. To better clarify their clinical meaning, the individual enzymes are discussed relative to the organ in which they are clinically most important. Overlap may occur for this classification because the same enzyme may be used for investigating disease in several organs.

MUSCLE ENZYMES

Enzymes in this category include creatine kinase and aldolase.

Creatine Kinase

Creatine kinase (EC 2.7.3.2; adenosine triphosphate:creatine *N*-phosphotransferase; CK) is a dimeric enzyme (82 kDa) that catalyzes the reversible phosphorylation of creatine (Cr) by ATP.

Creatine + Adenosine triphosphate ⇌ Phosphocreatine (creatine phosphate) + Adenosine diphosphate + $H^{\oplus}$

(forward: pH = 9.0; CK, Mg_2^+; reverse: pH = 6.7)

Creatine: $^{\ominus}O(O=)C{-}CH_2{-}N(CH_3){-}C(=NH)NH_2$

Phosphocreatine: $^{\ominus}O(O=)C{-}CH_2{-}N(CH_3){-}C(=NH){-}NH{-}PO_3^{2\ominus}$

Adenosine triphosphate: $AMP{-}P(=O)(O^{\ominus}){-}O{-}P(=O)(O^{\ominus}){-}O^{\ominus}$

Adenosine diphosphate: $AMP{-}P(=O)(O^{\ominus}){-}O^{\ominus}$

Physiologically, when muscle contracts, ATP is converted to adenosine diphosphate (ADP), and CK catalyzes the rephosphorylation of ADP to ATP using creatine phosphate (CrP) as the phosphorylation reservoir.

Optimal pH values for the forward (Cr + ATP → ADP + CrP) and reverse (CrP + ADP → ATP + Cr) reactions are 9.0 and 6.7, respectively. At neutral pH, the formation of ATP is favored; a pH of 9.0 is optimal for the formation of CrP, another high-energy compound. Mg^{2+} is an obligate activating ion that forms complexes with ATP and ADP. The optimal concentration range for Mg^{2+} is narrow, and excess Mg^{2+} is inhibitory. Many metal ions, such as Mn^{2+}, Ca^{2+}, Zn^{2+}, and Cu^{2+}, inhibit enzyme activity, as do iodoacetate and other sulfhydryl-binding reagents. Activity is inhibited by excess ADP and by citrate, fluoride, nitrate, acetate, iodide, bromide, malonate, and L-thyroxine.[4] Urate and cystine are potent inhibitors of the enzyme in serum. Even chloride and sulfate ions inhibit activity, and the concentrations of these ions should be kept low in any enzyme assay system based on the CrP + ADP (reverse) reaction.

The enzyme in serum is relatively unstable, activity being lost as a result of sulfhydryl group oxidation at the active site of the enzyme. Activity can be partially restored by incubating the enzyme preparation with sulfhydryl compounds, such as *N*-acetylcysteine, dithiothreitol (Cleland reagent), and glutathione. The agent of choice in current assays is *N*-acetylcysteine, which has the advantage of being a very soluble substance used at a final concentration of 20 mmol/L in the assay reagent.

Creatine kinase activity is greatest in striated muscle and heart tissue, which contain some 2500 and 550 U/g of protein, respectively. Other tissues, such as the brain and the smooth muscle of the gastrointestinal tract and the urinary bladder, contain significantly less activity, and the liver and erythrocytes are essentially devoid of activity (Table 29.3).

Creatine kinase is a dimer composed of two subunits, each with a molecular weight of about 40 kDa. These subunits (B and M) are the products of loci on chromosomes 14 and 19, respectively. Because the active form of the enzyme is a dimer, only three different pairs of subunits can exist: BB (or CK-1), MB (or CK-2), and MM (or CK-3). The Commission on Biochemical Nomenclature has recommended that isoenzymes be numbered on the basis of their electrophoretic mobility, with the most anodal form receiving the lowest

TABLE 29.3 Approximate Concentrations of Tissue Creatine Kinase (CK) Activity (Expressed as Multiples of CK Activity Concentrations in Serum) and Cytoplasmic Isoenzyme Composition

Tissue	Relative CK Activity	ISOENZYMES, %		
		CK-BB	CK-MB	CK-MM
Skeletal muscle (type I, slow twitch, or red fibers)	50,000	<1	3	97
Skeletal muscle (type II, fast twitch, or white fibers)	50,000	<1	1	99
Heart	10,000	<1	22	78
Brain	5000	100	0	0
Gastrointestinal tract smooth muscle	5000	96	1	3
Urinary bladder smooth muscle	4000	92	6	2

CK-BB, Creatine kinase isoenzyme BB; *CK-MB,* creatine kinase isoenzyme MB; *CK-MM,* creatine kinase isoenzyme MM.

number. Accordingly, the CK isoenzymes are numbered CK-1, CK-2, and CK-3. The distribution of these isoenzymes in the various tissues of humans is shown in Table 29.3. All three of these isoenzyme species are found in the cytosol of the cell or are associated with myofibrillar structures. However, there exists a fourth isoenzyme that differs from the others both immunologically and by electrophoretic mobility. This isoenzyme (CK-Mt) is located between the inner and outer membranes of mitochondria and occurs in two different oligomeric forms, dimers and octamers, that are readily interconvertible. Their molecular weights are about 80 and 370 kDa, respectively. CK-Mt constitutes, in the heart for example, up to 15% of total CK activity. The gene for CK-Mt is located on chromosome 15.

Creatine kinase activity may also be found in macromolecular form—the so-called macro-CK. It exists in two forms: types 1 and 2. Type 1 is a complex of CK, typically CK-BB, and an immunoglobulin, often IgG, but other complexes have been described, such as CK-MM with IgA. Macro-CK type 1 is not of pathologic significance, but it can be the cause of increased CK results and also interfere with the assay of CK-MB by some immunoinhibition methods, resulting in diagnostic confusion and leading to unnecessary further investigation. Prevalence has been estimated as between 0.8% and 2.3%, but this is dependent on the population studied.[5] In a 10-year retrospective study, more than 80% of those positive for macro-CK type 1 (immunoglobulin bound) were female.[6] Macro-CK type 2 is oligomeric CK-Mt, with a reported prevalence of between 0.5% and 2.6% in hospitalized patients. It is found predominantly in adults who are severely ill with malignancy or liver disease and in children who have notable tissue distress. The appearance of this isoenzyme in serum is usually associated with a poor prognosis. Macro-CK can be detected as abnormally migrating bands by electrophoretic methods (Fig. 29.3). If electrophoretic separation is not available, the polyethylene glycol (PEG) 6000 precipitation method can be used (see the Amylase section later in this chapter).

Both M and B subunits have a C-terminal lysine residue, but only the former can be hydrolyzed by the action of carboxypeptidases present in blood. Carboxypeptidases B (EC 3.4.17.2) and N (arginine carboxypeptidase; EC 3.4.17.3) sequentially hydrolyze the lysine residues from CK-MM to produce two CK-MM isoforms: CK-MM_2 (one lysine residue removed) and CK-MM_1 (both lysine residues removed). Loss

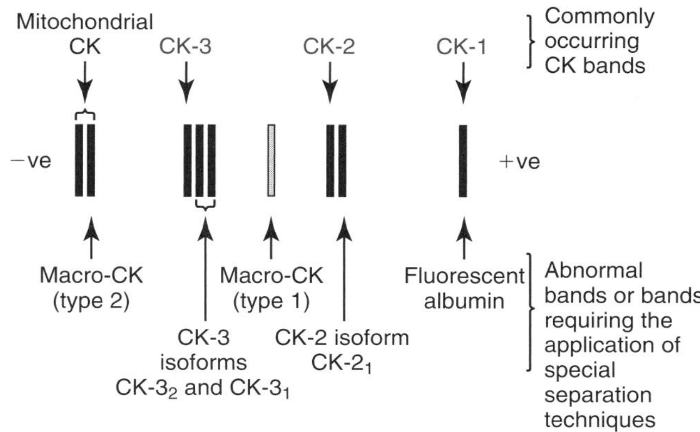

FIGURE 29.3 A diagrammatic representation of the electrophoretic pattern of creatine kinase (CK) isoenzymes (some of which are seen, in blood, only in disease) and some of the reported anomalous forms.

of the positively charged lysine produces a more negatively charged CK molecule with greater anodic mobility at electrophoresis. Because CK-MB has only one M subunit, the dimer coded by the M and B genes is named CK-MB_2 and the lysine-hydrolyzed dimer is named CK-MB_1.[7]

Clinical Significance

Creatine kinase determination is the preferred laboratory test in case of suspected muscle damage. Serum CK is increased in nearly all patients when injury, inflammation, or necrosis of skeletal or heart muscle occurs.

Increase of serum CK activity may be the only sign of subclinical neuromuscular disorders.[8] In case series, 30% to 44% of asymptomatic subjects with persistently elevated CK up to fivefold the upper reference limit (URL) have myopathy. Serum CK activity is greatly elevated in all types of muscular dystrophy. In progressive muscular dystrophy (particularly Duchenne sex-linked muscular dystrophy), enzyme activity in serum is highest in infancy and childhood (7–10 years of age) and may be increased long before the disease is clinically apparent. Serum CK activity characteristically falls as patients get older and as the mass of functioning muscle diminishes with progression of the disease. About 50% to 80% of asymptomatic female carriers of Duchenne dystrophy show three- to sixfold increases in CK activity.

High values of CK (up to 50-fold the URL in active disease) are noted in viral myositis, polymyositis, and other inflammatory myopathies. However, in neurogenic muscle diseases, such as myasthenia gravis, multiple sclerosis, poliomyelitis, and parkinsonism, serum enzyme activity is not increased. Very high activity is also encountered in malignant hyperthermia, an inherited life-threatening condition characterized by high fever and brought on by administration of inhalation anesthesia (usually halothane) to the affected individual. Molecular genetic investigations have confirmed the skeletal muscle type ryanodine receptor to be the major malignant hyperthermia locus with more than 70% of families carrying a mutation in this gene.[9]

Skeletal muscle that is diseased or chronically damaged (eg, by extreme exercise) may contain significant proportions of CK-MB owing to the phenomenon of "fetal reversion," in which fetal patterns of protein synthesis (in the case of CK, the B monomer) reappear. Thus, serum CK-MB isoenzyme may increase in such circumstances. This explanation may also account for the increased CK-MB values sometimes observed in chronic renal failure (uremic myopathy).

In acute rhabdomyolysis caused by crush injury, with severe muscle destruction, serum CK activities exceeding 200 times the URL may be found. In this condition, a very high serum CK, mirroring myoglobinuria and its haem-induced mechanism of renal injury, has been associated with the risk of development of acute renal failure. If the CK remains below 5000 U/L (≈30 times the URL) during the first 3 days after the insult, the probability of developing renal failure appears to be low.[10] Serum CK can also be mildly increased by other direct trauma to muscle, including intramuscular injection and surgical intervention. Finally, a number of drugs, when given at pharmacologic doses, can increase serum CK activities. The drugs principally responsible are statins, fibrates, antiretrovirals, and angiotensin II receptor antagonists. The clinical spectrum of statin-induced myotoxicity includes asymptomatic rise in serum CK activity, myalgia, myositis, and rhabdomyolysis (0.02%).[11] Routine monitoring of CK in asymptomatic patients is not recommended; however, CK must be assessed in patients presenting with muscle pain and weakness and statin treatment stopped if values rise to more than fivefold the URL.[12]

Changes in serum CK and its MB isoenzyme after acute MI have been the mainstay of diagnosis for many years. However, it is now more advantageous to use more cardiac-specific nonenzymatic markers, such as cardiac troponin I or T. CK-MB determination (measured by mass assays) can still be used with some success to estimate the extent of myocardial necrosis to assist with assessment of infarct prognosis.[13] When peak CK-MB is compared with estimates of infarct size, good correlations can be obtained (Table 29.4). A problem with using CK-MB for this purpose is the requirement for frequent sampling to ensure that peak CK-MB values are correctly identified.

Hypothyroidism is a common cause of endocrine myopathy. About 60% of hypothyroid subjects show an average increase of CK activity fivefold greater than the URL. The major isoenzyme present is CK-MM, suggesting muscular involvement.

During normal childbirth, a sixfold increase in maternal total serum CK activity occurs. Surgical intervention during labor further increases the activity of CK in serum. CK-BB may be increased in neonates, particularly in brain-damaged or very low birth weight newborns. The presence of CK-BB in blood, usually at low concentrations, may, however, represent a physiologic finding in the first days of life.

TABLE 29.4 Decision Limits of Creatine Kinase-MB Mass Peak for Infarct Size Definition

Microscopic MI (focal necrosis)	<10 μg/L
Small MI (<10%LV)	10–60 μg/L
Medium MI (10%–30% LV)	60–225 μg/L
Large MI (>30% LV)	>225 μg/L

LV, Left ventricle; *MI,* myocardial infarction.

Methods for Determination of Creatine Kinase Activity

Numerous photometric, fluorometric, and coupled enzyme methods have been developed for the assay of CK activity using the forward (Cr → CrP) or the reverse (Cr ← CrP) reaction. Currently, all commercial assays for total CK are based on the reverse reaction, which proceeds about six times faster than the forward reaction.

$$\text{Creatine phosphate} + \text{ADP} \xrightarrow[\text{pH 6.7}]{CK} \text{Creatine} + \text{ADP}$$

$$\text{ADP} + \text{glucose} \xrightarrow{HK} \text{Glucose-6-phosphate} + \text{ADP}$$

$$\text{Glucose-6-phosphate} + \text{NADP}^{\oplus} \xrightarrow{G6PD} \text{6-Phosphogluconate} + \text{NADPH} + \text{H}^{\oplus}$$

Creatine kinase catalyzes the conversion of CrP to Cr with concomitant phosphorylation of ADP to ATP. The ATP produced is measured by hexokinase (HK)/glucose-6-phosphate dehydrogenase (G6PD)–coupled reactions that ultimately convert $NADP^+$ to NADPH, which is monitored spectrophotometrically at 340 nm. Szasz and colleagues optimized the assay by adding *N*-acetylcysteine to activate CK, ethylenediaminetetraacetic acid (EDTA) to bind calcium and to increase the stability of the reaction mixture, and adenosine pentaphosphate (Ap_5A) in addition to AMP to inhibit adenylate kinase (AK).[14] A reference method based on this previous experience was developed by the International Federation of Clinical Chemistry and Laboratory Medicine (IFCC) for the measurement of CK at 37°C.[15]

Specimens for CK analysis include serum and heparin plasma. Anticoagulants other than heparin should not be used in collection tubes because they inhibit CK activity. CK activity in aliquoted serum is relatively unstable and is rapidly lost during storage. Average stabilities are less than 8 hours at room temperature, 48 hours at 4°C, and 1 month at −20°C. Therefore, the serum specimen should be chilled to 4°C if the serum is not analyzed immediately and stored at −80°C if analysis is delayed for longer than 30 days. A moderate degree of hemolysis is tolerated because erythrocytes contain no CK activity. However, severely hemolyzed specimens (free hemoglobin concentration >20 g/L) are unsatisfactory because enzymes and intermediates (AK, ATP, and G6P) liberated from the erythrocytes may affect the lag phase and side reactions occurring in the assay system.

For a single laboratory, the analytical specifications for desirable performance of CK assays, derived from biologic variation of the enzyme, are as follows: imprecision (as coefficient of variation [CV]) of 11.4% or less, bias of ±11.5, and total error of ±30.3%.[16] In an international study assessing the accuracy of CK results from six diagnostic companies, all of the evaluated assays showed statistically significant bias when compared with the IFCC reference procedure. Given the low assay imprecision, more than 95% of participating laboratories were, however, expected to comply traceability to the IFCC procedure within the biologically derived total error budget.[17]

Reference Intervals

Serum CK activity is subject to a number of physiologic variations. It is influenced by sex, age, race, muscle mass, and physical activity. The distributions of CK activity are notably skewed with a tail toward higher values in reference populations. Males have higher values than females, and blacks have higher values than nonblacks. However, there is a CK decline with aging in males. In white subjects, the reference interval was found to be 46 to 171 U/L for men and 34 to 145 U/L for women when measured with an assay traceable to the IFCC 37°C reference procedure.[18] Newborns generally have higher CK activity (up to 10 times the URL in adults) resulting from skeletal muscle trauma during birth. Serum CK in infants decreases to the adult reference interval by 6 to 10 weeks of age.

CK activity in the serum of healthy people is due almost exclusively to CK-MM activity (although small amounts of CK-MB may be present) and is the result of physiologic turnover of muscle tissue. Exercise, particularly if unaccustomed, and muscle trauma can increase serum CK activity, which may ascend as high as 10 times the URL within 24 hours of activity.[19]

Methods for Separation and Quantification of Creatine Kinase Isoenzymes

Even if not routinely used, electrophoretic methods are useful for separation of all CK isoenzymes. The isoenzyme bands are visualized by incubating the support (eg, agarose, cellulose acetate) with a concentrated CK assay mixture using the reverse reaction. NADPH formed in this reaction is then detected by observing the bluish-white fluorescence after excitation by long-wave (360 nm) ultraviolet light. NADPH may be quantified by fluorescent densitometry, which is capable of detecting bands of 2 to 5 U/L. The mobility of CK isoenzymes at pH 8.6 toward the anode is BB >MB >MM, with the MM remaining cathodic to the point of application. The discriminating power of electrophoresis also allows the detection of abnormal bands (eg, macro-CK) (see Fig. 29.3). Disadvantages of electrophoresis include that the turnaround time is relatively long, the procedure is highly labor intensive and is not adaptable to clinical chemistry analyzers, and interpretative skills are required.

Immunochemical methods are applicable to the direct measurement of CK-MB. Immunoinhibition techniques measuring the catalytic activity of the B subunit of CK dimer were first introduced. Currently, the most common approach is to measure concentrations of the CK-MB protein ("mass") by using immunoassays with monoclonal antibodies (see Chapter 22).[20] Measurements use the "sandwich" technique in which one antibody specifically recognizes only the MB dimer. The sandwich technique ensures that only CK-MB is estimated because neither CK-MM nor CK-BB reacts with both antibodies. Mass assays are more sensitive than activity-based methods with a limit of detection for CK-MB usually less than 1 µg/L. Other advantages include sample stability, noninterference with hemolysis, anticoagulants or other catalytic activity inhibitors, full automation, and fast turnaround time. With CM-MB mass assays, the URL for males is 5.0 µg/L, with values for females being less than male values, although many laboratories use a single reference limit (male).

Aldolase

Aldolase (EC 4.1.2.13; D-fructose-1,6-bisdiphosphate D-glyceraldehyde-3-phosphate-lyase; ALD) is a tetrameric enzyme (160 kDa) that catalyzes the splitting of D-fructose-1,6-diphosphate to D-glyceraldehyde-3-phosphate (GLAP) and dihydroxyacetone-phosphate (DAP), an important reaction in the glycolytic breakdown of glucose to lactate.

Aldolase is a tetramer with subunits determined by three separate gene loci. Only two of these loci, those producing A and B subunits, appear to be active simultaneously in most tissues, so the most common isoenzyme pattern consists of various proportions of the components of a five-member set of isoenzymes, of which two members correspond to the A and B homopolymers. The locus that determines the structure of the C subunit is active in brain tissue, as is the A locus, so this tissue contains ALD A and C, together with the three corresponding heteropolymers.

Aldolase is probably present in all cells, although it occurs in particularly large quantities in muscle, liver, and brain. The primary isoenzyme in normal serum is the A homomer.

Clinical Significance

Serum ALD determinations have been of some clinical interest in primary diseases of skeletal muscle, such as progressive muscular dystrophy and polymyositis. Some researchers believe that increased ALD activity is useful in distinguishing neuromuscular atrophies from myopathies in combination with the CK-to-AST (aminotransferase) ratio.[21] In general, however, measurement of ALD activity in the serum of subjects with suspected muscle disease does not add information to that available more readily from measurement of other enzymes, especially CK.[22] Accordingly, ALD measurement within clinical laboratories should be discouraged.

Methods for Measurement of Aldolase Activity

All assay methods are based on the forward ALD-catalyzed reaction. In the analytical approach on which all commonly used procedures and kits are based, the ALD reaction is coupled with two other enzyme reactions. Triosephosphate isomerase (EC 5.3.1.1) is added to ensure rapid conversion of all GLAP to DAP. Glycerol-3-phosphate dehydrogenase (EC 1.1.1.8) is added to reduce DAP to glycerol-3-phosphate, with NADH acting as hydrogen donor. The decrease in NADH concentration is then measured.

Aldolase activity in serum is quite stable. Activity is unchanged at ambient temperatures for up to 48 hours and at 4°C for several days. Hemolyzed specimens should not be used; plasma is preferred over serum because of the possible release of platelet enzyme during the clotting process.

Reference Intervals

The reference interval for the activity of ALD in adults is 2.5 to 10 U/L, measured at 37°C. However, a definite sex difference has been noted, with men having higher values. Serum ALD activity in neonates is fourfold that seen in adults, and in children, is twice that in adults. Adult values are attained by the time the child reaches puberty.[23]

LIVER ENZYMES

Enzymes in this category include alanine and aspartate aminotransferases, glutamate dehydrogenase, alkaline phosphatase, 5′-nucleotidase, GGT, and glutathione S-transferase. The aminotransferases, alkaline phosphatase and GGT, are widely used and available on automated analyzers. They have long been mistakenly considered as a part of "liver function tests." They are not, of course, tests of liver function, but the habit sometimes persists. The others have not been adopted as widely.

The most common alterations in liver enzyme activities encountered in clinical practice is divided into two major pathophysiology subgroups—hepatocellular damage (increased transaminase and glutamate dehydrogenase activities) and cholestasis (increased alkaline phosphatase, 5′- nucleotidase, and GGT activities), although certain liver diseases may display a mixed biochemical picture (Fig. 29.4).

Aminotransferases

The aminotransferases constitute a group of enzymes that catalyze the interconversion of amino acids to 2-oxo-acids by transfer of amino groups. Aspartate aminotransferase (EC 2.6.1.1; L-aspartate:2-oxoglutarate aminotransferase; AST) and alanine aminotransferase (EC 2.6.1.2; L-alanine:2-oxoglutarate aminotransferase; ALT) are examples of aminotransferases that are of clinical interest.

The 2-oxoglutarate/L-glutamate couple serves as one amino group acceptor and donor pair in all amino-transfer reactions; the specificity of the individual enzymes derives from the particular amino acid that serves as the other donor of an amino group. Thus, AST catalyzes the following reaction:

$$\underset{\text{L-Aspartate}}{^{\ominus}OOC\text{-}CH(NH_2)\text{-}CH_2\text{-}COO^{\ominus}} + \underset{\text{2-Oxoglutarate}}{^{\ominus}OOC\text{-}C(=O)\text{-}CH_2\text{-}CH_2\text{-}COO^{\ominus}} \xrightleftharpoons{AST,\ P\text{-}5'\text{-}P} \underset{\text{Oxaloacetate}}{^{\ominus}OOC\text{-}C(=O)\text{-}CH_2\text{-}COO^{\ominus}} + \underset{\text{L-Glutamate}}{^{\ominus}OOC\text{-}CH(NH_2)\text{-}CH_2\text{-}CH_2\text{-}COO^{\ominus}}$$

ALT catalyzes the analogous reaction as follows:

$$\underset{\text{L-Alanine}}{^{\ominus}OOC\text{-}CH(NH_2)\text{-}CH_3} + \underset{\text{2-Oxoglutarate}}{^{\ominus}OOC\text{-}C(=O)\text{-}CH_2\text{-}CH_2\text{-}COO^{\ominus}} \xrightleftharpoons{ALT,\ P\text{-}5'\text{-}P} \underset{\text{Pyruvate}}{^{\ominus}OOC\text{-}C(=O)\text{-}CH_3} + \underset{\text{L-Glutamate}}{^{\ominus}OOC\text{-}CH(NH_2)\text{-}CH_2\text{-}CH_2\text{-}COO^{\ominus}}$$

The reactions are reversible, but the equilibria of the AST and ALT reactions favor formation of aspartate and alanine, respectively.

Pyridoxal-5′-phosphate (P-5′-P) and its amino analog, pyridoxamine-5′-phosphate, function as coenzymes in in vivo amino-transfer reactions. The P-5′-P is bound to the inactive apoenzyme and serves as a true prosthetic group. P-5′-P bound to the apoenzyme accepts the amino group from the first substrate, aspartate or alanine, to form enzyme-bound pyridoxamine-5′-phosphate and the first reaction product, oxaloacetate or pyruvate, respectively. The coenzyme in amino form then transfers its amino group to the second substrate, 2-oxoglutarate, to form the second product, glutamate. P-5′-P is thus regenerated.

Both coenzyme-deficient apoenzymes and holoenzymes may be present in serum. Therefore, addition of P-5′-P under measurement conditions that allow recombination with the enzymes usually produces an increase in aminotransferase activity. For clinical assays, in accordance with the principle that all factors affecting the rate of reaction must be optimized and controlled, the addition of P-5′-P in aminotransferase methods is recommended to ensure that all enzymatic activity is measured.

Transaminases are widely distributed throughout the body. Whereas AST is found primarily in the heart, liver, skeletal muscle, and kidney, ALT is found primarily in the liver and kidney, with lesser amounts in heart and skeletal muscle (Table 29.5). ALT is exclusively cytoplasmic, but both mitochondrial and cytoplasmic forms of AST are found in cells. These are genetically distinct AST isoenzymes with a dimeric structure composed of two identical polypeptide subunits of about 400 amino acid residues. About 5% to 10% of the activity of total AST in serum from healthy individuals is of mitochondrial origin.[24]

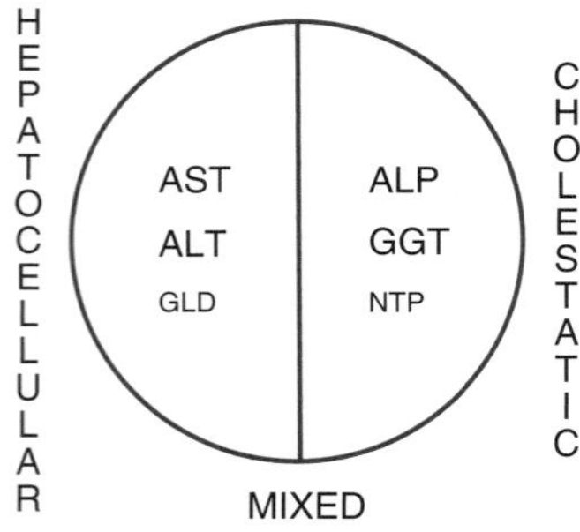

FIGURE 29.4 Liver enzymology patterns. *ALP,* Alkaline phosphatase; *ALT,* alanine aminotransferase; *AST,* aspartate aminotransferase; *GGT,* γ-glutamyltransferase; *GLD,* glutamate dehydrogenase; *NTP,* 5′-nucleotidase.

Clinical Significance

Liver disease is the most important cause of increased transaminase activity in serum and represents the indication for their requesting (see Chapter 61). Although serum activities of both AST and ALT become increased whenever disease processes affect liver cell integrity, ALT is the more

TABLE 29.5 Transaminase Activities in Human Tissues, Relative to Serum as Unity

	AST	ALT
Heart	7800	450
Liver	7100	2850
Skeletal muscle	5000	300
Kidneys	4500	1200
Pancreas	1400	130
Spleen	700	80
Lungs	500	45
Erythrocytes	15	7
Serum	1	1

ALT, Alanine aminotransferase; *AST,* aspartate aminotransferase.
From King J. *Practical clinical enzymology.* London: D. Van Nostrand Co Ltd; 1965.

liver-specific enzyme. Serum increases of ALT activity are rarely observed in conditions other than parenchymal liver disease.[25] Moreover, increases of ALT activity persist longer than do those of AST activity. Thus, the incremental benefit of routine determination of AST, in addition to ALT, may be limited. Ideally, laboratories reporting abnormal ALT results (ie, >2 URL) should offer AST as a reflex test and calculate the AST-to-ALT ratio (AAR) because it provides useful diagnostic and prognostic information.

In most types of liver disease, ALT activity is higher than that of AST; exceptions may be seen in alcoholic hepatitis, hepatic cirrhosis, and liver neoplasia. In viral hepatitis and other forms of liver disease associated with acute hepatic necrosis, serum AST and ALT activities are increased even before the clinical signs and symptoms of disease (eg, jaundice) appear. Activities for both enzymes may reach values as high as 100 times the URL, although 10-fold to 40-fold increases are most frequently encountered. The most efficient aminotransferase threshold for diagnosing acute liver injury lies at seven times the URL (sensitivity and specificity >95%). In acute viral hepatitis, peak values of transaminase activity occur between the 7th and 12th days; activities then gradually decrease, reaching physiologic concentrations by the 3rd to 5th week if recovery is uneventful.[26] Peak activities bear no relationship to prognosis and may fall with worsening of the patient's condition, perhaps because of a lack of further functional hepatocytes to continue enzyme release.

Persistence of increased ALT for longer than 6 months after an episode of acute hepatitis is used to diagnose chronic hepatitis. Most patients with chronic hepatitis have maximum ALT less than seven times the URL. ALT may be persistently normal in 15% to 50% of patients with chronic hepatitis C, but the likelihood of continuously normal ALT decreases with an increasing number of measurements. In patients with acute hepatitis C, ALT should be measured periodically over the next 1 to 2 years to determine if it becomes and stays normal.[26]

The picture in toxic hepatitis is different from that in infectious hepatitis. In acetaminophen-induced hepatic injury, the transaminase peak is more than 85 times the URL in 90% of cases—a value rarely seen with acute viral hepatitis. Furthermore, AST and ALT activities typically peak early and fall rapidly.[26]

Nonalcoholic fatty liver disease (NAFLD) is the most common cause of aminotransferase increases other than viral and alcoholic hepatitis. NAFLD includes a spectrum of liver pathology, from simple steatosis to nonalcoholic steatohepatitis (NASH), in which inflammatory changes and focal necrosis may progress to liver fibrosis, cirrhosis, and hepatic failure. NAFLD is now considered to be an additional feature of the "metabolic syndrome." Indeed, serum aminotransferase elevation in NAFLD is associated with higher body mass index, waist circumference, serum triglycerides, and fasting insulin and lower high-density lipoprotein (HDL) cholesterol—all features characteristic of this syndrome.

Aminotransferase activities observed in cirrhosis vary with the status of the cirrhotic process and range from the URL to four to five times higher, with an AAR greater than 1. This appears to be attributable to a reduction in ALT production in a damaged liver, associated with reduced clearance of AST in advancing liver fibrosis. An AAR of 1 or greater has an approximately 90% positive predictive value for diagnosing the presence of advanced fibrosis in patients with chronic liver disease. Furthermore, the amount of increase in the AAR can reflect the grade of fibrosis in these patients.

Two- to fivefold increases of both enzymes occur in patients with primary or metastatic carcinoma of the liver, with AST usually being higher than ALT, but activities are often normal in the early stages of malignant infiltration of the liver. Slight or moderate increases of AST and ALT activities have been observed after administration of various medications, such as nonsteroidal antiinflammatory drugs, antibiotics, antiepileptic drugs, statins, or opiates. Over-the-counter medications and herbal preparations are also implicated. In patients with increased transaminases, negative viral markers, and a negative history for drugs or alcohol ingestion, the workup should include less common causes of chronic hepatic injury (eg, hemochromatosis, Wilson disease, autoimmune hepatitis, primary biliary cirrhosis, sclerosing cholangitis, celiac disease, α_1-antitrypsin deficiency).[27]

After acute MI, increased AST activity appears in serum, as might be expected from the high AST concentration in heart muscle. AST activity also is increased in progressive muscular dystrophy and dermatomyositis, reaching concentrations up to eight times normal; they are usually normal in other types of muscle disease, especially in those of neurogenic origin. Pulmonary emboli can increase AST to two to three times normal, and slight to moderate increases are noted in acute pancreatitis, crushed muscle injury, and hemolytic disease.

Several authors have described AST linked to immunoglobulins, or macro-AST. Typical findings include a persistent increase in serum AST activity with normal ALT concentrations in an asymptomatic subject, with absence of any demonstrable pathology in organs rich in AST. Increased AST activity might reflect decreased clearance of the abnormal complex from plasma. Macro-AST has no known clinical relevance. However, identification is important to avoid unnecessary diagnostic procedures in these subjects. Laboratory procedures for the demonstration of macro-AST include electrophoresis with specific enzyme stain (atypical origin band) and differential precipitation with PEG 6000 (see the Amylase section later in this chapter).[28]

POINTS TO REMEMBER

Testing of AST in addition to ALT should be limited because:

- ALT is the more liver-specific enzyme. Moreover, increases of ALT activity persist longer than AST.
- The incremental benefit of routine determination of AST, in addition to ALT, is limited.
- Laboratories reporting abnormal ALT results (ie, greater than twice the URL) should offer AST as a reflex test and calculate the AST-to-ALT ratio because it provides useful diagnostic and prognostic information.

Methods for Measurement of Transaminase Activity

The assay system for measuring transaminase activity contains two amino acids and two oxo-acids. Because no convenient method is available for assaying amino acids, formation or consumption of the oxo-acids is measured. Continuous-monitoring methods are commonly used to measure transaminase activity by coupling transaminase reactions to specific dehydrogenase reactions. The oxo-acids formed in the transaminase reaction are measured indirectly by enzymatic reduction to corresponding hydroxy acids, and the accompanying change in NADH concentration is monitored spectrophotometrically. Thus oxaloacetate, formed in the AST reaction, is reduced to malate in the presence of malate dehydrogenase (MD).

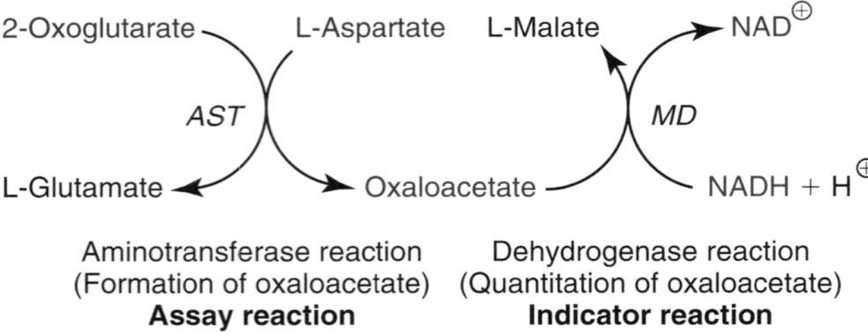

Pyruvate formed in the ALT reaction is reduced to lactate by lactate dehydrogenase (LDH). The substrate, NADH, and an auxiliary enzyme, MD or LDH, must be present in sufficient quantity so that the reaction rate is limited only by the amounts of AST and ALT, respectively. As the reactions proceed, NADH is oxidized to NAD^+. The disappearance of NADH is followed by measuring the decrease in absorbance at 340 nm for several minutes, either continuously or at frequent intervals. The change in absorbance per minute (ΔA/min) is proportional to the micromoles of NADH oxidized and in turn to micromoles of substrate transformed per minute. A preliminary incubation period is necessary to ensure that NADH-dependent reduction of endogenous oxo-acids in the sample is completed before 2-oxoglutarate is added to start the transaminase reaction. After a brief lag phase, the change in absorbance (ΔA) is monitored. As already mentioned, supplementation with P-5′-P ensures that all transaminase activity of the sample is measured.

Because of the large numbers of AST and ALT activity measurements performed daily in clinical laboratories throughout the world, standardization of transaminase measurements is a priority need for patient care. As discussed in Chapter 22, the reference system approach, based on the concepts of metrologic traceability and the hierarchy of analytical measurement procedures, gives clinical laboratories and the medical community universal means of creating and ensuring the comparability of results. In this system, the IFCC reference measurement procedure forms the highest metrologic level and thereby constitutes the definition of the respective measurable enzyme quantity.[16] Primary IFCC procedures for the measurement of catalytic activity concentrations of AST and ALT at 37°C have been published.[29,30] Values assigned to the manufacturer's product calibrators and measurement results of lower metrologic levels, including those used in daily clinical practice, should be traceable to these top-level reference measurement procedures, thus improving the accuracy and comparability of transaminase results. It should be remembered that the concept of the reference system is valid only if the reference procedure and corresponding routine procedures have identical, or at least very similar, specificities for the measured enzyme. Thus, it will not be possible to calibrate procedures for aminotransferases that do not incorporate P-5′-P using a procedure that does, such as the IFCC reference procedure, because the ratio of preformed holoenzyme to apoenzyme differs among specimens.

AST activity in serum is stable for up to 48 hours at 4°C. Specimens have to be stored frozen if they are to be kept longer. ALT activity should be assayed on the day of sample collection because activity is lost at room temperature, 4°C, and −25°C. ALT stability is better maintained at −70°C. Hemolyzed specimens should not be used, especially when AST is measured, because of the large amount of this enzyme present in red cells.

Biological variation data suggest that imprecision (CV) of less than 6.2%, bias of ±6.5%, and total error of ±16.7% for AST and imprecision (CV) of less than 9.7%, bias of ±11.5%, and total error of ±27.5% for ALT, respectively, are required for clinical use of aminotransferase determinations.[31] In general, the imprecision target is easily met using current aminotransferase methods. In an international study, the desirable accuracy of ALT results was obtained by the great majority (≥90%) of participating laboratories, but for AST, a bias often exceeding the desirable goal was shown.[17] A more recent experience has confirmed these data, attributing the poor trueness of AST results to the frequent lack of P-5′-P addition in the commercial reagents that are used.[32]

Reference Intervals

Using methods traceable to the IFCC reference procedure and a careful selection of healthy individuals, the AST URL for adults, calculated as the 97.5th percentile of the reference distribution, was 35 U/L, with no significant sex-related differences.[33] Conversely, a clear difference in ALT activities has been noted between men and women. Corresponding ALT URLs are 60 U/L and 42 U/L, respectively.[33] ALT does not reveal a distinct age dependency during childhood, but serum AST activity in neonates and in children younger than 3 years old is twice that in adults. Adult values are attained by the time the child reaches puberty.[34] A circadian variation has been observed in ALT activity, and serum concentrations of both aminotransferases tend to increase in the winter.[35]

Glutamate Dehydrogenase

Glutamate dehydrogenase (EC 1.4.1.3; L-glutamate: NAD[P]$^+$oxidoreductase, deaminating; GLD) is a mitochondrial enzyme found mainly in the liver, heart muscle, and kidneys, but small amounts occur in other tissue, including brain and skeletal muscle tissue, and in leukocytes.

Glutamate dehydrogenase is a zinc-containing enzyme that consists of six polypeptide chains and has a molecular weight of about 350 kDa. Larger polymers are also found. The enzyme catalyzes the removal of hydrogen from L-glutamate to form the corresponding ketimino-acid, which undergoes spontaneous hydrolysis to 2-oxoglutarate.

$$\text{L-Glutamate} + NAD^{\oplus} \xrightleftharpoons{\text{Glutamate dehydrogenase}} \text{Ketimino acid} + NADH + H^{\oplus}$$

$$\text{Ketimino acid} + H_2O \xrightarrow{\text{Spontaneous}} \text{2-Oxoglutarate} + NH_3$$

Although NAD$^+$ is the preferred coenzyme, NADP$^+$ also acts as the hydrogen acceptor. GLD is inhibited by metal ions, such as Ag^+ and Hg^+, by several chelating agents, and by L-thyroxine.

Clinical Significance

Glutamate dehydrogenase is increased in the serum of patients with hepatocellular damage.[36] Four- or fivefold increases are seen in chronic hepatitis; in cirrhosis, increases are only up to twofold. Very large rises in serum GLD occur in halothane toxicity, and notable increases are seen in response to some other hepatotoxic agents.

Glutamate dehydrogenase potentially offers differential diagnostic potential in the investigation of liver disease, particularly when interpreted in conjunction with other enzyme test results. The key to this differential diagnostic potential is to be found in the intraorgan and intracellular distribution of the enzyme as discussed earlier in this chapter. As an exclusively mitochondrial enzyme, GLD is released from necrotic cells; therefore, compared with hepatic disorders with extensive necrosis, release is less in diffuse inflammatory processes, and in these conditions, the release of cytoplasmic enzymes, such as ALT, is quantitatively more pronounced. GLD can therefore be of value in estimating the severity of liver cell damage.

Glutamate dehydrogenase is more concentrated in the central areas of the liver lobules than in the periportal zones. This pattern of distribution is the reverse of that of ALT. Pronounced release of GLD therefore is to be expected in conditions in which centrilobular necrosis occurs (eg, as a result of ischemia, in halothane toxicity).

Methods for Determination of Glutamate Dehydrogenase Activity

Continuous-monitoring methods have been developed for determination of GLD using both forward and reverse reactions. The equilibrium favors the formation of glutamate, and higher reaction rates are observed when 2-oxoglutarate is used as a substrate. Serum is added to a solution of NADH, an ammonium salt, and ADP in buffer at a pH of 7.5, and the reaction is initiated by the addition of the substrate, 2-oxoglutarate. The rate of decrease in absorbance at 340 nm is measured. The German Society for Clinical Chemistry has published optimum reaction conditions for 37°C.[37] Oxamate is incorporated into the reaction mixture because this acid inhibits LDH activity, avoiding the critical consumption of NADH by this enzyme in serum. There is no international reference measurement procedure for GLD.

Glutamate dehydrogenase activity in serum is stable at 4°C for 48 hours and at −20°C for several weeks.

Reference Intervals

The GLD URLs are 6 U/L (women) and 8 U/L (men) when a method optimized at 37°C is used.

Alkaline Phosphatase

Alkaline phosphatase (EC 3.1.3.1; orthophosphoric-monoester phosphohydrolase [alkaline optimum]; ALP) catalyzes the alkaline hydrolysis of a large variety of naturally occurring and synthetic substrates.

Alkaline phosphatase activity is present in most organs of the body and is especially associated with cell surfaces located in the mucosa of the small intestine and the proximal convoluted tubules of the kidney, in bone (osteoblasts), liver, and placenta, anchored on the cell membrane by glycosylphosphatidylinositol ("ectoenzyme"). Although the exact metabolic function of the enzyme is not yet understood, it appears that ALP is associated with lipid transport in the intestine and with the calcification process in bone.

Alkaline phosphatase exists in multiple forms (molecular weight ranges from 70 to 120 kDa), some of which are true isoenzymes, encoded at separate genetic loci (Fig. 29.5).[38] Bone, liver, and kidney ALP forms share a common primary structure coded for by the same genetic locus, but they differ in carbohydrate content.

Some divalent ions, such as Mg^{2+}, Co^{2+}, and Mn^{2+}, are activators of the enzyme, and Zn^{2+} is a constituent metal ion. The correct ratio of Mg^{2+} to Zn^{2+} ions is necessary to avoid displacement of Mg^{2+} and to attain optimal activity. Phosphate, borate, oxalate, and cyanide ions are inhibitors of ALP activity. Variations in Mg^{2+} and substrate concentrations change the pH optimum. The type of buffer present (except at low concentrations) affects the rate of enzyme activity. Buffers can be classified as inert (carbonate and barbital), inhibiting (glycine and propylamine), or activating (2-amino-2-methyl-1-propanol [AMP], tris [hydroxymethyl] aminomethane [TRIS], and diethanolamine [DEA]).

The ALP activity present in the sera of healthy adults originates mainly in the liver, with most of the rest coming from

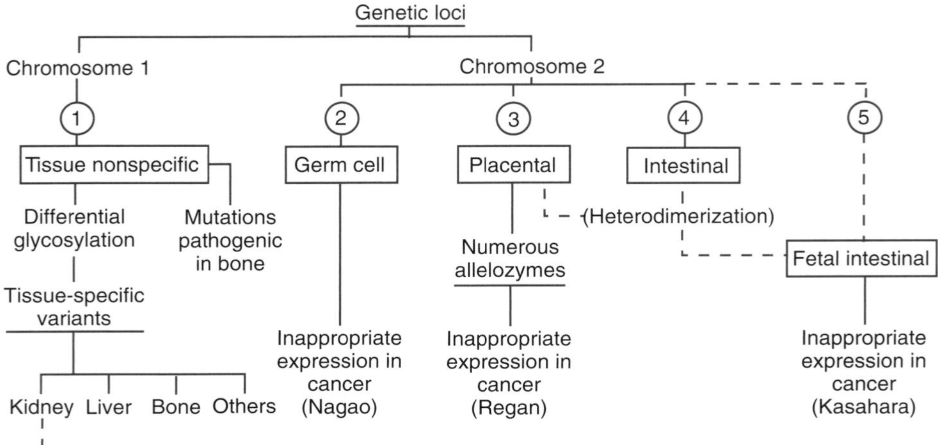

FIGURE 29.5 Identities, chromosomal assignments, and main physiologic and pathologic expression of genes encoding human alkaline phosphatases. The gene names (and gene symbols) are alkaline phosphatase, liver, bone, and kidney (ALPL); alkaline phosphatase, intestinal (ALPI); alkaline phosphatase, placental (ALPP); and alkaline phosphatase, placental-like 2 (ALPPL2). *Broken lines* show two alternative proposed origins of the fetal intestinal ALP; the sequence of a cDNA is reportedly identical to that of adult intestinal ALP. All isoenzymes and isoforms are glycoproteins, imposing a further level of microheterogeneity. Different processes of cleavage or preservation of the membrane-anchoring domain can generate additional isoforms. (Modified from Moss DW. Perspectives in alkaline phosphatase research. *Clin Chem* 1992;38:2486-92.)

the skeleton. The respective contributions of these two forms to the total activity are age dependent. Minimal amounts of intestinal ALP may also be present, particularly in the sera of individuals of blood group B or O (ie, those who are secretors of blood group substances). Because intestinal ALP activity in serum may increase after a meal, ALP should be measured preferentially in fasting sera.

Clinical Significance

Increases in serum ALP activity commonly originate from one or both of two sources: liver and bone. Consequently, serum ALP measurements are of particular interest in the investigation of two groups of conditions: hepatobiliary disease and bone disease associated with increased osteoblastic activity (see the Bone Enzymes section later in this chapter; for more discussion on bone disease, see Chapter 64).

Serum ALP was the first enzyme to be used for the investigation of hepatic disease. The response of the liver to any form of biliary tree obstruction induces the synthesis of ALP by hepatocytes. The newly formed ectoenzyme is released from cell membrane by the action of bile salts and enters the circulation to increase the enzyme activity in serum.[39] Increase tends to be more notable (greater than fourfold the URL) in extrahepatic obstruction (eg, by stone, by cancer of the head of the pancreas) than in intrahepatic obstruction and is greater the more complete the obstruction. Serum enzyme activities may reach 10 to 12 times the URL and usually return to baseline on surgical removal of the obstruction. A similar increase is seen in patients with advanced primary liver cancer or widespread secondary hepatic metastases. ALP increase (greater than twofold the URL) can predict outcomes (liver transplantation or death) of patients with primary biliary cirrhosis.[40]

Liver diseases that principally affect parenchymal cells, such as infectious hepatitis, typically show only moderately (less than threefold) increased or even normal serum ALP activities. Increases may also be seen as a consequence of a reaction to drug therapy and ALT/ALP-based criteria to discriminate the type of liver injury in drug-induced hepatic toxicity have been recommended (Table 29.6). Intestinal ALP isoenzyme, an asialoglycoprotein normally cleared by the hepatic asialoglycoprotein receptors, is often increased in patients with liver cirrhosis.

An increase of up to two to three times URL is observed in women in the third trimester of pregnancy, with the additional enzyme being of placental origin. This makes ALP an unreliable marker of hepatobiliary disease in pregnancy. Reports have also described a benign familial increase in serum ALP activity caused by increased concentrations of intestinal ALP.[41] Transient, benign increases in serum ALP may be observed in infants and children, with changes often more than 10 times the URL. Increases in both liver and bone forms are seen. These changes seem to reflect a reduction in

TABLE 29.6 Enzyme-Based Criteria for Drug-Induced Liver Toxicity (Enzyme Values Expressed as Multiples of the Upper Reference Limit in Serum)

Injury Type	ALT	ALP	ALT/ALP Ratio
Hepatocellular	>2 URL	<URL	≥5
Cholestatic	<URL	>2 URL	≤2
Mixed	>2 URL	>2 URL	2–5

ALP, Alkaline phosphatase; *ALT,* alanine aminotransferase; *URL,* upper reference limit.
Data from the Council of International Organizations of Medical Sciences; 1990.

the removal of ALP from blood caused by transient modifications of enzyme glycosylation.[42] Mutations in the tissue-nonspecific ALP gene are associated with hypophosphatasia, a rare inherited disorder characterized by poor bone mineralization and low serum ALP activity.

A result of the application of techniques of isoenzyme analysis to the characterization of ALP in serum was the discovery that forms of the enzyme essentially identical to the normal placental isoenzyme appear in the sera of some patients with malignant disease. These carcinoplacental isoenzymes (eg, Regan isoenzyme) appear to result from de-repression of the placental ALP gene. As described later, the presence of these isoenzymes can be readily detected in serum by their stability at 65°C. Tumors have also been found to produce ALPs that appear to be modified forms of non-placental isoenzymes (Kasahara isoenzyme).

Methods for Determination of Alkaline Phosphatase Activity

Numerous methods have been developed for determining ALP activity. In general, methodologic developments have been directed toward increasing the speed and sensitivity of the assay by selecting readily hydrolyzed substrates and phosphate-accepting buffers and toward the use of continuous-monitoring methods based on "self-indicating" substrates.

The most popular of the chromogenic or self-indicating substrates for ALP is 4-nitrophenyl phosphate (usually abbreviated 4-NPP, or PNPP from the older name, *p*-nitrophenyl phosphate). This ester is colorless, but the final product is yellow at the pH of the reaction:

The enzyme reaction is continuously monitored by observing the rate of formation of the 4-nitrophenoxide ions. With improvement in reaction conditions, this reaction forms the basis of current recommended and standard methods of ALP assay. Other self-indicating substrates include phenolphthalein monophosphate, thymolphthalein phosphate, and α-naphthyl phosphate. With the ALP methods discussed, the liberated phosphate group is transferred to water. The rate of phosphatase action is enhanced, however, if certain amino alcohols are used as phosphate-accepting buffers. Among these activators are compounds such as AMP, DEA, TRIS, ethylaminoethanol (EAE), and *N*-methyl-D-glucamine (MEG). Enzyme activity in the presence of optimal concentrations of these buffers is two- to sixfold greater than in the presence of a nonactivating buffer, such as carbonate.

Alkaline phosphatase catalyzes the hydrolysis of 4-NPP, forming phosphate and free 4-nitrophenol (4-NP, PNP), which in dilute acid solutions is colorless. Under alkaline conditions, 4-NP is converted to the 4-nitrophenoxide ion, which has a very intense yellow color. The rate of formation of 4-NP by the action of the enzyme on 4-NPP at 37°C is then monitored at 405 nm with a recording spectrophotometer. The IFCC-recommended method uses 4-NPP as the substrate and AMP as the phosphate-acceptor buffer. It includes Mg^{2+} and Zn^{2+}, optimal concentrations of which are controlled by the addition of Mg^{2+} and Zn^{2+}, and the chelating agent *N*-hydroxyethylethylenediaminetriacetic acid (HEDTA). Although Zn^{2+} ions are present in a total concentration of 1 mmol/L, most are bound to HEDTA, leaving only a small, experimentally determined optimal concentration of free ions. A similar situation exists for Mg^{2+} ions. Thus, HEDTA acts as a metal ion buffer, maintaining optimal concentrations of both ions.[43]

Serum or heparinized plasma, free of hemolysis, should be used. Complexing anticoagulants—such as citrate, oxalate, and EDTA—must be avoided because they bind cations, such as Mg^{2+} and Zn^{2+}, which are necessary cofactors for ALP activity measurement. Blood transfusion (containing citrate) causes a transient decrease in serum ALP through a similar mechanism. Freshly collected serum samples should be kept at room temperature and assayed as soon as possible but preferably within 4 hours after collection. In sera stored at a refrigerated temperature, ALP activity increases slowly (2%/d). Frozen specimens should be thawed and kept at room temperature for 18 to 24 hours before measurement to achieve full enzyme reactivation.

Desirable analytical specifications for ALP determination are imprecision (CV) of less than 3.0%, bias of ±5.5%, and total error of ±14%.[44] As for other clinically important enzymes, the current emphasis is on the standardization and traceability of the commercial assays to the IFCC reference measurement system for ALP. A preliminary experience has shown, with some exceptions, a fairly good harmonization among ALP results obtained with eight of the most popular chemistry systems.[45]

Reference Intervals

Alkaline phosphatase activities in serum vary with age and gender. Infants and peripubertal children show higher ALP activity (up to threefold) than healthy adults as a result of the leakage of bone ALP from osteoblasts during bone growth. However, activities in growing children are highly variable and the decrease in ALP activity to typical adult ranges is known to differ from subject to subject, occurring on average 2 years earlier in females than in males. Using a method traceable to the IFCC reference procedure, the following reference intervals (central 95th percentiles) have been established in adult individuals: 33 to 98 U/L for premenopausal women (18–49 years) and 43 to 115 U/L for men (≥20 years).[43] For women, a progressive increase of both lower and URL after menopause is described.[46]

Methods for Separation and Quantification of Alkaline Phosphatase Isoenzymes

Assays for ALP isoenzymes are needed when (1) the source of an increased ALP in serum is not obvious and should be clarified, (2) the main clinical question is concerned with

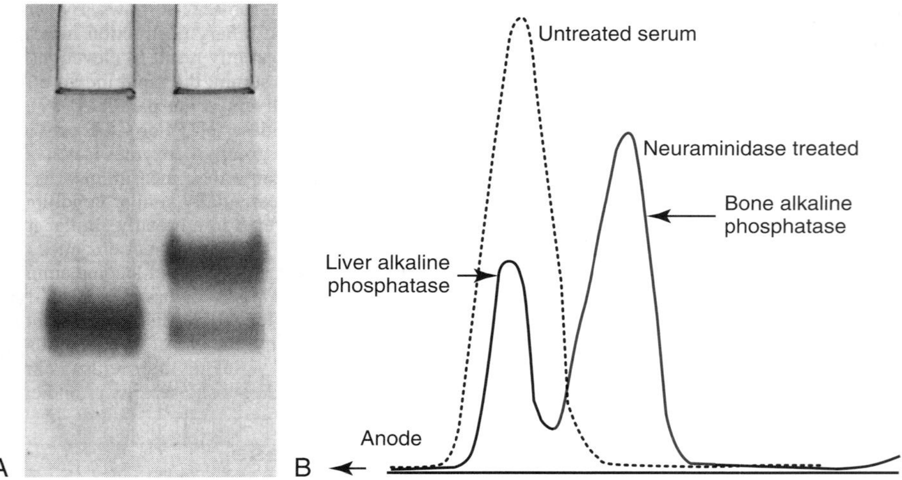

FIGURE 29.6 A, Polyacrylamide-gel electrophoresis of bone and liver alkaline phosphatases in human serum. *Left,* Mixture of two sera containing, respectively, entirely bone phosphatase and entirely liver phosphatase. *Right,* Mixture of the same two sera after each has been treated with neuraminidase for 10 minutes at 37°C. The anodal direction is downward. The more anodal zone is liver phosphatase. **B,** Densitometric scans of electrophoretic patterns shown in **A**. *Broken line,* Scan of mixture of untreated sera; *solid line,* scan of mixture of sera treated briefly with neuraminidase. (From Moss DW, Edwards RK. Improved electrophoretic resolution of bone and liver alkaline phosphatases resulting from partial digestion with neuraminidase. *Clin Chim Acta* 1984;143:177-182.)

detecting the presence of liver or bone involvement separately, or (3) it is important to ascertain any modifications in the activity of osteoblasts to monitor disease activity and the effects of appropriate therapies in the case of metabolic bone disorders.

Criteria that have been used to differentiate the isoenzymes and other multiple forms of ALP include (1) electrophoretic mobility, (2) stability to denaturation by heat or chemicals, (3) response to the presence of selected inhibitors, (4) affinity for specific lectins, and (5) immunochemical characteristics.[47]

The same electrophoretic techniques are used for the separation of ALP isoenzymes in serum as for separation of serum proteins. After electrophoresis, ALP zones are made visible by incubating the gel in a solution of buffered substrate (eg, 1-naphthyl phosphate, to which a chromogenic system, usually represented by a diazonium salt, is added; in the case of electrophoresis on cellulose acetate, the strips are covered with an agar gel layer containing the staining system). The liver ALP typically moves most rapidly toward the anode. Bone ALP, which typically gives a more diffuse zone than the liver form, has slightly reduced anodal mobility, although the two zones usually overlap to some extent. Whereas intestinal ALP migrates more slowly than the bone enzyme, the placental isoenzyme commonly appears as a discrete band overlying the diffuse bone fraction. An additional band, which is frequently present in the serum of patients with various hepatic diseases, contains a high molecular weight form of ALP but is also strongly negatively charged. Therefore, it moves slowly in starch gel or may even fail to enter polyacrylamide gel, but it migrates more anodally than the main liver zone on nonsieving media, such as cellulose acetate. Investigations of this form have revealed that it corresponds to the main liver form attached to the membrane moiety (membrane particle [fragment] ALP).

Complexes between ALP and immunoglobulins, or macro-ALP, occur occasionally in serum, giving rise to abnormally migrating bands in the γ-globulin zone; however, they do not provide specific diagnostic information in the present state of knowledge. PEG precipitation (see the Amylase section later in this chapter) may represent a suitable alternative for macro-ALP detection.

A sample pretreatment approach can be used to improve the electrophoretic separation between bone and liver ALPs, exploiting differences in the carbohydrate portions of the two forms of ALP. Serum is treated briefly (ie, for 15 minutes at 37°C) with neuraminidase to remove a portion of the terminal sialic acid residues. Because the sialic acid residues of bone ALP are more readily attacked than those of liver ALP, the electrophoretic mobility of the bone form is reduced more than that of liver ALP. The improved separation allows quantitative estimates to be made by densitometric scanning (Fig. 29.6).[48] As an alternative to electrophoretic fractionation of ALP, measurement of GGT, which is increased in liver disease but not in bone disease, may be a useful rapid tool to distinguish between the two diseases as the explanation for an increased serum ALP.

Prolonged (overnight) incubation of the serum sample with neuraminidase is used to confirm the presence of intestinal ALP. This treatment reduces the anodal mobility of all ALP isoenzymes except that of intestinal origin, which is neuraminidase resistant because terminal sialic acid residues are not present in the molecule. Because placental ALP is heat stable, incubation of the serum sample at a temperature as high as 65°C for 30 minutes provides a convenient test for the presence of this isoenzyme. Immunologic methods provide the best quantitative measurements of intestinal or placental ALPs. Much more difficult is the production of antibodies that selectively react with different products of the tissue-nonspecific ALP gene, including liver- and bone-derived isoforms, because these antibodies should recognize specific sugar sidechains instead of a particular amino acid sequence. Until now, no monoclonal antibodies have fully discriminated between liver and bone ALPs. Despite lack of complete specificity, commercially available immunoassays of bone ALP may offer some advantages, but their value has not been convincingly demonstrated, partly because measurements of total ALP provide the required clinical information in many situations.

5′-Nucleotidase

5′-Nucleotidase (EC 3.1.3.5; 5′-ribonucleotide phosphohydrolase; NTP) is a phosphatase that acts only on nucleoside-5′-phosphates, such as adenosine-5′-phosphate (AMP) and adenylic acid, releasing inorganic phosphate.

Adenosine-5′-monophosphate (AMP) + H_2O → (Nucleotidase, pH 6.6 to 7.0) Adenosine + $HOPO_3^{2-}$

5′-Nucleotidase is a glycoprotein that is widely distributed throughout the tissues of the body and is principally localized in the cytoplasmic membrane of the cells in which it occurs ("ecto-5'-nucleotidase"). Its pH optimum is between 6.6 and 7.0.

Clinical Significance

Despite its ubiquitous distribution, serum NTP activities appear to reflect hepatobiliary disease with considerable specificity. NTP is increased three- to sixfold in those hepatobiliary diseases in which there is interference with the secretion of bile. This may be due to extrahepatic causes (a stone or tumor occluding the bile duct), or it may arise from intrahepatic conditions, such as cholestasis caused by chlorpromazine, malignant infiltration of the liver, or biliary cirrhosis. When parenchymal cell damage is predominant, as in infectious hepatitis, serum NTP activity is only moderately increased.

The assay of NTP activity has been considered of value as an addition to measurement of nonspecific total ALP in patients with suspected hepatobiliary disease, and increased NTP activity is routinely interpreted as evidence of a hepatic origin of increased ALP activity in serum. However, approximately half of individuals in whom liver ALP activity is increased in serum may simultaneously show a normal NTP. On the other hand, increased NTP in the serum of patients with normal liver ALP is very often associated with the presence of liver disease. Thus, the frequent dissociation of the two enzyme activities supports the usefulness of determining both (liver) ALP and NTP to enhance diagnostic efficiency in patients with suspected liver disease.[49]

Methods for Determination of 5′-Nucleotidase Activity

The substrates most generally used in measuring the activity of NTP are AMP and IMP (inosine-5′-phosphate). However, these substrates are organic phosphate esters and thus can be hydrolyzed to an appreciable degree by other nonspecific (alkaline) phosphatases, even at a pH as low as 7.5, which is the pH assumed optimal for NTP activity. Methods for the estimation of NTP in serum therefore must incorporate some means for correcting for the hydrolysis of the substrate by the nonspecific phosphatases.

In a commercially available assay, serum NTP catalyzes the hydrolysis of IMP to yield inosine, which is then converted to hypoxanthine by purine-nucleoside phosphorylase (EC 2.4.2.1). Hypoxanthine is oxidized to urate with xanthine oxidase (EC 1.2.3.2). Two moles of hydrogen peroxide are produced for each mole of hypoxanthine liberated and converted to uric acid. The formation rate of hydrogen peroxide is monitored by a spectrophotometer at 510 nm by the oxidation of a chromogenic system. The effect of ALPs on IMP is inhibited by β-glycerophosphate. This material is substrate for ALP but not for NTP, and by forming substrate complexes with the former enzyme, it reduces the proportion of total ALP activity that is directed to the hydrolysis of the NTP substrate, IMP.[50] There is no international reference procedure for NTP measurement in serum.

5′-Nucleotidase activity in serum or plasma heparin is stable for at least 4 days at 4°C and 4 months at −20°C.

Desirable analytical specifications for NTP determination are imprecision (CV) of less than 2.1%, bias of ±2.9%, and total error of ±8.3%.[44]

Reference Interval

The reference interval for NTP activity at 37°C is from 3 to 9 U/L, with no sex-related differences.

γ-Glutamyltransferase

Peptidases are enzymes that catalyze the hydrolytic cleavage of peptides to form amino acids or smaller peptides. They constitute a broad group of enzymes of varied specificity, and some individual enzymes act as amino acid transferases and catalyze the transfer of amino acids from one peptide to another amino acid or peptide. γ-Glutamyltransferase (EC 2.3.2.2; γ-glutamyl-peptide:amino acid γ-glutamyltransferase; GGT) catalyzes the transfer of the γ-glutamyl group from peptides and compounds to an acceptor.[51] The γ-glutamyl acceptor is the substrate itself, some amino acid or peptide, or even water, in which case simple hydrolysis takes place. The enzyme acts only on peptides or peptide-like compounds containing a terminal glutamate residue joined to the remainder of the compound through the terminal (-γ-) carboxyl. Glycylglycine is five times more effective as an acceptor than is glycine or the tripeptide (gly-gly-gly), but little is known about the optimal properties of the acceptor cosubstrate. The peptidase transfer reaction is considerably faster than the simple hydrolysis reaction. An example of a reaction catalyzed by the enzyme is shown here:

γ-Glutamyl-*p*-nitroanilide
Substrate (donor)
+
Glycylglycine
Acceptor
γ-*Glutamyltransferase*
pH 8.2
p-Nitroaniline
Donor residue
+
p-Glutamylglycylglycine
Transfer product

GGT is present (in decreasing order of abundance) in proximal renal tubule, liver, pancreas, and intestine. The enzyme is present in cytoplasm (microsomes), but the larger fraction is located in the cell membrane and may transport amino acids and peptides into the cell across the cell membrane in the form of γ-glutamyl peptides. GGT is critical for the maintenance of adequate intracellular concentrations of reduced glutathione, a major antioxidant agent.[52]

GGT activity in serum comes primarily from the liver, where it is predominantly found in the biliary pole of the hepatocyte. However, it is also found in both the cytosol and the smooth endoplasmic reticulum (where it is susceptible to induction). The enzyme in serum is heterogeneous with respect to both net molecular charge (eg, shown by electrophoresis) and size. These forms appear to derive from post-translational modifications of a single type of enzyme molecule rather than resulting from the existence of true isoenzymes. For example, high molecular weight forms may represent the release of cell membrane fragments into the circulation. Despite numerous investigations, clear correlations between patterns of multiple forms and particular diseases cannot be discerned.

Clinical Significance

Even though renal tissue has the highest concentration of GGT, the enzyme present in serum appears to originate primarily from the hepatobiliary system. GGT is a sensitive indicator of the presence of hepatobiliary disease, being increased in most subjects with liver disease regardless of cause, but its usefulness is limited by lack of specificity. Similar to ALP, it is highest in cases of intrahepatic or posthepatic biliary obstruction, reaching activities some 5 to 30 times the URL. High increases of GGT are also observed in patients with primary or secondary (metastatic) liver neoplasm and other hepatic space-occupying lesions, presumably caused by intrahepatic obstruction. Moderate increases (two to five times the URL) occur in infectious hepatitis. Small increases in GGT activity are observed in more than 50% of patients with NAFLD, and similar but transient increases are noted in cases of drug intoxication. In acute and chronic pancreatitis and in some pancreatic malignancies (especially if associated with hepatobiliary obstruction), enzyme activity may be 5 to 15 times the URL.

Increased activities of GGT are found in the sera of patients with alcoholic hepatitis and in the majority of sera from people who are heavy drinkers. GGT is also increased with increased body weight and obesity, and the effect of alcohol is more marked in these groups. Increased concentrations of the enzyme are also found in the serum of subjects receiving anticonvulsant drugs such as phenytoin and phenobarbital. Such an increase in GGT activity in serum may reflect induction of new enzyme activity by the action of the alcohol and drugs or their toxic effects on microsomal structures in liver cells.

In acute MI, GGT activity is usually normal. If there is a rise, it occurs at about the fourth day, reaches a maximum value in another 4 days, and probably implies liver damage secondary to cardiac insufficiency.

Unlike ALP, serum GGT is not increased in conditions in which osteoblastic activity is increased, so the enzyme measurement can be useful in differentiating the source of ALP activity increase in serum, whether it is of bone or liver origin.

Epidemiologic evidence has shown that serum GGT activity possesses an independent prognostic value for cardiovascular morbidity and mortality.[53] Indeed, experimental work has documented that active enzyme is present in atherosclerotic plaques, and this appears related to the ability of GGT to mediate redox/pro-oxidant reactions at a cellular level.[54] In a recent metaanalysis of 29 prospective cohort studies, the pooled fully adjusted risk ratio (95% confidence interval) for cardiovascular disease was 1.23 (1.16–1.29) for a 1–standard deviation change in baseline log concentrations of GGT.[55]

Methods for Determination of γ-Glutamyltransferase Activity

Early GGT assays used L-γ-glutamyl-*p*-nitroanilide (GGPNA) as the substrate, with glycylglycine serving as the γ-glutamyl residue acceptor. However, GGPNA has limited solubility in the reaction mixture, and it is therefore difficult to obtain saturating substrate concentrations. The *p*-nitroaniline produced in the reaction is determined by its yellow color, which is monitored at 405 nm.

Derivatives of GGPNA are also available and have been used in other methods. With these derivatives, various groups have been introduced into the benzene ring to increase solubility in water. The most useful of these substrates is L-γ-glutamyl-3-carboxy-4-nitroanilide, which is readily soluble in water and is split by GGT at a rate comparable with that observed with GGPNA. In the IFCC reference measurement procedure for GGT, L-γ-glutamyl-3-carboxy-4-nitroanilide serves as the substrate, with glycylglycine serving as an acceptor. Buffering is provided by glycylglycine itself. The temperature of the reaction is 37°C, and the wavelength of measurement of the reaction product, 5-amino-2-nitrobenzoate, is 410 nm.[56] This is a slightly longer wavelength than is used for the non-carboxylated substrate because the carboxy derivative has a higher absorbance than the noncarboxylated substrate, and the longer wavelength reduces the blank absorbance.

γ-Glutamyltransferase activity is stable for at least 1 month at 4°C and for 1 year at −20°C. Nonhemolyzed serum is the preferred specimen, but EDTA plasma has also been used. Heparin may produce turbidity in the reaction mixture; citrate, oxalate, and fluoride depress GGT activity by 10% to 15%.

Desirable analytical specifications for GGT determination are imprecision (CV) of less than 3.7%, bias of ±11.8%, and total error of ±22.2%.[16,44] Currently, there is an international standardization effort requiring the manufacturers of in vitro diagnostic medical devices to meet the metrologic traceability of values assigned to their calibrators by using the IFCC primary reference procedure and suitable reference materials.[16] In 2006, a pilot study involving 70 European laboratories assessed GGT assays from six manufacturers for traceability to the IFCC reference procedure, and only one company system fully complied.[17] Eight years later, a substantial improvement in analytical performance of marketed GGT assays has been demonstrated, showing that the harmonization effort of manufacturers was successful in terms of implementation of IFCC traceable results.[32]

Reference Intervals

In adults, the URL for GGT activity in serum is 40 U/L for females and 70 U/L for males, when measured with an assay traceable to the IFCC reference procedure.[33] Reference limits are approximately twofold higher in people of African ancestry. In normal full-term neonates, GGT activity at birth is approximately six to seven times the adult reference interval. The activity then declines, reaching adult values by the age of 5 to 7 months.[57]

Glutathione S-Transferase

Cytosolic glutathione S-transferases (EC 2.5.1.18; GST) are dimeric enzymes that catalyze the nucleophilic addition of glutathione to the electrophilic centers of a wide variety of chemical structures, accomplishing detoxification reactions. In addition, GSTs exert part of the glutathione peroxidase activity and have an important function in intracellular binding and transport of a wide variety of both endogenous and exogenous compounds. The family of human enzymes is divided into four main classes: α, μ, π, and θ.[58]

α-GST is found at high concentrations in the human liver and is released quickly and in large quantities from damaged hepatocytes into the bloodstream.

Clinical Significance

Unlike aminotransferases, which are found predominantly in the periportal hepatocytes, α-GST is evenly distributed across the liver acinus and therefore is released in all types of hepatocyte injury. In liver transplant recipients, α-GST was found to be more valuable than AST in detecting early rejection episodes postoperatively and less susceptible to the confounding effects of infection. The follow-up studies on α-GST have, however, yielded inferior sensitivity and accuracy than preliminary studies, clearly questioning the clinical utility of this marker.

Methods for Determination of Glutathione S-Transferase

Several problems have been associated with GST activity measurements. First, normal plasma activity is low and difficult to measure. Second, GST binds a number of anions, such as bile salts and bilirubin, that inhibit enzyme activity. Immunoassays have been described that allow the precise and specific measurement of α-GST concentrations. The only methodologic problem relates to the assay turnaround time, which takes several hours.

Reference Interval

Using a commercially available enzyme immunoassay for α-GST, the URL was 11.4 μg/L.[59]

PANCREATIC ENZYMES

The most commonly used serum biomarkers for investigation of pancreatic disease, and more specifically acute pancreatitis, are digestive enzymes. Assays of lipase, (P-type) amylase, and trypsin are applied. Pancreatic function and pathology are discussed in Chapter 62.

Lipase

Human pancreatic lipase (EC 3.1.1.3; triacylglycerol acylhydrolase; LIP) is a single-chain glycoprotein with a molecular weight of 48 kDa and an isoelectric point of about 5.8. The LIP gene resides on chromosome 10. LIP concentration in the pancreas is about 5000-fold greater than in other tissues, and the concentration gradient between the pancreas and serum is approximately 20,000-fold.[60] For full catalytic activity and greatest specificity, the presence of bile salts and a cofactor called *colipase,* which is a small molecular weight protein of 10,000 kDa secreted by the pancreatic acinar cells, are required. Human LIP can be fully activated in vitro by colipases from other species (eg, porcine colipase); this property is used in analytical formulations of the LIP assay.[61]

Lipases are defined as enzymes that hydrolyze glycerol esters of long-chain fatty acids. Only ester bonds at carbons 1 and 3 (α-positions) are attacked, and products of the reaction include 2 moles of fatty acids and 1 mole of 2-acylglycerol (β-monoglyceride) per mole of substrate. The latter is resistant to hydrolysis, probably because of steric hindrance, but it can spontaneously isomerize to the α-form (3-acylglycerol). This isomerization permits the third fatty acid to be split off but at a much slower rate. A scheme for the steps in complete hydrolysis of a molecule of triglyceride to glycerol and three fatty acids is shown here:

$H_2C{-}OFA(1)$ / $HC{-}OFA(2)$ / $H_2C{-}OFA(3)$ Triglyceride $\xrightarrow[H_2O,\ OH^-]{Lipase}$ $H_2C{-}OH$ / $HC{-}OFA(2)$ / $H_2C{-}OFA(3)$ α,β-Diglyceride + FA(1)OH (Fatty acid I) $\xrightarrow[H_2O,\ OH^-]{Lipase}$ $H_2C{-}OH$ / $HC{-}OFA(2)$ / $H_2C{-}OH$ β-Monoglyceride + FA(3)OH (Fatty acid III)

Isomerization → $H_2C{-}OH$ / $HC{-}OH$ / $H_2C{-}OFA(2)$ α-Monoglyceride $\xrightarrow[H_2O,\ OH^-]{Lipase}$ $H_2C{-}OH$ / $HC{-}OH$ / $H_2C{-}OH$ Glycerol + FA(2)OH (Fatty acid II)

LIP acts only when the substrate is present in an emulsified form at the interface between water and the substrate. The rate of LIP action depends on the surface area of the dispersed substrate. Bile acids ensure that the surface of the dispersed substrate remains free of other proteins, including lipolytic enzymes, by lining the surface of the insoluble substrate and the aqueous medium. LIP seems to gain access to the substrate surface in the following manner: Colipase attaches to a micelle of bile salts, thus forming a colipase–bile salt complex that reconfigures the structure of colipase with exposure of a site with high affinity and high specificity for LIP, which therefore attracts LIP and anchors it to the substrate surface, allowing enzyme action to proceed. The control of secretion of LIP and its associated factors appears to be driven by gastrointestinal luminal content, particularly the presence of acid or digested proteins and fats in the duodenal lumen. Secretion of colipase, bile acids, and LIP is driven by cholecystokinin and secretin release.[62]

Most LIP activity found in serum derives from pancreatic acinar cells, but some is secreted by gastric, pulmonary, and intestinal mucosa. LIP is a small enough molecule to be filtered through the glomerulus. It is totally reabsorbed by the renal tubules, and it is not physiologically detected in urine. Evidence suggests that pancreatic LIP may exist in at least two isoforms, although the exact nature of these is unknown.[60] Complete absence of LIP has been reported. Such congenital absence results in fat malabsorption and severe steatorrhea.

Clinical Significance

LIP measurement of serum is the recommended biochemical test to diagnose acute pancreatitis. The clinical sensitivity is 80% to 100% depending on the selected diagnostic cutoff, and the clinical specificity is 80% to 100% depending on the mix of the patient population studied. After an attack of acute pancreatitis, serum LIP activity increases within 4 to 8 hours, peaks at about 24 hours, and decreases within 7 to 14 days. Increases between 2 and 50 times the URL have been reported. The increase in serum LIP activity is not necessarily proportional to the severity of the attack.[61]

Acute pancreatitis is sometimes difficult to diagnose because it must be differentiated from other acute intraabdominal disorders with similar clinical findings, such as perforated gastric or duodenal ulcer, intestinal obstruction, or mesenteric vascular obstruction. In differential diagnosis, increase of serum LIP activity to greater than three times the URL, in the absence of renal failure, is a more specific diagnostic finding than increases in serum α-amylase activity.[63] Furthermore, LIP concentrations remain increased longer than those of α-amylase do, which is another advantage over α-amylase measurement in patients with delayed presentation (Fig. 29.7). Therefore, it is recommended that LIP should replace α-amylase as the initial diagnostic test for acute pancreatitis in the emergency department; obtaining both serum α-amylase and LIP levels is not warranted.[64]

Obstruction of the pancreatic duct by a calculus or by carcinoma of the pancreas may increase serum LIP activity, depending on the location of the obstruction and the amount of remaining functioning tissue. In patients with a reduced glomerular filtration rate, serum LIP activity is increased. Thus, care should be exercised in the interpretation of increased serum LIP values in the presence of renal disease. Although rare, inaccuracies in serum LIP estimation have also been shown to arise from the presence of macroforms of LIP, consisting of enzyme bound to IgG. Finally, investigation of the biliary tract by endoscopic retrograde pancreatography or treatment with opiates (which causes the sphincter of Oddi to contract) may increase serum LIP activity.

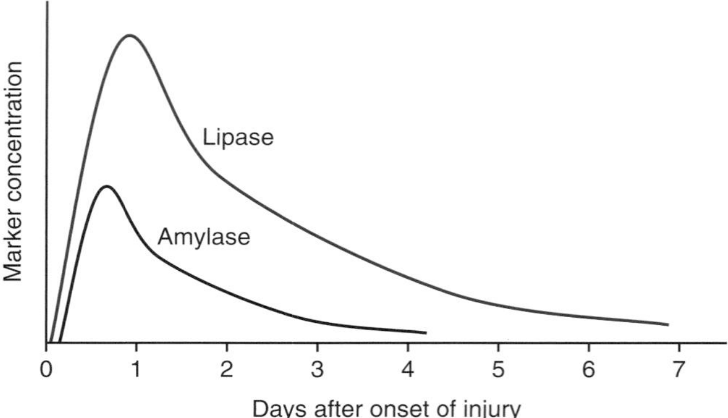

FIGURE 29.7 Time-dependent changes in serum amylase and lipase after acute pancreatitis.

Methods for Measuring Lipase Activity

Many LIP methods have been described; they have used both triglyceride and nontriglyceride substrates and titrimetric, turbidimetric, spectrophotometric, fluorometric, and immunologic techniques. In general, long-chain triglyceride (and some diglyceride) substrates have demonstrated correlation of results with the clinical state that is superior to that seen with methods using other substrates.[65]

In titrimetric methods, LIP catalyzes the hydrolysis of fatty acids from an emulsion of olive oil or oleic acid. The fatty acids liberated are titrated with dilute alkali. Kinetic versions use an automated potentiometric titrator (an instrument commonly referred to as a "pH-stat"). The amount of alkali used is recorded as a function of time and serves as a measure of fatty acid produced during the reaction.

In the turbidimetric method, LIP catalyzes the hydrolysis of fatty acids from an emulsion of oleic acid with a simultaneous decrease in the turbidity of the reaction mixture. Absorbance at 340 nm is read, and the ΔA/min is taken as a measure of LIP activity. Turbidities have occasionally been observed to increase rather than decrease during the reaction period. Such increases have frequently been observed in specimens containing rheumatoid factor. The method linearity (approximately three times the URL) is limited, with many clinical samples needing to be diluted.

Numerous substrates and complex auxiliary and indicator systems are used in spectrophotometric methods. They have the advantage of minimum sample volume requirements (<25 μL), good precision, wide dynamic range, and ease of automation. In the Ortho Clinical Diagnostics spectrophotometric reaction rate LIP slide method, the (synthetic) substrate is 1-oleoyl-2,3-diacetylglycerol, and the emulsifier is dodecylbenzene sulfonate. LIP activity is measured by a complex auxiliary and indicator enzyme system to produce a colored dye detectable at 540 nm. However, the substrate is likely to be more specific for intestinal than pancreatic LIP and may be subject to interference by postheparin lipase and pancreatic carboxylesterase.

In the enzymatic reaction rate diglyceride assay for LIP, the following sequence of indicator and auxiliary enzymes is used:

$$\text{1,2-Diacylglycerol} + H_2O \xrightarrow[\textit{pH 8.7}]{\textit{Pancreatic lipase, Colipase}} \text{2-Monoacylglycerol} + \text{Fatty acid}$$

$$\text{2-Monoacylglycerol} + H_2O \xrightarrow{\textit{Monoglyceride lipase}} \text{Glycerol} + \text{Fatty acid}$$

$$\text{Glycerol} + \text{ATP} \xrightarrow{\textit{Glycerol kinase}} \text{L-}\alpha\text{-glycerophospate} + \text{ADP}$$

$$\text{L-}\alpha\text{-glycerophospate} + O_2 \xrightarrow{\textit{L-}\alpha\textit{-glycerophospate kinase}} \text{Dihydroxyacetone phosphate} + H_2O_2$$

$$2\ H_2O_2 + \text{4-Aminoantipyrine} + \text{TOOS} \xrightarrow{\textit{Peroxidase}} \text{Quinonediimine dye (colored)} + 2\ H_2O$$

TOOS is sodium *N*-ethyl-*N*-(2-hydroxyl-3-sulfopropyl)-m-toluidine, and its oxidation produces an intensely colored dye detectable at 550 nm.

More recently, a synthetic substrate (1,2-O-dilauryl-rac-glycero-3-glutaric acid-[4-methyl-resorufin]-ester) consisting of two glycerol ether bonds and one ester bond has been proposed, and assays based on its use are currently gaining widespread use. LIP hydrolyzes the ester bond in an alkaline medium to an unstable dicarbonic acid ester that spontaneously hydrolyzes to yield glutaric acid and methylresorufin; this is a bluish-purple chromophore with peak absorption at 580 nm.

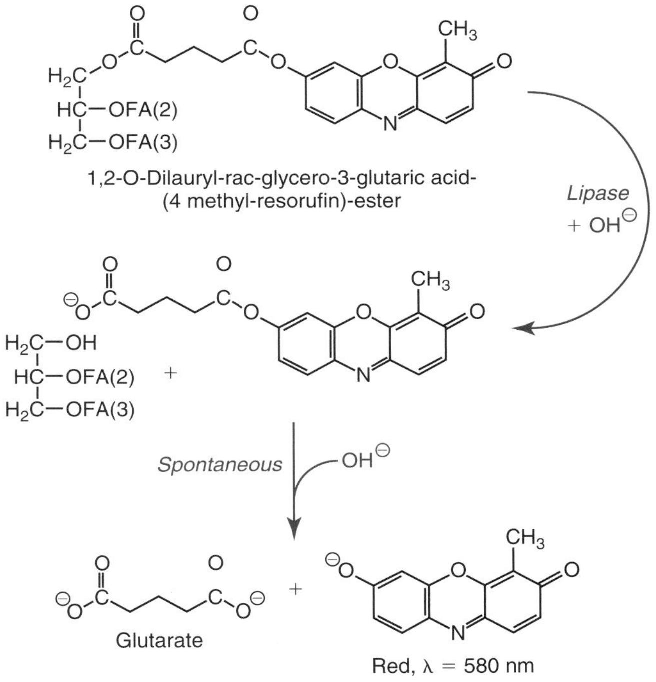

The rate of methylresorufin formation is directly proportional to the LIP activity of the sample. Compared with previous LIP spectrophotometric methods, this assay principle is based on a direct reaction and appears to have increased specificity for pancreatic LIP.[66]

LIP is among the more poorly standardized laboratory tests, so misdiagnosing acute pancreatitis is a real possibility, especially if clinicians receive results from different analytical systems. Commercial methods use different measurement principles that may reflect differences in analytical specificity.[67] Because of these issues, the IFCC has started to debate on a concept for the development of a reference procedure for LIP using spectrophotometry as the measurement technique.[68] The proposed substrate for LIP is the 1,2-dioleoylglycerol and the increase of NADPH after a complex reaction scheme using four auxiliary reactions is spectrophotometrically recorded in the indicator reaction of the method.[69]

$$\text{1,2-Dioleoylglycerol} + H_2O \xrightarrow{\text{LIP}} \text{2-Monooleoylglycerol} + \text{oleic acid}$$

$$\text{2-Monooleoylglycerol} + H_2O \xrightarrow{\text{monoacylglycerol lipase}} \text{Glycerol} + \text{oleic acid}$$

$$\text{Glycerol} + \text{ATP} \xrightarrow{\text{glycerol kinase}} \text{ADP} + \text{glycerol-3-phosphate}$$

$$\text{ADP} + \text{glucose} \xrightarrow{\text{ADP-dependent hexokinase}} \text{Glucose-6-phosphate} + \text{AMP}$$

$$\text{Glucose-6-phosphate} + \text{NADP} \xrightarrow{\text{glucose-6-phosphate dehydrogenase}} \text{6-Phospho-glucono-1,5-lactone} + \text{NADPH}$$

LIP activity in serum is stable at room temperature for 1 week; sera may be stored for 3 weeks in the refrigerator and for several years if frozen.

Biological variation data suggest that imprecision (CV) of less than 16.1%, bias of ±11.3%, and total error of ±37.9% for LIP measurements are required for clinical use.[31]

Reference Intervals

Reference intervals for LIP activity are largely method dependent. For the enzymatic reaction rate diglyceride assay, the suggested URL is 45 U/L at 37°C. The URL is 64 U/L at 37°C for methylresorufin assay. There are no gender- or age-related differences.

Amylase

α-Amylases (EC 3.2.1.1; 1,4-α-D glucan glucanohydrolase; AMY) are enzymes of the hydrolase class that catalyze the hydrolysis of 1,4-α-glucosidic linkages in polysaccharides. Both straight-chain (linear) polyglucans, such as amylose, and branched polyglucans, such as amylopectin and glycogen, are hydrolyzed but at different rates. In the case of amylose, the enzyme splits the chains at alternate α-1,4-hemiacetal (–C–O–C–) links, forming maltose and some residual glucose; maltose, glucose, and a residue of limit dextrins are formed if branched-chain polyglucans are used as substrate. The enzyme does not attack the α-1,6-linkages at the branch points. AMYs are calcium metalloenzymes, with the calcium essential for functional integrity. However, full activity is displayed only in the presence of various anions—such as chloride, bromide, nitrate, cholate, or monohydrogen phosphate—with chloride and bromide being the most effective activators. AMYs in human serum have a moderately sharp pH optimum at 6.9 to 7.0.

AMYs normally occurring in human plasma are small molecules with molecular weights varying from 54 to 62 kDa. The enzyme is thus small enough to pass through the glomeruli of the kidneys, and AMY is the only plasma enzyme normally found in urine. AMYs are present in a number of organs and tissues. The greatest concentration is noted in the salivary glands, which secrete a potent AMY (S-type) to initiate hydrolysis of starches while the food is still in the mouth and esophagus. The action of the S-AMY, once referred to as *ptyalin,* is terminated by acid in the stomach. In the pancreas, the enzyme (P-type) is synthesized by acinar cells and then is secreted into the intestinal tract by way of the pancreatic duct system. In the intestinal tract, effective action of pancreatic and intestinal AMY is favored by mildly alkaline conditions in the duodenum. Intestinal maltase then further hydrolyzes maltose to glucose. AMY activity is also found in extracts from semen, testes, ovaries, fallopian tubes, striated muscle, lungs, and adipose tissue. The enzyme is present in colostrum, tears, and milk. Epithelial tumors of the lung and ovary may also contain considerable AMY activity. Ascitic and pleural fluids may contain AMY as a result of the presence of a tumor or pancreatitis.

The enzyme present in normal serum and urine is predominantly of pancreatic (P-AMY) and salivary gland (S-AMY) origin. These isoenzymes are products of two closely linked loci on chromosome 1. AMY isoenzymes also undergo posttranslational modification of deamidation, glycosylation, and deglycosylation to form a number of isoforms. Indeed, nonenzymic deamidation appears to be the mechanism for "aging" that occurs when AMY is sequestered (eg, pancreatic pseudocysts) or subjected to prolonged in vitro storage. Although P-AMY is not glycosylated, S-AMY may exist in both glycosylated and deglycosylated forms; these isoforms can be separated in both serum and urine using isoelectric focusing or electrophoresis. Individuals with isolated P-AMY deficiency, a rare condition, have carbohydrate maldigestion resulting in abdominal distention, flatulence, loose stools, and poor weight gain.

Clinical Significance

Blood AMY activity is physiologically low and constant and greatly increases in acute pancreatitis and salivary gland inflammation. In acute pancreatitis, a rise in serum AMY activity occurs within 5 to 8 hours of symptom onset; activities typically return to baseline by the third or fourth day. A four- to sixfold increase in AMY activity above the URL is usual, with maximal concentrations attained in 12 to 72 hours (see Fig. 29.7). The magnitude of the increase of serum enzyme activity is not related to the severity of pancreatic involvement; however, the greater the rise, the greater the probability of acute pancreatitis. A portion of the clearance of AMYs from the circulation occurs via renal excretion into the urine, and increased serum activity is reflected in an increase in urinary AMY activity. Compared with serum AMY, urine AMY reaches higher concentrations and persists for longer periods. The specificity of AMY for the diagnosis of acute pancreatitis is low (20% to 60%, depending on the mix of the patient population studied) because increased values are also found in a number of acute intraabdominal disorders and in several extrapancreatic conditions (Table 29.7).

Lack of specificity of total AMY measurement has led to interest in the direct measurement of P-AMY instead of total enzyme activity for the differential diagnosis of patients with acute abdominal pain. By applying the best decision limit (an activity equal to threefold the URL), the specificity of P-AMY for the diagnosis of acute pancreatitis was greater than 90%.[70] Sensitivity in late detection of this condition is also notably improved with P-AMY. P-AMY values remain increased in 80% of patients with uncomplicated pancreatitis 1 week after onset, when only 30% still show increased total AMY activity. This long-standing increase in P-AMY activity in serum also makes redundant the traditional measurement of total AMY in urine—a test performed to achieve better diagnostic sensitivity in the late phase of pancreatitis.

Biliary tract diseases, such as cholecystitis, cause up to a fourfold increase in serum P-AMY activity as a result of primary or secondary pancreatic involvement. Various intraabdominal events can lead to a significant increase in serum P-AMY activities, up to a fourfold increase and sometimes beyond. Such increases may be caused by leakage of P-AMY from the intestine into the peritoneal cavity and then into the circulation.

In renal insufficiency, serum AMY activity is increased in proportion to the extent of renal impairment (usually, no more than five times the URL). Hyperamylasemia also occurs in neoplastic disease.[71] Tumors of the lung and serous and mixed (serous and mucinous) carcinomas of the ovary can produce hyperamylasemia (with an S-type isoenzyme mobility) with increases as high as 50 times the URL. Cases of AMY-producing multiple myeloma have been described. The AMY isoenzyme in cases of ruptured ectopic pregnancy is not

TABLE 29.7 Causes of Hyperamylasemia

Pancreatic disease	Pancreatitis, any cause (P-AMY↑)*
	Pancreatic trauma (P-AMY↑)
Intraabdominal diseases other than pancreatitis	Biliary tract disease (P-AMY↑)
	Intestinal obstruction (P-AMY↑)
	Mesenteric infarction (P-AMY↑)
	Perforated peptic ulcer (P-AMY↑)
	Gastritis, duodenitis (P-AMY↑)
	Ruptured aortic aneurysm
	Acute appendicitis (perforated)
	Peritonitis
	Trauma
Genitourinary disease	Ectopic, ruptured tubal pregnancy
	Salpingitis (S-AMY↑)
	Ovarian malignancy (S-AMY↑)
	Renal insufficiency (mixed)
Miscellaneous	Salivary gland lesions (S-AMY↑)
	Acute alcoholic abuse (S-AMY↑)
	Diabetic ketoacidosis (S-AMY↑)
	Macroamylasemia (S-AMY↑ or P-AMY↑)
	Septic shock (S-AMY↑)
	Cardiac surgery (S-AMY↑)
	Tumors (usually S-AMY↑)
	Drugs (usually S-AMY↑)

*Predominant isoenzyme type is shown in parentheses: *P-AMY,* pancreatic; *S-AMY,* salivary; *mixed,* either or both isoenzymes may be present.

well characterized. In severe cases presenting late, the increased isoenzyme may be P-AMY (from pancreatic involvement related to peritonitis) despite the fact that S-AMY is present in fallopian tube.

In 1% of the population, macroamylases are present in sera and may cause hyperamylasemia; these are complexes of ordinary AMY (usually S-type) and IgG or IgA. These macroamylases cannot be filtered through the glomeruli of the kidneys because of their large size (>200 KDa molecular weight) and are thus retained in the plasma, where their presence may increase AMY activity some two- to eightfold above the URL, typically stable over time. No clinical symptoms are associated with this disorder, but some cases have been detected during investigation of abdominal pain.

A decrease in serum P-AMY activity (less than the lower reference limit) is highly specific for an exocrine pancreatic insufficiency and can make intubation tests for pancreatic function unnecessary. If, however, P-AMY is normal, reduced pancreatic function cannot be excluded.[72]

POINTS TO REMEMBER

Pancreatic enzymes in acute pancreatitis:

- The diagnostic performance of pancreatic enzymes is greatly improved by restricting their use to a population with suspected disease.
- Lipase measurement is superior to P-AMY in terms of diagnostic performance.
- It is recommended that lipase replace P-AMY as initial test for acute pancreatitis; measuring both serum P-AMY and lipase is not warranted.
- The measurement of total AMY should be considered obsolete.

Methods for Determination of α-Amylase Activity

Historically, saccharogenic, amyloclastic, and chromolytic starch methods were the assays of choice for determining AMY activity. These assays have been completely displaced in favor of ones with well-defined substrates with shorter glucosyl chains. The use of defined AMY substrates and auxiliary and indicator enzymes in the AMY assay has improved the reaction stoichiometry and has led to more controlled and consistent hydrolysis conditions. Substrates used include small oligosaccharides and 4-nitrophenyl (4-NP)-glycoside substrates.

When hydrolyzed by AMY, small oligosaccharide substrates have been found to give better defined products than do starches. For example, both maltopentaose and maltotetraose showed good stability, consistent hydrolysis products, and unambiguous reaction stoichiometry. Several variations of the reaction rate formulation have been devised.[73]

4-Nitrophenyl (4-NP)-glycoside substrates are prepared by bonding 4-NP to the reducing end of a defined oligosaccharide. If the oligosaccharide is maltoheptaose (G7), the substrate is then 4-NP-G7. AMY splits this substrate to produce free oligosaccharides (G5, G4, and G3) and 4-NP-G2 (9%), 4-NP-G3 (31%), and 4-NP-G4 (60%). P-AMY hydrolyzes the substrate at a greater rate than does S-AMY in the ratio 1.8 : 1. G6, G1, 4-NP-G6, and 4-NP-G5 are not produced in appreciable quantities. In the original assay, the result of combined hydrolysis by AMY in the specimen and by the reagent α-glucosidase (EC 3.2.1.20; maltase) is that more than 30% of the product is free NP. Free NP is detected by its absorbance at 405 nm. α-Glucosidase does not react with any oligosaccharide containing more than four glucose molecules in the chain; G4 is hydrolyzed only very slowly.[74] Problems arose with the use of the 4-NP-glycoside assay with regard to the poor stability of the reconstituted assay mixture because of slow hydrolysis of the 4-NP-glycoside by α-glucosidase. This effect has been reduced by covalently linking a "blocking" group (ie, a 4,6-ethylidene group; ethylidene-protected substrate [EPS]) to the nonreducing end of the molecule. The blocked substrate also shows a different and more advantageous hydrolysis pattern. Thus, the ethylidene-4-NP-G7 substrate fragments approximately as 4-NP-G2 (40%), 4-NP-G3 (40%), and 4-NP-G4 (20%). Therefore, liberation of 4-NP is increased; however, the reaction rate is reduced in proportion, so these two effects compensate for each other.[75] A novel-type α-glucosidase is also available (recombinant enzyme AGH-211) that completely hydrolyzes nitrophenylated substrates. As a result, cleavage of one α-glucosidic linkage by AMY results in the release of one molecule of 4-NP:

$$\text{5 Ethylidene-4-NP-G}_7 + 5\,H_2O \xrightarrow{\alpha\text{-Amylase}} \text{2 Ethylidene-G}_5 + \text{2 4-NP-G}_2 + \text{2 Ethylidene-G}_4 + \text{2 4-NP-G}_3 + \text{Ethylidene-G}_3 + \text{4-NP-G}_4$$

$$\text{2 4-NP-G}_2 + \text{2 4-NP-G}_3 + 10\,H_2O \xrightarrow{\alpha\text{-Glucosidase}} \text{4 4-NP} + \text{10 G}$$

The IFCC has optimized this method at 37°C, recommending it as a reference measurement procedure for AMY.[76]

With the exception of heparin, all common anticoagulants inhibit AMY activity because they chelate calcium; citrate, EDTA, and oxalate inhibit it by as much as 15%. Therefore, AMY assays should be performed only on serum or heparinized plasma. AMY is quite stable; activity is fully retained during storage for 4 days at room temperature, for 2 weeks at −4°C, for 1 year at −25°C, and for 5 years at −75°C.

Biologic variation data suggest that AMY measurements require an imprecision (CV) of less than 4.4%, maximum bias of ±7.4%, and a total error lower than ±14.6% for good quality.[16] In a study, the performance of commercial assays was assessed using an approach in which this maximum allowable error was applied in evaluating assay trueness.[17] Measurement of AMY showed major drawbacks, suggesting the need for improvement in implementing traceability to higher order references. Manufacturers are still marketing (and laboratories still using) AMY assays that do not comply with the IFCC recommended procedure. The lack of result comparability among different assays adds another hindrance to the effective use of total AMY as a diagnostic tool.

Reference Interval

Using the IFCC recommended method at 37°C, the serum AMY reference interval in whites was 31 to 107 U/L.[76] Ethnoracial differences have been reported with higher AMY values in Asians.

Analytical Methods and Reference Intervals for Amylase Isoenzymes

Methods for AMY isoenzymes based on electrophoresis, ion-exchange chromatography, isoelectric focusing, selective inhibition of the S-AMY by a wheat germ inhibitor, immunoprecipitation by a monoclonal antibody, and immunoinhibition have been introduced. However, only methods based on selective isoenzyme inhibition by monoclonal antibodies have shown sufficient precision, reliability, practicability, and analytical speed to allow the introduction of P-AMY determination into clinical practice.

A double monoclonal antibody assay is commercially available that uses the synergistic action of two immunoinhibitory monoclonal antibodies to S-AMY.[77] After the S-AMY activity is inhibited by the addition of antibodies, uninhibited P-AMY activity is measured using EPS-4-NP-G7 as a substrate. It is an attractive convenience to have this more specific assay available in full automation today on clinical chemistry platforms with reagent costs similar to total AMY, which permits laboratories to abandon the latter.[70]

False-positive P-AMY results have been reported in subjects with macroamylasemia, in whom immunoglobulin complexed to AMY forms diminishes or voids the ability of monoclonal antibodies included in the test to efficiently inhibit S-AMY. Upon electrophoresis, macro-AMY usually forms a broad migrating band, clearly different from the homogeneous bands that are produced by AMY isoenzymes present in serum (Fig. 29.8). If electrophoretic separation is not available, precipitation of the macrocomplex by a PEG 6000 solution (240 g/L) represents a good alternative. Residual AMY activity of less than 30% in the supernatant is indicative of macroamylasemia.[78]

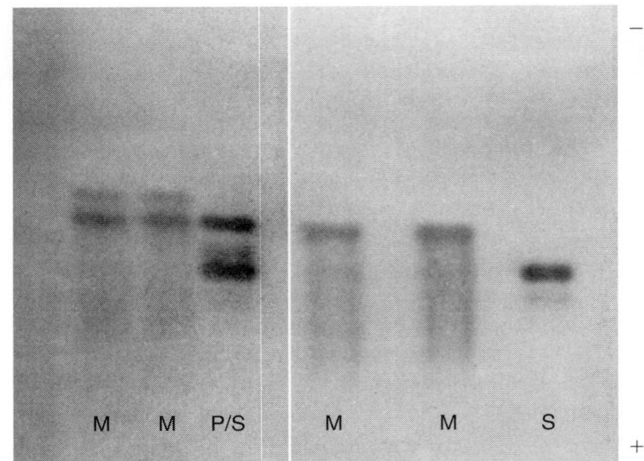

FIGURE 29.8 Electrophoretic separation of amylase isoenzymes. *M,* Macroamylasemia; *P/S,* mixture of two samples containing, respectively, pancreatic juice and saliva; *S,* saliva.

In healthy adults, P-AMY represents approximately 40% to 50% of total AMY activity in serum. Using the immunoinhibition method at 37°C, the reference interval for P-AMY activity in sera from adults was 13 to 53 U/L.[79] Serum P-AMY activity is not demonstrable in most children younger than 6 months, but activity rises slowly thereafter to reach adult concentrations at 5 years of age, reflecting the postnatal development of exocrine pancreatic function. As a consequence, use of this enzyme for the diagnosis of acute pancreatitis in young children should be avoided.

Trypsin

Trypsin (EC 3.4.21.4; no systematic name; TRY) is a pancreas-specific serine protease characterized by the presence at the active site of serine and histidine, both of which participate in the catalytic process. TRY hydrolyzes peptide bonds formed by the carboxyl groups of lysine or arginine with other amino acids, although esters and amides involving these amino acids are actually split more rapidly than peptide bonds.[80]

The acinar cells of the human pancreas synthesize two major trypsins (1 and 2) in the form of the inactive proenzymes (or zymogens), trypsinogens-1 and -2, with a third form (trypsinogen-3) making up less than 10% of the total. These zymogens are stored in zymogen granules and are secreted into the duodenum under the stimulus of the vagus nerve or the intestinal hormone cholecystokinin-pancreozymin. The two trypsinogens represent approximately 19% of the total protein in pancreatic juice; normally, the pancreas secretes trypsinogen-1 at about two- to fourfold the concentration of trypsinogen-2, but in pancreatic disease, the ratio of trypsinogen-1 and -2 is reversed. In the intestinal tract, the trypsinogens are converted to the active enzyme TRY by the duodenal enzyme enterokinase or by preformed TRY (autocatalysis) (Fig. 29.9). When trypsinogens are converted to active TRY, a small peptide is cleaved from the *N*-terminal region of trypsinogen (trypsinogen activation peptide [TAP]).

TRY-1 is also described as cationic and TRY-2 as anionic because of their differing electrophoretic mobility; the cationic form predominates and is the better documented enzyme. TRY-1 and TRY-2 have molecular weights of 25,800

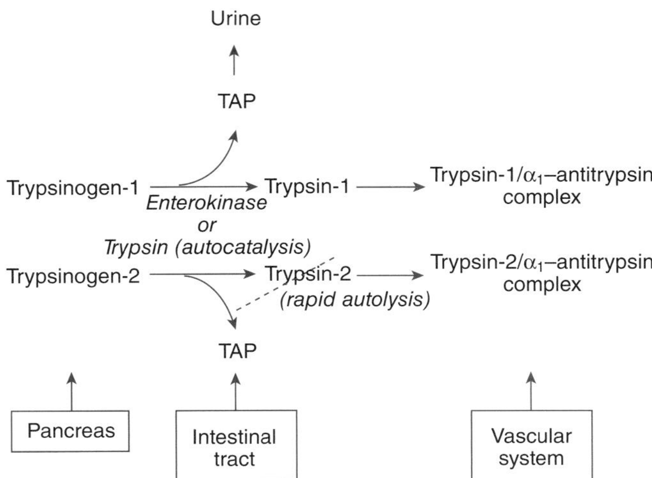

FIGURE 29.9 A comprehensive representation of the human trypsin system. *TAP,* Trypsinogen-activation peptide.

and 22,900 Da and pI values of 4.6 to 6.5 and greater than 6.5, respectively. TRY-2 differs from TRY-1 in that it rapidly undergoes autolysis at neutral or alkaline pH values, and calcium does not stabilize it against autolysis. Because the two trypsins show little immunologic cross-reactivity, a specific immunoassay for each of them is possible.

Materials such as soybeans, lima beans, and egg whites contain natural TRY inhibitors—small polypeptides such as α_1-antitrypsin (α_1-protease inhibitor) and α_2-macroglobulin—that combine irreversibly with TRY and inactivate it by blocking the active center. Similar nondialyzable TRY inhibitors (eg, pancreatic secretory trypsin inhibitor [PSTI]) are present in the pancreas, pancreatic juice, serum, and urine. These inhibitors protect plasma and other proteins against hydrolysis by TRY and other proteases if for some reason any appreciable quantity of the enzyme enters the vascular system.[80] The absence of α_1-antitrypsin is associated with an increased tendency toward panlobular emphysema in early life; this example illustrates the effects of uninhibited proteases on organ function.

Clinical Significance

Trypsin-1 (Cationic Trypsin). In healthy individuals, free trypsinogen-1 is the major form found in serum. After an attack of acute pancreatitis, serum TRY-1 rises in parallel with serum AMY activity to peak values ranging from 2 to 400 times the URL. The distribution of the different forms of TRY-1 appears to be related to the type and severity of acute pancreatitis. Thus, in the mildest form of acute pancreatitis, 80% to 99% of TRY-1 exists as free trypsinogen-1, with smaller proportions existing as bound TRY-1. In the more severe forms, in which the mortality rate ranges from 20% to more than 50%, the proportion of free trypsinogen-1 may be as low as 30% of the total, with appreciable proportions existing as the α_1-antitrypsin– and α_2-macroglobulin–bound TRY-1.[81]

TRY-1 in serum is increased in chronic renal failure, as are serum AMY and LIP. Thus, renal failure must be ruled out when increased concentrations are interpreted. In chronic pancreatitis without steatorrhea, plasma concentrations of TRY-1 do not differ from those found in health; when steatorrhea is present, however, fasting concentrations are extremely low. In the relapsing phase of chronic pancreatitis, plasma TRY may be considerably increased. In carcinoma of the pancreas, TRY concentrations may be high, normal, or even low.

In comparison with P-AMY and LIP measurements, TRY-1 is a more difficult test to perform, with an assay turnaround time of several hours. Because TRY estimation has no distinct role in the routine management of patients with acute pancreatitis, this test is considered of limited clinical value.

Cystic fibrosis is a genetic disorder that primarily affects the lungs and digestive system, resulting in the production of thick mucus that blocks ducts in the pancreas, preventing normal transport of trypsinogen. In this condition, plasma TRY concentrations have been reported to be high in neonates; as the disease progresses, activity falls. Newborn screening is done by the measurement of immunoreactive trypsinogen-1 in dried blood specimens. Infants who have a high TRY concentration on initial testing undergo further assessment via a repeat test 1 to 3 weeks later, or by analysis of the initial blood spot for specific DNA mutations.

Trypsin-2 (Anionic Trypsin). Serum trypsinogen-2 increases more than trypsinogen-1 in acute pancreatitis, the concentrations of the former being on average about 10-fold those of the latter.[82] Consequently, larger amounts of trypsinogen-2 are excreted into urine. Urinary trypsinogen-2 measurement has shown high sensitivity and negative predictive value for the diagnosis of acute pancreatitis on admission to the hospital. However, the positive predictive value of this test is low.

Methods for Determination of Trypsin

Early studies used catalytic assays, but it was soon recognized that other proteolytic enzymes present in serum could also hydrolyze the same substrates. A major advance has been the development of commercial immunoassays to specifically quantify TRY in blood. In the case of TRY-1, immunoassays detect trypsinogen-1, TRY-1, and the TRY-1–α_1-antitrypsin complex. They do not detect the TRY-1–α_2-macroglobulin complex, for which different assays are necessary. Free TRY-1 is not usually found in serum; it is always complexed. Because no assay standardization is available, reference intervals are method dependent.

A rapid (5-minute) urinary trypsinogen-2 test strip is available, which is based on the use of immunochromatography with monoclonal antibodies. The test is considered positive at urinary trypsinogen-2 concentrations greater than 50 μg/L.

BONE ENZYMES

Bone enzymes are direct products of active osteoblasts (bone ALP) and osteoclasts (tartrate-resistant acid phosphatase) (see Chapter 64).

Alkaline Phosphatase (Bone Isoform)

Bone, liver, and kidney isoforms of ALP are posttranslational modifications of the same gene product and are identified by their unique carbohydrate content (see Fig. 29.5). They were described previously in the section on liver enzymes. Bone ALP (BAP) is produced by the osteoblast and has been demonstrated in matrix vesicles deposited as "buds" derived from the cell's membrane. The enzyme therefore is an excellent indicator of global bone formation activity. Genetic inability to produce tissue-nonspecific ALP, including bone isoform, a rare inherited disorder known as hypophosphatasia, results in severe bone disease and impaired bone growth.

Clinical Significance in Bone Disease

Advantages of using BAP concentrations in serum as bone formation markers in clinical practice include low diurnal variability and lack of renal function concerns. Among the bone diseases, the highest concentrations of BAP are encountered in Paget disease (osteitis deformans) as a result of the action of osteoblastic cells as they try to rebuild bone that is being resorbed by uncontrolled activity of osteoclasts. Values from 10 to 25 times the URL are not unusual, and in broad terms, the increase reflects the extent of disease. The correlation coefficient of this relationship is around 0.7, meaning that approximately 50% of the variance in ALP can be explained by disease extent; the remaining 50% is explained by disease "activity."[83] It is worth commenting that, in the right clinical setting, mostly measurement of total ALP is sufficient for assessing bone turnover and monitoring Paget disease. In vitamin D deficiency (osteomalacia and rickets), concentrations two to four times the URL may be observed, and these fall slowly to baseline on treatment. Primary hyperparathyroidism and secondary hyperparathyroidism are associated with slight to moderate increases of BAP in serum, with the existence and degree of increase reflecting the presence and extent of skeletal involvement. Very high enzyme concentrations are present in patients with osteogenic bone cancer. Increased BAP indicates bone metastasis in 70% of prostate cancers and its use has been included in the European Association of Urology guidelines for staging this neoplasia.[84] The 2012 Kidney Disease: Improving Global Outcome (KDIGO) clinical practice guideline for the evaluation and management of chronic kidney disease recommends to evaluate associated mineral and bone disorders by measuring total ALP activity together with serum calcium, phosphate, and parathyroid hormone (PTH), at least once in adults with glomerular filtration rate (GFR) less than 45 mL/min/1.73 m^2.[85] The level of evidence for recommending specific BAP measurement instead of total ALP has been considered inadequate by the guideline extensors.[86] BAP can be slightly increased in osteoporosis, but individuals with osteoporosis are not clearly distinguished from age-matched control participants even if, over the entire population, concentrations are inversely correlated with bone mineral density. Transient increases may be found during healing of bone fractures. Physiologic bone growth increases BAP in serum, and this accounts for the fact that in the sera of growing children, the enzyme concentration is 1.5 to 7 times that in healthy adult serum, the maximum being reached earlier in girls than in boys.

Methods for Determination of Bone Alkaline Phosphatase

In general, separation of tissue-nonspecific ALP forms (ie, bone and liver) is difficult because of structural similarity. At present, BAP in serum can be measured by electrophoretic and immunochemical methods (see the section on liver enzymes). Immunoassays for BAP, which measure enzyme activity or mass, are commercially available; cross-reactivity with the liver isoform, however, has been established:

Assay	Type	Cross-Reactivity, %
Beckman Coulter Tandem-R-Ostase	Mass-based IRMA	12.7–16.5
Beckman Coulter Tandem-MP-Ostase	Mass-based ELISA	8.1–16.2
Quidel MicroVue BAP	Activity-based EIA	5.9–20.0

EIA, Enzyme immunoassay; *ELISA,* enzyme-linked immunosorbant assay; *IRMA,* immunoradiometric assay.

This general limitation should be borne in mind when test results are interpreted.

With the use of immunoassays measuring serum BAP concentrations, the enzyme is said to be stable at −20°C for 2 years.

Biologic variation data suggest that imprecision (CV) of less than 3.3%, bias of ±9.1%, and total error of ±20.5% for BAP measurements are desirable.[87] However, available data for BAP immunoassays show that the imprecision goal is generally not achieved, and the intermethod variation is quite large with a significant potential impact on clinical decision making.[88]

Reference Intervals

When the electrophoretic procedure is used, the reference interval for BAP activity in healthy adults is 10 to 50 U/L. For subjects older than 50 years, the BAP activity in women is significantly higher than in men (URL: 54 vs. 45 U/L, respectively). For children 4 to 15 years old, the reference interval is 54 to 369 U/L.[46]

The reference interval for adult men for BAP concentrations in serum does not change with age (7.5 to 26.1 µg/L), but menopause increases BAP concentrations in women (URL: 22.7 µg/L in premenopausal and 31.6 µg/L in postmenopausal women, respectively).[89] Prepubertal concentrations of BAP are six- to sevenfold higher than in healthy adults.

Acid Phosphatase (Tartrate-Resistant 5b Isoform)

Under the name of acid phosphatase (EC 3.1.3.2; orthophosphoric-monoester phosphohydrolase [acid optimum]; ACP) are included all phosphatases with optimal activity below a pH of 7.0.

ACP is present in lysosomes, which are organelles present in all cells with the possible exception of erythrocytes. Extralysosomal ACPs are also present in many cells. The greatest concentrations of ACP activity occur in prostate, bone (osteoclasts), spleen, platelets, and erythrocytes. The lysosomal and prostatic enzymes are strongly inhibited by dextrorotatory tartrate ions, but the erythrocyte and bone isoenzymes are not. Most of the normally low ACP activity of (unhemolyzed) serum is of a tartrate-resistant type (TR-ACP) and probably originates mainly in osteoclasts. Activities of this fraction are increased physiologically in growing children and pathologically in conditions of increased osteolysis and bone remodeling.[90]

At least four ACP-determining genes have been identified and mapped. The erythrocyte ACP gene is located on chromosome 2 and is polymorphic, and a further gene on chromosome 19 encodes the TR-ACP expressed in osteoclasts and other tissue macrophages, such as alveolar macrophages and Kupffer cells (type 5 ACP). Isoenzyme 5 consists of two structurally related isoforms that differ by their carbohydrate content: TR-ACP 5a, which derives mainly from macrophages and dendritic cells, and type 5b, a more specific marker of osteoclastic activity sialic-acid free. Genes encoding the tartrate-inhibited lysosomal and prostatic ACPs, mapped to chromosomes 11 and 13, respectively, exhibit considerable homology.[91]

Acid phosphatases are unstable, especially at temperatures above 37°C and at a pH above 7.0. Some of the enzyme forms in serum are particularly labile, and more than 30% of ACP activity may be lost in 3 hours at room temperature. Acidification of the serum specimen to a pH below 6.5 aids in stabilizing the enzyme activity.

Clinical Significance

TR-ACP is a potentially useful marker of conditions with a marked osteolytic component. Slight or moderate increases in serum TR-ACP activity often occur in Paget disease, in hyperparathyroidism with skeletal involvement, and in the presence of malignant invasion of the bones by cancers such as breast cancer in women (see Chapter 64).[92] Increased concentrations of the osteoclast-derived ACP are also present in serum in osteoclastoma (giant cell tumor), an osteoclastic neoplasm, and in osteopetrosis (marble bone disease) in which the osteoclasts fail to resorb bone. High concentrations of TR-ACP in the serum of these patients are proportional to the osteoclast number, suggesting that changes in osteoclast function and number do not always go hand in hand.[93] TR-ACP appears to show relatively small dynamic changes in comparison with other markers of bone resorption (eg, those related to type I collagen metabolism). This may be attributable to the fact that the enzyme is released into the sealed osteoclast microenvironment, rather than directly into the circulation.

Unlike blood concentrations of other markers of bone resorption (eg, C-telopeptide of type I collagen), TR-ACP is not affected by renal dysfunction. The only nonbone condition in which increased activities of TR-ACP are found in serum is Gaucher disease of the spleen, a lysosomal storage disorder. Its source in this disease is the abnormal macrophages in the spleen and other tissues, which overexpress this normal macrophage constituent. The hairy cells of hairy cell leukemia (leukemic reticuloendotheliosis) also express the osteoclast-type ACP, providing a useful histologic marker. However, in this condition, the isoenzyme does not enter the plasma in increased amounts.

Although once widely used to detect or monitor carcinoma of the prostate, determination of ACP (tartrate-inhibited) activity in serum has now been replaced by prostate-specific antigen (PSA).

Methods for Determination of Tartrate-Resistant Acid Phosphatase

Continuous-monitoring methods for assay of TR-ACP activity are based on the principle introduced by Hillmann in which α-naphthol released from its phosphate ester forms a colored product with the stabilized diazonium salt of 2-amino-5-chlorotoluene-1,5-naphthalene disulfonate (Fast Red TR). Alcohols, such as 1,5-pentanediol, accelerate the reaction and increase sensitivity by acting as phosphate acceptors in transfer reactions. The addition of sodium tartrate inhibits the sensitive isoenzymes (ie, prostatic and lysosomal ACPs) if they are present in the sample.

Immunoassays for serum TR-ACP have been developed that preferentially detect isoform 5b and are now commercially available. A first method uses a monoclonal antibody to bind serum TR-ACP in a solid-phase format. After the capture, osteoclastic enzyme (type 5b) is specifically determined by measuring its activity at an optimal pH of 6.1. Another assay uses two monoclonal antibodies generated against purified bone TR-ACP 5b. One of the antibodies captures active intact isoform, and the second eliminates interference of inactive 5b fragments in serum. After the immunoreaction, binding TR-ACP 5b activity is measured (fragments absorbed immunocapture enzymatic assay [FAICEA]). There is, however, the reality that both immunoassays are not entirely bone specific.[94]

Serum should be immediately separated from erythrocytes and stabilized by the addition of 50 μL of acetic acid (5 mol/L) per milliliter of serum to lower the pH to 5.4, at which the enzyme is stable. Under these conditions, TR-ACP activity is maintained at room temperature for several hours, for up to 1 week if the serum is refrigerated, and for 4 months if stored at −20°C. Hemolyzed serum specimens are contaminated with considerable amounts of the erythrocyte tartrate-resistant isoenzyme and should be rejected.

Biologic variation of TR-ACP indicates that imprecision (CV) of less than 5.4%, bias of ±4.3%, and total error of ±16% are needed for suitable enzyme measurements.[87]

Reference Intervals

In the sera of healthy adults, the reference interval for TR-ACP activity, measured at 37°C, is 1.5 to 4.5 U/L. Children show higher TR-ACP activities (3.4 to 9.0 U/L).

MISCELLANEOUS ENZYMES

Lactate Dehydrogenase

Lactate dehydrogenase (EC 1.1.1.27; L-lactate: NAD$^+$ oxidoreductase; LDH) is a hydrogen transfer enzyme that catalyzes the oxidation of L-lactate to pyruvate with the mediation of NAD$^+$ as a hydrogen acceptor.

$$\underset{\text{L-Lactate}}{CH_3-CH(OH)-COO^{\ominus}} + NAD^{\ominus} \underset{\text{pH 7.4 to 7.8}}{\overset{\text{Lactate dehydrogenase, pH 8.8 to 9.8}}{\rightleftharpoons}} \underset{\text{Pyruvate}}{CH_3-C(=O)-COO^{\ominus}} + NADH + H^{\oplus}$$

As indicated, the reaction is reversible, and the reaction equilibrium strongly favors the reduction of pyruvate to lactate (P → L)—the "reverse reaction."

The pH optimum for the lactate-to-pyruvate (L → P) reaction is 8.8 to 9.8, and an assay reaction mixture, optimized for LDH-1 at 37°C, contains NAD$^+$, 9 mmol/L, and L-lactate, 80 mmol/L. For the P → L assay, at 37°C, the optimum pH is 7.4 to 7.8, NADH is 300 μmol/L, and pyruvate is 0.85 mmol/L. The optimal pH varies with the predominant isoenzymes in the sample and depends on the temperature and on substrate and buffer concentrations. The specificity of the enzyme extends from L-lactate to various related 2-hydroxyacids and 2-oxo-acids. The catalytic oxidation of 2-hydroxybutyrate, the next higher homolog of lactate, to 2-oxobutyrate is referred to as 2-hydroxybutyrate dehydrogenase (HBD) activity. LDH does not act on D-lactate, and only NAD^+ serves as a coenzyme.

The enzyme has a molecular weight of 134 kDa and is composed of four peptide chains of two types: M (or A) and H (or B), each under separate genetic control. The structures of LDH-M and LDH-H are determined by loci on human chromosomes 11 and 12, respectively. The subunit compositions of the five isoenzymes, in order of decreasing anodal mobility in an alkaline medium, are LDH-1 (HHHH; H_4), LDH-2 (HHHM; H_3M), LDH-3 (HHMM; H_2M_2), LDH-4 (HMMM; HM_3), and LDH-5 (MMMM; M_4). A different, sixth LDH isoenzyme, LDH-X (also called LDH_C), composed of four X (or C) subunits, is present in postpubertal human testes. A seventh LDH, called LDH-6, has been identified in the sera of severely ill patients.

LDH is inhibited by reagents with reactivity against thiol groups, such as mercuric ions and *p*-chloromercuribenzoate, the inhibition being reversed by the addition of cysteine or glutathione. Borate and oxalate inhibit by competing with lactate for its binding site on the enzyme; similarly, oxamate competes with pyruvate for its binding site. Both pyruvate and lactate in excess inhibit enzyme activity, although the effect of pyruvate is greater. Inhibition by either substrate is greater for the H form than for the M form, and substrate inhibition decreases with increases in pH. EDTA inhibits the enzyme perhaps by binding Zn^{2+}; however, the postulated activator role for zinc ions is not fully established.

LDH activity is present in many cells of the body and is invariably found only in the cytoplasm of the cell. Enzyme concentrations in various tissues are about 1500 to 5000 times greater than those physiologically found in serum. Therefore, leakage of the enzyme from even a small mass of damaged tissue increases the observed serum activity of LDH to a significant extent. Different tissues show different isoenzyme composition. In the heart, kidneys, and erythrocytes, the electrophoretically faster-moving isoenzymes LDH-1 and LDH-2 predominate; in the liver and skeletal muscle, the more cathodal LDH-4 and LDH-5 isoenzymes predominate, although skeletal muscle damage may also result in anodic LDH patterns. Isoenzymes of intermediate mobility account for the LDH activity from many sources (eg, spleen, lungs, lymph nodes, leukocytes, platelets).

Clinical Significance

Because of its wide tissue distribution, serum LDH increases occur in a variety of clinical conditions, including MI, hepatitis, and hemolysis, as well as disorders of the kidneys, lung, and muscle. Serum LDH measurement is, however, relevant only in hematology and oncology.[95]

Hemolytic anemias significantly increase LDH concentrations in serum. Marked increases of LDH activity—up to 50 times the URL—have been observed in the megaloblastic anemias. These anemias, usually resulting from the deficiency of folate or vitamin B_{12}, cause the erythrocyte precursor cell to break down in the bone marrow (ineffective erythropoiesis), resulting in the release of large quantities of LDH-1 and LDH-2 isoenzymes. These increases rapidly return to normal after appropriate treatment. For monitoring purposes, LDH is relevant in predicting disease activity in leukemia, and the survival rate (probability of survival) and duration in Hodgkin disease and non-Hodgkin lymphoma.

Patients with malignant disease often show increased LDH activity in serum; up to 70% of patients with liver metastases and 20% to 60% of patients with other nonhepatic metastases (eg, lymph nodes) have increased LDH activity. Notably elevated LDH-1 is observed in germ cell tumors (≈60% of cases) such as teratoma, seminoma of the testis, and dysgerminoma of the ovary.[96] The percentage of patients with increased LDH depends on the stage of the disease. LDH appears to be a useful predictor of outcome in patients with testicular nonseminomatous germ cell tumors, melanoma, and small cell lung cancer.

Increases of LDH activity (predominant LDH-4 and LDH-5 isoenzymes) are observed in liver disease, but their clinical use in a liver profile appears limited and would not appear to add significantly to the aminotransferase activity investigation. LDH measured in pleural fluid (better if in combination with serum LDH) aids in distinguishing exudative from transudative effusions.[97]

Macro-LDH, usually because of the formation of an autoantibody–enzyme complex that leads to a persistent increase in the amount of circulating enzyme, has been estimated to occur in fewer than 1 in 10,000 people. Documentation of a macro-LDH (eg, by the presence of an abnormally migrating band at electrophoresis) should be established in suspected individuals to avoid additional follow-up investigation or unnecessary treatment.

Methods for Determination of Lactate Dehydrogenase Activity

Laboratory methods for quantitation of total LDH activity use kinetic spectrophotometry to measure the interconversion of the coenzyme NAD^+ and NADH at 340 nm. The most widely used procedures employ the L → P reaction because it is claimed that there is less dependence on the NAD^+ and lactate concentrations and less contamination of NAD^+ with inhibiting products. A reference method based on this reaction has been developed by the IFCC for LDH at 37°C.[98]

Serum is the preferred specimen for measuring LDH activity. Plasma samples may be contaminated with platelets, which contain high concentrations of LDH. Serum should be separated from the clot as soon as possible after the specimen has been obtained. Hemolyzed serum must not be used because erythrocytes contain 4000 times more LDH activity than does serum. The different isoenzymes vary in their sensitivity to cold, LDH-4 and LDH-5 being especially labile. Activity of LDH-4 and LDH-5 is lost if the samples are stored at −20°C. Thus serum specimens should be stored at room temperature, at which no loss of activity occurs for at least 3 days.

The specifications for desirable performance of LDH assays, derived from biologic variation of the enzyme, are as follows: imprecision (CV) of 4.3% or less, bias of ±4.3%, and total error of ±11.4%.[16,31] Comparability of LDH measurements still has major drawbacks: This is mainly the result of using methods with different analytical specificity for this enzyme, obtaining results that may not be traceable to the internationally accepted reference measurement system.[32] The assay manufacturers can play a pivotal role in paving the road to harmonization of LDH measurements by recalibrating biased methods with suitable calibration materials.[99]

Reference Intervals

The reference interval for LDH activity in adult white subjects, determined at 37°C with a procedure traceable to the IFCC reference method, was found to be 125 to 220 U/L.[100] LDH reference intervals are higher in children, with a gradual decrease noted over the whole childhood period.[34]

Methods for Separation and Quantification of Lactate Dehydrogenase Isoenzymes

Electrophoretic separation on agarose gels or cellulose acetate membranes is the procedure most commonly used to demonstrate LDH isoenzymes. After the isoenzymes have been separated by electrophoresis, a reaction mixture is layered over the separation medium (typically D,L-lactate, 500 mmol/L, and NAD^+, 13 mmol/L, often dissolved in a suitable pH 8.0 buffer). The NADH generated over the LDH zones is detected by its fluorescence, when excited by long-wave ultraviolet light (365 nm), or by its reduction of a tetrazolium salt to form a colored formazan.

Using an agarose gel technique with fluorometric quantitation of generated NADH, the following reference intervals for isoenzymes were obtained (expressed as percent of total LDH): LDH-1, 14% to 26%; LDH-2, 29% to 39%; LDH-3, 20% to 26%; LDH-4, 8% to 16%; and LDH-5, 6% to 16%.

Cholinesterase

Two related enzymes have the ability to hydrolyze acetylcholine. One is acetylcholinesterase (EC 3.1.1.7; acetylcholine acetylhydrolase), which is called *true cholinesterase* or *choline esterase I*. True cholinesterase is found in erythrocytes, the lungs and spleen, nerve endings, and the gray matter of the brain. It is responsible for the prompt hydrolysis of acetylcholine released at the nerve endings to mediate transmission of the neural impulse across the synapse. Degradation of acetylcholine is required for depolarization of the nerve, so that it is repolarized in the next conduction event.

The other cholinesterase is acylcholine acylhydrolase (EC 3.1.1.8; acylcholine acylhydrolase; CHE), also called pseudocholinesterase, serum cholinesterase, butyrylcholinesterase, or choline esterase II, which is found in the liver, pancreas, heart, white matter of the brain, and serum. Although CHE activity in the human body is about threefold higher than acetylcholinesterase activity, its exact biologic role is unknown. A physiologic role for CHE in deactivation of octanoyl ghrelin, a hormone that stimulates feeding and promotes weight gain through its metabolic actions, has been proposed.

The type of reaction catalyzed by both cholinesterases is shown:

$$\underset{\text{Acetylcholine bromide}}{Br^{\ominus}\ (CH_3)_3N^{\oplus}{-}CH_2{-}CH_2{-}O{-}C(=O){-}CH_3} + H_2O \xrightarrow{\text{Cholinesterase}} \underset{\text{Acetate}}{CH_3{-}COO^{\ominus}} + \underset{\text{Choline bromide}}{Br^{\ominus}\ (CH_3)_3N^{\oplus}{-}CH_2{-}CH_2OH} + H^{\oplus}$$

The two enzymes differ in specificity toward some substrates while behaving similarly toward others. The serum enzyme acts on benzoylcholine but cannot hydrolyze acetyl-β-methylcholine; the red blood cell (RBC) enzyme acts on the latter but not on the former. The RBC enzyme splits only choline esters; aryl and alkyl esters are not attacked. The RBC enzyme is inhibited by its substrate, acetylcholine, if present at about 10^{-2} mol/L; the serum enzyme is not inhibited by this substrate.

The two enzymes are inhibited by the alkaloids prostigmine and physostigmine, both of which contain quaternary nitrogen (present in choline) in their structures. These two compounds are typical competitive inhibitors, competing with the choline residue of acetylcholine for its binding site on the enzyme surface. Some organic phosphorous compounds, such as diisopropyl fluorophosphate, irreversibly inhibit both enzymes. The phosphoryl group binds very tightly to the enzyme site at which binding of the acyl group normally occurs, thus preventing attachment of the acetylcholine. Both enzymes are also inhibited by a large variety of other compounds, including morphine, quinine, tertiary amines, phenothiazines, pyrophosphate, bile salts, citrate, fluoride, and borate.

CHE in normal sera is separated by electrophoresis into 7 to 12 bands, the number depending on the experimental technique used. The forms of CHE differ in molecular size and appear to be aggregates of different numbers of the same basic unit. Of greater interest are the atypical (genetic) variants of the enzyme, characterized by diminished activity against acetylcholine and other substrates, which are found in the sera of a small fraction of apparently healthy people.

The gene on chromosome 3 controlling the synthesis of CHE can exist in many allelic forms. Four of the most common forms are designated as E^u, E^a, E^f, and E^s. These four allelic genes can be combined to form one normal and nine abnormal genotypes. At least 40 other forms exist, and another gene locus is recognized (E_2). The normal, most common phenotype is designated as E^uE^u, or UU (u for *usual*). The gene E^a is referred to as the *atypical* gene; the sera of people homozygous for this gene (E^aE^a = AA) are only weakly active toward most substrates for CHE and demonstrate increased resistance to inhibition of enzyme activity by dibucaine. The E^f gene (f for *fluoride resistant*) gives rise to a weakly active enzyme but with increased resistance to fluoride inhibition. The E^s gene (s for *silent*) is associated with the absence of enzyme or the presence of a protein with minimal or no catalytic activity. Mutations that give rise to the atypical and fluoride-resistant CHE variants involve a change in the structure of the active center. The variant enzymes (allelozymes) are less effective catalysts than the usual form; the affinity of the enzymes for the substrates is reduced (ie, K_m is increased), and affinity for competitive inhibitors, such as dibucaine or fluoride, is similarly decreased. This gives rise to the characteristic dibucaine- or fluoride-resistant properties of the genetic variants that are exploited in their characterization.

Homozygous forms, AA and FF, are found in 0.3% to 0.5% of the white population; their incidence among blacks is even lower. Inheritance of increased CHE activity has been reported in a few families. This is apparently due to increased production of the usual allelozyme.

Clinical Significance

Measurements of CHE activity in serum are used (1) as a test of liver function, (2) as an indicator of possible insecticide poisoning, and (3) for the detection of patients with atypical forms of the enzyme who are at risk for prolonged responses to certain muscle relaxants used in surgical procedures.[101]

Measurement of serum CHE activity can serve as a sensitive indicator of the synthetic capacity of the liver. In the absence of genetic causes or known inhibitors, any decrease in CHE activity reflects impaired synthesis of the enzyme by the liver. Serial measurement of CHE has been promoted as an indication of prognosis in patients with liver disease and for monitoring liver function after liver transplantation. Although the retesting interval for disease monitoring has not been defined, a reference change value of approximately 20% to assess significance of changes in serial CHE results has been proposed.[102]

Among the organic phosphorous compounds that inhibit cholinesterase activity are many insecticides, such as parathion, sarin, and tetraethyl pyrophosphate. Workers in agriculture and in organic chemical industries may be subject to poisoning by inhalation of these materials or by direct contact with them. Obviously, if enough material is absorbed to inactivate all the acetylcholinesterase of nervous tissue, death will result. Both cholinesterases are inhibited, but the activity of the serum enzyme falls more rapidly than does that of the erythrocyte enzyme. A 40% drop in CHE activity occurs before the first symptoms are felt, and a drop of 80% is required before neuromuscular effects become apparent. Near-zero concentrations of enzyme activity require emergency treatment with enzyme reactivators such as pyridine-2-aldoxime. Upon retesting, in 3 to 5 days, CHE activity should increase by 15% to 20% if a significant organophosphate-induced inhibition has occurred previously.

Succinyldicholine (suxamethonium) and mivacurium, muscle relaxant drugs used in surgical procedures to aid in endotracheal intubation, are hydrolyzed by CHE, and their pharmacologic effect normally persists only long enough to meet the needs of the surgical procedure. In patients with low enzyme activities or in those with a weakly active variant, destruction of the drug will not occur rapidly enough, and the patient may enter a period of prolonged paralysis of the respiratory muscles (apnea) requiring mechanical ventilation until the drug effects gradually wear off. Preoperative screening of CHE activity has been advocated to identify patients in whom suxamethonium administration may lead to complications; however, in many countries, this is not recommended because all individuals undergoing surgery are considered to be potentially at risk. The degree of drug sensitivity varies with the phenotype of the patient. Total CHE activity is highest in individuals who are homozygous for the usual allele and progressively lower in those who are heterozygous for the usual and a variant allele, those who are homozygous or heterozygous for variant alleles, and those in whom two "silent" alleles are paired and no activity is detected. Whereas subjects who possess one normal allele (ie, who are heterozygous for the normal and a variant allele) usually produce enough enzyme to protect themselves against suxamethonium sensitivity, patients with paired variant alleles (as homozygotes or heterozygotes) show various degrees of sensitivity. The phenotypes most susceptible to apnea after succinylcholine administration include AA, AS, FF, FS, SS, AF, and to some extent UA. Measurements of total CHE activity and determination of the "dibucaine number" and "fluoride number" are needed to fully characterize CHE variants. The latter values indicate the percentage inhibition of enzyme activity toward specified substrates in the presence of standard concentrations of dibucaine or fluoride. Mutation genotyping may confirm CHE gene abnormalities.

Methods for Determination of Serum Cholinesterase Activity

Many of the contemporary methods use acylthiocholine esters as substrates. The iodide salts of acetylthiocholine, propionylthiocholine, butyrylthiocholine, benzoylthiocholine, and succinylthiocholine all have been used. These substrates are hydrolyzed at approximately the same rate as choline esters, and the thiocholine formed can be measured by reaction with chromogenic disulfide agents, such as 5,5′-dithio-bis(2-nitrobenzoate) (DTNB) (Ellman's reagent). The reaction of the thiocholine product with colorless DTNB forms colored 5-mercapto-2-nitro-benzoic acid, which is measured spectrophotometrically at 410 nm. The clinical question being asked may influence the choice of substrate suitable for measuring the enzyme. Measuring CHE activity using succinyldithiocholine is the method of choice to diagnose succinylcholine sensitivity, purely based on the enzyme activity recorded in serum. This method is also well suited for other clinical applications of the test.[103] At present, however, most automated instruments prefer the use of butyrylthiocholine as substrate for determining the CHE activity.

Kalow and Genest, using benzoylcholine as a classic substrate, demonstrated the qualitative difference in CHEs. Based on differences such as sensitivity to inhibition by the local anesthetic dibucaine, they developed a simple test to classify the type of CHE as usual, intermediate, or atypical. With 10^{-5} mol/L dibucaine ("dibucaine number"), the usual CHE is inhibited by 80%, but atypical CHE is inhibited by only 20%. Subjects heterozygous for the normal and atypical gene show about 60% inhibition of CHE. To differentiate other genotypes, sodium fluoride can be used as a CHE inhibitor. Molecular biologic methods that can be used to identify various CHE genetic defects have been developed and are being used increasingly in clinical laboratories.

Serum is the sample of choice. Enzyme activity in serum is stable for several weeks if the specimen is stored under refrigeration and for several years if stored at −20°C. Moderate hemolysis does not interfere if separated serum has been centrifuged to remove red blood cell ghosts.

Desirable analytical specifications for CHE determination are imprecision (CV) of 3.1% or less, bias of ±4.8%, and total error of ±9.8%.[31]

Reference Intervals

Using the succinyldithiocholine/DTNB method at 37°C, the reference interval for healthy adults with the usual CHE genotype was estimated to be 33 to 76 U/L for women and 40 to 78 U/L for men, respectively. The median activity in individuals with heterozygous genotype was 22 U/L (range, 5–35 U/L), and for atypical homozygotes 1.5 U/L (range, 1–4 U/L).[104] A value less than 23 U/L was approximately five times as likely to occur in a succinyldicholine-sensitive individual as in a normal one.[103] At birth, CHE activity is lower than adult values by about 50%. It increases during the next 3 to 6 years to exceed adult values by about 30%. From the fifth year of life, the activity starts to decrease before it stabilizes at the adult value, which is reached at puberty. The significant CHE decrease (30%) during pregnancy and early puerperium is explained by hemodilution.

CHE phenotyping, based on determination of dibucaine (DN) and fluoride (FN) numbers, has been established:

Phenotype	DN Range	FN Range
UU	≥77	≥55
UF	72–76	≥53
UA	48–72	≥44
AF	45–59	<44
FF	64–69	<44
AA	<35	*

*Redundant for AA phenotype attribution.

Lipoprotein-Associated Phospholipase A_2

Lipoprotein-associated phospholipase A_2 (EC 3.1.1.47; platelet-activating factor [PAF] acetylhydrolase; Lp-PLA_2), a 45,400-Da monomeric protein, is a calcium-independent member of the phospholipase A_2 superfamily. It is produced mainly by monocytes, macrophages, T lymphocytes, and mast cells and has been found to be upregulated in atherosclerotic lesions, especially in complex plaque prone to rupture. Lp-PLA_2 has proatherogenic properties by promoting modification of oxidized low-density lipoproteins (LDLs). In particular, the enzyme cleaves oxidized phosphatidylcholine components of the lipoprotein particle, generating two potent proinflammatory and proatherogenic mediators, namely, lysophosphatidylcholine (lysoPC), and oxidized free fatty acids. LysoPC serves as a potent chemoattractant for T cells and monocytes, promotes endothelial dysfunction, and stimulates macrophage proliferation, thus enhancing lesion progression.[105]

Clinical Significance

Several prospective epidemiologic studies have reported an association between increased plasma concentrations of Lp-PLA_2 and future coronary and cerebrovascular events.[106] The strength of association varies and is generally modest (hazard ratios <2). However, because some controversy persists as to its independence from LDL cholesterol, no clear recommendation on the clinical usefulness of Lp-PLA_2 can be given until definitive data document its incremental value above and beyond traditional cardiovascular risk factors. Furthermore, no data show that Lp-PLA_2 reduction per se improves clinical outcomes. Unlike other emerging cardiovascular risk markers, Lp-PLA_2 is not an acute-phase reactant and thus is unaffected by systemic inflammatory processes.

Methods for Determination of Lipoprotein-Associated Phospholipase A_2

Risk estimates were similar, whether the mass concentration or the activity of the enzyme was measured.[107] A manual enzyme-linked immunosorbant assay (ELISA) method for Lp-PLA_2 mass concentration has received US Food and Drug Administration clearance for use as an aid in cardiovascular risk prediction. An immunoturbidimetric method that uses the same monoclonal antibodies has become commercially available, allowing the assay to be run on automated chemistry analyzers. A panel of national experts has recommended that an Lp-PLA_2 concentration above 200 μg/L be used as the threshold for higher risk of cardiovascular events. Lp-PLA_2 variability across gender (10% higher in males) and ethnicity (15% higher in whites than African Americans or Hispanics) has been reported.

EDTA plasma is the recommended sample for measuring Lp-PLA_2. Samples should be analyzed within 1 hour. For laboratories that cannot immediately process samples, these should undergo separation and freezing at −70°C before analysis.

SELECTED REFERENCES

For a full list of references for this chapter, please refer to ExpertConsult.com.

8. Morandi L, Angelini C, Prelle A, et al. High plasma creatine kinase: review of the literature and proposal for a diagnostic algorithm. *Neurol Sci* 2006;**27**:303–11.
16. Infusino I, Schumann G, Ceriotti F, et al. Standardization in clinical enzymology: a challenge for the theory of metrological traceability. *Clin Chem Lab Med* 2010;**48**: 301–7.
25. Kim WR, Flamm SL, Di Bisceglie AM, et al. Serum activity of alanine aminotransferase (ALT) as an indicator of health and disease. *Hepatology* 2008;**47**:1363–70.
26. Dufour DR, Lott JA, Nolte FS, et al. Diagnosis and monitoring of hepatic injury. II. Recommendations for use of laboratory tests in screening, diagnosis, and monitoring. *Clin Chem* 2000;**46**:2050–68.
36. Schmidt ES, Schmidt FW. Glutamate dehydrogenase: biochemical and clinical aspects of an interesting enzyme. *Clin Chim Acta* 1988;**43**:43–56.
38. Moss DW. Perspectives in alkaline phosphatase research. *Clin Chem* 1992;**38**:2486–92.
52. Whitfield JB. Gamma glutamyl transferase. *CRC Crit Rev Clin Lab Sci* 2001;**38**:263–355.
55. Kunutsor SK, Apekey TA, Kahn H. Liver enzymes and risk of cardiovascular disease in the general population: a meta-analysis of prospective cohort studies. *Atherosclerosis* 2014;**236**:7–17.
63. Tenner S, Baillie J, DeWitt J, et al. American College of Gastroenterology guideline: management of acute pancreatitis. *Am J Gastroenterol* 2013;**108**:1400–15.
64. Phillip V, Steiner JM, Algül H. Early phase of acute pancreatitits: assessment and management. *World J Gastrointest Pathophysiol* 2014;**5**:158–68.
70. Panteghini M, Ceriotti F, Pagani F, et al., for the Italian Society of Clinical Biochemistry and Clinical Molecular Biology (SIBioC) Working Group on Enzymes. Recommendations for the routine use of pancreatic amylase measurement instead of total amylase for the diagnosis and monitoring of pancreatic pathology. *Clin Chem Lab Med* 2002;**40**:97–100.
91. Moss DW, Raymond FD, Wile DB. Clinical and biological aspects of acid phosphatase. *CRC Crit Rev Clin Lab Sci* 1995;**32**:431–67.
93. Henriksen K, Tanko LB, Qvist P, et al. Assessment of osteoclast number and function: application in the development of new and improved treatment modalities for bone diseases. *Osteoporos Int* 2007;**18**:681–5.
95. Huijgen HJ, Sanders GT, Koster RW, et al. The clinical value of lactate dehydrogenase in serum: a quantitative review. *Eur J Clin Chem Clin Biochem* 1997;**35**:569–75.

101. McQueen MJ. Clinical and analytical considerations in the utilization of cholinesterase measurements. *Clin Chim Acta* 1995;**237**:91–105.
103. Mosca A, Bonora R, Ceriotti F, et al. Assay using succinyldithiocholine as substrate: the method of choice for the measurement of cholinesterase catalytic activity in serum to diagnose succinylcholine sensitivity. *Clin Chem Lab Med* 2003;**41**:317–22.
106. Vittos O, Toana B, Vittos A, et al. Lipoprotein-associated phospholipase A2 (Lp-PLA2): a review of its role and significance as a cardiovascular biomarker. *Biomarkers* 2012;**17**:289–302.

30

Enzymes of the Red Blood Cell

Wouter W. van Solinge and Richard van Wijk

ABSTRACT

Background

Red cell metabolism provides the cell with energy to pump ions against electrochemical gradients, maintain its shape, keep iron from hemoglobin in the reduced form, and maintain enzyme and hemoglobin sulfhydryl groups. The main source of metabolic energy comes from glucose. Glucose is metabolized through the Emden-Meyerhof glycolytic pathway and through the hexose monophosphate shunt, producing adenosine triphosphate and nicotinamide-adenine dinucleotide (NADH). 2,3-Bisphosphoglycerate, an important regulator of the oxygen affinity of hemoglobin, is also generated during glycolysis. The hexose monophosphate shunt oxidizes glucose-6-phosphate, thereby generating nicotinamide adenine dinucleotide phosphate (NADPH). NADPH serves the red cell to maintain high concentrations of reduced glutathione (GSH). The red cell lacks the capacity for de novo purine synthesis but has a salvage pathway that permits synthesis of purine nucleotides from purine bases.

Content

Hereditary red blood cell (RBC) enzymopathies are genetic disorders affecting genes encoding RBC enzymes involved in red cell metabolism. They cause a specific type of anemia designated hereditary nonspherocytic hemolytic anemia (HNSHA). HNSHA is a normocytic normochromic hemolytic anemia. In contrast to other hereditary red cell disorders such as membrane disorders or hemoglobinopathies, morphologic abnormalities of the RBC are absent. The diagnosis is based on detection of reduced specific enzyme activity and molecular characterization of the defect on the DNA level. The most common enzyme disorders are deficiencies of glucose-6-phosphate dehydrogenase and pyruvate kinase. However, there are a number of additional enzyme disorders, rarer and often much less known, causing HNSHA.

31

Tumor Markers

Catharine Sturgeon

ABSTRACT

Background

Tumor markers are substances present in and produced by a tumor or produced by the host in response to a tumor. Measured qualitatively or quantitatively by chemical, immunological, genomic, or proteomic methods, tumor markers can be used to identify the presence of a cancer and/or to differentiate a tumor from normal tissue. Tumor markers can contribute to cancer management as screening tests for malignancy in asymptomatic patients, diagnostic aids, prognostic indicators, therapy predictors, and/or posttreatment monitoring. Reflecting the heterogeneous nature of cancer, tumor markers encompass a variety of tumor-derived or tumor-associated molecular species. Tumor markers can be produced by different tumor types. Few are organ-specific and few are specific for a particular malignancy. Tumor markers range from simple molecules (eg, catecholamines) through relatively well-characterized proteins (eg, hormones, enzymes, and gene products) to very large heterogeneous glycoproteins and mucins (eg, CA125), which may be defined by the antibodies used to measure them. Although their structures vary widely, the same general principles apply to all tumor markers currently used in clinical practice.

Content

This chapter provides a brief overview of cancer, highlighting its variability and some of the current clinical challenges this important family of diseases poses to laboratory medicine. These are linked with chronological developments in tumor marker applications, from the early recognition of the importance of Bence Jones proteins in myeloma through to molecular and genetic assessment of mutations in solid tumors. Requirements of the "ideal" tumor marker are considered before reviewing the general principles that guide the effective use of tumor markers (ie, requirements that must be met in the preanalytical, analytical, and postanalytical phases of laboratory provision). The tumor markers most frequently used in routine practice are reviewed, and requirements for provision of an optimal tumor marker service are considered.

Tumor markers are substances that may be present in abnormally high concentrations in body fluids or tissue from patients with cancer.[1] Tumor markers can aid cancer management in a number of ways, including screening, diagnosis, prognostic assessment, therapy prediction, and/or posttreatment monitoring. Reflecting the heterogeneous nature of cancer, tumor markers encompass a variety of molecular species, which may be tumor-derived or tumor-associated. Many tumor markers are produced by a variety of different tumors, and few tumor markers are organ-specific or specific for a single type of malignancy.

Tumor markers range from simple molecules (eg, catecholamines) to relatively well-characterized proteins (eg, hormones, enzymes, and gene products) to much more heterogeneous glycoproteins and mucins (eg, CA125), which may be defined by the antibodies used to measure them. Several important tumor markers (eg, α-fetoprotein [AFP], carcinoembryonic antigen [CEA], and human chorionic gonadotropin [hCG]) are oncofetal antigens, which are present in the fetus in normal pregnancy but are expressed at high concentrations in tissue or body fluids of adults with some cancers. Tumor markers are present in cells, tissues, or body fluids and can be measured either qualitatively or quantitatively using chemical, immunologic, or molecular biological methods. While their structures and properties vary widely, the broad principles underpinning their evidence-based clinical application are common to all tumor markers.

This chapter provides a brief overview of cancer and a history of tumor marker development, followed by a comprehensive review of these broad principles. Clinically relevant tumor markers for a number of malignancies are then discussed in detail, considering current practice and future requirements.

CANCER: AN OVERVIEW

Cancer is the name given to a collection of heterogeneous but related diseases that can start in most parts of the body and that are characterized by uncontrolled division of cells that ultimately may spread into surrounding tissues.[2] It is rarely clear what leads to this autonomous growth in individual patients, with causative factors likely to be multifactorial as well as dependent on the organ involved. Factors that have been implicated include exposure to carcinogens, which may be physical (eg, radiation), chemical (eg, polycyclic hydrocarbons), or biological (eg, viral). Exposure to such agents may cause cancer by direct genotoxic effects on deoxyribonucleic acid (DNA) (eg, as with radiation) or by increasing cell proliferation (eg, by a hormone) or both (eg, through use of tobacco). Excess weight, physical inactivity, and poor nutrition may also contribute to the development of some cancers.

Genetic predisposition to some cancers is increasingly identifiable due to advances in molecular techniques. However, simple genetic analysis of mutations within cancerous cells may be too simplistic to explain a complex process. Sophisticated interaction and communication of cancer cells with their surrounding cellular microenvironment are likely to be essential for both survival and dissemination of cancer cells.[3] Improved understanding of such interactions is already leading to more finely targeted therapies.

For the present, cancer remains a leading cause of death in the United States, second only to heart disease, although death rates have decreased significantly over the last three decades. American Cancer Society figures show that for all cancers the 5-year relative survival rate* for cancers diagnosed from 2004–2010 was 68% as compared to only 49% from 1975–1977.[4] Such figures suggest that early detection and more effective treatment combined with prevention (eg, decreased smoking, improved diet) could reduce the future mortality rate for cancer. However, the identification of smaller more indolent cancers with newer techniques and screening programs may also be contributing to the perceived increase in survival.

Death rates for individual cancers vary markedly (Table 31.1).[2,268] On comparing the number of deaths per year with the number of new cases, it is clear that lung and bronchus cancer, colon and rectum cancer, and non-Hodgkin lymphoma are the most lethal (71.4%, 37.5%, and 27.5%, respectively). Although the annual numbers of newly diagnosed lung cancer and prostate cancer cases are similar, there are nearly six times more deaths from lung cancer, demonstrating both the heterogeneity of different cancers and the need for good understanding of their natural history, including at the molecular level.

Also evident from Table 31.1 are the considerable advances in treatment over recent decades. Many patients survive for much longer than previously. Although surgical removal of a primary tumor is the only curative therapy for almost all cancers, new chemotherapeutic and biological therapies that prevent progression are increasingly available (Table 31.2). It has been suggested that some relatively indolent cancers should be considered to be chronic diseases like diabetes, to be controlled rather than cured. Breast and prostate cancers are among the best examples. However, for these and other cancers, distinguishing cancers that are likely to progress rapidly from those that are slow-growing or indolent is critical for treatment selection. This distinction remains a challenge for many cancers.

Early detection of malignancy optimizes any opportunities for curative surgery for some in situ cancers. Unfortunately most cancers do not produce symptoms until tumors are too large to be removed surgically or until cancerous cells have spread to other tissue either by invading local lymph nodes or by distant spread (metastasis) to other organs. Systemic treatments (chemotherapy, endocrine therapy, or immunotherapy) are then usually the only options but are not curative. Any residual viable cancerous cells remaining after treatment may proliferate, develop resistance to further therapy, and ultimately cause the death of the patient.

*Relative cancer survival rates compare observed survival with that expected for people without the cancer. This helps to correct for deaths that are not cancer-related and provides a more accurate estimate of the effect of cancer on survival. Relative survival rates are at least as high as overall survival and usually higher.

TABLE 31.1 Estimated Number of New Cancer Cases and Deaths in the United States for Some Common Cancers (2015 Figures)

Cancer	Incidence	Number of Deaths	Number of Deaths as a Percentage of Incidence
Bladder	74,000	16,000	21.6%
Breast	234,190	40,730	17.4%
Cervix	12,900	4100	31.8%
Colorectal (colon, rectum, anorectal)	139,970	50,710	36.3%
Gastric	24,590	10,720	43.6%
Hepatocellular carcinoma	35,660	24,550	68.8%
Lung and bronchus	221,200	158,040	71.8%
Melanoma	73,870	9940	13.5%
Ovarian	21,290	14,180	66.6%
Pancreatic	48,960	40,560	82.8%
Prostate	220,800	27,540	12.5%
Testicular	8430	380	4.5%
Thyroid	62,450	1950	3.1%
Unknown	31,510	43,840	Near 100%

NOTE: Lack of specificity in recording the underlying cause of death on death certificates and/or an undercount in the case estimate probably accounts for figures suggesting more deaths than cases.

Data for incidence and deaths from the American Cancer Society. *Cancer facts and figures 2015.* American Cancer Society, 2015. Estimated new cases are based on 1995–2011 incidence rates reported by the North American Association of Central Cancer Registries. Estimated deaths are based on 1997–2011 US mortality data from the National Center for Health Statistics, Centers for Disease Control and Prevention.

HISTORICAL BACKGROUND

The timeline shown in Fig. 31.1 illustrates how closely introduction of new tumor markers has mirrored developments in analytical techniques and more recently has been influenced by the availability of new therapies, many of which are effective only in subsets of cancer patients.[5] Precipitation of a protein from acidified boiled urine in 1847 heralded the identification of Bence Jones protein, the first tumor marker to be used clinically.[6] Characterized more than a century later by the Nobel Prize–winning studies of Porter, Edelman, and Poulik[7] as the monoclonal light chain of immunoglobulin secreted by tumor plasma cells, measurement of Bence Jones protein (paraproteins or M-protein) still forms the basis of many diagnoses of multiple myeloma. (See Chapter 28.)

In the first half of the twentieth century, the presence or absence of several hormones, enzymes, and isoenzymes[8] and

TABLE 31.2 Treatment Options for Malignancies

Treatment	Relevant Malignancies*
Active surveillance	Prostate cancer
Curative surgery (curative only in early-stage disease for most malignancies)	Early-stage bladder, breast, cervical, colorectal, gastric, germ cell, GIST, GTD, HCC, liver, lung, melanoma, ovarian, prostate, thyroid, and other cancers
Hepatic resection	Advanced colorectal cancer
Liver transplant	Advanced hepatocellular carcinoma
Palliative surgery	Advanced colorectal cancer
Radiotherapy	Bladder, breast, cervical, colorectal, gastric, germ cell, lung, prostate, and thyroid cancers
Brachytherapy	Prostate cancer
Radioiodine	Thyroid cancer
Chemotherapy	Bladder, breast, cervical, colorectal, germ cell, GTD, HCC, lung, ovarian, prostate, and other cancers
Ablative therapy (alcohol, radiofrequency, microwave, chemoembolization)	Hepatocellular carcinoma
Endocrine therapy	Breast and prostate cancer
Immunotherapy	Bladder, breast, colorectal, gastric, GIST, lung, melanoma, and non–small cell lung cancers

*Treatment of testicular cancers as for germ cell tumors. Treatment of cancers of unknown primary dependent on immunohistochemistry.
GIST, Gastrointestinal stromal tumors; *GTD,* gestational trophoblastic disease; *HCC,* hepatocellular carcinoma.

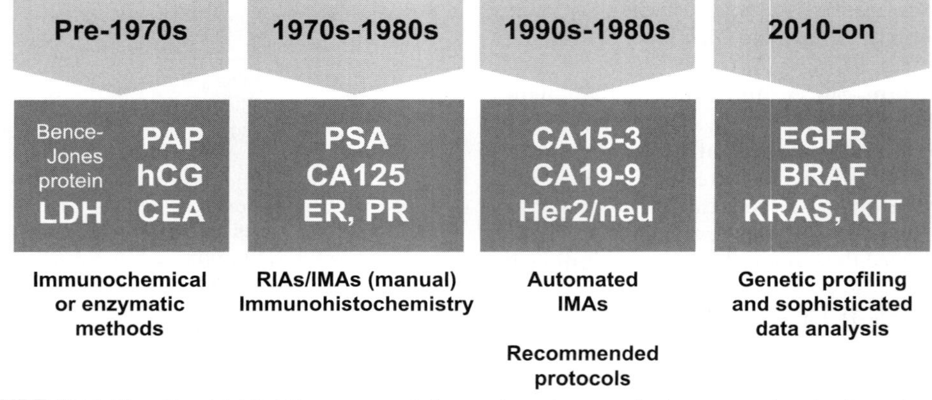

FIGURE 31.1 Timeline highlighting some of the major advances in tumor marker testing since the early identification of Bence Jones proteins and their association with hematological malignancy in the 19th century.

blood group antigens were recognized to be associated with malignancy, but it was not until the development of the technique of radioimmunoassay (RIA) in the 1960s[9] that these observations could be translated into routine clinical practice. The application of RIA to the measurement of previously identified oncofetal antigens, including AFP, hCG, and CEA, facilitated their clinical use.[10] Monoclonal antibody technology[11] subsequently enabled the development of two-site immunoradiometric assays (IRMA) of complex cancer-associated mucins identified primarily by their reactivity with given monoclonal antibody pairs (eg, the carbohydrate or cancer-associated antigens CA125 and CA15-3). The radiolabels initially used were soon replaced with less hazardous nonisotopic labels, providing immunoenzymatic assays (IEMA), immunochemiluminescent assays (ICMA), and immunofluorescent (IFMA) assays that were much more readily automated than, and rapidly replaced, assays requiring isotopic labels (see Chapter 23). As a consequence, tumor marker measurements, which had previously generally been provided in specialist laboratories, became widely available.

Advances in molecular genetics using monoclonal antibodies and molecular probes to detect chromosome or protein alterations, including the study of oncogenes, suppressor genes, and genes involved in DNA repair, have led to rapid understanding and use of tumor markers at both molecular and cellular levels, particularly in high-risk individuals. Estrogen, progesterone, and epidermal growth factor receptor measurements are now routinely performed for breast cancer patients to enable identification of optimal treatment, while establishing the presence or absence of the breast cancer susceptibility genes *BRCA1* and *BRCA2* provides additional prognostic information.

Mass spectrometry is also increasingly used both as a discovery and a diagnostic tool, albeit with limited success thus far in translating new tumor marker tests into clinical practice[12,13] (see Chapter 21). These developments, for which sophisticated bioinformatics support (eg, neural networks, support vector machines, and other algorithms) is essential,[14] are encouraging the use of multiparametric analysis for cancer diagnosis, prognosis, and therapy prediction. The last is becoming increasingly important, with the advent of new and expensive immunotherapies that are effective only in relatively small subsets of patients whose tumors fulfill certain well-defined molecular criteria.[5]

GENERAL PRINCIPLES GUIDING THE USE OF ALL TUMOR MARKERS

Tumor markers are surrogate indicators that can help to increase or decrease the clinical suspicion that a future clinically important event, such as the development of a new or secondary cancer, recurrence, progression, or death will or will not occur, and/or that a specific treatment will reduce that risk.[15] Tumor markers can help make or confirm a cancer diagnosis, monitor treatment effectiveness and the course of disease, estimate prognosis, and/or predict whether a specific therapy is likely to be successful (Table 31.3). Their measurement should permit more efficient application of therapies by ensuring that these are applied only to those patients most likely to benefit and reducing exposure to unnecessary toxicity for those patients unlikely to benefit.[5,16] Tumor markers should be measured only after careful consideration of whether the result is likely to provide information that may improve outcome for the individual patient[17] or if required as part of a clinical trial.

In order to achieve optimal use of tumor markers, an evidence-based approach to clinical decision making is essential.[18] As discussed later in this chapter, careful consideration must be given to whether an individual tumor marker can fulfill requirements for each use (see Table 31.3). In practice, most are appropriate only in selected clinical circumstances. Many guidelines on tumor marker use (Table 31.4), including those of the American Society for Clinical Oncology (ASCO)

TABLE 31.3 Current Clinical Applications of Tumor Markers

Clinical Application	Requirements	Examples
Screening for cancer	An acceptable test for a disease that poses an important health problem, for which the natural history is well understood, the test identifies treatable early-stage cancers, and early intervention with effective treatment improves outcome.[39] High clinical sensitivity (few false negatives) and specificity (few false positives) are essential prerequisites because the population screened is asymptomatic.	*Population screening*: Fecal occult blood testing for colorectal cancer.[20,269] *Screening of high-risk groups:* Serum hCG testing for choriocarcinoma in women who have had a molar pregnancy.[38]
Diagnosing cancer	High clinical sensitivity and specificity as for screening. Most serum tumor markers are not cancer-specific and/or organ-specific and are raised in different cancers and/or in nonmalignant disease, severely limiting their use in diagnosis.	*As a diagnostic aid in high-risk groups:* Serum AFP testing as an adjunct to ultrasound for hepatocellular carcinoma (HCC) in patients with cirrhosis who are at high risk of developing HCC.[270] *Differential diagnosis:* CA125 contributes (with menopausal status and ultrasound findings) to calculation of the "risk of malignancy index," which is used to differentiate patients with benign and malignant pelvic masses.[204]
Assessing prognosis	A test that can provide a probability estimate of outcome (risk of relapse or disease progression) and/or differentiate indolent from aggressive disease for a heterogeneous population of patients, thereby influencing treatment decisions.[5]	Serum AFP, hCG, and lactate dehydrogenase (LDH) measurements are mandatory for determining prognosis and selection of chemotherapy in patients with metastatic nonseminomatous germ cell tumors.[271] Microsatellite instability (MSI) occurs when germline alleles of microsatellites (short stretches of DNA that are repeated at multiple locations throughout the genome) lose or gain a repeat unit due to failure of mismatch repair. Presence of MSI is associated with good prognosis in colorectal cancer patients, especially in Stage II or III disease,[123] and their presence, associated with other established prognostic factors, may obviate the need for adjuvant chemotherapy in patients with Stage II disease.[5] Gene expression profiles such as the Oncotype Dx test, which measures expression of 21 genes in breast tumor tissue, enable calculation of a recurrence score that predicts the risk of distant disease at 10 years in a specific subset of breast cancer patients.[272]

Continued

TABLE 31.3 Current Clinical Applications of Tumor Markers—cont'd

Clinical Application	Requirements	Examples
Prediction of treatment response	A test that can identify whether or not a potential treatment is likely to be effective and of benefit to the patient.	Measurement of estrogen receptors (ER) is mandatory for all newly diagnosed invasive breast cancers[92,99] to predict response to treatment with antiestrogen therapy (ie, aromatase inhibitors and tamoxifen). The additional measurement of progesterone receptors (PR) can improve the accuracy of prediction.[21,99] Measurement of human epidermal growth factor receptor 2 *(HER2)* is essential to identify patients with *HER2*-positive breast cancer who are likely to benefit from treatment with anti-*HER2* monoclonal antibody therapy (eg, trastuzumab).[97,99]
Monitoring response during and/or shortly after treatment	A test that assesses whether the tumor is responding to treatment, enabling withdrawal and/or change of ineffective treatment.	In patients receiving treatment for ovarian cancer, a reduction of at least 50% in CA125 concentrations from a pretreatment sample has been defined as a response, provided it is confirmed and maintained for at least 28 days and if a pretreatment CA125 concentration was greater than twice the upper limit of the reference interval and measured within 2 weeks of the start of chemotherapy.[273] Biological response to systemic chemotherapy, as assessed by serial measurement of serum CEA and CA19-9 in patients receiving chemotherapy for colorectal cancer with liver metastases, agrees with response as assessed by radiology in over 94% and 91% of patients, respectively,[130] suggesting that this could decrease the need for imaging studies, such as computerized tomography (CT), which require exposure of patients to significant doses of radiation.
Monitoring disease posttreatment to detect progression	A test that reliably indicates earlier than clinical symptoms whether disease is progressing in patients with no evidence of disease posttherapy and/or in patients with detectable disease. Whether this information is helpful crucially depends on whether alternative therapies are available.	Inclusion of CEA measurements in intensive follow-up strategies for patients with nonmetastatic colorectal cancer following curative surgery has been shown to improve overall survival and increase the detection of asymptomatic recurrences and hence the frequency of curative surgery attempted at recurrence.[274] Such follow-up is also associated with earlier detection of recurrence.

TABLE 31.4 Selected Expert Groups That Have Developed Guideline Recommendations Relevant to Tumor Marker Use

Abbreviation	Name of Organization	Website
ASCO	American Society for Clinical Oncology	http://jco.ascopubs.org/site/misc/specialarticles.xhtml
EGTM	European Group on Tumor Markers	http://www.egtm.eu/
ESMO	European Society for Medical Oncology	http://www.esmo.org/Guidelines
NACB	National Academy of Clinical Biochemistry	https://www.aacc.org/community/national-academy-of-clinical-biochemistry
NCCN	National Comprehensive Cancer Network	http://www.nccn.org/professionals/physician_gls/f_guidelines.asp
NICE	National Institute for Health and Care Excellence	https://www.nice.org.uk/guidance
SIGN	Scottish Intercollegiate Guideline Network	http://www.sign.ac.uk/

and the European Society for Medical Oncology (ESMO), focus primarily on clinical management, with relatively little mention of tumor marker or other laboratory tests.

Guidelines published by the National Comprehensive Cancer Network (NCCN) in the United States include patient pathways that clearly indicate which tumor markers should be measured and when. Complementing these clinically oriented guidelines, those published by the National Academy of Clinical Biochemistry (NACB) and the European Group on Tumor Markers (EGTM) focus on the use of tumor markers, considering in detail requirements for their appropriate use in all phases of both the patient pathway and laboratory provision, helpfully comparing recommendations made with those of other groups. Recommendations relating to tumor marker use for specific malignancies are summarized later in this chapter.

While there have been many reports on tumor markers in the last fifty years—the number of publications on "neoplastic antigens" increasing from about 260 in 1973 in *Index Medicus*[10] to more than 223,000 in 2015 in *PubMed*—the number of tumor markers with established roles in clinical practice has remained rather low. Only a few new serum and tissue markers have been introduced into routine practice in the last 25 years,[13,19] although there have been major developments in fecal testing for colorectal cancer.[20] (See the section on colorectal cancer.) Well-established and commonly requested serum tumor markers whose measurement is generally available in most large clinical laboratories are listed in Table 31.5, along with some of their properties and the cancers with which they are primarily associated. Some less commonly requested serum tumor markers with an established clinical role are shown in Table 31.6. Table 31.7 lists some of the tissue markers whose measurement enables informed decisions regarding selection of endocrine and immunotherapy in individual patients. Some of the many other tumor markers that have not found clinical application are tabulated elsewhere.[10,21,22]

The broad principles guiding the validation of any new tumor marker and its subsequent introduction into routine clinical practice are essentially similar and are considered in detail in the following sections. Early in the evaluation of a promising new tumor marker, critical aspects include rigorous validation of analytical performance and clinical utility and demonstration of clinical value.[23] While in the past tumor markers may have been prematurely introduced into clinical use without appropriate evaluation,[17] objective assessment of the potential clinical value of a proposed new tumor marker, together with an estimate of the magnitude of its benefit, including effect on patient outcome, is now a prerequisite for introducing a new test into routine practice. Three key issues in tumor marker evaluation are clinical utility, magnitude of effect, and reliability.[24] Only when these have been established and regulatory requirements fulfilled should the tumor marker be adopted into routine clinical practice. It is then essential to ensure that the test is requested appropriately, that those requesting the test are aware of any preanalytical

TABLE 31.5 Properties and Applications of Commonly Requested Serum Tumor Markers

Tumor Marker	Biochemical Properties	Molecular Weight	Main Clinical Applications
Alkaline phosphatase	Phosphohydrolase	Variable	Raised activities associated with presence of liver and/or bone metastases
Alpha-fetoprotein (AFP)	Glycoprotein, ~4% carbohydrate; considerable homology with albumin	~70 kDa	Diagnosis and monitoring of primary hepatocellular carcinoma, hepatoblastoma, and germ cell tumors. Prognosis of germ cell tumors.
Cancer antigen 125 (CA125)	Mucin identified by monoclonal antibodies OC125 and M11; developed from serous cystadenocarcinoma cell line	~200 kDa	Monitoring ovarian carcinoma. Measurement required for determination of the "Risk of Malignancy index" (RMI) for ovarian carcinoma.
Carcinoembryonic antigen (CEA)	Family of glycoproteins, 45% to 60% carbohydrate	~180 kDa	Monitoring colorectal adenocarcinomas
ConfirmMDx	A multiplex epigenetic assay	Not applicable	Reducing unnecessary repeat prostatic biopsies in men who have had at least one negative biopsy
Human chorionic gonadotropin (hCG)	Glycoprotein hormone consisting of two noncovalently bound subunits (α and β). α-Subunit similar to LH, FSH, and TSH; β-subunit considerable homology with LH	~36 kDa	Diagnosis, prognosis, and monitoring germ cell tumors and gestational trophoblastic neoplasia
Lactate dehydrogenase (LDH)	Enzyme of the glycolytic pathway	Variable	Diagnosis, prognosis, and monitoring of germ cell tumors. Used to monitor a wide range of malignancies, including hematological malignancies.
Paraproteins	Monoclonal immunoglobulins	Variable	See Chapter 28.
Prolactin	Pituitary hormone	~22 kDa, but high molecular forms also exist	See Chapter 65.
Prostate-specific antigen (PSA)	Glycoprotein; member of the kallikrein family with serine protease activity; circulates as free enzyme or complexed to α_1-antichymotrypsin (measurable) or α_2-macroglobulin (not detected by most immunoassays)	~30 kDa (free enzyme)	Diagnosis, risk assessment, and monitoring of prostate carcinoma. Lower concentrations of free PSA relative to complexed PSA (ie, free: total ratio) found in prostatic cancer as compared with benign prostatic hypertrophy.

TABLE 31.6 Properties and Applications of Less Commonly Requested Serum Tumor Markers

Tumor Marker	Properties	Molecular Weight	Main Clinical Applications
Calcitonin	32-amino acid peptide	~3.5 kDa	Monitoring medullary carcinoma of the thyroid
Cancer antigen 15.3 (CA15.3), BR 27.29	Mucin (MUC-1 glycoprotein peptide) identified by monoclonal antibodies	>250 kDa	Monitoring breast cancer
Cancer antigen 19.9 (CA19.9)	Glycolipid carrying the Lewis[a] blood group determinant	~1000 kDa	Monitoring pancreatic carcinoma following curative resection
Catecholamines	Biogenic amines	~0.2 kDa	See Chapter 63
Chromogranin A	Member of the granin family of acidic secretory glycoproteins	~49 kDa	Monitoring neuroendocrine tumors
CYFRA 21-1	Fragments of cytokeratin 19	~30 kDa	Monitoring lung carcinoma
Gut hormones	Small peptide hormones, including vasoactive intestinal peptide (VIP), pancreatic polypeptide (PP), somatostatin, gastrin	—	See Chapter 62
Human epididymis protein 4 (HE4)	Product of the WFDC2 (HE4) gene that is overexpressed in patients with ovarian carcinoma	~25 kDa	Monitoring ovarian cancer. Potentially an aid in diagnosis as part of the risk of malignancy algorithm (ROMA) (207). Under evaluation.
Inhibin A (α-β_A) Inhibin B (α-β_B)	Heterodimeric glycoproteins composed of an α- and a β-subunit. There are several forms of the β-subunit, as indicated	32 kDa	Monitoring of ovarian granulosa cell tumors and testicular Sertoli and Leydig tumors
β_2-microglobulin	Component polypeptide chain of the HLA antigen complex	~11 kDa	Providing prognostic information for patients with multiple myeloma
Neuron-specific enolase (NSE)	Dimer of the enzyme enolase	~87 kDa	Monitoring small cell lung carcinoma, neuroblastoma, and neuroendocrine tumors
Placental alkaline phosphatase (PLAP)	Heat-stable isoenzyme of alkaline phosphatase	~86 kDa	Monitoring of germ cell tumors (seminomas)
Pro-gastrin releasing peptide (proGRP)	More stable precursor of gastrin releasing peptide	~16 kDa	Monitoring small cell lung carcinoma
Prostate cancer gene 3 protein (PCA3)	Protein product of PCA3 gene in urine of prostate cancer patients	~86 kDa	Potentially an aid to diagnosis of prostate cancer, particularly in biopsy-negative men. Under evaluation.
Prostate marker algorithm Phi	Not applicable	Not applicable	An algorithm combining serum measurements of total PSA, free PSA, and proPSA in serum
Prostate marker algorithm 4K	Not applicable	Not applicable	An algorithm combining serum measurements of free and total PSA, human kallikrein 2, and intact PSA
Squamous cell carcinoma antigen (SCC)	Serine protease inhibitor isolated from glycoprotein subfraction of tumor antigen TA-4	~48 kDa	Monitoring squamous cell carcinomas (eg, cervix)
S100 proteins	Family of proteins characterized by two calcium-binding sites that have helix-loop-helix conformations	~20 kDa	Monitoring malignant melanoma
Thyroglobulin (Tg)	Glycoprotein dimer of two identical subunits	~670 kDa	Monitoring differentiated thyroid cancer
Tissue polypeptide antigen (TPA)	Fragments of cytokeratins 8, 18, and 19	~22 kDa	Monitoring bladder and lung carcinoma

TABLE 31.7 Tissue Markers Whose Measurement Informs Selection of Endocrine and Immunotherapy in Individual Patients

Tumor Marker	Biochemical Properties	Molecular Weight	Main Clinical Applications
Anaplastic lymphoma receptor tyrosine kinase *(ALK)*	Enzyme encoded by the *ALK* gene	~176 kDa	Predicting response to the thymidine kinase inhibitor (TKI) crizotinib in non–small cell lung cancer
BRA mutation	Proto-oncogene that encodes the serine/threonine protein kinase B-Raf	~87 kDa	Predicting response to inhibitors of BRAF-mutated protein, including vemurafenib and dabrafenib in melanoma
Estrogen receptor (ER)	Nuclear transcription factor	~5 kDa	Predicting response to endocrine therapy in breast cancer
Human epidermal growth factor receptor-2 (*HER2* or c-erb2)	Transmembrane glycoprotein encoded from *HER2*/neu oncogene	~185 kDa	Predicting response to Trastuzumab (Herceptin) in breast cancer. Predicting response to tyrosine kinase inhibitors (TKIs) in non–small cell lung cancer.
KRAS mutation	Guanosine-nucleotide-(GTP)-binding protein	~23 kDa	Predicting response to tyrosine kinase inhibitors (TKIs) in non–small cell lung cancer and reducing need for testing for *HER2* and *ALK* alterations
Progesterone receptor	Nuclear transcription factor	A form ~4 kDa B form: ~120 kDa	Predicting response to endocrine therapy in breast cancer

requirements, that these are met in routine practice, that analytical performance is reliable as confirmed by rigorous internal quality control and proficiency testing, and that post-analytical reporting of results to clinical users is both informed and informative.

Tumor Marker Validation

The steps required to take a new tumor marker into routine use—from the research laboratory to the specialist laboratory and then into routine clinical practice—have been described in detail.[13,25] A position statement from the European Group on Tumor Markers provides detailed recommendations about the essential steps in the validation of a tumor marker.[23] Criteria for the use of omics-based predictors in clinical trials have also been published by a panel convened by the US National Cancer Institute.[26,27] Assuming there is preliminary evidence that the marker has clinical potential, there are six requirements for validation prior to introduction into routine use.

Protocols for Sample Collection and Processing

Availability of clinical specimens (eg, serum, plasma, tissue) that have been collected, processed, and stored following validated standard operating procedures (SOP) that take account of potentially confounding factors, including those described below, is essential.[23,28] The panel should include samples from patients with a variety of malignant and nonmalignant conditions. Specimens from biobanks may be appropriate provided their provenance is well documented.[29-31]

Analytical/Technical Validation

Each specific assay that will be used in the clinic must be developed and validated,[13] having regard to the requirements described below (see the section on analytical requirements). Metrological requirements were established at the Stockholm Conference in 1999[32] and have recently been updated.[33,34] These incorporate assessments in which components of biological variation of the marker are taken into account where feasible. Detailed guidance on analytical requirements for tumor markers is available for serum-based immunoassays[15] and immunohistochemical tests.[35]

Clinical Validation

Defining the specific context in which the tumor marker is to be used is an essential first step that will identify the population to be used in the clinical validation step (ie, the type of specimens required from carefully defined groups of subjects), the informative statistics, and the acceptability criteria.[23] Clinical validation should be reported in terms of diagnostic accuracy for tests intended for use in diagnosis, as described in Tables 31.8 and 31.9.[267] Pitfalls in clinical validation include study bias, overfitting of data, and multiplicities (statistical problems that may occur—for example, with disease subset analysis or the use of several different endpoints). The risk of these can be decreased by strict adherence to a written protocol and reporting of all planned steps and all work completed.[36] The European Group on Tumor Markers has proposed a four-phase model for tumor marker monitoring trials that is analogous to those used for the investigation of new drugs.[37] Biomarker kinetics and correlation with tumor burden are assessed in Phase I, while in Phase II, the ability of the marker to identify, exclude, and/or predict a change in disease status is evaluated. In Phase III the effectiveness of intervention based on trends in tumor marker concentration is assessed by measuring patient outcome in randomized trials, while Phase IV involves clinical evaluation of long-term effects following incorporation of the tumor marker into routine clinical care. The first two phases are also applicable to tumor markers intended to be used solely for screening or diagnosis.[37]

Demonstration of Clinical Value

Strong evidence that the test will benefit the patient (eg, by increasing overall survival or leading to fewer invasive procedures or hospital visits) is now mandatory for introduction of new tests into most health care systems. Ideally this

TABLE 31.8 Parameters Used to Describe and Validate the Clinical Performance of a Tumor Marker

Parameter	Description	Calculation
Clinical sensitivity	How successfully the test identifies individuals who have the condition	TP/(TP + FN)
Clinical specificity	How successfully the test excludes individuals who do not have the condition	TN/(TN + FP)
Prevalence	How common the condition is in the study cohort	(TP + FN)/(TP + FN + TN + FP)
Positive predictive value (PPV) or positive likelihood ratio	How much more likely the test is to be positive in a patient with the condition than in a person without it	TP/(TP + FP)
Negative predictive value (NPV) or negative likelihood ratio	How much more likely the test is to be negative in a patient without the condition than in a person with it	TN/(TN + FN)
Accuracy	How likely it is that the test will correctly identify the presence or absence of a cancer	(TP + TN)/(TP + TN + FP + FN)
Receiver operating characteristic (ROC) curve (see Figure 31.3)	Graphical representation of test performance over a range of test concentrations	
Area under the (ROC) curve (AUC)	Numerical means of comparing different tests	

TP, True positive; *TN,* true negative; *FP,* false positive; *FN,* false negative.

TABLE 31.9 Example of Calculations for Data From 100,000 Women Post–Hydatidiform Mole Using Human Chorionic Gonadotropin to Detect Choriocarcinoma

	Positives	Negatives	Totals
HCG positive	7920 (TP)	920 (FP)	8840 (TP + FP)
HCG negative	80 (FN)	91,080 (TN)	91,160 (FN + TN)
Totals	8000 (TP + FN)	92,000 (TN + FP)	100,000 (All)

Sensitivity = TP/(TP + FN) = 99%
Specificity = TN/(TN + FP) = 99%
Prevalence = (TP + FN)/(TP + FN + TN + FP) = 8%
Positive predictive value = TP/(TP + FP) = 89.6%
Accuracy = (TP + TN)/(TP + TN +FP + FN) = 99%

Modified from Roulston JE, Leonard RCF. *Serological tumour markers.* Edinburgh: Churchill Livingstone; 1993. Used with permission.

should be high-level evidence from a prospective or retrospective randomized clinical trial or systematic review of the literature.[23]

Achieving Regulatory Approval

Requirements vary in different countries but in the United States involve either clearance approval by the U.S. Food and Drug Administration (FDA) and evaluation in a CLIA-certified laboratory[25] or by a laboratory-developed test (LDT) pathway.

Postmarket Evaluation

Analytical performance of the test in the routine clinical setting should be subject to continued evaluation, best achieved through implementation of rigorous internal quality control (IQC) and proficiency testing procedures. Ongoing clinical audit to ensure that the marker retains its clinical value and that it is being used in the setting in which it was originally validated is also essential.[13] When a newly introduced tumor marker replaces an earlier one, it is essential to ensure that the first test is discontinued.

"Ideal" Tumor Marker

In view of the above, it is helpful to consider requirements of an "ideal" tumor marker, which include the following:

1. Detectable only in a given malignancy and absent in the healthy population or in nonmalignant conditions (ie, with clinical specificity and clinical sensitivity approaching 100%).
2. Present in a readily acquired biological matrix (eg, serum, urine, tumor tissue).
3. Present at concentrations proportional to tumor burden.
4. Conveniently measured by a readily available, simple, reproducible, and inexpensive procedure.
5. Beneficial to clinical care with a measurable effect on patient outcome.

No such tumor marker has yet been identified. However, measurement of hCG approaches ideal in the screening and monitoring of women who have had a molar pregnancy and are at risk of developing gestational trophoblastic neoplasia (choriocarcinoma)[38] (see the section on screening for cancer). Other tumor markers can also contribute usefully to patient management provided they are used intelligently and with regard to requirements of the clinical application (see Table 31.3) as outlined below.

Clinical Applications of Tumor Markers

Screening for Cancer

Screening for disease differs fundamentally from diagnosis or "case finding" because the aim of screening is to detect unsuspected disease in asymptomatic subjects (see Table 31.3). The World Health Organization (WHO) criteria for screening programs originally proposed by Wilson and Jungner in 1968[39] remain valid. Table 31.10 compares how well these criteria are met by a long-established national

TABLE 31.10 WHO Criteria for Screening and How Well These Are Met by Established Screening Programs

WHO Requirements[39]	Example: Screening for Choriocarcinoma in a Selected Population (Already Est. in the UK[40])	Example: Screening for Prostate Cancer (Under Evaluation Nationally and Internationally)
Disease		
Should be an important health problem	Accounts for 0.02% of cancer deaths, in women of childbearing age	Second leading cause of cancer deaths among men in some Western countries
Should be serious	Fatal if not treated	Mortality rate significant if not treated
Should have a recognizable early (premalignant) stage	Previous partial or complete hydatidiform mole in previous pregnancy. (Screening restricted to women who have had such a pregnancy.)	None identified. (PSA may be increased in benign prostatic hyperplasia, which is not precancerous.)
Should have a natural history that is well understood	Steps in progression reasonably well documented	Natural history reasonably understood, but what differentiates aggressive from indolent tumors unknown. Significant risk of overdetection.
Test or Examination		
Should be accurate and reliable	hCG assays have ~99% specificity and sensitivity for the disease. (hCG is not detectable in serum in healthy nonpregnant subjects.)	In a population of 63-year-old men at a cutoff point of 4.0 μg/L, PSA had a sensitivity of 46% and a specificity of 91% for identifying prostate cancer that was clinically important within the next 10 years
Should be acceptable to the population being screened	Screening test can be performed on urine specimens that can be conveniently collected at home by the patient and sent by mail to the screening center	Blood sampling acceptable to most patients
Should be part of an ongoing surveillance system	A national registration system can be established for patients at risk	Recall systems likely to be complex to administer
Should be repeated at intervals if desirable (depending on the natural history of the disease)	Lifetime follow-up recommended because disease can recur years later	Benefit of repeat testing still being assessed
Relating to Treatment of Identified Disease		
Early intervention should be of more benefit than treatment started at a later stage	Prompt treatment with chemotherapy is highly desirable	Benefit of treatment not proven yet except in men with localized disease who are candidates for radical prostatectomy. In these men the absolute reduction in the risk of death after 10 years is small, but the reduction in the risks of metastasis and local tumor progression are substantial. Watchful waiting in some patients is as appropriate as active intervention.
There should be an acceptable and effective treatment for patients with recognized disease	Chemotherapy is highly effective	Radical prostatectomy may be curative in disease confined to the prostate. See above comment also.
There should be appropriate facilities for diagnosis and treatment	Three specialist centers undertake testing in the United Kingdom, with all patients referred for treatment to Charing Cross Hospital, London	Significant requirements for additional diagnostic imaging, urologists, counselors, and so on
There should be an agreed policy about whom to screen and treat	All women with a previous history of a molar pregnancy should be screened	General agreement that men over 50 years old (or younger if family history) may benefit from screening. How to select those who will benefit from treatment not known.
The chance of physical or psychological harm should be less than the chance of benefit	Treatment is lifesaving	Physical side effects of surgical and/or radiation treatment include incontinence and impotence in a significant number of patients. Psychological anxiety associated with a positive test and the uncertainty about whether screening reduces the risk of death from prostate cancer.

Continued

TABLE 31.10 WHO Criteria for Screening and How Well These Are Met by Established Screening Programs—cont'd

WHO Requirements[39]	Example: Screening for Choriocarcinoma in a Selected Population (Already Est. in the UK[40])	Example: Screening for Prostate Cancer (Under Evaluation Nationally and Internationally)
Cost of Screening Program		
Should be balanced against the benefits it provides	Costs of the screening test and program are relatively low compared with the social cost avoided per life saved	Accurate cost analysis not yet available but likely to be considerable; should include costs of patient education, advertising for screening, PSA test, biopsy, pathology, staging, definitive therapy, secondary therapy, monitoring, and treatment of complications.

TABLE 31.11 Effect of Prevalence of the Predictive Value of a Positive Test

	POSITIVE PREDICTIVE VALUE	
Disease Prevalence (%)	Test Sensitivity and Specificity = 95%	Test Sensitivity and Specificity = 99%
0.02	0	2.0
0.1	1.9	9.0
1.0	16.1	50.0
2.0	27.9	66.9
5.0	50.0	83.9
8.0	62.2	89.6
50.0	95.0	99.0

Modified from Roulston JE, Leonard RCF. *Serological tumour markers*. Edinburgh: Churchill Livingstone; 1993. Used with permission.

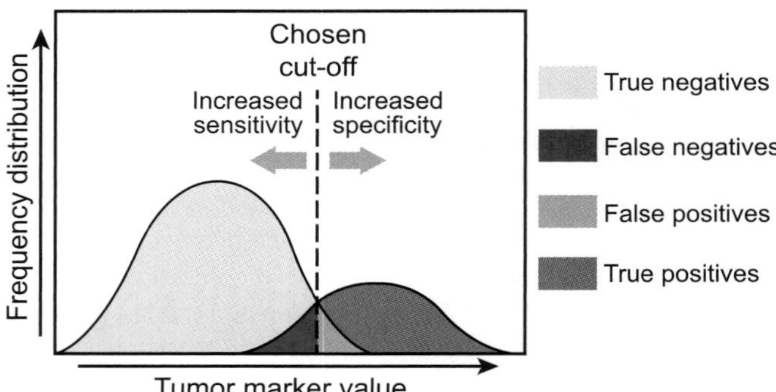

FIGURE 31.2 The effect of tumor marker cutoff concentration on sensitivity and specificity (proportion of true negatives) and sensitivity (proportion of true positives) in diseased and disease-free populations.

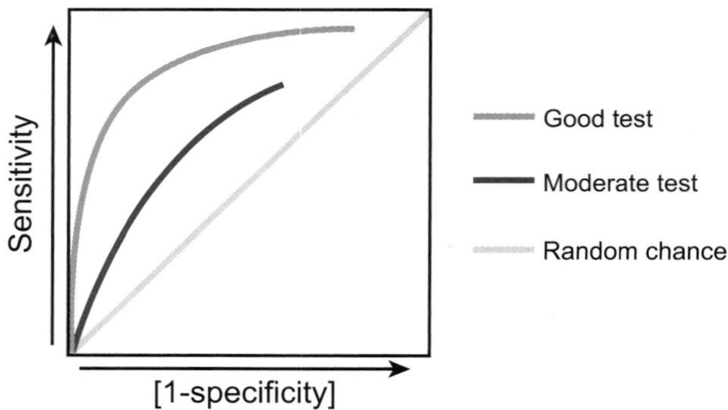

FIGURE 31.3 Receiver operating characteristic (ROC) plot from which assay performance is assessed by plotting sensitivity as a function of (1 − specificity). A highly discriminatory test will give a curve of steep slope from the origin, while a random test will give a straight line as indicated. (Modified from Roulston JE, Leonard RCF. *Serological tumour markers*. Edinburgh: Churchill Livingstone; 1993.)

screening program for choriocarcinoma in high-risk women and by proposed screening programs for prostate cancer.[40] High sensitivity and high specificity of the test for the target disease are essential. Also fundamental to the success of the choriocarcinoma screening program is the high prevalence of the condition (estimated as 3% to 10%) in the high-risk population being screened, yielding a positive predictive value of approximately 92%. The important effect of prevalence of disease on positive predictive value is further illustrated in Table 31.11.

The relevant test parameters described in Table 31.8 are depicted schematically in Fig. 31.2. Diagnostic accuracy is established by studying test performance at different decision (cutoff) concentrations in appropriately selected diseased and disease-free populations. The relationship between these parameters is most conveniently depicted graphically by a receiver operating characteristic (ROC) plot (Fig. 31.3). Changing the decision concentration selected alters both sensitivity and specificity but cannot improve both concurrently. These parameters define the characteristics of the test and, together with the prevalence of the disease in the population studied, yield the positive predictive values (Box 31.1). The low prevalence of the majority of cancers, even in age groups most at risk, together with the low sensitivity and specificity of most tumor markers, generally precludes their use in screening. However, successful population screening for early colorectal cancer using a fecal immunochemical test for hemoglobin (FIT) is routine in some countries.[20] The efficacy of screening patients at high risk of hepatocellular carcinoma (HCC) and ovarian cancer is being actively investigated, and there is continuing debate about whether to screen for prostate cancer. The possibility of implementing genetic screening for some conditions is also being considered. These issues are

BOX 31.1 Example Calculation Showing the Effect of Prevalence on Positive Predictive Value for Choriocarcinoma Detection With a Previous Molar Pregnancy

Assuming a Disease Prevalence of 8%

Of 1000* women screened:

Number with disease = 80 (0.08 × 1000), so with a specificity of 99%, **79.2** (80 × 0.99) cases correctly identified (true positives)

Number without disease = 920 (0.92 × 1000), so with a sensitivity of 99%, **9.2** [920 × (1.0 – 0.99)] negative cases are incorrectly identified as having the disease (false positives)

The positive predictive value (probability) of obtaining a positive result in a patient with choriocarcinoma is therefore [79.2/(79.2 + 9.2)] × 100 = **89.6** (An excellent test)

Assuming a Disease Prevalence of 1%

Of 1000* women screened:

Number with disease = 10 (0.01 × 1000), so with a specificity of 99%, **9.9** (10 × 0.99) cases correctly identified (true positives)

Number without disease = 990 (0.99 × 1000), so with a sensitivity of 99%, **9.9** [990 × (1.0 – 0.99)] negative cases are incorrectly identified as having the disease (false positives)

The positive predictive value (probability) of obtaining a positive result in a patient with choriocarcinoma is therefore [9.9/(9.9 + 9.9)] × 100 = **50.0** (Still a good test but not as good as the case when the prevalence is higher)

*In 1000 women, assuming test specificity and sensitivity are both 99%.

Modified from Roulston JE, Leonard RCF. *Serological tumour markers*. Edinburgh: Churchill Livingstone; 1993. Used with permission.

considered in more detail in the organ-specific sections in this chapter.

Diagnosis of Cancer

The same limitations of lack of sensitivity and specificity that apply to the use of tumor markers for screening also apply to diagnosis and case finding (see Table 31.3). Tumor markers are not helpful for diagnosis in patients with nonspecific symptoms and cannot replace a biopsy for establishing the primary diagnosis of cancer.[41] However, in carefully selected undiagnosed patients who are at high risk of malignancy, raised concentrations of tumor markers may be informative and facilitate diagnosis (eg, when the patient is unable or unwilling to undergo more invasive testing such as colonoscopy).[41] In general, the higher the serum tumor marker value, the greater the likelihood of malignancy, but conversely it is essential to remember that results within the reference interval never necessarily exclude malignancy. The NACB recommends that requests for panels of tumor marker measurements be actively discouraged, together with inappropriate requests for PSA in women or CA125 in men, because these are unlikely to lead to improved patient outcomes.[15]

Assessing Prognosis

Prognostic markers predict the likely outcome of disease with respect to risk of relapse or disease progression (see Table 31.3). They are generally most useful at the time of initial diagnosis, when a marker of good prognosis is suggestive of prolonged survival and/or the possibility of cure. A marker of poor prognosis indicates an increased probability of early recurrence. Prognostic markers can help identify patients with aggressive tumors that require further treatment (eg, with systemic adjuvant chemotherapy following surgery) while minimizing the risk of overtreatment of patients with indolent disease that is unlikely to progress. It is important to note that prognostic markers provide a probability estimate of outcome for a heterogeneous population of patients and that no prognostic marker can accurately predict outcome for an individual patient.[5]

Although many tumor markers have been reported to have prognostic significance, with more than 20,000 references relating to cancer prognostic markers in PubMed, fewer than 10 are regularly used in clinical practice.[5] Possible reasons for this include inadequate study design, use of inappropriate statistical tests and overoptimistic reporting, failure of a marker to provide independent prognostic information adding to that from established prognostic factors (eg, tumor size, grade, and lymph node involvement), and inadequate validation. Most prognostic markers are measured in tissue, but as indicated in Table 31.3, measurement of AFP, hCG, and LDH following primary surgery in patients with nonseminomatous germ cell tumors is essential. These markers provide strong independent prognostic information complementing that of conventional prognostic factors and have been well validated. Additionally, although prognostic markers may be of limited use unless there is a therapy that can change the course of the disease, some patients and caregivers may find prognostic information helpful.

Prediction of Treatment Response

The heterogeneous nature of cancer means that even cancers of the same histological type may vary widely in response to a particular treatment, and for most cancers only a subset of patients will respond (see Table 31.3).[5] Predictive markers that can identify those who will respond are therefore critical in treatment planning so that treatment can be offered to patients who will benefit and so alternative treatment can be offered to those who will not, also sparing them unnecessary side effects. With the development and use of new and costly molecularly targeted treatments, predictive markers (most of which are measured in tissue rather than serum) are increasingly both a clinical and an economic necessity.[5] Several important predictive markers for breast cancer are already well established in clinical use. Further promising predictive markers are now available for breast cancer, colorectal cancer, glioma, melanoma, and non–small cell lung cancer, while others are being investigated. (See the sections on specific cancers.)

Monitoring Response During and/or Shortly After Treatment

While the use of predictive tumor markers is increasingly important, the main application of most serum tumor markers is in monitoring the course of disease. For most diagnosed cancer patients, it is helpful to measure the relevant tumor marker pretreatment in order to provide a baseline for subsequent interpretation, and for some cancers, measurements made during and immediately after treatment are also desirable. In general, a decrease in marker concentrations to within expected population (ie, "normal") limits following treatment is a favorable sign. In some cases subnormal or absent posttreatment values should be achieved (eg, for PSA postprostatectomy or thyroglobulin following thyroid ablation). Measurement of AFP and hCG is mandatory for germ cell tumors prior to surgical excision because the pretreatment concentration is required to calculate the half-life of tumor marker decline following chemotherapy. Similarly, in ovarian cancer, measurement of CA125 and the extent of its decline during primary treatment may provide helpful prognostic information. (See the sections on specific cancers.)

Monitoring Disease Posttreatment to Detect Progression or Recurrence

Serial monitoring of tumor marker concentrations posttreatment provides early indication of disease recurrence, often months before there are clinical signs and symptoms. Whether early detection is of benefit depends crucially on whether a rising tumor marker concentration will prompt clinical action (eg, early ultrasound, CT or MRI scanning), whether an alternative treatment is available for the individual patient, and/or whether that treatment can be implemented without scan evidence of progression if none is available. If none of these apply and if the patient is not enrolled in a clinical trial, the patient should be made aware of the potential implications of having the test done, and whether tumor marker monitoring is likely to be of benefit should be seriously considered and discussed.[41,42]

QUALITY REQUIREMENTS FOR TUMOR MARKER USE IN THE CLINIC

While tumor marker results provide objective information that can facilitate clinical management, their appropriate selection and measurement are essential. The clinical laboratory should provide readily available information to those requesting tumor markers to encourage selection of the correct test or tests (and, more important, to discourage inappropriate requesting) and to ensure that specimen timing is appropriate and other preanalytical requirements are met. Ensuring that results are analytically correct and that accurate and informative reports are returned to the requesting clinician are also laboratory responsibilities.[15,43] Laboratory-oriented guidelines for tumor markers that outline quality requirements for provision of a high-quality tumor marker service have been developed by the NACB[15] and the European Group on Tumor Markers and form the basis of the following discussion.

Pre-Preanalytical Requirements

Although numerous serum tumor markers can be measured (see Tables 31.5 and 31.6), only those listed in Table 31.5 are commonly requested from the clinical laboratory. Table 31.12 summarizes the current recommendations of the NACB for their appropriate clinical use,[21,22] while typical clinical presentations that might prompt a request are described in Table 31.13.

Requests for tumor markers received in the clinical laboratory fall into three main categories: those for diagnosed cancer patients who have already been referred to specialist centers and are being or have been treated, those for patients who have been referred to a hospital for investigation of suspected malignancy and further investigation, and those requested by a family doctor or other primary care health professionals for patients who have presented with symptoms that could raise the suspicion of malignancy.[44] Requests in the first category are likely to be made to monitor response to treatment (with a baseline measurement prior to therapy always desirable) or to detect recurrence and are most likely to be appropriate.

Nonspecialist users, whether in primary or secondary care, should always consider carefully whether a tumor marker result is likely to be helpful before the request is made. Requestors should be aware of the lack of sensitivity of most tumor markers, particularly for early-stage disease, their lack of specificity for a particular cancer, and the numerous non-malignant conditions in which they may be increased (see Table 31.13). Nonspecialist users should also be aware that increased tumor marker concentrations do not necessarily indicate malignancy. Attempting to identify the reason for an increased tumor marker that should not have been requested and that is not associated with malignancy can be an expensive and time-consuming process, as well as psychologically stressful for the patient. Conversely, nonspecialist users should be reminded that whatever the malignancy or tumor marker, a result within the reference interval never necessarily excludes malignancy or progressive disease.[41] Clinical biochemists should also think carefully before requesting additional tests that might lead to a diagnosis of malignancy and should seek the agreement of the clinician caring for the patient before doing so.

Unfocused requests such as "tumor marker screen" or "malignancy?" from emergency departments and other receiving units should be actively discouraged and met with offers of educational support. Reviewing requests prior to analysis is no longer feasible in most laboratories, but it can be helpful to provide readily available advice about appropriate test selection at the time of the request, together with reminders of their low sensitivity and specificity. This should be reasonably readily implemented when electronic requesting is available. Through the Pathology Harmony initiative in the United Kingdom, general advice that can be readily disseminated to nonspecialist users has been prepared.[45,46]

Preanalytical Requirements

Specimen Timing

Timing of specimens within the day for tumor marker measurement is not usually critical because there is little evidence of diurnal variation for most markers. A pretreatment specimen is always helpful when interpreting subsequent results. Specimens should be taken before some procedures that may transiently release tumor markers into the circulation (eg, CA125 following abdominal surgery, CEA following colonoscopy, and PSA after prostatic biopsy or digital rectal examination). Awareness of benign conditions that may cause transient increases in tumor marker concentrations (Table 31.14) and avoidance of inappropriate timing, if possible (eg, measurement of CA125 in a woman who is menstruating, PSA in a man with an active urinary tract

TABLE 31.12 Most Frequently Requested Serum Tumor Markers and National Academy of Clinical Biochemistry (NACB) Recommendations for Their Appropriate Clinical Use.[21,22]

		CURRENTLY RECOMMENDED CLINICAL APPLICATIONS				
	Relevant Cancer	Screening or Early Detection	Diagnosis or Case Finding	Prognosis (With Other Factors)	Detecting Recurrence	Monitoring Therapy
Alpha-fetoprotein (AFP)	Germ cell/testicular tumor		√	√	√	√
	Hepatocellular carcinoma	√*	√†	√	√	√‡
Calcitonin	Medullary thyroid carcinoma		√		√	√
Cancer antigen 125 (CA125)	Ovarian cancer	√§	√‖	√	√	√¶
Cancer antigen 15-3 (CA15-3)	Breast cancer				√#	√**
Cancer antigen 19-9 (CA 19-9)	Pancreatic cancer		√††	√	√	√‡‡
Carcinoembryonic antigen (CEA)	Colorectal cancer			√	√‡	√‡
Human chorionic gonadotropin (hCG)	Germ cell and testicular cancers; gestational trophoblastic neoplasia§§		√	√	√	√
Paraproteins (M protein/Bence Jones protein) (also measured in urine)[275]	Multiple myeloma		√		√	√
Prostate-specific antigen (PSA)	Prostate cancer		√	√	√	√
Thyroglobulin	Thyroid cancer (follicular or papillary)				√	√

*Only for subjects in high-risk groups (eg, with chronic HBV, HCV, or cirrhosis) and only in conjunction with ultrasound (impact on mortality unclear).
†In conjunction with liver imaging, AFP levels greater than 200 μg/L are regarded as virtually diagnostic of HCC in patients with hypervascular lesions.
‡Especially for disease that cannot be evaluated by other modalities.
§Only for women at high risk of ovarian cancer and only in conjunction with transvaginal ultrasound.
‖Only for differential diagnosis of pelvic masses, especially in postmenopausal women.
¶Preliminary results of a randomized trial show no survival benefit from early treatment based on a raised serum CA125 level alone,[276] so this recommendation may be modified to exclude asymptomatic patients.
#Postsurgery when it may provide lead time for early detection of metastasis but clinical value unclear.
**Especially in patients with nonevaluable disease (for which CEA is also recommended) in carefully selected patients.
††In patients where pancreatic disease is strongly suspected, CA19-9 may complement other diagnostic procedures.
‡‡Especially after chemotherapy and in combination with imaging.
§§Use of hCG in screening for gestational trophoblastic neoplasia, a rare malignancy that usually develops after a molar pregnancy, provides an excellent example of "best practice" in screening.
Modified from Sturgeon CM, Lai LC, Duffy MJ. *Serum tumour markers: how to order and interpret them. BMJ* 2009;339:b3527. Used with permission. Further information is available from the Trophoblastic Tumour Screening and Treatment Centre, Department of Medical Oncology, Charing Cross Hospital, London W6 8RF, UK (Tel: +44 (0) 20 8846 1409) or at http://www.hmole-chorio.org.uk/.

infection, or CA19-9 in a subject with cholestasis), reduce the risk of misinterpreting spuriously raised results that may cause undue distress to the patient and also decrease confidence in laboratory testing.

Specimen Handling

Serum or plasma is usually (but not always) equally appropriate for tumor marker measurements, although gel tubes may not be suitable for some assays. Requirements should always be checked in the product information supplied with the reagents and/or from other sources. Tumor markers are generally stable, but serum or plasma should be separated from the clot and stored at 4°C (short-term) or below −30°C as soon as possible, following relevant guidelines where available. For longer-term storage, specimens should be stored at −70°C. Heat treatment (eg, to deplete serum complement components or to inactivate human immunodeficiency virus [HIV]) should be avoided, particularly for hCG (which may dissociate at increased temperature to form its free α- and β-subunits) and PSA. Potential influence of transit time on analyte results should be considered when samples are exposed to increased temperatures. Standardized conditions of specimen collection and fixation are crucial for immunohistochemical analyses.[47]

Analytical Requirements

Assay Validation

Prior to their introduction into routine clinical practice, both immunoassays and immunohistochemical methods must be validated as described above by defined and well-characterized protocols that meet regulatory guidelines (eg, FDA approval in the United States and CE marking in Europe). Individual laboratories should verify analytical performance prior to introduction into routine use.[48]

TABLE 31.13 **Clinical Presentations That Might Prompt Requests for the Most Frequently Used Tumor Markers**

Tumor Marker*	Relevant Cancer	Typical Clinical Presentation	Other Cancers in Which the Marker May Be Raised†
Alpha-fetoprotein (AFP)	Germ cell/ testicular tumor	Diffuse testicular swelling; hardness	Gastric, colorectal, biliary, pancreatic, lung
	Hepatocellular carcinoma	Ascites, encephalopathy, jaundice; upper abdominal pain; weight loss; early satiety in high-risk subjects (ie, hepatitis B or C–related cirrhosis)	As above
Cancer antigen 125 (CA125)	Ovarian cancer	Pelvic mass; persistent, continuous, or worsening unexplained abdominal or urinary symptoms; bloating	Breast, endometrial, cervix, peritoneal, uterus, lung, pancreas, hepatocellular, non-Hodgkin lymphoma
Cancer antigen 19-9 (CA19-9)	Pancreatic cancer	Progressive obstructive jaundice with profound weight loss and/or pain in the abdomen or midback	Colorectal, gastric, hepatocellular, esophageal, ovary
Carcinoembryonic antigen (CEA)	Colorectal cancer	Intermittent abdominal pain, nausea, vomiting, or bleeding; palpable abdominal mass	Breast, gastric, lung, mesothelioma, esophageal, pancreatic
Human chorionic gonadotropin (hCG)	Germ cell/ testicular tumor	Diffuse testicular swelling, hardness, and pain	Lung cancer
	Gestational trophoblastic neoplasia	Symptoms leading to x-ray showing cannonball secondaries; previous history of hydatidiform mole (see also Table 31.10)	Lung cancer
Paraproteins (M protein/Bence Jones protein) (also measured in urine)[275]	Multiple myeloma	Combination of symptoms including some/all of the following: anemia; back pain; weakness or fatigue; osteopenia; osteolytic lesions; raised ESR or globulins; spontaneous fractures; recurrent infections	
Prostate-specific antigen (PSA)	Prostate cancer	Frequency, urgency, nocturia, dysuria; acute retention; back pain, weight loss, anemia	None

*Tumor markers are often not helpful in diagnosis.

†This list is not comprehensive. The marker may be raised in other cancers.

Modified from Sturgeon CM, Lai LC, Duffy MJ. Serum tumour markers: how to order and interpret them. *BMJ* 2009;339:b3527. Used with permission.

Internationally recognized guidelines for the performance of immunohistochemical tests should be adopted where these are available. If appropriate high-quality reference materials are not available, it is essential that methods for immunohistochemistry are described in detail.

Internal Quality Control

As for any laboratory tests, robust procedures for internal quality control (IQC) should be established. Within-run variability less than 5% and between-run variability less than 10% should be readily achievable for automated tumor marker methods. Some newer techniques may perform significantly better than this, although manual and/or research assays may be less precise.[49] Appropriate action should be taken immediately if an assay run fails to meet objective criteria for assay acceptance so no potentially erroneous results are reported. Criteria for acceptance should be predefined and preferably based on logical criteria such as those of Westgard.[50] The number of IQC specimens included per run should allow identification of an unacceptable run with a given probability appropriate to the clinical application.[51] Given the long-term monitoring involved in cancer care, assay stability should be ensured over prolonged periods.

Quality control (QC) material not provided by the method manufacturer is preferable because kit controls may provide an overly optimistic impression of performance.[49,52] At least one authentic serum matrix control from an independent source should be included in addition to any QC materials provided by the method manufacturer. Negative and low positive controls should be included for all tumor markers and should include concentrations close to important decision points (eg, 0.1 and 3 or 4 μg/L for PSA; 4–7 μg/L for AFP; 5 U/L for hCG).[49] The broad concentration range should be covered, and ideally a high concentration control should occasionally be included to check the accuracy of dilution, whether manual or onboard.

Proficiency Testing/External Quality Assessment

Proficiency testing (PT) specimens should ideally be prepared from authentic patient sera, which for tumor markers may require dilution of high-concentration patient sera into a normal serum base pool.[53,54] As for IQC, specimens prepared by spiking purified analyte into serum base pools is likely to provide an overly optimistic impression of between-method performance.[52] PT specimens should be commutable with patient specimens to ensure valid between-method

TABLE 31.14 Nonmalignant Conditions That Can Increase Serum Tumor Marker Concentration, Which May Lead to Incorrect Interpretation

Clinical Condition	Tumor Markers*
Acute cholangitis	CA19-9
Acute hepatitis	CA125, CA15-3
Acute and/or chronic pancreatitis	CA125, CA19-9
Acute urinary retention	CA125, PSA
Arthritis/osteoarthritis/rheumatoid arthritis	CA125
Benign prostatic hyperplasia (BPH)	PSA
Cholestasis	CA19-9
Chronic liver diseases (eg, cirrhosis, chronic active hepatitis)	CEA, CA125, CA15-3, CA19-9
Chronic renal failure	CA125, CA15-3, CEA, hCG
Colitis	CA125, CA15-3, CEA
Congestive heart failure	CA125
Cystic fibrosis	CA125
Dermatological conditions	CA15-3
Diabetes	CA125, CA19-9
Diverticulitis	CA125, CEA
Endometriosis	CA125
Heart failure	CA125
Irritable bowel syndrome	CA125, CA19-9, CEA
Jaundice	CEA, CA19-9
Leiomyoma	CA125
Liver regeneration	AFP
Menopause	HCG
Menstruation	CA125
Mesothelioma	CEA
Nonmalignant ascites	CA125
Ovarian hyperstimulation	CA125
Pancreatitis	CA125, CA19-9
Pericarditis	CA125
Peritoneal inflammation	CA125
Pregnancy	AFP, CA125, hCG
Prostatitis	PSA
Recurrent ischemic strokes in patients with metastatic cancer	CA125
Respiratory diseases (eg, pleural inflammation, pneumonia)	CA125, CEA
Sarcoidosis	CA125
Systemic lupus erythematosus	CA125
Urinary tract infection	PSA

*This list is not comprehensive; these markers may be raised in other nonmalignant conditions.

comparisons.[55,56] Concentrations should assess performance over the working range and should include assessment of linearity on dilution, baseline security, and stability of results over time.[53]

It is the responsibility of the PT provider to ensure that specimens are stable in transit. The target values (usually consensus means for heterogeneous analytes such as the tumor markers) should be accurate and stable as demonstrated by assessment of their accuracy (eg, recovery of known amounts of added analyte), stability (ie, reproducibility on repeat distribution of the same pool), and linearity on dilution (ie, by issuing different dilutions of the same patient specimen).[53] Because tumor markers are often monitored over long periods, regular assessment of reproducibility and stability of results over time is highly desirable. Reproducibility of results at low concentration is particularly important for AFP and hCG in germ cell tumors and PSA in patients following prostatectomy because treatment may be instituted solely on the basis of a small increase in tumor marker concentration.

Occasional specimens should ideally be distributed to assess whether interference is observed in different methods (eg, from heterophilic and other antibodies, high-dose hooking). Evaluation of interpretation and technical results is required for PT of immunohistochemical tests and can also be provided for quantitative tests through interpretative exercises and surveys of practice. These can make a powerful contribution to national audit by highlighting differences in reference intervals, reporting practice, and interpretation of clinical results, particularly when the ethos of the PT scheme is educational rather than regulatory.

Standardization

Major international efforts continue to be directed toward encouraging manufacturers to calibrate their methods accurately in terms of the established relevant International Standard (IS) or Reference Reagents (Table 31.15). While availability of such standards does not guarantee improvement in between-method agreement, a reference material (provided its commutability can be demonstrated) provides a benchmark against which the accuracy of calibration can be assessed.[57] Following adoption of the first IS for PSA by most providers of PSA assays, the mean between-laboratory CVs observed in the UK National External Quality Assessment Service (UK NEQAS) PT scheme for PSA decreased by approximately twofold, from more than 20% in 1995 to approximately 9.5% in 2005.[58] Encouraging use of equimolar methods for PSA (ie, PSA methods that recognize free and complexed PSA equally well) contributed to this improvement.

Improved understanding of what is being measured in an assay for a heterogeneous tumor marker is critical if improved comparability is to be achieved, as illustrated by the number of hCG-related molecules in Table 31.15. Some further progress has been made by organizing collaborative workshops to identify the more clinically appropriate antibody specificities,[59,60] and discussions are in progress about how to improve between-method comparability for the complex CA tumor markers for which no ISs have been established (see Table 31.15). It is helpful if manufacturers provide clear information about the specificity of the antibodies used in their methods and data on cross-reactivity that is readily comparable with that of other methods so users are aware of the differences.

Despite these efforts to improve comparability, the molecular heterogeneity of most tumor markers means that results obtained using different methods are not interchangeable, and considerable care is required in the interpretation of serial results obtained in more than one method.

Clinically Relevant Interferences

Tumor marker measurements are subject to the same interferences as all immunoassays[61] (see Chapter 23), but clinical

TABLE 31.15 WHO International Standards and Reference Reagents for Major Tumor Markers

Tumor Marker	Code	Year Established	Description	Reference
AFP	IS 72/225	1972	Crude cord serum (50%)	277
CA125	—	—	No IS established	—
CA15-3	—	—	No IS established	—
CA19-9	—	—	No IS established	—
CA72-4	—	—	No IS established	—
CEA	IRP 73/601	1973	CEA purified from liver metastases to primary colorectal cancer	278
hCG	IS 07/364	2009	hCG, highly purified from human urine	279
hCGα	IRP 75/569	1975	α-subunit of hCG from human urine	280
hCGβ	IRP 75/551	1975	β-subunit of hCG from human urine	280
hCG	IRR 99/688	2001	hCG, free from nicked forms and free subunits, highly purified from human urine	281
hCGn	IRR 99/642	2001	Nicked hCG, partially degraded, missing peptide bonds in the hCGβ-40-50 region, highly purified from human urine	281
hCGα	IRR 99/720	2001	α-subunit of hCG, dissociated from hCG	281
hCGβ	IRR 99/650	2001	Highly purified dissociated urinary hCGβ, free from intact dimeric hCG, hCGα, and hCGβn	281
hCGβn	IRR 99/692	2001	Partially degraded nicked hCGβ, missing peptide bonds in the hCGβ-40-50 region	281
hCGβcf	IRR 99/708	2001	Residues hCGβn-6-40, joined by disulphide bonds to hCGβn-55-92	281
PSA	IRR 96/670	2000	90:10 ratio of bound:free PSA	282
fPSA	IRR 96/668	2000	Purified free PSA	282

International Standards and Reference Reagents are available from the National Institute for Biological Standards and Control, Potters Bar, Herts, UK. Available at *http://www.nibsc.ac.uk/catalog/standards/preps/sub_endo.html.*
hCG, Human chorionic gonadotropin; *hCGα,* hCG β-subunit; *hCGβ,* hCG β-subunit; *hCGn,* nicked hCG; *hCGβn,* nicked hCG β-subunit; *hCGβcf,* hCG β-core fragment; *IRP,* International Reference Preparation; *IRR,* International Reference Reagent; *IS,* International Standard; *PSA,* prostate-specific antigen; *fPSA,* free prostate-specific antigen.

biochemists need to be aware of several that are of particular relevance.[62]

High-Dose "Hooking." Because tumor marker concentrations can range over several orders of magnitude, protocols enabling identification of high-dose "hooking" are essential to minimize the risk of reporting erroneously low results, particularly in patients for whom markers are being measured for the first time. An example is shown in Fig. 31.4. The risk of "hooking" can be reduced by using solid-phase antibodies of higher binding capacity, by using sequential assays that include a wash step, and by assaying specimens at two dilutions. Methods vary in their vulnerability to this interference.

Specimen Carryover. Specimen carryover is possible whenever high-concentration specimens are assayed, so it is desirable to check periodically for this possibility. Tumor markers such as hCG can range over five orders of magnitude, so carryover of 1/10,000 can still lead to a false-positive result in the following sample.

Interference From Heterophilic or Human Antimouse Antibodies. Some patient sera contain antiimmunoglobulin antibodies (most often IgG) that may react with some antibodies used as reagents in immunoassays. High concentrations of human antimouse antibodies (HAMAs) may also be present in serum from cancer patients who have received treatment with mouse monoclonal antibodies for imaging or therapeutic purposes. If either type is present, results may be falsely high or low. Identifying the presence of interfering antibodies requires a high degree of clinical suspicion that a tumor marker result is not correct, which may be aided by having relevant clinical details available. Once suspected, possible interference can be investigated by assaying the specimen at several dilutions, by reassaying after treatment with a commercially available blocking agent, by adding further nonimmune mouse serum to the reaction mixture and reassaying, and/or by reassaying the specimen using a different method provided by a different manufacturer (using different

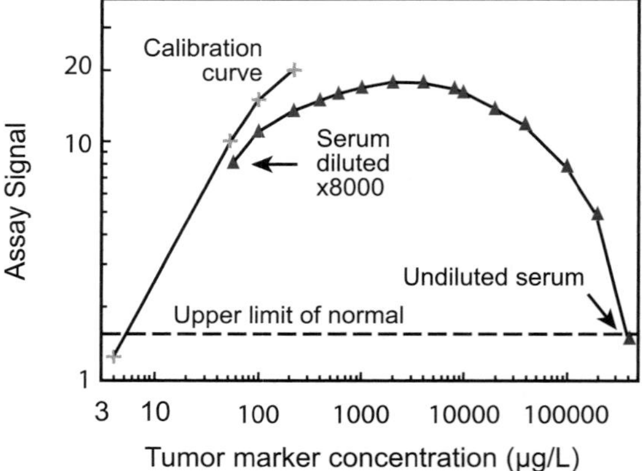

FIGURE 31.4 High-dose hooking in tumor marker immunoassays. The extremely high tumor marker concentration blocks antibody binding sites in the immunoassay such that the apparent result "hooks" back onto the calibration curve and an erroneously low result may be reported.

antibodies) and preferably using a different methodology (eg, radioimmunoassay).[61] Caution should be applied in interpretation. For example, linear dilution does not always exclude the presence of HAMA, while nonlinear dilutions may be more informative.

Postanalytical Requirements

Brief clinical information about the source of the suspected or diagnosed malignancy and the treatment stage (eg, preoperative, postoperative, prechemotherapy) is highly desirable. This information should be recorded both in the laboratory computer and on the laboratory report, which should include cumulative and, if possible, graphical reporting of serial results because trends in tumor marker results are generally more informative than single results. Such reporting facilitates interpretation of results and can also help to identify occasional errors in requesting or in the laboratory (eg, incorrect sample identification or missampling on an analyzer). Cumulative or graphic display of results also highlights unexpected results (eg, sudden changes that are out-of-accord with the clinical picture) that require confirmation and further investigation. Brief comments relating to interpretation of the analytical results (eg, whether or not an increase is likely to be clinically significant) and helpful advice about the frequency of monitoring and the need for confirmatory specimens are also desirable.

Urgent results that may be required for immediate patient management should be identified by the reporting biochemist so as to ensure that they reach the relevant clinician promptly (eg, by telephone if appropriate). These include tumor marker results that can be used to diagnose advanced disease in critically ill but treatable patients (eg, AFP in hepatoblastoma, hCG in choriocarcinoma, AFP and hCG in nonseminomatous germ cell tumors, and PSA in men with advanced prostate cancer that may respond to endocrine therapy). The consequences of failure to report such results by telephone can be severe.[62,63]

In view of the method-related differences discussed above, the method used should be stated on the clinical report so any changes in method are readily identifiable. If there has been a method change, it is highly desirable that the laboratory indicates whether this is likely to influence interpretation of the trend in results. There should be a defined protocol if methods are changed, and the likely effect should be communicated to clinical users prior to the change. Managing the change may necessitate analyzing the previous specimen by the new method or by requesting a further specimen to re-establish the baseline and/or confirm the trend in marker concentrations. If the results are likely to be significantly affected by the change in method, as should be clear from the initial validation, it may be desirable to run old and new methods in parallel for a defined changeover period, an approach that also helps clinicians become accustomed to the new values.

Reference intervals should be derived using an appropriate healthy population and should be specific to the method used (see Chapter 8). They are usually most relevant for cancer patients pretreatment. Subsequently, the patient's individual "baseline" results provide the most important reference point for most marker results, and application of reference intervals derived in healthy populations can be misleading. For example, at least six weeks postprostatectomy, a confirmed PSA concentration of 2.0 μg/L suggests persistent or progressive disease, although this concentration is well within reference intervals for healthy individuals. Provided "baseline" marker concentrations are well established in diagnosed patients posttreatment, sustained increases even within the reference interval or other decision limits may be significant and should be treated as possible relapse, provided the measurement procedure is the same.[64]

Reporting critical increases in tumor marker concentrations, taking into account the analytical performance of the test, biological variation (where possible), and the individual reference intervals, helps to contribute to an earlier diagnosis of relapse. The percentage increase or decrease that constitutes a significant change should be defined and should take account of analytical and biological variation,[65,66] as well as the expected rate of change in benign and malignant conditions and the time between samples. For tumor markers, differences in the magnitudes of their biological variation contribute significantly to these percentages.[67-69] A confirmed increase or decrease of ±25% is frequently considered to be of clinical significance,[67] but more work is required in this area.[68]

Laboratories should be able to provide calculated tumor marker half-lives or doubling times for markers for which these are relevant (eg, AFP and hCG). Half-lives are defined as the time to 50% reduction of circulating tumor marker concentration following complete removal of tumor tissue. Their calculation may be irrelevant if a 50% reduction does not represent a significant change. (See the section on germ cell tumors for calculation details.)

Proactive provision of a high-quality tumor marker service helps to encourage good communication between laboratory and clinical staff and is likely to encourage appropriate use of tumor marker tests as well as early identification of any results that are not in accord with the clinical picture and require investigation. An example of a laboratory report that fulfills many of these requirements is shown in Fig. 31.5.

Use of Tumor Markers in Specific Malignancies

International and national guidelines on the clinical management of most cancers are regularly updated (see Table 31.4). Modified versions of these guidelines are also frequently adopted and adapted for regional or local use and are similarly readily accessible. Increasing numbers of patients are enrolled in clinical trials with well-defined protocols that may include tumor marker measurements, sometimes as surrogate endpoint indicators.

The optimal use of serum tumor markers for assessing prognosis, monitoring therapy, and detecting recurrence has been studied in greatest detail for choriocarcinoma and germ cell tumors, relatively rare diseases for which tumor marker measurement is mandatory. Serum tumor marker measurements also contribute significantly to the management of more common cancers (eg, colorectal, ovarian, and prostate) and are less widely used for others (eg, bladder, breast, and lung). In contrast, measurement of several tissue tumor markers is mandatory for management of breast cancer and is becoming increasingly important in other cancers (eg, lung and melanoma). The extent to which tumor markers currently contribute to the management of a number of important malignancies is briefly reviewed in the following sections.

ST ELSEWHERE HOSPITAL

PATIENT:	Test patient	PATIENT:	123456789Z
DOB:	01/02/03	CONSULTANT/GP:	Dr John Smith
WARD/PRACTICE:	Medical centre 1	HOSPITAL:	

← Standard patient demographics including patient number

ADDITIONAL DETAILS:

← Space for recording relevant information

← Possibility of graphical reporting - log scale or not

← Relevant clinical decision limit

LAB/SPECIMEN/METHOD	DATE	TUMOUR MARKER (<4.0 units)	CLINICAL DETAIL
Lab A 244374 Method 1	03.03.1999		Post-surgery
Lab A 578221 "	04.05.2000	2.5 units	
Lab B 613365 Method 2	15.06.2000		For change of treatment?
Continued...			

← Cumulated results across hospitals and including method and clinical details

COMMENTS:

Confirms recent increase. [Reprt copied to Urology and Oncology, as requested.]

← Comments - selected from presented choices depending on marker, concentration and age of patient

FIGURE 31.5 Desirable clinical laboratory report for tumor markers that fulfills current reporting recommendations. (Modified from Sturgeon CM, Lai LC, Duffy MJ. Serum tumour markers: how to order and interpret them. *BMJ* 2009;339:b3527. Used with permission.)

POINTS TO REMEMBER

Cancer and Tumor Markers

- Cancer is a heterogeneous disease that is a leading cause of death, although death rates for individual cancers vary markedly, and considerable advances in treatment have been made over recent decades.
- Tumor markers are surrogate indicators that can help make or confirm a cancer diagnosis, monitor treatment effectiveness and the course of disease, estimate prognosis, and/or predict whether a specific therapy is likely to be effective.
- Optimal use of tumor markers requires an evidence-based approach to clinical decision making and knowledge of the limitations of these tests particularly in relation to clinical sensitivity and specificity.
- Tumor marker results are rarely diagnostic and cannot replace biopsy for the primary diagnosis of cancer.
- Tumor marker measurements are not recommended for patients with vague symptoms when the population likelihood of cancer is low.
- A raised tumor marker result never necessarily indicates malignancy, and, conversely, a result within the reference interval never necessarily excludes malignancy.
- In diagnosed patients a pretreatment result is essential and provides the baseline against which subsequent results can be assessed.
- Tumor marker results should always be confirmed on a repeat specimen if decisions about therapy depend on the result.
- Tumor marker results should always be interpreted in the context of all available information and the possible influence of other factors (eg, medication, analytical effects) should be carefully considered.

Bladder Cancer

Approximately 600,000 Americans are currently affected by bladder cancer, with 74,000 new cases diagnosed each year.[70] The most common symptom of bladder cancer is intermittent hematuria, which is present in 80% to 85% of patients. Presenting symptoms may also include voiding problems or dysuria. Transitional cell carcinomas account for the majority of bladder cancers, but adenocarcinomas, squamous cell carcinomas, and sarcomas also occur. Diagnosis is usually established by cystoscopic evaluation. Cytology of cells shed into the urine is very effective in identifying high-grade bladder cancers but misses many papillary urothelial neoplasms of low malignant potential. The majority of bladder cancer patients are diagnosed with nonmuscle invasive tumors. Primary treatment is complete surgical resection, usually by transurethral resection with or without intravesical treatments with bacille Calmette-Guèrin immunotherapy or intravesical chemotherapy.[22,71] Radiotherapy may also be required. Even when resection is considered to be complete, there is a high risk of recurrence, and 50% to 70% of patients will develop tumor recurrence within 5 years, depending on the stage of disease. Lifelong surveillance is therefore required.

Tumor Markers Relevant to Bladder Cancer. Markers evaluated for bladder cancer include nuclear matrix proteins (NMPs), human complement factor H-related protein, fibronectin, telomerase, cytokeratins, and survivin. NMPs make up the internal structure of the nucleus and contribute to the regulation of some of the key functions that occur in the nucleus, including DNA replication and RNA synthesis. Some studies suggest that NMPs released by cancer cells may differ from those in normal cells and that different types of cells may have different NMPs.[72]

The FDA has approved an ELISA for the measurement of nuclear mitotic apparatus protein, a component of the nuclear matrix that is overexpressed in bladder cancer. Approved uses of the NMP-22™ test are as an aid in the diagnosis of symptomatic patients or those with risk factors suggesting transitional cell carcinoma (TCC) and in the management and monitoring of patients with TCC. A qualitative point-of-care version of the test is available as an aid in monitoring patients with a history of bladder cancer.

The bladder tumor–associated antigens (BTA), human complement factor H-related protein, and related proteins are involved in the regulation of the alternative pathway of complement activation that prevents complement-mediated damage to healthy cells.[73] It has been suggested that BTA may allow tumor cells to evade the host immune system by preventing tumor cell lysis by immune cells. The BTA-Trak and BTA-Stat tests have been approved by the FDA for use as an aid in conjunction with cystoscopy in the management of bladder cancer patients.

None of the currently available urine tumor markers for bladder cancer are sensitive enough to eliminate the need for cystoscopy, and cytology remains integral to the detection of occult bladder cancer. However, results of an evaluation in which sensitivity and specificity ranges were compared for seven commercially available tumor marker assays suggest that because these tests have relatively high sensitivities, their measurement could be used to extend the period between cystoscopies during surveillance of patients with TCC.[74] This is broadly in accord with the conclusions of an International Consensus Panel on bladder tumor markers that found the most practical use of noninvasive tests is to monitor bladder cancer recurrence, thereby reducing the number of surveillance cystoscopies performed each year.[75] The Panel also concluded that markers may be useful in the screening of high-risk individuals for early detection of bladder cancer but that more prospective studies would be needed to strengthen this argument. Current National Comprehensive Cancer Network (NCCN) recommendations are that use of urinary tumor markers for bladder cancer is optional.[71] Tumor marker use should be reserved for follow-up of patients who have received adjuvant treatment for cancers staged as cTa (high grade; confined to the mucosa) or cT1 (low and high grade; superficially invading the *lamina propria*).[71]

Breast Cancer

Breast cancer is the most common cancer in women worldwide, affecting 10% to 12% of women. In symptomatic women, the main presenting features include a lump in the breast, nipple change, or discharge and skin contour changes. More than 1.2 million new cases are detected each year, with approximately 500,000 deaths.[76] Worldwide the incidence appears to be increasing, but in some Western countries, mortality rates are declining. This decrease has been attributed to earlier detection by systematic screening with mammography, greater awareness among women of early signs of breast cancer, and the availability of adjuvant treatment for newly diagnosed cases. In the United States, where breast cancer represents 14% of all new cancer cases, it is estimated that there will be about 231,840 new cases of breast cancer in 2015 and 40,290 deaths from the disease,[77] with nearly 3 million women living with the disease in the United States. While 5-year relative survival rates increased from 75.2% in 1975 to 89.7% in 2003, survival rates have not changed significantly since then.[77] For the approximately 60% of breast cancer patients in the United States who have localized disease at diagnosis (ie, confined to the primary site), the 5-year survival rate is 98.6%, compared with 25.9% for the 6% of patients who have distant metastases at diagnosis.

Primary treatment for localized breast cancer is either breast-conserving surgery and radiation or mastectomy.[1,78] Following primary treatment, most women with invasive breast cancer receive systemic adjuvant therapy such as chemotherapy, hormone therapy, or immunotherapy, or a combination of these. Depending on estrogen receptor status and other factors, not all patients with breast cancer require adjuvant treatment.

Tumor Markers Used in the Management of Breast Cancer. Tissue tumor marker measurements that are essential for the management of breast cancer include those for receptors for estrogen, progesterone, and *HER2* (see Table 31.7). CA15-3 and the closely related BR27.29 (see Table 31.6) are the serum markers of choice for breast cancer. Measurement of CEA (see Table 31.5) may also be helpful in patients with metastatic breast cancer. In early-stage disease, concentrations of CA15-3 may be similar to those found in healthy women or women with benign breast disease.

Screening and Diagnosis. Early detection undoubtedly improves 5-year survival, but the low specificity and sensitivity of currently available serum tumor markers, especially in early-stage disease, precludes their use in screening for breast cancer. In practice, x-ray imaging with mammography is the only screening modality. Whether the benefits of such screening outweigh the harms associated with overdiagnosis and exposure to radiation is subject to continuing debate.[79] Results of clinical trials conducted over long periods of time may be influenced by confounding factors not originally accounted for during trial design—for example, introduction of more effective therapies.

An independent review commissioned by Cancer Research UK and the English Department of Health concluded in 2013 that the UK breast screening programs confer significant benefit and should continue.[80] Review of older randomized controlled trials and more recent observational studies suggested a 20% reduction in mortality in women invited to screening. This corresponded to one breast cancer death avoided for every 235 women invited to screening, and one death avoided for every 180 women who attend screening.[80] In contrast, authors of a Cochrane review evaluated results of seven trials involving 600,000 women in the age range 39 to 74 years who were randomly assigned to receive screening mammograms or not.[81] The studies with the most reliable information showed that screening did not reduce breast cancer mortality. Assuming screening reduces breast cancer mortality by 15% after 13 years of follow-up, and overdiagnosis and overtreatment is at 30%, the authors concluded that for every 2000 women invited for screening over 10 years, one will avoid dying of breast cancer, 10 healthy women who would not have been diagnosed without screening will be treated unnecessarily, and more than 200 women will experience significant ongoing psychological distress because of false-positive findings.[81] In a complementary study, Surveillance, Epidemiology and End Results (SEER) data were used to examine trends in breast cancer incidence from 1976 through 2008.[82] The authors estimated that in 2008, breast cancer was overdiagnosed in more than 70,000 women in the United States (31% of all breast cancers diagnosed that year) and that despite the substantial increase in early breast cancers detected, screening is having at best only a small effect on the rate of death from breast cancer. The authors cautioned that the question "Should I be screened for breast cancer?" is not answered by their study, but clearly there is a need to inform women considering screening of the advantages and disadvantages. The Cochrane review includes an evidence-based leaflet for laypeople.[81]

Women who are at increased risk of breast cancer because of a strong family history of breast cancer (eg, relatives diagnosed at a young age) or because they are carriers of the *BRCA1*, *BRCA2*, or *TP53* genetic mutations are likely to benefit from additional screening with magnetic resonance imaging (MRI). This is the current policy in the United Kingdom.[83]

Definitive diagnosis of breast cancer requires biopsy and histology. Serum tumor markers do not contribute to this, but preoperative measurements of CA15-3 and/or CEA are desirable if either marker is going to be used for posttreatment monitoring. A high CA15-3 concentration (eg, >40–50 kU/L) in a patient with apparently localized breast cancer should prompt further investigation to exclude the possibility of metastatic disease.[76]

Prognosis. Accurate assessment of prognosis is essential for optimal management of breast cancer patients to avoid undertreatment of patients with advanced disease and overtreatment of patients with indolent disease. The extracellular serine protease urokinase plasminogen activator (uPA) and its endogenous inhibitor plasminogen activator inhibitor 1 (PAI-1) are the best-validated tissue prognostic markers for breast cancer.[5,84] Both uPA and PAI-1 promote tumor progression and metastasis at concentrations found in tumor tissue. Several retrospective and prospective studies have shown that increased concentrations of the two markers are statistically independent and potent predictors of poor patient outcome, including in the subset of patients with lymph node–negative disease.[84] The latter has been confirmed in two independent studies, one a randomized prospective clinical trial in which tumor marker evaluation was the primary purpose of the trial and the other a pooled analysis of data from retrospective and prospective trials.[84] Measurement of uPA and PAI-1 by ELISA requires a relatively large amount of fresh or freshly frozen tissue. Because tissue is usually formalin-fixed and their measurement is therefore precluded in small tumors, they are not widely used in clinical practice. Their use may be encouraged in the following situations:

- when measured by immunohistochemistry on formalin-fixed paraffin-embedded tissue, as is now feasible,[85] results are found to predict patient outcome as accurately as those obtained by ELISA
- if they can be reliably measured in core needle biopsies, as has also been reported[85]

Multigene Profiling in Prognosis. Several gene expression profiles or multigene panels have been proposed for determining prognosis in breast cancer patients. The Oncotype DX test, originally developed for lymph node–negative ER–positive patients receiving adjuvant tamoxifen, measures the expression of 16 cancer-associated and 5 control genes in breast tumor tissue at the RNA level.[86] A recurrence score (RS) between 0 and 100, calculated from the expression levels of these genes, predicts the risk of distant disease recurrence at 10 years. Newly diagnosed patients with invasive breast cancer can then be divided into those at low (RS <18), medium (RS 18–31), or high (RS >31) risk of recurrence.[86] The prognostic impact of the Oncotype DX test is independent of standard factors, including patient age, lymph node status, tumor grade, and tumor size, and it has been shown to be prognostic in additional patient groups (eg, ER-positive patients receiving treatment with aromatase inhibitors).[87] Performance of Oncotype DX is recommended by several expert groups, especially for predicting risk of disease recurrence in ER-positive lymph node–negative patients receiving tamoxifen and for identifying the patients in this group who might benefit from adjuvant chemotherapy.[21,78,88,89]

Other gene profiles are available, including the MammaPrint test that measures the expression of 70 genes involved in signal transduction pathways responsible for breast cancer metastasis.[90] MammaPrint is approved by the FDA to assist in the assignment of women with ER-positive or ER-negative breast cancer into high- or low-risk groups for recurrence. Prospective randomized clinical trials are currently addressing the use of Oncotype DX and MammaPrint as predictive and/or prognostic tools in populations of women with early-stage lymph node–negative breast cancer.[78]

A validated serum tumor marker that provided prognostic information independent of the standard prognostic factors mentioned above would clearly also be desirable. A number of studies have shown that high preoperative serum concentrations of CA15-3 predict shortened disease-free or overall survival in breast cancer patients.[76] Although heterogeneous in design, almost all studies demonstrated that CA15-3 provided additional independent prognostic information in total patient populations as well as in subgroups of patients with lymph node–positive or –negative disease and those with ER-positive or -negative disease. This may be because the marker is detecting micrometastases or occult disease that is not clinically evident.[76] Only the European Group on Tumor Markers currently recommends measurement of CA15-3 for determining prognosis in patients with early breast cancer.[91] Because CA15-3 measurement is relatively convenient and inexpensive, it may be appropriate to use it when planning optimal treatment of newly diagnosed patients with breast cancer[76] but further evaluation is required.

Therapy Prediction. Measurement of ER, the longest-established molecular marker for breast cancer, is mandatory in all newly diagnosed invasive breast cancer patients to determine whether antiestrogen endocrine therapy is likely to be effective.[92] Patients with ER-positive tumors tend to respond to hormonal therapy, while those with ER-negative tumors will be treated using other therapies (eg, chemotherapy). Aromatase inhibitors (eg, anastrozole, letrozole, and exemestane), which inhibit estrogen synthesis, have largely replaced selective estrogen receptor modulators (eg, tamoxifen) for first-line endocrine therapy in postmenopausal women.[93] The negative predictive value of ER is high; that is, patients who are ER-negative are very unlikely to benefit from endocrine therapy.[94] However, in both early and advanced breast cancer, the positive predictive value is less accurate. Only about 50% of ER-positive patients with advanced breast cancer show objective response following treatment with hormone therapy, and almost all eventually develop recurrence. The risk of recurrence in ER-positive patients with early breast cancer who receive adjuvant hormone therapy is significantly reduced, but approximately 30% will have relapsed after 15 years.

Highlighting the importance of ER measurement in breast cancer patients, authors of a recent study of the effects of screening and systemic adjuvant therapy on ER-specific breast cancer mortality in the United States concluded that for ER-positive breast cancers, adjuvant endocrine therapy made a higher relative contribution to breast cancer mortality reduction than screening.[95] For ER-negative cases the relative contributions were similar for screening and adjuvant treatment.

Patients with breast cancers that overexpress the *HER2* gene are candidates for treatment with the humanized monoclonal antibody trastuzumab (Herceptin) and other anti-*HER2* therapies (eg, lapatinib) developed subsequently.[93] Because amplification of the *HER2* gene occurs in only 20% of patients with invasive breast cancers, it is important to identify these to avoid use of the therapies in patients unlikely to respond. Lapatinib, a low molecular weight compound that blocks tyrosine kinase activity of both *HER2* and epidermal growth factor receptor (EGFR), can be given orally and has less toxicity than trastuzumab. A number of anti-*HER2* therapies have now been cleared by the FDA for clinical use.

Detailed recommendations and good practice guidelines for measurement of ER and progesterone receptors (PR),[92] *HER2*,[96] and EGFR[97] have been published by the American Society for Clinical Oncology (ASCO) and the College of American Pathologists (CAP) and endorsed by the NCCN.[78]

Monitoring. Most women who have been treated for breast cancer, with or without adjuvant therapy and/or curative surgery, are subsequently evaluated at regular intervals with history, physical examination, and annual mammography. The aim of follow-up is to identify early recurrence or metastatic disease on the assumption that early intervention will improve survival.[98] If serum tumor markers are measured, CA15-3, CEA, and/or BR27.29 are the markers of choice, and the quality requirements described above must be met.

The clinical value of serial measurements of CA15-3 and other tumor markers is unclear, although they are used for postoperative monitoring in some countries. Such regular determination can provide a lead time of 5 to 6 months, but it is still unclear whether early intervention based on tumor marker increase alone results in improved outcome or better quality of life.[76] Only the European Group on Tumor Markers currently recommends routine tumor marker measurement in postoperative surveillance of women with breast cancer.[89] The NACB states that tumor markers can be measured in certain situations (eg, in monitoring therapy in patients with advanced disease where other methods of evaluation are not possible), but their routine measurement is not currently recommended by the European Society for Medical Oncology (ESMO) or the NCCN.[21,76] However, the NCCN includes rising tumor markers (CA15-3, CEA, and BR27.29) in its definition of disease progression and states that marker increases raise the suspicion of tumor progression, while cautioning that such increases may be seen in responding disease.[78] ASCO states that CEA, CA15-3, and the closely related CA27-29 may be used as adjunctive assessments, but not alone, to contribute to decisions regarding therapy in women with metastatic breast cancer.[99]

The evidence on which the above recommendations are based is primarily from two prospective randomized trials in the early 1990s, both of which concluded that intensive follow-up programs did not improve patient outcome.[76] Since then, however, a number of more effective and less toxic therapies have become available, and supportive care therapies have also improved. Despite the challenges involved in designing and performing the necessary trials to demonstrate effectiveness of intensive follow-up,[98,100] the Southwest Oncology Group, in collaboration with members of the National Cancer Institute's Clinical Trials Network, is undertaking such a prospective clinical trial. The aim of the trial is to evaluate the impact of serial testing of tumor markers in patients with stage II and III breast cancer to determine whether early initiation of therapy at the time of tumor marker–detected relapse can result in an improvement in overall survival.[98] As well as evaluating the impact of serial tumor marker measurements on outcome, the results of such trials may provide important information about late effects of cancer diagnosis and treatment, including long-term physical and emotional consequences and the impact on quality of life.[101]

Cervical Cancer

Cervical cancer is the fourth most common cancer in women worldwide and a leading cause of cancer death in women in the developing world, where 85% of cases occur. In the United States 12,360 new cases were diagnosed in 2014, and 4020 patients died of the disease. The most important factor in the development of cervical cancer and other anogenital cancers (eg, vaginal, vulvar, anal, penile, and oropharyngeal) is persistent infection with human papilloma viruses (HPV), the most frequent sexually transmitted viruses. Primary prevention is therefore feasible with prophylactic vaccination.[102,103]

There are more than 130 strains of HPV, 40 of which affect the anogenital area and at least 15 of which are oncogenic. These high-risk viruses are associated with cervical intraepithelial neoplasia (CIN), squamous cell carcinoma, and adenocarcinoma of the cervix, with strains 16 and 18 accounting for 70% of cervical cancers. While 90% of genital HPV infections clear within 2 years, persistence of strains 16 and 18 is more common than for other strains. Persistence is also longer in immunosuppressed women (eg, women with HIV) who are at higher risk of developing precancerous lesions and invasive cervical cancer, as are women who have had an organ transplant or who have inflammatory bowel disease.

Most women are asymptomatic and are frequently diagnosed only after abnormal cervical cytology is identified in a screening program using cervical cytology.[104,105] Introduction of widespread screening in the United States has decreased the incidence of cervical cancer from 14.8 per 100,000 women in 1975 to 6.6 per 100,000 in 2008, with a similar reduction in mortality.[104,105] HPV screening or testing is not presently used in routine practice, but the potential benefits of including HPV screening or testing in existing screening programs have been described, and it is being gradually introduced in a number of countries.[105] Following successful trials, HPV testing is incorporated into the UK NHS Cervical Screening Programme.[106] If a sample taken during the cervical screening test shows low-grade or borderline cell abnormalities, the sample is automatically tested for HPV. Women with higher-grade abnormalities are referred immediately for colposcopy. Other countries, including Australia,[107] are considering similar introduction of HPV screening.

Nonspecific symptoms that may be associated with cervical cancer include intermenstrual, postcoital, or postmenopausal bleeding, blood-stained vaginal discharge, and pelvic pain or dyspareunia. Treatment planning of patients with cervical cancer is primarily determined by the clinical stage of the disease and histological type (squamous cell carcinoma, approximately 85%; adenocarcinoma, approximately 10% to 15%; and adenosquamous carcinoma, approximately 3%). Early-stage disease can be treated by radical hysterectomy and pelvic lymphadenectomy or radiotherapy. For more advanced disease, chemoradiation or neoadjuvant chemotherapy may also be required.

Tumor Markers Used in the Management of Cervical Cancer. Squamous cell carcinoma antigen (SCCA) is the serum tumor marker of choice for squamous cell cervical carcinoma, while CEA and CA125 may have possible utility in patients with cervical adenocarcinoma.[22] Serum SCCA concentrations correlate with tumor stage, tumor size, residual tumor posttreatment, recurrent or progressive disease, and survival in patients with squamous cell cervical carcinoma. They may be used to individualize treatment planning, particularly for patients with low-stage squamous cell cervical cancer, and an increased pretreatment concentration has been found to be an independent risk factor for poor survival in several studies. However, whether serum SCCA measurements are useful in clinical practice remains uncertain. There is no evidence that earlier detection of recurrent disease through tumor marker monitoring influences treatment outcome or prognosis after treatment.[108] Consequently, no currently available serum tumor markers are recommended for routine clinical use in patients with cervical cancer.

Colorectal Cancer

Colorectal cancer is the second leading cause of cancer-related death both worldwide[109] and in the United States, where it is also the fourth most frequently diagnosed cancer.[110] Typical symptoms at presentation include altered bowel habit, weight loss, anemia, and fecal occult blood. The natural history of the disease is reasonably well understood, involving a slow multistage process from mucosal cell hyperplasia to adenoma formation, growth, and dysplasia, followed by malignant transformation and invasive cancer. Approximately 70% of newly diagnosed colorectal cancer patients already have lymph node involvement (Union for International Cancer Control [UICC] Stage III or IV) and consequently poor prognosis.[109] In the United States, 5-year survival is approximately 90% for locally confined tumors, approximately 70% for those that have spread regionally, but only approximately 10% if distant metastases are present,[111] emphasizing the importance of detecting early-stage disease.

Tumor Markers Used in the Management of Colorectal Cancer. Carcinoembryonic antigen (CEA), an oncofetal antigen first identified as being associated with colorectal cancer in the 1960s, remains the most relevant serum tumor marker for colorectal cancer. However, in recent years, a variety of other markers have become increasingly important in the diagnosis and management of colorectal cancer, as described below.

Screening for Colorectal Cancer Using Tumor Markers. Several randomized controlled trials have shown that population-based screening using fecal occult blood testing (FOBT) can reduce mortality from colorectal neoplasia, with an average reduction in mortality of at least 16%.[112] Based on this evidence, a number of countries have introduced screening for colorectal cancer, replacing the early guaiac-based tests (which detect the pseudo-peroxidase activity of hemoglobin) with newer fecal immunochemical tests (FIT) (which detect the globin component of hemoglobin).[20] Because both types of test lack specificity for colorectal cancer, follow-up colonoscopy is required for positive tests.

Typically patients can collect fecal samples at home and mail the sample to a central testing laboratory for either test, but FITs have a number of advantages over guaiac tests. FITs are easier to use and can be automated, they can provide quantitative rather than qualitative results with adjustable cutoff points, they are less vulnerable to interference (eg, due to diet or drugs), they have greater analytical specificity and better clinical sensitivity for cancers and advanced adenomas, and they are cost-effective.[20,112,113] Ease of use is particularly important because the success of any screening program depends on its acceptability to the population being screened and consequently its uptake. For colorectal cancer screening programs, uptake is significantly lower than the 75% desirable goal set by the American Cancer Society for similar adult preventive programs.[114,115]

Analysis of genetic and/or epigenetic markers in fecal material forms the basis of an automated DNA screening test for colorectal cancer that has been approved by the FDA.[116] Tumor-specific DNA changes in aberrant methylated BMP3 and NDRG4, a mutant form of KRAS, beta-actin, and hemoglobin are detected. The sensitivity of the test was superior to FIT for detection of both colorectal cancer and advanced precancerous lesions, but FIT was more specific, resulting in fewer false-positive results. Further refinement of DNA tests is likely, with blood-based measurements an attractive possibility for future population screening.

Individuals with a family history of colorectal cancer (eg, a first-degree relative diagnosed before the age of 45 years), nonpolyposis colon cancer (hereditary nonpolyposis colorectal cancer [HNPC] or Lynch syndrome), or familial adenomatous polyposis (FAP) are at high risk of developing colorectal cancer and should be referred for risk assessment and endoscopic screening according to agreed protocols.[117-119] Mismatch repair (MMR) gene mutations associated with these conditions (eg, *MLH1, MSH2, PMS2,* and *MSH6*) may result in microsatellite instability (MSI) and predispose carriers to colorectal, endometrial, stomach, and small bowel cancers. Determination of MSI or MMR mutation or hypermethylation is therefore recommended as a prescreen for Lynch syndrome in patients with colorectal cancer and may also provide helpful prognostic information in all colorectal cancer patients as discussed below.[119] Genetic counseling and germline gene testing for Lynch syndrome should be offered to patients in whom MSI is present or in whom MMR function loss is detected. Those patients with MSI-high tumors that are negative for *MLH1* mutation should be considered for *BRAF* mutation and/or *MLH* promoter methylation testing.

Diagnosis. CEA is the serum tumor marker of choice for colorectal cancer, but its low clinical sensitivity, particularly for early-stage disease, precludes its use in diagnosis. Depending on the cutoff point chosen, serum CEA will be increased in only 30% to 50% of patients at the time of diagnosis, and it cannot be used in isolation to diagnose even advanced disease. Because it can also be increased in nonmalignant liver and renal disease, as well as in other malignancies (see Tables 31.13 and 31.14), the specificity of CEA is low for patients with primary localized colorectal cancer. However, clearly increased concentrations can assist in diagnosis in certain clinical circumstances. Markedly increased concentrations are suggestive of metastatic disease (generally to the liver) but do not necessarily indicate a colorectal primary source.

Prognosis, Staging, and Therapy Prediction. A number of studies have shown that increased preoperative CEA concentrations at the time of initial presentation of patients with colorectal cancer are associated with adverse outcome.[120] Several of these studies showed CEA to be an independent prognostic marker in the total cohort studied, as well as in patients with Stage II and/or III disease, and that CEA predicted outcome in Stage II disease. It is therefore generally recommended that CEA be measured preoperatively in newly diagnosed colorectal cancer patients to provide both prognostic information and a baseline value for interpreting subsequent concentrations.[120,121] Studies comparing the prognostic value of CEA with newer prognostic markers such as MSI status and gene expression profiling (eg, for MMR mutations) would also be desirable because CEA measurement is likely to be considerably simpler and less expensive than measurement of tissue-based molecular markers. Inclusion of CEA for risk stratification in clinical trials evaluating new adjuvant systemic treatments for patients with colorectal cancer would be desirable to establish whether CEA can be used to select patients who would benefit from such therapy.[120]

Several studies have shown that MSI and/or MMR status may have prognostic value in colorectal cancer patients, with the presence of MSI or defective MMR activity (dMMR) associated with a favorable outcome.[122,123] The European Group on Tumor Markers states that these measurements should be made in patients with Stage II colon cancer who are being considered for adjuvant 5-fluorouracil-based therapy because patients with MSI/dMMR may not require such therapy.[120] Inclusion of CEA for risk stratification in clinical trials evaluating new adjuvant systemic treatments for patients with colorectal cancer would be desirable to establish whether CEA can be used to select patients who would benefit from such therapy.[120]

Patients with advanced colorectal cancer may be treated with antiepidermal growth factor (EGFR) monoclonal antibodies such as cetuximab and panitumumab, which bind to the extracellular domain of EGFR. Early clinical trials suggested response rates in unselected patients of only 10% to 15% with antibody treatment, whether alone or with chemotherapy. However, retrospective analysis of data from randomized controlled trials has shown that patients with specific mutations, usually in codons 12 of the *K-RAS* gene, almost never benefit from such treatment, but 15% to 20% of patients with wild-type *K-RAS* show an objective response with antibody alone, and 35% to 40% do so when treated with cetuximab and irinotecan.[120] Illustrating the complexity of genetic testing, there is some evidence that patients with a specific mutation at codon 13 of the *K-RAS* gene do benefit from antibody treatment. While requiring further investigation, modeling studies suggest that administering anti-EGFR antibody treatment only to patients with wild-type *K-RAS* would result in significant net cost savings.[124]

Monitoring. Metaanalyses of a number of randomized controlled trials designed to compare intensive follow-up with either control or minimal follow-up of patients with colorectal cancer who have undergone curative resection have demonstrated that intensive follow-up improves overall survival.[125] Two of these metaanalyses concluded that overall survival was significantly improved only when CEA testing was included in the intensive follow-up arm.[126,127] It is now generally agreed that CEA testing should be performed every 3 to 6 months for 5 years following curative surgery for colorectal cancer.[120,125,128] CEA results within the reference interval do not exclude recurrence.

An increase in CEA should prompt referral for early investigation of possible recurrence, but prior to undertaking further investigations, any increase should be confirmed by a second sample taken within approximately 1 month. Rechecking CEA and considering more frequent testing in patients at high risk of recurrence may be desirable.[128] This should not be regarded as overuse but as follow-up of abnormal results. What constitutes a significant increase in CEA is not yet well established. The European Group on Tumor Markers regards a significant increase as being an elevation at least 30% over that of the previous concentration.[120] Smaller consecutive increases (eg, 15% to 20%) observed on at least three successive occasions with minimal intervals of 2 weeks between them may also prompt intervention. In a randomized, controlled multicenter prospective study in 11 Dutch hospitals, an intensified follow-up schedule was introduced. This consisted of CEA measurements every 2 months during the first 3 years postsurgery, with imaging undertaken in patients with two CEA rises.[129] An increase of 20% compared with the previous CEA (provided CEA was >2.5 μg/L) was considered to be significant. The intensified protocol based on CEA rise detects recurrences earlier than standard protocols, resulting in an increase in the curable recurrence rate, but whether it will result in higher disease-specific and overall survival, be cost-effective, and maintain acceptable quality of life has yet to be established.[129]

Resection of metastatic deposits in the liver is an option that can prolong survival for a small but increasing number of patients with Dukes Stage B or C disease, provided they are detected early, before symptoms develop. It is therefore recommended that CEA be measured every 3 months for at least 3 years following surgery in patients with Dukes Stage B or C disease who would be candidates for liver resection. Measurement of CEA following liver resection provides a helpful indication of its success.

Measurement of CEA is also recommended during chemotherapy for metastatic disease, although care in interpretation is required because CEA concentrations may be affected by factors other than tumor progression (eg, liver damage). Confirmed increases during treatment can inform decisions to change treatment or withdraw ineffective treatment. CEA-defined responses agree well with radiologic responses (the "gold standard") in over 90% of cases, enabling the conclusion that use of CEA is as accurate as CT imaging for assessing the response of colorectal cancer liver metastases to chemotherapy.[130]

As discussed previously, monitoring of colorectal cancer outside a clinical trial should only be undertaken if it is likely to benefit the patient. CEA concentrations in individual patients should be monitored using the same methods because the results obtained in two methods may not be the same. If a change of method is unavoidable, rebaselining may be necessary as described above. Coordination of follow-up monitoring should ideally be supported by an automatic computer system such as that developed for CEA monitoring by surgeons in the Netherlands.[131]

Gastric Cancer

Gastric cancer is relatively rare, although it is the second most common gastrointestinal cancer worldwide. Approximately 25,000 new cases are diagnosed in the United States each year, more than 60% of which will have already spread to regional lymph nodes or metastasized.[132] Survival is closely related to stage at diagnosis, with 5-year survival approximately 65% for localized disease and less than 5% for patients with distant metastases.

Tumor Markers Used in the Management of Gastric Cancer. Although CEA and CA19-9 are increased in 20% to 50% of patients with advanced disease and AFP in 20% to 25%, these markers are increased in fewer than 20% of patients with early-stage disease and consequently cannot be used for screening or diagnosis of gastric cancer. Measurement of serum CEA or CA19-9 may provide early indication of recurrence in a proportion of patients, but their use is not recommended because there is currently no evidence that this improves clinical outcome.

This may change with the availability of more effective systemic treatment as 10% to 25% of patients overexpress *HER2*. Because patients with advanced *HER2*-positive gastric tumors benefit from treatment with the anti-*HER2* antibody,[133] if such patients are being considered for systemic therapy,[120,134] *HER2* measurement should be performed and scored using immunohistochemistry and/or fluorescent in situ hybridization (FISH) as per recent recommendations.[135] Multiple biopsies may be necessary to minimize the risk of inappropriate interpretation due to the heterogeneity of expression of *HER2* in gastric cancer.[136,137]

Gastrointestinal Stromal Tumors

Gastrointestinal stromal tumors (GISTs) present predominantly in middle-aged and older individuals and, although rare, are the most common mesenchymal tumors of the gastrointestinal tract, occurring in the stomach, small bowel, large bowel, esophagus, and omentum. Increased awareness of this tumor type since the 1990s has led to appropriate pathological diagnoses, with incidence estimated as between 0.68 to 1.5 per 100,000 population in several Western countries.[138]

Tumor Markers Used in the Management of GIST. Molecularly, over 95% of GISTs are characterized by the presence of KIT protein (also known as CD117 antigen), whose measurement in serum is recommended by a number of expert groups.[120] Mutations in the *KIT* gene occur in approximately 80% to 85% of all cases, while mutations in the homologous *PDGFRA* gene are found in 5% to 10% of GIST patients. While not a replacement for histopathology in the diagnosis of GISTs, immunostaining for KIT protein is recommended as a diagnostic aid, with the provisos that it may also be present in some nonabdominal tumors and its absence does not necessarily exclude GIST.[120,139]

The outcome for patients with GISTs has been dramatically improved in recent years with the use of imatinib and sunitinib, tyrosine kinase inhibitors that block KIT and PDGFRA as well as BCR-ABL. Response to these drugs depends on the mutational status of the *KIT* gene with patients, so *KIT* and *PDGFRA* mutational analysis is also recommended prior to prescribing imatinib to patients with GISTs.[120]

Germ Cell Tumors

Although representing only 1% of all male tumors, germ cell tumors (GCTs) are the solid tumor most frequently diagnosed in men between the ages of 20 and 34 years and account for about 95% of malignant tumors arising in the testes.[140] They also occur elsewhere, particularly along the "midline," ie, from the coccyx to the perineal gland, including the mediastinum and the retroperitoneum. The incidence of GCTs has increased over the last few decades, with 8430 new cases predicted in the United States in 2015.[141] Risk factors include positive family history, cryptorchidism, testicular dysgenesis, Klinefelter syndrome, and a prior history of GCT.

Although GCTs are usually aggressive, they respond well to treatment with surgery and, where appropriate, adjuvant chemotherapy and/or radiotherapy. Anticipated 5-year survival rates are now 98% in the United States, although 5-year survival rates in patients presenting with advanced disease are 50% to 60%. Delay in diagnosis results in higher stage at presentation. There are well-established national and international guidelines relating to the management of patients with GCTs. The established standard therapy must be closely followed at all stages of management to maximize the chance of cure.[140] Treatment in specialist centers is advantageous, and all patients should be discussed at multidisciplinary team meetings at which a clinical biochemist is present.

Tumor Markers Used in the Management of Germ Cell Tumors. Measurements of hCG, AFP, and LDH are integral to the management of patients with GCTs. Tumor marker results should be reviewed together with histological immunostaining and radiological results and any inconsistencies noted when treatment decisions are considered.

Screening. The low prevalence of GCTs in the general population, together with the relatively low sensitivity and specificity of AFP, hCG, and LDH, preclude the use of tumor markers in screening.

Diagnosis. Although rare, the possibility of a GCT should be considered in any patient with a poorly defined epithelial malignancy, especially young individuals with midline masses. Plasma concentrations of AFP and hCG should be measured in any male with a suspicious lump in the testes and in any patient with malignancy of unknown origin. Hyperthyroidism may be a presenting feature if the hCG concentration is very high because hCG shares structural similarities with TSH. If patients with clinical findings consistent with GCTs (eg, testicular lump, lung metastases, abdominal mass) have markedly increased serum concentrations of AFP and/or hCG, they should be urgently discussed with physicians responsible for managing GCTs at the regional cancer center. Referral for immediate chemotherapy may be appropriate before later surgery to remove residual tumor.

Measurement of serum tumor markers is essential for the differential diagnosis of GCTs because treatment differs according to whether the GCT is seminomatous, nonseminomatous (NSGCT) (with yolk sac elements), or a combined tumor with both seminomatous and nonseminomatous elements. Serum or plasma concentrations of AFP and/or hCG are increased in 80% to 85% of men with NSGCT, while less than 25% of those with seminomas have raised hCG and none have raised AFP. Nonseminomas are more clinically aggressive, so tumors with both elements are managed as for nonseminomas. Increased AFP precludes a diagnosis of seminoma. Marker measurements can sometimes modify histopathological diagnoses. Increased AFP in a patient diagnosed with seminoma suggests that the AFP may not be related to the tumor (eg, may be of liver origin) or that yolk sac elements were overlooked.

Measurement of hCG and AFP is essential before surgery for a suspected GCT in order to allow the rate of fall of the markers to be monitored posttreatment. Some patients with pure seminoma histologically may have mildly increased preoperative AFP concentrations of 6 to 36 μg/L (5–30 kU/L) that remain stable postsurgery. Such AFP concentrations may be considered to be "normal" for that patient and unrelated to the tumor provided they are unchanged before and after orchiectomy and remain stable when rechecked 4 weeks after surgery.

As for all tumor markers, it is important to remember that concentrations within the reference interval do not necessarily exclude malignancy. Only a small proportion of seminomas or dysgerminomas (the female equivalent of seminomas) produce hCG, and up to 25% of NSGCT do not produce AFP or hCG.

A significant proportion of hCG secreted by seminomas may be present as the free beta-subunit of hCG (hCGβ), so, as for other oncology applications, an hCG method that recognizes both intact hCG and the free subunit is required. hCG increases have to be interpreted with caution because hypogonadism and marijuana use may cause benign serum increases. Some immunoassay methods for hCG may be vulnerable to interference from heterophilic antibodies, and high-dose "hooking" is always a possibility (see the earlier section on interferences). Both AFP and hCG can be increased in nonmalignant diseases and other malignancies, and both are significantly raised in pregnancy.

Prognosis. The lowest tumor marker concentration reached postsurgery, the primary tumor site, and the sites of metastatic disease all contribute to the prognostic classification of GCTs. The criteria developed by the International Germ Cell Cancer Collaborative Group (IGCCCG)[283] are shown in Table 31.16. Treatment depends on whether the tumor is classified as having good, intermediate, or poor prognosis. It is important to note that the tumor marker concentrations in Table 31.16 are following primary surgery. Whether measurements made before primary surgery are prognostic is debatable because some patients with large primary tumors may have very high AFP and hCG concentrations that return to normal following surgery.

Monitoring. Tumor markers should be measured before and after surgical excision of GCTs because calculation of the tumor marker half-life provides helpful information about the success of treatment. Provided that disease is confined to the testis or ovary, serum AFP and/or hCG should decline to normal with apparent half-lives of 5 to 6 days for AFP and 1 to 2 days for hCG. Fig. 31.6 shows the decrease in AFP observed in a patient with widespread metastatic disease who had a complete radiological and marker response to chemotherapy. The equation used to calculate the apparent half-life ($t_{1/2}$) of the tumor marker is

$$t_{1/2} = \frac{-0.3t}{\log_{10}\dfrac{[M]_T}{[M]_{TO}}}$$

where $[M]_T$ and $[M]_{T0}$ are tumor marker concentrations at time T and T_0, respectively, and t is the difference in days between T and T_0. Further treatment with chemotherapy or radiation is required if AFP or hCG remain increased following surgery or if imaging identifies residual or metastatic disease.

Long-Term Surveillance. Following treatment, tumor markers should be measured regularly following defined clinical protocols. Time intervals will depend on both prognostic category and treatment. Clearly any significant increases in tumor markers must be reported immediately to the relevant clinical team. The importance of careful monitoring of tumor markers is illustrated in Fig. 31.7. After an initially very good response to a number of different chemotherapy regimes, the patient required surgery, further chemotherapy, and ultimately a successful bone marrow transplant.

Seminoma patients who remain well for 5 years after treatment and who are at low risk of recurrence can be discharged from follow-up, as can NSGCT patients who have remained well for 10 years. Because there is increasing evidence that chemotherapy with platinum-based drugs can increase the risk of cardiovascular events, separate long-term monitoring for this may be desirable.

Gestational Trophoblastic Disease

Gestational trophoblastic disease (GTD) forms a group of rare and previously fatal diseases of pregnancy.[142] Now highly curable, they develop in the trophoblast cells that surround the embryo immediately after conception. They may occur following a molar pregnancy, a nonmolar pregnancy, or a live birth. The possibility of GTD should be considered in any

TABLE 31.16 Metastatic Germ Cell Tumor Classifications

	Primary and Metastatic Features		Tumor Marker Concentrations	5-Year Progression-Free Survival	5-Year Survival
Prognostic Categories for Nonseminomas					
Good prognosis nonseminomas (56% of nonseminomas)	Testis or retroperitoneal primary ***and*** No nonpulmonary visceral metastases	***AND***	Good marker concentrations—ie, all of AFP <1000 μg/L (ie, <830 kU/L) ***and*** hCG <5000 U/L ***and*** LDH <1.5 times the upper limit of normal	89%	92%
Intermediate prognosis nonseminomas (28% of nonseminomas)	Testis or retroperitoneal primary ***and*** No nonpulmonary visceral metastases	***AND***	Intermediate marker concentrations—ie, any of AFP ≥1000 μg/L (ie, ≥830 kU/L) ***or*** ≤10,000 μg/L (ie, ≤8,300 kU/L) ***or*** hCG <5000 U/L and <50,000 U/L ***or*** LDH ≥1.5 times and ≤10 times the upper limit of normal	75%	80%
Poor prognosis nonseminomas (16% of nonseminomas)	Mediastinal primary ***or*** Nonpulmonary visceral metastases	***OR***	Poor marker concentrations—ie, any of AFP >10,000 μg/L (ie, >8,300 kU/L) ***or*** hCG >50,000 U/L ***or*** LDH >10 times the upper limit of normal	41%	48%
Prognostic Categories for Seminomas					
Good prognosis seminomas (90% of seminomas)	Any primary site ***and*** No nonpulmonary visceral metastases	***AND***	Normal AFP, any hCG and any LDH concentrations.	82%	86%
Intermediate prognosis seminomas (10% of seminomas)	Any primary site ***and*** Nonpulmonary visceral metastases	***AND***	Normal AFP, any hCG and any LDH concentrations.	67%	72%
Poor prognosis seminomas (None)	No seminomas classified as having poor prognosis				

AFP, α-Fetoprotein; *hCG,* human chorionic gonadotropin; *hCGβ,* human chorionic gonadotropin β-subunit; *LDH,* lactate dehydrogenase; *N,* upper limit of normal; *PFS,* progression-free survival.
Modified from International Germ Cell Consensus Classification: a prognostic factor-based staging system for metastatic germ cell cancers. International Germ Cell Cancer Collaborative Group. *J Clin Oncol* 1997;15:594–603.

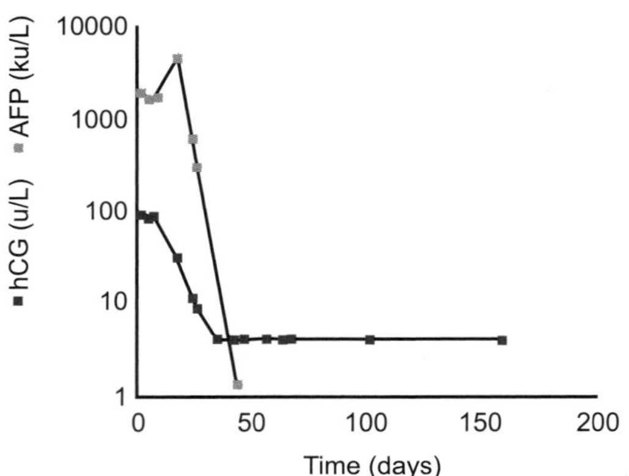

FIGURE 31.6 Tumor marker responses in a patient with widespread metastatic disease who had a complete radiological and marker response to chemotherapy.

woman who develops hyperemesis, excessive uterine enlargement, persistent irregular vaginal bleeding after pregnancy, and/or early failed pregnancy.[38] More rarely, women may present with hyperthyroidism, early-onset preeclampsia, or abdominal distension due to theca lutein cysts. Very rarely, women likely to have metastatic disease present with respiratory failure or neurological symptoms such as seizures. A urine pregnancy test for hCG should be performed in any woman presenting with such symptoms (see subsequent text). Ultrasound scanning provides helpful information, but diagnosis requires histological examination of the products of conception following surgical evacuation. If there is any evidence of persistence of GTD, which is most commonly defined as a persistent increase of serum hCG, the condition is referred to as gestational trophoblastic neoplasia (GTN).[143]

In the United Kingdom, the comprehensive guidelines for management of GTN developed by the Royal College of

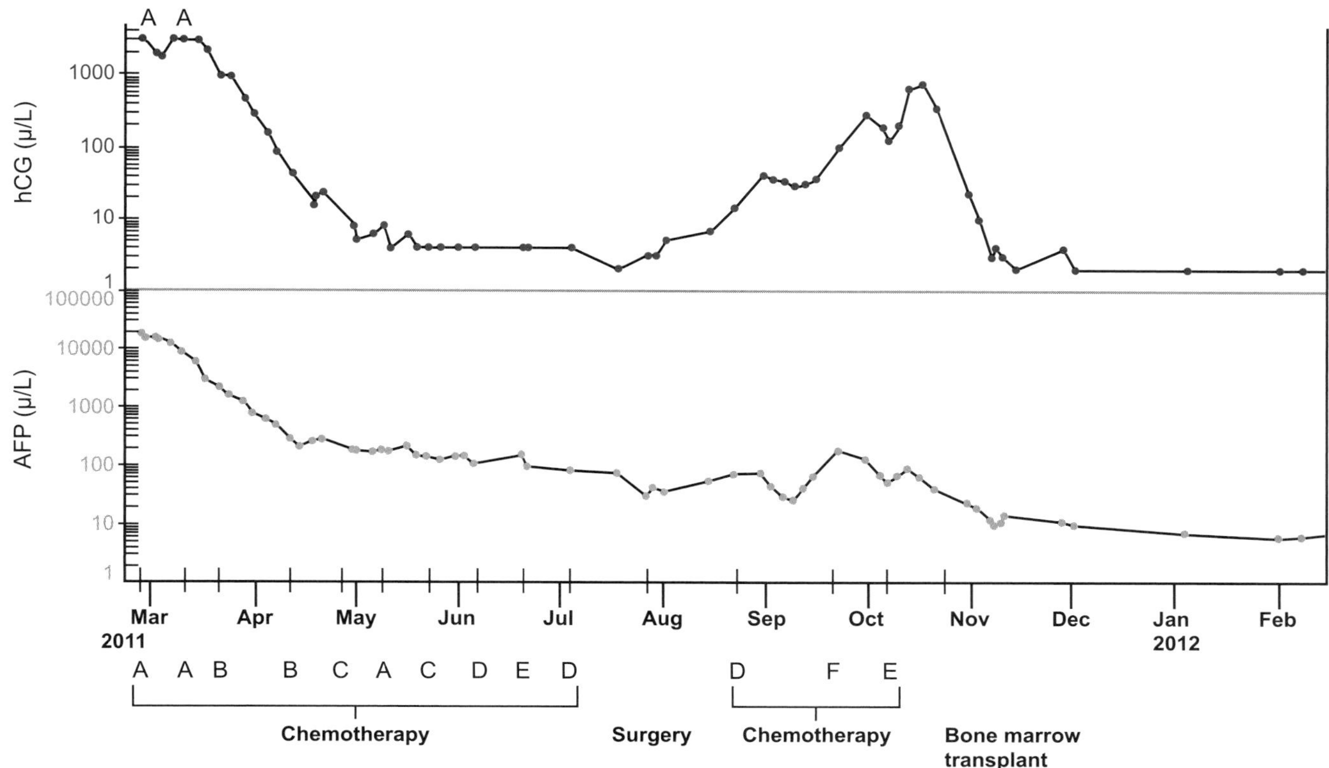

FIGURE 31.7 Tumor marker monitoring of a patient who required a number of chemotherapy treatments prior to surgery, further chemotherapy, and a bone marrow transplant.

Obstetrics and Gynaecology are followed.[143] These, together with an effective registration and treatment program for GTD, have contributed to the impressively high cure (98% to 100%) and low chemotherapy (5% to 8%) rates observed in the United Kingdom.[38] Characteristics of the main forms of GTD are briefly described below.

Hydatidiform Moles. Hydatidiform moles (commonly termed "molar pregnancies") are nonviable products of conception. They are the most common form of GTD and are themselves nonmalignant. They may develop when a sperm fertilizes an "empty" egg that contains no nucleus or DNA (a "complete" mole) or when two sperm fertilize a normal egg ("partial" mole). Because all of the genetic material comes from the father in complete moles, fetal tissue is not present. In appearance, both types of moles grow in clusters like bunches of grapes, each of which is a villi swollen with fluid. Following initial surgery to evacuate the mole, few patients with partial hydatidiform mole require further treatment, and these moles rarely become malignant. Approximately 20% of patients with complete moles will require further surgery or chemotherapy, and a small proportion of these moles will become malignant, developing into choriocarcinoma.

Invasive Moles. Following surgical removal of a complete mole by curettage of the lining of the uterus, about 20% of women develop invasive moles. These penetrate the myometrium (the muscular wall of the uterus), sometimes resulting in heavy bleeding. The tumor metastasizes to other sites (most frequently the lung) in about 15% of patients. The risk of metastasis is increased if more than 4 months elapse between cessation of periods and treatment, if the uterus has become very large, if the woman is over 39 years old, or if she has had a previous GTD.

Choriocarcinoma. Choriocarcinoma most frequently develops from a complete hydatidiform mole but can occur after normal pregnancy or after early fetal loss in pregnancy. Metastasis to distant organs is more likely than for invasive moles but can be treated highly effectively with chemotherapy.

Placental Site Trophoblastic Tumors. These rare forms of GTD develop if the placenta remains attached to the uterus after a normal pregnancy or abortion. The tumors must be completely removed surgically and are not sensitive to chemotherapy, but they do not usually metastasize.

Tumor Markers in Gestational Trophoblastic Disease. Successful clinical management of gestational trophoblastic disease depends on accurate measurement of hCG, which has approximately 99% specificity and sensitivity for this disease in the clinical setting described above, achieving almost ideal tumor marker performance in this application (see Table 31.10). Measurement of hCG using a method that recognizes both hCG and its free beta-subunit (hCGβ) is recommended for this and all other oncology applications.[144-146]

hCG in Screening for GTD. Screening of women at high risk of developing GTD (ie, women who have had a partial or complete hydatidiform mole in a previous pregnancy) is conveniently performed by measuring hCG in urine collected by the patient in her own home and sent by mail to the screening center (see Table 31.10). In the United Kingdom there is a well-established registration form that enables the lifetime follow-up that is recommended because the disease can occur years after the affected pregnancy. Three specialist centers provide hCG testing in urine, with all patients referred for treatment to a specialist unit in London. Costs of the program are relatively low compared with the social cost avoided per life saved.[38]

hCG as an Aid to Diagnosis of GTD. As described above, definitive diagnosis requires histological examination of the products of conception. Estimation of hCG serum concentrations may be helpful in diagnosing molar pregnancies because values greater than two multiples of the median for the gestational date are suggestive of GTD.[143]

hCG in Prognosis. Prognosis is assessed according to the International Federation of Gynaecology and Oncology staging system for GTN,[142] which includes pretreatment hCG concentration as one of the eight prognostic factors used for scoring. Women with scores of 7 or higher are at high risk of recurrence and are treated with intravenous multiagent chemotherapy until the hCG concentration has returned to normal and then for a further 6 consecutive weeks. (Following complete and partial molar pregnancies, approximately 15% and 0.5% of women, respectively, require chemotherapy.[143])

Monitoring. Posttreatment monitoring is essential in the follow-up of molar pregnancy and involves serial measurements of hCG in either blood or urine. A urinary pregnancy (hCG) test should be performed 3 weeks after medical management of failed pregnancy if products of conception are not sent for histological examination. Following a diagnosis of GTD and surgical evacuation, if hCG has reverted to normal within 56 days, then follow-up will be for 6 months from the date of uterine evacuation. If hCG has not reverted to normal within 56 days, then follow-up will be for 6 months from normalization of the hCG concentration. In the United Kingdom, women who had GTD in a previous pregnancy are requested to notify the screening center following any future pregnancies, whatever the outcome of the new pregnancy. hCG concentrations are then checked 6 to 8 weeks after the end of that pregnancy to exclude disease recurrence.[143]

Hepatocellular Carcinoma (Primary Liver Cancer)

The eleventh most commonly diagnosed cancer in the United States, hepatocellular carcinoma (HCC) is the sixth most common cause of cancer death.[147] Worldwide, however, HCC is the second leading cause of cancer death and the fifth most frequently diagnosed cancer, with an incidence that has increased exponentially in recent decades.[148] Asian countries account for approximately 78% of the 600,000 new cases of HCC reported annually.[149] Risk factors are generally the same as those for liver cirrhosis. In China, Southeast Asia, and sub-Saharan Africa, the major causative factors are chronic infection with hepatitis B virus (HBV) and ingestion of food contaminated with aflatoxin B, a fungal toxin that is both genotoxic and carcinogenic. Nonviral causes associated with increased risk for HCC are more common in Western countries and include alcoholic cirrhosis, inherited errors of metabolism (relatively rare and including hereditary hemochromatosis, porphyria *cutanea tarda*, and α_1–antitrypsin deficiency), Wilson disease, and Stage IV primary biliary cirrhosis.[150] The increasing incidence of HCC in Europe probably reflects the increased frequency of chronic hepatitis C infection and liver cirrhosis, both of which are strong predisposing factors for HCC.[22] Patients with metabolic syndrome or diabetes mellitus who have nonalcoholic fatty liver steatohepatitis (NASH) also appear to be at increased risk of HCC, although to a lesser extent than those with cirrhosis due to hepatitis C (HCV) infection.[151] (See Chapter 61.)

Signs and symptoms of HCC at presentation may include jaundice, hepatomegaly, ascites, peripheral edema, pruritus, bleeding esophageal varices, and right upper quadrant pain. In some cases biopsy confirmation of a diagnosis may not be required (eg, if liver nodules are larger than 1 cm in size and there are at least two classic enhancements on either of the recommended imaging modalities [three-phase contrast-enhanced CT or MRI]).[150] If there are only one or two enhancements by either modality, a core needle biopsy or fine needle aspiration biopsy is required for diagnosis. Several staging systems are available, but because the characteristics of HCC vary geographically, none is universally used. However, the Barcelona Clinic Liver Cancer (BCLC) staging system is widely accepted and is being used in many clinical trials.[152] The NCCN guidelines broadly categorize patients as those who are potentially resectable or transplantable and have preserved liver function, those with unresectable disease, those who are inoperable due to performance status or comorbidity with local disease only, and those with metastatic disease.[150]

Potentially curative treatment options include liver transplantation (for which only about 5% of patients are suitable), surgical resection (which requires very good liver function and has a recurrence rate of 50% to 60% after 5 years), ablative therapy (with alcohol, radiofrequency, and/or microwaves), chemoembolization, and chemotherapy. Eligibility for these treatments depends on diagnosis of early-stage disease. The 5-year survival rate for patients with disease confined to the liver is about 43% but is only about 11% for those with spread to regional lymph nodes and less than 5% for those with metastatic disease at presentation.[147] Unfortunately, early-stage disease is often asymptomatic, and in developed countries only 30% to 40% of HCC patients are diagnosed early enough for curative treatment.

Tumor Markers for Hepatocellular Carcinoma. Many tumor markers are increased in HCC, but α-fetoprotein (AFP) is at present the most clinically useful. As described previously (see the section on germ cells), AFP is an oncofetal antigen that is appropriately increased in pregnant women and most frequently inappropriately increased in patients with germ cell tumors and HCC. It may also be chronically or intermittently increased in some benign conditions, particularly those associated with liver damage and/or liver regeneration. Serum AFP concentrations may range from within the reference interval to as high as 10×10^6 μg/L (8.3×10^6 kU/L). However, it is important to note that pretreatment serum AFP may not be increased in up to 20% of patients with HCC, especially in early-stage disease, and that concentrations may be transiently raised in regenerating nodules during recovery from viral hepatitis.

Screening for HCC in High-Risk Groups Using AFP. There is increasing evidence that early detection of HCC through screening of high-risk populations can improve clinical outcome by enabling potentially curative therapies.[153,154] In this context, high-risk patients include men and women with established cirrhosis due to HBV or HCV infection or genetic hemochromatosis, men with alcohol-related cirrhosis who are abstinent from alcohol or likely to comply with treatment, and men with cirrhosis due to primary biliary cirrhosis. The primary screening modality is abdominal ultrasound.

Guideline recommendations are inconsistent regarding AFP measurement, as outlined below. Additionally, when screening programs have been implemented, the uptake has sometimes been insufficiently high to enable reliable interpretation of the data.

In a large randomized controlled trial in China in which 18,816 men and women with HBV infection or a history of chronic hepatitis were screened with ultrasound scanning (USS) and AFP, the detection rate was 84% for ultrasound alone, 69% for AFP alone, and 92% for AFP and ultrasound.[155] Both ultrasound and AFP have limitations: While ultrasound is highly operator dependent, AFP has limited sensitivity and specificity for HCC. The American Association for the Study of Liver Diseases (AASLD) currently does not recommend inclusion of AFP in screening protocols for HCC.[152] However, other groups recommend screening patients at high risk for HCC with both USS and AFP every 3 to 6 months (eg, Asian Oncology Summit[149]) or every 6 to 12 months (eg, NCCN[150]). Results of several studies suggest that inclusion of AFP increases the sensitivity of screening, especially in detecting early-stage HBV-related HCC[156] and HCC in patients with cirrhosis.[157]

Studies suggest that patterns of serial AFP test results (rather than the most recent single value) can more accurately identify those patients with HCV and advanced fibrosis or cirrhosis who are most likely to develop HCC,[158] although the patterns of increase may be complex.[159] Use of longitudinal AFP screening algorithms has been shown to lead to earlier detection of HCC in high-risk groups when compared with the single-threshold approach.[160] If serum AFP is rising or if a liver mass nodule is identified on ultrasound, the NCCN recommends additional imaging with a three-phase CT scan or an MRI.[150] According to the NACB, AFP concentrations of 20 μg/L or higher (ie, ≥17 kU/L) and rising should prompt further investigation even if ultrasound is negative.[22]

Successful screening programs require excellent organization with standardized screening tests, protocols, and algorithms, as well as reliable recall procedures and quality control systems, but a number of reports suggest that this is often not the case for HCC screening.[161-164] Although a large proportion of patients with cirrhosis are seen only by their primary care provider, when 1000 primary care providers in North Carolina were surveyed by questionnaire, only 45% of the 391 respondents screened for HCC.[163] Only 6.2% of 12,485 gastroenterology and hepatology providers in the United States who were sent a 21-question electronic survey responded. Even in the group of respondents, who are likely to be engaged and informed about HCC surveillance, surveillance imaging practices largely deviated from practice guidelines.[161] Establishing more clinically effective screening programs requires agreed protocols, including AFP decision points and algorithms, together with greater physician awareness of guidelines and the availability of potentially effective therapies.[162-164] Although the economic efficiency of screening varies according to the etiology of cirrhosis, authors of a UK study concluded that screening for HCC with AFP and ultrasound is both clinically effective and cost-effective.[165]

AFP as an Aid to Diagnosis. The same caveats that apply to the use of AFP for screening apply to its use as an aid to diagnosis, where its measurement in conjunction with ultrasound may aid in early detection of HCC and guide further management. Generally USS-detected nodules of less than 1 cm should be monitored every 3 months, but 1 to 2 cm nodules in cirrhotic livers should be investigated by two imaging modalities (eg, CT and MRI) and treated as HCC if imaging results are consistent with this. For liver lesions more than 2 cm in size where USS results are typical of HCC and AFP is greater than 200 μg/L (i.e, approximately 170 kU/L), a diagnosis of HCC can be made without proceeding to biopsy.[22] The AASLD guidelines no longer recommend AFP testing as part of diagnostic evaluation because AFP concentrations may be raised in nonmalignant conditions (see Table 31.14) and may be within normal limits in a substantial number of HCC patients, and because imaging is more definitive,[152] as is also recognized by the NCCN.[150] However, the NCCN recommends additional CT or MRI imaging for patients with a rising serum AFP in the absence of a liver mass.[150] If no mass is detected, AFP testing and liver imaging should be continued every 3 months.

AFP in Prognosis. In combination with other factors, AFP concentrations may provide prognostic information in untreated HCC patients and in those being considered for liver resection or transplantation, with high concentrations generally associated with poor prognosis.[22,166] Preoperative AFP decision limits ranging from 200 to 1000 μg/L (ie, approximately 170–830 kU/L)[†] have been suggested to predict outcome after liver transplantation, but there is no international agreement about the decision concentration.[166] In some studies, AFP concentrations of less than 400 μg/L (ie, approximately 330 kU/L) have been used together with tumor size and number to select patients for liver transplantation after downstaging protocols, while in others, dynamic changes in AFP concentrations greater than 15 μg/L (ie, approximately 12 kU/L) are considered to be the most relevant preoperative predictor of recurrence and overall survival after transplantation. In the United Kingdom, current NHS Blood and Transplant guidelines state that measurement of AFP, CEA, and CA19-9 are required when assessing patients prior to possible transplant and that patients with serum AFP greater than 1200 μg/L (ie, >1000 kU/L) should be deselected from eligibility for transplant.[168]

A study using the Organ Procurement and Transplant Network (OPTN) database concluded that serum AFP greater than 400 μg/L (ie, >330 kU/L) and tumor volume less than 115 cm^3 could distinguish patients who are likely to have poor outcome from those who should have an acceptable outcome.[169] Although decision limits differ, there is general agreement that AFP concentrations add prognostic information in HCC patients and may be used for decisions regarding transplantation in combination with imaging criteria.[166] They may also be helpful in decision making before and after downstaging prior to treatment. Biomarkers other than AFP are not helpful.

Periodic measurement of AFP in patients on transplant waiting lists is also recommended at the same time as imaging procedures (eg, dynamic CT, dynamic MRI, or contrast-enhanced ultrasonography) because a rise in AFP is associated with poorer outcome.[166]

[†]1 μg/L of AFP is approximately equivalent to 0.83 kU/L.[167] This factor applies for most current immunoassays, but Instructions for Use provided by the manufacturer should always be consulted to confirm this.

AFP in Posttreatment Monitoring. Measurement of AFP at follow-up visits is recommended by the NACB, NCCN, and others to monitor disease status after liver resection or liver transplantation, for detection of recurrence or after ablative therapies, and/or during palliative treatment.[22,150,166] This reflects the general consensus that earlier identification of disease may enable alternative treatments to be instituted or entry in a clinical trial. Current practice suggests monitoring patients with AFP every 3 months for 2 years and then every 6 to 12 months. Rising AFP concentrations should be confirmed with a repeat specimen within 3 months. Reevaluation, including AFP measurement, should be instituted earlier if there is clinical suspicion of disease recurrence.

Lung Cancer

Lung cancer has been the most common cancer in the world for several decades, with an estimated 1.8 million new cases in 2012, 58% of which occurred in less-developed regions.[170] It is also the most common cause of death from cancer worldwide, accounting for nearly 20% of all cancer deaths. The highest estimated incidence rates are in central and eastern Europe and in eastern Asia. In the United States, the lifetime risk of developing lung cancer is about 6.6%, and the 5-year survival rate is 17.4%.[171] Trends in incidence and mortality generally reflect smoking habits and/or exposure to other environmental or occupational carcinogens. Public health campaigns to discourage smoking and to minimize other risk factors should ultimately reduce incidence.

Early symptoms are nonspecific and include dyspnea, cough, and thoracic pain, with hemoptysis often indicating advanced disease. Patients with suspected lung cancer are investigated with CT and/or MRI, bronchoscopy, and biopsy. Histological differentiation and staging of lung cancer is essential for therapeutic stratification because there are two major histological types with different clinical behaviors and sensitivity to chemotherapy and radiotherapy.

About 75% to 85% of lung cancers are primarily non–small cell lung cancers (NSCLC) (squamous cell carcinoma, adenocarcinoma, and large cell carcinoma) and require surgery as first-line treatment, with subsequent adjuvant radiotherapy and/or chemotherapy if appropriate. Several new biological therapies are also available, including the tyrosine kinase inhibitors, which target EGFR, and bevacizumab, which targets the angiogenic factor VEGF.[5,172] The remaining 15% to 25% are small cell lung cancers (SCLC), which often have neuroendocrine components (see Chapter 63) and are primarily treated with chemotherapy and/or radiotherapy. Small cell lung cancers are aggressive tumors that are characterized by rapid doubling time and metastasize early. Many lung cancers are mixed tumors and include both small cell and non–small cell components.

Five-year relative survival rates depend strongly on tumor stage at diagnosis, with about 55% of patients with localized disease surviving for 5 years, compared with only 4.2% of patients with distant disease at presentation.[171] The US Preventive Services Task Force therefore recommends annual screening for lung cancer with low-dose CT in adults aged 55 to 80 years who have smoked heavily within the past 15 years.[173] There is uncertainty about potential harms of screening,[174] and other options are being investigated.

Tumor Markers in the Management of Lung Cancer. A number of serum tumor markers have been investigated for lung cancer, but those most frequently associated with SCLC are neuron-specific enolase (NSE) and progastrin-releasing peptide (ProGRP). Cyfra 21-1 and CEA are primarily associated with NSCLC. Squamous cell carcinoma antigen (SCCA) may be raised in the subset of NSCLC patients with squamous cell carcinoma. Properties of these markers are summarized in Table 31.6.

Screening and as Aids to Diagnosis. No serum tumor markers are sufficiently sensitive or specific, whether singly or in combination, for use in screening for lung cancer, even in specific high-risk groups such as smokers. The patterns of increased serum concentrations of CEA, Cyfra 21-1, NSE, SCC, and ProGRP may reflect the histological subtype present, but further validation is required.[175] In patients in whom inoperable lung cancer is suspected but for whom histology is not available, clearly increased serum NSE and/or ProGRP would support a diagnosis of SCLC, while clearly raised serum SCC concentrations are consistent with squamous cell cancer.

Prognosis. There are numerous studies of potential prognostic factors in lung cancer.[176] Measurements of Cyfra 21-1, CEA, and/or LDH may provide prognostic information for NSCLC, while NSE and LDH can be used similarly in SCLC.

Therapy Prediction. Serum tumor markers cannot be used to predict therapy response in lung cancer patients. However, as for colorectal cancer, anti-EGFR therapy is available for treatment of patients with NSCLC. The mechanism differs, however, because inhibition of EGFR in NSCLC is usually achieved with tyrosine kinase inhibitors (TKIs), particularly the quinazoline derivatives gefitinib and erlotinib, rather than with monoclonal antibody targeting as in colorectal cancer.[5] In addition gefitinib and erlotinib bind to an intracellular domain, selectively inhibiting mutant EGFR TKI activity, while in colorectal cancer, cetuximab and panitumumab both bind to the extracellular domain of wild-type EGFR.

Disease response was only observed in approximately 10% of advanced NSCLC patients in early trials of anti-EGFR TKIs in unselected patients.[5] Subsequent trials have demonstrated that (when compared to chemotherapy) improved response rates, longer progression-free survival, and better quality of life are achieved by treating patients with specific activating mutations in EGFR with either gefitinib or erlotinib. Patients without the relevant activating mutations generally do not benefit from TKIs.

In addition, in 3% to 7% of NSCLC patients, fusion of the anaplastic lymphoma receptor tyrosine kinase *(ALK)* and echinoderm microtubule associated protein-like 4 *(EML4)* genes occurs as a result of an inversion on chromosome 2. The fusion leads to continuous activation of *ALK* activity, which in turn gives rise to enhanced cell proliferation and decreased cell survival.[177] Crizotinib, a tyrosine kinase inhibitor, induces tumor regression and prolongs survival in patients with advanced NSCLC whose tumors have an *ALK* translocation. Because *ALK* translocations are present in only approximately 5% of NSCLC patients, molecular testing is essential for successful use of crizotinib.

The American Society of Clinical Oncology (ASCO) has updated its recommendations for managing care in patients with early- and late-stage lung cancer, endorsing guidelines issued by the College of American Pathologists (CAP), the International Society for the Study of Lung Cancer (IASLC), and the Association for Molecular Pathology on the molecular testing of patients with lung cancer.[178] The guidelines focus on EGFR and ALK testing, including when and how to do the testing, which is recommended for all patients with lung adenocarcinoma or mixed lung cancer (both primary and metastatic) with a component of adenocarcinoma. The ASCO guidelines add a caveat to the previous guidelines in recommending that squamous or small cell lung cancer should be tested for *EGFR* and *ALK* in those who never smoked because the tumors may have an unusual pathology.

ASCO recommends that testing for KRAS mutations be performed initially because the presence of a KRAS mutation eliminates the need to probe for *EGFR* and *ALK* alterations, which are mutually exclusive with KRAS. Testing for other molecular biomarkers is not recommended, and ASCO cautions that although testing in early-stage disease enables more rapid treatment of some patients, this needs to be balanced against the extra cost for patients who do not have a recurrence. The need for frequent updating of guidelines in this fast-moving field is clearly evident.[179]

Monitoring. In view of the limited treatment options available and the often aggressive nature of the disease, serial monitoring of individual lung cancer patients with serum tumor markers is controversial and is not mentioned in most published clinical guidelines. Serial determinations of the appropriate marker following surgery may provide an indication of the completeness of tumor removal and early indication of subsequent recurrence. The latter is only likely to benefit the patient if alternative treatment is available.

Although reliable criteria for assessment of "biochemical remission" have yet to be developed, tumor marker measurements may assist in evaluating the response (or lack of response) to therapy in patients receiving systemic treatment, enabling discontinuation and/or modification of ineffective treatment. As yet there is no evidence to suggest that tumor marker monitoring improves patient outcome.

Melanoma

Melanoma is a skin cancer that can occur anywhere on the body but is most common in skin that is frequently exposed to sunlight. Malignant cells form in the melanocytes, which are derived from the neural crest and are found throughout the lower part of the dermis. The incidence of melanoma has steadily increased over the last 30 years.[180] Surgery is curative in early-stage disease, but the prognosis is poor in metastatic disease. Signs of melanoma include changes in the appearance of moles or pigmented areas of the skin. Five-year relative survival in the United States is greater than 98% in localized disease but falls to 16% to 17% in metastatic disease.[180]

Tumor Markers Used in the Management of Melanoma. Diagnosing malignant melanoma in pathological specimens involves staining with antibodies to S100, a family of multifunctional proteins with regulatory roles in a number of cellular processes (see Table 31.6). S100 is increased in serum in patients with malignant melanoma, but further studies are required to establish its clinical utility. S100B lacks sensitivity in early disease. Rising concentrations are specific and sensitive for progression in patients with advanced disease, but its measurement is only appropriate if further treatment options are available. Although very nonspecific, LDH can be used to monitor patients with melanoma and may have prognostic value in advanced disease.

Therapy Prediction. Mutations of the *BRAF* gene (v-raf murine sarcoma viral oncogene homolog B1), which encodes a protein with serine/threonine kinase activity, are present in approximately 50% of skin melanomas occurring on intermittently sun-exposed skin and in 30% of those on skin chronically exposed to sun.[5] Most *BRAF* mutations (~80%) are V600E, with V600K and V600D *BRAF* mutations representing a smaller group. The mutations lead to activation of downstream MAPK signaling, which then drives the growth and progression of skin melanomas.

The *BRAF*-mutated protein can be selectively targeted by a number of inhibitors, including vemurafenib and dabrafenib, both of which are very effective in patients with *BRAF* mutation-positive advanced melanomas. Commercially available predictive biomarker assays have now been cleared by the FDA for the identification of patients with metastatic or unresectable melanoma who are likely to benefit from these drugs.

Neonatal and Pediatric Tumors

In children under 15 years old, cancer is the second leading cause of death, but advances in treatment mean that over 70% of children diagnosed with cancer are cured. Tumor markers can contribute significantly to the management of childhood tumors, including childhood neuroblastomas, malignant hepatic tumors, and germ cell tumors. The general principles are the same as for adult patients, but there are some additional points that need to be noted.

Tumor Markers Used in the Management of Childhood Malignancies. AFP and hCG are the tumor markers most frequently used in childhood malignancies. When interpreting AFP, it is essential to remember that plasma AFP is markedly increased at birth and then declines steadily to adult concentrations by 6 to 12 months. AFP is higher in preterm infants and may remain increased for longer in children with delayed development. Appropriate gestational and age-related reference data are therefore required. Serial measurements are often more useful than isolated results, particularly in neonates in whom acute hepatocellular damage may result in marked increases in AFP concentrations.

It is important to note that age-related reference intervals must be applied when interpreting AFP results in neonates and infants under 12 months old. Although generally AFP concentrations fall sharply after birth, even in the most premature babies, they may still be very high in healthy babies, even at 30 days of life. A comprehensive early study reported mean and standard deviations for 12 age ranges (from premature to 8 months old) in helpful tabular form. AFP concentrations in 11 premature babies were high and variable (mean 134,735 μg/L, standard deviation 41,444 μg/L) (Table 31.17).[181] AFP concentrations in infants reached adult values by 8 months of age. This is not entirely in accord with a later study that found that by the age of 2 years, adult serum AFP concentrations had still not been achieved,[182] although reported reference intervals were broadly in accord with those of the first study. The much wider age ranges considered in the more recent Caliper study make comparison of the reference intervals reported difficult.[183] In addition, results for infants less than 1 month old are reported only as "greater than 2000 μg/L" in the Caliper study.

Additional care must be taken to avoid reporting results that are inappropriately low due to high-dose "hooking"

TABLE 31.17 Indicative and Approximate Pediatric Reference Intervals for AFP in Infants and Babies

Age	No. of Subjects	Mean ± Standard Deviation (μg/L)*
Premature	11	134,734 ± 41,444
Newborn	55	48,406 ± 34,718
Newborn to 2 weeks	16	33,113 ± 32,503
2 weeks to 1 month	43	9452 ± 12,610
1 month	12	2654 ± 3080
2 months	40	323 ± 278
3 months	5	88 ± 87
4 months	31	74 ± 56
5 months	6	46.5 ± 19
6 months	9	12.5 ± 9.8
7 months	5	9.7 ± 7.1
8 months	3	8.5 ± 5.5

*Results in μg/L should be multiplied by 0.83 to obtain kU/L.
Data from Wu JT, Book L, Sudar K. Serum alpha fetoprotein (AFP) levels in normal infants. *Pediatric Research* 1981;15:50–52.

because tumor marker concentrations may be very high in some childhood cancers. Considerable care is also required to ensure that dilutions of serum are made and recorded correctly. Because AFP and hCG requests for young children are relatively infrequent, it is highly desirable that all such samples be routinely assayed at more than one dilution.

Childhood Germ Cell Tumors. Measurement of AFP and hCG is mandatory because either or both are frequently increased at the time of diagnosis. Yolk sac tumors are the most common "pure" germ cell tumors in childhood. Dysgerminomas are the most common pure malignant germ cell tumor occurring in the ovary and central nervous system in girls who may present with precocious puberty. Infants or young boys rarely present with seminomas.

Hepatoblastoma. Hepatoblastoma and HCC are the most frequent malignant hepatic tumors in childhood, and differential diagnosis is essential. More than 80% of children with hepatoblastoma and about 50% of those with HCC have tumors that produce AFP, often to extremely high concentrations (eg, 1.2×10^6 μg/L [1.0×10^6 kU/L]). Children with hepatoblastomas that secrete hCG may develop precocious puberty. Complete surgical resection is the treatment of choice, with adjuvant chemotherapy also important. Overall survival rates are greater than 80% if complete resection is achieved and greater than 60% otherwise.

Children with hepatoblastomas may have positive hepatitis B serology and/or other laboratory abnormalities, including anemia and hyperbilirubinemia. Complete surgical resection is the optimal treatment for HCC. Unfortunately, aggressive chemotherapy has not significantly improved outcome, and most children with HCC die within 12 months of diagnosis.

Neuroblastoma. Neuroblastomas are malignant embryonal tumors that may exhibit extremely malignant behavior or may regress spontaneously. They account for 8% to 10% of childhood cancers, with about 80% of cases occurring in children less than four years old. Treatment includes surgery, chemotherapy, and radiotherapy. The diagnosis can be confirmed, and the success of treatment monitored, by measuring urinary catecholamines, which are increased in more than 90% of cases (see Chapter 63). Poorer outcome is generally seen if NSE, LDH, and/or ferritin are increased.

Ovarian Cancer

Ovarian cancer is relatively rare (approximately 12.1 new cases per 100,000 women per year in the United States) and is most frequently diagnosed in women between 55 and 64 years old.[184] Women with a family history of ovarian cancer are at increased risk of the disease, for which early detection is key to improving survival. Five-year survival rates are higher than 90% for women diagnosed with localized disease (ie, confined to the ovary) but fall to approximately 28% for women in whom the disease has already metastasized at diagnosis. Including all disease stages, the 5-year survival figure for women diagnosed in the United States in 1975 was 33.7%. Despite improvements in treatment (usually surgical cytoreduction or "debulking" followed by platinum and taxane-based chemotherapy) for women diagnosed in 2007, this figure only increased to 44.1%, probably because fewer than 15% of ovarian cancers are localized at diagnosis. Early detection is difficult due in part to the relative rarity and heterogeneity of the disease (in the United Kingdom the average general practitioner will see a patient with a new ovarian cancer only once every 5 years), and to the absence of specific symptoms.[185] It is estimated that as many as 30% of women with ovarian cancer may present for the first time at the Emergency Department.[186]

Most malignant ovarian tumors (80% to 85%) are surface epithelial carcinomas, which occur in five distinct histological subtypes: serous (approximately 70%), mucinous (approximately 10%), endometrioid (approximately 5%), clear cell (approximately 3%), and transitional (approximately 2%); the remaining 10% are termed unclassified or undifferentiated. Borderline tumors are very slow growing and of low malignancy potential. When evaluating the clinical utility of tumor markers in ovarian cancer, the different clinical behavior and patterns of tumorigenesis and gene expression of the different subtypes must be taken into consideration. Germ cell tumors account for about 15% of malignant ovarian tumors (see the germ cell section) or sex cord stromal tumors, two-thirds of which are granulosa cell tumors.

Tumor Markers Used in the Management of Ovarian Cancer. CA125 (see Table 31.5) is the most widely used serum tumor marker for all epithelial ovarian cancers but is most sensitive for serous adenocarcinomas. Because many benign conditions are associated with increased CA125, careful interpretation of results in the clinical context is paramount. For example, occasional and sometimes transiently raised concentrations of CA125 greater than 5000 kU/L may be seen in patients with nonmalignant ascites (see Table 31.14). CA125 is also increased in other malignancies, particularly adenocarcinomas (see Table 31.13). Method-related differences in results can lead to misinterpretation of serial results, and some methods are vulnerable to interference, particularly from heterophilic antibodies (see the section on analytical requirements and Chapter 23). In addition, there are clinically significant differences in individual patient characteristics in healthy postmenopausal women (including age, race, and previous gynecological history) that are particularly relevant to the use of CA125 in screening.[187]

Human epididymal protein 4 (HE4), which is a member of the "four disulfide core" family of proteinase inhibitors, has recently emerged as a promising serum tumor marker that is upregulated in epithelial ovarian cancers and could potentially complement or replace measurement of CA125 in ovarian cancer patients.[188,189] Serum HE4 is less sensitive than CA125 for detecting early-stage ovarian cancers among asymptomatic women but has better sensitivity and specificity for differentiating malignant from nonmalignant pelvic masses, especially in premenopausal patients.[190] HE4 is not increased during menstruation but significantly increases in renal failure and with advancing age.

The serum markers of choice for ovarian germ cell tumors are AFP, hCG, and LDH (see the section on germ cell tumors), while for granulosa cell tumors, inhibin is the appropriate tumor marker. An inhibin method that detects all forms of inhibin, including A, B, and pro-αC, is required.

Screening for Ovarian Cancer. In view of the need for early diagnosis, a reliable screening test could make a major difference to survival of patients with ovarian cancer because most patients with advanced disease die of it. Assuming a disease prevalence of 40 per 100,000 in women over 50 years old, very high specificity (99.7%) is required to achieve an acceptable positive predictive value of 10% for ovarian cancer. The feasibility of screening women over 50 years of age has been investigated extensively in several large major randomized controlled trials.

The Prostate, Lung, Colorectal, and Ovarian Cancer (PLCO) trial in the United States included 78,216 women aged between 55 and 74 years who were recruited into the trial between 1993 and 2001 and followed up for a maximum of 13 years for cancer diagnoses and death.[191] The simultaneous screening with CA125 and transvaginal ultrasound in this trial did not reduce ovarian cancer mortality when compared with usual care, but diagnostic evaluation following a false-positive screening test result was associated with complications.[191] Subset analysis of results from a cohort of women in the PLCO trial identified high-risk categories for predicting risk of cancer in women with abnormal CA125, transvaginal ultrasound scan, or both, at initial and subsequent screens.[192] This could provide guidance for clinical decisions regarding the need for surgery in these women, but the authors caution that conclusions from their descriptive analysis are not definitive and validation and refinement of their results in other populations of postmenopausal women are required.

Annual screening with ultrasound and CA125 in a single-arm prospective study carried out at the University of Kentucky included 37,293 women over 50 years old and women over 25 years with a documented family history of ovarian cancer.[193] Comparison of outcome with that of a historic control group demonstrated a decrease in stage at detection as well as an increase in 5-year survival of 20% (74.8% ± 6.6% compared with 53.7% ± 2.2%). However, these results may reflect a combination of lead time of screen detection and a healthy volunteer effect.[194]

A two-stage strategy was employed in a single-arm prospective study of postmenopausal women conducted in Texas[195] and using the Risk of Ovarian Cancer (ROCA) algorithm.[196] ROCA compares an individual's serial profile with that of cases and controls to estimate the risk of having ovarian cancer, thereby using CA125 velocity rather than a single threshold cutpoint. In the study, 4051 women were triaged to their next annual CA125 (low-risk group), repeat CA125 in 3 months (intermediate-risk), or transvaginal ultrasound and referral to a gynecologic oncologist (high-risk).[195] Specificity for ovarian cancer in the study population of 4051 women of average risk for the disease was 99.9% with a positive predictive value of 40%.

Similar results were reported in the much larger United Kingdom Collaborative Trial of Ovarian Cancer Screening (UKCTOCS), in which CA125 was measured annually for 202,638 postmenopausal women and then interpreted using a risk of ovarian cancer algorithm (ROC).[197] Patients were then triaged as in the study above to return to "normal risk" (return to annual screening), intermediate risk (repeat CA125), or "elevated risk" (repeat CA125 and transvaginal ultrasound). Women with persistently increased risk were then clinically assessed. The number of screen-detected primary invasive epithelial ovarian or tubal cancers was double the number that would have been detected using a fixed cutoff, supporting the use of velocity-based algorithms in cancer screening strategies that use blood biomarkers.[197] Survival data from this trial are not yet available.

The situation is different for women who are *BRCA1* or *BRCA2* mutation carriers. Respectively, 1% to 2.5% and 0.4% to 0.8% of these women will develop ovarian cancer each year.[198] The American College of Obstetricians and Gynecologists recommends that risk-reducing salpingo-oophorectomy (ie, total removal of the ovaries and fallopian tubes) should be offered by age 40 years for these women.[199] For women who decline this operation, the National Comprehensive Cancer Network (NCCN) view is that while there may be circumstances where offering screening with transvaginal ultrasound and/or CA125 may be helpful, data do not yet support routine ovarian screening, but this can be considered at the clinician's discretion.[200] These recommendations may change when outcome data are available from two large clinical trials. Preliminary results from the United Kingdom Familial Ovarian Cancer Screen Study (UK FOCSS), which involves annual screening with CA125 and transvaginal ultrasound of 3563 women at greater than 10% risk of ovarian or fallopian tube cancer, suggest that a clinically meaningful stage shift (ie, earlier detection) occurred in women who were screened according to protocol as opposed to those who underwent delayed screening.[201] Results from the UK FOCSS study and those from a prospective study undertaken by the Gynecologic Oncology Group and including longitudinal CA125 screening among women at increased risk of ovarian cancer should help to clarify whether screening could be a viable alternative to risk-reducing surgery for women at genetic risk for ovarian and fallopian tube cancers.[202]

Diagnosis. CA125 measurement in isolation is not recommended for diagnosis due to its low sensitivity and specificity for ovarian cancer. A level within the reference interval does not necessarily exclude ovarian cancer because CA125 is not increased in more than 50% of women with early-stage cancers or in 20% to 25% of women with advanced-stage cancers. Similarly an increased concentration does not necessarily indicate ovarian cancer, particularly in premenopausal women (see Table 31.14). Nevertheless, extremely high CA125 values may be helpful in evaluating premenopausal women provided other potential causes are considered (see Tables 31.13 and 31.14), prompting referral to a gynecologic

TABLE 31.18 **Risk of Malignancy Algorithms Used for Ovarian Cancer**

Risk of Malignancy Index (RMI): Calculated as U × M × [CA125] where U, M, and [CA125] are as defined in the table below	
Ultrasound characteristics that are scored (one point each)	Multinodular cyst, evidence of solid areas; evidence of metastases; presence of ascites; presence of bilateral lesions.
Score assigned for ultrasound score, **U**	**U** = 0 for ultrasound characteristics score of 0 **U** = 1 for ultrasound characteristics score of 1 **U** = 3 for ultrasound characteristics score of 2–5
Score assigned for menopausal status, **M**	**M** = 1 if premenopausal **M** = 3 if postmenopausal
Score assigned for tumor marker level, **CA125**	**CA125** = the serum CA125 concentration in kU/L (or U/mL)
Interpretation when triaging women with ovarian cysts	High RMI (>250): Operation performed by gynecological oncologist in a cancer center. Moderate RMI (25–250): Operation performed by a lead clinician in a cancer center. Low RMI (<25): Operation performed by a general gynecologist if conservative management is not appropriate.
Risk of Malignancy Algorithm	
ROMA calculation	The algorithm can be embedded in specialist software and combines serum concentrations of human epididymis protein 4 (HE4) (pmol/L) and CA125 (kU/L or mU/mL) with menopausal status to generate a single numerical score that correlates with the likelihood of malignancy being seen at surgery.[207] It is independent of ultrasound.

Modified from Sturgeon CM, Duffy MJ, Walker G. The National Institute for Health and Clinical Excellence (NICE) guidelines for early detection of ovarian cancer: the pivotal role of the clinical laboratory. *Ann Clin Biochem* 2011;48:295–99.

oncologist, particularly if associated with ascites or evidence of metastasis.[199]

In postmenopausal women with a pelvic mass, CA125 measurement can help in differentiating malignant from nonmalignant masses. CA125 concentrations greater than 95 kU/L in postmenopausal women can discriminate such masses with a positive predictive value of 95%.[203] This can be further refined by using either of two well-established "risk of malignancy" (RMI) algorithms that incorporate an ultrasound score, a menopausal score, and CA125 concentration in kU/L.[204,205] Using the RMI scoring system and a cutoff RMI value of 200, the positive predictive value for malignancy is about 80%. A further "assessment of different neoplasias in the adnexa" algorithm (ADNEX) has been developed.[206]

The commonly used RMI scoring system is shown in Table 31.18, together with the more recently developed "risk of malignancy algorithm" (ROMA) scoring system that includes CA125, HE4, and menopausal status.[207] The ROMA performs similarly to the RMI[208] and has been further refined in the "Copenhagen Index" (CPH-I), which includes serum HE4, serum CA125, and age without menopausal status or ultrasound.[209] The ROMA and CPH-I algorithms do not include ultrasound. However, because routine investigations for suspected ovarian cancer usually include ultrasound, cost savings are unlikely. Caution is also essential when applying any of these algorithms because they perform best in patients with high-grade serous histology and less well in patients with Stage I disease where clear cell and endometrioid histologies predominate.[210]

It has recently been recognized that calling ovarian cancer the "silent" cancer is a misconception because women may develop symptoms several months before diagnosis of early-stage disease.[199] Reflecting this, the UK National Institute for Health and Clinical Excellence (NICE) guidelines for the early detection of ovarian cancer recommend that general practitioners should measure serum CA125 in women presenting with persistent, frequent (>12 times a month), and continuous symptoms suggestive of ovarian cancer, which include abdominal bloating or distention, early satiety and/or loss of appetite, pelvic or abdominal pain, and/or increased urinary urgency and/or frequency.[211] If CA125 is 35 kU/L or higher, an ultrasound scan of the abdomen should be arranged to enable calculation of the RMI. Women with an RMI score of greater than 250 should then be referred to a specialist multidisciplinary team. Clearly there are significant drawbacks to the first-line use of CA125 in the early detection of ovarian cancer, but it is the best serum marker available.[186] According to the American College of Obstetricians and Gynecologists, the best way to detect ovarian cancer is through a high index of suspicion for a diagnosis.[199] Rigorous implementation of the NICE recommendations should promote this and facilitate timely referral. Clinical audit will be required to demonstrate whether the approach is cost-effective.[186]

Prognosis. CA125 measurements can indirectly reflect tumor burden in patients with epithelial ovarian cancer and provide some indication of likely clinical outcome, with higher preoperative concentrations generally associated with worse prognosis. Five-year survival rates in patients with a preoperative CA125 concentration greater than 65 kU/L have been found to be significantly lower than those for patients with CA125 less than 65 kU/L.[212] Reliable prediction prior to cytoreductive surgery of its likely success would be desirable to help select patients who could be spared from futile surgical procedures.[213] A metaanalysis of serum CA125 concentrations greater than 500 kU/L was associated with poor surgical outcomes, positive and negative likelihood ratios too low for clinical utility, and preoperative serum CA125 concentrations unable to reliably predict surgery success in advanced epithelial ovarian cancer.[213] However, values greater than 500 kU/L may predict the likelihood of difficult or complex surgery, potentially aiding treatment planning. Preliminary studies suggest that preoperative CA125 may be useful in stratifying patients for neoadjuvant chemotherapy.

Following primary treatment with surgery and/or chemotherapy, a nadir CA125 concentration (eg, to ≤5 kU/L[214]) and a more rapid rate of decrease (eg, ≥50% during the initial two cycles of platinum-based chemotherapy[215]) are generally associated with more favorable prognosis.[213] Several factors may influence CA125 concentrations, particularly following surgery, and these, together with sample timing, must be taken into account to minimize the risk of misinterpretation of results. The natural half-life of CA125 is approximately 5 days, so its clearance postsurgery can take up to 25 days. In addition, CA125 concentrations often fall following tumor debulking and/or drainage of ascites, while peritoneal injury often increases CA125 concentrations transiently. Generally, a prolonged CA125 half-life and/or failure to fall to within reference limits is predictive of poor response to treatment and a higher rate of relapse. However, these observations have yet to be validated prospectively.

Monitoring. CA125 measurements are used to monitor subgroups of patients with ovarian cancer, many of whom are included in clinical trials, during treatment and follow-up. Criteria used to evaluate changes in CA125 during first-line trials in ovarian cancer are included in the "Response Evaluation Criteria in Solid Tumors" (RECIST). Provided that the pretreatment concentration is at least twice the upper limit of the reference interval, a CA125 response is defined as a 50% decrease from the pretreatment concentration provided that the decrease is maintained for at least 28 days.[216] Failure to respond to treatment is defined as doubling of the nadir value in patients with increased CA125 that never normalizes or an increase to greater than 70 kU/L for patients whose increased pretreatment concentrations normalized on first-line chemotherapy. The RECIST criteria enable objective assessment of response that can influence decisions to continue effective treatment or change ineffective treatment. Generally, after cytoreductive surgery and combination chemotherapy, persistent increase of CA125 correlates with persistent disease in 90% of cases, and CA125 concentrations track tumor volume with up to 90% accuracy.[217] However, up to 50% of patients with normal concentrations of CA125 following chemotherapy have been found to have small volumes of persistent disease at second look operation, a procedure that is now largely discontinued.

Following completion of treatment, standard practice has been to monitor women with ovarian cancer for potential increases in CA125 prior to clinical signs of relapse (median lead time approximately 4 to 5 months). The UK-based Medical Research Council/European Organisation for Research and Treatment of Cancer (MRC-EORTC) conducted a randomized trial to evaluate the utility for such monitoring of CA125. Those enrolled had completed platinum-based chemotherapy and had a normal CA125 concentration. During this international multicenter trial, for which recruitment was completed after 9 years, CA125 was measured every 3 months, with the results not revealed to clinicians or patients.[218] An increase in CA125 to greater than 70 kU/L prompted random assignment either to the early- or the delayed-treatment arm. Patients in the early-treatment arm were notified of the rising concentrations and started chemotherapy 4 weeks later. In the delayed-treatment arm, patients continued on follow-up and only started chemotherapy if clinical signs or symptoms of relapse occurred. Results of the trial indicated that early intervention based on CA125 conferred no survival advantage but resulted in earlier deterioration in quality of life.[218] It was concluded that the value of routine measurement of CA125 in the follow-up of patients with ovarian cancer who attain a complete response after first-line treatment is not proven and that these patients should be told that routine CA125 monitoring is not necessary until or unless they are worried or develop any signs that indicate tumor relapse.

The results of the MRC-EORTC trial challenge the existing assumptions about the benefit of monitoring with CA125 and have generated considerable debate.[219,220] Aspects of the study that have been questioned include a perceived lack of detailed definition of primary treatment, the appropriateness of 70 kU/L as a decision limit, absence of information about how many asymptomatic recurrences were treated, and whether the second-line chemotherapy treatments used were optimal throughout the trial and reflect current best practice.[220,221] The European Society of Gynaecological Oncology (ESGO) issued a consensus statement advising that the use of CA125 should not be universally abandoned in the routine follow-up of all patients with ovarian cancer.[222] Current ESGO recommendations are that CA125 follow-up should be continued in patients after complete response on primary treatment for epithelial ovarian cancer if they have been or are being treated as part of a clinical trial and/or if they are being considered for further studies on second-line treatment and/or if they will not have routine (quarterly) follow-ups, including regular imaging, and/or if they would be eligible for secondary surgery at recurrence.[220,222] ESGO further recommends that appropriate follow-up with CA125 should be continued in all cases of nonepithelial cancer and that CA125 doubling of the posttreatment nadir should be used instead of doubling of the upper limit of reference when assessing response.[220] These recommendations are broadly in line with those of other groups, most of which recommend that the pros and cons of monitoring with CA125 should be objectively discussed with the patient.[221,223-225] This is in accord with the views of the MRC-EORTC trial coordinator, who also provides patients with the option of having CA125 measurements made but not being told the results, an option potentially particularly helpful for patients in a clinical trial where routine CA125 measurements are mandated.[218]

The ongoing discussion and dilemmas prompted by the results of the MRC-EORTC study are common to other serum tumor markers for which there is little evidence that measurement influences outcome and/or is of benefit to the patient. Some of the challenges of implementing an evidence-based medicine approach are illustrated by the results of a small survey relating to the MRC-EORTC trial results. A large majority of ovarian cancer patients stated that they would not alter their views on being monitored with CA125 based on the study results, even though almost all respondents (97%) believed the study results.[226]

Pancreatic Cancer

Pancreatic cancer is the twelfth most common cancer in the United States, representing 3% of all new cancer cases, and the fourth leading cause of cancer death.[227,228] Although the

5-year survival rate has doubled since 1975, it was on average only 7.2% from 2005–2011, in part reflecting the difficulty of diagnosing the disease, which is more common with increasing age (median age at diagnosis is 71 years) and affects more men than women. Most patients present with symptoms that, in order of frequency, commonly include jaundice, weight loss, abdominal pain, nausea or vomiting, and pruritus.[229] The 60% to 70% of pancreatic ductal adenocarcinomas are located in the head of the pancreas and often present with jaundice or exocrine insufficiency due to common bile duct and/or pancreatic duct obstruction, respectively. They consequently tend to be diagnosed at an earlier stage than the 20% to 25% of tumors located in the body or tail of the pancreas. Only 9% of patients with pancreatic cancer are diagnosed when the tumor is still localized and resectable.[227] In a recent review of 1000 patients who had undergone pancreatectomy in a single institution, 25% were found to have diabetes preoperatively.[229] Initial evaluation of a patient with suspected pancreatic cancer should include a detailed medical and family history because 5% to 10% of patients with pancreatic cancer have familial disease.

Tumor Markers Used in the Management of Pancreatic Cancer. A number of serum tumor markers have been studied in pancreatic cancer, but the best-validated and most clinically useful is CA19-9, a sialylated Lewis a antigen (Le^a) commonly produced in pancreatic and hepatobiliary disease but also increased in many other conditions (see Table 31.14). It is important to be aware that CA19-9 is undetectable (usually <1.0 kU/L) and therefore uninformative in Le^a-negative individuals who constitute 5% to 10% of the general population.[229,230]

Screening and Diagnosis. The low positive predictive value of CA19-9 means it cannot be used in screening, but in symptomatic patients, it contributes to diagnosis with sensitivity of 79% to 81% and specificity of 82% to 90%.[230] However, it should only be measured in patients in whom pancreatic cancer is suspected and with the usual caveats that a result within the reference interval does not exclude pancreatic malignancy and vice versa. Because CA19-9 may be increased in biliary infection (cholangitis), inflammation, or biliary obstruction (of any etiology), the NCCN recommends that it is best measured after biliary decompression is complete and bilirubin is normal.[230] False increases are frequently observed in patients with biliary obstruction due to benign pancreatobiliary and other conditions.

Prognosis. Preoperative CA19-9 concentrations correlate with both American Joint Cancer Committee (AJCC) staging and disease burden, so they can complement information from imaging, laparoscopy, and biopsy when assessing whether a pancreatic tumor is resectable.[229,230] In patients without biliary obstruction, a high CA19-9 concentration is used in some centers as an indication for staging laparoscopy, with concentrations greater than 130 kU/L found in one center to be strongly associated with the identification of subradiographic unresectable disease.[231] A prospective analysis of CA19-9 concentrations in patients treated with adjuvant chemoradiotherapy has also demonstrated a significant survival difference favoring patients with postoperative CA19-9 values less than 180 kU/L.[232] Low postoperative CA19-9 concentrations at 3 months and before adjuvant chemotherapy have also been shown to be independent prognostic factors.[233] In the same study, the 11 patients with postadjuvant therapy CA19-9 concentrations less than 37 kU/L survived for longer than the 8 patients with higher CA19-9 values, suggesting possible prognostic value. Similar results have been observed elsewhere, with normalization of CA19-9 following neoadjuvant therapy associated with longer median survival among both nonresected and resected groups of patients.[234]

Therapy Prediction. Postoperative CA19-9 concentrations may help to predict the benefit of adjuvant therapy (usually gemcitabine-based). In one study, patients with CA19-9 concentrations of 90 kU/L or less who received gemcitabine-based adjuvant therapy had a longer disease-free survival than those who did not (26 months vs. 16.7 months), but patients with CA19-9 concentrations greater than 90 kU/L did not appear to benefit from adjuvant treatment.[233]

Gemcitabine is a prodrug that is taken into cells via a nucleoside transporter. There is increasing evidence that human equilibrative nucleoside transporter (hENT1) may be an excellent predictive marker of survival in pancreatic cancer patients treated with adjuvant gemcitabine-based chemotherapy postoperatively,[230] although the results of a number of studies have been inconclusive, possibly reflecting the lack of a commercial source of the antibody and no CLIA-approved testing. However, results of a metaanalysis of 11 clinical studies involving a total of 851 pancreatic cancer patients suggested that high hENT1 expression may be associated with improved overall survival and disease-free survival of pancreatic cancer patients and that further study is warranted.[235]

Monitoring. Rising CA19-9 concentrations suggest progression and can be used, together with radiographic and clinical data, to influence decisions to initiate palliative treatment in a patient whose disease progresses after surgery or to change (or discontinue) chemotherapy in patients progressing during treatment.[229,230] Obtaining a CA19-9 measurement immediately before each therapeutic intervention is essential in order to have a baseline with which to compare subsequent results.[230] ASCO does not recommend the routine use of serum CA19-9 alone to monitor response to treatment but states that in advanced disease, CA19-9 can be measured at the start of treatment for locally advanced metastatic disease and every 1 to 3 months during active treatment.[121] An increase may indicate progression and should prompt confirmation with other modalities.

It is also particularly important that the same CA19-9 method be used for serial monitoring because the results are not interchangeable among methods (see earlier discussion). (Measurement of CEA or possibly CA125 to monitor progression of pancreatic cancer may be considered provided they are increased at diagnosis and if the tumor does not produce CA19-9, which is the marker of choice.[229])

Prostate Cancer

Prostate cancer is most frequently diagnosed in men aged 65 to 74 years old. It accounted for approximately 13.3% of all new cancer cases in the United States in 2015, but for only 4.7% of all cancer deaths.[236] While many more men with prostate cancer die with, rather than of, their cancer, some prostate cancers are lethal. Developing a reliable and noninvasive means of differentiating aggressive cancers from indolent cancers remains the major challenge for diagnosis of prostate cancer. Common symptoms at presentation include frequency, urgency, nocturia, dysuria, acute retention,

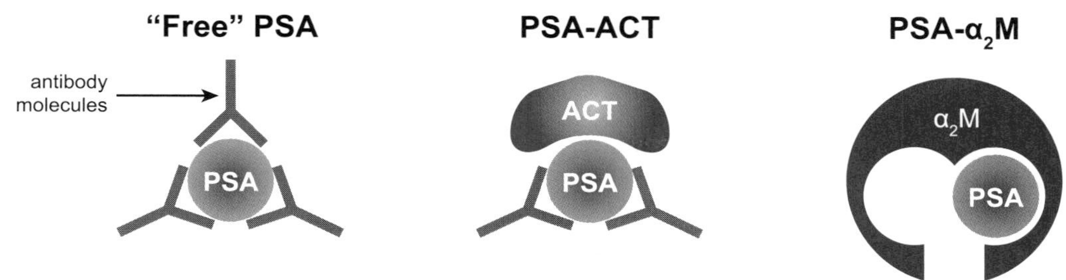

FIGURE 31.8 Schematic depiction of free and complexed PSA. *ACT,* α-Antichymotrypsin; *α-M,* α-macroglobulin.

prostatic enlargement, back pain, weight loss, and anemia. Further complicating diagnosis, the first six of these symptoms may be associated with benign prostatic hyperplasia or hypertrophy, a nonmalignant condition associated with natural increase in size of the prostate with advancing age. The last three symptoms tend to be symptomatic of more advanced prostate cancer.

According to data for 2005 to 2011 from the United States, 98.9% of patients survived for 5 years, with 5-year relative survival of 100% in the 80% of prostate cancer patients with localized disease.[236] Even for men diagnosed with distant metastases at presentation, the 5-year relative survival was 28.2%. There is uncertainty about what constitutes optimal treatment of early-stage disease confined to the prostate. Options include curative surgery (prostatectomy), brachytherapy, and radiotherapy. "Active surveillance" without intervention is also a realistic option. In advanced disease that has metastasized (usually to bone), endocrine therapy to suppress testosterone (eg, with antiandrogens such as Zoladex) is effective because prostate cancers are dependent on testosterone. Ultimately many advanced cancers become "castration resistant" (ie, no longer respond to traditional androgen-reducing treatments), and other treatment options, including chemotherapy, are required.

Widespread measurement of serum prostate specific antigen (PSA), which in both asymptomatic and symptomatic patients can identify potential prostatic disease and inform decisions to proceed to prostatic biopsy, is likely to account for increases in the apparent incidence of prostate cancer. However, many of the cancers identified will be indolent, and overdiagnosis is recognized as a major issue for health systems. By the age of 80 years, autopsy studies have shown that approximately 80% of men will have some cancer cells in their prostate,[237,238] although fewer than 5% of men will die from the disease.

Tumor Markers Used in the Management of Prostate Cancer

Prostate-Specific Antigen. Optimal treatment of patients with prostate cancer depends on PSA, the most important serum tumor marker for this disease. Unlike many other tumor markers, PSA is essentially organ-specific. However, PSA is not cancer-specific because increased serum concentrations occur in men with benign prostatic disease and/or urinary tract infections and following intervention involving the prostate. Prostatic biopsy is therefore required for definitive diagnosis of malignancy.

A member of the kallikrein serine protease family and the enzyme responsible for dissolving the seminal coagulum, 70% to 90% of immunoreactive PSA protein in blood is bound to protease inhibitors, primarily alpha-1-antichymotrypsin (ACT). The remaining 10% to 30% of the immunoreactive protein circulates in a free or unbound form, thought to be biologically inactive and known as "free PSA" (Fig. 31.8). Multiple forms of free PSA and its precursor forms (eg, proPSA) exist in serum and have been proposed as new markers for prostate cancer. In clinical practice, methods measuring total PSA (ie, free PSA and the PSA-ACT complex) are most often used. Several strategies to improve the diagnostic accuracy of PSA with the primary aim of decreasing the number of unnecessary biopsies are available as described below.

Age-Related Reference Intervals. Prostate size (ie, volume) can increase with age, particularly in men with benign prostatic hyperplasia (BPH), and may be associated with increased serum PSA values. Historically, a single PSA reference interval of less than 4.0 μg/L has been used. Higher PSA reference intervals in older men (eg, <5.0 or <6.0 μg/L) could decrease unnecessary biopsies (ie, increase specificity) in this age group, while lower reference intervals in younger men (eg, <2.5 or <3.0 μg/L) could increase cancer detection (ie, improve sensitivity). Race-specific reference ranges have similarly been suggested because PSA tends to be higher in some populations (eg, African Americans).[239] However, equivocal results have been reported in the literature, and the value of age- or race-related reference intervals remain unclear.[240] The NHS Prostate Cancer Screening Management Programme currently recommends use of age-related reference intervals,[241] but other groups, including the NCCN,[240] make no recommendations regarding their routine use.

Percent-Free PSA ("Free to Total" Ratio). The ratio of free PSA to total PSA is lower in prostate cancer patients than in men with BPH and those without prostatic disease. Determination of the ratio may therefore enable better discrimination of prostatic cancer and BPH. Measurement of percent-free PSA is likely to be most informative when total PSA is between 3 or 4 and 10 μg/L (the so-called "diagnostic gray zone") and is most often determined in patients with normal digital rectal examinations (DREs) who have previously undergone prostate biopsy.[21,240,242] While measurement of percent-free PSA has been shown to reduce the number of unnecessary biopsies by 25% to 40%, some cancers may be missed, in part due to the difficulty of selecting an optimal cutpoint. Values reported in the literature range from 8% to 25%, although most are between 15% and 20%. Men with percent-free PSA less than 10% have a greater than 50% probability of being diagnosed with prostate cancer, while those with percent-free PSA greater than 25% have a less than 10% chance of having prostate cancer. Men in the first group would generally be advised to go forward for biopsy. Whether men in the second group would find this likelihood sufficiently low not to undergo a biopsy is debatable.[243]

Preanalytical requirements for measurement of free PSA are more rigorous than for total PSA. Its half-life in blood is much shorter than that of total PSA (about 2.5 hours vs. 3 to 4 days), so rapid transfer to the laboratory is required.[239,244] Later addition of the test to a stored sample may therefore be inappropriate. It is also essential that free PSA and total PSA measurements are made using paired kits from the same supplier.

Complexed PSA. Direct measurement of complexed PSA (cPSA) is possible, so by determining the ratio of complexed PSA to total PSA, information analogous to that for percent-free PSA can be obtained. However, although approved (in conjunction with DRE) as an aid in the detection of prostate cancer in men aged over 50 years, cPSA has not gained widespread use in clinical practice.[240]

PSA Density. Assessment of PSA density potentially identifies men who have high serum PSA due to a large prostate rather than to prostate cancer. PSA density is estimated by dividing serum PSA (in μg/L) by prostate volume (in cc) as determined by transrectal ultrasound (TRUS).

Results of some studies suggest that such correction improves PSA specificity in men with larger prostates and improves test sensitivity in men with smaller glands, but other studies have not shown any benefit. Lack of precision due to variations in prostate shape, poor reproducibility of ultrasound volume measurements, and age-related variation in the ratio of prostate epithelium to stroma may account for these different conclusions. PSA density is rarely used in clinical practice but may be considered in evaluating patients, for whom prostate volume has previously determined by TRUS.[240]

PSA Velocity. PSA velocity (PSAV), the rate of change of PSA over time, has been suggested to reflect aggressiveness of prostate cancer, with higher rates of change associated with greater risk of prostate cancer death. There are a number of caveats to the use of PSAV.[240] The predictive value of PSAV can be influenced by PSA concentration, and it is not useful in patients with PSA values greater than 10 μg/L. PSAV may be influenced by prostatitis, urinary tract infection, and catheterization, all of which can cause rapid transient increases in PSA. PSAV may be affected by measurement fluctuations due either to analytical interassay variability or to individual biological variability. These factors, together with likely differences in how PSAV is calculated (eg, the number of measurements and time frame required for assessment), are likely to account for different study conclusions that make it difficult to know how best to implement use of PSAV in clinical practice.[245]

Other Tumor Markers for Prostate Cancer. Tests that are not at present widely used in clinical practice include PCA3 (a noncoding, prostate tissue–specific RNA measured in urine), phi (an algorithmic combination of total PSA, free PSA, and proPSA measured in serum), 4K score (an algorithmic combination of free and total PSA, human kallikrein 2, and intact PSA measured in serum), and ConfirmMDx (a multiplex epigenetic assay) (see Table 31.6).

PSA in Screening for Prostate Cancer. Screening asymptomatic men for prostate cancer with PSA is highly controversial for a number of reasons (see Table 31.10).[243,246] Probably the most important of these is the inability of PSA to differentiate aggressive prostate cancers that require treatment from indolent cancers that will not progress. Consequently, there are significant risks of overdiagnosis and overtreatment of some men.

The feasibility of screening with annual PSA measurements has been investigated in two large randomized controlled prospective clinical trials and three smaller trials that were the subject of a recent Cochrane systematic review.[247] A total of 341,342 participants were included in the five trials. Three of these trials used methodology that was assessed by the Cochrane group as posing a high risk of bias and did not meet the inclusion criteria. The two large studies, the European Randomized Study of Screening for Prostate Cancer (ERSPC)[248] and the US Prostate, Lung, Colorectal, and Ovarian (PLCO) Cancer Screening Trial,[249] were both assessed as posing a low risk of bias but reported contradictory results.

The ERSPC study was the only one of the five trials to report a significant (21%) reduction in prostate cancer–specific mortality in a prespecified subgroup of men aged 55 to 69 years after 13 years of follow-up.[248] After the same length of follow-up, the PLCO study found no evidence of a mortality benefit for organized annual screening as compared with opportunistic screening, which forms part of standard care.[249] An analysis of the reasons for differences in screening outcomes in the eight countries represented in the ERSPC study concluded that the balances of benefits and harms in prostate cancer screening have not yet been adequately characterized.[250] Authors of both studies conclude that population screening should not be implemented at present.[248,249] In accord with existing recommendations, asymptomatic men requesting PSA measurement should be objectively informed of the risks of overdiagnosis and overtreatment and potential adverse side effects before undergoing the test.[238,251,252]

PSA as an Aid to Diagnosis of Prostate Cancer. Men with symptoms suggestive of prostate cancer should be offered a PSA test and a DRE before referral for specialist care. A PSA result within the reference interval does not necessarily exclude prostatic disease, and an increased PSA does not necessarily indicate malignancy. In general, however, the higher the PSA result, the greater the likelihood of prostate cancer, providing prostatitis, urinary tract infection, catheterization, and other possible confounding factors have been excluded.[15,239] Results above the upper limit of the reference interval but less than 10 μg/L are considered to be within a "gray zone" where additional testing (eg, percent free PSA) may be implemented in some centers before proceeding to biopsy. A second specimen to confirm a raised PSA result is always desirable. Whether PSA velocity can helpfully contribute to diagnosis remains controversial.[245,253-255] After recent reviews of available evidence, it has been concluded that high PSA velocity is not an indication for biopsy and that men with an indication for biopsy (ie, PSA above the relevant threshold) should be biopsied irrespective of PSA velocity.[245] Men with PSA below biopsy thresholds but with high PSA velocity should be offered repeat PSA measurement at a shorter time interval.

In most cases diagnosis requires prostatic biopsy and pathological confirmation, but this may not be essential if clinical suspicion of malignancy is high, there is evidence of bone metastases, and the PSA concentration is clearly increased (eg, >100 μg/L). Prior to any prostatic biopsy, the benefits and potential side effects and the caveats associated with PSA measurement should be discussed with the patient, and individual risk factors (eg, age and ethnicity) and comorbidities should be carefully considered.

PSA in Prognosis and Therapy Prediction of Prostate Cancer. In patients with immunohistochemically confirmed prostate cancer, treatment depends on whether the disease is confined to the prostate or has spread to other organs, so accurate pretreatment staging is crucial. The pretreatment serum PSA value correlates with the risk of extraprostatic extension, seminal vesicle invasion, and lymph node involvement and is an independent predictor of response to all forms of treatment.[256] Predictive tables or nomograms are available that combine pretreatment PSA concentrations with information on clinical stage and the immunohistochemical Gleason score, which assesses the degree of cellular differentiation in the prostate tissue examined and ranges from 2 in well-differentiated tumors to 10 in completely anaplastic tumors.

Such nomograms can provide a reasonable indication of whether disease is localized to the prostate and aid in predicting treatment outcome. For example, a patient with a PSA of less than 10 μg/L and a Gleason score of 6 or lower is unlikely to have metastatic disease, so pelvic lymph node dissection may not be necessary,[256] and treatment options will include radical prostatectomy, localized radiotherapy, or active surveillance, as described above. It is important to note that if the algorithm includes both total PSA and free PSA measurements, these results must be obtained using paired methods, as described above. Algorithms may also be method-specific, in which case it is also essential to ensure that the algorithm used is appropriate.

Pretreatment PSA concentrations can also be used to assess whether bone, CT, and/or MRI scans are likely to be helpful for staging asymptomatic men with localized prostate cancer. Bone scans are generally not necessary in patients with newly diagnosed prostate cancer who have a PSA of less than 20.0 μg/L, unless history or clinical examination suggests bony involvement and/or if the patient has a Gleason score of greater than 8 or Stage T3 or higher prostate cancer.[256] Similarly, although supporting evidence is sparse, CT is rarely positive when the pretreatment PSA concentration is less than 20.0 μg/L, unless disease is locally advanced or the Gleason score is 8 or higher.[256]

Following radical prostatectomy, PSA should decrease to and remain at undetectable concentrations, with measurable concentrations indicative of residual disease or possibly the presence of benign glands. The American Urological Association (AUA) defines biochemical recurrence as an initial postprostatectomy PSA value of 0.2 μg/L or higher, followed by a subsequent confirmatory value but cautions that a cutpoint of 0.4 μg/L may be better for predicting the risk of metastatic relapse.[256] However, because the median interval from PSA recurrence to cancer death is between 5 and 12 years (depending on the Gleason score and PSA velocity), such an increase indicates risk of recurrence but not necessarily need for initiation of treatment. The utility of "ultrasensitive" PSA methods is not yet established, in part due to considerable variation in results at very low concentrations.

The rate of fall is likely to be slower in patients who have received radiotherapy, and PSA rarely falls to less than 0.2 μg/L because not all prostate tissue is ablated. However, the level should remain stable. The American Society for Therapeutic Radiation and Oncology (ASTRO) has concluded that any rise in PSA value to 2.0 μg/L or higher and above the nadir predicts true failure with great sensitivity and specificity after both external beam radiotherapy and interstitial prostate brachytherapy whether or not accompanied by androgen deprivation.[256] Establishing "target PSA" concentrations is challenging, especially following interstitial prostate brachytherapy, after which PSA concentrations may continue to decline for more than 5 years. The ASTRO endpoints also cannot be readily compared with results in surgical series.

In patients receiving hormonal therapy, a low nadir after treatment has prognostic significance and can be quantitatively linked to survival. Patients failing to achieve a PSA nadir of less than 4.0 μg/L 7 months after initiation of therapy are associated with very poor prognosis (median survival approximately 1 year), while those achieving a nadir of less than 0.2 μg/L have relatively good prognosis (median survival >6 years).[257] Similar survival differences have been reported in patients with no radiological evidence of metastases who received hormonal therapy in response to a PSA rise following radiological prostatectomy or radiotherapy. Those for whom the PSA nadir is greater than 0.2 μg/L within 8 months of endocrine therapy have a 20-fold greater risk of cancer-specific mortality than those with a PSA nadir of less than 0.2 μg/L.[258]

PSA in Monitoring of Prostate Cancer. A major clinical role for PSA is in evaluating the efficacy of treatment in patients following treatment, with sustained increases in PSA providing objective evidence of disease progression, often months before other diagnostic procedures. Consistently rising PSA usually, although not always, indicates recurrence. There is continuing debate about the magnitude and number of increases required to define biochemical recurrence that are influenced by the type of treatment.[256] An increase in PSA should always be confirmed, taking into account intraindividual biological variation in PSA of up to 20% to 30% before concluding an increase is clinically significant. For patients in whom it can be calculated (ie, those for whom multiple PSA determinations that are unaltered by secondary therapy and separated by sufficient time), PSA doubling time can provide valuable information about the likely time to progression.[259] Patients with a PSA doubling time of greater than 15 months have a low likelihood of prostate cancer–specific mortality over a 10-year period.[260] A stable PSA concentration does not necessarily exclude progression if clinically suspected. In some patients, knowledge of increasing PSA concentrations may have adverse psychological consequences, and monitoring with PSA may be undesirable, particularly if effective alternative treatments are not available.

Testicular Cancer

Germ cell tumors, which are described above, account for more than 90% of testicular tumors in adults. Leydig and Sertoli cell tumors develop in the stroma, the hormone-producing tissue of the testicles, and represent 4% of adult testicular tumors and 20% of childhood tumors. Leydig cell tumors normally produce androgens. They usually do not spread beyond the testicle and can be cured by surgical removal. Those that do spread are usually resistant to both chemotherapy and radiation. Tumors of the Sertoli cells, which normally support sperm-producing cells, are very similar to Leydig cell tumors and are also difficult to treat if they spread beyond the testes. As for granulosa cell tumors of the ovary, the marker of choice for both Sertoli and Leydig cell tumors is inhibin, and the same analytical requirements apply.

Thyroid Cancer

Thyroid cancers represent approximately 2% to 4% of cancers in all age groups, with women more than three times more likely to be affected. There are four histological types: papillary, follicular, and anaplastic thyroid cancer and medullary thyroid carcinoma (MTC). The diagnosis is often made when a patient presents to the thyroid clinic with a painless neck lump. Because the major differential diagnosis required is between benign and malignant thyroid nodules, the reader is referred to Chapter 67 for more detailed discussion. The use of the relevant tumor markers is described briefly here.

Tumor Markers Used in the Management of Thyroid Cancers. Papillary and follicular thyroid cancers are differentiated thyroid cancers and can be monitored posttreatment by measuring serum concentrations of thyroglobulin. A large complex glycoprotein synthesized by the follicular cells of the thyroid and stored in the colloid space (see Table 31.6), thyroglobulin is present in benign and malignant thyroid tissue. Its production is stimulated by thyroid-stimulating hormone (TSH), either from the pituitary or by injection of recombinant human TSH. In patients with an intact thyroid, thyroglobulin reflects thyroid volume and injury and also TSH receptor stimulation. It should be undetectable in serum in the absence of thyroid cells.

MTC is a rare and challenging malignancy that often presents as a lump in the neck, with or without metastasis, dysphagia, or systemic effects such as diarrhea or flushing. The 10-year survival is approximately 75%, but patients may survive for many more years, even with a significant tumor burden. Most appropriately managed in specialist centers, medullary thyroid carcinoma has a hereditary component in about 25% of cases and can be associated with multiple endocrine neoplasia (MEN 2b) (see Chapter 63). Germline testing for the RET proto-oncogene distinguishes hereditary from sporadic MTC and should be offered to all patients with a family history consistent with MEN2 or familial MTC. Prophylactic thyroidectomy may be indicated in children, and screening for other endocrine tumors (eg, pheochromocytoma, pituitary, parathyroid) is essential. Calcitonin, a 32-amino acid polypeptide produced by the C cells of the thyroid, is an excellent tumor marker for MTC. CEA is also a very good marker of tumor burden in MTC.

Screening, Diagnosis, and Prognosis. Serum thyroglobulin measurement is not helpful in screening for or diagnosis of thyroid cancer and has no value as a prognostic marker. Basal calcitonin measurements can contribute to the diagnosis of C-cell hyperplasia and MTC. CEA should also be measured preoperatively.

Monitoring. Thyroglobulin has an important role in monitoring patients with papillary or follicular thyroid cancer after treatment with surgery and/or radioiodine. Following either of these treatments, TSH is usually kept suppressed by adjusting the replacement dose of thyroxine in order to minimize the risk of stimulating the growth of any remaining thyroid cancer cells. If TSH is suppressed, serum thyroglobulin should be undetectable following complete ablation, and a rising thyroglobulin over time suggests recurrence. More sensitive assessment of the presence of residual or recurrent tumor can be achieved by measuring plasma thyroglobulin concentration after administering recombinant TSH or withdrawal of thyroxine replacement, although the use of newer thyroglobulin assays with lower analytical sensitivity may avoid the need for these interventions.

Calcitonin and CEA should be measured before surgery and 6 weeks postsurgery. Any increase should be confirmed with an early repeat determination using the same analytical method. Provided the concentrations fall to within reference limits following treatment, annual monitoring may be adequate after the first year.

Analytical and Reporting Requirements for Thyroglobulin. There are several potential pitfalls in thyroglobulin measurement. Analytically, radioimmunoassay and immunometric methods for thyroglobulin are vulnerable to interference from antithyroglobulin autoantibodies that may be present in some patient sera. Results obtained may be falsely low or falsely high, with immunometric methods being particularly prone to giving falsely low results. Appropriate cautions should be added to reports.

Cancers of Unknown Primary

When cancer is found in one or more metastatic sites but the primary site of origin cannot be determined, the diagnosis made is of cancer of unknown primary or occult primary cancer.[261,262] Such cancers account for 2% to 3% of all new cancer diagnoses, with approximately 31,000 cases diagnosed per year in the United States.[263] Symptoms vary according to the sites of metastases and may include swollen lymph nodes, abdominal mass, shortness of breath, pain in the chest or abdomen, bone pain, skin tumors, anemia, weakness, fatigue, poor appetite, and/or weight loss. The average survival time is about 9 to 12 months after diagnosis.

Routine clinical investigations to demonstrate the organ of origin are generally unproductive, with an approximate 30% rate of identification that has not been associated with significant improvement in survival.[262] However, for a small subset of patients with cancer of unknown primary (possibly <1%), tumor marker measurements can contribute to diagnosis of an unsuspected but potentially treatable malignancy that has presented in an atypical manner.[262] These include gestational choriocarcinoma, germ cell tumors of the testis or ovary, prostate cancer, ovarian cancer, and breast cancer.

Tumor Markers Used in the Management of Cancers of Unknown Primary. Measurement of AFP and hCG is recommended in patients with midline metastatic disease (mediastinal nodes or presence of a retroperitoneal mass) to assess the possibility of a germ cell tumor.[264-266] CA125 measurement is recommended in women with symptoms that could be consistent with an occult non–germ cell ovarian malignancy, together with a gynecologic-oncologic consultation if indicated.[264,266] Men presenting with bone metastases or multiple sites of involvement should have PSA levels assessed.[264-266] Chromogranin A measurement is recommended by ESMO in patients with features of neuroendocrine tumors.[265] Measurement of estrogen and progesterone receptors may identify hormone-sensitive tumors amenable to specific therapy.[265] In patients with suspected origin of malignancy in the pancreas, measurement of CA19-9 is recommended by the NCCN.[266] The usual caveats apply to the use of these tumor markers in diagnosis. If their measurement identifies a likely primary source of malignancy (eg, a germ cell tumor), then monitoring protocols, if required, should be according to protocols previously described for these cancers and tumor markers.

POINTS TO REMEMBER

Tumor Markers

- Carefully used, tumor markers can contribute usefully to patient management, but awareness of their limitations is essential.
- Measurement of tissue markers, including *ALK, BRAF, HER2, KRAS,* and the estrogen and progesterone receptors, informs selection of endocrine and immunotherapy in individual patients in non–small cell lung cancer, melanoma, and/or breast cancer.
- In the management of germ cell tumors, AFP and hCG measurement in serum is mandatory.
- Measurement of CEA in serum is recommended for postoperative follow-up of Stages II and III colorectal cancer patients if further treatment is an option.
- PSA measurement in serum contributes to diagnosis of prostate cancer and may be used for detecting recurrence and monitoring therapy.
- Measurement of serum AFP, CA125, or CA19-9 may, respectively, aid early detection of hepatocellular carcinoma, ovarian cancer, or pancreatic cancer in appropriately selected high-risk patients.
- Opportunistic screening with panels of tumor markers is not helpful.
- Serial results are nearly always more useful than single isolated results because the main application of tumor markers is in monitoring.
- Excellent communication between clinical and laboratory colleagues is essential for optimal use of tumor markers.

CONCLUSION

Tumor marker measurements contribute significantly to the management of cancer patients, but considerable care is required to ensure that their use is appropriate. The clinical laboratory should proactively encourage correct test selection, sample handling, analysis, reporting, and interpretation of tumor marker results, taking particular care to remind users of the caveats associated with these tests. This is essential not only for the well-established tumor markers but also for the new generation of molecular and genetic tumor markers on which clinicians increasingly will rely to provide optimal care. Involvement of laboratorians in developing clinical pathways that will enable optimal use of tumor markers—both the well-established and the newly developing—in routine practice provides new and exciting challenges that clinical laboratories are well positioned to meet.

SELECTED REFERENCES

For a full list of references for this chapter, please refer to ExpertConsult.com.

21. Sturgeon CM, Duffy MJ, Stenman UH, et al. National Academy of Clinical Biochemistry laboratory medicine practice guidelines for use of tumor markers in testicular, prostate, colorectal, breast, and ovarian cancers. *Clin Chem* 2008;**54**:e11–79.
22. Sturgeon CM, Duffy MJ, Hofmann BR, et al. National Academy of Clinical Biochemistry Laboratory Medicine Practice Guidelines for use of tumor markers in liver, bladder, cervical, and gastric cancers. *Clin Chem* 2010;**56**: e1–48.
23. Duffy MJ, Sturgeon CM, Sölétormos G, et al. Validation of New Cancer Biomarkers: A Position Statement from the European Group on Tumor Markers. *Clin Chem* 2015;**61**: 809–20.
27. McShane LM, Cavenagh MM, Lively TG, et al. Criteria for the use of omics-based predictors in clinical trials: Explanation and elaboration. *BMC Med* 2013;**11**:220.
37. Sölétormos G, Duffy MJ, Hayes DF, et al. Design of tumor biomarker-monitoring trials: a proposal by the European Group on Tumor Markers. *Clin Chem* 2013;**59**:52–9.
41. Sturgeon CM, Lai LC, Duffy MJ. Serum tumour markers: how to order and interpret them. *BMJ* 2009;**339**:b3527.
88. Harris L, Fritsche H, Mennel R, et al. American Society of Clinical Oncology 2007 Update of Recommendations for the Use of Tumor Markers in Breast Cancer. *J Clin Oncol* 2007;**25**:5287–312.
98. Henry NL, Hayes DF, Ramsey SD, et al. Promoting quality and evidence-based care in early-stage breast cancer follow-up. *J Natl Cancer Inst* 2014;**106**:dju034.
113. Allison JE, Fraser CG, Halloran SP, et al. Population screening for colorectal cancer means getting FIT: the past, present, and future of colorectal cancer screening using the fecal immunochemical test for hemoglobin (FIT). *Gut Liver* 2014;**8**:117–30.
120. Duffy MJ, Lamerz R, Haglund C, et al. Tumor markers in colorectal cancer, gastric cancer and gastrointestinal stromal cancers: European group on tumor markers 2014 guidelines update. *Int J Cancer* 2014;**134**:2513–22.
156. Sinn DH, Yi J, Choi MS, et al. Serum alpha-fetoprotein may have a significant role in the surveillance of hepatocellular carcinoma in hepatitis B endemic areas. *Hepatogastroenterology* 2015;**62**:327–32.
162. Dalton-Fitzgerald E, Tiro J, Kandunoori P, et al. Practice patterns and attitudes of primary care providers and barriers to surveillance of hepatocellular carcinoma in patients with cirrhosis. *Clin Gastroenterol Hepatol* 2015;**13**:791–8 e1.
177. Duffy MJ, Crown J. Companion biomarkers: paving the pathway to personalized treatment for cancer. *Clin Chem* 2013;**59**:1447–56.
178. Rekhtman N, Leighl NB, Somerfield MR. Molecular testing for selection of patients with lung cancer for epidermal growth factor receptor and anaplastic lymphoma kinase tyrosine kinase inhibitors: American Society of Clinical Oncology endorsement of the College of American Pathologists/International Association for the Study of Lung Cancer/Association for Molecular Pathology Guideline. *J Oncol Pract* 2015;**11**:135–6.
185. Sundar S, Neal RD, Kehoe S. Diagnosis of ovarian cancer. *BMJ* 2015;**351**:h4443.
200. National Comprehensive Cancer Network (NCCN) Clinical Practice Guidelines in Oncology: Genetic/familial high-risk assessment: Breast and ovarian. Version 2. 2015. <http://www.nccn.org/professionals/physician_gls/PDF/genetics_screening.pdf>.
239. Price CP, Allard J, Davies G, et al. Pre-and post-analytical factors that may influence use of serum prostate specific

antigen and its isoforms in a screening programme for prostate cancer. *Ann Clin Biochem* 2001;**38**: 188–216.

256. Carroll P, Albertsen PC, Greene K, et al. *AUA University. PSA testing for the pre-treatment staging and post-treatment management of prostate cancer: 2013 revision of 2009 Best Practice Statement., Vol.* Linthicum, Maryland: American Urological Association; 2013.

275. Rajkumar SV, Dimopoulos MA, Palumbo A, et al. International Myeloma Working Group updated criteria for the diagnosis of multiple myeloma. *Lancet Oncol* 2014;**15**: e538–4.

32

Kidney Function Tests

*Edmund J. Lamb and Graham R.D. Jones**

ABSTRACT

Background
The functional unit of the kidney is the nephron. In nearly all types of renal disease, impaired function of the kidneys is attributed to a diminished number of functioning nephrons rather than to compromised function of individual nephrons. Because glomerular filtration is the initiating phase of all nephron functions, quantitative or qualitative assessment of the glomerular filtration rate (GFR), or some variable that bears a reasonably constant relationship to it, together with assessment of the integrity of the filtration barrier, generally provides the most useful indices for physicians to assess the severity and progress of kidney damage.

Content
This chapter describes tests that have proved the most practical and useful for screening for and diagnosing impaired kidney function in clinical laboratories and for assessing the severity and monitoring the course and management of chronic kidney disease (CKD). Classification of CKD is primarily based upon measures of GFR and proteinuria/albuminuria and of acute kidney injury (AKI) upon serum creatinine and urine output. This chapter discusses the contemporary use of kidney function tests to facilitate diagnosis and classification, including their biochemistry and physiology, analytical procedures, and clinical utility.

INTRODUCTION

The functional unit of the kidney is the nephron, with each kidney containing between 0.4 and 1.2 million nephrons. In nearly all types of renal disease, impaired function of the kidneys is attributed to a diminished number of functioning nephrons rather than to compromised function of individual nephrons. Because glomerular filtration is the initiating phase of all nephron functions, quantitative or qualitative assessment of the glomerular filtration rate (GFR)—or some variable that bears a reasonably constant relationship to it—and assessment of the integrity of the filtration barrier generally provide the most useful indices for physicians to assess the severity and progress of kidney damage.

Defects or changes in particular functions of the nephrons can also be identified and evaluated. For example, assessment of the maximum concentrating capacity of the kidneys gives an estimate of vasopressin (antidiuretic or ADH)-controlled reabsorption of solute-free water in the distal portion of the tubule. Pinpoint defects, caused by genetic deficiencies of specific tubular transport systems or ion channels that give rise to characteristic biochemical disorders, are considered in Chapter 59.

This chapter discusses the tests that have proved most practical and useful for screening and diagnosing impaired kidney function in clinical laboratories and for monitoring the course and management of progressive chronic kidney disease (CKD). In general, where blood markers are discussed, either heparinized plasma or serum can be used for most of these tests. The term *serum* is used throughout the chapter. The classification systems for both CKD and acute kidney injury (AKI) are described in detail in Chapter 59. Classification of CKD is primarily based upon measures of GFR and proteinuria/albuminuria and of AKI upon serum creatinine and urine output. This chapter describes the contemporary use of kidney function tests to facilitate diagnosis and classification, including their biochemistry and physiology, analytical procedures and clinical utility. The chapter starts with the commonly used urine reagent strip tests, then describes the individual analytes often measured for assessment of renal function, and finally concludes with a description of ways to determine the GFR.

URINE ANALYSIS

Examination of the urine is often the first step in the assessment of a patient suspected of having or confirmed as having deterioration in kidney function. The appearance (color and odor) of urine itself can be helpful; a darkening from the pale normal straw color indicates more concentrated urine or the

*Data on current creatinine method usage in the United Kingdom were provided by Finlay Mackenzie from the United Kingdom National External Quality Assessment Scheme, Birmingham, United Kingdom. Further information about the UKNEQAS estimated GFR scheme may be found at www.bimingh amquality.org.uk. We are grateful to the College of American Pathologists and the Royal College of Pathologists of Australasia Quality Assurance Program for data on current creatinine method usage and performance in the United States and Australasia, respectively. We also acknowledge the input of Professor Christopher Price to previous editions of this chapter.

presence of another pigment. Hemoglobin and myoglobin can give a pink-red-brown coloration, depending on the concentration. Turbidity in a fresh sample may indicate infection but also may be due to fat particles in a patient with nephrotic syndrome or, rarely, chyluria. Excessive foaming of urine when shaken suggests proteinuria. Very unusual colors may be seen in response to treatment with some medications or in certain diseases (eg, black urine in alkaptonuria). Urine is often evaluated via point-of-care testing either using reagent strips or via microscopic examination.

Reagent Strip ("Dipstick") Testing

Over the years, many tests of renal significance have been adapted for use on strips of cellulose or pads of cellulose or strips of plastic that have been coated or impregnated with reagents for the analyte in question. This type of analytical test is commonly known as a "dipstick" test. A reagent strip may contain reagents for just one test per stick or reagents for multiple tests on a single stick. With this type of test, the different methods detect substances that may overflow from plasma into the urine, such as glucose, ketones, bilirubin diglucuronate, and urobilinogen, changes in the concentration of which reflect a change in organ systems in the body. These tests can also detect changes in constituents that are linked to alterations brought about by a pathological condition affecting the kidney or urinary tract. These include tests for urine protein or albumin, pH, nitrite, specific gravity, and hemoglobin. Urine samples for reagent strip testing should be collected in sterile containers, and testing should be performed on the fresh urine unless delayed measurement has been validated. As with all laboratory tests, the preanalytical factors of timing of collection, patient preparation, and sample handling must be considered.[1] Reagent strips should be used only if they have been stored properly desiccated because they can deteriorate in a matter of hours. Specific attention to timing and assessment of color change must be monitored; timing can significantly differ between analytes (eg, from 30 seconds to 2 minutes). Reagent strips are available from a number of different manufacturers: Concentrations associated with the semiquantitative results determined from the color charts supplied with the strips are not always comparable among manufacturers, which can make direct comparison of performance difficult.

In addition to manual reading of reagent strips, automated readers have come into routine use, including devices designed for use at the point of care and within the laboratory.[2] These automated instruments may have additional features such as cell and other particle counting facilities based on flow cytometry (see Chapter 25) or automated microscopy.[3]

The use of an automated reader can reduce interoperator variability and improve diagnostic accuracy,[4-7] as well as perform calculations based on the result (eg, calculate a protein to creatinine ratio). Additionally, some automated readers provide results on a continuous scale as opposed to the semiquantitative results that are obtained from visual reading of reagent strips. The manual and automated methods use the same reagent strips (strips and readers must come from the same manufacturer); therefore, the understanding of testing methodology and limitations is the same, irrespective of the reading mechanism. However, with laboratory-based analysis the stability of the sample for each of the tests must be considered.

Examples of the method principles and comments on the performance of tests pertinent to the assessment of kidney function are given in the following sections.

Total Protein

Proteinuria is a cardinal sign of kidney disease. Although not all patients with CKD will have proteinuria, it is a common finding in those patients, and its presence suggests a poorer prognosis in a concentration-dependent manner.[8-12] Use of a reagent strip assay has been considered an important initial test in any patient suspected of having renal disease. Among patients with suspected or proven CKD, including reflux nephropathy, and early glomerulonephritis, and those with hypertension or previously detected asymptomatic hematuria, annual urinalysis for proteinuria has been accepted as a useful way of identifying patients at risk of progressive kidney disease. Often the findings of proteinuria and/or hematuria are incidental when urine is being subjected to testing by multitest reagent strip devices for another purpose (Fig. 32.1). Currently no proven role has been identified for reagent strip protein analysis in the screening of unselected populations.[13,14] For many years, reagent strip testing for proteinuria was deemed inadequate for the detection of CKD among patients with diabetes, in whom urinary albumin loss should be measured specifically (see later). Growing consensus suggests that reagent strip testing is also inadequate in other clinical scenarios. Clinical interpretation of urinary protein measurements, including by reagent strip devices, is discussed later in this chapter (see the "Quantitative Assessment of Proteinuria" section).

The reagent strip test for total protein includes a cellulose test pad impregnated with tetrabromphenol blue and a citrate buffer (pH3). The reaction is based on the "protein error of indicators" phenomenon by which certain chemical indicators demonstrate one color in the presence of protein and another in its absence. Thus tetrabromphenol blue is green in the presence of protein at pH 3 but yellow in its absence. The test has a lower detection limit of 150 to 300 mg/L, depending on the type and proportions of protein present. The reagent is most sensitive to albumin and less sensitive to globulins, Bence Jones protein, mucoproteins, and hemoglobin.[15-17] Indeed, it is confusing to note that one commercial application of this principle has been manufactured as Albustix, although the chemical principle underlying this test is identical to those of devices that claim to measure "protein."[15]

A creatinine test pad (using the peroxidase-like activity of transition metal creatinine complexes) has been added to some reagent strip systems that, with the appropriate automated device, can enable a protein-to-creatinine ratio (PCR) to be reported, thereby reducing the within-subject variation seen with random urine collections. An evaluation of one such device (Multistix PRO 10LS; Siemens Medical Solutions, Tarrytown, New York) read semiquantitatively on the Clinitek Status automated strip reader (Siemens) in a renal outpatient setting concluded that the test was suitable for ruling out significant proteinuria (>0.3 g/day).[18]

Albumin

Reagent strip methods are available for the more specific detection of albumin at low concentrations (ie, in the approximate range 20–200 mg/L). Both colorimetric and immunological methods for detecting albumin have been described

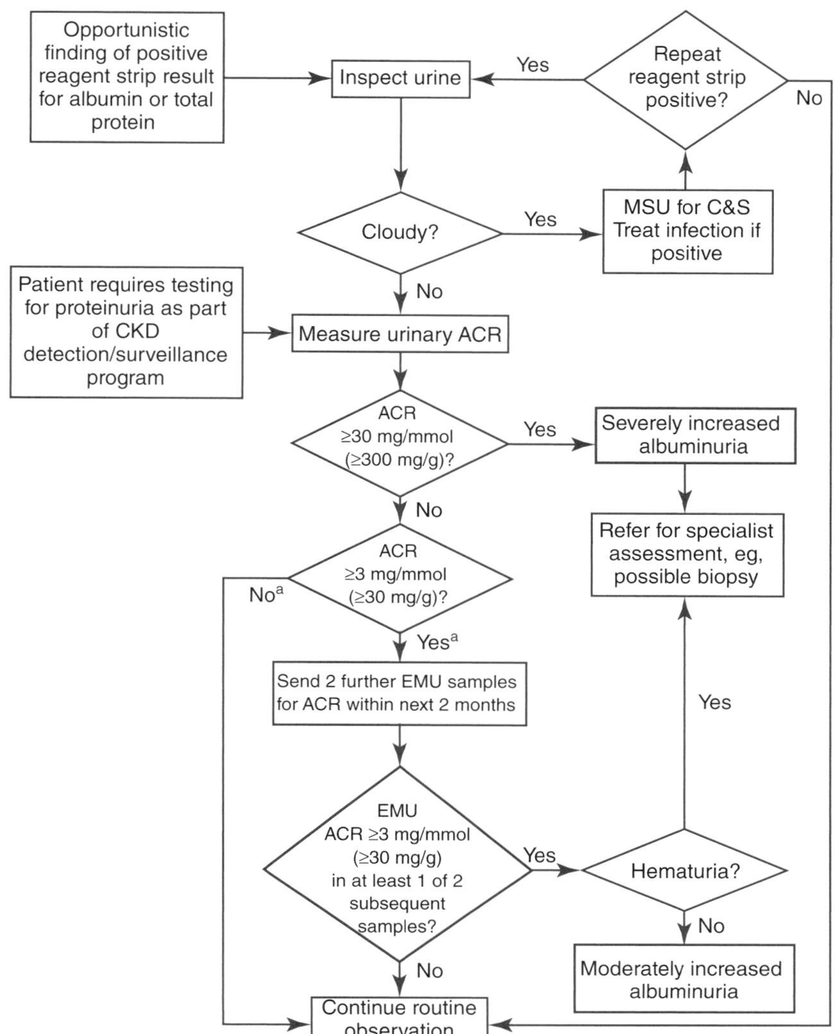

FIGURE 32.1 Suggested protocol for the further investigation of an individual demonstrating a positive reagent strip test for albuminuria/proteinuria or quantitative albuminuria/proteinuria test. Reagent strip device results should be confirmed using laboratory testing of the albumin-to-creatinine ratio (ACR) on at least two further occasions. Patients with two or more positive (≥3 mg albumin/mmol creatinine) tests on early morning samples 1 to 2 weeks apart should be diagnosed as having persistent albuminuria. (The possibility of postural proteinuria should be excluded by the examination of an early morning urine.) Protein-to-creatinine ratio (PCR) measurement can be substituted for the ACR but is insensitive in the detection of moderately increased albuminuria/proteinuria: Approximate PCR equivalent to an ACR of 30 mg/mmol is 50 mg/mmol. [a]Consider other causes of increased ACR (eg, menstrual contamination, uncontrolled hypertension, symptomatic urinary tract infection, heart failure, other transitory illnesses and strenuous exercise), especially in the case of type 1 diabetes present for less than 5 years. The presence of hematuria may indicate nondiabetic renal disease. *Note:* US guidelines express albuminuria or proteinuria as mg/g creatinine, whereas other guidelines use mg/mmol creatinine. An approximate conversion factor of 0.1136 can be used to convert results in mg/g to mg/mmol. However, for clarity and pragmatism, recent guidelines have accepted decision points that are approximately equivalent: hence, when using this protocol in the US, 300 mg/g should be substituted for 30 mg/mmol and 30 mg/g for 3 mg/mmol.[57] *ACR,* Albumin-to-creatinine ratio; *C&S,* culture and sensitivity; *CKD,* chronic kidney disease; *EMU,* early morning urine; *MSU,* midstream urine.

for use with urine samples, the former based on binding of bis(3′,3″-diiodo-4′,4″-hydroxy-5′,5″-dinitrophenyl)-3,4,5,6-tetrabromosulfonephthalein (DIDNTB) at pH 1.5.[19] Examples include the Clinitek Microalbumin reagent strip read on a Clinitek Status analyzer (both Siemens), which produces semiquantitative albumin and albumin-to-creatinine ratio (ACR) results, and the Micral reagent strip (Roche Diagnostics), which provides a visual result for albumin alone. Other point-of-care devices that provide a similar service are available, although they use technology other than the usual reagent strips—for example, the DCA Vantage (Siemens) and the Afinion (Axis Shield) devices, which are capable of reporting fully quantitative ACR results. Reasonable analytical performance has been demonstrated.[20-22] Diagnostic performance has been reported in several settings.[23] Sensitivity of the Clinitek semiquantitative device for albuminuria detection does not achieve the 95% level deemed acceptable by the American Association for Clinical Chemistry and the American Diabetes Association,[24] whereas the fully quantitative DCA device achieves this criterion.[23,25,26]

Hemoglobin

The presence of hemoglobin in the urine may be due to glomerular, tubulointerstitial, or postrenal disease, although the latter two causes are the more common. The presence of blood in the urine can be detected by using a phase contrast microscope to determine the presence of red cells in the urine sediment or by using a reagent strip test. Chemical detection of hemoglobin in urine depends on the peroxidase activity of the protein employing a peroxide substrate and an oxygen acceptor.

For this test, the reagent pad is impregnated with buffered tetramethyl benzidine (TMB) and an organic peroxide. The method depends on detection of the peroxidase activity of hemoglobin, which catalyzes the reaction of cumene hydroperoxide and TMB. The color change ranges from orange to pale to dark green, and red cells or free hemoglobin are detected together with myoglobin. Two reagent pads are used for the low hemoglobin level; if intact red cells are present, the low-level pad will have a speckled appearance, with a solid color indicating hemolyzed red cells. The presence of intact red cells is consistent with a source of bleeding in the urinary tract, although the survival of intact red cells is dependent on the tonicity of the urine. Free hemoglobin can be seen with intravascular hemolysis as well as bleeding in the renal tract. The detection limit for free hemoglobin is 150 to 600 μg/L or 5 to 20 intact red cells/μL. The test is equally sensitive to hemoglobin and myoglobin, and thus a negative result excludes myoglobinuria. Water must not be used as a negative control with this test because of the matrix requirements of the assay: A false-positive result will be obtained.

The presence of free hemoglobin or red cells in the urine indicates the presence of renal or bladder disease. Hematuria can be present in a range of kidney diseases, including glomerular nephritis, polycystic kidney disease, sickle cell disease, vasculitis, and a range of infections. A spectrum of urologic diseases may also give rise to hematuria, including bladder, prostate, and pelvic and/or ureteral malignancy, kidney stones, trauma, bladder damage, and ureteral stricture. The presence of persistent hematuria is a marker of potential CKD. At present, reagent strips are the only routine method for determining hematuria. While requests for urine ACR are recommended for investigation and staging of CKD, the use of reagent strips for hemoglobin in this context is less common.

Glucose

Glucose appears in urine when the tubular maximal resorptive capacity is exceeded; typically this occurs at a blood glucose concentration of approximately 180 mg/dL (10 mmol/L), although this is highly variable. The test can therefore provide an indication of the presence of hyperglycemia during the time the urine was produced. However, while a positive result for urine glucose supports a diagnosis of diabetes mellitus, it plays no role in the diagnostic criteria for the disease. Due to variability in the tubular resorption of both water and glucose, urine glucose cannot be used to estimate plasma glucose concentration.

For glucose measurements, the reagent pad is impregnated with glucose oxidase, peroxidase, potassium iodide, and a blue dye. The reaction employs glucose oxidase and peroxidase to produce hydrogen peroxide, which is subsequently reduced with concurrent oxidation of potassium iodide to release iodine. The free iodine blends with the background color to produce a range of colors from green to dark brown. The detection limit of this method is in the range of 72 to 127 mg/dL (4–7 mmol/L), with an upper limit of 2018 mg/dL (111 mmol/L).

Leukocytes and Nitrite

The presence of leukocyte esterase is indicative of pyuria (ie, the presence of white blood cells in the urine; significant pyuria is normally defined as a urinary white cell count of 10 leukocytes/mL or greater). The detection of nitrite is indicative of the presence of bacteria that degrade nitrate excreted in the urine. The combination of the two tests is valuable in patients with urinary tract infections (UTI). The absence of both constituents is a valuable test to "rule out" UTI, thereby reducing the number of samples sent to the laboratory for additional tests.[27,28] The nitrite test may be less helpful in young children, in whom the urine remains in the bladder for less time, thereby limiting the time for nitrite production.

The reagent strip test for leukocytes uses an absorbent cellulose pad impregnated with a buffered mixture of derivatized pyrrole amino acid ester and diazonium salt. Granulocytic leukocytes contain esterases, which catalyze the hydrolysis of the derivatized pyrrole amino acid ester to liberate 3-hydroxy-5-phenylpyrrole. This pyrrole then reacts with a diazonium salt to produce a purple product. The test is claimed to have a detection limit of 5 to 15 cells/μL in urine, and the darkest color block is equivalent to 500 cells/μL or greater. A decrease in the true test result may occur in samples with increased glucose concentration, high specific gravity, or in the presence of cephaloxin, cephalothin, tetracycline, or high concentrations of oxalic acid.

To measure nitrite, the reagent pad is impregnated with *p*-arsanilic acid and tetrahydro-benzo(h)quinolin-3-ol. The reaction is based on arsanilic acid in the presence of nitrite converting to a diazonium salt, which couples with the quinolol to produce a pink color. The detection limit of the test is 61 to 103 μg/dL (13–22 μmol/L) nitrite in urine with a normal specific gravity. The test is less sensitive with urine that has a high specific gravity. At urine ascorbic acid concentrations above approximately 25 mg/dL (1.4 mmol/L), a false-negative result may occur at low nitrite values (81 μg/dL [13 μmol/L] or less). The test measures only nitrite and is claimed to detect populations of bacteria at a level of 10^5/mL or more.

Specific Gravity

The specific gravity test correlates with osmolality and can provide a bedside indication of the concentration of urine. The test device for specific gravity consists of an absorbent cellulose pad impregnated with bromthymol blue, polymethylvinyl ether, and/or maleic anhydride and sodium hydroxide. The test depends on the apparent pK_a change of the pretreated polyelectrolyte in relation to ionic strength; the hydrogen ions released are detected by the pH indicator. The color changes from a dark blue at low specific gravity (1.000) to yellow-green at a specific gravity of 1.030. While specific gravity performed on routine clinical samples using a laboratory analyzer shows a high correlation with urine osmolality, a urine reagent strip result, with either automated or triplicate visual reading, showed only limited correlation with the laboratory test.[29] Laboratory-based testing showed different responses to different solutes,[30] especially with devices that detect ionic species and lead to an underestimation of specific gravity in the presence of glucose. Caution with interpretations should also be considered for urine collected after intravenous administration of iodine-containing radiopaque compounds for radiologic studies that could give extraordinarily high values.[30] Glucose and protein may also contribute substantial increments to the density of urine, and semiquantitative determination of these substances is necessary for valid interpretation or correction of urine specific gravity measurements. Diabetic patients with uncontrolled hyperglycemia and glucosuria may have high urine specific gravity even when the normal renal concentrating function is seriously impaired. For assessment of urine concentration, measurement of osmolality is the preferred method.

pH

Measurement of urine pH can be helpful in the assessment of patients with renal tubular acidosis and in stone formers, although evaluation using a pH electrode may be more informative. To measure the pH of a sample, the test pad is impregnated with indicators, one example being a mixture of methyl red and bromthymol blue. Methyl red in a diluted form is red at pH values below 4.2 and yellow at values above 6.2. Bromthymol blue is yellow at pH values below 6.0 and blue at values above 7.6. At pHs within these values, the indicators give shades of orange and green, respectively. Thus the reagent blocks are compared with a color chart where the lowest pH block at 5.0 is orange in color and the highest at 8.5 is blue. It is important to recognize that the pH of urine as well as the color of the testing strip can change after collection; therefore careful adherence to the recommended procedure is important.

Microscopic Examination of Urine

Microscopic examination of the sediment obtained from the centrifugation of a fresh urine sample shows the presence of a few cells (erythrocytes, leukocytes, and cells derived from the kidney and urinary tract), casts (composed predominantly of Tamm-Horsfall glycoprotein [THG]), and possibly fat or pigmented particles. An increase in red cells or casts implies hematuria possibly caused by glomerular disease; white cells or casts imply the presence of white cells in the tubules. Inflammation of the upper urinary tract may result in polymorphonuclear leukocytes and various types of casts; in lower urinary tract inflammation the casts are not present. In acute glomerulonephritis, hematuria may lead to coloration of the urine and the presence of large numbers of red cells and white cells; as the duration of the disease increases, the amount of sediment diminishes. Nephrologists often describe urine as "bland" or as having an "active urinary sediment." Having an active urinary sediment means that red blood cells, white blood cells, and casts associated with active kidney inflammation can be detected when urine is examined under the microscope.

New Instrumental Techniques

Flow cytometry and flow imaging systems have been developed for the characterization of erythrocytes in the differential diagnosis of hematuria and as a means of improving the recognition of other particulate material in urine. This form of analysis can be used to discriminate between and quantify the particulate matter in a defined volume of urine, bringing the added benefit of better standardization of the technique.[31] Thus the flow imaging method can identify red blood cells, white blood cells, white blood cell clumps, hyaline casts, pathological casts, squamous epithelial cells, nonsquamous epithelial cells, yeast, crystals, and sperm. As stated earlier, these have been combined with automated readers, and these systems have the potential to replace urinary microscopy because they offer better discriminatory power and quantitation, while providing closer agreement among laboratories.[32] The principles of flow cytometry are described in Chapter 25. A flow imaging analyzer, such as the Iris iQ200 (Iris Diagnostics, Chatsworth, California), analyzes unspun urine by aspirating the sample through a flowcell positioned in a microscope. A digital camera captures the images, and neural network-based particle image recognition software is used to identify and count the particles present from five hundred 884 × 680 μm fields with 0.68 μm resolution. The number of particles for the volume scanned is then calculated. Flow image analysis has been shown to be more accurate than the flow cytometric approach, and it helps to improve workflow and save valuable technologist time by reducing the number of manual microscopic examinations required.[33,34] However, it has been suggested that manual microscopy may still be required for the assessment of crystals.[35]

Proton nuclear magnetic resonance (NMR) has also been investigated as a means of characterizing low molecular weight molecules.[36] Metabolic profiles have been generated, and with the use of sophisticated computer analysis, distinctive patterns of molecules have been associated with damage to specific parts of the nephron. It is expected that this technique will be used to identify individual molecules for which selective assays can then be developed.[36]

QUANTITATIVE ASSESSMENT OF PROTEINURIA: TOTAL PROTEIN AND ALBUMIN

Higher molecular weight proteins are retained within the circulation by the glomerular filter, and lower molecular weight proteins are freely filtered and reabsorbed and catabolized within the tubular cells. Consequently, the appearance of notable amounts of protein in the urine suggests renal disease. The association between kidney disease and proteinuria dates to at least as far back as the early 19th century, when Bright first described albuminous nephritis.[37] Proteinuria can be classified as either tubular or glomerular, depending on the pattern of proteinuria observed (see Chapter 59). A third category, overflow proteinuria, is also recognized in which filtration of excessive amounts of low molecular weight protein exceeds the tubular capacity for reabsorption (Table 32.1). Examples of the latter include Bence Jones proteinuria and myoglobinuria. Proteinuria is a potent risk marker for progressive kidney disease, and reduction of protein excretion is a therapeutic target. This section considers the analytical approach and the rationale used in the quantitation of

TABLE 32.1 Characterization of Proteinuria

Type of Proteinuria	Causes	Examples of Proteins Seen
Glomerular	Increased glomerular permeability	Progressively increasing loss of higher molecular weight proteins as permeability increases (eg, albumin, IgG)
Overflow	Increased plasma concentration of relatively freely filtered protein	Bence Jones protein Lysozyme Myoglobin
Tubular	Proximal tubular damage: decreased tubular reabsorptive capacity and/or release of intracellular components (eg, due to nephrotoxic drugs)	α_1-microglobulin β_2-microglobulin Retinol binding protein Enzymuria (eg, *N*-acetyl-β-d-glucosaminidase, alkaline phosphatase, α-glutathione-S-transferase)
	Decreased nephron number: increased filtered load per nephron	As above
	Distal tubular damage	Tamm-Horsfall glycoprotein π-glutathione-S-transferase

urinary proteins, with emphasis on total protein and albumin measurement.

Sample Collection for Total Protein and Albumin Measurement

Extensive discussion is provided in the literature about the appropriate urine sample to use for the investigation of urinary protein loss. It is generally recognized that a 24-hour sample is the definitive means of demonstrating and quantifying the presence of proteinuria. However, overnight, first void in the morning (early morning urine [EMU]), second void in the morning, or random sample collections have also been used. Because creatinine excretion in the urine is fairly constant throughout the 24-hour period, measurement of the ACR or PCR allows the use of a spot sample, with correction for variations in urinary concentration in an individual,[38,39] but with the addition of some between-person variability due to the rate of creatinine production (see later).

Several authors have recommended use of the PCR on a spot sample based on its excellent diagnostic performance and the good correlation that has been demonstrated with the 24-hour collection.[4,40-47] Ginsberg and colleagues studied this issue in detail and found little variation in the ratio during the daytime, indicating that the first void and either of the two subsequent collections can give a reliable indication of the 24-hour urine protein loss.[41] Newman and colleagues demonstrated a significant reduction in the within-subject variation (CV_I[†]) in the PCR compared with the protein concentration in random urines collected throughout the day (a mean reduction from 96% to 39%).[48] In a systematic review, random urine PCR was shown to perform better as a test for ruling out significant proteinuria than as a rule-in test; the authors suggested that positive PCR results may still require confirmation with a 24-hour collection.[49]

[†]CV_I values are used throughout this chapter to indicate relative within-subject variation of markers. It should be noted, however, that in many instances, and particularly at higher CV_I values, the distribution is not Gaussian.

A body of literature also supports the use of ACR as a suitable alternative to timed measurement of urine albumin loss.[50-55] However, a recent metaanalysis of the diagnostic performance of urinary ACR and urinary albumin concentration in random urine samples from patients with diabetes, both compared against albumin loss as measured in a 24-hour collection, found no advantage to using the ACR compared to albumin concentration in the spot sample.[56]

Although the gold standard is the accurately timed 24-hour specimen, it is widely accepted that this is a difficult procedure to control effectively, and inaccuracies in urinary collection may contribute to errors in estimation of protein losses. For most purposes, spot urine ACRs (or PCRs) are used in place of 24-hour collections.[57-59] An EMU sample is preferred because it correlates well with 24-hour protein loss and is unaffected by orthostatic (postural) proteinuria.[13] However, a random urine sample is acceptable if no EMU sample is available with a low result excluding proteinuria. If required, daily albumin or protein loss (in mg) can be estimated by multiplying the ACR or PCR (measured in mg/mmol) by a factor of 10 because, although daily excretion of creatinine depends on muscle mass, an average value of 10 mmol creatinine per day can be assumed.[39,60] Some authors have suggested that adjusting ACR for variations in creatinine excretion by taking into account the influence of age, gender, and race improves the ability of ACR to estimate albuminuria[61] (see later). Multiple forms of result presentation may occur due to the use of varying sample types, units, and reporting of ratios, as well as analyte concentrations; it is essential to ensure that the correct reference interval or clinical decision point is applied to results and that there is awareness of the relevant uncertainties when using decision points from one sample type to another (eg, when switching from EMU to a random spot urine or 24-hour sample).

The diagnosis of albuminuria requires the demonstration of increased albumin loss (either increased ACR or increased albumin loss in a timed collection) in at least two out of three urine samples collected in the absence of infection or an acute metabolic crisis (see Fig. 32.1). This recommendation is suggested to avoid errors due to short-term clinical changes in the patient, as well as a response to the very high CV_I in urine albumin and urine protein (for more discussion on biological variability, see Chapter 7).

Establishing the diagnosis of albuminuria or proteinuria has both prognostic and management implications. In the setting of diabetes, the best possible metabolic control should be achieved before patients are examined for albuminuria, and patients should not be screened during other transitory illnesses. Screening should commence 5 years after diagnosis in patients with type 1 diabetes mellitus and at diagnosis in patients with type 2 diabetes without proteinuria, and should continue on an annual basis up to the age of 75 years. Patients demonstrating an ACR of 3.0 mg/mmol or greater should have urine samples sent to the laboratory on two other occasions (ideally within 2 months) for albumin estimation.[57] Patients demonstrating increased ACRs in one or both of these additional samples have persistent albuminuria. It is important to consider other causes of increased albumin loss, including upright posture (orthostatic proteinuria),[62,63] menstrual contamination, vaginal discharge, uncontrolled hypertension, symptomatic UTI,[64] heart failure, and strenuous exercise.[65] Diabetic nephropathy is uncommon in patients who have had type 1 diabetes for less than 5 years, and other causes of kidney disease should be considered.

Samples for urinary albumin (or total protein) measurement may be analyzed fresh, stored at 4°C for up to 1 week, or stored at −70°C for longer periods. Freezing at −20°C appears to result in loss of measurable albumin and is not recommended. For analysis, stored samples should be allowed to reach room temperature and thoroughly mixed prior to testing.[66]

Analytical Methods: Total Protein

Numerous methods can be used for the measurement of protein in urine, including the original Lowry method,[67] turbidimetry after mixing with trichloroacetic or sulfosalicylic acid,[68] turbidimetry with benzethonium chloride (benzyl dimethyl {2-[2-(*p*-1,1,3,3-tetramethyl butylphenoxy) ethoxy]ethyl} ammonium chloride),[69] and dye binding with Coomassie Brilliant Blue,[70] pyrogallol red molybdate,[71] and pyrocatecholviolet-molybdate, which is used in dry-slide applications.

Total protein measurement is more difficult in urine than in serum. The concentration of urinary protein is normally low (100–200 mg/L); large sample-to-sample variation in the amount and composition of proteins is common. The concentration of nonprotein potentially interfering substances is high relative to the protein concentration and is highly variable, and the inorganic ion content is high. All these factors affect the precision and accuracy of the various methods.

Concerns about different responses to different proteins have led to many variants of the published methods. Because of the need for automation, the benzethonium chloride and dye-binding methods have become the most popular in current clinical use.[72] The analytical range of the turbidimetric assays has been of concern, with the equivalent to an "antigen excess" equivalence point being apparent when high protein concentrations give a lower signal because an inadequate amount of denaturant is present relative to protein. This limitation can be overcome by monitoring the rate of turbidity formation.

As with urine reagent strip analysis, turbidimetric and dye binding methods do not provide equal analytical specificity and sensitivity for all proteins. Most approaches tend to react more strongly with albumin than with globulin and other nonalbumin proteins,[68,73,74] although incorporating sodium dodecyl sulfate (SDS) in pyrogallol red reagent is claimed to reduce this issue.[75] Additionally, between-method variation in response to low molecular weight proteins is quite marked, and this may contribute to differences at low total urine protein concentrations.[76] Significant interferences include aminoglycosides,[77] nonvisible hematuria,[78] and infused modified gelatin solutions used as plasma expanders,[79] all of which may falsely increase measured urinary total protein concentration.

Traceability of Urinary Total Protein Measurement

A key difficulty with urine protein assays lies with the different analytical specificity of the assays and consequently the definition of the measurand. As different methods are responding to different properties of proteins and the abundance of these properties varies between the proteins found in urine, the "quantity intended to be measured" is not the same for different assays. In this setting, metrological traceability and standardization of the different assays is not possible. For those reasons, a reference measurement procedure is not listed by the Joint Committee for Traceability in Laboratory Medicine (JCTLM, http://www.bipm.org/jctlm/), and a standardized reference material for urinary total protein is not available. The variety of methods in use means that significant between-laboratory variation is inevitable.[80] This variation tends to diminish at higher concentrations of urinary total protein, presumably in part as albumin becomes the predominant protein and thus reduces the relative between-sample variation. In addition to the methodologic differences between various protein assays, calibration differences have been found to be one of the major determinants of inter-method variability.[72,81,82] Improvements in assay comparability are possible with the use of a "urine protein" calibrator but nonlinearity of the material in different assays and variation in sample protein composition limit this approach.[82] These methodological problems are a major reason why urine albumin is a preferred analyte for assessment of proteinuria.

Analytical Methods: Albumin

Urinary albumin has been measured using immunoassay since the 1960s when the first such assays became available.[83] Urinary albumin is predominantly measured using quantitative immunoturbidimetric or nephelometric approaches capable of detecting albumin at low concentrations. Commercial assays typically have lower limits of quantitation of between 2 and 5 mg/L. Considerable disagreement has been reported between different commercial urinary albumin assays.[84] Due to the wide range of concentrations that may be observed for urine albumin (greater than 100-fold), immunological light scattering methods are falsely low due to a high-dose hook or prozone effect.[85] Solutions to such issues include retesting samples with high total protein concentration and the use of antigen addition protocols.[86]

Dry chemistry systems have been developed for the quantitation of albumin in urine.[87,88] For example, in one such device, the urine albumin laterally flows along a porous matrix through an area containing gold particle–labeled antibodies to albumin. In the presence of albumin, these antibody molecules are neutralized and pass through a portion of the

TABLE 32.2 Characteristics of Some Clinically Important Urinary Proteins

Protein	Mr (kDa)	Free Plasma Concentration (g/L)	Diameter (nm)	pI	Glomerular Sieving Coefficient	Filtered Load >(mg/L)*	Urinary Concentration (mg/L)†	% Reabsorbed
IgG	150	10	5.5	7.3	0.0001	1	0.1	99
Albumin	66	40	3.5	4.7	0.0002	8	5	99
α_1-Microglobulin	31	0.025	2.9	4.5	~0.3	7.5	5	99
Retinol-binding protein	22	0.025	2.1	4.5	~0.7	17.5	0.1	99
Cystatin C	12.8	0.001	3.0	9.2	~0.7	0.7	0.1	99
β_2-Microglobulin	11.8	0.002	1.6	5.6	0.7	1.1	0.1	99

*Concentration in the glomerular filtrate.
†Typical concentrations observed in health.

matrix containing immobilized albumin to a detection zone, where they appear as a pink coloration.[87] Point-of-care testing devices for urinary albumin have been discussed earlier (see the Reagent Strip ["Dipstick"] Testing section).

Traceability of Urinary Albumin Measurement

As for total protein, no JCTLM listed reference measurement procedure or higher order reference material is currently available. A candidate liquid chromatography tandem mass spectrometry (LC/MS-MS) reference measurement procedure and urinary albumin and creatinine reference materials have been developed and are undergoing validation (for additional discussion on LC/MS-MS, see Chapter 17).[89] To date, most urinary albumin assays have been standardized against a serum-based calibrant (ERM-DA-470k/IFCC) distributed by the Institute for Reference Materials and Measurements of the European Commission, as has been recommended by Kidney Disease Improving Global Outcomes (KDIGO).[90] In a recent comparison of 17 commercial assays, the average bias compared with the candidate reference method was generally within ± 20% at 30 mg/L and ± 10% at 300 mg/L.[84] The differences between results from these assays are due to a combination of nonlinearity, imprecision, and some differences in analytical specificity. However, because bias is the major error component, improvements can be achieved by using appropriate reference material. Although intuitively standardization issues should be more easily addressed than those for total protein measurement, albumin is known to undergo polymerization and fragmentation on storage, when freeze-thawed, and when lyophilized.[66,91] Some data have suggested that a significant proportion of albumin present in urine may be nonimmunoreactive,[92-95] although later studies would appear to have refuted this hypothesis as being caused by coeluting proteins in size exclusion high-performance liquid chromatography (HPLC).[96-98]

Reference Intervals, Definitions of *Proteinuria* and *Albuminuria*, and Biological Variability

There is no consistent definition of *proteinuria*. The upper limit of the reference interval‡ for urinary total protein loss varies between 150 and 300 mg/d, depending on the laboratory.[99] Given average daily creatinine excretion of about 10 mmol (0.11 g), an upper limit of normal protein loss of 150 mg/d is equivalent to a urinary PCR of approximately 15 mg/mmol (130 mg/g). The protein in the urine of healthy individuals is made up of albumin (<30 mg/d) and some smaller proteins, together with proteins secreted by the tubules, of which THG (Tamm-Horsfall glycoprotein) predominates (for more discussion on THG, see Chapter 59).[100] Typical concentrations of proteins found in urine are listed in Table 32.2. Readers should note that the units of expression used for ACR and PCR differ depending on whether it is inside or outside the United States.§

Proteinuria is often detected at the point of care using urine reagent strip devices, and clinical proteinuria has sometimes been defined as equivalent to a color change of "+" or greater on the relevant pad on the strip. This equates to approximately 300 mg/L of total protein or a PCR of 50 mg/mmol, or protein loss of approximately 500 mg/d (assuming an average urine volume of 1.5 L/day). Indeed, the limits for proteinuria and albuminuria are best described as clinical decision points because they are generally described or defined by expert groups rather than as the product of formal reference interval studies. For example, although formal reference interval studies have been performed for urine albumin and ACR, the results have been shown to be highly dependent on age, gender, hypertension, obesity, and triglyceride concentration.[101] Additionally population studies demonstrate that urine albumin and the ACR have highly skewed distributions, with the median less than one-fifth the value of the 97.5th percentile, a situation where a large uncertainty would be expected in an estimate of the upper reference interval.

Among patients with diabetes, the classification of diabetic nephropathy has traditionally been based on concentrations of albuminuria (commonly expressed as an ACR). Exact definitions of albuminuria differed among national societies[55] and by gender.[102] For a variety of reasons that will be discussed, this concept has now been simplified and extended to nondiabetic kidney disease. In the international classification

‡Laboratories should verify that these ranges are appropriate for use in their own settings.

§US guidelines express albuminuria or proteinuria as mg/g creatinine, whereas other guidelines use mg/mmol creatinine. A conversion factor of 0.1136 can be used to convert ACR or PCR results in mg/g to mg/mmol (eg, 200 mg/g = 23 mg/mmol, 30 mg/g = 3.4 mg/mmol).

of kidney disease (see Chapter 59), three categories of albuminuria, expressed as an ACR, are recognized: A1 normal to mildly increased, less than 3.0 mg/mmol (approximately equivalent to <30 mg/g); A2 moderately increased, 3 to 30 mg/mmol (approximately equivalent to 30–300 mg/g); and A3 severely increased, greater than 30 mg/mmol (approximately equivalent to ≥300 mg/g).[57] This classification has been broadly accepted in other national guidelines, although in Australasia, gender-specific cut-points of less than 2.5 mg/mmol for men and less than 3.5 mg/mmol for women have been retained.[58,59] The gender differences relate to differences in average creatinine excretion between men and women; however, these differences are small when compared against the considerable within-subject variation (see later).

The KDIGO categories are approximately equivalent to what would have formerly been considered normoalbuminuria, microalbuminuria, and macroalbuminuria (sometimes referred to as "clinical" or "significant" proteinuria), respectively. *Microalbuminuria* is a term that has been widely used to describe an increase in urinary albumin loss above the reference interval for healthy nondiabetic subjects but at a level that is not generally detectable by less sensitive clinical tests such as reagent strips designed to measure total protein. The term *microalbuminuria* is somewhat misleading in that the albumin being measured is identical in form to that circulating in plasma, and the so-called microalbuminuric range refers to increased, not "micro-," albumin losses.[55] Current guidelines do not support the continuing use of this term,[57,59] and the term *albuminuria* is used in this chapter.

The rate of albumin loss is affected by a variety of physiological factors (eg, exercise, posture, time of day), and the variability is such that reliance cannot be placed upon a single estimation.[103] A variety of estimates of the within-person biological variability (CV_I) of urinary albumin loss have been reported, ranging from 4% to 103% (median 33%) when expressed as an ACR. In most studies the CV_I for ACR was lower than other measures of albuminuria.[55,104-109] Howey and colleagues reported that the variability was lowest in EMU samples and could be reduced by expressing the concentration relative to creatinine concentration.[110] It should be noted that reports of the biological variability of total proteinuria are similar to those of albumin. Indeed, the biological variability of ACR explains most of the variability in PCR.[111] Recent studies of the cubulin gene suggest that genetically determined variability in the tubular handling of albumin may contribute to individual variability.[112]

Creatinine excretion is affected by a variety of nonrenal influences, including age and gender; therefore it follows that different cutoffs for ACR (and PCR) may be required in different individuals.[113,114] For example, as creatinine excretion falls with age, ACR rises in the absence of any change in the rate of albumin loss. While it has been suggested that age-related decision points could be used, the lower creatinine is itself a risk predictor and carries some of the prognostic information in the ACR;[115] such limits are not generally used in clinical practice. Similarly, extremes of body muscularity can affect the ACR and PCR, leading to low-range, false-positive results for subjects with very low muscle mass and vice versa. At the population level systematic differences in creatinine excretion with age and sex can affect prevalence estimates, and at the individual level extremes of muscularity can affect diagnosis.

Clinical Significance

The physiology and pathophysiology of renal protein handling and the clinical significance of proteinuria in specific clinical situations are discussed in more detail in Chapter 59; more general considerations follow. Proteinuria may be detected and measured using reagent strip devices or laboratory measurements of either total protein or albumin.

Like most analytes in urine, protein excretion displays considerable biological variability. Because standard urine reagent strips rely on estimation of protein concentration, this in turn depends on hydration or how concentrated the urine sample is; these tests can give only a rough indication of the presence or absence of pathological proteinuria. Ralston and colleagues observed poor specificity for reagent strip analysis in detecting protein loss of 300 mg/d in a rheumatology outpatient population.[44] A pooled analysis of six studies undertaken in obstetric patients reported positive and negative likelihood ratios for "+" protein or greater on reagent strip analysis for predicting 300 mg/d proteinuria as 0.6 (95% CI: 0.5–0.8) and 3.5 (1.7–7.3), respectively,[116] suggesting that reagent strips are not good at ruling in or ruling out significant proteinuria during pregnancy. KDIGO and the National Institute for Health and Care Excellence (NICE) advise against the use of reagent strips to detect proteinuria.[57,59] An evidence-based systematic review undertaken by the US National Academy of Clinical Biochemistry (NACB) recommended against the use of reagent strips when undertaking proteinuria screening.[117] Academy reviewers found no evidence that the use of urine reagent strip testing for proteinuria at the point of care improved patient outcomes; they described significant evidence of a high false-negative rate and poor negative predictive value compared with laboratory testing. The National Kidney Foundation Kidney Disease Outcomes Quality Initiative (NKF-KDOQI), NACB, and NICE concur that these devices may give false-negative results when the urine is dilute.[13,117,118] Most authors agree that positive tests require confirmation by laboratory measurement of the PCR or ACR on an early morning or random urine sample.[13] A suitable protocol for the further investigation of patients found to have proteinuria at screening is given in Fig. 32.1.

In the setting of preeclampsia, proteinuria is generally defined as greater than 300 mg/d or a PCR greater than 30 mg/mmol.[45] Currently there is insufficient evidence to substitute urine albumin measurement for total protein in this setting.[46]

Most commonly, proteinuria reflects albuminuria. Several groups have suggested that urinary total protein measurement can be replaced by urine albumin measurement.[119-122] Strong evidence has linked urinary albumin loss to cardiovascular mortality and kidney disease progression in diabetes.[123] Other evidence suggests that urinary albumin is a more sensitive test to enable detection of glomerular pathology associated with some other systemic diseases, including hypertension and systemic sclerosis.[124,125] In health, relatively small amounts of albumin (<30 mg/d) are lost in the urine. Because of this, and because total protein assays are imprecise at low concentrations, relatively large increases in urine albumin loss can occur without a significant measurable increase in urinary total protein. In a methodologic study of urine from patients attending renal transplant, general nephrology and medicine and obstetric clinics, Newman and colleagues observed increased albumin losses (defined here as ≥25 mg/d) in 63% of samples that were classified as not having increased total protein loss (defined here as ≥250 mg/d).[120] Changes in albumin loss may also reflect overall changes in vascular permeability and therefore may not indicate explicit deterioration in renal function.[126] Concern has been expressed that replacing urinary total protein measurement with albumin measurement may cause tubular proteinuria to be missed.[13,27] Counter to this, it is known that in most situations, tubular proteinuria is also accompanied by albuminuria[121,127] and, furthermore, that an increased PCR in the presence of normal albumin loss may represent a false-positive signal.[128]

Increased urinary albumin loss has been considered a clinically important indicator of deteriorating renal function in diabetic subjects for many years.[129,130] Both European and US diabetes societies recommend regular screening of urinary albumin loss when monitoring type 1 and type 2 diabetes.[102,131-135] This recommendation came as a consequence of the widespread availability of sensitive assays for urinary albumin measurement and effective treatments, validated in large multinational trials, along with detailed cost-benefit analyses in the vanguard of evidence-based medicine. Because large numbers of clinical studies have been performed, guidelines for albuminuria screening in diabetes are now well-established.[102,131,136] The management of albuminuria in the setting of diabetic nephropathy is discussed in Chapter 59.

Increased urinary albumin loss is common among the general population and is not solely attributable to the presence of diabetes. Epidemiological data from the Third National Health and Nutrition Examination Survey (NHANES III) in the United States suggest that the population prevalence of albuminuria is 7.8%.[137] Similar estimates have been reported from population surveys in Australia (6.8%)[138] and the Netherlands (7.2%).[139] In the Netherlands study, after individuals with diabetes and hypertension were excluded, the population prevalence was 6.6%. Among patients with risk factors for CKD, prevalences were notably higher. For example, in the NHANES III study, 28.8% of people with diabetes and 16% of those with hypertension had albuminuria.[137]

In the last decade, strong evidence has emerged linking albuminuria to cardiovascular and noncardiovascular morbidity and mortality in nondiabetic individuals,[139-146] including in the general population,[147] among older people,[148] people with kidney disease,[149] and among others with hypertension.[150] Albuminuria also predicts the development and progression of kidney disease,[151-155] the requirement for renal replacement therapy,[156] and the risk of AKI.[157] Some of the most powerful data comes from metaanalyses undertaken by the CKD Prognosis Consortium demonstrating continuous associations between increasing ACR and subsequent risk of all-cause and cardiovascular mortality,[158] kidney failure, AKI and CKD progression in the general population, and in populations with increased risk for cardiovascular disease; these associations extend down to concentrations of albuminuria previously considered normal (Fig. 32.2).[159-161] These data have provided a powerful stimulus to the classification of kidney disease based on concentrations of albuminuria.[57] In contrast to the situation among the diabetic population, however, little information is currently available concerning the risks and benefits of intervention (eg, with angiotensin-converting-enzyme [ACE] inhibitors or angiotensin receptor blockers [ARBs]) in albuminuric nondiabetic individuals.

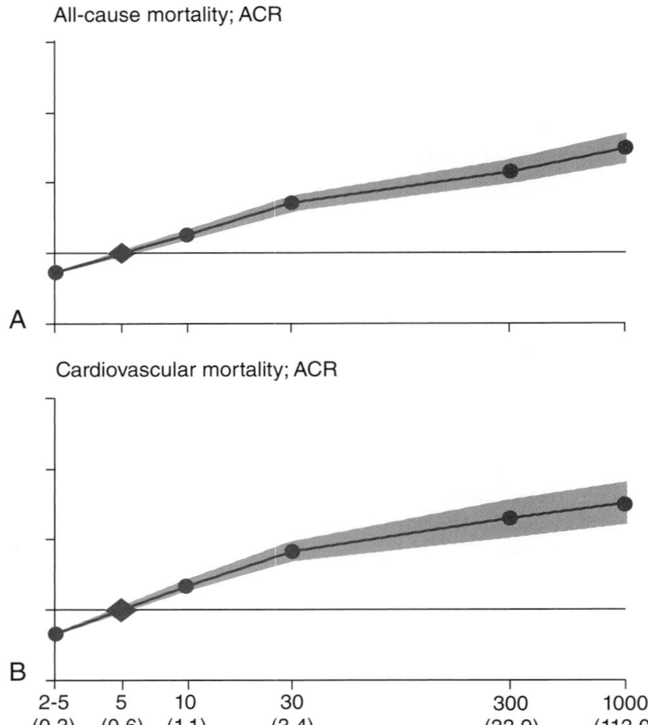

FIGURE 32.2 Relationship of albuminuria with mortality. Hazard ratios (HR) and 95% CIs for all-cause **(A)** and cardiovascular mortality **(B)** according to albumin-to-creatinine ratio (ACR). The horizontal line crosses the *y*-axis at an HR of 1.0, with the axis being plotted on a doubling scale (ie, 1, 2, 4, and 8). HRs *(circles)* and 95% CIs *(shaded areas)* are adjusted for age, gender, ethnic origin, history of cardiovascular disease, systolic blood pressure, diabetes, smoking, and total cholesterol and spline estimated glomerular filtration rate (eGFR). The reference *(diamond)* was ACR 0.6 mg/mmol (5 mg/g). To convert ACR in mg/g to mg/mmol, multiply by 0.113. Approximate conversions to mg/mmol are shown in parentheses. (Reprinted with permission from Matsushita K, van der Velde M, Astor BC, et al. Association of estimated glomerular filtration rate and albuminuria with all-cause and cardiovascular mortality in general population cohorts: a collaborative meta-analysis. *Lancet* 2010;375:2073–81.)

POINTS TO REMEMBER

Urinary Albumin

- Albumin (Mr 66 kDa) is predominantly retained in the circulation by the glomerular basement membrane due to its size and negative charge.
- In health, only small amounts of albumin are filtered. This is largely reabsorbed in the proximal tubule.
- Albuminuria may arise due to both glomerular (increased filtration) and tubular (decreased resorption) disease.
- Albumin is the predominant urinary protein in the setting of proteinuria.
- Due to high biological variability and nonrenal influences, albuminuria should be confirmed on at least two occasions.
- Measurement of the albumin-to-creatinine ratio (ACR) allows the use of a spot sample with correction for variations in urinary concentration in an individual.

QUANTITATIVE ASSESSMENT OF PROTEINURIA: OTHER URINARY PROTEINS

Bence Jones Proteinuria

The presence of immunoglobulin light chains (Bence Jones proteins, 22 kDa) in the urine is an important indication of the presence of myeloma and, in approximately 20% of cases, may occur in the absence of a paraprotein band in the serum.[162] The pathological significance of these proteins is considered in greater detail in Chapter 59. A variety of tests have been used for the detection of Bence Jones protein, including the classic heat test and the Bradshaw test. To date, electrophoresis supplemented by immunofixation has been the most reliable approach.[162,163] Quantitation of Bence Jones protein excretion may be required when patients with light chain only myeloma are monitored. This has generally been achieved by using a combination of electrophoresis and densitometry,[162] but immunoassays for kappa and lambda serum-free light chains may play a role in this setting (see Chapter 59).

Myoglobinuria

Myoglobin is a small (17.8 kDa), heme-containing protein normally catabolized by endocytosis and proteolysis in the proximal tubule following glomerular filtration. Typically, only 0.01% to 5.0% of filtered protein appears in the urine. However, following rhabdomyolysis, large amounts of myoglobin are released into the plasma, saturating the tubular reabsorptive mechanism. This results in the appearance of notable quantities of myoglobin in the urine (which may color the urine red-brown). Further, myoglobin is directly toxic to the renal tubules and can cause acute tubular necrosis with AKI.[164] Myoglobin will give a positive reaction with hemoglobin reagent strip tests, and basic methods of detection have relied on this principle following removal of hemoglobin (eg, by ammonium sulfate precipitation or filtration with 20,000 Mr cutoff), although false-negative and false-positive results were common.[165] Urinary myoglobin is better measured by immunochemical means, although preconcentration of urine may be required.[166] However, for most purposes, evidence that rhabdomyolysis has occurred is better provided by an increase in serum creatine kinase activity not attributable to a cardiac source.[165] There is no strong evidence demonstrating that urinary myoglobin measurement provides useful prognostic information in this setting.[167]

Tubular Proteinuria, Including Markers of Acute Kidney Injury

The integrity of the renal tubule can be assessed indirectly through measurement of functional change and detection of tissue damage. The most common approach has been the measurement of urinary concentrations of low molecular weight proteins using immunoassay technology. These are freely filtered at the glomerulus and then are reabsorbed and catabolized within the proximal tubule. Consequently, the appearance of notable quantities of these proteins in the urine reflects failure of tubular reabsorptive mechanisms (see Table 32.1). There has been considerable study of urinary β_2-microglobulin and retinol binding protein (RBP) in this context;[168] however, both markers are hampered by pH-dependent instability.[169,170] α_1-Microglobulin (Mr 31 kDa), also referred to as protein HC because of its human complex-forming capacity with IgA, is synthesized by the liver, and the free form is readily filtered at the glomerulus; it is also widely used as a marker of tubular damage.[171] For the identification of tubular damage, urinary RBP may be more sensitive than α_1-microglobulin, but the higher concentration and excellent stability of the latter in human urine ex vivo facilitates its use as a marker of tubular damage in clinical studies.[172,173] Cystatin C, generally measured in serum as a marker of GFR (see later), can also be measured in urine as a marker of proximal tubular damage.[174-176] THG, located in the thick ascending limb of the loop of Henle,[177] has been used as a marker of more distal tubular damage.[178]

Tubular damage results in the release of intracellular components into the urinary tract, and the measurement of these components reflects the functional integrity of the tubule. A large number of enzymes have been measured in urine. *N*-acetyl-β-D-glucosaminidase (NAG) is stable in urine and has been used as a marker of tubular integrity. The measurement of NAG has been undertaken in a variety of diseases associated with renal injury, including hypertension, drug nephrotoxicity, transplantation, idiopathic membranous nephropathy,[179] and diabetic nephropathy.[180] However, although it is a sensitive marker of kidney damage, it has not generally been shown to provide a unique benefit over other markers of tubular proteinuria. Measurement of α- and π-glutathione-S-transferase (EC 2.5.1.18) isoenzymes has been proposed to discriminate between proximal and distal tubular damage, respectively, but the role of these markers in clinical practice has yet to be established.[181] An evaluation of several of these biomarkers in patients presenting to hospital with nonoliguric acute tubular necrosis suggested that urinary cystatin C and α_1-microglobulin were the best predictors of an unfavourable outcome as reflected by the requirement for renal replacement therapy.[182]

AKI (discussed in detail in Chapter 59) is characterized by an abrupt decline in kidney function. Most definitions of AKI are based upon recognition of changes in serum creatinine concentration.[183,184] However, serum creatinine is known to be a poor biomarker for AKI, underestimating the early stages of disease, failing to identify sepsis-induced AKI, and contributing to incorrect assessment of treatment efficacy. The need for better biomarkers of AKI has long been appreciated,[185] and the last few years have seen many newer biomarkers emerge as a result of proteomic discovery studies.[186] Paramount among these have been plasma and urinary neutrophil gelatinase–associated lipocalin (NGAL)[187-192] and kidney injury molecule-1 (KIM-1).[193,194] More recently, interleukin-18 (IL-18) and tissue inhibitor of metalloproteinases-2 (TIMP-2) have been proposed.[195] In contrast to serum creatinine concentration, changes in concentrations of these newer biomarkers appear to occur more rapidly (within hours) of onset of AKI. KIM-1 is a type-1 transmembrane protein that normally is not present in urine but is expressed on the proximal tubule apical membrane in response to injury.[193] Renal expression of NGAL is increased following kidney injury, and, in an emergency care setting, urinary NGAL has been found to be a better predictor of the presence of AKI than urinary NAG, α_1-microglobulin, α_1-acid glycoprotein, or serum creatinine concentration.[188] Most reports have demonstrated reasonable short- and long-term stability of NGAL and KIM-1 in urine at 4°C and −80°C, respectively.[196] In the clinical setting, urine is not always easily obtained; measurement of plasma NGAL has also been found to be useful in predicting AKI.[189,197] The biological variation of urinary NGAL, KIM-1, and IL-18 have been reported to be 71%, 69%, and 68%, respectively, among healthy subjects.[198]

Characterization of Proteinuria

As glomerular damage increases, the permeability of the membrane also increases, with an increasing proportion of higher molecular weight proteins appearing in the urine. The relative clearance of a range of proteins can be measured to assess the selectivity of the membrane and to provide an assessment of glomerular damage. The protein selectivity index is generally considered to be of limited value. A commercial semiautomated sodium dodecyl sulfate-agarose gel electrophoresis system (Hydragel, Sebia Electrophoresis, Norcross, Georgia) has been introduced for qualitative analysis of urinary proteins. This separates proteins on the basis of their molecular size, enabling visualization of glomerular, tubular, and mixed patterns of proteinuria. This approach has also been used for the detection and quantitation of Bence Jones proteinuria.[199] Panels of protein measurements, including albumin, α_1-microglobulin, IgG, and α_2-macroglobulin, have been employed in the differential diagnosis of prerenal and postrenal disease.[200] This general strategy was extended with the inclusion of reagent strip tests for hematuria, leukocyturia, and proteinuria in the development of an expert system achieving 98% concordance with clinical diagnosis.[201]

Analytical Methods: Individual Urinary Proteins

Immunoassay is the preferred method for the accurate and sensitive quantitation of individual proteins (see Chapter 23). A variety of approaches have been used, including immunodiffusion immunoassay, electroimmunoassay, light-scattering assay with particle enhancement, and labeled immunometric assays, but light-scattering immunoassay, with turbidimetric or nephelometric detection of immunoaggregate formation, is the most popular approach.

Automated measurement of NGAL in urine[202] and plasma (The NGAL Test, BIOPORTO Diagnostics, Denmark) has been described, and a routine method for urine on a specific automated immunoassay platform is available (Abbott Laboratories, Maidenhead, Berkshire, UK). Measurement in whole blood using a point-of-care testing device (Triage Biosite, Alere Inc., Waltham, Massachusetts) is also available. Substantial intermethod variability exists between NGAL assays, most likely due to a combination of standardization and epitope-recognition issues.[203] For example, some assays may preferentially detect the dimeric form of NGAL, which is produced by neutrophils, compared to the monomeric form resulting from renal damage.[204] The reference interval for urinary NGAL concentration is influenced by age and gender,[205] in addition to leukocytouria[206] and CKD.[207]

Enzymuria can be measured using a variety of enzyme assay approaches. For example, one method used for the assay of NAG employs the substrate 4-methylumbelliferyl-N-acetyl-β-D-glucosaminide with fluorometric measurement of the methylumbelliferone released by the enzyme.[208] Alternative substrates generating products capable of being detected in the visible spectrum have also been described.[209]

CREATININE

Biochemistry and Physiology

Creatine, the immediate precursor of creatinine, is synthesized in the kidneys, liver, and pancreas by two enzymatically mediated reactions. In the first, transamidation of arginine and glycine forms guanidinoacetic acid; in the second, methylation of guanidinoacetic acid occurs with S-adenosylmethionine as the methyl donor. Creatine is then transported in blood to other organs such as muscle and brain, where it is phosphorylated to phosphocreatine, a high-energy compound.

Interconversion of phosphocreatine and creatine is a particular feature of the metabolic processes of muscle contraction. A proportion of free creatine in muscle (thought to be between 1% and 2%/d) spontaneously and irreversibly converts to its anhydride waste product, creatinine. Thus the amount of creatinine produced each day in an individual is fairly constant and is related to the muscle mass. In health, the blood concentration of creatinine is also fairly constant although it may be influenced by diet (see later). Creatinine (Mr approximately 113 Da) is present in all body fluids and secretions and is freely filtered by the glomerulus. Although it is not reabsorbed to any great extent by the renal tubules, a small but notable tubular secretion is present, as well as concentration-related losses in the gut. Creatinine production also decreases as the circulating concentration of creatinine increases; several mechanisms for this have been proposed, including feedback inhibition of the production of creatine, reconversion of creatinine to creatine, and conversion to other metabolites.[210,211]

Sample Collection

Creatinine in serum, plasma, or diluted urine is stable for at least 7 days at 4°C, and serum creatinine is stable during long-term frozen storage (at −20°C and below) and after repeated thawing and refreezing.[212-214] However, it should be noted that delayed separation (beyond 14 h) of serum from erythrocytes leads to a significant increase in apparent serum creatinine concentration using some kinetic Jaffe (but not enzymatic) assays, possibly as the result of release of noncreatinine chromogens from the red cells (see later).[215,216] Posture, length of tourniquet application, and fist clenching are not associated with changes in creatinine measurements.[217]

Bacterial contamination, which can occur in samples stored for long periods of time, has been reported to falsely lower creatinine values measured using the Jaffe reaction, purportedly as the result of bacterial production of a substance that retards the reaction.[218] Creatinine concentration increases in blood after meals containing cooked meat, because of the conversion of creatine to creatinine. Ideally blood for serum creatinine measurement should be obtained in the fasting state.[219-223] While the effect is dependent on the amount and type of meat consumed and time of sampling, the effect can be to increase the creatinine concentration by 25%,[223] with consequent similar reduction in estimates of GFR based on the result. Use of creatine ethyl ester, a component of some nutritional supplements, has also been shown to cause an increase in serum creatinine concentration following its conversion to creatinine within the gastrointestinal tract.[224]

Analytical Methods

Serum creatinine is measured in virtually all clinical laboratories as a test of kidney function. Most laboratories use adaptations of the same assay for measurements in both serum and urine. Both chemical and enzymatic methods are used to measure creatinine in body fluids.

Chemical Methods: The Jaffe Reaction

Most chemical methods for measuring creatinine are based primarily on the reaction with alkaline picrate. In this reaction, first described by Jaffe in 1886, creatinine reacts with picrate ion in an alkaline medium to yield an orange-red complex. Despite considerable literature on the subject, the reaction mechanism and the structure of the product remain unclear.[225]

The Jaffe reaction is not specific for creatinine. Many compounds have been reported to produce a Jaffe-like chromogen, including protein,[226,227] glucose, ascorbic acid,[228] ketone bodies,[229] pyruvate,[228] guanidine, hemoglobin F,[227] blood-substitute products,[230] streptomycin,[231] and cephalosporins;[232] the reader is referred to comprehensive reviews.[233,234] The degree of interference from these compounds is dependent on the precise reaction conditions chosen. It is therefore important to be aware that different versions of the Jaffe reaction used by different manufacturers will respond in variable ways to interferences—that is, there are many Jaffe assays with different performance characteristics (see later for more details). Among the interferences, the effects of ketones and ketoacids are probably of the greatest significance clinically, although the effect is method dependent. Thus reports on acetoacetate interference vary from a negligible increase to an increase of 3.5 mg/dL (310 μmol/L) in the apparent creatinine concentration at an acetoacetate concentration of 8 mmol/L. Bilirubin is a negative interferent with the Jaffe reaction. The addition of buffering ions such as borate and phosphate, along with surfactant, has been used to minimize the effects of this interference. A popular maneuver in this context has been the addition of ferricyanide (O'Leary method), which oxidizes bilirubin to biliverdin, thus reducing its interference.[235,236] Noncreatinine chromogens do not generally interfere with urinary creatinine measurements.

Historically, several approaches have been used in an attempt to improve the general specificity of the Jaffe reaction. These have included absorption of creatinine into hydrated aluminium silicate (Fuller's earth, Lloyd's reagent), with subsequent elution, acid blanking, the use of ion-exchange resins[229] or solvent extraction, and oxidation of interferents with compounds such as cerium sulfate; generally these modifications have not proved practical and are no longer used.

The greatest success in terms of common usage and specificity has come from the use of a kinetic measurement approach in combination with careful choice of reactant concentrations and the time of reading the change in optical absorption. Although manual methods have traditionally been equilibrium methods, with 10 to 15 minutes allowed for color development at room temperature, kinetic assays were developed in a quest both for specificity and for faster and automated analyses. Early studies of interferences in kinetic methods identified two types of noncreatinine chromogens: those whose rates of adduct formation were very rapid in the first 20 seconds after mixing of reagent and sample (eg, acetoacetate) and those whose rates did not become rapid until 80 to 100 seconds after mixing (eg, protein). The "window" between 20 and 80 seconds, therefore, was a period in which the rate signal being observed could be attributed predominantly to the creatinine-picrate reaction (some investigators found 60 seconds as the upper limit of this window). Thus improved specificity in kinetic assays was achieved by selecting times for rate measurements 20 to 80 seconds after initiation of the reaction (mixing). This approach has been implemented on various automated instruments, and kinetic assays are now the most widely used approach to creatinine measurement. Extensive literature exists on the choice of reactant concentrations and reading interval and on the choice of wavelength and reaction temperature.

Picrate Concentration. The Jaffe reaction is pseudo-first order with respect to picrate up to 30 mmol/L picrate, with most methods employing a concentration between 3 and 16 mmol/L. At concentrations greater than 6 mmol/L, the rate of color development becomes nonlinear, so a two-point fixed interval rather than a multiple data point approach is required.

Hydroxide Concentration. The initial rate of reaction is pseudo-first order with respect to hydroxide concentrations above 0.5 mmol/L; however, at 500 mmol/L, degradation of the Jaffe complex is increased. Furthermore, at hydroxide concentrations greater than 200 mmol/L, the blank absorbance increases notably.

Wavelength. Although the absorbance maximum of the Jaffe reaction is between 490 and 500 nm, improved method linearity and reduced blank values have been reported at other wavelengths, the choice varying with hydroxide concentration.

Temperature. The rate of Jaffe complex formation and the absorptivity of the complex are temperature dependent, with measurable differences being observed even between 25°C and 37°C. Consequently, temperature control is an important component of assay reproducibility. A higher temperature (41°C) was used in one Jaffe assay by Beckman Coulter (Beckman Coulter, High Wycombe, UK) to reduce bilirubin interference. This required an instrument with assay-specific temperature control, which is not a feature of most chemistry analyzers.[237]

Rate Blanking. The effect of bilirubin on absorbance in the assay environment commences after addition of the sample and before the addition of the picrate reagent. This has been exploited by measuring the rate of change in absorbance prior to picrate addition and subtracting this from the rate of absorption after addition. Good resistance from bilirubin interference has been demonstrated using this approach.[238]

Compensation. In an attempt to adjust for reaction with noncreatinine chromogens, some manufacturers have introduced so-called *compensated* Jaffe assays, in which a fixed concentration is automatically subtracted from each result. For example, Roche Diagnostics Ltd. (Lewes, Sussex, UK) has realigned its assays on the Cobas Integra and Hitachi systems by −0.20 mg/dL and −0.32 mg/dL (−18 and −28 μmol/L), respectively. Such assays produce results more closely aligned with isotope dilution mass spectrometry (IDMS) reference measurement procedures.[239,240] However, they make an assumption that the noncreatinine chromogen interference is a constant between samples. This is clearly an oversimplification, especially when adult and pediatric samples are compared.[227]

Other chemical approaches to the measurement of creatinine have been tried, including reaction with 1,4-naphthoquinone-2-sulphonate; use of *o*-nitrobenzaldehyde to convert creatinine to methylguanidine and its reaction with α-naphthol and sodium hypochlorite under alkaline conditions;[241] and reaction with 3,5-dinitrobenzoic acid.[242] None of these reactions is widely used in clinical laboratories.

The purpose of describing these approaches to assay design is not to suggest that clinical laboratories should make these adjustments to assays. Rather, these have been developed by manufacturers who are then responsible for ensuring the total performance of the assay, including precision, reagent stability, linearity, and analytical range, after making these modifications to improve analytical specificity. It is, however, incumbent on laboratorians to understand the mechanisms of action of the assays in their laboratory to facilitate troubleshooting in the event of assay failure. For example, interpretation of an assay reaction curve or possible points of assay failure requires an understanding of the underlying assay mechanism.

Enzymatic Methods

Enzymes from several metabolic pathways have been investigated for the enzymatic measurement of creatinine. All of the methods involve a multistep approach leading to a photometric end-point. Primarily three approaches are used; they are described in the subsequent paragraphs (Fig. 32.3).

Creatininase. The enzyme creatininase (EC 3.5.2.10; creatinine amidohydrolase) catalyzes the conversion of creatinine to creatine. Creatine is then detected with a series of enzyme-mediated reactions involving creatine kinase, pyruvate kinase, and lactate dehydrogenase, with monitoring of the decrease in absorbance at 340 nm (Fig. 32.3A). Initiating the reaction with creatininase allows for the removal of endogenous creatine and pyruvate in a preincubation reaction. The kinetics of the reaction is poor, and a 30-minute incubation is required to allow the reaction to reach equilibrium. This shortcoming can be overcome by a kinetic approach but with a further reduction in sensitivity. The approach has not been popular, in part because of poor sensitivity, poor precision, and the relatively high cost of reagents.

Creatininase and Creatinase. An alternative, more popular approach has used the enzyme creatinase (EC 3.5.3.3; creatine amidinohydrolase), which yields sarcosine and urea, the former being measured with additional enzyme-mediated steps using sarcosine oxidase (EC 1.5.3.1; yielding glycine, formaldehyde, and hydrogen peroxide) and peroxidase (Fig. 32.3B).[243,244] Hydrogen peroxide can be detected through a variety of methods. Care must be taken to watch for interference (eg, by bilirubin) in the final reaction sequence. This problem has been approached with the addition of potassium ferricyanide (with limited success) or bilirubin oxidase. The potential interference caused by ascorbic acid can be overcome by inclusion of ascorbate oxidase. The influence of endogenous intermediate creatine and urea can be overcome by a preincubation step, initiating the reaction with creatininase. This system has been incorporated in a point-of-care testing device using polarographic detection.[245] An alternative detection system involves measurement of the reduction of nicotanimide adenine dinucleotide by formaldehyde in the presence of formaldehyde dehydrogenase (Fig. 32.3C).[246]

Creatinine Deaminase. Creatinine deaminase (EC 3.5.4.21; creatinine iminohydrolase) catalyzes the conversion of creatinine to N-methylhydantoin and ammonia.[247] Early methods concentrated on the detection of ammonia using either glutamate dehydrogenase or the Berthelot reaction.[248] An alternative approach involves the enzyme N-methylhydantoin amidohydrolase (Fig. 32.3D).[249]

Dry Chemistry Systems. Several multilayer dry reagent methods have been described for the measurement of creatinine using enzyme-mediated reactions. An early "two-slide" approach employed creatinine deaminase, with the ammonia diffusing through a semipermeable and optically opaque layer to react with bromophenol blue to obtain an increase in absorbance at 600 nm. A second multilayer film lacking the enzyme was used to quantitate endogenous ammonia, enabling blank correction.[250] A later, more precise single-slide method used the creatininase-creatinase reaction sequence.[251] Lidocaine metabolites have been reported to interfere with this method.[252] The creatinine deaminase system described previously has been used and adapted for use as a point-of-care testing device (see Fig. 32.3D).[253] In all cases, the color produced in the film is quantitated by reflectance. A dry chemistry system has been described in which a nonenzymatic approach was used, based on the reaction with 3,5-dinitrobenzoic acid.[254]

Other Methods

The JCTLM lists isotope dilution (ID) GCMS and LCMS as reference procedures for measurement of creatinine in serum and urine. GCMS was developed in the 1980s[255,256] and was accepted as the method of choice for establishing the true concentration of creatinine in serum because of its excellent specificity and low imprecision (see later).[256,257] In these procedures, creatinine must be derivatized before GC analysis because of its polarity. In addition, a cation-exchange cleanup step before GC analysis is necessary because creatine is derivatized into the same chemical species as creatinine. A method coupling HPLC with IDMS for the direct quantification of creatinine has been reported.[258] This method offers simplicity and improved speed of analysis because only a simple protein precipitation without derivatization is required and equivalent performance can be obtained from GC and LC methods.[259]

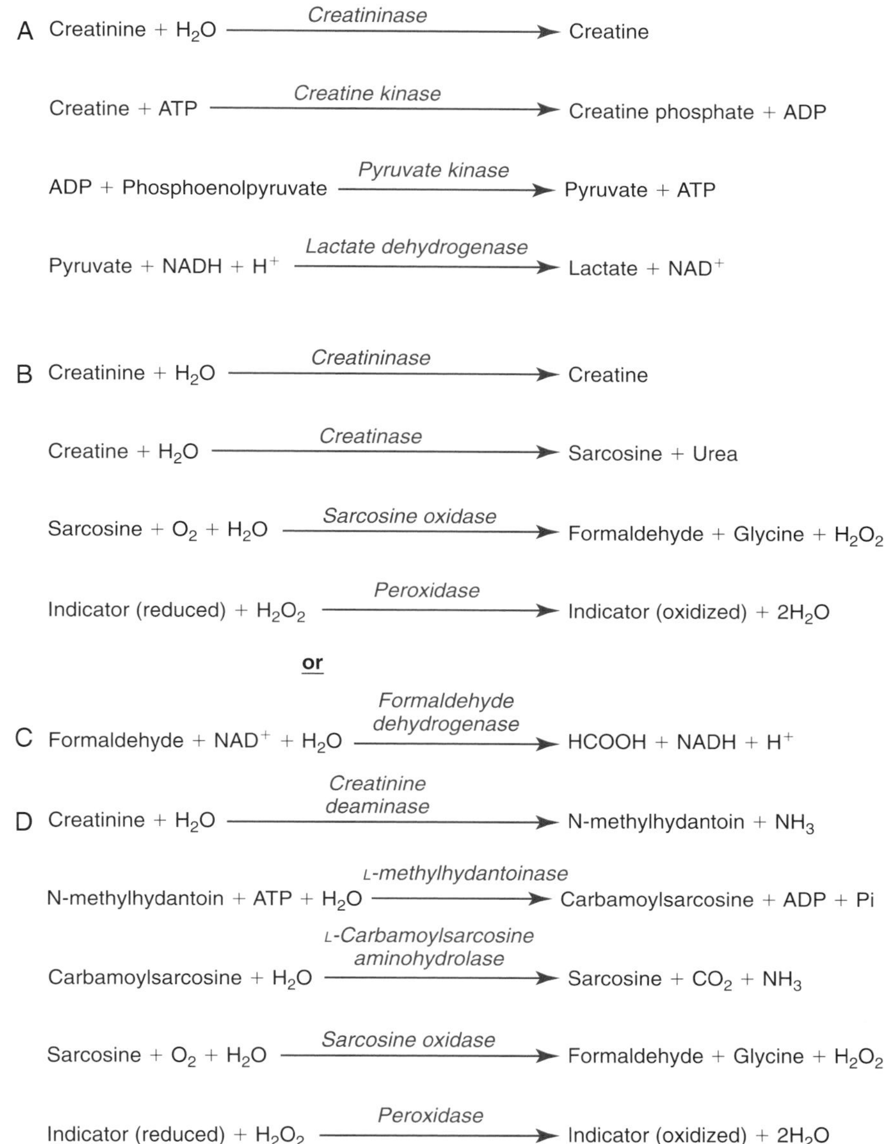

FIGURE 32.3 Determination of creatinine using a variety of enzymatic methods. For additional details, see text.

Sensitive and specific approaches to creatinine measurement using HPLC have been described using both cation-exchange[260-262] and reversed-phase techniques.[263,264] Separation is followed by quantitation using an on-stream Jaffe reaction,[260] native absorbance of creatinine at approximately 230 nm,[261-266] or enzymatic detection.[267] All HPLC approaches are reported to be rapid, specific, and precise, and several have been proposed as candidate reference methods.[261,267,268] Thienpont and colleagues reported between-day and within-run imprecision of less than 1%, with deviation from GC-IDMS target values of +0.1%.[268] HPLC appears to provide an excellent designated comparison method for in-house use by manufacturers.[269]

A capillary electrophoresis approach to serum creatinine measurement using diode array detection has been described.[270] A high-performance capillary electrophoresis method[271] and a reagent-free midinfrared method[272] for urinary creatinine measurement also have been described.

Quality Issues to Consider With Creatinine Methods

Methodologic aspects of creatinine measurements are complex by virtue of the large number of variants of the Jaffe and enzymatic reactions in use. Due to lower costs, Jaffe assays are far more widely used globally and remain the predominant method type in most developed countries (see later). Although enzymatic methods are more expensive, they are used in dry chemistry systems (with their lower reagent requirement), including some point-of-care testing devices. None of the methods, including enzymatic assays, are free from interferences, and laboratorians assessing a new creatinine method (eg, as part of an analyzer purchase) should review the data for interference due to bilirubin, protein, glucose, and ketones/ketoacids; bilirubin will also be particularly important in enzymatic procedures that generate hydrogen peroxide. Despite criticism of the Jaffe methods, good correlation has generally been noted between them and enzymatic procedures, with average differences likely to be due as much to calibration as to interference.

Historically, as a result of reaction with noncreatinine chromogens, Jaffe methods have often overestimated true serum creatinine concentrations by up to 20% compared with HPLC or IDMS methods at physiologic concentrations.[226,273-275] Variation in bias was largely related to differences in the calibration of creatinine assays,[276] which may include effects due to different concentrations of noncreatinine chromogens in the calibrator compared with patient samples. There is evidence of overall improvement in bias following widespread adoption of international standardization in 2009, coupled with a shift away from traditional ("uncompensated") kinetic Jaffe assays. Of 346 participants in the United Kingdom National External Quality Assessment Scheme (UKNEQAS) for serum creatinine in November 2014, at a creatinine concentration of 0.84 mg/dL (74.5 μmol/L) (mean of enzymatic methods), the overall between-laboratory CV was 6.0% and the overall all laboratory mean was 0.84 mg/dL (74.4 μmol/L). Similar data from the Royal College of Pathologists of Australasia Quality Assurance Programme (RCPAQAP) in 2014 for native serum samples showed between-laboratory CVs of 5.4% and 4.7% at 0.78 and 0.96 mg/dL (69 and 85 μmol/L), respectively (144 laboratories, data with permission). It should be noted that these results were obtained with assays produced by multinational companies meeting European and US regulations with assays traceable to IDMS. The US National Kidney Disease Education Programme (NKDEP) defined desirable performance standards for creatinine in terms of effect on error of GFR estimates, stating that the desirable total error goal should be less than 7.6% at a serum creatinine concentration of 1.0 to 1.5 mg/dL (88 and 133 μmol/L).[269] However, analytical performance still requires improvement. In two recent European studies, Jaffe methods have failed to meet these performance goals, and they have been met by enzymatic methods, including when both assays types are from the same manufacturer.[277,278] Generally, interlaboratory and within-laboratory agreement is best at supraphysiological creatinine concentrations and deteriorates as serum creatinine concentrations become lower. Due to the hyperbolic relationship between serum creatinine and GFR, imprecision at lower creatinine concentrations contributes to greater error in GFR estimation than at higher creatinine concentrations. Creatinine-based estimates of GFR (see later) will clearly vary, depending on how accurate the creatinine measurement is that is used in their calculation. The more a method overestimates "true" creatinine, the greater will be the underestimation of GFR, and vice versa. The performance requirements for measurement of pediatric samples are more difficult to meet due to the lower concentrations and changes in background noncreatinine chromogens. One recommendation is for the use of enzymatic assays for pediatric measurements.[227,279] Similar considerations will also apply to samples taken from pregnant women, where creatinine concentrations will also be lower.

In the early 2000s, it was the appreciation of CKD as a major public health issue[13,90,118] and of its identification using GFR-estimating equations that led to increased focus on the measurement of creatinine and ultimately to the development of a standardized reference material for universal application.[13,269,280] A significant factor in these improvements was the work of the Laboratory Working Group of the NKDEP. During the first decade of the 21st century, this group of laboratory scientists and clinicians worked with international manufacturers to seek their engagement in producing assays traceable to IDMS, and by 2009, all major manufacturers involved in the process had complied with this request. This process cost many millions of dollars for each company to meet regulatory and marketing costs, in addition to the scientific and manufacturing costs of adjusting assay calibration. Standardization, however, will not solve the problem of different reactivity with noncreatinine chromogens across different individual patient samples, which can be resolved only by the use of highly specific creatinine methods. Wider adoption of enzymatic methods could further improve between-laboratory agreement in creatinine measurement, although even enzymatic assays are subject to certain interferences.[228] Furthermore, enzymatic methods are used by a minority of laboratories at present. Of 346 participants in the UKNEQAS for serum creatinine in November 2014, 61% used a "compensated" kinetic Jaffe assay, 4% used traditional kinetic Jaffe reactions, and 35% used an enzymatic assay (including the Vitros dry-slide enzymatic method; Ortho Clinical Diagnostics, Raritan, New Jersey). In the United States, of 5375 laboratories in the College of American Pathologists Survey in 2015, 58% used kinetic Jaffe reactions, 10% used "rate-blanked" kinetic Jaffe assays, 2% used an endpoint Jaffe method, and 30% used an enzymatic assay (including Vitros dry-slide users).

Traceability of Serum Creatinine Measurement

Standardized serum matrix reference materials (SRM 967) with known creatinine concentrations (0.80 mg/dL [71 μmol/L] and 4.00 mg/dL [354 μmol/L]) and validated commutability have been prepared by the National Institute of Standards and Technology (NIST) and included in the JCTLM list of standardized reference materials, along with pure creatinine preparations and other matrix matched materials. Most clinical laboratory methods adjusted their calibration to be traceable to SRM 967 and an IDMS reference measurement procedure by 2009.[281,282] Several IDMS methods, linked to either LC or GC, have been approved by the JCTLM as reference measurement procedures for serum/plasma creatinine (see earlier). Thus with JCTLM-listed reference materials, procedures, and reference measurement services (laboratories), a full reference system is in place to define the top of calibration hierarchies for creatinine measurement in serum and urine. While the term *IDMS traceable* has been used as shorthand for a traceable assay, the top of the calibration hierarchy is the pure material, with values transferred through the reference method performed in a reference laboratory. The preferred role of the matrix-matched material, such as SRM 967, is to validate the accuracy after performance of the assay standardization. For additional discussion on standardization issues, refer to Chapter 6.

For traceable results in the routine laboratory, there is the need for the accuracy of the reference measurements to be passed to the field method with minimal increase in bias or uncertainty. This has been a major contributor to method biases in Jaffe assays because the noncreatinine chromogens in patient samples may be different from those in the calibration material, giving biased results even if the creatinine concentration in the calibrator is accurately assigned. The use of aqueous calibrators for Jaffe assays is an obvious example of the use of noncommutable materials in the calibration hierarchy. "Compensated" assays are an example where this issue is recognized and addressed. A key issue for laboratories is that, particularly for Jaffe assays, the calibrator, together with its value assignment, must match the specific assay. In practice this means purchasing assays kits from manufacturers that provide reagents and calibrators and ensure traceability. In many parts of the developing world, creatinine assays are sold without calibrators or with aqueous calibrators, where bias in the clinical result is highly likely.

Reference Intervals and Biological Variability

Given the earlier discussion, prior to the introduction of standardized "IDMS-traceable" methods, published reference intervals for serum creatinine were method dependent (see Chapter 8). A systematic review of creatinine reference intervals in which studies were included only when their calibration was traceable to the reference IDMS procedure proposed adult reference intervals of 0.72 to 1.18 mg/dL (64–104 μmol/L) in men and 0.55 to 1.02 mg/dL (49–90 μmol/L) in women.[283] These data were derived using an enzymatic (Roche Diagnostics Ltd., Basel, Switzerland) assay. Reference interval data for children may be found in the same publication. Serum creatinine concentration is generally very stable from age 18 to about 60 years old, after which time there is a significant increase in many, but not all, of the population. In the adult population, consideration of reference intervals has perhaps taken less of a priority due to the increasing use of GFR estimating equations based on serum creatinine to assess kidney function. Due to its high between-person variability, serum creatinine is also commonly interpreted against previous results from the same patient rather than against the reference interval, and clinically significant changes can occur with all results remaining within the reference interval. For more discussion on biological variability, see Chapter 7. Among children, however, GFR estimating equations are less commonly used, and reference intervals are therefore of greater clinical utility. Particularly among children, reference intervals based on enzymatic creatinine assays should be used.[283,284] For additional information on creatinine reference intervals in males and females at different age groups, refer to the Appendix.

Urinary creatinine excretion is higher in men (14–26 mg/kg/d, 124–230 μmol/kg/d) than in women (11–20 mg/kg/day, 97–177 μmol/kg/day). Following reduction in muscle mass, creatinine excretion decreases with age: Typically, for a 70-kg man, creatinine excretion will decline from approximately 14.5 to 9.1 mmol/d with advancing age from 30 to 80 years.[285] Measurement of urinary creatinine excretion can be a useful, if approximate, indication of the completeness of a timed urine collection. Creatinine excretion is often used as a method of normalizing the urinary excretion of analytes; that is, the concentration of the test analyte (in mmol or grams) is divided by the total amount of creatinine (in mmol or grams) excreted in the same urine specimen. This method is a rough correction for volume differences between patient specimens. Similarly, expressing the concentration of a substance as a ratio to the creatinine concentration is a useful method of adjusting for urinary concentration differences in random ("spot") urine samples. The benefits of this approach in reporting urinary total protein and albumin measurements have been discussed above.

An early study demonstrated a CV_I in healthy volunteers for serum creatinine of 4.1%.[286] Subsequently, across a variety of settings, the reported CV_I of creatinine has ranged from 5.3% to 6.4%.[287] Within-person biological variability of urinary creatinine excretion is reported as 11% (see www.westgard.com).

Clinical Significance

The clinical utility of creatinine measurement is considered later in this chapter, together with other GFR markers.

POINTS TO REMEMBER

Creatinine

- Creatinine is produced at a fairly constant rate within an individual as a result of breakdown of creatine within muscle tissue.
- Creatinine is freely filtered at the glomerulus and also secreted in the tubules to a lesser extent.
- Because it is predominantly excreted by the kidneys, plasma creatinine concentration is inversely proportional to GFR (halving the GFR approximately doubles the serum creatinine).
- In addition to GFR, other factors related to creatinine production affect plasma creatinine concentration, including age, gender, race, muscularity, certain drugs, diet, and nutritional status.
- Estimated GFR using the $\text{CKD-EPI}_{\text{creat}}$ equation is recommended for clinical use unless there is evidence of a superior equation.

CYSTATIN C

Biochemistry and Physiology

Cystatin C has come to clinical attention with regard to renal function due to the use of serum measurements for the estimation of GFR. Cystatin C is a low molecular weight (12.8 kDa) protein synthesized by all nucleated cells whose physiologic role is that of a cysteine protease inhibitor.[288] The gene has been sequenced, and the promoter region has been identified as that of the housekeeping type, with no known regulatory elements, and, consequently, the rate of cystatin C release into the circulation was initially considered to be constant.[289] Over time a number of factors have been identified that can affect cystatin C production and thus the circulating concentration. These include a correlation of production with thyroid hormone concentration[290-292] and with obesity.[293] Positive associations have also been made with diabetes, cigarette smoking, C-reactive protein, and white cell count and an inverse relationship with serum albumin.[294,295] More important, muscle mass does not have a major effect on cystatin C concentration.[296,297]

Cystatin C is removed from the circulation by the kidneys with no known extrarenal routes of elimination.[298-300] Due to its small size and high isoelectric point (pI 9.2), it is more freely filtered than some other putative protein markers of GFR.[298] Following filtration, cystatin C is essentially fully resorbed and broken down in the tubules usually leading to very low concentrations in the urine. However, in the setting of renal tubular damage, urinary cystatin C concentrations rise, which may provide a test for this condition.[174-176,182,301]

In addition to renal function and pathophysiological factors, serum cystatin C concentrations are also affected by age, gender, pregnancy, weight, and height.[294,295,302] The influences of age and gender are taken into account with some cystatin C–based GFR estimating equations (see later). Evidence has emerged of a genetic influence on circulating cystatin C concentration, independent of renal function,[303] although the impact on CKD classification based on cystatin C measurement was modest.[304]

Analytical Methods

Historically, cystatin C was has been measured by immunodiffusion or rocket electroimmunoassay. While these methods have been replaced in current practice, immunoassay remains the detection method for all available assays. Given the clinical need for rapid results, the most practical approaches described are to use particle-enhanced turbidimetric or nephelometric immunoassay, which can run on automated chemistry analysers or specific nephelometers.[305-308] Using these assays, a between-day imprecision of CV 3% to 6% can be expected at the upper limit of the reference interval (≅1.00 mg/L) and less than 3% at higher values. Given the known values of within-subject biological variation (CV_I) for cystatin C of about 5%, it would be beneficial to improve the precision of routine assays. The use of immunoassays makes cystatin C relatively free of the interferences that affect Jaffe creatinine assays. However, typically the reagents are markedly more expensive than creatinine assays measured using either Jaffe or enzymatic techniques. In addition to current wet-chemistry methods, there is the potential for dry-chemistry point-of-care devices based on sandwich immunoassays using monoclonal antibodies.[309]

Traceability of Cystatin C Measurement

The early stages of cystatin C research paralleled that of serum creatinine with assay differences making comparison of results from different assay manufacturers problematic.[310] There were also drifts in assays from the same manufacturer over time, again making direct comparison of results difficult.[311,312] To address these issues, an international standard was developed by an International Federation of Clinical Chemistry and Laboratory Medicine (IFCC) working party.[313,314] The material, known as ERM-DA471/IFCC Cystatin C in human serum, has verified commutability and is listed on the JCTLM database. Most manufacturers have restandardized their assays against this material, and the use of these traceable assays in research and in the routine laboratory is recommended to allow direct comparability of results.

Reference Intervals and Biological Variability

While single reference intervals for adult males and females of all ages are commonly used, it is now well established that cystatin C concentrations are higher in males than females and climb throughout adult life, reaching concentrations 50% or more above young adult values in the elderly.[315-317] This change with age is not a surprising finding because there is typically a fall in GFR with advancing age in most populations; however, this challenges the utility of population reference intervals in elderly patients. An unselected population interval will normalize the decline in renal function with age, whereas a health-associated interval will first need to define kidney health for the reference population on which to base the intervals. Again, in a similar manner to serum creatinine, the clinical decisions based on cystatin C are more likely to be made using estimated GFR values derived from cystatin C than on the serum cystatin C concentration itself, making the reference interval less relevant as a decision support tool. Cystatin C concentrations are higher than adult values during the first year of life, starting approximately 50% higher than adult concentrations and falling gradually to near adult values by the end of the first year of life. These studies also demonstrated even higher cystatin C concentrations in preterm infants.[318,319]

As stated previously, only reference interval studies performed using assays with validated traceability to the reference material ERM-DA471/IFCC should be used. If a single young adult interval is to be used, 0.6 to 1.1 mg/L would be reasonable, based on the subjects aged 23 to 50 years old in the study by Voskoboev and colleagues.[317]

Reported values of CV_I for serum cystatin C in healthy volunteers have varied between 4.5%[320] and 8.6%,[321] with a value listed in the Ricos Database of 5.0% (www.westgard.com).

Clinical Significance

Because cystatin C is produced at a relatively constant rate, freely filtered at the glomerulus and neither secreted nor reabsorbed intact in the proximal tubule, its concentration in serum can serve as a marker of GFR. Kyhse-Andersen and colleagues,[322] using receiver operator analysis, were the first to demonstrate the superiority of cystatin C measurement compared with creatinine for the detection of kidney disease. This has been confirmed by many others,[298,322-324] including metaanalyses.[325,326]

In a similar manner to serum creatinine, equations have been developed to estimate GFR based on serum cystatin C with or without added demographic variables; some of these equations are given in Table 32.3. Given the nature of cystatin C clearance, the equations are generally modifications of the concept that GFR is related to the reciprocal of serum cystatin C. Only equations developed using results traceable to the reference material ERM-DA471/IFCC and with high-quality formal GFR measurements as the reference standard are considered here; earlier equations should not be used. In 2012 KDIGO recommended the use of the Chronic Kidney Disease-Epidemiology Collaboration (CKD-EPI) cystatin C equation ($CKD\text{-}EPI_{cys}$) for standardized cystatin C results.[57,327] An equation combining results for both creatinine and cystatin C ($CKD\text{-}EPI_{creat\text{-}cys}$) has also been recommended by KDIGO.[327] Combined equations also exist for pediatric subjects.[328]

The process of refining and revising GFR estimating equations is ongoing, and newer equations are being developed all the time. One example is the CAPA (Caucasian, Asian, pediatric, and adult) equation, which is derived from diverse populations producing a simple equation without factors for race or gender[329]; another is the Berlin Initiative Study 2 (BIS2) equation using both creatinine and cystatin C and focusing on the elderly.[330,331] A different approach is to perform cystatin C and creatinine-based GFR estimations separately and consider the presence of an interfering factor in one of the equations if the results are not concordant.[332] It is the role of the laboratory, together with nephrologists, to assess the most appropriate equation based on the evidence available and discussion with the relevant clinical groups.

TABLE 32.3. **Representative GFR Estimating Equations for Use in Adults**

Abbreviation	GFR Equation
Cockcroft and Gault[469]	$([(140 - \text{age}) \times \text{weight})] \times 1.23)/(\text{Scr}) \times 0.85$ (if female)
MDRD (ID-MS traceable)[475]	GFR (mL/min/1.73 m^2) = $175 \times (\text{Scr} \times 0.01131)^{-1.154} \times (\text{age})^{-0.203} \times$ (1.210 if patient is black) $\times$ (0.742 if patient is female)
CKD-EPI$_{creat}$[481]	$141 \times \min(\text{Scr} \times 0.01131/\kappa, 1)^{\alpha} \times \max(\text{Scr} \times 0.01131/\kappa, 1)^{-1.209} \times 0.993^{\text{age}} \times 1.018$ [if female] $\times$ 1.159 [if black], where Scr is serum creatinine, κ is 0.7 for females and 0.9 for males, α is −0.329 for females and −0.411 for males, min indicates the minimum of Scr/κ or 1, and max indicates the maximum of Scr/κ or 1.
CKD-EPI$_{cys}$[327]	$133 \times \min(\text{Scys}/0.8, 1)^{-0.499} \times \max(\text{Scys}/0.8, 1)^{-1.328} \times 0.996^{\text{Age}} \times 0.932$ [if female], where min indicates the minimum of Scys/κ or 1, and max indicates the maximum of Scys/κ or 1.
CKD-EPI$_{creat-cys}$[327]	$135 \times \min(\text{Scr} \times 0.01131/\kappa, 1)^{\alpha} \times \max(\text{Scr} \times 0.01131/\kappa, 1)^{-0.601} \times \min(\text{Scys}/0.8, 1)^{-0.375} \times \max(\text{Scys}/0.8, 1)^{-0.711} \times 0.995^{\text{Age}} \times 0.969$ [if female] $\times$ 1.08 [if black], where Scr is serum creatinine, Scys is serum cystatin C, κ is 0.7 for females and 0.9 for males, α is −0.248 for females and −0.207 for males, min indicates the minimum of Scr/κ or 1, and max indicates the maximum of Scr/κ or 1.
BIS1[330]	$3736 \times (\text{Scr} \times 88.4)^{-0.87} \times \text{age}^{-0.95} \times 0.82$ [if female]
BIS2[330]	$767 \times \text{Scys}^{-0.61} \times \text{Scr}^{-0.40} \times \text{age}^{-0.57} \times 0.87$ [if female]
CAPA cystatin C equation[329]	$130 \times \text{cystatin C}^{-1.069} \times \text{age}^{-0.117} - 7$

Age is given in years, serum creatinine in μmol/L, serum cystatin C (Scys) in mg/L, and weight in kilograms.
BIS, Berlin Initiative Study; *CAPA,* Caucasian, Asian, Pediatric, and Adult; *CKD-EPI,* Chronic Kidney Disease–Epidemiology Consortium; *ID-MS,* isotope dilution-mass spectrometry; *MDRD,* modification of diet in renal disease; *Scr,* serum creatinine; *Scys,* serum cystatin C.

The above discussion is based on the ability of cystatin C or combined cystatin C-creatinine equations to estimate GFR. Generally the use of cystatin C equations provides some, albeit modest, improvement over equations based on serum creatinine alone. An increasing body of evidence suggests that the use of cystatin C GFR-estimating equations gives improved risk prediction of death and kidney failure unrelated to the accuracy of the GFR estimation[333-335]; this improved predictive ability may relate to non-GFR determinants of serum cystatin C concentration.[336] Partly as a consequence of its predictive ability, a recommended clinical role for estimating GFR from cystatin C has come from KDIGO, which suggest, if confirmation of CKD is required, measuring cystatin C in adults who have creatinine-estimated GFR between 45 and 59 mL/min/1.73 m^2 and who do not have markers of kidney damage.[57] If eGFR$_{cys}$ or eGFR$_{creat-cys}$ is also less than 60 mL/min/1.73 m^2, the diagnosis of CKD is confirmed. If eGFR$_{cys}$ or eGFR$_{creat-cys}$ is 60 mL/min/1.73 m^2 or greater, the diagnosis of CKD is not confirmed. This approach has also been recommended in the United Kingdom.[59]

POINTS TO REMEMBER

Cystatin C

- Cystatin C is a low molecular weight protein (12.8 kDa) produced at a fairly constant rate from most body cells.
- A modest increase in production is seen in obesity, hyperthyroidism, and inflammation.
- Cystatin C is removed from the circulation by the kidneys. It is freely filtered at the glomerulus and largely destroyed in the tubules.
- The clinical utility of cystatin C can be improved with a GFR estimating equation—for example, the CKD-EPI$_{cys}$ equation.

UREA

Biochemistry and Physiology

Urea ($CO[NH_2]_2$, Mr 60 Da) is the major nitrogen-containing metabolic product of protein catabolism in humans, accounting for more than 75% of the nonprotein nitrogen eventually excreted. During the process of protein catabolism, nitrogen derived from amino acids enters the urea cycle via intermediates, which include aspartate and ammonia. The biosynthesis of urea is carried out exclusively in the liver by the enzymes of the urea cycle (Fig. 32.4). The rate of production of urea is dependent on the rate of protein catabolism from both dietary sources and endogenous protein, which is largely derived from muscle tissue. After production, urea is distributed evenly throughout the total body water due to its ability to diffuse through most cell membranes facilitated by urea transporter proteins.[337] Urea is therefore described as having a volume of distribution equal to the total body water.

Renal excretion accounts for more than 90% of urea removal from the body, with losses through the gastrointestinal tract and skin accounting for most of the remainder. Urea is freely filtered at the glomerulus and is neither actively reabsorbed nor secreted by the tubules. However, as part of normal kidney function, 40% to 70% of urea moves passively out of the renal tubule and into the renal interstitium, ultimately to reenter plasma. The back-diffusion of urea is also dependent on urine flow rate, with less entering the interstitium in high-flow states (eg, pregnancy) and more with low-flow situations (eg, prerenal reduction in GFR due to fluid losses). Because water is resorbed to a far greater extent than the urea back-diffusion, urea is markedly concentrated during the process of urine formation, being present in urine at about 20 to 100 times the plasma concentration. Urinary urea is the major contributor to urine osmolality, and the daily amount of urea excreted in the urine is directly related to the rate of urea production and therefore to the rate of protein

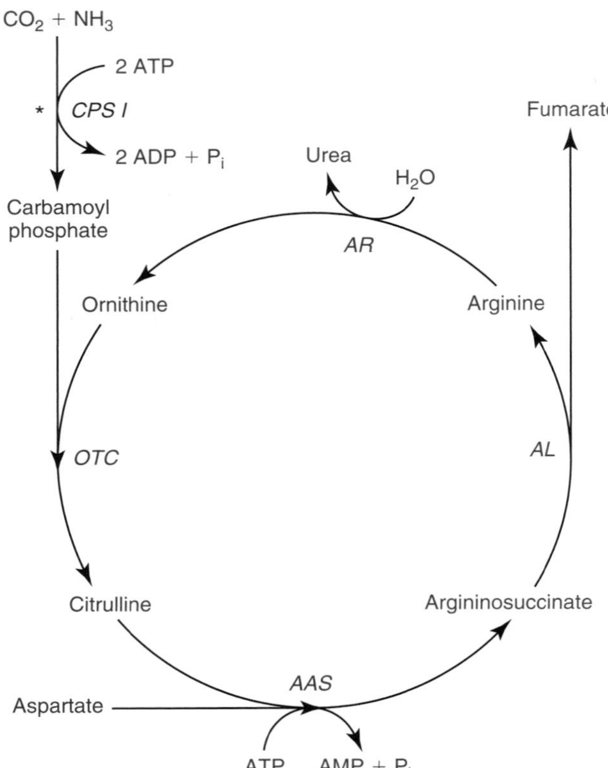

FIGURE 32.4 The urea cycle pathway. *AAS,* Argininosuccinate synthetase; *AL,* argininosuccinate lyase; *AR,* arginase; *ADP,* adenosine diphosphate, *ATP,* adenosine triphosphate; *CPS I,* carbamyl phosphate synthetase I (*N-acetylglutamate as positive allosteric effector); *OTC,* ornithine transcarbamylase; P_i, inorganic phosphate.

breakdown. The role of urea in the functioning of the kidney is complex, involving specific urea transporters under the action of vasopressin.[338,339]

Analytical Methods

Chemical methods based on direct reactions with urea and enzymatic methods with urea as the enzyme substrate are the two principal approaches that have been used to quantify urea in body fluids. Although once widely used, chemical methods have been almost universally superseded by enzymatic approaches. For a more detailed description of direct chemical urea measurement, the reader is referred to Taylor and Vadgama.[340]

Enzymatic Methods

The vast majority of urea measurements in clinical laboratories are undertaken using enzymatic methods based on preliminary hydrolysis of urea with urease (urea amidohydrolase, EC 3.5.1.5; main source jack bean meal) to generate ammonium ion, which then is quantitated. This approach has been used in end-point, kinetic, conductimetric, and dry chemistry systems.[340]

$$\underset{\text{Urea}}{(H_2N)_2C{=}O} + 2\,H_2O \xrightarrow{\text{Urease}} 2\,NH_4^{\oplus} + CO_3^{\ominus\ominus}$$

Spectrophotometric approaches to ammonium quantitation include the Berthelot reaction and the enzymatic assay with glutamate dehydrogenase [l-glutamate:NAD(P) oxidoreductase (deaminating), EC 1.4.1.3].[341] This latter approach was proposed as a reference method in 1980[342] and adapted to a range of analytical platforms.

$$NH_4^{\oplus} + \text{2-Oxoglutarate} \xrightarrow[\text{NADH} + H^{\oplus} \rightarrow NAD^{\oplus}]{\text{Glutamate dehydrogenase}} \text{Glutamate} + H_2O$$

For serum assays, the reaction system is usually formulated with urease, so the addition of sample containing urea starts the reaction. A decrease in absorbance resulting from the glutamate dehydrogenase reaction is monitored at 340 nm. In another example of a coupled-enzyme assay system for urea, ammonia produced from urea by urease then reacts with glutamate and adenosine triphosphate in the presence of glutamine synthetase (EC 6.3.1.2). Adenosine diphosphate produced in this second enzymatic reaction is then quantitated in third and fourth steps using pyruvate kinase (EC 2.7.1.40) and pyruvate oxidase (EC 1.2.3.3), respectively, thus generating peroxide. In the final step, peroxide reacts with phenol and 4-aminophenazone, catalyzed by peroxidase (EC 1.11.1.7), to yield a quinone-monoamine dye that can be quantitated spectrophotometrically.[343]

Methods for the measurement of urea using dry chemistry systems using the urease approach and a range of detection methods have been described.[344,345] It is also possible to measure urea using a conductimetric method in which sample and a urease-containing reagent are incubated in a conductivity cell with the rate of change of the conductivity being monitored as the urea is converted to an ionic species. In a potentiometric approach, an ammonium ion-selective electrode is employed, and urease is immobilized on a membrane.[346-348] A similar approach has been used to enable real-time monitoring of dialysis efficiency.[349] An alternative enzymatic approach to the measurement of urea has been described by Morishita and colleagues, using a system incorporating leucine dehydrogenase (EC 1.4.1.9), in addition to urease, which eliminates interference from endogenous ammonium.[350]

The analytical specificity of all of the methods is good, particularly for the urease-glutamate dehydrogenase procedure; however, endogenous ammonia interference must be expected when the protocol employs the sample to initiate the reaction. This may be relevant in aged samples, in some urines, and in particular metabolic disorders. Typically, within-run CVs of less than 3.0% with between-day values of less than 4.0% are achievable in the concentration range of 14 to 20 mg/dL (5 to 7 mmol/L). Given the high intrinsic biological variation of serum urea (see later), this is well within desired standards of analytical performance.[340]

Traceability of Urea Measurement

Reference methods based on IDMS are available for urea measurement and are listed by the JCTLM.[351] The JCTLM database also lists pure and serum matrix-matched reference materials and reference measurement services based on this IDMS technology. A study of routine assays from major suppliers in 2008 indicated that for most methods the average method bias was 10% or less,[352] although there were many method groups where the bias was both statistically and clinically different from the reference method values.

Reference Intervals and Biological Variability

Serum urea concentrations are higher in men than in women, and there is an increase in the upper reference limit throughout adult life by a factor of about 50% from the 20s to the 70s.[353,354] It is likely that this is largely mediated by the expected decline in renal function with age. Additionally, population differences are expected based on average protein intake. Pregnancy is associated with lower urea concentrations compared with age-matched nonpregnant women due to the associated glomerular hyperfiltration.[355] In the pediatric age range, from after the first 2 weeks, the first year of life is associated with low serum urea, followed by a rise to slightly above adult concentrations to age about 10 years and then falling to young adult values by the late teens.[356]

A reference interval for serum urea in healthy adults is 2.1 to 7.1 mmol/L (6–20 mg/dL expressed as urea nitrogen). In adults older than 60 years of age, a higher reference interval (eg, 2.9–8.2 mmol/L [8–23 mg/dL]) may be used. Determined reference intervals will depend on the age, diet, and gender balance of the reference population, and decisions are required about partitioning in implementing a reference interval for routine use. The use of age-, gender-, and population-specific reference intervals will make serum urea more sensitive to the disease-related changes (see later). For more information on urea reference intervals in males and females at different age groups, refer to the Appendix.

Although the term *blood urea nitrogen* (BUN) continues to be used in some countries for ordering serum urea tests with results reported as mg/dL of BUN, this terminology is incorrect and obsolete because blood is rarely analyzed for nitrogen (rather, the true measurand is urea in serum). The long-established habit of reporting and expressing results of a urea assay in units of urea nitrogen appears to be strongly entrenched in the United States, although the SI system recommends the use of urea, expressed in mmol/L. Because urea contains two nitrogen atoms (each Mr 14) out of a total Mr of 60, the mass concentration of urea in a sample is 60/28 (2.14) times the urea nitrogen concentration. To convert this to molar units, and allowing for the change in the denominator from dL to L, 1 mg/dL BUN = $10 \times 2.14/60$ = 0.357 mmol/L urea.

On an average protein diet, urinary urea excretion expressed as urea nitrogen is 12 to 20 g/d (430 to 710 mmol/d). The balance in the physiological rates of production and removal discussed earlier produce a within-subject biological variation for serum urea described by a CV_I of about 12% (see https://www.westgard.com/biodatabase-2014-update.htm), with a CV_I for 24-hour urinary urea excretion of about 18%.[357]

Clinical Significance

Measurement of blood and serum urea has been used for many years as an indicator of kidney function. However, it is generally accepted that creatinine measurement provides better information in this respect. Serum and urinary urea measurement may still provide useful clinical information in particular circumstances. The measurement of urea in dialysis fluids is widely used in assessing the adequacy of renal replacement therapy (see Chapter 59).

Urea concentration in serum is affected by the rate of production as well as the rate of removal. This both limits its value as a test of kidney function and allows its use for a range of other factors. For example, plasma urea production, and therefore plasma concentration, is increased by a high-protein diet, increased endogenous protein catabolism, reabsorption of blood proteins after gastrointestinal hemorrhage, and treatment with cortisol or its synthetic analogues.

Urea removal from the circulation can be reduced due to any cause of reduced glomerular filtration, including prerenal, renal, or postrenal factors, and its differential response relative to creatinine can be useful diagnostically. In obstructive postrenal conditions (eg, malignancy, nephrolithiasis, and prostatism), both serum creatinine and urea concentrations will be increased, although in these situations the increase in serum urea is greater than in creatinine because of increased back-diffusion. These considerations give rise to the main proposed clinical use of serum urea—namely, its measurement in conjunction with that of serum creatinine and subsequent calculation of the urea to creatinine ratio (also referred to as the BUN to creatinine ratio).[358] This can be used as a crude discriminator between prerenal and intrinsic azotemia. For a normal individual on a normal diet, the reference interval for the ratio is between about 49 and 81 mmol urea/mmol creatinine (12 and 20 mg urea/mg creatinine). In the setting of known AKI, a raised urea to creatinine ratio (>81 mmol/mmol) is thought to be more indicative of a prerenal cause than an intrinsic renal cause, such as acute tubular necrosis. The rationale is that the urea resorption from the urine is higher with the slow flow rates of reduced renal perfusion and lower in the setting of tubular damage. A recent assessment of this tool has found it to be inaccurate in many cases, but it did identify higher in-hospital mortality in AKI patients with a urea to creatinine ratio greater than 80 mmol/mmol.[359]

Urea is increased in chronic heart failure, leading to an increased urea to creatinine ratio, which is considered a poor prognostic indicator.[360] The observed increase in urea is greater than expected based on reduced renal filtration alone, and it is thought to be mediated by neurohormonal activation.[361] Urea is widely used as part of a clinical risk prediction score, CURB-65 (consisting of assessment of confusion, urea, respiratory rate, blood pressure, and age greater than/less than 65 years), in the stratification of patients presenting to hospital with pneumonia.[362]

A low serum urea concentration occurs in the setting of low protein intake—for example, starvation or anorexia nervosa. This is less commonly seen among hospital inpatients who, although often do not consume adequate nutrients, do not exhibit a low serum urea due to the presence of significant catabolism of endogenous protein. Low serum urea concentration can also be seen with end-stage liver disease due to decreased urea synthesis.

Due to tubular back-diffusion, a measured urea clearance underestimates GFR, making it a poor clinical tool for this purpose. Previously the average of urea clearance and creatinine clearance, which under- and overestimate the actual GFR, respectively, has been suggested as a routine tool for GFR estimation, but this practice is no longer recommended due to poor performance.[363] Measurement of urinary urea provides a crude index of overall nitrogen balance and may be used as a guide to replacement in patients receiving parenteral nutrition.[364]

URIC ACID (URATE)

Biochemistry and Physiology

In humans, uric acid (2,6,8-trihydroxypurine) is the major product of catabolism of the purine nucleosides, adenosine and guanosine (Fig. 32.5). Purines from the catabolism of dietary nucleic acid are converted to uric acid directly. The bulk of purines excreted as uric acid arise from degradation of endogenous nucleic acids. The daily synthesis rate of uric acid is approximately 400 mg; dietary sources contribute another 300 mg. In men consuming a purine-free diet, the total body pool of exchangeable uric acid is estimated at 1200 mg; in women it is estimated to be 600 mg. By contrast, patients with gouty arthritis and tissue deposition of uric acid may have uric acid pools as large as 18,000 to 30,000 mg.

Overproduction of uric acid may result from increased synthesis of purine precursors. Synthesis and metabolism of the major precursors are illustrated in the outline in Fig. 32.5. The second enzymatic step in the synthetic pathway (Fig. 32.5A), formation of 5′-phosphoribosylamine, is the first irreversibly committed step in purine biosynthesis. The intracellular concentration of the substrate phosphoribosylpyrophosphate (PRPP) regulates de novo purine synthesis. The enzyme PRPP-amidotransferase is controlled through feedback inhibition by the purine nucleotides that are the final products of the biosynthetic pathway. The first purine nucleotide formed by ring closure is inosine monophosphate (IMP); adenosine and guanosine monophosphates are derived from IMP through enzymatically mediated interconversions. Adenine and guanine nucleotides may then be used as precursors for the corresponding nucleosides that are the building blocks of deoxyribonucleic acid and ribonucleic acid, or, when further phosphorylated, these nucleotides become carriers of high-energy bonds in the form of ATP and guanosine triphosphate.

Catabolism of the nucleotides (Fig. 32.5B) begins with removal of their ribose-linked phosphate, a process catalyzed by purine 5′-nucleotidase. Removal of the ribose moiety of inosine and guanosine by the action of purine-nucleoside phosphorylase forms hypoxanthine and guanine, both of which are converted to xanthine. Xanthine is converted to uric acid through the action of xanthine oxidase.

Reutilization of the major purine bases, adenine, hypoxanthine, and guanine, is achieved through "salvage" pathways (Fig. 32.5C), in which phosphoribosylation of the free bases leads to resynthesis of the respective nucleotide monophosphates. Adenine is converted to adenosine monophosphate through the action of adenine phosphoribosyl transferase (APRT), hypoxanthine, and guanine to their monophosphates through hypoxanthine-guanine phosphoribosyl transferase (HGPRT, EC 2.4.2.8). The HGPRT pathway is quantitatively more important than the APRT pathway.

Lower primates and mammals other than humans carry purine metabolism one step further with the formation of allantoin from uric acid, a step mediated by uricase ([urate:oxygen] oxidoreductase, EC 1.7.3.3). In humans, approximately 75% of uric acid excreted is lost in the urine; most of the remainder is secreted into the gastrointestinal tract, where it is degraded to allantoin and other compounds by bacterial enzymes.

Renal handling of uric acid is complex and involves four sequential steps: (1) glomerular filtration of virtually all the uric acid in capillary plasma entering the glomerulus; (2) reabsorption in the proximal convoluted tubule of about 98% to 100% of filtered uric acid; (3) subsequent secretion of uric acid into the lumen in the distal portion of the proximal tubule; and (4) further reabsorption in the distal tubule. The net urinary excretion of uric acid is 6% to 12% of the amount filtered.

The physicochemical properties of uric acid are important in considering uric acid concentrations in the circulation, in tissue, and in the kidneys. The first pK_a of uric acid is 5.75; above this pH, uric acid exists chiefly as urate ion, which is more soluble than uric acid. At a urine pH below 5.75, uric acid is the preponderant form. On the basis of the ionization form in the circulation it has been proposed that *urate* should be the preferred term rather than *uric acid* when describing serum measurements.

Analytical Methods

Phosphotungstic acid (PTA), uricase, and HPLC-based methods have been described for measuring uric acid.[365] PTA methods are now rarely used: the reader is referred to a review for additional details.[365]

Uricase Methods

The enzyme uricase ([urate:oxygen] oxidoreductase; EC 1.7.3.3; main sources *Aspergillus flavus*, *Candida utilis*, *Bacillus fastidiosus*, and hog liver) is used as a single step or as the initial step to oxidize uric acid. Uricase methods became feasible and popular as a result of the availability of high-quality, low-cost preparations of the bacterial enzyme. Preliminary precipitation of protein is not required. Generally, only guanine, xanthine, and a few other structural analogs of uric acid act as alternative substrates, and then only at concentrations improbable in biological fluids, thus giving these methods excellent analytical specificity.

Uricase acts on uric acid to produce allantoin, hydrogen peroxide, and carbon dioxide.

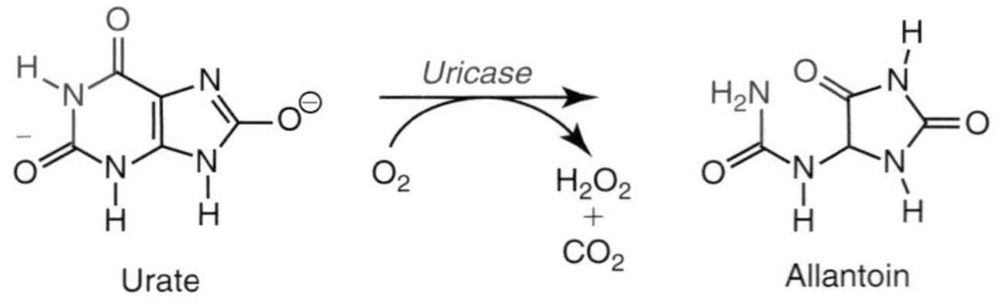

$$\text{Urate} + O_2 \xrightarrow{\text{Uricase}} \text{Allantoin} + H_2O_2 + CO_2$$

The reaction can be observed in either the kinetic or the equilibrium mode. The *Bacillus fastidiosus* enzyme has the highest Michaelis constant (10×10^{-5} mol/L), and the hog liver has the lowest (1.7×10^{-5} mol/L); the choice of enzyme influences the incubation period required to reach equilibrium and the conditions for a pseudo first-order kinetic approach. The decrease in absorbance as urate is converted may be monitored by a spectrophotometer at 293 nm.[366] However, at this wavelength, most of the absorbance is due to serum proteins. Therefore there is a high signal-noise ratio that can compromise the precision of the method. A high-quality spectrophotometer with narrow bandpass is necessary, and this is rarely satisfied with automated analyzers.

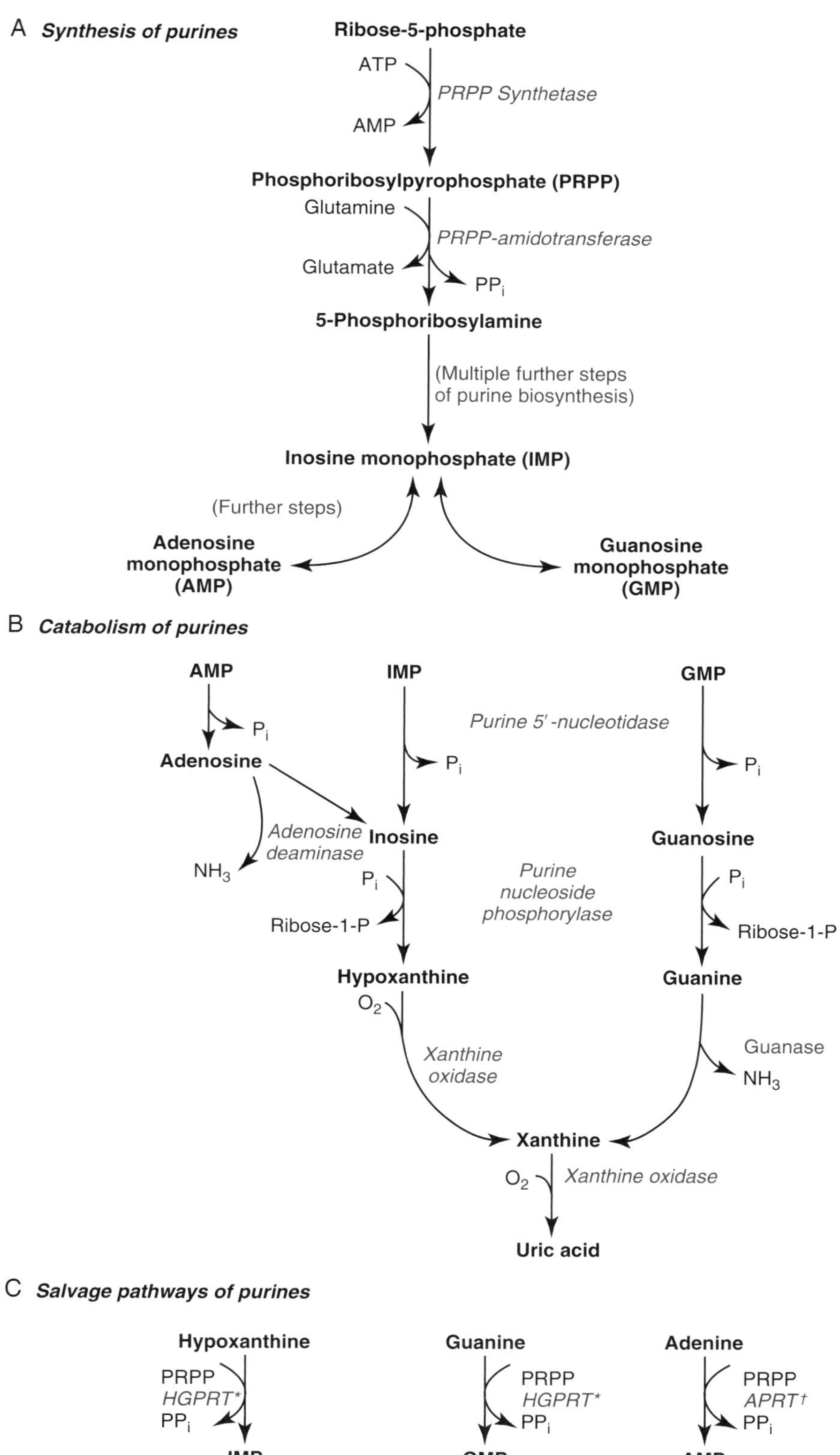

*Hypoxanthine-guanine phosphoribosyl transferase.
†Adenine phosphoribosyl transferase.

FIGURE 32.5 Metabolism of purines: **A,** Synthesis. **B,** Catabolism. **C,** Salvage pathways.

Most current enzymatic assays for serum urate involve a peroxidase system coupled with one of a number of oxygen acceptors to produce a chromogen.[367,368] The step for quantitation of the hydrogen peroxide produced is sometimes referred to as a Trinder reaction. One popular method measures hydrogen peroxide with the aid of horseradish peroxidase (donor:hydrogen-peroxide oxidoreductase; EC 1.11.1.7) and an oxygen acceptor to yield a chromogen in the visible spectrum.[369] Its popularity is probably due to the use of less expensive enzymes and greater analytical sensitivity. The most common oxygen acceptor used is 4-aminophenazone, together with phenol or a substituted phenol. The benefit of using substituted phenols is the enhanced molar absorptivity, as follows: phenol $\approx 5.5 \times 10^3$ L • mol/cm, tribromo-phenol $\approx 23.6 \times 10^3$ L • mol/cm, and tribromo-3-hydroxybenzoic acid $\approx 30.0 \times 10^3$ L • mol/cm. Alternative oxygen acceptors include 3-methyl-1-benzothiazoline hydrazone (MBTH), 2,2′-azino-di-(3-ethyl-benzothiazoline)-6-sulfonate (ABTS), and *o*-dianisidine.

Although many combinations of oxygen acceptor and phenol have been described, the choice should be guided by minimization of interference and sufficient absorbance to ensure good precision. The use of a substituted phenol yielding a highly absorbing product helps to reduce the potential interference by reducing the sample volume requirement. The major interferants to minimize are ascorbic acid and bilirubin. In general it is necessary to employ ascorbate oxidase (L-ascorbate:oxygen oxidoreductase; EC 1.10.3.3) in uric acid methods.[370] Aminophenazone with a substituted phenol or the addition of ferrocyanide[369,371] has been used to minimize bilirubin interference. Alternatively, use of the oxygen acceptor azure-D2 (3,7-diamino-5-pheno-thiazine [thionine] derivative), which can be monitored at 600 nm, reduces the spectral but not the chemical[372] interference caused by hyperbilirubinemia.[373] It has also been shown that unknown metabolites in the serum of patients with kidney failure, thought to be phenolic compounds, will interfere by competing with the reagent phenol, giving a low recovery of urate.[374] This interference can be overcome by using a phenolic derivative, thereby generating a higher-absorbing product and reducing the sample volume.

Although many methods for the quantitation of uric acid are described in the literature, the most popular methods today employ the uricase-mediated reaction; however, the measurement of the rate of the reaction may be compromised by the choice of detector reaction, owing to an interfering enzyme or a molecule that competes in the final color generation step. Today reactions that generate a visible end product are preferred because of the higher color yield; however, care should be taken that interference caused by ascorbate (eg, intravenous vitamin C), bilirubin, and unspecified interferents in serum from patients with kidney failure is minimized.

Dry Chemistry Systems

Devices that use uricase in a dry reagent format to measure uric acid have been described. For example, a multilayer film system employs uricase and peroxidase separated by a semipermeable membrane from a leuco dye that is oxidized to form a colored product.[375] A cellulose matrix pad system employs uricase, peroxidase, and MBTH as oxygen acceptors; the system uses a diluted serum sample, which helps to reduce interferences, although ascorbic acid was shown to be a significant interferant.[376] A third system incorporates separation of serum from red cells and uricase, peroxidase, and a substituted phenol to measure urate.[377] All three systems use a reflectance meter system to facilitate accurate and precise quantitation of the color change.

Several electrochemical and biosensor systems have been described for the measurement of uric acid. In most cases uricase is employed, being linked in examples to an oxygen electrode[378] or to a metal-organic probe whose fluorescence is quenched by oxygen.[379] Detection of uric acid has also been demonstrated as part of a multianalyte array.[380] A nonenzymatic approach has been described on a microchip, based on chemiluminescence microflow injection analysis.[381]

HPLC Methods

HPLC methods using pellicular ion-exchange or reversed-phase columns have been used to separate and quantify uric acid. The column effluent is monitored at 293 nm to detect the eluting uric acid. HPLC methods are specific and fast, mobile phases are simple, and the retention time for uric acid is less than 6 minutes, reasonable conditions that recommend these methods for reference use.[382]

Traceability of Uric Acid Measurement

The JCTLM lists pure substance and matrix matched certified reference materials for uric acid as well as IDMS reference methods and reference measurement services for analysis in serum and urine.[257,383-385]

The performance of commonly used methods in over 6000 laboratories was assessed by the College of American Pathologists, using a commutable sample and reference method determination. The medians of the majority of instrument groups were within 3% of the target, and all of the laboratories were within the minimal total error standard based on within-subject and within-group biological variation, suggesting that most routine methods are meeting clinical needs.[352]

Preanalytical Factors and Interferences

Urate is not normally affected by tube additives such as heparin, ethylenediaminetetraacetic acid (EDTA), separation gels, or procoagulants, but it is recommended that laboratories supply collection requirements for their clients based on their specific assay. Serum and lithium heparin plasma have been reported to produce equivalent results, and urate is stable in uncentrifuged blood at room temperature for at least 24 hours.[386] It has also been reported that urate is stable in serum for 48 hours at room temperature, 14 days at 4°C, and 4 months at −20°C.[387] In lithium heparin tubes with separator gel, urate is stable for at least 7 days after centrifugation.[388]

Rasburicase is a urate-consuming enzyme (urate oxidase) used to treat patients with tumor lysis syndrome. Rasburicase can lower serum urate concentrations in blood collection tubes ex vivo unless both whole blood and serum are cooled before and after separation or treated by acidification.[389,390]

Traditionally, urinary uric acid excretion is determined in a 24-hour urine sample. If analysis is not undertaken promptly, alkalinization of the sample is recommended to maintain uric acid in solution.[391] Samples at low pH and high uric acid concentrations may be more prone to uric acid precipitation if alkalinization is not performed.[392]

Reference Intervals and Biological Variability

The serum urate concentration increases gradually with age, rising about 10% between the ages of 20 and 60 years (see Appendix). A significant rise is seen in women after menopause, reaching concentrations similar to those found in men. Additionally, higher concentrations of serum urate are found with increases in waist circumference, body mass index, and other components of the metabolic syndrome.[393] Thus a population reference interval may require partitioning on the basis of gender and age and will be affected by the metabolic status of the population. It can be argued that a clinical decision point for the relevant clinical question (see later) may be more useful than a population reference interval given the interaction with common comorbidities. A reference interval for serum urate has been reported to be 3.5 to 7.2 mg/dL (0.21–0.43 mmol/L) for males and 2.6 to 6.0 mg/dL (0.16–0.36 mmol/L) for females.[394]

During pregnancy, serum urate concentrations fall during the first trimester and until about 24 weeks' gestation, when values begin to rise and eventually exceed nonpregnant concentrations.[395,396] Reference intervals at 32, 36, and 38 weeks' gestation have been reported as 1.9 to 5.5 mg/dL (0.11–0.32 mmol/L), 2.0 to 5.8 mg/dL (0.12–0.34 mmol/L), and 2.7 to 6.5 mg/dL (0.16–0.38 mmol/L), respectively.[396]

Urinary uric acid excretion in individuals on a diet containing purines is 250 to 750 mg/d (1.5–4.5 mmol/d). Excretion may decrease by 20% to 25% on a purine-free diet to less than 400 mg/d (2.4 mmol/d).

Biologic variability for serum urate has been reported as a CV_I of 8.6% and for 24 hours urinary uric acid as a CV_I of 16.8% (www.westgard.com). For further discussion on biological variability, see Chapter 7. A seasonal variation has been described with serum urate concentration about 5% to 7% higher in the summer months,[397] as well as a small diurnal variation, generally not exceeding 0.5 mg/dL (0.03 mmol/L);[398] these factors have not led to recommendations with regard to timing of sample collection.

Clinical Significance

The most common clinical use for urate assessment is risk assessment for gout and determination of therapy adequacy. Other clinical conditions where serum urate measurements have potential utility include cardiovascular risk assessment and diagnosis of preeclampsia. Urine uric acid measurements may play a role in assessing the cause of hyperuricemia and assessing risk of renal stone formation.

Hyperuricemia

The major causes of hyperuricemia are summarized in Box 32.1. Asymptomatic hyperuricemia is frequently detected through biochemical screening, although there is an absence of evidence for clinical benefit resulting from this practice.

Gout. Gout occurs when monosodium urate precipitates in joints and tissues from supersaturated body fluids. These deposits of urate are responsible for the clinical signs and symptoms. Gouty arthritis is caused by urate crystal formation in joint fluid and may be associated with deposits of crystals (tophi) in tissues surrounding the joint. The deposits may occur in other soft tissue as well, and wherever they occur they elicit an intense inflammatory response consisting of polymorphonuclear leukocytes and macrophages. The first metatarsophalangeal joint (big toe) is the classic site for gout.

BOX 32.1 Causes of Hyperuricemia

Increased Formation

Primary

Idiopathic
Inherited metabolic disorders

Secondary

Excess dietary purine intake
Increased nucleic acid turnover (eg, leukemia, myeloma, radiotherapy, chemotherapy, trauma)
Psoriasis
Altered ATP metabolism
Tissue hypoxia
Preeclampsia
Alcohol

Decreased Excretion

Primary (Idiopathic)

Secondary

Acute or chronic kidney disease
Increased renal reabsorption
Reduced secretion
Lead poisoning
Preeclampsia
Organic acids (eg, lactate and acetoacetate)
Salicylate (low doses)
Thiazide diuretics
Trisomy 21 (Down syndrome)

Gout is a condition characterized by occasional attacks and long periods of remission. It is important to appreciate that the serum uric acid concentration is often normal during an acute attack and is not a component of the diagnostic criteria. Demonstration of uric acid crystals in joint aspirate fluid is the pathognomonic for gout. For details on the diagnostic criteria and associated evidence base, readers are referred to the European League Against Rheumatism (EULAR) guidelines.[399] This report also provides information on the risk factors for the development of gout, which represent those for increasing concentrations of serum uric acid; of these, the major ones are male gender, CKD, hypertension, and obesity.

Gout may be classified as primary or secondary. *Primary* gout is associated with essential hyperuricemia, which has a polygenic basis. In more than 99% of cases, the cause is uncertain, but the condition is probably due to a combination of metabolic overproduction of purines (25% of patients have increased PRPP amidotransferase activity), decreased renal excretion (80% of patients show decreased renal tubular secretion of uric acid), and increased dietary intake. Very rarely, primary gout is attributable to inherited defects of enzymes in the pathways of purine metabolism.

Secondary gout is a result of hyperuricemia attributable to several identifiable causes. Renal retention of uric acid may occur in CKD of any type or as a consequence of administration of drugs; diuretics, in particular, are implicated in the latter instance. Organic acidemia caused by increased acetoacetic acid in diabetic ketoacidosis or to lactic acidosis may interfere with tubular secretion of urate. Increased nucleic acid turnover and a consequent increase in catabolism of purines may be encountered in rapid proliferation of tumor cells and in massive destruction of tumor cells on therapy with certain chemotherapeutic agents.

Management of an acute attack of gout can be divided into broad strategies: management of the attack and prevention of subsequent attacks. The main focus for acute management is pain relief, generally involving the use of nonsteroidal antiinflammatory drugs (NSAIDs). Avoidance of subsequent attacks is based on lifestyle and pharmacotherapy to reduce plasma urate. Patients should be advised to avoid foods that have high purine content (eg, liver, kidneys, red meat, and sardines) and drugs that affect urate excretion (thiazide diuretics and salicylates). Specific pharmacologic interventions include the use of uricosuric drugs (eg, probenecid and sulfinpyrazone), which enhance renal excretion of uric acid by blocking the carriers in the tubular cells that mediate reabsorption, or the xanthine oxidase inhibitor allopurinol. Historically measurement of urinary uric acid excretion has been described as an aid in separating overproduction from underexcretion and thus in selecting appropriate treatment in this context but is not now recommended as part of routine investigation for patients with gout.[400,401] An evidence-based treatment target for prevention of gout recurrence is a serum urate concentration less than 0.36 mmol/L.[400]

Kidney Disease. Kidney disease associated with hyperuricemia may take one or more of several forms: (1) gouty nephropathy with urate deposition in renal parenchyma, (2) acute intratubular deposition of urate crystals, and (3) urate nephrolithiasis.[402]

Kidney Stones. Uric acid kidney stones occur in approximately one in five patients with clinical gout. Although serum and urinary uric acid should be measured in stone formers, many uric acid stone formers do not demonstrate hyperuricuria or hyperuricemia. However, this may reflect the use of reference intervals derived in a purine-rich, westernized society.[403] The cause of uric acid stone formation also involves the passage of a persistently acid urine with loss of the postprandial alkaline tide.[402] Undissociated uric acid (pK_a 5.57) is relatively insoluble, whereas urate at pH 7.0 is greater than 10 times more soluble. Thus in patients with urinary pH persistently less than 6.0, normal urinary concentrations of uric acid will produce supersaturation. Measurement of urinary pH throughout the day may be useful.[403] Pure uric acid stones account for approximately 8% of all urinary tract stones and, unlike many of the calcium-containing stones, are radiolucent. Allopurinol is the mainstay of treatment of uric acid stones. Hyperuricuria has long been considered a risk factor for calcium stone formation (see Chapter 59), although this has been questioned.[404] Consequently, attempts to increase urinary pH with potassium alkali salts may be counterproductive as a result of increased calcium stone formation.

Preeclampsia. Preeclampsia is pregnancy-induced hypertension associated with proteinuria (>0.3 g/d) and often edema and may become life-threatening for the mother or the fetus (see Chapter 69). Treatment involves management of the hypertension and delivery as soon as it is safe to do so. It is also characterized by increased serum uric acid concentration, which may contribute to the pathogenesis of the condition.[405] Possible clinical roles for serum urate measurement in preeclampsia include use as a predictive tool prior to the onset of hypertension, or as a tool to guide management, particularly the decision on timing of delivery. There does not appear to be sufficient evidence for the former role, and there is uncertainty in the latter. There is supporting evidence for the use of urate measurements,[406] and measurement recommendations appear in some guidelines[407] but not others.[408] If assessing urate concentrations in this setting, it is important to use pregnancy-specific reference intervals.

Inherited Diseases. Hyperuricemia can be a feature of several inherited disorders of purine metabolism, most of which are rare, and the diagnosis requires support from a specialist purine laboratory. Some brief details follow, but readers are referred to specialist textbooks for further information. The Lesch-Nyhan syndrome is characterized by a complete deficiency of HGPRT, the major enzyme of the purine salvage pathways. This X-linked genetic disorder is manifested clinically by mental retardation, abnormal muscle movements, and behavioral problems (self-mutilation and pathologic aggressiveness). Patients may, in the first weeks of life, have symptoms of crystalluria, AKI, and gout. Hyperuricemia, hyperuricuria, and markedly decreased concentrations of HGPRT are present in erythrocytes, fibroblasts, and other cells. Intracellular concentrations of PRPP and rates of purine synthesis are increased. Neurologic symptoms of this syndrome may be related to decreased availability of purines to the developing brain, which has limited capacity for de novo purine synthesis and therefore relies on the purine salvage pathways to supply it with most of the purine nucleotides it requires. DNA technology has been applied to prenatal diagnosis in the first trimester, using chorionic biopsy material. HGPRT assays on cultured fibroblasts obtained by amniocentesis may be used in the second trimester. Partial deficiency of HGPRT (severe X-linked gout) presents in adolescence or early adulthood as early gout, kidney failure, or nephrolithiasis. Increased levels of intracellular PRPP production with consequent increased uric acid concentrations can also occur owing to mutations in PRPP synthetase (EC 2.7.6.1) (PRPP synthetase superactivity), which is also inherited as an X-linked recessive trait. An autosomal dominant familial juvenile hyperuricemic nephropathy has been recognized. Glucose-6-phosphatase deficiency leads to hyperuricemia as a result of both overproduction and underexcretion of uric acid.

Hypouricemia

Hypouricemia, often defined as serum urate concentrations less than 2.0 mg/dL (0.12 mmol/L), is much less common than hyperuricemia. It may be secondary to any one of a number of underlying conditions. Severe hepatocellular disease with reduced purine synthesis or xanthine oxidase activity is one possibility. Another is defective renal tubular reabsorption of uric acid. Defective reabsorption may be congenital, as in generalized Fanconi syndrome, or acquired. The reabsorption defect may be acquired acutely because of injection of radiopaque contrast media or chronically because of exposure to toxic agents. Overtreatment of hyperuricemia with allopurinol or uricosuric drugs and cancer chemotherapy with 6-mercaptopurine or azathioprine (inhibitors of de novo purine synthesis) may also cause hypouricemia. Very rarely, hypouricemia may occur as the result of an inherited metabolic defect. Hypouricemia in combination with xanthinuria is rarely encountered and suggests a deficiency of xanthine oxidase, either in isolation or as part of combined molybdenum cofactor deficiency (sulfite oxidase/xanthine oxidase deficiency). Purine nucleoside phosphorylase (EC 2.4.2.1) deficiency and other inherited defects have also been described.

Cardiometabolic Outcomes and Urate

Recent publications have highlighted positive associations between serum urate concentrations and a range of important cardiovascular and health outcomes that are generally associated with the metabolic syndrome. These associations include the presence of obesity and insulin resistance,[393] development of hypertension and renal disease,[409] cardiovascular disease,[410] type 2 diabetes,[411] and all cause and cardiovascular mortality.[412] More important, as well as indicating risk for patients with hyperuricemia, these relationships occur within the usually described "normal range" with the higher urate values associated with increasing risk. While these associations appear to be robust, it is less clear whether or not there is a causal association[413] or whether urate-lowering therapy may be beneficial. Recently prospective trials have been published using allopurinol in hyperuricemic patients with diabetes or polycystic kidney disease, with the aim of slowing or reversing the rate of GFR reduction.[414,415] Uric acid is generally seen as a metabolic waste product. However, it also has antioxidant properties in the circulation, with beneficial effects on endothelial function, in contrast to a pro-oxidant action intracellularly.[416] The role of measurement of urate in the routine laboratory, validated clinical decision points, and appropriate management of patients based on the results remains to be determined; however, it is likely that there will be more roles for this analyte in the future.

POINTS TO REMEMBER

Urate

- Urate (uric acid) is the major end product of catabolism of the purine nucleosides.
- Excretion of urate is predominantly renal.
- Reference intervals for urate are influenced by many factors, including age, gender, menopausal status, diet, and waist circumference.
- Gout occurs when monosodium urate precipitates in joints and tissues from supersaturated body fluids, eliciting an intense inflammatory response.
- When treating gout, a target urate concentration of less than 6 mg/dL (<0.36 mmol/L) is used.

MEASUREMENT OF METABOLITES RELATED TO KIDNEY STONE FORMATION

Kidney stones are discussed in detail in Chapter 59. Details are given here of the measurement of three metabolites commonly assessed as risk factors in the evaluation of patients with kidney stones—namely, urinary oxalate, citrate, and cystine. Urate metabolism in this context has been discussed earlier (see Uric Acid, Kidney Stones).

Oxalate

Ideally, urine for oxalate analysis should be collected into acid to prevent the crystallization of calcium oxalate crystals. Acidification also prevents ex vivo formation of oxalate from ascorbate, a cause of factitious hyperoxaluria in individuals ingesting excessive amounts of vitamin C.[417] A number of approaches for the measurement of urinary oxalate have been employed, including HPLC, enzymatic and capillary electrophoretic methods.[418-420] The enzymatic methods employ the enzyme oxalate oxidase (EC 1.2.3.4. oxalate:oxygen oxidoreductase). With this method, the sample of urine is initially acidified to pH 1.8 (typically with 2 mmol/L HCl) to ensure complete solubilization of any calcium oxalate crystals. The oxalate is oxidized to carbon dioxide and hydrogen peroxide by oxalate oxidase, and the hydrogen peroxide is detected with horseradish peroxidase and coupled with an oxygen acceptor reagent such as 3-dimethyl aminobenzoic acid and 3-methyl-2-benzothiazolinone hydrazone to yield an indamine dye that absorbs at 590 nm. A charcoal column pretreatment step to remove interferents from the urine has been used,[421] although this may not be necessary.[420] An alternative approach to the detection of hydrogen peroxide using catalase has also been described. The oxalate oxidase is specific for oxalate; however, the peroxide detection reaction may suffer from interferences (eg, turbidity in the catalase-mediated reaction, ascorbic acid, and other reducing agents in the peroxidase-mediated reaction). The choice of oxygen acceptor will determine the potential for interference from compounds such as ascorbic acid.

Citrate

Citrate is measured by GC, capillary electrophoresis,[418] or an enzyme-mediated reaction. While methods using aconitase (EC 4.2.1.3) and isocitrate dehydrogenase (EC 1.1.1.42), or citrate lyase (EC 4.1.3.6) and oxaloacetate decarboxylase (EC 4.1.1.3) have been described, a method using the lyase together with malate dehydrogenase (EC 1.1.1.37) and lactate dehydrogenase (EC 1.1.1.27) is preferred. The combination of the two dehydrogenase pathways has been proposed to ensure that any oxaloacetate ion enzymatically decarboxylated is also measured. The enzyme-mediated decarboxylase pathway is less favored because of the poor stability of the enzyme. Using a reaction sequence that involves incubation of the sample with all constituents except the citrate lyase ensures that all endogenous oxaloacetate and pyruvate are removed. Analysis of serum involves a deproteinization step, while urine should be titrated to pH 8.0 before analysis. A typical incubation period is 10 to 15 minutes, and the citrate can be quantitated from the decrease in the absorbance at 340 nm. A cheap, rapid, automated adaptation of this procedure, which does not require a deproteinizing step, has been described.[422]

Cystine

Cystine, a dimer of cysteine, can be measured in urine using the cyanide-nitroprusside test, thin layer chromatography, by quantitative amino acid analysis using either ion exchange or LC techniques or MS. In the cyanide-nitroprusside test, cystine is split into two molecules of cysteine by cyanide. Sodium nitroprusside reacts with the free sulfide groups to give a magenta color. The test is hazardous and will give false-negative results in acidified or infected urines, in patients receiving D-penicillamine therapy, or if the sodium nitroprusside solution is not fresh. Further, it cannot distinguish between cystine and homocystine. It is not useful when monitoring the treatment of known cystinurics, who require quantitation of their urinary cystine output or concentration (see Chapter 70). In practice, amino acid analysis (see Chapters 28 and 70) allows simultaneous quantitation of the dibasic amino acids, which may be helpful for characterizing the clinical phenotype. However, cystine concentration does not necessarily equate directly with cystine *solubility*, which will vary at different urinary pHs. A novel approach, cystine capacity, has been developed that directly measures the ability of a patient's urine to solubilize or precipitate cystine.[423]

ASSESSMENT OF KIDNEY FUNCTION: ESTIMATION OF GLOMERULAR FILTRATION RATE

The GFR is widely accepted as the best overall measure of kidney function, enabling a statement of the complex functions of the kidney in a single numeric expression.[13] A decrease in GFR precedes kidney failure in all forms of progressive disease. Different kidney pathologic conditions can progress to renal failure and dialysis dependency at rates varying from weeks to several decades.[424,425] Symptoms accompanying progressive kidney disease (see Chapter 59) and their correlation with GFR will be influenced by this rate of progression. Measuring GFR in established disease is useful in targeting treatment, monitoring progression, and predicting the point at which renal replacement therapy will be required. It is also used as a dosage guide to prevent toxicity by drugs excreted by the kidneys. Several methods are used to measure the GFR; most involve the ability of the kidneys to clear an exogenous or endogenous marker. Improving methods and the discovery of new markers of GFR and glomerular or tubular damage will continue to provide important contributions to the early diagnosis of renal disease.

The Concept of Clearance

Most of the clinical laboratory information used to assess kidney function is derived from or related to measurement of the clearance of some substance by the kidneys. Renal clearance of a substance is defined as the volume of plasma from which the substance is completely cleared (removed) by the kidneys per unit of time.

Provided a substance *S* is freely filtered in the glomerulus and neither secreted nor resorbed intact into the bloodstream from the tubules, the renal clearance of *S* is equal to the GFR, and carries the same unit dimension (volume/time). Furthermore, provided substance *S* is also in stable concentration in the plasma and is physiologically inert, freely filtered at the glomerulus, and not secreted, reabsorbed, synthesized, or metabolized by the kidney tubules, the amount of that substance filtered at the glomerulus is equal to the amount excreted in the urine (ie, the amount of *S* entering the nephrons must exactly equal the amount leaving it). The amount of *S* filtered at the glomerulus equals GFR multiplied by plasma *S* concentration: GFR × PS. The amount of *S* excreted equals the urine *S* concentration (US) multiplied by the urinary flow rate (V, volume excreted per unit time).

Because filtered *S* = excreted *S*,

$$\mathrm{GFR} \times \mathrm{PS} = \mathrm{US} \times \mathrm{V} \quad (1)$$

$$\mathrm{GFR} = (US \times V)/PS \quad (2)$$

where:

GFR = the flow rate in mL per minute of plasma through the glomerular membranes estimated as a *clearance* in units of mL of plasma cleared of a substance per minute

US = urinary concentration of the substance

V = volumetric flow rate of urine in mL per minute

PS = plasma concentration of the substance (in the same units as the urinary concentration of the substance)

The term (US × V)/*PS* is defined as the clearance of substance *S* and is an accurate estimate of GFR provided the aforementioned criteria are satisfied. Inulin satisfies these criteria and has long been regarded as the most accurate (gold standard) estimate of GFR (see later). The formula for clearance given above is specified in mL/min. This is the most commonly used unit for GFR and is recommended for universal adoption to avoid confusion from the use of different units, although recognizing that the use of minute rather than second is not a strict use of the Systeme Internationale (SI).

Kidney size and GFR are roughly proportional to body size. It is conventional to adjust clearance estimates to a standard body surface area (BSA) of 1.73 m^2, even though this may not be the average BSA of the population. For the sake of uniformity, the use of this format is also preferred over expressing normalization per meter squared ($mL.min^{-1}.m^{-2}$). It is common to use the formula devised by Du Bois and Du Bois in 1916 when estimating BSA, even though the data used to establish this equation were very limited.[426]

$$\mathrm{BSA} = \mathrm{Weight\ (kg)}^{0.425} \times \mathrm{Height\ (cm)}^{0.725} \times 7.2 \times 10^{-3} \quad (3)$$

A variety of exogenous (radioisotopic and nonradioisotopic) and endogenous markers have been used to estimate clearance (Table 32.4). Measurement of clearance may require accurate measurements of both serum and urinary concentrations of the marker used plus a reliable urine collection. For a reliable serum measurement, the substance must have reached a steady-state concentration and must not be rapidly changing. For reliable urine collection, the urine flow must be adequate (several mL/min), the collection period long enough, and complete bladder emptying achieved; this is problematic.

Exogenous Markers of Glomerular Filtration Rate

Reference determination of GFR is considered to be that measured using exogenous markers, although practical limitations restrict their widespread use. The "gold standard" approach is considered to be urinary clearance of inulin (see later).[427]

GFR measurements may be based on the urinary or plasma clearance of the marker. In selecting a marker for accurate measurement of GFR when using either urinary or plasma clearance methods, it is essential that (1) renal tubular secretion or reabsorption does not influence elimination of the marker, (2) plasma protein binding of the marker is negligible, and (3) no extrarenal elimination of the marker occurs. Incomplete bladder emptying may also contribute to inaccuracy in urinary clearance approaches. For research purposes, in patients with low (<30 mL/min) GFR and in patients with ascites or edema, measurement is best performed using a urinary clearance method.[428] From a clinical management perspective, in most patients either urinary or plasma clearance approaches are acceptable.

TABLE 32.4 Markers of Glomerular Filtration Rate in an Approximate Hierarchical Arrangement

Hierarchy	Marker	Advantages*	Disadvantages
Gold standard	Inulin (sinistrin) continuous infusion urinary clearance	• Gold standard: closest known ideal filtration marker	• Exogenous compound • Time-consuming/complex procedure requiring a timed urine collection • Requires urinary catheterization or is prone to errors due to incomplete bladder emptying • Complex laboratory analysis
Silver standard	Inulin (sinistrin) single bolus plasma clearance	• Closest known ideal filtration marker • Acceptable agreement with urinary inulin clearance • No requirement for urine collection	• As above, plus some extrarenal clearance (0.083 mL/min/kg)
	^{125}I-iothalamate urinary clearance	• Radioisotopic[†](simple measurement) • Acceptable agreement with urinary inulin clearance	• Exogenous compound • Radioisotopic[†] (risks of ionizing radiation) • Time-consuming/complex procedure • Not available in all countries • Reports of allergic reactions • Slight positive bias to urinary inulin clearance, probably due to tubular secretion
	^{125}I-iothalamate single bolus plasma clearance	• Radioisotopic[†] (simple measurement) • No requirement for urine collection	• As above
	^{51}Cr-EDTA urinary clearance	• Radioisotopic (simple measurement) • Acceptable agreement with urinary inulin clearance • Widely available in Europe but not available in United States	• Exogenous compound • Radioisotopic (risks of ionizing radiation) • Time-consuming/complex procedure • Probable tubular reabsorption • ^{51}Cr less readily available than ^{99m}Tc
	^{51}Cr-EDTA single bolus plasma clearance	• As above, but no requirement for urine collection	• As above, plus some extrarenal clearance (0.079 mL/min/kg)
	Iohexol urinary clearance	• Nonradioisotopic • Widely available • Inexpensive • Acceptable agreement with urinary inulin clearance	• Exogenous compound • Time-consuming/complex procedure • Complex measurement requiring ID-MS or HPLC • Reports of allergic reactions
	Iohexol single bolus plasma clearance	• As above, but no requirement for urine collection • Acceptable agreement with urinary inulin clearance	• As above, plus some extrarenal clearance (0.087 mL/min/kg)
	^{99m}Tc-DTPA urinary clearance	• Radioisotopic (simple measurement) • Short half-life • Widely available • Acceptable agreement with urinary inulin clearance	• Exogenous compound • Radioisotopic (risks of ionizing radiation) • Time-consuming/complex procedure • Protein binding of ^{99m}Tc leading to GFR underestimation • Variable dissociation of ^{99m}Tc from DTPA causing imprecision and bias
	^{99m}Tc-DTPA single bolus plasma clearance	• As above, but while agreement with urinary inulin clearance is not validated, acceptable agreement with other silver standards	• Unacceptable agreement with urinary inulin clearance
	^{99m}Tc-DTPA renal imaging	• Radioisotopic (simple measurement) • Short half-life • Allows determination of split kidney function	• As above • Poor accuracy

Continued

TABLE 32.4 Markers of Glomerular Filtration Rate in an Approximate Hierarchical Arrangement—cont'd

Hierarchy	Marker	Advantages*	Disadvantages
Bronze standard	Cystatin C (serum or plasma)	• Endogenous • Not secreted/reabsorbed by kidney • Less influenced by physiological variation in relationship with GFR than creatinine • Unaffected by recent meat intake • Internationally standardized assays • Incorporated in GFR estimating equations	• More expensive than creatinine • Influenced by thyroid function and obesity • Possible genetic influences on plasma concentration
	Creatinine (serum or plasma)	• Endogenous • Inexpensive • Internationally standardized assays • Incorporated in GFR estimating equations	• Analytical interferences • Physiological/racial/pathological variation in GFR/creatinine relationship • Affected by diet/meat intake • Variable tubular secretion, affected by certain drugs • Variable intestinal losses
Of uncertain clinical use at present	β-trace protein (serum or plasma)	• Endogenous • Incorporated in GFR estimating equations	• Further evaluation required • No international assay standardization • Assays not readily available • Genetic and inflammatory influences on plasma concentration
	SDMA (plasma)	• Endogenous • Close relationship with GFR	• Further evaluation required • No international assay standardization • Not tested in GFR equations • Assays not readily available
	RBP (serum or plasma)	• Endogenous • Not secreted/reabsorbed by kidney	• Nonrenal influences on production rate
	α_1-Microglobulin (serum or plasma)	• Endogenous • Not secreted/reabsorbed by kidney	• Nonrenal influences on production rate • Less freely filtered than RBP
	β2-microglobulin	• Endogenous	• Nonrenal influences on production rate
	Creatinine urinary clearance	• Endogenous • Inexpensive	• Requires a timed urine collection • Variable tubular secretion • Analytical interferences • Less accurate than GFR estimating equations
	Urea (serum or plasma)	• Endogenous • Inexpensive	• Poor sensitivity and specificity

*Comparisons against urinary inulin clearance are based on the systematic review of Soveri and colleagues.[427]

†Nonradioisotopic iothalamate methods are also available, but measurement of nonradioactive iothalamate is complex.

EDTA, Ethylenediaminetetraacetic acid; *DTPA*, diethylenetriaminepentaacetic acid; *ID-MS*, isotope dilution-mass spectrometry; *HPLC*, high performance liquid chromatography; *RBP*, retinol binding protein; *SDMA*, symmetric dimethylarginine.

Constant infusion or single bolus injection methods may be used to administer an exogenous marker. In the constant-infusion technique, the fasting subject is required to drink 500 mL of water 1 hour before the study begins, after which he or she is required to take 200 mL every half hour until the end of the study. The subject remains supine throughout the study. An intravenous loading dose of the marker selected is then followed by a constant infusion of a given quantity of marker per minute for 3 hours. After equilibration for 1 hour, blood is drawn and urine samples are collected hourly for 3 hours. This technique can be used with any exogenous marker, the dosage being all that will vary between molecules. For example, for inulin, an intravenous loading dose of 2.3 g would be followed by a constant infusion of 18.1 mg/min for 3 hours.

Single-bolus plasma clearance methods have obvious practical advantages compared with the complex continuous-infusion methods. A single dose of the marker (eg, inulin, 70 mg/kg; iohexol, 5 mL, Ominipaque 300 mg iodine/mL [Nycomed AS, Oslo, Norway]; or ^{51}Cr-EDTA, 50 to 100 μCi) is injected, and venous blood samples are collected at timed intervals (eg, typically 120, 180, and 240 minutes after the start of the injection for ^{51}Cr-EDTA). A later sampling time is required to reduce error in the case of individuals with GFR less than 30 mL/min.[429] The GFR is calculated using knowledge of the amount of marker injected and the decrease in marker concentration (activity) as a function of time. Elimination of the marker is described by a two-compartment model that comprises an initial equilibration or distribution phase while the marker mixes between the vascular and extravascular spaces and is being cleared from the plasma by the kidney. This gives rise to a biexponential clearance curve (Fig. 32.6). The first sample should be taken no earlier than 2 hours after injection to avoid inclusion of the fast exponential in the GFR calculation.[429]

GFR is normally calculated using single-exponential analysis by plotting log marker concentration against time and using slope-intercept analysis. The half-life is calculated from the slope (k) and the volume of distribution (C_0) of the marker just after injection.

$$\text{GFR} = k \times C_0 \quad \textbf{(4)}$$

Because this model ignores the distribution phase, GFR is overestimated. Various corrections are used to adjust for this (eg, those proposed by Chantler and Barrett[430] and Brochner-Mortensen[431]). For additional details, see Blake and colleagues.[432]

Formal measurements of GFR are not without error, due to both controllable and noncontrollable factors. Factors that are inherent to the procedures are the patient's biological variation, uncertainties regarding the timing of the samples, measurements of the marker, and measurement of the administered dose. Controllable errors include minimization of the uncertainties associated with the listed factors and error avoidance (eg, "tissued" intravenous line when injecting ligand, mistiming of sample collections, insufficient time for prolonged collections in subjects with low GFR, and errors in the calculations). Measurement of GFR should be seen as a specialist activity and as such are performed better in centers that perform larger numbers of tests. Strict adherence to agreed protocols is required to ensure optimal performance. This remains an important area of further research.[427]

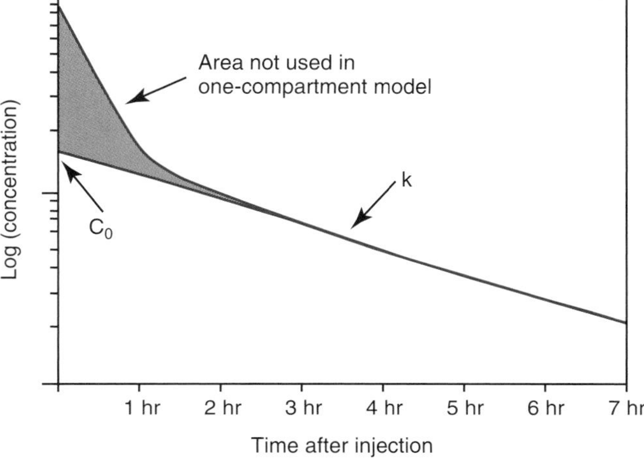

FIGURE 32.6 Semilog plot used in a single compartmental analysis of the plasma disappearance curve of a glomerular filtration rate (GFR) marker. In this simplified representation of contrast agent elimination, the distribution phase (hatched area) is neglected, which leads to underestimation of the true area under the curve.

Nonradiosotopic Markers

Nonradioactive compounds used to measure GFR include inulin and iohexol.[433]

Inulin Clearance. The fructose polymer inulin (approximately 5000 Da Mr) satisfies the criteria as an ideal marker of GFR. Inulin clearance using a constant-infusion urinary clearance approach has long been regarded as the gold standard measure of GFR. Acceptable single-bolus plasma clearance approaches have also been evaluated.[434] However, lack of availability of simple laboratory methods of measurement remains an impediment to universal usage. Early methods for the measurement of inulin were based on the hydrolysis of inulin with concentrated sulfuric acid and condensation with anthrone to give a green product that could be read at 620 nm. More recent methods have been based on the enzyme inulinase (EC 3.2.17), which converts inulin to fructose; the fructose can then be determined with the aid of sorbitol dehydrogenase (EC 1.1.1.14) according to the following reaction sequence.[435]

$$\text{Inulin} \xrightarrow{\text{Inulinase}} \text{Fructose} + \text{NADH} \xrightarrow{\text{Sorbitol dehydrogenase}} \text{Sorbitol} + \text{NAD}$$

The amount of inulin present can be determined from the reduction of nicotinamide-adenine dinucleotide, reduced form (NADH), measured as a decrease in absorbance at 340 nm. The method can be calibrated with inulin or fructose; endogenous fructose in each sample is measured by incubation with an inactivated inulinase reagent. Urine samples require predilution (typically 1 in 40) before analysis. Typical between-run imprecision of less than ±2% for serum and less than ±4% for urine can be obtained with an automated assay.

An alternative method for detecting the fructose produced involves the use of fructokinase (EC 2.7.1.4), phosphoglucose isomerase, and glucose-6-phosphate dehydrogenase (EC 1.1.1 .49) measuring in this case the nicotinamide-adenine dinucleotide phosphate, reduced form (NADPH) produced.[436,437]

Iohexol Clearance. Clearance of the nonradioactive x-ray contrast agent iohexol has been proposed as a simpler alternative to inulin clearance in the assessment of GFR.[438-442] Serum iohexol can be measured by HPLC,[439,443] capillary electrophoresis,[444,445] and LC/MS-MS.[446,447] Single-bolus plasma clearance of iohexol demonstrates good agreement with constant-infusion urinary inulin clearance.[427] The nonradioisotopic and stable nature of iohexol enables analysis of samples to be delayed and common reference centers to be used for multinational studies. An outpatient procedure based on filter paper blood spots has been described.[448]

Radioisotopic Markers

Radiopharmaceuticals that have been used include ^{51}Cr-EDTA,[430,432,449-451] ^{99m}Tc-diethylenetriaminepentaacetic acid (DTPA), and ^{125}I-iothalamate. The relative merits of these markers have been reviewed.[452] ^{51}Cr-EDTA is widely used in clinical practice in the United Kingdom, while ^{125}I-iothalamate is widely used in the United States.[428] Compared to urinary clearance of inulin, a recent systematic review concluded that "renal clearance of ^{51}Cr-EDTA or iothalamate and plasma clearance of ^{51}Cr-EDTA or iohexol are sufficiently accurate methods to measure GFR."[427] There was insufficient evidence to make a strong recommendation regarding plasma clearance of ^{99m}Tc-DTPA in this respect.[427,453]

Endogenous Markers of Glomerular Filtration Rate

Although the clearance of infused markers is generally considered an accurate assessment of GFR, to date these procedures have generally been considered too costly and cumbersome for high-volume clinical use, particularly when GFR must be assessed on a regular basis (eg, when patients are receiving nephrotoxic drugs or when making other drug-dosing decisions). Recognition of CKD as a major public health issue has focused attention on the need for simple and readily available markers of GFR.[13,118] Creatinine and certain low molecular weight proteins (eg, cystatin C) have been used as endogenous markers of GFR. The use of urea in this context is of limited value[454] and is not discussed further. Endogenous markers obviate the necessity for injection and require only a single blood sample, simplifying the procedure for the patient, the clinician, and the laboratory. The most widely used endogenous marker of GFR is creatinine, expressed as its serum concentration or as renal clearance. The use of creatinine as a marker of GFR was developed in 1926 by Rehberg,[455] who exogenously administered creatinine. This led to the work of Popper and Mandel,[456] who in 1937 developed the use of endogenous creatinine clearance.

Creatinine

Most commonly, GFR is assessed by measuring serum creatinine. Serum creatinine concentration is a product of the rate of release into the circulation as well as the rate of removal. Awareness of the influence of both of these factors is required for an understanding of the use of creatinine measurements. Creatinine is freely filtered at the glomerulus, and its concentration is inversely related to GFR—that is, for the same creatinine production, a halving of the GFR will lead to an approximate doubling of the serum creatinine concentration. Creatinine is convenient and cheap to measure. However, its production is affected by age, gender, race, muscle mass nutritional status, and various other preanalytical and analytical influences discussed earlier (see the "Creatinine" section).[234,285] Further, a small (but significant) and variable proportion of the creatinine appearing in the urine is derived from tubular secretion. Typically 7% to 10% is due to tubular secretion,[458] but this amount is increased in the presence of renal insufficiency and inhibited by certain drugs (eg, cimetidine,[457] trimethoprim[459]). Perhaps most important, serum creatinine can remain within the reference interval until notable kidney function has been lost (Fig. 32.7).[285]

Because plasma creatinine is derived from creatine and phosphocreatine breakdown in muscle, the reference interval encompasses the range of muscle mass observed in the reference population used. This limitation contributes to the insensitivity of creatinine as a marker of diminished GFR. Additionally, in patients with CKD, extrarenal clearance of creatinine becomes important when caused by degradation as a result of bacterial overgrowth in the small intestine, further blunting the anticipated increase in plasma creatinine in response to falling GFR.[13] Consequently, serum creatinine measurement will not detect people with mildly reduced GFR

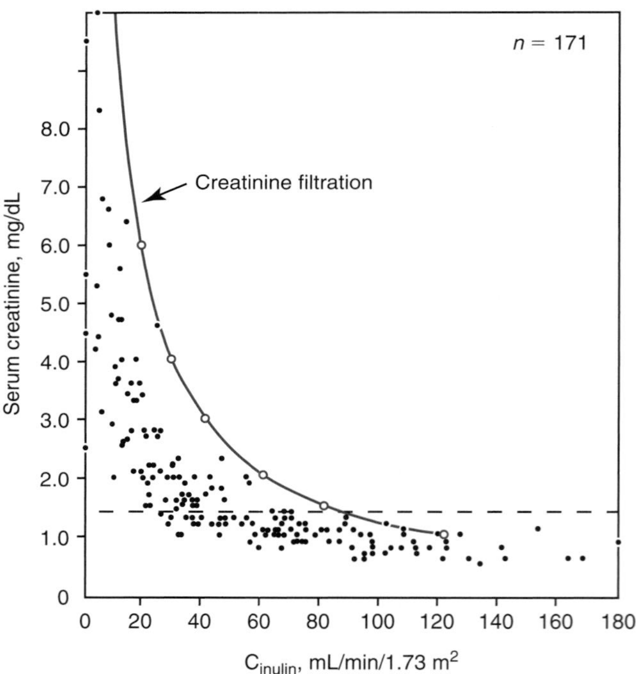

FIGURE 32.7 The relationship between serum creatinine concentration and glomerular filtration rate (GFR), measured as the clearance of inulin, in 171 patients with glomerular disease. The hypothetical relationship between GFR and serum creatinine is shown as a *continuous line*, assuming that only filtration of creatinine takes place. The *dashed horizontal line* represents an upper limit of normal for serum creatinine (1.4 mg/dL, 124 μmol/L) widely used at the time of publication. Because of creatinine secretion and/or a creatinine deficit through gut excretion, the serum creatinine consistently overestimates the GFR. (From Shemesh O, Golbetz H, Kriss JP, Myers BD. Limitations of creatinine as a filtration marker in glomerulopathic patients. *Kidney Int* 1985;28:830–8.)

(60–89 mL/min/1.73 m^2) and will fail to identify many patients with CKD and category 3A GFR (45–59 mL/min/1.73 m^2). Thus, although an increased serum creatinine concentration generally equates with impaired kidney function, a normal serum creatinine does not necessarily equate with normal kidney function. Because of all these limitations, it is recommended that serum creatinine measurement alone is not used to assess kidney function.[13,57] However, while interpretation of creatinine concentration against population-based decision points is insensitive for the detection of CKD, changes in serum creatinine within an individual may be used as a sensitive tool for detecting changes in kidney function, whether the results are within or outside population reference intervals. In this setting, changes greater than expected by chance (ie, that due to biological and analytical variation) are likely to indicate a significant change in GFR in a patient.[460]

Creatinine Clearance

Because creatinine is endogenously produced and released into body fluids at a reasonably constant rate within an individual, its clearance can be measured as an indicator of GFR.[285] Creatinine clearance in the past has been seen as more sensitive for detection of renal dysfunction than serum creatinine measurement. However, it requires a timed urine collection, which introduces its own inaccuracies.[461-463] In adults, the within-subject day-to-day CV for repeated measures of creatinine clearance exceeds 25%.[464] Although tubular secretion undermines the theoretical value of creatinine as a marker of GFR, in the context of creatinine clearance, this has historically been offset to some extent by the use of nonspecific methods to measure serum creatinine, which have led to an overestimation of serum but not urine concentration. The use of IDMS-traceable enzymatic assays or "compensated" Jaffe methods has removed this possibly fortuitous offset (see discussion earlier under "Creatinine, Analytical Methods"). Consequently, creatinine clearance measurements today overestimate GFR, usually equating or exceeding inulin GFR in adults by a factor of 10% to 40% at clearances above 80 mL/min. However, as GFR falls, tubular secretion rises disproportionately, and creatinine clearance can reach nearly twice that of inulin.[465] Tubular reabsorption of creatinine has been reported at low GFRs but may represent diffusion of creatinine through gap junctions between tubular cells or directly through the tubular epithelial cells, down a concentration gradient.[285] Whatever the mechanism, this further devalues the use of creatinine clearance. Thus, at best, creatinine clearance only provides a crude index of GFR, and it is generally considered unsuitable for this purpose,[427] although it remains in common use in recommendations for drug-dosing decisions (see later).

Estimating Glomerular Filtration Rate

The approximate mathematical relationship between serum creatinine and GFR (GFR α 1/SCr) can be improved by correcting for some of the confounding variables that influence this relationship. Many different equations have been derived that estimate GFR using serum creatinine corrected for some or all of gender, body size, race, and age.[13,466] These generally produce a better estimate of GFR than serum creatinine alone or measured creatinine clearance,[13,465-468] and professional societies throughout the world have recommended that such estimates should be used in preference to, or in association with, serum creatinine.[13,57,59,279] In adults, several such equations have been widely used, including the Cockcroft and Gault equation, the Modification of Diet in Renal Disease (MDRD) Study equations, and the CKD-EPI equations.

The Cockcroft and Gault equation is one of the earliest of these equations (see Table 32.3).[469] It remains widely used, particularly in the context of assessing drug dosages for patients with kidney impairment (see later). However, in addition to several theoretical objections to the use of the equation (eg, females were not included in the original derivation of the equation, creatinine clearance rather than a reference GFR method was used, and the traceability of the creatinine assay was not defined), the requirement for measurement of body weight has been a major practical impediment to the use of the equation in wider clinical practice.

The era of GFR estimation as a widely used simple clinical tool across both primary and secondary care really began with publication of the MDRD Study equation in 1999. The original equation was developed in 1628 predominantly middle-aged patients enrolled in the MDRD Study, a study of chronic renal insufficiency. It was validated against an iothalamate clearance estimate of GFR, and the reported GFR is already corrected for BSA. It is suitable for use in black African Americans with the use of a factor, and there is no requirement for knowledge of patient weight. The original version of the MDRD equation used age, gender, race (black or white), serum creatinine, urea, and albumin as covariables.[363] An abbreviated version of the equation, sometimes referred to as the "four-variable equation," was subsequently published that did not require albumin or urea.[470]

The creatinine assay used to derive the MDRD equation was a kinetic Jaffe method with a positive bias compared with reference creatinine assays. Many publications subsequently highlighted the critical susceptibility of the MDRD equation to the bias of the creatinine assay used.[240,471-473] Increasing use of IDMS-traceable creatinine assays would have added a systematic bias to the results.[281,282] Subsequently, therefore, the four-variable equation was indirectly restandardized against an IDMS assay, using a Roche enzymatic assay as the designated comparison method.[474,475] In practice, this was achieved by the substitution of a different constant factor (175 instead of 186) (see Table 32.3). Use of the IDMS-standardized version of the MDRD equation was widely endorsed by national organizations.[118,269,476,477] Generally, the MDRD equation was found to provide a more accurate assessment of GFR than the Cockcroft and Gault equation,[478,479] although the differences were somewhat marginal and not universally observed.[466] The most important advantage of the MDRD equation, however, was its practical advantage of reliance only on data readily available in the laboratory computer system, allowing automatic reporting of the estimated GFR with the results for serum creatinine.

However, the MDRD equation has limitations. Accuracy of GFR estimating equations is commonly expressed as the P_{30}, the percentage of estimated GFR values within 30% of true (measured) GFR. This metric captures aspects of imprecision (measurement error), bias (systematic over- and/or underestimation), and individual scatter in the relationship between measured and estimated GFR. The MDRD equation has been reported to significantly underestimate GFR (particularly in individuals with GFR ≥60 mL/min/1.73 m^2),[479-481] and its precision is poor:[478] reported P_{30} values typically range between 73% and 93%.[482] Because of its poorer performance at higher levels of GFR, several national societies and expert groups recommended that numerical values of GFR should be reported only up to 60 mL/min/1.73 m^2 using the MDRD equation.[269,476,477,483]

In 2009 the Chronic Kidney Disease Epidemiology Collaboration described an equation including log serum creatinine (modeled as a two-slope linear spline with gender-specific knots at creatinine concentrations of 0.9 and 0.7 mg/dL [80 and 62 μmol/L] in males and females, respectively), gender, race, and age on the natural scale (CKD-EPI_{creat}) (see Table 32.3).[481] In most studies that have undertaken head-to-head comparisons, P_{30} values for the CKD-EPI_{creat} equation are slightly superior to those of the MDRD equation, particularly at higher levels of GFR (>60 mL/min/1.73 m^2).[482] KDIGO have recommended that the CKD-EPI_{creat} equation should be used to estimate GFR, unless an alternative equation can be demonstrated to improve accuracy.[57] The format of the equation with the flatter relationship between creatinine and GFR for creatinine concentrations below the gender-specific knots has a number of effects in this range. First, it makes the result less sensitive to the effect of assay imprecision. Second, while it improves estimation of GFR in this range at the population level, it changes the within-person link of (approximately) halving the GFR with a doubling of the serum creatinine concentration.

Because the relationship between creatinine and kidney function varies among individuals, disease conditions, and populations, no GFR equation to date has found universal applicability. This remains an intense area of ongoing research.[484] Some brief comments in relation to age and ethnicity follow. Generally the CKD-EPI_{creat} equation demonstrates slightly superior performance to the MDRD equation in older white populations.[330,485,486] The Berlin Initiative Study (BIS) Group published equations with claimed superior performance in older people (see Table 32.3),[330] although external validations have been equivocal.[331,487] There are little data in black elderly populations.

The relationship between creatinine and GFR varies among some ethnicities, presumably due to differences in muscularity and dietary pattern. The original MDRD and CKD-EPI_{creat} equation publications showed a clear distinction between African American and non–African Americans.[363,481] However, the black ethnicity coefficient developed in America for use among African Americans in both the MDRD and CKD-EPI_{creat} equations may not be transferable to other populations of African ancestry in other locations.[488-490] Different coefficients may lead to significant improvements in other populations (eg, Japanese,[491-492] black South African,[492] and Thai[493]). The use of the CKD-EPI_{creat} equation without a race coefficient has, however, been validated to provide acceptable performance in many different racial groups (eg, indigenous Australians,[494] Chinese,[495] Hispanic and Europeans,[492] Brazilian,[496] and mixed Asian populations[497]).

Assessment of the possible requirement to adjust GFR estimating equations for race is a major practical limitation to their global application. Issues involved include the differential effects of race (genetics) and environment (diet, exercise, muscularity); the definition of race both for study purposes and application at an individual level; and approach to individuals of mixed parentage. Assessing the effects of race in the published literature is also difficult due to differences and limitations in the individual studies of interest. These factors include accuracy of creatinine measurement (now largely solved with IDMS traceable assays), differences in measured GFR (see Exogenous Markers of Glomerular Filtration Rate), and different populations in studies (eg, due to age, gender, body composition and distribution, and causes of reduced renal function). The ideal study to assess racial effects is one where all aspects of the comparison are the same, with the single difference being the race of the subject. This criterion was satisfied by the original MDRD study.[363] It is important to recognize that equations developed within a study will have optimal performance within the study data set, making it imperative to assess equations with a validation as well as a training set, and ideally to confirm any differences using a completely different set of data, as was done with the CKD-EPI equations. These difficulties support the approach of the KDIGO to use the CKD-EPI_{creat} equation unless there is good evidence to support another equation.[57] From a practical point of view, there is also a benefit to all laboratories in a country or region using the same equation (or equations) to provide uniform information to requesting doctors.

It is likely that one of the major factors affecting the performance of creatinine-based GFR estimating equations is variability in creatinine production due to the amount of muscle mass. The added variables in equations (ie, age, gender, African American ancestry), although derived empirically, are generally related to the expected differences in muscle mass of the person. More correctly for the CKD-EPI_{creat} and MDRD equations, this is the difference in muscle mass relative to body size (expressed as the BSA). The equations then assume a constant relationship between muscularity and BSA for all subjects meeting the conditions for the equation. This raises the possibility that other relatively simple measurements of body composition may provide an improvement in GFR estimation. However, this has proved somewhat disappointing, with only modest improvements based on the inclusion of weight[498] or other measures of body composition.[499] This may indicate that the relationship between muscle mass and creatinine production is less close than has been considered or that these approaches have been inadequate to accurately add to the estimation of the muscle effect. In practical terms the routine use of equations with factors not included in the laboratory computer system is less satisfactory as automatic reporting is more difficult.

Serum creatinine is an imperfect marker of GFR; therefore it is not altogether surprising that equations based predominantly upon it are imperfect. Their use cannot circumvent the very significant spectral interferences affecting serum creatinine measurement (ie, hemolysis, icterus, and lipemia) and the other factors that influence creatinine measurements. The equations are also unsuitable for use in patients with AKI, in whom serum creatinine concentrations may change rapidly. Note that these factors affect all assessments based on serum creatinine, including creatinine alone, creatinine clearance, and all creatinine-based equations. In situations where the normal relationship between muscle mass and body size is disturbed, the equations will be inaccurate (eg, among bodybuilders, amputees, and people with muscle wasting disorders), and the equations are also not suitable for patients on dialysis and for use during pregnancy. Notwithstanding this, in general, equations improve the estimation of GFR compared with serum creatinine alone. Both the CKD-EPI and

BIS groups have also published equations combining creatinine and cystatin C; these are discussed earlier (see Cystatin C, Clinical Significance).

Selected Other Markers of Glomerular Filtration

In addition to cystatin C (see earlier), many other proteins with molecular weights of less than 30 kDa are primarily cleared from the circulation by renal filtration and can be considered to be relatively freely filtered at the glomerulus. Such proteins are reabsorbed (and metabolized) in the proximal tubule or excreted into the urine: thus they are entirely eliminated from the circulation by the kidney. Therefore they have the potential to meet the criteria for use as a marker of GFR, and the value of some of these proteins, including α_2-microglobulin, RBP, α_1-microglobulin, and β-trace protein (BTP), has been explored. The relationship between circulating concentrations of these proteins shows the same hyperbolic form as serum creatinine. In the same manner as creatinine, variation in production is a potential confounding factor in these other markers. For example, serum concentrations of most of these proteins have been found to be influenced by other, nonrenal factors such as inflammation (α_2-microglobulin) and liver disease (RBP, α_1-microglobulin).[500]

BTP, also known as prostaglandin-D2 synthase, is synthesized in the glial cells of the central nervous system, and as a GFR marker appears to have similar performance characteristics to cystatin C.[501] BTP has been incorporated in several published GFR estimating equations.[502-506] However, BTP assays are less readily available on automated platforms than those for cystatin C, and there is no international standardization. Furthermore, the biological variability of BTP appears higher than for cystatin C,[507] and there is evidence that BTP concentrations are affected by the inflammatory state[508] and by genetic polymorphism.[509] A potential use for BTP, with a molecular weight of 25,200 Da, is estimation of residual GFR in dialysis patients provided the dialysis membrane does not allow molecules of this size to pass.[510]

Dimethylarginines are produced in all nucleated cells as a result of methylation of arginine residues in proteins and subsequent release of free methylarginines following proteolysis.[511] It is known that both asymmetric dimethylarginine (ADMA) and symmetric dimethylarginine (SDMA) accumulate in the blood of patients with kidney failure.[512,513] ADMA is mainly metabolized through enzymatic degradation in both the liver and kidney involving dimethylarginine dimethylaminohydrolase (DDAH). Consequently, the relationship between ADMA and GFR will be confounded by hepatic function. Conversely, SDMA is mainly eliminated from the body by renal excretion,[514] and it is a promising marker of GFR, demonstrating a strong relationship with measured GFR.[515-517] SDMA has also been shown to be an early and sensitive marker of abrupt change in kidney function following kidney donation.[518] However, at the present time SDMA measurement is not readily available in clinical laboratories.

Reference Intervals and Biological Variability of GFR

An average GFR of approximately 125 mL/min/1.73 m^2 is often assumed in young, healthy adults.[57] As early as 1950, Davies and Shock[519] demonstrated that GFR was influenced by age. They undertook urinary inulin clearance in 70 males aged between 24 and 89 years old. Average GFR in the third decade of life was approximately 125 mL/min/1.73 m^2, falling to approximately half that value in octogenarians. Given the obvious need therefore to have representative numbers of subjects across all ages and the complexity of reference GFR assessments, most studies on healthy individuals have been somewhat limited in size.[438,520] Some of the strongest data come from evaluation of potential living kidney donors, who commonly undergo a formal GFR measurement as part of their assessment and in many other ways may be considered a "healthy" population (eg, hypertension, diabetes, and preexisting kidney disease will have been excluded). Poggio and colleagues reported urinary ^{125}I-iothalamate clearances in 1057 prospective donors, stratified by age, gender, and race.[521] In non–African American males and females aged 18 to 25 years old, median GFR was 110 mL/min/1.73 m^2 (5th to 95th percentiles, 90–136 mL/min/1.73 m^2) and 112 mL/min/1.73 m^2 (91–148 mL/min/1.73 m^2), respectively. In the cohort overall, GFR was slightly higher in females than in males, but no differences were observed between African Americans and non–African Americans. GFR declined at a rate of approximately 4 mL/min/1.73 m^2 per decade in individuals younger than age 45 and 8 mL/min/1.73 m^2 per decade in individuals aged 45 and older.[521]

GFR itself, as with any physiological measurement, has an intrinsic biological variability that must be taken into account in any consideration of disease-related change. Using a variety of exogenous reference markers, values (coefficient of variation, CV%) ranging between 5.5% and 11.6% have been reported for the biological variation of GFR.[432,441,464,522-525] The biological variability of estimated GFR will, of course, reflect the variability of the endogenous marker being used (eg, creatinine, cystatin C, or BTP, as discussed earlier), with adjustment for the coefficients in the respective equation. Because age generally only changes slightly among measurements, the variation in estimated GFR results is dependent on the variability of the biological marker, and because the estimated GFR is close to proportional to 1/(marker concentration) (ie, marker concentration^{-1}), the CV_I of the marker is transferred to the CV_I of the estimated GFR result produced, with the exact effect depending on the power coefficient applied to the marker. For example, using creatinine data, Selvin and colleagues calculated the CV_I of estimated GFR using the MDRD equation to be 9.6% compared to 6.6% when calculated using the CKD-EPI$_{creat}$ equation, with a CV_I for creatinine estimated at 7.6%.[507] This reflects the power coefficient in the MDRD equation (−1.154) and the data from the CKD-EPI$_{creat}$ equation using results from above and below the gender-specific knots (−1.209 above the knot and −0.329 and −0.411 for females and males, respectively). The variabilities of both measured and estimated GFR are less than half that reported for creatinine clearance.[464] For additional discussion on biological variability, see Chapter 7.

GFR Measurement and Estimation: Future Considerations

Evaluation of kidney function remains an essential component of medical practice, and research into new and better markers of kidney function will continue. The ideal GFR estimating equation would require only demographic variables routinely supplied to laboratories in addition to easily and cheaply measured biomarkers amenable to standardization and that satisfy the criteria of an ideal GFR marker. Such an equation would achieve a P_{30} greater than 90% across a range of populations and clinical situations. To date, such an equation does not exist, but there are GFR equations that are adequate, if not perfect, for clinical purposes in many settings. Critically, there is an increasing realization that not all GFR reference methods are equivalent[526] and that imprecision in reference measurements may limit the accuracy ultimately achievable by estimating equations.[525] This realization has been matched by a shift in emphasis of much research toward the prognostic value of equations and markers as compared to accuracy in GFR assessment.[334,335,527-530] In the next era, proteomic, metabolomic,[531] and genomic[532] studies are likely to further illuminate our understanding of the relationship between GFR markers and GFR itself.

Assessment of Kidney Function at the Extremes of Age

As discussed earlier in this chapter, current widely used markers of GFR are imperfect, and the limitations of these tests are accentuated in both pediatric and older populations. At birth, serum creatinine concentrations approximate those of the maternal circulation. Serum creatinine concentration rises rapidly in the first 48 hours of life, especially in premature infants.[533] It then gradually falls during the neonatal period, with slower falls observed in premature infants.[534] By 3 weeks, serum creatinine concentrations are approximately half the birth values, and a further slower fall to a nadir occurs after about 3 months.[535,536] Serum creatinine concentrations are lower in infants than in adults, despite their lower GFR, reflecting the lower muscle mass (decreased creatinine production rate). From about 6 months of age until later teenage years, there is a continual linear rise in serum creatinine, reflected in age-specific reference intervals.[283] Because the absolute GFR (in mL/min) is also rising during this time period, the rise in serum creatinine indicates a more rapid growth in creatinine production. Of note, the GFR expressed relative to the BSA (in mL/min/1.73 m^2) rises to adult values by about age 2 years and then remains stable.[537] The percentage of measured creatinine due to noncreatinine chromogen interference in Jaffe methods is proportionally increased in children, and compensatory adjustments applied to adult samples are probably inappropriate in children and pregnancy, because of their lower total protein concentrations.[227] In the setting of pediatric intensive care medicine, the usefulness of serum creatinine may be further limited by analytical interferences caused by high concentrations of bilirubin and competition with creatinine for tubular secretion by commonly used antibiotics (eg, trimethoprim, cimetidine). By contrast, serum cystatin C concentrations in infants appear to more closely reflect GFR, being increased in the first 3 months of life and then falling to approximate adult concentrations by age 1 year (Fig. 32.8).[318,538]

Further, the diagnostic accuracy of cystatin C for reduced GFR is superior to that of creatinine in children.[539,540] As in adults, equations have been developed to enable GFR estimation in children based predominantly on height and serum creatinine measurement.[541,542] The Schwartz equation has been updated for use with an IDMS-traceable enzymatic creatinine assay. Further, a newly developed "CKiD" study equation has been developed that includes both serum cystatin C and creatinine, in addition to urea, height, and gender.[328] This equation appears to be more accurate than either version of the original Schwartz equations. Specifically adult GFR estimating equations should not be used, even in subjects close to 18 years of age, because the age factors would predict these subjects to have more muscle mass than young adults, an uncommon finding at this stage of growth.

Serum creatinine concentrations in healthy older people are not dissimilar to those in younger people, except among nonagenarians and centenarians, despite the decrease in GFR that occurs, on average, with aging (see Reference Intervals and Biological Variability of GFR).[519,521,543] Possible reasons for this include reduced muscle mass and poorer nutrition. Whatever the reason, the same level of serum creatinine may indicate very different degrees of kidney function in younger and older people, and a normal serum creatinine concentration cannot exclude significant renal impairment. In two large primary care studies,[544,545] estimated GFRs less than 50 mL/min were common in patients with normal serum creatinine. This was most pronounced in older age groups (eg, discordance between normal serum creatinine and reduced GFR was observed in 47% of patients aged greater than or equal to 70 years or older, compared with 1.2% of patients aged 40 to 59 years,[544] and the sensitivity of serum creatinine for detecting severely reduced GFR (<30 mL/min/1.73 m^2) was only 46%.[545] As observed in children, serum cystatin C, however, does appear to reflect the age-related decline in kidney function[546,547] and appears to be more sensitive than serum creatinine for detection of reduced GFR.[548,549] By taking into account the differing relationship between creatinine and GFR with age, GFR-estimating equations allow for improved detection of reduced kidney function in older people.

Assessment of Kidney Function for Drug-Dosing Decisions

A common indication for assessing kidney function is to assist with drug-dosing decisions. Drugs that are cleared from the body by renal filtration will accumulate in the circulation when kidney function is decreased, leading to an increased risk of toxicity. There are many drugs where a reduced dose, or a prolonged dosing interval, is recommended in this setting. Additionally, nephrotoxic drugs should be avoided or used at reduced doses in the setting of preexisting renal impairment. As with other indications for assessments of renal function, an estimate of GFR is generally used to assist with these decisions; however, there are some important considerations for GFR estimation for this purpose.

Drug-dosing guidance is provided by the manufacturer on the drug product label after approval by the US Food and Drug Administration (FDA) and may also be found from other sources such as textbooks and expert clinical guidelines. These sources will indicate if a change in dosing is required in the presence of renal impairment and the nature of the required change. It is beyond the scope of this textbook to cover all aspects of drug dosing in kidney disease, and readers are referred to expert recommendations for further information.[550]

As discussed in this chapter, there are several ways to assess kidney function, and it is necessary to understand the strengths and limitations of these for good prescribing

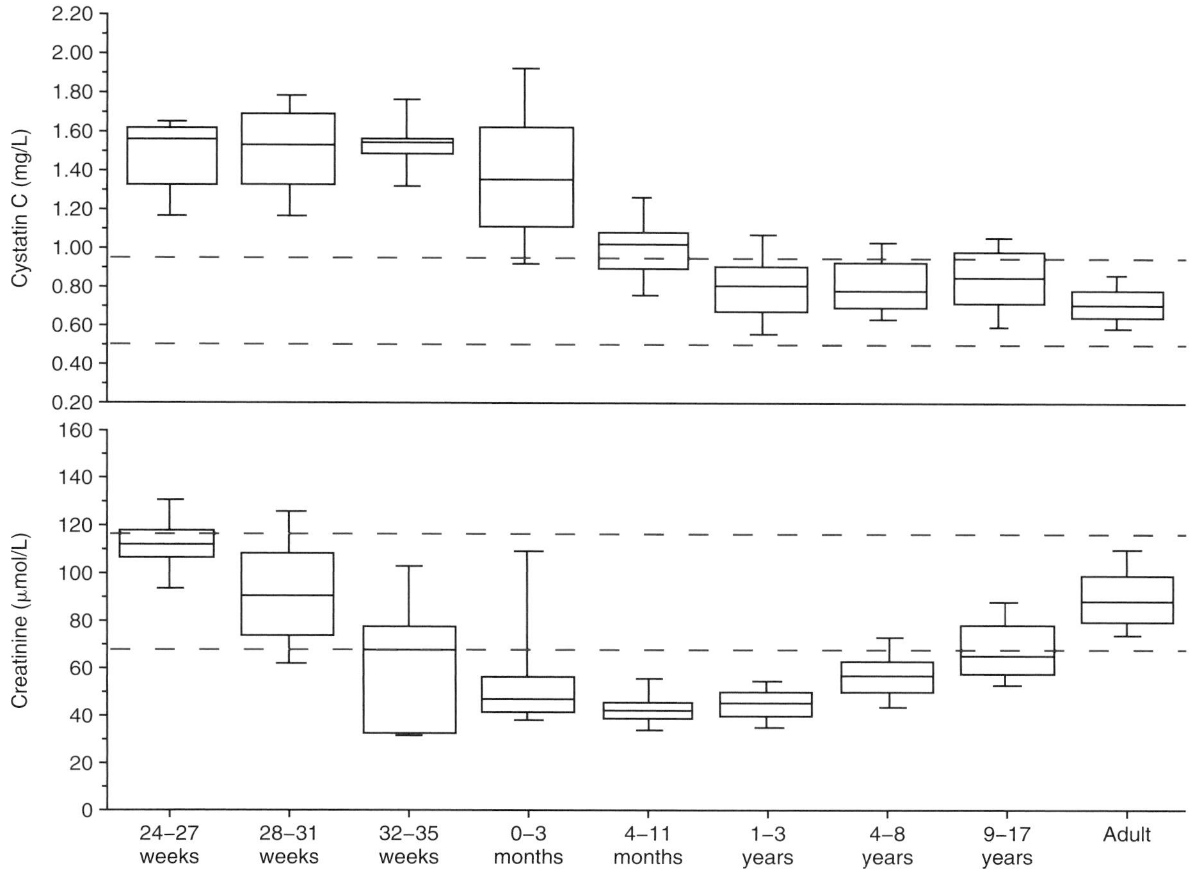

FIGURE 32.8 Age-related changes in cystatin C and creatinine superimposed upon the reference interval (horizontal dashed lines). Box and whiskers plot: The box represents the 25th to 75th percentiles with a horizontal line at the median; the whiskers extend to the highest and lowest values. Note that the changes are representative only as the intervals were produced prior to cystatin C assay standardization. (From Newman DJ. Cystatin C. *Ann Clin Biochem* 2002;39:89–104.)

practices. As well as understanding the kidney function measurement, it is also necessary to know the degree of accuracy required for dosing decisions. For many drugs the options are coarse, such as doubling or halving the dose (eg, ½, 1, or 2 tablets), while dose adjustment for some drugs may require greater accuracy. The dose adjustment advice provided on the drug product label may also indicate the coarseness of the decision—for example, for digoxin, there are three recommended starting protocols based on GFR greater than 50 mL/min, 10 to 50 mL/min, and less than 10 mL/min.[551]

Reduced kidney function can affect drug metabolism in several different ways. The most obvious is a reduction in clearance, but there may also be effects from changes in the volume of distribution, organic acid accumulation, reduced serum albumin concentration, and changes in tubular handling. Additionally a drug may be only partially cleared by the kidneys, described as having a fractional excretion less than one. Whereas with drugs that are fully cleared by the kidney, a rule of thumb may be to halve the dose with a halving of the GFR, a smaller reduction may be required with a smaller fractional excretion.

Historically, drug-dosing recommendations have been based on either the measured creatinine clearance or the estimated creatinine clearance, with the latter usually calculated with the Cockcroft and Gault equation.[469] This situation has arisen because these approaches (1) were used in most pharmacokinetic studies of drugs during their development; (2) are recommended in the medicines product information, which is based on guidance from the FDA;[552] and (3) are supported by long clinical experience. Another relevant factor is the reporting of the results in mL/min, as described later.

More recently, GFR estimated with the MDRD or CKD-EPI equations has become commonplace, with the advantages of ready availability on clinical laboratory reports and demonstrable improved accuracy compared with the Cockcroft and Gault equation. Despite these apparent advantages, the use of estimated GFR for drug-dosing decisions has been highly controversial.[553,554] The main concerns over MDRD and CKD-EPI estimated GFR relates to the fact that these approaches were not used in the primary studies on which dosing advice has been based and the fact the results are reported in mL/min/1.73 m^2—that is, adjusted for BSA.

Estimation of GFR by different methods (eg, CKD-EPI equations vs. Cockcroft and Gault estimated creatinine clearance) in the same patient may produce, often quite markedly, different results,[555] an unsurprising finding given the inherent imprecision and accuracy issues discussed earlier. In some cases the differences are large enough to contribute to a different drug-dosing decision. If Cockcroft and Gault was the estimate used in the original studies, there are clear arguments that this method should be preferred. However, as stated previously, due to creatinine standardization, there is no guarantee that a Cockcroft and Gault result today matches one produced in a clinical study prior to the mid-2000s. An alternative view would be that the gold standard for GFR is a formal measurement with exogenous substances. Using this approach, a landmark study by Stevens and colleagues in 2009, comparing FDA dosing guidance for 15 drugs in the setting of renal impairment, demonstrated that more drug-dosing decisions using the MDRD equation (78%) would match those made with a formal GFR measurement than if the Cockcroft and Gault equation was used (73%).[551] More important, these authors used estimated GFR with BSA adjustment removed (see later).

GFR can be reported as an estimate of the amount of fluid filtered per unit time, with the units of mL/min, or this can be adjusted to a standard BSA, typically 1.73 m^2 (see The Concept of Clearance) and expressed as mL/min/1.73 m^2. The latter reporting format is recommended for CKD diagnosis and classification, or smaller patients would have a higher rate of CKD than larger patients and vice versa. However, the amount of drug removed from a patient through the kidneys is related to the actual filtration rate rather than the BSA adjusted rate, leading to a preference for the use of results in mL/min for drug-dosing decisions. A particular concern is the smaller, older person where a BSA-adjusted GFR estimate may be normal, but without the BSA adjustment, the result is reduced, leading to a reduction in the recommended dose of some drugs. The solutions to this problem are either to retain the use of creatinine clearance or Cockcroft and Gault–estimated creatinine clearance for drug-dosing decisions, because the results are produced directly in mL/min, or to remove the BSA adjustment from estimated GFR results when required.[554]

When GFR estimates are adjusted to a BSA of 1.73 m^2, it follows that the formula to remove BSA normalization is GFR (mL/min) = (BSA/1.73) × GFR (mL/min/1.73 m^2). The removal of the BSA adjustment leads to a higher GFR "number" in larger people (BSA above 1.73 m^2) and vice versa. A person with a BSA near 1.73 m^2 has negligible change following removal of the BSA adjustment. A patient in the range 60 to 70 kg (132–154 lbs), unless extremely tall or short, will have a BSA within 10% of 1.73 m^2.[556] It has been suggested that, as a bedside estimate, patients who are lighter or heavier than this should have the BSA adjustment removed.[557]

The NKDEP supports this general approach with the following suggestions: (1) utilize estimated GFR or estimated creatinine clearance for drug dosing; (2) if using estimated GFR in very large or very small patients, adjust for BSA; (3) consider assessing kidney function using alternative methods such as measured creatinine clearance or measured GFR, using exogenous filtration markers when prescribing drugs with narrow therapeutic indices, or for individuals in whom estimated GFR and estimated creatinine clearance provide different estimates of kidney function, or for individuals in whom any estimates based on creatinine are likely to be inaccurate.[558] To this could be added the use of therapeutic drug monitoring with dosing based on blood concentrations where this is available. Drugs with predominant renal clearance where drug measurements are recommended include digoxin, gentamicin, vancomycin, and lithium.

SELECTED REFERENCES

For a full list of references for this chapter, please refer to ExpertConsult.com.

23. McTaggart MP, Newall RG, Hirst JA, et al. Diagnostic accuracy of point-of-care tests for detecting albuminuria: a systematic review and meta-analysis. *Ann Intern Med* 2014;**160**:550–7.
49. Price CP, Newall RG, Boyd JC. Use of protein:creatinine ratio measurements on random urine samples for prediction of significant proteinuria: a systematic review. *Clin Chem* 2005;**51**:1577–86.
55. Miller WG, Bruns DE, Hortin GL, et al. Current issues in measurement and reporting of urinary albumin excretion. *Clin Chem* 2009;**55**:24–38.
57. Kidney Disease Improving Global Outcomes. Clinical Practice Guideline for the Evaluation and Management of Chronic Kidney Disease. *Kidney Int* 2013;**3**:1–150.
59. National Institute for Health and Care Excellence. Chronic kidney disease. Early identification and management of chronic kidney disease in adults in primary and secondary care. 2014:<http://www.nice.org.uk/nicemedia/live/13712/66658/.pdf>.
84. Bachmann LM, Nilsson G, Bruns DE, et al. State of the art for measurement of urine albumin: comparison of routine measurement procedures to isotope dilution tandem mass spectrometry. *Clin Chem* 2014;**60**:471–80.
121. Lamb EJ, Mackenzie F, Stevens PE. How should proteinuria be detected and measured? *Ann Clin Biochem* 2009;**46**: 205–17.
138. Atkins RC, Briganti EM, Zimmet PZ, et al. Association between albuminuria and proteinuria in the general population: the AusDiab Study. *Nephrol Dial Transplant* 2003;**18**:2170–4.
159. Matsushita K, van der Velde M, Astor BC, et al. Association of estimated glomerular filtration rate and albuminuria with all-cause and cardiovascular mortality in general population cohorts: a collaborative meta-analysis. *Lancet* 2010;**375**: 2073–81.
184. Bellomo R, Ronco C, Kellum JA, et al. Acute renal failure—Definition, outcome measures, animal models, fluid therapy and information technology needs: the Second International Consensus Conference of the Acute Dialysis Quality Initiative (ADQI) Group. *Crit Care* 2004;**8**:R204–12.
191. Haase-Fielitz A, Haase M, Devarajan P. Neutrophil gelatinase-associated lipocalin as a biomarker of acute kidney injury: a critical evaluation of current status. *Ann Clin Biochem* 2014;**51**:335–51.
228. Greenberg N, Roberts WL, Bachmann LM, et al. Specificity characteristics of 7 commercial creatinine measurement procedures by enzymatic and jaffe method principles. *Clin Chem* 2012;**58**:391–401.
269. Myers GL, Miller WG, Coresh J, et al. Recommendations for improving serum creatinine measurement: a report from the Laboratory Working Group of the National Kidney Disease Education Program. *Clin Chem* 2006;**52**:5–18.
283. Ceriotti F, Boyd JC, Klein G, et al. Reference intervals for serum creatinine concentrations: assessment of available data for global application. *Clin Chem* 2008;**54**:559–66.
314. Grubb A, Blirup-Jensen S, Lindstrom V, et al. First certified reference material for cystatin C in human serum ERM-DA471/IFCC. *Clin Chem Lab Med* 2010;**48**:1619–21.

327. Inker LA, Schmid CH, Tighiouart H, et al. A new equation to estimate glomerular filtration rate from standardized creatinine and cystatin C. *N Engl J Med* 2012;**367**:20–9.
333. Peralta CA, Shlipak MG, Judd S, et al. Detection of chronic kidney disease with creatinine, cystatin C, and urine albumin-to-creatinine ratio and association with progression to end-stage renal disease and mortality. *JAMA* 2011;**305**: 1545–52.
427. Soveri I, Berg UB, Bjork J, et al. Measuring GFR: a systematic review. *Am J Kidney Dis* 2014;**64**:411–24.
481. Levey AS, Stevens LA, Schmid CH, et al. A new equation to estimate glomerular filtration rate. *Ann Intern Med* 2009;**150**: 604–12.
482. Earley A, Miskulin D, Lamb EJ, et al. Estimating equations for glomerular filtration rate in the era of creatinine standardization: a systematic review. *Ann Intern Med* 2012;**156**:785–95.
485. Kilbride HS, Stevens PE, Eaglestone G, et al. Accuracy of the MDRD (Modification of Diet in Renal Disease) study and CKD-EPI (CKD Epidemiology Collaboration) equations for estimation of GFR in the elderly. *Am J Kidney Dis* 2013;**61**: 57–66.
494. Maple-Brown LJ, Hughes JT, Lawton PD, et al. Accurate assessment of kidney function in indigenous Australians: the estimated GFR study. *Am J Kidney Dis* 2012;**60**:680–2.
497. Teo BW, Xu H, Wang D, et al. Estimating glomerular filtration rates by use of both cystatin C and standardized serum creatinine avoids ethnicity coefficients in Asian patients with chronic kidney disease. *Clin Chem* 2012;**58**: 450–7.
530. Matsushita K, Mahmoodi BK, Woodward M, et al. Comparison of risk prediction using the CKD-EPI equation and the MDRD study equation for estimated glomerular filtration rate. *JAMA* 2012;**307**:1941–51.

33

Carbohydrates

*David B. Sacks**

ABSTRACT

Background
Carbohydrates are widely distributed in plants and animals. They perform numerous functions, ranging from structural components of DNA to serving as sources of energy. Glucose is derived from breakdown of carbohydrates in the diet and in body stores. In addition, glucose can be synthesized from protein or triglyceride.

Content
This chapter describes the chemistry and metabolism of carbohydrates. Carbohydrates in the diet are digested and absorbed in the gastrointestinal tract. Blood glucose concentration is regulated by the action of several hormones, including insulin. Measurement of glucose, one of the most commonly performed analytical procedures, is described in detail. Hyperglycemia, which is caused by diabetes mellitus, is the most frequent disorder of carbohydrate metabolism. Hypoglycemia is uncommon except in patients with diabetes. Inborn errors of carbohydrate metabolism and glycogen storage diseases are also addressed.

Carbohydrates, including sugars and starches, are widely distributed in plants and animals. They perform multiple functions, ranging from being structural components of deoxyribonucleic acid (DNA) and ribonucleic acid (RNA) (*ribose* and *deoxyribose* sugars) to serving as sources of energy *(glucose)*. Glucose is derived from the breakdown of carbohydrates in the diet (grains, starchy vegetables, and legumes) and in body stores (glycogen), and by endogenous synthesis from protein or from the glycerol moiety of triglycerides. When energy intake exceeds expenditure, the excess is converted to fat and glycogen for storage in adipose tissue and liver or muscle, respectively. When energy expenditure exceeds calorie intake, endogenous glucose formation occurs from the breakdown of carbohydrate stores and from noncarbohydrate sources (eg, amino acids, lactate, glycerol).

The glucose concentration in the blood is maintained within a fairly narrow interval under diverse conditions (feeding, fasting, or severe exercise) by hormones, such as insulin, glucagon, or epinephrine (also called *adrenaline*).

Measurement of glucose is one of the most commonly performed analytical procedures. The most frequently encountered disorder of carbohydrate metabolism is high blood glucose concentrations caused by diabetes mellitus, which is estimated to affect over 415 million of the world adult population. The incidence of hypoglycemia (low blood glucose) is unknown, but, excluding patients who use exogenous insulin to control blood glucose, it is low.

*The author gratefully acknowledges the original contributions by Drs. Wendell T. Caraway and Nelson B. Watts, on which portions of this chapter are based.

CHEMISTRY OF CARBOHYDRATES

Carbohydrates are aldehyde or ketone derivatives of polyhydroxy (more than one —OH group) alcohols, or compounds that yield these derivatives on hydrolysis. The term *carbohydrate* refers to hydrates of carbon and is derived from the observation that empirical formulas for these compounds contain approximately one molecule of water per carbon atom. Thus glucose, $C_6H_{12}O_6$, and lactose, $C_{12}H_{22}O_{11}$, can be written as $C_6(H_2O)_6$ and $C_{12}(H_2O)_{11}$, respectively. These compounds are not hydrates in the usual chemical sense, however, and noncarbohydrate compounds, such as lactic acid, $CH_3CH(OH)COOH$ or $C_3(H_2O)_3$, can have similar empirical formulas.

Monosaccharides

Monosaccharides, or simple sugars, consist of a single polyhydroxy aldehyde or ketone unit and cannot be hydrolyzed to a simpler form. The backbone is made up of several carbon atoms. Sugars containing three, four, five, six, and seven carbon atoms are known as *trioses, tetroses, pentoses, hexoses,* and *heptoses,* respectively. One of the carbon atoms is double bonded to an oxygen atom to form a carbonyl group. An *aldehyde* has the carbonyl group at the end of the carbon chain, whereas if the carbonyl group is at any other position, a *ketone* is formed (Fig. 33.1). The simplest carbohydrate is glycol aldehyde, the aldehyde derivative of ethylene glycol. The aldehyde and ketone derivatives of glycerol are, respectively, glyceraldehyde and dihydroxyacetone (see Fig. 33.1). Monosaccharides are termed *aldose* or *ketose,* according to the position of the carbonyl group (Fig. 33.2).

Compounds that are identical in composition and differ only in spatial configuration are called *stereoisomers.* The

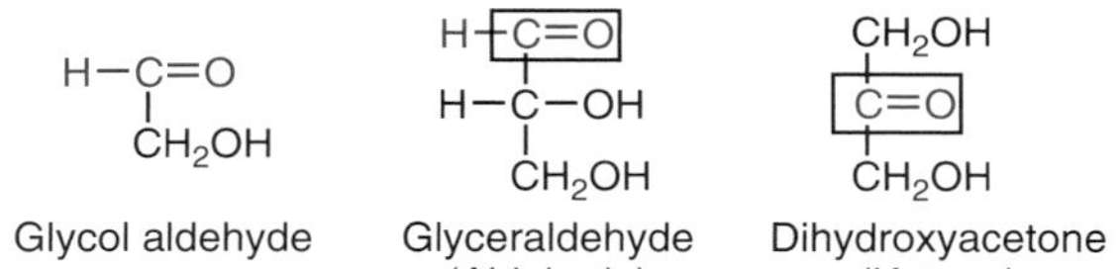

H–C=O	H–C=O	CH_2OH
CH_2OH	H–C–OH	C=O
	CH_2OH	CH_2OH
Glycol aldehyde	Glyceraldehyde (Aldehyde)	Dihydroxyacetone (Ketone)

FIGURE 33.1 Two- and three-carbon carbohydrates.

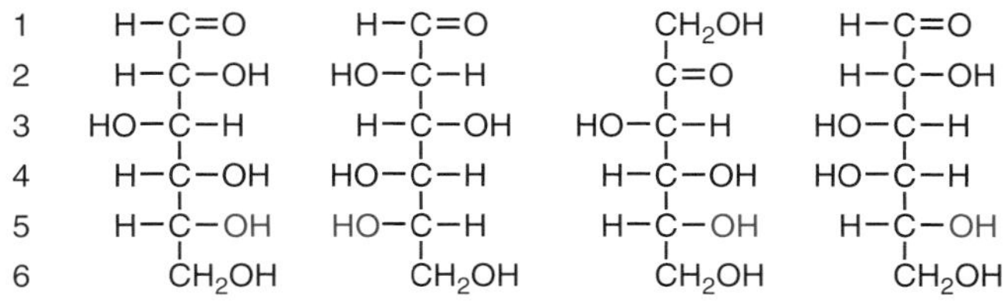

1	H–C=O	H–C=O	CH_2OH	H–C=O
2	H–C–OH	HO–C–H	C=O	H–C–OH
3	HO–C–H	H–C–OH	HO–C–H	HO–C–H
4	H–C–OH	HO–C–H	H–C–OH	HO–C–H
5	H–C–OH	HO–C–H	H–C–OH	H–C–OH
6	CH_2OH	CH_2OH	CH_2OH	CH_2OH
	D-Glucose (Aldose)	L-Glucose (Aldose)	D-Fructose (Ketose)	D-Galactose (Aldose)

FIGURE 33.2 Typical six-carbon monosaccharides.

carbon atoms in the unbranched chain are numbered, as shown by the numbers at the left of the formula for D-glucose (see Fig. 33.2). The designation D or L refers to the position of the hydroxyl group on the carbon atom adjacent to the last (bottom) CH_2OH group. In general, the designation of D or L for a sugar molecule refers to the stereoisomeric forms of the highest-numbered asymmetric carbon atom.* By convention, the D-sugars are written with the hydroxyl group on the right, and the L-sugars are written with the hydroxyl group on the left (see Fig. 33.2). Most sugars in the human body are of the D-configuration. Several different structures exist, depending on the relative positions of the hydroxyl groups on the carbon atoms.†

The formula for glucose can be written in the form of aldehyde or enol, a short-lived reactive species. Shift to the enol anion is favored in alkaline solution.

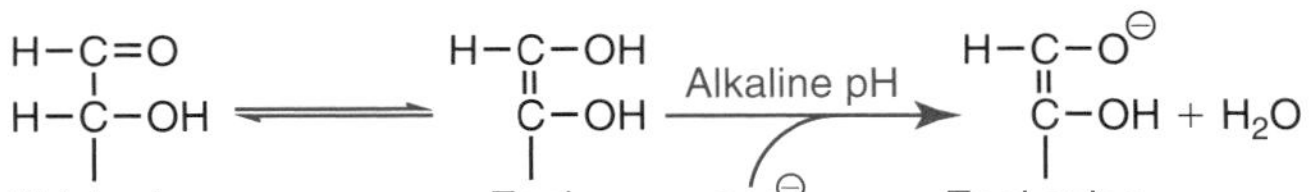

H–C=O / H–C–OH (Aldehyde) ⇌ H–C–OH / C–OH (Enol) —Alkaline pH, $OH^{\ominus}$→ H–C–$O^{\ominus}$ / C–OH (Enol anion) + H_2O

The presence of a double bond and a negative charge in the enol anion makes glucose an active reducing substance that is oxidized by relatively mild oxidizing agents, such as cupric (Cu^{2+}) and ferric (Fe^{3+}) ions. Glucose in hot alkaline solution readily reduces cupric ions to cuprous ions, and the carbonyl carbon is oxidized to carboxylic acid. The color change has been used as a presumptive indication for the presence of glucose, and for many years, blood and urine glucose were measured this way. Other sugars reduce cupric ions in alkaline solution.

Aldehyde and alcohol groups react to form hemiacetals. In the case of glucose, the aldehyde group reacts with the

†Although the D and L designations are retained in this chapter, readers should be aware that in the Cahn-Ingold-Prelog system, a series of sequence rules determine configurations. In this system, the symbols R and S are used to designate configurations instead of D and L.

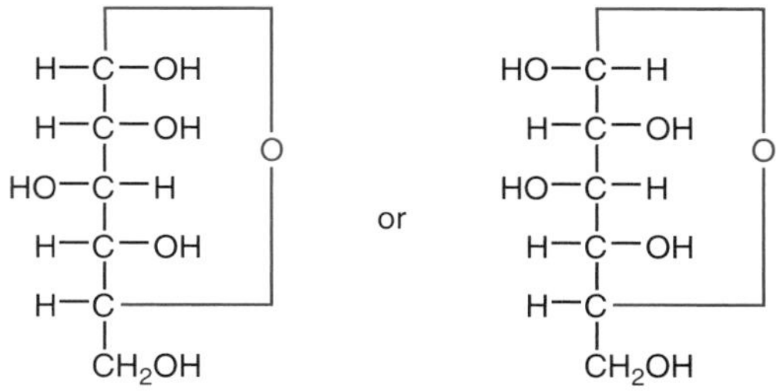

α-D-Glucose		β-D-Glucose
H–C–OH		HO–C–H
H–C–OH		H–C–OH
HO–C–H (O)	or	HO–C–H (O)
H–C–OH		H–C–OH
H–C		H–C
CH_2OH		CH_2OH

FIGURE 33.3 Structure of D-glucose (hemiacetal form).

hydroxyl group on carbon 5 (Fig. 33.3). Note that this ring structure contains an additional asymmetric carbon atom and exists in two stereoisomeric forms. By convention, the form with the hydroxyl group on the right of the first carbon atom is called α-D-glucose, and the form with the hydroxyl group on the left is called β-D-glucose. The common anhydrous crystalline glucose is in the α-D-form. The β-D-form is obtained by crystallization from acetic acid. The two forms differ with respect to optical rotation of polarized light. The specific rotation—$[\alpha]_D^{25\,°C}$—for the α-D-form is +113 degrees, and for the β-D-form it is +19.7 degrees. As a result of mutarotation, either form in aqueous solution gives rise to an equilibrium mixture that has a specific rotation of +52.5 degrees. The equilibrium established at room temperature is such that about 36% of glucose exists in the α-form and 64% in the β-form; only a trace remains in the free aldehyde form. The enzyme glucose oxidase reacts only with β-D-glucose. For this reason, calibrating solutions to be used in glucose oxidase methods for glucose determinations should be permitted to stand at least 2 hours to obtain equilibrium comparable with that in the test samples to be analyzed.

From the ring structures shown in Fig. 33.3, it is not apparent why the aldehyde group should react with the distant hydroxyl group on carbon 5. The spatial arrangement of the atoms is better represented by a symmetric ring structure, depicted by the Haworth formula, in which glucose is considered as having the same basic structure as pyran (Fig. 33.4). In this formula, the plane of the ring is considered to be perpendicular to the plane of the paper, with heavy lines pointing toward the reader. Hydroxyl groups in position 1 are then below the plane (α-configuration) or above the plane (β-configuration). A six-member ring sugar, containing five carbons and one oxygen, is a derivative of pyran and is called a *pyranose.* When linkage occurs with formation of a five-member ring, containing four carbons and one oxygen, the sugar has the same basic structure as furan and is called a *furanose.* Representative formulas are shown in Fig. 33.4. Fructose is shown in two cyclic forms. Fructopyranose is the configuration of free sugar, and fructofuranose occurs whenever fructose exists in combination in disaccharides and polysaccharides, as in sucrose and inulin.

Disaccharides

Two monosaccharides join covalently by an *O-glycosidic bond,* with the loss of a molecule of water, to form a disaccharide. The chemical bond between the sugars always involves the aldehyde or ketone group of one monosaccharide joined to an alcohol group (eg, maltose) or to an

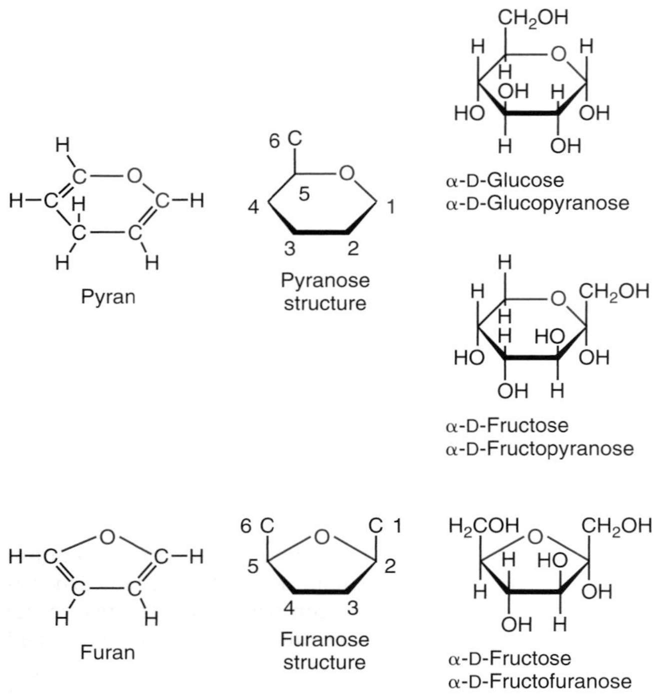

FIGURE 33.4 The Haworth formula for monosaccharides.

aldehyde or ketone group (eg, sucrose) of the other monosaccharide. The most common disaccharides are the following:

Maltose = Glucose + Glucose
Lactose = Glucose + Galactose
Sucrose = Glucose + Fructose

Several conventions are followed in the nomenclature of disaccharides (Fig. 33.5). The compound is written with the nonreducing end to the left. An *O* precedes the name of the first (left) monosaccharide, emphasizing that the linkage occurs by an oxygen atom. The configuration of the anomeric (carbonyl) carbon is designated α or β. Five- (furanosyl) and six- (pyranosyl) membered rings are distinguished, and carbon atoms joined by the glycosidic bond are identified. Because sucrose has no reducing end, it is written as *O*-α-D-glucopyranosyl-(1 → 2)-β-D-fructofuranose or *O*-β-D-fructofuranosyl-(2 → 1)-α-D-glucopyranose. If the linkage between two monosaccharides is between the aldehyde or ketone group of one molecule and a hydroxyl group of another molecule (as in maltose and lactose), one potentially free ketone or aldehyde group remains on the second monosaccharide. Consequently, the second glucose residue can be oxidized (thus the disaccharide is a reducing sugar) and is capable of existing in α- or β-pyranose form. The reducing power, however, is only approximately 40% of the reducing power of the two single monosaccharides added together, primarily because one of the reducing groups is not available. On the other hand, if the linkage between two monosaccharides involves the aldehyde or ketone groups of both molecules (as in sucrose), a nonreducing sugar results because no free aldehyde or ketone group remains.

Lactulose is a synthetic disaccharide formed from fructose and galactose through isomerization of lactose. Lactulose is nondigestible and can be used as an osmotic laxative as well as in laboratory investigations of intestinal malabsorption.

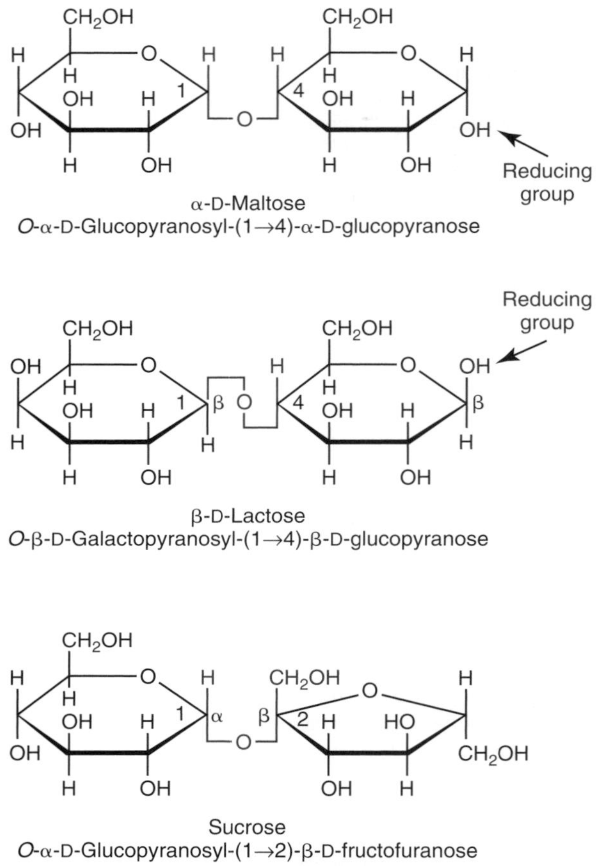

FIGURE 33.5 Structural formulas of disaccharides.

Polysaccharides

The linkage of multiple monosaccharide units results in the formation of polysaccharides. The major storage carbohydrates are starch in plants and glycogen in animals, both of which form granules inside cells. The suffix *-an* attached to the name of a monosaccharide indicates the main type of sugar present in the polysaccharide. Starch and glycogen, for example, are glucosans, because they are composed of a series of glucose molecules. Inulin, a polysaccharide found in the tubers of certain plants, consists largely of fructose units and is known as a *fructosan.*

Nearly all starches consist of a mixture of two types of glucosans called *amyloses* and *amylopectins.* The relative proportions of these two glucosans in a starch vary from approximately 20% amylose and 80% amylopectin in wheat, potato, and ordinary corn starch to nearly 100% amylopectin in the starch of waxy corn. On the other hand, a few corn starches are known to contain as much as 75% amylose. Both amylose and amylopectin consist of glucose residues, but their structures exhibit one significant difference. Amylose consists of one long unbranched chain of glucose units linked together by α-1,4-linkages, with only the terminal aldehyde group free (Fig. 33.6). In amylopectin, most of the units are similarly connected with α-1,4-links, but α-1,6-glycosidic bonds are present every 24 to 30 residues, producing sidechains (see Fig. 33.6). Amylopectin contains up to 1 million glucose residues. The structure of glycogen is similar to that of amylopectin, but branching is more extensive in glycogen and occurs every

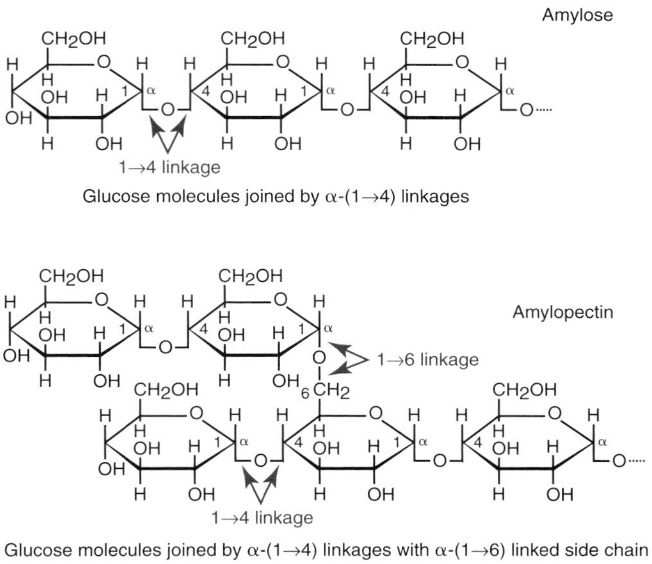

Amylose

1→4 linkage

Glucose molecules joined by α-(1→4) linkages

Amylopectin

1→6 linkage

1→4 linkage

Glucose molecules joined by α-(1→4) linkages with α-(1→6) linked side chain

FIGURE 33.6 Structures of the polysaccharides amylose and amylopectin.

O-linked

Thr

Protein chain

N-linked

Asn

Protein chain

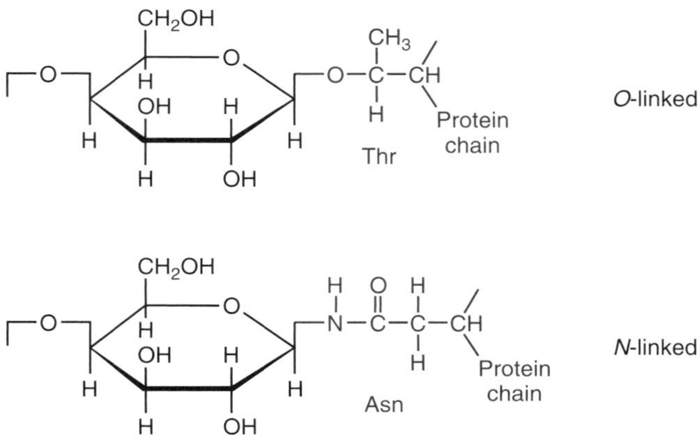

FIGURE 33.7 Glycosidic linkages between oligosaccharides and protein.

8 to 12 glucose residues. These branches enhance the solubility of glycogen and allow the glucose residues to be mobilized more readily. Glycogen is most abundant in liver and is found in skeletal muscle as well. The most favorable conformation for α-1,4-linked polymers of D-glucose, such as starch or glycogen, is a tightly coiled helical structure.

The difference in structure between amylose and amylopectin is important when the appropriate starch substrate is selected for amylase determinations (see Chapter 22). The rate of hydrolysis is affected by structural differences in the starch. α-Amylase from the pancreas hydrolyzes internal α-1,4-glycosidic linkages. This hydrolysis results initially in the production of some maltose and a mixture of dextrins, which subsequently are hydrolyzed to maltose. The β-1,6-linkages are not attacked by α-amylase, and relatively large molecules of so-called residual (limit) dextrins are left after the action of the enzyme on amylopectin. *Dextrins* are the products of partial hydrolysis of starch. They are a complex mixture of molecules of different sizes. Those formed from amylose are unbranched chains, whereas amylopectins produce branched chains of glucose molecules. *Cellulose,* an important structural polysaccharide in plants, is an unbranched polymer of glucose residues joined by β-1,4-linkages. The β-configuration facilitates the formation of long straight chains, producing fibers of high tensile strength. The β-1,4-linkages are not hydrolyzed by α-amylases. Because humans do not have *cellulases,* they are unable to digest vegetable fiber.

Chitin, the principal component of the exoskeleton of arthropods (insects and crustacea), consists of *N*-acetyl-D-glucosamine residues in a β-1,4-linkage. The only chemical difference from cellulose is that the substituent at C-2 is an acetylated amino group instead of a hydroxyl group.

Glycoproteins

Glycosylation is one of the most frequent enzymatic modifications of proteins. Many integral membrane proteins have oligosaccharides covalently attached to the extracellular region, forming *glycoproteins.* In addition, most proteins that are secreted, such as antibodies, hormones, and coagulation factors, are glycoproteins. The number of attached carbohydrates varies among proteins, comprising 1% to 70% of the weight of the glycoprotein. The oligosaccharides are attached by *O*-glycosidic linkages to the sidechain oxygen of serine and/or threonine residues or by *N*-glycosidic linkages to the sidechain nitrogen of asparagine residues (Fig. 33.7).

One of the biological functions of the carbohydrate chains is to regulate the life span of proteins. For example, removal of sialic acid residues from the end of oligosaccharide chains on erythrocytes results in the disappearance of red blood cells from the circulation. Carbohydrates have also been implicated in cell-cell recognition, and in secretion and targeting of proteins to specific subcellular domains. Defects in protein glycosylation have been linked to several very rare forms of congenital muscular dystrophy that are associated with brain abnormalities.[1]

METABOLISM OF CARBOHYDRATES

Carbohydrate metabolism provides glucose, a major energy source for the human body. After digestion of carbohydrates and absorption of glucose, blood glucose concentration is controlled by the action of several hormones. Glucose is synthesized de novo or stored in the tissue as glycogen.

Digestion and Absorption

Ingested starch and glycogen are partially digested by the action of salivary amylase in the mouth to form intermediate dextrins and maltose (see Chapter 62). The acid pH of the stomach inhibits amylase activity, but alkaline pancreatic secretions increase the pH in the small intestine, allowing pancreatic amylase to complete digestion to oligosaccharides, preponderantly maltose. Maltose, along with any ingested lactose and sucrose, is hydrolyzed by the appropriate disaccharidase (*maltase, lactase,* or *sucrase*) from the intestinal mucosa to glucose, galactose, and fructose.

These monosaccharides are absorbed across the wall of the duodenum and ileum by an active, energy-requiring, carrier-mediated transfer process. The rate of absorption for glucose and galactose is several times greater than for similar molecules absorbed by passive diffusion (eg, xylose). Some conversion of fructose to glucose may occur during the process of absorption, and the interconversion can be visualized in terms of the enediol form common to both (Fig. 33.8). Fructose is absorbed more slowly than glucose and galactose by a carrier-mediated process different from glucose and galactose transport mechanisms. The monosaccharides are then transported by the portal vein to the liver.

Intermediary Metabolism

The metabolism of hexoses proceeds according to the body's requirements. This results in (1) energy production by conversion to carbon dioxide and water, (2) storage as glycogen in the liver or conversion to triglyceride in the liver and subsequent storage in adipose tissue, or (3) conversion to keto acids, amino acids, or protein.

Some steps in the intermediary metabolism of glycogen and hexoses are shown in Fig. 33.9. Each step is catalyzed by enzymes. In some cases, different enzymes are responsible for the forward and reverse reactions. For example, the initial phosphorylation of glucose is mediated by glucokinase, but the reverse reaction depends on glucose-6-phosphatase.

Various inborn errors of metabolism (Table 33.1) result from deficiencies or absence of some of the enzymes listed in Fig. 33.9. Some of these are discussed later in the chapter. The relationship of carbohydrate metabolism to the production of lactate, ketone bodies, and triglycerides is also depicted in Fig. 33.9. The pentose phosphate pathway, also known as the *hexose monophosphate shunt,* is an alternative pathway for glucose metabolism that generates the reduced form of nicotinamide-adenine dinucleotide phosphate (NADPH), which is used in maintaining the integrity of red blood cell membranes, in lipid and steroid biosynthesis, in hydroxylation reactions, and in other anabolic reactions. The complete picture of intermediary metabolism of carbohydrates is complex and is interwoven with the metabolism of lipids and amino acids. For details, readers should consult a biochemistry textbook.

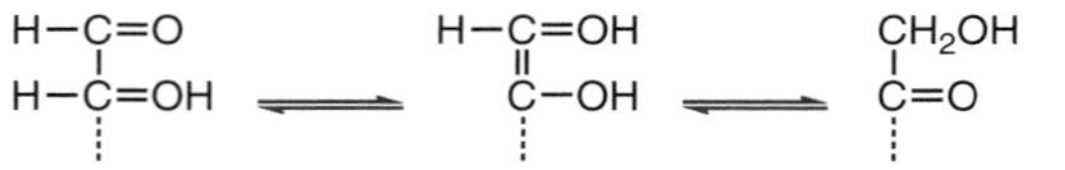

H–C=O / H–C–OH ⇌ H–C–OH ‖ C–OH ⇌ CH_2OH / C=O

D-Glucose Enediol D-Fructose

FIGURE 33.8 Interconversion of glucose and fructose.

TABLE 33.1 Inborn Errors of Carbohydrate Metabolism

Enzyme Deficiency	Disease State
Glucose-6-phosphatase (9)*	Type I GSD (von Gierke disease)
Muscle phosphorylase	Type V GSD (McArdle disease)
Liver phosphorylase	Type VI GSD (Hers disease)
Galactose-1-phosphate-uridyl transferase (2)	Galactosemia
Galactokinase (1)	Galactosemia
Uridine diphosphate-galactose-4-epimerase (3)	Galactosemia
Fructokinase (19)	Essential fructosuria
Fructose-1-phosphate aldolase (20)	Hereditary fructose intolerance
Pyruvate kinase (23)	Hemolytic anemia
Glucose-6-phosphate dehydrogenase (10)	Hemolytic disease

*Numbers in parentheses refer to enzymes in Fig. 33.9.
GSD, Glycogen storage disease.

Regulation of Blood Glucose Concentration

The concentration of glucose in the blood is regulated by the complex interplay of multiple pathways, modulated by several hormones. *Glycogenesis* is the conversion of glucose to glycogen. The reverse process—namely, the breakdown of glycogen to glucose and other intermediate products—is termed *glycogenolysis.* The formation of glucose from noncarbohydrate sources, such as amino acids, glycerol, or lactate, is termed *gluconeogenesis.* The conversion of glucose or other hexoses into lactate or pyruvate is called *glycolysis.* Further oxidation to carbon dioxide and water occurs through the Krebs (citric acid) cycle and the mitochondrial electron transport chain coupled to oxidative phosphorylation, generating energy in the form of adenosine triphosphate (ATP). Oxidation of glucose to carbon dioxide and water also occurs through the hexose monophosphate shunt pathway, which produces NADPH. Discussion of the hormones that regulate blood glucose is provided in Chapter 46.

HYPOGLYCEMIA

Hypoglycemia is a blood glucose concentration below the fasting value, but it is difficult to define a specific limit.[2] The most widely suggested cutoff is 50 mg/dL (2.8 mmol/L), but some authors suggest 60 mg/dL (3.3 mmol/L).[3] A transient decline may occur 1.5 to 2 hours after a meal, and it is not uncommon for a plasma glucose concentration as low as 40 mg/dL (2.8 mmol/L) to be observed 2 hours after ingestion of an oral glucose load. Similarly, extremely low fasting blood glucose values may occasionally be noted without symptoms or evidence of underlying disease. Hypoglycemia is rare in patients who do not have drug-treated diabetes mellitus.[4]

Symptoms of hypoglycemia vary among individuals, and none is specific. Epinephrine produces the classic signs and symptoms of hypoglycemia: trembling, sweating, nausea, rapid pulse, lightheadedness, hunger, and epigastric discomfort. These autonomic (neurogenic) symptoms are nonspecific and may be noted in other conditions, such as hyperthyroidism, pheochromocytoma, or even anxiety. Although controversial, it has been proposed that a rapid decrease in blood glucose may trigger the symptoms even though the blood glucose itself may not reach hypoglycemic values, whereas gradual onset of hypoglycemia may not produce symptoms.[5]

The brain cannot store or produce glucose, and in resting adults the central nervous system (CNS) consumes approximately 50% of the glucose used by the body.[6] Very low concentrations of plasma glucose (<20 or 30 mg/dL; <1.1 or 1.7 mmol/L) cause severe CNS dysfunction. During prolonged fasting or hypoglycemia, ketones may be used as an energy source. The broad spectrum of symptoms and signs of CNS dysfunction range from headache, confusion, blurred vision, and dizziness to seizures, loss of consciousness, and even death; these symptoms are known as *neuroglycopenia.*

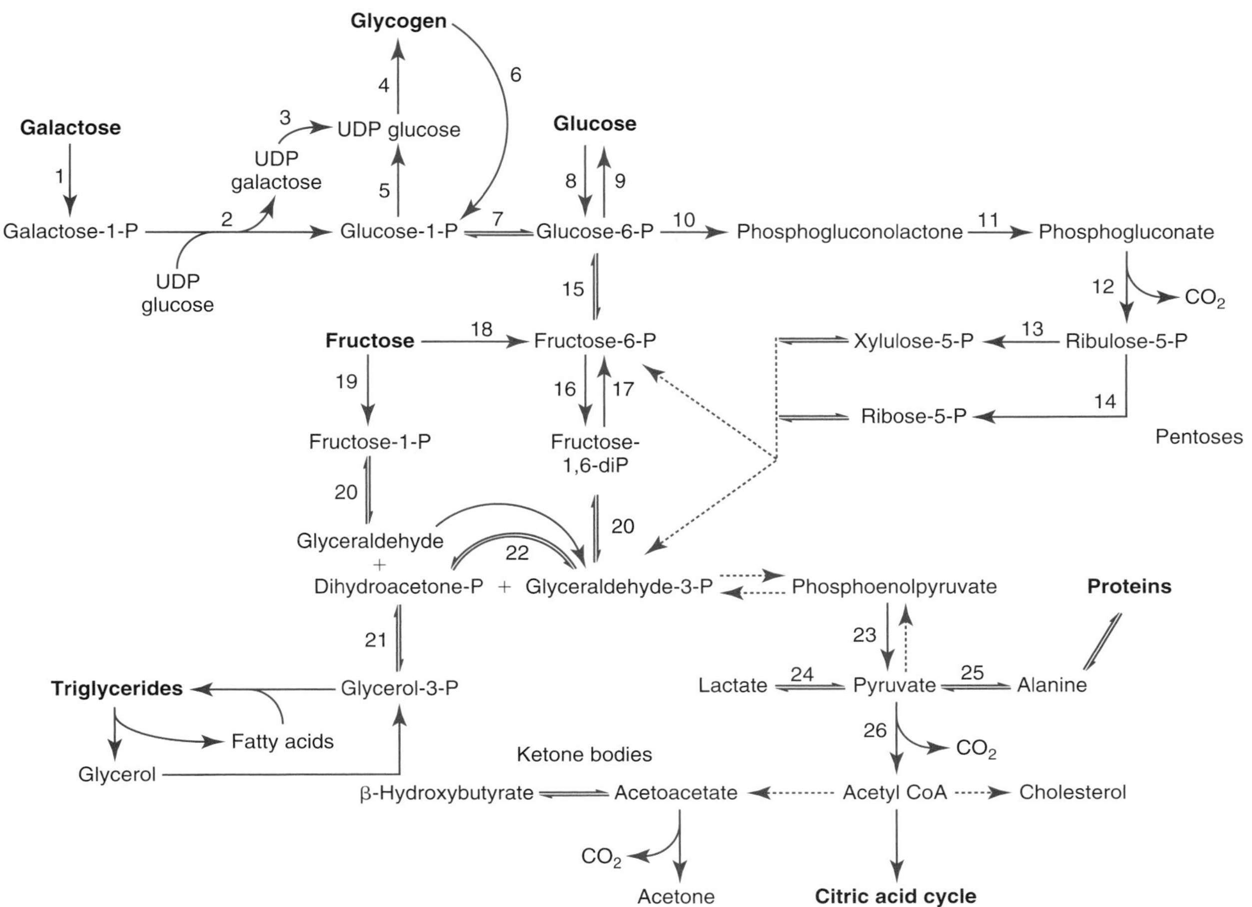

FIGURE 33.9 Major steps in the intermediary metabolism of carbohydrates. Numbers shown refer to specific enzymes. (- - - - - - - - -), Multistep pathway; (————), single-step pathway.

1. Galactokinase
2. Galactose-1-P-uridyl transferase
3. UDP-galactose-4-epimerase
4. Glycogen synthetase (plus branching enzyme)
5. UDP-glucose pyrophosphorylase
6. Glycogen phosphorylase
7. Phosphoglucomutase
8. Glucokinase (and hexokinase)
9. Glucose-6-phosphatase
10. Glucose-6-phosphate dehydrogenase
11. 6-Phosphogluconolactonase
12. 6-Phosphogluconate dehydrogenase
13. Ribulose-5-P-epimerase
14. Ribose-5-P-isomerase
15. Phosphohexose isomerase
16. Phosphofructokinase
17. Fructose-1,6-diphosphatase
18. Hexokinase (extrahepatic)
19. Fructokinase
20. Aldolase
21. Glycerol phosphate dehydrogenase
22. Triose-P-isomerase
23. Pyruvate kinase
24. Lactate dehydrogenase
25. Alanine aminotransferase
26. Pyruvate dehydrogenase

BOX 33.1 Causes of Hypoglycemia

Neonates
Small for gestational age/prematurity
Respiratory distress syndrome
Maternal diabetes mellitus
Toxemia of pregnancy
Other (eg, cold stress, polycythemia)

Infants
Ketotic hypoglycemia
Congenital enzyme defects
Glycogen storage disease
Deficiency of gluconeogenic enzymes
Galactosemia
Hereditary fructose intolerance
Leucine hypersensitivity
Endogenous hyperinsulinism
Reye syndrome
Idiopathic

Adults
Ill or Medicated Individual
Drugs
- Insulin or insulin secretagogue
- Alcohol
- Others (quinine, indomethacin)

Critical illness
- Hepatic, renal, or cardiac failure
- Sepsis (including malaria)
- Inanation

Hormone deficiency
- Cortisol
- Glucagon and epinephrine

Seemingly Healthy Individual
Endogenous hyperinsulinism
Insulinoma
Functional β cell disorders
- Noninsulinoma pancreatogenous hypoglycemia
- Post gastric bypass hypoglycemia
- Insulin autoimmune hypoglycemia
- Antibody to insulin
- Antibody to insulin receptor
- Insulin secretagogue
- Other

Accidental, surreptitious, or malicious hypoglycemia

Restoration of plasma glucose usually produces a prompt recovery, but irreversible damage may occur.

The age of onset of hypoglycemia is a convenient way to classify the disorder (Box 33.1), but it is important to remember that some overlap can occur among the various groups. For example, some glycogen storage disorders may present in the third decade of life, and hormone deficiencies occur in childhood.

Hypoglycemia in Neonates and Infants

Neonatal blood glucose concentrations are much lower than adult concentrations (mean <35 mg/dL; <2.0 mmol/L), and they decline shortly after birth when liver glycogen stores are depleted. Glucose concentrations as low as 30 mg/dL (1.7 mmol/L) in a term infant and 20 mg/dL (1.1 mmol/L) in a premature infant may occur without clinical evidence of hypoglycemia. The more common causes of hypoglycemia in the neonatal period include prematurity, maternal diabetes, gestational diabetes mellitus (GDM), and maternal eclampsia (see Box 33.1; for review, see reference 7). These are usually transient. Hypoglycemia with onset in early infancy is usually less transitory and may be due to inborn errors of metabolism or ketotic hypoglycemia; it usually occurs after fasting or a febrile illness.

Fasting Hypoglycemia in Adults

Hypoglycemia may result from a *decreased* rate of hepatic glucose production or an increased rate of glucose use. Symptoms suggestive of hypoglycemia are fairly common, but hypoglycemic disorders are rare. However, true hypoglycemia usually indicates serious underlying disease and may be life threatening. A precise threshold for establishing hypoglycemia is not always possible, and values as low as 30 mg/dL (1.7 mmol/L) may be encountered in healthy premenopausal women after a 72-hour fast.[8] Symptoms usually begin at plasma glucose concentrations below 55 mg/dL (3.1 mmol/L), and impairment of cerebral function begins when glucose is less than 50 mg/dL (2.8 mmol/L).

More than 100 causes of hypoglycemia have been reported. Some of the more common conditions are listed in Box 33.1. Drugs are the most prevalent cause,[9] and a wide variety, including pentamidine, gatifloxacin, and quinine, can produce hypoglycemia. Oral hypoglycemic agents, which have a long half-life (35 hours for chlorpropamide), are the most frequent cause of drug-induced hypoglycemia. Sulfonylureas stimulate secretion of insulin, proinsulin, and C-peptide, and may mimic an insulinoma. Differentiation is made by demonstration of the drug in blood or urine. Surreptitious administration of insulin can be detected by finding low C-peptide concentrations with increased insulin concentrations.

Ethanol produces hypoglycemia by inhibiting gluconeogenesis, and this is aggravated by malnutrition (low glycogen stores) in patients with chronic alcoholism. Decreased glucose production in hepatic failure (eg, viral hepatitis, toxins) caused by impaired gluconeogenesis or glycogen storage may result in hypoglycemia. Because dysfunction of more than 80% of the liver is necessary for hypoglycemia to develop, evidence of liver disease is invariably present. Deficiency of growth hormone (especially with coexistent ACTH deficiency), glucocorticoids, thyroid hormone, or glucagon may also produce hypoglycemia. Although a deficiency of glucocorticoids (eg, Addison disease) is most consistently associated with hypoglycemia, most glucocorticoid-deficient adults are not hypoglycemic. Hormonal deficiency causes hypoglycemia in children more frequently than it does in adults.

Demonstration of a low plasma glucose concentration in the presence of an abnormally high plasma insulin value is highly suggestive of an insulin-producing pancreatic islet cell tumor.[10] Because insulin concentrations exhibit a wide range in normal people, absolute hyperinsulinemia occurs in fewer than 50% of patients with insulinomas. Serum insulin concentrations that are inappropriately high for concurrent plasma glucose have been proposed to increase diagnostic accuracy. Critical diagnostic findings include a plasma insulin concentration of at least 18 pmol/L, plasma C-peptide concentrations greater than or equal to 0.2 nmol/L, and plasma proinsulin concentrations of at least 5.0 pmol/L when fasting plasma glucose is below 55 mg/dL (3.1 mmol/L). Ratios employing insulin and glucose alone have less diagnostic value. Provocative tests (glucagon,[11] tolbutamide,[12] calcium,[13]) or suppression tests (infusion of insulin and measurement of C-peptide), although strongly recommended in the past, generally are not necessary. Intra-arterial calcium stimulation with right hepatic vein sampling for insulin gradients appears to be a sensitive preoperative test for localizing insulinoma, although advances in imaging are making this approach far less common.[14]

Spontaneous production of antibodies to insulin may produce hypoglycemia (these antibodies are distinct from those elicited by insulin therapy and from the antibodies detected in certain patients with type 1 diabetes). Anti-insulin antibodies that cause hypoglycemia have been reported in Graves disease, multiple myeloma, systemic lupus erythematosus, and rheumatoid arthritis. This disorder is reported primarily among persons of Japanese or Korean ancestry and is less frequent among whites.[4] Patients exhibit postprandial hyperglycemia and fasting hypoglycemia.[15] Laboratory analysis demonstrates low plasma C-peptide and very high plasma insulin concentrations during hypoglycemia. The high insulin concentrations are believed to be an assay artifact caused by the antibody, and diagnosis is usually made by demonstrating high-titer serum insulin antibodies.

Nonpancreatic neoplasms that cause hypoglycemia are often extremely large mesenchymal neoplasms that appear to overuse glucose but may also have an inhibitory effect on glucose mobilization. Tumors of epithelial origin may cause hypoglycemia, frequently by producing insulin-like growth factor (IGF) 2.[16,17]

Hypoglycemia caused by septicemia should be relatively easy to diagnose[18] The mechanism is not well defined, but depleted glycogen stores, impaired gluconeogenesis, and increased peripheral use of glucose may be contributing factors. Glucose tolerance is commonly depressed in renal disease, and hypoglycemia may occur in end-stage renal failure.

Some of the conditions producing fasting hypoglycemia are readily apparent, but others require a lengthy diagnostic workup. Once hypoglycemia is demonstrated, specific tests should be performed to establish the underlying cause. The oral glucose tolerance test (OGTT) is not an appropriate study for evaluating a patient suspected of having hypoglycemia.[4]

Postprandial Hypoglycemia

Several drugs and a group of disorders may produce hypoglycemia in the postprandial (fed) state.[19] These include antibodies to insulin or the insulin receptor, and inborn errors (eg, fructose-1,6-diphosphatase deficiency). Also included is *reactive hypoglycemia* (referred to as *functional hypoglycemia*), which has been the subject of much debate.[3] Many commentaries and editorials have been published regarding the existence of reactive hypoglycemia (Hofeldt[1] and references listed therein). The general consensus is that no scientific evidence supports the existence of "functional hypoglycemia." It has been proposed that for individuals with vague symptoms after food ingestion, the preferred terminology should be *idiopathic reactive hypoglycemia*[19] or *idiopathic postprandial syndrome*.[2]

At the Third International Symposium on Hypoglycemia,[20] reactive hypoglycemia was defined as a clinical disorder in which the patient has postprandial symptoms suggesting hypoglycemia that occur in everyday life and are accompanied by a blood glucose concentration less than 45 to 50 mg/dL (2.5 to 2.8 mmol/L) as determined by a specific glucose measurement on arterialized venous or capillary blood, respectively. Patients complain of autonomic symptoms occurring approximately 1 to 3 hours after eating and seem to obtain relief, lasting 30 to 45 minutes, by food intake. These symptoms are rarely due to low blood glucose concentrations (eg, diabetes mellitus, gastrointestinal dysfunction, hormonal deficiency states). Most of these individuals have postprandial autonomic symptoms without neuroglycopenia in the postprandial state. Some experts in the field state that no true hypoglycemic disorder is characterized solely by autonomic symptoms.[2] A 5- or 6-hour glucose tolerance test was the standard procedure to establish the presence of postprandial hypoglycemia, but its use has been discredited.[3] The test is not reproducible in any particular individual, and low values for plasma glucose may be noted in the absence of symptoms, whereas symptoms may occur with normal glucose concentrations.[21] In addition, patients who have low blood glucose concentrations with autonomic symptoms 3 or 4 hours after an oral glucose load may have identical symptoms with normal blood glucose values after a mixed meal.[2] This may be due in part to anxiety provoked by the stressful environment during the glucose tolerance test. Demonstration of increased plasma epinephrine concentrations at the glucose nadir during an OGTT was reported to differentiate patients with reactive hypoglycemia,[22] but patients studied were identified on the basis of autonomic symptoms and signs, and only 25% demonstrated hypoglycemia. The OGTT should not be used in the diagnosis of reactive hypoglycemia.[23]

Postprandial hypoglycemia is infrequent, and demonstration of hypoglycemia during spontaneously occurring symptomatic episodes is necessary to establish the diagnosis.[15] If this is not possible, a 5-hour meal tolerance test[21] (which simulates the composition of a normal diet) or a *hyperglucidic* (high-glucose) breakfast test[3] has been proposed. A protocol for a mixed-meal test can be found in Cryer and associates.[4]

A diagnosis of hypoglycemia has been used to explain a wide variety of disorders that appear unrelated to blood glucose abnormalities.[24] These nonspecific symptoms include fatigue, muscle spasms, palpitations, numbness, tingling, pain, sweating, mental dullness, sleepiness, weakness, and fainting. Behavior abnormalities, poor school performance, and delinquency have been incorrectly attributed to low blood glucose concentrations. Widespread use of the insensitive and nonspecific 5-hour glucose tolerance test caused overdiagnosis of hypoglycemia and led the American Diabetes Association (ADA) to publish a statement to discourage the inappropriate use of the OGTT for the diagnosis of hypoglycemia.[23] Lay publications[25] have supported this recommendation, but it is still important for the medical community to reassure such patients that low blood glucose is not the cause of their symptoms and to deal with specific abnormalities that might underlie patients' complaints or problems. A diagnosis of hypoglycemia should not be made unless a patient meets the criteria of Whipple's triad of low blood glucose concentration with typical symptoms alleviated by glucose administration.

Demonstration of a plasma glucose concentration greater than 70 mg/dL (3.9 mmol/L) during a symptomatic episode indicates that the symptoms unequivocally are not the result of hypoglycemia.

Hypoglycemia in Diabetes Mellitus

Hypoglycemia occurs frequently in both type 1 and type 2 diabetes,[26,27] and it is the limiting factor in glycemic management of diabetes. Patients using insulin experience approximately one to two episodes of symptomatic hypoglycemia per week, and severe hypoglycemia (ie, requiring assistance from others or associated with loss of consciousness) affects about 10% of this population per year. In patients practicing intensive insulin therapy (eg, multiple injections, continuous subcutaneous insulin infusion), these figures are increased twofold to sixfold. The chief adverse event associated with intensive therapy in the Diabetes Control and Complications Trial (DCCT) was a threefold increase in the incidence of severe hypoglycemia.[28] An estimated 2% to 4% of people with type 1 diabetes die from hypoglycemia.[4] Similarly, hypoglycemia occurs in patients with type 2 diabetes (caused by oral hypoglycemic agents or insulin) but is less frequent than in type 1 diabetes. Recent evidence suggests that severe hypoglycemia may have long-term sequelae, including dementia and death from cardiovascular disease. Two pathophysiologic mechanisms contribute to hypoglycemia in patients with diabetes.

Defective Glucose Counterregulation

Counterregulatory responses become impaired in patients with type 1 diabetes,[26] increasing the risk of hypoglycemia. The response of glucagon to hypoglycemia is impaired by an unknown mechanism early in the course of type 1 diabetes. Epinephrine secretory response to hypoglycemia becomes deficient later in the course of the disease. These defects are selective because other stimuli continue to elicit glucagon and epinephrine secretion. Glucose counterregulation does not appear to be defective in patients with type 2 diabetes.

Hypoglycemia Unawareness

Up to 50% of patients with long-standing (more than 30 years) type 1 diabetes do not experience neurogenic warning symptoms and are prone to more severe hypoglycemia. The mechanism is thought to be associated with a decreased epinephrine response to hypoglycemia. Intensively treated patients with type 1 diabetes require lower plasma glucose concentrations to elicit symptoms of hypoglycemia. Some authors have claimed that human insulin results in an increased incidence of hypoglycemia unawareness, but analysis of 45 studies revealed no significant differences in hypoglycemic episodes between insulin from different species.[29]

Evaluation of Hypoglycemia

The Endocrine Society issued guidelines in 2009 for the evaluation of adult hypoglycemic disorders.[4] These guidelines were cosponsored by the American Diabetes Association, the European Association for the Study of Diabetes, and the European Society of Endocrinology. Patients should be evaluated for hypoglycemia only if Whipple triad—symptoms and/or signs of hypoglycemia, low plasma glucose concentration, and resolution of symptoms or signs after plasma glucose is raised—is documented.

POINTS TO REMEMBER

Disorders of Glucose Homeostasis

- Hyperglycemia (increased blood glucose concentration), caused by diabetes mellitus, is the most frequently encountered disorder of carbohydrate metabolism.
- Hypoglycemia is a blood glucose concentration below the fasting value.
- The symptoms of hypoglycemia vary among individuals, and none is specific.
- Symptoms suggestive of hypoglycemia are fairly common, but true hypoglycemia is rare in individuals who do not have drug-treated diabetes mellitus.
- Hypoglycemia occurs frequently in patients with diabetes and is the limiting factor in glycemic management.
- True hypoglycemia usually indicates serious underlying disease.

The classic diagnostic test is the prolonged fast, which should be conducted in a hospital.[4] During the fast, the patient should be allowed to drink calorie-free fluids. All nonessential medications should be discontinued, and patients should be active when awake. Blood should be drawn every 6 hours for analysis of plasma glucose, insulin, C-peptide, proinsulin, and β-hydroxybutyrate. When plasma glucose concentration is less than 60 mg/dL (3.3 mmol/L), sampling should be performed every 1 to 2 hours. Samples for plasma insulin, C-peptide, and proinsulin should be analyzed only in those samples in which the glucose concentration is less than 60 mg/dL (3.3 mmol/L). The fast should be concluded when plasma glucose concentration falls to less than 45 mg/dL (2.5 mmol/L) and the patient has symptoms and/or signs of hypoglycemia. If this does not occur, the fast should be terminated after 72 hours. At the conclusion of the fast, blood should be collected for analysis of glucose, insulin, C-peptide, proinsulin, β-hydroxybutyrate, and oral hypoglycemic agents. Then 1 mg of glucagon should be injected intravenously and plasma glucose concentration measured 10, 20, and 30 minutes later. This concludes the protocol, and the patient can be fed. Insulin antibodies should be measured, but not necessarily during hypoglycemia. When a deficiency is suspected, plasma cortisol, growth hormone, or glucagon should be measured at the beginning and end of the fast. A gender difference is observed in plasma glucose concentrations during prolonged fasting, with women exhibiting significantly lower concentrations than men. Low plasma glucose is necessary, but not sufficient, to establish the diagnosis. Absence of symptoms or signs of hypoglycemia during the fast excludes the diagnosis of a hypoglycemic disorder. Symptoms, signs, or both, combined with concentrations of glucose less than 55 mg/dL (3.1 mmol/L), insulin of at least 18 pmol/L, C-peptide of at least 0.2 nmol/L, and proinsulin of at least 5.0 pmol/L document endogenous hyperinsulinism. If β-hydroxybutyrate is 2.7 mmol/L or less and glucose is increased by at least 25 mg/dL (1.4 mmol/L) after intravenous glucagon (the latter indicating preserved hepatic glycogen stores), hypoglycemia is mediated by insulin or IGF.

Tolbutamide Tolerance Test

Tolbutamide [1-butyl-3-(*p*-tolylsulfonyl)urea] (Orinase) stimulates the normal pancreas to produce insulin. The response of the pancreas to intravenous tolbutamide has been used in the investigation of fasting hypoglycemia. Blood specimens are obtained for glucose and insulin before intravenous injection of 1 g of a water-soluble form of tolbutamide and at 2, 15, 30, 60, 90, and 120 minutes afterward. Healthy people have a decrease in plasma glucose concentration to about 50% of the fasting value by 30 minutes, with a return to baseline at 120 minutes. Patients with fasting hypoglycemia exhibit a lower glucose nadir, with hypoglycemia persisting up to 2 hours. The insulin response provides further diagnostic information. The peak insulin concentration at 2 minutes is normally less than 150 μIU/mL (900 pmol/L). This value is increased in patients with islet cell tumors, and an increased insulin concentration at 60 minutes is reported to be the most reliable discriminator.[30] In various conditions such as liver disease, malnutrition, or renal insufficiency, plasma glucose responses to tolbutamide are indistinguishable from those seen with islet cell tumors, but only patients with insulinoma exhibit exaggerated plasma insulin concentrations.

DETERMINATION OF GLUCOSE IN BODY FLUIDS

Many analytical procedures are used to measure blood glucose concentrations. In the past, analyses were often performed with relatively nonspecific methods that could produce falsely increased values. Today, almost all common methods are enzymatic (eg, hexokinase,[31,32] glucose oxidase), and older methods, such as photometric or oxidation reduction techniques, are rarely used. The glucose assays most widely used in the United States may be determined by inspecting proficiency testing surveys conducted by the College of American Pathologists (CAP). Results from 5775 laboratories (18% from outside the United States) reported in a survey conducted in 2014 are displayed in Table 33.2 (see e-Table 33.2 at ExpertConsult.com for the data in SI units). These data show that automated hexokinase methods are used in 74% of participating laboratories. Glucose oxidase is the only other method that is widely used. The most significant change in the past 30 years is the disappearance of the *o*-toluidine method, which was used in the SMA 12/60 Autoanalyzer. It must be emphasized that these data apply only to this CAP survey and are weighted to laboratories participating on a voluntary basis or in compliance with regulatory agencies. Furthermore, testing performed in physicians' offices is not included. Many kits are commercially available for measuring glucose and are widely used, especially in smaller laboratories. Reference to CAP surveys reveals that all glucose oxidase or hexokinase methods exhibit coefficients of variation (CVs) less than or equal to 3.3% for glucose values on lyophilized serum. The method of glucose measurement does not influence the result. Comparison of pooled serum samples measured by approximately 6000 clinical laboratories shows that mean glucose concentrations measured by the hexokinase and glucose oxidase methods are essentially the same.[33] However, when evaluated against a reference measurement procedure, significant biases of up to 13% are observed among different methods.

Specimen Collection and Storage

In individuals with a normal hematocrit, fasting whole blood glucose concentration is approximately 10% to 12% lower than plasma glucose. Although glucose concentrations in the water phase of red blood cells and plasma are similar (the erythrocyte plasma membrane is freely permeable to glucose), the water content of plasma (93%) is approximately 11% higher than that of whole blood. In most clinical laboratories, plasma or serum is used for most glucose determinations; methods for self-monitoring of glucose use whole blood samples but may measure the glucose concentration in the plasma phase. Venous plasma is recommended for diagnosis of diabetes.[34,35] Although older methods of analysis reported that glucose concentrations in plasma were 5% lower than in serum,[36] a 2004 study indicated that glucose values measured in serum and plasma are essentially the same.[37] During fasting, capillary blood glucose concentration is only 2 to 5 mg/dL (0.1 to 0.3 mmol/L) higher than that of venous blood. After a glucose load, however, capillary blood glucose concentrations are 20 to 70 mg/dL (1.1 to 3.9 mmol/L) (mean ≈30 mg/dL (1.7 mmol/L); equivalent to 20% to 25%) higher than concurrently drawn venous blood samples.[38,39]

Glycolysis decreases serum glucose by approximately 5% to 7% in 1 hour (5 to 10 mg/dL; 0.3 to 0.6 mmol/L) in normal uncentrifuged coagulated blood at room temperature.[40,41] The rate of in vitro glycolysis is higher in the presence of leukocytosis or bacterial contamination, but others have observed a slight decrease.[42] In separated, nonhemolyzed

TABLE 33.2 Methods of Glucose Analysis in 5775 Laboratories (Traditional Units)*

Method	Number†	Percent of Total	Mean, mg/dL	SD	CV, %
Hexokinase					
Photometric (visible)	410	7	119.1	3.6	3.0
Photometric (ultraviolet)	3860	67	116.3	3.4	2.9
Glucose Oxidase					
Photometric	956	17	116.2	2.6	2.2
Oxygen electrode	512	9	116.1	2.1	1.8
Glucose Dehydrogenase	26	<1	117.8	5.0	4.3

*Results are based on 2014 CAP Survey, Set C-C, Specimen CHM-12 (Copyright 2014 College of American Pathologists; data used with permission). See text for discussion of methods.

†*Number* indicates how many laboratories use the indicated method/type.

CV, Coefficient of variation for all results by all methods of the indicated method/type from all manufacturers. It may include a component of variation attributable to differences in calibrators and to matrix effects.

sterile serum, the glucose concentration is generally stable as long as 8 hours at 25°C and up to 72 hours at 4°C; variable stability is observed with longer storage periods.[43] Plasma, removed from the cells after moderate centrifugation, contains leukocytes that also metabolize glucose, although cell-free sterile plasma has no glycolytic activity.

Glycolysis has been found to be inhibited and glucose stabilized for as long as 3 days at room temperature by adding sodium fluoride (NaF) or, less commonly, sodium iodoacetate to the specimen. Fluoride ions prevent glycolysis by inhibiting enolase, an enzyme that requires Mg^{2+}. This inhibition is due to the formation of an ionic complex consisting of Mg^{2+}, inorganic phosphate, and fluoride ions; this complex interferes with the interaction of enzyme and substrate. Fluoride is also a weak anticoagulant because it binds calcium; however, clotting may occur after several hours. It is therefore advisable to use a combined fluoride-oxalate mixture, such as 2 mg of potassium oxalate ($K_2C_2O_4$) and 2 mg NaF/mL of blood, to prevent late clotting. Other anticoagulants (eg, EDTA, citrate, heparin) can also be used. Fluoride ions in high concentration inhibit the activity of urease and certain other enzymes; consequently, the specimens are unsuitable for determination of urea in procedures that require urease and for direct assay of some serum enzymes. $K_2C_2O_4$ causes loss of cell water, thereby diluting the plasma. Therefore samples collected in these tubes should not be used for measurement of analytes other than glucose. Although fluoride maintains long-term blood glucose stability, the rate of decline in the first hour after sample collection is not altered, and glycolysis may continue for up to 4 hours.[40] A 2009 study showed that acidification of blood using citrate buffer inhibits in vitro glycolysis more effectively than fluoride.[44] When available, tubes containing citrate buffer, sodium fluoride, and EDTA may be an effective and practical method to stabilize glucose. If these tubes are not available, the cells should be removed within minutes to minimize glycolysis. Alternatively, the tube should be placed in ice-water slurry and the cells separated within 30 minutes.[35] Neither of these approaches is practical in routine analysis. It may not be necessary to use a fluoride-containing tube if plasma is separated from cells within 30 minutes of blood collection. However, inhibitors of glycolysis are required in patients with greatly increased leukocyte counts (eg, blast crisis) because differences of up to 65 mg/dL (3.6 mmol/L) have been observed between glucose values with and without glycolytic inhibitors after 1 to 2 hours of contact with the blood cells.

Cerebrospinal fluid (CSF) may be contaminated with bacteria or other cells and should be analyzed immediately for glucose. If a delay in measurement is unavoidable, the sample should be subjected to centrifugation and stored at 4°C or at −20°C. For more details on glucose measurement in body fluids, see Chapter 43.

In 24-hour collections of urine, glucose may be preserved by adding 5 mL of glacial acetic acid to the container before starting the collection. The final pH of the urine is usually between 4 and 5, which inhibits bacterial activity. Other preservatives that have been proposed include 5 g of sodium benzoate per 24-hour specimen, or chlorhexidine and 0.1% sodium nitrate ($NaNO_2$) with 0.01% benzethonium chloride. These may be inadequate, and urine should be stored at 4°C during collection. Urine samples may lose as much as 40% of their glucose after 24 hours at room temperature.[45]

POINTS TO REMEMBER

Measurement of Glucose

- Measurement of glucose is one of the most commonly performed analytical procedures.
- Glucose may be measured in blood, urine, or cerebrospinal fluid.
- Almost all common methods are enzymatic.
- The glucose concentration in whole blood is 10% to 12% lower than the plasma glucose concentration.
- Glycolysis occurs in whole blood in a test tube, and delay in separating cells from plasma (or serum) can significantly decrease the glucose concentration.

Methods

Hexokinase and glucose oxidase are the two main types of methods used to measure glucose in body fluids.

Hexokinase Methods

Glucose is phosphorylated by ATP in the presence of hexokinase and Mg^{2+}. The glucose-6-phosphate formed is oxidized by glucose-6-phosphate dehydrogenase (G6PD) to 6-phosphogluconate in the presence of nicotinamide-adenine dinucleotide phosphate (NADPH). The amount of NADPH produced is directly proportional to the amount of glucose in the sample and is measured by absorbance at 340 nm. G6PD derived from yeast is used in the assay with $NADP^+$ as the cofactor. The oxidized form of nicotinamide-adenine dinucleotide (NAD^+) is the cofactor if bacterial *(Leuconostoc mesenteroides)* G6PD is used, and the NADH produced is measured at 340 nm.

$$\text{Glucose} + \text{ATP} \xrightleftharpoons{\textit{Hexokinase}} \text{Glucose-6-phosphate} + \text{ADP}$$

$$\text{Glucose-6-phosphate} \xrightleftharpoons{\textit{G-6-PD}} \text{6-Phosphogluconate}$$

$$\text{NADP}^{\oplus}\ (\text{or NAD}^{\oplus}) \rightarrow \text{NADPH} + \text{H}^{\oplus}\ (\text{or NADH})$$

A reference method based on this principle has been developed and validated.[59] Serum or plasma is deproteinated by adding solutions of barium hydroxide ($Ba[OH]_2$) and zinc sulfate ($ZnSO_4$). The clear supernatant is mixed with a reagent containing ATP, NAD^+, hexokinase, and G6PD, incubated at 25°C until the reaction is complete, and NADH is measured. Calibrators and blanks are carried through the entire procedure, including the deproteination step. Detailed specifications are given for the equipment, materials, and reagents, including tests of enzyme reagent adequacy.

Although highly accurate and precise, the reference method is too exacting and time-consuming for routine use in a clinical laboratory. An alternative approach is to apply the reaction directly to serum or plasma and use a specimen blank to correct for interfering substances that absorb at 340 nm.[46] Because almost all methods are automated and rely on commercially prepared reagents supplied in lyophilized form, only a general discussion of the procedure is presented here.

Serum may be used if separated promptly. NaF containing plasma with an anticoagulant such as EDTA, heparin, or oxalate may be used, although citrate is preferred. Hemolyzed specimens containing more than 0.5 g hemoglobin/dL are unsatisfactory because phosphate esters and enzymes released from red blood cells interfere with the assay. Other sources of interference include drugs, bilirubin, and lipemia (triglycerides ≥500 mg/dL [5.65 mmol/L] cause positive interference). A sample blank is therefore recommended for lipemic and icteric samples. This blank is prepared by adding 10 μL of sample to isotonic saline or buffer instead of reagent. The absorbance of this mixture, read against water at 340 nm, is subtracted. Although fructose interferes in the assay, normal fasting serum has low fructose concentrations. After ingestion of fructose 0.75 g/kg of body weight, serum fructose concentration increases up to 2.5 mg/dL (0.7 mmol/L) within 1 hour, and an increase persists for 2 hours. Solutions administered during glucose tolerance testing therefore should not contain any fructose.

Absorbance of sample or calibrator reaction mixtures is measured after the reactions have continued to completion (equilibrium reaction). Although glucose concentrations may be calculated directly, based on the molar absorptivity of NADPH or NADH, inclusion of a set of calibrators is recommended to detect possible deterioration of enzymes, ATP, $NADP^+$, or NAD^+, all of which are unstable. Reagents may also contain substances that react with the coenzymes. The presence of these substances can be evaluated by measuring the increase in absorbance observed in a reagent blank. Reagents are unsuitable for use if the absorbance at 340 nm exceeds 0.35, using water as the blank. The highest calibrator provides a check on the linearity of response and the adequacy of the enzyme reagent. The procedure is linear from 0 to 500 mg/dL (0 to 27.8 mmol/L). Glucose concentrations that exceed 500 mg/dL (27.8 mmol/L) should be diluted with isotonic saline and reassayed.

Hexokinase procedures in which indicator reactions produce colored products are available, enabling absorbance to be measured in the visible range.[47] An oxidation reduction system containing phenazine methosulfate (PMS) and a substituted tetrazolium compound, 2-(*p*-iodophenyl)-3-*p*-nitrophenyl-5-phenyltetrazolium chloride (INT), is reacted with NADPH formed in the reaction. The reduced INT is colored with maximum absorbance at 520 nm. The PMS-INT color developer must be refrigerated when not in use and must be protected from exposure to light to retard autoreduction.

Glucose Oxidase Methods

The enzyme glucose oxidase catalyzes the oxidation of glucose to gluconic acid and hydrogen peroxide (H_2O_2):

$$\text{Glucose} + 2H_2O + O_2 \xrightarrow{\text{Glucose Oxidase}} \text{Gluconic Acid} + 2\,H_2O_2$$

Addition of the enzyme peroxidase and a chromogenic oxygen acceptor, such as *o*-dianisidine, results in the formation of a colored compound that is measured:

$$\underset{\text{(Colorless)}}{\text{o}-\text{Dianisidine}} + H_2O_2 \xrightarrow{\text{Peroxidase}} \underset{\text{(Colored)}}{\text{Oxidized o}-\text{Dianisidine}} + 2H_2O$$

Glucose oxidase is highly specific for β-D-glucose. As noted earlier, 36% and 64% of glucose in solution are in α- and β-forms, respectively. Complete reaction of glucose therefore requires mutarotation of the α- to the β-form. Some commercial preparations of glucose oxidase contain an enzyme —mutarotase—that accelerates this reaction. Otherwise, extended incubation time allows spontaneous conversion.

The second step, which involves peroxidase, is much less specific than the glucose oxidase reaction. Various substances, such as uric acid, ascorbic acid, bilirubin, hemoglobin, tetracycline, and glutathione, inhibit the reaction (presumably by competing with the chromogen for H_2O_2), producing lower values. Incorporation of potassium ferrocyanide significantly decreases interference by bilirubin. Most interfering substances can be eliminated by the use of a Somogyi filtrate. Acid filtrates cannot be used because peroxides, which cause falsely increased results, may be released. Most modern methods omit the preparation of protein-free filtrates to make the procedure faster and simpler. Some glucose oxidase preparations contain catalase as a contaminant; catalase activity decomposes peroxide and decreases the final color obtained. Calibrators and unknowns should be analyzed simultaneously under conditions in which the rate of oxidation is proportional to the glucose concentration.

In some methods, the final mixture is acidified slightly to stop the reaction, and the intensity of the yellow chromophore is measured at 400 nm. In stronger acid solution, the color becomes pink, with maximum absorbance at 540 nm, and both sensitivity and stability are improved. Other approaches to measure the H_2O_2 produced include the peroxide-mediated oxidative coupling of 3-methyl-2-benzothiazolinone hydrazone (MBTH) with *N*,*N*-dimethylaniline (DMA) catalyzed by peroxidase,[32] or the oxidative coupling of *p*-aminophenazone (PAP) to phenol.[48] Both procedures have been automated. The MBTH-DMA and PAP procedures are not affected by high concentrations of creatinine, uric acid, or hemoglobin and are performed directly on serum. The chromogen 2-amino-4-hydroxybenzenesulfonic acid produces a yellow color in the presence of peroxidase and H_2O_2.[49] Additional components are not required to produce the color, and the assay can be performed on as little as 2 μL of serum.

Glucose oxidase methods are suitable for measuring glucose in CSF but not in urine because urine contains high concentrations of substances that interfere with the peroxidase reaction (such as uric acid), producing falsely low results. The glucose oxidase method therefore should not be used for urine. A method in which the urine is first pretreated with an ion-exchange resin to remove interfering substances has been described.

Modified Glucose Oxidase Methods

Some instruments use a polarographic oxygen electrode that measures the rate of oxygen consumption after the sample is added to a solution containing glucose oxidase.[50] Because this measurement involves only the first reaction shown earlier, interferences encountered in the peroxidase step are eliminated. To prevent formation of oxygen from H_2O_2 by catalase present in some preparations of glucose oxidase, H_2O_2 is removed by two additional reactions:

$$H_2O_2 + C_2H_5OH \xrightarrow{\text{Catalase}} CH_3CHO + 2H_2O$$

$$H_2O_2 + 2H^+ + 2I^- \xrightarrow{Molybdate} I_2 + 2H_2O$$

The latter reaction is effective even when catalase activity has diminished on storage of reagents. The procedure can be applied directly to urine, serum, plasma, or CSF. However, this approach cannot be used for the determination of glucose in whole blood because blood cells consume oxygen.

In the YSI Model 23A (Yellow Springs Instrument Co., Yellow Springs, Ohio), glucose oxidase is immobilized in a thin layer of resinous material sandwiched between two membranes. When a buffered sample is introduced, glucose diffuses through the first polycarbonate membrane and reacts with the enzyme to produce H_2O_2. This diffuses through the second, smaller-pore cellulose acetate membrane and is oxidized at a platinum anode. The current generated is directly proportional to the glucose concentration in the diluted sample.

$$H_2O_2 \rightarrow 2H^+ + O_2 + 2e^-$$

The circuit is completed at a silver cathode, where oxygen is reduced to water.

$$4H^+ + O_2 + 4e^- \rightarrow 2H_2O$$

Any H_2O_2 diffusing back into the sample chamber is destroyed by catalase to prevent interference with the analysis. Determinations may be performed on 25 µL of plasma, serum, or whole blood. Good precision and correlation with an oxygen consumption rate analyzer have been reported.[17]

The Vitros System (Ortho-Clinical Diagnostics, Raritan, N.J.) uses dry multilayer films for chemical analyses.[51] Glucose is measured by a glucose oxidase procedure. A 10-µL sample of serum, plasma, urine, or CSF is placed on a porous film on top of the layer containing the reagents. Glucose diffuses through the film and reacts with the reagents to produce a colored end product or dye. The intensity of this dye is measured through a lower transparent film by reflectance spectrophotometry. Advantages of this system include small sample size, absence of liquid reagents, and improved stability on storage.

Glucose Dehydrogenase Methods

The enzyme glucose dehydrogenase (β-D-glucose: NAD oxidoreductase; EC 1.1.1.47) catalyzes the oxidation of glucose to gluconolactone. Mutarotase is added to shorten the time necessary to reach equilibrium. The amount of NADH generated is proportional to the glucose concentration.

Glucose dehydrogenase for this assay is isolated from *Bacillus cereus*. The reaction (1) appears to be highly specific for glucose, (2) shows no interference from common anticoagulants and substances normally found in serum, and (3) provides results in close agreement with hexokinase procedures. However, products containing maltose, icodextrin (which is converted to maltose), or galactose spuriously increase results obtained with point-of-care glucose meters that use glucose dehydrogenase pyrrolo-quinoline quinine (GDH-PQQ). Maltose is found in some intravenous immune globulins, and icodextrin is a glucose polymer present in some peritoneal dialysis solutions. These substances do not interfere with glucose measuring systems that use glucose dehydrogenase with NAD as a cofactor. Glucose dehydrogenase methods have been adapted to continuous-flow analyzers,[52] including the use of immobilized enzyme,[53] and to a centrifugal analyzer.[54]

Reference Intervals

Although glucose is assayed by several different analytical procedures, reference limits do not vary significantly among methods. The following values should apply to virtually all currently used glucose assays.[‡]

	Sample Fasting Glucose, mg/dL
Plasma/Serum	
Adults	74–99 (4.1–5.5 mmol/L)
Children	60–100 (3.3–5.6 mmol/L)
Premature neonates	20–60 (1.1–3.3 mmol/L)
Term neonates	30–60 (1.7–3.3 mmol/L)
Whole blood	65–95 (3.6–5.3 mmol/L)
CSF	40–70 (2.2–3.9 mmol/L) (60% of plasma value)
Urine	
24 hour	1–15 mg/dL (0.1–0.8 mmol/L)

Note that the ADA[55] and WHO criteria[35] of fasting glucose of 126 mg/dL (7.0 mmol/L) or greater—not the reference interval—is used for the diagnosis of diabetes. Moreover, the threshold for diagnosis of hypoglycemia is variable and is considerably less than the lower limit of the reference interval. There is no sex difference. Plasma glucose values increase with age from the third to the sixth decade: fasting, approximately 2 mg/dL (0.1 mmol/L) per decade; postprandial, 4 mg/dL (0.2 mmol/L) per decade; and after a glucose challenge, 8 to 13 mg/dL (0.4 to 0.7 mmol/L) per decade.[56] Fasting plasma glucose does not increase significantly after age 60, but glucose concentrations after a glucose challenge are substantially higher in older individuals.[57] Evidence of an association of increasing insulin resistance with age is inconsistent, and visceral obesity appears to be responsible for the reported decrease in glucose tolerance in middle age.[58]

CSF glucose concentrations should be approximately 60% of plasma concentrations and must always be compared with concurrently measured plasma glucose for adequate clinical interpretation.

Measurement of Glucose in Urine

Examination of urine for glucose is rapid, inexpensive, and noninvasive and has been used to screen large numbers of samples. The older screening tests detect sugars that reduce copper, producing a color.[59] Unfortunately, these tests react with reducing substances other than glucose (Box 33.2). Qualitative, semiquantitative, and quantitative methods are available for measuring glucose in urine and have essentially replaced the nonspecific tests in adults. *Note:* A reducing sugar method rather than an enzymatic method specific for glucose must be used when screening neonates and infants for inborn errors of metabolism that result in the appearance of reducing sugars other than glucose (eg, galactose, fructose) in the urine.

Qualitative Method

In one such method, using Benedict reagent (cupric ion complexed to citrate in alkaline solution), reducing substances

BOX 33.2 Reducing Substances in Urine

Fructose	Ketone bodies
Lactose	Sulfanilamide
Galactose	Oxalic acid
Maltose	Hippuric acid
Arabinose	Homogentisic acid
Xylose	Glucuronic acid
Ribose	Formaldehyde
Uric acid	Isoniazid
Ascorbic acid	Salicylates
Creatinine	Cinchophen
Cysteine	Salicyluric acid
Glucose	

convert cupric to cuprous ions, forming yellow cuprous hydroxide or red cuprous oxide.

Semiquantitative Methods

Convenient paper test strips are commercially available from a number of manufacturers (Clinistix and Diastix, Siemens Healthcare Diagnostics; and Chemstrip, Roche Diagnostics). All of the strips use the glucose-specific enzyme glucose oxidase in a chromogenic assay. For example, Clinistix has filter paper impregnated with glucose oxidase, peroxidase, and the dye *o*-toluidine. Other dyes, such as tetramethylbenzidine (TMB) have been used. The test end of the strip is moistened with freshly voided urine and examined after 10 seconds. A blue color develops if glucose is present at a concentration of 100 mg/dL (5.6 mmol/L) or greater. Results are read by comparing the test color with a standard color chart. Automated urinalysis systems capable of analyzing 300 strips per hour are commercially available. The test is more sensitive for glucose than the copper reduction test (Clinitest), which has a detection limit of 250 mg/dL (13.9 mmol/L). Despite these claims, evaluation of dipsticks reveals high imprecision at low urine glucose concentrations.[60] Clinitest was reported to detect glucose only when it was above 1 g/L (55.6 mmol/L), and only Chemstrip μG could differentiate urine glucose at 300 mg/L (16.7 mmol/L) (upper limit of reference interval) from 600 mg/L (33.3 mmol/L).[61] The sensitivity of the strip has been adjusted to take into account the presence of enzyme inhibitors normally present in urine. Thus a positive test result is obtained with lower concentrations of glucose in water than in urine. For the same reason, misleading high results may be obtained with very dilute specimens.

False-positive results may be produced by contamination of urine with H_2O_2 or a strong oxidizing agent, such as hypochlorite (bleach). Exposure of dipsticks to air gives false-positive readings after 7 days.[62] False-negative results may occur with large quantities of reducing substances, such as ketones, ascorbic acid, and salicylates. Several antibiotics contain ascorbic acid as a preservative, which is excreted essentially unchanged. For routine examinations, a negative result by the strip test is usually interpreted to mean that the urine specimen is negative for glucose.

Other strip tests (Keto-Diastix, Siemens Healthcare Diagnostics; and DiaScreen 2GK, Arkray) are designed for the semiquantitative estimation of both glucose and ketone bodies. The glucose portion of the strip uses the glucose oxidase-peroxidase method. The hydrogen peroxide produced oxidizes iodide to iodine, yielding various intensities of brown that correspond to the concentration of glucose in urine. The detection limit is 100 mg/dL (5.6 mmol/L). The Diastix glucose test is reported to be less inhibited by ascorbic acid than Clinistix. Chemstrip now has an iodate-impregnated mesh layer that is stated to virtually eliminate interference from ascorbic acid.

Quantitative Methods

Applications of various procedures for quantitative determination of glucose in urine were discussed earlier in this chapter under "Determination of Glucose in Body Fluids." Hexokinase or glucose dehydrogenase procedures are recommended for greatest accuracy and specificity. Glucose oxidase procedures that depend only on the consumption of oxygen or the production of H_2O_2 are also reliable. Glucose oxidase procedures that include the H_2O_2-peroxidase reaction are not acceptable.

LACTATE AND PYRUVATE

Lactic acid, an intermediate in carbohydrate metabolism (see Fig. 33.9), is derived predominantly from white skeletal muscle, brain, skin, renal medulla, and erythrocytes. The blood lactate concentration depends on the rate of production in these tissues and the rate of metabolism in the liver and kidneys. Approximately 65% of total basal lactate production is used by the liver, particularly in gluconeogenesis. The *Cori cycle* consists of the conversion of glucose to lactate in the periphery and the reconversion of lactate to glucose in the liver. Extrahepatic removal of lactate occurs by oxidation in red skeletal muscle and the renal cortex. A moderate increase in lactate production results in increased hepatic lactate clearance, but uptake by the liver is saturable when plasma concentrations exceed 2 mmol/L. For example, during strenuous exercise, lactate concentrations may increase significantly, from an average concentration of about 0.9 mmol/L to more than 20 mmol/L within 10 seconds. There is no uniformly accepted concentration for the diagnosis of lactic acidosis, but lactate concentrations exceeding 5 mmol/L and pH less than 7.25 indicate significant lactic acidosis.

Under certain conditions, the ratio of lactate to pyruvate is an indicator of redox status. For example, by rearranging the equation for the equilibrium constant for the reaction catalyzed by lactate dehydrogenase (EC 1.1.1.27), the ratio of lactate to pyruvate is shown to be proportional to the ratio of NADH to NAD^+.

Clinical Significance

Pyruvate is one of the critical metabolites in cells, most of which originates from glycolysis.[63] It is further metabolized by four enzyme systems: alanine aminotransferase (alanine production), pyruvate carboxylase (the major regulatory enzyme in gluconeogenesis), lactate dehydrogenase (lactate formation), and pyruvate dehydrogenase (see Fig. 33.9). The last is a complex of enzymes that decarboxylate pyruvate in the presence of oxygen to acetyl coenzyme A (CoA), allowing entry into the citric acid cycle. Measurement of pyruvate is useful in the evaluation of patients with inborn errors of metabolism who have increased serum lactate concentrations. A lactate-to-pyruvate ratio less than 25 suggests a defect in gluconeogenesis, whereas an increased ratio ($\geq$35) indicates reduced intracellular conditions found in hypoxia. Inborn errors associated with an increased lactate-to-pyruvate ratio include pyruvate carboxylase deficiency and defects in oxidative phosphorylation.[64] A high lactate-to-pyruvate ratio appears to be a sensitive test for detecting mitochondrial muscle toxicity of zidovudine therapy.[65] Pyruvate is also measured in clinical studies evaluating reperfusion after myocardial ischemia. Patients with Alzheimer's disease were reported to have higher CSF pyruvate concentrations than control subjects, and concentrations correlate with the severity of dementia.[66]

Lactic acidosis occurs in two clinical settings: type A (hypoxic), which is associated with decreased tissue oxygenation, such as shock, hypovolemia, and left ventricular failure; and type B (metabolic), which is associated with disease (eg, diabetes mellitus, neoplasia, liver disease), drugs and/or toxins (eg, ethanol, methanol, salicylates), or inborn errors of metabolism (eg, methylmalonic aciduria, propionic acidemia, fatty acid oxidation defects). Lactic acidosis is not uncommon and occurs in approximately 1% of hospital admissions. It has a mortality rate greater than 60%, and approaches 100% if hypotension is also present. Type A is much more common.

The mechanism of type B lactic acidosis is not known but is speculated to be a primary defect in mitochondrial function with impaired oxygen use. This leads to reduced stores of ATP and NAD^+, with accumulation of NADH and H^+. In the presence of decreased liver perfusion or liver disease, lactate removal from the blood is reduced, thereby aggravating the lactic acidosis.

Measurement of serum lactate in trauma patients on admission to the emergency department does not identify patients at risk of death, but it may be useful for identifying those patients at low risk of death.[67] Evidence obtained in 2008 from a multicenter trial supports measurement of lactate in fetal scalp blood during labor in the management of intrapartum fetal distress to prevent severe acidemia at birth.[68]

An uncommon and often undiagnosed cause of lactic acidosis is D-lactic acidosis.[69] It was thought that D-lactate was not produced in human metabolism, but normal individuals have a large capacity to metabolize D-lactate.[69] Moreover, absorption and accumulation of D-lactate from abnormal intestinal bacteria may cause systemic acidosis. This occurs after jejunoileal bypass surgery and manifests as altered mental status (from mild drowsiness to coma) with increased blood concentrations of D-lactate. Virtually all commonly used laboratory assays for lactate use L-lactate dehydrogenase, which does not detect D-lactate. D-Lactate can be measured by gas-liquid chromatography or, more easily, by using a specific D-lactate dehydrogenase (Sigma) from *Lactobacillus leishmanni*.[70] The enzyme assay can be readily automated. Lactate in CSF normally parallels concentrations in the blood, but not in children.[71] With biochemical alterations in the CNS, however, CSF lactate values change independently of blood values. Increased CSF lactate concentrations are noted in cerebrovascular accidents, intracranial hemorrhage, bacterial meningitis, epilepsy, inborn errors of the electron transport chain, and other CNS disorders. In aseptic (viral) meningitis, lactate concentrations in CSF are not usually increased; hence, CSF lactate has been used to help discriminate between viral and bacterial meningitis,[72] but the clinical utility has been questioned. In a few children with inherited metabolic disease, CSF lactate concentrations may be increased despite plasma lactate in the reference interval.[71]

Methods for Measuring Lactate and Pyruvate in Body Fluids

Determination of Lactate in Whole Blood

Principle. Lactate is oxidized to pyruvate by lactate dehydrogenase in the presence of NAD^+. The NADH formed in this reaction is measured by a spectrophotometer at 340 nm and serves as a measure of the lactate concentration.[73,74,75,76]

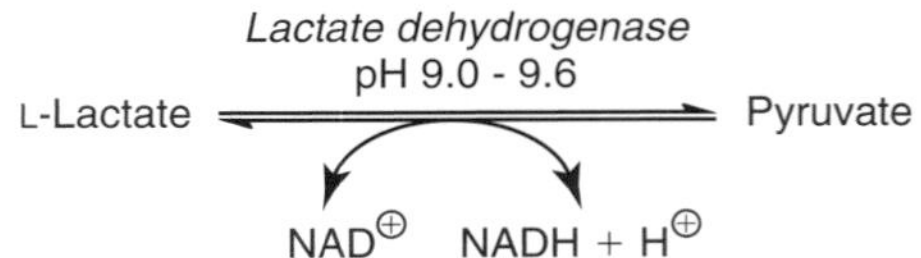

The equilibrium of the reaction normally lies far to the left. However, by using a pH of 9.0 to 9.6 and an excess of NAD^+, and by trapping the reaction product pyruvate with hydrazine, the equilibrium can be shifted to the right. Pyruvate can also be removed by reacting it with L-glutamate in the presence of alanine aminotransferase. Use of tris(hydroxymethyl)-aminomethane (TRIS) buffer results in more rapid completion of a side reaction between NAD^+ and hydrazine and prevents the "creeping" of blank values observed when glycine buffer is used.[74]

Because of its high specificity and simplicity, the enzymatic method is the method of choice for measuring lactate, although other methods may also be used (eg, gas chromatography,[77] photometry). The Vitros Analyzer (Ortho-Clinical Diagnostics) uses an assay in which lactic acid is oxidized to pyruvate by lactate oxidase. The H_2O_2 generated oxidizes a chromogen system, and absorbance of the resulting dye complex, measured by a spectrophotometer at 540 nm, is directly proportional to the lactate concentration in the specimen. Each mole of lactate oxidized produces 0.5 mole of dye complex.

$$L-\text{Lactate}+O_2 \xrightarrow{\text{Lactate Oxidase}} \text{Pyruvate}+H_2O_2$$

$$2H_2O_2+\text{4-aminoantipyrine}+\text{1,7-dihydronapthalene} \xrightarrow{\text{Peroxidase}} \text{red dye}$$

Reference Intervals. The reference intervals[78] for lactate in adults are as follows:

LACTATE

Specimen	mmol/L	mg/dL
Venous Blood		
At rest	0.3–2.0	2.7–18
Arterial Blood		
At rest	0.3–1.5	2.7–13.5

Patients in the hospital exhibit a wider range of lactate concentrations, with lactic acidosis occurring when blood lactate concentrations exceed 45 mg/dL (5 mmol/L). Vigorous exercise dramatically increases lactate concentrations (up to 10-fold), and even movement of leg muscles by patients at bed rest may result in significant increases. Plasma values are about 7% higher than those in whole blood, although differences depend on the procedure used. CSF values are usually similar to blood concentrations but may change independently in CNS disorders. Age-related reference intervals for CSF lactate (and lactate-to-pyruvate ratios) have been established in children.[79] The upper limit of the reference interval (90th percentile) for CSF lactate in children in the hospital from birth to 15.5 years varies continuously from 16 to 17 mg/dL (1.78 to 1.88 mmol/L).[79] Normal 24-hour urine output of lactate is 5.5 to 22 mmol/d.

Determination of Pyruvate in Whole Blood

Principle. The reaction involved in the determination of pyruvate is essentially the reverse of the reaction used in the lactate procedure.

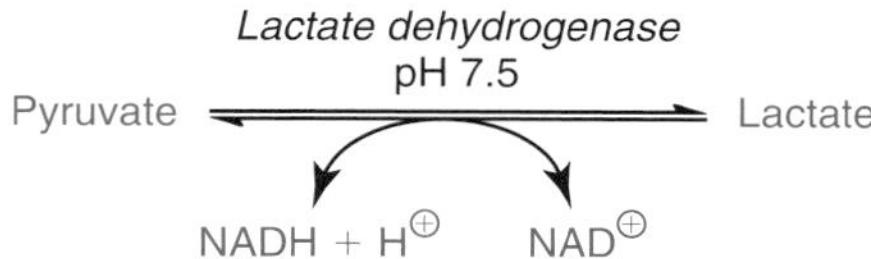

At about pH 7.5, the equilibrium constant strongly favors the reaction to the right. The method is very specific, and 2-oxoglutarate, oxaloacetate, acetoacetate, and β-hydroxybutyrate do not interfere, as with photometric methods.

Reference Intervals. Fasting venous blood, drawn with a patient at rest, has a pyruvate concentration of 0.3 to 0.9 mg/dL (0.03 to 0.10 mmol/L). Arterial blood contains 0.2 to 0.7 mg/dL (0.02 to 0.08 mmol/L). Values for CSF are 0.5 to 1.7 mg/dL (0.06 to 0.19 mmol/L).[80] Age-related reference intervals in CSF have been established in children.[77] Urine output of pyruvate is normally 1 mmol/d or less.

INBORN ERRORS OF CARBOHYDRATE METABOLISM

Deficiency or absence of an enzyme that participates in carbohydrate metabolism may result in accumulation of monosaccharides, which is measured in the urine (see Table 33.1 and Fig. 33.9). Most of these conditions are inherited as autosomal recessive traits. Sugars frequently appear in the urine as a result of excessive consumption without underlying disease.

Disorders of Galactose Metabolism

Galactose is derived from milk in the diet. It resembles glucose in structure, but the hydroxyl group on the fourth carbon has a different spatial arrangement (see Fig. 33.2). A deficiency of any of the enzymes that participate in the conversion of galactose to glucose results in *galactosemia.*

Galactose-1-Phosphate Uridyl Transferase Deficiency

Infants with this deficiency (prevalence 1/30,000 to 1/60,000) fail to thrive on milk because half of the milk sugar—lactose—is galactose. Within a few days of milk ingestion, neonates manifest vomiting and diarrhea. Failure to thrive, liver disease, cataracts, and mental retardation develop later. Hypoglycemia may occasionally develop. The diagnosis should be considered when the urine demonstrates the presence of a reducing substance that does not react in a glucose oxidase test. Early detection and treatment (withholding galactose from the diet) are necessary to prevent irreversible changes. Because other reducing sugars may give similar results, galactose should be identified by paper chromatography (discussed later). Diagnosis is suggested by detecting galactose and galactose-1-phosphate in blood and is confirmed by direct assaying of red blood cell transferase activity. A spot test is also available. Screening of neonates is performed in many countries. Treatment with a galactose-free diet is usually effective.

Uridine Diphosphate Galactose-4-Epimerase Deficiency

Uridine diphosphate galactose-4-epimerase deficiency (estimated prevalence in the United States is approximately 1/7,000 in African Americans and 1/70,000 in whites)[81] exhibits clinical findings similar to those of transferase deficiency.

Galactokinase Deficiency

Galactokinase deficiency is a milder condition (estimated prevalence is approximately 1/100,000 to 1/150,000) manifested predominantly by cataracts in the early weeks of life caused by galactitol deposits in the lens. The diagnosis is confirmed by demonstrating normal transferase activity and no galactokinase in red blood cells.

Disorders of Fructose Metabolism

Fructose may appear in the urine after fruit, honey, or syrup is eaten, but it has no significance in these circumstances. Three disorders of fructose metabolism, inherited as autosomal recessive traits, produce fructosuria.

Essential Fructosuria

This rare and harmless defect is due to a lack of fructokinase. Affected persons are asymptomatic, and the condition is usually detected by the presence of a reducing substance in routine urinalysis. The amount of fructose in the urine depends on the amount of fructose and sucrose ingested.

Hereditary Fructose Intolerance

A deficiency of fructose-1-phosphate aldolase produces this disorder with hypoglycemia and liver failure. Although the incidence of this disorder is unknown, it may be up to 1/20,000 in the United Kingdom.[82] Fructose ingestion inhibits glycogenolysis and gluconeogenesis, producing severe hypoglycemia. Early detection is important because this condition responds to a diet devoid of sucrose and fructose.

Hereditary Fructose-1,6-Diphosphatase Deficiency

Patients with this deficiency (incidence is unknown) have episodes of apnea and hyperventilation and hypoglycemia, ketosis, and lactic acidosis caused by severe impairment of gluconeogenesis. The condition is diagnosed by demonstrating the enzyme defect in liver biopsy specimens or by mutational analysis.

Disorders of Pentose Metabolism

Alimentary Pentosuria

Pentoses may be present in the urine after large quantities of fruits such as cherries, plums, grapes, or prunes are eaten.

Essential Pentosuria

This is a harmless inborn error (estimated incidence 1/40,000 to 1/50,000 in the United States) caused by a deficiency of L-xylulose reductase, an enzyme involved in the glucuronic acid oxidation pathway. The glucuronic acid oxidation pathway has no essential function in humans. Affected individuals excrete 1–4 g L-xylulose in urine per 24 hours.

Other Urinary Sugars

Lactose is sometimes detected in the urine of women during lactation and occasionally toward the end of pregnancy. Patients with lactase deficiency, a common disorder caused by a congenital or acquired deficiency of intestinal lactase, exhibit abdominal pain, diarrhea, and lactose in the urine. Maltose has on rare occasions been detected in the urine of some patients.

Many reducing substances other than sugars may be found in urine (see Box 33.2). Ascorbic acid (vitamin C) may be ingested in large quantities or may be present in antibiotic preparations administered intravenously. In either case, excess concentrations usually appear in the urine and contribute significantly to the total reducing substances present.

Methods for Measuring Individual Sugars

Qualitative Tests for Glucose

Techniques for separating and identifying sugars have included fermentation, optical rotation, osazone formation with phenylhydrazine, specific chemical tests, and paper or thin-layer chromatography. The availability of glucose oxidase test strips, specific for glucose, has greatly simplified the differentiation of glucose from other reducing substances. For practical purposes, the urinary sugars of clinical interest are glucose and galactose. Urine from infants and children should be tested routinely by both glucose oxidase and copper reduction tests to identify individuals with inborn errors of metabolism. Reducing substances other than glucose should be further identified by chromatographic procedures.

Qualitative Tests for Urinary Sugars Other Than Glucose

Fructose (Selivanoff Test). Hot HCl converts fructose to hydroxymethyl furfural (HMF), which links with resorcinol to produce a red compound. To make the reagent, dissolve 50 mg of resorcinol in 33 mL of concentrated HCl, and then dilute it to 100 mL with water. Add 0.5 mL of urine to 5 mL of reagent in a test tube and bring it to a boil. Fructose produces a red reaction within 30 seconds. The test is sensitive to 100 mg fructose/dL, provided there is no excess glucose. A 2-g/dL solution of glucose produces about the same color as 100 mg/dL of fructose after 30 seconds of boiling. A solution of fructose (0.5 g/dL) should be used as a control. With high concentrations of fructose, a red precipitate forms.

Pentoses (Bial Test). By heating with HCl, pentoses are converted to furfural, which reacts with orcinol to form green compounds. Dissolve 300 mg of orcinol in 100 mL of concentrated HCl, and add 0.25 mL of ferric chloride solution (10 g/dL). Glucose, if present in the urine, should be removed by fermentation with yeast. Add 0.5 mL of urine to 5 mL of reagent in a test tube, and bring to a boil. Pentoses produce a green reaction. The detection limit of the test is 100 mg pentose/dL. A solution of xylose (0.5 g/dL) should be used as a control. Glucuronates produce a similar color if the boiling is prolonged. As with Selivanoff reagent, fructose produces a red reaction.

Identification of Urinary Sugars by Paper Chromatography

Sugars can be separated by ascending or descending chromatography on paper and located after color development with dinitrosalicylic acid. Variable rates of migration depend on the solubility of the sugars in the particular solvent system. Presumptive identification is made by comparing the migration (R_f) value of the unknown to those of reference compounds. One procedure may be performed conveniently in a 6 × 18-inch Pyrex jar with a tightly fitting cover.

Identification of Urinary Sugars by Thin-Layer Chromatography

Urine sugars can be identified by thin-layer chromatographic techniques as described by Young and Jackson.[83] When frequent chromatographic separations are necessary, this method is preferred over paper chromatography because of the shorter time required. If such studies are performed infrequently, paper chromatography is simple, is adequate for most separations, and requires little actual working time.

GLYCOGEN STORAGE DISEASE

Glycogen, although present in most tissue, is stored principally in the liver and skeletal muscle. During fasting, liver glycogen is converted to glucose to provide energy for the whole body. In contrast, skeletal muscle lacks glucose-6-phosphatase, and muscle glycogen can be used only locally for energy. Glycogen storage disease is a generic name encompassing at least 12 rare inherited disorders of glycogen storage in tissue (see Table 33.1). The different forms of glycogen storage disease are categorized by numeric type in the chronological sequence in which these defects were identified. Each form is due to a deficiency of a specific enzyme in glycogen metabolism, producing a quantitative or qualitative defect of glycogen storage. Numerous mutations have been identified in patients with these conditions (http://www.ncbi.nim.nih.gov/omim/). The most common mutations are listed in Table 33.3. Because liver and skeletal muscle have the highest rates of glycogen metabolism, these are the structures most affected. The liver forms (types I, III, IV, VI, and IX), which comprise approximately 80% of the total, are marked by hepatomegaly (caused by increased liver glycogen stores) and hypoglycemia (caused by inability to convert glycogen to glucose). Hypoglycemia is manifested by autonomic clinical symptoms (sweating, shakiness, and lightheaded feeling), growth retardation, and laboratory findings of decreased insulin and increased glucagon concentrations in the blood. The muscle forms (types II, V, and VII), in contrast, have mild symptoms that usually appear in young adulthood during strenuous exercise, owing to the inability to provide energy for muscle contraction. Other muscle disorders may exhibit similar symptoms but are readily differentiated by evaluation of glycogen stores. The specific diagnosis of each type is made directly by demonstrating the enzyme defect in tissue. A very brief overview is provided here; for a more detailed description, readers should consult Chen.[84]

Type I (Glucose-6-Phosphatase Deficiency)

Type I is the most common and severe form, and patients have an accumulation of glycogen of normal chemical structure in the liver. The disease is characterized by massive hepatomegaly, growth retardation, fasting hypoglycemia, increased lactic acid concentrations in the blood (caused by excessive glycolysis), hyperuricemia (caused by competitive inhibition by lactate of renal tubular urate secretion and increased uric

TABLE 33.3 Common Mutations in Glycogen Storage Disease

Nucleotide Change	Amino Acid Change	Frequency	Ethnic Background
GSD Ia			
c.247C→T	p.Arg83Cys	32%	White
c.247C→T	p.Arg83Cys	93% to 100%	Jewish
c.248G→A	p.Arg83His	38%	Chinese
c.378_379dupTA	p.130X	50%	Hispanic
c.648G→T	Splicing	88%	Japanese
c.648G→T	Splicing	36%	Chinese
c.562G→C	p.Gly188Arg	21%	White
GSD Ib			
c.352T→C	p.Trp118Arg	50%	Japanese
c.1042_1043delCT	p.400X	50%	White
c.1015G→T	p.Gly339Cys	50%	White
GSD II			
c.32.13T→G	Aberrant splicing	75%	Italian
c.1935C→A	p.Asp645Glu	—	Taiwanese
c.2560C→T	p.Arg854X	—	African American
GSD III			
c.16C→T	p.Gln66X	25%	White
c.17delAG	p.25X	75%	White
c.2590C→T	p.Arg864X	10%	White
c.3682C→T	p.Arg1228X	5%	White
c.3965delT (3964delT)	p.1348X	7%	African American and white
c.4455delT	p.1503X	100%	North African Jewish
GSD V			
C→A	p.Arg50X	50–80%	
G→A	p.Gly204Ser	10%	
GSD VII			
G→A	Deletion	65%	Ashkenazi

Modified in part from Pyhtila BM, Shaw KA, Neumann SE, Fridovich-Keil JL. Newborn screening for galactosemia in the United States: looking back, looking around, and looking ahead. JIMD Rep. 2015;15:79–93. doi: 10.1007/8904_2014_302. Epub 2014 Apr 10.

acid production), and hypertriglyceridemia (increased lipolysis caused by decreased glucose). Glucagon and epinephrine do not produce hyperglycemia but result in increased lactate concentrations. The failure of blood glucose to increase in response to galactose administration (oral or intravenous) is diagnostic. Galactose is normally converted to glucose (see Fig. 33.9), but in these patients glucose-6-phosphate cannot be hydrolyzed to glucose. Treatment includes partaking of frequent meals and nasogastric feeding at night to maintain blood glucose concentrations. Glucose-6-phosphatase activity can be assayed in a liver biopsy. Two main subtypes have been identified: type Ia and type Ib.[81] Type 1a (also called *von Gierke disease*) is caused by a deficiency of the glucose-6-phosphatase catalytic subunit, whereas type Ib is due to a defect in the glucose-6-phosphatase transport system. Another form, termed type 1c, was originally attributed to a defect in microsomal phosphate transport, but it is likely that types Ib and Ic represent a single disease.[85] Many mutations have been described in types Ia and Ib.[85]

Individuals with type I glycogen storage disease exhibit decreased availability of liver glycogen demonstrated by decreased or absent blood glucose response to epinephrine administration. An assay based on this phenomenon is known as the *epinephrine tolerance test.* With it, an intramuscular injection of 1 mL of a 1/1000 (1 g/L) solution of epinephrine hydrochloride is given, and blood samples are taken at 30, 45, 60, 90, and 120 minutes. Healthy people increase blood glucose by 35 to 45 mg/dL (1.9 to 2.5 mmol/L) in 40 to 60 minutes, with a return to the fasting concentration within 2 hours. This test is rarely used because the diagnosis of von Gierke disease is based on failure to increase blood glucose in response to galactose administration, with confirmation by direct assay of glucose-6-phosphatase activity.

Type II (Acid α-Glucosidase Deficiency)

Type II is an autosomal recessive disorder that affects predominantly the heart and skeletal muscle, producing muscle weakness and cardiomegaly. Liver function is normal, and patients do not have hypoglycemia. The two forms are infantile *(Pompe disease),* which usually presents in the first few months of life (presenting symptoms include weakness and respiratory difficulties, and patients usually die from cardiac failure within 1 year), and a juvenile form that is milder and may present in the second or third decade of life with difficulty in walking. More than 200 mutations in the acid α-glucosidase gene are known (http://www.pompecenter.nl). The diagnosis is made by measuring α-glucosidase (acid maltase) activity in skeletal muscle biopsy, peripheral blood cells, or cultured skin fibroblasts. Enzyme replacement therapy with recombinant human acid α-glucosidase was approved in the United States in 2006.

Type III (Amylo-1,6-Glucosidase Deficiency)

Deficiency of glycogen debranching enzyme results in storage of an abnormal form of glycogen (also called *limit dextrinosis*, *Cori disease*, or *Forbes disease*). Both liver and muscle are usually affected (type IIIa), producing hepatomegaly and muscle weakness. Approximately 15% of patients have only liver involvement, without apparent muscle disease (type IIIb). Clinical and biochemical features resemble those of type I disease. Differentiation from type I is seen by a hyperglycemic response to galactose, lower concentrations of urate and lactate in the blood, and increased serum transaminase and creatine kinase activities. Enzyme deficiency can be demonstrated in muscle or liver and occasionally in erythrocytes.

Type IV (Branching Enzyme Deficiency)

Type IV (also called *Andersen disease* or *amylopectinosis*) is an extremely rare disorder manifested by production of an abnormal form of unbranched glycogen in all tissues. Patients exhibit hepatosplenomegaly with ascites and liver failure. Abnormal glycogen can be identified in the tissues and muscles; leukocytes or cultured fibroblasts can be used to demonstrate the enzyme deficiency.

Type V (Muscle Phosphorylase Deficiency)

Type V, also called *McArdle disease,* usually presents in the second or third decade with muscle cramps after exercise. Moderate exercise can be sustained, and patients get a "second wind" when symptoms disappear if exercise is continued. Increased plasma creatine kinase activities at rest, failure of ischemic exercise to increase serum lactate concentrations while producing an exaggerated increase in ammonia, myoglobinuria, and diminished activity of muscle phosphorylase establish the diagnosis. Patients respond to oral glucose administration or injections of glucagon.

Type VI (Liver Phosphorylase or Phosphorylase Kinase Deficiency)

Type VI, or *Hers disease,* is a heterogeneous group of diseases arising from a deficiency of liver phosphorylase or one of the subunits of phosphorylase kinase. It is a rare and relatively benign disorder manifested as hepatomegaly caused by increased deposits of normal glycogen in the liver. Diagnosis is made by measuring enzyme activity in the liver or in red or white blood cells.

Type VII (Muscle Phosphofructokinase Deficiency)

Patients with this rare autosomal recessive disorder (also known as *Tarui disease*) have deposits of abnormal glycogen in muscle. Exercise intolerance, unresponsiveness to glucose administration, and hemolysis (caused by decreased glycolysis in erythrocytes) are noted clinically, producing hyperbilirubinemia, pigmenturia, and reticulocytosis. The specific enzyme defect can be demonstrated.

REFERENCES

1. Martin-Rendon E, Blake DJ. Protein glycosylation in disease: new insights into the congenital muscular dystrophies. *Trends Pharmacol Sci* 2003;**24**:178–83.
2. Service FJ. Hypoglycemic disorders. *N Engl J Med* 1995;**332**: 1144–52.
3. Brun JF, Fedou C, Mercier J. Postprandial reactive hypoglycemia. *Diabetes Metab* 2000;**26**:337–51.
4. Cryer PE, Axelrod L, Grossman AB, et al. Evaluation and management of adult hypoglycemic disorders: an Endocrine Society Clinical Practice Guideline. *J Clin Endocrinol Metab* 2009;**94**:709–28.
5. DeFronzo RA, Hendler R, Christensen N. Stimulation of counterregulatory hormonal responses in diabetic man by a fall in glucose concentration. *Diabetes* 1980;**29**:125–31.
6. Gerich JE. Physiology of glucose homeostasis. *Diabetes Obes Metab* 2000;**2**:345–50.
7. Haymond MW. Hypoglycemia in infants and children. *Endocrinol Metab Clin North Am* 1989;**18**:211–52.
8. Merimee TJ, Tyson JE. Stabilization of plasma glucose during fasting: normal variations in two separate studies. *N Engl J Med* 1974;**291**:1275–8.
9. Seltzer HS. Drug-induced hypoglycemia: a review of 1418 cases. *Endocrinol Metab Clin North Am* 1989;**18**:163–83.
10. Fajans SS, Vinik AI. Insulin-producing islet cell tumors. *Endocrinol Metab Clin North Am* 1989;**18**:45–74.
11. Kumar D, Mehtalia SD, Miller LV. Diagnostic use of glucagon-induced insulin response: studies in patients with insulinoma or other hypoglycemic conditions. *Ann Intern Med* 1974;**80**: 697–701.
12. Service FJ, Dale AJ, Elveback LR, et al. Insulinoma: clinical and diagnostic features of 60 consecutive cases. *Mayo Clin Proc* 1976;**51**:417–29.
13. Kaplan EL, Rubenstein AH, Evans R, et al. Calcium infusion: a new provocative test for insulinomas. *Ann Surg* 1979;**190**: 501–7.
14. Doppman JL, Chang R, Fraker DL, et al. Localization of insulinomas to regions of the pancreas by intra-arterial stimulation with calcium. *Ann Intern Med* 1995;**123**: 269–73.
15. Palardy J, Havrankova J, Lepage R, et al. Blood glucose measurements during symptomatic episodes in patients with suspected postprandial hypoglycemia. *N Engl J Med* 1989;**321**: 1421–5.
16. Daughaday WH. The possible autocrine/paracrine and endocrine roles of insulin-like growth factors of human tumors. *Endocrinology* 1990;**127**:1–4.
17. Shapiro ET, Bell GI, Polonsky KS, et al. Tumor hypoglycemia: relationship to high molecular weight insulin-like growth factor-II. *J Clin Invest* 1990;**85**:1672–9.
18. Miller SI, Wallace RJ Jr, Musher DM, et al. Hypoglycemia as a manifestation of sepsis. *Am J Med* 1980;**68**:649–54.
19. Hofeldt FD. Reactive hypoglycemia. *Endocrinol Metab Clin North Am* 1989;**18**:185–201.
20. Lefebvre PJ, Andreani D, Marks V. *Statement on "post-prandial" or reactive hypoglycemia. Hypoglycemia*. Serono Symposium: Raven Press; 1987. p. 79.
21. Charles MA, Hofeldt F, Shackelford A, et al. Comparison of oral glucose tolerance tests and mixed meals in patients with apparent idiopathic postabsorptive hypoglycemia: absence of hypoglycemia after meals. *Diabetes* 1981;**30**:465–70.

22. Chalew SA, McLaughlin JV, Mersey JH, et al. The use of the plasma epinephrine response in the diagnosis of idiopathic postprandial syndrome. *JAMA* 1984;**251**:612–15.
23. Special report: Statement on hypoglycemia. *Diabetes* 1973;**22**:137.
24. Cahill GF Jr, Soeldner JS. A non-editorial on non-hypoglycemia. *N Engl J Med* 1974;**291**:905–6.
25. The fad disease. Hypoglycemia is being diagnosed too often. Time April 7, 1980:71.
26. Cryer PE, Fisher JN, Shamoon H. Hypoglycemia. *Diabetes Care* 1994;**17**:734–55.
27. Gerich JE. Lilly lecture 1988. Glucose counterregulation and its impact on diabetes mellitus. *Diabetes* 1988;**37**:1608–17.
28. DCCT. The effect of intensive treatment of diabetes on the development and progression of long-term complications in insulin-dependent diabetes mellitus. *N Engl J Med* 1993;**329**: 977–86.
29. Richter B, Neises G. "Human" insulin versus animal insulin in people with diabetes mellitus. *Cochrane Database Syst Rev* 2002;(3):CD003816.
30. Boehm TM, Lebovitz HE. Statistical analysis of glucose and insulin responses to intravenous tolbutamide: evaluation of hypoglycemic and hyperinsulinemic states. *Diabetes Care* 1979;**2**:479–90.
31. Burrin JM, Price CP. Measurement of blood glucose. *Ann Clin Biochem* 1985;**22**(Pt 4):327–42.
32. Passey RB, Gillum RL, Fuller JB, et al. Evaluation and comparison of 10 glucose methods and the reference method recommended in the proposed product class standard (1974). *Clin Chem* 1977;**23**:131–9.
33. Miller WG, Myers GL, Ashwood ER, et al. State of the art in trueness and interlaboratory harmonization for 10 analytes in general clinical chemistry. *Arch Pathol Lab Med* 2008;**132**: 838–46.
34. Standards of medical care in diabetes—2014. *Diabetes Care* 2014;**37**(Suppl. 1):S14–80.
35. World Health Organization. Definition and Diagnosis of Diabetes Mellitus and Intermediate Hyperglycermia: Report of a WHO/IDF Consultation. Geneva: World Health Org, 2006.
36. Ladenson JH, Tsai LM, Michael JM, et al. Serum versus heparinized plasma for eighteen common chemistry tests: is serum the appropriate specimen? *Am J Clin Pathol* 1974;**62**: 545–52.
37. Miles RR, Roberts RF, Putnam AR, et al. Comparison of serum and heparinized plasma samples for measurement of chemistry analytes. *Clin Chem* 2004;**50**:1704–5.
38. Kuwa K, Nakayama T, Hoshino T, et al. Relationships of glucose concentrations in capillary whole blood, venous whole blood and venous plasma. *Clin Chim Acta* 2001;**307**: 187–92.
39. Larsson-Cohn U. Differences between capillary and venous blood glucose during oral glucose tolerance tests. *Scand J Clin Lab Invest* 1976;**36**:805–8.
40. Chan AY, Swaminathan R, Cockram CS. Effectiveness of sodium fluoride as a preservative of glucose in blood. *Clin Chem* 1989;**35**:315–17.
41. Weissman M, Klein B. Evaluation of glucose determinations in untreated serum samples. *Clin Chem* 1958;**4**:420–2.
42. Sazama K, Robertson EA, Chesler RA. Is antiglycolysis required for routine glucose analysis? *Clin Chem* 1979;**25**: 2038–9.
43. Boyanton BL Jr, Blick KE. Stability studies of twenty-four analytes in human plasma and serum. *Clin Chem* 2002;**48**: 2242–7.
44. Gambino R, Piscitelli J, Ackattupathil TA, et al. Acidification of blood is superior to sodium fluoride alone as an inhibitor of glycolysis. *Clin Chem* 2009;**55**:1019–21.
45. Lott JA, Turner K. Evaluation of Trinder's glucose oxidase method for measuring glucose in serum and urine. *Clin Chem* 1975;**21**:1754–60.
46. Neese JW. Glucose, direct hexokinase method: selected methods. *Clin Chem* 1982;**9**:241–8.
47. Wright WR, Rainwater JC, Tolle LD. Glucose assay systems: evaluation of a colorimetric hexokinase procedure. *Clin Chem* 1971;**17**:1010–15.
48. Trinder P. Determination of glucose in blood using glucose oxidase with an alternative oxygen acceptor. *Ann Clin Biochem* 1969;**6**:24–7.
49. Reljic R, Ries M, Anic N, et al. New chromogen for assay of glucose in serum. *Clin Chem* 1992;**38**:522–5.
50. Kadish AH. A new and rapid method for the determination of glucose by measurement of rate of oxygen consumption. *Clin Chem* 1968;**14**:116–31.
51. Curme HG, Columbus RL, Dappen GM, et al. Multilayer film elements for clinical analysis: general concepts. *Clin Chem* 1978;**24**:1335–42.
52. Bush JL, Campbell J, Sanderson JA. Performance of a glucose procedure based on the glucose dehydrogenase reaction on Technicon continuous flow equipment. *Clin Chem* 1981; **27**:1050.
53. Sundaram PV, Blumenberg B, Hinsch W. Routine glucose determination in serum by use of an immobilized glucose dehydrogenase nylon-tube reactor. *Clin Chem* 1979;**25**: 1436–9.
54. Lutz RA, Fluckiger J. Kinetic determination of glucose with the GEMSAEC (ENI) centrifugal analyzer by the glucose dehydrogenase reaction, and comparison with two commonly used procedures. *Clin Chem* 1975;**21**:1372–7.
55. American Diabetes Association. Diagnosis and classification of diabetes mellitus. *Diabetes Care* 2010;**33**(Suppl. 1):S62–9.
56. O'Sullivan JB. Age gradient in blood glucose levels. Magnitude and clinical implications. *Diabetes* 1974;**23**:713–15.
57. DECODE. Consequences of the new diagnostic criteria for diabetes in older men and women. DECODE Study (Diabetes Epidemiology: Collaborative Analysis of Diagnostic Criteria in Europe). *Diabetes Care* 1999;**22**:1667–71.
58. Sacks DB, Arnold M, Bakris GL, et al. Guidelines and recommendations for laboratory analysis in the diagnosis and management of diabetes mellitus. *Clin Chem* 2011;**57**:e1–47.
59. Horrocks RH, Manning GB. Partition chromatography on paper: identification of reducing substances in urine. *Lancet* 1949;**1**:1042–5.
60. Froom P, Bieganiec B, Ehrenrich Z, et al. Stability of common analytes in urine refrigerated for 24 h before automated analysis by test strips. *Clin Chem* 2000;**46**:1384–6.
61. Bandi ZL, Myers JL, Bee DE, et al. Evaluation of determination of glucose in urine with some commercially available dipsticks and tablets. *Clin Chem* 1982;**28**:2110–15.
62. Cohen HT, Spiegel DM. Air-exposed urine dipsticks give false-positive results for glucose and false-negative results for blood. *Am J Clin Pathol* 1991;**96**:398–400.
63. Pithukpakorn M. Disorders of pyruvate metabolism and the tricarboxylic acid cycle. *Mol Genet Metab* 2005;**85**:243–6.

64. Robinson BH. Lactic acidemia (disorders of pyruvate carboxylase, pyruvate dehydrogenase). In: Shriver CR, Beaudet AL, Sly WS, et al., editors. *The metabolic and molecular bases of inherited disease*. New York: McGraw-Hill; 1995. p. 1479–99.
65. Chariot P, Monnet I, Mouchet M, et al. Determination of the blood lactate:pyruvate ratio as a noninvasive test for the diagnosis of zidovudine myopathy. *Arthritis Rheum* 1994;**37**: 583–6.
66. Parnetti L, Gaiti A, Polidori MC, et al. Increased cerebrospinal fluid pyruvate levels in Alzheimer's disease. *Neurosci Lett* 1995;**199**:231–3.
67. Hung KK. Best Evidence Topic report. BET 2. Serum lactate as a marker for mortality in patients presenting to the emergency department with trauma. *Emerg Med J* 2009;**26**:118–19.
68. Wiberg-Itzel E, Lipponer C, Norman M, et al. Determination of pH or lactate in fetal scalp blood in management of intrapartum fetal distress: randomised controlled multicentre trial. *BMJ* 2008;**336**:1284–7.
69. Uribarri J, Oh MS, Carroll HJ. D-lactic acidosis. A review of clinical presentation, biochemical features, and pathophysiologic mechanisms. *Medicine (Baltimore)* 1998;**77**: 73–82.
70. Ludvigsen CW, Thurn JR, Pierpont GL, et al. Kinetic enzymic assay for D(-)-lactate, with use of a centrifugal analyzer. *Clin Chem* 1983;**29**:1823–5.
71. Hutchesson A, Preece MA, Gray G, et al. Measurement of lactate in cerebrospinal fluid in investigation of inherited metabolic disease. *Clin Chem* 1997;**43**:158–61.
72. Bailey EM, Domenico P, Cunha BA. Bacterial or viral meningitis? Measuring lactate in CSF can help you know quickly. *Postgrad Med* 1990;**88**:217–19, 23.
73. Astles R, Williams CP, Sedor F. Stability of plasma lactate in vitro in the presence of antiglycolytic agents. *Clin Chem* 1994;**40**:1327–30.
74. Livesley B, Atkinson L. Accurate quantitative estimation of lactate in whole blood [Letter]. *Clin Chem* 1974;**20**:1478.
75. Lubran M. Measurement of lactic and pyruvic acid in biological fluids. In: Sunderman FW, Sunderman FW Jr, editors. *Laboratory diagnosis of endocrine diseases*. St. Louis: Warren H. Green; 1971. p. 401–8.
76. Marbach EP, Weil MH. Rapid enzymatic measurement of blood lactate and pyruvate. Use and significance of metaphosphoric acid as a common precipitant. *Clin Chem* 1967;**13**:314–25.
77. Savory J, Kaplan A. A gas chromatographic method for the determination of lactic acid in blood. *Clin Chem* 1966;**12**: 559–69.
78. Toffaletti JG. Blood lactate: biochemistry, laboratory methods, and clinical interpretation [Crit Rev]. *Clin Lab Sci* 1991;**28**(4): 253–68.
79. Benoist JF, Alberti C, Leclercq S, et al. Cerebrospinal fluid lactate and pyruvate concentrations and their ratio in children: age-related reference intervals. *Clin Chem* 2003;**49**: 487–94.
80. Pryce JD, Gant PW, Sau KJ. Normal concentrations of lactate, glucose, and protein in cerebrospinal fluid, and the diagnotic implications of abnormal concentrations. *Clin Chem* 1970;**16**: 562–5.
81. Pyhtila BM, Shaw KA, Neumann SE, et al. Newborn screening for galactosemia in the United States: looking back, looking around, and looking ahead. *JIMD Rep* 2015;**15**:79–93. doi:10.1007/8904_2014_302. [Epub 2014 Apr 10].
82. James CL, Rellos P, Ali M, et al. Neonatal screening for hereditary fructose intolerance: frequency of the most common mutant aldolase B allele (A149P) in the British population. *J Med Genet* 1996;**33**(10):837–41.
83. Young DS, Jackson AJ. Thin-layer chromatography of urinary carbohydrates: a comparative evaluation of procedures. *Clin Chem* 1970;**16**:954–9.
84. Chen Y-T. Glycogen storage diseases. In: Scriver CR, Beaudet AL, Sly WS, et al., editors. *The metabolic and molecular bases of inherited disease*, vol. 8. New York: McGraw-Hill; 2001. p. 1521–51.
85. Koeberl DD, Kishnani PS, Bali D, et al. Emerging therapies for glycogen storage disease type I. *Trends Endocrinol Metab* 2009;**20**:252–8.

34

Lipids, Lipoproteins, Apolipoproteins, and Other Cardiovascular Risk Factors

*Alan T. Remaley, Thomas D. Dayspring, and G. Russell Warnick**

ABSTRACT

Background
Lipid metabolism is central to normal physiology and important in understanding the pathogenesis of cardiovascular disease, a major worldwide cause of morbidity and mortality. Increases in the plasma concentrations of cholesterol on certain lipoprotein fractions can result in the increased deposition and retention of cholesterol in the vascular wall, leading to atherosclerosis. Other pathological processes, such as inflammation, also contribute to the development of cardiovascular disease.

Content
This chapter first describes the basic pathways in lipid and lipoprotein metabolism, as well as genetic and acquired disorders in these pathways. Next, the pathophysiology of the development of coronary heart disease, in regard to lipoprotein metabolism and inflammation, is discussed and how the various lipid and lipoprotein tests can be used in adult and pediatric populations for predicting cardiovascular disease risk. Issues related to the measurement and the standardization of various lipid and lipoprotein biomarkers are reviewed, as well as other cardiovascular risk biomarkers, such as CRP.

Lipids are ubiquitous in the body tissue and play a vital role in virtually all aspects of life, providing a source of metabolic fuel and energy storage, serving as hormones or precursors of hormones, acting as functional and structural components in cell membranes, and forming insulation to allow nerve conduction or to prevent heat loss. This chapter discusses the basic biochemistry, biology, clinical significance, and analytical considerations of lipids, with a special emphasis on those involved in cardiovascular disease.

BASIC BIOCHEMISTRY

Much attention has been focused on certain lipids and the lipoproteins that transport them in the circulation, mainly because of their strong association with coronary heart disease (CHD). As a consequence, use of the term lipids in clinical chemistry and laboratory medicine has virtually become synonymous with lipoprotein metabolism and atherosclerosis—a key step in the pathogenesis of CHD. In the early 1980s, findings from the landmark Coronary Primary Prevention Trial first demonstrated that treatments that lower plasma cholesterol result in a reduction in the incidence of CHD. Subsequently, several primary and secondary prevention trials, using diet or drugs to lower blood cholesterol, have also shown a reduction in cardiovascular death and/or atherosclerotic clinical events. Based on these trials and other evidence, the National Heart, Lung, and Blood Institute in the 1980s established the National Cholesterol Education Program (NCEP) to increase public awareness about cholesterol; devise strategies for the diagnosis and treatment of hypercholesterolemia in adults, children, and adolescents; and improve the laboratory measurement of lipids. Many other international and national organizations have subsequently established similar programs to address these issues.

Basic Lipid Biochemistry

The general term lipid applies to a class of hydrophobic molecules that are synthesized by the condensation of thioesters or isoprene units, which are soluble in organic solvents but nearly insoluble in water. Chemically, lipids are usually enriched in carbon and hydrogen and after hydrolysis typically yield fatty acids or complex alcohols, which are usually esterified with fatty acids. Some lipids are more complex, containing other chemical groups, such as sialic, phosphoryl, amino, or sulfate groups. The presence of these charged or polar groups makes these lipids amphipathic, which gives them the property of having an affinity for both water and organic solvents; this is an important feature in their ability to form cell membranes. Lipids can be broadly subdivided into five groups based on their chemical structure (Box 34.1).

*The authors gratefully acknowledge the contributions by Drs. Nader Rifai, John Albers, and Paul Bachorik, on which portions of this chapter are based. Additional portions have been adapted from Rifai N, Kwiterovich PO Jr.: Disorders of lipid and lipoprotein metabolism in children and adolescents. In Soldin SJ, Rifai N, Hick JMB, eds: Biochemical basis of pediatric diseases, 3rd edition. Washington, DC: AACC Press, 1998.

BOX 34.1 Classification of Clinically Important Lipids

Sterol Derivatives
Cholesterol and cholesteryl esters
Steroid hormones
Bile acids
Vitamin D
Noncholesterol sterols

Fatty Acids
Short chain (2 to 4 carbon atoms)
Medium chain (6 to 10 carbon atoms)
Long chain (12 to 26 carbon atoms)
Prostaglandins

Glyceryl Esters
Triglycerides, diglycerides, and monoglycerides (acylglycerols)
Phosphoglycerides

Sphingosine Derivatives
Sphingomyelin
Glycosphingolipids

Terpenes (Isoprene Polymers)
Vitamin A
Vitamin E
Vitamin K

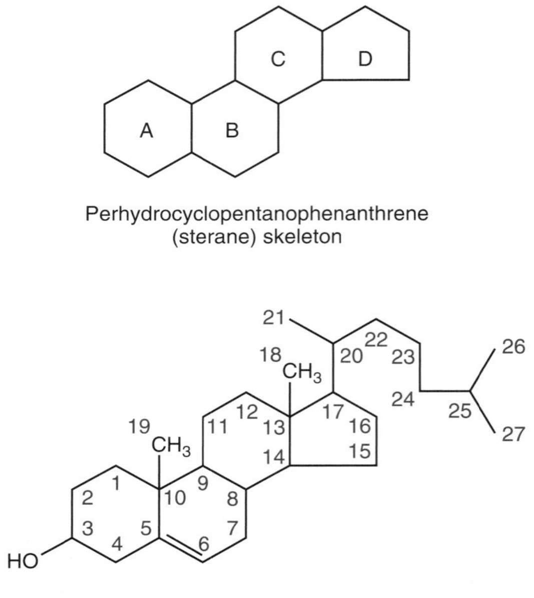

FIGURE 34.1 Structure of cholesterol.

Cholesterol

Every living organism has been found to contain cholesterol or, in the case of plants, cholesterol-like molecules called phytosterols.[1] Cholesterol (386.65 g/mol) is a sterol that has a tetracyclic perhydrocyclopentanophenanthrene skeleton and contains one unsaturated carbon double bond and one primary alcohol, thus making it an amphipathic lipid. Altogether it contains 27 carbon atoms ($C_{27}H_{46}O$), numbered as shown in Fig. 34.1. Knowledge of its structure and numbering system is important not only to clinical chemists but also to practicing clinicians because cholesterol is the starting point in many different metabolic pathways. These include vitamin D synthesis (see Chapter 64), steroid hormone synthesis (see Chapter 36), and bile acid metabolism (see Chapter 61). In addition, because enzymes that modify cholesterol or its derivatives are known by their site and type of reaction (eg, 21-hydroxylase in cortisol synthesis), the nomenclature of many diseases (eg, 21-hydroxylase deficiency in adrenogenital syndrome) depends on a knowledge of the structure of cholesterol.

Cholesterol Absorption. Cholesterol enters the intestinal lumen from three sources: the diet, bile, and the intestine. Animal products—especially meat, egg yolk, seafood, and dairy products—provide the bulk of dietary cholesterol. Although dietary cholesterol intake varies considerably, the average American diet contains approximately 300 to 450 mg of cholesterol per day and 200 to 250 mg of phytosterols. A much larger amount of cholesterol enters the gut from biliary secretion (3 to 10 times higher than what is ingested from food.[2] Additional quantities arise from the turnover of intestinal mucosal cells (~300 mg) and from direct intestinal secretion.[3] Practically all cholesterol in the intestinal lumen is present in the unesterified or free form. Esterified cholesterol, which is approximately 15% to 20% of dietary cholesterol, is rapidly hydrolyzed in the intestine to free cholesterol and free fatty acids by cholesterol esterases secreted from the pancreas and small intestine. Because the majority of the intestinal pool of cholesterol is from endogenous and not exogenous sources, there is a relatively poor relationship between dietary cholesterol and coronary atherosclerosis.[4] Consistent with this observation, the AHA/ACC guideline in 2013 on the treatment of blood cholesterol stated that there is insufficient evidence that lowering dietary cholesterol can have a major impact on plasma cholesterol levels.[5]

To be absorbed, unesterified cholesterol first must be solubilized by emulsification. This occurs through the formation of mixed micelles that contain unesterified cholesterol, phytosterols, stanols (saturated sterols), fatty acids, monoacylglycerides (derived from dietary triglycerides), lysophospholipids, and conjugated bile acids. Formation of mixed micelles promotes cholesterol absorption in brush border of the proximal small intestine by both solubilizing cholesterol and facilitating its transport to the surface of the luminal cell, where it is absorbed by an active process involving an enterocyte membrane sterol influx protein called Niemann Pick C1 Like 1 protein (NPC1L1).[6] Loss of function of the *NPC1L1* gene is associated with both reduced plasma cholesterol concentrations and reduced risk of coronary heart disease. NPC1L1, which is also expressed at the hepatobiliary border, is the drug target for the cholesterol absorption inhibitor ezetimibe.[6] NPC1L1 has a sterol-sensing domain that acts with other proteins, including the A2 adaptor protein and clathrin to facilitate sterol internalization. Because of their strong detergent-like effects, bile acids are the most important factor in micelle formation. In the absence of bile acids, digestion and absorption of both cholesterol and triglyceride are severely impaired, leading to fat malabsorption. In healthy individuals, the degree of cholesterol absorption can vary widely, but on average about 50% of intestinal cholesterol is absorbed.[7]

Absorption of cholesterol and phytosterols is limited by the presence of a sterol efflux transporter called the ATP binding cassette transporter G5/G8, which is a heterodimer of G5 and G8. The ABCG5/G8 transporter is located at the luminal and biliary borders, respectively, of enterocytes and hepatocytes and effluxes excess sterols and stanols back into the gut lumen or biliary tree for return to the gut.[7] Polymorphisms that cause partial loss of function of ABCG5 or ABCG8 result in hyperabsorption of cholesterol and mild to moderate degrees of phytosterolemia. Total loss of function of either ABCG5 or ABCG8 results in an autosomal recessive variant of familial hypercholesterolemia originally called sitosterolemia, but now often termed *phytosterolemia* or *xenosterolemia*. It is characterized by a marked increase in plasma and tissue concentrations of cholesterol and phytosterols, such as sitosterol, campesterol, and stigmasterol, and an increased risk of cardiovascular disease.[7]

The ability of cholesterol to form micelles is also influenced by the quantity of dietary fat but not by its degree of saturation. Increased amounts of fat in the diet results in expansion of mixed micelles, which in turn allows more cholesterol to be solubilized and absorbed. As lipid absorption occurs in the small intestine, the micelles break up, and the bile acids are either reabsorbed at the ileum or excreted. Any cholesterol not absorbed is also excreted either as free cholesterol or as coprostanol or cholestanol after conversion by gut microbes.[8]

After its absorption into enterocytes, cholesterol and phytosterols have several possible fates. Acyl-coenzyme A:cholesterol acyltransferases (ACAT) esterifies cholesterol to cholesteryl ester (CE). Free sterols can also be effluxed or pumped out of enterocytes by the ATP binding cassette transporters A1 (ABCA1) onto small HDL particles. In fact, about a third of high-density lipoprotein-cholesterol (HDL-C) is formed by the gut by this process. In addition to acting as a lipid absorption organ, the intestine can also act as a secretory organ by returning cholesterol, stanols, phytosterols, and free cholesterol back to the gut lumen via ABCG5/G8 transporters. Because of the combined actions of NPC1L1 and ABCG5/G8 transporters, relatively small amounts of phytosterols and stanols ever reach the systemic circulation. This allows absolute concentrations or phytosterols and stanols or their ratios to total cholesterol to be used as biomarkers of cholesterol absorption.[9,10]

Lipids, including triglycerides (TG), phospholipids (PL), free and unesterified sterols, and a number of specific apoproteins, with the help of microsomal transfer protein (MTP) and apolipoprotein (apo) B-48, are assembled into a large lipoprotein called chylomicron (see section on lipoprotein metabolism, intestinal pathway). Patients with a rare deficiency in this process develop a disease called chylomicron retention disorder, which is characterized by excess lipid accumulation in enterocytes and fat malabsorption. Chylomicrons are secreted into the lymphatics and eventually into the thoracic duct, which connects to the systemic venous circulation at the junction of the left subclavian vein and the left internal jugular vein.

Cholesterol Synthesis. In addition to dietary sources, cholesterol can also be synthesized by all tissues from acetate (Fig. 34.2). Knowledge of this biochemical pathway, which took decades to elucidate, has acquired great significance, because drug agents for lowering plasma cholesterol are based on the rate-limiting step in this pathway—namely, HMG-CoA reductase. The necessity for understanding the fundamental biochemistry of this pathway was originally underscored by the triparanol disaster of 1960. Triparanol is a drug that inhibits the final step in the endogenous cholesterol synthetic pathway—the conversion of desmosterol to cholesterol—but it does not inhibit HMG-CoA reductase (see Fig. 34.2). When triparanol was used to treat hypercholesterolemia, the drug caused tissue accumulation of desmosterol, resulting in the development of cataracts, alopecia, and accelerated atherosclerosis.

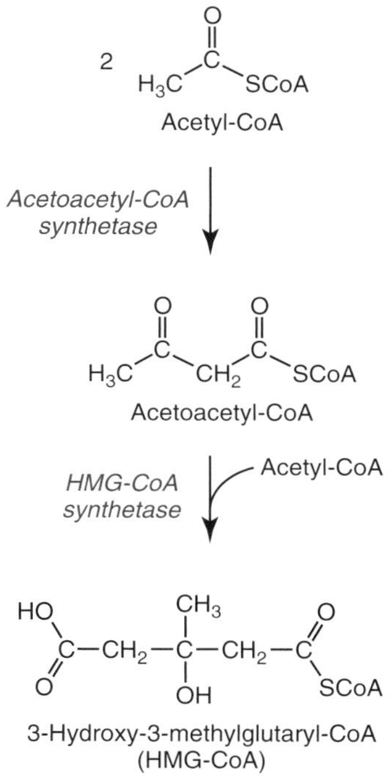

FIGURE 34.2 Cholesterol biosynthesis (stage 1).

Although both the liver and the small intestine play a major regulatory role in cholesterol homeostasis, all cells have the capacity to synthesize cholesterol (10 mg/day/kg) from acetate and/or acetyl-CoA. Extrahepatic tissues are responsible for greater than 80% of total cholesterol production.[11,12] Cholesterol biosynthesis can be conceptualized as occurring in three stages (Figs. 34.2 through 34.4). In the first stage, acetyl-CoA, a key metabolic intermediate that can be derived from carbohydrates, amino acids, and fatty acids, forms the six-carbon thioester HMG-CoA. In the second stage, HMG-CoA is reduced by HMG-CoA reductase to mevalonate, which is then decarboxylated to form five-carbon isoprene structure. These isoprenes are condensed to form first a 10-carbon (geranyl pyrophosphate) and then a 15-carbon intermediate (farnesyl pyrophosphate). Two of these C_{15} molecules combine via the enzyme squalene synthetase to form the final product of the second stage: squalene, a 30-carbon acyclic hydrocarbon. The second stage is important because it contains the regulatory enzyme HMG-CoA reductase, as well as the enzyme geranyl transferase, the second important site of cholesterol regulation. At this step there is the regulated diversion of farnesyl pyrophosphate from the synthesis of cholesterol for the production of other physiological lipids,

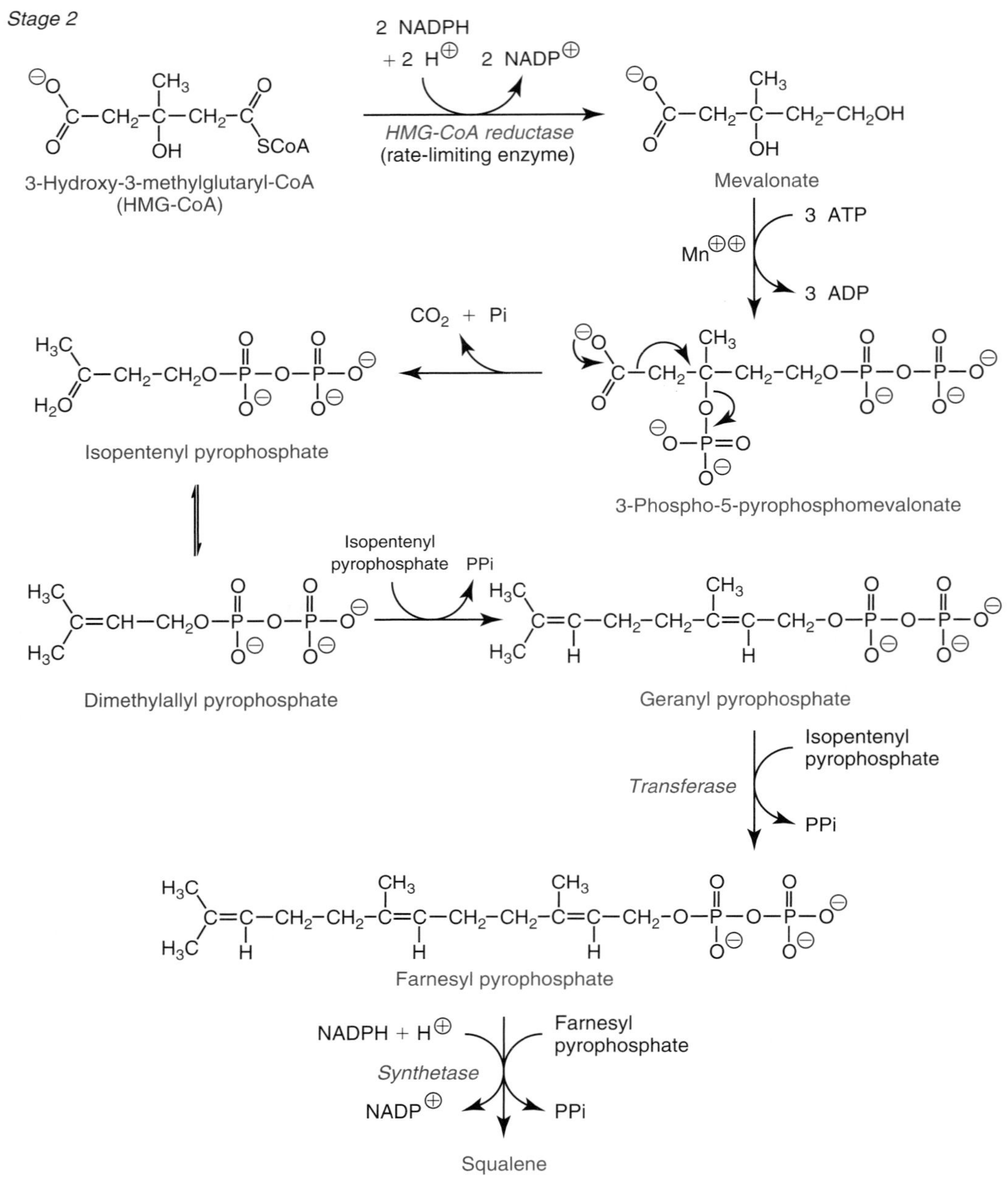

FIGURE 34.3 Cholesterol biosynthesis (stage 2).

such as dolichol or the modification (prenylation) of important membrane anchored proteins, such as Ras with farnesyl or geranylgeraniol groups.

The third and final stage of cholesterol synthesis occurs in the endoplasmic reticulum, with many of the lipid intermediate products being bound to a specific carrier protein. Squalene, after initial oxidation, undergoes cyclization to form lanosterol, a four-ring, 30-carbon intermediate. Lanosterol then undergoes several transitions either by the Kandutsch-Russell or Bloch pathways to become cholesterol with lathosterol and desmosterol, respectively, as the penultimate intermediates. The enzyme that dictates which pathway is used is determined by the stage at which the double bond at position C24 of the aliphatic side chain is reduced.[13] Defects of enzymes in these pathways can lead to desmosterolosis, lathosterolosis, Smith-Lemli-Opitz, and other malformation syndromes.[14] The most common biomarkers used to assess cholesterol synthesis are absolute concentrations of desmosterol and lathosterol or their ratios to total cholesterol.[15]

Cholesterol Esterification. The majority of cholesterol in the body is stored in cells or is transported in lipoprotein cores as hydrophobic cholesteryl ester (CE) molecules. The fatty acids most frequently esterified to the hydroxyl group of cholesterol are the 16-carbon unsaturated palmitic acid or the 19-carbon monounsaturated oleic acid, creating cholesteryl palmitate or oleate, respectively. Several intracellular enzymes (esterases) exist that can convert CE back to free cholesterol.

Almost all of the cholesterol in plasma is bound to lipoproteins, such as very low-density lipoprotein (VLDL),

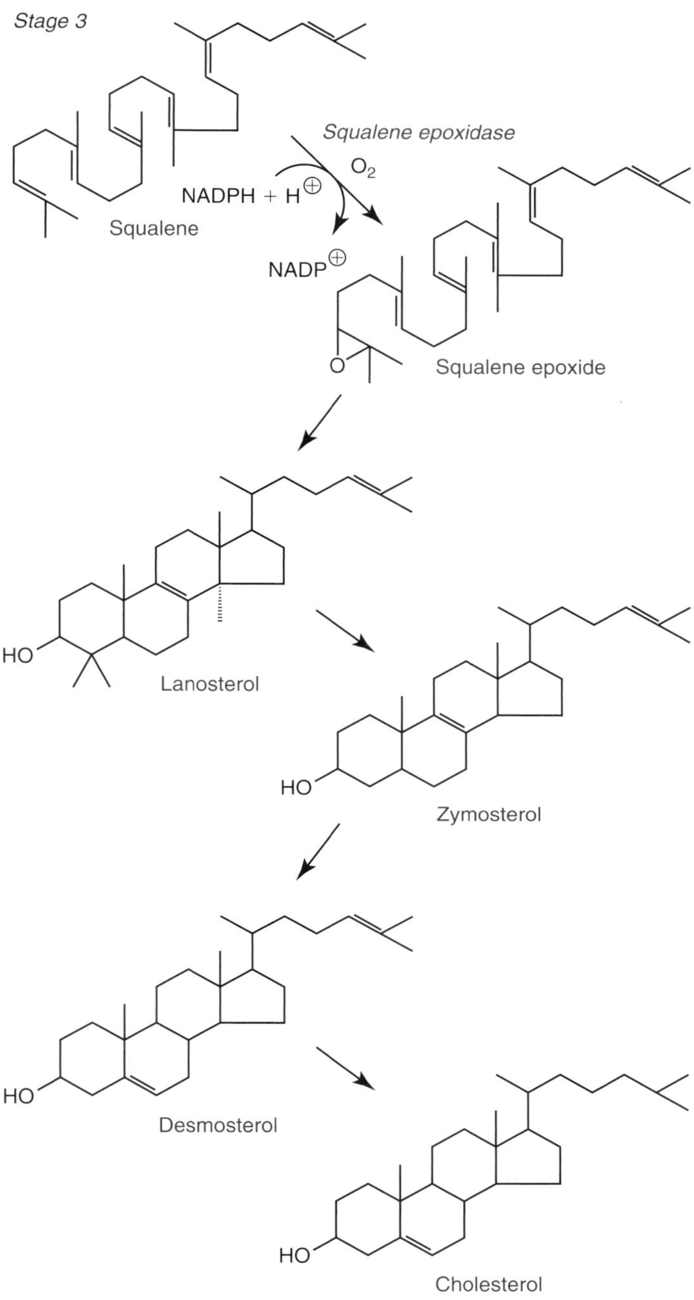

FIGURE 34.4 Cholesterol biosynthesis (stage 3; Bloch pathway).

intermediate-density lipoprotein (IDL), or low-density lipoprotein (LDL), or is effluxed to high-density lipoprotein (HDL) (see section on lipoprotein metabolism, hepatic pathway). The major apoprotein found in VLDL, IDL, and LDL is apo B-100, a large protein that contains over 4500 amino acids. The apo B-48 protein is found on chylomicrons and is a truncated version of apo B-100. It is produced in the intestine by a posttranscriptional editing step, which introduces a stop codon at about the middle of the apo B-100 mRNA transcript, thus resulting in a protein that is about 48% the length of the full-length apo B-100 protein.

The esterification of cholesterol is critical because it serves to enhance the lipid-carrying capacity of lipoproteins and prevents intracellular toxicity by free cholesterol. In the plasma, the reaction is catalyzed by lecithin-cholesterol acyltransferase (LCAT) and in the cell by acylcholesterol acyltransferase (ACAT). ACAT is an energy-requiring enzyme, and the initial reaction (Fig. 34.5) involves activation of a fatty acid with thio-coenzyme A (Co-ASH) to form an acyl-CoA, which in turn reacts with cholesterol to form cholesteryl ester. In contrast, the LCAT reaction does not require CoASH and transfers a fatty acid transfer from the second carbon position of phosphatidylcholine (lecithin) to the hydroxyl group on the A-ring of cholesterol (see Fig. 34.5). Cholesteryl esters account for about 70% of the total cholesterol in plasma, and LCAT is responsible for the formation of most

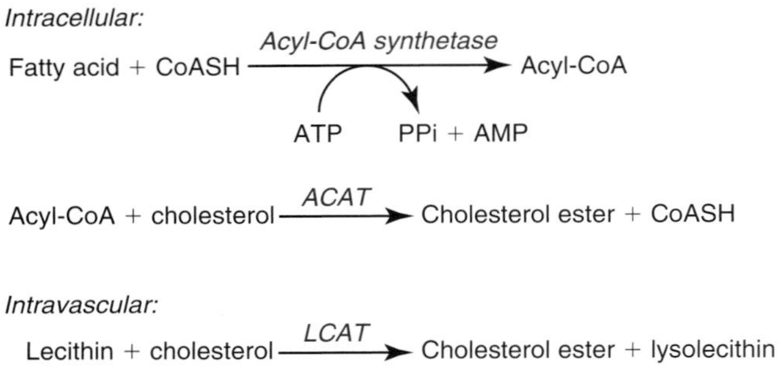

Intracellular:

Fatty acid + CoASH —(*Acyl-CoA synthetase*; ATP → PPi + AMP)→ Acyl-CoA

Acyl-CoA + cholesterol —(*ACAT*)→ Cholesterol ester + CoASH

Intravascular:

Lecithin + cholesterol —(*LCAT*)→ Cholesterol ester + lysolecithin

FIGURE 34.5 Intracellular and intravascular esterification of cholesterol mediated by ACAT and LCAT, respectively.

of it, with the residual being produced by ACAT and released into the circulation by the secretion of lipoproteins. Two different LCAT activities have been described, with α-LCAT esterifying the free cholesterol of HDL and β-LCAT activity occurring on apoB-containing lipoproteins.[16] LCAT is synthesized in the liver and released into the circulation; it primarily resides on HDL and to a lesser degree on LDL and is activated by apo A-I (see section on apolipoproteins). The esterification of cholesterol by LCAT on the polar hydroxyl group of cholesterol makes cholesteryl ester more hydrophobic than cholesterol. This causes the cholesterol on the surface of lipoproteins, once esterified, to partition into the more hydrophobic core of lipoproteins, where triglycerides are also located. This is especially important in the maturation or enlargement of HDL particles, allowing the surface to accommodate more free cholesterol from cellular efflux.

Cholesterol Catabolism. Once a lipoprotein enters the cell, its cholesteryl esters and glycerol esters are hydrolyzed in lysosomes by lysosomal acid lipase (LAL), which is encoded by the gene *LIPA*. Partial or complete lack of this enzyme results in a lysosomal storage disorder, resulting in the intracellular accumulation of cholesteryl esters and triglycerides, particularly in the liver. The partial loss of LAL results in the late-onset form of the disease and produces a clinical disorder known as *cholesteryl ester storage disease* (CESD).[17] CESD should be suspected in adult with dyslipidemia associated with elevated transaminases, LDL-C, and reduced HDL-C. Unlike other forms of dyslipidemia, less than 50% of patients with this disease have increased plasma TG levels. The almost complete loss of activity of this enzyme presents usually shortly after birth as *Wolman disease*, which often results in liver failure from lipid accumulation. A recombinant human LAL known as sebelipase alfa is being investigated in clinical trials as a potential therapy.[17]

Cholesterol reaching the liver may be secreted unchanged into bile as free cholesterol, metabolized to bile acids, or incorporated into and secreted back into the circulation on lipoproteins. Approximately one-third of the daily production of cholesterol, or about 400 mg/d, is converted into bile acids (Fig. 34.6). Conversion of cholesterol to cholic and chenodeoxycholic acids, the major bile acids in humans, involves shortening of the cholesterol sidechain and hydroxylation of the sterol nucleus. The first step, which is also the rate-limiting step, is hydroxylation of the 7-position, catalyzed by the enzyme 7α-hydroxylase. The bile acids are made even more polar after conjugation with glycine or taurine and then are excreted into the bile, where they play an active role in fat absorption, as discussed previously. Some of the bile acids are deconjugated by bacteria and converted into secondary bile acids. Cholic acid is converted to deoxycholic acid, and chenodeoxycholic acid is metabolized to lithocholic acid. Except for lithocholic acid, about 90% of the bile acids are reabsorbed in the lower third of the ileum and returned to the liver by the portal vein by the enterohepatic pathway (see also Chapter 61).

A significant amount of cholesterol and phytosterols are also excreted from enterocytes and hepatocytes via the ABCG5/G8 transporter back into the gut lumen or bile, where they are resolubilized with bile salts and phospholipids. If the amount of cholesterol in bile exceeds the capacity of these solubilizing agents, the excess cholesterol can precipitate, forming cholesterol gallstones, which account for about 80% of gallstones in Western societies. It is important to note that except for the liver and a few endocrine tissues (adrenal gland and gonads), most cells cannot further catabolize or modify cholesterol. Because of this and its limited aqueous solubility, cholesterol tends to accumulate, leading in cells to apoptosis or to extracellular crystals, both of which can contribute to the development of atherosclerosis. As discussed below, cells have the ability to rid themselves of excess cholesterol to HDL via active sterol efflux pumps or by free diffusion to lipoproteins, erythrocytes, or albumin.[18]

Fatty Acids

Fatty acids, one of the simplest lipid-type molecules, are generically indicated by the chemical formula RCOOH, where "R" stands for an alkyl chain. Fatty acid chain lengths vary and are commonly classified according to the number of carbon atoms present. Three somewhat arbitrarily defined groups of fatty acids are those containing 2 to 4 carbon atoms (short chain), 6 to 12 carbon atoms (medium chain), and 14 to 26 carbon atoms (long chain). Those of importance in human nutrition and metabolism are long-chain fatty acids and typically contain an even number of carbon atoms.

Fatty acids are further classified according to their degree of saturation. Saturated fatty acids have no double bonds between carbon atoms, whereas monounsaturated fatty acids contain one double bond, and polyunsaturated fatty acids contain more than one double bond (Fig. 34.7). The double bonds in polyunsaturated fatty acids of both animal and plant origin are usually 3 carbon atoms apart. Some fatty acids from marine fish living in deep, cold waters (eg, salmon), which form liquid oils at room temperature, possess numerous (up to 6) unsaturated bonds and are typically more than 20 carbon atoms in length. These fatty acids are prone to oxidation, which occurs at the sites of unsaturation. Labeling of carbon atoms in fatty acids can take place from the carboxyl terminal (Δ-numbering system) or from the methyl terminal (η- or ω-numbering system; Table 34.1). In addition, carbon atoms may be labeled with Greek symbols, with α being adjacent to the carboxyl group and ω being the farthest away. In the Δ-system, fatty acids are abbreviated according to the number of carbon atoms, the number of double bonds, and the position(s) of double bond(s). For example, linoleic acid, which contains 18 carbons and 2 unsaturated bonds between carbons 9 and 10 and between carbons 12 and 13, is written as $C_{18}:2.^{9,12}$ Using the η- or ω-system, linoleic acid would be abbreviated to C_{18}:2n-6, where only the first carbon forming the unsaturated pair is written. The *Geneva*

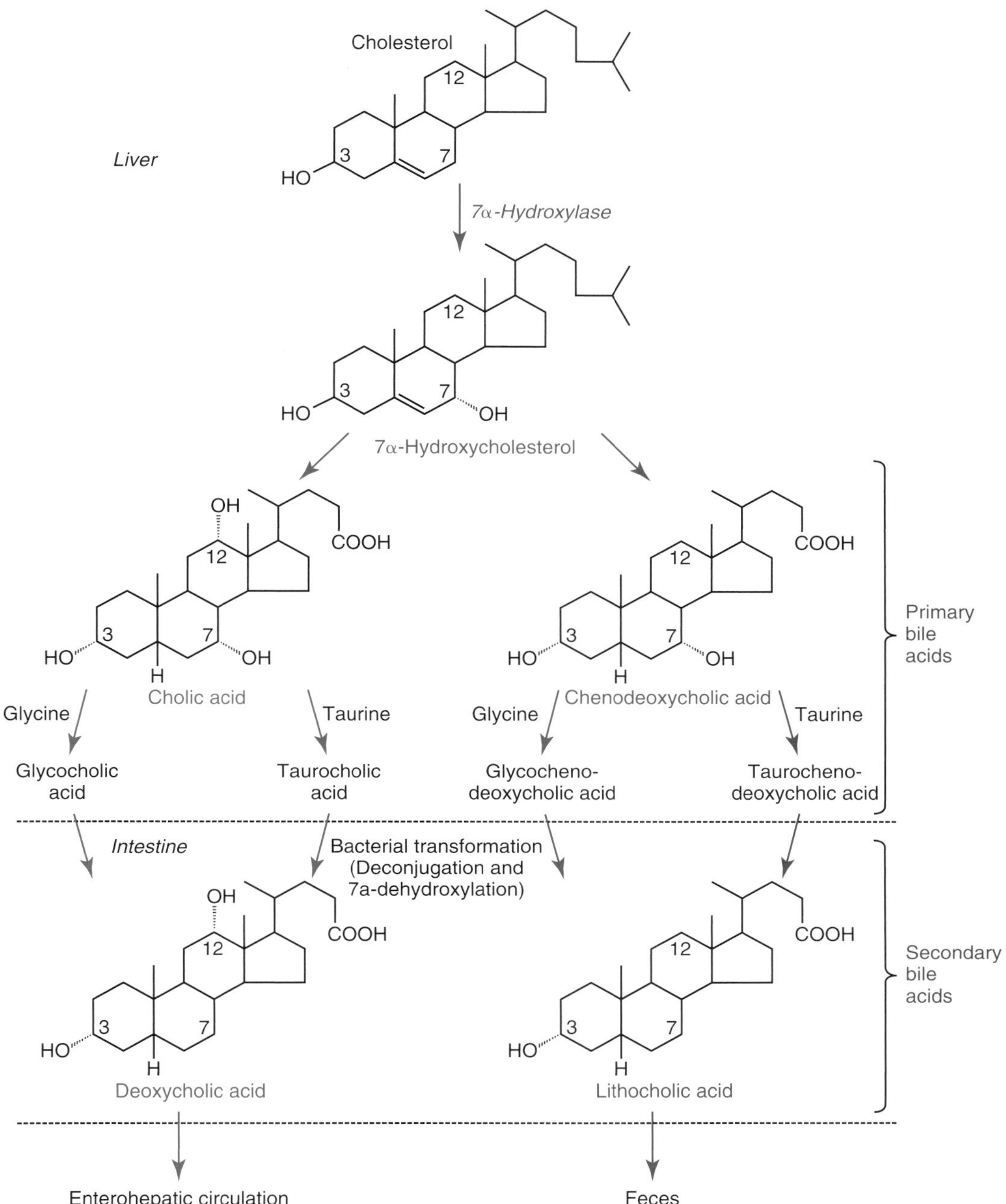

FIGURE 34.6 Bile acid synthesis.

or *systematic* classification is a third system for naming fatty acids (see Table 34.1). Depending on the number of double bonds, fatty acids can be termed as –anoic (none), -dienoic (two), –trienoic (three), and so on.

In saturated fatty acids, the acyl chain is extended and flexible (ie, the carbon atoms rotate freely around the longitudinal axis), and each internal carbon atom is fully saturated or, in other words, is covalently linked to two hydrogen molecules. Cis-unsaturated fatty acids have a fixed 30-degree bend in their acyl chains at each double bond because two hydrogen molecules are missing from the same side of the carbon double bond, thus causing the bend. Lipids containing cis-unsaturated fatty acids, such as triglycerides or phospholipids, have more complex spatial structures and lower melting points because these lipids cannot interact and pack as tightly by van der Waals interactions. As a consequence, lipids containing cis-unsaturated fatty acids, such as olive oil and other plant oils, are usually liquids at room temperature. In mammals, all naturally occurring unsaturated fatty acids are of the cis variety. Trans unsaturated fatty acids result from a chemical process called *catalytic hydrogenation,* a process used to "harden" unsaturated fats from plant sources in the manufacture of certain foods, such as margarine. Trans fats are artificially altered alkyl-molecules where cis-dienes are chemically hydrogenated into a trans-diene configuration, creating fatty acid isomers with very different physical properties. Although trans fatty acids are still unsaturated, one hydrogen is missing from each side of the carbon double bond, making these fatty acids resemble more the linear configuration of the acyl chain of saturated fatty acids. This accounts for why lipids made with trans fatty acids form solids at room temperature. Epidemiologic and experimental studies have shown that trans fatty acids may promote CHD, and an effort is under way to reduce the use of catalytic hydrogenation in food processing and to lower the overall consumption of trans fatty acids.[19]

The average diet in Western societies contains up to 40% fat, 90% of which is in the form of fatty acids conjugated to glycerol, as in the case of triglycerides or phospholipids, or to cholesterol (CE). In addition, humans can synthesize most fatty acids, including saturated, monounsaturated, and some polyunsaturated fats. In contrast, linoleic (C_{18}:$2^{9,12}$) acid, a plant-derived fatty acid, and linolenic (C_{18}:$3^{9,12,15}$) acid cannot be synthesized and must be obtained from the diet and are termed *essential fatty acids.* Linoleic acid is converted to arachidonic acid, which has an important role in prostaglandin synthesis and in myelinization of the central nervous system.

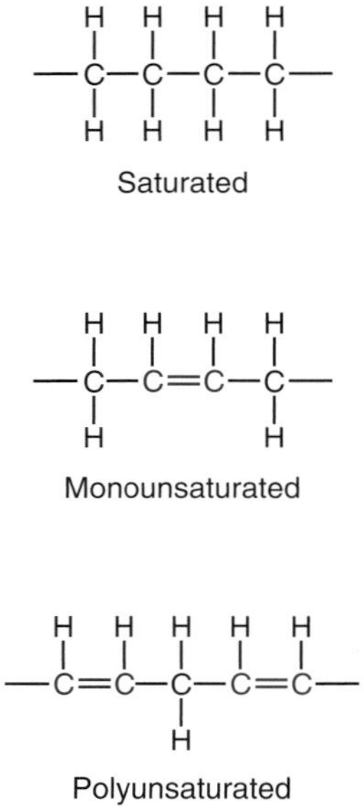

Saturated

Monounsaturated

Polyunsaturated

FIGURE 34.7 Saturated and unsaturated fatty acids.

The fatty acid carboxyl group has a pK_a of approximately 4.8, so free fatty acid molecules in both plasma and intracellular fluid exist primarily in an ionized form. Although most fatty acids in the plasma are esterified, relatively small amounts are also transported as free fatty acids bound to albumin. One albumin molecule can carry as many as 20 molecules of fatty acid. The normal concentration of free fatty acids in human blood is relatively low at 0.30 to 1.10 mmol/L, or about 8 to 31 mg/dL of plasma. The flux, however, of free fatty acids through the plasma is very large and is sensitive to physiologic energy demands (exercise and physical work), the availability of blood glucose, and psychological stresses that cause the liberation of epinephrine.

Fatty Acid Catabolism. Long-chain fatty acids are oxidized in the mitochondria and produce energy by a series of reactions that operate in a repetitive manner to shorten the fatty acid chain by two carbon atoms at a time from the carboxy (—COOH) terminus in a process known as β-oxidation. For example, 1 mole of C_{16} fatty acid is converted to 8 moles of acetyl-CoA. Acetyl-CoA does not normally accumulate in the cell but is enzymatically condensed with oxaloacetate, derived largely from carbohydrate metabolism (Fig. 34.8), to yield citrate, a major component of the tricarboxylic acid cycle or *Krebs cycle.* The Krebs cycle serves as a common pathway for the final oxidation of nearly all food material, whether derived from carbohydrate, fat, or protein. It is important to note that the efficiency of the Krebs cycle depends on the availability of sufficient oxaloacetate to serve as an acceptor for acetyl-CoA.

Complete oxidation of a single fatty acid molecule produces a relatively large quantity of energy. For example, the complete oxidation of 1 mole of palmitic acid to carbon dioxide and water produces 16 moles of CO_2, 16 moles of H_2O, and 129 moles of adenosine triphosphate, or 2340 Cal.[†] Thus the standard free energy for oxidation of palmitic acid is 2340 Cal, whereas the free energy liberated by hydrolysis of 129 moles of ATP is only 940 Cal, indicating that the efficiency of energy conservation in fatty acid oxidation is approximately 40% under standard conditions.

[†]The unit used in discussing the energy value of food is the calorie (Cal), equal to 1000 calories or 1 kilocalorie (kcal). In the SI system, the unit of energy is the joule (J), and 1 calorie equals 4.1868J.

TABLE 34.1 Fatty Acids Commonly Found in Human Tissue

Common Name	Systematic Name	Δ-Numbering	η-(ω) Numbering
Lauric	Dodecanoic	12:0	12:0
Myristic	Tetradecanoic	14:0	14:0
Palmitic	Hexadecanoic	16:0	16:0
Palmitoleic	9-Hexadecenoic	$16{:}1^{9}$	16:1n-7
Stearic	Octadecanoic	18:0	18:0
Oleic	9-Octadecenoic	$18{:}1^{9}$	18:1n-9
Linoleic*	9,12-Octadecadienoic	$18{:}2^{9,12}$	18:2n-6
Linolenic*	9,12,15-Octadecatrienoic	$18{:}3^{9,12,15}$	18:3n-3
Arachidic	Eicosanoic	20:0	20:0
Arachidonic	5,8,11,14-Eicosatetraenoic	$20{:}4^{5,8,11,14}$	20:4n-6
Eicosapentaenoic	5,8,11,14,17-Eicosapentaenoic	$20{:}5^{5,8,11,14,17}$	20:5n-3
Docosahexaenoic (Cervonic)	4,7,10,13,16,19-Docosahexaenoic	$22{:}6^{4,7,10,13,16,19}$	22:6n-3

*Essential fatty acids.

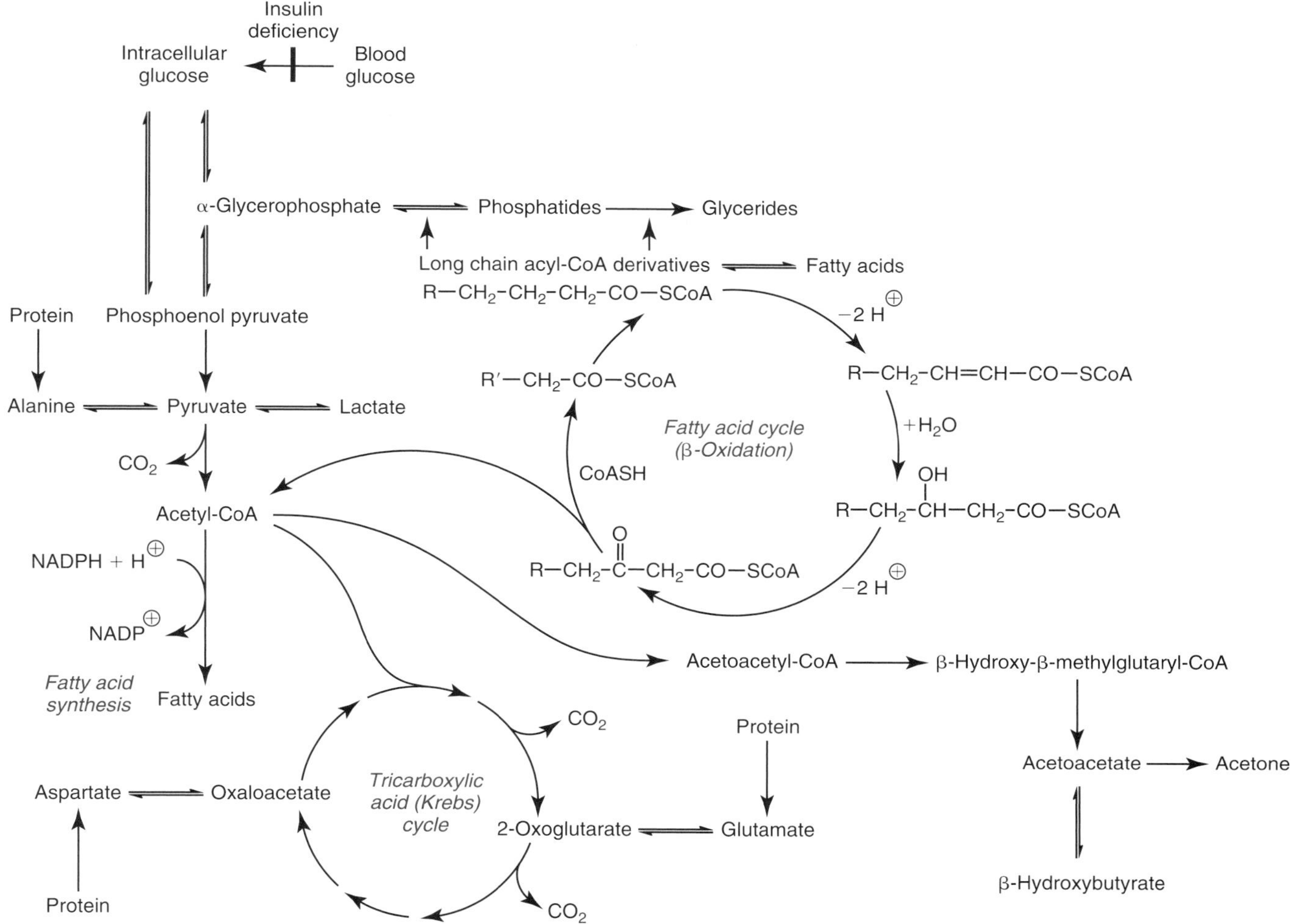

FIGURE 34.8 Metabolic relations among intermediates of carbohydrate, fat, and protein metabolism. Note that acetyl-CoA is produced from both carbohydrate and fat. The glucogenic amino acids, derived from protein metabolism, enter glycolytic paths as α-keto acids. Ketogenic amino acids enter as acetyl-CoA.

By means of suitable enzyme reactions, the chemical energy stored in fatty acids can be released for metabolic processes or stored in the form of high-energy compounds, such as ATP. Triglycerides that contain three fatty acid molecules are an efficient storage form for metabolic energy. The amount of energy produced by metabolizing 1 mole of palmitic acid (16 carbon atoms) is approximately twice that produced by metabolizing an equivalent amount (2.5 mole) of glucose (6 carbon atoms per molecule). Carbohydrate storage also requires water for hydration; triglyceride storage does not. In addition to their high intrinsic energy content, the storage of triglycerides in subcutaneous fat deposits provides insulation for the body.

Ketone Formation. During prolonged starvation, or whenever carbohydrate metabolism is severely impaired, as in uncontrolled diabetes mellitus (see Chapter 57) or intentionally induced nutritional ketosis from carbohydrate restriction, the formation of acetyl-CoA exceeds the supply of oxaloacetate. The abundance of acetyl-CoA results from excessive mobilization of fatty acids from adipose tissue and their conversion by β-oxidation in the liver. The resulting excess acetyl-CoA is diverted to an alternative pathway in the mitochondria to form acetoacetic acid, β-hydroxybutyric acid, and acetone—three compounds known collectively as *ketone bodies*. Increased ketone bodies is a frequent finding in severe, uncontrolled diabetes mellitus, but much lower levels can also result from nutritionally induced ketosis.[20] As shown in Fig. 34.9, the first product, acetoacetyl-CoA, condenses in the mitochondria with a third molecule of acetyl-CoA to yield HMG-CoA. This pool of HMG-CoA in the mitochondria is distinct from the pool in the cytosol, which is used for cholesterol biosynthesis. The HMG-CoA produced in the mitochondria is cleaved enzymatically to yield acetoacetate and acetyl-CoA. Some of the acetoacetate formed in liver cells is usually reduced to β-hydroxybutyrate. Because acetoacetate is unstable, a further portion decomposes to form carbon dioxide and acetone, the third ketone body found in high concentrations in pathologic ketotic states like severe, untreated diabetes mellitus. Ketosis, therefore, develops from excessive production of acetyl-CoA because the body attempts to derive necessary energy from stored fat in the absence of an adequate supply of carbohydrate metabolites

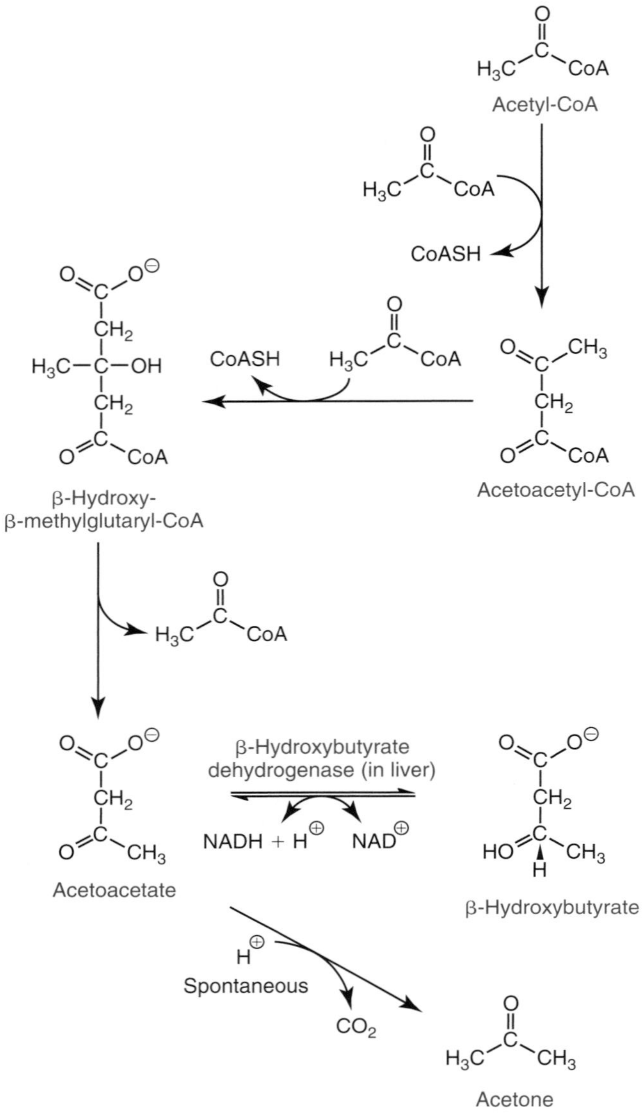

FIGURE 34.9 Formation of ketone bodies.

(see Chapter 33). In nutritional ketosis, the ketones serve as a physiologic energy supply and are sometimes associated with increased LDL-C.[21]

Inadequate incorporation of acetyl-CoA into the Krebs cycle may be further aggravated by inhibition of the oxaloacetate-generating enzyme system through excess accumulation of palmitic-CoA and other long-chain fatty acid–CoA derivatives in the liver. Skeletal muscle and the heart (and the brain in prolonged fasting) use ketone bodies by resynthesizing their CoA derivatives and subsequently oxidizing them for the production of energy. Although liver cells are largely responsible for generating ketones, they cannot metabolize acetoacetate because the liver lacks 3-ketoacid CoA transferase, the enzyme required for transferring CoA from succinyl-CoA.

The entire process of pathologic ketosis is reversed by restoring adequate metabolism of carbohydrate. In starvation, restoration consists of adequate carbohydrate ingestion. In diabetes mellitus, ketosis can be reversed by insulin administration, which permits circulating blood glucose to be taken up by the cells. With restored concentrations of oxaloacetate, acetyl-CoA can then enter the Krebs cycle, thus restoring the normal pathway for energy metabolism. Eventually, the release of fatty acids from adipose tissue slows down and is finally reversed. A graphic view of these metabolic reactions is outlined in Fig. 34.8, which shows the overall interrelationship between carbohydrate, fatty acid, and protein metabolism.

Prostaglandins. Prostaglandins and related compounds are derivatives of long chain fatty acids, such as arachidonate. This group consists of prostaglandins, thromboxanes, some hydroperoxy— and hydroxy—fatty acid derivatives, and leukotrienes. As described below, these lipids are known to affect a wide variety of biological functions. They are also relatively short lived and extremely potent, producing physiologic actions at concentrations as low as 1 μg/L.

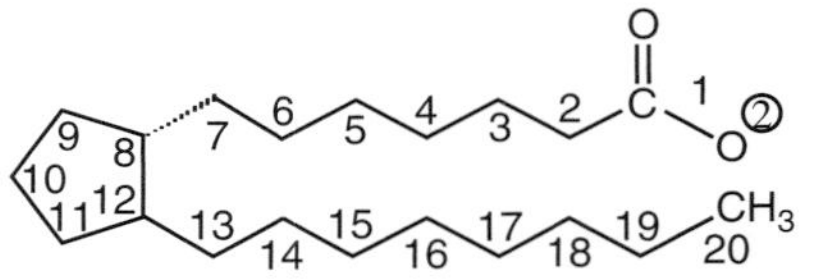

The prostaglandins are a series of C_{20} unsaturated fatty acids containing a cyclopentane ring; the parent fatty acid has been given the trivial name *prostanoic acid.* The seven-carbon chain linked to C-8 of prostanoic acid (R_1) projects below the plane of the ring, whereas the eight-carbon chain attached to C-12 (R_2) projects above the ring. By convention, prostaglandins are abbreviated *PG,* with the class designated by a capital letter (A, B, E, F, G, H, and I), followed by a number and then in some cases a Greek letter (Fig. 34.10). With the exception of PGG and PGH, which have the same ring structure (cyclopentane endoperoxide), the letters refer to different ring structures. PGA and PGB have keto groups at C-9, with the A series having a double bond between C-10 and C-11, and the B series having a double bond between C-8 and C-12. PGE also has a C-9 keto bond but a hydroxyl group at C-11. The F series has hydroxyl groups at both C-9 and C-11. The difference between PGG and PGH, which have identical ring structures, occurs in the sidechain at C-15 in R_2. The G series has a peroxide group, whereas the H series has a hydroxyl group. The I series has a double-ring formation, with the C-9 of the cyclopentane ring linked to C-6 of the sidechain by an oxygen molecule to form a second five-sided ring (see Fig. 34.10). The endoperoxide PGs (G and H series) are intermediates in the formation of other PGs.

The number after the capital letter is usually written as a subscript and is used to designate the number of unsaturated bonds in the PG sidechains and not within the ring structure itself. In PGE_1, for example, a double bond exists between C-13 and C-14. In the 2 series (PGE_2), which are more common, a double bond exists between C-13 and C-14 and between C-5 and C-6; in the 3 series (PGE_3), an additional double bond occurs between C-17 and C-18. The bond between C-13 and C-14 is always trans, whereas bonds between C-5 and C-6 and between C-17 and C-18 are always cis. At C-15, all naturally occurring prostaglandins have a hydroxyl group that projects below the plane of the ring. Use of the Greek letter (α or β) applies only to the F series and refers to the hydroxyl group found at C-9. In the α-series, the hydroxyl group projects below the ring plane in the same

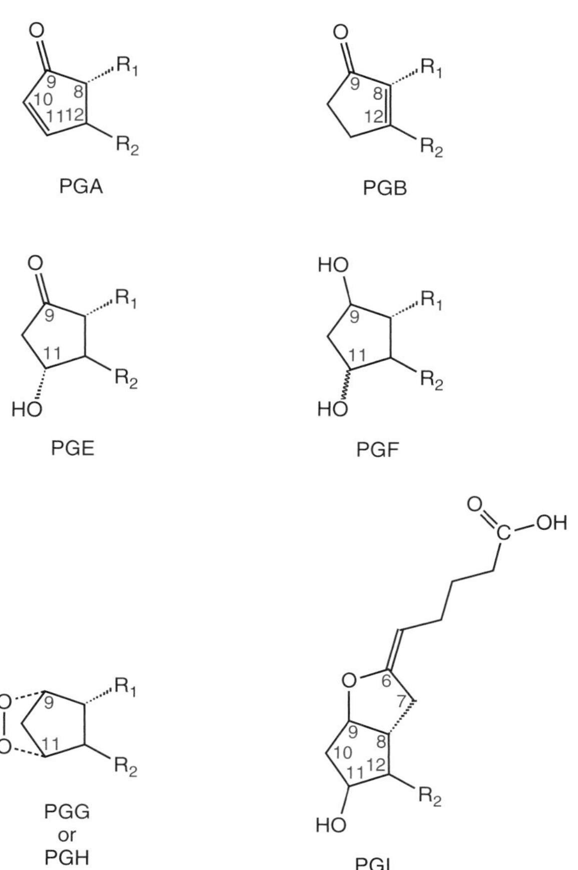

FIGURE 34.10 Major prostaglandin classes (series). R_1 and R_2 are prostaglandin side chains.

TABLE 34.2 Naturally Occurring Prostaglandins

Primary Prostaglandin	Other Prostaglandins
PGE_1	PGA_1
$PGF_{1\alpha}$	PGA_2
PGE_2	19α-$OHPGA_1$
$PGF_{2\alpha}$	19α-$OHPGA_2$
PGG_2	PGB_1
PGH_2	PGB_2
PGI_2	19α-$OHPGB_2$
Thromboxane A_2	PGE_3
Thromboxane B_2	$PGF_{3\alpha}$

direction as the C-11 hydroxyl group, whereas the β-series denotes that the hydroxyl at C-9 is above the plane of the ring. Over 16 naturally occurring prostaglandins have been described (Table 34.2), but only 7, along with 2 thromboxanes, are commonly found throughout the body, and they are termed the *primary prostaglandins.*

Although prostaglandins have hormone-like actions, they are different from most other hormones in that they are synthesized at the site of action and are made in almost all tissues. Linoleic acid ($C_{18}:2^{9,12}$) is the precursor of two of the three 20-carbon fatty acids that form prostaglandins; linolenic acid ($C_{18}:2^{9,12,15}$) is the other precursor. Both of these

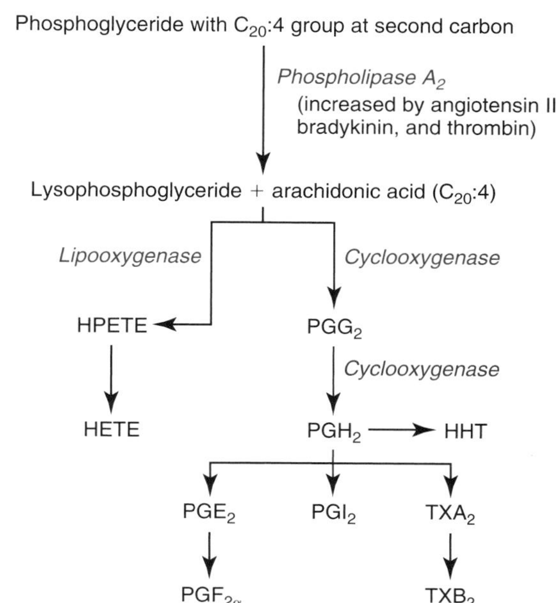

FIGURE 34.11 Synthesis of prostaglandins from arachidonic precursor. *HPETE, HETE, HHT,* 12-l-Hydroxy-5,8,10-heptadecatrienoic acid; *PG,* prostaglandin; *TX,* thromboxane.

fatty acids are considered essential because they cannot be synthesized in the body and therefore must be present in the diet. The three C_{20} fatty acids subsequently formed are $C_{20}:3^{5,8,11}$ (eicosatrienoic acid), $C_{20}:4^{5,8,11,14}$ (eicosatetraenoic or arachidonic acid), and $C_{20}:5^{8,11,14,17}$(eicosapentanoic acid). These three fatty acids form the PG_1, PG_2, and PG_3 series, respectively.

Once formed, prostaglandins exert very short-lived effects and are rapidly catabolized to inactive forms within a few seconds. Inactivation of prostaglandin appears to be mediated by two enzymes: 15 α-hydroxy-prostaglandin dehydrogenase and Δ^{13}-prostaglandin reductase. Prostaglandins are not stored; instead, precursor C_{20} fatty acids are present in tissue attached to the C-2 position (see later section in this chapter on glycerol esters) of phosphoglycerides. When necessary, the C_{20} precursor is hydrolyzed by phospholipase A_2. Release of the C_{20} fatty acid appears to be the rate-limiting step in prostaglandin synthesis and is stimulated by many different agents, such as bradykinin, thrombin, or angiotensin II.

Although it is probable that all prostaglandins follow a similar synthetic pathway, $C_{20}:4$ (arachidonic acid) has been the most intensively studied and is used to illustrate the pathway (Fig. 34.11). Once released, arachidonic acid follows one of two pathways. The lipoxygenase route produces 12-L-hydroperoxy-5,8,10,14 eicosatetraenoic acid (HPETE); HPETE then spontaneously decomposes to 12-L-hydroxy-5,8,10,14 eicosatetraenoic acid (HETE). The alternative pathway is mediated by cyclooxygenase (COX) to produce the endoperoxides PGG_2 and PGH_2. The latter can be degraded to 12-L-hydroxy-5,8,10-heptadecatrienoic acid. What controls the entry into a specific pathway remains speculative; however, it is known that nonsteroidal antiinflammatory drugs (NSAIDs; aspirin, ibuprofen, and indomethacin) inhibit the COX, thereby decreasing prostaglandin synthesis. Two isoforms of COX are known: COX-1 and COX-2. The COX-1 enzymes are constitutively expressed, whereas COX-2

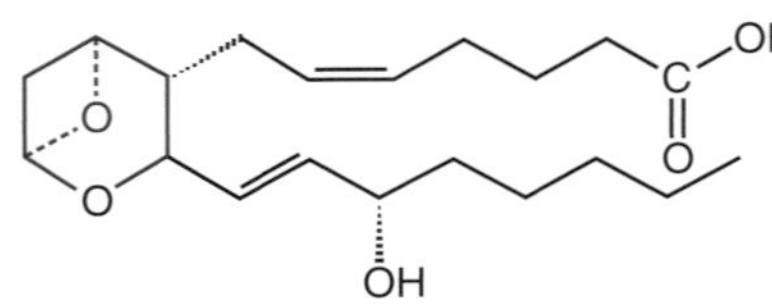

Thromboxane A_2 (TXA_2)

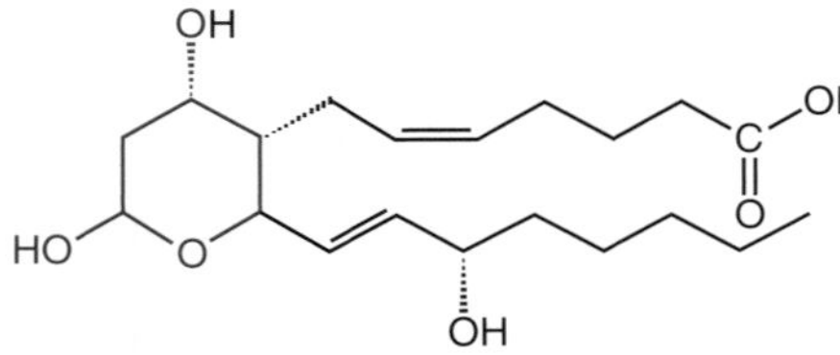

Thromboxane B_2 (TXB_2)

FIGURE 34.12 Structures of thromboxanes.

TABLE 34.3 Prostaglandin-Mediated Effects

Site of Action	Physiologic Response
Arterial smooth muscle	Alters blood pressure
Uterine muscle	Induces labor, therapeutic abortion
Lower gastrointestinal tract	Increases motility
Bronchial smooth muscle	Bronchospasm
Platelets	Increases coagulability
Capillaries	Increases permeability
Stomach	Enhances gastric acid secretion
Adipose tissue	Inhibits triglyceride lipolysis

is induced in response to inflammation. Certain drugs that inhibit both COX enzymes have nephrotoxic and ulcerogenic side effects. Therefore newer NSAIDs have been developed that preferentially inhibit COX-2 to reduce side effects, but they have been found to also be associated with an increased incidence of cardiovascular disease.[22]

Prostaglandin I_2, or prostacyclin, is also derived from arachidonic acid (see Fig. 34.11) in the vascular endothelium. It has a powerful vasodilatory action, especially on the coronary arteries, and is responsible for inhibiting platelet aggregation. Thromboxane A_2 is also synthesized from arachidonic acid but is produced by platelets. It has the opposite effect of prostacyclin (ie, it stimulates the contraction of arterial smooth muscle and enhances platelet aggregation). It has a very short half-life—about 30 seconds—and is rapidly converted to its inactive metabolite, thromboxane B_2. The thromboxanes are differ from other prostaglandins in that they contain six-sided rings of five carbon atoms and one oxygen atom (Fig. 34.12). Table 34.3 lists some reported functions of the various prostaglandins.

Glycerol Esters (Acylglycerols)

As already described, almost all complex lipids contain fatty acids, and in most cases they are covalently linked to a backbone containing an alcohol. One of the most common

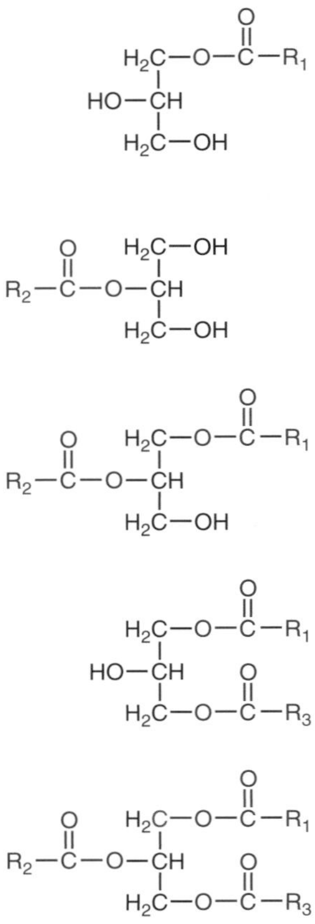

1-Monoglyceride

2-Monoglyceride

1,2-Diglyceride

1,3-Diglyceride

Triglyceride

FIGURE 34.13 Structure and classification of glycerol esters (acylglycerols). R_1, R_2, and R_3 are fatty acids of varying chain length.

alcohols found in lipids is glycerol, a three-carbon molecule containing three hydroxyl groups.

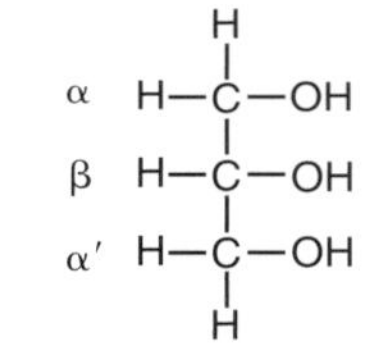

$$
\begin{array}{ll}
 & \mathrm{H} \\
\alpha & \mathrm{H-C-OH} \\
\beta & \mathrm{H-C-OH} \\
\alpha' & \mathrm{H-C-OH} \\
 & \mathrm{H}
\end{array}
$$

The two terminal carbon atoms in the molecule are chemically equivalent and are designated α and α′. The center carbon is labeled β. A common alternative labeling system uses the stereospecific numbering system with sn-1, sn-2, and sn-3, respectively, relating the numeral 1 for the α-carbon, 2 for the β-carbon, and 3 for the α′-carbon. The class of acylglycerol (glyceride) is determined by the number of fatty acyl groups present: one fatty acid, monoacylglycerols (monoglycerides), two fatty acids, diacylglycerols (diglycerides), and three fatty acids, triacylglycerols (triglycerides). In a monoacylglycerol, the fatty acid may be linked to any of the three carbon atoms. By convention, the number system is used to indicate the carbon position (eg, 1-monoglyceride indicates a fatty acid attachment to the α- or sn-1 carbon). This numbering system applies to all acylglycerols, including the phosphoglycerides, as shown later. Diglycerides may be 1,2- or 1,3-diglycerides (Fig. 34.13).

Triglycerides (TG) are the most prevalent glycerol esters encountered in the body and constitute 95% of tissue storage fat; they also form the core lipid component of lipoproteins and are the predominant form of glyceryl ester found in plasma. The types of fatty acids found in monoglycerides, diglycerides, or triglycerides vary considerably and usually include combinations of the long-chain fatty acids shown in Table 34.1. Thus a TG formed from just five different fatty acids can exist as 105 different molecular TG species and therefore a wide variety of molecular weights.[23] Triglycerides from plants (eg, corn, sunflower seed, safflower oils) tend to have large quantities of *cis*-unsaturated fatty acids, such as C_{18}:2 or linoleic acid, and are liquid at room temperature. Triglycerides from animals, especially ruminants, tend to have C_{14}:0 through C_{18}:0 fatty acid residues (saturated fats) and are solids at room temperature. Rarely, some plant triglycerides, such as coconut oil, are highly saturated and form solids at room temperature.

Triglycerides are digested (hydrolyzed) in the duodenum and the proximal ileum. Through the action of pancreatic and intestinal lipases and in the presence of bile acids, which activate lipases, they are hydrolyzed to glycerol, monoglycerides, and fatty acids. After absorption, triglycerides are reassembled from glycerol, monoglycerides, and fatty acids in intestinal epithelial cells and are combined with cholesterol and apo B-48 to form chylomicrons.

Another major class of glyceryl esters, the phospholipids or phosphoglycerides, contains phosphoric acid at the third (α′) carbon atom (Fig. 34.14). In their simplest form, the A group is an H atom, so the molecule is called a *diacylphosphoglyceride.* Usually, however, the A is an alcohol-derived group, such as choline, serine, inositol, or ethanolamine (see Fig. 34.14). If A is choline, the molecule is referred to as phosphatidylcholine; if it is ethanolamine, it is referred to as phosphatidylethanolamine; and so on. The term lecithin, which is an older designation, is still commonly used for phosphatidylcholines. Because of the wide variety of fatty acid residues at positions R_1 and R_2 (see Fig. 34.14), many different types of phospholipids can be formed. These phospholipids are named according to the fatty acid acyl ester attached at C-1 and C-2 of the glycerol. Saturated fatty acids are typically attached to the C-1 position, whereas (poly)unsaturated fatty acids are often present at the C-2 position. A phospholipid that has lost one of its O-acyl groups is called a lysophospholipid. In inner mitochondrial membranes, more complex phosphoglycerides known as *cardiolipins* can be found. They are derived from two phosphoglyceride molecules joined by a glycerol bridge. Enzymes that deesterify or hydrolyze phospholipids are termed *phospholipases* or *lysophospholipases.*

Sphingolipids

Sphingolipids, a fourth class of lipids found in humans, are derived from the amino alcohol sphingosine (Fig. 34.15). This dihydric 18-carbon alcohol contains an amino group at C-17. A fatty acid containing 18 or more carbon atoms can be attached to the amino group through an amide linkage to form *ceramide.* This is an intermediary step in the formation of three important sphingolipids—namely, sphingomyelin, galactosylceramide, and glucosylceramide (see Fig. 34.15). The sugar-containing ceramides can also have a sulfate group attached (usually on the 2-position of the galactose residue) to form the sulfatides. The glycosyl ceramides can have additional monosaccharide moieties, such as galactose, *N*-acetylgalactosamine, and *N*-acetylneuraminic acid to form complex globosides and gangliosides. These complex sphingolipids form the major lipids of cell membranes, particularly in the central nervous system. Gangliosides, for example, are particularly prevalent in the gray matter of the brain, whereas membrane glycosphingolipids have major roles in cellular interactions, growth, and development. Some glycolipids on red cells form blood group antigens, while others have been found to be tumor antigens.

Terpenes

Terpenes are polymers of the five-carbon isoprene unit and form the backbone structure of vitamins A, E, and K (see

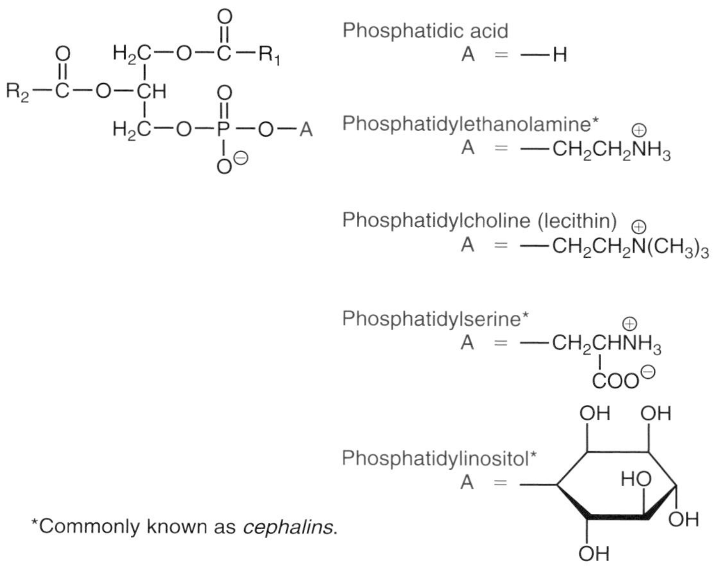

Phosphatidic acid
A = —H

Phosphatidylethanolamine*
A = $—CH_2CH_2NH_3^{\oplus}$

Phosphatidylcholine (lecithin)
A = $—CH_2CH_2N^{\oplus}(CH_3)_3$

Phosphatidylserine*
A = $—CH_2CH(COO^{\ominus})NH_3^{\oplus}$

Phosphatidylinositol*
A = (inositol ring: OH, OH, HO, OH, OH)

*Commonly known as *cephalins.*

FIGURE 34.14 Structures of phosphoglycerides and common alcohol groups associated with them. R_1 and R_2 are fatty acid(s) of varying carbon atom lengths.

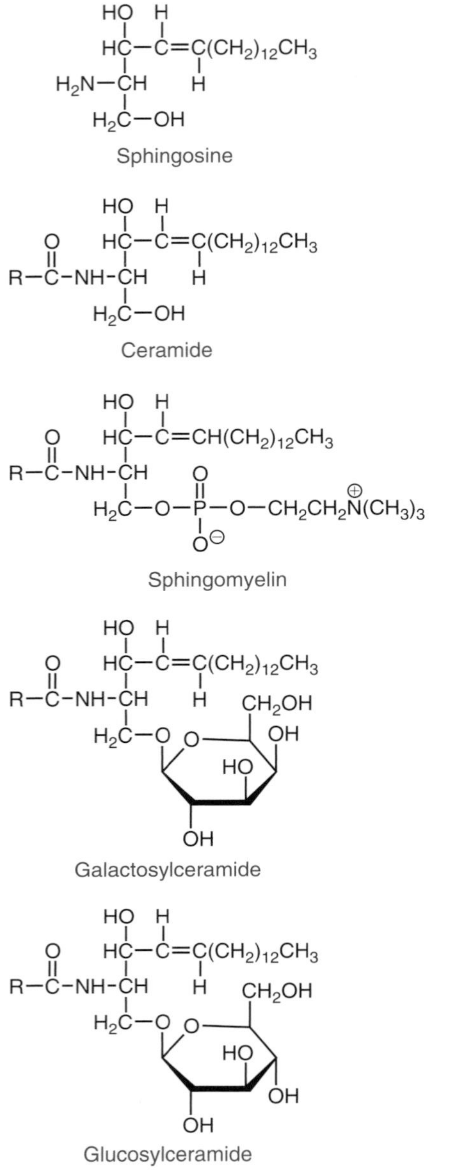

Sphingosine

Ceramide

Sphingomyelin

Galactosylceramide

Glucosylceramide

FIGURE 34.15 Structures of sphingolipids.

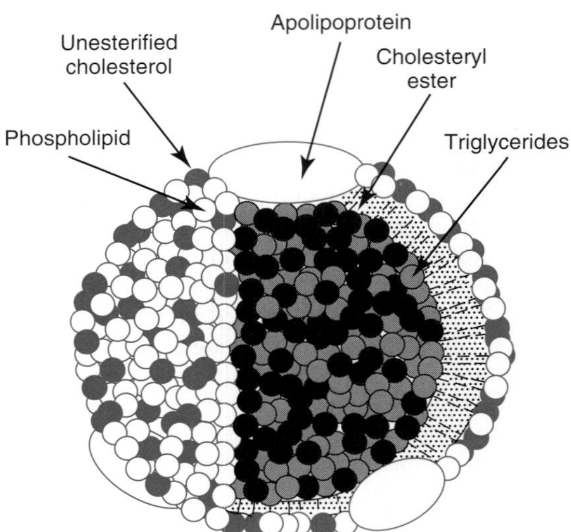

FIGURE 34.16 Structure of a typical lipoprotein particle.

Chapter 37) and the dolichols, which play an important role in protein glycosylation.

Lipoproteins

Lipids, whether synthesized or absorbed from the diet, must be transported to various tissues to accomplish their metabolic functions. Because of their relative aqueous insolubility, they are transported in the plasma in macromolecular complexes called *lipoproteins.* Lipoproteins are typically spherical particles with more hydrophobic nonpolar lipids (triglycerides and cholesteryl esters) in their core and more polar or amphipathic lipids (phospholipids and free cholesterol) oriented on the surface as a single monolayer like a micelle. They also contain one or more specific proteins, called *apolipoproteins,* which usually are also located on their surface (Fig. 34.16).[24] This arrangement of core lipids with the overlying phospholipid, cholesterol, and a protein coat is stabilized by noncovalent forces, mostly through hydrogen bonding and van der Waals forces. This binding is loose enough to allow the rapid spontaneous exchange of cholesterol, which is more water soluble than the other lipids, between plasma lipoproteins and cell membranes, including erythrocytes. The other more hydrophobic lipids require specific transfer proteins to exchange between lipoproteins, such as cholesteryl ester transfer protein (CETP), which exchanges triglycerides and cholesteryl esters between lipoproteins. Another important transfer protein is the phospholipid transfer protein (PLTP), which promotes the transfer of phospholipids between lipoproteins.

Lipoproteins have different physical and chemical properties (Table 34.4) because they contain different proportions of lipids and proteins (Table 34.5). Historically, lipoproteins have been categorized on the basis of their hydrated densities, as determined by ultracentrifugation or electrophoretically by their charge and size. The major lipoprotein fractions include chylomicron, VLDL, IDL, LDL, HDL, and lipoprotein(a) [Lp(a)]. Among these major lipoproteins, they can be further subdivided, depending on the technology, to even more subclasses.

Lp(a) is a unique lipoprotein (see Table 34.4) that is structurally related to LDL, containing one apo B-100 per particle and a similar lipid composition.[25,26] Lp(a) also contains a carbohydrate-rich protein called apolipoprotein(a) [apo(a)], which is covalently bound to apo B-100 through a disulfide linkage. Apo(a) has significant sequence homology with plasminogen, but unlike plasminogen, it is not an active protease. Apo(a) contains a high degree of variation in its polypeptide chain length because of a variable number of kringle domains (Fig. 34.17). Plasminogen contains five kringle domains, but apo(a) only contains kringle types 4 and 5. There are 10 distinct classes of kringle 4–like domains that differ from one another in amino acid sequence. Kringle 4 type 1 and kringle 4 types 3 to 10 are present as a single copy, but kringle 4 type 2 is present in variable numbers of repeats (3 to >40) (see Fig. 34.17).[27] Thus there are different-sized isoforms of apo(a) classically described as large, high molecular weight (HMW) or small, low molecular weight (LMW) forms. Paradoxically, due to ease of hepatic production and secretion of the LMW isoforms as compared to HMW isoforms,

TABLE 34.4 Characteristics of Human Plasma Lipoproteins

Variable	Chylomicron	VLDL	IDL	LDL	HDL	Lp(a)
Density, g/mL	<0.95	0.95–1.006	1.006–1.019	1.019–1.063	1.063–1.210	1.040–1.130
Electrophoretic mobility	Origin	Pre-β	Between β and pre-β	β	α	Pre-β
Approximate Molecular weight, Da	$0.4–30 \times 10^9$	$5–10 \times 10^6$	$3.9–4.8 \times 10^6$	2.75×10^6	$1.8–3.6 \times 10^5$	$2.9–3.7 \times 10^6$
Diameter, nm	>70	27–70	22–24	19–23	4–10	27–30
Lipid-lipoprotein ratio	99:1	90:10	85:15	80:20	50:50	75:27–64:36
Major lipids	Exogenous triglycerides	Endogenous triglycerides	Endogenous triglycerides, cholesteryl esters	Cholesteryl esters	Phospholipids	Cholesteryl esters, phospholipids
Major proteins	A-I	B-100	B-100	B-100	A-I	(a)
	B-48	C-I	E	—	A-II	B-100
	C-I	C-II	—	—	—	—
	C-II	C-III	—	—	—	—
	C-III	E	—	—	—	—

HDL, High-density lipoprotein; *IDL*, intermediate-density lipoprotein; *LDL*, low-density lipoprotein; *Lp(a)*, lipoprotein(a); *VLDL*, very low-density lipoprotein.

TABLE 34.5 Chemical Composition (%) of Normal Human Plasma Lipoproteins*

	SURFACE COMPONENTS			CORE LIPIDS	
	Cholesterol	Phospholipids	Apolipoproteins	Triglycerides	Cholesteryl Esters
Chylomicrons	2	7	2	86	3
VLDL	7	18	8	55	12
IDL	9	19	19	23	29
LDL	8	22	22	6	42
HDL_2	5	33	40	5	17
HDL_3	4	25	55	3	13

*Surface components and core lipids given as percentage of dry mass.
HDL, High-density lipoprotein; *IDL*, intermediate-density lipoprotein; *LDL*, low-density lipoprotein; *VLDL*, very low-density lipoprotein.
From Havel RJ, Kane JP. Introduction: Structure and metabolism of plasma lipoproteins. In: Scriver CR, Beaudet AL, Sly WS, Valle D, editors. *The metabolic and molecular bases of inherited diseases*. 7th ed., vol. II. New York: McGraw-Hill; 1995:1841–50. Reproduced with permission of The McGraw-Hill Companies.

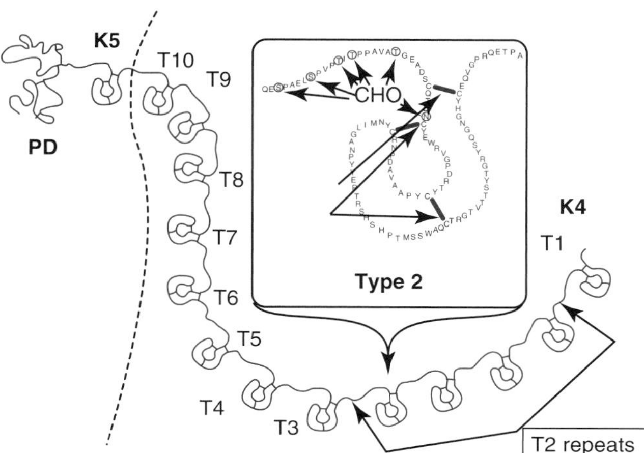

FIGURE 34.17 Structure of apolipoprotein(a). *K*, Kringle type; *T*, kringle subtype; *PD*, protease domain.

there can be significant discordance between Lp(a) mass and Lp(a) particle concentrations (Lp(a)-P). At the same Lp(a) mass, those with LMW isoforms will have a higher Lp(a)-P concentration than those with HMW isoforms. It is believed that LMW isoforms are more atherogenic than HMW, but this may be mostly related to their greater Lp(a)-P concentration than to anything inherent in the particle. Further confusing the picture is the codominant type of inheritance that occurs with Lp(a), with patients frequently having two different types of apo(a)-size isoforms. Lp(a) is now widely recognized as one of the most proatherogenic lipoproteins because it has some of the same features of an LDL particle but also has other functions that can promote atherogenesis, such as modulating fibrinolysis and the tissue factor pathway, and it is one of the main carriers of oxidized phospholipids.[28]

Although all lipoproteins, even in the fasting state, transport some triglycerides, most plasma triglycerides are present in VLDL. In the postprandial state, chylomicrons appear transiently and contribute significantly to the total plasma triglyceride concentration. In contrast, LDL normally carries about 70% of total plasma cholesterol but relatively small amounts of triglyceride (see Table 34.5). HDL contains about

TABLE 34.6 **Classification and Properties of Major Human Plasma Apolipoproteins**

Apolipoprotein	Molecular Weight, Da	Chromosomal Location	Function	Lipoprotein Carrier(s)
Apo A-I	29,016	11	Cofactor LCAT	Chylomicron, HDL
Apo A-II	17,414	1	Not known	HDL
Apo A-IV	44,465	11	Activates LCAT	Chylomicron, HDL
Apo B-100	512,723	2	Secretion of triglyceride from liver binding protein to LDL receptor	VLDL, IDL, LDL
Apo B-48	240,800	2	Secretion of triglyceride from intestine	Chylomicron
Apo C-I	6630	19	Activates LCAT Inhibits clearance of chylomicrons	Chylomicron, VLDL, HDL
Apo C-II	8900	19	Cofactor LPL	Chylomicron, VLDL, HDL
Apo C-III	8800	11	Inhibits clearance of chylomicrons	Chylomicron, VLDL, LDL HDL
Apo E	34,145	19	Facilitates uptake of chylomicron remnant and IDL	Chylomicron, VLDL, LDL HDL
Apo(a)	187,000-662,000	6	Unknown	Lp(a)

HDL, High-density lipoprotein; *IDL,* intermediate-density lipoprotein; *LCAT,* lecithin cholesterol acyltransferase; *LDL,* low-density lipoprotein; *Lp(a),* lipoprotein(a); *LPL,* lipoprotein lipase; *VLDL,* very low-density lipoprotein.

20% to 30% of plasma cholesterol and also only a small amount of triglycerides. In pathologic states characterized by hypertriglyceridemia, both LDL and HDL, however, acquire increased core triglycerides, which promotes their lipolyis and the generation of smaller, denser forms of LDL and HDL.

Lipoproteins can also be separated electrophorectically according to charge, size, or both, on agarose or on other solid support material, such as cellulose acetate, paper, or polyacrylamide gels.[29] At a pH of 8.6, HDL migrates with the α-globulins, LDL with the β-globulins, and VLDL and Lp(a) between the α- and β-globulins, in the pre–β-globulin region. IDL forms a broad band between β- and pre–β-globulins. Chylomicrons remain at the point of application. This forms the basis for the following common classification of lipoproteins: pre–β-lipoprotein, VLDL; β-lipoprotein, LDL; and α-lipoprotein, HDL.

Apolipoproteins

Apolipoproteins are the protein components of lipoproteins, and their physical characteristics and main functions are summarized in Table 34.6. Each class of lipoprotein has a variety of apolipoproteins in differing proportions, with the exception of LDL, which contains mostly apo B-100. Apo A-I is the major protein in HDL. Apo C-I, C-II, C-III, and E are present in various proportions in all lipoproteins. Apolipoproteins collectively have three major physiologic functions: activating important enzymes in the lipoprotein metabolic pathways, maintaining the structural integrity of the lipoprotein complex, and facilitating uptake of lipoprotein into cells through their recognition by specific cell surface receptors.[30] Besides these main apolipoproteins, lipoproteins have been found to weakly bind a large number of other plasma proteins, but their relevance to lipoprotein metabolism is not fully understood at this time.[31]

Apolipoprotein A

Most apolipoproteins, including those in the apo A family, contain a structural motif called an *amphipathic helix.* It is an α-helix with approximately half the amino acid residues comprising hydrophobic amino acids, which face toward the neutral lipid core when bound to a lipoprotein particle. The other side of the helix faces outward toward the surface of a lipoprotein particle and contains polar or charged amino acids. In general, the binding of amphipathic helices to lipoproteins is relatively weak, thus allowing apolipoproteins to readily exchange between different lipoproteins during their metabolism.

Together, apolipoprotein A-I and apo A-II constitute about 90% of total HDL protein. The ratio of apo A-I to A-II in HDL is about 3 : 1.[32] In addition to being an important structural component of HDL, apo A-I is a ligand for the major cellular membrane sterol efflux protein, ATP binding cassette transporter A1 (ABCA1).[33] It is also a cofactor for LCAT, the enzyme responsible for esterifying free cholesterol, a crucial step in the maturation and remodeling of HDL.[34] Apo A-I can be present in from one to five copies per HDL particle, and it is the degree of twisting of apo A-I around the HDL particle surface that modulates particle size.[35] Apo A-I on spherical HDL particles has been proposed to exist in a trefoil configuration when three copies are present, but it can accommodate more copies in a similar structural arrangement.[35] A relatively small amount of Apo A-I has also been described on highly atherogenic, ultra-small, highly oxidized LDL particles.[36]

The exact role of apo A-II is unclear, but there is some evidence that it inhibits LCAT and activates hepatic triglyceride lipase. Apo A-II can also delay the lipolysis of large TG-rich lipoproteins by interfering with lipoprotein lipase.[37] Apo A-IV, which is found in the apo A-I/C-III/A-IV gene cluster on chromosome 11, is synthesized in the intestine and is secreted as a component of chylomicrons. Chylomicrons may contain a variable number of apo A-IV proteins, which may allow it to exist in a wide spectrum of sizes. Apo A-IV may also contribute to the lipolysis of lipoproteins by facilitating the release of apo C-II from either HDL or VLDL.[38,39] Other potential functions of apo A-IV are activation of LCAT,[40] promoting intestinal lipid absorption as well as satiety through a hypothalamic effect.[38] Another recently recognized apolipoprotein is Apo A-V.[41] It is relatively low in abundance compared with other apolipoproteins and appears to modulate triglyceride concentrations by several mechanisms, including modulating VLDL secretion. Apo A-V, as part of TG-rich lipoprotein, also traffics with the particle and binds to glycosylphosphatidylinositol-anchored high-density lipoprotein binding protein 1, thus facilitating its interaction with lipoprotein lipase.[41,42] Several polymorphisms of apo A-V have been associated with hypertriglyceridemia.[43]

Apolipoprotein B

As already discussed, apolipoprotein B exists in two forms: apo B-100 and apo B-48.[30] In the fasting state, most of the apo B in plasma is apo B-100. Apo B-100, a single polypeptide of more than 4500 amino acids, is the full-length translation product of the *APOB* gene. In humans, apo B-100 is made in the liver and is secreted into plasma as part of VLDL, IDL, or LDL.[44] Apo B-100 is also the major apolipoprotein of LDL and its measurement can serve as a surrogate for LDL particle concentration (LDL-P).[45] Unlike other apolipoproteins, however, apo B-100 is not transferable and cannot move from one lipoprotein particle to another because in addition to amphipathic helices, it has β-sheets[46]—a structural motif with much higher affinity for lipids. It is for this reason that apo B-100 remains bound with VLDL as it is transformed by lipolysis into LDL.

Apo B-48 contains 2152 amino acids and is identical to the amino-terminal portion of apo B-100. Apo B-48 results from posttranscriptional modification of internal apo B-100 messenger ribonucleic acid, in which a single base substitution produces a stop codon corresponding to residue 2153 of apo B-100. Apo B-48 is made in the intestine and is the major apo B component of chylomicrons. Both apo B-100 and apo B-48 play important roles in the secretion of VLDL and chylomicrons, respectively. Apo B-100 is recognized by the LDL receptor in hepatic and peripheral tissues; it allows the LDL receptor-mediated internalization of LDL[47] (see sections on lipoprotein metabolism, endogenous and exogenous pathways). Apo C-III and apo(a) can camouflage the LDL receptor binding domain, hindering the LDL receptor mediated clearance of apo C-III–containing particles and Lp(a), respectively.[44,48]

Apolipoprotein C

The apolipoprotein C family mainly consists of three closely related proteins—apo C-I, apo C-II, and apo C-III—that are mostly made by the liver and, to a lesser degree, in the intestine. Another member of this family—apo C-IV—does not appear to be present in significant amounts in human serum. Apolipoproteins C-I and C-II are associated with all lipoproteins except LDL, whereas apo C-III is also found on LDL. Apo C-I, the smallest of the C apolipoproteins with 57 amino acids, has been reported to activate LCAT and is also known to inhibit LPL, hepatic lipase (HL), phospholipase A2, and CETP.[49] In fact, it accounts for most of the CETP-inhibitory activity found in human plasma HDL. Apo C-II, consisting of 78 amino acids, plays an important role in the metabolism of triglyceride-rich lipoprotein (VLDL and chylomicrons) by acting as an activator of lipoprotein lipase.[50] Because of differences in sialic acid content, apo C-III, a 79 amino acid glycoprotein, exists in at least three different isoforms termed 0, 1, and 2. Apo C-III_1 and apo C-III_2 correlate more with TG levels than apo C-III_0, and apo C-III_2 is also associated with generation of small LDL.[51] Recent studies reveal that apo C-III stimulates VLDL assembly and secretion and interferes with VLDL receptor, LDL-receptor–related protein (LRP), and LDL receptor uptake of lipoproteins but does not, as previously thought, decrease lipolysis by direct inhibition of LPL.[52] In hypertriglyceridemia, most VLDL is secreted with apo C-III but without apo E, and such particles are not cleared until they lose apo C-III during lipolytic conversion to dense LDL.[44] LDLs that contain apo C-III were particularly atherogenic in the CARE study Physicians Health Study and Women's Health Study.[53,54] Apo C-III is also implicated in several inflammatory pathways. Mendelian randomization studies have shown loss-of-function mutations in *APOCIII* to be linked to favorable lipid profiles and lower incidence of coronary artery disease. Antisense therapy with oligonucleotides that interfere with apo C-III synthesis are in clinical trials.[55]

Apolipoprotein E

Apolipoprotein E is a 34-kDa plasma glycoprotein containing 299 amino acids. It is synthesized primarily by the liver but is also produced locally by many other tissues and cell types, such as in the brain and by macrophages. ApoE is found on all lipoproteins, but only a small amount is on LDL. Removal of apo E–bearing lipoproteins is mediated by several different cellular receptors that recognize a cluster of positively charged amino acids in a specific region of apo E. It regulates lipoprotein uptake in the liver through the interaction of a wide variety of receptors, such as the chylomicron remnant receptor, the LDL receptor-related protein, and the LDL receptor. It also promotes the interaction of lipoproteins with proteoglycans.[30]

Three common apo E isoforms, designated E_2, E_3, and E_4, can be separated by isoelectric-focusing electrophoresis. These isoforms have amino acid substitutions at residues 112 and 158. Apo E_2 has cysteine residues in both positions, and apo E_4 has arginine residues in both positions, whereas apo E_3 has cysteine and arginine at positions 112 and 158, respectively. Apo E_2 has reduced binding affinity for the B and/or E remnant receptor compared with apo E_3, which can result in the accumulation of apo E–containing lipoprotein in the circulation.[56] In contrast, apo E_4–containing lipoproteins are cleared more rapidly than those containing apo E_3. These isoforms are coded for by three alleles of the apo E gene: ε2, ε3, and ε4. The ε3 allele is most frequent, although relative proportions of the three alleles vary among populations.[57-59] These apo E alleles have been shown to contribute significantly to the variability of LDL-C and apo B-100 concentrations within populations.[60] Individuals with at least one ε2 allele tend to have lower concentrations of apo B-100 and LDL-C than do those who are homozygous for the ε3 allele, whereas individuals with at least one ε4 allele tend to have higher concentrations of apo B-100 and LDL-C. This most likely occurs because increased hepatic uptake of lipoproteins in the presence of the ε4 allele leads to an increase in hepatic cholesterol and downregulation of the LDL receptor. Apo E_4 is also associated with increased cholesterol absorption. In the distant past, this may have offered a selective evolutionary advantage for humans on calorie-restricted and low-fat diets, but it now appears to be a disadvantage in regards to CHD risk with our current diets. Statin hyporesponsiveness has often been noted in apo E4 patients, which may be related to

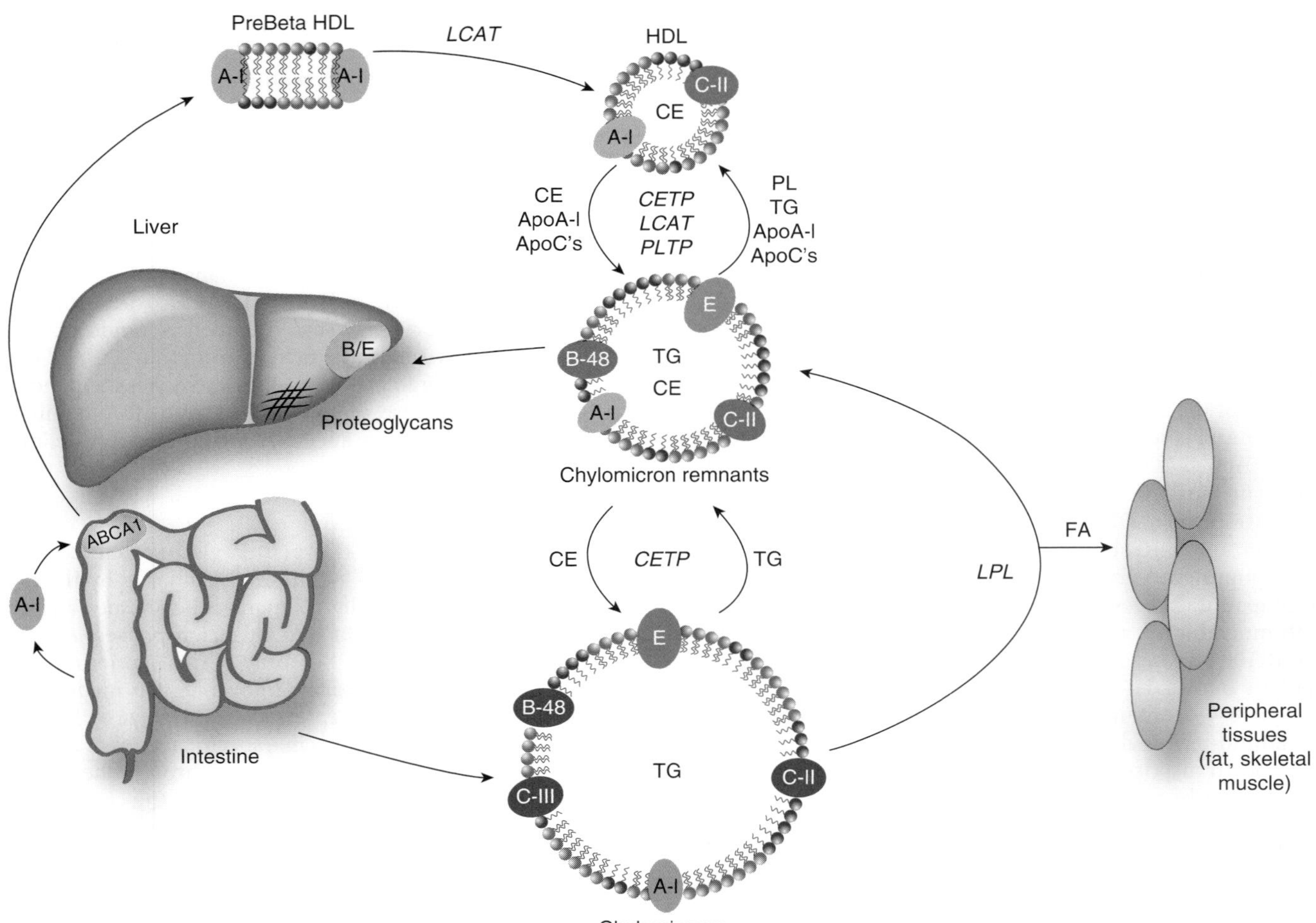

FIGURE 34.18 Intestinal (exogenous) lipoprotein metabolism pathway. *A-1,* Apolipoprotein A-I; *ABCA1,* ATP binding cassette transporter A1; *B-48,* apolipoprotein B-48; *B/E,* ApoB- and ApoE-dependent receptors; *C-II,* apolipoprotein C-II; *CE,* cholesterol ester; *CETP,* cholesterol ester transfer protein; *E,* apolipoprotein E; *FA,* fatty acid; *FC,* free cholesterol; *HDL,* high-density lipoprotein; *LCAT,* lecithin:cholesterol acyltransferase; *LPL,* lipoprotein lipase; *PL,* phospholipid; *PLTP,* phospholipid transfer protein; *TG,* triglyceride.

the lesser efficacy of statins in patients who hyperabsorb cholesterol.[3] A metaanalysis of 24 trials, however, suggested there was little clinical utility for APOE genetic testing for guiding treatment with statins.[61] In addition, patients with APOE 4 alleles have also been reported to respond to fish oil supplementation, with a paradoxical increase in LDL-C, but this also has not held up in larger studies.[62]

Epidemiologically, the apo E_4 allele has been strongly associated with Alzheimer's disease and other neurologic diseases,[63] but newer data suggest that risk is not isoform dependent but rather apo E concentration related.[64,65] This association is likely related to the role of apo E in modulating lipid metabolism in the brain, but the exact connection between apo E_4 and neurologic disease is not known.

Lipoprotein Metabolism

The various pathways of lipoprotein metabolism are complex and intersect at several points. They include the intestinal or hepatic pathways, which are based on whether the lipoprotein involved in these pathways transport lipids from dietary (exogenous) or hepatic (endogenous) origin (Figs. 34.18 and 34.19). Other key pathways are the intracellular LDL receptor pathway (Fig. 34.20) and the HDL-mediated cholesterol (reverse cholesterol transport) pathway (Fig. 34.21).

Intestinal (Exogenous) Pathway

The primary function of the intestinal pathway has been described to be the absorption of dietary lipid and its delivery, particularly triglyceride, to peripheral tissues and the liver. This pathway begins when nascent chylomicrons are assembled from dietary triglycerides and cholesterol in the enterocytes and stored in secretory vesicles in the Golgi apparatus. Chylomicrons are released by exocytosis into the extracellular space and enter the circulation by way of lymphatic ducts. The lipid content of nascent chylomicrons consists mainly of triglycerides (90% by mass) and only a small amount of protein, mostly apo B-48 and the A apolipoproteins (2% by mass).[66] Shortly after secretion, these lipoprotein particles quickly acquire the C apolipoproteins and apo E from circulating HDL (see Fig. 34.18). Apo C-II on

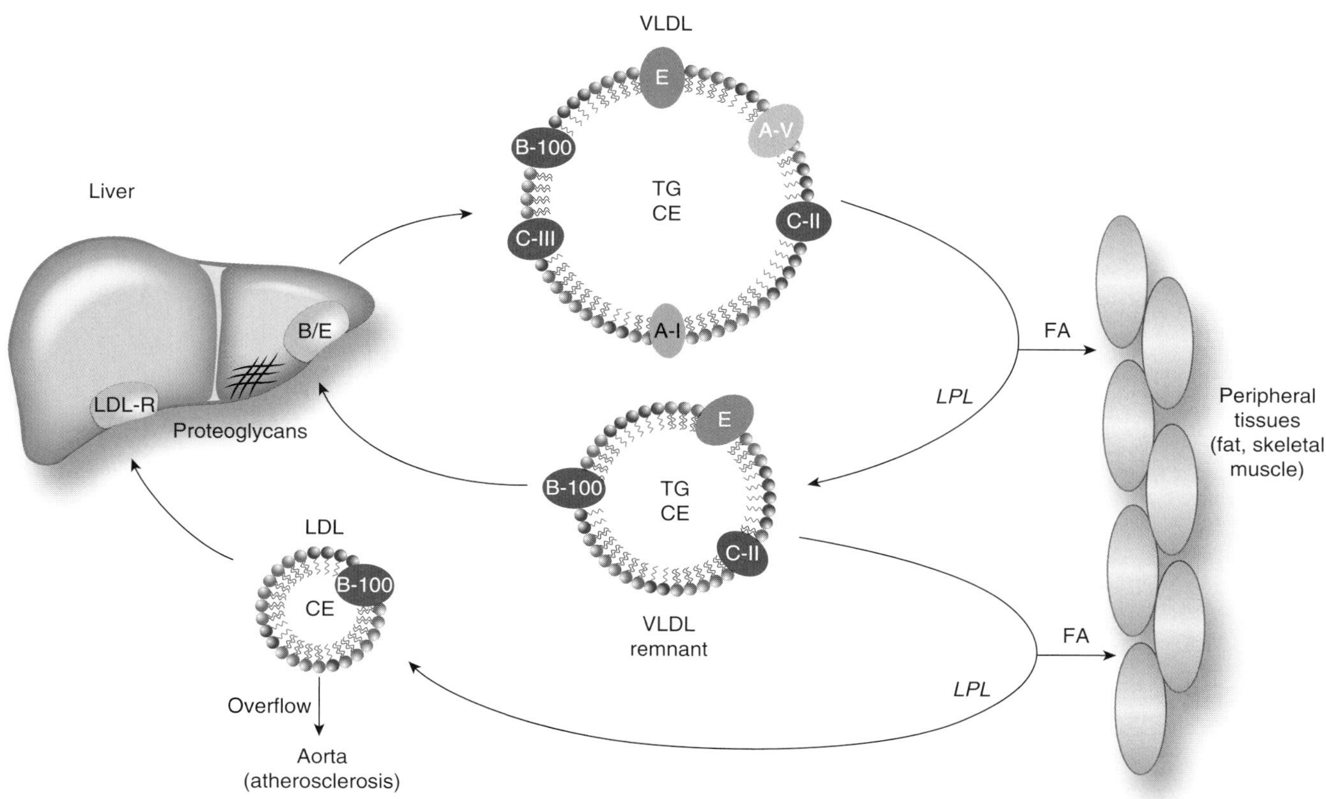

FIGURE 34.19 Hepatic (endogenous) lipoprotein metabolism pathway. *A-1,* Apolipoprotein A-I; *A-V,* apolipoprotein A-V; *B-100,* apolipoprotein B-100; *B/E,* ApoB- and ApoE-dependent receptors; *C,* apolipoprotein C-II; *CE,* cholesterol ester; *E,* apolipoprotein E; *FA,* fatty acid; *FC,* free cholesterol; *HDL,* high-density lipoprotein; *IDL,* intermediate-density lipoprotein; *LCAT,* lecithin cholesterol acyltransferase; *LDL,* low-density lipoprotein; *LDLR,* low-density lipoprotein receptor; *LPL,* lipoprotein lipase; *PL,* phospholipid; *TG,* triglyceride; *VLDL,* very low-density lipoproteins.

the surface of chylomicrons promotes lipolysis of TG by activation of lipoprotein lipase (LPL), which is mostly attached to the luminal surface of endothelial cells. The released fatty acids generated by lipolyis associate with albumin and can be taken up by muscle cells as an energy source or into adipose cells for storage. Simultaneously, some of the phospholipids on chylomicrons are transferred back to HDL during this process. The partially lipolyzed chylomicrons, called the chylomicron remnants, are smaller and contain 10% to 20% less triglyceride than the original nascent chylomicron. Because of the presence of apo B-48 and apo E on their surface, chylomicron remnants are recognized by specific hepatic remnant receptors and are quickly internalized within hours by receptor-mediated endocytosis and are further hydrolyzed within the lysosomes. Proteoglycans in the hepatic sinusoids also contribute to the uptake of lipoproteins. Cholesterol that enters hepatocytes can be used in bile acid synthesis, incorporated into newly synthesized lipoprotein, effluxed to apo A-I particles, secreted directly into the bile, or stored as cholesteryl ester. Furthermore, cholesterol from chylomicron remnant uptake downregulates HMG-CoA reductase, the rate-limiting enzyme of cholesterol biosynthesis (see earlier section on cholesterol synthesis).

With respect to cholesterol, the vast majority (85% to 90%) of cholesterol that enters the intestinal lumen is from endogenous, not dietary (exogenous), sources.[67] Large amounts of endogenously produced cholesterol enters the gut lumen via hepatobiliary delivery; direct intestinal secretion routes, termed *transintestinal cholesterol efflux* (TICE); or enterocyte membrane shedding of cholesterol.[67] After absorption, cholesterol is used in chylomicron formation or in the formation of nascent HDL by a process dependent on the ABCA1 transporter. Further complicating the issue about the source of cholesterol is that intestinally absorbed, exogenous fatty acids of exogenous origin, which are first incorporated into enterocyte as TG in chylomicrons, immediately after entering the circulation start exchanging TG by the cholesteryl ester transfer protein with other lipoproteins. In this way the endogenously produced lipoproteins produced by the liver (VLDL, IDL, LDL, and HDL) rapidly acquire and traffic exogenous lipids as well.

Hepatic (Endogenous) Pathway

The hepatic pathway is involved with the delivery of lipids that are packaged in the liver to peripheral cells (see Fig. 34.19). As discussed previously, however, chylomicrons also deliver endogenously produced cholesterol, and much of the lipoprotein transport of lipids is not only to peripheral cells but also back to the gut or liver. When dietary cholesterol acquired from the receptor-mediated uptake of chylomicron

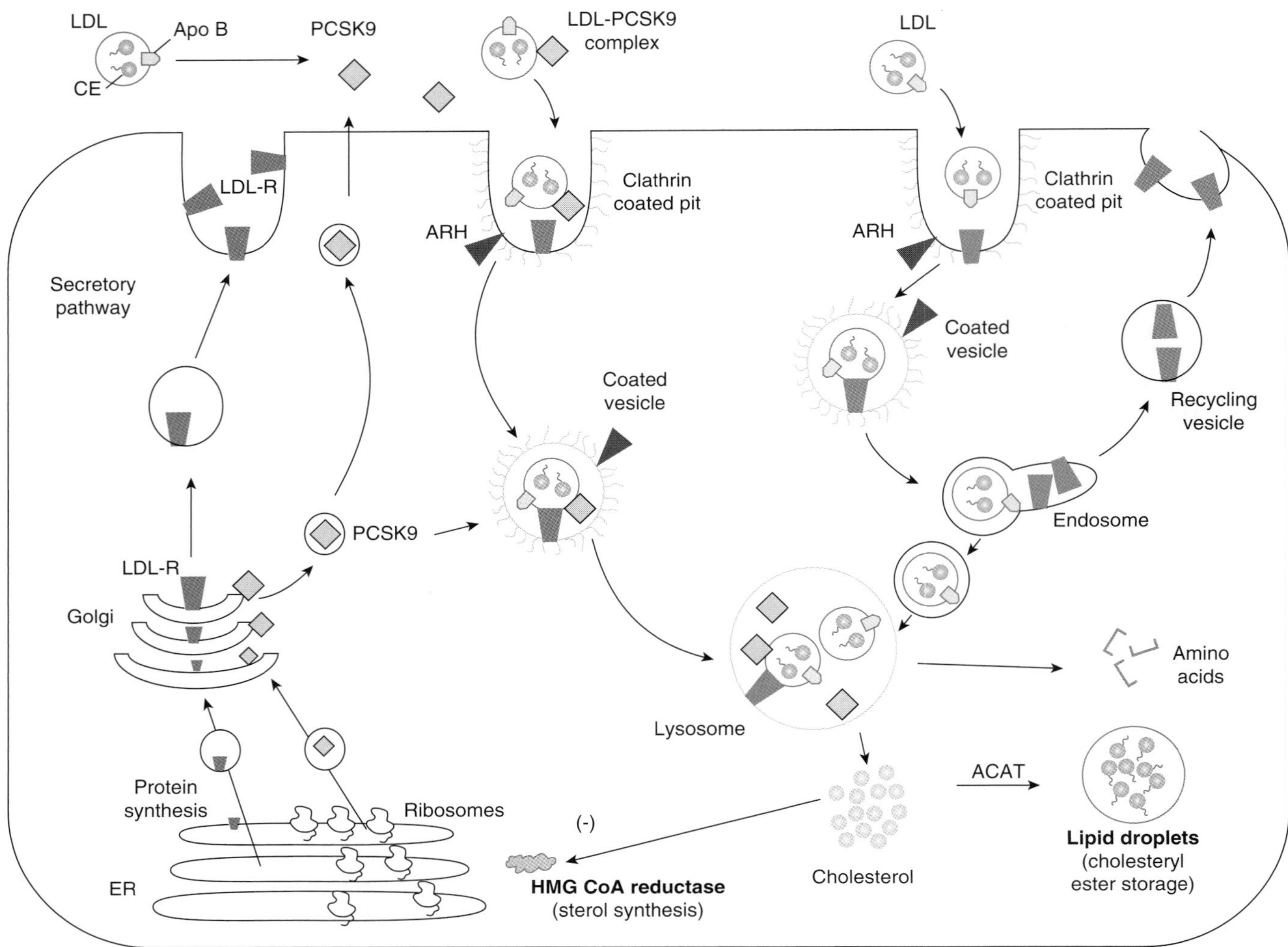

FIGURE 34.20 Low-density lipoprotein receptor pathway. *ACAT,* Acyl-CoA cholesterol acyltransferase; *Apo B,* apolipoprotein B-100; *ARH,* autosomal recessive hypercholesterolemia adaptor protein, *HMG-CoA reductase,* 3-hydroxy-3-methylglutaryl coenzyme A reductase; *LDL,* low-density lipoprotein; *LDL-R,* low-density lipoprotein receptor; *PCSK9,* proprotein convertase subtilisin/kexin type 9.

remnants is insufficient, hepatocytes can also synthesize their own cholesterol by increasing the activity of HMG-CoA reductase or acquire cholesterol via internalization of LDL particles or through the delipidation of HDL particles when it interacts with the scavenger receptor B1 (SR-BI). Endogenously made triglycerides and acquired or synthesized cholesterol are packaged along with apo B-100 into VLDL particles in the endoplasmic reticulum in a step involving the microsomal transfer protein. A total loss of function of the microsomal transfer protein results in the inability to secrete apo B–containing lipoproteins and is referred to as *abetalipoproteinemia.* VLDL is a triglyceride-rich particle (55% by mass) that contains apo B-100 and variable amounts of apo E and C apolipoproteins. The liver may also directly secrete a small amount of IDL and LDL with or without apo E and C-III.[44] Additional C apolipoproteins may be transferred from HDL to VLDL after it enters the circulation. As in the case of chylomicron metabolism, apo C-II present on the surface of VLDL activates LPL on endothelial cells, which leads to the hydrolysis of VLDL triglycerides and the release of free fatty acids. During lipolysis, the particle reduces in size, and excess surface phospholipids may be removed by the phospholipid transfer protein and transferred to HDL. It is important to note, however, that the rate of hydrolysis of VLDL triglyceride is significantly lower than that of chylomicron triglyceride. The much larger chylomicrons have many more copies of apo C-II per particle than do VLDLs, thus enhancing its binding to LPL and enhancing its clearance. The average residence time of VLDL triglyceride is 15 to 60 minutes, compared with only 5 to 10 minutes for chylomicron triglyceride.

During lipolytic catabolism of VLDL, as surface PL and core TG are hydrolyzed and CETP mediates the exchange of core TG for CE with other lipoproteins, the VLDL reduces in size allowing the C and other apolipoproteins to transfer to HDL, resulting in smaller CE-rich remnant VLDL remnants that can be taken up by the liver or continue down the lipolytic cascade where they are converted to smaller, denser IDL particles, which can be removed by hepatic remnant receptors that recognize apoE. Alternatively, VLDL remnants can be removed from the circulation after interaction with hepatic proteoglycans and then can be directly internalized by cells

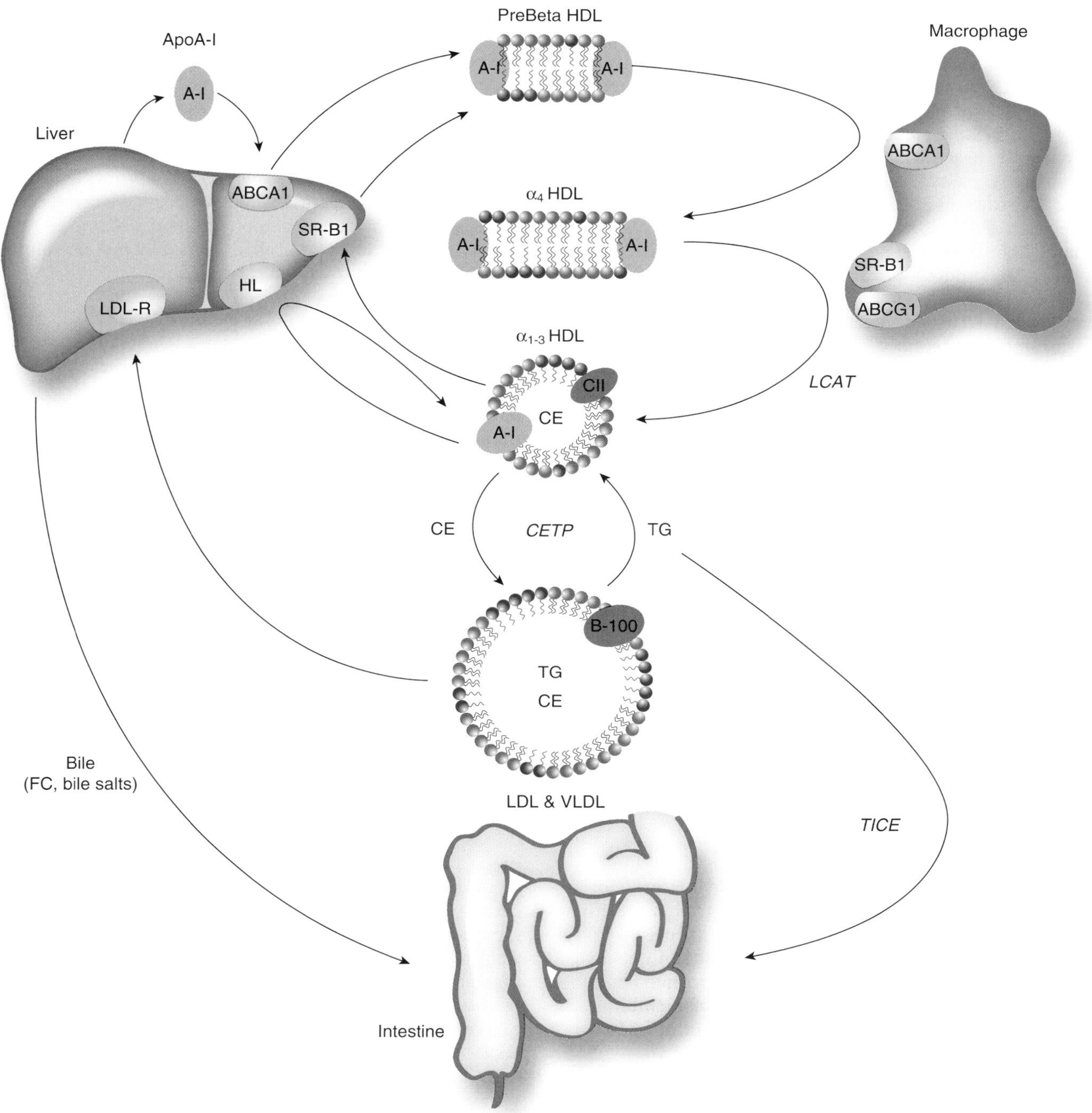

FIGURE 34.21 Reverse-cholesterol transport pathway. *ABCA1,* ATP binding cassette transporter A1; *ABCG1,* ATP binding cassette transporter GI; *A-I,* apolipoprotein A-1; *B,* apolipoprotein B-100; *CE,* cholesterol ester; *CETP,* cholesteryl ester transfer protein; *FC,* free cholesterol; *HL,* hepatic lipase; *HDL,* high-density lipoprotein; *LCAT,* lecithin cholesterol acyltransferase; *LDL,* low-density lipoprotein; *LDL-R,* LDL receptor; *SR-B1,* scavenger receptor B-I; *TG,* triglyceride; *TICE,* transintestinal cholesterol excretion; *VLDL,* very low-density lipoproteins.

or possibly transferred to hepatic remnant receptors for uptake. Both VLDL remnants and IDL contribute to the return of cholesterol to the liver in a process termed *indirect reverse cholesterol transport.* The lipolytic fates of VLDL and IDL are highly dependent on their content of apo C-III and E.[44] As VLDL and IDL are depleted of core triglycerides, excess surface components, such as phospholipids, free cholesterol, and apolipoproteins, are transferred to existing HDL or are used in the generation of de novo HDL particles when they form complexes with lipid-free apo A-I.

CE molecules are also transferred from HDL to LDL by cholesteryl ester transfer protein (CETP) in exchange for triglyceride and this exchange can be inhibited by lipid transfer inhibitory protein or apolipoprotein F.[68] This transfer of neutral lipids from apo A-I to apo B particles is termed *heterotypic exchange* in contrast to the homotypic exchange that occurs between different apo A-I particles or between different apo B particles. The net result of the coupled lipolysis and CE exchange reaction is the replacement of much of the triglyceride core of the original VLDL with CE. In humans, about half of IDL is removed by the liver, and the other half undergoes further hydrolysis, leading to the generation of LDL. Most LDL and its cholesterol content are eventually returned to the liver or intestine by the LDL receptor or by nonreceptor-mediated clearance,[69,70] but when present in excess, LDL particles, independent of size, infiltrate into the vessel wall, where they accumulate and can cause atherosclerosis.

Low-Density Lipoprotein Receptor Pathway

The mechanism by which LDL is removed from the circulation is reasonably well understood and primarily occurs via both the LDL receptor and nonreceptor pathways.[70] Compared with VLDL and chylomicrons, LDL has a relatively long residence time in the circulation of about 3 days.[71] Specific receptors present on plasma membranes recognize and bind apo B-100 or apo E when present on LDL (see Figs. 34.19 and 34.20). LDL in the circulation can acquire a hepatic secreted protein called proprotein convertase subtilisin kexin type 9 (PCSK9).[72] LDL particles (with or without PCSK9) bind to membrane-expressed LDL receptors via the LDL-receptor binding domain on apo B-100 and then are internalized in clathrin-coated pits and fuse with endosomes, which are mediated by a protein called the autosomal recessive hypercholesterolemia (ARH) clathrin adaptor protein. If PCSK9 is present on the complex, it directs the LDL receptor to a catabolic pathway, and the receptor is degraded. Without PCSK9, the lipids are catabolized, but the LDL-receptor protein is recycled back to the cell membrane, allowing for more efficient removal of LDL from the circulation.[72] Once LDL is delivered to the lysosome, apo B-100 is degraded into small peptides and amino acids. CE is hydrolyzed to free cholesterol, making it available for the synthesis of cell membranes, steroid hormone synthesis in endocrine tissues, or bile acid synthesis in hepatocytes.

Cells have multiple pathways for regulating their cholesterol content, most likely because of the cytotoxicity of excess cholesterol. Oversupply of unesterified cholesterol (1) decreases the rate of endogenous cholesterol synthesis by inhibiting the rate-limiting enzyme HMG-CoA reductase; (2) increases the formation of CE from unesterified cholesterol, catalyzed by ACAT; and (3) inhibits the synthesis of new LDL receptors by suppressing transcription. Many different intracellular pathways are also available for coordinated gene regulation of cholesterol metabolism, but the sterol regulatory element-binding protein (SREBP) transcription factors, which sense intracellular cholesterol concentrations, appear to play the most central role.[73]

Under normal circumstances some LDL is taken up by extrahepatic tissue, mostly steroidogenic tissue and adipocytes, through LDL receptors, scavenger receptors B1, or non-receptor-mediated pinocytosis. Non-receptor-mediated uptake becomes important as plasma LDL concentrations increase, as in familial hypercholesterolemia (FH). Nonreceptor-mediated uptake is not saturable and is not regulated and is probably largely due to the interaction of LDL with hepatic proteoglycans. Scavenger receptor A is also unregulated, and some recognize LDL that has been modified in various ways, such as by oxidation. Scavenger receptors A are largely found in macrophages; this probably accounts for the accumulation of lipid that occurs in these cells in atherosclerotic plaque. Macrophages that become engorged with cholesteryl esters are called *foam cells* and are found in xanthomas and in atherosclerotic plaques.

Reverse Cholesterol Transfer Pathway

The traditional concept of reverse cholesterol transport (RCT) pathway has recently undergone radical rethinking and might be better described as HDL-mediated trafficking of cholesterol. Historically, RCT was thought to help the body maintain cholesterol homeostasis by removing excess cholesterol from peripheral cells and delivering it to the liver for excretion. It was believed to be mediated mostly by HDL, thus accounting for its antiatherogenic property.[74] Recent evidence shows that this pathway is a much more complicated, dynamic process involving every other lipoprotein, including LDL, the intestine, and other organs and pools of cholesterol. Total RCT is the sum of direct and indirect pathways, which ultimately relocates or rids the body of unneeded sterols.[18]

This pathway begins when lipid-poor apolipoprotein A-I (apo A-I) is secreted from the liver or the small intestine. Apo A-I rapidly acquires phospholipid and cholesterol from cells by the ATP binding cassette transporter 1 (ABCA1).[74] ABCA1 is believed to pump excess cholesterol and other lipids to the outer surface of the plasma membrane, where apo A-I, in a detergent-like extraction process, removes phospholipid and cholesterol and forms nascent HDL. The form of HDL produced in this process is discoidal in shape and is named preβ-HDL based on its electrophoretic migration. Preβ-HDL forms a flat phospholipid disc in a bilayer-like configuration because it is relatively deplete in neutral core lipids like triglycerides and cholesteryl esters. Two molecules of apo A-I stabilize preβ-HDL by wrapping around the sides of the phospholipid bilayer. Although the majority of HDL formed by this process occurs in the liver and intestine, ABCA1 is also present in peripheral cells and enables them to efflux excess cholesterol to HDL. This is believed to result in the generation of a larger discoidal species of HDL called $alpha_4$-HDL. Because the majority of cholesterol within HDL is of hepatic origin, the particles have to be performing more than just RCT back to the liver, so the concept has recently emerged that HDLs traffic cholesterol in numerous directions and help the body equilibrate cholesterol among the various tissue pools. Hepatic lipase and SR-BI are believed responsible for regenerating smaller spherical forms of HDL and preβ-HDL, respectively, from mature HDL to restart this cycle.

As HDL acquires cholesterol, lecithin-cholesterol acyltransferase (LCAT-α) esterifies cholesterol by transferring fatty acids from the sn-2 position of neighboring phospholipids (PL), generating lysophospholipid and the much more hydrophobic CE.[34] CE then moves to the core of HDL, thereby transforming it from a discoidal to a spherical shape, which is the shape found in mature HDL. Lysolecithin is removed from the surface of lipoproteins by binding with albumin.

The larger spherical forms of HDL, which are sometimes called $alpha_{1-3}$-HDL based on its electrophoretic migration, can also acquire additional cholesterol by other cellular membrane transporters, such as by ABCG1 and the bidirectional sterol membrane CE transporter, scavenger receptor-B1 (SR-B1). As it matures, HDL can also acquire surface PL from phospholipid transfer protein, and smaller HDL particles can fuse, creating even larger species.[75] Large HDL particles can also acquire unesterified cholesterol from cells via free diffusion[76] or from other lipoproteins, erythrocyte membranes, or albumin-trafficked cholesterol. During this process, numerous serum proteins and other lipid moieties can also attach to various subsets of HDL particles, which may contribute in some way to its antiatherogenic function.[77]

With respect to cardioprotection, the likely most important cholesterol-related function of HDL is delipidation of arterial wall sterol-laden macrophages called foam cells. This process, termed *macrophage reverse cholesterol transport*, is accomplished by both free diffusion and the ABCA1 and G1 and SR-B1 mediated efflux.[76] Interestingly, although the amount of cholesterol effluxed is related to benefit, the amount of cholesterol removed in this process is so small that it has a negligible effect on the total pool of HDL-C, thus limiting its use as a marker of this process.[78]

Circulating cholesterol-rich, PL-rich, TG-poor HDLs have several options in dispensing their lipid cargo. CE can be transferred to other lipoproteins in exchange for TG via CETP. In this process, HDL particles can transfer CE to apo B–containing particles in a process called *heterotypic exchange* or to other HDL species in a process called *homotypic exchange*.[79] Because it is by far the most numerous apo B–containing particle, much of the CE-TG exchange comes between HDLs and LDLs. Potent CETP-inhibitors, which not only dramatically raise HDL-C but also significantly reduce LDL-C, suggest that a substantial number of the cholesterol molecules within LDLs derive from HDLs.[80,81] Modulation of the CETP-mediated exchange between LDL and HDL may occur by apolipoprotein F.[68] After receiving CE from HDL, LDL and other apo B–containing particles can traffic it to the liver or intestine in a pathway called indirect RCT. Additional options for HDL trafficking of cholesterol is direct delivery by SR-B1–mediated uptake to the liver or steroidogenic tissues or adipocytes, which serve as a cholesterol storage organ. HDL particles may also participate in direct RCT by other putative hepatic-located receptors, such as the holoparticle or mitochondrial-produced ATP synthase β-subunit,[82] or by apo E receptor–mediated removal.

The liver has many options for the "directly or indirectly" acquired cholesterol: use it in its cell membranes, convert it to bile acids, lipidate the newly forming VLDL, efflux it to apo A-I, or directly excrete it to the biliary system via ATP binding cassette transporters G5 and G8 (ABCG5, ABCG8). The intestine can also promote cholesterol excretion by a new pathway called *transintestinal cholesterol efflux* (TICE).[67] The exact pathway by which TICE promotes cholesterol excretion into the intestine is not known but is thought to involve the direct transfer of cholesterol from either HDL or apo B–containing lipoproteins to the enterocyte, which then excretes it into the intestinal lumen.

As mature HDLs acquire TG via CETP exchange, they are subject to increased lipolysis by hepatic lipase and endothelial lipase. In this process, the larger HDLs are converted to smaller subspecies, which can break apart releasing apo A-I, leading to its renal catabolism by the megalin-cubilin complex.[83] Other, smaller HDLs can then reenter the lipidation cycle. Although LDL is the major product from the lipolysis of VLDL, surface materials from TG-rich particles are transferred to the small circulating HDL_3 and subsequently esterified by LCAT to create the larger cholesteryl ester–rich HDL_2. HDL_2 contains twice as many cholesterol molecules per unit of apolipoproteins as does HDL_3. HDL_2 can be converted back to HDL_3 by hepatic lipase.[84]

HDL nomenclature has been continually evolving and can be quite confusing.[84] As preβ-HDL species mature, they may evolve into what a recent expert committee has labeled very small, small, medium, large, and very large particles. Historically, the small particles have been called HDL_3 (subtypes a, b, and c, with a being the largest), and the large particles have been called HDL_2 (subtypes a and b, with b being larger). NMR spectroscopic separation also refers to small, medium, and large particles called H1 to H5, with H5 being the largest. Two-dimensional electrophoretic separation with apo A-I staining classifies HDLs into preβ and α species, with α-4 being the smallest and α-1 being the largest.[84]

Reference Lipid, Lipoprotein Cholesterol, and Apolipoprotein Concentrations

At birth, the typical plasma cholesterol concentration is about 66 mg/dL (1.7 mmol/L) and is roughly equally distributed among LDL and HDL, with only a small amount in VLDL. Typical triglyceride concentration in newborns is only about 36 mg/dL (0.41 mmol/L).[85] Cord blood apo A-I, apo B-100, and Lp(a) have mean concentrations of about 80, 33, and 4 mg/dL, respectively.[86,87] Lipid, lipoprotein cholesterol, and apolipoprotein concentrations then rise sharply during the first few months of life, with LDL becoming the predominant carrier of plasma cholesterol, and remain relatively unchanged until puberty. A profile consisting of total cholesterol of about 155 mg/dL (4.0 mmol/L), LDL-C of 90 mg/dL (2.3 mmol/L), HDL-C of 53 mg/dL (1.7 mmol/L), TG of 55 mg/dL (0.62 mmol/L), apo B of 86 mg/dL, and apo A-I of about 130 mg/dL is typical for a normal prepubertal subject. After puberty, triglycerides, LDL-C, and apo B-100 all increase in both sexes. HDL-C and apo A-I are stongly influenced by androgen levels, and it is the reason they are usually lower in men. After puberty, lipids levels continue to increase throughout adult life, with total and LDL-C and apo B being higher in men than in women up to age 55.[88] Thereafter, women have higher total and LDL-C and apo B levels than their age-matched male counterparts.[89] In contrast to the other lipid parameters, Lp(a) concentration increases slowly and gradually to reach Lp(a) adult values after the third year of life.[86] In women, as estrogen levels fall during menopause, Lp(a) can further increase.

Plasma lipid and lipoprotein reference intervals based on Lipid Research Clinics (LRC) population are presented in Tables 34.7 through 34.10.[‡] Reference intervals for apo A-I and B-100 are from the Framingham Heart Study, using

‡Laboratories should verify that these ranges are appropriate for use in their own settings.

TABLE 34.7 Population Distributions for Total Cholesterol, mg/dL*

	MALE								FEMALE						
	PERCENTILES								PERCENTILES						
Age, y	5	10	25	50	75	90	95	Age, y	5	10	25	50	75	90	95
0–4	114			155			203	0–4	112			156			200
5–9	125	131	141	153	168	183	189	5–9	131	135	150	164	177	189	197
10–14	124	132	144	161	173	191	204	10–14	125	131	142	159	171	191	205
15–19	118	123	135	152	168	183	191	15–19	119	126	140	157	176	198	208
20–24	118	126	142	159	179	197	212	20–24	121	132	147	165	186	220	237
25–29	130	137	154	176	199	223	234	25–29	130	142	158	178	198	217	231
30–34	142	152	161	190	213	237	258	30–34	133	141	158	178	197	215	227
35–39	147	157	176	195	222	248	267	35–39	139	149	165	186	209	233	249
40–44	150	161	179	204	229	251	260	40–44	146	156	172	193	220	241	259
45–49	163	171	188	210	234	255	275	45–49	148	162	182	204	213	256	268
50–54	156	158	189	211	234	262	274	50–54	163	171	188	214	240	267	281
55–59	161	172	188	214	236	260	280	55–59	167	182	201	229	251	270	294
60–64	163	170	191	215	237	262	287	60–64	172	186	207	226	251	282	300
65–69	166	174	192	213	250	275	288	65–69	167	179	212	233	259	282	291
70+	144	160	185	214	236	253	265	70+	173	181	196	226	249	268	280

*To convert to mmol/L, multiply by 0.0259.

From Lipid Research Clinics Program Epidemiology Committee. Plasma lipid distributions in selected North American population: the Lipid Research Clinics Program prevalence study. *Circulation* 1979;60:427–39; and Lipid Metabolism Branch, Division of Heart, Lung, and Blood Institute. The Lipid Research Clinics population studies data book, volume I. The prevalence study. NIH Publication No. 80-1527. Bethesda, Md: National Institutes of Health, 1980.

TABLE 34.8 Population Distributions for Triglycerides, mg/dL*

	MALE								FEMALE						
	PERCENTILES								PERCENTILES						
Age, y	5	10	25	50	75	90	95	Age, y	5	10	25	50	75	90	95
0–4	29			56			99	0–4	34			64			112
5–9	28	34	39	48	58	70	85	5–9	32	37	45	57	74	103	126
10–14	33	37	46	58	74	94	111	10–14	39	44	53	68	85	104	120
15–19	38	43	53	68	88	125	143	15–19	36	40	52	64	85	112	126
20–24	44	50	61	78	107	146	165	20–24	37	42	60	80	104	135	168
25–29	45	51	67	88	120	141	204	25–29	42	45	57	76	104	137	159
30–34	46	57	76	102	142	214	253	30–34	40	45	55	73	104	140	163
35–39	52	58	80	109	167	250	316	35–39	40	47	61	83	115	170	205
40–44	56	69	89	123	174	252	318	40–44	45	51	66	88	116	161	191
45–49	56	65	88	119	165	218	279	45–49	44	55	71	94	139	180	223
50–54	63	75	94	128	178	244	313	50–54	53	58	75	103	144	190	223
55–59	60	70	85	117	167	210	261	55–59	59	65	80	111	163	229	279
60–64	56	65	84	111	150	193	240	60–64	57	66	78	105	143	210	256
65–69	54	61	78	108	164	227	256	65–69	56	64	86	118	158	221	260
70+	63	71	87	115	152	202	239	70+	60	68	83	110	141	189	289

*To convert to mmol/L, multiply by 0.0113.

From Lipid Research Clinics Program Epidemiology Committee. Plasma lipid distributions in selected North American population: the Lipid Research Clinics Program prevalence study. *Circulation* 1979;60:427–39; and Lipid Metabolism Branch, Division of Heart, Lung, and Blood Institute. The Lipid Research Clinics population studies data book, volume I. The prevalence study. NIH Publication No. 80-1527. Bethesda, Md: National Institutes of Health, 1980.

approved World Health Organization (WHO)/International Federation of Clinical Chemistry and Laboratory Medicine (IFCC) calibrators.[90,91] They are also available from the National Health and Nutrition Examination Survey III (NHANES III) (Tables 34.11 and 34.12).[92] Because NHANES was designed to reflect the US population, data for the distribution of these proteins in the main American ethnic groups are available (Table 34.13). Using this information, apo B-100 cut points similar to those recommended for LDL-C can be developed; apo B-100 values that correspond to desirable, borderline high risk, high risk, and very high risk are 88, 115, 132, and 152 mg/dL, respectively; apo A-I values

TABLE 34.9 Population Distributions for Low-Density Lipoprotein Cholesterol, mg/dL*

MALE								FEMALE							
	PERCENTILES								PERCENTILES						
Age, y	**5**	**10**	**25**	**50**	**75**	**90**	**95**	**Age, y**	**5**	**10**	**25**	**50**	**75**	**90**	**95**
5–9	63	69	80	90	103	117	129	5–9	68	73	88	98	115	125	140
10–14	64	83	82	94	109	123	133	10–14	68	73	81	94	110	126	136
15–19	62	68	80	93	109	123	130	15–19	59	73	78	93	110	129	137
20–24	66	73	85	101	118	138	147	20–24	57	65	82	102	118	141	159
25–29	70	75	96	116	138	157	165	25–29	71	75	90	108	126	148	164
30–34	78	88	107	124	144	166	185	30–34	70	77	91	109	129	146	156
35–39	81	92	110	131	154	176	189	35–39	75	81	96	116	139	161	172
40–44	87	98	115	135	157	173	186	40–44	74	84	104	122	146	165	174
45–49	97	106	120	140	163	185	202	45–49	79	89	105	127	150	173	186
50–54	89	102	118	143	162	185	197	50–54	88	94	111	134	160	186	201
55–59	88	103	123	145	168	191	203	55–59	89	97	120	145	168	199	210
60–64	83	107	121	143	165	188	210	60–64	100	105	126	149	168	191	224
65–69	98	104	125	146	170	199	210	65–69	92	99	125	151	184	205	221
70+	88	100	119	142	164	182	186	70+	96	108	126	147	170	189	206

*To convert to mmol/L, multiply by 0.0259.

From Lipid Research Clinics Program Epidemiology Committee. Plasma lipid distributions in selected North American population: the Lipid Research Clinics Program prevalence study. *Circulation* 1979;60:427–39.

TABLE 34.10 Population Distributions for High-Density Lipoprotein Cholesterol, mg/dL*

MALE								FEMALE							
	PERCENTILES								PERCENTILES						
Age, y	**5**	**10**	**25**	**50**	**75**	**90**	**95**	**Age, y**	**5**	**10**	**25**	**50**	**75**	**90**	**95**
5–9	38	43	49	55	64	70	75	5–9	36	38	48	52	60	67	73
10–14	37	40	46	55	61	71	74	10–14	37	40	45	52	58	64	70
15–19	30	34	39	46	52	59	63	15–19	35	38	43	51	61	68	74
20–24	30	32	38	45	51	57	63	20–24	33	37	44	51	62	72	79
25–29	31	32	37	44	50	58	63	25–29	37	39	47	55	63	74	83
30–34	28	32	38	45	52	59	63	30–34	36	40	46	55	64	73	77
35–39	29	31	36	43	49	58	62	35–39	34	38	44	53	64	75	82
40–44	27	31	36	43	51	60	67	40–44	34	39	48	56	65	79	88
45–49	30	33	38	45	52	60	64	45–49	34	41	47	58	68	82	87
50–54	28	31	36	44	51	58	63	50–54	37	41	50	62	71	84	92
55–59	28	31	38	46	55	64	71	55–59	37	41	50	60	73	85	91
60–64	30	34	41	49	61	69	74	60–64	38	44	51	61	75	87	92
65–69	30	33	39	49	52	74	75	65–69	35	38	49	62	73	85	96
70+	31	33	40	48	56	70	75	70+	33	38	45	60	71	82	92

*To convert to mmol/L, multiply by 0.0259.

From Lipid Research Clinics Program Epidemiology Committee. Plasma lipid distributions in selected North American population: the Lipid Research Clinics Program prevalence study. *Circulation* 1979;60:427–39.

that correspond to low and high are 114 and 154 mg/dL, respectively.[92] Until Lp(a) assays are better standardized, the development of absolute reference intervals for Lp(a) is problematic and cut points are instead often based on the 80th percentile population distribution for a given assay.[26]

CLINICAL SIGNIFICANCE

The clinical significance of lipid and lipoprotein testing is primarily associated with atherosclerotic vascular diseases of the aorta and coronary, intra- and extracranial, renal, intestinal, and peripheral arteries. Major morbidities from the development of atherosclerosis include myocardial infarction, ischemic events, stroke, revascularizations, and heart failure.

Association With Coronary Heart Disease

As early as 1910, Windaus first described cholesterol in the lesions of diseased arteries. Subsequently, many studies confirmed that free and esterified cholesterol accumulates in the aorta, coronary arteries, and cerebral vessels, and that the rate of accumulation varies among individuals. The association

TABLE 34.11 Serum Apo A-I Concentrations in Persons Aged ≥4 Years by Sex and Age: Means and Selected Percentiles, United States, 1988–91

	APO A-I*, mg/dL								
			PERCENTILES						
Age, y	Mean, (SEM)†	SD	5th	10th	25th	50th	75th	90th	95th
Males‡									
4–5	135 (2)	19	109	112	122	132	149	159	172
6–11	142	20	111	117	126	141	150	168	177
12–19	129	19	99	106	116	128	141	153	165
≥20	136	22	106	111	121	133	147	164	176
20–29	135	21	105	112	121	132	145	164	173
30–39	135	20	105	111	122	132	145	161	173
40–49	136 (2)	25	103	108	119	133	149	164	178
50–59	136 (2)	21	107	111	121	134	147	167	173
60–69	140 (2)	23	111	116	123	136	153	172	184
≥70	138	23	109	114	122	134	150	167	180
Females‡									
4–5	131	18	104	111	118	130	140	155	163
6–11	136	17	110	117	125	135	145	157	166
12–19	136	23	105	111	120	132	146	165	180
≥20	151	27	113	120	132	147	166	186	202
20–29	148 (2)	30	111	117	128	143	164	185	209
30–39	145	24	110	115	126	143	160	173	189
40–49	149 (2)	24	115	122	134	145	165	181	195
50–59	156 (2)	29	117	123	134	152	173	199	211
60–69	157 (2)	28	120	125	138	154	171	191	205
≥70	155 (2)	26	118	124	137	153	171	189	199

*Combined data for total population, including all three ethnic groups.
†All SEMs were 1 mg/dL unless otherwise indicated. To convert to μmol/L, divide by 2.81.
‡Estimates based on 400 to 800 subjects in each age and sex subgroup.
Modified from Bachorik PS, Lovejoy KL, Carroll MD, Johnson CL. Apolipoprotein B and AI distributions in the United States, 1988–1991: results of the National Health and Nutrition Examination Survey III (NHANES III). *Clin Chem* 1997;43:2364–78.

between serum cholesterol and atherosclerosis in humans was first suggested in 1938 when Muller and Thanhauser each demonstrated familial aggregation of hypercholesterolemia and CHD.[93,94] Additional studies showed that when the total cholesterol concentration is high, the incidence and prevalence of CHD are also high, although the association with total mortality is not as strong.[95] In the 1960s, Fredrickson and colleagues noted that all lipid disorders (hyperlipidemia and dyslipidemia) can be classified into distinct lipoprotein disorders—hyperbetalipoproteinemia (increased LDL-C) or hypoalphalipoproteinemia (low HDL-C)—which at the time provided a better mechanistic explanation of lipid-related disorders than did total lipid concentrations.

The overall relationship between cholesterol and atherosclerotic coronary disease is curvilinear.[11] According to the Multiple Risk Factor Intervention Trial (MRFIT), if a risk ratio of 1.0 is arbitrarily assigned at a cholesterol value of 200 mg/dL (5.2 mmol/L), the risk ratio increases to 2.0 at 250 mg/dL (6.5 mmol/L) and to 4.0 at 300 mg/dL (7.76 mmol/L) (Fig. 34.22). Pathologic studies have helped to explain this curvilinear relationship. When 60% of the surface of coronary arteries is covered with plaque, one enters a critical phase in which any increase in serum cholesterol will markedly increase coronary disease risk. Results of the LRC-Coronary Primary Prevention Trial (CPPT) show that use of the concentration at the 95th percentile of a population distribution is inappropriate to define hypercholesterolemia. Data from this and other studies suggest that risk disproportionately increases as cholesterol concentrations increase; at concentrations of 200 to 240 mg/dL (5.2–6.2 mmol/L), the risk begins to accelerate at a greater rate. On average, each 1% reduction in cholesterol (2 to 3 mg/dL) (0.05–0.08 mmol/L) results in about a 2% reduction in CHD incidence—a relationship of considerable clinical and public health significance. In addition, the Cholesterol-Lowering Atherosclerosis Study (CLAS) demonstrated the benefit of cholesterol lowering in people with established disease and even in those with normal or moderately increased total cholesterol, as defined at the time of the study as 185 to 240 mg/dL (4.78–6.21 mmol/L).[96] More recent statin studies utilizing intravascular coronary ultrasound have shown that individuals with preexisting disease may actually show some reversal of existing atherosclerosis if they are aggressively treated so they achieve LDL-C below 70 mg/dL (1.8 mmol/L).[97,98]

Many epidemiologic and clinical studies have shown that other lipids and lipoproteins besides LDL, such as HDL and lipoprotein subfractions, are also useful for predicting CHD risk.[99] In the case of LDL, many studies have suggested that small, dense LDL subfractions may be better correlated with CHD risk than large, less dense LDL subfractions.[100,101]

TABLE 34.12 Serum Apo B-100 Concentrations in Persons Aged ≥4 Years by Sex and Age: Means and Selected Percentiles, United States, 1988–91

	APO B-100*, mg/dL								
			PERCENTILES						
Age, y	Mean, (SEM)†	SD	5th	10th	25th	50th	75th	90th	95th
Males‡									
4–5	79	14	58	0.62	69	79	89	98	103
6–11	79	16	56	0.61	69	76	89	99	105
12–19	78	17	55	0.58	67	75	85	98	110
≥20	107	25	66	0.74	89	106	122	138	150
20–29	91	22	59	0.66	76	88	103	117	130
30–39	106	24	63	0.73	89	107	122	136	143
40–49	112 (2)	24	71	0.82	97	111	126	140	152
50–59	116 (2)	26	75	0.84	98	116	133	149	160
60–69	117 (2)	23	81	0.89	101	116	133	148	156
≥70	110	24	73	0.81	95	109	123	142	152
Females‡									
4–5	82	14	58	0.64	72	82	91	99	104
6–11	82	17	57	0.61	70	81	90	101	113
12–19	81	20	53	0.58	67	79	92	104	119
≥20	103	28	66	0.71	83	99	119	140	153
20–29	91	23	63	0.67	74	86	102	119	132
30–39	93	23	59	0.68	76	89	107	123	132
40–49	99	21	70	0.75	84	96	114	129	136
50–59	116 (2)	29	75	0.84	96	114	133	156	168
60–69	119 (2)	31	75	0.82	98	118	135	156	173
≥70	118	28	79	0.84	98	116	135	152	168

*Combined data for total population, including all three ethnic groups.
†All SEMs were 1 mg/dL unless otherwise indicated. To convert to μmol/L, divide by 55.0.
‡Estimates based on 400 to 800 subjects in each age and sex subgroup.
Modified from Bachorik PS, Lovejoy KL, Carroll MD, Johnson CL. Apolipoprotein B and AI distributions in the United States, 1988–1991: results of the National Health and Nutrition Examination Survey III (NHANES III). *Clin Chem* 1997;43:2364–78.

TABLE 34.13 Age-Adjusted* Mean Apo A-I and Apo B Concentrations in Persons Aged ≥4 Years by Sex and Age Group, United States, 1988–91

	MEAN (SEM)† CONC, mg/dL					
	APO A-I			APO B		
Age, y	White	Black	Mexican-American	White	Black	Mexican-American
Males						
All	134	145	135 (2)	99	96	101
4–11	140 (2)	145	139 (2)	79	79	79
12–19	127	139 (2)	131 (3)	78	78	79
≥20	135	146	135 (2)	106	102	109
Females						
All	146	151	144 (2)	97	96	98
4–11	133	142 (2)	132	82	82	81
12–19	122 (2)	144 (2)	140 (4)	80	82	83
≥20	151	154	147 (2)	103	101	105

*Age-adjusted by the direct method to the 1980 US Census population.
†All SEMs were 1 mg/dL unless otherwise indicated. To convert to μmol/L: for APO A-I, divide by 2.81; for APO B, divide by 55.0.
Modified from Bachorik PS, Lovejoy KL, Carroll MD, Johnson CL. Apolipoprotein B and AI distributions in the United States, 1988–1991: results of the National Health and Nutrition Examination Survey III (NHANES III). *Clin Chem* 1997;43:2364–78.

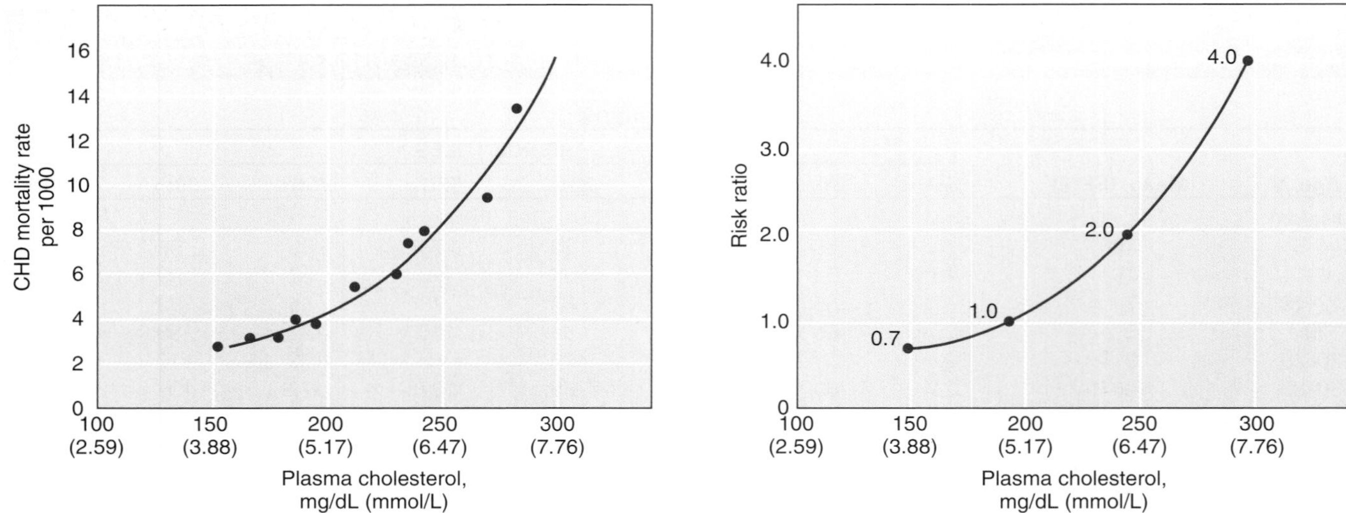

FIGURE 34.22 Relationship between cholesterol concentration and coronary heart disease mortality, expressed by yearly rate per 1000 and risk ratios (Multiple Risk Factor Intervention Trial [MRFIT] participants).

Triglyceride is also viewed in the Adult Treatment Panel III (ATP III) reports[102] as a risk factor, but the newest ACC/AHA Guidelines have minimized the importance of TG for CHD risk prediction or managment.[5] Chylomicron and VLDL remnants and IDL, the products of the breakdown of triglyceride-rich lipoprotein, are now also increasingly recognized as important players in atherogenesis and may account for the stronger association of nonfasting TG than fasting TG with cardiovascular events.[103] These apo B–containing lipoproteins may promote atherosclerosis when their concentrations in plasma are high or when their presence in circulation is prolonged by adversely affecting endothelial cell function, inflammation, blood viscosity, and coagulation forces.

In the early 1970s, Alaupovic first suggested that apolipoproteins could be considered as risk markers when the contribution of lipids and lipoproteins to the development of atherosclerotic disease is evaluated.[104] Several studies showed that in people with CHD, changes in serum concentrations of apo A-I and apo B-100 are similar to those for HDL and LDL, respectively. Apo B-100 values were increased and apo A-I values were decreased in people with CHD compared with those without disease. In several studies, apo A-I and apo B-100 were better discriminators of people with CHD than the cholesterol concentration of the corresponding lipoprotein,[105-107] at least in univariate analyses. Furthermore, these two apolipoproteins were shown to correlate better with the degree of coronary stenosis than LDL-C and HDL-C.[108] It has been shown that only 14.5% of patients with myocardial infarction younger than the age of 60 years have LDL-C above the 95th percentile. In contrast, 35% of these patients have apo B-100 above the 95th percentile.[109] The measurement of apo B-100 provides information regarding the number of apo B-100–containing particles because only one apo B molecule is present per lipoprotein particle. If the concentration of LDL-C is low, normal, or slightly increased, but apo B-100 or total LDL-P is greatly increased, it is likely explained by cholesterol-depleted particles—either small LDL or TG-rich, CE-depleted LDL of any size. Increased serum apo B-100 and decreased apo A-I concentrations were also found in children of parents with premature atherosclerotic disease.[110] Overall, these and other findings suggest that apolipoproteins and other measures of particle number may be superior as cardiovascular risk markers, but they are not recommended by most guidelines as screening tests[5] and are mostly used at this point in deciding therapy in patients with intermediate cardiovascular disease risk.[111]

Although CHD is often not manifested clinically until the fourth decade of life, atherosclerosis is a process that begins early in life and progresses silently for many decades. Genetic disorders—for example, gain of function of PCSK9 or loss of function of NPC1L1—result in only modest reductions in LDL-C, but they are lifelong and result in marked reductions in cardiovascular disease.[112-114] Autopsies performed on young American soldiers killed in action in Korea[115] and Vietnam[116] revealed the presence of subclinical atherosclerotic lesions. Coronary artery lesions were also found in aortas of children as young as the age of 3[117] and in 10-year-olds in the International Atherosclerosis Project.[118] In the Pathobiological Determinants of Atherosclerosis in Youth (PDAY) study, intimal lesions appeared in all examined aortas and in more than half of the right coronary arteries of the youngest age group (15 to 19 years); they increased in prevalence and extent with age through the oldest age group (30 to 34 years).[119] This study also showed that some regions of the arteries were lesion prone and others were lesion resistant, and the propensity to develop raised or advanced lesions differed among right coronary artery, abdominal aorta, and thoracic aorta. Findings from the Bogalusa Heart Study[120] showed a correlation between systolic blood pressure, higher total and LDL cholesterol, and lower HDL cholesterol concentrations and the degree of coronary and aortic atherosclerosis in children and adolescents. In the PDAY study, postmortem cholesterol and thiocyanate, a marker for cigarette smoking, predicted the extent of coronary and aortic atherosclerosis, respectively, in autopsies of those aged 14 to 34.[121] Therefore a direct relationship between determinant risk factors and the extent of atherosclerotic lesions in youth seems to exist and suggests that the identification and treatment of children and young adults who may be at high risk for developing CHD offer the possibility of preventing or delaying development of this disease.

Disorders of Lipoprotein Metabolism

Lipid disorders can be diagnosed by the measurement of total lipids, as well as lipoprotein-based biomarkers. These disorders have been traditionally defined in terms of arbitrary cut points for lipids and lipoproteins, but increasingly their definition is based on the relationship between lipoprotein concentrations and risk for CHD.

Primary Versus Secondary Hyperlipoproteinemia

When hyperlipidemia is first evaluated, it should be determined whether it is from a primary lipoprotein disorder or is secondary to a wide variety of metabolic diseases. The diagnosis of primary hyperlipidemia is made after secondary causes have been ruled out (Table 34.14). The most commonly seen secondary causes in the first year of life are glycogen storage disease and congenital biliary atresia. Hypothyroidism, nephrotic syndrome, and diabetes mellitus are more prevalent later in childhood. Of course, lipid and lipoprotein concentrations are also influenced by exogenous factors, such as dietary and alcohol intake and numerous pharmacologic agents, such as steroids, isotretinoin, β-blockers, and antiretroviral agents (see Table 34.14).

TABLE 34.14 Causes of Secondary Hyperlipidemia and Dyslipoproteinemia

Disorder	Cause
Exogenous	Drugs: corticosteroids, isotretinoin (Accutane), thiazides, anticonvulsants, beta-blockers, anabolic steroids, oral estrogens, HAART (antiretroviral therapy), various antipsychotic medications
	Alcohol
	Obesity
Endocrine and metabolic	Acute intermittent porphyria
	Diabetes mellitus
	Hypopituitarism
	Hypothyroidism
	Lipodystrophy
	Polycystic ovary syndrome (PCOS)
	Pregnancy
Storage disease	Cystine storage disease
	Gaucher disease
	Glycogen storage disease
	Juvenile Tay-Sachs disease
	Niemann-Pick disease
	Tay-Sachs disease
Renal	Chronic renal failure
	Hemolytic-uremic syndrome
	Nephrotic syndrome
Hepatic	Benign recurrent intrahepatic cholestasis
	Congenital biliary atresia
Acute and transient	Burns
	Hepatitis
	Acute trauma (surgery)
	Myocardial infarction
	Bacterial and viral infections
Others	Anorexia nervosa
	Starvation
	Idiopathic hypercalcemia
	Klinefelter syndrome
	Progeria (Hutchinson-Gilford syndrome)
	Systemic lupus erythematosus
	Werner syndrome

Familial Dyslipoproteinemias

Historically, lipoprotein phenotypes reflecting lipoprotein metabolic disorders were first classified into one of five patterns (types I to V), according to Fredrickson and colleagues, based on an electrophoretic separation scheme. However, not all lipid disorders fit nicely into these phenotypes, and there is also great overlap in their phenotypes. Currently, outside of specific genetic disorders, there is no well-accepted lipoprotein disorder classification scheme, although de Graaf and colleagues described a logistical algorithm for diagnosing disorders based on apo B particles.[122] Defects leading to lipoprotein disorders may be related to increased production of lipoproteins, abnormal intravascular processing (eg, enzymatic hydrolysis of triglyceride), and defective cellular uptake of lipoproteins. A significant decrease/increase in production or a decrease/increase in removal/production of lipoproteins can lead to marked abnormalities in lipid and lipoprotein concentrations. Multiple diseases, the most common of which are described in the next section, alter the various steps in the metabolic pathway of lipoproteins.

Deficiency in Lipoprotein Lipase Activity. This disorder is characterized by marked hyperchylomicronemia and a corresponding increase in triglycerides, which are often over 1000 mg/dL (11.3 mmol/L) and can reach as high as 10,000 mg/dL (113 mmol/L).[123] As discussed previously, LPL is essential for the hydrolysis of triglyceride during the conversion of chylomicrons to chylomicron remnants. VLDL cholesterol can also be elevated, but the concentrations of HDL-C and LDL-C cholesterol are usually low (type I pattern). Furthermore, the concentration of apo C-II, the activator of LPL, is normal. This disorder is usually expressed in childhood. It appears that those patients with low to absent LPL activity present with symptoms at an earlier age, whereas those with a partial deficiency become symptomatic later in life. This disease is usually detected after recurrent episodes of severe abdominal pain and repeated attacks of pancreatitis, which is the greatest source of morbidity in these patients. Eruptive xanthomas and lipemia retinalis are usually present when plasma triglyceride concentrations exceed 2000 and 4000 mg/dL (22.6 and 45.2 mmol/L),[123] respectively. The acuteness of the symptoms is directly proportional to the degree of hyperchylomicronemia. It is important to note that patients with this disorder do not appear to be predisposed to atherosclerotic disease. The diagnosis is made by finding a TG-to-cholesterol ratio of 10:1 and very low or undetectable levels of LPL activity in plasma after heparin treatment, which is used to displace LPL bound to proteoglycans on endothelial cells. This autosomal recessive disorder is extremely rare (one per million individuals), but more than 40 insertions and deletions in the LPL gene have been described. Acquired LPL deficiency typically occurring later in life due to the formation of a blocking autoantibody has also been described.

Deficiency in Apolipoprotein C-II. Deficient or defective apo C-II, the required activator for LPL, reduces the activity of this enzyme, impairs chylomicron catabolism, and increases plasma triglycerides (homozygotes: from 1000 to 10,000 mg/dL) (11.3–113 mmol/L). Those affected by this rare autosomal recessive disorder typically have less than 10% of the normal concentration of apo C-II.[124] Total cholesterol tends to vary considerably (150–890 mg/dL; 3.88–23 mmol/L) in these patients, but the TG-to-cholesterol ratio in homozygotes is 10:1. HDL and LDL cholesterol concentrations are often below the 5th percentile. Furthermore, plasma apo A-I, A-II, and B-100 concentrations are also decreased, whereas apo C-III and E concentrations can be increased. Heterozygotes may have normal TG levels despite reduced apo C-II concentrations. Although the clinical symptoms are similar to those seen in patients with LPL deficiency, they are usually milder and are often expressed at a later age. The predominant symptom is usually recurrent abdominal pain caused by attacks of pancreatitis. As with LPL deficiency, patients with apo C-II deficiency do not appear to be predisposed to atherosclerosis.

The diagnosis is made upon documentation of low-LPL activity in postheparin plasma that is restored to near-normal levels by the addition of normal apo C-II to the assay mixture. In another approach, the absence of apo C-II can be recognized by using an immunoassay for apo C-II. However, the latter approach may not distinguish between normal subjects and those with normal concentrations of a nonfunctional form of apo C-II. The defective apo C-II disorder is inherited in an autosomal recessive mode but at an even lower frequency than LPL deficiency.

Mimicking LPL and apo C-II deficiency are even rarer causes of hypertriglyceridemia, such as defects in the glucosylphosphatidylinositol-anchored high-density lipoprotein-binding protein 1 (GPIHBP1),[125] lipase maturation factor (LMF),[126] or mutations in apo A-V.[43]

Familial Combined Hyperlipidemia. About 10% to 15% of patients with premature CHD have familial combined hyperlipidemia (FCHL), thus making it one of the more common forms of dyslipidemia.[127] This disorder is recognized by carefully studying patients over time because their lipid phenotype can vary.[11] Patients with FCHL can have multiple lipoprotein abnormalities, including increased plasma concentrations of total and LDL cholesterol (type IIa) or triglyceride (type IV), or both (type IIb). In almost all cases, their apo B-100 concentrations are increased (>90th percentile).[128] First-degree relatives of patients with FCHL frequently also have at least two lipid abnormalities.

FCHL appears to be caused by overproduction of VLDL and apo B-100 and can be affected by obesity, but the underlying molecular defect is not known. Kinetic studies have shown that the rate of flux of apo B-100 from VLDL in FCHL is approximately twice that of normal subjects.[129,130] This causes apo B-100 to be increased (by more than 125 mg/dL), even in subjects with normal LDL-C. Because of the decreased lipid-to-protein ratio in these patients, both VLDL and LDL particles tend to be small and dense. When increased, LDL-C is about 190 mg/dL (4.91 mmol/L), but it is lower than that typically seen in heterozygous familial hypercholesterolemia. Triglyceride concentrations are usually between 200 and 400 mg/dL (2.26 and 4.52 mmol/L) but can be significantly higher. HDL-C is often low, particularly in the presence of hypertriglyceridemia. Xanthomas and other clinical symptoms of hyperlipidemia are not very common in these patients and if present should suggest an alternative diagnosis. The association of FCHL with CHD incidence, however, is very high. In addition to increased IDL, the presence of high concentrations of small, dense LDL and low concentrations of HDL-C might explain the increased risk for CHD in this disorder.

Although the gene mutation(s) responsible for FCHL remain unknown, it is thought to have a prevalence of about 1 in 100 persons. The expression of FCHL is often delayed until adolescence, although young children from families with premature CHD can sometimes present with increased cholesterol or triglyceride, or both.[131]

Hyperapobetalipoproteinemia. This disorder is characterized by increased LDL–apo B-100 (LDL-P) concentrations but with normal or only moderately increased concentrations of LDL-C.[132,133] The ratio of LDL cholesterol to apo B-100 is therefore reduced in these patients (≤1.2). Total cholesterol and triglyceride may be normal but are usually increased, and HDL-C and apo A-I are usually low. This disorder, strongly associated with insulin resistance, appears to be caused by overproduction of VLDL and apo B-100 in the liver, which leads to the formation of small dense pro-atherognic LDL particles. The exact mode of inheritance and the prevalence of this disorder remain unclear, however, about one third of children of a parent with premature CHD or hyperapobetalipoproteinemia will have this disorder.[134] Hyperapobetalipoproteinemia and FCHL share many features, suggesting a metabolic and genetic association between these two disorders.

Familial Hypertriglyceridemia. The TG concentrations in this disorder are typically 200 to 1000 mg/dL (2.26–11.3 mmol/L) unless other metabolic issues exacerbate the TG level. The production of large VLDL with abnormally high triglyceride content appears to be responsible for familial hypertriglyceridemia (FHTG).[135] There is overproduction of VLDL in the liver, leading to saturation of lipolysis by LPL and TG accumulation. The cholesterol content of VLDL is also increased, but plasma LDL-C and apo B-100 concentrations are usually normal. This finding suggests that the conversion of VLDL to LDL is not increased in these patients. Furthermore, plasma HDL-C in FHTG is often dramatically decreased, probably secondary to the hypertriglyceridemia.

The cause of the overproduction of VLDL triglyceride is unknown, but obesity is commonly found in many of these patients. Administration of estrogen and corticosteroids aggravates hypertriglyceridemia and sometimes can lead to acute pancreatitis. The diagnosis of FHTG requires study of other family members to differentiate this disorder from FCHL. This disorder appears to be polygenic, often is not expressed until adulthood, and has an estimated frequency in the population of about 1:500 persons. About one in five children born to affected parents manifest the phenotype early in life.[136] Coronary disease is not common unless the metabolic syndrome is also present.[137]

Type V Hyperlipoproteinemia. This disorder, which still gets its name from the old Fredrickson classification, is characterized by an increase in both chylomicrons and VLDL and has an incidence of about 1 in 500. It is most commonly seen as a transient phenotype and is frequently found in association with diabetes mellitus. Although the exact molecular cause of this disorder is not known, the metabolic defect appears to be increased production or decreased removal of VLDL, or a combination of both. The activity of LPL in these patients may be normal or low, and the plasma concentration of apo C-II is normal.[131]

Although this disorder is not usually expressed in childhood, several affected preadolescents have been described.[131] Clinical presentations in adult patients include eruptive xanthomas, lipemia retinalis, pancreatitis, and abnormal glucose tolerance with hyperinsulinism. Premature atherosclerotic complications are not as commonly seen. This heterogeneous syndrome appears to be inherited in an autosomal dominant mode, but its genetic basis has not yet been fully elucidated.

Dysbetalipoproteinemia (Type III). This autosomal recessive disorder is caused by a primary genetic defect in the removal of lipoprotein remnants of both intestinal and hepatic origin.[30] As indicated earlier, apo E present on the surface of lipoprotein remnants interacts with specific hepatic receptors and facilitates the removal of lipoproteins from the circulation. Patients with dysbetalipoproteinemia may be homozygous for a rare mutation in apo E or may be homozygous for the apo E_2 allele.[56] However, the APOE 2-2 genotype is seen in only about 16% of patients, and type III can be present with any of the other apo E genotypes.[138] Overt type III hyperlipoproteinemia also only occurs in a small minority—less than 5% of patients homozygous for apo E_2—indicating that occurrence of the defective alleles is necessary but not sufficient to produce this disease.[139] The altered forms of apo E that occur in this disorder cannot typically as efficiently bind specific hepatic receptors, leading to the accumulation of lipoprotein remnants. These particles are cholesterol enriched with a density less than 1.006 g/mL and are commonly referred to as β-VLDL or floating β-lipoprotein.

The disease is thought to require a "second hit" to manifest in addition to the genetic propensity, and they include the use of exogenous estrogen, alcohol, obesity (especially related to carbohydrate loading), diabetes, hypothyroidism, and renal disease. The phenotype is characterized by increased plasma cholesterol and triglycerides, and the concentrations of the two lipids are about the same when expressed in milligrams per deciliter. β-VLDL present in type III has been shown to contain both apo B-100 and B-48, and therefore is related to triglyceride-rich lipoprotein remnants from both hepatic and intestinal origin. Apo B levels are not usually elevated and LDL-P is not usually high. Sniderman developed an algorithm using lipid and apo B concentrations to facilitate this diagnosis.[122]

This disorder has a late onset and is rarely manifested in childhood.[85] The most distinctive clinical presentation of dyslipoproteinemia is the presence of palmar xanthomas, yellow deposits that occur in the creases of the palms.[140] Tuberous and tuberoeruptive xanthomas also occur but are not unique to this syndrome. Premature atherosclerosis develops in up to half of these patients, particularly in the lower extremities.[141] Because of the familial nature of this disorder and the predisposition of these patients to premature atherosclerotic disease, family members should be carefully evaluated. This disorder has a fairly high frequency (0.2% in adult women and 0.4% to 0.5% in adult men), but it is often missed due to lack of awareness and due to infrequent use of definitive diagnostic tests, such as lipoprotein electrophoresis.[138]

Familial Hypercholesterolemia. The disease familial hypercholesterolemia (FH) is most often caused by a defect in the LDL receptor gene. However, the term now encompasses a wide variety of other inherited lipid disorders, most of which affect the LDL receptor pathway, although some, like phytosterolemia, do not always present with a marked elevation of total cholesterol. As discussed earlier, the LDL receptor is a cell surface receptor and is responsible for the recognition and removal of LDL from the circulation.[142] The defects seen in patients with FH include reduced LDL binding because of defective or absent LDL receptors. In another variant of this disorder, a person may make a receptor that binds LDL normally but cannot efficiently internalize LDL particles.[47]

FH is characterized clinically by increased plasma LDL cholesterol and cholesterol deposition in skin, tendons, and arteries. The type of transmission varies with each specific FH disorder, but the most common is transmitted in an autosomal dominant manner, so the disease is expressed in the heterozygous, compound heterozygous and homozygous states. Heterozygous FH is one of the most commonly seen genetic metabolic disorders, with an incidence of at least 1 in 500 persons in the United States and higher in other populations. The prevalence of homozygous FH is about one in a million persons. Now that sophisticated genetic testing is becoming more available, many of these suspected homozygous genotypes patients turn out to be compound heterozygotes.[143] Mean plasma LDL-C in children and adult heterozygotes is usually two to three times that of normal, whereas mean plasma LDL-C of homozygotes is four to six times that of normal subjects. Although the number of LDL particles is increased in these patients, their lipid composition and lipid-to-protein ratio are usually normal.[144] Apo B-100 is increased in proportion to LDL-C. Triglyceride concentration may be normal or only slightly increased, and HDL-C concentration is slightly decreased in both heterozygotes and homozygotes. Elevations of Lp(a) are common in FH patients, especially in those with CVD[145] and are associated with aortic calcification and stenosis.[146]

Hypercholesterolemia is present at birth in most FH patients and persists throughout life. In heterozygotes, xanthomas appear toward the end of the second decade of life, and clinical manifestations of atherosclerotic disease appear during the fourth decade.[147] In homozygotes, the unique yellow-orange cutaneous xanthomas develop in early infancy and sometimes are even present at birth.[148] Tendon xanthomas and atherosclerotic complications begin during childhood. Death from myocardial infarction can occur in homozygotes before the end of the third decade and even earlier, but the prospect for these patients are much better with aggressive lipid-lowering therapy.[131]

Although increased plasma LDL cholesterol is indicative of the heterozygous form of FH, it is not sufficient to make the diagnosis; it is now common practice to confirm the diagnosis by sequencing the gene for the LDL receptor. More than 150 different mutations in the LDL receptor gene or in molecules affecting its normal function have been shown to disrupt the normal process of LDL removal from the circulation.[149] Other genetic mutations, such as PCSK9, can lead to an autosomal dominant form of FH.[150] PCSK9 is a protease that increases LDL receptor catabolism, and gain of function mutations can lead to increased concentrations of circulating LDL by decreasing expression of the LDL receptor and is the basis for a new type of therapy involving a monoclonal antibody against PCSK9.[151] A rare autosomal recessive disorder involving a clathrin adaptor protein (ARH) has also been described. ARH is a chaperone protein that appears to be necessary for proper recycling of the LDL receptor on the plasma membrane and when defective leads to an autosomal recessive form of FH.[152]

Familial Defective Apolipoprotein B-100. This disorder results from a mutation in the apo B-100 gene rather than the LDL receptor itself, usually from a mutation leading to a single substitution of glutamine for arginine at residue 3500 of apo B-100. This substitution reduces the positive charge of apo B-100 and decreases its affinity for the LDL receptor.[153] Other, rarer mutations in apo B affecting its binding to the LDL receptor have also been described. Plasma LDL cholesterol in heterozygotes of this disorder can range from normal to greatly increased because of inadequate removal of LDL particles by LDL receptors.[154] Those with increased LDL cholesterol have an increased incidence of CHD, but often the disease appears to be less aggressive than FH. Triglyceride and HDL cholesterol concentrations are not usually affected. It is often difficult to differentiate these patients from heterozygous FH patients, but because the management of these two disorders is similar, the distinction may not be that clinically important. The frequency of this mutation is fairly common at 1 : 500 to 1 : 600 in hypercholesterolemic persons in populations of European descent,[155] but the mutation is much rarer in non-European populations.

Hypoalphalipoproteinemia. This group of disorders is characterized by relatively normal total lipids, but HDL-C is reduced to below the 5th percentile,[156] and it can be associated with an increased incidence of CHD.[157] Several known molecular defects can lead to hypoalphalipoproteinemia. Rarely, patients can have mutations in apo A-I, the main protein component of HDL, which can lead to profoundly low concentrations of HDL.[131] These patients typically have corneal clouding and xanthomas, and they are at increased risk for development of premature CHD. Heterozygotes exhibit no clinical signs but have about half the normal concentrations of HDL-C and apo A-I. Mutations such as a rearrangement at the apolipoprotein gene locus that inactivates both apo A-I and C-III, deletion of the entire locus, and an insertion in the apo A-I gene have all been described.[158,159]

Tangier disease, so named because it was first observed in patients from Tangier Island in Chesapeake Bay (Eastern United States), is characterized by severely reduced plasma HDL-C, abnormal HDL subfraction distribution, and an accumulation of cholesteryl esters in many tissues throughout the body.[156,160,161] Kinetic studies have demonstrated that increased catabolism of HDL, rather than a defect in biosynthesis, is the cause of Tangier disease.[162] Tangier disease is caused by mutations in the *ABCA1* (ATP-binding cassette A1) gene on chromosome 9q31 and is inherited in an autosomal dominant fashion. As already mentioned, the ABCA1 transporter is a key protein for the efflux of cholesterol from hepatocytes, enterocytes, and peripheral cells, particularly from macrophages, and it is important in the biogenesis of HDL.[33] After lipid-free or lipid-poor apo A-I enters the plasma compartment via secretion from hepatocytes or enterocytes, or by dissociation from a lipoprotein particle, it must acquire additional lipid by the ABCA1 transporter, or it will be quickly catabolized by filtration in the kidney. Plasma cholesterol is usually decreased to about 70 mg/dL (1.8 mmol/L) in homozygotes and to about 160 mg/dL (4.14 mmol/L) in heterozygotes. Triglyceride can sometimes be modestly increased and may depend on the diet.[160] In homozygotes, plasma HDL-C and apo A-I concentrations are often undetectable; apo A-II is present at less than 10% of its normal concentration and is often found in apo B-100–containing lipoprotein.[163] Heterozygotes are characterized by half-normal concentrations of HDL-C, apo A-I, and apo A-II.

Clinical symptoms of Tangier disease result from the deposition of cholesteryl esters in various tissues in the body. The three major clinical signs are hyperplastic orange tonsils enriched in cholesteryl esters, splenomegaly, and peripheral neuropathy. Other clinical signs that may be seen include hepatomegaly and corneal opacities. Severely reduced HDL-C and enlarged orange tonsils (mostly seen in children) are pathognomonic for this disorder. Current evidence suggests that these patients have an increased incidence of CHD,[156] but they are seemingly less affected than would be expected from their low HDL, which has been attributed to the fact that patients also often have reduced concentrations of LDL.

Mutations in the gene for LCAT, which esterifies cholesterol, can also result in hypoalphalipoproteinemia.[164] As already discussed, LCAT is important in the proper maturation of HDL. In the absence of LCAT, the primary form of HDL that is found is pre–β-HDL, which is the nascent discoidal form of HDL that is phospholipid rich but cholesterol poor. Because of its small size, this form of HDL is rapidly catabolized, leading to the low overall concentration of HDL in these patients. This is an autosomal recessive disorder, but patients with some mutations with partial activity on LDL develop only cloudy corneas from cholesterol deposition and have a disorder called Fish Eye disease. In contrast, familial LCAT deficiency subjects have almost complete absence of LCAT activity on both HDL and LDL and develop not only cloudy corneas but also a mild hemolytic anemia, splenomegaly, and glomerulosclerosis, which is the main cause of morbidity in these patients. It is believed that patients develop renal disease, which first starts as severe proteinuria because of the presence of Lp-X. This is an abnormal lipoprotein particle that also sometimes accumulates in liver disease and appears to be trapped by mesangial cells in the glomerulus, leading to lipid deposition and eventually to glomerulosclerosis. Unlike other lipoprotein particles, which have a single layer of phospholipids on their surface, Lp-X has a phospholipid bilayer–like structure and can even form multilamellar vesicles with an aqueous core. It is believed that such structures are formed when neutral lipid, such as cholesteryl esters, is insufficient to form the neutral lipid core in lipoproteins. Patients with LCAT deficiency appear to possibly have a modestly increased risk for CHD. Similar to Tangier disease subjects, they may be protected because they often have low LDL cholesterol concentrations as much of the cholesterol on LDL is ultimately derived from HDL as a consequence of the reverse cholesterol transport pathway.

Diagnosis of Lipoprotein Disorders

On the basis of findings from many different clinical trials, such as MRFIT and the LRC-CPPT,[165,166] hypercholesterolemia in adults is recognized by all guidelines as a

TABLE 34.15 ATP III Classification of LDL, Total, and HDL Cholesterol, mg/dL*

LDL cholesterol	<100	Optimum
	100–129	Near or above optimum
	130–159	Borderline high
	160–189	High
	≥190	Very high
Total cholesterol	<200	Desirable
	200–239	Borderline high
	≥240	High
HDL cholesterol	<40	Low
	≥60	High

*To convert to mmol/L, divide by 38.66.
ATP, Adult Treatment Panel; *HDL,* high-density lipoprotein; *LDL,* low-density lipoprotein.
Modified from National Heart, Lung, and Blood Institute. Third report of the Expert Panel on Detection, Evaluation, and Treatment of High Blood Cholesterol in Adults (Adult Treatment Panel III, or ATP III). (NIH Publication No. 02-5215). Washington, D.C. 2002.

TABLE 34.16 Categories of Risk for LDL Cholesterol Goals

Risk Category	LDL Goal, mg/dL†
CHD and CHD risk equivalents	<100
Multiple (2+) risk factors*	<130
0–1 risk factor	<160

*Refer to Box 34.2 for list of risk factors.
†To convert to mmol/L, divide by 38.66.
CHD, Coronary heart disease.
Modified from National Heart, Lung, and Blood Institute. Third report of the Expert Panel on Detection, Evaluation, and Treatment of High Blood Cholesterol in Adults (Adult Treatment Panel III, or ATP III). (NIH Publication No. 02-5215). Washington, D.C. 2002.

TABLE 34.17 Clinical Identification of the Metabolic Syndrome

Risk Factor	Defining Level
Abdominal obesity (waist circumference)	
Men	>102 cm (>40 in)
Women	>88 cm (>35 in)
Triglycerides	≥150 mg/dL*
High-density lipoprotein cholesterol	
Men	<40 mg/dL
Women	<50 mg/dL
Blood pressure	≥130/≥85 mm Hg
Fasting glucose	≥100 mg/dL

*To convert to mmol/L, divide by 86.96.
Modified from National Heart, Lung, and Blood Institute. Third report of the Expert Panel on Detection, Evaluation, and Treatment of High Blood Cholesterol in Adults (Adult Treatment Panel III, or ATP III). (NIH Publication No. 02-5215). Washington, D.C. 2002.

BOX 34.2 Major CHD Risk Factors (Exclusive of LDL Cholesterol)

Cigarette smoking
Hypertension (blood pressure ≥140/90 mm Hg or on antihypertensive medication)
Low HDL cholesterol (<40 mg/dL)*
Family history of premature CHD (CHD in male first-degree relative <55 years; CHD in female first-degree relative <65 years)
Age (men ≥45 years; women ≥55 years)

*To convert to mmol/L, divide by 38.66.
Modified from executive summary of the third report of the National Cholesterol Education Program (NCEP) Expert Panel on Detection, Evaluation, and Treatment of High Blood Cholesterol in Adults (Adult Treatment Panel III). *JAMA* 2001;285:2486–97.

major atherosclerosis risk factor. The National Institutes of Health, which sponsored the National Cholesterol Education Program (NCEP), has issued over the years three different Adult Treatment Panel (ATP) reports (ATP I to III) for the detection, evaluation, and treatment of hypercholesterolemia. In ATP I, strategies for primary prevention of CHD in subjects with LDL-C of 160 mg/dL (4.14 mmol/L) or greater, or of 130 to 159 mg/dL (3.36–4.11 mmol/L) and multiple risk factors (two or more) were first addressed.[167] ATP II added new features, such as for subjects with existing CHD, a lower LDL-C goal of 100 mg/dL (2.59 mmol/L) or less was established, and the use of the HDL-C test was given greater prominence.[168] The ATP III report built on the earlier recommendations and expanded the indications for intensive cholesterol lowering (Table 34.15).[102] ATP III called for intensive LDL-C lowering in several other groups of high-risk patients. It also recommended lipid screening starting at age 20, to be repeated every 5 years, and for those with two or more risk factors, recommended Framingham Risk Scoring (Table 34.16). In addition to LDL-C, other risk determinants, presented in Box 34.2, were used to assess risk and determine goals and modalities of LDL-C–lowering therapy. The highest category of risk consists of those with CHD or CHD risk equivalents (other forms of atherosclerotic disease, such as peripheral arterial disease, abdominal aortic aneurysm, and symptomatic carotid artery disease, diabetes, or multiple risk factors that confer a 10-year Framingham risk for CHD >20%). Although the primary target of risk reduction therapy is LDL-C, the ATP III recognized the metabolic syndrome, a constellation of several risk factors (increased triglycerides, decreased HDL-C, obesity, hypertension, and insulin resistance), as a secondary target of therapy. By definition, those with three or more of these risk factors are considered to have the metabolic syndrome.[102] Specific criteria for clinical identification of the metabolic syndrome are listed in Table 34.17.

For the pediatric population, the American Academy of Pediatrics[169,170] defined "high cholesterol" in children and adolescents from families with hypercholesterolemia or premature vascular disease as concentrations greater than the 95th percentile for total and LDL cholesterol in unaffected children (Table 34.18). "Borderline" total and LDL cholesterol concentrations are defined as values between the 75th and 95th percentiles. More recently, the NHLBI recommended universal screening for dyslipidemia by the age of 9 to 11 years and subsequently at an age of 17 to 21 years.[171] Lipid screening should be performed with either a fasting lipid panel (total cholesterol, HDL-C, TG, non–HDL-C, LDL-C) or a nonfasting lipid panel (total cholesterol, HDL-C, non–HDL-C).

TABLE 34.18 NCEP Classification of Total and LDL Cholesterol in Children and Adolescents*

Category	Total Cholesterol	LDL Cholesterol
Desirable	<170	<110
Borderline	170–199	110–120
High	≥200	≥130

*All values are in mg/dL; to convert to mmol/L, multiply by 0.0259.

The Bogalusa Heart Study found that by using the selective screening approach, only 50% of white children and only 20% of black children with high LDL-C concentrations (>95th percentile) were detected.[120] Furthermore, it has been shown that self-reported cholesterol values among parents are an ineffective means of identifying children with high cholesterol.[172] In fact, more than 90% of children with total cholesterol greater than the 75th or 95th percentile were missed when physicians relied on cholesterol values reported by the parents. The universal screening approach is now advised for children on the basis of these findings.

In 2013, NHLBI passed the mission of cardiovascular guideline production to a new task force from the American College of Cardiology/American Heart Association (ACC/AHA), which recently issued new recommendations on the *Treatment of Blood Cholesterol to Reduce Atherosclerotic Cardiovascular Risk in Adults,*[5] on *The Assessment of Cardiovascular Risk,*[173] and *For the Management of Overweight and Obesity in Adults.*[174] The new statement, which for the most part only considered Level I evidence from randomized, blinded, clinical trials and not expert opinion, eliminated numerical treatment targets for LDL-C and non-high-density lipoprotein cholesterol (non–HDL-C) and introduced a new pooled risk calculator for treatment initiation decisions based on cardiovascular disease, which includes not only coronary heart disease but also stroke and peripheral vascular disease. The new risk calculator also has a separate algorithm for African Americans. Patients deemed to be at high risk for CHD, including those with an LDL-C greater than 190 mg/dL (4.91 mmol/L), are advised to initiate lifestyle changes and drug therapy, defined as high-dose statins, in an attempt to reduce LDL-C by 50% from the baseline (Fig. 34.23). Other high-risk groups who are potential candidates for high-dose statins (or moderate-dose if they cannot tolerate high-dose statins) are patients with preexisting CVD and diabetic patients (ages 40–75). Primary prevention patients between ages 40 and 75 who do not fall into one of these high-risk categories should have their 10-year CVD risk calculated and should be treated with high- or moderate-dose statins if it is greater than 7.5% and moderate-dose statins if their risk falls between 5% and 7.5%. Primary prevention patients with a 10-year risk of less than 5% or if they fall outside the age range for the risk calculator (<40 years or >75 years) are generally not recommended for statin therapy but could be considered for lifestyle changes combined with statin therapy, depending on other considerations, such as a strong family history of premature CVD or the results of ancillary testing, such as CRP. Compared to the previous ATP guidelines, it is estimated that significantly more patients will be now treated with statins by the new ACC/AHA guidelines, but some younger patients who would appear to be at risk based on the older guidelines would no longer be treated. Follow-up laboratory testing is recommended by the new guidelines only to judge compliance and to ensure that at least 50% reduction in LDL-C is achieved. Specific cholesterol treatment goals for LDL-C and non–HDL-C are no longer advised. Overall, use of nonstatin therapies is also discouraged by these new guidelines, although this may change in the future with new information, such as the recent clinical trials that show that ezetimibe added to statin was more efficacious compared to statin monotherapy in reducing CV events in an acute coronary syndrome setting.[175] There was no specific guidance on the management of patients with moderate to high triglycerides or increased lipoprotein(a). The ACC/AHA statement also took no position for or against utilizing apolipoprotein B, LDL-particle number, or lipoprotein(a). However, other national and international organizations have included other CVD biomarkers in their lipid and lipoprotein recommendations, particularly for patients at intermediate risk.[176] Because of some of the major differences between the new ACC/AHA guidelines and the previous ATP guidelines, several organizations, such as the National Lipid Association and American Association of Clinical Endocrinology, do not currently endorse the ACC/AHA guidelines and/or have published their own guidelines.[111,177]

Management of Lipoprotein Disorders

Management of Hypercholesterolemia in Adults

According to ATP III, the central element in the clinical prevention of CHD was founded on a public health approach that entailed lifestyle changes, such as a low-fat diet, increased physical activity, and weight control. Although this therapeutic lifestyle approach offered the opportunity for reducing the morbidity and mortality of CHD in the entire population, more intensified preventive measures for higher-risk individuals were indicated.[178] The primary goal was to reduce one's long-term (>10 years) and short-term (<10 years) risks; the target LDL-C value depends on the person's absolute risk (Table 34.19). A more aggressive approach was recommended for those individuals who have already suffered a coronary event and for those with established CHD or those at very high risk of CHD, such as persons with diabetes. Specific models for therapeutic lifestyle changes and how to integrate drug therapy in the primary prevention of CHD were recommended (Fig. 34.24). A combination approach of weight reduction, increased physical activity, and appropriate control of lipid concentrations is recommended for the management of patients with metabolic syndrome.

A wide variety of pharmacologic agents were noted to be available for cholesterol lowering in adults,[179] including bile acid–binding resins (cholestyramine and colestipol), niacin, gemfibrozil, fenofibrate, ezetimibe, and HMG-CoA reductase inhibitors (statins). These drugs can be used individually or in combination. As noted above, the current ACC/AHA cholesterol management statement[5] is prioritized on similar lifestyle advice as ATP III but emphasizes the use of only statins for those patients above a certain CVD risk threshold and do not recommend target treatment goals for LDL-C.

Management of Hypercholesterolemia in Children and Adolescents

To lower serum cholesterol concentration in children and adolescents, current pediatric guidelines have adopted

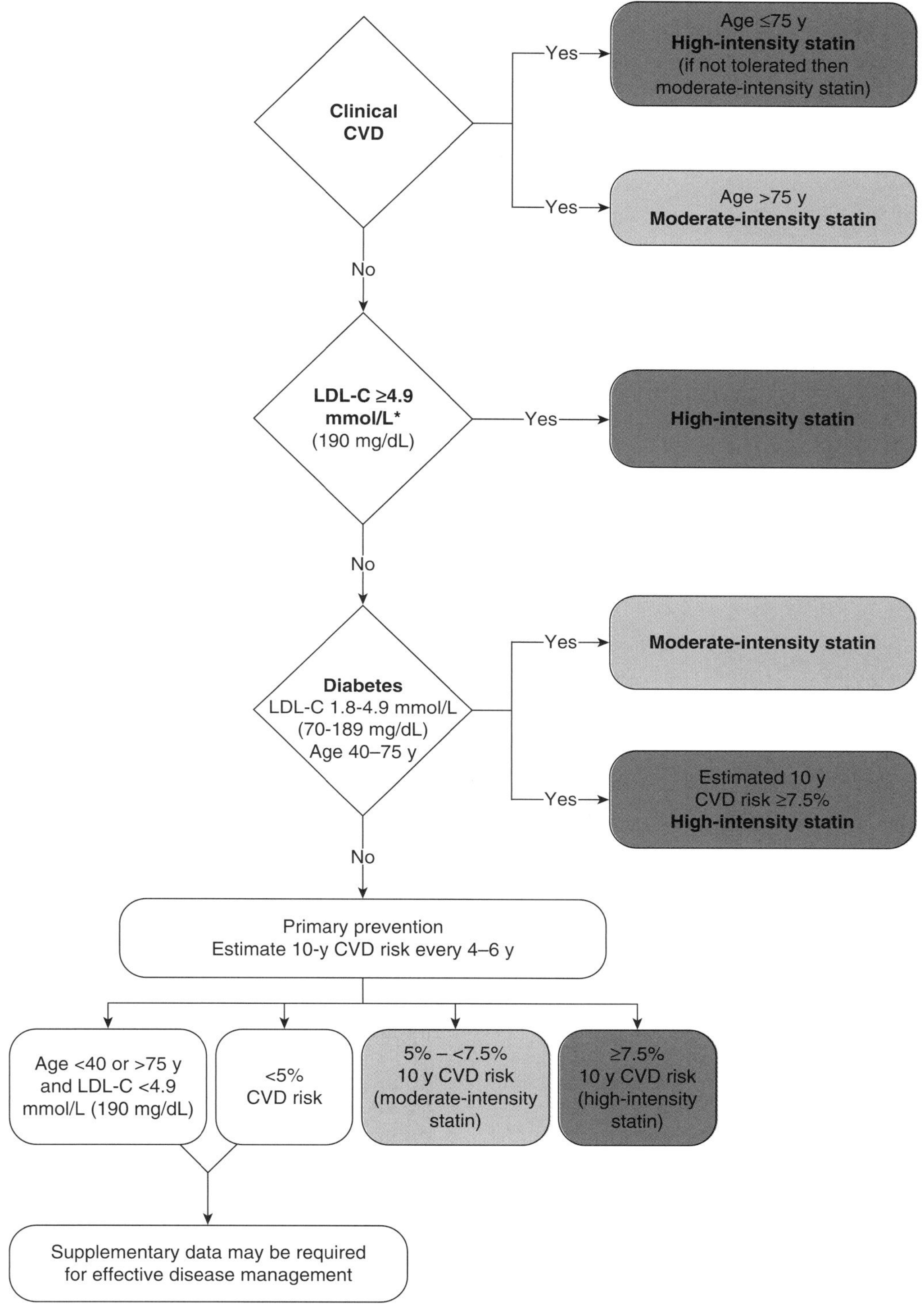

FIGURE 34.23 Algorithm from the ACC/AHA 2013 guidelines on the assessment and treatment of cardiovascular disease risk in adults. *To convert to mmol/L, divide by 38.66. (Modified from 2013 ACC/AHA guideline on the treatment of blood cholesterol to reduce atherosclerotic cardiovascular risk in adults: a report of the American College of Cardiology/American Heart Association Task Force on Practice Guidelines. *Circulation* 2014;129[suppl 2]:S1-S45).

TABLE 34.19 LDL Cholesterol Goals and Cut Points for Therapeutic Lifestyle Changes and Drug Therapy in Different Risk Categories

Risk Category	LDL Goal, mg/dL*	LDL Level at Which to Initiate Therapeutic Lifestyle Changes, mg/dL	LDL Level at Which to Consider Drug Therapy, mg/dL
CHD or CHD risk equivalents (10-year risk >20%)	<100	≥100	≥130 (100–129: drug optional)
2+ risk factors (10-year risk ≤20%)	<130	≥130	10-year risk 10% to 20%: ≥130 10-year risk <10%: ≥160
0–1 risk factor (10-year risk <10%)	<160	≥160	≥190 (160–189: LDL-lowering drug optional)

*To convert to mmol/L, divide by 38.66.

CHD, Coronary heart disease; *LDL,* low-density lipoprotein.

Modified from National Heart, Lung, and Blood Institute. Third report of the Expert Panel on Detection, Evaluation, and Treatment of High Blood Cholesterol in Adults (Adult Treatment Panel III, or ATP III). (NIH Publication No. 02-5215). Washington, D.C. 2002.

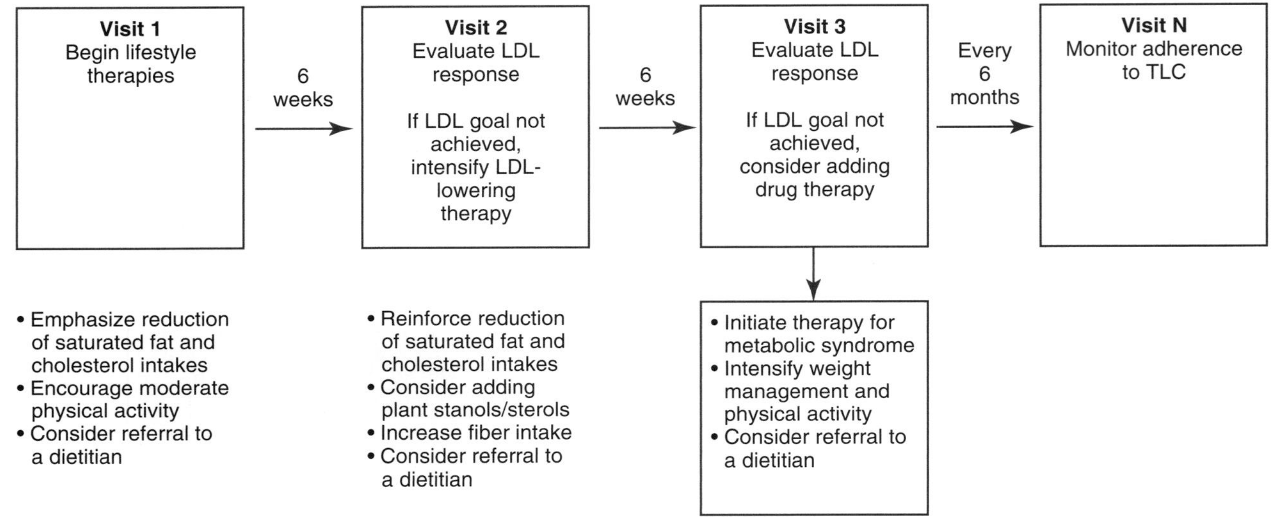

FIGURE 34.24 Model of steps in therapeutic lifestyle change. *LDL,* Low-density lipoprotein. (Modified from Executive summary of the third report of the Expert Panel on Blood Cholesterol Levels in Children and Adolescents, National Cholesterol Education Program. Lipid Metabolism Branch, Division of Heart, Lung, and Blood Institute. NIH Publication No. 01-3670. US Department of Health and Human Services, Public Health Service, National Institutes of Health. Bethesda, Md: National Institutes of Health, 2003)

strategies that combines two complementary approaches: a population approach and an individualized approach.

Population Approach. The population approach attempts to lower the mean cholesterol concentration by instituting population-wide modifications in nutrient intake and eating habits. Genetic studies have shown that even a modest decrease in mean cholesterol concentration in children and adolescents, if carried into adulthood, is likely to have a significant impact on lowering the incidence of CHD. The population approach is also critical from a public health standpoint because the focus of treating most aggressively those patients at the greatest risk for CVD does not take into account the fact that the majority of patients who do go on to develop CVD are in the middle of the distribution for total cholesterol or LDL-C and may not appear to be at high risk, using the guidelines developed for the individualized approach.

In regard to children with hypercholesterolemia, it is thought that intake of total fat can be safely limited to 30% of total calories. It is recommended that saturated fat intake be limited to 7% to 10% of calories and that dietary cholesterol be limited to 300 mg/day. However, fat intake for infants younger than 12 months should not be restricted without medical indication.[171]

Individualized Approach. The latest NHLBI guidelines in 2011 for the management of children at risk for cardiovascular disease are aimed at primary care physicians and are integrated guidelines that make age-specific recommendations on the multiple risk factors that contribute to cardiovascular disease.[180] An algorithm on how to use these guidelines is shown in Fig. 34.25. Unlike previous pediatric guidelines, which largely recommended identifying at-risk children based on family history of CHD or dyslipidemia, the current guidelines recommend univeral screening by lipid testing at specific ages. Because it is more convenient, particularly for children, a nonfasting sample is adequate for screening, and criteria based on non–HDL-C, which is simply total cholesterol minus LDL-C, is used for making the initial decisions on managment. If non–HDL-C is greater than 145 mg/dL (3.75 mmol/L), a fasting sample should be analyzed for lipids.

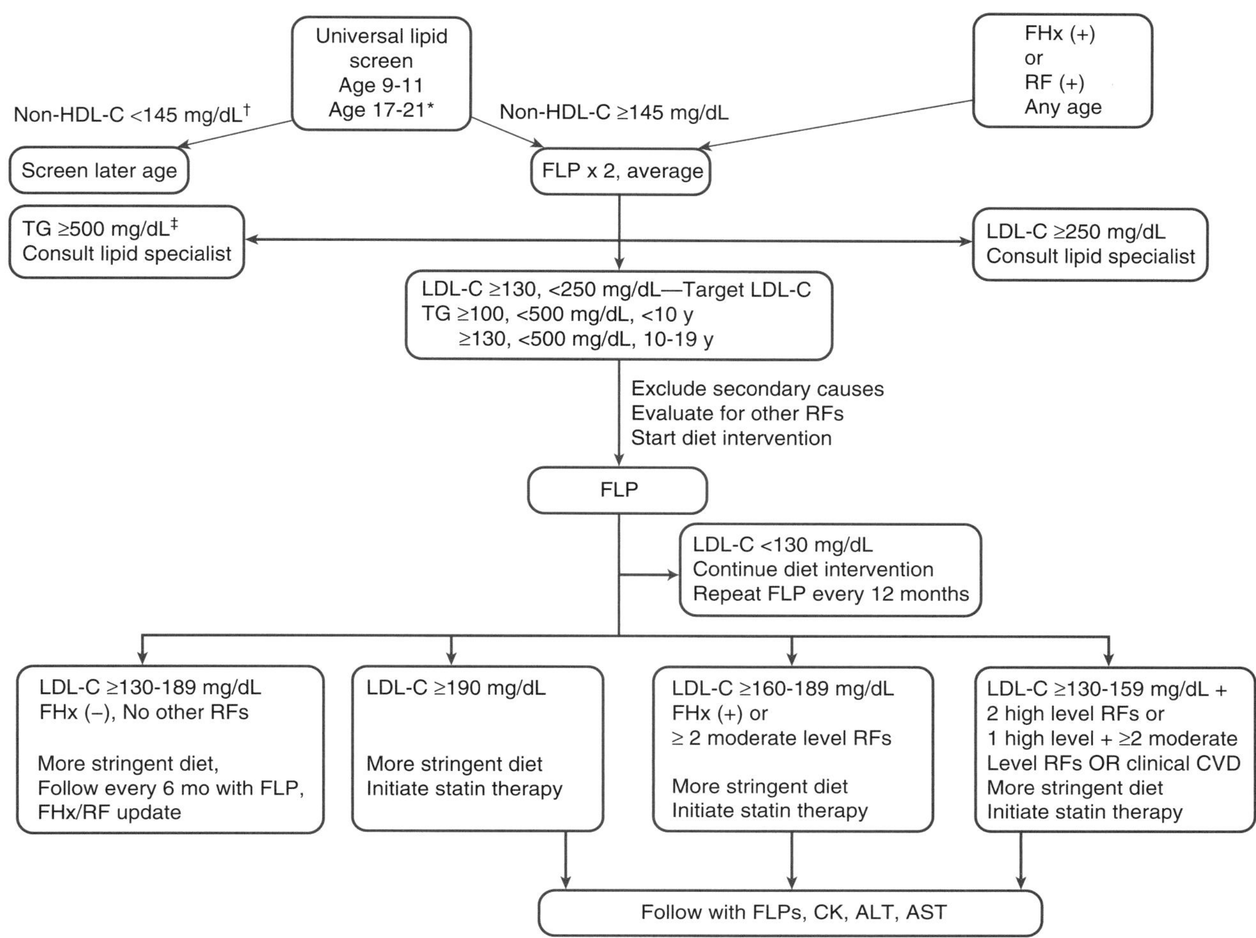

FIGURE 34.25 Algorithm for the assessment of coronary heart disease (CHD) risk in children based on lipid screening. *For ages 19 to 21, non–HDL-C >90 mg/dL is the recommended cut point. †For HDL-C and LDL-C, to convert to mmol/L, divide by 38.66. ‡To convert to mmol/L, divide by 86.96. *FHx(+),* Positive family history; *RF,* risk factor; *FLP,* fasting lipid profile; *ALT,* alanine aminotransferase; *AST,* aspartate aminotransferase; *CK,* creating kinase. (Modified from Expert Panel of Integrated Guidelines for Cardiovascular Health and Risk Reduction in Children and Adolescents. Summary report. *Pediatrics* 2011;128:S1–S44.)

Children with a TG of 500 mg/dL (5.65 mmol/L) or higher, or an LDL-C of 250 mg/dL (6.47 mmol/L) or higher likely have a genetic lipid disorder and should be referred to a lipid specialist.

Like adults, recommended interventions for children are calibrated to the degree of CHD risk, and lifestyle changes are the first line of therapy for all patients. The most common type of dyslipidemic pattern in children is a moderate to severe increase in triglycerides, with a moderate increase in LDL-C and a low HDL-C. This type of dyslipidemia is often found in obesity and typically shows a good response to diet changes and weight loss. Because there is less long-term safety and effectiveness data on drug therapy for children than adults, there is greater concern on using drugs, like statins, in this population. Nevetheless, it is well understood that the process of atherosclerosis often begins at an early age and that CHD risk factors in children, such as dyslipidemia and obesity, often persist into adulthood. For children with heterozygous familial hypercholesterolemia, earlier treatment has clearly been shown to lead to reduced cardiovascular disease. Statin therapy is advised for those aged 10 years or older with an LDL cholesterol of 190 mg/dL (4.91 mmol/L) or greater after a 6-month trial of lifestyle management. As described in Fig. 34.25, children with an LDL less than 130 mg/dL (3.36 mmol/L) may also be candidates for statin therapy, depending on their other risk factors and family history. If children are placed on statin therapy, unlike adults, they should be started with the lowest possible dose, and hepatic transaminases and creatine kinase should be carefully monitored.

Management of Hypertriglyceridemia

ATP-III guidelines, using evidence-based findings, reported triglycerides to be an independent risk factor for CHD in both men and women and placed greater emphasis on management of patients with TG disorders. Subsequently, this has been sustained by triglyceride position statements from the AHA, AACE, and European Atherosclerosis Society Consensus Panel.[181,182] Cardiovascular-related risk for TG begins at concentrations greater than 100 mg/dL (1.13 mmol/L) and becomes substantial at levels greater than 150 to 200 mg/dL (1.7–2.26 mmol/L). The different organizations classify elevated TG somewhat differently, with the AHA listing levels greater than 200 mg/dL (2.26 mmol/L) as high and greater than 500 mg/dL (5.66 mmol/L) as very high, whereas the Endocrine Society lists moderate concentrations as 200 to 999 mg/dL (1.7–11.3 mmol/L), severe as 1000 to 1999 mg/dL (11.3–22.6 mmol/L), and very severe as greater than 2000 mg/dL (22.6 mmol/L).

In the general population, several conditions and factors are associated with increased triglyceride concentrations, including obesity, pregnancy, cigarette smoking, physical inactivity, and excess alcohol intake, as well as several diseases (eg, type 2 diabetes, chronic renal failure), drugs (eg, corticosteroids, estrogens, retinoids, antipsychotics, antiretoviral), and genetic disorders (eg, FCHL, FHTG). NCEP ATP-III emphasized that hypertriglyceridemia is often associated with the metabolic syndrome in association with reduced HDL-C, insulin resistance, hypertension, and increased waist size. Triglyceride-rich lipoproteins, which include remnant lipoproteins; TG-rich LDL; and small, dense LDL, are currently recognized to be atherogenic. In practice, VLDL-C (measured or calculated as TG/5) is often used as a measure of these atherogenic lipoproteins. Therefore ATP III suggested the addition of non–HDL-C (total cholesterol − HDL-C) as an indicator for all atherogenic lipoproteins (mainly LDL and remnant VLDL).[178] Non–HDL-C is used as a secondary target of therapy in persons with triglycerides of 200 mg/dL (2.26 mmol/L) or greater by NCEP and the NLA lipid recommendations but not the ACC/AHA guidelines.[5] The goal for non–HDL-C in those with increased triglycerides is 30 mg/dL (0.78 mmol/L) above that set for LDL-C. The treatment of hypertriglyceridemia depends on the cause of the increase and the severity. Those with triglycerides less than 200 mg/dL (2.26 mmol/L) are treated with weight reduction and increased physical activity; for those at 200 to 499 mg/dL (2.26–5.63mmol/L), drug therapy is also considered (statins and fibrates, specifically fenofibrate). In the latter group, the non–HDL-C goal becomes a secondary target of therapy (Table 34.20). Those with triglycerides greater than 500 mg/dL (5.65 mmol/L) usually are at increased risk of pancreatitis and are treated with a low-fat diet (≤15% of calorie intake), weight reduction, increased physical activity, and triglyceride-lowering drugs (fibrates, statins, high-dose omega-3 fatty acids, and possibly niacin).

TABLE 34.20 Comparison of LDL Cholesterol and Non–HDL Cholesterol Goals for Three Risk Categories

Risk Category	LDL Goal, mg/dL*	Non-HDL Goal, mg/dL
CHD and CHD risk equivalent (10-year risk for CHD >20%)	<100	<130
Multiple (2+) risk factors and 10-year risk ≤20%	<130	<160
0–1 risk factor	<160	<190

*To convert to mmol/L, divide by 38.66.

CHD, Coronary heart disease; *HDL,* high-density lipoprotein; *LDL,* low-density lipoprotein.

Modified from National Heart, Lung, and Blood Institute. Third report of the Expert Panel on Detection, Evaluation, and Treatment of High Blood Cholesterol in Adults (Adult Treatment Panel III, or ATP III). (NIH Publication No. 02-5215). Washington, D.C. 2002.

MEASUREMENT OF LIPIDS, LIPOPROTEINS, AND APOLIPOPROTEINS

Lipoproteins and their lipid and apolipoprotein constituents have become increasingly important in characterizing the risk of cardiovascular disease and in the diagnosis and management of lipoprotein disorders. In recent decades, our knowledge of such disorders has evolved from an essentially descriptive association between elevated plasma lipids and increased risk for CVD to a much broader understanding of the underlying biochemistry, physiology, and genetic interactions. Remarkable advances have also been made in our understanding of the contribution of lipoproteins to the development and progression of arterial lesions. Advances have also been made in the analytical techniques and methods used for measuring lipids, lipoproteins, and apolipoproteins. In this section, we begin with a brief historical perspective on the development of measurement technology, which is followed by a more detailed discussion of pertinent methods.

Historical Perspective and Background

The causal relationship between increased plasma concentrations of LDL and risk of CHD and the efficacy of LDL lowering to reduce risk was widely acknowledged by the mid-1980s.[95] Awareness of the importance of intervention emphasized the necessity for uniform means of defining hyperlipidemia and CHD risk. Previous practice had been to use arbitrarily defined cutoffs based on prevailing lipid and lipoprotein concentrations in the general population or in local populations of "normal patients." Because of the relative nonspecificity of early chemical methods for cholesterol measurement and the different types of methods then in use, significant biases sometimes existed between values obtained in different laboratories, and it was not uncommon for "normal" reference intervals to be laboratory specific. Quantitation of the relationship between total or LDL-C concentration and risk for CHD, demonstration of the efficacy of treatment, and development of reference methods and Centers for Disease Control and Prevention (CDC) standardization programs for lipids and lipoproteins[183] made possible the use of risk-related cutoff points used in the earlier ATP-III guidelines (see Tables 34.15 and 34.18). This led to the necessity for uniform definitions of hyperlipidemia based on commonly accepted risk-based lipid and lipoprotein cutoffs and the availability of accurate lipid and lipoprotein measurements.

Consensus Guidelines From Expert Panels

Beginning in the mid-1980s, the NCEP convened several expert panels to develop guidelines for diagnosis and treatment of hypercholesterolemia and for reliable lipid and lipoprotein measurements. Two laboratory panels issued recommendations for blood lipids and lipoproteins. The first, the NCEP Laboratory Standardization Panel, focused on measurement of total cholesterol[184]; the second, the NCEP Working Group on Lipoprotein Measurement, addressed measurements of triglycerides, HDL-C, and LDL-C.[185] In 2009, expert recommendations for apo B and LDL-P were published.[105] Here we summarize the principal considerations and recommendations for clinical lipid and lipoprotein measurements.

Basic Issues

In developing recommendations for lipid and lipoprotein measurement, the different NCEP panels considered several basic issues. First, in most of the large-scale clinical and epidemiologic studies that established (1) relationships between lipids and lipoproteins, (2) risk for CHD, and (3) efficacy of cholesterol lowering, measurements were made in standardized laboratories in which the accuracy of measurements was traceable to CDC reference methods. This included studies such as the National Diet Heart Study in the 1960s, various LRC program studies (early 1970s to 1990), Specialized Centers of Research in Atherosclerosis studies (early 1970s to the present), and several NHANES studies conducted between 1960 and 1994.[183] Second, various methods used in laboratory or nonlaboratory settings should be capable of similar accuracy (ie, the reliability of the measurements should be independent of how, where, or by whom they were made). Ideally, it should be possible to consider all lipid measurements made in the United States (and eventually globally) as if they had been made in a single laboratory. This premise does *not* require that all laboratories use the same methods, but it does require methods that are capable of providing values equivalent to those on which the relationships between lipids, lipoproteins, and the risk for CHD were established. Third, as new methods are developed, particularly those that may be more accurate and precise for various lipoproteins or lipoprotein subfractions, the particular lipoprotein included in the measurement should be specified. This is done to ensure that new methods can be linked to those that were used to establish the known lipoprotein–CHD risk relationships. To achieve these aims, development of reference methods that could be used as accuracy targets for lipid and lipoprotein measurements was required; also, guidelines for analytical performance were established.

Analytical Challenges

Plasma lipoproteins are heterogeneous and polydisperse macromolecular complexes that vary considerably in size, composition, and function, and consequently present exceptional analytical challenges (see Table 34.4). Traditionally, lipoprotein concentrations have been expressed in terms of their cholesterol content. This approach simplified the methods used to determine lipoproteins because the lipoprotein fractions of interest have only to be separated from one another; the other plasma proteins do not have to be removed. Analytically, cholesterol has a known molecular structure and can be accurately and precisely measured with appropriate chemical or biochemical methods.

Triglycerides and the lipoproteins themselves, however, are not unique chemical entities (eg, triglycerides consist of many possible fatty acyl groups covalently attached to three positions on a glycerol backbone through ester linkages) (see Fig. 34.13). Fatty acyl groups vary in chain length and degree of saturation, leading to a mixture of triglycerides of different molecular weights. Consequently, triglyceride methods usually measure the glycerol backbone, and triglyceride concentration is then stated only in terms of molar concentration. In the United States, however, lipids have been traditionally expressed in terms of mass concentration (milligrams per deciliter), which is an approximation requiring an assumption about the average molecular weight of triglycerides. Because palmitate, stearate, and oleate are the major fatty acids in plasma triglycerides and have similar molecular weights, the conversion between molar and mass concentration usually assumes an average triglyceride molecular weight of 885 Da, the molecular weight of tri-oleyl glycerol (olein).

The situation for the accurate measurement is even more complicated for LDL and HDL. For example, LDL consists of a population of multiple subparticles varying in size and lipid composition, each containing apo B-100 as the major apolipoprotein component. Thus LDL has neither a unique molecular weight nor consistent lipid or protein composition. HDL is even more heterogeneous, consisting of at least 12 subclasses, differing in composition, function, and even CHD risk relationships.[186] Because of these characteristics, the exact concentration and composition of a fraction identified as LDL or HDL may vary, depending on how the fraction is isolated. Once isolated, however, the cholesterol content can be measured accurately. A major consideration, therefore, was to define the lipoproteins in a uniform way to afford a common basis for standardization and the assessment of accuracy without inhibiting the development of new methods or necessitating use of the same methods in all laboratories.

Analytical Approach

For more than 50 years, the CDC has maintained reference methods for cholesterol, triglycerides, and HDL-C and has provided standardization programs targeted for the research laboratories. In addition, these reference methods were used to establish the accuracy of lipid and lipoprotein measurements in several population studies, including the LRC and CPPT studies, and several NHANES studies conducted by the National Center for Health Statistics since the 1960s.[187] From these studies, cut points for risk characterization in patients were derived. Because the standardization programs were already accepted as authoritative by the general laboratory and research communities, the NCEP laboratory panels recommended the CDC reference methods as the basis for defining "accuracy" in the context of recommendations for reliable lipid and lipoprotein measurements. Use of this approach had several advantages. First, it established the same basis for accuracy that had been used in developing the relationships between lipid and lipoprotein concentration and CHD; second, it provided a reference point by which the accuracy of existing or newly developed methods could be assessed.

Lipids and Lipoproteins

Various technologies have been used to separate and measure plasma lipids and lipoproteins and lipoprotein subfractions, including enzymatic, immunochemical, and chemical precipitation reagents, and physical methods, such as ultracentrifugation, electrophoresis, column chromatography, and others.[188] Moreover, although different methods of lipoprotein separation may produce similar lipoprotein fractions, they usually do not produce identical fractions, giving rise to systematic biases among methods that purport to measure the same component. The present discussion focuses primarily on accepted reference methods and procedures commonly used in clinical practice for lipid and lipoprotein measurements.

Reference Methods

Reference methods are the "gold standards" or accuracy targets that have been developed for the more common analytes, such as cholesterol, triglycerides, and LDL and HDL cholesterol.[189] The reference method for cholesterol is fully validated and credentialed through the Joint Committee for Traceability in Laboratory Medicine. The other methods, although not formally credentialed, have been accepted by consensus.

Cholesterol. The original CDC reference method for cholesterol[190-192] is based on a chemical method devised by Abell and colleagues. The method exhibits an approximate 1.6% positive bias compared with isotope dilution mass spectrometry, which is considered to be the highest-order method for cholesterol and was developed and applied by the National Institute of Standards and Technology.[191] Cholesterol may be expressed in terms of molar (millimoles per liter) or mass (milligrams per deciliter) concentration. Molar concentration is converted to mass concentration using the following equation:

$$\text{mg/dL} = \text{mmol/L} \times 38.7 \qquad \textbf{34.1}$$

The CDC reference method, demonstrated to be readily transferable to other laboratories,[190] has been widely adopted by reference laboratories and diagnostic manufacturers as the accuracy target and the basis for calibration in cholesterol measurements.

Triglycerides. As for cholesterol, the original CDC reference procedure for triglycerides[183,185,189] was a chemical method. It depended on the extraction and alkaline hydrolysis to produce glycerol, which was then oxidized with periodate and reacted with chromotropic acid to generate a chromagen in the following reaction:

$$\text{Triglycerides} + \text{KOH} \rightarrow \text{Fatty acids} + \text{Glycerol} \qquad \textbf{34.2}$$

$$\text{Glycerol} + \text{Periodate} \rightarrow \text{Formic acid} + \text{Formaldehyde} \qquad \textbf{34.3}$$

$$\text{Formaldehyde} + \text{Chromotropic acid} \rightarrow \text{Chromogen} \qquad \textbf{34.4}$$

Results may be expressed in terms of molar concentration (millimoles per liter) or mass concentration (milligrams per deciliter). The following equation is used to convert mmol/dL to mg/dL:

$$\text{mg/dL} = \text{mmol/L} \times 88.5 \qquad \textbf{34.5}$$

The equation assumes an average molecular weight of 885 g/mol (triolein) for plasma triglycerides. To facilitate standardization of triglyceride measurements, a designated comparison method (DCM) has been developed by the Cholesterol Reference Method Laboratory Network (CRMLN), involving similar extraction steps followed by more robust enzymatic quantitation of the triglyceride-derived glycerol.[193] This DCM, established in other reference laboratories, is expected to become the secondary accuracy target for triglycerides. In 2011, because the original reference method of the CDC was complex and not robust, a new reference method was developed for triglyceride based on gas chromatographic isotope dilution mass spectrometry (GC-IDMS). In this new method, all glycerides (triglycerides, diglycerides, and monoglycerides), as before, are chemically reduced to glycerol, which then is measured by GC-IDMS.

High-Density Lipoprotein Cholesterol. Both a reference method and a designated comparison method have been developed to measure HDL cholesterol.

Reference Method. Because HDL consists of several populations of particles that vary somewhat in their cholesterol content, HDL is commonly defined in terms of the method used to prepare the HDL-containing fraction. The CDC reference method[89,189] uses a combination of ultracentrifugation and polyanion precipitation to isolate HDL. The cholesterol in this fraction is then quantitated using the CDC reference method for cholesterol. In this method, VLDL and chylomicrons, if present, are first removed by ultracentrifugation of an accurately measured volume of serum for 16.2 hours at 33,700 rpm in a Beckman-type 50.4 rotor. Under these conditions, VLDL and any chylomicrons accumulate as a floating layer at the top of the ultracentrifuge tube (d = 1.006 g/mL). A tube-slicing technique is used to remove the VLDL fraction. The infranatant, which contains IDL, LDL, Lp(a), HDL, and the other serum proteins, is recovered quantitatively. The apo B-100–containing lipoproteins in 2 mL of this fraction are precipitated by adding 80 μL of injectable heparin (5000 USP units/mL of 0.15 mol/L NaCl in water) and 100 μL of 1.0 mol/L manganese chloride to water. The precipitate is removed by centrifugation, and cholesterol in the clear supernatant is measured. HDL cholesterol may be expressed in molar or mass concentration; molar concentration is converted to mass concentration using Eq. 34.1.

Heparin-$MnCl_2$ was selected as the precipitation reagent primarily for historical reasons because it was the method most commonly used in early studies to establish the relationship between HDL cholesterol concentration and risk for CHD. The ultracentrifugation step was included to prevent interference with sedimentation of the apo B-100–containing lipoproteins by the lighter triglyceride-rich lipoproteins, VLDL, and chylomicrons.

Designated Comparison Method. Only a few routine diagnostic laboratories have an ultracentrifuge and the experience required to reliably perform the CDC reference method for HDL cholesterol. Furthermore, ultracentrifugation is expensive and necessitates obtaining an impractically large specimen volume, typically 5.0 mL. As a practical alternative, the CRMLN laboratories developed and validated a modified dextran sulfate (50,000 Da) procedure as a DCM to provide results approximately equivalent to those of the CDC reference method (RM), while avoiding ultracentrifugation.[194] The $MgCl_2$ concentration in the precipitant reagent was decreased slightly from that used in the previously published primary method to increase HDL-C values slightly, achieving closer agreement with the CDC reference method.

Low-Density Lipoprotein Cholesterol. The CDC has also defined a reference method for LDL-C based on the similar techniques already described for HDL-C.[195] After ultracentrifugation to remove the VLDL and any chylomicrons present, the bottom fraction (d = 1.006) is subjected to precipitation by heparin and manganese, as described previously. After measurement of cholesterol in the d = 1.006 fraction and in the heparin-Mn^{2+} supernatant solution, LDL-C is calculated by difference. It should be noted that the LDL fraction as measured by this reference method, which is commonly called β-quantification, is a so-called "broad-cut fraction" and includes not only LDL but also IDL and Lp(a).

POINTS TO REMEMBER

LDL

- LDL cholesterol is a causative factor of CVD.
- Apo B-100 is the main protein in LDL.
- LDL is removed from circulation by LDL receptors.
- LDL cholesterol concentrations are estimated using the Friedewald calculation or can be directly measured using homogeneous methods.
- HMG-reductase inhibitors (statins) are the most effective drugs in reducing LDL cholesterol concentrations.

Application of Reference Methods to Standardization

Background. Early efforts in the mid-1980s to achieve general standardization of methods used by clinical laboratories began with a fairly traditional approach with secondary reference materials provided to the laboratory community. The reference materials consisted of lyophilized serum pools with target values assigned on the basis of replicate measurements, using the reference methods. However, problems were recognized with this approach, primarily from the confounding effects of matrix changes in the reference materials, making them noncommutable with native clinical samples.[196] Secondary reference materials prepared from pooled serum spiked with artificial analytes and subjected to freezing and freeze-drying are not always commutable and did not behave like fresh patient specimens with some routine methods. In several notable cases, diagnostic manufacturers used the secondary reference materials to assign presumably reliable targets to their calibrators but subsequently found that results on patient specimens became inaccurate. The problem was compounded by national proficiency testing programs, which, in an attempt to improve accuracy, began to report reference method target values with similarly prepared survey materials. Laboratories were adjusting calibration to achieve apparent accuracy on the survey materials; however, in some instances, results on actual patient specimens were made inaccurate.

Recognition of these problems focused attention on the issues of "analyte" and "matrix" effects in reference materials.[196] Procedures commonly used in preparing secondary reference materials were inducing changes in the analytes themselves and in the other constituents and fluids surrounding the analytes that made their analyses no longer comparable with measurements in authentic fresh patient specimens. After considerable study and deliberation, the conclusion was reached that the only universally reliable means of transferring accuracy from the reference methods to diagnostic manufacturers and individual laboratories was through direct comparison studies on fresh, representative patient specimens.[197] As a consequence, the CDC and other groups cooperated to organize a network of reference laboratories to provide the reference methods and fresh sample comparison studies.

The Cholesterol Reference Method Laboratory Network. Because the CDC standardization laboratory maintaining the reference methods did not have the capacity to perform all necessary comparison studies directly, it was obvious that the reference laboratory capability would have to be expanded to accommodate the needs of the industry and the laboratory community. To this end, the CDC and several other interested laboratories cooperated to establish the Cholesterol Reference Method Laboratory Network (CRMLN). Each participating network laboratory underwent stringent protocols to transfer the CDC reference methods and to maintain comparability with the CDC. In turn, the network laboratories performed comparison studies using fresh patient sera with the diagnostic manufacturers and with individual laboratories. Throughout the 1990s, the network was large and active to accommodate the demands of comparison studies. As standardization has steadily improved in subsequent years, the concentration of activity has declined, and the number of domestic US network laboratories has decreased. However, at the same time, the network laboratory program has expanded to include additional international laboratories.

The network offers protocols, based on Clinical and Laboratory Standards Institute guidelines, whereby diagnostic manufacturers ensure accuracy by completing comparison studies using the reference methods. A measurement system qualifies for certification by demonstrating agreement within specified limits for total cholesterol, HDL-C, and LDL-C and for triglycerides. Based on comparison results, calibrator set points are adjusted if necessary to bring performance into agreement with the reference methods. Diagnostic manufacturers and distributors and instrument partners are encouraged to certify their systems at least every 2 years and to ensure that every production lot is calibrated to maintain traceability to the accuracy targets; this can be accomplished through ongoing participation in the CDC and/or CRMLN program. The CDC website (http://www.cdc.gov/labstandards/crmln.html/) provides details of the program, protocols for comparison studies, contact information for the CDC and/or CRMLN, and a listing of commercial methods that have qualified for certification.

Routine Methods

Reference methods are complex, typically time-consuming, and at least partially manual, and they require a high degree of expertise for reliable operation. Consequently, simpler and more practical methods have evolved for routine clinical use.

Cholesterol. Enzymatic methods for cholesterol measurement are precise, accurate when calibrated appropriately, and easily adapted for use with modern analyzers. Commercially available cholesterol reagents commonly combine all of the enzymes and other required components into a single photometric reagent. The reagent usually is mixed with a few μL of serum or plasma and incubated under controlled conditions for color development, and absorbance is measured in the visible portion of the spectrum, generally at about 500 nm. The reagents typically use a bacterial cholesteryl ester hydrolase to cleave cholesteryl esters.

$$\text{Cholesteryl ester} + H_2O \xrightarrow{\text{Cholesteryl ester hydrolase}} \text{Cholesterol} + \text{Fatty acid} \quad (34.6)$$

The 3-OH group of cholesterol is then oxidized to a ketone in an oxygen-requiring reaction catalyzed by cholesterol oxidase.

$$\text{Cholesterol} + O_2 \xrightarrow{\text{Cholesterol oxidase}} \text{Cholest-4-en-3-one} + H_2O_2 \quad (34.7)$$

H_2O_2, one of the reaction products, is measured in a peroxidase catalyzed reaction that forms a colored dye:

$$H_2O_2 + \text{Phenol} + \text{4-Aminoantipyrine} \xrightarrow{\text{Peroxidase}} \text{Quinoneimine dye} + 2\,H_2O \quad \textbf{34.8}$$

These methods may be subject to interference from other colored compounds or those that compete with the oxidation reaction or react with peroxide, such as bilirubin, ascorbic acid, and hemoglobin. Assays are usually linear up to about 1000 mg/dL (25.9 mmol/L). Reagents have been refined by adding substances, such as bilirubin oxidase and dual-wavelength readings, to minimize the effects of hemolysis; interference from bilirubin generally is not an issue now in concentrations below 5 mg/dL (85.5 umol/L).[192,198] Enzymatic reagents are not entirely specific for cholesterol because β-hydroxy sterols and plant sterols (eg, sitosterol) can also react. In human serum or plasma, however, this is not a major problem because these interfering sterols are generally present in relatively low concentrations.

In practice, reagent formulations vary from manufacturer to manufacturer. In most cases, the reagent from a particular manufacturer will have been optimized for use with one or several specific instruments and calibration materials—usually those sold by that manufacturer. Over the past few years, most manufacturers have been supplying calibration materials with assigned values that are traceable to the CDC reference method; this has helped reduce interlaboratory variation. Thus cholesterol methods are best thought of as "measurement systems" composed of reagent, calibrator (cholesterol standard), and instrument. When a reagent-calibrator-instrument system from a single manufacturer is used, cholesterol measurements in the laboratory usually are accurate within 1% to 3% of reference values, and such systems are routinely operated with coefficients of variation less than 2.5%. In some cases, however, a reagent from one manufacturer might be used with an instrument from another. In this instance, the responsibility is on the user rather than the manufacturer to ensure that reagent and sample volumes, time and temperature of incubation, and the calibration produce precise and accurate measurements. Although the cholesterol oxidase reagent described previously in this chapter is by far the most common, reagents have been developed for using cholesterol dehydrogenase, which may have advantages in some instances.[199] In addition, other highly sensitive enzymatic methods have been described for specialized applications.[200] Free or unesterified cholesterol can be readily quantified by deleting the cholesterol esterase from the reagent.

Triglycerides. Triglycerides are also commonly measured with enzyme reagents directly in plasma or serum. Reagents combining all required enzymes, cofactors, and buffers are available from various manufacturers. As for cholesterol, such reagents are optimized for use with particular instrument-calibrator systems. Several different enzyme reactions have been used. In all methods, the first step is the lipase-catalyzed hydrolysis of triglycerides to glycerol and fatty acids:

$$\text{Triglyceride} + 3\,H_2O \xrightarrow{\text{Lipase}} \text{Glycerol} + 3\text{ fatty acids} \quad \textbf{34.9}$$

Glycerol then is phosphorylated in an ATP-requiring reaction catalyzed by glycerokinase:

$$\text{Glycerol} + \text{ATP} \xrightarrow{\text{Glycerokinase}} \text{Glycerophosphate} + \text{Adenosine diphosphate (ADP)} \quad \textbf{34.10}$$

In the most commonly used methods, glycerophosphate is then oxidized to dihydroxyacetone and H_2O_2 in a glycerophosphate oxidase–catalyzed reaction,

$$\text{Glycerophosphate} + O_2 \xrightarrow{\text{Glycerophosphate oxidase}} \text{Dihydroxyacetone} + H_2O_2 \quad \textbf{34.11}$$

and the H_2O_2 formed in the reaction is measured as described in reaction (8).

Alternatively, glycerophosphate can be measured in a reduced form of nicotinamide-adenine dinucleotide (NADH)-producing reaction, and NADH is measured by a spectrophotometer set at 340 nm or in a diaphorase-catalyzed reaction to form a reaction product whose absorbance is measured at 500 nm:

$$\text{Glycerophosphate} + \text{Nicotinamide-adenine dinucleotide (NAD)} \xrightarrow{\text{Glycerophosphate dehydrogenase}} \text{Dihydroxyacetone phosphate} + \text{NADH} + H^+ \quad \textbf{34.12}$$

$$\text{NADH} + \text{Tetrazolium dye} \xrightarrow{\text{Diaphorase}} \text{Formazan} + \text{NAD}^+ \quad \textbf{34.13}$$

Other methods measure the ADP produced in reaction (10), as shown in Eqs. 34.14 and 34.15:

$$\text{ADP} + \text{Phosphoenol pyruvate} \xrightarrow{\text{Pyruvate kinase}} \text{ATP} + \text{Pyruvate} \quad \textbf{34.14}$$

$$\text{Pyruvate} + \text{NADH} + H^+ \xrightarrow{\text{Lactate dehydrogenase}} \text{Lactate} + \text{NAD}^+ \quad \textbf{34.15}$$

Loss of NADH is photometrically measured at 340 nm.

Enzymatic triglyceride methods are fairly specific in that they do not detect glucose or phospholipids. Most are linear in the concentration range up to about 1000 mg/dL (11.3 mmol/L), and when automated, they are operated with coefficients of variation up to approximately 3%. The methods are usually calibrated with reference solutions of pure glycerol or with serum-based secondary calibrators. However, because all methods measure the glycerol component, any free glycerol in the sample contributes to the apparent amount of triglyceride. With routine methods, the decision must be made whether to correct for free glycerol by using a method that corrects for the free glycerol blank.

Triglyceride Blanks (Correction for Endogenous Glycerol). Glycerol concentrations in freshly collected serum or plasma in healthy subjects are usually less than 5 to 10 mg/dL (543–1086 umol/L). Because this small amount is medically insignificant, the triglyceride blank is usually ignored. Glycerol, however, can be higher in samples with increased triglyceride concentrations and from patients with conditions such as diabetes or those receiving total parenteral nutrition, but even in these conditions, the free glycerol concentration does not generally substantially affect the interpretation. Rarely, glycerol can be markedly increased by 50- to 100-fold in a rare disorder called *hyperglycerolemia,* which is the result of a deficiency in glycerokinase.[201] This is sometimes called pseudohypertriglyceridemia and can result in improper CV risk assessment and treatment.[202]

Although triglyceride blanks in most cases can be ignored in clinical measurements, they can dramatically affect conclusions about method accuracy.[203] Triglyceride blanking usually requires a separate analysis of glycerol, expressed in terms of equivalent triglyceride concentration, and the measured blank value is subtracted from the total triglyceride measurement.[204] Free glycerol can be measured enzymatically using reactions such as those shown in Eqs. 34.10 and 34.11 with a reagent that is identical to the triglyceride reagent but lacking lipase—an approach designated as *two-cuvette blanking.* An alternative to the two-step approach carried out in a single cuvette first consumes any free glycerol to produce a colorless product in a preliminary reaction before a lipase enzyme is added to cleave and measure the triglyceride-derived glycerol.

Triglyceride blanking by either of these approaches increases the time and cost of triglyceride analysis. A more common practice, designated *calibration blanking,* which is used by some manufacturers, involves adjusting calibrator set points to compensate for the average amount of free glycerol in specimens. This is accomplished through a comparison study on actual patient specimens versus the reference method or an accurate equivalent. The calibration blanking approach will underestimate the blank in a few specimens but will give a better and reasonably reliable estimation for most specimens.

Traditionally, triglycerides have been determined on fasting samples obtained from patients after a 10- to 12-hour fast—a practice based on the historical practice in epidemiology studies to achieve a uniform metabolic state. However, patients do not routinely present to physicians' offices in the fasting state, and studies have suggested that triglyceride values measured on nonfasting samples may be more predictive of CHD risk.[205] Postprandial collections are more likely to include remnant lipoproteins that are more atherogenic and reflective of the patient's usual metabolic state. Some national guidelines, particulary in children, have been modified to recommend nonfasting collections as an acceptable alternative, and in the future, nonfasting may replace fasting collections. A disadvantage of this approach is that it will preclude the use of calculating LDL-C with the Friedewald equation because of the presence of chylomicrons and elevated triglycerides.

POINTS TO REMEMBER

Triglycerides

- Triglycerides are independently and positively associated with CVD.
- Markedly increased triglycerides can cause pancreatitis.
- Triglycerides are mostly transported on chylomicrons in a postprandial sample and on VLDL in a fasting sample.
- Total triglycerides can be measured in a plasma or serum, using enzymatic assays.

Phospholipids. Quantitative measurement of phospholipids is rare in routine clinical practice but more common in research studies. The choline-containing phospholipids lecithin, lysolecithin, and sphingomyelin, which account for at least 95% of total phospholipids in serum, are readily measured by an enzymatic reaction sequence using phospholipase D, choline-oxidase, and horseradish peroxidase.[206,207] Kit methods with this enzymatic sequence are available commercially. Before enzymatic reagents became available, the common quantitative method involved extraction and acid digestion with analysis of the total lipid-bound phosphorus.[208]

High-Density Lipoprotein Cholesterol. Under current recommendations for characterizing the cardiovascular disease risk in patients, measurement of the two major cholesterol-carrying lipoproteins, HDL and LDL, is critical for CVD risk assessment. HDL is classically defined in terms of its density range (1.063–1.21g/mL) obtained by ultracentrifugation, which has been used as the standard by which the accuracy of other HDL methods is judged. However, the density range of Lp(a) (1.04–1.08 g/mL) overlaps that of HDL (see Table 34.4), so in patients with high Lp(a) concentrations, ultracentrifugation at 1.063 g/mL would overestimate the true HDL concentration. As a consequence, the CDC reference method, described previously, uses precipitation to separate HDL, similar to the approach used for many research determinations.[209] Most routine laboratories now use the newer direct or homogeneous assays, which became available beginning in the early 1990s. The homogeneous assays have advantages in terms of efficiency and convenience because they are capable of full automation. However, homogeneous assays have been shown to lack specificity, especially on specimens from patients with unusual lipoprotein distributions (see later). Because pretreatment precipitation methods were the standard for decades and preceded the currently more common homogeneous assays, these methods will be reviewed first.

Precipitation Methods. In earlier years, HDL-C was most commonly measured (Box 34.3) in supernatant solutions after precipitation of the apo B-100–containing lipoproteins (VLDL, IDL, Lp[a], LDL, and, when present, chylomicrons)

BOX 34.3 Methods for HDL Separation/Quantification

Precipitation (First Generation)

Heparin-Mn^{2+}
- 0.46 mmol/L (LRC method)
- 0.92 mmol/L (recommended for EDTA plasma)

Dextran sulfate (50 kDa) Mg^{2+} (AACC Selected Method and DCM)

Phosphotungstate-Mg^{2+}

Facilitated Separation (Second Generation)

Magnetic with/dextran sulfate-Mg^{2+}

Homogeneous (Third Generation)

Antibody four-reagent method (International Reagents Corp.)

Polyethylene glycol modified enzymes w/cyclodextrin (Kyowa Medex)

Synthetic polymer/detergent (Daiichi)

Antibodies (Wako)

Catalase (Denka Seiken)

directly from plasma or serum, using agents such as polyanions in the presence of divalent cations.[89] As indicated earlier, LDL and HDL are the largest contributors to total cholesterol in healthy people, with LDL accounting for about two-thirds and HDL for about one-third of the total cholesterol. On average, IDL and Lp(a) each account for only about 2 to 3 mg/dL (0.05–0.078 mmol/L) of the total cholesterol, although their concentrations can be considerably higher in some individuals. Polyanions bridge positively charged groups on lipoproteins, and their action is facilitated in the presence of divalent cations, which interact with negatively charged groups, causing aggregation and precipitate formation. Precipitation is usually complete within 10 to 15 minutes at room temperature; at 2° to 4°C, a 30-minute incubation period is preferred. The precipitate is then sedimented by centrifugation, typically for 45,000 g-min (ie, the equivalent of 1500 × g for 30 minutes). Centrifugation at higher g-forces (eg, 10,000 × g) accelerates sedimentation and can improve complete removal of apo B–containing particles. HDL-C is then enzymatically measured in the clear supernatant.

Of several polyanion-divalent cation combinations, heparan sulfate with $MnCl_2$ was the most common and eventually used in the CDC reference method. With the transition to enzymatic cholesterol assays, residual Mn^{2+} was found, however, to interfere, giving artifactually high results. Techniques were then devised to reduce this interference, but additional manipulations were required, making them inconvenient for routine use (eg, the chelator ethylenediaminetetraacetic acid [EDTA] added to the cholesterol reagent to complex residual manganite),[210] or carbonate was added in a second precipitation step to precipitate excess Mn^{2+}.[211] Most laboratories avoided these tedious approaches and adopted alternative precipitants, such as dextran sulfate or phosphotungstate with Mg^{2+}.[212] A method that used dextran sulfate with molecular weight of 50 kDa was developed during the 1980s and became the most commonly used precipitation reagent.

The precipitability of lipoproteins with polyanions and divalent cations depends on the lipid and protein compositions of the particles.[213] Thus various precipitants differ in their ability to precipitate apo B-100–containing lipoprotein while leaving HDL in solution,[185] resulting in potential biases between reagents. With modern reagent-instrument-calibrator systems, conditions generally are optimized to produce values that closely approximate and are traceable to reference method values. Also, the precipitation methods can be inaccurate under certain conditions, such as with high concentrations of triglyceride-rich lipoproteins. Also, any residual turbidity in the supernate indicates inadequate sedimentation of the apo B-100–containing lipoprotein, resulting in overestimation of HDL cholesterol. Samples with high triglyceride concentrations (generally those above 400 mg/dL [4.52 mmol/L]) frequently produce turbid supernatants because the triglycerides can reduce the density of the lipoprotein-precipitating reagent complex to the point that some of the complex remains unsedimented. In cases of extremely high triglyceride concentrations, some of the precipitate may even form a floating layer over a clear or turbid supernatant, in addition to the usual precipitate at the bottom of the centrifuge tube.

Such supernates require additional treatment by one of several techniques. Before precipitation, the sample can be ultracentrifuged and the triglyceride-rich lipoproteins removed as described previously for the reference method. Alternatively, a turbid supernatant sometimes can be cleared by centrifuging for a longer time or at higher g-forces.[214] Or more commonly, the sample can be diluted twofold with saline to reduce the concentration of triglyceride-rich lipoproteins before the precipitant is added. A fourth approach is to pass the turbid supernatant through a 0.45-μm filter to remove the unsedimented precipitate before cholesterol in the filtrate is measured.[214]

HDL-C determination can also be affected by sample matrix effects, which arise from the unusual nature of the sample itself, processing effects, or the addition of anticoagulants or preservatives.[196] For example, HDL-C measurements can be inaccurate and usually are more variable when obtained from lyophilized samples than from fresh or frozen sera. Additives including anticoagulants, such as citrate and fluoride, can have large osmotic effects that cause water to shift from the cells to the plasma. This dilutes the lipoprotein by 10% or more and produces erroneously low values. EDTA, earlier the preferred anticoagulant for lipoprotein measurements, causes a slight dilution but has been used because it also inhibits certain oxidative and other changes that can affect some lipoprotein or apolipoprotein measurements. Lipid and lipoprotein concentrations in EDTA plasma tend to be about 3% lower than in serum. EDTA, however, complexes some of the Mn^{2+} in the heparin-Mn^{2+} method, and it has been found necessary to use a higher concentration of $MnCl_2$ (0.092 mol/L, final concentration in the reaction system) when the procedure is used with EDTA plasma than with serum (0.046 mol/L). Heparin, by virtue of its high molecular weight, and when present in concentrations used for anticoagulation, has no measurable effect on lipid or lipoprotein concentration, and it does not affect HDL-C measurements. A variation of the precipitation method, involving the use of magnetic beads complexed with dextran sulfate, helped reduce interference from high triglyceride samples,[215,216] but it is no longer commercially available.

Homogeneous Assays. A major breakthrough in HDL determination was reported in 1994[217] with publication of the first of a series of so-called homogeneous methods for lipoproteins (Box 34.4). Compared with earlier precipitation methods requiring manual pretreatment steps, homogeneous methods were much better suited for the automated systems used in the modern clinical laboratory. Elimination of manual pretreatment was timely because laboratories were under pressure to reduce operating costs. The fully automated homogeneous methods also improved precision through more consistent pipetting of smaller specimen volumes and precise temperature control and reaction timing, which facilitated achieving the NCEP analytical performance goals.

The first homogeneous assay for HDL-C required four successive reagent additions (International Reagents Corp., Kobe, Japan). The first reagent contained polyethylene glycol, resulting in aggregation of the apo B-100–containing chylomicrons, VLDL, and LDL. The second reagent protected or blocked the aggregated lipoproteins with antibodies to apo B-100 and apo C. The cholesterol reaction enzymes (cholesterol esterase, cholesterol oxidase, and peroxidase) were added in the third reagent, which acted only on the unprotected HDL-C. The fourth reagent stopped the color reaction and solubilized the aggregates with guanidine salts, clearing the

BOX 34.4 Methods for LDL Separation/Quantification

β-Quantification

Ultracentrifugation at density 1.006 kg/L to float and remove VLDL and any chylos

Measurement of total cholesterol in bottom fraction (LDL-C + HDL-C)

Precipitation of bottom fraction with heparin/Mn^{2+} to remove LDL

Measurement of total cholesterol in supernatant, which equals HLD-C

LDL is calculated by subtracting HDL-C from total cholesterol in bottom fraction; most commonly used by specialty lipid laboratories

Calculation Using Friedewald Formula

(LDL chol) = (Total chol) − (HDL chol) − (Triglyceride)/5*

Homogeneous Reagents

LDL solubilization (Kyowa Medex)

LDL protected/deprotected by surfactants (Daiichi)

LDL protected/catalase (Wako)

Non-HDL catalase/LDL azide (Denka Seiken)

LDL protected by calixarene/cholesterol dehydrogenase (International Reagents Corp.)

*When values are in mg/dL.

reaction mixture for measurement of color. This breakthrough method, even though not suited for all analyzers because of the multiple reagent additions, was capable of full automation, paving the way for subsequent simpler two-reagent homogeneous methods.

In 1995, a second homogeneous method[218] became available (Kyowa Medex Co., Tokyo, Japan; Roche Diagnostics, Indianapolis, Indiana) that used sulfated α-cyclodextrins together with Mg^{2+} to selectively block but not precipitate chylomicrons and VLDL, providing selectivity without the necessity for precipitation. Second, covalently linked polyethylene glycol molecules enhanced the specificities of the enzymes cholesterol esterase and cholesterol oxidase toward the cholesterol in HDL. Polyethylene glycol having an MW of 6000 Da was thought to optimize the specificities at concentrations lower than those used previously to precipitate lipoproteins, implying that modified enzymes were able to distinguish lipoprotein classes on the basis of their size and/or charge. The result was a fully automated homogeneous assay with only two reagent additions applicable for general use. The original kit included the second enzyme-containing reagent in lyophilized form, necessitating reconstitution, but a modification introduced in mid-1998 included both reagents in liquid form.[111] A third modification decreased the Mg^{2+} concentration, apparently to reduce carryover in pipetting.

A synthetic polymer, together with a polyanion to block the non-HDL lipoproteins, was used in a third homogeneous assay (Daiichi Pure Chemicals Co., Tokyo; Genzyme Corp., Cambridge, Massachusetts).[215,219,220] A detergent was added that exposes only cholesterol in HDL to the enzymes, giving specificity for HDL-C. This method required two reagent additions: the first with the polyanion and polymer-blocking agents and the second with detergent, enzymes, and substrates. A subsequent modification provided both reagents in liquid form with other changes to improve specificity and decrease potential interference.[221-223] A third modification without Mg^{2+} has been reported.[224,225]

A fourth early homogeneous assay was based on immunoinhibition and included two reagents (Wako Pure Chemicals Industry, Osaka, Japan).[226,227] The first reagent contained an antibody to human apo B-100 that reacted with apo B-100–containing lipoproteins, chylomicrons, VLDL, and LDL, blocking their reaction to enzymes added in the second reagent. The current formulation included both reagents in liquid form.

A fifth homogeneous method (Denka Seiken Co., Niigata, Japan; Polymedco Inc., Cortlandt Manor, New York; Randox Laboratories Limited, Crumlin, United Kingdom) allowed cholesterol esterase and oxidase to react with lipoproteins other than HDL, generating peroxidase, which in turn was scavenged by the enzyme catalase.[227,228] An inhibitor of catalase and a surfactant in a second reagent specifically reacted with HDL-C, producing color through the usual peroxidase sequence. In subsequent years, the various homogeneous reagents have undergone many additional modifications in attempts to improve their convenience and specificity. Currently, at least seven separate reagent formulations are available.

At least one instrument application for each of the homogeneous assays discussed previously in this chapter has qualified for certification by the CRMLN, implying at least the capability to achieve agreement with the reference method. However, conditions, and especially calibration, may be different on various instrument applications, and many have not been evaluated. Thus certification for the reagents cannot be considered universally applicable to all distributor versions, instrument applications, and lots. Similarly, published evaluation studies have confirmed that these methods can be accurate but may not be so in every commercial application.[183] Laboratories choosing to adopt homogeneous assay applications that have not been certified by the CRMLN are encouraged to confirm that their particular systems are accurate. In addition, an evaluation of all current homogeneous HDL-C and LDL-C assays revealed that many of these assays lack ruggedness because of lack of lipoprotein specificity, especially on specimens with unusual lipoprotein composition.[209]

Specificity and Interference. The accuracy of measuring HDL-C in each individual specimen is a function not only of mean bias or overall inaccuracy of a method related to calibration but also its specificity for HDL-C and absence of interference by other lipoproteins and constituents of the specimen matrix. CRMLN certification studies and many published evaluation studies undertaken to assess accuracy included only samples from relatively normal subjects. Most studies did not determine performance in samples from patients with extreme hyperlipidemias, such as type III or other conditions such as liver and kidney disease, which often result in unusual lipoproteins with atypical separation characteristics. Only a few studies have included such extreme specimens and have raised questions about the specificity of the homogeneous reagents.[209,229,230] Most studies of interference have used fairly traditional spiking designs; they have been relatively modest in scope and have not properly addressed abnormal lipoprotein composition.[216,222,228,231,232] Hemoglobin below 2 g/L and bilirubin less than 10 mg/dL

(1086 umol/L) do not interfere appreciably with any of the homogeneous methods.

Considerations in Choosing a High-Density Lipoprotein Method. Laboratories have had to consider the alternatives in deciding whether to replace a conventional pretreatment method with a homogeneous reagent: improved efficiency on the one hand versus occasional discrepant results on the other. Routine clinical laboratories tend to choose the fully automated methods, often because of unavoidable pressures to improve efficiency. Laboratories performing research and supporting lipid clinics, on the other hand, often choose to retain a conventional precipitation method. An important factor in the latter choice is that a laboratory supporting long-term studies cannot tolerate potential changes and shifts in results that may have occurred because of frequent modifications to the homogeneous reagents.

POINTS TO REMEMBER

HDL

- HDL cholesterol is inversely related to CVD risk.
- HDL cholesterol can be directly measured using a homogeneous assay or measured in a fasting plasma sample as cholesterol in the supernatant after precipitation of LDL and VLDL.
- Apo A-I is the main protein in HDL.
- The causal link between HDL cholesterol and CVD is uncertain.

Low-Density Lipoprotein Cholesterol. Methods for LDL-C generally quantitate a so-called broad-cut fraction, including not only the primary LDL species in the 1.019 to 1.063 kg/L density range but also IDL, density 1.006 to 1.019 kg/L, and Lp(a).[233] Therefore the usual convention for total cholesterol on a fasting sample without cholesterol is based on the following formula:

$$\text{Total cholesterol (chol)} = \text{VLDL chol} + \text{LDL chol} + \text{HDL chol} \qquad \textbf{34.16}$$

LDL-C can be measured using both indirect and direct methods, and either approach has been used in major studies that established the relationship between LDL-C concentration and risk for CHD.

Indirect Methods. Indirect methods for measuring LDL-C are based on measuring a number of lipid-related analytes, followed by their use in calculating the LDL-C content of a specimen. This includes use of the Friedewald equation and the β-quantification method.

The Friedewald Equation. In the most widely used indirect method (see Box 34.4), cholesterol, triglyceride, and HDL-C are measured and LDL-C is calculated from primary measurements using the following empirical equation developed by Friedewald and colleagues:[234]

$$(\text{LDL chol}) = (\text{Total chol}) - (\text{HDL chol}) - (\text{Triglyceride})/5 \qquad \textbf{34.17}$$

where all concentrations are given in mg/dL (triglyceride/2.22 is used when units are expressed in mmol/L). The factor (triglyceride)/5 is an estimate of VLDL-C and is based on the average ratio of triglyceride to cholesterol in VLDL. Several investigators have evaluated the accuracy of Eq. 34.17. For example, DeLong and colleagues[235] recommended use of the expression 0.16 × (triglyceride) as a better estimate of VLDL-C. Other factors have been suggested for particular populations,[185] but no single factor has been accurate under all circumstances. However, when the original factor (triglyceride)/5 was compared with a combined ultracentrifugation-polyanion precipitation method in about 5000 samples, errors in LDL-C cholesterol estimated by equation were found to be symmetrically distributed about zero.[236] On balance, the NCEP recommended use of the original factor (triglyceride/5) for estimating LDL cholesterol with the Friedewald equation.[185]

In practice, the Friedewald calculation is reasonably accurate, but under several well-known circumstances, it cannot be used. First, the calculation is precluded in samples that have triglyceride concentrations above 400 mg/dL (4.52 mmol/L) or in those that contain increased quantities of chylomicrons (nonfasting specimens). At high triglyceride concentrations, the factor (triglyceride)/5 as an estimate of VLDL-C is not appropriate because such samples also contain chylomicrons, chylomicron remnants, or VLDL remnants, all of which have higher triglyceride/cholesterol ratios. Under these circumstances, use of the factor (triglyceride)/5 would overestimate VLDL-C and therefore underestimate LDL-C. The Friedewald equation has been found to be most accurate in samples with triglyceride concentrations below 200 mg/dL (2.26 mmol/L),[236] and the error becomes unacceptably large (ie, >10%) at triglyceride concentrations greater than 400 mg/dL (4.52 mmol/L).

The opposite error can occur if the Friedewald equation is used in patients with type III hyperlipoproteinemia, which is characterized by the presence of β-VLDL not normally present in the blood. Biochemically, as its name implies, β-VLDL occurs in the VLDL density range but has β mobility on electrophoresis and is much richer in cholesterol than the usual VLDL, with a ratio of triglyceride to cholesterol on the order of 3:1. Application of the factor (triglyceride)/5 in patients with type III hyperlipidemia would underestimate VLDL-C and overestimate LDL-C. Fortunately, both of these conditions are uncommon. The 95th percentile for fasting plasma triglycerides in the United States is below 300 mg/dL (3.39 mmol/L), indicating that only a small percentage of specimens will exceed the 400-mg/dL (4.52 mmol/L) cutoff. Plasma from fasting subjects does not normally contain chylomicrons; even if present, chylomicrons can be observed visually as a floating "cream" layer in samples that have been allowed to stand undisturbed at 4°C overnight. Finally, the prevalence of type III hyperlipoproteinemia in the general population is only about 1 to 2 per 1000 persons.[166] On the other hand, as treatments for hyperlipidemia become more effective and more common, patients with very low triglyceride concentrations are encountered. In this instance, the calculation may be distorted and LDL-C overestimated.[283] Nevertheless, because of the ease of the calculation and its reasonable accuracy, calculation of LDL-C has persisted as the most common approach to determining LDL-C.

β-Quantification (Ultracentrifugation-Polyanion Precipitation). This method is the precursor to the reference methods developed for HDL and LDL and may be used in samples for which the Friedewald equation is unreliable. β-quantification follows the procedure adopted from the NIH

Laboratory that was used in the LRC Program, combining preparative ultracentrifugation and polyanion precipitation.[89] An accurately measured aliquot of plasma at native density of 1.006 g/mL is first ultracentrifuged at 105,000 × g for 18 hours at 10°C. VLDL and, if present, chylomicrons and/or β-VLDL float over the infranatant containing primarily LDL and HDL, plus any IDL and Lp(a) that may be present. The floating layer, removed with the aid of a tube slicer, is sometimes analyzed as a check on recovery and may be saved for electrophoretic analysis to determine the presence of β-VLDL. The infranatant solution is remixed and reconstituted to known volume, and its cholesterol content is measured. HDL-C is usually measured in a separate aliquot of plasma, but when necessary, an aliquot of the d 1.006 g/mL infranatant can be treated to remove the apo B-100–containing lipoproteins (IDL, LDL, and Lp[a]); HDL-C is then measured in the clear supernatant. VLDL and LDL cholesterol are calculated as follows:

$$(\text{VLDL chol}) = (\text{Total chol}) - (d > 1.006\ \text{g/mL chol}) \quad \mathbf{34.18}$$

$$(\text{LDL chol}) = (d > 1.006\ \text{g/mL chol}) - (\text{HDL chol}) \quad \mathbf{34.19}$$

LDL-C measured in this way is unaffected by the presence of chylomicrons or other triglyceride-rich lipoproteins, or by β-VLDL. VLDL-C is usually calculated from Eq. 34.18 rather than measured directly in the ultracentrifugal supernatant because it can be difficult to recover this fraction quantitatively, particularly when triglyceride concentrations are high.

Lipoproteins Included in the "LDL Cholesterol" Measurement. In this context, the term *LDL cholesterol* includes cholesterol in IDL and Lp(a) fractions, as well as the core LDL. Although IDL and Lp(a) cholesterol usually contribute only a few mg/dL to the "total LDL cholesterol" measurement, their contributions can be significant in patients with increased high IDL or Lp(a) concentrations. For example, assuming that cholesterol (ie, sterol nucleus) constitutes about 30% of the mass of Lp(a), it can be calculated that the Lp(a) cholesterol concentration would contribute about 12 mg/dL (0.31 mmol/L), or about 12%, to the LDL-C measurement in a patient with an Lp(a) concentration of 40 mg/dL and an apparent LDL-C concentration of 100 mg/dL (2.59 mmol/L). It has been suggested that a more specific measure of LDL-C measurement could be obtained by correcting the measured LDL-C value for the contribution of Lp(a) cholesterol,[237,238] and a similar argument might be made for IDL. However, both IDL and Lp(a) contribute to increased risk for CHD (see section on Lp[a]); therefore, although such correction will increase the specificity of methods for LDL-C, per se, it might also give LDL-C values that underestimate cardiovascular risk. Moreover, this might occur more frequently with patients with CHD or those who are at risk for CHD based on their "LDL cholesterol" concentrations. Consequently, the NCEP Working Group on LDL Cholesterol Measurement suggested that LDL-C values should *not* be corrected for the contribution of other atherogenic lipoproteins; this group also recommended that further research should be conducted to establish the individual contributions of IDL, Lp(a), and LDL-C to CHD risk. NCEP guidelines published in 2001 expand on this concept by introducing the term *non–HDL cholesterol,* which includes all of the apo B–containing atherogenic lipoproteins, including not only cholesterol on Lp(a) and IDL but also VLDL, remnant lipoproteins, and chylomicrons for nonfasting samples.[178]

Diagnosis of the Type III Lipoprotein Pattern. The ratio of VLDL cholesterol to plasma triglyceride, expressed in terms of mass, is 0.2 or lower in normal samples and in those from patients with lipoprotein disorders other than type III hyperlipidemia or dysbetalipoproteinemia. In type III hyperlipoproteinemia, the ratio is 0.3 or higher because of the presence of β-VLDL; the elevated ratio can persist even after treatment. In addition, β-VLDL can be observed directly by subjecting the VLDL fraction to agarose gel electrophoresis, where it migrates electrophoretically with LDL rather than VLDL (see Fig. 34.26). The combination of a VLDL cholesterol/plasma triglyceride ratio of 0.3 or higher and the observation of β-VLDL in the ultracentrifugal supernatant is considered diagnostic of the type III lipoprotein pattern.[138]

Direct Methods. Both selective precipitation and homogeneous immunoassay methods have been used to measure LDL-C.

Selective Precipitation. Several direct methods reported for LDL-C measurement are based on selective precipitation with polyvinyl sulfate or heparin at low pH.[239-241] LDL-C is then calculated as the difference between total cholesterol and that in the supernatant, or in another variation, directly in the LDL precipitate. It is not clear whether atherogenic lipoproteins other than LDL itself are also detected; these methods might be expected to be subject to similar sources of error as those encountered with precipitation methods for HDL separation. A more specific method used a mixture of polyclonal antibodies to apo A-I and apo E linked to a resin to bind VLDL, IDL, and HDL, with LDL-C measured in a filtrate by the usual methods. This method was reasonably precise and was in good agreement with ultracentrifugation-polyanion precipitation.[239,242-244] The reagent was in commercial distribution for several years, but because it required a separate pretreatment step, it was eventually superseded by a new class of direct homogeneous reagents patterned after the homogeneous reagents for HDL-C.

Homogeneous Assays. Following approaches similar to those used with homogeneous methods for HDL-C, homogeneous assays have also been developed to measure LDL-C. For example, at least seven homogeneous LDL-C methods are commercially available (see Box 34.4), which differ by containing different detergents and other chemicals, allowing specific blocking or solubilization of lipoprotein classes to achieve specificity for LDL. Most suppliers offer kits with two reagents; these are readily adaptable to most clinical chemistry analyzers.

Sugiuchi and colleagues developed the first homogeneous method for measuring LDL-C,[245] a reagent distributed by Kyowa Medex (Tokyo, Japan) and Roche Diagnostics (Indianapolis, Indiana). With this method, LDL-C was directly measured by suppressing the other lipoproteins (other methods suppressed LDL first and reacted with other lipoproteins before determining LDL-C). The method was formulated in two reagents. The first had $MgCl_2$, dye, buffer (pH 6.75), and α-cyclodextrin sulfate,[218] which has a highly concentrated negative charge to mask cholesterol in chylomicrons and VLDL in the presence of magnesium ions.[245] The second reagent included the enzymes cholesterol oxidase and cholesterol esterase, peroxidase, dye, buffer (pH 6.75), and a

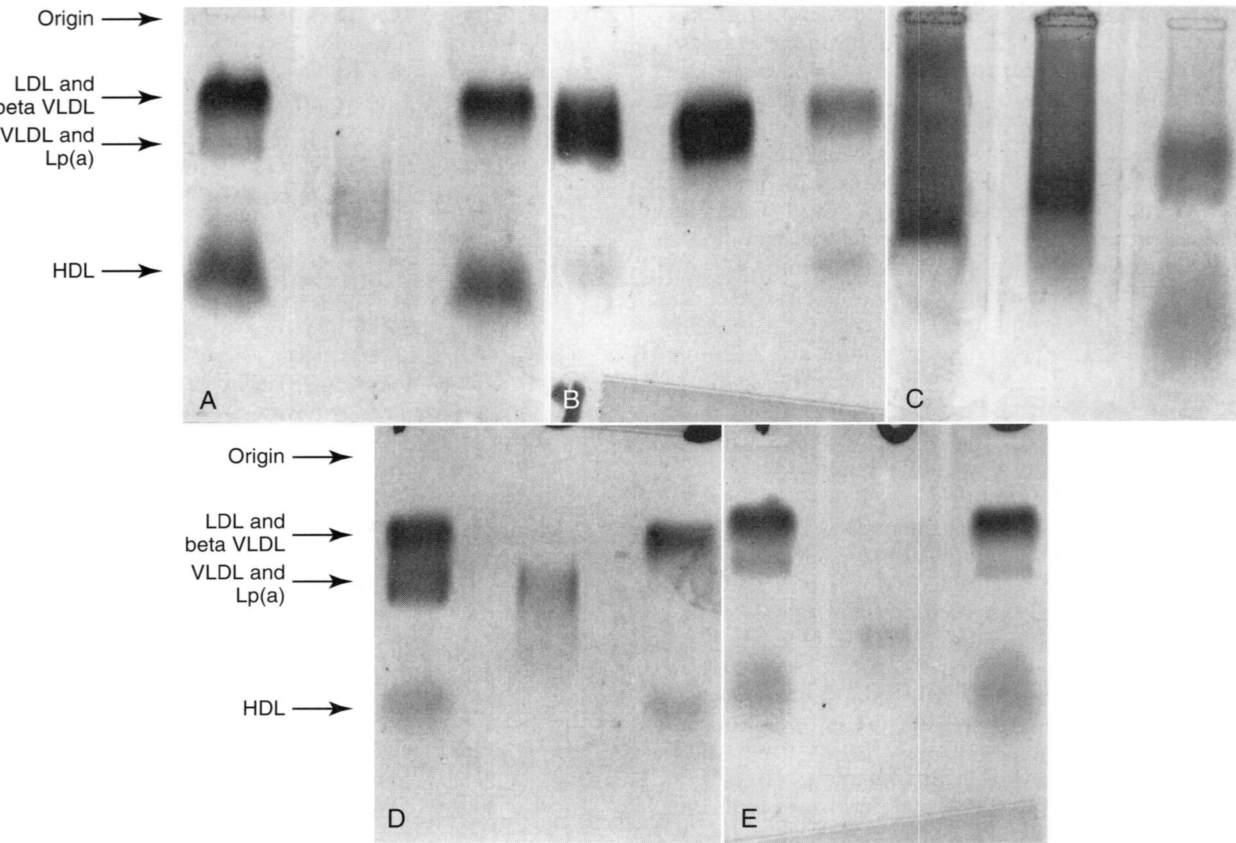

FIGURE 34.26 Agarose gel electrophoresis of plasma lipoprotein. In each photograph, the samples were applied in the following order, reading from left to right: unfractionated plasma, ultracentrifugal density 1.006 g/mL supernatant solution, ultracentrifugal infranatant solution. **A,** Pattern seen in normal samples and samples with high LDL cholesterol concentrations. **B,** Type III hyperlipoproteinemia pattern. **C,** Severe hypertriglyceridemia, triglyceride = 3840 mg/dL. Note chylomicrons at origin. **D,** Pattern observed in samples with moderately elevated triglyceride, triglyceride = 281 mg/dL, LDL cholesterol = 145 mg/dL. Note absence of chylomicrons. **E,** Pattern observed in patients with high concentrations of Lp(a). Note presence of Lp(a) in infranatant solution. This sample had an Lp(a) concentration of 77 mg/dL. *LDL,* Low-density lipoprotein; *Lp(a),* lipoprotein(a); *HDL,* high-density lipoprotein; *VLDL,* very low-density lipoprotein.

polyoxyethylene-polyoxypropylene polyether (POE-POP) to block cholesterol, especially in HDL. The molecular mass of POP in the POE-POP molecule and the hydrophobicity index determine selectivity to LDL; 3850 Da was demonstrated to be optimum.

A second method by Sekisuie Medical Co. (Tokyo, Japan; formerly Daiichi Pure Chemicals) was also a two-reagent system. The first reagent contained ascorbic acid oxidase, 4-aminoantipyrine, peroxidase, cholesterol oxidase, cholesterol esterase, buffer (pH 6.3), and a detergent, which solubilized all non-LDL lipoproteins, allowing reaction of their cholesterol with the esterase and oxidase enzymes, forming a colorless product. The second reagent contained N,N′-bis-(4-sulfobutyl)-m-toluidine Na_2 (DSBmT), buffer (pH 6.3), and a detergent to specifically release LDL cholesterol. The resulting hydrogen peroxide reacted with N,N′-bis-(4-sulfobutyl)-M-toluidine disodium salt to generate a colored product.

A third method (Wako Pure Chemicals) included a reagent with Good's buffer (pH 6.8) (N-[2-hydroxy-3-sulfopropyl]-3,5-dimethoxyaniline, sodium salt); cholesterol esterase; cholesterol oxidase; catalase; polyanions; and amphoteric surfactants, the last selectively protecting LDL from enzymatic reaction. The non–LDL cholesterol reacted with esterase and oxidase, producing hydrogen peroxide, which was consumed by catalase. The second reagent included Good's buffer (pH 7.0), 4-aminoantipyrene, peroxidase, sodium azide, and a deprotecting reagent, which removed the protecting agent from LDL, enabling the specific reaction of cholesterol esterase and cholesterol oxidase with its cholesterol, producing hydrogen peroxide and a blue color complex.[246,247]

Non–LDL cholesterol was removed by a fourth method (Denka Seiken, Niigata, Japan; Polymedco Inc., Cortlandt Manor, New York) via a selective reaction with cholesterol oxidase and cholesterol esterase, with the resulting peroxide by-product eliminated by reaction with catalase (CAT). In this two-reagent method, the first reagent contained $MgCl_2$, cholesterol esterase, cholesterol oxidase, catalase, N-(2-hydroxy-3-sulfopropyl)-3,5-dimethoxyaniline sodium salt, and Emulgen 66 (polyoxyethylene compound; Kao) and Emulgen 90 (both nonionic surfactants) in Good's buffer (PIPES; 100 mmol/L; pH 7.0). Its second reagent contained

TABLE 34.21 Analytical Performance of Homogeneous LDL-C Assays

			RECOVERY, %			ACCURACY	
	Imprecision, CVs	Dynamic Range, mg/L	LDL	VLDL	IDL	Bias, %	Bias, mg/L
Kyowa	0.7–3.1	2–4100	97–105	16	52–64	0.8–11.2	−60 to −80
Daiichi	<3.1	4–10,000	87	19	31–47	3.9–5.1	−48 to −80
Wako	≤1.2	10–3000	—	—	—	0.4	−15
Denka	<1.8	70–5500	95	10	31	—	—
IRC	≤0.6	?–4000	—	—	—	—	—

peroxidase, 4- aminoantipyrine, sodium azide (to inhibit the catalase), and Triton X-100 in Good's buffer. The hydrophilic/lipophilic balance of the detergents was chosen to obtain appropriate selectivity to the lipoproteins.[248]

In a fifth method (International Reagents Corp., Kokusai-Kobe, Japan), its first reagent contained the detergent calixarene, which converts LDL to a soluble complex. Cholesterol esters of HDL-C and VLDL-C were preferentially hydrolyzed by a cholesterol esterase (chromobacterium), cholesterol oxidase, and hydrazine, which divert the accessible cholesterol to cholestenone hydrazone. A second reagent with deoxycholate broke up the LDL-calixarene complex, allowing LDL-C to react with the esterase, a dehydrogenase, and β-NAD to yield cholestenone and β-NADH.

Analytical Performance of LDL Methods. Evaluations of LDL homogeneous assays indicate that CVs are generally less than 3% and consistently within the NCEP performance target of less than 4% CV (Table 34.21). By contrast, CVs for the Friedewald calculation have been estimated to approximate 4% in expert laboratories but may be higher in routine clinical laboratories.[233] With regard to accuracy, all of the homogeneous assays have qualified for certification through the CRMLN program, suggesting agreement with reference methods, at least in relatively normal specimens. Nevertheless, as indicated previously for HDL-C methods, many different instrument applications are available, and not all have been evaluated for bias. Factors, such as lot-to-lot differences, unique calibrations by distributors, different calibrations from country to country, and reformulations of reagents might affect actual biases.[209] In a 2002 study, four homogeneous assays were compared with the LDL RM; unacceptable total error was found, and the authors recommended caution in adopting the methods.[249] A 2010 study of all current homogeneous assays for LDL-C found that these assays work relatively on normolipidemic samples but found frequent discordant results compared with the reference β-quantification procedure for patients with dyslipidemias.[230] Overall, these studies suggest that homogeneous assays interact unequally with different components of the "broad-cut LDL": LDL subclasses, IDL, Lp(a), and Lp-X. A 2002 study of two homogeneous reagents using isolated lipoprotein fractions confirmed the lack of specificity for VLDL and LDL subclasses.[249] The two homogeneous methods included about 20% of isolated VLDL. Also, the reagents missed about 30% of IDL and up to 50% of isolated LDL fractions, especially the important smaller and more atherogenic subclasses. Through compensating errors, the inclusion of some VLDL could offset the loss of LDL fractions, so the overall lack of specificity may not be obvious in relatively normal specimens. However, lack of specificity for lipoprotein subclasses and differences among reagents can cause substantial errors in some specimens, depending on the particular lipoprotein profile and the particular reagent characteristics.[230]

Spiking studies, in which potential interfering substances are added to a sample, have demonstrated that these methods are not subject to significant interference from bilirubin and hemoglobin. However, higher concentrations of triglycerides have been shown to interfere, thus increasing apparent LDL-C; this is not surprising given the reported lack of specificity for LDL and the inclusion of some VLDL in the measurement.[248,250,251] On the other hand, the sulfated α-cyclodextrin used in the Sugiuchi assay to block VLDL-C appeared to cause underestimation of LDL-C.[245,247,252]

A major potential advantage of homogeneous methods over the Friedewald calculation is the ability to use nonfasting specimens, which are convenient in managing patients. Results, judged by mean differences between paired fasting and nonfasting specimens, were promising, but patient classifications were poorer with nonfasting specimens.[248,252,253] Lipoprotein composition is affected by recent diet; changes have been observed even with the more robust ultracentrifugation method. However, the changes are relatively small, and the convenience of being able to use nonfasting specimens may offset minor effects on accuracy. A prospective analysis suggested that LDL-C may not be as predictive of CHD risk in nonfasting specimens,[254] but more comprehensive studies will be needed to address this question.

Other Considerations in Adopting a Homogeneous LDL Method. Clinical laboratories are faced with the decision of whether to implement fully automated homogeneous methods for LDL-C, either replacing or supplementing the traditional Friedewald calculation. The considerations are certainly not as compelling for homogeneous LDL methods as for HDL. Even given the technical disadvantages of the Friedewald method—that is, the necessity for fasting, poor precision from cumulative variations in the three underlying measurements, and well-known limitations in certain patients—it is firmly entrenched in routine practice and likely will be displaced only if homogeneous methods can demonstrate clear advantages. Substantially better analytical performance or overall improved cost-effectiveness in characterizing or monitoring patients has yet to be shown for homogeneous LDL methods. A 2002 review suggests that homogeneous assays can be recommended only to supplement calculation for those patients with elevated triglycerides or other conditions precluding calculation.[233]

Oxidized LDL. In 1983, Brown and Goldstein reported that circulating LDL must undergo some structural modification before it becomes fully proatherogenic.[142] Patients who completely lack LDL receptors accumulate large amounts of cholesterol in their macrophages and form foam cells. The receptors, which recognize the modified LDL, were termed the scavenger receptors.[255] Currently, several modifications that enhance the uptake of LDL by macrophages in vitro have been described, such as glycation, self-aggregation, immune complex formation, hydrolysis, and oxidation; the latter has received the greatest attention.[256]

LDL is oxidized in microdomains in the arterial wall, where it is sequestered by proteoglycans and other extracellular matrix constituents and is protected from plasma antioxidants. This process is a free radical–driven lipid peroxidation chain reaction that is initiated by the free radical attacking the double bond associated with polyunsaturated fatty acids (PUFAs), leading to the generation of malonedialdehyde and 4-hydroxynonenal.[257] These intermediate compounds then bind to apo B-100, giving it an increased net negative charge and rendering it unrecognizable by native LDL receptors.

Oxidized LDL (oxLDL) has several proatherogenic properties, including rapid uptake by macrophages to form foam cells, chemoattraction for circulating monocytes, promotion of the differentiation of monocytes into tissue macrophages, and inhibition of the motility of resident macrophages.[256] It is cytotoxic to several types of cells and is immunogenic. Laboratory, clinical, and epidemiologic studies have shown that this oxidation also occurs in vivo. LDL extracted from human atherosclerotic lesions was shown to be oxidatively modified; circulating anti-oxLDL antibodies were detected in serum, with titers correlating with progression of atherosclerotic lesions; the use of various antioxidants (vitamin E and probucol among others) delayed the progression of atherosclerotic lesions.

Several commercial assays specific for various epitopes of oxLDL are currently available (eg, Mercodia, Uppsala, Sweden).[258] However, at the present time, the clinical relevance of oxLDL assays has not been established; therefore, its routine measurement is not recommended.

Total Lipoproteins and Lipoprotein Subclasses. Several approaches have been used to quantitate all of the lipoproteins and, in some cases, lipoprotein subclasses in a single procedure. Among the earliest methods for characterization of lipoprotein subclasses was analytical ultracentrifugation; however, the method is tedious and is not widely used except for research studies.[259] Subsequently, other, more practical methods were developed. In one of these procedures, samples are loaded onto a gel and are subjected to an electrical field, causing the negatively charged lipoproteins to move into the gradient and achieving separation based on particle mobility and/or size. The electropherogram is stained and scanned densitometrically, and areas under the various lipoprotein peaks are reported, usually in relative percents. Relative values can be converted to equivalent lipoprotein cholesterol or apo B concentrations, using assumed average compositions for the particles. Electrophoresis, usually in agarose, for determination of major lipoprotein classes in unfractionated samples is relatively easy to perform but has limited clinical application, such as for detecting β-VLDL in type III hyperlipidemia.[260] Resolution adequate for determination of lipoprotein subclasses can be achieved in gradient gels of polyacrylamide,[261] but this approach is technically more demanding and is performed by only specialized reference laboratories.

Density gradient ultracentrifugation is also used to characterize lipoprotein subclasses; it is performed in a vertical rotor with measurement of cholesterol continuously in fractions eluted from the gradient.[262-264] Mathematical curve deconvolution derives the component lipoprotein profiles and allows calculation of their concentrations in terms of cholesterol or other constituents. The method can determine concentrations of VLDL, IDL, LDL, Lp(a), and HDL cholesterol. LDL cholesterol subclasses can be expressed separately or can be combined to obtain a measurement similar to that provided by the Friedewald equation or by β-quantification. A disadvantage is that the procedure is technically demanding and requires instrumentation not usually available in routine clinical laboratories.

Nuclear magnetic resonance (NMR) spectroscopy[265,266] detects protons in lipoprotein-associated fatty acyl methyl or methylene groups. Signals from subfractions of VLDL, LDL, and HDL vary by particle size and can be resolved mathematically through deconvolution based on calibration samples with values reported in terms of numbers of lipoprotein particles. A sample can be analyzed quickly using a small volume of serum or plasma. The method was recently automated and is now available as a routine clinical laboratory analyzer. The different-size lipoprotein fractions can be aggregated to calculate LDL-P and HDL-P, which in several studies have been shown to be superior to LDL-C and HDL-C as CVD risk biomarkers.[267,268] Recently, a new mass spectrometry technique based on airborne ion mobility has also been developed for measuring total lipoprotein subfractions.[269] An automated method for determining the small, dense fraction of LDL has also been described.[270,271] Although some of these new tests based on univariate analysis appear to be superior to conventional lipid and lipoprotein tests for CVD risk prediction, more studies are needed to determine how to best integrate these new tests into the current guidelines, and more effort is needed to improve the standardization of these total lipoprotein particle and subclass methods.[272]

Intermediate-Density (Remnant) Lipoproteins. Remnant lipoproteins include the lipolytic products of catabolism of the triglyceride-rich lipoproteins, VLDL and chylomicrons, occurring in the VLDL and LDL ranges. A traditionally defined fraction at the lighter end of the LDL density range, the IDL portion comprises the 1.006 to 1.019 g/mL fraction, which is obtained by sequential ultracentrifugation for quantitation, generally in terms of cholesterol content. Clinically, remnant lipoproteins have been shown to be predictive of CHD risk.[273] A method used to measure cholesterol in remnant-like particles (RLPs) has become commercially available, using specific antibodies to separate a fraction of lipoprotein remnants. This fraction seems to be particularly indicative of conditions conferring increased CHD risk.[274,275] A fully automated method was recently reported for determination of lipoprotein remnants. However, measurement of triglycerides in nonfasting samples includes the remnant fraction and seems to supersede the need for independent measurement of remnants.[276]

Sources of Variation in Lipid and Lipoprotein Measurements

Lipid and lipoprotein concentrations vary within individuals when measured on several occasions over time. Sources of variation can be broadly categorized as analytical and physiologic or preanalytical. Analytical variations are inherent in the measurements themselves and arise from sample collection procedures, volume measurements, instrument function, reagent formulations, uncertainty in the assignment of values to calibration materials, and other such factors. Normal physiologic variation occurs independently of analytical error and reflects actual changes in concentration that occur through the course of normal, day-to-day living. Such variations result from factors such as change in posture, which causes the redistribution of water between vascular and nonvascular spaces, thereby changing the concentrations of nondiffusible plasma components.[277,278] Recent food intake produces transient increases in plasma triglycerides of 50% or greater and decreases of up to 10% to 15% in LDL and HDL cholesterol, depending on the fat content of the meal.[279-281] Seasonal changes in lipids and lipoproteins have also been observed, probably resulting from changes in dietary and exercise patterns throughout the year.[282,283] Normal physiologic variations tend to occur in both directions, causing lipid or lipoprotein concentrations to vary somewhat about a mean value for a particular patient. Other kinds of physiologic conditions cause changes from the patient's usual steady-state concentrations—for example, acute illness or stress, pregnancy, dietary changes that result in weight loss or gain, changes in saturated fat intake, or the effects of treatment with lipid-lowering medications. In these cases, changes tend to occur in one direction, and they are not considered normal physiologic fluctuations. Lipoprotein concentrations eventually return to original steady-state concentrations when the patient recovers, or a new steady state is achieved.

Because normal physiologic variations occur, it is difficult to evaluate a patient based on a single measurement that applies only to the current sample. It is more appropriate to consider the patient's usual range of concentrations and his or her average steady-state concentration. From the laboratory's standpoint, the aim is to provide accurate measurements in the particular sample being measured. For this reason, the laboratory is primarily concerned with minimizing analytical error. From the physician's standpoint, however, the goal is to establish the patient's usual range of concentration for purposes of diagnosis and judge the effects of treatment. This aim is affected primarily by physiologic variation because physiologic variation contributes the larger proportion of the sample-to-sample variation observed in serial samples from the same patient. Some sources of physiologic variation, such as posture during blood sampling, can be controlled; other factors that cannot be controlled, such as pregnancy, should be considered in interpreting laboratory results.

Analytical Variation

Table 34.22 illustrates the current overall variation of lipid and lipoprotein measurements in more than 100 laboratories participating in an accuracy-based survey conducted by the College of American Pathologists. In this survey, fresh frozen serum is sent to participating laboratories, and the results are compared with the reference method when available. Results from total cholesterol meet the NCEP error goal for bias and imprecision.[185] The average bias was in the range of −01.18% to 0.29%, and CVs were less than 3%. These numbers represent the totals of within- and among-laboratory components of variation and suggest that reliable cholesterol measurements can be provided by most clinical laboratories. Similarly, the overall bias and precision of various triglyceride assays were relatively good. For HDL-C, most participants used one of the current direct assays, and the average bias slightly exceeded the NCEP-recommended bias of 5% or less; the mean CV of the assays also slightly exceeded the 4% or less goal for imprecision. Results for LDL-C are not shown because freezing of the serum was found to affect the commutability of the material, but the performance of the direct LDL-C assay is comparable with that of the direct HDL-C assay, suggesting the need for improvement. It is important to note that the performance of direct HDL-C and LDL-C assays may not be as good in patients with dyslipidemias or other conditions that may affect the specificity of assays for the lipoprotein being measured.[230]

TABLE 34.22 Analytical Variation of Lipid and Lipoprotein Measurements*

Analyte	ABL-01/ 2009	ABL-02/ 2009	ABL-03/ 2009
Cholesterol			
Number of laboratories	135	135	134
Mean, mg/dL	150.8	179.2	244.9
CV, %	2.1	2.2	1.8
CDC value	152.6	180.0	244.2
% Bias	−1.18	−0.44	0.29
HDL-C			
Number of laboratories	134	133	135
Mean, mg/dL	31.7	56.6	49.2
CV, %	4.6	3.8	4.7
CDC value	33.9	56.8	49.3
% Bias	−6.49	−0.35	−0.20
	ABL-04/ 2008	**ABL-05/ 2008**	**ABL-06/ 2008**
Triglyceride			
Number of laboratories	142	141	142
Mean, mg/dL	88.8	204.8	225.7
CV, %	3.2	2.4	2.3
CDC value	91	202.5	223.6
% Bias	−2.42	1.14	0.94

*Bias calculated as: (Test mean − CDC value/CDC value) × 100.
CDC, Centers for Disease Control and Prevention measurement done with reference method; *CV,* coefficient of variation; *HDL-C,* high-density lipoprotein cholesterol.
Data from College of American Pathologists Chemistry Survey, Northfield, Ill, 2009.

Physiologic Variation

The normal physiologic component of variation is calculated from the total variation of measurements in serial specimens from the same patients, after adjustment for analytical variation.[284-288] Such estimates differ somewhat from study to study, but after an extensive review of the literature, the NCEP panels concerned with lipid and lipoprotein measurement assumed average physiologic CVs (Table 34.23). A wide variety of factors contribute to physiologic variations (Table 34.24). Physiologic variations observed for cholesterol,

HDL-C, and LDL-C are similar. Physiologic variation for triglyceride is considerably higher because fasting triglyceride concentrations can vary widely within an individual. Because the analytical CVs for these assays are relatively small, it can be calculated that, on average, physiologic variations contribute about 70% to 98% of the overall variance of lipid and lipoprotein concentrations (see Table 34.23). For this reason, a patient's usual lipid or lipoprotein concentration cannot be reliably established from a single measurement. NCEP guidelines recommend that for cholesterol, the average of measurements in two serial samples obtained at least 1 week apart should be used; two to three serial specimens are recommended, if feasible, for triglyceride and for HDL-C and LDL-C.

TABLE 34.23 Physiologic Variation in Lipid and Lipoprotein Concentrations in Serial Specimens From the Same Individual

Component	Physiologic Variation, % CV	Percentage of Variance Contributed by Physiologic Variation*
Total cholesterol	6.5	91
Triglyceride	23.7	98
HDL cholesterol	7.5	69
LDL cholesterol	8.2	81

*Assuming the following analytical CVs: total cholesterol, 2%; triglyceride, 3%; HDL cholesterol, 5%; LDL cholesterol, 4%.

NCEP Recommendations for Lipid and Lipoprotein Measurements

The following information has been summarized from the NCEP recommendations for lipid and lipoprotein measurement:[184,185]

1. Database linkage. Laboratories that provide lipid and lipoprotein measurements should maintain linkage with existing epidemiologic databases relating lipid and lipoprotein concentration to risk for CHD. Because these databases have been established largely on the basis of CDC standardized methods, the methods used for cholesterol, triglycerides, HDL-C cholesterol, and LDL-C should give results with accuracy traceable to those used to establish those databases. Accordingly, CDC reference methods for cholesterol, triglycerides, and HDL-C serve as the basis for judging the accuracy of other methods.
2. Reference methods. Reference methods should provide serum equivalent values.
3. Routine methods. In most cases, lipid and lipoprotein measurements can be made using specimens of serum or plasma. Measurements in EDTA plasma can be converted to serum-equivalent values using the following equation:

$$\text{Equivalent serum value} = \text{Plasma value} \times 1.03 \qquad \textbf{34.20}$$

TABLE 34.24 Representative Preanalytical Sources of Variation (Including Biological)

	TC	HDL-C	TG	LDL-C
Intraindividual biological variation of healthy individuals (coefficient of variation)	6.5%	7.5%	23.7%	8.2%
Sampling				
Nonfasting	NC	–	++	–
Prolonged total fasting	++	–	+	+
Posture from standing to:				
Supine	–	—	—	—
Sitting	–	–	–	–
Anticoagulants from serum:				
Plasma	–	–	–	–
Behavioral				
Diet				
Saturated fatty acids (palmitic acid)	+	NC	+	+
Monounsaturated fatty acids	–	NC	–	–
Polyunsaturated fatty acids	—	–	NC	—
Cholesterol intake	+	NC	NC	+
Fish oil	NC	NC	–	NC
Obesity	+	–	++	+
Smoking	+	–	++	+
Exercise (strenuous)	–	+	–	–
Alcohol intake	+	+	++	–
Clinical Sources				
Myocardial infarction				
24 hours	NC	NC	NC	NC
6 weeks	–	–	NC	–
Stroke	–	NC	NC	–
Hypertension diuretics	+	–	++	+
Nephrosis	++	NC	++	++
Diabetes (insulin resistance)	+	–	++	++
Infections	–	–	++	–
Pregnancy, second trimester	+	NC	++	+
Transplantation				
Cyclosporine	++	–	+	++
Prednisone	+	–	++	+

HDL-C, High-density lipoprotein cholesterol; *LDL-C,* low-density lipoprotein cholesterol; *NC,* essentially no change or trend; *TC,* total cholesterol; *TG,* triglycerides; +, minimal to moderate increase; ++, moderate to high increase; –, minimal to moderate decrease; —, moderate to high decrease.

Data from Cooper GR, Myers GL, Smith SJ, Schlant RC. Blood lipid measurements: variation and practical utility. *JAMA* 1992;267:1652–60.

4. Cholesterol measurements. In practice, a fasting or a nonfasting sample is used for cholesterol measurements. Triglycerides, HDL-C, and LDL-C measurements should preferably be made in samples collected after a 12-hour fast. As a convenience to the patient, such measurements are made after a 9-hour fast without introducing unduly large errors into the measurements.
5. Blood samples. Blood samples should be collected in the seated position whenever possible. If this is not feasible, the patient should be sampled in the same position on each occasion.
6. Specimen storage. Serum or plasma should be removed from cells within 3 hours of venipuncture. Specimens can be stored for up to 3 days at 4°C; up to several weeks at −20°C in a non–self-defrosting freezer; and at −70°C or lower for longer periods.
7. Serial samples. Using the mean of several serial measurements for clinical decisions is recommended to average out the effects of physiologic and analytical variation. Measurements therefore should be made in at least two serial samples collected at least 1 week apart, with the values averaged. Three serial samples are preferred for measurement of triglycerides, HDL-C, and LDL-C, but two serial specimens can be used if necessary.
8. Glycerol blanking. The NCEP Working Group on Lipoprotein Measurement originally recommended the use of glycerol blanking for triglyceride measurement, but at this time it is not a common practice because only a limited number of commercial assays of these types are available.
9. Goals for analytical performance. The NCEP goals for analytical performance differ slightly from CDC standardization criteria because NCEP goals are stated in terms of total error, which reflects both bias and imprecision,[184] whereas CDC standardization criteria consider each separately. NCEP recommendations for total error are shown in Table 34.25.

These guidelines were established after consideration of degrees of accuracy and imprecision that are achievable in well-controlled research and clinical laboratories.[9] A laboratory can approximate its conformance to the total error recommendations using the following equation:

$$\text{Total error} = \%\ \text{Bias} + 1.96\ \text{X}\ (\text{CVa}) \qquad \textbf{34.21}$$

where % bias is the mean laboratory difference between the measured value for a commutable serum control pool and the reference value for the pool, and CVa is the overall analytical CV for the pool, including within- and among-run variations, and calculated as follows:

$$\frac{\text{Standard deviation}}{\text{Laboratory mean}} \times 100 \qquad \textbf{34.22}$$

Bias should be calculated as the difference from reference values rather than from manufacturers' stated values when these differ.

The individual biases and CVs shown in Table 34.25 should be viewed as examples of conditions under which the total error criteria can be met. A laboratory with less bias can tolerate slightly greater imprecision without exceeding the total error criteria. Conversely, imprecision must be lower if bias increases. For example, a laboratory operating with a bias of 3% and a CV of 3% for cholesterol would have a total error of 3% + (1.96 ∞ 3%), or 8.9%. If, however, bias is only 1%, the CV could be as high as 4% without exceeding the criteria for total error [1% + (1.96 ∞ 4%) = 8.8%]. (In practice, many laboratories can achieve total errors under 6%, assuming a bias of 2% and a CV of 2%.) It is important to note that the NCEP panel considered that the physician usually does not distinguish between lipid and lipoprotein measurements on the basis of the method used to make the measurements. For this reason, NCEP guidelines do not distinguish among measurements made in the laboratory and those made in alternative settings with desktop analyzers or other methods.

As mentioned previously, CDC standardization criteria consider bias and imprecision separately. For this reason, each of the two criteria must be met to achieve standardization. Current CDC standardization criteria are shown in Table 34.26. NCEP guidelines are directed primarily to laboratories and users of laboratory measurements. The reader is referred to the original reports for more extensive discussion of these issues.[184,185] The NCEP panels have made many other recommendations to improve lipid and lipoprotein measurements, only several of which are mentioned here. First, it was recommended that manufacturers of calibration materials, control pools, and analytical systems calibrate their materials and methods to provide values with accuracy traceable to reference method values. Many manufacturers are now doing this,

TABLE 34.25 National Cholesterol Education Program Recommendations for Analytical Performance of Lipid and Lipoprotein Measurements

	Total Error, %	CONSISTENT WITH Bias, %	CV, %
Cholesterol	8.9	≤±3	≤3
Triglycerides	≤15	≤±5	≤5
HDL cholesterol*	≤13	≤±5	≤4
LDL cholesterol	≤12	≤±4	≤4

*When HDL-C <42 mg/dL, the CV criterion is SD ≤1.7.
CV, Coefficient of variation; *HDL*, high-density lipoprotein; *LDL*, low-density lipoprotein.

TABLE 34.26 CDC Standardization Criteria for Lipid and Lipoprotein Measurement

	Bias,*† %	CV,‡ %
Cholesterol	≤±3	≤3
Triglycerides	≤±5	≤5
HDL cholesterol*	≤±5	≤4

*With respect to reference values.
†Maximum allowable.
‡CVs shown apply at HDL cholesterol concentrations >42 mg/dL. At lower concentrations, precision criteria are based on standard deviation (SD ≤1.7).
CDC, Centers for Disease Control and Prevention; *CV*, coefficient of variation; *HDL*, high-density lipoprotein.

which probably accounts for the relatively small interlaboratory biases for total and HDL-C, as reflected in Table 34.22.

Apolipoproteins

Apolipoproteins are measured by a wide variety of immunoassays, including radioimmunoassay (RIA), ELISA, immunoturbidimetric assay, and immunonephelometric assay. The concentration of a particular apolipoprotein usually determines the immunotechnique used for its measurement.

Apolipoproteins A-I and B-100

Immunoturbidimetry and immunonephelometry are widely used to measure apo A-I and apo B-100, which are present at relatively high concentrations. According to the CAP Proficiency Testing Survey, all clinical laboratories in the United States that measure apo A-I and apo B-100 use one of these two approaches. Alternatively, more sensitive techniques, such as ELISA, are perhaps more suitable for those apolipoproteins present at much lower concentrations, such as apo C-I and apo C-II. The following paragraphs discuss some unique analytical issues that pertain to apolipoprotein testing.[289]

Presence of a Given Apolipoprotein on Different Lipoproteins. Apolipoprotein B-100, for example, is present on LDL, IDL, VLDL, and Lp(a) particles, which vary significantly in size and composition. To correctly determine the concentration of total apo B-100, the anti–apo B-100 antibody used must be able to recognize apo B-100 present on various lipoprotein classes equally and must display similar kinetic patterns with all of them.[290]

"Masking" Phenomenon. Unlike other plasma proteins, apolipoproteins circulate in the bloodstream as part of a lipoprotein complex. As discussed earlier, lipoprotein particles are heterogeneous spheres consisting of lipids and apolipoproteins. The antigenic sites of these proteins are often covered by lipids.[291,292] To have a maximal antigen-antibody interaction, these epitopes must be unmasked. Nonionic detergents such as Tween 20 or Tween 80 are usually added to the assay buffer to disrupt the lipoprotein particles and make all of the antigenic sites on the apolipoproteins accessible to the antibodies.

Suitable Antibodies (Polyclonal vs. Monoclonal). Polyclonal antibodies are widely used in clinical laboratories for the measurement of plasma protein concentrations. However, immunoassays are often sensitive to the nature of the antibody used.[292] The development of polyclonal antibodies is affected by several factors, such as the purity and dose of the antigen used, the species of host animal, and the immunization procedure. Monoclonal antibodies are viewed as a viable alternative to alleviate these problems. However, expression of particular epitopes varies with the lipoprotein particles and among individuals; in addition, the apolipoproteins themselves are polymorphic in nature. Therefore a single monoclonal antibody might not detect a particular variant. If a monoclonal antibody is used to determine an apolipoprotein, it should be directed to an epitope that is expressed on all polymorphic forms of that particular apolipoprotein. Furthermore, the epitope should be equally reactive to the antibodies, regardless of which lipoprotein class contains it. Alternatively, a mixture of monoclonal antibodies directed at different epitopes of the apolipoprotein may be used. Such mixtures are referred to as *panmonoclonal* antibodies.

Availability of Primary Calibrators. In general, to standardize a particular protein, a purified form of that protein is used as a primary calibrator. However, the purified preparation must express the same immunoreactivity as the native protein. Unfortunately, once removed from its natural milieu, apo B-100 is insoluble in aqueous buffers. This phenomenon is attributed to the very hydrophobic nature of apo B-100. An LDL preparation with density of 1.030 to 1.050 g/mL, often referred to as *narrow-cut* LDL, is generally used as the primary standard for apo B-100. The protein concentration of the purified preparation is determined by amino acid analysis. In contrast, freshly purified apo A-I is soluble in aqueous buffers and is suitable as a primary standard.

As indicated earlier, several immunotechniques are used for the quantification of apo A-I and apo B-100. These techniques are affected differently by the analytical issues discussed previously. RIA and ELISA, for example, are normally used for the determination of analytes present at these very low concentrations (nanograms per milliliter). Therefore large dilutions (up to 40,000-fold) are required when these techniques are applied to apo A-I or apo B-100 measurement, which can result in a substantial analytical error. In addition, these assays are relatively time-consuming and are not easily automated, and RIA requires the use of isotopes. However, the techniques permit the use of monoclonal or polyclonal antibodies and primary or secondary calibrators and are less affected by the matrix of the specimen, thus permitting the determination of protein concentration in the presence of lipemia. An advantage of immunoturbidimetric and immunonephelometric assays are that they are fully automated and thus highly precise and can use polyclonal or multiple monoclonal antibodies. However, they can be affected by the background turbidity of the specimen (eg, in samples with high triglyceride concentrations). The addition of detergents to the assay buffers reduces nonspecific light scattering; this has helped to diminish this problem.

Considerable effort has been expended over the past decade by national and international organizations in overcoming the problems of apo A-I and B-100 standardization.[293] The Committee on Apolipoproteins of the IFCC embarked on an ambitious international collaborative study aimed at developing secondary serum reference materials that can be used, without influence of matrix bias effects, as master calibrators for all current commercial assays.[294] This program has now been successfully completed.[295,296] A lyophilized serum preparation for apo A-I, designated SP1-01, and a liquid-stabilized serum preparation for apo B-100, designated SP3-07, have been approved as international reference materials by the World Health Organization (WHO). An apo A-I value of 150 mg/dL was assigned to SP1-01 by a highly standardized RIA calibrated with purified apo A-I for which the mass value had been determined by amino acid analysis.[296] An accuracy-based apo B-100 value of 122 mg/dL was assigned to SP3-07 using a nephelometric method that was calibrated with freshly isolated LDL, for which the apo B-100 mass value was determined by a standardized sodium dodecyl sulfate–Lowry protein procedure.[295]

The WHO and the IFCC have appointed the CDC to be the repository for the WHO-IFCC First International Reference Reagents for Apolipoproteins A-I and B-100. Northwest Lipid Research Laboratories (NWLRL) in Seattle uses an IFCC calibration protocol to conduct the standardization and distribution program for manufacturers of instruments and reagents. This protocol involves establishing the linearity of dose response, the parallelism of kinetic responses of standards and calibration sera, and the equality of intercepts for the reference materials and an analysis of fresh frozen sera. NWLRL can be contacted for standardization services and the distribution of apolipoprotein reference materials. These reference materials are also available for reference laboratories in countries where standardized commercial methods are not readily available. It has been shown that through the use of these international reference materials, the analytical performance of apo A-I and apo B-100 measurement, in terms of accuracy and precision, is superior to that of HDL and LDL cholesterol.[295,296] This effort has demonstrated that the use of certified reference materials can significantly reduce the bias of apo A-I and apo B-100 measurements by different immunotechniques. However, an external quality assurance program using fresh or fresh frozen samples and WHO-IFCC–based value assignments is indispensable in monitoring the performance of clinical chemistry laboratories and manufacturers to ensure that accurate apolipoprotein measurements are made. The NWLRL conducts a quarterly standardization program or Reference Lipoprotein Analysis Basic Survey, which provides the accuracy base for cholesterol, triglyceride, HDL-C, LDL-C, and apo A-I and apo B-100. To minimize matrix effects, the survey uses fresh human serum and leads to certification of traceability to the national reference system for cholesterol and to the WHO-IFCC International Reference Reagents for apo A-I and apo B-100.

Apolipoprotein measurements have been shown to further aid in the detection of CHD risk and the diagnosis of hyperlipoproteinemia. For example, measurement of apo B-100 provides a reliable clinical tool by which to identify subjects with increased risk for CHD who may not be readily identified by conventional cholesterol or lipoprotein cholesterol measurements (eg, subjects with a borderline elevation of LDL-C, subjects with hypertriglyceridemia without an LDL cholesterol elevation). In addition, apo B-100 measurements can assess whether lipid-lowering drugs are effective in lowering the number of atherogenic apo B–containing lipoproteins. However, for apolipoprotein measurements to be used in routine clinical practice, clinically meaningful cutoff values for clinical decision making need to be established, and more information regarding their clinical utility is needed. The use of cutoff values for apo A-I and apo B-100, similar to those recommended by the NCEP for HDL and LDL cholesterol, respectively, has been suggested.[90,91] An apo A-I concentration less than 120 mg/dL may be associated with increased risk of CHD, whereas apo A-I of 160 mg/dL or greater may be protective. Apo B-100 cut points of 100 and 120 mg/dL approximately correspond to the LDL cholesterol cut points of 130 and 160 mg/dL (3.36–4.14 mmol/L), which fall at approximately the 50th and 75th percentiles, respectively. Alternatively, Sniderman and Cianflone have suggested that apo B-100 values greater than the 75th percentile should be regarded as high risk and a value greater than the 50th percentile as moderate risk.[109]

Lipoprotein(a)

The structural heterogeneity of Lp(a) as a consequence of apo(a) size heterogeneity has important implications for the accurate measurement of Lp(a) in human plasma.[26,297-300] Repeated antigenic determinants are present in variable numbers in different Lp(a) particles, and the immunoreactivity of the antibodies directed to these repeated epitopes can vary as a function of apo(a) size. As a consequence, immunoassays using polyclonal antibodies or monoclonal antibodies specifically directed to kringle 4 type 2 epitopes will tend to underestimate apo(a) concentration in samples with apo(a) of smaller size than the apo(a) present in the assay calibrator and will tend to overestimate the apo(a) concentration in samples with larger apo(a). A detailed evaluation of the effect of apo(a) size heterogeneity on measurement of Lp(a) has been reported.[299] Monoclonal antibody–based assays have the theoretical advantage that the antibodies can be immunochemically characterized and preselected on the basis of their specificity to single epitopes (eg, those not located in kringle 4 type 2 domain).

Assays are used to measure Lp(a) in turbidimetric, nephelometric, radiometric, and enzymatic methods. Most of these assays, except for the enzyme immunoassay (ELISA), are based on the use of polyclonal antibodies from various animal species. Commercially available, direct-binding, sandwich-type ELISAs are usually based on the use of a combination of monoclonal and polyclonal antibodies. One approach takes advantage of the presence of both apo(a) and apo B in Lp(a) particles. In this approach, Lp(a) particles are "captured" using a polyclonal or monoclonal antibody to apo(a), and an enzyme-conjugated antibody to apo B-100 is used as the detection antibody. An ELISA method based on this approach has been described and is commercially available.[301] In another approach, both capture and detection antibodies are specific for apo(a). At present, it is not clear which approach would be better with respect to estimating the risk for CHD or stroke because the pathogenic mechanisms involved have not yet been elucidated. Thus it is not known whether the risk is associated simply with an increased number of Lp(a) particles in the circulation (as measured using an anti–apo B antibody) or is also related to the presence of polyforms of a particular size (as might be detected more readily with anti-apo(a) detection antibodies). It is likely that both factors influence the risk.

Historically, Lp(a) concentrations have been reported in terms of total Lp(a) particle mass[302] or, alternatively, in terms of Lp(a) protein.[297] If the aim is to provide Lp(a) values that are independent of apo(a) size, it is recommended that the Lp(a) assay use antibodies directed to an apo(a) domain other than kringle 4 type 2 or to the apo B-100 component of Lp(a). This would allow the values to be expressed in nanomoles per liter. Panmonoclonal mixtures of antibodies to kringle 4 type 2 may be preferred if particular sizes of polyforms contribute to the risk.

At present, Lp(a) measurements are not well standardized, and most Lp(a) assays have not been evaluated for their apo(a) size sensitivity. As a result, Lp(a) values reported in clinical studies are difficult to compare. Despite this a value of about 30 mg/dL of total Lp(a) particle mass has traditionally been used as a cutoff, above which elevated concentrations of Lp(a) are associated with increased risk of CHD. Lp(a) concentrations can also be expressed in terms of particle number and mass of apo(a), apo B-100, or Lp(a) cholesterol. At present, Lp(a) values are most commonly expressed in terms of total Lp(a) mass. In view of the current lack of reference methods or standardization procedures for Lp(a), it is difficult to define precise cutoffs that can be used to make clinical decisions. Although less than ideal, one approach would be to establish a reference interval for each assay and report individual results in terms of percentile values within these intervals. In whites, patients with Lp(a) values above the 80th percentile can be considered at increased risk for coronary atherosclerosis. However, because Lp(a) values can vary among ethnic groups, reference values need to be population based. Furthermore, such cutoffs may have to be racially specific. For example, African Americans in general have significantly higher Lp(a) concentrations than whites,[303] but they do not manifest a higher incidence of CHD. An IFCC committee, using an approach similar to that of the apo A-I and B-100 committee, developed reference materials that can be used with all commercially available Lp(a) methods.[304,305] As expected, the use of a common calibrator led to improved harmonization of Lp(a) results but not complete standardization. Only when appropriate antibodies are used can standardization be achieved.

Virtually all retrospective case-control studies in whites have reported a strong association between increased Lp(a) and the risk of CHD. In contrast, prospective studies have provided contradictory results, with four of them finding an association between high Lp(a) concentrations and CHD, and three finding no association. Several studies have suggested that apo(a)-size isoforms may be related to a high prevalence of CHD (see earlier discussion). The procedure with the greatest resolution and sensitivity for determination of apo(a) phenotypes involves separation of apo(a) on agarose gel electrophoresis, immunoblotting with a specific antibody, and detection with ^{125}I-labeled protein A. This approach identifies at least 34 apo(a) polymorphs. It can be used to express apo(a) size in terms of kringle number and is consistent with observations on the size variation of the apo(a) gene obtained by pulsed-field gel electrophoresis and genomic blotting.[306]

Apolipoprotein E

As discussed earlier, homozygosity for apo E_2 is characteristic of type III familial hyperlipoproteinemia. Homozygosity for apo E_2 is a necessary but not sufficient condition for expression of the type III hyperlipoproteinemia; a second gene defect or condition appears to be required to cause the characteristic hyperlipidemia. Heterozygosity for some rare apo E mutants may also be associated with type III hyperlipoproteinemia.[307] The study of apo E variants has assumed greater importance in the last few years because of the association between the apo E_4 allele and Alzheimer's disease and dementia.[63]

Traditionally, the determination of apo E isoforms was assessed by isoelectric focusing (IEF) techniques that permit identification of charge variations of the different isoforms. In early studies, IEF was performed on VLDL that had been extracted to remove the lipids. The separated proteins were then stained for protein.[308] This approach is not used as frequently today because it requires a relatively large volume of plasma and because of the expensive and time-consuming step of ultracentrifugation to isolate VLDL. Apo E phenotypes are now assessed by IEF of a small volume of plasma, followed by immunoblotting with specific antibodies to apo E. This approach can be applied in the clinical laboratory and is well adapted to large-scale population studies. However, it is important that the samples are analyzed fresh or, if stored, that they are kept at −70°C before analysis to minimize the introduction of artifacts. Misclassification can occur because of posttranslational modifications or nonenzymatic glycation of apo E, the presence of rare variants that have the same charge as the common isoforms, overlooked faint apo E_4 bands, and false-positive apo E_2 bands. Interpretation of the patterns requires significant experience in the use of the technique.

The availability of techniques based on the polymerase chain reaction (PCR) permits an analysis of the variation in the nucleotide sequence of the apo E gene (Fig. 34.27). One approach for apo E genotyping uses oligonucleotides to amplify apo E gene sequences containing amino acid positions 112 and 158; the amplified products are digested with *Hha*I and are subjected to electrophoresis on polyacrylamide gels.[309] Alternatively, allele-specific oligonucleotide (ASO) primers can be used to specifically amplify E_2, E_3, and E_4 polymorphic sequences of the apo E gene.[310]Another approach, the amplification refractory mutation system (ARMS), is based on the strictness of the PCR primer for the 3′ end mismatch and is simple, rapid, and nonisotopic. Reagent costs for the ARMS assay are, however, higher than for the restriction isotyping assay. The single-strand conformation polymorphism (SSCP) method has also been used for apo E genotyping.[311] It can detect unknown apo E mutations but is not very convenient because it requires radiolabeled primers. Because restriction isotyping is rapid, requiring only 1 hour to digest the PCR product and several hours for electrophoresis, and does not require radioactive reagents, it may be the most practical method for apo E genotyping in the diagnostic clinical laboratory. Because of potential errors in interpretation or unpreventable artifacts in the apo E phenotype method, apo E genotyping is more reliable for determining the common apo E alleles and would be the method of choice if DNA or whole blood is available. However, most apo E genotyping methods do not detect rare mutations. Discrepancies of 5% to 20% between results of phenotyping and genotyping have been reported.

OTHER CARDIAC RISK FACTORS

Despite the strong association of lipid concentrations with CHD risk, it has long been recognized that half of all myocardial infarctions occur among individuals without overt hyperlipidemia. In the Women's Health Study (WHS), for example, 77% of future cardiovascular events occurred among those with LDL cholesterol concentrations less than 160 mg/dL (4.14 mmol/L), and 46% occurred among those with LDL cholesterol less than 130 mg/dL (3.36 mmol/L).[312] Furthermore, in a 2003 analysis of more than 120,000 patients, approximately 20% of all coronary events occurred in the absence of any of the major classical risk factors: hyperlipidemia, hypertension, diabetes, and smoking.[313] Another large study showed that 85% to 95% of participants with CHD had at least one conventional risk factor, but so too did those participants without CHD, despite follow-up for as long as 30 years.[314] Part of the discordance between lipid concentrations and events can be explained by measuring other markers

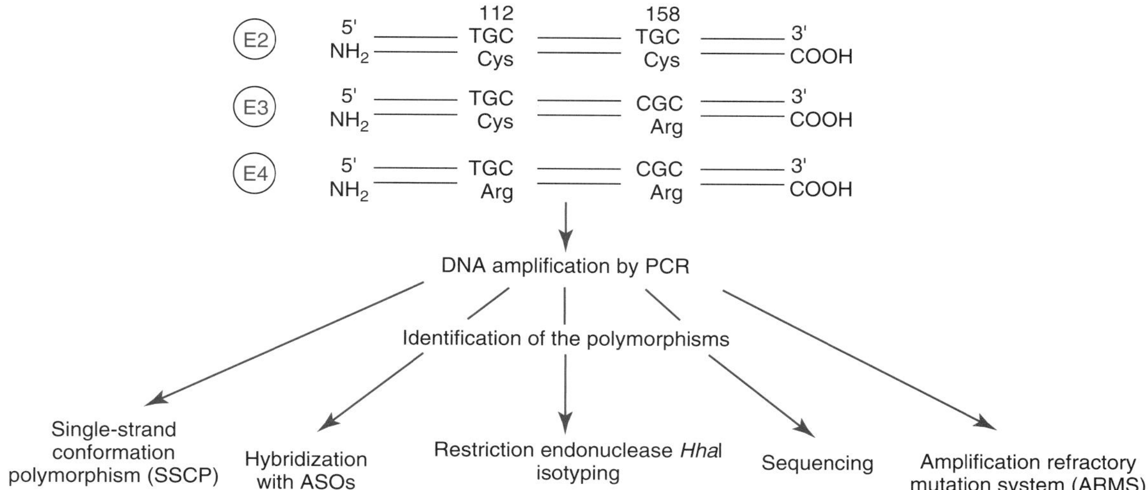

FIGURE 34.27 Different methods for investigating apolipoprotein E polymorphism at the genomic level. *ASO,* Allele-specific oligonucleotide; *PCR,* polymerase chain reaction. (From Siest G, Pillot T, Regis-Bailly A, et al. Apolipoprotein E: an important gene and protein to follow in laboratory medicine. *Clin Chem* 1995;41:1068–86.)

such as apoB and LDL-P,[315] and thus raise the question whether only traditional risk factors are adequate to identify all individuals at increased risk of CHD.

A wide variety of nonlipid biochemical markers have also been suggested in an effort to better identify those individuals at increased CHD risk, including markers of fibrinolytic and hemostatic function (tissue-type plasminogen activator antigen, plasminogen activator inhibitor-1, fibrinogen, von Willebrand, D-dimer, thrombin-antithrombin III complex, and factors V, VII, and VIII), homocysteine, and markers of inflammation (high-sensitivity C-reactive protein [hsCRP], lipoprotein-associated phospholipase A2 [Lp-PLA_2], myeloperoxidase, serum amyloid A, interleukins, adhesion molecules, heat shock proteins, and matrix metalloproteases). NT-proBNP and high-sensitivity troponin I have all emerged as predictors of risk, even in primary prevention settings. Clinically, use of most of these markers in screening is of limited value for one or more of the following reasons:

1. Lack of standardization among available methods
2. Inconsistent findings from prospective epidemiologic studies regarding their ability to independently predict future CHD risk (see discussion on homocysteine later in this chapter)
3. Inability to significantly improve prognostic value when added to traditional lipid screening or existing global risk prediction algorithms, such as the Framingham risk score
4. Unavailability of an appropriate interventional modality that not only modulates the concentration of the biomarker but also reduces the risk associated with increased concentration of that biomarker

A 2009 expert panel of the National Academy of Clinical Biochemistry (NACB) stated in its report on Laboratory Medicine Practice Guidelines for Emerging Biomarkers for Primary Prevention of Cardiovascular Disease that of all examined novel markers, only hsCRP met the previously mentioned criteria for acceptance as a biomarker of risk in the primary prevention setting.[316] These recommendations were consistent with those stated in the earlier report of the American Heart Association (AHA) and the CDC (AHA/CDC).[317] For this reason, hsCRP is discussed in greater detail in this section. A brief discussion of homocysteine, for historical reasons, is also presented.

High-Sensitivity C-Reactive Protein

Tillet and Francis in 1930 described a substance that was present in the sera of acutely ill patients and was able to bind the cell wall C-polysaccharide of *Streptococcus pneumoniae* and to agglutinate the organisms. In 1941, the substance was shown to be a protein and was given the name *C-reactive protein (CRP).* CRP was subsequently shown to be an acute-phase reactant that was important in the nonspecific host defense against inflammation, especially infection; it is routinely monitored as an indication of infection and autoimmune disease, using methods that have detection limits of 3 to 8 mg/L.

Chronic inflammation is an important component in the development and progression of atherosclerosis, and numerous epidemiologic studies have demonstrated that increased serum CRP concentrations are positively associated with the risk of future coronary events, such as coronary artery disease, cerebrovascular disease, or peripheral arterial disease.[318-320] It has also been shown to be predictive of future events in patients with acute coronary syndromes and in those with stable angina and coronary artery stents.

The use of CRP for these purposes requires the use of hsCRP assays that have detection limits less than 0.3 mg/L.[321] Several automated immunoturbidimetric and immunonephelometric assays are commercially available and are capable of sensitive and precise measurements at low concentrations of CRP. The analytical performance of several of these assays has been evaluated.[321] In this section, we summarize the basic biochemistry, clinical significance, and analytical considerations of the measurement of hsCRP. Additional information is presented in Chapter 28.

Biochemistry

CRP consists of five identical, nonglycosylated polypeptide subunits noncovalently linked to form a disk-shaped cyclic polymer with a molecular weight of approximately 115 kDa. It contains little or no carbohydrate and is synthesized primarily in the liver. Its production is controlled by interleukin-6, and it binds to polysaccharides present in many bacteria, fungi, and protozoal parasites and polycations, such as histones.

Clinical Significance

Of the markers mentioned previously in this chapter, only hsCRP has fulfilled the required criteria for a novel marker of CHD risk according to the expert panels of the AHA/CDC[317] and the NACB.[316] Here we discuss the roles of hsCRP in CHD, the metabolic syndrome, diabetes, and hypertension, and its possible role in atherogenesis. We conclude with a discussion of possible preventive measures in those individuals with increased concentrations of hsCRP. Comprehensive reviews on this subject have been published.[322,323]

Cardiovascular Disease. Prospective epidemiologic studies have consistently shown that a single assay result for hsCRP is a strong predictor of myocardial infarction,[312,318,324] stroke,[312] peripheral vascular disease,[319] and sudden cardiac death[325] in individuals without a history of heart disease. The association between hsCRP and future CHD reflects the current understanding of vascular biology because it is known that chronic inflammation plays a pivotal role in atherogenesis. This association has been observed in studies from around the world involving middle-aged and elderly persons and high- and usual-risk populations.[318,324,325] The association is apparent even in studies with follow-up periods up to 20 years, as seen in the Honolulu Heart Study.[326] In a direct comparison of traditional and novel biochemical markers of CHD risk, hsCRP was the strongest predictor of future coronary events.[320]

In general, those individuals with hsCRP values in the top quartile of the sample distribution are two to three times more likely to experience a future vascular event than those in the bottom quartile. The association between hsCRP and future vascular events is linear and is independent of age, smoking, hypertension, dyslipidemia, and diabetes. For example, 8-year follow-up data from the Physicians' Health Study and the WHS showed that after adjustment for traditional risk factors, an increase in future cardiovascular risk of 26% was noted for men and 33% for women for each quintile increase in baseline hsCRP.[320]

Although most of the available data on hsCRP and incident CHD have been derived from nested case-control studies, event-free survival data from large cohorts have been published,[312,327] thus enabling estimation of absolute risks rather than relative risks of disease. Data from the WHS, for example, showed hsCRP to be a stronger predictor of risk than LDL cholesterol (Fig. 34.28) and demonstrated that event-free survival was poorest for persons with increases in both LDL cholesterol and hsCRP; the best survival was observed for those with low values of both measures.[312] Event-free survival was significantly worse for those with high hsCRP and low LDL cholesterol as compared with those with high LDL cholesterol and low hsCRP (Fig. 34.29).

Because hsCRP values minimally correlate with lipid concentrations, and because lipid parameters account for less than 3% to 5% of the variance in hsCRP measurement, measurement of hsCRP does not replace but instead complements the evaluation of lipids and other classical CHD risk factors in primary prevention settings.[327] Data from the WHS show that hsCRP adds prognostic information not only at all concentrations of the risk defined by current LDL cut points of the NCEP, but also at all concentrations of the risk specified by the Framingham risk score algorithm—an observation of significant public health implications.[327] Contemporary algorithms were developed for the assessment of global cardiovascular risk in approximately 11,000 men and 25,000 women followed for a median period longer than 10 years (Reynolds risk score).[328,329] Initially, the model was developed in women using 35 different variables, of which only the addition of hsCRP and family history of cardiovascular disease to the traditional Framingham risk components led to improved accuracy in classification; 40% to 50% of women at intermediate risk (5% to 20%, estimated 10-year risk) were reclassified into higher- or lower-risk categories.[328] Similar

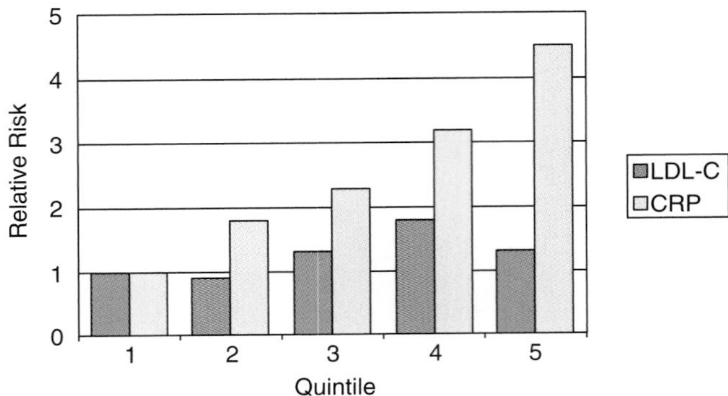

FIGURE 34.28 Head-to-head comparison of LDL cholesterol and hsCRP in their ability to predict future vascular events. *hsCRP,* High-sensitivity C-reactive protein; *LDL,* low-density lipoprotein cholesterol. (From Ridker PM, Rifai N, Rose L, Buring JE, Cook NR. Comparison of C-reactive protein and low-density lipoprotein cholesterol levels in the prediction of first cardiovascular events. *N Engl J Med* 2002;347:1557–65.

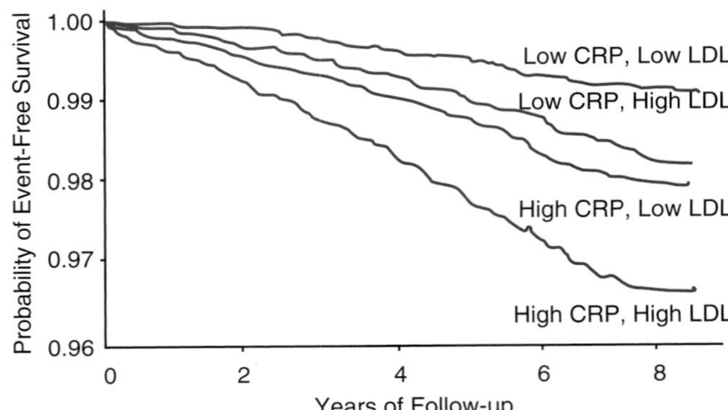

FIGURE 34.29 Cardiovascular event-free survival according to baseline levels of hsCRP and LDL cholesterol. (From Ridker PM, Rifai N, Rose L, Buring JE, Cook NR. Comparison of C-reactive protein and low-density lipoprotein cholesterol levels in the prediction of first cardiovascular events. *N Engl J Med* 2002;347:1557–65.)

findings were seen in men, with about 20% of those in intermediate risk being reclassified into higher- or lower-risk categories.[329] However, a 2009 report has cautioned about extending to other ethnic groups the use of algorithms developed in primarily a white population.[330]

Metabolic Syndrome, Diabetes, and Hypertension. Studies have demonstrated a significant association between hsCRP and future risk of metabolic syndrome, diabetes, and hypertension—conditions that confer increased cardiovascular risk. hsCRP values are positively correlated not only with components of the metabolic syndrome that are commonly assessed in clinical practice, such as increased triglycerides, reduced HDL cholesterol, obesity, high blood pressure, and high fasting glucose, but also with other components that are not easily captured in such settings, such as fasting insulin, microalbuminuria, and impaired fibrinolysis.[331] Data from the WHS show that hsCRP measurement improves the cardiovascular risk prediction beyond that of metabolic syndrome status as assessed in clinical practice;[332] those women with metabolic syndrome and hsCRP greater than 3 mg/L were at twice the risk of future coronary events compared with those with metabolic syndrome and hsCRP less than 3 mg/L. Similar results were observed in the West of Scotland Coronary Prevention Study (WOSCOPS).[333]

Increased hsCRP concentrations have also been implicated in the development of type 2 diabetes mellitus. Prospective studies have found strong, graded relationships between hsCRP and incident diabetes, which in many instances persisted after adjustment for body mass index and other covariates.[334] In WOSCOPS, the top quintile of hsCRP was associated with a threefold risk of incident diabetes over a 5-year period compared with the lowest quintile,[335] and in the WHS, the top quartile of hsCRP was associated with a fourfold risk during 4 years of follow-up compared with the lowest quartile.[334] These data support the hypothesis that inflammation, atherothrombosis, and diabetes are tightly interrelated disorders of the immune system.

Accumulating data also suggest a link between blood pressure and vascular inflammation, perhaps mediated by angiotensin II.[336] For example, angiotensin II infusion activates nuclear factor-κB and leads to increased interleukin-6 expression in human vascular smooth muscle cells.[337] Moreover, cross-sectional studies show graded linear relationships between interleukin-6 and intercellular adhesion molecule-1 and both systolic and diastolic blood pressure.[338] The relationship between blood pressure, hsCRP, and incident cardiovascular events was assessed in the WHS.[339] Despite their strong correlation, hsCRP and blood pressure were independent determinants of future cardiovascular events during an 8-year follow-up period, and hsCRP retained incremental prognostic value at all concentrations of blood pressure. Compared with women with blood pressures lower than 120/75 mm Hg and hsCRP values less than 3 mg/L, those with blood pressures of 160/95 mm Hg or greater and hsCRP values of 3 mg/L or greater were more than eight times as likely to experience a future cardiovascular event. hsCRP also predicts incident hypertension itself. In the same cohort, after adjustment for multiple potential confounders, those women in the highest quintile of hsCRP were at a 50% higher risk of developing hypertension compared with those in the lowest quintile.[340] Moreover, high hsCRP concentration was associated with an increased risk of incident hypertension at all baseline blood pressures and among individuals without traditional CHD risk factors. On the basis of these data, it has been hypothesized that hsCRP may play a critical role in the development of hypertension. Whether or not blood pressure reduction leads to reduced hsCRP values is uncertain and is being tested in an ongoing clinical trial.

Possible Role of CRP in Atherogenesis. It is not clear at present whether CRP is a marker that reflects systemic or vascular inflammation or is an actual participant in atherogenesis. However, findings from pathologic and in vitro studies are increasingly supporting the latter. Recent reports have shown CRP to enhance expression of local endothelial cell surface adhesion molecules,[341] monocyte chemoattractant protein-1,[341] endothelin-1,[342] and endothelial plasminogen activator inhibitor-1;[343] reduce endothelial nitric oxide bioactivity[342]; increase the induction of tissue factor in monocytes[344] and LDL uptake by macrophages[345]; and colocalize with the complement membrane attack complex within atherosclerotic lesions.[346] In addition, it has been demonstrated that expression of human CRP in CRP-transgenic mice directly enhances intravascular thrombosis in both arterial injury and photochemical injury models of endothelial disruption.[346] For a more complete discussion of the possible role of CRP in atherogenesis, as determined by vascular biology experimental studies, refer to the review by Devaraj and colleagues.[347] Investigators in two studies in which the mendelian randomization approach was used concluded that hsCRP is not a causal factor in cardiovascular disease.[348,349] Critics of such an approach, however, indicate that when findings from mendelian randomization analysis are positive, they strongly suggest causality, but the opposite is not always true. It is important to remember that whether or not CRP is a causative factor will not preclude or affect its utility as a marker of cardiovascular disease.

Role in Disease Intervention. Although many behavioral interventions known to reduce the risk of clinical cardiovascular events have been linked to lower hsCRP values, it is not definitely known at present whether lowering of hsCRP will necessarily lead to a reduction in vascular events. For example, a reduction not only in hsCRP but also in several proinflammatory cytokines and adhesion molecules was seen in obese premenopausal women assigned to a weight-loss program as compared with women in the control group.[350] Whether these effects translate into reduced risk of subsequent cardiovascular events has not yet been elucidated.

Although no specific drugs are known to lower hsCRP concentrations, several pharmacologic agents have demonstrated cardioprotective ability, such as aspirin and statins, with the latter having the ability to reduce hsCRP values. In the Physicians' Health Study, a large primary prevention trial, reduction in the risk of future myocardial infarction associated with assignment to aspirin was 56% among those with baseline hsCRP concentrations in the highest quartile, and this value declined proportionately with hsCRP values until a reduction of only 14% was noted among those in the lowest quartile, suggesting that aspirin may prevent ischemic events through antiinflammatory and antiplatelet effects.[351] The effect of aspirin on lowering hsCRP concentrations is uncertain at present.

The ability of statins to lower hsCRP was first described for pravastatin using data accumulated in the Cholesterol and

Recurrent Events (CARE) trial.[352,353] These data were initially highly controversial because they suggested that statins have both lipid-lowering and antiinflammatory effects. However, confirmatory work rapidly showed the effect of statins on hsCRP to be a consistent and important class effect. Studies of atorvastatin, cerivastatin, lovastatin, pravastatin, and simvastatin have shown that median hsCRP concentrations typically decline by 15% to 25% as early as 6 weeks after initiation of therapy.[354] It is important to note that the magnitude of LDL cholesterol reduction caused by statin therapy is minimally correlated with the magnitude of hsCRP reduction.[354]

Data from two large 5-year randomized trials suggest that cardiovascular risk reduction attributable to statin therapy may be most marked for those with increased hsCRP concentrations at baseline. In the CARE trial, the proportion of recurrent events prevented by pravastatin was 54% among persons with increased hsCRP values but only 25% among persons with lower hsCRP values, even though baseline lipid concentrations were nearly identical in those with and without evidence of inflammation.[353] Similarly, in the Texas Air Force Coronary Atherosclerosis Prevention Study, lovastatin therapy was associated with a 42% reduction in first cardiovascular events among participants with low LDL cholesterol concentrations (<149 mg/dL) (3.85 mmol/L) but high hsCRP values (>1.6 mg/L).[327] As a result of these provocative findings, JUPITER, a clinical trial specifically designed to test the efficacy of statins in reducing clinical cardiovascular events among persons with hsCRP of 2 mg/L or greater and LDL cholesterol less than 130 mg/dL (3.36 mmol/L), who make up an estimated 25% of the US population, was launched.[355] Approximately 18,000 subjects with such a phenotype were randomized to 20 mg of rosuvastatin per day or placebo and followed for a period of 4 years for the occurrence of myocardial infarction, stroke, arterial revascularization, hospitalization for unstable angina, or death from cardiovascular disease (primary end point).[355] However, the safety and efficacy board of the trial terminated it ahead of schedule because its continuation was deemed unethical based on the overwhelmingly positive results. Findings revealed a reduction in the primary trial end point of 44% in those who received rosuvastatin compared with those on placebo (Fig. 34.30).[356] The number of subjects with this phenotype who have to be treated with statin to prevent a single coronary event was 25, a number that is similar to those seen in hyperlipidemia trials. Furthermore, using hsCRP less than 2 mg/L and LDL cholesterol less than 70 mg/dL (1.8 mmol/L) as dual target goals for statin therapy, a reduction of 65% in cardiovascular events was seen; a reduction of 80% in cardiovascular events was noted in those who achieved that concentration of LDL cholesterol but hsCRP less than 1 mg/L (see Fig. 34.30).[357] The concept of dual target goals, using both LDL cholesterol and hsCRP, to optimize statin therapy in patients with acute coronary syndrome has been explored and has been shown to be beneficial (see Fig. 34.30).[201,358,359] Based on much of the above data, the National Lipid Association recommended routine CRP measurement in those patients who had intermediate risk defined as a 5% to 20% Framingham Score (FRS) to be considered for those with CHD or CHD-equivalents and reasonable for those with family history of CHD or who have had recurrent events. It was not advised for low risk (<5% FRS).[360]

POINTS TO REMEMBER

CRP

- CRP is an acute phase plasma protein and can be markedly increased in various infections and inflammatory diseases.
- Modest increases in CRP may also occur with low-level chronic inflammation such as that which occurs in CVD.
- CRP is positively associated with CVD and may be useful in assessing patients with intermediate CVD risk.
- Sensitive immunoassays of CRP (hsCRP) are used for assessing CVD risk.

ANALYTICAL CONSIDERATIONS

To measure the concentrations required for use in vascular disease assessment, high-sensitivity methods were developed for CRP. Of the various techniques used by investigators and manufacturers to improve the sensitivity of CRP assays, the most successful approach has been to amplify the light-scattering properties of the antigen-antibody complex by covalently coupling latex particles to a specific antibody—a procedure that is easily automated using standard laboratory instrumentation. More than 30 hsCRP assays, most of which use this approach, are now commercially available.[361] In a study of nine such assays, all achieved a lowest detection limit of 0.3 mg/L or less, and five had within-laboratory analytical imprecision less than 10% (ie, reproducibilities greater than 90%).[321] However, hsCRP assays from different laboratories showed significant discrepancies in reported results, underscoring the need for additional standardization.

Standardization

Agreement among hsCRP methods is essential because an individual patient's result will be interpreted within the context of nationally established cut points, or patients will be treated to a target value. A standardization program led by the CDC was initiated in 2002 to address this issue.[362] In Phase I, a suitable common calibrator was identified, and in more recently published findings from Phase II, this common calibrator was shown to harmonize patients' results in most commercially available assays.[363]

Biological Variability of CRP

Despite being an acute-phase reactant, hsCRP exhibits a relatively low degree of intraindividual variability in clinically stable patients. In a study of such patients, the use of two independent measurements of hsCRP taken 90 days apart enabled the classification of 90% of participants into the exact or immediately adjacent biomarker tertile, a percentage comparable with that observed for cholesterol (Fig. 34.31).[361,364] Furthermore, the age-adjusted correlation between two hsCRP measurements from blood samples drawn 5 years apart was 0.6, a value comparable with that of cholesterol and other lipid parameters.[352] Other groups of investigators reported a 3-year, age-adjusted reliability coefficient of 0.52.[365] Although findings from this epidemiologic study of initially healthy middle-aged men suggest that three independent measurements should be taken to maximize the biomarker's predictive ability,[365] whether serial assessment of hsCRP provides incremental clinical benefit is uncertain. Provided that a value less than 10 mg/L is obtained,

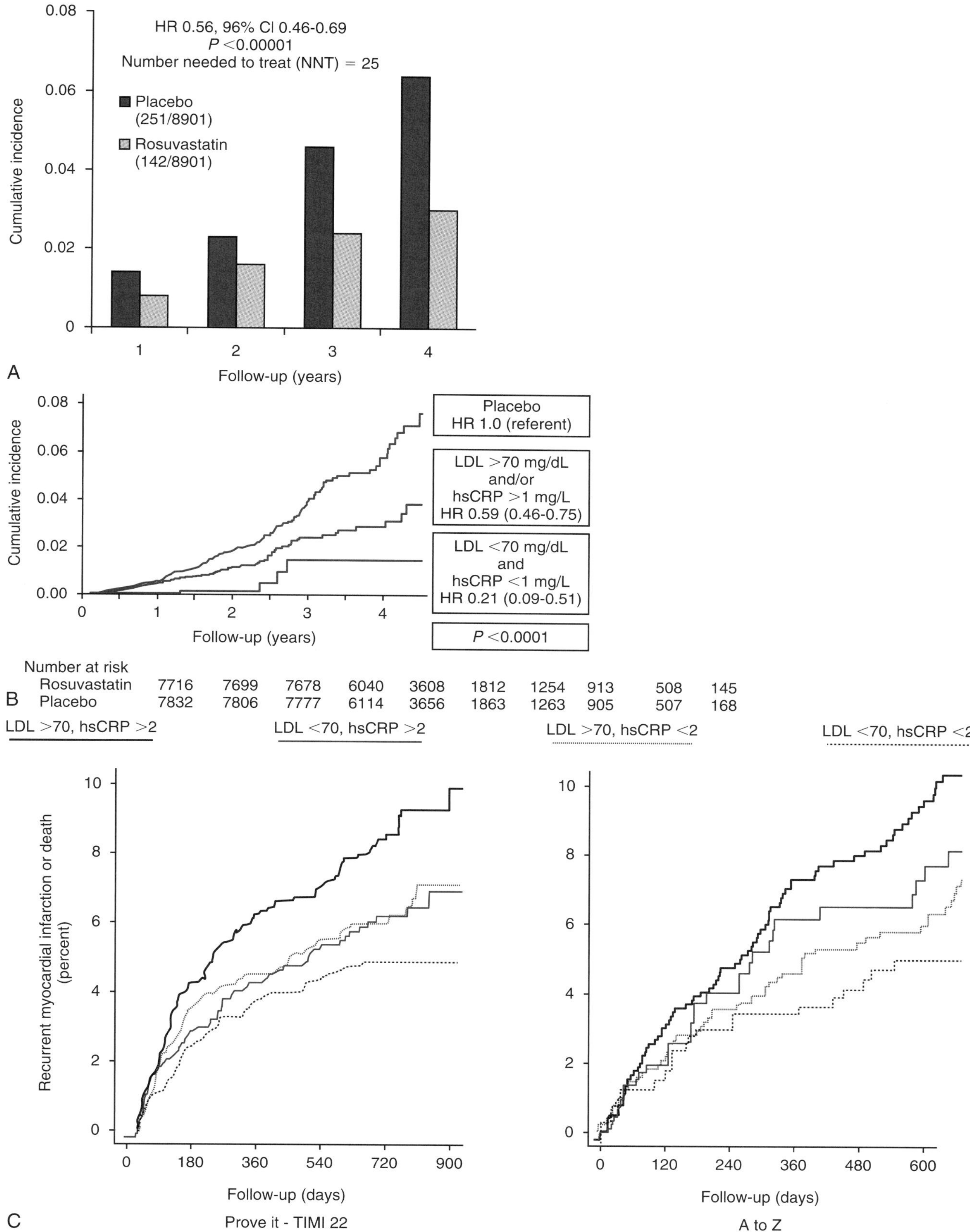

FIGURE 34.30 A, Cumulative incidence of cardiovascular events in the JUPITER trial. **B,** Cumulative incidence of cardiovascular events in JUPITER in placebo and statin groups according to achieved LDL cholesterol and hsCRP. **C,** Cumulative incidence of cardiovascular events in PROVE IT and A to Z in placebo and statin groups, according to achieved LDL cholesterol and hsCRP. (**A** Data from *N Engl J Med* 2008;359:2195–207; **B** data from *Lancet* 2009;373:1175–82; **C** from *Circulation* 2006;114:281–8; *N Engl J Med* 2005;352:20–8.)

TABLE 34.27 Population Distributions of CRP, mg/L

Population	PERCENTILE						
	5th	10th	25th	50th	75th	90th	95th
American women*	0.2	0.3	0.6	1.5	3.5	6.6	9.1
American men	0.3	0.4	0.8	1.5	3.2	6.1	8.6
European women*	0.3	0.4	0.9	1.7	3.4	6.2	8.8
European men	0.3	0.6	0.8	1.6	3.3	6.5	8.6

*Only women not taking hormone replacement therapy.
Data from Rifai N, Ridker PM. Population distributions of C-reactive protein in apparently healthy men and women in the United States: implication for clinical interpretation. *Clin Chem* 2003;49:666–9; Imhof A, Frohlich M, et al. Distributions of C-reactive protein measured by high-sensitivity assays in apparently healthy men and women from different populations in Europe. *Clin Chem* 2003;49: 669–72.

TABLE 34.28 Distributions of CRP Among Men, mg/L

	PERCENTILE						
	5th	10th	25th	50th	75th	90th	95th
White American	0.2	0.4	0.7	1.6	3.4	6.7	12.3
African American	0.1	0.2	0.7	1.7	3.9	8.2	13.2
Mexican American	0.2	0.4	0.6	1.6	3.2	6.3	9.8
Japanese	—	<0.3	0.4	1.6	3.5	7.8	—

Data from Ford ES, Giles WH, Myers GL, et al. Population distribution of high-sensitivity C-reactive protein among US men: findings from National Health and Nutrition Examination Survey 1999–2000. *Clin Chem* 2003;49:686–90; Yamada S, Gotoh T, Nakashima Y, et al. Distribution of serum C-reactive protein and its association with atherosclerotic risk factors in a Japanese population: Jichi Medical School Cohort Study. *Am J Epidemiol* 2001;153:1183–90.

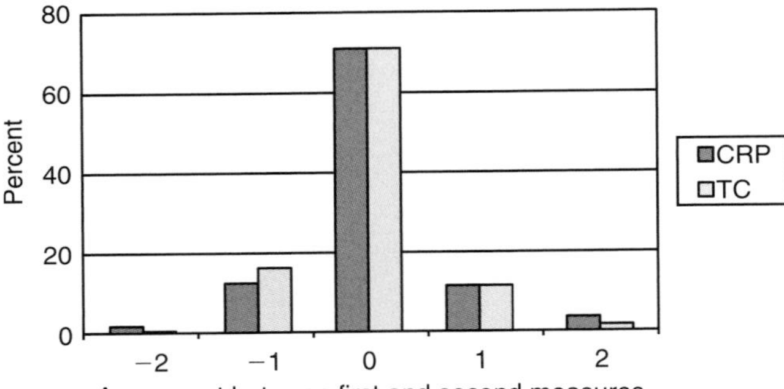

FIGURE 34.31 Within-person variability: comparison of hsCRP with total cholesterol. (From Ledue TB, Rifai N. Preanalytic and analytic sources of variations in C-reactive protein measurement: implications for cardiovascular disease risk assessment. *Clin Chem* 2003;49:1258–71.)

the AHA/CDC panel recommends the use of two hsCRP measures taken 2 or more weeks apart, with the average value used to estimate vascular risk.[317] Because hsCRP may reflect subclinical infection, values greater than 10 mg/L should be disregarded initially and the test repeated when the patient has stabilized. Similar recommendations were issued by the NACB expert panel. Furthermore, because hsCRP values are unaffected by food intake and exhibit almost no circadian variation,[229,364] measurements can be made without regard for fasting status or time of day.

Reference Values

Data from several large US and European cohorts indicate that the distribution of circulating hsCRP concentrations appears comparable among men and women not using postmenopausal hormone replacement therapy (HRT),[366,367] with the 50th percentile for both genders being about 1.5 mg/L (Table 34.27). hsCRP concentrations are higher in women who use oral HRT than in women who do not, and increased hsCRP from oral HRT has been associated with increased risk of thrombotic events.[368]

Information on the distribution of hsCRP concentrations in nonwhite populations is sparse. In the nationally representative NHANES data set, no significant differences were noted in the distribution of hsCRP concentrations among white, black, and Mexican-American men (Table 34.28).[369] Moreover, a comparable hsCRP distribution was seen in Japanese men.[370] Although additional studies on the distribution and prognostic ability of CRP in nonwhite populations are clearly necessary, existing data are insufficient to support the exclusion of any racial or ethnic group from current guidelines for CRP testing.

Most studies have reported only a modest relationship between age (range, 18 to 88 years) and serum hsCRP concentrations. In the WHS, for example, median hsCRP concentrations for individuals aged 45 to 54, 55 to 64, 65 to 74, and 75 years or older were 1.31, 1.89, 1.99, and 1.52 mg/L, respectively.[367] Reference values of less than 1, 1 to 3, and greater than 3 mg/L, which correspond to approximate tertiles of the CRP distribution in healthy adults, are recommended for classification of individuals into low, moderate, and high cardiovascular risk groups in primary prevention settings by AHA/CDC and NACB expert panels.[316,317] Because of the prognostic additive effect of hsCRP to the lipid screen, an algorithm combining hsCRP and LDL cholesterol using the NCEP cut points has been proposed (Fig. 34.32).[367] According to the AHA/CDC and NACB recommendation, hsCRP should be part of the global risk assessment of CHD in the primary prevention setting, and individuals with intermediate risk as determined by the Framingham risk score will benefit the most from its measurement.[316,317]

Homocysteine

Many disorders are associated with increased concentrations of total homocysteine.[371] In this section, the basic biochemistry, clinical significance, and measurement of total homocysteine (tHcy) are summarized.

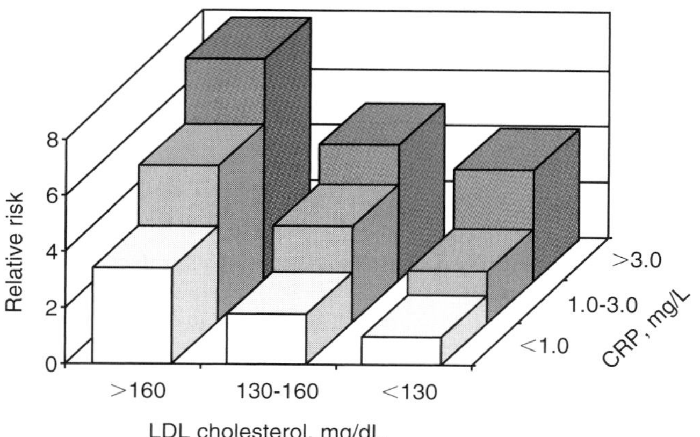

FIGURE 34.32 Algorithm for risk assessment of CHD risk employing CRP and LDL cholesterol. (From Rifai N, Ridker PM. Population distributions of C-reactive protein in apparently healthy men and women in the United States: implication for clinical interpretation. *Clin Chem* 2003;49:666–9.)

Basic Biochemistry

Homocysteine is a sulfur-containing amino acid, with each molecule of homocysteine containing one atom of sulfur. It is formed during the metabolism of methionine and requires folic acid as a cofactor (Fig. 34.33). At low concentrations, homocysteine may be anabolized back to methionine in a cycle that involves tetrahydrofolate or catabolized to cysteine by enzymes that require vitamin B as a cofactor. Consequently, a deficiency of folic acid or vitamins B_6 and B_{12} can result in increased concentrations of homocysteine (see Chapter 37).[372] Homocysteine does not normally accumulate in plasma because it is very unstable in aqueous solution and, when present in excess, undergoes oxidation to homocysteine.

Clinical Significance

Numerous studies have suggested an association between elevated concentrations of circulating homocysteine and various vascular and cardiovascular disorders.[371,373] Clinically, the measurement of tHcy is also important to diagnose homocystinuria and to identify individuals with or at a risk

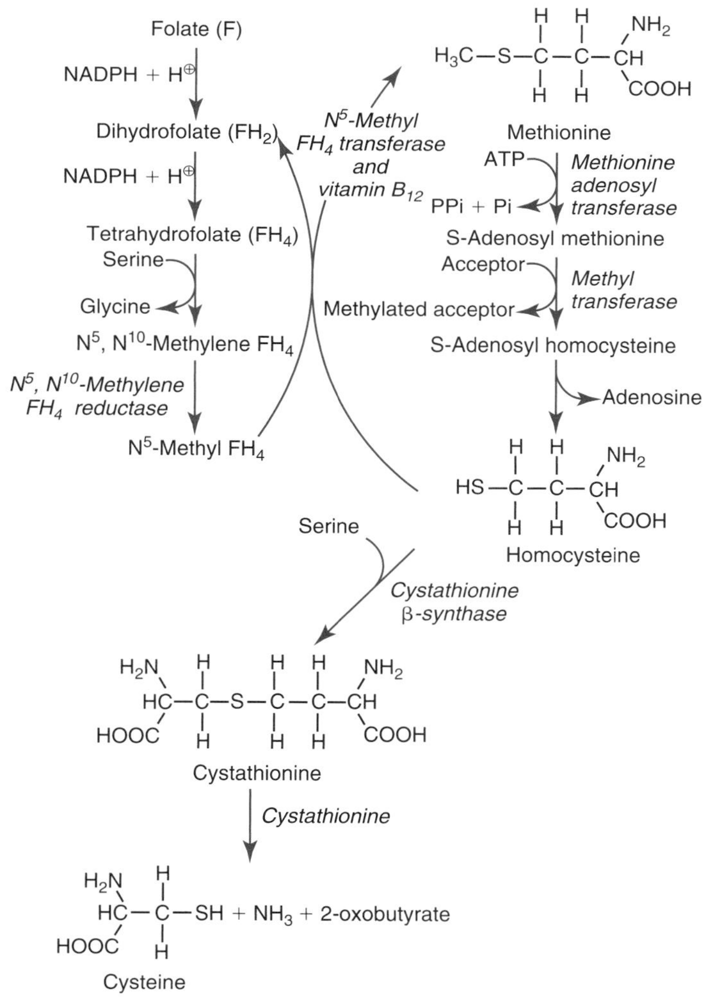

FIGURE 34.33 Biochemical pathways of the conversion of methionine to homocysteine and cysteine.

of developing cobalamin or folate deficiency.[371] Although numerous studies have demonstrated a causal relationship between tHcy and CVD, controversy continues about the clinical significance of this relationship because (1) the methylenetetrahydrofolate reductase 677C>T polymorphism is a strong risk factor for increased tHcy but not for CVD; (2) an apparent discrepancy has been noted between prospective and retrospective case-control studies; and (3) data from controlled clinical trials are lacking.[371] Because of this concern over the clinical significance of the causal relationship between tHcy and CVD, Refsum and colleagues developed the following recommendations:[371]

- Measurement of tHcy in the general population to screen for CVD risk is not recommended.
- In young CVD patients (<40 years), tHcy should be measured to exclude homocystinuria.
- In patients with CVD or persons at high risk for CVD events, a high tHcy concentration should be used as a prognostic factor for CVD events and mortality.
- CVD patients with tHcy greater than 15 µmol/L belong to a high-risk group; it is especially important for them to follow a healthy lifestyle and to receive optimal treatment for known causal risk factors.
- Increased tHcy combined with low vitamin concentrations should be handled as a potential vitamin deficiency. Other causes of increased tHcy should be considered.

Measurement of Total Homocysteine

Physiologically, homocysteine exists in reduced, oxidized, and protein-bound forms.[374] Methods for tHcy first introduced in the mid-1980s resolved the problems related to the presence of multiple unstable Hcy species in plasma by converting all Hcy species into the reduced form, HcyH, which is measured as an indication of tHcy content.[375] Consequently, modern methods require pretreatment of plasma or serum specimens with a reducing agent such as dithioerythritol, dithiothreitol, mercaptoethanol, tributyl phosphine, or tris(2-carboxyl-ethyl) phosphine that converts all Hcy species into the reduced form.

More recent tHcy methods include enzyme immunoassays and chromatography-based methods.[376] In practice, immunoassays[377] are used most often for most routine purposes. Chromatographic assays include amino acid analysis; high-performance liquid chromatography (HPLC) with ultraviolet, fluorescence, or electrochemical detection,[378-381] capillary electrophoresis with fluorescence detection; gas chromatography-mass spectrometry (GC-MS); and liquid chromatography with tandem MS (MS-MS).[382] The different tHcy methods give comparable results,[383,384] but more standardization of the tHcy assay is necessary.[376]

To obtain accurate results, it is generally recommended that specimens be refrigerated and quickly centrifuged to remove cells.[374] If unspun specimens are allowed to stand at room temperature, glycolysis can double homocysteine concentrations. Addition of fluoride or specific *S*-adenosylhomocysteine hydrolase inhibitors will prevent problems caused by glycolysis.[374] Short-term (1 month) within-person biological variability of plasma homocysteine has been reported to be approximately 7%; thus only a single measure of homocysteine is commonly done.[385] Homocysteine values do not show much long-term variability, but they can change in response to diet or treatment with folate.[385] Reference intervals for fasting homocysteine concentrations have been reported to be 13 to 18 µmol/L for serum[380,386] and 10 to 15 µmol/L for plasma.[59] The reference interval for total homocysteine in pediatric patients has been reported to be 3.7 to 10.3 µmol/L.[387]

SELECTED REFERENCES

For a full list of references for this chapter, please refer to ExpertConsult.com.

4. Kidambi S, Solca C, Patel S. Tracking the dietary cholesterol molecule. *Future Lipidol* 2006;**1**:357–68.
5. Stone NJ, Robinson JG, Lichtenstein AH, et al. 2013 ACC/AHA guideline on the treatment of blood cholesterol to reduce atherosclerotic cardiovascular risk in adults: a report of the American College Of Cardiology/American Heart Association Task Force on practice guidelines. *Circulation* 2013;**129**:S1–45.
11. Grundy SM. Cholesterol and coronary heart disease. *JAMA* 1986;**256**:2849.
37. Brewer HB. Hypertriglyceridemia: changes in the plasma lipoproteins associated with an increased risk of cardiovascular disease. *Am J Cardiol* 1999;**83**:3–12.
38. Kohan AB, Wang F, Lo C-M, et al. Apoa-iv: current and emerging roles in intestinal lipid metabolism, glucose homeostasis, and satiety. *Am J Physiol Gastrointest Liver Physiol* 2015;**308**:G472–81.
45. Cromwell WC, Barringer TA. Low-density lipoprotein and apolipoprotein b: clinical use in patients with coronary heart disease. *Curr Cardiol Rep* 2009;**11**:468–75.
46. Segrest JP, Jones MK, De Loof H, et al. Structure of apolipoprotein b-100 in low density lipoproteins. *J Lipid Res* 2001;**42**:1346–67.
77. Toth PP, Barter PJ, Rosenson RS, et al. High-density lipoproteins: a consensus statement from the National Lipid Association. *J Clin Lipidol* 2013;**7**:484–525.
78. Cuchel M. Macrophage reverse cholesterol transport: key to the regression of atherosclerosis? *Circulation* 2006;**113**:2548–55.
84. Rosenson RS, Brewer HB, Chapman MJ, et al. HDL measures, particle heterogeneity, proposed nomenclature, and relation to atherosclerotic cardiovascular events. *Clin Chem* 2011;**57**:392–410.
98. Nissen SE, Nicholls SJ, Sipahi I, et al. Effect of very high-intensity statin therapy on regression of coronary atherosclerosis. *JAMA* 2006;**295**:1556.
102. Expert Panel on Detection E, Treatment of High Blood Cholesterol in A. Executive summary of the third report of the national cholesterol education program (ncep) expert panel on detection, evaluation, and treatment of high blood cholesterol in adults (adult treatment panel iii). *JAMA* 2001;**285**:2486–97.
111. Jacobson TA, Ito MK, Maki KC, et al. National lipid association recommendations for patient-centered management of dyslipidemia: part 1 – executive summary. *J Clin Lipidol* 2014;**8**:473–88.
151. Abifadel M, Elbitar S, El Khoury P, et al. Living the pcsk9 adventure: from the identification of a new gene in familial hypercholesterolemia towards a potential new class of anticholesterol drugs. *Curr Atheroscler Rep* 2014;**16**.
195. Myers GL, Kimberly MM, Waymack PP, et al. A reference method laboratory network for cholesterol: a model for

standardization and improvement of clinical laboratory measurements. *Clin Chem* 2000;**46**:1762–72.

201. Ridker PM, Cannon CP, Morrow D, et al. C-reactive protein levels and outcomes after statin therapy. *NEJM* 2005;**352**:20–8.
288. Marcovina SM, Gaur VP, Albers JJ. Biological variability of cholesterol, triglyceride, low- and high-density lipoprotein cholesterol, lipoprotein(a), and apolipoproteins a-i and b. *Clin Chem* 1994;**40**:574–8.
300. Marcovina SM. Report of the National Heart, Lung, and Blood Institute workshop on lipoprotein(a) and cardiovascular disease: recent advances and future directions. *Clin Chem* 2003;**49**:1785–96.
312. Ridker PM, Rifai N, Rose L, et al. Comparison of c-reactive protein and low-density lipoprotein cholesterol levels in the prediction of first cardiovascular events. *NEJM* 2002;**347**: 1557–65.
316. Myers GL, Christenson RHM, Cushman M, et al. National Academy of Clinical Biochemistry laboratory medicine practice guidelines: emerging biomarkers for primary prevention of cardiovascular disease. *Clin Chem* 2008;**55**: 378–84.

35

Electrolytes and Blood Gases

Emily I. Schindler, Sarah M. Brown, and Mitchell G. Scott

ABSTRACT

Background
Electrolyte balance within the human body is essential for maintenance of health. Dysregulation of electrolytes affects water homeostasis and acid-base status, and often results in overt clinical signs and symptoms. The laboratory is tasked with aiding the clinician by providing accurate, timely results to narrow or confirm a diagnosis. In challenging cases in which the clinical context is lacking or conflicting, it is even more important for the laboratory to provide reliable data.

Content
This chapter compares methods and describes their advantages, disadvantages, and pitfalls in the analysis of electrolytes (including detailed discussions on sodium [Na], potassium [K], chloride [Cl], and bicarbonate [HCO_3^-]) and blood gases. Sweat Cl testing, which plays a central role in the diagnosis of cystic fibrosis (CF) and is known to be technically challenging, is also discussed.

Maintenance of water homeostasis is paramount to life for all organisms. In humans, the maintenance of water homeostasis in various body fluid compartments is primarily a function of the four major electrolytes, Na^+, K^+, Cl^-, and HCO_3^-. These electrolytes also have a role in acid-base balance and heart and muscle function, and serve as cofactors for enzymes. Abnormal electrolyte concentrations may be the cause or the consequence of a variety of medical disorders. Because of their physiologic and clinical inter-relationships, this chapter discusses determination of (1) electrolytes, (2) osmolality, (3) sweat testing, (4) blood gases and pH, and (5) oxygen hemodynamics.

ELECTROLYTES

Electrolytes may be classified as *anions,* which are negatively charged ions that move toward an anode, or *cations,* which are positively charged ions that move toward a cathode. Important physiologic electrolytes include Na^+, K^+, calcium (Ca^{2+}), magnesium (Mg^{2+}), Cl^-, HCO_3^-, phosphates ($H_2PO_4^-$, HPO_4^{2-}), and sulfate (SO_4^{2-}), and some organic anions, such as lactate. Although amino acids and proteins in solution also carry an electrical charge, they are usually considered separately from electrolytes. Proteins in serum are usually anions, and albumin accounts for most of the difference between the commonly measured cations (Na^+, K^+) and anions (Cl^-, HCO_3^-), which is also known as the anion gap. Hydrogen ion (H^+) concentration is routinely measured as pH, but its concentration is so low relative to other ions (10^{-9} vs. 10^{-3} mol/L) that its role as an electrolyte is negligible for clinical purposes. The major electrolytes (Na^+, K^+, Cl^-, HCO_3^-) occur primarily as free ions, whereas significant amounts (>40%) of Ca^{2+}, Mg^{2+}, and trace elements are bound by proteins, mainly albumin. Determination of body fluid concentrations of the four major electrolytes (Na^+, K^+, Cl^-, and HCO_3^-) is commonly referred to as an electrolyte profile.

Specimens for Electrolyte Determination

Serum and plasma are the usual specimens analyzed for electrolytes. Capillary blood, collected in microsample tubes or capillary tubes, or applied directly from a fingerstick to some point-of-care devices, is another common sample. Arterial or venous heparinized whole blood specimens obtained for blood gas and pH determinations may also be used with direct ion-selective electrodes (ISEs). Differences in values between serum and plasma and between arterial and venous samples have been documented (for details see Chapter 5), but the difference between serum and plasma K^+ is considered clinically the most significant. Heparin, either lithium (Li^+) or ammonium salt, is required if plasma or whole blood is assayed. Use of plasma or whole blood has the advantage of shortening the turnaround time, because it is not necessary to wait for the blood to clot. Furthermore, plasma or whole blood provides a distinct advantage in determining K^+ concentrations, which are invariably higher in serum depending on platelet count.[1,2] Grossly lipemic blood can be a source of analytical error (see the section on Electrolyte Exclusion Effect), with some methods requiring ultracentrifugation of lipemic serum or plasma before analysis. Hemolysis of red blood cells will cause erroneously high K^+ results; this problem is usually undetected when whole blood is analyzed. In addition, unhemolyzed specimens that are not promptly processed may have increased K^+ concentrations because of K^+ leakage from red blood cells when whole blood is stored at 4°C.

Urine collection for Na^+, K^+, or Cl^- assays should be done without the addition of preservatives. Body fluid aspirates, feces, or gastrointestinal (GI) fluid samples may also be submitted for electrolyte analysis. (The reader is referred to Chapter 43 for an in depth discussion of body fluid analysis.)

Sodium

Sodium is the major cation of extracellular fluid. Because it represents approximately 90% of the approximately 154 mmol of inorganic cations per liter of plasma, Na^+ is responsible for almost one-half the osmotic strength of plasma. It therefore plays a central role in maintaining the normal distribution of water and the osmotic pressure in the extracellular fluid compartment (ECF). The daily diet of the adult male in the United States contains 3 to 6 g (90–250 mmol) of Na^+ (7–14 g of NaCl), which is nearly completely absorbed from the GI tract.[3] The body requires only 1 to 2 mmol/day, and the excess is excreted by the kidneys, which are the ultimate regulators of the amount of Na^+ (and thus water) in the body.

Sodium is freely filtered by the kidney glomeruli. Seventy percent to 80% of the filtered Na^+ load is then actively reabsorbed into the proximal tubules, with Cl^- and water passively following in an iso-osmotic and electrically neutral manner. Another 20% to 25% is reabsorbed in the loop of Henle, along with Cl^- and more water. In the distal tubules, interaction of the adrenal hormone aldosterone with the coupled Na^+-K^+ and Na^+-H^+ exchange systems results directly in the reabsorption of Na^+, and indirectly of Cl^-, from the remaining 5% to 10% of the filtered load. It is the regulation of this latter fraction of filtered Na^+ that primarily determines the amount of Na^+ excreted in the urine. These processes are discussed in detail in Chapter 60.

Specimens

Serum, plasma, and urine may be stored at 4°C or may be frozen. Erythrocytes contain only one-tenth of the Na^+ present in plasma, so hemolysis does not cause significant errors in serum or plasma Na^+ values. Lipemic samples should be ultracentrifuged and the infranatant analyzed unless a direct ISE is used (see the section on Electrolyte Exclusion Effect).

Fecal and GI fluid specimens require preparation before assay. Because significant electrolyte loss in feces only occurs when stools are liquid, only liquid stool samples may be justified for analysis. Immediately after collection, liquid stool specimens should be clarified of particulate matter by filtration through gauze or filter paper and by centrifugation. If not analyzed immediately, fecal and GI fluids should be stored frozen to prevent microbial growth.

Determination of Sodium in Body Fluids

Sodium may be determined by (1) atomic absorption spectrophotometry (AAS), (2) flame emission spectrophotometry (FES), (3) electrochemically with an Na^+ ISE, or (4) spectrophotometrically. FES, now very rarely performed, was the original method of Na^+ determination. ISE methods are by far the most common used today. Excellent trueness and imprecision with coefficients of variation of less than 1.5% are readily achieved with modern equipment. Because Na^+ and K^+ are routinely assayed together, methods for their analysis are described together later in this chapter.

Reference Intervals

A typical reference interval for serum Na^+ is 136 to 145 mmol/L.[4,5] The central 95% of Na values from more than 16,000 subjects in the National Health and Nutrition Examination Survey III (NHANES III) was 136 to 146 mmol/L.[6] The interval for premature newborns at 48 hours is 128 to 148 mmol/L, and the value for umbilical cord blood from full-term newborns is approximately 127 mmol/L (see Appendix on Reference Intervals for additional newborn ranges). Laboratories should verify that these ranges are appropriate for use. Further guidance is provided in Chapter 8.

Urinary Na excretion varies with diet, but for an adult male consuming 7 to 14 g of NaCl per day, an interval of 120 to 240 mmol/day is typical.[3] A large diurnal variation in Na^+ excretion has been noted, with the rate of Na^+ excretion during the night being only 20% of the peak rate during the day. The Na^+ concentration of cerebrospinal fluid is 136 to 150 mmol/L.[7] Mean fecal Na^+ excretion is less than 10 mmol/day.[8]

Potassium

Potassium is the major intracellular cation. In tissue cells, its average concentration is approximately 150 mmol/L, and in erythrocytes, the concentration is approximately 105 mmol/L. High intracellular concentrations are maintained by the Na^+, K^+ adenosine triphosphate (ATP)ase pump, which continually transports K^+ into the cell against a concentration gradient. Diffusion of K^+ out of the cell into the ECF and plasma occurs whenever pump activity is decreased because of (1) depletion of metabolic substrates such as glucose, (2) competition for ATP between the pump and other energy-consuming activities of the cell, or (3) slowing of cellular metabolism (as occurs with refrigeration). The importance of these considerations for sample integrity for analysis of K^+ is discussed later.

The body requirement for K^+ is satisfied by an average dietary intake of 2.4 to 4.4 g/day (60–120 mmol/day). K^+ absorbed from the GI tract is rapidly distributed, with a small amount taken up by cells, and most excreted by the kidneys. K^+ filtered through the glomeruli is almost completely reabsorbed in the proximal tubules and is then secreted into the distal tubules in exchange for Na^+ under the influence of aldosterone. Aldosterone enhances K^+ secretion and Na^+ reabsorption in the distal tubules by a Na^+-K^+ exchange mechanism. The kidneys respond to K^+ loading with an increase in K^+ output, so that urine collected during or after a period of high K^+ intake may have K^+ concentrations as high as 100 mmol/L. In contrast, the tubular response to conserve K^+ is slow in the initial stages of depletion. Unlike the prompt response to conserve Na^+ in deficit states, it can take up to 1 week for the tubules to reduce K^+ excretion to 5 to 10 mmol/day from the typical 50 to 100 mmol/day.

Factors that regulate distal tubular secretion of K^+ include intake of Na^+ and K^+, mineralocorticoid concentration, and acid-base balance. Because renal conservation mechanisms are slow to respond, K^+ depletion can be an early consequence of restricted K^+ intake or loss of K^+ by extrarenal routes (eg, diarrhea). A diminished glomerular filtration rate is typical of renal failure, and the consequent decrease in distal tubular flow rate is an important factor in the retention of K^+ associated with chronic renal failure.

Specimens

Comments made earlier on specimens for Na^+ analysis are generally applicable to those for K^+ analysis, with some caveats. K^+ concentrations in plasma and whole blood are 0.1 to 0.7 mmol/L lower than those in serum, and most reference intervals for serum K^+ are 0.2 to 0.4 mmol/L higher than those for plasma K^+. The extent of this difference depends on the platelet count, because additional K^+ in serum is primarily a result of platelet rupture during clotting.[1,2] This variability in the amount of additional K^+ in serum makes plasma the specimen of choice.

Specimens for determining K^+ concentrations in serum or plasma must be collected by methods that minimize hemolysis, because release of K^+ from as few as 0.5% of erythrocytes can increase K^+ values by 0.5 mmol/L. An increase in K^+ of 0.6% has been estimated for every 10 mg/dL of plasma hemoglobin (Hb) caused by hemolysis.[9] Thus, slight hemolysis (Hb ≈ 50 mg/dL) can be expected to raise K^+ values by approximately 3%, marked hemolysis (Hb ≈ 200 mg/dL) by 12%, and gross hemolysis (Hb >500 mg/dL) by as much as 30%. Use of correction factors based on a hemolysis index have been suggested for estimating K^+ in hemolyzed samples,[10] but their use has been questioned.[11] Regardless, it is imperative that any visible hemolysis be noted when reporting K^+ values with a comment that results are falsely elevated whether an estimate of the extent of elevation is provided[10] or not.[11] If K^+ concentrations are determined by ISE on whole blood specimens using a blood gas instrument or a point-of-care device, increases in K^+ concentrations caused by hemolysis will often be overlooked. When hemolysis is suspected, a portion of the specimen should be centrifuged and visually inspected.

Clinically significant preanalytical errors can occur for K^+ determinations if blood samples are not processed expediently. As mentioned earlier, maintenance of the intracellular–extracellular K^+ gradient depends on the activity of the energy-dependent Na^+-K^+-ATPase. If a whole blood specimen is maintained at 4°C versus 25°C before separation, glycolysis is inhibited, and the energy-dependent Na^+-K^+-ATPase cannot maintain the Na^+/K^+ gradient. An increase in plasma K^+ will occur as a result of K^+ leakage from erythrocytes and other cells. The increase of K^+ in serum is on the order of 0.2 mmol/L by 1.5 hours at 25°C, and, in contrast, is as high as 2 mmol/L after 4 hours at 4°C.[12]

A falsely decreased K^+ value can be observed if an unseparated sample is stored at 37°C, because glycolysis occurs and K^+ shifts intracellularly. Even at room temperature, extreme leukocytosis can initially cause falsely decreased K^+ concentrations. The extent of this decrease depends on leukocyte count, temperature, and glucose concentrations, but it has been reported to be as much as 0.7 mmol/L at 37°C.[13] In addition to causing pseudohypokalemia, samples from leukemic patients with very high white blood cell (WBC) counts (>300 × 10^9 cells/L) can result in a pseudohyperkalemia due to WBC rupture.[14] Taken together, the recommendation for reliable K^+ determinations is to collect blood with heparin and to maintain it near 25°C, then to separate the plasma within minutes by high-speed centrifugation. In practical terms, separation within 1 hour when samples are maintained at room temperature is unlikely to introduce great error.

Finally, skeletal muscle activity causes K^+ efflux from muscle cells into plasma and can cause a marked elevation in plasma K^+ values. A common example occurs when an upper arm tourniquet is not released before beginning to draw blood after a patient clenches his or her fist repeatedly. The plasma K^+ values can artificially increase as much as 2 mmol/L because of the muscle activity.[15]

Reference Intervals

Reported reference intervals for the serum of adults vary from 3.5 to 5.1 mmol/L and from 3.7 to 5.9 for newborns.[4] For plasma, a frequently cited interval is 3.3 to 4.9 mmol/L for adults (for more information refer to the Appendix on Reference Intervals). The central 95% of plasma K^+ values from more than 16,000 subjects in the NHANES III were from 3.4 to 4.7 mmol/L.[6] Laboratories should verify that these ranges are appropriate for use in their own settings. Further guidance is provided in Chapter 8.

Cerebrospinal fluid concentrations are approximately 70% those of plasma.[7] Urinary excretion of K^+ varies with dietary intake, but a typical observed range is 42 to 86 mmol/day for males and 33 to 70 mmol/day for females.[3] In severe diarrhea, GI loss may be as much as 60 mmol/day.[8]

POINTS TO REMEMBER

Potassium

- K^+ is susceptible to several causes of preanalytical error.
- Improper phlebotomy techniques can cause falsely elevated K^+ values.
- Storing whole blood at 4°C will cause falsely elevated K^+ values.
- Ex vivo hemolysis will cause falsely elevated K^+ values.
- Different K^+ reference intervals should be used for plasma and serum.

Methods for the Determination of Sodium and Potassium

Although AAS, FES, or spectrophotometric methods have been used for Na^+ and K^+ analyses in the past, most laboratories now use ISE methods. For example, in 2015, of the laboratories reporting proficiency data for Na^+ and K^+ to the College of American Pathologists (CAP), more than 99% were using ISE methods.[16]

Flame Emission Spectrophotometry. Although at one time it was the most common method for Na^+ and K^+ analyses, FES is no longer a common laboratory method. Samples are diluted in a diluent containing known amounts of Li^+ and are aspirated into a propane air flame. Na^+, K^+, and Li^+ ions, when excited, emit spectra at specific unique wavelengths. The Li^+ emission signal is used as an internal standard against which the Na^+ and K^+ signals are compared. Limitations of this method are detailed in Chapter 14.

Ion-Selective Electrodes. Analyzers fitted with ISEs usually contain Na^+ electrodes with glass membranes and K^+ electrodes with liquid ion exchange membranes that incorporate valinomycin. Potentiometry is the determination of change in electromotive force (E; potential) in a circuit between a measurement electrode (the ISE) and a reference electrode because the selected ion interacts with the membrane of the ISE. In instrument applications, the measuring system is calibrated by the introduction of calibrator solutions containing defined amounts of Na^+ and K^+. The potentials of the calibrators are determined, and the $\Delta E/\Delta$ log concentration responses are stored in the microprocessor memory for calculating unknown concentration when E of the unknown is measured. The response of potentiometric electrodes to analytes is a complex process that depends on the composition and thermodynamic and kinetic properties of the sensor membrane, bathing solution, and interface zone between the membrane and the analyte and between the membrane and the bathing solution.[17] For simplicity, E is described as the sum of the boundary potential *(EPB1)* at the sample/ion-sensitive film boundary and *EPB2* at the membrane/internal contact boundary, and by the diffusion potential *(ED)* inside the membrane itself. A constant, *C*, is added to account for potential at the internal sensor and/or contact interface.[17]

Frequent calibration, initiated by the user or by microprocessor-controlled uptake of the calibrator, is typical of most current ISE systems. Some instruments are designed to measure Na^+ and K^+ in whole blood, particularly point-of-care testing (POCT) devices and blood gas analyzers.

Two types of ISE methods are in use and must be distinguished (refer also to Chapter 14 for detail). With indirect ISE methods, the sample is introduced into the measurement chamber after mixing with a large volume of diluent. Indirect ISEs are the most commonly used methods on current automated high-throughput clinical chemistry systems.[16] Indirect methods were developed early in the history of ISE technology, when dilution was necessary to present a small sample in a volume large enough to adequately cover a large electrode and to minimize the concentration of protein at the electrode surface. With direct ISE methods, the sample is presented to the electrodes without dilution. This approach became possible with the miniaturization of electrodes. Direct ISEs are used in blood gas analyzers and point-of-care devices where whole blood is directly presented to the electrodes.

Errors observed in the use of ISEs fall into three categories. First are errors caused by lack of selectivity. For instance, many Cl^- electrodes lack selectivity against other halide ions.[18] Second are errors introduced by repeated protein coating of the ion-sensitive membranes, or by contamination of the membrane or salt bridge by ions that compete or react with the selected ion and thus alter the electrode response. Such errors in ISE measurements necessitate periodic changes of the membrane as part of routine maintenance. Finally, the electrolyte exclusion effect, which applies only to indirect methods and is caused by the solvent-displacing effect of lipid and protein in the sample, results in falsely decreased values.[19] Chapter 14 explains the differences and pitfalls of indirect versus direct ISEs in more detail.

Spectrophotometric Methods. Spectrophotometric methods are based on Na^+- or K^+-specific enzyme activation. However, the cost of reagents for these methods and the fact that few problems exist with ISE methods have resulted in "niche" use of these methods, primarily with smaller instruments used in physicians' offices, and more recently "isolation" laboratories for patients with emerging infectious diseases.[20]

Kinetic spectrophotometric assays for Na^+ are based on activation of the enzyme β-galactosidase by Na^+ to hydrolyze *o*-nitrophenyl-β-D-galactopyranoside.[21] The rate of production of *o*-nitrophenol (the chromophore) is measured at 420 nm.

$$o\text{-Nitrophenyl-}\beta\text{-D-galactopyranoside} \xrightarrow[\beta\text{-Galactosidase}]{Na^{\oplus}} \text{Galactose} + o\text{-Nitrophenol } (\lambda_{max} = 420\text{ nm})$$

K^+-specific enzyme activation assays are illustrated by methods using pyruvate kinase, which is one of several K^+-enhanced enzymes that ultimately leads to increased nicotinamide adenine dinucleotide via lactate hydrogenase.[22]

Electrolyte Exclusion Effect

The electrolyte exclusion effect describes the exclusion of electrolytes from the fraction of the total plasma volume that is occupied by solids.[19] The volume of total solids (primarily protein and lipid) in an aliquot of plasma is approximately 7%, so that approximately 93% of plasma volume is actually water. The main electrolytes (Na^+, K^+, Cl^-, HCO_3^-) are confined to the water phase. When a fixed volume of total plasma (eg, 10 µL) is pipetted for dilution before flame photometry or indirect ISE analysis, only 9.3 µL of plasma water that contains the electrolytes is added to the diluent. Thus a concentration of Na^+ determined by flame photometry or indirect ISE to be 140 mmol/L is the concentration in the total plasma volume, *not* in the plasma water volume. If the plasma contains 93% water, the concentration of Na^+ in plasma water is $[140 \times (100/93)]$, or 150 mmol/L. This negative "error" in plasma electrolyte analysis has been recognized for many years.[19] Although it is the electrolyte concentration in plasma water that is physiologic (the Na^+ concentration of normal saline is 150 mmol/L), it was assumed that the volume fraction of water in plasma was sufficiently constant that this difference could be ignored. All electrolyte reference intervals are based on this assumption and actually reflect concentrations in total plasma volume and not in water volume. Virtually all concentrations measured in the clinical chemistry laboratory are related to the total sample volume rather than to the water volume. This electrolyte exclusion effect becomes problematic when pathophysiologic conditions are present that alter the plasma water volume, such as hyperlipidemia or hyperproteinemia. In these settings, falsely low electrolyte values are obtained whenever samples are diluted before analysis, as in flame photometry or with indirect ISE methods[19] (Fig. 35.1).

Indirect ISE methods dilute the sample in a diluent of fixed high ionic strength so that for Na^+, the activity coefficient approaches a value of 1. Under these circumstances, the measurement of activity (a), where $a = \gamma$ (concentration) and γ is the activity coefficient, is tantamount to the measurement of concentration. It is the dilution of total plasma volume and the assumption that plasma water volume is constant that render both indirect ISE and flame photometry methods equally subject to the electrolyte exclusion effect. In certain settings, such as ketoacidosis with severe hyperlipidemia[23] or multiple myeloma with severe hyperproteinemia,[24] the negative exclusion effect may be so large that laboratory results lead clinicians to believe that electrolyte concentrations are normal or low when the concentration in the water phase may actually be high or normal, respectively. In severe

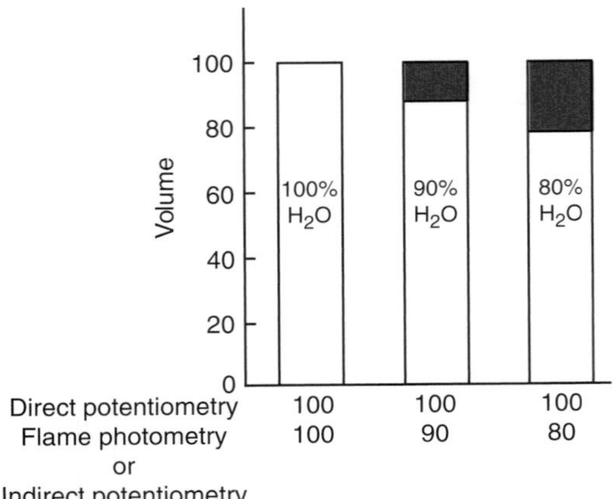

FIGURE 35.1 Predicted influence of water (H_2O) content on sodium measurements for a 100-mmol/L sodium chloride solution by direct ion-selective electrode versus flame emission photometry or indirect ion-selective electrode. *Red areas* represent nonaqueous volumes, which could consist of lipids, proteins, or even a slurry of latex or sand particles. (Modified from Apple FS, Koch DD, Graves S, Ladenson JH. Relationship between direct-potentiometric and flame-photometric measurement of sodium in blood. *Clin Chem* 1982;28:1931–5.)

hypoproteinemia, the effect works in reverse, resulting in falsely high (2% to 4%) Na^+ or K^+ values. Direct ISE methods still determine the concentration relative to activity but do not require sample dilution. Because there is no dilution, activity is directly proportional to the concentration in the water phase, not the concentration in the total volume. To make results from direct ISEs equivalent to those from flame photometry and indirect ISEs, most direct ISE methods actually operate in what is commonly referred to as the "flame mode." In this mode, the directly measured concentration in plasma water is multiplied by the average water volume fraction of plasma (0.93). Although the latter may vary widely, as long as the activity of the specific ion is constant, the concentration of the ion in the water phase becomes independent of the relative proportions of water and total solids if the ion is not bound by proteins. Therefore, direct ISE methods are free of electrolyte exclusion effects, and the values determined by direct ISE methods—even in the flame mode—are directly proportional to activity in the water phase and define electrolyte concentrations in a more physiological and physicochemical sense. For this reason, most clinical chemists and physicians have reached the conclusion that direct ISE methods for electrolyte analysis are the methods of choice. However, it is clear that results from direct methods will continue to be converted to total plasma volume concentrations using flame mode, which is good because more than 80% of laboratories use indirect ISE methods.[16]

POINTS TO REMEMBER

Electrolyte Exclusion Effect

- Lipemic samples and those with high lipid concentrations will have artificially low electrolyte values with indirect ISE methods.
- Hyperproteinemic samples will have artificially low electrolyte values with indirect ISE methods.
- Direct ISE methods are not subject to the electrolyte exclusion effect.

Chloride

Chloride is the major extracellular anion. Therefore, Cl^-, similar to Na^+, is significantly involved in the maintenance of water distribution, osmotic pressure, and anion–cation balance in the ECF. In contrast to its high ECF concentrations (≈103 mmol/L), the concentration of Cl^- in the intracellular fluid of erythrocytes is 45 to 54 mmol/L, and in the intracellular fluid of most other tissue cells, it is only approximately 1 mmol/L. In gastric and intestinal secretions, Cl^- is the most abundant anion.

Cl^- ions are almost completely absorbed from the intestinal tract. They are filtered from plasma at the glomeruli and are passively reabsorbed, along with Na^+, in the proximal tubules. In the thick ascending limb of the loop of Henle, Cl^- is actively reabsorbed by the Cl^- pump, which promotes passive reabsorption of Na^+. Loop diuretics such as furosemide and ethacrynic acid inhibit the Cl^- pump. Cl^- concentrations are not homeostatically controlled and passively reflect the concentration of the major ions, Na^+ and HCO_3^-, as well as falling when pathological concentrations of other anions (eg, ketoacids and lactate) are present.

Methods for Determination of Chloride in Body Fluids

Chloride is determined largely by ISE, with some laboratories performing coulometric-amperometric titration (see also Chapter 14) for analyses requiring a broad range, such as sweat Cl^- testing.

Specimens. Chloride most often is measured in serum or plasma, urine, and sweat. Cl^- is stable in serum and plasma. Hemolysis does not significantly alter serum or plasma Cl^- concentration because the erythrocyte concentration of Cl^- is approximately half of that in plasma. Because very little Cl^- is protein bound, change in posture, stasis, and the use of tourniquets have little effect on its plasma concentration. Measurement of Cl^- in gastric aspirates or intestinal drainages is an adjunct to parenteral replacement therapy. Fecal Cl^- determination may be useful for the diagnosis of congenital hypochloremic alkalosis with hyperchloridorrhea (increased excretion of Cl^- in stool).

Coulometric-Amperometric Titration. The general principles of coulometry and amperometry are described in Chapter 14. Reactions in coulometric-amperometric determinations of Cl^- depend on the generation of silver (Ag^+) from a Ag^+ electrode at a constant rate and on the reaction of Ag^+ with Cl^- in the sample to form insoluble AgCl[25]:

$$Ag^+ + Cl^- \rightarrow AgCl$$

After the stoichiometric point is reached, excess Ag^+ in the mixture triggers the shutdown of the Ag^+ generation system. A timing device records elapsed time between the start and stop of Ag^+ generation. Because the time interval is proportional to the amount of Cl^- in the sample, the concentration of Cl^- can be calculated using Faraday's law:

$$Q = it = nFN$$

where Q is the charge passed for time t at the constant current i; n is the number of electrons involved in the electrochemical reaction; F is Faraday's constant (96,485 coulombs/mol); and N is the number of moles of analyte in the sample.[26]

Applications of the coulometric-amperometric principle (often called the Cotlove chloridometer technique)[25] are the most precise methods for measuring Cl^- over the entire range of concentrations found in body fluids. This method is subject to interferences by other halide ions, by cyanate (CN^-) and thicyanate (SCN^-) ions, by sulfhydryl groups, and by heavy metal contamination. Maintenance of the systems is crucial for proper operation. Today, none of 5135 laboratories report Cl^- results by using coulometry,[16] but some laboratories maintain these instruments for sweat analysis (see later section in this chapter).

Ion-Selective Electrode Methods. Solvent polymeric membranes that incorporate quaternary ammonium salt anion exchangers, such as tri-*n*-octylpro-pylammonium Cl^- decanol, are used to construct Cl^--selective electrodes in clinical analyzers. Although they are by far the most common methods for measuring Cl^- in clinical laboratories, these electrodes have been described as having membrane instability and lot-to-lot inconsistency in terms of selectivity to other anions.[18] Anions that tend to be problematic include other halides and organic anions, such as SCN^-, which can be particularly problematic because of their ability to solubilize in the polymeric organic membrane of these electrodes.

More than 99% of 5135 laboratories reporting in a 2015 CAP proficiency test survey for Cl^- used indirect ISE methods.[16]

Reference Intervals

Reported reference intervals[4] for Cl^- in the serum or plasma vary from 98 to 107 mmol/L to 100 to 108 mmol/L.[4,5] The central 95% of Cl^- values from more than 16,000 subjects in NHANES III was 98 to 111 mmol/L.[6] For more data in various age groups, refer to the Appendix on Reference Intervals. Laboratories should verify that these ranges are appropriate for use in their own settings. Further guidance is provided in Chapter 8.

Serum values vary little during the day. Spinal fluid Cl^- concentrations are approximately 15% higher than those in serum.[7] Urinary excretion of Cl^- varies with dietary intake, but an interval of 110 to 250 mmol/day is typical. Fecal excretion of Cl^- (for eight healthy subjects) has been reported as 3.2 ± 0.7 mmol/day (SEM).[8]

Bicarbonate (Total Carbon Dioxide)

Total carbon dioxide (CO_2) is used here to describe the quantity that is measured most often in automated clinical chemistry analyzers by acidification of a serum or plasma sample, and measurement of CO_2 released by the process, or by alkalinization and measurement of total HCO_3^-. Under certain conditions of collection and specimen handling, total CO_2 values determined in this manner will be almost identical to values for the calculated concentration of total CO_2 obtained in blood gas analysis (see later section in this chapter on Application of the Henderson-Hasselbalch equation).

Specimens

The same sample types used for Na^+ or K^+ may be assayed. Given a specimen in a vacuum-draw tube, the concentration of total CO_2 is most accurately determined when the assay is done as promptly as possible after collection and centrifugation of the blood occurs in a fully filled unopened tube. Ambient air contains far less CO_2 than does plasma, and gaseous dissolved CO_2 will escape from the specimen into the air, with a consequent decrease in the CO_2 value of up to 2 to 3 mmol/L in the course of 1 hour. In practical terms, the logistics of high-volume processing and automated analysis of specimens almost ensures that most CO_2 measurements are done on specimens that have lost some dissolved gaseous CO_2, simply because preservation of anaerobic conditions is not practical between the time plasma is placed on an instrument and the time it is sampled. Thus, the term bicarbonate may be preferable to total CO_2.

Methods for Determination of Serum or Plasma Total Carbon Dioxide

One of the earliest methods for determining total CO_2 was the manometric method for total CO_2 content, using the Natelson microgasometer,[27] but it has been supplanted in clinical laboratories by automated methods.

The first step in automated methods is acidification or alkalinization of the sample. Acidifying the sample converts the various forms of CO_2 in plasma to gaseous CO_2 by dilution with an acid buffer. Alkalinizing the sample converts all CO_2 and carbonic acid to HCO_3^-. Methods for total CO_2 measurement with today's automated instruments may be electrode-based or enzymatic. In indirect electrode-based methods, the amount of released gaseous CO_2 after acidification is determined by a partial pressure of CO_2 (PCO_2) electrode in the reaction chamber of the CO_2 module. Approximately 16% of laboratories reporting CAP data used an indirect ISE method in 2015, with the remainder using enzymatic methods.[16] Direct ISE methods for total CO_2 are no longer common on automated analyzers due to problems with specificity.[28]

In enzymatic methods for CO_2, the specimen is first alkalinized to convert all CO_2 and carbonic acid to HCO_3^-. The enzymatic reactions are as follows:

$$\text{Phosphoenolpyruvate} + HCO_3^- \xrightarrow{\text{Phosphoenolpyruvate carboxylase}} \text{Oxaloacetate} + P_i$$

$$\text{Oxaloacetate} + \text{NADH} + H^+ \xrightarrow{\text{Malate dehydrogenase}} \text{Malate} + \text{NAD}^+$$

Decreased absorbance of nicotinamide adenine dinucleotide hydride at 340 nm is proportional to the total CO_2 content.

Reference Intervals

The reference interval for total CO_2 in adults is 22 to 28 mmol/L but can be instrument dependent.[4,5] For more information, refer to the Appendix on Reference Intervals. The central 95% of CO_2 values from more than 16,000 subjects in NHANES III was 21 to 35 mmol/L.[6] Laboratories should verify that these ranges are appropriate for use in their own settings. Further guidance is provided in Chapter 8.

Reference intervals are influenced by physiological changes throughout life.[29] Through childhood, from the age of 6 to 12 months to 18 years of age, there is a steady increase in serum HCO_3^- (by 5–7 mmol/L), which is attributed to the fall in respiratory rate and subsequent increase in PCO_2. In tandem with this gradual increase in HCO_3^-, a modest increase in serum Na^+ (2–3 mmol/L) and decrease in serum Cl^- (2–3 mmol/L) are observed. In pregnancy, HCO_3^- levels are decreased by 2 to 3 mmol/L (due to progesterone, which is known to increase respiratory activity in pregnancy).[29]

Principles of Osmotic Pressure and Osmosis

Osmometry is a technique for measuring the concentration of solute particles that contribute to the osmotic pressure of a solution. Osmotic pressure governs the movement of solvent (water in biological systems) across membranes that separate two solutions. Different membranes vary in pore size and thus in their ability to select molecules of different size and shape. Examples of biologically important selective membranes are those enclosing the glomeruli and capillary vessels that are permeable to water and to essentially all small molecules and ions, but not to large protein molecules. Differences in the concentrations of osmotically active molecules that cannot cross a membrane cause those molecules that can cross the membrane to move to establish an osmotic equilibrium. This movement of solute and permeable ions exerts what is known as osmotic pressure.

As an example, consider an aqueous solution of sucrose placed within a sac made up of a membrane permeable only to water, with an open vertical glass tube (a crude manometer) attached to the sac. If the sac is placed into a beaker of distilled water, water will move from the beaker across the membrane into the sucrose solution. The pressure of this solvent movement will cause the sucrose solution to rise up the tube. At equilibrium, the gravitational pressure of the column of solution in the tube equals the osmotic pressure and prevents further net movement of water from the beaker. The height of the rise of the sucrose solution in the manometer tube is a measure of the osmotic pressure of the sucrose solution. This is the pressure that would have to be exerted on the sucrose side of the membrane to prevent the flow of water across the membrane.

Osmosis is the process that constitutes the movement of solvent across a membrane in response to differences in osmotic pressure across the two sides of the membrane. Water migrates across the membrane toward the side containing more concentrated solute.

If the sucrose solution in the aforementioned membrane sac were replaced with a NaCl solution of the same molarity, the solution in the manometer would reach equilibrium at a point almost twice as high as that observed with sucrose, because NaCl dissociates into two ions per molecule. If ion activity is unrestricted, the NaCl solution would have twice as many osmotically active particles (osmoles) for the same molar concentration as the sucrose solution. In reality, the number of active particles is less than this (≈0.93 for NaCl), as explained later in this chapter. The total number of individual (solute) particles present in a solution per given mass of solvent, regardless of their molecular nature (ie, nonelectrolyte, ion, or colloid), determines the total osmotic pressure of the solution. In blood plasma, for example, nonelectrolytes such as glucose and urea, and to a much lesser extent, proteins, contribute to the osmotic pressure.

Colligative Properties

In addition to increasing osmotic pressure when the solute is added to the solvent, the vapor pressure of the solution is lowered below that of the pure solvent. As a result of the change in vapor pressure, the boiling point of the solution is raised above and the freezing point of the solution is lowered below that of the pure solvent.

These four properties of solutions—(1) increased osmotic pressure, (2) lowered vapor pressure, (3) increased boiling point, and (4) decreased freezing point—are called *colligative properties.* All are directly related to the total number of solute particles per mass of solvent. For instance, a 1-molal solution in water boils at a temperature 0.52°C higher and freezes at a temperature 1.858°C lower than pure water. The vapor pressure of this solution is 0.3 mm Hg lower than the vapor pressure of pure water , which is 23.8 mm Hg at 25°C. The osmotic pressure of the same solution is increased from zero to 17,000 mm Hg (22.4 atmospheres). The term *osmolality* expresses concentrations relative to mass of the solvent (1 osmolal solution is defined to contain 1 Osmol/kg H_2O), whereas the term *osmolarity* expresses concentrations per volume of solution (1 osmolar solution is defined to contain 1 Osmol/L solution). Osmolality (Osmol/kg H_2O) is a thermodynamically more exact expression because solution concentrations expressed on a weight basis are temperature independent, whereas those based on volume vary with temperature. Although the term osmolarity is often used in the medical literature, osmolality is what the clinical laboratory measures.

An electrolyte in solution dissociates into two (in the case of NaCl) or three (in the case of $CaCl_2$) particles; therefore, the colligative effects of such solutions are multiplied by the number of dissociated ions formed per molecule. However, because of incomplete electrolyte dissociation and associations between solute and solvent molecules, many solutions do not behave in the ideal case, and a 1-molal solution may give an osmotic pressure lower than theoretically expected. The osmotic activity coefficient is a factor used to correct for deviation from the "ideal" behavior of the system:

$$\text{Osmolality} = \text{osmol} / \text{kg H}_2\text{O} = \Phi nC$$

where Φ = osmotic coefficient; n = number of particles into which each molecule in the solution potentially dissociates; and C = molality in moles per kilogram of H_2O. A table of osmotic coefficients of most solutes of biological interest has been compiled.[30]

Glucose has an osmotic coefficient of 1.00, whereas the Φ for NaCl is 0.93 at the concentrations found in serum and the derivation of $1.86 \times Na^+$ (millimoles) in the formula to calculate plasma osmolality (NaCl potentially contributes two osmotically active particles times 0.93 = 1.86). Ethanol has an osmotic coefficient of 0.83. The total osmolality or osmotic pressure of a solution is equal to the sum of the osmotic pressures or osmolalities of all solute species present. The electrolytes Na^+, Cl^-, and HCO_3^-, which are present in relatively high concentrations, make the greatest contributions to serum osmolality. Nonelectrolytes such as glucose and urea, which are present normally at lower molal concentrations, contribute less, and serum proteins contribute less than 0.5% of the total serum osmolality because even the most abundant protein is present at millimolar concentrations.

Determination of Plasma and Urine Osmolality

Determination of plasma and urine osmolality can be useful in the assessment of electrolyte and acid-base disorders. Comparison of plasma and urine osmolalities can determine the status of water regulation by the kidneys in settings of severe electrolyte disturbances, which might occur in diabetes insipidus or the syndrome of inappropriate antidiuretic hormone. The reader is referred to Chapter 60 for further information on water balance.

The major osmotic substances in normal plasma are Na^+, Cl^-, glucose, and urea; therefore, expected plasma osmolality can be calculated from the following empirical equation:

$$\text{mOsmol / kg} = 1.86[\text{Na}^+(\text{mmol / L})] + \text{Glucose (mmol / L)} + \text{Urea (mmol / L)} + 9$$

or

$$\text{mOsmol / kg} = 1.86[\text{Na}^+(\text{mmol / L})] + \text{Glucose (mg / dL)} / 18 + \text{Urea (mg / dL)} / 2.8 + 9$$

The 9 mOsmol/kg added to the previous equation represents the contributions of other osmotically active substances in plasma, such as K^+, Ca^{2+}, and proteins, and 1.86 is two times the osmotic coefficient of Na^+, reflecting the contributions of both Na^+ and Cl^-. Some versions of this equation do not include the plus 9 mOsmol/kg factor.

$$\text{mOsmol / kg} = 2 \times \text{Na (mmol / L)} + \text{Glucose (mmol / L)} + \text{Urea (mmol / L)}$$

or

$$2 \times \text{Na (mmol / L)} + \text{Glucose (mg / dL)} / 18 + \text{Urea (mg / dL)} / 2.8$$

The reference interval for plasma osmolality is 275 to 300 mOsmol/kg.[4] Comparison of measured osmolality versus calculated osmolality can reveal the presence of an osmolal gap, which can be important in determining the presence of exogenous osmotic substances. Comparison of calculated and measured osmolalities can also confirm or rule out suspected pseudohyponatremia caused by the electrolyte exclusion effect. Most clinical laboratories use freezing point depression as a basis for the measurement of osmolality because of its simplicity and the fact that vapor pressure osmometers will not detect volatile substances such as methanol. Furthermore, freezing point depression, unlike vapor pressure, is independent of changes in ambient temperature.

Freezing Point Depression Osmometer. The instrument used is a freezing point depression osmometer, often referred to simply as an osmometer. The components of a freezing point depression osmometer (Fig. 35.2) are as follows:

1. A thermostatically controlled cooling bath or block maintained at −7°C.
2. A rapid stir mechanism to initiate (or "seed") freezing of the sample.

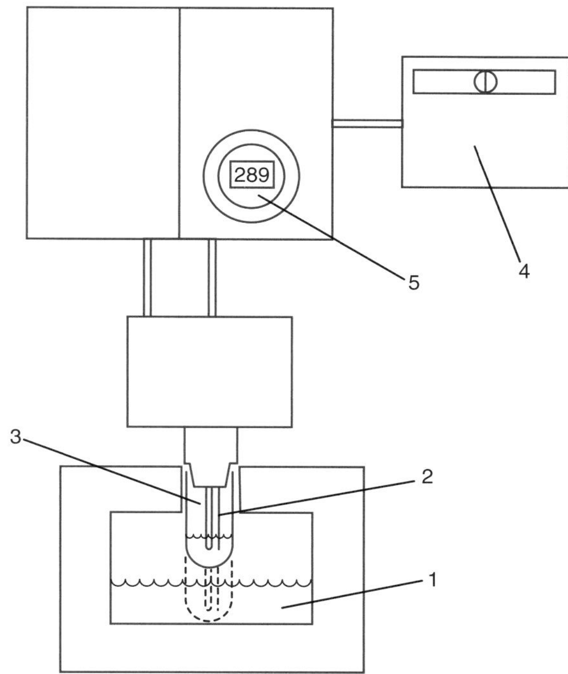

FIGURE 35.2 Block Diagram of a Freezing Point Depression Osmometer. The test tube is shown above the liquid in the cooling bath *(solid line)* and inside the cooling liquid *(dashed line)*. *1,* Cooling fluid; *2,* stirring rod; *3,* thermistor; *4,* galvanometer; *5,* potentiometer with direct readout.

3. A thermistor probe connected to a circuit to measure the temperature of the sample. (The thermistor is a glass bead attached to a metal stem whose resistance varies rapidly and predictably with temperature.)
4. A galvanometer that displays the freezing curve and that is used as a guide when the measuring potentiometer is used.
5. A measuring potentiometer.

In most instruments today, components 4 and 5 are replaced by a light-emitting diode (LED) display that indicates the time course of the freezing curve and the final result.

During analysis, the sample, in which the thermistor probe and the stirring wire are centered, is lowered into the bath, and with gentle stirring, is super cooled to a temperature several degrees below its freezing point (−7°C). When the LED display (or galvanometer) indicates that sufficient super cooling has occurred, the sample is raised to a point above the liquid in the cooling bath, and the wire stirrer is changed from a gentle rate of stir to a momentarily vigorous amplitude, which initiates freezing of the super cooled solution. This freezing occurs only to the slush stage, with approximately 2% to 3% of the solvent solidifying. The released heat of fusion initially warms the solution, and then the temperature plateaus and remains stationary, indicating the equilibrium temperature at which both freezing and thawing of the solution occur. At the end of the equilibrium temperature plateau, the galvanometer again indicates decreasing temperature as the sample freezes further toward a complete solid. An example of the calculation to obtain osmolality is as follows: if the observed freezing point is −0.53°C, then

$$\text{mosmol / kg H}_2\text{O} = \frac{-0.53}{-1.86} \times 1000 = 285$$

where −1.86°C = molal freezing point depression of pure H_2O.

Day-to-day imprecision of ±2 mOsmol/kg H_2O should be attainable by current osmometers. More than 99% of laboratories in the 2015 CAP surveys use freezing point depression osmometers.[16]

POINTS TO REMEMBER

Osmolality

- Osmolality reflects the total number of individual (solute) particles present in a solution per given mass of solvent, regardless of their molecular nature (ie, nonelectrolyte, ion, or colloid) and is independent of the molecular weight of the particle.
- An increased number of solute particles affects the colligative properties of a solution by increasing osmotic pressure.
- Lowering vapor pressure.
- Increasing the boiling point.
- Decreasing the freezing point.
- Only freezing point osmometers should be used clinically because they can detect volatile solutes (eg, ethanol and methanol).

SWEAT CHLORIDE

Analysis of Cl^- ion concentration in sweat is used to confirm the diagnosis of CF. CF is caused by dysfunction of the CF transmembrane conductance regulator (CFTR), a Cl^- channel in the ABC transporter superfamily. Functional abnormalities in CFTR result in impaired electrolyte transport in secretory and absorptive epithelia, including the reabsorptive duct of the sweat gland. This leads to high salt loss via the sweat gland in patients with CF. Electrolyte abnormalities in sweat were first described in 1953,[31,32] after many CF patients presented to the hospital with heat prostration following a heat wave in New York in 1948. The first clinical measurements of sweat Cl^- were from sweat collected after thermal induction of sweating. Patients were wrapped in plastic and placed in a room controlled at 90°F and 50% humidity for 30 to 90 minutes, and sweat was collected from filter paper placed on the patients' backs.[33] This practice was both cumbersome and dangerous. Gahm and Shwachman, who founded the thermal sweat collection procedure, proposed a screening method in which the patient's hand or foot was imprinted on an agar plate infused with K^+ chromate. If "considerable" Cl^- was present on the hand or foot, a white-yellow discoloration would appear.[34] In 1959, Gibson and Cooke introduced a method for localized sweating[35] that remains the basis of sweat analysis today (see the following).

In 1989, the *CFTR* gene was identified as the genetic basis of CF. Although more than 1900 mutations in the 168 kb gene are known today, most mutations are not associated with CF, and mutational analysis is often insufficient for diagnosis.[36,37] Quantitative analysis of Cl^- in sweat remains the gold standard for diagnosis of CF.[38]

Quantitative Analysis of Sweat Chloride

Instrumentation used for measuring Cl^- in sweat should be able to detect concentrations as low as 10 mmol/L on unadulterated sweat. ISEs are usually too imprecise at the low concentration typically found in normal subjects. Cl^- concentration in sweat is best determined by coulometric titration (see earlier section of this chapter).

Sweat Collection

Sweat collection is a two-step procedure involving (1) localized sweating produced by iontophoresis of the cholinergic drug pilocarpine nitrate into an area of the skin, and (2) collection of sweat from the stimulated area. Iontophoresis uses a small electric current to deliver pilocarpine into the sweat glands from the positive electrode, and an electrolyte solution at the negative electrode completes the circuit. There are two methods for pilocarpine iontophoresis and sweat collection, using filter paper or gauze, or using plastic microbore tubing. The filter paper/gauze method, sometimes referred to as the Gibson-Cooke method, is the original method. Iontophoresis is achieved with electrodes over reagent-soaked gauze, followed by collection of sweat from the collection site into clean gauze. Alternatively, electrodes attached to pilocarpine-containing agar disks can be used for stimulation and sweat collected into plastic capillary tubing, such as the Macroduct system.[39] The inner flexor surface of the forearm is the preferred site for sweat testing. Sweat stimulation can be performed on the inner thigh; however, this site yields lower sweat volume.[40]

Reference Intervals for Sweat Chloride

Reference intervals for Cl^- in sweat were established from more than 7200 sweat tests performed from 1959 to 1966.[41] Results from newborn screening initiatives led the Cystic Fibrosis Foundation (CFF) to recommend stratifying intervals by patient age; however, a 2011 study reported that only 30% of CFF centers follow this recommendation.[42]

Infants

For infants up to and including 6 months of age, the following diagnostic thresholds are recommended based on sweat Cl^- test results[43]:

- ≤29 mmol/L: CF unlikely
- 30 to 59 mmol/L: intermediate probability of CF
- ≥60 mmol/L: indicative of CF

Beyond Infancy

For individuals older than 6 months of age, the following diagnostic thresholds are recommended[43]:

- ≤39 mmol/L: CF unlikely
- 40 to 59 mmol/L: intermediate probability of CF
- ≥60 mmol/L: indicative of CF

The functional upper limit for sweat Cl^- is 160 mmol/L.[44] Sweat Cl^- concentrations greater than 160 mmol/L can represent specimen contamination or analytical error. A normal sweat Cl^- concentration alone is insufficient to rule out the diagnosis; it should be interpreted in light of the clinical picture and with the knowledge that "normal" concentrations have been associated with CF. Some mutations of the CF gene are associated with intermediate or normal sweat Cl^- concentrations.[38] For example, according to the CFF registry, 3.5% of CF patients had sweat Cl^- concentrations less than 60 mmol/L, and 1.2% had concentrations less than 40 mmol/L.[45] Clinical practice regarding follow-up of intermediate sweat Cl^- results varies widely. The CFF recommends a repeat sweat Cl^- test within 2 months of the intermediate result. Other laboratory tests include analysis of CFTR, fecal elastase evaluation, and pulmonary cultures.[42]

Reasons for Falsely Elevated Chloride in Sweat

The most common cause of falsely elevated sweat Cl^- is evaporation. The 2007 CFF guidelines[45] for sweat testing were established with the goal of reducing preanalytical variations in sweat testing. Testing procedures should minimize the opportunity for evaporation and contamination of the sweat sample. Sweat samples should be analyzed soon after collection on the same day. However, the laboratory can store the sweat samples if necessary. If sweat is collected into gauze, it should be reweighed promptly and can be stored with a tightly fitting lid up to 72 hours at 4°C.[43] If sweat is collected in microbore tubing coils, it should be transferred to a 0.2-mL microcentrifuge tube with a tight-fitting cap and stored for up to 72 hours. The sweat should not be stored or transported in the microbore tubing.[43] Other causes of falsely elevated sweat Cl^- include (Box 35.1) malnutrition, hypothyroidism, pan-hypopituitarism, glycogen storage disease, untreated adrenal insufficiency, atopic dermatitis, ectodermal dysplasia, familial cholestasis, familial hypoparathyroidism, vasopressin-resistant diabetes insipidus, and type I fucosidosis.[46] Edema, hypoproteinemia, and administration of mineralocorticoids can decrease sweat electrolytes.[47,48]

Critical Issues Associated With Sweat Collection

Sufficient Sample Collection

The CFF requires 75 mg or 15 μL of sweat, if collected by Gibson-Cooke or Macroduct, respectively.[45] This is based on a theoretical but unsubstantiated sweat rate. Recent studies have shown that there is no correlation between sweat weight and Cl^- concentration, and a specimen volume requirement should be based on analytical sensitivity and not specimen volume.[40,49] Regardless, CFF accredited centers must adhere to CFF guidelines for the number of "quantity not sufficient" (QNS) specimens. On average, the percentage of insufficient samples should not exceed 5% for patients older than 3 months of age and 10% for patients younger than 3 months of age. Insufficient sweat samples can be the result of several factors, such as age, race, and skin condition. Collecting an adequate amount of sweat can be more challenging in patients younger than 1 month of age.[50] For this reason, it is recommended that sweat testing in asymptomatic individuals be performed when the infant is at least 2 weeks of age, is more than 36 weeks' gestation at birth, and weighs more than 2 kg.[38] To increase the chances of an adequate sample volume, two sites can be stimulated at one patient encounter. If the laboratory collects sweat from two sites (bilateral testing),[51] the collection is considered QNS only when both sites are inadequate. The forearm is preferred over the inner thigh as a site for sweat stimulation in patients of all ages because this site produces more sweat after iontophoresis.[40]

BOX 35.1 Reported Diseases or Conditions Other Than Cystic Fibrosis Associated With an Elevated Sweat Electrolyte Concentration[43]

- Anorexia nervosa
- Atopic dermatitis
- Autonomic dysfunction
- Celiac disease
- Environmental deprivation
- Familial cholestasis
- Fucosidosis type 1
- Glycogen storage disease type 1
- Hypogammaglobulinemia
- Keratitis, ichthyosis, deafness *(KID)* syndrome
- Mauriac's syndrome (malnutrition of)
- Protein-calorie malnutrition
- Pseudohypoaldosteronism
- Psychosocial failure to thrive
- Systemic lupus erythematosus
- Trioesphosphate isomerase *(TPI)* deficiency
- Untreated adrenal insufficiency
- Untreated hypothyroidism

Quality of Sweat Collection and Analysis

Sweat collection is a manual process with many opportunities for error. Most errors result in QNS collections (QNS by CFF guidelines). Quality of sweat collection can be maintained by having a sufficient test volume to maintain competency, and limiting the testing personnel to a few number of well-trained individuals. All CFF accredited CF Centers in the United States are required to follow Clinical and Laboratory Standards Institute (CLSI)-C34-A2 guidelines for sweat collection and analysis.[43,45] Other evidence-based guidelines include the Guidelines for the Performance of the Sweat Test for the Investigation of Cystic Fibrosis.[52]

The Centers for Disease Control and Prevention does not list sweat as a potentially infectious material unless it is visibly contaminated with blood.[53] However, laboratory personnel should practice the same standard precautions they would use with any other body fluid. All equipment used in iontophoresis should be disinfected between patients in accordance with procedures consistent with the institution's infection control policies. Disinfectants must not contain bleach, which could contaminate the sweat sample.

Patient Education

Sweat testing is one of the few clinical chemistry tests involving direct patient contact. Patients and their parents often have questions about the sweat test that their physicians may not have answered. Also, it is important to have the patient physically prepared for the sweat collection. The patient should be physiologically and nutritionally stable, well hydrated, free of acute illness, and not receiving mineralocorticoids. The patient should avoid using lotions on the skin before sweat collection. Possible adverse events during sweat collection include redness and itching at the stimulation site. Pilocarpine urticaria associated with sweat testing is rare but has been reported. Burns to the patient's skin after iontophoresis are extremely rare but can occur.

Sweat Conductivity Screening

Sweat conductivity might be used as a screening test for CF. Compared with sweat Cl^- analysis, sweat conductivity is easier to perform and requires a smaller sample (minimum

BOX 35.2 Diagnostic Algorithm for Cystic Fibrosis (CF) After Newborn Screening[38]

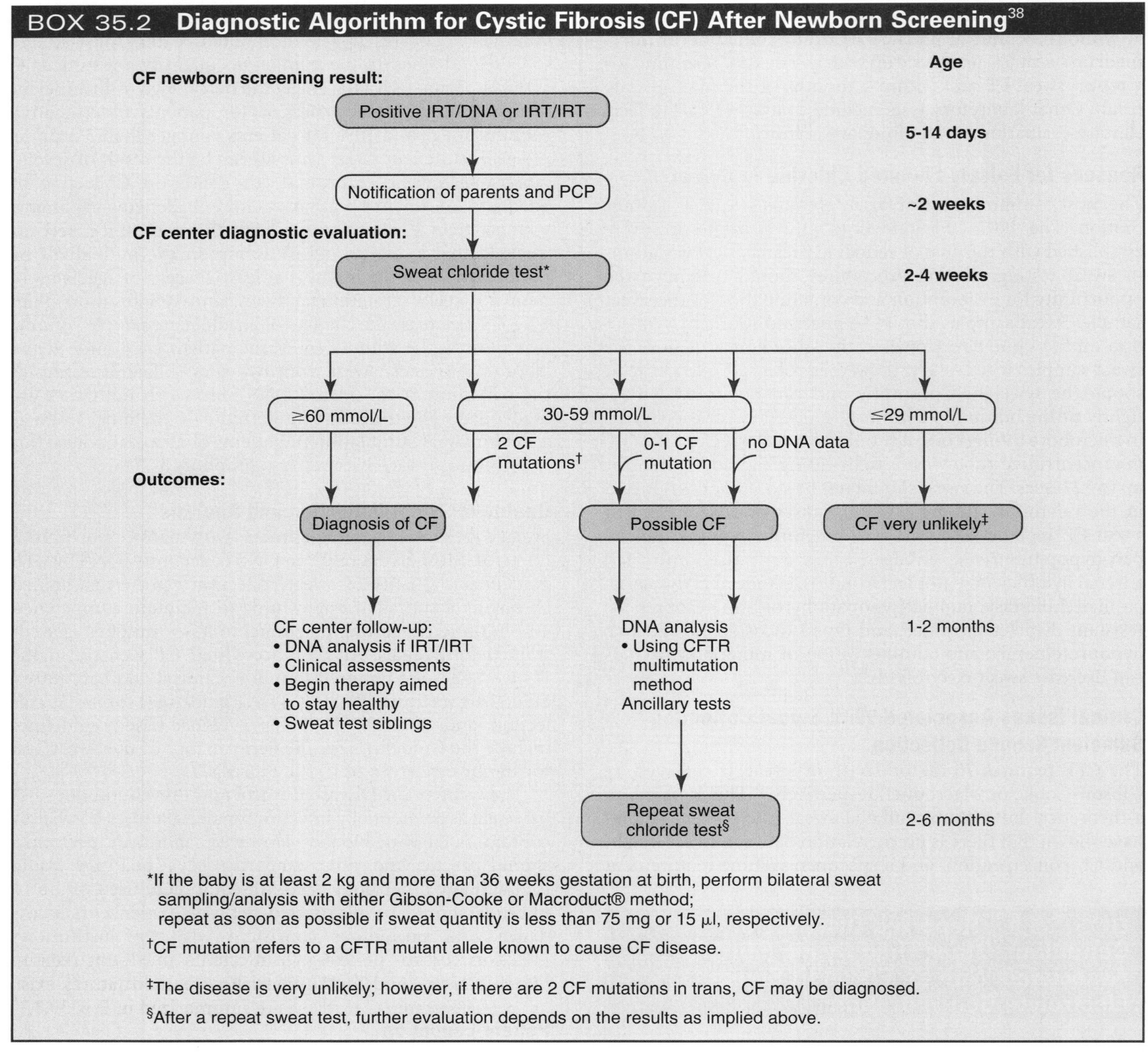

*If the baby is at least 2 kg and more than 36 weeks gestation at birth, perform bilateral sweat sampling/analysis with either Gibson-Cooke or Macroduct® method; repeat as soon as possible if sweat quantity is less than 75 mg or 15 μl, respectively.

†CF mutation refers to a CFTR mutant allele known to cause CF disease.

‡The disease is very unlikely; however, if there are 2 CF mutations in trans, CF may be diagnosed.

§After a repeat sweat test, further evaluation depends on the results as implied above.

of 6 μL). Sweat conductivity is measured by comparing electrical conductance of sweat to that of NaCl standard solutions. Sweat conductivity is expressed as millimoles per liter (equivalent NaCl), a unit that represents the molar concentration of a solution of NaCl that has the same conductivity as the sweat sample at the same temperature and does not represent the actual Na^+ or Cl^- concentration in the sweat sample.[54] Sweat conductivity is not diagnostic for CF. The CFF has approved the Macroduct Sweat-Chek for screening at clinical sites such as community hospitals, using sweat conductivity of ≥50 mmol/L as the cutoff for referral to an accredited CF care center.[54]

Newborn Screening for Cystic Fibrosis

Screening tests for CF is part of newborn screening programs (NBS) in all 50 states of the United States. NBS for CF is predominated by two algorithms (Box 35.2), which both start with measuring immunoreactive trypsinogen (IRT) from a dried blood spot and followed by either a second IRT measurement (IRT/IRT) or DNA mutation analysis (IRT/DNA). IRT is a pancreatic enzyme that is elevated in patients with CF. There is no standardized cutoff for IRT. The IRT/IRT algorithm requires a second specimen for the second IRT measurement. These results can be confounded by natural decreases in IRT during the newborn stage; there is a risk of a biologic false negative.[55,56]

IRT/DNA algorithms have the advantage of not requiring a second specimen and improved positive predictive value. Mutations on NBS panels vary from state to state in the United States, with some states only screening for the ΔF508 mutation.[57] The American College of Medical Genetics recommends a 25 mutant allele panel for screening based on

BOX 35.3 Conversion Factors, Prefixes, Symbols, and Descriptors Used in Discussions of Gases Measured in Blood and Expired Air*[63]

Conversion Factors

1 mm Hg = 0.133 kPa

1 kPa = 7.5 mm Hg

kPa: 1 kilopascal = 1000 pascal. The pascal is the standard international derived unit of pressure; it equals 1 Newton/m^2

General Prefixes

P: partial pressure or tension

Usage: PO_2, PCO_2, PH_2O

Alternative: pO_2

S: saturation fraction

Usage: SO_2

Alternative: sO_2

c: substance concentration

Usage: ctO_2 for concentration of total O_2

Usage: $ctCO_2$ for concentration of total CO_2

Usage: $cHCO_3^-$ for concentration of bicarbonate

d: dissolved gas, used with substance concentration *(c)*

t: total, used with substance concentration *(c)*, thus

$$ctCO_2 = cHCO_3^- + cdCO_2$$

Specimen origin is indicated by lower case letters. Whole blood and plasma are distinguished by capitals.

a: arterial B: blood

v: venous P: plasma

c: capillary

Usage: PO_2(aB), for partial pressure of O_2 in arterial blood

Prefixes Associated With External Respiration

V: volume of air or blood (unit, L)

$\dot{V}$: volume rate (unit, L/min)

F: substance fraction, also called mole fraction

E: expired air

I: inspired air

A: alveolar air

Usage: $\dot{v}$(A) means alveolar ventilation; $\dot{v}$(B) cardiac output; FO_2(I) fraction of O_2 in inspired air; PO_2(A) partial pressure of O_2 in alveolar air; and PCO_2(E) partial pressure of CO_2 in expired air.

Other Descriptors

BTPS: *Body Temperature* (37°C or 310.16 K) and ambient *Pressure*, fully *Saturated* (PH_2O = 47 mm Hg or 6.25 kPa)

STPD: *Standard Temperature* (0°C or 273.16 K) and standard *Pressure* (760 mm Hg or 101.08 kPa) of *Dry* gas

Amb: ambient atmosphere (unit is atm, atmosphere)

B: barometric (atmospheric)

BTPS: Usage: *P*(amb), *P(Amb)*

SVP: *Saturated Vapor Pressure*, the vapor pressure of water. SVP_T means SVP at a specified temperature (eg, $SVP_{37°C}$ = 47 mm Hg; PH_2O[saturated])

ATPS: *Ambient Temperature* and *Pressure*, *Saturated* with water vapor

*This list is not complete but is presented to facilitate interpretation of terms used in the text and to illustrate various forms that may be encountered in the literature.

PCO_2, Partial pressure of carbon dioxide; *PH_2O*, partial pressure of water; *PO_2*, partial pressure of oxygen.

prevalence in the general population. Included are alleles occurring at frequencies greater than 0.1% and correlated with clinical presentation of CF.[58] Increasing the number of mutations on NBS increases the sensitivity of the screen but also increases the number of carriers identified.[59] Carriers of *CFTR* mutations are more likely to have intermediate sweat Cl^- results.[60] A survey of CFF accredited CF care centers demonstrated that 70% of centers provide genetic counseling to patients to help reduce carrier misconceptions.[42] (See Chapter 49 for more genetic screening information.)

Infants with a positive NBS should also have a quantitative sweat Cl^- analysis, even when two disease-causing mutations are found.[61] However, NBS programs differ in which combination of positive tests in the screen should be used to refer to sweat analysis. Positive NBS should not be followed by sweat conductivity.

BLOOD GASES AND PH

Clinical management of respiratory and metabolic disorders often depends on rapid, accurate measurements of O_2 and CO_2 in blood. Vigorous measures to support life in patients with cardiopulmonary impairment depend largely on assisted ventilation using mixtures of gases that are tailored in response to laboratory blood gas results. Determination of blood gases also plays an important part in the detection of acid-base imbalances. Modern instruments for blood gas determination are simple to operate, and with meticulous maintenance and quality control, are capable of rapid, reliable laboratory data. Details of the pathophysiology of blood gases in relation to respiration and acid-base disorders are discussed in detail in Chapter 60.

Nomenclature for this area of analysis has been recommended by the CLSI,[62] but alternative nomenclatures exist and are in common use; these are summarized in Box 35.3.[63]

Behavior of Gases

Determination of gas pressures in expired air or blood depends on the application of certain physical principles (Table 35.1). The partial pressure (tension) of a gas dissolved in blood is by definition equal to the partial pressure of the gas in an imaginary ideal gas phase in equilibrium with the blood. At equilibrium, the partial pressure of a gas is the same in erythrocytes and plasma, so that the partial pressure of a gas is the same in whole blood and plasma. The partial pressure of a gas in a gas mixture is defined as the substance fraction of gas (mole fraction) times the total pressure.

Various spaces where gases are present include the ambient environment (room air), the bronchial tree and alveoli of the patient, and the measuring chamber of a laboratory instrument. In all these spaces, atmospheric (barometric) pressure, *P*(Amb), is the prevailing pressure, and partial pressures of each of the gases present in these spaces must add up to the value of *P*(Amb), which will vary with altitude and barometric

TABLE 35.1 Physical Principles Applied in Blood Gas Measurements

Boyle's law: The volume of an ideal gas at a constant temperature varies inversely with the pressure exerted to contain it.	$V \propto 1/P$
Charles' (Gay-Lussac's) law: The volume of an ideal gas at a constant pressure varies directly with its absolute temperature.	$V \propto T$
Avogadro's hypothesis: Equal volumes of different ideal gases at the same temperature and pressure contain the same number of molecules.	$n_i/V_i = n_j/V_j$
Dalton's law: The total pressure exerted by a mixture of ideal gases is the sum of the partial pressures of each of the gases in the mixture.	$P = \Sigma P_i$
Henry's law: The amount of a sparingly soluble gas dissolved in a liquid is proportional to the partial pressure of the gas over the liquid.	$c = \alpha \times P$

pressure. Scientific convention reduces measurements of gas volumes made at P(Amb) to standard temperature (0°C or 273.16 K) and pressure (760 mm Hg or 101.325 kPa) for dry gas (STPD) to make experimental data transferable. However, in blood gas work, the standard is that measurements of partial pressure are always made at body temperature (usually 37°C), at P(Amb), and in the presence of saturated water vapor (PH_2O = 47 mm Hg) (BTPS). Use of this BTPS convention (see Box 35.3) has the following practical effects:

1. It relates laboratory data for blood gases strictly to the geographic location of the patient, so that reference intervals become altitude dependent.
2. It assumes a standard body temperature of 37°C and that the measuring device also holds the sample of blood at exactly 37°C. This assumption requires special concern for thermal stability of the instrument. Just as important, it implies that in circumstances such as imposed hypothermia, when a patient's temperature is not 37°C, blood gas values determined at 37°C might need to be corrected to the actual body temperature to obtain an estimate of blood gas partial pressures in the patient.
3. It recognizes that partial pressures of measured gases in the blood coexist with a constant and standard saturated vapor pressure (SVP), which is identical for both the calibration conditions of the instrument and the measurement conditions of the blood sample.

Boyle's and Charles' laws and Avogadro's hypothesis are combined in what is called the general gas equation:

$$P = (nRT)/V$$

where P = pressure in units of millimeters of mercury (mm Hg) or kilopascals (kPa); V = volume in liters in which an ideal gas is contained; T = temperature in degrees kelvin (0°C = 273.16 K); n = number of moles of gas; and R = gas constant.

The standard international (SI) unit of P is the pascal. However, millimeters of mercury (also called torr) have continued to remain popular in some countries (see Box 35.3 for conversion factors). Use of SI units does have a practical advantage, in that 1 atm almost equals 100 kPa (1 atm = 101.325 kPa). Partial pressures expressed in kilopascals therefore are close estimates of percentages of the gases in the mixture at 1 atm. Pressure, P (or p), may mean total pressure, as in the expression P(Amb) for the mixture of gases in ambient air, or partial pressure in arterial blood, as in partial pressure of oxygen (PO_2[aB]). Numerical values and units of R differ depending on the units used for P, so that:

$$R = 62.36 \text{ mm Hg} \times \text{L°} \times \text{K}^{-1} \times \text{mol}^{-1}$$

or

$$R = 8.31 \text{ kPa} \times \text{L°} \times \text{K}^{-1} \times \text{mol}^{-1}$$

After terms are rearranged and n is evaluated as 1 mol and P as 760 mm Hg, the volume of 1 mol of a pure ideal gas at 0°C (no water vapor) is 22.4 L. The general gas equation is the justification for accepting partial pressures of gases in blood as estimators of their concentrations. However, PO_2 is related only to the concentration of dissolved O_2 (cdO_2) in the blood and PCO_2 to the concentration of dissolved CO_2 ($cdCO_2$) in the blood (see Henry's law, Table 35.1). The total concentration of O_2 in blood (ctO_2) is the sum of concentrations of dissolved O_2 and of O_2 bound to Hb, with cdO_2 being a small component of tO_2 (see later section on Hemoglobin Saturation). The total concentration of CO_2 ($ctCO_2$) is defined operationally as the sum of concentrations of dissolved CO_2, carbonic acid, HCO_3^-, undissociated HCO_3^-, and carbonate ion.

Dalton's law (see Table 35.1) may be written for room air as follows:

$$P(\text{amb}) = PO_2 + PCO_2 + PN_2 + PH_2O + PX$$

where PX = that of any other gas in the air sample. However, for gases in solution, Dalton's law does not apply because the sum of partial pressures of all dissolved gases may be lower than, equal to, or higher than the measured pressure of the solution. For instance, if the sum of gas tensions is significantly higher than the pressure of the solution, bubbles may form, as they do in the blood of divers surfacing from deep water (giving rise to a condition known as "the bends") or in a cold blood sample being warmed for analysis.

Dalton's law of partial pressures remains important for calibration and control of the measuring devices. Consider a calibrator gas certified to contain 15% O_2 (L/L or mol/mol) and 5% CO_2, the remainder being nitrogen (N_2). The mole fractions (or F) of the gases in the dry mixture are 0.15, 0.05, and 0.80, respectively. This mixture, after saturation with water vapor at 37°C (to mimic a patient's blood or alveolar air), is introduced into a blood gas instrument's measuring chamber (held at 37°C to mimic a patient's body temperature) for the purpose of calibrating the instrument for subsequent measurements of gases in patients' samples. If the local barometric pressure, P(Amb), on this occasion is 747 mm Hg, then humidified calibrator gas is present in the chamber at ambient barometric pressure, such that

$$P(\text{amb}) = 747 \text{ mm Hg} = PO_2 + PCO_2 + PN_2 + PH_2O$$

To set the instrument to the PO_2 and PCO_2 of the calibrator gas, first PH_2O at 37°C must be accounted for, which is equal to the SVP of water, 47 mm Hg. Therefore,

$$\begin{aligned} 747 \text{ mm Hg} - PH_2O &= PO_2 + PCO_2 + PN_2 \\ &= 747 - 47 \\ &= 700 \text{ mm Hg} \end{aligned}$$

If P(Amb) corrected for PH_2O represents the sum of partial pressures for the dry gases whose mole fractions are known, the exact PO_2 and PCO_2 values for the calibrator gas can be calculated, under circumstances of measurement, and then these calibrator values can be entered into the instrument.

The law of partial pressure is also applied in defining gas mixtures used to determine $PO_2(0.5)$ (P_{50}) and other derived quantities, and to control instrumentation with tonometered samples. Henry's law predicts the amount of dissolved gas in a liquid in contact with a gaseous phase (see Table 35.1).

The coefficient for O_2 in blood, αO_2, is 0.00140 (mol/L)/mm Hg (the corresponding coefficient for the volume–volume relationship is 31 µL/L/mm Hg). Therefore, when arterial PO_2 is normal (≈100 mm Hg), the cdO_2 in arterial blood is 0.140 mmol/L, which is a small proportion of the ctO_2 content in blood (≈9 mmol/L), the bulk of which is O_2 bound by Hb. Increasing the O_2 fraction of inspired air to 100% or increasing the pressure of inspired air, as in a hyperbaric chamber, forces more O_2 into a solution. In therapy with pure O_2, when PO_2 may rise to 640 mm Hg, the cdO_2 could be as high as 0.9 mmol/L. In hyperbaric treatment, an arterial PO_2 of 2500 mm Hg (≈3.2 atm) is equivalent to a cdO_2 of 3.5 mmol/L. Prediction of concentrations of cdO_2 in these therapies is useful because tissue oxygenation by dissolved O_2 becomes increasingly important when Hb-mediated O_2 delivery is impaired.

The $cdCO_2$ can be calculated in the same way: αCO_2 at 37°C in plasma = 0.0306 mmol/L/mm Hg. Thus, at a PCO_2 of 40 mm Hg, the $cdCO_2$ = 40 × 0.0306 = 1.224 mmol/L. In the determination of blood gases, PCO_2 is determined along with blood pH. As will be explained in the following, these two parameters in conjunction with the Henderson-Hasselbalch equation permit the calculation of HCO_3^-, as follows:

$$\log cHCO_3^- = \text{pH} - pK' + \log[PCO_2 \times \alpha CO_2(\text{P})]$$

The antilog is then taken to derive $cHCO_3^-$.

Application of the Henderson-Hasselbalch Equation in Blood Gas Measurements

Carbon dioxide and water react to form carbonic acid, which in turn dissociates to H^+ ions and HCO_3^-.

$$CO_2 + H_2O \xrightleftharpoons{K_{hydration}} H_2CO_3 \xrightleftharpoons{K_{dissociation}} H^{\oplus} + HCO_3^{\ominus}$$

Thus, the $ctCO_2$, the concentration of bicarbonate ($cHCO_3^-$), the $cdCO_2$, and the H^+ ion concentration (cH^+) are interrelated. The constant K for the hydration reaction is 2.29 × 10^{-3} (pK = 2.64 at 37°C), whereas the constant K for the dissociation of carbonic acid is 2.04 × 10^{-4} (pK = 3.69).

In the classic formulation, Henderson (1908), using concentrations for HCO_3^-, CO_2, and H^+, and assuming the concentration of H_2O to be constant, combined these two reactions and incorporated the constant K' with a value of 4.68 × 10^{-7}, and thus a pK' of 6.33 at 37°C:

$$K' = \frac{cH^+ \times cHCO_3^-}{cdCO_2}$$

The $cdCO_2$ includes the small amount of undissociated (dissolved) carbonic acid. It can be expressed as $cdCO_2 = \alpha \times PCO_2$, where α is the solubility coefficient for CO_2. $cHCO_3^-$ then represents $ctCO_2$ minus $cdCO_2$, which includes carbonic acid. The HCO_3^- concentration by this definition includes undissociated $NaHCO_3^-$, carbonate ($NaCO_3$), and carbamate (carbamino-CO_2; $RCNHCOO^-$), which are present in exceedingly small amounts in plasma. If the Henderson equation is rearranged and $cdCO_2$ is replaced by $\alpha \times PCO_2$, the following equation results:

$$cH^+ = K' \times \frac{\alpha \times PCO_2}{cHCO_3^-}$$

In 1916, Hasselbalch showed that a logarithmic transformation of the equation was a more useful form and used the symbols pH (= −log cH^+) and pK' (= −log K'). pH is defined as the negative log of the activity of H^+ (aH^+), which is the entity actually measured with pH meters. The resulting Henderson-Hasselbalch equation becomes

$$pH = pK' + \log \frac{cHCO_3^-}{\alpha \times PCO_2}$$

or

$$pH = pK' + \log \frac{ctCO_2 - (\alpha \times PCO_2)}{\alpha \times PCO_2}$$

K' is the apparent overall (combined) dissociation constant for carbonic acid. It is apparent because concentrations are used rather than activities and overall because both the $cdCO_2$ and the concentration of carbonic acid are used. K' depends not only on the temperature but also on the ionic strength of the solution.

For blood at 37°C, the normal mean value is pK'(P) = 6.103, with a normal biological SD of approximately ±0.0015, which is mainly caused by variations in ionic strength. The solubility coefficient for CO_2 gas, α, also varies with the composition of the solution. For pure water at 37°C, the solubility coefficient α = (0.0329 mmol) × (L^{-1}) × (mm Hg^{-1}), and for normal plasma at 37°C, it is (0.0306 mmol) × (L^{-1}) × (mm Hg^{-1}). When pK' and α for normal plasma at 37°C are inserted, the Henderson-Hasselbalch equation takes the following form:

$$pH = 6.103 + \log \frac{cHCO_3^-}{0.0306 \times PCO_2}$$

or

$$pH = 6.103 + \log \frac{ctCO_2 - 0.0306 \times PCO_2}{0.0306 \times PCO_2}$$

where PCO_2 is measured in millimeters of mercury and $cHCO_3^-$ and $ctCO_2$ are measured in millimoles per liter. By taking the antilogarithm, combining the constants, and expressing $[H^+]$ in nanomoles per liter, the equation becomes

$$cH^+ = 24.1 \times \frac{PCO_2}{cHCO_3^-}$$

If normal values are substituted in the equation:

$$cH^+ = 24.1 \times \frac{40}{24.1}\ \text{nmol/L} = 38.0\ \text{nmol/L}$$

Clearly, by measuring any two of the four parameters—PCO_2 or $cdCO_2$, pH, $ctCO_2$, and $cHCO_3^-$—and by using the Henderson-Hasselbalch equation with the preceding values for pK' and α, the other two parameters may be calculated. Although used as constants, these values must be recognized as means and are susceptible to biological variation. Changes in ionic strength of ±20% cause changes in pK' between 6.08 and 6.12. Variations in pK' of plasma also occur with temperature (pK will decrease by 0.0026 per 1°C increase and will decrease slightly with increasing pH). For most clinical purposes, these variations of pK' can be ignored. However, in pathological cases with markedly deviant ionic strength, the change in pK' may be significant. The value of α is affected by the presence of increased salts or proteins in solution (value decreases) or lipids (value increases). For instance, in lipemic plasma, the value of α may be 0.033 or even higher. Thus, parameters calculated on the assumption that pK' and α are invariant may have an error under certain pathologic circumstances, and several authors have suggested caution in using values calculated from blood gas analyzers in extremely ill patients and in children.[64,65]

For instance, one study showed that in 17 of 51 adult intensive care unit patients, calculated and measured tCO_2 values differed by more than 10%,[64] whereas another study showed differences of more than 20% in 27 of 107 pediatric intensive care unit patients.[65] The same holds true for comparison of 74 patient blood samples between calculated tCO_2 (using pH and PCO_2) of whole blood by a modern POCT device and measured tCO_2 using an automated analyzer on arterial plasma.[66] Finally, microprocessor algorithms use HCO_3^- values to calculate base excess.[67] Base excess is defined as the amount of acid required to return the blood pH of a patient to 7.4.

Oxygen in Blood

The ctO_2 of a blood sample is the sum of the concentrations of Hb-bound O_2 and of dissolved O_2. At a blood ctO_2 of 9 mmol/L, the O_2 associated with Hb as oxyhemoglobin (O_2Hb) is 8.86 mmol/L. The O_2Hb is defined as erythrocyte Hb with O_2 reversibly bound to iron of its heme group. Each mole of Hb-iron binds 1 mol of O_2. In erythrocytes, Hb exists as a tetramer (64,456 g/mol), but when Hb concentration is expressed in moles per liter, it is reported as the concentration of the monomer (16,114 g/mol). Thus 1 L of blood with a normal Hb concentration (cHb) of 9.3 mmol/L (≈15 g/dL or 150 g/L) carries 9.3 mmol of O_2 at STPD if all Hb is in the form of O_2Hb.

Thus, 1 g of Hb is capable of binding 1.39 mL (0.062 mmol) of O_2 at STPD. This value is referred to as the specific O_2-binding capacity of Hb A (Hb A, the normal adult gene product). Hb A reversibly binds O_2 at its heme moiety and binds biological effectors at other allosteric sites. Methemoglobin (MetHb), carboxyhemoglobin (COHb), sulfhemoglobin (SulfHb), and cyanmethemoglobin are forms of Hb that are not capable of reversible binding of O_2 because of chemical alterations of the heme moiety (see Chapter 38). These chemically altered Hbs are collectively termed dyshemoglobins. Another group of abnormal Hbs have genetically determined changes in their amino acid sequence that can alter their O_2 affinity. These Hbs are collectively referred to as Hb variants or hemoglobinopathies. More than 900 Hb variants have been described; only a small fraction are clinically significant (see Chapter 38).

Uptake of O_2 by the blood in the lungs is governed primarily by the PO_2 of alveolar air and by the ability of O_2 to diffuse freely across the alveolar membrane into the blood. At the PO_2 normally present in alveolar air (≈102 mm Hg) and with a normal membrane and normal Hb A, more than 95% of Hb will bind O_2. At a PO_2 more than 110 mm Hg, more than 98% of normal Hb A binds O_2. When all Hb is saturated with O_2, a further increase in the PO_2 of alveolar air simply increases the concentration of cdO_2 in the arterial blood. Delivery of O_2 by the blood to the tissue is governed by the large gradient between PO_2 of the arterial blood and that of the tissue cells, and by the dissociation of O_2Hb in the erythrocytes at the lower PO_2 of the blood–tissue cell interface.

Three properties of arterial blood are essential to ensure adequate O_2 delivery to the tissue:

1. Arterial PO_2 must be sufficiently high (≈90 mm Hg) to create a diffusion gradient from the arterial blood to the tissue cells. Low arterial PO_2 (hypoxemia) results in tissue O_2 starvation (hypoxia).
2. The O_2-binding capacity of the blood must be normal (ie, the concentration of Hb capable of binding and releasing O_2 must be normal). Decreased Hb concentration will cause anemic hypoxia.
3. Hb must be able to bind O_2 in the lungs yet release it at the tissue. In other words, the affinity of Hb for O_2 must be normal. Too great an affinity of Hb for O_2 may cause "affinity-based" tissue hypoxia, in which O_2 is not released at the capillary–tissue interface.

The PO_2 at the venous end of the capillaries should stay at approximately 30 to 45 mm Hg; thus the normal arteriovenous difference in PO_2 is 50 to 60 mm Hg.

Hemoglobin Oxygen Saturation

Before the factors that affect Hb affinity for O_2 are discussed, it is important to define the concept of Hb O_2 saturation (SO_2):

$$SO_2 = \frac{\text{Oxygen Content}}{\text{Oxygen Capacity}}$$

This is the fraction (percentage) of functional Hb that is saturated with O_2 and is essentially an indirect means of estimating the PO_2. However, at least three different approaches exist for determining O_2 "saturation," and although each is distinct, they are often used interchangeably to determine O_2 saturation. These three terms—Hb SO_2, fractional oxyhemoglobin (FO_2Hb), and estimated O_2 saturation (O_2Sat)—have distinct definitions set by the CLSI.[62] Ambiguous use of these terms occurs because in healthy subjects with normal amounts of normal Hb, the values for all three entities are very similar. However, these assumptions can lead to erroneous conclusions in seriously ill patients and those with dyshemoglobins or Hb variants.

Spectrophotometric methods are used to determine O_2Hb and HHb,[68] and SO_2 is calculated according to:

$$SO_2 = \frac{cO_2Hb}{cO_2Hb + cHHb}$$

where cO_2Hb is the concentration of oxyhemoglobin; *c*HHb is the concentration of deoxyhemoglobin; and the sum of oxyhemoglobin and deoxyhemoglobin represents all Hb capable of reversibly binding O_2. SO_2 is usually expressed as a percent in the United States, but it may also be expressed as a decimal fraction of 1.00.

SO_2 most often is determined by simple pulse oximetry, a spectrophotometric approach that can determine oxyhemoglobin and reduced Hb (HHb) but not COHb, MetHb, or SulfHb. These devices measure absorbance at 660 and 940 nm, for which O_2Hb and HHb have unique absorbance patterns.[69] These are bedside monitors used for monitoring Hb SO_2, and they serve this purpose extremely well. However, use of SO_2 in the initial evaluation of a patient with dyshemoglobins can be misleading. For instance, in a comatose patient with 15% COHb, the SO_2 by simple pulse oximetry might read 0.95, whereas the fraction of oxyhemoglobin in reality would be only 0.80. Thus, it seems reasonable to assess for the presence of dyshemoglobins before SO_2 is used for clinical purposes. The reference interval for SO_2 from healthy adults is 0.94 to 0.98 (94%–98%). For more information, refer to the Appendix on Reference Intervals.

Another expression of SO_2 is FO_2Hb, which is calculated as:

$$FO_2Hb = (cO_2Hb/cO_2Hb + cHHb + cCOHb + cMethHb + cSulfHb)$$

This value requires determination of all Hb species and can be performed on a co-oximeter present in modern blood gas analyzers. These instruments prepare a hemolysate from whole blood by sonication, and spectrophotometrically determine the total amount of Hb and the percent of each of the aforementioned species. This is accomplished by using monochromatic light at 6 to 128 fixed wavelengths between 535 and 670 nm and measuring absorbance at each of the wavelengths. Newer co-oximeters use a diode array and 128 wavelengths. Because each species of Hb has its own absorbance pattern, a microcomputer can calculate the percent of each one. The reference interval for FO_2Hb is 0.90 to 0.95 (90% to 95%).

Finally, the microprocessors of blood gas instruments estimate the SO_2 from measured pH, PO_2, and Hb using empirical equations.[70] This value should be clearly referred to as an estimated SO_2, but it frequently is reported as and referred to as *O_2Sat.* Calculated values such as O_2Sat should be interpreted with reservation because the algorithm assumes normal O_2 affinity of the Hb, normal 2,3-diphosphoglycerol (2,3-DPG) concentrations, and the absence of dyshemoglobins. Such calculated estimates have been found to vary by as much as 6% saturation from measured values.[71]

Decreases in arterial FO_2Hb may indicate a low arterial PO_2 or an impaired ability of Hb to bind O_2. The amount of O_2 that the blood can carry is determined by three major factors: (1) the PO_2, which reflects how much O_2 is dissolved in the blood; (2) the amount of normal Hb available in erythrocytes; and (3) the affinity of available Hb for O_2. Decreases in PO_2 indicate a reduced ability of O_2 to diffuse from alveolar air into the blood. This may be due to hypoventilation or to increased venoarterial shunting that is secondary to cardiac or pulmonary insufficiency, resulting in a right-to-left shunting of blood that has not reached equilibrium with alveolar air. This results in a decreased PO_2 and an increased PCO_2. Decreases in the concentration of total Hb can result from a decreased number of erythrocytes that contain a normal concentration of Hb (normochromic anemia) or a decreased mean cell concentration of Hb in the erythrocytes (hypochromic anemia). Decreased FO_2Hb hemoglobin can also occur as a result of poisonings that convert part of the Hb into the species COHb, MetHb, SulfHb, or cyanmethemoglobin, which cannot properly bind or exchange O_2. Clinically, it is important to distinguish between arterial hypoxemia (decreased arterial PO_2 and decreased FO_2Hb caused by decreased availability of O_2) and cyanosis (decreased FO_2Hb caused by abnormally high concentrations of reduced Hb or chemically altered Hb incapable of carrying O_2). In the setting of cyanosis, measurement of SO_2 or an O_2Sat could be normal if cyanosis is due to the presence of MetHb or COHb.[69] The O_2 concentration of blood (ctO_2) is the sum of O_2 bound to Hb and cdO_2. Blood gas analyzers determine ctO_2 by the following calculation[62]:

$$ctO_2(\text{mL}/\text{dL}) = FO_2Hb \times bO_2 \times ctHb(\text{g}/\text{dL}) + (\alpha O_2) \times (PO_2)$$

where $bO_2 = 1.39$ mL/g Hb and α, the solubility coefficient of O_2 at 37°C; and STPD = 0.00314 (mL/dL)/mm Hg = 0.00140 (mmol/L)/mm Hg. This calculation is based on FO_2Hb and *ct*Hb. If SO_2 is used, it is necessary to use the effective Hb concentration (ie, to subtract the concentration of any dyshemoglobins present from the concentration of *ct*Hb).

Hemoglobin-Oxygen Dissociation

The degree of association or dissociation of O_2 with Hb is determined by PO_2 and the affinity of Hb for O_2. When the SO_2 of blood is determined over a range of PO_2 and is plotted against PO_2, a sigmoidal curve called the O_2 dissociation curve is obtained. The shape of the curve is affected by the increasing efficiency with which HHb molecules bind more O_2 once some O_2 has been bound (cooperativity; see also Chapter 38). The location of the curve relative to the PO_2 required to achieve a particular concentration of SO_2 in the blood is a function of the affinity of Hb for O_2.

The affinity of Hb for O_2 depends on five factors: temperature, pH, PCO_2, concentration of 2,3-DPG, and the presence of minor Hbs such as COHb and MetHb. Dissociation of O_2 in relation to 2,3-DPG concentration and abnormal Hb proteins, such as fetal Hb (Hb F), thalassemias, and other hemoglobinopathies, are discussed in Chapter 38. Increases in 2,3-DPG shift the SO_2–PO_2 relationship to the right. This chapter describes the effects of temperature, pH, and PCO_2 on dissociation behavior.

Fig. 35.3 shows the effect of plasma pH on the O_2 dissociation curve (the Bohr effect). Similar graphs can be made for

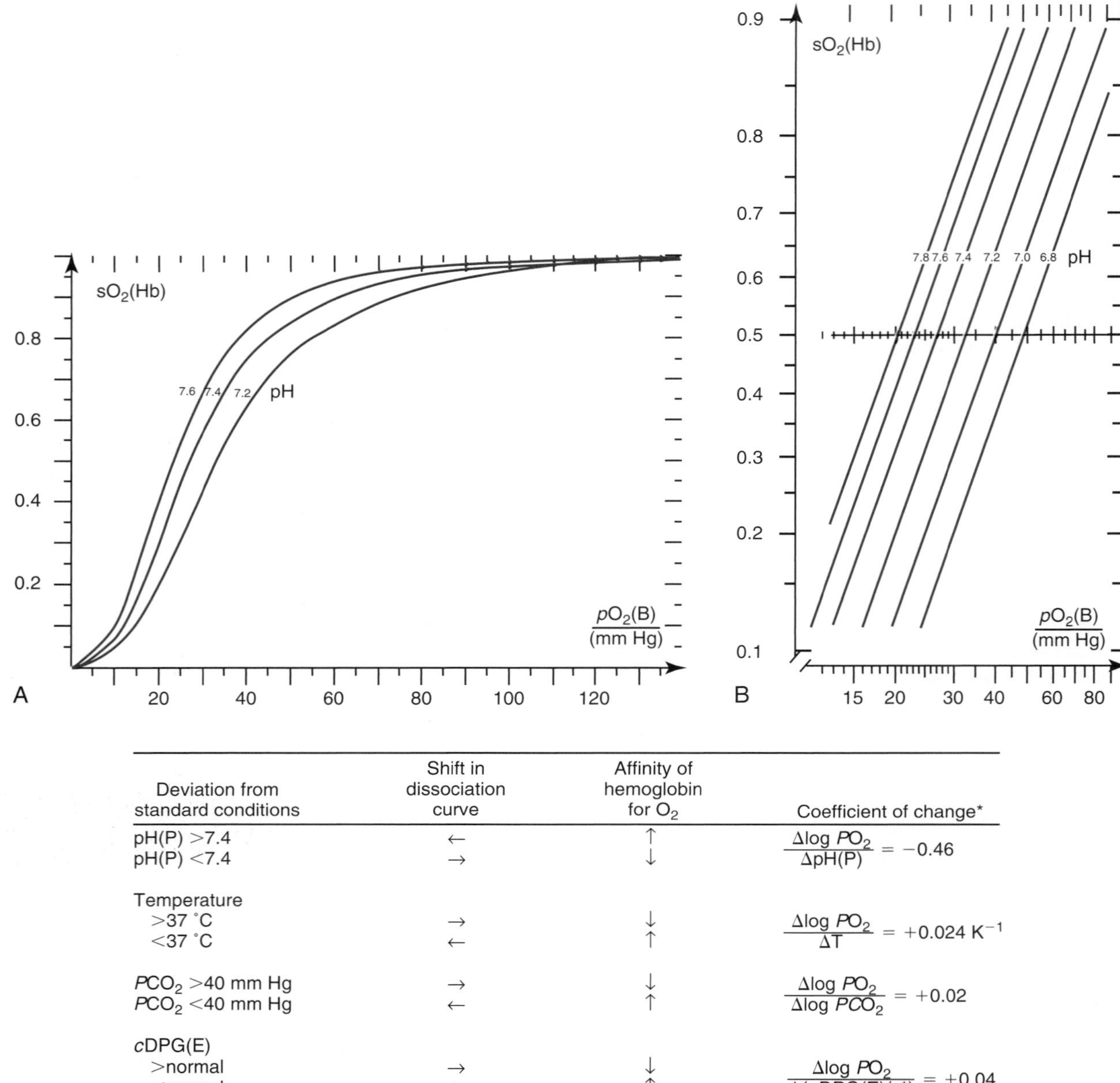

Deviation from standard conditions	Shift in dissociation curve	Affinity of hemoglobin for O_2	Coefficient of change*
pH(P) >7.4 pH(P) <7.4	← →	↑ ↓	$\frac{\Delta \log PO_2}{\Delta pH(P)} = -0.46$
Temperature >37 °C <37 °C	 → ←	 ↓ ↑	$\frac{\Delta \log PO_2}{\Delta T} = +0.024\ K^{-1}$
PCO_2 >40 mm Hg PCO_2 <40 mm Hg	→ ←	↓ ↑	$\frac{\Delta \log PO_2}{\Delta \log PCO_2} = +0.02$
*c*DPG(E) >normal <normal	 → ←	 ↓ ↑	$\frac{\Delta \log PO_2}{\Delta (cDPG(E)/c^*)} = +0.04$

FIGURE 35.3 A, Oxygen dissociation curves for human blood with different plasma pH but constant partial pressure of carbon dioxide (PCO_2) of 40 mm Hg, a 2,3-diphosphoglycerol (2,3-DPG) concentration in erythrocytes of 5.0 mmol/L, and temperature at 37°C. **B,** A hill plot. Conditions are the same as in **A.** The coefficients given in this chart form the basis for the correction of measured partial pressure of oxygen (PO_2). The effect of pH(P) to shift the dissociation curve is called the Bohr effect; the coefficient above for $\Delta \log PO_2/\Delta pH(P)$ applies to conditions when the PCO_2 is 40 mm Hg, and changes in pH(P) are due to changes in concentrations of noncarbonic acids and bases. If, however, the changes in pH(P) are being caused by changes in PCO_2, then the absolute value of the coefficient is greater (ie, $\Delta \log PO_2/\Delta pH[P] = -0.49$). The coefficients for the Bohr effect are specified for PO_2 of whole blood but use the pH of plasma, pH(P). The coefficient for the 2,3-diphosphoglycerol *(DPG)* effect is based on the DPG concentration in the erythrocytes, *c*DPG(E). $c^* = 1$ mmol/L.

variations of PCO_2 and temperature. The Hill logit-log transform (illustrated as the Hill plot; Fig. 35.3B) converts the curvilinear dissociation function into a linear function.

The linear transformations of the dissociation curves have allowed linear coefficients of change (see Fig. 35.3) to be determined for each of the factors that shift dissociation curves, and hence the lines on the Hill plot. These coefficients find applications for correcting measured PO_2 or calculated P_{50} for the effects of different body temperatures, PCO_2, pH, and 2,3-DPG concentrations.

Determination of $\mathbf{P_{50}}$. P_{50} is defined as the PO_2 at which the Hb of the blood is half saturated with O_2. The measured value of P_{50} differs from the standard value of P_{50} by some amount determined by the extent that pH differs from 7.40, PCO_2 differs from 40 mm Hg, temperature differs from 37°C, and 2,3-DPG differs from 5.0 mmol/L. The value of P_{50} therefore becomes a measure of the change of Hb affinity because of the factors that affect it. A procedure for determining P_{50} uses the principle that:

$$\log P_{50} = \log PO_2 - \text{logit}\ SO_2 / 2.7$$

where logit SO_2 = $\log[SO_2/(1 - SO_2)]$; and 2.7 = Hill slope.[72,73]

The P_{50} reference interval for adults, measured at 37°C and corrected to pH(P) of 7.4, is 25 to 29 mm Hg. For newborn infants, the interval is 18 to 24 mm Hg because of the presence of Hb F.

Clinical Significance. Increased values for P_{50} indicate displacement of the O_2 dissociation curve to the right (ie, decreased affinity of Hb for O_2). The chief causes are hyperthermia, acidemia, hypercapnia, high concentrations of 2,3-DPG, and the presence of a Hb variant with decreased O_2 affinity. The physiologic effects of decreased affinity of Hb are small. The affinity is still sufficient to bind adequate amounts of O_2 in the lungs, and the low affinity facilitates dissociation of O_2Hb at the peripheral tissues. In anemia, low affinity (as a result of increases in 2,3-DPG) is a desirable compensatory mechanism. The compensatory responses in healthy individuals to alter the P_{50} can be remarkable. For instance, in fully acclimatized (70 days) high-altitude climbers (eg, Mt. Everest), full cognition was maintained without supplemental O_2 at an altitude of 8400 m and an average PaO_2 of only 25 mm Hg.[74]

Low values for P_{50} signify displacement of the O_2 dissociation curve to the left (ie, increased affinity of Hb). The main causes are hypothermia, acute alkalemia, hypocapnia, low 2,3-DPG, and variant Hb. The physiologic consequence of increased affinity of Hb for O_2 is less efficient dissociation of O_2Hb at the peripheral tissue and lower tissue PO_2.

Tonometry

Tonometry is the process of exposing a sample to a gas phase in such a way that each gas in the gaseous phase partitions to an equilibrium between the liquid and gas. Equilibration by tonometry uses gases of known fractional composition, humidified at 37°C to give a saturated water vapor pressure of 47 mm Hg. The PCO_2 or PO_2 of such gases is calculated according to Dalton's law (see section on behavior of gases). Tonometry is used to treat blood samples for various special studies that are rarely requested in most hospital settings and to prepare quality control material in whole blood. Direct determination of P_{50} and of standard HCO_3^- are two applications of tonometry. Great detail on tonometry can be found in the second edition of this textbook.[75]

Determination of Partial Pressure of Carbon Dioxide, Partial Pressure of Oxygen, and pH

The instruments used for determination of PCO_2, PO_2, and pH are highly automated. Proper specimen collection and handling are critical for accurate determinations.

Specimens

Whole blood is the most likely specimen for a clinical laboratory to receive for gas analysis. Differences in measured blood gas values between arterial and venous blood are most pronounced for PO_2. PO_2 is the only clinical reason for arterial collections. PO_2 is generally approximately 60 mm Hg lower in venous blood after O_2 is released in the capillaries, whereas PCO_2 is 2 to 8 mm Hg higher in venous blood. pH generally is only 0.02 to 0.05 pH units lower in a venous sample.

Proper specimen collection is of paramount importance in obtaining accurate results for blood analysis for gases and pH. Placement of indwelling catheters with heparin locks for short- and long-term intravenous therapies is common. Failure to flush the lock properly has unpredictable effects on measured quantities and is often indicated by bizarre, nonphysiologic results.

Arterial or venous specimens are collected anaerobically with lyophilized heparin anticoagulant in 1- to 3-mL sterile syringes. Lyophilized heparin is preferable to liquid heparin because liquid heparin, which has atmospheric PO_2 and PCO_2 values, dilutes the sample, with the effect being the greatest when the syringe is not completely filled. An increasing ratio of liquid heparin to blood can have an increasingly marked effect on measured PCO_2 and the parameters calculated from it. In one study, dilution with 10% volume of liquid heparin having an atmospheric PCO_2 of 0.25 mm Hg led to a 10 to 20 mm Hg decrease in blood PCO_2.[76]

Anaerobic technique for collection means no exposure of blood to atmospheric air. The PCO_2 of air is approximately 0.25 mm Hg; this is much less than that of blood (≈40 mm Hg). Thus, the CO_2 content and PCO_2 of blood exposed to air will decrease, and blood pH, which is a function of PCO_2, will rise. The PO_2 of atmospheric air (≈155 mm Hg) is approximately 60 mm Hg higher than that of arterial blood and approximately 100 mm Hg higher than that of venous blood. Therefore, blood from patients breathing room air that is exposed to atmospheric air gains O_2, and blood with PO_2 more than 150 mm Hg, which occurs in patients undergoing O_2 therapy, loses O_2. Blood can also be exposed to air simply from the air in the needle and the syringe hub dead space. Error will be minimal if the resulting bubble is ejected immediately after drawing by holding the syringe tip up and ejecting a small drop of blood. The potential effect of small bubbles on blood gas results was clearly demonstrated in one study in which a 100-μL bubble of room air was added to 10 2-mL blood samples with PO_2 values between 25 and 40 mm Hg. In these samples, PO_2 increased an average of 4 mm Hg in only 2 minutes, whereas PCO_2 decreased 4 mm Hg.[77] Before analysis, mixing of the sample by vigorously rolling the syringe between the palms should be done to establish a homogeneous sample.

Arterialized capillary blood is sometimes an acceptable alternative to arterial blood when an arterial cannula is not available or when repeated arterial puncture must be avoided. Freely flowing cutaneous blood originates in the arterioles and corresponds closely to arterial blood in composition. However, arterialized capillary blood is not acceptable when systolic blood pressure is less than 95 mm Hg. Capillary puncture should be preceded by warming of the selected skin puncture site for 10 minutes to achieve vasodilation and adequate blood flow. For collection from the finger of a child or an adult, or from an infant's heel, warming may be accomplished by immersing the arm or leg in water warmed to 42°C. The first blood drop to appear should be wiped away, and subsequent free-forming drops should be taken up in a capillary collection tube containing lyophilized heparin. Only free-flowing blood provides a satisfactory sample, and collecting the drops as soon as they form minimizes aerobic exposure. Transport and analysis of specimens should be prompt. However, delayed analysis of up to 1 hour will have a minimal effect on reported values from most samples.[78] The pH of freshly drawn blood decreases on standing at a rate of 0.04 to 0.08 pH unit/hour at 37°C, 0.02 to 0.03/hour at 22°C, and less than 0.01/hour at 4°C. The decrease in pH is accompanied by a corresponding decrease in glucose and an equivalent increase in lactate. PCO_2 increases by approximately 5 mm Hg/hour at 3°C, by 1 mm Hg/hour at 22°C, and by only approximately 0.5 mm Hg/hour at 2°C to 4°C. The primary cause of these changes is glycolysis by leukocytes, platelets, and reticulocytes. In freshly drawn blood with a normal PO_2 that is maintained anaerobically, cell respiration causes PO_2 to decrease at a rate of approximately 2 mm Hg/hour at room temperature and 5 to 10 mm Hg/hour at 37°C. Adverse effects of glycolysis and respiration on pH, $ctCO_2$, PO_2, and PCO_2 of blood can best be prevented by analysis within 30 to 60 minutes after collection. If analysis must be delayed longer than 30 minutes, the syringe should be immersed in a mixture of ice and water until analysis. Under these conditions, changes are negligible because glycolysis is inhibited. With current blood gas instrumentation, introduction of a chilled sample carries little risk of a low-temperature effect on measurements because thermal equilibration to 37°C is rapid and complete.

The aforementioned small changes in values that can be expected with delays in analysis are true only when the WBC count is normal or only slightly elevated. Glycolysis and the resulting effects on pH, PO_2, and PCO_2 increase dramatically with markedly elevated WBC, such as occurs in leukemia. Experiments have shown that PO_2 decreases by 20 mm Hg in 2 minutes and by 40 mm Hg in only 5 minutes with WBC values more than 100,000/μL.[79,80] For samples with these types of WBC values, it is very difficult to overcome this effect. Even after the sample is immersed in ice, thermal equilibrium takes several minutes, allowing significant PO_2 loss before the contents reach 4°C. The only alternative to obtaining accurate blood gas values in such patients is immediate analysis performed at the point-of-care.

Instrumentation

Reference methods for blood gas and electrolyte determinations have been described in detail by the International Federation for Clinical Chemistry and Laboratory Medicine (IFCC).[63] A schematic diagram characteristic of a typical instrument is shown in Fig. 35.4. Electrochemical principles and structural features of electrodes are discussed in Chapter 14.

Operation of a traditional blood gas instrument begins with the operator presenting a blood specimen at the sample probe. The sample is taken through the probe by a peristaltic pump that loads the chamber with 60 to 150 μL of the sample. The sample then resides in the chamber long enough to allow thermal equilibration and completion of measurements. On completion of measurement, the pump pushes the sample to waste.

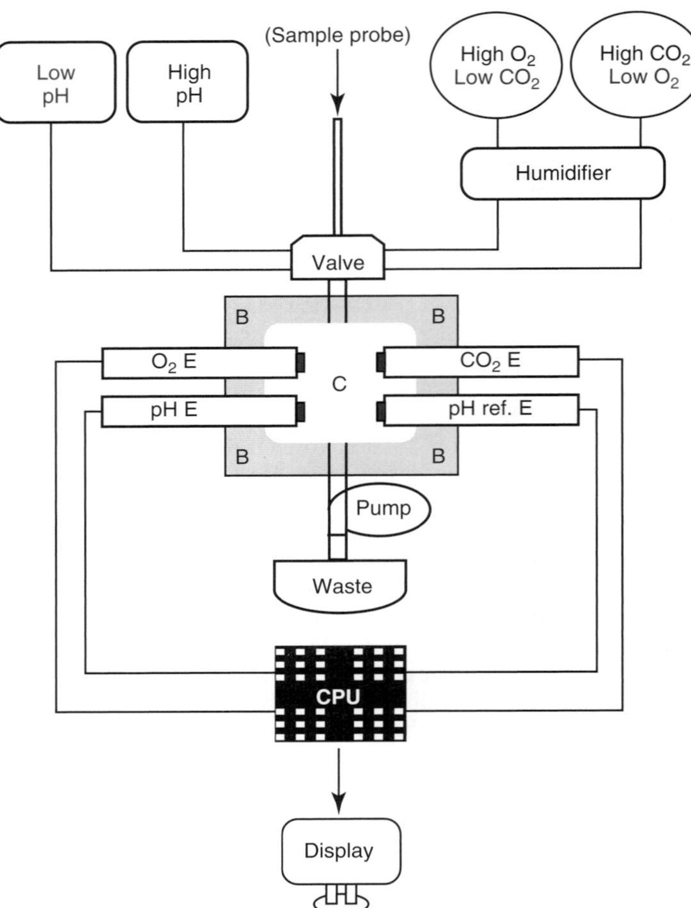

FIGURE 35.4 Diagram of Blood Gas Instrumentation. E (electrodes), pH, and gas standards are shown at the *top* of the diagram. *B,* Constant temperature bath at 37°C; *C,* chamber; *CO_2,* carbon dioxide; *CPU,* computer; *O_2,* oxygen.

Because electrodes are not stable over long periods of time, frequent calibration of pH, PCO_2, and PO_2 is required. The instrument (see Fig. 35.4) is designed so that a manually actuated or a microprocessor-actuated valve (self-calibrating) admits calibrator gases, standard buffers, or a sample to a small chamber (C) maintained at 37 ± 0.1°C. Most instruments contain a barometer so that barometric pressure *P*(Amb) is always known to the microprocessor during calibration. Other instruments perform point-of-care or bedside testing. Almost all manufacturers now produce small, portable, stand-alone, easy-to-operate instruments designed for "satellite lab" operations; several hand-held devices that use disposable electrodes are also available.[81] Readers are referred to Chapter 27 for a discussion of point-of-care testing.

Electrodes. The tip of the pH measuring electrode is made of H^+-sensitive glass (see Chapter 14), and aside from miniaturization, most pH measuring and reference electrodes differ little from those of free-standing pH meters. The membrane of the PCO_2 electrode usually consists of Teflon or silicone rubber approximately 25 μm thick. The electrolyte solution is a thin film containing NA HCO_3^- at 0.005 mol/L and NaCl at 0.1 mol/L saturated with AgCl. A spacer of nylon net or cellophane lies between the solution and the H^+-sensitive glass of the measuring element proper. As CO_2 diffuses from the sample into the electrolyte solution, the slight rise in (H^+) from its hydration reaction is measured as ΔpH by an especially sensitive potentiometer and is transformed electronically to Δlog PCO_2. The membrane of a PO_2 electrode in a standard blood gas analyzer is usually approximately 20-μm-thick polypropylene. The electrolyte solution is a thin film of phosphate buffer saturated with AgCl but also containing KCl; it is in contact with the polarized platinum cathode and the Ag/AgCl anode. As O_2 diffuses into the electrolyte, it reacts with the cathode to cause current to flow, which is measured.

Maintenance of Instrumentation. Sophistication of contemporary equipment and availability of high-quality calibrator materials have made reliable and accurate determination of blood pH and gases primarily a matter of meticulous maintenance, adherence to the manufacturer's recommended procedures, and control of the equipment and proper collection and handling of specimens. Software programs of the instrument's microprocessor often provide display warnings and diagnostic routines that alert the operator and assist in troubleshooting. The manufacturer's suggested maintenance schedule should be considered a minimum guideline, with reliance on experience to indicate maintenance frequency.

Cleanliness of the sample chamber and path is especially important. Automatic flushing to cleanse the sample chamber and path after each blood sample measurement is a feature of most instruments without disposable electrodes. Despite proper flushing, however, complete or partial clogging of the chamber or path, or both, may occur. Fibrin threads and small clots may be present in the specimen or may form while the sample resides in the warm chamber. If allowed to remain, they can affect subsequent measurements or calibrations by interfering with the contact of blood, buffers, or gases with electrode membranes. Visibility of the path through the heat sink is helpful for detecting clogs, dirt, and bubbles. Bubbles that fail to rinse out can be a particular problem if they settle on an electrode.

Quality Assurance and Quality Control

Elements of good quality assurance of blood gas and pH measurements include (1) proper maintenance of the instrument, (2) use of control materials, (3) verification of electrode linearity, (4) checking of barometer accuracy, and (5) accurate measurement of temperature.

External quality assurance (proficiency testing) mandated by federal law in the United States (Clinical Laboratory Improvement Amendments [CLIA] 1988) has assumed new importance for quality control of blood gas analysis. These rules became effective in January 1991 and set criteria for satisfactory interlaboratory performance, which are as follows: pH, target value ±0.04; PO_2, target value ±3 SD; and PCO_2, target value ±8% or ±5 mm Hg, whichever is greater. The significance of proficiency testing and the penalties for failure place strong incentives on consistent performance of internal control measures and effective response to failures of quality control. At the same time, pressures to control costs have raised the question of how many concentrations of control materials are necessary to monitor intralaboratory performance effectively and how often this should be done. Per CLIA 1988, the answer is one concentration of control every 8 hours, with the entire range of control concentrations covered in every 24-hour period. The CAP requires at least two concentrations of controls every 8 hours. In many laboratories, however, the practical answer is to run on every instrument in use, at least once per shift, three concentrations of control for pH, PO_2, and PCO_2, always on completion of maintenance and troubleshooting procedures. Newer analyzers, particularly the smaller satellite laboratory and point-of-care instruments, frequently have an *auto quality control* (QC) feature or use *electronic QCs*.[82] Auto QC consists of onboard QC material that is automatically analyzed by the instrument at designated intervals that fulfill regulatory requirements. Electronic QC, which is most common in devices with disposable electrode cartridges, consists of cartridges that verify the electronic specification of the instruments. For further discussion of these issues, see Chapter 27 on POCT.

Blood- and Fluorocarbon-Based Control Materials. Commercial blood-based control material usually consists of tanned human erythrocytes suspended in buffered medium and sealed in vials with a gas mixture of known O_2 and CO_2 content. Non-blood fluorocarbon materials with O_2-carrying properties similar to those of blood are also available. These products usually are made at three concentrations of pH, PCO_2, and PO_2. Unopened, these types of control materials have the advantages of a long shelf life in the refrigerator—20 to 28 days for tanned erythrocytes and even longer for the others.

Aqueous Fluid Control Materials. These materials consist of a buffered medium sealed in vials with gas mixtures; the fluid is equilibrated with the gas by vigorous shaking by hand immediately before the vial is opened, and a sample is admitted to the instrument. Coefficients of variation of 0.1% for pH, 2.5% for PCO_2, and 3.2% for PO_2 are common for these types of materials. The disadvantages of aqueous controls stem from their dissimilarity to blood. Lower viscosity and surface tension confer different washout characteristics and impair their ability to reflect clogging. Greater electrical conductivity reduces their effectiveness in detecting inadequate grounding, and lower thermal coefficients make them slower to detect failures of temperature control. Nevertheless, aqueous commercial controls are far and away the most common.

Sources of Analytical Error. General causes of analytical error include calibration of the instrument with incorrect set points for pH buffers or calibrator gases, degraded calibration materials, failure of temperature control of the measurement chamber, and a dirty sample chamber or path. Incorrect calibration may arise from wrong entries made for buffer or gas values into the microprocessor, from incorrect manual calculations of PCO_2 and PO_2 values by Dalton's law for calibrator gases, or from using gases that are dry because the humidification device is not working properly. Measurements of PO_2 are particularly sensitive to temperature error. To keep systematic error to 1% to 2%, the temperature control at 37°C must be within ±0.1°C. Built-in barometers can be checked by contacting nearby meteorologic stations. Gases other than O_2 present in a blood sample may affect performance of the PO_2 electrode. The anesthetic gases halothane and nitrous oxide have a direct effect because both can be reduced at the polarized cathode in competition with O_2. Under most circumstances, however, these effects are small and can be ignored.

Reference Intervals

Reference intervals for arterial blood PO_2, SO_2, PCO_2, and pH are extensively described in Chapter 60. Values for

PO_2 and PCO_2 will decrease with increasing altitude, but compensatory mechanisms keep pH values the same. The P_{50} corrected to pH 7.40 is 18 to 24 mm Hg for newborns and 24 to 29 mm Hg for adults. For more information, refer to the Appendix on Reference Intervals.

Temperature Correction of Measured pH, Partial Pressure of Carbon Dioxide, and Partial Pressure of Oxygen

In the Henderson-Hasselbalch equation, pK' and α are used as constants for a temperature of 37°C. The temperature-controlled sample chamber of an instrument is specified to be 37 ± 0.1°C, and it is at that temperature that all measurements of pH and partial pressure of gases are made. The body temperature of a febrile patient may be elevated to 40 to 41°C, or a patient may be made hypothermic for certain surgeries and have a temperature as low as 23°C. Most blood gas instruments on keyboard entry of a patient's actual temperature can calculate and present temperature-corrected pH and PCO_2. Correction of pH and PCO_2 to the actual temperature of the patient is usually omitted in states of hyperthermia. However, significant disagreement exists with respect to hypothermic states.[83]

The equation shown in Table 35.2 illustrates the complexity of the calculation used to correct PO_2 to the patient's body temperature.[62] Complexity is unavoidable because at PO_2 less than 100 mm Hg (SO_2 ≤0.95), the Hb–O_2 dissociation curve is shifted to the left by the decrease in temperature and by the concomitant rise in pH (see Fig. 35.4). For temperature corrections of PO_2 between 100 and 400 mm Hg, accurate formulas become even more complicated.

Continuous and Noninvasive Monitoring of Blood Gases

Obtaining arterial, venous, or capillary blood is an invasive procedure, and test results reflect conditions pertaining only to a single point in time. Repetitive sampling in intensive or acute care management carries risks, including infection and vascular complications. In premature infants particularly, repeated sampling imposes an undesirable blood loss. Decisive action during intensive cardiopulmonary care or cardiac surgery often demands continuous monitoring or discrete real-time data for blood gases.

Extensive discussion of noninvasive and continuous modes of monitoring is beyond the purview of this text. However, laboratorians must be aware of them, because blood samples and standard analytical equipment remain the reference for monitoring the effectiveness of such devices, and because responsibility for quality assessment and review for them is often assigned to the clinical laboratory. Some agencies, such as the CAP, have developed guidelines for laboratory oversight of "alternative test systems" that include transcutaneous and in vivo monitoring devices. Such guidelines state that "in some cases traditional approaches to management, quality control, etc. may not be directly applicable but that systems must be in place to ensure that accurate results are generated."

TABLE 35.2 Temperature Correction Formulas Recommended by the Clinical and Laboratory Standards Institute[62]

pH	$pH(T) = pH(37°C) - [0.147 + 0.0065 \times (pH(37°C) - 7.40)] \times [(T - 37°C)]$
PCO_2	$PCO_2\ (T) = PCO_2\ (37°C) \times 10^{[0.019 \times (T - 37°C)]}$
PO_2	$pO_2(T) = pO_2(37\ °C) \times 10^{\left(\frac{5.49 \times 10^{-11} \times pO_2^{3.88} + 0.071}{9.72 \times 10^{-9} \times pO_2^{3.88} + 2.30}\right) \times (T \cdot 37\ °C)}$

PCO_2, Partial pressure of carbon dioxide; *PO_2*, partial pressure of oxygen.

Pulse oximeters that continuously monitor SO_2Hb are common and are generally reliable.[69] Older pulse oximeters were susceptible to error depending on placement and motion, but technology has made these devices very reliable. Transcutaneous monitoring of PCO_2 and PO_2 is a noninvasive continuous monitoring approach that has been around for longer than 30 years and has had particular value and general success in neonatal and pediatric care.[84] These devices consist of gel-encased self-adhesive electrodes that heat the skin to 43 to 44°C to arterialize the capillaries and facilitate diffusion of O_2 through the skin.[85]

Transcutaneous monitoring of PO_2 can vary widely depending on whether the site of application reflects arterial, capillary, or venous blood flow. However, because there is little difference between arterial and venous PCO_2, transcutaneous monitoring of PCO_2 is less problematic, and pulse oximeters can often serve as a surrogate for PO_2. Transcutaneous monitoring works best in areas of thin skin, thus its popularity in neonates and in settings of euvolemia. In addition, hypovolemia can make pulse oximeter devices less reliable.[86] Nevertheless, their correlations with arterial co-oximetry are reasonable (r values ranging from 0.7 to 0.8), and they have been recommended for trending and monitoring. Transcutaneous monitoring can also be used to monitor local tissue perfusion after certain surgical procedures and trauma.[85]

In addition to monitoring PO_2 and PCO_2, new inline devices that also monitor pH, electrolytes, glucose, and hematocrit have been introduced to the market.[87] These consist of a single-use inline cartridge consisting of six conventional electrodes. The cartridge is attached to an arterial line and upon operator command withdraws approximately 1.5 mL of blood into the cartridge, where analysis takes place. The analytical time is approximately 60 seconds, after which the blood is returned via the arterial line. Cartridges undergo two-point calibration before they are placed in service, and a single-point calibration is used to flush the sensors after each analysis. Analysis can be repeated every 5 minutes, and it is claimed that cartridges can be used for up to 72 hours. In a multicenter study, results from 1414 paired sample measurements showed good agreement and correlation for results from an inline monitor compared with traditional laboratory methods.[87] The future of such devices will likely depend on costs versus benefits for patient care and outcomes.

SELECTED REFERENCES

For a full list of references for this chapter, please refer to ExpertConsult.com.

2. Nijsten MW, de Smet BJ, Dofferhoff AS. Pseudohyperkalemia and platelet counts. *N Engl J Med* 1991;**325**:1107.
7. Watson MA, Scott MG. Clinical utility of biochemical analysis of cerebrospinal fluid. *Clin Chem* 1995;**41**:343–60.

10. Zou J, Nolan DK, LaFiore AR, et al. Estimating the effects of hemolysis on potassium and LDH laboratory results. *Clin Chim Acta* 2013;**421**:60–1.
11. Mansour MM, Azzazy HM, Kazmierczak SC. Correction factors for estimating potassium concentrations in samples with in vitro hemolysis: a detriment to patient safety. *Arch Pathol Lab Med* 2009;**133**:960–6.
15. Don BR, Sebastian A, Cheitlin M, et al. Pseudohyperkalemia caused by fist clenching during phlebotomy. *N Engl J Med* 1990;**322**:1290–2.
20. Hill CE, Burd EM, Kraft CS, et al. Laboratory test support for Ebola patients within a high-containment facility. *Lab Med* 2014;**45**:e109–11.
24. Ladenson JH, Apple FS, Aguanno JJ, et al. Sodium measurements in multiple myeloma: two techniques compared. *Clin Chem* 1982;**28**:2383–6.
29. Sikaris KA. Physiology and its importance for reference intervals. *Clin Biochem Rev* 2014;**35**:3–14.
34. Gahm N, Shwachman H. Studies in cystic fibrosis of the pancreas; a simple test for the detection of excessive chloride on the skin. *N Engl J Med* 1956;**255**:999–1001.
36. Baker MW, Atkins AE, Cordovado SK, et al. Improving newborn screening for cystic fibrosis using next-generation sequencing technology: a technical feasibility study. *Genet Med* 2016;**18**:231–8.
38. Farrell PM, Rosenstein BJ, White TB, et al. Guidelines for diagnosis of cystic fibrosis in newborns through older adults: Cystic Fibrosis Foundation consensus report. *J Pediatr* 2008;**153**:S4–14.
40. DeMarco ML, Dietzen DJ, Brown SM. Sweating the small stuff: adequacy and accuracy in sweat chloride determination. *Clin Biochem* 2015;**48**:443–7.
43. Clinical and Laboratory Standards Institute (CLSI). *C34-A3. Sweat testing: sample collection and quantitative chloride analysis: approved guideline*. 3rd ed. Wayne, PA: CLSI; 2009.
61. Wagener JS, Zemanick ET, Sontag MK. Newborn screening for cystic fibrosis. *Curr Opin Pediatr* 2012;**24**:329–35.
64. Natelson S, Nobel D. Effect of the variation of pk' of the Henderson-Hasselbalch equation on values obtained for total CO2 calculated from pCO2 and pH values. *Clin Chem* 1977;**23**:767–9.
69. Haymond S, Cariappa R, Eby CS, et al. Laboratory assessment of oxygenation in methemoglobinemia. *Clin Chem* 2005;**51**: 434–44.
72. Kwant G, Oeseburg B, Zijistra WG. Reliability of the determination of whole-blood oxygen affinity by means of blood-gas analyzers and multi-wavelength oximeters. *Clin Chem* 1989;**35**:773–7.
74. Grocott MP, Martin DS, Levett DZ, et al. Arterial blood gases and oxygen content in climbers on Mount Everest. *N Engl J Med* 2009;**360**:140–9.
78. Andersen OS. Sampling and storing of blood for determination of acid-base status. *Scand J Clin Lab Invest* 1961;**13**:196–204.
80. Hess CE, Nichols AB, Hunt WB, et al. Pseudohypoxemia secondary to leukemia and thrombocytosis. *N Engl J Med* 1979;**301**:361–3.
81. Erickson KA, Wilding P. Evaluation of a novel point-of-care system, the i-stat portable clinical analyzer. *Clin Chem* 1993;**39**:283–7.
83. Bisson J, Younker J. Correcting arterial blood gases for temperature: (when) is it clinically significant? *Nurs Crit Care* 2006;**11**:232–8.

36

Hormones

Timothy J. Cole

ABSTRACT

Background

Hormones are a diverse group of compounds that circulate in body fluids at low variable concentrations, performing important signaling and communication roles between cells and tissues. Accurate measurement of hormone concentrations in patient samples is critical for accurate clinical diagnosis of acute illness and chronic disease.

Content

Endocrine hormones are chemical messengers that communicate between cells and tissues. They regulate development of the embryo, energy balance and integrated cellular metabolism, maintenance of homeostasis, cognition, and reproductive events throughout life. Hormones are classified into three major classes: polypeptide hormones, amino acid–derived hormones, and steroid- and vitamin-derived hormones. The synthesis and release of hormones from specialized endocrine cells and organs are tightly controlled. Each hormone is released for a specific purpose, has a defined half-life in circulation, and can negatively feedback to regulate subsequent hormone synthesis and release. Hormones act on target cells by binding to and activating specific protein receptors that are either imbedded in the cell plasma membrane or reside intracellularly. The two largest groups of cell surface receptors are the G-protein–coupled receptors (GPCRs) and the enzyme-coupled receptor families of proteins. Intracellular hormone receptors comprise the nuclear receptor (NR) superfamily. Receptor activation initiates intracellular signal transduction pathways that result in hormone-directed cellular and physiological change. Accurate monitoring of systemic hormonal status is critical for the clinical diagnosis of illness and disease caused by abnormal hormone concentrations or defective receptor-signaling interactions.

BACKGROUND

Hormones are chemical messengers synthesized and secreted by endocrine glands, organs, or isolated cells that have specific regulatory effects on the activity of target cells.[1] As a component of the endocrine system, hormones are produced at one site in the body, and in general, exert their action(s) at distant sites. Some hormones exert actions locally (paracrine), and other hormones exert their action on their cell of origin, regulating their own synthesis and secretion (autocrine). Classic endocrine hormones include insulin, thyroxine, and cortisol; neurotransmitters and neurohormones are examples of paracrine hormones, and certain growth factors that stimulate synthesis and secretion of other hormones from the same cell are examples of autocrine hormones. Table 36-1 lists hormones that are commonly measured in the clinical laboratory. Other hormones listed illustrate concepts and/or mechanisms of hormone action. Biochemical, clinical, and analytical information for specific hormones may be found in Chapters 42 and 57–72.

CLASSIFICATION OF HORMONES

Hormones are classified as (1) polypeptides or proteins, (2) derivatives of amino acids, and (3) steroids or vitamin derivatives.

Polypeptide or Protein Hormones

Adrenocorticotropic hormone (ACTH), insulin, and parathyroid hormone are examples of polypeptide or protein hormones. They are water soluble and circulate freely in plasma as the secreted complete molecule or as active or inactive fragments. The half-life of these hormones in plasma is relatively short (≤10–30 minutes), and their concentrations may vary dramatically depending on specific physiological and pathological states. These hormones initiate cellular responses by binding to a vast array of cell surface membrane receptors on target cells and activate intracellular signal-transduction pathways that lead to a specific action or changes within the target cell.[1,2] For example, insulin when released from pancreatic β-cells, binds to cell-surface insulin receptors at target tissues, such as the adipose and muscle, to promote the uptake of glucose from the bloodstream.

Amino Acid–Derived Hormones

Thyroid hormone such as thyroxine and the catecholamines are examples of hormones that are derived from amino acids; in both of these cases they are derived from tyrosine. They are water soluble and circulate in plasma bound to specific transport proteins (thyroxine) or circulate freely (catecholamines).[3,4] Thyroxine binds avidly to three specific binding proteins, transthyretin, thyroid-binding globulin,

Text continued on page 631

TABLE 36.1 Frequently Measured Hormones, Including Precursor Hormones and Cytokines

Endocrine Organ and Hormone	Hormone Type	Major Sites of Action	Principal Actions
Hypothalamus			
Thyrotropin-releasing hormone	Peptide (3aa, Glu-His-Pro)*	Anterior pituitary	Release of thyroid-stimulating hormone (TSH) and prolactin (PRL)
Gonadotropin-releasing hormone (Gn-RH)	Peptide (10aa)	Anterior pituitary	Release of luteinizing hormone (LH) and follicle-stimulating hormone (FSH)
Corticotropin-releasing hormone	Peptide (41aa)	Anterior pituitary	Release of adrenocorticotrophic hormone (ACTH) and β-lipotropic hormone (LPH)
Growth hormone-releasing hormone (GH-RH)	Peptides (40, 44aa)	Anterior pituitary	Release of growth hormone (GH)
Neuropeptide Y	36aa peptide released mainly from paraventricular neurons	Hypothalamus, thalamus, hippocampus, and gastrointestinal tract	Increased food intake, energy storage, reduced anxiety, and stress
Somatostatin[†] (SS) or growth hormone-inhibiting hormone (GH-IH)	Peptides (14, 28aa)	Anterior pituitary	Suppression of secretion of many hormones (eg, GH, TSH, gastrin, vasoactive intestinal polypeptide (VIP), gastric inhibitory polypeptide (GIP), secretin, motilin, glucagon, and insulin)
Prolactin-releasing peptide	Peptide (20aa)	Anterior pituitary	Release of PRL
Prolactin-releasing/inhibiting factor	Dopamine	Anterior pituitary	Suppression of synthesis and secretion of PRL
Kisspeptin	Peptide (54aa precursor cleaved to 13 and 14aa active peptides)	Gn-RH hypothalamic neurons	Stimulation of Gn-RH release via the G protein-coupled receptor GPR54
Anterior Pituitary Lobe			
Thyrotropin or TSH	Glycoprotein, heterodimer[‡] (α, 92aa; β, 112aa)	Thyroid gland	Stimulation of thyroid hormone formation and secretion
FSH	Glycoprotein, heterodimer[‡] (α, 92aa; β, 117aa)	Ovary	Growth of follicles with LH, secretion of estrogens, and ovulation
		Testis	Development of seminiferous tubules; spermatogenesis
LH	Glycoprotein, heterodimer[‡] (α, 92aa; β, 121aa)	Ovary	Ovulation; formation of corpora lutea; secretion of progesterone
		Testis	Stimulation of interstitial tissue; secretion of androgens
PRL	Peptide (199aa)	Mammary gland	Proliferation of mammary gland; initiation of milk secretion; antagonist of insulin action
GH or somatotropin	Peptide (191aa)	Liver	Production of insulin-like growth factor (IGF-1) (promoting growth)
		Liver and peripheral tissues	Anti-insulin and anabolic effects
Corticotropin hormone or ACTH	Peptide (39aa)	Adrenal cortex	Stimulation of adrenocortical steroid biosynthesis and secretion
β-Endorphin[†,§]	Peptide (31aa)	Brain	Endogenous opiate; raising of pain threshold and influence on extrapyramidal motor activity
Chorionic gonadotropin (CG) or choriogonadotropin	Glycoprotein, heterodimer[‡] (α, 92aa; β, 145aa)	Placenta	Maintenance of the corpus luteum (ovary) during pregnancy
α-Melanocyte-stimulating hormone (α-MSH)	Peptide (13aa)	Skin	Dispersion of pigment granules, darkening of skin
Leu-enkephalin (LEK)[†,§] and met-enkephalin (MEK)[†,§]	Peptide (5aa)	Brain	Same as β-endorphin

Continued

TABLE 36.1 Frequently Measured Hormones, Including Precursor Hormones and Cytokines—cont'd

Endocrine Organ and Hormone	Hormone Type	Major Sites of Action	Principal Actions
Posterior Pituitary Lobe			
Vasopressin or antidiuretic hormone	Peptide (9aa)	Arterioles Renal tubules	Increase of blood pressure; water reabsorption
Oxytocin	Peptide (9aa)	Smooth muscles (uterus, mammary gland)	Contraction; action in parturition and in sperm transport; ejection of milk
Pineal Gland			
Serotonin or 5-hydroxytryptamine (5-HT)	Indoleamine	Cardiovascular, respiratory, and gastrointestinal systems; brain	Neurotransmitter; stimulation or inhibition of various smooth muscles and nerves
Melatonin	Indoleamine	Hypothalamus	Suppression of gonadotropin and GH secretion; induction of sleep
Thyroid Gland			
Thyroxine (T_4) and triiodothyronine (T_3)	Iodoamino acids	General body tissue	Stimulation of oxygen consumption and metabolic rate of tissue
Calcitonin or thyrocalcitonin	Peptide (32aa)	Skeleton	Uncertain in humans
Parathyroid Gland			
Parathyroid hormone (PTH) or parathyrin	Peptide (84aa)	Kidney	Increased calcium reabsorption, inhibited phosphate reabsorption; increased production of 1,25-dihydroxycholecalciferol
		Skeleton	Increased bone resorption
Adrenal Cortex			
Aldosterone	Steroid	Kidney	Salt and water balance
Androstenedione[‖]	Steroid	Hormone precursor	Converted to estrogens and testosterone
Cortisol	Steroid	Many	Metabolism of carbohydrates, proteins, and fats; anti-inflammatory effects; others
Dehydroepiandrosterone (DHEA) and dehydroepiandrostenedione sulfate (DHEAS)	Steroids	Hormone precursors	Converted to estrogens and testosterone
17-Hydroxyprogesterone	Steroid	Hormone precursor	Converted to cortisol
Adrenal Medulla			
Norepinephrine and epinephrine	Aromatic amines	Sympathetic receptors	Stimulation of sympathetic nervous system
Epinephrine	Aromatic amines	Liver and muscle, adipose tissue	Glycogenolysis Lipolysis
Ovary			
Activin A	Peptides[¶] 2 β_A subunits	Pituitary, ovarian follicle	Stimulates release of FSH; enhances FSH action; inhibits androgen production by theca cells
Activin B	Peptides[¶] 2 β_B subunits	See activin A above	See activin A above
DHEA and DHEAS	Steroids	Hormone precursors	Converted to androstenedione
Estrogens	Phenolic steroids	Female accessory sex organs	Development of secondary sex characteristics
		Bone	Control of skeletal maturation
Follistatin	Peptides (288aa, 315aa)	Pituitary, ovarian follicles	Inhibits FSH synthesis and secretion by binding activin
Inhibin A	Peptide (α subunit and β_A subunit)	Hypothalamus, ovarian follicle	Inhibits FSH secretion; stimulates theca cell androgen production

TABLE 36.1 Frequently Measured Hormones, Including Precursor Hormones and Cytokines—cont'd

Endocrine Organ and Hormone	Hormone Type	Major Sites of Action	Principal Actions
Inhibin B	Peptide (α subunit and β_B subunit)	See inhibin A above	See inhibin A above
Progesterone	Steroid	Female accessory reproductive structure	Preparation of the uterus for ovum implantation, maintenance of pregnancy
Relaxin	Peptide[#]	Uterus	Inhibition of myometrial contraction
Testis			
Inhibin B	See above	Anterior pituitary, hypothalamus	Control of LH and FSH secretion
Testosterone	Steroid	Male accessory sex organs	Development of secondary sex characteristics, maturation, and normal function
Placenta			
Estrogens	See above	See above	See above
Progesterone	See above	See above	See above
Relaxin	See above	See above	See above
Chorionic gonadotropin (CG) or choriogonadotropin	Glycoprotein, heterodimer[‡] (α, 92aa; β, 145aa)	Same as LH	Same as LH; prolongation of corpus luteal function
Placental growth hormone	Peptides (22 and 26 kDa)	Same as GH	Same as GH
Chorionic somatomammotropin or placental lactogen	Peptide (191aa)	Same as PRL	Same as PRL
Pancreas			
Amylin	Peptide (37aa)	Pancreas	Inhibits glucagon and insulin secretion
Glucagon	Peptide (29aa)	Liver	Glycogenolysis
Insulin	Peptide[**]	Liver, fat, muscle	Regulation of carbohydrate metabolism; lipogenesis
Pancreatic polypeptide	Peptide (36aa)	Gastrointestinal tract	Increased gut motility and gastric emptying; inhibition of gallbladder contraction
SS[§]	Peptide (14aa)	Pancreas	Inhibition of secretion of insulin, glucagon
Gastrointestinal Tract			
Gastrin[§]	Peptide (17aa)	Stomach	Secretion of gastric acid, gastric mucosal growth
Ghrelin[§]	Peptide (28aa)	Anterior pituitary	Secretion of GH
Secretin	Peptide (27aa)	Pancreas	Secretion of pancreatic bicarbonate and digestive enzymes
Cholecystokinin-pancreozymin[§]	Peptide (33aa)	Gallbladder and pancreas	Stimulation of gallbladder contraction and secretion of pancreatic enzymes
Motilin	Peptide (22aa)	Gastrointestinal tract	Stimulation of gastrointestinal motility
VIP[§]	Peptide (28aa)	Gastrointestinal tract	Neurotransmitter; relaxation of smooth muscles of gut and of circulation; increased release of hormones and secretion of water and electrolytes from pancreas and gut
GIP	Peptide (42aa)	Gastrointestinal tract	Inhibition of gastric secretion and motility; increase in insulin secretion
Glucagon-like peptide-1	Peptide (30-31aa)	Gastrointestinal tract	Increase insulin and decrease glucagon secretion; inhibit gastric emptying
Bombesin[§]	Peptide (14aa)	Gastrointestinal tract	Stimulation of release of various hormones and pancreatic enzymes, smooth muscle contractions and hypothermia, changes in cardiovascular and renal function

Continued

TABLE 36.1 Frequently Measured Hormones, Including Precursor Hormones and Cytokines—cont'd

Endocrine Organ and Hormone	Hormone Type	Major Sites of Action	Principal Actions
Neurotensin[§]	Peptide (13aa)	Gastrointestinal tract and hypothalamus	Uncertain
Substance P[§]	Peptide (11aa)	Gastrointestinal tract and brain	Sensory neurotransmitter, analgesic; increase in contraction of gastrointestinal smooth muscle; potent vasoactive hormone; promotion of salivation, increased release of histamine
Kidney			
1,25-$(OH)_2$ cholecalciferol	Sterol	Intestine Bone	Facilitation of absorption of calcium and phosphorus; increase in bone resorption in conjunction with PTH
		Kidney	Increase in reabsorption of filtered calcium
Erythropoietin	Peptide (165aa)	Bone marrow	Stimulation of red cell formation
Renin-angiotensin-aldosterone system	Peptides (renin, 297aa; Ang I, 10aa; Ang II, 8aa, produced from Ang I by angiotensin-converting enzyme)	Renin (from kidney) catalyzes hydrolysis of angiotensinogen (from liver, 485aa) to Ang I in the intravascular space	Ang II increases blood pressure and stimulates secretion of aldosterone (see adrenal)
Liver			
IGF-1, formerly called somatomedin	Peptide (70aa)	Most cells	Stimulation of cellular and linear growth
IGF-2	Peptide (67aa)	Most cells	Insulin-like activity
Thymus			
Thymosin and thymopoietin	Peptides (28, 49aa)	Lymphocytes	Maturation of T lymphocytes
Heart			
Atrial natriuretic peptide (atriopeptin)	Peptide with an intrachain disulfide bond (28aa)	Vascular, renal, and adrenal tissues	Regulation of blood volume and blood pressure
B-type natriuretic peptide	Peptide with an intrachain disulfide bond (32aa)	Vascular, renal, and adrenal tissues	Regulation of blood volume and blood pressure
Adipose Tissue			
Adiponectin	Peptide oligomers of 30 kDa subunits	Muscle Liver	Increases fatty acid oxidation Suppresses glucose formation
Leptin	Peptide (167aa)	Hypothalamus	Inhibition of appetite, stimulation of metabolism
Resistin	Peptide (94aa)	Liver	Insulin resistance
Tissue necrosis factor-α	157aa secreted protein	Adipose in an autocrine or paracrine fashion	Pluripotent cytokine with a wide-range of actions.
Apelin	55aa protein	Adipose in an autocrine or paracrine fashion	Promotes angiogenesis locally in adipose tissue. Metabolic actions in adipose and muscle
Bone			
Osteocalcin	49aa	Bone, pancreas adipose tissue	Bone mineralization and calcium homeostasis, systemic metabolism
Osteopontin	314aa	Bone, pancreas, neutrophils	Bone remodeling, immune functions, chemotaxis
Osteonectin	285aa	Bone, paracrine action	Bone mineralization

TABLE 36.1 Frequently Measured Hormones, Including Precursor Hormones and Cytokines—cont'd

Endocrine Organ and Hormone	Hormone Type	Major Sites of Action	Principal Actions
Skeletal Muscle			
Myostatin	109aa monomer, active as a dimer	Skeletal muscle; paracrine actions	Inhibition of muscle differentiation and growth
Myonectin (CTRP15)	340aa	Adipose, liver	Promotes lipid uptake
Irisin (FNDC5)	112aa	White adipose tissue (WAT)	Conversion of WAT to Brown adipose tissue, increased thermogenesis
Multiple Cell Types			
Estrogens	See above	See above	See above
Galanin	Peptide (30aa)	Brain, pancreas, gastrointestinal tract	Regulates food intake, memory, and cognition; inhibits endocrine and exocrine secretions of pancreas; delays gastric emptying; prolongs colonic transport times
Parathyroid hormone-related peptide (PTH-RP)	Peptides (139, 141, 173aa)	Kidney, bone	Physiologic function conjectural; PTH-like actions; tumor marker
Growth factors (eg, epidermal growth factor, fibroblast growth factor, transforming growth factor family, platelet-derived growth factor, nerve growth factors)	Peptides	Many	Stimulation of cellular growth
Monocytes/Lymphocytes/Macrophages			
Cytokines (comprising; interleukins 1–37, Chemokines 1–48, type I, II, and III interferons, tumor necrosis factors, and lymphokines such as granulocyte macrophage colony-stimulating factor, granulocyte colony-stimulating factor	Peptides/small proteins	Many target cells and tissues	Stimulation or inhibition of cellular growth, plus other varied roles

**aa,* Amino acid residues.
†Also produced by gastrointestinal tract and pancreas.
‡Glycoprotein hormones composed of two dissimilar peptides. The α-chains are similar in structure or identical; the β-chains differ among hormones and confer specificity.
§Also produced in the brain.
‖Androstenedione is also produced in the ovary and testis.
¶Each activin and inhibin is found in multiple forms.
#Two chains linked by two disulfide bonds: α, 24aa; β, 29aa.
**Two chains linked by two disulfide bonds: α, 21aa; β, 30aa.

and albumin, and has a half-life of approximately 7 to 10 days; free-circulating catecholamines such as epinephrine have a short half-life of a minute or less. The catecholamines interact with a family of nine closely related cell surface adrenergic receptors[5] and initiate intracellular second messenger signal-transduction systems, whereas thyroid hormones move freely across the cell membrane to activate two specific intracellular NRs, thyroid hormone receptor-α and -β.

Steroid and Vitamin-Derived Hormones

Endogenous steroid hormones such as cortisol, estrogen, and testosterone are synthesized from cholesterol, are hydrophobic, and insoluble in water. These hormones circulate in plasma, reversibly bound to specific transport plasma proteins (eg, cortisol-binding globulin, sex hormone-binding globulin) with only a small fraction unbound that is freely circulating to exert physiological action. The half-life of circulating steroid hormones is 30 to 90 minutes. Free steroid hormones at their sites of action, because of their hydrophobicity, enter the cell by passive diffusion and bind with intracellular NRs in the cytoplasm or the nucleus.[6,7]

SYNTHESIS, RELEASE, AND GENERAL ACTION OF HORMONES

The physiological functions of hormones can be broadly categorized as those (1) affecting growth, development, and maturation; (2) control of systemic homeostasis, energy balance, and integrated metabolism; and (3) regulation of reproduction.

Synthesis and Release of Hormones

Many hormones are synthesized in specialized endocrine cells within specific endocrine glands. These include the polypeptide hormone insulin, which is synthesized in the β-cells of the pancreas; estradiol, which is synthesized in the granulosa cells of the ovary; and epinephrine (or adrenalin), which is synthesized by the medullary chromaffin cells of the adrenal gland. Some hormones require biosynthesis via complex enzymatic pathways, such as the cardiovascular hormone aldosterone, which is synthesized from precursor cholesterol in the outer zona glomerulosa cell layer of the adrenal cortex. Other hormones require simpler modification of a precursor compound such as vitamin D. All hormones attain a structural specificity that allows them to bind strongly to and activate specific receptors on target cells. In general, hormones are released from endocrine cells when they are required, either from intracellular stores or by induction of rapid biosynthesis. The biosynthetic pathways of hormones are critical to maintain homeostasis. Defects in those pathway enzymes can lead to debilitating endocrine disease, such as the genetic condition of congenital adrenal hyperplasia (CAH), which is a disease caused by mutations in the steroid biosynthetic enzymes of the adrenal cortex, which are required for production of cortisol, aldosterone, and androgen precursors from cholesterol.[8] The loss of end-product hormone production or the inappropriate buildup of steroid precursors can lead to complex cardiovascular and reproductive development dysfunction and gender ambiguity.[9] Examples of the three broad functional categories of hormone action are presented in the following and illustrate specific aspects on the synthesis, release, turnover, and action of endocrine hormones.

Growth, Development, and Maturation

Normal embryonic development and postnatal growth of the whole human organism is dependent on the complex integrative function of many hormones, including growth hormone, insulin-like growth factor-1 (IGF-1), thyroxine, the gonadal steroids (estrogen and androgen), and cortisol. Several pituitary hormones are responsible specifically for the growth and development of other endocrine glands, such as the adrenal, gonads, and thyroid; therefore, these hormones are responsible for control of synthesis and secretion of many secondary hormones. These hormones provide important negative feedback control on the secretion of the pituitary hormones. Other regulators of secretion of the pituitary hormones include circadian rhythms and the hypothalamic pulse generator that controls the pulsatile secretion of gonadotropins. Examples of hormones from the anterior pituitary gland that are important for growth and development include the following:

- Growth hormone is synthesized and secreted by pituitary somatotroph cells and stimulates the production and release of hepatic IGF-1. Both factors then have broad somatic growth actions, particularly in bone and cartilage.
- ACTH derived from the proopiomelanocortin precursor protein regulates growth of the adrenal glands and the synthesis and secretion of adrenal gland steroid hormones such as cortisol and androgen precursors (see Chapters 66 and 68).
- Pituitary thyrotroph-derived, thyroid-stimulating hormone (TSH) regulates the growth of the thyroid gland and the iodination of tyrosine residues in thyroglobulin to eventually produce the thyroid hormones triiodothyronine and thyroxine (see Chapter 65 and 67).

Energy Homeostasis and Integrated Metabolism

Energy homeostasis and the activity of many metabolic pathways in cells are tightly regulated by a diverse number of systemic and locally released hormones. There is a continual change in demand for energy use and storage during states such as feeding, exercise, starvation, infection, injury and/or trauma, or emotional stress. These states initiate the release and action of many hormones to regulate energy use and nutrient metabolism, modulate energy storage, and regulate physical and behavioral responses to stress. These hormonal activated pathways in cells are complex and may involve hormones from different organs. In general, systemic nutrient uptake, appetite, energy storage, and release are under neurological control via actions of specific hypothalamic and neuroendocrine hormones (eg, leptin and neuropeptide Y).[10]

The following are examples to illustrate the feedback control of hormone secretion and action, which is critical for homeostasis:

- Regulation of blood glucose concentrations: in response to a glucose load, insulin is promptly released from the pancreatic β-cells, which regulate the uptake of glucose into peripheral metabolic tissues (fat, muscle, liver, and brain) for the metabolism necessary to produce energy from glucose (see Chapter 33). As circulating glucose concentrations return to preload concentrations, insulin secretion slows. Several counter-regulatory hormones come into play to further regulate this process to ensure that blood glucose concentrations do not become too low. These include glucagon, cortisol, epinephrine, and growth hormone. Recent attention has focused on a group of gastrointestinal hormones termed "incretins" (see Chapter 62) that are released during eating and stimulate insulin secretion from the pancreas in advance of any measurable increase in blood glucose. Incretins also affect the rate of absorption of nutrients from the gut by slowing down the rate of gastric emptying. Another mechanism by which incretins have a role in the regulation of blood glucose is by delaying release of the counter-regulatory hormone glucagon from the α cells of the pancreatic islets. The most studied incretins are glucagon-like peptide-1 and gastric inhibitory peptide.[11]
- Regulation of serum calcium (see Chapter 64): the calcium-sensing receptor on the parathyroid gland

recognizes the ambient concentration of ionized calcium, which in turn regulates the synthesis and secretion of the hormone PTH. When ionized calcium concentrations fall (so imperceptibly that most analytical methods cannot detect the change), PTH synthesis and secretion are stimulated. Increased plasma concentrations of PTH will restore serum ionized calcium by enhancing renal tubular reabsorption of calcium and calcium efflux from bone. PTH also catalyzes the synthesis of the renal hormone calcitriol (1, 25-dihyroxycholecalciferol), which acts on the gut to increase intestinal absorption of calcium. These rapid responses of PTH and calcitriol quickly restore ionized calcium to concentrations in which the calcium-sensing receptor is no longer activated, and PTH and calcitriol synthesis and secretion return to basal levels.

- Water and electrolyte homeostasis is regulated by the steroid hormone aldosterone released from the adrenal gland, renin from the kidney, and vasopressin (antidiuretic hormone) from the posterior pituitary gland (see Chapters 60, 65, and 66).

Endocrine Control of Reproduction

The gonadotropin hormones luteinizing hormone (LH) and follicle-stimulating hormone (FSH) are released from pituitary gonadotroph cells in response to hypothalamic gonadotropin-releasing hormone to regulate the development, growth, and functions of the ovary and testis (see Chapter 68). In turn, the ovarian and testicular hormones estradiol and testosterone, respectively, initiate and regulate the following: pubertal growth; development and maintenance of secondary sex characteristics; the growth, development, and maintenance of the skeleton and muscles; and in part, the distribution of body fat.

CELL SIGNALING MECHANISMS OF HORMONE RECEPTORS

The specific action of an endocrine hormone on its target cell or tissue is a function of the interaction between the hormone and its cognate receptor. As discussed previously, several types of hormone-receptor interactions occur with cells and an individual cell may express and contain hundreds of different receptors that may be responding to multiple specific hormones at any given time.[1,12] The hormone-receptor complex provides the strong specificity of the hormone's action, eliciting a target tissue response. Many endocrine hormones circulate in picomolar or nanomolar concentrations (10^{-9} to 10^{-12} mol/L) but elicit specific and strong responses in specific target cells. Hormone receptors may be present on the cell surface imbedded in the plasma membrane or reside intracellularly within the cytoplasm or nucleus.

Cell Surface Hormone Receptors

Polypeptide or hydrophilic hormones bind to cell surface receptors, and the conformational change or the protein–protein interactions initiated resulting from this binding activates an effector system within the cells, which is responsible for the downstream actions of the hormone (Fig. 36-1).[12] For many peptide and polypeptide hormones, the intracellular effector that is activated by the hormone–receptor interaction is a specific intracellular G-protein (guanylnucleotide–binding protein),[12-14] and the cell surface receptors are called GPCRs (Fig. 36-2). GPCRs are the largest family of cell surface receptors, with approximately 830 genes coding for human GPCRs.[15] GPCRs are large proteins with seven membrane-spanning domains, an amino-terminal, a hormone-binding domain that is extracellular,

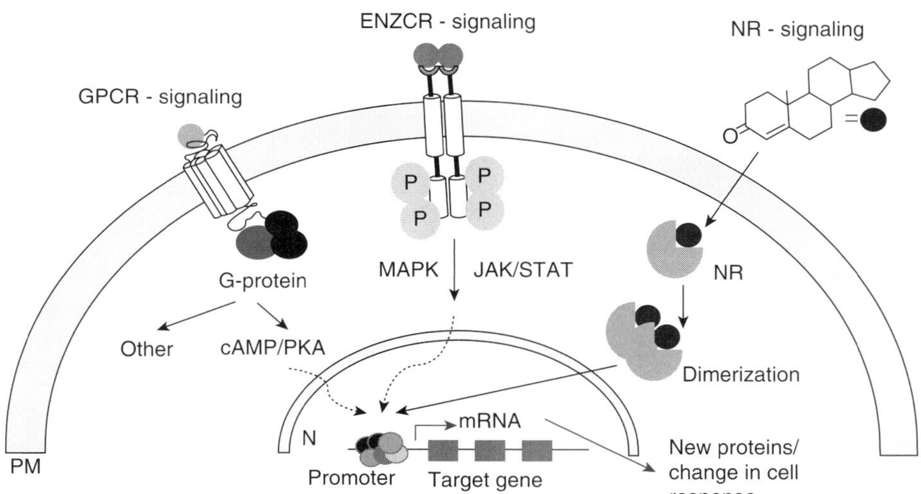

FIGURE 36.1 Endocrine Cell Signaling Is Mediated by Both Cell Surface and Intracellular Hormone Receptors. Cell surface receptors comprise two main classes of proteins called G-protein–coupled receptors *(GPCR)* and enzyme-coupled receptors *(ENZCR)*, whereas intracellular hormone receptors form the nuclear receptor *(NR)* superfamily of proteins. Cell surface receptors bind a circulating hormone using a specific extracellular protein domain and transduce a signal to the interior of the cell. In contrast, receptors for lipophilic hormones (eg, a steroid hormone) reside within the cell, in many cases in the cytoplasm in an inactive complex of proteins. The activated NR is then targeted to the nucleus. *cAMP*, Cyclic adenosine monophosphate; *JAK/STAT*, Jak kinase/STAT pathway; *MAPK*, MAP kinase pathway; *N*, nucleus; *P*, phosphate; *PKA*, protein kinase A; *PM*, plasma membrane.

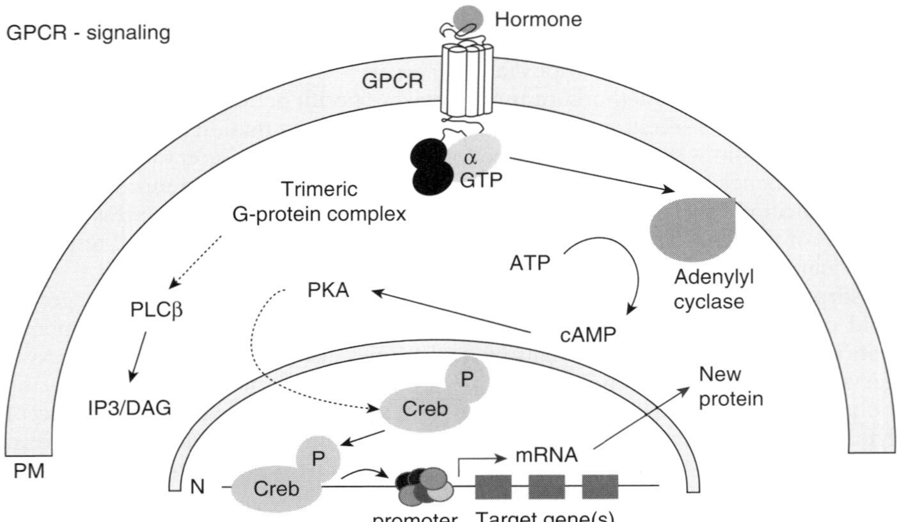

FIGURE 36.2 Endocrine Signaling via Cell Surface G-Protein–Coupled Receptors *(GPCRs)*. Binding of a hormone to the extracellular domain of a GPCR initiates a conformation change within the seven-transmembrane GPCR that promotes binding to an intracellular trimeric G-protein complex. Activation of the G-protein α subunit leads to stimulation of downstream effector proteins (eg, the enzyme adenylate cyclase) that produces cyclic adenosine monophosphate *(cAMP)*, a potent second messenger. cAMP activates protein kinase A *(PKA)*, which is then able to initiate other phosphorylation cascades within the cell, such as activation in the nucleus of the cAMP-response element binding protein *(Creb)*. Activation of other G-proteins (such as G_q) leads to stimulation of the effector enzyme phospholipase C-β *(PLCβ)* and the production of the second messengers inositol 1,4,5-trisphosphate *(IP_3)* and diacylglycerol *(DAG)*, which activate other pathways, such as activation of protein kinase C *(PKC)*.

and an intracellular carboxy-terminal tail of loop domains. The major structural groups of GPCRs have been identified and include four main classes, each of which contains receptors for specific subsets of hormones (see Table 36-1).[15] The class A GPCRs contain the Rhodopsin-like receptors that include receptors for olfactory compounds and melatonin; class B represents the secretin-like GPCRs (receptors for secretin, glucagons, and vasoactive intestinal polypeptide); class C, the largest by number, contains the metabotropic glutamate and/or pheromone receptors; and the class D contains fungal mating pheromone receptors. Stimulation of a G-protein initiates the specific intracellular signal transduction pathways that characterize the specific actions of the hormone. G-proteins are composed of α, β, and γ subunits, and are classified according to the α subunit, 20 of which have been identified to date. The many classes of GPCRs and G-proteins briefly described in this section provide some insight into the mechanisms responsible for the specificity of hormone action. The second major class of cell surface hormone receptors is the enzyme-coupled receptors (Fig. 36-3). These receptors have been divided into six subfamilies of receptors, of which the most well-characterized family is the receptor tyrosine-kinase (RTK) group of receptors, which mediate the actions of many common hormones and growth factors, such as insulin, IGF-1, epidermal growth factors, and fibroblast growth factors.[16] These receptors are characterized by initiating intracellular kinase cascades and regulating cell growth and metabolism, and are common targets for mutation in tumor cells.[17]

Intracellular Nuclear Receptors

Lipid-soluble steroid hormones (eg, estradiol) are primarily transported bound to plasma proteins such as albumin, with only a small fraction of the hormone circulating free or unbound. Free hormone enters the cell via passive diffusion and in most cases binds to intracellular NRs in the cytoplasm, or in some cases the nucleus (Fig. 36-4). NRs are characterized by a hormone or ligand-binding domain, a central DNA-binding domain, and an amino-terminal variable domain that contributes to recruitment of nuclear proteins such as transcriptional coactivators.[18] In a similar way to activated cell surface receptors, a change in the conformation of the NR is caused by binding of a lipid-soluble hormone to the ligand-binding domain. This conformational change, or activation of the receptor, enables the cytosolic hormone-receptor complex to move to the nucleus and bind to specific regulatory DNA sequences of a target gene, which permits a change in specific gene expression (see Fig. 36-4).

POSTRECEPTOR INTRACELLULAR SIGNAL TRANSDUCTION PATHWAYS

Receptors at the cell surface and intracellular NRs initiate a variety of different postreceptor cellular responses by activating complex intracellular signal transduction pathways. This is shown schematically in Fig. 36-1 for three classes of hormone receptors. Binding of the hormone or ligand to the receptor initiates activation of the receptor and initiation of

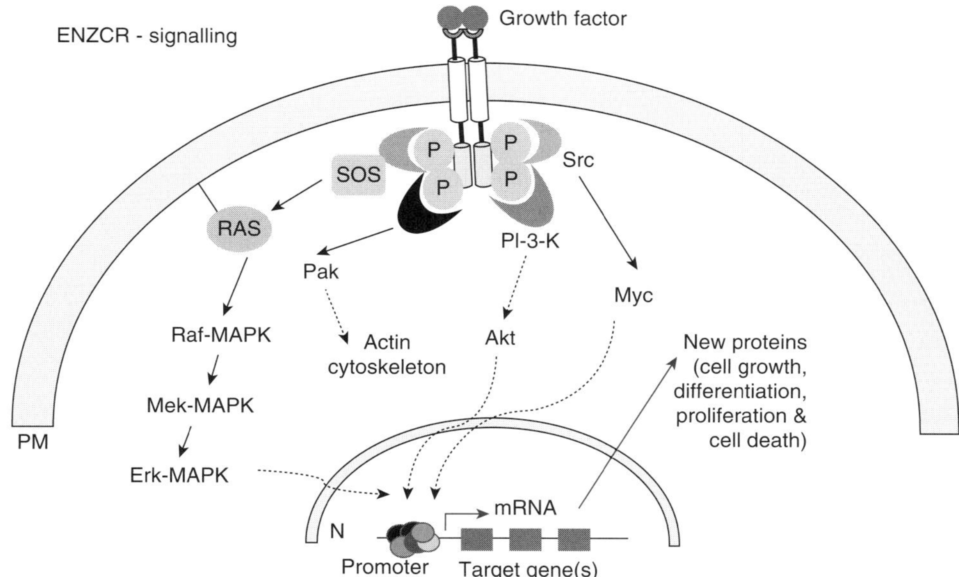

FIGURE 36.3 Endocrine Signaling via Cell Surface Enzyme-Coupled Receptors *(Enzcrs).* Binding of a circulating growth factor protein to an ENZCR promotes receptor dimerization and the autophosphorylation of the intracellular domains of the receptors by intrinsic kinase catalytic domains. Phosphorylated residues act as docking sites for SH2-domain–containing proteins that bind and transmit receptor activation via a variety of signaling cascades that involve the Ras/MAP kinase pathway *(MAKP)*, the phosphoinositol-3-kinase pathway *(PI-3-K)*, activation of c-Myc, and cytoskeletal changes via the kinase Pak. These activated pathways lead to cellular changes that include cell proliferation, differentiation, and cell death, and specific changes in nuclear gene expression programs. Raf, Mek, and Erk are members of the MAPK kinase pathway. Akt is a downstream mediator of the PI-3-kinase pathway. *SOS,* Son of sevenless.

downstream signaling that cause cellular changes both in the cytoplasm and the nucleus. Each of these three receptor-activated intracellular signaling pathways is described in more detail in the following.

SIGNAL TRANSDUCTION FROM CELL SURFACE G-PROTEIN–COUPLED RECEPTORS

The GPCRs are seven transmembrane proteins that are activated by a variety of hormones that include amino acids, small peptides, polypeptides, lipids, and odorant and/or taste compounds.[15] The intracellular C-terminal tail of the activated GPCR interacts directly with members of the G-proteins that are organized in a trimeric complex of an α, β, and γ G-protein subunit. Active G-protein subunits initiate signaling cascades via activation of specific enzymes, generating molecules that serve as potent second messengers to mediate the hormone response within the cell. The best known effector enzyme is adenylyl cyclase, which generates the second messenger cyclic adenosine monophosphate (cAMP), and phospholipase C, which generates both inositol 1, 4, 5-trisphosphate (IP_3) and diacylglycerol (see Fig. 36-2) from inositol phospholipids. The binding of a small number of hormone molecules on the cell surface leads to the production of a larger number of second messenger molecules, thus amplifying the signal initiated by the hormone. The cAMP-dependent protein kinases are a family of enzymes that, in the presence of cAMP, phosphorylate a number of intracellular enzymes and other proteins to activate or inactivate the function of these enzymes and proteins, thereby regulating their function. Phospholipase Cβ (see Fig. 36-2) acts on inositol phospholipids within the cell membrane to produce IP_3, which opens up ion channels to facilitate entry of calcium into the cytoplasm, where it acts as a messenger, and diacylglycerol, which modulates protein kinase C activity. Because hormones largely serve regulatory functions, many self-limiting steps are involved in more proximal biosynthetic processes. Without such self-limiting processes, hormone action would continue unabated. For cAMP, cessation of hormone action involves the inactivation of G-protein stimulation of adenylate cyclase by guanosine triphosphatase (GTPase). In the absence of hormone interaction with the GPCR (basal or unstimulated state), the G-protein is bound to guanosine diphosphate (GDP). Once the hormone is bound to the receptor, GDP is released from the G-protein and is replaced by GTP, and the G-protein–GTP complex activates adenylate cyclase. The G-protein–GTP complex is inactivated by GTPase, restoring the G-protein–GDP state, which cannot stimulate formation of cAMP until further hormone binding to the GPCR takes place. Within a few minutes (or less) of hormone–GPCR interaction and the initiation of hormone action, the receptor is phosphorylated by protein kinase A and protein kinase C. This phosphorylation of the hormone receptor permits internalization of the complex from the cell surface into the cytoplasm where dephosphorylation occurs, permitting degradation of the hormone and recycling of the GPCR to its original transmembrane location, awaiting coupling with more hormone.

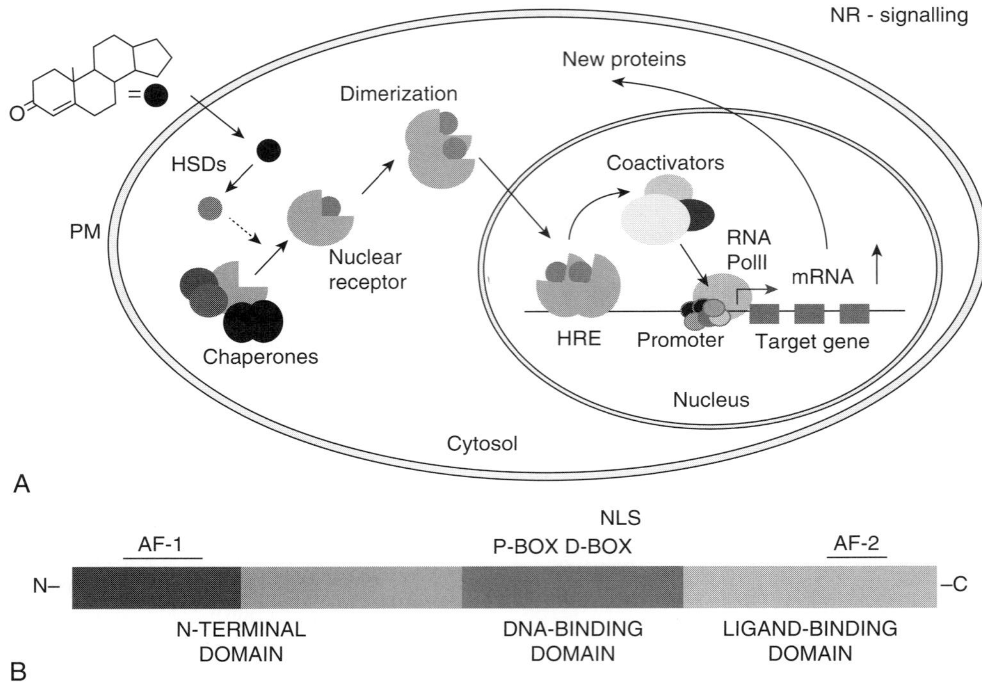

FIGURE 36.4 Endocrine Signaling by Intracellular Nuclear Receptors *(NRs).* **A,** NR signaling pathway in eukaryotic cells. Signaling is shown for a steroid hormone that enters the cell by passive diffusion. A number of steroids are converted to their active form from inactive precursors by enzymes such as hydroxysteroid dehydrogenases *(HSDs).* The bioactive steroid binds to the ligand-binding domain *(LBD)* of the NR, disrupting associated chaperone proteins, and triggers a conformational change in the NR that reveals a nuclear localization sequence *(NLS),* and promotes NR dimerization and nuclear translocation. In the nucleus, the NR dimer binding to specific hormone response elements *(HREs)* in the genomic DNA recruits co-activator or repressor proteins that enable direct interaction with target gene promoters to recruit RNA polymerase II *(RNA Pol II),* and modulation of the rate of gene transcription. **B,** Schematic domain structure of the nuclear receptor superfamily of proteins. Important functional protein domains are depicted for the nuclear receptor superfamily from the N- to C-terminus. *AF-1,* Activation function domain 1; AF-2, activation function domain 2; D-Box, sequence critical for receptor dimerization; *P-box,* sequence critical for DNA binding.

SIGNAL TRANSDUCTION FROM CELL SURFACE ENZYME-COUPLED RECEPTORS

The insulin receptor is a member of the second major class of cell surface hormone receptors, called the enzyme-coupled receptors. These have been classified into six subfamilies of enzyme-coupled receptors, with the best characterized being the RTKs.[16] These receptors mediate the actions of many common growth factor hormones such as the epidermal, fibroblast, platelet-derived, and vascular endothelial growth factors. RTKs are single transmembrane spanning proteins that dimerize upon hormone binding, an event that initiates intracellular signaling responses (see Fig. 36-3). The receptor dimer is then auto-phosphorylated by intrinsic C-terminal tyrosine kinase catalytic domains. The phosphorylated Tyr residues act as specific binding sites for effector proteins, such as phosphoinositol-3-kinase (PI-3-kinase) and phospholipase C-γ, which then transmit the signal within the cell (see Fig. 36-3). These effector proteins contain SH2 domains that specifically recognize phosphotyrosine residues on the activated receptor.[19] MAP–kinase pathway activation results in subsequent gene activation, as well as cell proliferation and differentiation.[20] These pathways do not use second messengers but involve activated enzyme cascades. RTKs and downstream signaling components are often mutated in cancer cells that then acquire a high proliferative phenotype. Gene mutations often produce constitutively active receptors or signaling effectors such as RAS and PI-3-kinase.[17]

SIGNAL TRANSDUCTION FROM INTRACELLULAR NUCLEAR RECEPTORS

In general, lipid-soluble hormones bind and activate the ligand-binding domain of intracellular NRs that then signal specific changes to the nucleus (see Fig. 36-4).[3] The human genome contains a group of 48 NR genes that encode the NR superfamily of receptors and are activated by a range of lipophilic steroid, dietary lipids, vitamins, fatty acid, and special small molecule ligands (eg, thyroid hormone). A large number of these receptors are still classified as orphan receptors with no known hormone ligand, and little is understood of their functional role in human biology and in clinical disease. Hormone binding initiates a conformational change that enables the hormone-receptor complex to localize to the nucleus and bind specific regulatory DNA hormone response elements (HREs) near to specific target genes.[3,21,22] Hormone translocation of the cytoplasmic NRs to the nucleus, once activated, is mediated by a conformational change in the receptor that exposes a nuclear localization sequence normally located within the DNA-binding domain. The binding specificity of the activated NR for specific HREs near the target gene is determined by the first zinc finger in the receptor's DNA-binding domain. Binding of the hormone-receptor complex to HREs promotes recruitment of a co-activator, and sometimes, co-repressor proteins that ultimately mediate activation or repression of gene transcription. Messenger RNA levels of target genes can be enhanced up to 1000-fold, leading to large changes in the synthesis of specific proteins that then drive cellular and physiological change. In addition to these nuclear gene expression changes, many NRs can be activated to produce rapid so-called "non-genomic" effects in the cytoplasm or at the cell membrane.

CLINICAL DISORDERS OF HORMONE ACTION

Although several chapters of this textbook detail a variety of endocrine disorders, a brief introduction to endocrine disorders is given here. In general, endocrine diseases may result from a deficiency or an excess of a single hormone or several hormones, or from resistance to the action of hormones in target cells. Hormone deficiency can be congenital (genetically inherited) or acquired, and hormone excess can result from endogenous overproduction (from within the body) or from exogenous overmedication. Hormone resistance can occur at several levels but can most simply be characterized as receptor-mediated, postreceptor-mediated, or at the level of the target tissue. The clinical manifestations will depend on the hormone system affected and the type of abnormality.

Metabolic Endocrine Disorders

Diabetes mellitus (DM) is an example of an endocrine metabolic disorder; it is the most common endocrine disorder in Western countries (see Chapter 57). It is classified as either type 1 or type 2. DM type 1 results from failure of the pancreas to secrete insulin although the pancreas is otherwise normal. Type 2, the most common form of DM, results from end-organ resistance to the action of insulin, which, in this case, is secreted from the pancreas in abundant amounts and circulates at high concentrations. Secondary DM occurs when a nonendocrine disease, such as pancreatitis, destroys the pancreas, including the insulin-secreting cells. The biochemical hallmark of DM is hyperglycemia. In contrast to diabetes, there are uncommon, insulin-producing tumors of the pancreas (insulinomas) in which the production of insulin is not regulated by the blood glucose concentration and the biochemical hallmark of the tumors is hypoglycemia. Thus, hyperglycemia can be present when there is insulin deficiency or insulin excess, and insulin excess can accompany both hyperglycemia and hypoglycemia. This simple illustration underscores the homeostatic and/or regulating nature of the endocrine system.

Reproductive Disorders: Congenital Adrenal Hyperplasia

Steroid hormone production in the adrenal cortex is critical for postnatal life. The adrenal gland is able to biosynthesize the steroids cortisol, aldosterone, and androgen precursors using a complex series of enzymatic reactions that modify the substrate cholesterol. Deficiencies in any of these important steroid biosynthetic enzymes can lead to defects in adrenal steroid production and lead to the clinical condition of CAH.[8,9] The most common genetic deficiency that affects young children is the loss of the enzyme 21-hydroxylase and is characterized by glucocorticoid (cortisol) and mineralocorticoid (aldosterone) deficiency associated with genital virilization and hyperandrogenism in females.[9] Clinical treatment of CAH relies on replacement of cortisol and aldosterone, sodium supplements, and reducing excess androgen secretion via blocking of ACTH secretion.

MEASUREMENT OF HORMONES AND RELATED ANALYTES

Hormones are measured by a variety of analytical techniques, including bioassay, receptor assay, immunoassay, and instrumental techniques, such as mass spectrometry interfaced with liquid or gas chromatography. A general overview of these techniques is given here. Analytical details for individual hormones using such techniques are found in the discussion of the individual hormones in their respective chapters.

Bioassay Techniques

Bioassays are based on observations of physiological responses specific for the hormone being measured. In vivo bioassays usually involve the injection of test materials (such as blood or urine from a patient) into suitably prepared animals; target gland or organ responses such as growth or steroidogenesis are then measured. In vitro bioassays involve the incubation of tissue samples, membranes, dispersed cells, or permanent cell lines in a defined culture medium, with subsequent measurement of an appropriate hormone response. Most in vitro bioassays measure responses proximal or distal to a second messenger such as stimulation of cAMP formation. Bioassays tend to be imprecise and are now rarely used in clinical medicine.

Receptor-Based Binding Assays

Receptor assays depend on the in vitro interaction of a hormone with its biological receptor. In this type of assay, unlabeled hormone displaces trace amounts of radioactively labeled hormone from specific receptor sites. A second approach is to measure a response, such as production of cAMP, when a test sample is added to a preparation that includes the receptor and the necessary co-factors. In general, receptor-binding assays are simpler to perform and have greater sensitivity than bioassays. Receptor-binding assays also have an advantage over immunoassays in that they reflect the biological function of a hormone, namely, the capacity to combine with specific receptors. By contrast, immunoassays may measure active hormone and inactive prohormone, hormone polymer, and metabolites when all share the common antigenic determinant or set of determinants of the assay antibody. In general, receptor-binding assays are not as sensitive as immunoassays, and proteolytic enzymes in the biological specimen may sometimes degrade the receptor or destroy the labeled tracer. The added complexity and lability of receptor preparations also contribute to the limited application of these assays in the routine clinical laboratory.

Immunoassay Techniques

Enzyme-linked immunosorbent assays or standard immunoassays that use specific antibodies are widely used to quantify hormones (see Chapter 23). Currently labeled antibody (immunometric) assays with nonisotopic labels are the method of choice for measuring concentrations of most hormones, especially peptides and proteins. Immunometric assays use saturating concentrations of two or more antibodies (often monoclonal) that are prepared against different epitopes of the protein molecule. One of the two antibodies is usually attached to a solid phase separation system and extracts the hormone from the serum specimen. The second antibody is linked to a signal molecule, which is then measured. The resultant signal is used to quantify the bound hormone.

Instrumental Techniques

Mass spectrometry coupled with gas and liquid chromatographs (see Chapters 16–21) are powerful qualitative and quantitative analytical tools that are widely used to measure hormone concentrations.[23-26] Technical advancements in mass spectrometry have resulted in the development of matrix-assisted laser desorption and/or ionization and electrospray ionization techniques that allow sequencing of peptides and mass determination of picomole quantities of analytes. Compared with older methods, tandem mass spectrometry offers greater analytical sensitivity, accuracy, and speed, and may allow simultaneous determination of multiple hormones related to a clinical condition.[26]

Specimen Requirements

To prevent preanalytical variation, appropriate protocols must be followed when sending samples to the laboratory for hormone measurement. Some hormones are directly affected by food (eg, insulin) or by circadian variability (eg, cortisol). In many clinical circumstances, the metabolic environment plays a crucial role in hormone production, and it is essential to obtain a simultaneous sample for measurement of both the hormone and the molecule(s) regulated by that hormone. An isolated measurement of plasma insulin without concurrent knowledge of the plasma glucose, or measurement of PTH independent of serum calcium, is of little, if any value. When a patient is evaluated for possible hormone deficiency or hormone excess, it is often necessary to perform a stimulation or suppression test. Most hormone assays can be performed on plasma or serum, and many can be performed on urine samples, usually a 24-hour collection. Increasingly, saliva has become a convenient body fluid for hormone analysis, particularly for hormones secreted in a diurnal rhythm (eg, cortisol). Unlike blood sampling, which requires the patient to present to a blood drawing facility, patients can be provided with salivary collection material so they can provide specimens to the laboratory collected at multiple times during the day or at unusual (but biologically relevant) times such as 11 PM—a commonly used time for obtaining a specimen for measurement of cortisol. For additional information on preanalytical and biological variability, see Chapters 4 and 5, respectively.

POINTS TO REMEMBER

- Hormones provide communication and regulation of activities between cells and tissues of the body
- Hormones are a diverse group of lipid-based, amino acid-derived and polypeptide molecules
- Hormones bind and activate specific protein receptors at target cells
- Hormone receptors are located both at the plasma membrane and in the cytoplasm of the cells
- Hormones trigger complex intracellular signaling cascades to bring about cellular changes

37

Vitamins and Trace Elements

*Norman B. Roberts, Andrew Taylor, and Ravinder Sodi**

ABSTRACT

Background

An adequate supply of vitamins and trace elements is critical for maintaining optimum health. Measurements of vitamin and trace element concentrations are frequently helpful in nutritional assessment and may be a requisite in suspected deficiency or toxicity, and in the management of patients with cystic fibrosis, patients undergoing bariatric surgery, and for those on nutritional support in the intensive or critical care unit. There is also great public interest in and many misconceptions regarding vitamins and trace elements.

Content

This chapter describes the chemistry, dietary sources, absorption, transport, metabolism, excretion, functions, and recommended intakes of the essential vitamins and trace elements required in humans. These include: the fat-soluble vitamins A, E, and K with the exception of vitamin D; the water-soluble vitamins B_1, B_2, B_6, B_{12}, C, folate, biotin, niacin, and pantothenic acid; and the trace elements chromium (Cr), cobalt (Co), copper (Cu), iodine (I), manganese (Mn), molybdenum (Mo), selenium (Se), and zinc (Zn). Free radicals, their measurement, and the trace elements fluoride (F^-), boron (B), silicon (Si), and vanadium (V) are briefly discussed. The causes and effects of vitamin and trace element deficiency and toxicity are outlined, and the laboratory assessment of the status, preanalytical variables that affect methods, and the suggested reference intervals are critically evaluated. Some illustrative cases are included. For methodologic details, readers are invited to access the original references listed online at ExpertConsult.com.

HISTORICAL PERSPECTIVE

Ancient Egyptians knew that eating ox liver could cure night blindness.[1] During ocean voyages to discover new lands and trade, sailors endured prolonged periods without fresh fruits and vegetables that resulted in vitamin deficiencies.[2] In 1747, the Scottish surgeon James Lind discovered that citrus fruits could prevent scurvy, a disease that caused poor wound healing, bleeding of gums, and a typical perifollicular hemorrhagic rash among others symptoms in sailors.[3] He recommended using lemons and limes, which was adopted by the British Royal Navy, which led to the nickname "Limey" for their sailors. In parts of Asia where polished white rice is a staple food, lack of vitamin B_1 resulted in beriberi. In 1884, a Japanese navy physician, Takaki Kanehiro, made the observation that beriberi was endemic in low-ranking crews who only ate rice.[4] With the support of the Japanese Navy, he undertook experiments using two crews; one fed only white rice and the other a mixed diet, and observed that the former had a higher incidence of beriberi. Unfortunately, he concluded that insufficient protein was the cause. It was not until 1897, when Christiaan Eijkman discovered that feeding unpolished rice rather than the polished variety to chickens, helped prevent beriberi in them.[5] Hopkins and Eijkman were awarded the Nobel Prize for Physiology or Medicine in 1929 for their discovery of several vitamins.[6] Around the turn of the 20th century, it was recognized that nutritional deficiencies caused diseases in addition to the then prevailing germ theory of disease.[7] Until the 1930s, when the first commercial yeast extract vitamin B complex and synthetic vitamin C tablets were first sold, vitamins were obtained solely through food. Today, vitamin and food supplements are a multibillion dollar industry, but it has been argued that they offer little benefit beyond consuming a healthy, balanced diet.[8] There is an increasing need for improved regulation in the vitamin industry, which is also plagued with false medical claims.[9] Specialist clinical laboratories have expanded their test repertoire to include the measurement of vitamins and trace elements. In this chapter, the biochemistry and clinical application of the commonly measured vitamins and trace elements are discussed. For a list of suggested reading on vitamins and trace elements, see Box 37.1.

VITAMIN AND TRACE ELEMENT STATUS

An adequate supply of micronutrients (vitamins and trace elements) is critical for maintaining health. There is increasing public awareness that good nutrition, including supplementation with vitamins and trace elements, is necessary to maintain quality of life. Evidence for regular use of micronutrient supplements is only available from randomized trials in a few selected groups. The general principle regarding assessment of nutritional status is to determine the

*The authors gratefully acknowledge the contributions of Donald B. McCormick, Harry L. Green, George G. Klee, David R. Milne, Malcolm Baines, and Alan Shenkin, on which portions of this chapter are based. They also thank Dr. Dinesh Talwar and the Scottish Trace Element & Micronutrient Reference Laboratory for advice on vitamin measurements.

BOX 37.1 Suggested Reading

1. Shenkin A. The role of vitamins and minerals. *Clin Nutr* 2003;22:S29–32.
   An important account of the historical and scientific context in which vitamins and minerals were incorporated into clinical practice.
2. Bates CJ. Vitamin analysis. *Ann Clin Biochem* 1997;34: 599–626.
   A good and timeless reference for the measurement of vitamins.
3. Taylor A. Detection and monitoring of disorders of essential trace elements. *Ann Clin Biochem* 1996;33:486–510.
   An authoritative and comprehensive description of the clinical indications and measurement of essential trace elements.
4. Frausto da Silva JJR, Williams RJP. *The biological chemistry of the elements: the inorganic chemistry of life.* 2nd ed. Oxford, UK: Oxford University Press; 2001.
   A classic text in simple prose that elegantly describes the role of the inorganic elements in nature and their evolution.
5. Valko M, Leibfritz D, Moncol J, Cronin MT, Mazur M, Telser J. Free radicals and antioxidants in normal physiological functions and human disease. *Int J Biochem Cell Biol* 2007;39:44–84.
   One excellent review of free radical theory, measurement, and associations with disease states.
6. Rosenfeld L. Vitamine—vitamin. The early years of discovery. *Clin Chem* 1997;43:680–685.
   An account of the history of vitamin research describing contributions of the early pioneers.
7. Battersby AR. How nature builds the pigments of life: the conquest of vitamin B_{12}. *Science* 1994;264:1551–1557.
   Although every vitamin has a fascinating story of discovery, intrigue, and delineation of function, the story of cobalamin may be resonant because of the current developments regarding the investigation of vitamin B_{12} deficiency. This paper gives a glimpse into the history of how one vitamin was conquered.
8. Ayling R, Marshall WD. *Nutrition and laboratory medicine.* London: ACB Venture Press; 2007.
   An authoritative textbook of the assessment of nutritional status.

extent to which the metabolic demand for nutrients has been or is currently being met by the supply. In clinical practice, this requires balancing supply and demand.

Accurate assessment of supply and intake is a complex process. In practice, a crude estimate of intake is obtained from a careful clinical history obtained by an experienced practitioner or from a food frequency questionnaire that summarizes the content of the individual's diet over several days, depending on how frequently particular typical foods are consumed.[10] A more accurate quantitative assessment usually requires a minimum of 3 days' recording of a complete dietary diary, which is subsequently analyzed using a computer program with reference tables of the nutritional contents of most foods.[10] Unfortunately, estimates of portion size, amounts consumed, and actual nutritional composition of the food consumed may be inaccurate. In addition, disease processes affect the amount actually consumed and absorbed, further reducing the accuracy of the estimate of nutritional intake.

Requirements for most nutrients, including the micronutrients to maintain health, have been characterized and made available in reports from the Institute of Medicine (IOM) of The National Academies.[11,12] However, the effects of disease may increase demands. For example, hypermetabolism, as a result of trauma or infection, increases the need for protein, energy, and micronutrients.[13] Increased losses from the gut, kidney, and skin, or through dialysis, may also increase the overall demand for these nutrients.[14]

An estimate of supply is also obtained from a careful dietary history, together with knowledge of any artificial nutritional supplements or therapy that may have been provided enterally or intravenously. Table 37.1 summarizes the Recommended Dietary Allowance (RDA)[11,12] used in the United States and the Population Reference Intakes[15] (from the European Union) for micronutrients. These amounts are expected to be present in the normal diet of healthy adults. Table 37.1 also summarizes the amounts present in 2000 kcal of most tube feeds used in nutritional support. It is clear that the amounts used enterally are greater than the oral amounts recommended in health to meet the increased needs that result from preexisting deficiencies and due to the disease process itself. The amounts recommended for supply during intravenous nutrition (IVN) are also summarized in Table 37.1. For the trace elements, these amounts are generally less than the oral and/or enteral requirements to allow for reduced absorption enterally. For the vitamins, these are usually greater than the oral and/or enteral requirements to allow for the effects of disease.

In an attempt to improve accuracy of assessing nutritional status, clinicians turn to the laboratory for a measurement that may reflect the net balance of supply and demand.[14,16-19] Laboratory scientists need to be aware of when such tests are useful, their limitations, especially in acutely ill patients, and how to interpret results in the context of the clinical situation.

Nutritional assessment in health and disease is considered in detail in Chapter 56. Measurements of micronutrient concentrations are undertaken as part of the nutritional assessment.

Although requirements for vitamins and trace elements in health are known (see Table 37.1), the effects of illness on these requirements are poorly understood and quantified. However, as depletion becomes more severe, biochemical or physiologic consequences pass through a series of subclinical stages. The metabolic or physiologic penalty of suboptimal nutritional status usually is not clear, but the assumption remains that suboptimal metabolism is likely to have detrimental effects (eg, subclinical deficiency of folic acid is associated with an increase in serum homocysteine concentration, which has been proposed to be an independent risk factor for coronary artery disease, although folate supplements do not reduce this risk).[20] Similarly, subclinical deficiency of Cr may be associated with impaired glucose tolerance and diabetes.[21]

The time course for development of a subclinical deficiency state varies for each individual vitamin and trace element, and depends on the nature and quantity of body stores. Moreover, the extent of depletion necessary before significant changes occur is poorly characterized. The consequences of

TABLE 37.1 Oral and Intravenous Micronutrient Intakes for Adults

	RDA (USA)	PRI (Europe)	Some Natural Food Sources*	Amount in 2000 kcal Tube Feed†	IV Intake‡
Vitamins					
A (μg)	900 (men); 700 (women)	700	Liver, yellow/orange fruits, leafy vegetables, fish, soya milk, milk	1000–2160	1000
E (mg)	15	0.4/g PUFA	Fruits and vegetables, meats, vegetable oils, unprocessed cereals, nuts, and seeds	20–64	9.1
K (μg)	120 (men); 90 (women)	100–200	Leafy green vegetables, especially spinach, eggs, liver	150	
B_1 (mg)	1.2 (men); 1.1 (women)	1.1	Brown rice, vegetables, potatoes, liver, eggs	1.4–3.4	6
B_2 (mg)	1.3 (men); 1.1 (women)	1.6	Vegetables, such as green beans and asparagus, bananas, dairy products	2–6	3.6
B_6 (mg)	1.3 (men and women <50 yrs); 1.7 (men >50 yrs); 1.5 (women >50 yrs)	1.5	Meat, bananas, vegetables, nuts	2–13.8	6
B_{12} (μg)	2.4	1.4	Meat and animal products	3–15	5
Folate (μg)	400	200	Leafy vegetables, cereal especially if fortified, bread, pasta, liver	340–880	600
C (mg)	90 (men); 75 (women)	45	Fruits especially citrus fruits and vegetables	100–300	200
Biotin (μg)	30§	15–100	Eggs, liver, kidney, pancreas, yeast, milk	100–660	60
Niacin (mg)	16 (men); 14 (women)	18	Meat, fish, eggs, vegetables, mushrooms, nuts	18–45	40
Pantothenic acid (μg)	5§	3–12ǁ	Meat, vegetables like broccoli, avocadoes, grains	7–20	15
Trace Elements					
Zinc (mg)	11 (men); 8 (women)	9.5	Red meats and some seafood	13–36	3.2–6.5
Copper (mg)	0.9	1.1	Organ meats, seafood, nuts, seeds, grains, cocoa products	2–3.4	0.3–1.3
Selenium (μg)	55	55	Organ meats, seafood, nuts, vegetables (dependent of soil selenium content)	30–130	40–100
Chromium (μg)	35 (men); 25 (women)§	30–200	Cereals, meats, fish	10–20	
Molybdenum, (μg)	45§	74–240	Legumes, grains, and nuts	19	
Manganese (mg)	2.3 (men); 1.8 (women)§	1–10ǁ	Nuts, legumes, tea, grains	2.4–8	0.05–0.2

Reference intakes for infants and children are age- and weight-dependent and are summarized in various sources[11,101]

For information regarding vitamin D, see Chapter 64.

*National Academies Press. Dietary reference intakes: vitamins. https://www.nationalacademies.org/hmd/~/media/Files/Activity%20Files/Nutrition/DRIs/DRI_Vitamins.pdf; and National Academies Press. Dietary reference intakes: elements. http://nationalacademies.org/hmd/~/media/Files/Activity%20Files/Nutrition/DRIs/New%20Material/6_%20Elements%20Summary.pdf.

†Shenkin A. Adult micronutrient requirements. In: Payne-James J, Grimble G, Silk D, editors. *Artificial nutrition support in clinical practice.* London: GMM; 2001:193–212.

‡Helphingstine CJ, Bistrian BR. New Food and Drug Administration requirements for inclusion of vitamin K in adult parenteral multivitamins. *JPEN J Parenter Enteral Nutr* 2003;27:220–4; Shenkin A, Allwood MC. Trace elements and vitamins in adult intravenous nutrition. In: Rombeau JL, Rolandelli RH, editors. *Clinical nutrition: parenteral nutrition.* Philadelphia: WB Saunders; 2001:60–79; and American Medical Association Department of Foods and Nutrition. Working conference on parenteral trace elements. *Bull N Y Acad Med* 1984;60:1115–212.

§Adequate intake.

ǁAcceptable range.

PRI, Population reference intake (Europe)[15]; *PUFA,* polyunsaturated fatty acid; *RDA,* recommended dietary allowance (United States).[11,12]

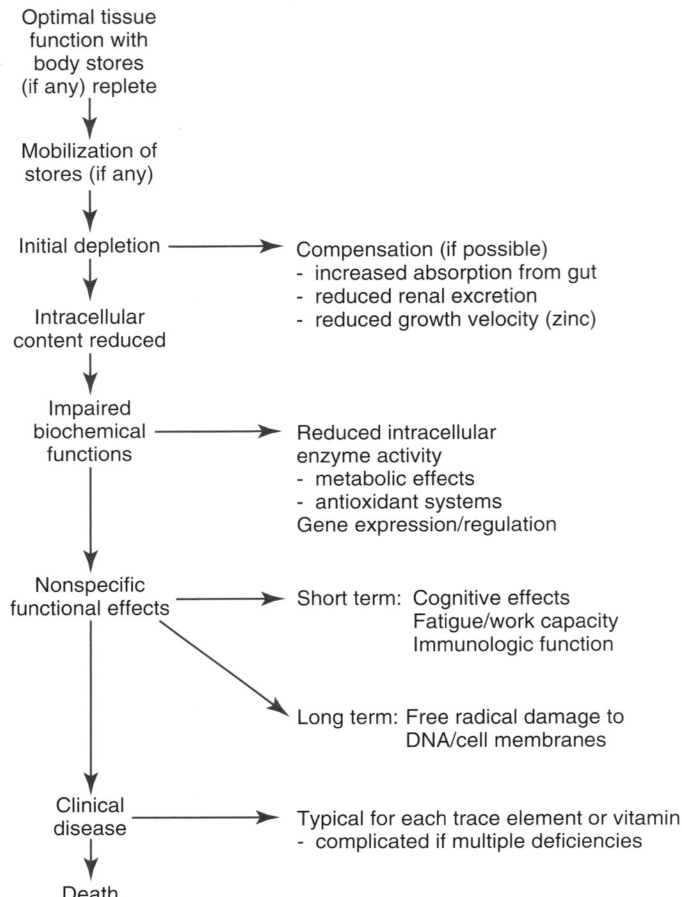

FIGURE 37.1 **Consequences of Inadequate Mineral or Trace Element Intake.** (From Shenkin A, Allwood MC. Trace elements and vitamins in adult intravenous nutrition. In: Rombeau JL, Rolandelli RH, editors. *Clinical nutrition: parenteral nutrition.* Philadelphia: Saunders, 2001:60–79.)

an inadequate intake are illustrated in Fig. 37.1 for a variety of biochemical and nonspecific physiologic effects. Fig. 37.1 shows a progression from optimal tissue status through a period of initial depletion until a period of subclinical deficiency is reached. In some cases, certain nonspecific histological changes may put the individual at risk of tissue damage or neoplastic change. With persistent mismatch of intake and demand, a full blown clinical deficiency state could develop.

GENERAL CONSIDERATIONS IN THE ANALYSES OF VITAMINS

Reference Intervals and Biological Variation

As for all laboratory tests, interpretation of tests of nutritional status requires access to relevant reference intervals and an understanding of factors that may alter them. Different laboratories and methods will inevitably have different reference intervals. It is important to note that reference intervals are only a guide and must be considered in the clinical context because deficiencies might still be present. Variables such as age, gender, ethnicity, and geographic location might affect the choice of typical diet and its chemical composition, thereby varying the concentration of vitamins. These factors introduce both within- and between-subject biological variation.[22] Seasonal variations may also alter the reference intervals of vitamins (eg, vitamins D[23] and A[24]).

Enzymes as Surrogate Markers of Vitamin Status

Several enzymes are dependent upon specific vitamins for functionality and may therefore be used as a surrogate measure of the vitamin's status.[25] These include erythrocyte enzymes such as transketolase, which is a marker of thiamine status, glutathione reductase, which is a marker for riboflavin, or transaminase which is a marker for pyridoxine. Glutathione peroxidase (GSHP) measured in plasma or erythrocytes may be used as an index of Se status. These are discussed further in the following sections.

Plasma Concentrations

Concentrations of vitamins and trace elements are measured most often in plasma or serum; this provides a reliable index of status for only a few of them (for example, vitamin B_{12} and vitamin D).[25] For others (eg, folate), their concentrations may reflect only the adequacy of recent intake. For some vitamins and trace elements, serum measurement is of limited value, especially in seriously ill patients. In part, this is a result of the lack of correlation between the amount of nutrient in the plasma compartment and the amount within the intracellular compartment in most body tissue. For example, substantial stores of particular vitamins or trace elements may be present in individual tissue (eg, vitamin A in the liver), but mobilization into the plasma is affected by the availability of appropriate binding proteins or by altered metabolism during the acute phase of an illness. Also, differences in the content of individual vitamins have been noted among tissues, but this may not be reflected in serum concentrations.

Tissue Concentrations

Tissue concentrations of vitamins or trace elements are rarely measured in nutritional assessment because this involves biopsy; however, when such tissue is available, measurement may be helpful (eg, Cu analysis of a liver biopsy of patients with suspected Wilson disease).[26] More commonly, certain types of cells may be obtained from blood samples and can provide useful information. For example, red cell folate is often used as a marker of folate status,[27] and leukocyte ascorbic acid is considered to be a better indicator of body stores than plasma ascorbate, but its use has not been widely adopted because of the large sample volume requirement, the difficulty involved in automating the analysis, the influence of fluctuating leukocyte numbers, and the relative difficulty of the analysis.[28,29]

Urine Measurements

For most vitamins, their measurements in urine are rarely helpful because most are not under homeostatic control, and excretion may be a direct reflection of recent intake rather than active retention in the face of whole body deficiency. Urine measurements indicate loss particularly of water-soluble, low-molecular-weight complexes (free or nonprotein-bound) and may be more useful in assessing overall removal and or exposure. High concentrations of excretion of certain water-soluble vitamins or trace elements may indicate ingestion of large quantities of supplements and not necessarily be a reflection of a deficiency or toxicity. However, pantothenic acid is measured primarily in urine.[30] Some metabolites of vitamin metabolism may be measured in urine (eg, the assessment of niacin status has been based on measurement of the two urinary metabolites, *N*′-methylnicotinamide and *N*′-methyl-2-pyridone-5-carboxamide).[31] Urinary excretion of biotin and 3-hydroxyisovaleric acid also appear to be better indicators of biotin status than blood concentrations alone.[32] The presence of low urinary iodide indicates iodide intake from a poor diet and is recommended by the World Health Organization (WHO) as a marker of iodine status.[33]

Effect of Inflammation on Vitamins

The concentration in plasma of various vitamins and trace elements can alter significantly when a systemic inflammatory response syndrome (SIRS) (previously known as the acute-phase response) results from trauma or infection.[34,35] This usually occurs independently of tissue stores.[34,36] The associated changes may be a result of variations in the binding proteins in plasma, such as albumin or retinol-binding protein (RBP), which decrease as part of SIRS. Studies in patients with SIRS as categorized on the basis of increased C-reactive protein (CRP) concentrations have documented decreases in vitamin A,[37,38] E,[35,37,39] B_2,[37] B_6,[40] C,[39,41] D,[42] carotenoids,[38] and changes in the concentrations of many trace elements.

In patients who are relatively stable, with minimal SIRS after injury, infection, or other inflammatory disease, it may be possible to interpret the plasma concentrations of trace elements or of vitamins.[41] One study in 1303 patients whose samples were referred to the Scottish Trace Element and Micronutrient Reference Laboratory for assessment of their micronutrient status examined the effect of the magnitude of SIRS on plasma micronutrient concentrations with the aim of providing guidance on the interpretation of results.[35] The findings are shown in Table 37.2. The study concluded that the degree of inflammatory response affected the interpretation of plasma micronutrient concentrations and demonstrated that a reliable clinical assessment could only be made if the CRP was less than 10 mg/L for vitamins A and D or less than 5 mg/L for vitamins B_6 and C.[35] There have been guidelines issued on nutrition support by national bodies such as the National Institute for Health and Care Excellence in the United Kingdom that recommend the monitoring of micronutrient concentrations in patients who receive total parenteral nutrition (TPN);[43] therefore, when implementing these guidelines, it is important to take the effect of SIRS into account when deciding on nutritional support (Table 37.2).[16] Also see Box 37.2 for illustrative case.

FREE RADICALS AND ANTIOXIDANTS

A free radical is any chemical species (atom, ion, or molecule) capable of independent existence that has an unpaired electron in an orbit, in most cases rendering them highly reactive. The hydrogen atom is the simplest radical because it contains only one electron. Free radicals can be formed by the loss or gain of a single electron from a nonradical, for example, the superoxide species (O_2^-) generated during the reduction of molecular oxygen (O_2) that occurs in the electron transport chain. Reactive O_2 species are chemically reactive molecules containing O_2, for example, hydrogen peroxide (H_2O_2), which is formed by the dismutation of O_2^- or direct reduction of O_2. Free radicals can be formed endogenously in the body by external stimuli such as irradiation, chemicals from air pollutants, or as byproducts of cellular metabolism. Most O_2 radicals are generated in the mitochondria by the electron transport chain. Several heme proteins generate O_2^- in the presence of O_2 catalyzed by transition metal ions, particularly iron (Fe) or Cu.

Free radicals have important functions in the body:

- Defense against microorganisms: phagocytic cells such as macrophages and neutrophils use free radicals to destroy infective agents.[46]
- Signal transduction: free radicals have been shown to act in numerous signaling pathways such as the nuclear factor-κβ signaling pathways, which are crucial for immunity, cell development, and growth.[47]
- Mitogenic effects: gene expression has also been shown to be altered by free radicals in both a deleterious and desirous manner.[48]

Free radicals have been implicated in various diseases, including atherosclerosis, cancer, diabetes mellitus, and neurological conditions such as Parkinson disease and Alzheimer disease.[46,49] Mechanisms involved in these diseases include damage to DNA strands,[50] lipid peroxidation,[51] and protein degradation.[52]

Organisms have evolved intricate ways of combating free radical damage. These include enzymatic and nonenzymatic antioxidants.[46] An antioxidant is a substance produced in sufficient quantity that neutralizes the lone electron of free radicals. Enzymatic antioxidants include peroxidases (eg, GSHP, catalase, and superoxide dismutase). Nonenzymatic

TABLE 37.2 Median Plasma Vitamin Concentrations According to C-Reactive Protein (CRP) Concentrations[35]

CRP concentration (mg/L)	Vitamin A (μmol/L)	Vitamin D (nmol/L)	Vitamin B_6 (μmol/L)	Vitamin C (μmol/L)
≤5	2.0	34	48	23
>5–10	2.0	33*	27*	18
>10–20	1.8*	31*	32*	17*
>20–40	1.6*	27*	24*	8*
>40–80	1.4*	23*	18*	6*
>80	1.0*	20*	15*	5*

Conversion factors for traditional units: Vitamin A: divide by 0.0349 to micrograms per deciliter; vitamin D: divide by 2.496 to nanogram per milliliter; vitamin B_6: divide by 4.046 to nanogram per milliliter; and vitamin C: divide by 56.78 to milligram per deciliter.
*Significant ($P < 0.05$) decrease compared with CRP category ≤5 mg/L.

BOX 37.2 Case: A 45-Year-Old Man With Low Vitamins and Trace Metals in the Intensive Trauma Unit[44]

A 45-year-old man, who had been previously fit and well, was admitted to the intensive trauma unit (ITU) after a car accident that resulted in multiple fractures and a subdural hematoma. He underwent craniotomy and decompression. He remained hemodynamically stable over the next few days with continuous ventilation. He was fed enterally via a nasogastric tube. He had no history of alcohol or recreational drug use and no significant past medical history. After 5 days in ITU, a micronutrient screen together with routine blood tests were ordered. The results for vitamins and selected trace elements were as follows:

Micronutrient	Result (Local Reference Interval)	Result (Local Reference Interval)
Vitamin A	0.5 µmol/L (1.0–2.8)	14 µg/dL (29–80)
Vitamin E	10 µmol/L (15–40)	0.4 mg/dL (0.6–1.7)
Vitamin C	10 µmol/L (15–90)	0.17 mg/dL (0.26–1.6)
Vitamin B_6	13 nmol/L (20–140)	3.2 ng/mL (5–35)
Beta carotene	0.6 µmol/L (1.6–5.8)	34 µg/L (90–310)
Zinc	8 µmol/L (12–18)	52 µg/dL (78–118)
Selenium	0.3 µmol/L (0.8–2.0)	24 µg/L (63–157)
Total protein	45 g/L (60–80)	4.5 g/dL (6.0–8.0)
Albumin	16 g/L (35–50)	1.6 g/dL (3.5–5.0)
CRP	120 mg/L (<3)	120 mg/L (<3)

Commentary

There was a significant decrease in the plasma concentration of all the measured vitamins and trace elements, which might suggest the patient developed a deficiency of micronutrients. C-reactive protein (CRP) is a positive acute-phase reactant and rises with acute inflammation or infection.[34,37] Albumin is a negative acute phase reactant, and most patients in the ITU tend to have a low concentration.[34] These results indicate the presence of a systemic inflammatory response and have important implications for interpreting vitamin and trace element results. Most trace elements and vitamins are negative acute-phase reactants, and therefore, when measured in the presence of acute inflammation, they will be low and may be interpreted to indicate micronutrient deficiency.[35] In inflammation, there is an increase in capillary permeability that results in leakage of albumin into the extracellular space. Because many macronutrients are bound to albumin and other circulating proteins, there is a transient fall in the measured concentration. On full recovery, there is normalization of micronutrient concentrations. Other causes of low micronutrients during the inflammatory response include sequestration in the liver and other organs, increased use in the catabolic state, and increased renal excretion.[37,45] The short duration of acute illness in the patient in this case was not sufficient to result in micronutrient deficiency, especially because of his apparent healthy state before the accident. In this case supplementation was not indicated.

Modified with permission from Murphy MJ, Srivastava R, Gaw A. *Case studies in clinical biochemistry*. Glasgow, UK: SA Press, 2012:103–4.

antioxidants include ascorbic acid (vitamin C), α-tocopherol (vitamin E), glutathione, carotenoids, flavanoids, urate, and proteins (eg, albumin, transferrin, and ceruloplasmin). The balance between free radical and antioxidant activity is crucial because both have important physiological roles.[53] It is also possible that the reducing agent (antioxidant) may facilitate pro-oxidant activity by regenerating the oxidized forms involved in the reduction process (eg, the production of H_2O_2 and hydroxyl radicals in the presence of Fe^{3+}). Similarly, it has been proposed that Se toxicosis exerts pro-oxidant activity due to methyl-selenide formation with the production of superoxide radicals and induction of oxidative stress.[54]

Measuring Free Radical Activity

Because it is not possible to measure all the active antioxidants in human samples, the concept of a "global" assessment of antioxidant capacity has been used.[55] The main approaches to measurement include: (1) quenched or delayed production of a stable, measurable radical species, for example, the total radical-trapping antioxidant parameter assay, which uses the stable radical species 2,2′-azinobis(3-ethylbenzthiazoline sulfonate) assay[56]; (2) the use of reduction properties of antioxidants against a radical cation or a metal ion, for example, the ferric-reducing ability of plasma[57]; or (3) the assessment of products of oxidative metabolism as a measure of the functional adequacy of vitamins and trace elements involved in antioxidant pathways (eg, malondialdehyde and F_2 isoprostanes, both of which give an indication of oxidation of polyunsaturated fatty acids within cells).[58] Measurements of total antioxidant capacity are usually standardized with the water-soluble vitamin E analog Trolox.[56] It has been suggested that more than one method should be used to validate any analysis because different methods give varying results.[59] Vitamins that contribute to plasma antioxidant capacity include ascorbate (up to 24% of measured capacity) and α-tocopherol (up to 10%).

A disadvantage of many methods of total antioxidant capacity measurement is the variable contribution of common plasma constituents, particularly albumin and urate, to the measured concentration.[60] Changes in circulating concentrations of these molecules caused by acute-phase changes or changes in renal function can alter measured values without reflecting changes in antioxidant vitamin concentration. This problem is typically resolved by using the antioxidant gap, which is a derived value that subtracts the Trolox equivalence of albumin and urate from the measured total antioxidant capacity.[61]

Few clinical studies have demonstrated any significant benefit from the provision of increased quantities of antioxidants.[62] One recent randomized control trial concluded that the early provision of antioxidants or glutamine did not improve clinical outcomes but was associated with an increase in mortality among critically ill patients with multiorgan failure.[63] In general, most studies have shown that antioxidant supplementation, usually with vitamin C and/or vitamin E, had no beneficial effect and may have been harmful when given at levels substantially above those normally found in the diet.[64-67]

VITAMINS

The word vitamin was coined in 1912 by the polish biochemist Casimir Funk and was derived from "vitamin" or "vital amine" meaning the "amine of life," as it was believed at the time that the disease-preventing constituents in food were amines, a fact that was true for thiamine, but not for other vitamins.[68] Vitamins are organic compounds required in trace amounts (microgram to milligram quantities per day) in the diet for health, growth, and reproduction, which is small in contrast to the relatively large amounts of such macronutrients as proteins, lipids, and carbohydrates.

Vitamin groups have historically been classified using a letter of the alphabet followed by an Arabic numeral in subscript to designate structural and functional similarity, for example, A_1 (retinol) and A_2 (3-dehydroretinol), or to indicate the approximate order in which they were first identified as members of the B-complex, for example, B_1 (thiamine) and B_2 (riboflavin). Common or generic chemical names give a better indication of the types of compounds involved. These often reflect the presence of some specific atom (*thia*mine), the prime functional group (pyridox*amine*), a larger portion of the molecular structure (phyllo*quinone*), or reflect the vitamin's functional properties (chole*calciferol*).

Another classification refers to the relative solubility of vitamins. Those of the fat-soluble group include vitamins A, D, E, and K, which are more soluble in organic solvents, whereas B-complex group vitamins and vitamin C are water soluble. The fat-soluble vitamins are absorbed, transported, and stored for longer periods of time and in a manner similar to fat, and this has implications for supplementation and deficiency as discussed in the following. Water-soluble vitamins function as coenzymes for several important enzymatic reactions in both mammals and microorganisms; in contrast, fat-soluble vitamins generally do not function as coenzymes and are rarely used by microorganisms.

The term vitamer refers to chemical compounds that generally have a similar molecular structure and that belong to a particular common or generic vitamin group. For example, vitamin A includes the vitamers carotenoids (α-carotene, β-carotene, γ-carotene, and the xanthophyll β-cryptoxanthin), retinoic acid, retinol, and retinal. Typically, vitamers serve similar functions, but they have varying potency that is dependent on differences in absorption and interconversions from one form to another. Table 37.3 gives a list of 13 known vitamins and vitameric groups essential to humans.

Vitamin A

Vitamin A serves an important role in vision, is required for gene expression, embryonic development, for immune and reproductive functions, and is an antioxidant. An illustrative case of vitamin A deficiency has recently been reported.[69] Also see Box 37.3 for illustrative case.

Chemistry

Vitamin A is the nutritional term for the group of compounds with a 20-carbon structure containing a methyl-substituted cyclohexenyl ring (β-ionone ring) and an isoprenoid side chain (Fig. 37.2), with a hydroxyl group (retinol), an aldehyde group (retinal), a carboxylic acid group (retinoic acid), or an ester group (retinyl ester) at the terminal C15.

Retinol, the principal vitamin A vitamer, can be oxidized reversibly to retinal—which shares all the biological activity of retinol—or further oxidized to retinoic acid, which shows some of its biological activity. The principal storage forms of vitamin A are retinyl esters, particularly palmitate. The term retinoids refers to retinol, its metabolites, and synthetic analogs with similar structure. Some dietary carotenoids (C40 polyisoprenoid compounds) are included in the vitamin A family and are classified as provitamin A because they are cleaved biologically to yield retinol. Although approximately 1000 compounds with carotenoid structure have been identified,[76] only approximately 50 possess provitamin A activity, with the principal dietary compounds being β-carotene, α-carotene, and β-cryptoxanthin. Vitamin A compounds are yellowish oils or low-melting-point solids (depending on isomeric purity) that are practically insoluble in water but are soluble in organic solvents and mineral oil. Vitamin A is sensitive to O_2 and to ultraviolet light, which induces a greenish fluorescence with an absorbance peak at 325 nm. The structure for the most common and effective provitamin A, β-carotene, is illustrated in Fig. 37.2. This compound is an orange-to-purple, water-insoluble solid that is oxidized in air to inactive products. The other carotenes, cryptoxanthin and β-apocarotenals, are asymmetric with only one β-ionone ring and yield less vitamin A activity.

Dietary Sources

Preformed vitamin A is obtained from animal-derived foods, such as liver, offal, and fish oils. Other sources are full cream milk, butter, and fortified margarines. The provitamin A carotenoids are obtained from yellow to orange fruits and vegetables, and from green leafy vegetables. Good sources are pumpkin, carrots, tomatoes, apricots, grapefruit, lettuce, and most green vegetables. The US National Health and Nutrition Examination Survey indicated that approximately 25% of the vitamin A requirement was provided by carotenoids and approximately 75% was provided by preformed retinol.[77]

Absorption, Transport, Metabolism, and Excretion

Preformed vitamin A, most often in the form of retinyl esters or carotenoids, is subject to emulsification and mixed micelle formation by the action of bile salts before they are transported into the intestinal cell. The retinyl esters are moved across the mucosal membrane and hydrolyzed to retinol within the cell to be then re-esterified by cellular RBP II and packaged into chylomicrons, which then enter the mesenteric lymphatic system and pass into the systemic circulation.[78] A small amount of the ingested retinoid is converted into retinoic acid in the intestinal cell. The efficiency of absorption of preformed vitamin A is high (70%–90%).[79]

Carotenoids, also in micellar form, are absorbed into the duodenal mucosal cells by passive diffusion. The efficiency of absorption of carotenoids is much lower than that for vitamin A (9% and 22%),[80] and is subject to more variables, including the carotenoid type, the amount in the meal, matrix properties, nutrient status, and genetic factors. Once inside the mucosal cell, β-carotene is principally converted to retinal by the enzyme β-carotene-15,15′-dioxygenase. Retinal is converted by retinal reductase to retinol and esterified. Beta-carotene can also be cleaved eccentrically to β-apocarotenals,

TABLE 37.3 Vitamins Required by Humans

Common or Generic Name	Vitamer or Common Chemical Name	Function	Symptoms and Causes of Deficiency or Associated Diseases	Currently Used Methods
Fat-Soluble Vitamins				
Vitamin A	Retinol, retinal, retinoic acid, carotenoids	Powerful antioxidant, important role in vision, required for gene expression, embryonic development, and immune and reproductive functions	Nyctalopia (night blindness), Bitot spot, xerophthalmia, keratomalacia. Common in infants and children, especially in less developed countries; due to fat malabsorption, cystic fibrosis, and may occur due to retinol-binding protein deficiency as a result of protein malnutrition, liver disease, and Zn deficiency	HPLC, LC-MS/MS
Vitamin E	Tocopherols, tocotrienols	Vitamin E is an antioxidant (prevents the peroxidation of unsaturated fatty acids), role in gene transcription, immunity, inhibits platelet aggregation, recently been implicated in bone physiology	Lipid peroxidation, red blood cell fragility causing hemolytic anemia, especially in premature infants. May occur due to fat malabsorption, cystic fibrosis	HPLC, LC-MS/MS
Vitamin K	Phylloquinones (K_1), menaquinones (K_2), menadiones (K_3)	Coagulation, bone metabolism	Increased clotting time, hemorrhagic disease of the newborn. Also due to fat malabsorption, cystic fibrosis, liver disease.	Prothrombin time, PIVKA, HPLC, LC-MS/MS
Water-Soluble Vitamins				
Vitamin B_1	Thiamine, aneurin	Forms the coenzyme thiamine pyrophosphate required for decarboxylation reactions involved in carbohydrate metabolism, and nerve function	Beri-beri, Wernicke-Korsakoff syndrome in alcoholics, rare thiamine-responsive IOM	Erythrocyte transketolase, HPLC, LC-MS/MS
Vitamin B_2	Riboflavin	Essential component of coenzymes involved in reduction-oxidation (redox) reactions in the body	Angular stomatitis, dermatitis, photophobia, riboflavin-dependent IOM	Erythrocyte glutathione reductase, HPLC, LC-MS/MS,
Vitamin B_3	Niacin, nicotinic acid, nicotinamide	Coenzyme or cosubstrate in many biological redox reactions, and thus for energy metabolism.	Pellagra (dermatitis, dementia, diarrhea). Seen in communities with corn-based staple diets, in carcinoid syndrome (precursor tryptophan diverted to serotonin formation), Hartnup disease (unable to absorb tryptophan), and medications such as isoniazid.	HPLC and LC-MS/MS for urine metabolite, nicotinamide coenzymes

Vitamin B_5	Pantothenic acid, panthenol, pantethine	General metabolism, acetyl and acyl transfer	Burning feet syndrome	Microbiological, CPB, HPLC, LC-MS, GC-MS
Vitamin B_6	Pyridoxine, pyridoxal, pyridoxamine	The active form pyridoxal phosphate is required for synthesis and catabolism of various amino acids	Epileptiform convulsions, dermatitis, anemia, medications such as penicillamine and isoniazid decrease it, pyridoxine-responsive IOM notably homocystinuria, and hyperhomocysteinemia (together with vitamin B_{12} and folate deficiencies)	Aspartate transaminase, HPLC, LC-MS/MS
Vitamin B_7	Biotin, vitamin H	Coenzyme for carboxylation reactions involved in gluconeogenesis, lipogenesis and catabolism of branched-chain amino acids; roles in cell signaling, epigenetic regulation of genes, and chromatin structure	Dermatitis, developmental delay. Seen with excessive raw egg consumption, those on parenteral nutrition and IOM, notably biotinidase deficiency	Microbiological, CPB, carboxylases, avidin binding, urinary metabolites
Vitamin B_9	Pteroylglutamic acid, folic acid, folate	Required for the interconversions of amino acids such as homocysteine to methionine and the biosynthesis of purines and pyrimidines, required for DNA synthesis	Megaloblastic anemia, neural tube defects. Caused by gut sterilization, malabsorption, decreased intake, increased requirements (eg, pregnancy), medications (eg, methotrexate, anticonvulsants). Deficiency linked to hyperhomocystinemia, cancer, and stroke	Red blood cell and serum folate, CPB, microbiological, homocysteine
Vitamin B_{12}	Cyanocobalamin, hydroxocobalamin, methylcobalamin	Required for erythropoiesis, methylation processes necessary for DNA and cell metabolism, and is a cofactor for various enzymes, notably those involved in the metabolism of methylmalonic acid and homocysteine	Pernicious and megaloblastic anemia, peripheral neuropathy. Caused by decreased intake (vegetarians), short bowel syndrome (loss of distal ileum), malabsorption syndromes, medications (N_2O, phenytoin, methotrexate, and proton pump inhibitors), and Imerslund-Grasbeck syndrome. Deficiency results in methylmalonic aciduria and homocysteinemia	CPB, immunometric, microbiological, methylmalonate, homocysteine, holotranscobalamin
Vitamin C	Ascorbic acid	Connective tissue formation, antioxidant	Scurvy, infantile scurvy (Barlow disease). Linked with osteoporosis, anemia, diabetes mellitus, cancer	Spectrophotometric-enzymatic methods, HPLC

For information regarding vitamin D, see Chapter 64.

CPB, Competitive protein binding; *HPLC,* high-performance liquid chromatography; *IOM,* inborn errors of metabolism; *LC-MS/MS,* liquid chromatography-tandem mass spectrometry; *PIVKA,* protein induced by vitamin K absence or antagonism; *RIA,* radioimmunoassay; *Zn,* zinc.

BOX 37.3 Case: A 13-Year-Old Boy With Fussy Eating Habits and Blindness[70]

A 13-year-old boy was referred by his primary care physician to the local hospital with a few months history of progressively "fuzzy" vision, particularly at night. Apart from a history of "fussy eating" habits, his medical history was unremarkable. On preliminary assessment, he was systemically well and interacted appropriately; clinical examinations were all normal. His height and weight were in the 50th centile for his age. On ophthalmologic examination, he was found to have reduced visual acuity in the left eye with no perception of light. He had normal vision in the right eye. A magnetic resonance imaging brain scan showed normal appearances of the optic nerves and chiasm. Electrodiagnostic testing was carried out and an electroretinogram demonstrated a complete absence of rod function but nearly normal cone function. This pattern was consistent with that seen in vitamin A deficiency. Selected blood tests results are shown in the following. An extremely low vitamin A concentration of less than 0.3 umol/L (normal 0.9–2.5 μmol/L) was found. Other routine blood test results not shown were all within reference limits. His dietary history was evaluated. The patient had an extremely selective eating pattern, consuming only potato chips, French fries, custard, and diluted juice since the age of 2 years. He was commenced on oral vitamin A supplementation and is showing continued improvement in his degree of visual loss. Ongoing care issues include improving nutritional status with dietetic and psychological input and repeat ophthalmology and electrodiagnostic testing to monitor progress.

	Result (Local Reference Interval)	
Vitamin A	<0.3 μmol/L (0.9–2.5)	<8.6 μg/dL (26–72)
α-carotene	<0.2 μmol/L (0.3–1.1)	<10 μg/L (14–60)
Vitamin B_{12}	176.8 pmol/L (190–900)	241 pg/mL (259–1227)
Vitamin D	61 nmol/L (25–170)	24 ng/mL (10–68)
Vitamin E	14 μmol/L (13–24)	0.6 mg/dL (0.56–1.0)
Adjusted calcium	2.14 mmol/L (2.20–2.70)	8.6 mg/dL (8.8–10.8)

Commentary

Blindness secondary to vitamin A deficiency is common in developing countries.[71] However, sporadic cases can occur in developed countries due to nutritional insufficiency secondary to food faddism in otherwise healthy children.[72] The condition has a variable course. Permanent visual damage is possible in cases of prolonged or severe visual loss.[73] Rod function appears to recover most quickly and completely. and central cones, if affected (as in this case), have slower recovery.[74,75] This case highlights the importance of checking for visual problems in fussy eaters and those at risk of nutritional deficiencies, thereby ensuring that appropriate management is undertaken to prevent permanent visual loss.

We are grateful to Dr Salma Rashid Ali and colleagues for permission to use this case. Patient consent was received, and this case has previously been presented as a poster.

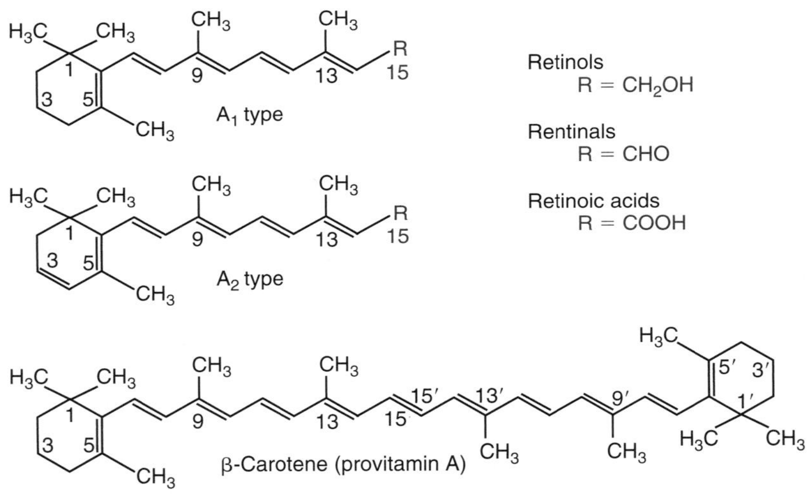

Retinols
R = CH_2OH

Rentinals
R = CHO

Retinoic acids
R = COOH

A_1 type

A_2 type

β-Carotene (provitamin A)

FIGURE 37.2 Vitaminic Forms of A_1, A_2, and β-Carotene.

which can be further degraded to retinal or retinoic acid. The newly synthesized retinyl esters, from both preformed vitamin A and carotenoids, along with exogenous lipids and nonhydrolyzed carotenoids, then pass with chylomicrons via the lymphatic system to the liver, where uptake by parenchymal cells again involves hydrolysis. In the liver, retinol is bound with RBP (molecular weight [MW] ≅ 21,000 Da) and transthyretin (thyroxine-binding prealbumin) (MW ≅ 55,000 Da) in a 1 : 1 : 1 complex of sufficient size to prevent loss by glomerular filtration and is returned to the circulation, or stored as esters within the stellate cells. Delivery of retinol to the tissue is controlled by the availability of the vitamin A–protein complex in the circulation, although this control mechanism can be bypassed by large doses of retinol.

Retinoic acid from the intestinal mucosa is transported bound to serum albumin via the portal vein. Retinoic acid cannot be significantly reduced to retinal, but it is rapidly metabolized in tissue, such as liver, to yield more polar catabolites (eg, 5,6-epoxyretinoic acid) and conjugates, such as retinoyl β-glucuronide, which are excreted. A small amount

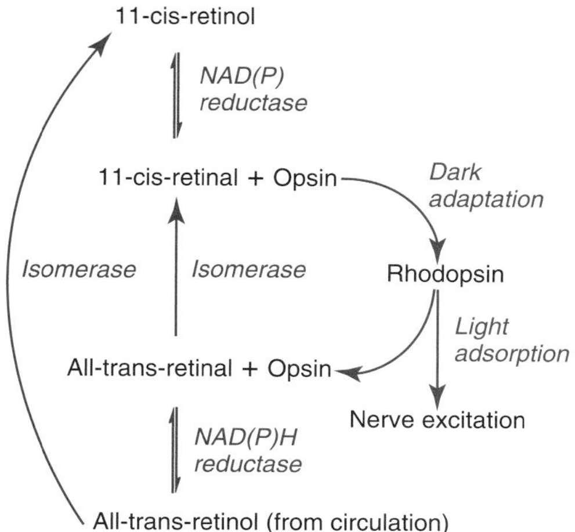

FIGURE 37.3 Participation of a Vitamers in the Visual Cycle. *NAD(P)H,* Nicotinamide-adenine dinucleotide phosphate.

of retinoic acid undergoes enterohepatic circulation after intestinal hydrolysis of the glucuronide, which is excreted in bile.

Functions

The participation of retinal in vision is considered the most important physiological function of vitamin A. All-*trans*-retinol is the predominant circulating form of vitamin A. Cells of the retina isomerize this to the 11-*cis* alcohol that is reversibly dehydrogenated to 11-*cis* retinal. This sterically hindered geometrical isomer of the aldehyde combines as a lysyl-linked Schiff base with suitable proteins (eg, opsin) to generate photosensitive pigments, such as rhodopsin.[81] Illumination of such pigments causes photoisomerization and the release of all-*trans*-retinal and the protein, a process that couples the large conformational change with ion flux and optic nerve transmission. The all-*trans*-retinal is isomerized to the 11-*cis* isomer, which combines with the liberated protein to reconstitute the photo pigment in a visual cycle (Fig. 37.3). The pyridine nucleotide–dependent dehydrogenase (reductase) can also reduce the all-*trans*-retinal to all-*trans*-retinol.[81]

Other functions of vitamin A include its role in reproduction,[82] growth,[83] embryonic development,[84] and immune function.[85] Many of these functions are mediated through the binding of retinoic acid to specific nuclear receptors that regulate genomic expression. In normal growth, and in maintenance of the integrity of epithelial cells, retinoic acid acts through the activation of retinoic acid receptors and retinoid X receptors[83] in the nucleus to regulate various genes that encode for structural proteins, enzymes, extracellular matrix proteins, RBPs, and receptors. Vitamin A deficiency impairs innate immunity by impeding normal regeneration of mucosal barriers damaged by infection and by diminishing the function of neutrophils, macrophages, and natural killer cells. Vitamin A is also required for adaptive immunity and plays a role in the development of both T-helper cells and B cells. Retinol and its metabolites and synthetic retinoids provide protective effects against the development of certain types of cancer by blocking tumor promotion, inhibiting proliferation, inducing apoptosis, inducing differentiation, or by performing a combination of these actions.[86,87] Finally, synthetic retinoids have been used successfully, both topically and systemically, to treat severe acne and other skin disorders of abnormal keratinization.[88] However, caution is required regarding the use of vitamin A or β-carotene supplements in the general population because they have been shown to be teratogenic.[89]

Requirements and Reference Nutrient Intakes

In the older system of international units, which is now largely redundant, a ratio for equivalence of activity of 1:2:4 for retinol/β-carotene/other provitamin A carotenoids was used, but this was superseded in 1967 by the retinol equivalent, which was devised by a Food and Agriculture/WHO Expert Committee that proposed an equivalence ratio of 1:6:12. However, studies using stable isotopes of β-carotene[90] led the Food and Nutrition Board of the US IOM to recommend the retinol activity equivalent (RAE) as the basis of calculation of retinol intake. In this system, 1 RAE = 1 μg retinol, 12 μg β-carotene, or 24 μg carotenoids. With this system, current RDAs for vitamin A are the following: 900 μg RAE for men 19 years and older; 700 μg RAE for women 19 years and older, with up to 770 μg RAE/day in pregnancy and up to 1300 μg RAE/day in lactation; 300 to 900 μg RAE for children 1 to 18 years, dependent on age and gender; and an adequate intake (AI) of 400 μg RAE at 0 to 6 months and 500 μg RAE from 7 to 12 months for infants.[11]

Intravenous Supply

The recommended provision of vitamin A to adults during IVN, whether this is partial or TPN, is 1000 μg retinol. This is usually provided as retinol palmitate and may be supplied with other fat-soluble vitamins in a mixture dissolved in a fat emulsion for intravenous feeding, or may be designed to be compatible with a mixture of all vitamins suitable for addition to other water-soluble nutrients.[91,92]

Deficiency

Vitamin A deficiency primarily affects infants and children, and its prevalence is subject to WHO surveillance.[93] Risk factors include poverty, low birth weight, poor sanitation, malnutrition, infection, and parasitism. Because hepatic accumulation of vitamin A occurs during the last trimester of pregnancy, preterm infants are relatively vitamin A deficient at birth.

Neonatal vitamin A supplementation has been a matter of some controversy due to mixed results in trials that have studied various populations.[94] Evidence from one systematic review of randomized trials showed benefit of vitamin A supplementation for children aged 6 to 59 months, which reduced all-cause mortality by 23% to 30%.[95] However, in children younger than 6 months, the results have been mixed—ranging from no benefit to possible harm—prompting calls for further large trials.[96,97] To address this issue, WHO, supported by the Bill & Melinda Gates Foundation, commissioned three large, double-blind, placebo-controlled, randomized trials in selected localities in India,[98] Ghana,[99] and Tanzania[100] to examine the effects of neonatal vitamin A supplementation using a standardized protocol. These three studies randomly assigned 99,938 newborn babies to receive one dose of 50,000 IU of vitamin A or placebo within 72 hours of birth. The results were somewhat mixed and showed some evidence of benefit for survival to 6 months of age in India (risk ratio [RR]: 0.90; 95% confidence interval [CI]: 0.81–1.00), but no benefit for survival in Tanzania or Ghana. There was a suggestion of increased risk of mortality by 6 months of age in the African countries (in Tanzania: RR: 1.10, 95% CI: 0.95–1.26; P = 0.193; in Ghana: RR: 1.12; 95% CI: 0.95–1.33; P = 0.183).[99,100] In addition, there was evidence of increased risk of bulging fontanelle in vitamin A–supplemented neonates. A closer examination of the data revealed that evidence of maternal vitamin A deficiency might be an important factor; in India almost 25% of all women studied were vitamin A deficient. In Ghana, this was less than 3%, and in Tanzania, this was 5% to 8%.[96] It may be inferred from this that maternal deficiency may be a potential predictor for neonatal supplementation, but at the present time, there is no strong evidence for a global policy for neonatal vitamin A supplementation.

In general, providing a daily oral intake of vitamin A that meets the RDA of 400 µg RAE is sufficient. Infants with birth weights of less than 1500 g (those at <30 weeks' gestation) have virtually no hepatic vitamin A stores and are at risk of vitamin A deficiency. Various researchers have observed that: (1) bronchopulmonary dysplasia, a debilitating, chronic lung disease that mimics some histologic features of vitamin A deficiency, is common in premature infants; (2) intramuscular injections of 630 µg RAE every 2 days can reduce the incidence of bronchopulmonary dysplasia; (3) blood concentrations of vitamin A decline during TPN, often reaching concentrations of 10 to 15 µg/dL (normal: 20 to 65 µg/dL) unless adequate supplements are given; and (4) vitamin A (retinol) delivered in TPN solutions may be absorbed into the inner walls of plastic administration sets; however, this loss can be minimized by using ethylene vinyl acetate rather than polyvinyl chloride.[101]

Fat malabsorption, particularly caused by celiac disease or chronic pancreatitis, and protein-energy malnutrition predispose to vitamin A deficiency. Liver disease diminishes RBP synthesis, and ethanol abuse leads to both hepatic injury and competition with retinol for alcohol dehydrogenase, which is necessary for the oxidation of retinol to retinal and retinoic acid.[102] Vitamin A deficiency may lead to anemia, although the precise mechanism is not known.[103]

Clinical features of vitamin A deficiency include degenerative changes in the eyes and skin and poor dark adaptation or night blindness (nyctalopia),[93] followed by degenerative changes in the retina. Xerophthalmia occurs when the conjunctiva becomes dry with small gray plaques with foamy surfaces (Bitot spots).[104] These lesions are reversible with vitamin A administration. More serious effects of deficiency are known as keratomalacia and cause ulceration and necrosis of the cornea, which lead to perforation, prolapse, endophthalmitis, and blindness. Usually, associated skin changes include dryness, roughness, papular eruptions, and follicular hyperkeratosis. The general change consists of atrophy of certain specialized epithelia, followed by metaplastic hyperkeratinization.

Toxicity

Toxic effects of hypervitaminosis A occur mainly as a result of ingestion of excess vitamin or as a side effect of inappropriate therapy.[105] Hypervitaminosis A occurs after liver storage of retinol, and its esters exceeds 3000 µg/g tissue, with ingestion of more than 30,000 µg/day for months or years, or if plasma vitamin A concentrations exceed 140 µg/dL (4.9 µmol/L). Older adults are more susceptible to vitamin A toxicity at lower doses because exposure to retinyl esters is longer because of delayed postprandial clearance of lipoproteins.[106]

Symptoms of acute toxicity present as abdominal pain, nausea, vomiting, severe headaches, dizziness, sluggishness, and irritability, followed within a few days by desquamation of the skin and recovery. Long-term toxicity from moderately high doses taken for protracted periods is characterized by bone and joint pain, hair loss, dryness and fissures of the lips, anorexia, benign intracranial hypertension, weight loss, and hepatomegaly. Administration of doses up to threefold the RDA for several years resulted in classic histological changes of hepatotoxicity in 41 patients.[107] In addition, it has been shown that osteoporosis and hip fracture are associated with vitamin A intakes that are only twice the RDA.[105] Infants given excess vitamin A over months to years can develop intracranial features, typically bulging fontanelle, and skeletal abnormalities at doses of 5500 to 6750 µg/day.[108]

Epidemiologic and experimental evidence has supported the view that high vitamin A intake in humans, acting via 13-*cis*-retinoic acid, is teratogenic.[89,109] The critical period of susceptibility is the first trimester of pregnancy, and primary abnormalities derive from the cranial neural crest cells. A 1995 study of almost 23,000 pregnant women found that those who ingested more than 4500 µg/day of preformed vitamin A were at greater risk of delivering infants with malformations of cranial neural crest cell origin than women who consumed less than 1500 µg/day.[110] A further intriguing association, supported in part by epidemiologic studies, is the one that has been observed between excessive vitamin A intake and reduction in bone mineral density (BMD). Studies of Scandinavian women showed that consistent loss of BMD at four sites was associated with increased intake of preformed vitamin A,[111] whereas other studies showed no increase in bone mineral loss with preformed vitamin A intakes of up to 2000 µg/day.[112] Hypervitaminosis A is also a known cause of hypercalcemia, especially in chronic kidney disease.[113,114]

Carotenemia results from long-term excessive intake of carotene-rich foods, principally carrots, and is usually reported in infants and children. This condition, in which yellowing of the skin is observed, is benign because the excess carotene is deposited rather than converted to vitamin A.[115] There is a role for the measurement of β-carotene in the differential diagnosis of specific cases of jaundice in children.[116] There have been reports of impaired activity of the enzyme β-carotene-15,15′-dioxygenase in children that leads to accumulation of β-carotene, especially when consuming carotene-rich foods, but it is a benign condition. Carotenemia has also been linked to amenorrhea, but the mechanism behind this association remains unknown.[117] Increased concentrations have also been found in hypothyroid patients, in whom conversion to vitamin A is decreased, and in patients with hyperlipemia that is associated with diabetes mellitus.[115]

Laboratory Assessment of Status

Although measurement of the plasma concentration of vitamin A is the most convenient and widely used assessment of vitamin A status, it is not an ideal indicator because it does not decline until liver stores become critically depleted, which is believed to occur at a concentration of approximately 20 μg/g liver.[71]

Vitamin A status is assessed by the measurement of retinol concentration. Retinol circulates in plasma as a 1 : 1 : 1 complex with RBP and transthyretin (TTR), forming a complex that prevents glomerular filtration.[118] The circulating concentration of RBP is determined by dietary protein and Zn, which are necessary for RBP synthesis. Thus, protein malnutrition, liver disease, and Zn deficiency resulting in RBP deficiency will lead to hypovitaminosis A.[118] In contrast, renal failure resulting in decreased excretion of RBP has been reported to result in hypervitaminosis A.[119] As previously discussed, another confounding factor in the assessment of vitamin A status is the effect of inflammation.[34,35,37,120] Both RBP and TTR are negative acute-phase proteins; thus inflammatory changes will result in transient falls in both proteins and plasma retinol. To distinguish inflammatory from nutritional causes of reduced plasma retinol concentrations, it may be necessary to measure CRP.[35]

Early chemical methods that are rarely used include the Carr-Price photometric method, which uses antimony trichloride in chloroform as the reagent, and the later Neeld-Pearson method, which uses trifluoroacetic acid to produce a blue pigment with the conjugated double bonds of vitamin A (and the carotenoids).[121] To improve specificity and sensitivity, later methods used high-pressure liquid chromatography (HPLC) after solvent extraction and other separation techniques, with fluorometric or spectrophotometric detection.[25,122,123] HPLC has brought enhanced specificity, lowered limits of detection, improved accuracy using primary standards, reference materials, and quality assurance schemes, and made acceptable reproducibility achievable (between batch coefficients of variation (CV) of less than 15% for both vitamin A and β-carotene). Both normal and reverse-phase HPLC have been used. In the normal-phase HPLC, compounds to be separated are adsorbed to microparticulate silica gel and are eluted in the order of least polar to most polar. Acceptable separation and quantitative yields of neutral and charged retinoids are obtained. Reverse-phase HPLC is preferable for acid-sensitive compounds (eg, 5,6-epoxyretinoic acid). Photometric, electrochemical, and mass spectrophotometric detectors have all been used. Refer to Chapter 16 for general principles of chromatography and extraction. Briefly, serum is deproteinized with ethanol that contains internal standards, centrifuged, and extracted with hexane. This is followed by evaporation to dryness, and the residue is redissolved in tetrahydrofuran. An aliquot of this solution is injected into a silica-coated (C_{18}) reverse-phase chromatographic column and detected photometrically with the absorbance measured at 325 nm for vitamin A and 450 nm for carotenes. Peak height ratios are used for quantification, with normalization using the internal standards.[123] HPLC-mass spectrometry methods have also been developed and are increasingly being used because of the widespread adoption of this technique by clinical laboratories.[124]

Because circulating retinol concentrations do not always correlate with total body stores of vitamin A, indirect tests have been used to assess these stores. The relative dose–response test, described first by Loerch and associates,[125] requires two blood samples to be collected—one before and one 5 hours after a physiologic dose of vitamin A. In vitamin A–depleted subjects, a rapid, large, and sustained rise in serum retinol concentration contrasts with a lower rise in vitamin A–sufficient subjects. A modified relative dose–response test using 3,4-didehydroretinyl acetate rather than retinyl acetate, and measuring the 3,4-didehydroretinyl/retinol ratio after 5 hours has been used by other workers to assess the vitamin A status.[126,127] The quantitative assessment of total body stores of vitamin A can also be undertaken using deuterated retinol dilution techniques, but this is rarely necessary.[128]

Recent advances in vitamin measurement involve the use of supported liquid extraction methodology for sample preparation using modified diatomaceous earth (natural fossilized biominerals containing high silica content) packed into columns or 96-well plates.[129] The method is similar to the traditional liquid–liquid extraction, but instead of two immiscible phases, the aqueous phase is immobilized onto an inert diatomaceous earth-based support material, and the solvent immiscible organic phase flows through the support. This method can be used for the extraction of a range of analytes, including fat- and water-soluble vitamins from aqueous samples such as blood. It provides excellent recovery, lower limits of quantification, and has good analytical sensitivity. It also has good reproducibility, removes matrix interferences such as proteins and phospholipids, and has improved throughput, with good amenability for automation with hyphenation to immunoassay, HPLC, and tandem mass spectrometry methods.[129-131]

Preanalytical Variables

Plasma, serum, or whole blood specimens are all suitable for retinol measurements. Fasting samples are recommended, especially if a patient is taking oral or parenteral vitamin A supplementation. A sample should be taken at least 8 hours after supplementation if fasting is not possible. Vitamin A samples are light sensitive and should be protected from light as much as possible by wrapping in foil.[132] Vitamin A showed good stability in whole blood collected into tubes containing lithium (Li) heparin for up to 48 hours at room temperature and without light protection.[133] Another study reported that vitamin A was stable for up to 72 hours in whole blood samples kept at 32°C and up to 14 days in serum stored at 11°C.[134]

Reference Intervals

Guidance reference intervals for serum vitamin A are 20 to 40 μg/dL (0.70–1.40 μmol/L) for 1- to 6-year-old children, 26 to 49 μg/dL (0.91–1.71 μmol/L) for 7- to 12-year-old children, 26 to 72 μg/dL (0.91–2.51 μmol/L) for 13- to 19-year-old adolescents, and 30 to 80 μg/dL (1.05–2.80 μmol/L) for adults.[135] Values more than 30 μg/dL (1.05 μmol/L) are associated with appreciable reserves in the liver and correlate well with vitamin A intake. Within the reference interval, values for men are generally approximately 20% higher than those for women.[132] By HPLC, with ultraviolet detection, the reference interval for serum α-carotene is 14 to 60 μg/L (26–112 nmol/L), β-carotene is 90 to 310 μg/L (167–577 nmol/L), lutein is 80 to 200 μg/L (140–352 nmol/L), and lycopene 100 to 300 μg/L (186–559 nmol/L).[132] However, it must be borne in mind that reference intervals will be dependent on the local population diet. For more information, refer to the Appendix on Reference Intervals. Laboratories should verify that these ranges are appropriate for use in their own settings.

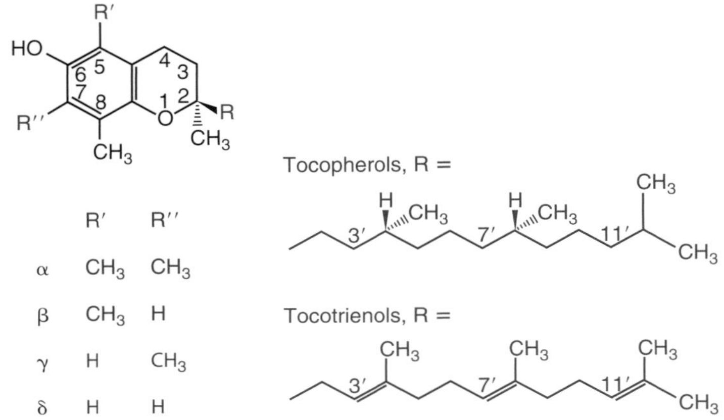

FIGURE 37.4 Vitaminic Forms of Vitamin E.

Vitamin D

As discussed in Chapter 64, vitamin D plays an essential role as a hormone in the control of calcium and phosphorous metabolism and bone physiology.

Vitamin E

Vitamin E is an antioxidant that acts to prevent the peroxidation of unsaturated fatty acids by free radicals. It also has a role in gene transcription, immunity, inhibits platelet aggregation, and has recently been implicated in bone physiology.

Chemistry

Vitamin E is the nutritional term for the group of tocopherols and tocotrienols that have biological activity similar to the naturally occurring form RRR-α-tocopherol (formerly D-α-tocopherol).[136] Both groups have a common 6-chromanol nucleus substituted with methyl groups at positions 2 and 8, and with a phytyl tail of isoprenoid units at position 2. The isoprenoid chain is saturated in the tocopherols, but it is unsaturated at positions 3′, 7′, and 11′ for tocotrienols (Fig. 37.4). The Greek letter prefixes α, β, γ, and δ indicate the presence or absence of methyl groups at positions 5 and 7. The tocopherols have three asymmetric carbon atoms in the isoprenoid chain, giving eight optical isomers. The naturally occurring tocopherols occur as the RRR forms, whereas the synthetic compounds found in foods and supplements are of various racemic forms (RRR-, RSR-, RRS- and RSS-α-tocopherol) and are less biologically active. Tocopherol and tocotrienols are viscous oils at room temperature, soluble in fat solvents, and insoluble in aqueous solutions, although a water-soluble analog (Trolox-6-hydroxy-2,5,7,8-tetramethylchroman-2-carboxylic acid) does exist. Also, tocopherol and tocotrienols are stable with acid and heat in the absence of O_2, but are labile to O_2 in alkaline solutions and to ultraviolet light.

Dietary Sources

The principal sources of dietary vitamin E are oils and fats, particularly wheat germ oil and sunflower oil, grains, and nuts. Meats, fruits, and vegetables contribute little vitamin E. Gamma-tocopherol is the major form of vitamin E in many plant seeds in the US diet, but it is present at only one-quarter to one-tenth of the concentration of α-tocopherol in human plasma.[137]

Absorption, Transport, Metabolism, and Excretion

In the presence of bile, vitamin E is absorbed from the small intestine. Most forms of vitamin E are absorbed nonselectively and are secreted in chylomicron particles, along with triacylglycerol and cholesterol. Some of this chylomicron-bound vitamin E is transported and delivered to the peripheral tissue (mainly adipose tissue) with the aid of lipoprotein lipase. The liver takes up the chylomicron remnants where α-tocopherol is incorporated into very-low-density lipoproteins by α-tocopherol transfer protein (α-TTP), enabling further distribution of α-tocopherol throughout the body. Plasma vitamin E is further delivered to the tissue by low-density lipoprotein and high-density lipoprotein. The specificity of α-TTP for α-tocopherol is probably responsible for its preferential storage in most tissue. Vitamin E is excreted via the bile, in urine as tocopheronic acid and its beta-glucuronide conjugate, as carboxyethyl hydroxychromans, and by other unknown routes.[138]

Functions

The inhibition of free radical mediated lipid peroxidation is the main role for vitamin E.[139] This occurs mainly within the polyunsaturated fatty acids of membrane phospholipids. Tocopherols and tocotrienols inhibit lipid peroxidation largely because they scavenge lipid peroxyl radicals faster than the radical can react to adjacent fatty acid sidechains or membrane proteins. The resultant tocopheryl or tocotrienyl radicals may then react with additional peroxyl radicals to produce tocopherones (nonradicals), or they may be regenerated by transfer of an electron to ascorbate to form the ascorbyl radical. Thus, vitamins E and C act synergistically to reduce lipid peroxidation (Fig. 37.5).[140] Some epidemiologic surveys have shown an association between reduced vitamin E intake (and other dietary factors) and increased incidence of chronic disease, particularly cardiovascular disease and cancer, although intervention studies have produced mixed results.[66,141-143] The Women's Antioxidant Cardiovascular Study[144] confirmed the lack of effect of antioxidants on cardiovascular events and also in slowing the rate of cognitive decline.[145] Vitamin E has also no proven effect in reducing the incidence of various cancers.[64,146]

Beyond its antioxidant properties, α-tocopherol inhibits protein kinase C and 5-lipoxygenase and activates protein phosphatase 2A and diacylglycerol kinase. Some genes

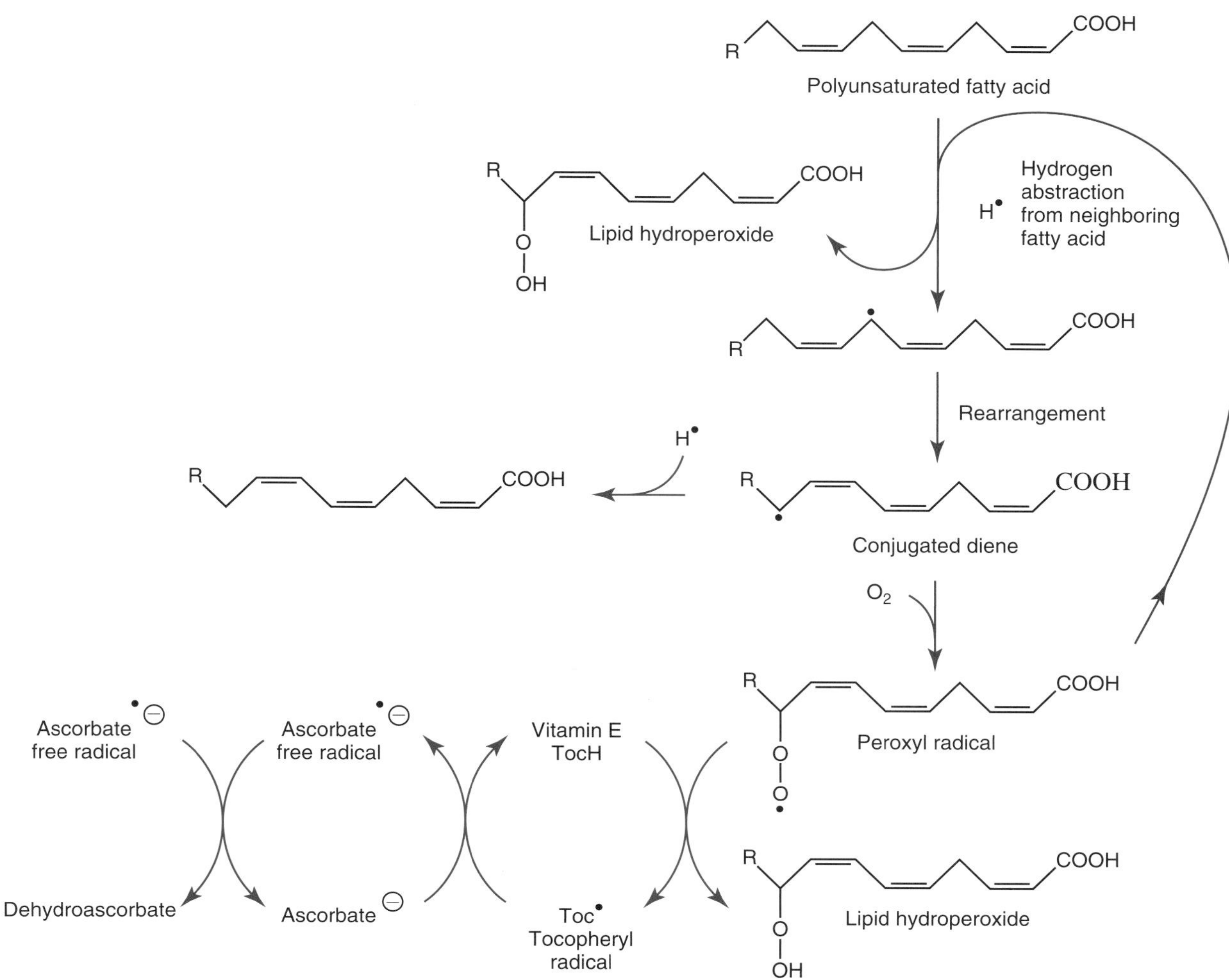

FIGURE 37.5 Lipoperoxidation and Synergistic Action of Vitamins E and C.

(coding for CD36, α-TTP, α-tropomyosin, and collagenase) are affected by α-tocopherol at the transcriptional level. Alpha-tocopherol also induces inhibition of cell proliferation, platelet aggregation, and monocyte adhesion, which are believed to be the result of direct interaction of α-tocopherol with cell components.[147,148] There is some evidence that vitamin E may have anti-inflammatory properties.[137]

A recent study showed that serum vitamin E is a determinant of bone mass by stimulating osteoclast fusion.[149] In that study, mice deficient in α-TTP (Ttpa$^{-/-}$), a mouse model of genetic vitamin E deficiency, had high bone mass as a result of a decrease in bone resorption. The authors showed that vitamin E could stimulate osteoclast fusion via an intricate mechanism, resulting in loss of bone mass.[149] The authors suggested that because of the widespread use of vitamin E, a large, randomized-controlled trial examining the effect of vitamin E on human bone mass may be warranted.

Requirements and Reference Nutrient Intakes

The requirement for vitamin E is related to the polyunsaturated fatty acid content of cellular structures and therefore depends on the nature and quantity of dietary fat that affect such composition.[150] Hence, the minimum adult requirement for vitamin E is not certain, but is probably not more than 3 to 4 mg (4.5–6 IU) of RRR-α-tocopherol per day for those who ingest a diet containing the minimum of essential fatty acids (3% of calories). Because vitamin E activity is derived from a series of tocopherols and tocotrienols in usual mixed diets, the α-tocopherol equivalent is used based on the abundance and activity relative to the biologically most active RRR-α-tocopherol. The α-tocopherol equivalent is the sum of α-tocopherol, β-tocopherol (multiplied by a factor 0.5), γ-tocopherol (multiplied by 0.1), and α-tocotrienol (by 0.3). It has been estimated that a range of 7 to 13 mg of α-tocopherol equivalents (10–20 IU) can be expected in balanced diets supplying 1800 to 3000 kcal. This intake will maintain plasma concentrations of total tocopherols within the reference interval of 0.5 to 1.2 mg/dL (12–28 μmol/L), which ensures an adequate concentration in all tissue.[151] Some investigators claim that the ratio of circulating α-tocopherol to total lipids (or triglycerides or β-lipoproteins) is a more accurate indicator of tissue vitamin E status than circulating α-tocopherol alone.[152]

In 2000, the RDA for vitamin E for both male and female adults was increased by 50%, from 10 to 15 mg/day (35 μmol/day or 21 IU), by the US Food and Nutrition Board.[11] Most European reference intakes are related to the polyunsaturated fatty acid intake.[153] Critics have argued that without supplementation, this amount could not be met by the usual North American diet.[154] There has also been concern raised that because of the antiaggregatory effect of vitamin E on platelets, the widespread use of aspirin may have an additive effect and result in increased incidence of bleeding and hemorrhagic stroke.[154,155] Another departure in the newer recommendations was that the daily requirement must be met by RRR-α-tocopherol alone, because the other forms of vitamin E are not converted to α-tocopherol and are poorly recognized by the α-tocopherol transfer protein in the liver.[67]

Intravenous Supply

The recommended amount of vitamin E to be supplied intravenously to adults as α-tocopherol is 9.1 mg/day or 10 IU/day.[156,157] This is lower than the oral dose but accounts for complete delivery into the bloodstream.

Deficiency

Premature and low birth weight infants are particularly susceptible to vitamin E deficiency because placental transfer is poor and infants have limited adipose tissue where much of the vitamin is normally stored.[151] Signs of deficiency include (1) irritability, (2) edema, and (3) hemolytic anemia. Anemia reflects the shortened life span of erythrocytes with fragile membranes; it does not respond to Fe therapy, which may aggravate the condition. Although symptoms of vitamin E deficiency are rare in children and adults, deficiency can occur in some conditions (eg, fat malabsorption states, including cystic fibrosis and chronic cholestasis[158] in children), and can cause neuropathy[159] and hemolytic anemia.[160] The genetic disorder abetalipoproteinemia (vitamin E is transported on lipoproteins) can also confer vitamin E deficiency.[161] Mutations of the gene coding for α-TTP lead to low plasma α-tocopherol concentrations and can cause neurologic symptoms, including cerebellar ataxia,[162] which requires treatments with large amounts (up to 2 g/day or 3 IU) of vitamin E. Hypovitaminosis E may be present asymptomatically and only manifest acutely as a result of oxidative stress, as in major trauma or SIRS.[157]

Toxicity

Vitamin E toxicity only results from excessive supplementation. Such supplementation is contraindicated in subjects with coagulation defects caused by vitamin K deficiency and in those receiving anticoagulant drugs.[154] The US Food and Nutrition Board has recommended a tolerable upper limit of 1000 mg/day (1430 IU/day) of vitamin E for adults 19 years and older, based on the absence of hemorrhagic toxicity in animal models.[11] However, this has been challenged on the grounds that in those who regularly take aspirin, this intake may be high and may be associated with an increased risk of bleeding.[154] A comprehensive review of tolerance and safety of vitamin E suggested that intakes up to 3000 mg/day (4285 IU/day) were safe, and reversible side effects of gastrointestinal symptoms, increased creatinuria, and impairment of blood coagulation are seen at intakes of 1000 to 3000 mg/day (1430–4285 IU/day).[163] However, as noted earlier, long-term use of intakes more than 400 mg/day (572 IU/day) may cause increased mortality.[66]

Laboratory Assessment of Status

Assessment of vitamin E status has been achieved by functional methods such as (1) protection of erythrocyte hemolysis on addition of peroxide,[164] (2) inhibition of formation of lipid peroxidation products (malondialdehyde, thiobarbituric acid–reactive substances [ethane or pentane]),[165] or (3) direct measurement of vitamin E concentration in tissues (erythrocytes, lymphocytes, or platelets) or serum.[122,123] Early direct methods used photometric or fluorometric measurement often based on the Emmerie-Engel procedure, in which tocopherol is oxidized to tocopheryl quinone by Fe chloride ($FeCl_3$), and the resultant Fe^{2+} is coupled with α,α′-dipyridyl to form a red color.[25] Later, chromatographic methods were used, including thin layer and gas liquid chromatography, which had the ability to separate the tocopherols and the tocotrienols, but these methods were labor intensive and time consuming.[25] HPLC is currently the method of choice for quantification of tocopherols in serum, because it offers the advantages of accuracy (through the use of primary standards) and reproducibility (between-batch CVs of <5%), and the ability to quantitate multiple analytes, including vitamin A and some carotenoids, in a single analytical run.[122,123] Both α- and γ-tocopherols are the principal vitamers seen, although others may be detected with minor modifications to the analytical conditions. HPLC-mass spectrometry methods have also been developed and are increasingly being used because of the widespread adoption of this technique by clinical laboratories.[124]

Preanalytical Variables

Plasma, serum, or whole blood specimens are all suitable, but it is recommended that local laboratories should be consulted for their preferred sample type. Vitamin E is light-sensitive and samples should be protected from light as much as possible by wrapping in foil.[132] Vitamin E showed good stability in whole blood collected in Li heparin tubes for up to 48 hours at room temperature and without light protection,[133] whereas another study reported that vitamin E was stable for up to 72 hours in whole blood samples kept at 32°C and up to 14 days in serum stored at 11°C.[134]

Reference Intervals

Guidance reference intervals for serum or plasma (heparin) vitamin E are 0.1 to 0.5 mg/dL (2.3–11.6 μmol/L) for premature neonates, 0.3 to 0.9 mg/dL (7–21 μmol/L) for children (1–12 years),[135] 0.6 to 1.0 mg/dL (14–23 μmol/L) for adolescents (13–19 years), and 0.5 to 1.8 mg/dL (12–42 μmol/L) for adults.[166] Because vitamin E circulates mainly bound to lipoproteins, it has been shown that correcting for the concentration of cholesterol gives a better reflection of vitamin E status. As a ratio of cholesterol, the reference interval is 3.5 to 9.5 μmol/mmol cholesterol.[132] For more information refer to the Appendix on Reference Intervals. Laboratories should verify that these ranges are appropriate for use in their own settings.

Vitamin K

Vitamin K has important roles in coagulation and bone metabolism.

Chemistry

Vitamin K is the common generic name for a group of compounds with a methylated naphthoquinone structure (2-methyl-1,4-napthoquinones) that is substituted with side chains at carbon 3. Phylloquinone (K_1 type), which is synthesized in plants, and menaquinones, (K_2 type), which is of bacterial origin, are the two principal natural classes of vitamin K (Fig. 37.6). The principal vitamin K_1 (phylloquinone) bears a saturated, phytol, 20-carbon side chain derived from four isoprenoid units; this is the main K vitamin produced by plants and is the major dietary form for humans.[167,168] K_2 shows greater variation, but an all-*trans*-farnesylgeranylgeranyl, 35-carbon chain of 7 isoprenoid units is typical; these are produced in humans by large bowel bacteria, although their contribution to vitamin K status remains a matter of dispute.[168] Several synthetic analogs and derivatives have been used in human nutrition; most relate to or derive from menadione (K_3), which lacks a side chain substituent at position 3, but can be converted to menaquinone (MK) (eg, MK-4, where 4 is the number of isoprenoid side chains) through addition of the side chain in the liver.[169] The K vitamins are insoluble in water, but they do dissolve in organic fat solvents. They are destroyed by alkaline solutions and reducing agents, and are sensitive to ultraviolet light.

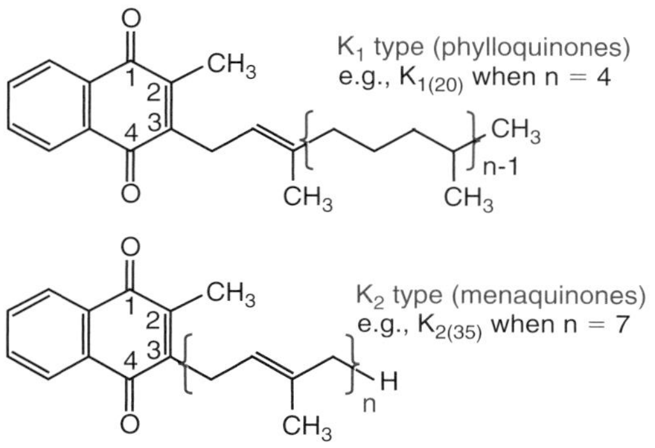

FIGURE 37.6 Vitaminic Forms of Vitamin K.

Dietary Sources

The main dietary sources of the phylloquinones are green vegetables, margarines, and plant oils, whereas some MKs can be obtained from cheese, other milk products, and eggs.[170]

Absorption, Transport, Metabolism, and Excretion

As for other fat-soluble vitamins, the absorption of natural vitamin K from the small intestine into the lymphatic system is facilitated by bile. The efficiency of absorption varies from 15% to 65%, as reflected by recovery in lymph within 24 hours. Vitamins K_1 and K_2 are bound to chylomicrons for transport from mucosal cells to the liver. K_3 is more rapidly and completely absorbed from the gut before entering the portal blood. In the liver, intracellular distribution is seen mostly in the microsomal fraction, where phenylation of K_3 to form K_2 occurs. Release of vitamin K to the bloodstream allows association with circulating β- lipoproteins for transport to other tissue. Significant concentrations of vitamin K have been noted in the spleen and skeletal muscle.

Within metabolically active and vitamin K–dependent tissue, especially the liver, a microsomal vitamin K cycle exists (Fig. 37.7). The vitamin (quinone) is normally reduced by a thiol-sensitive flavoprotein system to hydroquinone, which then can couple to O_2 and carbon dioxide with the use of γ-carboxylation of glutamyl residues in specific proteins (eg, prothrombin).[171] The 2,3-epoxide of vitamin K that is subsequently formed is reduced to the starting vitamin K quinones—a process that can be antagonized by vitamin K antagonists such as warfarin.

Only traces of metabolites of vitamins K_1 and K_2 appear in urine; a considerable portion of vitamin K_3 is conjugated at the hydroquinone concentration to form β-glucuronide and sulfate esters, which are excreted.[172]

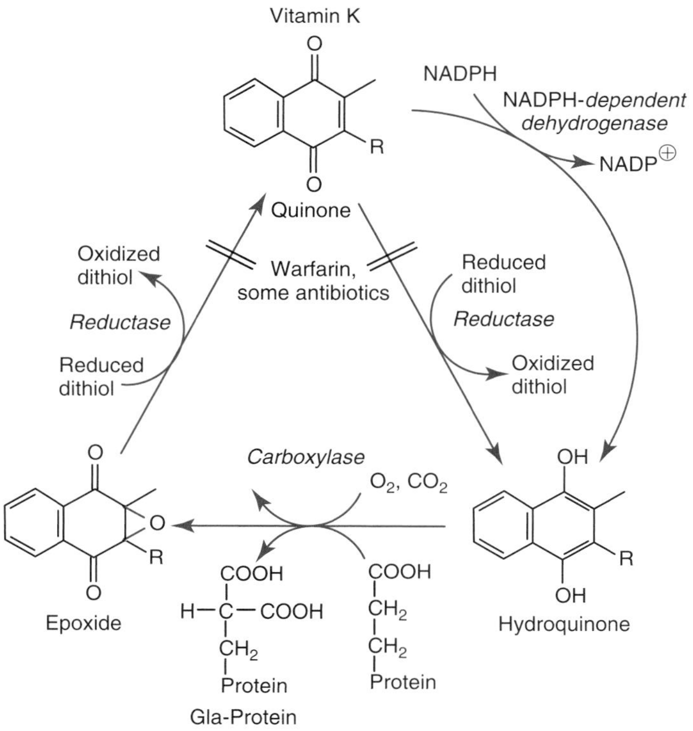

FIGURE 37.7 Metabolic Cycling of Vitamin K, the Effect of Warfarin, and the Formation of γ-Carboxyglutamyl (Gla) Proteins. *NAD(P)H*, Nicotinamide-adenine dinucleotide phosphate.

Functions

The essential and most thoroughly defined role of vitamin K is as a cofactor to vitamin K–dependent carboxylase, an enzyme necessary for the post-translational conversion of specific glutamyl residues in target proteins to γ-carboxyglutamyl (Gla) residues. This γ-carboxylation increases the affinity of these proteins for calcium.[173,174] The antihemorrhagic function of vitamin K depends on the formation of the Gla proteins prothrombin (factor II), proconvertin (factor VII), plasma thromboplastin component (factor IX), and Stuart factor (factor X), which, together with two other hemostatic vitamin K–dependent proteins, proteins C and S, and calcium, initiate a process to form thrombin that then catalyzes the conversion of fibrinogen to a fibrin clot.[174] See Chapter 71 for further discussion on hemostasis.

Proteins that contain γ-carboxyglutamyl are also abundant in bone tissue, with osteocalcin accounting for up to 80% of the total γ-carboxyglutamyl content of mature bone. Epidemiologic studies have shown an association between low vitamin K intakes and hip fracture risk.[175] Intervention studies have shown that vitamin K_1 can increase BMD in osteoporotic patients and can reduce fracture rates.[176] Evidence indicates that vitamins K and D may act synergistically in maintaining bone density.[171]

A further major Gla protein, matrix Gla protein (MGP), which contains five residues of γ-carboxyglutamic acid, is found in vascular smooth muscle, bone, and many soft tissues (heart, kidney, and lungs).[174,177] It is believed that MGP accumulates at sites of calcification, including calcified aortic valves and bone, and is a potent inhibitor of calcification. In experimental studies with mice lacking the gene coding for MGP, calcification of the arteries was observed that led to hemorrhagic death of the animals as a result of blood vessel rupture.[178] Several other Gla proteins have been identified, and putative roles have been assigned.[170]

Requirements and Reference Nutrient Intakes

Although the human gut bacteria synthesize large quantities of MKs, and such compounds are found in the liver in concentrations up to 10 times those of phylloquinones, absorption of these compounds has been difficult to demonstrate, and dietary restriction of vitamin K leads to evidence of inadequacy, as demonstrated by under-carboxylation of vitamin K–dependent proteins.[168] Thus, dietary reference intakes for vitamin K have been revised by the Food and Nutrition Board of the US IOM. Current recommendations are 120 μg/day for men older than 18 years, 90 μg/day for women older than 18 years (including those pregnant or lactating), 30 to 75 μg/day for children 1 to 18 years (dependent on age), 2.0 μg/day for infants up to 6 months, and 2.5 μg/day for infants between 7 and 12 months, with the latter requirements met by breast milk.[11]

Intravenous Supply

In the United States, it remains controversial whether vitamin K should be included in preparations of vitamins for use in TPN. Although this has been standard in Europe for many years,[18] the long-standing recommendation from the American Medical Association was not to include vitamin K, because this would complicate the provision of adequate warfarin therapy in those patients who require anticoagulation.[179] However, the 2003 requirements of the US Food and Drug Administration (FDA) specified that vitamin K should be included in vitamin supplements for both infants and adults, making the judgment that the physiologic and practical benefits of regular provision outweigh any problems in readjusting warfarin dosage.[156] The recommended intravenous (IV) adult dose is 150 μg/day, which is provided as phytonadione.

Deficiency

Although vitamin K deficiency in the adult is uncommon, the risk is increased with fat malabsorption states such as (1) bile duct obstruction, (2) cystic fibrosis, and (3) chronic pancreatitis and liver disease.[180,181] Risk is also increased by the use of drugs that interfere with vitamin K metabolism, such as the coumarin anticoagulants (eg, warfarin) and antibiotics containing the *N*-methylthiotetrazole side chain (eg, cephalosporin).[168] Other at-risk groups are hospitalized patients with poor nutrient intakes or those receiving TPN, when fat-soluble vitamin supplements may not fully meet requirements. Conversely, ingestion of supraphysiologic doses of vitamins A and E has been reported to induce vitamin K deficiency, probably through competitive mechanisms.[171] Defective blood coagulation and demonstration of abnormal noncarboxylated prothrombin are currently the only well-established signs of vitamin K deficiency.

Hemorrhagic disease of the newborn[182,183] can develop readily because of (1) poor placental transfer of vitamin K, (2) hepatic immaturity leading to inadequate synthesis of coagulation proteins, and (3) the low vitamin K content of early breast milk. Prothrombin concentrations during this period are only approximately 25% of adult concentrations. Severe diarrhea and antibiotics used to suppress diarrhea readily exacerbate the situation, so prothrombin concentrations can drop below 5% of the adult concentration, and bleeding can occur. This condition is routinely prevented by the prophylactic administration of 0.5 to 1.0 mg of phylloquinone intramuscularly, or 2.0 mg given orally, immediately after birth.

Toxicity

The use of high doses of naturally occurring vitamin K (K_1 and K_2) appears to have no known toxic effect; however, K_3 treatment can lead to the formation of erythrocyte cytoplasmic inclusions known as Heinz bodies and hemolytic anemia.[184] With severe hemolysis, increased bilirubin formation and undeveloped capacity for its conjugation may produce kernicterus in the newborn.

Because no adverse effects associated with vitamin K consumption from food or supplements have been reported in humans or animals, the US IOM has reported that a quantitative risk assessment cannot be performed, and thus an upper limit cannot be derived for vitamin K.[11]

Laboratory Assessment of Status

A wide range of biochemical and functional tests are available for vitamin K status.[25] Because of its relatively low plasma concentration (approximately 50 times lower than vitamin D and at least 10^3 times lower than vitamin A or E), vitamin K has long presented an analytical challenge. For this reason, vitamin K status has traditionally been assessed by functional methods, primarily by its effect on clotting time. The prothrombin time is assessed by adding a portion of tissue thromboplastin to recalcified plasma and measuring the clotting time against a normal control sample (see Chapter 71). In vitamin K deficiency, the prothrombin rises at least 2 seconds beyond the control time and may rise above 30 seconds (normal, 10–14 seconds). Attempts at cross-laboratory standardization led to the introduction of the international normalized ratio (INR), by which prothrombin time can be expressed as a fraction of the control time.

A more sensitive (1000-fold) assessment of vitamin K status with respect to prothrombin can be made by the immunoassay of des-γ-carboxy prothrombin, or under-carboxylated prothrombin, which is protein induced by vitamin K absence or antagonism (PIVKA-II).[185,186] PIVKA-II has proved to be a useful marker of subclinical vitamin K deficiency. Another measurement of deficient γ-carboxylation, plasma under-carboxylated osteocalcin, has been shown to correlate individually with PIVKA-II and plasma phylloquinone concentrations, and has a better correlation with plasma phylloquinone than PIVKA-II.[187] In this study of biochemical indexes of vitamin K nutritional status in a healthy adult population, the urinary γ-carboxyglutamic acid/creatinine ratio was measured by derivatization, HPLC separation, and fluorometric detection, and was shown to be sensitive to changes in dietary phylloquinone intake. This marker may have advantages in epidemiologic surveys as a less invasive sample.

Direct measurement of plasma phylloquinone is probably the best indicator of vitamin K status and has been shown to correlate with intake.[188] HPLC methods are the mainstay of vitamin K measurement[189-191] and typically require 0.2 to 2.0 mL of serum or plasma. Protein precipitation and lipid extraction (often into hexane), followed by solvent evaporation, preparative HPLC (to isolate vitamin K from other lipids), re-evaporation of the vitamin K–rich fraction, dilution in the mobile phase, and further HPLC with electrochemical or fluorometric detection, often after postcolumn reduction,[192,193] are required. HPLC-mass spectrometry methods have also been developed.[194] In general, typical between-batch imprecision values are CVs of 11% to 18% with limits of detection of less than 50 pmol/L. An External Quality Assessment Scheme is available.[195]

Preanalytical Variables

Plasma, serum, or whole blood specimens are all suitable, but it is recommended that local laboratories should be consulted for their preferred sample type. Vitamin K is light-sensitive, and samples should be protected from light as much as possible by wrapping in foil.[132] Vitamin K showed good stability in whole blood collected into tubes containing a clot activator for up to 72 hours at room temperature and without light protection.[133]

Reference Intervals

Because plasma vitamin K concentration is influenced by plasma triglyceride due to the association of circulating vitamin K_1 with very low density lipoproteins, it is expressed as a ratio of the triglyceride concentration.[196] It is also affected by the acute phase response in SIRS, which is likely as a result of the inflammation-dependent plasma lipid redistribution.[37] The suggested reference interval for plasma vitamin K is 0.2 to 2.2 nmol/mmol triglyceride.[132,196] For more information, refer to the Appendix on Reference Intervals. Laboratories should verify that these ranges are appropriate for use in their own settings.

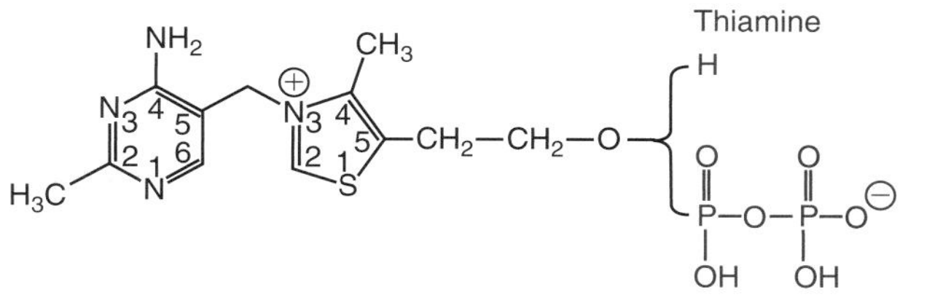

FIGURE 37.8 Thiamine and the Pyrophosphate Coenzyme.

Vitamin B_1

Vitamin B_1, which is also known as thiamine or aneurin, forms the coenzyme thiamine pyrophosphate (TPP). It is required for the essential decarboxylation reactions catalyzed by the pyruvate and 2-oxoglutarate complexes.

Chemistry

The structure of thiamine [3-(4-amino-2-methyl-pyrimidyl-5-methyl)-4-methyl-5-(β-hydroxyethyl)thiazole] is that of a pyrimidine ring, bearing an amino group, linked by a methylene bridge to a thiazole ring (Fig. 37.8). The thiazole has a primary alcohol side chain at C5, which can be phosphorylated in vivo to produce thiamine phosphate esters, the most common of which is TPP (also known as thiamine diphosphate [cocarboxylase]). Monophosphate and triphosphate esters also occur. The basic vitamin is isolated or synthesized and handled as a solid thiazolium salt (eg, thiamine chloride hydrochloride). Thiamine is somewhat heat labile, particularly in alkaline solutions, where base attacks occur at C2 of the thiazolium ring.

Dietary Sources

Small amounts of thiamine and its phosphates are present in most plant and animal tissues, but more abundant sources include unrefined cereal grains, liver, heart, kidney, and lean cuts of pork. The enrichment of flour and derived food products, particularly breakfast cereals, has considerably increased the availability of this vitamin.

Absorption, Transport, Metabolism, and Excretion

Thiamine absorption occurs primarily in the proximal small intestine[198] by a saturable (thiamine transporter) process at a low concentration (≤1 μmol/L) and by simple passive diffusion beyond that, although percentage absorption diminishes with an increased dose. Absorbed thiamine undergoes intracellular phosphorylation, mainly to the pyrophosphate, but at the serosal side, 90% of transferred thiamine is present in the free form.[199] Thiamine uptake is enhanced by thiamine deficiency and is reduced by thyroid hormone, diabetes, and ethanol ingestion. The gene for the specific thiamine transporter has been identified, and the transporter has been cloned.[200] Thiamine is carried by portal blood to the liver. The free vitamin is present in plasma, but the coenzyme, TPP, is the primary cellular component. Approximately 30 mg is stored in the body, with 80% as pyrophosphate, 10% as triphosphate, and the rest as thiamine and its monophosphate. About half of body stores are found in skeletal muscle, with much of the remainder in the heart, liver, kidneys, and nervous tissues (including the brain, which contains most of the triphosphate).

The three tissue enzymes known to participate in the formation of phosphate esters are (1) thiaminokinase (a pyrophosphokinase), which catalyzes formation of TPP and adenosine monophosphate (AMP) from thiamine and adenosine triphosphate (ATP); (2) TPP-ATP phosphoryltransferase (cytosolic 5′-adenylic kinase), which forms the triphosphate and adenosine diphosphate from TPP and ATP; and (3) thiamine triphosphatase, which hydrolyzes TPP to the monophosphate. Although thiaminokinase is widely distributed in the body, phosphoryl transferase and the membrane-associated triphosphatase are found mainly in nervous tissue.[201]

With the use of labeled thiamine probes, a study of thiamine metabolism at normal loads produced an estimated half-life of thiamine of 9.5 to 18.5 days, and showed a large number of breakdown products in the urine.[202] Several of these urinary catabolites are shown in Fig. 37.9.

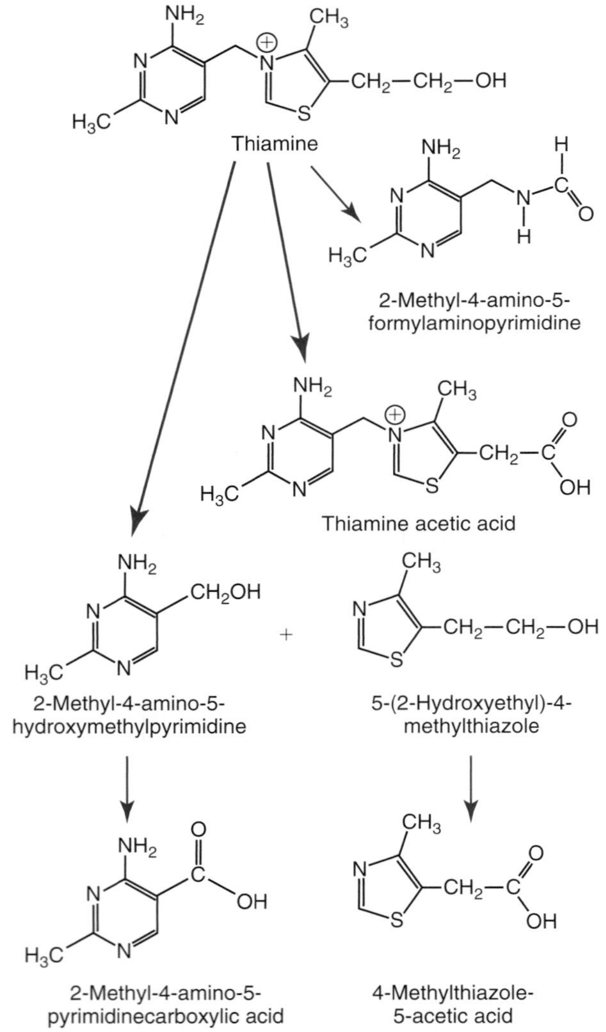

Functions

Thiamine is required by the body as the pyrophosphate (TPP) in two general types of reactions: (1) the oxidative decarboxylation of 2-oxo acids catalyzed by dehydrogenase complexes; and (2) the formation of α-ketols (ketoses) as catalyzed by transketolase and as the triphosphate (TTP) within the nervous system. TPP functions as the magnesium (Mg)-coordinated coenzyme for the active aldehyde transfers in multienzyme dehydrogenase complexes that affect decarboxylative conversion of α-keto (2-oxo) acids to acyl-coenzyme A (acyl-CoA) derivatives, such as pyruvate dehydrogenase and α-ketoglutarate dehydrogenase. These are often localized in the mitochondria, where efficient use in the Krebs tricarboxylic acid (citric acid) cycle follows.

Three types of subunit proteins constitute such dehydrogenase complexes: (1) a TPP-dependent decarboxylase, which converts the 2-oxo acid to an α-hydroxyalkyl–TPP complex; (2) a transacylase core, which contains lipoyl residues that are acylated by the α-hydroxyalkyl–TPP; and (3) a flavin adenine dinucleotide (FAD)-dependent dihydrolipoyl dehydrogenase, which re-oxidizes the reduced lipoyl residues produced after transfer of their acyl functions to reduced CoA. In addition to energy and an ultimate ATP supply derived from reactions in the Krebs cycle, the initial pyruvate dehydrogenase–catalyzed step provides acetyl-CoA as a biosynthetic precursor to other essential compounds, such as lipids and acetylcholine of the parasympathetic nervous system.

Transketolase is a TPP-dependent enzyme found in the cytosol of many tissues, especially liver and blood cells, in which the principal carbohydrate pathways exist. In the pentose phosphate pathway, which additionally supplies reduced nicotinamide-adenine dinucleotide phosphate (NADPH) necessary for biosynthetic reactions, this enzyme catalyzes the reversible transfer of a glycoaldehyde moiety from the first two carbons of a donor ketose phosphate to the aldehyde carbon of an aldose phosphate.

Although thiamine as its pyrophosphate contributes to nervous system composition and function in such essential reactions as energy production and biosynthesis of lipids and acetylcholine, a further specific, non-cofactor role for thiamine has been proposed in excitable cells. Here, TTP is believed to be involved in the regulation of ion channels, specifically, chloride channels of large unitary conductance (the "maxi-chloride channels").[203,204] TTP may also have more basic metabolic functions, including acting as a phosphate donor for the phosphorylation of proteins, suggesting a potential role in cell signaling. A subacute necrotizing encephalomyelopathy has been seen in patients with Leigh syndrome, resulting from the presence of an inhibitor of TPP-ATP phosphoryl transferase and a consequent reduction in TTP concentration.[205]

FIGURE 37.9 Principal Urinary Catabolites of Thiamine.

Requirements and Reference Nutrient Intakes

Because thiamine is necessary mainly for the metabolism of carbohydrates, fats, and alcohol, a direct correlation has been noted between physiologic requirements and the amount of metabolizable food intake. A greater requirement is present under situations in which metabolism is increased (eg, in normal conditions of increased muscular activity, pregnancy, and lactation, and in abnormal cases of protracted fever, post-trauma, and hyperthyroidism). Clinical signs of deficiency in adults can be prevented with intakes of thiamine of more than 0.15 to 0.2 mg/1000 kcal, but 0.35 to 0.4 mg/1000 kcal may be closer to a concentration necessary to maintain urinary excretion and TPP-dependent erythrocyte transketolase activity within normal reference intervals.[11,25] With further consideration of average caloric intakes and activities in different age groups, the most recent recommendations of RDA are 1.2 mg/day for men 19 years and older and 1.1 mg/day for women 19 years and older.[11] The requirement for pregnant women increases early in pregnancy and then remains constant; 1.4 mg/day is recommended.[11] The lactating woman secretes 0.1 to 0.2 mg of thiamine/day in milk, so 1.4 mg/day is suggested.[11] Based on the thiamine content of human milk and with an increment considered to provide a margin of safety, 0.2 mg/day is the allowance for infants up to 6 months, and 0.3 mg/day for infants 7 to 12 months. For children, due to growth, 0.5 mg/day is suggested for up to 3 years of age, and between 4 and 8 years, 0.6 mg/day is suggested.[11]

Intravenous Supply

Traditionally, the intravenous recommendation was 3 mg/day for adults, usually provided as thiamine hydrochloride, but also as thiamine mononitrate or tetrahydrate. In the 2000 FDA recommendations, this was increased to 6 mg/day, with recognition of the likelihood of increased demands for thiamine caused by hypercatabolism in such patients and the serious potential complications of deficiency.[206,207]

Deficiency

For an illustrative case of vitamin B_1 deficiency see Box 37.4. Causes of thiamine deficiency include inadequate intake caused by diets largely dependent on milled, nonenriched grains such as rice and wheat, or the ingestion of raw fish containing thiaminases,[208] which hydrolytically destroy the vitamin in the gastrointestinal tract. Tea may also contain anti-thiamine factors.[209,210] Chronic alcoholism often leads to thiamine deficiency caused by reduced intake, impaired absorption, impaired use, and reduced storage,[211] and may lead clinically to the Wernicke-Korsakoff syndrome.[207,212] Other at-risk groups include those who receive parenteral nutrition without adequate thiamine supplementation,[213] older adult patients taking diuretics,[214] and patients undergoing long-term renal dialysis.[215]

Beriberi (origin: Sinhalese from a word meaning weakness) is the disease that results from thiamine deficiency.[216,217] Clinical signs of thiamine deficiency primarily involve the nervous and cardiovascular systems. In the adult, the most frequently observed symptoms include mental confusion, anorexia, muscular weakness, ataxia, peripheral paralysis, ophthalmoplegia, edema (wet beriberi), muscle wasting (dry beriberi), tachycardia, and an enlarged heart. In infants, symptoms appear suddenly and severely, often involving cardiac failure and cyanosis. Commonly, the distinction between wet (cardiovascular) and dry (neuritic) manifestations of beriberi relate to duration and severity of the deficiency, the degree of physical exertion, and caloric intake. The wet or edematous beriberi[218] results from severe physical exertion and high carbohydrate intake, whereas the dry or polyneuritic beriberi[219,220] stems from relative inactivity with caloric restriction during a long-term deficiency. The three major physiologic derangements that typically involve the cardiovascular system are peripheral vasodilatation leading to a high-output state, biventricular myocardial failure, and retention of sodium (Na) and water, leading to edema. Nervous system involvement includes peripheral neuropathy, Wernicke encephalopathy, and the amnesic psychosis of Korsakoff syndrome. More rarely, but especially in seriously ill patients in hospitals, an acute form of cardiac failure has been described (Shoshin beriberi), which may be fatal, but can be successfully and rapidly reversed with high-dose intravenous thiamine.[206,221]

Several thiamine-responsive disorders are caused by genetic mutation. In thiamine-responsive megaloblastic anemia, the gene has been mapped and cloned, and designated as *SLC19A2* as a member of the solute carrier gene superfamily.[200] Mutations of this gene, the product of which is a membrane protein that transports thiamine with submicromolar affinity, have been found in all thiamine-responsive megaloblastic anemia kindreds studied. Thiamine-responsive pyruvate dehydrogenase complex deficiency, which presents with lactic acidosis, can be caused by a point mutation within the TPP-binding region,[222] and a thiamine-responsive, branched-chain keto acid dehydrogenase complex deficiency, which presents as a form of maple syrup urine disease, is caused by mutations in the E1 α-subunit of the enzyme complex.[223] Therapeutic doses of 5 to 20 mg/day of thiamine have proved beneficial in these cases.

Toxicity

Because no reports have described adverse effects from consumption of excess thiamine from food and supplements (supplements of 50 mg/day are widely available without prescription), and because the data are inadequate for a quantitative risk assessment, no tolerable upper intake levels has been defined for thiamine.[11] However, because stimulators of transketolase enzyme synthesis, such as thiamine, support the high rate of nucleic acid ribose synthesis necessary for tumor cell survival, chemotherapy resistance,

BOX 37.4 Case: Agitation, Opthalmoplegia, and Vitamin B_1 Deficiency as a Result of Losing Weight by Prolonged Dietary Restriction[197]

A 38-year-old white Scottish man with mild learning difficulties presented with a 3-day history of diplopia and agitation, after 7 days of presumed viral gastroenteritis. On admission, he was agitated, mildly confused, tachycardic, and tachypnoeic. There were no chest signs or peripheral edema. He had complete bilateral sixth cranial nerve palsies and horizontal nystagmus, with dilated, slowly reacting pupils. Limb movements were clumsy, with moderate cerebellar signs and dysdiadochokinesis, but he had no tremor. He was clinically jaundiced. Electrocardiography (ECG) showed inferolateral T-wave inversion. His heart size was at the upper limit of normal on chest radiography. On specific questioning, he gave a history of lifelong avoidance of alcohol, but had 34 kg weight loss over the preceding 3 months. This information was corroborated by his parents and practice nurse. At an initial weight of 127 kg (body mass index 42.4 kg/m^2), he had received dietary advice from his practice

Continued

BOX 37.4 Case: Agitation, Opthalmoplegia and Vitamin B_1 Deficiency as a Result of Losing Weight by Prolonged Dietary Restriction—cont'd

nurse. He proceeded to lose weight, which fell rapidly from 123 kg at 4 weeks, to 110 kg at 8 weeks, 104 kg at 11 weeks, and finally 93 kg (body mass index 31 kg/m^2) on admission. More recently, pursuing greater weight loss, he had eliminated all bread, cereals, and fats, on a diet considered starvation by his parents, without nutritional supplements. Selected biochemical, hematologic, vitamin, and trace element results available on the stated days are shown:

Test	Reference Range (Conversion Factor to Traditional Units)	DAY				
		1	2	3	4	50
Calcium (adjusted)	2.10–2.60 mmol/L (1 mmol/L = 4 mg/dL)	2.67				2.52
Magnesium	0.70–1.00 mmol/L (1 mmol/L = 2 mEq/L)	0.94				0.89
Ferritin	10.0–275.0 μg/L (1 μg/L = 2.25 pmol/L)	224				25.0
CRP	<10 mg/L (1 mg/L = 9.52 mmol/L)	11	13	12	6.7	2.7
Albumin	32–45 g/L	40	37	38	37	41
Bilirubin	<20 μmol/L (1 μmol/L = 0.06 mg/dL)	48	38	35	24	16
Alkaline phosphatase	40–150 U/L (1 U/L = 0.02 μcat/L)	140	126	130	116	93
Aspartate aminotransferase	<40 U/L (1 U/L = 0.02 μcat/L)	34				17
Alanine aminotransferase	<50 U/L (1 U/L = 0.02 μcat/L)	70	57	59	62	18
γ-glutamyltransferase	<70 U/L (1 U/L = 0.02 μcat/L)	111	86	87	74	
Hemoglobin	130–180 g/L	152	149	153	144	139
Vitamin B_1	275–675 ng/g hemoglobin	132				453
RBC vitamin B_2	1.0–3.4 nmol/g hemoglobin	1.6				2.9
RBC vitamin B_6	250–680 pmol/g hemoglobin	139				619
Vitamin B_{12}	200–900 pg/mL (1 pg/mL = 0.74 pmol/L)	481				328
Folate	3.1–20.0 ng/mL (1 ng/mL = 2.27 nmol/L)	1.4				3.3
Vitamin C	15–90 μmol/L (1 μmol/L = 0.02 mg/dL)	3				27
Vitamin A	1–3 μmol/L (1 μmol/L = 28.65 μg/dL)	0.5				0.9
Vitamin E	15–45 μmol/L (1 μmol/L = 0.04 μg/dL)	20				20
Copper	10.0–22.0 μmol/L (1 μmol/L = 6.37 μg/dL)	14.4				17.1
Manganese	70–280 nmol/L (1 nmol/L = 0.05 μg/L)	182				176
Selenium	0.8–2.0 μmol/L (1 μmol/L = 78.74 μg/L)	0.66				0.74
Zinc	10.7–18.0 μmol/L (1 μmol/L = 6.54 μg/dL)	15.1				10.8

Commentary

Because of the presence of agitation and cerebellar signs, the most likely cause of the ophthalmoplegia and electrocardiographic manifestation is Wernicke encephalopathy as a result of acute vitamin B_1 (thiamine) deficiency. Praising the patient for losing weight inadvertently motivated him to try harder, which inevitably led him to starvation and consequently malnutrition. The classic triad of Wernicke encephalopathy is ophthalmoplegia, ataxia, and mental confusion. Low concentrations of red blood cell (RBC) thiamine diphosphate (TDP), the active form of thiamine, confirmed the diagnosis. TDP reflects body thiamine stores and correlates with transketolase functional testing (discussed in the following). Vitamins A, C, B_6, folate, and selenium were all low without a marked systemic inflammatory response, as evidenced by the only marginally raised C-reactive protein (CRP). Vitamin B_1 deficiency causes inhibition of carbohydrate metabolism and accumulation of acetaldehyde, which affects astrocytes within cranial nerve nuclei. Magnesium is required for vitamin B_1 action. Despite deficiencies in other vitamins, there were no associated features. The immediate treatment for thiamine deficiency in alcoholics or malnourished patients is intravenous thiamine, commonly administered with water-soluble vitamins B and C as Pabrinex (thiamine 250 mg) before switching to oral thiamine supplementation (refer to local guidance for dosing regimens). Ophthalmoplegia usually resolves rapidly with treatment. The most important learning point is that without thiamine repletion, carbohydrate administration would precipitate Wernicke-Korsakoff syndrome and permanent anterograde amnesia. Magnesium repletion is also required to allow thiamine to function.

The signs of cardiomegaly and ECG abnormalities indicated wet beri-beri in addition to the classic neurological signs of dry beri-beri, which are both as a result of thiamine deficiency. If left untreated, this condition progresses to high output heart failure, which is a reported cause of sudden death from starvation or anorexia nervosa. This is discussed in the text.

Obstructive jaundice and ultrasonography showed several small gallstones within the gallbladder. Symptomatic cholelithiasis is a recognized complication of consuming a low-fat diet or of extreme weight loss.

The patient was treated with 5-mL intravenous Pabrinex, which contains anhydrous glucose (1 g), ascorbic acid (500 mg), nicotinamide (160 mg), pyridoxine hydrochloride (50 mg), riboflavin (4 mg), and thiamine hydrochloride (250 mg) 3 times daily for 3 days, resumed normal feeding, and made a good recovery with eventual normal findings on ECG, chest radiography, echocardiography, and normal neurological signs.

We are grateful to Dr. Dinesh Talwar for highlighting this illustrative case.

From McKenna LA, Drummond RS, Drummond S, Talwar D, Lean MJ. Seeing Double: the low carb diet. *BMJ* 2013;346:f2563.

and proliferation, some concern has been expressed that thiamine supplementation of common food products may contribute to increased cancer rates in the Western world.[224] However, little evidence is available to support this assumption. Individuals given high-dose intravenous thiamine in the treatment of beriberi rarely develop anaphylaxis (frequency of approximately 1 : 100,000).

Laboratory Assessment of Status

As thiamine deficiency develops, rapid loss of the vitamin is seen from all tissues except the brain. The decrease of TPP in the erythrocyte roughly parallels the decrease of this coenzyme in other tissue.[225] During this time, thiamine concentrations in urine fall to near zero; urinary metabolites remain high for some time before decreasing.

Historically, assessment of thiamine status was performed using an animal bioassay (correction of bradycardia in thiamine-deficient rats). Later, it was performed by microbiological assays; some bacterial microbiological assays are still in use in the food industry. Early chemical methods were often based on the production of a fluorophore, thiochrome, when thiamine is oxidized with ferricyanide in alkaline solution—a property that is used in some modern chromatographic methods.[25]

Because the basic biological function of thiamine is to act as the pyrophosphate cofactor in a number of enzyme systems, two differing approaches to assessment of status have become available. The analyte, free or phosphorylated, can be measured directly in a suitable body fluid or tissue, or its properties as an enzymatic cofactor can be exploited in a functional assay. Both approaches have their advantages and disadvantages, and consensus as to which is the more useful has not been achieved; the two are probably complementary, each supplying some, but not all, of the information necessary to assess thiamine adequacy (Table 37.4).

The most commonly used enzyme for the functional assay is transketolase. Transketolase catalyzes two reactions in the pentose phosphate pathway (Fig. 37.10). As an enzyme within the erythrocyte, transketolase is independent of nonspecific changes in the extracellular plasma. As vitamin B_1 deficiency becomes more severe, (1) thiamine becomes limited in the body cells, (2) the amount of the coenzyme is depleted, and (3) transketolase activity subsequently diminishes. The TPP effect measures the extent of depletion of the transketolase enzyme for coenzyme by assaying enzyme activity before and after TPP supplementation.[226] The percent increase in activity is defined as the TPP effect (or the activation coefficient). Several methods are available to measure transketolase activity. In the Brin procedure,[227] activities of holo forms and apo forms of transketolase in erythrocyte hemolysates are measured before and after addition of TPP, by spectrophotometric determinations of the amount of ribose-5′-phosphate used or the hexose-6-phosphate formed. This method is reliable but time-consuming. In an alternative method, the rate of formation of glyceraldehyde-3-P is measured indirectly by a coupled reaction in a system containing excess triosephosphate isomerase, glycerolphosphate dehydrogenase, and NADH. Glyceraldehyde-3-P is converted by triosephosphate isomerase to dihydroxyacetone-P, which, in the presence of glycerolphosphate dehydrogenase and NADH, is reduced to glycerol-1-P. The rate of NADH oxidation, measured at 340 nm, is proportional to the transketolase activity. Kinetic methods such as these have been automated with consequent improvements in throughput and precision.[25]

The transketolase activation test basically consists of two tests: (1) measurement of basal activity, and (2) assessment of the degree to which basal activity can be increased by exogenous TPP; each may be influenced by different factors. There is some evidence that long-term deficiency states of thiamine may down-regulate synthesis of the apoenzyme.[228] In comparison studies against erythrocyte TPP concentrations, better correlations were obtained with basal activity rather than the activation coefficient.[229]

Other potential disadvantages of the transketolase test include reductions in apoenzyme synthesis in diseases other than thiamine deficiency, such as diabetes,[230] liver disease,[231] reduced apoenzyme-to-coenzyme binding with apotransketolase variants,[232] lack of stability relative to TPP on processing and storage,[233] lack of a standard or External Quality Assessment Scheme, and variations in published upper limits

TABLE 37.4 Relative Merits of Direct (Erythrocyte Thiamine Pyrophosphate) or Functional (Erythrocyte Transketolase Activation) Measurements in Assessing Thiamine Status

	Erythrocyte Thiamine Pyrophosphate	Erythrocyte Transketolase Activation
Advantages	Pure standard available	May correlate better with clinical conditions in repleted patients
	Precise and robust method	Large database established
	More stable when frozen	
	Depletes at rates similar to other organs	
	Method (HPLC) allows measurement of other forms of thiamine	
	Can detect tissue accumulation	
Disadvantages	May normalize early with parenteral treatment	Depletion of apoenzyme may be non-nutritional related (eg, liver disease, diabetes)
		Variants may have abnormal binding
		May be influenced by cofactor deficiencies (eg, magnesium)
		Difficult to standardize, less robust
		Derived activation coefficient reduces precision

HPLC, High-performance liquid chromatography.

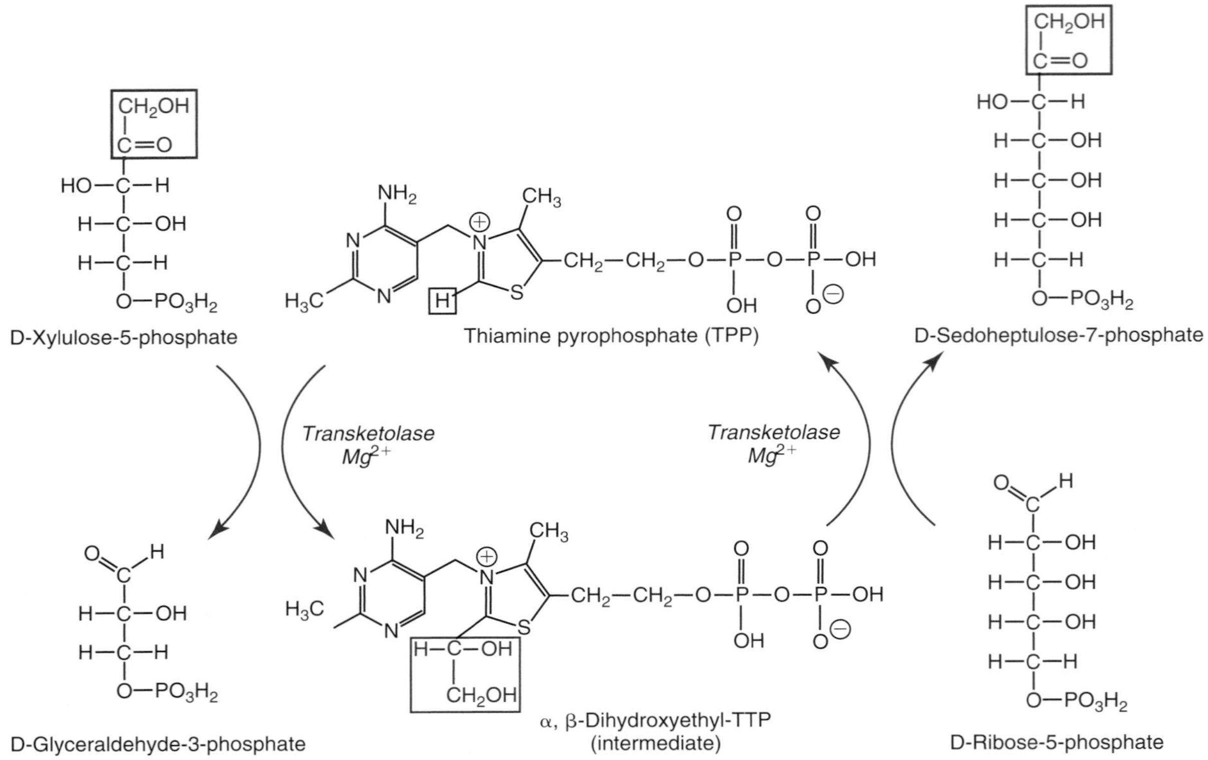

FIGURE 37.10 The Transketolase Reaction.

for the activation coefficient from 15.5% to 40%. The main advantages of the transketolase test are that it is widely used, has a relatively large database and body of experience, and is claimed to correlate better with clinical conditions in alcoholic patients being repleted with thiamine.[234]

Circulating thiamine concentration may be directly measured in plasma, erythrocytes, or whole blood. The plasma (or serum) concentration is believed to reflect recent intake and is mainly unphosphorylated thiamine at low concentrations (approximately 10–20 nmol/L). Because the erythrocyte contains approximately 80% of the total thiamine content of whole blood[235] (mainly as the pyrophosphate) and erythrocyte thiamine stores deplete at a similar rate as other major organs, HPLC measurement of TPP in erythrocytes is a good indicator of body stores. Typical HPLC methods include a protein precipitation step, pre- or postcolumn formation of the fluorophore, thiochrome (usually with alkaline ferricyanide), and isocratic separation.[236] The method is easily standardized with pure TPP; it has good precision (CVs of <5%) and acceptable limits of detection (≈10 nmol/L), and the analyte is stable at −70°C for at least 7 months and at room temperature for 48 hours.[229] Whole blood samples may be analyzed in a similar manner to washed erythrocytes and may provide the advantage of simpler sample handling, but they are subject to variable plasma dilution. However, a good correlation has been obtained between erythrocyte and whole blood TPP concentrations, particularly when whole blood TPP includes a correction for hemoglobin (Hb). A rapid HPLC method for measuring both thiamine and its phosphate esters has been described.[237]

Determination of the urinary excretion of thiamine in a 4-hour specimen, especially with comparison of excretion before and after a test load, is helpful in differentiating among extremes of thiamine status. However, as with most assessments based on the quantity of water-soluble vitamins in urine, excretion can be influenced considerably by dietary intake, absorption, and other factors. Measurements of certain urinary metabolites, notably thiamine acetic acid, have been suggested as reflecting thiamine status but are not routinely requested.[202]

Preanalytical Variables

Whole blood collected into containers with the preservatives Li heparin or ethylenediaminetetraacetic acid (EDTA) is recommended, but local laboratories should be consulted for their preferred sample type. A recent study using HPLC with fluorimetric detection[133] reported that vitamin B_1 showed good stability up to 72 hours at room temperature.

Reference Intervals

Reference intervals for thiamine and its esters depend on whether: (1) erythrocytes, whole blood, or plasma is used as a sample; (2) cellular concentrations are expressed per liter of packed red cells or grams of Hb; and (3) mass or SI units are used. Some guidance intervals are as follows: for erythrocyte transketolase activity, 0.75 to 1.30 U/g Hb (48.4–83.9 kU/mol Hb) is used; for percent TPP effect (activation), 0% to 15% is normal, 16% to 25% is marginally deficient, and more than 25% is severely deficient with clinical signs. For direct TPP concentration measurements, typical intervals are 173 to 293 nmol/L for erythrocytes and 90 to 140 nmol/L for whole blood,[238] 280 to 590 ng/g Hb in erythrocytes, and 275 to 675 ng/g Hb in whole blood with less than 150 ng/g Hb indicating clinical deficiency.[132,236] For more information, refer to the Appendix on Reference Intervals. Laboratories should verify that these ranges are appropriate for use in their own settings.

Vitamin B_2

Vitamin B_2, also known as riboflavin, is an essential component of coenzymes that are involved in reduction-oxidation (redox) reactions in the body.

Chemistry

Flavins are a family of yellow-colored compounds with the basic structure of 7,8-dimethyl-10-alkylisoalloxazine.[239] Riboflavin, commonly known as vitamin B_2, is the precursor of all biologically important flavins, notably flavin mononucleotide (FMN) (riboflavin-5′-phosphate) and flavin adenine dinucleotide (FAD) (Fig. 37.11). Riboflavin and its related metabolites act as cofactors to several redox enzymes. FMN is formed from riboflavin by flavokinase-catalyzed phosphorylation, and FAD is formed from FMN and ATP by the action of FAD synthetase, also called pyrophosphorylase. FAD is further converted by covalent bonding to form various tissue flavoproteins.[240] Flavins are stable during exposure to heat but are decomposed by light, which causes photodegradation of the D-ribitol side chain at position 10 of the isoalloxazine ring system to ultimately yield lumiflavin (7,8,10-trimethylisoalloxazine) under alkaline conditions and lumichrome (7,8-dimethylalloxazine) at all pH values, especially in neutral-to-acidic solutions. Flavins are chemically and biologically reduced to nearly colorless compounds that rapidly re-oxidize on exposure to air (O_2).

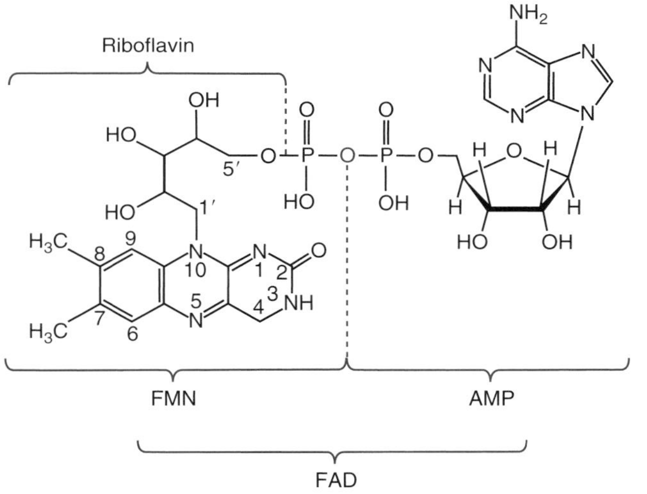

FIGURE 37.11 Riboflavin and Flavin Mononucleotide *(FMN)* as Components of Flavin Adenine Dinucleotide *(FAD)*. *AMP*, adenosine monophosphate.

Dietary Sources

Rich sources of the coenzyme forms of the vitamin include liver, kidney, and heart. Many vegetables are also good sources, but cereals are low in flavin content. Current practices of fortification and enrichment of cereal products have made these significant contributors to the daily requirement. Milk from cows and from humans is a good source of the vitamin and probably the main source in western diets,[241,242] but considerable loss can occur from exposure to light during pasteurization and bottling, or as a result of irradiation to increase vitamin D content.

Absorption, Transport, Metabolism, and Excretion

Most dietary riboflavin is taken in as a complex of proteins with the coenzymes FMN and FAD. These coenzymes are released from noncovalent attachment to proteins as a consequence of gastric acidification. Nonspecific action of pyrophosphatase and phosphatase on the coenzyme occurs in the upper gut.[243] The vitamin is primarily absorbed in the proximal small intestine by a saturable transport system that is rapid and proportional to intake before leveling off at doses near 27 mg/day of riboflavin/day.[244] Bile salts appear to facilitate uptake, and a modest amount of the vitamin circulates via the enterohepatic system.[245] Active transport at lower concentrations of intake was believed to be Na ion–dependent and to involve phosphorylation, although later work suggested that uptake is independent of Na ions.[239,246] The transport of flavins in human blood involves loose binding to albumin and tight binding to numerous globulins, with major binding noted to several classes of immunoglobulins (IgA, IgG, and IgM).[247] Pregnancy increases the concentration of carrier protein for riboflavin, which results in a higher rate of riboflavin uptake at the maternal surface of the placenta.[248] Uptake of riboflavin into the cells of organs such as the liver is facilitated, possibly requiring a specific carrier at physiologic concentrations, but it can occur by diffusion at higher concentrations.[249] Metabolic interconversions of flavins at the cellular concentration are outlined in Fig. 37.12.

Conversion of riboflavin to coenzymes occurs within the cellular cytoplasm of most tissues but particularly in the small intestine, liver, heart, and kidney. The obligatory first step is

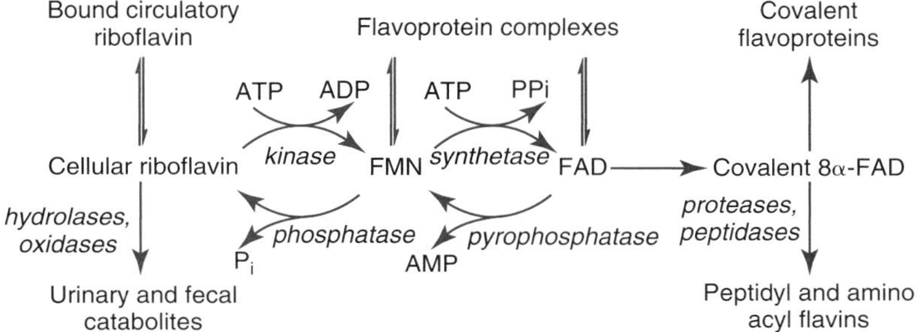

FIGURE 37.12 Cellular Interconversions of Flavins. *ADP*, Adenosine diphosphate; *AMP*, adenosine monophosphate; *ATP*, adenosine triphosphate; *FAD*, flavin adenine dinucleotide; *FMN*, flavin mononucleotide; *PPi*, pyrophosphate.

the ATP-dependent phosphorylation of the vitamin catalyzed by flavokinase. The FMN product can be complexed with specific apoenzymes to form several functional flavoproteins, but the larger quantity is further converted to FAD in a second ATP-dependent reaction catalyzed by FAD synthetase (pyrophosphorylase). Biosynthesis of flavocoenzymes, particularly at the flavokinase step, is likely tightly regulated. Thyroxine and triiodothyronine stimulate FMN and FAD synthesis in mammalian systems.[250,251] FAD is the predominant flavocoenzyme present in tissue, where it is complexed mainly with numerous flavoprotein dehydrogenases and oxidases. Some FAD (<10%) can become covalently linked to any of five specific amino acid residues of a few important apoenzymes.[252] Examples include 8α-*N*(3)-histidyl FAD within succinate dehydrogenase and 8α-*S*-cysteinyl FAD within monoamine oxidase, both of mitochondrial localization. Turnover of covalently attached flavocoenzymes requires intracellular proteolysis, and further degradation of the coenzymes involves nonspecific pyrophosphatase cleavage of FAD to FMN and AMP, and further action by nonspecific phosphates on FMN and AMP. Because there is little storage of riboflavin as such, urinary excretion reflects dietary intake. Milk contains reasonable quantities of the vitamin and lesser amounts of coenzyme, principally FMN. Smaller quantities of side chain degradation products such as lumichrome, 10-formylmethylflavin and 10-(2′-hydroxyethyl)flavin, and ring-altered compounds are excreted; this may largely result from the action of intestinal microorganisms.[253] Traces of 8α-flavin peptides and catabolites are found in urine and feces.

Functions

Riboflavin and its coenzyme derivatives are involved in a large variety of chemical reactions. These derivatives are capable of one- and two-electron transfer processes and play a pivotal role in coupling the two-electron oxidation of most organic substrates to the one-electron transfer of the respiratory chain,[254] thus becoming involved in energy production. They also function as electrophiles and nucleophiles, with covalent intermediates of flavin and substrate frequently involved in catalysis. Flavoproteins catalyze dehydrogenation reactions, hydroxylations, oxidative decarboxylations, deoxygenations, and reductions of O_2 to H_2O_2.[242,255] The chemical versatility of the flavoproteins is clearly controlled by specific interactions with the proteins with which they are bound.[254] Other major functions of riboflavin include drug metabolism in conjunction with the cytochrome P450 enzymes and lipid metabolism.

Flavins also have pro-oxidative and antioxidative functions. They are believed to contribute to oxidative stress through their ability to produce superoxide and to catalyze the production of H_2O_2.[254] As an antioxidant, FAD is a coenzyme to glutathione reductase in the regeneration of reduced glutathione from oxidized glutathione, which is necessary for the removal of lipid peroxides.[46] Riboflavin deficiency is associated with increased lipid peroxidation.[256] Flavins have also been linked with apoptosis[254] and have homocysteine-lowering properties[257]; FAD is a cofactor to methylenetetrahydrofolate reductase (MTHFR) in the remethylation of homocysteine.[257] An interaction between folate, riboflavin, and the genotype of MTHFR is apparent, especially in colorectal cancer.[258] Other possible therapeutic uses of riboflavin include prophylaxis of migraine attacks[259] and treatment of lactic acidosis caused by the use of nucleoside reverse transcriptase inhibitors in patients with AIDS[260] or by genetic defects in the mitochondrial respiratory chain, as seen in Leigh disease.[261] Riboflavin is also effective in treating the lipid storage myopathy associated with mutations of the *ETFDH* (electron-transferring flavoprotein dehydrogenase) gene.[262] Antagonism of riboflavin metabolism has been used as an anti-infective agent, notably in malaria treatment.[263,264]

Requirements and Reference Nutrient Intakes

Riboflavin status has been assessed on the basis of the relationship of dietary intake to overt signs of hyporiboflavinosis, urinary excretion of the vitamin, erythrocyte riboflavin content, and erythrocyte glutathione reductase activity. Calculations have been based on protein allowances, energy intakes, and body size, but these do not differ significantly because they are interdependent. At least 0.5 mg of riboflavin/1000 kcal is required by adults, and 0.6 mg/1000 kcal constitutes the allowance suggested for all ages. Based on considerations such as these, the current RDA has been set at 1.3 mg/day for men 19 to 70 years of age and older, and 1.1 mg/day for women in the same age group. Children 1 to 3 years old have an RDA of 0.5 mg/day, which increases to 0.6 mg/day up to age 8 years. From 8 to 18 years, RDAs progressively approach adult concentrations. Because pregnant women tend to excrete less riboflavin as pregnancy progresses and additionally exhibit FAD stimulation of erythrocyte glutathione reductase activity, recommended allowances call for an additional 0.3 mg/day during pregnancy. During lactation, between 18 and 80 μg of riboflavin is secreted daily into every 100 mL of human milk.[265] If it is assumed that an infant will ingest an average of 750 mL of milk per day during its first 6 months and 600 mL/day for the next 6 months, this secretion rate translates into an ingestion of between 100 and 600 μg of riboflavin per day/day. Furthermore, if it is assumed that 70% of maternally ingested riboflavin is used for milk production, these data suggest that the present RDA for lactating women should be increased by an additional 400 to 500 μg/day. Accordingly, the RDA for lactating women has been set at 1.6 mg/day.[11]

Intravenous Supply

The recommended intravenous supply of riboflavin in adults is 3.6 mg/day.[18,179] Riboflavin in TPN mixtures may be subject to degradation under exposure to ultraviolet light, so bags containing riboflavin should contain fat emulsion or should be covered to provide protection from light.[18]

Deficiency

Although riboflavin has a wide distribution in foodstuffs, many people live for long periods on low intakes; consequently, minor signs of deficiency are common in many parts of the world. In addition to poor intake, functional deficiency can be induced by diseases such as hypothyroidism[250] and adrenal insufficiency,[266] which inhibit the conversion of riboflavin to its coenzyme derivatives, by drugs such as chlorpromazine, imipramine, and amitriptyline,[267] which have a similar tricyclic structure to riboflavin, by the anticancer drug doxorubicin[268] and the antimalarial quinacrine.[264] Excess ethanol ingestion interferes with both digestion and absorption of riboflavin.[269]

Because flavin coenzymes are widely distributed in intermediary metabolism, the consequences of deficiency may be widespread. Riboflavin coenzymes are involved in the metabolism of vitamin B_{12} and folic acid (irreversible reduction of 5,10-methylenetetrahydrofolate to 5-methyltetrahydrofolate [5-MTHF]), and therefore, are a determinant of plasma homocysteine concentration, pyridoxine (conversion to pyridoxal 5-phosphate) and niacin (conversion of 5-hydroxytryptamine to tryptophan, which is required for niacin synthesis).[242,255] Therefore, deficiency will affect enzyme systems other than those requiring flavin coenzymes per se. With increasing riboflavin deficiency, tissue concentrations of FMN and FAD will fall, as does flavokinase activity, thus further decreasing FMN concentrations. FMN concentrations are decreased proportionately more than FAD concentrations. Decreases in the activities of enzymes requiring FMN generally follow the fall in tissue concentrations, whereas FAD-dependent enzymes are more variably affected.

The deficiency syndrome is characterized by (1) sore throat, (2) hyperemia, (3) edema of the pharyngeal and oral mucous membranes, (4) cheilosis, (5) angular stomatitis, (6) glossitis (magenta tongue), (7) seborrheic dermatitis, and (8) normochromic, normocytic anemia associated with pure red blood cell (RBC) aplasia of the bone marrow.[242,255,270] However, some of these symptoms, such as glossitis and dermatitis, when encountered in the field, may be seen to have resulted from other complicating deficiencies.

Because riboflavin-derived cofactors are essential for the function of numerous dehydrogenases, they have been linked to genetic defects such as Brown-Vialetto-Van Laere and Fazio-Londe syndromes.[271] Mutations in the electron transferring flavoprotein genes *(ETFA/ETFB)* and its dehydrogenase (ETFDH) are causative for multiple acyl-CoA dehydrogenase deficiency.[272] Mutations in ACAD9, which encodes the acyl-CoA dehydrogenase 9 protein, were recently reported in mitochondrial disease with respiratory chain complex I deficiency.[271] These conditions are responsive to riboflavin therapy.

Toxicity

No adverse effects have been associated with ingestion of riboflavin appreciably above RDA amounts probably because of its limited solubility and limited gastric absorption. One study reported no short-term side effects in 49 patients treated with 400 mg/day of riboflavin with meals for at least 3 months.[259] Because of lack of data for risk assessment, no tolerable upper intake amount has been proposed for riboflavin.[11]

Laboratory Assessment of Status

Riboflavin status can be assessed by (1) determination of urine riboflavin excretion, (2) by a functional assay measuring the erythrocyte glutathione reductase activation coefficient, which is the ratio between enzyme activity determined with and without the addition of the cofactor, FAD, or (3) direct measurement of riboflavin or its metabolites in plasma or erythrocytes. The advantages and disadvantages of functional and direct methods were discussed in the section on thiamine.

Urinary riboflavin has been measured using fluorometric and microbiological procedures,[25] but for specificity, HPLC combined with fluorometric detection is the method of choice.[253,273] Under conditions of adequate intake (AI), the amount excreted per day is more than 120 µg or 80 µg/g creatinine. The rate of excretion expressed as micrograms per gram creatinine is greater for children than for adults. Conditions that cause negative nitrogen balance and the administration of antibiotics and certain psychotropic drugs (phenothiazine derivatives) increase urinary riboflavin as a consequence of tissue depletion and displacement. A load return test may augment reliability but is more cumbersome.

Riboflavin status is commonly assessed by the determination of FAD-dependent glutathione reductase activity in freshly lysed erythrocytes.[273,274] This enzyme-based assay has been chosen for most surveys of riboflavin status. Most methods measure the rate of change of absorbance at 340 nm caused by the oxidation of NADPH and have been automated to give rapid throughputs and CVs of less than 2% within the run, although some have used fluorescence detection with increased sensitivity.[275] Potential problems include that (1) in long-standing riboflavin deficiency, apoenzyme activity may be reduced, possibly leading to a misleading activation coefficient calculation, and (2) in patients with glucose-6-phosphate deficiency, a misleadingly low activation coefficient may be measured, which is possibly caused by enhanced binding of FAD to the apoenzyme.[276] Thus, methodologic variation can lead to substantial differences in results.

Direct measurement of riboflavin, FMN, and FAD in plasma or erythrocytes is undertaken by HPLC, usually with fluorescence detection after protein precipitation,[275] or by capillary zone electrophoresis with laser-induced fluorescence detection.[277] In a study of riboflavin status, with FMN and FAD concentrations in plasma and erythrocytes from older adult subjects at baseline and after low-dose riboflavin supplementation obtained using activation coefficient measurements and capillary zone electrophoresis with laser-induced fluorescence detection, it was concluded that concentrations of all B_2 vitamers, except plasma FAD, are potential indicators of vitamin B_2 status, and that plasma riboflavin and erythrocyte FMN may be useful in assessment of vitamin B_2 status in population studies.[278] In critically ill patients, plasma albumin-bound FAD may decrease as a result of the systemic inflammatory response and due to redistribution of FAD because of the increased tissue requirement; red cell FAD is unaffected.[40,274,279] Therefore, the measurement of red cell FAD is more sensitive and recommended, especially in critically ill patients.

Preanalytical Variables

Whole blood collected into containers with the preservatives Li heparin or EDTA is recommended, but local laboratories should be consulted for their preferred sample type. Ideally, a fasting sample should be collected, especially if the patient is receiving oral or parenteral vitamin B_2 supplementation. Otherwise, sampling should be undertaken at least 8 hours post-supplementation.[132] Because vitamin B_2 is light-sensitive, samples should be protected from light by wrapping with foil. However, a recent study using HPLC with fluorimetric detection[133] reported that vitamin B_2 showed good stability up to 72 hours at room temperature.

Reference Intervals

Guidance reference intervals for the activation coefficient of erythrocyte glutathione reductase by FAD are 1.20

(adequacy), 1.21 to 1.40 (marginal deficiency), and 1.41 and above (deficiency).[25] The reference interval for erythrocyte riboflavin using a fluorometric method has been suggested to be 10 to 50 μg/dL (266–1330 nmol/L).[280] The reference interval for serum or plasma concentrations of riboflavin has previously been quoted as 4 to 24 μg/dL (106–638 nmol/L); however, lower intervals have been reported using liquid chromatography with tandem mass spectrometry[281] or using the established HPLC with fluorometric detection method.[273] One group that studied 119 apparently healthy individuals using HPLC with fluorometric detection[274] obtained the following results (median [range]: plasma FAD: 101 nmol/L (57–170); plasma FMN: 6.3 nmol/L (3.3–14.1); plasma riboflavin: 11 nmol/L (4–34); erythrocyte FAD: 1.9 pmol/g Hb (0.7–3.8); erythrocyte FMN: 0.11 pmol/g Hb (0.04–0.44); and erythrocyte riboflavin: 0.02 pmol/g Hb (0.01–0.13). For the recommended test of vitamin B_2 sufficiency (erythrocyte FAD) using HPLC with fluorometric detection, the suggested reference interval is 1.0 to 3.4 nmol/g Hb.[132,274] For more information, refer to the Appendix on Reference Intervals. Laboratories should verify that these ranges are appropriate for use in their own settings.

Vitamin B_6

Pyridoxine (pyridoxol), pyridoxamine, and pyridoxal are the three natural forms of vitamin B_6. They are converted to the active form pyridoxal phosphate, which is required for synthesis, catabolism, and interconversions of various amino acids.

Chemistry

The vitamin B_6 group is composed of three natural forms: pyridoxine (pyridoxol), pyridoxamine, and pyridoxal (PL), which are 4-substituted 2-methyl-3-hydroxyl-5-hydroxymethyl pyridines (Fig. 37.13). During metabolic conversion, each vitamer becomes phosphorylated at the 5-hydroxymethyl substituent. Although both pyridoxamine-5′-phosphate (PMP) and pyridoxal-5′-phosphate (PLP; P-5′-P) interconvert as coenzyme forms during aminotransferase (transaminase)-catalyzed reactions, PLP is the coenzyme form that participates in a large number of B_6-dependent enzyme reactions.

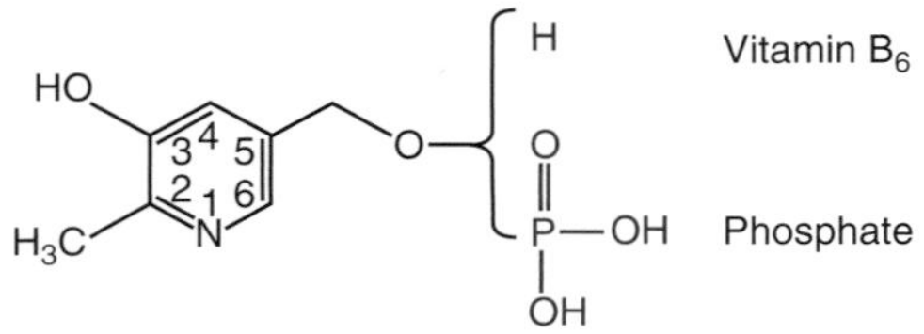

FIGURE 37.13 Free and Phosphorylated Forms of Vitamin B_6.

Dietary Sources

Vitamin B_6 is widely distributed in animal and plant tissues, where the phosphorylated forms, particularly PLP, predominate. Meats, poultry, and fish are good sources, as are yeast, certain seeds, bran, and bananas; somewhat more limited sources are milk, eggs, and green leafy vegetables.[282] In the United States and in some other countries, fortified ready-to-eat cereals are the main dietary source of vitamin B_6. The common commercial form of the vitamin is pyridoxine hydrochloride, which is a water-soluble, white crystalline solid. Solutions of B_6 vitamers are decomposed by light, especially in the ultraviolet region, at neutral to alkaline pH, and there is significant loss during thermal processing of foods.

Absorption, Transport, Metabolism, and Excretion

Food sources of animal origin contain mainly PLP with some PMP, whereas plant sources also contain pyridoxine-5′-glucoside, which is absorbed in a different manner. The phosphorylated sources are hydrolyzed by the intraluminal action of intestinal alkaline phosphatase, but pyridoxine-5′-glucoside is less effectively hydrolyzed by nonspecific glycosidase within cells, and some pyridoxine-5′-glucoside can be absorbed intact and hydrolyzed in various tissues.[283] The nonphosphorylated vitamers are readily absorbed by the mucosal cells through a process of passive diffusion, which does not appear to be limited by load, although a carrier mechanism may also exist.[284] Here, as in other cells requiring vitamin B_6, the unphosphorylated vitamers may be "metabolically trapped" as phosphorylated forms by cytoplasmic PL kinase, which is responsible for catalyzing the ATP-dependent phosphorylation of all three vitamin forms. Transport to the liver via the portal vein is done by the unphosphorylated form.

Fig. 37.14 shows the intracellular metabolism of vitamin B_6. Most cells contain a cytosolic FMN-dependent, pyridoxine

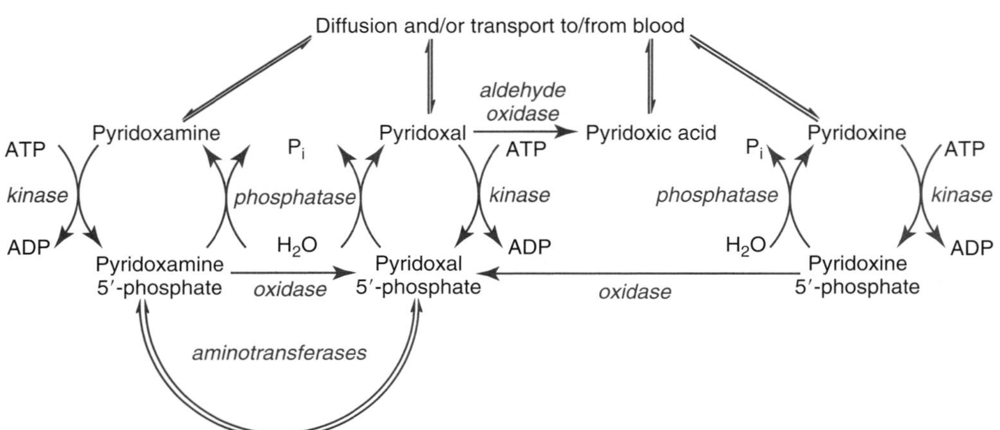

FIGURE 37.14 Metabolism of Vitamin B_6. *ADP,* Adenosine diphosphate; *ATP,* adenosine triphosphate.

(pyridoxamine)-5′-phosphate oxidase responsible for catalyzing the O_2-dependent conversion of pyridoxine phosphate and pyridoxamine phosphate to PLP (and H_2O_2). PLP can enter directly into subcellular organelles such as hepatocyte mitochondria and can bind for catalytic function with numerous specific apoenzymes throughout the cell. In addition, the erythrocyte traps PLP as a conjugate Schiff base with Hb. Vitamin B_6 in muscle accounts for 80% of body stores, mostly as PLP bound to glycogen phosphorylase.[285] Total body stores of vitamin B_6 are believed to be approximately 1 mmol.

Release of free vitamin, mainly PL, occurs when physiologic nonsaturating concentrations of vitamin are absorbed. The phosphates are hydrolyzed by nonspecific alkaline phosphatase located on the plasma membrane of cells. Some PLP is released into the circulation by the liver. PLP is the principal tissue form of vitamin B_6, whereas PL constitutes much of the circulating vitamin. The main catabolite excreted in urine is 4-pyridoxic acid (4-PA), which is formed by the action of the FAD-dependent general liver aldehyde oxidase, and NAD-specific aldehyde dehydrogenase, which is found in most tissues.[286,287]

Functions

As coenzyme PLP, vitamin B_6 functions in more than 100 reactions that embrace the metabolism of macronutrients, such as proteins, carbohydrates, and lipids.[288] PLP-dependent enzymes that are involved in amino acid metabolism are especially diverse. Because PLP is able to condense its 4-formyl substituent with the α-amino group of an amino acid to form an azomethine (Schiff base) linkage, a conjugated double-bond system extending from the α-carbon of the amino acid to the pyridinium nitrogen in PLP results in reduced electron density about the α-carbon. This configuration potentially weakens each of the bonds from the amino acid α-carbon to the adjoined hydrogen, carboxyl, and side chain functions. A given apoenzyme then locks in a particular configuration of the coenzyme-substrate compound, such that maximal overlap of the bond to be broken will occur with the resonant, coplanar, electron-withdrawing system of the coenzyme complex. Aminotransferases affect breaking of the α-hydrogen bond with the ultimate formation of a 2-oxo acid and pyridoxamine-5′-phosphate; this reversible reaction provides an interface between amino acid metabolism and that of ketogenic and glucogenic reactions (see Chapter 29).

Other examples of PLP-requiring enzymes are the amino acid decarboxylases that lead to formation of amines, including several that are functional in nervous tissue (eg, epinephrine, norepinephrine, serotonin, γ-aminobutyrate): cysteine desulfhydrase and serine hydroxymethyltransferase, which use PLP to effect the loss or transfer of amino acid side chains; phosphorylase, which catalyzes phosphorolysis of the α-1,4-linkages of glycogen; and cystathione β-synthase in the trans-sulfuration pathway of homocysteine. In addition, the biosynthesis of heme depends on the early formation of 5-aminolevulinate from PLP-dependent condensation of glycine and succinyl-CoA, followed by decarboxylation. An important role in lipid metabolism is the PLP-dependent condensation of L-serine with palmitoyl-CoA to form 3-dehydrosphinganine, a precursor of sphingomyelins. Therapeutically, vitamin B_6 has been used for the treatment of some intractable seizures in neonates and infants and for the treatment of other vitamin B_6–responsive inborn errors of metabolism,[289] as well as carpal tunnel syndrome.[290]

Requirements and Reference Nutrient Intakes

Requirements for vitamin B_6 are complicated by (1) differences in protein intake, (2) the probable provision of a fraction of the necessary quantity through bacterial synthesis in the intestinal tract, (3) the use of alcohol and oral contraceptives, and (4) the infrequent cases in which extra requirements are apparent.[291,292] Estimates of requirements with some margin of safety have been based on the production and cure of clinical signs of deficiency but occur more often on biochemical parameters. The latter include determination of the urinary excretion of vitamin B_6 and 4-PA or xanthurenic acid after a tryptophan load test, plasma concentrations of PLP, and RBC transaminase activity.[11] A ratio of 0.016 mg of vitamin B_6 per gram of protein intake has been suggested for normal adults and may be extrapolated to children and adolescents. Recent recommendations have proposed RDAs of 0.5 mg/day for children 1 to 3 years, 0.6 mg/day for children 4 to 8 years, 1.0 mg/day for children 9 to 13 years, 1.3 mg/day for boys 14 to 18 years, 1.3 mg/day for men to age 50 years, and 1.7 mg/day for men older than 50 years. Girls 14 to 18 years of age have an RDA of 1.2 mg/day; women aged 19 to 50 years have an RDA of 1.3 mg/day; and women older than 50 years have an RDA of 1.5 mg/day.[11] An addition of 0.6 mg B_6 per day is suggested for pregnant women to match the increased protein allowance that occurs during gestation. During lactation, 2.0 mg/day is recommended to accommodate for extra protein intake and to provide a concentration of 0.10 to 0.25 mg/L of the vitamin in milk, which is adequate for breast-fed infants.[11]

Intravenous Supply

The recommended intravenous supply of vitamin B_6 for adults has been increased from 4 to 6 mg/day to ensure adequate amounts in patients who sometimes receive large amino acid intakes.[156] This is usually provided as pyridoxine hydrochloride.

Deficiency

Vitamin B_6 deficiency in isolation is rare; it is more usual in association with deficits in other vitamins of the B-complex. As with other water-soluble vitamins that function as coenzymes, the relative affinity of the coenzyme for a given apoenzyme and the extent to which a particular holoenzyme-catalyzed reaction is essential are reflected in the progressive symptoms of deficiency of the vitamin. Investigations into the consequences of vitamin B_6 deficiency in the human patient use diets deficient in the vitamin and/or diets containing an antagonist, usually 4′-deoxypyridoxine.[293] However, in some instances, drug interactions have led to hypovitaminosis of B_6.[293-295] The antituberculosis drug isoniazid (isonicotinic acid hydrazide) forms hydrazones with PL and PLP. As with other carbonyl reagents, not only do such compounds cause loss by displacement and urinary excretion, but the Schiff bases formed with PL inhibit PL kinase,[296] and the PLP Schiff bases may additionally inhibit some PLP-dependent enzymes.[297] Penicillamine (β-dimethyl cysteine), which is used in the treatment of patients with Wilson disease in an attempt to decrease the damaging concentrations of Cu found in the liver, inactivates PLP by forming a thiazolidine derivative.[294]

Other drugs that can cause vitamin B_6 deficiency include the antiparkinsonian drugs benserazide and carbidopa, which react by forming hydrazones, and theophylline.[295,298]

Several vitamin B_6–responsive inborn errors of metabolism[299,300] are known. Pyridoxine-responsive epilepsy that presents in cases of infantile convulsions occurs, as a result of the apoenzyme for glutamate decarboxylase having poor affinity for the coenzyme or due to pyridoxine 5'-phosphate oxidase deficiency. This prevents the active form of vitamin B_6 from being synthesized from dietary or supplemented pyridoxine. There is also a type of chronic anemia in which the number, but not the morphologic abnormality, of erythrocytes is improved by pyridoxine supplementation. Xanthurenic aciduria occurs as a result of the decreased affinity of the mutant enzyme kynureninase for PLP, whereas primary cystathioninuria is caused by defective cystathionase. Finally, homocystinuria, which is caused by deficiency of the enzyme cystathionine β-synthetase (or synthase) or due to the enzyme's decreased activity as a result of vitamin B_6 deficiency, both result in the accumulation of plasma homocysteine spilling over into urine (homocystinuria). In all of these metabolic derangements, high-dose (200 to 1000 mg/day) vitamin B_6 may be necessary.[300] Low vitamin B_6 status (together with low vitamin B_{12} and folate status) in humans has been linked to hyperhomocysteinemia and is an independent risk factor for cardiovascular disease,[301,302] although clinical trials have been inconclusive.[303]

Biochemical markers of vitamin B_6 deficiency occur early and become more marked as the deficiency progresses.[304] Plasma concentrations of PLP and urinary output of B_6 and 4-PA are decreased within 1 week of removal of the vitamin from the diet. Because liver kynureninase activity is decreased, xanthurenic acid is increased in urine. Aminotransferase activity in serum and RBCs also decreases. Clinically, electroencephalographic abnormalities appear within 3 weeks, and epileptiform convulsions are a common finding in young vitamin B_6–deficient subjects. In addition, skin changes occur, including dermatitis with cheilosis and glossitis. Hematologic manifestations may include a decrease in the number of circulating lymphocytes and possibly a normocytic, microcytic, or sideroblastic anemia.[287,305]

Toxicity

Although no adverse effects have been observed with high intakes of vitamin B_6 from food sources, high oral supplemental doses have been found to have neurotoxic and photosensitive effects. The first reported cases in humans were a series of seven patients who had taken between 2 and 6 g/day of pyridoxine for up to 40 months.[306] Four of these patients were unable to walk, and all showed severe sensory neuropathy of the extremities, although most of the symptoms were reversed on stopping the pyridoxine. None of the subsequent studies showed any evidence of sensory nerve damage at intakes at less than 200 mg/day. Based on the end point of development of sensory neuropathy, 1998 recommendations have set a tolerable upper intake amount of 100 mg/day for adults.[11]

Laboratory Assessment of Status

As with the other B vitamins that act as coenzymes, biochemical assessment of vitamin B_6 can be made by direct chemical analysis of the vitamer or its metabolites, or by functional means. Measurements that have been used are PLP in plasma or red cells, its metabolite 4-PA in urine or plasma, the activity and activation coefficient of the red cell aminotransferases (aspartate and alanine), and the tryptophan load metabolite excretion test.[25] Because no single marker adequately reflects status, a combination of these markers offers the best approach.

Direct assessment was originally performed by microbiological techniques using specific strains of *Saccharomyces carlsbergensis* for all three natural vitamers, *Enterococcus faucium* for PL and pyridoxamine, and *Lactobacillus casei* for PL. Concentrations of 20 μg vitamin B_6 per gram creatinine in urine are considered indicative of marginal or inadequate dietary intake of the vitamin. Plasma PLP and plasma or urine 4-PA are most commonly measured by HPLC; PLP is measured with fluorescence detection following precolumn fluorophore formation as a semicarbazone[307,308] or a pyridoxic acid phosphate,[309] and 4-PA is measured with its natural fluorescence. During deficiency, the concentration of 4-PA will drop well below the normal concentration of at least 0.8 mg/day in urine. Using ion-pair, reversed-phase chromatography,[310] plasma vitamin B_6 vitamers (PLP, PL, PN, PMP, PM, and 4-PA) were measured in 90 patients who underwent coronary angiography before and after treatment with pyridoxine 40 mg/day for up to 84 days. PLP, 4-PA, and to a lesser degree PL, were found to be the predominant B_6 metabolites in pretreatment plasma. After treatment, PN was also detectable, and PN and PL showed the largest increases in concentration. Increases in plasma concentrations of PLP, PL, and 4-PA occurred within 3 days of supplementation and were steady for the remainder of the study period. In critical illness, plasma PL and PLP are low, and the relationship between them is disturbed, whereas this is less pronounced in red and white blood cells, suggesting that intracellular PLP concentrations are more reliable than plasma measurements in such patients.[311] Other direct measurements have used recombinant enzyme technology. A homogeneous, nonradioactive recombinant enzymatic method for PLP has been described that uses 5 μL of plasma, has a detection limit of 5 nmol/L, and may be applicable to adaptation to an automated analyzer.[312]

Functional assessment of vitamin B_6 status may be made by measuring the activity of red cell aspartate (or alanine) aminotransferase and its activation coefficient on incubation with PLP, although because the apoenzyme is highly unsaturated with PLP, the results obtained have greater variability than those derived by corresponding methods for vitamins B_1 and B_2 and thus are considered less useful.[25] Activation coefficients of less than approximately 1.5 for aspartate aminotransferase and 1.2 for alanine aminotransferase are considered normal, but this may depend somewhat on the assay method used. Measurement of urinary tryptophan metabolites, particularly xanthurenic acid, following an oral load (2–5 g) of L-tryptophan, is one of the most common indices used in studies of vitamin B_6 nutriture, because changes can be recognized early and measurements are relatively easy.[313] Amounts of xanthurenate well above normal (≈25 mg/day) are seen in vitamin B_6 deficiency. Concentrations of other metabolites, such as kynurenic acid and 3-hydroxykynurenine, are increased. A method describing the simultaneous determination of tryptophan and its metabolites, including kynurenic and xanthurenic acids, by liquid chromatography with diode array, fluorescence, and tandem mass spectrometry detection systems has been published.[314]

Preanalytical Variables

Whole blood collected into containers with the preservatives Li heparin or EDTA is recommended, but local laboratories should be consulted for their preferred sample type. Ideally, a sample should be collected after fasting, especially if the patient is receiving oral or parenteral vitamin B_6 supplementation. Otherwise, sampling should be undertaken at least 8 hours post-supplementation.[132] Because vitamin B_6 is light-sensitive, samples should be protected from light by wrapping with foil. However, a recent study using HPLC with fluorimetric detection reported that vitamin B_6 in whole blood significantly and gradually increased by a mean of 9.9% over basal concentration in 24 hours when kept at room temperature.[133] It is therefore recommended that if delay in transportation is anticipated, erythrocytes should be prepared by centrifugation, and removal of plasma and the white cells in the buffy layer and the cells should be stored frozen until dispatch. It was suggested that this may be the result of increased instability caused by light exposure[308] or due to release from erythrocytes as a result of hemolysis.[133]

Reference Intervals

Vitamin B_6 is affected by SIRS as shown in Table 37.2, which lists the magnitude of change in vitamin B_6 with increasing CRP concentrations. A guidance reference interval given by one source for plasma PLP was 9.5 to 24 ng/mL (39–98 nmol/L), and plasma concentrations less than 5 ng/mL (20 nmol/L) were judged deficient.[25] Another study in 126 apparently healthy individuals derived a reference interval of 5.2 to 34 ng/mL (21–138 nmol/L), whereas for erythrocyte PLP, the reference interval given was 250 to 680 pmol/g Hb, with a concentration of less than 200 pmol/g Hb indicating being at risk of deficiency.[132,308] For more information, refer to the Appendix on Reference Intervals. Laboratories should verify that these ranges are appropriate for use in their own settings.

Vitamin B_{12}

Vitamin B_{12}, also known as cyanocobalamin, is a water-soluble vitamin that is required for erythropoiesis, for methylation processes necessary for DNA and cell metabolism, and is a cofactor for various enzymes, especially those involved in the metabolism of methylmalonic acid (MMA) and homocysteine.

Chemistry

Vitamin B_{12} is one of the most structurally complex small molecules produced by nature, and the only known carbon–metal bond (involving Co) found in a biologically active molecule.[315] The generic term vitamin B_{12} refers to a group of physiologically active substances chemically classified as cobalamins or corrinoids. They are composed of tetrapyrrole rings surrounding central Co atoms and nucleotide side chains attached to the Co atoms. The cobalamin tetrapyrrole ring, exclusive of Co and other side chains, is called a corrin. All compounds containing this corrin nucleus are corrinoids. The Co–corrin complex is termed cobamide. In cobalamins, 5,6-dimethylbenzimidazole riboside is bound to the Co atom by one of its imidazole nitrogens, and its 2′-ribose carbon is linked with an ester of aminoisopropanol and propionic acid to the corrin ring (Fig. 37.15).

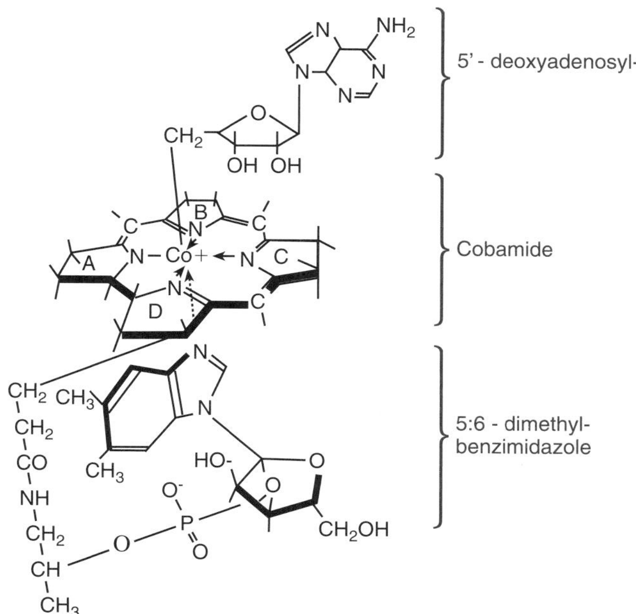

FIGURE 37.15 The Structure of 5′-Deoxyadenosyl Cobalamin.

Cobalamins differ in the nature of additional side groups bound to Co. Examples include methyl (methylcobalamin), 5′-deoxyadenosine (deoxyadenosyl [short form, adenosyl], cobalamin, or coenzyme B_{12}), hydroxyl (hydroxocobalamin), water (aquocobalamin, or vitamin B_{12b}), and cyanide (cyanocobalamin). Cyanocobalamin is a stable compound that forms dark red, needle-like crystals; it is the reference compound for measuring serum cobalamin concentration. Less stable serum cobalamins may be converted to this compound for quantification. The predominant physiologic form of cobalamin in serum is methylcobalamin, whereas that in the cytosol is adenosylcobalamin. It is recommended that the term vitamin B_{12} be used as the generic descriptor for all corrinoids that qualitatively exhibit the biological activity of cyanocobalamin.[316] Cyanocobalamin has a MW of 1355 Da and a solubility of 12 g/L in water at 20°C. It is soluble in lower alcohols and aliphatic acids, but it is insoluble in acetone, ether, and chloroform. It is gradually destroyed on exposure to light.[316] Aqueous solutions of cyanocobalamin exhibit a distinctive absorption spectrum with maxima at 278, 361, and 550 nm, and with absorptivity coefficients of 115, 207, and 63, respectively, at these maxima. The spectrum is independent of pH but changes when cyanocobalamin binds to the intrinsic factor (IF). Because of its stability in aqueous solutions and its distinct absorption spectrum, accurate concentrations of cyanocobalamin are prepared and used as calibrators for the measurement of serum cobalamin concentrations.

Dietary Sources

Because plants do not use the vitamin, the main dietary sources are meat and meat products, dairy products, fish and shellfish, and fortified ready-to-eat cereals.[11]

1. Adenosylcobalamin-dependent, L-methylmalonyl–CoA mutase reaction

L-methylmalonyl-CoA ⇌ Succinyl-CoA

2. Methylcobalamin-dependent, methionine synthase reaction

CH_3-Cob(III)alamin + homocysteine → Cob(I)alamin + methionine

Cob(I)alamin + 5-methyltetrahydrofolate → CH_3-Cob(III)alamin + tetrahydrofolate

FIGURE 37.16 Participation of Cobalamin Coenzymes in Human Metabolism. *CoA,* coenzyme A.

Absorption, Transport, Metabolism, and Excretion

The uptake of vitamin B_{12} from the intestine into the circulation is a complex mechanism, involving vitamin B_{12}–binding molecules, receptors, and transporters.[317-319] Vitamin B_{12} is tightly bound to proteins and must be released from food by stomach acid and pepsin. The synthetic form is free and therefore readily available for metabolism. Thus, acid-blocking drugs such as proton pump inhibitors (eg, omeprazole) can cause vitamin B_{12} deficiency.[320] The free vitamin B_{12} molecule is bound to haptocorrin (HC) (R protein) and travels with it into the duodenum, where the HC is digested by pancreatic enzymes. Liberated vitamin B_{12} then binds to the IF,[321] a glycoprotein with a MW of approximately 50 kDa that is produced by the gastric parietal cells in the fundus and body of the stomach. One molecule of IF binds one molecule of vitamin B_{12}. Gastric secretion of IF is stimulated by food, histamine, and gastrin produced by the antrum portion of the stomach; it is inhibited by vagal blockade.[316,321,322] When the vitamin B_{12}–IF complex reaches the distal ileum, it is bound by specific receptors known as the cubam complex, which consists of two subunits, namely, cubilin and amnionless[323-325] on the surface of mucosal epithelial cells, and it is internalized. The vitamin B_{12}–IF complex is dissociated within the mucosal epithelial cells by lysosomes and released into blood.

In circulation, vitamin B_{12} then binds to two circulating binding proteins, HC (referred to as holohaptocorrin when bound to vitamin B_{12} and previously known as transcobalamin I)[326] and transcobalamin (TC; holotranscobalamin when bound to vitamin B_{12} and previously known as transcobalamin II)[327]; however, only the TC-bound fraction has receptor-mediated cellular uptake as described previously, and therefore, it is the bioactive fraction. The function of HC, which is released by granulocytes, is currently unknown, and low HC concentrations, found in approximately 15% of persons with low serum cobalamin, could be one of the most common causes of low cobalamin concentrations.[328] HC accounts for 80% to 94% of endogenous plasma vitamin B_{12}, whereas TC accounts for the remainder,[329] but the latter is the more important vitamin B_{12} transport protein in plasma. TC is a β-protein synthesized mainly in the liver and has a MW of approximately 43 kDa; it has a single vitamin B_{12}–binding site per molecule.[330] TC transports vitamin B_{12} to receptors on cell membranes throughout the body. Binding is rapid: if TC–vitamin B_{12} is injected intravenously, it is almost completely cleared in one passage through tissue, mostly by the liver.[331] The TC–vitamin B_{12} complex enters the cell by pinocytosis. Lysosomal proteolysis degrades TC and releases vitamin B_{12}. Unbound vitamin B_{12} can enter the tissue cells, but the process is inefficient.[331]

As previously discussed, only vitamin B_{12} bound to TC is capable of cellular uptake,[329,332] and as a result, malabsorption of TC-bound vitamin B_{12} leads to deficiency in a large proportion of cases.[333] Almost all vitamin B_{12} (bound to TC) is taken up by hepatocytes as the blood in the portal vein passes through the liver, where it is stored and subsequently released in blood to meet physiologic demands. If the quantity of vitamin B_{12} exceeds the capacity of hepatocyte receptors, most of the excess is excreted by the kidneys. Normally, approximately 1 mg of vitamin B_{12} is stored in the liver, which is a quantity equivalent to the daily metabolic requirement for 2000 days.[334] Thus, when the dietary supply of vitamin B_{12} is interrupted or mechanisms of absorption are impaired, vitamin B_{12} deficiency does not become evident for several years.[329]

Vitamin B_{12} is continually secreted in the bile, but most is reabsorbed and is available for metabolic functions. If circulating vitamin B_{12} concentrations exceed the binding capacity of the blood, the excess will be excreted in the urine, but in most circumstances, the highest losses of vitamin B_{12} occur through the feces.

Functions

Vitamin B_{12} is a cofactor or coenzyme for various enzyme systems.[335] In humans, it is required in adenosylcobalamin, a coenzyme to L-methylmalonyl-CoA mutase in the conversion of L-methylmalonyl CoA to succinyl-CoA (Fig. 37.16). The conversion of L-methylmalonyl-CoA to succinyl-CoA links propionyl-CoA, which is formed from branched-chain amino acids such as valine, isoleucine, and methionine with the tricarboxylic acid cycle. Congenital defects of mutase synthesis or inability to synthesize adenosylcobalamin results in life-threatening methylmalonic aciduria and metabolic ketoacidosis.[336] It is also required in methylcobalamin, a coenzyme to methionine synthase in the conversion of homocysteine to methionine. In this reaction (see Figs. 37.16 and 37.17), methylcobalamin serves as an intermediate in the transfer of a methyl group from 5-MTHF to homocysteine for the formation of methionine. Methionine is required for protein synthesis and as the methyl donor, *S*-adenosylmethionine. Congenital defects in methionine synthase or the synthesis of methylcobalamin results in severe hyperhomocysteinemia.[336] As discussed under the section on vitamin B_6, defects in the enzyme cystathionine β-synthase or its cofactor vitamin B_6 also result in hyperhomocysteinemia. Vitamin B_{12} is also vital for erythropoiesis; deficiency leads to macrocytosis characterized by an increased mean corpuscular volume of more than 98 fL (as seen in the complete/full blood count) and megaloblastic anemia, which is characterized by immature, large, and nucleated RBCs as a result of defective DNA

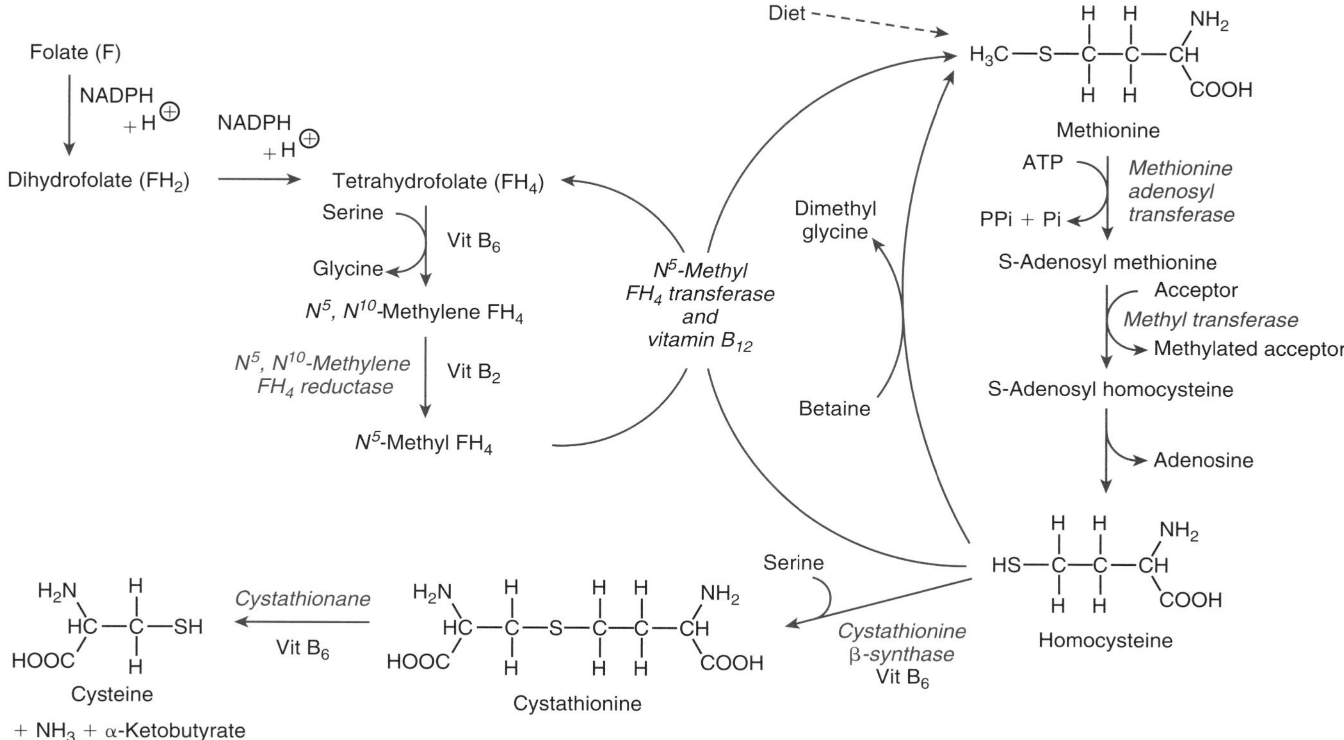

FIGURE 37.17 **Metabolism of Homocysteine and Methionine.** Note that N^5-methyl FH_4 is referred to as 5-MTHF and FH_4 as THF in the text. *ATP,* Adenosine triphosphate; *NADPH,* nicotinamide-adenine dinucleotide phosphate; *Pi,* inorganic phosphate; *PPi,* pyrophosphate.

synthesis that relies on adequate concentrations of vitamin B_{12} (and folate). As shown in Fig 37.17, on the left the remethylation pathway is shown whereby homocysteine is converted to methionine catalyzed by methionine synthase (N^5-methyl FH_4 transferase) which requires vitamin B_{12}. This pathway links the folate cycle to homocysteine metabolism. On the right the transmethylation pathway is depicted showing the metabolism of methionine to homocysteine, which is then converted to cysteine in the transsulphuration pathway.

Requirements and Reference Nutrient Intakes

Total body stores of vitamin B_{12} are estimated to be between 2 and 5 mg in adult men,[334] of which approximately 1 mg is in the liver and a smaller amount in the kidney. A daily obligatory loss of vitamin B_{12} of approximately 0.1% of the body pool is believed to occur, irrespective of size,[337] suggesting that a daily requirement to maintain stores would be 2 to 5 µg. The daily Western diet contains between 5 and 30 µg of vitamin B_{12}, with average ingestion of 7 to 8 µg/day by adult men and 4 to 5 µg/day by adult women. Additional small amounts may be available from vitamin B_{12} synthesis by intestinal microorganisms. Of the amount ingested, between 1 and 5 µg is absorbed.[329]

The RDA for vitamin B_{12} is based on the amount necessary for maintenance of hematologic status and normal serum vitamin B_{12} concentrations; it assumes 50% absorbance of ingested vitamin B_{12}. The RDA for adults (19–50 years) has been set at 2.4 µg/day, with an increase to 2.6 µg/day in pregnancy and to 2.8 µg/day in lactation. RDAs for children are 0.9 µg/day at 1 to 3 years, 1.2 µg/day at 4 to 8 years, 1.8 µg/day at 9 to 13 years, and 2.4 µg/day at 14 to 18 years.

Because 10% to 30% of older persons may be unable to absorb naturally occurring vitamin B_{12}, it is recommended that those older than 50 years meet their RDA mainly by consuming foods fortified with vitamin B_{12} or with a vitamin B_{12}–containing supplement.[11]

Intravenous Supply

The recommended intravenous intake for adults is 5 µg/day as cyanocobalamin—an amount in excess of the oral recommendation that will more than meet requirements.[179]

Deficiency

Deficiency of vitamin B_{12} in humans is associated with macrocytosis, megaloblastic anemia, and neuropathy. The most common cause of vitamin B_{12} deficiency is pernicious anemia, an autoimmune disease in which chronic atrophic gastritis in the fundus and body region of the stomach results from autoantibodies to gastric parietal cells directed against gastric parietal cell H^+/K^+-ATPase, which is responsible for secreting acid (H^+) in exchange for potassium (K^+).[338] Loss of parietal cells also leads to decreased production of IF. In addition to IF deficiency, blocking autoantibodies that bind the vitamin B_{12}–binding sites of IF prevent the formation of the vitamin B_{12}–IF complex required for recognition by the cubam complex in the distal ileum.[339,340] One population study showed that 1.9% of persons older than 60 years have undiagnosed pernicious anemia,[338] although the diagnosis is made most commonly in young to middle-aged black women and in middle-aged to older adult whites.[341] Pernicious anemia may also occur in children because of failure of IF secretion or secretion of biologically inactive IF.[342] Other groups at risk for vitamin B_{12} deficiency include those (1) older than 65 years of age, (2) with malabsorption, (3) who are vegetarians or vegans, (4) with autoimmune disorders (pernicious anemia usually occurs as part of the autoimmune polyglandular syndrome type 3B that includes autoimmune thyroiditis), and (5) taking prescribed medication known to interfere with vitamin absorption or metabolism, including nitrous oxide (also known as laughing gas, which inactivates vitamin B_{12} by oxidizing its Co atom), phenytoin, dihydrofolate reductase inhibitors, metformin, and proton pump inhibitors, as well as (6) infants with suspected metabolic disorders.[343]

Intestinal malabsorption of vitamin B_{12} may be caused by gastrectomy or ileal resection, with an inverse relationship noted between the length of ileum resected and absorption of vitamin B_{12}. Other causes of malabsorption include tropical sprue, inflammatory disease of the small intestine, intestinal stasis with overgrowth of colonic bacteria, which consume vitamin B_{12} ingested by the host, and HIV infection.[344] Another cause of vitamin B_{12} malabsorption is failure to extract cobalamin from food. Cobalamin bound to food is not absorbed in some patients, whereas absorption of non–food-bound cobalamin in the Schilling test (see the following) is unimpaired. This is particularly a problem in patients with compromised gastric status or early in the course of development of pernicious anemia.[338,343]

Vegetarians have a lower intake of vitamin B_{12} than omnivores, and although clinical signs of deficiency are uncommon, biochemical markers of status indicate functional vitamin B_{12} deficiency. In a study of 66 lactovegetarians or lacto-ovovegetarians, 29 vegans, and 79 omnivores, the incidence of low holotranscobalamin II was 77%, 92%, and 11%, respectively, in the three groups; increased MMA occurred in 68%, 83%, and 5%, respectively, and increased total homocysteine was found in 38%, 67%, and 16%, respectively.[345]

A large number of disorders are associated with cobalamin deficiency in infancy or childhood. Of these, the most commonly encountered is the Imerslund-Grasbeck syndrome,[346] a condition that is characterized by inability to absorb vitamin B_{12}, with or without IF, and proteinuria. It appears to be due to an inability of intestinal mucosa to absorb the vitamin B_{12}–IF complex as a result of mutations in cubilin or amnionless.[347] The second most common of these is congenital deficiency of gastric secretion of IF.[342] Rarely, a congenital deficiency of vitamin B_{12} in a breast-fed infant is due to deficiency of vitamin B_{12} in maternal breast milk resulting from unrecognized pernicious anemia in the mother.[348] This is rare because most women with undiagnosed and untreated pernicious anemia are infertile.[329,338] Methylmalonic acidemias (acidurias) and homocysteinemias may be caused by vitamin B_{12} deficiency, and depending on the underlying mutation, may or may not be responsive to supplementation with the vitamin.[349]

The hematologic effects of vitamin B_{12} deficiency are indistinguishable from those of folate deficiency. Classical morphologic changes in the blood, in approximate order of appearance, are hypersegmentation of neutrophils, macrocytosis, anemia, leukopenia, and thrombocytopenia, with megaloblastic changes in bone marrow accompanying the peripheral blood changes. The cause of the hematologic abnormalities is believed to be an imbalance of decreased DNA synthesis and adequate RNA synthesis caused by the secondary block in folate metabolism caused by vitamin B_{12} deficiency.[343] Many immature cells die in the bone marrow, possibly by apoptosis, leading to the release of bilirubin and lactate dehydrogenase into the blood. This is termed ineffective erythropoiesis. All bone marrow lesions can be reversed by vitamin B_{12} treatment.

In addition to hematologic changes, vitamin B_{12} deficiency can lead to a demyelinating disorder of the central nervous system in humans. Serious and often irreversible neurologic disorders can occur, such as burning pain or loss of sensation in the extremities, weakness, spasticity and paralysis, confusion, disorientation, and dementia. This condition has been given the name "subacute combined degeneration of the spinal cord." Neurologic symptoms may occur without any discernible hematologic changes in the blood[350]; an intriguing inverse relationship between the hematologic and the neurologic has been observed. The incidence of neurologic complications is between 75% and 90% of all individuals with clinically observable vitamin B_{12} deficiency; in approximately 25% of cases, these may be the only clinical manifestation of deficiency.[317,343] The mechanism of the disorder is uncertain, although indirect evidence suggests that disorders of both enzyme systems requiring vitamin B_{12} coenzymes are necessary before neurologic symptoms occur. The response of neurologic symptoms to vitamin B_{12} replacement is often dependent on the duration of the symptoms. Vitamin B_{12} deficiency may be associated with other mainly gastrointestinal complications, such as glossitis of the tongue, appetite and weight loss, flatulence and constipation, mental changes, and infertility.[329,338,343] The neurological and cognitive manifestation of vitamin B_{12} deficiency is increasing, but data remain inconclusive, although there is some evidence that supplements of vitamin B_{12} and folate may normalize homocysteine concentrations.[351,352]

Toxicity

No adverse effects have been associated with excess vitamin B_{12} intake from food or supplements in healthy people. Daily oral doses of up to 2 mg of cyanocobalamin have been used for treatment of deficiency in those who tolerate oral supplementation.[353] Data in the literature are insufficient to propose a tolerable upper intake amount for vitamin B_{12}.[11]

Laboratory Assessment of Status

Both direct and indirect (functional) methods are available for assessment of vitamin B_{12} status. Indirect tests include assays for urinary and serum concentrations of MMA, plasma homocysteine, the deoxyuridine suppression test, and the vitamin B_{12} absorption test. Cytochemical staining of RBC precursors and the test for IF-blocking antibodies are other ancillary methods of assessing vitamin B_{12} status.

A comprehensive review of methods for measuring vitamin B_{12} in various biological samples has been published.[354] Microbiological, competitive protein binding (CPB), and immunometric assays have been used for quantification of serum vitamin B_{12}. Microbiological assays have largely been replaced by other, more convenient and precise methods, although they remain reference methods for the determination of biologically active vitamin B_{12}.[355] The most widely used procedures use *Euglena gracilis, Lactobacillus leishmannii,* or a mutant of *Escherichia coli,* although each of these organisms is susceptible to growth inhibition by antibiotics or other drugs, such as methotrexate, that may be present in a patient's serum. Furthermore, these assays require at least 24 hours for the establishment of adequate growth of these microorganisms. However, use of microtiter enzyme-linked immunosorbent assay plate technology has enhanced the usefulness of some microbiological assays.[356]

Commercial kits are available for CPB assays of vitamin B_{12}. The vitamin B_{12} binder used is often nonhuman IF, usually obtained from a hog stomach. If the IF is not highly purified, it may contain R proteins, which bind not only vitamin B_{12} but also related metabolically inactive compounds, yielding higher values. Therefore, IF must be highly purified or must have cobinamide (a vitamin B_{12} analog) added to the IF to saturate all binding sites on the R proteins. Cobinamide is not bound by IF.

In a widely used CPB assay, vitamin B_{12} (cobalamin) competes with ^{57}Co-labeled cobalamin for a limited number of binding sites on IF. Some assays require a preliminary step in which the specimen is boiled in a buffered solution containing dithiothreitol, potassium cyanide (KCN), and ^{57}Co-labeled tracers to release vitamin B_{12} from endogenous binding proteins. Alternatively, other procedures irreversibly denature endogenous binding proteins by increasing the pH from 12 to 13 and then readjusting the pH to 9.3 before the binding reagent is added. Subsequent separation of bound and free folate and vitamin B_{12} is achieved by contact with dextran-coated charcoal, which absorbs the free (unbound) molecules, leaving protein-bound vitamin B_{12} in the solution.

Most immunometric methods use solid-phase separation by immobilizing the IF binder on beads or magnetic particles. The free vitamin B_{12} then remains in the supernatant, and the bound analytes become part of the solid-phase suspension. For simultaneous folate/vitamin B_{12} measurement, a γ-scintillation counter that discriminates between the energy levels of ^{57}Co (for vitamin B_{12}) and ^{125}I (for folate) must be used.

Multiple automated and semiautomated systems are available for measuring vitamin B_{12} and folate; for example, chemiluminescence is used as a signal. The precision of automated systems allows specimens to be analyzed in singlet, where CVs less than those found for the mean of duplicates of radioimmunoassays are maintained.

Indirect tests assess the functional adequacy of vitamin B_{12}. Serum MMA concentration is increased when lack of adenylcobalamin causes a block in the conversion of methylmalonyl-CoA to succinyl-CoA. It is a sensitive test of status, and is often the first analyte to be raised in subclinical vitamin B_{12} deficiency.[343,357] It has a further advantage in that it is unaffected by folate deficiency. Early methods for MMA lacked sensitivity and specificity; this situation has been resolved by the adoption of gas chromatographic–mass spectrometric methods following derivatization for both urine and serum[358,359] or liquid chromatographic–mass spectrometric methods.[360] Unfortunately MMA is increased by renal insufficiency and in persons aged older than 65 years.[329,361] Plasma total homocysteine concentration is also a sensitive indicator of vitamin B_{12} status because methylcobalamin is required for the remethylation of homocysteine to methionine, but it is not specific because it is elevated in deficiencies of folate, vitamin B_{12}, vitamin B_2, and vitamin B_6.[317,362] Plasma concentrations of total homocysteine can be reliably measured by HPLC with fluorescent or electrochemical detection, and with enzymatic and capillary gas chromatography–mass spectroscopy methods.[363] Plasma samples for homocysteine analysis must be obtained soon after venipuncture to reduce preanalytical increases that may occur on standing, although these can be minimized by using a fluoride–EDTA tube.[363] Increased screening of plasma total homocysteine concentrations as an independent risk factor for cardiovascular disease may lead to identification of additional cases of subclinical vitamin B_{12} deficiency.[302,363]

The measurement of holotranscobalamin is potentially useful as a specific marker of biologically available vitamin B_{12}, because it is the only vitamin B_{12} moiety that is specifically available for uptake by all cells and has been shown to have the best diagnostic accuracy for vitamin B_{12} deficiency.[329,333] However, assays for holotranscobalamin are not widely available at present.[317] Other methods have been described for the measurement of holotranscobalamin in serum, using an immobilized monoclonal antibody to human TC, followed by measurement of released cobalamin by CPB[364] or an automated assay by enzyme immunoassay termed active B_{12}.[365] Another method uses magnetic beads coated with cobalamin to precipitate apotranscobalamin, followed by measurement of holotranscobalamin in the supernatant by an enzyme-linked immunosorbent assay.[366] Although these methods claim to be precise and simple to perform, their interpretation has been questioned,[367] and their sensitivity and specificity in the diagnosis of vitamin B_{12} deficiency remains to be established.

The deoxyuridine suppression test[368] measures the effects of the previous addition of deoxyuridine on uptake of radiolabeled thymidine into the DNA of cultured bone marrow cells, peripheral blood lymphocytes, or whole blood. Normal samples that contain vitamin B_{12} can convert deoxyuridine to thymidine and therefore do not take up as much thymidine. Samples from patients who are deficient in vitamin B_{12} show less suppression than those from normal patients. Because it is relatively time-consuming, the deoxyuridine suppression test is not widely available for use as a diagnostic test.

The Schilling test[369] is primarily a test of vitamin B_{12} absorption and not of status, but it permits differentiation of causes of vitamin B_{12} deficiency (pernicious anemia or intestinal malabsorption). The proportion absorbed from orally administered ^{57}Co- or ^{58}Co-labeled vitamin B_{12} is measured by determining radioactivity in feces, urine, or serum, or by externally scanning the liver. The usual procedure is to measure radioactivity in a 24-hour urine sample, which is collected after oral administration of 0.5 µg of radioactive Co-labeled vitamin B_{12} after an overnight fast. In normal individuals, 8% or more of the dose administered is excreted in the urine, whereas in people with pernicious anemia, less than 7% (often 0%–3%) is excreted. A confirmatory test for lack of IF requires ingestion of vitamin B_{12} and IF.

Preanalytical Variables

Spurious increases in vitamin B_{12} have been reported in patients with pernicious anemia when using automated analyzers based on the competitive binding of serum vitamin B_{12} with reagents using IF. This has been attributed to the high concentrations of IF-blocking autoantibodies in these patients, which interferes with the assay.[370-372] Up to 70% of patients with pernicious anemia have IF-blocking antibodies.[338] Assay manufacturers are aware of this problem and have taken steps to inactivate the IF-blocking antibodies.[370] However, at the present time, the scale of the problem is unknown, and alternative methods should be used if in doubt, including the measurement of IF-blocking antibodies.

For vitamin B_{12}, whole blood collected into container with a clot activator to obtain serum is recommended, but local laboratories should be consulted for their preferred sample type. Ideally, a fasting sample should be collected, especially if the patient is receiving oral or parenteral vitamin B_{12} supplementation. One recent study that used a radioimmunoassay method[133] reported that vitamin B_{12} showed good stability up to 72 hours at room temperature, corroborating similar data reported earlier using an enzyme immunoassay-based method.[134] There are no special requirements for MMA, but delayed freezing should be avoided.

Regarding homocysteine, the recommendations are to collect a fasting sample because a high protein meal may increase it. It is decreased in the supine position because it is bound to albumin; more than 3 minutes duration of venous stasis may increase it. However, these factors are not necessarily crucial because they are unlikely to affect the interpretation of the results. EDTA tubes are the most widely used, but use of serum, or citrated or heparinized rather than EDTA plasma, will not greatly influence the results. Blood samples should be centrifuged within 1 hour or kept cold by collecting on ice until centrifugation.[363,373]

Reference Intervals

Depending on the laboratory and the procedure used, reference intervals vary widely. A recent WHO consultation defined a serum vitamin B_{12} concentration of less than 203 ng/L (150 pmol/L) as deficient.[355] Changes in serum vitamin B_{12} concentration as a function of age in healthy adults have been the subject of contradictory reports. Data from a study population in the United States (Framingham Study) showed an increased prevalence (40.5% of 222 subjects) of low serum vitamin B_{12} concentration (<258 pmol/L) in older adults in comparison with a control group of younger subjects (17.9% incidence).[374] Vitamin B_{12} concentrations within the reference interval may not necessarily reflect adequate vitamin B_{12} status, because serum concentrations may be maintained at the expense of tissue stores. Conversely, low serum vitamin B_{12} concentrations may not be indicative of vitamin B_{12} deficiency. Most of the vitamin B_{12} in serum is bound to HC, which is released by granulocytes and has no functional role in the transport of vitamin B_{12} to cells.[326,328] Low serum vitamin B_{12} concentration may be due to a reduction in HC as a consequence of low total granulocyte mass. This has been observed in benign neutropenia, multiple myeloma, and leukemic reticuloendotheliosis, and may be expected in other conditions in which the bone marrow is hypoplastic, aplastic, or replaced by malignant cells.

Increased MMA and low holotranscobalamin may be found in patients with normal vitamin B_{12}; hence, holotranscobalamin is a better predictor of B_{12} than total B_{12}.[375] Serum MMA concentrations less than 376 nmol/L have been considered acceptable in an older adult US population,[374] as have concentrations less than 320 nmol/L in a group of older Dutch subjects.[376] MMA is increased by renal insufficiency and age.[329,361] Reference intervals for holotranscobalamin have been variable, but are in the range of 19 to 134 pmol/L[365] and are age- and sex-dependent.[377] Homocysteine levels less than 15 µmol/L, or if the individual is older than 65 years, less than 20 µmol/L are considered acceptable.[363] For more information, refer to the Appendix on Reference Intervals. Laboratories should verify that these ranges are appropriate for use in their own settings.

Folic Acid

Folic acid, also known as folate, pteroylglutamic acid, or vitamin B_9, serves as a carrier of one-carbon groups in many metabolic reactions. It is necessary for the interconversions of amino acids, such as homocysteine to methionine, and the biosynthesis of purines and pyrimidines, which are required for DNA synthesis.

Chemistry

Folate and folic acid are generic terms for a family of compounds that function as coenzymes in the processing of one-carbon units and that are derived from pteroic acid (*Pte*), to which one or more molecules of glutamic acid are attached. Pteroic acid is composed of a pteridine ring joined to a *p*-aminobenzoic acid residue (Fig. 37.18). In basic solution, this substance has absorption maxima at 256, 282, and 365 nm, and is fluorescent. When pteroic acid is conjugated with one molecule of L-glutamic acid, pteroylglutamic acid (PteGlu) is formed; this can be reduced to dihydrofolic acid (H_2PteGlu or DHF/FH_2) with hydrogens in positions 7 and 8, or to tetrahydrofolate (H_4PteGlu or THF/FH_4) with hydrogens in positions 5, 6, 7, and 8. Only the reduced forms are biologically active. Other folate derivatives have multiple glutamic acid residues ($H_4PteGlu_n$), where n, the number of glutamate residues, may be 1 to 7. Biochemically, these polyglutamates are similar to monoglutamates, but the former function as the natural coenzymes. Multiple forms of folic acid occur with substitutions of functional groups, such as methyl, formyl, methylene, hydroxymethyl, and others at nitrogen atoms in the pteroic acid residue, usually N^5 or bridging N^5 and N^{10}. Although various forms of folic acid are normally present in human serum and other body fluids, the principal form is 5-MTHF (N^5-Methyl FH_4). This is slowly oxidized in alkaline solution, but the process is reversed by adding ascorbic acid. It is relatively stable in acid solutions, but it is unstable when exposed to light.

Dietary Sources

The principal food sources of folate are liver, dark green leafy vegetables such as spinach, legumes such as kidney and lima beans, and orange juice,[11] although in countries where cereal fortification with folate is established, cereal is often the major source of dietary folate.[355,378]

Absorption, Transport, Metabolism, and Excretion

Folate is absorbed from dietary sources such as those listed previously, mainly as reduced methyl- and formyl-tetrahydropteroylpolyglutamates. The bioavailability of folate from food sources is variable and is dependent on factors such as incomplete release from plant cellular structure, entrapment in the food matrix during digestion, inhibition of deglutamation by other dietary constituents, and possibly the degree of polyglutamation.[379] The bioavailability of supplemental folic acid is greater than that of food folate and may be as high as 100% for folic acid supplements taken

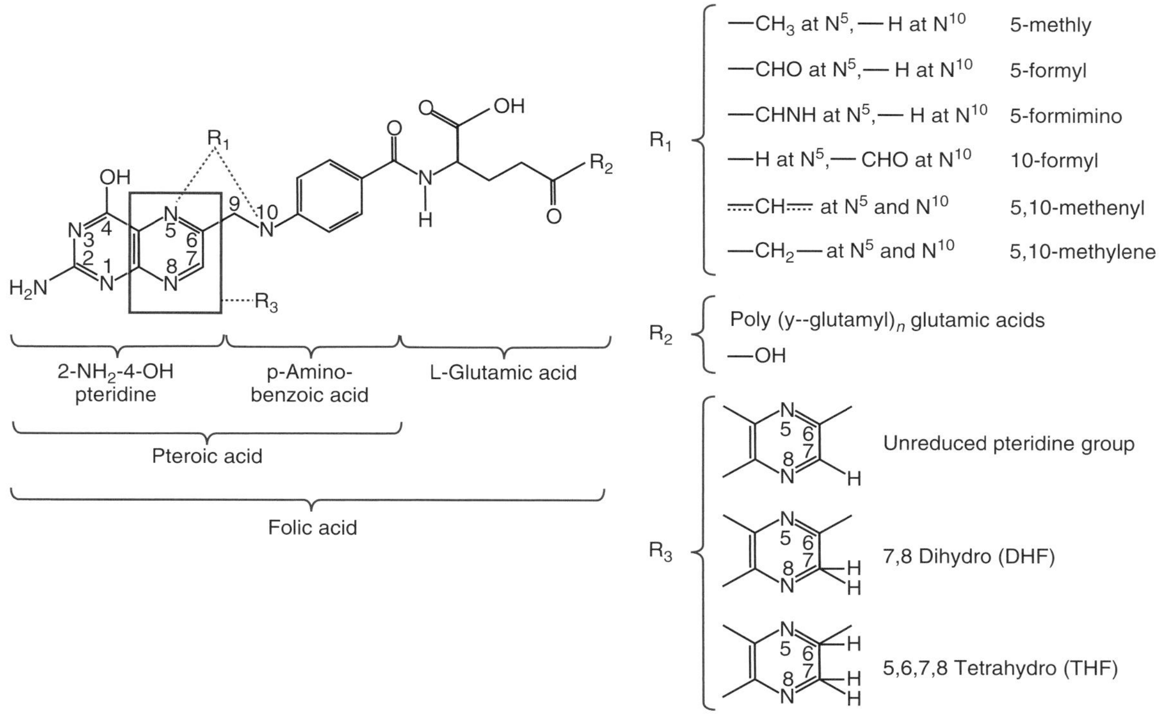

FIGURE 37.18 Structure and Relationships of Folic Acid and Its Derivatives.

on an empty stomach compared with approximately 50% for food folates.[11] Polyglutamate forms of folate present in food are first converted to monoglutamates by pteroylpolyglutamate hydrolase in the intestinal mucosa. Absorption of monoglutamyl folates at low concentration occurs through a saturable transport process with an acidic pH optimum (pH ≈ 5), with an additional, apparently nonsaturable absorption mechanism when intestinal folate concentrations exceed 5 to 10 µmol/L.[380,381] After cellular uptake, most of the folate is reduced and methylated, and enters the circulation as THF, circulating loosely bound to albumin or to a lesser degree to a high-affinity folate-binding protein. Uptake by certain cells (kidney, placenta, and choroid plexus) occurs by membrane-associated folate-binding proteins that act as folate receptors, and the reduced folate carrier, a member of the SLC19 family, facilitates uptake by most tissue.[382] Once within the cell, THF is demethylated and converted to the polyglutamyl form by folylpolyglutamate synthase, which helps to retain folate within the cell. For release into the circulation, the polyglutamates are reconverted to monoglutamates by polyglutamate hydrolase.

Folic acid and vitamin B_{12} metabolism are linked by the reaction that transfers a methyl group from 5-MTHF to cobalamin. In cases of cobalamin deficiency, folate is "trapped" as 5-MTHF and is "metabolically dead" (also known as the methyl-trap hypothesis).[383] It cannot be recycled to the active form, which is THF and back into the folate pool to serve as the main one-carbon unit acceptor for many biochemical reactions. Eventually, cellular depletion of 5,10-MTHF ensues (see Fig. 37.17), causing a reduction in purine and pyrimidine synthesis and hence DNA, which results in megaloblastic anemia and neuropathies. This concept is supported by the fact that THF corrects megaloblastic anemia in patients with congenital methylmalonic aciduria and homocystinuria, whereas it is not corrected with 5-MTHF. However, some investigators have suggested that vitamin B_{12} is required for the conversion of folic acid to the formyl form, and that formyltetrahydrofolates are natural substrates for forming folate polyglutamates.

Protein-free plasma folate is filtered at the glomerulus, and most is reabsorbed by the proximal renal tubules. Consequently, intact urinary folate represents only a small percentage of intake. Folate is predominantly excreted by catabolism following cleavage of the C^9-N^{10} bond to produce *p*-aminobenzoylpolyglutamates, which then are hydrolyzed to monoglutamates and *N*-acetylated before excretion. Biliary excretion of folate has been estimated at approximately 100 µg/day, but much of this is reabsorbed in enterohepatic circulation. Fecal losses have been studied by radiolabeling and have been found to be similar in type and quantity to urinary losses.[384]

Functions

Folate coenzymes, together with coenzymes derived from vitamins B_{12}, B_6, and B_2, are essential for one-carbon metabolism. Biochemically, a carbon unit from serine or glycine is transferred to THF to form 5,10-MTHF, which then is (1) used in the synthesis of thymidine (and incorporation into DNA), (2) oxidized to formyl-THF for use in the synthesis of purines (precursors of RNA and DNA), or (3) reduced to 5-MTHF, which is necessary for the methylation of homocysteine to methionine. Much of this methionine is converted to *S*-adenosylmethionine, a universal donor of methyl groups to DNA, RNA, hormones, neurotransmitters, membrane lipids, and proteins.[385] Some of these reactions are illustrated in Fig. 37.19. Different folates are involved in these reactions, depending on the chemical state of the single carbon fragments transferred (Table 37.5).

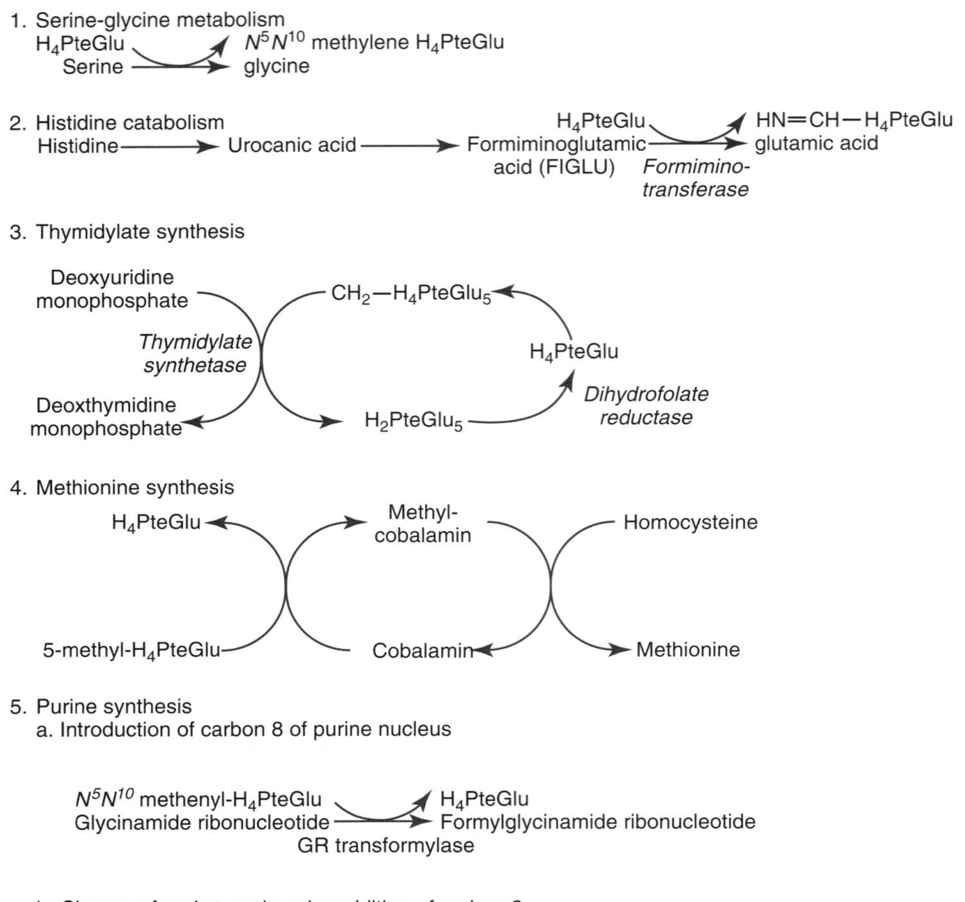

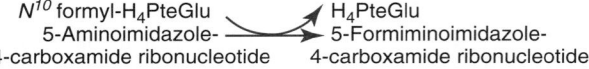

FIGURE 37.19 **The Five Major Metabolic Functions of Folate in Human Cells.** Note that H_4PteGlu is also referred as THF and N^5,N^{10} methylene H_4PteGlu as 5,10-MTHF in the text. *GR,* glycinamide ribonucleotide; *PteGlu,* pteroylglutamic acid.

Interconversions of these forms of folic acid take place through various electron transfer reactions facilitated by specific enzyme systems and coenzymes, such as reduced forms of flavin-adenine dinucleotide and NADPH. Conversion between the N^5-, N^{10}-methylene form and N^{10}-formyl forms is readily reversible, but the reduction of methylene to methyl and the reduction of free THF to formyltetrahydrofolate are essentially irreversible. Conversion of 5-MTHF back to THF requires cobalamin (see Fig 37.17).

Requirements and Reference Nutrient Intakes

Based on folate concentrations in liver biopsy samples, and because the liver contains approximately half of all body stores, total body stores of folate are estimated to be between 12 and 28 mg.[386] Kinetic studies that show both fast turnover and slow turnover folate pools indicate that approximately 0.5% to 1% of body stores are catabolized or excreted daily,[387] suggesting a minimum daily requirement of between 60 and 280 µg to replace losses. In calculating nutritional requirements, the concept of dietary folate equivalents (DFEs) has been used to adjust for the nearly 50% lower bioavailability

TABLE 37.5 Folic Acid Derivatives Formed From One-Carbon Reactions Involving Folate as Coenzyme

Reaction	Group Transferred	Folic Acid Derivative
Serum/glycine metabolism	Methylene (–CH_2–)	N^5,N^{10}-methylene THF/FH_4
Histidine catabolism	Formimino (–CHNH)	N^5-formimino THF/FH_4
Thymidylate synthesis	Methylene (–CH_2–)	N^5,N^{10}-methylene THF/FH_4
Methionine synthesis	Methyl (–CH_3)	N^5-methyl THF/FH_4
Purine synthesis	Methenyl (–CH–)	N^5,N^{10}-methyenyl THF/FH_4
	Formyl (–CHO)	N^{10}-formyl THF/FH_4

of food folate compared with supplemental folic acid, such that 1 DFE = 1 μg of food folate = 0.6 μg of folic acid from fortified food or as a supplement consumed with food = 0.5 μg folic acid supplement taken on an empty stomach.[11] Before the fortification program of cereal grains with folic acid was conducted between 1988 and 1994, the median intake of folate from food in the United States was approximately 250 μg/day; this figure is expected to increase by approximately 100 μg/day after fortification. Recommendations on dietary reference intakes made in 1998 by the US IOM have shifted the emphasis away from prevention of deficiency toward the concept of optimal health.[11] Current RDAs of the US IOM are 400 μg/day DFEs for adults 19 years and older and for adolescents between 14 and 18 years, 300 μg/day DFEs for children 9 to 13 years, 200 μg/day DFEs for children 4 to 8 years, and 150 μg/day DFEs for children 1 to 3 years. Adequate intake for infants 0 to 6 months is set at 65 μg/day DFEs, and for infants 7 to 11 months, 80 μg/day DFEs. Based on maintenance of erythrocyte folate concentrations during pregnancy, the RDA for pregnant women of all ages is set at 600 μg/day DFEs, and for lactating women of all ages, the RDA is 500 μg/day DFEs.[11,388]

Intravenous Supply

The previous adult recommendation for an intravenous supply of folic acid of 400 μg/day has been increased to 600 μg/day as part of the requirements set by the FDA.[11,156]

Deficiency

Deficiency of folate may result from (1) absence of intestinal microorganisms (gut sterilization), (2) poor intestinal absorption (eg, after surgical resection, in celiac disease or sprue), (3) insufficient dietary intake (including chronic alcoholism), (4) excessive demands (as in pregnancy, liver disease, and malignancies), (5) administration of antifolate drugs (eg, methotrexate), and (6) anticonvulsant therapy (which increases folate requirements, especially during pregnancy).[389] Inadequate folate intake leads first to decreased serum folate concentration, then to a decrease in RBC folate concentration and an increase in plasma homocysteine, and then to megaloblastic changes in the bone marrow and other tissues. Megaloblastic anemia (characterized by large, abnormally nucleated erythrocytes in the bone marrow) is the major clinical manifestation of folate deficiency, although sensory loss and neuropsychiatric changes may also occur. Deficiencies of folate and Fe may coexist in malnourished people, in which case the latter may mask the expected macrocytic and megaloblastic changes.

Pregnancy brings increased demand to folate stores because of increased DNA synthesis, and one-carbon transfer reactions and low serum folate concentrations in pregnancy are associated with adverse outcomes, including preterm delivery, infant low birth weight, and fetal growth retardation.[390] In addition, many observational studies have confirmed a reduction in risk of neural tube defects (NTDs) with periconceptual folic acid supplementation.[391,392] In a large controlled intervention trial, conducted in two regions of China, that involved approximately 250,000 women, a daily supplement of 400 μg of folic acid taken at least 80% of the time was associated with an 85% risk reduction of NTDs in an area of high baseline frequency of the NTD and a 40% reduction in an area of low baseline frequency.[393] Current suggestions are that women planning pregnancy should take at least 400 μg/day until the 12th week of pregnancy, although a daily intake of 5 mg of folic acid is recommended, especially for those with a history of NTDs.[394,395] Since the US FDA program of fortification of all grain products with folic acid (140 μg/100 g) began in 1996, study populations have shown a doubling of mean plasma folate concentrations and significant falls in total homocysteine concentrations, with a substantial reduction in the incidence of NTDs.[396] A recent study designed to determine the optimal RBC folate concentration required to prevent NTDs with 400 μg/day analyzed data from two regions in nonfortified populations of China.[397] The results showed an inverse dose–response relationship of NTDs with RBC folate concentrations, with women with the lowest RBC folate concentration having the highest risk of NTDs. The threshold optimal RBC folate concentration for the prevention of NTDs was found to be 1000 nmol/L.[397] These data will help to guide policy decisions with regard to voluntary versus mandatory folate fortification of foods.

Although the cause of NTDs is probably multifactorial, involving more than one aspect of folate use,[398] one factor that contributes to this and other folate-requiring conditions is genetic polymorphism. The most extensively studied polymorphic alleles are those of 5,10- MTHFR,[399] the enzyme responsible for the irreversible reduction of 5,10-MTHF to 5-MTHF, the methyl donor of homocysteine to methionine. Recent metaanalyses have strongly suggested a significant association of the variant MTHFR C677T and a suggestive association of other polymorphisms with increased risk of NTDs.[400,401] A single-point C-to-T mutation at base pair 677 (C677T), which causes substitution of valine for alanine, leads to a thermolabile protein with reduced enzymatic activity. The homozygous T/T enzyme has an incidence of approximately 12% in Asian and white populations with a 50% loss of enzyme activity; the heterozygous C/T variant has an incidence of up to 50% in some populations, with a lesser degree of enzyme inactivity.[402] Although plasma and RBC folate and homocysteine concentrations are associated with MTHFR genotype, with those with MTHFR T/T showing lower folate and high homocysteine concentrations, one trial that undertook supplementation with folic acid doses of 100 μg/day or 4000 μg/week did not reduce high homocysteine concentrations in those with the MTHFR T/T genotype.[403]

The role of folic acid in the metabolism of homocysteine has received much interest.[404] Elevation of plasma homocysteine concentration has been postulated to be an independent risk factor for coronary artery disease[302,303,405] and cerebrovascular disease.[406,407] The involvement of folate in its coenzyme forms with homocysteine and methionine metabolism is shown in Fig. 37.17. Folate is the principal micronutrient determinant of homocysteine status,[408] and supplementation with folate (0.5–5.0 mg/day) has been used as a treatment modality to reduce circulating homocysteine concentrations.[409,410] However, the most recent Cochrane metaanalyses of trials of homocysteine-lowering therapy with folate, vitamins B_6 or B_{12} given alone or in combination have not shown a reduction in cardiovascular disease.[411] A recent trial of folate among adults with hypertension in China without a history of stroke or myocardial infarction studied the combined use of enalapril and 0.8 mg folic acid, compared with enalapril alone, and found that it significantly reduced the risk of first stroke.[412] This study showed that targeting individuals with low baseline folate and choosing primary endpoints in trials carefully provided better insight into the intricate interplay of nutrients and disease processes.

Folate appears to have a protective effect on colorectal cancer development,[413] but it is associated with increased risk of gastric cancer[414] and prostate cancer,[415] and may be associated with lung cancer.[416] One metaanalysis of 10 randomized controlled trials showed a borderline significant increase in frequency of overall cancer in the folic acid–supplemented group compared with the control group,[415] whereas another showed that cancer incidences were higher in the folic acid–supplemented groups than the non-folic acid-supplemented groups (relative risk:1.21; 95% confidence interval: 1.05–1.39). Another metaanalysis showed that fortification of foods to prevent NTDs was not associated with increased cancer incidence during the first 5 years of treatment because the doses used for fortification were a magnitude lower than those used in clinical trials.[417] Even so, it has been suggested that folic acid supplementation trials should be performed with careful monitoring (of cancer incidence) to help guide future policy decisions.[395]

Lower than normal serum folate concentrations have been reported in patients in psychiatric disorders, but treatment with folate has given mixed results.[418] Limited evidence suggests that folate may have a role as a supplement to other treatments for depression.

Toxicity

No adverse effects have been reported from the consumption of folate-fortified foods, thus any signs of toxicity are associated with supplemental folate. Most of the limited evidence suggests that excessive folate supplementation, typically in doses up to 10 mg/day (although some have given 500 mg/day), can precipitate or exacerbate neuropathy in vitamin B_{12}–deficient subjects, and it is this endpoint that has been used to set a tolerable upper intake concentration of 1 mg/day from fortified foods or supplements for adults.[11] One recognized complication of folate supplementation is that it "masks" vitamin B_{12} deficiency, because the associated anemia responds to folate alone. This may delay treatment of the deficiency, allowing neurologic abnormalities to progress.[419] It has been recommended that if a low serum folate is present concomitantly with low vitamin B_{12}, the latter should be corrected first. In addition, serum folate, rather than RBC folate, is the preferred marker for folate status in the presence of vitamin B_{12} deficiency (discussed further in the following).[419]

Laboratory Assessment of Status

Folate status may be reliably assessed by direct measurement of serum and RBC or whole blood concentrations, and its metabolic function as a coenzyme may be assessed by metabolite concentrations such as plasma homocysteine. Serum folate concentrations are considered indicative of recent intake and not of tissue stores, but serial measurements have been used to confirm AI. Whole blood and RBC folate concentrations are more indicative of tissue stores over the lifetime of RBCs and are therefore a better indicator of longer term folate status than serum folate. Because folate is taken up only by the developing RBC in the bone marrow and not by the mature cell, RBC concentrations reflect folate status over the 120-day life span of the cell. However, a pathology benchmarking review concluded that serum and RBC folate provide equivalent information regarding folate status.[27] Urine folate excretion is not a recommended indicator of folate status.[419]

CPB assays have now largely replaced microbiological procedures for the measurement of serum, whole blood, or RBC folate, although the use of microtiter 96-well plates has enabled a microbiological assay using *Lactobacillus casei* to be partially automated.[420] The binder used in the CPB folate assay is a protein that occurs naturally in milk, called β-lactoglobulin or milk folate binder; it is commonly used together with a radioactive ^{125}I-folate label, although nonisotopic fluorescence and bioluminescence labels are becoming more popular. One commercial assay uses selective protein binding coupled with ion capture, followed by fluorescence assay. A comparison of frequently used laboratory analyzers showed marked variation.[421] However, because problems of standardization and inter-method agreement persist with CPB assays, more specific analytical techniques have been developed, including HPLC with electrochemical or mass-spectrometric detection.[25]

Several analytes are known to be indicative of folate metabolism. Plasma homocysteine is considered a sensitive indicator of folate status and is strongly correlated with serum folate concentration in the lower range, which is less than 10 nmol/L (4.5 μg/L).[419] A homocysteine concentration more than 15 μmol/L is indicative of folate deficiency.[419] However, because the concentration of homocysteine is dependent on age, sex, renal function, genetic factors, and the status of other vitamins (B_6 and B_{12}), it is not a specific marker of folate status.[363] Similarly, the methylation of DNA is dependent on adequate MTHFR. A sensitive new method for the rapid detection of abnormal methylation patterns among global DNA patterns has been reported and may have promise as a functional marker,[422] as may measurement of the degree of uracil incorporation into DNA, with 5,10-methylene THF required for the conversion of deoxyuridine monophosphate to deoxythymidine monophosphate by thymidylate synthetase.[423,424]

Preanalytical Variables

Whole blood collected into containers with the preservatives Li heparin or EDTA is the required sample type for RBC folate, whereas tubes containing clot activators are required for serum folate. Local laboratories should be consulted for their preferred sample type. Ideally, a fasting sample should be collected, especially if the patient is receiving folate supplementation. A recent study using a radioimmunoassay method reported that RBC folate collected into containers with EDTA showed good stability up to 48 hours when stored at room temperature.[133] However, serum folate significantly and progressively decreased over time with a maximum decrease of 26.8% compared with a basal concentration at 72 hours when kept at room temperature,[133] and was consistent with a previous report that analyzed serum folate using a microbiologic assay.[134] Due to the instability of folate in serum, it is therefore recommended that if delay in transportation is anticipated, serum should be separated from RBCs by centrifugation and stored frozen until analysis. Because there is a significant amount of folate in RBCs, hemolysis invalidates serum folate results.[425]

Reference Intervals

Because of methodologic differences, reference intervals for folate are method dependent. Data collected from the National Health and Nutritional Examination Survey (NHANES) of 1988 to 1994 in the United States, in which almost 3000 blood samples were analyzed, revealed reference intervals of 2.6 to 12.2 μg/L (6.0–28.0 nmol/L) for serum folate and 103 to 411 μg/L (237–945 nmol/L) for RBC folate.[426] However, a recent analysis conducted since mandatory supplementation of cereal grain products began, yielded age-, sex-, and ethnicity-specific reference intervals for both serum and RBC folate.[378] This demonstrates the importance of establishing local, or at least national, reference intervals. Biochemical deficiency has been defined as a concentration of less than 3 μg/L (7.0 nmol/L) for serum folate and less than 150 μg/L (340 nmol/L) for RBC folate.[419] For more information, refer to the Appendix on Reference Intervals. Laboratories should verify that these ranges are appropriate for use in their own settings.

Vitamin C

Vitamin C (L-ascorbic acid) serves as a reducing agent in several important hydroxylation reactions in the body. An illustrative case of vitamin C deficiency has recently been reported.[69]

Chemistry

The term vitamin C refers to all molecules that exhibit antiscorbutic properties (derived from Latin word for scurvy, scorbutus) in humans and includes both ascorbic acid and its oxidized form, dehydroascorbic acid (DHA) (Fig. 37.20). The vitamin C redox system comprises these molecules and the free radical intermediate, monodehydroascorbic acid, the product of one-electron oxidation of ascorbic acid. L-ascorbic acid is the enol form of 2-oxo-L-gulofuranolactone, the enolic hydroxyl on ring carbon 3 having a pK_a of 4.2 and conferring its acidic nature. The vitamin is a white, crystalline solid that is readily soluble in water. Acidic solutions (below pH 3) show that the absorption maximum is 245 nm, whereas solutions of the ionized material (above pH 5) have an absorption peak at 265 nm. Ascorbic acid is a relatively strong reductant with an E'_0 (pH 7) of +0.58 V. The DHA form is more labile than the reduced form to hydrolytic ring opening to yield 2,3-diketo-L-gulonic acid, which is not antiscorbutic.[427]

Dietary Sources

Plants and most animals possess the ability to synthesize the vitamin from D-glucose via the lactones of D-glucuronic and L-gulonic acids; however, some mammals, including humans, lack L-gulonolactone oxidase, the enzyme that catalyzes the formation of 2-keto-L-gulonolactone from D-glucose, which then spontaneously tautomerizes to L-ascorbic acid. Excellent sources of the vitamin include citrus fruits, berries, melons, tomatoes, green peppers, broccoli, brussel sprouts, and leafy green vegetables.[11] Losses during processing, especially with heat and aerobic conditions, can be considerable.

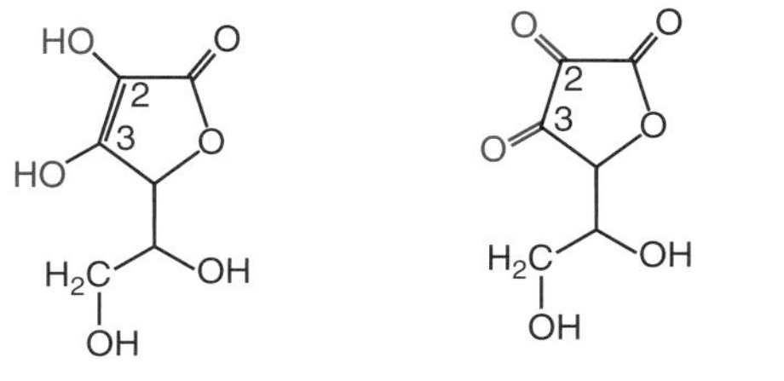

L-Ascorbic acid Dehydroascorbic acid

FIGURE 37.20 L-Ascorbic and Dehydroascorbic Acids.

Absorption, Transport, Metabolism, and Excretion

Gastrointestinal absorption of ascorbic acid occurs throughout the ileum via a combination of Na-dependent active transport at low concentrations and simple diffusion at high concentrations.[428,429] Between 70% and 90% of a usual dietary intake of ascorbic acid (up to 180 mg/day) is absorbed, falling to 50% or less at loads greater than 1 g/day.[430] The absorbed ascorbic acid moves rapidly from the intestinal cell into the blood through a process of facilitated diffusion modulated by glucose. In one study, DHA was shown to cross the apical membrane by facilitated diffusion, whereas ascorbate transport was mediated by a Na-dependent electrogenic process modulated by glucose.[431] One review surmised that ascorbate uptake by cells is mediated by specific transporters—the Na-dependent transporters, SVCT 1 and SVCT 2—whereas DHA is mediated via the facilitated-diffusion glucose transporters GLUT 1, 3, and 4.[432]

Vitamin C is found in most tissues, including the brain, but glandular tissues, such as pituitary, adrenal cortex, corpus luteum, and thymus, have the highest amounts, and the eye lens has 20 to 30 times the plasma concentration.[433] DHA, once transported intracellularly, is reduced to ascorbate; in plasma, vitamin C exists predominantly as the ascorbate ion. Many cells, particularly hepatic cells, neutrophils, mononuclear phagocytes, osteoblasts, and erythrocytes, are capable of DHA uptake and recycle it to ascorbate, which maintains a human body pool of up to 2 g.[430] The biological half-life of vitamin C in an individual ranges from 8 to 40 days, with an average of approximately 16 days.[430] Vitamin C is inversely related to the dose consumed and is conserved during periods of low intake, with absorption becoming maximum with minimum urinary excretion.[430] Excretion of unchanged ascorbate occurs increasingly with increased dosage, with almost all of an injected dose of more than 500 mg excreted over 24 hours.[434] DHA that is not recycled may be irreversibly delactonized to 2,3-diketogulonic acid and further degraded to oxalic acid for urine excretion. Other catabolic products of 2,3-diketogulonic acid are L-lyxonic acid, L-xylose, and L-threonic acid.

Functions

Ascorbic acid, working in synchrony with vitamin E, is one of the most effective water-soluble antioxidants in biological fluids[140,427,435] and is capable of scavenging physiologically important reactive O_2 species and reactive nitrogen species. Both ascorbate and the ascorbyl radical have low reduction potentials and react with most other biologically relevant radicals.[46] The ascorbyl radical is relatively stable because of resonance stabilization of the unpaired electron. Ascorbate can regenerate other small molecule antioxidants, including α-tocopherol, reduced glutathione, urate, and β-carotene, from their respective radical species, and therefore may prevent oxidative damage to biological macromolecules, including DNA, lipids, and proteins.[46] Vitamin C has been shown to also exhibit pro-oxidant properties,[436] and although pro-oxidants tend to have deleterious effects, pharmacologic doses of ascorbate may have beneficial pro-oxidant activity in the treatment of certain diseases, especially cancer.[437] It has recently been proposed that the balance between antioxidant and pro-oxidant activity is important for health and too much antioxidant might actually be harmful.[53] However, this has been disputed by other investigators.[438] It has also been recognized that DHA has important intracellular properties that are different from, but sometimes complementary to, those of ascorbate.[439]

Ascorbic acid acts as a cofactor for a number of mixed function oxidases in hydroxylation processes in which it promotes enzyme activity by maintaining metal ions in their reduced form (particularly Fe and Cu). Vitamin C has a functional role in the formation of collagen by acting as a cofactor for protocollagen hydroxylase, the enzyme responsible for hydroxylation of prolyl and lysyl residues within nascent peptides in connective tissue proteins.[440] Among these are collagen and related proteins, which make up the intercellular material of cartilage, dentin, and bone.

Ascorbate is also involved in (1) carnitine biosynthesis, serving as a cofactor to 6-*N*-trimethyl-L-lysine hydrolase; (2) γ-butyrobetaine hydrolase, which converts γ-butyrobetaine to carnitine; (3) degradation of tyrosine via 4-OH phenylpyruvate dioxygenase; (4) synthesis of adrenal hormones via dopamine β-hydroxylase; (5) biosynthesis of corticosteroids and aldosterone; (6) hydroxylation of cholesterol in the formation of bile acids; and (7) folate metabolism and leukocyte functions.[427,435]

Vitamin C also has an important role in the intestinal absorption of non-heme Fe, by maintaining it in its reduced ferrous form.[441] More recently identified functions include nucleic acid and histone dealkylation and proteoglycan deglycanation.[435]

Requirements and Reference Nutrient Intakes

The amount of vitamin C sufficient to alleviate and cure the clinical signs of scurvy is only 10 mg/day, which is probably near the minimum requirement in humans. However, this amount is not adequate to maintain near saturation of tissue in the adult human male, who has a body pool of 1.5 to 2 g and shows clinical symptoms of deficiency when this total pool falls below approximately 300 mg.[442] Acknowledgment of functions of vitamin C beyond the antiscorbutic and antioxidant has led to the development of the concept of the optimal nutrition state, along with the intake required to achieve this. Current recommendations of the US IOM regarding estimated average requirements and RDAs have reflected this approach.[11] The RDA for adult males older than 19 years and older than 70 years is 90 mg/day, and the corresponding RDA for women is 75 mg/day. To provide for fetal needs, an additional 10 mg/day is recommended for pregnant women to offset the decrease in plasma vitamin C concentration during pregnancy. A lactating woman should receive an additional 45 to 50 mg/day because an average of 18 to 22 mg may be secreted in 600 to 700 mL of milk. Children 1 to 3 years of age have an RDA of 15 mg/day; those 4 to 8 years old have an RDA of 25 mg/day. Boys aged 9 to 13 have an RDA of 45 mg/day, and those 14 to 18 years have an RDA of 75 mg/day. Corresponding values for girls are 45 and 65 mg/day, respectively. No RDA is given for infants up to 1 year old; instead, AI amounts of 40 mg/day up to 6 months and 50 mg/day from 7 to 12 months are recommended. Some special groups, such as smokers, should take an additional 35 mg/day.[11,443]

Intravenous Supply

The recommended IV intake for adult patients receiving TPN was 100 mg for many years,[179] but this has been increased to 200 mg/day.[156] This change reflects the expected increased requirements for wound healing and for antioxidant activity.

Deficiency

Scurvy results due to deficiency of vitamin C and still occurs in developed countries, albeit rarely, either as part of general malnutrition or in isolation. Those most at risk of the disease include: (1) older adult men, particularly those who live alone; (2) those with alcohol dependence and smokers; (3) those taking unbalanced diets, especially populations who have limited access to fresh fruits and vegetables either due to weather conditions or disasters both natural and manmade; (4) some mentally ill patients; (5) renal failure patients undergoing peritoneal dialysis or hemodialysis; (6) those with increased requirements such as the sick and pregnant women; and (7) some patients with cancer.

Lack of vitamin C or scurvy[444] causes an inability to form adequate intercellular cement substance in connective tissue, bones, and dentin, which often results in swollen, tender, and often bleeding or bruised loci at joints and in other areas where structurally weakened tissue cannot withstand stress. Bone formation is usually impaired, causing poor growth and lesions. Infantile scurvy, also known as Barlow disease,[445] exhibits a bayonet-rib syndrome. The gums are livid and swollen, cutaneous bleeding often begins on the lower thighs as perifollicular hemorrhages, and large spontaneous bruises (ecchymoses) may arise almost anywhere on the body. This condition may be misconstrued as child abuse.[446] Ocular hemorrhages, drying of salivary and lacrimal glands, parotid swelling, femoral neuropathy, edema of the lower extremities, and psychologic disturbances have also been described. Some scorbutic patients may develop anemia, display radiologic changes characteristic of osteoporosis, or die suddenly from heart failure.[427]

Diseases of vitamin C deficiency that might reflect its role as an antioxidant include increased risk of coronary heart disease, as demonstrated in a cohort of Finnish men,[447] and increased risk of death by stroke in a cohort of older adult British individuals.[448] An important metaanalysis showed that dietary vitamin C intake, but not vitamin C from supplements, correlated inversely with coronary heart disease, suggesting that benefit is derived from other components of a healthy diet.[449]

Vitamin C deficiency has also been linked to anemia, diabetes mellitus, various types of cancer, cataract formation, and osteoporosis; however, there is no clear evidence for a causal link.[427,435,450] A recent metaanalysis of randomized placebo-controlled trials investigated the effect of vitamin C supplementation (>200 mg/day) on the common cold and found that regular vitamin C supplementation did not significantly reduce the incidence of the common cold in the general population (pooled risk ratio from 24 trials involving 10,708 participants: 0.97; 95% confidence interval: 0.94–1.00).[451] Most trials used 1 g/day of vitamin C. One critique of the trials was that in most of them, common colds were self-diagnosed, and no clear criteria were used to adjudicate the severity or duration of the common colds reported. Even so, the same metaanalysis found that there was some merit in vitamin C supplementation in those engaging in short periods of intensive exercise or sport.

Toxicity

Vitamin C is generally well tolerated by healthy individuals, and ingestion of supplements of 2 to 4 g/day—as taken by some for prevention or amelioration of the common cold—is usually without hazard, although gastrointestinal irritation has been reported.[452] Other potential but rare adverse effects include increased oxalate excretion and kidney stone formation,[453] increased uric acid excretion, excess Fe absorption, lowered vitamin B_{12} concentrations, systemic conditioning and "rebound" scurvy, and pro-oxidant effects in the presence of free Fe^{3+} or Cu^{2+} ions. Ingestion of amounts of vitamin C of more than 200 mg/day shows little increase in plasma steady-state concentrations, which suggests that overload of vitamin C is unlikely because excess is usually excreted because of the inverse relationship between vitamin C dose and absorption.[430] Consideration of such data has led the Food and Nutrition Board of the US IOM to propose a tolerable upper intake amount for vitamin C of 2 g/day for adults older than 19 years.[11,450]

Laboratory Assessment of Status

At present, no useful functional tests of vitamin C adequacy are available; thus laboratory assessment of status is made by direct measurement of plasma, urine, or tissue concentrations of ascorbic acid, total vitamin C, or (rarely) metabolite. Because ascorbic acid is readily oxidized by dissolved O_2 at a neutral pH, plasma samples should be treated with a metal-chelating and protein-precipitating acid (eg, metaphosphoric acid) soon after a phlebotomy followed by prompt freezing.[454,455] Samples so treated may be stored at −80°C for several years.[25] Plasma ascorbate concentration is considered a reliable indicator of vitamin C intake[450] and has been measured photometrically by oxidation with 2,4-dinitrophenylhydrazine to form the red *bis*-hydrazone, or with 2,4-dichlorophenol-indophenol, which is reduced to a colorless form.[25] A more specific approach is to use the enzyme ascorbate oxidase to convert ascorbate to dehydroascorbate, which then is coupled with *o*-phenylene diamine to form a product that is measured fluorometrically[25] or at 340 nm on an automated analyzer.[456] A spectrophotometric method for measuring ascorbic acid in methanol/trichloroacetic acid extracts prepared from human plasma after enzymatic oxidation of ascorbic acid to DHA by ascorbate oxidase has also been published. The kinetics of the concentration-dependent absorbance changes of DHA is monitored with phosphate-citrate-methanol buffers.[457]

HPLC methods offer the potential advantage of specificity but generally are time-consuming. Detection may be done by precolumn derivatization to the fluorescent quinoxaline, or by electrochemical or coulometric means. Care must be taken during the analysis to prevent oxidation of the ascorbate before detection by using dithiothreitol or homocysteine added to the sample and mobile phase.[25] With suitable sample preparation, ascorbic acid, total vitamin C, and, by difference, DHA, may be measured together with HPLC[455,458] or gas chromatography–mass spectrometry.[459,460]

Leukocyte ascorbic acid is considered to be a better indicator of body stores than plasma ascorbate, but its use has not been widely adopted because of the large sample volume requirement, the difficulty involved in automating the analysis, the influence of fluctuating leukocyte numbers, and the relative difficulty of the analysis.[29] Urinary excretion and RBC concentrations have not been found to be specific and useful indices of vitamin C status; however, urinary concentrations of ascorbic acid, especially after a load test, can be helpful in the clinical diagnosis of scurvy.[29]

Preanalytical Variables

Blood collected into containers with the preservatives Li heparin or EDTA is the required sample type for vitamin C, but local laboratories should be consulted for their preferred sample type. Ideally, a fasting sample should be collected, especially if the patient is receiving vitamin C supplementation. Vitamin C is unstable in plasma, and samples must be treated within 4 hours of collection with 6% metaphosphoric acid (1 : 1 ratio of sample and acid) and stored frozen until analysis.[132,455] Dithiothreitol may also be used as a preservative.[461] A recent study using a HPLC with an electrochemical detection method reported that vitamin C collected into clot activator tubes (serum) without prompt acid treatment on collection decreased rapidly with an average of more than 50% disappearing after 24 hours.[133] By contrast, blood collected into Li heparin containers with sulphosalicylic acid treatment at the time of collection, centrifuged promptly, and stored at −20°C showed good stability up to 48 hours.[133] Vitamin C in plasma or serum is known to be readily degraded by oxidation caused by high temperature, light, neutral pH, pro-oxidant material such as certain enzymes, and interaction with Fe or Cu.[25,462] Li heparin has been shown to be the best anticoagulant for vitamin C stability.[133,462]

Reference Intervals

Interpretation of results in seriously ill patients with SIRS is limited by the acute fall in plasma and leukocyte ascorbic acid seen in injury, infection, or after surgery.[41,463] One recent study showed that plasma ascorbic acid concentration significantly decreased by 74% within 48 hours of injury and remained low even after adjustment for albumin.[463] The decrease in vitamin C due to SIRS had been attributed to transient redistribution, increased urinary excretion, and increased use in neutralizing free radicals and in regenerating tocopherol (vitamin E). Table 37.2 shows the magnitude of change in vitamin C with increasing CRP concentrations.

With AI of vitamin C, plasma concentrations of the total vitamin (ascorbic acid plus DHA) are between 0.4 and 1.5 mg/dL (23–85 μmol/L). This range is similar to values reported by an automated method (0.46–1.49 mg/dL, 26.1–84.6 μmol/L)[456] and HPLC with electrochemical detection (0.26–1.59 mg/dL, 15.0–90.0 μmol/L).[132] Concentrations at or near the lower limit value may be seen in some cases with subclinical vitamin C deficiency and in older individuals. A value less than 0.2 mg/dL (≈10 μmol/L) is considered deficient.[132] The guidance reference interval for vitamin C concentration is 20 to 53 μg/10^8 leukocytes (1.14–3.01 fmol/leukocyte). A value of less than 10 μg/10^8 leukocytes (0.57 fmol/leukocyte) is considered deficient. For more information, refer to the Appendix on Reference

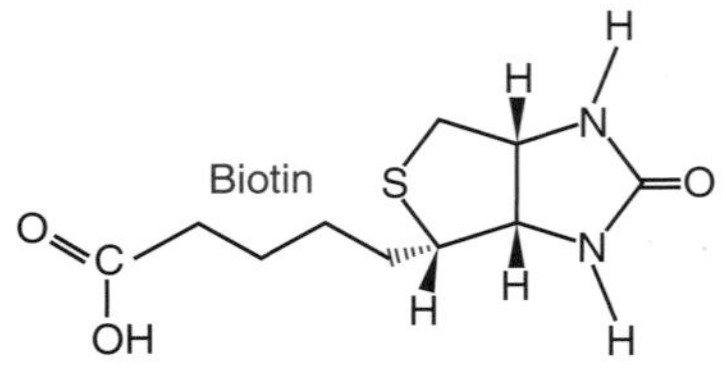

FIGURE 37.21 Structure of Biotin.

Intervals. Laboratories should verify that these ranges are appropriate for use in their own settings.

Biotin

Biotin (also known as vitamin H or B_7) is a water-soluble vitamin that serves as a coenzyme for a number of carboxylation reactions (eg, pyruvate, acetyl-CoA, propionyl Co-A, decarboxylases) involved in gluconeogenesis, lipogenesis, and catabolism of branched-chain amino acids. Biotin also has roles in cell signaling, epigenetic regulation of genes, and chromatin structure.

Chemistry

Biotin is *cis*-tetrahydro-2-oxothieno[3,4-*d*]-imidazoline-4-valeric acid (Fig. 37.21) and occurs mainly bound to protein. The ε-amino group of the lysyl side chain of the protein is linked via an amide function involving the carboxyl group of the valeryl side chain of biotin. In addition, some biotin is linked noncovalently as a complex with avidin, a protein in egg whites. The ureido ring and the ionizable carboxyl group of biotin allow modest solubility of the white crystalline solid in aqueous solution, especially at an alkaline pH. Oxidizing agents convert the thioether to sulfoxides and sulfones, which lack biotin activity.

Dietary Sources

Mammals cannot synthesize biotin, and therefore, depend on dietary intake for supply. Good sources of biotin include eggs, liver, kidney, pancreas, yeast, and milk. Cereal grains, fruits, most vegetables, and meat are poor sources.[11]

Absorption, Transport, Metabolism, and Excretion

Biotin in the diet is largely linked to lysine residues on protein, and digestion of these proteins by gastrointestinal proteases and peptidases produce biocytin (ε-*N*-biotinyl lysine) and biotinyl peptides, and the latter may be further hydrolyzed by intestinal biotinidase to release biotin.[464] Avidin, a protein found in raw egg whites, binds biotin tightly and prevents its absorption; therefore, raw egg consumption can lead to biotin deficiency.[465] The peptide biocytin (ε-*N*-biotinyl lysine) is resistant to hydrolysis by proteolytic enzymes in the intestinal tract but together with biotin is readily absorbed. Biotinidase is found in intestinal secretions and the brush-border membrane of the intestine.

A biotin carrier, the Na-dependent multivitamin transporter[466] for which pantothenic acid and lipoate compete, is located in the intestinal brush-border membrane and transports biotin against a Na ion concentration gradient. At higher biotin doses (>25 μmol/L), there is passive diffusion across cell membranes. By contrast, transport of biotin across the basolateral membrane is Na-independent and electrogenic.[467] Biocytinase (biotin amidohydrolase) in plasma and erythrocytes catalyzes the hydrolysis of biocytin to yield free biotin. Biotin is cleared from the circulating blood more rapidly in deficient than in normal mammals; it is taken up by such tissues as liver, muscle, and kidney, and is localized in cytosolic and mitochondrial carboxylases. Covalent attachment of biotin to apoenzymes involves ATP-dependent conversion of the vitamin to biotinyl-5′-adenylate, followed by condensation of the biotinyl moiety with ε-amino groups of specific lysyl residues in apoenzymes preformed from subunits. The enzymes responsible for catalyzing the formation of the ε-*N*-biotinyl-L-lysyl (biocytinyl) moiety of proteins are holoenzyme synthetases.[464]

Approximately one-half of absorbed biotin is excreted as the metabolites bisnorbiotin, which occurs from β-oxidation of the valeric acid side chain, and biotin sulfoxide, which occurs from oxidation of sulfur in the heterocyclic ring.[464] Circulating plasma and urinary excretion patterns show a ratio of 3:2:1 for biotin, bisnorbiotin, and biotin sulfoxide. Minor metabolites are bisnorbiotin methyl ketone and biotin sulfone. Balance studies in humans, in whom only 1 mg is the usual total body content, showed that urinary excretion of biotin often exceeds dietary intake, and that in all cases, fecal excretion was as much as three to six times greater than dietary intake because of microfloral biosynthesis.

Functions

The principal biochemical function of biotin in humans is as a cofactor for carboxylation reactions. Five carboxylases are currently found in human tissue; one of these, an acetyl-CoA carboxylase, is inactive and may act as a storage vehicle for biotin.[468] The others are carboxylases for acetyl-CoA, propionyl-CoA, β-methylcrotonyl-CoA, and pyruvate. These enzymes operate via a common mechanism, which involves phosphorylation of bicarbonate by ATP to form carbonyl phosphate, followed by transfer of the carboxyl group to the sterically less hindered nitrogen of the biotin moiety. The resulting *N*(1)-carboxybiotinyl enzyme can then exchange the carboxylate function with a reactive center in a substrate. With cytosolic acetyl-CoA carboxylase, the product is malonyl-CoA, which is used for fatty acid biosynthesis. In mitochondria, pyruvate carboxylase catalyzes the formation of oxaloacetate, which, together with acetyl-CoA, forms citrate. The other carboxylases are involved in the metabolism of odd-numbered fatty acids and branched-chain fatty acids.[467,468]

Recent advances have implicated biotin in the epigenetic regulation of gene expression.[469] It has been shown that biotin attaches to histones (DNA-binding proteins) via an amide bond and that the reversible biotinylation of histones is important in regulating gene expression or repression.[470]

Requirements and Reference Nutrient Intakes

At present, scientific data are insufficient to allow recommendations of RDAs for biotin. Intestinal microfloras are likely to contribute significantly to the body pool of available biotin, making determination of the dietary requirements difficult. Mean urinary excretion, which is reflective of dietary intake, varies from 6 to 50 μg/day for adults who ingest 28 to 100 μg/day. Consideration of urinary excretion of both biotin and the metabolite 3-hydroxyisovalerate[32] has led to recommendations of AI, rather than RDAs.[11] The suggested AI for adults 19 years and older is 30 μg/day. For adolescents 14 to 18 years, it is 25 μg/day; for children 9 to 13 years, the AI

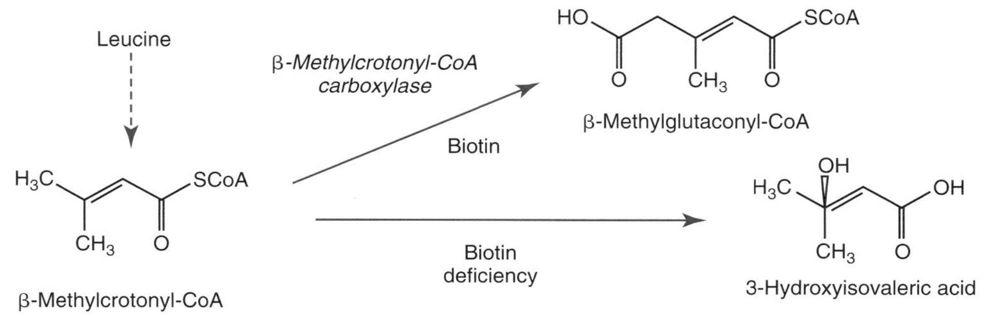

Leucine

β-Methylcrotonyl-CoA carboxylase

Biotin

Biotin deficiency

β-Methylcrotonyl-CoA

β-Methylglutaconyl-CoA

3-Hydroxyisovaleric acid

FIGURE 37.22 Formation of 3-Hydroxyisovaleric Acid Under Conditions of Biotin Deficiency. *CoA*, Coenzyme A.

is 20 μg/day; for children 4 to 8 years, the AI is 12 μg/day; for children 1 to 3 years, it is 8 μg/day; and for infants younger than 1 year, it is 0.7 μg/kg of body weight. An additional 5 μg/day is recommended for lactating mothers. Those undergoing hemodialysis or peritoneal dialysis, or with a biotinidase deficiency, would require additional amounts.

Intravenous Supply

The recommended supply of biotin for adults during TPN is 60 μg/day.[179]

Deficiency

Biotin deficiency is uncommon but may be seen (1) with prolonged consumption of raw egg whites, which contains the protein avidin that binds biotin in the intestines, and which prevents absorption, (2) in those on TPN without biotin supplementation,[471] and (3) in those with inborn errors of biotin metabolism. The first two situations may be complicated by effects on gut flora that produce biotin.[464,467]

Symptoms of biotin deficiency include anorexia, nausea, vomiting, glossitis, pallor, conjunctivitis, ataxia, hypotonia, depression, dry scaly dermatitis, and developmental delay in infants and children. Based on urinary excretion pattern of the biotin metabolite, 3-hydroxyisovaleric acid (Fig. 37.22), concerns have been expressed about marginal biotin deficiency in pregnancy because this has been shown to be teratogenic in fetuses.[472,473] Studies have shown that approximately one-half of pregnant women in the United States are marginally biotin deficient despite normal intake, and that this has important health policy implications.[474] However, because a causal link between maternal biotin deficiency and deleterious effects on the fetus or mother have not been clearly established, the jury is still out regarding biotin supplementation in pregnancy.[465] Significantly lowered urinary excretion or circulating blood concentrations have been found in alcoholic individuals, in patients with achlorhydria, and among older adults and some athletes.[464] Biotin has also been linked to immune function, lipid metabolism consistent with roles for biotin-dependent acetyl-CoA and propionyl-CoA carboxylases, and encephalopathies.[464]

The inborn errors of biotin metabolism include: (1) deficiency of biotinidase, which leads to the inability to use protein-bound biotin in the diet or to recycle endogenous biotin from holocarboxylases; (2) deficiency of biotin-dependent holocarboxylase synthetase, which leads to the inability to attach biotin to lysine residues of enzymes (ie, conversion of apocarboxylases to holocarboxylases); and (3) biotin transporter dysfunction (reported in a single case to date).[464,475] These causes all lead to isolated or multiple biotin-dependent carboxylase deficiency. The characteristic manifestation is metabolic acidosis due to abnormal organic acid excretion, associated with neurological abnormalities and skin changes. Biotinidase deficiency presents in the neonatal period, dependent on the availability of free biotin in the diet, whereas holocarboxylase synthetase deficiency can variably present at birth or up to the age of 8 years. Treatment is with biotin supplementation and clinical support as required. Finally, an autosomal recessive condition known as biotin-responsive basal ganglia disease has been reported that presents in childhood with subacute episodes of encephalopathy usually triggered by febrile illnesses; it disappears without neurological manifestations if biotin is given.[476]

Toxicity

No adverse effects of biotin in doses up to 300 times normal dietary intake have been reported, which has been administered to patients with biotinidase deficiency.[464] Tolerable upper intake amounts for biotin have not been set because the data are insufficient.[11]

Laboratory Assessment of Status

Traditionally, biotin has been measured in biological samples by microbiological assays, in which whole blood is first digested with papain or acid hydrolysis to release free biotin, samples of which are added to a biotin-deficient medium inoculated with a test organism such as *Lactobacillus plantarum*.[477] Other methods for unbound biotin include avidin-binding assays, in which a competitive protein-binding radioassay is set up with ^{3}H-labeled biotin, and nonradioactive enzyme-linked sorbent assays, using streptavidin as the binding agent.[478] Generally, the biotin content of RBCs is similar to that of plasma for a given method, but agreement between methods is often poor, which may relate to the specificity of the methods used.[477] Urinary excretion of biotin and 3-hydroxyisovaleric acid appear to be better indicators of biotin status than blood concentrations.[32] This was shown in a study of experimental biotin deficiency, when both urinary biotin and metabolites, measured by HPLC separation followed by an avidin-binding assay, and urinary 3-hydroxyisovaleric acid, measured by gas chromatography–mass spectrometry, showed significant changes, whereas serum biotin concentration did not. Functional markers of biotin status are being increasingly investigated. Lymphocyte propionyl-CoA carboxylase has been shown to be an early and sensitive indicator of biotin deficiency in marginal biotin deficiency[479] in patients on prolonged TPN without biotin[480] and in children with protein-energy malnutrition.[481]

Biotinidase is measured by quantitating the release of p-aminobenzoic acid from N-biotinyl-p-aminobenzoate. The mean ± SD of normal biotinidase activity is 5.8 ± 0.9 nmol p-aminobenzoate liberated per minute per milliliter of serum.[482,483]

Preanalytical Variables

There are no specific preanalytical factors that affect biotin measurement.

Reference Intervals

Typical reference interval values for whole blood biotin by a microbiological method are 0.5 to 2.20 nmol/L (mean of 1.31 nmol/L).[477] Deficiency is considered likely when less than 0.5 nmol/L. For more information, refer to the Appendix on Reference Intervals. Laboratories should verify that these ranges are appropriate for use in their own settings.

Niacin

Niacin (nicotinamide and nicotinic acid amide) is a precursor of the ubiquitous pyridine nucleotide coenzymes nicotinamide-adenine dinucleotide $(NAD)^+$ and nicotinamide-adenine dinucleotide phosphate $(NADP)^+$, which are required as coenzyme or cosubstrate in many biological redox reactions, and thus for energy metabolism. Niacin has been used therapeutically for dyslipidemia at pharmacological doses.

Chemistry

The term niacin (also known as niacinamide or vitamin B_3) refers to nicotinic acid (pyridine-3-carboxylic acid), its amide nicotinamide, and derivatives that show the same biological activity as nicotinamide. However, there is a distinction between the two primary vitamin forms with regard to some aspects of their metabolism and especially their different pharmacological actions at high doses. Structures of both vitamers and the two coenzyme forms containing the nicotinamide moiety are shown in Fig. 37.23.

Free forms of the vitamin are white, stable solids that are soluble in water. Oxidized coenzymes are labile to alkali, whereas reduced (dihydro) coenzymes are labile to acid. Reduction of oxidized coenzymes commonly occurs through the addition of a hydride ion to the *para* (4) position of the nicotinamide ring, with simultaneous formation of a solvated proton. NADH and NADPH (but not NAD and NADP) absorb light in the near-ultraviolet region (339 nm). This forms the basis for many biochemical assays.

Dietary Sources

NAD (diphosphopyridine nucleotide) and NADP (also termed triphosphopyridine nucleotide) represent most of the niacin activity found in good sources, which include meat, fish, eggs, vegetables, mushrooms, nuts, and yeast.[11] Milk, canned salmon, and several leafy green vegetables contribute lesser amounts but are still sufficient to prevent deficiency. In countries where fortification of processed cereals is practiced, this may provide up to 20% of niacin intake. In addition, some plant foodstuffs, especially cereals, such as corn and wheat, contain niacin bound to various peptides and sugars in forms that nutritionally are not readily available (niacinogens or niacytin).[484]

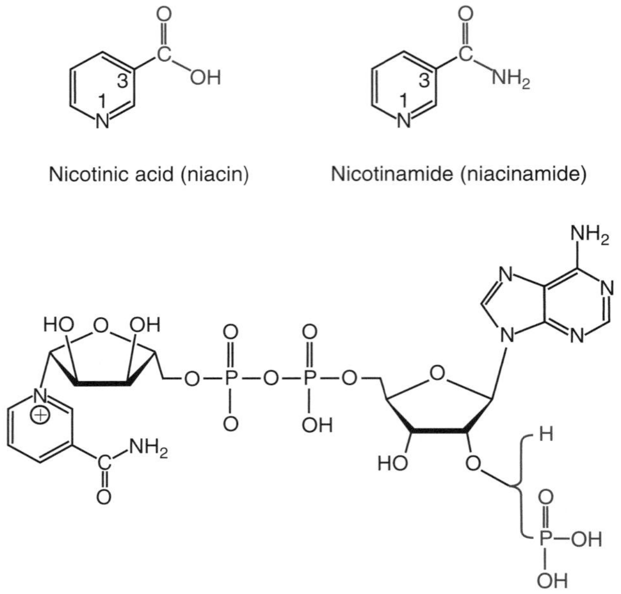

FIGURE 37.23 Niacin, Niacinamide, and Coenzyme.

Tryptophan is a precursor of niacin. Thus, proteins in diet provide a considerable proportion of the niacin requirements. As much as two-thirds of niacin required by adults can be derived from tryptophan metabolism via nicotinic acid ribonucleotide to NAD and NADP. It has been shown that 60 mg of tryptophan can provide the equivalent of 1 mg of niacin in the adult.[485]

Absorption, Transport, Metabolism, and Excretion

Dietary NAD and NADP are hydrolyzed by enzymes, such as NAD glycohydrolase, in the intestinal mucosa to release nicotinamide, which, together with any nicotinic acid, is rapidly absorbed in the stomach and the intestine by Na^+-dependent facilitated diffusion at low concentrations and passive diffusion at higher concentrations.[486] Nicotinamide is the main circulating form in the plasma postabsorption or following release from hydrolyzed liver NAD; it can be taken up by most tissues requiring NAD by simple diffusion.

Once inside blood, kidney, brain, and liver cells, both nicotinic acid and nicotinamide are converted to coenzyme forms. The first step involves the cytosolic phosphoribosyltransferase-catalyzed reaction of nicotinate or nicotinamide with 5-phosphoribosyl-1-pyrophosphate to form pyrophosphate and nicotinic acid ribonucleotide or nicotinamide ribonucleotide, respectively. An additional source of nicotinic acid ribonucleotide is the action of quinolate phosphoribosyltransferase on quinolinate formed from tryptophan.[485] The efficiency of this pathway is under nutritional and hormonal regulation, with deficiency of vitamin B_6 (riboflavin) and Fe slowing the conversion; protein, tryptophan, energy, and niacin restriction increase the efficiency.[487] Nicotinic acid ribonucleotide from whatever source is converted to deamido-NAD by an adenylyltransferase-catalyzed attachment of the AMP moiety from ATP; the deamido compound subsequently reacts with glutamine and a cytosolic ATP-dependent synthetase step to yield NAD, glutamate, and phosphate. Nicotinamide mononucleotide is directly converted by adenylyltransferase to NAD. NADP is formed by kinase-catalyzed phosphorylation of NAD. In the tissue, most of the vitamin is present as nicotinamide in NAD and NADP, although the liver may contain a significant fraction of free vitamin.[488,489] Little storage of niacin as such occurs.[486]

Excess niacin is excreted mainly as the *N*-methylnicotinamide (NMN) after methylation in the liver and as the two oxidation products of NMN, *N*-methyl-2-pyridone-5-carboxamide, and *N*-methyl-4-pyridone-carboxamide.[490,491]

Functions. Niacin is essential because the coenzymes NAD and NADP in which nicotinamide acts as an electron acceptor or a hydrogen donor function in a large number of redox reactions. Many enzymes function as dehydrogenases and catalyze such diverse reactions as the conversion of alcohols (often sugars and polyols) to aldehydes or ketones, hemiacetals to lactones, aldehydes to acids, and certain amino acids to keto acids.[489] The common mechanism of operation involves the stereospecific abstraction of a hydride ion from substrate, with *para* addition to one or the other side of carbon 4 in the pyridine ring of the nucleotide coenzyme. The second hydrogen of the substrate group oxidized is concomitantly removed as a proton and ultimately is exchanged as a hydronium ion. Most dehydrogenases using NAD or NADP function reversibly. Glutamate dehydrogenase, for example, favors the oxidative direction, whereas others, such as glutathione reductase, preferentially catalyze reduction.

In addition to redox reactions, NAD is a substrate for three classes of enzymes that cleave the β-*N*-glycosylic bond of NAD to free nicotinamide and catalyze the transfer of adenosine diphosphate (ADP)-ribose.[492] One such enzyme, poly (ADP-ribose) polymerase-1 , is involved in base excision repair and is believed to be important for genomic stability.[493]

Nicotinic acid, when used as a pharmaceutical agent, has important antiatherogenic properties. It effectively lowers triglycerides, raises high-density lipoprotein cholesterol, and shifts low-density lipoprotein particles to a less atherogenic phenotype.[494,495]

Requirements and Reference Nutrient Intakes

Requirements for niacin are expressed as niacin equivalents, which take into account the contributions of tryptophan derived from protein (1 mg of niacin = 60 mg of tryptophan).[496,497] Earlier estimates of niacin requirements were based on energy expenditure, reflecting the biological function of niacin coenzymes in the oxidation of fuel molecules. However, current recommendations merely reflect the fact that different age groups and sexes demonstrate different energy expenditures, and no directly relevant studies have linked energy intake or expenditure with niacin requirements.[11] The average US diet supplies between 0.7 and 1.1 g of tryptophan per day.[77] Based on niacin metabolite excretion data, current RDAs for men 19 years to older than 70 years are 16 mg/day of niacin equivalents, and for women of the same age, 14 mg/day is the RDA. An increase of 4 mg/day during pregnancy is recommended, and an increase of 3 mg/day for lactation will offset the preformed niacin lost in milk. Human milk contains approximately 0.17 mg of niacin and 22 mg of tryptophan per deciliter (or 70 kcal); these amounts are adequate to meet the niacin needs of the infant. Adequate intakes of 2 mg/day of preformed niacin and 4 mg/day have been extrapolated from adult requirements for infants 0 to 6 months and 7 to 12 months, respectively. RDAs are set at 6 mg/day for children 1 to 3 years, 8 mg/day for children 4 to 8 years, 12 mg/day for boys and girls 9 to 13 years, 14 mg/day for girls 14 to 18 years, and 16 mg/day for boys 14 to 18 years.[11]

Intravenous Supply

The recommended supply for adult patients receiving TPN is 40 mg/day in the form of nicotinamide.[179] This is above the oral recommendations and will ensure AI to match increased energy expenditure.

Deficiency

Pellagra is the classic deficiency disease in humans that has been most often found among those who subsist chiefly on corn (maize), which is low in both niacin and tryptophan concentrations.[444] Although its pathogenesis has been attributed to a deficiency of these two factors, other associated complicating factors include lack of pyridoxal-5-phosphate (vitamin B_6), FAD, and Fe, which are required in the conversion of tryptophan to niacin, and the presence of mycotoxins elaborated by mold infestations, mainly by *Fusarium*.[498] Niacin deficiency, and therefore, pellagra may occur in: (1) people who consume corn-based staple diets in less developed countries, although this is now rare except during war or famine[499]; (2) carcinoid syndrome, in which up to 60% of tryptophan is catabolized to 5-hydroxytryptophan and serotonin, which results in niacin deficiency[500]; (3) Hartnup disease, an autosomal recessive disorder in which several amino acids, including tryptophan, are poorly absorbed in the intestines, which results in inadequate niacin for body requirements[501]; and (4) treatment with the antituberculous drug isoniazid, which competes with pyridoxal-5-phosphate (vitamin B_6), which is required as a cofactor in the conversion of tryptophan to niacin.[502]

The typical presentation of pellagra is that of a chronic wasting disease associated with dermatitis, dementia, and diarrhea.[503] The characteristic erythematous dermatitis is bilateral and symmetric, and occurs on skin areas exposed to sunlight. Mental changes include fatigue, insomnia, and apathy, all of which precede an encephalopathy characterized by confusion, disorientation, hallucination, loss of memory, and eventually, frank organic psychoses. Diarrhea, when it occurs, reflects widespread inflammation of the intestinal mucous surfaces, including a bright red tongue; other gastrointestinal manifestations include achlorhydria, glossitis, stomatitis, and vaginitis.

Toxicity

Although no toxic effects have been associated with niacin intake from naturally occurring foods, the use of supplements and of pharmacological doses of niacin has produced adverse effects in some patients. In disorders of reduced tryptophan availability, such as Hartnup disease and carcinoid syndrome, daily niacin doses of 40 to 200 mg may be required, and in the treatment of dyslipidemias, nicotinic acid in doses up to 6 g/day may be used. Such doses are commonly associated with vascular dilation or "flushing," a burning, tingling sensation of the face (that may be reddened), arms, and chest that is believed to be mediated by prostaglandins. This may be reduced by gradual increments of the drug and by taking it with meals. Other side effects of high-dose niacin treatment are pruritus, nausea, vomiting, and diarrhea, although these symptoms often abate with continued therapy. Additional effects include abnormal glucose tolerance, hyperuricemia, peptic ulcer, hepatomegaly, jaundice, and increased serum aminotransferases. In a study of 814 patients taking a combination extended-release niacin preparation (maximum dose, 2 g), flushing caused intolerance in 10% of those studied, hepatotoxicity was seen in 0.5%, and myopathy was not reported.[504] The symptoms of flushing have been taken as an endpoint sign in the formulation of a tolerable upper intake amount for niacin. This has been set at 35 mg/day for adults 19 years and older, with lower amounts for children and adolescents.[11]

Laboratory Assessment of Status

At present, no blood markers are commonly used as indicators of niacin status. Most assessments of niacin nutriture have been based on measurement of the two urinary metabolites, *N'*-methylnicotinamide and *N'*-methyl-2-pyridone-5-carboxamide.[31] Normally, adults excrete 20% to 30% of their niacin in the form of methylnicotinamide and 40% to 60% as the pyridone. An excretion ratio of pyridone to methylnicotinamide of 1.3:4.0 is thus normal, but latent niacin deficiency is indicated by a value below 1.0. As depletion occurs, pyridone is absent for weeks before clinical signs are noted, and methylnicotinamide excretion falls to a minimum at about the time that clinical signs become evident.

HPLC-based methods are currently the methods of choice for analysis,[505] although some capillary electrophoresis methods have been developed.[506] However, measurement of 2-pyridone and *N'*-methylnicotinamide concentrations in plasma may provide a more reliable metabolite ratio than urine measurements. Another approach that may prove valuable is the ratio of erythrocyte niacin coenzymes NAD to NADP.[496,500] NAD concentrations respond to the niacin status, whereas NADP concentrations remain relatively constant under different conditions of niacin status. The niacin number is NAD/NADP × 100; a niacin number less than 130 is indicative of risk of developing niacin deficiency.

Preanalytical Variables

There are no specific preanalytical variables that affect the measurement of niacin or its metabolites.

Reference Intervals

Based on HPLC methods,[506,507] a guidance reference interval for the excretion rate of N^1-methylnicotinamide is 2.4 to 6.4 mg/day (17.5–46.7 μmol/day) or 1.6 to 4.3 mg/g creatinine (11.7–31.4 μmol/g creatinine). For more information, refer to the Appendix on Reference Intervals. Laboratories should verify that these ranges are appropriate for use in their own settings.

Pantothenic Acid

Pantothenic acid is a water-soluble vitamin required primarily as a component of CoA, which is required for the metabolism of fat, protein, and carbohydrate via the citric acid cycle.

Chemistry

Pantothenic acid, which is also known as vitamin B_5 (name derived from Greek *pantothen*, meaning from everywhere), is of ubiquitous occurrence in nature, where it is synthesized by most microorganisms and plants. It is the amide formed by the linkage between pantoic acid (D-2,4-dihydroxy-3,3-dimethylbutyric acid) derived from L-valine, and β-alanine derived from L-aspartate. Addition of cysteamine at the C-terminal end and phosphorylation at C4 of pantoic acid form 4'- phosphopantetheine, which serves as a covalently attached prosthetic group of acyl carrier proteins; when attached to ribose 3'-phosphate and adenine, CoA is formed, as shown in Fig. 37.24. Pantothenic acid is a hygroscopic, viscous oil that is easily destroyed by heat, especially at extremes of pH. The most common commercial synthetic form is the calcium salt.

Dietary Sources

Pantothenic acid is widely distributed in foods, mostly within CoA-containing compounds, and is particularly abundant in animal sources, legumes, and whole grain cereals. Excellent food sources (100–200 μg/g dry weight) include egg yolk, kidney, liver, and yeast. Fair sources (35–100 μg/g) include broccoli, lean beef, skimmed milk, sweet potatoes, and molasses.[11] More than one half of the pantothenate in wheat may

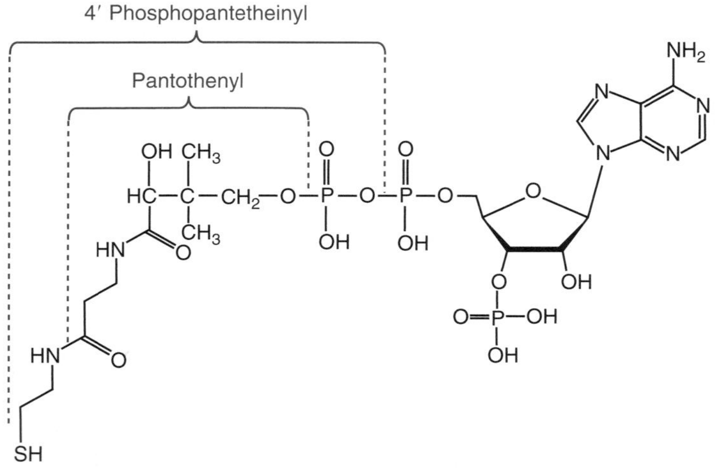

FIGURE 37.24 Pantothenate and 4′-Phosphopantetheine as Components of Coenzyme A.

be lost during manufacture of flour, and up to one-third is lost during cooking of meat.

Absorption, Transport, Metabolism, and Excretion

Pantothenic acid is taken in as dietary CoA compounds and 4′-phosphopantetheine and is hydrolyzed by pyrophosphatase and phosphatase in the intestinal lumen to dephospho-CoA, phosphopantetheine, and pantetheine, which are further hydrolyzed to pantothenic acid.[508,509] The vitamin is primarily absorbed as pantothenic acid through a saturable process at low concentrations and through simple diffusion at higher ones. The saturable process is facilitated by a Na-dependent multivitamin transporter, for which biotin and lipoate compete.[510] After absorption, pantothenic acid enters the circulation and is taken up by cells in a manner similar to its intestinal adsorption. The synthesis of CoA from pantothenate is regulated by pantothenate kinase, which itself is subject to negative feedback from the products CoA and acyl-CoA.[509] Pantothenic acid is excreted in the urine after hydrolysis of CoA compounds by enzymes that cleave phosphate and the cysteamine moieties. Only a small fraction of pantothenate is secreted into milk and even less into colostrum.

Functions

Pantothenic acid has two major metabolic roles—the first as part of CoA, and the second as the prosthetic group of the acyl-carrier protein (ACP). In the former role, CoA is primarily involved in acetyl and acyl transfer reactions in catabolic processes of carbohydrate, lipid, and protein chemistry. Examples of these are the acetylation of sugars, phospholipid, isoprenoid, and steroid biosynthesis and protein acetylation.[508] Acetyl-CoA that derives from the metabolism of carbohydrates, fats, and amino acids can acetylate compounds, such as choline and hexosamines, to produce essential biochemicals; it can also condense with other metabolites, such as oxaloacetate, to supply citrate and cholesterol. As the 4′-phosphopantetheine moiety of ACP, the phosphodiester-linked prosthetic group uses the sulfhydryl terminus to exchange with malonyl-CoA to form an ACP-S malonyl thioester, which can chain elongate during fatty acid biosynthesis.[508] Pantothenic acid used pharmaceutically may provide the benefits of lowering cholesterol, enhancing athletic performance, and relieving symptoms of rheumatoid arthritis.[508,509,511]

Requirements and Reference Nutrient Intakes

Urinary excretion of pantothenic acid in a typical American diet averages 2.6 mg/day,[512] but may vary from 2 to 7 mg/day in adults consuming 5 to 7 mg/day and is strongly dependent on intake; another 1 to 2 mg/day is lost in feces. There are no RDAs established for pantothenic acid, and the primary criterion used to estimate AI is whether intake is adequate to replace urinary excretion. It has been set at 5 mg/day for adolescents 14 to 18 years and for adults.[11] Children 1 to 3 years, 4 to 8 years, and 9 to 13 years have AIs set at 2, 3, and 4 mg/day, respectively, extrapolated from adult values, and infants up to 6 months and between 7 to 12 months have AIs reflecting intake from human milk, set at 1.7 and 1.8 mg/day, respectively. An additional 1 mg/day is suggested in pregnancy, and an additional 2 mg/day is suggested for lactating mothers.[11]

Intravenous Supply

The recommended intravenous supply for adults is 15 mg/day of dexpanthenol.[179]

Deficiency

The widespread availability of pantothenic acid in food is commensurate with its many roles and makes dietary deficiency of pantothenate unlikely in humans. Symptoms have been produced in a few volunteers who received ω-methylpantothenic acid as an antagonist[513] and in people fed semisynthetic diets virtually free of pantothenate.[514] Subjects became irascible, and developed postural hypotension and rapid heart rate on exertion, epigastric distress with anorexia and constipation, numbness and tingling of the hands and feet, hyperactive deep tendon reflexes, and weakness of finger extensor muscles. The eosinopenic response to adrenocorticotropic hormone was impaired. More severe deficiency in animals leads to adrenal cortical failure. Historically, pantothenic acid deficiency has been associated with the "burning feet syndrome," which was also reported by prisoners in the second World War in Asia and relieved only by pantothenic acid supplementation—not by other B-group vitamins that have also been linked to it.[515,516]

Toxicity

No reports have described adverse effects, with the exception of occasional mild diarrhea, with oral pantothenic acid given in doses as high as 20 g/day.[509] In the absence of evidence of toxicity, a tolerable upper intake amount has not been derived for pantothenic acid.[11]

Laboratory Assessment of Status

No convenient or reliable functional tests of pantothenic acid status are currently available; thus, assessments are made by direct measurement of whole blood or urine pantothenic acid concentrations. Urine measurements are perhaps the easiest to conduct and interpret, and concentrations are closely related to dietary intake. Whole blood measurements are preferred to plasma, which contains only free pantothenic acid and is insensitive to changes in pantothenic acid intake. Concentrations of pantothenic acid in all of the fluids already described can be measured by microbiological assay, most commonly using *Lactobacillus plantarum*.[517,518] Some assays have relied on enzymes such as pantothenase to release pantothenic acid from CoA.[519,520] Methods that have been used to measure pantothenic acid in human samples include radioimmunoassay,[521] liquid chromatography coupled to mass spectrometry,[30] gas chromatography–mass spectrometry,[522] and a stable isotope dilution assay based on liquid chromatography-mass spectrometry.[523] CoA and ACP have been measured by enzymatic methods.[509]

Preanalytical Variables

There are no specific preanalytical variables that affect the measurement of pantothenic acid.

Reference Intervals

Urinary excretion of less than 1 mg/day of pantothenic acid is considered abnormally low. Suspicion of inadequate intake is further supported if whole blood concentrations are less than 100 μg/L. A guidance reference interval for pantothenic acid in whole blood or serum is 344 to 583 μg/L

(1.57–2.66 μmol/L),[524] and for urinary excretion 1 to 15 mg/day (5–68 μmol/day).[521] For more information, refer to the Appendix on Reference Intervals. Laboratories should verify that these ranges are appropriate for use in their own settings.

POINTS TO REMEMBER

Vitamins

- Vitamin A: Antioxidant; important role in vision
- Vitamin E: Antioxidant; multiple functions, including bone metabolism
- Vitamin K: Coagulation; bone metabolism
- Vitamin B_1: Coenzyme for decarboxylation and transketolation reactions; involved in carbohydrate metabolism
- Vitamin B_2: Prosthetic group for oxidation-reduction reactions
- Vitamin B_3: Hydrogen acceptors (as NAD and NADP) in many oxidation-reduction reactions
- Vitamin B_5: CoA required for metabolism of carbohydrates, fats, and proteins
- Vitamin B_6: Coenzyme for enzymes involved in metabolism of various amino acids
- Vitamin B_7: Coenzyme for carboxylation reactions involved in gluconeogenesis and lipogenesis
- Vitamin B_9: Required for the interconversions of amino acids and the biosynthesis of purines and pyrimidines
- Vitamin B_{12}: Required for erythropoiesis, methylation processes necessary for DNA metabolism, and is a cofactor for various enzymes
- Vitamin C: Connective tissue formation; antioxidant

SPECIAL CASES FOR VITAMIN AND TRACE ELEMENT MEASUREMENT

In addition to high-risk groups with vitamin deficiencies or those with specific conditions that require measurement of specific micronutrients as part of investigations, these are some special scenarios in which vitamins and trace metals are a requisite in the management of these cases, as discussed in the following. Also see the section on Clinical Applications under Trace Elements for further details.

Cystic Fibrosis

Cystic fibrosis (CF) is a multiorgan disorder that involves lung disease and exocrine pancreatic insufficiency due to mutations in the CF transmembrane regulator on the apical membranes of epithelial cells acting as a chloride channel.[525] As a result of pancreatic insufficiency, which affects up to 90% of patients with CF,[526] malabsorption of fat-soluble vitamins is common and is associated with poor outcomes if not corrected by supplementation. The CF Foundation guidelines (United States),[527] Cystic Fibrosis Trust (United Kingdom),[528] and other national organizations all recommend (with some minor variations) the supplementation of vitamins A, D, E, and K, and Zn in infants younger than 2 years of age, together with monitoring vitamins A, D, E. If there is liver disease, prothrombin time should also be monitored 2 months after commencing supplementation, and yearly thereafter or more frequently if values are abnormal. A similar regimen in terms of vitamin supplementation and monitoring is recommended in adults.[529] The vitamin(s) dose is adjusted according to the measured plasma concentrations as necessary. A critical Cochrane review concluded that there was insufficient evidence to show whether vitamin A supplementation in patients with CF was beneficial, because to date there have been no placebo-controlled randomized controlled trials.[530] The same is likely to be true of the other fat-soluble vitamins, and until well-powered trials can provide the data, the recommendations and protocols of national CF bodies should be followed. See Box 37.5 for illustrative case.

Post-Bariatric Surgery Micronutrient Monitoring

Obesity continues to be a major public health problem globally, with some estimates suggesting that 1.1 billion adults and 10% of children are obese, as defined by a body mass index (BMI) ≥30 kg/m^2.[531] Obesity is associated with increased mortality and significant medical and psychological comorbidity, and may be considered a bona fide disease state.[532] Both nonsurgical management and bariatric surgery can result in weight loss that translates to improved health and wellbeing. There are clear indications for bariatric surgery for patients with clinically severe obesity, especially if they also have type 2 diabetes mellitus. Patients who have undergone bariatric surgery have shown improved outcomes.[533,534] Because of the potentially increased need for bariatric surgery as a treatment for obesity, clinical practice guidelines have been published regarding classification of obesity, indications for treatment modalities, pre- and post-bariatric surgery monitoring, and general patient management.[532,535] Obesity is discussed further in Chapter 56. All bariatric procedures affect nutritional intake and absorption to varying degrees. There is also increasing awareness that patients who have undergone bariatric surgery show marked micronutrient deficiencies, and there is evidence that this may be a delayed effect after surgery and could become progressively worse over time.[536-543] Thus, supplementation is inevitable, and macronutrient monitoring may be required. Guidelines delineating which vitamin and trace metal to measure and when have been published, and minor modifications may have been implemented by national and local bodies.[532]

Critical Care Patients

Critically ill patients have increased requirements for micronutrients as a result of the SIR. Patients in the intensive or critical care unit (or other hospital ward) tend to be on nutritional support, either enteral or parenteral, and as such, will receive micronutrients. In special circumstances, it may be necessary to measure the vitamin and trace element status, and to monitor changes using various protocols.[43] However, as discussed in earlier sections, the effects of SIR on micronutrients must be appreciated (see Table 37.2). Nutritional assessment is discussed in Chapter 56. Various national guidelines are available on which micronutrients to measure, including the frequency and between-testing duration.[43]

TRACE ELEMENTS

The term trace element was originally used to describe the residual amount of inorganic analyte quantitatively determined in a sample. More sensitive methods allow accurate determination of most inorganic micronutrients present at low concentrations in body fluids and tissue. However,

BOX 37.5 Case: A Typical Teenager With Cystic Fibrosis and Fat-Soluble Vitamin Deficiencies

A 16-year-old female with cystic fibrosis genotyped homozygous for the delta F508 mutation had a current forced expiratory volume in 1 second of 3.37 L (117%). This patient had obesity, liver disease, impaired glucose tolerance (glycosylated hemoglobin, 48 mmol/mol; fasting plasma glucose, 5.5 mmol/L; 2-hour post-oral glucose load, 10.5 mmol/L), pancreatic insufficiency, and nasal polyps. This patient is on multivitamins (vitamin C 15 mg; nicotinamide 7.5 mg; riboflavin 500 μg; thiamine 1 mg; vitamin A, 2500 U; vitamin E, 100 mg/day, vitamin D_3, 9600 IU/day (240 nmol/day), ursodeoxycholic acid (1200 mg/day), azithromycin (500 mg, 3 times per week), and enzyme replacement (Creon [pancrelipase] 25,000 lipase units with 3 meals and 2 snacks). Selected results for vitamins at her annual reviews are summarized in the table in the following:

Fat-Soluble Vitamin	Vitamin A	Vitamin E	Vitamin E/Cholesterol	Vitamin D
Reference interval (U)	0.9–2.5 μmol/L	13–24 μmol/L	3.5–9.5 μmol/mmol	25–170 nmol/L
2012	1.6	19	4.7	<18
2013	1.3	11	3.5	
2014	1.6	11	2.9	<8
2015	1.2	8	2.6	30

Commentary

Lung function as assessed by spirometry was good. Fat-soluble vitamins were below the reference interval at diagnosis (data not shown). Despite regular annual review and supplementation as per agreed guidelines and local protocols, this case demonstrates that these patients need careful monitoring for adherence, vitamin dose adjustment if deemed deficient, and constant motivation. This case also highlights the importance of measuring vitamins in these patients, and in the view of the author, they should be considered as therapeutic drug monitoring (TDM).

We are grateful to Miss Gillian Smith, Pediatric Dietitian, NHS Lanarkshire for highlighting this case, which is included here with written informed patient consent.

those present in body fluids (micrograms per liter) and in tissue (milligrams per kilogram) are still widely referred to as "trace elements," and those found at nanograms per liter or micrograms per kilogram levels are known as "ultratrace elements." The corresponding dietary requirements are quoted in milligrams per day or micrograms per day, respectively.

The biologic effects of deficiency disease define the essential trace elements. An element is considered essential when signs and symptoms induced by a deficient diet are uniquely reversed by an adequate supply of the particular trace element under investigation.

There are good clinical examples of reversible deficiency disease for Fe, I, Co (as cobalamins), Se, Cu, and Zn. Enough is known about the biochemical functions of these elements to explain their importance in human nutrition. For others, such as Mn, Cr, Mo, and V, although they have known biologic functions, usually as enzyme cofactors, their importance in clinical practice remains to be determined. Other elements, such as bromine (Br), fluorine (F), cadmium (Cd), lead (Pb), strontium (Sr), Li, and tin (Sn), have been claimed by at least one investigator to be essential for one or more animal species, as demonstrated by dietary deprivation studies. It should be noted that all of these elements are toxic at higher concentrations (see Chapter 42).

The clinical importance of trace elements extends beyond considerations of being essential in maintaining health and in toxicology. Pharmacological applications are associated with a number of both essential and nonessential elements. Trace elements in this category include F, which is used for protection against dental caries; Li salts, which is used to treat depression; and Sr (as the citrate or ranelate salt), which is used for the treatment of osteoporosis. Dosages required for a beneficial pharmacological effect tend to greatly exceed the amounts of these elements normally found in food.

For some trace elements, continued suboptimal dietary intake—in the presence of physiologic, nutritional, or other metabolic stress—may eventually have a detrimental effect. Additional dietary supplementation may then have a "health restorative" effect. Examples include the effects of B in the presence of vitamin D depletion[544] and the need for increased V with an experimentally induced deficient or excessive supply of dietary I.[545] The possible role of supplements in preventing cancer is discussed in the following sections on the individual elements.[546,547]

Dose–Effect Relationships

Deficiency disease may be seen with low intake of recognized essential trace elements. With an increasing dietary supply, a plateau region of optimal supply can be reached. Higher intakes result in adverse toxic effects. The concentration window separating beneficial dietary intake from toxic intake varies depending on the element in question and on the nature of the chemical species present in the diet. This is similar to the dose–effect relationship described for organic micronutrients (Fig. 37.25). Therefore, the RDAs are set at amounts that are sufficient to prevent deficiency. A tolerable upper intake value that prevents toxicity has been proposed for the inorganic micronutrients of known importance to human health.[12]

Reversal of clinical signs and symptoms by supplementation with a single trace element or with micronutrient mixtures has been used as indirect evidence of a preexisting deficiency. Growth velocities in children, regaining lean body mass, rate of wound healing, resistance to infection, and

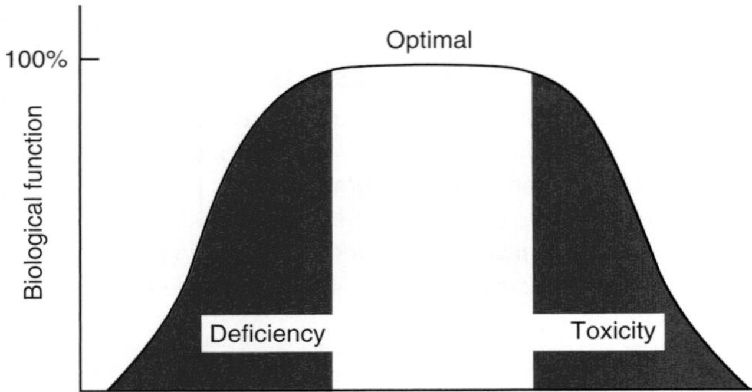

FIGURE 37.25 Model of the Relationship Between Tissue Concentration and Intake of an Essential Nutrient and Dependent Biological Function.

alterations in cognitive function can be assessed. However, many confounding factors, in particular, the presence of disease, SIR, or other nutritional deficits, can affect the interpretation of changes in these indices.

Reductions in metalloenzyme activity induced by the deficiency may be partially or wholly restored by effective treatment. Reversal of hematologic and immunologic function abnormalities, as well as hormonal changes induced by the deficiency can all be addressed by adequate supplementation and/or dietary modifications.

Chemistry and Metal Interactions

To improve understanding of essential trace elements and how they function, it is necessary to consider the ionic forms, relative solubilities, possible organo-complex formation, and resultant speciation. This approach will provide a proper basis from which to understand physiologic function and the relevant approaches to measurement.

Trace elements interact with available ligands, mainly the electron donors nitrogen, sulfur, and O_2, to form a wide variety of chemical complexes or species. Some metals such as Fe, Cu, Mo, and Cr are stable in more than one valence state and participate in biologically important oxidation–reduction reactions. The transition metals (eg, Fe, Cu, and Co) with an incompletely filled 3d orbital coordinate with a large number of groups to form stable complexes. Zn, which lies at the end of the first transition series in the periodic table, Zn^{2+}, with a complete 3d electron shell, is a particularly stable ion with unique biological functions. Reviews of the biological chemistry of the essential elements are elegantly described by Frausto da Silva and Williams.[548]

Bioavailability from foods and drinks primarily depends on solubility and the presence of other dietary components that either promote or inhibit absorption. The formation of soluble complexes with citric and other organic acids is also important.[549,550] Absorption of these organo-metallic complexes will be facilitated through organic acid transporters.[551] Fe, in the form of heme-Fe derived from meat products, is more readily absorbed than inorganic Fe.[552] However, other dietary components can inhibit absorption by reducing solubility. Mo ion can form insoluble Cu-molybdate (MoO_4^{2-}) complexes in the intestine, limiting absorption. Phytate and fiber form insoluble complexes with Zn with well-described deficiency as a consequence.[553] Interelement interactions are less well recognized, but it is known that increasing dietary Zn reduces Fe uptake and vice versa.[554] However, the species of the element and presumably its solubility are also important, because different salts of Zn have different effects. An excessive intake of Zn induces synthesis of intestinal metallothionein (MT) that traps the metal in the cell, which is eventually shed into the lumen. Because MT also strongly binds Cu, this is also lost, and the body load can become severely depleted.

Synergistic interactions occur in other tissues and can have important biological and clinical consequences. For example, the interaction between Se and I has been investigated. The deiodinase enzymes that remove I from thyroxine (T_4) to produce the biologically active triiodothyronine (T_3) are selenoproteins. Also, the selenoprotein GSHP is active in the thyroid gland to decrease excess H_2O_2 formation. Therefore, Se is important in thyroid hormone metabolism. In certain areas of the world, combined Se and I deficiency occurs, and provision of Se may be necessary to correct hypothyroidism, but this may also precipitate its onset.[555]

Se deficiency in experimental animal studies is exacerbated by vitamin E depletion. The antioxidant properties of tocopherol and GSHP are similar, and can, to some extent, overlap, although this is highly species dependent.[556]

Zn and vitamin A are interrelated, and it appears that Zn depletion limits the bioavailability of vitamin A. With insufficient Zn, RBP synthesis is reduced, leading to reduced vitamin A transport and intake.[557] Controlled studies found that combined Zn and vitamin A supplementation is more effective clinically than vitamin A alone or Zn alone in controlling diarrhea and minimizing respiratory infection.[558] Further discussion of the concepts raised here is included in the sections on individual elements in the following.

Biochemistry and Homeostasis

Most aspects of intermediary metabolism require essential trace elements in the form of metalloenzymes that have a number of catalytic properties. Specific metalloproteins are required for the transport and safe storage of reactive metal ions such as Fe^{3+} or Cu^{2+}. Examples include MT (Cu, Zn), transferrin, ferritin, and hemosiderin (Fe), and ceruloplasmin (Cu).

Because dietary intakes vary, homeostatic controls are required to regulate the supply of essential trace elements to cells. These involve regulation of intestinal absorption, specific transport systems in peripheral blood, uptake and storage mechanisms in tissue, and control of excretion. The principal excretory route for some important trace metals is in feces, both by regulation of initial absorption and by re-secretion into the intestinal tract in bile and other intestinal fluids.[559]

For other elements, urinary excretion is the primary route for elimination. Loss of trace elements by other routes, such as in hair and/or nails, by skin cell desquamation, and in sweat, is generally minor; published studies have reported such measured losses.[560] However, menstrual Fe loss or seminal fluid Zn loss can be important.

In addition to poor dietary intake, overt deficiency may result from intestinal malabsorption and increased excretory losses may be a result of disease, injury, and infection. Liver disease, inflammatory bowel disease, and renal disease will affect trace element absorption and excretion to a variable extent and may cause an acquired deficiency disease.

Catabolic responses to injury, infection, and malignant disease can result in increased essential trace element losses in feces and in urine. Severe burn injuries cause extensive loss in exudates through the damaged skin.[561]

Postsurgical patients, especially those with short bowel syndrome, require prolonged periods of nasogastric tube feeding or intravenous feeding, and if treated with nutrient regimens lacking sufficient inorganic micronutrients, they will develop symptomatic deficiency disease. Clinical cases of trace element deficiency have been described for Cu, Zn, Se, and Cr.[562]

Inborn Errors

Although genetic defects in the metabolism of trace elements are rare, they are nonetheless important because of the information they provide for homeostatic control mechanisms. This information has led to the development of effective therapeutic strategies. The most commonly investigated disorders are those that affect Fe (hemochromatosis), Cu (Wilson disease and Menkes syndrome), Zn (acrodermatitis enteropathica), and Mo (Mo cofactor disease). These are reviewed in relevant sections of this chapter.

Clinical Applications

Nutritional Support

The importance of trace elements to normal health and well-being is discussed in the chapter on Nutrition (see Chapter 56). RDAs for healthy individuals should be obtained from a balanced diet and are discussed in the subsequent sections that describe individual elements. Other considerations regarding trace element status that may be clinically relevant include increased exposure, feeding difficulties (enteral and parenteral nutrition or reduced absorption, eg, short bowel, celiac disease, and so on), genetic disorders, post-bariatric surgery, and prophylactic supplementation.

Increased exposure, with a risk of toxicity, can occur where there is contamination of food, drinking water, or other beverages. Tragic situations involving elements such as arsenic and mercury have been described, but essential elements are also harmful when exposure is excessive; for example, poisoning with Se and Zn can occur. A more unusual source of Zn is dental fixatives. Individuals with poorly fitting dentures are liable to use more than the recommended amount of fixative and can ingest large amounts of Zn as a consequence. The response is increased synthesis of MT that binds Zn and Cu in the enteral cells. With continued liberal use of the fixative, these individuals become Cu deficient and can develop anemia and myeloneuropathy.[563]

Trace element support to patients who receive enhanced enteral or parenteral nutrition is common practice. Monitoring patients is considered necessary to ensure that sufficient essential elements are being absorbed but also to avoid excess accumulation[564] or undue exposure to contaminants such as aluminium.[565] Protocols for monitoring are suggested by competent authorities (eg, American Society for Parenteral and Enteral Nutrition, European Society of Pediatric Gastroenterology, Hepatology and Nutrition; see Chapter 56 for details). Individuals with real or potentially impaired gastrointestinal absorption may be similarly monitored depending on the severity of the underlying clinical condition.

Various diseases with a genetic component are relevant to the clinical chemistry of trace elements. Acrodermatitis enteropathica, with impaired absorption of Zn, is successfully treated by oral supplementation using soluble Zn. However, the condition that features an inability to absorb and use Cu, Menkes disease, fails to respond to replacement, and is invariably fatal. Wilson disease, in which Cu is absorbed but not incorporated into ceruloplasmin, is a Cu toxicity disorder. Depending on the actual gene affected, the symptoms displayed by patients vary from almost none to acute liver failure in childhood. Therefore, biochemical diagnosis can be complicated and involve measuring Cu concentrations in serum, urine, and liver biopsy, ceruloplasmin in serum, excretion of Cu after a chelation challenge, and in difficult cases, ^{65}Cu absorption.[566] Treatment involves the use of chelating agents to remove Cu from tissues and/or large oral doses of Zn to block absorption in the gut.[26] Therefore, measurements of Cu and Zn concentrations in serum and urine are appropriate from time to time to assess whether chelation is causing Zn deficiency or whether oral supplementation is excessive. Treatment of phenylketonuria and other disorders of amino acid metabolism may require highly refined or restricted diets, with a potential for insufficient trace elements. Regular assessment of Se status, in particular, is commonly practiced throughout childhood.

Bariatric surgery has developed into a well-used approach to treat morbid obesity, and the number of patients who have received such treatment is steadily increasing.[567] From a metaanalysis of publications between 1980 and 2013,[536] it was concluded that serum Zn and Cu concentrations decrease after surgery. Experience from laboratories and from other workers[568] indicate that Se concentrations are also reduced but usually return to normal without active intervention. As with parenteral nutrition, guidelines on monitoring have been produced by a number of organizations, such as British Obesity and Metabolic Surgery Society.[569]

Recommendations for increasing the intake of trace elements without evidence of deficiencies impinge on the realm of fringe medicine. Elite athletes routinely include micronutrient supplements with their diets, although there is little evidence that this does anything other than replace whatever is lost during training and competition. Products containing Cr are widely advertised as promoting muscle performance, but carefully planned trials were unable to show any benefit.[570,571] A thorough review of studies of trace elements and other minerals concluded that although deficiency may impair performance, supplementation with Ca, Mg, Fe, Zn, Cu, and Se does not enhance performance in well-nourished athletes, and that although Cr, B, and V have been studied as potential anabolics by potentiating the effects of insulin or testosterone, there are no beneficial effects on body composition or muscular strength and endurance.[572,573]

As suggested earlier, there is no rationale for increasing the intake of trace elements when there is no evidence of deficiency. One group who may benefit from supplements is older adults in whom Zn intake, absorption, and serum concentrations are lower than other groups. Immune and neurological functions in older adults are reported to positively respond to oral Zn supplementation.[574-576] Some work has suggested that increased daily intake of Se reduced the incidence of some cancers[577,578]; however, other studies have failed to confirm these initial observations, and a Cochrane review of 55 prospective observational studies pointed to the limitations of the work and concluded that there was no convincing evidence that Se supplementation reduces the incidence of cancer in humans.[579]

Does regular consumption of essential trace elements help to maintain good health or prevent disease? There is a common claim that Zn supplements will help avoid catching the common cold. After looking at a Cochrane review of 14 therapeutic trials and 2 trials of prophylactic use in1781 patients across 5 countries, it was concluded that Zn decreased the mean duration of symptoms when administered within 24 hours of symptom onset in both a lozenge and syrup form, from 7.5 to 6.75 days and from 5.9 to 5.1 days, respectively.[580] The likely mechanism(s) of action remains unclear, but influences on the immune response occur with inhibition of rhinovirus replication.[581]

Prostheses and Implants

Metallic components of orthopedic devices and other implants represent a source of internal exposure because surface reactions such as corrosion and wear cause release into surrounding tissue and into circulation. A recent concern is metal-on-metal hip prostheses. A proportion of patients have experienced failure of the device and present with pain and poor functionality. When the hip is opened at surgical revision, tissue is discolored and inflamed, and structures sometimes called "pseudo-tumors" are evident. Some investigations of possible implications of these devices were performed during the 1970s with measurements of Cr and Co concentrations in blood and urine.[582] The incidence of failure increased considerably during the mid-2000s after the introduction of newer designs of prostheses, which together with the superior detection limits of inductively coupled plasma mass spectrometry, stimulated further work. In addition to Cr and Co, other elements, such as titanium, nickel, Mo, and Zn have been measured in blood, urine, and tissue specimens.[583-586]

Investigations have been directed toward two primary questions: (1) is the release of metal associated with functional failure of the implant; and (2) is there any toxicity associated with the release of these metals?

Concentrations of Cr and Co in blood and other fluids are considerably increased when there is undue wear from metal-on-metal joints. Authorities in Australia, the United States, the United Kingdom, and Europe have recommended that these measurements be used to guide surgeons as to the intensity of postsurgical follow-up.[587-589] Interpretation of results depends on whether there has been a total hip replacement or a resurfacing; in the former, titanium concentrations are also useful.

It is uncertain as to whether the metals released from joints present a toxic threat to the patient. Both Cr and Co have been defined as carcinogens, and Co is responsible for a number of systemic symptoms, including impaired hearing and visual disturbances.[590]

Pharmacological Uses

From the early days of pharmacology, practitioners sourced their remedies from mineral salts and metal ores alongside those from plants and their extracts. A formulation consisting of gold dissolved in *aqua regia*, neutralized by the addition of chalk, was recommended by Roger Bacon in the thirteenth century, as a cure for leprosy,[591] while drinking or bathing in mineral waters at spa resorts has long been held to relieve rheumatism, gout, diabetes, dermatitis, and many other diseases. Such preparations and beliefs are still in use and held. Ethnic and patent medicines containing heavy metals are sold among many cultures claiming to cure various ailments.[592]

Metal-containing drugs have an impressive pedigree within more conventional pharmacology. Li is effective for the treatment of depressive illness and is widely used throughout the world.[593] Gold compounds have been used for several decades. A proportion of patients with rheumatoid arthritis respond well to chrysotherapy, although with untoward complications in a proportion of subjects and development of newer drugs, it is now prescribed infrequently.[594] Co salts were found to induce an impressive hemopoietic response in patients with refractory anemia,[595] but with the advent of erythropoietin, this approach is no longer practiced. It is in the treatment of neoplastic disease that metallo-drugs are now of greatest interest. Platinum compounds are administered to patients with a wide range of tumors with improved survival rates for testicular, bladder, ovarian, and colorectal cancer.[596] Developments of other metal-containing anticancer agents (eg, ruthenium) have been reported.[597] Clinical chemists may be called upon to advise on or measure trace element concentrations when there is a therapeutic range in blood or where there are issues of possible toxicity.

As with other agents, metals or metal salts have also been used for more disreputable purposes such as murder, suicide, and procurement of abortion. Such events may then require determination of trace element concentrations in body fluids, tissues, and other materials as part of forensic investigations.

Investigating mechanisms of action and monitoring therapeutic response in relation to concentration of a drug (or a metabolite) require accurate and specific measurements.[598] In addition to simple measurement of concentrations in body fluids and tissues, studies using stable isotopes are especially valuable. Stable isotopes serve as tracers that can be administered with safety and followed to investigate aspects of the physiology of elements.[599] Pb isotope ratios have the potential to identify sources of exposure in poisoning episodes.[600]

Laboratory Assessment of Trace Element Status

As understanding of underlying biochemical intracellular mechanisms increases for a particular trace element, the determination of active species becomes of increased importance.[601] Furthermore, the ability to study metal complexes to explore the properties of a potential "active species" and uncover the details associated with their specific composition and geometry are likely to be important to understanding their action.[602]

For I, assays of the thyroid hormones and of their control and feedback systems have largely replaced direct determination of the element. Cobalamin (vitamin B_{12}) is measured in body fluids by immunoassay rather than by a nonspecific Co determination. This practice is gradually being extended to other trace elements, in which metalloenzymes and protein species are proposed as additional indices of Fe, Zn, Cu, and Se status.

Biological parameters have been thoroughly described for assessing Fe status, but biomarkers for Zn and Cu are not routinely used.[603] Nonetheless, some new markers are being identified (eg, Zn-induced MT monocyte mRNA relates to low Zn intake).[604]

For several of the ultratrace elements (Cr, Mo, and V), insufficient information is currently available as to the critical molecular species underlying their biological actions.[605] Direct methods of determining total trace element concentrations in biological samples are therefore required. This can pose severe analytical difficulties and requires specialist laboratory facilities, with use of appropriate techniques to reduce sample contamination.

Assessment of trace element status also includes the various procedures to determine dietary intakes such as duplicate diets, food diaries, and balance studies.[606] The latter approach is facilitated by the availability of stable isotopes that may be used as tracers.[607] Recommended dietary intakes given in the following sections refer to those given in Chapter 56.

Many reference intervals for concentrations of trace elements in biological fluids have been published.[608,609] Those given in the following sections are taken from the tables in the Appendix to this book or from recent well-conducted studies. It should be noted that intervals can be influenced by factors such as age and diet. The reference intervals presented here are for guidance.

General Considerations in the Analyses of Trace Elements

Analytical factors to be considered in the measurement of trace elements include specimen requirements, preanalytical factors, collection equipment, and analytical methods.

Specimen Requirements

Trace element concentrations are usually determined in whole blood, blood plasma or serum, and urine, but many other specimen types, including leukocytes, saliva, cerebrospinal fluid, breast milk, and sweat may be analyzed. Tissue samples may be obtained by needle biopsy (liver, bone) or after an autopsy. Analysis of hair and nail samples offers a noninvasive means of sampling tissue and is used to assess toxic metal exposure. Measurements of hair and nails for essential elements may be of value on a group basis during studies of severely depleted populations, but these are of limited value in the investigation of individual subjects. Problems of external contamination from environmental pollution, cosmetics, shampoos, and other sources are difficult to control.[610]

Concentrations of the relevant carrier proteins transferrin (Fe), albumin (Zn), ceruloplasmin (Cu), and selenoprotein P (Se) provide useful additional information.

Measuring essential trace elements in leukocytes or platelets affords a direct measure of intracellular trace element concentrations. However, separation of different types of white cells and platelets in whole blood requires large sample volumes and is subject to serious problems of contamination before trace element analysis.[611] Moreover, studies show considerable inconsistency and fail to usefully discriminate between healthy and patient groups.[612,613]

Preanalytical Factors

Numerous variables can affect trace element concentrations, and these require careful control.[614] Guidelines outlining sample collection procedures and limitations are available for essential and toxic trace elements.[615,616] Age, sex, ethnic origin, time of sampling in relation to food intake, time of day and year, history of medication, tobacco use, and other factors should be recorded and are especially important when reference intervals are to be established from healthy control populations.[614,616]

When investigating patients, the SIR must be considered.[34] The acute-phase reaction causes increased permeability of capillaries and transfer of certain plasma carrier proteins and their trace metals into the interstitial space (Se and Zn). Hepatic synthesis of some plasma proteins, the so-called acute-phase proteins, is also induced, so that these proteins increase in concentration in plasma, together with any metals that they carry (Cu). In addition, marked changes in kinetics occur with altered rates of transfer to and from the tissue. Knowledge of the effect of disease on metal kinetics and distribution is therefore essential.

Collection

The choice of specimen container is important to avoid contamination. Trace metal-free tubes are commercially available and are essential for elements such as aluminum, Cr, Mn, and Zn. For blood plasma collection, Li heparin as an anticoagulant is suitable for most analyses. For blood serum, containers with gel clotting agents must be avoided for most elements. When there is any concern over contamination, special arrangements may have to be made to collect blood via plastic cannulas or silanized steel needles with the sample then placed into containers that are free from contamination. To avoid contamination from the needle during venous sampling, it is recommended that samples for trace elements are drawn last (assuming a minimum sample collection of three), because this will provide washout of the needle.

Zn, Mg, and Mn are at much greater concentration in red cells than in plasma, and therefore, separation of plasma or serum from the cells should be completed within approximately 6 hours. Blank tubes should always be checked before any collection system is used. If samples are to be referred to a specialist laboratory for analysis, it is useful to include a blank tube together with the specimen(s).

A plain plastic container with no added preservative is suitable for random urine or tissue biopsy specimens. For 24-hour urine collections, polyethylene bottles with no chemical additives are used. On receipt in the laboratory, the sample volume should be measured, and aliquots should be stored at 4°C or −15°C until analysis.[617] It is important that urine should not be collected into disposable fiber or stainless steel containers.

For additional details and advice, local specialist laboratories should be consulted (see Box 37.6 for addresses of some organizations that may provide further information and direction). For additional discussion on sample collection and preanalytical variation, refer to Chapters 4 and 5.

Analytical Methods for Measuring Trace Elements

An analytical method used for determination of trace and ultratrace elements in biological specimens must be sensitive, specific, precise, accurate, and relatively fast. The detection limits of such methods are important because concentrations of trace or ultratrace elements in some samples are in the nanograms per gram to micrograms per gram range. Ideally, the detection limit of the method should be at least 10 times

BOX 37.6 Organizations Providing Proficiency Testing and Quality Assurance Programs for Vitamin or Trace Element Testing Laboratories*

Vitamins

The College of American Pathologists
325 Waukegan Road
Northfield, IL 60093-2750
USA
Contact: Survey Coordinator
www.cap.org
Phone: (800) 323-4040

Societe Francaise de Biologie Clinique (SFBC)
Secretariat Technique
4, avenue de l'observatoire
75006 Paris
France
www.sfbc.asso.fr
Phone: (33) 156 81 85 68

SKML–Dutch Foundation for Quality Assessment in Clinical Chemistry
SKML CFB
Mercator 1
Toernooiveld 214
NL-6525
EC Nijmegen
The Netherlands
www.skml.nl
Phone: (31) 24 361 66 37

INSTAND e.V. - Gesellschaft zur Förderung der Qualitätssicherung in medizinischen Laboratorien e.V. (vormals Hämometerprüfstelle) D-40223
Düsseldorf - Ubierstr. 20 - Postfach 250211
Germany
www.instand-ev.de
Phone: (49) 211 159213 0

United Kingdom National External Quality Assurance Scheme (UK NEQAS)
UK NEQAS Office
UK NEQAS Birmingham Quality
Queen Elizabeth Medical Centre
PO Box 3909
Birmingham
B15 2UE
www.ukneqas.org.uk

Trace Elements

Laboratoire de Toxicologie Humaine
Institute National de Sante Publique du Quebec
945, Ave Wolfe, Sainte-Foy Quebec G1V 5B3
Canada
www.inspq.qc.ca
Phone: (418) 650-5115

UKNEQAS for Trace Elements
SAS Trace Element Centre
15 Frederick Sanger Road, Guildford
Surrey, UK
GU2 7YD
www.surreyeqas.org.uk/trace-elements-teqas
Phone: (44) 1483 689022

New York State Department of Health
Wadsworth Centre
PO Box 509
Albany, NY 12201-0509
USA
www.wadsworth.org/clep
Phone: (518) 485-5378

*Addresses correct as of September 2016. This list is not exhaustive.

lower than the concentrations in the specimens, thus ensuring sufficient accuracy and precision.

Analytical techniques used for clinical trace metal analysis include spectrophotometry, atomic absorption spectrophotometry, inductively coupled plasma optical emission (ICP-OES), and inductively coupled plasma mass spectrometry (ICP-MS). Other techniques, such as neutron activation analysis (NAA) and x-ray fluorescence spectrometry, and electrochemical methods such as anodic stripping voltammetry, are used less commonly. NAA requires a nuclear irradiation facility and is not readily available, and anodic stripping voltammetry requires time-consuming complete mineralization of samples for analysis.

Because these techniques are described in other chapters (Chapters 13, 17, and 42), only features that are particularly relevant to the analysis of clinical samples are mentioned here.

Spectrophotometry

Spectrophotometric methods are based on a color-forming reagent. They are rarely specific for a particular metal, are subject to sample matrix interferences, and are sensitive enough for only the more abundant trace elements, such as Fe, Zn, and Cu. Methods for Zn and Cu have been described,[618,619] and reagent kits are available commercially.

Atomic Absorption Spectrometry

Flame atomic absorption spectrophotometry (AAS) is widely used to determine concentrations of Zn and Cu in serum. Electrothermal (graphite furnace) AAS affords the sensitivity to measure other elements of clinical interest. Applications of AAS to clinical pathology have been reviewed.[620]

Inductively Coupled Plasma Mass Spectrometry

Inductively coupled plasma mass spectrometry has become the method of choice for analysis of clinical specimens, providing ease of use, low detection limits, and high throughput.[621,622]

Because ICP-MS can be used to determine stable isotopes, it is applicable for stable isotope tracer experiments and isotope dilution analysis. An interesting example was the measurement of isotopes used to analyze samples from the

Franklin expedition to the Arctic. The pattern of Pb isotopes found was inconsistent with the theory that the explorers experienced Pb poisoning from their canned food.[623] The principles of mass spectrometry are discussed in Chapter 17. Clinical applications of ICP-MS have been described and reviewed.[624]

Other Techniques

Other techniques applied to trace element analysis are largely exploited for research investigations. The relationship among metals, their cellular disposition, chemical properties, interactions with cellular components, and mechanisms of action are now described under the heading of metallomics.

Using either laser ablation ICP-MS or x-ray fluorescence spectrometry, two- or even three-dimensional images of how trace elements are distributed within biological materials can be produced with low micrometer spatial resolution. Speciation refers to techniques to determine the molecular species of an element within a tissue or fluid. Approaches such as HPLC, coupled with ICP-MS, are frequently adopted. A typical application involves locating metalloproteins, separated by electrophoresis or similar methods, followed by extraction from the gel for further analysis. Results from these studies provide insight as to the metabolism of an element and how different species might interact with other molecules. For example, the extent of platinum binding to DNA can be shown to influence the outcome of cancer therapy. Therefore, these approaches allow investigations of the disposition of metals and metalloproteins in various diseases and how these relate to underlying cellular processes.[625-628]

Quality Assurance Considerations

As with all clinical laboratory measurements, quality assurance procedures are essential for trace element analysis. Unlike many other areas of laboratory medicine, a number of certified reference materials that contain trace elements are available for biological fluids and tissues.

It is recommended that laboratories measuring trace elements should participate in one or more proficiency testing or external quality assessment schemes. Organizations that provide such schemes are listed in Box 37.6. For additional discussion on quality control, please refer to Chapter 6.

Trace Elements

Trace elements discussed in this chapter include Cr, Co, Cu, I, Mn, Mo, Se, and Zn. F, B, Si, and V are also briefly discussed. Fe is discussed in Chapter 38.

Chromium

Chromium occurs naturally in various materials. It has many industrial uses and is discharged into the environment as industrial waste. The function and biochemistry of Cr have been reviewed.[629,630]

Chemistry. Chromium (atomic number 24, atomic weight 51.99) is a transition metal that occurs in biology with valence 3^+ or 6^+, which each have markedly different properties. Trivalent Cr^{3+} is a d^3 cation that usually forms octahedral complexes with slow ligand exchange. It is considered an essential trace element that enhances the action of insulin.[631] The element has no redox or acid-base properties, but in the hexavalent (Cr^{6+}) form it is a strong oxidant that can cause tissue damage,[632,633] although toxic Cr^{6+} is normally rapidly reduced to Cr^{3+} during contact with foodstuffs and gastric contents.

There is a biologically active form of Cr^{3+} found in brewer's yeast, known as the glucose tolerance factor.[634,635] The structure of the Cr^{3+} bioactive molecule is believed to be an octahedral Cr complex, with two molecules of nicotinic acid having four coordination sites linked to glutamic acid, glycine, and cysteine; however, attempts to isolate and purify the substance have not been successful. It is not clear whether glucose tolerance factor in brewer's yeast is better used than inorganic Cr in relation to insulin activation.

Dietary Sources. Estimates of the amount of Cr in foodstuffs vary, in part because of analytical difficulties, but also because of contamination caused by contact with stainless steel during food processing, storage, and cooking. Processed meats, whole grain products, green beans, broccoli, and some spices are relatively good sources, but fruit and dairy products are not. Foodstuffs with high amounts of sucrose or fructose are intrinsically low in Cr; furthermore, these sugars may promote urine loss. The estimated dietary intake for adults in the United States varies from 20 to 30 μg/day. Supplements containing Cr are taken by approximately 8% of adults in the United States; the NHANES III survey estimated that this adds another 23 μg Cr/day.[636,637]

Absorption, Transport, Metabolism, and Excretion. Intestinal absorption of Cr^{3+} is low, ranging from 0.4% to 2.5%, so fecal output mainly consists of unabsorbed dietary Cr. In a 2001 study, 1.7% of a Cr^{3+} dose was absorbed as the chloride, whereas Cr^{6+} (chromate) fractional absorption was from 3.9% to 12.0%. This variation was probably related to lack of conversion of Cr^{6+} to the Cr^{3+} form, and the rapid appearance of both Cr^{3+} and Cr^{6+} in the blood suggests that both must be absorbed from the stomach and from the intestine.[630,638-640]

Absorption is increased marginally by ascorbic acid, amino acids, oxalate, and other dietary factors. After absorption, Cr binds to plasma transferrin with an affinity similar to that of Fe.[639] It then concentrates in human liver, spleen, other soft tissue, and bone.[641] Urine Cr output is approximately 0.1 to 2.0 μg/day (1.9–38.4 nmol/day); the amount excreted to some extent is dependent on intake. Paradoxically, urine output appears to be relatively increased at low dietary amounts. Thus, 2% is lost in urine at an intake of 10 μg/day (190 nmol/day), but only 0.5% at an intake of 40 μg/day (770 nmol/day).[642] Running and resistive exercises increase urine Cr excretion.[643,644]

Functions. Severely Cr-deficient rats showed impaired growth, reduced life span, corneal lesions, and alterations in carbohydrates, lipids, and protein metabolism. Supplementation with inorganic Cr restored glucose tolerance in these animals. Repetition of laboratory studies on experimental animals by other groups yielded inconsistent results. Claims of benefit from Cr supplementation in diabetic patients, in older adults, and in malnourished children were published but were not confirmed by others. It was later realized that Cr concentrations measured by earlier methods were orders of magnitude too high because of contamination of samples before analysis. Also ineffective background optical correction was used in the graphite furnace AAS systems that were available.[645] However, many of the important biological observations made in those early investigations have since been confirmed using more accurate analytical techniques.[646]

The biochemical mechanism that allows Cr to potentiate the actions of insulin receptors on cell membranes has been intensively investigated.[647] It is now suggested that a low MW intracellular octapeptide (LMWCr), also known as chromodulin, binds Cr^{3+} and enhances the response of insulin receptors. Chromodulin binds four Cr^{3+} ions and then locates on cell membranes near the site of insulin receptors. The structure of chromodulin has been examined by a variety of advanced spectroscopic techniques, and the complex has been shown to possess a unique type of multinuclear assembly, with Cr centers having an octahedral coordination with O_2-based ligands.[648]

Chromodulin, which was first described in the 1980s, has been isolated from liver, kidney, and other tissues in several species of experimental animals. Its proposed mode of action consists of the following: (1) inactive insulin receptors on cell membranes are converted to an active form by binding circulating insulin; (2) this binding stimulates movement into cells of Cr bound to plasma transferrin; (3) Cr then binds to apoLMWCr, converting it to an active form that then binds to the insulin receptors and potentiates kinase activity; and (4) as plasma glucose and insulin fall to normoglycemic concentrations, the LMWCr factor is released from the cell to terminate its effects.[629] It is believed that released chromodulin is the naturally occurring form of Cr in urine.[649]

Requirements and Reference Nutrient Intakes. Because evidence has been insufficient to set an estimated average requirement, an AI based on estimated intakes has been set at 35 μg/day for adult men and 25 μg/day for adult women with lower levels for children and higher levels in pregnancy and during lactation.[12] No tolerable upper limit has been set for dietary Cr^{3+} intake.[12]

Intravenous Supply. It is now advised that patients on short-term TPN (<1 to 3 months) should receive Cr at doses of 10 to 15 μg/day. Those on long-term TPN who are clinically and biochemically stable may be receiving enough Cr via contamination of their nutrients.[650]

Commercial multielement intravenous additives usually contain approximately 10 to 30 μg of Cr. When high concentrations of glucose (20%–50%) are given intravenously as the main energy source, increased loss of Cr in urine may occur. Urinary losses could be monitored (although this is rarely done) and input increased, especially if signs of unexplained glucose intolerance are seen. However, reports have indicated that excessive amounts of Cr may have been given to children and adults during TPN, with possible detrimental effects on renal function.[651,652]

Deficiency. Clinical signs of human Cr deficiency were clearly described first in patients who received parenteral nutrition for a prolonged period using a nutritional regimen that did not supply sufficient Cr.[650] Only a few case histories have been published.[653] All patients had similar presentations, with previously stable patients developing insulin-resistant glucose intolerance, weight loss, and in some cases, neurologic deficits. Addition of substantial amounts of Cr^{3+} to the intravenous regimen (150–200 μg/day) reversed glucose intolerance and reduced insulin requirements with eventual improvement in neurologic symptoms.[21,654-658]

These cases, although rare, influenced the US Food and Nutrition Board to designate Cr as an essential trace element.[12] It is not clear why so few cases of clinical Cr deficiency have been reported in comparison with Zn, Cu, and Se, but this fact might be related to Cr contamination of infusion fluids, especially in the amino acid mixture.[659]

Clinical Significance. Chromium is believed to play a role in impaired glucose tolerance, diabetes, and cardiovascular disease.[21,654-658]

Impaired Glucose Tolerance and Diabetes. More than 15% of adults aged 40 to 74 years are believed to have impaired glucose tolerance; it has been suggested that poor Cr nutritional status may be a factor.[21,654-658] Tissue Cr concentrations of patients with diabetes tend to be lower than in control subjects.[660] However, the variability of dietary Cr intake and the lack of an easily usable laboratory or clinical marker to identify those patients with poor Cr status create difficulties. A controlled trial of higher doses (250 and 1000 μg of Cr) given as Cr-picolinate was conducted in China on 180 subjects with type 2 diabetes.[21] This trial reported improvements in glucose handling and reduction in glycosylated Hb. Benefit was also found in previous studies on populations of malnourished children in Jordan, Nigeria, and Turkey. It is possible that other interacting dietary depletions may aggravate Cr deficiency in these populations.[646]

It has been suggested that a short-term dosage of less than 1000 μg/day may be a useful additional treatment for type 2 diabetes. Not all patients respond to Cr supplements—clinical response correlates with baseline insulin sensitivity, fasting glucose, and glycated Hb[661]—but in such patients, insulin resistance is improved.[660] Monitoring of kidney function and clinical assessment of dermatologic changes have been advised.[662] One group maintains that Cr supplementation has been shown to improve glucose handling in all the main types of diabetes,[663] but this is not a widely held view.[664] Cr therapy in the control and prevention of diabetes remains of considerable interest and is the subject of much controversy. However, recommendations of the American Diabetes Association state that "at the present, benefit from Cr supplementation in persons with diabetes has not been conclusively demonstrated."[665]

Glucose Intolerance in Older Adults. Glucose intolerance is age-related, and Cr supplementation trials in older adults have been conducted with variable results.[658,666] An inability to determine which of the older adult subjects were initially Cr-depleted makes it difficult to interpret the findings. If the observations can be confirmed, and if an age-related decrease is seen in Cr concentrations in hair, sweat, and blood serum, additional studies on older adults are needed.[667] In a study of free-living older adult French subjects with good dietary habits and who consumed well-balanced diets, daily Cr intakes were dramatically lower than the French recommendations, mainly due to the low Cr density of foods.[668] A negative correlation between Cr intakes and insulin, body mass index, and leptin was observed, suggesting implications in poor glucose control.

Cardiovascular Disease. Chromium depletion has long been believed to be associated with increased cardiovascular risk.[660,669,670] A double-blind, 12-week study of 23 healthy adult men showed that 200 μg of Cr (as chromium chloride [$CrCl_3$]) increased high-density lipoprotein cholesterol and decreased insulin concentrations.[671] Other reports of favorable lipid responses to Cr supplementation have also been published.[672] Abnormal lipid profiles have been found in patients with type 2 diabetes and may be associated with increased risk of cardiovascular disease. However, additional larger-scale studies are necessary to confirm the effects of Cr on risk factors for cardiovascular disease.

Studies in animal models showed that intramuscular injection of Cr reduced the size of lipid deposits in the coronary vasculature of hypercholesterolemic rabbits.[673] Lipid deposits in the ascending aorta were similarly reduced, as were serum cholesterol concentrations. In another study with rabbits, $CrCl_3$ resulted in a significant decrease in coronary and aortic lipid deposits, as well as serum cholesterol concentrations, whereas the kidney function tests and histopathology remained normal.[674] These findings suggest that high Cr may be beneficial as a treatment option for removal of atherosclerotic lesions in human patients, a hypothesis that has not been tested yet.

Toxicity. Hexavalent Cr (Cr^{6+}) is a recognized carcinogen, and industrial exposure to fumes and dusts containing this metal is associated with increased incidence of lung cancer,[632] dermatitis,[675] skin ulcers, and hypersensitivity reactions.[676] Environmental health risks arise from soil contamination by Cr^{6+} waste disposal sites left by the leather tanning and dyestuff industries. Hexavalent Cr is more efficiently absorbed than Cr^{3+}, and its toxicity and carcinogenic effects involve reduction of Cr^{6+} to Cr^{3+} by cysteine, with formation of intracellular DNA adducts.[677] Trivalent Cr species are relatively nontoxic in part because of their poor intestinal absorption and rapid excretion in urine.[647]

However, Cr-picolinate is a widely used dietary supplement, and this compound has been reported to cause renal and hepatic damage when used at high doses.[678] Patients with preexisting renal or liver disease may be at particular risk for adverse effects. Others have shown that Cr-picolinate has a different intracellular pathway compared with other forms of Cr^{3+}.[679] There have been reports of benefits from Cr-picolinate related to diabetes control,[21] but claims that this supplement can promote body fat loss and muscle mass gain have not been substantiated.[679]

Markedly increased concentrations (up to 1000-fold) have been observed in both plasma (12 μg/L; 230 nmol/L) and urine (50 μg/L; 2600 nmol/L) in patients with problem hip prostheses (as discussed previously).[680]

Laboratory Assessment of Status. A beneficial response of glucose-intolerant patients to Cr supplementation is presently the only means of confirming Cr deficiency. No practicable method of assessing intracellular Cr depletion is yet available, and no consistently reliable animal model has been identified for Cr deficiency. Furthermore, it has been known from early animal experiments that circulating Cr is not in equilibrium with physiologically important reserves.[646]

A possibly useful test has been proposed that uses radioactive $^{51}Cr^{6+}$ to label red cells. The ion is then reduced to Cr^{3+}, and the amount bound to cell membranes is dependent on the amount of Cr^{3+} initially present, which, in turn, is a reflection of the adequacy of Cr nutritional status. The test was applied to 25 patients with type 2 diabetes and 35 control subjects. No difference was found, and it was concluded that Cr nutrition had only a minor role in this condition.[681]

Direct determination of Cr in the diet, in oral and intravenous nutritional support regimens, and in blood plasma or serum can be carried out only if great care is taken to prevent contamination before and during analysis. Specialist trace element laboratories using ICP-MS and stable Cr isotopes now offer improved analytical sensitivity and allow tracer methods for metabolic studies.[607]

Detection of increased amounts of Cr in urine provides confirmation of recent occupational or environmental exposure to excess Cr. It also may be useful for monitoring urine Cr in trials that use pharmacologic dosages of Cr, both to confirm compliance and to detect potential toxicity. This is possible using available graphite furnace AAS or ICP-MS.[682]

Reference Intervals. Low reference intervals are now considered to be normal for serum (0.1–0.2 μg/L; 2–3 nmol/L) and for urine (0.1–2.0 μg/L; 1.9–38.4 nmol/L). Thus, detection of deficiency by direct analysis is difficult.[645] For more information, refer to the Appendix on Reference Intervals. Laboratories should verify that these ranges are appropriate for use in their own settings.

Cobalt

Cobalt is essential for humans only as an integral part of vitamin B_{12} (cobalamin). No other function for Co in the human body is known. Details of vitamin B_{12} biochemistry and function were discussed earlier. The microflora of the human intestine cannot use Co to synthesize physiologically active cobalamin. The human vitamin B_{12} requirement must be supplied by the diet. Free (non-vitamin B_{12}) Co does not interact with the body vitamin B_{12} pool. In Europe, the recommended supplementation during TPN is 0 to 1.67 μg/day.

Co status is usually assessed through measurement of vitamin B_{12} or cobalamin. Normal values in plasma are less than 1 μg/L (<17 nmol/L); for urine, the values are 1 to 3 μg/L (17–34 nmol/L).[683] Increased exposure from industrial uses, particularly with hard metal drilling and cutting blades, leads to high urinary Co concentrations. Increases are also associated with hip prostheses (discussed earlier), for which concentrations can be markedly raised with no apparent clinical evidence of overt toxicity.[684,685] However, there are anecdotal accounts of Co toxicity with metal-on-metal hip prostheses.[590]

Erythropoiesis can be stimulated by inorganic Co ions.[595] Previously, $CoCl_2$ was administered at daily doses of 25 to 300 mg for this purpose and was proved to be effective in stimulating erythropoiesis in both nonrenal and renal anemia.[595] The mode of action is that the Co^{2+} ion stabilizes the hypoxia-inducible transcription factors that increase the expression of the erythropoietin gene (*EPO*). Because erythropoietin treatment is now used to treat anemia, Co therapy to treat anemia is no longer practiced, but because Co was not a substance normally tested for, its use gained some credibility among athletes and the horse racing fraternity. There are side effects associated with long-term Co exposure affecting the gastrointestinal tract, thyroid, heart, and the sensory systems.[685-687] Concentrations in biological fluids and tissues can be determined by ICP-MS.

Copper

Copper is an important trace element that is associated with a number of metalloproteins. It is present in biological systems in both 1^+ and 2^+ valence states.

Chemistry. Copper (atomic number 29, atomic weight 63.54) has Cu^{1+} and Cu^{2+} oxidation states in biological systems; facile exchange between these ions gives the element important redox properties. Because of their high electron affinities, of all essential trace metals these ions are most strongly bound to organic molecules. Cu in biological material is complexed with proteins, peptides, and other organic ligands. An elaborate series of binding and transport proteins inside cells protects the genome from Cu-generated free radical attack.[688] This keeps the concentration of free Cu in the cytoplasm low ($\cong 10^{-15}$ mol/L). Cu bioinorganic chemistry evolved concurrently with that of molecular O_2.[548] Numerous blue-colored Cu-containing proteins, most of which are oxidases, are located outside the cytoplasm on the surface of cell membranes or in vesicles. However, the Cu metalloenzyme superoxide dismutase (SOD) protects against random free radical damage both in the cytoplasm and in blood plasma. Paradoxically, it was the ability of Cu ions to generate free radicals that led to the evolutionary development of the extracellular matrix by polymerization and crosslinking of low MW substrates. This allowed the formation of collagen, chitin, and other structural proteins essential for the development of multicellular life forms.[548]

Dietary Sources. The Cu content of food is variable and can be affected by application of Cu-containing fertilizers and fungicidal sprays. Also, the use of Cu-containing cooking vessels contributes to total intake, notably in the case of Indian childhood cirrhosis, which is believed to be due to consuming milk that is stored in Cu vessels.[689,690] The metal is most plentiful in organ meats, such as liver and kidney, with relatively high amounts also found in shellfish, nuts, whole grain cereals, bran, and all cocoa-containing products. Lesser amounts of Cu are found in white meats and in dairy products, especially cow's milk. The median intake of Cu in the United States is approximately 1.0 to 1.6 mg/day. Intake mainly from meat and vegetables in the older adult (older than 60 years) is prone to be low, particularly among low-income groups and those with less education. Continual assessment of the nutriture is needed in this group.[691]

Absorption, Transport, Metabolism, and Excretion. Copper absorption occurs mainly in the small intestine, although gastric uptake has been shown to occur to a lesser extent.[692,693] Some Cu may be incorporated by inhalation and skin absorption. The extent of intestinal Cu absorption varies with dietary Cu content and is approximately 50% at low Cu intakes (<1 mg/day of Cu) but only 20% at higher intakes (>5 mg/day of Cu).[693] Cu intestinal uptake is pH dependent and relatively efficient. Absorption is reduced by other dietary components such as Zn (which induces MT that binds Cu^{2+}),[694] vitamin C (which converts Cu^{2+} to Cu^{+} that is insoluble and therefore not absorbed),[695,696] MoO_4^{2-}, and Fe, and is increased by amino acids and by dietary Na.[692,693]

Absorbed Cu is transported to the liver in portal blood bound to albumin, where it is incorporated by hepatocytes into cuproenzymes and other proteins, and then is exported in peripheral blood to tissue and organs. Although two-thirds of the 80 to 100 mg of total body Cu content is located in the skeleton and muscle, the liver is the key organ in Cu homeostasis.[693] Using a tracer (^{65}Cu), up to 68% of plasma Cu was shown to be bound to ceruloplasmin, and 4.1 ± 0.8% of total body Cu was predicted to be in plasma.[697]

The ceruloplasmin molecule contains six to eight atoms of Cu per molecule with six atoms of Cu involved in the protein's ferroxidase and free radical scavenging activities. The other one to two atoms of Cu are termed "labile" and may allow ceruloplasmin to act as a Cu transporter, with a pool of Cu being exchanged between albumin, transcuprein, and the labile sites of ceruloplasmin.[698-700] Thus, up to 90% of Cu exported from the liver into peripheral blood is in the protein bound form either to ceruloplasmin, transcuprein, and/or MT.

Ceruloplasmin is a positive acute-phase reactant that is increased during infection and after tissue injury.[34] The protein is also increased in concentration during pregnancy and during use of oral contraceptives, leading to a rise in serum Cu concentration.[701] A smaller amount of Cu in plasma (<10%) is bound to albumin by specific peptide sequences, and this Cu is in equilibrium with plasma amino acids. This fraction may be important for cellular uptake.

An overview of Cu metabolism is illustrated in Fig. 37.26. Between 0.5 and 2.0 mg/day of Cu (8–31 µmol/day) is excreted via bile into feces. Patients with cholestatic jaundice or other forms of liver dysfunction therefore are at risk for Cu accumulation caused by failure of excretion. Cu losses in urine and sweat account for less than 3% of dietary intake. Urine Cu output is normally less than 60 µg/day (<1 µmol/day).[693,702,703]

Functions. Copper, a catalytic component of numerous enzymes, is also a structural component of other important proteins in humans, animals, plants, and microorganisms. Some of those considered of potential importance in human biochemistry are briefly described in the following sections. Only small amounts of Cu are present in biological fluids, and essentially none of it exists as the free ion. These properties and the low redox potential of Cu dictate special structural and mechanistic features in Cu transporters.[704]

Energy Production. Cytochrome c oxidase is a multisubunit complex containing Cu and Fe. Located on the external face of mitochondrial membranes, the enzyme catalyzes four-electron reduction of molecular O_2, establishing a high-energy proton gradient across the inner mitochondrial membrane that is necessary for ATP production. Cytochrome c and cytochrome c oxidase are essential for oxidative phosphorylation that serves as the basis of intracellular energy production.[705]

Connective Tissue Formation. Protein-lysine 6-oxidase (lysyl oxidase) is a cuproenzyme that is essential for stabilization of extracellular matrixes, specifically for enzymatic crosslinking of collagen and elastin. Complex mechanisms involve the deamination of lysine and hydrolysine residues at specific extracellular sites. The enzyme is highly associated with connective tissue and is located in the aorta, dermal connective tissue, fibroblasts, and cytoskeleton of many other cells.[706]

Iron Metabolism. Copper-containing enzymes, namely ferroxidase I (ceruloplasmin), and ferroxidase II, and hephaestin in the enterocyte oxidize ferrous Fe to ferric Fe. This allows incorporation of Fe^{3+} into transferrin and eventually into Hb. Ferroxidase II is a yellow protein, the importance of which in Fe metabolism is not as well characterized as that of ceruloplasmin.[707]

Central Nervous System. Dopamine mono-oxygenase is an enzyme that requires Cu as a cofactor and uses ascorbate as an electron donor. This enzyme catalyzes the conversion of dopamine to norepinephrine, an important neurotransmitter. Soluble and membrane-bound forms of the enzyme are present, with the latter found in chromaffin granules of the adrenal cortex. Monoamine oxidase, one of the numerous amine oxidases, is a Cu-containing enzyme that catalyzes the

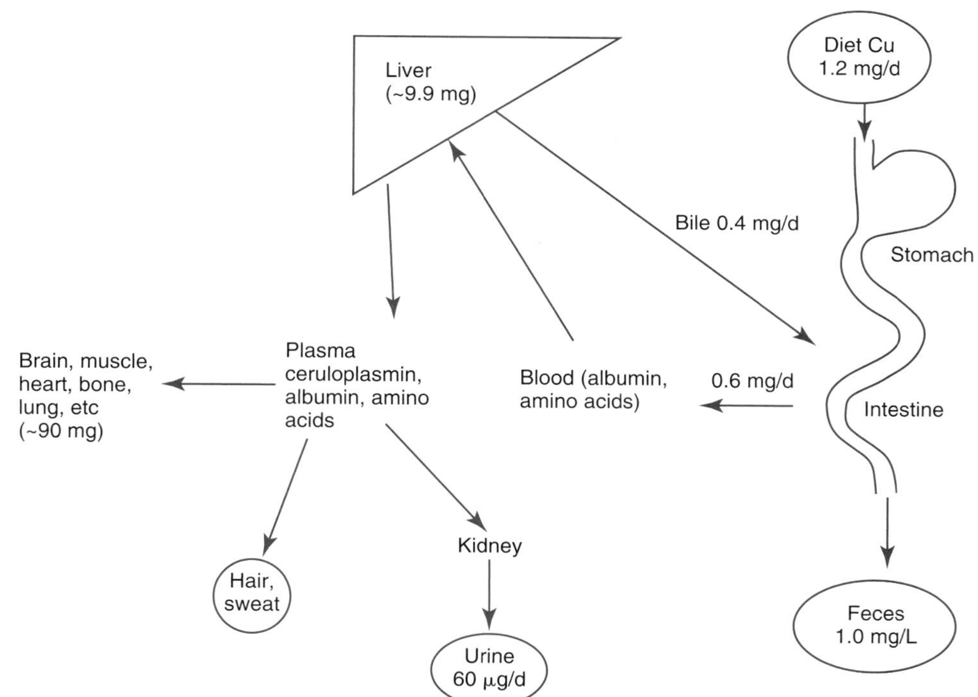

FIGURE 37.26 Metabolism of Copper. (Modified from Harris ED. Copper. In: O'Dell BL, Sunde RA, editors. *Handbook of nutritionally essential mineral elements.* New York: Marcel Dekker, 1997:231–73.)

degradation of serotonin in the brain and is also involved in the metabolism of catecholamines.[708]

Formation of the phospholipids necessary for myelin sheath formation is affected by cytochrome c oxidase depletion. It is now known that the prion protein binds Cu^{2+} and may be involved in Cu regulation within the brain.[709] Also, a dysfunction in Cu homeostasis has been shown in Alzheimer disease, with an excess of fragmentation of ceruloplasmin in cerebrospinal fluid. This has been related to increased proteolysis of ceruloplasmin, indicating an inflammatory process rather than a causative effect of Cu on Tau protein precipitation.[710]

Melanin Synthesis. Tyrosinase is a Cu-containing enzyme that is present in melanocytes and catalyzes the synthesis of melanin. Starting with L-dopa as a substrate, tyrosinase catalyzes multiple oxidative steps to produce the melanin biopigments pheomelanin and eumelanin.[711]

Antioxidant Functions. Both intracellular and extracellular SODs are Cu- and Zn-containing enzymes that are able to convert superoxide radicals to H_2O_2, which can be removed subsequently by catalase and other antioxidant defenses. The plasma protein ceruloplasmin also binds Cu ions and thus prevents oxidative damage from free Cu ions, which can generate hydroxyl radicals.[48]

Regulation of Gene Expression and Intracellular Copper Handling. Copper-dependent proteins act as transcription factors for specific genes, such as those regulating SOD and catalase. MT synthesis is controlled by Cu-responsive transcription factors. This protein is important in regulating the intracellular distribution of Cu.[712] Additional specialized proteins act as "chaperones" to deliver Cu to intracellular sites and to prevent oxidative damage by free Cu ions.[713]

Cells tightly regulate Cu homeostasis through three Cu transporters: Ctr1, ATP7A, and ATP7B. Ctr1 imports Cu and the platinum-based compounds such as cisplatin, carboplatin, and oxaliplatin into the cell. ATP7A and ATP7B are Cu exporters that eject the Cu and platinum-based compounds from cytoplasm. Cells that overexpress ATP7B show increased efflux of cisplatin and carboplatin from the cytoplasm and reduced accumulation of these compounds. These findings suggest that high concentration of extracellular Cu/platinum is detectable by the cell, which causes Ctr1 to rapidly withdraw from the membrane into the cytoplasm, where Ctr1 is quickly degraded. This negative feedback mechanism reduces the uptake of Cu/platinum and reduces its toxicity.[714]

In addition, both apo- and Cu^{I}-Atox1, the Cu chaperone, react faster with *trans*-platinum complexes than with cisplatin; however, less protein aggregation is observed in the reaction of *trans*-platinum complexes. These results indicate that the roles of Atox1 in the regulation of cellular trafficking of platinum drugs are dependent on the coordination configurations of Cu. Thus, the role of Cu control is increasingly important in understanding how the cytotoxic platinum compounds are regulated.[715]

Inborn Errors of Copper Metabolism. Menkes syndrome is an X-linked condition caused by a defective gene that regulates the metabolism of Cu in the body.[716] Wilson disease is inherited as an autosomal recessive trait, which leads to a defect in Cu metabolism, with accumulation of Cu in the liver, brain, kidney, cornea, and other tissues.[26] Investigation of these rare genetic defects has been of great value in uncovering details on the control of Cu transport. Cu-transporting P-type ATPases, known as ATP7A and ATP7B, are essential factors in maintaining Cu balance.[717,718]

Impaired intestinal transport of Cu caused by a mutation in the *ATP7A* gene leads to the severe Cu deficiency disease seen in Menkes syndrome. Defects in the *ATP7B* gene affect both incorporation of Cu into ceruloplasmin and Cu excretion via bile. This results in a toxic accumulation of Cu and forms the basis of Wilson disease.

Another genetic defect results in failure of hepatic synthesis of ceruloplasmin (aceruloplasminemia), which is a neurodegenerative disease. Retinal damage, secondary Fe overload, and insulin-dependent diabetes present in the fourth to fifth decade of life.[719]

Angiogenesis. Copper plays an essential role in promoting angiogenesis, as was shown in the stimulation of blood vessel formation in the avascular cornea of rabbits.[720] On X-ray fluorescence microscopy, highly vascularized ductal carcinomas showed Cu clustering in putative neoangiogenic areas.[721]

Various clinical trials have established that Cu privation by diet or by Cu chelators diminishes a tumor's ability to mount an angiogenic response. These data have shed new light on the functional role of Cu in microvessel development, and of equal importance, have stimulated new nutritional models of cancer therapeutic intervention. The use of tetrathiomolybdate can directly and reversibly downregulate Cu delivery to secreted metalloenzymes, which suggests that proteins involved in metal regulation might be fruitful drug targets.[722] Initial observations in animal models of breast cancer were encouraging,[723] but later studies showed no benefit at least in neuroglioblastoma.[724]

Requirements and Reference Nutrient Intakes. The recommended dietary intake of Cu for adults is 0.9 mg/day.[12] This is close to the lower limit of 1.0 mg/day found in dietary surveys and has led to suggestions that marginal Cu depletion could be likely in the US population.[725] The tolerable upper limit is 10 mg/day.[12]

Intravenous Supply. The usual adult supply of Cu given intravenously varies from 0.3 to 1.3 mg/day (5–20 μmol/day), with higher amounts required in those patients with preexisting depletion or biliary losses, and lower amounts in those with cholestasis.

Deficiency

Malnourished Infants. When malnourished infants with a history of chronic diarrhea were rehabilitated using a formula based on cow's milk, they developed Fe-resistant anemia, neutropenia, and other hematologic disorders, as well as bone lesions. Cu supplementation of milk reversed these abnormalities, and the addition of 2.5 mg/day of Cu is now advised.[726]

Premature Infants. Most of the accumulation of Cu in the fetal liver occurs in the last 3 months of pregnancy, and premature infants fed formula lacking sufficient Cu are at risk of deficiency disease because they lack adequate liver Cu stores. Hematologic abnormalities and easily fractured brittle bones have been described.[727] Radiographic changes in infants with Cu deficiency include osteopenia and metaphyseal spurs.[728] As noted earlier, formulas based on cow's milk require Cu supplementation. Monitoring of plasma Cu is advisable, and results should be related to postnatal age: at 4 weeks, mean values are 42 μg/dL (6.6 μmol/L), rising to 55 μg/dL (8.7 μmol/L) by 14 weeks.[729]

Nutritional Support. Adults and children fed intravenously without the addition of sufficient Cu to the nutrient regimen develop symptomatic Cu deficiency. Hematologic changes of hypochromic anemia and neutropenia are reversed by Cu supplementation.[730,731] Similar effects have been reported during prolonged enteral feeding via jejunostomy.[732] Children may develop the typical bone changes mentioned previously.

Menkes Syndrome. History and aspects of the diagnosis and therapy of this condition have been reviewed.[716,733,734] It is a rare condition (1/100,000 live births), the mutation is X-linked, and it typically occurs in male infants at 2 to 3 months. Such infants present with loss of previously normal development, hypotonia, seizures, and failure to thrive. Physical changes in the hair (pili torti) and in facial appearance, as well as neurologic abnormalities, suggest the diagnosis. Low concentrations of Cu in plasma, liver, and brain occur because of impaired intestinal Cu absorption. First-line tests would provide findings of plasma Cu less than 65 μg/dL (<10 μmol/L) and ceruloplasmin less than 220 mg/L, along with demonstration of pili torti by microscopic examination of the hair. Additional tests can demonstrate failure of isotopic Cu egress from cultured fibroblasts and show plasma catecholamine abnormalities.[735] Placental Cu measurement and direct mutation analysis are additional investigative procedures. Deficiency of the Cu enzyme dopamine monooxygenase in cerebrospinal fluid is believed to be an important finding that allows early diagnosis. The effectiveness of therapy with parenteral Cu histidine is debatable, although success has been claimed in less severely affected cases, especially if treatment is started early.

Malabsorption Syndromes. Patients at risk include those with celiac disease, tropical sprue, CF, and short bowel syndrome. Excessive intake of oral Zn supplements can cause anemia and hematologic abnormalities in the absence of occult blood loss.[736] Cu deficiency is caused by Zn induction of MT in the intestinal mucosa, which then sequesters dietary Cu, blocking its absorption.

Cardiovascular Disease. Animal studies show that severe Cu deficiency causes cardiac damage, but the abnormality differs from that seen in human cardiovascular disease. The myocardium is hypertrophied and may rupture in animal models. Coronary artery pressure is decreased, but in human ischemic disease, it is increased.[737] The role of Cu in human cardiovascular disease is controversial, although much supporting evidence for a positive link with low dietary Cu intake has been published.[725]

Epidemiologic surveys have shown that increased plasma Cu values are a positive cardiovascular risk factor. A US study of 4400 adult men and women found that those with plasma Cu values in the two highest quartiles had the greatest risk of dying from cardiovascular disease.[738] An increase in plasma ceruloplasmin and hence plasma Cu may be a nonspecific response to the inflammation of arteries found in arteriosclerosis. It is known that the ceruloplasmin hepatic mRNA increases during inflammation, and that this is induced by interleukin-6.[739] Insulin is also known to be involved in the transcriptional regulation of ceruloplasmin synthesis.[740]

Anemia. Copper deficiency is an established cause of hematologic abnormalities, but it is frequently misdiagnosed. Patients with Cu deficiency can present with a combination of hematologic and neurologic abnormalities that may masquerade as a myelodysplastic syndrome. Usual hematologic features include anemia, leucopenia, and rarely, thrombocytopenia.[538] Review of records between 1970 and 2005 of patients (excluding any with Wilson disease) whose plasma Cu concentrations were less than 69 μg/dL (10.9 μmol/L) and with normal plasma Zn identified various hematologic abnormalities on bone marrow examination, including vacuoles in myeloid precursors, Fe-containing plasma cells, and a decrease in granulocyte precursors and ring sideroblasts.[741] Thus, Cu deficiency is a rare but treatable cause of hematologic abnormalities.

Neuropathy. Copper deficiency is an increasingly recognized cause of gait unsteadiness. A case report of Cu deficiency due to celiac disease suggested that ataxia associated with celiac disease was likely to be due to a Cu-deficiency myeloneuropathy.[742]

A case of Cu deficiency–associated myeloneuropathy has been described, in which the patient was malabsorbing Cu and had a low plasma Cu concentration of 2.4 μg/dL (0.37 μmol/L), probably as a result of excess Zn intake (plasma Zn 225 μg/dL [34.4 μmol/L]). Reference intervals are 70 to 140 and 80 to 120 μg/dL (11–22 and 12–18 μmol/L) for Cu and Zn, respectively.[743] For more information, refer to the Appendix on Reference Intervals. Laboratories should verify that these ranges are appropriate for use in their own settings.

Toxicity. As mentioned previously, Wilson disease is a genetic disorder of Cu metabolism that causes an increase in Cu to toxic concentrations.[26] Problems of diagnosis and appropriate laboratory investigations have been reviewed.[744,745] It has been suggested that ceruloplasmin oxidase activity and serum free Cu concentration should be monitored in patients on long-term Cu-chelation therapy to prevent iatrogenic Cu deficiency.[746]

The incidence of Wilson disease is estimated to be 1 of 30,000 live births with a carrier frequency of 1 of 90 in the general population. The presentation is highly variable, so adolescents or young adults with otherwise unexplained liver disease or neurologic symptoms should be screened, especially when a family history of suspected Wilson disease is reported. Initial investigations should include plasma Cu and ceruloplasmin, which usually will be less than 50 μg/dL (8 μmol Cu/L) and less than 200 mg/L ceruloplasmin. Although the total plasma Cu is decreased, the non–ceruloplasmin-bound fraction is increased, allowing deposition of Cu in the brain, eyes, and kidneys.

Slit-lamp eye examination may detect Cu deposits in the eye (Kayser-Fleischer rings), and abnormalities in liver function tests may be noted with an increased urine Cu output of more than 500 μg/L (>8 μmol/L). Liver biopsy for Cu analysis is useful in suspected cases, and results more than 250 μg/g Cu dry weight are usually found (normal, 8–40 μg/g Cu dry weight). Failure of Cu incorporation into plasma ceruloplasmin can be demonstrated using an oral dose of stable ^{65}Cu isotope.[566] This may be helpful in excluding Wilson disease when other tests are equivocal. Gene tracking and mutation detection are now possible, but because several hundred mutations exist, this may not be informative.

Diagnosis can be difficult in patients with Wilson disease who present with acute liver failure.[747,748] Prompt diagnosis is important because urgent liver transplantation may be required.[749] In these cases, greatly increased plasma Cu will be found but without an appropriately increased ceruloplasmin. The unbound plasma Cu fraction can increase to more than 80% of total plasma Cu (normal, 5%–10%). Excess Cu is released from the necrotic liver and causes intravascular hemolysis and renal failure.[750]

The chronic form of Wilson disease is treated by oral chelating agents, such as penicillamine and trientine, which remove excess Cu from tissue and increase urine excretion, and the oral administration of Zn salts or ammonium MoO_4^{2-}, which blocks Cu intestinal absorption.[26] However, use of ammonium tetrathiomolybdate has been shown to cause pituitary atrophy in animals treated for Cu overload. This was believed to be a result of significant accumulation of total Mo in the pituitary, so care must be used in administration of this therapy.[751]

Toxicity can also arise directly from Cu contamination of diet and water supplies. Quality standards regarding Cu in drinking water have been published by WHO.[752] Guidelines for the maximum Cu content of drinking water have been suggested and vary from approximately 1 to 3 mg/L. Some children may be genetically sensitive to Cu in drinking water and may develop chronic liver disease,[753] which has been found in Indian children.[689,690] Acute poisoning has been recorded after accidental or intentional ingestion of Cu sulfate. Environmental aspects of Cu toxicity and its impact upon human health have been reviewed.[754,755]

Release of Cu from intrauterine devices has also been reported to cause Cu toxicity in numerous reports, but this does not appear to be a current major public health problem.[702,756,757]

Laboratory Assessment of Status. Several well-controlled dietary deprivation studies have demonstrated the usefulness of the clinical laboratory in providing measures of Cu status. For example, plasma Cu and ceruloplasmin assays are convenient and widely used to confirm severe Cu deficiency. However, they are not sensitive indicators in marginal Cu depletion.[758] Interpretation of results should take the SIR or acute-phase reaction into account.

Because approximately 90% of plasma Cu is bound to ceruloplasmin, factors that increase the hepatic synthesis of ceruloplasmin, such as an acute-phase response or estrogen-containing oral contraceptive pills, will increase plasma Cu independently of dietary Cu intake.[739,759] In premature infants with liver immaturity and low ceruloplasmin synthesis, plasma Cu values less than 30 μg/L (<5 μmol Cu/L) suggest the necessity for increased Cu input.

Dietary depletion studies that used low Cu diets demonstrated a decrease in plasma Cu and then a return upon dietary supplementation; however, plasma Cu values remained largely within the reference interval.[693] It has been suggested that the ratio of immunologically to enzymatically measured ceruloplasmin might be a useful index of marginal Cu depletion. This ratio, which is the specific activity of ceruloplasmin, will be low in marginal Cu depletion. Apoceruloplasmin increases in blood serum during Cu depletion; this will contribute to the total ceruloplasmin assay. The enzymatic activity decreases even in marginal Cu depletion. The specific activity of ceruloplasmin is therefore sensitive to Cu status and is not affected by age, sex, or hormonal influences. In a study of Cu depletion, 12 postmenopausal women were fed a low Cu diet (0.57 mg/day) for 35 days, followed by supplementation for 35 days (2 mg/day).[760] Responsive markers were red cell SOD, platelet cytochrome oxidase, red cell GSHP, and clotting factor VIII. Although of potential value for detecting marginal Cu depletion, these measurements are not in widespread use because of sample instability and lack of standardized methods. It has been suggested that interpretation of a Cu value can be properly assessed only by an adjusted Cu/ceruloplasmin ratio.[761]

However, this procedure is fraught with problems, not least of which is caused by the inaccuracy in the ceruloplasmin assay. To assay the free fraction, a chelating agent (EDTA) was used to dissociate Cu from albumin and transcuprein while not affecting the atoms of Cu firmly located within the ceruloplasmin protein. The subsequent analysis was referred to as exchangeable Cu (ExCu). It was argued that this ExCu is the Cu available to most cells or the bioavailable (free) portion of plasma Cu, and monitoring of this should enable better identification of individuals at risk of toxicity and/or deficiency.[762,763] Urinary Cu excretion is decreased during dietary deprivation, but the change from an already low basal value is small, and difficulties in reliable collection and with sample contamination make this of limited use.

Reference Intervals. For adults, plasma Cu is usually in the reference interval of 70 to 140 µg/dL (11–22 µmol/L). Values in women of childbearing age and especially in pregnancy are higher. For adults, a plasma Cu level less than 50 µg/dL (8 µmo/L), and for infants less than 30 µg/dL (5 µmol/L), indicates probable Cu deficiency. Adjusting the Cu concentration to account for variations in ceruloplasmin is unfortunately problematic, because it depends on the accuracy of the immunoassay. In some cases, the calculation can produce apparently negative values for free Cu.[761]

The most reliable procedure to determine free Cu is probably plasma ultrafiltration; a reference interval of 0 to 10 µg/dL (0–1.6 µmol/L) was reported in 137 healthy adult (20–59 years) blood donors.[762] The ultrafilterable (free) Cu concentrations for patients diagnosed with Wilson disease were at least sixfold greater than the upper limit.

Urine Cu excretion is normally less than 60 µg/day (<1.0 µmol/day), and values of more than 200 µg/day (3 µmol/L) are found in Wilson disease. A Cu concentration in a liver biopsy sample of more than 250 µg/g Cu dry weight (normally 8–40 µg/g dry weight) is indicative of Wilson disease, in the absence of other causes of cholestatic disease.

Excretion of Cu in urine, in response to an oral penicillamine test, of more than 25 µmol/day was shown to be diagnostic of Wilson disease in children. However, a later study found post-penicillamine Cu greater than this value in 29 of 38 patients with Wilson disease and also in 4 of 60 control subjects, which indicated that the test is valuable in the diagnosis of Wilson disease with active liver disease, but is unreliable in excluding the diagnosis in asymptomatic siblings.[764] For more information, refer to the Appendix on Reference Intervals. Laboratories should verify that these ranges are appropriate for use in their own settings.

Iodine

Iodine is the heaviest of all the essential elements. The association between goiter and areas with low iodine concentrations in the soil revealed the essentiality of the element to human health. Its biological role, as a component of the thyroid hormones, is discussed in Chapter 67.

Chemistry. Iodine (atomic number 53, atomic weight 126.9) is a halogen lying within period 5 of the periodic table. The solid sublimes at normal or slightly increased temperatures, a property shared by few other elements, giving a purple vapor. The element normally exists in the environment as the iodide (I^-) anion, which if left within the atmosphere, will slowly oxidize to the diatomic molecule, I_2.

Dietary Sources. The primary sources of dietary I are usually dairy products, especially milk. Other important foods include seafood and plants grown on I-rich soil. Deficiency is common where concentrations are low in soils and food products. Fortification programs, with I added to table salt, are established in many countries. An exception is the United Kingdom, which, coupled to reduction in salt intake to prevent hypertension, has led to some concern that females of childbearing age may have suboptimal I status.[765] After I fortification programs have been implemented, some cases of I-induced hyperthyroidism have been observed.[766]

Absorption, Transport, Metabolism, and Excretion. Absorption of dietary I^- is not entirely understood. The Na^+/I^- symporter (NIS) on the apical surface of enterocytes of the small intestine is responsible for uptake into vesicles within the cell, but movement into the circulation is not clear.[767,768] Under normal circumstances, 90% to 95% of the intake is absorbed. Subsequent transport, movement into thyroid cells (which also involves an NIS), synthesis of thyroid hormones, and release are discussed in Chapter 67. I is primarily excreted in the urine.

Functions. The essential function for I relates to thyroid physiology (see Chapter 67). Although I is concentrated in thyroid tissue and hormones, approximately 70% of the body's I is distributed in other tissues, including mammary glands, eyes, gastric mucosa, fetal thymus, cerebrospinal fluid and the coroid plexus, arterial walls, the cervix, and salivary glands. Its role in mammary tissue relates to fetal and neonatal development, but its role in the other tissues is partially unknown.

Requirements and Reference Nutrient Intakes. The daily dietary reference intake recommended by the US IOM is 110 to 130 µg for infants up to 12 months, 90 µg for children up to 8 years, 120 µg for children up to 13 years, 150 µg for adults, 220 µg for pregnant women, and 290 µg for lactating mothers.[12] Similar values are cited by authorities in other countries.

The thyroid gland requires up to 70 µg/day to synthesize adequate amounts of thyroid hormones. The higher RDAs provide for optimal function of other body systems, including lactating breast, gastric mucosa, salivary glands, oral mucosa, and arterial walls.

Intravenous Supply. Recommendations from the American Society for Clinical Nutrition, European Society for Pediatric Gastroenterology, Hepatology, and Metabolism, and the European Society for Clinical Nutrition and Metabolism are summarized in a statement from the Iodine Global Network.[769,770] These recommendations propose daily I intakes of 70 to 170 µg in adults and 1 µg/kg for infants and children. It has been suggested that these amounts may be inadequate in infants, but that dermal absorption from topical iodinated disinfectants will prevent deficiency at a particularly vulnerable stage of life. However, with the wider use of noniodinated antiseptics, preterm infants being parenterally fed may become I deficient.[770,771]

Clinical Deficiency. Deficiency of I is a major health problem throughout the world.[772] It occurs in regions where the soil and groundwater are deficient in the element, and if crops are grown in these soils, they will be low in I concentration. Deficiency may also develop after prolonged use of special diets that may have a low I content.[773]

Low dietary I causes increased secretion of thyroid stimulating hormone (TSH) by the pituitary gland. This in turn increases I^- uptake by the thyroid gland, leading to reduced renal clearance and urinary excretion. TSH also stimulates thyroglobulin breakdown and increases 3,5,3'-triiodothyronine (T_3) production relative to T_4. In chronic I deficiency, hyperplasia of thyroid epithelial cells can occur, which in severe situations, may be clinically evident as goiter.[774]

The most serious adverse effect of I deficiency is impaired development of nervous tissue in the fetus.[775] Thyroid hormones are required for neuronal migration and myelination of the fetal brain. Severe maternal I deficiency during pregnancy increases the risk of stillbirths and congenital abnormalities. A decrease in intelligence quotient points has been shown in children who are I deficient.[776]

The enzymes responsible for synthesis of thyroid hormones require Se and the implications of Se deficiency on thyroidal function are of current interest.[777]

Toxicity. Iodine is a strong oxidizing agent and acts as an acid corrosive. I vapor irritates the eyes, skin, and mucous membranes.

There is a high tolerance to ingested I with a wide margin of safety. I intakes of up to 1100 μg/day are well tolerated by most adults,[12] although in children long-term intakes of 500 μg/day or more are associated with mild thyroid enlargement.

Causes of acute toxicity include accidental or deliberate ingestion of I, which results in corrosive damage to the gastrointestinal tract, cardiovascular collapse, and renal failure. In the presence of starch, blue I^- salts form, and blue emesis is characteristic of I poisoning. Common causes of long-term toxicity are liberal use of I to open wounds, large injections of I-containing radio-contrast media, and amiodarone treatment for cardiac arrhythmias.

Iodine toxicity causes a rapid decrease in release of T_4 and T_3 from thyroglobulin, decreased uptake of I^- by the thyroid gland, and hence, decreased synthesis of the thyroidal hormones. This culminates in acute hypothyroidism with low plasma T_4 and T_3 and high TSH concentrations.

Laboratory Assessment of Status. Urine is the matrix of choice for suspected I toxicity and for the assessment of recent I intake. For epidemiological studies, such as population-based surveys, the median urinary I concentration can be used to classify that population's I status. Adequate I status is indicated by a population median urinary I concentration of more than 0.79 μmol/L (100 μg/L). However, the urine I test is not an appropriate test to diagnose I deficiency in individuals. A common mistake is to assume that all individuals with a random urinary I concentration of less than 0.79 μmol/L (100 μg/L) are I deficient. Urine I levels have a low predictive value in an individual because urinary I concentration varies substantially between days and seasons, as well as within a day (up to threefold) as a consequence of circadian rhythm and due to differences in fluid intake. Because the thyroid gland can store large amounts of I (12–16 mg in an I-sufficient individual), a low urine I concentration does not indicate I deficiency any more than a low urinary Na indicates Na deficiency. However, it is recommended that I status can be

TABLE 37.6 Epidemiological Criteria for Assessing Iodine Status

MEDIAN URINARY IODINE			
(μmol/L)	(μg/L)	Iodine Intake	Iodine Status
Children >6 Years Old and Adults			
<0.16	<20	Insufficient	Severe deficiency
0.16–0.39	20–49	Insufficient	Moderate deficiency
0.39–0.78	50–99	Insufficient	Mild deficiency
0.79–1.57	100–199	Adequate	Adequate nutrition
1.58–2.36	200–299	Above requirements	May pose a slight risk of more than adequate
≥2.36	≥300	Excessive	Risk of adverse health consequences
Pregnant Women			
<1.18	<150	Insufficient	
1.18–1.96	150–249	Adequate	
1.96–3.93	250–499	Above requirements	
≥3.93	≥500	Excessive	
Lactating Women and Children <2 yrs			
<0.79	<100	Insufficient	
≥0.79	≥100	Adequate	

reliably estimated if 10 repeat random urine samples are collected, but clearly, the large number of samples required is a major limitation.[778]

Reference Intervals. WHO-recommended urinary concentrations for various population groups are given in Table 37.6.[779] In 24-hour urine collections, the expected excretion of I is 0.60 to 4.30 μmol/L (76–546 μg/L). I concentration in serum or whole blood provides no useful information relevant to I nutritional status. For more information, refer to the Appendix on Reference Intervals. Laboratories should verify that these ranges are appropriate for use in their own settings.

Manganese

Manganese is present in biological systems bound to protein in the 2^+ or 3^+ valence state. It is associated mainly with the formation of connective and bony tissue, with growth and reproductive functions, and with carbohydrate and lipid metabolism.

Chemistry. Maganese (atomic number 25, atomic weight 54.94) is a first transition series metal ($3d^5s^2$) and is next to Fe in the periodic table. Of its 11 oxidation states, only Mn^{2+} and Mn^{3+} are found in biological systems, most often bound to protein. The Mn^{2+} ion with an unpaired electron is paramagnetic and can be detected in tissue by magnetic resonance imaging. The bioinorganic chemistry of Mn is complex, and detailed accounts have been published.[548]

Dietary Sources. Manganese-rich sources include whole grain foods, nuts, leafy vegetables, soy products, and teas.

Average intake in the United States is approximately 2 mg/day, with median values for adult men of 2.2 mg/day (range, 0.3–8.3 mg/day); for women, it is 1.8 mg/day (range, 0.3–5.9 mg/day) (NHANES III),[780] and in a British survey, the average household intake was 3.4 mg/day.[781] Vegetarian diets containing large quantities of whole grains and nuts can supply more than 10 mg/day.

Absorption, Transport, Metabolism, and Excretion. Dietary Mn is absorbed from the small intestine by mechanisms that may have a common pathway with that of Fe. Mn absorption is increased at low dietary intakes and is decreased at higher intakes, with tracer studies suggesting absorption efficiencies of 2% to 15%. Diets high in Fe, Ca, Mg, phosphates, fiber, phytic acid, oxalate, and tannins from tea can reduce the absorption of Mn.[782]

Once absorbed, Mn is transported in portal blood to the liver bound to albumin. It is exported to other tissues bound to transferrin and possibly to α_2-macroglobulin. Excretion of Mn occurs primarily via bile into feces, with urine output being very low and not sensitive to dietary intake.[783,784]

Functions. Manganese, which is a constituent of many important metalloenzymes, acts as a nonspecific enzyme activator. Mn^{2+} ions can be replaced by Mg^{2+}, Co^{2+}, and other cations during the activation of some enzymes.[19,784] Some important Mn-dependent enzymes are discussed in the following sections.

Superoxide Dismutase. Manganese-dependent SOD is a mitochondrial enzyme that is an important factor in limiting O_2 toxicity; it is one of the most studied enzymes in human biochemistry. The enzyme catalyzes the breakdown of the superoxide radical O_2^- to H_2O_2, which is then removed by catalase and GSHP.[785]

Pyruvate Carboxylase. This enzyme acts in combination with phosphoenol pyruvate carboxykinase, an enzyme that is activated by Mn ions. These enzymes are required to catalyze the formation of phosphoenol pyruvate, from pyruvate, a key reaction in the hepatic synthesis of glucose.

Arginase. Arginase is the terminal enzyme in the urea cycle, which hydrolyzes L-arginine to urea and ornithine, and completes the deamination of amino acids. Arginase is most concentrated in the liver, but it is also found in other tissues. The structure of the enzyme isolated from rat liver shows that it has a unique binuclear Mn cluster.[786] The activity of arginase affects the production of nitric oxide by limiting the availability of L-arginine required for synthesis of nitric oxide synthetase. This relationship has been investigated in a number of diverse diseases, including asthma and schizophrenia.[787]

Glycosyl Transferases. These enzymes are responsible for the sequential addition of carbohydrate molecules to proteins to form proteoglycans, and ultimately, connective tissue and cartilage. Therefore, they are important for the structural integrity of bone and skin, and for normal wound healing.

Requirements and Reference Nutrient Intakes. Because of lack of information on Mn dietary requirements, the US Food and Nutrition Board has set an AI amount for adults at 2.3 mg/day for males and 1.8 mg/day for females.[12] A tolerable upper intake limit of 11 mg/day was set for adults based on no observed effect for Western diets. For infants, the upper limit could not be set because of lack of data.[12] Concern has arisen about the potential toxicity of Mn in infants whose immature hepatic development reduces the biliary excretion of excess Mn. Therefore, the only dietary source of Mn in the age group (0–12 months) should be a normal diet or a formula. In addition, because Mn in drinking water and supplements may be more bioavailable than that obtained from food, caution should be taken when using Mn supplements, especially in individuals with liver disease who may be susceptible to the toxic effects of excess Mn.[12] The recommended supplementation during TPN is 0.06 to 0.1 μg/day.

Deficiency. Overt Mn deficiency has not been documented in humans eating natural diets. However, in numerous animal studies, signs of experimentally induced Mn deficiency include impaired growth and reproductive function, skeletal abnormalities, impaired glucose tolerance, and impaired cholesterol synthesis.[788-790] Seven young men fed experimental diets low in Mn developed skin lesions and low plasma cholesterol.[791]

Prolidase deficiency in infants is a rare genetic disorder that causes skin ulceration, mental retardation, increased urinary excretion of iminodipeptides, recurrent infections, and splenomegaly. It is known to be associated with abnormalities of Mn biochemistry, with one study suggesting less than one-half of normal arginase activity due to a defect in the supply of Mn for enzyme activation.[792]

Various unrelated medical conditions have been observed to be associated with lowered serum or whole blood Mn. These include osteoporosis, diabetes mellitus, and epilepsy.[793]The clinical relevance of these observations remains unclear.

Toxicity. The occupational health hazard from prolonged exposure to Mn-containing dust or fumes is well recognized. Neurologic symptoms resembling Parkinson disease develop slowly over a period of months or years.[793]

Of concern is the possibility that patients with severe liver disease may have neurologic and behavioral signs of Mn neurotoxicity resulting from failure to excrete Mn in bile.[794] Mn deposition in the globus pallidus during liver failure results in T_1-weighted magnetic resonance signal hypersensitivity. By causing deficits in neurotransmitter production, Mn ions may be partially responsible for symptoms of postsystemic hepatic encephalopathy. Deposition of Mn in the brain has been demonstrated in children with biliary atresia[795] and in adult cirrhotic patients.[796]

Patients receiving Mn intravenously during TPN, especially those with cholestasis, have shown evidence of Mn retention and deposition in the midbrain and brain stem. Typical symptoms include a Parkinsonian-like tremor and abnormalities of gait.[797] Children have been observed to accumulate Mn in the globus pallidus and brain stem, but with nonspecific symptoms.[798] A study in adults that compared the effects of increasing doses of Mn in patients receiving home parenteral nutrition showed a good correlation between blood Mn, magnetic resonance imaging intensity, and T_1 values in the globus pallidus.[799] A dose of 55 μg/day revealed no abnormalities on magnetic resonance imaging, and blood Mn remained within the reference interval.

In a study of 30 patients who received long-term home IVN, concentrations of Mn were increased in whole blood (>11.6 μg/L, 210 nmol/L) in 26 patients, and in plasma (>4 μg/L; 23 nmol/L) in 23 patients. No patients had signs of neurologic disease. In a control group of patients with cholestatic disease, but who were not receiving IVN, whole blood Mn was within the reference interval.[800] This suggests that cholestasis alone will not lead to increased blood Mn, and the main reason for high blood concentrations in patients on IVN is excess provision; however, this may be exacerbated by cholestasis. Infants (0–12 months) who require IVN are at particular risk because of immature hepatic function. In a group of 57 children who received IVN, 11 had both cholestasis and increased blood Mn, and 1 had a movement disorder. Four of these 11 patients died, and whole blood Mn was found to be very high (34–101 μg/L; 615–1840 nmol/L) among the 7 survivors. Mn supplements were reduced or withdrawn, and after 4 months, blood Mn had declined to 35 μg/L (643 nmol/L). During the same period, serum bilirubin declined significantly.[564] The long-term outcome of Mn deposition was investigated in two children on long-term TPN who initially had abnormalities on magnetic resonance imaging and increased whole blood Mn. After reduction of Mn input, they were followed for a 3-year period with improvement in the abnormalities seen on magnetic resonance imaging and a fall in whole blood Mn concentrations. No neurologic signs were found, and the children developed normally thereafter.[801] It is now recommended that only 1 μg/kg of Mn should be administered during TPN in infants[564] and no more than 55 to 110 μg/day in adults.[802]

All patients who require prolonged IVN, especially those who have cholestasis, should be monitored for evidence of Mn retention. However, the data in the literature are conflicting about the method for assessing Mn stores in humans as a definitive biomarker of Mn exposure or in whom induced neurotoxicity has yet to be identified. The biomonitoring of Mn relies on the analysis of whole blood Mn concentrations, which are highly variable among the human population and are not strictly correlated with Mn-induced neurotoxicity. Alterations in dopaminergic and catecholaminergic metabolism have been studied as predictive biomarkers of Mn-induced neurotoxicity. Because of these limitations, various approaches for biomonitoring Mn exposure and neurotoxic risk need to be assessed, particularly if patients are on TPN for longer than 30 days.[803]

Laboratory Assessment of Status. It is necessary to balance the need for adequate Mn nutrition against potential risk from toxicity.[793] This necessitates monitoring of Mn status in at-risk patients. Whole blood Mn concentrations are not responsive to dietary depletion, but measurements of serum Mn, lymphocyte Mn SOD activity, and blood arginase are potentially useful when possible nutritional depletion is assessed, although these are rarely performed in clinical practice. Whole blood Mn and serum Mn in combination with brain magnetic resonance imaging scans and neurologic assessment are used to detect excessive exposure. Mn in whole blood and plasma or serum can be determined by standard graphite furnace AAS (GFAAS)[804] or by ICP-MS.[805]

Plastic cannulas should be used for phlebotomy, and hemolysis should be prevented during sample separation. Whole blood has approximately 10 times as much Mn as plasma or serum, and is not as affected by contamination from steel needles during sample collection.

Whole blood values are used to indicate long-term exposure related to the RBC cycle, whereas plasma concentrations, although lower, will increase in response to acute exposure typical of changes after absorption and/or infusion.

Reference Intervals. The reference interval for serum Mn is 0.5 to 1.3 μg/L (9–24 nmol/L). The reference interval for whole blood Mn is 5 to 15 μg/L (90–270 nmol/L). Increases in serum Mn to more than 1.6 μg/L (>30 nmol/L) or in blood Mn to more than 20 μg/L (>360 nmol/L) are indices of Mn retention. For more information, refer to the Appendix on Reference Intervals. Laboratories should verify that these ranges are appropriate for use in their own settings.

Molybdenum

The essential need for Mo by animals and humans is based on its incorporation into metalloenzymes. In plants, Mo is part of the nitrogen fixation and nitrate assimilation process, and therefore, is fundamental to life. The functional chemical species is the MoO_4^{2-} ion, and its production in the environment is the rate-limiting factor.[806]

Chemistry. Molybdenum (atomic number 42, atomic weight 96.4) is a metal in the second transition series. The element can have a number of oxidation states, but the most stable in biological systems is Mo^{6+} as found in MoO_4^{2-}. Mo has the highest atomic number of the essential trace metals. A close parallel can be seen between Mo, tungsten, and V chemistry. Molybdenum enzymes are ecologically vital, facilitating important carbon, nitrogen, and sulfur cycles.[548]

Dietary Sources. Legumes, such as peas, lentils, and beans, are good sources of Mo, along with grains and nuts, whereas meats, fruits, and many vegetables are relatively poor sources. Average dietary intake for US adults is 76 to 109 μg/day.

Absorption, Transport, Metabolism, and Excretion. Mo is efficiently absorbed over a wide range of dietary intakes, mainly as MoO_4^{2-}, although competitive inhibition of absorption by sulfate reduces intestinal uptake. Concentrations in whole blood are approximately 1.0 μg/L (10 nmol/L), and up to 90% or more of Mo in whole blood is bound to RBC proteins. Transport of small amounts in blood plasma may involve α_2-macroglobulin. Urine output directly reflects the dietary intake of Mo, with stable isotope studies at high and low concentrations of intake indicating renal homeostatic regulation.[807,808]

Functions. Several important mammalian enzymes, such as sulfite oxidase, xanthine dehydrogenase, and aldehyde oxidase, require Mo as a cofactor.[809] This organic component is a molybdopterin complex. Sulfite oxidase is probably the most important enzyme in relation to human health. This enzyme catalyzes the last step in the degradation of sulfur amino acids, oxidizing sulfite to sulfate and transferring electrons to cytochrome c. Xanthine dehydrogenase and aldehyde oxidase hydroxylate numerous heterocyclic substances, such as purines, pteridines, and others.[810,811]

Requirements and Reference Nutrient Intakes. The RDA for Mo has been set at 45 μg/day for adults, which is below the estimated average dietary intake. In children up to 1 year, an AI is between 2 and 3 μg/day, whereas between 1 and 13 years, the RDA varies between 17 and 34 μg/day. In pregnancy and during lactation, 50 μg/day is recommended.[12] In Europe, the recommended supplementation during TPN is 10 to 25 μg/day.

Deficiency. Mo deficiency has not been observed in healthy people consuming a normal diet. A single case report described a patient who received prolonged parenteral nutrition during treatment for severe Crohn's disease who developed an intolerance to intravenous amino acids, especially L-methionine.[812] Clinical signs included tachycardia, visual defects, neurologic irritability, and eventually coma. Symptoms improved on discontinuation of amino acid infusion. Biochemical abnormalities included high plasma methionine and low plasma uric acid concentrations. Increased urinary sulfite and thiosulfate, and other abnormalities of urinary sulfur output were reported, with low excretion of uric acid and xanthine metabolites, suggesting defects in sulfite oxidase and xanthine oxidase. Treatment with ammonium MoO_4^{2-} (300 μg/day) improved the clinical and biochemical abnormalities.

Lack of additional reports of this nature suggests that for most patients, sufficient Mo is present as a contaminant in TPN fluids. Nonetheless, it is now common to include a small amount of Mo (19 μg/day; 0.2 μmol/day) in trace element additive mixtures.

Rare recessive inherited diseases result from defects in the biosynthesis of the Mo cofactor, and in most cases, they lead to early childhood death. First symptoms include failure to thrive and seizures; in later stages, lens dislocations are noted, together with cerebral atrophy. Disease-causing mutations have been located, and the possibility of gene therapy is being investigated.[813,814]

Biochemical diagnosis is made by detection of excess sulfite in urine using the Merckoquant Sulfite Dipstick test (Merck KGaA, Darmstadt, Germany).[815] Samples should not be evaluated until at least 10 days after birth and should be tested within 10 minutes of collection. Mo cofactor deficiency can also be identified by finding a low plasma uric acid. Specialized centers offer biochemical prenatal diagnosis on chorionic villous samples.[811]

Toxicity. Mo compounds have low toxicity in humans. Reports have described increased blood uric acid in those with occupational exposure and in Armenian populations that have an abnormally high dietary intake (10–15 mg/day). A single report of acute toxicity from self-administration of 300 to 800 μg/day with a cumulative total of 13.5 mg over 18 days led to acute psychosis and seizures,[816] but it is inconsistent with another study in healthy men who were given as much as 1500 μg/day for 24 days, with no adverse effects reported.[807]

Excess Mo intake induces Cu deficiency in ruminants by blocking absorption through formation of an insoluble thiomolybdate-Cu complex. This is the basis for the use of ammonium MoO_4^{2-} in the management of Wilson disease.[817] Speculation suggests that blockade of Cu absorption using MoO_4^{2-} may influence new blood vessel formation (angiogenesis) during tumor growth.[818]

Laboratory Assessment of Status. Whole blood and serum or plasma Mo concentrations are too low to be used to detect deficiency. However, urinary output is responsive to increases or decreases in input. Measuring urate or sulfite in the urine is the most valuable means of confirming Mo cofactor disorder or possible Mo deficiency by detecting changes in sulfur and purine metabolism. Until recently, only NAA had sufficient sensitivity to measure Mo in biological samples.[819] With the availability of ICP-MS, studies using stable Mo isotopes are now possible. This technique has been used to investigate absorption and excretion of Mo during depletion and repletion studies.[807]

Reference Intervals. Approximately 0.5 μg/L (5 nmol/L) is present in plasma or serum, together with approximately 1 μg/L (10 nmol/L) in whole blood using NAA.[819] Urine Mo concentrations determined by ICP-MS vary from 40 to 60 μg/L (416–625 nmol/day), dependent upon recent dietary intake.[820] For more information, refer to the Appendix on Reference Intervals. Laboratories should verify that these ranges are appropriate for use in their own settings.

Selenium

Selenium is a constituent of the enzyme GSHP and is considered an essential element for humans; it is believed to be closely associated with vitamin E in its functions.

Chemistry. Selenium (atomic number 34, atomic weight 78.96) is a nonmetal that has several chemical forms and valences. Se is in group VI of the periodic table; therefore, it has a bioinorganic chemistry that is related to sulfur.[548,821] The most important biologically active compounds contain selenocysteine, where Se is substituted for sulfur in cysteine. Considered to be the twenty-first amino acid, selenocysteine is incorporated into proteins by the specific codon UGA, which was previously believed to be solely a stop codon.[822] Selenomethionine is synthesized by plants but not in animals or humans. Because it is biologically identical to methionine and shares the same metabolic pathways, selenomethionine is nonspecifically incorporated into the general protein pool and is present in major proteins such as albumin and Hb. Se in selenomethionine makes up approximately one-half of the total dietary intake and is made available for selenocysteine synthesis when the methionine pathways catabolize selenomethionine. Ingested Se compounds, selenate, selenite, selenocysteine, and selenomethionine, are metabolized largely via selenide, which may be associated with a chaperone protein before being converted to selenophosphate, which is an important precursor in the synthesis of selenocysteine proteins (Fig. 37.27).[821,823]

Dietary Sources. Selenium enters the food chain mainly as selenomethionine from plants that take the element up from the soil but do not appear to use it. The soil content of Se is highly variable and can be low in volcanic soils when soluble salts are leached out by ground water. Soils in parts of China and New Zealand are particularly low in Se. Acid soils, where insoluble Se complexes can be formed with Fe and aluminum occur in some parts of Europe, resulting in low available soil Se. The geographic source of plant and animal foodstuffs determines the amount of dietary intake. In the United States and Canada, wheat and other cereal products are a good source of Se. Average intakes in North America are 93 μg/day in women and 134 μg/day in men, whereas in Europe, average dietary intake is approximately 40 μg/day.[821] Intakes in China are as low as 11 μg/day and in New Zealand 28 μg/day, but importation of high Se wheat may have improved intakes recently.[824]

Absorption, Transport, Metabolism, and Excretion. Intestinal absorption of various dietary forms of Se is efficient but is not regulated. The inorganic salts selenite and selenate used as dietary supplements and in food fortification are almost completely absorbed, but much of the selenate ion is rapidly excreted in urine.[825] Se from inorganic salts is more rapidly incorporated into GSHP and other selenoproteins than Se from organic sources containing selenomethionine. However, Se-enriched yeast containing the organic forms is considered less toxic and is widely used as a dietary supplement.[12]

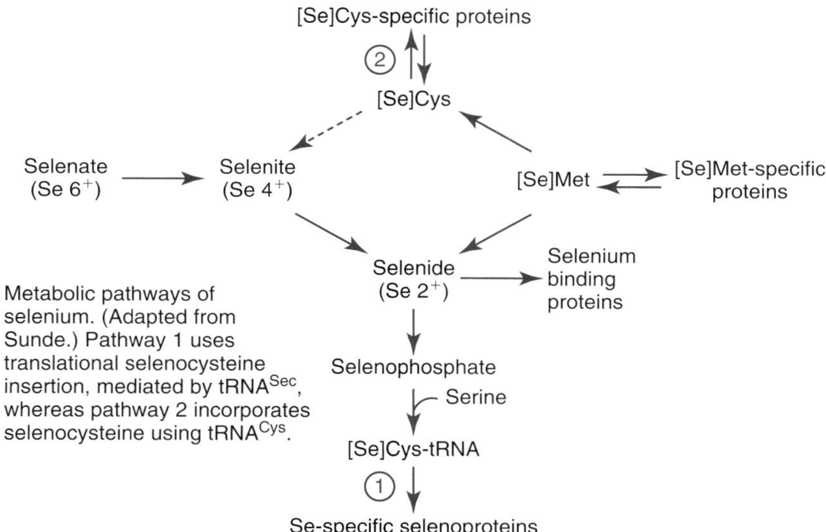

FIGURE 37.27 Metabolic Pathways of Selenium.

Contradictory data have indicated that increased Se concentration is correlated with the amount of selenomethionine administered but not the selenite, and neither GSHP activity nor selenoprotein P concentration respond to Se supplementation.[826] Also, plasma Se seems to reflect the selenomethionine, and Se in the form of selenomethionine was much better absorbed than selenite. This would suggest that a yeast complex is the better supplement. This study also suggested that a Se intake greater than 800 μg/day for at least 16 weeks was safe because no adverse events were reported.[826]

Whole body Se is approximately 15 mg, as estimated by direct tissue analysis and radioisotope techniques, with the tissue concentration of Se being highest in the kidney and the liver, followed by the other organs. Radioisotope-labeled Se accumulates initially in the liver, kidneys, and lungs. Se present in some selenocysteine proteins appears to be a functional reserve. When dietary Se is limited, synthesis of GSHPx-1 is downregulated, making Se available for synthesis of other proteins.[827]

The concentrations of Se in whole blood and in plasma and/or serum are related to dietary intake. Approximately 50% to 60% of total plasma Se is present as the protein selenoprotein P, a highly basic protein that has multiple histidine residues and approximately 10 atoms of Se per molecule. Approximately 30% of plasma Se is present as GSHPx-3; the remainder is incorporated into albumin as selenomethionine.[828]

Urinary output of Se is the major route of excretion and reflects recent dietary intake. The concentrations excreted vary widely, ranging from less than 20 μg/L (0.25 μmol/L) to more than 1000 μg/L (12.7 μmol/L), depending on intake and the geographic origins of the food, which reflects the Se content of soil.[824,829]

Functions. More than 30 biologically active selenocysteine-containing proteins have been identified; more than 15 have been purified, and their biological functions have been investigated.[823,830] Some of these are discussed in the following.

Glutathione Peroxidase. This enzyme has four isoforms: GSHPx-1 in RBC cytosol, GSHPx-2 in gastrointestinal mucosa, blood plasma GSHPx-3, and GSHPx-4 located in the cell membrane phospholipids. These enzymes use the reducing power of glutathione to remove an O_2 atom from H_2O_2 and lipid hydroperoxides. They may also be involved in regulation and formation of arachidonic metabolites derived from hydroperoxides.[831]

Iodothyronine Deiodinase. Type I (Dio1), II (Dio2), and III (Dio3) isoforms of this enzyme are responsible for conversion of the precursor hormone T_4 to the active hormone T_3. Type I, thyroxine-5-deiodinase, is located in the thyroid, liver, kidney, and muscle, and is responsible for more than 90% of plasma T_3 production. Pituitary, brain, and brown adipose tissue contain the type II and III deiodinases.[823,830]

Thioredoxin Reductases. Three isoforms catalyze the NADPH-dependent reduction of thioredoxin and are important in maintaining the intracellular redox state.

Selenophosphate Synthetase. This enzyme is required for the intracellular synthesis of selenoproteins via a monoselenium phosphate intermediate.

Selenoprotein P. This protein is the major Se-containing protein in blood plasma; it may be a transport protein for the element, and it has an antioxidant function.[832]

Other Selenoproteins. These include selenoprotein tungsten, sulfur, nitrogen, and a 15-kDa selenoprotein (SEP15), which all have varying functions, including anti-inflammatory effects, antiapoptotic roles linked to glucose metabolism and insulin sensitivity, calcium mobilization for muscle development, and others.[821,823]

Requirements and Reference Nutrient Intakes. It is proposed that the RDA for Se should be set at 55 μg/day for adults.[12] On this basis, dietary surveys in North America do not indicate that Se deficiency is likely in the general population, and moreover, surveys estimate that 50% of Americans take dietary supplements. However, in Europe, intakes are suboptimal, and supplementation may be warranted.[821]

Intravenous Supply. Uncertainty continues about the most appropriate intake, but given the previous figures for dietary requirement, intravenous requirement is unlikely to be less than 40 μg/day and in many adult patients, especially the more seriously ill, it may be 100 μg/day or more. In most patients who receive parenteral nutrition at home or after surgery, 60 to 100 μg/day will meet their requirements. Patients who commence parenteral nutrition already depleted in Se may require more. Critically ill patients or those with severe burns may have higher requirements. There is good evidence that up to 400 μg/day is beneficial in burn patients, but the evidence is inconclusive regarding the benefit of high-dose Se in severe sepsis.[833]

Deficiency. The role of Se in human medicine has been extensively reviewed.[777,821,834] Animal studies in the 1950s demonstrated the nutritionally beneficial effects of Se by showing that there was Se-responsive liver necrosis in vitamin E–deficient rats. Important Se-dependent diseases are seen in farm animals, such as white muscle disease in sheep and cattle, and myopathy of cardiac and skeletal muscle in lambs and calves. In these animals, some cause of oxidative stress, such as increased physical activity or vitamin E deficiency, together with dietary Se deficiency, is required to elicit the disease.

Severe Deficiency. Symptomatic Se deficiency has been well characterized in Keshan disease, and nutritional depletion in hospital patients.

Keshan Disease. Conclusive evidence of a role for Se in human nutrition came with publication of the results of large-scale trials in China that showed the protective effects of Se supplementation in children and young adults who experienced endemic cardiomyopathy. Increased virulence of the Coxsackie virus as a result of Se deficiency has been implicated as a cause of the myocarditis. This was observed in areas of the country (Keshan region) with low soil Se concentrations.[835]

Kashin-Beck Disease. A type of severe arthritis is described in parts of China and neighboring areas of Russia where soil Se is particularly low. Se supplementation in Se-deficient areas has been shown to prevent this disease. However, Se supplementation in some areas showed no significant effect, proving that deficiency of Se may not be the dominant cause in Kashin-Beck disease; other unidentified factors may be involved.[836]

Nutritional Depletion in Hospital Patients. Selenium was one of the last essential trace elements to be accepted as nutritionally important, with more attention previously given to its potential toxicity. Initially, inadequate Se provision in specialized diets was used to treat inborn errors,[837] and during long-term parenteral nutrition[838] and it led to cases of deficiency. Symptomatic cases continue to be reported, although the need for Se supplementation with monitoring during nutritional support is now well established.[833] Symptoms of severe deficiency include muscle weakness.[839] Cases involving cardiomyopathy, which is usually fatal and resembles Keshan disease,[840] and macrocytosis and pseudo-albinism in children,[841] have been described.

Marginal Deficiencies. Marginal Se deficiencies have been reported to have effects on thyroid function, immune function, fertility, mood, inflammatory conditions, cardiovascular disease, viral virulence, type 2 diabetes mellitus, and have implications for cancer chemoprevention.

Thyroid Function. Selenium and other trace elements are necessary for normal thyroid function because the important deiodinase enzymes are selenoproteins.[777] Three children with biochemical and clinical signs of hypothyroidism were successfully treated with oral Se therapy.[842] Although the deiodinases are not believed to be significantly affected in marginal Se depletion, it has been observed that endemic goiter in Sri Lanka, which is resistant to iodine supplementation, occurs in areas with low soil Se.[843] Similarly, endemic thyroid disease in Zaire may be related to the combination of I and Se depletion. Care must be taken because the stimulation of thyroid hormone metabolism may induce hypothyroidism.

The low T_3 syndrome observed after major trauma may also be related to changes in Se status affecting the activity of iodothyronine deiodinase, with Se supplements reversing most of the biochemical abnormalities found in thyroid function tests.[844]

However, the exact role of Se in thyroid function continues to be controversial. A study of a New Zealand population with both marginal Se status and mild I deficiency showed that additional Se improved GSHP activity but not the thyroid hormone status of older New Zealanders.[845] Also, no significant treatment effects were found for TSH, free T_3, free T_4, or the ratio of T_3 to T_4. It was concluded that no synergistic action of Se and I occurs. A study in the United Kingdom reached a similar conclusion—that Se supplementation had no effect on thyroid status.[846]

Immune Function. Deficiency of Se is accompanied by loss of immunocompetence, and this is related to the reduction of selenoproteins in the liver, spleen, and lymph nodes. Both cell-mediated immunity and B-cell function are impaired.[821]

Considerable Se losses in wound exudates after severe burns have been recorded, and supplementation with a mixture of Se, Zn, and Cu leads to a reduction in respiratory infection.[847] Supplementation, even in apparently Se-adequate individuals, has some immune function stimulatory effects, including improvement in natural killer cell activity and increases in interleukin-2 receptor expression.[821,834] It has been speculated that the increased infection rates in patients with AIDS may be related to Se depletion, and this may even influence the progression from HIV positivity to the AIDS syndrome.[848]

It has been suggested that antioxidant nutrient deficiencies may hasten the progression of HIV disease by impairing antioxidant defenses; it was shown that well-nourished subjects are able to mount a compensatory antioxidant response to HIV infection.[849] However, the role of Se in particular was equivocal in that among 913 HIV-infected pregnant women from Tanzania, Se supplements (selenomethionine) given during and after pregnancy did not improve HIV disease progression, although it reduced the risk of mortality in children older than 6 weeks.[850]

Fertility and Reproduction. Adequate Se supply is necessary for successful reproduction in a variety of farm animals. Various studies have looked at the situation in humans. Male fertility could be affected by Se depletion in so far as it is necessary for testosterone synthesis and for maintenance of sperm viability.[821,834]

Mood. The brain is reportedly prioritized with regards to supply of Se during dietary depletion and/or repletion studies in animals, and the turnover of neurotransmitters is altered. This led to extensive studies on the role of Se and other antioxidants in senility of the older adults, in epilepsy in children, and in Alzheimer disease. Marginal Se depletion has been associated with anxiety, confusion, and hostility, and improvements have been claimed after supplementation.[821,834]

Inflammatory Conditions. Many conditions associated with inflammation and increased oxidative stress could be influenced by Se status. Positive effects from supplementation studies in arthritis and in pancreatitis have been reported. Low serum Se values are found in asthma, and some limited clinical trial studies have shown benefits from supplementation.[821,834] In a trial in patients in intensive care with SIRS, high-dose Se supplements over 9 days were associated with reduced mortality in the most severely ill.[851] However, these results have not been confirmed in all studies[852]; hence, definitive recommendations regarding high-dose supplements in intensive care cannot yet be made.[853]

Cardiovascular Disease. The protective role of Se against cardiovascular disease has been extensively investigated, but with no conclusive findings.[821,834] The low soil Se concentration in Finland resulted in low Se content in locally grown food. This, together with concerns about the high incidence of coronary disease in parts of the country, led to Se fortification of agricultural fertilizers. Although an impressive decline in coronary disease mortality was found between 1972 and 1992, the benefits have been linked primarily to other major diet and lifestyle changes.[854]

Viral Virulence. It is now considered possible that an unusually virulent strain of the Coxsackie virus is part of the cause of cardiomyopathy in Se-depleted regions of China. This is consistent with marked seasonal variations in the incidence of the disease.[835]

It is known that nutritional depletion will impair immune responses and will increase the lethality of viruses and other infectious agents. A series of experimental studies on mice have shown that a nonlethal form of Coxsackie B (CVB 3/O) converted to a virulent strain when inoculated into Se-deficient mice.[855] Inoculation of Se-adequate mice with the mutated virus then caused myocarditis. Sequencing of DNA from the altered virus showed that six nucleotide changes corresponded to nucleotide sequences in the genome of a virulent strain of the virus. Further evidence came from experiments with GSPHx knockout mice. More than half of these mice infected with the nonlethal CVB/3O virus developed myocarditis, but none of the wild-type controls were affected. The virus recovered from these affected mice showed genome changes similar to those seen in virulent strains of the virus. It is believed that the Se-deficient host altered the viral pathogen, probably involving oxidative stress in the tissue of depleted animals. Additional animal studies have demonstrated that a mild strain of influenza virus exhibits increased virulence when given to Se-deficient mice.[856]

It is speculated that a similar process occurs in regions of the world, such as parts of Africa, where the human population has depletions of Se and other micronutrients, and is intermittently exposed to viral disease, but no direct evidence has been forthcoming. However, an epidemic of optic and peripheral neuropathy in Cuba that affected more than 50,000 individuals was shown to be associated with deficiencies of several micronutrients, including Se.[857] Supplementation of the population with a multicomponent micronutrient mixture coincided with subsidence of the disease.

Cancer Chemoprevention. Although it is not primarily a nutritional issue, interest in the role of Se supplementation in the prevention of certain types of cancer continues. Experimental work on animals shows that chemical carcinogenesis is modified by Se.[821] Epidemiologic surveys have also found a link between cancer incidence and soil Se content, suggesting a higher incidence of certain cancers in individuals with a low Se intake.[858] Large-scale trials in China, conducted on more than 130,000 individuals, compared one township (n = 20,847) at high risk for viral hepatitis B and liver cancer with four control townships in the same area. The high-risk population received Se-enriched table salt, and in an 8-year follow-up, the average incidence of liver cancer was reduced by 35%. No reduction in incidence was seen in control populations. Studies on 226 people with chronic hepatitis B found that a controlled trial of Se-enriched yeast reduced the development of liver cancer during a 2-year follow-up.[859]

For some years, it was hoped that Se supplementation above the minimum dietary requirement might have a role in cancer prevention, particularly in relation to prostatic cancer.[577] This was based essentially on secondary analyses of randomized controlled trials,[858,860] and supportive epidemiologic and preclinical data indicated the potential of Se and vitamin E for preventing prostate cancer and other cancers (eg, lung, colorectal). The mechanism was not established, but in Se-adequate subjects, it was suggested that excess Se may produce a low MW methylated Se compound that has chemopreventive properties. However, the large Se and vitamin E cancer prevention study known as the Selenium and Vitamin E Cancer Prevention Trial (SELECT) concluded that Se or vitamin E, alone or in combination at the doses and formulations used, did not prevent prostate cancer in this population of relatively healthy men.[861]

Toxicity. Areas of China and the United States have large amounts of Se in the soil, and locally produced food contains excess Se. Clinical signs of selenosis include garlic odor on the breath, hair loss, nail damage, nervous system and skin disorders, poor dental health, and paralysis in extreme cases.[862] The tolerable upper limit has been set at 400 μg/day for adults and less than 280 μg/day for children.[12] Cases of toxicity from self-administered dosages have been reported. Because of a manufacturing error, 13 individuals taking supplements containing 27.3 mg per tablet (27,300 μg) showed clinically significant Se toxicity that resulted in selenosis symptoms, including nausea, abdominal pain, diarrhea, peripheral neuropathy, fatigue, irritability, and hair and nail changes.[863]

Symptoms of Se toxicity vary among individuals and are dependent on a number of factors, such as dose, type, and form of Se ingested, and length of time the product was used. Symptoms of Se poisoning can include significant hair loss, muscle cramps, nausea, vomiting, diarrhea, joint pain, fatigue, fingernail changes, and blistering skin. Patients have reported that symptoms typically occur within 5 to 10 days after daily ingestion of these supplements begins. After use of the product is discontinued, symptoms of Se toxicity may last for several weeks, but they should improve eventually without treatment for the poisoning. Nail changes are the most common sign of long-term Se poisoning.[864] The nails become brittle, and white spots and longitudinal streaks appear on the surface. Fragile nails and similar changes obviously are not specific for selenosis; other causes include fungal infection, psoriasis, and arsenic exposure. As yet, no proven antidote for Se poisoning is known.

Laboratory Assessment of Status. Early animal studies and human population surveys used whole blood as the main indicator of Se status, but plasma or serum concentrations are now more commonly measured. Samples can be analyzed using a fluorometric method after acid digestion.[865] The more convenient GFAAS assay[866] and ICP-MS are the preferred procedures in routine laboratories.[867]

The main components of plasma Se are extracellular GSHPx-3 and selenoprotein P. RBC GSPHx-1 and plasma GSPHx-3 are assayed by enzymatic methods using a variety of peroxide substrates, with tertiary-butyl peroxide being a commonly used substrate because it is not as affected by catalase as is H_2O_2. The values obtained are dependent on the substrate used and the reaction conditions. During Se supplementation studies, the plateau reached in plasma GSPHx-3 activity has been used to assess minimum dietary requirements.[868-870]

The effects of different forms of inorganic and organic Se supplementation on GSPHx activity in blood lymphocytes, granulocytes, platelets, and erythrocytes were described in a trial on 45 human volunteers.[871] Some changes were acute and transient, whereas cytosolic GSHPx activity (GSHPx-1) increased gradually in both treatment groups over 28 days. The time course for development of deficiency and repletion of enzyme activity has been studied in patients who received TPN at home.[872] After 1 year on TPN without Se supplements, all patients had low plasma Se and RBC GSHPx, and cellular metabolism of exogenous H_2O_2 was impaired. With replacement of Se as selenious acid, a rapid increase in GSHPx-3 was seen within the first 24 hours, and normal concentrations were reached within 1 to 2 weeks. Platelet GSHPx also returned to normal in 1 to 2 weeks, whereas polymorph GSHPx was more variable but normalized in approximately 3 weeks. RBC GSHPx took 3 to 4 months to recover, consistent with the need for formation of these cells in the presence of Se.

The major Se-containing plasma protein selenoprotein P can be determined by immunologic methods.[873] The production of monoclonal antibodies to selenoprotein P has been described and used to study the structure and function of the protein and to quantify it.[874] It is also possible to separate selenoprotein P from other plasma proteins by heparin affinity chromatography followed by GFAAS Se analysis.[828] Selenoprotein P concentration in plasma responds rapidly to supplementation and has been used in nutritional studies of Chinese populations to confirm the adequacy of intake.[875]

Plasma selenoprotein P, plasma GSPHx-3, and total plasma Se concentration are all lowered by the acute-phase response to injury or infection.[876] This effect should be considered when plasma Se values are interpreted in postoperative patients or those with infection or inflammatory disease. Hair and nail Se analysis can be useful as a measure of long-term dietary Se intake. Because Se is a sulfur analog, it is incorporated into the sulfur-rich keratin of hair and nails. One study showed a correlation between toenail Se, blood Se, and dietary intake.[877] In a study of a 10-year-old child receiving TPN who developed Se-responsive muscle weakness, hair analysis was used to help assess Se dosage.[878] An analytical method using microwave-assisted acid digestion of hair and nails, followed by GFAAS Se analysis, was described.[879] In a small study using this procedure, values for hair and nail Se in healthy people in the United Kingdom were found to be 0.32 to 0.76 μg/g (n = 25) and 0.17 to 0.66 μg/g (n = 27), respectively. However, for population studies, use of Se-containing hair preparations will affect hair Se results, and this would have to be carefully assessed and controlled.

Urine Se output is mainly a reflection of recent dietary input and has not been extensively used in population surveys.[829]

In summary, many possible markers for Se status have been identified. In practice, measurement of plasma Se or GSHPx provides a good estimate of status as well as the adequacy of recent intake in particular, provided that these values are interpreted with knowledge of changes in the acute-phase response. For a better index of long-term intake, platelet, RBC, or neutrophil GSHPx, or hair or nail Se can also be measured. The value of various biological parameters in assessing Se status has been systematically reviewed; these parameters were shown to change in response to Se treatment, although no single parameter was regarded as optimal.[880]

Reference Intervals. The reference interval for Se in whole blood, plasma or serum, hair, and nails should be established locally, because these indices are affected by dietary Se intake. Plasma Se adult values are in the interval 63 to 160 μg/L (0.8–2.0 μmol/L). Values less than 40 μg/L (0.5 μmol/L) indicate probable Se depletion.

Values in children are lower, and in the United Kingdom are as follows: 16 to 71 μg/L (0.2–0.9 μmol/L) for those younger than 2 years old; 40 to 103 μg/L (0.5–1.3 μmol/L) for 2 to 4 year olds; and 55 to 134 μg/L (0.7–1.7 μmol/L) for 4 to 16 year olds.[881] Values of less than 8 μg/L (0.1 μmol/L) in neonates are strongly suggestive of Se depletion. Increased plasma values are found in suspected Se toxicity, and results of more than 5 μmol/L (400 μg/L) are an indication of excess intake.

In cases of toxicity (selenosis), serum concentrations were as high as 1400 μg/L (17.7 μmol/L) with no obvious effects, and acute fatal poisonings were seen with Se up to 30,000 μg/L (380 μmol/L).[864] However, the nature of the Se compound is important, because most reports that describe acute Se poisoning involve ingestion of inorganic compounds such as selenious acid, which is found in gun-bluing agents, and fatalities that occur within the first day are associated with postmortem blood Se concentrations greater than 1400 μg/L (17.7 μmol/L). In an earlier study of patients with selenosis from eating vegetables containing grossly elevated Se contents, blood concentrations were 1300 to 7500 μg/L (16.5–95 μmol/L).[882]

RBC GSHPx-1 activity in adults varies from 13 to 25 U/g Hb, whereas values in children are slightly lower.[881] The use of local age-related reference intervals is recommended. For more information, refer to the Appendix on Reference Intervals. Laboratories should verify that these ranges are appropriate for use in their own settings.

Zinc

The discovery of a variety of Zn-related clinical disorders has directly demonstrated the importance of Zn in human nutrition. It is second to Fe as the most abundant trace element in the body.

Chemistry. Zinc (atomic number 30, atomic weight 65.37) is at the end of the first transition series. Zn^{2+}, with a filled 3d electron shell, is a particularly stable ion. The bioinorganic chemical features of Zn, which underlie the diverse biological functions of this trace metal, include its relatively high abundance compared with other trace elements.[548] Zn has fast ligand exchange kinetics and flexible coordination geometry, and it is a good electron acceptor (strong Lewis acid) with no redox reactions. It has been hypothesized that Zn ions, present in the cytoplasm at 10^{-11} moles and in equilibrium with numerous Zn metalloenzymes and transcription factors, can act as a "master hormone," particularly in relation to cell division and growth.[548] No naturally colored Zn complexes have been identified; this may have delayed recognition of the biological importance of Zn until suitable atomic spectroscopic methods were developed that could be applied to biological samples and used as probes to identify and study metalloproteins.

Dietary Sources. Zn is widely distributed in food mainly bound to proteins. The bioavailability of dietary Zn is dependent on the digestion of these proteins to release Zn and allow it to bind to peptides, amino acids, phosphate, and other ligands within the intestinal tract. The most available dietary sources of Zn are red meat and fish, whereas white meat and flesh from young animals provide less Zn. Wheat germ and whole bran are good sources, but their Zn content is reduced by milling and food processing. The median intake for men in the United States is approximately 14 mg/day, and for women, it is 9 mg/day.[77]

The intake distribution from various foods showed that intake was potentially poor in those older than 60 years because of a diet deficient in legumes and meat.

Absorption, Transport, Metabolism, and Excretion. The net intestinal uptake of Zn is regulated by control of absorption efficiency in the face of variable dietary Zn input and varies from 20% to 50% of the dietary content. At an intake of 12.2 mg/day, fractional absorption was 26%, but at the low intake of 0.23 mg/day, this increased to 100%. These and other measurements were made on 12 male volunteers using a stable ^{67}Zn tracer to assess Zn homeostasis and plasma Zn kinetics.[883] Estimates of Zn absorption have also been compared using four different stable isotope techniques.[884] It was concluded that a double isotopic tracer ratio method is accurate and is recommended as a practicable procedure. When this method was used, the fraction of dietary Zn absorbed was equivalent to 30 ± 10%. Fine control of net absorption is attained by secretion of endogenous Zn into the intestinal lumen from pancreatic fluid and other intestinal fluids.[559] Such losses range from less than 1 mg/day on a low Zn diet to more than 5 mg/day on a Zn-rich diet. The ability to conserve dietary Zn by limiting intestinal loss can allow a positive metabolic balance, even at low dietary Zn intakes. Interaction with other dietary constituents, such as phytate, calcium, and Fe, reduces the net absorption of Zn significantly, so that diets high in phytate and calcium reduce the growth rate of young rats. In essence, the greater the intake, the greater the overall excretions, but with increasing overall retention.[559]

New insights into mammalian Zn metabolism have been acquired through the identification and characterization of Zn transporters. These proteins all have transmembrane domains and are encoded by two solute-linked carrier (SLC) gene families: *ZnT (SLC30)* and *ZIP (SLC39)*. At least 9 ZnT and 15 ZIP transporters are present in human cells. They appear to have opposite roles in cellular Zn homeostasis. ZnT transporters reduce intracellular Zn availability by promoting Zn efflux from cells or into intracellular vesicles; ZIP transporters increase intracellular Zn availability by promoting extracellular Zn uptake, and perhaps, vesicular Zn release into the cytoplasm. Both ZnT and ZIP transporter families exhibit unique tissue-specific expression, differential responsiveness to dietary Zn deficiency and excess, and differential responsiveness to physiologic stimuli via hormones and cytokines.[885]

A study of patients who underwent ileostomy confirmed regulated expression of plasma membrane Zn transporters in the human intestine and suggested that regulated control of Zn uptake is dependent on body status.[886] In human diets, leavening of bread and exposure of cereals to wet heat lower the phytate content, thus increasing Zn availability. Other factors, such as dietary fiber and a constituent of beans, also lower Zn intestinal absorption, but to a lesser extent.[559,887] Fe at supplemental dosages (up to 65 mg/day) may decrease Zn absorption, so that pregnant and lactating women taking Fe may require Zn supplementation.[888] The effects of Zn and Fe on their relative intestinal absorption have been reviewed.[889]

Absorbed Zn is transported to the liver by the portal circulation, where active incorporation into metalloenzymes and plasma proteins, such as albumin and α_2-macroglobulin, occurs. Blood plasma contains less than 1% of the total body content of Zn and lies within a narrow concentration interval (80–120 μg/dL; 12–18 μmol/L). Approximately 80% of plasma Zn is associated with albumin, and most of the rest is tightly bound to α_2-macroglobulin.[890] The Zn on albumin is in equilibrium with plasma amino acids (mostly histidine and cysteine), and this small (<1%) ultrafilterable fraction may be important in cellular uptake mechanisms (Fig. 37.28).[887]

The total adult body content of Zn is approximately 2 to 2.5 g, and the metal is present in the cells of all metabolically active tissues and organs. Approximately 55% of the total is found in muscle, and approximately 30% in bone.[559,887] The prostate, semen, and the retina have particularly high local concentrations of Zn. Almost all Zn in RBCs is present in the form of carbonic anhydrase, so that RBC Zn concentration is approximately 10 times higher than that in plasma. Hemolysates normally have approximately 50 μg/g Hb, and total leukocyte Zn is normally approximately 100 ± 25 μg/10^{10} cells.

Fecal excretion includes both unabsorbed dietary Zn and Zn resecreted into the gut. The total amount normally equals the total dietary intake and is on the order of 10 to 15 mg/day in healthy populations. In contrast, urine output of Zn is normally only approximately 0.5 mg/day (7.6 μmol/day), but this can increase markedly during catabolic illness. The release of intracellular contents from skeletal muscle has been established as the source of excess urinary Zn in the postoperative period, as assessed by a labeled Zn radiotracer. Two patients took an oral dose of 5 μCi radioactive ^{65}Zn about a month before elective surgery for total hip replacement, allowing incorporation of the tracer into skeletal muscle. Urine output of radioactive Zn, total Zn, and total nitrogen was measured before operation and daily for 3 weeks after surgery. A large increase in the excretion of all of these was observed, with peaks occurring at 10 days. Good correlation was noted between the radioactive Zn and total Zn in the urine of both patients, suggesting skeletal muscle as the source.[891] Urine Zn also increases more than threefold during short-term total starvation, as a result of release from skeletal muscle and excretion of ketone bodies.[892]

Dietary intakes of Zn are lower in older adults because of reduced energy requirements; it is not clear whether aging influences adaptive homeostatic mechanisms or how aging affects the function, expression, or gene regulatory responses

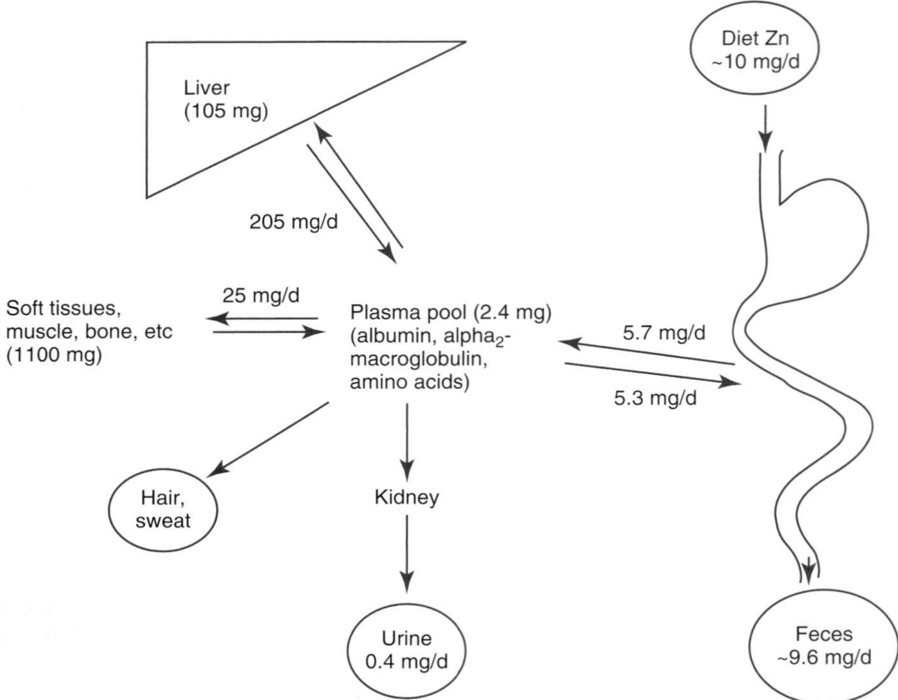

FIGURE 37.28 Summary of Zinc Metabolism.

to Zn of Zn transporters.[893] However, in a study of aged mice, Zn supplementation reversed some age-related thymic defects, indicating that this may be of considerable benefit in improving immune function and overall health in older adult populations.[894] Furthermore, advancing age, particularly very old age, is associated with an increase in the percentage of cells with short telomeres, resulting in cells that have a tendency toward premature apoptosis. These observations have been related to impaired production of Zn MT and possibly Zn deficiency, and therefore, are of significance as prognostic factors in age-related disease.[895]

Functions

General. More than 300 Zn metalloenzymes occur in all six categories of enzyme systems. Important examples in human tissue include carbonic anhydrase, alkaline phosphatase, RNA and DNA polymerases, thymidine kinase carboxypeptidases, and alcohol dehydrogenase.[896] The key roles of Zn in protein and nucleic acid synthesis explain the failure of growth and impaired wound healing observed in individuals with Zn deficiency. In some enzymes, such as Cu and Zn SOD, structural stability is ensured by Zn protein binding and the catalytic activity of the enzyme by the active Cu site. Classifications of Zn enzymes and their structure and mode of action have been detailed in various texts.[548,887] Proteins can form domains able to bind tetrahedral Zn atoms by coordination with histidine and cysteine to form folded structures that have become known as "Zn fingers." These biologically active molecules have important roles in gene expression by acting as DNA-binding transcription factors; they play a key role in developmental biology and in the regulation of steroid, thyroid, and other hormone synthesis.[897,898] Zn binding to the metal response factor MTF1 activates MT expression. This multifunctional, low MW protein (9000–10,000 Da) has a high content of cysteine and reversibly binds Zn. MT is important in intracellular Zn trafficking and helps to maintain intracellular Zn concentrations. Hepatic synthesis of MT is induced by interleukin-1, interleukin-6, and glucocorticoids in response to infection, trauma, and other stressors.[887,899]

Prostate Function. Secretion by the prostate of large amounts of Zn (resultant concentration 65.4–130.8 mg/L; 1–2 mmol/L) is required for the functioning of sperm, to maintain both vitality and an antibacterial environment.[900] The mechanism of this aspect of Zn function is regulation of motility through interaction of Zn^{2+} ions with semenogelin during semen coagulum formation at ejaculation and during liquefaction of the coagulum in the female reproductive tract.[901] However, the determination of Zn in seminal plasma does not discriminate on the basis of actual sperm fertility. Nevertheless, other studies have implicated seminal Zn with parameters of semen quality, in that decreased seminal Zn can be a risk factor for sperm abnormality and idiopathic male infertility; smokers in particular are susceptible to Zn deficiency in their seminal fluid.[902,903] These data suggest that poor Zn nutrition may be an important risk factor for low quality of sperm and idiopathic male infertility. Routine determination of Zn concentrations during infertility investigation is therefore recommended.

Seminal plasma Zn concentrations are virtually normal in chronic prostatitis and adenoma, whereas with prostatic neoplasm, a highly significant decrease (100-fold) in Zn secretion has been noted.[904] Prostate cancer cells do not secrete Zn because of a reduced capacity for accumulation of intracellular Zn caused by the decrease in ZIP1 protein expression and the intracellular redistribution of intracellular transporter ZIP3.[905] These neoplastic cells are extremely sensitive to the Zn^{2+} ion; direct tumor injection causes marked cell death, and therefore, may represent a possible chemo prevention therapy.[906]

Requirements and Reference Nutrient Intakes. In the United States, the dietary reference intake (DRI) for Zn is 11 mg/day for men and 8 mg/day for women. Infants and young children need smaller amounts. Increased amounts are required during pregnancy and lactation.[12] Strict vegetarians may need as much as 50% more Zn per day because of increased phytic acid and fiber in their diet.

Intravenous Supply. Stable adult patients require 2.5 to 5.0 mg/day but in those who are depleted or who have increased gastrointestinal losses, the requirement is approximately 6 mg/day.

Clinical Deficiency. As might be expected from the multiple biochemical functions of Zn, the clinical presentation of deficiency disease is varied, nonspecific, and related to the degree and duration of depletion.[907] Signs and symptoms include depressed growth with stunting, increased incidence of infection (possibly related to alterations in immune function), diarrhea, altered cognition, defects in carbohydrate use, reproductive teratogenesis, skin lesions, alopecia, eyesight defects, and other adverse clinical outcomes.

Effects on Growth. It has been claimed that dietary Zn deficiency is prevalent in countries worldwide where a cereal-based diet high in phytate and fiber but low in animal protein is common.[908] This condition could affect as many as two billion people and may be a major public health issue comparable with recognized deficiencies of Fe and I. In children, reduced growth rates and other developmental abnormalities are reversible by Zn supplementation. A metaanalysis of 37 intervention trials showed that Zn supplementation had a significant effect on linear growth and weight regain.[909] Studies also showed that lean tissue retention and protein synthesis are increased if Zn is added to therapeutic regimens used in famine relief, especially when soya-based formulations with a high phytate content are used as a protein source.[910]

It is known that the Zn in human breast milk is efficiently absorbed because of the presence of factors such as picolinate and citrate. However, the total quantity of Zn in breast milk is related to maternal nutritional status, and a physiologic decline in the Zn content of "mature milk" is noted after approximately 6 months' lactation. Although cases of symptomatic Zn deficiency have been reported in breast-fed infants,[911] the need for Zn supplementation for women in low-income countries during pregnancy is controversial. Reduction of neonatal morbidity and incidence of infection has been reported in some studies, but the large-scale introduction of Zn supplementation for pregnant women requires more controlled trials.[912]

Acrodermatitis Enteropathica. Acrodermatitis enteropathica is characterized by periorificial and acral dermatitis, alopecia, and diarrhea.[887] Patients with this disorder have abnormally low blood Zn concentrations (<30 μg/dL; 4.6 μmol/L); symptoms are reversed by oral Zn supplementation, with this being diagnostic. This formerly fatal condition is an autosomal recessive inborn error affecting Zn absorption from the intestinal mucosa. The gene defect involves ZIP4, a Zn transporter that plays an important role in Zn homeostasis.[913,914]

Parenteral Nutrition. When clinical techniques were developed for TPN in the 1960s and 1970s, early sources of amino acids were based on whole protein hydrolysates that had Zn and other trace elements present as contaminants. When these were replaced by mixtures of synthetic amino acids in the 1980s, this necessitated the addition of trace element additives. Some patients who require intravenous feeding after surgery are likely to be significantly Zn depleted because of poor oral intake before and after surgery. They also may have increased Zn losses from the intestinal tract via diarrhea and in urine from catabolism of muscle during periods of negative nitrogen balance. Diarrhea, mental depression, dermatitis, delayed wound healing, and alopecia are seen during the anabolic period of weight regain when Zn is insufficient in the nutritional regimen to support tissue repair.[915] Provision of adequate Zn intravenously to achieve a positive Zn balance is associated with improvement in nitrogen balance.[916] Routine provision of 6.5 mg/day in the parenteral nutrition regimen is normally adequate in stable patients,[917] but increased amounts of Zn and other micronutrients are required in the most severely injured patients.[13]

Infectious Disease. Zn depletion impairs immunity[907,918] and has a direct effect on the gastrointestinal tract;[559] this increases the severity of enteric infections. A placebo-controlled trial of Zn supplementation (10–20 mg/day) of 1240 children aged 6 to 30 months was conducted in North India.[919] A substantial reduction in the incidence of severe and prolonged diarrhea was reported in the treated group. A review of controlled trials of Zn supplementation of children in low-income countries found significant clinical benefits.[920] Six of nine trials claimed improvement in cases of persistent diarrhea; a lower rate of infection was described in five trials of respiratory disease. Some caution is required with the doses of Zn used. In a study of severely malnourished children, those treated with doses of 3 to 6 mg/kg of Zn had significantly increased mortality compared with those given 1.0 to1.5 mg/kg of Zn.[921] Interaction with vitamin A is important; in populations at risk of Zn and vitamin A deficiency, provision of Zn alone increased the incidence of respiratory infection, but when vitamin A was added, respiratory infections were decreased.[557]

Other Conditions. Other groups of individuals are considered to be at risk from a marginal dietary deficiency or from an acquired deficiency secondary to disease. These groups include female adolescents during pregnancy and lactation. Patients with malabsorption syndrome, inflammatory bowel disease, alcoholic liver disease, and anorexia nervosa may also be affected.[559,887,907] A significant proportion of cases of sickle cell anemia have clinical signs and symptoms, together with some laboratory abnormalities of Zn deficiency. These patients apparently respond well to Zn supplementation.[922]

Subclinical Effects of Deficiency. When Zn deficiency is not severe enough to cause clinical signs and symptoms, it may have a subclinical affect on immune function, the synthesis and action of hormones, and neurologic function.

Immune Function. Patients with Zn deficiency in the Middle East were known to die before the age of 25 years because of various infections and parasitic disease. In Zn deficiency, a reduction in the activity of serum thymulin, the thymus-specific hormone involved in T-cell function, and an imbalance between Th1 and Th2 helper cells have been reported. The lytic activity of natural killer cells also decreases. Moreover, Zn is necessary for intracellular binding of tyrosine kinase to the T-cell receptors CD4 and CD8, which are required for T-lymphocyte activation. These complex changes result in impairment of cell-mediated immunity and may serve as the basis for increased infection rates seen in marginal Zn depletion.[923]

Lowering of plasma Zn in the acute-phase response associated with inflammatory conditions is believed to be related to increased intake into tissue. For example, in the liver, this occurs by upregulation of the Zn transporter ZIP4. Thus, Zn deficiency is frequently observed during autoimmune disease, indicating that modulating Zn homeostasis could be a promising approach by which to counteract inflammation and autoimmunity.[924]

It has been suggested that Zn supplements may be beneficial in reducing the severity or duration of the common cold. Studies have been inconsistent, putative benefits small, and because of the doses of Zn used, a high incidence of side effects was encountered.[580]

Hormones. Zn is believed to have a role in the synthesis and actions of many hormones via Zn transcription factors. Zn depletion is associated with low circulating concentrations of testosterone, free T_4, insulin-like growth factor, and thymulin.[923,925] Both plasma insulin-like growth factor and growth velocity are increased in children who are given Zn.[926] Production of testosterone has been shown to be improved in patients given Zn supplements when initial plasma concentrations indicated Zn deficiency.[927] Hence, Zn may play an important role in modulating serum testosterone concentrations in normal men.

Neurologic Effects. Severe Zn deficiency is known to affect mental well-being, with varying degrees of confusion and depression consistent with Zn enzymes having important activity in brain development and function. The history of Zn in relation to the brain and possible relevance to human disease has been reviewed.[928]

Zn has been shown to be a neurosecretory product or cofactor and is highly concentrated in the synaptic vesicles of a specific contingent of neurons, called Zn-containing neurons.[929] Zn in the vesicles probably exceeds 1 mmol/L in concentration and is only weakly coordinated with any endogenous ligand. Zn-containing neurons are found almost exclusively in the forebrain, where in mammals they have evolved into a complex and elaborate associational network that interconnects most of the cerebral cortices and limbic structures. Alterations in Zn homeostasis may be associated with brain dysfunction, including brain inflammatory status.[930] Zn ion dyshomeostasis may also play a role in the aging neuron through deterioration of synapses.[931]

Toxicity. Clinical effects of ingestion of a Zn-contaminated diet include abdominal pain, diarrhea, nausea, and vomiting. Single doses of 225 to 450 mg of Zn can induce vomiting, with milder forms of gastrointestinal upset reported at 50 to 150 mg/day (dosages that were initially used in therapy). More than 60 mg/day of Zn can result in Cu depletion by causing intestinal blockade of intestinal absorption. The US IOM has set the tolerable upper amount of intake for adults at 40 mg/day.[12]

It is also important to note that Zn^{2+} ions themselves may be toxic, as shown from cell culture experiments with neurones,[932] which indicated the importance of the compartmentalization of Zn within cells. Apparent lack of toxicity in vivo may be related to cellular protection afforded by extra production of the Zn-complexing protein MT.[933]

Laboratory Assessment of Status. Although plasma Zn determination is insensitive to dietary Zn intake and is subject to a variety of influences, it remains the most widely used laboratory test to confirm severe deficiency and to monitor adequacy of Zn provision, especially when interpreted together with changes in serum albumin and the acute-phase response. No practicable laboratory procedures have been established for clearly identifying populations with marginal Zn depletion. Clinical and biochemical responses to Zn supplementation therefore are used to postulate a marginally Zn-depleted state. Thus, in contrast to Fe, for which a number of indicators of metabolism and/or function are available, an effective measure to assess the functional Zn status of humans has remained elusive. Nevertheless, various factors have been used, such as MT, Zn transporter proteins, and cytokine gene expression (as transcript abundance), in which Zn supplementation in human subjects indicated enhanced production.[934]

A systematic review confirmed that among healthy individuals, plasma and urinary and hair Zn are reliable biomarkers of Zn status in suitable samples.[604]

Serum/Plasma Zinc. It was once claimed that plasma samples are preferred to serum for Zn analysis because of possible Zn contamination from erythrocytes, platelets, and leukocytes during clotting and centrifugation, but this has not been confirmed in other studies. All of the preceding analytical methods have sufficient sensitivity to measure concentrations of Zn. Spectrophotometric methods are available for use on main chemistry platforms but are subject to various interferences.

A study using stable Zn isotope tracers during experimental induction of acute Zn depletion (0.23 mg/day) found that the plasma Zn concentration took 5 weeks to decline to 65% of baseline values, and that the observed fall was caused by a reduction in Zn release from the slowest Zn pool.[883] Care has to be taken in controlling numerous preanalytical factors that will lower plasma Zn independently of dietary intake. These include collection of samples in relation to meals, time of day, and use of steroid-based medications, such as the contraceptive pill. Any cause of hypoalbuminemia will also lower plasma Zn. Plasma albumin is a negative acute-phase reactant that is redistributed into the interstitial space from the plasma pool during infection, after trauma, and in chronic disease. The induction of hepatic MT synthesis during the acute-phase response and subsequent sequestering of Zn further lower the plasma concentration.[34] It is therefore essential to consider plasma Zn results along with plasma albumin and plasma CRP or another marker of the acute-phase response.

Knowledge of bioavailable Zn is of fundamental importance. Five cases of hyperzincemia (between 5 and 10 times the upper limit of normal) were recorded in patients with apparent Zn deficiency, indicating extremely low bioavailable free Zn.[935] Presentation signs included recurrent infections, hepatosplenomegaly, arthritis, anemia, and persistently raised CRP. A binding protein that effectively sequestered functional Zn was identified as calprotectin, and the observations were subsequently explained as a new disease entity of dysregulation of calprotectin.

Blood Cell Zinc. Some investigators have suggested that the Zn content of white cells and platelets better reflects tissue Zn.[936] The Zn content of neutrophils, lymphocytes, and platelets has been shown to decline more rapidly than plasma Zn in experimental studies of Zn depletion in humans.[907] However, the relatively large volume of blood required and problems with contamination make large-scale application to patients in hospital or to population surveys difficult, especially in studies involving children. Erythrocyte Zn has been suggested as an alternative; however, in a study of low-income black women (n = 580) stratified by total daily Zn intake during pregnancy, no changes in erythrocyte Zn were found, although plasma Zn increased with intake.[937]

Zinc in Hair. Low levels of Zn in hair has been associated with poor growth in children, and has been used as a criterion for initiating supplementation studies. However, variables such as hair growth rate and external contamination from hair dyes and cosmetics can cause inconsistent results. Results from individual patients are difficult to interpret.[604,614,938]

Zinc-Dependent Enzymes. Despite the large number of Zn metalloenzymes that have been identified, no single enzyme assay has yet found acceptance as an indicator of Zn status. This may be a result of avid retention of Zn by these enzymes, even in the face of dietary Zn depletion, and of difficulties with reproducible measurements of activity. However, bone-specific alkaline phosphatase, extracellular SOD, and lymphocyte and plasma 5-nucleotidase appear to be responsive to Zn intake.[939]

Metallothionein. Determination of MT in RBCs and MT mRNA in circulating monocytes is considered of probable value because MT falls in Zn deficiency. However, clinical use of these measurements has not yet been confirmed by large-scale investigations of depleted populations.[939]

Urine Zinc. A slight fall in the urine excretion of Zn has been noted during dietary deficiency. Difficulties of sample contamination during collection make this of limited practical value. However, increased urine Zn is an important source of loss in the severely injured catabolic patient, although measurement is rarely required except in research studies.[891] Urine output increases with amino acid infusion given during TPN.

Reference Intervals. Serum and/or plasma Zn concentrations exhibit both circadian and postprandial fluctuations. Concentrations are decreased after food and are higher in the morning than in the evening.

A reference interval for clinical guidance is 80 to 120 μg/dL (12–18 μmol/L). Fasting morning values of plasma Zn less than 70 μg/dL (10.7 μmol/L) on more than one occasion require further investigation. Results less than 30 μg/dL (5 μmol/L) suggest likely deficiency. Urine Zn excretion lies in the range from 0.2 to 1.3 mg/24 hours (3–21 μmol/24 hours). For more information, refer to the Appendix on Reference Intervals. Laboratories should verify that these ranges are appropriate for use in their own settings.

Other Possibly Essential Elements

More than 15 additional trace elements are considered by some investigators to have a potentially important role in human medicine. Reviews by Nielsen consider these in detail and discuss emerging concepts of "essentiality."[605,940] The clinical laboratory will consider some, such as Pb, Cd, arsenic, aluminum, and nickel, primarily as toxic elements (see Chapter 42). Others, such as Li and F, are classified as pharmacologically beneficial, and monitoring of dosages may be required.

For a few elements (B, Si, and V), circumstantial evidence for their essentiality is available, and measurable responses in humans have been observed during variations in their dietary intake. These elements are discussed in the following. These and other elements have been promoted by the supplement industry, and the clinical chemist may be asked for advice and possibly for monitoring of dosages in cases of suspected toxicity. Methods using AAS, ICP-OES, and ICP-MS can be applied for the determination of most of these elements in biological samples.[614]

Contamination of TPN solutions by small amounts of metals, such as aluminum, Pb, Cd, and nickel, could also be a problem, as could the lack of others, such as Si, B, and V, when long-term nutritional support is required.[940]

POINTS TO REMEMBER

Trace Elements

Boron: Has a role in boron neutron capture therapy for brain cancer
Chromium: Required for insulin and glucose metabolism
Cobalt: Active factor in vitamin B_{12}
Copper: Metabolism perturbed in Wilson disease
Fluoride: Reduces tooth decay
Iodine: Extensive deficiency in many countries
Manganese: Symptoms of toxicity resemble Parkinson disease
Molybdenum: Required for sulfite oxidase activity
Selenium: Dietary intakes vary considerably depending on concentrations in the soil
Silicon: Important in the synthesis of collagen and bone
Vanadium: Potential role in the treatment of diabetes
Zinc: Deficiency leads to a large number of symptoms

Fluoride

Fluoride is the most widely used of the "pharmacologically beneficial trace elements" in the area of public health. Dental caries has been described as the last major epidemic of preventable bacterial disease, and dental decay leads to tooth loss, nutritional problems, and systemic infection. National bodies have provided guidelines regarding the fluoridation of water to prevent dental caries in the general population.[941]

Dietary Sources. Many studies over the past 50 years have established that the addition of F^- to drinking water reduces the incidence of tooth decay; more than 60% of the US population now uses fluoridated water. Clinical studies from 1950 to 1980 in 20 different countries found that adding F^- to community water supplies, within the reference interval of 0.7 to 1.2 mg/L, reduced the incidence of caries in both primary (infant) and permanent teeth. The subject is controversial, and there has been opposition to mass medication with fluoride. Systematic reviews of the benefits and risks associated with the use of F^- are available.[942,943]

F^- supplementation of salt, sugar, and milk has been used in areas where F^- is not added to water supplies. F^- is also added to toothpastes, and systematic reviews suggest that they do confer protection from dental caries.[944]

In Europe, the recommended supplementation during TPN is 0.57 to 1.45 mg/day.

Absorption, Transport, Metabolism, and Excretion. Fluoride ions are absorbed from both the stomach and the small intestine. Soluble salts are efficiently absorbed, and a peak increase of F^- occurs in blood plasma within 1 hour of ingestion. Ions are rapidly cleared from plasma into tissue in exchange with anions, such as hydroxyl, citrate, and carbonate. At least 95% of the 2.6 g of total body F^- is located in bones and teeth. Almost 90% of excess F^- is excreted in urine.[945]

Functions. The F^- ion can be exchanged for hydroxyl in the crystal structure of apatite, a main component of skeletal bone and teeth. This stabilizes the regenerating tooth surface. F^- is present in saliva and may be released from dental plaques at low pH.[946] Initially, benefit was considered to involve only the erupting teeth of children, but topical effects on adult teeth are now believed to reduce decay.[943,944]

Initial evidence from small studies suggests that pharmacological doses of F^- may reduce the incidence of bone fracture in patients with osteoporosis. However, a metaanalysis of F^- therapy from 11 controlled studies on 1429 subjects found that although this increased lumbar bone density, the incidence of vertebral fracture was not significantly decreased.[947] Another study showed that NaF was more effective than etidronate at increasing lumbar bone mass, but no differences were observed in the incidence of fracture.[948] The problem with F^- is the potential for excess, and monitoring was believed to be essential; a higher incidence of side effects, mainly gastrointestinal symptoms and lower extremity pain syndrome, was observed in the F^- group.

Toxicity. Dental fluorosis, the mottling of enamel in the erupting teeth of children, is now estimated to affect approximately 20% of the population. This can be a disfiguring condition, and it occurs in a greater proportion of children than initially expected.[949] The risk for and severity of dental fluorosis depends on the amount, timing, frequency, and duration of the exposure to F^-.[941] Because children tend to be prone to ingesting toothpaste, it has been suggested that "pediatric" toothpastes with lower F^- content should be made available in areas where fluoridation of the water supply exists.

Occupational exposure to inhaled F^- dusts among cryolite workers during aluminum refining has resulted in severe bone abnormalities, but safety equipment now limits such exposure. No cases of skeletal fluorosis are attributed to the use of controlled fluoridation of water supplies. However, skeletal fluorosis may occur in areas of the world where naturally occurring drinking water has high concentrations of F^-, such as China and the Indian subcontinent. It is believed that exposure to F^- intakes of 10 to 25 mg/day for 10 years or longer may result in skeletal fluorosis, but other nutritional factors may make these populations more susceptible.[950,951]

Although numerous adverse effects have been attributed to water fluoridation, investigators have found no convincing evidence of increased rates of cancer, heart disease, kidney disease, liver disease, presenile dementia, birth defects, or Down syndrome.

Laboratory Assessment of Status. Laboratory analysis of drinking water may be required to assess possible F^- excess in natural well waters, and may also be necessary during incidents of failure of the equipment used to treat drinking water. Determination of F^- in urine can be used to assess exposure to different sources of F^-.[952] Direct determination using a F^--specific electrode is used for drinking water and urine. For food, feces, and tissue, previous separation of F^- from the sample matrix is required, using a Conway diffusion procedure.[953] The combination of the F^- electrode with flow injection has allowed the use of a rapid and sensitive method for serum and urine F^- analysis.[954]

Reference Intervals. Concentrations of F^- in body fluids and tissue vary widely, depending on the F^- content of drinking water and input from diet, toothpaste, and mouth rinses. For urine, a guideline interval is 0.2 to 3.2 mg/L (10.5–168 μmol/L). For more information, refer to the Appendix on Reference Intervals. Laboratories should verify that these ranges are appropriate for use in their own settings.

Boron

Boron has not been officially designated as essential to human health, although it is considered an essential macronutrient for plants.

Dietary Sources. It is believed that the acceptable safe range of intake is from 1 to 13 mg/day, and evidence suggests that some people are consuming less than 1 mg/day. Plant foods, especially fruits, leafy vegetables, nuts, and legumes are good sources, whereas meat, fish, and dairy products are not.[605,955]

Absorption, Transport, Metabolism, and Excretion. Dietary B is efficiently absorbed as boric acid $B(OH)_3$ and is efficiently excreted into urine, with approximately 85% to 100% of an oral dose of borate appearing in urine over a 5- to 7-day period. The oral toxicity of B is relatively low; it has been estimated that safe population mean intakes are less than 13 mg/day, and that individuals are at risk of toxicity when intakes continually exceed 100 mg/day for up to 6 days. The richest food sources are nuts and dried fruits (15–30 mg/kg) and wine (8.5 mg/L). The use of $B(OH)_3$ food additives is now prohibited, except for caviar at 4000 mg/kg. Thus, a toxic intake of B could be provided by 200 g of nuts plus 20 g of caviar, or by 25 g of low-fat crisps plus 12 L of wine.

Functions. Boron is normally present in living organisms such as the borate ion (BO_3^{3-}), which has essential properties in plants that affect cell wall integrity.[956] However, it is still not known to have any specific physiologic function in humans, although various studies have suggested that it may be a bioactive beneficial element.[957] In vitro, animal, and human experiments have shown that B beneficially affects bone growth and central nervous system function, alleviates arthritic symptoms, facilitates hormone action, and is associated with a reduced risk for some types of cancer. Several findings suggest that this influence is through the formation of boroesters in biomolecules containing *cis*-hydroxyl groups. These biomolecules include those that contain ribose (eg, S-adenosylmethionine, diadenosine phosphates, and nicotinamide adenine dinucleotide). In addition, B may form boroester complexes with phosphoinositides, glycoproteins, and glycolipids that affect cell membrane integrity and function. Both animal and human data indicate that an intake of less than 1.0 mg/day inhibits the health benefits of B.[957,958]

Some of these effects were more evident when dietary Cu was marginal and Mg inadequate. Further research is needed to clarify the role of B in human and animal physiology, and to firmly establish optimal dietary requirements.[959]

Laboratory Assessment of Status. Problems with contamination and loss of volatile B compounds during sample preparation have limited the reliable documentation of B concentrations in human tissue and body fluids.[960] A complex technique that involved a porous graphite column (inductively coupled plasma atomic emission spectrophotometry and an inductively coupled plasma time-of-flight mass spectrometer) has been developed for investigation of B neutron capture in cancer therapy.[961] Adaptation of this method for nutritional studies of B should be possible.

Reference Intervals. Normal concentrations in plasma of 19.5 to 78.9 μg/L (1.8–7.3 μmol/L) was established by ICP-MS.[962] Excretion in urine is normally less than 1 mg/day and up to 5 mg/L with B intake of 0.65 to 4.34 mg/day.

Silicon

Silicon is a nonmetal that has an atomic weight of 28; it is a member of the group IV series of elements. Similar to elements in this group, it forms tetrahedral types of complexes and a multitude of polymers. Silica is used to refer to the naturally occurring materials composed principally of Si dioxide. The term silicone refers to any of a large group of siloxane polymers that do not occur naturally and are based on the structure of alternating O_2 and Si (...-Si-O-Si-O-Si-O-...), with organic side groups attached to the four-coordinate Si atoms. In some cases, organic side groups can be used to link two or more of these -Si-O- backbones together. By varying -Si-O- chain lengths, side groups, and crosslinking, silicones can be synthesized with a wide variety of properties and compositions. These compounds have a variety of uses from parchment coatings to sealant and breast implants. Si is widely distributed in nature and is the second most abundant element, accounting for approximately 28% of the earth's crust. Si is always found in nature as the oxide silica or as a silicate, and it plays an important role in cell structural organization.

Dietary Sources. Soluble silica (orthosilicic acid) is ubiquitous in the diet (20–50 mg/day) and in natural waters (0.8–44 mg/L),[963] and unlike crystalline silica (quartz), it has no associated toxicity. Si is widely distributed in plants and is an essential element for structural integrity. Amorphous silica is incorporated as an anticaking agent at concentrations up to 2% in a variety of foods. Beer can also be rich in Si, with up to 20 mg/L content.[964] No values have been suggested for the recommended intake of Si.

Absorption, Transport, Metabolism, and Excretion. The absorption of Si seems to be dependent on its polymeric nature; the smaller the molecule (ie, monomeric orthosilicic acid), the more effective is absorption, whereas the larger polymer forms are poorly absorbed.[963] Passive nonfacilitated transport appears to occur and is probably based on size-related simple diffusion. The efficiency of absorption is up to 60% of an ingested load, with most excreted renally within 24 hours of exposure. As yet, little evidence suggests retention in any tissue-specific site.

Functions. In veterinary and laboratory animals, Si has been shown to be important in the synthesis of collagen and bone. The few supplementation studies in humans have indicated associated increases in trabecular bone volume and BMD.[965] Silica deprivation experiments in the 1970s in growing chicks and rats suggested that silica is essential for normal growth and development, although this remains to be confirmed. It has been suggested that soluble silica is essential for living organisms, because it binds endogenous aluminum and thereby prevents its toxicity, although this remains unproven.[966] The use of Si in IVN has also been advocated.[955]

Laboratory Assessment of Status. Normal fasting plasma concentrations of Si are less than 33 μg/dL (12 μmol/L).[967] These are raised in renal failure, particularly in patients on hemodialysis, up to more than 420 μg/dL (150 μmol/L) and can be higher, depending on the content of dialysis water.[968] Urine Si excretion depends on intake and varies from 2.8 to 28 mg/day (100–1000 μmol/day). Toxicity from Si has never been reported, although increased urinary concentration was determined in a patient with magnesium silicate renal stones.[969]

Vanadium

Vanadium, a group V trace element that belongs to the first transition series of elements, is ubiquitously distributed. It can exist in four valency states—2, 3, 4, and 5; thus, its chemistry is complex. V occurs in neutral solutions as metavanadate, the predominant species in body fluids, and enters cells by an anion transport system. Exogenously administered vanadyl sulfate and ammonium vanadate have been found to bind serum transferrin tightly, indicating that this protein may serve as a V transporter. Although the V requirement of a few organisms has been established, the essentiality in humans remains to be proven.[970] The importance of V in man has been reviewed.[970,971]

Although most foods contain low concentrations of V (<1 ng/g), food is the major source of exposure to V for the general population; however, absorption of V salts from the gastrointestinal tract is poor. Excretion by the kidneys is rapid, with a biological half-life of 20 to 40 hours. Estimated daily intake of the US population ranges from 10 to 60 μg. Vanadyl sulfate is a supplement that is commonly used to enhance weight training in athletes at doses up to 60 mg/day. In general, the toxicity of V compounds is low. Most of the toxic effects of V compounds result from local irritation of the eyes and upper respiratory tract, rather than from systemic toxicity.

Functions. Vanadium plays a limited role in biology. Nevertheless, a V-containing nitrogenase is used by some nitrogen-fixing microorganisms. Clinical interest in the vanadate compounds involves their potential role in the treatment of diabetes. Various studies have suggested that these compounds reduce the requirement for insulin by activating the cellular response without the presence of insulin, in effect mimicking its action.[972] Different oxidation states for vanadate (V^{5+}) and vanadyl (V^{4+}; ie, vanadyl sulfate) mimic the rapid responses of insulin through alternative signaling pathways not involving insulin receptor activation. The insulin-like effects of V may be initiated by inhibiting phosphotyrosine phosphatases and stimulating protein tyrosine kinase activity, implying that cells (adipose cells in particular) contain distinct vanadyl (V^{4+})-sensitive and vanadate (V^{5+})-sensitive phosphotyrosine phosphatases. However, in a previous study of type 2 diabetes ($n = 16$), no dose relationship was noted between the drug administered and glucose regulation after administration of vanadyl sulfate.[973]

Amounts given in such trials are much greater than the suggested normal intake, suggesting that V compounds are more likely to work as alternative therapies, rather than indicating the essential function of the element. The value of V compounds in cancer treatment has been reviewed.[974]

Laboratory Assessment of Status. Plasma and urine concentrations are usually measured by GFAAS or ICP-AES. Use of ICP-MS revealed a number of urinary V compounds in healthy volunteers ($n = 95$) at concentrations of 1 to 10 μg/L (20–200 nmol/L).[962] Measurement of the V^{5+}-ion concentration using size exclusion chromatography coupled with ICP-MS yielded serum concentrations at approximately the detection limit of the assay at less than 0.05 μg/L (<1 nmol/L). Studies with high-resolution ICP-MS also showed whole blood concentrations of less than 0.05 μg/L (<1 nmol/L), indicating that careful sampling techniques are required for confident use of analyzed concentrations.[682]

SELECTED REFERENCES

For a full list of references for this chapter, please refer to ExpertConsult.com.

11. National Academies Press. Dietary reference intakes: vitamins. <https://www.nationalacademies.org/hmd/~/media/Files/Activity%20Files/Nutrition/DRIs/DRI_Vitamins.pdf>.
12. National Academies Press. Dietary reference intakes: elements. <http://nationalacademies.org/hmd/~/media/Files/Activity%20Files/Nutrition/DRIs/New%20Material/6_%20Elements%20Summary.pdf>.
16. Shenkin A. Biochemical monitoring of nutrition support. *Ann Clin Biochem* 2006;**43**:269–72.
35. Duncan A, Talwar D, McMillan DC, et al. Quantitative data on the magnitude of the systemic inflammatory response and its effect on micronutrient status based on plasma measurements. *Am J Clin Nutr* 2012;**95**:64–71.
46. Valko M, Leibfritz D, Moncol J, et al. Free radicals and antioxidants in normal physiological functions and human disease. *Int J Biochem Cell Biol* 2007;**39**:44–84.
77. Block G, Dresser CM, Hartman AM, et al. Nutrient sources in the American diet: quantitative data from the NHANES II survey. I. Vitamins and minerals. *Am J Epidemiol* 1985;**122**:13–26.
234. Howard JM. Assessment of vitamin B(1) status. *Clin Chem* 2000;**46**:1867–8.
303. Wald DS, Wald NJ, Morris JK, et al. Folic acid, homocysteine, and cardiovascular disease: judging causality in the face of inconclusive trial evidence. *BMJ* 2006;**333**:1114–17.
317. Stabler SP. Clinical practice. Vitamin B12 deficiency. *N Engl J Med* 2013;**368**:149–60.
338. Toh BH, van Driel IR, Gleeson PA. Pernicious anemia. *N Engl J Med* 1997;**337**:1441–8.
406. Hankey GJ. Is plasma homocysteine a modifiable risk factor for stroke? *Nat Clin Pract Neurol* 2006;**2**:26–33.
475. Baumgartner MR. Vitamin-responsive disorders: cobalamin, folate, biotin, vitamins B1 and E. *Handb Clin Neurol* 2013;**113**:1799–810.
532. Mechanick JI, Youdim A, Jones DB, et al. Clinical practice guidelines for the perioperative nutritional, metabolic, and nonsurgical support of the bariatric surgery patient–2013 update: cosponsored by American Association of Clinical Endocrinologists, the Obesity Society, and American Society for Metabolic & Bariatric Surgery. *Endocr Pract* 2013;**19**:337–72.
548. Frausto Da Silva JJR, Williams RJP. *The biological chemistry of the elements. The inorganic chemistry of life*. 2nd ed. Oxford, UK: Oxford University Press; 2001.
589. Hannemann F, Hartmann A, Schmitt J, et al. European multidisciplinary consensus statement on the use and monitoring of metal-on-metal bearings for total hip replacement and hip resurfacing. *Orthop Traumatol Surg Res* 2013;**99**:263–71.
628. Crans DC, Woll KA, Prusinskas K, et al. Metal speciation in health and medicine represented by iron and vanadium. *Inorg Chem* 2013;**52**:12262–75.
694. Prasad AS, Brewer GJ, Schoomaker EB, et al. Hypocupremia induced by zinc therapy in adults. *JAMA* 1978;**240**:2166–8.
746. Mak CM, Lam CW. Diagnosis of Wilson's disease: a comprehensive review. *Crit Rev Clin Lab Sci* 2008;**45**:263–90.
765. Vanderpump MP, Lazarus JH, Smyth PP, et al. Iodine status of UK schoolgirls: a cross-sectional survey. *Lancet* 2011;**377**:2007–12.
821. Rayman MP. Selenium and human health. *Lancet* 2012;**379**:1256–68.

38

Hemoglobin, Iron, Bilirubin

*M. Domenica Cappellini, Stanley F. Lo, and Dorine W. Swinkels**

ABSTRACT

Background

Hemoglobin (Hb), iron (Fe), and bilirubin are analytes that may be viewed collectively in terms of a manufacturing process in which the raw material (Fe) is incorporated with other raw materials in a multistage complex process leading to a finished product (Hb). This finished product has a limited life span, after which degradation into the waste product (bilirubin) occurs.

Content

This chapter describes the processes involved in Hb synthesis and degradation. These processes can be disrupted by a deficiency in the supply of raw material, lack or disruption of regulatory or synthesis mechanisms, excessive loss of the finished product, or excessive conversion to or deficiency in the elimination of waste products. Defects in these processes that become manifest in clinical disorders are described. They include Fe deficiency anemias (IDAs), liver disease, and various genetic diseases, including Fe overload or distributions disorders, Crigler-Najjar and Gilbert syndromes, hemoglobinopathies, and thalassemias. Reliable analytical methods for the measurement of the analytes involved were among the first to be developed for routine use in the clinical laboratory. Recently, because of important discoveries in the underlying biological processes, new Fe biomarkers have been added to this laboratory toolbox. This chapter illustrates that laboratory analysis has contributed significantly to the understanding of the (patho)physiologic roles of these analytes and has allowed the design of novel algorithms and diagrams for the management of these disorders. The challenges ahead are described, and include further standardization of parameters to increase their usefulness for both public health and clinical practice.

HEMOGLOBIN

Hemoglobin is a hemoprotein whose primary function is to transport oxygen from the lungs to the body tissue. It was first isolated in 1849, and was the first oligomeric protein to be characterized by ultracentrifugation and to have (1) its molecular mass accurately determined, (2) its physiologic function described, and (3) after the 25-year study of Perutz and colleagues in Cambridge, its structure defined by x-ray crystallography.[1] In 1949, Pauling and colleagues[2] showed that Hb from patients with sickle cell disease differed from normal Hb because it has two to four additional net positive charges. Later, the reasons for the charge difference were elucidated by locating the single amino acid difference between Hb from normal individuals and Hb from those with sickle cell disease.[3-6]

Biochemistry

Hemoglobin is a globular protein with a diameter of 6.4 nm and a molecular mass of approximately 64,500 Da. As shown in Fig. 38.1, Hb consists of four globin subunits (two α- and two non–α-, β-, γ-, or δ-chains), with each looped about itself to form a pocket or cleft in which the heme group nestles. Normally, this heme pocket is formed entirely by nonpolar (hydrophobic) amino acids. The heme moiety (see Fig. 38.1) is suspended within this pocket by an attachment of its Fe atom to the imidazole group of the proximal histidine (position 92 of the β-chain [β92] or position 87 of the α-chain [α87]). The imidazole group of the distal histidine (β63 or α58) is also in contiguity with the Fe of heme, but it appears to swing into and out of this position to permit the passage of oxygen into and out of the Hb molecule. The four Fe atoms are in the divalent state, whether Hb is oxygenated or deoxygenated.

Globin Structure of Normal and Fetal Hemoglobin

In normal human adults, Hb A is composed of two normal α- and two normal β-polypeptide chains and is represented symbolically as $\alpha_2\beta_2$; it represents at least 96% of the total Hb contained in a sample of whole blood. Hb A_2 is typically approximately 2.5% to 3.0% of total Hb; it contains two α- and two δ-chains, and is designated as $\alpha_2\delta_2$. HbA2′ is considered a variant of Hb A_2 and is the result of a glycine-to-arginine substitution in the 16th position of the δ-chain; it occurs in 1% to 2% of African Americans. It rarely forms more than 3% of the total Hb. Fetal Hb (Hb F) predominates during fetal life but rapidly diminishes during the first year of postnatal life. In normal adults, less than 1% of Hb is Hb F. It consists of two α- and two γ-chains ($\alpha_2\gamma_2$).

In early embryonic life, the yolk sac produces the globin chains ζ and ε. These globin chains combine to form the

*The authors gratefully acknowledge the contributions of Trefor Higgins, MSc, John H. Eckfeldt, MD, PhD, James C. Barton, MD, and Basil T. Doumas, PhD, upon which portions of this chapter are based.

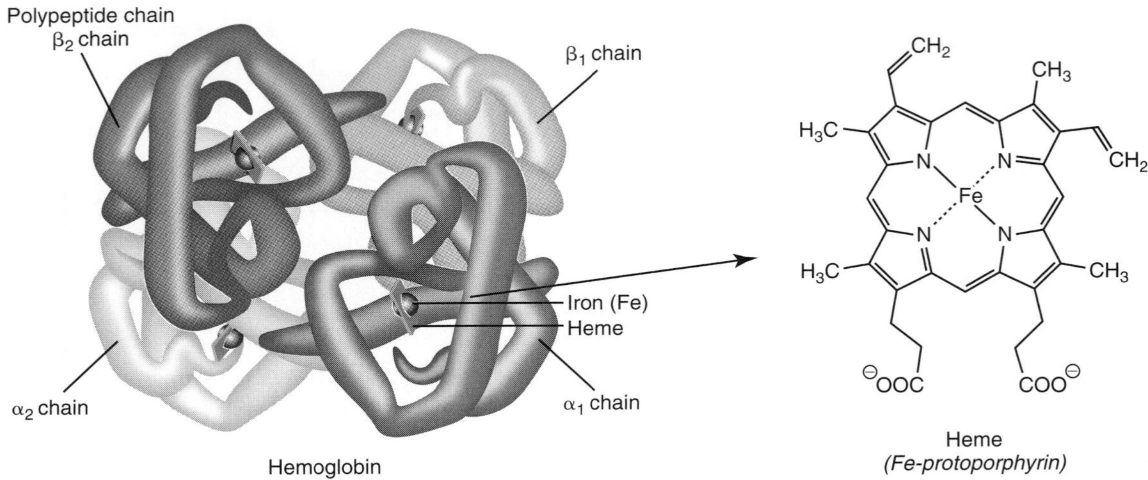

FIGURE 38.1 Model of the Hemoglobin Tetramer With the α-Chain Subunits Facing the Reader. Each subunit contains a molecule of heme attached to an atom of iron.

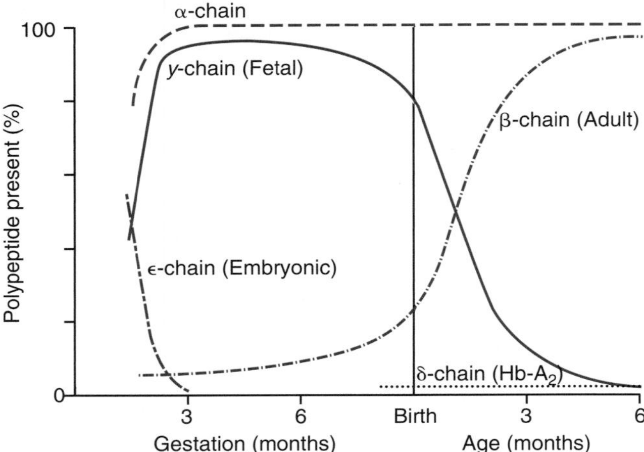

FIGURE 38.2 Changes in Relative Proportions of Globin Chains at Various Stages of Embryonic, Fetal, and Postnatal Life. *Hb-A₂,* Glycosylated hemoglobin (Reprinted from Huehns ER, Dance N, Beaven GH, Hecht F, Motulsky AG. Human embryonic hemoglobins. *Cold Spring Harbor Symp Quant Biol* 1965;29:327–331.)

major embryonic Hbs, Hb Gower 1 ($\zeta_2\varepsilon_2$) and 2 ($\alpha_2\varepsilon_2$), and Hb Portland 1 ($\zeta_2\gamma_2$) and 2 ($\zeta_2\beta_2$). Production of the ζ-chain ceases at the gestational age of approximately 4 months.

Production of α- and γ-chains starts at approximately 6 weeks' gestation, with Hb F ($\alpha_2\gamma_2$) increasing in concentration to become the major Hb found in the fetus (Fig. 38.2). Glycine or alanine may be found at position 136 of the γ-chain in the fetus, giving rise to two distinct γ-chains designated Gγ and Aγ, respectively. Formation of Hb A ($\alpha_2\beta_2$) commences at approximately 28 weeks' gestation, and at birth it can form up to 15% of the total Hb, with the remainder of the Hb consisting mainly of Hb F with a small amount of Hb A_2. Production of the γ-chain declines after birth, and normal adult Hb F concentrations are usually obtained by 1 year of age, but may be elevated until 2 years of age.

Protein Structure. As with all proteins, the function of Hb is dictated by its primary, secondary, tertiary, and quaternary structures.

Primary Structure. The α- and non–α-globin chains of Hb are 141 and 146 amino acid residues in length, respectively. Some sequence homology has been noted, with 64 individual amino acid residues in identical positions in both α- and β-chains. The β-chain differs from the δ- and γ-chains by 39 and 10 residues, respectively. The amino terminal of the β-globin chain is the site of attachment of glucose (HbA_{1c}), urea, and salicylate.[7] The carboxy terminal amino acid of the β-chain is tyrosine and can function as a part of salt bridges. Although no disulfide bonds are present, six SH groups have been noted (from cysteine at positions α104, β93, and β112). The γ-chain has a glycine amino terminal, and the alkali resistance of Hb F is attributed to the presence of threonine and tryptophan at positions 112 and 130 of the γ-chain, respectively. The γ-chain is unique in that it is the only globin chain to be highly susceptible to acetylation, and acetylated Hb F is a prominent feature in cord and neonatal blood, and may form as much as 25% of the total Hb. The N-terminal valine of the β-globin chain of HbA_{1c} can also be acetylated to a smaller degree (<1%–3%), for example, in alcoholic liver disease.[7]

Secondary Structure. Approximately 75% to 80% of polypeptide chains of the α- and non–α-chains are arranged in helices, with the remainder forming nonhelical turns. The β-chain of Hb A is arranged into eight helices identified as A through H. In contrast, the α-chain is missing an equivalent of the D helix and has only seven helices. Nomenclature within the helices identifies the helix and the position within the helix of the amino acid residue (eg, F3 is the third amino residue in the F helix). Amino acid residues in the peptide chains that join adjacent helices are described by the identification of two adjacent helices and the position of residues within the joining peptide. For example, EF3 would be the third residue in the peptide joining the E and F helices.

Tertiary Structure. The tertiary structure of Hb refers to the arrangement of helices into a three-dimensional, pretzel-like structure. The heme group, located in a crevice between

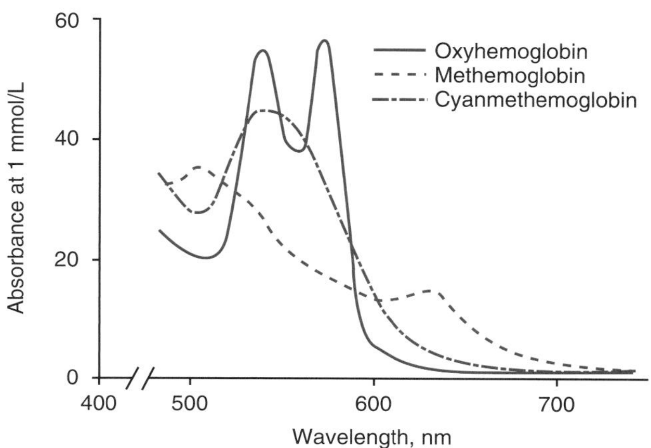

FIGURE 38.3 Spectrophotometric Absorption Curves for Oxyhemoglobin, Methemoglobin, and Cyanmethemoglobin. Oxyhemoglobin and cyanmethemoglobin are used in measuring the concentration of hemoglobin *(Hb)*. The peak at 630 nm, which is distinctive for methemoglobin, is abolished by addition of cyanide, and the resultant decrease in absorbance is directly proportional to the methemoglobin concentration. All heme proteins exhibit their maximum absorbance in the Soret band region of 400 to 440 nm. Because the absorbance of Hb in the Soret region is approximately 10 times the absorbance at 540 nm, the Soret peaks have been omitted from this diagram. The absorbance curve for methemoglobin is greatly influenced by small changes in pH. The curve given here was obtained at a pH of 6.6.

the E and F helices, is attached to histidine residues in each globin chain. This attachment is essential to maintaining the secondary and tertiary structure of the globin chains.

Quaternary Structure. The quaternary structure of Hb results from the attachment of the four globin chains to each other. Strong $\alpha_1\beta_1$ and $\alpha_2\beta_2$ dimeric bonds hold the molecule in a stable form. The tetrameric $\alpha_1\beta_2$ and $\alpha_2\beta_1$ bonds make significant contributions to the stability of the structure. Shifting, rotation, and sliding in the quaternary structure result in a number of physiologic effects, including the sigmoid-oxygen dissociation curve and the Bohr effect (described in greater detail later in this chapter).

Modified Hemoglobins

In addition to the Hbs discussed previously, carboxyhemoglobin, methemoglobin, and sulfhemoglobin are other Hbs whose structure has been environmentally or chemically modified.

Each of the modified Hbs has a characteristic spectral pattern, as shown in Fig. 38.3. These spectral characteristics form the basis of analysis in the many co-oximeters and blood gas analyzers that provide, in a single analysis, the simultaneous quantitative measurement of carboxyhemoglobin, methemoglobin, and sulfhemoglobin. The spectral scans are performed using multidiode arrays covering a number of wavelengths, followed by patented calculations that discriminate between normal and modified Hbs.

Carboxyhemoglobin. Carboxyhemoglobin is formed by the preferential attachment of carbon monoxide instead of oxygen to Hb. Carboxyhemoglobin concentrations (usually expressed as a carboxyhemoglobin saturation) have been known to reach 20% in individuals who are exposed to significant workplace concentrations of carbon monoxide. For example, police directing traffic at busy intersections and workers in radiator and welding shops have high carboxyhemoglobin concentrations at the end of the working day. The ability to perform heavy manual work or complex tasks is impaired at carboxyhemoglobin concentrations of 10% or less.[8] Faulty home furnaces and automobile exhaust systems have been known to produce large amounts of carbon monoxide, sometimes with tragic results. Carboxyhemoglobin saturation that varies from 15% to 25% may be associated with dizziness, headaches, and nausea, and greater than 50% saturation is considered life threatening.[9] After removal of the exposed individual from the carbon monoxide source, a slow decline in carboxyhemoglobin saturation occurs, in keeping with the half-life of 4 to 5 hours at sea level.[10]

Methemoglobin. The Fe of heme is normally in the reduced ferrous state (Fe^{2+}). Under alkaline conditions, the Fe is oxidized to the ferric state (Fe^{3+}) by toxic agents, such as nitrates (found in some well waters), aniline dyes, chlorates, drugs (eg, quinones, phenacetin, and sulfonamides), or local anesthetics (eg, procaine, benzocaine, and lidocaine). This oxidation converts the heme to hematin[11] and the Hb to methemoglobin. Patients with methemoglobin are cyanotic because methemoglobin is unable to reversibly bind oxygen. Methemoglobin is normally reduced to Hb in the cell by the reduced form of the nicotinamide-adenine dinucleotide–cytochrome reductase system.

Hereditary methemoglobinemia is a rare condition that was first described in Europeans, but was later found in individuals of many racial backgrounds. Familial methemoglobinemia in an autosomal recessive mode of transmission is due to a deficiency in the enzyme nicotinamide-adenine dinucleotide–cytochrome b5 reductase. Hb variants, Hb M Saskatoon, Hb Freiburg, and Hb St. Louis stabilize the ferric Fe state and are associated with an autosomal dominant familial methemoglobinemia. Methemoglobinemia is treated by the administration of ascorbic acid or methylene blue.

Sulfhemoglobin. Sulfhemoglobin is produced by the reaction of sulfur-containing compounds with heme to form an irreversible chemical alteration and oxidation of Hb by the introduction of sulfur in one or more of the porphyrin rings. The most common cause of sulfhemoglobinemia is exposure to drugs,[12] such as phenacetin and sulfonamides. Sulfhemoglobin cannot transport oxygen, and cyanosis is noted at low concentrations.

Biosynthesis

The biosynthesis of Hb requires the biosynthesis of both heme and the globin polypeptide chains.

Heme Biosynthesis. Heme, ferrous protoporphyrin IX, consists of four pyrrole rings surrounding an Fe atom with four of the six electron pairs of Fe attached to the nitrogen atoms in the pyrrole rings (see Chapter 39). One of the remaining electron pairs attaches to a histidine residue in a globin chain, and the other pair is available for binding and transporting an oxygen molecule. The latter electron pair is protected from oxidation by the surrounding nonpolar amino acid residues of the globin chain. Hemin results from the relatively easy oxidation of the Fe of heme from the ferrous to the ferric state.[11] To remain electrically neutral, a halide molecule, usually chloride, becomes attached to hemin. In

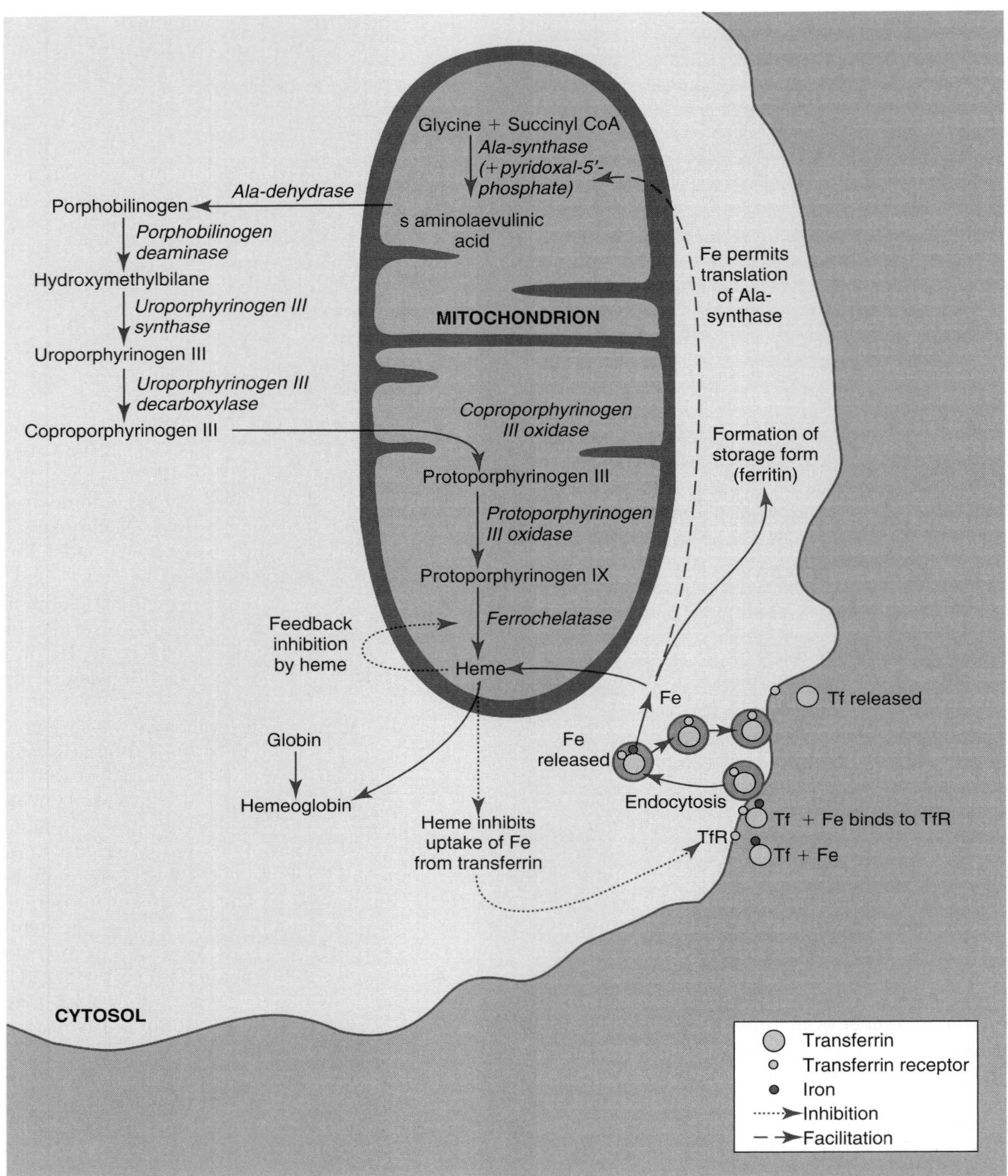

FIGURE 38.4 Heme Synthesis. *CoA*, Co-enzyme A; *Fe*, iron; *TfR*, transferrin receptor. (From Bain BJ. *Haemoglobinopathy Diagnosis*. London: Blackwell, 2001.)

alkaline solution, hematin is formed by the replacement of the halide atom of hemin by a hydroxyl group.

The biosynthesis of heme, shown schematically in Fig. 38.4, takes place primarily in the bone marrow and the liver, and is an eight-step process, with each step involving a different genetically controlled enzyme. Details of this process are given in Chapter 39.

Heme synthesis is controlled by a regulatory negative feedback loop in which heme inhibits the activity of ferrochelatase and the acquisition of Fe from the transport protein transferrin. The decrease in Fe acquisition leads to a decrease in Fe uptake into the cell, with a subsequent decrease in δ-aminolevulinic acid and heme production. Fe deficiency and increased erythropoietin synthesis lead to the combination of the Fe regulatory proteins with the Fe-responsive elements in the transferrin receptor protein messenger ribonucleic acid (mRNA). This combination in turn leads to protection of the mRNA from degradation with subsequent increased uptake of Fe into erythroid cells caused by the increased expression of transferrin receptors on the cell membrane.

Globin Synthesis. The genes that control the α-like and ζ-globin chains are located in a cluster on chromosome 16 at position 16p13.3, which is near the chromosome 16 telomere

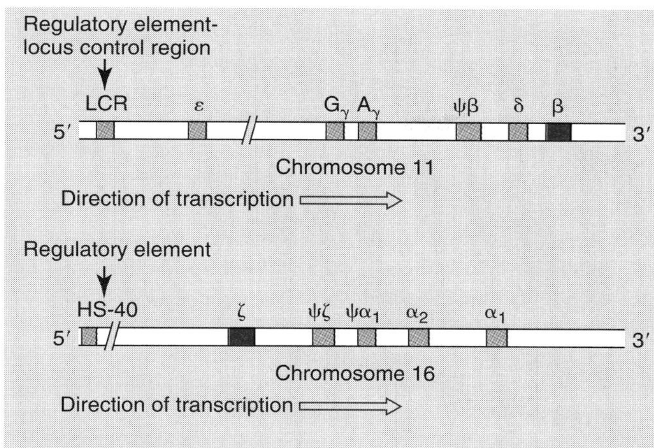

FIGURE 38.5 Globin α- and β-Gene Clusters. (From Bain BJ. *Haemoglobinopathy Diagnosis*. London: Blackwell, 2001.)

(Fig. 38.5). The α-like gene extends more than 28 kb, and contains, reading from the upstream (5′) end to the downstream (3′) end of the DNA segment, an embryonic α-like, ζ-globin gene, a hypervariable region, a pseudo(ψ)–ζ-gene, a pair of pseudo (ψ)–α-genes, a pair of functional α-globin genes, an unexpressed α-like θ gene, and finally, another hypervariable region. Alpha-thalassemia arises from the deletion of one or more α-globin genes or point mutations. Deletion of all four genes, with subsequent production of Hb Bart, is incompatible with life.

The β-, γ-, and δ-globin genes are clustered closely together on chromosome 11. Reading from the 5′ end, the gene sequence is an ε-gene followed by two γ-genes (designated Gγ and Aγ, respectively), a pseudo–ψβ-gene, a δ-gene, and another β-gene. Therefore, two genes determine the γ-chain, with one gene each determining the δ- and β-chains. Substantial variability is seen between individuals and groups with the α- and β-genes, with the most frequent being multiples of the ζ-, ψζ-, and α-genes. The β-globin locus has the locus control region (LCR) at the upstream region of the globin genes. The LCR consists of several DNase I hypersensitive sites that contain binding motifs for transcription activators and functions as an enhancer to regulate the spatio-temporal transcription of the globin genes. When the globin gene is actively transcribed, the LCR hypersensitive sites are positioned in close proximity to the active gene, forming a chromatin loop.

In common with all genes, the globin genes consist of introns (intervening noncoding sequences) and exons (coding sequences) with codons (triplets of nucleotides) coding for specific amino acids. The globin genes have three exons and two introns with a promoter region (specific for the globin chain) at the 5′ end of each gene. This structure has been highly conserved throughout evolution. The upstream regions flanking the first exon contain a number of sequence motifs that are necessary for specifying correct transcriptional initiation. A TATA box is found at the 30-bp upstream of the initiation site, together with one or more CCAAT sites at 70 bp upstream. The gene promoters also contain a CACCC or CCGCCC box that binds erythroid Krüppel-like factor 1, and some have binding sites for erythroid transcription factor GATA-1. In model systems, mutations introduced into such sequences lead to reduction in the level of transcription.[13]

Physiological Role

The Fe of heme is in the ferrous state and is able to combine reversibly with oxygen to act as the major oxygen-carrying moiety. The term *cooperativity* is used to describe the interaction of globin chains in such a way that oxygenation of one heme group enhances the probability of oxygenation of the other heme group. The *Bohr effect* refers to reduction of oxygen affinity, with a decrease in pH from the physiologic range (7.35–7.45) to 6.0 and is another result of this cooperativity. Because the pH of the tissue decreases as a result of the presence of the end products of anaerobic metabolism, carbon dioxide (CO_2) and carbonic acid, the delivery of oxygen to the exercising tissue is enhanced. The oxygen dissociation curve of normal blood Hb is sigmoidal (Fig. 38.6). Physiologically, the CO_2 reversibly combines with the amino terminal groups of Hb to form carbamated Hb, which facilitates the removal of approximately 10% of the CO_2 that forms because of metabolism in the tissue to the lungs. Removal and transport of CO_2 from the tissue are enhanced by the preference for the attachment of more CO_2 by carbamated Hb.

Clinical Significance

The thalassemia syndromes and hemoglobinopathies are clinical disorders related to Hb pathophysiology. Although they may have some similar clinical manifestations,[19] they form two distinct disease groups of genetic origin. The thalassemias originate from insufficient or absent globin chain production due to gene deletion or nonsense mutations, which are mutations that affect the transcription or stability of mRNA products. The name *thalassemia* is derived from the Greek word for "sea," *thalassa,* because early cases of β-thalassemia were described in children of Mediterranean origin.

Hemoglobinopathies, the most common single gene disorder in the world, are structural Hb variants arising from mutations in the globin genes, which result in substitutions or disruptions in the normal amino acid residue sequence in one or more of the globin chains of Hb.

Thalassemia Syndromes

Thalassemias are identified by the globin chain in which a production deficiency occurs. For example, α- and β-thalassemias result from a deficiency in α- or β-globin chain production, respectively (Box 38.1). They are further clinically classified depending on the extent of globin chain production and the resultant severity of the anemia. All the thalassemias have a similar pattern of inheritance: in most cases the gene defects are transmitted in a Mendelian autosomal fashion. Thus, the severe symptomatic varieties result from the interaction of more than one genetic determinant. The inheritance of α-thalassemia is more complicated because it involves the products of the linked pairs of α genes (αα).

Alpha-Thalassemias. The α-thalassemias arise from deficiencies in production of the α-globin chains and are caused by deletions or (less frequently) point mutations in one or more of the four α-globin genes.There are two major classes of α thalassemias: α^0 in which both α genes are inactivated (−−/), and α^+ thalassemias, in which only

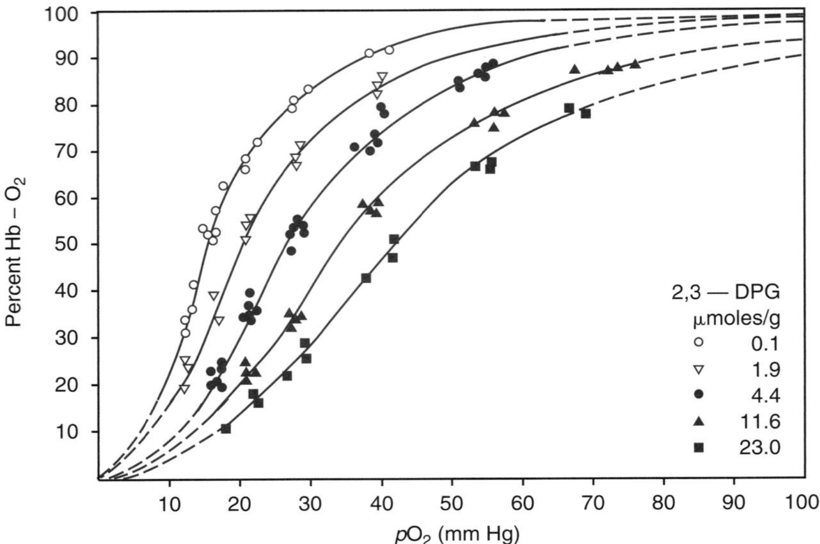
100
90
80
70
60
50
40
30
20
10
Percent Hb – O2
10 20 30 40 50 60 70 80 90 100
pO2 (mm Hg)
2,3 — DPG
μmoles/g
0.1
1.9
4.4
11.6
23.0

FIGURE 38.6 Normal Oxygen Dissociation Curve of Hemoglobin *(Hb)*. Changes in 2,3-diphosphoglycerate *(2,3-DPG)* concentration in the erythrocyte greatly influence the position of the curve. As the concentration of 2,3-DPG increases, the curve shifts to the right. pO_2, Partial pressure of oxygen. (From Duhm J. The effect of 2,3-DPG and other organic phosphates on the Donnan equilibrium and the oxygen affinity of human blood. In: Roth M, Astrup P, eds. Oxygen affinity of hemoglobin and red cell acid base status [Alfred Benzon Symposium, IV]. Copenhagen, Denmark: Alfred Benzon Foundation, 1972.)

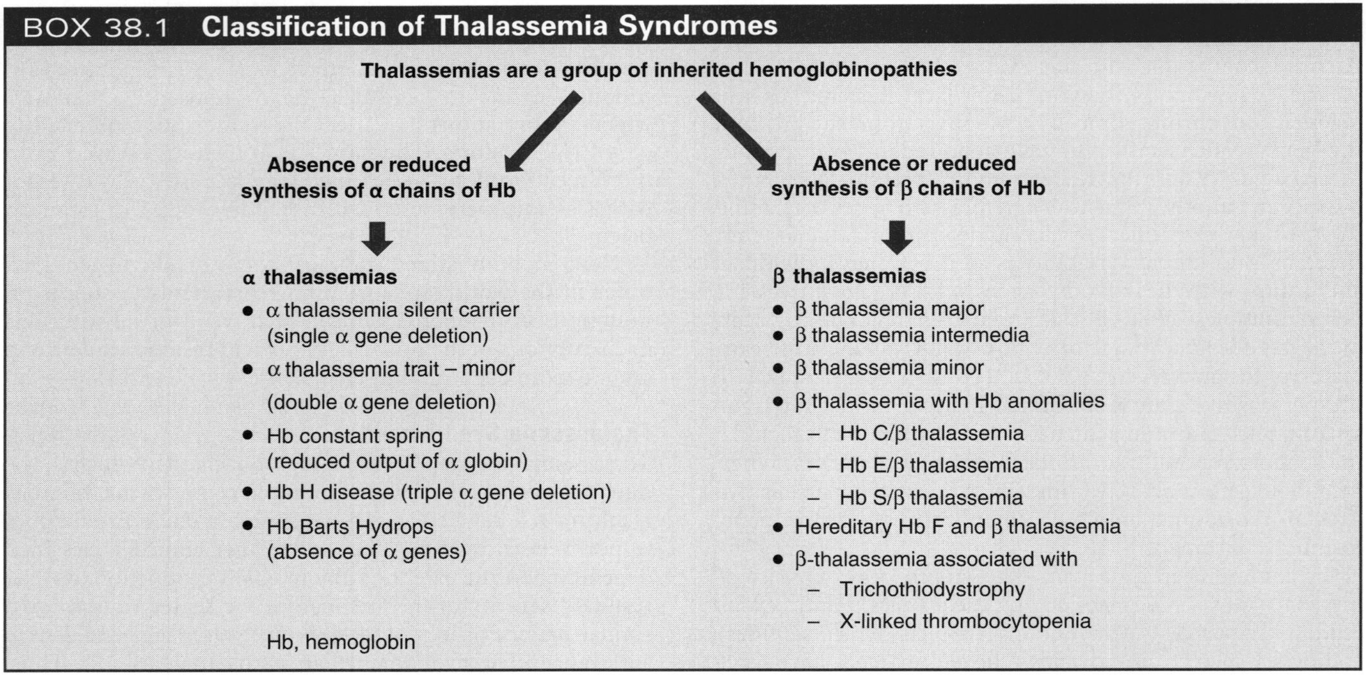
BOX 38.1 Classification of Thalassemia Syndromes
Thalassemias are a group of inherited hemoglobinopathies
Absence or reduced synthesis of α chains of Hb
Absence or reduced synthesis of β chains of Hb
α thalassemias
• α thalassemia silent carrier (single α gene deletion)
• α thalassemia trait – minor (double α gene deletion)
• Hb constant spring (reduced output of α globin)
• Hb H disease (triple α gene deletion)
• Hb Barts Hydrops (absence of α genes)
β thalassemias
• β thalassemia major
• β thalassemia intermedia
• β thalassemia minor
• β thalassemia with Hb anomalies
– Hb C/β thalassemia
– Hb E/β thalassemia
– Hb S/β thalassemia
• Hereditary Hb F and β thalassemia
• β-thalassemia associated with
– Trichothiodystrophy
– X-linked thrombocytopenia
Hb, hemoglobin

one of the pair is defective either due to α deletion or to α mutation. Point mutations are much less frequent. The conventional nomenclature for the point mutations of an α-gene is "$\alpha^T\alpha$," and for deletion, it is "–α." The clinical spectrum of α thalassemias correlates well with the number of the affected α-genes (ie, from normal to the loss of all four genes). The inheritance of a normal allele (αα) with one of the α^+or α^0 results, most frequently, in a "α-thalassemia minor" (– –/αα; –α/αα;–α^T/αα;$\alpha^T\alpha$/–α;–α/–α). In general, carriers of such genotypes have lower levels of total Hb, mean corpuscular volume (MCV), and mean cell Hb (MCH), but they also have a higher red blood cell (RBC) count than normal. The greatest differences are seen in MCH, which is usually less than 26 pg. The peripheral blood smear is quite variable, showing various degrees of hypochromia with some target cells and occasional poikilocytes. In carriers of α^0 thalassemia

TABLE 38.1 The Alpha-Thalassemias

Condition	Affected Number of Alpha-Globin Genes	Phenotype
Silent carrier	One gene affected	Asymptomatic or occasional low red blood cell indexes
Alpha-thalassemia trait	Two genes affected	Mild microcytic and hypochromic anemia
Hb H disease	Three genes affected	Mild-to-moderate anemia, splenomegaly, jaundice
Alpha-thalassemia major/Hb Bart's hydrops	Four genes affected	Most severe form Hb Bart's hydrops Death in utero or at birth

Hb, Hemoglobin.
Data from Vichinsky EP. Alpha thalassemia major–new mutations, intrauterine management, and outcomes. *Hematology Am Soc Hematol Educ Program.* 2009:35–41.

(−−/αα), it is possible to observe in a few red cells inclusions, which are β_4 tetramers that are due to an excess of free β chains. The carriers of nondeletional forms ($\alpha\alpha^T/\alpha\alpha$) show slightly more marked hematological changes than those carriers of deletional forms. The Hb concentration in adult carriers of α^+ or α^othalassemia is indistinguishable from normal, but the percentage of Hb A_2 is slightly lower. Traces of Hb Bart (γ_4) in the neonatal period are detectable in a large proportion of neonates with α-thalassemia, and they decline during the first 6 months after birth. Alpha-thalassemias are common in areas where β-thalassemia is also found at a high frequency. Thus, the coinheritance of α–and β-thalassemia traits may occur and even ameliorate the hematological parameters. In some cases for genetic counseling in families in whom α- and β-thalassemias are present, genotype determination is essential. The unstable mutant Hb^{CT} causes a severe reduction in α_2 globin expression from the affected chromosome; therefore, the carriers, but particularly the homozygotes, have a more severe phenotype than α-thalassemia minor, but it is not as severe as most cases of Hb H disease (Table 38.1).

The α-thalassemias occur worldwide and are particularly prevalent in South East Asia, Southern China, Mediterranean countries (particularly Greece and the Greek Cypriot part of Cyprus), India, the Middle East, and the islands of the South Pacific. Individual types of α-thalassemias are discussed in the following sections and reviewed in the literature.[14]

Hemoglobin Bart's. Hemoglobin Bart's results from deletion of all four α-globin genes, with the subsequent inability to produce any α-globin chains, leading to failure of synthesis of Hb A, F, or A_2. In the fetus, an excess number of γ-globin chains join together to form unstable tetramers known as Hb Bart's (γ^4). Mothers who carry a fetus with Hb Bart's usually present clinically between 20 and 26 weeks' gestation with pregnancy-induced hypertension and polyhydramnios. Ultrasound of the fetus shows hydrops. Severe anemia (Hb usually <80 g/L) is noted on a fetal blood sample obtained by cordocentesis. It is important to rule out other causes for the hydropic fetus by performing serologic testing for toxoplasmosis, rubella, cytomegalovirus, and herpes simplex testing.

High-performance liquid chromatography (HPLC) analysis of a cordocentesis blood sample shows one or two very sharp and narrow peaks at the injection point on the chromatogram (Fig. 38.7A). The major band is Hb Bart's with a smaller band attributed to Hb Portland. Complete absence of Hb F is noted. Alkaline electrophoresis shows a band migrating at or close to the solvent front (Hb Bart's), with another band in the Hb A position (Hb Portland).

Hb Bart hydrops fetalis is almost invariably fatal,[15] with some fetuses dying in utero, and others surviving a few hours after birth. Treatment using intrauterine transfusion has had very limited success, with potential complications in the children of growth retardation and severe brain damage, which may be related to long-standing intrauterine anemia.

Laboratory investigation of the parents of fetuses with Hb Bart's shows a normal HPLC pattern with normal Hb F and A_2 quantification. Parental analysis typically shows a decreased concentration of Hb and decreased MCH and MCV, with the blood smear showing hypochromic, microcytic red cells. The Hb H test may be positive in one or both parents. A two α-gene *cis*-deletion (−/αα) or a three gene deletion (−/−α) is seen in genetic testing of both parents. This requirement restricts the incidence of Hb Bart's to a much smaller population than would be expected based on the worldwide distribution of two α-gene deletions because the presence of *trans* deletions in both parents would not give rise to a four gene deletion in the offspring. Hb Bart's is relatively common in South East Asia, particularly in Thailand, the Philippines, and Hong Kong, where there is a high prevalence of the –SEA deletion.

Hemoglobin H Disease. This disorder is usually caused by a three α-globin gene deletion (−−/−α) and is characterized by a chronic anemia of variable severity.[16] Individuals with nondeletional Hb H disease ($\alpha^T\alpha/--$) are usually more severely affected and are more likely to require transfusion therapy than those with deletional Hb H disease. Significant underproduction of α-globin chains occurs with subsequent joining of free β-globin chains to form the insoluble β-globin chain tetramer Hb H. HPLC analysis of a hemolysate from an individual with Hb H disease shows two bands with low retention times forming a doublet together with a normal Hb A band. Hb F and Hb A_2 concentrations are within the reference interval (see Fig. 38.7D). Electrophoresis at alkaline pH shows a fast moving band together with a band in the Hb A position that possibly has reduced staining compared with other samples run concurrently. The complete blood count (CBC) (Table 38.2) shows a moderately reduced concentration of Hb and markedly reduced MCV and MCH, increased red cell distribution width (RDW), and slightly raised RBC count. Fe studies are normal, although the ferritin concentration may be elevated. Blood film after staining RBC with brilliant cresyl blue shows many cells with inclusion bodies (Fig. 38.8). Hb H disease, according to a recent clinical classification, can be considered a nontransfusion-dependent thalassemia.[17] Fe therapy is not indicated, and transfusion therapy is usually unnecessary except for acute illness in pregnancy. Genetic counseling is recommended to prospective parents who have Hb H disease.

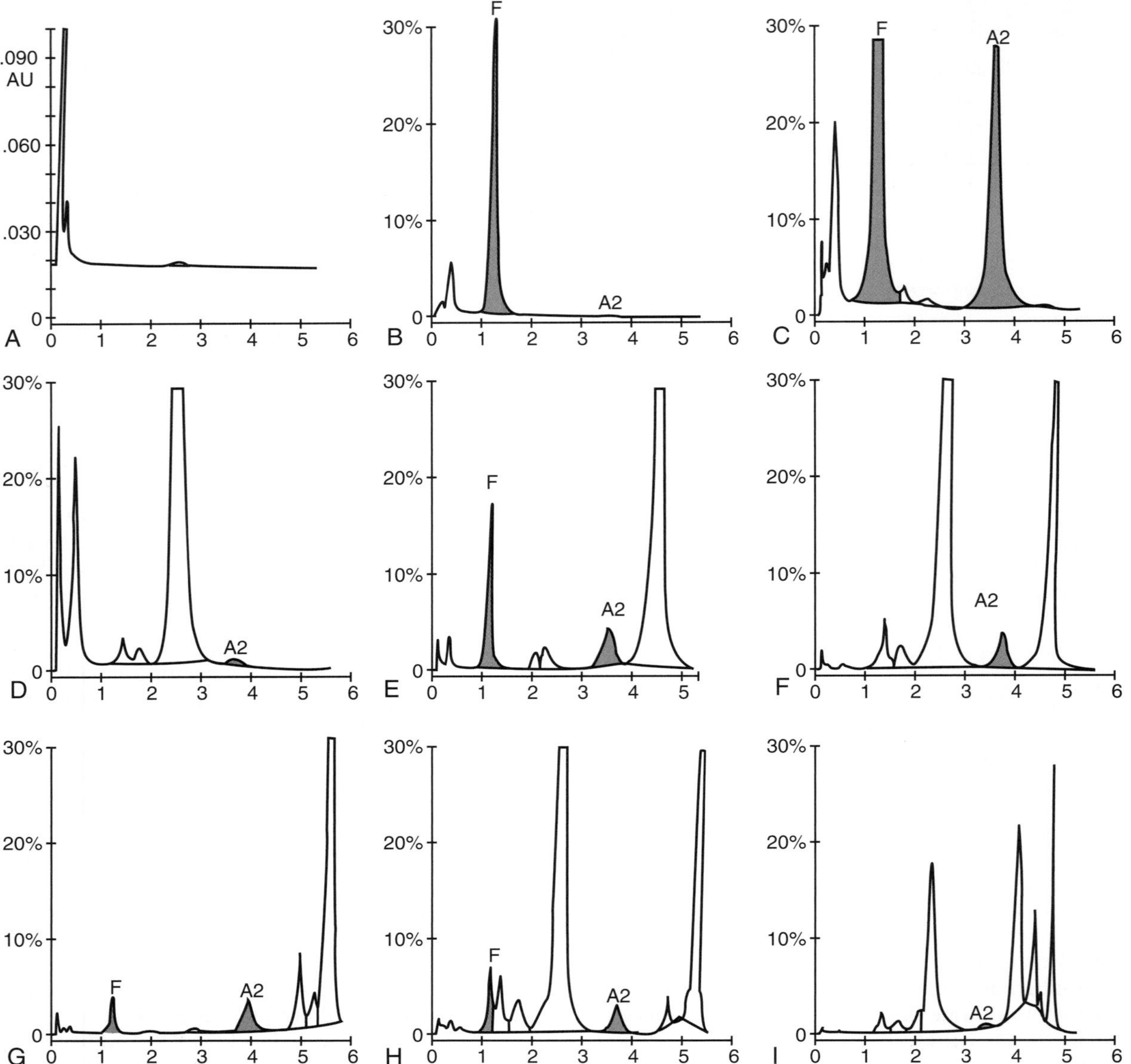

FIGURE 38.7 High-Performance Liquid Chromatography Chromatograms Obtained on the Bio-Rad Variant β-Thal Short Program for **(A)** Hemoglobin *(Hb)* Bart's; **(B)** β0-Thalassemia Major; **(C)** B+-Thalassemia Homozygous E; **(D)** Hb H; **(E)** Homozygous S; **(F)** S Trait; **(G)** Homozygous C; **(H)** C Trait; and **(I)** Hb S-Hb G Philadelphia. (From Clarke GM, Trefor N, Higgins TN. Laboratory investigation of hemoglobinopathies and thalassemias: review and update. *Clin Chem* 2000;46:1284–90.)

Alpha-Thalassemia Minor. Alpha-thalassemia minor is the result of two α-chain gene deletions. These deletions may be seen on the same gene (−−/αα,α°–thalassemia), described as a *cis* deletion, or on different genes (−α/−α, α^{+}–thalassemia), described as a *trans* deletion. The CBC of affected individuals shows a mildly reduced Hb with low MCV and MCH. HPLC analysis shows no abnormal Hb peaks, and Hb F and Hb A_2 concentrations are within the reference intervals. The blood film may show a rare cell with punctate inclusions. Fe studies are normal. In the routine clinical laboratory, the diagnosis of α-thalassemia minor is based on exclusion criteria rather than definitive tests. The presence of thalassemic indexes in a patient with normal Hb A_2 and Hb F quantification is often the only basis for many diagnoses of α-thalassemia minor, particularly in the setting of a positive family history. Reliable diagnosis of an α-thalassemia trait (α+ or α°thalassemia) can only be achieved by DNA analysis using different methods (Gap-polymerase chain reaction [PCR], multiplex ligation-dependent probe amplification [MLPA], allel specific oligonucleotide hybridization [ASO] sequencing). Molecular diagnosis is required in couples at risk for Bart hydrops fetalis syndrome, which results from a deletion of all four α-globin genes.[18] With the availability of genetic testing, a photometric enzyme-linked immunosorbent assay (ELISA) test for the identification of adult carriers of the (SEA) α°thalassemia deletion, used for screening purposes, has become obsolete.[19]

Alpha-Thalassemia Silent. An α-thalassemia trait describes a single α-globin chain gene deletion or mutation (−α/αα; $\alpha^{T}\alpha/\alpha\alpha$). A single α-globin gene deletion or mutation is frequently clinically and hematologically silent.

TABLE 38.2 Definition of the Parameters That Constitute a Complete Blood Count

Parameter	Definition
White blood cell count (WBC)	The number of WBCs in the blood
WBC differential count	The number (or percentage) of each type of WBC present in the blood
Red blood cell (RBC) count	The number of RBCs in the blood
Hematocrit (Hct)	The Hct is the proportion of blood volume that is occupied by RBCs.
Hemoglobin (Hb)	The protein molecule in RBCs that carries oxygen
Mean cell volume (MCV)	The MCV is the average volume of an RBC
Mean cell Hb	The average amount of Hb in the average RBC
Mean cell Hb concentration	The average concentration of Hb in a given volume of blood
Red cell distribution width	A measurement of the variability of RBC size
Platelet count	The calculated number of platelets in a volume of blood

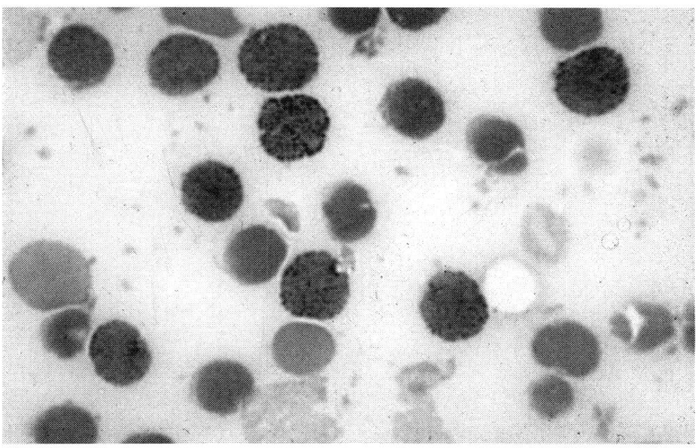

FIGURE 38.8 Hemoglobin H Preparation Showing Punctate Inclusions on a Patient With Hemoglobin H Disease.

A CBC of an individual with this trait shows a normal or marginally decreased Hb concentration, MCV, and MCH. Fe studies are normal, and no abnormal Hb peaks are seen on HPLC analysis.

The effects of various α-thalassemias on the percentage of β-chain Hb variants are shown in Table 38.3.[20] In general, the percentage of the Hb variant decreases as a percentage of total Hb as the number of α-chain deletions increases.

Beta-Thalassemias. The β-thalassemias result from a reduction in the synthesis of the β-globin chain[21] and are commonly found in (1) the Mediterranean region, (2) Africa, (3) the Middle East, and (4) South East Asia, especially the southern provinces of China, including Hong Kong, the Indian subcontinent, the Malay peninsula, Myanmar (Burma), and

TABLE 38.3 Effects of a Thalassemia on the Percentage of Beta-Chain Variant Hemoglobin in Heterozygotes

	AS	AC	AE
αα/αα	41.0 ± 1.8	43.8 ± 1.5	30.0 ± 1.5
αα/α–	35.4 ± 1.6	37.5 ± 1.4	27.0 ± 2.0
α^{-}/α^{-} or $\alpha\alpha/^{-}$	28.1 ± 1.4	32.2 ± 0.8	22.0 ± 2.0

AS, Carrier of hemoglobin (Hb) S; *AC*, carrier of Hb C; *AE*, carrier of HbE.

Modified from Bunn HF, Forget BG, eds. *Hemoglobin: Molecular Genetic and Clinical Aspects.* Philadelphia: Saunders, 1986.

Indonesia.[22] Frequency of gene distribution is estimated at 3% to 10% in some populations. The high frequency of β-thalassemia in the tropics is believed to reflect an advantage of heterozygotes against *Plasmodium falciparum* malaria. With increasing migration, β-thalassemia, once considered a rare genetic disease in Northern Europe, Australia, and North America, is now becoming more common all over the world. More than 250 β-thalassemia mutations have been described; however, in each ethnic group, a relatively small number of mutations account for most cases (the ratio most often quoted is that ≤20 mutations account for ≥80% of cases). Most are point mutations within the gene or its immediate flanking sequence. A few β-thalassemia mutations that segregate independently of the β-globin gene cluster have been described, presumably involving *trans*-acting regulatory factors. An updated list of these mutations is accessible at the Globin Gene Server Website (http://globin.cse.psu.edu). Simple deletions of the β-globin gene are rare, ranging in size from 290 bp to more than 60 Kb. The 619 bp deletion at the 3′ end of the β gene is relatively common among Sindhi and Punjabi populations in India and Pakistan. The remaining deletions are restricted to single families, are necessarily β^0 thalassemias, and interestingly, they are associated with an unusual high level of Hb A_2 in heterozygotes. Large deletions that affect the entire β-globin gene cluster $(\epsilon\gamma\gamma\delta\beta)^{o}$are rare and restricted to single families. Finally, some highly unstable β-chain variants may manifest as a dominant form of β-thalassemia.

The clinical classification of β-thalassemia includes: thalassemia major (TM; transfusion-dependent), thalassemia intermedia (TI; of intermediate severity, nontransfusion-dependent) and thalassemia minor (asymptomatic). The severity of the clinical manifestations correlates well with the degree of imbalance of globin chains, depending on the β-globin gene defects and their interaction. The production of β-globin chains is quantitatively reduced to different degrees, whereas the synthesis of α-globin continues as normal, resulting in accumulation of excess unmatched α-globin chains in the erythroid precursors. Clinical manifestations of β-thalassemia range from mild anemia to severe life-threatening disease that requires lifelong transfusions (Fig. 38.9).

Beta°-Thalassemia (Beta-Thalassemia Major). This is sometimes called Cooley anemia, after the physician who first described the condition in 1925 in the children of Italian and Greek immigrants in New York by noting that these children (1) failed to grow, (2) had frequent infections, (3) appeared

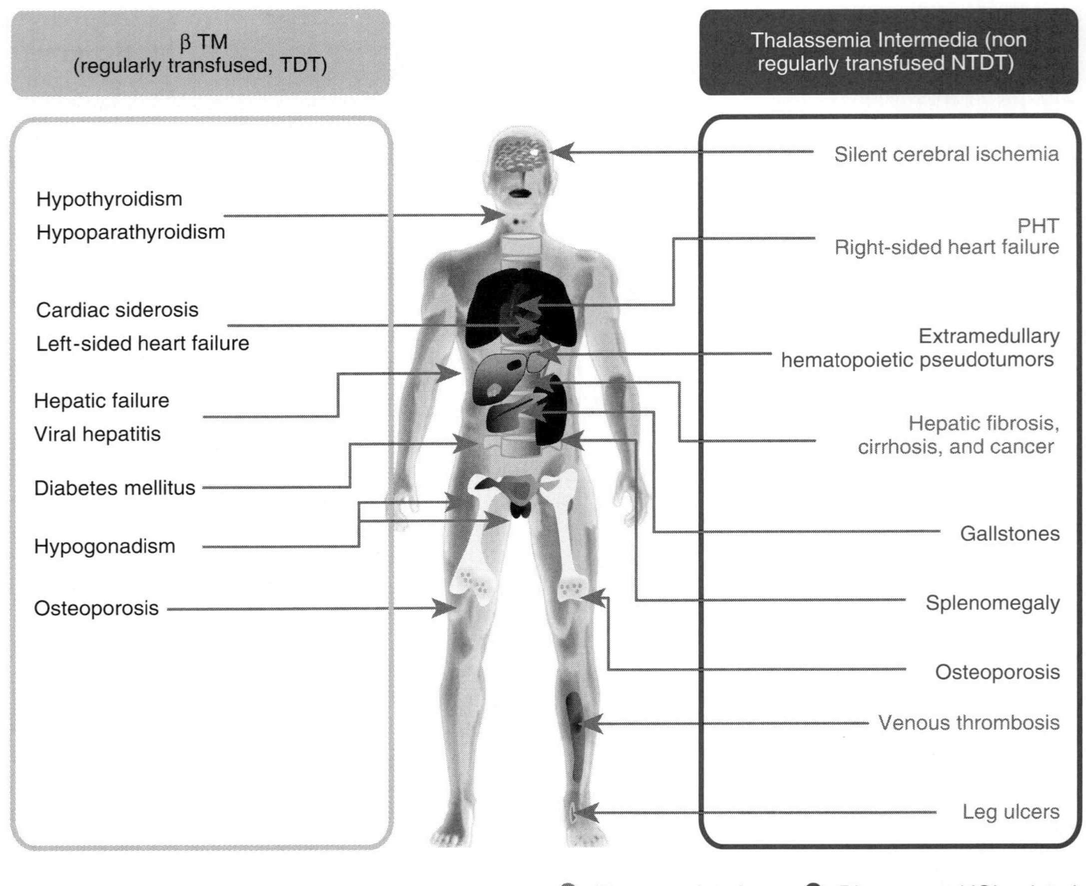

FIGURE 38.9 Clinical Complications in Thalassemia Major and in Thalassemia Intermedia. *β-TM*, β thalassemia major; *IOL*, iron overload; *PHT*, pulmonary hypertension; *TDT*, transfusion-dependent thalassemia. (Modified from Musallam K, Rivella S, Vichinsky E, Rachmilewitz EA. Non-transfusion-dependent thalassemias. *Haematologica* 2013;98:833–844.)

pale and malnourished, (4) had splenomegaly, and (5) had facial bone changes.

Beta-TM results from mutations that interfere with translation or are involved in the initiation, elongation, or termination of globin chain synthesis. Mutations that interfere with translation account for almost 50% of all β-thalassemia mutations. Included in this are frame shift or nonsense mutations that produce premature termination codons, which result in incomplete translation of the β-globin gene and nonproduction of the β-globin chain, leading to β°-thalassemia.

Clinical presentation usually occurs at younger than 1 year of age, with features such as small size for age, abdominal girth expansion, and failure to thrive. Physical examination of the patient may reveal frontal bossing[23] (an unusually prominent forehead) caused by thickening of the cranial bones, pallor, and prominence of the cheek bones, which in older children obscures the base of the nose and exposes the teeth. These features are a result of marrow expansion (up to a 30-fold increase) caused by ineffective erythropoiesis with production of highly unstable α-globin tetramers, leading to a sequence of events responsible for bone marrow expansion, anemia, hemolysis, splenomegaly, and increased Fe absorption.

Typical CBC results include severe anemia with Hb concentration between 30 and 65 g/L, MCV of 48 to 72 fL, and MCH of 23 to 32 pg. A characteristic markedly abnormal RBC morphology is noted on the peripheral blood smear; this includes a large number of microcytes and/or macrocytes, numerous target cells, which may have a bridge joining the central and peripheral pigment zones, polychromasia, and occasional spherocytes, schistocytes, and nucleated red cells. When a patient's RBCs are of unequal size (anisocytosis), the diameter of the RBC varies from 3 to 15 μm with little pigment; shape distortion is noted, along with prominent basophilic stippling. RBC osmotic fragility is frequently observed. Typical peripheral blood on a patient with β° thalassemia is shown in Fig. 38.10.

White blood cell (WBC) and platelet counts are usually normal. Nucleated red cells can be present and inappropriately counted as WBCs. Ferritin is usually within the upper half of the reference interval, and total bilirubin is mildly elevated, with a borderline elevation in the conjugated fraction. Urinalysis frequently shows increased urobilinogen or urobilin concentration, and urine is often dark brown to black because of the presence of dipyroles and mesobilifuscin. The latter features reflect ineffective hematopoiesis with intramedullary red cell destruction. HPLC analysis (see Fig.

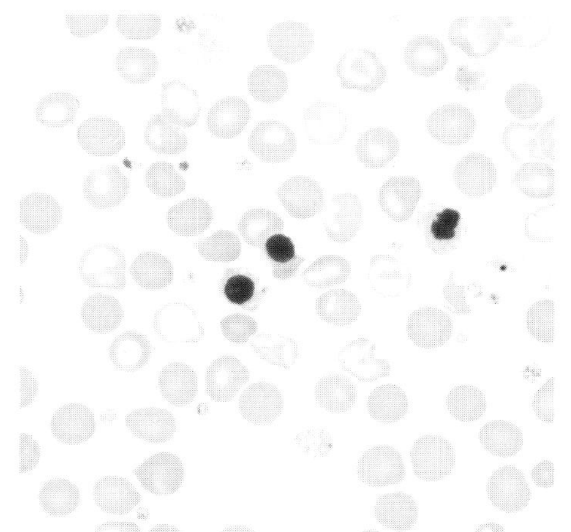

FIGURE 38.10 Peripheral Blood Smear of an Individual With β0-Thalassemia. (From Rodak BF, Carr JH. *Clinical Hematology Atlas.* 5th ed. Philadelphia: Elsevier; 2017.)

38.7B) shows a major Hb F peak with absence of an Hb A peak and variable Hb A_2 (reference interval, 1–5.9%; mean, 1.7%) peak. Electrophoresis at alkaline and acid pH shows a dominant band in the F position on both gels.[24]

Family studies on both parents and siblings should be performed, and the classical β-thalassemia minor pattern, described later in the chapter, should be found in the parents. Siblings may be normal or may have β-thalassemia minor. A family case history is seen in Fig. 38.11.

The conventional treatment for TM patients includes regular transfusion therapy and Fe chelation. Many patients with TM require splenectomy because of hypersplenism. However, optimal clinical management may delay or even obviate the need for splenectomy, which was common in the past. After splenectomy, inclusion bodies consisting of denatured α-chains can be observed in the blood smear after staining with methyl violet. Fe overload is an inevitable and serious complication of long-term blood transfusion therapy that requires adequate treatment to prevent early death mainly from Fe-induced cardiac disease. Puberty is often delayed, incomplete, or completely absent. In boys, active spermatogenesis may occur, and Leydig cell function is normal. The quality and duration of life of TM patients has

TEST/REF	INDEX PAT 7 MO F	MOTHER 33 YRS	FATHER 40 YRS	SIBLING 3 YR F
Hb	¯72 G/L	¯114	¯132	122
REF	105-135	120-160	135-175	115-135
RBC	¯3.23 (10^{12}/L)	5.19	↑6.61	4.42
REF	3.70-5.30	4.10-5.20	4.50-6.00	3.90-5.30
MCV	¯69 fL	¯68	¯63	80
REF	70-86	80-100	80-100	75-87
MCH	¯22 pg	¯22	¯20	28
REF	26-35	26-35	26-35	26-35
HbA	¯0.00	0.94	↑0.93	0.96
REF	0.94-0.98	0.94-0.98	0.94-0.98	0.94-0.98
HbA2	0.030	↑0.054	↑0.058	0.030
REF	<0.03	<0.03	<0.03	<0.03
HbF	0.97	<0.01	<0.01	<0.01
REF	<0.10	<0.01	<0.01	<0.01

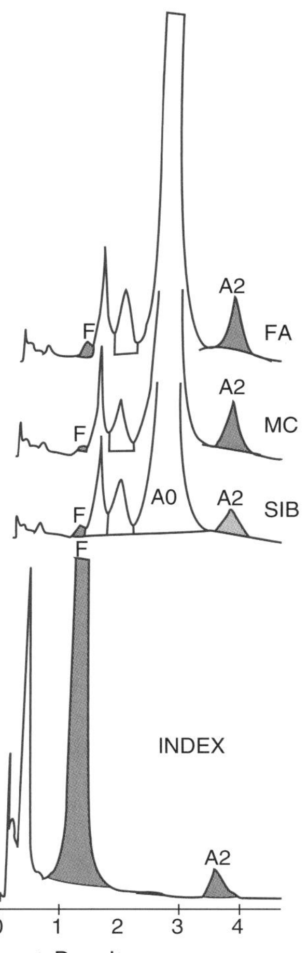

FIGURE 38.11 High-Performance Liquid Chromatograms and Complete Blood Count Results From a Family Study of a Child With β0-Thalassemia. *Hb*, Hemoglobin; *MCH*, mean cell hemoglobin; *MCV*, mean corpuscular volume; *RBC*, red blood cell. (From Berendt HL, Blakney GB, Clarke GM, Higgins TN. A case of β-thalassemia major detected using HPLC in a child of Chinese ancestry. *Clin Biochem* 2000;33:311–313.)

been transformed over the last 10 years, with life expectancy increasing well into the third and fourth decades. Many children who are adequately transfused and are fully compliant with Fe chelation therapy develop normally, enter puberty, and become sexually mature. The availability of oral Fe chelators, such as Deferiprone (ApoPharma, Toronto, Canada) and Deferasirox (Novartis, Basel, Switzerland), has significantly improved the adherence to chelation, which has affected survival.[25] Nevertheless, prolongation of life is accompanied by several complications, partly due to the underlying disorder and partly as a consequence of the treatment with blood transfusions and Fe overload, such as diabetes mellitus, hypothyroidism, hypoparathyroidism, and liver disease.[25]

Allogeneic hemopoietic stem cell transplantation is currently the only method available to cure transfusion-dependent TM; it has been used worldwide.[26] Gene therapy and other innovative therapeutic modalities for the cure of TM are under investigation.[27]

Beta-Thalassemia Intermedia. Thalassemia intermedia is a clinical term used to describe patients with anemia and splenomegaly, but who do not have the full spectrum of clinical severity found in TM. The clinical phenotypes of TI lie between those of thalassemia minor and major, encompassing a wide clinical spectrum. Mildly affected patients are almost completely asymptomatic until adult life, experiencing only mild anemia and spontaneously maintaining Hb levels between 7 and 10 g/dL (70–100 g/L). Patients with more severe TI generally present between the ages of 2 and 6 years, and although they are able to survive without regular transfusion therapy, growth and development can be retarded. Most TI patients are homozygotes or compound heterozygotes for mild-to-moderate β-gene mutations (β^+/β^+; β^o/β^+), less commonly, only a single β-globin gene is affected. Because the clinical severity of the disease is dictated by the different extent of globin chain imbalance, at least three different mechanisms may promote the mild clinical characteristics of TI compared with TM: inheritance of mild or silent β-gene mutations; coinheritance of determinants associated with increased γ-chain production that contributes to neutralizing the large proportion of unbound α-chains; and coinheritance of α-thalassemia that reduces the synthesis of α-chains, thereby reducing the α/non–α-chain imbalance. Three main factors are responsible for the clinical sequelae in TI patients: rate of ineffective erythropoiesis, chronic anemia, and Fe overload.

TI is clinically labeled as nontransfusion-dependent thalassemia because the affected patients do not require lifelong regular transfusions for survival, although they may require occasional or even frequent blood transfusions in particular situations such as pregnancy, surgery, and infections. Nontransfusion-dependent thalassemia also includes Hb E/β-thalassemia (mild and moderate forms) characterized by clinical symptoms similar to β-TI. Hb E is caused by a G to A substitution in codon 26 of the β-globin gene; Hb E is synthesized at a reduced rate and behaves like a mild β-thalassemia mutation. Patients with Hb E/β-thalassemia coinherit a β-thalassemia allele from one parent and the structural variant (Hb E) from the other. The resulting clinical phenotype could be severe, similar to TM, or moderate, similar to TI.[28]

HPLC analysis shows a variable Hb F peak with a reduced Hb A peak. Hb A_2 is above the reference interval at concentrations greater than those associated with β-thalassemia minor. Bands in the A and F positions are seen on electrophoresis at both alkaline and acid pH. Hb is significantly reduced to values between 6 and 10 g/dL (60–100 g/L). The peripheral blood smear shows the same features seen in β^o-thalassemia, including anisocytosis, hypochromia, target cells, basophilic stippling, and nucleated RBCs.

Beta-Thalassemia Minor (Beta-Thalassemia Trait). Patients with β-thalassemia minor are often asymptomatic, except at times of hematopoietic stress, such as infection or pregnancy, when they can become more anemic. The CBC on patients with a β-thalassemia trait shows low normal or decreased Hb concentration and hematocrit (Hct), decreased MCV (<80 fL) and MCH (<25 pg), and variable RDWs. The discriminant factor is less than 60 pg (see the Analytical Methods section for definition). However, for patients with liver disease and β-thalassemia, MCV and MCH may be at the low end of the reference interval. The peripheral blood smear shows microcytic RBCs with occasional hypochromia, poikilocytosis, and target cells.

The diagnosis of β-thalassemia minor, with appropriate indexes in the CBC, is dependent on the finding of a raised Hb A_2 (>3.3%). Hb A_2 and Hb A_2' should be added together to obtain an accurate Hb A_2 value for the investigation of β-thalassemia minor. Hb A_2 may be elevated in HIV-positive women without hypochromic microcytic indexes,[29] those with hyperthyroidism or megoblastic anemia, and individuals with some unstable Hbs.[30] Fe-depleted individuals should become Fe replete before a definitive diagnosis of β-thalassemia is made, because Hb A_2 may be falsely low. HPLC is the preferred method for this quantification; densitometric scanning of the Hb A_2 band on an alkaline electrophoresis gel is not recommended because of its poor precision and accuracy.[30] In 30% to 40% of all cases of β-thalassemia minor, Hb F could be mildly elevated (1%–2%). The life span of the RBC may be reduced, and individuals with diabetes may show a lower HbA_{1c} compared with normal individuals with equivalent glycemic control. The β-thalassemia mutations may be identified preferentially by direct sequencing or by gap–PCR.

Delta-/Beta-Thalassemia. The δβ-thalassemias are the result of deletions that affect various parts of the β-globin locus. These deletions are partially compensated by an increased expression of the γ genes that raises the level of Hb F. The length of deletion accounts for different forms of δβ-thalassemia, including both $^G\gamma$ and $^A\gamma$ genes or only $^A\gamma$, and vary from 9 to 100 Kb. Hb Lepore is a hybrid of δ- and β-chains that result from a crossover between the two misaligned genes; this Hb is synthesized inefficiently and gives rise to a form of δβ-thalassemia.

Both heterozygous and homozygous conditions have been described. It is found in a variety of ethnic groups, but it is most prevalent in Eastern Mediterranean countries, especially Greece and Italy. CBC analysis shows a reduced concentration of Hb (8–13.5 g/dL; 80–135 g/L) with reduced MCV and MCH, and sometimes an increased RDW. HPLC analysis shows an Hb A peak with a normal or reduced Hb A_2 concentration and a raised Hb F concentration (between 5% and 20%), with the highest Hb F concentration seen in the Sardinian type of δβ-thalassemia.

Hereditary Persistence of Fetal Hemoglobin. The term hereditary persistence of Hb F (HPFH) is used to describe a group of genetic conditions in which the concentration of Hb

F is increased above the upper limit of the reference interval because of a reduction in β-globin synthesis and a compensatory increase in δ-globin synthesis. However, deletions of δ and β genes are also the molecular basis for many forms of HPFH that usually have higher levels of compensatory Hb F production than the δβ-thalassemias. Several deletional variants of HPFH have been described, including Greek, Indian, Italian, Corfu, and black. In black HPFH, the Hb F is raised to between 10% and 36% of the total Hb with normal Hb A_2 concentrations. Hb, MCV, and MCH are within the reference intervals. This condition is clinically innocuous and asymptomatic. Similarly, no clinical abnormalities are associated with Greek HPFH, although the concentration of Hb F is in the range of 15% to 25%.

Other HPFHs are due to point mutations in the promoter region upstream from the transcription start site in either the $^{G}\gamma$ and $^{A}\gamma$ genes, which alter the binding of one or more transcription factors; these are known as "nondeletion HPFHs."

The increase in Hb F in these forms is distributed heterogeneously among the red cells in otherwise normal individuals. The Hb F concentration varies between 1% and 13% of total Hb heterozygotes and between 19% and 21% of homozygotes. No clinical or hematologic abnormalities are noted.

Hemoglobinopathies

If only single point mutations are considered, 1695 possible Hb variants are known; 733 were identified by mid-2007.[31] Currently, more than 900 hemoglobinopathies have been described, but only 9 have some clinical significance. Recent migration from regions with a high frequency of hemoglobinopathies (South East Asia or Africa) to regions that had low frequencies (Western Europe, Central and South America, and Canada) has increased the incidence of hemoglobinopathy in these areas to such an extent that some western European countries have introduced neonatal testing for Hb variants. The incidental finding of a hemoglobinopathy during HPLC analysis for HbA_{1c} has increased both the number and the incidence of Hb variants.[32,33] Several Hb variants (eg, Hb Rambam, Niigata, Camden) interfere with HPLC methods for quantifying HbA_{1c} (for a more extensive list, see Elder and colleagues[34]), and one Hb variant was found to be the result of interference in pulse oximetry measurements.[35]

Nomenclature. Hemoglobin variants are named using (1) letters (Hbs S, D, E, and so on), (2) the family name of the index case (Hb Lepore), (3) the place of discovery of the variant or place of origin of the propositus (Hb Edmonton), or (4) the name of the river (Hb Saale) flowing through the city in which the propositus lived. In some cases, both a letter and a name are used, as in Hb J-Baltimore, indicating that the Hb is classified as having electrophoretic mobility similar to that of other J Hbs but differs from them in amino acid sequence, and was originally discovered in Baltimore. The term *AS trait* (sometimes abbreviated to *S trait*) is used to describe a heterozygous state in which one of the β-globin chains is S and the other is A. In instances in which no normal β-globin chain is present (eg, Hb SD), the β-globin chain present in the higher concentration is usually, although not always, placed first. A systematic nomenclature system is now used alongside the variant name to describe the affected chain and location on the chain and the amino acid substitution. For example, Hb Spanish Town [$\alpha 27(\beta 8)^{Glu \rightarrow Val}$], a Hb variant named after a district in Kingston, Jamaica, and found in Jamaicans of African descent, results from a substitution of valine for glutamic acid in position 27 of the α-globin chain, which is located in position 8 of the B helix of the α-chain.

Classification of Hemoglobin Variants. Hemoglobin variants are classified according to the type of mutation.[20] Single point mutations in α-globin chains give rise to substitution of one amino acid residue. As an example, Hb San Diego [$\beta 109(G11)^{Val \rightarrow Met}$] has a methionine residue instead of the normal valine at position 109 of the β-chain. Hb C Harlem [$\beta 6(A3)^{Glu \rightarrow Val}$; $\beta 73(E17)^{Asp \rightarrow Asn}$] is an example of an Hb variant in which two amino acid residues are substituted, namely, valine replaces glutamic acid at position 6 and asparagine replaces aspartic acid at position 73 of the β-chain. Hb C Harlem is electrophoretically similar to Hb C but behaves like Hb S in every other aspect, including clinical manifestation. Deletion Hb variants arise from the deletion of one to five amino acid residues in the globin chain. Hb Vicksburg [$\beta 75(E19)^{Leu \rightarrow 0}$] is an example of this category, having a deletion of leucine in position 75 of the β-chain. Insertion Hbs arise from insertion of one to three amino acid residues into the globin chain. Hb Grady is an example of this category, with an insertion of a three amino acid residue sequence (glutamine-phenylalanine-threonine) between positions 118 and 119 of the α-chain. Deletion–insertion Hbs arise from the deletion of a portion of the normal amino acid residue sequence and the insertion of another sequence, with resultant lengthening or shortening of the globin chain. An example of this type of Hb variant is Hb Montreal, in which the three normal amino acid residues between positions 72 and 76 of the β-globin chain are replaced with a four amino acid residue sequence. Elongation Hbs result from a single bp mutation or frameshift at the 3′ end of exon 3 or the 5′ end of exon 1 of the α_2- or the β-globin chain. The elongation Hb, Hb Constant Spring (named after an ethnic Chinese family from the Constant Spring district of Jamaica), has an additional 31 amino acid residues joined at position 142 (the carboxy terminal) of the α-chain. Fusion Hbs result from the fusion of an α- or β-globin chain with a portion of another globin chain. Hb Lepore-Hollandia results from the fusion of the first 22 amino acid residues of the δ-chain with the amino acid sequence from position 50 onward of normal β-globin. For the latter four categories, the systematic name is long and cumbersome, prompting universal use of the variant name rather than the systematic nomenclature.

Types of Hemoglobin Variants. In α-chain variants, the variant usually forms less than 25% of the total Hb (Hb G Philadelphia is an exception) because the mutation typically occurs in only one of the four genes that code for the α-globin chain. For β-chain variants in the heterozygous state, the variant forms more than 25% but less than 50% of the total Hb. Based on the mutation of only one of the β-globin chain genes, the β-chain variant should form 50% of total Hb. However, if the amino acid substitution results in a net negative charge to the β-variant chain, then the variant chain competes more effectively for α-chains and the percent of the Hb variant is greater than Hb A (eg, Hb N-Baltimore). The converse is true; a decrease in negative charge results in a percent of the variant Hb being less than Hb A (eg, Hb S). This information can be used to categorize an unknown Hb variant as an α- or β-globin chain variant and in preliminary Hb variant identification.

Hb VarDatabase is a relational database of Hb variants and thalassemia mutations and may be accessed at http://globin.cse.psu.edu/hbvar/menu.html.

Laboratories should maintain a bank of hematologic and chromatographic data for Hb variants found in their facilities.

Hemoglobin S. Hemoglobin S [$\beta 6(A3)^{Glu \rightarrow Val}$] in the heterozygous or homozygous state is the most widespread of the Hb variants and arises from a substitution of valine for glutamic acid at position 6 in the A helix of the β-globin chain. Hb S is found frequently in West and North Africa, the Middle East (especially Saudi Arabia), and the Indian subcontinent. Approximately 8% of African Americans are heterozygous for Hb S, and homozygous Hb S is found in 1 in 500 newborns in this group. Four haplotypes originating from different geographic locations have been described. The widespread distribution of the single point gene mutation responsible for the synthesis of Hb S in areas where *P. falciparum* malaria is endemic is due to protection of Hb S heterozygotes from the worst manifestations of this malaria.

Homozygous Hemoglobin S. In homozygous Hb S (Hb SS), a valine for glutamic acid substitution occurs on both β-globin chains because of the inheritance of mutated β-globin chain genes from both parents. This condition is described as "sickle cell anemia" or "sickle cell disease" because of the sickle-shaped RBCs that occur when a sickle cell crisis occurs. It sometimes is written as $\beta^S\beta^S$.[36]

HPLC analysis (see Fig. 38.7E) of a hemolysate of an individual homozygous for Hb S shows no Hb A peak and a small Hb A_2 peak. The apparent Hb A_2 concentration may be falsely increased because of the presence of glycated Hb S. Hb S forms 85% to 90% of the total Hb. The Hb F concentration is variable, with females having higher concentrations than males, and is somewhat, although not exclusively, haplotype-dependent. The highest Hb F concentrations (10%–25%) are found in individuals from the Middle East and the Indian subcontinent with the Arab-Indian haplotype. Low Hb F concentrations (5%–6%) are found in the West African Cameroon (sometimes called Senegal) haplotype. The remaining haplotypes, the Benin and Bantu, have Hb F concentrations in the range of 6% to 7%. Increased concentrations of Hb F mitigate the clinical manifestations of sickle cell anemia to some extent. Electrophoresis (Fig. 38.12) at both alkaline and acid pH shows a single large band in the Hb S position with small bands at the Hb A_2 and Hb F positions. The sickle cell screen test is positive.

CBC analysis of an individual homozygous for Hb S indicates a moderate to a major decrease in Hb concentration (60–100 g/L), with normal to increased MCV and MCH. In individuals with a concurrent thalassemia, the Hb is further decreased, and both MCV and MCH are lowered. In the neonate, the peripheral blood smear shows occasional sickle and target cells and Howell-Jolly bodies. As a patient's age increases, these features of hyposplenism become increasingly evident. In the adult, the percentage of sickle cells observed can be as great as 30% to 40%. In the setting of a sickle cell crisis, fewer sickle cells may be present than when individuals are clinically well. Howell-Jolly bodies, target cells, Pappenheimer bodies, boat-shaped cells, and nucleated RBCs are noted. The platelet count and neutrophil counts are elevated. Sometimes blister cells, in which the Hb appears to be present in only one half of the cell, are observed.

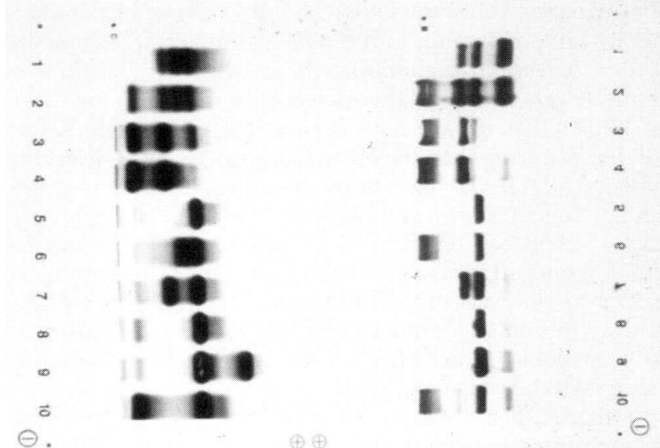

FIGURE 38.12 Alkaline *(Left)* and Acid *(Right)* Electrophoresis of Various Hemoglobinopathies. Lane 1, hemoglobin *(Hb)* S, Hb FA control. Lane 2, HB S, Hb F, HbCA control. Lane 3, transfused SC disease. Lane 4, SC disease. Lane 5, Hb A (normal). Lane 6, Hb Presbyterian. Lane 7, Hb S. Lane 8, raised Hb A2 (β-thalassemia trait). Lane 9, Hb J Baltimore. Lane 10, Hb C.

Treatment of children with homozygous Hb S includes the use of hydroxyurea, with an increase in the quantity of Hb F, sometimes to 25%. In adults, transfusion or erythroexchange are needed to keep Hb S at less than 40%.

Heterozygous Hemoglobin S (Hemoglobin S Trait). High-performance liquid chromatography analysis (see Fig. 38.7F) of a hemolysate of a blood sample from an individual who is heterozygous for Hb S shows peaks in the Hb A and S positions, with 40% of the total Hb found in the Hb S peak. Hb S concentrations less than 30% are suggestive of coinheritance of α-thalassemia. Hb F concentration is variable. Electrophoresis (see Fig. 38.12) at both alkaline and acid pH shows bands in the A and S positions.

CBC analysis from an individual who is heterozygous for Hb S shows a slightly decreased concentration of Hb, and sickle cells are not typically seen on the peripheral blood film. Patients are often asymptomatic, and the first time an individual is diagnosed as heterozygous for Hb S (sickle cell trait) is often when an HbA_{1c} analysis is requested for the individual or when a family study is initiated for genetic counseling. In the United States, neonatal screening programs are designed specifically to detect both heterozygous and homozygous Hb S in newborns. Although individuals with the sickle cell trait are clinically asymptomatic, genetic counseling should be considered because coinheritance of two β-globin gene abnormalities may contribute to a sickle cell disorder. Alpha- and β-thalassemia can be coinherited with heterozygous Hb S.

Hemoglobin SC (Hemoglobin SC Disease). Hemoglobin SC disease arises when both β-globin chains are substituted at position 6 with valine (Hb S) or lysine (Hb C). On HPLC and capillary electrophoresis, analysis peaks are noted in the S and C positions, with the S peak forming most of the Hb present.

Electrophoresis (see Fig. 38.12) at both alkaline and acid pH shows bands in the S and C positions, and the sickling test is positive.

Hemoglobin SD. Hemoglobin S may be coinherited with Hb D (SD disease). Individuals with this disease have similar but milder clinical presentation compared with that of sickle cell disease (Hb SS). HPLC analysis shows two peaks—one in the Hb S position that forms approximately 38% to 42% of the total Hb, and the other in the Hb D position that forms 43% to 45% of the total Hb. The Hb F concentration is usually within the reference interval, although concentrations as high as 14% have been observed in some individuals with SD disease. Alkaline electrophoresis shows a band in the S position. Acid electrophoresis shows bands in the S and A positions. The sickling test is positive. CBC analysis shows a greatly decreased concentration of Hb, with normal to slightly elevated MCV. Target, boat-shaped, nucleated, red, and sickle cells—together with anisocytosis and poikilocytosis—are noted on the peripheral blood smear.

Hemoglobin S/O Arab. Coinheritance of Hb S and Hb O Arab presents a similar or somewhat milder clinical presentation to sickle cell disease and is found in the Middle East and North Africa.

Hemoglobin S/G Philadelphia. One or more abnormal α-globin chains can combine with Hb S. In African Americans and West Africans, the combination of Hb G Philadelphia [α68(E17)$^{Asn \rightarrow Lys}$] with Hb S is prevalent. HPLC analysis (see Fig. 38.7I) of blood samples from these individuals shows at least two major peaks and two smaller peaks. The two major peaks are due to combinations of the normal α-chain with the normal β-chain and the abnormal α-chain with the normal β-chain. The two smaller peaks are due to combinations of the normal α-chain with the abnormal β-chain and the abnormal α-chain with the abnormal β-chain. Electrophoresis at alkaline pH shows major bands in the A and S positions, with a minor band in the C position. At acid pH, bands are seen in the A and S positions. CBC analysis gives a slightly decreased Hb concentration with normal MCV and MCH. Alpha- or β-thalassemia can be coinherited with Hb G Philadelphia and Hb S. In these cases, CBC analysis results in markedly decreased MCV and MCH with reduced Hb concentration.

Double heterozygosity Hb G Philadelphia/Hb S occurs in 1 in 125,500 African Americans. On HPLC of patients with the Hb G Philadelphia/Hb S trait, four bands are noted, representing four different Hb species, namely, normal α-chain with normal β-chain, abnormal α-chain with normal β-chain, normal α-chain with abnormal β-chain, and abnormal α-chain with abnormal β-chain. Hb electrophoresis at alkaline pH shows bands in the A, S, and C positions. At acid pH, bands are noted in the A and S positions. In African Americans, the Hb G Philadelphia mutation occurs with an α-chain deletion, which is *cis* to the mutated alle ($\alpha^G/\alpha\alpha$). This results in a change in the amount of mutated α-chain (α^G) from the usual 25% to approximately 30%. No clinical or hematologic manifestations are noted with Hb G Philadelphia/Hb S.

Hemoglobin C [β6(A3)$^{Glu \rightarrow Lys}$]. Hemoglobin C arises from a substitution of lysine for glutamic acid at position 6 of the β-globin chain. Hb C may be found in the homozygous (Hb C disease, $\beta^C\beta^C$) or heterozygous (Hb C trait) state. Hb C is commonly found in West Africa and the Caribbean. It is the second most commonly studied of all the Hb variants after Hb S. HPLC analysis (see Fig. 38.7G) of samples from individuals with homozygous Hb C shows a large peak in the C position, with Hb C forming 90% to 95% of the total Hb. Hb F concentrations are variable. Glycated Hb C is found as a small peak eluting before the Hb C peak. The ratio of the elution times of glycated Hb C to Hb C is the same as that of HbA_{1c} and Hb A. Electrophoresis at alkaline and acid pH shows a single band in the C position.

Mild to moderate anemia is the most common clinical presentation. CBC analysis shows normal or slightly decreased Hb concentrations with a normochromic and normocytic red cell morphology. An increase in polychromasia may be present, and the reticulocytes may contribute to an increase in the MCV. The peripheral blood smear shows numerous target cells, with occasional nucleated RBCs and characteristic irregular contracted red cells (sometimes called pyknocytes). Hb C crystals may be seen, and bilirubin concentrations may be slightly elevated. Red cell survival and osmotic fragility are decreased.

Heterozygous Hemoglobin C (Hemglobin C Trait). High-performance liquid chromatography analysis (see Fig. 38.7H), capillary electrophoresis, and electrophoresis at both alkaline and acid pH (see Fig. 38.12) on blood samples from individuals who are heterozygous for Hb C reveal bands in the A and C positions, with Hb C forming 38% to 45% of the total Hb. CBC analysis may show target cells and is generally normochromic, with the MCV near the lower limit of the reference interval.

Heterozygous Hb C individuals are usually asymptomatic. Genetic counseling may be useful when prospective parents have abnormalities in the β-globin gene.

Hb C may be coinherited with both α- and β-thalassemias, and the concentration of Hb C is related to the number of functioning α-genes. With only two functioning α-genes, the Hb C concentration can fall to 32% of the total Hb. Coinheritance of Hb C with β^0- or β^+-thalassemia results in moderately severe anemia with splenomegaly. The Hb F concentration is often increased.

Hemoglobin D Punjab [β121(GH4)$^{Glu \rightarrow Gln}$]. Hemoglobin D Punjab is an Hb variant in which glutamic acid at position 121 of the β-globin chain is replaced with glutamine. The names Hb D Los Angeles and Hb D Punjab are used to describe this variant, with the former name used more often in North America and the latter in the United Kingdom. Hb D Punjab is found in the Punjab region of the Indian subcontinent, especially in Sikhs from the Lycus Valley. Large-scale immigration from this area to the United Kingdom, the United States, and Canada has widened the distribution of Hb D Punjab. Hb D Punjab is also found in Caucasians whose foreparents lived in the Indian subcontinent at the time of the British Raj. Hb D Punjab is found in both heterozygous (Hb D Punjab trait) and homozygous (Hb D Punjab disease, $\beta^D\beta^D$) states.

HPLC analysis of blood from an individual with homozygous Hb D Punjab shows normal or marginally raised Hb F and Hb A_2 peaks, with a large peak in the Hb D position forming more than 90% of the total Hb. Electrophoresis at alkaline pH shows a band in the S position, which migrates to the A position in acid electrophoresis. CBC analysis shows a mild decrease in Hb concentrations, MCV, and MCH, with target cells observed in the blood smear. Patients present clinically with mild anemia.

HPLC analysis of individuals with the Hb D Punjab trait shows two peaks—one at the A position and the other at the D position—with Hb D forming 30% to 40% of the total Hb. The Hb F and Hb A_2 concentrations are within or slightly above the reference intervals. Electrophoresis at alkaline pH shows two bands—one in the A position and the other in the S position. On electrophoresis at acid pH, a single band in the A position is noted. HPLC is the preferred method for identification of Hb D because a similar electrophoretic pattern, on both alkaline and acid pH, is seen with Hb G. CBC analysis is unremarkable except for the presence of target cells on the blood smear.

Individuals with Hb D Punjab trait are clinically asymptomatic.

Coinheritance of Hb D Punjab (both heterozygous and homozygous states) with β-thalassemia is common. CBC analysis of these patients shows decreased concentrations of Hb with markedly decreased MCV and MCH. Target and irregular contracted cells, together with hypochromia and anisocytosis, are seen on the blood smear. Quantification of Hb A_2 in individuals with coinheritance of Hb D Punjab and β-thalassemia presents a challenge to the laboratory because HPLC analysis underestimates the Hb A_2 concentration due to an unstable rising baseline in these individuals. Although not normally recommended, quantification of Hb A_2 by densitometry on alkaline electrophoresis may be the only method available to many laboratories. CBC analysis shows a greatly decreased concentration of Hb with low MCV and MCH. The blood smear shows target cells (erythrocytes with an increased surface area-to-volume ratio that appear as a target with a bull's eye) and contracted cells with hypochromia and anisocytosis.

Individuals with coinheritance of Hb D Punjab and β-thalassemia present with a notable compensated anemia.

Hemoglobin D Iran [b22(B4)$^{Glu \rightarrow Gln}$]. Hemoglobin D Iran is a β-globin chain variant in which glutamine replaces glutamic acid at position 22 of the β-globin chain.

On HPLC analysis, peaks are seen in the A and A_2 positions with quantification for Hb A_2 far above what is normally expected. Alkaline electrophoresis shows two bands—one in the A position and the other in the S position. On acid electrophoresis, a single band in the A position is noted. Individuals with Hb D Iran are asymptomatic.

Hemoglobin E [b26(B8)$^{Glu \rightarrow Lys}$]. Hemoglobin E is a β-chain variant with lysine replacing glutamic acid at position 26 of the β-globin chain. More individuals have the Hb variant Hb E than any other variant. Hb E is found in both homozygous and heterozygous states and may be combined with β-thalassemia. It is widespread in the Far East, including Southern China, Cambodia, Thailand, and Laos. Hb E has been increasingly found in the United States and Canada, which is caused by emigration from these areas. It may be believed of as the "thalassemic variant" because some of the features of the CBC resemble thalassemia, especially in the homozygous state.

HPLC analysis of blood from individuals with homozygous Hb E (Hb E disease, $\beta^E\beta^E$) shows a single peak (>90% of the total Hb) coeluting with Hb A_2. Hb F is within or marginally above the reference interval. On alkaline electrophoresis, a single band is noted in the C position, which migrates to the A position in acid electrophoresis. CBC analysis shows normal to marginally decreased Hb concentrations with low MCV and MCH. Target cells are noted in the peripheral blood smear. Fe studies are normal.

Homozygous Hb E individuals are usually asymptomatic, although slight anemia may be present.

HPLC analysis of blood from individuals with heterozygous Hb E reveals two peaks—one in the A position and the other in the A_2 position. Hb E forms approximately 30% of the total Hb. Capillary electrophoresis resolves Hb E from Hb A_2. Hb A_2 is higher in patients with Hb E than in patients without a Hb variant or thalassemia because of decreased synthesis of the abnormal β-globin chain, which allows for increased binding between the excess α-globin and δ-globin chains producing Hb A.[37,38] CBC analysis shows normal Hb concentrations and occasionally low MCV. Target cells are noted in the peripheral blood smear. Fe studies are normal.

Heterozygous Hb E individuals are usually asymptomatic, although slight anemia may be present.

Coinheritance of Hb E and thalassemia produces an anemia of variable severity. HPLC of a patient with coinheritance of β-thalassemia and homozygous E is shown in Fig. 38.7C. Coinheritance of homozygous Hb E and β-thalassemia leads to a severe anemia, with greatly reduced Hb concentrations, MCV, and MCH with increased Hb F concentration. Numerous target cells are noted on the peripheral blood smear, together with microcytosis, anisocytosis, hypochromia, and a few nucleated red cells. Fe studies are normal. In the most severe cases, the clinical presentation is similar to that of β^0-thalassemia, and transfusion may be the only therapy. Coinheritance of heterozygous Hb E with α-thalassemia produces a less severe anemia with low Hb, MCV, and MCH. Target cells are noted on the peripheral blood smear, together with microcytosis and hypochromia. Patients who are pregnant may need to be monitored closely, although transfusion is not usually required.

Quantification of Hb A_2, which is important in the diagnosis of possible coinheritance of β-thalassemia with Hb E, provides a challenge to the laboratory, in that Hb E and Hb A_2 coelute. Molecular studies are the only satisfactory method by which to establish coinheritance of Hb E and β-thalassemia, although the severity of the disease, family studies, and increased Hb F may lead to suspicion of coinheritance.

Hemoglobin O Arab [b121(GH4)$^{Glu \rightarrow Lys}$]. Hemoglobin O Arab is a β-chain variant with lysine replacing glutamic acid at position 121 of the β-globin chain. Hb O Arab is found in a wide variety of ethnic groups in North Africa and Eastern Europe, and is not confined, nor is it even common, among Arab populations. Hb O Arab has been found in both heterozygous and homozygous states.

HPLC analysis of blood from an individual with homozygous Hb O Arab shows a single band between the S and C positions, with Hb O Arab forming more than 90% of the total Hb. Electrophoresis at alkaline pH shows a band close to the C position. On electrophoresis at acid pH, a band is seen between the A and S positions (but closer to A). CBC analysis shows a normal or marginally low Hb concentration, MCV, and MCH. The peripheral blood smear shows slight microcytosis.

No unusual hematologic features are noted in individuals with heterozygous Hb O Arab. HPLC analysis of blood from these individuals shows two peaks—one in the A position and the other eluting close to the C position and forming 30% to 40% of the total Hb. Electrophoresis at alkaline electrophoresis shows bands in the A position and close to the C position. On acid electrophoresis, two bands are noted—one in the A position and the other in a position between the A and S positions.

Hybrid Hemoglobins. Hybrid Hbs, or crossover Hbs, describe a group of Hb variants in which one of the globin chains is a hybrid of amino acid sequences of two other globin chains. The term crossover Hb is sometimes used because there is a point in the amino acid sequence at which there is crossover from the amino acid sequence of one globin chain to another globin chain. Individuals with these hybrid Hb variants present with clinical features and laboratory findings, particularly in their CBCs, which are similar to those of thalassemia. Production of the hybrid globin chain is reduced. Hb Lepore is the prototypical hybrid Hb.

Hemoglobin Lepore. Hemoglobin Lepore is classified as a δβ-hybrid Hb variant on the basis that the non–α-chain is a hybrid of δ- and β-globin chains. It is unique in that it is the only hemoglobinopathy named after the family name of the index case. Delta-/beta-hybrid Hbs arise because there are deletions of part of the 3′ portion of the δ-globin gene and in the 5′ portion of the β-globin chain, with resultant formation of a δβ-fusion gene. Three distinct variations of Hb Lepore have been described. In Hb Lepore-Hollandia (δβ-hybrid [δ through 22; β from 50]), a variant found in Canada and Papua New Guinea, fusion occurs at the first 22 amino acid residues of the δ-globin chain, with the amino acids from position 50 onward of the β-globin chain. In Hb Lepore-Baltimore (δβ-hybrid (δ through 50: β from 86]), which is found mainly in individuals of Spanish ancestry, the first 50 amino acid residues of the δ-globin chain are fused with amino acid residues from position 86 of the β-globin chain. In Hb Lepore-Boston-Washington (δβ-hybrid [δ through 87; β from 116]), the most common Hb Lepore, the first 87 amino acid residues of the δ-globin chain are fused with amino acid residues from position 116 onward of the β-globin chain. Hb Lepore-Boston-Washington, sometimes called Hb Lepore-Boston, is found mainly in individuals of Italian descent, although it has been found in individuals from Eastern Europe.

HPLC analysis of blood from individuals with Hb Lepore shows greatly elevated Hb A_2 concentration with marginally reduced Hb A. The Hb A_2 concentration is usually greater than 10% of the total Hb and is falsely increased because of the coelution of Hb A_2 and Hb Lepore. Electrophoresis at alkaline pH shows a band in the S position for Hb Lepore-Boston-Washington and in a position between the A and S positions for the other Hb Lepore variants. At acid pH, a single band is present in the A position for all Hb Lepore variants. Hb A_2 and Hb Lepore are resolved on capillary electrophoresis.

CBC analysis shows greatly reduced concentrations of Hb, MCV, and MCH in Hb Lepore homozygotes. Hematologic findings are similar to those of β-TM or β-TI. CBC analysis of heterozygotes shows slightly reduced MCV and MCH. Hematologic findings are similar to those of the β-thalassemia trait. Fe studies are normal in both heterozygotes and homozygotes. The similarity of the hematology in Hb Lepore and in β-thalassemia makes careful review of HPLC and electrophoretic analysis essential. A greatly elevated Hb A_2 by HPLC analysis and a small band in the S position on electrophoresis at alkaline pH suggest Hb Lepore.

Elongation Hemoglobins. Elongation Hbs, of which there are 13 (7 α-chain and 6 β-chain variants) result from lengthening of the C or N terminus of either globin chain. The most important, from a clinical perspective, are the five C-terminal, α-chain variants in which the terminal codon TAA is changed and an amino acid sequence is added. The prototypical elongation Hb is Hb Constant Spring. In this variant, the C-terminal TAA codon is changed to CAA in the α_2-gene, and a 31 amino acid sequence is added at the C-terminal end to give an α-globin chain length of 173 amino acid residues, rather than the normal 142 residue length. This increase in length results in instability of the Hb variant, and synthesis of this elongated globin chain is reduced. Hb Constant Spring is found in South East Asia, especially in Vietnam, Cambodia, and Laos, and is found in both the heterozygous and homozygous states.

Patients with Hb Constant Spring present with slightly reduced Hb, MCV, and MCH, with hypochromia and microcytosis in the peripheral blood smear. Fe studies are often normal.

The instability of Hb Constant Spring presents a challenge to the laboratory diagnosis of this variant. The blood used for analytical procedures should be as fresh as possible. Samples older than 24 hours should not be used. HPLC analysis of blood from individuals with Hb Constant Spring demonstrates a small peak in the C position, which forms approximately 4% to 6% of the total Hb in the homozygote and 1% to 3% in the heterozygote. On electrophoresis at alkaline pH, a small band migrating cathodally to the application point may be seen. This electrophoretic mobility is unique because it is the only Hb variant that moves toward the cathode rather than the anode.

Hb Constant Spring is commonly found in combination with α^0-thalassemia, especially the (–SEA) mutation. The clinical presentation of this combination results in a severe form of Hb H disease.

Analytical Methods

The laboratory plays a crucial role in detection and characterization of the hemoglobinopathies and thalassemias, as discussed in the next sections.[39] Several recommendations have been put forth for laboratory investigations of abnormal Hbs and thalassemias.[40-42] For example, in 1978, the International Committee for Standardization in Hematology expert panel on abnormal Hbs published recommendations for the laboratory investigation of these conditions.[43] In its initial investigation, (1) a CBC, (2) electrophoresis at pH 9.2, (3) tests for solubility and sickling, and (4) quantification of Hb A_2 and Hb F were recommended. If an abnormal Hb was found as a result of these initial tests, further tests, including electrophoresis at pH 6.2, globin chain separation, and isoelectric focusing, were recommended by the panel. If the presence of an unstable Hb or Hb with altered oxygen affinity was suspected, then heat and isopropanol stability tests were recommended. Although new techniques have replaced some of these tests, the approach of using multiple assays in the initial investigation of hemoglobinopathies and thalassemias is an accepted practice that is used in many laboratories involved in the investigation of these disorders. In addition to these tests, the Fe status of the patient should be ascertained by measurement of ferritin or by the Fe/total Fe-binding capacity/saturation index. Information on the ethnicity and/or nationality of the patient, when allowed under patient confidentiality rules, may provide useful information because thalassemias (eg, β-thalassemia in individuals of Mediterranean origin) and certain hemoglobinopathies (eg, Hb S trait and homozygous S in African Americans) are associated with particular ethnic and/or national groups.

The 2010 guidelines of the British Committee for Standards in Haematology[44] for the laboratory diagnosis of hemoglobinopathies recommend that qualification for genetic counseling requires identification of Hbs S, C, D Punjab, O Arab, E, Lepore, and H, and the detection of carriers of α^0-thalasssemia and β-thalasssemia traits. To accomplish this, it is recommended that "all ethnic groups" be screened for the β-thalassemia trait when the mean cell (or corpuscular) Hb (MCH) is less than 27 pg. All ethnic groups, except for Northern European Caucasians, should be screened for Hb variants. Selected ethnic groups should be screened for α^0-thalassemia trait when the MCH is less than 25 pg. Recommended methods include HPLC and Hb electrophoresis for identification of Hb variants, and HPLC and microcolumn chromatography for quantification of Hb A_2. Electrophoresis is not recommended for the quantification of Hb A_2. In addition, it is recommended that two methods, based on different analytical principles, be used to establish a presumptive identification of the Hb variant. A flowchart (Fig. 38.13) is suggested for identification of α^0-, β-, and δβ-thalassemia traits and Hb variants.

Preferred Specimen

The preferred blood sample for use in detection and characterization of the hemoglobinopathies is one collected with potassium or sodium salts of ethylenediaminetetraacetic acid as the anticoagulant. To minimize the formation of degradation products, which are especially noticeable as small bands eluting with similar retention time as HbA_{1c} and Hb F on HPLC analysis, testing should be performed within 5 days of collection, and samples should be stored at 4°C.

Techniques

Analytical techniques used to measure RBCs and their indexes, Hb, and related compounds include (1) determination of CBC, (2) electrophoresis, (3) immunoassay, (4) separation techniques such as HPLC, capillary electrophoresis, and mass spectrometry, (5) molecular techniques such as DNA analysis, and (6) specific tests for specific variants.

Complete Blood Count. A CBC of a whole blood sample consists of (1) numbers of RBCs (erythrocytes), (2) numbers of WBCs, (3) numbers of platelets, (4) a measure of Hb, (5) estimates of red cell volume, and (6) estimation of WBC subtypes (see Table 38.2). (Note: A CBC is also known as a full blood count, a full blood examination, or a blood panel.) Knowledge of red cell indexes[45,46] and the information obtained from microscopic examination of a peripheral blood film is vital to the diagnosis of both α- and β-thalassemias. Hemoglobinopathies have a lesser impact on red cell indexes, but may present abnormal red cell morphology on peripheral blood films. In thalassemias, the Hb concentration and the MCV, an index of cell size, are decreased, sometimes markedly, whereas in hemoglobinopathies, both are often normal. One study recommends that an MCV of less than 72 fL (reference interval ≈80–100 fL)[47] is maximally sensitive and specific for the presumptive diagnosis of thalassemia. However, an MCH less than 27 pg (reference interval ≈26–35 pg)[47] has been recommended as the decision point for further investigation for IDA and thalassemia. The rationale for the selection of MCH over MCV as the decision point for further investigation is the potential increase of up to 5 fL in MCV in samples older than 24 hours.

The RBC count may be in the upper half of or above the reference interval in thalassemias but within the reference interval in most hemoglobinopathies without a coinherited thalassemia. In contrast, the RBC count is low in IDA and anemia of chronic disease (ACD) and is proportionally related to the decrease in Hb concentration. The RDW, a measure of variation in the size of the RBC (anisocytosis), tends to be above the reference interval in IDAs and other microcytic anemias. The RDW in thalassemias is usually within or close to the reference interval, reflecting the uniformity of red cell size. However, in Hb H disease and δβ-thalassemia, the RDW is moderately increased. Some authors have suggested the use of the ratio between the percentage of microcytes and the percentage of hypochromic cells (M/H ratio) in the differentiation between IDA and the β-thalassemia trait. This ratio has been found to be higher for β-thalassemia traits than for IDA.[48]

In thalassemias, the RBCs in the peripheral blood smear are hypochromic and microcytic. Characteristic sickle- or crescent-shaped RBCs are seen (Fig. 38.14) in the peripheral blood smear of patients who are homozygous for Hb S (sickle cell disease), and targets are seen in blood smears from patients who are homozygous for Hb E (see Fig. 38.14) and Hb C. In addition, microspherocytes (erythrocytes whose diameter is less than normal, but whose thickness is increased) and crystalline inclusions (Hb C cells) have been found in peripheral blood smears from individuals who are homozygous for Hb C. These findings are less uniformly present than the typical morphologic features of sickle cell disease.

Several algorithms or discriminant indexes, based on conventional and more innovative parameters from the CBC, have been developed and evaluated for the differentiation between Fe deficiency from thalassemia[47,49-52] (Table 38.4).[53]

A recent meta-analysis of the most frequently used discriminant indexes has demonstrated high variation in the performance of these parameters for distinguishing the thalassemia trait from IDA.[53] In general, the newer indexes seem to be able to make this distinction better than the more traditional formulas. The M/H ratio was shown to be superior over other discriminant indexes. Notwithstanding its high performance, even the M/H ratio cannot be used for making a final diagnosis of the thalassemia trait. Its value lies in screening of microcytic individuals, to select those in whom additional laboratory investigations are warranted for confirming the presence of thalassemia. Although the CBC parameters are often the first indication that the patient might have a thalassemia or a hemoglobinopathy, these data are not sufficient to allow the final diagnosis. In addition, the Fe status of the patient, as measured with ferritin or Fe/Fe-binding and/or saturation index tests (see the next section), helps in differentiating IDA from ACD and thalassemia. However, ferritin is elevated in acute-phase reactions, and Fe deficiency can mask an underlying thalassemia (see also Chapter 72 on the differential diagnosis of various forms of anemia).

An algorithm based on MCV, MCH, Hb A_2, and Hb F quantifications has been advocated to better discriminate among β-thalassemia minor, Fe deficiency, δβ-thalassemia, and HPFH[54] (see Chapter 72 for an MCV-based algorithmic

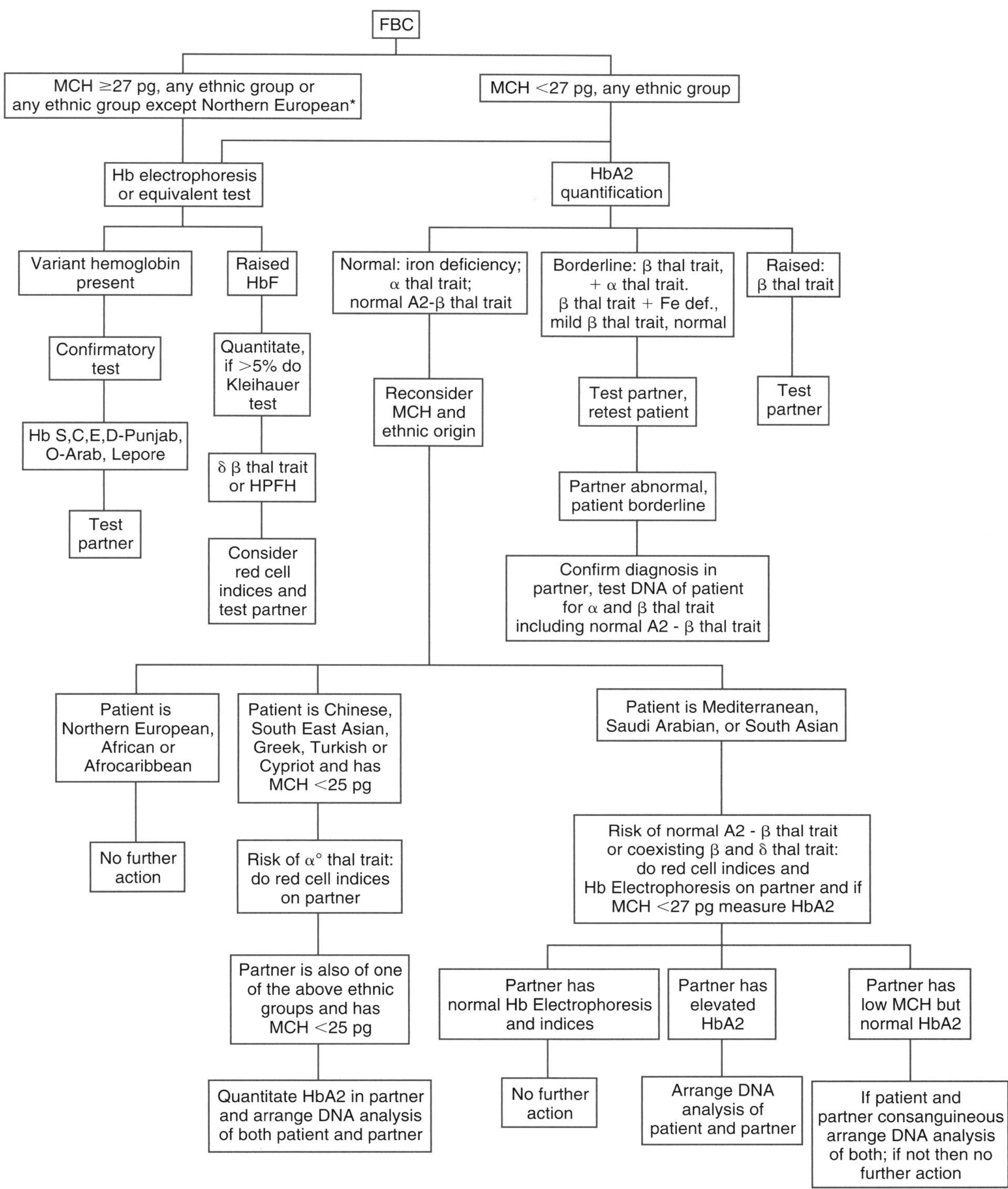

FIGURE 38.13 **Flowchart Demonstrating Procedures for Diagnosis of α^0-, β-, and *β-Thalassemia Traits and Clinically Significant Hemoglobin Variants in Pregnant Women ("Patients") and Their Partners.** Selective screening is acceptable in low-incidence areas but only if accurate information on ethnic origin is available. *FBC,* Full blood count; *Hb,* hemoglobin; *Hb S, C, E, D, F, Punjab, Arab, Lepore,* various types of hemoglobin; *MCH,* mean cell hemoglobin; *thal,* thalassemia. (Modified from Laboratory diagnosis of haemoglobinopathies. *Br J Haematol* 1998;101:783–792.)

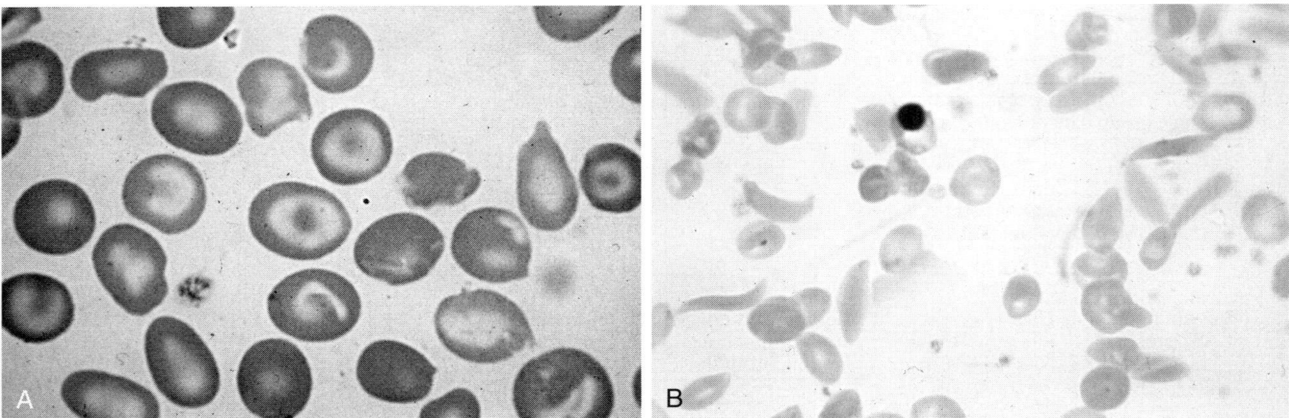

FIGURE 38.14 Peripheral Blood Smear From Patients With **(A)** Homozygous Hemoglobin *(Hb)* E and **(B)** Homozygous Hb S.

TABLE 38.4 Discriminant Indexes for Distinguishing Thalassemia Trait From Iron Deficiency Anemia in Patients With Microcytic Red Blood Cells

Discriminant Index	Calculation	Cutoff Value*
England and Fraser	MCV – RBC – (5 Hb) – 3.4	0
RBC	RBC	5.0
Mentzer	MCV/RBC	13
Srivastava	MCH/RBC	3.8
Shine and Lal	MCV^2 × MCH	1.53
Bessman	RDW	15
Ricerca	RDW/RBC	4.4
Green and King	MCV^2 × RDW/100 Hb	65
Jayabose (RDW index)	MCV/(RBC × RDW)	220
Sirdah	MCV – RBC – (3 Hb)	27.0
M/H ratio	Microcytic RBC %/ hypochromic RBC %	3.7
Ehsani	MCV – (10 RBC)	15

*Cutoff values transformed into general used units: Hb in grams per deciliter; RBC in 10^{12}/L; MCV in femtoliter; MCH in picograms; and RDW in percentage.

Hb, Hemoglobin; *MCH*, mean cell Hb; *MCV*, mean cell volume; *RBC*, red blood cell; *RDW*, red cell distribution width.

Data from Hoffmann JJ, Urrechaga E, Aguirre U. Discriminant indices for distinguishing thalassemia and iron deficiency in patients with microcytic anemia: a reply. *Clin Chem Lab Med* 2015;53:1883–1894.

approach to anemia diagnosis). For more information on the clinical usefulness of these CBC parameters and discriminative algorithms, and for conditions leading to microcytic anemia, the reader is referred to the literature.[49-53]

Electrophoresis. Electrophoresis (see Chapter 15) under alkaline conditions (pH 9.2) is the most common initial screening method for the detection and preliminary identification of hemoglobinopathies.[55] Several media, including paper and cellulose acetate, have been used, although agarose[56] is now the medium of choice and the one usually supplied commercially. A pH 9.2 barbital buffer is the most common buffer system. Visualization of separated Hb bands is achieved by using a protein-binding stain, such as Amido Black or Ponceau S. Hb bands stain blue with Amido Black and reddish pink with Ponceau S. After clearing of excess stain, Hb bands on the agarose media are clearly seen against the clear background. The *left panel* of Fig. 38.12 shows an alkaline electrophoresis gel stained with Amido Black. Quantification by densitometry of Hb A_2 and F bands on alkaline electrophoresis, although commonly performed by laboratories, is not recommended by the College of American Pathologists in the hemoglobinopathy survey critiques[57] because of high analytical imprecision resulting from limitations of densitometry in quantifying faint bands. Scanning densitometry is not adequate for Hb A_2 quantification because the precision requirement is 10 times greater than what is needed for Hb variant quantification and cannot be met by densitometric methods.[30]

At alkaline pH, Hbs migrate according to electrical charge, with Hb H moving the fastest (closest to the anode). The order of migration (fastest to slowest) is Hb H, Hb N, Hb I, Hb J, Hb A, Hb F, Hb S, and Hb C. Hb D and Hb G comigrate with Hb S, and Hb E, Hb O, and Hb A_2 comigrate with Hb C. Hb Constant Spring migrates slightly toward the cathode. An easy way to remember the sequence is Hb A goes to the anode, whereas Hb C migrates to the cathode. Hb F and Hb S follow after Hb A in alphabetical order.

Electrophoresis at pH 6.4 using a citrate buffer is performed when an abnormal band is noted on alkaline Hb electrophoresis. Agarose is the preferred medium, with acid violet as the preferred stain. The same Hb variants performed on agarose electrophoresis at pH 6.4 and stained with acid violet are shown in the *right panel* of Fig. 38.12. The order of migration (cathode to anode, fastest to slowest) is Hb F, Hb A, Hb S, and Hb C. Hb D, Hb G, Hb I, Hb J, Hb O, Hb A_2, and Hb E comigrate with Hb A.

Based on positions of the bands in acid and alkaline electrophoresis, a presumptive identification of the Hb variant may be made. For example, bands are found on alkaline electrophoresis in both A and C positions. On acid electrophoresis, if bands are found in the A and C positions, then a presumptive identification of the Hb C trait may be made because this pattern is characteristic. However, if a band is found only in the A position on acid electrophoresis, then a presumptive identification of Hb E may be made. If

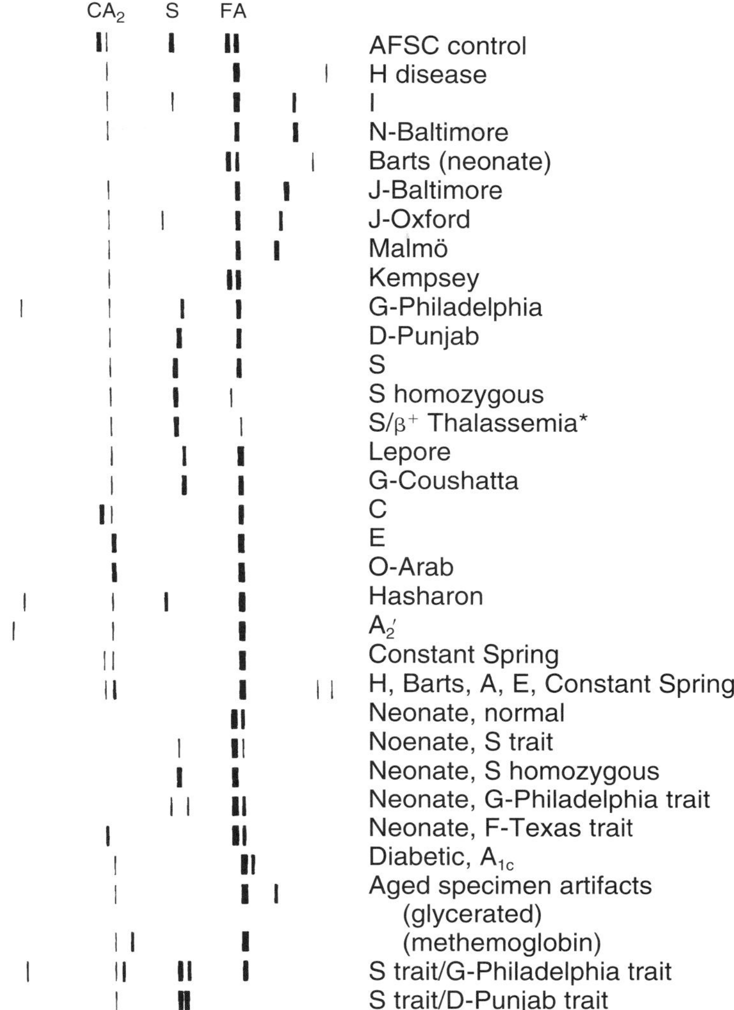

FIGURE 38.15 A Diagram of Isoelectric Focusing Patterns for a Variety of Hemoglobin *(Hb)* Variants. The conditions shown represent heterozygotes (traits), unless otherwise indicated. The width of the bars approximates the relative density of the bands observed. The acid anodic (pH 6) side is to the *right*, and the alkaline cathodic (pH 8) side is to the *left*. The same pattern is observed in homozygous patients with Hb S disease who have received Hb A by transfusion.

bands are found in the C position on alkaline electrophoresis and between the S and A positions on acid electrophoresis, then a presumptive identification of Hb O may be made. Further testing is required to determine whether the Hb O is Hb O Arab, Hb O Indonesia, or Hb O Padova. Fairbanks[58] described a numbering system for the most common Hb bands on alkaline electrophoresis (Hb H is position 1, Hb A is position 5, Hb S is position 9, and Hb C is position 13) that allowed the position of a band to be described more exactly than the commonly used descriptive term "between S and A positions." Unfortunately, this system has not found universal acceptance. Laboratories should keep a bank of obtained electrophoretic data to help future identification of unusual Hb variants.

Specific types of electrophoresis that are used for Hb analysis include isoelectric focusing, electrophoresis, and capillary electrophoresis.

Isoelectric Focusing Electrophoresis. Isoelectric-focusing electrophoresis (IEF)[59] has greater resolving power than conventional electrophoresis, but it is more expensive, time-consuming, and technique-dependent to perform (see Chapter 15). Commercial IEF gels are made of cellulose acetate or polyacrylamide with the pH gradient produced by the inclusion of amphoteric materials of different pHs in bands in the gel. Locations of the Hb bands are identified using stains similar to those used in conventional electrophoresis. The bands or zones produced by IEF (Fig. 38.15) are more clearly defined than with those seen with conventional electrophoresis, and reliable quantification of separated Hbs may be made at high concentrations using densitometry. However, quantification of Hb A_2 and Hb F at low concentrations is imprecise and is not recommended. The Hb elution pattern in IEF is similar to that of alkaline Hb electrophoresis, except that Hb D and Hb G are resolved from each other and from Hb S. Historically, IEF has been used extensively to identify and characterize Hb variants; however, it is currently less frequently used because of the previously mentioned limitations.

Capillary Isoelectric Focusing Electrophoresis. Capillary IEF[60-64] combines the detection sensitivity of capillary electrophoresis (see Chapter 15) with the resolution qualities and existing extensive data on Hb variant separation by immunoelectrophoresis and the automated sampling and digital data acquisition techniques developed for chromatography. With this approach, the hemolysate is introduced into the capillary chamber using low-pressure injection and then is focused at high voltage (typically ≈30 kV and 0.5–1.5 μA), during which it is essential to maintain adequate cooling. The separated Hbs are then eluted, using low-pressure and simultaneous voltage, past a single-wavelength spectrophotometric detector set to read at 415 nm or a dual-wavelength detector set at 415 and 450 nm. In routine use, the Hbs are typically separated within 15 minutes, but the elution time may be extended if the presence of an abnormal Hb is suspected. Hb variants[62] are identified by comparison of isoelectric point values and migration times of the unknown, using Hb A as the reference peak, with known controls and published data. Quantification is based on integration of the measured absorbance of the bands, and accurate results have been obtained for Hb A_2 and Hb F concentrations.

Capillary Electrophoresis. The introduction of commercial capillary electrophoresis instrumentation for the separation of Hbs has made this technique available to clinical laboratories.[61] Separation in an alkaline buffer at a specific pH using high voltages is based on charge difference, electrolyte pH, and electro-osmotic flow. Hb measurement is commonly performed at a wavelength of 415 nm, and identification is based on retention time. All common Hb variants are separated, and quantification of Hb F and Hb A_2 is performed in a single analytical run.[60,65,66] Cotton and colleagues[60] initially described the application of this technique for the identification of Hb variants and quantification of Hb A_2; others have described the usefulness of the technique in the clinical laboratory.[37,67,68] Advantages of capillary electrophoresis over HPLC include quantification of Hb A_2 in the presence of Hb E (due to incomplete resolution of Hb A_2 from Hb E in HPLC), quantification of Hb H, and identification of Hb Lepore.

High-Performance Liquid Chromatography. High-performance liquid chromatography using a column packed with cation-exchange resin[69-71] provides, in a single analytical protocol, the quantification of Hb F and Hb A_2 (see Chapter 16 for a detailed discussion of HPLC). With it, the initial identification of an Hb variant on the basis of elution time may be made. It has also been used to detect α-thalassemia phenotypes.

After injection and subsequent adsorption onto the particles of a cation-exchange resin, molecules of Hb are eluted using gradient elution. Detection of eluted Hbs is achieved by monitoring the effluent solvent stream using a dual-wavelength photometer (usually set to measure at wavelengths of 415 and 690 nm). The technique is precise for the quantification of both Hb F and Hb A_2, and presumptive identification of the common Hb variant may be made. These features have made HPLC the method of choice for hemoglobinopathy and thalassemia screening for many laboratories, including those that perform neonatal hemoglobinopathy screening. Fig. 38.7 shows the separation on a commercial system of nine Hb variants.

Several commercial methods are available but lack the resolution achieved by noncommercial methods. A noncommercial HPLC method has been described, with the retention time and relative concentration of 40 common Hb variants listed.[71] This system (1) requires a longer time for analysis, (2) provides superior resolution, and (3) overcomes the problem of coelution of several Hb variants that occurs with commercial systems. For example, with one commercial system, Hb E, Hb Osu-Christianborg, Hb G-Coushatta, Hb Lepore, and Hb G-Copenhagen coelute with Hb A_2, making Hb A_2 quantification and definitive identification of the Hb variants impossible.[72,73]

Other chromatographic problems, such as rising baseline, have resulted in falsely low Hb A_2 concentration in Hb D patients.[74,75] This may be corrected mathematically to produce a more accurate result. Patients with Hb S have falsely increased Hb A_2 concentrations; this was originally believed to be caused by the coelution of glycated Hb S with Hb A_2.[76] Subsequent studies have shown that the increase in Hb A_2 in patients with Hb S is due to coelution of carbamylated Hb S species.[77] Diagnosis of coinheritance of β-thalassemia with Hb S may be compromised by this false increase in Hb A_2. However, knowledge of the concentration of Hb A_2 is not essential in making the diagnosis of β^0- or β^+-thalassemia in these patients. In the case of β^0-thalassemia (β-TM), no δ-globin chain is produced, and the electrophoretic pattern and HPLC analysis closely resemble those of a homozygous Hb S patient (large Hb F and Hb S peaks with no Hb A peak). In β^+-thalassemia (β-TI), the concentration of Hb S is greater than that of Hb A, a situation that otherwise is seen only in recently transfused patients who have sickle cell disease. Coinheritance of β-thalassemia minor and Hb S may be diagnosed in these patients by setting the upper limit of the reference interval at 5.0%.[78] Capillary zone electrophoresis and microcolumn methods have been described that eliminate the interference of glycated Hb S with Hb A_2 quantification.

The use of relative elution time rather than absolute elution time in initial identification of an unknown Hb variant is useful and recommended. The reference Hb ideally is one that is found in low concentrations in most individuals. In this regard, Hb A_2 is probably most useful as a reference point despite the number of coeluting Hb variants.

The elution time of the Hb may change slightly with increasing Hb variant concentration. For example, Hb F concentrations obtained by HPLC are often lower than those obtained from alkaline denaturation and/or spectrophotometric methods that are often quoted in standard hematology texts and used for the diagnosis of juvenile myelomonocytic leukemia and monosomy 7 syndrome. Caution should be used in interchanging Hb F concentrations obtained by HPLC with those obtained by other methods.

It should be noted that hemoglobinopathies may interfere with glycated Hb analysis because results may be falsely increased or decreased, depending on the particular method and the hemoglobinopathy.[7,55,79] Hb variants that cannot be separated from Hb A or HbA_{1c} will produce spuriously increased or decreased results by ion-exchange HPLC (see also Chapter 57 on Diabetes Mellitus).

Electrospray Mass Spectroscopy

Electrospray mass spectrometry (see Chapter 17) is becoming the method of choice[80] for the complete characterization of newly discovered Hb variants.[31-33,56,73,77,81-83] By using this method, the mass of the variant, whether it is an α- or a β-chain variant, as well as the possible location and identity of the amino acid residue substitution and the quantity of variant present, can be derived.

To analyze a sample with this technique, the globin chains first are separated and then are isolated by semipreparative HPLC. The isolated fractions are further concentrated using a variety of techniques, including membrane filtration. The fraction containing the mutant globin chain is digested using specific endopeptidases that selectively cut at certain amino acid residues of the globin chain. The resultant digested peptide fragments are further separated by preparative HPLC, and the mutant peptide is sequenced using Edman degradation. Another portion of the digested globin chains is entered into the electrospray mass spectrometer, and the resultant mass spectrum provides information on the mass of the mutant globin chain, which can be used to provisionally identify the substituted amino acid. For Hb Rambam,[56] the mass spectrum of the β-globin chain shows the mass of the normal β-chain to be 15,867 Da and the mass of the mutant β-chain to be 15,925 Da. The increase in the mass of 58 in the mutant β-globin chain may be attributed to a change in amino acid residue from glycine (75 Da) to aspartic acid (133 Da).

Tandem mass spectroscopy has been used for newborn screening for sickle cell disease[84,85] and for the characterization of Hb A_2.[86]

DNA Analysis

DNA analysis is used in the investigation of thalassemias and hemoglobinopathies to identify specific individuals at risk and those who may benefit from genetic counseling in populations with a known high incidence of disease. For example, DNA analysis has been used to do the following:

1. Diagnose α^0- and α^+-thalassemia.[87-89]
2. Investigate potentially life-threatening disorders of Hb synthesis in the fetus; it is performed at less than 10 weeks' gestation on chorionic villus[54] samples.
3. Characterize the β-thalassemia genotype.[90-93]
4. Screen at-risk populations for clinically significant Hb variants.[90,94]
5. Distinguish between conditions that have similar laboratory and clinical presentations but are the result of different genetic conditions.

The Southern blot analysis of genomic DNA using α- and ζ-primers is widely used in the investigation of α-thalassemias, especially in the identification of individuals with α^0-thalassemia. PCR, which uses allele-specific primers, is used by reference laboratories in the identification of common β-thalassemia mutations and some hemoglobinopathies. Gene sequencing information may supplement these techniques in some cases.

Specific Tests

Tests that are used to measure Hbs and related analytes include those for Hb H, Hb S, unstable Hbs, and globin chains.

Determining Hemoglobin H. Hemoglobin H, an insoluble tetramer consisting of four β-globin chains, arises in α-thalassemia, in which decreased production of α-globin chains is caused by nonexpression of three of the four α-globin genes and a subsequent excess of β-globin chains. If these tetramers are oxidized, precipitation occurs, which may be viewed microscopically. In the laboratory, this oxidation is achieved by staining unfixed cells with freshly prepared methylene blue or brilliant cresyl blue at 37°C. Inclusion of positive and negative controls with each batch of Hb H preparations is essential because substantial batch-to-batch variability is seen in the dye.[95] Controversy is ongoing regarding the necessity to perform this test on freshly collected blood, and whether the test should be performed in all suspected α-thalassemia cases.

In Hb H disease, 30% to 100% of the red cells contain inclusions, which have been described as looking like golf balls. In α-thalassemia silent (one functional α-gene), as few as 1 cell with inclusions per 1000 to 10,000 red cells may be seen, and the diagnosis of α-thalassemia silent or minor cannot be made definitively in the absence of Hb H inclusions. The presence of Hb H inclusions may serve as confirmation of a presumptive diagnosis of α^0-thalassemia (α-TM) or Hb H disease.

Precipitate patterns resembling Hb H inclusions may arise from staining of reticulin and Howell-Jolly bodies and other protein and nucleic acid entities. Hb H inclusions may be very rare and difficult to detect when reticulocytosis is increased.

Hb H detection by this method is laborious to perform and is subjective. However, for detection of the two α-gene *cis* deletion (–/αα) of α^0-thalassemia, the test is reported to have a clinical sensitivity of 0.47 and a specificity of 0.99.[19]

Use of molecular tests in selected groups with suspected α-thalassemia (eg, females of childbearing age) is becoming the standard, rather than use of the Hb H preparation, in all age groups.

Sickling and Hemoglobin S Solubility Tests. Sickling tests are useful in confirming the presence of Hb S in a sample after initial electrophoresis at alkaline pH. When Hb S is oxygenated, it is fully soluble. When Hb S is deoxygenated, polymerization occurs, forming deformed red cells with a characteristic rigid sickle shape. In the laboratory, deoxygenation and lysis of RBCs is achieved using a solution of sodium metabisulfite in a phosphate buffer. Addition of the sodium metabisulfite reagent to an Hb S–containing blood sample induces the typical sickle shape of RBCs (which is the basis of the sickling test by microscopic investigation of the blood film preparation), and it also causes turbidity (which is the basis of the solubility test). In the Hb S solubility test, this turbidity is visualized by holding a lined card or a card with writing on it behind the reaction test tube (Fig. 38.16). In positive samples, lines or letters cannot be seen, whereas in negative samples, lines or letters are clearly visible. Both a positive and a negative control should be used with each test. The hematocrit (Hct) of the blood sample to be tested should be measured, and if it is less than 15%, the amount of blood used in the test should be doubled because low Hb concentration is a cause of falsely negative sickling screens. Lipemic samples and samples with a monoclonal protein (M-protein) may give a false-positive result. Hb C Harlem and Hb Memphis [$\alpha 23(B4)^{Glu\psi Gln}$] also give a positive result in this procedure; therefore, it is essential to identify the Hb in all positive tests by other techniques. The test is subjective, and the combination of two identification techniques, such as HPLC and alkaline electrophoresis, may eliminate the necessity to perform this test on a routine basis.

Tests for Unstable Hemoglobins. These tests use heat or isopropanol to precipitate the unstable Hb and must be performed on fresh blood. More than 100 unstable Hbs are

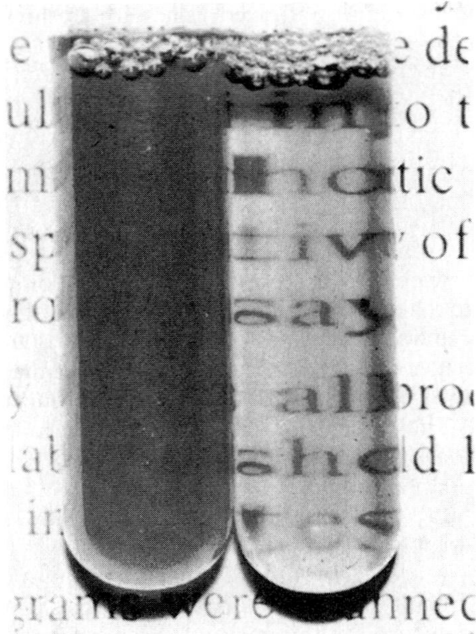

FIGURE 38.16 Solubility Test for Hemoglobin *(Hb)* S. Deoxyhemoglobin S *(left tube)* is insoluble in 2.3 mol/L phosphate buffer. In contrast, normal hemolysate *(right tube)* is sufficiently transparent that print can easily be read through it.

mainly the result of the interchange of nonpolar amino acid residues for polar amino acid residues in positions in the α- or β-globin chain associated with the heme cleft. Hb Hasharon $[\alpha47(CD)^{Asp\psi His}]$, an Hb variant found in Ashkenazi Jews, results from substitution of the nonpolar amino acid residue histidine for the polar aspartic acid residue at position 47 of the α-chain. In conventional nomenclature, Hb Hasharon should be written as $\alpha47(CE5)^{Asp\psi His}$; however, to maintain uniformity with β-, γ-, and δ-globin chains, the term *CD* is used to designate the corresponding interhelical segment of the α-chain, which does not have a D segment.

Nonpolar isopropanol weakens the internal bonds within Hb, decreasing the stability of the Hb molecule. Normal Hb (Hb A) precipitates within 40 minutes at 37°C in the presence of a 17% solution of isopropanol with a pH 7.4 Tris buffer. Unstable Hbs usually precipitate within 5 minutes under these conditions. Both a positive and a negative control should be included with each analysis, although a positive control may not always be readily available. An umbilical cord blood or neonatal sample, not fresh, may be an acceptable alternative as a positive control. At the time of reading, the negative control should be clear, and the positive control should have some flocculation.

Normal Hb is stable when heated to 50°C. However, unstable Hbs precipitate to varying extents when similarly treated. A hemolysate of the sample in a pH 7.4 Tris-phosphate buffer is divided into two aliquots. One is stored at 4°C, the other is heated at 50°C for 2 hours. Both samples are centrifuged, and Hb quantification is performed on each supernatant. Quantification of the unstable Hb is calculated using the following formula:

$$\%\ \text{Unstable hemoglobin} = \frac{\text{Hb}\,(4\,°\text{C}) - \text{Hb}\,(50\,°\text{C})}{\text{Hb}\,(4\,°\text{C})} \times 100$$

Frequently, both heat and isopropanol stability tests are performed when a suspected unstable Hb variant is investigated. Unstable Hb variants may not appear on HPLC or electrophoresis, especially if the variant is unstable enough to precipitate before analysis by these techniques.

Globin Chain Analysis. Globin chain analysis by electrophoresis and HPLC has been replaced by mass spectroscopy; however, the techniques used to dissociate the globin chains—urea and dithiothretiol treatment—are still used.

IRON

Iron is involved in the function of all cells. It is able to accept and donate electrons, depending on its oxidation state: ferrous iron (Fe[II]) or ferric iron (Fe[III]). Fe is mostly locked into Fe protoporphyrin (heme) and Fe–sulphur clusters, which serve as enzyme cofactors. Hemoproteins are involved in numerous biological functions, such as oxygen binding and transport (Hbs), oxygen metabolism (catalases, peroxidases), cellular respiration, and electron transport (cytochromes).[96] Proteins containing nonheme Fe are important for fundamental cellular processes such as DNA synthesis, cell proliferation and differentiation (ribonucleotide reductase), gene regulation, drug metabolism, and steroid synthesis.[96] However, Fe can also cause damage, because Fe(II) catalyzes the generation of highly reactive hydroxyl radicals (•OH) from hydrogen peroxide (H_2O_2) ($Fe^{2+} + H_2O_2 \rightarrow Fe^{3+} + HO^- + HO^{\cdot}$), which is called the "Fenton reaction."[97] These hydroxyl radicals damage cellular membranes, proteins, and DNA. A large number of scavenger molecules protect cells against Fe-mediated tissue damage. Proteins sequester Fe to reduce this threat. Fe circulates bound to plasma transferrin, which is needed to offer the highly insoluble Fe(III) to cells via the transferrin receptor. Fe can safely be stored within cells in the form of ferritin and hemosiderin.[98] Under normal circumstances, only small amounts of Fe exist outside this physiologic sink, although stored Fe can be mobilized for reuse. Many diseases arise from imbalances in Fe homeostasis. Too much Fe accumulates in hereditary hemochromatosis (HH) and in the Fe-loading anemias, which are often aggravated by multiple transfusions. In IDA, insufficient amounts of Fe are available for heme synthesis. In ACD, Fe is redistributed to macrophages to promote resistance to infections.[99]

Iron Metabolism

Systemic and Cellular Iron Regulation

The control of Fe homeostasis acts at both the cellular and the systemic level, and involves a complex system of different cell types, transporters, and signals. To maintain systemic Fe homeostasis, communication between cells that absorb Fe from the diet (duodenal enterocytes), consume Fe (mainly erythroid precursors), and store Fe (hepatocyte and tissue macrophages) must be tightly regulated. Each of these cell types plays an essential role in the homeostatic Fe cycle. The β-defensin–like antimicrobial peptide hepcidin is believed to be the long-anticipated regulator that controls Fe absorption and macrophage Fe release.[100] Hepcidin is synthesized in the liver upon changes in body Fe needs, anemia, hypoxia, and inflammation, and is secreted in the circulation. It counteracts the function of ferroportin, a major cellular Fe exporter protein in the membrane of macrophages and the basolateral site of enterocytes, by inducing its internalization

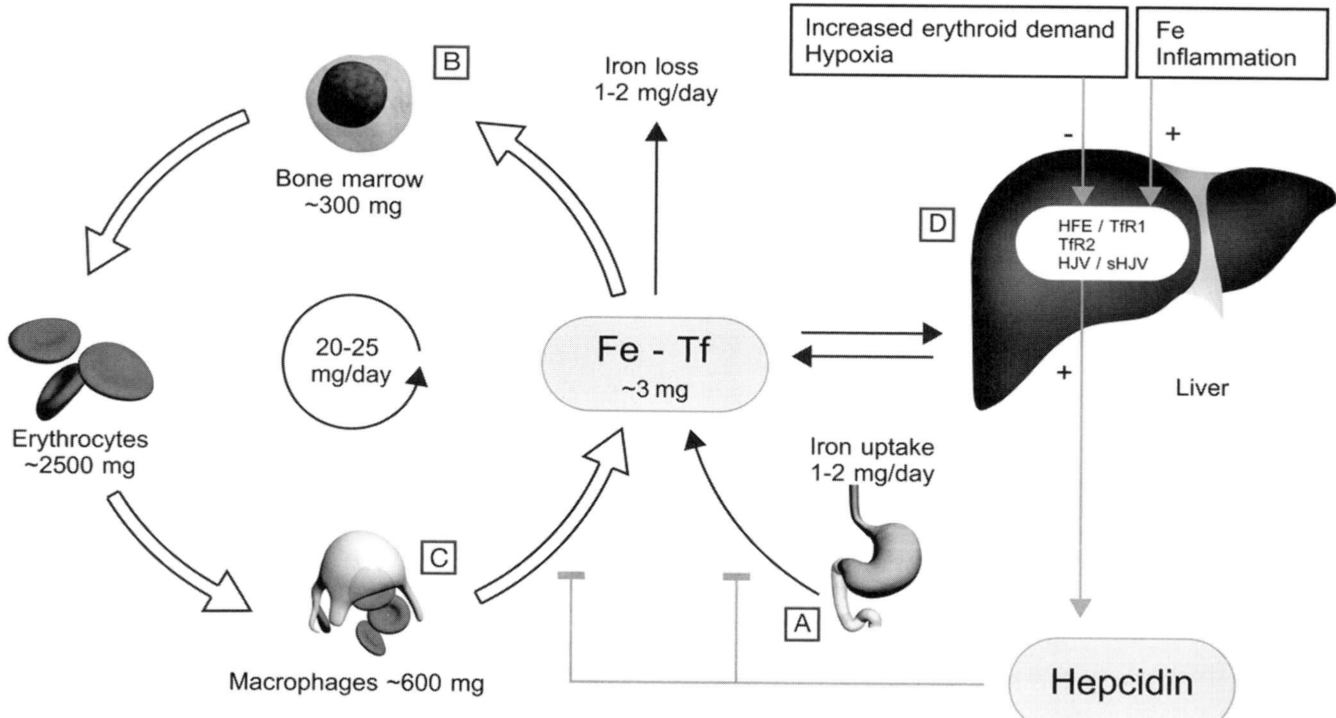

FIGURE 38.17 Systemic Iron *(Fe)* Homeostasis. The largest flux of Fe takes place in the recycling of Fe from senescent erythrocytes out of *(A)* macrophages to incorporation in *(B)* erythroid precursors in the bone marrow. Values for the different tissues and fluxes are approximate. The *(D)* liver and *(C)* reticuloendothelial macrophages function as major iron stores. Only 1 to 2 mg Fe is absorbed and lost every day. Importantly, the total amount of Fe in the body can only be regulated by absorption, whereas Fe loss occurs only passively from sloughing of skin and mucosal cells, as well as from blood loss. Hepcidin, a recently identified antimicrobial, β-defensin–like peptide secreted by the liver, decreases the plasma Fe concentration by inhibiting Fe export by ferroportin from *(A)* duodenal enterocytes and *(C)* reticuloendothelial macrophages.[101] As a consequence, an increase in hepcidin production results in a decrease in plasma Fe levels (reviewed in references 102,110,117,118,125). Hepcidin expression of the hepatocyte is regulated by circulating and stored Fe levels, inflammatory stimuli, the erythroid Fe demand, and hypoxia, by pathways involving expression of *HFE, TFR2,* hemojuvelin *(HJV),* and *TMPRSS6* genes.[117] In HFE-, transferrin receptor (TfR)-2, and HJV-related hereditary hemochromatosis, hepcidin production is low despite increased liver Fe, which results in inappropriately increased Fe absorption.[218] Defects in the *TMPRSS6* gene, encoding for matriptase-2, result in Fe refractory iron deficiency anemia.[183,185,186] The letters *A, B, C,* and *D* refer to sites with special functions in iron metabolism. (From Swinkels DW, Janssen MC, Bergmans J, Marx JJ. Hereditary hemochromatosis: genetic complexity and new diagnostic approaches. *Clin Chem* 2006;52:950–968.)

and degradation.[101,102] Background information on these major pathways of Fe exchange and the role of hepcidin in Fe regulation is provided in Fig. 38.17.

Cells involved in Fe homeostasis are duodenal enterocytes, hepatocytes, macrophages, and erythroid precursors. Fig. 38.18 displays these key sites in Fe homeostasis and their function in more detail to illustrate the description of the pathophysiology for the different Fe disorders. The Fe enters the body through the diet. Most Fe absorption takes place in the duodenal and proximal jejunum enterocytes in different phases. In the luminal phase, Fe is solubilized and converted from trivalent Fe into bivalent Fe by duodenal cytochrome B. During the mucosal phase, Fe is bound to the brush border and transported into the mucosal cell by the Fe transporter divalent metal transporter (DMT1). In the cellular phase, Fe is either stored in cellular ferritin or transported directly to the opposite side of the mucosal side. In the last phase of Fe absorption, Fe^{2+} is released into the portal circulation by the basolateral cellular exporter ferroportin. Enterocytic Fe export requires hephaestin, a multicopper oxidase homologous to ceruloplasmin, which oxidases Fe^{2+} to Fe^{3+} for loading onto transferrin. This cellular efflux of Fe is inhibited by the peptide hormone hepcidin by binding to ferroportin and subsequent degradation of the ferroportin-hepcidin complex.

The hepatocyte serves as the main storage for Fe surplus (most body Fe is present in erythrocytes and macrophages). Furthermore, this cell, as the main producer of hepcidin, largely controls systemic Fe regulation. The signal transduction pathway runs from the membrane to the nucleus, where the bone morphogenetic protein receptor, the membrane protein hemojuvelin (HJV), the HFE protein, transferrin receptors (TfR)-1 and -2, and matriptase-2 play an essential role. Through intracellular pathways, a signal is given to hepcidin transcription. The membrane-associated protease

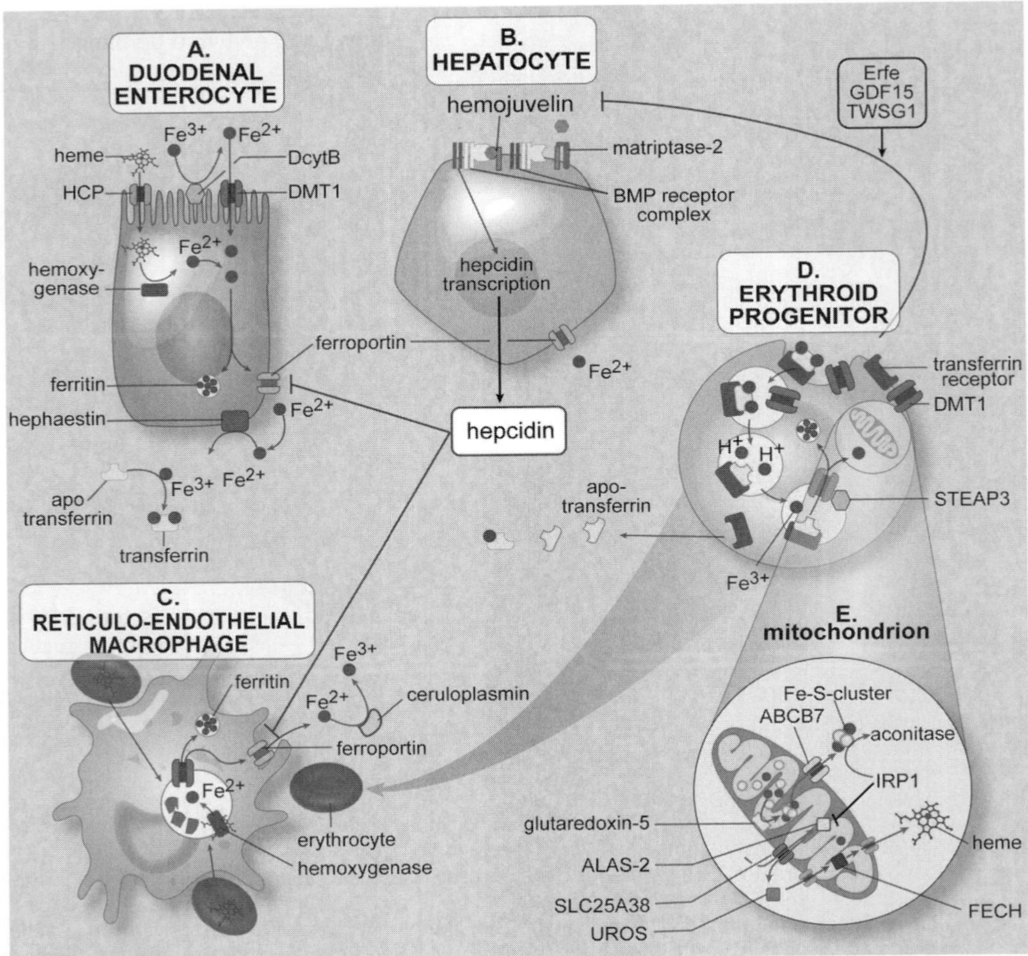

FIGURE 38.18 Cells and Proteins Involved in Iron Homeostasis and Heme Synthesis. **A,** The enterocyte. **B,** The hepatocyte. **C,** The macrophage. **D,** The erythroid progenitor. **E,** The mitochondria of the erythroid progenitor. *ALAS2,* δ-Aminolevulinic acid synthase; *BMP,* bone morphogenetic protein; *CP,* ceruloplasmin; *DCytB,* duodenal cytochrome B; *DMT1,* divalent metal transporter; *Erfe,* erythroferrone; *FECH,* ferrochelatase; *GLRX5,* glutaredoxin-5; *HCP,* heme carrier protein 1, a low affinity heme transporter; *HJV,* hemojuvelin; *MHB,* hydroxymethylbilane; *PPIX,* protoporhyrin IX; *TfR1,* transferrin receptor 1; *UROS,* uroporhyrinogen III synthase. (From Donker AE, Raymakers RA, Vlasveld LT, van Barneveld T, Terink R, et al. Practice guidelines for the diagnosis and management of microcytic anemias due to genetic disorders of iron metabolism or heme synthesis. *Blood* 2014;123:3873–3886 and based on the work reviewed in references 96, 117, 118, 125, 186, 218, and 236.)

matriptase-2 (encoded by *TMPRSS6*) detects Fe deficiency and blocks hepcidin transcription by cleaving HJV. The macrophage belongs to the group of reticuloendothelial cells and breaks down senescent RBCs. During this process, Fe is released from heme proteins. This Fe can either be stored in the macrophage as hemosiderin or ferritin, or may be delivered to the erythroid progenitor as an ingredient for new erythrocytes. The Fe exporter ferroportin is responsible for the efflux of Fe^{2+} into the circulation. In both hepatocytes and macrophages, this transport requires the multicopper oxidase ceruloplasmin, which oxidases Fe^{2+} to Fe^{3+} for loading unto transferrin.

In the erythroid progenitor cell, transferrin with Fe molecules is endocytosed via the TfR1. After endocytosis, Fe is released from transferrin, converted from Fe^{3+} to Fe^{2+} by the ferroreductase six-transmembrane epithelial antigen of prostate 3 (STEAP3), and transported to the cytosol by DMT1, where it is available mainly for the heme synthesis. The apotransferrin is transported back to the cell surface and released, ready to transport additional Fe. Erythropoiesis has been reported to communicate with the hepatocyte by the proteins growth differentation factor 15 (GDF15), twisted gastrulation 1 (TWSG1), and erythroferrone (ERFE), which inhibit signaling to hepcidin. In the mitochondria of the erythroid progenitor, the heme synthesis and Fe-sulfur cluster synthesis takes place. In the first rate-limiting step of heme synthesis, 5-aminolevulinic acid (ALA) is synthesized from glycine and succinyl-coenzyme A by the enzyme δ-aminolevulinic acid synthase (ALAS2) in the mitochondrial matrix. The protein SLC25A38 is located in the mitochondrial membrane and is probably responsible for the import of glycine into the mitochondria and may also export ALA to the cytosol. In the heme synthesis pathway, the uroporhyrinogen III synthase (UROS) in the cytosol is the fourth enzyme. It is responsible for the conversion of hydroxymethylbilane to uroporphyrinogen III, a physiologic precursor of heme. In the last step, ferrochelatase located in the mitochondrial intermembrane space is responsible for the last step (ie, the incorporation of Fe^{2+} in protoporhyrin IX to form heme). GATA-binding factor I (GATA 1) is critical for normal erythropoiesis, globin gene expression, and megakaryocyte development, and among others, it regulates expression of uroporhyrinogen III synthase and ALAS2 in erythroblasts. The enzyme glutaredoxin-5 plays a role in the synthesis of the Fe-sulfur clusters, which are transported to the cytoplasm, probably via the transporter ABCB7.

Human hepcidin is predominantly produced by hepatocytes as an 25-amino acid peptide (molecular weight: 2789.4 Da)[100,103,104] that is secreted into the circulation. Subsequent amino-terminal processing of the 25-amino acid form can result in the appearance of three main smaller hepcidin forms of 24, 23, 22, and 20 amino acids.[105,106] These hepcidin peptides form a hairpin structure, with four intramolecular disulfide bridges.[107] Much is still unknown about the origin of the smaller isoforms. They are believed to arise due to degradation of the full-length hepcidin in the circulation or the urine. The cleavage of hepcidin also occurs during sample storage at room temperature.

Under physiologic conditions, the smaller hepcidin isoforms are present in the urine, but not, or at low concentrations, in the serum.[108,109] These smaller hepcidin isoforms only occur in serum in diseases that are associated with increased concentrations of hepcidin-25, such as sepsis and chronic kidney disease (reviewed in Kroot and colleagues[110] and Girelli and colleagues[111]). Only the full-length, 25-amino acid hepcidin is biologically active and induces significant hypoferremia.[112,113]

Hepcidin is bound to α2-macroglobulin, but the percentage amount of hepcidin that freely circulates varies between 11% and 98% among reports.[114-116]

Several physiologic and pathologic processes regulate the synthesis of hepcidin.[100,110,117-119] These functional signaling routes by which (1) Fe status, (2) erythropoietic activity, (3) hypoxia, and (4) inflammation affect hepcidin expression are increasingly being investigated. These routes comprise four highly interconnected regulatory pathways (Fig. 38.19). Situations that demand circulating Fe to be increased (particularly erythropoietic activity) elicit a decrease in hepatocellular hepcidin synthesis. These conditions include Fe deficiency, hypoxia, anemia, and conditions characterized by increased erythropoietic activity. A decrease in hepcidin results in the release of stored Fe and an increase in dietary Fe absorption. In contrast, infection or inflammation causes an increase in hepcidin synthesis. This leads to a deficiency of Fe available for erythropoiesis and is considered the mechanism that underlays the reticuloendothelial Fe sequestration and intestinal Fe absorption impairment; low serum Fe concentrations are characteristic of ACD.

Intracellular Iron Regulation

The expression of proteins involved in Fe uptake, storage, and release of Fe from the cell is determined by the Fe need of the cell and regulated at the posttranscriptional level by the Fe responsive protein and Fe regulatory element (IRP/IRE) network.[120] In the cell, the IRP1 and IRP2 interact with the IRE on the mRNA and affect the translation to protein. In conditions of high cellular Fe levels, the IRPs are inactive. In contrast, low cellular Fe levels increase IRP activity. In the latter condition, IRPs bind to the IRE and inhibit mRNA translation (in the case of ferritin and ferroportin) or increase mRNA stability (in the case of cellular Fe importers, such as TfR1 and DMT1). The result is that more Fe enters the cell, and less Fe is stored in ferritin or leaves the cell via ferroportin. In conditions of low cellular Fe, there is also less synthesis of ALAS-2, the first enzyme in the heme synthesis and less production of hypoxia-inducible factor (HIF)-2α in the kidney fibroblasts, resulting in a decrease in erythropoetin (EPO) production. As such, the body decreases the heme and RBC synthesis in case of Fe scarcity, which results in microcytic anemia (see also Chapter 72). Thus, although key aspects of systemic Fe metabolism are regulated transcriptionally (hepcidin expression) and posttranslationally (ferroportin function by hepcidin), intracellular Fe homeostasis is largely controlled by a posttranscriptional mechanism involving the IRP1/IRP2 network.

Body Iron Distribution

Most of the body Fe (3–5 g) is found in heme-containing oxygen transport and storage proteins, including Hb (>2.5 g) and myoglobin (≈130 mg). Small amounts (≈150 mg) are incorporated into enzymes, with active sites containing heme or Fe-sulfur clusters, including peroxidases, catalases, ribonucleotide reductase, and enzymes of the Krebs cycle and the electron transport chain. Most nonheme Fe (≈1 g in adult men) is stored as ferritin or hemosiderin in macrophages and hepatocytes. Only a small amount (≈3 mg) of Fe is bound to the circulating serum protein transferrin. An estimate of the average amount of Fe contained in each of these compartments for an average man is presented in Table 38.5 and in the literature.[121-125]

The total volume of red cells in an average man is approximately 2.5 L, with each milliliter containing approximately 1 mg of Fe (1 g Hb contains 3.4 mg Fe). Therefore, the body contains approximately 2.5 g of Fe incorporated into Hb (see Table 38.5).[122,124] Cellular Fe in excess of immediate needs is stored as an Fe oxide within the nanocavity of ferritin and a partially degraded form of ferritin known as hemosiderin.[126]

Ferritin is a protein, which was first isolated in 1937 from the spleen of the horse by the French scientist Laufberger.[127] In later years, ferritin was found to be an evolutionary conserved, ubiquitous protein that can accommodate up to 4500 Fe atoms. In humans, ferritin is a heteropolymer of 24 subunits of two types, heavy/heart (H) and light/liver (L), which assemble to make a hollow spherical shell, which can take up atoms of Fe stored as ferric oxyhydroxide phosphate.[126,128] The ferroxidase activity of H-ferritin converts Fe^{2+} to Fe^{3+}, which is necessary for Fe deposition into the nanocage. L-ferritin induces Fe nucleation. L-ferritin is predominant in Fe-storing tissues (liver, reticuloendothelial), whereas H-ferritin is preferentially expressed in cells with significant antioxidant activity (brain, heart).[128] Different proportions of ferritin subunits give rise to the heterogeneity of the holoprotein in various tissue types.

Fe^{2+} is delivered to ferritin by cystoplasmatic chaperones.[129] The release of Fe from ferritin is mediated by multiple mechanisms,[128] among which are authophagy and lysosomal degradation of ferritin.[130,131] Physiologically, degradation of ferritin is coupled to the supply of metabolic Fe availability

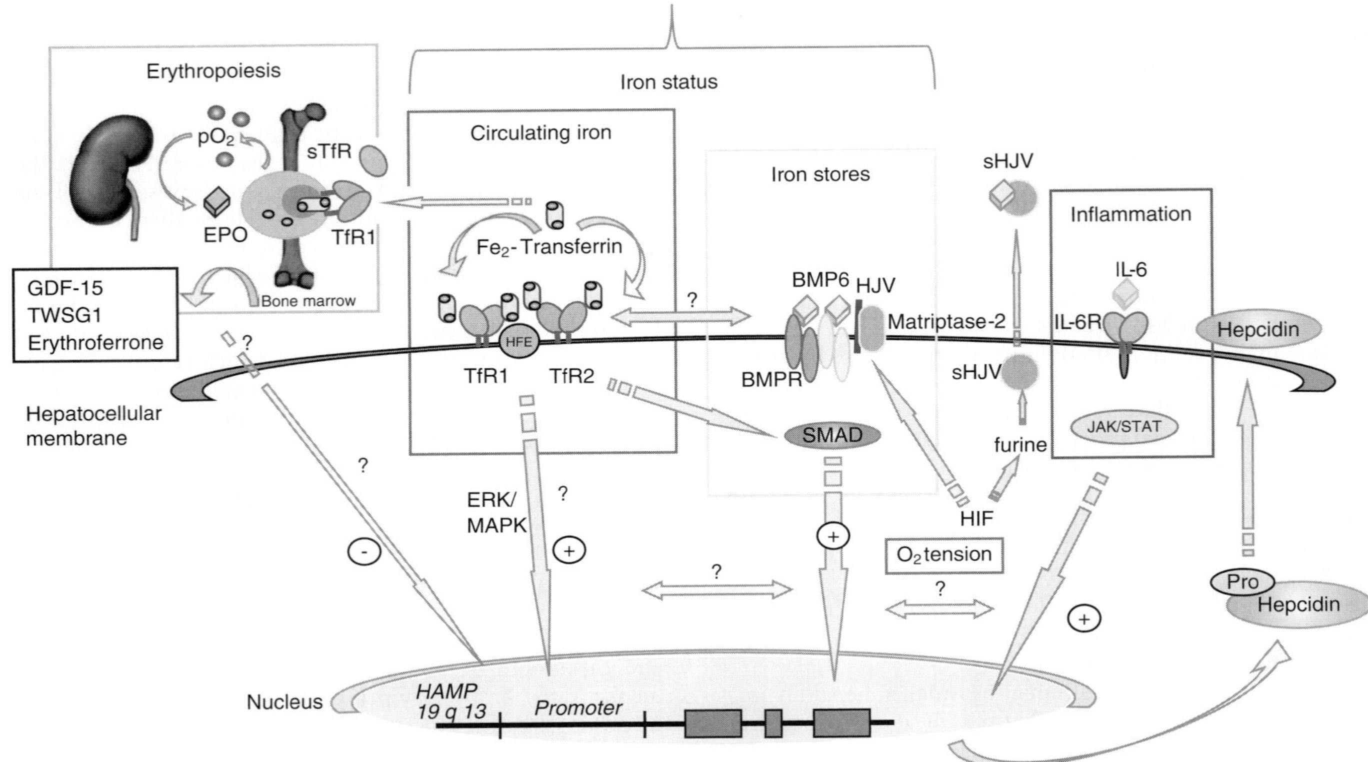

FIGURE 38.19 Regulation of Hepcidin Synthesis of the Hepatocyte. Four functionally defined hepcidin regulatory pathways are depicted: erythropoiesis, iron status, oxygen (O_2) tension, and inflammation. Increased erythropoiesis is associated with decreased hepcidin expression by mechanisms that remain to be defined. Candidate signaling molecules from the marrow include growth differentiation factor-15 (GDF-15), twisted gastrulation protein homolog 1 (TWSG1), and erythroferrone (ERFE). Increased body iron status increases hepcidin expression through two mechanisms: a circulating iron signal provided by ferri-transferrin and a cellular iron stores signal provided by bone morphogenetic protein 6 (BMP-6). The ferri-transferrin signal acts through transferrin receptors 1 and 2 and is modulated by the hemochromatosis protein HFE. The BMP-6 signal acts through its receptor and is modulated by the BMP coreceptor hemojuvelin (HJV) and by neogenin. Decreased O_2 tension leads to decreased hepcidin expression by increasing the transcription of two genes, matriptase-2 and furin, which are responsive to hypoxia-inducible factor (HIF). Matriptase-2 cleaves HJV from the cell surface, preventing its function as a coreceptor. Furin cleaves HJV during processing to produce a soluble form that serves as a BMP-6 decoy. Infections and other forms of inflammation increase hepcidin expression by the cytokine interleukin (IL)-6. *BMPR,* Bone morphogenetic protein receptor; *HAMP,* hepcidin gene; *EPO,* erythopoietin; *ERK,* extracellular signal-regulated kinases; *JAK-STAT,* Janus-associated kinase–signal transducers and activators of transcription; *MAPK,* mitogen-activated protein kinases; *pO*$_2$ partial pressure of oxygen; *TfR1,* transferin receptor 1. (Modified from Kroot JJ, Tjalsma H, Fleming RE, Swinkels DW. Hepcidin in human iron disorders: diagnostic implications. *Clin Chem* 2011;57:1650-1669; Fleming RE, Ponka P. Iron overload in human disease. *N Engl J Med* 2012;366:348–359; and reviewed in references 110,117,118.)

TABLE 38.5 Iron Content of Compartments in an Average Male

Compartment	Iron Content (mg)
Hemoglobin	2500
Storage iron*	1000
Myoglobin	130
Other cellular iron containing proteins	150
Transport (transferrin)	3
Total	3000–5000

*Sum of parenchymal and reticuloendothelial iron stored in ferritin or hemosiderin.
Data from several references.[121-124, 468]

under Fe-limiting conditions.[132] Ferritin is present in nearly all cells of the body and provides a reserve of Fe that is readily available for formation of Hb and other heme proteins. Fe bound to ferritin is shielded from body fluids and thus is unable to cause oxidative damage, which would occur if it were in a free ionic form. In men, the total body content of stored Fe, mostly as ferritin, is approximately 1000 mg; in healthy premenopausal women, Fe stores are typically lower.[124] The expression of ferritin is tightly regulated at the transcriptional and posttranscriptional level by a variety of factors, including Fe, cytokines, hormones, and oxidative stress.[98,128]

After the development of the first immunoassays for the measurement of ferritin in serum in the 1970s, ferritin levels were shown to reflect body Fe stores by studies that used quantitative phlebotomy, radio-Fe retention, and bone marrow aspirate.[133-135] In particular, it is now widely accepted that 1 μg/L of serum ferritin corresponds to approximately 8 to 10 mg of stored Fe.[135-137] However, when comparing individuals of widely differing body weight, the conversion of 120-μg serum ferritin per kilogram tissue storage Fe is preferable because ferritin is a concentration measurement.[122] Serum ferritin differs from tissue ferritin in that it is glycosylated, contains mostly L-chains, and is Fe-poor (mostly apoferritin).[138] Serum ferritin reflects both reticuloendothelial and parenchymal Fe stores.[137] However, despite its long history of use in the assessment of body Fe stores, the source and detailed secretory pathway of serum ferritin from cells are not completely understood, although animal studies suggest that macrophages contribute significantly to serum ferritin concentrations.[139] Also, the receptor interactions and the cellular effects of serum ferritin are unclear and topics of active debate.[138]

Hemosiderin is an aggregated and partially deproteinized ferritin that is formed when ferritin is partially degraded.[140] In contrast to ferritin, hemosiderin is insoluble in aqueous solutions—a difference that has been used traditionally to distinguish these two Fe storage compounds. Fe is only slowly released from hemosiderin, possibly because it occurs in relatively large aggregates and therefore has a much smaller surface-to-volume ratio. Like ferritin, hemosiderin is found predominantly in cells of the liver, spleen, and bone marrow.

Myoglobin closely resembles a single Hb subunit. Because myoglobin does not form tetramers, it lacks the allosteric oxygen-binding properties of Hb.

Fe in the circulation is bound to free sites on the plasma Fe-transport protein transferrin. Transferrin keeps Fe nonreactive in the circulation and extravascular fluid, and delivers it to cells with transferrin receptors. Transferrin was discovered by the Americans Schade and Caroline[141] as a saturable Fe-binding component in human plasma that is capable of inhibiting growth of *Shigella dysenteriae*. Transferrin is a glycoprotein with an approximate molecular mass of 80 kDa[142] and two homologous high-affinity binding sites for the ferric (Fe^{3+}) Fe.[143-146] Each site can bind one atom of trivalent Fe together with one ion of HCO_3^-. The Fe atoms are incorporated one at a time and appear to bind randomly at either or both of the two sites. The functional differences between the two binding sites led to the Fletcher-Huehns hypothesis, according to which, the two sites of transferrin behaved differently, the one delivering Fe preferentially to erythroid cells, and the other to nonerythroid tissues.[147] Transferrin experts in the 1970s and 1980s were obsessed with this hypothesis, and currently, the physiologic importance of the presence of different binding sites is still not fully clear.

The apotransferrin-Fe^{3+} complex is called monoferric or diferric (=holo) transferrin. Because the transferrin Fe-binding capacity normally largely exceeds plasma Fe concentrations, transferrin-bound Fe is the only physiologic source available to most cells. High transferrin saturation facilitates parenchymal Fe disposition. Cells regulate the intake of transferrin bound Fe by altering the expression of surface TfR1. TfR1 is a transmembrane glycoprotein composed of a 190-kDa (under nonreducing conditions) homodimer that binds two holotransferrin molecules with high affinity or monoferric transferrin with a lower affinity, one by each subunit.[148] Its rate of synthesis is elevated in case of increased requirements of the cell for Fe. In patients in whom transferrin becomes highly saturated, as in patients with Fe-loading anemias (see section on Disorders of Erythroid Maturation), untreated hemochromatosis, other severe Fe overload disorders, patients who have received multiple blood transfusions, or patients who are supplemented with a high-dose oral Fe due to Fe deficiency, additional Fe released into the circulation is bound to low-molecular-weight compounds (eg, citrate).[149-151] This so-called nontransferrin bound Fe (NTBI) is readily taken up by certain cell types, including hepatocytes and cardiomyocytes, and contributes to oxidant-mediated cellular injury. A fraction of the circulating NTBI is redox-active and designated labile plasma Fe.[152] Although there are methods for measuring serum NTBI and labile plasma Fe, insufficient standardization and clinical correlation currently limit clinical use of these measurements.[149,153,154]

Clinical Significance

Iron deficiency, Fe overload, and ACD are the most prevalent disorders of Fe metabolism. Fe disorders may be classified (1) according to pathophysiology (Table 38.6), (2) heritability (genetic or acquired), or (3) as being a "primary," (eg,

TABLE 38.6 Features of Iron Metabolism Disorders

Disorder	Gene	Inheritance	Age at Presentation	Systemic Iron Overload	Anemia	Ferritin	TSAT
Impaired Hepcidin-Ferroportin Axis[118,218,469]							
HH type 1	*HFE*	AR	Adult	Variable	No	Variable	High
HH type II A	*HAMP*	AR	Child	Yes	No	High	High
HH type II B	*HJV*	AR	Child to young adult	Yes	No	High	High
HH type III	*TfR2*	AR	Young adult	Yes	No	High	High
HH type IVA [220,221,224]	*SLC40A1* (LOF*)	AD	Adult	Yes	Sporadically	High	Normal
HH type IV B[220,221]	*SLC40A1* (GOF)	AD	Adult	Yes	No	High	High

Continued

TABLE 38.6 Features of Iron Metabolism Disorders—cont'd

Disorder	Gene	Inheritance	Age at Presentation	Systemic Iron Overload	Anemia	Ferritin	TSAT
Iron Transport Disorder[186,241]							
Low Iron Availability for Erythropoiesis							
IRIDA[183,185]	*TMPRSS6*	AR/AD		No	Yes	Low–normal	Low
Aceruloplasminemia[230,231]	*CP*	AR		Yes	Yes	High	Normal/low
Anemia of chronic disease[199]	NA	NA	Variable	No*	Yes	Normal–high	Low
Defect in iron acquisition of erythroid progenitor cells							
Hypotransferrinemia [245]	*Tf*	AR		yes	Yes	High	100%
Microcytic anemia with iron loading [241]	*DMT1*	AR		Yes	Yes	Variable	High
Erythroid Dysmaturation[186,470]							
Nontransfusion-dependent thalassemias (β-thalassemia intermedia; Hb H disease)[239]	Globin	AR	Variable	Yes	Yes	High	High
Sideroblastic Anemia Congenital[186,242,470]							
X-linked sideroblastic anemia	*ALAS-2*	XL	Child	Variable	Mild/no anemia	Variable	Variable
Sideroblastic anemia	*SLC25A38*	AR	Child	Yes	Severe	High	High
Sideroblastic anemia	*GLRx5*	AR	Adult	Yes	Mild	High	High
Sideroblastic anemia with ataxia	*ABCB7*	XL	Child	No	Mild	Normal	Normal
Myelodysplastic syndrome (RA, RARS)[243]	NA	NA	Adult	Variable	Variable	Variable	Variable
Congenital dyserythopoietic anemia Type Ia, Ib, II, III, IV[244]	*CDAN1, C15ORF41, SEC23B, KIF23, KLF1*	Variable	Child	Variable	Yes	Variable	High
Other Iron Disorders							
Localized iron overload [249,250]							
Neurodegeneration with brain iron accumulation							
Neonatal hemochromatosis[246,247]	NA	NA	Neonate	Yes	No	Yes	Yes
Iron overload in sub-Saharan Africa[225,226]	Unclear	Unclear	Adult	Yes	No	Yes	Yes
Hyperferritinemia-cataract syndrome[228,468]	*FTL*-IRE	AD	Variable	No	No	High	Normal
Chronic liver disease[232,233] Metabolic syndrome Steatohepatitis Cirrhosis	NA	NA	Variable	No/mild	Variable	Variable/high	Variable
Parenteral iron loading/chronic erythrocyte transfusion[240,252]	NA	NA	Variable	Yes	No	High	High
Iron deficiency (anemia)[155]	NA	NA	Variable	No	Variable	Low	Low

*Often referred to as "ferroportin disease."
GOF, Gain of function mutation; *HH*, hereditary hemochromatosis; *IRE*, iron response element; *IRIDA*, iron refractory iron deficiency anemia; *LOF*, loss of function mutation; *RA*, refractory anemia; *RARS*, refractory anemia with ringed sideroblasts; *TSAT*, transferrin saturation.

resulting from a defect in an Fe metabolism–related protein) or "secondary" (eg, the consequences of defects in other proteins).

Iron Deficiency

Iron deficiency and IDA, defined when anemia and Fe deficiency coexist, are global health problems and common medical conditions seen in everyday clinical practice.[155-159] Fe deficiency accounts for approximately one-half of the approximately 1 billion subjects with anemia worldwide.[156,159,160] Prevalence of anemia is highest in South Asia and Central, West, and East Sub-Saharan Africa.[156] The Fe-amenable share of anemia burden is highest where few other causes of anemia exist (ie, in Central Asia [65%], South Asia [55%], and Andean Latin America [62%]).[156]

Fe deficiency is particularly a disorder of children and premenopausal women in low- and middle-income countries, but it can also occur in men, and in developed countries and people of all ages.[155,157,161] In children, Fe deficiency is frequently caused by the increased physiologic needs for dietary Fe for growth and development.[157] In adults, and especially premenopausal women, Fe deficiency is almost always the result of chronic blood loss or childbearing.[161]

IDA is associated with impaired quality of life,[162] work productivity,[163] aerobic exercise capacity,[164,165] and fatigue,[166] and there is also a relationship between Fe status and depression and cognitive functioning.[167,168] Fe deficiency also affects immune function and the susceptibility to infections.[169,170] Furthermore, Fe deficiency is a predictor of mortality in patients with nondialysis chronic kidney disease[171] and heart failure,[172] and treating Fe deficiency in patients with heart failure improves quality of life.[173]

Because Fe does not only play a key role as an oxygen carrier in the heme group of Hb, but is also found in cytochromes and myoglobin, this might explain why Fe deficiency has effects beyond that of anemia. This was appreciated already in the nineteenth century.[174,175] More recently, several studies showed that Fe supplementation reduces fatigue in nonanemic women with low ferritin levels.[176,177] In addition, there are reports that showed the effects of Fe deficiency without anemia on deficits and attention spans leading to learning and problem solving difficulties in children.[178] Hence, diagnosing and treating Fe deficiency with or without anemia is a major issue in clinical practice.

Fe deficiency was recognized as "chlorosis," a term derived from the Greek word meaning green, by Johannes Lange in 1554.[121,174,179] This condition became well known as the green sickness, probably because of the greenish pallor occurring in teenage "virgineus" girls. The disease preoccupied many clinicians between the middle of the seventeenth century and the end of the nineteenth century, and yet is not seen today. Therefore, currently most people believe that chlorosis resulted from a combination of factors affecting adolescent girls: the demands of growth and the onset of menses, an inadequate diet, and a legacy of poor Fe stores from early childhood. In the early 1830s, anemia, hypochromia, and lack of Fe in the blood were linked to this disorder.[179] Other distinguishing clinical features ascribed to a lack of Fe at that time were epithelial changes involving the tongue and nails, and achlorhydria. Currently, anemia most often affects women with poor diets, multiple pregnancies, or menstrual irregularities. In 1832, the French physician Pierre Blaud described the response of chlorosis to his famous pills (ferrous sulfate plus potassium carbonate). However, the use of Fe in the treatment of chlorosis received a major setback when the chemist Bunge in 1902 ascribed the effect of Fe as a placebo effect. All doubt was resolved in 1932 in a publication by Heath and colleagues,[180] who found that Hb levels increased upon intramuscular and subcutaneous injections with Fe.[174] Until today, ferrous sulfate remains a cornerstone of modern treatment of Fe deficiency.

IDA is generally an acquired condition due to blood losses, malabsorption, insufficient Fe intake, or a combination of these.[155] Some patients with chronic disease are especially vulnerable to develop absolute Fe deficiency (eg, patients with gastrointestinal tumors because of blood losses). Patients with advanced chronic kidney disease also have a negative Fe balance as a result of reduced dietary intake, impaired absorption from the gut, and increased Fe losses.[181] In addition, patients with chronic kidney disease also often have a functional Fe deficiency because the available circulating Fe cannot keep pace with the requirements of erythropoiesis stimulated with erythropoiesis stimulating agents.[182]

Recently, the elucidation of systemic Fe homeostasis has also led to the discovery of a rare (autosomal recessive) inherited disorder, Fe refractory IDA (IRIDA), which is an IDA that does not improve with oral Fe supplementation. IRIDA is caused by mutations in *TMPRSS6*, the gene encoding matriptase-2, which inhibits the signaling pathway that activates hepcidin.[155,183-191] To date, *TMPRSS6* defects have been identified in more than 60 IRIDA families of different ethnic origin.[186] Typical findings include marked microcytosis, extremely low transferrin saturation (TSAT), and low to normal ferritin and high hepcidin levels for the low body Fe levels. The diagnosis is confirmed by bi-allelic pathogenic defects in the *TMPRSS6* gene. Rarely, monoallelic defects have also been described to cause the disorder. IRIDA is a rare disease and is likely to be overlooked. Knowledge of this condition is valuable because it prevents unnecessary, invasive, and expensive diagnostic procedures and forms an indication for intravenous Fe treatment. Population studies and studies in Tmprss6-haploinsufficient mice suggest an association of variants in *TMPRSS6*, with susceptibility to develop Fe deficiency and anemia, especially in the presence of other risk factors such as blood loss, inflammation, and infection.[187-189] IRIDA due to a defect in matriptase-2 should be distinguished from other causes of IDA refractory to Fe supplementation, among which are disorders of the gastrointestinal tract, such as *Helicobacter pylori* infection and (partial or total) gastrectomy and gastric bypass (bariatric) surgery.[190,191]

An emerging cause of Fe deficiency is obesity. It has been largely attributed to functional Fe deficiency associated with low-grade, inflammation-induced hepcidin levels and a subsequent hepcidin-mediated decrease of Fe uptake from food and less release from reticuloendothelial system stores.[192]

Many different measurements have been advocated for the diagnosis of Fe deficiency. Originally, emphasis was placed on the RBC indexes; hypochromic and microcytemic anemias were generally considered to be a synonym for Fe deficiency in the first half of the twentieth century.[193] Subsequently, techniques such as staining of marrow with Perls' Prussian Blue to allow visualization of ferric Fe and measurement of (1) serum Fe, (2) Fe-binding capacity (and later transferrin), (3)

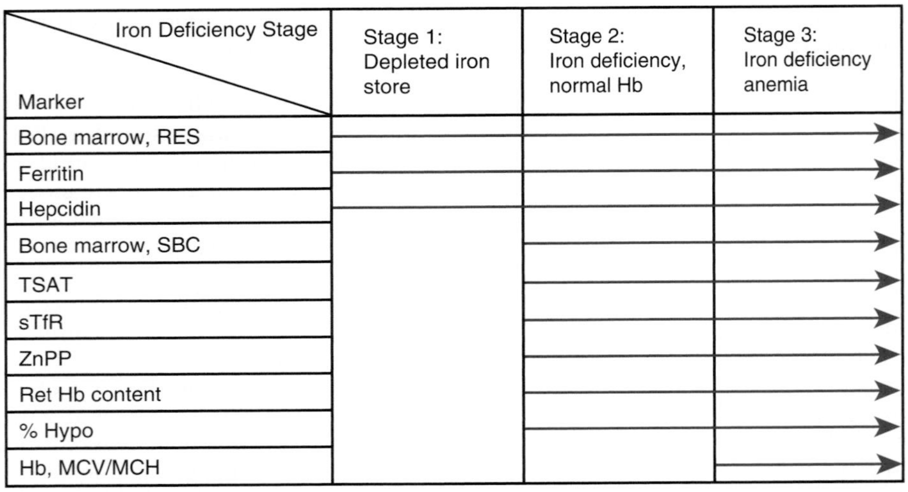

Marker \ Iron Deficiency Stage	Stage 1: Depleted iron store	Stage 2: Iron deficiency, normal Hb	Stage 3: Iron deficiency anemia
Bone marrow, RES	→	→	→
Ferritin	→	→	→
Hepcidin	→	→	→
Bone marrow, SBC		→	→
TSAT		→	→
sTfR		→	→
ZnPP		→	→
Ret Hb content		→	→
% Hypo		→	→
Hb, MCV/MCH			→

FIGURE 38.20 Alterations in Biochemical and Hematological Parameters at Different Stages of Iron Deficiency. In detecting different stages, the various tests efficiently complement each other to characterize the severity of iron deficiency in the individual patient. Iron deficiency stage 1: bone marrow hemosiderin within reticuloendothelial (RES) cells and ferritin assess the iron stores and allow the diagnosis of iron depletion. In this stage, hepcidin is low (mostly undetectable) to increase maximal iron uptake from the diet and release from the reticuloendothelial system stores. Iron deficiency stage 2: pathological values of transferrin saturation *(TSAT)*, bone marrow sideroblast count *(SBC)*, soluble transferrin receptor *(sTfR)*, zinc protoporphyrin *(ZnPP)*, reticulocyte hemoglobin *(Ret-Hb)* content, percentage of hypochromic cells (% Hypo) indicate that iron-deficient erythropoiesis has already developed. Iron deficiency stage 3: Hb below normal values defines iron deficiency anemia, which is accompanied by low red cell indexes. *MCH*, Mean cell Hb; *MCV*, mean cell volume. (Modified from Hastka J, Lasserre JJ, Schwarzbeck A, Reiter A, Hehlmann R. Laboratory tests of iron status: correlation or common sense? *Clin Chem* 1996;42:718–724.)

serum ferritin, (4) erythrocyte Zn-protoporphyrin (ZnPP), (5) soluble transferrin receptor (sTfR), (6) the percentage of hypochromic red cells and reticulocyte Hb content, and (7) hepcidin were reported and used for their usefulness in diagnosing Fe deficiency. Although most of these parameters readily identify severe, uncomplicated Fe deficiency, the large number of tests advocated for the diagnosis of Fe deficiency reflects the fact that none of them are sufficient to detect mild Fe deficiency or Fe deficiency in a clinically complex setting, or in populations exposed to malaria, HIV, tuberculosis, and other infections.[155,158,194,195] Interpretation and definition of common clinical decision limits and development of guidelines is further complicated by (1) lack of standardization of many parameters (ie, for ferritin, sTfR, ZnPP, reticulocyte-Hb content parameters, and hepcidin), and (2) reliance on original studies performed in different clinical settings and populations. As a result, studies, and expert and international guidelines differ in the conclusions that they draw regarding the advantages of one method over another, and overall diagnostic strategies. Overall, a low ferritin level is a sensitive and specific indicator of Fe deficiency uncomplicated by other diseases. A TSAT (<15%–20%) indicates an Fe supply that is insufficient to support normal erythropoiesis. However, simple correlations between the various tests of Fe status do not exist.[196] Therefore, in determining Fe status, it is important to consider the whole picture rather than relying on single tests (Table 38.7). For the diagnosis of Fe-deficient states, plotting the different biochemical markers and erythrocyte parameters has been proposed, but this alternative approach is not widely used in clinical practice.[197,198] In less complex clinical settings, the diagnosis of Fe deficiency can be defined in three progressive stages, each characterized by its own combination of test results (Fig. 38.20).[196]

Anemia of Chronic Disease

Anemia of chronic disease, also named anemia of inflammation, is an Fe distribution disorder. Although the global prevalence of ACD is unknown, country-level studies suggest it is common.[156,199] It is often observed in patients with infectious and inflammatory diseases, among whom are patients with chronic kidney disease, inflammatory bowel disease, chronic heart failure, malignancies, and hepatic diseases.[172,182,199,200] The pathogenesis comprises three principal abnormalities: shortened erythrocyte survival, impaired marrow response, and disturbances in Fe metabolism. The disturbances in Fe metabolism are characterized by maldistribution of body Fe stores, with ample reticuloendothelial Fe contents relative to parenchymal Fe stores, with low circulating Fe (hypoferremia) and subsequent Fe–restricted erythropoiesis.[199,201,202] Thus, whereas in IDA the Fe supply depends on the amount of Fe stores, in ACD, the supply depends on its rate of mobilization. The pathophysiology of these Fe-related aspects in ACD can be attributed to a cytokine-induced increase in hepcidin synthesis.[199,203,204] A more specific descriptive but rarely used designation for the disease that refers to these aspects is therefore "hypoferremic anemia with reticuloendothelial siderosis."

The disease may lead to "functional Fe deficiency," a state of Fe-resticted erythropoiesis, in which there is insufficient Fe mobilization from the (otherwise adequate) body Fe stores to meet the Fe demands of the erythroid precursors. This is especially the case in conditions with increased erythroid Fe demands (eg, in some subjects with chronic kidney disease after treatment with erythropoiesis-stimulating agents).[182] Since the widespread introduction of erythropoiesis-stimulating agents, it has been recognized that supplemental Fe is necessary to optimize Hb response and allow minimization of the erythropoiesis-stimulating agent dose for both economic reasons and recent concerns about safety.

ACD is a typically normocytic, normochromic anemia. It is diagnosed when serum Fe concentrations are low despite adequate Fe stores, as evidenced by serum ferritin that is not low. In the setting of inflammation, it may be difficult to differentiate ACD from IDA, and the two conditions may coexist.

POINTS TO REMEMBER

Anemia of Chronic Disease

- ACD is typically normocytic and normochromic.
- The pathogenesis of ACD includes shortened erythrocyte survival, impaired marrow function, and disturbances of Fe metabolism.
- ACD is an acquired Fe distribution disorder with relatively low circulating Fe levels, despite the presence of adequate total body Fe stores.
- In ACD, the release of Fe from cells to the circulation is inadequate to support heme formation.
- In ACD, Fe is sequestered in reticuloendothelial macrophages.
- Patients with ACD have anemia, low Fe, low transferrrin, low TSAT, normal or moderately elevated ferritin, elevated hepcidin, and mostly normal sTfR concentrations.

Iron Overload

Iron overload disorders are typically insidious, causing progressive and sometimes irreversible tissue damage before clinical symptoms develop (see also Chapter 42 section on Iron Overload). However, with a high awareness, the consequences of Fe toxicity can be attenuated or prevented. Fe overload disorders can be categorized according to whether the underlying pathophysiological defect is in the hepcidin-ferroportin axis, erythroid maturation, or in Fe transport.[118] There are also some less common disorders that do not fit into one of these categories (see Table 38.6). Fe overload may also develop as a consequence of multiple RBC transfusions and parenteral Fe supplementation.

Disorders of the Hepcidin-Ferroportin Axis. Each of the six disorders in this group has a primary form of Fe overload and is a subtype of HH (primary) (see Table 38.6). HH was first described at the end of the nineteenth century by von Recklinghausen, but also by Trousseau and Troisier. It was von Recklinghausen who originally introduced the term hemochromatosis. In 1935, Sheldon wrote his classic review in which hemochromatosis was regarded as a rare disease that results from excess total body Fe and organ failure attributable to Fe toxicity.[174] By the 1980s, a higher prevalence was suggested, probably because of the widespread availability of serum Fe, Fe-binding capacity, and ferritin assays by that time. In the 1970s, hemochromatosis was recognized as an autosomal recessive disorder linked to the short arm of chromosome 6, which contains the gene that encodes HLA-A.[205] However, in 1996, Feder and colleagues[206] identified the hemochromatosis *(HFE)* gene (previously called the HLA-H gene). These authors attributed the most common form of HH to homozygosity for the p.Cys282Tyr (C282Y) sequence variation of this gene.

Five of the six different HH disorders may lead to a classical HH phenotype: normal Hb, elevated ferritin and TSAT, and tissue Fe overload (see Table 38.6). The pathophysiology of these five conditions is similar, with an increased Fe absorption exceeding the needs of the body, which leads to increased Fe stores due to inadequate hepcidin-mediated down-regulation of ferroportin. This leads to Fe deposition in parenchymal organs (eg, the liver and the pancreas).

Initial clinical symptoms of tissue Fe overload of these disorders are often nonspecific and vague—fatigue and joint pain. In later stages, disease manifestations may include diabetes mellitus, hypogonadism and other endocrinopathies, liver cirrhosis, cardiomyopathy, skin pigmentation, and in cirrhotic patients, increased susceptibility of liver cancer.[207-209] Early diagnosis and therapeutic phlebotomy can prevent the development of tissue damage, reduce morbidity and mortality, and provide long-term survival similar to the general population.[207,209,210]

Phlebotomy remains the mainstay of treatment for HH. One unit of blood of 500 mL contains approximately 200 to 250 mg Fe, depending on the Hb concentration, and should be removed once per week as tolerated. Each phlebotomy should be preceded by measurement of the Hct or Hb to avoid anemia. TSAT usually remains elevated until Fe stores are depleted, whereas ferritin, which may initially fluctuate, eventually begins to fall progressively with Fe mobilization, and is reflective of depletion of Fe stores. Therefore, serum ferritin is recommended to monitor treatment, and its analysis should be performed after every 10 to 12 phlebotomies (≈3 months) in the initial stages of treatment. It can be confidently assumed that excess Fe stores have been mobilized when the serum ferritin drops to between 50 and 100 μg/L. As the target range of 50 to 100 μg/L is approached, testing may be repeated more frequently to preempt the development of overt Fe deficiency. Development of Fe deficiency should be avoided. Once Fe depletion has been achieved, the aim is to prevent re-accumulation. The advocated standard practice is to maintain the serum ferritin at 50 to 100 μg/L.[207,209]

Of the white population, approximately 1 in 200 are *HFE* C282Y homozygotes, and approximately 1 in 10 carries the mutation. Another common mutation in *HFE* includes His63Asp (H63D). In patients with Fe overload and of European ancestry, nearly 80% have been found to be homozygous for the C282Y mutation in *HFE*. A smaller proportion (5%) are compound heterozygous for the C282Y/H63D mutation.[206] Although 38% to 76% of C282Y homozygous people have been found to develop raised serum Fe parameters,[211] such as ferritin and TSAT, disease penetrance is 2% to 38% in men and less (1%–10%) in women, presumably because menstrual blood loss and childbearing protects them from Fe overload.[212,213] Also, both disease severity and clinical expression correlate well with the degree of Fe overload, but are heterogenous among patients, depending not only on the age of diagnosis but also on other genetic and dietary modifiers that remain still largely unknown. Among C282Y/H63D compound heterozygotes, the risk of disease progression is low, and documented Fe overload disease is rare.[214,215] Furthermore, C282Y/H63D compound heterozygous hemochromatosis patients with clinical disease expression frequently have additional risk factors for Fe overload or liver disease.[216] Thus, although C282Y/H63D compound heterozygosity is a risk factor for slightly higher serum Fe parameters and mildly increased hepatic Fe stores, guidelines from the European Molecular Genetics Quality Network consider the genotype itself to be insufficient to cause hemochromatosis.[216] Likewise, homozygosity for H63D is also rarely associated with hemochromatosis and is also not considered a disease-associated genotype.[216] Most patients with HFE-associated HH do not present until middle age (and women not until after menopause).

Since the discovery of the hemochromatosis *(HFE)* gene, our understanding of Fe regulation, transport, and storage molecules has remarkably increased with the description of hepcidin, HJV, TfR2, and ferroportin proteins, in which alterations can lead to various types of HH.[217,218]

Mutations in *TfR2* cause a more severe form of HH, with a presentation in young adults (HH type 3). Juvenile forms of HH are due to mutations in genes encoding HJV (HH type 2a), or in rare cases, hepcidin (HH type 2b). Juvenile forms of HH are generally characterized by its early onset and a particularly severe phenotype, with patients typically presenting before the age of 30 years with severe systemic Fe overload, heart failure, and hypopituitarism as common clinical manifestations.[219]

Another form of classical HH is caused by mutations in *SLC40A1* (ferroportin) that interfere with the regulation by hepcidin.[220,221] Because this causes excessive ferroportin-mediated intestinal Fe uptake, these mutations are described as gain-of-function mutations. The phenotype of this so-called HH type 4B or atypical HH in affected patients is similar to that in patients with HFE-hemochromatosis.[222,223] In contrast, Fe overload in subjects with loss-of-function ferroportin mutations (a condition referred to as "ferroportin disease"[220]) is restricted to the reticuloendothelial system, which leads to the combination of high ferritin concentrations, a normal TSAT percent, and (rarely) Fe-restricted erythropoiesis with mild anemia or impaired tolerance of phlebotomy.[224] Patients rarely develop Fe-related disease symptoms. A polymorphism (Q248H) in the ferroportin gene is associated with African Fe overload (also designated Bantu siderosis), a condition that may be attributed to the combination of excess Fe intake from their traditional beer and minor changes in ferroportin function.[225,226]

Diagnosis of ferroportin disease is complex because it requires that all various conditions causing increased hyperferritinemia (combined with a normal TSAT percentage) are ruled out. Ferroportin disease should always be suspected in familial forms of hyperferritinemia or in sporadic cases of high ferritin in the absence of known secondary causes, such as infection, metabolic syndrome, inflammation, renal insufficiency, and malignancy.[138,227] Differential diagnoses should also include other disorders with elevated ferritin and a normal TSAT percentage—which is familial hyperferritinemia—a congenital cataract syndrome (HHCS) that is a rare disease without Fe overload but with high ferritin concentrations,[228,229] aceruloplasminemia, which manifests predominantly with neurologic symptoms,[230,231] and the increasingly prevalent metabolic syndrome present in obese, hypertensive, insulin-resistant, or dyslipidemic individuals.[232,233] Patients with the metabolic syndrome also often have body Fe overload, but in contrast to the Fe overload in HH, the Fe load is only mild to moderate and mostly in the macrophages, where tissue toxicity is likely to be lower.

POINTS TO REMEMBER

HFE-Related Hereditary Hemochromatosis

- HFE-HH is an autosomal recessive inherited Fe overload disorder.
- HFE-HH is associated with low hepcidin levels that lead to increased intestinal Fe absorption.
- Only a small portion of C282Y homozygous subjects develop clinical disease.
- Approximately 80% of Caucasians with documented Fe overload are C282Y homozygous.
- HFE-HH has a genetic prevalence of 1 in 200 Caucasians.
- Increased TSAT and ferritin are found in approximately one-half of C282Y homozygotes.
- Fe overload in patients with HFE-HH is characterized by an elevation of both the TSAT percentage and ferritin levels.
- Patients with compound heterozygosity for C282Y/H63D have a low risk of developing documented Fe overload; clinical disease progression can often be attributed to other risk factors.
- Fe overload in patients with HFE-related HH can be treated by phlebotomies.
- Phlebotomy is monitored by ferritin (aimed at levels between 50 and 100 μg/L) and Hb (preventing anemia).
- Striving for low-normal TSAT levels in these patients carries the risk of the development of IDA.

Disorders of Erythroid Maturation. This class of disorders represents forms of secondary Fe overload, and includes the Fe-loading anemias, among which are thalassemia syndromes (especially the β-thalassemias), sideroblastic anemias, and the congenital dyserythropoietic anemias.[234,235] These diseases are characterized by ineffective erythropoiesis (ie, by apoptosis of erythroid precursors), failure of erythroid maturation, and consequent expansion of the number of erythroid precursor cells in the bone marrow. Bone marrow–derived signaling molecules, such as GDF15, TWSG1 ERFE, are then believed to downregulate hepcidin.[236,237] This physiological mechanism by which the erythroid marrow expansion combined with ineffective erythropoiesis induces a positive Fe balance, which was originally introduced by Finch in 1994 as the "erythroid regulator" of Fe balance.[122] As a result, hepcidin in these diseases is inappropriately low for the body Fe stores, and as a consequence, (parenchymal) systemic Fe overload with an elevated TSAT percentage and serum ferritin levels develops. RBC transfusions further worsen the Fe burden in these disorders.

In patients with β-TM and β-TI, Fe overload is a major contributor to the morbidity in patients with severe forms, even when they do not receive regular transfusions.[238] Paradoxically, in these patients (low hepcidin–mediated) excess gastrointestinal Fe absorption persists despite massive increases in total body Fe load. Fe overload is more common in β-TI than in Hb H disease (the most severe nonfatal form of α-thalassemia), because in β-TI the erythropoietic signal more strongly suppresses Fe-loading–induced signaling to hepcidin.[239] To date, Fe overload in thalassemia is treated with Fe chelation.[240]

The sideroblastic anemias are heterogeneous disorders of heme and Fe-sulfur cluster synthesis, with inherited (primary), secondary (myelodysplastic syndrome with ringed sideroblasts), and syndromic and nonsyndromic forms.[186,241-243] The best-characterized inherited forms are caused by genes encoding for proteins involved in the heme or Fe-sulfur cluster synthesis in the mitochondria. Fe that would otherwise be incorporated in these end products accumulates in the mitochondria that produce the characteristic ring sideroblasts, which is a ring around the nucleus of the erythroid precursor cells in the bone marrow.

The congenital dyserythropoietic anemias are a group of rare hereditary disorders characterized by congenital anemia, ineffective erythropoiesis with distinct morphological features in the bone marrow late erythroblasts, and the development of secondary hemochromatosis.[244] Patients usually present with macrocytic or normocytic anemia, jaundice, splenomegaly, and low reticulocyte for the degree of anemia. Management may require repeated transfusions. Fe overload is treated with chelation.

Disorders of Iron Transport. The pathophysiologic feature that is shared by these disorders is insufficient delivery of transferrin-bound Fe to the bone marrow for heme synthesis despite Fe stores. The resulting Fe-restrictive erythropoiesis, anemia, and hypoxia all contribute to low hepcidin-induced Fe overload.

Hypotransferrinemia is a rare autosomal recessive disease in which transferrin levels are severely reduced and insufficient to bind all the Fe that enters the plasma.[245] The consequent levels of NTBI cannot be used for heme synthesis and cannot increase hepcidin synthesis. The ensuing anemia and low transferrin levels contribute to hepcidin levels that are low for the Fe overload (low hepcidin/ferritin ratio), leading to severe Fe overload.

Because ceruloplasmin catalyzes cellular efflux of Fe by oxidizing Fe^{2+} to Fe^{3+} for binding to transferrin, patients with aceruloplasminemia, among others, present with low transferrin saturation, with consequent Fe restrictive erythropoiesis and anemia in combination with Fe overload in parenchymal cells and macrophages, including the nervous system.[186,231]

Patients with defects in SLC11A2 (DMT1) mostly present in childhood with microcytic anemia and an elevated TSAT percentage. Serum ferritin levels vary from low to moderately increased, with some association with erythrocyte transfusions or intravenous Fe supplementation. Only seven patients have been described thus far.[186,241]

Other Forms of Iron Overload. Neonatal hemochromatosis is a severe form of an acquired and secondary severe Fe overload associated with newborn liver failure.[246] In most cases, it is allo-immune–mediated, that is, it is caused by transplacental maternal immunoglobulin-G directed against an as-yet-unidentified fetal liver antigen.[247]

Mutations in the frataxin gene are responsible for Friedreich ataxia, the most common form of inherited ataxias. Frataxin appears to be required for normal mitochondrial Fe export.[153,248] The Fe-mediated mitochondrial injury results in neurologic and cardiac manifestations. Several other heritable Fe disorders fall under the descriptive term "neurodegeneration with brain Fe accumulation." In most forms Fe accumulates in the basal ganglia, causing progressive extrapyramidal movement disorders.[249,250] In all these conditions, systemic Fe status remains unaffected.

Acquisition of Fe from nondietary sources in amounts that exceed the body's limited excretory capacity can cause acquired and secondary forms of Fe overload. Long-term erythrocyte transfusion is the most common cause.[240] In some patients with ineffective erythropoiesis and (probably) increased GDF15, TWSG1, and/or ERFE expression, transfusion exacerbates Fe overload due to increased absorption. This is especially prevalent in patients with β-TM. Among such patients, cardiac siderosis is the most common cause of death.[238] Transfusion Fe overload develops in many persons with sickle cell disease and causes clinical disease in some, but the pattern of hemosiderosis seems different to that described in thalassemia; in particular, most Fe loading occurs in the liver, with little cardiac Fe deposition.[251] Fe overload also occurs in persons with renal insufficiency as a result of the administration of excessive intravenous or intramuscular Fe supplements.[252] Long-term transfusion is usually the sole cause of Fe overload in persons treated for severe aplastic anemia, Blackfan-Diamond syndrome, Fanconi anemia, acute leukemia, autoimmune hemolytic anemias, and myelodysplasia without ringed sideroblasts.

Analytical Methods

Several methods are used to measure Fe and related analytes. These include methods for serum Fe, total Fe-binding capacity, transferrin, transferrin saturation, and serum ferritin, hepcidin, serum transferrin receptor, ZnPP, and RBC analytical parameters.

Methods for Serum Iron, Total Iron-Binding Capacity, Transferrin, and Transferrin Saturation

Principles. With serum Fe assays, Fe is (1) released from transferrin by decreasing the pH of the serum, (2) reduced from Fe^{3+} to Fe^{2+}, and (3) complexed with a chromogen such as bathophenanthroline or ferrozine. Such Fe-chromogen complexes have an extremely high absorbance in the visible region that is proportional to Fe concentration. The assay may be performed manually or in an automated fashion by any of several commercially available methods.

Transferrin can be measured directly using immunological techniques. Alternatively, transferrin can be quantified in terms of the amount of Fe it will bind, a measure called the total Fe-binding capacity (TIBC).[253] The TIBC can also be calculated after the measurement of unsaturated Fe binding capacity (UIBC), by adding UIBC to Fe concentration.

For TIBC, a practical and chemical way of its determination in serum or plasma was reported in 1957.[254] In 1978, this assay was refined by the International Committee for Standardization in Haematology, and described as a recommended procedure[255] that was (again) revised in 1990.[256] The measurement of TIBC consists of three steps. The first step involves addition of supraphysiological amounts of Fe(III)-chloride to saturate the free binding sites on transferrin; in the second step, unbound excess Fe is removed by adsorption onto solid magnesium carbonate, charcoal, or by an ion-exchange resin; and the third step is a colorimetric (or in the past radio-isotopic) determination of Fe that is dissociated from transferrin at acidic pH. More direct TIBC assays were developed in the 1990s.[257,258] Automated chemistry analyzers can also measure UIBC and calculate TIBC, rather than measure it directly.[259]

The first immunodiffusion method for transferrin was described in 1965.[260] This methodology was largely replaced by automated immunoturbidimetric or immunonephelometric procedures that were developed in the 1970s.[260-262]

The combination of total serum Fe and either TIBC or transferrin measurement allows the calculation of the saturation of transferrin with Fe (ratio of Fe concentration and TIBC multiplied by 100). Transferrin concentration can be used to derive TIBC, and indirectly, TSAT. Because 1 mol of transferrin (average molecular mass 79,570 Da[142] has the capacity to bind two atoms of Fe (atomic mass 55.84 Da), the theoretically derived formulas for calculating transferrin (and TSAT) from TIBC and vice versa are as follows[263]:

$$\text{Transferrin (g/L)} = 0.007 \times \text{TIBC } (\mu\text{g/L})$$

$$\text{TIBC } (\mu\text{g/dL}) = \text{transferrin (mg/dL)} \times 1.41 \text{ TIBC } (\mu\text{mol/L}) = \text{transferrin (g/L)} \times 25.2$$

$$\text{TSAT (\%)} = [(\text{Serum Fe } (\mu\text{g/dL})]/[\text{transferrin (mg/dL)}] \times 70.9 = [(\text{Serum Fe } (\mu\text{mol/L})]/[\text{transferrin (mg/dL)}] \times 398$$

These mathematical derivations have weaknesses that are described in the following (see Comments and Precautions).

Reference Intervals. The normal mean serum Fe value for men is approximately 120 μg/dL (21.8 μmol/L). The composite reference interval is approximately 70 to 200 μg/dL (13–36 μmol/L); however, values vary substantially from one laboratory to another.[121]

The TIBC averages 340 μg/L (61 μmol/L) in both men and women, with a composite reference interval of 250 to 435 μg/dL (45–78 μmol/L).

In contrast to TIBC, the release of new protein reference materials in 1994 (CRM 470 or ERM-DA470) enabled the definition of "interim" reference intervals for transferrin in 1996 as 2.0 to 3.6 g/L.[264,265] Because the establishment of new reference intervals would take considerable time, this reference interval was based on consensus informed by studies that had already been undertaken.[264,265] This has been accepted by the International Federation of Clinical Chemistry and Laboratory Medicine and many national scientific societies. Reference intervals have also been determined in a Japanese population using the same standardization.[266] The results obtained were more or less similar (1.90–3.20 g/L), suggesting that racial differences are not very pronounced.

The reference interval used for TSAT varies between laboratories. The approximate and mostly used reference interval is 15% to 45%.

Clinical Relevance. The serum Fe concentration refers to the Fe^{3+} bound to serum transferrin and does not include the Fe contained in serum as free Hb, ferritin, or bound to albumin, or low-molecular-weight molecules as citrate or oxalate. In clinical situations, serum Fe measurements are often combined with TIBC or transferrin, to calculate the TSAT that is considered more useful for clinical interpretation.[267]

Total Iron-Binding Capacity or Transferrin. Because only approximately one-third of the Fe-binding sites of transferrin are occupied by Fe^{3+} in normal subjects, serum transferrin has considerable reserve Fe-binding capacity. The serum TIBC or transferrin varies in disorders of Fe metabolism. In persons with Fe overload, such as patients with Fe-loading anemias and HH, the TIBC or transferrin is decreased. Transferrin is also decreased in conditions with impaired synthesis, such as chronic liver diseases and malnutrition, and in conditions with increased losses (eg, nephrotic syndrome). Transferrin is increased in persons with Fe deficiency, and because it is a negative acute phase protein, it is decreased in those with chronic inflammatory disorders or malignancies. Some therefore consider transferrin to be the best test to distinguish between IDA and ACD,[268] but in hospitalized patients, it is not very sensitive to detect Fe deficiency.[121,269]

Serum Iron and Transferrin Saturation. Serum Fe and TSAT are low in absolute and functional Fe deficiency and increased in Fe overload diseases, recent ingestion and absorption of Fe medication, acute hepatitis, or chronic liver failure. Erythropoietic response to specific therapies for anemias of other causes (eg, treatment of pernicious anemia with cyanocobalamin) decreases serum Fe concentration through increased efficiency of Fe incorporated into developing erythroblasts. The clinical situations in which TSAT are used are summarized in the following.

To detect Fe deficiency, the TSAT thresholds proposed by the various guidelines vary among 15%, 16%, and 20% for the general population.[121,182,200]

In patients with functional Fe deficiency and ACD, which are often observed in patients with autoimmune diseases, chronic kidney diseases, inflammatory bowel disease, and chronic heart failure, the reticuloendothelial system has abundant Fe, and serum ferritin is normal to high, but the release of this Fe to the circulation is inadequate to support heme formation. As a result, serum Fe decreases, and because serum Fe decreases more than transferrin, TSAT is also low. Similar to TSATs, the absolute amount of circulating Fe available for the tissues is lower in conditions when the transferrin levels are lower, as is the case for many patients with chronic (low grade) inflammatory disorders.

The detection of functional Fe deficiency is often used as guidance for treatment with erythropoiesis-stimulating agents. The treatment is costly, and it is effective only if Fe delivery to the developing erythrocytes is adequate. To detect this Fe deficiency in patients with these chronic diseases, the proposed cutoffs of TSAT are generally similar to those of patients with Fe deficiency (see Table 38.7),[172,182,200,270] although some guidelines use thresholds of 25% to 30% for patients with chronic kidney diseases.[182,270] In these guidelines, the proposed cutoff values for TSAT are often combined with proposed threshold values for ferritin.

Overall, the degree of reduction tends to be greater in patients with Fe deficiency than in those with ACD and functional Fe deficiency, but considerable overlap consists between these conditions. A value less than 5% is almost certain for IDA or IRIDA (see Table 38.7).

TSAT is useful for detecting impending Fe overload in patients with HH.[271] Although most patients with C282Y homozygosity have elevated serum Fe parameters,[211] especially TSAT, only a small proportion of them develop clinical disease.[212,213] Because the diurnal variation of TSAT is high, some studies and guidelines on HH recommend sampling for TSAT after an overnight fast[209,272] or recommend repeated testing on a fasting specimen if the initial screen is abnormal.[207,209,271] However, others have found that the TSAT of HFE-hemochromatosis patients at risk for organ Fe overload is elevated throughout the day, or that the use of fasting samples shows no improvement in the sensitivity and specificity in the detection of C282Y homozygotes, precluding the need for fasting sampling.[273-275] Thus, sampling after an overnight fast does not necessarily improve the reliability of the TSAT test for the diagnosis of HH. Over the years, different studies have used a variety of cutoff levels for TSAT to identify patients who are eligible for further testing. Some guidelines use a TSAT of more than 45% for women and more than 50% for men,[209] and others use 45% as the threshold for both sexes.[207]

In the monitoring of the Fe status of HH patients who are treated by phlebotomies, assessment of the TSAT is not useful because values fluctuate widely even when stores have been returned to normal, reflecting daily Fe absorption more than overall Fe balance. Striving for low TSAT levels in these patients carries the risk of developing IDA.

In conditions of hyperferritinemia, TSAT enables distinguishing predominant parenchymal Fe overload (elevated TSAT) from reticuloendothelial system overload (normal TSAT). In the presence of an elevated TSAT, patients tend to have a lower ferritin level for a given Fe burden than patients with normal and low TSAT.[151] For example, a ferritin level of 500 µg/L would therefore represent a more significant risk threshold for patients with a high TSAT than for patients with a TSAT within the reference interval.

TSAT percentage can also be used to test for acute Fe toxicity in (rare) situations of accidental or intended ingestion of Fe-containing pharmaceuticals.[276] For Fe toxicity, refer to Chapter 42.

In patients in whom transferrin becomes highly saturated, additional Fe is released into the circulation. This plasma NTBI and its labile (redox active) component (labile plasma Fe or LPI) are potentially toxic forms of Fe that contribute to oxidant-mediated cellular injury.[149,151,153]

At a population level, a higher TSAT (>50%) was reported to be associated with a higher mortality.[277] This relationship may be due to clinically unexpressed hemochromatosis, but high Fe availability from other causes may also be harmful.[278] However, in patients with nondialysis-dependent chronic kidney disease, a higher TSAT ratio is associated with lower mortality.[171]

Comments and Precautions

Preanalytical Aspects. Acute or recent hemorrhage, including that caused by blood donation, results in low serum Fe concentration. Except when atomic absorption spectroscopy is used, hemolysis has little effect on serum Fe assay results because native Hb binds Fe so tightly that, even with the acidic conditions of most dye-binding methods, little Hb-bound Fe is released under the serum Fe assay conditions. Consequently, Fe from in vitro hemolysis is simply not measured.[279] Partially denatured Hb seems to be more prone to increase the Fe measured by the dye-binding methods.[280]

Because intravenous Fe preparations and Fe chelators bind Fe much more loosely than do Fe-binding dyes, the chromogen-binding Fe assays usually also measure the Fe in the circulating Fe preparations and chelates, leading to falsely elevated Fe concentrations and TSAT percentages.[281-283]

Analytical Aspects. Studies from Eckfeldt and Witte[267] and Tietz and coworkers[279,284,285] in the 1990s questioned the reliability of the routine methods measuring low Fe concentrations at that time. They found that a low pH is crucial for reliable results to be obtained, and suggested that the reference method used was affected by high ferritin levels. From these studies, it also appeared that many commercially available methods underestimated the true value of serum Fe concentration by 25% or more, and some methods were considered unreliable at quantifying concentrations of serum Fe at less than 30 µg/dL (5 µmol/L). Methods that included deproteinization, by precipitation or by dialysis, consistently appeared to provide results that were substantially higher than those results obtained by methods that did not include a step of deproteinization. More recently, however, the use of mostly colorimetric assays on instruments from a restricted number of manufacturers, along with proficiency testing using commutable samples, has resulted in small between laboratory and methodology variations.[286]

Pros and Cons of Chemically Measured Total Iron-Binding Capacity Versus Immunochemically Measured Transferrin

1. Serum from patients with Fe overload may contain Fe bound loosely to other molecules than transferrin, such as citrate and albumin (and sometimes Fe chelators). This may result in (i) TIBC methods generally overestimating the Fe-binding capacity of transferrin, and (ii) TSAT calculated from immunochemically measured transferrin measurements to be more than 100%.
2. UIBC-based methods generally exhibit a significant negative bias compared with TIBC methods.[287]
3. The chemical methods for TIBC require a relatively large sample volume.
4. The TIBC assays are (i) sensitive to contamination of laboratory consumables with Fe,[288] and (ii) show a large variation; reference intervals differ by as much as 35% among commercial methods.
5. In contrast to TIBC, internationally accepted interim reference intervals are available for serum transferrin.
6. The introduction of the international CRM 470 in 1994 (later renamed ERM-DA470) protein reference material has led to a significant reduction in interlaboratory variation for transferrin measurements.[289,290] This new calibrator yielded transferrin concentrations that were 13% lower than those obtained with the older calibrator.[259] In 2008, a new serum protein reference material was produced and released (ERM-DA470k/IFCC) to reliably replace ERM DA470 for calibration purposes for 12 proteins, including transferrin[291] (see Box 38.2). The use of these transferrin-containing, protein-based calibrators for the primary calibration of the automated UIBC and TIBC methodologies allows for value assignment of UIBC and TIBC that are in better agreement with values obtained by immunologically measured transferrin assays.[287] Coefficients of variation for transferrin are low and lower than those for TIBC measurements.[292]

In view of these observations, especially the better reproducibility and better possibility for standardization, determination of transferrin concentration, rather than TIBC, is recommended.[263] However, in non-European populations characterized by a marked genetic variation in transferrin (transferrin BC and transferrin CD variants),[293,294] in certain cases, immunochemical determination of transferrin may lead to errors. In these populations, TIBC measurements may be preferred.

The Relation Between Chemically Measured Total Iron-Binding Capacity Versus Immunochemically Measured Transferrin. Although the correlation between TIBC and immunologically determined transferrin is generally considered good, conversion factors between the two analytes found in an Australian study from 1992 showed large differences.[292] The preceding mathematical derivations also have shortcomings.

The addition of excess amounts of Fe(III)-chloride in the TIBC assay results in nonspecific binding of Fe to albumin and other plasma proteins. This leads to overestimation of TIBC, especially in patients with hyperferritineima and with low transferrin concentrations (as for instance observed in liver diseases and in the nephrotic syndrome[295]), and to a nonlinear relationship between serum transferrin concentration and TIBC. Thus, contrary to the theory, the relationship between TIBC and transferrin is not fixed, especially when results are outside the reference interval.[261,287] This complicates the development of a universal formula for the conversion of transferrin values into TIBC.[296]

Developing such a formula is complicated because the molecular mass of transferrin varies due to glycation; for example, alcoholics often have higher amounts of desialylated forms of transferrin of lower molecular weight.[297,298] Because of the uncertainty as to the molecular mass of transferrin, the biases of the early TIBC and transferrin methodologies, and the variation in the TIBC-transferrin relation in some diseases, different TIBC to transferrin conversion factors are applied by different laboratories.[287,292] Therefore, a number of manufacturers recommend that the experimentally determined factor of 1.27 be applied instead of the theoretically derived 1.41.[296] This can be regarded as a mathematical compensation for the non-transferrin–bound Fe (which is included in the measurement in the TIBC assay but not in the transferrin immunoassay).

Biological Variation. Plasma Fe and TSAT display a large biological variation in healthy subjects.

The intraindividual day-to-day variation of Fe and TSAT is approximately 25% to 30%.[299-303] In contrast, TIBC (or transferrin values) show only a slight day-to-day variation or diurnal variation, with a variation for TIBC between 4.8% and 8.8%[299,302,303] and for transferrin, a variation of 3% (https://www.westgard.com/biodatabase-2014-update.htm). Also, variations in results obtained at the same time of the day on sequential days or weeks remain substantially greater than analytical variations, even when samples are taken after an overnight fast.[304]

Serum Fe concentrations and TSAT have significant diurnal variation, with highest values in the morning and lowest values in the evening[303,305,306] that are inversely related to serum hepcidin-25 concentration.[307-310] In contrast, some studies have shown Fe levels that are highest in the afternoon or evening.[302,311] These findings show that the time of blood sampling has an impact on the results for Fe and TSAT. The exact rhythm has not yet been established, probably due to between-subject variations in the timing of the circadian phase.[306] The influence of food intake on plasma Fe (and TSAT) is also controversial, and recommendations for blood sampling conditions for Fe parameters differ to a great extent. Although many laboratories recommend fasting plasma samples for Fe and TSAT, studies often lack adequate information on food intake,[312] and studies with direct comparisons between fasting and nonfasting conditions are lacking. Recommendations on blood sampling for Fe and TSAT measurements are contradictory. It has been argued that the practice of restricting blood collection for Fe and TSAT to a specific time of the day does not necessarily improve the reliability of the test.

Methods for Serum Ferritin

Principles. The presence of small amounts of ferritin in human serum was already appreciated several years after the discovery of ferritin in 1937.[137,313] However, the quantification of ferritin awaited the purification of ferritin and the development of sensitive immunoassay techniques. In 1972, using an immunoradiometric assay, Addison and colleagues demonstrated that ferritin could be reliably detected in human serum.[314] The early assays have since been supplanted by enzyme-linked immunoassays (ELISAs) that use colorimetric and fluorescent substrates or by antibodies with chemiluminescent labels. These assays are sandwich immunoassays in which one antibody is the "capture" antibody, and another antibody is the "detecting" antibody. The antibodies can be polyclonal and/or monoclonal, and they determine the epitope specificity of the assay. Numerous variations have been described, and to date, serum ferritin is included in the latest batch and random access automated analyzers for immunoassays from several manufacturers.

Reference Intervals. The published reference intervals and diagnostic cutoffs, recommended by the various manufacturers of ferritin immunoassays, and those used in the laboratories vary distinctly. This diversity is due to a broad range of thresholds and approaches to their definition. This can be attributed to:

1. Laboratories define reference intervals differently (eg, 2.5%–97.5% or 5%–95% or mean ± 1 or 2 SDs). Reference intervals are derived in samples from the community or from referral laboratories (with different populations), and values outside this interval are regarded as a pathologic Fe deficiency or overload rather than using cutoffs defined by their ability to detect pathologic states in properly designed diagnostic accuracy studies. For instance, some manufacturers and laboratories define a normal range as the ferritin concentration found in unselected, apparently normal subjects. However, a proportion of the normal population, particularly young women, have almost no storage Fe without being anemic. The normal range in young women will thus include ferritin concentrations found in Fe deficiency. In addition, with the emerging epidemic of obesity, this normal range will also include a proportion of the population that have elevated ferritin concentrations related to high body mass index. Thus, similarly to lipid concentrations, a reference interval for ferritin, based only on the adult population, may not be suitable, and it should be replaced by a lower and upper diagnostic cutoff value based on risk estimates. Using population-based reference intervals, this risk may be hidden in the outer portion(s) of the conventional reference interval.
2. Values that are compounded by variation and evolution in assay techniques and platforms and the limited use of WHO reference materials.[315] Ferritin standardization poses challenges because different laboratories assess different ferritin isoforms and use different antibodies and

standards in immunoassays, complicating and potentially misleading the interpretation and comparability of the results.[316]

3. Race/ethnicity factors (especially in Native Africans, African Americans, and Asians) are also associated with higher mean concentrations of serum ferritin than are typical of Caucasians, but the basis of this phenomenon is incompletely understood.[317]

Clinically, the heterogeneity in recommended and used ferritin reference intervals and diagnostic thresholds causes confusion for clinicians and patients, whereas for public health, these differences impair comparison and systematic reviewing of survey data, slow development of global estimates of the prevalence of Fe deficiency, and obscure estimates of the effectiveness and safety of nutrition interventions.[318]

Overall, reference intervals vary and depend on age and gender. Serum ferritin concentrations are normally within the range of 12 to 300 μg/L and are lower in children (especially after the age of 6 months) than adults. Mean values are lower in women before menopause than in men, reflecting women's lower Fe stores caused by the losses during menstruation and childbirth. The changes in serum ferritin concentration during development from birth to old age reflect changes in the amounts of Fe stored in tissues.

Most publications agree that ferritin concentrations of less than 12 to 30 μg/L identify absolute Fe deficiency. In populations exposed to infections and in patients with renal failure, inflammatory bowel diseases, chronic heart failure, or other (low grade) inflammatory diseases, threshold values indicating Fe deficiency are generally considered to be higher than in those without these diseases (see the following). In these situations, concentrations more than 100 μg/L generally exclude absolute Fe deficiency, and for concentrations between 30 and 100 μg/L, other parameters are needed to diagnose Fe deficiency. Values more than 200 and 300 μg/L are often applied, for women and men, respectively, to define Fe overload.

Clinical Relevance. The serum ferritin concentration roughly reflects the body Fe content in many subjects. It provides a more general assessment of Fe stores than does bone marrow aspiration, which involves the examination of reticuloendothelial cells in the marrow for Fe.[137,319] The serum ferritin concentration declines early in the development of Fe deficiency, long before changes are observed in blood Hb concentration, erythrocyte size, or serum Fe concentration. Accordingly, a low serum ferritin concentration is a sensitive indicator of Fe deficiency uncomplicated by other concurrent disease. Plasma ferritin concentration is increased in patients with body Fe overload of any cause and is used to gauge the effectiveness of phlebotomy therapy and Fe chelation therapy. Ferritin is also a positive acute-phase reactant in various inflammatory conditions.[320-322] As a result, hyperferritinemia is not synonymous with Fe overload, and many disorders result in increased serum ferritin concentration[137,313,323-325] that do not always correlate with elevation in body Fe content.

Plasma ferritin threshold values to diagnose Fe deficiency and Fe overload differ between guidelines of various authorities. Presently, the WHO defines Fe deficiency as serum or plasma ferritin of less than 15 μg/L in adults and less than 12 μg/L in children aged younger than 5 years, or less than 30 μg/L when inflammation is concurrent. In children aged older than 5 years, Fe deficiency is regarded as present when ferritin concentrations are less than 15 μg/L.[160,326] The WHO also concluded that Fe overload could be best defined as a ferritin concentration of more than 300 μg/L in male patients and more than 200 μg/L in female patients.[160] Although widely implemented and cited, these cutoffs are based on expert opinion and not on a systematic appraisal of published work. As such, these thresholds have not been universally adopted.

Ferritin data from 55 studies, published between 1972 and 1988, on the diagnostic accuracy of serum ferritin, measured by radio-immunoassay for the detection of IDA across an exhaustive population of anemic patients with and without inflammatory, liver, or neoplastic diseases, was systematically reviewed by Gyuatt and colleagues.[322] The study concluded that IDA could be ruled in at a ferritin decision cutoff of 15 μg/L, whereas it could be ruled out by adopting thresholds of 40 μg/L for the general population and 70 μg/L for patients with inflammatory and/or liver disease, respectively.[322,327]

Currently recommended cutoffs for the diagnosis of Fe deficiency are based on this systematic review and the previously mentioned older studies that have various forms of heterogeneity and bias. For example, the absence of international ferritin standards[328] and the consequent heterogeneity of the analytical performance of ferritin methods invalidate the calculation of summary estimates of diagnostic accuracy and the cutoff values derived from summary receiver-operating curves, and carry the risk of misclassifying patients. Nevertheless, all reviews from the 2000s and 2010s on the topic[329-332] and the 2011 guideline of the British Society of Gastroenterology[333] use the recommendations by Guyatt and colleagues on ferritin values to rule out Fe deficiency anemia in the general population without any critical assessment of the original studies or any further update. Using the second or third international ferritin standards from the 1990s, there have hardly been any studies that have also evaluated the diagnostic accuracy of ferritin in comparison with the gold standard.[327] The substantial amount of clinical evidence accumulated up to the 1990s, together with a report of the technical limitations of bone marrow aspirate evaluation,[334] supported the practical introduction of ferritin as a key biomarker for Fe deficiency detection without any further validation or criticism. However, by 2012, Ferraro and colleagues[327] recognized that using assays traceable to the second (or third) international standards for ferritin measurement made it impossible to find robust information for the revalidation of the diagnostic accuracy data (including recommended cutoffs).

Overall, guidelines since the 1990s have varied in proposed thresholds for the general population, women, and children. Most guidelines propose thresholds between 12 and 30 μg/L to identify Fe deficiency, but there are also some guidelines that use 45 to 50 μg/L or even 100 μg/L as a threshold to identify probable or possible Fe deficiency in the general population. Moreover, especially for the diagnosis of Fe deficiency, the preceding WHO definition is inadequate in many conditions in which increases in ferritin tend to overestimate Fe stores.[321] In these conditions (ie, patients with infections, inflammatory diseases, chronic kidney disease, and coronary heart failure), ferritin has shortcomings in guiding Fe therapy.[172,200,270,335-338] Due to the presence of inflammation, threshold values that indicate Fe deficiency are generally considered to be higher than values in the healthy population.

Serum ferritin concentrations of less than 100 μg/L in nondialyzed chronic kidney disease, coronary heart failure, and active inflammatory bowel disease, and less than 200 μg/L in long-term dialysis patients, are often cited as being associated with a high likelihood of Fe deficiency and a potentially good response to intravenous Fe therapy.[172,182,200,270] Proposed threshold concentrations below which functional Fe deficiency can be diagnosed in patients with renal failure treated with erythropoiesis-stimulating agents vary between 100 and 1200 μg/L.[182] However, most guidelines on patients with renal failure and inflammatory bowel disease cite that at values of more than 500 to 800 μg/L, there is a risk of exacerbating Fe overload with further therapy.[182,200]

For reasons of cost and practicality, plasma ferritin is considered the best biomarker of Fe status.[160,326] The WHO recommended ferritin for assessing the prevalence of Fe deficiency in a population, except when inflammation was present.[339] To improve monitoring the benefits of Fe intervention, algorithms have been developed that correct for the effect of inflammation on the serum ferritin value using several inflammatory markers.[195,321] These algorithms are not universally applicable in part because the markers vary with the type of inflammation and the stages of a particular disease.

Serum ferritin concentration is increased in patients with body Fe overload of any cause. However, when elevated, serum ferritin does not always correlate with elevations in liver Fe content, and the level of serum ferritin does not indicate whether Fe is stored in parenchymal cells or in the reticuloendothelial macrophages.[126,137] Parenchymal Fe storage is considered to be more toxic than reticuloendothelial system overload, as evidenced by the relatively mild Fe overload in loss of function ferroportin disease compared with the more severe Fe overload observed in HFE-hemochromatosis.[138,224,233] Moreover, for a certain degree of body Fe level, ferritin concentrations are higher in conditions in which Fe is preferentially distributed to the reticuloendothelial system (such as in transfused patients or patients with chronic inflammatory diseases) compared with diseases in which Fe is accumulated in parenchymal cells (hepatocytes) due to hyperabsorption (such as in HH, certain nontransfusion-dependent sideroblastic anemias, and β-TI).[340] High TSAT facilitates parenchymal Fe deposition; therefore, a combination of high TSAT and hyperferritinemia can be observed in patients with HH[341] and transfusion-induced Fe overload.[151]

As observed for Fe deficiency, threshold values to diagnose Fe overload also differ between guidelines. Reliable evidence on the diagnostic accuracy of ferritin is not available due to several limitations of studies, such as (1) lack of a universal definition of HH, (2) lack of comparison of ferritin to a reference standard for detecting HH, (3) adoption of different serum ferritin thresholds, ranging from 200 to 500 μg/L,[209,271,342] and (4) lack of traceability of ferritin assays.[327] Despite this lack of solid evidence for ferritin thresholds to diagnose Fe overload, validation studies, in which body Fe stores were assessed by phlebotomy (as a retrospective gold standard surrogate marker for storage Fe in HFE-HH[122,209]), showed that serum ferritin is a highly sensitive test for Fe overload in hemochromatosis. Most subjects who are homozygous for the HFE C282Y mutation have elevated TSAT, but only a fraction of them have elevated ferritin or documented Fe overload. For the detection of susceptibility to Fe overload, serum ferritin is a less sensitive screening test than TSAT (or UIBC). *HFE* mutation analysis confirmed that not all subjects with *HFE* gene mutations develop an elevated TSAT percentage and not all subjects with an *HFE* mutation-induced TSAT percentage develop raised ferritin. However, normal serum ferritin rules out Fe overload.

Ferritin is also used in the monitoring of Fe depletion treatment in HH patients. Although firm evidence is lacking, guidelines recommend ferritin treatment targets between 50 and 100 μg/L. Lower ferritin values carry the risk of the development of Fe deficiency. Moreover, because low ferritin concentrations are associated with low hepcidin levels, this exacerbates the release of Fe into the circulation, with an ensuing vicious circle that leads to the need for more frequent maintenance phlebotomies in these patients.[343]

Elevated ferritin has a low specificity for parenchymal Fe overload. In addition, low ferritin lacks sensitivity of Fe deficiency in the presence of concurrent diseases, and elevated ferritin observed in several disorders does not always correlate with body Fe stores. These disorders include infection, inflammatory disorders, hemophagocytotic lymphohistiocytosis, and related macrophage activation syndromes, Gaucher disease, adult-onset Still disease, hereditary hyperferritinemia–cataract syndrome, hyperthyroidism, tumors, liver and renal failure, cell necrosis, chronic alcohol consumption, nonalcoholic fatty liver disease, and/or the metabolic syndrome .[209,344-349] A clue to the cause of the elevation is often the accompanying clinical setting. For example, an isolated elevation of serum ferritin of 600 to 800 μg/L with a normal TSAT in the context of excessive alcohol consumption or obesity is a common presentation. In these conditions, the isolated elevated serum ferritin concentration often reflects increased total body Fe (largely) sequestered in the reticuloendothelial system, which clinically is of less concern.[138,233]

The serum ferritin test is also used for monitoring Fe overload in patients with chronic kidney disease, which may occur as a result of excessive Fe supplements given to optimize Hb content and to minimize the dose and costs of erythropoietin treatment. However, serum ferritin does not always correlate with the Fe content of the liver in these patients.[350,351]

Serum ferritin is often used for the assessment of Fe loading and to monitor Fe chelation therapy in patients with Fe-loading anemias, such as the thalassemia syndromes and sickle cell anemia. In these diseases, serum ferritin generally correlates with liver Fe concentrations as assessed by liver biopsy or magnetic resonance imaging (MRI) techniques.[340,352] At the same time, ferritin concentrations do not always accurately reflect (changes in) tissue Fe in individual patients, and trends in ferritin have been reported to be a worse predictor of changes in liver Fe stores in sickle cell disease than in thalassemia.[353] In nontransfusion-dependent thalassemia syndromes, such as β-TI and α-thalassemia (Hb H disease), ferritin is relatively low for the liver Fe concentration,[354] and thus underestimates the extent of Fe overload.[340,355] In these patients, Fe accumulates as a result of hyperabsorption in the parenchymal cells (hepatocytes).[340,356] In contrast, in transfused patients and patients with concomitant inflammation, Fe is preferentially distributed to the reticuloendothelial macrophages, leading to relatively high serum ferritin for the liver Fe concentration.[139,340] For example, because ferritin of 800 to 1000 μg/L represents a significant risk threshold in patients with β-TI (and HH and certain sideroblastic anemias), it is recommended to start chelation when ferritin concentrations reach the preceding values. However, in long-term transfused β-TM or sickle cell patients, these ferritin concentrations are generally considered acceptable.[340,354,356] In addition, hepatotoxic processes cause parallel increases in liver enzymes and serum ferritin as part of the acute phase response. These conditions are common in sickle cell disease and may contribute to the weaker association between ferritin and liver Fe concentration in this population.[353] Thus, for patients with Fe-loading anemias, trends in serum ferritin are helpful and inexpensive guides to monitoring the relative changes in body Fe stores. However, intersubject variability is quite high and ferritin values may change disproportionately from trends in total body Fe load over periods of several years.[353] Because of this variability, serum ferritin is best checked frequently (every 1–2 months) so that running averages can be calculated; this corrects for many of the transient fluctuations related to inflammation and liver damage.

Although serum ferritin trends can provide more rapid feedback on Fe status, anchoring of serum ferritin trends to gold standard assessments of Fe burden is desirable. Because liver biopsy is invasive and subject to sampling variability, annual liver Fe concentration measurement by MRI for all patients on long-term transfusion therapy is currently recommended.[357] Overall, in patient studies, increased plasma ferritin has been shown to be a strong predictor of premature death.[358] In the general population, moderately to markedly increased ferritin concentrations predict myocardial infarction, carotid plaques, and early death in a dose-dependent manner.[358-360] Because correction for markers of inflammation markedly attenuated the risk associated with hyperferritinemia in some reports,[361] prospective controlled studies are needed to assess if hyperferritinemia-associated risk merely represents a risk marker or is a risk factor.

Comments and Precautions

1. The analytical within-run coefficient of variation for the automated ferritin assay was reported to be 3.1%.[362]
2. Ferritin is a stable marker. It has a (nonsignificant) diurnal rhythm,[299,306,362] with highest levels occurring around noon. The day-to-day variation varies between 5.9% in a recent study and approximately 14% in older studies.[299,362] The cause of this day-to-day variation is not known, but presumably reflects fluctuations in intracellular protein synthesis and leakage of intracellular stored ferritin, which occurs in starvation, heavy exercise, and inflammation.[137]

Standardization. Since the 1970s, results from ferritin assays in blood have varied widely according to the isoferritin type of labeled ferritin,[328] the specificity of antibodies, and the type of ferritin used as a standard. For better comparability of analytical results and more meaningful interpretation of reported data, a project for the development of a reference material for ferritin was started in the 1980s.[363,364] This led to the release of three preparations, subsequently established as International Standards (IS) by the WHO.[365] The first IS for ferritin (human liver, code 80/602) was established in 1985.[363] It was superseded by the second IS (human spleen, code 80/578) in 1992. Unfortunately, because the value of this second IS was not traced to the first IS, a new traceability chain had to be established, making ferritin values 5% to 10% higher if the second IS was used for calibration.[316] The second IS was replaced by the third IS for ferritin (recombinant L-chain, code 94/572) in 1997.[364] At this time, the ferritin value assigned to the third IS traceable to the second IS, so that the continuity between the two materials is warranted, and the traceability chain remains unbroken. In 1999, requirements for assay traceability, as outlined in the European Community In Vitro Diagnostic Directive, prompted manufacturers to align their analytical systems to the higher-order third IS.[366] A comparison study in 2008 showed that commercial assays had reasonable agreement, but also that some assays still had not been calibrated to the current standard[316] (Box 38.2). The latter carries the risk of assay drift, and because most clinically useful cutoffs (especially for Fe deficiency) are based on old studies, this prevents the optimal use of ferritin in current clinical practice.[327]

POINTS TO REMEMBER

Serum Ferritin

- A low serum ferritin concentration is a sensitive indicator of Fe deficiency uncomplicated by other concurrent diseases.
- Low ferritin lacks sensitivity of Fe deficiency in the presence of some concurrent diseases.
- Serum ferritin concentration is increased in patients with body Fe overload of any cause.
- Elevated ferritin observed in several disorders does not always correlate with body Fe stores.
- Ferritin is an acute-phase reactant, and there is a positive correlation between inflammation and ferritin levels.
- Parenchymal Fe overload is considered to be more toxic than reticuloendothelial Fe overload.
- For a certain degree of body Fe levels, ferritin concentrations are higher in conditions in which Fe is preferentially distributed to the reticuloendothelial system, compared with diseases in which Fe is accumulated in parenchymal cells.
- Elevated ferritin has a low specificity for parenchymal Fe overload.
- A high TSAT facilitates parenchymal Fe overload.
- In combination with a high TSAT, hyperferritinemia carries a high risk of tissue Fe toxicity.
- Published cutoffs are often based on older studies that were conducted in the absence of international standards.

BOX 38.2 Standardization and Harmonization of Iron Parameters

- International standards and reference materials have been developed for ferritin, transferrin, and sTfR, but not for hepcidin and ZnPP.
- Not all current ferritin assays are calibrated against the international standard.
- For sTfR, commutability of the reference material has not been firmly established yet.
- For transferrin, the release of protein reference materials allowed the standardization of assays.
- Shortcomings in standardization preclude the definition of universal reference intervals and clinical decision limits for ferritin, sTfR, hepcidin, and ZnPP do not exist yet.

sTfR, Soluble transferrin receptor; *ZnPP*, zinc protoporphyrin.

Methods for Hepcidin

Principles. Currently, several in-house and commercial immunochemical assays and laboratory-developed mass spectrometry assays have been shown to provide reliable hepcidin results.[110] Some of the mass spectrometry assays have been thoroughly validated and are used in patient care, but most assays are labeled for "research use only."

Since the discovery of hepcidin in 2001,[100] there has been substantial interest in developing a reliable assay of the peptide in body fluids. Accurate determination of hepcidin concentrations in serum and urine has improved our understanding of Fe metabolism disorders and may provide a useful tool in the differential diagnosis and clinical management of such diseases. However, development of hepcidin assays has proven to be challenging. Hepcidin is a small, evolutionarily conserved peptide; therefore, it is difficult to generate antibodies against it.[100,107,110,367] Several early studies used a commercial serum-based immunoassay that measures the hepcidin precursor prohepcidin rather than the bioactive peptide.[368] The relevance of these studies is questionable because prohepcidin concentrations correlate with neither urinary and serum hepcidin concentrations, nor with relevant physiological responses (reviewed in Kroot and colleagues[110]). The first assays to measure bioactive hepcidin-25 were an immunodot assay in 2004,[369] and surface-enhanced laser desorption/ionization time-of-flight mass spectrometry assays (SELDI-TOF MS) in urine and serum[307,370,371] that were developed between 2005 and 2008. Unfortunately, these assays were only able to measure hepcidin in a semiquantitative manner. In the late 2000s, substantial progress was made by the introduction of hepcidin analogues and by using stable isotopes as internal standards to quantify hepcidin-25 in serum and urine by updated TOF-MS assays.[104,109] In these years, competitive (c)-ELISA tests for human serum hepcidin were also developed.[109,308] Since then, several groups and manufacturers have reported reliable plasma, serum, and urine hepcidin assays that represent two main methodologies: (1) mass spectrometry and (2) immunochemical assays, which include c-radioimmunoassay (c-radioimmunoassay, c-ELISA, c-ELISA using antibody mimetics,[372] and a 2-site ELISA).[373] At the time of this writing, some of the commercially available immunochemical research kits for serum hepcidin have been found to be suitable to differentiate between hepcidin concentrations in serum samples of control subjects and patients with various Fe disorders,[374,375] whereas several other commercial kits for human hepcidin have not unequivocally been confirmed to provide reliable results.[376,377]

Immunoassays may be more appropriate for large-scale quantitation due to its high throughput and relatively low costs compared with mass spectrometry–based assays. However, most immunochemical assays measure total hepcidin, without distinguishing the full-length hepcidin-25 from the smaller isoforms (hep20, hep22, hep23, and hep24).[110] The clinical relevance of specifically measuring hepcidin-25 is unclear. It is also not clear whether measurement of individual isoforms will be relevant for Fe disorders. Urinary hepcidin measurements roughly correlate with serum and/or plasma hepcidin measurements,[307] but measurement of urine hepcidin may pose several challenges, for example, the high concentration of smaller isoforms compared with the bioactive hepcidin-25, sensitivity to oxidation, significant (pre) analytical variation, and possible variations related to the glomerular filtration, tubular reabsorption, and production by tubular epithelial cells. These issues make measurement of hepcidin somewhat disadvantageous in urine compared with serum, which implies that for reliable interpretation of urinary hepcidin more information on renal hepcidin production and handling is needed as an alternative for serum concentrations.

Reference Intervals. Because hepcidin assays are not harmonized and standardized, there are no universal reference intervals or decision limits. Current variations in absolute hepcidin values between assays[378,379] preclude direct comparison of hepcidin results between studies. This implies that until harmonization is achieved, reference intervals and clinical decision limits for certain patient populations specific to the assay methods should be used.

Hepcidin concentrations are lower in premenopausal women than in postmenopausal women. In men, hepcidin concentrations are more constant with aging.[380] In physiological conditions, hepcidin is strongly associated with serum ferritin in men and women.[308,380,381] Hepcidin concentrations have not been consistently compared among races, and there are few studies in children and pregnant women.[374,382-384]

Because hepcidin is a hormone, hepcidin values should always be interpreted in the context of other indexes of Fe metabolism (eg, TSAT and ferritin) and inflammatory parameters. Therefore, ideally, reference intervals for hepcidin/TSAT and hepcidin/ferritin ratios should be defined. For instance, it is possible that normal concentrations of hepcidin in (1) IDA are inappropriately high for the TSAT, and perpetuate Fe restriction,[385] and (2) in HH are inappropriately low for the ferritin levels and cause unrestricted intestinal Fe absorption.[343,386]

Clinical Relevance. The measurement of hepcidin has provided important insights into the pathophysiology of Fe disorders, among which are HH, anemia of inflammation, and IRIDA.[110,387] Proof-of-principle studies highlight hepcidin as a promising diagnostic tool and therapeutic target in the management of Fe disorders. Most promising applications of hepcidin are in the diagnosis of IRIDA, in the differentiation between ACD and IDA, in the guidance of Fe supplementation therapy, and in assessing indication and monitoring of therapy with hepcidin agonists or antagonists, which are currently under development.[110,388-392] In addition, multiple studies have shown that serum hepcidin cannot be considered a valuable clinical tool in diagnosing and treating renal anemia, but that it might be a biomarker for cardiovascular disease.[393]

Comments and Precautions. The quantification of hepcidin has been found to be complicated by its tendency to aggregate[394] and to stick to laboratory plastics, necessitating implementation of robust laboratory procedures. It is unknown whether the current methodologies measure the free or a carrier protein-bound hepcidin and whether it is clinically relevant to distinguish between the free and bound fractions.[114-116] The presence of hepcidin-24, -23, -22, and -20 isoforms, which plays no role in the regulation of Fe metabolism, can interfere with the quantification of hepcidin-25 in immunoassays that use antibodies that react with all these hepcidin isoforms.

Hepcidin shows a circadian variation, with levels increasing during the course of the day,[307-310] and a considerable day-to-day variation.[309,395] For use in patient care and clinical studies, it is important to understand these limitations.

Two international "round robin" studies highlighted significant problems with hepcidin assay harmonization and standardization.[378,379] Although the correlation among multiple methods was high, the absolute hepcidin concentrations measured by individual assays were very different. The exact causes of these discrepancies are unknown, but they may be related to the use of multiple hepcidin standards, problems with oxidation or aggregation of the synthetic or native hepcidin, hepcidin binding to plasma proteins, and to a lesser extent, the presence of multiple hepcidin degradation products in body fluids. The second round robin study in 2012 included first efforts in the search for commutable samples, which was not successful.[379] Subsequent studies aiming at harmonization are ongoing (see Box 38.2).[396]

Method for Serum Transferrin Receptor

Cell membranes of developing erythroid cells, especially the erythroblasts, in bone marrow are rich in TfRs (TfR1) to which the Fe-transferrin complex binds. The number of transferrin receptors increases in the presence of high erythroid proliferation rates and low Fe supplies and decreases in bone marrow hypoplasia and suppression. These variations in the quantity of transferrin receptors in erythropoietic tissue are also reflected in changes in soluble or serum transferrin receptor (sTfR1 or sTfR), a truncated form of the transferrin receptor. sTfR was identified in 1986 and was shown to be a single polypeptide chain with a molecular mass of 84.9 KDa[397,398] that can be measured by a variety of standard immunoassay techniques.[399] In the years thereafter, sTfR was described to be helpful in the investigation of the pathophysiology of anemia, to distinguish IDA from ACD and to detect functional Fe deficiency.

Principles. Serum TfR concentrations were first determined by Kohgo and colleagues with a two-site immunoradiometric assay using a purified TfR protein from normal human placenta and two commercially available monoclonal antibodies against sTfR.[398] Then multiple ELISAs and immunoenzymatic assays were developed.[400] Subsequently, automated latex-enhanced immunoassays (nephelometry and turbidimetry) were introduced.[401] Using polystyrene-linked anti-sTfR monoclonal antibodies, these methods had distinctly better measurement precision in comparison to the more labor-intensive ELISA kits. The automated homogeneous immunoturbidimetric assay was characterized by a high sample throughput and excellent precision.[401,402] In addition, sTfR concentrations were also assessed by fluoroimmunoassays and immunofluorometric assays, which were based on immunoreactants labeled with fluorescent probes. The high sensitivity of fluorescence measurement combined with the sensitivity of the probe to changes in its environment offered the possibility of monitoring the concentration of sTfR directly in the reaction mixture.[403]

Reference Intervals. Current commercial methods for the assay of sTfR are characterized by different reference intervals. The different reference intervals have been attributed to differences in preparations of TfR used to raise antibodies and as a standard in the various assays. Therefore, no generic reference interval can be given.

Clinical Relevance. The level of sTfR is closely related to erythroid Fe demands and the erythroid proliferation rate. The most important determinant of sTfR levels appears to be marrow erythropoietic activity that can cause variations up to 8 times below and up to 20 times above average normal values.[397]

sTfR is increased in situations characterized by the following.

1. High erythroid proliferation rates, especially in combination with adequate Fe supply:

   sTfR levels are increased when erythropoiesis is stimulated in conditions with increased erythroid precursor cells (eg, hemolysis), treatment with erythrocyte-stimulating agents, and ineffective erythropoiesis (thalassemia syndromes).[404] The elevation of sTfR in response to erythrocyte-stimulating agents is higher in conditions of Fe overload than in normal conditions, when subjects are more prone to develop functional Fe deficiency.[405] Apparently, these situations of adequate Fe supply enable the erythroid precursor cells to further increase their Fe demands.
2. High erythroid Fe demands relative to Fe supply: because the rate of synthesis of TfR reflects the Fe demands of the erythroid precursors, sTfR will increase in conditions of absolute or functional Fe deficiency, especially when Fe availability is low.

sTfR concentrations are suppressed in situations characterized by diminished erythropoietic activity. This occurs in conditions with high levels of cytokines,[406-409] among which are hypoplastic anemia in renal failure, in patients with rheumatoid arthritis, or in patients with other forms of ACDs. sTfR levels may remain within the normal range even when Fe stores are depleted[407] because cytokines or other factors also suppress erythropoiesis directly or through inhibition of erythropoietin production.

Measurements of sTfR are helpful to:

1. Investigate the pathophysiology of anemia: measurements of STfR can be used to (i) quantitatively evaluate the absolute rate of erythropoiesis, (ii) assess the adequacy of marrow proliferative capacity for any given degree of anemia, and to (iii) monitor the erythropoietic response to various forms of therapy, which allows prediction of erythropoietic response early when changes in Hb are not yet apparent.[397]
2. Distinguish IDA from ACD: sTfR levels are considerably elevated in IDA but remain mostly normal in the anemia of inflammation, and thus may be of considerable help in the differential diagnosis of (microcytic) anemia.[197,333,397,410,411] This is particularly useful to identify concomitant Fe deficiency in a patient with inflammation because ferritin values are then generally normal. If Fe deficiency coexists in ACD, sTfR elevates proportionally to the degree of Fe deficiency.[412] This implies that the measurement of sTfR may be valuable in areas of the world where inflammation is prevalent, to detect individuals who require Fe replacement strategies, especially in children and women of childbearing age.[413] However, in some studies, IDA could not be distinguished from ACD based on sTfR.[268,414] For example, in patients with rheumatoid arthritis or other forms of anemia of chronic disorders, sTfR levels may remain within the normal range even when Fe stores are depleted[407] because cytokines or other factors also suppress erythropoiesis directly or through inhibition of erythropoietin production. In contrast, levels may be elevated even when

Fe stores are adequate[415] because marrow erythropoietic activity may be increased. This is exemplified by malaria. Active malaria is associated with changes in erythropoietic activity brought about by hemolysis (which would tend to increase sTfR levels) and inflammation (which would decrease sTfR levels). The predominant effect was shown to be suppression of erythropoiesis by inflammation in active malaria, which resulted in decreased sTfR levels[406] and an appropriate marrow response to mild anemia in asymptomatic infection, with elevated sTfR levels.[416] Thus, the diagnostic value of sTfR levels for Fe deficiency may be impaired in individuals living in highly endemic areas for malaria. Therefore, the relationship between Fe status and sTfR levels in patients with inflammation depends on the severity of inflammation, the degree of anemia, the adequacy of erythropoietin production, and the (suppressing) effect of cytokines on erythroid activity.[397]

3. Detect functional iron deficiency: elevated sTfR levels are also the characteristic feature of functional Fe deficiency, a situation defined by bone marrow Fe deficiency despite adequate Fe stores.[417] For example, this may occur after blood donation in patients or donors with adequate Fe stores. In these subjects, despite normal ferritin levels, sTfR increases as a result of functional bone marrow Fe deficiency to keep up with the increased erythroid demand to replace the donated RBCs. In other situations, it may be difficult to distinguish the respective influence of erythropoiesis and Fe deficiency. Serum TfR has been proposed as an indicator of adequate Fe supply to the erythron in patients with renal failure. However, these patients often have low sTfR concentrations as a result of erythroid hypoplasia,[404,418] and Fe deficiency is then associated with a relative elevation of sTfR concentrations that nevertheless remain within reference limits.[419] The interpretation of sTfR values can also be difficult in patients treated with erythropoiesis-stimulating agents. In these patients, levels of sTfR reflect more erythroid response to erythropoiesis-stimulating agents than to functional Fe deficiency.[409,420] In addition, in renal failure, sTfR increments correlate well with later hematocrit increases,[421] whereas levels are not different in patients with low or high ferritin,[422] and correction of Fe deficiency with oral Fe is associated with little changes.[338,420] Thus, sTfR should be considered to be predominantly a marker of erythroid response to erythropoiesis-stimulating agents. Consequently, in patients on erythropoiesis-stimulating agents, sTfR does not provide reliable information on tissue Fe levels because increased erythropoiesis itself raises the total erythroblast mass (and thus sTfR concentrations[423]).

Because of the reciprocal relationship between sTfR and ferritin concentrations, a combination of serum TfR and ferritin may be better to estimate Fe status. Cook and colleagues showed that the ratio of (the log of) sTfR/ferritin provides a good estimation of total Fe in population studies.[424] Moreover, the ratio sTfR/log ferritin was also shown to be a good predictor of absolute Fe deficiency in patients with chronic inflammation.[412] Use of this ratio to distinguish IDA from ACD with or without concurrent IDA has since then been promoted by various authors.[199,417] However, use of this ratio has not gained wide acceptance, and its use in areas with malaria has similar potential disadvantages as those described for sTfR.

Another shortcoming of sTfR (and its ratio with ferritin) as a marker of body Fe metabolism is that there is no international standardization of sTfR assays, and reference intervals of the various assays vary widely.[425] This began to change with the introduction of a WHO reference standard reagent in 2010[365] (see the following).

Standardization. The usefulness of sTfR assays for screening for Fe deficiency in the developing world is limited by their relatively high cost and lack of ISs.[158]

Several proteins have been used as reference materials in sTfR assays: sTfR, TfR isolated from placenta, and a receptor produced by genetically engineered methods. The use of TfR isolated from placenta as a standard for the determination of sTfR in serum may be invalid because of its differences in immunological activities with sTfR.[399,426] Because of the difficulties in purifying sufficient quantities of sTfR for use as a WHO reference reagent, the suitability of a lyophilized recombinant soluble transferrin receptor (WHO reference reagent 07/202) was evaluated for this purpose in 2010.[365] The recombinant sTfR was a few amino acids shorter than circulating sTfR. In common with sTfR, recombinant sTfR lacked the two interchain disulfides. The reagent showed acceptable overall parallelism to the manufacturers' in-house standards and the tested serum samples. The inclusion of the serum samples in the evaluation showed adequate commutability of the reagent. These proof-of-principle findings hold promise for future standardization of a sTfR assay that will allow significant reduction of intermethod variability. To firmly establish this new reference material, results of harmonization studies that include additional data collection on commutability by the Centers for Disease Control and Prevention, are currently awaited (see Box 38.2). Further improvement in standardization of various commercial sTfR immunoassays may require the selection of a reference method. Commercial standardization against the WHO reference reagent will then necessitate the recalibration and redefinition of reference intervals for the commercial assays.

Methods for Erythrocyte Zinc Protoporphyrin

Metal-free protoporphyrin (free erythrocyte protoporphyin) in erythrocytes has been associated with lead poisoning and Fe deficiency since the early clinical studies of porphyrins in the 1950s and 1960s.[427,428]

It is now known that many of these early reports were describing the metabolically formed protoporphyrin zinc chelate that was being converted to the metal-free protoporphyrin during sample processing. ZnPP received virtually no attention until 1974, when its presence in circulating erythrocytes was identified as a toxic response to lead,[429] a biochemical change that initially found widespread use in screening young children for long-term lead exposure. More information can be found at Chapter 39 on Porphyrias and Chapter 42 on Toxic Metals.

Principles. In the last step of the heme biosynthetic pathway (see also Chapter 39), the enzyme ferrochelatase catalyzes Fe and zinc chelation to protoporpyhrin. This secondary reaction occurs to a trace extent in the bone marrow during normal heme biosynthesis and cell maturation, whereas enhanced ZnPP accumulation appears in circulating erythrocytes during states of Fe deficiency in the marrow.[430,431] ZnPP remains bound within circulating erythrocytes during their life span.

The easiest available method to measure ZnPP is by its direct determination in a drop of whole blood or washed erythrocytes by hematofluorometry. The hematofluorometer, of which there are a few on the market, is a dedicated instrument that directly measures ZnPP fluorescence and heme (Hb) absorption in whole blood or in washed erythrocytes, and presents the result as a ratio of these two factors. Although the determination is simple and rapid, it is not without pitfalls. Fluorescent elements in plasma (mostly bilirubin) may result in falsely increased values. A common solution to eliminate this interference is by washing the erythrocytes free of plasma.[432] It is a measurement that can be performed in a finger stick capillary sample as a point-of-care test and has a relatively low price.

Reference Intervals. As a metabolic byproduct that forms during Hb synthesis in the developing erythrocyte, ZnPP is found in blood in healthy individuals at a ratio of approximately 50 ZnPP molecules per 1×10^6 heme molecules.[428] The minor nonheme porphyrins in healthy erythrocytes consist of approximately 95% ZnPP and 5% free erythrocyte protoporphyrin. Expression of results is recommended in standard international units (ie, millimoles of ZnPP per mole of heme). The ratio of metabolites is recommended in part to eliminate the effects of dilution by changes in plasma volume.

Reference intervals and cutoff points differ between studies as less than 30 to less than 80 ZnPP mmol/mol heme.[428,433] This variation can be attributed to the fact that (1) ZnPP lacks harmonization and standardization (see Box 38.2); (2) values are mostly taken from manufacturers' manuals for which the origin remains largely unknown; (3) values are derived from different populations; and (4) values serve different diagnostic and clinical purposes.

Clinical Relevance. The ZnPP ratio of the erythrocytes reflects Fe availability and use in the bone marrow. The level of free erythrocyte protoporphyrin or rather ZnPP increases dramatically in Fe deficiency and is a sensitive laboratory abnormality in this condition.[427,428] Clinically, ZnPP quantification is valuable as a tool for evaluating Fe nutrition and metabolism. Diagnostic determinations are applicable in a variety of clinical settings, including pediatrics, obstetrics, and blood banking.[428] In pediatrics, ZnPP has been described to enable detection of pre-anemic but Fe-depleted children, who would benefit from Fe supplementation.[434] In pregnant women, the ZnPP/heme ratio has the advantage of not being affected by dilution, thereby avoiding the misinterpretation of laboratory results that may occur with plasma volume change.[435]

For donor screening, ZnPP has the potential to detect the imbalance between bone marrow needs and supplies. ZnPP assessment in a drop of whole blood has been described to be a reliable assay to detect Fe deficiency and to protect blood donors from the development of IDA. It is relatively cheap and easy to perform by point-of-care testing in clinical blood bank practice.

ZnPP is also proposed as a useful screening test for Fe deficiency in field studies, particularly in children.[436]

Elevated ZnPP concentrations can also be found when the demands exceed the delivery of Fe to the bone marrow, for example, in ineffective erythropoiesis (thalassemia syndromes),[437] sideroblastic anemias,[242] ACDs,[438] and functional Fe deficiency.[439] As mentioned earlier, ZnPP is also increased in lead poisoning in urban and industrial settings, because lead impairs Fe use by immature erythrocytes, and ZnPP levels correlate with lead concentrations.[203,429,440]

In sum, ZnPP is increased in Fe deficiency and adds to the diagnostic armamentarium of Fe deficiency. However, ZnPP is also increased in other diseases. Its clinical usefulness is limited by the lack of harmonization and standardization, universal reference intervals, and cutoff points for decision-making.

Methods for Red Blood Cell Analytical Parameters

Fe is an essential part of Hb that resides in RBCs. RBCs are defined by three quantitative values: the proportion of the blood sample that is occupied by red cells or hematocrit (Hct), the concentration of Hb, and the red cell concentration per unit volume (RBC). Three additional indexes that describe average qualitative characteristics of the red cell population are also collected. These are MCV, MCH, mean corpuscular Hb concentration (MCHC), and RDW. Novel hematologic parameters have recently been developed, among which are Hb content of reticulocytes or percentage of hypochromic cells.

Changes in these values by disturbances in Fe metabolism can be routinely collected and calculated by automated hematology analyzers, largely replacing many of the previously used manual or semiautomated methods of RBC characterization. The use of hematology analyzers imparts a high degree of precision compared with manual measurements and calculations. These RBC indexes are defined and the methodology used to measure them are described, as well as their clinical relevance. For a more comprehensive description of these methods and related strengths and weaknesses, the reader is referred to hematology and clinical laboratory textbooks[121,441] and reviews[442,443] and to Chapter 73 on Automated Hematology.

Definition and Principle. Since the 1980s, instrumentation has virtually replaced manual cell counting. Hematology analyzers are marketed by multiple instrument manufacturers. These analyzers typically provide the eight standard hematology parameters (CBC, plus a three- or five-part differential leucocyte) count in less than 1 minute on 200 μL of whole blood. The various hematology analyzers rely on two basic principles of operation: electronic impedance (resistance) and optical scatter. Electronic impedance, or low-voltage direct current, was developed by Coulter in the 1950s, and is the most common methodology used.[443a,443b] Optical scatter or flow cytometry, using both laser and nonlaser light, is frequently used in today's hematology instrumentation.

In the hematology counters, RBCs per volume unit are counted after whole blood dilution in an isotonic solution. For the determination of Hb, most automated instruments use modifications of the cyanmet Hb assay. Another method involves the use of sodium lauryl sulfate to convert Hb to sodium lauryl sulfate-methemoglobin.

Hct is the proportion of the volume of a blood sample that is occupied by red cells. Hct may be determined manually by centrifugation of blood at a given speed and time as originally described by Wintrobe in 1929.[444] The height of the column of the red cells after centrifugation compared with the total blood sample volume yields the Hct. Macromethods (using 3-mm test tubes and high-speed centrifugation, or micromethods using capillary tubes and high-speed centrifugation) may also be used. Automated analyzers do not depend on centrifugation techniques to determine Hct, but instead calculate Hct by direct measurement of RBC number and red cell volume (Hct = red cell number per volume × mean red cell volume).

Reticulocyte counts reflect the number of reticulocytes or immature, non-nucleated RBCs that (still) retain RNA. Hematology analyzers evaluate reticulocytes based on optical scatter or fluorescence after the RBCs are treated with fluorescent dyes or nucleic acid stains to stain residual RNA in the reticulocytes.

The average volume of RBCs (MCV in femtoliters or 10^{-15} L) is usually measured directly with automated instruments, but it may also be calculated by dividing the Hct by the red cell count (10^{12}/L) and multiplying its quotient by 1000. Cells with low MCV are named "microcytic" cells.

MCH is a measure of the average Hb content per red cell and is expressed in picograms or 10^{-12} g, or in femtomole (1 fmol = 16.11 pg). Thus, the MCH is an expression of the Hb mass of RBCs. Cells with a low MCH are named "hypochromic" cells.

MCHC is the average concentration of Hb in a given red cell volume and is expressed in grams (or moles) of Hb per deciliter or liter of packed RBCs.

The RDW is a red cell measurement that quantitates cellular volume heterogeneity, reflecting the range of red cell sizes in a sample.

Next to these more traditional parameters, novel parameters emerged in the 1990s and 2000s, among which are measures based on increased hypochromia and measures of reticulocyte Hb content.[182,442,443]

The reticulocyte Hb content parameter, such as CHr (Siemens, Erlangen, Germany) and Ret-He (Sysmex, Kobe, Japan), is a measure of Hb content of reticulocytes expressed in picograms per cell (or femtomole per cell). It is a real-time parameter that reflects whether Fe availability has met the Fe need of the earliest released reticulocytes during the previous 3 to 4 days.[442,445]

The percentage of hypochromic cells parameter (hypochromic red blood cells [HRC], Hypo-He) can be regarded as a time-averaged marker of Fe-restricted erythropoiesis. Both the reticulocyte Hb content and the percentage of hypochromic cell parameters can be performed simultaneously during routine blood counts with relatively low incremental costs and no additional blood sampling. Several manufacturers of automated hematology equipment facilitate analysis of these innovative parameters.[182,442,443,446,447]

Clinical Relevance. Hemoglobin, Hct, MCV, MCH, and MCHC are (slightly) elevated in many persons with untreated HFE hemochromatosis. This is predominantly due to increased Fe delivery to developing erythroid cells in subjects whose TSAT with Fe is significantly elevated.[448,449]

In IDA, MCV, MCH, and reticulocyte Hb content are reduced, and the RDW and the percentage of hypochromic cells are increased. The percentage and absolute number of reticulocytes may be normal or slightly increased. MCV, MCH, the percentage of hypochromic cells, and reticulocyte Hb content are less readily affected in conditions of anemia of chronic inflammation.

MCV, MCHC, percentage of hypochromic cells, and reticulocyte content parameters all have (some) limitations in terms of sample stability, but differences between analyzers exist.[450,451] MCV and MCHC are also affected by the presence of reticulocytes, which exhibit increased MCV and decreased MCHC.

In contrast, MCH is invariable once the Hb synthesis is terminated during reticulocyte maturation, and as such, is the best indicator of the amount of Hb synthesized (and thus Fe availability) during erythroid differentiation.[333,443] Therefore, MCH is a useful red cell index for the diagnosis of Fe deficiency.

The percentage of hypochromic cells has been proposed as a parameter for the diagnosis of functional Fe deficiency in patients with chronic renal failure treated with erythropoiesis-stimulating agents.[452] However, because the percentage of hypochromic red cells is dependent on the size of the RBCs, it is strongly influenced by the time between sampling and analysis, and therefore, it is not that helpful in the real-life clinical setting and not recommended by the Kidney Disease Improving Global Outcomes Anemia guideline.[181]

Reticulocyte Hb content parameters provide insight into the adequacy of the Fe supply to erythroid precursor cells over the last few days.[442] Studies support the clinical usefulness of reticulocyte content parameters as:

1. An early marker for Fe-restricted erythropoiesis due to Fe deficiency before the development of anemia in adults and children[445,453,454] or to acute infection or inflammation[455,456];
2. A guidance for diagnosing functional Fe deficiency and optimizing intravenous Fe therapy in patients receiving erythropoietin for end-stage renal failure, although the evidence of reduction in erythropoiesis-stimulating agent use has been less convincing[338,439,457,458]; and
3. As an early marker of erythropoietic response to Fe supplementation.[459-461]

Because reticulocyte Hb content parameters are also affected by other factors, such as impairment of β-globin chain synthesis or by megaloblastosis, values should be interpreted in the context (pathophysiology) of the patient.

Overall, the promise of these novel parameters is restrained by the absence of clinically validated and standardized assays, and the absence of clinical decision limits. Further investigation is required to compare these parameters across different analytical platforms and to enable the development of software applications, including new algorithms for anemia discrimination and follow-up monitoring in case of therapy. For more details, refer to Chapter 73 on Automated Hematology.

Gold Standard Assessment of Body Iron

Bone Marrow Examination. The absence of stainable bone marrow Fe is the most commonly accepted reference standard index of Fe deficiency. One way of evaluating Fe stores is by examining a marrow aspirate for hemosiderin within reticuloendothelial cells.[319] Using this method, normal marrow is graded 1+ to 3+. In Fe deficiency, marrow hemosiderin is absent; in the anemia of chronic disorders, Fe is always present, most often of grade 2 or 3+, but sometimes 4 or 5+. Fe stores are greatly increased (5 to 6+) in TM and in sideroblastic anemias. However, this method for quantification of Fe stores may be misleading when Fe stores are not normally distributed between reticuloendothelial and parenchymal tissues as occurs in ACD. Another way of evaluating bone marrow Fe also includes evaluation of Fe in the erythroblasts, which represents the useable and functional

Fe stores.[462] Differentiation between functional Fe deficiency and quantitative deficiency of Fe stores is important, especially in areas of high infection pressure.[462]

Overall, bone marrow aspirates are invasive, although generally safe procedures. Methodological problems may limit interpretation of bone marrow Fe stores.[334,463,464] These include technical limitations, that is, few particles included in the slide, operator experience, interobserver error, and stain quality. Bone marrow examination for the sole purpose of assessing Fe stores is rarely justifiable. It may be helpful in the diagnosis of unexplained forms of anemia and if there are concerns that a high serum ferritin value is not a true reflection of body Fe stores.

Liver Biopsy and Magnetic Resonance Imaging Techniques. In Fe overload disorders, the liver Fe concentration represents the best single surrogate of changes in body Fe. Chemical analysis of liver Fe biopsy is considered the gold standard method used for the analysis of liver Fe concentration. However, it has high sampling variability, processing bias, potential major complications (estimated rate is ≈0.5 %), and poor patient acceptance.[465] As an alternative, MRI techniques have emerged as the dominant noninvasive modality for tissue Fe quantification.[466,467] However, it should be noted that hepatic MRI cannot distinguish between parenchymal (hepatocytes) and more benign reticuloendothelial (Kupffer cells) Fe overload, and can therefore be misleading for the assessment of Fe burden when Fe stores are not normally distributed.[181] Moreover, both liver biopsy and MRI measure a relevant, but not complete portion, of body Fe stores. Liver biopsy used to be the gold standard for the diagnosis of HH before HFE genotyping became available. Now that genetic testing is readily available, homozygosity for HFE C282Y in patients with increased body Fe stores with or without clinical symptoms is sufficient to make a diagnosis of HFE-HH. When there is hyperferritinemia with confounding cofactors, a liver biopsy may still be necessary in the diagnostic workup of HH to show whether Fe stores are increased.[209] In patients with Fe-loading anemias and/or patients on long-term transfusion therapy, liver biopsy and MRI techniques may be used as the gold standard assessment of Fe burden.[457] Liver biopsy also still has a role in assessing liver fibrosis and cirrhosis in patients with Fe overload.

BILIRUBIN

Bilirubin is the orange-yellow pigment derived from senescent RBCs. It is extracted and biotransformed mainly in the liver and is excreted in bile and urine. The chemistry, biochemistry, and analytical methods for bilirubin and related compounds are reviewed in this section.

Chemistry

Bilirubin was discovered by Virchow in 1849 in blood extravasates; he called the yellow pigment "hematoidin." The term *bilirubin* was coined by Stadeler in 1864, and in 1874, Tarchanoff demonstrated the direct association of bile pigments with Hb. In 1942, Fisher and Plieninger synthesized bilirubin IXα and proposed the structure shown in Fig. 38.21A. This linear tetrapyrrolic structure of the bilirubin molecule was accepted for longer than 30 years. However, important chemical properties of the bilirubin molecule are its insolubility in water and its solubility in a variety of nonpolar solvents. The solubility of bilirubin in nonpolar, lipid solvents is not predicted from this linear tetrapyrrole structure because the two propionic acid side chains would be expected to make the bilirubin molecule highly polar and therefore water soluble.

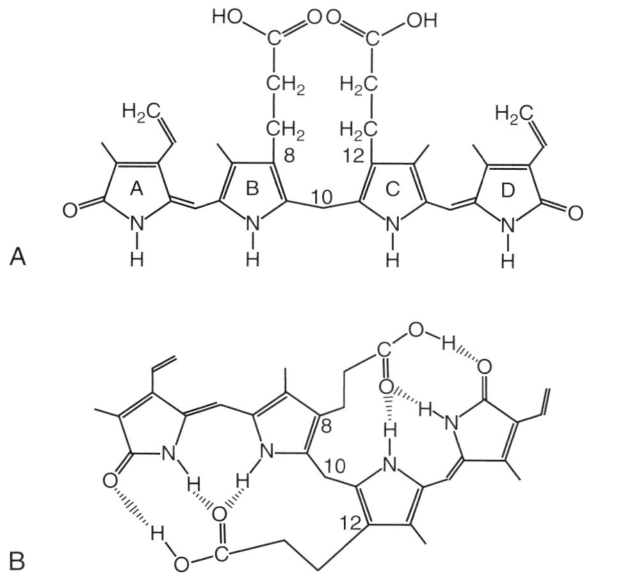

FIGURE 38.21 A, A Linear Molecular Representation of Unconjugated Bilirubin. B, The Preferred Structure of Unconjugated Bilirubin IXa, *Z,Z* Configuration. The folded ridge-tile structure is stabilized by six hydrogen bonds formed between the two carboxyl groups of the sidechains and the two carbonyl and four imino groups. The ridge involves carbon atoms 8 through 12. *CO,* Carbon monoxide; *Fe,* iron; *NADPH,* nicotinamide adenine dinucleotide phosphate reduced.

The overall chemical structure of bilirubin was established by x-ray crystallography.[472] According to this work, bilirubin assumes a ridge-tiled configuration stabilized by six intramolecular hydrogen bonds. Two additional important structural features have also been noted: (1) a so-called *Z-Z (trans)* conformation for the double bonds between carbons 4 and 5 and 15 and 16, and (2) an involuted hydrogen-bonded structure in which the propionic acid–carboxylic acid groups are hydrogen-bonded to the nitrogen atoms of the pyrrole rings (see Fig. 38.21B).[473] These bonds stabilize the *Z-Z* configuration of bilirubin and prevent its interaction with polar groups in aqueous media. When exposed to light, the *Z-Z* configuration is converted to the *E-E (cis)* conformation and to other combinations, namely, 4*E*-15*Z* and 4*Z*-15*E*. The *E-E* conformation and other *E*-containing isomers do not permit the degree of internal hydrogen bonding that occurs in the *Z-Z* conformation and therefore are more water soluble than in the *Z-Z* conformation. Thus, light-exposed forms of bilirubin are more water soluble and are readily excreted in the bile. This is the rationale for irradiating jaundiced newborns with 450-nm light.[474]

The bilirubin molecule in the crystalline state takes, as mentioned earlier, the form of a ridge tile rather than a linear tetrapyrrole, with the ridge being along the line C8-C10-C12. In this configuration, rings A and B lie in one plane and rings C and D in another, with a 98° angle between the two rings. The preferred conformation of bilirubin in aqueous solution at pH 7.4 is not known, but the occurrence of a hydrogen-bonded structure in aqueous solution would explain some of the unique chemical properties of bilirubin IXα. For example, the addition of hydrogen bond–breaking chemicals, such as caffeine, methanol, ethanol, urea, or surface active agents, is required for unconjugated bilirubin to react with diazo reagent. These reagents likely act by breaking the internal hydrogen bonds of the bilirubin molecule, allowing it to react with diazotized sulfanilic acid or other diazo compounds. In contrast, bilirubin IXα monoglucuronide and diglucuronide are soluble in water and react readily with diazo reagents. The bulky glucuronic acid moiety precludes conjugated bilirubin from undergoing internal hydrogen bond formation. Bilirubin glucuronides, which are water soluble, are readily excreted in the bile and urine, whereas unconjugated bilirubin is not.

Bilirubin derived from natural sources consists almost entirely (99%) of the isomer IXα. Bilirubins IXβ and IXδ, which arise from cleavage of the β- and δ-methene bridges, consist of less than 0.5% of bilirubin isolated from bile. However, bilirubin reference materials available from commercial sources and from the National Institute of Standards and Technology (Standard Reference Material 916a) contain variable quantities of IIIα and XIIIα isomers.[475] The two isomers are formed by cleavage of bilirubin IXα at the central methylene bridge; subsequent recombination of the two different dipyrrole units gives a mixture of the three isomers. This isomerization of bilirubin occurs in aqueous solution at acidic or neutral pH, but not when bilirubin is bound to albumin.[476]

Biochemistry

Bilirubin IXα is produced from the catabolism of protoporphyrin IX by a microsomal heme oxygenase.[477] The tetrapyrrolic product of the ring opening at the α-methene bridge is the green pigment biliverdin, which is subsequently reduced to bilirubin by the reduced form of nicotinamide adenine dinucleotide phosphate–dependent cytosolic enzyme biliverdin reductase (Fig. 38.22). For each mole of heme catabolized by this pathway, one mole each of carbon monoxide, bilirubin, and ferric Fe is produced. Daily bilirubin production from all sources in humans averages from 250 to 300 mg. Approximately 85% of the total bilirubin produced is derived from the heme moiety of Hb released from senescent erythrocytes that are destroyed in the reticuloendothelial cells of the liver, spleen, and bone marrow. The remaining 15% is produced from RBC precursors destroyed in the bone marrow (so-called ineffective erythropoiesis) and from the catabolism of other heme-containing proteins, such as myoglobin, cytochromes, and peroxidases.

In blood, bilirubin is bound to albumin ($K_d \approx 10^{-8}$ mol/L) and is transported to the liver.[478] Bilirubin then dissociates from albumin by an unknown process at the sinusoidal membrane of the hepatocyte. It is transported across the membrane (Fig. 38.23).

It is theorized the organic anion transport proteins (OATPs) 1A1 (OMIM*604843) and 1B3 (OMIM*605495), which are encoded on the solute carrier organic anion transporter (SLCO) superfamily of genes, are responsible for the uptake of bilirubin into the hepatocyte.[479] Once inside the liver cells, bilirubin is reversibly bound to soluble proteins known as ligandins or protein Y. Ligandins are cytosolic proteins of the glutathione-*S*-transferase gene family and include approximately 5% of the total protein of human liver cytosol.[479,480] Ligandin also binds a variety of other compounds, such as steroids, bromsulphthalein, indocyanine green, and some carcinogens. Ligandin likely plays an important role in the processing of these compounds; it may increase the net efficiency of uptake by retarding the reflux of these substances back to plasma.

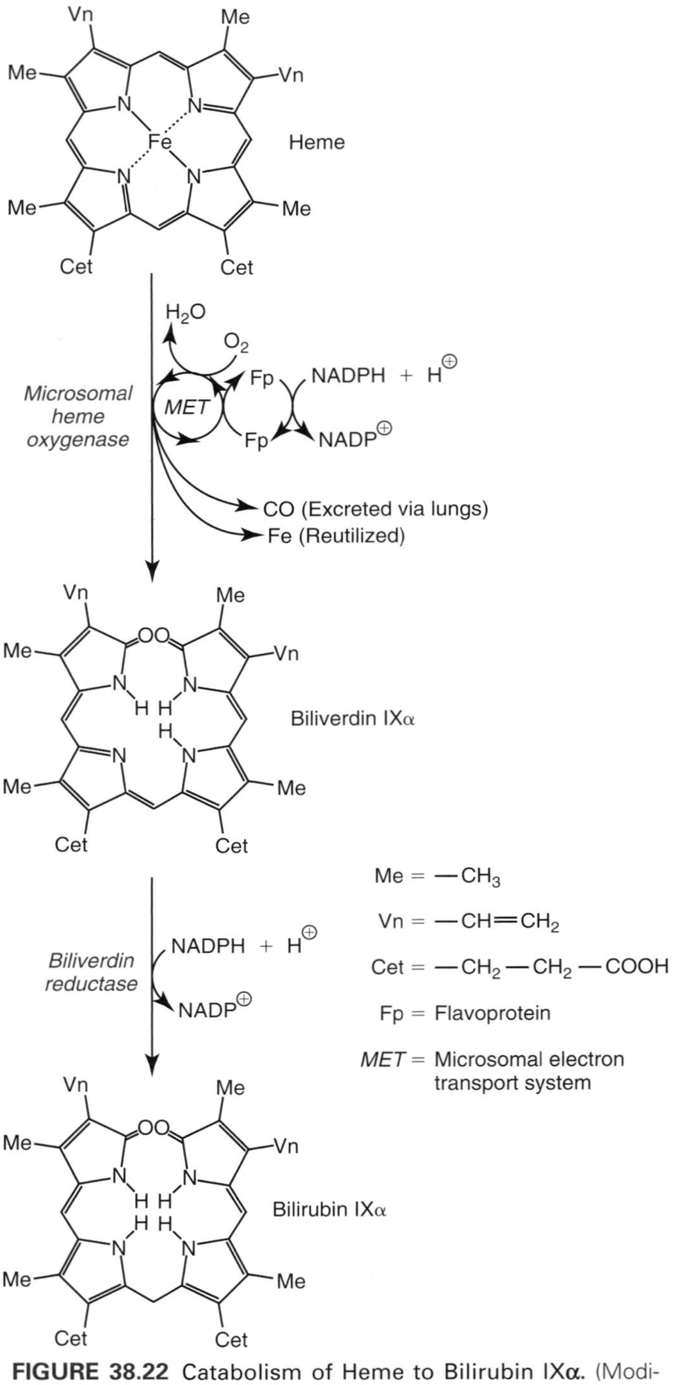

Inside the hepatocytes, bilirubin is rapidly conjugated with glucuronic acid to produce bilirubin monoglucuronide and

Me = $-CH_3$

Vn = $-CH{=}CH_2$

Cet = $-CH_2-CH_2-COOH$

Fp = Flavoprotein

MET = Microsomal electron transport system

FIGURE 38.22 **Catabolism of Heme to Bilirubin IXα.** (Modified from Tenhunen R, Marver HS, Schmid R. The enzymatic conversion of hemoglobin to bilirubin. *Trans Assoc Am Physicians* 1969;82:363–71.)

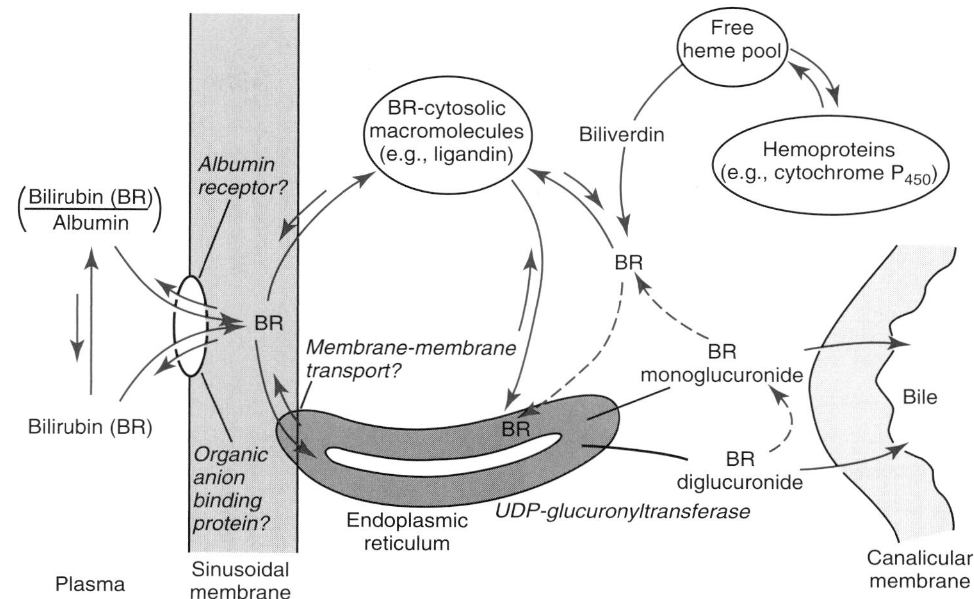

FIGURE 38.23 Bilirubin Uptake, Metabolism, and Transport in the Hepatocyte. (From Gollan JL, Schmid R. Bilirubin update: formation, transport, and metabolism. In: Popper H, Schaffner F, eds. *Progress in Liver Diseases*. Vol 7. Chapter 15. Philadelphia: WB Saunders, 1982.)

diglucuronide, which then are excreted into bile (see Fig. 38.23). The enzyme bilirubin uridine diphosphate (UDP)–glucuronyltransferase 1A1 (OMIM*191740) is a tetramer that catalyzes the formation of bilirubin monoglucuronide and diglucuronide. This is a transmembrane protein primarily localized to the smooth endoplasmic reticulum. A specific binding site exists for bilirubin and glucuronic acid.[481] It is speculated that the monomer catalyzes monoglucuronide formation and the tetramer is required for the diglucuronide conjugate at the luminal surface of the endoplasmic reticulum.[482] The bilirubin diglucuronide returns to the cytosol, likely through a transporter, and binds to ligandin where it will diffuse to either the canalicular pole for secretion into bile or the sinusoidal pole for secretion back into plasma. The process is mediated by an adenosine triphosphate–binding cassette transporter ABCC2, which was previously named multidrug-related protein 2 (MRP2), at the canalicular pole. Although other transporters exist for this function, such as ABCG2, most are removed by MRP2/ABCC2. At the sinusoidal pole, an ABCC3 transporter returns bilirubin into plasma where reuptake is possible by the OATP1B1 and OATP1B3 transporters.[483]

In adults, virtually all bilirubin excreted in bile is in the form of glycosidic conjugates; glucuronides account for approximately 95% of them, and glucosides and xylosides constitute the remainder. Of the glucuronides, diglucuronide is the major fraction (≈90%), and monoglucuronide is the minor fraction (≈10%).

Bilirubin glucuronides are not substantially reabsorbed in the intestine. Rather, they are hydrolyzed by the catalytic action of β-glucuronidase from the liver, intestinal epithelial cells, and bacteria. This unconjugated bilirubin is then reduced by anaerobic intestinal microbial flora to form a group of three colorless tetrapyrroles collectively called urobilinogens. In each of these three bilirubin reduction products, all bridge carbons are in the saturated (methylene) form. The urobilinogens differ from one another in the degree of hydrogenation of the vinyl sidechains and in the two end pyrrole rings. Urobilinogens contain 6, 8, or 12 more hydrogen atoms than does bilirubin and are named stercobilinogen, mesobilinogen, or urobilinogen, respectively. Up to 20% of the urobilinogen produced daily is reabsorbed from the intestine and enters the enterohepatic circulation. Most of the reabsorbed urobilinogen is taken up by the liver and is reexcreted in the bile; a small fraction (2%–5%) enters the general circulation and appears in urine. In the lower intestinal tract, the three urobilinogens are spontaneously oxidized at the middle methylene bridge to produce the corresponding bile pigments stercobilin, mesobilin, and urobilin, which are orange-brown and the major pigments of stool. Approximately 50% of the conjugated bilirubin excreted in bile is metabolized to products other than the urobilinogens. The detailed structure of these metabolites has not been characterized.

Clinical Significance

Jaundice is a condition characterized by hyperbilirubinemia and deposition of bile pigment in the skin, mucous membranes, and sclera, with a resulting yellow appearance of the patient; it is also called icterus. Defects in bilirubin metabolism resulting in jaundice can occur at each step of the metabolic pathway (see Fig. 38.23). The disorders are usually classified as inherited disorders of bilirubin metabolism and jaundice of the newborn. All of these disorders are characterized by elevations in conjugated or unconjugated bilirubin in the absence of other abnormal liver tests. Bilirubin fractionation is clinically useful only for these disorders.

Patients are occasionally seen with isolated elevations in bilirubin concentration. In most cases, this is due to inherited disorders of bilirubin metabolism, familial hyperbilirubinemia, or hemolysis. It is not difficult to establish hemolysis as the cause of hyperbilirubinemia because the patient with

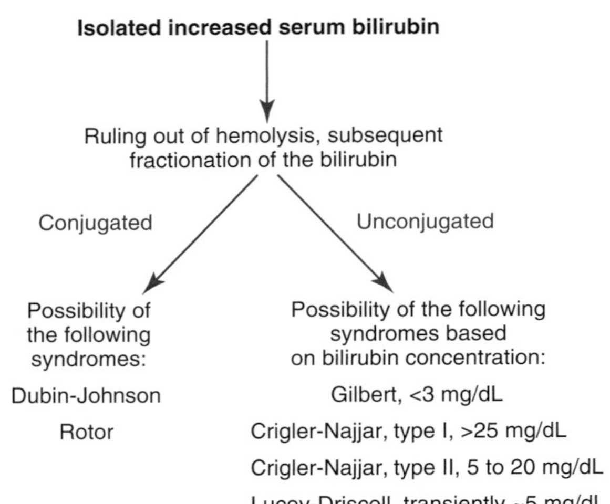

FIGURE 38.24 Algorithm for Differentiating the Familial Causes of Hyperbilirubinemia.

severe hemolysis will have many other disease manifestations. An algorithm for differentiating familial causes of hyperbilirubinemia is presented in Fig. 38.24.

Inherited Disorders of Bilirubin Metabolism

Inherited disorders of bilirubin metabolism include Gilbert, Crigler-Najjar (types I and II), Lucey-Driscoll, Dubin-Johnson, and Rotor syndromes.

Gilbert Syndrome. Gilbert syndrome is a benign condition manifested by mild unconjugated hyperbilirubinemia. This abnormality, which affects 3% to 10% of the population, is clinically important because it is often misdiagnosed as chronic hepatitis.[484] The serum concentration of bilirubin fluctuates between 1.5 and 4 mg/dL (26 and 70 μmol/L) and tends to increase with fasting. Hepatic glucuronyltransferase activity is low (≈30% of normal activity) because of a mutation in the bilirubin-UDP-glucuronosyltransferase (*UGT1A1*) gene located on chromosome 2. In most patients, this mutation is a repeat in the promoter, so that there are seven rather than the "normal" six ATs. Occasionally, subjects are encountered with five or eight repeats; the transcription of the gene is inversely proportional to the number of repeats,[485] so that bilirubin concentrations tend to be higher in those patients with the largest number of repeats in the promoter. In Asia, Gilbert syndrome is sometimes found to be caused by a single point mutation in exon 1 of the *UGT1A1* gene.[486] The Framingham Heart Study population was studied for subjects homozygous for the insertion of seven TA repeats in the promotor region of the *UGT1A1* gene (designated UGT1A1*28; genotype 7/7) and discovered higher bilirubin concentrations strongly associated with a lower risk of cardiovascular disease.[487] These findings support the concept of bilirubin possessing a protective antioxidant effect that leads to the prevention of low-density lipoprotein oxidation, thus lowering cardiovascular risk.[488] Additional protective effects have been suggested for diabetes and metabolic syndrome.[489,490] Gilbert syndrome is easily distinguished from chronic hepatitis by the absence of anemia and bilirubin in urine, and by normal liver function tests. The condition is probably inherited as an autosomal recessive trait. Despite the fact that total biliary bilirubin is reduced, the ratio of bilirubin monoglucuronide to diglucuronide is increased, suggesting that a defect is also present in the conversion of bilirubin monoglucuronide to diglucuronide.

Patients with Gilbert syndrome may be predisposed to acetaminophen toxicity because acetaminophen is primarily metabolized by glucuronidation. The diagnosis is usually made by chance on routine medical examination or when jaundice occurs after an intercurrent infection or fasting. Special diagnostic tests are occasionally necessary and include demonstrating a rise in bilirubin on fasting and a fall in bilirubin upon taking phenobarbital. No treatment is needed, but patients must be reassured that they do not have liver disease.

Crigler-Najjar Syndrome (Type I). Crigler-Najjar syndrome type I (OMIM* 218800),[491] a rare disorder caused by complete absence of UDP-glucuronyltransferase 1A1, is manifested by high concentrations of unconjugated bilirubin often exceeding 20 mg/dL (340 μmol/L). Because no glucuronidation occurs, conjugated bilirubin is not detectable. It is inherited as an autosomal recessive trait. Most mutations have been identified to exist in exons 2 to 5, and result in truncated proteins or amino acid substitutions resulting in little to no enzyme activity.[492] Most patients die of severe brain damage caused by kernicterus (encephalopathy related to increased serum bilirubin that leads to permanent brain damage) within the first year of life. Phlebotomy and plasmapheresis can reduce the serum bilirubin, but encephalopathy usually develops. Early liver transplantation is the only effective therapy.

Crigler-Najjar Syndrome (Type II). Crigler-Najjar syndrome type II (OMIM*606785)[493] is a rare autosomal dominant disorder characterized by a partial deficiency of UDP-glucuronyltransferase 1A1. Enzymatic activities are usually less than 10% of normal activity. Unconjugated bilirubin is usually 5 to 20 mg/dL (85–340 μmol/L). Unlike the Crigler-Najjar syndrome type I, type II responds dramatically to phenobarbital, and a normal life span is expected. Pregnant type II patients can be treated with phototherapy and phenobarbital without affecting either the mother or the fetus.[494]

Lucey-Driscoll Syndrome. Lucey-Driscoll syndrome,[495,496] also known as maternal serum jaundice or transient familial hyperbilirubinemia, is a familial form of unconjugated hyperbilirubinemia caused by a circulating inhibitor of bilirubin conjugation. The hyperbilirubinemia is mild and lasts for the first 2 to 3 weeks of life.

Dubin-Johnson Syndrome. Dubin-Johnson syndrome[497] is due to a rare autosomal recessive disorder and is characterized by jaundice with predominantly elevated conjugated bilirubin and a minor elevation of unconjugated bilirubin. Excretion of various conjugated organic anions and bilirubin, but not bile salts, into bile is impaired, reflecting the underlying defect in canalicular excretion. At least 20 mutations in the *ABCC2* gene on chromosome 10 have been identified to result in the Dubin-Johnson phenotype.[498] The transporter ABCC2 is responsible for the active transport of many organic anions, in addition to conjugated bilirubin, into the bile canaliliculus.[499]

Intravenous cholangiography does not show the gallbladder, but a ^{99m}technetium-hepatobiliary iminodiacetic acid (HIDA) scan does. A derangement in the excretion of urinary coproporphyrin occurs, and the normal ratio of coproporphyrin I to III is reversed. The liver has a characteristic greenish black appearance, and liver biopsy reveals a dark brown pigment in hepatocytes and Kupffer cells that looks like lipofuscin but probably is melanin. Serum alanine aminotransferase and alkaline phosphatase are usually normal, and pruritus is absent. The condition is benign, although patients may develop jaundice during pregnancy or while taking oral contraceptives.

Rotor Syndrome. Rotor syndrome[500-502] is another form of conjugated hyperbilirubinemia similar to Dubin-Johnson syndrome, but without pigment in the liver. Contrary to findings in Dubin-Johnson syndrome, the gallbladder is seen on intravenous cholecystography. Total urinary coproporphyrins are elevated, with approximately two-thirds being coproporphyrin I. The prognosis is excellent.

Jaundice in the Neonate

Disorders that cause jaundice in the neonate are classified as unconjugated or conjugated hyperbilirubinemia (Box 38.3).[503,504]

Unconjugated Hyperbilirubinemia. Unconjugated hyperbilirubinemia poses a risk for development of kernicterus (acute bilirubin encephalopathy), especially in low birth weight infants. Kernicterus refers to a neurologic syndrome that results in brain damage because of deposition of bilirubin in the basal ganglia and brain stem nuclei. In term infants, the early symptoms of kernicterus are poor feeding, lethargy, and vomiting; later, opisthotonos (backward arching of the trunk), and seizures; death may follow. Seventy percent of affected infants die within the first week, and those remaining have severe brain damage. This syndrome can be prevented by phototherapy and exchange transfusion in infants with elevated unconjugated bilirubin concentrations.

Causes of unconjugated hyperbilirubinemia in the neonate are physiologic jaundice of the newborn, hemolytic disease, and breast milk hyperbilirubinemia.

Guidelines for Assessing Risk. In 2004, the Subcommittee on Hyperbilirubinemia of the American Academy of Pediatrics (AAP) issued new guidelines for the management of jaundice in the neonate.[504] These guidelines became necessary because newborns are currently discharged between 36 and 72 hours after birth, and severe hyperbilirubinemia may not be present at discharge. The time-honored bilirubin concentration of 20 mg/dL (340 μmol/L), which was considered critical and required action (eg, phototherapy, exchange transfusion), is now being abandoned and replaced by monitoring the increase in bilirubin concentration from the time of birth until the time of discharge from the hospital. In practice, it is now recommended that a plot of bilirubin concentration (milligrams per deciliter or micromoles per liter) versus time (hours) is constructed and compared with the Bhutani predictive nomogram for hyperbilirubinemia found in the AAP guideline.[505] The nomogram is easily searchable on the internet. Others have chosen to create a numeric chart that indicates multiple hours of age, total bilirubin concentration, and risk.[506] Alternatively, websites have been developed to provide the hour-specific risk as described in the 2004 AAP

BOX 38.3 Physiologic Classification of Jaundice

Unconjugated Hyperbilirubinemia

Increased Production of Unconjugated Bilirubin From Heme

Hemolysis
- Hereditary
- Acquired

Ineffective erythropoiesis

Rapid turnover of increased red blood cell mass (in the neonate)

Decreased Delivery of Unconjugated Bilirubin (in Plasma) to Hepatocyte

Right-sided congestive heart failure

Portocaval shunt

Decreased Uptake of Unconjugated Bilirubin Across Hepatocyte Membrane

Competitive inhibition
- Drugs
- Others

Gilbert syndrome

Sepsis, fasting

Decreased Storage of Unconjugated Bilirubin in Cytosol (Decreased Y and Z Proteins)

Competitive inhibition

Fever

Decreased Biotransformation (Conjugation)

Neonatal jaundice (physiologic)

Inhibition (drugs)

Hereditary (Crigler-Najjar)
- Type I (complete enzyme deficiency)
- Type II (partial deficiency)

Hepatocellular dysfunction

Gilbert syndrome

Conjugated Hyperbilirubinemia (Cholestasis)

Decreased Secretion of Conjugated Bilirubin Into Canaliculi

Hepatocellular disease
- Hepatitis
- Cholestasis (intrahepatic)

Dubin-Johnson and Rotor syndromes

Drugs (estradiol)

Decreased Drainage

Extrahepatic obstruction
- Stones
- Carcinoma
- Stricture
- Atresia

Sclerosing cholangitis

Intrahepatic obstruction
- Drugs
- Granulomas
- Primary biliary cirrhosis
- Bile duct paucity
- Tumors

guidelines. For example, at http://bilitool.org, two options for determining risk are provided, each depending on the desired patient data for input. One requires the date and time of birth, date and time of draw, and the total bilirubin (milligrams per deciliter or micromoles per liter), whereas the other option requires the patient's age in hours and total bilirubin (milligrams per deciliter or micromoles per liter).

Interestingly, Trikalinos and colleagues and the US Preventative Services Task Force reported in 2009 that the benefits of implementing bilirubin screening did not provide evidence to decrease the incidence of kernicterus.[507,508] In contrast, a retrospective study by Kuzniewicz and colleagues of 360,000 term newborns showed a significant reduction in severe hyperbilirubinemia when bilirubin screening was implemented.[509] Consistent with these findings, a 5-year prospective study that involved more than 1 million infants showed universal bilirubin screening before discharge significantly reduced the incidence of severe hyperbilirubinemia with a small increase in phototherapy use.[510] Nevertheless, additional recommendations were made in 2009 that require universal predischarge bilirubin screening and a structured approach to management and follow-up based on the predischarge screening process.[511]

Clinical practice guidelines have been developed in several other countries, including Canada in 2001, the United Kingdom in 2008, Norway in 2011, and Australia in 2012.[512-515] Many recommendations are similar throughout these guidelines; however, there are notable differences.[516] For example, the United Kingdom guideline recommends interpreting bilirubin concentrations using a threshold table (not a nomogram) for infants at ≥38 weeks' gestation with hyperbilirubinemia. With the age determined in hours, and the bilirubin concentration, the table can be used to identify one of four follow-up procedures, such as repeating bilirubin measurement within 6 to 12 hours or starting phototherapy.

Physiologic Jaundice of the Newborn. Babies frequently become jaundiced within a few days of birth; this condition is known as physiologic jaundice of the newborn. Bilirubin concentrations reach a peak within 3 to 5 days of birth and remain elevated for less than 2 weeks. Bilirubin is usually less than 5 mg/dL (85 μmol/L), with 90% unconjugated. Factors contributing to physiologic jaundice include (1) an increased bilirubin load in the newborn because the RBCs have a shortened life span; (2) the appearance of "shunt" bilirubin, which is bilirubin derived from ineffective erythropoiesis or non-RBC sources; (3) decreased conjugation of bilirubin because of a relative lack of glucuronyl transferase (conjugating enzyme) in the first few days after birth; (4) increased absorption of bilirubin in the intestine caused by β-glucuronidase in meconium, which hydrolyzes bilirubin conjugates to unconjugated bilirubin that can be passively reabsorbed; and (5) exposure of breast-feeding infants to pregnanediol, nonesterified fatty acids, and other inhibitors of bilirubin conjugation present in breast milk.

Bilirubin concentrations of 13 mg/dL (222 μmol/L) or greater occurred in 6% of 2297 infants who weighed more than 2500 g.[517] Physiologic jaundice generally is not harmful, but bilirubin concentrations of more than 10 mg/dL (170 μmol/L), coupled with prematurity, low serum albumin, acidosis, and substances that compete for the binding sites of albumin (eg, ceftriaxone, sulfisoxazole, aspirin), may increase the risk for kernicterus. Physiologic jaundice of the newborn is treated with phototherapy; the infant is exposed to light of approximately 450 nm that disrupts intramolecular hydrogen bonds in the bilirubin molecule and yields several photoisomers that are more water soluble than the *Z,Z*-isomer and thus are excreted in the bile.[494] Exchange transfusions are rarely necessary.

Hemolytic Disease. Hemolytic disease of the newborn results from maternal–fetal incompatibility of Rhesus blood factors (Rh) in which the maternal Rh-negative blood becomes sensitized by a previous pregnancy with an Rh-positive fetus or an Rh-positive blood transfusion. The infant becomes jaundiced with unconjugated bilirubin in the first or second day of life and is susceptible to kernicterus. The diagnosis is confirmed by a Coombs' test with Rh-positive blood in the infant and Rh-negative blood in the mother. Other rare, inherited hemolytic anemias, such as glucose-6-phosphate dehydrogenase deficiency, may also lead to unconjugated hyperbilirubinemia (see Chapter 30 on Enzymes of the Red Blood Cell for more detail.)

Breast Milk Hyperbilirubinemia. This type of hyperbilirubinemia affects approximately 30% of breast-fed newborns. It is due to α-glucuronidase in breast milk, which hydrolyzes conjugated bilirubin in the intestine. The unconjugated bilirubin, being more lipophilic, is passively absorbed. The condition lasts for a few weeks and is treated by discontinuation of breast-feeding.

Conjugated Hyperbilirubinemias. These syndromes are characterized by hyperbilirubinemia in which conjugated bilirubin exceeds 1.5 mg/dL (26 μmol/L). The most important are idiopathic neonatal hepatitis and biliary atresia. Diagnosing the cholestatic syndromes may be difficult. The family history may be helpful in diagnosing α_1-antitrypsin deficiency, cystic fibrosis, galactosemia, hereditary fructose intolerance, and tyrosinosis. Serum tyrosine and α_1-antitrypsin concentrations should be obtained. If galactosemia is suspected, the diagnosis is confirmed by absence of the enzyme UDP galactose-1-phosphate uridyl transferase in cells and tissues, such as RBCs and liver. Serologic tests may be necessary for hepatitis A, B, and C, and for adenovirus, Coxsackie virus, cytomegalovirus, herpes simplex, rubella, and *Toxoplasma*. Liver biopsy may be performed, but the liver tends to look similar, with giant cells and extramedullary erythropoiesis dominating in hepatitis and cholestatic syndromes. The typical features of periportal red hyaline globules seen with periodic acid–Schiff stain that are characteristic for α_1-antitrypsin deficiency usually are not seen early in the course of the disorder. An HIDA isotope scan is essential for determining the patency of the biliary tree. Percutaneous or endoscopic cholangiography may be done in patients with equivocal HIDA scan results.

Conjugated hyperbilirubinemia is seen fairly often in the newborn as a complication of parenteral nutrition.

Idiopathic Neonatal Hepatitis

Approximately 75% of cases of hepatitis in the neonate are idiopathic giant cell hepatitis, a disorder of unknown origin characterized by cholestatic jaundice. A familial trend may reflect an autosomal recessive inheritance. Jaundice appears within the first 2 weeks. The child initially appears well and gains weight. The liver and spleen then become enlarged, and stools become pale. Serum aminotransferases are usually 400 U/L; the prothrombin time is prolonged. Liver biopsy reveals characteristic giant cells with hepatocyte acinar formation. Cholestasis is prominent. It is important to rule out extrahepatic biliary obstruction, such as occurs in biliary atresia, with an HIDA scan.

Treatment is supportive, with adequate nutrition and correction of hypoprothrombinemia. The prognosis is favorable, with 90% of infants surviving without sequelae.

Biliary Atresia

Biliary atresia is a heterogeneous group of acquired disorders that involve the extrahepatic or intrahepatic bile ducts. Possible causes include cytomegalovirus, reovirus III, Epstein-Barr virus, rubella virus, α_1-antitrypsin deficiency, Down syndrome, and trisomy 17 or 18.

Extrahepatic biliary atresia may involve all or part of the extrahepatic biliary tree. Also termed neonatal hepatitis, it is the most common cause for neonatal cholestasis and considered the most common reason for liver transplantation, accounting for 40% to 50% of all pediatric liver transplantations.[518] Obstruction due to either inflammation, fibrosis, or a mixed source results in biliary atresia. The frequency of disease changes with geographic region from 1 in 5600 in Taiwan[519] to 1 in 13,700 live births in the United States. Females are slightly more affected than males.[520] Symptoms begin within the first few months of life. The gallbladder is usually absent. Involvement of the hepatic or common duct leads to the characteristic syndrome of severe cholestatic jaundice. It occurs in 1 in 10,000 births, with females more commonly affected than males. Jaundice and pruritus usually appear in the first week. Stools are pale, and the urine is tea colored. Jaundice is deep, but the aminotransferases are only mildly elevated. If jaundice persists beyond 14 days of age, a direct or conjugated bilirubin measurement must be performed to exclude biliary atresia. If it is elevated, the urine should be tested for bile and the stool color inspected; if the stool is not green or yellow, biliary atresia is likely. Early identification of this condition is essential if these infants are to benefit from the operation of portoenterostomy, which should be performed no later than 60 days after birth.[521] If portoenterostomy is not successful, liver transplantation is the treatment of choice. Children rarely live beyond 3 years unless the lesion is surgically correctable.

More recently, clinical phenotypes have been developed based on the combination of clinical, pathological, and molecular features. The perinatal form is the most common clinical form. Approximately 80% of newborns fall into this phenotype. Characteristically, both jaundice and acholic stools develop after birth.[522] The embryonic form is found in 10% of affected newborns. Common features are associated with early onset injury, including the absence of extrahepatic bile ducts, and abnormalities of the spleen that may or may not be portal vein defects. When specific splenic and portal vein defects are observed, it is termed biliary atresia splenic malformation syndrome.[523] Patients with biliary atresia splenic malformation have poorer outcomes after hepatoportoenterostomy. Cystic biliary atresia is detected in approximately 8% of patients. In this phenotype, a cystic malformation is located near the obstructed site and has been correlated with improved bile drainage after hepatoportoenterostomy. Delaying portoenterostomy past 70 days of age will typically have a poorer response.[524,525] The last phenotype is cytomegalovirus-associated biliary atresia. Several studies have indicated that the presence of cytomegalovirus results in poor bile drainage and a high risk of death after hepatoportoenterostomy.[526] Staging of biliary atresia remains unclear because histopathology, molecular staging, and clinical outcome lack correlation. Numerous factors for the observed pathophysiology have been implicated, such as defective embryogenesis, genetic factors, environmental factors, viral infection, and autoimmunity. These factors have been classified into three broad categories of abnormal morphogenesis, environmental factors, and inflammatory dysregulation.[527] Research to improve the outcome of this disease has progressed substantially; however, much remains to be completed. Fortunately, large multicenter investigations will be facilitated by the European consortium of Biliary Atresia and Related Disease and the Childhood Liver Disease Research Network.[528,529]

Intrahepatic biliary atresia is characterized by a paucity of intrahepatic bile ducts. Jaundice usually appears within the first few days of life. Serum bilirubin is elevated, and serum cholesterol may be very high, leading to the formation of xanthomas. The hepatic histology is nonspecific, showing bile duct paucity, giant cells, inflammation, and fibrosis. Survival into adolescence is common, although growth is usually retarded.

A syndromic variant, Alagille syndrome,[530] has similar features, but it is an autosomal dominant condition with a characteristic triangular face, skeletal abnormalities, retinal pigmentation, and pulmonary stenosis.

Treatment of intrahepatic biliary atresia includes intramuscular replacement of vitamins A, D, and E. Medium-chain triglycerides that do not need bile acids for absorption provide calories in patients with partial atresia. Cholestyramine may relieve pruritus. Ursodeoxycholic acid reduces serum enzyme activities and relieves pruritus in some patients.

Analytical Methods

Several analytical techniques are used to measure bilirubin and metabolites in serum, urine, and feces. Measurement of bilirubin in amniotic fluid is discussed in Chapter 43 on Body Fluids.

Serum Bilirubin

The reaction of bilirubin with diazotized sulfanilic acid, known as the diazo reaction, discovered by Ehrlich in 1883 and applied to the measurement of bilirubin in serum and bile by van den Bergh and Muller in 1916, is the basis of the most widely used methods for measuring bilirubin. These researchers observed, in sera from jaundiced infants, the reaction was slow and required an accelerator to proceed, and that it was rapid in bile and in adult sera without addition of ethanol, which led to the terms indirect and direct bilirubin, respectively. The chemical nature of direct and indirect bilirubins was elucidated by Billing and colleagues in the mid-1950s.[531] By using open-column, reversed-phase chromatography on siliconized kieselguhr (cellite or diatomaceous earth), investigators isolated three bilirubin fractions—unconjugated bilirubin (indirect reacting fraction) and bilirubin monoglucuronide and diglucuronide (direct reacting fractions). Kuenzle and colleagues[532] were the first to successfully use an open-column chromatography technique that did not involve a deproteinization step. They obtained four bilirubin fractions—unconjugated bilirubin (α-bilirubin), monoconjugated bilirubin (β-bilirubin), diconjugated bilirubin (γ-bilirubin), and a fraction bound strongly to protein (δ-bilirubin). The last fraction was clearly distinct from the albumin-bilirubin complex that exists in serum.

Diazo Methods. The most widely used chemical methods for bilirubin measurement are those based on the coupling of bilirubin with a diazo compound.[533] In this reaction (Fig. 38.25), diazotized sulfanilic acid (the diazo reagent) reacts with bilirubin to produce two azodipyrroles (azopigments), which are reddish-purple at neutral pH and blue at low or high pH values. Van den Bergh and Muller[534] applied this reaction to the quantitation of bilirubin in serum. They described the fraction of bilirubin that reacted with the diazo reagent in the absence of alcohol as the direct bilirubin fraction and used the term indirect bilirubin for the difference between total bilirubin (found after the addition of alcohol to the reaction mixture) and the direct bilirubin fraction. Numerous variations of the van den Bergh and Muller method have been developed. All use one of a variety of "accelerators," which, like alcohol, facilitate the reaction of unconjugated (indirect) bilirubin with the diazo reagent; the most commonly used accelerators are caffeine,[535] dyphylline,[536] and several surface active agents. The diazo method of Malloy and Evelyn,[537] which uses methanol as an accelerator, has substantial matrix effects, negative interference by Hb, turbidity due to protein precipitation by methanol, and a long reaction time.[538] This method, which has been virtually abandoned, is mentioned here for historical reasons only.

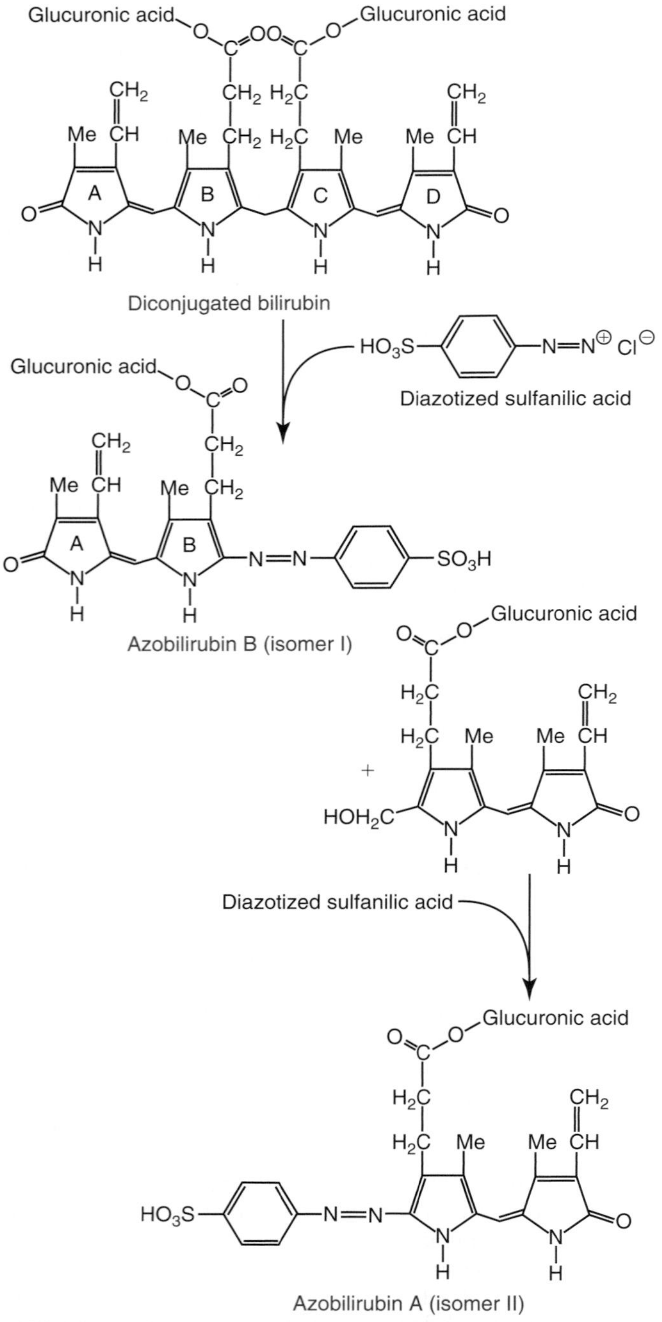

Glucuronic acid — Glucuronic acid — Diconjugated bilirubin — HO_3S–C₆H₄–$N{\equiv}N^{\oplus}\ Cl^{\ominus}$ Diazotized sulfanilic acid — Azobilirubin B (isomer I) — + — Diazotized sulfanilic acid — Azobilirubin A (isomer II)

FIGURE 38.25 The Reaction of Bilirubin Glucuronide With Diazotized Sulfanilic Acid to Produce Isomers I and II of Azobilirubin B. Unconjugated bilirubin reacts in the same way to produce isomers I and II of azobilirubin A.

The diazo method described by Jendrassik and Grof in 1938[535] and later modified by Doumas and colleagues[539] gives results for serum total bilirubin that are reproducible and reliable.[540-542] In this procedure, an aqueous solution of caffeine and sodium benzoate serve as the accelerators. Studies on the mechanism by which the caffeine-benzoate solution facilitates the reaction of unconjugated bilirubin with the diazo reagent have provided strong, albeit indirect, evidence that caffeine, and perhaps benzoate, displaces unconjugated bilirubin from its association sites on albumin. This occurs by (1) formation of hydrogen bonds between bilirubin and caffeine,[543,544] thus making bilirubin water soluble, or (2) complex formation and disruption of the bilirubin internal hydrogen bonds. With the use of samples prepared by addition of unconjugated bilirubin and authentic human diconjugated (with glucuronic acid) bilirubin to low-bilirubin pooled sera—and a nuclear magnetic resonance technique—Lo and Wu[545] have shown that the modified Jendrassik-Grof total bilirubin assay detects unconjugated and diconjugated bilirubin quantitatively (as unconjugated bilirubin equivalents). This method has acceptable transferability among laboratories[540,542,546] and is currently the method of choice.

Other methods for determining bilirubin include direct spectrophotometric measurement of total bilirubin in serum using analysis of a two-component system by measuring absorbance at two wavelengths and solving a system of two simultaneous equations. This approach is applicable to sera from healthy neonates because only unconjugated bilirubin is present in such sera. Correction for oxyhemoglobin is necessary because it is invariably present in sera from neonates.

Calibrators for Bilirubin Measurements. A number of instrument manufacturers use bovine serum, instead of human serum, as the protein base for preparing fluids for calibrating methods for total and direct bilirubin; the protein base is enriched with unconjugated bilirubin or ditaurobilirubin or both. Unconjugated bilirubin in human serum reacts completely with the reference method and with diazo methods available in commonly used clinical analyzers; however, its reaction in bovine serum from commercial sources is incomplete and unpredictable.[547] That makes the assignment of accurate bilirubin values to calibrators virtually impossible, the protein base of which is commercial bovine serum. In human serum, ditaurobilirubin was underestimated by two of seven clinical analyzers tested;

the calibrators of these two analyzers were made in bovine serum. Ditaurobilirubin in commercial bovine serum was underestimated by all analyzers and by the reference method; in human serum, it was underestimated by two analyzers only. The practice of using bilirubin calibrators in bovine sera should be abandoned because it compromises the accuracy of bilirubin measurements in jaundiced neonates. However, fresh bovine serum (obtained from a slaughterhouse) has only a small effect on the measurement of unconjugated bilirubin or ditaurobilirubin.

High-Performance Liquid Chromatography. High-performance liquid chromatography (HPLC) methods have been developed for relatively rapid separation and quantification of the four bilirubin fractions. HPLC has been helpful in separating and detecting the various bilirubin photoisomers produced during phototherapy in newborns and thus in elucidating the mechanism by which phototherapy lowers the concentration of bilirubin in newborn blood.[474,548] Several HPLC methods are available for analysis of bilirubin fractions. In the method of Blanckaert,[549] bilirubin conjugates, but not unconjugated bilirubin, are converted to the corresponding bilirubin methyl esters by base-catalyzed transesterification in methanol followed by extraction with chloroform. With this procedure, the α-, β-, and γ-bilirubin fractions are recoverable, but the δ-fraction (δ-bilirubin) remains in the denatured protein pellet that is produced by the chloroform extraction. In the HPLC method of Lauff and coworkers,[550] all four bilirubin fractions remain in solution after a step that involves salting out globulins with sodium sulfate. Both methods require the use of dim incandescent or yellow light to minimize photodegradation of the various bilirubin species. A simple and fast HPLC method has been published by Adachi and associates[551]; this method uses a Micronex RP-30 column (Sekisui Chemical Co., Mount Laurel, New Jersey), which does not require salting out of globulins or chemical transformation of bilirubin conjugates. This method separates serum bilirubin into five fractions; the fifth fraction eluted between the monoglucuronide and the unconjugated bilirubin is the *Z,E* or the *E,Z* photoisomer. The elution sequence is the same as in the procedure of Lauff and colleagues.[550] Osawa and associates have successfully developed an isocratic mobile phase.[552] The elution buffer includes 0.8% sodium ascorbate to maintain the stability of the bilirubin species. Isolation was improved with the addition of 1% Brij 35. This method strongly correlates with the HPLC method by Adachi and colleagues. Using the method by Osawa and colleagues, molar absorptivities for unconjugated bilirubin, bilirubin monoglucuronide, bilirubin diglucuronide, and δ -bilirubin were calculated at 450 nm, giving this method the potential for evaluating the accuracy of bilirubin assays.

Additional studies have indicated that the δ-bilirubin fraction consists of one or more bilirubin species that are covalently bound to albumin.[553] Existence of covalent linkage is supported by the fact that the associated bilirubin species are not released from the albumin fraction by treatment with strong acid or base, or a variety of strong denaturing agents, by hydrolysis with proteolytic enzymes, or by boiling in methanol. Delta-bilirubin reacts directly (without a promoter) with diazotized sulfanilic acid. The discovery of δ-bilirubin has solved the mystery of persistent high bilirubin concentrations that mostly direct react in patients with intrahepatic or obstructing jaundice long after hepatitis has subsided or obstruction has been relieved. It is the slowest fraction to clear from serum because it follows the catabolism of albumin, which has a half-life of approximately 17 to 19 days.

HPLC has been helpful in elucidating the nature of the bilirubin species that occur naturally in blood or are formed during phototherapy. Clinically, it offers little, if any, aid to the physician in the differential diagnosis of jaundice, because knowing the percentage of each of the bilirubin fractions in blood is of no diagnostic value. It cannot be considered as a reference method for measuring total bilirubin in blood because its accuracy and precision are inadequate. The method is calibrated with unconjugated bilirubin with the untested assumption that the other three bilirubin fractions have molar absorptivities identical to that of the calibrator,[554] when in fact this is not known. Furthermore, errors in measurement of the four species may be cumulative and may result in a large total error; also, the method is insensitive at total bilirubin concentrations of less than 1 mg/dL (17 μmol/L) and is too laborious for routine clinical analysis. Some of the δ-bilirubin may be lost during pretreatment of samples.

A capillary electrophoresis method for measuring the different types of bilirubin has been developed by Wu and his associates.[555]

Enzymatic Methods. Enzymatic methods for total and direct bilirubin and for bilirubin conjugates with glucuronic acid are based on the oxidation of bilirubin with bilirubin oxidase to biliverdin with molecular oxygen.[556] At a pH near 8, and in the presence of sodium cholate and sodium dodecylsulfate, all four bilirubin fractions are oxidized to biliverdin, which is further oxidized to purple and finally colorless products. The decrease in absorbance at 425 or 460 nm is proportional to the concentration of total bilirubin. Results obtained by the bilirubin oxidase method were in good agreement with those obtained by the Jendrassik-Grof procedure.[557] Direct bilirubin is measured at pH 3.7 to 4.5; at this pH range, the enzyme oxidizes bilirubin conjugates and δ-bilirubin, but not unconjugated bilirubin.[558,559] At pH 10, the enzyme selectively oxidizes the two glucuronides.[559,560] Delta-bilirubin is not oxidized at all, and only 5% of unconjugated bilirubin is measured as conjugates.[560]

Transcutaneous Measurement of Bilirubin. A noninvasive approach for measuring bilirubin was introduced in 1980 by Yamanouchi and colleagues.[561] The first bilirubinometer (icterometer) was a reflectance photometer, which used two filters to correct for the color of Hb and required measurements at eight body sites. Efforts to improve the accuracy of such measurements have been successful and led to the development of devices of acceptable performance. Reports indicate that at least one of these devices (Bili*Check* $SpectR_x$ Inc., Norcross, Georgia) provides results that are within ±2 mg/dL (34 μmol/L) of those obtained using a serum diazo procedure.[562,563] Another study found that the Bili*Check* underestimated serum bilirubin when its concentration was greater than 10 mg/dL (170 μmol/L).[564]

Although transcutaneous bilirubin measurements may not substitute for laboratory quantitative determinations, they provide instantaneous information, reduce the necessity for serum bilirubin determinations, spare infants the trauma of heelsticks, and save money.[565] Furthermore, they are useful in determining whether it is necessary to draw blood in a jaundiced infant before initiating treatment, such as phototherapy or exchange transfusion (currently, this is extremely rare). Another application is predicting those babies who require follow-up according to the "hour-specific" serum bilirubin nomogram developed by Bhutani and coworkers.[505]

See also the section on Guidelines for Assessing Risk earlier in this chapter.

Urine Bilirubin. Because only conjugated bilirubin is excreted in urine, its presence indicates conjugated hyperbilirubinemia. The most commonly used method for detecting bilirubin in urine involves the use of a dipstick impregnated with a diazo reagent. Dipstick methods are capable of detecting bilirubin concentrations as low as 0.5 mg/dL (9 μmol/L) .

A fresh urine specimen is required because bilirubin is unstable when exposed to light and room temperature, and it may be oxidized to biliverdin (which is diazo negative) at the normally acidic pH of the urine. If the test is delayed, the sample must be protected from light and stored at 2°C to 8°C for no longer than 24 hours. The reagent strip (ChemStrip, Roche Diagnostics, Indianapolis, Illinois; Multistix, Siemens Healthcare Diagnostics, Deerfield, Illinois) is immersed in the urine specimen for no longer than 1 second and is read 60 seconds later. During this time, bilirubin reacts with a diazo reagent, yielding a pink to red-violet color, the intensity of which is proportional to the bilirubin concentration. The reaction mechanism for urinary conjugated bilirubin is the same as that described in Fig. 38.25, except that 2,6-dichlorobenzene-diazonium-tetrafluoroborate is substituted for diazotized sulfanilic acid in the Chemstrip, and 2,4-dichloroaniline diazonium salt in the Multistix. Another commonly used test, more sensitive than the Multistix, is the Ictotest reagent tablet (Siemens Healthcare Diagnostics); in this semiquantitative procedure, the diazo reagent is *p*-nitrobenzenediazonium-*p*-toluenesulfonate.

Chemstrip and Multistix strips for bilirubin in urine are highly specific tests and have a low incidence of false-positive results. However, medications that color the urine red or that give a red color in an acid medium, such as phenazopyridine, can produce a false-positive reading. Large quantities of ascorbic acid or of nitrite also worsen the detection limit of the test. In practice, bilirubin is rarely measured in urine.

Urobilinogen in Urine and Feces

The measurement of urobilinogen in urine is of no diagnostic value in the assessment of liver disease. The same applies to the measurement of urobilinogen in fecal 72- or 96-hour specimens. Both tests are obsolete and are not presented here.

SELECTED REFERENCES

For a full list of references for this chapter, please refer to ExpertConsult.com.

14. Piel FB, Weatherall DJ. The α-thalassemias. *N Engl J Med* 2014;**371**:1908–16.
16. Fucharoen S, Viprakasit V. Hb H disease: clinical course and disease modifiers. *Hematology Am Soc Hematol Educ Program* 2009;**1**:26–34.
25. Borgna-Pignatti C, Marsella M. Iron chelation in thalassemia major. *Clin Ther* 2015;**37**:2866–77.
26. Baronciani D, Angelucci E, Potschger U, et al. Hemopoietic stem cell transplantation in thalassemia: a report from the European Society for Blood and Bone Marrow Transplantation Hemoglobinopathy Registry, 2000-2010. *Bone Marrow Transplant* 2016;**51**:536–41.
28. Musallam KM, Rivella S, Vichinsky E, et al. Non-transfusion dependent thalassemia. *Haematologica* 2013;**98**:833–44.
51. Schoorl M, Schoorl M, van Pelt J, et al. Application of innovative hemocytometric parameters and algorithms for improvement of microcytic anemia discrimination. *Hematol Rep* 2015;**7**:5843.
52. Brugnara C, Mohandas N. Red cell indices in classification and treatment of anemias: from M.M. Wintrobes's original 1934 classification to the third millennium. *Curr Opin Hematol* 2013;**20**:222–30.
111. Girelli D, Nemeth E, Swinkels DW. Hepcidin in the diagnostics of iron disorders. *Blood* 2016;**127**: 2809–13.
118. Fleming RE, Ponka P. Iron overload in human disease. *N Engl J Med* 2012;**366**:348–59.
138. Wang W, Knovich MA, Coffman LG, et al. Serum ferritin: past, present and future. *Biochim Biophys Acta* 2010;**1800**:760–9.
155. Camaschella C. Iron-deficiency anemia. *N Engl J Med* 2015;**372**:1832–43.
186. Donker AE, Raymakers RA, Vlasveld LT, et al. Practice guidelines for the diagnosis and management of microcytic anemias due to genetic disorders of iron metabolism or heme synthesis. *Blood* 2014;**123**:3873–86.
199. Weiss G, Goodnough LT. Anemia of chronic disease. *N Engl J Med* 2005;**352**:1011–23.
212. Beutler E, Felitti VJ, Koziol JA, et al. Penetrance of 845G–> A (C282Y) HFE hereditary haemochromatosis mutation in the USA. *Lancet* 2002;**359**:211–18.
215. Gurrin LC, Bertalli NA, Dalton GW, et al. HFE C282Y/H63D compound heterozygotes are at low risk of hemochromatosis-related morbidity. *Hepatology* 2009;**50**: 94–101.
322. Guyatt GH, Oxman AD, Ali M, et al. Laboratory diagnosis of iron-deficiency anemia: an overview. *J Gen Intern Med* 1992;**7**:145–53.
327. Ferraro S, Mozzi R, Panteghini M. Revaluating serum ferritin as a marker of body iron stores in the traceability era. *Clin Chem Lab Med* 2012;**50**:1911–16.
396. van der Vorm LN, Hendriks JC, Laarakkers CM, et al. Toward worldwide hepcidin assay harmonization: identification of a commutable secondary reference material. *Clin Chem* 2016;**62**:993–1001.
397. Beguin Y. Soluble transferrin receptor for the evaluation of erythropoiesis and iron status. *Clin Chim Acta* 2003;**329**: 9–22.
473. Lightner DA. Structure, photochemistry, and organic chemistry of bilirubin. In: Heirwegh KPM, Brown SB, editors. *Bilirubin Chemistry*. Boca Raton, FL: CRC Press; 1982. p. 1–58.
483. Erlinger S, Arias IM, Dhumeaux D. Inherited disorders of bilirubin transport and conjugation: new insights into molecular mechanisms and consequences. *Gastroenterology* 2014;**146**:1625–38.
504. Subcommittee on Hyperbilirubinemia. Management of hyperbilirubinemia in the newborn infant 35 or more weeks of gestation. *Pediatrics* 2004;**114**:297–316.

527. Asai A, Miethke A, Bezerra JA. Pathogenesis of biliary atresia: defining biology to understand clinical phenotypes. *Nat Rev Gastroenterol Hepatol* 2015;**12**: 342–52.

539. Doumas BT, Poon PKC, Perry BW, et al. Candidate reference method for determination of total bilirubin in serum: development and validation. *Clin Chem* 1985;**31**: 1779–89.

541. Lo SF, Jendrzejczak B, Doumas BT. Laboratory performance in neonatal bilirubin testing using commutable specimens: a progress report on a College of American Pathology study. *Arch Pathol Lab Med* 2008;**132**:1781–5.

39

Porphyrins and the Porphyrias

Michael N. Badminton, Sharon D. Whatley, Eliane Sardh, and Aasne K. Aarsand

ABSTRACT

Background

The porphyrias are a group of rare, mainly inherited metabolic disorders that result from decreased or, in one rare form of erythropoietic protoporphyria increased, activities of the enzymes of heme biosynthesis. Each porphyria is defined by the association of characteristic clinical features with a specific pattern of accumulation of heme precursors that reflects increased formation of the substrate of the enzyme that is partially deficient or becomes secondarily rate-limiting in that type of porphyria.

Content

This chapter describes the metabolic pathway and regulation of heme biosynthesis, the excretion of heme precursors, the different porphyrias, and abnormalities of porphyrin metabolism not caused by porphyria. Porphyrias can be classified as hepatic or erythropoietic according to the main site of overproduction of heme precursors. From a clinical viewpoint, porphyrias are usually classified as acute, in which acute neurovisceral attacks occur, or as nonacute. Acute porphyrias include 5-aminolevulinate (ALA) dehydratase deficiency porphyria, acute intermittent porphyria (AIP), variegate porphyria (VP), and hereditary coproporphyria (HCP). The nonacute porphyrias encompass porphyria cutanea tarda (PCT), congenital erythropoietic porphyria (CEP), and EPP. This chapter also covers the diagnostic approaches, with detailed information on biochemical and genetic analysis, and clinical management of the various forms of porphyrias.

The porphyrias are a group of uncommon, inherited disorders of heme biosynthesis.[1,2] Each porphyria results from a partial deficiency of one of the enzymes of the pathway converting ALA to heme, or in one disorder, increased activity of the rate-controlling enzyme of erythroid heme biosynthesis. Each functional abnormality is associated with a specific pattern of overproduction, accumulation, and excretion of pathway intermediates, which are excreted in excessive amounts in urine, feces, or both. The clinical consequences depend on the nature of the heme precursors that accumulate. In the acute porphyrias, excess porphyrin precursors (ALA and porphobilinogen [PBG]) are associated with potentially fatal acute neurovisceral attacks that most often are provoked by various commonly prescribed drugs or hormonal factors. In the nonacute porphyrias, and in those acute porphyrias in which skin lesions occur, accumulation of porphyrins results in photosensitization of sun-exposed skin. Diagnosis depends on laboratory investigations to demonstrate the pattern of heme precursor accumulation and excretion specific for each type of porphyria, and it requires examination of appropriate specimens for the key metabolites using adequately sensitive and specific methods. DNA analysis is rarely necessary for diagnosis of symptomatic cases, but it is the method of choice when investigating healthy at-risk relatives. Molecular analysis also continues to provide new information about the underlying pathophysiology. Abnormalities of porphyrin accumulation and excretion also occur in a wide variety of other disorders that are collectively more common than the porphyrias. Recognition of secondary porphyrin disorders is important to avoid diagnostic errors.

PORPHYRIN CHEMISTRY

Before porphyrin synthesis and disorders of porphyrin metabolism are discussed, porphyrin structure, nomenclature, and chemical characteristics are reviewed.

Structure and Nomenclature

The basic porphyrin structure consists of four monopyrrole rings connected by methene bridges to form a tetrapyrrole ring (Fig. 39.1).[1] Many porphyrin compounds are known, but only a limited number are of clinical interest. The porphyrin compounds of relevance to the porphyrias (Table 39.1) differ in the substituents occupying peripheral positions 1 through 8. Variation in the distribution of the same substituents around the peripheral positions of the tetrapyrrole ring gives rise to porphyrin isomers, which are usually depicted by Roman numerals (eg, I, II, III). The reduced form of a porphyrin, known as a porphyrinogen (see Fig. 39.1), differs by the absence of six hydrogens (four from the methylene bridges and two from ring nitrogens). Porphyrinogens are unstable in vitro and are spontaneously oxidized to the corresponding porphyrins. Under the lower oxygen tension of the cell, porphyrinogens are sufficiently stable to act as intermediates of the heme biosynthetic pathway; aromatization to protoporphyrin at the penultimate step requires an enzyme.

Chelation of Metals

The arrangement of four nitrogen atoms in the center of the porphyrin ring enables porphyrins to chelate various metal ions. Protoporphyrin that contains iron (Fe) is known as heme; ferroheme refers specifically to the Fe^{2+} complex and ferriheme to Fe^{3+}. Ferriheme associated with a chloride counter ion is known as hemin or as hematin when the counter ion is hydroxide.

Spectral Properties

Porphyrins were named from the Greek root for "purple" ("porphyra") and owe their color to the conjugated double-bond structure of the tetrapyrrole ring. The porphyrinogens have no conjugated double bonds, and therefore, are colorless. Porphyrins show particularly strong absorbance near 400 nm, often called the Soret band. When exposed to light in the 400-nm region, porphyrins display a characteristic orange-red fluorescence in the range of 550 to 650 nm. Absorbance and fluorescence are altered by substituents around the porphyrin ring and by metal binding. Zinc (Zn) chelation shifts the fluorescence emission peak of protoporphyrin to shorter wavelengths and reduces the fluorescence intensity. The strong binding of iron alters the character of protoporphyrin to the extent that heme lacks significant fluorescence.

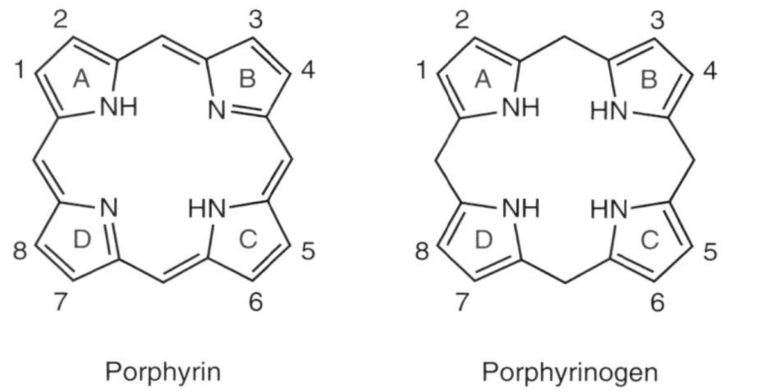

Porphyrin Porphyrinogen

FIGURE 39.1 **Porphyrin and porphyrinogen structures.** Numbers 1 to 8 represent various substituents, the nature and order of which determine the type of porphyrin or porphyrinogen (see Table 39.1). The numbering system and ring designations are based on the Fischer system. A revised system formulated by the International Union of Pure and Applied Chemistry–International Union of Biochemistry Joint Commission on Biochemical Nomenclature is appropriate for more complex needs. Because of increasing complexity, this Roman numeral designation is no longer recommended above IV.[190]

Solubility

Porphyrins are only marginally soluble in water. The differing solubilities of individual porphyrins are of importance not only in the design of analytical methods for their extraction and fractionation but in determining the route of excretion from the body. At pH 7, the carboxyl groups are ionized, and the molecule has a net negative charge. Below pH 2, the pyrrole nitrogens and the carboxyl groups become protonated so that the molecule has a net positive charge. At physiological pH, the solubility of a given porphyrin is determined by the number of substituent carboxyl groups. Uroporphyrin has eight carboxylate groups and is the most soluble porphyrin in aqueous media. Protoporphyrin has only two carboxylate groups and is essentially insoluble in water, but it dissolves readily in lipid environments and binds readily to the hydrophobic regions of proteins (eg, albumin). Coproporphyrin, with four carboxylate groups, has intermediate solubility.

Traditional extraction methods for porphyrins involve two steps, extraction into an acidified organic solvent, followed by a second or back extraction into aqueous acid. The initial extraction takes advantage of the fact that at pH 3 to 5 (near to their isoelectric point) porphyrins are less soluble in aqueous media and move into the organic phase. Coproporphyrin and protoporphyrin are readily extracted into diethyl ether, but the more carboxylated porphyrins (uroporphyrin and heptacarboxylate porphyrin) require a more hydrophilic solvent such as cyclohexanone or butanol. The back extraction induces porphyrin compounds to move back into the aqueous solution by decreasing the pH to less than 2, which causes protonation of the pyrrolenine nitrogen and carboxylate groups, thereby reversing the solubility characteristics of porphyrins. Compounds such as heme and chlorophyll, in which the pyrrole nitrogens are tightly bound to Fe and magnesium, respectively, remain uncharged at low pH and trapped in the organic layer.

HEME BIOSYNTHESIS

The complex tetrapyrrole ring structure of heme is built up in a stepwise fashion from the very simple precursors succinyl–coenzyme A (CoA) and glycine (Fig. 39.2).[3] The

TABLE 39.1 Substituents Around the Macrocycle in Porphyrins of Clinical Importance

Position	1	2	3	4	5	6	7	8
Uroporphyrin-I	C_m	C_{et}	C_m	C_{et}	C_m	C_{et}	C_m	C_{et}
Uroporphyrin-III	C_m	C_{et}	C_m	C_{et}	C_m	C_{et}	C_{et}	C_m
Heptacarboxylate porphyrin-III	C_m	C_{et}	C_m	C_{et}	C_m	C_{et}	C_{et}	Me
Hexacarboxylate porphyrin-III	Me	C_{et}	C_m	C_{et}	C_m	C_{et}	C_{et}	Me
Pentacarboxylate porphyrin-III	Me	C_{et}	Me	C_{et}	C_m	C_{et}	C_{et}	Me
Coproporphyrin-I	Me	C_{et}	Me	C_{et}	Me	C_{et}	Me	C_{et}
Coproporphyrin-III	Me	C_{et}	Me	C_{et}	Me	C_{et}	C_{et}	Me
Isocoproporphyrin	Me	Et	Me	C_{et}	C_m	C_{et}	C_{et}	Me
Dehydroisocoproporphyrin	Me	Vn	Me	C_{et}	C_m	C_{et}	C_{et}	Me
Deethylisocoproporphyrin	Me	H	Me	C_{et}	C_m	C_{et}	C_{et}	Me
Protoporphyrin	Me	Vn	Me	Vn	Me	C_{et}	C_{et}	Me
Pemptoporphyrin	Me	H	Me	Vn	Me	C_{et}	C_{et}	Me
Deuteroporphyrin	Me	H	Me	H	Me	C_{et}	C_{et}	Me
Mesoporphyrin	Me	Et	Me	Et	Me	C_{et}	C_{et}	Me

C_{et}, Carboxyethyl (–CH_2CH_2COOH); C_m, Carboxymethyl (–CH_2COOH); *Et,* ethyl (–CH_2CH_3); *Me,* methyl (–CH_3); *Vn,* vinyl (–CH=CH_2).

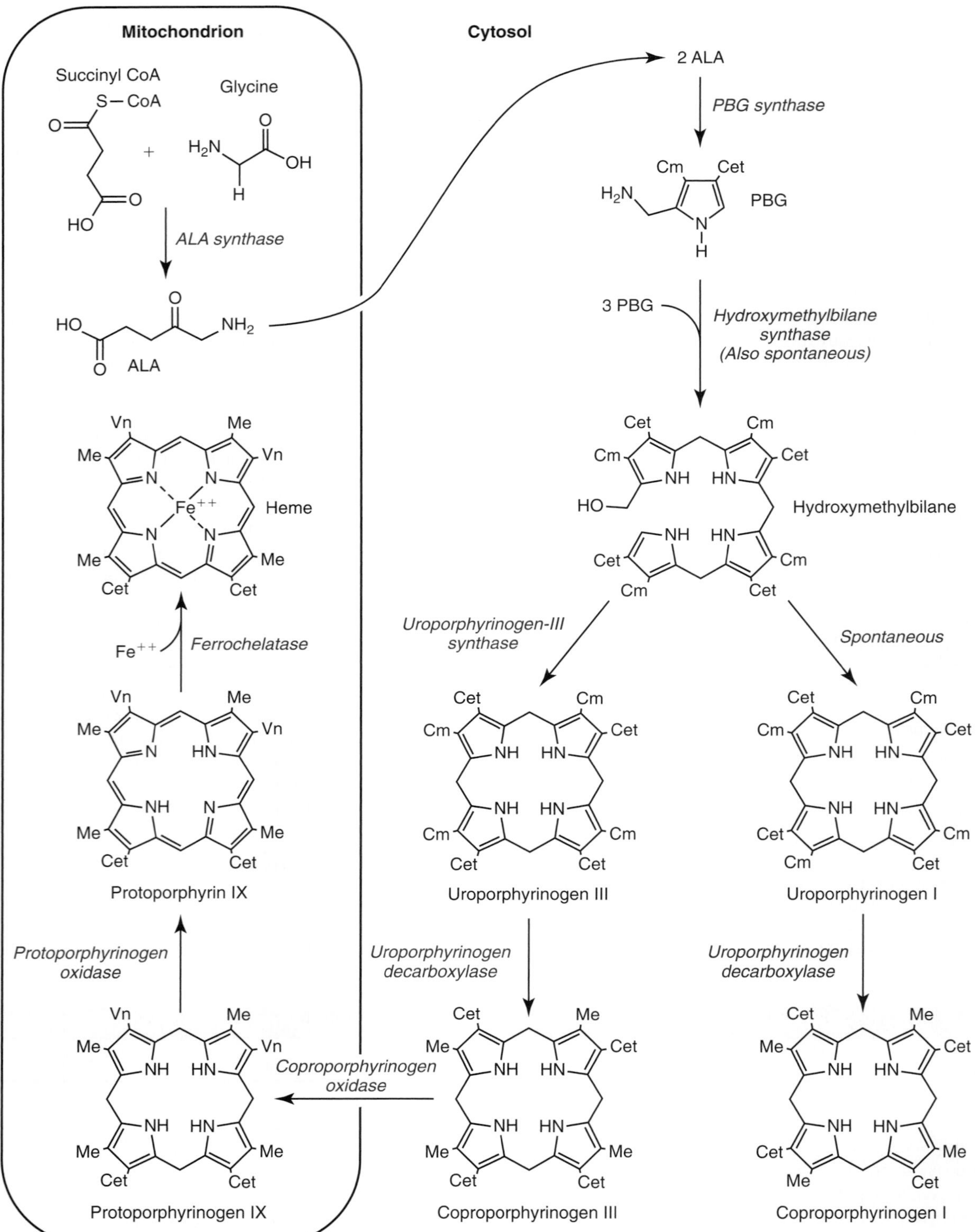

FIGURE 39.2 Biosynthetic pathway of porphyrins and heme. *C_{et}*, Carboxyethyl (–CH_2CH_2COOH); *C_m*, carboxymethyl (–CH_2COOH); *CoA*, coenzyme A; *Fe*, iron; *Me*, methyl (–CH_3); *Vn*, vinyl (–CH=CH_2); *PBG*, porphobilinogen.

TABLE 39.2 Human Enzymes and Genes of Heme Biosynthesis

Enzyme	Monomer Mol Mass*† (kDa)	Chromosomal Location of Gene	Gene Size (kb)	No. of Exons	Expression
ALAS1	70.6	3p21.2	17	12	Ubiquitous
ALAS2	64.6	Xp11.21	22	11	Erythroid cells
ALAD	36.3	9q32	13	13	Ubiquitous and erythroid-specific mRNAs
HMBS	37.0	11q23.3	10	15	Ubiquitous and erythroid-specific isoforms
UROS	29.5	10q26.1-q26.2	34	10	Ubiquitous and erythroid-specific mRNAs
UROD	40.8	1p34.1	3	10	Ubiquitous
CPOX	40.3	3q11.2-q12.1	14	7	Ubiquitous
PPOX	50.8	1q23.3	5	13	Ubiquitous
FECH	47.8	18q21.3	45	11	Ubiquitous

*5-Aminolevulinic acid dehydratase (ALAD) is a homo-octamer, and hydroxymethylbilane synthase (HMBS) and uroporphyrinogen-III synthase (UROS) are monomers; all other enzymes are homodimers.

†Molecular masses for 5-aminolevulinate synthase (ALAS)1, ALAS2, coproporphyrinogen oxidase (CPOX), and ferrochelatase (FECH) include presequences that are cleaved during mitochondrial import.

PPOX, Protoporphyrinogen oxidase; *UROD*, uroporphyrinogen decarboxylase.

pathway is present in all nucleated cells. From measurements of total bilirubin production,[4] it has been estimated that daily synthesis of heme in humans is 5 to 8 mmol/kg body weight. Of this, 70% to 80% occurs in the bone marrow and is used for hemoglobin synthesis. Approximately 15% is synthesized in other tissues, mainly in the liver, and is used to produce cytochrome P450, mitochondrial cytochromes, and other hemoproteins. The pathway is compartmentalized, with some steps occurring in the mitochondrion and others in the cytoplasm. Several carriers that transfer intermediates across the mitochondrial membrane have now been identified.[5-7] Although all are potential sites for pathogenic mutations, so far only one such mutation has been identified: a mutation in the erythroid-specific mitochondrial glycine transporter SLC25A38 that causes nonsyndromic autosomal recessive sideroblastic anemia.[5]

Enzymes of Heme Biosynthesis

The genes for all enzymes of human heme biosynthesis have been characterized (Table 39.2). The enzymes of the heme synthesis pathway listed by name and Enzyme Commission (EC) number are described in the following paragraph. The structures of human hydroxymethylbilane synthase (HMBS), uroporphyrinogen-III synthase (UROS), uroporphyrinogen decarboxylase (UROD), coproporphyrinogen oxidase (CPOX), ferrochelatase (FECH), bacterial 5-aminolevulinate synthase (ALAS), 5-aminolevulinic acid dehydratase (ALAD), and protoporphyrinogen oxidase (PPOX) have been determined by x-ray crystallography.[8-15]

5-Aminolevulinate Synthase (EC 2.3.1.37)

ALAS, the initial enzyme of the pathway, catalyzes the formation of ALA from succinyl-CoA and glycine. The enzyme is mitochondrial and requires a cofactor of pyridoxal phosphate, which forms a Schiff base with the amino group of glycine at the enzyme surface. The carbanion of the Schiff base displaces CoA from succinyl-CoA with the formation of α-amino-β-ketoadipic acid, which is then decarboxylated to ALA. The activity of ALAS is rate limiting as long as the catalytic capacities of other enzymes in the pathway are normal.

5-Aminolevulinic Acid Dehydratase (EC 4.2.1.24)

5-Aminolevulinic acid dehydratase (also known as PBG synthase) is a cytoplasmic enzyme that catalyzes the formation of the monopyrrole PBG from two molecules of ALA with elimination of two molecules of water. The enzyme requires Zn ions as a cofactor and reduced sulfhydryl groups at the active site; therefore, it is susceptible to inhibition by lead.

Hydroxymethylbilane Synthase (EC 2.5.1.61)

Hydroxymethylbilane synthase (also known as PBG deaminase) is a cytoplasmic enzyme that catalyzes the formation of one molecule of the linear tetrapyrrole 1-hydroxymethylbilane (HMB; also known as preuroporphyrinogen) from four molecules of PBG with the release of four molecules of ammonia.[16] The enzyme has two molecules of its own substrate: PBG, which is attached covalently to the apoenzyme as a prosthetic group.[17] The enzyme is susceptible to allosteric inhibition by intermediates farther down the heme biosynthetic pathway, notably coproporphyrinogen-III and protoporphyrinogen-IX.[18]

Uroporphyrinogen-III Synthase (EC 4.2.1.75)

Uroporphyrinogen-III synthase is a cytoplasmic enzyme that rearranges and cyclizes HMB to form uroporphyrinogen-III.[16] Each pyrrole ring of HMB contains a methylcarboxylate and an ethylcarboxylate substituent, which are in the same orientation. By the rotation of zero, one, or two alternate or two adjacent pyrrole rings, it is possible to arrive at four different isomers. Apart from closing the ring structure, the enzyme rotates the D-ring via a spirane intermediate,[19] producing the type III isomer, which is an essential reaction because only this isomer contributes to heme biosynthesis. HMB is unstable, and in those porphyrias in which excess HMB accumulates, cyclization occurs nonenzymatically with the formation of the type I isomer. Normally, only minimum amounts of uroporphyrinogen-I are formed.

Uroporphyrinogen Decarboxylase (EC 4.1.1.37)

This is the last cytoplasmic enzyme in the pathway, and it catalyzes the decarboxylation of all four carboxymethyl groups to form the tetracarboxylic coproporphyrinogen. The enzyme will use I and III isomers of uroporphyrinogen as substrate. Decarboxylation commences on ring D and proceeds stepwise through rings A, B, and C with formation of heptacarboxylate, hexacarboxylate, and pentacarboxylate intermediates at a single active site.[20] Decreased UROD activity causes accumulation of these intermediates in addition to its substrate, uroporphyrinogen. At high substrate concentrations, decarboxylation occurs by a random mechanism.[21]

Coproporphyrinogen Oxidase (EC 1.3.3.3)

Coproporphyrinogen oxidase, which is located in the intermembrane space of the mitochondria, catalyzes the sequential oxidative decarboxylation of the 2- and 4-carboxyethyl groups to vinyl groups to produce the more lipophilic protoporphyrinogen-IX, with formation of a tricarboxylic intermediate, harderoporphyrinogen.[22] Oxygen is required as the oxidant. The enzyme requires sulfhydryl groups for activity, making it a target for inhibition by metals.[23] The enzyme is specific for the type III isomer, so that metabolism of the I series of porphyrins does not occur beyond coproporphyrinogen-I. The product of the enzyme differs from the substrate in that replacement of two of the carboxyethyl groups by vinyl groups introduces a third substituent into the molecule. Therefore, the number of possible isomeric forms is increased, and conventionally the numbering system changes, so that the III isomer becomes the IX isomer. In UROD-deficient states, one of the ethylcarboxylate groups of the accumulated pentacarboxylate porphyrinogen is decarboxylated by CPOX to form the isocoproporphyrin series of porphyrins.

Protoporphyrinogen Oxidase (EC 1.3.3.4)

Protoporphyrinogen oxidase, a flavoprotein located in the inner mitochondrial membrane, catalyzes the removal of six hydrogens (four from methylene bridges and two from ring nitrogens) to form protoporphyrin-IX. This involves a three-step, six-electron flavin adenine dinucleotide–dependent oxidation that consumes molecular oxygen.[3] Nonenzymatic oxidation also occurs in vitro. However, under the low oxygen tension in the cell, PPOX is essential for oxidation to occur. The protoporphyrin produced is the only porphyrin that functions in the heme pathway. Other porphyrins are produced by nonenzymatic oxidation and represent porphyrinogens that have irreversibly escaped from the pathway.

Ferrochelatase (EC 4.99.1.1)

Ferrochelatase (also known as heme synthase) is an Fe-sulfur protein located in the inner mitochondrial membrane.[15] This enzyme inserts ferrous Fe into protoporphyrin to form heme. During this process, two hydrogens are displaced from the ring nitrogens. Other metals in the divalent state also act as substrates, yielding the corresponding chelate (eg, incorporation of zinc [Zn^{2+}] into protoporphyrin to yield Zn protoporphyrin). In Fe-deficient states, Zn^{2+} successfully competes with Fe^{2+} in developing red cells, so that the concentration of Zn protoporphyrin in erythrocytes increases. Some other dicarboxylic porphyrins also serve as substrates (eg, mesoporphyrin). Integration of the final stages of erythroid heme biosynthesis may be facilitated by interaction between FECH and proteins involved in Fe import.[24]

REGULATION OF HEME BIOSYNTHESIS

Heme supply in all tissues is controlled by the activity of mitochondrial ALAS, the first enzyme of the pathway. Two isoforms of ALAS are known. The ubiquitous isoform, ALAS1, is encoded by a gene on chromosome 3p21 and is expressed in all tissues. Because it has a half-life of approximately 1 hour, changes in its rate of synthesis produce short-term alterations in enzyme concentration and cellular ALAS activity. Synthesis of ALAS1 is under negative feedback control by heme.[25] In the liver, but not most other tissues, ALAS1 is induced by a wide variety of drugs and chemicals that induce microsomal cytochrome P450–dependent oxidases (CYPs). This effect is thought to be mediated mainly by direct transcriptional activation by drug-responsive nuclear receptors,[26] rather than occurring secondary to depletion of an intracellular regulatory heme pool as a consequence of use of heme for CYP assembly. Induction of ALAS1 is prevented by heme, which acts by destabilizing messenger RNA (mRNA) for ALAS1, by blocking mitochondrial import of pre-ALAS1, by increased proteolysis by Lon peptidase 1,[27] and possibly by inhibiting transcription.[28] In addition, ALAS1 activity is regulated by a transcriptional co-activator, PGC-1α, which is an effect that forms a link between the rate of hepatic heme synthesis and nutritional status.[29]

The erythroid isoform, ALAS2, is encoded by a gene on chromosome Xq21-22 and is expressed only in erythroid cells. Its activity is regulated by two distinct mechanisms.[30] Transcription is enhanced during erythroid differentiation by the action of erythroid-specific transcription factors, and mRNA concentrations are regulated by Fe. Fe deficiency in erythroid cells promotes specific binding of Fe regulatory proteins to an Fe-responsive element in the 5′ untranslated region of ALAS2 mRNA with consequent inhibition of translation.[31]

EXCRETION OF HEME PRECURSORS

Typically, only minute quantities of heme precursors accumulate in the body. The route of excretion largely depends on solubility. The porphyrin precursors ALA and PBG are water soluble and are excreted almost exclusively in urine. Uroporphyrinogen, with eight carboxylate groups, is readily water soluble and is also excreted via the kidney. The last intermediate of the pathway, protoporphyrin (and also protoporphyrinogen), which has only two carboxylate groups, is insoluble in water and is excreted in the feces via the biliary tract. The other porphyrins are of intermediate solubility and appear in both urine and feces. Coproporphyrinogen-I is taken up and excreted by the liver in preference to the III isomer, so that coproporphyrinogen-I predominates in feces and coproporphyrinogen-III in urine. All porphyrinogens in the urine or feces are slowly oxidized to the corresponding porphyrins. Reference intervals for porphyrins and their precursors in urine, feces, and blood are given in Table 39.3, Chapter 8, and in the Appendix on Reference Intervals.

Once in the gut, porphyrins are susceptible to modification by gut flora. The two vinyl groups of protoporphyrin are reduced to ethyl groups, hydrated to hydroxyethyl groups, or removed, giving rise to a variety of secondary porphyrins. Gut flora can also metabolize heme (whether dietary heme, as components from cells sloughed off from the lining of

TABLE 39.3 Adult Reference Intervals

Specimen	Analyte	Reference Interval (SI Units)	Reference Interval (Traditional Units)
Urine	Porphobilinogen	<1.5 µmol/mmol creatinine[130]	<3.0 mg/g creatinine
		<10 µmol/L[120]	<0.23 mg/dL
	5-aminolevulinic acid	<3.8 µmol/mmol creatinine[130]	<4.4 mg/g creatinine
		<50 µmol/L[130]	<0.66 mg/dL
	Total porphyrin	<35 nmol/mmol creatinine[130]	<216 µg/g creatinine
		20–320 nmol/L[120]	14–224 µg/L
	Uroporphyrin	0.8–3.1 nmol/mmol creatinine[32]	5.9–22.8 µg/g creatinine
	Heptacarboxylate porphyrin	<0.9 nmol/mmol creatinine[32]	<6.3 µg/g creatinine
	Coproporphyrin-I	1.2–5.7 nmol/mmol creatinine[32]	6.9–33.0 µg/g creatinine
	Coproporphyrin-III	4.8–23.8 nmol/mmol creatinine[32]	27.8–137.7 µg/g creatinine
	% Coproporphyrin-III*	68–86[32]	68–86
Feces	Total porphyrin	10–200 nmol/g dry wt[120]	6–117 µg/g dry wt
	Coproporphyrin-I	1.1–5.5 nmol/g feces[32]	0.7-3.6 µg/g feces
	Coproporphyrin-III	0.2–2.5 nmol/g feces[32]	0.1–1.6 µg/g feces
	Coproporphyrin-III/I ratio	0.3–1.4[139]	0.3–1.4
	Total dicarboxylate porphyrin	0.5–12.8 nmol/g feces[32]	0.3–7.2 µg/g feces
Erythrocytes	Total porphyrin	0.4–1.7 µmol/L erythrocytes[120]	25–106 µg/dL erythrocytes

Laboratories should verify that these ranges are appropriate for use in their own settings. Further guidance is provided in Chapter 8.
*Percentage of total coproporphyrin.
SI, Standard International.

TABLE 39.4 Main Types of Human Porphyria

Disorder	Defective Enzyme	Prevalence* (per million)	Neurovisceral Crises	Skin Lesions	Inheritance
Acute Porphyrias					
ADP	ALAD	–	+	–	AR
AIP	HMBS	5.9	+	–	AD
HCP	CPOX	0.9	+	+[†‡]	AD
VP	PPOX	3.2	+	+[†‡]	AD
Nonacute Porphyrias					
CEP	UROS	0.3	–	+[‡]	AR
PCT	UROD	40	–	+[‡]	Complex (20% AD)
EPP	FECH	9.2	–	+[§]	AR
XLEPP	ALAS2	0.15	–	+[§]	XL

*Estimated prevalence of clinically overt disease.[67,94,191]
†Skin lesions and neurovisceral crises may occur alone or together.
‡Fragile skin, bullae.
§Acute photosensitivity without fragile skin, bullae.
AD, Autosomal dominant; *ADP*, ALA dehydratase deficiency porphyria; *AIP*, acute intermittent porphyria; *ALA*, 5-aminolevulinate; *ALAD*, 5-aminolevulinic acid dehydratase; *ALAS*, 5-aminolevulinate synthase; *AR*, autosomal recessive; *CEP*, congenital erythropoietic porphyria; *EPP*, erythropoietic protoporphyria; *FECH*, ferrochelatase; *HCP*, hereditary coproporphyria; *HMBS*, hydroxymethylbilane synthase; *PCT*, porphyria cutanea tarda; *PPOX*, protoporphyrinogen oxidase; *UROD*, uroporphyrinogen decarboxylase; *UROS*, uroporphyrinogen-III synthase; *VP*, variegate porphyria; *XLEPP*, X-linked erythropoietic protoporphyria.

the gut or heme resulting from gastrointestinal bleeding) to produce a variety of dicarboxylic porphyrins.[32] In addition, some bacteria are capable of de novo synthesis of porphyrins.

PORPHYRIAS

The porphyrias are a group of metabolic disorders that result from decreased or, in one rare form of erythropoietic protoporphyria increased, activities of the enzymes of heme biosynthesis[1,2] (Table 39.4). All are inherited in monogenic patterns, apart from some forms of PCT and rare erythropoietic porphyrias associated with malignant myeloid disorders. Each type of porphyria is defined by the association of characteristic clinical features with a specific pattern of accumulation of heme precursors that reflects increased formation of the substrate of the enzyme that is partially deficient or becomes secondarily rate-limiting in that type of porphyria (Table 39.5). Defects that cause porphyria have been identified in all enzymes of the pathway except for ALAS1. Mutations that decrease ALAS2 activity cause nonsyndromic X-linked

TABLE 39.5 **Porphyrias: Patterns of Overproduction of Heme Precursors During Clinically Overt Phase of Disease**

Porphyria	Urine PBG/ALA	Urine Porphyrins	Fecal Porphyrins	Erythrocyte Porphyrins	Plasma Fluorescence Emission Peak
ADP	ALA	Copro-III	Not increased	ZPP	–
AIP	PBG>ALA	Mainly uroporphyrin from PBG	Normal or increased* Copro-III/I ratio normal	Not increased	615–622 nm†
CEP	Not increased	Uro-I, Copro-I	Copro-I	ZPP, Proto, Copro-I, Uro-I	615–620 nm
PCT	Not increased	Uro, Hepta‡	Isocopro, Hepta, Penta	Not increased	615–622 nm
HCP	PBG>ALA§	Copro-III, uroporphyrin from PBG	Copro-III, Copro-III/I ratio increased	Not increased	615–622 nm†
VP	PBG>ALA§	Copro-III, uroporphyrin from PBG	Proto IX>Copro-III‖ X-porphyrin Copro-III/I ratio increased	Not increased	624–628 nm
EPP	Not increased	Not increased	±Proto¶	Proto	626–634 nm#
XLEPP	Not increased	Not increased	±Proto	Proto, ZPP**	626–634 nm#

*Slight increase only unless uroporphyrin is present.[141]
†Not always increased.
‡Other methylcarboxylate-substituted porphyrins are increased to a smaller extent; uroporphyrin is a mixture of type I and III isomers; heptacarboxylate porphyrin is mainly type III.
§PBG and ALA may be normal when only skin lesions are present.
‖Coproporphyrin-III/I ratio increased, but usually less than in overt HCP.[140]
¶Not increased in approximately 40% of patients.
#Protoporphyrin (Proto) bound to globin. If hemolysis is present the peak shifts to the left (ie, at 626–628 nm or is quenched).
**Zn-protoporphyrin (ZPP) 20 to 60% of total protoporphyrin.
AIP, Acute intermittent porphyria; *ALA*, 5-aminolevulinate; *ALAD*, 5-aminolevulinic acid dehydratase; *CEP*, congenital erythropoietic porphyria; *EPP*, erythropoietic protoporphyria; *HCP*, hereditary coproporphyria; *PBG*, porphobilinogen; *PCT*, porphyria cutanea tarda; *UROD*, uroporphyrinogen decarboxylase; *UROS*, uroporphyrinogen-III synthase; *VP*, variegate porphyria; *XLEPP*, X-linked erythropoietic protoporphyria.

sideroblastic anemia[33]; those that increase activity cause an X-linked erythropoietic protoporphyria (XLEPP).[34]

The porphyrias are characterized clinically by two main features: skin lesions on sun-exposed areas and acute neurovisceral attacks, typically comprising (1) abdominal pain, (2) peripheral neuropathy, and (3) mental disturbance. The skin lesions are caused by porphyrin-catalyzed photodamage, of which singlet oxygen is the main mediator.[35] Acute attacks are associated with increased formation of ALA, and consequently, PBG from induced activity of hepatic ALAS1 and partial hepatic heme deficiency, often in response to induction of hepatic CYPs by drugs and other factors. The relationship of these biochemical changes to the neuronal dysfunction that underlines all clinical features of an acute attack is uncertain.[36,37] The observation that correction of the metabolic defect in the liver by transplantation is curative,[38] and that domino transfer of the affected organ to an unaffected recipient causes acute attacks indistinguishable from those suffered by the donor,[39] suggests that their primary cause is release of a neurotoxin, probably ALA,[40] formed in the liver.

In Table 39.4, the porphyrias are classified as acute, in which acute neurovisceral attacks occur, or as nonacute. Porphyrias are also classified as hepatic or erythropoietic, according to the main site of overproduction of heme precursors. The main hepatic porphyrias are AIP, HCP, VP, and PCT. Erythropoietic porphyrias include CEP and EPP. Porphyrias may also be classified as cutaneous or acute porphyrias; however, it should be noted that even with these classifications, some porphyrias are difficult to place.

Acute Porphyrias

The acute porphyrias include (1) ALA dehydratase deficiency porphyria (ADP), (2) AIP, (3) VP, and (4) HCP. These disorders are autosomal dominant, except for the very rare disorder, ADP, which is autosomal recessive.

Biochemistry and Molecular Genetics

The inherited defect in each of the autosomal dominant acute porphyrias (see Table 39.4) is a mutation that leads to complete or near complete inactivation of one of the pairs of allelic genes that encode the enzyme whose partial deficiency causes the disorder. Enzyme activities are therefore half of normal in all tissues in which they are expressed, reflecting the activity of the normal gene *trans* to the mutant allele. Heme supply is maintained at normal or near-normal concentration by upregulation of ALAS1, with a consequent increase in the substrate concentration of the defective enzyme. These compensatory changes vary among tissues; they are most prominent in the liver and are undetectable in most other organs. These changes also vary among individuals. Thus in all autosomal dominant acute porphyrias, some individuals show no evidence of overproduction of heme precursors, and others have biochemically manifest disease with or without clinical symptoms.

Low clinical penetrance (the frequency of expression of an allele when it is present in the genotype) is a prominent feature of all the autosomal dominant acute porphyrias.[1,2] Family studies indicate that many affected individuals are asymptomatic throughout life. Surveys of blood donors suggest that the AIP gene may be present in as many as 1 in 1675 of the population.[41] For all three disorders, the gene frequency is sufficiently high for rare "homozygous" variants of AIP, HCP, or VP to occur in individuals who are homozygotes or compound heterozygotes for disease-specific mutations,[22,42] and for the same person to have two separate types of porphyria.[43] Approximately 25% of patients with overt acute porphyria have no family history of the disease. Such sporadic presentation is a reflection of the high prevalence and low penetrance of mutations in the population; acute porphyria caused by de novo mutation is uncommon.

All the autosomal dominant acute porphyrias show extensive allelic heterogeneity. More than 393 disease-specific mutations have been identified in the *HMBS* gene in AIP, approximately 65 in the *CPOX* gene in HCP, and more than 170 in the *PPOX* gene in VP.[44] Approximately 5% of families with AIP have *HMBS* mutations that only impair expression of the ubiquitous isoform and therefore do not decrease activity in erythroid cells.[45] All other mutations in the autosomal dominant acute porphyrias affect all tissues. Most are restricted to one or a few families, but founder mutations are present in some populations and explain the high frequency of VP in South Africans of Dutch descent and of AIP in Sweden.[46,47]

Clinical Features

The life-threatening, acute neurovisceral attacks that occur in AIP, VP, and HCP are clinically identical.[1,2,48,49] Acute attacks are more common in women, usually occurring first between the ages of 15 and 40 years, and are rare before puberty. The main clinical features are summarized in Table 39.6. The clinical features of ADP, which has been reported in only six patients, are similar but may start in childhood.[2,50]

Acute attacks almost always start with abdominal pain that rapidly becomes very severe but is not accompanied by other signs of an acute surgical condition.[48,51] Pain may also be present in the back and thighs and may occasionally be most severe in these regions. Signs of autonomic neuropathy, such as vomiting, constipation, tachycardia, and hypertension, are frequent. When convulsions occur, they may be a consequence of hyponatremia or secondary to central nervous system involvement and may be associated with posterior reversible encephalopathy syndrome, a serious complication of long-standing attacks.[51,52] Pain may dissipate within a few days, but in severe cases, a predominant motor neuropathy develops that may progress to flaccid quadriparesis.[51] Persistent pain and vomiting may lead to weight loss and malnutrition. The acute phase may be accompanied by mental confusion with abrupt changes in mood, hallucinations, and other psychotic features. However, these mental disturbances disappear with remission. Persistent psychiatric illness is not a feature of the acute porphyrias, although mild anxiety or depression may be present in some patients.[53] Abdominal pain usually resolves within 2 weeks, but recovery from neuropathy may take many months, and is not always complete. Most patients have one or a few attacks followed by complete recovery and prolonged remission. Approximately 5% have repeated acute attacks, which in women may be premenstrual.[48]

Precipitating factors have been identified in approximately two-thirds of patients who present with acute attacks. The most important are drugs, alcohol (especially binge drinking), the menstrual cycle, calorie restriction, infection, and stress. Acute attacks may complicate a small proportion of pregnancies in affected patients. Drugs are frequent precipitants of acute attacks in VP, and hormonal factors appear to be more important in AIP.[48] Drugs known to provoke acute attacks include barbiturates, sulfonamides, progestogens, and some anticonvulsants, but many others have been implicated in the precipitation of acute attacks.[54]

Skin lesions similar to those of PCT and other bullous porphyrias are present in approximately 80% of patients with clinically manifest VP (see Table 39.4). Approximately 60% of patients with this condition present with skin lesions alone. The skin is less commonly affected in HCP; skin lesions without an acute attack are uncommon and usually are provoked by intercurrent cholestasis.

Long-term complications of acute porphyria include chronic renal failure, hypertension, and primary hepatocellular carcinoma.[1,2]

TABLE 39.6 Clinical Features of an Acute Neurovisceral Attack of Porphyria

Symptom/Sign	Percent of Acute Attacks
Abdominal pain	85–90
Nonabdominal pain	25–70
Vomiting and nausea	30–90
Constipation/diarrhea	50–80
Psychologic symptoms (insomnia, anxiety, depression, confusion, hallucinations)	20–85
Acute encephalopathy (headache, somnolence, seizures, altered consciousness)	2–20
Motor neuropathy (muscle weakness, pain, low/absent tendon reflexes)	10–90
Hemi/tetraparesis	30–40
Respiratory paralysis	10–55
Sensory neuropathy	10–40
Hypertension	40–75
Tachycardia (>80/min)	30–85
Hyponatremia (<135 nmol/L)	30–60

Data from Harper P, Sardh E. Management of acute intermittent porphyria. *Exp Opin Orphan Drugs* 2014;2:349–368.

Treatment

As soon as an attack of acute porphyria is suspected as the cause of illness, drugs and other potential provoking agents should be withdrawn, and supportive treatment should begin using drugs that are known to be safe.[2,48,55] Opiates are usually required to control pain and an antiemetic such as ondansetron may be required to control nausea and vomiting. Patients with acute porphyria are prone to severe hyponatremia and are particularly susceptible to cerebral edema. Therefore careful administration of any intravenous fluids, with avoidance of hypotonic solutions, is essential. If hyponatremia develops, it should be corrected slowly to avoid osmotic demyelination (for more details on hyponatraemia and its treatment, see Chapter 60). Adequate caloric intake must be maintained, preferably by giving carbohydrate-rich supplements orally or if necessary via a nasogastric tube. When vomiting prevents enteral administration, dextrose given intravenously as a 10% solution in saline should suffice initially. In prolonged acute attacks, total parenteral nutrition should be considered.

Unless the attack is mild and is clearly resolving, specific treatment with intravenous human hemin should be started as soon as the diagnosis has been established.[2,48,55] This treatment increases the concentration of heme in the liver, thus decreasing the activity of ALAS1 and the formation of ALA and PBG. The effect of treatment may be monitored by measuring these metabolites, but this is not essential because clinical improvement is the required endpoint. Heme administration will not reverse an established neuropathy. If heme preparations are not available, carbohydrate loading can ameliorate an acute attack, probably by decreasing ALA synthase activity,[29,56] but this treatment is less effective than intravenous heme.

Repeated attacks are difficult to control. Cyclic premenstrual attacks in women may be prevented by suppression of ovulation with gonadotropin-releasing hormone (gonadorelin) analogs, but many patients require repeated courses of intravenous heme.[1,2,55,57] Orthotopic liver transplantation leads to immediate and prolonged remission with restoration of PBG excretion to normal.[38]

Management of Families

Diagnosis of autosomal dominant acute porphyria should be followed by investigation of the patient's family to identify affected, often asymptomatic, relatives, so that they can be advised to avoid drugs and other factors known to provoke potentially fatal acute attacks.[54] Presymptomatic diagnosis also has the benefit that specific treatment can be started promptly if an attack does develop without a delay while a diagnosis is sought. Although attacks are rare before puberty, children should be tested at as young an age as is practicable to ensure that their status is known by the time they reach puberty and to enable the very low risk for affected children to be further reduced. Counseling to reduce the risk of an acute attack should include comprehensive information about the disease, including specific advice to guide selection of safe drugs as well as provision of jewelry, an identity card, or some other means to identify the individual as having an acute porphyria. Where available, patients should be made aware of the relevant national patient support group. A list of online resources for patients and professionals can be found in Box 39.1.

POINTS TO REMEMBER

Acute Porphyrias

- Present clinically after puberty.
- Low clinical penetrance means that there is often no family history.
- Clinical effects are due to autonomic, central, and motor neuropathy.
- Common precipitants are drugs, hormonal fluctuations, excess alcohol consumption, starvation, infection, and stress.
- Diagnosed by demonstrating increased PBG excretion in a random urine sample.
- Mild hyponatraemia is common.
- Specific treatment is with intravenous human hemin.

BOX 39.1 Online Resources

American Porphyria Foundation: http://www.porphyriafoundation.com. Provides information for patients and professionals, including a searchable drug database for acute porphyrias.

European Porphyria Network: http://www.porphyria.eu. A multilingual website providing information for patients and professionals. Provides contact details for porphyria specialist centers. Specific guidance for certain clinical areas or topics are covered, and a safe and unsafe drug list for acute porphyrias is available.

The Drug Database for Acute Porphyria: http://www.drugs-porphyria.com. The database is searchable and provides evidence-based monographs for each drug that has been assessed with regard to safety in acute porphyrias.

South African Porphyria Centre: http://www.porphyria.uct.ac.za. Provides information for patients and professionals. Section on prescribing in acute porphyrias includes advice on specific disorders, including malaria, tuberculosis, and HIV.

Nonacute Porphyrias

The nonacute porphyrias include PCT, CEP, and EPP.

Porphyria Cutanea Tarda

Porphyria cutanea tarda is by far the most common porphyria.[58] The annual incidence of new cases in the United Kingdom is between two and five per million of the population. The disease occurs at all ages in both sexes, with onset usually during the fifth and sixth decades.

Clinical Features. Lesions on sun-exposed skin, particularly the backs of the hands, the forearm, and the face, are present in all patients. These lesions are identical to those seen in the other bullous porphyrias (see Table 39.4). Increased mechanical fragility of the skin, with trivial trauma leading to erosions, is present in virtually all patients. Subepidermal bullae, milia, hypertrichosis of the face, and patchy pigmentation are also common. Erosions and bullae heal slowly to leave atrophic scars, milia, and depigmented areas. Patchy or diffuse sclerodermatous changes are less common and, unlike the other skin lesions, may affect areas of the trunk that are not exposed to sun.

Skin lesions are often the first sign of underlying liver cell damage. Clinically, overt liver disease is uncommon, but minor alterations in biochemical tests of liver function are present in more than 50% of patients. Needle biopsy of the liver reveals hepatic siderosis in most patients, usually accompanied by minor histopathologic abnormalities such as mild fatty infiltration, focal necrosis of hepatocytes, and inflammation of portal tracts. Cirrhosis is present in less than 15% of patients, but carries a high risk of hepatocellular carcinoma.

This combination of skin lesions with liver damage is strongly associated with alcohol abuse, estrogens, infection with hepatotropic viruses, particularly hepatitis C (HCV), and mutations in the hemochromatosis *(HFE)* gene.[58-60] PCT may also complicate HIV infection.[60] Hepatic Fe overload and at least one of the other associated factors are present in almost all patients. Studies have found that between 15%

and 92% of patients have antibodies to HCV.[61] Between 10% and 20% of PCT patients of Northern European descent are homozygous for the c.845G>A (p.Cys282Tyr) mutation in the *HFE* gene, although a few of them have other clinical signs or symptoms of Fe overload. However, increased serum ferritin concentrations and other biochemical indicators of Fe overload are common in PCT irrespective of the HFE genotype, suggesting that the origin of hepatic Fe overload is multifactorial. PCT may occur in association with other disorders, notably chronic renal failure, systemic lupus erythematosus, and hematologic malignancies. In addition, rare cases of a PCT-like syndrome resulting from production of porphyrins by primary hepatic tumors have been described.[62]

Pathogenesis and Molecular Genetics. PCT results from a decrease in activity of UROD in the liver, which leads to overproduction of uroporphyrin and other carboxymethyl-substituted porphyrinogens. These auto-oxidize to porphyrins, which accumulate in the liver and skin, where they act as photosensitizers and are excreted in urine and bile. Two main types of PCT can be identified by measurement of UROD activity in liver and extrahepatic tissue, and by analysis of the *UROD* gene. In most populations, approximately 80% of patients have the sporadic (type I) form of PCT, in which the enzyme defect is restricted to the liver, and the *UROD* gene appears to be normal. Typically, no family history of PCT is reported, but rare cases are clustered in families (type III PCT). The rest have familial (type II) PCT. In this form, mutation of one *UROD* gene leads to half-normal UROD activity in all tissues, which is inherited in an autosomal dominant manner. As with the other autosomal dominant porphyrias, clinical penetration of familial PCT is low with considerable allelic heterogeneity; each of the more than 120 mutations is described as present in only one or a few families, except in Norway, where the high prevalence of PCT has been attributed to a founder effect.[63] A rare variant of familial PCT, hepatoerythropoietic porphyria (HEP), in which *UROD* mutations, some of which have also been found in familial PCT, are present on both alleles, has been described.[42,58] PCT may also be caused by exposure to certain polyhalogenated aromatic hydrocarbons, such as hexachlorobenzene and 2,3,7,8-tetrachlorodibenzo-*p*-dioxin.[58]

In families with familial PCT, a decrease of 50% in enzyme activity is not by itself sufficient to cause clinically overt disease. Further inactivation of UROD in the liver seems to be required, and the process responsible for this inactivation also appears to be responsible for inactivation of hepatic UROD in sporadic PCT and in toxic PCT caused by chemicals. The inactivation process decreases catalytic activity without impairing enzyme concentration, is Fe dependent, and is reversible. Evidence from experimental models of PCT suggests that UROD is inactivated by a porphomethene inhibitor that is produced by Fe-dependent oxidation of a substrate of the UROD reaction, which is possibly mediated by hepatic CYPs, particularly CYP1A2.[64]

Treatment. In addition to protection of the skin from sunlight, two specific treatments may be used for PCT: depletion of hepatic Fe stores by repeated phlebotomy or other means and low-dose oral chloroquine.[65] In patients with chronic renal failure and PCT, hepatic Fe stores can be decreased by erythropoietin with or without phlebotomy. In end-stage renal failure and hemodialysis, renal transplantation should be considered.

Congenital Erythropoietic Porphyria

Congenital erythropoietic porphyria is the least common but most severe of the cutaneous porphyrias.[66] The prevalence is less than one per million in the United Kingdom.[67] This disorder is also known as Günther disease.

Clinical Features. The clinical features vary in severity from hydrops fetalis with death in utero—through onset in infancy of severe skin lesions with transfusion-dependent hemolytic anemia—to mild skin lesions, resembling PCT, that do not start until adult life. Late-onset cases may also develop in association with hematologic malignancy, particularly myelodysplasia.[68,69]

Most patients present in early infancy. Blisters on skin exposed to the sun or other sources of ultraviolet A (UVA) and near visible radiation and reddish-brown staining of diapers by urinary porphyrins are common early signs. The skin lesions resemble those of PCT but are more severe and persistent throughout life. With age, progressive scarring, particularly if erosions become infected, and atrophic changes lead to photomutilation with erosions of the terminal phalanges; destruction of ears, nose, and eyelids; and alopecia. Accumulation of porphyrin in bone is visible as erythrodontia—brownish-red teeth that fluoresce in UVA light. The skin changes are usually accompanied by hemolytic anemia and splenomegaly. Hemolysis may be fully compensated or mild, but in some patients, anemia is severe enough to require repeated transfusion.

Molecular Pathology. CEP is an autosomal recessive disease resulting from decreased UROS activity (see Table 39.2). Patients are homoallelic or heteroallelic for mutations in the *UROS* gene, or rarely, the *GATA1* gene, which encodes an erythroid transcription factor.[70-72] Decreased UROS activity leads to massive overproduction of uroporphyrinogen-I and other isomer-I series of porphyrins, mainly in the bone marrow. Porphyrins accumulate in erythroid cells and are released into the plasma as these cells die. Most patients are heteroallelic unless their parents are consanguineous. More than 49 separate mutations have been identified, with c.217T>C (p.Cys73Arg) being the most common.[71,73] Some correlation has been noted between genotype and severity of disease.[71,74] Patients who are homozygous for p.Cys73Arg have particularly severe disease; in compound heterozygotes, the effect of p.Cys73Arg is modified by the nature of the mutation on the other allele.

Treatment. Protection against sunlight and prevention of skin infection are essential. Reflectant sunscreen ointments may occasionally provide some benefit, but physical avoidance of UVA radiation is usually necessary. Blood hypertransfusion, hydroxyurea, and intravenous heme have been used to suppress erythropoiesis and porphyrin formation; oral activated charcoal has been used to decrease the enterohepatic circulation of porphyrin and antioxidant preparations to ameliorate the effects of porphyrin accumulation, but none have been shown to have a reliable long-term effect.[66,71,73] Hemolytic anemia may require repeated transfusion and infusion of deferoxamine or other procedures to prevent Fe overload.

At present, the only curative treatment is allogeneic bone marrow transplantation. Family donors are usually screened for *UROS* mutations, although the current evidence indicates that transplantation using a heterozygous carrier is effective. Gene therapy by introduction of a normal *UROS* gene into the patient's hematopoietic stem cells remains under development.[75]

Erythropoietic Protoporphyria and X-Linked Erythroietic Protoporphyria

The protoporphyrias are characterized by life-long acute photosensitivity caused by accumulation of protoporphyrin-IX in the skin.[76,77] The absence of fragile skin, subepidermal bullae, and hypertrichosis distinguish them clinically from all other cutaneous porphyrias.

Clinical Features. Patients present with acute photosensitivity characterized by burning pain. Symptoms normally start between birth and the age of 6 years, with median age of onset at 1 year, and both sexes are equally affected.[78] Diagnosis is often delayed; the median age at diagnosis is reported as 12 and 22 years in the United Kingdom and Sweden, respectively.[78,79] Onset after the age of 40 years is rare; most cases are associated with myelodysplasia and are caused by acquired somatic mutation of *FECH*.[80] Exposure to sun is followed, usually within 5 to 30 minutes, by an intensely painful, burning, prickling, itching sensation in the skin, most frequently on the face and the backs of the hands. Symptoms persist for several hours or occasionally for days, and are not relieved by shielding the skin from light. Patients characteristically seek relief by plunging their hands into water or covering their skin with wet towels. Young children may become distressed by the pain. The skin may appear normal throughout, although there is often erythema, which may be followed by edematous swelling with crusting. These changes usually subside within a few hours, so that by the time the child reaches the physician, nothing remains to be seen, and the episode may be dismissed as severe sunburn. Subsequent exposure to sunlight provokes a similar reaction. Recurrent episodes lead to chronic skin changes that are often minor and difficult to detect. Typical lesions are shallow linear scars over the bridge of the nose and elsewhere on the face; the skin may become thickened and waxy, especially over the knuckles. Seasonal palmar keratoderma is present in approximately 3% of patients.[81] Symptoms tend to be more severe during spring and summer, and may improve during pregnancy.

The most severe complication of protoporphyria is progressive hepatic failure that is caused by accumulation of protoporphyrin in the liver.[82] Approximately 20% of patients have abnormal biochemical tests of liver function, particularly increased aspartate aminotransferase, but only 2% to 5% of patients develop liver failure. Protoporphyria may also increase the risk of cholelithiasis, because the formation of gallstones is promoted by high concentrations of protoporphyrin in the bile. Erythropoiesis is impaired in all patients with a downward shift in hemoglobin concentration, so that approximately 50% of women and 30% of men have a mild microcytic anemia.[83] Biochemical evidence of vitamin D deficiency is present in up to 50% of patients.[84]

Molecular Pathology and Genetics. Protoporphyria is a clinical syndrome that results from increased formation of protoporphyrin mainly or exclusively in the bone marrow. The toxic effects of protoporphyrin on the skin and other tissues are directly responsible for its main clinical manifestations.[76] Accumulation of protoporphyrin in the liver is the result of failure of the liver to excrete the increased load it receives through release of protoporphyrin from erythrocytes and their immediate precursors.[82]

In most patients, overproduction of protoporphyrin results from decreased activity of FECH. FECH-deficient protoporphyria (EPP) is an autosomal recessive disease. In most families, photosensitive individuals are compound heterozygotes for a *FECH* mutation that abolishes or severely decreases FECH activity and a hypomorphic *FECH* c.315-48C (rs2272783) allele.[85-88] This allele (previously denoted as IVS3-48T>C) is a polymorphic *FECH* variant that shows marked variation in frequency among populations, ranging from less than 1% in West Africans to approximately 10% in Western Europeans to 56% in Japanese.[89] Substitution of a T nucleotide by a C nucleotide at a polymorphic site in intron 3 (c.315-48T>C) enhances use of an alternative splice site, leading to increased formation of an unstable, untranslated mRNA and reduction of *FECH* expression by approximately 30%.[86] Together, these two functional defects decrease FECH activity to below the threshold of approximately 35% of normal, at which protoporphyrin accumulation and clinical symptoms occur. In populations in whom the hypomorphic allele is common, EPP families show pseudodominant inheritance. In approximately 4% of families with FECH-deficient EPP, clinically affected individuals are heteroallelic or homoallelic for *FECH* mutations and tend to have lower enzyme activities than those in whom a *FECH* mutation is *trans* to the c.315-48C allele.[85] To date, all patients with seasonal palmar keratoderma have been found to have this form of EPP.[81] FECH-deficient EPP may show less allelic heterogeneity than other porphyrias,[87] but most mutations in *FECH* are restricted to one or a few families; more than 190 mutations have been identified.

In approximately 2% of families with protoporphyria, overproduction of protoporphyrin is caused by gain-of-function mutations in *ALAS2* (XLEPP), which leads to formation of protoporphyrin in excess of the amount required for hemoglobinization.[34] XLEPP is inherited in an X-linked pattern, with expression of disease in males and most females. The risk of liver disease appears to be substantially greater in XLEPP and in patients with dysfunctional *FECH* variants on both alleles, particularly those without palmar keratoderma, than in compound heterozygotes for the hypomorphic allele.[85] Among patients with *FECH* mutations *trans* to a c.315-48C allele, some evidence suggests an association between null mutations and severe liver disease, but this association is too weak to be of any practical use.[85]

Treatment. Acute photosensitivity has been controlled by avoidance of sunlight, suitable clothing, and reflectant sunscreens, if these are cosmetically acceptable.[90] Some patients are helped by production of a photoprotectant tan by measures such as narrowband ultraviolet B phototherapy or dihydroxyacetone ointment.[76,91] Oral β-carotene, which acts as a singlet oxygen quencher, may be effective in some patients, but little support for its use has been gained from clinical trials.[90] Doses should be sufficient to maintain a plasma concentration of 6 to 8 μg/L.[76] A new treatment that relies on a subcutaneous implant to deliver an α-melanocyte–stimulating hormone analogue, afemelanotide, which stimulates skin pigmentation, has recently been given market authorization in Europe.[92] Patients should be monitored for vitamin D deficiency.[84]

At present, no reliable method is known for predicting liver failure in protoporphyria. All patients should have at least annual biochemical tests of liver function. Persistent abnormalities should be investigated by liver biopsy and further treatment considered if even mild hepatocellular necrosis and fibrosis are present.[82] Once liver failure becomes irreversible, orthotopic liver transplantation is the only treatment, but protoporphyrin may reaccumulate in the transplanted liver.[82] Reaccumulation can be prevented by bone marrow transplantation.[93]

POINTS TO REMEMBER

Cutaneous Porphyrias

- Porphyrins absorb light with wavelengths at approximately 400 nm.
- The absorbed radiant energy is either:
  - released as red fluorescent light
  - interacts with molecular oxygen to create reactive oxygen species.
- The skin lesions are therefore caused by porphyrin-catalyzed photodamage.
- Photosensitivity can occur in any porphyria in which porphyrin ring structures accumulate; this includes all the porphyrias, except AIP and ADP.
- Symptoms manifest clinically as an immediate or delayed photosensitivity dependent on the type of porphyrins that accumulate and their localization within the skin.
- Protection of the skin from sunlight is essential to reduce symptoms.

Rare Variants

The porphyrias are common enough in the general population for patients with either two different porphyrias or homozygous and/or compound heterozygous forms of all the autosomal dominant porphyrias to have been reported. Although inheritance of null mutations on both alleles in any of the heme biosynthesis genes is embryonally lethal, homozygous or compound heterozygous mutations that allow for some residual enzyme activity have been reported. In general, there is increased representation of missense mutations in these patients.[94]

5-Aminolevulinate Dehydratase Deficiency Porphyria

Unlike the other acute porphyrias, ADP is an autosomal recessive disorder, although its presentation is similar with acute attacks of abdominal pain and neuropathy.[95] Biochemically, the patients have marked increases in urine ALA and coproporphyrin with normal or slightly increased urine PBG.[96] ADP is rare, with only five genetically confirmed patients described who are compound heterozygotes for a range of mutations in the *ALAD* gene.[96-100] The diagnosis of lead poisoning needs to be excluded because this leads to similar biochemical results. ADP can be confirmed either by enzymatic methods or by the identification of two mutations in the *ALAD* gene. Individuals who are heterozygous for mutations in the *ALAD* gene are asymptomatic, although they may be more susceptible to lead poisoning.[101]

Homozygous and/or Compound Heterozygous Autosomal Dominant Porphyrias

Rare cases of homozygous porphyrias have been reported. In the acute porphyrias, homozygous dominant AIP appears to be the most severe, with a phenotype comprising predominantly chronic progressive neurodegenerative disease and no acute attacks.[102] Homozygous dominant VP is more widely reported and manifests in infancy with photosensitive skin lesions, skeletal abnormalities, and mental retardation, but no neurovisceral crises.[94] Homozygous dominant HCP is described with two clinical presentations, either neonatal presentation with acute and cutaneous symptoms,[103] or skin lesions, hepatosplenomegaly, and neonatal hemolytic anemia, a condition also known as harderoporphyria. It is caused by missense mutations in exon 6 of the *CPOX* gene.[104]

Autosomal dominant PCT, also known as HEP, is a rare form of cutaneous porphyria. Skin lesions usually develop before 6 years of age, and when severely affected, resemble CEP. The biochemical patterns are similar to PCT, except that erythrocyte Zn protoporphyrin is also increased.[42]

Dual Porphyria

Patients are said to have a dual porphyria when they have deficiency of two enzymes in the heme biosynthetic pathway. Frequently, patients will have an enzyme deficiency of UROD together with another porphyria (HMBS or PPOX or CPOX or UROS deficiency).[43] Other coexistent porphyrias have also been found, for example, CPOX with UROS deficiency[105] or HMBS[106] or CPOX deficiency with ALAD deficiency.[107] These dual porphyrias can be a cause of much confusion in interpreting the biochemical findings. Molecular confirmation of defects in two genes may therefore be required before a diagnosis of dual porphyria can be confirmed.[108]

Abnormalities of Porphyrin Metabolism Not Caused by Porphyria

Abnormalities of porphyrin metabolism may occur in a number of diseases other than the porphyrias. These disorders are more often the cause of abnormal porphyrin metabolism than porphyria and need to be considered when data from patients in whom porphyria is suspected are interpreted.[109,110]

Lead and Other Heavy Metals

Lead exposure increases urinary ALA and coproporphyrin-III excretion, and causes accumulation of Zn-protoporphyrin (ZPP) in erythrocytes. The definitive test for lead toxicity is measurement of blood lead, but occasionally lead exposure is responsible for porphyria-like symptoms and may be an unexpected finding when patients are evaluated for suspected porphyria.[111] Increased ALA excretion occurs secondary to inhibition of ALAD caused by lead displacing Zn at its catalytic center. Two isoenzymes (ALAD1 and ALAD2) are produced from the *ALAD* gene by alternative splicing activated by two nontranslated codominant alleles 1 and 2.[112] The ALAD2 isoenzyme is more electronegatively charged than ALAD1, so that its affinity for lead is higher.[113] As a consequence, individuals with the ALAD2 genotype are more susceptible to lead toxicity.[101] In addition, individuals who are heterozygous for ALAD deficiency appear to be at increased risk from lead exposure.

CPOX requires sulfhydryl groups for activity and therefore is potentially a target for inhibition by lead, which results in increased coproporphyrin excretion. Increased concentrations of red cell ZPP associated with lead exposure are probably not caused by inhibition of *FECH* because inhibition of this enzyme requires higher lead concentrations than those usually encountered after lead exposure. Lead exposure may lead to an intramitochondrial deficiency of ferrous Fe, so that Zn replaces Fe as a substrate for FECH.[114] Once formed, erythrocyte ZPP remains elevated for the life of the red cell. Because the half-life of an erythrocyte is longer than that of blood lead, monitoring of lead workers requires both whole blood lead and ZPP testing. ZPP measurement also has the advantage that no interference from lead contamination occurs via the skin when the blood sample is collected, especially if a finger-prick sample is used. Coproporphyrinuria has also been reported after exposure to arsenic and other heavy metals.[110] For further details, see Chapter 42 on Toxic Elements.

Secondary Coproporphyrinuria: Hepatobiliary and Other Disorders

Coproporphyrinuria secondary to excess alcohol intake, liver dysfunction, or drugs is by far the most common abnormality of porphyrin excretion. Alcohol increases the excretion of coproporphyrin-III in normal individuals, and coproporphyrin excretion is frequently increased in chronic alcoholism.[115,116]

In cholestatic jaundice, hepatitis, and cirrhosis, impaired biliary excretion of coproporphyrin-I leads to its appearance in the urine with reversal of the normal coproporphyrin-isomer ratio so that the I isomer predominates.[110,116] Impaired biliary excretion is also probably the cause of the coproporphyrinuria that may accompany severe infections, other acute illnesses, and the administration of some drugs.

Coproporphyrinuria is also a feature of inherited forms of jaundice. In the Dubin-Johnson syndrome, overall urinary excretion of coproporphyrin is normal, but that of coproporphyrin-I is increased, and excretion of coproporphyrin-III is reduced.[117] In Rotor syndrome, urinary excretion of coproporphyrin-I is increased with normal coproporphyrin-III excretion, and in Gilbert syndrome, urinary excretion of both isomers is increased (see Chapter 38).[110]

Increased Fecal Porphyrin Concentration

The dicarboxylic porphyrin fraction of feces contains protoporphyrin and other dicarboxylic porphyrins derived from it by bacterial reduction or removal of vinyl side groups. Additional protoporphyrin and other dicarboxylic porphyrins have been formed by the action of gut flora on heme-containing proteins derived from the diet or from gastrointestinal hemorrhage.[32,118] Even minor gastrointestinal hemorrhage, particularly if it occurs high in the gut (which may not give rise to a positive occult blood test) can markedly increase the concentration of dicarboxylic porphyrins in feces. Porphyrins may come directly from the diet, and one report described consumption of brewer's yeast that produced a fecal porphyrin profile that was indistinguishable from VP.[119]

Increased Plasma Porphyrin Concentration: Renal and Other Disorders

Plasma porphyrin concentrations may be increased when hepatobiliary or renal excretion of porphyrins is impaired.[120] In end-stage renal failure, concentrations are often markedly increased; clearance of porphyrins by dialysis is inefficient.[121,122] Dermatologic problems are common in patients undergoing dialysis, and skin lesions may resemble those of PCT.[123] Concentrations of porphyrins in the plasma of dialysis patients, although often much higher than normal, rarely approach those found in patients with active skin lesions caused by PCT. It seems unlikely that the skin lesions are related to the increased porphyrin concentrations. However, PCT is itself an uncommon complication of end-stage renal failure. Because such patients are often anuric, careful evaluation of plasma and fecal porphyrins is required to distinguish PCT and those acute porphyrias in which skin lesions may occur, from the dermatosis of renal failure.[124] Although plasma porphyrin concentrations are usually higher in chronic renal failure with PCT than in renal failure alone, unequivocal diagnosis of PCT in this situation may be achieved by fractionation of plasma porphyrins by high-performance liquid chromatography (HPLC), or preferably, by fecal porphyrin analysis.[124]

Hematologic Disorders

In Fe deficiency anemia, Zn acts as an alternative substrate for FECH, leading to increased erythrocyte ZPP. Increased red cell protoporphyrin (mostly ZPP) may also occur in sideroblastic, megaloblastic, and hemolytic anemias.[109,125]

Hereditary Tyrosinemia Type I

Succinylacetone, which accumulates in this disease, has a structural resemblance to ALA and is therefore a competitive inhibitor of ALAD. Consequently, its substrate ALA accumulates, and excess amounts are excreted in urine. Patients with hereditary tyrosinemia suffer neurologic crises similar to attacks of acute porphyria, and some have been treated with heme infusions.[126] They are also at increased risk of hepatocellular carcinoma and renal failure.

LABORATORY DIAGNOSIS OF PORPHYRIA

Laboratory investigation is essential for identification of the porphyrias because none have clinical features that are sufficiently distinctive to allow diagnosis on clinical grounds alone. In patients with current symptoms caused by porphyria, it should always be possible to demonstrate excessive production of heme precursors. Diagnosis in symptomatic patients thus depends on demonstrating specific patterns of overproduction of heme precursors (see Table 39.5) and is usually straightforward, provided appropriate specimens are examined for the relevant intermediates using adequately sensitive techniques.[120,127-129] Although the porphyrias are uncommon disorders, the variability of the associated clinical features may make it necessary to consider them as differential diagnoses in many patients presenting with similar symptoms. Therefore, it is important to apply diagnostic strategies that not only allow for the diagnosis of a porphyria, but also adequately exclude the diagnosis. The full spectrum of porphyria-related analyses is usually only performed by specialist laboratories. If less specialized laboratories offer screening tests or single porphyria-related analyses, they must advise requesting physicians about the limitations of this approach and how to secure adequate diagnostics both for symptomatic patients and for those being investigated due to a family history of porphyria. Acute attacks of porphyria are always associated with excess excretion of PBG and/or ALA, and in patients with cutaneous symptoms caused by porphyria, increased accumulation or excretion of porphyrins is always evident. DNA and enzyme analyses give no information about disease activity, are rarely necessary to confirm the diagnosis in clinically overt porphyria, and are mainly of use for family studies in the autosomal dominant acute porphyrias and in protoporphyria.

Patients With Symptoms of Porphyria

Strategies for the laboratory investigation of patients suspected on clinical grounds of having porphyria depend on the mode of presentation.

Patients With Current or Past Symptoms Consistent With an Acute Neurovisceral Attack

In patients with acute neurovisceral symptoms, diagnostic strategies must be applied depending on the clinical setting, including (1) diagnosing or excluding acute porphyria as the cause of current symptoms, (2) differentiating among the different acute porphyrias, and (3) investigating possible acute porphyria in a patient who no longer has active symptoms. Failure to correctly diagnose an attack of acute porphyria not only delays appropriate life-saving treatment but may result in unnecessary surgery or administration of drugs that aggravate the attack, with potentially fatal consequences. Alternatively, a false diagnosis of porphyria may be just as serious because of delayed vital surgery or other treatment, and may also lead to analgesic (including opiate) misuse and dependency.

Investigation During a Suspected Acute Attack. The essential, first-line investigation in any patient with a suspected attack of acute porphyria is measurement of urinary PBG by an adequately sensitive and specific method.[120,130] Based on the currently available evidence, PBG excretion is always increased during an acute attack of AIP, HCP, or VP, usually to a concentration that exceeds 10 times the upper reference limit.[131] Normal PBG excretion, at a time when symptoms are present, provides strong evidence against any type of acute porphyria as their cause, except for the rare ADP. In ADP, PBG is normal or only slightly elevated, whereas ALA is markedly increased. In AIP, PBG excretion usually remains elevated for years after an attack.[132] However, in VP or HCP, PBG may rapidly return to normal (sometimes within days) once the attack starts to resolve.[133,134] Therefore, if a suspected attack is entering remission, or if clinical suspicion of acute porphyria persists, further investigations are advisable, even if PBG excretion is normal. Testing for ALA is often performed along with PBG, with ALA being increased to a lesser extent than PBG in acute porphyrias.[2,131] Measurement of ALA also allows lead poisoning and ADP to be detected. Patients using methenamine hippurate, a widespread prophylactic for urinary tract infection, may present with falsely low or negative ALA and PBG results.[135]

Increased urinary PBG requires careful evaluation, because although the patient clearly has an acute porphyria, the disease may not be the cause of current symptoms. In AIP, a high urinary PBG excretion increases the likelihood that porphyria is responsible for symptoms, but the final diagnosis should be made on clinical grounds. Some AIP patients who have never clinically expressed the disease may have increased PBG excretion in the absence of symptoms.[136] Poor correlation has been noted between urinary PBG concentration and symptoms, with no "threshold" above which symptoms appear. It is generally accepted that PBG excretion increases further from baseline during an acute attack in AIP, but there is substantial variation in urine PBG excretion due to natural biological variation.[137] Therefore detection and interpretation of a change in urine PBG excretion requires recent information about the patient's baseline excretion. Where this is available, a more than twofold increase in urine PBG excretion is likely to be related to the patient's symptoms and not caused by analytical and biological variation alone.[137]

If increased urinary PBG is found by a qualitative and/or semiquantitative screening test, confirmation by a specific, quantitative method, preferably using the same urine sample, is essential to exclude possible false positives. Measurement of urinary total porphyrin has no role in the screening for acute porphyria. Although in vitro polymerization of PBG to uroporphyrin usually increases the urinary porphyrin concentration when excess PBG is present, false negatives may occur, and secondary coproporphyrinuria is common.[138]

Differentiation Among the Acute Porphyrias. Management of the attack is the same regardless of the type of porphyria, so further investigation is not a matter of urgency. However, differentiation between the acute porphyrias is necessary for deciding which gene to examine by DNA analysis and for the selection of appropriate tests for use in family studies. The absence of skin lesions does not exclude VP or HCP (see Table 39.4).

Once the diagnosis of acute porphyria has been established by demonstration of an unequivocal increase in urinary PBG excretion, various strategies have been developed for distinguishing the different types of acute porphyria.[127-129,139] The most efficient diagnostic strategy uses plasma fluorescence scanning and fecal porphyrin fractionation with coproporphyrin III and I separation to differentiate among AIP, VP, and HCP.[139] In AIP and HCP, overlapping plasma fluorescence emission maximum wavelengths, usually 618 to 621 nm, are seen, whereas the finding of a plasma fluorescence emission maximum of 624 to 628 nm is diagnostic for VP (see Table 39.5).[140] In symptomatic VP patients, the plasma fluorescence peak is always present and typically persists years after remission of clinical symptoms, but its performance may be reduced with increasing age.[140] Based on data from 467 patients with AIP, VP, and HCP diagnosed by mutational analysis, the cutpoint of 623 nm can be used to distinguish VP from the other acute porphyrias.[139] In patients with AIP and HCP, the plasma fluorescence scan may also be normal.

Increased fecal total porphyrin excretion can be found in all three of these acute porphyrias, but high levels of excretions are typically only present in VP and HCP (see Table 39.5). The total fecal porphyrins may be increased in some patients with AIP, particularly if a method that extracts uroporphyrin in addition to ether-soluble porphyrins is used.[141] Fecal protoporphyrin (and other dicarboxylate porphyrins), and to a lesser extent, coproporphyrin-III, are increased in VP (see Table 39.5). In HCP, coproporphyrin-III and the coproporphyrin isomer-III:I ratio are elevated with protoporphyrin-IX only minimally raised or normal. In AIP, coproporphyrin-III excretion and the isomer ratio are normal (see Table 39.5).[139] The diagnosis of HCP thus depends on the demonstration of a high fecal coproporphyrin III/I ratio after exclusion of VP by plasma fluorescence scanning, and the diagnosis of AIP follows the exclusion of VP and HCP. If fecal porphyrin fractionation with coproporphyrin III and I separation is not available, the finding of normal total fecal porphyrin in combination with a negative plasma fluorescence scanning result or an emission peak maximum below 623 nm is diagnostic of AIP.

Analysis of urinary porphyrins has no role in differentiating between the acute porphyrias. Enzyme measurements are mainly of use in patients with atypical presentations that suggest the possibility of a homozygous variant. Enzyme assay of red cell HMBS activity is not sensitive enough and lacks specificity for the diagnosis of AIP.[131,139] Activities in patients with AIP may overlap those in normal individuals, particularly if the patient is acutely ill or in patients with changes in red cell turnover, and activities are normal in the 3% of patients with mutations that affect only the ubiquitous isoform. Assays of leukocyte coproporphyrinogen oxidase or protoporphyrinogen oxidase (the enzymes deficient in HCP and VP, respectively) are technically difficult and are no longer necessary for diagnosis.

AT A GLANCE

Diagnostic Strategy: Acute Porphyria

Diagnostic strategy for the three autosomal dominant acute porphyrias: patients presenting with current or recent symptoms consistent with an attack of acute porphyria and a negative family history.

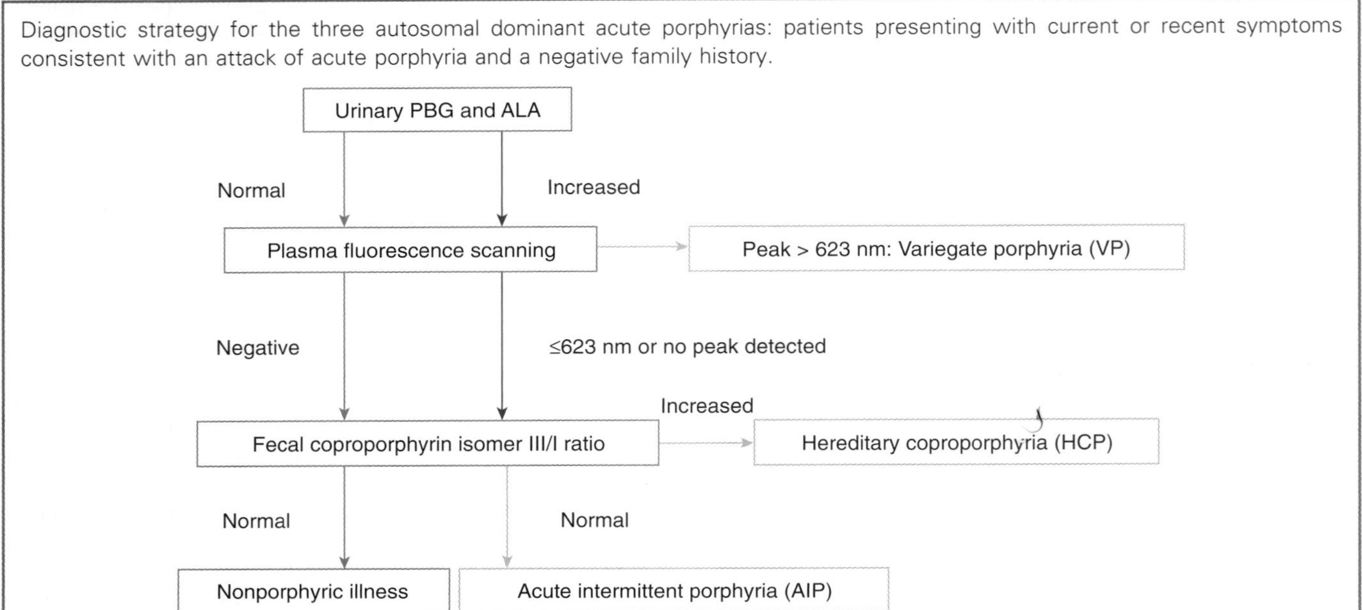

Investigation of an Asymptomatic Patient With Past Symptoms Consistent With an Acute Attack. Diagnosis may be less straightforward when a patient presents for investigation after all clinical symptoms have resolved. Appropriate investigations include measurement of urinary PBG and ALA by specific quantitative methods, plasma fluorescence scanning, and fecal porphyrin fractionation with coproporphyrin III and I separation to diagnose and differentiate among the acute porphyrias. In VP and HCP, excretion of PBG and ALA is usually normal in the absence of symptoms, but the plasma fluorescence scan in VP and the fecal coproporphyrin-isomer ratio in HCP remain abnormal for years after the onset of full clinical remission.[134,140,142] A recent report showed that ALA and PBG excretion remain increased in AIP patients for many years after an acute attack.[132] However, a retrospective study, based on data collected over three decades, reported that ALA and PBG concentrations were within the reference interval in approximately 10% to 20% of AIP patients in clinical remission.[131]

If all these tests are normal, the patient may have AIP in remission, but is most likely to have had a nonporphyric illness with symptoms mimicking those of acute porphyria. If clinical suspicion remains high, mutational analysis of *HMBS*, supplemented by assay of HMBS activity in mutation-negative patients, may help to distinguish these possibilities.[139] Mutational analysis of the *CPOX* and *PPOX* genes is rarely indicated.

Patients With Cutaneous Symptoms

Skin lesions of cutaneous porphyrias are always accompanied by overproduction of porphyrins.

Patients With Acute Photosensitivity Without Skin Fragility or Bullae. Often patients in this group will be children and will have protoporphyria or acute photosensitivity caused by a disorder other than porphyria. For suspected EPP, the essential investigation consists of measurement of erythrocyte protoporphyrin concentration using a sensitive fluorometric method. Screening tests using solvent extraction of blood or fluorescence microscopy of erythrocytes are unreliable. If the erythrocyte porphyrin concentration is within the reference interval, EPP is excluded. If the concentration is increased, it is important to determine whether the increase is caused mainly by free protoporphyrin, as in EPP, both free and ZPP as in XLEPP, or primarily by ZPP, as in Fe deficiency and lead toxicity.

In FECH-deficient EPP, ZPP is typically less than 15% of the total erythrocyte protoporphyrin. The combination of a markedly increased total protoporphyrin with more than 15% ZPP suggests XLEPP,[143] although individuals have been described with distributions of ZPP and free protoporphyrin similar to EPP.[143] The plasma porphyrin concentration is increased in all forms of EPP (see Table 39.5),[78] but not in lead poisoning, Fe deficiency, or other anemias associated with an increased total erythrocyte porphyrin concentration. Thus, plasma fluorescence scanning is a useful additional investigation, particularly in the uncommon patients with EPP in whom erythrocyte protoporphyrin concentrations are only marginally increased. However, some laboratories participating in external quality assessment schemes have reported (false) negative plasma fluorescence scanning results in EPP patients with low concentrations of free protoporphyrin.[144] Fecal protoporphyrin excretion may also be increased, but measurement has no role in the diagnosis (see Table 39.5). DNA analysis is required to confirm the diagnosis of XLEPP in patients with an increased percentage of ZPP or in patients with a family history suggestive of XLEPP. It is also the most reliable way to identify patients who have dysfunctional *FECH* variants, other than c.315-48C, on both alleles, and who may therefore have an increased risk of developing liver disease. Assay of FECH activity in lymphocytes has also been used for this purpose but is available in very few specialist laboratories.[86]

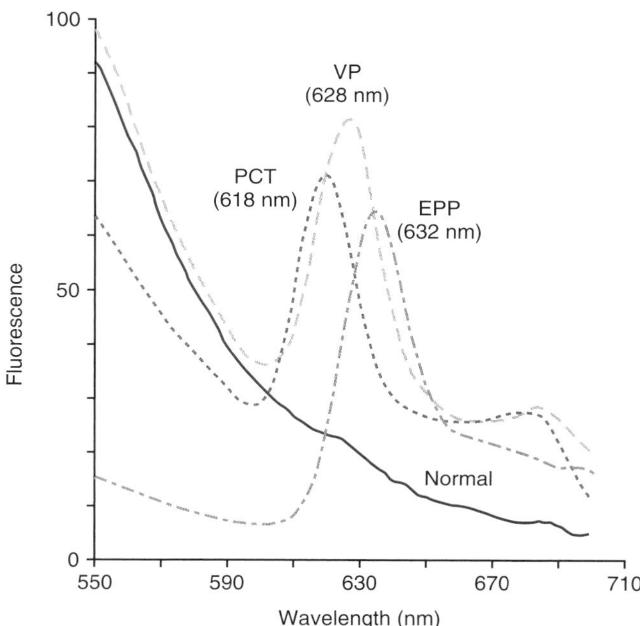

FIGURE 39.3 Fluorescence emission spectra (excitation, 405 nm) of dilutions in phosphate-buffered saline of plasma from a normal individual and from patients with various porphyrias. *EPP*, Erythropoietic protoporphyria; *PCT*, porphyria cutanea tarda; *VP*, variegate porphyria.

Patients With Bullae, Fragility, and/or Scarring. Clinically indistinguishable skin lesions occur in PCT, VP, HCP, CEP (see Table 39.4), HEP, and other rare variants.[42] In addition, identical skin lesions characterize the pseudoporphyria caused by some drugs and the use of sunbeds, in which porphyrin metabolism is normal.[110] Although there is little published evidence,[142] it is generally acknowledged that in patients with current cutaneous symptoms, plasma porphyrin fluorescence scanning is a highly sensitive method for identifying or excluding porphyria as a cause of the skin problem. However, a false negative result is possible if the patient is no longer symptomatic or if the fluorimeter used is not appropriately configured for porphyrin analysis.[144] Most patients with bullae and fragility caused by porphyria will have PCT or VP, with prevalence being affected by local founder effects. Initial investigations should include fluorescence emission spectroscopy of plasma and measurement of total urinary porphyrins.[120,142] A plasma emission peak at approximately 626 nm is diagnostic for VP (see Table 39.5 and Fig. 39.3), and no further investigations are necessary. Increased excretion of urinary total porphyrins and an emission peak at approximately 618 to 620 nm usually indicate PCT but are not specific for this disorder (see Table 39.5 and Fig. 39.3). PCT can be differentiated from the other bullous porphyrias, apart from HEP, by fractionation of urinary or fecal porphyrins, which allows identification of individual porphyrins (Fig. 39.4). In PCT, uro- and heptaporphyrins dominate in plasma and urine, and hepta-, penta-, and isocoproporphyrins dominate in feces.[145] Although inherited deficiency of UROD is an important risk factor for PCT, identification of familial PCT, either by analysis of UROD activity or mutation screening of the *UROD* gene is not essential for the management of individual patients. HCP rarely presents with skin symptoms alone but can be diagnosed on the basis of an increased fecal coproporphyrin isomer III/I ratio after exclusion of VP. In CEP, markedly increased concentrations of urinary porphyrins are evident,[71] mainly consisting of uro- and coproporphyrin type I isomers.[145] In feces, excretion of coproporphyrin type I isomers is usually also markedly increased, with type I isomers contributing more than 80% of the total coproporphyrin.[145,146] Accumulation of uroporphyrin I, coproporphyrin I, and both Zn and free protoporphyrin have been reported in erythrocytes. Confirmation of the diagnosis of CEP thus requires fractionation of urinary and fecal porphyrins using a technique that separates porphyrin isomers and measures erythrocyte porphyrins. Identification of *UROS* mutations may be helpful in confirming the diagnosis, in the assessment of prognosis, defining treatment, and allowing family studies.[147] Further differential diagnosis in young children with bulla and fragile skin are PCT and HEP, which can be differentiated by measurement of erythrocyte porphyrins, erythrocyte UROD activity, and by mutational analysis of *UROD*. Suspected homozygous VP and other rare cutaneous porphyrias similarly require intensive investigation.

Patients may present for investigation after their skin lesions have healed. In PCT, excretion and plasma porphyrin concentrations return to normal during remission, but the proportions of individual porphyrins in urine and feces may remain abnormal for longer than total porphyrin concentrations, and determination of individual porphyrins may suggest the diagnosis.[148] The plasma fluorescence scan in VP and fecal coproporphyrin-III excretion in HCP remain abnormal during clinical remission.

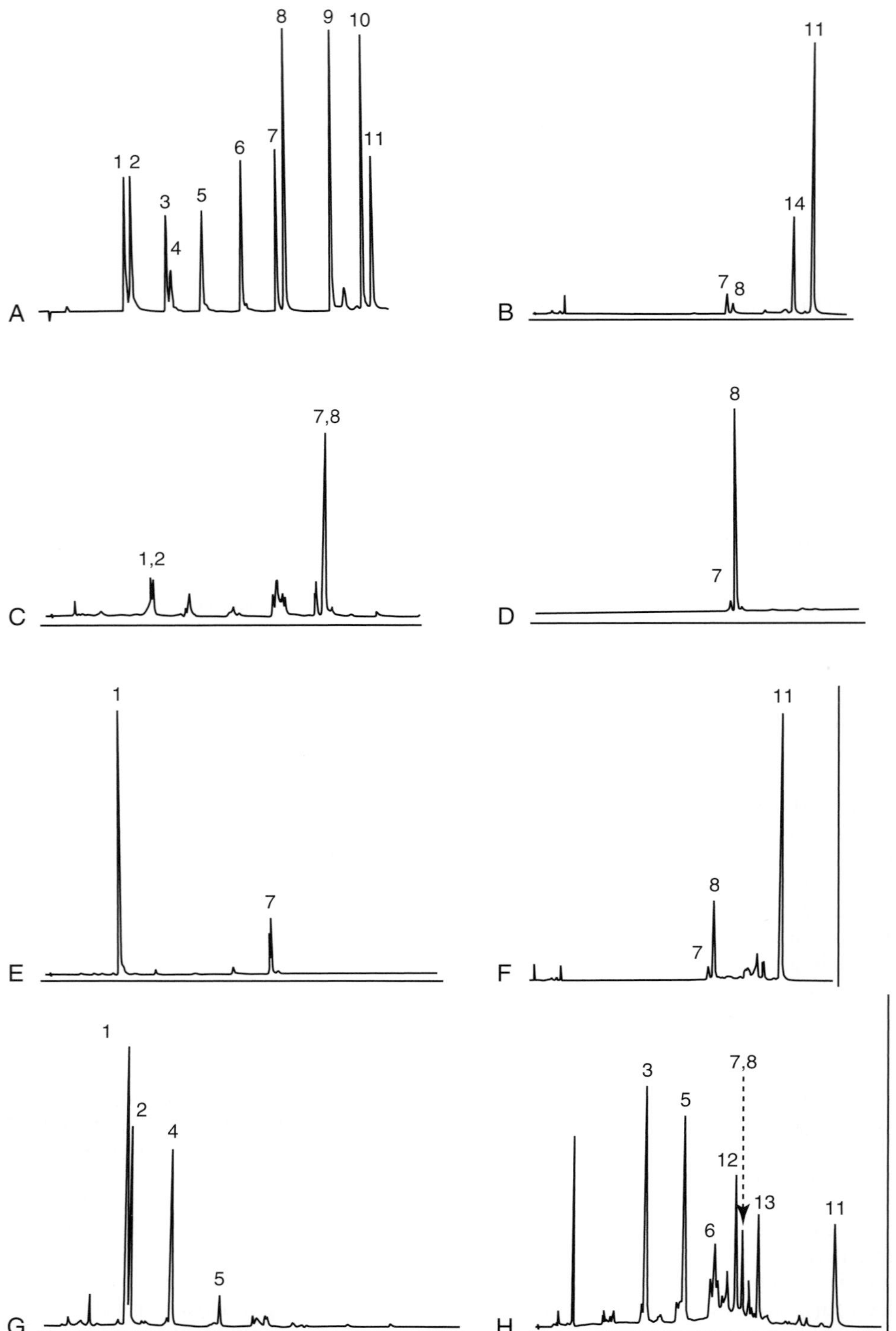

FIGURE 39.4 Representative high-performance liquid chromatography chromatograms for *(A)* working standard, *(B)* normal feces, *(C)* normal urine, *(D)* feces (hereditary coproporphyria), *(E)* urine (congenital erythropoietic porphyria), *(F)* feces (variegate porphyria), *(G)* urine (porphyria cutanea tarda), and *(H)* feces (porphyria cutanea tarda) chromatographic conditions. Peaks are *(1)* uroporphyrin-I, *(2)* uroporphyrin-III, *(3)* heptacarboxylate porphyrin-I, *(4)* heptacarboxylate porphyrin-III, *(5)* hexacarboxylate porphyrin, *(6)* pentacarboxylate porphyrin, *(7)* coproporphyrin-I, *(8)* coproporphyrin-III, *(9)* deuteroporphyrin-IX, *(10)* mesoporphyrin-IX, *(11)* protoporphyrin-IX, *(12)* hydroxyisocoproporphyrin, and *(13)* isocoproporphyrin.

AT A GLANCE

Diagnostic Strategy: Nonacute Porphyria

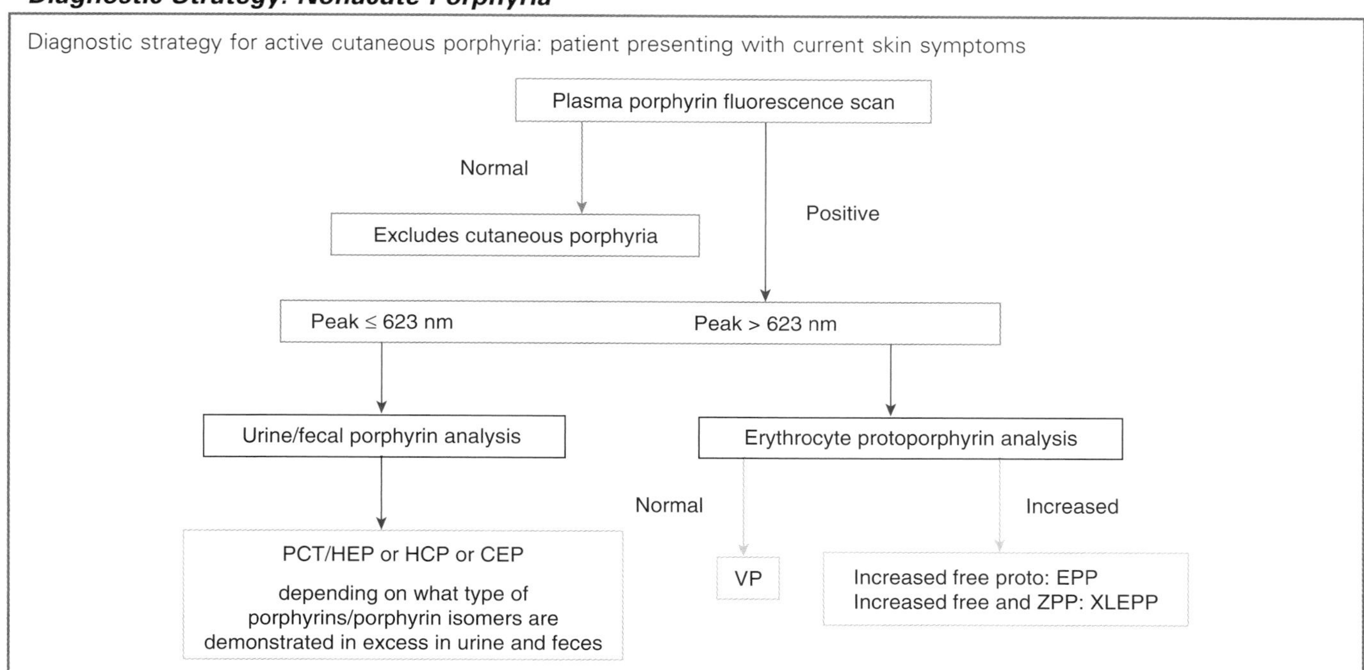

Asymptomatic Relatives of Patients With Porphyria

Depending on the type of porphyria, investigation of healthy at-risk relatives may be beneficial.

Presymptomatic Diagnosis of Autosomal Dominant Acute Porphyrias

Screening of family members to identify asymptomatic individuals who have inherited AIP, VP, or HCP and therefore are at risk for acute attacks is an essential part of the management of families with these disorders. Screening may be carried out by metabolite measurement, enzyme assay, and/or DNA analysis. Mutation detection by DNA analysis is the method of choice for family studies, unless a mutation cannot be identified in the proband, because it is more sensitive than biochemical methods[139] and allows asymptomatic disease to be excluded with certainty. The most sensitive metabolite assays for the presymptomatic diagnosis of each disorder are shown in Table 39.7. Metabolites are almost always normal before puberty, except in HCP.[149,150] Urinary PBG excretion in AIP and the plasma fluorescence scan in VP may also be normal in asymptomatic adults shown by DNA analysis to be affected.[131,151] Measurement of the activity of the defective enzyme is more sensitive, but diagnostic accuracy is limited by the overlap between activities in individuals with disease and in the normal population. In the few AIP families in which a mutation is not identified, erythrocyte HMBS assay may be helpful.

Erythropoietic Protoporphyria

In EPP caused by mutations in the *FECH* gene, testing of the unaffected parent for the presence of the hypomorphic *FECH* c.315-48C allele is helpful in assessing the risk that a future child will have clinically overt disease; the presence of this

TABLE 39.7 Presymptomatic Diagnosis of Autosomal Dominant Acute Porphyrias: Metabolite Measurements in Asymptomatic Individuals With Porphyria Proven by Mutational Analysis

Porphyria	Metabolite	No. of Individuals	Sensitivity	Specificity
AIP	Urine PBG*	98†	59%	100%
HCP	Fecal coproporphyrin isomer-III/I ratio‡	28§	96%	100%
VP	Plasma porphyrin fluorescence	112†	64%	100%

*Greater than 1.5 µmol/mmol creatinine.
†Aged 15 years or more.
‡Greater than 1.4.
§Aged 7 years or more.
AIP, Acute intermittent porphyria; *HCP*, hereditary coproporphyria; *PBG*, porphobilinogen; *VP*, variegate porphyria.

allele increases the risk from approximately 1 in 100 to 1 in 4.[152] In addition, asymptomatic individuals from EPP families may wish to know whether they have inherited a severe *FECH* mutation and thus have the potential to transmit the disease. FECH assay and/or mutation identification is required for this purpose; erythrocyte protoporphyrin concentrations are rarely unequivocally abnormal in such individuals. In XLEPP, mutational analysis of the *ALAS2* gene may be required to identify female carriers who show phenotypic and biochemical heterogeneity, reflecting the degree of X-chromosomal inactivation of the mutant gene.[153]

Other Porphyrias

Family investigation has a more limited role in the clinical management of other porphyrias. In PCT, the autosomal dominant familial form has been identified by erythrocyte UROD assay or mutational analysis, but as yet little evidence suggests that family studies are necessary unless requested by anxious relatives because the identification of a mutation does not alter the management of the patient.[63]

In the autosomal recessive porphyrias, CEP and ADP, screening of families for asymptomatic carriers is not normally helpful, because the low carrier frequency in the general population makes the risk of transmission to the next generation very low. For severe homozygous or compound heterozygous porphyrias, such as CEP, ADP, HEP, and homozygous dominant acute porphyrias, prenatal diagnosis may be indicated and has been reported for CEP[73] and HEP.[154]

LABORATORY ANALYSIS

The analytical methods used in conjunction with porphyrias are described here briefly.

Preanalytical Aspects: Specimen Collection and Stability

For porphyrin analysis, all samples must be protected from light because urinary porphyrin concentrations have been observed to decrease by up to 50% if kept in the light for 24 hours. Urinary porphyrins and PBG are best analyzed in fresh, random (10 to 20 mL) samples collected without preservative. Very dilute urine (creatinine <2 mmol/L) is unsuitable for analysis, and it may be helpful to request an early morning urine sample to ensure it is appropriately concentrated.

Urine often is of normal color in the nonacute porphyrias, except in CEP, when it is usually red, occasionally to such an extent that it is mistaken for hematuria. During an acute attack, urine may be a red-brown color because of the presence of uroporphyrin and other pigments formed by the nonenzymatic polymerization of PBG.

Twenty-four hour urine collections (1) offer little advantage, (2) delay diagnosis, and (3) increase the risk of losses during the collection period, and within-subject biological variation is significantly lower when estimated per millimole creatinine.[137] PBG and porphyrins are stable in urine in the dark at 4°C for up to 48 hours and for at least a month at −20°C. Specimens for ALA estimation should be promptly refrigerated. Urine specimens have been stored at 4°C in the dark for at least 2 weeks without significant loss of ALA,[155] and frozen specimens are stable for weeks, but repeated freeze–thawing should be avoided.[156] Although PBG is more stable at approximately pH 8 to 9, ALA is more stable at approximately pH 3 to 4, although more acidic environments notably reduce ALA stability.

Approximately 5- to 10-g wet weight of feces is adequate for porphyrin measurements. Diagnostically, important changes in concentration are unlikely to occur within 36 hours at room temperature, and samples are stable for many months at −20°C.

Blood anticoagulated with ethylenediaminetetraacetic acid shows no loss of protoporphyrin for up to 8 days at room temperature and for at least 8 weeks at 4°C in the dark.

Quality Management and External Quality Assessment

Few commercial methods are available for porphyrin-related analyses, and most methods are developed in-house. Both harmonization and standardization are lacking. Comparison of analyses between specialist laboratories has revealed differences in diagnostic strategies and analytical quality that may influence their ability to diagnose and monitor porphyria.[144] Participation in external quality assessment (EQA) schemes, preferably assessing the total testing process, and use of internal quality control (IQC) are therefore particularly important for porphyria-related analyses to ensure acceptable diagnostic performance. IQC is available commercially for urine analytes (porphyrin, ALA, and PBG), but not for fecal, plasma, or erythrocyte porphyrins. Porphyrin EQA schemes aimed at less specialized laboratories are also available in some countries and may accept participants from other countries. For laboratories undertaking fluorometric porphyrin analyses, participation in an expert EQA scheme is essential to avoid misdiagnosis. The European Porphyria Network[157] operates a clinical EQA scheme, assessing the total testing process for porphyria-related analyses in all sample types. The scheme is open to specialist laboratories throughout the world.[158] A specialized analytical EQA scheme covering all sample types is operated by the Royal College of Pathologists of Australasia[159] and is open to enrollment by any laboratory.

Methods for Porphyrins and Porphyrin Precursors in Urine and Feces

The water-soluble metabolites, PBG and ALA, are excreted by the kidney and usually are measured in the urine in the clinical laboratory. Both have been measured in plasma by HPLC–mass spectrometry and fluorometric enzyme assays.[127,160] Mass spectrometry is also being used to measure urinary ALA and PBG simultaneously,[161,162] as well as to identify patterns of urinary and fecal porphyrin excretion.[163,164] However limited knowledge on the diagnostic accuracy of these methods, small sample numbers, and equipment expense mean that these methods are not yet in widespread use.

Porphobilinogen

Most methods for PBG are based on the reaction of Ehrlich's reagent (dimethylaminobenzaldehyde in acidic solution) with the α-methene carbon of the pyrrole ring to form a colored product variously described as "rose red" or "magenta," which has a characteristic absorption spectrum, with a peak at 553 nm and a shoulder at 540 nm. Porphyrins do not contain any α-methene hydrogens and therefore do not react. Some other substances in urine may react with the reagent to give red products (eg, urobilinogen), may inhibit the reaction, or are pigmented themselves and so mask the red chromogen.[127,165] All need to be removed. This is best achieved by ion-exchange chromatography (first described by Mauzerall and Granick[166]), but methods for accurate quantification of PBG based on this procedure are time-consuming.

Qualitative screening tests in which urine reacts directly with Ehrlich's reagent and is assessed visually for the formation of red chromogen (eg, the Watson-Schwartz[167] and Hoesch[168] tests) have been criticized for poor detection limits and interferences, even when solvent extraction has been used to separate the PBG-Ehrlich compound from the urobilinogen-Ehrlich complex.[169,170] The Mauzerall-Granick method has been modified in attempts to produce an alternative that is acceptable for screening purposes. Buttery and Stuart[171] avoided the use of columns by employing batchwise treatment with resin, and visually compared the final color with that of a surrogate calibrator. Blake and colleagues[130] eliminated the centrifugation steps by using resin-filled syringes with detachable filters and compared the final color with a variety of artificial calibrators. These modifications reduced the time taken to perform the test to 10 minutes and produced a semiquantitative result.[172] If a qualitative or semiquantitative screening test is used, it is essential to include appropriate controls and to confirm all positive test results using a specific quantitative method.

Commercial methods for measurement of both PBG and ALA, based on that of Mauzerall and Granick,[166] are available (Bio-Rad Laboratories, Hercules, California; Recipe Clinical Diagnostics, Munich, Germany). In-house prepared ion-exchange resin columns can also be used. PBG in the resin eluate reacts with Ehrlich's reagent to form a colored product that is scanned in a spectrometer. Scanning the spectrum of the product is essential if interferences are to be identified. For example, imipenem often gives a peak at 580 nm with Ehrlich's reagent.[173] Urinary PBG that is raised at least two to three times the upper reference limit is diagnostic of an acute porphyria (suggested reference intervals are given in Table 39.3), but it is important that individual laboratories determine a cut point above which further investigation is required. False negative urine PBG results can be seen in patients on methenamine hippurate (Hiprex, Sanofi-Aventis, Bridgewater, New Jersey).[135]

5-Aminolevulinic Acid

It is possible to measure ALA directly,[127,160] but it is more usually converted into an Ehrlich-reacting pyrrole through condensation with a reagent such as acetylacetone after separation from PBG by two-stage, anion-exchange chromatography.[166] Commercial methods based on that of Mauzerall and Granick[166] are available (Bio-Rad Laboratories and Recipe Clinical Diagnostics). A photometric method has been proposed for more rapid testing. Several interferences have been observed,[135,173] including the acetylacetone derivatization step that forms a compound with penicillin that reacts with Ehrlich's reagent.[174]

Analysis of Porphyrins in Urine and Feces

Methods for porphyrin fractionation are complex and time-consuming and are not available in every laboratory. Consequently, simple qualitative screening tests are often used to differentiate the majority of specimens that do not require further investigation from the few that justify fractionation of the individual porphyrins. Screening tests in which extracts of urine or feces are examined visually for typical red-pink fluorescence of porphyrins are not sensitive analytically and should not be used.[170] Methods based on spectrophotometric scanning of acidified urine or fecal extracts for the presence of the Soret band are recommended and yield semiquantitative information.[120] Quantitative fluorometric methods are also available.[130]

All methods for the fractionation of porphyrins are based on varying solubilities of individual porphyrins caused by their different β-substituents and, to a lesser extent, on the substituent order around the macrocycle. Methods include (1) differential extraction with solvents, (2) paper and thin-layer chromatography, and (3) HPLC. Solvent extraction methods should not be used because they yield only limited and sometimes misleading information.[175] Reversed-phase HPLC, the current method of choice, separates all porphyrins of clinical interest, including isomers and metal chelates, without the need for previous methylation. Spectrophotometric or fluorometric detection has been used; the latter method is more sensitive and specific. Porphyrins in urine should be expressed as a ratio to creatinine concentration to correct for dilution. Suggested reference values for urine and feces total and individual porphyrins are given in Table 39.3.

Semiquantitative Method for Total Porphyrin in Urine

This simple method for total urine porphyrins[120] uses scanning spectrometry. A typical spectrum is shown in Fig. 39.5. This method is reproducible, but it is only semiquantitative. The detection limit depends on the amount of background absorbance, but concentrations of approximately 50 nmol/L should be detected in urine of normal color. Very occasionally, urine contains substances that produce high background absorbance, making identification of any peak in the 400-nm region difficult. Such samples require analysis by alternative methods, such as HPLC. Increased concentrations require further investigation to identify individual porphyrins; porphyria should not be diagnosed on the basis of increased total porphyrin alone.

Semiquantitative Method for Total Porphyrin in Feces

This simple method for total fecal porphyrins uses scanning spectrometry after extraction.[176] The expression of concentration on a dry weight basis corrects for the moisture content of feces. Total fecal porphyrin determined by this method, unlike most of those based on solvent extraction, includes uroporphyrin.[141] Very occasionally, feces contain substances that produce very high background absorbance, making identification of any peak in the 400-nm region difficult. Such samples require analysis by alternative methods, such as HPLC.

Increased total fecal porphyrin concentration requires further investigation by fractionation, identification, and quantification of individual porphyrins using a technique, such as reversed-phase HPLC, which resolves coproporphyrin-I and -III isomers. Porphyria should never be diagnosed on the basis of raised total fecal porphyrin alone.

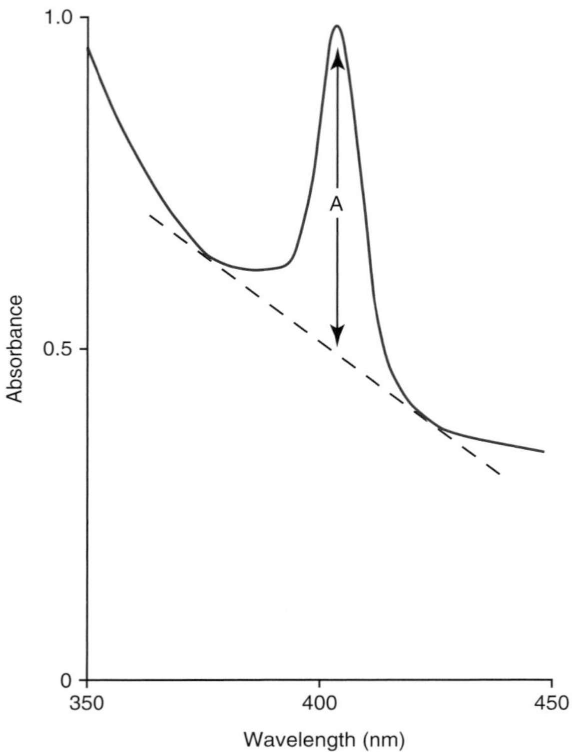

FIGURE 39.5 Absorption spectrum of acidified urine showing the procedure for measurement of corrected absorbance *(A)* of the porphyrin peak.

High-Performance Liquid Chromatography Fractionation of Porphyrins in Urine and Feces

This method for fractionation of urinary and fecal porphyrins uses sample preparation, HPLC separation, and fluorometric detection.[177] Samples are assayed with and without addition of a calibrator to assist with fluorometric peak identification.

Fig. 39.4 shows typical profiles from patients with various types of porphyria. For diagnostic purposes, quantification of individual porphyrins is rarely necessary, particularly if the concentrations are clearly elevated. Table 39.5 shows expected findings in the various types of porphyria, and reference intervals for individual porphyrin fractions are given in Table 39.3. Considerable variation is evident in the reference intervals quoted in the literature, probably as a consequence of difficulties in calibration.

The extraction method for fecal porphyrins results in some interference with the chromatography caused by dissolution of a proportion of the diethyl ether in the aqueous phase. As a result, an extra peak elutes just before the uroporphyrin position. This peak contains any uroporphyrin in the sample, up to 50% of the heptacarboxylate porphyrins, and smaller quantities of hexacarboxylate and pentacarboxylate porphyrins (see Fig. 39.4H).

Methods for Blood Porphyrins

The methods described here require a spectrofluorometer with a red-sensitive photomultiplier. If such equipment is not available locally, samples should be referred to a specialized laboratory. Erythrocyte and plasma measurements are rarely required for the urgent assessment of acutely ill patients.

Determination of Erythrocyte Total Porphyrin

The most widely used method for erythrocyte total porphyrin is based on double extraction and fluorometry.[130,178] Total erythrocyte porphyrin concentrations are increased in (1) EPP and XLEPP, (2) CEP, (3) the rare homozygous variants of the autosomal dominant porphyrias, (4) Fe deficiency, (5) hemolytic anemia, (6) some other forms of anemia, and (7) lead poisoning. A total porphyrin concentration within the reference interval excludes EPP. Suggested reference intervals are given in Table 39.3. Distinction between the protoporphyrias and other causes of increased erythrocyte total porphyrin concentration requires differentiation between protoporphyrin and its Zn chelate, because the acidic condition of this assay dissociates the Zn chelate and provides only a measure of total porphyrin.

Determination of Zinc-Protoporphyrin and Protoporphyrin

If erythrocyte (proto)porphyrin concentration is increased, it is important to differentiate between free protoporphyrin, as in EPP or ZPP, as in Fe deficiency and lead toxicity (Fig. 39.6). This requires extraction with a neutral solvent, such as ethanol[179] or acetone,[180] to prevent the demetalation caused by strong acids, followed by fluorescence spectroscopy or HPLC to distinguish free protoporphyrin from ZPP (fluorescence emission maxima 630 nm and 587 nm, respectively). The qualitative method for ZPP and protoporphyrin using extraction and fluorometry[179] can, with experience, be used to screen for EPP without the necessity for quantitative analysis. It is possible to quantify both ZPP and protoporphyrin by measuring the peak heights at 587 nm and 630 nm above a constructed baseline, if calibrator solutions of both protoporphyrins are prepared, provided allowance is made for a contribution of fluorescence from ZPP at the maximum wavelength for free protoporphyrin. A limitation of this method is that the efficiency of the extraction of ZPP is only approximately 50%. Hematofluorometers specifically designed to measure ZPP concentrations are unsuitable for measurement of the concentration of free protoporphyrin and should not be used to screen for EPP.

Analysis of Plasma Porphyrins

Plasma porphyrins may be determined by fluorescence emission spectroscopy of saline-diluted plasma[181] or deproteinized extracts, or by HPLC.[182] The fluorescence emission method, which offers the advantages of simplicity and inclusion of porphyrins that are bound covalently to plasma proteins, is detailed in the following section. The HPLC-based method has the advantage of fractionating plasma porphyrins and identifying specific porphyrias such as PCT.[182]

Fluorescence Emission Spectroscopy of Plasma Porphyrins

This method determines the fluorescence emission spectrum of saline-diluted plasma excited at 405 nm.[181] Fig. 39.3 shows typical fluorescence emission maximum wavelengths for various porphyrias. In VP, the plasma contains porphyrin covalently bound to protein with a fluorescence emission maximum at 624 to 628 nm.[140,181] In other porphyrias, porphyrin is noncovalently bound to albumin and hemopexin.[183] In freshly separated plasma, protoporphyrin has a fluorescence emission peak at approximately 632 nm. If separation

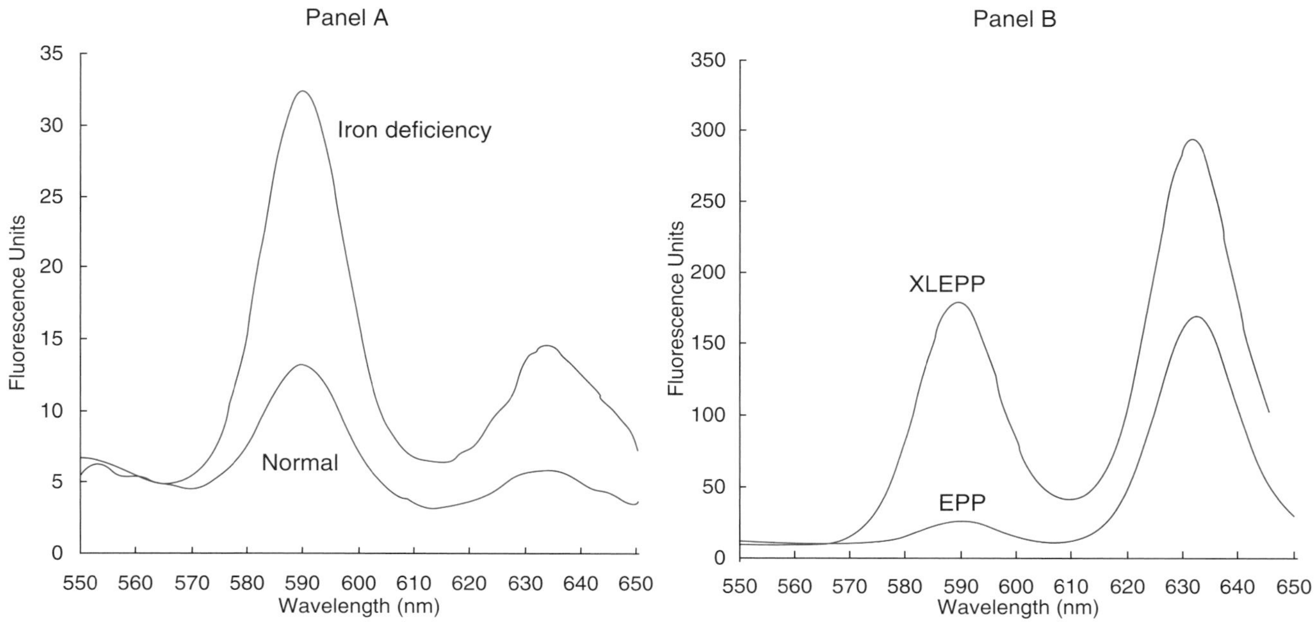

FIGURE 39.6 Fluorescence emission spectra (excitation at 405 nm) of ethanolic extracts of erythrocytes from a *(A)* normal individual and with iron deficiency and *(B)* from patients with erythropoietic protoporphyria *(EPP)* or X-linked erythropoietic protoporphyria *(XLEPP)*. Note that different scales are used.

is delayed, binding to globin released from red cells decreases the peak toward 626 nm. Apart from porphyrias (see Table 39.5), the plasma porphyrin concentration may be increased in conditions in which porphyrin excretion is impaired, such as renal failure and cholestasis.

POINTS TO REMEMBER

Diagnostics

- Identification of individual porphyrias usually requires analysis of urine, feces, and blood samples.
- All specimens must be protected from light.
- Symptomatic porphyria is always associated with increased production of porphyrins and porphyrin precursors.
  - Active acute autosomal dominant porphyria can be diagnosed by measuring increased PBG in a random urine sample.
  - Active cutaneous porphyrias can be diagnosed as a first step by finding a positive plasma porphyrin fluorescence emission screen in a freshly separated plasma sample.
- EPP cannot be diagnosed by urine porphyrin analysis; a blood sample for erythrocyte protoporphyrin analysis is essential.
- Fluorescent porphyrin analysis requires a red-sensitive photomultiplier for detection.
- Laboratories specializing in porphyria diagnosis must register with an appropriate EQA scheme.

Enzyme Measurements

Assay of individual enzymes of the heme biosynthetic pathway is rarely required for the assessment of patients with symptoms of porphyria. However, measurement of enzyme activities may be useful for family studies when it is not possible to identify the individual mutation or when DNA analysis is not available, and for the identification of uncommon subtypes such as nonerythroid AIP and "homozygous" forms of autosomal dominant porphyrias. Erythrocytes are a convenient source of cytoplasmic enzymes (ALAD, HMBS, UROS, and UROD), but assay of the mitochondrial enzymes (CPOX, PPOX, and FECH) requires nucleated cells such as lymphocytes, Epstein-Barr virus–transformed lymphoblasts, or cultured fibroblasts.[127] Assays for enzymes that use porphyrinogens as substrates are difficult because the substrate (1) is unstable, (2) has to be prepared fresh, particularly with protoporphyrinogen, and (3) undergoes nonenzymatic oxidation during the assay. However, erythrocyte HMBS measurement is relatively straightforward and has been the most widely used of these enzyme assays.

Assay of Erythrocyte Hydroxymethylbilane Synthase Activity

The enzymatic assay measures the rate of formation of porphyrinogens from PBG by hemolyzed erythrocytes. The reference interval (mean ± 2 SDs) is 20- to 42-nmol uroporphyrin per milliliter of erythrocytes per minute at 37°C.[184]

Measurement of erythrocyte HMBS activity discriminates between individuals with AIP and their unaffected relatives, with a likelihood ratio of 3.4.[131] Although activities are usually below the reference interval in AIP, some overlap is noted between activities in AIP and healthy individuals, and activities are within the reference interval in the uncommon nonerythroid form.[131,139] In addition, erythrocyte HMBS activity declines sharply with erythrocyte age and is markedly influenced by the proportions of reticulocytes and young cells in peripheral blood. Activity may increase in acutely ill patients, for example, during an acute attack of porphyria[185] and may also be increased or decreased in disorders other than porphyria, including liver disease and chronic alcohol abuse.[131] In France, the prevalence of abnormally low HMBS activities in the general population is approximately 1 in 800.[41]

DNA Analysis

DNA analysis is required in the porphyrias mainly (1) for family screening, (2) for identifying the pattern of inheritance in families with EPP, and (3) as an aid in assessing prognosis in CEP. Its use as a front-line diagnostic investigation is largely restricted to exclusion of an acute porphyria in patients without current symptoms or biochemical abnormalities, and to the investigation of rare atypical cases. Screening of families for porphyria by DNA analysis is a two-stage process. First, the mutation that causes porphyria in the family under investigation needs to be identified by analysis of DNA from a family member in whom the diagnosis of a specific type of porphyria has been established unequivocally. Second, that patient's relatives are then screened for the mutation. The first part of this process is the more complex. Because most mutations are restricted to one or a few families, identification of a mutation in a new family almost always requires analysis of all exons with their flanking intronic sequences and the promoter region. Only in those countries where founder mutations predominate, as with, for example, VP in South Africa[46] and AIP in Sweden,[47] is initial testing for a single mutation useful.

Analysis of a gene for the presence of a mutation is most commonly carried out using direct sequencing of genomic DNA. All laboratories offering a genetic testing service should take part in a relevant external quality control scheme such as that provided by the European Molecular Genetics Quality Network.[186] If no mutation is identified by direct sequencing, gene dosage analysis should be carried out to search for large deletions that are undetectable by standard sequencing protocols. Polymerase chain reaction–based methods for gene dosage analysis include quantitative fluorescent polymerase chain reaction, multiplex ligation probe amplification, and real-time quantitative polymerase chain reaction (see Chapter 47). Sufficient patients have now been identified with gross deletions in porphyria genes[139,187,188] to indicate that a method for gene dosage analysis should be included in routine protocols for mutation analysis. Unclassified variants continue to be identified in the porphyria genes, and these need to be assessed individually.[189] However, proof that a missense mutation causes disease may require expression and characterization of the mutant enzyme in a prokaryotic or eukaryotic vector. The use of a gene panel containing all porphyria genes without initial biochemical diagnosis of the type of porphyria may lead to confusion due to the presence of both unclassified variants and because of the high prevalence of nonpenetrant mutations.

Once the mutation that causes porphyria in a family has been identified, relatives are screened for its presence by direct sequencing of the region containing the mutation or by some other mutation-specific method (see Chapter 47). The *FECH c.315-48C* allele is readily identified by direct sequencing.

The clinical sensitivity of mutation detection in the acute porphyrias is high, provided gene dosage analysis is included in the analysis; for example, it is 98% for *HMBS*, 100% for *PPOX*, and 97% for *CPOX*.[139] Investigation of a large number of unrelated patients with EPP identified *FECH* or *ALAS2* mutations in 94% to 100% of them[87,143]; indirect evidence suggests that sensitivity for mutation detection in the *UROD* gene is approximately 95%.[63] At least 10% of mutant *UROS* alleles are undetected by current methods.[73]

POINTS TO REMEMBER

Genetic Testing in Acute Porphyria

- The main purpose is to identify family members who are at risk of an acute attack.
- The type of acute porphyria must be determined biochemically in the index case.
- The pathogenic mutation must be identified in the relevant gene.
- Family members should be appropriately counseled and offered testing for the presence of the familial mutation.
- After appropriate counseling and consent, testing of children is clinically justifiable.
- Patients with a predictive diagnosis of acute porphyria should be counseled on the avoidance of agents or behaviors that can trigger acute attacks.

SELECTED REFERENCES

For a full list of references for this chapter, please refer to ExpertConsult.com.

1. Anderson K, Sassa S, Bishop D, et al. Disorders of heme biosynthesis: X-linked sideroblastic anemia and the porphyrias. In: Scriver C, Beaudet A, Sly W, et al., editors. *The metabolic and molecular basis of inherited disease*. 8th ed. New York: McGraw-Hill; 2000. p. 2961–3062.
2. Puy H, Gouya L, Deybach JC. Porphyrias. *Lancet* 2010;**375**:924–37.
34. Whatley SD, Ducamp S, Gouya L, et al. C-terminal deletions in the ALAS2 gene lead to gain of function and cause X-linked dominant protoporphyria without anemia or iron overload. *Am J Hum Genet* 2008;**83**:408–14.
37. Meyer UA, Schuurmans MM, Lindberg RL. Acute porphyrias: pathogenesis of neurological manifestations. *Semin Liver Dis* 1998;**18**:43–52.
48. Hift RJ, Meissner PN. An analysis of 112 acute porphyric attacks in Cape Town, South Africa: evidence that acute intermittent porphyria and variegate porphyria differ in susceptibility and severity. *Medicine (Baltimore)* 2005;**84**: 48–60.
55. Stein P, Badminton M, Barth J, et al. Best practice guidelines on clinical management of acute attacks of porphyria and their complications. *Ann Clin Biochem* 2013;**50**:217–23.
58. Elder GH. Porphyria cutanea tarda and related disorders. In: Kadish K, Smith K, Guilard R, editors. *Medical aspects of porphyrias*, vol. 14. The porphyrin handbook. Amsterdam: Academic Press; 2003. p. 67–92.
64. Phillips JD, Bergonia HA, Reilly CA, et al. A porphomethene inhibitor of uroporphyrinogen decarboxylase causes porphyria cutanea tarda. *Proc Natl Acad Sci USA* 2007;**104**: 5079–84.
71. Desnick RJ, Astrin KH. Congenital erythropoietic porphyria: advances in pathogenesis and treatment. *Br J Haematol* 2002;**117**:779–95.
78. Holme SA, Anstey AV, Finlay AY, et al. Erythropoietic protoporphyria in the U.K.: clinical features and effect on quality of life. *Br J Dermatol* 2006;**155**:574–81.

120. Deacon AC, Elder GH. ACP Best Practice No 165: front line tests for the investigation of suspected porphyria. *J Clin Pathol* 2001;**54**:500–7.
132. Marsden JT, Rees DC. Urinary excretion of porphyrins, porphobilinogen and delta-aminolaevulinic acid following an attack of acute intermittent porphyria. *J Clin Pathol* 2014;**67**:60–5.
139. Whatley SD, Mason NG, Woolf JR, et al. Diagnostic strategies for autosomal dominant acute porphyrias: retrospective analysis of 467 unrelated patients referred for mutational analysis of the HMBS, CPOX, or PPOX gene. *Clin Chem* 2009;**55**:1406–14.
144. Aarsand AK, Villanger JH, Stole E, et al. European specialist porphyria laboratories: diagnostic strategies, analytical quality, clinical interpretation, and reporting as assessed by an external quality assurance program. *Clin Chem* 2011;**57**:1514–23.
152. Gouya L, Puy H, Robreau AM, et al. The penetrance of dominant erythropoietic protoporphyria is modulated by expression of wildtype FECH. *Nat Genet* 2002;**30**:27–8.
164. Danton M, Lim CK. Porphyrin profiles in blood, urine and faeces by HPLC/electrospray ionization tandem mass spectrometry. *Biomed Chromatogr* 2006;**20**:612–21.
166. Mauzerall D, Granick S. The occurrence and determination of delta-amino-levulinic acid and porphobilinogen in urine. *J Biol Chem* 1956;**219**:435–46.
177. Lim CK, Peters TJ. Urine and faecal porphyrin profiles by reversed-phase high-performance liquid chromatography in the porphyrias. *Clin Chim Acta* 1984;**139**:55–63.
182. Hindmarsh JT, Oliveras L, Greenway DC. Plasma porphyrins in the porphyrias. *Clin Chem* 1999;**45**:1070–6.
191. Elder G, Harper P, Badminton M, et al. The incidence of inherited porphyrias in Europe. *J Inherit Metab Dis* 2013;**36**:849–57.

40

Therapeutic Drugs and Their Management

*Michael C. Milone and Leslie M. Shaw**

ABSTRACT

Background
Therapeutic drug monitoring (TDM) is the traditional term used for the activity of measuring drug concentrations to tailor the dose of the medication to an individual. The use of monitored drug therapy is generally reserved for drugs with a narrow therapeutic index, with variable pharmacokinetic behavior, and for which the efficacy or toxicity is difficult to measure or detect early during therapy.

Content
In this chapter, we review the rationale for TDM, the fundamental principles of pharmacokinetics that are required to effectively use drug concentration data and preanalytical and analytical factors affecting concentration measurement. We also provide a broad overview of a selected group of commonly monitored drugs that includes some of the challenges and pitfalls to their monitoring.

The ability of medicines to both heal and hurt has been recognized since ancient times. Immortalized by the writing of the Renaissance Swiss-German physician, Paracelsus, over 500 years ago[1]:

> *All things are poison and nothing is without poison, only the dose makes that a thing is not a poison.*

The challenge in medicine is therefore to determine the optimal dose of medicine that will help a patient with limited associated harm.

Studies in the 1990s identified that adverse events associated with drug therapy rank within the top 10 causes of death in the United States.[2] Although many of the severe or fatal events may not be preventable, more than a third appear to be preventable.[3] In addition to the tragic life and death consequences of adverse drug events (ADEs), failed drug therapy also has a significant economic impact. The estimated cost of ADEs ranges from $17 to $29 billion in the United States alone.[4] Just examining hospital-associated ADEs, the average cost of treating each preventable event is estimated to be greater than $3000 in addition to the increased length of stay.[5] The causes of preventable drug-related adverse events vary; however, inadequate monitoring of therapy represents major sources of preventable ADEs, contributing to as much as 40% of these events.[2] Improving monitoring strategies is therefore likely to have an important impact on both health and its associated cost.

Drug therapy may be monitored in many ways. Clinical signs and symptoms of toxicity are often an effective way to detect toxicity or treatment failure. β-Blockers represent a typical example. Blood pressure and heart rate monitoring can be used to assess efficacy and toxicity of these drugs. Both are also easily measurable in the clinical setting and even at home. As a result, there is little need to perform monitoring beyond these straightforward clinical assessments.

The efficacy and toxicity of some drugs, however, can be much more difficult to monitor on clinical signs and symptoms alone. Insulin treatment in diabetes represents a case in point. The consequences of inappropriate insulin treatment are insidious, potentially life threatening, and very difficult to detect. Excessive insulin can lead to an acute decrease in blood glucose culminating in coma, permanent brain injury, and death. Inadequate insulin dosing, although not as acutely life threatening, leads over time to vascular disease, end-stage renal failure, blindness, and neuropathy that results in significant morbidity and mortality. Laboratory testing of blood glucose, a direct biomarker of insulin's mechanism of action, provides an ideal means to monitor insulin therapy and prevent these complications. It is so important in diabetes therapy that it has driven the commercial development of simple, point-of-care devices that patients can use to routinely monitor their therapy at home. Biomarkers of drug efficacy or toxicity such as blood glucose, while highly desirable, are not always available. In the absence of a useful biomarker of drug effect, measuring the drug itself provides a potential surrogate.

Therapeutic drug monitoring (TDM) is the traditional term used for the activity of measuring drug concentrations to tailor the dose of the medication to an individual. There is an implicit assumption in TDM of a relationship between drug concentrations and efficacy or toxicity outcomes. The use of TDM and *applied pharmacokinetics* to guide drug therapy began in the 1960s, coincident with the development of robust analytical techniques.[6-9] Since this time, TDM has

*The authors gratefully acknowledge the contributions by Christine L.H. Snozek, Gwendolyn A. McMillan, and Thomas P. Moyer on which this chapter is based.

become the standard of care for monitoring therapy with many drugs, including antiepileptic drugs (AEDs), immunosuppressive drugs (ISDs), and antibiotics. TDM is a complex process that involves several members of the health care team, including pharmacists, laboratory professionals, and physicians. To justify the costs associated with TDM, it must improve clinical outcome as well as reduce the overall cost of drug therapy. Prospective, randomized, concentration-controlled trials (RCCTs) of TDM are limited; however, some of these RCCTs show that concentration control can improve efficacy and reduce toxicity of drug therapy.[10-17] Cost-effectiveness of TDM is lacking for most drugs, but TDM has been shown to improve the costs of aminoglycoside therapy.[18] TDM also may aid in detection of nonadherence to drug therapy,[19-21] which represents a frequent and important cause of preventable ADEs.[3,22] This benefit may even extend to drugs not routinely monitored by traditional blood concentration monitoring.[23]

This chapter will focus on the general principles of pharmacology and their application to TDM with a discussion of the pharmacology and TDM of some commonly monitored drugs. It is difficult to provide a comprehensive review of TDM in a single chapter. Readers are therefore referred to textbooks dedicated to the subject of TDM and applied pharmacology for more in-depth information.

FUNDAMENTAL PRINCIPLES OF APPLIED PHARMACOKINETICS

Basic Concepts and Definitions

Pharmacology comprises the body of knowledge surrounding chemical agents and their effects on living processes. This is a broad field, and it has traditionally been confined to drugs that are useful in the prevention, diagnosis, and treatment of disease. *Pharmacotherapeutics* is the part of pharmacology concerned primarily with the application or administration of drugs to patients for the purpose of prevention and treatment of disease. For this aspect of medical practice to be effective, the *pharmacodynamic* and *pharmacokinetic* (PK) properties of drugs should be understood. *Toxicology* is the subdiscipline of pharmacology concerned with adverse effects of chemicals on living systems. Toxic effects and mechanisms of action may be different from therapeutic effects and mechanisms for the same drug. Similarly, at the high dose of drugs at which toxic effects may be produced, rate processes are frequently altered compared with those at therapeutic doses. For these reasons, the terms *toxicodynamics* and *toxicokinetics* are now applied to these special situations.

Pharmacodynamics

Pharmacodynamics encompasses the processes of interaction of pharmacologically active substances with target sites, and the biochemical and physiologic consequences leading to therapeutic or adverse effects. For many drugs, the ultimate effect or mechanism of action at the molecular level is poorly understood, if at all. A pharmacologic effect (ie, the therapeutic or toxic response to a drug) may be elicited by direct interaction of the drug with the receptor controlling a specific function or by a drug-mediated alteration of the physiologic process regulating the function. For most drugs, the intensity and duration of the observed pharmacologic effect are proportional to the concentration of the drug at the receptor. In a given tissue, the site at which a drug acts to initiate events leading to a specific biological effect is called the site of action of the drug.

The mechanism of action of a drug is the biochemical or physical process that occurs at the site of action. Drug action is usually mediated through a receptor. Cellular enzymes, as well as structural or transport proteins, are important examples of drug receptors. Nonprotein macromolecules also may bind drugs, resulting in altered cellular functions controlled by membrane permeability or DNA transcription. Some drugs are chemically similar to important natural endogenous substances and may compete for binding sites. In addition, some drugs may block formation, release, uptake, or transport of essential substances. Others may produce an effect by interacting with relatively small molecules to form complexes that actively bind to receptors. These and other examples of receptor binding are more completely discussed in pharmacology texts.[24-29]

Although the exact molecular interactions that give rise to the mechanism of action for many drugs remain obscure, numerous theoretical models have been developed to explain drug action. One concept postulates that a drug binds to intracellular macromolecular receptors through ionic and hydrogen bonds and van der Waals forces. This theoretical model further postulates that if the drug-receptor complex is sufficiently stable and able to modify the target system, an observable pharmacologic response will occur. As Fig. 40.1 illustrates, the response is concentration dependent until a maximal effect is reached. The plateau may be due to saturation at the receptor or overload of a transport process.

The utility of monitoring drug concentration is based on the premise that pharmacologic response correlates with the concentration of the drug at the site of action (receptor). Although attempts have been made to measure the concentration of drugs at the receptor site in a patient,[30] in general, this approach is technically impractical, if not impossible for most drugs. Studies have shown that for many drugs, a strong correlation exists between the serum drug concentration and the observed pharmacologic effect. In addition, years of relating blood concentrations to drug effects have demonstrated

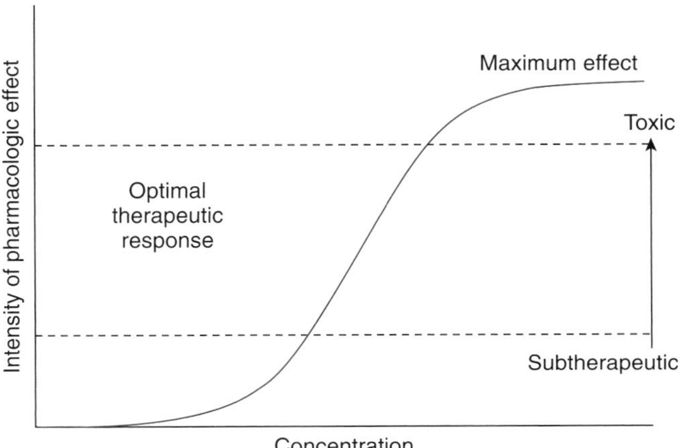

FIGURE 40.1 The dose-effect relationship. The probability of increasing pharmacologic response and risk for toxicity parallels concentration for most drugs. The plateau (maximum effect) is likely due to saturation at the receptor.

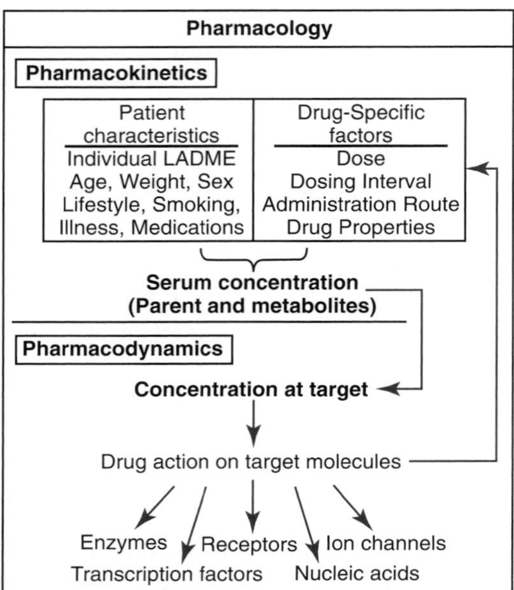

FIGURE 40.2 Conceptual relationship between pharmacodynamics and pharmacokinetics. Many drug- and patient-specific factors determine both the serum concentration of a therapeutic compound and its metabolites. Serum concentration in turn is related to the amount of drug present at the target site, resulting in effects on a variety of molecules (several examples shown) to induce a pharmacologic response. The efficacy and degree of response provide feedback to allow optimization of the dosing regimen for an individual patient. *LADME,* Liberation, absorption, distribution, metabolism, elimination.

the clinical utility of drug concentration information. One must nevertheless always keep in mind that a serum drug concentration does not necessarily equal the concentration at the receptor but rather merely reflects it.

Pharmacokinetics

Pharmacokinetics describes the processes of uptake of drugs by the body, the distribution of the drugs into tissue, the biotransformations (ie, metabolism) they undergo, and the elimination of the drugs and their metabolites from the body. Applied pharmacokinetics is the discipline that uses the principles of pharmacokinetics to enhance safety and effectiveness of a drug in an individual patient. It is this aspect of pharmacology that most strongly influences the interpretation of TDM results and that is dealt with in more detail in this chapter. Fig. 40.2 illustrates the conceptual relationship between pharmacodynamics and pharmacokinetics and the many factors affecting drug concentration and pharmacologic response.

CONSTANT CHANGE OF DRUGS IN THE BODY

A large number of factors are now recognized to have a profound influence on the pharmacokinetics of drugs and consequently on a patient's pharmacologic response (Box 40.1). For example, the consideration of the patient's history, with particular emphasis on his or her pathophysiologic state and adjunct drug therapy, is essential at the initiation of drug therapy and TDM because these important factors may affect absorption, distribution, metabolism, and excretion of a drug.

BOX 40.1 Factors That Affect Drug Distribution in Humans

Demographic Factors

Age
Weight
Gender
Race
Genetics (eg, metabolic enzyme polymorphisms)

Health-Related Factors

Liver disease (cirrhosis, hepatitis, cholestasis)
Kidney disease
Thyroid disease (hypothyroidism or hyperthyroidism)
Cardiovascular disease (arrhythmias, congestive heart failure)
Gastrointestinal disease (eg, sprue or other malabsorption, peptic ulcer disease)
Cancer
Surgery
Burns
Volume status (eg, dehydration)
Nutritional status (cachectic or anorexic)
Pregnancy or other factors affecting plasma proteins or body composition

Extracorporeal Factors

Hemodialysis
Peritoneal dialysis
Cardiopulmonary bypass
Hypothermia or hyperthermia

Chemical and Environmental Factors

Absorption of Drug

Food or coadministered drug affecting extent or rate of absorption
Immediate- or extended-release formulation

Distribution of Drug

Coadministered drugs affecting protein binding to plasma proteins or tissue

Metabolism of Drug

Food, herbs, or drugs competing for metabolism
Coadministration of drugs that induce metabolic enzymes (eg, phenobarbital)
Coadministration of drugs that inhibit metabolic enzymes (eg, cimetidine)

Excretion of Drug

Coadministration of drug competing for renal tubular secretory pathways (eg, probenecid, penicillin)
Coadministration of drugs enhancing renal tubular reabsorption

Absorption

Most drugs administered chronically to patients are administered extravascularly. Although intramuscular and subcutaneous routes are used, the oral route accounts for most of the extravascular doses administered. The absorption process depends on the drug's dissociating from its dosing form, dissolving in gastrointestinal fluids, and then diffusing across biological membrane barriers into the bloodstream. The rate and extent of drug absorption may vary considerably depending on the nature of the drug itself (eg, solubility, pK_a), on the matrix in which it is present, and on the physiologic environment (eg, pH, gastrointestinal motility, vascularity).

The fraction of a drug that is absorbed into the systemic circulation is referred to as its bioavailability. The bioavailability *(f)* of a given drug is usually calculated by comparing, in the same subjects, the area under the plasma concentration–time curve (AUC) of an equivalent dose of the intravenous form and oral form:

$$f = \frac{AUC_{oral}}{AUC_{iv}} \quad (1)$$

The bioavailability of a particular drug, if the drug is to be useful, must generally be great enough so that the active component can pass in sufficient amount and in a desirable time from the gut into the systemic circulation. Bioavailability of greater than 70% is most desirable for drugs to be orally useful. An exception would be a case in which the lumen of the gastrointestinal tract is the site of drug action (eg, antibiotics used to sterilize the gut such as oral vancomycin). Low bioavailability would then be considered advantageous.

Some drugs that are rapidly and completely absorbed nevertheless have low bioavailability to the systemic circulation. This is true of drugs with a high *hepatic extraction rate.* After oral administration, drugs that are absorbed in the lumen of the small intestine are carried by the portal vein directly to the liver. The liver may extensively metabolize a drug with a high hepatic extraction rate before it reaches the systemic circulation, leading to low oral bioavailability. This phenomenon is the first-pass effect.

In addition to the extent of absorption, the rate of absorption is also important. The absorption of a drug is generally considered a first-order process, and the absorption rate constant of a drug is usually much greater than its elimination rate constant. Efforts are now being made in the pharmaceutical industry to decrease the apparent rate of absorption of many drugs by manipulating their formulations (eg, theophylline, tacrolimus) to produce slow-release or sustained-release products. Formulations that provide sustained release permit drugs taken orally to be taken at less frequent intervals. Conditions that may influence the extent or rate of drug absorption include abnormal gastrointestinal motility, diseases of the stomach as well as of the small and large intestine, gastrointestinal infections, radiation, food, and interaction with other substances in the gastrointestinal tract. One should be particularly aware of coadministered drugs that directly affect gut absorption, such as antacids, kaolin, sucralfate, cholestyramine, and antiulcer medications.

Distribution

After a drug enters the vascular compartment, it interacts with various blood constituents and is carried by various transport processes to different body organs and tissues. The overall process is referred to as *distribution.* The factors determining the distribution pattern of a drug are binding of the drug to circulating blood components, binding to fixed receptors, passage of the drug through membrane barriers, and the ability to dissolve in structural or storage lipids. Molecular weight, pK_a, lipid solubility, and other physical and chemical properties of the drug are important determinants of distribution.

Once a drug enters the systemic circulation, it distributes and comes to equilibrium with many of the blood components, such as plasma proteins. An equilibrium exists between free and protein-bound drug. It is generally believed that only the free fraction of the drug is available for distribution and elimination. In addition, only the free drug is available to cross cellular membranes or to interact with the drug receptor to elicit a biological response. Therefore changes in the protein-binding characteristics of a drug can have a profound influence on the distribution and elimination of a drug, as well as on the manner in which total plasma or serum steady-state concentrations are interpreted. Each drug has its own characteristic protein-binding pattern that depends on its physical and chemical properties. As a general rule, however, acidic drugs are bound primarily to albumin and basic drugs primarily to globulins, particularly α_1-acid glycoprotein (AAG). Some drugs bind to both albumin and globulins.

Depending on its affinity for plasma proteins, a drug may be either tightly or loosely bound. A weakly bound drug can be displaced from its protein sites by a drug with a greater affinity for the plasma protein–binding sites. For example, phenytoin and valproic acid, drugs that are frequently coadministered for epilepsy, compete with each other as they bind to albumin. Because valproate is present at higher concentration, its mass causes a significant shift of phenytoin from bound to free form. Protein binding of a drug also depends on the physical characteristics of the plasma proteins and on the presence or absence of fatty acids or other drugs in the blood. Fatty acids can displace a drug from its protein-binding sites; tightly bound drugs are not displaced, but a weakly bound drug can be displaced quite rapidly by free fatty acids present in increased concentrations. It is important to recognize that even though the total drug concentration may remain unchanged, displacement of a drug from its plasma protein-binding sites increases free drug concentrations and can result in clinical toxicity. Remember that the free fraction is the form that crosses biological membranes and is available to bind to the receptor, so increasing the free fraction can produce significant toxicity.

Anything that alters the concentration of free drug in the plasma ultimately alters the amount of drug available to enter the tissues and interact with specific receptor systems. Disease states can alter free drug concentrations. For example, in uremia, the composition of plasma is altered by an increase in nonprotein nitrogen compounds, by acid-base and electrolyte imbalances, and often by a decrease in albumin; free drug concentrations are frequently increased. Patients may experience adverse effects that are a direct consequence of the increased free drug concentrations, especially if only total plasma drug concentration is monitored in these patients. For example, phenytoin is 90% bound and 10% free in healthy subjects. In uremic patients, 20% to 30% of the total plasma concentration of phenytoin may be free. In a healthy patient who has a total plasma phenytoin concentration of 15 μg/mL, the free phenytoin concentration is likely to be 1.5 μg/mL. If a uremic patient has a total concentration of 15 μg/mL, the free drug concentration may be 4.5 μg/mL. A free phenytoin concentration of 4.5 μg/mL is sufficient to precipitate severe phenytoin side effects, including lethargy and increased seizure frequency. In uremic patients, it is advisable to quantitate free phenytoin concentrations and adjust the drug dose to maintain free phenytoin concentration at approximately 2.0 μg/mL.

Alteration of protein concentration in response to acute stress can alter free drug concentration. For example, after myocardial infarction, there is a rapid rise in AAG concentration. Lidocaine is a commonly employed drug for control of arrhythmias secondary to acute myocardial infarction, but lidocaine is a basic drug that is highly bound to AAG. Doses of lidocaine adequate to control arrhythmia immediately after infarction are likely to become ineffective 48 to 72 hours later because the higher concentration of AAG that occurs after infarction diminishes the amount of free drug available to tissue.[31] The arrhythmia reappears, and because the total lidocaine plasma concentration necessary to control the arrhythmia seems to be in the toxic range, the lidocaine dose is decreased when in reality it should be increased to maintain the optimal free concentration.

Some drugs exhibit saturation of the available plasma protein–binding sites at optimal total drug concentrations. For example, disopyramide binding is concentration dependent and varies widely among patients. Consequently, its total concentration and the observed clinical responses vary markedly among patients. Valproic acid is also a drug that shows saturation at concentrations greater than 100 μg/mL. Thus an increase of total plasma valproate concentration from 100 to 125 μg/mL represents a significant increase in the free valproate concentration.

Any change in normal physiologic status can alter free drug concentrations and thus change the distribution of drugs between plasma and tissue. Geriatric patients often exhibit hypoalbuminemia with a marked decrease in protein-binding sites for drugs. In the elderly, the classic signs of drug intoxication usually are not apparent; instead, the clinical symptoms of drug intoxication are manifested as impaired cognitive function—particularly confusion, which is a common symptom in patients with dementia. Reduction of drug dose to decrease the free drug concentrations may result in dramatic improvements in cognitive function and behavior in these patients.

Estimation of the free drug concentration will continue to be of interest to TDM. Equilibrium dialysis represents the gold-standard method for measuring the free, unbound concentration of a drug. However, this method typically requires 16 to 18 hours of incubation to achieve equilibrium, which severely limits the turnaround time for testing. Ultrafiltration techniques are useful alternatives that usually can be accomplished in a fraction of the time. In ultrafiltration, a sample of serum or plasma is forced through a filter membrane with a low molecular weight cutoff value, typically by centrifugation, to yield a protein-free sample. Provided this process is done rapidly and under appropriate temperature control, ultrafiltration can provide a useful estimate of the free drug concentration in circulating blood.[32,33] Sample drawing, processing, and storage can modify dissociation equilibria for some drugs affecting both equilibrium dialysis and ultracentrifugation measurements. Measurement of drugs in oral fluid (ie, saliva) has been advocated as an alternative to plasma or serum testing because of the ease of collection and correlation with free drug concentration for some drugs. Despite these drawbacks, free drug estimations by ultrafiltration are superior to estimations of free drug concentration based on measurements in saliva. Few drugs show a strong correlation between salivary concentration and free drug concentration in plasma.[34] In addition, collection of saliva from acutely ill patients is often more difficult than blood collection.

Metabolism

The rate of the enzymatic process to metabolize a drug is usually characterized by the Michaelis-Menten equation

$$\frac{dC}{dt} = \frac{V_{max} \times C}{K_m + C} \tag{2}$$

where V_{max} is the maximum velocity of the reaction; K_m, the Michaelis-Menten constant, is the drug concentration at which the rate of metabolism is half of the maximum; and C is the drug concentration in blood.

Drugs are usually administered to achieve concentrations in the blood well below the K_m of a particular drug. Therefore if K_m is much greater than C, Eq. 40.2 can be simplified to

$$\frac{dC}{dt} = \left(\frac{V_{max}}{K_m}\right) \times C \tag{3}$$

and V_{max}/K_m can be written as the constant, K, such that

$$\frac{dC}{dt} = KC \tag{4}$$

where K is a simple first-order rate constant for the metabolic elimination. In other words the rate of drug elimination from blood is proportional to the concentration of drug. *First-order kinetics* are characteristic of the metabolism of most drugs.

In the event that concentrations significantly exceed the K_m for a particular drug, the rate of elimination of the drug becomes independent of concentration and thus descriptive of a *zero-order* process in which Eq. 40.2 can be approximated by:

$$\frac{dC}{dt} = V_{max} \tag{5}$$

Several drugs, notably phenytoin, salicylates, ethanol, and theophylline, cannot be characterized by simple first-order kinetics. Instead, the rate of metabolism of these compounds is said to be *capacity-limited* or *nonlinear,* meaning clearance or the apparent half-life changes with changes in concentration. Fig. 40.3 shows how the kinetics of elimination is linear (first order) until the capacity of clearance pathways is reached, which occurs at concentrations that approach the K_m of the enzymatic pathways mediating metabolism. At this point, the relationship between dose and steady-state concentration becomes nonlinear. It should be evident, therefore, that important clinical considerations arise when a patient is treated with a drug that displays nonlinear kinetics. First, changes in dosing result in disproportionate changes in steady-state drug concentrations so that titration to appropriate serum concentrations must be approached conservatively. Second, because both clearance and apparent half-life of the drug change with increasing drug concentration, the length of time required to reach a new steady-state concentration is prolonged.

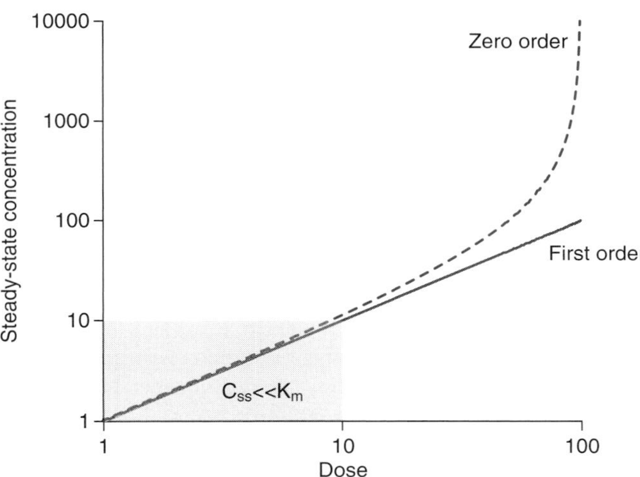

FIGURE 40.3 Nonlinear response to dose changes. Drugs with first-order kinetics *(solid black line)* display serum steady-state concentrations *(C)* that vary proportionately with dose. In contrast, for drugs with zero-order kinetics *(dotted red line)*, an increase in dose may result in a disproportionate increase in serum steady-state concentrations.

All of the equations previously described for predicting dose or concentration assume linear kinetic systems; they are therefore not adaptable to treatment with drugs that display nonlinear kinetics. Methods for predicting phenytoin dose and concentration and using a linearized Michaelis-Menten equation have been developed and applied to individualize drug dosing regimens.

Biotransformation

The liver is the principal organ responsible for xenobiotic metabolism. One of its major roles is to convert lipophilic nonpolar molecules to more polar water-soluble forms. The drug molecule (a xenobiotic) can be modified by phase I reactions, which alter chemical structure by oxidation, reduction, or hydrolysis; or by phase II reactions, which conjugate the drug (glucuronidation or sulfation) to water-soluble forms. Typically, both phase I and phase II reactions occur. Most drug metabolism takes place in the microsomal fraction of the hepatocytes, where many environmental chemicals and endogenous biochemicals (xenobiotics) are also processed and by the same mechanisms.

Enzymes of the hepatic microsomal system can be induced or inhibited. Enzyme induction and inhibition have greatest significance for drugs with low to moderate hepatic extraction fractions.

Microsomal enzyme induction leads to an increase in the activity of enzymes present, most commonly through increases in the quantity of the oxidizing enzymes. The many isoenzymes of cytochrome P450 are affected variably by different enzyme-inducing drugs. Two classic and clinically relevant enzyme inducers can be contrasted.

First, phenobarbital represents the type of enzyme inducer with broad induction effects. After a latency period, production of cytochrome P450, cytochrome P450 reductase, and related enzymes is increased. In addition, liver weight, hepatic blood flow, bile flow, and production of hepatic proteins also increase. This induction apparently increases the P450 isoenzyme mass for which debrisoquine is a substrate because the hepatic clearance of debrisoquin is increased after phenobarbital administration. This enzyme system is referred to as cytochrome P450-2D6. Phenobarbital induction has little effect on theophylline clearance, suggesting a different isoenzyme for theophylline metabolism.

Theophylline and polycyclic hydrocarbons in tobacco smoke (3-methylcholanthrene) represent a second type of enzyme inducer with broad induction effects. They induce cytochrome P45-1A in which no change in P45 reductase occurs, and a different terminal oxidase appears. After this type of induction, the clearance of theophylline but not that of antipyrine is increased. These substances have served as prototypes for the classification of enzyme inducers. Obviously, when patients are on a drug with a narrow therapeutic index (TI), their dosing regimen would need to be adjusted should a known enzyme-inducing drug be added to or deleted from their therapy.

Because the drug-metabolizing enzymes of the liver are nonspecific and interact with a wide variety of endogenous and exogenous substances, it is not surprising that the presence of one drug inhibits the metabolism of a second drug that is coadministered. Several general mechanisms have been proposed to describe these events. They include substrate competition, competitive or noncompetitive inhibition, product inhibition, and repression (where the amount of enzyme is reduced by either decreased synthesis or increased degradation). Most drug-drug interactions probably fall into the categories of substrate competition or competitive or noncompetitive inhibition. Examples of drugs that have been shown to significantly inhibit drug metabolism include chloramphenicol, cimetidine, valproic acid, allopurinol, and erythromycin. As with enzyme inducers, the addition or deletion of an inhibitory drug in a patient's drug therapy requires appropriate TDM and dose adjustment of the affected drug. TDM allows one to monitor these processes and adjust dosing accordingly.

The role of TDM becomes particularly apparent for drugs that undergo hepatic metabolism. Wide variability in the rate of metabolism of any given drug exists not only in different patients in the general population but also in the same patient at different times and in different circumstances. This variability is due to factors such as age, weight, gender, genetics, exposure to environmental substances, diet, coadministered drugs, and disease. Furthermore, unlike kidney function, in which creatinine provides a useful biomarker of function, there is no acceptable endogenous biochemical marker by which hepatic function, and consequently hepatic capability for drug clearance, can be routinely assessed before drug therapy is initiated.

The biotransformation of drugs may produce metabolites that are pharmacologically active. In such instances the metabolite should also be measured because it is contributing to the effect of the drug on the patient. Primidone and procainamide are examples of such drugs. If the metabolite is inactive, it need not be measured, but steps should be taken to ensure that it does not interfere in the analytical process. The latter problem of metabolite interference can cause significant problems for monitoring certain patients, such as transplant patients receiving the ISDs cyclosporine or tacrolimus, which have numerous active and inactive metabolites that cross-react to varying degrees with the antibodies used in immunoassays for these drugs.[35]

Excretion

Excretion of drugs or chemicals from the body can occur through biliary, intestinal, pulmonary, or renal routes. Although each of these represents a possible mechanism of drug elimination, renal excretion is a major pathway for the elimination of most water-soluble drugs or metabolites and is important in TDM. Alterations in renal function may have a profound effect on the clearance and apparent half-life of the parent compound or its active metabolite(s); decreased renal function causes increased serum drug concentrations and increases the pharmacologic response.

Kidney function, in contrast to liver function, is readily and reliably evaluated by estimation of creatinine clearance. Creatinine is a metabolic product of muscle metabolism and is produced at a constant rate by the body. It is primarily eliminated from the body by the kidneys through the glomerular filtration mechanism. Renal clearance of creatinine at 120 mL/min approximates the glomerular filtration rate of 90 to 130 mL/min (see Chapter 32). Therefore measurement of creatinine clearance on a routine basis provides an effective tool to evaluate kidney function. A strong correlation has been shown to exist between creatinine clearance and the total body clearance or elimination rate constant of those drugs primarily dependent on the kidneys for their elimination. Examples of drugs whose therapeutic use is adjusted to account for changes in creatinine clearance include gentamicin, tobramycin, amikacin, digoxin, vancomycin, and cyclosporine.

CHARACTERIZING DRUG EXPOSURE WITH MINIMAL ASSUMPTIONS: THE NONCOMPARTMENTAL ANALYSIS OF CONCENTRATION DATA OVER TIME

In pharmacokinetics, mathematical approaches are used to predict or describe certain events, usually for calculating a dosing regimen or predicting the serum drug concentration after a given drug dose. The mathematical tools most often used in clinical pharmacokinetics are compartmental models and model-independent relationships.

Model-independent relationships are becoming increasingly popular in clinical pharmacokinetics. The main advantages of model-independent relationships are fewer relationships to remember, fewer restrictive assumptions, a more general insight into elimination mechanisms, and easier computations. However, model-independent relationships are not without disadvantages; conceptualization of compartments or physiologic spaces may be lost, specific information that may be clinically relevant or pertinent to mechanisms of distribution or elimination can be lost, and the difficulty in constructing profiles of concentration versus time can be increased requiring greater numbers of samples to be collected.

The most frequently used model-independent, noncompartmental analysis approach for characterizing drug exposure uses algorithms to estimate the AUC after dosing of a drug. One of the simplest methods to estimate the AUC from timed concentration data uses the linear trapezoidal rule to divide the concentration-time curve of a drug into a series of trapezoids, the sum of which represents the AUC as diagrammed in Fig. 40.4. Accurate AUC estimation using the trapezoidal rule usually requires intense blood sampling during the dose interval.

In TDM, we are rarely concerned with a drug administered as a single, one-time intravenous bolus. Drugs are administered repetitively in the usual therapeutic situations. Fig. 40.5 shows that a drug repetitively administered at a fixed dosing interval will accumulate in the body until a steady-state condition exists. Note that a typical dosing cycle is once each half-life. *Steady state* can be defined as that point in the dosing scheme when the amount entering the circulation (governed by dosing rate) equals the amount eliminated (governed by elimination rate).

Theoretically, the AUC for the first dose of drug when time is extrapolated from time of zero to infinity should be equal to the AUC for a dose interval (τ) at steady state (see Fig. 40.4). The average drug concentration at steady state (C_{ss}) is

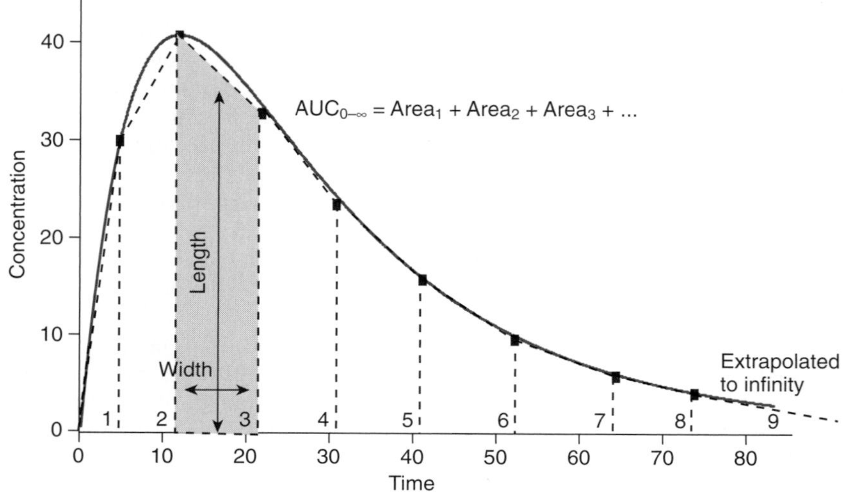

FIGURE 40.4 Determination of area under the curve (AUC) using the model independent trapezoidal rule for the extravascular (oral) route of administration.

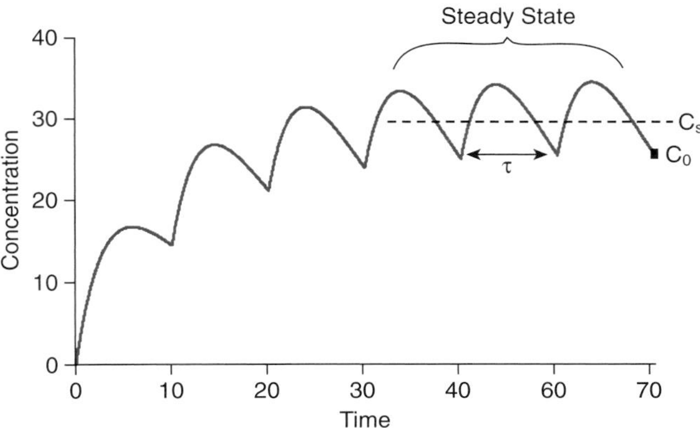

FIGURE 40.5 Concentration versus time curve for successive doses of a medication administered at constant dose interval (τ). At steady state the dose-time curves replicate.

a frequent concentration reported for many drugs, and may be calculated using the formula

$$C_{ss} = \frac{AUC}{\tau} \quad (6)$$

where τ represents the time duration of the dose interval. The maximum concentration (C_{max}) and minimum concentration (C_{min}) of a drug during a dose-interval are also frequently of interest because these concentrations may be associated with efficacy and/or toxicity of a drug. For most drugs, the C_{min} at steady state (also frequently referred to as the trough concentration) is the concentration obtained immediately before the dose at time of zero minutes (referred to as C_0); however, although generally the case, it is important to recognize that the C_{min} does not have to be equivalent to the C_0 concentration.

Clearance

Knowing the AUC of a drug after a defined dose allows calculation of the model-independent parameter of clearance, which provides a useful picture of the body's ability to eliminate a drug. Total body clearance (Cl_T or simply Cl) is defined as the theoretical total volume of blood, serum, or plasma completely cleared of drug per unit of time. It is usually expressed in units of mL/min, L/h, mL/min/kg, or L/h/kg. Cl is the sum total of all the clearances contributed by each elimination route (ie, $Cl = Cl_{kidney} + Cl_{liver} + Cl_{biliary} + \ldots$). Cl is typically calculated from the AUC using the formula

$$Cl = \frac{D_0 \times f}{AUC_{0\to\infty}} \quad (7)$$

where $AUC_{0\to\infty}$ is the AUC for the first dose integrated over time from zero to infinity. The variable f represents the bioavailable fraction of the drug, which is not generally known for orally administered drugs in a particular patient. Thus an apparent oral clearance (Cl_a) of a drug is calculated using

$$Cl_a = \frac{D_0}{AUC_{0\to\infty}} \quad (8)$$

Although Cl is model-independent, it can be related to model-dependent parameters such as the volume of distribution and elimination rate in a first-order, one-compartment model, as discussed in greater detail in the following section.

Hepatic Clearance

For drugs dependent solely on hepatic elimination, total body clearance (Cl_T) equals hepatic clearance (Cl_H). When the liver is considered from a purely physiologic perspective, the hepatic clearance is determined by the hepatic blood flow (Q) and the hepatic extraction fraction (E).

$$Cl = Q \times E \quad (9)$$

The hepatic extraction fraction of a drug reflects the affinity of a particular drug for hepatic microsomal enzymes; E can be found experimentally or calculated by the equation

$$E = \frac{C_a - C_e}{C_a} \quad (10)$$

where C_a is the concentration of the drug in blood entering the liver and C_e is the concentration of the drug in the hepatic venous effluent. For drugs that possess a high extraction fraction, hepatic clearance approaches hepatic blood flow (Q). The total body clearance of highly extracted drugs primarily depends on hepatic blood flow for their elimination. These drugs usually have low bioavailability because of the first-pass effect described earlier. Lidocaine is an example of such a drug. The clearance of low-extracted drugs is less dependent on blood flow and more dependent on the quantity and quality of the hepatic microsomal enzymes. Total body clearance of these drugs is affected by hepatic function, enzyme inducers and inhibitors, and changes in free drug concentration. Readers should recognize that this is a superficial view of a complex process. Several excellent reviews on this subject are available.[24,27,36]

PREDICTING DRUG CONCENTRATIONS USING A COMPARTMENTAL MODEL

Compartmental models are deterministic; that is, the drug concentration in blood and time data determine or define the model. The number and values of compartments assigned to the model have no true physiologic meaning or anatomic reality. The intravascular fluid compartment (blood) usually is the anatomic reference compartment. The advantage of intravascular fluid as the reference compartment is the ease with which it may be sampled to provide a definitive profile of blood concentration of drug versus time. The actual number of compartments can be quite extensive. However, for the sake of simplicity, one-, two-, and three-compartment models are most often used.

One-Compartment, First-Order Kinetic Model

In the simplest compartment model, the body is considered as a single compartment, as shown schematically in Fig. 40.6. It is assumed that after introduction of a drug, the substance is rapidly and uniformly distributed throughout the body, or said to be *kinetically homogeneous* within the compartment. Such a model is frequently applied to water-soluble antibiotics such as gentamicin. Fig. 40.7 illustrates graphically the relationship between log of concentration within the

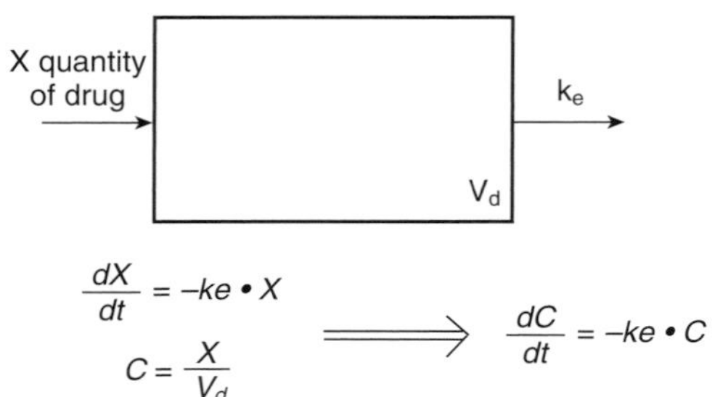

FIGURE 40.6 Schematic one compartment model and mathematical representation as discussed.

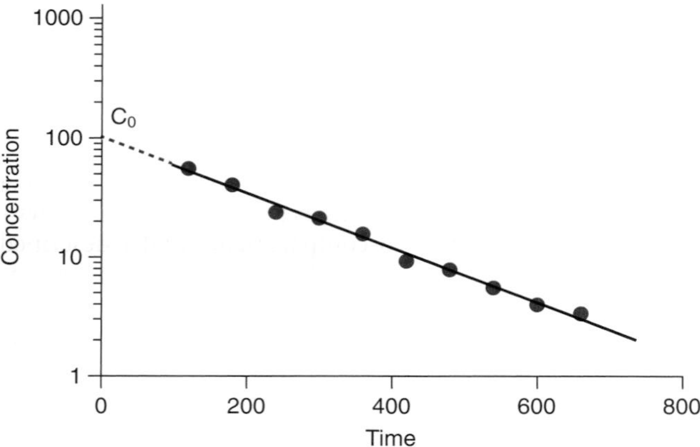

FIGURE 40.7 Semi-log plot of drug concentration *(C)* versus time extrapolated to time = 0 at which time, $C = C_0$, the theoretical initial concentration after a bolus administration.

compartment and time for a single-bolus injection of a drug. In the simple model of first-order elimination, the instantaneous change in quantity of drug within the compartment is proportional to the quantity (X) by the equation

$$\frac{dX}{dt} = -k_e X \quad \textbf{(11)}$$

Integration of this equation using Laplace transformation yields the equation

$$X_t = X_0 \times e^{-k_e t} \quad \textbf{(12)}$$

where X_0 is the initial quantity of the drug within the compartment, X_t is the blood concentration of the drug as a function of time, and k_e is the first-order elimination rate constant. From a practical perspective, the quantity of drug within the blood compartment cannot be easily measured. Instead, the concentration of drug within the compartment is the measured quantity. Dividing both sides of Eq. 40.12 by a volume of distribution (V_d) term converts this equation to

$$C_t = C_0 \times e^{-k_e t} \quad \textbf{(13)}$$

where C_0, the initial concentration after bolus administration (which cannot be easily measured), is estimated by extrapolating the line shown in Fig. 40.7 to zero time. From knowledge of C_0 and k_e, one can theoretically predict the concentration at any time (C_t). As shown later, most drugs are administered in repetitive doses rather than in a single bolus.

Volume of Distribution

For a drug that is assumed to be administered intravenously as a rapid bolus into a single, kinetically homogenous compartment, the C_0 is related to the compartment volume as follows:

$$C_0 = \frac{Dose}{V_d} \quad \textbf{(14)}$$

V_d is called apparent *volume of distribution* because it is not a real volume in the physiologic sense, but instead is a proportionality constant to translate the absolute amount of drug present in the compartment *(X)* into its concentration relative to a volume. The V_d for an orally administered drug can be determined easily from concentration data using the one-compartment model after correction for bioavailability, *f* by

$$V_d = \frac{Dose \times f}{C_0} \quad \textbf{(15)}$$

The units of V_d are usually liters (L). Although V_d is a mathematical term and not a real physiologic parameter, it is useful for contrasting degrees to which different types of drugs distribute. For instance, the polar hydrophilic drug gentamicin has a $V_d = 0.2$ L/kg of body weight, whereas the nonpolar lipophilic drug desipramine has a $V_d = 34$ L/kg of body weight. Gentamicin is concentrated in the blood, whereas desipramine is predominantly distributed into tissue.

Linear Kinetics of Elimination

Using the same assumptions of a one-compartment model as described earlier for calculation of the V_d, the first-order elimination rate constant can be determined by log transformation of Eq. 40.13 to give the natural logarithmic function:

$$\ln(C_t) = \ln(C_0) - k_e t \quad \textbf{(16)}$$

Given a zero time blood drug concentration (C_0), a nonzero time concentration *(C_t)*, and a defined time *(t)*, then k_e can be readily determined either algebraically or graphically. For example, in a plot of ln C_t versus *t*, the slope of the linear relationship is $-k_e$. The elimination rate constant k_e represents the fraction of drug removed per unit time and has units of reciprocal time (minute^{-1}, hour^{-1}, or day^{-1}).

Elimination Rate Constant and Half-Life

The elimination rate constant k_e can be related to another parameter, *half-life* ($t_{1/2}$), by the equation:

$$t_{1/2} = \frac{0.693}{k_e} \quad \textbf{(17)}$$

where $t_{1/2}$ is usually defined as the time required for the amount of drug in blood to decline to half of a measured value. The constant, 0.693, in the equation represents the natural logarithm of 2. Fig. 40.7 demonstrates how the half-life can be rapidly determined from a semi-log plot of drug concentration versus time. As few as two successive

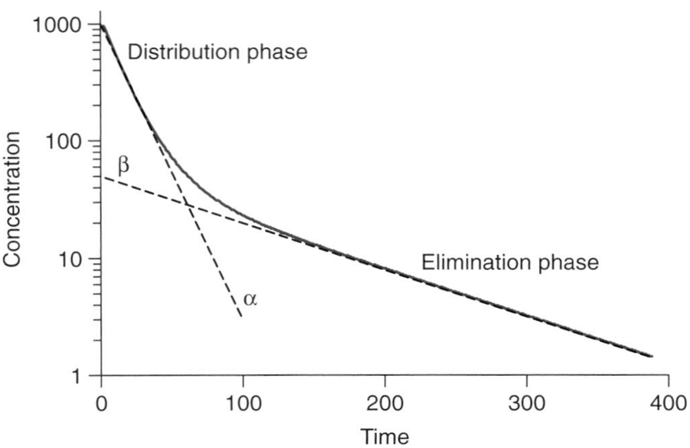

FIGURE 40.8 Drug concentration in plasma after administration of a dose for a two-compartment model. Decline from the original concentration (C_0) is affected by both the distribution phase (characterized by the constant α) and the elimination phase (characterized by the constant β) as described.

concentrations collected at times t_1 and t_2 are required for the estimate of k_e using the equation

$$k_e = \ln(C_{t1}) - \ln\left(\frac{C_{t2}}{t_2}\right) - t_1 \quad \textbf{(18)}$$

As discussed previously in the section on model-independent characterization of pharmacokinetics, *Cl* is a useful derived parameter for describing the elimination of a drug from the body. For a drug described well by a one-compartment, first-order kinetic model, *Cl* is mathematically related to V_d and k_e by the following relationship:

$$Cl = V_d \times k_e \quad \textbf{(19)}$$

It is important to recognize that the previous equations are relevant only in the context of intravenous bolus administration of a drug. More prolonged infusions of drugs and oral administration require additional model terms to characterize the infusion rates, duration, or absorption lag time into the pharmacokinetic models presented. Details on these more complex one-compartment models can be found in textbooks dedicated to pharmacokinetics.[36]

Two-Compartment and Multicompartment Models

Fig. 40.8 illustrates the more complex kinetics demonstrated by a two-compartment model. The curve is described by the following equation:

$$C_t = Ae^{-\alpha t} + Be^{-\beta t} \quad \textbf{(20)}$$

where the rate constant α is the slope of the curve during the phase in which the drug is being distributed, referred to as the *distribution phase.* β is the slope of the curve during the phase in which the drug is being eliminated by metabolism and excretion (assuming that distribution is complete) and is derived by extrapolating the *elimination phase* of the curve in Fig. 40.8 to time = 0 that would have existed if distribution had been immediate and complete. *A* is an estimate, using the method of residuals, of the theoretical plasma concentration

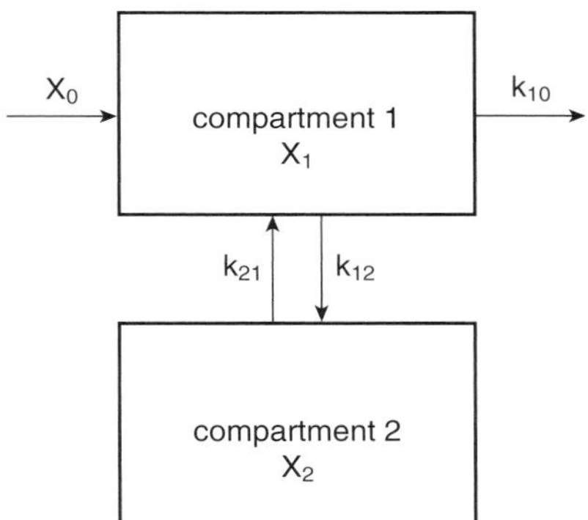

FIGURE 40.9 Two-compartment pharmacokinetic model. k_{21} and k_{12} are distribution rate constants, and k_{10} is the elimination rate constant for the central compartment, compartment 1 in this diagram.

at time = 0, immediately after intravenous injection of a bolus of the drug. *B* is derived by extrapolation of the terminal slope of the distributive phase line to time = 0. From a physiologic perspective, the two-compartment model described earlier accounts for the initial decline of drug concentration in the reference compartment (ie, the sampled plasma compartment) into a vascularized tissue compartment (the second compartment). A three-compartment model mimics a system like the two-compartment model with a third reservoir, such as adipose tissue or cellular nuclei, in which the drug resides over the long term. Fig. 40.9 depicts a two-compartment model, after an intravenous bolus administration of a drug. In these figures, X_0 represents the drug dose given and therefore the amount of drug in the system at zero time, X_1 the amount of drug in the central or reference compartment, and X_2 the amount of drug in the peripheral compartment in the case of the two-compartment model. k_{10} represents the elimination rate constant; that is, the rate at which the drug leaves the reference compartment and is lost from the system. k_{12} and k_{21} are transfer rate constants describing, for the two-compartment model only, rates at which the drug is exchanged between compartments within the system. Which model is the best for a particular drug is somewhat empirical and based on model-fitting statistics. For a more detailed discussion around model fitting, readers are referred to textbooks devoted to the subject.[37-40]

GENERAL CONSIDERATIONS FOR THE CLINICAL USE OF THERAPEUTIC DRUG MONITORING

There is no universal set of rules that determine whether a drug might benefit from TDM; however, numerous characteristics of a drug contribute to the need for TDM. TDM is most valuable when the drug in question is used chronically, has variable pharmacokinetics, and has a narrow TI. For drugs with a narrow TI, there is little if any window between blood (or serum for those drugs routinely measured in serum) concentrations associated with efficacy and those associated with toxic effects. The immunosuppressive calcineurin inhibitor drug tacrolimus provides a good example of a narrow TI drug with a wide variability in PK as shown in Fig. 40.10. The concentrations of tacrolimus that are associated with efficacy (ie, freedom from graft rejection) and those

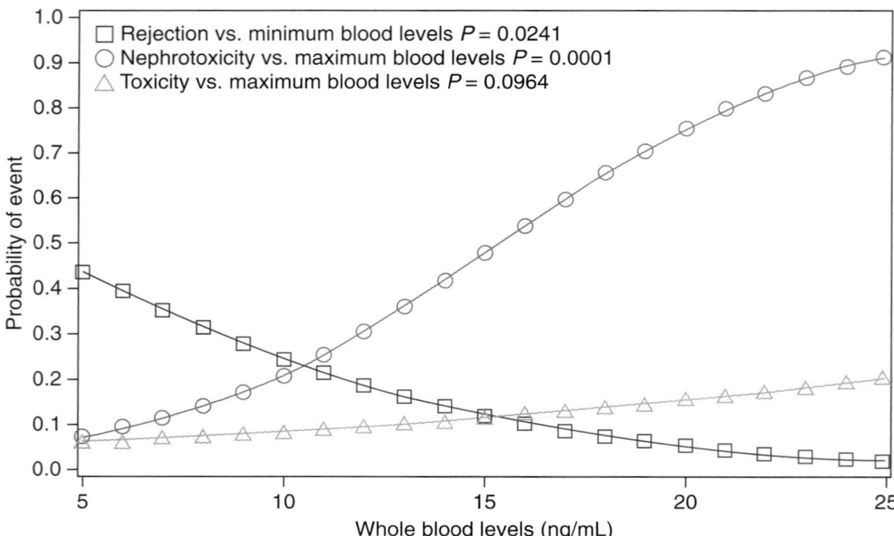

FIGURE 40.10 The pharmacodynamics of tacrolimus in renal transplantation. (Reprinted with permission from Venkataramanan R, Shaw LM, Sarkozi L, et al. Clinical utility of monitoring tacrolimus blood concentrations in liver transplant patients. *J Clin Pharmacol* 2001;41:542–551.)

associated with kidney toxicity overlap considerably. TDM helps navigate this tightrope. By itself, however, narrow TI is not necessarily sufficient to warrant TDM. Many narrow TI drugs are routinely used without monitoring, such as most cancer chemotherapy drugs. Additional factors therefore contribute to the need for TDM, such as the severity of failed drug therapy (eg, antimicrobials) or toxicity (eg, ISDs). Difficulty in recognizing efficacy or toxicity with use of these drugs can be life threatening. Many patients, especially those with chronic disease, also require prolonged drug therapy. The problem of compliance is particularly evident with patients who are characteristically free of pain or unusual discomfort, as with epilepsy, asthma, hypertension, mild heart disease, and transplantation. Patients may develop a sense that their disease has been cured and they no longer need the drug. The end result of noncompliance is exacerbation of the existing disorder and treatment failure. Drug concentration values provide positive feedback to physicians regarding complying and noncomplying patients.

For TDM to be useful, the concentration data must be accurate and precise. Numerous factors affect the measurement of drugs in blood. These factors, if not recognized, may lead to erroneous decision making that could negate any benefits of monitoring and might even lead to more harm than good from TDM.

Preanalytical Factors That Affect Therapeutic Drug Monitoring Results

To interpret a TDM result, it is critical that the dose of drug given to the patient is known. Dosage uniformity standards exist for drugs approved by the US Food and Drug Administration (FDA). Although most drug formulations are fairly consistent, the actual dose of a drug in a single tablet, suspension, or vial may vary. US Pharmacopeia (USP) standards dictate that the mean dose contained in a tablet must be within ±10% of the product labeling and no tested sample may fall outside of 75 and 125% of the mean. As a result, the dose content for a single dose theoretically could vary by as much as 25% and still fall within acceptable USP content uniformity limits. This is further compounded by inaccuracies introduced by manipulation of the dose (eg, splitting of scored tablets), failure to administer or consume the entire dose (eg, from vomiting). Drugs also may degrade over time or by storage method, leading to further inaccuracy of dose.

Beyond dose accuracy, pharmacokinetics is inherently time-based. Thus accurate timing of sample collection is often an important factor, especially when timed samples such as peak or trough samples are the primary means of monitoring. Vancomycin trough samples provide an example in which collection immediately before the next dose is recommended because of the relatively short half-life of this drug (~6 to 12 hours).[41] Premature sampling may lead to falsely increased concentrations that could alter decision-making given the generally narrow therapeutic range for this drug. In contrast, drugs with slow distribution but long half-life, such as digoxin, are optimally sampled in the postdistributive phase of longer than 6 hours after dosing. Sampling during steady state (generally more than four doses) is also an important assumption made for monitoring of many drugs, such as vancomycin.

Variation in collection and handling of samples for TDM also can affect the quality of concentration data. Although serum is the preferred sample for monitoring of many drugs, different collection tubes are available for generating serum that include plain glass or plastic tubes without additive (eg, red-stoppered BD Vacutainer tubes [Becton, Dickinson, Franklin Lakes, New Jersey]), as well as specialized serum separator tubes (eg, yellow-stoppered BD Vacutainer tubes) that contain a gel that separates serum from the cellular components after centrifugation. The latter tube may affect drug concentration because of adsorption of drug by the gel after prolonged contact. The adsorptive effects vary across drugs and have been shown to significantly reduce the concentration of some drugs such as phenytoin, particularly when the collection tubes are underfilled.[42] The stability of drugs after collection also may vary, with some drugs requiring prompt serum generation followed by freezing for optimal stability (eg, busulfan).

The importance of preanalytical factors in the accuracy and precision of TDM results should not be underestimated. TDM laboratories are part of a larger health care system. It is imperative that laboratories engage and work with the many parts of this system, including pharmacists, nursing staff, and the phlebotomy team. Each individual plays an important role in TDM, and the effective control of the many factors that affect TDM accuracy are key to success of this complex feedback control system.

POINTS TO REMEMBER

Preanalytic Factors Affecting Therapeutic Drug Monitoring Results

- Dose accuracy
- Appropriate sampling time
- Specimen collection and handling
- Physiologic changes in the patient (eg, serum albumin concentration)

Analytical Factors That Affect Monitoring Results

The laboratory, of course, plays a central role in the TDM process. Beyond the preanalytical factors affecting TDM results, analytical factors are important considerations in the interpretation of drug concentration data. Notable challenges in the analytical field include the availability of standardized reference material and the selectivity of methods for the drug of interest.

As discussed in Chapter 2, analytical error falls into two general categories, random error and systematic error. Random error is generally inherent to a particular method. Efforts to characterize and limit random error are a mainstay of the development and validation of most analytical methods. In contrast, systematic error or bias is often insidious. Determining whether a method gives accurate results over the long term and across laboratories is often a difficult task. This is generally accomplished by either comparing the results of testing against a definitive analytical method or using a certified reference material. The International Union of Pure and Applied Chemistry defines a definitive method as[43]:

> *A method of exceptional scientific status, which is sufficiently accurate to stand alone in the determination of a given property for the certification of a reference material. Such a method must have a firm theoretical foundation so that systematic error is negligible relative to the intended use. Analyte masses (amounts) or concentrations must be measured directly in terms of the base units of measurements, or indirectly related through sound theoretical equations. Definitive methods, together with Certified Reference Materials, are primary means for transferring accuracy—ie, establishing traceability.*

Definitive methods generally employ very time-consuming and expensive techniques (eg, isotope dilution mass spectrometry) to establish material purity and quantity that are not practical for general use in most clinical laboratories. The availability of certified reference material (also frequently referred to as standardized reference material) to which methods may be compared is a critical factor in helping control systematic error. Early studies of method comparability for AEDs demonstrated that concentrations varied greatly across laboratories as well as within laboratories over time. These data led to the development in the early 1980s by the National Institute for Standards and Technology (NIST) of a standard reference material of sufficient purity and accuracy to allow standardization of AED monitoring methods across different laboratories and manufacturers.[44] Unfortunately, this type of standardized reference material is unavailable for other monitored drugs.

The ability of a given method to detect a compound of interest among many potential substances present in a sample (referred to as method selectivity) represents another potential source of systematic error. Selectivity is particularly important for TDM tests because many drugs are structurally related, including to some endogenously produced compounds. Most drugs are also extensively metabolized through a number of different pathways of biotransformation. These metabolites are often similar to the parent compound in structure, but pharmacologic activity is variable. Tacrolimus provides a useful example. Antibodies directed against tacrolimus that are used for immunoassays demonstrate similar reactivity toward tacrolimus along with two of its metabolites, 15-desmethyl-tacrolimus and 31-desmethyl-tacrolimus. Although both metabolites are detected equally, the 15-desmethyl metabolite exhibits little immunosuppressive activity whereas the 31-desmethyl metabolite exhibits immunosuppressive activity similar to that of tacrolimus. These metabolites are generally low in abundance in most patients; however, alterations in metabolism secondary to liver dysfunction can lead to their accumulation, resulting in a systematic error that complicates test interpretation.[45,46] Selectivity often differs greatly across analytical platforms, and this important performance characteristic must be recognized when interpreting testing, especially when done by different laboratories that employ different testing methods (eg, immunoassay vs. liquid chromatography–tandem mass spectrometry (LC-MS/MS).

The Concept of a Therapeutic Range

The relationship between serum drug concentration and clinical outcome forms the basis for TDM, as depicted in Fig. 40.1. One of the most common interpretative errors encountered regarding TDM is the presumption that a concentration within a reported therapeutic range will ensure treatment success in the absence of toxicity, and concentrations outside this range will not. In reality, the probability of success and toxicity are a continuum across the concentration range. These probabilities are maximized and minimized, respectively, within the therapeutic range. Nevertheless, therapeutic success can certainly occur at concentrations below the therapeutic range. More importantly, success also may be achieved by concentrations above the therapeutic range without associated toxicity in some patients. Experienced users of TDM often recognize these relationships and weigh the risks and potential benefits of drug concentrations in the context of the clinical situation using the therapeutic range as a guide.

Similar to a reference interval for any laboratory test, therapeutic ranges are based on population data from drug therapy trials and in some instances confirmed or established by randomized concentration-controlled trials. The application of these population-based ranges to an individual therefore assumes similarity to the target population. Differences in metabolism, physiology, and/or the underlying disease process can alter these relationships, leading to unexpected and undesirable results. Phenytoin used for seizure control illustrates this limitation. A fairly good relationship between serum phenytoin concentration and seizure control exists. However, several factors have been shown to alter the dose-response relationships for phenytoin that might have an impact on the utility of defined therapeutic ranges. The presence of concomitant liver disease significantly alters the pharmacokinetics of phenytoin because of its high degree of binding to albumin, a protein that is significantly altered with moderate to severe liver disease. As a result, individuals with liver disease are at significantly higher risk for toxicity at total serum phenytoin concentrations that are otherwise appropriate for individuals without liver disease. The recognition of this problem led to the development of methods for measuring phenytoin that is unbound to albumin in serum (also known as free phenytoin) which also correlates with seizure control. Nevertheless, this example illustrates the need for caution in applying population-based relationships to individual patients who may not be represented by the population used for defining the therapeutic range.

Beyond Empiric Dosing: Model-Based Dosage Adjustment

Use of a single measured drug concentration such as a trough concentration to forecast drug dose is one of the most commonly employed approaches to dose adjustment because of the simplicity of obtaining this in a clinical setting. In the simplest method of applying concentration data in the clinic, a provider adjusts a dose empirically based on these single concentrations in an attempt to achieve the desired concentration at the next measurement. This approach, which is generally based on a model (eg, linear kinetics of elimination) and experience of the provider, will eventually yield the desired concentration in most patients; however, it may take long periods of monitoring to ultimately achieve the desired control. Beyond the costs, time is sometimes critical to treatment success such as with the use of antibiotics to treat life-threatening infections.

One of the major pitfalls to the use of a single, timed drug level for the adjustment of drug dosing is the potential error associated with an individual result. Patients are often treated with drugs during times when physiology is quite variable, such as the critically ill patient with an infection receiving an aminoglycoside antibiotic. Under these circumstances, a single concentration measurement usually does not possess sufficient information content to assess the adequacy of exposure or forecast future drug concentrations with dose changes.

To improve the precision of dose estimation based on a monitored drug concentration, several pharmacokinetic-based methods have been developed to estimate patient-specific pharmacokinetic parameters using two or more drug concentrations. The first described and most simple of these methods, often referred to as the Zaske-Sawchuk method,[47] was developed in the context of therapy with aminoglycoside antibiotics. In this method, multiple concentrations are obtained to estimate pharmacokinetic parameters for a specific patient that can be used to guide dosing.

Although the Zaske-Sawchuk method significantly improved the precision of therapy with aminoglycoside antibiotics and other drugs, numerous limitations still exist. Multiple concentration measurements are required for adequate confidence in parameter estimation. More importantly, they ignore prior information regarding parameter estimates that have been derived from population-based studies that could assist in the initial dosing of the patient. These methods also discard prior studies performed in a patient under evaluation that provide useful information regarding PK variability within an individual patient.

Improved methods of parameter estimation that use the Bayes theorem have therefore been developed in an attempt to overcome some of these limitations. Although beyond the scope of this chapter, the Bayes theorem provides a theoretical framework to relate the parameter estimates that are made from a set of concentration data to any prior information about these parameters. As a result, Bayesian methods permit incorporation of prior concentration and parameter information into the estimation process. Numerous studies have demonstrated the improvement in precision of concentration control for many drugs, often with less available data; however, the question of whether Bayesian methods improve clinical outcomes over simpler approaches remains.

POINTS TO REMEMBER

Analytical Factors That Affect Therapeutic Drug Monitoring Results

- Method selectivity for the target drug versus its metabolites
- Method precision relative to the desired therapeutic target range
- Availability of standardized reference material
- Interfering substances in the sample (eg, antibodies that react with assay reagents)

THERAPEUTIC DRUG MONITORING OF SPECIFIC DRUGS IN COMMON CLINICAL USE

Antiepileptic Drugs

A number of AEDs are used to treat seizures (Table 40.1). Most can be measured by chromatographic methods or individually analyzed by immunoassay. The advantage of chromatographic methods such as gas chromatography–mass chromatography (GC-MS) or LC-MS is the ability to simultaneously analyze multiple AEDs in a single assay, with some methods reported to detect more than 20 individual compounds.[48] Immunoassay procedures are less labor intensive and are usually quicker to perform than chromatographic methods for measuring a single analyte. As a result, immunoassays are the mainstay of monitoring for these drugs in most clinical laboratories.

Phenytoin

Phenytoin (diphenylhydantoin), most commonly available as Dilantin but also available in generic form, is used in the treatment of primary or secondary generalized tonic-clonic

TABLE 40.1 Pharmacokinetic Parameters of Antiepileptic Drugs

Drug	RECOMMENDED THERAPEUTIC RANGE		Mean Time to Steady State (d)	Observed Range of Half-life in Adults (h)	Mean Volume of Distribution (L/kg)	Mean Oral Bioavailability (%)	Protein Binding (%)	Important Metabolizing Enzymes
	μg/mL	μmol/L						
Carbamazepine	4–12	17–51	2–4	8–12	1.4	70	75	CYP3A4
Clonazepam	0.015–0.060	0.048–0.190	3–10	17–56	3.2	>90	85	CYP3A4
Ethosuximide	40–100	283–708	7–10	30–60	0.7	>90	0	CYP3A4
Felbamate	30–60	126–252	3–4	14–21	0.8	>90	25	CYP3A4
Gabapentin	2–12	12–70	1–2	5–9	0.9	Variable	0	NA
Lamotrigine	2.5–15	10–59	3–6	20–30	1.2	>90	55	NA
Levetiracetam	12–46	70–270	1–2	6–8	0.6	>90	0	NA
Phenobarbital	10–40	43–172	12–24	70–140	0.7	>90	50	CYP2C19
Phenytoin	10–20 (free: 1.0–2.0)	40–79	5–17	30–100	0.6	80	90	CYP2C9, 2C19
Primidone	5–10	23–46	2–4	3–22	0.7	>90	20	CYP2C9, 2C19
Topiramate	5–20	15–59	4–5	20–30	0.7	80	15	NA
Valproic acid	50–100	346–693	2–4	11–20	0.2	>90	90	CYP2C9,2C19, 2B6, 2E1, 2A6
Zonisamide	10–40	47–188	9–12	50–70	1.4	65	50	CYP2C9, 3A4

seizures, partial or complex-partial seizures, and status epilepticus. The drug is not effective for absence seizures. Phenytoin likely has many targets, but the most well-described mechanism of action is the modulation of voltage-gated sodium channels through prolonging channel inactivation, which reduces the ability of the neuron to respond at high frequency.[49,50] The physiologic effect of this action is reduction in central synaptic transmission, aiding in control of abnormal neuronal excitability.

Phenytoin is not readily soluble in aqueous solutions. When administered by intramuscular injection, most of the dose precipitates at the site of injection and is then slowly absorbed. The prodrug fosphenytoin (Cerebyx) was introduced as a therapeutic form of phenytoin to improve phentytoin's pharmacology. Fosphenytoin has increased aqueous solubility for intramuscular injection.[51] After injection, it is rapidly converted to phenytoin. Absorption of oral phenytoin is slow and sometimes incomplete. Variations in the drug preparation have been blamed for low bioavailability. Once absorbed, the drug is tightly bound to protein (90% to 95%). As with all drugs, the pharmacologic effect of phenytoin is directly related to the amount present in the free (unbound) state. Only free phenytoin is available to cross biological membranes and interact at biologically important binding sites. The degree of protein binding can be reduced by the presence of other drugs, anemia, and hypoalbuminemia, which can occur in the elderly. In these conditions, an increased effect is observed at the same total drug concentration as in plasma from normal patients.

The optimal therapeutic concentration for seizure control without side effects is 10 to 20 µg/mL (40 to 79 µmol/L). In a large population study, Buchthal and colleagues[52] found a 50% response rate in patients with plasma concentrations greater than 10 µg/mL (40 µmol/L) and an 86% suppression of seizure activity at concentrations exceeding 15 µg/mL (59 µmol/L). These concentrations also serve as reasonable guidelines when the drug is used as a cardiac antiarrhythmic agent. Free phenytoin concentration in the range of 1 to 2 µg/mL (1 to 8 µmol/L) is frequently considered optimal. This free phenytoin reference interval[†] is based largely on studies of total serum phenytoin and an assumed 10% unbound drug fraction; however, the free fraction of phenytoin has been reported to vary considerably in otherwise healthy individuals from as low as 3% to as high as 37% in some patients.[53] Total phenytoin concentrations in excess of 20 µg/mL (79 µmol/L) do not usually enhance seizure control and are often associated with nystagmus and ataxia. Total phenytoin plasma concentrations in excess of 35 µg/mL (139 µmol/L) have been shown to actually precipitate seizure activity. A side effect of phenytoin not related to plasma concentration is development of gingival hyperplasia.

Phenytoin is metabolized by hepatic microsomal hydroxylating enzymes. The principal metabolite is 5-(*p*-hydroxyphenyl)-5-phenylhydantoin, which is excreted principally as a glucuronide ester. Other minor metabolites are of minimal clinical importance. Hepatic metabolism of phenytoin may become saturated within the therapeutic range. Once metabolism is saturated, small dose increments result in large changes in blood concentration (see Fig. 40.10); this phenomenon partially explains the wide variation in dose among patients that is required to accomplish a therapeutic effect.[54] Because of this saturation phenomenon, first-order kinetics do not generally apply to total phenytoin at blood concentrations in excess of 5 µg/mL (20 µmol/L).

The time to collect the specimen is dictated by the reason for monitoring. If a patient displays any symptoms of intoxication, the peak blood concentration is of interest. This specimen is collected 4 to 5 hours after the dose, although the peak level may be delayed up to 8 hours if the drug is given in conjunction with substances that increase stomach acidity. If the principal question at hand is adequate therapy, the trough concentration is more useful and the specimen is collected just before the next dose is given.

A number of drug interactions result in alteration of the disposition of phenytoin. Alcohol, barbiturates, and carbamazepine induce oxidative enzymes; this induction results in increased metabolism of phenytoin, reduced serum concentration of both total and free phenytoin, and reduced pharmacologic effect. Drugs such as chloramphenicol, cimetidine, disulfiram, isoniazid, and dicumarol compete with phenytoin metabolism, resulting in increase of both total and free phenytoin concentrations and enhancement of the pharmacologic effect. Salicylate, valproic acid, phenylbutazone, sulfisoxazole, and sulfonylureas compete with phenytoin for serum protein-binding sites. The end result is diminished total serum concentration of phenytoin while the free phenytoin concentration and pharmacologic effect remain approximately the same. The interest in monitoring the free phenytoin concentration is in response to these altered disposition states.

Carbamazepine

Carbamazepine (Tegretol) is used in the treatment of generalized tonic-clonic, partial, and partial-complex seizures. It is also used for the treatment of pain associated with trigeminal neuralgia and as a mood-stabilizing drug in bipolar disorder. Like phenytoin, carbamazepine modulates the synaptic sodium channel, which prolongs inactivation, reducing the ability of the neuron to respond at high frequency.[50] The physiologic effect of this action is reduction in central synaptic transmission, aiding in control of abnormal neuronal excitability. The mechanisms of action in mood stabilization are less clear, but appear to work through effects on inositol metabolism and glycogen synthase kinase 3-b (GSK3-b), which is an essential part of the Wnt/b-catenin pathway.[55] This latter pathway has been shown recently to play a critical role in neuronal adhesion, plasticity, and survival, as well as brain development.[56] In addition, GSK3-β appears critical to the action of dopamine and serotonin on the brain affecting behavior,[57] likely explaining many of the effects of mood-stabilizing drugs such as carbamazepine that inhibit this pathway.

After oral administration, carbamazepine is slowly and erratically absorbed with wide individual variability. The drug is highly protein bound (80%). The elimination half-life early in therapy is approximately 24 hours. With chronic therapy, the enzymes responsible for metabolism are induced, and the elimination half-life is reduced to 15 to 20 hours. Because hepatic metabolism is the principal means by which drug is eliminated from plasma, any reduction in liver function results in drug accumulation.

[†]Laboratories should verify that these ranges are appropriate for use in their own settings.

The therapeutic concentration range for optimal pharmacologic effect of carbamazepine is 4 to 12 μg/mL (17 to 51 μmol/L); however, this range depends on concomitant use of other AEDs. Toxicity associated with excessive carbamazepine ingestion occurs at plasma concentrations in excess of 15 μg/mL (63 μmol/L) and is characterized by symptoms of blurred vision, paresthesia, nystagmus, ataxia, drowsiness, and diplopia. Side effects unrelated to plasma concentration include development of an urticarial rash, which usually disappears on discontinuation of the drug, and hematologic depression (leukopenia, thrombocytopenia, and aplastic anemia).

The active metabolite of carbamazepine is carbamazepine-10,11-epoxide. This metabolite has been found to accumulate in children to concentrations equivalent to carbamazepine. It may contribute to symptoms of intoxication in children who have a therapeutic plasma concentration of the parent drug. Because carbamazepine is metabolized through the hepatic oxidative enzyme system, drugs that induce this system (phenytoin, phenobarbital) increase the rate of clearance of carbamazepine.

Coadministration of phenobarbital, phenytoin, or valproic acid increases the rate of metabolism of carbamazepine, reducing the blood concentration. Erythromycin and propoxyphene interfere with metabolism, increasing carbamazepine concentrations.

Because of carbamazepine's relatively long half-life, the specimen yielding the most useful information is the one representing the trough concentration; however, in the case of suspected mild intoxication, the peak value of the plasma concentration correlates more closely with toxicity. The peak specimen should be collected 4 to 8 hours after the oral dose in the setting of immediate-release formulations of carbamazepine.

Valproic Acid

Valproic acid (Depakene or Depakote) is used for treatment of absence seizures. It also has been shown to be useful against tonic-clonic and partial seizures when used in conjunction with other AEDs such as phenobarbital or phenytoin. Beyond its use in the treatment of epilepsy, valproate also has mood-stabilizing effects that make it a useful agent, and alternative, in the treatment of bipolar disorder. The drug inhibits the enzyme γ-aminobutyric acid (GABA) transaminase, resulting in an increase in the concentration of GABA in the brain. GABA is a potent inhibitor of presynaptic and postsynaptic discharges in the central nervous system. Valproic acid also modulates the synaptic sodium channel by prolonging inactivation, which reduces the ability of the neuron to respond at high frequency.[50,58] Additional mechanisms of action have been reported, such as effects on inositol metabolism and GSK-3 activity that might explain its utility in mood disorders.[55,59,60]

Valproic acid is rapidly and almost completely absorbed after oral administration. Peak concentrations occur 1 to 4 hours after an oral dose. The principal metabolite, 2-*n*-propyl-3-ketopentanoic acid, has anticonvulsant activity comparable to that of valproic acid, although this metabolite does not accumulate in plasma. The single-dose half-life is 16 hours in healthy adults, but this reduces to 12 hours on chronic therapy and may be as short as 8 hours in children. In neonates and in hepatic disease, when metabolism is reduced, the half-life becomes prolonged. Valproic acid is highly protein bound (93%). In circumstances when competition for protein binding increases, such as in uremia, cirrhosis, or concurrent drug therapy, the percent of free valproic acid increases.

The minimum effective therapeutic concentration of valproic acid is 50 μg/mL (346 μmol/L). Concentrations in excess of 100 μg/mL (693 μmol/L) have been associated with hepatic toxicity and acute toxic encephalopathy.

Clearance of valproic acid is rapid, presenting a dosing dilemma. The dose must be adequate to provide a plasma concentration greater than 40 μg/mL (277 μmol/L) while avoiding concentrations in excess of 100 μg/mL (693 μmol/L). The ideal specimen for monitoring the blood concentration is that drawn just before the next dose, usually early in the morning, to confirm that an adequate dose has been prescribed before bedtime. Dosing is particularly problematic in young children, who might sleep for more than one complete half-life of the drug.

Valproic acid modulates the action of various other common AEDs. It inhibits the nonrenal clearance of phenobarbital, resulting in increased phenobarbital concentrations. It competes with phenytoin for protein-binding sites. The free phenytoin concentration remains approximately the same, but the total phenytoin in the plasma decreases. Because the free phenytoin concentration remains unchanged, the pharmacologic effect is retained. Other common antiepileptic drugs that induce hepatic oxidative enzymes result in increased valproic acid clearance; this increased clearance rate requires a higher dose to maintain effective therapeutic concentrations.

Ethosuximide

Ethosuximide (Zarontin) is used for the treatment of absence seizures characterized by brief loss of consciousness. Ethosuximide reduces the flow of calcium through T-type calcium channels in the synapse of thalamic neurons; because thalamic neurons are the main source of 3-Hz spike-wave rhythms in absence seizures, reduction of calcium flow slows the rate of these seizure-inducing pulses.

Ethosuximide is readily absorbed from the gastrointestinal tract. The drug is cleared mainly by metabolism as either the hydroxyethyl compound or the glucuronide ester of the hydroxyethyl metabolite with a half-life of approximately 33 hours, although this may be prolonged in adults. The trough specimen yields the most useful information regarding therapeutic efficacy. The optimal therapeutic concentration of ethosuximide is 40 to 100 μg/mL (283 to 708 μmol/L). Toxicity related to an excessive blood concentration of ethosuximide is rare. Symptoms of gastrointestinal distress, lethargy, dizziness, and euphoria may be encountered early in therapy, but patients usually become tolerant to these symptoms.

Topiramate

Topiramate (Topamax) is a sulfamate-substituted monosaccharide anticonvulsant also approved for use in migraine headache therapy. The mechanisms by which topiramate exerts these effects is not clearly established. It is proposed that several effects may contribute to topiramate's pharmacologic activity, including blockage of voltage-dependent sodium channels, augmentation of the neurotransmitter γ-aminobutyrate action at some of the subtypes of the GABA-A receptor, antagonism of the AMPA/kainite subtype of glutamate receptors, and inhibition of isozymes II and IV of carbonic anhydrase.[61]

Topiramate is indicated as initial monotherapy or in combination with other anticonvulsants in patients 2 years of age and older with partial-onset or primary generalized tonic-clonic seizures and also is effective in patients with seizures associated with Lennox-Gastaut syndrome and was originally approved for use as an anticonvulsant by the FDA in 1996.[62]

Topamax is generally well and rapidly absorbed after oral administration with a usual T_{max} between 2 and 4 hours and bioavailability of up to 95%. Coingestion of food can delay absorption by approximately 2 hours without effect on T_{max}. Average steady-state serum concentrations can fall by approximately 50% when either phenytoin or carbamazepine is coadministered.[63] The metabolism of topiramate is not well understood or described, but renal clearance of unchanged drug has been reported to account for the majority of clearance in the absence of coadministered inducing drugs such as phenytoin or carbamazepine. In the presence of the latter, the contribution of hepatic clearance increases. Thus, on introduction of one of these inducing drugs into the patient's regimen, or withdrawal, closer monitoring of serum concentrations of topiramate is warranted. In the presence of significant renal disease, lowering the dosage and judicious use of TDM is recommended. Topiramate is only weakly bound to plasma proteins such that circumstances that alter drug binding in serum do not affect topiramate clearance or steady-state concentrations.

Based on retrospective studies and a concentration-controlled study, the usual range of concentrations is 5 to 20 µg/mL (15 to 59 µmol/L). The majority of seizure patients treated with topiramate are maintained with good safety and efficacy at concentrations in the middle of this target range.[64,65]

Lamotrigine

Lamotrigine (Lamictal) is not a GABA analog, but binds to the GABA receptor; it is therefore considered a GABA-receptor agonist. Lamotrigine acts like phenytoin and carbamazepine, blocking repetitive nerve firings induced by depolarization of spinal cord neurons. Lamotrigine was approved by the FDA in 1994 for adjunctive therapy of partial seizures in adults. It has yet to be approved for use in children. Studies also suggest lamotrigine is effective against absence seizures.[66-68]

Lamotrigine is well tolerated and completely absorbed from the gastrointestinal tract after oral administration. It is 60% bound to plasma proteins. Optimal response appears to occur with blood concentrations in the range of 2.5 to 15 µg/mL (~10 to 60 µmol/L). However, dizziness, ataxia, diplopia, blurred vision, nausea, and vomiting are signs of toxicity that may occur when the blood concentration exceeds 10 µg/mL (40 µmol/L). Half-life ranges from 15 to 35 hours with monotherapy.[64] Elimination occurs through hepatic metabolism; the primary metabolite is the glucuronide ester. Coadministration with cytochrome P450–inducing drugs such as phenobarbital, phenytoin, or carbamazepine results in reduced lamotrigine concentrations—dosage increases of approximately 30% are required to maintain optimal blood concentrations.

Chromatographic methods for analysis of lamotrigine have been reported.[69] Commercially available immunoassays for lamotrigine also have been introduced.

Levetiracetam

Levetiracetam (Keppra) is an anticonvulsant drug approved in the United States for adjunctive therapy in patients with partial seizures. Levetiracetam belongs to the lactam class of molecules that share a five-member pyrrolidone ring, which includes piracetam and ethosuximide. The mechanism of action for levetiracetam, although not fully understood, appears to be by binding to the synaptic vesicle protein SV2A, leading to a reduction in the rate of synaptic vesicle release.[70]

Levetiracetam, available in both oral and intravenous formulations, is mostly absorbed (>95%) within the gastrointestinal tract. Food intake causes a modest delay in absorption with reduced peak serum concentrations; however, overall bioavailability is unaffected. Levetiracetam is metabolized to the inactive acetamide form by hydrolysis (~27% to 34%), with the majority of the drug excreted by the kidneys unchanged into urine. Clearance of the drug is therefore affected by kidney disease. An increase in levetiracetam clearance has been observed during the third trimester of pregnancy; however, this change in clearance is variable. Because there is no significant hepatic metabolism of levetiracetam, liver function does not affect the pharmacokinetics of this drug.[71]

Serum concentrations of levetiracetam appear to correlate linearly with dose within the typical dosing range. Although the optimal target range for serum concentration has not been fully defined, retrospective analysis of data from clinical trials of levetiracetam suggest that concentrations within the range of 12 to 46 µg/mL (70 to 270 µmol/L) are associated with efficacy.[72]

Felbamate

Felbamate (Felbatol) was approved by the FDA in 1993 for primary or adjunctive therapy of partial seizures. Its use is limited to patients who fail other drug treatments, because felbamate carries with it a substantial risk for aplastic anemia and liver failure that is not related to blood concentration. Biweekly monitoring of complete blood count, serum aminotransferases, and bilirubin is recommended to detect early onset of these side effects. Felbamate is particularly effective in control of Lennox-Gastaut syndrome.

Felbamate is completely absorbed from the gastrointestinal tract. The drug is 30% bound to plasma proteins, and optimal blood concentrations for felbamate, while poorly defined, have been suggested to range from 30 to 60 µg/mL (126 to 252 µmol/L).[73] It is eliminated by hepatic metabolism, with its half-life ranging from 14 to 21 hours. Felbamate saturates metabolism when the concentration exceeds 120 µg/mL (504 µmol/L); at that concentration, metabolism converts from first order to zero order. There are currently no commercially available immunoassays for felbamate. HPLC[74] and capillary electrophoresis[75] have been reported for felbamate analysis.

Phenobarbital

Phenobarbital is used in the treatment of all seizures except absence seizures, and is known by a wide variety of proprietary names and found in combination with many other drugs. It is particularly useful for treatment of generalized tonic-clonic, partial, focal motor, temporal lobe, and febrile seizures. It is also known to reduce synaptic transmission, resulting in decreased excitability of the entire nerve cell and a consequent sedating effect. Phenobarbital potentiates synaptic inhibition through action on the GABA-A receptor by increasing the duration of chloride flow into the synapse.[25] The end result is an increase in seizure threshold and inhibition of the spread of discharges from the epileptic foci.

Absorption of oral phenobarbital is slow but complete. The time at which peak plasma concentrations are reached is widely variable and ranges from 4 to 10 hours after the dose. Phenobarbital is 40% to 60% bound to plasma proteins. The elimination half-life is from 70 to 100 hours and is age dependent (children average 70 hours, geriatric patients 100 hours). Because hepatic metabolism is one of the prime routes of elimination, reduced liver function results in prolonged half-life.

The optimally effective therapeutic concentration of phenobarbital is between 15 and 40 μg/mL (66 to 177 μmol/L).[76] The predominant side effect observed in adults at blood concentrations greater than 40 μg/mL (177 μmol/L) is sedation, although tolerance to this effect develops with chronic therapy.

Phenobarbital is metabolized in the liver to *p*-hydroxy phenobarbital, which is largely excreted as the glucuronide or sulfate ester. When renal and hepatic functions are decreased, patients experience decreased clearance of the drug. Elimination of phenobarbital may be decreased in the presence of valproic acid and salicylate if reduction in urinary pH occurs. During chronic administration of either valproate or salicylate, the concentration of phenobarbital may increase 10% to 20% and a dose adjustment may be necessary to avoid intoxication. Phenobarbital induces mixed-function oxidative enzymes, resulting in increased metabolism of other xenobiotics after approximately 1 to 2 weeks of therapy.

Because of the long elimination half-life of phenobarbital, the blood concentration does not change rapidly. Therefore a serum specimen collected late in the dose interval (trough) is representative of the overall effect. Results from specimens collected 2 to 4 hours after the dose can be misleading because they may be construed to be the peak concentration when in actuality they precede the peak. Table 40.1 summarizes pharmacokinetic data of anticonvulsant drugs.

Primidone

Primidone (Mysoline) is effective in the treatment of tonic-clonic and partial seizures. The mechanism of action of this drug is similar to that described for phenobarbital, and the therapeutic effect is due partially to the accumulation of its major metabolite, phenobarbital. A second metabolite of primidone, phenylethylmalonamide, also has some antiepileptic activity.

Primidone is rapidly and completely absorbed after oral administration. Once absorbed, it is not highly protein bound and has a half-life of approximately 10 hours. Disposition of the drug is not known to be significantly altered by other disease states or other drugs.

The optimal therapeutic concentration of primidone has been established as 5 to 12 μg/mL (23 to 55 μmol/L). Because phenobarbital is an active metabolite of primidone, concurrent analysis of phenobarbital is required for complete result interpretation. The previously defined therapeutic range for phenobarbital applies to adequate primidone therapy. The phenobarbital concentrations rise gradually over a period of 1 to 2 weeks after therapy is initiated. Toxicity secondary to accumulation of primidone occurs at serum concentrations in excess of 15 μg/mL (69 μmol/L) and is usually associated with symptoms of sedation, nausea, vomiting, diplopia, dizziness, ataxia, and a phenobarbital concentration greater than 40 μg/mL (177 μmol/L). Specimen collection is dictated by the same rules that apply for phenobarbital; the trough concentration is most useful.

Coadministration of acetazolamide with primidone results in decreased gastrointestinal absorption of primidone and subsequent diminished plasma concentrations. Primidone administered in association with phenytoin produces a modest increase in the ratio of phenobarbital to primidone because phenytoin competes with the hepatic hydroxylating enzymes associated with phenobarbital's metabolism. Coadministration of valproic acid, for the same reasons outlined for phenobarbital, causes a modest increase in both primidone and phenobarbital serum concentrations.

Zonisamide

Zonisamide is the generic name used in the United States for a widely used seizure medication whose common brand name is Zonegran. The FDA approved zonisamide use in 2000, with the suggestion that it be used together with other anticonvulsants in the treatment of partial seizures in adults.[77] Mechanism of action studies in various in vitro neuronal culture systems indicate that zonisamide blocks repetitive firing of voltage-sensitive sodium channels and reduces voltage-sensitive T-type calcium currents without affecting L-type calcium currents, thereby suppressing overall excitation of nerve cells.[77]

Orally administered zonisamide is generally well absorbed, with little to no effect of concomitant food consumption, and this drug is only weakly bound to plasma proteins. Zonisamide is extensively metabolized by oxidative, acetylation, and other pathways and has essentially linear pharmacokinetics resulting in linearity for doses ranging from 10 to 15 mg/kg per day.[64] Concomitantly administered inducing drugs such as phenytoin or carbamazepine cause increased metabolism-based clearance and therefore a need for dose adjustment that can be aided by TDM of zonisamide. When concomitant therapy with an inducing drug is being withdrawn, adjustment of dosing of zonisamide using TDM is warranted.

A target TDM range of 10 to 40 μg/mL (47 to 188 μmol/L) has been recommended, based largely on retrospective studies, and, as with all other anticonvulsants, there is significant overlap of serum zonisamide concentrations between seizure-free patients and patients who do not respond to therapy with this drug and between patients who encounter side effects and those who do not. Thus finding an optimal therapeutic concentration within the individual patient is an essential need, not simply titrating the patient to be within the target therapeutic range.[77]

Antibiotics

Antibiotics that require TDM include aminoglycosides, chloramphenicol, sulfonamides, vancomycin, trimethoprim, β-lactams, and tetracyclines. Pharmacokinetic details of these antibiotics are summarized in Table 40.2.

Aminoglycosides

Aminoglycosides are polycationic agents that kill aerobic gram-negative bacteria. They act by binding to the 30S ribosomal subunit of bacterial mRNA, thereby inhibiting protein

TABLE 40.2 Pharmacokinetic Parameters of Commonly Monitored Antibiotics

Drug	Therapeutic Targets* μg/mL (μmol/L)	Half-life (h)	Volume of Distribution (L/kg)	Oral Bioavailability (%)	Protein Binding (%)
Aminoglycosides					
Amikacin	C_{max}: 25–35 (43–60) C_{min}: 1–8 (1.7–13.7)	2†	0.2–0.4	NA	<11
Gentamicin	C_{max}: 5–12 (10.5–25) C_{min}: <1 (<2)	2†	0.2–0.4	NA	<30
Tobramycin	C_{max}: 5–12 (11–25.7) C_{min}: <1 (<2)	2†	0.2–0.4	NA	<15
Glycopeptides					
Vancomycin	C_{min}: >10–15 (>6.9–10.4)	6–12‡	0.4–1	<1§	10–50
Other					
Chloramphenicol	C_{max}: 10–25 (31–77) C_{min}: 1–8 (3–25)	Adults: 1.5–4.1 Newborn: ≥24¶	0.2–3.1 mean: 0.6–1.0	70–80‖	60

*Target blood concentrations depend on the infection (eg, tissue compartment), organism, and its sensitivity to the antibiotic (ie, minimum inhibitory concentration).
†Clearance of aminoglycoside antibiotics depends on kidney function. The half-life shown is the average elimination phase half-life in healthy individuals; however, the half-life may be significantly prolonged in individuals with renal disease.
‡Vancomycin best conforms to a multicompartment (two or three compartment) pharmacokinetic model. The half-life shown represents the terminal, elimination half-life.
§Absorption of vancomycin from the gastrointestinal tract leading to toxic concentrations has been observed in individuals with pseudomembranous colitis.
¶Chloramphenicol clearance is reduced in neonates because of limited glucuronide conjugating activity of the liver. Half-life is generally >24 hours immediately after birth and decreases to ~10 hours by 2 weeks of age.
‖Bioavailability of chloramphenicol depends on the chemical form (succinate or palmitate).
NA, Not applicable.

synthesis. They are inactive under anaerobic conditions because an oxygen-dependent active transport mechanism is involved in the transfer of aminoglycosides across the bacterial cell wall. The aminoglycoside class of drugs includes amikacin, gentamicin, kanamycin, neomycin, netilmicin, sisomicin, streptomycin, and tobramycin.

The aminoglycosides are a very polar group of compounds and are thus poorly absorbed from the intestinal tract. They are routinely administered intravenously or intramuscularly to achieve a high degree of bioavailability. When administered directly into the blood, they rapidly distribute to the extracellular fluid but do not cross cell membranes or bind to plasma proteins; this behavior is consistent with their unusually low volume of distribution. Most tissues and nonrenal or hepatic secretions contain very small concentrations of aminoglycosides, the exceptions being the renal cortex, where the drug is concentrated, and bile, because of active hepatic secretion. The drugs are mainly excreted by glomerular filtration. Elimination half-lives are short, ranging from 2 to 3 hours. Because clearance is highly dependent on renal function, any impairment of glomerular filtration causes accumulation of these drugs.

Therapy with antibiotic agents such as the aminoglycosides differs from the approach used for most other drugs discussed in this chapter. The goal is to achieve a concentration in plasma such that the bacteria are killed but the host remains undamaged. Because the organisms treated are variable and can become resistant to certain drugs, treatment with specific aminoglycoside agents should always be directed by susceptibility testing.

Numerous studies, summarized by Schentag,[78] Zaske,[79] and Mandell and colleagues,[80] recommend a limit to the blood concentration of aminoglycosides, although considerable variability is reported regarding the relationship of blood concentration to later onset of toxicity. Renal tubular necrosis and degeneration of the auditory nerve are the side effects most frequently experienced after exposure to high concentrations of aminoglycosides.[81] Both peak and trough specimens are required to monitor toxicity. Table 40.2 identifies target maximum peak and trough serum concentrations; in this mode of monitoring, the intent of therapy should be to dose the patient in such a manner that the peak concentration does not exceed these limits. In a large surgical patient survey in which dosing was carried out under controlled conditions, limited nephrotoxicity was experienced when the peak serum concentration of gentamicin was maintained below 8 μg/mL (17 μmol/L).[79] Using similar guidelines, Keys and colleagues[81] reported a 40% incidence of mild nephrotoxicity using a sensitive index of renal clearance (iothalamate clearance) when trough values regularly exceeded the limits defined in Table 40.2.

Dose corrections must be made in patients with compromised renal function because these patients have prolonged half-life and slower elimination.[82,83] This should then be followed by quantification of the blood concentration and dose adjustment following the method outlined by Gilbert.[84]

Toxicity associated with aminoglycosides manifests as delayed-onset vestibular and cochlear sensory cell destruction and acute renal tubular necrosis. The degree and severity of cell damage are variable among the different drugs, but they all cause cell damage if the concentrations are high. Unfortunately, the therapeutic concentration guidelines identified in Table 4.2 do not guarantee the avoidance of toxicity; a small number of patients experience toxic effects regardless of the concentration. Fortunately, most patients reverse the toxic effects without direct intervention if the toxicity is associated with reasonable blood concentrations. Irreparable loss of vestibular, cochlear, or renal function usually correlates with administration of one of the aminoglycosides at increased blood concentrations for periods longer than 2 weeks.

In certain patients with adequate renal function (generally glomerular filtration rate >30 mL/min), an alternative dosing schedule of once-daily, high-dose aminoglycoside therapy can be used. This dosing schedule is based on the concentration-dependent antimicrobial effect of these drugs, in which peak concentrations achieved rather than the time above the minimum inhibitory concentration (MIC) is most closely correlated with antimicrobial effect.[85-87] Unlike efficacy, toxicity of aminoglycoside antibiotics appears to be correlated with both peak and trough concentrations.[88,89] Peak concentrations at or above the therapeutic target based on MIC are generally ensured with the once-daily strategy, and trough level concentration monitoring is used to reduce risk for toxicity. Based on several studies comparing once-daily dosing with conventional dosing with multiple-daily dosing and TDM, once-daily dosing appears to be equally as effective as multiple-daily dosing. The incidence of nephrotoxicity with once-daily dosing appears equal or lower compared to conventional dosing; however, the incidence of ototoxicity is less clear, with at least one study showing an increased risk for ototoxicity in pediatric patients using a once-daily regimen.[90-92]

Heparin has been implicated as a deactivator of gentamicin by formation of an inactive complex.[93] This complex, although biologically inactive, retains some structural resemblance to the initial aminoglycoside and cross-reacts with antibodies to the specific aminoglycoside. Heparin concentrations encountered in therapeutic antithrombotic therapy are less than 3 units/mL, making an in vivo complication unlikely. However, specimen collection tubes containing heparin (1000 units/mL) may lead to complex formation, a phenomenon that could interfere with some immunoassay procedures.

Before the 1980s, aminoglycoside antibiotics were analyzed by the bioassay technique. This method is variable and subject to significant interference by numerous drugs. Such assays should now be considered obsolete. Liquid chromatographic and immunochemical methods are available with enzyme immunoassay, fluorescence polarization immunoassay, or similar nonisotopic immunoassays, which are now considered the methods of choice for aminoglycoside analysis.

Chloramphenicol

Chloramphenicol (eg, Chloromycetin) is used as a bactericidal agent. It acts by binding to the 50S ribosomal subunit of bacteria mRNA and inhibits protein synthesis in prokaryotic organisms. Use of this drug depends on its relative toxicity against the microorganism versus the host. The drug is used against gram-negative bacteria such as *Haemophilus influenzae, Neisseria meningitidis, Neisseria gonorrhoeae, Salmonella typhi,* all *Brucella* species, *Bordetella pertussis, Vibrio cholerae,* and *Shigella.* These organisms all are susceptible to a concentration of 6 μg/mL (19 μmol/L). Organisms that require higher concentrations of 12 μg/mL (37 μmol/L) are *Escherichia coli, Klebsiella pneumoniae, Pseudomonas pseudomallei, Chlamydia,* and *Mycoplasma.*

Chloramphenicol is rapidly absorbed in the gastrointestinal tract. Peak serum concentrations occur 1 to 2 hours after the oral dose. In plasma, chloramphenicol is approximately 50% protein bound and is cleared with a half-life of 2 to 3 hours. Peak serum concentrations after administration of chloramphenicol palmitate or succinate occur 4 to 6 hours after the dose. Chloramphenicol distributes to all tissues, and it concentrates in the cerebrospinal fluid. The drug is actively metabolized by the liver by *N*-acetylation and glucuronidation. Thus chloramphenicol accumulates in cases of hepatic disease. Renal disease does not dramatically reduce clearance.

Host toxicity displayed after chloramphenicol therapy includes hematologic toxicity and cardiovascular collapse; both show a modest relationship to blood concentration. The blood concentration–related hematologic toxicities include anemia, characterized by maturation arrest in the marrow; cytoplasmic vacuolation of early erythroid and myeloid cells; reticulocytopenia; and increases in both serum iron and serum iron-binding capacity. These symptoms are associated with serum concentrations in excess of 25 μg/mL (77 μmol/L). Development of idiosyncratic aplastic anemia also has been observed, but this complication appears unrelated to dose or blood concentration. Cardiovascular collapse, which occurs primarily in newborns, has been related to a total serum chloramphenicol concentration in excess of 50 μg/mL (155 μmol/L). An oral dose of 50 mg/kg per day results in an optimal peak serum concentration of 10 to 25 μg/mL (31 to 77 μmol/L) in a healthy adult.

Procedures for the determination of chloramphenicol concentrations in blood serum include high-performance liquid chromatography (HPLC) and immunoassay. Methods for chloramphenicol determination must be able to differentiate between the prodrug forms, chloramphenicol palmitate or succinate, and their active metabolite, chloramphenicol.

Vancomycin

Vancomycin is a glycopeptide that is bactericidal against gram-positive bacteria and some gram-negative cocci. Vancomycin is used because of its activity against methicillin-resistant staphylococci and corynebacteria. It has thus become popular for treatment of endocarditis and sepsis caused by these organisms.

Although the drug is generally poorly absorbed when given orally, absorption leading to toxicity has been observed in patients with pseudomembranous colitis.[94] A 1-g dose given intravenously every 12 hours usually results in a peak blood concentration of 20 to 40 μg/mL (14 to 28 μmol/L) and a trough concentration of 5 to 10 μg/mL (4 to 7 μmol/L). It has an average elimination half-life of 5 to 6 hours. Blood concentration–related toxicity involves the auditory nerve. Concentrations less than 30 μg/mL (21 μmol/L) are rarely associated with this development.[95] Toxicities not related to dose or blood concentrations include fever, phlebitis, and pain at the infusion site. Erythema or flushing of the face, neck, and upper torso occurring within approximately 5 to 10 minutes after vancomycin infusion (sometimes referred to as "red man syndrome" or "red neck syndrome") also has been observed. This syndrome is due to acute, non–immunoglobulin E-mediated mast cell degranulation and is generally controlled by slow infusion and administration of antihistamines. In patients with impaired renal function, the serum concentration may increase to toxic concentrations because of reduced clearance. Immunoassay is the standard approach to monitoring concentrations; HPLC methods to monitor the serum concentration are available.

Antifungal Antibiotics

Over the past decade, increasing evidence has accumulated to support the use of TDM to enhance the therapeutic safety and efficacy of antifungal medicines. The azole class of antifungals has the most data supporting concentration monitoring. Data supporting the monitoring of flucytosine are limited. Studies of TDM for other classes of antifungal medicines, including the echinocandins (ie, caspofungin) and the polyenes (eg, amphotericin B), have generated data showing either no or limited value to monitoring these drugs.

HPLC and LC-MS methods for detection of multiple azoles have been described and represent the predominant methods used for clinical testing by reference laboratories. Although these methods are generally highly specific, it should not be assumed that results are transferable across laboratories. A recent review of proficiency testing data that evaluated 5 years of data from 57 different laboratories around the world demonstrated that a wide variation in results, especially at low concentrations, is common, leading to results that can deviate by more than 20%.[96] New immunoassays for voriconazole and posaconazole have been described, but experience with these is limited. The availability of reliable immunoassays for these antifungals could foster more widespread experience in the effectiveness of their monitoring. Metabolism of the drugs also can affect interpretation of concentration data as discussed in more detail later.

Antifungal Azoles

The azoles represent an important class of drugs with broad-spectrum antifungal activity toward both pathogenic yeast and dimorphic fungi such as *Aspergillus* species. These drugs consist of two main structural families, the imidazoles and triazoles. The former class, which includes clotrimazole and ketoconazole, while active after systemic administration, are currently used primarily in topical formulations because of their poor oral absorption and the significant toxicity associated with their systemic use. The safer, triazole class, which includes fluconazole, itraconazole, voriconazole, and posaconazole, are the primary azoles in use systemically for the treatment of serious, invasive fungal infections, and these are the drugs described further below. All of the azoles mediate their antifungal activity by preferentially inhibiting fungal 14α-demethylase (a cytochrome P450 enzyme), which is critical for the generation of ergosterol required for cytoplasmic membrane synthesis.

Fluconazole. Fluconazole is available in both intravenous and oral formulation. It is frequently used in prophylaxis against invasive candidiasis and in the treatment of invasive fungal infections by *Cryptococcus neoformans,* coccidiomycosis, and candidiasis. Fluconazole shows high bioavailability of approximately 90%, and this absorption appears unaffected by food or gastric pH. It shows low serum protein binding with wide tissue distribution required for its use in treating invasive systemic fungal infections. Fluconazole is primary cleared by the kidney, with an average half-life of approximately 32 hours.[97]

Due to the predominantly renal clearance of fluconazole, dosing requires adjustment according to estimated glomerular filtration rate.[98] There appears to be a pharmacodynamics dose-response relationship between exposure to fluconazole as assessed by the ratio of dose to the MIC of the organisms and efficacy.[99] Despite this relationship, TDM has not been generally recommended for fluconazole because of its linear pharmacokinetics[100] and generally good safety profile in adults and children.[101] However, evidence suggests that critically ill adults and children may not achieve adequate exposure based on commonly recommended doses. This may be particularly challenging in patients with central nervous system disease or patients with infections caused by organisms with a high MIC. Monitoring may therefore be warranted in some patients, but applying TDM to these settings is challenging because of the lack of appropriately defined target concentrations, which is likely to be affected significantly by the MIC of the organism.

Itraconazole. Itraconazole is a broad-spectrum antifungal agent with activity toward most clinically relevant organisms, including *Candida, Cryptococcus,* and *Aspergillus* species. Itraconazole is available in oral and intravenous (outside the United States) formulations. Unlike fluconazole, itraconazole exhibits much more variable bioavailability that appears to depend on the specific formulation used. Absorption is influenced by food and gastric pH for some formulations.[102,103] Itraconazole also displays nonlinear pharmacokinetics with slow clearance.[104-106] Due to the pharmacokinetic properties of itraconazole along with the appreciable gastrointestinal, neurologic, and liver toxicity,[107] TDM generally has been recommended for this drug.[108-111] The optimal target concentration for itraconazole will likely depend on the organism, its MIC, and its infection site, as suggested by experimental model systems[112,113]; however, retrospective studies suggest that concentrations above 0.5 μg/mL (0.7 μmol/L) are associated with the lowest risk for invasive fungal infections when used as prophylaxis in the setting of neutropenia.[114-116] Data on serum concentrations associated with efficacy in the treatment of invasive fungal infections is very limited, but most responding patients have concentrations greater than 0.6 to 1.0 μg/mL (0.9 to 1.4 μmol/L) on day 7 of treatment, suggesting that this may be a useful threshold to ensure efficacy.[117,118] The association between itraconazole concentration and toxicity also has been explored. Unfortunately, although a pharmacodynamic relationship appears to exist, these studies were performed using a bioassay for itraconazole that detects both the parent drug and the biologically active hydroxyitraconazole metabolite making it difficult to interpret the data when compared to concentrations obtained by HPLC or LC-MS, which are the methods generally used in the clinical setting.[119,120] Specific measurement of itraconazole alone also markedly underestimates the biologic activity of itraconazole in serum because of the presence of the hydroxylitraconazole metabolite, which may contribute as much as 80% of the biological activity in serum.[121]

Voriconazole. Voriconazole is a second-generation triazole with broad-spectrum antifungal activity, including enhanced potency against *Aspergillus* species, and is approved by the FDA for treatment of invasive aspergillosis, candidemia in nonneutropenic patients, esophageal candidiasis, disseminated candidiasis, and as salvage therapy for fungal infections caused by *Scedosporium apiospermum* and *Fusarium* species.

Therapy with voriconazole is generally initiated with a protocol-guided loading dose followed by empirically guided maintenance dosing. For patients who improve clinically from this treatment and who can tolerate orally administered drugs, empirically guided conversion to oral dosing of this antifungal can be achieved. The conversion from intravenous to oral voriconazole is made possible and effective as a result of the high bioavailability shown for adults[122]; however, bioavailability has been reported to vary significantly, especially in children,[123,124] with reported bioavailability as low as 60%.[125] Voriconazole, like itraconazole, displays saturable, nonlinear kinetics with variable clearance because of genetic and nongenetic variation in CYP450 metabolism, making prediction of concentration from dose difficult.

Based on the observed nonlinear pharmacokinetics and wide intersubject and intrasubject variability, the poor dose versus serum concentration relationship, narrow TI, and frequent drug-drug interactions, TDM has been advocated for voriconazole as a way to improve on both efficacy outcomes and toxicity.[126,127] Based on mostly retrospective study data, it has been recommended that voriconazole trough concentrations be maintained between target of 1 to 2 μg/mL (3 to 6 μmol/L) on the low end and 5 to 6 μg/mL (15 to 17 μmol/L) on the upper end to maximize efficacy and limit neurologic and possibly hepatic toxicity.[126] To provide stronger support for instituting TDM for these medicines, the conduct of scientifically rigorous randomized, prospective concentration-controlled trials is optimal to verify the results of retrospective study data. Fortunately, a recent prospective, concentration-controlled study of voriconazole dosing to achieve serum concentrations in the 1- to 5-μg/mL (3 to 15 μmol/L) range on day 4 of therapy demonstrated both an improvement in efficacy and reduction in toxicity of voriconazole therapy when compared with standard fixed dosing.[128] These data lend excellent support to the benefits of TDM for voriconazole and further validate the retrospectively defined target range for monitoring.

Posaconazole. Posaconazole is a broad-spectrum antifungal with structural similarity to itraconazole and activity toward *Candida, Aspergillus, Cryptococcus,* and *Mucor* species. It is currently available only in oral form. It is used in the treatment of invasive fungal infections and increasingly in the prophylaxis against infection in neutropenic patients. Posaconazole exhibits variable bioavailability. Absorption appears saturable and significantly affected by food and gastric pH. Administration with a high-fat meal increases exposure by as much as twofold to threefold compared to the fasting state.[129]

Posaconazole exhibits linear pharmacokinetics with a half-life of approximately 24 to 37 hours depending on the formulation. Due to the long half-life of this drug, steady-state concentrations are generally not reached until the end of the first week of dosing. The long elimination time also means that the concentrations change little over the typical 12-hour dose interval. Based on the variable pharmacokinetics observed with this drug, the presence of a concentration-response relationship in retrospective data,[130-132] and the risk for treatment failure, TDM has been advocated for posaconazole. No prospective data are available to guide selection of a therapeutic concentration range; however, a minimum concentration of 0.7 μg/mL (1 μmol/L) has been suggested for prophylaxis, based largely on analysis of phase III clinical trial data.[108] The minimum concentration for patients with invasive aspergillosis is suggested to be 1 μg/mL (1.4 μmol/L) based on the pharmacodynamics relationships identified in the retrospective analysis of concentrations in clinical trials[132]; however, as for the other antifungals, the organism and its sensitivity to the posaconazole as well as the tissue sites will likely influence the efficacy. Although hepatotoxicity has been observed with posaconazole, the pharmacodynamics relationship between serum concentration and toxicity, if any, is unclear.

5-Flucytosine

One of the first antifungals developed, the pyrimidine analog 5-fluocytosine, is a broad-spectrum agent that is coadministered with another fungicidal drug (typically amphotericin B) to prevent the emergence of resistant pathogen populations. Toxicity of 5-flucytosine is well correlated with serum concentrations greater than 100 μg/mL (775 μmol/L) and manifests with myelosuppression (eg, thrombocytopenia) or hepatic dysfunction evidenced by increased transaminases.[133]

5-Flucytosine bioavailability is excellent, but its renal elimination is variable and may be affected by nephrotoxicity associated with amphotericin B. 5-Flucytosine dose is therefore adjusted according to renal function as typically assessed by creatinine clearance.[133] Based on the seriousness of toxicity and the well-documented concentration-response relationships, TDM has long been recommended for this drug to prevent toxicity. Because of its short half-life, the drug is administered in multiple doses daily. It is recommended to draw TDM samples at peak serum concentrations, roughly 2 hours after a dose, and the first measurement should be made within the first 72 hours after initiation of treatment. Target concentrations for efficacy appear to vary with the pathogen and the extent of infection, and the relationships to efficacy have been much less defined. Based on the strong evidence that the risk for myelotoxicity rises significantly with peak serum concentrations above 100 μ/mL (775 μmol/L), peak concentrations of 50 to 100 μg/mL (388 to 775 μmol/L) have been recommended for most patients to minimize toxicity.[108]

Antineoplastic Agents

Methotrexate

Methotrexate has proved useful in the management of acute lymphoblastic leukemia in children; choriocarcinoma and related trophoblastic tumors in women; carcinomas of the breast, tongue, pharynx, and testes; maintenance of remission in leukemia; and treatment of severe, debilitating psoriasis. High-dose methotrexate administration followed by leucovorin rescue is effective in treatment of carcinoma of the lung and osteogenic sarcoma. Intrathecal administration is effective in treating meningeal leukemia or lymphoma. Table 40.3 lists pharmacokinetic parameters for methotrexate.

Methotrexate inhibits DNA synthesis by decreasing availability of pyrimidine nucleotides. Methotrexate competitively inhibits the enzyme dihydrofolate reductase, thus decreasing the concentrations of the tetrahydrofolate essential to the methylation of the pyrimidine nucleotides and consequently the rate of pyrimidine nucleotide synthesis. Leucovorin, a folate analog, is used to rescue host cells from methotrexate inhibition; as a synthetic substrate for dihydrofolate

TABLE 40.3 Pharmacokinetic Parameters for Commonly Monitored Antineoplastic Drugs

Drug	Minimum Effective Concentration	Minimum Toxic Concentration	Mean Half-Life (h)	Mean Volume of Distribution (L/kg)	Mean Protein Binding (%)	Metabolizing Enzymes
Busulfan, 6 h dosing	AUC: 900 μmol × min/L	AUC:1350 μmol × min/L	2.6	0.99	10	SULT
Busulfan, 24 h dosing	AUC: 2400 μmol × min/L	AUC: 6000 μmol × min/L	2.6	0.99	10	SULT
Methotrexate						
At 24 h	<10 μmol/L	>10 μmol/L	1.8	0.55	46	None
At 48 h	<1 μmol/L	>1 μmol/L	8.4	0.55	46	None
At 72 h	<0.1 μmol/L	>0.1 μmol/L	>10	0.55	46	None
Azathioprine	NA	NA	0.2	0.8	0	HGPRT, TPMT
6-mercaptopurine	NA	NA	0.9	0.56	19	TPMT

reductase, leucovorin administration allows resumption of tetrahydrofolate-dependent synthesis of pyrimidines and reinitiation of DNA synthesis. Methotrexate is a nonspecific cytotoxin, and prolongation of blood concentrations appropriate to killing tumor cells may lead to severe, unwanted cytotoxic effects such as myelosuppression, gastrointestinal mucositis, and hepatic cirrhosis.

Serum concentrations of methotrexate are commonly monitored during high-dose therapy (>50 mg/m^2) to identify the time at which active intervention by leucovorin rescue should be initiated. Criteria for blood concentrations indicative of a potential for toxicity after single-bolus high-dose therapy are as follows[134,135]:

1. Methotrexate concentration greater than 10 μmol/L 24 hours after dose
2. Methotrexate concentration greater than 1 μmol/L 48 hours after dose
3. Methotrexate concentration greater than 0.1 μmol/L 72 hours after dose

Characteristically, blood concentrations are monitored at 24, 48, and 72 hours after the single dose and leucovorin is administered when methotrexate concentrations are inappropriately high for a postdose phase. The route of elimination for methotrexate is primarily renal excretion. During the period of high blood concentrations, particular attention must be paid to maintaining output of a large volume of alkaline urine. The p*Ka* of methotrexate is 5.5; thus small decreases in urine pH result in significant reduction in its solubility. Keeping urinary pH alkaline diminishes the risks for intratubular precipitation of the drug and obstructive nephropathy during the treatment period. Monitoring blood concentrations therefore provides the basis for decisions for timing of initiation and continuance of leucovorin treatment and for managing urinary pH.

Methotrexate has been measured in biological specimens using a wide variety of techniques. Radioimmunoassay (RIA) and the folate reductase inhibition techniques have been used, but nonisotopic immunoassays are now the method of choice. Liquid chromatographic procedures have been developed to allow for co-analysis of the drug and its metabolites.[136]

Busulfan

Busulfan is a DNA alkylating agent available in both oral and intravenous formulation. High-dose busulfan is often used as part of the myeloablative preparative regimen for hematopoietic stem cell transplantation (HSCT). Clinical use of busulfan is complicated by significant interpatient variability in pharmacokinetic behavior, with reported coefficients of variation (CVs) of 23[137] and 25%[138] for the oral and intravenous formulations, respectively. Age, obesity, underlying disease, and organ dysfunction also exert a significant influence on observed clearance for busulfan. Children under the age of 6 years typically display more than twice the average clearance of 2.5 mL/min per kilogram reported for adults.[139,140] The observed variability in the pharmacokinetic behavior of busulfan is relevant because several studies have identified a pharmacodynamic relationship between exposure to busulfan and both its toxicity and efficacy. Exposure to busulfan is typically estimated by measurement of several plasma concentrations over a 6-hour dose interval. This exposure is generally expressed as either the AUC in μmol × min/L or mean steady-state concentration ($\bar{C}_{SS}$), which is easily derived from the AUC (in ng × min/mL) by dividing this quantity by the dose interval in minutes (t). The risk for toxicity caused by busulfan (venoocclusive disease or pulmonary toxicity) appears to rise significantly with a $\bar{C}_{SS}$ greater than 900 to 1025 ng/mL (3.65 to 4.16 μmol/L).[141-144] In contrast, the risk for relapse in patients undergoing HSCT for chronic myelogenous leukemia rises substantially with a $\bar{C}_{SS}$ of less than 917 ng/mL (3.72 μmol/L), indicating that a very narrow therapeutic range of exposure exists for this drug.[145]

Control of busulfan exposure within the apparent tight therapeutic range requires an accurate and precise estimate of exposure. To achieve this level of accuracy and precision, a pharmacokinetic study using extensive sampling is typically performed. Early approaches used noncompartmental analysis with estimation of AUC using the trapezoidal rule, which is required for the complex kinetics observed with oral busulfan. Although this approach was effective and can be used with intravenous formulations of busulfan, fitting the concentration data to a one-compartment, first-order pharmacokinetic model by nonlinear regression has become the preferred method for estimating the $\bar{C}_{SS}$ or AUC for a dose interval when using intravenous dosing of busulfan. Dosing of busulfan is usually every 6 hours over 4 days for a total of 16 doses. As a result, a study is typically performed after the first dose, and the results are promptly reported to effect a dose adjustment as early as possible in the course of the treatment regimen; however, the completion and reporting of a busulfan pharmacokinetic study is not a simple task. A variety of chromatographic methods are used for measurement of busulfan in plasma, with GC-MS and LC-MS/MS generally the preferred methods. Given the complexity of the analytical methodology, onsite testing is not always available. Sample extraction and analysis also usually require several hours to complete for a single patient. Nevertheless, using the previously described TDM approach with dose adjustment, exposures that are within less than 10% of the target exposure are possible and toxicity can be avoided without a compromise in efficacy.[141,142,144-146]

Thiopurines

Originally developed in the 1950s for their potent cytotoxic activity, the thiopurine drugs, 6-mercaptopurine (6-MP), azathioprine (AZA) (an azo precursor to 6-mercaptopurine), and 6-thioguanine (6-TG), represent a class of drugs used today to treat cancer (eg, acute lymphoblastic leukemia), rheumatologic disease, inflammatory bowel disease (IBD), and solid organ transplant rejection. These agents derive their potent pharmacologic activity from the dependence of normal and malignant lymphocytes on purine metabolism for proliferation and function. After the bioactivation of 6-MP and 6-TG through phosphoribosylation via hypoxanthine-guanine phosphoribosyltransferase (HGPRT) and conversion to 6-TG nucleotides, these thiol-containing nucleotides are readily incorporated into DNA. Cell death by apoptosis causes secondary to failure of base mismatch repair induced by the false nature of these thioguanine nucleotides. Incorporation into RNA and inhibition of purine biosynthesis are likely to further contribute to the cytotoxic effect of these compounds.[25]

Myelosuppression represents the most pronounced toxicity associated with the thiopurine drugs. The dose-dependence of myelosuppression is well recognized; however, some individuals are much more sensitive to the myelosuppressive effects of 6-MP and AZA than others. The pharmacokinetic behavior of 6-MP and AZA is characterized by poor oral bioavailability (<25%) with a relatively short half-life ($t_{1/2}$) of approximately 50 minutes. The clearance of 6-MP is variable and is mediated primarily via two enzymatic pathways: (1) oxidation to thiouric acid by xanthine oxidase and (2) S-methylation via thiopurine S-methyltransferase (TPMT). Xanthine oxidase contributes significantly to the poor bioavailability of 6-MP and AZA through first-pass metabolism within the intestines and liver. Inhibition of xanthine oxidase via allopurinol leads to a fivefold increase in 6-MP bioavailability. In contrast, allopurinol exhibits little effect on 6-MP pharmacokinetics in plasma, suggesting that the contribution of xanthine oxidase to metabolism once the drug is absorbed is negligible.[147]

The large interindividual variability in sensitivity to toxicity noted with these drugs has led to the search for genetic factors that might contribute to the pharmacokinetics and pharmacodynamic variation of these drugs. TPMT-mediated metabolism appears to be the principal mechanism for plasma clearance of 6-MP. Studies in the 1980s demonstrated that white individuals could be classified into three categories of TPMT activity based on enzymatic assays of TPMT in red blood cell (RBC) lysates with frequencies suggestive of a monogenic inherited trait in Hardy-Weinberg equilibrium.[148] Individuals with the lowest TPMT activity, approximately 0.3% of whites, exhibit approximately 10-fold higher erythrocyte 6-TG nucleotide concentrations than the majority of individuals with wild-type enzymatic activity after 6-MP therapy.[149] All individuals with the lowest TPMT phenotype experience toxicity associated with doses of 6-MP derived from population-based pharmacokinetics and pharmacodynamics studies. Individuals with intermediate activity (~11% in white populations) also demonstrate higher erythrocyte 6-TG nucleotide concentrations that are intermediate between those of individuals with wild-type and low activity. The pharmacodynamics effects of this intermediate phenotype are still relevant, with 30% to 60% of heterozygous individuals experiencing significant 6-MP–associated toxicity requiring dose reductions.[149,150] These findings support the importance of TPMT as the principal mechanism for 6-MP and AZA clearance, and they further indicate that pretreatment recognition of individuals in the reduced metabolism category will benefit from a dose-reduction in 6-MP or AZA. Although TPMT activity explains much of the toxicity associated with these drugs, TPMT may explain only approximately a third of the toxicity.[151] Additional polymorphisms in genes such as inosine triphosphate phosphorylase also appear to contribute to the toxicity of these drugs.[152]

The dependence of 6-TG on TPMT for methylation leading to inactivation suggests that 6-TG pharmacokinetics should be well correlated with TPMT phenotype.[153] Despite the expectation that 6-TG nucleotide concentrations should be correlated with clinical efficacy and toxicity, the results of clinical studies exploring this relationship in patients with IBD are mixed.[154-158] This in part may be explained by the complex nature of the metabolic pathways involved. In a study of IBD patients resistant to thiopurine therapy, Dubinsky and colleagues[159] demonstrated that patients who respond to an increase in 6-MP/AZA dose show a significant rise in 6-TG nucleotide concentrations.[159] Furthermore, those who failed to respond to dose escalation also failed to show a significant rise in 6-TG nucleotide concentrations. Instead, a skewing toward TPMT metabolism with a rise in 6-methylmercaptopurine (6-MMP) ribonucleotide concentrations was noted, and this is associated with increased risk for hepatotoxicity.[159,160] These data suggest serial monitoring of 6-TG nucleotide and 6-MMP concentrations alone may be able to identify patients at risk for therapeutic failure, perhaps as a result of preferential metabolism by TPMT. Based on a metaanalysis of studies in IBD, the suggested optimal concentrations of 6-TG nucleotide fall within the range of 230 to 260 pmol/8 $\times 10^8$ RBC range with concentrations above 400 pmol/8 $\times$ 10^8 RBCs associated with increased toxicity.[161,162] Measurement of 6-TG nucleotide concentrations may play their most useful role in identifying patients with poor adherence to thiopurine therapy.[163] This is relevant because Mantzaris and associates[164] reported that most patients with IBD exhibit some degree of therapy nonadherence. The role of monitoring 6-TG nucleotide concentrations in other settings such as other autoimmune diseases, transplantation, and oncology is less clear.

Immunosuppressive Drugs

Tacrolimus

Tacrolimus (Prograf), formerly called FK-506, is a macrolide antibiotic isolated from a strain of *Streptomyces*

TABLE 40.4 Immunosuppressive Regimens and Associated Tacrolimus Target Ranges Used at the Author's Institution

Organ	Immunosuppressive Regimen	Time After Transplant	TACROLIMUS THERAPEUTIC RANGE µg/L	TACROLIMUS THERAPEUTIC RANGE nmol/L
Kidney	Tacrolimus + MMF	0–1 mo	8–12	10.4–15.6
		2–3 mo	7–10	9.1–13
		4–6 mo	6–8	7.8–10.4
		7–12 mo	5–7 (6–8 for higher risk)	6.5–9.1 (7.8–10.4 for higher risk)
		>12 mo	4–6 (5–7 for higher risk)	5.2–7.8 (6.5–9.1 for higher risk)
Heart	Tacrolimus + MMF	0–3 mo	10–12	13–15.6
		4–6 mo	10	13
		6–12 mo	8–10	10.4–13
		>12 mo	5–8	6.5–10.4
Liver	Tacrolimus + steroids ± azathioprine or MMF	0–3 wk	8–12 (6–8 with renal insufficiency)	10.4–15.6 (7.8–10.4 with renal insufficiency)
		4–6 wk	6–10 (6–8 with renal insufficiency)	7.8–13 (7.8–10.4 with renal insufficiency)
		7 wk–9 mo	5–8	6.5–10.4
		10 mo–2 y	4–6 (6 for AIH; 3–4 with renal insufficiency if also on an antiproliferative agent)	5.2–7.8 (7.8 for AIH; 3.9–5.2 with renal insufficiency if also on an antiproliferative agent)
		>3 y	3–4 (6 for AIH)	3.9–5.2 (7.8 for AIH)
Lung	Tacrolimus + MMF + steroids	0–12 mo	8–12	10.4–15.6
		>12 mo	6–8	7.8–10.4
Bone marrow	Tacrolimus		5–15	6.5–19.5

AIH, Autoimmune hepatitis; *MMF*, mycophenolate mofetil.

tsukubaensis that has significant immunosuppressant properties.[165] Tacrolimus mediates its immunosuppressive action by entering the lymphocyte and binding to a receptor known as FK506-binding protein (FKBP). Once bound to FKBP, this drug-receptor complex interacts with, and blocks, the calcium-dependent phosphatase calcineurin, which is critical for the translocation of nuclear factor of activated T cells (NFAT) to the nucleus, where the latter regulates the transcription of cytokines and other genes important for T-cell activation, proliferation, and function. Calcineurin inhibition therefore leads to marked suppression of T cell–mediated immune responses such as those involved in solid organ transplant rejection and graft-versus-host disease after bone marrow transplantation. NFAT plays a role in other cell types, likely contributing to the toxic effects of tacrolimus.

Tacrolimus is administered predominantly orally in capsule form (Prograf) containing 0.5 mg, 1 mg or 5 mg of the drug. A sterile solution containing the equivalent of 1 mg/mL of tacrolimus for intravenous administration and an ointment containing 0.1% or 0.03% for topical use on skin are also available. Rapid but incomplete absorption is characteristic of standard oral tacrolimus formulations, with an average time to peak concentration of 1.6 to 2.3 hours and average oral bioavailability of 17% to 22%.[166] Several prolonged-release formulations of tacrolimus have been developed, with the first, Advagraf, now available commercially.[167] Extended-release formulations afford delayed maximal concentrations with improved bioavailability leading to a slight reduction in dose to achieve equivalent AUC.

There is a fairly good correlation between tacrolimus trough concentration, graft rejection, and toxicity.[168] The target range for tacrolimus blood concentrations depends on the concomitant use of other ISDs, the transplant type, and the time after transplantation. An example of the immunosuppressive regimens used at our institution with the associated tacrolimus target ranges are shown in Table 40.4. Recent trends have aimed toward reducing the exposure for the calcineurin inhibitors tacrolimus and cyclosporine A (CsA) because of the increased recognition of long-term nephrotoxicity associated with their use in all solid organ transplant types.[169] Neurotoxicity is another notable adverse effect of tacrolimus. Like nephrotoxicity, the severity of neurologic toxicity generally correlates with trough concentration, with most significant neurologic events occurring with tacrolimus concentrations above 15 ng/mL (19 nmol/L).[170] Because the application of IDSs to transplantation is continuously evolving and the pharmacodynamics relationships depend on concomitant ISDs, the target concentration ranges for tacrolimus must be regularly reviewed to ensure they reflect current standards of practice.

The steady-state trough concentration of tacrolimus per unit of dose varies widely within and among patients.[168,171,172] The between-subject variability of dose-normalized tacrolimus has been estimated to be fivefold.[171] Factors known to contribute to this variability are many and include hematocrit; plasma albumin concentration; patient age; genotypes of metabolizing enzyme CYP3A5; drug-drug, herb-drug, and food-drug interactions; and disease.[166,173] The influence of one or more of these factors in transplant patients explains the wide within- and between-subject variability of tacrolimus concentrations. This, taken together with the narrow TI and the requirement of contemporary practice to lower the tacrolimus dosing and target trough concentration during the first transplant year and beyond to limit nephrotoxicity, is the basis for the need for close concentration monitoring of this drug.

Due to the high binding of tacrolimus to FK506-binding proteins within cells, including erythrocytes, the plasma concentration of tacrolimus is typically 1.5% to 8% of whole blood. Methods for quantitative analysis of this drug therefore generally begin with cell lysis and protein precipitation of whole blood to liberate cell-bound tacrolimus to allow measurement of the total drug present within whole blood. The lysis step is most commonly performed as a manual step using a water-miscible solvent (eg, methanol) solution containing zinc sulfate ($ZnSO_4$) followed by centrifugation. Performance of this initial step is one of the critical points in tacrolimus analysis, and it represents an important source of potential error if not performed correctly or consistently.

Interferences in the measurement of tacrolimus include metabolites of the drug and other substances present in human blood such as antibodies that react with components of the assay (for additional discussion on interference in immunoassay, refer to Chapter 23).[174-176] The former represents the more frequent and challenging interfering substance. Tacrolimus undergoes extensive metabolism by the liver and gastrointestinal cytochrome P450 (CYP) enzyme system with less than 0.5% of the parent drug excreted unchanged in the feces and urine.[166] The CYP3A isoenzymes are the principle CYP enzymes involved in tacrolimus metabolism, with more than 15 different metabolites described. However, significant variability in metabolism has been reported because of both genetic factors and physiologic factors such as liver dysfunction.[177] Interference by metabolites represents a significant problem for the immunoassay methods. Evaluation of cross-reactivity for the most abundant metabolites of tacrolimus demonstrate that the M2 (31-desmethyl tacrolimus) and M3 (15-desmethyl tacrolimus) metabolites yield as much as 80% cross-reactivity with the antibodies used in some immunoassays.[178] M2 displays immunosuppressive activity equal to that of the parent compound, tacrolimus, in vitro, whereas M3 has minimal immunosuppressive activity. Hematocrit, and to a lesser extent albumin, have a significant impact on the measured concentration of tacrolimus. Several studies have demonstrated that a low hematocrit (<33%) leads to an increase in measured tacrolimus (upward bias) when compared with LC-MS/MS reference methods.[179,180] This bias is inversely related to the hematocrit, with as much as a 50% increase at a hematocrit of 20%. A similar bias is observed when albumin concentrations fall below 3 g/dL (4.4 μmol/L).

Cyclosporine

Cyclosporine (Sandimmune [Cyclosporin A or CsA] and Neoral) is a cyclic peptide composed of 11 amino acids, some of novel structure, isolated from the fungus *Trichoderma polysporum*. The compound has been shown effective in suppressing solid organ allograft rejection, graft-versus-host disease, and bone marrow transplantation. CsA is approved for use in renal, cardiac, hepatic, pancreatic, and bone marrow transplants.

CsA acts by a mechanism that is very similar to that of tacrolimus. After entry into the cell, CsA forms a complex with cytoplasmic receptors termed *cyclophilins* that are molecularly distinct from FKBP. These cyclosporine:cyclophilin molecular complexes interact with and inhibit the calcineurin phosphatase, preventing NFAT activation that is critical for lymphocyte proliferation and function.

Absorption of CsA in the form of Sandimmune is highly variable, ranging from 5% to 40%. There is a poor relationship between dose and blood concentration; however, the whole-blood concentration of CsA correlates with the degree of immunosuppression and toxicity.[181] A microemulsion form of CsA, Neoral, has more reproducible absorption, averaging 40%, and exhibits better correlation among dose, blood concentration, and clinical response.[182,183]

Immunosuppression requires trough whole-blood concentrations of at least 100 ng/mL (83 nmol/L).[181] Kahan and colleagues[184] found that trough whole-blood concentrations exceeding 600 ng/mL (499 nmol/L) were associated with hepatic, renal, neurologic, and infective complications. Shaw and colleagues[185] discussed strategies for reducing the toxicity of CsA and other ISDs.

Therapeutic trough blood concentrations of CsA for renal transplants are 100 to 300 ng/mL (83 to 250 nmol/L), whereas 200 to 350 ng/mL (166 to 291 nmol/L) is used as the target concentration for cardiac, hepatic, and pancreatic transplants[181,186]; however, concomitant immunosuppression used in combination therapy, similar to combined drug therapy in other situations such as AED therapy in epilepsy, significantly affects the range of concentrations that are effective. Simultaneous immunosuppression with low-dose prednisone and either AZA or mycophenolate mofetil (MMF) allows the patient to enjoy a good response to CsA at lower concentrations; some renal transplant patients obtain a satisfactory response with trough CsA concentration of 70 ng/mL (58 nmol/L).

CsA is slowly absorbed, and peak concentrations are reached in 4 to 6 hours. Like tacrolimus, CsA is also highly (~90%) protein bound and concentrated in erythrocytes.[187] The degree of concentration in erythrocytes is temperature dependent in vitro; thus measurement of plasma concentration requires strict attention to specimen temperature if reproducible results are to be obtained.[188] Because of this effect, the best specimen for analysis is whole blood. The elimination profile of CsA is biphasic. An early elimination phase with an apparent half-life that typically ranges from 3 to 7 hours is followed by a slower elimination phase with an apparent half-life ranging from 18 to 25 hours. The volume of distribution is 17 L/kg. Many of the 31 known metabolites of CsA are inactive.[189] One of the major metabolites, hydroxylated at the number 1 amino acid, retains approximately 10% of the immunosuppressive activity of the parent compound.

Several drugs alter the disposition of CsA. Ketoconazole, erythromycin, melphalan, amphotericin B, and aminoglycoside antibiotics all prolong metabolism of CsA sufficiently to increase the risk for nephrotoxicity.[190] Coadministration of phenytoin, phenobarbital, carbamazepine, and rifampin results in induction of cytochrome P450 enzymes, which increase the rate at which CsA is metabolized.[181] Intravenous administration of sulfadimidine and trimethoprim decreases CsA concentrations.

The first procedure available for analysis of CsA was an RIA developed by Sandoz Pharmaceuticals (Princeton, New Jersey), the producer of the drug. This immunoassay, like most antibody-based assays for CsA, exhibited cross-reactivity with inactive metabolites. Currently, nonisotopic immunoassays performed on whole blood are the most commonly employed methods for measurement of CsA; however, many laboratories use HPLC and LC-MS/MS methods, which are more specific and less subject to metabolite interference. It is therefore important to ensure consistency with TDM by following individuals with the same method over time and to interpret results within the context of the method used.

Sirolimus

Sirolimus, also known as rapamycin, is a macrocyclic antibiotic that is a fermentation product of the actinomycete *Streptomyces hygroscopicus* that was isolated from soil samples collected on Rapa Nui (Easter Island) after a search for novel antifungal agents. Structurally, sirolimus is a lipophilic macrocyclic lactone comprising a 31-membered macrolide ring. It demonstrates antifungal, antitumor, and immunosuppressive activity in animal model studies and is approved in the United States for the prophylaxis of acute rejection in renal transplant patients.

The complex of sirolimus and the intracellular immunophilin, FKBP12, modulates the immune response by combining with the specific cell-cycle regulatory protein called the mammalian target of rapamycin (mTOR) and inhibiting its activation. This inhibition results in suppression of cytokine-driven T-lymphocyte proliferation, inhibiting the progression from the G_1 to the S phase of the cell cycle.[191]

The metabolism of sirolimus by the human body is driven by oxidative metabolism via CYP3A in the gastrointestinal tract and liver. There are at least seven metabolites characterized as 41-O- and 7-O-demethyl; several hydroxy, hydroxy-demethylated; and didemethylated sirolimus.[192-194] Total sirolimus metabolites accounted for 48% to 70%, and no single metabolite accounted for more than 10% of sirolimus in trough whole blood from stable renal transplant patients[195]; however, the immunosuppressive activity of individual metabolites is reported to be lower than that of the parent drug.[196]

Sirolimus is available as both an oral solution and a tablet. It is rapidly absorbed from the gastrointestinal tract, with the average time to reach maximal concentration in whole blood of approximately 2 hours.[197,198] The average bioavailabilty of sirolimus is low, at 15%, and attributable to extensive intestinal and hepatic metabolism by CYP3A and counter-transport by the multidrug efflux pump P-glycoprotein in the gastrointestinal tract. This absorption barrier varies considerably across patients and within-patient. It is also the site of clinically important drug-drug and drug-food interactions.[199]

Sirolimus distributes extensively into blood cells as reflected by the average blood-to-plasma ratio of 36 : 1 in renal transplant patients. Approximately 95% distributes into RBCs, 3% in plasma, and 1% each in lymphocytes and granulocytes.[192] The extensive and avid binding of sirolimus to the ubiquitously distributed intracellular FKBP12 accounts for the high ratio of blood to plasma sirolimus concentration. Approximately 2.5% of the sirolimus within the plasma fraction is unbound, with the remainder bound to plasma proteins.[199]

The relationship between sirolimus whole-blood trough concentrations has been investigated in renal transplant patients who received concomitant full-dose CsA and corticosteroid therapy. According to these analyses, the minimum effective sirolimus concentration below which there is a significant increase in risk for acute rejection is 4 to 5 µg/L (4.4 to 5.5 nmol/L).[199,200] The threshold concentration of 13 to 15 µg/L (14 to 16 nmol/L) was identified, above which the risks for the concentration-related side effects are thrombocytopenia (<100,000 platelets/mm^3), leukopenia (<4000 leukocytes/mm^3), and hypertriglyceridemia (>300 mg/dL or 3.4 mmol/L serum triglycerides) increase significantly.[200] More studies are needed to define these relationships for other transplant populations and for different concomitant immunosuppressants.

Several chromatographic (ie, LC-MS, LC-MS/MS, HPLC) detection methods have been validated and are in use in laboratories worldwide.[201-206] A commercial, automated immunoassay also has been developed. This latter assay, while showing high precision, exhibits modest bias because of metabolite interference (~25%) when results are compared to chromatographic methods.[207]

Everolimus

In April, 2010, everolimus, a more water-soluble analog of sirolimus, was approved for use in CsA-sparing regimens, including the requirement for adjusting everolimus doses using target trough blood concentrations in renal transplant patients. The target ranges were established from earlier retrospective studies[208-211] and used prospectively to demonstrate equivalent acute rejection rates compared to the combination of standard dose CsA and empirical dose mycophenolate mofetil (MMF).[212] More recently, the use of everolimus has expanded with approval in liver transplantation in combination with low-dose tacrolimus.[213]

The mechanism of action and pharmacodynamic effects of everolimus are comparable to those of sirolimus. Similar to the other ISDs, wide pharmacokinetic variability of everolimus has been observed.[214] This variability is driven by the variable metabolism via CYP3A4/5 and *p*-glycoprotein along with frequent drug-drug interactions that are comparable to that observed for sirolimus. Everolimus trough concentrations show a significant, linear correlation with overall drug exposure as assessed by AUC with a coefficient (r^2) of 0.79. Similar degrees of correlation between everolimus trough concentration and thrombocytopenia, leucopenia, hypertriglyceridemia, or hypercholesterolemia have been observed in an investigation of 54 stable renal transplant patients (18 to 68 years).[215] Based on the robust correlation between trough concentration and both efficacy and toxicity, a trough concentration of 3 to 8 ng/mL (3.1 to 8.3 nmol/L) has been suggested as the optimal target range.[216]

The bioanalytical method used for measurement of everolimus concentration in the pharmacokinetic assessments and prospective TDM protocols of many clinical investigations is a validated LC-MS/MS method.[208,212] Use of this bioanalytical methodology provides for sensitive and selective measurement of everolimus, and this attribute is important for reliable measurement of blood concentrations at the low end of the recommended target concentration range (3 ng/mL [3.1 nmol/L]) in currently used immunosuppression protocols.[212,217] In the future, we can anticipate the availability of immunoassays for everolimus, and it will be essential to understand the comparison between these methods and the current chromatographic methods.

Mycophenolic Acid

Mycophenolic acid (MPA) is a product of *Penicillium* species that exhibits antitumor, antiviral, antifungal, antibacterial, and immunosuppressive activity. MPA is administered as its morpholinoethyl ester, MMF. MMF, also known as RS-61433, is considered a prodrug because its immunosuppressive activity is expressed only after its hydrolysis to MPA in the body. MPA inhibits inosine monophosphate dehydrogenase, an important enzyme in the purine metabolic pathway. T lymphocytes rely on this pathway for purine synthesis, whereas other cells use the hypoxanthine–guanosine ribosyl transferase salvage pathway for purine biosynthesis. Thus MPA selectively inhibits purine synthesis and thus transcription in T lymphocytes.[218] MPA is of interest clinically because it has immunosuppressive activity similar to the thiopurine AZA, but without many of its side effects.

MMF is completely absorbed and rapidly and completely metabolized to MPA, the active metabolite. The latter is metabolized in the liver by phase II enzymes to form the major metabolite mycophenolic acid glucuronide (MPAG). The elimination half-life of MPA averages 18 hours, the volume of distribution averages 4 L/kg, and typical serum concentrations range from a peak of 12 μg/mL (37.4 μmol/L) to a trough value of 2 μg/mL (6.24 μmol/L).[219] Studies of MPA pharmacokinetics has shown that exposure correlates poorly with the dose of the drug, and many patients on standard fixed dosing have subtherapeutic concentrations of MPA.[220-223] It has therefore been suggested that monitoring serum concentrations of MPA is useful to overcome the variable pharmacokinetic behavior of this drug.[224,225] A prospective, randomized concentration-controlled study in kidney transplant patients demonstrated a positive correlation between AUC and acute rejection.[226] This same study, however, failed to reveal a correlation between AUC and gastrointestinal toxicity, the primary adverse effect of MPA. Subsequent prospective studies exploring the utility of TDM in MMF therapy have had mixed results, which may in part be a result of differing study designs. In particular, one of the studies failing to show a benefit used trough concentration monitoring. Unfortunately, trough concentrations, although simpler to collect, show a relatively poor correlation to AUC, likely limiting their utility. Limited sampling strategies that use three or four concentrations during the first few hours after dosing have shown improved correlation with dose interval AUC, and these strategies may be a better alternative to trough monitoring when full dose interval sampling is not feasible for AUC determination. Based on the available studies, the optimal immunosuppression for MPA appears to be achieved with target AUCs in the range of 30 to 60 mmol*min/mL range. Although poorly correlated, this is approximated by trough serum concentrations in the range of 2 to 4 μg/mL (6.24 to 12.5 μmol/L).[227]

Various methods for measurement of MPA have been developed. Most clinical studies have used a reference HPLC or LC-MS/MS method. Commercial immunoassays for MPA determination are also available. These latter assays have slight positive bias, especially in patients with low glomerular filtration rate, likely the result of recognition of both MPA and its glucuronide-conjugated metabolite.[228]

Cardiac Glycosides

Digoxin

Digoxin (Lanoxin) is one of a group of cardiac glycosides obtained from digitalis plants (eg, *Digitalis lanata*). Although used with substantially less frequency than in the past because of newer drugs, digoxin is still used for treatment of supraventricular arrhythmias such as atrial fibrillation because of its activity on atrioventricular nodal conduction. Digoxin also acts as an inotropic agent restoring the force of cardiac contraction in congestive heart failure. However, this use has decreased substantially. The drug binds to the extracytoplasmic side of the α-subunit of membrane-bound Na^+,K^+-ATPase, inhibiting both cellular Na^+ efflux and K^+ influx in myocardial cells. This reduces the sodium/potassium gradient in the Purkinje fibers of the atrial, junctional, and ventricular myocardium, resulting in a decreased transmembrane potential. Inhibition of Na^+, K^+-ATPase is postulated to enhance movement of calcium ions in the cell, increasing calcium ion availability and improving cardiac contractility. In addition to direct effects on the excitable tissues within the heart through the Na, K-ATPase, digoxin also has been shown to alter autonomic activity within the heart to promote parasympathetic activity, which may further contribute to its mechanism of action.[229-231]

At low concentrations, digoxin causes the atrium to be less electrically excitable. Moderate concentrations of digoxin are required to reduce the rate of depolarization in the spontaneously depolarizing conductive fibers (Purkinje fibers), and toxic concentrations of digoxin are necessary to diminish depolarization of the ventricular myocardium. Disagreement over the clinical value of digoxin measurements and the failure of the digoxin concentration to correlate with clinical toxicity are usually related to aberrations in serum and tissue concentrations of sodium, potassium, magnesium, and calcium. Increased sensitivity to digoxin can be noted in states of hypokalemia, hypomagnesemia, and hypercalcemia, which make establishment of the true therapeutic concentration of digoxin difficult because all parameters are interactive.

Absorption of digoxin is variable and dependent on the drug formulation. The USP requires more than 65% of digoxin in tablet form to dissolve in 60 minutes. In plasma, digoxin is 25% protein bound. Digoxin is concentrated in tissues, and at steady state the concentration of digoxin in cardiac tissue is 15 to 30 times that of plasma. Accumulation of digoxin in tissue lags behind the plasma concentration; that is, although the peak plasma concentration is reached 2 to 3 hours after the oral dose, the peak tissue concentration occurs 6 to 10 hours after an oral dose. Although pharmacologic effects and toxicity correlate with tissue concentration rather than plasma concentration, the safe therapeutic plasma concentration of digoxin has been reported to range from 0.8 to 2.0 ng/mL (1 to 2.6 nmol/L).[232] This range is not determined at the peak plasma concentration but rather at the time of peak tissue concentration.[233] Thus, to ensure a correlation between plasma concentration and tissue concentration, the appropriate time to collect the specimen is 8 hours or more after the dose, at which time serum digoxin has reached distributional equilibrium with the drug in tissues. Results from specimens collected earlier than 8 hours after the dose are misleading because high concentrations may be misinterpreted as toxic concentrations, whereas they are more likely due to incomplete distribution.

Digoxin toxicity is characterized by nonspecific symptoms of nausea, vomiting, anorexia, and predominance of green/yellow visual distortion. Cardiac symptoms of intoxication include multiform premature ventricular contractions, ventricular bigeminy, ventricular tachycardia, and ventricular fibrillation. Combinations of decreased conduction and increased automaticity may result in paroxysmal atrial tachycardia with atrioventricular node block and nonparoxysmal junction tachycardia. These symptoms are frequently observed when the blood concentration exceeds 2 ng/mL (2.6 nmol/L) in adults. Children can tolerate higher concentrations and do not usually exhibit toxicity until the digoxin concentration exceeds 4 ng/mL (5.2 nmol/L).[234]

Significant controversy has surrounded the use of digoxin in the heart failure setting. A large prospective study of concentration-controlled digoxin in the 0.8 to 2 ng/mL (1 to 2.6 nmol/L) target range for the treatment of heart failure (the Digitalis Intervention Group [DIG]) demonstrated that the cohort of patients receiving digoxin therapy experienced a higher overall mortality compared to a placebo control, arguing against the use of digoxin in this setting.[235] A retrospective analysis of the DIG study data demonstrated that the overall mortality was correlated with serum digoxin concentration. The mortality in the patients with serum digoxin concentrations in the 0.5 to 0.8 ng/mL (0.6 to 1 nmol/L) range was in fact lower than in patients receiving the placebo control. Significantly increased mortality was observed in patients with serum digoxin concentrations greater than 1.2 ng/mL (1.5 nmol/L). This result indicates that the target concentration range of 0.8 to 2 ng/mL (1 to 2.6 nmol/L), suggested by the earlier pharmacodynamics studies of toxicity, is not optimal for balancing the effectiveness of digoxin with its toxicity in the heart failure population; lower concentrations of digoxin may be required to balance safety and efficacy.[236]

Elimination of digoxin follows first-order kinetics; 50% to 70% is excreted unchanged or in the form of digoxigenin monosaccharides or disaccharides in the urine. A small amount is metabolized to dihydrodigoxin and also excreted by the kidneys. The remainder is found in the stool as digoxigenin and its saccharides. As a result, digoxin toxicity develops more frequently and lasts longer in patients with renal impairment. Dose requirements are decreased in patients with renal disease. Bresnahan and Vlietstra[233] present a simple method for calculating dose, which is based on creatinine clearance. Coadministration of cyclosporine,[237] quinidine,[238] or verapamil[239] prolongs the rate of clearance of digoxin, requiring dose adjustment.

Decreased gastrointestinal absorption occurs with sprue and small intestinal resections, high-fiber diets, hyperthyroidism, and situations of increased gastrointestinal motility. Although seldom used, when quinidine is added to digoxin in the treatment of atrial fibrillation to convert patients to normal sinus rhythm, the concomitant administration of quinidine typically causes serum digoxin concentrations to increase twofold to threefold. The increase is probably due to decreased renal and extrarenal clearance. Studies have provided evidence that the *p*-glycoprotein multidrug transporter, responsible for export of digoxin from renal tubules to tubular lumen, is inhibited by drugs such as quinidine and verapamil.[240-242]

Currently, immunoassays remain the most widely used method for measurement of digoxin in serum and biological fluids.[243] For routine measurement of digoxin concentrations, several commercially available immunoassays are widely used, including RIA, fluorescence polarization, chemiluminescence, and enzyme immunoassays. The rich history of digoxin measurement methods and the overall improvements made over the past two decades has been reviewed and is beyond the scope of this chapter. More details can be found in the article by Jortani and Valdes.[244] Use of Digibind (GlaxoSmithKline, Middlesex, United Kingdom) or DigiFab (Protherics, West Conshohocken, Pennsylvania), digoxin-specific Fab fragments that neutralize the drug and are used in the setting of acute toxicity, can complicate digoxin measurement by many immunoassays. Results of digoxin monitoring after administration of Digibind should therefore be interpreted with caution.[245] Methods to eliminate the interference by therapeutic antidigoxin Fab therapy using ultrafiltration of serum to isolate free drug and remove the interfering Fab have been described, but these methods lack standardization.[246,247]

Drugs Used in Psychiatry

Lithium

Lithium (eg, Eskalith, Lithane, Lithonate) is administered as lithium carbonate and used for the treatment of the manic phase of affective disorders, mania, and manic-depressive illness. The mechanism of action for lithium is not entirely clear. Early research suggested that it acts by enhancing reuptake of catecholamines, thereby reducing their concentration in the neuronal junction and producing a sedating effect on the central nervous system. More recently, lithium along with other mood-affecting drugs, such as valproic acid, carbamazepine, and the tricyclic antidepressants (TCAs), have been shown to inhibit GSK3-β, a protein central to the Wnt/β-catenin signaling pathway that affects gene expression involved in many aspects of cellular behavior, neuronal polarity, plasticity and survival, and brain development.[56] GSK3-β appears critical in the action of dopamine and serotonin on the brain in affecting behavior.[57] At least two mechanisms account for lithium's effects on GSK3-β. Lithium directly competes with magnesium, which is an important cation for GSK3-β activity. It also indirectly affects GSK3-β by inhibiting a critical phosphatase normally required for its activation.[248] Although other mechanisms of action cannot be excluded, the mechanisms described previously are likely to account for many of lithium's effects on mood.

Absorption of lithium from the gastrointestinal tract is complete, with peak plasma concentration reached 2 to 4 hours after an oral dose. This cation does not bind to protein. Lithium elimination is biphasic; during the first phase, 30% to 40% of the dose of lithium is cleared, with an apparent half-life of 24 hours. During the second phase, the remainder of lithium incorporated into the cellular ion pool is cleared, exhibiting a half-life of 48 to 72 hours. Clearance is predominantly a function of the kidneys, where active reabsorption occurs. Reduced renal function causes prolonged clearance times.

The optimal therapeutic response to lithium has not been related to a specific serum concentration; however, toxicity is related to serum concentration. Serum lithium concentrations are monitored to ensure patient compliance and avoid intoxication. It is recommended that a standardized 12-hour post-dose serum lithium concentration be used to assess adequate therapy.[249] The interval of 1 to 1.2 mmol/L was identified as the optimal trough therapeutic concentration. Concentrations of 1.2 to 1.5 mmol/L signifies a warning range, and a concentration in excess of 1.5 mmol/L in a specimen drawn 12 hours after the dose indicates a significant risk for intoxication. Early symptoms of intoxication include apathy, sluggishness, drowsiness, lethargy, speech difficulties, irregular tremors, myoclonic twitching, muscle weakness, and ataxia. These symptoms, although not life threatening, are uncomfortable for patients and indicate that life-threatening seizures are imminent.

Lithium excretion parallels that of sodium. It readily passes the glomerular membrane and is reabsorbed in the proximal convoluted tubules. In situations in which patients are vulnerable to dehydration (fever, watery stools, vomiting, loss of appetite, hot weather), the potential for lithium intoxication is increased. In dehydration, the proximal tubular response to reabsorption of sodium (and lithium) is reduction of clearance. Increased reabsorption of lithium leads to increased blood concentration of lithium. Severe intoxication, characterized by muscle rigidity, hyperactive deep tendon reflexes, and epileptic seizures, is usually associated with lithium concentrations in excess of 2.5 mmol/L.

The concentration of lithium in serum, plasma, urine, or other body fluids can be determined by several methods, including flame emission photometry, atomic absorption spectrometry, ion-selective electrode, or inductively coupled plasma–mass spectrometry (ICP-MS) or optical emission spectrometry (ICP-OES). In contemporary clinical practice, automated methods are primarily used for routine measurement of lithium in serum using a chromophore (eg, a substituted porphyrin) that forms a colored product readily detected spectrophotometrically on binding to lithium.[250] The availability from NIST of a Standard Reference material (NIST SRM 3129a) provides manufacturers with the opportunity to prepare traceable calibrators and improve standardization of assays.[251]

Tricyclic Antidepressants

Although TCAs were originally developed in the 1950s and a number of newer antidepressant drugs have been developed, such as the selective serotonin reuptake inhibitors (SSRIs), TCAs continue to remain useful in the treatment of depression as well as anxiety disorders and chronic pain. TCAs work primarily by blocking the serotonin and norepinephrine transporters that mediate reuptake, resulting in increased synaptic concentrations of these neurotransmitters.[252] In addition to blocking serotonin and norepinephrine reuptake, TCAs also have been shown to bind and block a variety of neurotransmitter receptors with high affinity, including members of the serotonin (5-HT) receptor family,[253,254] α-adrenergic receptors,[253] and *N*-methyl-D-aspartate receptor NMDA receptors.[255] These interactions likely contribute to both the beneficial actions of TCAs along with their side effects.

TCAs are nearly completely absorbed from the gastrointestinal tract but undergo first-pass hepatic metabolism, so their ultimate bioavailability is variable. Because these drugs slow gastrointestinal activity and gastric emptying, their absorption also may be delayed, further contributing to variability. Once absorbed, they are highly protein and tissue bound, resulting in large apparent volumes of distribution. Peak plasma concentrations are reached from 2 to 12 hours after the oral dose. Metabolism is by *N*-demethylation and aromatic ring hydroxylation, followed by conjugation with glucuronic acid. If the drug administered is the tertiary tricyclic amine (amitriptyline, doxepin, imipramine), metabolism causes accumulation of the respective secondary amine (nortriptyline, nordoxepin, desipramine). These substances have generally equal pharmacologic activity and accumulate to concentrations approximately (but variably) equal to that of the parent drug. The hydroxylated metabolites have little pharmacologic activity. Taking these factors into consideration (ie, variable bioavailability, high volume of distribution, variable metabolic activity, and generation of pharmacologically active metabolites), it is not surprising that patient response to these drugs is widely variable. Determining the serum concentration gives the physician the assurance that a patient has been properly dosed.

Drugs such as cimetidine, chloramphenicol, haloperidol, methylphenidate, and phenothiazines inhibit hepatic oxidative enzymes. Inhibition of end-product metabolism of the tertiary TCAs results in a greater accumulation of the secondary amine metabolite (amitriptyline is metabolized to nortriptyline, doxepin to nordoxepin, imipramine to desipramine), because conversion to the aromatic ring hydroxylated metabolites is blocked. Coadministration of perphenazine with a TCA causes accumulation of the secondary amine to concentrations two to four times normal, with onset of toxicity occurring at the expected blood concentrations.

TCAs show a good correlation between therapeutic response and serum concentration. A linear relationship between clinical improvement and serum concentration is noted for most of these drugs, the exception being nortriptyline, which has a specific therapeutic window. A serum concentration of nortriptyline below or above the concentration range of 50 to 150 ng/mL (0.19 to 0.57 μmol/L) correlates with worsening of moods. The other antidepressants do not display this effect; the upper limit of the optimum blood concentration for these other antidepressants is limited by the onset of toxicity. Toxicity is expressed as dry mouth and perspiration, signs that may also occur with depression. Thus it is difficult to differentiate between mild toxicity from the drug and the disease that is being treated. More serious toxicity is expressed as atrioventricular node block, characterized by a widening of the electrocardiographic QRS interval. Onset occurs at serum concentrations ranging from 800 to 1200 ng/mL (3.0 to 4.6 μmol/L), and the severity of intoxication is related to the serum concentration.[256] The relationship between serum concentration and cardiac toxicity diminishes with time after intoxication as the drug is absorbed into tissues. Despite this toxicity, the TCAs remain useful drugs in the treatment of depression.

Numerous methods have been published for analysis of TCAs. These drugs present various problems to the clinical laboratory: (1) the therapeutic serum concentration is 10 to 100 times lower than that of other commonly monitored drugs, and thus to be clinically useful the method must be able to measure serum concentrations below 25 ng/mL (~0.09 μmol/L); (2) these drugs have metabolites that also must be measured; and (3) they are structurally similar to common sleep inducers, antihistamines, and many over-the-counter medications used for appetite suppression, which are potential interferences. Of the many hundreds of methods published, only a few have satisfactorily overcome these obstacles. Analysis by gas-liquid chromatography (GLC)-MS, using selected ion monitoring, was the historical reference method, using either the electron impact mode[257] or the chemical ionization mode.[258] HPLC with photodiode array detection has also been successfully used for analysis of TCAs[259]; however, LC-MS/MS is the preferred reference method because of the ability to measure multiple TCAs and their metabolites simultaneously.[260,261]

Others

Theophylline

Theophylline, available under many proprietary names, relaxes bronchial smooth muscles to relieve or prevent asthma. The therapeutic effect of theophylline is likely due to antagonism of adenosine receptors in smooth muscle, whereas the toxic effects are due to inhibition of cyclic nucleotide phosphodiesterase. With increased use of β-adrenergic agonists, and because of the considerable toxicity associated with it, theophylline is now considered a second-level approach used only in treatment of persistent asthma.[262]

Theophylline is readily absorbed after oral, rectal, or parenteral administration. If the drug is taken orally without food, the blood concentration peaks within 2 hours. If it is administered with food or as a slow-release formula, peak concentrations occur 3 to 5 hours after the dose. Once absorbed, it is 50% protein bound. The drug is rapidly cleared in adolescents and in adults who smoke because of its higher rate of metabolism secondary to increased levels of CYP1A2. In these individuals, the half-life ranges from 3 to 4 hours. Nonsmoking adults in good health have an elimination half-life of approximately 9 hours. The half-life in neonates and in adults with congestive heart failure can be prolonged to 20 to 30 hours, depending on the degree of liver immaturity or loss of liver function. Coadministration of cimetidine, ciprofloxacin, and ticlopidine leads to reduced clearance of theophylline.

The relationship between serum concentration and prevention of symptoms of chronic asthma has been well documented.[263] There is a proportional relationship between forced expiratory volume and theophylline concentration, with the optimum therapeutic effect occurring at concentrations ranging from 8 to 20 μg/mL (44 to 111 μmol/L). Suppression of exercise-induced bronchospasm in asthmatic patients occurs at concentrations exceeding 10 μg/mL (56 μmol/L) and is optimal at 15 μg/mL (83 μmol/L). Neonatal apnea treated with theophylline responds to slightly lower concentrations, ranging from 5 to 10 μg/mL (28 to 56 μmol/L).[264] Relaxation of bronchial smooth muscle is directly proportional to blood concentration and continues at concentrations greater than 20 μg/mL (111 μmol/L). When the blood level exceeds 20 μg/mL (111 μmol/L), the secondary side effects become significant.

Theophylline typically exhibits first-order kinetics of elimination when used in most patients with serum concentrations in the range of 5 to 15 μg/mL (28 to 83 μmol/L); however, at serum concentrations greater than 20 μg/mL (111 μmol/L), theophylline exhibits zero-order pharmacokinetics with small dose increases leading to disproportionately large increases in serum concentration and intoxication. Symptoms of theophylline toxicity include nausea, vomiting, headache, diarrhea, irritability, and insomnia. Transient central nervous system stimulation occurring at initial administration is not directly related to blood concentration. This effect diminishes with chronic use. Serious toxicity characterized by cardiac arrhythmias and seizures is usually associated with serum concentrations in excess of 30 μg/mL (167 μmol/L). Once seizure activity begins, the final prognosis is very poor. Morbidity is reported in nearly all patients, and mortality can be as high as 50%.[265]

Immunoassay is the standard method for determination of theophylline concentration. Theophylline, caffeine, and dyphylline can be measured simultaneously by HPLC.

Caffeine

A minor metabolite of theophylline in adults, caffeine has been shown to accumulate to significant concentrations in neonates. Caffeine itself is an effective inhibitor of apnea,[266] which may explain the lower therapeutic concentration required for control of neonatal apnea. Therapy with caffeine alone also has been demonstrated as effective in the treatment of neonatal apnea; it is gaining popularity because of caffeine's long half-life in neonates (>30 hours). The optimal therapeutic concentration of caffeine in this situation ranges from 8 to 14 μg/mL (41 to 72 μmol/L). Caffeine can be measured by HPLC or immunoassay.

SUMMARY AND CONCLUSION

The development of analytical techniques for drug measurement over the decades since TDM largely began in 1970s has dramatically increased our understanding of pharmacokinetics and the ways in which drugs are used, especially those with low TI. Although understanding pharmacokinetics is critical to successful drug therapy, it is also important to not forget the variation in the pharmacodynamics effects of many drugs. Laboratory tests for inosine-5′-monophosphate dehydrogenase (IMPDH) activity, the enzyme targeted by the ISD, mycophenolic acid, illustrate the potential of combined pharmacokinetic-pharmacodynamic modeling of drug therapy.[267] New technologies in the area of genomics and proteomics set the stage for increasing our understanding of the pharmacokinetic and pharmacodynamic behavior of many drugs. It is anticipated that TDM over the next decade will progress from traditional pharmacokinetic approaches to more integrated pharmacokinetic-pharmacodynamic monitoring approaches that fine tune a drug regimen through incorporation of newly identified genetic and protein biomarkers. The goals will remain the same: finding the right drug and regimen for a patient. The tools are simply evolving.

SELECTED REFERENCES

For a full list of references for this chapter, please refer to ExpertConsult.com.

18. Touw DJ, Neef C, Thomson AH, et al. Cost-effectiveness of therapeutic drug monitoring: a systematic review. *Ther Drug Monit* 2005;**27**:10–17.
33. Wright JD, Boudinot FD, Ujhelyi MR. Measurement and analysis of unbound drug concentrations. *Clin Pharmacokinet* 1996;**30**:445–62.
41. Rybak MJ, Lomaestro BM, Rotschafer JC, et al. Vancomycin therapeutic guidelines: a summary of consensus recommendations from the Infectious Diseases Society of America, the American Society of Health-System Pharmacists, and the Society of Infectious Diseases Pharmacists. *Clin Infect Dis* 2009;**49**:325–7.

48. Shibata M, Hashi S, Nakanishi H, et al. Detection of 22 antiepileptic drugs by ultra-performance liquid chromatography coupled with tandem mass spectrometry applicable to routine therapeutic drug monitoring. *Biomed Chromatogr* 2012;**26**:1519–28.
54. Richens A. Clinical pharmacokinetics of phenytoin. *Clin Pharmacokinet* 1979;**4**:153–69.
64. Patsalos PN, Berry DJ, Bourgeois BF, et al. Antiepileptic drugs: best practice guidelines for therapeutic drug monitoring. A position paper by the subcommission on therapeutic drug monitoring, ILAE Commission on Therapeutic Strategies. *Epilepsia* 2008;**49**:1239–76.
78. Schentag JJ. Aminoglycosides. In: Evans WE, Schentag JJ, Jusko WJ, editors. *Applied pharmacokinetics: principles of therapeutic drug monitoring*. San Francisco: Applied Therapeutics; 1980. p. xii, 708.
109. Chau MM, Kong DC, van Hal SJ, et al. Consensus guidelines for optimising antifungal drug delivery and monitoring to avoid toxicity and improve outcomes in patients with haematological malignancy, 2014. *Intern Med J* 2014;**44**: 1364–88.
134. Ferrari S, Sassoli V, Orlandi M, et al. Serum methotrexate (MTX) concentrations and prognosis in patients with osteosarcoma of the extremities treated with a multidrug neoadjuvant regimen. *J Chemother* 1993;**5**: 135–41.
145. Slattery JT, Clift RA, Buckner CD, et al. Marrow transplantation for chronic myeloid leukemia: the influence of plasma busulfan levels on the outcome of transplantation. *Blood* 1997;**89**:3055–60.
150. Evans WE, Hon YY, Bomgaars L, et al. Preponderance of thiopurine S-methyltransferase deficiency and heterozygosity among patients intolerant to mercaptopurine or azathioprine. *J Clin Oncol* 2001;**19**:2293–301.
177. Jusko WJ, Thomson AW, Fung J, et al. Consensus document: therapeutic monitoring of tacrolimus (FK-506). *Ther Drug Monit* 1995;**17**:606–14.
191. MacDonald A, Scarola J, Burke JT, et al. Clinical pharmacokinetics and therapeutic drug monitoring of sirolimus. *Clin Ther* 2000;**22**(Suppl. B):B101–21.
213. Keating GM, Lyseng-Williamson KA. Everolimus: a guide to its use in liver transplantation. *Biodrugs* 2013;**27**:407–11.
219. Staatz C, Tett S. Clinical pharmacokinetics and pharmacodynamics of mycophenolate in solid organ transplant recipients. *Clin Pharmacokinet* 2007;**46**:13–58.
234. Terra SG, Washam JB, Dunham GD, et al. Therapeutic range of digoxin's efficacy in heart failure: what is the evidence? *Pharmacotherapy* 1999;**19**:1123–6.
236. Rathore SS, Curtis JP, Wang Y, et al. Association of serum digoxin concentration and outcomes in patients with heart failure. *JAMA* 2003;**289**:871–8.
249. Bettinger TL, Crismon ML. Lithium. In: Burton ME, editor. *Applied pharmacokinetics & pharmacodynamics: principles of therapeutic drug monitoring*. Philadelphia.: Lippincott Williams & Wilkins; 2006. p. 789–812.
263. Hendeles L, Weinberger M. Theophylline: therapeutic use and serum concentration monitoring. In: Taylor WJ, Finn AL, editors. *Individualizing drug therapy: practical applications of drug monitoring*. New York, N.Y.: Gross, Townsend, Frank; 1981. p. 32–65.

41

Clinical Toxicology

Loralie J. Langman, Laura K. Bechtel, Brenton M. Meier, and Chris Holstege

ABSTRACT

Background

Toxicology is a broad multidisciplinary science whose goal is to determine the effects of chemical agents on living systems. Innumerable potential toxins can inflict harm, including pharmaceuticals, herbals, household products, environmental agents, occupational chemicals, drugs of abuse, and chemical terrorism threats. Each year millions of human exposure cases are reported worldwide (see http://www.aapcc.org/; http://www.worldlifeexpectancy.com/world-poison-report; and http://www.overdoseday.com/resources/facts-stats/).[1] The Centers for Disease Control and Prevention reported that poisoning (both intentional and unintentional) is one of the top 10 causes of injury-related death in the United States in all adult age groups. From the beginnings of written history, poisons and their effects have been well described. Paracelsus (1493–1541) correctly noted that "Alle Dinge sind Gift, und nichts ist ohne Gift; allein die Dosis macht, daß ein Ding kein Gift sei," which means, "Everything is a poison; there is nothing which is not. Only the dose differentiates a poison." As life in the modern era has become more complex, so has the study of poisons, their identification, and their treatments.

Content

This chapter provides a general overview of clinical toxicology and the laboratory services necessary to support the care of poisoned patients. Because a comprehensive discussion of all aspects of toxicology is beyond the scope of this chapter, the clinical significance and toxicity of only a select number of common drugs, drugs of abuse, and other chemicals are discussed.

BASIC INFORMATION

In practice, it is neither possible nor necessary to test for all of the hundreds or thousands of clinical toxins that may be encountered. In reality fewer than 25 substances account for 80% or more of cases of intoxication treated in most emergency departments.[2] Moreover, some drugs are encountered very infrequently in some locations but with relatively high frequency in others. For example, phencyclidine (PCP) use is almost nonexistent in some areas but is responsible for a relatively high number of intoxications in a few large metropolitan cities. Thus the scope of clinical toxicology testing provided by the laboratory will depend on the pattern of local drug use and the available resources of the institution and should be developed in consultation with the appropriate clinical staff.

The value of drug and substance testing (screening) is well established (1) in the workplace, (2) for some athletic competitions, (3) to monitor drug use during pregnancy, (4) to evaluate drug exposure and/or withdrawal in newborns, (5) to monitor patients in pain management and drug abuse treatment programs, and (6) to aid in the prompt diagnosis of toxicity for a select number of drugs or agents for which a specific antidote or treatment modality is required (Table 41.1). In many other instances of drug toxicity, the value of drug screening, especially on an emergency basis, is more controversial.[3-6]

Approaches to drug testing vary from the provision of just a few specific tests (eg, acetaminophen, salicylate, ethanol, digoxin, iron) to testing for additional targeted groups of drugs (eg, stimulant panel and coma panel) or to a more comprehensive general drug screen that might include 100 or so drugs and/or substances. For all of these situations, it is imperative that the laboratory communicate with the physician concerning the scope (and limitation) of the service and the proper timing and selection of specimens; when possible, the laboratory should assist with interpretation of results. At a minimum, the laboratory should clearly identify and indicate limit of detection for the drugs that it has the capability of detecting. Otherwise, the report of a negative result for a drug screen could be misleading.

Clinical Considerations

To operate effectively, the laboratory should be closely associated with the health care team directly managing the patient. Through close and collaborative work, clinical information provided will help guide appropriate ordering of tests and ensure that interpretation of results is complete and accurate. For example, the team caring for the patient should provide the following information with the laboratory request:

1. The time and date of the suspected exposure along with the time and date of sample collection.
2. History from the patient or witnesses that might aid in identification of the toxin.

TABLE 41.1 Antidote or Specific Treatment for Intoxication

Toxin	Potential Antidote and Treatment
Acetaminophen	*N*-Acetylcysteine
Aluminum	Deferoxamine
Anticholinergics	Physostigmine
Arsenic	2,3-Dimercaptosuccinic acid (DMSA), dimercaprol (BAL)
Barbiturates	Multiple-dose oral activated charcoal, sodium bicarbonate
Benzodiazepines	Flumazenil
β-Adrenergic blockers	Calcium, glucagon, high-dose insulin
Calcium channel blockers	Calcium, glucagon, high-dose insulin
Carbamates	Atropine
Carbamazepine	Multiple-dose oral activated charcoal, extracorporeal techniques
Cardiac glycosides	Anti–digoxin Fab fragments
Carbon monoxide	Oxygen (normobaric or hyperbaric)
Copper	D-Penicillamine
Cyanide	Hydroxocobalamin, nitrites, thiosulfate
Ethylene glycol	Fomepizole (4-methylpyrazole), ethanol, hemodialysis
Heparin	Protamine sulfate
Iron	Desferoxamine
Isoniazid	Pyridoxine
Lead	Ethylenediaminetetraacetic acid (EDTA), dimercaprol (BAL), 2,3-dimercaptosuccinic acid (DMSA), D-penicillamine
Mercury	Dimercaprol (BAL), 2,3-dimercaptosuccinic acid (DMSA), D-penicillamine
Methanol	Fomepizole (4-methylpyrazole) or ethanol, hemodialysis
Methemoglobin	Methylene blue, vitamin C
Methotrexate	Leucovorin
Opioids	Naloxone
Organophosphates	Atropine, pralidoxime
Sulfonylureas	Glucose, octreotide
Salicylates	Sodium bicarbonate, hemodialysis
TCAs	Sodium bicarbonate
Theophylline	Multiple-dose oral activated charcoal, extracorporeal techniques
tPA, streptokinase, urokinase	Aminocaproic acid
Warfarin	Phylloquinone (vitamin K_1), plasma

3. Assessment of the physical state of the patient at the time of presentation.

Such information is useful to guide test selection and interpretation of results.

Analytical Considerations

Because of the wide range of drugs of interest, no single analytical technique is adequate for broad-spectrum drug detection. Therefore several analytical approaches in combination are generally required. These may include simple, inexpensive, and rapid spot tests; immunoassays (see Chapter 23); and chromatographic and/or mass spectrometric techniques (see Chapters 16, 17, and 20), including thin-layer chromatography (TLC), high-performance liquid chromatography (HPLC), gas chromatography (GC), gas chromatography-mass spectrometry (GC-MS or GC-tandem MS [GC-MS/MS]), liquid chromatography-mass spectrometry (LC-MS, LC-MS/MS), and high-resolution mass spectrometry (HRMS, time of flight [TOF], orbitrap)[7-9] Currently, GC-MS is the most widely used definitive confirmatory procedure, although LC-MS/MS is increasingly used in clinical and forensic setting. Confirmatory testing is mandatory for forensic drug testing (eg, workplace drug testing).

Speed of analysis, or turnaround time, and availability are critical issues in clinical toxicology. A drug analysis that requires several hours to complete or that is not available at all hours of the day is of little value in a clinical emergency. Alternatively, a rapid test that provides false information could result in erroneous diagnostic and therapeutic decisions. For numerous agents, quantitative determinations guide management during a clinical emergency. These agents include acetaminophen (paracetamol), salicylate, ethanol, methanol, isopropanol, ethylene glycol, carbamazepine, phenytoin, valproic acid, phenobarbital, iron, lithium, theophylline, and digoxin, and in whole blood, carboxyhemoglobin, and methemoglobin. Results for these determinations should be available within 1 hour of specimen receipt.[10]

Proper selection of analytical methods and interpretation of results require knowledge of the pharmacology and pharmacokinetics of the toxins of interest. For example, the potential hepatotoxicity of acetaminophen is related to the concentration of unmetabolized drug. Conversely, Δ-9-tetrahydrocannabinol (THC)—a metabolite of marijuana—is measured in urine as an indication of marijuana use.

Clinical Evaluation

Primary Survey

When a health care team initially evaluates a patient who presents with a potential toxicologically induced health problem, the final diagnosis is often determined by (1) reviewing the history, (2) performing a directed physical examination, (3) using ancillary tests (eg, electrocardiogram [ECG], radiology), and (4) applying a rational and evidence-based approach to laboratory testing. Often no specific antidote or treatment is available for a poisoned patient and careful supportive care is the most appropriate intervention.[11]

All patients who present with potential toxicity should be thoroughly assessed, and it is imperative that clinicians follow a standard "ABC" approach with attention to airway, breathing, and circulation, respectively. The patient's airway should be open and unblocked and adequate ventilation ensured. If the patient's airway is not secure and endotracheal tube intubation is considered, the first diagnostic test that should be performed is a rapid bedside glucose concentration. Hypoglycemia can result in coma or new-onset seizures, thereby mimicking a toxic cause. In addition, numerous toxins are clinically associated with hypoglycemia (eg, sulfonylureas, ethanol, *Mentha pulegium*). Clinical effects induced by hypoglycemia can be rapidly reversed with intravenous glucose, thus preventing unnecessary and costly procedures and testing.

Too often, health care providers are lulled into a false sense of security when a patient presents with altered mental status and oxygen saturations on pulse oximetry that are adequate on high-flow oxygen. If the patient has inadequate ventilation or a poor gag reflex, the patient may be at risk for progressive carbon monoxide narcosis or aspiration, respectively, and yet may be maintaining adequate oxygen saturation on supplemental oxygen. Capnography (monitoring of the concentration or partial pressure of carbon dioxide in the respiratory gases) is an emerging technology that is becoming more available in health care facilities and should be considered for use in appropriate cases.[12] It is imperative that the health care team avoid the common complication of aspiration pneumonitis by ensuring that the airway is secured if necessary.[13,14] An arterial blood gas (ABG) value can rapidly aid the health care team in determining the need for intubation and mechanical ventilation. The ABG can also provide valuable information regarding the patient's acid-base status and can help the clinician begin to generate a differential diagnosis. For example, in the scenario of a febrile toxic patient who presents with an altered mental status, a normal ABG (lack of acidosis) eliminates the possibility of uncoupling of oxidative phosphorylation as a cause of that patient's fever. Finally, an ABG with cooximetry can rapidly assist in determining other toxic causes, such as carbon monoxide poisoning (depending on the timing of the blood draw in relation to the exposure) and methemoglobinemia.

The initial treatment of hypotension in all toxic patients consists of the administration of intravenous fluids.[15] The patient's pulmonary status should be closely monitored to ensure that pulmonary edema (a rare complication in poisoned patients) does not develop as fluids are infused. Symptomatic toxic patients should be placed on continuous cardiac monitoring with pulse oximetry, and the health care team must perform frequent neurologic checks to ensure continued protection of the airway. Acutely poisoned patients should receive a large-bore peripheral intravenous line, and all symptomatic patients should have a second line placed in the peripheral or central venous system, depending on the severity of their clinical status. At this time in patient care, blood can be drawn and sent for appropriate laboratory diagnostic testing. Placement of a urinary catheter should be considered early in the care of hemodynamically unstable poisoned patients to monitor urinary output as an indicator of adequate perfusion. A rapid bedside urine dipstick test can provide helpful information quickly as health care team members await further laboratory testing. For example, a urine specific gravity will give insight into the patient's initial hydration status, and the appearance of tea-colored urine positive for blood may indicate the presence of myoglobinuria in a comatose patient with rhabdomyolysis.

Secondary Survey

The secondary survey involves a thorough examination of the entire patient. For adequate access to a toxic patient, the patient must be completely undressed. Exposure of the patient ensures that a complete physical examination is performed.[11] If the patient is not completely undressed, an important diagnostic clue may be missed. For example, skin lesions consistent with pressure necrosis on the back of a comatose patient may indicate the need to obtain other testing, including a urine myoglobin concentration. A comatose drug abuser may have attached transdermal drug patches (eg, fentanyl, clonidine) in atypical locations (eg, gluteal sulcus) that when found can rapidly lead to a diagnosis, avoiding the need for further laboratory testing. Besides completing a thorough physical review of all organ systems, the secondary survey involves reviewing items brought with the patient (eg, medication bottles, drug paraphernalia). Searching carefully through the patient's clothing may assist in providing clues that change the plan for specific laboratory tests or explain specific laboratory findings. For example, the discovery of a cough and cold product in the patient's pocket that contains dextromethorphan (DXM) could explain the clinical presentation of an agitated patient with hyperreflexia whose initial urine toxicology screen was positive for PCP but later was found negative on confirmation.

Toxic Syndromes

Toxic syndromes ("toxidromes") are clinical syndromes that are essential for the successful recognition of poisoning patterns. A toxidrome is the constellation of clinical signs and symptoms that suggests a specific class of poisoning. An important component of the secondary survey is to determine whether a specific toxic syndrome is present.[11] The most commonly encountered toxidromes include (1) anticholinergic, (2) cholinergic, (3) opioid, (4) sedative-hypnotic, and (5) sympathomimetic (Table 41.2). Many toxidromes have several overlapping features. For example, anticholinergic findings are highly similar to sympathomimetic findings, with an exception being the effects on sweat glands: anticholinergic agents produce warm, flushed dry skin, but sympathomimetic agents produce diaphoresis. Toxidrome findings also may be affected by individual variability, comorbid conditions, and coingestants. For example, tachycardia associated with sympathomimetic or anticholinergic toxidromes may be absent in a patient who is concurrently taking β-antagonist medications. Additionally, although toxidromes may be applied to classes of drugs, one or more toxidrome findings may be absent for some individual agents within these classes. For instance, meperidine is an opioid analgesic, but it does not induce miosis, which helps to define the classic opioid toxidrome. When accurately identified, the toxidrome may provide invaluable information for diagnosis and subsequent treatment, although the many limitations impeding acute toxidrome diagnosis must be carefully considered.

Anticholinergic

Characteristics of the anticholinergic syndrome have long been taught using the old medical adage, "dry as a bone, blind as a bat, red as a beet, hot as a hare, and mad as a hatter," which corresponds with a symptomatic person's anhidrosis, mydriasis, flushing, fever, and delirium, respectively. Depending on the dose and time since exposure, various central nervous system (CNS) effects may manifest from an anticholinergic agent. Restlessness, apprehension, abnormal speech, confusion, agitation, tremor, picking movements, ataxia, stupor, and coma have been described after exposure to various anticholinergics. When manifesting delirium, the individual will often stare into space and mutter, fluctuating between occasional lucid intervals with appropriate responses and then descriptions of vivid hallucinations. Phantom behaviors, such as plucking or picking in the air or at garments, are characteristic. Hallucinations are prominent,

TABLE 41.2 Symptoms of the Important Toxidromes

Toxidrome	Symptom
Anticholinergic	Agitation
	Blurred vision
	Decreased bowel sounds
	Dry skin
	Fever
	Flushing
	Hallucinations
	Ileus
	Lethargy/coma
	Mydriasis
	Myoclonus
	Psychosis
	Seizures
	Tachycardia
	Urinary retention
Cholinergic	Diarrhea
	Urination
	Miosis
	Bradycardia
	Bronchorrhea
	Emesis
	Lacrimation
	Salivation
Opioid	Bradycardia
	Decreased bowel sounds
	Hypotension
	Hypothermia
	Lethargy/coma
	Miosis
	Shallow respirations
	Slow respiratory rate
Sedative-hypnotic	Ataxia
	Blurred vision
	Confusion
	Diplopia
	Dysesthesias
	Hypotension
	Lethargy/coma
	Nystagmus
	Respiratory depression
	Sedation
	Slurred speech
Sympathomimetic	Agitation
	Diaphoresis
	Excessive motor activity
	Excessive speech
	Hallucinations
	Hypertension
	Hyperthermia
	Insomnia
	Restlessness
	Tachycardia
	Tremor

and they may be benign, entertaining, or terrifying to the patient experiencing them. Exposed patients may have conversations with hallucinated figures and/or may misidentify persons they typically know well. Simple tasks typically performed well by the exposed person may become difficult. Motor coordination, perception, cognition, and new memory formation are altered.

Mydriasis causes photophobia. Impairment of near vision occurs because of loss of accommodation and reduced depth of field secondary to ciliary muscle paralysis and pupillary enlargement. Tachycardia and exacerbated heart rate responses to exertion are expected. Systolic and diastolic blood pressure may show moderate elevation. A decrease in capillary tone may cause skin flushing. Intestinal motility slows, resulting in nausea, vomiting, and decreased bowel sounds. All glandular cells become inhibited, resulting in dry mucous membranes of the mouth and inhibition of sweating with resultant dry skin. Urination may be difficult, and urinary retention may occur. The exposed patient's temperature may become elevated from an inability to sweat and dissipate heat. In warm climates, this may result in marked hyperthermia.

Numerous substances can cause the anticholinergic syndrome. More common agents include antihistamines, atropine, cyclic antidepressant drugs, phenothiazines, anti-Parkinson drugs, cyclobenzaprine, scopolamine, and several plants, such as *Datura stramonium* (Jimson weed).

Cholinergic

Acetylcholine is a neurotransmitter found throughout the CNS, including (1) the sympathetic and parasympathetic autonomic ganglia, (2) the postganglionic parasympathetic nervous system, and (3) the skeletal muscle motor end plate. Acetylcholine binds to and activates muscarinic and nicotinic receptors. Activating muscarinic receptors stimulates or inhibits cellular function in visceral smooth muscle, cardiac muscle, and secretory glands. Alternatively, nicotinic receptors are present at postsynaptic membranes in autonomic ganglia and at skeletal muscle motor end plates. The enzyme acetylcholinesterase (AChE) regulates the activity of acetylcholine within the synaptic cleft. Acetylcholine binds to the active site of AChE, where the enzyme rapidly hydrolyzes acetylcholine to choline and acetic acid. These hydrolyzed products rapidly dissociate from AChE, so that the enzyme is free to act on another molecule.

The respiratory effects of cholinergic poisoning tend to be dramatic and are considered to be the major factor leading to the death of its victims. Respiratory failure typically occurs as a triad of increased airway resistance, neuromuscular failure, and depression of central respiratory centers. Profuse watery nasal discharge, marked salivation, bronchorrhea, and bronchoconstriction result in a prolonged expiratory phase, cough, and wheezing. Because of the widespread presence of cholinergic receptors in the brain, cholinergic poisoning can produce great variation in neurologic signs and symptoms, including centrally mediated respiratory failure, coma, and seizures. Cholinergic cardiotoxicity can result in two clinical scenarios: a period of intense sympathetic activity that results in sinus tachydysrhythmias or a period of increased parasympathetic tone that leads to bradydysrhythmias, prolongation of the PR interval, and atrioventricular block. Muscular symptoms may be vague and may consist of muscular weakness and difficulty with ambulation that can progress to muscular fasciculations and subsequent paralysis. Cholinergic agents cause constriction of both the sphincter muscle of the iris and the ciliary muscle of the lens, as well as stimulation of the lacrimal gland, resulting in lacrimation and miosis. The dermal sweat glands are innervated by sympathetic muscarinic receptors. When these receptors are stimulated, profuse sweating occurs. Cholinergic gastrointestinal and genitourinary symptoms may result in nausea, vomiting, abdominal cramps, tenesmus, and involuntary defecation and urination. Two mnemonics have been developed to help recall cholinergic clinical effects: DUMB BELS (diarrhea, urination, miosis, bradycardia, and bronchorrhea-bronchoconstriction, emesis, lacrimation, sweating-salivation)[16] and SLUDGE (salivation, lacrimation, urination, defecation, gastrointestinal distress, emesis-eye findings, miosis).[17]

Agents that cause these cholinergic clinical effects include organophosphate and carbamate insecticides (cholinesterase inhibitors), certain species of mushrooms that contain muscarine, and nicotinic receptor agonists such as nicotine, lobeline, and conine.

Opioid

Opioids can induce coma, respiratory depression, bradycardia, hypotension, hypothermia, miosis, pulmonary edema, decreased bowel sounds, and decreased reflexes. Common causes of this syndrome, in which CNS depression and miosis are the two cardinal signs, include morphine, codeine, diacetylmorphine, oxycodone, hydrocodone, hydromorphone, and methadone. Meperidine and propoxyphene toxicity has been associated with mydriasis and not with miosis. Numerous drugs can mimic the opioid syndrome by inducing coma, respiratory depression, and miosis, including α_2 agonists (eg, clonidine, oxymetazoline) and the antipsychotics.

Sedative Hypnotic

Sedative-hypnotics are a broad class of drugs (eg, benzodiazepines, barbiturates, meprobamate, ethchlorvynol, zolpidem) that can induce sedation, respiratory depression, hypotension, hyporeflexia, nystagmus, dysarthria, staggering gait, apnea, and coma. Numerous sedative-hypnotics have been used to commit drug-facilitated crimes (see later), such as the solution of chloral hydrate in ethanol (called a "Mickey Finn"). Few diagnostic clinical features distinguish the drugs in this large class from one another.

Sympathomimetic

Norepinephrine is the neurotransmitter for postganglionic sympathetic fibers (adrenergic) that enervate skin, eyes, heart, lungs, gastrointestinal tract, exocrine glands, and some neuronal tracts in the CNS. Physiologic responses to activation of the adrenergic system are complex and depend on the type of receptor ($\alpha1$, $\alpha2$, $\beta1$, $\beta2$) activated; some are excitatory, and others have opposing inhibitory responses. Stimulation of the sympathetic nervous system produces CNS excitation (agitation, anxiety, tremors, delusions, and paranoia), tachycardia, hypertension, mydriasis, hyperpyrexia, and diaphoresis. In severe cases, seizures, cardiac arrhythmias, and coma may occur. Examples of drugs that produce a sympathomimetic response include amphetamines, cocaine, PCP, ephedrine, methcathinone, and pseudoephedrine.

Hyperthermic Syndromes

Toxin-induced hyperthermic syndromes are potentially devastating and require rapid management. Even though the patient's temperature is one of the vital signs, the temperature often is not obtained in clinical practice. Fever in a poisoned patient can be associated with several hyperthermic syndromes: sympathomimetic toxicity, uncoupling of oxidative phosphorylation, serotonin syndrome, neuroleptic malignant syndrome, malignant hyperthermia, anticholinergic poisoning, and withdrawal syndromes.[18] Sympathomimetics, such as amphetamines and cocaine, may produce hyperthermia as the result of excess serotonin and dopamine, leading to thermal deregulation.[19] Uncoupling of oxidative phosphorylation, as seen in severe salicylate poisoning, occurs when the process of oxidative phosphorylation is disrupted, leading to heat generation and a reduced ability to aerobically generate adenosine-5′-triphosphate (ATP).[20] Serotonin syndrome occurs when a relative excess of serotonin is present at both peripheral and central serotonergic receptors.[21] Patients may present with hyperthermia, alterations in mental status, and neuromuscular abnormalities (rigidity, hyperreflexia, clonus), although individual variability is noted in these findings.[22] Serotonin syndrome is associated with drug interactions such as those associated with the combination of monoamine oxidase inhibitors and meperidine, but it also may occur with single-agent therapeutic dosing or overdosing of serotonergic agents. Neuroleptic malignant syndrome is a condition caused by relative deficiency of dopamine within the CNS.[23] It has been associated with dopamine receptor antagonists and the withdrawal of dopamine agonists such as levodopa/carbidopa products. Malignant hyperthermia occurs when genetically susceptible individuals are exposed to specific depolarizing neuromuscular blocking agents or volatile general anesthetics. It clinically is associated with elevated temperature, tachycardia, muscle rigidity, and hypercarbia. Anticholinergic poisoning may result in hyperthermia through impairment of normal cooling mechanisms such as sweating. Withdrawal syndromes can produce excessive adrenergic responses (eg, sedative-hypnotic withdrawal, ethanol withdrawal) and subsequent heat generation. It should be noted that opioid withdrawal is not associated with fever or altered mental status. Overall, differentiating among the toxic hyperthermic syndromes may be challenging, and additional causes of hyperthermia such as heat stroke and infection should be explored.

ANCILLARY TESTS

Electrocardiogram

Interpretation of the electrocardiogram (ECG) in the poisoned patient can significantly facilitate appropriate laboratory testing, diagnosis, and management of the poisoned patient because numerous substances can cause ECG changes.[24] Despite the fact that drugs have widely varying indications for therapeutic use, many unrelated drugs share common cardiac electrocardiographic effects if taken at therapeutic doses or in overdose. Potential toxins can be placed into broad classes on the basis of their cardiac effects. For example, agents that block cardiac potassium efflux channels and agents that block cardiac fast sodium channels can lead to characteristic changes in cardiac indices consisting of QRS prolongation and QT prolongation, respectively. The recognition of specific ECG changes associated with other clinical data (toxidromes) can be potentially lifesaving.[25]

Radiographic Studies

Radiologic testing is sometimes used to diagnose complications associated with poisonings, such as aspiration pneumonitis and anoxic brain injury. The use of radiology also has been advocated to detect the presence of potentially radiopaque poisons. For example, O'Brien and associates[26] studied the detectability of 459 different tablets and capsules using plain radiography.[26] Investigators used a ferrous sulfate tablet as a control in grading the radiopacity of other tablets. Overall, of the wide variety of pills tested, only 6.3% were graded as having radiopacity the same as or greater than that of ferrous sulfate; 29.6% were regarded as having at least moderate opacity; and the largest remaining portion of pills (64%) was regarded as no more than minimally detectable. Based on this and other studies, the indiscriminate use of plain abdominal x-rays is not justified, and a negative film should not be relied on to rule out potential toxic pill ingestion, especially if enough time is given to allow the pills to dissolve.

Anion Gap

Obtaining a basic metabolic panel in all poisoned patients is recommended and is an important initial screening test. When low serum bicarbonate is discovered on a metabolic panel, the clinician should determine whether an elevated anion gap exists. The formula most commonly used for the anion gap (AG) calculation is as follows[27]:

$$AG = [Na^+] - [Cl^- + HCO_3^-]$$

This equation allows one to determine whether serum electroneutrality is being maintained. The primary cation (sodium) and anions (chloride and bicarbonate) are represented in the equation.[28] Other contributors to this equation are "unmeasured."[29] Other serum cations are not commonly included in this calculation because either their concentrations are relatively low (eg, potassium) or assigning a number to represent their respective contribution is difficult (eg, magnesium, calcium).[29] Similarly, a multitude of other serum anions (eg, sulfate, phosphate, organic anions) are also difficult to measure and quantify in an equation.[28,29] These "unmeasured" ions represent the anion gap calculated using the previous equation. The reference limit for this anion gap is accepted to be 8 to 16 mmol/L,[29] but it has been suggested that because of changes in the technique used to measure chloride, these limits should be lowered to 6 to 14 mmol/L.[28] Practically speaking, an increase in the anion gap beyond an accepted reference limit, accompanied by metabolic acidosis, represents an increase in unmeasured endogenous (eg, lactate) or exogenous (eg, salicylates) anions.[27] Clinically useful mnemonics for causes of high anion gap metabolic acidoses are the classic MUDPILES (representing methanol, uremia, diabetes, paraldehyde, iron (and isoniazid), lactate, ethylene glycol, and salicylate) and the more recently proposed GOLD MARK (glycols [ethylene and propylene], oxoproline, L-lactate, D-lactate, methanol, aspirin, renal failure, and ketoacidosis). For further discussion of these causes of high anion gap metabolic acidoses the reader is referred to Chapter 60.

It is imperative that clinicians who admit poisoned patients initially presenting with an increased anion gap metabolic acidosis investigate the cause of that acidosis. Many symptomatic poisoned patients may have an initial mild metabolic acidosis on presentation caused by processes resulting in elevated serum lactate (eg, transient hypoxia or hypovolemia). However, with adequate supportive care (eg, oxygenation and hydration), the anion gap acidosis should steadily improve. If, despite adequate supportive care, an anion gap metabolic acidosis worsens in a poisoned patient, the clinician should consider continued absorption of exogenous acids (eg, salicylate), formation of acidic metabolites (eg, ethylene glycol, methanol, toluene metabolites), and cellular ischemia with worsening lactic acidosis (eg, cyanide) as potential causes.

Osmolal Gap

The main osmotically active constituents of serum are sodium (Na^+), chlorine (Cl^-), bicarbonate (HCO_3^-), glucose, and urea. Several empirical formulas based on measurement of these substances have been used to estimate the serum osmolality.[30-37] In practice, one has not shown itself to be superior to the others, yet each equation demonstrates significant differences in the osmolal gap reference interval.[*,38] Therefore reference intervals must be validated on appropriate patient populations. Two commonly used formulas (in conventional and International System of Units [SI] units) are presented here:

$$\text{OSMc (mOsm/kg)} = 2\ \text{Na (mmol/L)} + \text{Glucose (mg/dL)}/18 + \text{Urea (mg/dL)}/2.8$$

$$\text{OSMc (mOsm/kg)} = 2\ \text{Na (mmol/L)} + \text{Glucose (mmol/L)} + \text{Urea (mmol/L)}$$

or

$$\text{OSMc (mOsm/kg)} = 1.86\ \text{Na (mmol/L)} + \text{Glucose (mg/dL)}/18 + \text{Urea (mg/dL)}/2.8 + 9$$

$$\text{OSMc (mOsm/kg)} = 1.86\ \text{Na (mmol/L)} + \text{Glucose (mmol/L)} + \text{Urea (mmol/L)} + 9$$

The difference between the actual osmolality (OSMm), measured by freezing-point depression, and the calculated osmolality (OSMc) is referred to as Δ-osmolality, or the osmolal gap (OSMg).

$$\text{OSMg} = \text{OSMm} - \text{OSMc}$$

Elevated OSMg implies the presence of unmeasured osmotically active substances. Volatile alcohols (ethanol, methanol, isopropanol, acetone, and ethylene glycol), when present at significant concentrations, increase serum osmolality, thus resulting in an increased OSMg. The calculation of OSMg is commonly used as a screen.[32] However, it is important to remember that volatile alcohols are not detected when osmolality is measured with a vapor pressure osmometer. Therefore, for the purpose of determining the OSMg, only osmolality measurements based on freezing point depression are acceptable.

*Laboratories should verify that these ranges are appropriate for use in their own settings.

What constitutes a normal OSMg is widely debated. Traditionally, a normal gap has been defined as 10 mOsm/kg or less. The original source of this value is an article by Smithline and Gardner,[39] which declared that this number was pure convention. A further clinical study has not shown this assumption to be correct. However, large variability is seen in the normal population. Researchers have found the OSMg to vary from −9 to +5 mOsm/kg,[40] from −13.5 to +8.9,[41] and from −10 to +20 mOsm/kg,[42] depending on the population studied. An important point to consider is that the day-to-day coefficient of variance of sodium was 1%. This analytical variance alone may account for the variation found in patients' OSMg.[42]

One would expect that each 100 mg/dL (21.7 mmol/L) of ethanol (molecular weight = 46.068 g/mol) in serum results in an approximate increase of 21.7 mOsm/kg.[43] However, this is not found to be the case. Applying a correction factor of 0.83 to the ethanol value will more closely approximate the contribution of ethanol to the OSMg.[32] By considering this effect of ethanol on the serum osmolality, it is possible to determine what portion of an increased OSMg is due to ethanol. The contribution of ethanol to the measured osmolality can be calculated (ethanol, mg/dL/4.6 × 0.83) and included in the preceding formula for Δ-osmolality calculation. However, it has been observed that ethanol and methanol do not follow a completely predictable relationship with OSMg. In severe ethanol and methanol intoxication, OSMg increases with increasing concentration, making it appear that something is present besides the alcohol.[31-34,44]

A significant residual OSMg (>10 mOsm/kg) would suggest the possible presence of isopropanol, methanol, acetone, or ethylene glycol. This information, in conjunction with the presence or absence of metabolic acidosis or serum acetone, is helpful to the clinician when specific measurements of alcohols other than ethanol and of ethylene glycol are not available on an emergency basis (Table 41.3). It must be realized that ketones and substances administered to patients such as polyethylene glycol (burn cream),[45] mannitol (osmotic diuretic), and propylene glycol (solvent for diazepam and phenytoin) may increase serum osmolality.

For the diagnosis of ethanol intoxication, OSMg has lost its usefulness because ethanol can be measured quickly on most chemistry analyzers. However, because other toxic alcohols can be measured only by chromatographic techniques, it is still useful. Unfortunately, OSMg as a screening method is insensitive to low, yet clinically significant, concentrations of ethylene glycol (<50 mg/dL) and methanol (<30 mg/dL).[43]

TABLE 41.3 Laboratory Findings Characteristic of Ingestion of Alcohols

Alcohol	Serum Osmolal Gap	Metabolic Acidosis With Anion Gap	Serum Acetone	Urine Oxalate
Ethanol	+	−	−	−
Methanol	+	+	−	−
Isopropanol	+	−	+	−
Ethylene glycol	+	+	−	+

SCREENING PROCEDURES FOR DETECTION OF DRUGS

Screening procedures are designed for the relatively rapid and generally qualitative detection of a particular drug or drug class or other toxic substances. In general, screening tests have adequate clinical sensitivity but may not be highly specific. Thus a negative result yielded by a screening procedure may rule out with reasonable certainty the presence of clinically significant concentrations of a particular analyte. However, because of possible interferences, a positive result should be considered "presumptive positive" and should be confirmed by an alternative procedure of greater specificity.

Spot Tests

Spot tests are less frequently employed now because some have been largely replaced by rapid immunoassays that may be performed at the point of care or in the central laboratory. For a more comprehensive description, refer to previous editions of this textbook.

Immunoassay

Different types of immunoassays are useful in screening specimens for drugs. In some cases, these assays are relatively specific for a single drug (eg, lysergic acid diethylamide [LSD]), but in others, several drugs of a similar class are detected (eg, opiates). The detection limit for various members of a class of drugs or the degree of cross-reactivity for similar drugs varies, and each manufacturer of immunoassay reagents should be consulted for specific information. These assays are easy to perform; many are available for use on automated instrumentation and may be able to provide semiquantitative results. For the vast majority of drugs of abuse, immunoassays are the methods of choice for initial screening. However, for a more comprehensive drug screening, chromatographic procedures complement immunoassays.

Point of Care

Numerous point-of-care (POC) drug test devices for urine (and oral fluid) are designed for easy, rugged, and portable use by nontechnical personnel. Although these devices are relatively simple to use, proper training of nonlaboratory users is important for optimal performance (see Chapter 27).[46,47] These noninstrumental immunoassay test devices are designed for use at the site of collection; results are available within minutes and are variously configured to detect only one drug or many drugs simultaneously. The spectrum of drugs tested commonly includes the traditional Substance Abuse and Mental Health Services Administration (SAMHSA) or National Institute on Drug Abuse (NIDA) 5 (amphetamine, cocaine, marijuana, opiates, and PCP), but also may include barbiturates, benzodiazepines, buprenorphine, methamphetamine, methadone, methylenedioxymethamphetamine (MDMA), oxycodone, and, tricyclic antidepressants (TCAs).

As previously cited, such devices are also available for measurement of acetaminophen and salicylate in serum or whole blood. Evaluations for some of these test devices for urine and oral fluid have been published.[48,49] A comprehensive review of onsite drug testing is also available.[50] The assay principles of these POC test devices include the following:

- Sequential competitive binding microparticle capture immunoassay

- Homogeneous microparticle capture immunochromatography
- Solid-phase competitive sequential enzyme immunoassay
- Latex-agglutination-inhibition immunoassay

A more detailed description of these methods can be found in Chapters 23 and 27 and in the package insert for each specific test kit.

Planar Chromatography

Planar chromatography, commonly known as TLC, is a versatile procedure that requires no instrumentation and thus is operationally relatively simple and inexpensive (see previous editions of this textbook). With this technique, a large number of drugs may be detected; it may be applied to the analysis of serum, gastric contents, or urine. Urine is the specimen of choice because most drugs and drug metabolites are present in urine in relatively high concentrations. However, application of TLC to drug screening requires considerable experience and skill to recognize drug and metabolite patterns and various color hues for detection; it has largely been replaced by other chromatographic techniques. For a more comprehensive description, refer to previous editions of this textbook.[51]

Gas Chromatography

Also known as gas LC, GC is relatively rapid, is capable of resolving a broad spectrum of drugs, and is widely used for qualitative and quantitative drug analysis.[52] Capillary columns, because of their high efficiency, are analytical columns commonly used for drug detection by GC. In many instances, nonderivatized drugs have good GC properties when capillary columns are used; in some instances, derivatization to a less polar or more volatile compound is necessary. Common detectors for drug detection by GC are flame ionization and alkali flame ionization (nitrogen phosphorus) detectors and mass spectrometers, which provide the greatest accuracy of identification. Numerous methods for general drug screening by GC-MS have been published, but one comprehensive method that can be adapted to multiple body fluids and tissues is described here.[52]

High-Performance Liquid Chromatography

The resolving power of HPLC (see Chapter 16) for separating widely divergent chemical constituents has been applied to the complex challenge of comprehensive drug screening in biological fluids. Advantages of HPLC over GC include the ability to analyze polar compounds without derivatization (eg, morphine, benzoylecgonine) and thermally labile drugs (eg, chlordiazepoxide). The advent of diode array detectors that provide a spectral scan of compounds as they elute from the column greatly increased the discriminatory power of this technique.[53-56] LC-MS or LC-MS/MS and high-resolution MS currently play a limited role in comprehensive screening, but are rapidly gaining in popularity.[8,57-62]

PHARMACOLOGY AND ANALYSIS OF SPECIFIC DRUGS AND TOXIC AGENTS

The toxic, pharmacologic, biochemical, and analytical characteristics of several individual drugs and toxins are discussed in this section.

Agents That Cause Cellular Hypoxia

Carbon monoxide and methemoglobin-forming agents interfere with oxygen transport, resulting in cellular hypoxia. Cyanide interferes with oxygen use and therefore causes an apparent cellular hypoxia.

Carbon Monoxide

Carbon monoxide is a colorless, odorless, tasteless gas that is a product of incomplete combustion of carbonaceous material. Common exogenous sources of carbon monoxide include cigarette smoke, gasoline engines, and improperly ventilated home heating units. Small amounts of carbon monoxide are produced endogenously in the metabolic conversion of heme to biliverdin.[63] This endogenous production of carbon monoxide is accelerated in hemolytic anemias.[64]

Toxic Effects. When inhaled, carbon monoxide combines tightly with the heme iron (Fe^{2+}) of hemoglobin to form carboxyhemoglobin. The binding affinity of hemoglobin for carbon monoxide is approximately 250 times greater than that for oxygen. Therefore high concentrations of carboxyhemoglobin limit the oxygen content of blood. Moreover, the binding of carbon monoxide to a hemoglobin subunit increases the oxygen affinity for the remaining subunits in the hemoglobin tetramer. Thus, at a given tissue PO_2 value, less oxygen dissociates from hemoglobin when carbon monoxide is also bound, shifting the hemoglobin-oxygen dissociation curve to the left. Consequently, carbon monoxide not only decreases the oxygen content of blood but also decreases oxygen availability to tissue, thereby producing a greater degree of tissue hypoxia than would result from an equivalent reduction in oxyhemoglobin caused by to hypoxia alone.[65,66] Carbon monoxide also may bind to other heme proteins, such as myoglobin and mitochondrial cytochrome oxidase a_3; this may limit oxygen use when tissue PO_2 is very low.[65,66]

The toxic effects of carbon monoxide are a result of tissue hypoxia. Organs with high oxygen demand, such as heart and brain, are most sensitive to hypoxia and thus account for the major clinical sequelae of carbon monoxide poisoning. It must be emphasized that the carboxyhemoglobin concentration, although helpful in diagnosis, does not always correlate with the clinical findings or prognosis.[67,68] Factors other than carboxyhemoglobin concentration that contribute to toxicity include length of exposure, metabolic activity, and underlying disease, especially cardiac or cerebrovascular disease. Moreover, low carboxyhemoglobin concentrations relative to the severity of poisoning may be observed if the patient was removed from the carbon monoxide–contaminated environment a significant time before blood sampling.[69]

An insidious effect of carbon monoxide poisoning is the delayed development of neuropsychiatric sequelae, which may include personality changes, motor disturbances, and memory impairment. These manifestations do not correlate with the length of exposure or the maximum blood carboxyhemoglobin concentration.[70]

Treatment for carbon monoxide poisoning involves removal of the individual from the contaminated area and administration of oxygen. The half-life ($t_{1/2}$) of carboxyhemoglobin in the body is variable, and attempts to determine the exact elimination $t_{1/2}$ for carbon monoxide based on the inhaled oxygen concentration have not been validated. In room air the approximate half-life is approximately

4 to 5 hours, and during hyperbaric oxygen therapy it is as short as 12 to 20 minutes.[71,72] The findings from randomized controlled human studies are not consistent regarding the benefit of hyperbaric oxygen for carbon monoxide–poisoned patients, and there is therefore no consensus regarding its role in treatment.[72,73]

Analytical Methods. Carbon monoxide may be released from hemoglobin and then measured by GC, or it may be determined indirectly as carboxyhemoglobin by spectrophotometry. GC methods are accurate and precise even for very low concentrations of carbon monoxide. Spectrophotometric methods are rapid, convenient, accurate, and precise, except at very low concentrations of carboxyhemoglobin (<2% to 3%).

GC methods measure the carbon monoxide content of blood. When blood is treated with potassium ferricyanide, carboxyhemoglobin is converted to methemoglobin and carbon monoxide is released into the gas phase. Measurement of the released carbon monoxide may be performed by GC using a molecular sieve column and a thermal conductivity detector.[74] A lower detection limit is achieved by incorporating a reducing catalyst (eg, nickel) between the GC column and the detector to convert carbon monoxide to methane. The methane may then be detected with a flame ionization detector.[75] A very low detection limit may be achieved with the use of a heated mercuric oxide reaction chamber between the GC column and an ultraviolet (UV) light detector. As carbon monoxide elutes from the column, it reacts with mercuric oxide to form mercury gas, which has a high molar absorptivity at 254 nm.[76] In practice, the carbon monoxide binding capacity is also determined after an aliquot of the blood specimen is treated with carbon monoxide to saturate the hemoglobin. The results are then expressed as percent of carboxyhemoglobin:

$$\%\,\text{HbCO} = \frac{\text{CO}_{\text{content}}}{\text{CO}_{\text{capacity}}} \times 100$$

GC methods are accurate and precise and are considered to be reference procedures. Reference intervals for carboxyhemoglobin in rural nonsmokers are approximately 0.5%; for urban nonsmokers, 1% to 2%; and for smokers, 5% to 6%.[77] Values may be increased by approximately 3% in cases of hemolytic anemia.[64]

Spectrophotometric methods rely on the characteristic spectral absorption properties of carboxyhemoglobin.[78,79] Among several such methods, the most popular are based on automated, multiwavelength measurements of several hemoglobin species. Automated, multicomponent spectrophotometric methods are most rapid and convenient for the determination of carboxyhemoglobin and other hemoglobin species. Spectrophotometric methods generally compare favorably with gas chromatographic procedures at carboxyhemoglobin concentrations greater than 2% to 3%, but their precision is poor below these concentrations.[76] Therefore they are sufficiently accurate and precise for measurement of carbon monoxide after exogenous exposure but are too insensitive to detect the increased endogenous production of carbon monoxide that occurs in hemolytic anemia.

Fetal hemoglobin has slightly different spectral properties than adult hemoglobin. Consequently, falsely high carboxyhemoglobin values of 4% to 7% may occur when blood from neonates is measured by some spectrophotometric methods using fewer wavelengths.[80] Moreover, erroneous results may occur with lipemic specimens, with bilirubin, and in the presence of methylene blue (see section on "Methemoglobin-Forming Agents").

Methemoglobin-Forming Agents

The heme iron in hemoglobin is normally present in the ferrous state (Fe^{2+}). When oxidized to the ferric state (Fe^{3+}), methemoglobin is formed and this form of hemoglobin cannot bind oxygen. Congenital methemoglobinemia may result from a deficiency of nicotinamide adenine dinucleotide (NADH)-methemoglobin reductase or, more rarely, from hemoglobin variants (hemoglobin M) in which heme iron is both more susceptible to oxidation and more resistant to reduction by the methemoglobin reductase system. (For more information on methemoglobinemia refer to Chapters 30 and 38).

Toxic Effects. An acquired (toxic) methemoglobinemia may be caused by various drugs and chemicals (Box 41.1). Additionally, oxides of nitrogen and other oxidant combustion products make smoke inhalation a potential cause of methemoglobinemia.[81] The normal percentage of methemoglobin is less than 1.5% of total hemoglobin. The severity of symptoms usually correlates with measured methemoglobin levels; methemoglobin percentages up to 20% may cause slate-gray cutaneous discoloration, cyanosis, and chocolate-brown blood. Percentages between 20% and 50% may cause dyspnea, exercise intolerance, fatigue, weakness, and syncope. More severe symptoms of dysrhythmias, seizures, metabolic acidosis, and coma are associated with methemoglobin percentages of 50% to 70%, and greater than 70% may be lethal.[82,83] All of these symptoms are a consequence of hypoxia associated with the diminished oxygen content of the blood, and with a decreased oxygen dissociation from hemoglobin species in which some, but not all, subunits contain heme iron in the ferric state (ie, shift of dissociation curve to the left). The PO_2 is normal in these patients and therefore so is the calculated hemoglobin oxygen saturation. Thus a normal PO_2 in a cyanotic patient is a significant indication for the possible presence of methemoglobinemia. Direct measurement of methemoglobin is important in these cases and may be performed by the manual spectrophotometric method of Evelyn and Malloy or by automated multiwavelength measurements with a cooximeter (see section on "Carbon Monoxide").

Specific therapy for toxic methemoglobinemia involves the administration of methylene blue, which acts as an electron transfer agent in the nicotinamide adenine dinucleotide phosphate (NADPH)-methemoglobin reductase reaction, thereby increasing the activity of this system several-fold.[82,84] Methylene blue and sulfhemoglobin cause spectral interference in the measurement of methemoglobin with some cooximeters[85,86] but not with the Evelyn-Malloy method.[87] Ascorbic acid can reverse methemoglobin by an alternative metabolic pathway but is of minimal use acutely because of its slow action.[81]

Analytical and Preanalytical Considerations. Methemoglobin can be measured in blood manually[86,87] or by automated multiwavelength measurements with a cooximeter.[88] Methemoglobin interferes with the noninvasive pulse oximetry method, measuring the absorbance of light at 660 nm (oxyhemoglobin) and 940 nm (deoxyhemoglobin). Because

BOX 41.1 Examples of Acquired Causes of Methemoglobinemia

Local Anesthetics
Benzocaine
Lidocaine
Prilocaine

Antimicrobials
Chloroquine
Dapsone
Primaquine
Sulfonamides
Trimethoprim

Analgesics
Phenazopyridine
Phenacetin

Nitrites and Nitrates
Ammonium nitrate
Amyl nitrite
Butyl nitrite
Isobutyl nitrite
Potassium nitrate
Sodium nitrate

Nitrogen Oxides
Nitric oxide
Nitrogen dioxide

Miscellaneous
Aminophenol
Aniline, *p*-chloraniline
Bromates
Chlorates
4-Dimethyl-amino-phenolate (4-DMAP)
Metoclopramide
Nitrobenzene
Nitroethane
Nitroglycerin
Phenazopyridine
Potassium permanganate
Propanil

methemoglobin is not stable at room temperature, specimens should be kept on ice or refrigerated but not frozen.[86] The stability of methemoglobin at 4°C has not been well studied. Some sources indicate significant decreases in methemoglobin concentration after 4 to 8 hours,[89] whereas others report little or no change after 24 hours.[86] Freezing results in an increase in methemoglobin concentration.[86]

Cyanide

Cyanide consists of one atom of carbon bound to one atom of nitrogen by three molecular bonds (C≡N). Inorganic cyanides (also known as cyanide salts) contain cyanide in the anion form *(*CN^-*)* and are used in numerous industries, such as metallurgy, photographic developing, plastic manufacturing, fumigation, and mining. Organic compounds that have a cyano group bonded to an alkyl residue are called nitriles. For example, methyl cyanide is also known as acetonitrile (CH_3CN). Hydrogen cyanide (HCN) is a colorless gas at standard temperature and pressure with an inconsistently reported bitter almond odor. Cyanogen gas, a dimer of cyanide, reacts with water and breaks down into the cyanide anion. Many plants, such as *Manihot* (cassava), *Linum, Lotus, Prunus, Sorghum,* and *Phaseolus* species, contain cyanogenic glycosides. Iatrogenic cyanide poisoning may occur during use of nitroprusside as a vasodilator given to reduce blood pressure and afterload. Each nitroprusside molecule contains five cyanide molecules, which are slowly released in vivo. If endogenous sulfate stores are depleted, as in the malnourished or postoperative patient, cyanide may accumulate even with therapeutic nitroprusside infusion rates (2 to 10 mcg/kg per minute).

Toxic Effects. Hydrocyanic acid binds to hemoglobin. The hydrocyanic acid bound in the erythrocyte is in equilibrium with free hydrocyanic acid in the serum at a ratio of 10:1. Cyanide in serum readily crosses all biological membranes and avidly binds to heme iron (Fe^{3+}) in the cytochrome a-a_3 complex within mitochondria.[90,91] When bound to cytochrome a-a_3, cyanide is a competitive inhibitor that causes decoupling of oxidative phosphorylation. Patients exposed to toxic concentrations of cyanide may exhibit rapid onset of symptoms typical of cellular hypoxia—flushing, headache, nausea and vomiting, anxiety, confusion, and collapse, initial hypertension, and tachycardia progressing to hypotension, cyanosis, bradycardia, and apnea, coma, seizures, complete heart block, and death if the dose is sufficiently large.[92,93]

Hydroxycobalamin or the cyanide antidote kit should be administered as soon as cyanide poisoning is suspected. Hydroxocobalamin, a vitamin B_{12} precursor, is a metalloprotein with a central cobalt atom that complexes cyanide, forming cyanocobalamin (vitamin B_{12}). Cyanocobalamin is eliminated in the urine or releases the cyanide moiety at a rate sufficient to allow detoxification by rhodanese. The cyanide antidote kit contains amyl nitrite, sodium nitrite, and sodium thiosulfate. Thiosulfate donates the sulfur atoms necessary for rhodanese-mediated cyanide biotransformation to thiocyanate. The mechanism of nitrite is less clear. The traditional rationale relies on the ability of nitrite to generate methemoglobin. Because cyanide has a higher affinity for methemoglobin than for cytochrome a_3, cytochrome oxidase function is restored.

Analytical Methods. Cyanide determination was traditionally performed by spectrometry after microdiffusion separation.[94-96] However, more recently chromatography has been employed. GC has used both headspace gas and direct injection sampling couple with electron capture, nitrogen selective, or mass spectrometric detection methods.[97-101] LC followed by fluorescences and mass spectrometric detection also have been described.[102,103]

Alcohols of Toxicologic Interest

Several alcohols are toxic and medically important; they include ethanol, methanol, isopropanol, acetone (also a metabolite of isopropanol), and ethylene glycol.

Ethanol

Ethanol is the most widely used and often abused chemical substance. Consequently, measurement of ethanol is one of the more frequently performed tests in the toxicology laboratory. Ethanol is considered a CNS depressant whose effects

TABLE 41.4 Stages of Acute Alcoholic Influence and Intoxication

Blood Alcohol Concentration (mg/dL)	Influence	Clinical Signs and Symptoms
0.01–0.05	Subclinical	Influence or effects not apparent or obvious Behavior appears normal Impairment detectable by special tests
0.03–0.12	Euphoria	Mild euphoria Increased sociability, talkativeness, self-confidence Decreased inhibitions Mild sensorimotor impairment Slowed information processing Loss of efficiency in finer performance tests Impairment of perception and memory
0.09–0.25	Excitement	Emotional instability, loss of critical judgment comprehension Decreased sensory response, increased reaction time Reduced visual acuity, peripheral vision, and glare recovery Sensorimotor incoordination, impaired balance Drowsiness
0.18–0.30	Confusion	Disorientation, mental confusion, dizziness Exaggerated emotional states (fear, rage, grief, etc.) Disturbances of vision (diplopia, etc.) and of perception of color, form, motion, dimensions Increased pain threshold Ataxia, dysarthria, apathy, lethargy
0.25–0.40	Stupor	General inertia, approaching loss of motor functions Markedly decreased response to stimuli Marked muscular incoordination, inability to stand or walk Vomiting, incontinence of urine and feces Impaired consciousness, sleep or stupor
0.35–0.50	Coma	Unconsciousness, coma, anesthesia Depressed or absent reflexes Subnormal temperature Impairment of circulation and respiration Possible death
0.45 +	Death	Possible death from respiratory arrest

Modified from Dubowski KM. Alcohol determination in the clinical laboratory. *Am J Clin Pathol* 1980;74:747-750.[939]

vary depending on the blood ethanol concentration (Table 41.4) but are also heavily influenced by an individual's tolerance. Symptoms vary from euphoria and decreased inhibitions, to increased disorientation and incoordination, and then to coma and death. A blood alcohol concentration of 80 mg/dL (0.08%) or less has been established as the statutory limit for operation of a motor vehicle in most countries.

Because of many factors, not all individuals experience the same degree of CNS dysfunction at similar blood alcohol concentrations. Moreover, the CNS actions of ethanol are more pronounced when the blood ethanol concentration is increasing (absorptive phase) than when it is declining (elimination phase), in part because of the phenomenon of acute tolerance.[104] In addition, heavy alcohol use leads to a more chronic form of tolerance. When consumed with other CNS depressant drugs, ethanol exerts a potentiation or synergistic depressant effect. This can occur at relatively low alcohol concentrations, and numerous deaths have resulted from combined ethanol and drug ingestion.[105]

The pharmacologic mechanisms for the CNS depressant actions of ethanol are complex and incompletely understood, but probably involve both enhancement of major inhibitory neurons and impairment of excitatory neurons. The principal CNS inhibitory neuronal system is mediated by the neurotransmitter γ-aminobutyric acid (GABA). When GABA binds to its postsynaptic receptor subtype $GABA_A$, this oligomeric ion-gated complex "opens" to allow inward flux of chloride, leading to membrane hyperpolarization and subsequent decreased electrical response. This GABA-mediated inhibitory response is enhanced by ethanol and sedative, hypnotic, and anesthetic agents, including barbiturates, benzodiazepines, and volatile anesthetics.[106] Neuronal nicotinic acetylcholine receptors also may be prominent molecular targets of alcohol.[107] Both enhancement and inhibition of nicotinic acetylcholine receptor function have been reported depending on receptor subunit concentration and the concentrations of ethanol tested. Ethanol also inhibits the function of the *N*-methyl-D-aspartate (NMDA)-receptor and kainate-receptor subtypes; (α-amino-3-hydroxy-5-methyl-4-isoxazole-propionic acid [AMPA]) receptors are largely resistant to alcohol.[108]

The aforementioned chronic tolerance to ethanol is considered to be mediated by ethanol-induced increased responsiveness and upregulation in the synthesis of NMDA receptors, attained by concomitant downregulation and desensitization through phosphorylation of $GABA_A$ and

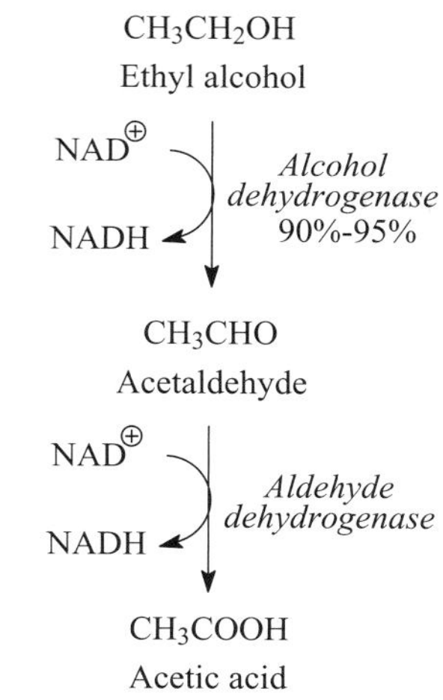

FIGURE 41.1 Metabolism of ethanol.

glutamate receptors.[106,109,110] Largely because of these adaptive changes, abrupt withdrawal from chronic, heavy ethanol use leads to a physical abstinence syndrome that has prominent features that are the opposite of those produced by intoxication. This includes features of CNS excitation, anxiety, irritability, insomnia, muscle tremor and cramps, hallucinations, and increased temperature, blood pressure, heart rate, and seizures.[111] This syndrome can be fatal if the patient is not monitored properly.

Ethanol is metabolized principally by liver alcohol dehydrogenase (ADH) to acetaldehyde, which is subsequently oxidized to acetic acid by aldehyde dehydrogenase (Fig. 41.1). The rate of elimination of ethanol from blood approximates a zero-order process. This rate varies among individuals, averaging approximately 15 mg/dL (3.2 mmol/L) per hour for males and 18 mg/dL (3.9 mmol/L) per hour for females.[112,113] At both low (<20 mg/dL, <4.3 mmol/L)[114] and high (>300 mg/dL, <65.1 mmol/L) ethanol concentrations, elimination more closely resembles first-order kinetics, and it is accelerated at high concentrations.[115] The elimination rate is also influenced by drinking habits (eg, alcoholics have increased elimination rates caused by enzyme induction).[116]

Methanol

Methanol is used as a solvent in several commercial products, as a constituent in windshield wiper fluid, copy machine fluids, fuel additives (octane boosters), paint remover or thinner, antifreeze, canned heating sources, deicing fluid, shellacs, and varnishes. It may be consumed intentionally by individuals as an ethanol substitute, accidentally when present as a contaminant in illegal whiskey, or inadvertently by children.

The CNS effects of methanol are substantially less severe than those of ethanol. Methanol is oxidized by liver ADH (at approximately one-tenth the rate of ethanol) to formaldehyde. Formaldehyde in turn is rapidly oxidized by aldehyde dehydrogenase to formic acid, which may cause serious acidosis and optic neuropathy, potentially resulting in blindness, CNS bleeds, or death.[117,118] The mainstay of therapy for methanol toxicity includes the administration of fomepizole or ethanol as a competitive ADH inhibitor, either folate or folinic acid, and hemodialysis when required.

Ethanol is a teratogen, and alcohol consumption during pregnancy can result in a baby with fetal alcohol spectrum disorder (FASD). FASD is an umbrella term that describes the variety of effects that can occur in an individual whose mother drank alcohol during pregnancy (see http://www.nofas.org). These effects may include physical, mental, behavioral, and/or learning disabilities with possible lifelong implications and are 100% preventable when a woman completely abstains from alcohol during her pregnancy.

Isopropanol and Acetone

Isopropanol is readily available to the general population as a 70% aqueous solution for use as rubbing alcohol, but also can be found in cleaners, disinfectants, antifreezes, cosmetics, solvents, inks, and pharmaceuticals. It has about twice the CNS depressant action as ethanol.[119] Isopropanol has a short $t_{1/2}$ of 2.5 to 3.0 hours[119] because it is rapidly metabolized by ADH to acetone, which is eliminated much more slowly ($t_{1/2}$, 3 to 6 hours).[120] Therefore concentrations of acetone in serum often exceed those of isopropanol during the elimination phase after isopropanol ingestion. Acetone has CNS depressant activity similar to that of ethanol, and because of its longer $t_{1/2}$, it may prolong the apparent CNS effects of isopropanol.[119,120] Supportive care is the mainstay of treatment, with rare reports of dialysis in severe intoxication. Isopropanol is a secondary alcohol (the hydroxyl group is attached to a central, rather than a terminal, carbon), consequently it is metabolized to a ketone, not an acid, and therefore ingestions do not cause significant metabolic acidosis.[121,122]

Ethylene Glycol

Ethylene glycol is present in antifreeze products, deicing products, detergents, paints, and cosmetics. It may be ingested accidentally or for the purpose of inebriation or suicide. Because it tastes sweet, some animals are attracted to it. Veterinarians are often familiar with ethylene glycol toxicity because of cases involving dogs or cats that drank radiator fluid.

Ethylene glycol itself has initial CNS effects resembling those of ethanol.[123] However, metabolism of ethylene glycol by ADH to glycoaldehyde, which is then metabolized to glycolic, glyoxylic, and oxalic acids.[123-125] Oxalate readily precipitates with calcium to form insoluble calcium oxalate crystals. Tissue injury is caused by widespread deposition of oxalate crystals and the toxic effects of glycolic and glyoxylic acids.[124,126,127] Serum concentrations associated with death from ethylene glycol ingestion have been observed to vary from 0.06 to 4.3 g/L,[125,128] (0.97 mmol/L to 69.3 mmol/L) highlighting the lack of correlation between ethylene glycol concentration and severity of toxicity. It is thus impossible to define a serum ethylene glycol concentration associated with a high probability of death, a result largely of the timing of the blood collection in relation to the ingestion and the amount that had already been metabolized to more toxic metabolites. However, the serum concentration of glycolic acid correlates more closely with clinical symptoms and mortality than does the concentration of ethylene glycol.[126,128] Because of the rapid elimination of ethylene glycol ($t_{1/2}$, 2 to 5 hours),[125] its serum concentration may be low or undetectable at a time when glycolic acid remains elevated.[126,128-130] Thus the determination of ethylene glycol and glycolic acid provides useful clinical and confirmatory analytical information in cases of ethylene glycol ingestion. The mainstay of therapy for ethylene glycol toxicity includes administration of ethanol or fomepizole as a competitive ADH inhibitor and dialysis.

Analysis

Ethanol

Serum, Plasma, and Blood Ethanol. Serum, plasma, and whole blood are suitable specimens for the determination of ethanol. Alcohol distributes into the aqueous compartments of blood; because the water content of serum is greater than that of whole blood, higher alcohol concentrations are obtained with serum than with whole blood. Experimentally, the ratio of serum to whole blood ethanol is 1.18 (1.10 to 1.35)[131] and varies slightly with hematocrit.[132] Therefore laboratories that perform alcohol determinations should make clear the choice of specimen.

Because of the volatile nature of alcohols, specimens should be kept capped to avoid evaporative loss. Blood may be stored, when properly sealed, for 14 days at room temperature or at 4°C, with or without preservative.[133] For longer storage or for nonsterile postmortem specimens, sodium fluoride should be used as a preservative to minimize changes in ethanol concentration.

To measure ethanol in serum and plasma, enzymatic analysis is the method of choice for many laboratories. In this method, ethanol is measured by oxidation to acetaldehyde with NAD, a reaction catalyzed by ADH. With this reaction, the formation of NADH, measured at 340 nm, is proportional to the amount of ethanol in the specimen[134]:

$$\text{Ethanol} + \text{NAD} \xrightarrow{\text{ADH}} \text{Acetaldehyde} + \text{NADH}$$

Under most assay conditions, ADH is reasonably specific for ethanol, with interferences by isopropanol, acetone, methanol, and ethylene glycol of typically less than 1%. As a precaution the venipuncture site is recommended to be cleansed with an alcohol-free disinfectant, such as aqueous benzalkonium chloride.

Spuriously increased results for ethanol have been described in the presence of high concentrations of lactate dehydrogenase (LDH) and lactate.[135,136] The basis of the lactate/LDH interference stems from increased blood concentrations of lactate in conjunction with increased concentrations of LDH. The increased lactate concentration may result from both clinical pathologic conditions and trauma, especially tissue hypoperfusion.[137] The following reaction describes the source of the interference:

$$\text{Lactate} + \text{NAD} \xrightarrow{\text{LDH}} \text{Pyruvate} + \text{NADH}$$

As NADH is measured in the assay, it is easy to see how increased lactate and LDH could result in a positive ethanol. However, not all ethanol assays are known to have this interference.[137] It is recognized that the lactate and LDH must hit some critical concentration for the interference to occur with those affected assays. It appears that a lactate concentration greater than 15 mmol/L (normal is 0.7 to 1.8 mmol/L) and an LDH concentration greater than 2000 IU/L (normal is less 170 IU/L) may be required for the interference to be observed, although variations in these numbers are also possible.[136] Theoretically other dehydrogenases and substrates may cause similar interference.[138]

In clinical laboratories serum (or plasma) is the most common specimen for ethanol analysis by ADH methods; this method also performs well with urine or oral fluid. Whole blood determinations can be made directly,[139] or a precipitation step may be required before analysis to avoid interference from hemoglobin.[140] Results from these methods generally compare closely with those from gas chromatographic methods.[139] For more information about these methods, see "Analysis of Volatile Alcohols" section, later.

Estimation of Blood Alcohol. During the early part of the twentieth century, Dr. Erik M. P. Widmark, a Swedish physician, did much of the foundational research regarding alcohol pharmacokinetics in the human body. In addition, he developed an algebraic equation that can be used to estimate the amount of alcohol consumed by an individual or the associated blood alcohol concentration when the values of the other variables are given.[141,142]:

$$N = W \bullet \rho \bullet [C_t + \beta \bullet t]/(d \bullet Z)$$

N = Number of drinks
W = Body weight (kg)
ρ (rho) = Volume of distribution (L/kg) (0.68 for males, 0.55 for females)
C_t = Blood alcohol concentration (kg/L)
β = Rate of ethanol elimination (0.15 g/L per hour)
t = Time since first drink (h)
d = Specific gravity of alcohol (0.8)
Z = Amount of ethanol alcohol per drink (L) (15 mL of ethanol in a standard drink)

Note that it may be necessary to convert the units from those more commonly reported. It is important to remember that this formula should be used only after completion of alcohol absorption and when equilibrium has been reached between blood and body tissue.

Frequently the time since the first drink is unknown; the formula can be modified to estimate the number of drinks in an individual's system at the time of the test.

$$N = W \bullet \rho \bullet [C_t]/(d \bullet Z)$$

The rate of elimination in the average person is commonly estimated at 0.015 g/100 mL per hour (range, 0.010 to 0.030 g/100 mL per hour).[143] Retrograde extrapolation is an estimation of a subject's alcohol concentration at a prior time, derived from a blood alcohol concentration measured at a later time. This process may be applied when certain assumptions are made concerning absorption rates, elimination rates, and patterns of alcohol consumption, including drinking duration and volume consumed. Unfortunately, to be forensically useful and scientifically valid, such extrapolations may require facts about the person and that person's alcohol consumption, as well as related information that often is not available. Consequently, significant legal debate surrounds the validity and accuracy of retrograde extrapolation.

Breath Ethanol. Statutory laws for driving under the influence of alcohol were originally based on the concentration of ethanol in venous whole blood. Because the collection of blood is invasive and requires intervention by medical personnel, the determination of alcohol in expired air (breath) has become the mainstay of evidential alcohol measurements.[144-146] Clinical interest in determination of breath alcohol at the point of care is growing. The fundamental principle for use of breath analysis is that alcohol in capillary alveolar blood rapidly equilibrates with alveolar air in a ratio of approximately 2100:1 (blood to breath). This blood-to-breath ratio may actually be closer to 2300:1 but is also very variable. Nevertheless, in the United States, evidential breath alcohol measurements are based on the ratio of 2100:1. The lower blood-to-breath ratio will predict a slightly lower than actual blood alcohol concentration; its use therefore is not prejudicial. To alleviate confusion and uncertainty surrounding the conversion from breath to blood alcohol concentration, the traffic laws in many countries specify per se limits for blood and/or breath.

Before breath alcohol analysis, a deprivation period of 15 minutes is required to allow for clearance of any residual alcohol that may have been present in the mouth (eg, very recent drinking, use of alcohol-containing mouthwash, vomiting of alcohol-rich gastric fluid). Duplicate tests, performed 5 to 10 minutes apart and within 20 mg/dL (0.02%, 4.3 mmol/L) are used as an additional safeguard against mouth alcohol contamination.

During the period of active alcohol absorption, generally 30 to 60 minutes depending on a variety of factors,[147,148] and before peak blood alcohol concentration is obtained, the alcohol concentration in arterial blood will be initially higher than that in peripheral venous blood, and the converse is true in the postabsorptive phase.[149] Because end-expiratory air equilibrates with pulmonary alveolar and capillary blood, the breath alcohol concentration more closely reflects that of arterial alcohol[150]; however, the difference between arterial and venous blood is within the analytical error of most assays.

Determination of ethanol in expired air requires specialized breath alcohol analyzers. Several commercial evidential breath alcohol measurement devices are available. Principles of measurement used in such analyzers include (1) infrared absorption spectrometry (most common), (2) dichromate-sulfuric acid oxidation-reduction (photometric), (3) GC (flame ionization or thermal conductivity detection), (4) electrochemical oxidation (fuel cell), and (5) metal oxide semiconductor sensors.[144,145] Breath alcohol devices also may be used for POC patient medical evaluation (eg, emergency department).

Oral Fluid Ethanol. Because oral fluid (saliva) may be easily and noninvasively collected, interest is growing in its use for ethanol measurements and detection of drugs, but it is not a frequently used sample for ethanol determinations (see later section on "Detection of Drugs of Abuse Using Other Types of Specimens").

Urine Ethanol. Urine has been used as an alternative, less invasive specimen for determination of alcohol use. During the postabsorptive phase after alcohol ingestion, the concentration of alcohol in urine is roughly 1.3 times that in blood.[151] However, the use of urine alcohol measurements to estimate blood concentrations is discouraged because the ratio of 1.3 is highly variable, and, perhaps more important, the urine alcohol concentration may better reflect an average of the blood alcohol concentration during the period in which urine is collected in the bladder. The detection of alcohol in urine represents ingestion of alcohol within the previous 8 to 12 hours.

Ethanol Biomarker. Ethyl glucuronide (EtG), ethyl sulfate (EtS) and phosphatidylethanols (PEths) are biomarkers of ethanol consumption. EtG and EtS are phase II metabolites of ethanol. EtG is a phase II metabolite of ethanol formed through the uridine diphosphate glucose–glucuronosyltransferase catalyzed conjugation of ethanol with glucuronic acid.[152] Ethyl sulfate is also formed directly by the conjugation of ethanol with sulfate group.[153] PEth are formed by phospholipase D in the presence of ethanol.[154]

Because EtG has a long urinary elimination time (≤80 hours), its specificity for ethanol exposure, and the low detection limits, EtG is used as a marker of recent ethanol intake in a variety of clinical and legal settings, including medical monitoring for relapse, emergency department patient evaluation, postmortem assessment, and transportation accident investigation.[155,156]

Monitoring both EtG and EtS in urine improves sensitivity when using ethanol biomarkers for monitoring recent drinking. EtG, but not EtS, can be produced after specimen collection in diabetics by glucose fermentation.[157] Whereas upper respiratory tract infections and β-glucuronidase hydrolysis may lower levels of EtG, they do not seem to affect EtS.[158] However, challenges associated with factors such as establishing appropriate cutoff concentrations capable of distinguishing between drinking and incidental exposure such as nonbeverage sources of ethanol exposure (ie, hand sanitizers, mouthwash),[159,160] nonuniform laboratory reporting limits, sample stability, and microbial activity may complicate interpretation of results.[155] However, some interpretive guides have been proposed. EtG greater than 1000 ng/mL may indicate heavy drinking in the previous 48 hours or light drinking the same day. An EtG from 500 to 1000 ng/mL may indicate heavy drinking in the previous 3 days, light drinking in the past 24 hours, or intense "extraneous exposure" within 24 hours. Values less than 500 ng/mL may indicate heavy drinking in the previous 3 days, light drinking in the past 36 hours, or recent extraneous exposure.[158]

PEths are a group of phospholipids with a common phosphoethanol head group with two fatty acid chains that differ in chain length and degree of unsaturation.[154] PEth is a promising marker because of its persistence in blood for as long as 3 weeks after even only a few days of moderately heavy drinking (approximately four drinks per day).[158,161,162] Therefore PEth may be used in conjunction with EtG and EtS to discriminate incidental ethanol exposure from moderate to heavy binge alcohol drinking.[163]

Volatile Alcohols (Methanol, Isopropanol, and Acetone). Methanol poisoning can be lethal if not recognized early. Unfortunately, in some instances, a latent period can be as long as 12 to 24 hours[147] before toxicity is recognized, making laboratory identification of this poisoning critical. Development of GC methods for volatiles in 1964[164,165] was a significant step in the recognition and treatment of ingestion of this very toxic alcohol.

Flame ionization GC remains the most common method for detection and quantitation of volatile alcohols in biological samples.[151] Not only does it distinguish among ethanol, methanol, isopropanol, and acetone, it has the capability to measure concentrations as low as 10 mg/dL (0.01%). Specimens are prepared by a variety of methods; the two most common are direct injection and headspace analysis. Direct injection involves injection of a sample prepared by diluting it with an aqueous solution of internal standard (thus reducing the amount of matrix introduced into the

GC). Repeated injection of biological aqueous matrix into the GC will cause buildup on the injector and front of the analytical column, requiring frequent maintenance and column replacement. This can be alleviated by the use of headspace injection. The volatility of the alcohols is used to separate them from the matrix. Specifically, the "Gas Law" states that at a given temperature, the amount of volatile substance in the air space above the liquid—headspace—is proportional to the concentration of the volatile alcohol in the solution. Therefore the sample in the headspace allows calculation of the concentration in the specimen.

Headspace GC analysis is another excellent method for measurement of methanol, isopropanol, acetone, and ethanol. In addition, an adaptation of this technique may be used to measure formate, the toxic metabolite of methanol, after esterification to methyl formate. Conversely, direct injection GC is the method of choice for ethylene glycol, because it has a higher boiling point and is not as amenable to headspace analysis. A modification of the GC procedure described in 2005 has the potential of combining both toxic alcohols in a single GLC analysis.[166] Assessment of ethylene glycol metabolites is a clinically useful method that allows the simultaneous determination of ethylene glycol and glycolic acid; such a method that is free from interference by propylene glycol (a diluent for parenteral drugs) or 2,3-butanediol (may be present in serum from some alcoholics) would be highly desirable.[130,167] Similar techniques are used to measure volatile alcohols in blood, serum, oral fluid, urine, other clinical specimens and postmortem specimens (eg, vitreous fluid, skeletal muscle).

Analgesics (Nonprescription)

Analgesics are substances that relieve pain without causing loss of consciousness. When used in excess, analgesics such as acetaminophen and salicylate can result in a toxic response.

Acetaminophen

Acetaminophen (*N*-acetyl-*p*-aminophenol) has analgesic and antipyretic actions. In common with the group of drugs referred to as nonsteroidal antiinflammatory drugs (NSAIDs; eg, aspirin, ibuprofen, indomethacin), the pharmacologic actions of acetaminophen are related to its competitive inhibition of cyclooxygenase (COX) enzymes. This results in decreased production of prostaglandins, which are important mediators of inflammation, pain (low to moderate), and fever.[168] Contrary to other NSAIDs, acetaminophen has very weak antiinflammatory activity—a consequence of its weak inhibition of peripheral tissue COX compared with that in the brain. In normal doses, acetaminophen is safe and effective, but it may cause severe hepatic toxicity or death when consumed in overdose quantities. Less frequently, nephrotoxicity with or without associated hepatotoxicity, also may occur.

Acetaminophen is normally metabolized in the liver to glucuronide (50% to 60%) and sulfate (≈30%) conjugates.[169] A smaller amount (≈10%) is metabolized by a cytochrome P450 mixed-function oxidase pathway that is thought to involve formation of a highly reactive intermediate (Fig. 41.2), *N*-acetyl-*p*-benzoquinone imine (NAPQI).[170] This intermediate normally undergoes electrophilic conjugation with glutathione and then subsequent transformation to cysteine

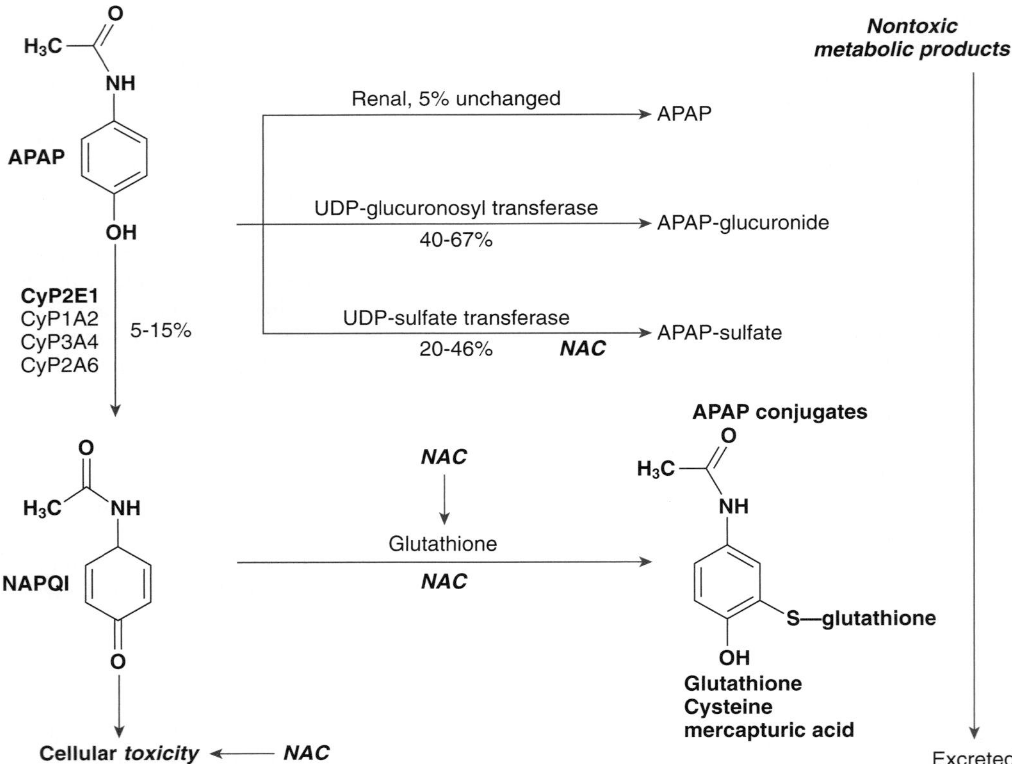

FIGURE 41.2 Pathways of acetaminophen metabolism APAP (*N*-acetyl-*p*-aminophenol/acetaminophen) NAPQI (*N*-acetyl-*p*-benzoquinone imine), NAC (*N*-acetyl-L-cysteine).

and mercapturic acid conjugates of acetaminophen. With acetaminophen overdose, the sulfation pathway becomes saturated; consequently, a greater portion is metabolized by the P450 mixed-function oxidase pathway. When the tissue stores of glutathione become depleted, arylation of cellular molecules by the benzoquinoneimine intermediate leads to hepatic necrosis.[170]

The initial clinical findings in acetaminophen toxicity can be absent of relatively mild and nonspecific symptoms (nausea, vomiting, and abdominal discomfort) and thus are not predictive of impending hepatic necrosis, which typically begins 24 to 36 hours after toxic ingestion and becomes most severe by 72 to 96 hours.[171] Although uncommon with severe overdose, coma and metabolic acidosis may occur before development of hepatic necrosis.[172]

Specific therapy for acetaminophen overdose is the administration of *N*-acetyl-L-cysteine (NAC), which probably acts as a glutathione substitute.[173] NAC may also provide substrate to replenish hepatic glutathione,[174] enhance sulfate conjugation,[175] or both. The time of administration of NAC is critical. Maximum efficacy is observed when NAC is administered within 8 hours, and efficacy declines with time; therefore it is most effective when administered before hepatic injury occurs, as signified by elevations of aspartate aminotransferase (AST) and alanine aminotransferase (ALT).[176] However, NAC treatment may provide beneficial effects even after liver injury has occurred, presumably through its ability to improve tissue oxygen delivery and use.[177]

The measurement of serum acetaminophen concentrations becomes paramount for proper assessment of the severity of overdose and for appropriate decision making for antidotal therapy. If serum acetaminophen results are not available locally within 8 hours of suspected ingestion, treatment with NAC should begin until levels are available. The Rumack-Matthew nomogram relates serum acetaminophen concentration and time after acute ingestion to the probability of hepatic necrosis (Fig. 41.3).[178]

Several qualifications pertain to the use of this nomogram. First, to use the nomogram, blood samples should not be obtained earlier than 4 hours after ingestion to ensure that absorption is complete. Second, the nomogram applies only to an acute single ingestion and not to chronic ingestion. Toxicity from chronic ingestion of acetaminophen or other drugs is cumulative and typically occurs at lower blood concentrations than in acute overdose. Third, the nomogram is not useful if the time of ingestion is unknown or is considered unreliable. In this case, when the exact time of ingestion is unknown, clinicians should err on the side of treating with NAC until the acetaminophen concentration is not detectable and no transaminase elevation is seen. Fourth, if acetaminophen is coingested with a substance that may delay absorption (ie, an anticholinergic agent), the patient should be clinically monitored for effects. If, for example, no anticholinergic signs or symptoms develop after the 4-hour acetaminophen concentration is measured, it may be assumed that absorption will not be delayed and the concentration can be plotted normally. If, however, the patient develops anticholinergic signs and symptoms, and the acetaminophen concentration is detectable, that patient should be treated with NAC because absorption is most likely delayed and the concentration should not be plotted. Fifth, alcoholic patients, fasting or malnourished patients, and patients on long-term

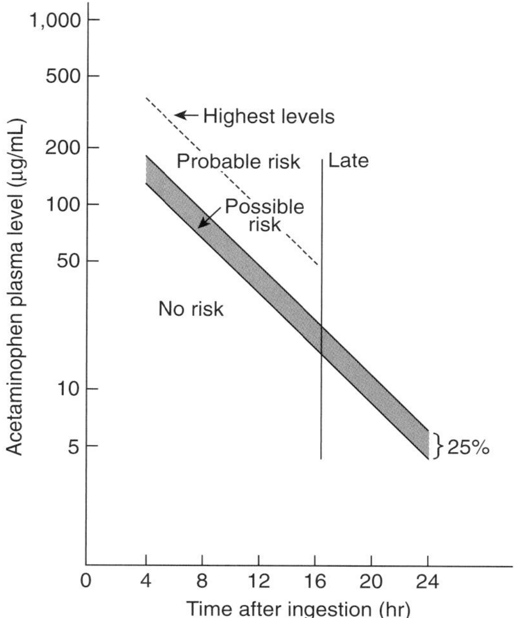

FIGURE 41.3 Rumack-Matthew nomogram. (From Rumack BA, Peterson RC, Koch GG, Amara IA. Acetaminophen overdose. 662 cases with evaluation of oral acetylcysteine treatment. *Arch Intern Med* 1981;141[3]:380–385.)

therapy with microsomal enzyme-inducing drugs (eg, phenobarbital) may have increased susceptibility to acetaminophen hepatotoxicity,[179-182] presumably as a result of induction of cytochrome P450 (see later) and, in the case of alcoholics or fasting patients, depletion of glutathione (see later). In these cases, it has been proposed that the decision line in the nomogram should be lowered by 50% to 70%.[181,183] Others do not advocate any change in the therapeutic decision line for such patients with acute ingestion. These risk factors may be more important in chronic acetaminophen poisoning. Although therapeutic guidelines for chronic acetaminophen poisoning have not been established, it is recommended to administer NAC if the transaminases are elevated or the acetaminophen level is greater than 10 µg/mL (66 µmol/L).[184] It is important to notice the units here are micrograms per milliliter and that care should be taken for this and any drug in interpreting quantitative results, because confusion may occur between mass and molar units, potentially resulting in adverse outcomes.

An area of some controversy is whether acetaminophen screening should be performed on all intentional overdose patients. One of the most worrisome aspects of acetaminophen poisoning is that initial clinical symptoms (eg, nausea, vomiting, abdominal pain) may be vague or even absent in the first 24 hours.[185] This possible delay in diagnosis is particularly problematic because the antidote, NAC, has been shown to be most effective when initiated within the first 8 hours.[176] Studies looking at the issue of universal acetaminophen screening recommend screening all patients with suicidal ingestion and those with altered mental status in whom ingestion is suspected.[186,187]

Analytical Methods. Many spectrophotometric methods are available for the determination of acetaminophen.[188,189] In general, these methods are relatively easy to perform but are subject to various interferences such as bilirubin or bilirubin by-products absorbing at similar wavelengths.[188,190] Some methods measure the nontoxic metabolites and parent acetaminophen and thus may produce especially misleading results. Therefore only methods specific for parent acetaminophen should be used.[191] Immunoassays are widely used for this purpose because they are rapid, easily performed, and accurate. A different spectrophotometric approach uses arylacylamide amidohydrolase to hydrolyze acetaminophen (but not conjugates) to *p*-aminophenol and acetate. Subsequent formation of the absorbing species depends on the reaction of generated *p*-aminophenol with 8-hydroxyquinoline[192] or o-cresol.[193] Arylacylamide amidohydrolase methods are susceptible to interference by NAC,[194] bilirubin, and immunoglobulin (Ig)M monoclonal immunoglobulins.[195] Most chromatographic methods are very accurate and are considered reference procedures.[196] A qualitative, one-step lateral flow immunoassay (cutoff of 25 μg/mL [165 μmol/L]) may be suitable for POC application, yet it has a low positive predictive value.[197]

Salicylate

Acetylsalicylic acid (aspirin) has analgesic, antipyretic, and antiinflammatory properties. These therapeutic benefits derive from its ability to inhibit biosynthesis of prostaglandins by acetylation of active site serine and subsequent irreversible inhibition of COX enzymes (COX-1; COX-2 isoenzymes).[168] Salicylate, the metabolite of aspirin, also reduces prostaglandin synthesis by uncertain mechanisms. Aspirin also interferes with platelet aggregation and thus prolongs bleeding time. The platelet inhibitory effect is a consequence of the ability of aspirin to acetylate and irreversibly inhibit platelet COX, thereby reducing the formation of thromboxane A_2, a potent mediator of platelet aggregation. Platelets have little or no capacity for protein synthesis; therefore the duration of this enzyme inhibition is the normal life span of the platelets (8 to 11 days).[198] Because of this platelet inhibitory activity, low-dose aspirin has been recommended as prophylactic therapy for some individuals at risk for thromboembolic disease.[199,200] An epidemiologic association has been noted between aspirin ingestion and Reye syndrome in children and adolescents with viral infection (eg, varicella, influenza).[201] Therefore aspirin use in these patients is done cautiously. However, because of the therapeutic benefits and the overall lack of serious side effects at normal doses in most patients, aspirin is widely available and frequently consumed.

Absorption of normal doses of regular aspirin from the gastrointestinal tract is generally rapid, with peak serum concentration achieved within 2 hours.[168] This peak value may be delayed for 12 hours or longer for enteric-coated or slow-release formulations.[202] Once absorbed, aspirin has a very short half-life ($t_{1/2}$ = 15 minutes) because of its rapid hydrolysis to salicylate. Salicylate is eliminated mainly by conjugation with glycine to form salicyluric acid and to a lesser extent with glucuronic acid to form phenol and acyl glucuronides.[203] A very small amount is hydroxylated to gentisic acid. These metabolic pathways may become saturated even at high therapeutic doses. Consequently, serum salicylate concentration may increase disproportionately with dosage. At high therapeutic or toxic doses, the salicylate elimination half-life is prolonged (15 to 30 hours vs. 2 to 3 hours at low dose) and a much larger portion of the dose is excreted in urine as salicylate.[168] Therapeutic serum salicylate concentrations are generally lower than 60 mg/L (0.4 mmol/L) for analgesic-antipyretic effects and 150 to 300 mg/L (1.1 mmol/L to 2.2 mmol/L) for antiinflammatory actions.[168]

Salicylates directly stimulate the central respiratory center and thereby cause hyperventilation and respiratory alkalosis. Additionally, salicylates cause uncoupling of oxidative phosphorylation. As a result, heat production (hyperthermia), oxygen consumption, and metabolic rate may be increased. Salicylates also enhance anaerobic glycolysis but inhibit the Krebs cycle and transaminase enzymes, which leads to accumulation of organic acids and thus to metabolic acidosis.[204]

The primary acid-base disturbance observed with salicylate overdosage depends on age and severity of intoxication. Respiratory alkalosis predominates in children over 4 years of age and in adults, except in very severe cases that may progress through a mixed respiratory alkalosis–metabolic acidosis to metabolic acidosis.[205] In children younger than age 4, the initial period of respiratory alkalosis may be brief and therefore may not be observed; in such cases, metabolic acidosis predominates.[204] CNS depression is more pronounced when acidemia is severe, which is a consequence of increased brain uptake of nonionized salicylic acid. Respiratory acidosis, a result of severe CNS depression or pulmonary edema, sometimes may occur and is indicative of a poor prognosis.

After acute salicylate overdose, patients initially may be asymptomatic, especially if that product is enteric coated. Salicylate-toxic patients may develop nausea, vomiting, abdominal pain, tinnitus, tachypnea, oliguria, and altered mental status ranging from agitation to lethargy to coma.[206] Toxic doses of aspirin may form concretions or bezoars and produce pylorospasm, thereby delaying absorption. Serum salicylate in such instances may not reach maximum concentration for 6 hours or longer.[207,208] Therefore a concentration drawn soon after the original ingestion may not be reflective of the potential peak concentration—an important consideration when assessment of the severity of toxicity is based on such measurements. Use of salicylate concentrations to guide management must be done cautiously and only in conjunction with careful evaluation of a patient's clinical status. Toxic concentrations alone are of poor prognostic value; however, certain clinical findings predict a poor prognosis, including pulmonary edema, fever, coma, and acidosis. Initial serial concentrations should be performed every 2 hours while the patient is monitored clinically. When the concentrations begin to decline and the patient's clinical status is improved, concentrations can be measured less frequently.

Interpretation of salicylate concentrations as a guide for clinical management decisions can be difficult. Perhaps the most well-known attempt at using salicylate concentrations to predict the severity of salicylate toxicity was the nomogram developed by Done.[207] After examining both the clinical symptoms and the salicylate concentrations in patients who had a single acute overdose, Done created a nomogram that predicts severity of poisoning based on the salicylate concentration drawn at a given time from ingestion. This tool has significant limitations, however. Because this nomogram as originally developed was based on only 38 pediatric patients, its utility for acute adult overdose is not known. One of the assumptions allowing the creation of this nomogram was that salicylates are eliminated by first-order kinetics. It has since been well established that some of the pathways for elimination of salicylates become saturated in overdose and follow zero-order kinetics.[209] One study demonstrated significant disagreement between the clinical severity predicted by the nomogram and the severity judged by physicians.[210] Therefore its use is not recommended for management of the salicylate-poisoned patient.

The need to screen all intentional overdose patients for salicylates is highly debated.[187,211,212] Diagnosis of salicylate poisoning based solely on clinical examination is not without pitfalls. Although large, acute ingestions are usually detected through history and clinical symptoms, whereas chronic salicylate toxicity often is more difficult to diagnose. Chronic intoxication can manifest in a fashion similar to that of acute exposures, yet such exposures typically are more insidious and therefore are often misdiagnosed.[208] In these cases, patients have presented with nonspecific symptoms such as fever, abdominal pain, and encephalopathy and subsequently been misdiagnosed with surgical abdomen, myocardial infarction, sepsis, encephalitis, and alcoholic ketoacidosis.[208,213-215]

Because products containing salicylates are readily available, the clinical effects of salicylate toxicity are nonspecific and lack of metabolic acidosis does not rule out the potential for salicylate toxicity; clinicians should have a low threshold for obtaining serum salicylate concentrations. Some suggest that in any patient with a history of salicylate ingestion or possessing characteristic signs or symptoms of salicylate poisoning, a serum salicylate concentration should be obtained. Early identification of salicylate toxicity can be lifesaving.

Treatment for salicylate intoxication is directed toward (1) decreasing further absorption, (2) increasing elimination, and (3) correcting acid-base and electrolyte disturbances. Activated charcoal binds aspirin and prevents its absorption. Elimination of salicylate may be enhanced by alkaline diuresis and in severe cases by hemodialysis.[204] Sodium bicarbonate may be given to alleviate metabolic acidosis. Indications for hemodialysis include serum salicylate value greater than 1000 mg/L (7.2 mmol/L), severe CNS changes, intractable metabolic acidosis, pulmonary edema, hepatic failure with coagulopathy, and renal failure.[216]

Analytical Methods. Classic methods for the measurement of salicylate in serum are based on the method of Trinder.[217] These procedures rely on the reaction between salicylate and Fe^{3+} to form a colored complex that is measured at 540 nm. To lessen endogenous background interference, a protein precipitation step or a serum blank is necessary. Nevertheless, blank readings equivalent to approximately 20 to 25 mg/L (0.1 mmol/L to 0.2 mmol/L) are generally observed. Moreover, interference by salicylate metabolites, endogenous compounds, and some drugs, especially structurally related drugs such as diflunisal (difluorophenyl salicylate),[218] may occur. Azide, present as a preservative in some commercial control sera, also causes interference. Despite these limitations, photometric methods continue to be successfully used to assess salicylate overdose. The Trinder method results agreed very closely with those of a reference HPLC procedure.[219] However, significant interference with the Trinder method was observed for one patient, who consumed an overdose of dichloralphenazone. Thus, for best interpretation of test results, as much information as possible should be obtained regarding drug ingestion history.

Other methods for salicylate quantitation include fluorescent polarization immunoassay[220] and salicylate hydroxylase–mediated photometric techniques.[221] These procedures are subject to some of the same interferences as the Trinder method, but the salicylate hydroxylase method is considered more specific[221] and has been adapted to automated analyzers. Gas and liquid chromatographic methods are the most specific methods for salicylate,[222,223] but their general availability, especially for emergency use, is limited. A qualitative, one-step lateral flow immunoassay (cutoff of 100 μg/mL [0.7 mmol/L]) is commercially available for POC application but has a low positive predictive value (0.47).[197]

The units reported with each concentration should be documented before management decisions are made. Laboratories may alternatively report concentrations in terms of milligrams per deciliter and milligrams per liter. This important distinction, which involves a 10-fold difference in concentration, is infamous for causing confusion. In extreme cases of these miscommunications, hemodialysis has been ordered for patients thought to have astronomically high salicylate concentrations that were later proved to be nontoxic.[224]

Agents Related to the Anticholinergic Toxidrome

TCAs, phenothiazines, and antihistamines have divergent therapeutic applications; however, in overdose, they often share similar anticholinergic and antihistaminic toxidromes as principal components of their overall toxic effects.

Tricyclic Antidepressants

TCAs, so named because of their three-ring structure (Fig. 41.4), represent a class of drugs frequently prescribed for the treatment of depression and neuropathic pain (see Chapter 40). The TCAs have been largely supplanted by the newer, less toxic selective serotonin reuptake inhibitors (SSRIs) and other atypical agents for depression, which now are accepted broadly as drugs of first choice, particularly for medically ill or potentially suicidal patients and for the elderly and the young.[225-229] Fatalities are much less common since modern antidepressants have widely replaced these drugs. However, because of their continued use and narrow therapeutic range, TCAs are frequently associated with severe or fatal toxicity after overdose.[230-232]

TCAs block neuronal uptake of serotonin and norepinephrine.[233] TCAs have many other pharmacologic actions that apparently do not contribute to the therapeutic effects but do contribute to the side effects. TCAs have at least moderate affinity for blockade of α_1-adrenergic receptors, much less for α_2, and virtually none for β-receptors,[234] leading to vasodilation and hypotension.[233] TCAs have sedative effects and potential for seizures related to antihistamine activity.[233] TCAs exert central and peripheral anticholinergic effects (dry skin and mouth, flushing, hyperpyrexia, dilated pupils, constipation, urinary retention, and decreased gastrointestinal motility) through their blockade of M1 muscarinic receptors,[233] TCAs inhibit GABA channels, resulting in an increased risk for seizures.

Cardiovascular effects, the most serious manifestation of TCA overdose, accounts for the majority of fatalities. Several mechanisms may contribute to cardiovascular toxicity, as follows[235]:

1. Anticholinergic effects and inhibition of neuronal reuptake of catecholamines result in tachycardia and potential for early hypertension.
2. Peripheral α-adrenergic blockade causes vasodilation and contributes to hypotension.
3. Cardiac fast sodium channel blockade and potassium efflux blockade result in QRS and QT prolongation,

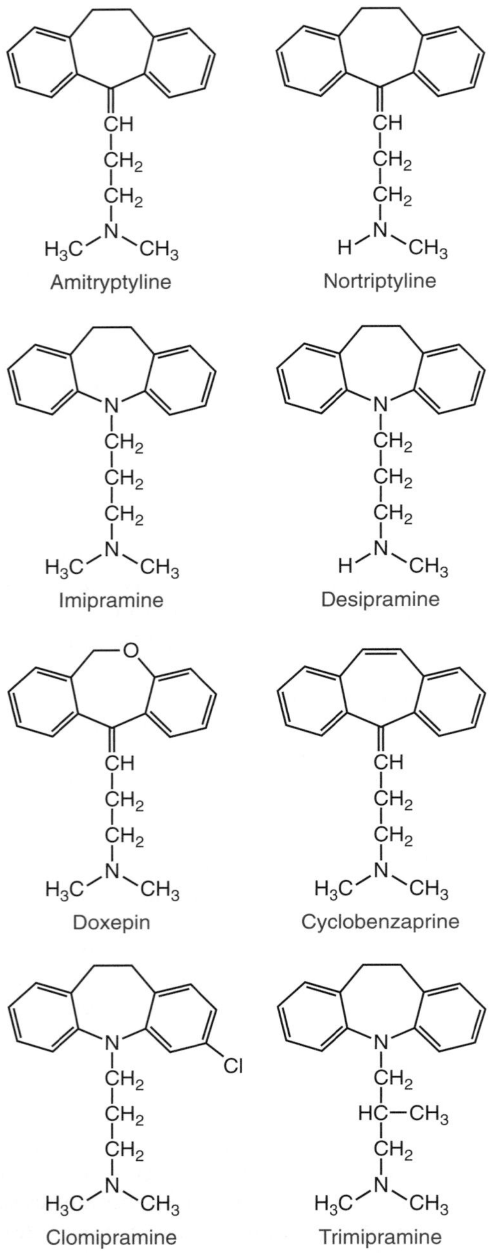

FIGURE 41.4 Structure of tricyclic antidepressants and related drugs.

respectively, and risk for decreased cardiac output and ventricular dysrhythmias.

4. Metabolic and/or respiratory acidosis that may further contribute to inhibiting the cardiac fast sodium channel.

Some tolerance to the sedative and autonomic effects of TCAs tends to develop with continued drug use.[234] Occasionally, patients show physical dependence, with malaise, chills, muscle aches, and sleep disturbance after abrupt discontinuation, particularly of high doses.[234] Some withdrawal effects may reflect increased cholinergic activity after its inhibition.[234] Some of these reactions have been confused with clinical worsening of depressive symptoms. Emergence of agitated or manic reactions has been observed after abrupt discontinuation of TCAs.[234]

In general, antidepressants are associated with several clinically important drug interactions (eg, serotonin syndrome),[236] and they potentiate the effects of alcohol and probably other sedatives.[234] TCAs are oxidized by hepatic cytochrome P450 microsomal enzymes, followed by conjugation with glucuronic acid.[234] The *N*-demethylated metabolites of several TCAs are pharmacologically active and may accumulate in concentrations approaching or exceeding those of the parent drug, to contribute variably to overall pharmacodynamic activity.

Analytical Methods. TCAs are measured by chromatographic or immunoassay methods. Immunoassays are rapid and relatively easy to perform but may be subject to interference by other drugs, such as chlorpromazine,[237] thioridazine,[238] cyclobenzaprine,[237] and diphenhydramine,[239] and are not able to necessarily identify which TCA is being quantitated. In cases of overdose, qualitative identification (serum or urine) is sufficient, because the severity of intoxication is more reliably indicated by an increase in the QRS interval than by the serum concentration.[240]

Cyclobenzaprine, a tricyclic amine structurally very similar to amitriptyline (see Fig. 41.4), is used as a centrally acting skeletal muscle relaxant. Similar to amitriptyline, cyclobenzaprine causes sedation, produces central and peripheral muscarinic blockade, and potentiates adrenergic actions. In overdose, cyclobenzaprine may cause a typical anticholinergic toxidrome and cardiac arrhythmias, hypotension, and coma. The analytical distinction between amitriptyline and cyclobenzaprine is often difficult. Cyclobenzaprine cross-reacts with immunoassays for TCAs and can coelute or comigrate with amitriptyline in HPLC and TLC. However, cyclobenzaprine and amitriptyline have different UV spectra; therefore they may be distinguished by HPLC using a diode array detector by multiwavelength scanning or dual-wavelength discrimination.[241,242] However, amitriptyline and cyclobenzaprine are well resolved using capillary column GC and may be distinguished by careful examination of their respective mass spectra.[243]

Antipsychotic Drugs

The antipsychotic drugs are generally used for primary psychiatric disorders such as (1) schizophrenia, (2) bipolar disorder, (3) schizoaffective disorder, and (4) psychotic depression. In addition to their psychotherapeutic effects, these drugs have a number of other actions, so that certain members of this group are used as antiemetics (prochlorperazine), as antihistaminics (promethazine),[244] and for sedation or potentiation of analgesia and general anesthesia.[234] Antipsychotic compounds are traditionally divided and subdivided according to their chemical structure (Table 41.5 and Fig. 41.5).[244,245]

The primary pharmacologic effect of all antipsychotic drugs is thought to be blockade of D_2 receptors in the CNS.[234,245,246] Studies show that classical antipsychotics reduce psychotic symptoms, and this correlates with their affinity for the D_2 receptor.[245] However, the drugs bind to many other receptors, including histamine (H_1, H_2), $GABA_A$, muscarinic receptors, α_1- and α_2-adrenoreceptors, and sodium and potassium voltage-gated ion channels.[247-250] The atypical antipsychotics on the other hand have a different mechanism that may involve other dopamine receptors, serotonin receptors, or both.[245]

TABLE 41.5 Examples of Classical and Atypical Antipsychotics

Antipsychotics	Examples[244,245,250,940]
Classical Antipsychotics	
Phenothiazines	Chlorpromazine
	Promethazine
	Trichlorperazine
	Perphenazine
	Fluphenazine
	Thioridazine
	Mesoridazine
	Trifluoperazine
Thioxanthines	Flupenthixol
	Zuclopenthixol
Dibenzoxazepine	Loxapine
Dihydroindoles	Molindone
Butyrophenones	Droperidol
	Haloperidol
Diphenylbutylpiperidines	Pimozide
Benzamides	Sulpiride
Atypical Antipsychotics	
Dibenzodiazepine derivatives	Clozapine
	Olanzapine
Benzothiazepine derivatives	Quetiapine
	Zotepine
Benzisoxazole derivatives	Risperidone
Benzoisthioazole piperazine	Ziprasidone
Imidazolindone derivatives	Sertindole

The principal manifestations of phenothiazine toxicity involve the CNS and the cardiovascular system.[234,251,252] The most common effects in significant phenothazine overdose include (1) sedation, (2) hypotension, (3) anticholinergic effects, and (4) ECG changes.[247,250] Phenothiazines are relatively safe and rarely cause death when ingested alone.

All of the neuroleptic drugs are metabolized in the liver. Many have active metabolites and complex metabolic pathways. The main enzymes involved in metabolism are cytochrome P450 enzymes, specifically CYP1A2, CYP2D6, and CYP3A4.[247,253,254] Many sources of variation are found in cytochrome P450–mediated metabolism; however, where multiple enzymes are involved, such variability has only a relatively small effect on clearance and drug concentrations.

Analytical Considerations. Toxicity is strongly correlated with peak serum concentrations and thus usually occurs within the first 4 to 6 hours after ingestion of these rapidly absorbed drugs.[250] Neuroleptics may be detected by chromatographic methods or by immunoassay. GC is the primary chromatographic method used to measure antipsychotic drugs, and nitrogen phosphorus, electron capture, and MS detectors are the detection systems of choice. However, HPLC, LC-MS, and LC-MS/MS methods are being used more commonly.

Antihistamines

Antihistamines are popular medications used by the general public for treatment of allergic reactions and as common sleep aids. Antihistamines are widely available, and many do not require a prescription.

Histamine is released from mast cells and plays an important physiologic role in immediate hypersensitivity and allergic responses. Histamine functions as a neurotransmitter in the CNS and stimulates gastric acid secretion. Antihistamine drugs currently available clinically antagonize H_1 and H_2 histamine receptors. First-generation lipophilic antihistamines, such as diphenhydramine (Benadryl), bind H_1 receptors and exhibit peripheral and CNS system effects; they also can bind to muscarinic and adrenergic receptors, resulting in their anticholinergic activity. H_1 and H_2 receptors are coupled via G-proteins to phospholipase C and adenylyl cyclase, respectively.[255] The principal H_2 receptor response is stimulation of gastric acid secretion, whereas other actions of histamine (eg, smooth muscle contraction, vasodilation, increased capillary permeability, pain, itching) are primarily mediated by H_1 receptors.

The broad binding affinities of H_1 receptor antagonists are attributed to a common substituted ethylene amine ($—CH_2CH_2NR_2—$) moiety found in H_1-receptor antagonists and in acetylcholine.[256] Second-generation antihistamines, such as fexofenadine (Allegra), are highly specific for peripheral H_1 receptors and do not penetrate the CNS. Therefore second-generation H_1-receptor antagonists display minimal sedative and anticholinergic effects.

The therapeutic actions of H_1 antagonists include (1) smooth muscle relaxation, (2) decreased bronchial secretions, (3) decreased allergic response, and (4) sedation. They are therefore used to treat immediate hypersensitivity reactions, as cold remedies, to suppress motion sickness, and for sedation. The H_2 antagonists are widely used to treat peptic ulcer disease. Overdose with first-generation H_1 antihistamines manifests clinically with CNS depression, stimulation, peripheral anticholinergic effects, and seizures.[255,257]

Analytical Considerations. Common clinically available antihistamines can be detected qualitatively and quantitatively in blood and urine specimens; this is done primarily by GC and MS or LC-MS/MS. Yet the clinical necessity of quantitative serum antihistamine concentrations is questionable. Poor correlation has been noted among patient age, dose, blood concentration, clinical effects, and death.[258-260] Antihistamines are detected by forensic laboratories as agents potentially used in facilitating sexual assault (see section "Drugs Used in Sexual Assault").

Although detection of antihistamines is not typically clinically relevant in the acutely toxic patient, it is important to note that very high concentrations of first-generation antihistamines, such as promethazine and diphenhydramine, have been documented to cross-react with urine drug immunoassay screen analyses. Therefore physicians and medical review officers should be aware of potential false-positive results from onsite drug testing devices, as well as immunoassay screens specifically documented in amphetamine,[261,262] propoxyphene,[263,264] and TCAs.[265-267]

Plants

Several plant and mushroom species contain antimuscarinic compounds that result in anticholinergic symptoms when ingested. These compounds are competitive antagonists at central and peripheral muscarinic receptors. Common centrally acting agents derived from plants are atropine and

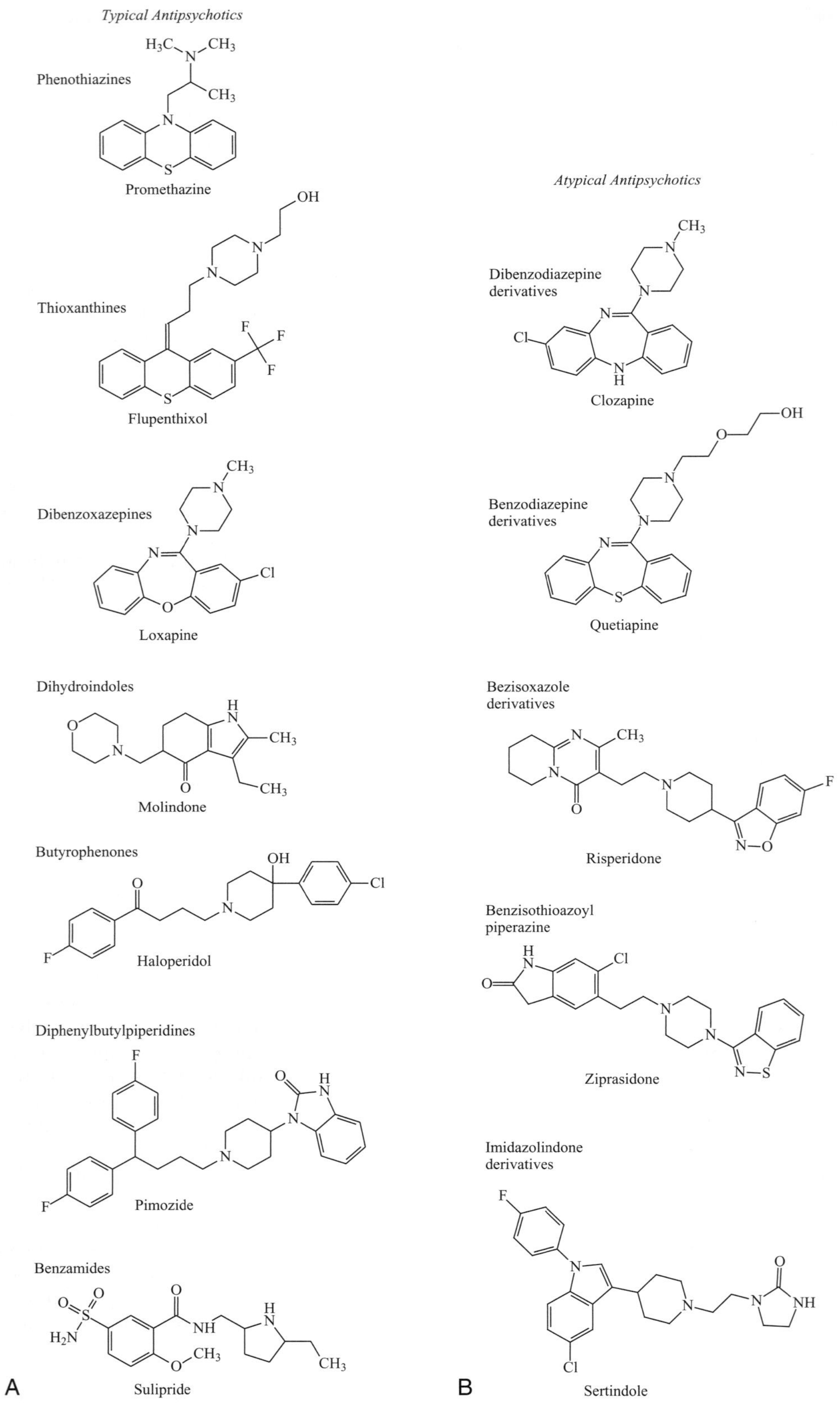

FIGURE 41.5 Classification and structure of select antipsychotic drugs.

scopolamine. These tropane alkaloid agents contain a tertiary amine structure permitting penetration of the CNS. These compounds have been isolated from numerous plants, such as *Atropa belladonna* (deadly nightshade) and *Datura stramonium* (Jimson weed), and are abused for their hallucinogenic potential. Patients are clinically managed on the basis of clinical presentation, rather than by identification of ingested plants or drug-specific testing.[268] Testing for atropine and scopolamine can be performed by LC-MS/MS and is available in some clinical laboratories. LC-MS/MS techniques are described to identify muscarine but are not readily available in clinical laboratories.[269]

Agents Related to Cholinergic Syndrome

Agents inducing cholinergic syndrome are diverse, but the commonality is their ability to produce uncontrolled acetylcholine transmission through inactivation of cholinesterase enzymes or direct stimulation of acetylcholine receptors. Acetylcholine is an essential neurotransmitter that affects parasympathetic synapses (autonomic and CNS), sympathetic preganglionic synapses, and the neuromuscular junction (see also previous section, "Toxic Syndromes" and Table 41.2). The duration of acetylcholine action is controlled by AChE and butyrylcholinesterase (pseudocholinesterase). AChE is found in red blood cells, nervous tissue, and skeletal muscle. Butyrylcholinesterase is found in plasma, liver, heart, pancreas, and brain. For more details the reader is referred to the cholinesterase section of Chapter 29 on serum enzymes.

Organophosphate and Carbamate Compounds

Organophosphate (eg, malathion, parathion, diazinon, chlorpyrifos [Dursban]) and carbamate (eg, Sevin, Furadan) insecticides (Fig. 41.6), as well as military nerve agents (eg, sarin [GB], soman [GD], tabun [GA], VX), exert their toxicity by inhibiting the action of AChE and thereby causing a pronounced cholinergic response.[17,270,271]

Organophosphate inhibition is a consequence of phosphorylation of the serine hydroxyl group at the active site of the cholinesterase enzyme catalytic triad (Ser-Glu-His). The partially electropositive phosphorus is attracted to the partially electronegative serine. Subsequent hydrolysis results in irreversible dealkylation ("aging") of the AChE.[272] Aging proceeds at variable rates depending on the size and branching of the alkyl groups (24 to 48 hours) to form a phosphoryl oxyanion serine bond that is completely resistant to even pharmacologically mediated hydrolysis.

Three neurologic sequelae of organophosphate poisoning may occur after the initial cholinergic crisis has responded to atropine and oxime therapy in what is referred to as intermediate syndrome.[273] Paralysis of proximal limb muscles, neck flexors, cranial nerves, and respiratory muscles may occur 24 to 96 hours after cholinergic resolution. Respiratory muscle paralysis may be severe enough to result in death. This phenomenon, caused by excessive nicotinic receptor stimulation, may result from redistribution of lipophilic organophosphates from adipose tissue or inadequate oxime therapy. In another syndrome, organophosphate-induced delayed neuropathy,[274] weakness of extremities, ataxia, and eventually paralysis may occur 1 to 3 weeks after severe intoxication. Respiratory muscles are not affected. It is believed that this peripheral neuropathy is the consequence of phosphorylation and inhibition of an axonal membrane enzyme that is designated neuropathy target esterase. Alternatively, phosphorylation and activation of a calcium (Ca^{2+})/calmodulin kinase may in turn enhance proteolysis of neuronal cytoskeletal proteins and cause structural changes in neurofilaments, resulting in impaired axonal transport.[274] Finally, extrapyramidal symptoms similar to those of Parkinson's disease have occurred very rarely several days after cholinergic crisis resolution. A favorable response was observed with an antiparkinsonian agent.[275]

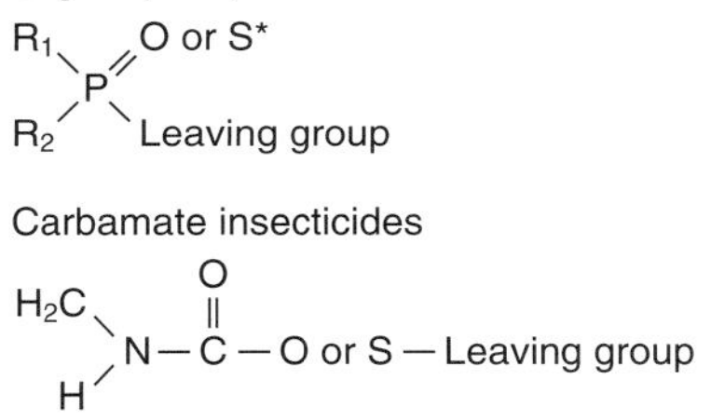

Organophosphate insecticides and nerve agents

R_1, R_2 — P (=O or S*) — Leaving group

Carbamate insecticides

H_3C–N(H)–C(=O)–O or S — Leaving group

FIGURE 41.6 General chemical structure for organophosphate, nerve gas, and carbamate insecticides.

Although carbamates are structurally different from organophosphates (see Fig. 41.6), carbamates exert their toxicity at the active site of AChE but inhibit enzyme activity through carbamylation rather than phosphorylation of the serine hydroxyl group. In contrast to the phosphoryl-serine bond, the carbamyl-serine bond undergoes spontaneous hydrolysis and regeneration of enzyme activity occurs in hours rather than days.[276] Carbamates exhibit poor CNS penetration and have a shorter duration of action; therefore neurotoxicity is usually less severe. Oximes are not recommended for carbamate toxicity and may exacerbate symptoms by stabilizing the carbamylation of AChE enzymes.[277]

Nerve agents are also organophosphorus inhibitors of AChEs, yet these agents are more potent than their pesticide counterparts.[278] Nerve agents share a similar structural backbone to that observed in organophosphate insecticides (see Fig. 41.6).

Excess synaptic acetylcholine stimulates muscarinic receptors (peripheral and CNS) and stimulates but then depresses or paralyzes nicotinic receptors. Activation of peripheral muscarinic receptors causes signs and symptoms described by the mnemonics SLUDGE or DUMB BELLS (see the section "Toxic Syndromes"). CNS neurotoxic effects include (1) restlessness, (2) agitation, (3) lethargy, (4) confusion, (5) slurred speech, (6) seizures, (7) coma, (8) cardiorespiratory depression, and (9) death. Stimulation or paralysis of nicotinic receptors at the neuromuscular junction causes muscle fasciculations, cramping, weakness, and respiratory muscle paralysis; stimulation of nicotinic receptors at sympathetic ganglia results in a sympathomimetic syndrome that includes hypertension, tachycardia, pallor, and mydriasis.

The actual signs and symptoms observed with these toxins depend on the balance of muscarinic and nicotinic receptor activation. Although miosis (muscarinic action) is most common, it may not always be present, and indeed mydriasis (nicotinic action) may occur. Likewise, tachycardia (nicotinic effect) may be present rather than bradycardia (muscarinic action). Death most commonly results from respiratory failure, a consequence of nicotinic receptor–mediated muscle paralysis, combined with muscarinic-facilitated bronchorrhea, bronchoconstriction, and intractable seizures that may be nonconvulsive because of paralysis.

Specific therapy for organophosphate and carbamate insecticide poisoning includes administration of atropine to block the muscarinic (but not nicotinic) actions of acetylcholine. In addition, pralidoxime is given to reactivate cholinesterase. Pralidoxime binds to the cholinesterase catalytic site and, through nucleophilic attack by its oxime group, dephosphorylates or decarbamylates the serine group. Administration of a site-directed nucleophile (pyridine-2-aldoxime chloride [2-PAM]) targets AChE reactivation during the transition state. Oxime antidotes such as 2-PAM contain a quaternary nitrogen that binds to the choline-binding site of AChE, positioning the oxime for nucleophilic attack, and by transferring the phosphoryl group from the serine hydroxyl group to itself, it releases free, active enzyme.[279,280] 2-PAM is not effective on aged AChE, so it must be administered as soon as possible after intoxication. Administration of pralidoxime may not be necessary in cases of carbamate insecticide poisoning because carbamylated cholinesterase spontaneously reactivates within a few hours. In fact, pralidoxime is considered contraindicated in these cases by some authors, because cholinesterase inhibition by carbaryl (Sevin), but not by other carbamates, may be enhanced by pralidoxime. Others administer pralidoxime in either case because the particular insecticide ingested may not be known.[17,271] A more potent bisquaternary oxime, obidoxime, is available outside the United States. Pralidoxime is ineffective in reactivating the "aged" form of the phosphorylated enzyme. Reactivation of aged AChE requires de novo cellular synthesis of enzyme (days).

Diagnosis of organophosphate and carbamate toxicity depends mainly on exposure history, physical presentation, clinical suspicion, and laboratory support. Treatment requires immediate attention and should not rely on laboratory confirmation. Yet cholinesterase activity is often monitored by clinicians in potential occupational exposure, after acute intentional and accidental exposure, and to determine response to therapy.

Cholinesterase activity is measured to assess exposure and to monitor reactivation during treatment. AChE and butyrylcholinesterase enzyme activity are typically monitored using Ellman colorimetric or Michel electrometric analyses using whole blood, plasma, serum, and dried blood spots.[281,282]

AChE activity present at nerve junctions is similar to that present in red blood cells and is an appropriate index of neurotoxicity.[283] This assay is more sensitive than serum cholinesterase activity and often is used to confirm exposure and to predict enzyme reactivation during treatment. A different cholinesterase, butyrylcholinesterase (pseudocholinesterase), is present in serum and is also inhibited by these insecticides. The activity of butyrylcholinesterase declines then returns to normal more rapidly than is observed for the red cell enzyme. Serum butyrylcholinesterase can be readily assessed on hemolyzed samples and in clinical laboratories without isolation of red blood cells. However, interindividual variability is high; therefore preexposure activities are optimal when butyrylcholinesterase activities are interpreted.[284] Because butyrylcholinesterases are synthesized in the liver, this assay is particularly sensitive to interferences such as pregnancy and liver disease (acute and chronic hepatitis, cirrhosis, malignancy).[285] Thus red cell cholinesterase activity theoretically should correlate more closely with the degree of neurotoxicity. In acute poisoning, symptoms generally begin when cholinesterase activity is inhibited by approximately 50% of the lower reference limits, and this degree of inhibition is of diagnostic value. However, the degree of cholinesterase inhibition generally does not correlate well with the clinical severity of poisoning. Interpretation of test results is made more difficult by considerable individual variability of normal activities (see also Cholinesterase section of Chapter 29 on Serum Enzymes). The presence of urinary organophosphate and carbamate metabolites is generally assessed by GC-MS[286] and GC-MS/MS.[287] These methods are labor intensive and are typically reserved for monitoring chronic occupational exposure to specific agents rather than for emergency management of acute toxicity.

Drugs of Abuse

Drug use and abuse are widespread in society, and public awareness has been heightened as to their impact on public safety and on lost productivity in industry. To resolve these issues, governmental, industrial, educational, and sports agencies are increasingly requiring drug testing of prospective and existing employees, students, and participants in professional and amateur athletics. Moreover, drug abuse during pregnancy is a matter of concern, both medically and socially.[288] Testing for drugs of abuse may be a medical requirement for (1) organ transplantation candidates, (2) pain management clinics, (3) drug abuse treatment programs, and (4) psychiatric programs.[289] Drug testing for these purposes represents a significant activity for toxicology laboratories.

Testing for drugs of abuse usually involves testing a single urine specimen for various drugs. It should be noted, however, that testing of a single random urine drug specimen detects only fairly recent drug use and it does not differentiate casual use from chronic drug abuse. The latter requires sequential drug testing and clinical evaluation. Moreover, urine drug testing alone cannot determine the degree of impairment, the dose of drug taken, or the exact time of use.[290,291] Because of these and other limitations of testing for drugs in urine, integrating the use of alternative biological specimens for drug testing is a matter of growing interest (see Chapter 43).

Amphetamine Type Stimulants

Several stimulants and hallucinogens chemically related to phenylethylamine are referred to collectively as amphetamine-type stimulants (ATSs). They are considered to be sympathomimetic drugs, meaning that they mimic endogenous transmitters in the sympathetic nervous system.[292]

Amphetamine and Methamphetamine. Amphetamine and methamphetamine (Fig. 41.7) are CNS stimulant drugs that have limited[293] legitimate pharmacologic use,[294] including in narcolepsy, obesity, and attention-deficit hyperactivity disorders. They produce an initial euphoria and have a high abuse potential. These drugs have a stimulating effect on both the central and peripheral nervous systems. In the brain, a primary action is to elevate the concentrations of extracellular monoamine neurotransmitters (dopamine, serotonin, norepinephrine) by promoting presynaptic release from the nerve endings.[295-297] Amphetamine and methamphetamine are substrates for the dopamine, serotonin, and norepinephrine transporters. Once in the cell, they interfere with the vesicular monoamine transporter and monoamine oxidase (MAO),[296,298] depleting synaptic vesicles of their

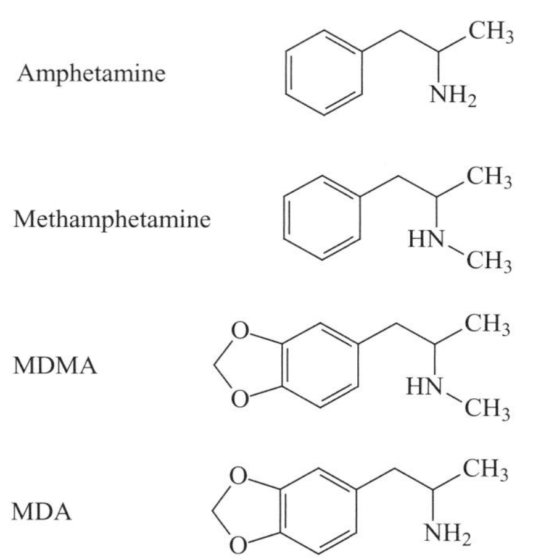

FIGURE 41.7 Select amphetamine-type stimulants. *MDA,* Methylenedioxyamphetamine; *MDMA,* methylenedioxymethamphetamine.

neurotransmitter content. As a consequence, concentrations of dopamine (or other transmitter amines) in the cytoplasm increase and quickly become sufficient to cause release into the synapse by reversal of the plasma membrane dopamine transporter (DAT). Normal vesicular release of dopamine consequently is decreased (because synaptic vesicles contain less transmitter), whereas nonvesicular release is increased. Similar mechanisms apply to other biogenic amines (serotonin and norepinephrine).[297,299]

Amphetamine cardiovascular activation is thought to be due to the release of norepinephrine from sympathetic nerve endings.[296] Stereotyped repetitive behavior and some aspects of locomotor activity induced by amphetamine probably are a consequence of the release of dopamine from dopaminergic nerve terminals, particularly in the neostriatum.[296] The anorectic effect and at least a component of its locomotor-stimulating action are mediated by release of norepinephrine.[296] With higher doses, dopamine release in the mesolimbic system and enhanced release of 5-hydroxytryptamine (5-HT; serotonin) in tryptaminergic neurons may be responsible for disturbances of perception and frank psychotic behavior.[296,300] High doses also lead to decreases in brain concentrations of the neurotransmitters dopamine and 5-HT, as well as a reduction in the activity of enzymes responsible for their synthesis (tyrosine dehydroxylase and tryptophan hydroxylase, respectively).[292]

Amphetamine and methamphetamine (1) increase blood pressure, heart rate, body temperature, and motor activity; (2) relax bronchial muscle; and (3) depress the appetite. Abuse of these drugs may lead to strong psychologic dependence, marked tolerance, and mild physical dependence associated with tachycardia, increased blood pressure, restlessness, irritability, insomnia, personality changes, and a severe form of chronic intoxication psychosis similar to schizophrenia. These unpleasant responses reinforce repetitive use of the drugs to maintain the "high." Tolerance and psychologic dependence develop with repeated use of amphetamines.[294] Long-term effects may include depression and impaired memory and motor skills, probably caused by a decrease in dopamine transporters and damage to dopaminergic and serotonergic neurons. Methamphetamine has greater CNS efficacy, most likely because of its greater ability to penetrate the CNS.[301]

The optical isomers of amphetamine and methamphetamine exhibit stereoselective pharmacologic properties. The CNS activity of S(+) amphetamine (D-amphetamine) is three to four times greater than that of R(−) amphetamine (L-amphetamine), but the latter drug has more potent cardiovascular effects than the former.[294,302] The CNS effects of S(+) methamphetamine (D-methamphetamine) are approximately 10 times greater than those of R(−) methamphetamine (L-methamphetamine), but the latter drug has greater vasoconstrictive properties than the former.[294,303] Because of minimal CNS activity and thus low abuse potential, R(−) methamphetamine is included in some nonprescription nasal inhalants (eg, Vick's) for its vasoconstrictive properties.

The main metabolic pathways of amphetamine and methamphetamine include (1) aromatic hydroxylation, (2) aliphatic hydroxylation, (3) *N*-demethylation, (4) oxidative deamination, (5) *N*-oxidation, and (6) conjugation of nitrogen.[304] Amphetamine itself is extensively metabolized to a variety of metabolites, including norephedrine and *p*-hydroxyamphetamine, both of which are pharmacologically active, and may be glucuronidated before excretion.[292] Amphetamine is metabolized in a stereoselective manner such that the elimination half-life for R(−) amphetamine may be as much as 40% longer than that for S(+) amphetamine.[305,306] Methamphetamine is metabolized in liver primarily by hydroxylation and, to a lesser extent, by *N*-demethylation to amphetamine. Overall metabolism, including formation of amphetamine, is enantioselective.[305,307] Thus, when racemic methamphetamine is ingested, urine specimens contain relatively more R(−) methamphetamine than S(+) methamphetamine, but a greater amount of S(+) amphetamine than R(−) amphetamine.[308,309]

In addition to hepatic metabolism, amphetamine is eliminated as unchanged drug in urine. Elimination is dependent on urine pH, and although typically approximately 30% of a dose is excreted unchanged, this may vary from as much as 74% in acidic urine to as little as 1% in alkaline urine.[302] Therefore elimination half-life (renal excretion and hepatic metabolism) also varies with urine pH from 7 to 14 hours at acidic pH to 18 to 34 hours at alkaline pH.[301] These effects of urine pH on the elimination of unchanged amphetamines are a consequence of tubular reabsorption of nonionized amphetamine (pK_a, 9.9). Methamphetamine is eliminated in urine in a pH-dependent manner similar to that for amphetamine.

Pharmacogenetics may play a role in the differences seen in the metabolism and elimination of these drugs. CYP2D6 is responsible for the 4-hydroxylation of amphetamine and methamphetamine and the *N*-demethylation of methamphetamine.[304,310-312] However, the effects of methamphetamine are not reliably predicted from serum concentrations.[313]

Designer Stimulants. The terms "designer drugs" and "club drugs" originated in the 1980s.[314] These drugs include phenylethylamine, benzylpiperazine, phenylpiperazine, pyrrolidinophenone, and cathinone and derivatives, and they have gained popularity and notoriety among people who participate in all-night dance parties (raves) and visit nightclubs.[315-317] Most designer drugs produce feelings of euphoria and energy and a desire to socialize[318]; they also promote social and physical interactions. They are used at these events to enhance energy for prolonged partying and/or dancing and to distort

BOX 41.2 Designer Drugs Related to Phenylethylamine, Benzylpiperazine, Phenylpiperazine, Pyrrolidinophenone, and Cathinone[317,328,923-926]

Phenylethylamines

3,4-Methylenedioxymethamphetamine (MDMA; ecstasy)
3,4-Methylenedioxyethylamphetamine (MDEA; "Eve")
3,4-Methylenedioxyamphetamine (MDA), which is also a metabolite of MDMA
Paramethoxyamphetamine (PMA)
Paramethoxymethamphetamine (PMMA)
2,5-Dimethoxy-4-methylamphetamine (DOM)
2,5-Dimethoxy-4-methylthioamphetamine (DOT)
4-Iodo-2,5-dimethoxyamphetamine (DOI)
2,5-Dimethoxy-4-bromo-amphetamine (DOB)
2,5-Dimethoxy-4-bromo-methamphetamine (MDOB)
3,4-(Methylenedioxyphenyl)-2-butanamine (BDB)
N-Methyl-1-(3,4-methylenedioxy-phenyl)-2-butanamine (MBDB)
6-Chloro-3,4-methylenedioxymethamphetamine (Cl-MDMA)
3,4-Methylenedioxymethcathinone
4-Bromo-2,5-diemethoxy-phenylethylamine (2C-B)
2,5-Dimethoxy-4ethylthio-phenylethylamine (2C-T-2)
2,5-Dimethoxy-4 propylthio-phenylethylamine (2C-T-7)

Benzylpiperazines

1-Benzylpiperazine (BZP)
1-(3,4-Methylenedioxybenzyl)-piperazine (MDBP)

Phenylpiperazines

1-(3-Trifluoromethylphenyl)piperazine (TFMPP)
1-(3-Chlorophenyl)piperazine (mCPP)
1-(4-Methoxyphenyl)piperazine (MeOPP)

Pyrrolidinophenone

α-Pyrrolidinopropiophenone (PPP)
4-Methoxy-α-pyrrolidinopropiophenone (MOPPP)
3,4-Methylenedioxy-α-pyrrolidinopropiophenone (MDPPP)
4-Methyl-α-pyrrolidinopropiophenone (MPPP)
4-Methyl-α-pyrrolidinohexanophenone (MPHP)

Cathinones

Beta-keto analogs of methamphetamine
- Methcathinone
- Mephedrone (4-MMC)
- Methylone (MDMC)
- Butylone (bk-MBDB)
- Ethylone
- 4-Methylethcathinone (4-MEC)
- 4-Fluoromethcathinone (3-FMC)
- 3-Fluoromethcathinone (4-FMC)
- Ethcathinone
- Methedrone
- Naphyrone

α-Pyrrolidinophenone-derived
- α-Pyrrolidinovalerophenone (α-PVP)
- α-Pyrrolidinopropiophenone (PPP)
- 4-Methoxy-α-pyrrolidinopropiophenone (MOPPP)
- 3,4-Methylenedioxy-α-pyrrolidinopropiophenone (MDPPP)
- 4-Methyl-α-pyrrolidinopropiophenone (MPPP)
- 4-Methyl-α-pyrrolidinohexanophenone (MPHP)
- 3,4-Methylenedioxypyrovalerone (MDPV)

or enhance visual and auditory sensations. The moniker "club drug" does not imply that recreational use is restricted to this social environment. In this context, designer drugs mistakenly have the reputation of being safe; several experimental studies in rats and humans and epidemiologic studies have revealed risks to humans such as life-threatening serotonin syndrome, hepatotoxicity, neurotoxicity, psychopathology, and the abuse potential of such drugs.[317-319]

Some of the more common designer amphetamines are listed in Box 41.2; however, only a few will be discussed here.

3,4-Methylenedioxymethamphetamine and 3,4-Methylenedioxyamphetamine. MDMA (also known as "ecstasy" and "molly") is categorized as a stimulant as a result of its sympathomimetic effects, including (1) peripheral vasoconstriction, (2) bronchodilation, (3) cardiorespiratory stimulation, (4) pupillary dilation, and (5) appetite suppression. The drug is a sympathomimetic; however, it has significantly fewer CNS stimulant properties than methamphetamine.[314] It also is categorized as an empathogen-entactogen.[314,320]

Similar to amphetamine and methamphetamine, MDMA causes release of biogenic amines by reversing the action of their respective transporters. It has a preferential affinity for the serotonin transporter and therefore most strongly increases the extracellular concentration of serotonin.[297] This release is so profound that marked presynaptic intracellular depletion occurs for 24 hours after a single dose. With repetitive administration, concentrations of 5-HT, 5-hydroxyindoleacetic acid (5-HIAA), tryptophan hydroxylase, and serotonin transporter density are reduced.[321] Some suggest that serotonin depletion may become permanent; this has triggered a debate on its neurotoxicity. Although direct proof from animal models for neurotoxicity remains weak, several studies have reported long-term cognitive impairment in heavy users of MDMA.[297]

MDMA is a chiral compound in which the S(+)-enantiomer possesses greater pharmacologic activity. MDMA undergoes demethylation to MDA,[322] with the rate of conversion of S(+)-MDMA to S(+)-MDA exceeding that of R(−)-MDMA to R(−)-MDA. Consequently, the concentrations in urine of R(−)-MDMA and S(+)-MDA are greater than those for S(+)-MDMA and R(−)-MDA subsequent to ingestion of racemic MDMA.[323,324]

MDMA is *N*-demethylated in humans to MDA, by CYP1A2 and CYP2D6.[314] Although extensive and poor MDMA metabolizers have been identified, the contribution of these polymorphisms to MDMA toxicity is unclear, because the metabolism may be saturable even at normal doses, resulting in greater dose-proportional excretion of the parent drug.[325] The saturable kinetics does, however, suggest that beyond a certain threshold, small increases in dose may result in larger increases in plasma concentration and consequently greater risk for toxicity.[314]

3,4-Methylenedioxyethylamphetamine. Methylenedioxyethylamphetamine (MDEA) is an empathogen-entactogen drug of the phenethylamine family that produces distinctive emotional and social effects similar to those of MDMA. On the street, it is known as "love." MDEA undergoes oxidative cleavage of the methoxy rings but also

N-deethylation.[304,326] MDEA undergoes deethylation to MDA, with the rate of conversion of S(+)-MDEA to S(+)-MDA exceeding that of R(−)-MDEA to R(—)-MDA.[327]

The MDEA enantiomers have different pharmacokinetic properties. They include *S*-MDEA, which produces elevated mood and impairment in conceptually driven cognition, and *R*-MDEA, which produces increased depression and enhanced visual feature processing[327]; a generally higher affinity toward *S*-MDEA than *R*-MDEA is seen.[327]

Paramethoxyamphetamine and Paramethoxymethamphetamine. Paramethoxyamphetamine (PMA) and paramethoxymethamphetamine (PMMA) are methoxylated phenylethylamine derivatives with effects similar to but more potent than those of MDMA; they are frequently sold on this basis.[328] PMA is a metabolite of PMMA,[329] but it is also an especially toxic designer amphetamine that has resulted in several deaths from its unsuspected ingestion as an ecstasy substitute.[330]

PMA is 10 times more active than MDMA in elevating brain serotonin concentrations and inhibiting serotonin uptake, but it has only a few effects on the dopamine system.[331-334] Inhibition of MAO A is a further pharmacologic property of PMA.[335] These pharmacologic properties are thought by some to be responsible for the higher rate of death seen with PMA compared with other substituted amphetamines.[336] Multiple deaths have been associated with its use; symptoms usually mimic serotonin syndrome and include hyperthermia, tachycardia, seizures, cardiac dysrhythmias, and coma.[337-339]

Cathinone and Derivatives. Cathinones are β-ketoamphetamines with structural similarity to those of dopamine, methamphetamine, MDMA, and pyrovalerone. Cathinone is a naturally occurring stimulant found in the leaves of the Khat plant *(Catha edulis)*. Synthetic derivatives of cathinone emerged as drugs of abuse in approximately 2003 and were sold on the internet and in head shops, smoke shops, and gas stations as "bath salts" and labeled as "not for human consumption." These compounds are frequently insufflated (snorted), but other routes of administration are also reported. As new designer cathinone derivatives are produced by clandestine laboratories, the US government attempts to schedule as many of these drugs as possible (Synthetic Drug Abuse Prevention Act of 2012, Synthetic Cathinones Control Act of 2013). The race continues to schedule synthetic drugs with high abuse potential and no known medicinal value. The more common cathinones are listed in Box 41.2. Cathinone derivatives are abused because of their psychostimulant and hallucinatory effects, but they also have been involved with human toxicity and fatality. Cathinones block dopamine and serotonin neurotransmitter reuptake, thereby prolonging the effects at peripheral and central neural junctions.[340] Common clinical presentations in patients are agitation, paranoia, auditory and tactile hallucinations, psychosis, myoclonus, and headaches. These symptoms can be severe and last for several days. Peripheral effects may include hyperthermia, hypertension, tachycardia, hyponatremia, nausea, vomiting, and chest pain, as seen during sympathomimetic toxidrome.

Ephedrine and Pseudoephedrine. Ephedrine and pseudoephedrine amines are diastereoisomers that possess two asymmetric carbon atoms and exist as four isomers designated as 1R,2S- and 1S,2R-ephedrine and 1R,2R- and 1S,2S-pseudoephedrine.[341] The 1R,2S-ephedrine (ephedrine) and 1S,2S-pseudoephedrine (pseudoephedrine) isomers occur naturally in various plants of the *Ephedra* genus.

Ephedrine and pseudoephedrine have been used as nasal decongestants, bronchodilators, and CNS stimulants and for treatment of obesity.[296,342] Ephedrine is both an α- and a β-adrenergic receptor agonist; in addition, it enhances the release of norepinephrine from sympathetic neurons and is considered a mixed-acting sympathomimetic drug.[296] Many dietary supplements contain ephedra, the herbal form of ephedrine. These products are widely marketed for energy enhancement or weight loss[343,344] and are used by some athletes to enhance performance. Adverse effects such as hypertension, tremors, myocardial infarction, seizures, and stroke have resulted in fatalities.[345-347] Because of this, the US Food and Drug Administration (FDA) banned the sale of dietary supplements containing ephedra in 2004.[296] However, herbal products containing ephedra remain in use in other countries.

Pseudoephedrine is used primarily as a decongestant because of its vasoconstrictive properties (α-adrenergic action).[348] Pseudoephedrine is used as a nasal decongestant and precursor for the illicit synthesis of methamphetamine. Because of this, the quantity per purchase of products containing these drugs is now restricted in many places.

Phenylpropanolamine. Phenylpropanolamine (PPA) was widely available in a number of nonprescription cold medications and diet control products. Adverse effects are similar to those described for ephedrine. In response to an FDA warning of increased risk for hemorrhagic stroke, especially in women, PPA has been withdrawn from the market by most manufacturers.[349] PPA is also a metabolite of ephedrine and pseudoephedrine.[344,348]

Phentermine. Phentermine is a sympathomimetic amine with less sympathomimetic and CNS stimulant activity than amphetamine.[302,350] Phentermine is currently approved for use as an anorectic agent.[351] The exact mechanism of action in treating obesity is not yet established, although it may involve other CNS actions or metabolic effects. However, because of its stimulant effects it can increase blood pressure.[350]

Methylphenidate (Ritalin). Methylphenidate (MPH) is a phenethylamine derivative with psychostimulant properties similar to those of S(+) amphetamine. It is commonly used to treat attention-deficit hyperactivity disorder and narcolepsy.[297,352] Its pharmacologic properties are essentially the same as those of the amphetamines.[296] Like many of its related amphetamine-type stimulants, it exists as an isomer, as (R,R)-methylphenidate (D-MPH), and as (S,S)-methylphenidate (L-MPH).[353] The pharmacologic actions of MPH are almost solely performed by the D-isomer.[353] Methylphenidate is rapidly metabolized, favoring L-MPH over D-MPH,[353] such that the more potent D-MPH has a half-life of approximately 6 hours and the less potent L-MPH has a half-life of approximately 4 hours.[296] Diversion and abuse of methylphenidate have been increasing among children and adults because of its stimulant and purported aphrodisiac properties. In overdose, the clinical effects of methylphenidate are similar to those of amphetamine and produce signs of generalized CNS stimulation that may lead to seizures.[297]

Analytical Methods for Amphetamine-Type Stimulants. The initial screening test for amphetamines and related drugs is typically immunoassay. For confirmation of a presumptive positive test, a quantitative drug measurement is commonly performed using GC-MS or LC-MS/MS.

Immunoassay. Most amphetamine immunoassays have been designed to detect amphetamine/methamphetamine; others have been designed to detect MDMA and MDA; and others to more broadly capture the ATS group—all with varying cross-reactivities.[354,355] Many older immunoassays lacked the ability to distinguish between the isoforms.[356] Currently, many use antibodies specific for S(+) amphetamine (D-amphetamine) and/or S(+) methamphetamine (D-methamphetamine). The degree of cross-reactivity of these antibodies varies, with antibodies raised to immunogenic protein (hapten) linked to the amphetamine molecule through the phenyl ring having better cross-reactivity than those linked through the side-chain.[314]

Not all amphetamine immunoassays were suitable for detection of the amphetamine-derived designer drugs PMA, PMMA, and MDEA[357-360] and especially not for the cathinone- and piperazine-derived substances.[361,362] Alternatively, other chemically related compounds such as pseudoephedrine and phentermine have been shown to produce positive results.[363] Additionally, many psychotropic medications have been reported to interfere with immunoassays.[301,364] Immunoassays from different manufacturers can have very different interference profiles, which the pathologist and the laboratory scientist must understand and relay to clinicians.

Regarding methylphenidate, it should be noted that its detection by urine drug immunoassay is problematic because it does not cross-react well with amphetamine immunoassays; detection of the parent drug is made difficult by its generally low concentration; and ritalinic acid, present in much higher concentration, is difficult to extract and analyze by GC; it is unstable upon storage even when frozen.[352]

Confirmatory Methods. All positive immunoassay results should be confirmed by a second independent method, but what may be more significant is that if other designer amphetamines (see Box 41.2) are suspected, a negative immunoassay screen cannot rule out the presence of these drugs. Fortunately, numerous GC- and LC-based methods for identification and quantitation of these drugs in biological samples have been put forth.[365-367]

Amphetamine-type stimulants are considered volatile and are lost during a dry-down or evaporation step, if this is part of the procedure. This loss is avoided by the addition of a small amount of hydrochloric acid during the evaporation step, or the addition of a less volatile "keeper" solvent such as dimethylformamide (DMF).[292] Also, because of their extreme volatility at the high temperatures encountered in GC-MS, derivatization before analysis lowers the limit of detection. Although many derivatives are available for GC-MS use, the most commonly used include heptafluorobutyric anhydride (HFBA), pentafluoropropionic anhydride (PFPA), trifluoroacetic anhydride (TFAA), and 4-carbethoxyhexfluorobutyryl chloride (4-CB). However, the 4-CB derivative in the presence of ephedrine or pseudoephedrine may generate methamphetamine,[368] which leads to the US Department of Health and Human Services rule to have amphetamine also detected to report a positive methamphetamine result.[301]

Methamphetamine is a prototypical basic drug (pK_a 9.9) that is readily extracted from biological material into organic solvents at alkaline pH. It is readily soluble in chloroform, *N*-butyl chloride, ethyl acetate, and diethyl ether and is extracted in most common protocols designed to isolate alkaloidal and basic drugs. It also readily extracts back into acid and back into organic solvents without significant loss.[292] Most published methods for analysis of members of the amphetamine class in urine, plasma, and blood use liquid-liquid extraction (LLE) or solid-phase extraction (SPE).[314]

Methamphetamine is readily analyzed by GC; this is the most popular method in use today for analysis of methamphetamine in biological material. Its poor UV absorption properties make it an unsuitable candidate for HPLC with UV detection, and it has no native fluorescence and no significant oxidative electrochemical properties at low voltages.[292] LC may be used for MDMA analysis and offers an advantage over GC in that MDMA and its polar metabolites can be quantified simultaneously without derivatization.[314]

The molecular weight of methamphetamine, the low intensity of its mass fragments in electron impact mode, and the structural similarity of many endogenous and exogenous compounds result in its mass spectrum not being highly characteristic.[292] The issue of lack of specificity of the methamphetamine mass spectrum is resolved by derivatization.[369] Many methods have been published for analysis of amphetamine, methamphetamine, and related compounds.[292,314,324,370-374]

Unfortunately, routine GC-MS also does not distinguish between the two isomers and necessitates the use of chiral chromatography to differentiate between them. Chiral discrimination of methamphetamine isomers may be necessary to distinguish the use of nonprescription nasal inhalants [R(−) methamphetamine] from the illicit use of methamphetamine [S(+) and R(−)] or other prescription medications, as indicated in Table 41.6. Some immunoassays have high specificity for S(+)isoforms. However, definitive enantiodiscrimination requires the use of a chiral derivatization reagent conventional GC-MS[393,308,375,376] or possibly chiral separation by LC-MS or LC-MS/MS. Also, care must be taken in interpreting the results. Several other prescription drugs available metabolized to amphetamine and/or methamphetamine are listed in Table 41.6. A careful review of the patient's prescription history and understanding of metabolic patterns will prevent misinterpretation as "street amphetamine" use.

Regarding methylphenidate, its confirmation by GC-MS is complicated by the fact that it does not form a stable *N,O*-di-trimethylsilyl derivative. However, after sequential reactions with MSTFA (*N*-methyl-*N*-[trimethylsilyl]trifluoroacetamide) and MBTFA (*N*-methyl-bis [trifluoroacetamide])

TABLE 41.6 Prescription Drugs That Are Metabolized to Amphetamine or Methamphetamine

Brand Name	Drug Name	Compounds Detected[292, 302, 941-943]
Adderall	Amphetamine	Amphetamine
Dexedrine	D-Amphetamine	D-Amphetamine
Desoxyn	D-Methamphetamine	D-Methamphetamine
Deprenyl	Selegiline	L-Methamphetamine L-Amphetamine
Vyvanse	Lisdexamfetamine	Amphetamine
Didrex	Benzphetamine	Methamphetamine Amphetamine

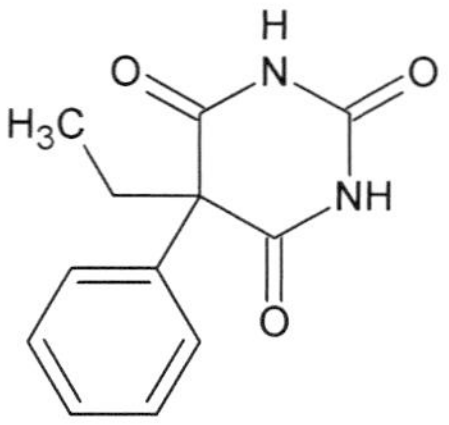

FIGURE 41.8 Structure of phenobarbital.

to form the *N*-trifluoroacetyl, *O*-trimethylsilyl ester,[377] it is possible to measure methylphenidate by GC-MS. Ritalinic acid may be isolated from urine using a dehydration procedure, then methylated with dimethylformamide dimethyl acetal, and the resulting methylphenidate analyzed by GC-MS. Finally, ritalinic acid may be analyzed directly by LC-MS/MS[378] or GC-MS, after sequential reactions with MSTFA and MBTFA to form the *N*-trifluoroacetyl, *O*-trimethylsilyl ester[377] or after methylation to re-form methylphenidate.

Barbiturates

Since antiquity, alcoholic beverages and potions containing laudanum (an alcoholic herbal preparation containing opium) and various herbals have been used to induce sleep. In the middle of the nineteenth century, bromide was the first agent to be introduced specifically as a sedative-hypnotic. The success of barbital in 1903 and phenobarbital (Fig. 41.8) in 1912[379] spawned the synthesis and testing of more than 2500 barbiturate derivatives, of which approximately 50 were distributed commercially. Today, approximately a dozen are in medical use. The barbiturates were so dominant that fewer than a dozen other sedative-hypnotics were marketed successfully before 1960.

The anxiolytic properties of the barbiturates are less than those exerted by the benzodiazepines.[379] Because of their low therapeutic index and high potential for abuse, they have been largely replaced by the much safer benzodiazepines. Phenobarbital is effective as an anticonvulsant drug (see Chapter 40), and short- and ultra-short-acting barbiturates are used for intravenous anesthesia. The classification of barbiturates as "ultra-short-acting," "short-acting," "intermediate-acting" and "long-acting" refers to the duration of effect and not to the elimination half-life (Table 41.7). The duration of action is determined by the rate of distribution into the brain and subsequent redistribution to other tissues.[379] Anesthetic doses of barbiturates, such as pentobarbital, are used to reduce intracranial pressure from cerebral edema associated with head trauma, surgery, or cerebral ischemia.[380] Therefore appropriate analytical methods are necessary to monitor serum pentobarbital concentrations in these circumstances.

Barbiturates continue to be, although much less frequently than in the past, subject to abuse. Because of their rapid onset and short duration of action, the short- to intermediate-acting barbiturates that are used as sedative-hypnotics (amobarbital, butabarbital, butalbital, pentobarbital, and secobarbital) are most commonly abused. The longer acting barbiturates (mephobarbital and phenobarbital), used primarily for their anticonvulsant properties, are rarely abused. The detection period in urine after ingestion of barbiturates varies with different assays and depends on the pharmacologic properties of the drugs. Short- to intermediate-acting barbiturates generally may be detected for 1 to 4 days after

TABLE 41.7 Half-Life and Significant Active Metabolites of Select Barbiturates

Drug	Half-Life[944]	Active Metabolite[944]
Ultra-Short-Acting		
Thiopental	6–46 h	Pentobarbital
Methohexital	1.2–2.1 h	
Thiamylal	0.6–0.8 h initial 12–34 h terminal	
Short-Acting and Intermediate-Acting		
Pentobarbital	15–48 h	
Secobarbital	22–29 h	
Butalbital	35–88 h	
Aprobarbital	14–34 h	
Amobarbital	15–40 h (dose dependent)	
Butabarbital	34–42 h	
Long-Acting		
Phenobarbital	2–6 d	
Mephobarbital	48–52 h	Phenobarbital

use; long-acting barbiturates, such as phenobarbital, may be detected for several weeks after long-term use.[381]

Barbiturates act throughout the CNS; nonanesthetic doses preferentially suppress polysynaptic responses, suppress CNS neuronal activity, and thus have sedative and hypnotic properties.[382] The site of inhibition occurs primarily at synapses where neurotransmission is mediated by GABA acting at $GABA_A$ receptors. This CNS suppression is a result of barbiturate-enhanced activation of the inhibitory GABAergic neuronal system.[379] Postsynatic $GABA_A$ receptors are multisubunit transmembrane chloride conductance channels that when activated by GABA open to allow flow of chloride into the neuron, with subsequent hyperpolarization and inhibition of electrical transmission. High doses of barbiturates increase neural chloride conductance independent of GABA.[379] Mechanisms underlying the actions of barbiturates on $GABA_A$ receptors appear to be distinct from those of GABA or the benzodiazepines, and they promote the binding of benzodiazepines.[379,383] In addition, barbiturates suppress excitatory glutamate-responsive AMPA ion-gated receptor subtypes. Taken together, the findings that barbiturates activate inhibitory $GABA_A$ receptors and inhibit excitatory AMPA receptors explain their CNS-depressant effects.[384]

The barbiturates produce varying degrees of CNS depression, ranging from mild sedation to general anesthesia. Barbiturates reversibly depress the activity of all excitable tissues. The CNS is exquisitely sensitive, and even when barbiturates are given in anesthetic concentrations, direct effects on peripheral excitable tissues are weak. However, serious deficits in cardiovascular and other peripheral functions occur in acute barbiturate intoxication.[379] Severe intoxication results in coma, hypothermia, hypotension, and cardiorespiratory arrest.[379] Pharmacodynamic (functional) and pharmacokinetic tolerance to barbiturates can occur. With long-term administration of gradually increasing doses, pharmacodynamic tolerance continues to develop over a period of weeks to months, depending on the dosage schedule, whereas pharmacokinetic tolerance reaches its peak in a few days to a week.

Tolerance to effects on mood, sedation, and hypnosis occurs more readily and is greater than tolerance to anticonvulsant and lethal effects; thus, as tolerance increases, the therapeutic index decreases.[379]

The barbiturates undergo extensive hepatic metabolism. The metabolic elimination of barbiturates is more rapid in young people than in the elderly and in infants, and half-lives are increased during pregnancy in part because of the expanded volume of distribution. Chronic liver disease, especially cirrhosis, often increases the half-life of the biotransformable barbiturates. Repeated administration, especially of phenobarbital, shortens the half-life of barbiturates that are metabolized as a result of induction of microsomal enzymes.[379] Oxidation of radicals at C5 is the most important biotransformation that terminates biological activity.[379] Oxidation results in the formation of alcohols, ketones, phenols, or carboxylic acids, which may appear in the urine as such or as glucuronic acid conjugates.[379] For phenobarbital and amobarbital, *N*-glycosylation is an important metabolic pathway. Other biotransformations include *N*-hydroxylation, desulfuration of thiobarbiturates to oxybarbiturates, opening of the barbituric acid ring, and *N*-dealkylation of *N*-alkylbarbiturates to active metabolites (eg, mephobarbital to phenobarbital). Except for the less lipid-soluble aprobarbital and phenobarbital, nearly complete metabolism and/or conjugation of barbiturates in the liver precedes their renal excretion.[379] As a result, only a relatively small amount of an administered barbiturate dose is excreted in urine as a parent drug; notable exceptions are phenobarbital and aprobarbital. Approximately 25% of phenobarbital and nearly all of aprobarbital is excreted unchanged in the urine. The renal excretion can be increased greatly by osmotic diuresis and/or alkalinization of urine.[379] Nevertheless, the parent drugs, rather than hydroxy or carboxylic acid metabolites, are targeted for detection in urine screening and confirmation procedures. This analytical approach is generally successful for barbiturates because these drugs are ingested in sufficiently high doses to allow detection of unmetabolized drug in urine.

Analytical Methods

Screening. Numerous commercial immunoassays for barbiturates are available. Most use antibodies directed toward secobarbital, and although the degree of cross-reactivity of other barbiturates varies with each assay, most have sufficient cross-reactivity to detect the major therapeutically used barbiturates.[385,386]

Confirmation Testing. Numerous confirmation methods for barbiturates have been described. These include GC with flame ionization detection,[387-389] nitrogen phosphorus detection[390] and MS,[391-397] capillary electrophoresis-UV,[398-400] LC using UV (LC-UV) detection,[401,402] LC-MS,[403,404] and MS.[405] GC-MS has merits attributable to high resolution and precise retention times with sharp peaks; however, the detection limit of GC-MS for barbiturates is compromised by adsorption at its NH group.[406] To overcome this problem, derivatization before injection is widely used, but this procedure is time-consuming.[391,395,397] On-column methylation is a rapid and sensitive method,[390] but phenobarbital cannot be distinguished from mephobarbital after methylation.

Benzodiazepines

Benzodiazepines are any of a group of compounds having a common molecular structure and acting similarly as depressants of the CNS. The term *benzodiazepine* refers to the portion of the structure composed of a benzene ring fused to a seven-membered diazepine ring and a phenyl ring attached to the five position of the diazepine ring.[379,385] The prototype benzodiazepines are diazepam and nordiazepam (*N*-desmethyl diazepam) (Fig. 41.9). The most common benzodiazepines in medical use are listed in Table 41.8.

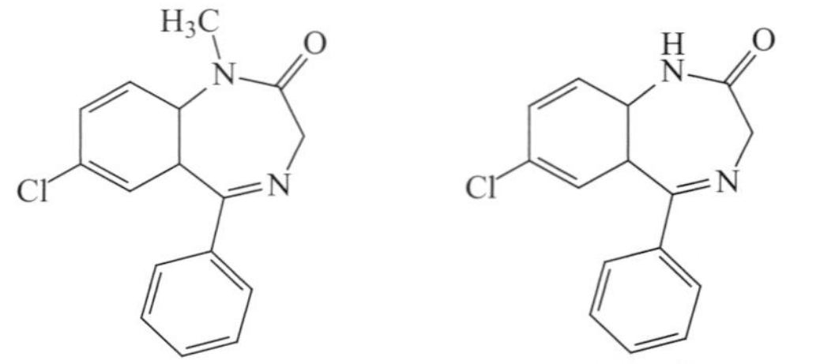

A Diazepam B Nordiazepam

FIGURE 41.9 Structure of **(A)** diazepam and **(B)** nordiazepam.

TABLE 41.8 Half-Life of Select Benzodiazepines

Drug	Half-Life (h)[944]	Significant Phase I Metabolites[944]
Short-Acting		
Midazolam	1–4	α-Hydroxy-midazolam
Estazolam	10–24	3-Hydroxy-estazolam
Flurazepam	1–3	Hydroxy-ethyl-flurazepam
	47–100 (*N*-desalkyl-flurazepam)	*N*-desalkyl-flurazepam*
Temazepam	3–13	Oxazepam
Triazolam	1.8–3.9	α-Hydroxy-triazolam
Intermediate-Acting		
Flunitrazepam†	9–25	7-Amino-flunitrazepam
Long-Acting Agents		
Diazepam	21–37	Nordiazepam* Oxazepam* Temazepam*
Quazepam	39–53	3-Hydroxy-quazepam *N*-Desalkyl-2-oxo-quazepam 2-Oxo-3-hydroxy-quazepam
Alprazolam	6–27	α-Hydroxy-alprazolam
Chlordiazepoxide	6–27	Nordiazepam* Oxazepam*
Clonazepam	19–60	7-Amino-clonazepam
Clorazepate‡	2	Nordiazepam*
	31–97 (nordiazepam)	Oxazepam*
Lorazepam	9–16	
Oxazepam	4–11	

*Active metabolite.
†Not available in the United States.
‡Converted to nordiazepam by gastric HCl.

Pharmacologic Response. As a class of drugs, benzodiazepines are among the most commonly prescribed drugs in the Western hemisphere because of their (1) efficacy, (2) safety, (3) low addiction potential, (4) minimal side effects, and (5) high public demand for sedative and anxiolytic agents. They have largely replaced barbiturates for sedative-hypnotic use because they have fewer side effects and liver enzyme inductions and are safer in overdose.[379,407-409]

Long-term benzodiazepine use poses a risk for the development of dependence and abuse,[410,411] particularly for those agents with the shortest half-life, the highest potency (alprazolam, triazolam), and the greatest lipophilicity (diazepam).[412,413] Regular use will produce tolerance to most of the adverse effects of benzodiazepines.[414] Consequently, some of the sedative and other adverse effects of benzodiazepines discussed earlier may wane with repeated drug use.[414] Tolerance may take weeks or months to develop, although this will depend on the dose of drugs used, the frequency of administration, and the pharmacokinetic half-life of the drug. Drugs with a short half-life are more likely to produce a quicker onset of tolerance.[414] Recent studies suggest an association of dementia with chronic benzodiazepine use.[415]

The benzodiazepines given by themselves or in combination with other drugs, particularly narcotic analgesics (opioids), are among the most widely abused drugs. Their ability to suppress or dampen withdrawal symptoms and boost the effects of heroin and other opioids has made them a favored drug type among the drug-using population.[414] They are also widely used by the cocaine-using population, especially clonazepam, to increase the seizure threshold.[414] They also are used in drug-facilitated crimes (see later section). [414]

Although the benzodiazepines exert qualitatively similar clinical effects, important quantitative differences in their pharmacodynamic spectra and pharmacokinetic properties have led to varying patterns of therapeutic application. Several distinct mechanisms of action are thought to contribute to the sedative-hypnotic, muscle relaxant, anxiolytic, and anticonvulsant effects of the benzodiazepines, and specific subunits of the $GABA_A$ receptor are responsible for specific pharmacologic properties of benzodiazepines.[379]

All the benzodiazepines are well absorbed, with the exception of clorazepate; this drug is decarboxylated rapidly in gastric juice to *N*-desmethyldiazepam (nordiazepem), which subsequently is absorbed.[379] Benzodiazepines are rapidly distributed to the CNS. Subsequently, benzodiazepines are more slowly redistributed from the CNS to more poorly perfused tissue, such as adipose tissue and muscle. The rate of this redistribution is an important determinant of the duration of action of benzodiazepines and, similar to that for gastrointestinal absorption, is largely determined by drug lipophilicity, with the more lipophilic drugs, such as midazolam and triazolam, having the shortest duration of action. These drugs cross the placental barrier and are secreted into breast milk.[379]

Benzodiazepines may be divided into four categories based on their elimination half-lives: (1) ultra-short-acting; (2) short-acting agents, with half-lives less than 6 hours; (3) intermediate-acting agents, with half-lives of 6 to 24 hours; and (4) long-acting agents, with half-lives greater than 24 hours.[379] These pharmacokinetic properties in part determine the primary clinical applications for some benzodiazepines. For instance, midazolam ($t_{1/2}$, 1 to 4 hours) is used for preanesthetic sedation or for sedation for endoscopic procedures because of its rapid onset and short duration of action. Benzodiazepines useful in treating anxiety generally have intermediate to long elimination half-lives (alprazolam and diazepam), and those primarily used as anticonvulsants (clonazepam) have the longest. Elimination half-life clearly is not the sole determinant of duration of action of benzodiazepines, and in some cases the rate of drug redistribution from the CNS may be a more important factor.[416]

Benzodiazepines undergo hepatic oxidation (phase I) and conjugation (phase II), often forming metabolites with pharmacologic activity (see Table 41.8). Cytochrome P450 enzymes, particularly CYP3A4 and CYP2C19, are frequently involved.[379] After these reactions, conjugation with glucuronic acid occurs; these glucuronidated metabolites constitute the major urinary products of benzodiazepines.[379,407,411,412,417] Inhibitors of CYP3A4 (erythromycin, clarithromycin, ritonavir, itraconazole, ketoconazole, nefazodone, and grapefruit juice) affect the metabolism of benzodiazepines.[418] However, benzodiazepines apparently do not significantly induce the synthesis of hepatic cytochrome P450 enzymes; their long-term administration usually does not result in accelerated metabolism of other drugs.

Nordiazepam is a major metabolite common to the biotransformation of diazepam, clorazepate, and prazepam; it is formed from chlordiazepoxide via an intermediate metabolite demoxepam.[379] Some benzodiazepines, such as oxazepam and lorazepam, are conjugated directly and do not undergo phase I metabolism. In some cases, metabolic transformations occur before the drug reaches significant concentrations in the systemic circulation. For example, clorazepate is decarboxylated to nordiazepam by stomach acid, and flurazepam and prazepam are converted to active metabolites by hepatic first-pass metabolism.[379,408]

Because active metabolites of some benzodiazepines are biotransformed more slowly than are the parent compounds, the duration of action of many benzodiazepines bears little relationship to the half-life of elimination of the drug that has been administered (see Table 41.8). For example, the half-life of flurazepam in plasma is 1 to 3 hours, but that of a major active metabolite (*N*-desalkylflurazepam) is 50 hours or longer.[419] Conversely, with benzodiazepines that lack active metabolites (oxazepam, lorazepam, temazepam, triazolam, and midazolam), the half-life is an important determinant of their duration of action. Additional factors that influence the duration of benzodiazepine action are hepatic metabolism and acute tolerance, resulting in decreased response to benzodiazepines with continued drug exposure.

Virtually all results of the pharmacologic effects of benzodiazepines are caused by their actions on the CNS. The most prominent of these effects are (1) sedation, (2) hypnosis, (3) decreased anxiety, (4) muscle relaxation, (5) anterograde amnesia, and (6) anticonvulsant activity. Only two effects of these drugs result from peripheral actions: (1) coronary vasodilation, seen after intravenous administration of therapeutic doses of certain benzodiazepines, and (2) neuromuscular blockade, seen only with very high doses. Ethanol increases both the rate of absorption of benzodiazepines and the associated CNS depression. Except for additive effects with other sedative or hypnotic drugs, reports of clinically important pharmacodynamic interactions between benzodiazepines and other drugs have been infrequent.

Benzodiazepines are believed to exert most of their effects by interacting with inhibitory neurotransmitter receptors directly activated by GABA. GABA receptors are membrane-bound proteins that are divided into two major subtypes: $GABA_A$ and $GABA_B$ receptors. The ionotropic $GABA_A$ receptors are responsible for most inhibitory neurotransmission in the CNS. Binding enhances GABA-mediated chloride transmembrane conductance, which results in hyperpolarization and diminished neural electrical discharge. Ultimately, this reduces the arousal of the cortical and limbic systems in the CNS.[414] Benzodiazepines also depress the electrical afterdischarge in the amygdala, hippocampus, and septum components of the limbic system that affect emotions.[414] In contrast are the metabotropic $GABA_B$ receptors. Benzodiazepines act at $GABA_A$ but not $GABA_B$ receptors by binding directly to a specific site that is distinct from that of GABA binding. Multiple $GABA_A$ receptors are known, and benzodiazepines seem to interact with many of these subtypes, which could account for the varied pharmacologic uses of these drugs.[385] Unlike barbiturates, benzodiazepines do not activate $GABA_A$ receptors directly but rather require GABA to express their effects as they only modulate the effects of GABA. Benzodiazepines modulate GABA binding, and GABA alters benzodiazepine binding in an allosteric fashion.[379] The remarkable safety of benzodiazepines compared with barbiturates is probably related to this effect.

New-generation sedative-hypnotics such as zolpidem (Ambien), eszopiclone (Lunesta), and zaleplon (Sonata) also modulate the $GABA_A$ receptor, yet they are structurally different, permitting unique physiologic properties that will be discussed in a subsequent section (see "Drugs Facilitated Crimes").

Benzodiazepines occasionally have paradoxical effects and sometimes cause garrulousness, anxiety, irritability, tachycardia, and sweating. Amnesia, euphoria, restlessness, hallucinations, and hypomanic behavior have been reported to occur during use of various benzodiazepines. The release of bizarre uninhibited behavior has been noted in some users, whereas hostility and rage may occur in others; collectively, these are sometimes referred to as *disinhibition* or *dyscontrol reactions.* Paranoia, depression, and suicidal ideation occasionally may accompany the use of these agents. Such paradoxical or disinhibition reactions are rare and appear to be dose related.[379] Valproate and benzodiazepines given in combination may cause psychotic episodes.[379]

Long-acting benzodiazepines (diazepam, chlordiazepoxide, and clorazepate) are given in relatively large doses and may be detected for several days to weeks or even months after long-term use. Short-acting benzodiazepines (alprazolam and triazolam) are used in lower doses and might be detected only for a few days. The treatment of benzodiazepine toxicity is primarily supportive. Flumazenil may be used in select cases and is a competitive inhibitor of the benzodiazepine site on the GABA complex. It finds its greatest utility in the reversal of benzodiazepine-induced sedation from minor surgical procedures. However, flumazenil should not be administered as a nonspecific coma-reversal drug and should be used with extreme caution after intentional benzodiazepine overdose because it has the potential to precipitate withdrawal in benzodiazepine-dependent individuals and/or to induce seizures in those at risk.

Analytical Methods. Benzodiazepines are measured using a variety of techniques. However, their structural diversity and wide variations in potency provide a challenge for laboratories to detect all relevant members in one analytical scheme. Reviews of analysis of benzodiazepines have been published.[420-422] These cover the range of techniques used both to screen for the presence of the class of drugs and to confirm the presence of one or more members.

Screening. Screening techniques using immunoassay kits will rarely be able to detect all members of the class because of differing immune reactivities among active drug and metabolites. This seems to apply to the more potent members (ie, lorazepam, triazolam, clonazepam).[420] Several commercial immunoassay systems are available for the detection of a wide variety of benzodiazepines and metabolites, but they differ somewhat in their ability to detect the various benzodiazepines, their metabolites, and glucuronide conjugates. Cross-reactivity in screening immunoassays of the various benzodiazepines and their metabolites varies considerably across manufacturers, and screening assays are not able to distinguish between the individual benzodiazepines. Most assays are calibrated to the common metabolite oxazepam, temazepam, or nordiazepam.[423] However, the large number of different functional groups that may be present on the benzodiazepine nucleus makes it difficult to detect all drugs in this class, and some compounds such as midazolam, chlordiazepoxide, and flunitrazepam may not be detected by many assays.[424-429] Nordiazepam is the benzodiazepine antagonist of flumazenil detected by most immunoassays for benzodiazepine. Other factors, such as low doses and short half-lives, make the detection of some benzodiazepines especially challenging. In the absence of sufficiently sensitive or specific immunoassays, direct analysis by a confirmatory method is warranted in suspected cases.

It should be noted that benzodiazepines may be identified and quantified in serum, but such quantitative information is not warranted in cases of benzodiazepine overdose because serum concentrations are not predictive of severity of intoxication.[408] However, a urine or serum immunoassay screening test for benzodiazepines is valuable in the evaluation of patients with an unknown cause of CNS depression.

Confirmation Testing. Analysts need to be aware that the specimen type will dictate the target substance. Blood analyses invariably will target the parent benzodiazepine and perhaps the major active metabolite (eg, nordiazepam for diazepam and other analogs metabolized to nordiazepam). This applies similarly to analyses targeted for saliva. In urine, a metabolite is often the required target species.[414]

Benzodiazepines and their metabolites have been extracted from biological specimens by LLE or SPE. When urine specimens are analyzed, a hydrolysis step is necessary to cleave the glucuronide conjugates.[385] Enzymatic hydrolysis is preferred over acid hydrolysis because some benzodiazepines are unstable and rearrange to form benzophenones.[385]

Many benzodiazepines are analyzed without derivatization by GC; these include diazepam, nordiazepam, flurazepam, and alprazolam. Drugs that are more polar, such as those with hydroxyl groups (oxazepam, temazepam, and lorazepam) or a nitro group (clonazepam, nitrazepam), display poor chromatographic characteristics and require derivatization.[385] Chlordiazepoxide is thermally unstable and may degrade at high temperatures in the GC.[385] Some consider GC-MS to be the definitive confirmation method[414]; however, LC with UV detection (240 nm) has been used to detect benzodiazepines and metabolites without derivatization. LC-MS and LC-MS/MS are becoming increasingly useful and popular methods for benzodiazepines.[405,430-435]

Cannabinoids

Naturally occurring cannabinoids are a group of C21 compounds found in the marijuana plant *Cannabis sativa.* Cannabis is the most extensively abused drug in the world.[436] Cannabis has been used as a medicinal and an illicit psychotropic agent for centuries. The main psychotropic effects are (1) euphoria, (2) distorted perceptions, (3) relaxation, and (4) a feeling of well-being.[437,438] Laws in each country vary regarding the regulation of marijuana internationally. In the United States, cannabis is listed as a Schedule I substance under the Controlled Substances Act of 1970 of the Federal government. However, since 1996, 23 individual states have legalized cannabis for medical conditions and four states have legalized marijuana for recreational use, with more in the process to follow.

THC, the primary psychoactive component of the *C. sativa* plant (Fig. 41.10), binds to endogenous cannabinoid receptors, CB1 (central) and CB2 (peripheral).[439-442] These

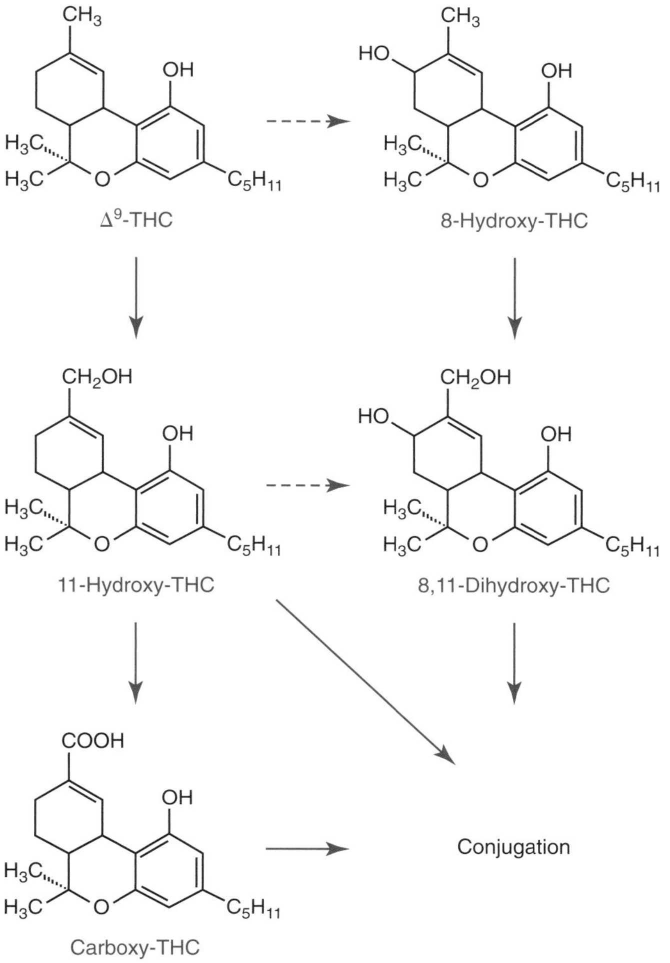

CH_3 OH H_3C H_3C O C_5H_{11} Δ^9-THC

HO CH_3 OH H_3C H_3C O C_5H_{11} 8-Hydroxy-THC

CH_2OH OH H_3C H_3C O C_5H_{11} 11-Hydroxy-THC

HO CH_2OH OH H_3C H_3C O C_5H_{11} 8,11-Dihydroxy-THC

COOH OH H_3C H_3C O C_5H_{11} Carboxy-THC

Conjugation

FIGURE 41.10 Principal metabolic route for Δ-9-tetrahydrocannabinol *(THC)* in humans.

transmembrane receptors are G-protein–coupled receptors that mediate signal transduction through inhibition of adenylate cyclase and calcium ions and activation of potassium ion channels.[443,444] The distribution pattern of CB1 receptors in the CNS accounts for most of the clinical effects of THC such as mood, memory, cognition, pain, and appetite.[445-447] CB2 may regulate immune and inflammatory processes. THC also acts on dopaminergic projections and has been shown to stimulate the reward pathways in the brain as is seen with other drug of abuse.[439]

THC is typically consumed by smoking the plant leaves, flower buds, and sometimes stems. THC also has been extracted from the glandular hairs of cannabis flowers and produced as a resin (hashish). Hashish is often a more potent form and has been mixed into foods, brewed as tea and then ingested, or smoked. Hemp oil has been extracted from cannabis seeds for use in soaps, body care products, and dietary supplements and is used because of its high essential fatty acid content but negligible THC content.

Pharmacologic Response. The effects of cannabis include feelings of euphoria and relaxation, altered time perception, lack of concentration, impaired learning and memory, and mood changes such as paranoia, psychosis, and panic attacks.[439] Although marijuana is the most frequently used illicit drug, it does have some limited legitimate medicinal use. Dronabinol (Marinol) contains synthetic THC and is used to treat anorexia and nausea in patients with acquired immunodeficiency syndrome (AIDS) and those with nausea and vomiting associated with chemotherapy, asthma, and glaucoma.[448]

When marijuana is smoked, THC rapidly diffuses into the plasma in seconds and is distributed multiphasically. First, it distributes to highly vascularized tissues in minutes because of its lipophilic nature.[449] THC then is redistributed back into the bloodstream, undergoes hepatic metabolism, and slowly accumulates into less vascularized and fatty tissues.[450,451] After cessation of marijuana smoking, THC and its metabolites are slowly released from fat stores.[452]

The main psychotropic effects after inhalation of marijuana occur within minutes and persist for several hours. The peak plasma concentration of THC depends on the dose, and numerous factors contribute to the variability in dose, such as (1) method of consumption, (2) depth of inhalation, (3) exposure frequency, and (4) cannabis potency.[439,453-455] Onset of clinical symptoms and peak plasma concentrations after oral ingestion of THC is slower than after inhalation, primarily as the result of first-pass hepatic clearance, and two THC peaks are frequently observed because of enterohepatic circulation.[439,456,457]

The concentration and ratio of THC and its metabolites has been used to estimate the time of exposure to marijuana.[458,459]

Analytical Methods. An immunoassay method is typically used to screen for potential cannabinoid use in workplace drug testing, athlete drug testing, and clinical specimens. A presumptive positive sample should be confirmed by quantitative GC-MS or LC-MS/MS. Confirmation of quantitative concentrations of the parent compound, THC, is typically reserved for forensic samples.

Screening. Legitimate concern has been raised concerning the potential for false-positive results from dietary sources and "passive inhalation" of sufficient side-stream marijuana smoke from nearby users, resulting in a positive urine cannabinoid test. Hemp seeds and oil are produced from the same *C. sativa* plant that is harvested for drug use. Hemp has been used to make soaps, lotions, rope, clothing, and as an ingredient in a wide variety of food products. In the mid-1990s several studies reported that ingestion of single or multiple doses of hemp products caused positive results in cannabinoid screens and confirmatory analyses. Since 1998, the US Federal Government has prohibited the importation of *C. sativa* seeds and oil containing greater than 0.3% THC to reduce human exposure to THC. The concentration of THC consumed in drug use is 2% to 20%.[453,460] Subsequent studies have suggested that these measures were successful in reducing potential positive cannabinoid drug screen results from dietary sources.[460] Yet, immunoassay screens and GC-MS analyses of urine specimens from volunteers exposed to very low doses of THC (0.39 mg/d) have tested positive for cannabinoids.[461,462]

Numerous studies have been conducted to investigate exposure to THC from second-hand smoke, concluding that the SAMHSA cutoff is sufficient to separate moderate passive exposure from first-hand inhalation exposure to THC. Several of these studies demonstrated that significant concentrations of TCH-COOH (<10 ng/mL) could be detected in passive inhalers housed in unventilated confined facilities, but most were below the assay cutoff.[463,464] Individuals that tested positive (>20 ng/mL cutoff, immunoassay) were exposed to multiple marijuana cigarettes in an unventilated car containing 3500 L or less of air.[465,466] Therefore it is improbable that a passive inhaler would be able to sustain exposure to significant THC concentrations long enough to produce a positive drug screen. Nevertheless, as a precaution against passive inhalations resulting in a positive test, some laboratories screen for urine cannabinoids at a cutoff concentration of 100 ng/mL THC-COOH equivalents. However, at this cutoff value, test sensitivity in one study was only 47% when compared with that for GC-MS (cutoff value, 15 ng/mL THC-COOH). Test sensitivity increased to 93% at a cutoff value of 20 ng/mL THC-COOH equivalents.[467] The US federally mandated screening cutoff was reduced from 100 ng/mL to 50 ng/mL THC-COOH equivalents (Table 41.9).[468] One study demonstrated that such a reduction in screening cutoff resulted in a 23% to 54% increase in test sensitivity, depending on the immunoassay, with only a slight decrease (1.0% to 2.6%) in test specificity.[469] A 1997 study suggests that consideration should be given to lowering the values listed for THC-COOH.[470]

THC is metabolized by CYP450 liver enzymes to greater than 100 metabolites. The main active metabolite, 11-hydroxy-Δ-9-THC, is further oxidized to the most abundant inactive THC-COOH (see Fig. 41.10).[455,471] Immunoassay screens have been designed to detect cannabis use in urine samples using antibody reagents developed against the inactive THC-COOH metabolite; these reagents cross-react with numerous other THC metabolites. Therefore the presence of multiple cannabinoid metabolites in a patient specimen will have an additive effect in immunoassay screen analyses. Quantitative results based on these metabolites are 1.5 to 8 times greater than the actual concentration of THC-COOH as determined by GC-MS.[472] Therefore immunoassay results are interpreted as THC-COOH equivalents.

A positive result from a urine cannabinoid screen or confirmation does not indicate intoxication or degree of exposure. The window of detection for the urine concentration of THC-COOH varies among casual (2 to 7 days)[455] and chronic abusers (up to 73 days)[473,474] of marijuana and is dose dependent. Variables affecting the duration of detection include (1) dose, (2) frequency of exposure, (3) route of exposure, (4) body composition, (5) fluid excretion, and (6) method of detection. Therefore monitoring of abstinence is particularly challenging. Dilution of urine because of normal biological fluctuations (hydration) or ingested adulterants has caused a negative result on one day and a positive on the next. To correct for hydration fluctuations, urine concentrations of THC-COOH per milligram creatinine are normalized for monitoring individuals who are resuming cannabis use. Some people suggest that using these normalized THC-COOH:creatinine concentrations, a ratio is calculated by comparing any normalized urine specimen (U2) with a previously collected normalized urine specimen (U1). "New use" is defined as a U2/U1 ratio of 0.5 to 1.5 or greater collected from urine specimens taken more than 24 hours apart and containing THC-COOH concentrations greater than 15 ng/mL.[475-477] Using the 1.5 cutoff rate results in decreased false-positive but increased false-negative decisions.[475]

Confirmation. A positive screening result for THC obtained by immunoassay is confirmed by GC-MS analysis of the urine specimen. In the United States, the Division of Workplace Programs in SAMHSA set the cutoff for confirming the presence of TCH-COOH metabolite at 15 ng/mL (GC-MS).[478]

Synthetic Cannabinoids. Synthetic cannabinoids are synthetically derived compounds originally developed as potential therapeutic compounds used to characterize cannabinoid receptors (CB-1 and CB-2). In 2004, John W. Huffman synthesized alkylindol cannabinoid agonists consisting of modified THC functional groups (JWH-018). These cannabinoid receptor ligands were used to identify moieties important for binding and activity.[479,480] Modification of JWH-018 resulted in synthesis of JWH-122, JWH-073, JWH-081. In 2006, halogenated moieties of the "AM series" of JWH analogs were synthesized (AM-2201). Subsequently clandestine laboratories continue to substitute functional moieties and synthesize new compounds (Box 41.3).

The US Drug Enforcement Administration (DEA) has scheduled numerous synthetic cannabinoids to support prosecution of illegal synthetic cannabinoid production and distribution. As a result, the number of newly synthesized compounds has grown in an attempt to outpace the legislation and analytical detection. As one product becomes illegal, its prevalence in the public realm decreases and a new synthetic cannabinoid takes its place.

Synthetic cannabinoids are commonly sprayed on dried plant material and typically smoked. The clinical effects of these agents have not been well defined, with most clinical reports based on patient history of what was taken versus what was truly present in the product abused. Clinical effects of synthetic cannabinoids may be similar to those of THC. Yet some reported effects, such as anxiety, agitation, psychosis, and suicidality, may be more prominent.

Screening and Confirmation. Enzyme-linked immunoassays are commercially available. No single immunoassay kit can detect all known synthetic cannabinoid compounds, and the binding affinity of the compounds may limit the detection of certain "spice" compounds. GC-MS, LC-MS/MS,

TABLE 41.9 **Suggested Cutoff Concentrations for Different Matrices**

	Urine (ng/mL)*	Oral Fluid, (ng/mL)†	Sweat (ng/patch)[478]	Hair (pg/mg)[478]
Initial Test				
THC		4	4	
THC metabolite	50			1
Cocaine and metabolites	150	15	25	500
Opiates			25	200
Codeine/morphine	2000	30		
Hydrocodone/hydromorphone	300	30		
Oxycodone/oxymorphone	100	30		
6-MAM	10	3		
PCP	25	3	20	300
Amphetamine/methamphetamine	500	25	25	500
MDMA/MDA/MDEA	500	25	25	500
Confirmatory Test				
THC parent		2	1	
Δ9-THC-COOH	15			0.05
Cocaine		8		500
Benzoylecgonine (BE)	100	8	25	50
Cocaethylene				50
Norcocaine				50
Morphine	2000	15	25	200
Codeine	2000	15	25	200
Hydrocodone	100	15		
Hydromorphone	100	15		
Oxycodone	50	15		
Oxymorphone	50	15		
6-MAM	10	2	25	200 Must contain morphine ≥200 ng/mg
PCP	25	2	20	300
Amphetamine	250	15	25	300
Methamphetamine	250		25 Must contain amphetamine ≥ limit of detection	300 Must contain amphetamine ≥50 pg/mg
MDMA	250	15	25	300
MDA	250	15	25	300
MDEA	250	15	25	300

*http://www.gpo.gov/fdsys/pkg/FR-2015-05-15/pdf/2015-11524.pdf.
†http://www.gpo.gov/fdsys/pkg/FR-2015-05-15/pdf/2015-11523.pdf.
6-MAM, 6-Monoacetylmorphine; *MDA,* 3,4-methylenedioxyamphetamine; *MDEA,* methylenedioxyethylamphetamine; *MDMA,* 3,4-met hylenedioxymethamphetamine; *PCP,* phencyclidine; *THC,* Δ-9-tetrahydrocannabinol.

LC-HRMS, or TOF may be used to screen for or confirm the growing release of new synthetic cannabinoids entering the black market. The metabolism of synthetic cannabinoids is complex, such that many of compounds have common metabolites (Table 41.10), and confirmatory testing should not only be able to detect the large number of metabolites but also be adaptable to accommodate the rapidly changing landscape of drugs being introduced.

Cocaine

Cocaine is an alkaloid found in *Erythroxylon coca,* which grows principally in the northern South American Andes and to a lesser extent in India, Africa, and Java.[481,482] In clinical medicine, it is used mainly for local anesthesia and vasoconstriction in nasal surgery, and to dilate pupils in ophthalmology. Sigmund Freud famously proposed its use to treat depression and alcohol dependence, but the realities of cocaine addiction quickly brought this idea to an end.[297] Cocaine abuse has a long history and is rooted in the drug culture in the United States.[482] Cocaine is still one of the most common illicit drugs of abuse, and according to the National Survey on Drug Use and Health, the rate of 2014 use for cocaine (powder and crack combined) among individuals aged 12 and older has remained relatively stable since 2002 (see http://www.samhsa.gov/data/population-data-nsduh/reports).

Cocaine is sold on the street in two forms: a hydrochloride salt (powder) and a free-base product known as "crack." The

BOX 41.3 Synthetic Cannabinoids[927-938]

Alkylnaphthylindoles
JWH-018, -019, -072, -081, -122, -203, -210, -250,- 398

Haloalkylnaphthylindoles
AM-2201
MAM-2201

Naphthylindole
JWH-200

Cyclopropylindole
UR-144

Adamantylindazole
AKB-48 (APINACA)

Tetramethylcyclopropylindole
XLR-11

Substitution of Naphthalene Group
PB-22
BB-22
RCS-4
5-Fluoro AB-PINACA
ADB-PINACA
ADBICA

Substitution of Naphthalene and Indole Groups
AM-694
AB-FUBINACA

hydrochloride salt form of cocaine is administered by nasal insufflation ("snorting") or, less frequently, intravenously. Crack is a free-base form that has not been neutralized by an acid to make the hydrochloride salt. It comes as a rock crystal that is heated and its vapors smoked. The term refers to the crackling sound heard when it is heated.[482]

It should be noted that the use of crack cocaine is not to be confused with "free-basing," which is a process in which the user purifies cocaine hydrogen chloride by mixing an aqueous solution of cocaine with baking soda or ammonia and adding diethyl ether, thereby extracting the free form of the drug into the organic solvent, which is then evaporated to dryness. The drug can then be smoked. However, because of the extremely flammable nature of diethyl ether, and therefore the risk for igniting any remaining ether, free-basing is no longer commonly practiced.[482]

Chemically, cocaine is methylbenzoylecognine (COC), an ester of benzoic acid and the amino alcohol (methylecognine) that contains a tropine moiety.[481] Its metabolism is complex (Fig. 41.11) and occurs via both nonenzymatic hydrolysis and enzymatic transformation in the plasma and liver, where it is rapidly metabolized to benzoylecgonine (BE) and ecogonine methyl ester, both of which are inactive.[482] COC contains two ester moieties; the alkyl ester is hydrolyzed to its major metabolite BE via spontaneous hydrolysis at physiologic and alkaline pH.[482] It has been shown that COC is also hydrolyzed to BE by liver carboxylesterases.[483] BE is considered to be a pharmacologically inactive metabolite, but because its half-life is longer than that of COC, it is the most commonly monitored analyte in urine for determination of COC use.

BE is further metabolized to minor metabolites such as m-hydroxybenzoylecgonine (m-HOBE) and *p*-hydroxybenzoylecgonine (*p*-HOBE).[481,484] Of these, m-HOBE has been shown to be an important metabolite in the meconium of cocaine-exposed babies.[485,486] Positive BE results in urine are sometimes challenged in legal and administrative proceedings on the grounds that the presence of BE is due to the addition of COC to the urine sample with subsequent in vitro hydrolysis to BE. However, m-HOBE is believed to arise exclusively by an vivo metabolism[487]; therefore its presence confirms COC use. Additionally, in adults, m-HOBE has a longer half-life and the potential to be detected for longer periods[484,488] than BE; it has been useful in the clinical management of patients because it expands the detection window. It should be noted that cocaethylene (CE) possesses the same CNS stimulatory activity as cocaine in experimental animals.

Norcocaine (NC) is an *N*-demethylated metabolite of COC produced by liver cytochrome P450; it is of clinical interest because of its conversion into hepatotoxic metabolites.[482,489,490] NC is subsequently metabolized to hydroxyl-NC and then to NC-nitroxide.[490] Although the mechanism for hepatotoxicity is not well understood, it appears to be related to one or more of the *N*-oxidative metabolites. In animals, these metabolites have been reported to inhibit mitochondrial respiration, leading to ATP depletion and subsequent cell death.[491] NC concentrations have been shown to be present in greater concentrations in cholinesterase-deficient subjects[492] and in simultaneous cocaine and ethanol users.[493]

Anhydroecgonine methyl ester (AEME; methyl ecgonidine) has been identified as a unique COC metabolite after smoked COC (crack) administration. Anhydroecgonine ethyl ester (AEEE; ethyl ecgonidine) has been identified in COC smokers who also use ethyl alcohol.[494-496]

Pharmacologic Response. Cocaine has cardiovascular effects and is a potent CNS stimulant that elicits a state of increased alertness and euphoria[482] with actions similar to those of amphetamine but of shorter duration.[497] These CNS effects are thought to be largely associated with the ability of cocaine to block dopamine reuptake at nerve synapses, thereby prolonging the action of dopamine in the CNS. It is this response that leads to recreational abuse of cocaine. Cocaine also blocks the reuptake of norepinephrine at presynaptic nerve terminals; this produces a sympathomimetic response (including an increase in blood pressure, heart rate, and body temperature). Cocaine is effective as a local anesthetic and vasoconstrictor of mucous membranes and therefore is used clinically for nasal surgery, rhinoplasty, and emergency nasotracheal intubation.

The CNS and cardiovascular effects of cocaine exhibit acute tolerance; its effects are more pronounced when the concentration of cocaine in blood is increasing than when it is at a similar but decreasing concentration.[498,499] Thus a clockwise hysteresis is observed when the blood concentration of cocaine is plotted against its CNS or cardiovascular effects over time. This phenomenon mitigates against attempts to correlate isolated blood concentration values with psychomotor effects. Because rate of change is probably more significant than absolute concentration, the psychomotor stimulant effects of cocaine dependent on both dose and route of administration, with intravenous administration

TABLE 41.10 Metabolism of Selected Synthetic Cannabinoids[927-938]

Naphthoylindoles	Significant Phase I Metabolites	Halogenated Compound	Significant Phase I Metabolites
JWH-018	JWH-018 N-pentanoic acid	AM-2201	AM-2201 pentanoic acid, AM-2201 N-(4-hydroxypentyl)
JWH-019	JWH 019 N-(6-hydroxyhexyl)		
JWH-073	JWH 073 N-butanoic acid		
JWH-081	JWH-81 N-(5-hydroxypentyl)		
JWH-122	JWH 122 N-(4&5-hydroxypentyl)	MAM-2201	MAM-2201 N-pentanoic acid, MAM-2201 N-(4-hydroxypentyl)
JWH-175			
JWH-176			
JWH-200	JWH 200 (5-hydroxyindole)		
JWH-210	JWH 210 N-N(5-hydroxypentyl)		
JWH-398	JWH 398 N-(5-hydroxypentyl)		
AM-694	AM-694 N-pentanoic acid, AM-694 N-(5-hydroxypentyl)		
Alkylnaphthylacetylindoles			
JWH-250	JWH 250 N-(5-hydroxypentyl)		
Phenylacetylindoles			
RCS-8	RCS-8 N-(5-hydroxypentyl)		
Dibenzopyrans			
HU-210			
Cyclopropylindoles		**Halogenated Compound**	
UR-144	UR-144 N-pentanoic acid, UR-144 N-(5-hydroxypentyl)	XLR-11	XLR-11 N-pentanoic acid, XLR-11 N-(4&5-hydroxypentyl)
Naphthoylpyrroles			
JWH-307			
Adamantylindazoles		**Halogenated Compound**	
AKB-48 (APINACA)	AKB-48 pentanoic acid, AKB-48 N-(4&5-hydroxypentyl)	5F-AKB-48	AKB-48 N-pentanoic acid
Substitutions of Naphthalene		**Halogenated Compound**	
PB-22	PB-22 (3-carboxyindole)	5F-PB-22	PB-22 (3-carboxyindole)
RCS-4	RCS-4 N-pentanoic acid, RCS-4 (4&5-hydroxypentyl)		
AB-PINACA	AB-PINACA N-pentanoic acid	5-Fluoro AB-PINACA	AB-PINACA N-pentanoic acid
ADB-PINACA	ADB-PINACA N-pentanoic acid		
APICA	APICA-hydroxypentyl	5F-APICA	APICA-hydroxypentyl
		AB-FUBINACA	AB-FUBINACA Carboxylic acid

and smoking resulting in the most rapid rates of increase in concentration.

Acute cocaine toxicity produces a sympathomimetic response that may result in (1) mydriasis, (2) diaphoresis, (3) hyperactive bowel sounds, (4) tachycardia, (5) hypertension, (6) hyperthermia, (7) hyperactivity, (8) agitation, (9) seizures, or (10) coma. Sudden death as a result of cardiotoxicity may occur after cocaine use. Death also may occur after the sequential development of hyperthermia, agitated delirium, and respiratory arrest. Excited delirium and extreme physical activity may lead to rhabdomyolysis, acute renal failure, and disseminated intravascular coagulopathy.

COC is frequently used with other drugs, most commonly ethanol. In simultaneous COC and ethanol use, liver methylesterase catalyzes the conversion of COC to BE and the transesterification of COC to CE in the presence of ethyl alcohol.[482,500,501] This reaction occurs approximately 3.5 times faster than hydrolysis to BE.[502] COC administered with ethanol has been found to produce greater euphoria and enhanced perception of well-being relative to COC.[482,503] CE appears to be equipotent to cocaine with regard to dopamine transporter affinity[500] but is less potent than cocaine pharmacologically.[504,505] As a consequence, large amounts of COC and ethanol may be ingested, placing users at greater risk for

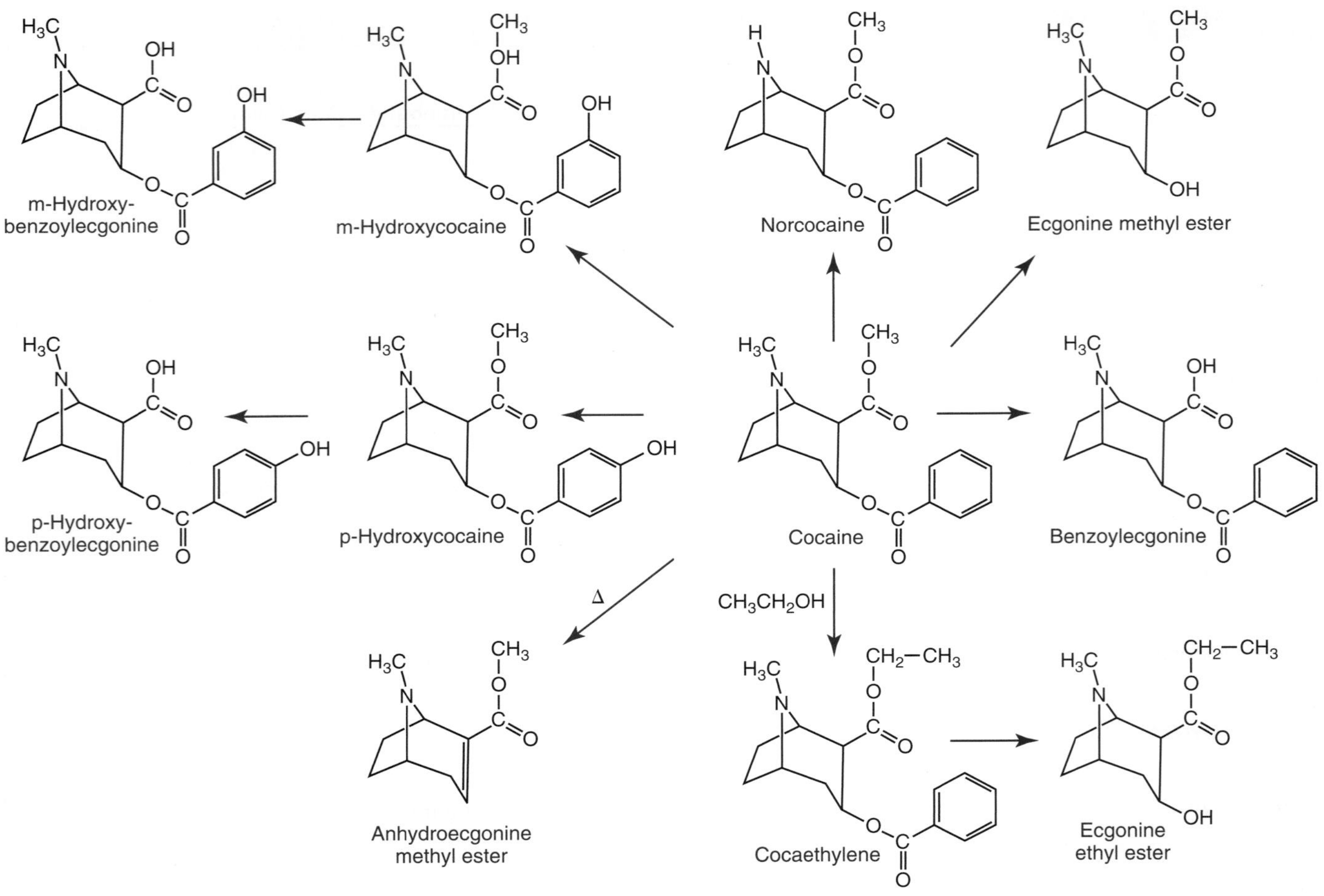

FIGURE 41.11 Metabolism of cocaine.

toxicity than if either drug were used alone. The elimination half-life for CE is longer than that for cocaine,[506,507] which may contribute to its toxicity. Additionally, with simultaneous administration of COC and ethanol, the production of NC may be increased, along with the potential for toxicity.[481,484,493] It has been suggested that simultaneous COC and ethanol use carries an 18- to 25-fold increase in risk for immediate death over COC alone[482,503,508,509]

Analytical Methods. The elimination half-life for cocaine ranges from 0.5 to 1.5 hours, for ecgonine methyl ester from 3 to 4 hours, and for BE from 4 to 7 hours.[5-7] The principal urinary metabolites are BE and ecgonine methyl ester. Only small amounts of cocaine are excreted in urine. The elimination half-life for cocaethylene is 2.5 to 6 hours,[19,218,221] which is considerably longer than for cocaine.

BE excretion is detectable for 1 to 3 days after cocaine use. However, for chronic heavy cocaine users, the detection time may extend to 10 to 22 days after the last dose,[510] apparently because of tissue storage of cocaine. Ordinarily, cocaine may be detected in urine by chromatographic methods for only approximately 8 to 12 hours after use, but in heavy chronic users, this detection period may last 4 to 5 days.[511] These facts should be considered when the results of urine drug testing for individuals in drug treatment programs are interpreted. A positive urine drug test for BE beyond 3 days after the last dose does not necessarily indicate continued use. For such purposes, it is better to monitor quantitatively the urinary excretion of benzoylecgonine, normalized to creatinine, over time.[512] Drug abstinence would be indicated by decreasing urinary excretion of cocaine metabolites. However, creatinine normalization may not always reliably indicate reuse.[513]

The initial screening test for cocaine (BE) is typically immunoassay. For confirmation of a presumptive positive, BE is quantified by GC-MS.

Screening. Because of the previously mentioned longer elimination half-life of BE, it is the analyte of choice in screening for cocaine use.[481] The initial screening test for BE is typically immunoassay, and screening immunoassays frequently have a cutoff of 300 ng/mL for it.

Confirmation. Most confirmation assays offer quantification of both the parent drug and metabolite. Numerous methods have been described for the measurement of COC and its metabolites. GC techniques for analysis of COC and its metabolites require derivatization, especially of polar metabolites. Early detection techniques have included flame ionization detection (FID), EC, and nitrogen-phosphorus detection (NPD).[514-519] GC-MS is the method of choice for many laboratories.[520-525] Some methods have included not only COC and BE but also clinically and forensically relevant secondary metabolites such as m-HOBE, CE, NC, AEME, and AEEE.[487,494,526,527] The use of LC-based separation techniques that detect COC, BE, and CE has been described previously, including LC-UV detection,[528-530] as well as LC–diode array detection (LC-DAD).[531] LC-MS/MS methods have been

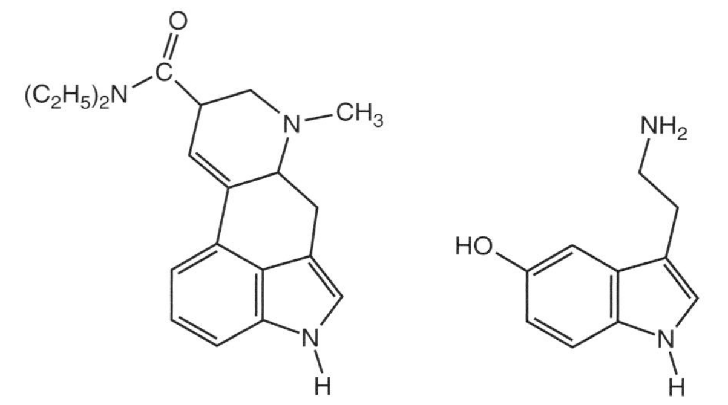

FIGURE 41.12 Chemical structure of lysergic acid diethylamide *(LSD)* and serotonin.

described, including COC, BE, and m-HOBE,[532-538] along with other relevant secondary metabolites such as CE, NC, AEME, and AEEE.[539] It has been suggested that AEME is not a truly unique indicator of smoked cocaine use, because it has been reported to be produced in the injector port of a GC[540-542] at high temperatures. However, less than 1% generation of AEME occurs if the injector port of the GC is maintained at 250°C.[494] In an LC method, high temperatures are not present in the injector or in any other part of the LC; therefore AEME is not generated and its presence identifies a smoked route of COC use.

Lysergic Acid Diethylamide

LSD shares structural features with serotonin (5-hydroxytryptamine; Fig. 41.12), a major CNS neurotransmitter and neuromodulator.[543,544] LSD is synthesized from D-lysergic acid, a naturally occurring ergot alkaloid found in the fungus *Claviceps purpurea,* which grows on wheat and other grains. During synthesis, some LSD epimerizes to iso-LSD, which is inactive.[256]

Pharmacologic Response. LSD is an extremely potent psychedelic ergot alkaloid derived from the fungus *C. purpurea.*[543] The drug LSD binds to serotonin receptors in the CNS and acts as a serotonin agonist. The principal psychologic effects of LSD are perceptual distortions of color, sound, distance, and shape; depersonalization and loss of body image; and rapidly changing emotions from ecstasy to depression or paranoia. These hallucinogenic actions of LSD are stereoselective, elicited only by the D-isomer. A resurgence has occurred in the use of LSD, previously popular as a drug of abuse during the 1960s. The US Department of Defense includes LSD among the drugs for which urine testing is required (see Table 41.9).

The physiologic effects of LSD are related to its sympathomimetic actions and include mydriasis (most frequent and consistent), tachycardia, increased body temperature, diaphoresis, and hypertension; at higher doses, parasympathomimetic actions may be observed (eg, salivation, lacrimation, nausea, vomiting [muscarinic actions]). Neuromuscular effects may include paresthesia, muscle twitches, and incoordination (nicotinic actions).[543,544]

The most common adverse effects of LSD are panic attacks. In addition, unpredictable recurrence of hallucinations (flashbacks) may occur weeks or months after last drug use, and LSD may elicit psychotic reactions (thought disorders, hallucinations, depression, and depersonalization). LSD is used illicitly because of its hallucinogenic effects. No evidence suggests that repeated LSD use results in dependence or withdrawal symptoms.[543,544]

Popular dosage forms include powder, gelatin capsule, tablet, and LSD-impregnated sugar cubes, filter paper, or postage stamps. The drug is rapidly absorbed from the gastrointestinal tract; the effects begin within 40 to 60 minutes, peak at approximately 2 to 4 hours, and subside by 6 to 8 hours. The elimination $t_{1/2}$ is approximately 3 hours. The metabolism of LSD in humans is incompletely understood, but 2-oxo-3-hydroxy-LSD is present in urine at concentrations 10- to 43-fold greater than LSD.[545-547] *N*-Demethyl-LSD is also present in urine specimens, but at concentrations approximately equivalent to those of LSD. The other metabolites are among those identified in animals, but as yet not conclusively identified in humans.[256] Iso-LSD is not a metabolite but is formed by nonenzymatic epimerization of LSD during synthesis or storage of urine at alkaline pH and elevated temperature.[548]

The clinical effects of LSD ingestion are usually benign and require no medical intervention. However, panic attacks may be severe and require treatment with diazepam; LSD-induced psychosis has been treated with haloperidol. Rare cases of massive overdose have resulted in life-threatening hyperthermia, rhabdomyolysis, acute renal failure, hepatic failure, disseminated intravascular coagulation, respiratory arrest, and coma. Few if any well-documented deaths directly related to LSD ingestion have been reported.

Analytical Methods. Because of the very high potency of LSD, and therefore a low typical dose (20 to 80 μg) and rapid and extensive metabolism, only approximately 1% to 2% of the drug is excreted unchanged in urine.[547] Thus detection of LSD presents an especially difficult analytical challenge. Even with sensitive assays, the detection window for LSD is generally only 12 to 24 hours.[547]

Immunoassays are targeted to detect LSD at the usual cutoff concentration of 500 pg/mL. Confirmation is typically performed by GC-MS[549,550] at the US Department of Defense established cutoff concentration of 200 pg/mL. Although the metabolites 2-oxo-3-hydroxy-LSD and *N*-demethyl LSD generally cross-react only when present at approximately 100 to 200 times the amount in LSD,[551] other metabolites may potentially account for some instances of nonconfirmed positive immunoassay response.[552,553] However, true false-positive results resulting from various therapeutic drugs may occur.[551,553,554] The detection window may be extended, perhaps twofold to threefold, by including 2-oxo-3-hydroxy-LSD in the confirmatory test, using sensitive techniques such as GC-MS/MS,[547] LC-MS/MS,[546] or LC-MS.[545,555] Likewise, detection of iso-LSD in addition to LSD may extend the detection interval.[556] Urine specimens should be protected from sunlight, bright fluorescent light, or elevated temperature at alkaline pH to avoid degradation of LSD[557] and 2-oxo-3-hydroxy-LSD or epimerization of LSD to iso-LSD.[548,557]

Opioids

The term *opioid* describes a wide range of compounds encompassing the natural and semisynthetic opiates—essentially variations on the structure of morphine—and fully synthetic opioids with minimal structural homology to the natural alkaloids (Fig. 41.13).[558] The defining characteristic of this

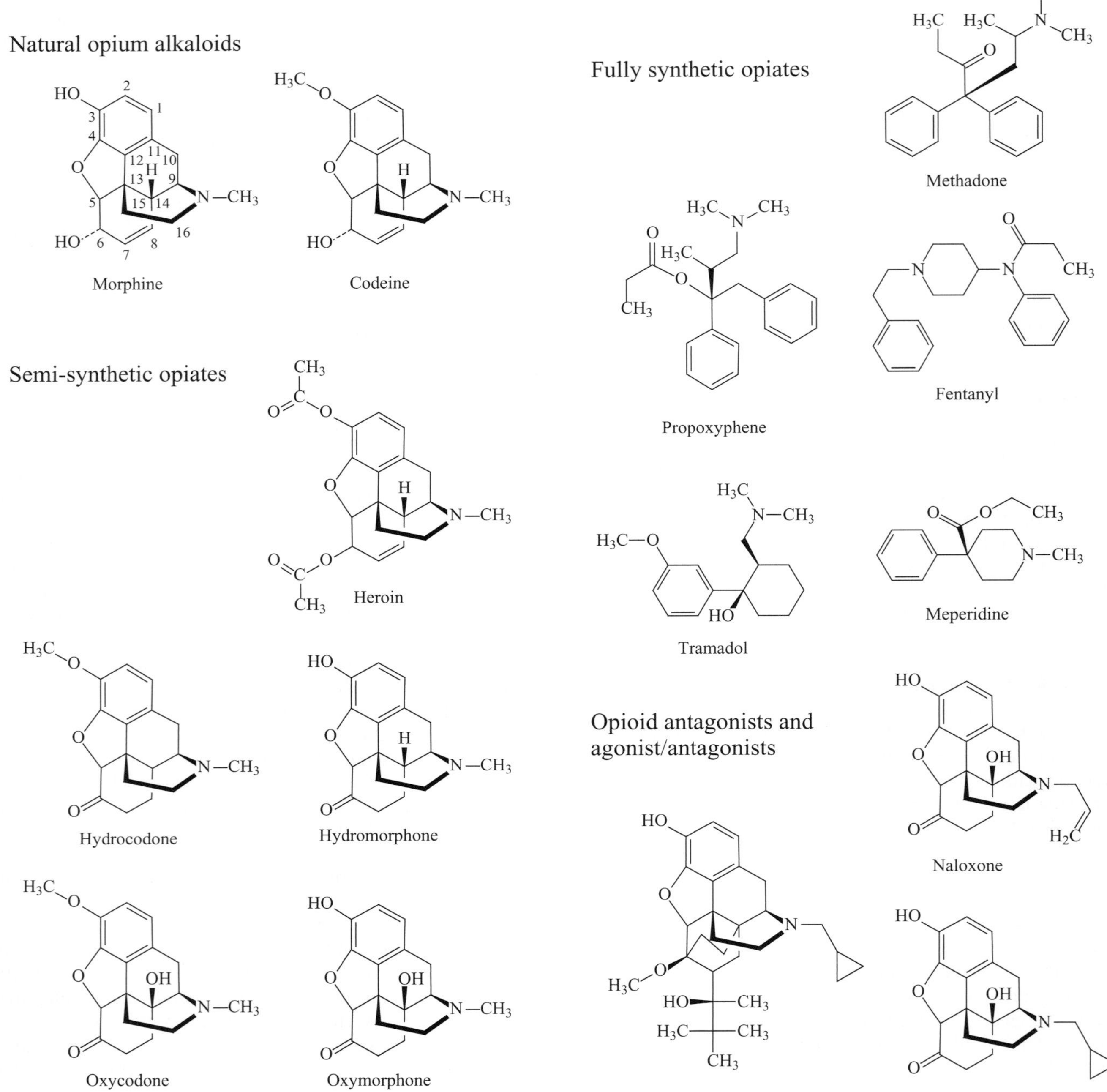

FIGURE 41.13 Structure and half-life of common opioids.

class of drugs is their morphine-like antinociceptive activity stemming from interaction with opioid receptors, which play a major role in pain perception.[559,560] Other compounds that are somewhat loosely referred to as opioids include receptor antagonists and mixed agonist/antagonists, as well as other opium-derived alkaloids such as papaverine that are not known to bind opioid receptors.[561]

Pharmacologic Response. For pain management, opioid therapy is a mainstay in treating acute needs such as postsurgical analgesia and in relieving moderate to severe chronic pain.[562] In the latter case, opioids are well accepted in the setting of cancer-related pain, but the propriety and effectiveness of their use in nonmalignant chronic pain are controversial.[562] Most opioids have both substantial addictive capacity and potentially life-threatening side effects; thus the benefits of their use in non–end-stage patients must be carefully weighed against the chance of rather serious consequences. In addition, the development of tolerance and the risk for prescription diversion complicate even further the process of monitoring long-term opioid therapy for compliance and efficacy.

The hallmark of opioids is their ability to interact with the family of opioid receptors that are variably distributed throughout the body; opioid receptor agonists typically produce analgesia, and antagonists block this response.[560,563] The biochemistry of opioid receptor binding, regulation, and signaling is complex and has been reviewed in detail elsewhere.[560,563,564] A general overview is presented here.

The classic opioid receptors are divided into the mu, delta, and kappa (μ, δ, and κ, or MOR, DOR, and KOR, respectively) subfamilies,[560] which exhibit considerable overlap in ligand specificity and downstream signaling.[560,563] A related protein, the ORL-1/nociceptin receptor, also has been described as an opioid receptor, although its characterization lags behind that of the other receptors.[565] Finally, the sigma receptor family will interact with some opioids but produces very different physiologic responses, including cardiac excitation and tachypnea; sigma receptors are now considered to be completely distinct from the classical opioid receptors.[563]

Opioids also have preferential or selective binding to one or more of the different receptor classes. It is possible for a compound to stimulate one opioid receptor subtype while inhibiting another, as with mixed agonist and antagonist compounds.[560,563] The effect of ligand binding varies across receptor classes. Morphine-like analgesia is thought to be mediated primarily through stimulation of MOR, although compounds with preferential binding to DOR or KOR also produce analgesia.[560,563] Other classic sequelae of opioid treatment are also attributable to MOR, including sedation and inhibition of respiratory function and gastrointestinal transit.[560,566,567] In contrast, neither DOR nor KOR is thought to affect respiration; DOR agonists do not produce sedation or reduce gastrointestinal motility.[560] KOR and its endogenous ligand dynorphin are implicated in response to addiction to numerous drugs such as opioids; KOR gene polymorphisms have been linked to susceptibility to alcohol dependence, supporting a role for this receptor in addictive behavior.[568-571]

In addition to undesirable side effects, a major concern in long-term opioid therapy is the development of tolerance.[560,563,572] Tolerant individuals may require many-fold increases in dose to achieve the same concentration of analgesia, which can greatly complicate interpretation of serum results and establishment of a therapeutic window. Tolerance to a particular opioid is thought to be a consequence of altered regulation of the opioid receptor(s) to which that compound binds; for this reason, cross-tolerance can occur when multiple drugs interact with the same receptor.[560,563,572,573] In addition, several of the enzymes involved in opioid metabolism (see later) display substrate-dependent alterations in activity. Although substrate inhibition and induction represent different phenomena than tolerance, the clinical effect can be similar and may necessitate modification of the therapeutic regimen.

The metabolism of opioids is varied, but numerous biotransformations are common to these drugs (Table 41.11). Several of the most commonly used opiates are formed in vivo by metabolism of other compounds, as is seen with codeine demethylation resulting in conversion to morphine.[560,574] This interconversion is a frequent source of confusion and must be considered when the results of opiate screens are interpreted; specific details will be outlined later for key opioids with active metabolites.

One of the more important CYP enzymes, CYP2D6, is particularly notable for its role in variable clinical response to opioids; it will be discussed in greater detail in a later section. Many additional CYP enzymes are involved in opioid metabolism, including CYP3A and CYP2C isoforms, among others.[574] It is important to note that several of these enzymes are subject to substrate inhibition and/or induction.[575] Substrate-dependent changes in metabolic activity are affected by other drugs, herbal supplements, or endogenous compounds that are substrates of the same enzyme. For example, methadone concentrations may be lower than expected in a patient taking St. John Wort—a noted CYP3A4 inducer—but higher in a patient ingesting a CYP3A4 inhibitor such as grapefruit juice.[575]

TABLE 41.11 Half-Life of Select Opiates

Drug	Half-Life[944]	Significant Phase I Metabolites
Natural Opium Alkaloids		
Morphine	1.3–6.7 h	
Codeine	1.2–3.9 h	Morphine
Semi-Synthetic Opiates		
Heroin	2–6 min	6-Monoacetylmorphine
Hydrocodone	3.4–8.8 h	Hydromorphone
Hydromorphone	3–9 h	
Oxycodone	3–6 h	Oxymorphone
Oxymorphone	4–12 h	

Opiates. Types of opiates include natural opium alkaloids, semisynthetic opiates, fully synthetic opioids, and opioid antagonists and mixed agonist and antagonists.

Natural Opium Alkaloids. Morphine and codeine are examples of natural opiates. The juice and seeds of the poppy plant are their primary source.

Opium is obtained from the unripe seed capsules of the poppy plant, *Papaver somniferum.* The milky juice is dried and powdered to make powdered opium, which contains several alkaloids. These alkaloids are divided into two distinct chemical classes: *phenanthrenes* and *benzylisoquinolines.* The principal phenanthrenes are morphine (10% of opium), codeine (0.5%), and thebaine (0.2%). The principal benzylisoquinolines are papaverine (1%), which is a smooth muscle relaxant, and *noscapine* (6%).[560] Only a few—morphine, codeine, and papaverine—have clinical usefulness.

Poppy seeds contain morphine and to a lesser extent codeine.[576] Ingestion of bakery products containing poppy seeds leads to excretion of morphine (and codeine) in urine.[577,578] Because of first-pass metabolism, no pharmacologic effect is experienced from poppy seed ingestion. Consumption of large amounts has been known to result in urine morphine concentrations up to 2000 ng/mL for a period of 6 to 12 hours after ingestion. In practice, it is obvious that caution is required when the results of a positive urine test for morphine and codeine are interpreted.

Morphine. The archetypical opiate, morphine, is used as the basis of comparison for relative characterizations of the opioid class. Morphine interacts primarily with MOR to mediate its effects, but it also shows some affinity for KOR.[560] Its major metabolites are glucuronide conjugates, including inactive morphine-3-glucuronide (M3G; ≈60%), active morphine-6-glucuronide (M6G; ≈10%), and a small amount of morphine-3,6-diglucuronide.[579,580] Free hydroxyl groups, such as the 3- and 6-hydroxy moieties of morphine, are frequently glucuronidated by enzymes of the uridine diphosphate glucuronyl transferase (UGT) family.[560,574] UGT2B7 is the isoform primarily responsible for morphine glucuronidation in humans[579]; other UGT enzymes such as UGT1A1 and UGT1A8 metabolize morphine in vitro, but their relevance in vivo remains uncertain.[581] Most morphine glucuronides are excreted in the feces, where substantial enterohepatic circulation of conjugated and intestinally deconjugated morphine occurs. The detection time for morphine is usually 48 hours, but this varies with individual differences in metabolism excretion and route and frequency of use.[582]

With long-term administration and when morphine concentrations are high, a minor fraction is converted to hydromorphone (up to 2.5% of the urine morphine concentration).[583] M6G has greater MOR agonist activity than morphine and appears to contribute less to unwanted side effects.[580,574,584] However, the relative importance of morphine and M6G in analgesia and adverse responses remains controversial.[580] The elimination half-life for glucoronides is longer than for morphine.[585] Therefore glucoronides accumulate in serum to greater concentrations than morphine, and in patients with renal insufficiency, morphine glucoronides are thought to significantly contribute to opioid toxicity, as patients are unable to excrete the water-soluble metabolites.[560,586]

Codeine. Because of its antitussive and analgesic properties, codeine is one of the most frequently prescribed opiates in the world; it is frequently combined with nonopiate analgesic agents such as aspirin and acetaminophen. Therefore detection of salicylate or acetaminophen along with codeine in the urine of patients who display an opiate toxidrome should lead to the measurement of salicylate or acetaminophen in serum to assess its toxicity. Alternatively, empirical quantitative serum acetaminophen and salicylate determinations are appropriate for patients with the opioid toxidrome. Codeine has only approximately one-tenth the analgesic potency of morphine and shows poor affinity for MOR, with only a fraction of the pain-relieving capacity of morphine; therefore it is generally considered a prodrug.[587] Analgesia is attributed to the small fraction (<10%) of codeine converted to morphine by CYP2D6 by *O*-demethylation, although some studies suggest that the predominant (≈80%) metabolite, codeine-6-glucuronide, may be capable of mediating CNS effects independently of morphine.[574] Both codeine and morphine may be detected in urine after codeine ingestion; however, after 30 hours only morphine may be detectable.[588] Codeine is also converted to an inactive metabolite, norcodeine (10%), and long-term high-dose administration leads to metabolism to the active compound hydrocodone (up to 11% of the urine codeine concentration).[574,589] During the early phase of excretion, codeine and conjugates predominate, but after this time, morphine conjugates are the major product. Approximately 3 days after codeine use, morphine and its conjugates are the only metabolites detected.[582,587]

Genetic variation may play a significant role in the metabolism of codeine and several other opioids. More than 100 alleles have been described for CYP2D6, with resultant enzymatic activity ranging from essentially zero, in the case of null alleles, to many times higher than normal, in the case of amplified alleles[590,591](see http://www.cypalleles.ki.se/cyp2d6.htm). Thus, at the same codeine dose, patients with minimal CYP2D6 activity (poor metabolizers) would likely receive inadequate analgesia because of lack of conversion to morphine; however, patients with very high CYP2D6 activity (ultra-rapid metabolizers) would be at risk for adverse responses to excessive morphine.[560,592] Without knowledge of the CYP2D6 genotype, these clinical presentations can be confusing; the possibility of pharmacogenetic effects is therefore important to consider when appropriate dosing, patient compliance, and potential diversion or illicit use is assessed. The pharmacokinetic pathway for codeine is shown in Fig. 54.3 and the pharmacogenetic aspects of codeine application are discussed in more detail in Chapter 54.

Semisynthetic Opiates. Heroin, hydrocodone, hydromorphone, oxycodone, and oxymorphone are examples of semisynthetic opiates.

Heroin. Heroin is a synthetic opiate that is made from morphine and is also called diacetylmorphine or diamorphine; it has an analgesic potency two to three times that of morphine[582] because of its better penetration across the blood-brain barrier. Heroin is no longer legally available in the United States, but it is still used elsewhere for fast-acting analgesia.[593] The two acetyl groups enhance CNS distribution,[594] providing a rapid effect when first-pass metabolism is bypassed (eg, intravenous administration). Heroin itself is rarely found in body fluids because of its extremely short half-life (2 to 6 minutes).[582,595] The metabolite, 6-acetylmorphine, is hydrolyzed to morphine,[595,596] and although it has a longer half-life (6 to 25 minutes),[595] it is detectable in urine for only approximately 8 hours after administration.[582] Both 6-acetylmorphine and morphine are pharmacologically active, with 6-monoacetylmorphine (6-MAM) being four to six times more potent than morphine.[582] Other than the presence of its unique metabolite 6-MAM, which is definitive for heroin use, the metabolic profile of heroin resembles that of morphine.[597] Given that acetylcodeine is a common contaminant of heroin, both morphine and low concentrations of codeine are frequently detected in urine after heroin use.

Hydrocodone. Hydrocodone has approximately six times the potency and greater oral bioavailability than codeine,[598] but it is thought to be more toxic than codeine.[599] Hydrocodone is *O*-demethylated to hydromorphone, *N*-demethylated to form norhydrocodone, and C6-keto–reduced to form approximately equal amounts of 6-α- and 6-β-hydrocol.[37,38] Similar to codeine, hydrocodone is metabolized by CYP2D6 to an active metabolite (hydromorphone) and therefore may be subject to pharmacogenetic variability in patients with abnormal CYP2D6 activity.[600]

It has been suggested that most of the pharmacologic effects of hydrocodone actually result from the hydromorphone formed during metabolism.[599] However, studies are somewhat contradictory. Hydrocodone may provide effective pain relief even in the absence of CYP2D6- mediated conversion to hydromorphone.[601,602] It remains unclear whether this is due primarily to the activity of hydrocodone itself or to that of other active metabolites.[601,603]

Hydromorphone. Oral hydromorphone is five to seven times more potent than morphine.[598] Although it is used as an analgesic in its own right with potency somewhat higher than that of hydrocodone,[602] hydromorphone is also a metabolite of hydrocodone.[583] Similar to morphine, hydromorphone is metabolized in large part to a 3-glucuronide by UGT2B7, but also to a lesser extent by UGT1A3.[604,605] Hydromorphone lacks a free hydroxyl group at the 6 position, thus there is no metabolite analogous to M6G.[604,605] Two minor metabolites of hydromorphone—dihydromorphine and dihydroisomorphine—have demonstrated pharmacologic activity, but their contribution may be minimal because of the small amount formed.[598,599]

Oxycodone. Oxycodone is a potent analgesic with high oral bioavailability[560,606] that is frequently formulated in combination with aspirin or acetaminophen. Therefore the detection of salicylate or acetaminophen along with oxycodone in the urine of patients who display an opiate toxidrome should lead to measurement of serum salicylate or acetaminophen concentration to assess toxicity. Noncombination oxycodone is also available in immediate- and extended-release dosage forms. The latter (OxyContin) is a very effective oral analgesic for patients with chronic pain (eg, cancer patients). The pills may be chewed, crushed, snorted, or solubilized for intravenous injection to permit immediate availability of the entire dose, which is intended for extended release over a 12-hour period. This practice has led to widespread misuse, more frequent emergency department visits, and increased mortality in the United States.[599]

Although its own strong analgesic activity precludes oxycodone from being considered a prodrug, it is converted to a highly active metabolite, oxymorphone, through the activity of CYP2D6.[607] This conversion appears to be less of a concern for CYP2D6 poor metabolizers, in whom oxycodone itself still provides analgesia, than for ultra-rapid metabolizers, who could be at increased risk for adverse effects.[608]

Oxymorphone. Oxymorphone provides potent analgesia with minimal interaction with CYP enzymes, although it is also a substrate for CYP2C9 and CYP3A4.[609] The majority of oxymorphone is metabolized by UGT2B7 to the 3-glucuronide; a minor metabolite, 6-hydroxyoxymorphone, is an active analgesic with a steady-state area under the curve (AUC) similar to that of the parent compound. Oxymorphone is a metabolite of oxycodone that is formed via CYP2D6.[604,605]

Fully Synthetic Opioids. Fentanyl, meperidine, methadone, propoxyphene, and tramadol are examples of fully synthetic opioids.

Fentanyl. Fentanyl is an alipophilic drug with numerous routes of administration that is used in applications ranging from anesthesia to rapid management of breakthrough pain.[610] Fentanyl has a rapid onset and short duration of effect. Fentanyl provides the structural backbone for a number of related, ultra-short-acting opioids, including remifentanil and sufentanil. Norfentanyl, the primary metabolite, is generated by CYP3A and is inactive[611]; the high potency of fentanyl and the clinical insignificance of its metabolites make it a preferred analgesic for patients with major organ failure.[610] Transdermal fentanyl patches are used for longer term administration and are gaining popularity among drug abusers, although nonstandard application of the patch (eg, chewing, extraction) carries substantial risk for overdose.[612]

The designer drug acetylfentanyl is an illicit structural analog of fentanyl. Acetylfentanyl emerged in early 2013 when a regional upswing in heroin overdose deaths was recognized.[613,614] Unknown to the user, heroin may be laced with acetylfentanyl. Acetylfentanyl is at least five times stronger than heroin and may require higher doses of naloxone as an antidote.

Meperidine. Originally synthesized as an anticholinergic, meperidine has analgesic potency comparable with or somewhat lower than that of morphine.[615] One major metabolite, normeperidine, also has analgesic activity; normeperidine is thought to be responsible for the serotonergic toxicity of meperidine, particularly in patients receiving concomitant monoamine oxidase inhibitors.[560,615] Meperidine use has declined in recent years in favor of alternatives such as fentanyl.

Methadone. A relatively long-acting opiate, methadone is used both for analgesia and in the treatment of opioid addiction.[560] It is thought to provide (1) milder withdrawal, (2) somewhat lower potential for abuse, and (3) reduced exposure to the risks of illicit intravenous drug use.[616] Methadone has affinity for both MOR and DOR,[617] the latter of which may explain its apparent utility in patients whose pain no longer responds to other opioids.[618] Substantial interindividual and intraindividual variability in metabolism and elimination has been noted; both urine pH and seemingly self-inducible metabolism substantially influence the pharmacokinetics of this compound, as do commonly coadministered drugs such as benzodiazepines and antiretrovirals.[560] Although a large fraction of methadone is excreted unchanged, measurement of a metabolite such as 2-ethylidene-1,5-dimethyl-3,3-diphenylpyrrolidine (EDDP) in the setting of addiction treatment provides evidence for patient compliance rather than an exogenously spiked sample.[619-621] EDDP excretion is less pH dependent than is clearance of the parent drug.[560,582,622] Use of the methadone-to-EDDP ratio to assess compliance has been suggested but is complicated by the pharmacokinetic variability already described.[619-621]

Propoxyphene. A relatively weak analgesic, propoxyphene is less potent than codeine but carries the significant risk for atypical adverse effects such as cardiac arrhythmia and seizure. The incidence of such negative responses is particularly high in the elderly.[623] In July 2009, the FDA required manufacturers to strengthen the black box warning to address the increased risk for overdose (see http://www.fda.gov/NewsEvents/Newsroom/PressAnnouncements/ucm170769.htm). However, its nonmedical abuse remains common.[624]

Tramadol. Unlike the majority of opioid agonists, tramadol has low abuse potential and therefore is unscheduled.[625] It has low affinity for opioid receptors and mediates analgesia through opioid-independent regulation of neurotransmitter uptake; however, its main active metabolite (*O*-desmethyltramadol, or M1) is a potent opioid receptor agonist.[574] These mechanisms are thought to work synergistically to provide greater total pain relief than the sum of each individual component. Metabolism to M1 occurs via CYP2D6; thus opioid-like effects are subject to genetic variability, as with codeine.[625] However, because of its effects on neurotransmission, tramadol has the potential to cause serotonergic toxicity even in patients lacking CYP2D6.[574] In fact, several synthetic phenylpiperidine opioids (tramadol, methadone, DXM, and propoxyphene) have been associated with increased risk for serotonin toxicity caused by weak reuptake inhibition of monoamines when used in combination with SSRIs, monoamine oxidase inhibitors, and amphetamine-type stimulants.[626-629]

Opioid Antagonists and Mixed Agonists and Antagonists. These clinically useful compounds produce very different physiologic responses, depending on the situation. For example, in opioid-naïve patients, mixed agonists and antagonists (MAAs) provide MOR-mediated analgesia with less risk for an adverse reaction, but the same dose in an opioid-tolerant patient may precipitate immediate withdrawal. In medical usage, coadministration of low-dose antagonists or MAAs alleviates minor opioid-induced side effects and appears useful in preventing opioid tolerance. In opioid addiction treatment, the addition of a low-dose antagonist to maintenance therapy seems to minimize subjective "feel-good" effects without substantially worsening withdrawal symptoms.

Buprenorphine, naloxone, and naltrexone are examples of opioid antagonists and mixed agonists and antagonists.

Buprenorphine. A semisynthetic derivative of thebaine, buprenorphine is a MOR partial agonist and a KOR antagonist. Low doses provide analgesia through MOR activation, but unlike full agonists, pain relief has a maximal threshold, or ceiling effect.[630] Buprenorphine is available as sublingual tablets (with or without naloxone) for the treatment of opioid dependence and as a transdermal patch.[624] Buprenorphine is metabolized via *N*-dealkylation by CYP3A4 to the active compound, norbuprenorphine, both of which can be further conjugated to inactive glucuronides by UGT1A1.[602,605] CYP3A4 and UGT1A1 are subject to environmental and genetic variability, although the effects of these factors on buprenorphine are not well characterized.[560] Sublingual formulation of the drug is eliminated primarily in feces, with only a small amount in urine, and is usually detectable for 1 to 3 days.[582]

Naloxone. The prototypical opioid antagonist naloxone binds nonspecifically to all three receptor types, with the greatest effect at MOR and the least effect at DOR.[560,631] Its efficacy is much greater by intravenous administration than by oral and sublingual routes.[624,632] This characteristic is advantageous in deterring misuse of prescribed opioids: oral or sublingual opioid/naloxone formulations provide the desired benefit when taken properly, but when diverted for intravenous use cause opioid antagonism and may precipitate withdrawal.[624,632] When buprenorphine/naloxone formulations are properly administered, naloxone is *N*-demethylated to noroxymorphone, and the metabolite may be detected in random urine specimens.

Naloxone is commonly used in comatose patients as a therapeutic and diagnostic agent. The standard dosage regimen is 0.4 mg administered slowly, preferably intravenously, with the dose increased until the desired end point is achieved—namely, restoration of respiratory function, ability to protect the airway, and improved concentration of consciousness. Naloxone has been known to precipitate profound withdrawal symptoms in opioid-dependent patients. Its clinical efficacy lasts for as little as 45 minutes. Therefore patients are at risk for recurrence of narcotic effect. This is particularly true for patients exposed to opioids with long elimination half-lives, such as methadone and sustained-release opioid products. Patients should be observed for resedation for at least 4 hours after reversal with naloxone. Because naloxone is renally eliminated, patients with renal dysfunction may have delayed resedation past the 4 hours and should therefore be observed for a longer period.

Naltrexone. Commonly used for the treatment of alcoholism, naltrexone is a potent antagonist of all three opioid receptors.[631] Its combined formulation with opioid agonists is less common than naloxone/opioid combinations; however, the greater oral bioavailability of naltrexone suggests that it may be useful in applications in which poor oral delivery limits the utility of naloxone.[624]

Analytical Methods. Many different immunoassay methods are used to screen for opiates. GC-MS has historically been the gold standard for confirmation of a positive screening test. LC-MS/MS is commonly used for confirmation in clinical and forensic specimens.

Screening Assays. Given their relatively rapid turnaround time and ability to identify several opiates, immunoassays are the methods of choice to screen urine samples for opiate content. For clinical application, a cutoff of 300 ng/mL morphine (or morphine equivalents) is commonly used to distinguish negative from positive urine specimens, whereas a cutoff of 2000 ng/mL is mandated by SAMHSA for workplace drug screening. Antibodies in opiate abuse screens commonly target morphine, because commercial immunoassay development has largely been driven by detection of illicit heroin use. Wide variability in cross-reactivity to other congeners has been noted; thus some opiates or opioids (see Fig. 41.13) with high abuse potential such as oxycodone are often poorly detected.[386,633,634] To address this problem, several immunoassays are commercially available for individual synthetic opioids, such as fentanyl. Finally, analytical interferences are also a problem with opiate immunoassays.[633,635-639] Other general opiate screening methods are available, including TLC, but these techniques are more labor intensive and may not provide adequate turnaround time for STAT or emergency testing. In this setting, point-of-care devices are being used more frequently.[640-642]

In pain management programs, urine drug testing is often used to monitor compliance or substitution for prescribed drugs. Based on the results of such tests, an individual may be dismissed from the program. It is important for drug-testing laboratories to communicate relevant aspects regarding testing method limitations as well as the metabolic interconversion of opiates to physicians responsible for these programs. As an example, monitoring compliance for oxycodone in pain management programs is problematic because of the low cross-reactivity of oxycodone in most opiate immunoassays. In this instance, a false-negative opiate immunoassay test may lead to an accusation of oxycodone diversion. Oxycodone immunoassay tests are available, but determination of oxycodone and its metabolite(s) by a confirmatory method (GC-MS, LC-MS, LC-MS/MS) may be more appropriate to monitor compliance for this drug.

Confirmation Testing. For compound-specific confirmation assays, GC-MS has historically been considered the method of choice. Analysis of specific opioids is typically performed using GC or LC. GC generally results in longer run times and is often incompatible with larger metabolites such as glucuronide conjugates. A wide variety of detectors are available for both GC and LC; MS or MS/MS is often preferred for the structural and mass-specific information provided. Analytical and technical considerations are discussed in detail later.

Sample Preparation and Extraction. The matrix and rationale for opioid testing influences the choice of method. Analysis of urine requires hydrolysis to recover glucuronide- or sulfate-conjugated metabolites of various opioids. Hydrolysis is performed by acidification (eg, concentrated hydrochloric acid at 115 to 120°C for 15 minutes)[578,643,644] or by enzymatic treatment with β-glucuronidase alone[645-647] or in combination with arylsulfatase.[648] Acid hydrolysis is simpler and more rapid and typically provides greater recovery than enzymatic methods, although a few studies have shown better recovery of some analytes with glucuronidase.[649] Acidification, however, destroys the metabolite 6-MAM, preventing conclusive determination of heroin use; it also partially degrades morphine.[650] For this reason, drugs-of-abuse testing for opiates typically employs enzymatic hydrolysis, regardless of its generally poorer analytical performance.

Serum analysis is performed with or without a hydrolysis step; if a hydrolysis step is included, results reflect the sum of parent drug and metabolites, that is, "total" drug concentration. For detection of illicit drug use, total concentrations are typically sufficient. However, omitting hydrolysis to preserve conjugated metabolites can be useful, for example, when both the parent and the metabolite are active compounds, as with morphine and M6G.

Methods of analysis from serum or urine were initially developed using LLE,[644,646,647,651-654] although SPE[648,655-658] is now often preferred. Some methods do not derivatize before GC analysis,[659,660] but this typically results in poor chromatographic properties. Although the number of derivatizing agents described in the literature is relatively limited, great variability in experimental conditions has been noted.[577,578,644,646-648,653,661-665]

Gas Chromatography. Several GC-MS methods have been developed to quantitate various combinations of morphine, other opiates, and their metabolites from extracts of human urine.[643,666,667] GC-MS is considered the reference method for determination of most natural and semisynthetic opiates, particularly in forensic settings, although other detectors are available and have been used for GC applications. Various GC-MS methods have been described for the identification and determination of opiates. Some investigators use chemical ionization,[668-671] but electron impact mode is more common. The GC is typically equipped with a 12- or 15-m fused-silica capillary column with a polar stationary phase of cross-linked dimethylsilicone, phenyl methyl silicone, or 95% dimethyl-5% polysiloxane.[646,648,662,664,672] Because of structural similarities between many opiates, particularly natural and semi-synthetic opiates, assays must be evaluated for interference from metabolites and congeners. The degree of overlap is such that the fragmentation patterns of various opioids can resemble one another greatly, as is seen with the mass spectra of the trimethylsilane (TMS) derivatives of hydromorphone, morphine, and norcodeine.[673] Chromatographic resolution of these compounds must be carefully optimized to provide reliable characterization, particularly because many structurally related opiates are commercially available and are part of the same metabolic pathways.

Although acetyl derivatives have the advantage of being stable for up to 72 hours when stored at room temperature in ethyl acetate, incomplete derivatization may occur when acetyl-donating agents are used.[646,664] Both morphine and 6-MAM are converted to diacetylmorphine (heroin); thus acetyl derivatization does not permit distinction among morphine, 6-MAM, and heroin. In addition to diacetylmorphine, a small amount of 3-monoacetylmorphine (3-MAM) is formed by acetylating agents; although clinically insignificant, 3-MAM shares the mass-to-charge ratio *(m/z)* 285 ion with deuterated (d3) d3-acetylcodeine and interferes with analysis of these compounds.[661]

In contrast to acetylating agents, TMS creates single derivatives for most opiates, although TMS derivatives are sensitive to moisture.[662] Several analytical interferences are associated with TMS; codeine and norcodeine derivatives coelute on GC, whereas 6-MAM produces an additional peak that coelutes with morphine and increases with room temperature storage.[674] Like with TMS, PFP derivatives are moisture-sensitive; however, no breakdown products are detected after storage for 24 hours.[661] The addition of pentafluoropropanol (PFPOH) improves the yield of PFP derivatives and allows morphine and 6-MAM to be clearly distinguished.[655,664]

Liquid Chromatography. Despite the long-standing role of GC in opiate analysis, LC methods are common and are often analytically advantageous. One notable example is that LC provides the ability to analyze glucuronide-conjugated metabolites as well as parent compounds. In addition, LC methods are able to measure polar metabolites without prior derivatization,[675] and on-column extraction is possible with some LC systems. As with GC, a variety of detectors are available for LC. For example, HPLC methods for opioid analysis have been described using fluorescence, UV-visible, electrochemical, and DAD detection, alone and in various combinations. In addition, several analytical methods for morphine and its glucuronide metabolites exist for LC-MS or LC-MS/MS with different MS interfaces.[676-688]

Analytical methods also include common opioids such as methadone[689] or buprenorphine[690] or other nonopioid drugs of abuse such as cocaine, amphetamines, and LSD.[675,691,692] Ultra-high-performance chromatographic methods using MS/MS or HRMS are gaining utility when comprehensive assays are necessary to monitor multiple drug classes with various polar characteristics in pain management populations. This population requires lower levels of quantitation than regulated drug cutoffs and broad analytical measurement range. Assays should test for illicit, prescribed, and nonprescribed drugs for monitoring compliance, misuse, and potential drug diversion.

For TDM testing, recent reports have focused on quantitation of multiple opioids used therapeutically (eg, in palliative care). For example, in one study, an LC-MS/MS method was developed that was capable of measuring 11 opioids and 5 metabolites, namely, buprenorphine, codeine, fentanyl, hydromorphone, methadone, morphine, oxycodone, oxymorphone, piritramide, tilidine, and tramadol, with the metabolites bisnortilidine, morphine glucuronides, norfentanyl, and nortilidine.[693] In another study, a combination screening and confirmation method was developed to identify fentanyl, alfentanil, remifentanil, and sufentanil and their respective *N*-dealkylated or deesterified metabolites using LC-MS/MS.[694] Metabolite profiling is another growing area in TDM testing, especially for compounds with known active metabolites such as tramadol.[695]

Mitragynine (Kratom). Mitragynine is an alkaloid found in the leaves of the South East Asian tree *Mitragyna speciosa.* Kratom leaves are chewed, smoked, or consumed in tea.[696] Leaves from this tree have traditionally been used for both their stimulant properties and as an opium substitute. Mitragynine is a potent and selective μ-opioid agonist.[697] It has been shown that the antinociceptive effects are mediated by its action on the supraspinal μ- and δ-opioid, whereas its psychoactive effects may be mediated by central opioid receptors.[698] Case reports of toxicity and death have been reported in polydrug exposure, including mytragynine.[699] Although widespread use of kratom has not been documented in the United States, its use has been increasing in some locations.

Screening and Confirmation. Mitragynine does not cross-react with commercially available immunoassays for opiates. However, it has been identified in patient samples by LC with UV[700,701] or LC-MS/MS[702-704] and direct analysis in real-time-MS.[705]

Phencyclidine and Ketamine

On the street, PCP and ketamine are sold under a variety of names. They are available as a colorless, odorless liquid, or as a white powder. Either form can be easily disguised in a beverage, or they can be added to marijuana or tobacco and smoked.

Pharmacologic Effects. PCP is listed as a Schedule II drug in the US Federal Controlled Substance Act and is not approved for human use. Ketamine is a Schedule III drug used as an anesthetic in pediatric medicine for short surgical procedures. Both drugs have been used illicitly in human cases of drug abuse, as well as in cases of drug-facilitated crimes.

Ketamine and PCP share similar structural features[256] and pharmacologic actions. They are classified as dissociative anesthetics because they produce rapid-acting dissociation of perception, consciousness, movement, and memory.[706-708] The effects are dose dependent and vary across individuals. Some individuals experience effects similar to the psychosis observed in schizophrenia.[709,710] An anesthetic dose produces profound analgesia, in which the individual is awake yet incapacitated, with limited voluntary limb movement. Both PCP and ketamine have been associated with psychologic disturbances.

The mechanism of action for these compounds consists of complex integration of neurologic pathways. They bind and antagonize the excitatory glutaminergic system by binding to NMDA receptors. They also decrease GABA transmission, disrupt cortical activity, and increase dopamine and norepinephrine synaptic reuptake. These actions can produce clinical effects such as euphoria, elevated blood pressure, tachycardia, and bronchodilation, all of which are consequences of inhibition of dopamine and norepinephrine synaptic reuptake.[708,711] At a higher dose, GABA-ergic and central nicotinic actions may produce sedation, lethargy, coma, and respiratory depression. Additionally, central and peripheral muscarinic and nicotinic responses may cause miosis or mydriasis, diaphoresis, increased salivation, bronchorrhea, blurred vision, and urinary retention.

Phencyclidine. PCP was synthesized in 1926 and was used clinically as a general anesthetic. Because of adverse side effects experienced by some individuals, such as acute psychosis and dysphoria during emergence from PCP-induced anesthesia, clinical use was discontinued. PCP is used recreationally for its mind-altering "out of body" experience. Recreational use of PCP declined in the 1980s but has reemerged in recent years. Presentation of adverse effects such as dysphoria, ataxia, nystagmus, agitation, anxiety, paranoia, amnesia, seizures, muscle rigidity, hostility, delirium, delusions, and hallucinations is unpredictable. Evidence of flashbacks have been documented with PCP use. Known dose thresholds or frequency of PCP use has not been correlated with flashback occurrences.

The onset of action for PCP is fast for intravenous and inhalation routes (2 to 5 minutes) and slower after oral administration (30 to 60 minutes).[712,713] Clinical effects typically last 4 to 6 hours, yet psychotic episodes have been reported to last a month.[709,710] The relationships among dosage, clinical effects, and serum concentrations are not a reliable predictor of the degree of PCP intoxication.[708] PCP has a pK_a between 8.5 and 9.4, is highly lipophilic, and distributes to the brain and fat tissues. An ion-trapping phenomenon occurs after oral, intravenous, or inhalation dosing. PCP enters acidic gastric fluid after oral administration, where concentrations may be 20 to 50 times greater than in serum, then undergoes gastroenterohepatic recirculation.[544] Ion trapping also occurs in cerebrospinal fluid (CSF), causing it to cross back into the blood; CSF may accumulate to concentrations 6 to 9 times greater than those observed in serum.[714] These properties may contribute to the waxing and waning of clinical effects and prolonged excretion. PCP has a large V_d of 5 to 7 L/kg, a long elimination $t_{1/2}$ (20 to 50 hours), a long duration of action (24 to 48 hours), and prolonged urinary excretion after the last dose (1 to 2 weeks; longer with long-term use).[544]

With repeated use of PCP, psychologic dependence may develop, but tolerance or withdrawal syndrome is not profound. A sense of superhuman strength coupled with lack of pain perception may lead to excessive physical exertion and accidental or intentionally induced trauma. Thus PCP-related deaths most often are secondary to these adverse behavioral drug effects. Treatment of PCP toxicity is supportive. Severe agitation or seizures may respond to diazepam; severe psychoses may require a neuroleptic drug, such as haloperidol. For the most serious cases, continuous nasogastric suction to help remove PCP may be beneficial; urine acidification to hasten elimination has been advocated by some but is controversial.[708]

Ketamine. Ketamine was discovered during subsequent studies characterizing PCP analogs. Liquid ketamine is rapidly injected intramuscularly. The liquid or powder form can be easily disguised in a victim's beverage; this has resulted in its use in DFSA.[715,716] Ketamine powder can even be sprinkled onto marijuana or tobacco and smoked.

Ketamine produces effects similar to those of PCP. Onset of clinical effects is rapid and depends on dose and route of administration. Anesthesia effects via intramuscular injection take as little as 20 to 30 seconds, oral ingestion approximately 30 minutes,[717] and nasal insufflation approximately 10 minutes.[718-720] Its hallucinatory effects may be short-acting (<1 hour) but so intense that the victim may have trouble discerning reality.[716] Ketamine has approximately one-tenth the potency of PCP, a shorter duration of action, and less prominent emergence reactions, especially in children.

Ketamine has a $t_{1/2}$ of 2 to 3 hours.[721] Ketamine is metabolized to norketamine, which has approximately one-third the activity of ketamine, and to dehydronorketamine, which also may be active.[256] Duration of anesthetic effects is dose dependent (usually <1 hour), and effects on the senses, judgment, and coordination can have a longer duration (≈6 to 24 hours). At higher doses, ketamine causes delirium, amnesia, dissociative anesthesia, hallucinations, delirium, hypersalivation, nystagmus, impaired motor function, hypertension, and potentially fatal respiratory problems. Effects on blood pressure and respiratory depression are significantly enhanced when coingested with alcohol.

Screening and Confirmation. Initial screening is typically done by immunoassay.[722] PCP is required to be included in US government–regulated drug abuse screening programs (see https://www.transportation.gov/odapc/part40). Whether PCP and ketamine are included in a general urine drug screen depends on applicable regulations and on the prevalence of use in the local community. In some locations, the prevalence of PCP or ketamine use may be too low to warrant routine screening.

Immunoassays are generally reliable; however, false-positive results for PCP have been reported because of high concentrations of DXM,[723,724] diphenhydramine,[725] and thioridazine.[726,727] Immunoassay-positive specimens should be confirmed using GC-MS[728,729] or LC-MS analyses.[730]

Specimen Validity Testing

Drug testing results for nonmedical purposes may provide the sole evidence for punitive action or denial of individual rights. Therefore this testing should be considered a forensic toxicology activity, requiring the highest standards of analytical methods, specimen security, and documentation.[731] Moreover, laboratories engaged in this testing in the United States should be appropriately certified by SAMHSA of the US Department of Health and Human Services (DHHS) or the Forensic Urine Drug Testing program sponsored jointly by the American Association for Clinical Chemistry and the College of American Pathologists.

Several techniques are used by persons attempting to mask or adulterate drugs to avoid detection. These tactics may include the exchange of urine from a drug-free individual or dilution of the urine specimen by excessive consumption of water, use of a diuretic, or simple addition of water to the specimen to reduce drug concentrations to below cutoff limits. Also, readily available adulterants, such as detergent, bleach, salt, alkali, ammonia, tetrahydrozoline, or acid, may be added to the specimen after collection in an attempt to interfere with immunoassay screening procedures. Other, more sophisticated adulterants specifically marketed to avoid drug detection include glutaraldehyde (Urine Aid, Clear Choice), nitrite (Klear, Whizzies), chromate (Urine Luck, Sweet Pee's Spoiler), and a combination of peroxide and peroxidase (Stealth). These adulterants also interfere with immunoassays to variable degrees, and the oxidizing agents (nitrite, chromate, peroxide/peroxidase) may result in destruction of morphine, codeine, and the principal metabolite resulting from marijuana use, thus interfering with their GC-MS confirmation and with immunoassays.[732]

Direct observation of urine collection is the most stringent means to guard against specimen exchange or adulteration. However, an individual's right to privacy and dignity must be weighed against the need for the highest degree of certainty of specimen integrity. Alternative measures to prevent specimen adulteration include (1) limitations on clothing or other personal belongings allowed in the specimen collection area, (2) addition of coloring agent to toilet water, and (3) inactivation of the hot water tap. In addition, several validity checks for specimen integrity may be made at the collection site and at the testing site. Validity testing criteria have been established by the DHHS for the drug testing program mandated for US federal employees (see https://www.transportation.gov/odapc/part40). Numerous commercial reagents for validity testing are available in both test strip and liquid forms.

Urine should be collected in tamper-proof specimen cups and a chain of custody maintained to identify all individuals involved in specimen collection, transfer, and testing. Specimens that test positive should be stored frozen for a minimum of 1 year. Detailed information on the collection and processing of specimens for drug testing has been presented in the federal rules for employee drug testing (see *Federal Register* 49 CFR Part 40, Procedures For Transportation Workplace Drug And Alcohol Testing Programs. https://www.transportation.gov/odapc/part40)[731] and in the federal regulations promulgated by the Department of Transportation and the Nuclear Regulatory Commission (see http://www.nrc.gov/reading-rm/doc-collections/cfr/part026).

Workplace drug testing generally is restricted to alcohol and a few drugs that have high abuse potential, some of which are illicit (see https://www.transportation.gov/odapc/part40). Depending on the nature of the testing program, testing may be provided for a select number of the following drug classes: *amphetamines,* barbiturates, benzodiazepines, *cannabinoids, cocaine,* LSD, *opiates,* synthetic opioids, and *PCP* (drugs in italics are required for testing by the National Institute of Drug Abuse and are known as the NIDA five). Testing programs for participants[675] engaged in athletic competition typically are much more extensive and include assays for a larger group of drugs, including stimulants, β-blockers, diuretics, and anabolic steroids (see https://www.wada-ama.org/). See "Athletes and Drug Testing" section for more detail.

Initial screening tests for the previously listed drugs are typically immunoassays. These assays are calibrated at established cutoff concentrations. Specimens yielding responses greater than the cutoff (threshold) value are considered positive, whereas values below the cutoff are considered negative. Cutoff values are not synonymous with assay detection limits. Instead, the cutoff is established higher than the detection limit (to ensure reliable measurement) but low enough to detect drug use within a reasonable time frame.

Immunoassays may demonstrate limited specificity within certain drug classes. Similar drugs may result in a positive test; for example, pseudoephedrine, present in cold medications, may produce a positive response in immunoassays designed to detect amphetamine and methamphetamine. Therefore it is imperative that positive screening tests be confirmed by an alternative, more definitive test. The most widely accepted method for drug confirmation is GC-MS. LC-MS/MS is also used for rapid detection and confirmation of drugs of abuse.[733,734]

For confirmation, quantitative drug measurements are performed using selective ion monitoring with GC-MS. Cutoff values for confirmation are established at or generally below cutoff values for the initial screening tests (see https://www.transportation.gov/odapc/part40). The result may be reported as positive or negative relative to the cutoff value. However, the actual concentration may be helpful when morphine and codeine results are interpreted and when individuals enrolled in drug treatment programs are monitored. In the latter case, subjects who test positive but who have decreasing values on sequential testing may be judged abstinent, whereas those whose values suddenly increase are likely noncompliant. For this purpose, it is essential to normalize the drug concentration to urine creatinine concentration (nanograms of drug per milligram of creatinine). This will help compensate for fluctuations in absolute drug concentration related to physiologic variation in urine dilution or concentration.[735,736]

Chain of Custody

Clinical drug testing can be readily distinguished from forensic drug testing because clinical specimens are not collected using a documented chain of custody. Chain of custody procedures are outside the scope of this chapter so will not be discussed in detail. Briefly, it refers to the documentation that unequivocally identifies the donor of a specimen and chronologically tracks handling of the samples from the collection to the completion of testing, reporting, and disposal. It is particularly important in criminal cases; the concept is also applied in civil litigation and sometimes more broadly in drug testing of athletes.

Drug-Facilitated Crimes

Drug-facilitated crimes is defined as voluntary or surreptitious use of alcohol, drugs, and/or chemical agents to incapacitate an individual and facilitate a criminal act. This includes drug-facilitated sexual assault.[737] In addition to alcohol, the drugs that have been implicated in drug-facilitated crimes include (1) chloral hydrate, (2) benzodiazepines, (3) nonbenzodiazepine sedative-hypnotics, (4) γ-hydroxybutyric acid (GHB), (5) dextramethorphan, (6) ketamine, (7) PCP, and nonprescription medications such as (8) antihistamines and (9) anticholinergics. The Society of Forensic Toxicologists Drug-Facilitated Crimes Committee has recommended analytical cutoff for testing of commonly encountered compounds (see http://soft-tox.org/files/SOFT_DFC_Rec_Det_Limits_1-2014.pdf). These drugs share similar characteristics that are desired by an assailant, such as fast onset, lack of color and taste, and easy access. Similar clinical effects permit the victim to be easily incapacitated. They include impaired judgment, confusion, reduced inhibitions, sedation, hypnosis, loss of muscle coordination, and sometimes anterograde amnesia. These effects are intensified when they are coadministered willingly or involuntarily with other psychotropic medications that produce CNS depression. This is a common occurrence in reported cases of sexual assault or rape.[738,739]

Studies performed in the United States indicated that ethanol, not surprisingly, was the most common drug involved. Following that were cannabis and benzodiazepines (diazepam and alprazolam), and less frequently reported were zolpidem, stimulants, opiates, diphenhydramine, citalopram, quetiapine, carisoprodol, GHB, methadone, DXM, tramadol, and methylone.[740,741] Some of the drugs not previously discussed are elaborated on in the following section.

Chloral Hydrate

Anecdotal reports concerning assailants dosing beverages with incapacitating compounds to assault their victims date back to the early nineteenth century. An infamous example is the saloon proprietor Mickey Finn. He was alleged to have drugged his customers with the addition of chloral hydrate to their ethanol-based beverages and subsequently robbed them.

Chloral hydrate is classified as a nonbarbiturate hypnotic. It is an inexpensive transparent crystalline compound that easily dissolves in beverages. It was first synthesized in 1832 and was one of the original "depressants" developed for the specific purpose of inducing sleep. This drug is still used today in pediatric medicine for sedating children before diagnostic procedures. Abuse and misuse of this drug and subsequent introduction of newer sedatives (barbiturates and benzodiazepines) led to its decline for medicinal purposes and therefore is very infrequently identified.

Pharmacologic Effects. The clinical diagnosis of chloral hydrate intoxication is difficult to differentiate from alcohol, benzodiazepine, and barbiturate intoxication, as all share similar clinical effects. Although the exact mechanism of action of chloral hydrate has not been determined, it is a general CNS depressant that has sedative effects with minimal analgesic effects when administered independently. At low doses, symptoms may include relaxation, dizziness, slurred speech, confusion, disorientation, euphoria, irritability, and hypersensitivity rash. At higher doses, chloral hydrate causes hypotension, hypothermia, hypoventilation, tachydysrhythmias, nausea, vomiting, diarrhea, headache, and amnesia.[719] Onset of action is rapid (10 to 20 minutes). The elimination half-life of chloral hydrate is 4 to 12 hours.[719,742] If coingested with alcohol, the metabolism of chloral hydrate may be seriously impaired. Because both ethanol and chloral hydrate are metabolized by CYP2E1 and ADH, coingestion may not only exacerbate their clinical effects but also prolong their duration of action.[742,743]

Analytical Methods. Chloral hydrate is not detected on routine, commercially available drug screens. Quantification of chloral hydrate and its metabolites trichloroethanol (TCE), TCE-glucuronide, and trichloroacetic acid is detected in plasma using HPLC-MS and capillary GC with electron-capture detection (GC-ECD),[405,744,745] or GC-FID.[746] Typical therapeutic concentrations are 2 to 12 μg/mL. Chloral hydrate metabolites have been detected as low as 10 ng/mL using GC-ECD.[745]

Benzodiazepines

It is estimated that 8% of sexual assault cases are positive for benzodiazepines.[738,739,747,748] Many benzodiazepines that have been reported in sexual assault victims are diazepam, triazolam, temazepam, tetrazepam, and clonazepam.[749-753] However, it has recently been shown that diazepam and alprazolam are the most frequently identified.[741]

The benzodiazepine flunitrazepam (Rohypnol), because of its potent sedative-hypnotic action, especially in combination with alcohol, and its ability to induce short-term (anterograde) amnesia, has gained notoriety for drug-facilitated crimes, even though its identification is uncommon compared with that of other benzodiazepines. Flunitrazepam is categorized as a Schedule I drug in the United States. Because it is still licensed for use in Europe, Asia, and Latin America for sedation and treatment of insomnia, the drug can be obtained through illegal trafficking.[754]

Pharmacologic Effects. Flunitrazepam is more potent than diazepam because of its slower dissociation from the GABA receptor.[755-757] It is rapidly absorbed and distributed into tissues upon oral administration. Onset of its sedative, amnesic, hypnotic, and disinhibitory effects can occur within 20 to 30 minutes.[755] Flunitrazepam has a long half-life (≈26 hours), permitting an extended window of detection in blood and urine. Although the effects of flunitrazepam occur rapidly when it is used alone, it is often coingested with alcohol, which amplifies its effects.[758,759] Initial symptoms may consist of dizziness, disorientation, lack of coordination, and slurred speech, all of which mimic alcohol intoxication. Another unique effect is anterograde amnesia as early as 15 minutes after oral administration.[760] Large doses (>2 g) have produced aspiration, muscular hypotonia, hypotension, bradycardia, coma, and death.[715,751,753]

Analytical Methods. The detection of flunitrazepam is especially challenging because of the low therapeutic and illicit doses and the varying degree of cross-reactivity with most immunoassays with the principal urinary metabolite 7-aminoflunitrazepam.[426,427,761] As with other benzodiazepines, prior glucuronidase hydrolysis may improve immunoassay detection. Enzyme-linked immunosorbent assay (ELISA) methods with high selectivity for 7-aminoflunitrazepam and low limits of detection have been developed.[428,429] Direct analysis or confirmation of 7-aminoflunitrazepam by GC-MS or LC-MS/MS is indicated in suspected cases of flunitrazepam ingestion.[429,762,763] Because of the development and implementation of specific toxicologic tests in response to increased public awareness, laboratories specializing in drug-facilitated crime cases routinely check for this drug and its metabolite.[739,764-767] Flunitrazepam metabolites are detectable as early as 7 days in hair samples (HPLC-MS/MS).[753] Deposition and stability of a drug in hair samples are variable, depending on the route of exposure and the chemical characteristics.

Nonbenzodiazepine Sedative-Hypnotics

Zopiclone, zolpidem, and zaleplon belong to a new generation of sedative-hypnotics that are structurally different from benzodiazepines (Fig. 41.14). Similar to benzodiazepines, these drugs modulate the $GABA_A$ receptor chloride channel by binding to the benzodiazepine (BZ) receptors, otherwise known as the $omega_1$ (ω_1) receptors, in the brain[768] without binding to peripheral BZ receptors.[769,770] Therefore these drugs have fewer muscle relaxant properties.[770]

Most of the nonbenzodiazepine sleep aids are available through a prescription as a Schedule IV drug and are readily prescribed, shared, and sold illegally. The rapid onset and amnesic properties of this class of drugs can result in disinhibition, passivity, and retrograde amnesia, making it a favored drug in drug-facilitated sexual assault. These drugs require only a low dosage to cause an effect and are rapidly metabolized. Because of the amnesic properties of these drugs, victims are often confused after the event and may be delayed in reporting their sexual assault. Commonly used drug screens do not test for these substances.

Use of these new-generation sleep aids in potentially facilitating sexual assault has been reported in the United States, the United Kingdom, and France for over a decade.[715,738,739,771,772] Yet only two published reports in the United States tested sexual assault victims for the presence of zolpidem.[773,774]

All may produce additive CNS-depressant effects when coadministered with other psychotropic medications such as anticonvulsants, antihistamines, ethanol, and drugs that produce CNS depression.

Pharmacologic Effects. Examples of nonbenzodiazepine sedative-hypnotics include (1) zolpidem, (2) zaleplon, (3) and zopiclone/eszopiclone.

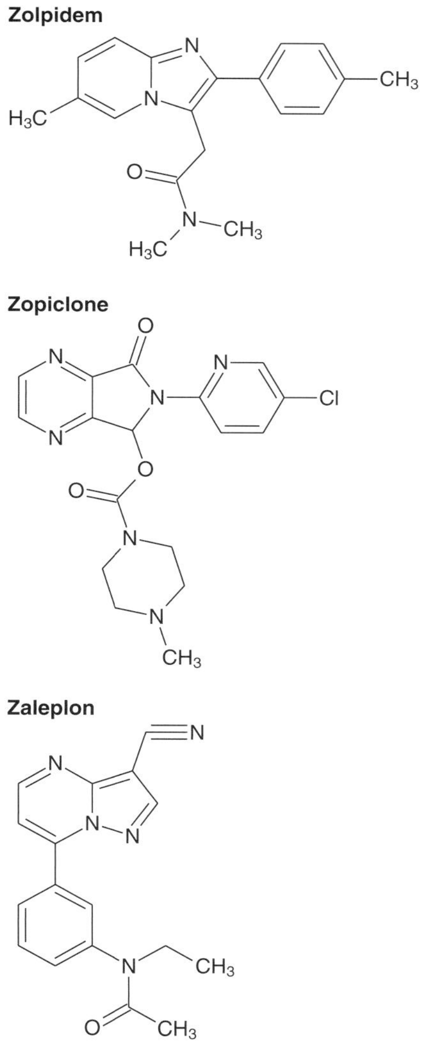

Zolpidem

Zopiclone

Zaleplon

FIGURE 41.14 Chemical structures of the nonbenzodiazepine sedative-hypnotics (zolpidem, zopiclone, zaleplon).

Zolpidem. The pharmacologic effects of zolpidem (Ambien) are believed to result from its interaction with a specific subtype of $GABA_A$ receptor complex consisting of α_1-subunits.[775] It is available as an immediate- or extended-release tablet. An average oral dose of 5 to 10 mg has a rapid onset of clinical symptoms between 10 and 30 minutes. Clinical effects peak at approximately 1.5 hours for immediate release, duration is approximately 6 to 8 hours for both immediate- and extended-release preparations, and the $t_{1/2}$ is approximately 2.5 hours.[776] Evidence of minimal respiratory depression is noted when used as a single agent, but it may produce additive CNS-depressive effects and death when coadministered with other sedatives.[777]

Zaleplon. Zaleplon (Sonata) is available as an immediate-release tablet or capsule. An average oral dose of 10 mg has a rapid onset of clinical symptoms of approximately 10 to 30 minutes. Although the $t_{1/2}$ for zaleplon is approximately 1 hour, the duration of clinical effects may persist for longer than 6 hours. This may be due to the higher affinity of zaleplon for specific α_2- and α_3-subunits of the GABA receptor, in contrast to zolpidem or zopiclone.[778] At higher doses its use may cause increased CNS effects and impaired motor skills.[719]

Zopiclone. Zopiclone exists as two stereoisomers; the active stereoisomer is S-zopiclone (eszopiclone). The exact mechanism of action of eszopiclone (Lunesta) is unknown, but its effect is believed to result from interaction with $GABA_A$ receptor complexes containing α_1- to α_5-subunits.[775] A dose of 7.5 mg[775a] has a rapid onset of clinical symptoms in approximately 30 minutes. Both immediate- and extended-release forms are available. The clinical effects of eszopiclone are longer in duration than those of zopiclone or zolpidem, with a $t_{1/2}$ of 6 hours.[769]

Analytical Methods. Because of the amnesic properties of these drugs, victims often may not report their sexual assault for several days. Therefore sensitive analytical techniques are necessary to detect these drugs and their metabolites in urine or hair samples after a single dose. Although these drugs do not cross-react with most benzodiazepine immunoassays, specific reagent systems (ELISA) directed against the nonbenzodiazepine hypnotics are available.[779] Screening and confirmation are performed by GC-MS or LC-MS/MS.

γ-Hydroxybutyrate, 1,4-Butanediol, and γ-Butyrolactone

γ-Hydroxybutyrate (GHB) and its synthetic precursor compounds, 1,4-butanediol (1,4-BD) and γ-butyrolactone (GBL), are Schedule I agents in the United States, and availability is restricted in numerous other countries. GHB is illegally purchased as an odorless and colorless liquid form or as an off-white powder that easily dissolves in liquids. When ingested, GHB stimulates dopamine release, leading to pleasurable effects such as euphoria, muscle relaxation, and heightened sexual desire.[780,781] It also has CNS depressant effects, resulting in sedation and hypnosis. Because GHB was reported to enhance growth hormone release, it has been used by body builders and athletes as a steroid alternative. Athletes have used GHB as a sleep aid because they believe it promotes rapid recovery from vigorous repetitive competition. These properties and the availability of GHB in dietary supplements have led to growing recreational abuse of the drug. GHB has become popular as a euphorigenic club drug, most often used in combination with alcohol, and also with MDMA or cocaine, to "mellow" their adverse stimulant properties. Its rapid onset and hypnotic and short-term amnestic properties have resulted in the use of GHB for drug-facilitated sexual assault (date rape drug).[715,716,772,782] It has been estimated that 4% of alleged sexual assault cases in the United States are positive for GHB.[715,739,766,783]

GHB is a naturally occurring substance produced in the brain. GHB is reversibly metabolized to GABA through multiple endogenous enzymes (Fig. 41.15).[784-786] Illicit consumption of GHB, or the synthetic GHB precursor compound 1,4-BD or GBL, will promote GABA activity.[786] In addition to increased metabolism to GABA, GHB has direct effects on the CNS by binding GHB-specific receptors and $GABA_B$ receptors.[787-789] The latter are G-protein–coupled receptors distinct from the $GABA_A$ receptors for depressant drugs, such as benzodiazepines and barbiturates. Of note, patients with GHB overdose do not respond to the opioid antagonist naloxone or to the benzodiazepine antagonist flumazenil. Fomepizole, an inhibitor of ADH, is likely beneficial for patients who ingest 1,4-butanediol.[790] GHB is suggested to increase dopamine concentrations in the substantia nigra, to potentiate the endogenous opioid system, and to mediate GABA transmission.[786]

Pharmacologic Effects. Onset of GHB effects occurs in approximately 15 to 30 minutes, depending on the dose (average, 1 to 5 g) and the chemical purity. The duration of response is short, typically 1 to 3 hours for normal dose and 2 to 4 hours with excessive doses. The clinical effects are dose dependent and typically last 3 to 6 hours. A low dose (<1 g) produces mild symptoms such as CNS depression, amnesia, hypotonia, and reduced inhibitions (similar to alcohol). Larger doses (1 to 2 g) cause increased somnolence, drowsiness, dizziness, bradycardia, and bradypnea. High doses (>2 g) often interfere with motor coordination and balance and may induce significant respiratory depression and bradypnea, Cheyne-Stokes respiration, nausea, and vomiting, diminished cardiac output, seizures, coma, and death.[777,791,792] Periods of agitation may be interspersed between times of apnea and unresponsiveness. It is uncertain whether this agitation is a direct GHB effect or a consequence of coingested stimulant drugs. Deaths have been reported but are almost always associated with coingestion of alcohol or other drugs.

Analytical Methods. GHB is metabolized rapidly ($t_{1/2}$ ≈30 minutes) and currently is not detected on immunoscreens. It is identified in urine and serum specimens using GC-FID or GC-MS.[783,793,794] Because GBH is metabolized rapidly, timely sample collection is an important facet of GBH assay; plasma samples should be collected within 6 to 8 hours after ingestion and urine samples within 10 to 12 hours. Urine and plasma concentrations may exhibit endogenous concentrations of GHB within 8 to 12 hours after ingestion (<1 mg/dL in urine; <4 mg/L in blood/plasma).[795] Samples approaching endogenous concentrations make it difficult to legally associate GHB doping in sexual assault cases. Exogenous concentrations of GHB have been detected in hair samples at 7 days after intoxication.[772] Timely presentation of the patient for medical attention and physician recognition of GHB symptoms presented by sexually assaulted victims are essential for prosecution of sexual offenders.

Dextromethorphan

DXM is structurally related to the opioids, but it does not bind to opioid receptors at normal dose and thus is devoid of analgesic activity.[796] The (–) isomer of DXM, levorphan (not available in the United States), is a potent opioid analgesic and is an example of the stereoselective nature of opioid receptor binding. DXM lacks analgesic activity but does have antitussive activity comparable with that of codeine. At high doses, DXM binds opioid receptors to produce miosis, respiratory depression, and CNS depression. High doses also may cause lethargy, agitation, ataxia, nystagmus, diaphoresis, and hypertension.[797-799]

DXM is present in various over-the-counter (OTC) cough medications, often in combination with antihistamines, nasal decongestants, guaifenesin, aspirin, and acetaminophen. Potential toxicity from OTC combination medications must be considered when DXM is consumed in large doses to achieve euphoric effects.[800,801] Abuse of DXM, especially by adolescents and teenagers, who refer to it as "dex, robos, and skittles," has become widespread. Abusers describe feelings of euphoria, dissociative effects such as a sense of floating, and hallucinations. Discontinuation of the drug is frequently followed by dysphoria and depression.

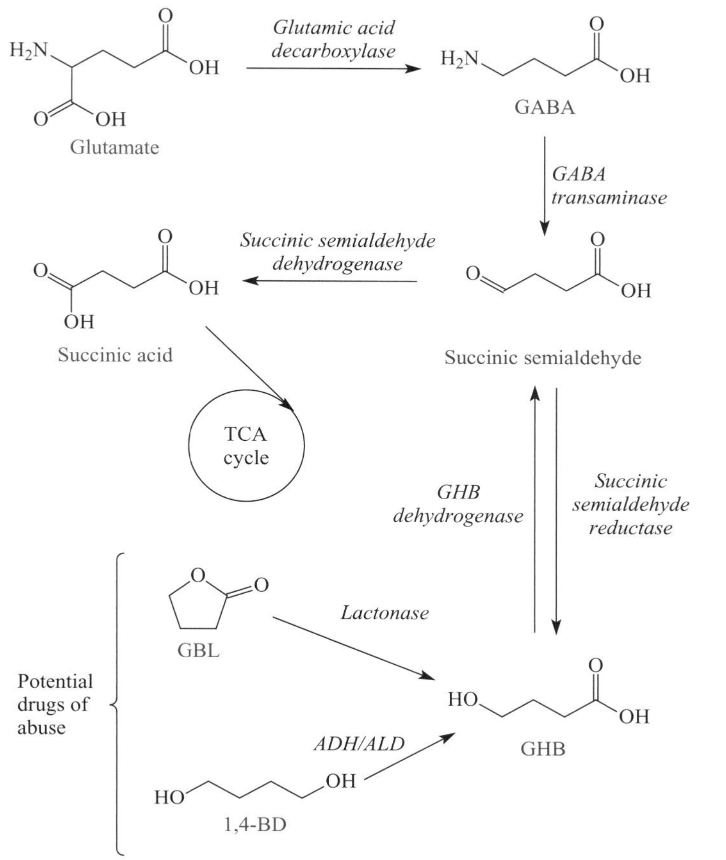

FIGURE 41.15 Metabolism of γ-hydroxybutyrate *(GHB)* and its synthetic precursor compounds; 1,4-butanediol (1,4-BD) or γ-butyrolactone *(GBL)* are often used illicitly. These drugs are endogenously metabolized to γ-aminobutyric acid *(GABA)*. GHB and GABA mediate GABA receptors. *TCA,* Tricarboxylic acid cycle.

Pharmacologic Effects. DXM is metabolized to dextrorphan[256] by the cytochrome P450 isoenzyme 2D6 (CYP2D6), which exhibits genetic polymorphisms. Dextrorphan may be responsible for the more pleasant psychotropic effects of high-dose DXM, whereas the parent drug may cause dysphoria, sedation, and ataxia.[799] Thus poor metabolizers (deficient in CYP2D6 activity) may be less prone and extensive metabolizers more prone to continue the abuse of DXM. Dextrorphan and to a lesser degree DXM bind to the PCP- and ketamine-binding site on the NMDA receptor, causing sedation; this may account for their similar dissociative psychotropic actions[796] (see "Phencyclidine and Ketamine" section).

Analytical Methods. Clinically approved doses of DXM are not detected by most clinical opiate immunoassays,[802] but larger doses may cross-react.[635] More recently developed ELISA assays are available to detect DXM and its major metabolite, dextrorphan.[803] Because most preparations contain DXM as the bromide salt, excessive ingestion of DXM may result in bromide poisoning and in a negative serum anion gap consequent to the disproportionate response to bromide with common methods of chloride analysis.[804] The presence of DXM or dextrorphan in a sample is confirmed by GC-MS or LC-MS/MS.

Dextrorphan is the enantiomer of levorphanol, a potent opioid agonist available in the United States (Levo-Dromoran). Unless chiral analytical techniques are used, these enantiomers are not resolved. Drug testing laboratories that use conventional chromatographic techniques should not report a finding of levorphanol only, but should instead report dextrorphan/levorphanol, with a comment on their isomeric relationship and on the origin of dextrorphan. This is especially important for pain management drug screening, in which a false report of levorphanol may result in dismissal from the program. This report duality is advisable even when parent DXM is also detected. Savvy abusers of levorphanol conceivably may coingest DXM to conceal use of levorphanol. If such is suspected, chiral resolution of dextrorphan and levorphanol would then be necessary.

Pain Management: The Epidemic of Chronic Pain and Substance Abuse in the United States

Urine drug testing (UDT) is an essential tool in the field of pain medicine. In the late 1990s, awareness grew about the personal and economic costs of poorly controlled pain. Billions of dollars were being spent each year to treat between 30 and 80 million Americans with debilitating, chronic pain.[805] Congress reacted by passing into law the Decade of Pain Control and Research. Overnight, pain became the fifth vital sign and the successful treatment of pain synonymous with quality of care.[806,807]

Prominent physicians and professional organizations at local, national, and international levels supported judicious opioid use to address not only acute and cancer-related pain, but society's pain at large.[808-812] In the United States, health care providers with little training in opioid management and addiction were empowered with a DEA license to incorporate opioid therapy into daily practice. Between 1997 and 2007, the retail sales of opioids nearly doubled, with a disproportionate increase in methadone, oxycodone, and fentanyl.[813,814] With only 5% of the world's population, the United States dominated the opioid scene, consuming 99% of the hydrocodone, 80% of the oxycodone, and 49% of the fentanyl worldwide.[436,815]

In short order, the negative consequences of widespread opioid use surfaced. Since 1999, the number of opioid-related deaths in the United States has more than doubled and now exceeds the number of deaths related to heroin and cocaine abuse combined.[813,814,816] In 2012, drug overdose was the leading cause of injury death, surpassing that from motor vehicle crashes between the ages 25 and 64.[817] For every one death from opioid abuse, there are 35 emergency department visits, 161 cases of abuse, and 461 cases of misuse, contributing to more than $55 billion in society and work-related costs.[818]

In an effort to curb the opioid epidemic, pain societies began to offer workshops on safe opioid prescribing at national meetings and provide consensus statements to guide the selection and monitoring of patients on long-term opioid therapy. State and federal government have made efforts to improve the monitoring and transparency of opioid prescribing and prosecute health care providers who operate outside safe practices for personal gain or other reasons.

The fruits of these efforts are foundational in clinical pain medicine and include the following:

1. Awareness of terminology related to opioid use such as tolerance, misuse, abuse, addiction, and diversion.
2. Appreciation of risk factors that are barriers to successful opioid therapy. These include sociodemographic factors, comorbid health and psychiatric factors, environmental factors, genetics and family history, and alcohol and other substance abuse history.[819,820]
3. Development and validation of opioid screening tools.
4. Expansion of prescription monitoring programs.
5. Support for opioid treatment agreements and opioid prescribing contracts.
6. Exploration of objective measures, such as UDT, to facilitate appropriate prescribing practices and patient adherence to the prescribed treatment plan.

Much of this chapter is devoted to understanding the science of urine toxicology and UDT. The methodologic details that determine whether a urine sample is consistent or inconsistent with prescribed medications are beyond the scope of most pain physicians. Yet, the pain physician must act on this information in a way that preserves the patient-doctor relationship; upholds the ethical principles of autonomy, beneficence, nonmalfeasance and justice; and complies with federal law.[821,822] This is no small task.

Urine Drug Testing

UDT in clinical practice is fundamentally different from forensic drug testing. Forensic testing follows chain of custody, and the expectation is that the results for illicit and controlled substances will be negative. In virtually all clinic practices, no chain of custody exists, and one hopes that prescribed medications will be found. The absence of prescribed medications is as much of a professional and ethical conundrum as the presence of illicit or unexpected controlled substances. Additionally, the pain physician must be keenly aware that a urine sample yielding consistent results ensures only that the expected parent compound and metabolites are present; not that the patient is using the medication as prescribed. This point cannot be overlooked because medication nonadherence in the chronic pain population is between 30% and 50%.[823]

Despite wide spread agreement that treating chronic pain with opioids can be risky and requires commitment to monitoring, controversy in pain medicine exists as to the type and frequency of UDT. This controversy likely stems from the paucity of high-quality research demonstrating that UDT significantly reduces the risks for misuse, abuse, and diversion.[824] Additionally, evidence exists that inconsistent UDTs do not necessarily alter prescribing practices.[825] Coincident are concerns about conflicts of interest and physician enticement because UDT is now a multibillion-dollar industry that has a history of incentivizing physicians to frequently order testing.[814,822,826]

UDT includes screening tools, such as POC and laboratory-based immunoassay testing, as well as confirmatory testing. POC testing is advantageous because results can be obtained during the clinic visit, but it has been under fire because it is costly and data for meaningful use in pain medicine are lacking.[827] No concrete evidence exists for when to use it or for whom it is appropriate. However, expert panels identify a unique role at the initial visit, where inconsistent results or finding illicit substances could influence the decision on whether to initiate opioid therapy.[828] Changes in Medicare reimbursement for POC testing has made it less attractive in the private setting and will likely curb its use.[827] More comprehensive, laboratory-based enzyme immunoassays (EIAs) should be considered instead of POC testing for routine monitoring.

Laboratory-based immunoassays have moderate sensitivity and low specificity.[815] They provide information about the general drug classes present in the urine but cannot distinguish among drugs within the same class. Immunoassays may completely miss semi-synthetic or synthetic opioids and therefore should be interpreted carefully based on the known limitations of the specific immunoassay used.

Confirmatory testing with GC and/or LC should be considered when screening results are inconsistent with prescribed medications and incorporated as a random part of routine monitoring. The high cutoff values inherent to most immunoassays result in high false-negative rates and may cause the physician to miss aberrant use of prescription medication or to lead to falsely accusing a patient of diversion. However, in some settings, confirmatory testing can cost in excess of $100 per drug class, so restraint should be used.

Confirmatory testing for only prescribed medications is less costly and fulfills the minimum requirements of a typical opioid prescribing contract. On the other hand, some physicians feel it is their obligation to "do no harm" by identifying those patients in whom concurrent use of other substances—prescription, recreation, or illicit—increases the risk for side effects or death.[815,822,829] UDT for THC is particularly complex. THC use is a risk factor for using other illicit substances and misusing opioids.[830] However, in recent years, THC has been legalized by more than 20 US states.[831] When and how to test for THC will likely evolve with the changing regulatory landscape.

Recently, numerous algorithmic approaches to UDT in pain medicine have been suggested. Although finer details differ, there are a few clear messages, as follows[814,815,818,819,828]:

1. UDT should be used to monitor all patients on chronic opioid therapy.
2. The patient should be informed of and willing to participate in random UDT as documented at the initiation of therapy, in the opioid prescribing contract.
3. Random UDT testing is preferred to scheduled testing because patients can and will modify usage if told in advance.
4. UDT before the initial consultation or POC testing during the initial visit might aid in the decision to initiate opioid therapy.
5. It is important to stratify patient risk into categories of low and high or low, medium, and high based on initial screening, comorbid conditions, previous drug/alcohol abuse, and family history.
6. At a minimum, UDT should be performed once per year.
7. More frequent UDT is recommended for patients who are at medium to high risk.
8. All unexplained results based on urine drug screening should undergo confirmatory testing.
9. Confirmatory testing should be performed at least once per year.
10. Urine temperature, pH, creatinine content, and specific gravity also should be tested to help identify adulterated samples.
11. Inconsistent or unexplained results should be discussed with the performing laboratory and then with the patient in an open, truthful manner.
12. In the event that misuse, abuse, or diversion is suspected, the physician must choose to continue the current treatment plan, take corrective action in an attempt to retain the patient, or dismiss the patient from practice.
13. Corrective actions include counseling, decreasing the time interval between appointments, limiting the number of pills, and referring to an addiction specialist.
14. Dismissing a patient from practice should be based on a prewritten policy that is reviewed with the patient.

Conclusions

UDT is an important tool in clinical pain medicine. The current epidemic of prescription medication abuse underscores the need for a consistent approach to monitoring that uses both subjective and objective measures. Although some advocate that routine UDT should include all testable substances with abusive potential, such practices are costly and likely unnecessary in many cases. High-risk patients, classified using validated clinical screening tools, require more careful and more frequent monitoring. POC and other EIA screening methods cannot differentiate among medications within the same drug class and may completely miss semisynthetic and synthetic opioids. For this reason, confirmatory testing with GC and/or LC should be performed at least annually and on all inconsistent samples. If misuse, abuse, or diversion is suspected, the physician must act in a way that promotes patient health and safety, while abiding by state and federal law. Such actions should be openly discussed and explicitly written in the opioid prescribing contract, signed at the initiation of every opioid treatment plan.

Detection of Drugs of Abuse Using Other Types of Specimens

The collection of biological samples for the purpose of determining exposure to various agents is dominated by blood and urine. Blood is considered invasive, and the collection of urine may require some invasion of privacy and loss of dignity; urine specimens are subject to adulteration or manipulation to evade detection. For these reasons, alternative biological specimens have been investigated.[832] Cutoff values have been proposed[478] for some of the matrices and are listed in Table 41.9. However, current guidelines for Federal Workplace Drug Testing have determined that urine will continue to be the only biological fluid approved for testing.[731] An additional review conducted by DHHS is expected.

Meconium, oral fluid, hair, and sweat have been investigated as alternative types of samples for drug analysis.

Meconium

Illicit drug use during pregnancy is a major social and medical issue. Drug abuse during pregnancy is associated with significant perinatal complications, including a high incidence of (1) stillbirth, (2) meconium-stained fluid, (3) premature rupture of the membranes, (4) maternal hemorrhage (abruptio placentae or placenta previa), and (5) fetal distress.[833] In the neonate, the mortality rate and morbidity (eg, asphyxia, prematurity, low birth weight, hyaline membrane disease, infection, aspiration pneumonia, cerebral infarction, abnormal heart rate and breathing patterns, drug withdrawal) are increased.[833]

Unfortunately, identification of the drug-exposed mother or her neonate is not easy. Maternal admission of the use of drugs is often inaccurate principally because of denial about addiction or fear of the consequences stemming from such admission. Likewise, many infants who have been exposed to drugs in utero may appear normal at birth and show no overt manifestations of drug effects. Thus identification of the drug-exposed mother or her infant requires a high index of suspicion. Drug testing, on the other hand, is an objective means of determining drug exposure in both mother and infant. In infants, drug testing is necessary to document proof of the infant's exposure to illicit drugs. Urine testing of the mother or newborn can detect only recent drug use (within a few days before birth), and urine collection from newborns may be problematic.

The first intestinal discharge from newborns is meconium, which is a viscous, dark green substance composed of intestinal secretions, desquamated squamous cells, lanugo hair, bile pigments, and blood. Meconium also contains pancreatic enzymes, free fatty acids, porphyrins, interleukin-8, and phospholipase A_2 primary bile acids, with a small quantity of secondary bile acids. Water is the major liquid constituent, making up 85% to 95% of meconium.[834] Meconium is derived from the Greek word *mekonion,* meaning poppy juice or opium. Aristotle is credited with noting the relationship between the presence of meconium in amniotic fluid and a sleepy fetal state in utero.[834] Meconium begins to form during the second trimester and continues to accumulate until birth; drugs taken by the mother can be detected in the meconium of the newborn.[835]

The disposition of drug in meconium is not well understood. The proposed mechanism is that the fetus excretes drug into bile and amniotic fluid. Drug accumulates in meconium by direct deposition from bile or through swallowing of amniotic fluid.[835,836] The first evidence of meconium in the fetal intestine appears at approximately the 10th to 12th week of gestation; meconium slowly moves into the colon by the 16th week of gestation.[834] Therefore the presence of drugs in meconium has been proposed to be indicative of in utero drug exposure up to 5 months before birth—a longer historical measure than is possible by urinalysis.[835]

Meconium has been used for detection of prenatal drug use, showing an improved drug detection rate compared with urine.[835,837-839] The collection of meconium is noninvasive, making sample collection easy,[840] and is more successful than urine collection.[841] The amount collected is usually sufficient for complete analysis, including confirmation. Meconium testing does have some limitations. Meconium is usually passed by full-term newborns within 24 to 48 hours, after which transition from a blackish-green color to a yellow color indicates the beginning of passage of neonatal stool. Infants with low birth weight (<1000 g) have been shown to pass their first meconium at a median age of 3 days. Thus meconium collection is missed because of delayed passage, and meconium may not be available soon after birth for early detection of intrauterine drug exposure.

In the clinical laboratory, meconium is an unfamiliar matrix; it is a sticky material that is more difficult to work with than urine. Meconium drug screening has been adapted to various analytical techniques, including radioimmunoassay (RIA), EIA, and fluorescence polarization immunoassay (FPIA). Urine drugs-of-abuse screening assays frequently use meconium extracts and therefore must be investigated for possible effects of matrix on accuracy, precision, and assay linearity. However, some other immunoassay screening methods have been used.

RIA, FPIA, EMIT, and ELISA have been used for detection of drugs in meconium, but ELISA is rapidly becoming the method of choice for screening.[842] The sample preparation for the ELISA screen is usually a simple buffer extraction versus a lengthy and more laborious sample preparation procedure for the other immunoassay methods.

As with any immunoassay-based drug screen, confirmation by MS is critical. Confirmation assays for meconium are more difficult than those for urine. Recovery of drugs from meconium is sometimes low (30% to 50%). A variety of GC-MS, LC-MS, and LC-MS/MS methods and their advantages and disadvantages have been described elsewhere[485,485,838,842] and will not be discussed here.

Many questions remain to be answered about the disposition of drugs in meconium. Some debate continues as to which are the most appropriate drug analytes to measure in meconium; Table 41.12 attempts to summarize the current knowledge. Meconium drug testing is growing but is far less standardized than UDT. Assay cutoff limits and units (nanogram per gram meconium or nanogram per milliliter of extract) may vary; suitable reference or control materials are not yet available.

Meconium should be sent to the laboratory for processing as soon as it is collected to prevent possible loss of drugs. Meconium allowed to stand at room temperature for 24 hours showed a decrease in cocaine and cannabinoid concentrations.[833] However, suspending meconium in an organic solvent, such as buffered methanol, may prevent decreases for as long as 72 hours.[833] For prolonged storage, meconium should be frozen. Drugs are stable in meconium, frozen at −15°C, for as long as 9 months.[833]

TABLE 41.12 Drugs and Metabolites of Significance in Meconium

Drug Class	Confirmation Compound[485,486,836,945]
Cocaine	Cocaine
	Benzoylecgonine
	Cocaethylene
	M-Hydroxybenzoylecgonine
Opiates	Morphine
	Codeine
	6-MAM
	Hydromorphone
	Hydrocodone
	Oxycodone
Cannabinoids	9-Carboxy-11-nor-Δ-9-THC
	11-Hydroxy-delta-9-tetrahydrocannabinol
	8,11-Dihydroxy-Δ9-tetrahydrocannabinol
Amphetamines	Amphetamine
	Methamphetamine
	MDMA
	MDA
	MDEA
Ethanol	Fatty acid ethyl esters
PCP	PCP

6-MAM, 6-monoacetylmorphine;
MDA, 3,4-methylenedioxyamphetamine;
MDEA, methylenedioxyethylamphetamine;
MDMA, 3,4-methylenedioxymethamphetamine;
PCP, phencyclidine; *THC,* Δ-9-tetrahydrocannabinol.

Overinterpretation of meconium data is a dangerous practice. It is clear that matrix effects are associated with the analysis of meconium, as they are with each biological fluid or tissue sample.[486] Another important confounding factor is possible contamination of the meconium specimen by urine. Numerous reports have described the specificity and sensitivity of different analytes with the use of different testing methods.[833,841,843-845] A tremendous and potentially inappropriate value has been placed on a meconium result. On occasion, decisions about treatment or custody of the infant have been based solely on meconium drug screen results. It is critical to remember that a positive test could indicate intrauterine drug exposure. However, a negative result does not rule it out. It is clear that additional work is necessary to address these important issues and to improve our understanding of the disposition of drugs in meconium.[486]

Oral Fluid

Reports concerning the appearance of organic solutes in saliva have been included in the scientific literature for longer than 70 years.[846] Analysis of saliva for drugs was first used almost 30 years ago for the purpose of therapeutic drug monitoring.[847] It has since been evaluated for use in forensic toxicology, with recognition of its advantages over other biological matrices. Most studies on saliva in humans use whole saliva.

The term *oral fluid* is preferred for the specimen collected from the mouth. Oral fluid is a complex fluid consisting not only of secretions from the three major pairs of salivary glands (parotid, submandibular, and sublingual), but also secretions from the minor glands (labial, buccal, and palatal), bacteria, sloughed epithelial cells, gingival fluid, food debris, and other particulate matter.[848] The concentration of drug from each secretion and the relative contributions of the various glands to the final fluid may vary.[846]

Clearly, before any drug circulating in plasma can enter the oral fluid, it must pass through the capillary wall, the basement membrane, and the membrane of the salivary gland epithelial cells. However, this fluid is not a simple ultrafiltrate of plasma, as has sometimes been suggested, but rather a complex fluid formed by different mechanisms, including ultrafiltration through pores in the membrane, active transport against a concentration gradient, and passive diffusion.[848-855]

Ethanol was the first drug of abuse to be investigated in oral fluid[856]; since then, many additional studies have expanded our knowledge of this drug in it. Ethanol appears to reach a higher peak concentration in oral fluid than in peripheral blood. Because distribution of ethanol in the body is considered to occur by passive diffusion, under equilibrium conditions, ethanol content will depend on the water content of the fluid or tissue being measured. The content in saliva therefore will be higher than that found in blood or serum. On a theoretical basis, the ratio of saliva to blood ethanol should be 1.17; however, lower ratios have been found in the postabsorption phase.[857,858]

In recent years, great interest has been expressed in the use of oral fluid testing for roadside drug screening, for monitoring the compliance of individuals on drug maintenance programs, and for workplace drug testing (see Table 41.9). Low concentrations of drugs and metabolites necessitate sensitive screening methods, which typically are immunoassays.[859] Again, the low concentrations of drugs have necessitated that confirmatory methods be equally sensitive. Many confirmatory methods have been developed for oral fluid testing of abused drugs, including GC-MS, LC-MS, and LC-MS/MS.[860-874] Specimens can be monitored for cannabinoids, cocaine, opiates, amphetamines, PCP, methadone, barbiturates, and benzodiazepines. Interpretation of the presence and concentrations of these drugs in saliva and information on their use have been extensively reviewed elsewhere.[875-877]

Several advantages are associated with monitoring oral fluid as contrasted with monitoring plasma or serum concentrations.[878] Collection of oral fluid is considered to be a noninvasive procedure, and some of the risks associated with the drawing of blood are avoided. Furthermore, for the patient, fear, anxiety, and discomfort that may accompany the drawing of blood are diminished. Although some training and explanation are necessary to ensure proper gathering of oral fluid samples, the level of training needed for blood sampling is not required. In principle, oral fluid drug concentration is related to plasma free drug concentration, except when buccal contamination may have occurred because of oral ingestion, smoking, or snorting of the drug. Therefore oral fluid has the potential to show a relation between behavior and impairment and drug concentration, making it a possible medium for monitoring drug intoxication or conducting therapeutic drug management.[859,879] On a related note, one significant disadvantage of oral fluid is that the window of detection is approximately equivalent to that of blood or serum and is short compared with that in urine.[873,878] Another disadvantage is the small volume of sample collected. The problem of small sample size can be overcome by using methods that simultaneously extract multiple drug groups.[859,880]

Hair

For more than 30 years, hair has been analyzed for trace metals, including lead, arsenic, and mercury. This was achieved using atomic absorption spectroscopy (see Chapters 13 and 42). At first, the examination of hair for organic substances, specifically drugs, was not possible because the analytical methods were not sensitive enough.[881] Baumgartner and associates in 1979[882] published the first report on the detection of morphine in the hair of heroin abusers using RIA. Since that time, interest in analysis of hair for the purpose of detecting drug use has increased.[883-886]

It is generally accepted that drugs enter hair by at least three mechanisms: (1) from blood that supplies the growing hair follicle, (2) through sweat and sebum, and (3) via the external environment.[881,887] The exact mechanism by which chemicals are incorporated into hair is not known. It has been suggested that passive diffusion may be augmented by binding of the drug to intracellular components of hair cells such as the hair pigment melanin. Specific binding of basic drugs to hair components is likely to involve both electrostatic attraction and weaker forces, such as van der Waals attraction. Neutral and acidic drugs presumably bind through weaker forces and possibly by other mechanisms.[888]

Factors that may affect how efficiently drugs are incorporated into hair are not well established but may include rate of hair growth, anatomic location of hair, hair color (melanin content), and hair texture (thick or fine, porous or not); these are determined by genetic factors and by the effects of various hair treatments.[881] For example, substantially higher binding was found in vitro with hair from black men than with hair from blonde white men, suggesting that melanin pigment plays an important role in drug binding.[889] Studies have demonstrated that after the same dosage is given, black hair incorporates much more of the drug than is incorporated by blond hair.[890-892] This may lead to bias in hair testing for drugs of abuse, and the possible genetic variability of drug deposition in hair and is still under evaluation.

Drugs, when deposited in hair, are generally present in relatively low concentrations (picogram, nanogram, microgram, milligram); thus sensitive analytical techniques are required for detection. Immunoassay procedures have been modified for use with hair.[881] Although GC-MS is generally the method of choice,[893] various GC-MS/MS or LC-MS/MS methods may be used for targeted analysis of low-dose compounds such as fentanyl, buprenorphine, and flunitrazepam.[894-898] These methods are also useful in the detection of some drugs or metabolites that typically appear in hair at trace concentrations, such as THC-COOH,[899,900] or in retrospective detection of drugs administered as single doses.[793,901-903]

As mentioned, external exposure to drugs causes them to be detected in hair, and because it is unlikely that anyone would intentionally or accidentally apply drugs of abuse to his or her own hair, the most crucial issue facing hair analysts today is technical and evidentiary false-positive findings.[881] False-positive results may be caused during or after collection. Externally deposited substances easily contaminate the hair because of its high surface-to-volume ratio. Substances deposited in hair from the environment are loosely bound to the surface of the hair and thus are removed by appropriate decontamination procedures. These usually involve a washing step.[881,883] It is fundamental to be able to distinguish between passive exposure (environmental contamination) and active consumption; consequently, decontamination procedures for hair are compulsory.[904] Needless to say, hair analysis is a complex scientific undertaking, and comprehensive reviews on this topic have been published.[905]

Hair is advantageous as a biological specimen because it is easily obtained, with less embarrassment; it is not easily altered or manipulated to avoid drug detection. Once deposited in hair, drugs are very stable, and analysis can be performed even after centuries.[906]

Hair also differs from other human materials, such as blood or urine, used for toxicologic analysis because of its substantially longer detection window (months to years). Hair grows at a relatively constant rate. The average rate of hair growth is usually stated to be 0.44 mm/d (range, 0.38 to 0.48 mm/d) for men and 0.45 mm/d (range, 0.40 to 0.55/d) for women in the vertex region of the scalp.[907] The rate of hair growth depends on anatomic location, race, gender, and age. Scalp hair grows faster than pubic or axillary hair (≈0.3 mm/d), which in turn grow faster than beard hair (≈0.27 mm/d).[904] It is generally accepted that sectional hair analysis can be used to prove drug history.[904] Numerous forensic applications in which hair analysis was used to document the case have been described in the literature; these include (1) differentiation between a drug dealer and a drug consumer, (2) chronic poisoning, (3) crime under the influence of a drug, (4) child sedation and abuse, (5) suspicious death, (6) child custody, (7) abuse of drugs in jail, (8) body identification, (9) survey of drug addicts, (10) chemical submission, (11) obtaining a driver's license, and (12) doping control.[908-910]

Sweat

Drugs may be excreted in sweat, with the parent drug generally present in a greater amount than metabolites.[877,884] Moreover, sweat excretion may be an important mechanism by which drugs enter hair.[911]

Sweat patch collection devices that resemble an adhesive bandage may be worn for several days to several weeks; during this time, drug, if present, accumulates in the absorbent pad in the patch, while water vapor escapes through the semipermeable covering.[912] Thus sweat drug testing offers the possibility of monitoring drug use over extended periods without the need for frequent collection of urine.[913] Sweat drug testing would be particularly advantageous for monitoring drug use in correctional institutions or in drug rehabilitation programs.[914]

Athletes and Drug Testing

"Doping" in athletic competitions has a history of abuse in a variety of sports for centuries. Regulation of performance-enhancing substances was initiated in 1967 in response to the death of Danish cyclist Knud Jensen at the 1960 Olympic Games in Rome. After decades of reform between universal governments and sporting agencies, the World Anti-Doping Agency (https://www.wada-ama.org/) was established in 1999. Currently, only a few facilities around the world are accredited by the International Organization for Standardization for detecting drug use among competitive athletes.[915] Prohibited drugs are substances or methods that conform to two of three criteria: (1) performance enhancing, (2) may endanger the athlete's health, or (3) go against the spirit of the sport. "In-competition" testing was established to detect drugs (stimulants, narcotics, cannabinoids, glucocorticosteroids) taken at the time of a competition to temporarily enhance performance. "Out-of-competition" testing is performed to detect substances and methods such as anabolic-androgenic steroids, hormones, hormone modulators, oxygen transfer enhancement, blood doping, and gene transfer, whose performance-enhancing effects have a gradual onset to allow for more intense and efficient training; they can be abruptly discontinued before competition.[915,916]

Most testing for prohibited substance abuse is performed by GC-MS. Specialized testing such as isoelectric focusing ("double blotting") was implemented at the 2002 Salt Lake City Olympics to discriminate between endogenous and recombinant forms of erythropoietin.[917] Erythrocyte phenotyping by flow cytometry is used to detect homologous blood transfusions.[918-920] Limited windows of detection and individual biological variability for specific substances (especially hormones) are challenges faced when novel analytical methods are developed and validated. Tracking of specific clinical biomonitors (eg, hormone or hormone-responsive protein concentrations) over an athlete's performance career, termed *biological passport* and *longitudinal profiling,* is currently under investigation.[921,922]

POINTS TO REMEMBER

- A toxidrome is the constellation of clinical signs and symptoms that suggests a specific class of poisoning
- Proper selection of analytical methods and interpretation of results require knowledge of the pharmacology and pharmacokinetics of the toxins of interest.
- Screening procedures are designed for the relatively rapid and generally qualitative detection of a particular drug or drug class or other toxic substances. Screening tests have adequate clinical sensitivity but may not be highly specific.
- Testing for drugs in a single random urine sample detects only fairly recent drug use and does not differentiate casual use from chronic drug abuse. It also cannot determine the degree of impairment, the dose of drug taken, or the exact time of use.

SELECTED REFERENCES

For a full list of references for this chapter, please refer to ExpertConsult.com.

2. Nice A, Leikin JB, Maturen A, et al. Toxidrome recognition to improve efficiency of emergency urine drug screens. *Ann Emerg Med* 1988;**17**:676–80.
8. McMillin GA, Slawson MH, Marin SJ, et al. Demystifying analytical approaches for urine drug testing to evaluate medication adherence in chronic pain management. *J Pain Palliat Care Pharmacother* 2013;**27**:322–39.
11. Erickson TB, Thompson TM, Lu JJ. The approach to the patient with an unknown overdose. *Emerg Med Clin North Am* 2007;**25**:249–81, abstract vii.

15. Holstege CP, Dobmeier SG, Bechtel LK. Critical care toxicology. *Emerg Med Clin North Am* 2008;**26**:715–39, viii–ix.
36. Krahn J, Khajuria A. Osmolality gaps: diagnostic accuracy and long-term variability. *Clin Chem* 2006;**52**:737–9.
52. Jones G. Post-mortem toxicology. In: Moffat A, editor. *Clarke's analysis of drugs and poisons*. 3rd ed. London, UK: Pharmaceutical Press; 2004. p. 95–108.
66. Tomaszewski C. Carbon monoxide. In: Flomenbaum NE, Goldfrank LR, Hoffman RS, et al., editors. *Goldfrank's toxicologic emergencies*. 8th ed. New York: McGraw Hill; 2006. p. 1689–704.
72. Olson KR. Poisoning. In: Olson KR, editor. *Current medical diagnosis & treatment*. 6th ed. McGraw-Hill; 2015.
105. Levine B, Caplan YH. Pharmacology and toxicology of alcohol. In: Caplan YH, Goldberger BA, editors. *Garriott's medicolegal aspects of alcohol*. 6th ed. Tucson AZ: Lawyers & Judges Publishing; 2015. p. 25–48.
112. Dubowski KM. Absorption, distribution and elimination of alcohol: highway safety aspects. *J Stud Alcohol* 1985;**10**: 98–108.
131. Payne JP, Hill DW, Wood DG. Distribution of ethanol between plasma and erythrocytes in whole blood. *Nature* 1968;**217**:963–4.
132. Winek CL, Carfagna M. Comparison of plasma, serum, and whole blood ethanol concentrations. *J Anal Toxicol* 1987;**11**: 267–8.
157. Helander A, Olsson I, Dahl H. Postcollection synthesis of ethyl glucuronide by bacteria in urine may cause false identification of alcohol consumption. *Clin Chem* 2007;**53**: 1855–7.
170. Mitchell JR, Thorgeirsson SS, Potter WZ, et al. Acetaminophen-induced hepatic injury: protective role of glutathione in man and rationale for therapy. *Clin Pharmacol Ther* 1974;**16**:676–84.
177. Hung OL, Nelson LS. Acetaminophen. In: Tintinalli JE, Stapczynski JS, Ma OJ, et al., editors. *Tintinalli's emergency medicine: a comprehensive study guide*. 7th ed. New York, NY: McGraw-Hill; 2011.
204. Veltri JC, Thompson MIB. Salicylates. In: Skoutakis VA, editor. *Clinical Toxicology of Drugs: Principles and Practice*. Philadelphia: Lea & Febiger; 1982. p. 227–43.
205. Chapman BJ, Proudfoot AT. Adult salicylate poisoning: deaths and outcome in patients with high plasma salicylate concentrations. *Q J Med* 1989;**72**:699–707.
234. Baldessarini R. Drug therapy of depression and anxiety disorders. In: Brunton LL, Lazo JS, Parker KL, editors. *Goodman & Gilman's the pharmacological basis of therapeutics*. 11th ed. McGraw-Hill; 2006.
256. Porter WH. Clinical toxicology. In: Burtis CA, Ashwood ER, Bruns DE, editors. *Tietz textbook of clinical chemistry and molecular diagnostics*. 4th ed. St. Louis, MO: Saunders; 2006. p. 1287–369.
282. Perez JW, Pantazides BG, Watson CM, et al. Enhanced stability of blood matrices using a dried sample spot assay to measure human butyrylcholinesterase activity and nerve agent adducts. *Anal Chem* 2015;**87**:5723–9.
296. Westfall TC, Westfall DP. Adrenergic agonists and antagonists. In: Brunton LL, Lazo JS, Parker KL, editors. *Goodman & Gilman's the pharmacological basis of therapeutics*. 11th ed. McGraw-Hill; 2006.
297. Lüscher C. Drugs of abuse. In: Katzung BG, editor. *Basic & clinical pharmacology*. 11th ed. McGraw-Hill; 2009.
314. Logan BK, Cooper FA. 3,4-Methylenedioxymethamphetamine: effects on human performance and behavior. *Forensic Sci Rev* 2003;**15**:11–28.
317. Maurer HH, Kraemer T, Springer D, et al. Chemistry, pharmacology, toxicology, and hepatic metabolism of designer drugs of the amphetamine (ecstasy), piperazine, and pyrrolidinophenone types: a synopsis. *Ther Drug Monit* 2004;**26**:127–31.
379. Charney DS, Mihic SJ, Harris RA. Hypnotics and sedatives. In: Brunton LL, Lazo JS, Parker KL, editors. *Goodman & Gilman's the pharmacological basis of therapeutics*. 11th ed. McGraw-Hill; 2006.
439. Huestis MA. Cannabis. In: Levine B, editor. *Principles of forensic toxicology*. 2nd ed. Washington DC: AACC Press; 2010. p. 269–303.
479. Wiley JL, Marusich JA, Huffman JW. Moving around the molecule: relationship between chemical structure and in vivo activity of synthetic cannabinoids. *Life Sci* 2014;**97**: 55–63.
543. Babu KM, Ferm RP. Hallucinogens. In: Flomenbaum NE, Goldfrank LR, Hoffman RS, et al., editors. *Goldfrank's toxicologic emergencies*. 8th ed. New York: McGraw-Hill; 2006. p. 1202–11.
560. Gutstein HB, Akil H. Opioid analgesics. In: Brunton LL, Lazo JS, Parker KL, editors. *Goodman & Gilman's the pharmacological basis of therapeutics*. 11th ed. McGraw-Hill; 2006.
731. *Federal Register* 49 cfr part 40. Procedures for transportation workplace drug and alcohol testing programs (updated as of August 31, 2009).
833. Ostrea EM Jr. Understanding drug testing in the neonate and the role of meconium analysis. *J Perinat Neonatal Nurs* 2001;**14**:61–82, quiz 105–6.
876. Drummer OH. Pharmacokinetics of illicit drugs in oral fluid [Review]. *Forensic Sci Int* 2005;**150**:133–42.
886. Kintz P. *Drug testing in hair*. Boca Raton, FL: CRC Pres; 1996.
944. Baselt RC, editor. *Disposition of toxic drugs and chemicals in man*. 10th ed. Seal Beach, CA: Biomedical Publications; 2014.

42

Toxic Elements

Frederick G. Strathmann and Lee M. Blum

ABSTRACT

Background
Elements have been recognized as toxins for centuries. Some elements are essential for life, but if an individual's exposure exceeds a certain threshold, toxicity may develop. When identified early, disease caused by elemental exposure is readily treatable with good outcomes. Conversely, if exposure is not identified and reduced, serious and sometimes irreparable damage to the nervous, renal, and cardiovascular systems can occur. The laboratory plays a key role in this process, and appropriate specimen collection coupled with accurate analysis can make a major difference in correct diagnosis.

Content
This chapter explores toxic elements and the role of the clinical laboratory in diagnosing and monitoring toxicity associated with exposure. A general overview of diagnostic and treatment options for the poisoned patient is followed by detailed descriptions for 23 elements most commonly associated with toxicity. Each section highlights the following areas: (1) sources of exposure, (2) toxicokinetics and toxicodynamics, (3) clinical presentation and treatment, (4) preanalytical and analytical aspects, (5) regulatory and occupational exposure aspects, and (5) areas of research. Each section concludes with recommendations for appropriate use and interpretation of test results. For a summary of the indication for use and interpretations of results for each element, see Table 42.1.

Elements have been recognized as toxins for centuries. For example, arsenic poisoning was a favored way to dethrone royalty in the Renaissance era, and mercury poisoning was common in eighteenth-century Europe, where it was associated with the generation of felt from beaver pelts to make the popular top hat and was the origin of the phrase "mad as a hatter." This chapter explores these and other toxic elements and the role of the clinical laboratory in diagnosing and monitoring toxicity associated with exposure.

CLASSIFICATION

Some elements are essential for life, but if an individual's exposure exceeds a certain threshold, toxicity may develop. Some nonessential elements are toxic even at low concentrations. Review of the periodic table provides some insight into the determination of an element's potential toxicity (Fig. 42.1).

Elements in rows 3 and 4 of groups 1 and 2 of the periodic table are essential elements. The gastrointestinal (GI) tract and the dermis are very effective at regulating the body burden of these compounds—patients rarely experience toxicity from one of these elements unless the element is injected directly into the vascular system. Elements in groups 6 through 12 in row 4 of the periodic table are essential for life but are required at low concentrations; many are protein cofactors required for enzymatic activity. The GI tract and the dermis regulate intake to some degree, but overload will induce passive diffusion that can lead to excessive concentrations and toxicity. Elements in rows 5 and below are classified as nonessential (or if essential, are required at picomolar concentrations or less). As one moves from right to left across the periodic table, the elements become more prevalent and therefore have greater potential to induce toxicity. Elements in groups 13 through 16 in rows 4 through 6 are of particular interest as toxins, because they have electron configuration that allows them to bond covalently with sulfur. Later in this chapter this characteristic is identified as a significant factor in the mechanism of action of this group of elements. These include arsenic, cadmium, lead, mercury, and thallium, all toxins of considerable concern. Elements in group 17 (halides) are essential for life but are toxic when present in excess. The inert elements that constitute group 18 are toxic in the gas phase because they can cause anoxia and their inert characteristic is the very cause of their toxicity.

POINTS TO REMEMBER

Elemental Toxicity

- Elements in rows 3 and 4 of groups 1 and 2 of the periodic table are essential elements.
- As one moves from right to left across the periodic table, the elements become more prevalent and therefore have greater potential to induce toxicity.
- Elements in groups 13 through 16 in rows 4 through 6 are of particular interest as toxins, because they have electron configuration that allows them to bond covalently with sulfur.

TABLE 42.1 Indications for Use and Interpretation of Results for Included Toxic Elements

Element	Indications for Use	Interpretation of Results
Aluminum	Urine aluminum may be useful for monitoring aluminum exposure and is preferred in the assessment of chronic exposure. Serum aluminum may be useful in the assessment of aluminum toxicity because dialysis and is the preferred test for routine screening.	Urine aluminum does not correlate well with degree of exposure. Serum aluminum >50 μg/L (1.9 μmol/L) is consistent with overload and may correlate with toxicity.
Antimony	Blood is useful for detecting recent exposure to antimony. Urine is useful for detecting chronic exposure to antimony.	Blood concentrations of antimony in unexposed individuals rarely exceed 10 μg/L (0.08 μmol/L). The form of antimony greatly influences distribution and elimination. Trivalent antimony readily enters red blood cells, has an extended half-life on the order of weeks to months and is eliminated predominantly through the bile. Pentavalent antimony resides in the plasma, has a relatively short half-life on the order of hours to days, and is eliminated predominantly through the kidneys. Reported symptoms after toxic antimony exposure vary based on route of exposure, duration, and antimony source and may include abdominal pain, dyspnea, nausea, vomiting, dermatitis, and eye irritation. Clinical presentation is similar to that of inorganic arsenic exposure. Urinary antimony levels predominantly reflect chronic exposure. Urine concentrations in unexposed individuals rarely exceed 1 μg/L (0.008 μmol/L), and urine antimony concentrations >10 μg/L (0.08 μmol/L) are indicative of significant and potentially toxic antimony exposure. The form of antimony greatly influences elimination with ~50% of the pentavalent and 10% of the trivalent form present in the urine within 24 h after exposure.
Arsenic	Blood arsenic is used for the detection of recent poisoning only. Blood arsenic levels in healthy subjects vary considerably with exposure to arsenic in the diet and the environment. A 24-h urine arsenic value is useful for detection of chronic exposure. If low-level chronic poisoning is suspected, the μg/g creatinine ratio may be a more sensitive indicator of arsenic exposure than the total arsenic concentration.	Potentially toxic ranges for blood arsenic: ≥600 μg/L (8 μmol/L). The ACGIH Biological Exposure Index (BEI) for arsenic in urine is 35 μg/L (0.5 μmol/L) based on the sum of inorganic and methylated species.
Beryllium	Direct measurement of beryllium in serum, plasma or urine can be used to confirm an exposure to beryllium but is not a useful indicator in determining time since exposure or the extent of an exposure.	The beryllium lymphocyte proliferation test is a more reliable indicator of beryllium sensitization and/or chronic beryllium disease.
Cadmium	Urine cadmium levels can be used to assess cadmium body burden. Blood cadmium levels can be used to monitor acute toxicity. For occupation exposure monitoring, a panel that includes cadmium in blood and urine as well as β_2-microglobulin in urine is preferred.	In chronic exposures, the kidneys are the primary target organ. Symptoms associated with cadmium toxicity vary based on route of exposure and may include tubular proteinuria, fever, headache, dyspnea, chest pain, conjunctivitis, rhinitis, sore throat, and cough. Ingestion of cadmium in high concentration may cause vomiting, diarrhea, salivation, cramps, and abdominal pain.

Continued

TABLE 42.1 Indications for Use and Interpretation of Results for Included Toxic Elements—cont'd

Element	Indications for Use	Interpretation of Results
Chromium	Chromium urine levels can be used to monitor short-term exposure. The preferred test for evaluating metal ion release from metal-on-metal joint arthroplasty is chromium in serum or chromium in blood. Metal ion testing of joint fluid chromium may be complementary to serum testing but is not recommended.	The form of chromium greatly influences distribution. Trivalent chromium resides in the plasma and is usually not of clinical importance. Hexavalent chromium is considered highly toxic. Symptoms associated with chromium toxicity vary based on route of exposure and dose and may include dermatitis, impairment of pulmonary function, gastroenteritis, hepatic necrosis, bleeding, and acute tubular necrosis. The ACGIH Biological Exposure Index for daily exposure of hexavalent chromium is an increase of 10 µg/g (192 nmol/g) creatinine between preshift and postshift urine collections. The ACGIH Biological Exposure Index for long- and short-term hexavalent chromium is a concentration of 30 µg/g (577 ng/g) creatinine and the end of shift at the end of the workweek. Concentrations of chromium may exceed 100 µg/L (1923 nmol/L) in fluid collected from an affected joint.
Cobalt	Serum or blood cobalt concentration can be used in the assessment of occupational exposure or toxic ingestion. Serum or blood is an acceptable specimen type for evaluating metal ion release from metal-on-metal joint arthroplasty.	Serum cobalt concentrations may be increased in asymptomatic patients with metal-on-metal prosthetics and should be considered in the context of the overall clinical scenario. Symptoms associated with cobalt toxicity vary based on route of exposure, and may include cardiomyopathy, allergic dermatitis, pulmonary fibrosis, cough and dyspnea.
Copper	Tests for the diagnosis of Wilson's disease include serum copper and ceruloplasmin and may include direct assessment of nonceruloplasmin bound copper. Urinary copper may be useful in chronic copper overload, in the assessment of significant exposure, or in monitoring chelation therapy.	Individuals with symptomatic Wilson's disease usually excrete more than 100 µg copper per day. Other conditions associated with elevated urine copper include cholestatic liver disease, proteinuria, some medications, and contaminated specimens. Elevated hepatic copper is seen with chronic biliary obstruction and cholestatic conditions. Results inconsistent with other findings may reflect heterogeneity in hepatic copper distribution. Serum copper may be elevated with infection, inflammation, stress, and copper supplementation. In females, elevated copper may also be caused by oral contraceptives and pregnancy (concentrations may be elevated up to 3 times normal during the third trimester).
Gadolinium	Not routinely monitored in the clinical setting.	High concentrations are most often the result of gadolinium-containing contrast agents. Avoid exposure to gadolinium-containing contrast agents for 48 hr before specimen collection. Prolonged excretion of gadolinium-containing contrast agents in individuals with renal insufficiency will require a longer postexposure duration before urine collection for trace and toxic element assessment by ICP-MS.
Iron	Acute iron overload is largely a clinical diagnosis, but laboratory testing can be used to determine severity and success of treatment. Serum iron concentration and transferrin saturation are the most common noninvasive tests for suspected chronic iron overload. Iron liver is useful in confirming hepatic iron overload, particularly in individuals with hemochromatosis and no common *HFE* gene mutations. Initial approach to diagnosis for hemochromatosis should include iron and iron-binding capacity	Serum iron <500 µg/dL (90 µmol/L) is typically not associated with toxicity. Serum iron >1000 µg/dL (179 µmol/L) has been associated with severe toxicity.

TABLE 42.1 Indications for Use and Interpretation of Results for Included Toxic Elements—cont'd

Element	Indications for Use	Interpretation of Results
Lead	Lead in blood is the preferred method to detect and confirm exposure to lead.	Blood lead of 5-9.9 μg/dL (0.2 μmol/L to 0.5 μmol/L): Adverse health effects are possible, particularly in children under 6 yr of age and pregnant women. Discuss health risks associated with continued lead exposure. For children and women who are or may become pregnant, reduce lead exposure. Blood lead of 20-70 μg/dL (1 μmol/L to 3.4 μmol/L): Removal from lead exposure and prompt medical evaluation are recommended. Consider chelation therapy when concentrations exceed 50 μg/dL (2.4 μmol/L) and symptoms of lead toxicity are present.
Manganese	Manganese in blood is a useful indicator of recent, active exposure and provides a modest indicator for distinguishing exposed from nonexposed individuals. Manganese in blood is recommended for monitoring potential accumulation with total parenteral nutrition. Urine has limited utility in the assessment of manganese toxicity. Manganese in red blood cells may be useful in the assessment of long-term, low-dose manganese exposure.	Whole-blood manganese concentrations >14 to 18 μg/dL (255 to 328 μmol/L) are indicative of manganism. Urine manganese values do not correlate well with exposure or adverse effects.
Mercury	Urinary mercury levels predominantly reflect acute or chronic elemental or inorganic mercury exposure. Urine mercury levels may be useful in monitoring chelation therapy. Blood mercury levels predominantly reflect recent exposure and are most useful in the diagnosis of acute poisoning as blood mercury concentrations rise sharply and fall quickly over several days after ingestion.	Urine mercury concentrations in unexposed individuals are typically <10 μg/L (50 nmol/L). 24-hr urine concentrations of 30 to 100 μg/L (150 to 499 nmol/L) may be associated with subclinical neuropsychiatric symptoms and tremor, whereas concentrations >100 μg/L (499 nmol/L) can be associated with overt neuropsychiatric disturbances and tremors. Blood mercury concentrations in unexposed individuals rarely exceed 20 μg/L (100 nmol/L). Dietary and nonoccupational exposure to organic mercury forms may contribute to an elevated total mercury result. Clinical presentation after toxic exposure to organic mercury may include dysarthria, ataxia, and constricted vision fields with mercury blood concentrations from 20-50 μg/L (100-249 nmol/L).
Molybdenum	Urine molybdenum is the preferred specimen for the assessment of molybdenum toxicity. Plasma molybdenum is reflective of dietary intake.	High dietary and occupational exposures to molybdenum have been linked to elevated uric acid in blood and an increased incidence of gout. Plasma molybdenum concentration has been shown to correlate with dietary intake.
Nickel	Urine nickel is the preferred specimen for the determination of exposure. Serum nickel may be informative in the investigation of toxic exposure. Measurement of nickel is not recommended in asymptomatic individuals or individuals with a low likelihood of exposure.	Elevations in nickel urine or serum should be interpreted with caution in individuals without potential exposure risks and may indicate contamination of the specimen. Serum nickel >10 μg/L (170 nmol/L) may be consistent with toxicity.
Platinum	Measurement of platinum in serum may be useful in determining the cause of renal impairment in patients exposed to platinum-containing compounds.	A definitive correlation between platinum in serum and degree of exposure is not known. Mild elevations in platinum may be observed for prolonged periods after platinum-containing antineoplastic administration.

Continued

TABLE 42.1 Indications for Use and Interpretation of Results for Included Toxic Elements—cont'd

Element	Indications for Use	Interpretation of Results
Selenium	Urine is the preferred specimen type in the assessment of selenium toxicity. Urine selenium levels can be used to assess nutritional status and monitor excretion. Plasma and serum contains 75% of the selenium measured in whole blood and reflects recent dietary intake.	Acute oral exposure to extremely high levels of selenium may produce gastrointestinal symptoms (nausea, vomiting, and diarrhea) and cardiovascular symptoms such as tachycardia. Chronic exposure to very high levels of selenium can cause dermal effects, including diseased nails and skin and hair loss, as well as neurologic problems such as unsteady gait or paralysis.
Silicon	Silicon is rarely measured in the clinical setting but may be conducted in exposure monitoring or investigation.	Silicon concentrations are influenced by diet, especially vegetable intake.
Silver	Measurement of silver is limited to monitoring of individuals treated with silver sulfadiazine or silver-containing nasal decongestants.	The typical concentration of serum silver is <2 ng/mL (18.5 nmol/L). Silver concentrations observed in serum of unaffected patients during treatment range up to 300 ng/mL (2781 nmol/L), with urine output as high as 550 μg/day (5 μmol/d).
Thallium	Blood thallium is useful as a biomarker of acute thallium exposure. Urine thallium is useful as a biomarker of chronic thallium exposure.	Blood thallium concentrations >100 μg/L (489 nmol/L) are considered toxic and >300 μg/L (1467 nmol/L) indicate severe ingestion. Urinary thallium levels may reflect recent or chronic exposure and the presence of thallium in urine after acute exposure may persist for up to several weeks. Urine thallium concentrations <5 μg/L (24.5 nmol/L) are unlikely to cause adverse health effects while concentrations >500 μg/L (2446 nmol/L) have been associated with clinical poisoning. Peripheral neuropathy and alopecia are well-documented effects of acute and chronic thallium exposure.
Titanium	No current recommendations exist regarding the assessment of titanium in patients with metal-on-metal prosthetics. Serum is the preferred specimen for monitoring titanium exposure.	Increased titanium concentrations in serum have been associated with wear of metal-on-metal prosthetic devices. Serum titanium concentrations >10 μg/L (209 nmol/L) have been associated with metal-on-metal prosthetic device wear.
Uranium	Urine is the preferred specimen type for occupational monitoring of uranium.	The ACGIH recommends a biological exposure index (BEI) for uranium of 200 μg/L (0.8 μmol/L) in an end of shift urine sample.
Vanadium	Vanadium in urine is the preferred mechanism for monitoring toxicity in the occupational setting. Assessment of vanadium in serum is not recommended for asymptomatic individuals with metal-on-metal or ceramic-on-ceramic prosthetics.	Serum vanadium concentrations >5.0 ng/mL (98 nmol/L) indicate probable exposure. Urine vanadium concentrations >14 μg/L (0.3 μmol/L) have been associated with reduced neurobehavioral abilities.

PREVALENCE OF ELEMENTAL TOXICITIES

At this point in our understanding of medical science, one might expect that elemental toxicities would be thoroughly known and avoidable. However, humans frequently still encounter elemental toxins and chronic, low-concentration exposures occur more frequently in particular individuals than in large population groups. Concern continues regarding low-concentration exposure to lead and the effect such exposure has on nervous system development in the young. Arsenic is common in our environment, and individuals are occasionally exposed because of a lack of knowledge of the household products they are using. Many insecticides contain arsenic as an active ingredient, and careless use of these products has led to significant exposure. Arsenic is frequently identified as the cause of peripheral neuropathy among patients who have been unknowingly exposed. Ground water contaminated with arsenic in the Bengal basin of Bangladesh presents a serious health risk to the large population living in that region. Cadmium is used to manufacture brightly colored paint pigments, and painters who fail to use adequate respiratory protection can experience significant exposure. Cadmium is also significantly present in tobacco products.[1] Studies indicate that apoptotic pathways are initiated by elements such as

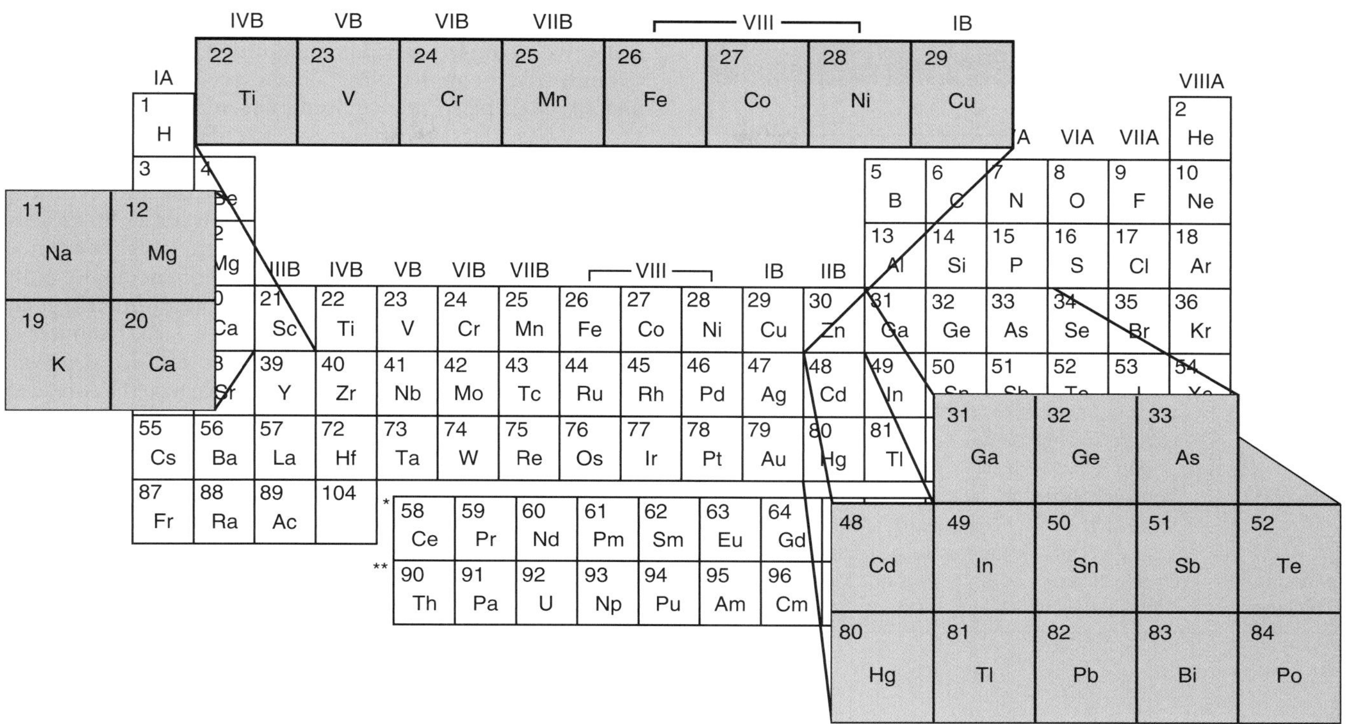

FIGURE 42.1 Periodic table, with emphasis on toxic elements.

arsenic, cadmium, nickel, beryllium, and possibly lead, antimony, and cobalt.[2]

The incidence of elemental poisoning across large populations attributable to arsenic, cadmium, lead, or mercury poisoning appears to be of the same scale as the more common inborn errors of metabolism, such as neonatal hypothyroidism and phenylketonuria, and is the same order of magnitude as the incidence of adult-onset hemochromatosis. Screening for these latter diseases is indicated because they are treatable, and treatment significantly reduces long-term morbidity. The same also may be true for elemental toxicities. When identified early, disease caused by elemental exposure is readily treatable with good outcomes. Conversely, if exposure is not identified and reduced, serious and sometimes irreparable damage to the nervous, renal, and cardiovascular systems can occur.

POINTS TO REMEMBER

- The incidence of elemental poisoning across large populations attributable to arsenic, cadmium, lead, or mercury poisoning appears to be of the same scale as the more common inborn errors of metabolism.
- When identified early, disease caused by elemental exposure is readily treatable with good outcomes.

DIAGNOSING TOXICITY

Confirming the diagnosis of elemental toxicity is difficult because signs and symptoms are similar to those of many non–element-dependent diseases. Diagnosis of elemental toxicity requires demonstration of all of the following factors: (1) a source of elemental exposure must be evident, (2) the patient must demonstrate signs and symptoms typical of the element, and (3) abnormal element concentration in the appropriate tissue must be evident. If one of these features is absent, a conclusive diagnosis of elemental toxicity cannot be made. The laboratory plays a key role in this process and appropriate specimen collection coupled with accurate analysis can make a major difference in correct diagnosis.

In clinical practice, analysis of toxic elements always should be considered in the clinical workup of the patient with (1) renal disease of unexplained origin, (2) bilateral peripheral neuropathy, (3) acute changes in mental function, (4) acute inflammation of the nasal or laryngeal epithelium, or (5) a history of exposure. Certain elements should be considered as the active, causative, or deficient agent in specific circumstances (Table 42.2).

TREATMENT

Route of exposure is an important aspect to elemental toxicity that can influence treatment and clinical outcomes. The clinical approach to elemental exposure comprises one of the following treatments: (1) Removal from exposure if the source is known, (2) decontamination, (3) enhanced elimination, or (4) antidotal treatment.

Removal from the source of exposure can be complicated if the element responsible is unknown or the source of exposure is in question. For less extreme cases of exposure or if evidence to support more invasive treatments is lacking, removal, often in conjunction with supportive care, may be the only form of treatment available.

Decontamination strategies may include gastric lavage, activated charcoal, and supportive therapies to maintain the ABCs (airway, breathing, blood circulation), as well as

TABLE 42-2 Conditions That Involve Metal Toxicity

Metal	Condition
Aluminum	Dialysis, encephalopathy, or dementia
Arsenic	Bilateral pain radiating from feet to legs, peripheral neuropathy, or unexplained impaired renal function
Cadmium	Impaired renal function in aerosol painters
Copper	Wilson's disease
Gadolinium	Nephrogenic systemic fibrosis
Iron	Hereditary hemochromatosis
Lead	Children younger than 2 years living in older homes or unexplained gastric upset, anemia, or impaired renal function at any age
Mercury	Acute changes in behavior, impaired speech, visual field constriction, hearing loss, and somatosensory disorders
Manganese	Onset of parkinsonism younger than age 50
Thallium	Acute hair loss

attention to water, electrolyte balance, and neurologic complications.[3] Prevention of absorption in the GI tract is one mechanism for treating the chronic copper overload seen in patients with Wilson's disease.[4]

Enhancement of elimination can be done through diuresis, biliary excretion, hemodialysis, or exchange transfusion.[3] Distribution of the element once absorbed has an impact of the utility of each of these approaches, and for several elements there is a lack of supporting data demonstrating improved outcomes after their use.

Antidotal treatments range from highly specific (eg, deferoxamine for iron and aluminum) to considerably less specific (eg, ethylenediaminetetraacetic acid [EDTA] for most divalent cations). The intent is to counteract the detrimental effects of the toxic element or to sequester it in a less toxic form. Although it is a highly useful method for treating elemental toxicity, the down side to chelation therapy is the potential for depletion of essential elements. The five most commonly used chelators are dimercaprol (British anti-Lewisite [BAL]), dimercaptosuccinic acid (DMSA or succimer), dimercaptopropane sulfonate (DMPS), EDTA, and D-penicillamine.[5]

POINTS TO REMEMBER

Diagnosing Elemental Toxicity

- Confirming the diagnosis of elemental toxicity is difficult because signs and symptoms are similar to those of many non–element-dependent diseases.
- Route of exposure is an important aspect to elemental toxicity that can influence treatment and clinical outcomes.

OVERVIEW OF ANALYTICAL TECHNIQUES

Analytical techniques used to measure elements in biological fluids include (1) atomic absorption spectrometry with flame (AA-F) or electrothermal atomization furnace (AA-ETA), (2) inductively coupled plasma emission spectroscopy (ICP-ES), (3) inductively coupled plasma mass spectrometry (ICP-MS), and (4) high-performance liquid chromatography (HPLC)-LC-ICP-MS. These techniques are specific and sensitive, and they provide the clinical laboratory with the capability to measure a broad array of elements at clinically significant concentrations. For example, ICP-MS is used to measure several elements simultaneously with the introduction of reactive cells and collisions cells further enhancing the utility of ICP-MS in the clinical laboratory.[6,7] Photometric assays have been used in the past but require large volumes of sample and have limited specificity. Spot tests are also available but should be considered obsolete because they are error prone, often yielding false-positive results. For more detailed discussion of these analytical techniques the reader is referred to Chapters 17 and 37.

SPECIFIC ELEMENTS

Aluminum (Al)

Aluminum or, alternatively, aluminium (Al), with the atomic number 13 and relative atomic mass of 26.9815, is a silvery, nonmagnetic, ductile metal in period 3, group 13, with one naturally occurring and stable isotope. In 1972, Alfrey and colleagues[8] first described an encephalopathy that was observed in patients undergoing prolonged hemodialysis for renal failure. The disease was characterized by abnormal speech, myoclonic jerks, and seizures. Patients with these signs also showed a predominance of osteomalacic fractures. Subsequently, it was found that exposure of patients in renal failure to (1) Al-laden dialysis water, (2) Al-containing oral phosphate binders, and (3) Al-laden albumin administered during dialysis is the primary cause of these signs of Al toxicity. Al is also a developmental toxicant if administered parenterally.[9]

Sources of Exposure

Under normal physiologic conditions, the usual daily dietary intake of Al is 5 to 10 mg, which is completely excreted. This excretion is accomplished by avid filtration of Al from the blood by the glomerulus of the kidney. Patients in renal failure lose this ability and are candidates for Al toxicity. The dialysis process is not highly effective at eliminating Al and also can be a significant source of exposure. Furthermore, it is common practice to administer Al-based gels orally to patients in renal failure to reduce the amount of phosphate absorbed from their diet to avoid excessive phosphate accumulation.[10] A small fraction of this Al may be absorbed, and patients in renal failure can accumulate this. After dialysis, albumin may be administered to replace that which is removed during dialysis. Some albumin products have high Al content resulting from the pharmaceutical purification process of passing the product through Al silicate filters.

Toxicokinetics and Toxicodynamics

The solubility of the Al compounds affects its toxicokinetics and subsequent health risks.[11] In general, inhaled soluble particles (eg, aluminum sulfate, hydrated aluminum chloride, and aluminum nitrate) are rapidly absorbed from the lungs, while the less or sparsely soluble particles (eg, aluminum metal, aluminum oxide, aluminum hydroxide, aluminum phosphate, and aluminum silicate) are retained in the lungs and then slowly released into the systemic circulation. Al accumulates in blood if not filtered by the kidney; avidly binds to proteins, such as transferrin; and rapidly distributes throughout the body. Deposition of it in bone interrupts physiologic calcium exchange; the calcium in bone becomes unavailable for resorption into blood, a process under the physiologic control of parathyroid hormone (PTH) and 1,25-dihydroxy vitamin D. The normal physiologic action of PTH on bone is blunted in patients with renal failure because their proximal tubular cells are not synthesizing the 1,25-dihydroxy vitamin D required for normal PTH action. It is typical for patients in renal failure to have high serum PTH values and normal or low serum calcium; this represents secondary hyperparathyroidism, the normal physiologic response to vitamin D deficit. Deposition of Al at the bone mineralization front and binding to parathyroid calcium receptors interfere with this physiologic process. The usual parathyroid response to these conditions decreases secretion of PTH. The result is lower than expected serum PTH concentration for the degree of renal disease present.

Clinical Presentation and Treatment

A biochemical profile that characterizes Al overload disease has been defined.[12] In human subjects with normal renal function, serum Al concentration is typically lower than 6 μg/L (0.2 μmol/L), but patients in renal failure invariably have serum Al concentrations significantly higher. Clinical guidelines published in 2006 suggest that patients with no signs or symptoms of osteomalacia or encephalopathy are likely to have serum Al concentrations less than 20 μg/L (0.74 μmol/L) and intact PTH concentrations of 150 to 300 ng/L (16.5 to 33 nmol/L), typical for secondary hyperparathyroidism associated with renal failure.[13] Patients with signs and symptoms of osteomalacia or encephalopathy typically have serum Al concentrations greater than 60 μg/L (2.2 μmol/L) and PTH concentrations less than 65 ng/L (7.15 nmol/L), indicative of Al-related bone disease. Patients with serum Al concentrations greater than 20 and less than 60 μg/L (>0.7 and <2.2 μmol/L) were identified as candidates for likely onset of Al-related bone disease; these patients required aggressive efforts to reduce their daily Al exposure. Efforts to reduce Al intake include (1) switching from Al-containing phosphate binders to calcium-containing phosphate binders, (2) ensuring that dialysis water contains less than 10 μg/L (0.4 μmol/L) of Al, and (3) ensuring that albumin used during postdialysis therapy is Al-free.

Al-related bone disease has been diagnosed and treated with deferoxamine, an avid chelator of both iron and Al.[14] The deferoxamine infusion test is useful for the ultimate diagnosis of Al overload disease, and the drug has demonstrated utility for treating acute Al overload.[14,15]

Adverse health effects in workers occupationally exposed to Al compounds have included pneumoconiosis (aluminosis) and fibrosis of the lungs and toxicity of the central nervous system, including balance disorders, difficulties with memory and concentration, impaired cognitive abilities, irritability, depression, and decreased psychomotor performances.[11] Although rare, contact sensitization of the skin by Al is also possible.

Preanalytical and Analytical Aspects

Preanalytical considerations related to collection of specimen for Al analysis are significant. Most of the common evacuated blood collection devices used in phlebotomy today have rubber stoppers made of Al silicate. Puncture of the rubber stopper for blood collection is sufficient to contaminate the sample with Al and produce an abnormal concentration of Al. Typically, blood collected in standard evacuated blood tubes will be contaminated by 20 to 60 μg/L (0.7 to 2.2 μmol/L) of Al; this is readily demonstrated by collecting blood from a healthy volunteer into a standard evacuated phlebotomy tube. Special evacuated blood collection tubes are required for Al testing.[16] These tubes are readily available from commercial suppliers and always should be used. Failure to pay attention to this issue can result in the generation of abnormal results because of sample contamination, which leads to misinterpretation and misdiagnosis.

Analysis of Al is routinely performed by ICP-MS. Alternatively, atomic absorption spectrometry with electrothermal atomization may be employed, but considerable attention must be paid to matrix interferences.

Regulatory and Occupational Exposure Aspects

Occupational exposure to Al compounds primarily occurs through inhalation of airborne particles in dusts and fumes. The solubility of the Al compounds affects its toxicokinetics and subsequent health risks.[11] In general, inhaled soluble particles (eg, aluminum sulfate, hydrated aluminum chloride, and aluminum nitrate) are rapidly absorbed from the lungs, while the less or sparsely soluble particles (eg, aluminum metal, aluminum oxide, aluminum hydroxide, aluminum phosphate, and aluminum silicate) are retained in the lungs and then slowly released into the systemic circulation.[11,17] The amount of Al absorbed by inhalation also appears to be related to particle size. Al fumes are absorbed more readily than dust particles,[18] and ultrafine nanoparticles of aluminum oxide can penetrate cell membranes.[19]

Biological monitoring of occupational exposure to Al can be determined by analysis of blood, serum, or urine. The concentration of Al in these specimens can be affected by both the intensity of a recent exposure and the Al body burden. Studies of aluminum welders indicate a fair correlation between Al in serum and urine[11,20,21]; however, in workers with normal kidney function, urinary Al concentrations are a more sensitive indicator of occupational Al exposure than serum Al levels.[11,22] After exposures to low-level airborne Al, urinary Al levels are increased, whereas serum concentrations are generally within the range of control subjects.[11,21-23] In chronically exposed welders, the Al concentration in urine collected after 1 or 2 exposure-free days (eg, after a weekend of no exposure) is likely a good indicator for determining the magnitude of the Al stored in the body; whereas in newly exposed workers, the urinary Al level is probably more influenced by recent exposures than by the body burden.[11,22]

Reference values for nonoccupationally exposed populations are generally less than 10 μg/L (0.4 μmol/L) in serum and less than 30 μg/g (1.1 μmol/g) creatinine in urine,[22] although studies from several countries have shown these upper limits of reference values could be less in some populations.[18,24] Guidance values for biological monitoring of occupational exposures to Al have been recommended and should be used in conjunction with workplace air monitoring and medical surveillance assessments. The Finnish Institute of Occupational Health (FIOH) set a biomonitoring action concentration for Al and its inorganic compounds at 81 μg/L (3.0 μmol/L; corrected to relative density of 1.021) in a morning urine specimen collected before the working shift on the first day after the weekend.[24] This value reflects exposure to Al during the few preceding days and gives an indication of the body burden and health risk involved. The reference limit for the nonexposed FIOH population is 16 μg/L (0.6 μmol/L). In Germany, the Commission for the Investigation of Health Hazards of Chemical Compounds in the Work Area (DFG) assigned a biological tolerance value (BAT) for Al in urine as 60 μg/g creatinine (2.2 μmol/g creatinine) in urine with a noncritical collection time.[25] In welders, urine Al levels of 81 μg/L (3 μmol/L) corresponded to serum Al concentrations of 5.7 μg/L (0.21 μmol/L).[11]

Areas of Research

Interest in the role of Al in Alzheimer disease (AD) was raised when Perl and Brody[26] observed that Al accumulates in the neurofibrillary tangle of patients with AD. He concluded that the focal accumulation of Al had an association with neurofibrillary degeneration in the hippocampal neurons that might play a role in the development of AD. Although a cause-and-effect relationship between accumulation of Al in brain and AD has yet to be conclusively demonstrated,[27,28] studies have clearly shown an increased concentration of Al in the brain.[29] It is possible that accumulation of Al in the neurofibrillary tangle of patients with AD is a secondary finding associated with the disease but not directly related to the cause. Also, the neurofibrillary tangle has a higher than normal affinity for Al that may explain increased accumulation of Al in brain tissue of Alzheimer patients.

Antimony (Sb)

Antimony (Sb), with the atomic number 51 and relative atomic mass of 121.760, is a lustrous gray metalloid in period 5, group 15, with two stable isotopes. Sb compounds have been known since ancient Egyptian times and were used as cosmetics by the women of that era. In the sixteenth century, Sb preparations were thought to be wonder drugs and in the nineteenth century were prescribed for various conditions.

Sources of Exposure

Pure metallic Sb is very brittle; however, alloys of Sb are used in various fields of technology. For example, addition of Sb to lead, tin, and copper increases the hardness of these elements when used as electrodes, bullets, type metal for printing, and ball bearings. Other uses include fire-resistant chemicals, pigments, and dyes.

Before the introduction of the antihelmintic drug praziquantel, several Sb-containing compounds were used in the treatment of leishmaniasis[30] and schistosomiasis, a parasitic disease carried by fresh water snails infected with one of the five varieties of the parasite *Schistosoma*.

Toxicokinetics and Toxicodynamics

Toxic effects of Sb are similar to those of arsenic; however, the majority of information specific to Sb toxicity has been obtained from the use of organic species for pharmacologic purposes.[31] Sb exists predominately in a pentavalent or trivalent state, with the trivalent form having inherently higher toxicity. Trivalent Sb is concentrated in red blood cells and the liver, whereas the pentavalent state predominates in the serum. Both forms are excreted in urine and feces; however, urine excretion predominates for pentavalent Sb and fecal elimination predominates for trivalent Sb.[32]

Sb has been shown to accumulate in organs and tissues with a high degree of vascularization such as the kidney and liver. Limited metabolism by glutathione-mediated reduction or methylation has been demonstrated for Sb, indicating a lessened detoxification process compared to that of arsenic.[31] Genotoxicity of Sb-containing compounds is complicated by the frequent coexposure to arsenic-containing compounds.[33] Data exist that demonstrate genotoxicity for trivalent Sb but not for pentavalent Sb, with limited evidence of mechanism or clinical relevance.[34]

Cardiovascular effects of Sb toxicity are related to the administration of Sb-containing drugs for clinical purposes and include increased blood pressure and altered electrocardiogram readings.[35]

Clinical Presentation and Treatment

Symptoms of acute exposure include a metallic taste, headache, nausea, and dizziness and, after a short interval, vomiting, diarrhea, and intestinal spasms. In chronic intoxication, adverse health effects include cardiac arrhythmias, upper respiratory tract and ocular irritation, spontaneous abortion, premature birth, and dermatitis.[36] Lymphocytosis, eosinophilia, and a reduction in leukocyte and platelet counts are also seen and indicate liver and spleen damage. Evidence supports increased risk for the development of lung cancer in Sb smelter workers, but the effect may be multifactorial and may be due, for example, to the presence of arsenic in the work environment. It is important to remember that when intoxication occurs with metallic Sb, the effect is caused not only by Sb but also by the lead, arsenic, and other elements that may accompany it.

Preanalytical and Analytical Aspects

Careful selection of specimen tube is important for Sb blood collection because the plastic in tubes other than certified trace element–free tubes may contain elevated concentrations of Sb. Preservation of collected urine has been shown to be unnecessary for the analysis of Sb for up to 65 days as demonstrated by fortification of 24-hour urine samples.[37] ICP-MS is typically used for Sb detection because of its increased sensitivity over that of other instrumentation. Historic methods for Sb measurements in blood have used time-consuming heated acid digestion for achieving better sensitivity, and simplified sample preparations measurements have been published more recently.[38]

Regulatory and Occupational Exposure Aspects

For purposes of biological monitoring after exposure to Sb, urine samples are preferable over blood.[39] Furthermore, studies of workers exposed to Sb have shown an increase over control subjects in the urinary excretion of Sb.[40-42] Urinary Sb concentrations were correlated to the intensity of airborne exposure in nonferrous smelter producing antimony pentaoxide and sodium antimonite ($r = 0.086$).[43] This correlation estimated an average increase of 35 μg/g (0.3 μmol/g) creatinine in the urine Sb concentration during the shift after an 8-hour exposure to 0.5 mg/m^3 Sb and average increase of

7 μg/g (0.06 μmol/g) creatinine after 8 hours of 0.1 mg/m^3 Sb.[41] In a study of glass manufacturing workers where the urine Sb concentrations correlated with airborne Sb levels ($r^2 = 0.068$), an air concentration of 0.5 mg/m^3 Sb corresponded to urine levels of 49 μg/L (0.4 μmol/L) and 0.1 mg/m^3 airborne level to 20 μg/L (0.02 μmol/L) Sb in urine.[42] Workers producing starter batteries exposed to antimony trioxide and antimony hydride also showed a correlation between airborne Sb levels and end of shift–end of workweek urinary Sb concentrations (r = 0.75)[43]; however, the corresponding urine levels to 0.5 mg/m^3 and 0.1 mg/m^3 air concentrations were higher, at 260 μg/g (2.1 μmol/g) creatinine and 60 μg/g (0.5 μmol/g) creatinine, respectively. The disparity noted in the urine Sb levels estimated from identical air concentrations likely results from the exposure to different Sb species (pentavalent antimony, antimony trioxide, and antimony hydride); the use of specimens collected at different times, in one case in which the urinary Sb concentrations were measured during the shift and in the other case the end of shift–end of week samples were tested; and, finally, the errors associated with extrapolating from the low measured airborne levels to the designated threshold air value of 0.5 mg/m^3.[43,44]

The American Conference of Governmental Industrial Hygienists (ACGIH) classifies antimony trioxide as a group A2 suspected human carcinogen. In Germany, the DFG designates Sb and its inorganic compounds (inhalable fraction) except for stibine (antimony hydride) as category 2 carcinogens, that is, substances that are considered to be carcinogenic for humans because sufficient data from long-term animal studies or limited evidence from animal studies substantiated by evidence from epidemiologic studies indicate that they can contribute to cancer risk.[45] No exposure equivalent for carcinogenic substances (EKA) correlations were established for antimony (III) oxide. The FIOH[46] has no established biomonitoring action limit for Sb, but recommends biological monitoring for Sb in a postshift urine specimen at the end of the workweek or exposure period. In pregnant women, the urine Sb concentration cannot exceed the reference limit for the nonexposed Finnish population at 1.1 μg/L (0.009 μmol/L) (corrected to relative density of 1.021).

Areas of Research

Reduced exposure to Sb has been studied in conjunction with the use of "green" ammunition as an alternative to conventional ammunition for indoor shooting ranges.[47] Metagenomic approaches have been published investigating potential of microbes with the ability to biotransform Sb to less toxic species for use in heavily contaminated soils.[48]

Arsenic (As)

Arsenic (As), with atomic number 33 and relative atomic mass of 74.9216, exists as gray, yellow, and black metalloids in period 4, group 15 and is monoisotopic. It is perhaps the best known of the elemental toxins, having gained notoriety from its extensive use by Renaissance nobility as an antisyphilitic agent and an antidote against acute As poisoning. Long-term administration of low As doses protects against acute poisoning by massive doses—a historic example of hepatic enzyme induction. This agent was memorably used in the well-known tale *Arsenic and Old Lace* as a means of terminating undesirable acquaintances. Currently, As is still a dangerous toxicant, as evidenced by the Bangladesh incident in which several hundred persons were poisoned by drinking ground water contaminated with As leaching from bedrock.[49] As is listed as the No. 1 toxicant on the Agency for Toxic Substances and Disease Registry (ATSDR) 2013 Substance Priority List of Hazardous Substances based on a combination of frequency, toxicity, and potential for human exposure.[50] Despite their inherent toxicity, As-containing compounds are used for therapeutic reasons. For example, As compounds have been used for decades in the management of protozoal infections such as trypanosomiasis. A preparation of arsenic trioxide called Fowler's agent was used in the nineteenth century as a health tonic and for a variety of ailments ranging from skin disease to leukemia. Arsphenamine was used intravenously to treat syphilis, yaws, and some protozoal infections.

Sources of Exposure

Nontoxic forms of As are present in many foods with arsenobetaine and arsenocholine, the two most common forms.[51] The foods that most commonly contain significant concentrations of organic As are shellfish and other predators in the seafood chain (eg, cod, haddock). In a large US population study, for all participants aged over 6 years of age, dimethylarsinic acid (DMA) and arsenobetaine had the greatest contribution to the total urinary As. Arsenobetaine was the primary contributor to high total urinary As concentrations.[52]

Toxicokinetics and Toxicodynamics

As exists in numerous toxic and nontoxic forms.[53] The toxic forms include (1) the inorganic species arsenite As^{3+}, also denoted as As(III); (2) arsenate As^{5+}, also known as As(V), and their less toxic metabolites; (3) monomethylarsonic acid (MMA); and (4) DMA. Detoxification occurs in the liver as As^{5+} is reduced to As^{3+} and then is methylated to MMA and DMA. As a result of these detoxification steps, As^{3+} and As^{5+} are found in the urine shortly after ingestion, whereas MMA and DMA are the species that predominate longer than 24 hours after ingestion. Urinary As^{3+} and As^{5+} concentrations peak in urine at approximately 10 hours and return to normal 20 to 30 hours after ingestion. Urinary MMA and DMA concentrations normally peak at approximately 40 to 60 hours and return to baseline 6 to 20 days after ingestion.[54,55] In a large US population study, for all participants older than 6 years of age, DMA and arsenobetaine had the greatest contribution to the quantity of total urinary As. Arsenobetaine was the primary contributor to high total urinary As concentrations.[52,56,57] Arsenic excretion in healthy people who have ingested arsenobetaine-containing foods is greater than 120 μg/24-h specimen.

The half-life of inorganic As in blood is 4 to 6 hours, and the half-life of the methylated metabolites is 20 to 30 hours. Blood concentrations of As are elevated for only a short time after administration, after which As rapidly disappears into the large body phosphate pool. Abnormal blood As concentrations in the 5 to 50 ng/mL (0.07 to 0.7 μmol/L) range are detected after exposure.[58] The structures of these and related As species are shown in Fig. 42.2.

The toxicity of As is due to three different mechanisms, two of which are related to energy transfer. Arsenic avidly binds to dihydrolipoic acid, a necessary cofactor for pyruvate dehydrogenase. Absence of the cofactor inhibits the conversion of pyruvate to acetyl coenzyme A—the first step in

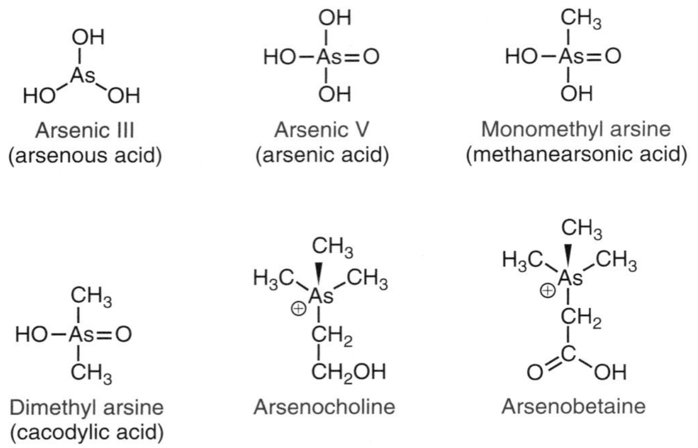

Arsenic III (arsenous acid)

Arsenic V (arsenic acid)

Monomethyl arsine (methanearsonic acid)

Dimethyl arsine (cacodylic acid)

Arsenocholine

Arsenobetaine

FIGURE 42.2 Structures of arsenic species.

gluconeogenesis. As competes with phosphate for reaction with adenosine diphosphate (ADP), resulting in formation of the lower-energy adipic acids rather than adenosine triphosphate (ATP). As also binds with any hydrated sulfhydryl group on protein, distorting the three-dimensional configuration of the protein, thus causing it to lose activity. This suggests that the primary mechanism of action of the toxicity of As is related to sulfhydryl binding. As also interferes with the activity of several enzymes of the heme biosynthetic pathway.[59] As is a known carcinogen as evidence suggests increased risk for bladder, skin, and lung cancers, as well as lung cancer associated with smoking, and after consumption of water with high As contamination.[60,61]

Clinical Presentation and Treatment

The symptoms of As toxicity may be nonspecific and often overlap with symptoms of other toxicants. Acute As toxicity can be characterized by GI distress, including vomiting and diarrhea, and cardiac arrhythmias.[62] Chronic toxicity may be characterized by renal failure, cardiac arrhythmias, liver dysfunction, and peripheral neuropathy.[63,64] Transverse white bands on the fingernails (Mees' lines) and hypopigmented macules on the skin have been documented after As exposure.[65,66]

As has been shown to interfere with the activity of several heme biosynthetic enzymes, including aminolevulinate synthase, porphobilinogen deaminase, uroporphyrinogen III synthase, uroporphyrinogen decarboxylate, coproporphyrinogen oxidase, ferrochelatase, and heme oxygenase.[59] Observed alterations in urine porphyrins include increases in copro/uro and copro I/III ratios.[67] Interestingly, the madness of King George III historically attributed to acute hereditary porphyria has been hypothesized to instead be a case of arsenic-induced porphyria based on retrospective analyses of hair.[68]

BAL is an effective antidote for treating As intoxication; the active agent in BAL is dimercaprol, a sulfhydryl-reducing agent. BAL was originally developed during World War II in response to the use of Lewisite, an As-based chemical warfare agent.[69] Other dimercaprol derivatives are available for treatment, including DMSA (succimer) and dimercapto-1-propanesulfonic acid (DMPS), the latter currently not approved for As chelation therapy in the United States despite past evidence of its utility in treating As toxicity.[70]

Preanalytical and Analytical Aspects

To distinguish among toxic inorganic species, HPLC techniques that separate the various species of As in biological fluids and tissues have been developed.[52] A typical finding in a urine specimen with total 24-hour excretion of As of 350 μg/24 h is that more than 95% is present as the organic nontoxic seafood species and less than 5% is present as the inorganic toxic species. Such a finding indicates that the elevated total As concentration was likely due to ingestion of seafood. Despite the availability of HPLC-ICP-MS methods for As speciation, it is noted that the use of a screening method for total As before speciation is of outstanding utility in reducing unnecessary costs.[71]

Hair analysis is frequently used to document time of As exposure. As circulating in the blood will bind to protein by formation of a covalent complex with sulfhydryl groups of the amino acid cysteine. Because As has a high affinity for keratin, which has high cysteine content, the As concentration in hair or nails is greater than in other tissues. Several weeks after exposure, transverse white striae, called Mees' lines, may appear in the fingernails; this event is caused by denaturation of keratin by elements such as As, cadmium, lead, and mercury. Because hair grows at a rate of approximately 1 cm/mo, hair collected from the nape of the neck can be used to document recent exposure. Axillary or pubic hair is used to document long-term (6 months to 1 year) exposure. Hair As greater than 1 μg/g dry weight indicates excessive exposure. In one study, the highest hair As observed was 210 μg/g dry weight in a case of chronic exposure that was the cause of death.[72]

Blood is the least useful specimen for identifying As exposure. Blood As concentrations are elevated for only a short time after administration[58] and rapidly disappear into the large body phosphate pool, because the body treats As like phosphate, incorporating it wherever phosphate would be incorporated. Absorbed As is rapidly circulated and distributed into tissue storage sites. Abnormal blood As concentrations are detected for only a few hours (<4 hours) after ingestion. This test is useful only to document an acute exposure when the As is likely to be greater than 20 ng/mL (0.3 μmol/L) for a short period. Typically, serum As is less than 40 ng/mL (0.5 μmol/L).

As has been accurately analyzed by ICP-MS. Mass response from the argon plasma is monitored for As (mass-to-charge ratio *[m/z]*, 75); however, the method must reduce the potential for interference from argon chloride (*m/z* 75) with the use of a dynamic reaction cell or collision cell with kinetic energy discrimination. Urine is the sample of choice for As analysis because of As is excreted predominantly by the kidney.[71]

Regulatory and Occupational Exposure Aspects

Workers potentially exposed to arsine (arsenic trihydride) include metal smelter and refiners, metallurgists, solderers, lead platers, battery makers, semiconductor manufacturers and recyclers, or any other occupation in which hydrogen comes in contact with As.[73-75] After an acute occupational exposure to arsine, the urinary As compounds detected in a worker were MMA, DMA, trivalent and pentavalent As, and arsenobetaine.[76] Because arsine is very toxic and has a strong odor, occupational exposures are likely to be very low, resulting in exposures similar to the background level of other As compounds.

Cardiovascular diseases and cerebrovascular effects are associated with chronic exposures to inorganic As compounds in the workplace.[77] Inhalation exposures to inorganic As compounds have been correlated to an increased incidence of lung cancer.[77,78] The ACGIH classifies As and its inorganic compounds as A1 carcinogens, confirmed human carcinogens. The recommended ACGIH Biological Exposure Index (BEI) for inorganic As plus methylated metabolites is 35 μg/L (0.5 μmol/L) in an end of workweek urine sample after the exposure to As and soluble inorganic compounds (excluding gallium arsenide and arsine).[79] After exposures to poorly soluble inorganic compounds, such as gallium arsenide, the urinary As concentration is more representative of the amount absorbed rather than to the total dose inhaled or ingested.[22]

Areas of Research

Cardiovascular injury secondary to inorganic As exposure has received increased attention, including the inclusion of increased risk for cardiovascular disease as a noncancer end point of interest by the US Environmental Protection Agency.[80] A clear mechanism of action remains to be determined; however, reports of oxidative damage to endothelial cells have been published.[81,82] Epigenetic changes as a result of As exposure have been identified, but the biological significance remains to be determined.[83]

Beryllium (Be)

Beryllium (Be), with the atomic number 4 and relative atomic mass of 9.0122, is a brittle, steel gray metal in period 2, group 2 and is monoisotopic. Be is an alkaline earth metal found in the earth's crust at an approximate concentration of 3 to 5 mg/kg; it is poisonous and is not necessary for human health. Be alloys are lightweight, stiff, and highly electrically conductive. Be metal and alloys and Be ceramics are used in a wide range of applications, including dental appliances, golf clubs, nonsparking tools, wheelchairs, satellite and spacecraft manufacture, circuit board production, and nuclear power and in weapons as a neutron modulator.

Sources of Exposure

The general population is exposed to low concentrations of Be through food and drinking water, but these exposures are not of clinical concern. The major route by which Be enters the body is by the respiratory tract, and industrial exposure usually occurs from inhalation and ingestion of Be dust. Acute exposure to Be is rare and is usually caused by an industrial accident or explosion.[84]

Toxicokinetics and Toxicodynamics

Inhaled Be compounds are cleared very slowly from the lungs. Soluble compounds are absorbed to a much greater degree than others such as Be oxide, which are much less soluble. Be salts are strongly acidic when dissolved in water, and this is thought to have a major toxic effect on human tissue. Absorbed Be accumulates in the skeleton, and renal clearance is very slow. Be inhibits a variety of enzyme systems, including alkaline phosphatase, acid phosphatase, phosphoglycerate mutase, hexokinase, and lactate dehydrogenase.[61]

Clinical Presentation and Treatment

Chronic Be exposure in the workplace has led to occupational health concerns because of its potential to cause a progressive and potentially fatal respiratory condition called chronic beryllium disease. This disease, also known as berylliosis, is characterized by the formation of granulomas resulting from an immune reaction to Be particles in the lung.[85] To reduce the number of workers currently exposed to Be in the course of their work at the US Department of Energy (DOE) facilities or among its contractors, the DOE has established a chronic beryllium disease prevention program to minimize the concentrations of, and the potential for exposure to, Be and has put forth medical surveillance requirements to ensure early detection of the disease.[86]

Studies have suggested that the size of the Be particles affects not only the site of deposition but also the amount deposited. This in turn may influence the clearance rate and thus the time of contact between the immune cells and Be.[87]

Preanalytical and Analytical Aspects

Several years ago, researchers noted that blood and lung cells from patients with chronic beryllium disease proliferated when exposed to Be in culture. This assay has been refined and is offered as the beryllium lymphocyte proliferation test (BeLPT). Unfortunately, because of the nature of the test and the variability across laboratories, the BeLPT has been known to produce false-negative and problematic results.[85,88] Efforts are under way by several groups to standardize the assay. Despite these issues, the BeLPT in bronchoalveolar cells is part of the current gold standard diagnosis for chronic beryllium disease.[89] Quantification of Be in serum or urine is not useful in making this diagnosis. Air analysis using the threshold limit value (TLV) is the preferred method of exposure evaluation.[90]

Regulatory and Occupational Exposure Aspects

The dose, particle size, and solubility of the Be compounds are critical factors affecting the deposition and clearance in the lungs.[91] Studies indicate that soluble compounds, such as beryllium chloride, have a pulmonary half-life of 20 days, with at least a third transferred to the systemic circulation.[92] Insoluble Be compounds, such as beryllium oxide, can be retained longer in the lungs and have an estimated pulmonary half-life of approximately 1 year. Inhaled Be exhibits multiphasic clearance from the lungs into blood.[93] Absorbed Be is mainly eliminated through the urine.

Although dermal absorption of Be probably contributes little to the body burden of occupationally exposed workers,[91] skin contact with Be can cause allergic reactions.[94]

Be and its compounds cause two types of Be-induced lung diseases, acute and chronic. Acute Be disease is caused by the inhalation of relatively high concentrations of Be dust and metal fumes, especially from soluble Be salts, which can result in an acute inflammation of the respiratory airways and lungs.[91] The occurrence of acute Be disease is relatively rare because of improved use of industrial hygiene practices. Chronic beryllium disease (or berylliosis) can develop after the inhalation of primarily insoluble Be compounds, such as beryllium oxide.[91] This disease, which is often fatal, is a cell-mediated immune reaction characterized by the formation of pulmonary masses or nodules (granulomas) that may take anywhere from a few months to many years to develop. It is believed that workers exposed to Be can become sensitized to Be, leading to the development of this disease.[95] The BeLPT is used to identify sensitized workers even if they are asymptomatic of disease. Because the predictability and reliability of screening by BeLPT have yet to be substantiated, the DFG in Germany has not recommended this test as an effective parameter.[91] Approximately 1 to 16% of exposed workers tested with the blood BeLPT were sensitized to Be.[96]

The Internal Agency for Research on Cancer IARC classifies Be and its compounds as a group 1 human carcinogen. Be and its compounds are designated as human carcinogens by the ACGIH (A1) and the German DFG (category 1). However, some investigators do not support the causal association between occupational exposure to Be and the risk for cancer and suggest further evaluation into the carcinogenicity of Be.[97,98]

Areas of Research

Be exposure and lung disease remains a continued focus of the American Thoracic Society, with a recent publication aimed at increased awareness.[99] Recent publications have reported on the increased incidence of chronic beryllium disease in men and women with human leukocyte antigen (HLA)-DPB1 mutations and Be exposure.[100,101]

Cadmium (Cd)

Cadmium (Cd), with the atomic number 48 and relative atomic mass of 112.414, is a soft, bluish-white metal in period 5, group 12, with 8 naturally occurring isotopes. An appreciation for the toxicity of Cd extends back to 1858 and the observed GI and respiratory effects after exposure to Cd-containing polishing agents. Famously, Cd toxicity was at the center of itai-itai disease (Japanese for "Ouch-Ouch"), a bone disease associated with fractures and severe pain that was identified after World War II in Japan. No biological function has been identified for Cd in humans; however, Cd serves as a metal cofactor of Cd-carbonic anhydrase in diatoms.[102]

Sources of Exposure

Cd is a by-product of zinc and lead smelting. It is used in industry in electroplating, in the production of rechargeable batteries, as a common pigment in organic-based paints, and in tobacco products. Spray painting of organic-based paints without the use of a protective breathing apparatus is a common source of chronic exposure. Auto repair mechanics are a work group that has significant opportunity for exposure to Cd.[103]

Toxicokinetics and Toxicodynamics

Cd toxicity is expressed via formation of protein-Cd adducts that change the conformational structure of the protein, causing it to denature. This protein denaturation occurs at the site of highest concentration—in the alveoli if exposure is due to dust inhalation, and in the proximal tubule of the kidney because this is a major route of excretion.[104] Once absorbed, nearly 80% of Cd is found in red blood cells.[103] Cd in plasma is transported to the liver bound to albumin, where Cd-induced synthesis and binding of the low molecular weight metallothionein becomes the transport system to the kidney tubules.[105]

The cellular effects of Cd include disruption of cell cycle progression, proliferation, differentiation, DNA replication and repair, and apoptosis.[106] Curiously, at low concentrations Cd has been shown to promote DNA synthesis and cell growth.[107] Indirect oxidative stress is a likely mechanism involved in Cd oxidative damage because Cd does not donate or accept electrons under physiologic conditions.[108]

Clinical Presentation and Treatment

The toxicity of Cd resembles that of As, Hg, and Pb in that it damages the kidney. Chronic exposure to Cd causes accumulated renal damage.[56] Breathing the fumes of Cd vapors leads to nasal epithelial deterioration and pulmonary congestion resembling chronic emphysema. Renal dysfunction with proteinuria of slow onset (over a period of years) is the typical presentation. Normal blood Cd concentration is less than 5 ng/mL (44 nmol/L), with most concentrations in the interval of 0.5 to 2 ng/mL (4 to 18 nmol/L). Moderately increased blood Cd (3 to 7 ng/mL or 27 to 62 nmol/L) may be associated with tobacco use.[1] Acute toxicity is observed when the blood concentration exceeds 50 ng/mL (444 nmol/L). Usual daily excretion of Cd is less than 3 μg/d (0.03 μg/d). Cd concentrations also increase with age and may be involved with senescence.[109]

Preanalytical and Analytical Aspects

Collection of urine samples using a rubber catheter has been known to result in elevated results because rubber contains trace amounts of Cd that are extracted as urine passes through it. Brightly colored plastic urine collection containers should be avoided because the pigment in the plastic may be Cd-based. Cd is usually quantified by atomic absorption spectrometry, but can be accurately quantified by ICP-MS.[103]

Regulatory and Occupational Exposure Aspects

Inhalation is the primary route of Cd exposure in the occupational setting, and the amount absorbed from the lungs depends on the solubility of the Cd compound and particle size. Absorption through the GI tract can occur from the clearance of particles deposited in the lungs and from contaminated hands and food. After chronic low-level exposures, approximately half of the Cd body burden is stored in the liver and kidneys. Urine is the main route of elimination, and thus urinary Cd levels are widely used to biomonitor chronic exposures in workers. However, because of the high binding capacity for Cd in the body, a urine level may provide no information about exposure in someone newly exposed to Cd. The lag time needed before the urinary Cd concentration correlates with exposure, depends on the intensity of the integrated exposure.[92] Until sufficient time of chronic Cd exposure has passed before urine testing can be used appropriately (~1 year), blood testing is suggested for newly exposed workers or when changes in exposure occur, because blood levels primarily reflect recent exposures.

The exposure assessment of Cd in OSHA Cadmium Standard is part of an overall periodic environmental, medical, and biological monitoring program. The biomonitoring requires testing in urine for both Cd and β_2-microglobulin with standardization to grams of creatinine for each component (μg/g creatinine); and in blood for Cd with standardization to liters of whole blood (μg/L). To convert μg/L to nmol/L or μg/g to nmol/g, multiply by 8.897. Table 42.3 shows the guidelines used in assessing the urine and blood tests and the actions to be taken with the results.

TABLE 42-3 Current Occupational Safety and Health Administration Guidelines for Cadmium

Biological Measurement	Normal Levels	Elevated Levels, Nonmandatory Removal	Highly Elevated Levels, Nonmandatory Removal	Highly Elevated Levels, Mandatory Removal
Cadmium in urine (μg/g creatinine)	≤3	>3 and ≤7	>7	>7
Cadmium in blood (μg/L)	≤5	>5 and ≤10	>10	>10
β_2- Microglobulin (μg/g creatinine)	≤300	>300 and ≤750	>750	>750
Trigger level	All three measurements at normal levels	Any one measurement at an elevated level	Any one measurement at a highly elevated level	After confirmed follow-up testing within 90 days, either CdU or CdB remains at a highly elevated level, or β_2MU remains at a highly elevated level and either CdU or CdB is at an elevated level.
Risk at this level	Negligible or relatively low risk for renal tubular proteinuria (ie, consistent with the background rate among the general population).	Elevated risk for renal tubular proteinuria (ie, above the background level experience by the general population).	Elevated, and perhaps highly elevated, risk for renal tubular proteinuria (ie, above the background level experienced by the general population). Risk may not be abnormal if β_2MU is highly elevated and CdU and CdB are at normal levels.	Highly elevated risk for renal tubular proteinuria
Actions	Provide annual biological monitoring and biennial medical examinations.	Provide semiannual biological monitoring and annual medical examination until all measurements return to normal levels.	If medically removed from job: Provide quarterly biological monitoring and semiannual medical examination until physician decides to return employee to job or permanently remove the employee from job. If not medically removed from job: Provide quarterly biological monitoring and semiannual medical examinations until all measurement return to normal levels.	Mandatory medical removal required. Provide quarterly biological monitoring and semiannual medical examinations until physician decides to return employee to job or permanently remove the employee from job.

From Occupational Safety and Health Administration. Medical evaluation of renal effects of cadmium exposures. *OSHA Brief.* Available at https://www.osha.gov/Publications/OSHA_3675.pdf.

Areas of Research

Cd toxicity continues to be of outstanding concern regarding environmental accumulation and the effect on both plants and animals. Of particular interest is the investigation of Cd exposure and increased risk for cardiovascular disease,[110] with a more recent publication proposing endoplasmic reticulum stress and impaired energy homeostasis in cultured cardiomyocytes.[111]

Chromium (Cr)

Chromium (Cr), with the atomic number 24 and relative atomic mass of 51.996, is a lustrous, hard, and brittle steely-gray metal in period 4, group 6, with 3 naturally occurring isotopes. Cr, from the Greek word *chroma* ("color"), makes rubies red and emeralds green. Among its many uses, it is most known for its application in making stainless steel, which is resistant to corrosion and discoloration. The requirement of Cr for sugar and lipid metabolism has resulted in considerable debate on its potential role in insulin resistance.[112,113] Homeostasis and functions of Cr are discussed in Chapter 37. Of late, Cr continues to make headlines as one of several metal ions released with wear because of highly publicized recalls of misaligned and accelerated failure rates of specific metal-on-metal (MoM) prosthetics.[114]

Sources of Exposure

Occupational exposure to Cr represents a significant health hazard.[115,116] Cr is used extensively (1) in the manufacture of stainless steel, (2) in chrome plating, (3) in the tanning of leather, (4) as a pigment in paints and dye for printing and textile manufacture, (5) as a cleaning solution, and (6) as an anticorrosive in cooling systems. The toxic form of Cr is hexavalent Cr^{6+} (Cr[VI]), and a strong oxidizing environment is required to convert the common form trivalent Cr^{3+} (Cr[III]) to Cr^{6+}, as might be found when Cr^{3+} is exposed to high temperatures in the presence of oxygen or during high-voltage electroplating.

Considerable attention has been given to Cr toxicity after release of Cr ions during normal and abnormal wear of MoM prosthetics after significant quality concerns with specific devices.[114] Although the idea of metal ion release is not a new concept,[117] the increased use of MoM prosthetic devices and attention given to poorly positioned and abnormally high failure rate of specific devices renewed interest in the potential for Cr toxicity.[118] However, the vast majority of Cr released from MoM prosthetics has been shown to be in the trivalent form, which is considerably less toxic than hexavalent Cr.[119] In May 2011 the US Food and Drug Administration (FDA) issued orders for postmarket surveillance studies to manufacturers of MoM hip replacement systems in response to an increasing concern over failed implant devices reported in Europe.[120] In the United States, no guidelines have been established for the assessment of metal ions in asymptomatic patients because of lack of knowledge regarding the prevalence of adverse events in the US population and no clear threshold levels associated with an adverse event. Internal exposure to metallic components of orthopedic devices and other implants is also discussed in the "Prostheses and Implants" section of Chapter 37.

Toxicokinetics and Toxicodynamics

Cr exists primarily as Cr^{3+} or Cr^{6+}, with Cr^{6+} being considerably more toxic than Cr^{3+}. Cr^{6+} is highly lipid soluble and readily crosses cell membranes, whereas Cr^{3+} is rather insoluble and does not readily cross membranes. Cr^{+6} compounds are powerful oxidizing agents and are more toxic systemically than Cr^{+3} compounds, given similar amounts and solubilities. At physiologic pH, Cr^{+6} forms CrO_4^{2-} and readily passes through cell membranes because of its similarity to essential phosphate and sulfate oxyanions. Intracellularly, Cr^{+6} is reduced to reactive intermediates, producing free radicals and oxidizing DNA, both potentially inducing cell death.[115] Severe dermatitis and skin ulcers can result from contact with Cr^{+6} salts. Clinically, monitoring biological specimens for Cr^{6+} is neither practical nor clinically useful to detect Cr toxicity, because the instant it enters a cell, it is reduced to nontoxic Cr^{3+}.[115] Inhalation of the vapors of Cr^{6+} causes erosion of the epithelium of the nasal passages and produces squamous cell carcinomas of the lung.[121]

Clinical Presentation and Treatment

Symptoms associated with Cr toxicity vary based on route of exposure and dose and may include dermatitis, impairment of pulmonary function, gastroenteritis, hepatic necrosis, bleeding, and acute tubular necrosis.[122] In the case of failing MoM prosthetics, elevated Cr in serum or blood is rarely the initial finding and instead is preceded by more telling physical symptoms such as reduced range of motion, swelling and inflammation around the joint, and general discomfort or pain. Although offered by many laboratories, measurement of Cr in joint fluid has relatively little clinical utility.[114]

Preanalytical and Analytical Aspects

Use of a plastic cannula for blood sampling was shown to be unnecessary in the assessment of Cr; however, sporadic contamination from stainless steel needles was observed.[123] Quantification of total Cr in urine can be used to assess exposure to total Cr. The presence of Cr in erythrocytes is suggestive of exposure to Cr^{6+} within the past 120 days, because Cr^{6+} crosses biological membranes but Cr^{3+} does not.[124] Increased serum Cr concentrations are observed in association with orthopedic implants made from Cr alloys.[125,126] ICP-MS is the preferred technology for quantification of Cr in body fluids but suffers from considerable interference because of polyatomics. Use of dynamic reactive cell technology or a collision cell with kinetic energy discrimination is required for reproducible and accurate measurements. For more details on the ICP-MS technology and Cr measurement the reader is referred to Chapter 37.

Regulatory and Occupational Exposure Aspects

Industrial exposures with Cr can be to the trivalent and hexavalent forms, which exhibit different toxicokinetics and toxicities in the body. Urine Cr levels are the most useful biomarker for assessing occupational exposure to water-soluble hexavalent Cr compounds[79]; however, other nonoccupational sources of both trivalent and hexavalent Cr from the diet, supplements, and the environment can have an impact on the total Cr concentration in urine. Furthermore, because Cr has been shown to accumulate in the body, urine Cr levels can be affected by both recent and past workplace exposures.[127-129] The measurement of Cr in erythrocytes has been used to gauge the intensity of exposure to hexavalent Cr[130-135]; however, insufficient data are available to determine a relationship for erythrocyte Cr levels with risks associated with exposures.[135]

Occupational exposures to hexavalent Cr compounds can cause respiratory irritation and tissue damage of the nose, throat, and lungs after inhalation and can cause irritation, burns, and ulcers on the skin with contact.[136,137] Hexavalent Cr has been associated with cancers of the lungs, nose, and nasal sinuses and classified as a human carcinogen by the Internal Agency for Research on Cancer.[138] Hexavalent Cr compounds are categorized as human carcinogens by the ACGIH (A1) and the DFG in Germany (category 1). The ACGIH suggests testing total Cr in urine for workplace exposure to hexavalent Cr (water-soluble fumes). The recommended BEI is 25 µg/L (481 nmol/L) of total Cr in an end-of-shift at end of workweek urine sample or an increase of 10 µg/L (192 nmol/L) during the shift by comparing preshift and postshift urine samples.[79]

Areas of Research

Recent investigations into contact dermatitis in children and adults have implicated Cr leaching from mobile phones as one potentially underappreciated source.[140]

Cobalt (Co)

Cobalt (Co), with the atomic number 27 and relative atomic mass of 58.9332, is a lustrous, hard, silver-gray metal in period 4, group 9, with 1 naturally occurring stable isotope. The word cobalt is derived from the German *kobalt* meaning "goblin" because of its superstitious reputation among miners. Co is widely distributed in the environment, is the essential cofactor in vitamin B_{12}, and has been widely used throughout history for decorative accents to glass and ceramics.

Sources of Exposure

Although relatively rare, Co is widely distributed in nature and is found in green vegetables, animal foods, and seafood.[141] Of Co in the body, 85% is in the form of cyanocobalamin or vitamin B_{12}, a Co complex similar in structure to that of porphyrins.[142] Co is used in alloys in which the presence of Co results in high melting point, strength, and resistance to oxygen. The addition of Co in MOM prosthetics adds resistance to surfaces undergoing heavy wear, and the release of Co from failed prosthetics remains of outstanding concern.[114] Co is found in rechargeable batteries and provides color to plastics, inks, glass, and paint.

Toxicokinetics and Toxicodynamics

Co in the form of cyanocobalamin is not toxic, whereas many other Co-containing compounds demonstrate a range of toxicities based on route of administration. Ingestion or inhalation of large doses may lead to pathologic disorders, and GI absorption varies considerably.[143] Acute toxicity manifests as pulmonary edema, nausea, vomiting, and hemorrhage. Long-term exposure affects several target organs, including the thyroid gland, lungs, immune system, and kidneys.[141] The mechanisms of Co toxicity include binding of sulfhydryl groups, resulting in enzyme inhibition; disruption of intracellular calcium homeostasis; and generation of reactive oxygen species. In the blood, Co partitions into red blood cells and has been demonstrated to bind to the globin moiety and does not displace iron at the center of heme.[144]

Accumulation of Co in the myocardium has been observed postmortem in lethal cases, and cardiac dysfunction has been noted in association with nonlethal occupational exposures[145] and in cases of MoM prosthetic failure.[146]

Clinical Presentation and Treatment

Co is not highly toxic, but large exposures will produce pulmonary edema, allergy, nausea, vomiting, hemorrhage, and renal failure. Occupational exposure occurs during production and machining of these metal alloys and has been known to result in interstitial lung disease. Cardiomyopathy and renal failure are symptomatic of acute Co exposure; this was exemplified by an incidence of mass population exposure to Co when beer contaminated with cobalt salts was consumed.[147] Chronic exposure may cause pulmonary syndrome, skin irritation, allergy, GI irritation, nausea, cardiomyopathy, hematologic disorders, and thyroid abnormalities. Co exposure alone may not lead to toxicity and must be considered within the context of exposure to multiple elements.[148]

Serum Co concentrations are increased above normal (>1 μg/L or >17 nmol/L) in patients with well-positioned and functioning orthopedic implants made from Co alloys.[125,126] Considerable attention has been given to Co toxicity in the context of failed MoM prosthetics, with several case reports of severe neurologic and cardiac abnormalities described.[146] In the case of failing MoM prosthetics, elevated Co in serum or blood is rarely the initial finding and instead is preceded by more telling physical symptoms such as reduced range of motion, swelling and inflammation around the joint, and general discomfort or pain. Although offered by many laboratories, measurement of Co in joint fluid has relatively little clinical utility.[114]

Preanalytical and Analytical Aspects

Quantification of active vitamin B_{12} is the usual way to assess nutritional status; quantification of serum, blood, or urine Co concentration is not typical for assessing vitamin B_{12} status. Co deficiency has not been reported in humans. Quantification of urinary Co is quantified in biological tissues by atomic absorption spectrometry or by ICP-MS.

Regulatory and Occupational Exposure Aspects

Absorption of Co through the lungs from inhalation of dust and fumes is the primary route of exposure in occupational settings, but absorption from dermal contact can occur.[137,149] Pulmonary absorption of the inhaled Co depends on the particle size and its solubility, with smaller particles deposited in the lower respiratory tract, where they dissolve or are phagocytized and translocated.[137] After inhalation, Co is eliminated from the body in several phases with a relatively rapid initial phase having a half-life ranging from hours to a few days and subsequent slower phases with half-lives ranging from months to years. Cobalt concentrations in urine increase proportionally more than that in the blood for workers during Co exposures, and Co concentrations in urine are primarily affected by recent exposures, but increase through the workweek under stable exposure conditions.[92]

The skin and respiratory tract are the two main target organs in workers exposed to cobalt metal, cobalt salts, and cobalt containing dusts.[150] Contact of Co with the skin can cause mild irritation and allergic reactions.[150,151] Inhaled cobalt dust and fumes can cause shortness of breath. Respiratory symptoms after chronic inhalation of Co can range from cough to respiratory hypersensitivity, progressive dyspnea, decreased pulmonary function, permanent disability, and death.[151] Pathogenic lesions in the parenchymal regions of the lungs known as "hard metal disease" can lead to severe alveolitis that progresses to end-stage pulmonary fibrosis.[150] In the hard metal industry, the coexposure of tungsten with Co has proved to be more toxic than the metallic Co alone.

The ACGIH BEI recommendations for the biological monitoring of Co are for Co and inorganic compounds, including cobalt oxides, but not combined with tungsten carbide, are 15 μg/L (255 nmol/L) in a urine sample collected at the end of shift, end of workweek; for Co with tungsten carbide, no specific exposure limit value is suggested, but biological monitoring should continue using an end-of-shift, end of workweek urine sample.[79] The DFG has an EKA for air concentrations of 0.01, 0.025, 0.050, 0.100, and 0.500 mg/m^3, with urine Co levels of 6, 15, 30, 60, and 300 μg/L (102, 255, 509, 1018, and 5091 nmol/L), respectively, in a specimen with a noncritical collection time. A "skin" notation is also assigned by the DFG for Co and Co compounds designating danger from percutaneous absorption. For these compounds, air monitoring alone is not enough to prevent adverse health effects; consequently, biological monitoring is also suggested to fully assess workplace exposures.[25]

Areas of Research

The effects of Co on voltage-dependent Na^+ channels in neurons has been investigated in rat skeletal muscle,[152] as well as reports of optic and auditory neuropathy in rabbits.[153] Cardiovascular toxicity continues to remain an intriguing line of investigation as a result of Co exposure.[154]

Copper (Cu)

Copper (Cu), with the atomic number 29 and relative atomic mass of 63.546, is a ductile metal with high electrical and thermal conductivity in period 4, group 11, with 2 naturally occurring stable isotopes. The use of Cu throughout history is well documented, with its first use estimated around 9000 BC. Bacteria will not grow on Cu, and for this reason Cu-containing alloys are often seen in areas such as doorknobs and hand rails. Homeostasis and analysis of Cu are discussed in Chapter 37.

Sources of Exposure

Cu ingestion has been known to cause serious toxicity,[155] and exposure may be caused by common pesticides. Copper arsenate is one of the active agents in marine antifouling paints and in the wood preservative used with green "treated" wood; copper arsenate wood products have been taken off the market in the United States because of this concern. Exposures to Cu have occurred from contaminated beverages and drinking water, as well as through the use of Cu-containing cookware.[156] Intentional ingestion of a toxic dose of copper sulfate has been used to commit suicide. Unintentional Cu toxicity has been reported after its use as an emetic and after ingestion of large quantities of coins.[156] Exposure to copper fume can occur during welding or refining processes.[157]

Toxicokinetics and Toxicodynamics

Cu is predominately absorbed in the small intestine, with minimal absorption occurring in the stomach. As the amount of dietary Cu increases, absorption decreases and this balance is regulated by an active transport system at low dietary levels (mediated by solute carrier family 3 transporters[158] with passive diffusion occurring at high dietary levels.[159] Cu absorption is reduced in the presence of elevated zinc as a result of metallothionein induction, and this relationship forms the basis for oral zinc therapy in genetic Cu imbalance.[160]

Cu is shuttled by chaperone proteins intracellularly with efflux into circulation regulated by P-type transport ATPases.[161] Once in circulation, Cu is transported to the liver bound to albumin with the majority of Cu leaving the liver bound to ceruloplasmin. Surprisingly, the genetic disease aceruloplasminemia does not severely disrupt Cu metabolism but does result in iron overload, indicating that other compensatory mechanisms of Cu transport exist.[162]

In the liver, Cu is incorporated into Cu-containing enzymes and proteins involved in a wide array of cellular functions, including electron transfer, iron oxidation, antioxidant defense, neurotransmitter regulation, clotting, and metal sequestration.[162] Although the majority of Cu stores are extrahepatic, the liver is the primary site for Cu metabolism.

In normal physiology, excess Cu that reaches the liver is exported into the bile while a minor amount is excreted renally. In Cu overload, tubular reabsorption is exceeded and urine Cu levels are considerably elevated.[159] The half-life of Cu in normal individuals is on the order of several weeks.[157,159]

Clinical Presentation and Treatment

Ingestion of Cu produces severe GI pain with erosion of the epithelial layer of the GI tract, hemolytic anemia, centrilobular hepatitis with jaundice, and renal damage. The classic presentation of Cu toxicosis is represented by the genetic disease of Cu accumulation known as Wilson's disease.[163] This disease is typified by hepatocellular damage (increased transferases) and/or changes in mood and behavior caused by accumulation of Cu in central neurons. Evaluation of serum and urine Cu concentration is useful in diagnosing Wilson's disease (see Chapters 37 and 61 for more detail). Increased serum Cu is observed in patients prescribed estrogen. Excess Zn ingestion interferes with absorption of Cu and leads to Cu deficiency, which is characterized by myeloneuropathy.[164]

Treatment of acute Cu toxicity is largely supportive based on symptoms, with relatively little guidance available regarding the use of the available chelating agents.[156] The overall treatment plan primarily includes fluid and electrolyte replacement, with chelation therapy used in severe ingestions.[165] Life-long drug therapy is the mainstay for individuals diagnosed with Wilson's disease and includes the use of Cu chelators such as D-penicillamine or oral zinc administration. After initial chelation therapy to remove excess Cu from the blood, low-dose chelation or ingestion of zinc salts is required regardless of the reduction in symptoms.[160,165]

Preanalytical and Analytical Aspects

Acute Cu overload is largely a clinical diagnosis, but laboratory testing can be used to determine severity and success of treatment. Elevations of serum Cu have been described in severe ingestions, but urine Cu levels are of limited utility.[156,159]

Laboratory results from patients presenting with symptoms consistent with Wilson's disease typically include low serum ceruloplasmin, elevated urinary Cu excretion, and liver function abnormalities. Although not always required for diagnosis, Cu concentration value in a liver biopsy from a patient with Wilson's disease will most often exceed 250 μg/g or 4 μmol/g.[160] Two recent guidelines are available that discuss diagnostic strategies for Wilson's disease.[4,166] Both highlight the calculation of non–ceruloplasmin bound Cu using concentrations of serum Cu and serum ceruloplasmin as potentially useful; however, both list concerns over the performance of necessary methods and the potential for overestimation of ceruloplasmin saturation.

Measurement of Cu is most often done using atomic absorption or atomic emission spectroscopy. In addition, Cu is readily measured by ICP-MS. For the laboratory assessment of Cu status see Chapter 37.

Regulatory and Occupational Exposure Aspects

Occupational inhalation of Cu dust causes respiratory irritation including coughing, sneezing, thoracic pain, and nasal discharge.[167] However, it is only on rare occasions that inhalation of Cu fumes may be associated with metal fume fever, an acute self-limiting illness characterized by shaking chills, fever, and body aches a few hours after inhalation exposure to the fumes of some metals.[168,169] Although Cu fumes may cause irritation to the upper respiratory tract after inhalation, no chronic damage to the pulmonary system has been observed from exposure to Cu dusts or fumes.[170] Even with an airborne exposure limit of 0.1 mg/m^3, no respiratory effects are expected to Cu dust and inorganic Cu compounds.[171] The occupational disease known as "vineyard sprayer's lung" observed in vineyard workers is considered to be caused by inhalation of the Cu component in an antimildew agent.[172] From the radiographic images, this disease resembles silicosis with micronodular disease in the early stages and progressive massive fibrosis in the later stages that eventually results in end-stage lung disease. Patients exhibit respiratory failure and an increased incidence of bronchogenic carcinoma compared to the general population.[173]

Studies of occupational exposures with Cu air levels up to approximately 1 mg/m^3 provide no clear or dose-dependent elevation in blood Cu concentrations in workers.[174] The lack of sufficient data pertaining to the relationship of occupational exposure, internal dose, and effect precludes the establishment of biological limit values.[92]

Areas of Research

Clinical methods for the direct measure of non–ceruloplasmin-bound Cu are available,[175] but discussion of their utility in current guidelines is absent. In addition, alternative assessments of Cu status such as relative, exchangeable Cu[176] are of unknown utility.

Gadolinium (Gd)

Gadolinium (Gd), with the atomic number 64 and relative atomic mass of 157.25, is a silver-white, malleable, and ductile metal in period 6 of the lanthanide series, with 6 stable isotopes. In the trivalent state, Gd has the greatest number of unpaired electrons providing increased signal intensity when used as a contrast agent in magnetic resonance imaging (MRI).

Sources of Exposure

Gd is a chemical element found in image contrast agents that are used during MRI and magnetic resonance angiography procedures. These agents have come under scrutiny by the FDA[177] because gadolinium-based contrast agent (GBCA) is thought to be involved in nephrogenic systemic fibrosis (NSF).

Toxicokinetics and Toxicodynamics

Because GBCA is excreted by the kidney, exposure is prolonged in patients with renal insufficiency,[178] it is thought that extended exposure permits transmetallation to occur; this allows free Gd to come in contact with proteins and other cellular components. Gd accumulates in tissues affected by NSF,[179] but it is not detectable in the tissue of patients with normal renal function.

Clinical Presentation and Treatment

Development of NSF because of GBCA is a debilitating disorder characterized by edema, plaques, discoloration, and severe thickening of the skin, resulting in contractures and immobility. In addition to GBCA exposure, other proposed contributing factors and associations with NSF include renal insufficiency, pharmaceutical erythropoietin usage, hypocalcemia acidosis, low serum albumin concentrations, and high serum ferritin concentrations.[180,181] Exposure to GBCA during a condition of low glomerular filtration rate appears to be the most consistent risk factor.[182,183] Although several different attempted therapies have been administered, some leading to moderate disease regression, no known cure is uniformly effective.[184]

Preanalytical and Analytical Aspects

Measurement of Gd is not routinely conducted in the clinical laboratory. However, laboratories using ICP-MS in the assessment of other elements should monitor Gd in all urine assays. Excess Gd in the urine of patients recently exposed to Gd-containing contrast agents may suppress elements of interest and may even saturate the detector, resulting in a loss of linearity and inaccuracy. For this reason, urine should not be collected or submitted for trace and toxic element assessment until after 48 hours after exposure to Gd-containing contrast agents.

Regulatory and Occupational Exposure Aspects

Industrial exposures to Gd compounds can occur through dermal contact where these substances are produced or used.[185] Animal studies indicate that Gd is taken up by the bone, liver, spleen, GI cells, and capillaries found mainly in the lungs and kidneys.[186-188]

Gd administered to animals displays prolonged prothrombin time and thrombocytopenia.[188] Gd affects various enzyme functions, including reduced total microsomal P_{450} activity and acts as a calcium antagonist.[186,187,189] It exhibits toxicity to the liver, spleen, and gastric mucosa.[188] Lanthanides in general are irritating to the eyes and abraded skin. Animal studies have shown that lanthanide chlorides and oxides can cause pulmonary toxicities such as bronchitis, pneumonitis, and granulomatous lesions, but there were no indications for development of pneumoconiosis, chronic pulmonary reactions, or cancer. Chronic exposures to dusts of lanthanides are a likely cause of pneumoconiosis in humans.[186]

Iron (Fe)

Iron (Fe), with the atomic number 26 and relative atomic mass of 55.845, is a soft, gray-black metal with 4 naturally occurring stable isotopes. Fe is the least energetically favorable fusion product formed in dying stars and is the most common element by mass and fourth most common by abundance in the environment. The use of Fe is highly integrated throughout history, the redox properties of Fe are essential in the Fe carrying capacity in vertebrates, and Fe is at the center of numerous enzymes from cellular respiration to drug metabolism. The homeostasis and analysis of Fe are reviewed in Chapter 38.

Sources of Exposure

For adults, a common cause of unintentional exposure is ingestion of high-dose Fe supplements, and in children chewable vitamin preparations are of concern. Blister packs and limitations on the number of pills dispensed have dramatically reduced the incidence of Fe overload in adults. Similarly, the reduced Fe content in children's vitamins has reduced the likelihood of Fe toxicity.[190] Finally, patients with renal failure and chronic anemia can be at risk for Fe overload from parenteral nutrition.

The three most common causes of chronic Fe overload include excess dietary intake, repeated blood transfusions and hereditary hemochromatosis. Regardless of the cause, the pathologic consequences of chronic Fe overload are analogous. There are numerous categories of hemochromatosis (see Chapter 61) and anemias (see Chapter 72) that lead to chronic Fe overload and are categorized as primary (inherited) or secondary syndromes.[191] Primary syndromes include HFE (a protein that modulates the expression of hepcidin [discussed later]) and non–HFE-related hemochromatosis (type 1), juvenile hemochromatosis (type 2), transferrin receptor 2 hemochromatosis (type 3), and ferroportin disease (type 4). Secondary Fe overload syndromes include Fe-loading anemias, chronic liver disease, treatment-induced and unclassified syndromes such as aceruloplasminemia, African iron overload, or neonatal iron overload. For more information on iron and iron overload syndromes, the reader is referred to Chapter 38.

Toxicokinetics and Toxicodynamics

The healthy body is greatly proficient at retaining and recycling absorbed Fe but has no regulated mechanism for Fe excretion. As a result, only 1 mg/day required to replace Fe lost in urine, biliary excretions, sloughing of gut cells, or menstruation.[192] Absorption of Fe starts in the gut, with acid hydrolysis of proteins to liberate bound Fe and the conversion of ferric iron (Fe^{+3}) to the more soluble ferrous (Fe^{+2}) form. Organic or heme Fe is absorbed at a fairly constant rate, whereas inorganic or nonheme Fe has a dynamically regulated mechanism for fine-tuning Fe absorption that includes a divalent metal transporter (DMT1) at the apical membrane and ferroportin at the basolateral membrane of enterocytes.[193]

The toxicity of free Fe is a consequence of its extensive redox chemistry, with the formation of hydroxyl radicals from the nonenzymatic reaction of Fe^{+2} and hydrogen peroxide of significant importance in cellular oxidative stress.[194] Because of this, the regulation of Fe transport involves several proteins to sequester Fe for storage, excretion, or transport, including transferrin (transport) and ferritin (storage). The majority of Fe is transported from enterocytes to target organs or cells by transferrin. Fe not immediately required in the synthesis of Fe-containing proteins is stored safely after incorporation into intracellular ferritin.[192]

During the absorption, distribution, and storage processes, Fe undergoes several interconversion events between Fe^{+2} and Fe^{+3}. Once delivered to target organs and cells, Fe is incorporated into a wide variety of proteins and enzymes, including hemoglobin, cytochromes, peroxidases, and other oxidases.[190] A majority of recycled Fe comes from the breakdown of protoporphyrin IX in senescent erythrocytes in the reticuloendothelial cells of the liver, spleen, and bone marrow by heme oxygenase.

Fe has no regulated mechanism for excretion. Excess Fe absorbed in enterocytes is stored in ferritin and eliminated from the body as the GI mucosal cells are sloughed.[190]

Clinical Presentation and Treatment

Acute ingestion can cause severe GI damage leading to increased uptake of Fe by nonspecific means, with distribution and damage to most major organs. Acute toxicity occurs within hours of ingestion and is often categorized into five clinical stages[195] but is of limited benefit in practical management. Depending on the severity of ingestion, symptoms can include abdominal pain, diarrhea and vomiting with cyanosis, metabolic acidosis, seizure, coma, and cardiac collapse, among the more concerning and severe complications. Ingestion of more than 0.5 g of Fe has been known to produce severe irritation of the epithelial lining of the GI tract, resulting in hemosiderosis, which may eventually develop into hepatic cirrhosis. The presence of Fe greater than 350 μg/dL (63 μmol/L) in serum corroborates this diagnosis.[196] Whole-bowel irrigation can be an effective decontamination procedure for acute Fe toxicity because absorption to activated charcoal is poor and the efficacy of gastric lavage can be limited because of the poor solubility of Fe tablets and their propensity for mass formation.

A hallmark of chronic Fe overload is the increased deposition of Fe in organs such as the liver and heart. The "classic triad" of bronzing skin, cirrhosis of the liver, and diabetes mellitus are present in a subset of individuals with severe Fe overload.[192] Chronic elevations in Fe result in hemosiderosis as ferritin degrades to hemosiderin and excess Fe is stored as less chemically active forms of Fe. Hemochromatosis is the deposition of excess Fe into tissues, often resulting in fibrosis.

Phlebotomy remains the most effective and safe treatment for chronic Fe overload and continues on a routine basis until serum ferritin is below 50 ng/mL (112 pmol/L). Careful monitoring of hemoglobin is often warranted if the risk for anemia is high.[197] An undesirable side effect of phlebotomy is an increase in non–transferrin bound iron and has been hypothesized as a potential complication for miscellaneous diseases not primarily categorized as Fe overload with speculation of the efficacy of oral chelation therapy as an alternative.[198] In both acute and chronic Fe overload, deferoxamine is the chelator of choice.

Preanalytical and Analytical Aspects

Acute Fe overload is largely a clinical diagnosis, but laboratory testing can be used to determine severity and success of treatment. Serum Fe concentration can be useful; however, interferences can confound interpretation during chelation treatment unless an atomization method such as atomic absorption is used. One might expect that total iron-binding capacity (TIBC) would be helpful because Fe concentrations less than the TIBC would be less likely to have excess unbound Fe. In reality, TIBC has been proved inaccurate and falsely elevated in acute Fe overdose.[199] Anion-gap metabolic acidosis and an elevated lactate may be found in severe ingestions.[190]

Serum Fe concentration and transferrin saturation are the most common noninvasive tests for suspected chronic Fe overload. In addition, ferritin and markers of acute liver injury such as alanine and/or aspartate aminotransferase can be helpful in determining the need for further clinical intervention. The need for liver biopsies in establishing a diagnosis in Fe-overload conditions has been reduced through the development of noninvasive methods such as genetic testing where applicable and imaging analyses. Liver biopsies do remain important in the evaluation of hepatic damage and unclassified genetic causes.[200]

Fe is most often measured on automated instrumentation; however, the measurement of Fe in tissue requires digestion of the tissue biopsy and is most often measured using ICP-MS. Isotopes of Fe may interfere with the assessment of other elements, such as nickel and typically require correction equations. In addition, the relative high abundance of Fe compared to manganese can result in inaccuracy if mass resolution is not adequate.

Regulatory and Occupational Exposure Aspects

Although Fe and Fe salts have varying degrees of solubility,[201] workplace exposures in the mining and processing of Fe involves exposures to other hazardous substances such as radioactivity, other metals, gases, and pyrolysis products. In mining operations, miners are exposed to radon and radon daughters that are often present in underground mines; to ore contaminated with toxic metals, including nickel and chromium; to silica and silicon containing dusts; and to diesel exhaust fumes from the use of motorized generators and vehicles. In the production of iron and steel, other hazardous exposures can include carbon monoxide from the blast furnaces; fluorine-containing gases from the use of fluorspar; airborne exposures of other elements used as alloys, such as chromium, nickel, tungsten, and vanadium, among others; and arsine and phosphine gases from Fe-containing arsenic and phosphorus.[201] Coexposures to silica occur in the foundry and steel industries from the production and use of ferrosilicon alloys.[202] Airborne polycyclic aromatic hydrocarbons are also present from the burning of carbonaceous materials, as are other chemicals from the use of organic binders such as phenol, formaldehyde, isocyanates, and various amines. Exposures to airborne refractory ceramic fibers from furnace insulation can occur in production and maintenance work.[203]

Inhalation of iron dust or fumes can result in pulmonary siderosis, in which Fe is incorporated and stored in the pulmonary interstitium. Pulmonary siderosis is a type of pneumoconiosis with minimal pulmonary reaction even with a heavy dust load.[204] The clinical course is benign and pulmonary function tests and blood gases are within normal reference intervals because fibrosis is not caused by Fe dust inhalation. Siderosis can regress after cessation of exposure. Iron foundry workers were also observed to have an increased incidence of bronchial obstruction. A study of iron foundry workers affected by small airway obstruction, found that 43 of the 99 subjects reexamined 30 months later had abnormal test results, indicating total airway obstruction. Deterioration of lung function even occurred in a subpopulation of nonsmokers.[205]

Epidemiologic studies of workers in the iron ore mines, foundries, and the iron and steel industry have shown an increased risk for developing lung cancers; however, the carcinogenicity of iron oxide cannot be readily discerned because of the coexposures to other toxicants in these workplaces. The International Agency for Research on Cancer (IARC) has found sufficient evidence in humans for the carcinogenicity of occupational exposures during iron and steel founding to classify these exposures as carcinogenic to humans (group 1).[206]

Iron pentacarbonyl (or iron carbonyl) is a strong reducing agent used in the chemical industry.[201] Vapors of iron pentacarbonyl form explosive mixtures with air and therefore should be stored under carbon monoxide, carbon dioxide, or nitrogen gas. It is highly toxic and warrants special handling in well-ventilated work areas by specially trained individuals. The German DFG assigned a skin notation to iron pentacarbonyl in recognition of the danger of its percutaneous absorption.[207]

Areas of Research

Copper plays an important and often overlooked role in Fe homeostasis through constant interactions during absorption, transport, and Fe recycling. As noted previously, a genetic lack of ceruloplasmin (aceruloplasminemia) is a secondary syndrome of Fe overload because ceruloplasmin and the associated copper ion cofactor is the major iron oxidation protein.[197]

Hepcidin has become a central theme in a majority of the primary Fe overload syndromes. Hepcidin, a protein produced predominantly by hepatocytes, counteracts the function of ferroportin by inducing its degradation, resulting in a subsequent decrease in circulating Fe. The entry of hepcidin into routine clinical assessment has been hampered by analytical obstacles inherent to the protein itself and a lack of harmonization of available assays.[208]

A growing area of interest is the presence of non–transferrin bound iron in diseases not primarily categorized as Fe overload, such as alcoholic liver disease, diabetes, and end-stage renal failure.[198]

Lead (Pb)

Lead (Pb), with the atomic number 82 and relative atomic mass of 207.2, is a soft, malleable bluish-white metal in period 6, group 14, with 4 stable isotopes. Pb has been used extensively throughout history, but use has been drastically reduced in the last few decades as a result of a better appreciation for its toxicity, especially during early childhood development. Turning Pb into gold was an obsession by ancient alchemists and today is possible using a particle accelerator, an immense supply of energy, and acceptance of very little yield for a lot of work.[209]

Sources of Exposure

Pb is present at high concentration (up to 35% w/w) in many paints manufactured before 1972. The Pb content of paints intended for household use was limited to less than 0.5% in 1978, but Pb is still found in paint products intended for nondomestic use and in artists' pigments. Ceramic products for use in homes available from noncommercial suppliers (eg, local artists) have been known to contain significant amounts of Pb; Pb is leached from the ceramic by weak acids such as vinegar and fruit juices. Leaded crystal contains up to 10% Pb, which is leached during long-term storage of fluids such as fruit juice, wine, and spirits.[210] Pb is also found in dirt from areas adjacent to homes painted with Pb-based paints and on highways, where it has accumulated from the use of leaded gasoline in automobiles. Use of leaded gasoline has diminished significantly since the introduction of unleaded gasoline, which has been required in personal automobiles in the United States since 1978. Pb is also found in soil near abandoned industrial sites where Pb may have been used. Water transported through Pb or Pb-soldered pipe contains some Pb, with higher concentrations found in water that is weakly acidic. Some foods (eg, moonshine distilled in Pb pipes) and some traditional home medicines also contain Pb.[211] Exposure to Pb from any of these sources by ingestion, inhalation, or dermal contact has been known to cause significant toxicity.

Toxicokinetics and Toxicodynamics

A typical diet in the United States contributes approximately 3 μg of Pb per day, of which 1 to 10% is absorbed; children may absorb as much as 50% of the dietary intake. The fraction of Pb absorbed is enhanced by nutritional deficiency. Most of the daily intake is excreted in the stool after direct

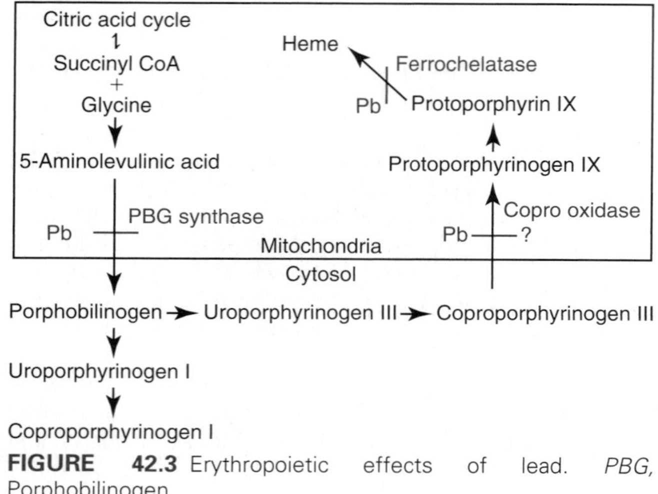

FIGURE 42.3 Erythropoietic effects of lead. *PBG,* Porphobilinogen.

passage through the GI tract. Although a significant fraction of the absorbed Pb is rapidly incorporated into bone and erythrocytes, Pb is ultimately distributed among all tissues. Lipid-dense tissues, such as the central nervous system, are particularly sensitive to organic forms of Pb. Erythrocyte turnover of Pb occurs within approximately 120 days. Pb is ultimately excreted in bile or urine.

Pb expresses its toxicity by several mechanisms that are described graphically in Fig. 42.3. Specifically, lead decreases heme biosynthesis by inhibiting δ-aminolevulinic acid dehydratase (ALAD) and ferrochelatase activity (see Chapter 30). Anemia caused by lack of heme is frequently observed in Pb toxicity. Pb also is an electrophile that avidly forms covalent bonds with the sulfhydryl group of cysteines in proteins. Thus proteins in all tissues exposed to Pb will have Pb bound to them. Keratin in hair contains a high fraction of cysteine relative to other amino acids and avidly binds Pb; hair analysis for Pb is a good marker for exposure. Some proteins become labile as Pb binds with them because Pb causes the tertiary structure of the protein to change; cells of the nervous system are particularly susceptible to this effect. Some Pb-bound proteins change their tertiary configuration sufficiently that they become antigenic; renal tubular cells are particularly susceptible to this effect because they are exposed to relatively high Pb concentrations during clearance.[56]

Clinical Presentation and Treatment

The development of Pb toxicity follows a progressive pattern. Fig. 42.4 describes this progression through a series of symptoms.[212]

The finding that Pb contributes significantly to decreased intellectual capability in the very young is of particular concern.[213,214] Young children are particularly prone to the effects of Pb because they have greater opportunity for exposure.[215] Children tend to spend a lot of time on the floor. In older homes that have been previously treated with Pb-based paints, Pb-laden paint chips and dust accumulate on the floor, which children are likely to ingest.

The World Health Organization (WHO) has defined blood Pb concentrations greater than 30 μg/dL (1.5 μmol/L) in adults as indicative of significant exposure.[216] Pb concentrations above 60 μg/dL (2.9 μmol/L) require chelation therapy. Similar to the situation seen in children, adult blood

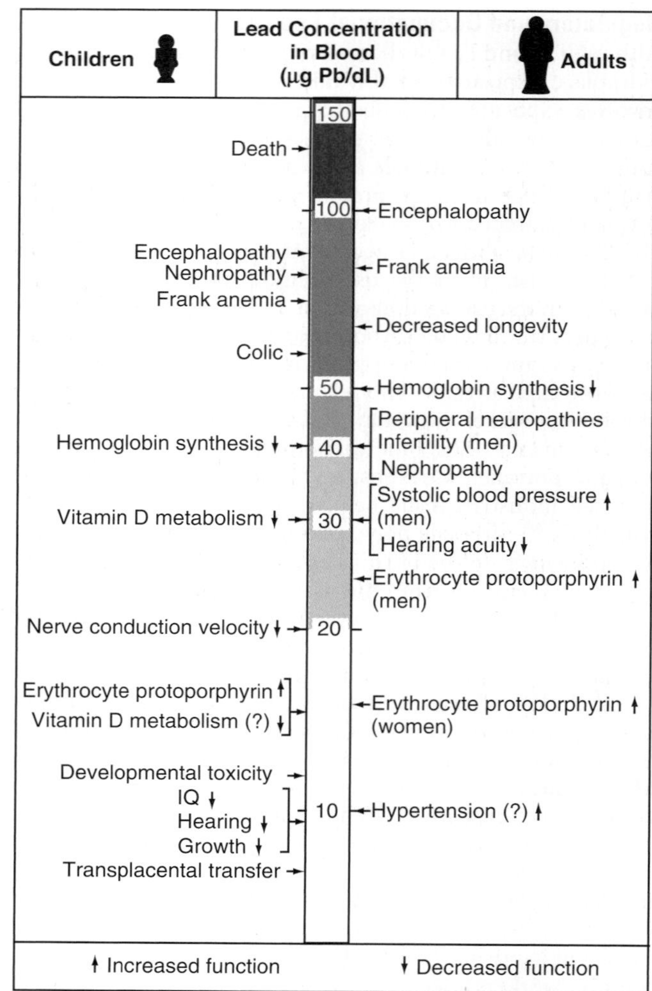

FIGURE 42.4 Effects of inorganic lead on children and adults (lowest observable adverse effect concentrations). (Reprinted with permission from Royce SE, Needleman HL, editors. *Case studies in environmental medicine: lead toxicity.* Washington, DC: US Public Health Service, Agency for Toxic Substances and Disease Registry; 1990.)

Pb concentrations have dropped to a mean value of 1.4 μg/dL (0.07 μmol/L) for ages 20 to 49 and a mean value of 1.9 μg/dL (0.09 μmol/L) for ages 50 to 69.[217] Given the decreasing blood Pb concentrations in adults, it may be important to revisit the recommendations regarding Pb exposure. Studies have shown a number of adverse health effects in adults exposed to Pb at concentrations below existing regulatory exposure limits. These include hypertension, adverse reproductive outcomes, and subtle central nervous system problems.[218]

Avoidance of continued exposure to Pb is paramount when blood Pb concentrations exceed acceptable reference intervals. Oral dimercaprol has become a standard therapy and is being used in the outpatient setting for all except those with the most severe Pb poisoning.[219] Although chelation therapy is effective in reducing blood Pb concentrations, a 2003 study indicated that chelation therapy given to preschool children with Pb concentrations in the range of 20 to 44 μg/dL (1 to 2.1 μmol/L) showed no beneficial effect on tests of cognition or behavior.[220] Thus prevention is the best therapeutic option.

Preanalytical and Analytical Aspects

The definitive test for Pb toxicity is measurement of blood Pb.[221] Over the past three decades, studies have shown an inverse relationship between blood Pb concentrations and children's IQ at increasingly lower Pb concentrations. In response, the CDC has continued to lower the suggested limit of normal for children and is now recommending 5 μg/dL (0.24 μmol/L) based on the 97.5% percentile of nonexposed children.[222] In addition, the term *blood lead level of concern* has been abandoned in favor of the viewpoint that all Pb is potentially harmful and therefore unsafe.[222] It is important to note that the median blood Pb concentration in children fell from 15 μg/dL (0.7 μmol/L) in 1978 to 2 μg/dL (0.1 μmol/L) in 1999.[220]

Although erythrocyte protoporphyrin concentrations are not a sensitive indicator of low-concentration Pb exposure, they are definitive markers for Pb overdose. For example, an erythrocyte protoporphyrin concentration greater than 60 μg/dL (1.1 μmol/L) is a significant indicator of Pb exposure (see Chapter 39). Serum ALAD concentrations are also a useful indicator for medium to high concentrations of Pb exposure; however, they do not correlate with low concentrations of Pb exposure. Serum Pb analysis is of very limited utility because Pb concentrations are abnormal for only a short time after exposure.[223] The National Health and Nutrition Examination Survey (NHANES) reported a median urine excretion as 0.37 μg/L or 0.40 μg Pb/g creatinine.[223a] Quantification of urine excretion rates before or after chelation therapy has been used as an indicator of Pb exposure.[224] Normally, the hair Pb content is lower than 5 μg/g (0.02 μmol/g); hair Pb concentration greater than 5 μg/g (>0.02 μg/g) indicates significant Pb exposure. Blood Pb concentrations have the strongest correlation with toxicity.

Analysis of Pb is routinely performed by ICP-MS,[6] electrothermal atomic absorption spectrometry,[225] or anodic stripping voltammetry.[226] Because Pb is concentrated in the erythrocytes, EDTA-anticoagulated blood is the specimen of choice for Pb analysis. Sodium heparin may also be used; however, samples that are not analyzed within 48 hours are frequently clotted and must be rejected. Care must be taken when obtaining capillary blood. Surface contamination, insufficient collection volume, or inadequate mixing with EDTA results in frequent sample rejection. Urinalysis also can be performed; urine quantification correlates with exposure.

If ICP-MS is used to measure Pb concentrations, it is essential to sum the masses of 206, 207, and 208 *m/z* to account for the natural isotopic variation of Pb in the environment. Failure to sum masses will skew results above or below the actual concentration because the isotopic abundance of a particular mass in the calibrator might not match the sample. However, this isotopic variation has been exploited to determine the source of Pb exposure. By determining the relative abundances of Pb in blood and of potential sources of exposure (eg, paint chips, soil), it is possible to identify a matching pattern. The exposure source with the same ratio of major Pb isotopes as that of the blood should then be avoided or removed from the patient's environment.

Regulatory and Occupational Exposure Aspects

The primary route of occupational exposure to Pb is by inhalation of fumes and dusts. The absorption of Pb is affected by the particle size and solubility of the Pb compound.[212] The larger particles (>2.5 μm) deposited in the airways can be transferred to the GI tract by mucociliary transport. Once in the blood, Pb is mostly bound to erythrocytes, is distributed to soft tissues, and accumulates in the bone. Pb readily passes through the blood–brain barrier and across the placental barrier. The main route of elimination for absorbed Pb is in the urine.

Biomarkers of exposure and biomarkers of effect have been used in assessing occupational Pb exposures. The direct measurement of Pb in blood reflects the concentration of the Pb in the soft tissues at steady state and therefore is an indicator of recent exposures. Most of the Pb body burden is stored in bones, so the bone Pb concentrations are a good indicator of cumulative or long-term exposures.[212,227] X-ray fluorescence techniques are used to measure Pb levels in bone.[227-229]

Exposures to Pb have been found to cause encephalopathy, peripheral neuropathy, neurologic and neurobehavioral effects, renal effects, hypertension, and reduced fertility.[212] Because of these adverse effects, the Occupational Health and Safety Administration (OSHA) has enacted standards to assess inorganic Pb exposure in the workplace.[230] The OSHA Standards for General Industry (CFR 1910.1025) and Construction (CFR 1926.62) applies to workers exposed to airborne Pb levels 30 μg/m^3 or greater time-weighted average and requires the removal of workers if a periodic and follow-up blood Pb level is 60 μg/dL (2.9 μmol/L) or greater, 50 μg/dL (2.4 μmol/L) or greater for construction, or the average blood Pb level of all tests over a 6-month period (or if there are fewer than three tests over a 6-month period, the average of three consecutive tests) is 50 μg/dL (2.4 μmol/L) or greater. Workers with a single blood Pb level meeting the numerical criteria for medical removal must have their blood Pb level retested within 2 weeks. If a worker is medically removed, a new blood Pb level must be measured monthly during the removal period. Workers are permitted to return to work when their blood Pb level is 40 μg/dL (1.9 μmol/L) or less.

The CDC/NIOSH reference interval for blood Pb level for adults is 5 μg/dL or 0.24 μmol/L,[231] and the geometric mean of the US population in 2011–2012 for blood Pb level in the adult population (≥20 years of age) is 1.09 μg/dL or 0.06 μmol/L.[223a] Because adverse health effects have been associated with Pb exposures resulting in blood concentrations less than 40 μg/dL (1.9 μmol/L), the current occupational standards may not be sufficiently protective and alternative workplace medical surveillance programs have been proposed.[232] The OSHA Standards give the examining physician flexibility in customizing protective procedures for individual workers; therefore the most current guidelines for managing Pb exposures should be implemented.[231]

According to the OSHA Lead Standards, a zinc protoporphyrin (ZPP) is required on each occasion a blood Pb level measurement is made. OSHA recommends a hematocrit determination whenever a confirmed ZPP of 50 μg/100 mL (0.8 μmol/L) whole blood is obtained to exclude anemia. ZPP levels in excess of 100 μg/100 mL (80 μmol/L) are considered elevated. However, ZPP is an insensitive biomarker for blood Pb levels less than approximately 20 μg/dL or 1 μmol/L.[233,234]

In a notice for intended changes, the new recommended ACGIH BEI for Pb in blood is 200 μg/L (1 μmol/L) with a notation for women of childbearing potential with blood Pb levels exceeding 50 µg/L (0.24 µmol/L) at risk for delivering a child with a blood Pb level over 50 µg/L (0.24 µmol/L).[79] For Pb and its compounds (except lead arsenate, lead chromate, and alkyl lead compounds), the DFG assigned a BLW (Biologischer Leit-Wert [Biological Reference Limit]) value of 300 µg/L (1.5 µmol/L) blood Pb for men and women older than 45 years, and a BAR (Biologischer Arbeitssoff-Referenzwerte [Biological Substance Reference Value]) value of 70 µg/L (0.3 µmol/L) blood Pb for women.[235] The FIOH recommends a biomonitoring action limit of 29 µg/dL (1.4 µmol/L) blood for monitoring inorganic Pb exposure.[46] According to the Finnish government a worker whose blood Pb concentration exceeds 49 µg/dL (2.4 µmol/L) must not work in a job that entails exposure to Pb. If the blood Pb concentration of one of the workers in a workplace exceeds 39 µg/dL (1.9 µmol/L), the "employer must specially monitor the workplace air Pb concentration, and the eventual health effects of exposure to Pb. In pregnant women, the blood Pb level is not to exceed the nonexposed reference interval in Finland of 1.9 µg/dL (0.09 µmol/L).

Areas of Research

Continued interest in determining the effects of even low blood Pb concentrations has resulted in numerous studies. These studies assessed intellectual impairment in children with Pb concentrations below 10 µg/dL (0.5 µmol/L). Data have revealed an inverse relationship between Pb concentrations and a child's IQ even at blood Pb concentrations less than 10 µg/dL (0.5 µmol/L).[213,214] Measurements of Pb in available blood supplies suggested the potential need to segregate low Pb blood products for neonatal transfusion.[236]

Manganese (Mn)

Manganese (Mn), with the atomic number 25 and relative atomic mass of 54.938, is a silvery metal in period 4, group 7, with 1 naturally occurring and stable isotope. Mn ions have a wide range of oxidation states and colors, making Mn an important constituent in pigments. Important in a wide variety of enzyme functions, severe Mn toxicity is most notably associated with irreversible neurologic damage. Mn homeostasis and function and the laboratory assessment of Mn status are described in Chapter 37.

Sources of Exposure

Mn is ubiquitous in the environment and is used as a binding agent in red brick, an anticorrosive in most steel alloys, a cleaning agent for glassware, and a common pigment in paints and glazes. The majority of Mn is used in the production of steel, where it is used as an alloy constituent as well as a deoxidizing and desulfurizing additive.[237] Mn is also found as an additive to gasoline in the form of methylcyclopentadienyl manganese tricarbonyl (MMT) and is released during the combustion process.[238] Outside of occupational exposure, the majority of Mn exposure occurs from food.

Toxicokinetics and Toxicodynamics

Absorption of Mn is primarily inhalation or oral, with dermal absorption being insignificant. Mn absorption in the GI tract is influenced by iron, calcium, phosphorus, fiber, and phytate, with transport in the gut occurring through common divalent metal transporters.[239] In blood, the Mn oxidation state influences binding to transferrin (trivalent) or α-macroglobulin (divalent). Absorbed Mn is rapidly eliminated from the blood and concentrates in the liver, with minor amounts transported to the bone and brain.[240]

Acute toxicity after Mn exposure is rare because of its relative lack of toxicity compared to those of other elements, with only a handful of nonoccupational cases being reported.[241,242] The only known case study of acute Mn toxicity resulting in death was published in 1941; however, it remains uncertain if Mn exposure was the sole reason for the associated symptoms and toxicity.[237]

The use of total parenteral nutrition (TPN) and Mn toxicity is well known, with several reports describing an association among TPN, increased whole-blood Mn, and accumulation of Mn in the brain.[243] For more information on TPN-related Mn retention and deposition refer to Chapter 37. Individuals with liver disease or impaired biliary excretion are at risk for Mn toxicity because this represents the major route for Mn excretion.[244]

The majority of available information regarding Mn toxicity is on the neurologic effects after chronic exposure. Unlike the damage found in the substantia nigra of patients with Parkinson's disease, Mn accumulates in the globus pallidus, the striatum of the basal nuclei,[245] and the substantia nigra.[246] Mn transport into the brain has been proposed to be mediated by divalent metal transporter proteins and transferrin receptors but remains controversial.[247] Neurotoxicity has been associated with Mn-induced oxidative stress and disruption of neurotransmitter synthesis and metabolism in the GABAergic and glutamatergic systems.[248]

Clinical Presentation and Treatment

Most of the Mn in daily diets is not absorbed. Humans exhibit toxicity to Mn when exposed to large quantities of dust containing the metal, which occurs in mining, ore crushing, machining of Mn alloys, and construction and destruction of brick. Mn exposure during metal welding has been suggested to cause neurologic disease, but this finding was not substantiated in a large study.[249] Mn toxicity is also a concern in newborns and children receiving long-term parenteral nutrition.[250] Neurologic findings associated with Mn toxicity are similar to those from patients with Parkinson's disease.[245] Mn madness includes nervousness, irritability, aggression, and compulsive behaviors such as laughing or crying.[251]

Reversal of more subtle symptoms such as headache and dizziness disappear after decontamination and removal from the source whereas the more severe neurologic symptoms do not.[237] Antiparkinsonian drugs have been used to reverse some of the neuromuscular signs associated with manganism; however, research suggests that the sites of Mn-induced toxicity in the brain are unique to those observed in idiopathic Parkinson's disease.[245]

Preanalytical and Analytical Aspects

Blood Mn concentration is a good indicator of exposure.[252] Commonly cited adult reference intervals for blood Mn are 0.4 to 1.1 ng/mL (7.0 to 20.0 nmol/L) for serum or plasma and 7.7 to 12.1 ng/mL (140 to 220 nmol/L) for whole blood. Typical daily excretion of Mn in urine varies from 0.2 to 0.5 µg/d (3.5 to 9.1 nmol/L). However, approximately 5% of healthy individuals excrete up to 2 µg of the element per day.

Because Mn-containing dust is common, contamination of urine with the metal occurs easily. Trace contamination of acid preservatives used for stabilizing the urine has been observed; however, acid stabilization has been shown to be unnecessary.[37] Mn is quantified by electrothermal atomization atomic absorption spectrometry and ICP-MS. Historic methods for Mn measurements in blood have used time-consuming heated acid digestion for sensitivity, however, simplified sample preparations measurements have been more recently published.[38]

Regulatory and Occupational Exposure Aspects

Exposures to Mn in the workplace are primarily from inhalation of dusts and fumes.[252] Absorption from inhalation depends on particle size and solubility. Smaller particles containing Mn are deposited in the lower respiratory tract and mainly absorbed into the blood and lymph nodes. Larger particles or nanosized particles trapped in the nasal mucosa may be transferred directly to the brain through the olfactory or trigeminal nerves. A significant fraction of the inhaled Mn particles are cleared from the respiratory system by the mucociliary transport mechanism and swallowed. The absorption of relatively soluble forms of Mn, such as manganese chloride, is expected to be higher than for the less soluble forms, such as manganese oxides. Mn is mostly bound to erythrocytes and transferrin in blood.[22] It is primarily distributed to the liver, kidneys, and brain. The elimination of Mn occurs mainly in the feces, with only a small amount present in the urine. The absorption and elimination of Mn in the body is tightly controlled by homeostatic mechanisms.[253]

The BAR reference interval in Germany used to compare occupationally exposed workers for Mn and its compound against nonoccupationally exposure population is 15 μg/L (273 nmol/L) in blood samples collected after the end of exposure or the end of the shift and with long-term exposure after several shifts.[254]

No biomonitoring action limit has been established by the FIOH for Mn and inorganic Mn compounds[46]; however, urinary Mn in a postshift urine specimen at the end of the workweek or exposure period can be used for biological monitoring of Mn exposure. According to the FIOH, the average urinary Mn concentration among welders of Mn-containing steels and in the manufacture of Mn batteries is usually below 2.7 μg/L (50 nmol/L) in urine corrected to relative density of 1.021. The reference interval in the nonexposed Finnish population in urine is 0.55 μg/L (10 nmol/L).

Areas of Research

A major focus of current research studies into Mn toxicity is further elucidation of the mechanisms underlying the neurologic damage.[246] The roles that glial cells play in Mn-mediated neurotoxicity are of considerable interest,[255] with investigations into astrocytes yielding intriguing insights.[256,257]

Mercury (Hg)

Mercury (Hg), with the atomic number 80 and relative atomic mass of 200.592, is a silver liquid at room temperature in period 6, group 12, with 7 stable isotopes. Its elemental symbol, Hg, is derived from the Greek word *hydrargyros*, meaning "water silver," and as is commonly referred to as quicksilver. Hg is one of only two elements that are liquid at standard temperature and pressure, (the other is bromine). The various forms of Hg have remarkably different toxicity profiles from largely benign unless inhaled (elemental Hg) to highly toxic (Hg salts and organic forms). Once commonplace in devices from thermometers to light bulbs, the potential toxicity of Hg has begun to overshadow its utility. The term "Mad as a hatter" was first used in reference to the Hg-induced dementia seen in workers with chronic exposure to Hg in the production of felt for hats.

Sources of Exposure

Hg is widely found in the environment[258] and occurs both naturally and as the result of industrial processes, with the single largest source of Hg being its natural out-gassing from granite rock.[259] Hg is also found in deposits throughout the world, mostly as cinnabar (mercuric sulfide), which is the source of the red pigment vermilion.

In the past, Hg was extensively used in the manufacture of devices such as thermometers, barometers, manometers, and sphygmomanometers. However, concerns about its toxicity have resulted in the phasing out of Hg-based instruments, which have been replaced with alcohol-filled, digital, or thermistor-based ones. It is still used as a dental amalgam and in lighting as mercury vapor lamps, although these are being replaced by sodium vapor bulbs. Hg is used in the pulp and paper industry as a whitener, as a catalyst in the synthesis of plastics, and as a potent fungicide in antifouling and latex paints.

Chemically, it is possible to convert Hg from its elemental state to its ionized state; in industry, this is frequently accomplished by exposing Hg^0 to a strong oxidant, such as chlorine. Elemental Hg is also bioconverted to both Hg^{2+} and alkyl Hg by microorganisms that exist both in the normal human gut and in the bottom sediment of lakes and rivers. When Hg^0 enters bottom sediment, it is absorbed by bacteria, fungi, and related microorganisms; these organisms metabolically convert it to Hg^{2+}, CH_3Hg^+, $(CH_3)_2Hg$, and similar species. Consequently, the methyl mercurials are accumulated in the aquatic food chain and reach their highest concentrations in predatory fish.[260,261] As a consequence of accumulation of methylmercury in the aquatic food chain, most human exposure to Hg happens through the eating of contaminated fish, shellfish, and sea mammals. For example, commercially distributed fish considered safe for consumption contain less than 0.3 μg/g (1.5 nmol/L), but some game fish contain more than 2 μg/g (10 nmol/L) and, if consumed on a regular basis, contribute to significant body Hg loads.

In the late 1980s, the public became concerned about exposure to Hg from dental amalgams.[258,262] However, later studies have failed to confirm a causal relationship.[263,264] Basic to the initial concerns was the fact that restorative dentistry used a Hg-silver amalgam for approximately 90 years as a filling material. In 1989, Hahn and colleagues[265] showed that a small (2 to 20 μg/d or 10 to 100 nmol/L) release of Hg^0 from amalgam occurs when it is mechanically manipulated, such as by chewing. The normal bacterial flora present in the mouth converts a fraction of Hg^{2+} to CH_3Hg^+; the latter has been shown to be incorporated into body tissue. In addition, the habit of gum chewing can cause release of Hg from dental amalgams at concentrations greatly above normal. Hansen and colleagues[264] noted in 1991 the release of up to 100 μg/d (499 nmol/d) of Hg in several human subjects who had the typical placement of dental amalgams (weighing ~800 mg each) after chewing gum for 8 hours. In 2010, the FDA issued rules that classify dental amalgam, reclassify dental mercury, and specify special controls for dental amalgam, mercury, and amalgam alloy.[266]

Concerns have been raised about the possible relationship between Hg exposure from vaccines and autistic disorders. In the United States, the prevalence of autism has risen from 1 in approximately 2500 in the mid-1980s to 1 in approximately 300 children in the mid-1990s.[267,268] Some investigators believe that this rise occurs because of the Hg that is present in vaccines as the preservative thimerosal (sodium ethyl mercury thiosulfate).[269-271] However, this causality has been questioned by numerous other studies, which have not been able to confirm this relationship.[272] In 2001, the Committee on Immunization Safety Review of the Board on Health Promotion and Disease Prevention of the Institute of Medicine initiated a study to review the connection between Hg-containing vaccines and neurodevelopmental disorders, including autism. The Committee has issued several reports; in its eighth and final report, put forth in 2004, the Committee reported that the hypothesis was biologically plausible, but that evidence was insufficient to accept or reject a causal connection. At that time, the Committee recommended a comprehensive research program.[273] The findings of this report have been challenged,[271] and thimerosal has been removed from most vaccines in the United States. The evidence linking Hg exposure from vaccines with autistic disorders has been highly criticized and resulted in the journal *Lancet* retracting the article linking autism to measles, mumps, and rubella (MMR) vaccines.[274-276]

Historically, Hg-containing compounds have been used for therapeutic reasons. For example, Hg has been used in medications that were touted as cures for syphilis and dysentery, to treat constipation, and as diuretics.[277] Intriguingly, the use of Hg-containing laxatives, termed "Thunder Clappers," on the Corps of Discovery Expedition with Lewis and Clark has left a discoverable trail of their movements, in more ways than one!

Toxicokinetics and Toxicodynamics

Hg is essentially nontoxic in its elemental form (Hg^0). In the absence of any chemical or biological system that chemically alters Hg^0, it is possible to consume it orally with no significant side effects. However, once Hg^0 is chemically modified to the ionized, inorganic species, Hg^{2+}, it becomes toxic. Further bioconversion to an alkyl Hg, such as methylmercury (CH_3Hg^+), yields a very toxic species of Hg that is highly selective for lipid-rich tissue, such as the neuron.[278] The relative order of toxicity is $Hg^0 \lll Hg^{2+} \ll CH_3Hg^+$ or $(CH_3)_2Hg$.

Hg toxicity is expressed in three ways. First, Hg^{2+} avidly reacts with sulfhydryl groups of protein, causing a change in the tertiary structure of the protein with subsequent loss of the biological activity associated with that protein; because Hg^{2+} becomes concentrated in the kidney during regular clearance processes, this is the target organ that experiences the greatest toxicity. Second, with the tertiary change noted previously, some proteins become immunogenic, eliciting a proliferation of β-lymphocytes that generate immunoglobulins to bind the new antigen (collagen tissues are particularly sensitive to this). Third, alkyl Hg species, such as CH_3Hg^+, are particularly lipophilic and avidly bind to proteins in lipid-rich tissue, such as neurons; myelin is particularly susceptible to disruption by this mechanism.[261] Hg also has been found to alter porphyrin excretion patterns.[279]

Clinical Presentation and Treatment

Each form of Hg manifests differently after a toxic exposure. For elemental Hg, poor absorption in the GI system reduces toxicity but can result in GI distress with prolonged contact or deposition.[280] With repeated injections of elemental Hg, seen in suicide attempts or psychiatric patients, the presentation was predominantly pleuritic chest pain, with other classic Hg-associated symptoms being absent.[281,282]

Experience with inorganic Hg poisoning has been gained from investigation of the 1951 to 1963 industrial dumping of Hg-laden waste sludge into Minamata Bay, Japan. Fish in Minamata Bay became heavily laden with Hg through the food chain. The local human population, whose diet depended on fish from the bay, exhibited symptoms of methylmercury poisoning, which include ataxia, impaired speech, visual field constriction, hearing loss, and somatosensory change, characterized histologically by cerebral cortex necrosis. Collectively, these symptoms have become known as Minamata disease.[283] Common target organs with inorganic Hg poisoning include the GI system, kidneys, and brain.

In adults, cases of methylmercury poisoning are characterized by the focal degeneration of neurons in regions of the brain such as the cerebral cortex and the cerebellum. Depending on the degree of in utero exposure, methylmercury may result in effects ranging from fetal death to subtle neurodevelopmental delays. Consequently, because pregnant women, women of child-bearing age, and young children are particularly at risk, the FDA recommends that they avoid eating shark, swordfish, mackerel, and tilefish.[284]

Preanalytical and Analytical Aspects

Analysis of blood, urine, and hair for Hg concentrations is used to determine exposure. The quantity of Hg found in blood and urine correlates with the degree of toxicity, and hair analysis has been used historically to document the time of peak exposure. However, it should be noted that hair analysis for elements in general is difficult because of contamination. Normal whole-blood Hg concentration is usually lower than 10 µg/L (49 nmol/L). Individuals who have mild occupational exposure (eg, dentists) may routinely have whole-blood Hg concentrations up to 15 µg/L (75 nmol/L).[275] Significant exposure is indicated when the whole-blood Hg concentration is greater than 50 µg/L (249 nmol/L) (if exposure is to methylmercury) or greater than 200 µg/L (997 nmol/L) (if exposure is to Hg^{2+}). The WHO safety standard for daily exposure of Hg is 45 µg/d; daily urine excretion exceeding 50 µg/d (249 nmol/d) indicates significant exposure. Normally, hair contains less than 1 µg/g (5 nmol/g) of Hg; greater amounts indicate increased exposure. Treatment with BAL or penicillamine will mobilize Hg, allowing for its excretion in the urine. Therapy is usually monitored by following urinary excretion of Hg; therapy may be terminated after the daily urine excretion rate falls below 50 µg/L (249 nmol/L).

Regulatory and Occupational Exposure Aspects

In industry, elemental Hg is present in the air as a vapor and its inorganic salts are there as aerosols.[22] Inhalation is the primary route of uptake from occupational exposures to Hg, although dermal absorption also can occur. Once absorbed, some elemental Hg is oxidized to the divalent form, which can bind to sulfhydryl groups in proteins such as albumin and metallothionein.[285,286] Elemental Hg is mainly distributed to the kidney and brain, while inorganic Hg salts are mostly delivered to the kidney. Hg is eliminated primarily through the feces and urine. Initially after exposure, more Hg may be eliminated in the feces than in the urine.[22] This may be due to the presence of binding sites in the kidneys.[285] The half-life of Hg in urine is approximately 40 days.[22] Therefore the Hg levels in urine do not necessarily reflect recent exposures in newly exposed workers.

Urinary Hg concentrations are primarily used to monitor long-term exposures to elemental Hg and its inorganic salts, whereas blood Hg concentrations are mainly useful for short-term, higher level exposures of these compounds.[287] Although studies of workers have shown good correlation between airborne Hg levels and blood concentrations,[288] urine is the preferred specimen for biological monitoring of workplace exposure to elemental Hg and its inorganic compounds because Hg levels in blood can be affected by the presence of organic Hg compounds from the consumption of dietary fish.[25,79] Studies examining the relationship between airborne Hg concentrations and urine levels in workers have shown variability in the urine Hg concentrations after workplace exposures.[289-292]; however, this variability may have been due to the methods used for air monitoring in the general work area compared with the microenvironments to which the workers were actually exposed.[293] Because biological monitoring in urine reflects long-term Hg exposures, the airborne exposure levels and urinary Hg concentration can be correlated, provided the exposures are relatively constant over a sufficiently long period and sample collection is standardized.[291,292]

Adverse effects on the nervous system and the kidneys are the main health concerns after Hg exposure. Workers exposed to Hg have shown various neuropsychomotor effects such as cognitive effects, impaired motor coordination and reaction time, deficits in attention and memory, and tremors.[294-297] Although some of these effects are reversible with the cessation of exposure, others can persist for many years. The kidneys are another target organ of Hg toxicity. Inorganic Hg is taken up by and accumulates in the kidneys.[285] The most vulnerable portion of the nephron to Hg is the pars recta of the proximal tubule. The binding for Hg with sulfhydryl groups in albumin, metallothionein, glutathione, and cysteine are implicated in the interactions of Hg with the kidney, including toxicity. Kidney cells are damaged as a result the toxic effects, leading to increased elimination of enzymes and proteins in the urine.[285,298] Urinary biomarkers are not adequately reliable as indicators of renal disease after Hg exposure[299]; however, patterns of biomarker excretion are shown to be sensitive to Hg intoxication.[299,300]

As previously mentioned, the biological monitoring for occupational exposure to elemental Hg and its inorganic compounds typically measures Hg concentrations in urine; however, there is a latent period before a steady state is reached when the urine determination reflects the exposure. Therefore urine measurements represent long-term Hg exposures and workers should be occupationally exposed to Hg for at least 6 months before implementing biomonitoring in urine. For the biological monitoring of elemental Hg exposure in the workplace, the ACGIH BEI recommends a urine Hg level of 20 μg/g (100 nmol/g) creatinine collected in a preshift specimen.[79] The DFG assigned a BAT value of 25 μg/g (125 nmol/g) creatinine for Hg and its inorganic compounds in a urine sample with the time of collection not critical.[25] The FIOH established biological action limits for Hg and inorganic Hg compounds in blood and urine samples.[46] The biological action limit in blood determined as inorganic Hg is 10 μg/L (50 nmol/L) in a specimen collected at any time. In this analysis, the inorganic and organic Hg are separated. For pregnant women, the inorganic Hg level in blood must not exceed the reference limit for the nonexposed Finnish population of 2 μg/L (10 nmol/L). The biomonitoring action limit in urine is 28 μg/L (140 nmol/L), measured as total Hg in a morning specimen collected toward the end of the workweek or exposure period and corrected to relative density of 1.021. The urine total Hg level is not to exceed the nonexposed reference interval in Finland of 4 μg/L (20 nmol/L) in pregnant women.

Areas of Research

Hg released from dental amalgams and its potential role in numerous disease states continues to be proposed and debated.[301] The potential for Hg-induced cardiomyopathies is of interest,[154] as is the utility of less conventional specimen types to assess in-utero Hg exposure.[302]

Molybdenum (Mo)

Molybdenum (Mo), with the atomic number 42 and relative atomic mass of 95.95, is a hard, silver-white metal in period 6, group 5, with 6 naturally occurring and stable isotopes. Mo has a rich history in weaponry because its addition to steel provides increased strength at higher temperatures. It was used for making Japanese samurai swords in the 14th century and later by the Germans in World War I to reinforce the "Big Bertha" gun. It was known as "moly be damned" by Midwestern miners in the United States.[303] Chapter 37 describes in detail the metabolism, function, and laboratory assessment of Mo status.

Sources of Exposure

Most Mo is used for the production of alloys, as well as catalysts, corrosion inhibitors, flame retardants, smoke depressants, lubricants, and Mo blue pigments. Mo is an essential trace element with the importance of organic-containing compound biological systems identified over 80 years ago.[304]

Toxicokinetics and Toxicodynamics

Between 25% and 80% of ingested Mo is absorbed predominately in the stomach and small intestine,[305] with the majority of absorbed Mo retained in the liver, skeleton, and kidney. In blood, Mo is extensively bound to α_2-macroglobulin and red blood cell membranes.[304] Mo can cross the placental barrier, and high levels of Mo in the diet of the mother can increase the Mo in the liver of the neonate.[306]

The metabolism of Mo is related to copper and sulfur because their absorption is inhibited by Mo.[307] Although not the primary treatment, Mo in the form of tetrathiomolybdate has shown utility in the treatment of copper overload in patients with Wilson's disease.[308] Very limited data on dose-response relationships are available for Mo, but toxicity correlates to solubility, with sparingly soluble compounds such as molybdenum metal and disulfide less toxic than highly soluble forms such as ammonium molybdate.[307]

Mo is rapidly eliminated in both urine and bile, with urine excretion predominating when intake is high.[304]

Clinical Presentation and Treatment

Mo toxicity is rarely reported because there are few known cases of human exposure to excess Mo. High dietary and occupational exposures to Mo have been linked to elevated uric acid in blood and an increased incidence of gout.[305]

Because of the inhibition of Cu absorption by Mo, Cu deficiency is a potential though not definitive symptom of Mo toxicity.[307] Inhaled Mo has been reported to damage the lungs, with pneumoconiosis reported in a small number of exposures.[309] Aching joints, inflammation, redness, discomfort, and limited range of movement are symptoms commonly reported in gout and symptoms reported in documented Mo exposures.[310]

Preanalytical and Analytical Aspects

Mo concentrations are measured by ICP-MS and graphite furnace atomic absorption. Semi-quantitative screening methods,[311] as well as quantitative methods in milk,[312] blood, and urine have been published.[313]

Regulatory and Occupational Exposure Aspects

Industrial exposures mainly result from the inhalation of dust and fine particles. Absorption occurs through the lungs and GI tract, but it depends on the chemical form and the route of exposure.[314] Water-soluble forms of Mo are absorbed through the lungs, and lesser soluble forms such as molybdenum trioxide and calcium molybdenum are retained in the lungs relatively longer. Insoluble species of Mo such as molybdenum disulfide are not absorbed from the GI tract, but the more soluble forms are. Once absorbed, the clearance of Mo from the plasma is biphasic.[315] Elimination of Mo is mostly in the urine.[304,315]

Workers chronically exposed to Mo in mines and processing plants showed a high incidence of weakness, fatigue, headache, irritability, lack of appetite, epigastric pain, joint and muscle pain, weight loss, red and moist skin, tremor of the hands, sweating, and dizziness.[314] Occupational exposures may cause an increase in serum uric acid and ceruloplasmin levels, as well as a rise in serum bilirubin and α-immunoglobulins.[314,316] Although these studies identified symptoms and changes in clinical chemistry as a result of Mo exposures, there are not enough data to identify a minimal effect level.[314] A direct effect on the lungs from chronic Mo exposure was reported in one study of 19 workers exposed to Mo and molybdenum trioxide for 3 to 7 years.[314] Three of the workers in this study displayed signs and symptoms suggestive of pneumoconiosis. Animal studies have shown molybdenum trioxide increased the incidence of tumors in mice.[317]

Although urine levels likely reflect recent exposures to soluble Mo compounds,[92] the information relating occupational exposure, internal dose, and effect is insufficient to determine biological limit values. However, workers occupationally exposed to Mo dust exhibited an increase in Mo plasma and urine concentrations.[316] The FIOH recommends testing for Mo in a postshift urine specimen collected at the end of the workweek or exposure period, but establishes no biomonitoring action limit.[46] They report a reference interval in a nonexposed Finnish population as 129 μg/L (1340 nmol/L) in urine corrected to a relative density of 1.021.

Nickel (Ni)

Nickel (Ni), with the atomic number 28 and relative atomic mass of 58.6934, is a silvery-white lustrous, hard, and ductile metal in period 4, group 10, with 5 naturally occurring and stable isotopes. Found in coins since the mid-19th century, Ni remains valuable for its corrosion resistance in plating but often is found at the center of reports involving hypersensitivity and allergic reactions to a wider range of products from cell phones to belt buckles.

Sources of Exposure

Ni is frequently used in the production of metal alloys (which are popular for their anticorrosive and hardness properties), in Ni-based rechargeable batteries, and as a catalyst in the hydrogenation of oils. Ni alloyed with transition metals is considered nontoxic, except that it will induce inflammation at the point of contact. Nickel carbonyl ($Ni[CO]_4$), used in petroleum refining, is one of the most toxic chemicals known to humans.[318]

In nonindustrial settings, Ni is found in a wide variety of consumer products, including utensils, jewelry, eyeglass frames, clothing buttons, braces, orthopedic implants, and some varieties of cell phones.[319] Despite its incorporation into MoM prosthetics and increased concern with failed MoM devices (see earlier section on "Chromium"), Ni has not been implicated as a significant contributor to the associated clinical presentation.[320]

Toxicokinetics and Toxicodynamics

The Ni species greatly influence the toxicity profile, as does the route of exposure and dose. Nickel oxides and sulfides and aqueous solutions of Ni in the oxidation state of 1^+, 2^+, or 3^+ are considered group I carcinogens.[321,322] Nickel carbonyl is absorbed after inhalation, readily crosses all biological membranes, and noncompetitively inhibits ATPase and RNA polymerase. Ni binds tightly to specific proteins in blood, including albumin, L-histidine, and α_2-macroglobulin.[323]

Ni binds to DNA with relatively weak affinity; however, considerably higher affinity binding is seen with DNA-associated proteins such as histones resulting in DNA hypermethylation, inhibition of histone acetylation, and ultimate gene silencing.[324] In addition, Ni has been demonstrated to inhibit DNA repair.[325]

The attempt to excrete Ni-protein complexes is the basis for Ni allergy resulting in tissue inflammation.[326] The main route of excretion is urine regardless of the route of ingestion.[327]

Clinical Presentation and Treatment

Contact dermatitis is the symptom often associated with Ni exposure in the nonoccupational setting. Ni allergy is the most common contact allergen in women because of its ubiquitous use in jewelry and cosmetic products.[328] Patch test studies have demonstrated a strong dose-response relationship between degree of exposure and severity of symptoms.[329]

Patients exposed to Ni carbonyl exhibit rapid onset of pulmonary congestion and inability to oxygenate hemoglobin, followed by development of lesions of the lung, liver, kidney, adrenal glands, and spleen.[330] Patients undergoing dialysis are exposed to Ni and accumulate Ni in blood and other organs.

Preanalytical and Analytical Aspects

Use of a plastic cannula for blood sampling was shown to be unnecessary in the assessment of Ni; however, sporadic contamination from stainless steel needles was observed.[123]

Regulatory and Occupational Exposure Aspects

Workplace exposures to various forms of Ni occur in a variety of industrial processes. Exposure to sparingly soluble Ni compounds such as nickel sulfide, nickel oxide, nickel carbonate, and nickel sulfidic ores generally occurs during the mining of nickel ores, the smelting and refining processes, and the grinding and welding of Ni-containing alloys.[331] The electroplating industry is usually the main source of workplace exposures to soluble forms of Ni such as nickel acetate, nickel chloride, nickel hydroxide, and nickel sulfate.[331] Exposure to nickel carbonyl (or nickel tetracarbonyl), an easily absorbed and highly toxic form of Ni, likely occurs in Ni refining, nickel coatings, plating glass, and as a catalyst in chemical reactions.[332]

Occupational Ni exposure mainly occurs by inhalation of dusts from sparingly soluble Ni compounds, aerosols from soluble Ni solutions, or gaseous Ni generally from nickel carbonyl.[22] Skin contact to airborne Ni and Ni-containing solutions is also possible, as is oral ingestion in facilities with poor industrial hygiene practices and workers who practice poor personal hygiene. The solubility of the Ni compound will affect the toxicokinetics of the Ni in the body. Soluble Ni compounds are more rapidly absorbed and eliminated compared to the poorly soluble forms. Inhaled particles of sparingly soluble Ni compounds can be retained in the lung tissue and regional lymph nodes, where they can accumulate and gradually be released over time.[333] The major elimination route for absorbed Ni is through the urine.

The toxicities of most significance after occupational exposure to Ni are the allergenic and carcinogenic effects. Ni exposure can cause sensitization of the skin (eg, contact dermatitis) and respiratory tract.[333] Occupational exposure to Ni compounds also can increase the risk for lung and nasal cancer in workers. The IARC classifies Ni compounds as human carcinogens (group 1).[334] Biological monitoring of Ni concentrations in body fluids after occupational Ni exposure has been extensively studied in workers,[331,334-345] and Ni concentrations in body fluids were found to be affected by the chemical species of the exposing Ni and the time of sample collection. In general, except for exposure to nickel carbonyl, in which where Ni urine levels can be useful in assessing the severity of the poisoning, elevated Ni concentrations in body fluids may not be directly correlated to exposure levels or risk for disease and only provides information about Ni uptake.[333-336]

Although a urine sample is the preferred specimen for biomonitoring Ni exposures, serum concentrations can be used to verify an elevated urine value.[331,333,346] The exposure equivalent correlations assigned by the DFG in Germany for Ni (nickel metal, nickel oxide, nickel carbonate, nickel sulfide, and sulfidic ores) with air concentrations of 0.10, 0.30 and 0.50 mg/m^3 are 15, 30, and 45 μg/L, respectively, in urine samples collected after long-term exposure, after several shifts. The exposure equivalents correlated to Ni (easily soluble Ni compounds, eg, nickel acetate and similar soluble salts, nickel chloride, nickel sulfate) air levels of 0.025, 0.050, and 0.100 mg/m^3 are 25, 40, and 70 μg/L (256, 681, 1192 nmol/L), respectively, in urine samples collected after long-term exposure, after several shifts. The BAR reference interval in Germany used to compare occupational exposed workers for Ni and its compounds against nonoccupationally exposed population is 3 μg/L (51 nmol/L) in urine samples collected after long-term exposure, after several shifts.[25]

Areas of Research

Ni has been included as one of the bivalent cationic metals classified as potential metalloestrogens capable of estrogen receptor activation and a possible role in breast cancer.[347] However, it remains controversial if the observed in vitro correlation with breast cancer after Ni exposure accurately translates into real-world risks after exposure.[348] The reproductive toxicology of Ni salts is interesting, including its role in calcium mimicry and potential effects on hormone dysregulation.[349]

Platinum (Pt)

Platinum (Pt), with the atomic number 78 and relative atomic mass of 195.084, is a dense, malleable, ductile, unreactive gray-white metal in period 6, group 10, with 6 naturally occurring isotopes. Pt is considered extremely rare, with the highest production currently from South Africa. A Nobel Prize in chemistry was awarded to Gerhard Ertl for work using Pt as a catalyst in the conversion of carbon monoxide to carbon dioxide. Most likely a result of its rarity, Pt has become synonymous with higher privilege as evidenced by "platinum" status award programs to music sales.

Sources of Exposure

The durability and underactivity of Pt has resulted in its use in jewelry and even aspects of laboratory testing, including Pt cones for ICP-MS. Pt salts are used in the preparation of sulfuric acid and petroleum, but the vast majority of Pt is used in automobile catalytic converters.[350]

A variety of Pt-containing antineoplastic agents are used in chemotherapy, typified by cisplatin (*cis*-dichlorodiammineplatinum dihydrate).[351,352] The year 2015 marked the 50th anniversary of the discovery of Pt-based chemotherapeutics,[353,354] with approval by the FDA for use in cancer treatment in 1978. Despite the significant side effects of Pt-based chemotherapeutics, a majority of cancer treatments include their use. One of many examples regarding the significant impact these compounds have had is the 10-year survival rates for testicular cancer at nearly 100% compared to 10% before their use.[355]

Toxicokinetics and Toxicodynamics

Pt-containing antineoplastic agents have some nephrotoxicity related to the concentration of Pt circulating in the blood.[356] Each antineoplastic agent demonstrates differing degrees of protein binding with *cis*-platinum 85% protein bound and carboplatin 30% protein bound. Pt distributes widely into various tissue compartments, and the various antineoplastics display divergent incorporation into red blood cells,[357] with the half-life equivalent to that of the red blood cell compartment.[358]

The antineoplastic effects of Pt-containing agents is due to the inhibition of DNA synthesis by the formation of DNA crosslinks, denaturation of DNA, and covalent binding to DNA bases.[359] DNA-protein adducts and platinated proteins also have been implicated in their antineoplastic and toxic effects.[360] Pt-compound binding to metallothionein has been suggested to play a significant role in the development of resistance to Pt-containing treatments.[361-363]

Carboplatin is excreted in the urine predominantly unchanged[357]; cisplatin excretion involves a more complex secretion and reabsorption process.[364] The majority of Pt salts are excreted within several days after exposure in both feces and urine, whereas Pt-containing compounds demonstrate biphasic excretion.[365]

Clinical Presentation and Treatment

Although it is not common to measure Pt concentrations in all patients receiving cisplatin therapy, quantification of Pt concentrations in patients with reduced renal function helps identify whether Pt is the cause of the compromised renal function. Peak serum concentrations greater than 1 μg/mL (5 μmol/L) but less than 1.5 μg/mL (7.7 μmol/L) correlate with little nephrotoxicity and good therapeutic response.[366]

Side effects of the Pt-containing antineoplastics include central and peripheral neurotoxicity, cardiotoxicity, nephrotoxicity, and severe GI complications, including nausea, vomiting, constipation, and diarrhea.[367] Sensitization to Pt after exposure was initially termed platinosis but is currently referred to as platinum salt sensitivity[368]; it is associated with watery eyes, sneezing, tightness of chest, difficulty breathing, coughing, skin lesions, and mucous membrane inflammation.[365]

Preanalytical and Analytical Aspects

Both AA-ETA and ICP-MS are used to measure Pt; however, highly sensitive methods have been published using ICP-MS for the detection of Pt in plasma ultrafiltrates and serum,[369] although at considerably lower concentrations than typical for acute exposures.

Regulatory and Occupational Exposure Aspects

Inhalation of Pt-containing vapors and particles is the main route of workplace exposures to Pt and its compounds; however, Pt also can be absorbed by oral ingestion and possibly through the skin.[370,371] Animal studies indicate that the rate of Pt absorption from the lungs depends on the water solubility of the compound with the water-soluble platinum (IV) sulfate removed from the lungs more rapidly than metallic Pt or platinum (IV) oxide.[370,372] After inhalation exposure in rats, the highest concentration of Pt was found in the lungs, trachea, kidneys, and bone. Pt is eliminated in the urine and feces.[372]

Metallic Pt is generally considered nontoxic[370]; however, sensitizing and allergic reactions can occur to the skin and respiratory tract after occupational exposures to Pt compounds, especially those containing halogens such as hexachloroplatinates, tetrachloroplatinates, and platinum halide salt complexes.[373] Hypersensitivity symptoms consists of urticaria and eczema typically in places of skin exposure; tearing and burning of the eyes; rhinitis, coughing, wheezing, tightness in the throat; and shallow breathing.[370] Pt salts are also considered to be causative agents of occupational asthma.[374] The risk for acquiring respiratory allergies after exposures to Pt is increased in smokers.[375,376]

Although it is difficult to determine a dose-effect relationship, studies of workers have shown a higher risk for developing allergies to Pt salts in those who are exposed to higher concentrations.[370] No biological threshold limits relating workplace exposure levels to internal dose and adverse health effects have been recognized for Pt and its compounds; however, biological monitoring of Pt has been suggested to evaluate individual Pt exposures in an attempt to prevent the allergic effects of Pt salts.[373] Urine samples collected after exposure or the next morning are the preferred specimen for biomonitoring exposure to Pt and its compounds and can reflect recent exposures.[377] However, even after several years past cessation of exposure, employees from a platinum refinery and catalyst production company had increased urinary Pt concentrations.[378]

Areas of Research

Ongoing areas of research include the effects of long-term Pt retention after chemotherapy.[379] Increased awareness has been raised regarding the possible contribution of residual Pt to cardiovascular disease, pulmonary dysfunction, and secondary neoplasms even decades after initial exposure.[380] Continued interest exists in attempts at harnessing the good while removing the bad aspects of Pt-based chemotherapeutics.[381] An appreciation for the role of platinated proteins in the observed toxicities is continuing to evolve.[360]

Selenium (Se)

Selenium (Se), with the atomic number 34 and relative atomic mass of 78.971, is a red or black nonmetal in period 4, group 16, with 5 naturally occurring and stable isotopes. In the 1930s Se was considered a toxic element; in the 1940s, a carcinogen; in the 1950s, it was declared an essential element; and since the 1960s and especially the 1970s, it has been viewed as an anticarcinogen. Glutathione peroxidase (in the form of selenocysteine) is part of the cellular antioxidant defense system against free radicals,[305] and Se is also involved in the metabolism of thyroid hormones[382] (eg, deiodinase enzymes and thioredoxin reductase).[383] Se homeostasis, physiologic function, and laboratory assessment of Se status are further described in Chapter 37.

Sources of Exposure

Most processed Se is used in the electronics industry; however, other uses include nutritional supplements, pigments, pesticides, rubber production, antidandruff shampoos, and fungicides.[383]

Toxicokinetics and Toxicodynamics

Se is well absorbed from the GI tract (~50%). Se exposure occurs primarily from food but can be found in drinking water, usually in the form of inorganic sodium selenate or sodium selenite. Se homeostasis is largely achieved by excretion by urine and feces. Other routes or elimination include sweat and, at very high intakes, exhalation of volatile forms of Se.[383]

Se toxicity is often discussed in the context of As toxicity because both are considered metalloids, different oxidation states dictate the severity of toxicity, and each element on opposite ends of the concentration spectrum can cause or treat cancer.[384] Se excess generates reactive oxygen species,[385] and several studies have associated Se excess with diseases such as amyotrophic lateral sclerosis,[386] diabetes,[387] chronic kidney disease,[388] and a potential but controversial role in cardiovascular disease.[389]

Urine is the primary route of excretion under most conditions. After high dose exposure, respiratory excretion as methylated species has been measured,[390] and urinary excretion continues to play an important role. Increased concentrations of Se in blood, urine, and hair have been documented after toxic exposures.[383] The interaction of Se with numerous other elements has been well studied, with both positive and negative effects observed.

Clinical Presentation and Treatment

Acute oral exposure to extremely high levels of Se may produce GI symptoms (nausea, vomiting, and diarrhea) and cardiovascular symptoms such as tachycardia. Chronic exposure to very high levels can cause dermal effects, including diseased nails and skin and hair loss, as well as neurologic problems such as unsteady gait or paralysis.[383] In 1984, 12 cases of Se toxicity were reported to the FDA and CDC because of the ingestion of Se supplements containing levels almost 200 times higher than stated on the label. The most common symptoms reported in these cases were nausea and vomiting, nail changes, hair loss, fatigue, abdominal cramps, watery diarrhea, and garlicky breath. No abnormalities of blood chemistry were seen in 67% of the victims, and renal and liver functions were normal.[391]

The EPA has determined that one specific form of Se, selenium sulfide, is a probable human carcinogen. Selenium sulfide is a very different chemical from the organic and inorganic Se compounds found in foods and in the environment.[392] In Hubei Province (China) during 1961 through 1964, almost half of the population of many villages died from chronic selenosis. The most common signs of Se poisoning were loss of hair and nails, skin lesions, tooth decay, and abnormalities of the nervous system.[393]

Preanalytical and Analytical Aspects

Urine is the predominate specimen required for the assessment of Se toxicity as the majority of Se is excreted in the urine.[383]

Regulatory and Occupational Exposure Aspects

The primary compound involved in most industrial exposures is selenium dioxide. The oxide is formed when Se is heated in air. Selenium dioxide reacts with water, including perspiration on the skin to form selenious acid, which can cause irritation. Industrial airborne Se compounds likely include elemental Se and selenium dioxide dusts and hydrogen selenide gas.[392] Adverse effects after occupational exposures to Se dusts or Se compounds mainly involve the respiratory tract; however, effects on the GI (nausea and vomiting), cardiovascular (elevated pulse rate and lowered blood pressure), and nervous (headache and malaise) systems and irritation to the eyes and skin can occur. Acute inhalation exposure to high levels of elemental Se and selenium dioxide dusts can produce irritation of the mucous membranes in the nose and throat, and cause coughing nosebleed, dyspnea, bronchial spasms bronchitis, and chemical pneumonia. The autopsy findings of a man occupationally exposed to Se for 50 years who suffered an acute myocardial infarction showed indications for generalized coronary atherosclerosis; severe passive congestion of the lungs, spleen, and liver; numerous perivascular noncaseating granulomas; and abnormally high levels of Se in the peribronchial nodes, lungs, hair, and nails.[394]

The available data relating occupational Se air concentrations, blood and urine levels, and risk for disease are limited. A worker in a photocopy machine manufacturing company exposed to a selenium alloy reported hair loss after 6 months of work that eventually deteriorated to complete body hair loss.[395] His measured blood Se concentration was 500 μg/L (6.3 μmol/L). Workers exposed to Se in a copper refinery had significantly lower Se plasma concentrations than a control group, while the urine levels were not significantly different between the two groups.[396] The investigators attributed the lower plasma Se concentrations in the exposed group to the increase in the urinary elimination of Se. Serum Se levels from 20 workers at a rubber tire repair shop averaged 148 ± 56 μg/L (1.9 ± 0.7 μmol/L) with a range of 70 to 296 μg/L (0.9 to 3.8 μmol/L), and the mean of the control group was 100 ± 18 μg/L (1.3 ± 0.2 μmol/L) with a range of 70 to 127 μg/L (0.9 to 1.5 μmol/L).[397] In this study, the shop workers showed no signs of selenosis, which is the adverse health effects associated with Se toxicity, including brittle hair, deformed nails, and loss of feeling and control in the legs and arms.[392]

Areas of Research

The association of Se with neurologic diseases such as amyotrophic lateral sclerosis remains an intriguing line of investigation.[398] The possible roles of Se in cardiovascular disease continue to be actively debated as does the possible role of Se toxicity in diabetes.[389]

Silicon (Si)

Silicon (Si), with the atomic number 14 and relative atomic mass of 28.08, is a lustrous gray metalloid in period 3, group 14, with 3 stable isotopes. Si is the second most abundant element in the earth's environment and constitutes 26% of the earth's crust. The use of Si in integrated circuits is arguably the most critical use of Si despite its widespread use in clay, silica sand, and stone for building and synthetic silicone polymers. Because of its similar valence of four with carbon, speculations of Si-based lifeforms have been extensively explored in science fiction. See also Chapter 37 for further discussion of Si metabolism and function.

Sources of Exposure

From the toxicologic viewpoint, several forms of Si are of interest, including asbestos (amorphous oxides of Si) and methylated polymers of Si (eg, silicone). Si is a necessary component to electronic applications in the form of Si wafers, in which its semiconducting properties are required. Alloys of Si are used in casts in the automobile industry.[399] Methylated polymers of Si are used in breast implants,[400] contact lenses,[401] explosives, and pyrotechnics. Injection of Si in the form of silicone has been used for body enhancement procedures because of its inert nature, durability, and thermal stability.

Toxicokinetics and Toxicodynamics

Inhalation of asbestos-containing dust leads to deposition of asbestos fibers in the pulmonary alveoli.[402,403] These fibers are needle-shaped spicules approximately 150 μm in length and up to 15 μm in diameter. When these fibers are inhaled, they deposit in the alveoli, where they are surrounded by macrophages and become coated with protein and mucopolysaccharide to form asbestos bodies. The diagnosis of asbestosis is made by interpretation of a chest radiograph by a qualified radiologist, demonstration of asbestos in sputum, and documentation of asbestos bodies in a lung biopsy sample by electron microscopy.[404] Direct analysis of lung tissue for Si is not useful because all lung tissue is infiltrated with Si, most of which is not asbestos. Thus direct analysis for Si cannot distinguish asbestosis from normal background Si.

Clinical Presentation and Treatment

Si, in the form of silicone, has been associated with toxicity after rupture of breast implants, leading to calcification, hematoma, necrosis, and capsular contracture.[405] Injection of silicone for body augmentation has been reported to cause potentially serious complications such as respiratory distress, liver dysfunction, and ultimately multiorgan failure.[406,407]

Preanalytical and Analytical Aspects

Si is rarely measured in the clinical setting. Exposure to Si as amorphous oxides or methylated polymers is most often investigated using imaging technology such as chest radiography, thin-section computed tomography, and knowledge of past history of cosmetic procedures.[128] If samples are collected for testing, it is imperative that glass containers are not used throughout the entire collection and storage processes.

Regulatory and Occupational Exposure Aspects

Inhalable silica particles are created from workers chipping, cutting, drilling, grinding, or processing items containing silica in mining and nonmining industries and in agricultural operations.[408,409] Inhaled particles are characterized by their size and aerodynamic properties.[202] Most particles greater than 5 μm are deposited in the tracheobronchial airways. Respirable particles have an aerodynamic diameter of less than 3 to 4 μm and are capable of penetrating into the alveolar spaces of the lungs. Inhaled silica particles are primarily cleared from the respiratory system through mucociliary action, lymphatic drainage, and phagocyte activity.[410] Given that crystalline silica is only slightly soluble in bodily fluids, it is not readily absorbed or distributed.[202] It can accumulate in lung tissue and lymph nodes.[411] Since crystalline silica is cytotoxic to macrophages, it can interfere with macrophage-medicated clearance from the lungs, resulting in minimal clearance of these particles at high concentrations. Amorphous silica is typically cleared from the lungs more rapidly than crystalline silica, which likely may be due to its higher solubility.[410,412] Most silica is not absorbed and is eliminated nonmetabolized in the feces.[410]

The disease most associated with respirable crystalline silica exposure is silicosis.[410] Acute silicosis may develop a short time after exposure to high concentrations of respirable crystalline silica. Chronic silicosis may result after years of exposure to relatively low concentrations of respirable crystalline silica. Potential sequelae of silicosis may be severe mycobacterial or fungal infections, which can result in pulmonary tuberculosis, and the development of cor pulmonale. Chronic obstructive pulmonary disease, including bronchitis and emphysema, is also associated with occupational exposures to respirable crystalline silica. Autoimmune, autoimmune-related, and renal diseases are other disorders observed in workers exposed to silica or with silicosis. Although the pathogenesis of these diseases is not readily apparent, the nephropathies seen after silica exposures may be through direct nephrotoxicity as well as the induction of autoimmune disease.[413] Amorphous silica is generally considered less toxic than crystalline silica, probably because it is more readily cleared from the lungs.[410,412]

Occupational exposures to respirable silica have been associated with an increased risk for developing lung cancer in workers.[408] The IARC classifies crystalline silica and cristobalite dust as carcinogenic to humans (group 1), whereas the carcinogenicity in humans of amorphous silica is not classifiable (group 3).[412] Crystalline silica is categorized as a human carcinogen (category 1) by the DFG in Germany and as a suspected human carcinogen (A2) by the ACGIH.[79,414]

Although the relationship between exposure to respirable silica dust and silicosis is established,[408] there is no biomarker available to assess the risk for developing silicosis. The cellular response to silica leading to fibrosis and silicosis is complicated and has not been fully elucidated. Factors such as particle size, worker susceptibility, crystalline surface, percentage of silica in total dust, and contributions of different polymorphs may affect the risk for disease development.[410] A review of studies investigating blood, serum, sputum, bronchoalveolar lavage samples, and gene patterns of exposed workers or those with silicosis has been inconclusive in determining a biomarker.[408]

Areas of Research

Si-containing microspheres and nanospheres have shown promise in the field of theranostics,[415] with continued investigation into potential toxicities of the nanoparticles.[416] Alternatives to Si-based polymers have been investigated for use in cosmetic procedures.[405] Porous Si microparticles are being developed for use in wound healing applications[417] and drug delivery devices.[418]

Silver (Ag)

Silver (Ag), with the atomic number 47 and relative atomic mass of 107.8682, is a soft, white, lustrous metal in period 5, group 11, with 2 naturally occurring and stable isotopes. Ag is the most electrically conductive metal on earth but is less commonly used for this purpose because of its relatively higher cost compared to that of copper. Ag has been used in coins, jewelry, photography, and even as an antibiotic.

Sources of Exposure

Ag is primarily used in electrical applications such as conductors, switches and contacts; soldering, brazing, or plating; and nonindustrial applications such mirrors, batteries, coins, jewelry, and utensils.[419] Ag may be used as a disinfectant[420] or woven into fibers to reduce odors and bacterial growth.[421] Ag is found in low concentrations in marine organisms[422] and is released from Ag utensils and dental amalgams.[423]

Toxicokinetics and Toxicodynamics

Soluble Ag compounds are more readily absorbed in comparison to metallic or insoluble Ag, with nearly 10% absorbed and 2 to 4% retained in tissues.[419] Ag deposits in many organs, including the subepithelium of the skin and mucous membranes, producing a syndrome called argyria (graying of the skin). Argyria is associated with growth retardation, hemopoiesis, cardiac enlargement, degeneration of the liver, and destruction of renal tubules. Neurologic effects are uncommon; however, case reports do exist describing myoclonic seizures as a result of Ag toxicity.[424] Ag is not known to be carcinogenic or toxic to the immune, cardiovascular, nervous, or reproductive systems.[425,426]

The deposition of Ag in tissues has been proposed to be a result of complex formation with RNA, DNA, protein sulfhydryl, amino, carboxyl, phosphate, and imidazole groups with light triggering the photoreduction to metallic Ag and eventual oxidization to insoluble silver sulfide.[419] Chelation therapy is ineffective in removing Ag as is dermabrasion.[427]

Ag is primarily eliminated in feces but can be measured in urine and blood. Blood is the preferred specimen type for occupational assessment and determination of toxic exposure.[428]

Clinical Presentation and Treatment

Acute symptoms of Ag toxicity include decreased blood pressure, diarrhea, stomach irritation, and decreased respiration.[419] Chronic exposure results in irreversible pigmentation of the tissue near the site of exposure or deposition and discoloration systemically into the skin, nails, mucous membranes, and internal organs if ingested. The differential diagnosis for Ag intoxication leading to argyria includes methemoglobinemia, polycythemia, Addison's disease, Wilson's disease, carcinoid syndrome, hemochromatosis, and non–Ag containing ingestions of other metals.[429]

Clinical interest in Ag analysis is limited to two applications: monitoring burn patients treated with Ag sulfadiazine and monitoring patients treated with Ag-containing nasal decongestants. The assessment of Ag in skin may be of interest to confirm past exposure if an adequate exposure history is unavailable. Because relatively little ingested Ag is excreted in the urine, assessment of Ag in this specimen type is of little clinical utility.

Preanalytical and Analytical Aspects

The typical concentration of serum Ag is less than 2 ng/mL (18.5 nmol/L). Ag concentrations observed in serum of unaffected patients during treatment range up to 300 ng/mL (2781 nmol/L), and their urine output has been found to be as high as 550 μg/day (5 μmol/d).[430]

Regulatory and Occupational Exposure Aspects

The primary occupational exposures to Ag occur by inhalation of dusts and fumes and by contact with the skin.[419,431] The absorption of Ag depends on the solubility of the Ag compound with soluble compounds more readily absorbed than metallic Ag or insoluble Ag compounds. Mucociliary action clears some of the inhaled Ag particles from the lungs. Absorbed Ag is distributed and deposited throughout the body. Once in the body, Ag can be reduced to metallic Ag and then oxidized to silver sulfide or silver selenide, resulting in a blue-gray pigment. The elimination of Ag is mainly through the feces, with minimal quantities excreted in the urine. Several Ag compounds seem to be absorbed through intact skin, although the amount absorbed is considered low.[431]

Irritation of the respiratory tract, skin, and eyes can result from exposure to Ag or Ag compounds by the release of Ag ions from metallic Ag or strong anions from some inorganic Ag compounds such as silver nitrate in the presence of moisture.[432] Exposures to metallic Ag and many Ag compounds can increase the risk for developing contact allergy and delayed hypersensitivity reactions.

Most occupational exposures are reported from soluble Ag compounds.[419] Studies have shown higher health risks associated with workers exposed to soluble Ag compounds such as silver nitrate compared to metallic Ag or sparingly soluble compounds, including silver halide and silver sulfate.[419,432] Chronic inhalation of soluble Ag compounds may cause a permanent pigmentation of the skin (argyria) and/or eyes (argyrosis), resulting in a bluish-gray or ash-gray discoloration. Exposure to soluble Ag compounds also may lead to irritation of the respiratory and GI tracts, skin, and eyes; damage to the liver and kidneys; and changes in blood cells. Staining of alveoli and bronchial tissue also may occur after inhalation of Ag compounds.[419] Bronchitis, emphysema, and reduced pulmonary volume have been reported in silver workers exposed to metallic Ag and other metals.[419,433,434] Animal studies involving inhalation of metallic Ag nanoparticles demonstrated a decrease in lung function and increased inflammatory changes and small granulomatous lesions in the lungs.[435] A study of workers manufacturing silver nanomaterials showed no significant findings in their health status.[436]

Several approaches to biological monitoring of silver in the workplace have been considered. Elevated urinary Ag concentrations were observed after occupational exposures[437,438]; however, the analysis of urine samples may be useful only after exposure to high levels of Ag because of urinary elimination is much lower than by the biliary route.[428] The determination of Ag fecal concentrations has been proposed as a measure of body burden,[439] but has been discounted because of the impracticality of sample collection.[428] The use of whole-blood samples has been suggested for biomonitoring Ag exposures in the workplace,[428] and increased Ag concentrations in whole-blood measurement have been observed in workers exposed to Ag.[437,440] However, there are insufficient data available to propose any biological threshold limits.[92] Whole-blood Ag levels in 98 workers from various occupational groups working with Ag, including bullion and jewelry production, cutlery and chemical manufacture, and Ag reclamation, were found to range from 0.1 to 23 μg/L (0.9 to 213 nmol/L) in the exposed group compared to between less than 0.1 and 0.2 μg/L (<0.9 and 1.9 nmol/L) in the reference population.[428]

Areas of Research

Ag-containing compounds continue to be of interest for antimicrobial applications, targeted delivery systems after surgery,[441] as well as numerous other medicinal applications.[442,443] Evidence for the toxic effects of Ag-containing compounds on the brain, cardiovascular system, and reproductive system remains controversial.[426]

Thallium (Tl)

Thallium (Tl), with the atomic number 81 and relative atomic mass of 204.385, is a soft gray metal in period 6, group 13, with 2 naturally occurring stable isotopes. Tl is often referred to as the "poisoner's poison" because it is nearly tasteless and highly toxic in low doses. Isotopes of Tl are used in diagnostic imaging[454] and were once used medicinally to treat ringworm.[445]

Sources of Exposure

Tl is a by-product of zinc and lead smelting and cadmium production. Interest in Tl derives primarily from its former use as a rodenticide, with accidental exposure the most likely reason for toxicity. Acute and often fatal poisoning has been reported after criminal and suicide attempts.[446,447] Additionally, environmental concerns are growing because Tl is a waste product of coal combustion and the manufacturing of cement. Tl is used in photoelectric cells, lamps, semiconductors, and scintillation counters.[448]

Toxicokinetics and Toxicodynamics

Tl is rapidly absorbed by ingestion, inhalation, and skin contact. It is considered to be as toxic as lead and mercury and has similar sites of action. Detectable concentrations of Tl have been reported as quickly as 1 hour after ingestion.[449] The mechanism of Tl toxicity consists of (1) competition with potassium at cell receptors to affect ion pumps, (2) inhibition of DNA synthesis, (3) binding to sulfhydryl groups on proteins in neural axons, and (4) concentration in renal tubular cells to cause necrosis.

Fecal elimination is the major route of excretion, although measured decrease in urine concentration coincides with the reduction in toxic symptoms and may persist for several months after exposure.[448]

Tl is cytotoxic and highly poisonous in acute oral doses. Tl intoxication has been described in four phases: immediate, intermediate, late, and residual.[450,451] In the immediate phase, GI symptoms such as nausea, vomiting, and abdominal pain can be observed. After a latency period of 3 to 7 days, the target organ is the nervous system. Injury to the peripheral nervous system results in severe neuralgic pain, particularly in the lower limbs. Adverse effects of the central nervous system, including encephalopathy and disturbances of the cranial nerves with ptosis, ophthalmoplegia, or facial paralysis, are also observed in severe poisoning. The late phase, occurring at 2 to 4 weeks, is characterized by areflexia and loss of sensation in the lower extremities and possibly the arms and alopecia. The recovery from Tl poisoning may require several months, and it may not be complete, leaving residual neurotoxic effects. Symptoms of chronic Tl toxicity may be similar to those described for acute poisoning; however, they may be nonspecific and not suspected until the appearance of alopecia.[450] The initial symptoms of chronic exposures may be excitation and insomnia, with subsequent pains in the joints, weakness, and polyneuritis occurring after weeks and months of exposure.

Clinical Presentation and Treatment

The clinical presentation of Tl toxicity varies based on dose, age, and acute or chronic exposure. Patients exposed to high doses of Tl (>1 g) demonstrate alopecia (hair loss), peripheral neuropathy, seizures, and renal failure. Peripheral neuropathy of the feet and less commonly the hands occurs within 1 week after exposure, and hair loss begins and continues for several weeks.[447] GI symptoms, including pain, diarrhea, and constipation have been reported in acute ingestion[452] in addition to myalgias, pleuritic chest pain, insomnia, optic neuritis, hypertension, cardiac abnormalities, Mees' lines, and liver injury.[447]

Preanalytical and Analytical Aspects

Typical serum concentrations are less than 10 ng/mL (49 nmol/L), and daily urine excretion is less than 10 μg/d (49 nmol/d). Exposed patients have been observed to have serum concentrations as high as 50 μg/mL (245 nmol/L), with urine output in excess of 500 μg/d (2446 nmol/d).[447] Tl is routinely measured by ICP-MS in blood and urine.

Regulatory and Occupational Exposure Aspects

One hundred twenty-eight male workers (ages 16 to 62 years) from three cement factories that were exposed to Tl for an average duration of 19.5 years (range, 1 to 42 years) had a median Tl concentration in spot urine samples of 0.8 μg/g creatinine (3.9 nmol/g) with a range of less than 0.3 to 6.3 μg/g creatinine (<1.5 to 31 nmol/L) compared to the range of Tl values measured in a reference group of less than 0.3 to 1.1 μg/g creatinine (<1.5 to 5.4 nmol/L).[453] In this investigation, none of the workers exhibited clinical symptoms associated with Tl toxicity. Evaluation of kidney function in 684 current and former lead workers exposed to multiple elements were found to have a median urinary Tl concentration of 0.39 μg/g creatinine (1.9 nmol/L) with a range of 0.07 to 1.60 μg/g creatinine (0.3 to 7.8 nmol/L).[454] In this study, the urine Tl levels were associated with serum creatinine and cystatin-C–based glomerular filtration measures in a direction opposite of that expected for renal toxicity. The authors also observed that the effects on the kidneys were attenuated because of the coexposure with the other metals and suggested that the risk assessments associated with low-level urine concentrations may be more complicated than originally thought, especially with multielement exposures.

Urine is the suggested specimen for biological monitoring of Tl.[22,451] Although there is insufficient information available correlating occupational exposure levels and urinary Tl concentrations to establish a threshold value, the biological monitoring of Tl in urine can assist in assessing the effectiveness of workplace control measures, especially because the ACGIH gives Tl and Tl compounds a "skin" notation designating the potential for a significant contribution to the overall exposure by the cutaneous route.[79] For exposures to Tl and inorganic Tl compounds, the FIOH has no established biomonitoring action limit but recommends testing for Tl in a postshift urine specimen.[46] The reference interval in the nonexposed Finnish population is 1 μg/L (5 nmol/L) in urine corrected to a relative density of 1.021.

Areas of Research

The use of Tl isotopes in imaging studies of the cardiovascular system continues to be reported.[444] Environmental contamination of Tl is a major focus, as is the continued study of the mechanisms of its toxicity.

Titanium (Ti)

Titanium (Ti), with the atomic number 22 and relative atomic mass of 47.867, is a lustrous silvery metal in period 4, group 4, with 5 naturally occurring and stable isotopes. Ti is the ninth most abundant element in the earth's crust by mass, and its light weight and high strength are useful in alloys for diverse applications. Military applications of Ti have been known for decades. Titanium dioxide is a common ingredient found in sunscreen formulations, and Ti use in recreational goods across numerous sports is widespread.

Sources of Exposure

Average daily oral intake through food consumption is 0.1 to 1 mg/d, which accounts for more than 99% of exposure. Ti-containing alloys are used in artificial joints, prosthetic devices, and implants. Titanium dioxide allows osseointegration between an artificial medical implant and bone providing increased strength to the prosthetic joint. Despite their wide use, exposure to these materials has not been linked to toxicity or sensitivity.[455] However, as implant wear occurs, a significant increase in detectable serum Ti becomes evident.[456]

Toxicokinetics and Toxicodynamics

In part because of the propensity to form titanium oxide, the element is considered nontoxic. GI absorption of Ti is low (~3%), and most ingested Ti is rapidly excreted in the urine and stool. Once absorbed, transferrin has been implicated in the transport of Ti throughout the body.[457] The total body burden of Ti is usually in the range of 9 to 15 mg, a significant portion of which is contained in the lung. Ti dust entering the respiratory tract is nonirritating and is almost completely nonfibrogenic in humans.[458] Suppression of osteoblast function has been observed in vitro with the in vivo significance unclear.[459]

Excretion of absorbed Ti is predominantly fecal, although measurable increases in urinary output have been reported after documented exposures.[460]

Clinical Presentation and Treatment

Increased serum Ti has been documented in patients with cementless Ti-alloy knee replacements and has been proposed as a marker of component wear.[461] Additionally, elevated concentrations of serum Ti were reported 10 years after MoM hip arthroplasty compared to baseline concentrations.[462] However, routine clinical assessment of Ti in the context of metal prosthetic device failure is not currently recommended.

Preanalytical and Analytical Aspects

Although Ti concentrations are not a measure of toxicity, they are useful in determining whether implant breakdown is occurring.[463] Serum Ti less than 1.0 ng/mL (21 nmol/L) suggests that a prosthetic device is in good condition. Serum concentrations greater than 3 ng/mL (63 nmol/L) in a patient with a Ti-based implant suggest prosthesis wear. An increased serum Ti concentration in the absence of corroborating clinical information does not independently predict prosthesis wear or failure. Ti is measured by ICP-MS and inductively coupled plasma–optical emission spectrometry. Of interest, measurement of Ti by ICP-MS is complicated by the presence of numerous polyatomic species, high susceptibility to oxide formation, and formation of interfering species in conventional reaction cells. Triple quadrupole ICP-MS applications have been proposed to provide a suitable alternative for Ti assessment.

Regulatory and Occupational Exposure Aspects

Workplace Ti exposures can result from inhalation of fumes, vapors, dusts, and particles and from contact with the skin.[464] A review of the literature revealed no studies pertaining to the absorption of titanium tetrachloride[464]; however, particles detected in an animal study after exposure to titanium tetrachloride aerosol were presumed to be titanium dioxide. Metallic titanium and titanium dioxide are insoluble forms of Ti.[465] Deposited titanium dioxide particles in the lungs are removed from the respiratory tract by mucociliary clearance and then swallowed.[466] The particles reaching the alveoli are eliminated by macrophage-mediated clearance and then transferred to the lymph nodes. The absorption of titanium dioxide from the GI system depends on particle size, with the smaller particles absorbed more rapidly. Studies on the dermal absorption of titanium dioxide particles demonstrate no penetration of particles through the skin.[466] Soluble forms of inorganic Ti compounds are absorbed and metabolized in the body.[465]

Titanium tetrachloride, used in the production of titanium dioxide among other things, can cause serious injuries to the respiratory tract, skin, and eyes. Titanium tetrachloride hydrolyzes on contact with water or moisture in the air, forming hydrochloric acid, titanium oxychloride, and heat that produce pulmonary injuries ranging from mild irritation to chemical bronchitis or pneumonia.[464] The reaction of titanium tetrachloride with the moisture of the skin (as perspiration) and eyes can cause severe burns.[467,468] Although there are case reports of pulmonary injuries from occupational exposures to titanium tetrachloride,[469] a study of 969 workers in titanium oxide production facilities showed no correlation between titanium tetrachloride exposures and an increased risk for cancer or other pulmonary diseases.[470] A study of 209 employees in a metal production plant exposed to titanium tetrachloride, titanium oxychloride, and titanium dioxide, found a reduction in lung function and the presence of pleural disease in subjects associated with their duration of work in Ti manufacturing.[471] However, the conclusions of this study were difficult to interpret because of limited information regarding past asbestos exposures in the plant. Excluding ultrafine particles, there are no indications of any adverse health effects after occupational exposures to titanium dioxide.[472,473] Although there is no evidence for an increased risk for lung cancer after long-term exposure,[472,473] the carcinogenicity of titanium dioxide remains in question.[466]

Areas of Research

Continued focus on failed and even adequately performing MoM prosthetic devices has prompted investigation into numerous areas, including metal toxicity during pregnancy.[474] Increased use of Ti-containing nanoparticles has sparked interest in the potential for genotoxicity resulting from reactive oxygen species.[475]

Uranium (U)

Uranium (U), with the atomic number 92 and relative atomic mass of 238.0289, is a silvery-white metal in period 7 of the actinide series, with 3 naturally occurring and stable isotopes. Widely known for its use in nuclear energy and weapons after enrichment, U ushered in the beginning of our understanding of radioactivity and gave us the SI unit for radioactivity, the becquerel.

Sources of Exposure

U is used for the commercial nuclear power industry and for military purposes such as fuel for naval ships and weapons manufacture.[476,477] It is also used in the chemical industry. Depleted U (a by-product of ^{235}U enrichment process) is a highly dense material and is used to produce military munitions and armaments, guidance equipment, aircraft stabilizers, and protective materials in radiation use. Occupational exposures occur in mining and milling U, converting and enriching processes, fabricating fuel, and manufacturing weapons.[476] The hazards in U mining not only include alpha-particle radiation from the U ore but also exposure to radon and its alpha-emitting daughters RaA and RaC.[477] Although some beta and gamma exposures to RaB, RaC, and Ra can occur, they are considered relatively insignificant. In the production of U metal, exposures occur from dusts of intermediates containing uranium trioxide and uranium tetrafluoride, and from gaseous uranium hexafluoride, which can form uranyl fluoride and hydrofluoric acid as a result of its reaction with moisture in the air.[477] Radiation hazards also exist from exposures to enriched uranium ^{235}U.

Toxicokinetics and Toxicodynamics

Only a small fraction of inhaled U is absorbed.[476] Based on urinary excretion of U, absorption from inhaled dust particles ranges from 0.76% to 5%. The amount absorbed depends on the solubility of the U compound, with soluble forms including uranium hexafluoride, uranyl fluoride, uranium tetrachloride, and uranyl nitrate hexahydrate and the less soluble forms, uranium tetrafluoride and uranium trioxide, while sparingly soluble forms such as uranium dioxide and triuranium octaoxide likely remain in lung tissue for a relatively long period. Small amounts of uranyl nitrate have been shown to be absorbed through intact skin with absorption efficiencies increased if the skin is damaged.[478] Once in the circulating blood, U is mostly distributed to the bone, liver, and kidney.[476] Elimination of absorbed U is mainly through the kidneys and then released in the urine.

Clinical Presentation and Treatment

The adverse health effects of exposure to natural and depleted U are primarily due to chemical toxicity; however, the retention of sparingly soluble compounds in the lungs also may involve a radiologic component.[286] Toxicities after exposures to more radioactive U isotopes, such as ^{232}U and ^{233}U, and combined ^{234}U and ^{235}U in enriched uranium are a result of both chemical and radiologic effects, which may be additive or potentiated in some instances. The critical organs of toxicity for U appear to be mainly the lungs, with exposure to sparingly soluble U compounds and the kidneys with the more soluble U compounds.[479]

Preanalytical and Analytical Aspects

Assessment of U typically involves the determination of the ratio between ^{238}U and ^{235}U. The concentrations of U isotopes can be measured by ICP-MS, thermal ionization MS, or secondary ion MS.[480] Other methods have employed isotope ratios measured by a single-detector magnetic sector-field ICP-MS instrument fitted with an ultrasonic nebulizer providing a very high level of accuracy.[481]

Regulatory and Occupational Exposure Aspects

The carcinogenic effects of U from occupational exposures is difficult to assess because of coexposures with radon, enriched uranium, plutonium, asbestos, and other chemical toxicants in the workplace.[477] However, U and its hardly soluble inorganic compounds are assigned to category 2 by the DFG as substances that are considered carcinogenic in humans based on long-term animal studies and/or epidemiologic studies.[25] Soluble U compounds are designated category 3B carcinogens in which in vitro or animal studies have shown evidence of carcinogenic effects. The ACGIH categorized both soluble and insoluble natural U compounds as A1, confirmed human carcinogens.[79]

The correlation between airborne U concentrations in the workplace and urinary U levels in exposed workers is weak. Only a minimal relationship was demonstrated between lung dose estimates from air monitoring and doses based on urine analysis.[482] No correlation is observed between exposure concentrations and urinary U levels in workers exposed to poorly soluble U compounds.[483] However, in an exposure to the soluble U compound uranium hexafluoride, an association was found in workers exposed to air concentrations of 10 to 500 μg/m^3 with urine concentrations ranging from 25 to 1000 μg/L (0.1 to 4.2 μmol/L) at the end of the workweek.[483] Recent exposures to soluble U compounds can be evaluated by measuring U in urine,[92] but the interpretation of the U results requires knowledge of the preexposure U levels and its dependence on nonoccupational exposures.[483-485] Geographic differences are found in the environmental background of U, resulting in regional variation in natural exposures to U, including dietary intake. Also, large individual daily fluctuations are seen in urinary U elimination levels. Therefore reliable evidence of occupational exposure to U can be determined if the average preexposure U concentration is measured, ideally using 24-hour urine samples.[483] It has been proposed that best practice is to test exposures by using the ratio of ^{234}U to ^{238}U and/or total U activity in occupational settings in which the enrichment of the likely exposure is known.[485]

The ACGIH recommends a BEI for U of 200 μg/L (0.8 μmol/L) in an end-of-shift urine sample.[79] This BEI should be used after at least several months of occupational exposure. Even though no BAR reference values are established, the German DFG suggests testing urine samples collected at a noncritical time for exposures to U and its sparingly soluble inorganic compounds and to soluble U compounds and using urine values between 25 and 60 ng/L (0.1 and 0.3 nmol/L) as guideline ranges for background exposures, provided no representative samples are available.[25,483] A skin notation is assigned by the DFG for U and its soluble and hardly soluble inorganic compounds[25] designating a warning about percutaneous absorption. For these compounds, air monitoring alone is inadequate to prevent adverse health effects; therefore, biological monitoring is also recommended to assess workplace exposures. Although no biomonitoring action limit has been established by the FIOH,[46] the analysis for U in a postshift urine specimen collected at the end of the workweek is recommended for the biological monitoring of exposure to U and U compounds. The urine U reference limit for the nonexposed Finnish population is 0.03 μg/g creatinine (0.13 nmol/g).

Areas of Research

A significant amount of research is ongoing regarding U in the potential impact on the environment because of its past and increasing uses both in energy production and military applications. The mechanism of U toxicity is still under investigation, including its effects on the kidneys,[486] exacerbation of traumatic brain injury,[487] and a considerable amount of literature using several model organisms.

Vanadium (V)

Vanadium (V), with the atomic number 23 and relative atomic mass of 50.9415, is a silvery gray, ductile, and malleable metal in period 4, group 5, with 1 naturally occurring and stable isotope. The role of V in humans is poorly defined but is known to be essential for certain bacteria and microorganisms. The controversial role of V in human biology extends from a proposed mechanism for increased insulin sensitivity to its use as a bodybuilding supplement. For more information on V see Chapter 37.

Sources of Exposure

V is recovered from minerals or is derived as a by-product of iron, titanium, and uranium refining. V compounds are used in dyes, photography, and ceramics and in the production of special glasses. V is also a component of many fiber mesh prosthetic devices. Approximately 85% of V is used in the production of alloys, specifically in aerospace applications.[488]

The main source of V intake for the general population is food, with an estimated daily intake of 20 μg, of which most is not absorbed but excreted in the feces. Concentrations of V are highest in whole grains, seafood, meats, parsley, dry mushrooms, and oysters.[488]

V has been recognized as an occupational hazard for many years. Elevated atmospheric V concentration can result from burning fossil fuels with a high V content. Inhalation and ingestion are the primary exposure routes.

Toxicokinetics and Toxicodynamics

Inhalation is the most effective route of absorption because less than 2% of ingested V is absorbed in the GI tract. V exists in numerous oxidation states and can readily form polymers.[489] Absorbed vanadate is transported by transferrin that is metabolized to vanadyl and in turn is transported by albumin. Transport across cell membranes has been proposed to be mediated by phosphate-transport mechanisms with bone widely demonstrated to be a site of V accumulation.[490] The toxicity of V has historically focused on its ability to inhibit the Na^+/K^+-ATPase enzyme.[491] Intracellularly, V binds to numerous entities, including proteins, amino acids, nucleic acids, phosphates, glutathione, citrate, oxalate, lactate, and ascorbate.[489] The clearance half-life is not well documented, but it appears to be on the order of several days.

Clinical Presentation and Treatment

V exposure can result in a metallic taste and so-called green tongue. Sensitization has been known to result in asthma or eczema. V compounds used controversially in the treatment for type 1 and type 2 diabetes have caused GI distress, weight loss, and toxicity of the liver and kidney.[492] Individuals chronically exposed to V have shown neurobehavioral complications in visuospatial abilities and attention.[493,494] A recent publication reported severe metallosis as a result of V toxicity after ceramic-on-ceramic prosthetic failure.[495] A case report of fatal V exposure in the form of ammonium vanadate reported abdominal pain, nausea, vomiting, diarrheas, hypoglycemia, and acute renal failure within 12 hours after ingestion. At autopsy, the V blood concentration was determined to be 6.22 mg/L (0.12 mmol/L) or approximately 6000 times higher than unexposed individuals.[496]

Preanalytical and Analytical Aspects

Because the kidney is primarily responsible for V elimination, increased serum concentrations are observed in dialysis patients and those with compromised renal function. Serum V values less than 1.0 ng/mL (20 nmol/L) are typical; values greater than 5.0 ng/mL (10 nmol/L) indicate probable exposure. Elevated serum V concentrations have been observed in patients with joint replacement; concentrations are likely to be increased above the reference interval in patients with metallic joint prosthesis.[497] A modest increase (1 to 2 ng/mL or 20 to 39 nmol/L) in serum V concentration is likely to be associated with a prosthetic device in good condition. Serum concentrations greater than 5 ng/mL (10 nmol/L) in a patient with a V-based implant suggests significant prosthesis wear. Increased serum trace element concentrations in the absence of corroborating clinical information do not independently predict prosthesis wear. Measurement of V is often done by graphite furnace atomic absorption or ICP-MS using reactive cell technology or collision cell with kinetic energy discrimination because of the high abundance of polyatomic interferences.

Regulatory and Occupational Exposure Aspects

Occupational exposures to V, especially vanadium pentoxide, generally occur in the workplace through inhalation of dust and aerosols.[498] These exposures can cause irritation to the respiratory tract, leading to cough, wheezing, chest pain, rhinitis, and sore throat. A green discoloration of the tongue is another manifestation associated with vanadium pentoxide exposure.[499] These clinical effects are generally reversible after the cessation of exposures. Inhalation of vanadium pentoxide has been observed to initiate bronchial hyperreactivity and asthma in the workplace.[499,500] Of 40 workers, 12 were found to have bronchial hyperreactivity as a result of exposure to vanadium pentoxide, with no significant changes observed in their baseline lung function.[500] This hyperreactivity was found to persist for up to 23 months after exposure ended. Vanadium dust exposures also can result in eye irritation, conjunctivitis, and increases in skin rashes.[498]

In a study on the genetic stability in 52 production workers it was observed that vanadium pentoxide inhalation causes oxidation of DNA bases, affects DNA repair, and increases formation of micronuclei, nucleoplasmic bridges, and nuclear buds, suggesting an increased risk for cancer and other diseases related to DNA stability in exposed workers.[501] The carcinogenicity of vanadium pentoxide investigated in a 2-year inhalation study showed evidence for an increased incidence of alveolar and bronchiolar neoplasms in both male and female mice, and although there were also increases in male rats, the findings of carcinogenic activity in female rats were equivocal.[317] The IARC classifies vanadium pentoxide as possibly carcinogenic to humans (group 2B).

Urine samples are more suitable than blood for biological monitoring of V in the workplace.[22] Since the German DFG assigned V and its inorganic compounds to category 2 carcinogens, EKA exposure equivalents are derived by correlating air concentrations of 0.025, 0.050, and 0.100 mg/m^3 with 35, 70, and 140 μg/g creatinine (0.7, 1.4, 2.7 μmol/g), respectively, in urine samples collected at the end of exposure or end of the workweek.[207] The biomonitoring action limit from the FIOH for V and V compounds is 30 μg/L (600 nmol/L) in a postshift urine specimen collected at the end of the workweek or exposure period and corrected to a relative density of 1.021.[46] For pregnant women, the workplace urine V concentration must not exceed the reference interval in the nonexposed Finnish population of 0.26 μg/L (7 nmol/L). Normal urinary V concentrations are considered to be less than 1 μg/g creatinine (0.02 μmol/g)[502] or approximately 0.51 μg/L (10 nmol/L) or less.[503]

Areas of Research

A complete understanding of the toxicity of V has remained elusive, second only to its confounding roles in normal human biology. Continued interest in V has led to its potential implication in cytokine-mediated inflammation, cytotoxic effects on neuronal and glial cells, and proposed genotoxicity.[504] V complexes are of interest for their potential therapeutic roles in several diseases, including a continued association with glucose regulation.[505]

SELECTED REFERENCES

For a full list of references for this chapter, please refer to ExpertConsult.com.

2. Pulido MD, Parrish AR. Metal-induced apoptosis: mechanisms. *Mutat Res* 2003;**533**:227–41.
3. Kazantzis G. Diagnosis and treatment of metal poisoning: general aspects. In: Nordberg GF, Fowler BA, Nordberg M, et al., editors. *Handbook on the toxicology of metals, Vol.* 3rd ed. San Diego, CA: Elsevier; 2007. p. 303–18.
5. Sears ME. Chelation: Harnessing and enhancing heavy metal detoxification: a review. *ScientificWorldJournal* 2013;**219840**.
6. Forrer R, Gautschi K, Lutz H. Simultaneous measurement of the trace elements Al, As, B, Be, Cd, Co, Cu, Fe, Li, Mn, Mo, Ni, Rb, Se, Sr, and Zn in human serum and their reference ranges by ICP-MS. *Biol Trace Elem Res* 2001;**80**:77–93.
7. Michalke B. Element speciation definitions, analytical methodology, and some examples. *Ecotoxicol Environ Saf* 2003;**56**:122–39.
16. Moyer TP, Mussmann GV, Nixon DE. Blood-collection device for trace and ultra-trace metal specimens evaluated. *Clin Chem* 1991;**37**:709–14.
31. Gebel T. Arsenic and antimony: comparative approach on mechanistic toxicology. *Chem Biol Interact* 1997;**107**:131–44.
37. Bornhorst JA, Hunt JW, Urry FM, et al. Comparison of sample preservation methods for clinical trace element analysis by inductively coupled plasma mass spectrometry. *Am J Clin Pathol* 2005;**123**:578–83.
38. Haglock-Adler CJ, Strathmann FG. Simplified sample preparation in the simultaneous measurement of whole blood antimony, bismuth, manganese, and zinc by inductively coupled plasma mass spectrometry. *Clin Biochem* 2015;**48**:135–9.
51. Heinrich-Ramm R, Mindt-Prufert S, Szadkowski D. Arsenic species excretion after controlled seafood consumption. *J Chromatogr B Analyt Technol Biomed Life Sci* 2002;**778**: 263–73.
54. Vahter M. What are the chemical forms of arsenic in urine, and what can they tell us about exposure? *Clin Chem* 1994;**40**:679–80.
186. Wells WH, Wells VL. The lanthanides: rare earth elements. In: Bingham E, Cohrssen B, Patty FA, editors. *Patty's toxicology*. 6th ed. Hoboken, N.J: John Wiley & Sons; 2012. p. 817–40.
191. Siddique A, Kowdley KV. The iron overload syndromes [Review]. *Aliment Pharmacol Ther* 2012;**35**:876–93.
197. Moyer TP, Highsmith WE, Smyrk TC, et al. Hereditary hemochromatosis: laboratory evaluation. *Clin Chim Acta* 2011;**412**:1485–92.
220. Rogan WJ, Ware JH. Exposure to lead in children: how low is low enough? *N Engl J Med* 2003;**348**:1515–16.
314. Sarmiento-Gonzalez A, Marchante-Gayon JM, Tejerina-Lobo JM, et al. High-resolution ICP-MS determination of Ti, V, Cr, Co, Ni, and Mo in human blood and urine of patients implanted with a hip or knee prosthesis. *Anal Bioanal Chem* 2008;**391**:2583–9.
321. Newton AW, Ranganath L, Armstrong C, et al. Differential distribution of cobalt, chromium, and nickel between whole blood, plasma and urine in patients after metal-on-metal (MoM) hip arthroplasty. *J Orthop Res* 2012;**30**:1640–6.
380. Brouwers EE, Huitema AD, Beijnen JH, et al. Long-term platinum retention after treatment with cisplatin and oxaliplatin. *BMC Clin Pharmacol* 2008;**8**:7.
448. Ibrahim D, Froberg B, Wolf A, et al. Heavy metal poisoning: clinical presentations and pathophysiology. *Clin Lab Med* 2006;**26**:67–97, viii.
478. McDiarmid MA, Gaitens JM, Squibb KS. Uranium and thorium. In: Bingham E, Cohrssen B, Patty FA, editors. *Patty's toxicology*. 6th ed. Hoboken, N.J: John Wiley & Sons; 2012. p. 769–816.

43

Body Fluids

Darci R. Block and Christopher M. Florkowski

ABSTRACT

Background

Body fluids are collected and analyzed either to gain insight into the processes that contribute to the accumulation of that fluid within a body compartment or to provide diagnostic information to investigate pathophysiologic processes.

Content

In the preanalytical phase, the route, equipment, and mechanism for obtaining and transporting the body fluid specimen (including required collection device, volume, temperature, and timeliness of transport to the laboratory) should be communicated and standardized.

In the analytical phase, body fluids often do not have manufacturer's performance claims or laboratory-developed test validation criteria. These include pleural, peritoneal, pericardial, and synovial fluids, as well as amniotic fluid and cervicovaginal secretions, saliva, sweat, semen, stool, pancreatic cysts fluid, fine needle aspiration biopsy (FNAB) washings, and some aspects of cerebrospinal fluid testing. These alternative specimen types may contain matrix interferences that may unknowingly produce inaccurate results that could negatively affect patient outcomes. Recommendations are under development for more robust validation approaches in many of these areas.

In the postanalytical phase, decision limits are available (eg, Light's criteria for discriminating a pleural exudate from a transudate),[1] although the major limitation is the paucity of methodologic detail from historical studies and that such criteria may not be applicable across all fluid types. For a clear understanding of how body fluid tests may leverage important decisions, it is critical that there is a good clinician-laboratory interface to communicate the limitations of body fluid analysis and that those results should always be interpreted in full clinical context.

SECTION IV

Molecular Diagnostics

Exam questions, case studies, and additional resources are available on ExpertConsult.com.
*Full versions of these chapters are available electronically on ExpertConsult.com.

44

Principles of Molecular Biology

John Greg Howe

ABSTRACT

Background
Molecular diagnostics and its parent field, molecular pathology, examine the origins of disease at the molecular level, primarily by studying nucleic acids. Deoxyribonucleic acid (DNA), which contains the blueprint for constructing a living organism, is the centerpiece for research and clinical analysis. Molecular pathology is an outgrowth of the enormous amount of successful research in the field of molecular biology that has discovered over the last seven decades the basic biological and chemical processes of how a living cell functions. The success of molecular biology, as noted by the large number of Nobel prizes awarded for its discoveries, is now used for clinical diagnosis and the development and use of therapeutics.

Content
The following chapters are devoted to describing this field and the specific applications currently being used to characterize and help treat patients with a variety of ailments, including hereditary genetic diseases, cancer neoplasms, and infectious diseases. In this chapter the fundamentals of molecular biology are reviewed, followed by a focus on genomes and their variants in Chapter 45. In Chapters 46 and 47 techniques for isolating and analyzing nucleic acids are discussed. The clinically important subdivisions of molecular diagnostics are then reviewed and include microbiology in Chapter 48, genetics in Chapter 49, solid tumors in Chapter 50, and hematopoietic malignancies in Chapter 51. Chapters 52 and 53 are devoted to the molecular diagnostic analysis of circulating tumor cells and circulating nucleic acids. Finally, pharmacogenetics and identity assessment are the focus of Chapters 54 and 55.

HISTORICAL DEVELOPMENTS IN GENETICS AND MOLECULAR BIOLOGY

Molecular diagnostics would not be possible without the many significant pioneering efforts in genetics and molecular biology. Earlier observations in genetics began with the discovery of the inheritance of biological traits made by Gregor Mendel in 1866 and the observation in 1910 that genes were associated with chromosomes by Thomas Morgan. The initial findings that contributed to determining that DNA was the transmittable genetic material were performed by Griffith in 1928 and Avery, McLeod, and McCarty in 1944.[1,2] The definitive studies, published by Hershey and Chase in 1952, demonstrated that radiolabeled phosphate incorporated into the DNA of a bacteriophage was found in newly synthesized DNA containing bacteriophage instead of radiolabeled sulfur in protein, which showed that DNA and not protein was the genetic material.[3]

Deciphering the structure of DNA required several crucial findings. These included the observation by Erwin Chargaff that the quantity of adenine is generally equal to the quantity of thymine, and the quantity of guanine is similar to the amount of cytosine[4] and the pivotal x-ray crystallography results produced by Rosalind Franklin and Maurice Wilkins.[5,6]

Molecular biology has historically traced its beginnings to the first description of the structure of DNA by James Watson and Francis Crick in 1953.[7,8] The description of the DNA structure initiated the dramatic increase in the knowledge of the biology and chemistry of our genetic machinery. The impact of the Watson and Crick discovery was so significant that it is considered one of the most important scientific discoveries of the 20th century.[9]

One reason the work of Watson and Crick had such a dramatic impact on scientific discovery was that they not only described the structure of DNA, but hypothesized about many of its properties, which took decades to confirm experimentally.[7,8,10] One of those properties was the replication of DNA, which was shown to be semiconservative by Meselson and Stahl[11] in 1958. At the same time, DNA polymerase, which replicates the DNA, was discovered by Arthur Kornberg.[12] Deciphering the genetic code was vital for understanding the information stored in DNA, and cracking the code in 1965 required many scientists, most prominently Marshall Nirenberg.[13] Additional studies described the transcription and translation processes and uncovered several startling findings. One finding was the isolation of reverse transcriptase, an enzyme that synthesizes DNA from ribonucleic acid (RNA), which demonstrates that genetic information can be transferred in part in a bidirectional manner.[14,15] Another finding showed that the eukaryotic gene structure was composed of alternating non–protein-encoding introns and protein-encoding exons.[16,17] Along with the discovery of the basic biology of genes and their expression, many important techniques were invented. For example, the isolation of restriction enzymes[18] and DNA ligase allowed for the construction of recombinant DNA,[19] which could be transferred from one organism to another, leading to the cloning of DNA[20] and the emergence of genetic engineering. The Southern blot method, which identified specific electrophoretically separated pieces of DNA, participated in many discoveries and was one of the first molecular diagnostics methods to be used to test for genetic diseases.[21] DNA sequencing technologies were invented[22,23] and further advances in these technologies led to the first large biological science research undertaking, the Human Genome Project. Along with DNA sequencing, further technical discoveries, including the polymerase chain reaction in 1986[24] and microarray technology in 1995,[25] became methodologic foundations for molecular diagnostics.

MOLECULAR BIOLOGY ESSENTIALS

Whether it is a bacterium, virus, or eukaryotic cell, the genetic material located in these organisms dictates their form and function. For the most part the genetic material is DNA, which is composed of two strands of a sugar-phosphate backbone that are bound together by hydrogen bonds between two purines and two pyrimidines attached to the sugar molecule, deoxyribose, in a double helix (Figs. 44.1 and 44.2). DNA in human cells is wrapped around histone proteins and packaged into nucleosome units, which are compacted further to form chromosomes (Fig. 44.3). There are 23 pairs of chromosomes, two of which are the sex chromosomes, X and Y. Each chromosome is a single length of DNA with a stretch of short repeats at the ends called telomeres and additional repeats in the centromere region. In humans, there are two sets of 23 chromosomes that are a mixture of DNA from the mother's egg and father's sperm. Each egg and sperm is therefore a single or haploid set of 23 chromosomes and the combination of the two creates a diploid set of human DNA, allowing each individual to possess two different sequences, genes, and alleles on each chromosome, one from each parent. Each child has a unique combination of alleles because of homologous recombination between homologous chromosomes during meiosis in the development of gametes (egg and sperm cells). This creates genetic diversity within the human population. If a child has a random DNA sequence change or mutation, the child's genotype is different from that inherited from either of the parents (de novo variant). If the child's genotype leads to visible disease, the child has acquired a different phenotype from the parents.

Human cells have a limited lifespan and die through a process called apoptosis. Therefore most cells replace themselves as they progress naturally through their cell cycle. As a cell moves through phases of the cell cycle, its DNA doubles during the synthesis phase when the double-stranded DNA molecule separates. Each strand of DNA is used as a template to make a complementary strand by DNA polymerase in a process called DNA replication. Eventually during the cell cycle, two cells are created from one during the final mitotic phase.

DNA is composed of genes that code for proteins and RNA. For DNA to convert its store of vital information into functional RNA and protein, the DNA strands need to separate so that RNA polymerase can bind to the start region of the gene. With the help of transcription factors that bind upstream to promoters, the RNA polymerase produces single strands of RNA that are further processed to remove the introns and retain the protein-encoding exons. The mature, processed RNA molecule, the messenger RNA (mRNA), migrates to the cytoplasm, where it is used in the production of protein.

To start the process of protein synthesis or translation, the mRNA is bound by various protein factors and a ribosome, which contains ribosomal RNA (rRNA) and protein. The

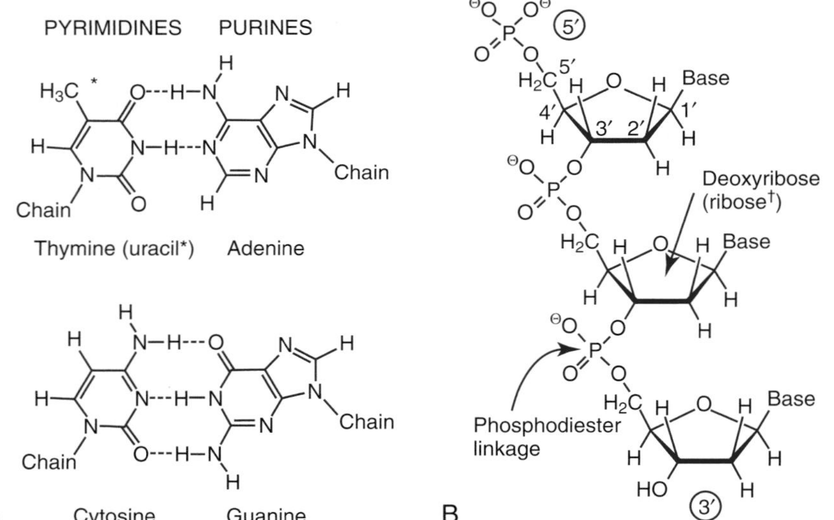

FIGURE 44.1 A, Purine and pyrimidine bases and the formation of complementary base pairs. *Dashed lines* indicate the formation of hydrogen bonds. (*In RNA, thymine is replaced by uracil, which differs from thymine only in its lack of the methyl group.) **B,** A single-stranded DNA chain. Repeating nucleotide units are linked by phosphodiester bonds that join the 5′ carbon of one sugar to the 3′ carbon of the next. Each nucleotide monomer consists of a sugar moiety, a phosphate residue, and a base. (†In RNA, the sugar is ribose, which adds a 2′-hydroxyl to deoxyribose.)

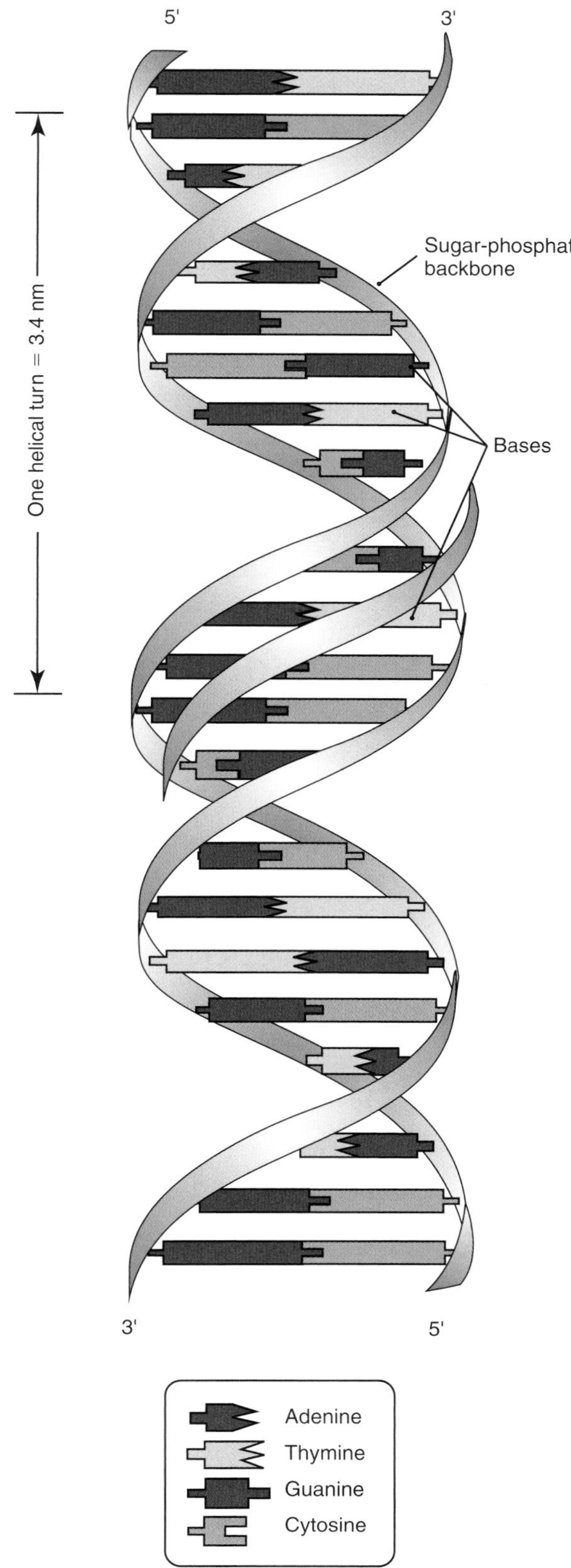

FIGURE 44.2 The DNA double helix, with sugar-phosphate backbone and pairing of the bases in the core-forming planar structures. (From Jorde LB, Carey JC, Bamshad MJ, editors: *Medical genetics*. 4th ed. Philadelphia: Mosby; 2010.)

mRNA-bound ribosome begins to produce a polypeptide chain by binding a methionine-bound transfer RNA (tRNA) to the mRNA's initiating AUG codon or triplet code. The conversion of the nucleic acid triplet code to a polypeptide is accomplished by the tRNA, which contains a nucleic acid triplet code (anticodon) in its RNA sequence that is specific for an amino acid bound to one end of the tRNA molecule. After synthesis, the protein migrates to its functional location and eventually is removed and degraded.

NUCLEIC ACID STRUCTURE AND FUNCTION

DNA is a rather simple molecule with a limited number of components compared to those of proteins. DNA is composed of a deoxyribose sugar, phosphate group, and four nitrogen-containing bases. Deoxyribose is a pentose sugar containing five carbon atoms that are numbered from 1′ to 5′, starting with the carbon that will be attached to the base in DNA and progressing around the ring until the last carbon that is not part of the ring structure. The bases consist of the purines, adenine and guanine and the pyrimidines, cytosine and thymine; an additional base, uracil, replaces thymine in RNA. A basic building block is the nucleotide, which consists of a deoxyribose sugar with an attached base at the 1′ carbon and a phosphate group at the 5′ carbon. The triphosphate nucleotide is the building block for making newly synthesized DNA. Newly synthesized DNA forms a polynucleotide chain that connects the individual nucleotides through the 5′ and 3′ carbons of each deoxyribose sugar via phosphodiester bonds.

Structure of Deoxyribonucleic Acid

DNA is double stranded, and the two strands bind to one another through hydrogen bonds between the bases on each strand. Hydrogen bonding is augmented by hydrophobic attraction (stacking) between bases on adjacent rungs of the DNA ladder. Both hydrogen bonds and base stacking are not covalent, but are weak bonds that can be broken and reestablished. This important property is exploited by many of the methods that are used in molecular diagnostics. The composition of DNA is equal quantities of guanine and cytosine and equal quantities of adenine and thymine, because, in general, guanine binds to cytosine and adenine binds to thymine.[4,7] There are two hydrogen bonds between adenine (A) and thymine (T) and three hydrogen bonds between cytosine (C) and guanine (G), and because of this difference in the number of hydrogen bonds, separating a guanine-cytosine (G-C) pair takes more energy than an adenine-thymine (A-T) pair (see Fig. 44.1).

Each of the two DNA strands is formed by a phosphate sugar backbone that starts at the 5′ phosphate and ends at a 3′ hydroxyl group with the complementary bases binding to one another between the two phosphate sugar backbones. Each strand is therefore a polar opposite of the other (see Fig. 44.2). When the two strands are bound to one another they progress in opposite 5′ to 3′ directions in an antiparallel configuration. By convention, the DNA sequence is denoted in a 5′ to 3′ direction. As discussed later, both the replication of new DNA and the transcription of DNA to RNA progress in the 5′ to 3′ direction. In addition, the conversion of RNA to protein, a process called translation, proceeds from the 5′ end of the RNA to the 3′ end. The combination of the base pairing

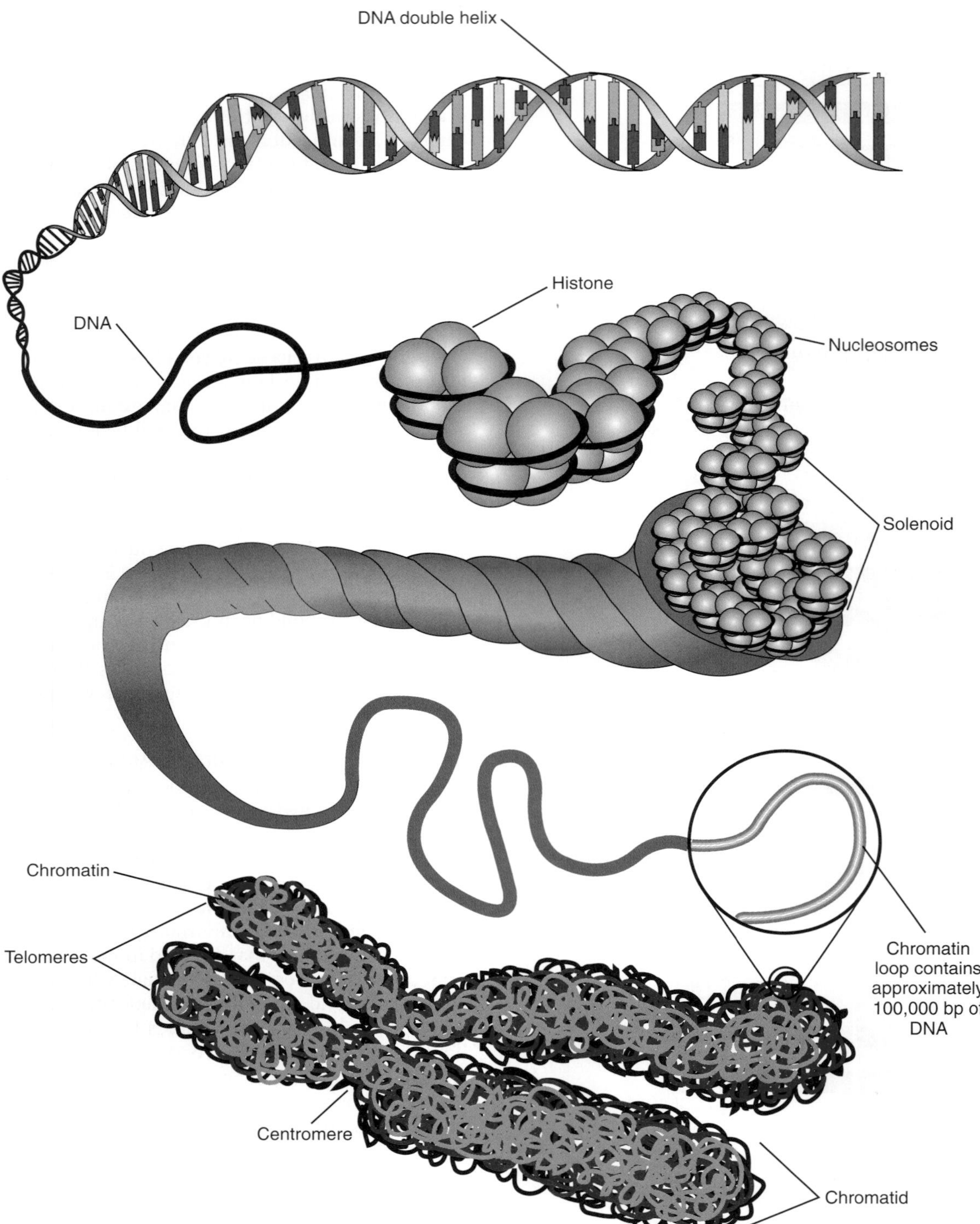

FIGURE 44.3 Structural organization of human chromosomal DNA. Double-stranded DNA is wound around the octamer core of histone proteins to form nucleosomes, which are further compacted into a helical structure called a solenoid. Nuclear DNA in conjunction with its associated structural proteins is known as chromatin. Chromatin in its most compact state forms chromosomes. The primary constriction of a chromosome is the centromere, and the chromosome's ends are the telomeres. (From Jorde LB, Carey JC, Bamshad MJ, editors. *Medical genetics.* 4th ed. Philadelphia: Mosby; 2010.)

and the directionality of the two DNA strands allows for the deciphering of the DNA sequence of one strand of DNA when the other complementary strand sequence is known.

Types of Deoxyribonucleic Acid

Double-stranded DNA in living cells is generally found as the right-handed B-DNA helical structure, which has specific dimensions. Each turn of the helix is 3.4 nm long and consists of 10 bases. The DNA sugar-phosphate backbone is on the outside of the helix, and the bases of each strand are inside bound to their complement on the other strand by hydrogen bonds. Other conformational structures of DNA occur, mostly associated with DNA sequences that are repeated. These non-B DNA forms include a left-handed Z-form, A-motif, tetraplex G-quadruplex, i-motif, hairpin, cruciform, and triplex and are abundant in the human genome because a large percentage of the genome contains various repeats. Non-B DNA is associated with many biological processes, including transcriptional control. However, these structures also can create genetic instability, which can lead to various diseases such as neurologic disorders.[26]

Molecular Composition of Ribonucleic Acid

The composition of RNA is similar to that of DNA because it contains four nucleotides linked together by a phosphodiester bond, but with several important differences. RNA consists of a ribose sugar with a hydroxyl group at the 2′ carbon instead of the hydrogen atom in DNA. The bases attached to the ribose sugar are adenine, cytosine, and guanine, but not thymine because RNA uses another pyrimidine—uracil—as a substitute for thymine.

Structure of Ribonucleic Acid

One significant difference between DNA and RNA is that RNA does not normally exist as two strands bound to one another, although a single strand can bind internally to itself creating functionally important secondary structures. Although in the past several decades the complexity and number of different RNAs has greatly expanded, the majority of cellular RNA is composed of a rather small number of RNA types. These include mRNA, rRNA, and tRNA.

Ribonucleic Acids Associated With Protein Production

mRNA is the most diverse group of the three major types of RNAs, but constitutes only a small percentage of the total RNA. mRNAs are transcribed from DNA that codes for proteins and therefore are used as the template for the translation of proteins. In the case of prokaryotes the mRNA is colinear with the protein that is translated; however, in eukaryotes the mRNA begins as a precursor RNA called premessenger or heterogeneous nuclear RNA (hnRNA) that includes untranslated intron and translated exon regions. After transcription the hnRNA is spliced into mature mRNA lacking the introns. The mature mRNA contains only exons and can be further modified by the addition of a 7-methylguanosine cap at the 5′ end, which protects the mRNA from degradation, and a polyadenosine (polyA) sequence at the 3′ end. In eukaryotes the production and processing of the hnRNA to mRNA takes place in the nucleus, and the final form of the mRNA is then transported to the cytoplasm to be translated.

rRNA is associated with ribosomes, which are the primary structures that produce protein through the biological process of translation. rRNA, unlike mRNA, does not code for proteins. The ribosome is composed of two structures, the 50S and 30S subunits found in prokaryotes and the 60S and 40S subunits found in eukaryotes. The "S" stands for Svedberg units and is determined by the centrifugal sedimentation rate. The Svedberg unit measures the mass, density, and shape of an object. The ribosome is a mixture of RNA and protein. In eukaryotes there are four major rRNAs: the 18S rRNAs found in the 40S subunit and the 28S, 5.8S, and 5S rRNAs found in the 60S subunit. In prokaryotes, the 50S subunit contains the 23S and 5S rRNAs and the 30S subunit contains the 16S rRNA. Synthesis of eukaryotic rRNA occurs as a large 45S precursor RNA that is enzymatically cleaved to form all the rRNAs except the 5S RNA, which is transcribed separately. Ribosomal RNAs have secondary and tertiary structures that are well conserved with various loops, stem loops, and pseudoknots that contribute to their function. Ribosomal RNA and protein, as the components of ribosomes, function to carry out the translation of proteins. The sequence of the 16S rRNA has alternating conserved and divergent regions that can be used to identify microorganisms. The structure of the ribosome is now known, and the rRNA is more important than ribosomal proteins in ribosome functioning. The RNA acts as a catalytic agent called a ribozyme.[27,28]

Another important group of RNAs are the tRNAs, which function as key molecules that act as a bridge between the nucleic acids and the proteins. They have a unique cloverleaf secondary structure, with the 3′ end covalently attached to the amino acid by specific aminoacyl tRNA synthetases. In the middle of the tRNA structure is the anticodon sequence that binds to a specific homologous codon in the mRNA. Therefore the codon directs the binding of a specific tRNA linked to its corresponding amino acid. The genetic code, which consists of a 64 3-base code, specifies the appropriate amino acid to be attached to the growing polypeptide chain (see Figs. 44.7 and 44.8, later in the chapter). There are several different classes of aminoacyl tRNA synthetases, but there is at least one aminoacyl tRNA synthetase for each of the 20 amino acids. There is also at least one tRNA for each amino acid; however, there can be more depending on the species.[29]

Besides the three major types of RNAs, other RNAs include nuclear, nucleolar, and cytoplasmic small RNAs, signaling RNAs, telomerase RNA, and micro-RNAs.[30] This list appears to be growing with each passing year. Some of the first characterized small RNAs, the nuclear and nucleolar small RNAs, are involved with the processing of precursor RNAs to mature RNAs, including splicing of hnRNA to mRNA and precursor rRNA to mature rRNAs. More recently a large number of microRNAs have been discovered that partly function in the regulation of translation. In addition, there are many other noncoding RNAs whose functions are just beginning to be understood.

Human Chromosome

Human double-stranded DNA that is contained in the sperm or egg is a single copy or haploid amount of DNA made up of approximately 3 billion base pairs (bp). To be more precise, the Human Genome Project consensus sequence of the human genome was 2.91×10^9 bp[31] and the first human to be sequenced, Craig Venter, had a genome size of 2.81×10^9 bp,[32]

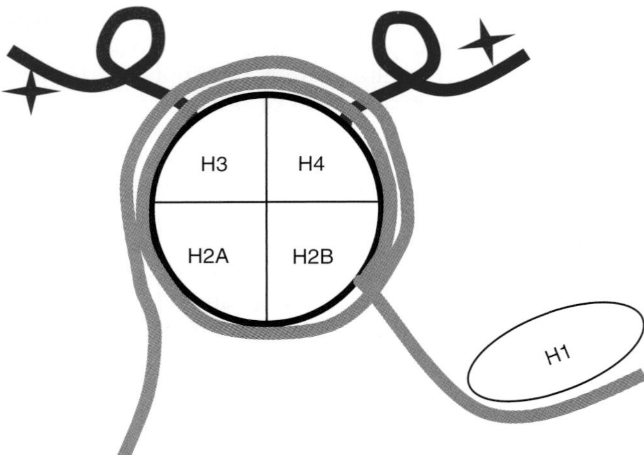

FIGURE 44.4 Schematic illustration of a nucleosome unit. A segment of DNA is wound around a nucleosome core particle consisting of an octamer of two each of the histone proteins H2A, H2B, H3, and H4. Tails with modifications (indicated by a *red star*) are shown to protrude from H3 and H4. Adjacent nucleosomes are separated by a segment of linker DNA and the linker histone, H1.

not including remaining gaps of highly repetitive sequences, many near centromeres and telomeres (see Chapter 45). The DNA in the cell is bound by many proteins to form chromatin (see Fig. 44.3). The proteins in chromatin consist of histones, which are bound in precise amounts per a length of DNA, and other proteins called nonhistone proteins that are bound more irregularly and in widely varying amounts. The histone proteins consist of eight proteins (two copies each of H2A, H2B, H3, and H4) that bind as a unit to 147 bp of DNA to make up a nucleosome, and the protein, H1, that binds between the nucleosomes (Fig. 44.4). The nucleosomes are the basic structure to which many other proteins interact and modify to regulate gene expression. For example, the access to DNA by transcription factors is controlled by proteins that remodel the histone proteins through phosphorylation, acetylation, and methylation. The nucleosomes are condensed into filaments and even more compact structures to form a chromosome (see Fig. 44.3). There are 23 pairs of chromosomes; 22 autosomal chromosomes and 2 sex chromosomes, X and Y, with an XX pair denoting female and an XY pair denoting male. The DNA in chromosomes is continuous for each chromosome and can be as much as several hundred million base pairs in length for the largest chromosomes.

From a cytogenetic viewpoint, regions of the chromosomes can be classified by their transcriptional activity. The more condensed heterochromatin DNA is transcriptionally inactive and stains with Giemsa, a mixture of several dyes that bind to AT-rich regions of DNA. The less condensed euchromatin DNA is transcriptionally active and does not stain with Giemsa. The ends of the chromosomes, called telomeres, contain a repeat sequence, such as TTAGGG that is found in humans and shortens with age. The centromeres, at the center of most chromosomes, are important for linking sister chromatids during mitosis and contain various satellite DNAs, such as α-satellite tandem repeats (171 bp) that are over several million base pairs (Mb) in length.

Surprisingly, most of the human DNA does not code for the expression of protein. As much as 50% of human DNA consists of many types of interspersed repeat sequences, such as satellites, telomeres, microsatellites, minisatellites, short and long interspersed nuclear elements (SINES, LINES), and retrovirus elements.[31] Like other eukaryotes, human genes are in pieces with the protein-encoding regions, exons, alternating with the introns, which do not code for protein sequence and occupy more than a quarter of the human DNA.[33] Other regions around the genes, such as the promoter regions and the 3′ untranslated regions are also not translated into proteins. After all the noncoding sequences are removed, the protein-coding DNA sequence spans only approximately 1.2 to 1.5% of human DNA. Even though most human DNA is not associated with protein-producing genes, the Encyclopedia of DNA Elements (ENCODE) project has shown that much of the non–protein-encoding DNA is transcribed into noncoding RNAs, most with unknown function.

CENTRAL DOGMA OF MOLECULAR BIOLOGY

Francis Crick originated the concept of the central dogma of biology, which describes the transfer of genetic information into functional macromolecules.[34] This was generally depicted to show the movement of genetic information from DNA to RNA via transcription using RNA polymerase and further translated into protein via ribosomes and various factors. This is a simplistic version of the original concept, which took into consideration every possible transfer of information even though no evidence existed at the time. However, since the original publication a number of other postulated transfers have been described. DNA can enzymatically replicate itself by DNA polymerase, and RNA can be made into DNA using reverse transcriptase.[35] Many of these enzymes are used in molecular diagnostics assays.

Deoxyribonucleic Acid Replication

A general principle underlying the synthesis or replication of new DNA is that it uses one of the two DNA strands as a template to make a new homologous strand. This is termed semiconservative replication and was first theorized by Watson and Crick.[7] DNA replication begins at an adenine and thymine (AT)-rich structure called an origin of replication. In bacteria there is generally only one origin of replication, but in eukaryotic cells there are thousands. Since DNA can be supercoiled into more structures, a topoisomerase is required to first unwind this structure so that the DNA is accessible. A DNA helicase binds to the double-stranded DNA and separates the two strands, providing two single-stranded DNA templates. Replication progresses in a 5′ to 3′ direction; therefore one strand, the leading strand, is synthesized as one continuous strand using the 3′ to 5′ template and the other strand, called the lagging strand, is synthesized in small segments called Okazaki fragments from the 5′ to 3′ template. Because the DNA polymerase requires a primer, small RNA primers are made by a primase enzyme on the 5′ to 3′ template and the Okazaki fragments are synthesized starting from the primer. Okazaki fragments are finally linked by a ligase (Fig. 44.5).[36]

DNA polymerases of various types have been identified and they function in many different roles, the most important being the replication of new DNA and the repair of

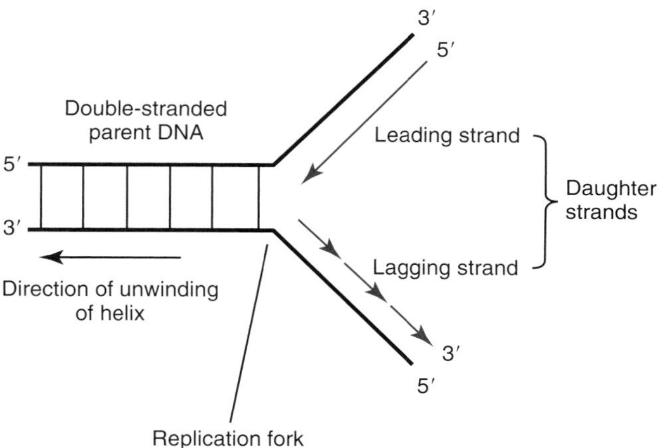

FIGURE 44.5 DNA replication. Double-stranded DNA is separated at the replication fork. The leading strand is synthesized continuously, whereas the lagging strand is synthesized discontinuously but is joined later by DNA ligase.

existing DNA. Using the template strand as a guide, the DNA polymerase binds a nucleotide triphosphate to the primer at a free 3′ hydroxyl group, releasing pyrophosphate. The specific nucleotide selected depends on the base on the template strand; for example, an adenine nucleotide is used if a thymine nucleotide is in the template strand. In summary, a complementary sequence is synthesized opposite the template strand. The insertion of the correct nucleotide does not always occur. Mistakes occur approximately every 100,000 nucleotides; therefore a major function of a DNA polymerase is error correction or proofreading and is accomplished by an intrinsic 3′ to 5′ exonuclease activity. DNA polymerases are important in molecular diagnostics because they are used in the polymerase chain reaction (PCR) and DNA sequencing.

DNA replication is part of the cell cycle and occurs during the synthesis phase. The rest of the cell cycle is the interphase, further divided into the first growth phase (G_1) and the second growth phase (G_2), along with the DNA replication or synthesis (S) phase that lies between G_1 and G_2. The mitosis phase, which involves the splitting of one cell into two cells, occurs after the G_2 phase. Mitosis is divided into six subphases: prophase, prometaphase, metaphase, anaphase, telophase, and cytokinesis.

At important control points in the cell cycle the cell will commit significant resources to proceed further. One of these control points is between the G_1 and S phase, just before it begins DNA replication. The G_1/S boundary control point is disrupted in many cancers. It is common for neoplasms to have mutations in the retinoblastoma gene *(RB1)*, whose protein product regulates cell cycle progression from G_1 to S. Another control point is between G_2 and M, just as the cell commits to creating two cells from one.

Deoxyribonucleic Acid Repair

The integrity of DNA is damaged in a variety ways that culminate in changes or mutations in the DNA sequence. DNA bases may be damaged, removed, cross-linked or incorrectly paired with one another, and single- or double-stranded breaks may also occur.[37,38] When the cell senses that its DNA has become damaged, it stops the progression of its cell cycle and initiates DNA repair processes.[39] Cells repair these lesions by employing multiple DNA repair mechanisms that are specific for the type of DNA lesion and include base excision repair, nucleotide excision repair, mismatch repair, and homologous recombination repair.

Mechanisms

Base excision repair removes bases that are damaged by deamination, oxidation, and alkylation. Deamination of guanine, cytidine, and adenine converts them into structures that will incorrectly base pair, creating transition mutations, which are changes between similar nitrogenous bases such as a purine to a purine. A transversion mutation is a change from a purine to a pyrimidine or vice versa. DNA glycosylases, such as uracil-DNA-glycosylase, cleave the damaged base, and a 5′-deoxyribose phosphate lyase removes the nucleotide upstream of the removed base. DNA polymerase and ligase then add a new nucleotide repairing the damage. One of the inherited disorders associated with this repair process that leads to a predisposition to various neoplasms is caused by mutations in *MUTYH,* a DNA glycosylase gene.[38,40]

Nucleotide excision repair removes base modifications that change the helical structure of DNA, including bulky DNA distortions and covalently bound structures that may be created by ultraviolet radiation and certain cancer drugs. The damage is recognized by global and transcription-mediated repair processes. After the repair is initiated, the transcription factor, TFIIH, binds to a complex of proteins and makes an incision. The damaged DNA is unwound, and the gap is filled by DNA polymerase and finally sealed by DNA ligase. Mutations in the nucleotide excision repair genes cause xeroderma pigmentosum, which leaves affected individuals susceptible to specific tumors.[38,41]

Mismatch repair recognizes base incorporation errors and base damage. DNA polymerase has a 3′ to 5′ editing exonuclease with a proofreading function that is not completely effective and allows some mismatches to occur that can lead to mutations after DNA replication. The mismatched nucleotides must be repaired on the newly synthesized strand of DNA, which in prokaryotes is recognized by its unmethylated state. In eukaryotes the mechanism is different, and it is proposed that proteins associated with the replication apparatus, specifically the proliferating cell nuclear antigen protein determines the appropriate DNA strand for repair.[38] These mutations are corrected with DNA mismatch repair proteins, which identify the mismatches by their methylation patterns, excise the surrounding sequence, and then repair the excision with new sequence. Mutations in the human mismatch repair genes are associated with Lynch syndrome (hereditary nonpolyposis colorectal cancer).

Double-stand breaks are a very destructive form of DNA damage that destabilizes the genome, sometimes resulting in gross chromosomal changes, such as translocations that are frequently found in cancer. Double-stranded breaks are caused by several processes, including ionizing radiation and chemotherapy drugs, and are repaired by either homologous recombination or nonhomologous end joining.[38,41] The homologous recombination repair pathway is initiated by recognition of a double-stranded break, followed by resection using exonucleases to create a 3′ single-stranded overhang. With the assistance of many proteins, RAD51 is bound to the single-stranded DNA, which invades the intact homologous double-stranded DNA of the sister chromatid and uses it as a template for new double-stranded DNA repair.[38]

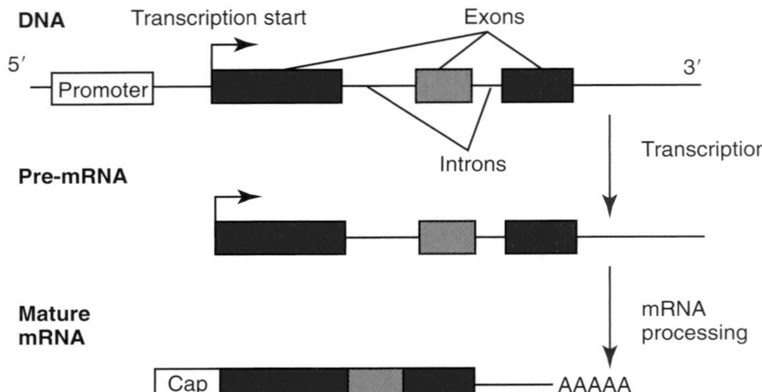

FIGURE 44.6 DNA transcription and messenger RNA processing. A gene that encodes for a protein contains a promoter region and variable numbers of introns and exons. Transcription commences at the transcription start site. Premessenger RNA or heterogeneous nuclear RNA (hnRNA) is processed by capping, polyadenylation, and intron splicing and becomes a mature messenger RNA.

DNA repair mechanisms operate independently to repair simple lesions. However, the repair of more complex lesions involves multiple DNA processing steps regulated by the DNA damage response pathway. When single- and double-stranded DNA breaks occur, a cascade of responses is initiated that culminates in either DNA repair, stopping the cell cycle, or programmed cell death. After DNA damage has occurred, the DNA damage response pathway activates the protein kinases ATM (ataxia telangiectasia mutated) and ATR (ataxia telangiectasia and Rad3-related protein) to phosphorylate signaling proteins, such as p53, which eventually leads to cell cycle arrest at the G_1/S boundary. This gives time for the DNA repair mechanism to repair the damaged DNA; however, if the damage is too extensive, the cell initiates apoptosis or cell death.[39]

Deoxyribonucleic Acid Modification Enzymes

There are two groups of nucleases, the endonucleases that cut through the sugar-phosphate backbone and exonucleases that digest the ends of DNA. The commercially important restriction endonucleases, which bacteria have acquired to protect themselves from viral infections, are used to cleave DNA at a specific nucleotide sequence or restriction sites.[42] Several thousand restriction endonucleases have been characterized and are used extensively to manipulate DNA in molecular biology and molecular diagnostics. Recent work has described new nucleases, such as the RNA-guided engineered nuclease, CRISPR/Cas system, that can precisely cleave genomic DNA.[43]

DNA glycosylases are a family of enzymes associated with base excision repair that are used in the first step of DNA repair to remove the damaged base, without disrupting the sugar-phosphate backbone. An important member of that family, uracil DNA glycosylase, repairs the most common mutation found in humans, the spontaneous deamination of cytosine to uracil, by removing the uracil base.

Gene Structure

The structure of prokaryotic genes is straightforward; almost all of the gene sequence is used to make protein; however, this is not the case with eukaryotic genes. One of the unique hallmarks of eukaryotic genes is that the protein-coding DNA is interspersed with regions that do not code for DNA, an observation made by Richard Roberts and Phillip Sharp in 1977. A mature mRNA retains only the protein-coding sequences called exons, and the sequences between the exons are non–protein-encoding sequences called introns that are removed during mRNA maturation (Fig. 44.6).[44]

In addition to introns and exons, eukaryotic genes consist of regulatory regions, such as promoters and enhancers, and 3′ regions that contain termination and polyadenylation signals. The regulation of the expression of eukaryotic genes can occur at all levels from transcription to splicing to translation to degradation; however, most gene regulation occurs at the initiation of transcription by various promoters and enhancers.[45] There are two groups of regulatory elements: one is close to the transcriptional start site and is made up of the core promoter and ancillary promoters slightly further away from the start of transcription. The other group of regulatory elements can be much further away, not only upstream but also downstream from the gene. This second group is made up of enhancers, silencers, insulators, and locus-specific control regions.[45,46] These regulatory elements contain specific sequences that bind to transcription factors that can upregulate or downregulate the expression of a gene. There are only several thousand human transcription factors, much less than the number of human genes; therefore each gene has many regulatory elements to provide the needed complexity to function in 200 different human cell types.[45]

A surprising property of human genes is that there are so few compared to less complex species. Humans have approximately 20,000 genes, many fewer than found in rice and only slightly more than found in the roundworm, *Caenorhabditis elegans*.[47-49] Recently, results from the ENCODE project have challenged the concept of "one gene, one protein."[50] Their studies show that the exon of one gene can be spliced into the exon of another gene.[51] This result, along with alternative splicing, demonstrates that one gene can make multiple proteins and is probably the reason humans have such a small number of genes.

Ribonucleic Acid Transcription and Splicing

RNA transcription involves synthesizing an RNA strand using DNA as a template. This requires many different proteins, the most important being the RNA polymerases, of which there are three types in eukaryotic cells. RNA polymerase I is specific for the rRNAs, 28S, 18S, and 5.8S, which are initially transcribed as a single primary transcript of 45S. RNA polymerase II transcribes all genes that encode proteins and the small nuclear RNA (snRNA) genes. RNA polymerase III transcribes a variety of small RNAs, including the 5S rRNA, and tRNA. Additional proteins called transcription factors function in combination to recognize and regulate transcription of different genes.[52]

The synthesis of RNA proceeds in a 5′ to 3′ direction using DNA as a template and a specific DNA sequence acts as a transcription start site. Transcription progresses through three phases: initiation, elongation, and termination. The initiation phase includes the binding of transcription factors to promoters upstream from the start site and includes the core promoter immediately upstream and the ancillary promoters further away. However, some of the small RNA gene promoters are in the middle of the gene. Transcription factors binding to upstream promoters act as regulators of the transcription of genes. These factors generally bind in pairs or dimers and have several functional domains. One functional domain of the transcription factor binds to a specific promoter DNA sequence via several structures, such as the helix-turn-helix, zinc finger, and leucine zipper structures. Another domain binds to the other transcription factor of the dimer pair, and a third domain may bind to the RNA polymerase complex that carries out transcription.[46] Even though promoters and the transcription factors binding to them are far away from the transcription initiation complex, the promoter DNA folds back on itself to allow for the transcription factors to interact with the RNA polymerase complex.[53]

Important recurring sequences are found in the core promoter. For example, the core promoter of an RNA polymerase II gene contains a TATAAA sequence, called a TATA box located upstream 25 to 40 nucleotides from the transcriptional start site. Only 20% to 30% of eukaryotic promoters contain TATA boxes, but they are highly regulated compared to those without TATA boxes that are mostly housekeeping genes.[45,54,55]

The first step in mRNA transcription is the binding of transcription factor IID (TFIID) to the TATA box, which in turn promotes the binding of other transcription factors (TFIIA, TFIIB, TFIIE, TFIIF, and TFIIH), RNA polymerase II, and proteins attached to the upstream promoter sites. To form a functional transcription complex, the promoter region's doubled-stranded DNA separates and the transcription complex moves away from the core promoter region.[45] Once started, the RNA polymerase adds nucleotides to the 3′ free hydroxyl group in a manner similar to that of DNA replication. Transcription is eventually terminated by one of several termination mechanisms. In bacteria a termination factor bound to the RNA polymerase recognizes a DNA sequence termination signal. In the case of genes transcribed by RNA polymerase II, termination is coupled with the polyadenylation step (see Fig. 44.6).

Two posttranscriptional processing events are performed on the newly formed hnRNA, one at each end of the RNA. At the 5′ end, the hnRNA is capped with a 7-methyl guanosine molecule to help protect the hnRNA from degradation. At the 3′ end, a polyadenosine (poly A) stretch is added by poly A polymerase after the RNA sequence AAUAAA is synthesized. Some transcribed mRNAs are not polyadenylated, such as histone mRNAs.[56]

Transcription initially produces an hnRNA that contains both exons and introns, which needs to be processed or spliced into mature mRNA for it to be properly translated into protein. RNA splicing involves cleavage and removal of intron RNA segments and splicing of exon RNA segments. The process uses consensus splice site sequences located at both the 5′ (GU) and 3′ (AG) ends of the intron and an internal intron sequence. Splicing requires the effort of a number of proteins and small RNAs that come together to form a spliceosome, which directs the splicing of exons and removal of introns.[57] Splicing begins with the binding of the U1 small nuclear ribonucleic protein (snRNP) to the donor splice site and the U2 snRNP to the internal intron sequence, followed by the binding of U4, U5, and U6 snRNPs, resulting in excising the intron and joining (splicing) of the ends of the two exons on either side of the excised intron (see Fig. 44.6).[57]

An important modification of the splicing process, alternative splicing, allows for the generation of different mRNAs from the same primary RNA transcript by the cutting and joining of the RNA strand at different locations. Among the types of alternative splicing are exon skipping, alternative 3′ and 5′ splice sites, and intron retention. It is estimated that 92% to 95% of all human genes are alternatively spliced.[58,59]

The movement of cellular signals from the surface of a cell to the nucleus is called signal transduction, and one of the eventual targets is the modification (eg, phosphorylation) of transcription factors, which can modulate the binding of other transcription factors to DNA and their dimerization, thereby controlling gene expression.[60] A common cascade of signaling begins with the activation of a receptor on the cell surface, such as a tyrosine kinase receptor. The tyrosine kinase receptor in the form of a dimer can be activated by binding to a hormone or growth factor, for example, which causes a dimerization and autophosphorylation of the tyrosine receptor protein kinase. This in turn activates a cytoplasmic protein, such as the guanine nucleotide exchange factor that activates the G-protein Ras, which can then modify another G-protein, Raf, which propagates the signal to a common signaling pathway, the mitogen-activated protein (MAP) kinases. The final enzyme in the pathway can then act on downstream targets, including other protein kinases, and transcriptional factors. Some mutations in the tyrosine kinase receptor or Ras protein switches them to an unregulated "on" position, which can lead to uncontrolled growth of the cell and eventually to cancer.[60]

Translation

The final phase of the transfer of information from DNA is to proteins, the structural and functional molecules that make up the majority of a living organism, such as the human body. Proteins are long single strands of various amino acids and are synthesized by a process called translation, which requires the functioning of many protein factors, tRNAs, and ribosomes.

Amino acids have a common structure consisting of a carbon atom bound to amino and carboxylic acid groups and a unique side chain. There are 20 amino acids each with a different side chain that give them their unique properties. The side chains can be divided into four types: nonpolar (hydrophobic), polar (hydrophilic uncharged), and negative

First Letter	Second Letter: U		C		A		G		Third Letter
U	UUU	Phenylalanine	UCU	Serine	UAU	Tyrosine	UGU	Cysteine	U
	UUC		UCC		UAC		UGC		C
	UUA	Leucine	UCA		UAA	Stop Codon	UGA	Stop Codon	A
	UUG		UCG		UAG	Stop Codon	UGG	Tryptophan	G
C	CUU	Leucine	CCU	Proline	CAU	Histidine	CGU	Arginine	U
	CUC		CCC		CAC		CGC		C
	CUA		CCA		CAA	Glutamine	CGA		A
	CUG		CCG		CAG		CGG		G
A	AUU	Isoleucine	ACU	Threonine	AAU	Asparagine	AGU	Serine	U
	AUC		ACC		AAC		AGC		C
	AUA		ACA		AAA	Lysine	AGA	Arginine	A
	AUG	Methionine	ACG		AAG		AGG		G
G	GUU	Valine	GCU	Alanine	GAU	Asparatic Acid	GGU	Glycine	U
	GUC		GCC		GAC		GGC		C
	GUA		GCA		GAA	Glutamic Acid	GGA		A
	GUG		GCG		GAG		GGG		G

FIGURE 44.7 Genetic code. Translation of messenger RNA to amino acids during protein synthesis.

and positively charged. Nonpolar (hydrophobic) amino acids include alanine, leucine, isoleucine, valine, proline, methionine, phenylalanine, and tryptophan. The uncharged polar (hydrophilic) amino acids include glycine, serine, threonine, cysteine, tyrosine, glutamine, and asparagine. The negatively charged (acidic) amino acids are aspartic acid and glutamic acid, and the positively charged (basic) amino acids are arginine, histidine, and lysine. A protein's amino acid makeup and sequence in the polypeptide chain determine the overall structure and function of the protein. Some amino acids have a more significant presence than others. For example, proline, which disrupts secondary structure, and cysteine, which can cross-link to another cysteine through disulfide bonds, can change the structure of a protein.

Protein structures are grouped into four different classes. The primary structure is the sequence of the amino acids in the protein. There are several common types of secondary structure, such as β-pleated sheets and α helixes. Proteins can be constructed with a combination of these different types of secondary structures. Tertiary structure applies to the folding of the polypeptide chain into a three-dimensional form. Quaternary structure is the structural relationship of more than one polypeptide/protein joining together, such as in immunoglobulin molecules, that contains light and heavy proteins bound together by cysteine residues.

Once proteins are synthesized, they can be modified in various ways. One of the most common modifications is phosphorylation of the amino acids serine, threonine, and tyrosine, which can regulate protein activity. Other modifications include proteolytic cleavage, such as removal of the signal transport sequence, and acetylation of the N-terminus of most eukaryotic proteins that helps to prevent degradation. Glycosylation of secreted and membrane proteins on asparagine, serine, and threonine residues and formation of disulfide bonds via cysteine cross-linking are additional modifications.

Taking into consideration these posttranslational modifications and alternatively spliced forms mentioned in an earlier section, the total number of proteins in the more than 200 human cell types is estimated to range from 250,000 to several million.[61]

The genetic code, which was deciphered in the early 1960s, is required to convert a nucleic acid sequence into an amino acid sequence.[13] It was reasoned that if there are 20 amino acids, a code of at least 3 nucleotides was necessary to have enough combinations. A 3-nucleotide code gives 64 combinations, and therefore one hallmark of the genetic code is that it is redundant, meaning that there are several codes for one amino acid. That is the case for most amino acids, but not all; for example, methionine and tryptophan have only one code. The redundancy is usually in the third base of the code. All of the 64 3-nucleotide codon possibilities code for an amino acid, except 3 that serve as stop codons (UAA, UGA, and UAG) (Fig. 44.7).

Protein synthesis or translation occurs in the cytoplasm and proceeds in three steps: initiation, elongation, and termination. The process requires tRNA and rRNA molecules, as well as ribosomes and initiation, elongation, and termination factors. One of the most important groups of molecules are the tRNAs, which are recognized by aminoacyl tRNA synthetase enzymes that attach amino acids to the 3′ end of specific tRNA molecules. Each tRNA has a 3-base sequence (anticodon) that facilitates the specific recognition and interaction with a codon in the mRNA.

The initiation step of protein synthesis is the most complex and begins with the binding of initiation factor 4E to the cap structure on the 5′ end of the mRNA and binding of poly-adenosine–binding protein (PABP) to the 3′ PABP

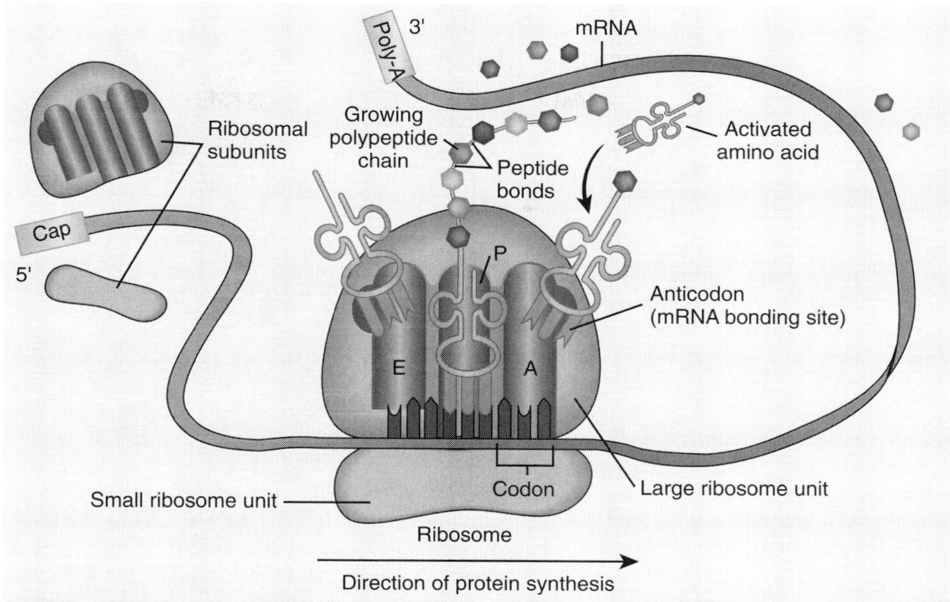

FIGURE 44.8 Translation. Shown is a ribosome bound to a messenger RNA converting the messenger RNA triplet code (codon) via a specific amino acid–bound transfer RNA containing a complementary anticodon sequence. There are three transfer RNA positions. A new amino acid–bound transfer RNA first arrives on the ribosome at the *A* or acceptor site at the front of the moving ribosome and then moves to the *P* or peptidyl site where the amino acid on the newly arrived transfer RNA combines with the growing polypeptide chain. Finally the now empty transfer RNA moves to the *E*, or exit site, where it prepares to leave the ribosome. (Modified from Huether SE, McCance KL. *Understanding pathophysiology*. 6th ed. St. Louis, Elsevier; 2017.)

polyadenosine tail. The binding of initiation factor 4G to both initiation factor 4E and PABP circularizes the mRNA and prepares it for binding to the preinitiation complex containing the 40S ribosomal subunit, initiation factor 2, and methionine tRNA. The preinitiation complex then scans the mRNA until it finds a methionine start codon (AUG), at which point the 60S ribosomal subunit binds forming the 80S initiation complex and initiates translation elongation.[62] This is a simplistic description of the initiation process because over a dozen additional initiation and auxiliary factors are involved.

Ribosomes have at least three structural positions where tRNAs can bind, the acceptor (A), peptidyl (P), and exit (E) sites. The acceptor site binds the incoming aminoacyl-tRNA. The peptidyl site holds the peptidyl-tRNA that is covalently linked to the growing polypeptide chain, and the exit site binds to the outgoing empty tRNA that carries no amino acid.[62,63]

The first codon (AUG) always codes for methionine; therefore to initiate translation the methionine tRNA binds to the aminoacyl-tRNA binding site of the ribosome. The tRNA specific for the next 3-base codon—for example, lysine—binds to the acceptor site of the ribosome and with the help of elongation factors (eg, eEF2), the amino acid in the peptidyl site is bound to the amino acid in the acceptor site by the formation of a peptide bond. A peptide bond is created between the amino group of one amino acid and the carboxyl group of the next amino acid through condensation releasing water. At the same time the tRNA shifts positions, with the methionine tRNA shifting to the exit site and the tRNA containing the growing chain of amino acids shifting to the peptidyl site. At the same time, the ribosome moves forward one codon and the next tRNA specific for the next codon through its anticodon binds in the acceptor site, and the process is repeated until a termination codon is reached (Fig. 44.8). Termination factors then bind and stop the translation process.[62] Protein synthesis occurs in the eukaryotic cytoplasm in the endoplasmic reticulum where multiple ribosomes called polyribosomes are involved in translating an individual mRNA.

Regulation of translation is not as extensive as that for transcription. However, there is global regulation of eukaryotic translation at the initiation step with phosphorylation of initiation factor 2B by four different protein kinases. This occurs when the cells are under stress, such as amino acid starvation or DNA damage.[64] In addition, mRNA-specific translational regulation can occur through binding to specific sequences located in the 5′ and 3′ untranslated regions. Furthermore, there are over 1000 microRNAs in humans,[65] many of which regulate transcription. The microRNA genes are transcribed as precursor RNA and then processed into a mature 22-nucleotide form by the processing enzymes Dicer and Drosha. The mature form of microRNAs can bind to specific sites on mRNA while associated with the Argonaute protein and either reversibly inhibit translation or degrade the mRNA.[62,66] For example, microRNAs Mir 15a/16-1 are deleted in chronic lymphocytic leukemia, thereby increasing Bcl2 expression and inhibiting apoptosis or cell death to prolong the life span of the cell.[67]

After proteins are synthesized there are two major processes to remove excess or damaged proteins. One process degrades the proteins ingested and uses nonspecific proteases,

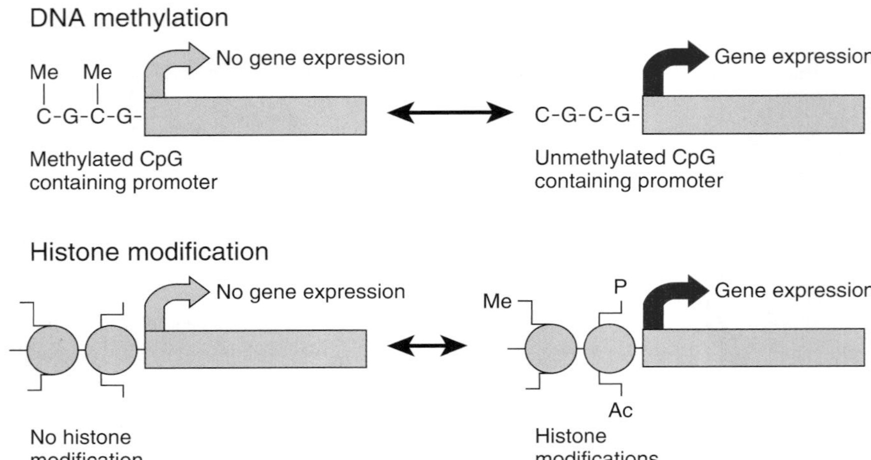

FIGURE 44.9 Epigenetics. *Top,* DNA methylation of CpG island regions indicated by *Me* in and around gene promoters is associated with loss of gene expression and silencing of the gene. When *CpG* islands are unmethylated, shown by absence of Me, gene expression is unaffected. *Bottom,* Modifications of the tails of histone proteins, such as methylation, acetylation, and phosphorylation, shown as *Me, Ac, and P,* respectively, can increase gene expression. (Modified from Zaidi SK, Young DW, Montecino M, van Wijnen AJ, Stein JL, Lian JB, et al. Bookmarking the genome: maintenance of epigenetic information. *J Biol Chem* 2011;286:18355–18361.)

such as pepsin and trypsin, to digest proteins associated with foodstuff in the gut into amino acids so they can be absorbed. The second process digests extracellular and intracellular proteins by either general proteinases within lysosomes or by protein degradation via ubiquination. With the latter mechanism, proteins are tagged for degradation by binding to ubiquitin, which is recognized by a large multiprotein structure, the proteasome that degrades the ubiquinated proteins by proteolysis.[68]

EPIGENETICS

Although the original meaning of epigenetics encompassed all molecular pathways that affect the expression of genes, over time the definition has focused on the regulation of gene expression by heritable modifications that do not change the DNA sequence.[69] More recently this has been broadened to include nonheritable modifications.[70-73] Currently there are three major areas of epigenetic modifications or marks: (1) DNA methylation; (2) chromatin conformation regulation through histone modifications, including ATP-dependent remodeling enzymes and histone variants; and (3) noncoding RNAs.[74]

Deoxyribonucleic Acid Methylation

DNA methylation is a well-known epigenetic change that is important in X chromosome inactivation, gene imprinting (eg, Prader-Willi, Angelman syndromes), and cancer. The most common methylation event is the methylation of cytosine to form 5-methylcytosine. DNA methylation typically occurs at cytosines directly upstream of guanines, or CpG dinucleotides. Cytosine is both methylated and demethylated by a variety of enzymes. The initial methylation state is catalyzed by one type of DNA cytosine-5-methyltransferase, whereas the maintenance of the methylated state is performed by another type of DNA cytosine-5-methyltransferase and occurs during each cell division after being established in early embryonic development.[75]

Demethylation involves three members of the ten-eleven translocation (TET) family of dioxygenases, which catalyze the conversion of 5-methylcytosine to other modified forms, such as 5-hydroxymethylcytosine during demethylation.[76] 5-Hydroxymethylcytosine is found in high amounts in neural cells and is postulated to regulate gene expression.[76]

Gene expression is altered by methylation via several mechanisms. The most direct effect is through altering the ability of transcription factors to bind to promoters. Methylation decreases the affinity of transcription factors to a DNA promoter and enhances the binding of methylation-specific transcription factors (Fig. 44.9). Additionally, methylation compacts the chromatin structure, thus reducing the access of transcription factors to a promoter.[77] Cancer is the most common human disease associated with aberrant DNA methylation.[78] Interestingly, the overall level of 5-methylcytosine in cancer cells is 60% less than in normal cells; however, certain promoter-specific CpG islands are hypermethylated.[78] Other human diseases that are associated with methylation include lupus and many neurologic diseases.

Chromatin Conformation Regulation

Many basic cellular functions require proteins to interact with DNA. However, DNA is generally not freely accessible but is wound around histones to form nucleosomes and further condensed or compacted into heterochromatin that decreases gene expression. The cell requires the DNA to be accessible to carry out DNA replication, repair, and transcription.[74,79] The chromatin, therefore, is a very dynamic structure; at any one point in time portions of the DNA are being exposed and other portions are being covered. The mechanisms that control chromatin conformation include histone modifications, histone variants, and ATP-dependent remodeling enzymes.

Specific histones are reversibly and posttranslationally modified at their N-terminal tails and globular regions to change the chromatin from a euchromatin state to a heterochromatin state and back (see Fig. 44.9). These modifications include acetylation of lysine residues at the N-terminal tails of H2A, H3, and H4 by histone acetyltransferases (HATs) and deacetylation by histone deacetylases (HDACs). Histone acetylation removes the positive charge on the lysine residue, leaving the lysine less attracted to the negatively charged DNA phosphate backbone and thereby opening the DNA.[77]

Histone methylation of lysine and arginine residues occurs mostly on histone protein H3, but also histone protein H4, and is carried out by histone methyltransferases (HMTs) and histone demethylases (HDMs). The effect of methylation on chromatin structure ranges from active to poised to repressed. Histone lysine and arginine residues can be mono-, di-, and tri-methylated, but the positive charge is unchanged.[39,79] Histone methylation is found associated with DNA transcription, replication, and repair.

Histones are phosphorylated at serine, threonine, and tyrosine residues and are associated with DNA repair and transcription. The addition of a negatively charged phosphate group to the histone will repel the histone away from the negatively charged DNA and loosen up the chromatin structure.[80] Other modifications include poly(ADP-ribosyl)ation, ubiquitination, SUMOylation, and glycosylation.[81]

Histone variants have been known for decades, but many of their functions are not well established. Histone protein variants H3.3 and H2A.Z are the most well-known and are shown to function in regulation of gene expression.[82] Histone variant H3.3 incorporates into chromatin independent of replication and is associated with active chromatin.[83,84]

ATP-dependent remodeling enzymes use the energy from the hydrolysis of ATP to change the structure of chromatin.[84,85] ATP-dependent remodeling enzymes are grouped into four families including SWItch/Sucrose NonFermentable (SWI/SNF), imitation switch (ISWI), inositol requiring 80 (INO80), and chromodomain (CHD).[79,85]

The remodeling enzymes have similar properties, including (1) specific interaction with nucleosomes, (2) attraction to the modified histone tail residues found in nucleosomes, (3) contain an ATPase domain, (4) ATPase regulatory function, and (5) ability to interact with transcription factors and chromatin-associated proteins.[81,85] The primary role of the enzymes is to remodel the chromatin structure. The SWI/SNF proteins function in the sliding and ejecting of nucleosomes, but do not function in chromatin assembly. The IWSI family of enzymes changes the nucleosome spacing through sliding that is necessary after DNA replication. This family interacts with unmodified histone tails and functions to regulate transcription. The CHD family functions to slide and eject nucleosomes, by which it regulates transcription. The INO80 family of proteins has an insertion in the middle of its ATPase domain and functions in promoting transcription and DNA repair. A mammalian member of this family, SWR1, can exchange histones to facilitate DNA repair.[81,85-87]

Noncoding Ribonucleic Acids

Most of the expressed RNA in a cell is not translated into protein. Only the mRNAs are translated into protein, and they represent only 1% to 5% of the total RNA depending on cell type. Much of this noncoding RNA is known and includes rRNA and tRNAs. However, over the last several decades two large groups of noncoding RNAs have been discovered, the short and long noncoding RNAs. The ENCODE project tested for the expression from DNA not associated with genes by using probes that overlapped one another regardless of the location of genes. Over 80% of the human DNA could be assigned a biochemical function, although biochemical function was liberally defined.[88] Nonetheless, it was determined that the bulk of the human genome is expressed into RNA.[89]

The short noncoding RNAs consist of microRNAs, small interfering RNAs and piwi interacting RNAs.[90,91] MicroRNAs regulate gene expression by binding to a specific sequence of the mRNA and inhibiting its translation. Small interfering RNAs (siRNA) inhibit translation by also binding to a region of the mRNA, but do so by initiating the degradation of the mRNA by the associated Argonaute protein. Piwi interacting RNAs (piRNA) function in the repression of transposons and are important in the development of gametes in many multicellular eukaryotic species.

The long RNAs are arbitrarily designated to be greater than 200 nucleotides while the short RNAs are between 20 and 200 nucleotides.[92] Only recently has the extent of long noncoding RNAs been appreciated.[89] The diversity of the long noncoding RNAs is predicted to be in the hundreds of thousands in vertebrates and their expression pattern is highly regulated during the development of an organism. A well-described example of a long noncoding RNA is XIST, which associates with the Polycomb group complex 2 and inactivates the X chromosome by inducing heterochromatin formation and repressing gene expression.[93] Examples such as XIST and a similarly acting protein, HotAir, have given rise to the possibility that the noncoding regions of the human genome have important functions.[92]

The function of most noncoding RNAs is unknown, but it is speculated that coding and noncoding RNAs, referred to as competing endogenous RNAs (ceRNAs), are in competition for shared microRNA binding sites in untranslated regions of mRNAs, thereby regulating their expression. The ceRNA hypothesis proposes a new layer of regulation of gene expression that could help explain the function of the large percentage of the human genome that expresses non–protein-coding RNA.[94-96]

UNDERSTANDING OUR GENOME

Genomics is recognized as a unique field since the first free-living organisms were completely sequenced in the 1990s. With the publication of the first draft of the human genome in 2001 and the final results of the Human Genome Project in 2004, the genomics field started to impart greater influence on biomedical research and its application to medicine.[31,97] Genomics is characterized by the comprehensive nature of its collection of data and the technical development necessary to obtain, analyze, store, and make available such large amounts of data. There are also ethical, legal, and social implications of the research and clinical application of genomics.[98]

Large research projects that were initiated during the latter years of the Human Genome Project produced comprehensive biological catalogs of genetic variants, important DNA functional sequences, and expressed products from not only humans but also many other organisms.[98]

Single nucleotide variants (SNVs) are the most common DNA differences found in the human population, and they number in the millions, with each individual differing on average by 1 in 1000 nucleotides. Human SNVs (including both benign polymorphisms and causative mutations) are cataloged in the SNP database (http://www.ncbi.nlm.nih.gov/SNP).

Genome-wide association studies employ microarray tests that use large numbers of SNVs to find associations between genetic variations and diseases. DNA variants are often clustered into regions by genetic recombination during the formation of sperm and eggs that are inherited as a unit, such that a unique SNV pattern or haplotype can be passed from generation to generation. The International HapMap Project also uses SNVs to investigate haplotype associations and disease.

The 1000 Genomes Project complements the previously mentioned projects by sequencing a large number of diverse human samples from around the world. The goal is to build a comprehensive catalog of the most common human genetic variants, which includes single nucleotide variants, as well as insertions, deletions, and copy number variants that are found in the population at greater than 1%. The Exome Aggregation Consortium (ExAC) has sequenced over 60,000 exomes to delineate common genetic variation within human exomes. The SNP database, International HapMap Project, 1000 Genomes Project, ExAC, and genome-wide association studies have helped to define genetic variability within individuals and populations to understand the basis of many genetic diseases.[98]

A more fundamental biology project is the encyclopedia of DNA elements, or ENCODE, whose goal is a catalog of the functional elements of the genomes of humans and other species. The functional elements include the genes and all their expressed RNA forms and epigenetic modifications.[51] One of the most important findings is the discovery that much of the human genome is expressed into RNA.

With the introduction of the first massively parallel DNA sequencing instrument in 2005 and subsequent instruments from 2006 onward, the current technologic era of genomics has progressed over the last decade to make significant inroads into applying genomics to patient care.[99] Along with the technologic innovation in DNA sequencing, there has been innovation in bioinformatics, which is required to manage and interpret the large amount of information generated by massively parallel DNA sequencing instruments.

Although the Human Genome Project is a significant feat, it was not the first whole genome to be sequenced. Whole genome sequencing initially focused on infectious pathogens, because of their impact on human health and also their size. The first free-living organism to be sequenced was *Haemophilus influenzae* in 1995.[100] Subsequently, many species from a cross-section of living organisms have been sequenced. The first individual human to have their whole genome sequenced was Craig Venter, who led one of the two groups that first sequenced the human genome. The second person to have their whole genome sequenced was James Watson, whose genome was the first to be sequenced by using massively parallel DNA sequencing.

An important clinical application of genomics is cancer diagnostics (see Chapters 50 and 51); however, the diversity and complexity of cancer requires a significant amount of basic biological information to interpret molecular diagnostic testing results of patient samples. The first whole genome sequencing of a cancer was an acute myeloid leukemia in 2008,[101] and many others have subsequently been sequenced. The Cancer Genome Atlas project includes large numbers of the most common cancers to identify all their associated mutations. For example, a recent study describes mutational data for 12 of the most common cancers.[102] The significant amount of basic information now available on human cancers and the availability of new therapeutics targeting specific cancer-associated genes allow the clinical use of molecular profiling in cancer patients.[103]

With the increasing use of genetic and genomic information to characterize a patient's disease, an interesting convergence of electronic medical records and genomics is emerging. The implementation of electronic medical records throughout the United States will allow for greater access to the large amount of genomic data that will be available on patients, which will eventually be a source for scientific research and discovery. The Electronic Medical Records and Genomics Network is currently developing tools and conditions under which genomic research can be pursued using electronic medical records.[104]

All of the previously discussed advances have made the field of molecular diagnostics an important and exciting area that is going to have an even greater impact on medicine in the future. As an increasing number of diseases are characterized at the molecular (eg, nucleic acid and protein) level, new therapeutics and diagnostics specifically targeting these molecular changes will continue to emerge.

POINTS TO REMEMBER

- The two strands of DNA are bound together by hydrogen bonds and stacking forces that can be broken and reformed without permanent damage to the DNA. This important property is exploited by many of the methods that are used in molecular diagnostics. This is a requirement for most of the DNA diagnostic assays.
- Even though human DNA has approximately 20,000 genes, this is far less than what would be expected given the number of proteins in a human cell. The higher number of proteins results from alternative splicing, which occurs in more than 95% of human genes.
- Only 1.2% to 1.5% of the human genome is translated into protein; however, much more of the genome is made into RNA.
- The conversion of DNA information into protein is facilitated by aminoacyl tRNA synthetases and their ability to create amino acid–specific tRNAs.
- The genetic code is redundant; the 3-base code can have 64 different combinations, but only 20 amino acids are recognized.

SELECTED REFERENCES

For a full list of references for this chapter, please refer to ExpertConsult.com.

7. Watson JD, Crick FH. Genetical implications of the structure of deoxyribonucleic acid. *Nature* 1953;**171**:964–7.

13. Nirenberg M, Leder P, Bernfield M, et al. RNA codewords and protein synthesis. VII. On the general nature of the RNA code. *Proc Natl Acad Sci USA* 1965;**53**:1161–8.
31. Venter JC, Adams MD, Myers EW, et al. The sequence of the human genome. *Science* 2001;**291**:1304–51.
35. Crick F. Central dogma of molecular biology. *Nature* 1970;**227**:561–3.
36. O'Donnell M, Langston L, Stillman B. Principles and concepts of DNA replication in bacteria, archaea, and eukarya. *Cold Spring Harb Perspect Biol* 2013;**5**:a010108.
38. Iyama T, Wilson DM 3rd. DNA repair mechanisms in dividing and non-dividing cells. *DNA Repair (Amst)* 2013;**12**:620–36.
44. Sharp PA. The discovery of split genes and RNA splicing. *Trends Biochem Sci* 2005;**30**:279–81.
45. Maston GA, Evans SK, Green MR. Transcriptional regulatory elements in the human genome. *Annu Rev Genom Hum Genet* 2006;**7**:29–59.
57. Wahl MC, Will CL, Luhrmann R. The spliceosome: design principles of a dynamic RNP machine. *Cell* 2009;**136**:701–18.
59. Kornblihtt AR, Schor IE, Allo M, et al. Alternative splicing: a pivotal step between eukaryotic transcription and translation. *Nat Rev Mol Cell Biol* 2013;**14**:153–65.
62. Jackson RJ, Hellen CU, Pestova TV. The mechanism of eukaryotic translation initiation and principles of its regulation. *Nat Rev Mol Cell Biol* 2010;**11**: 113–27.
68. Reinstein E, Ciechanover A. Narrative review: protein degradation and human diseases: the ubiquitin connection. *Ann Intern Med* 2006;**145**:676–84.
75. Schubeler D. Function and information content of DNA methylation. *Nature* 2015;**517**:321–6.
77. Zhang G, Pradhan S. Mammalian epigenetic mechanisms. *IUBMB Life* 2014;**66**:240–56.
88. ENCODE Project C. An integrated encyclopedia of DNA elements in the human genome. *Nature* 2012;**489**:57–74.
89. Djebali S, Davis CA, Merkel A, et al. Landscape of transcription in human cells. *Nature* 2012;**489**:101–8.
90. Castel SE, Martienssen RA. RNA interference in the nucleus: roles for small RNAs in transcription, epigenetics and beyond. *Nat Rev Genet* 2013;**14**:100–12.
97. International Human Genome Sequencing C. Finishing the euchromatic sequence of the human genome. *Nature* 2004;**431**:931–45.
98. Green ED, Guyer MS, National Human Genome Research Institute. Charting a course for genomic medicine from base pairs to bedside. *Nature* 2011;**470**:204–13.
99. Wheeler DA, Wang L. From human genome to cancer genome: the first decade. *Genome Res* 2013;**23**:1054–62.

45

Genomes and Variants

Carl T. Wittwer and Jason Y. Park

ABSTRACT

Background

One of the defining achievements of the early 21st century is the sequencing and alignment of more than 90% of the human genome. Of course, there is not a single human genome: individuals differ from each other by about 0.1% and from other primates by about 1%. Variation comes in many different forms, including single base changes and copy number changes in large segments of DNA. Even more challenging than sequencing the whole genome is documenting and understanding the clinical significance of human sequence variation. We are still very early in our understanding of the human genome.

Content

Beginning with a historical perspective, the structure of the human genome is described in detail followed by comparison to other interesting species. Then different types of genomic variation are covered, including single base changes (substitutions, deletions, insertions), copy number variations, translocations and fusions, short tandem repeats of different size and number, and larger repetitive segments, some of which can hop around the genome as transposons. The function of different genomic elements is considered along with many different classes of RNA transcribed from the DNA. How to name all the different genes, variants, and elements is a daunting task, and accepted nomenclature is presented. Many databases are available to mine accumulated genomic information. We end with a description of basic informatics tools that provide a pipeline from the raw data of massively parallel DNA sequencing to finished sequence with annotations on the variations that are observed.

It is easy to be carried away by the detectable peculiarities and to forget that much underlying variability is still hidden from view until some new technical device discloses the finer structure of chromosomes ...

Lionel Penrose, Chicago, Ill., Third ISCN Consensus Conference, 1966[1]

INTRODUCTION

In 1966 it was recognized that the effort to characterize human cytogenetic variation was only the tip of the iceberg in terms of our understanding of genetic detail and that many more types of variation would be revealed with advancing technology. Since the time when DNA was discovered as the major molecule for genetic inheritance, there has been a need to understand how DNA variations affect growth, development, and disease. Even after 50 years of advances in DNA technology, many types of DNA variation have yet to be identified, named, cataloged, and studied.

HUMAN GENOME

The word *genome* signifies the collection of genes in an organism and is believed to have been coined by the German botanist Hans Winkler in the 1920s.[2] The human genome encompasses all of the information needed for growth, development, and heredity. This information is copied in the nucleus of every cell in the body.[3]

Throughout the 1990s, there was an international effort to sequence the human genome. The first draft was released in 2001[4,5] followed by a more complete version in 2004.[6] The 2004 version contains 2.85 billion nucleotides (bases) and is considered 99% complete for euchromatic (actively transcribed) DNA. The overall size of the genome, including both euchromatic and heterochromatic sequences (tightly compact DNA found at centromeres and telomeres), is estimated to be 3.08 billion nucleotides. Thus, the total overall genome is only 92.5% complete. Within the 2.85 billion nucleotides of euchromatic DNA are 19,438 known genes and an additional 2188 predicted genes. The total number of nucleotides encoding protein is approximately 34 million (1.2%) of the genome. This portion of the genome encoding proteins is also known as the *exome*.

The 2004 genome contains 341 gaps in heterochromatic regions.[6] These regions could not be sequenced because of the presence of DNA that is difficult to sequence (eg, repetitive elements, GC-rich sequence) by existing technology or because no clone or template could be made for sequencing. The 2004 genome provides the reference sequence for most subsequent sequencing projects. A reference is required because commonly used DNA sequencing technologies require a scaffold on which sequence fragments are pieced together.[7]

The first human reference sequences were assembled by the University of California at Santa Cruz (UCSC) and were numbered starting with "hg1" in May 2000. The National Center for Biotechnology Information (NCBI) produced its own genome builds starting in December 2001 as NCBI build 28 (equivalent to hg10 from UCSC) as the genome was further refined. This led to the publicly available 2004 version of the human genome becoming known as NCBI35/hg17. This template or reference sequence has subsequently undergone continuous improvement under the international Genome Reference Consortium (GRC),[7] producing GRCh37/hg19. In the future, only one designation will be given, such as the currently released GRCh38.[3]

Ten years after the 2004 genome publication, efforts are underway to create "platinum genomes" that address the missing information (gaps) and improve the quality of data.[8] One group has sequenced several previous gaps by using DNA from a haploid cell line.[9] Another group has combined several long-read sequencing technologies to create a de novo assembly that does not require the use of a reference genome.[10] This approach dramatically improves the mapping of sequences generated and can be combined with data from short-read sequencing instruments.[10] Thus, hybrid sequencing methods are emerging that combine the advantages of short-read sequencing for single nucleotide base accuracy with the advantages of long-read sequencing for de novo assembly without a reference genome.[10] Ongoing improvements in sequencing technology are predicted to further decrease the gaps in human genome data and reveal new mechanisms of human variation. Genomic terms and definitions used in this chapter are given in Box 45.1.

Each human cell contains two copies of the 3.08-billion-nucleotide genome divided into 46 chromosomes. Table 45.1 summarizes statistics for the human genome and the types of variations that are important in clinical diagnostics. Three quarters of human DNA is intergenic or between genes. More than 60% of this intergenic sequence consists of "parasitic" DNA regions of mostly defective transposable elements 100 to 11,000 bases in length. Between 2 and 3 million of these "retrotransposons" are present in each copy of the genome. They contribute to genetic recombination and chromosome structure and provide an evolutionary record of sequence variation and selection.

Segmental duplications constitute 5.3% of the human genome. They are more than 1 kilobase (1000 bases or Kb) in length, have a sequence identity of at least 90%, and are not transposable. Segmental duplications are common in the human genome and are prone to deletion or rearrangement (or both), often with medical consequences. Intergenic DNA also carries most of the simple sequence repeats (SSRs) present in the genome. A subset of SSRs, the short tandem repeats (STRs) have repeat units of 1 to several bases that may be repeated up to thousands of times. STRs have played a large role in genetic linkage studies and in forensic and medical identity testing. They are formed by slippage during replication and are highly polymorphic among individuals. The most common STRs are dinucleotide repeats, such as ACACAC and ATAT. On average, one STR occurs every 2000 bases.

Approximately 2% of DNA is required to maintain the structure of chromosomes and is located at chromosome centers (centromeres) and ends (telomeres), making up heterochromatic DNA. Centromeric DNA includes many tandem copies of nearly identical 171 base pair (bp) repeats encompassing 0.24 to 5.0 Mb per chromosome. Each chromosome end is capped with several Kb of the telomeric 6 base repeat TTAGGG. Although intergenic DNA does not code for protein and was originally considered "junk," much of this DNA is transcribed to RNA, producing a complex "transcriptome" network of RNA control elements whose function and mechanics are active areas of investigation.[11]

One quarter of the human genome consists of genes. There are 19,438 known genes in addition to 2188 predicted genes in the human genome. The average gene covers 27,000 bases, but only about 1300 of these bases code for amino acids. The primary RNA transcript is processed by splicing to retain exons that are interspersed throughout the gene and have a higher GC content than noncoding regions. On average, 95% of a gene is excised as introns, retaining a mean of 10.4 exons, of which on average 9.1 are translated into proteins. Exons make up only 1.9% of the total genome, with 1.2% of the genome coding for proteins. Some important genes are present in many copies, so that overall protein expression is not affected if a chance variation occurs in one copy. If extra copies of genes lose their function, they are known as pseudogenes. At least as many pseudogenes as functional genes are present in the human genome. It is important to distinguish pseudogenes from functional genes because variants in pseudogenes are seldom of clinical importance, and they often complicate DNA diagnostic assays.

POINTS TO REMEMBER

Human Genome

- Contains approximately 3 billion bases
- Protein coding nucleotides are about 1% (30 million bases)
- Noncoding sequence has important regulatory roles

VARIATIONS IN SPECIFIC POPULATIONS

Large-scale human genome sequencing projects have cast a wide net across many diverse populations. These projects have provided a wealth of knowledge of the genetic diversity that exists in humans. An alternative approach to human genetic diversity is to examine more homogenous populations. Several studies have examined the genetics of a large number of individuals from Iceland. A recent whole-genome sequencing study of 2636 Icelanders observed 20 million single nucleotide variations (SNVs) and 1.5 million insertions/deletions (indels).[12] The data from this whole genome sequencing study were combined with a previous data set of 104,220 Icelanders who had been SNV typed at 676,913 locations. By applying whole-genome sequencing data from only a small subset of individuals, the full genetics could be inferred for a larger set of more than 100,000 individuals who had only had SNV typing.

Another interesting result of the Icelandic whole-genome study was the identification of 6795 loss of function single nucleotide variants, insertions, or deletions in 4924 genes.[13] Loss of function changes (homozygous or compound heterozygous) were found in 7.7% of the individuals sequenced. In essence, this study identified a surprisingly high percentage of individuals with "knocked-out" or functionally silenced genes.

BOX 45.1 Genomic Terms and Definitions

Annotation: Biologic information attached to genomic sequence.

Annotation Track: Optional metadata in a genome browser that allows viewing of genes, exons, SNVs, repeats, etc.

Assembly: Reconstruction of short sequence reads on a scaffold of reference DNA.

Binary alignment nap (BAM): After alignment to a reference genome, the aligned data for each read produces a sequence alignment map (SAM file). The BAM file is the binary equivalent of the SAM file, and allows for efficient random access of the data.

Browser extensible data (BED): A tab delimited text file that defines the data lines in an annotation track, including the chromosome name, the starting and the ending positions.

Contig: A linear stretch of consensus sequence assembled from smaller overlapping sequence fragments.

Copy number polymorphism (CNP): A copy number variant present at more than 1% in a population.

Copy number variant (CNV): A structural variant of a large region of the genome that has been deleted or duplicated.

Deletion: A DNA sequence that is missing in one sample compared to another. Deletions may be as small as one nucleotide or as large as an entire chromosome.

***De novo* assembly:** Formation of a contig without using a reference sequence.

FASTA File: A nucleotide sequence text file.

FASTQ file: A text output file of sequencing reads in a run, along with the quality scores of each position.

Fusion: A translocation, inversion, large deletion or large duplication resulting in a hybrid gene formed from originally separate genes.

Indel: Originally referred to a unique class of sequence variants that included both an insertion and a deletion resulting in an overall change in the number of base pairs. Today more commonly refers to either insertions or deletions or a combination thereof.

Insertion: An extra DNA sequence that is present in one sample compared with a reference sequence.

Heteroplasmy: A mixture of more than one type of mitochondrial sequence in one cell.

Intergenic: DNA sequence between genes.

Missense: A nucleotide substitution that changes a codon to the code for a different amino acid. Although these sequence changes are commonly referred to as missense "mutations," this is strictly a misnomer because missense variants may be benign and cause no disease.

Mutation: A disease-causing sequence variation. Historically, the term has been interchangeable with variant to describe any change in DNA sequence regardless of relation to disease causation. For current clinical descriptions or reporting, the use of mutation is reserved for the scenario when disease causation is known.

Nonsense: A nucleotide substitution that results in a stop codon, prematurely terminating the protein.

Nonsynonymous: Nucleotide substitutions that are predicted to change the amino acid coding. These substitutions include both missense and nonsense substitutions.

Oligonucleotide: A short single-stranded polymer of nucleic acid.

Phred score: Estimate of the error probability for a base called in DNA sequencing. It is represented as a Q-score; the higher the number, the higher the probability of a correct call.

Plasmid: An extrachromosomal ring of double-stranded, closed DNA found in bacteria.

Pseudogene: A genetic element that does not code for a functional gene product, usually because of accumulated sequence variations.

Sequence alignment map (SAM file): A file generated by alignment of sequence data to a reference genome. This file type is often converted to a BAM file to save space.

Short tandem repeat (STR): A simple sequence repeat that is 1–13 bases long.

Simple sequence repeat (SSR): A sequence from 1-500 bases that is repeated end to end. If the repeat unit is 1-13 bases, it is a microsatellite or STR. If the repeat is 14-500 bases it is a minisatellite.

Single nucleotide polymorphism (SNP): A benign single nucleotide variant (substitution, deletion, or insertion) that occurs in a population at a frequency of at least 1%.

Single nucleotide variation (SNV): A single nucleotide variant (substitution, deletion, or insertion). SNVs may be benign or may cause disease.

Structural variation: A region of DNA greater than 1000 bases in size that is inverted, translocated, inserted, or deleted.

Synonymous variant: A nucleotide change that results in no change to the predicted amino acid sequence. Although synonymous variants are typically considered to be benign since there is no protein coding change, there is the possibility of pathogenicity by changes in splicing, gene expression or mRNA stability.

Transposon: A mobile genetic element that can delete and insert itself variably into the genome.

Variant call format (VCF): After aligning all reads onto a reference sequence, variants that are different from the reference genome at a given nucleotide position are stored in a text file in a specific format.

Variation: A change in DNA sequence. It may be benign or may cause disease.

NONHUMAN GENOMES

Before the human genome was completed, other genomes of smaller size were sequenced, enabling advancements in technology and logistical organization to sequence the human genome.[14,15] Different genomes are varied in size, and the complexity can be surprising. One of the largest known genomes is the white spruce tree *(Picea glauca)* at 26.9 billion bases. On the opposite end of the spectrum is porcine circovirus-1, a single-stranded DNA virus with a genome that is less than 2000 bases. There is overlap in genome size among eukaryotes (animals, plants, fungi), viruses, and bacteria (Table 45.2 and Fig. 45.1).

Primates

Comparison of the chimpanzee genome with the human genome shows a genome-wide difference of only 1.23%.[16] This approximate 1% difference translates to 35 million

TABLE 45.1 The Human Genome and Its Sequence Variation

The Human Genome	
3.08 billion base pairs in 24 chromosomes	
23 chromosome pairs (46–244 million base pairs per chromosome)	
75% Intergenic Sequences	
Transposable elements	45%
Segmental duplications	5%
Simple sequence repeat	3%
Structural (centromeres, telomeres)	2%
Other	20%
25% Genes That Code for Proteins	
Introns	23%
Exons	1.9%
• Coding segments	1.2%
• Untranslated regions	0.7%
Number of genes	19,438 known 2,188 predicted
Average gene	27,000 base pairs 10.4 exons 9.1 transcribed exons 1340 exonic bases 446 amino acids
Sequence Variants	
99.9% identity (one difference every 1250 bases between randomly selected haploid genomes)	
Single-Nucleotide Variants (SNVs): Identified Every 75 Bases on Average	
Noncoding	97%
Average number within a gene	126
Average number within the coding region of a gene	5
Copy Number Variants (CNVs): Involves 5%–12% of the Genome	
Disease-Causing Variants	
SNVs	68%
• Missense (amino acid substitution)	45%
• Nonsense (termination)	11%
• Splicing	10%
• Regulatory	2%
Small insertions or deletions (or both)	24%
Structural variants (copy number variations, inversions, translocations, rearrangements, repeats)	8%
Epigenetic Alterations	
Variable initiation and alternative splicing	
Cytosine methylation	
Histone phosphorylation, methylation, acetylation	

Data from Lander et al,[4] Venter et al,[5] and International Human Genome Sequencing Consortium.[6]

TABLE 45.2 *Homo Sapiens* in Comparison to Other Genomes

Organism/Name	Group	Size (Mb)
Human *(Homo sapiens)*	Animals	3080
White spruce tree *(Picea glauca)*	Plants	26,900
Migratory locust *(Locusta migratoria)*	Animals	5760
Mouse *(Mus musculus)*	Animals	~2500
Rat *(Rattus norvegicus)*	Animals	~2750
Apple tree *(Malus domestica)*	Plants	742
Roundworm *(Caenorhabditis elegans)*	Animals	97
Aspergillus fumigatus	Fungi	~30
Baker's yeast *(Saccharomyces cerevisiae)*	Fungi	12.3
Haemophilus influenzae	Bacteria	1.8
Human immunodeficiency virus (HIV) 1	Viruses	0.0092
Porcine circovirus-1	Viruses	0.00173

Data from the National Center for Biotechnology Information. http://www.ncbi.nlm.nih.gov/genome.

nucleotides and 5 million insertion/deletion differences. There are also differences at the level of proteins between humans and chimpanzees: Only 29% of proteins are identical at the amino acid level, and proteins that are different only differ by an average of two amino acids.[16]

Two orangutan species have been sequenced.[17] Their genome sizes are similar to humans at approximately 3 billion bases. During evolutionary development, the number of structural rearrangements in orangutans has been less than the human and chimpanzee branches.[17] For example, the number of genome rearrangements greater than 100 Kb was 38 in the orangutan but 85 and 54 in the chimpanzee and human, respectively.

An example of non–protein-coding variation between primates is the number and types of DNA insertions. A comparison of five primate genomes (chimpanzee, gorilla, orangutan, gibbon, and macaque) identified regions of human DNA that were absent in nonhuman primates.[18] More than 200,000 human-specific DNA insertions were identified; the majority of these were less than 10 nucleotides in length and were eliminated from further study. There were 5582 genes identified that contained larger insertions; 2450 of these genes were expressed in brain tissue. Many of the human-specific insertions were transposable elements and long terminal repeats.[18]

Rodents

The mouse genome is 14% smaller than the human genome (2.5 billion bases compared with the human size of approximately 3 billion bases).[19] In comparison, the rat *(Rattus norvegicus)* genome is in between the size of the human and mouse (2.75 billion bases).[20] The number of genes is similar between the mouse and the human. About 40% of the rat, mouse, and human genomes are all in alignment. Another 30% of the rat and mouse genomes match each other but not the human genome.

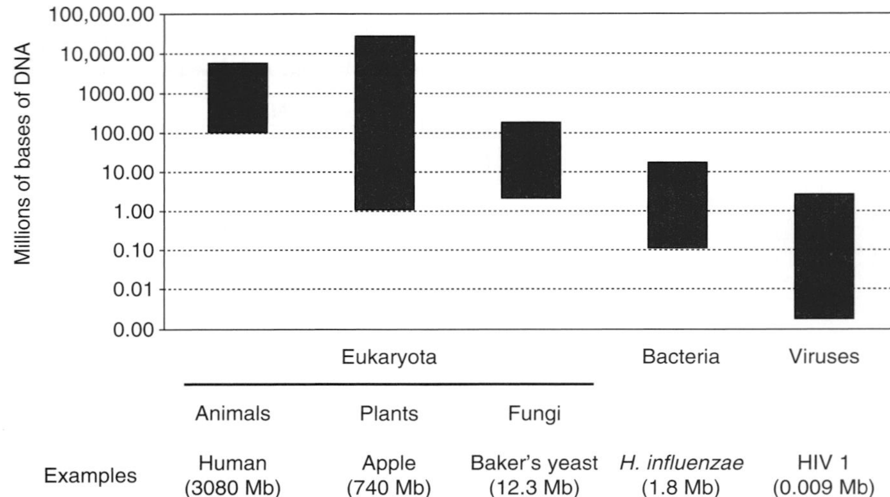

FIGURE 45.1 Range of genome sizes. Among different organisms, there is wide variation in genome size. In this plot of publicly available genomes, the *y*-axis is in megabases, and the *x*-axis lists various organisms: Eukaryota (animals, plants, fungi), bacteria, and viruses. On average, Eukaryota have larger genomes compared with bacteria and viruses; however, there are exceptions in which virus genomes are larger than bacteria or Eukaryota. The difference between the smallest and largest known genomes is more than 6 orders of magnitude. Several specific genome sizes are illustrated in Mb (megabases, million). (Data extracted from the National Center for Biotechnology Information. http://www.ncbi.nlm.nih.gov/genome.)

Fungi

Fungi are eukaryotes and their genomes are less complex than the human genome. Common fungi that cause human disease have genome sizes of 7.5 to 30 million bases and 8 to 16 chromosomes, as well as mitochondrial genomes. Some fungi have diploid genomes, and others have haploid genomes. Many of their genes have introns. For instance, *Aspergillus fumigatus* (a fungus that causes allergic reactions and systemic disease with a high mortality rate) has a haploid genome of about 30 million bases with more than 9900 predicted genes on eight chromosomes. Its genes are smaller than human genes, with an average length of 1400 bp and 2.8 exons per gene.

The first eukaryotic genome sequenced was *Saccharomyces cerevisiae* (baker's yeast).[15] This fungal genome has 12 million bases arranged into 16 chromosomes. In addition to the importance of yeast in baking breads and brewing alcohol, yeast is an important model organism and pathogen. With the identification of the approximately 6000 genes within the *S. cerevisiae* genome, systematic alteration of each gene or combination of genes can now be explored to examine the role of genes in yeast as well as higher organisms.

Bacteria

Bacterial genomes are considerably less complex than human or fungal genomes. Common bacteria have only one chromosome, usually a circular DNA double helix of 4 to 5 million base pairs, about 1000 times less than the amount of DNA in a human cell. About 90% of the DNA in bacteria codes for protein. There are no introns, but there are multiple small intergenic regions of repetitive sequences that are dispersed throughout the genome. *Escherichia coli*, a common bacterium in the human intestinal tract, has about 4300 genes.

In addition to the large circular chromosome that carries essential genes, bacteria also carry accessory genes in smaller circles of double-stranded DNA (dsDNA) known as plasmids. Plasmids range in size from 1000 to more than 1 million base pairs. Plasmids are important in molecular diagnosis of bacterial infections because they often encode pathogenic factors and antibiotic resistance.

The bacterial repertoire of DNA can be altered by (1) gain or loss of plasmids; (2) single-base changes, small insertions and deletions as in eukaryotic genomes; and (3) large segmental rearrangements, including inversions, deletions, and duplications. Some genes, such as those for ribosomal RNA, are present in many copies, making them good targets for molecular assays to identify the species of bacteria. In addition, the intergenic repetitive sequences serve as multiple targets for oligonucleotide probes, enabling the generation of unique DNA profiles or fingerprints for individual bacterial strains.

The first genome sequenced by random fragmentation and computational assembly was the pathogenic bacteria, *Haemophilus influenzae*.[14] The genomic DNA was fragmented into 19,687 templates inserted into plasmids and bacteriophages. A total of 24,304 sequences were successfully generated over 3 months. The sequencing data required 30 hours of computational time to be assembled. A total of 11 million bases of DNA were sequenced and used to generate the 1.8 million bases of the *H. influenzae* genome. In addition to being the first genome solved by shotgun sequencing, it was also the first bacterial genome sequenced. Multiple strains of *H. influenzae* have been subsequently sequenced. These additional genomes have revealed heterogeneity in the number of genes between different strains. Of the approximately 3000 genes identified, only 1461 are common to all strains.[21] The differences in genes among different strains may be associated with differences in the infectious pathogenicity of *H. influenzae*.[21] The success in sequencing the first *H. influenza* genome highlighted the importance and possible

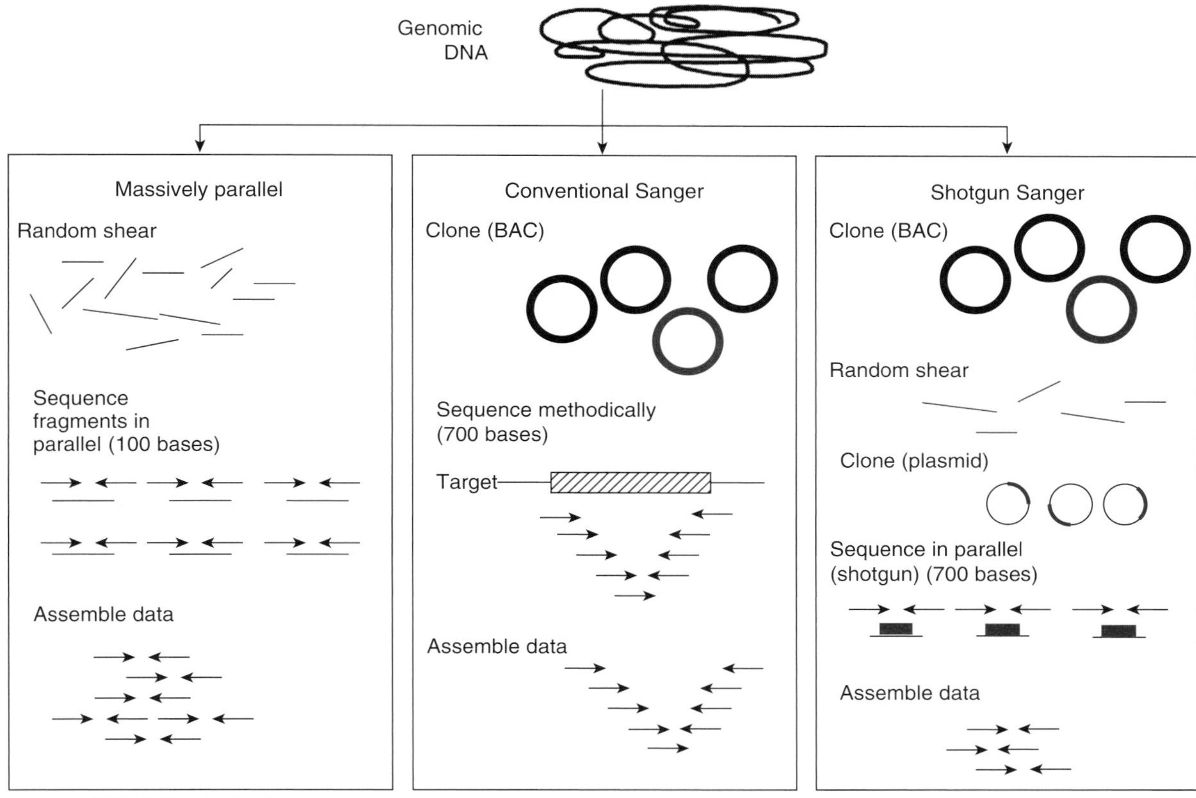

FIGURE 45.2 Genome sequencing approaches. Massively parallel sequencing *(left panel)* is the current technology used for genome sequencing, but it evolved out of earlier conventional Sanger *(middle panel)* and shotgun Sanger *(right panel)* sequencing methods. See text for details. *BAC,* Bacterial artificial chromosomes.

use of shotgun sequencing. Shotgun sequencing became an important technology for the successful completion of the human genome project. The project had begun otherwise, with the orderly "conventional" sequencing of large (150-Kb) fragments of DNA that were divided among members of the consortium and methodically sequenced.

Fig. 45.2 contrasts different sequencing approaches. Massively parallel sequencing is the current technology used for genome sequencing, but it developed out of earlier sequencing methods. When genomic DNA is sequenced by massively parallel sequencing, the basic steps include random DNA shearing (fragmentation), sequencing in parallel reactions, and data assembly *(left panel)*. The randomly sheared fragments are end modified with oligonucleotides that aid in the identification, immobilization, and sequencing of the fragments; this step is referred to as library creation. In the case of whole-genome sequencing, this "library" of modified fragments is then sequenced. However, if only a subset of genes is of interest or if only the coding nucleotides are of interest (exome), the specific targets can be hybridized and "captured" after the library step. Targeted capture of regions of interest is a key step in exome sequencing. More than 1 million sequencing reactions occur in parallel, generating more than 100 bases of data per reaction. After sequencing, the short reads of DNA are assembled based on a reference genome (eg, GRCh38).

In comparison, the conventional sequencing of genomes was the technology used for the initiation of the Human Genome Project (*middle panel* of Fig. 45.2). This method started with the genome cloned into large molecules such as Yeast Artificial Chromosomes (YAC) and later Bacterial Artificial Chromosomes (BAC). These larger molecules, which carried genomic inserts greater than 150 Kb in size, were then divided among the members of the genome sequencing consortium and methodically sequenced in 700 base reactions. Each round of sequencing depends on the sequencing data from the prior round. The assembly of data is not as computational intensive as massively parallel or shotgun sequencing.

Finally, shotgun sequencing was key to the speedy completion of the Human Genome Project (*right panel* of Fig. 45.2). Rather than methodically sequence targets of interest, the method relied on random shearing of DNA and subcloning the fragments into plasmids. The plasmids were then sequenced in parallel (separate) reactions. The evolutionary roots of massively parallel sequencing technology can be followed back to shotgun sequencing.

Viruses

Viral genomes are considerably less complex than bacterial genomes. Common viruses that infect humans vary in size from about 5000 to 250,000 bases, or 20 to 1000 times less than the amount of nucleic acid in *E. coli*. Because viruses use the host's cellular machinery, they do not need as many genes as bacteria. Small viruses may encode only several genes, but the larger viruses can encode hundreds. The viral genome consists of either DNA or RNA, and the nucleic acid may be single stranded or double stranded, linear or circular, with one or multiple fragments or copies per viral particle. As in bacteria, there are no introns. In fact, in some viruses the exons overlap with different reading frames coding different products from the same nucleic acid sequence. Noncoding regions are usually present at the terminal ends of linear genomes. Repeat segments are often found as terminal or internal repeats and may be inverted.

Sequence alterations in viruses are common. Areas of high sequence variation may be interspersed between conserved domains. Higher frequencies of variation correlate with lower polymerase fidelity and may allow escape from antibody recognition and antiviral drugs. Common sequence variants in viruses include single base changes, insertions, and deletions. Sequence diversity within a viral species may be so great that consensus sequences for molecular typing are difficult to find.

DNA THAT CODES FOR RNA BUT NOT PROTEIN

Even though 99% of the genome does not code for protein, most of it is transcribed into noncoding RNA. At least 93% of the genome is transcribed,[11] producing more than 10 times the amount of RNA than is produced from the coding segments of genes.[22] Both strands of DNA may be transcribed, and long noncoding transcripts may overlap coding regions, producing a complex transcriptome of functional RNA molecules that may variably regulate transcription of coding regions, RNA processing, mRNA stability, translation, protein stability, and secretion. In addition to long noncoding RNA, ribosomal RNA, and transfer RNA, specific classes of noncoding RNAs include small nuclear RNAs critical for splicing, small nucleolar RNAs that modify rRNA, telomerase RNA for maintenance of telomeres, small interfering RNAs, and microRNAs (miRNAs) that regulate gene expression.[23-25] In a recent review on RNA, 54 different categories were identified.[26] Some of the more important types of RNA are listed in Table 45.3.

TABLE 45.3 Some Common, Interesting, and Important Types of RNA

Abbreviation	Description
mRNA	Messenger RNA is translated to protein by the ribosome.
rRNA	Ribosomal RNA is a major component of ribosomes.
tRNA	Transfer RNA pairs an amino acid with its anticodon in protein synthesis.
ncRNA	Noncoding RNA is not translated to protein.
lncRNA	Long noncoding RNA is greater than 200 bases and is not translated to protein.
hnRNA	Heterogeneous nuclear RNA is the initial RNA transcript that includes introns.
Ribozyme	RNA that has catalytic activity.
Riboswitch	RNA that switches between 2 conformations under certain conditions (ligand exposure).
Telomerase RNA	Structural part of telomerase that also provides a hexamer template.
Xist RNA	X-inactive–specific transcript RNA inactivates one X chromosome in females.
snRNA	Small nuclear RNA is found in the eukaryotic nucleus.
snoRNA	Small nucleolar RNA are intron fragments essential for pre-rRNA processing.
siRNA	Small interfering RNA can cleave perfectly complementary target RNA.
gRNA	Guide RNA pairs with a RNA target and guides proteins for cleavage and so on.
miRNA	MicroRNA affects target mRNA regulation or decay.

MicroRNAs (or miRNAs) are particularly interesting as potential markers for disease. For example, circulating miRNAs have been correlated to many different types of cancer.[27] MicroRNAs are noncoding but functional single-stranded RNAs that are 21 to 22 bases long and are expressed in a tissue-specific manner. They are initially transcribed as longer precursors that undergo two rounds of truncations as they are transported from the nucleus to the cytoplasm in the cell. The mature miRNA is then integrated into a protein complex called the *RNA-induced silencing complex*, which regulates translation of mRNA. MicroRNAs hybridize to a 6 to 8 base sequence in the 3′ untranslated region of target mRNAs and inhibit mRNA expression either by mRNA degradation if the bases are perfectly complementary or by blocking of translation if they are imperfectly complementary. Currently for humans, there are 1881 precursor miRNAs and 2588 mature miRNAs cataloged in miRBase.[28] Despite the promise of miRNAs as tumor markers, the literature is often contradictory and inconsistent with few accepted conclusions.[29]

VARIATION IN THE HUMAN GENOME

If the DNA of any two individuals is compared, on average, one difference is noted every 1250 bases (ie, approximately 99.9% of the sequence is identical between randomly chosen copies of the human genome). However, copy-number variants involve a greater amount of the genome, with 0.5% of the genome differing on average between two individuals when copy-number variants greater than 50 Kb are considered.[30] That is, between individuals, at least five times as many bases are affected by copy number changes as by small sequence differences.

Most human genetic material is present in two copies, with the exception of the unpaired sex chromosome in males and mitochondrial DNA. The presence of only single gene copies on the X and Y chromosome in males leads to well-known sex-linked disorders. In contrast, the 16,500-bp mitochondrial genome is present in multiple copies per cell, constituting about 0.3% of human DNA, depending on the tissue source. Allele fractions may vary over a wide range when all mitochondria in a cell are considered. That is, sequence variations in mitochondrial DNA are heteroplasmic, meaning that the ratio of the wild-type allele to a variant allele can vary almost continuously, sometimes resulting in a wide range of symptoms even when only one sequence variant is involved.

Any sequence change from a reference sequence is called a sequence variant or variation. Many variations do not affect human health and are benign or silent. For example, most (1) copy-number variations, (2) SNVs, and (3) STRs found between genes are seldom associated with disease.

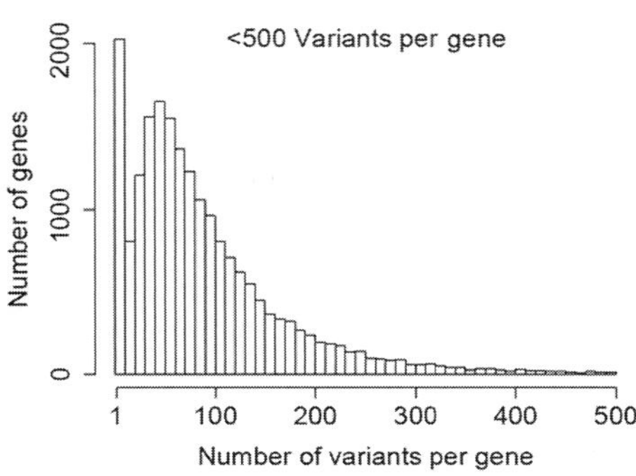

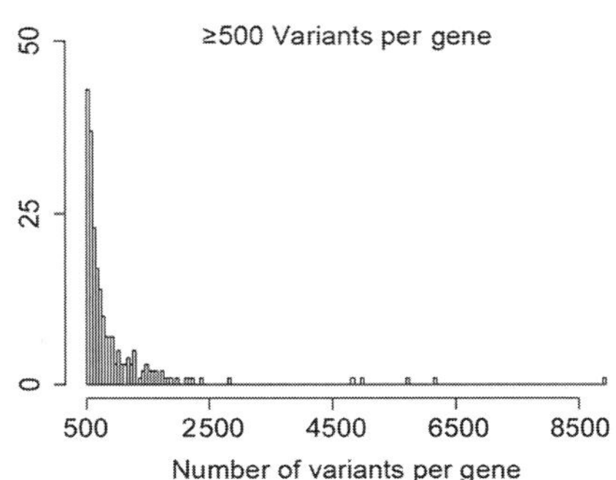

FIGURE 45.3 High number of variants per gene. In an examination of allelic heterogeneity, the Leiden Open Variation Database (LOVD) was queried for the number of unique alleles (variants) per gene. In the *left panel* are the genes with fewer than 500 variants per gene, and in the *right panel* are the genes with 500 or more variants per gene. The panels clearly demonstrate that there are currently thousands of genes with hundreds of variants and dozens of genes with thousands of variants. This high number of variants per gene is important in considering that the majority of variants are of unknown clinical significance. (From Cutting GR. Annotating DNA variants is the next major goal for human genetics. *Am J Hum Genet* 2014;94:5-10.)

Single Nucleotide Variants

The most common sequence variations are single base changes, also known as SNVs. More than 40 million SNVs have been described, and many new SNVs continue to be reported. Some SNVs are common in the population, with allele frequencies of 0.1 to 0.5 (ie, present in 10–50 of every 100 copies studied), but other single base changes are very rare. The vast majority of SNVs (97%) occur in noncoding regions; only 3% of SNVs are associated with exons. Similarly, most of the SNVs within introns, except for splicing and regulatory variants, are not known to affect gene function. In addition, some of the SNVs within exons are silent alterations that do not code for a change in amino acid sequence because of the redundancy in the genetic code. Still other SNVs in exons code for amino acid changes that do not affect protein function. However, some silent SNVs may affect DNA splicing, and others are of interest as genetic markers.

The international 1000 Genomes Project has a goal of sequencing approximately 2500 individuals representing populations from Europe, East Asia, South Asia, West Africa, and the Americas.[31] A report from this project on 1092 individuals from 14 populations mapped 38 million single nucleotide variants, 1.4 million short insertions and/or deletions, and more than 14,000 large deletions.[32] Individuals were found to have on average 3.6 to 3.9 million variants, of which 2300 to 2700 were nonsynonymous. Variants classified as disease causing were more than 10 per individual.

Another examination of SNVs revealed that there can be thousands of variants in each gene. These variants may or may not cause disease. In the current age of genomics, the lack of understanding of disease causation based on variant identification is referred to as an "interpretive gap."[33] In the Leiden Open Variation Database (LOVD), there are currently hundreds to thousands of variants identified for each gene (Fig. 45.3). However, the disease classification of these variants (eg, benign or pathogenic) lags far behind the ability to discover these variants.[33] Sequence alterations that are known to cause disease are often called *mutations, pathogenic variants,* or *disease-causing variants.* About 68% of known disease-causing variants involve only a single base change. Most of the remaining disease-causing variants (24%) are small insertions or deletions. The remainder (8%) includes more complex structural variations (see Table 45.1).

Most SNVs that cause disease are missense and result in an amino acid substitution; significantly fewer are nonsense variants that result in a termination codon and premature polypeptide chain termination. Approximately 10% of disease-causing variants are SNVs that affect splicing sites and result in altered concatenation of coding sequences. Finally, fewer than 2% of known disease-causing variants are SNVs that affect the regulatory efficiency of transcription by altering promoter and/or enhancer regions in introns or the stability of the RNA transcript.

Small insertion and/or deletion variants account for 24% of variants that cause disease. An insertion refers to the presence of extra bases, and deletion implies the absence of certain bases in comparison with a reference sequence. Insertions and deletions often cause a shift of the codon reading frame, resulting in altered amino acid sequence downstream of the variation—commonly followed by chain termination from a nonsense codon.

The remaining 8% of variants that relate to health and disease are mostly structural variants, including (1) duplications or deletions of entire exons or genes; (2) gene fusions, including chromosomal translocations and inversions; (3) STR expansions (eg, an increased number of trinucleotide repeats); (4) gene rearrangements (eg, rearrangements of immunoglobulin genes in B cells that are required for production of antibodies); (5) complex polymorphic loci related to health and disease (eg, human leukocyte antigens); and (6) copy number variants (CNVs).

Copy Number Variation (Gains and Losses)

Although SNVs are the most common sequence variant, CNVs cover more of the genome than SNVs. Examples of large gains or losses in genomic DNA have been known for many years with, for example, syndromic diseases. However, an examination of phenotypically normal individuals by array-based comparative genomic hybridization revealed an average of 12.4 large copy number variations per individual.[34] Some variants reached 2 million bases of DNA in phenotypically normal individuals. CNVs may be duplicated in tandem or may involve complex gains or losses of homologous sequences at multiple sites in the genome. CNV regions exist in every chromosome and involve 5% to 12% of the human genome.[30,35]

High-resolution comparative genomic hybridization has now revealed the presence of deletions across hundreds of additional individuals.[36-39] In total, these studies revealed more than 1000 unique deletions. Some deletions are in regions without known genes; however, hundreds of known or predicted genes exist at the site of the observed deletions. Interest in CNVs in relation to disease has increased recently as the extent of variation has become clear.[40] CNVs can involve genes or contiguous sets of genes. When the normal dosage of the gene is two but more than two functional copies of a gene are present, then the gene is "amplified." If a dosage-sensitive gene, such as HER2 *(ERBB2)* is amplified, it usually leads to overexpression of mRNA and protein, resulting in cellular abnormalities and possible progression to diseases such as cancer. When the normal gene dosage is two and loss of one of the functional copies of the gene occurs, disorders such as mental retardation and developmental delay may result. Structural variants can be determined by cytogenetic techniques, including karyotyping, fluorescent in situ hybridization, comparative genomic hybridization, and virtual karyotyping by SNV microarrays.

Fusions

Gene fusions arise by deletions, duplications, inversions, and translocations and are commonly found in cancer.[41] Often they arise by balanced translocations, whereby a chimeric protein is created by the fusion of two coding regions. Gene fusions promote tumor proliferation by either activating an oncogenic driver or inactivating a tumor suppressor. Although translocations are rare outside of cancer, massively parallel sequencing now allows insight into the myriad of translocations that occur in both hematologic and solid tumors. By identifying gene fusions that act as primary oncogenic drivers, the hope is that targeted therapies may be available for precision treatment.

Short Tandem Repeats

Short tandem repeats are DNA motifs that are defined by 1 to several bases that are repeated many times in tandem. STRs have been implicated in more than 40 genetic diseases.[42] In the case of fragile X, an expansion of a CGG repeat results in disruption of protein expression of the *FMR1* gene. For Huntington disease, an expansion of a CAG repeat results in abnormal protein expression of the *HTT* gene. Many massively parallel sequencing platforms use short reads of information that are less than 200 bases in length, and these short reads have made the analysis of repetitive sequences difficult. Thus, the current contribution of repetitive DNA to human variation and disease is probably underestimated. There is speculation that sequencing technology with longer reads of information in the thousands of bases will reliably detect repetitive DNA elements. In addition to advances in sequencing technology, there are promising informatics tools for characterizing repetitive DNA elements in standard massively parallel sequencing data sets.

One group proposes a "thesaurus" approach in which an extensive catalog of repetitive DNA elements is used within the existing analysis framework.[43] The catalog contains almost 3 billion entries that are representative of the variety of repetitive elements seen in a human genome. This approach was successful in detecting novel variants without extensive changes to typical analysis approaches. Massively parallel sequencing technology and informatics are limited in the amount of STR data that is sequenced and analyzed. A recent informatics tool, lobSTR, can accurately genotype STRs from massively parallel sequencing datasets.[44] When lobSTR was applied across whole-genome datasets from the 1000 Genomes Project, 700,000 STR loci were catalogued, and 350,000 STR loci were found per individual.[42] Some STR loci were common with 300,000 having a mean allele frequency of more than 1%, and 2237 were located within 20 bases of an exon–intron junction.[42] The high frequency of STR loci and their proximity to coding DNA suggest a larger role for STR variants in influencing growth, development, and disease.

Transposable Elements and Their Genetic Fossils

Transposable elements are composed of repetitive DNA that could originally facilitate homologous recombination or create deletions, duplications, inversions, and translocations.[45] Most of these elements are no longer active and are categorized as retrotransposons, including long terminal repeats (LTRs), long interspersed nuclear elements (LINEs), and short interspersed nuclear elements (SINEs). In a conservative estimate not including repeat-rich regions such as centromeres, these elements were found to comprise 30% to 50% of the total DNA in mammals. In comparison, the genomes of birds were less than 10% derived from transposable elements.[45]

In one human study, repetitive DNA including transposable elements and their nonfunctional descendants were estimated to consume 66% to 69% of the human genome.[46] In humans, active transposable elements include a subset of L1 LINEs and *Alu* (a type of SINE).[47] These active elements have de novo germline insertions ranging from 1 in 20 to 1 in 916 births.[47] The insertion of these elements has multiple possible effects on the transcriptional regulation of genes, including disruption of the open reading frame, creation of a novel promoter, alternative splicing, an alternative poly(A) tail, disruption of transcription factor bindings sites, and changes in small RNA regulation.[47] Common repeat sequences in the human genome are cataloged in Table 45.4. Their distribution in humans and other species is shown in Fig. 45.4.

Human Epigenetic Alterations[48]

In addition to the sequence variants considered, epigenetic alterations, including alternative splicing and methylation, affect gene expression. Even though the number of genes may be limited to less than 25,000, variable transcription initiation and exon splicing produce about 90,000 unique mRNA transcripts and protein products.

Methylation of cytosine to 5-methylcytosine occurs frequently; about 70% of CpG dinucleotides in the human genome are methylated. Although not inherited, interest in this "fifth base" has increased as correlations with cancer have been reported. CpG islands are about 1000 bases in length and are often found near the 5′ end of genes. These regions consist of clusters of CG dinucleotides that are usually not methylated in normal cells. However, CpG methylation correlates with condensed chromatin structure and promoter inactivation;

TABLE 45.4 Repeat Sequences in the Human Genome

Type	Abbreviations	Size	Copies (Thousands)	Genome (%)
Retrotransposons				
Long interspersed elements	LINEs	900 bp	850	21
	L1		516	16.9
	L2		315	3.22
	L3		37	0.31
Short interspersed elements	SINEs	100–400 bp	1500	13
	Alu	350 bp	1090	11
	MIR		393	2.2
	Ther2/MIR3		75	0.34
Long terminal repeats	LTRs	1.5–11 Kb	450	8
	ERV		112	2.89
	ERV(K)		8	0.31
	ERV(L)		83	1.44
	MaLR		240	3.65
Segmental Duplications		>1000 bp		5.3
Structural Repeat and Gene Clusters				
	Centromeres	171 bp		3-6
	Telomeres	6 bp		<0.1
	Ribosomal			0.41
DNA Transposons		80–3000 bp	300	3
Simple Sequence Repeats	SSRs	1–500 bp		3
Short Tandem Repeats	STRs	1–13 bp		
		1		0.17
		2		0.53
		3		0.10
		4		0.34
		5		0.27
		6		0.14
		7		0.09
		8		0.11
		9		0.09
		10		0.16
Processed Pseudogenes		~1300	20	1.2

Data extracted from Lander et al.,[4] Venter et al,[5] International Human Genome Sequencing Consortium,[6] Richard et al.,[70] Stultz et al.,[71] and Torrents et al.[72]

an important example occurs in tumor-suppressor genes. Other epigenetic targets include nucleosome histone phosphorylation, acetylation, and methylation that can all affect gene expression.

ENCODE Project

ENCODE (Encyclopedia of DNA Elements) is a project that was initiated by the National Human Genome Research Institute in 2003 to examine all functional elements in the human genome.[49] The functional elements defined were not only the discrete genome areas that encode a product such as protein but also any genome area that had a reproducible biologic effect on processes such as transcription or chromatin structure. These genome areas include both exons as well as non–protein-coding areas such as promoters, enhancers, and silencers. The genome areas that do not encode protein have significant contributions to human variation.[50] From a survey of 150 genome-wide association studies using SNVs to identify genes linked to disease, 465 unique disease-associated SNVs were identified.[51] Of these 465 variants, 88% ($n = 407$) were present in the regions between genes (intergenic) or within introns. These results suggest the importance of noncoding variants in disease. Thus, the initial analysis from ENCODE has revealed that genome variation in noncoding regions is significant in inherited diseases and cancer.[52]

POINTS TO REMEMBER

Variations

- Small variants such as single nucleotide changes are the easiest to correlate to human disease.
- Most of the genome is repetitive, noncoding sequences with functions just now being uncovered by massively parallel sequencing.

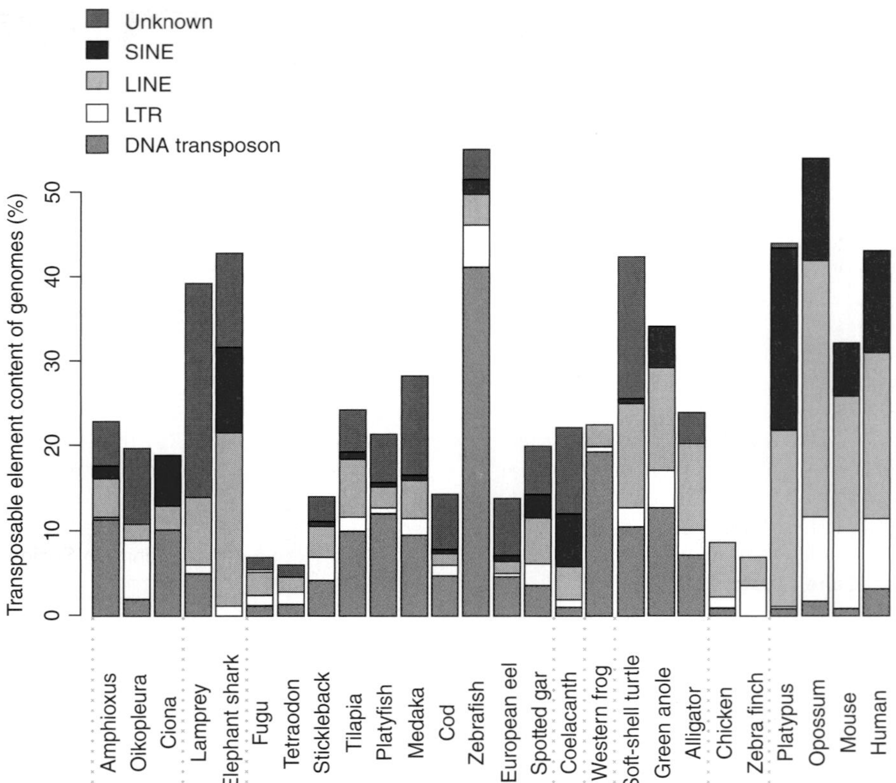

FIGURE 45.4 Transposable element diversity among species. A summary of the contribution of transposable elements to various genomes, including both retrotransposons and active transposons, is illustrated. The percentage of inactive retrotransposons (SINE, LINE, LTR) and active DNA transposons is shown for each organism. The organisms are organized into nonvertebrates (eg, Amphioxus), nonbony vertebrates (eg, lamprey), actinopterygian fish (eg, Fugu), lobe-finned fish (eg, Coelacanth), amphibians (eg, Western frog), nonbird reptiles (eg, soft-shell turtle), birds (eg, chicken), and mammals (eg, platypus). The figure clearly illustrates that in mammals, transposable elements contribute to more than 30% of the total genome. In comparison, in other organisms such as chicken and fugu, transposable elements are less than 10% of the genome. (From Chalopin D, Naville M, Plard F, et al. Comparative analysis of transposable elements highlights mobilome diversity and evolution in vertebrates. *Genome Biol Evol* 2015;7:567-580. This figure was reproduced by permission from Oxford University Press on behalf of the Society for Molecular Biology and Evolution and Dr. Jean-Nicolas Volff.)

NOMENCLATURE

Amino acid variations were associated with human disease long before DNA variation.[53] Amino acid variants were found first because techniques for amino acid sequencing matured before DNA sequencing. Advances in DNA technology enabled the investigation of DNA variations associated with disease. For example, the characterization of amino acid variants in the globin gene products (*HBB* and *HBA*) preceded the descriptions of DNA variation in the globin genes.

Small Variants

More than 20 years ago, the need for a database of human variants associated with disease was recognized. In 1996, the Mutation Database Initiative was sponsored by the Human Genome Organization (HUGO).[53] In 2001, the HUGO Mutation Database Initiative became the Human Genome Variation Society (HGVS).[54] In addition to the documentation and collection of variant information, the HGVS created a nomenclature system for standardizing the reporting of variations. An early recommendation proposed a hybrid model in which traditional disease alleles such as hemoglobin S for sickle cell disease and Z allele for α_1-antitrypsin deficiency would retain their historic nomenclature and new disease alleles would use the new nomenclature system.[55] The current HGVS nomenclature system has features that can be found in this early proposed system (Box 45.2).[56] In the HGVS system, disease alleles are described at the DNA level rather than as amino acid changes. Preferred terminology does not ascribe disease potential to the naming of a variant. For example, all variants are not disease-causing mutations. The preferred terms include sequence variant, CNV, and single nucleotide variant. Hemoglobin variants were initially named by a combination of letters (hemoglobin A, B, S, C, and F) and the city of discovery. Hematologists continue to use the traditional nomenclature (Table 45.5) that does not distinguish between variants from β-globin *(HBB)* and α-globin *(HBA)*. In addition to the hemoglobin genes, other

BOX 45.2 The Human Genome Variation Society Nomenclature for Naming Small Sequence Variants

The position of single nucleotide substitutions can be referenced to the genome (g.), amino acids in the protein (p.), or nucleotide bases in the cDNA transcript (c.). In all cases, the genome build and the sequence accession number should be specified.

For genomic coordinates, specify the chromosome and the base position followed by the base change. For example: GRCh37/hg19 Ch17: g.3424566C>T. Genomic coordinates are the only option for all intergenic variants, as well as deep intronic variants.

When the variant is within the protein coding region of a gene and protein coordinates are preferred, give the gene name followed by the number of the amino acid affected starting with the initiating methionine as 1. The wild-type amino acid is listed to the left of the number, and the variant amino acid is listed to the right. For example: *CYBB* p.T42R (or *CYBB* p.Tyr42Arg) for the 1 letter and 3 letter codes for amino acids, respectively. The protein coordinates best specify the phenotype, but it is a challenge to convey the results of frameshifts and the exact nucleotide change is often ambiguous.

When the variant is in or near the exons of a gene, you can use the cDNA coordinates. In this case, give the gene name followed by the base number using the A in the ATG initiation codon as 1 and then the base change. For example: *CYBB* c.125C>G. If the base change is in an intron (eg, a splice site mutation), you count from the nearest intron–exon boundary. For example: *CYBB* c.141+2T>C or c.142-12C>T. If the variant is 3′ of the ATG initiation sequence, you count down using negative numbers (*CYBB* c.-64C>T), or if it is 5′ of the last exon, you count up (*CYBB* c.*67G>A). With c. coordinates, you know the exact base change even though it may not change the amino acid sequence.

Nomenclature for insertions and deletions are also specified by the Human Genome Variation Society.

TABLE 45.5 Describing Hemoglobin Variants by Different Systems

Traditional Name	Disease Associated	Gene	Amino Acid Change (Traditional)*	Amino Acid Change (HGVS)	HGVS Nucleotide Change (mRNA Transcript)†	Genomic Coordinate (GRCh37/hg19)‡
Hemoglobin SS	Sickle cell anemia	*HBB*	Gln6Val	p.Gln7Val	c.20A>T hom (NM_000518.4)	Chr11:g.5248232
Hemoglobin CC	Hemolytic anemia	*HBB*	Glu6Lys	p.Glu7Lys	c.19G>A hom (NM_000518.4)	Chr11:g.5248233
Hemoglobin Austin	None	*HBB*	Arg40Ser	p.Arg41Ser	c.123G>T het (NM_000518.4)	Chr11:g.5247999
Hemoglobin G Philadelphia	None	*HBA2*	Asn68Lys	p.Asn69Lys	c.207C>A het (NM_000517.4)	Chr16:g.223235

*The amino acid change for hemoglobin diseases was characterized by amino acid sequencing before the advent of DNA sequencing. The first amino acid, methionine, was not included, resulting in the Gln to Val change in sickle cell anemia described as the "6" position rather than the "7" position.

†The "c." annotation is based on a reference transcript (NM number).

‡The HGVS nucleotide position is from 5′ to 3′ on the strand. However, the genomic coordinates are not oriented to the gene. The nucleotide position based on mRNA transcript may increase while the genomic position increases or decreases, depending on the orientation of the gene on the chromosome.

Data formatted according to den Dunnen JT, Antonarakis SE. Mutation nomenclature extensions and suggestions to describe complex mutations: a discussion. *Hum Mutat* 2000;15:7-12.

genes have both a traditional nomenclature system and the HGVS nomenclature. The basics of the HGVS nomenclature system for SNVs are introduced in Box 45.2.

Large Structural Variants

The determination of 46 chromosomes in humans occurred in 1956.[57] The following years were marked by increased activity in human cytogenetics, but with this rapid growth in knowledge it became apparent was that there was no coordination of how findings were named or classified.[1] Beginning in 1960, a consensus meeting of laboratories (Denver Conference) established basic guidelines for naming large chromosomal variations. The findings from multiple subsequent consensus conferences were unified in a single document, "An International System for Human Cytogenetic Nomenclature (1978)."

Some of the basic concepts of chromosomes are described in ISCN 1978: Autosomes are numbered from 1 to 22 in descending order of length. The sex chromosomes are named X and Y. The symbols p and q designated the short and long arms of the chromosomes, respectively. A chromosome band is the part of the chromosome that is clearly distinguishable from adjacent segments that are darker or lighter in appearance. G-bands are the bands resulting from Giemsa dye staining. In addition to describing the normal state of chromosomal features, ISCN 1978 considered the naming of chromosomal rearrangements such as inversions, deletions, and translocations.

In more recent times, the ISCN 2013 version introduced new features such as the term "hg" for "human genome build or assembly" and a chapter titled "Microarrays," which is devoted to naming changes identified by oligonucleotide microarrays. Of note, there is a separate consortium focused on microarrays known as ISCA (The International Standard for Cytogenomic Arrays). ISCA is focused on microarray testing quality improvement by projects such as variant databases linked to clinical data.[58]

Naming Genes

As significant as the naming of DNA variants, the naming of genes has also become standardized over the past thirty years.[59] The basic components of gene names include the gene name, which may include information on gene function, and the gene symbol, which is a short abbreviation in upper case Latin letters and Arabic numbers that are both italicized. The currently accepted gene naming system is by the HUGO Gene Nomenclature Committee (HGNC).[60] As with all standardization activities, there is a tradeoff. The more familiar historic names are established in the literature and used by practitioners in the specialty concerned with that gene. However, for a particular disease-associated gene, communication outside of the specialized field of knowledge may by difficult and lead to errors. Especially in the current era with genomic tests examining hundreds to tens of thousands of genes, a common gene naming system is necessary. In reporting specific genes, a hybrid approach that uses both the consensus nomenclature and the traditional name may be useful. A current database of recommended gene names and symbols as well as traditional names can be found on the HGNC online database. The HGNC database currently contains information on 18,990 protein-coding genes.

POINTS TO REMEMBER

Nomenclature

- The HGVS has created a systematic nomenclature for variants, including single nucleotide changes and small deletions and insertions.
- The Human Gene Nomenclature Committee provides a listing of accepted gene names.
- Within a specific field, common traditional names of genes and variants may be more familiar but communication outside of the field is best conducted with modern consensus nomenclature.

BOX 45.3 Human Genomic Databases

Comprehensive

NCBI (National Center for Biotechnology): ncbi.nlm.nih.gov/genome

Ensembl: ensembl.org/index.html

UCSC (University of California Santa Cruz): genome.ucsc.edu/

Genes and Disease

OMIM (Online Mendelian Inheritance in Man): ncbi.nlm.nih.gov/omim

ClinVar: ncbi.nlm.nih.gov/clinvar/

Decipher: decipher.sanger.ac.uk/index

Sequence Databanks

NCBI GenBank: ncbi.nlm.nih.gov/Genbank/

EMBL (European Molecular Biology Laboratory)-Bank: www.ebi.ac.uk/embl

DDBJ (DNA Data Bank of Japan): ddbj.nig.ac.jp/

MicroRNAs

miRBase: mirbase.org

General Variation Databases

Leiden Open Variation Database: lovd.nl/3.0/home

Human Genome Mutation Database: www.hgmd.cf.ac.uk/ac/index.php

Short Genetic Variations (dbSNP): ncbi.nlm.nih.gov/projects/SNP/

1000 Genomes: www.1000genomes.org/

Exomes (ExAC): exac.broadinstitute.org/

Specialized Variant Databases

Database of Genomic Structural Variation (dbVar): ncbi.nlm.nih.gov/dbvar

Database of Genomic Variants (DGV): dgv.tcag.ca/dgv/app/home

Retrotransposons: dbrip.brocku.ca/

Haplotypes (HapMap): hapmap.org/

Nomenclature

HUGO (Human Genome Organization) Gene names: genenames.org

HGVS (Human Genome Variation Society) Sequence variants: www.hgvs.org/mutnomen

DATABASES

Databases of DNA variations may be locus or disease specific (LSDB; eg, HbVar) or general databases that seek to capture information on all variants. Some of the commonly used general databases include dbSNP (Database of Single Nucleotide Polymorphisms), OMIM (Online Mendelian Inheritance in Man), HGMD (Human Gene Mutation Database), and ClinVar (Clinical Variant). Common databases and their web accessions are given in Box 45.3.

A systematic catalog of SNVs including small insertions and deletions was created as the dbSNP in 1998 as a collaboration between the NCBI and the National Human Genome Research Institute (NHGRI).[61] The reference identifier for variants in dbSNP begins with the prefix "rs." There are separate databases for structural variants known as dbVAR (Database of Genomic Structural Variation—NCBI) and DGV (Database of Genomic Variation—European Molecular Biology Laboratory [EMBL]). The prefix is either "nsv" for structural variants originating from dbVAR of the NCBI and "esv" for structural variants originating from DGV of EMBL.[62]

OMIM is manually curated by a team of professionals located at Johns Hopkins University.[63] It was started by the geneticist Victor McKusick in the 1970s as "Mendelian Inheritance in Man," first a series of published books and later an online resource. By design, the OMIM is not a comprehensive catalog of every variant ever described with disease but rather a catalog of genes and variants representative of a disease type. As of early 2015, 5461 diseases or syndromes were described in OMIM. However, of the approximately 20,000 protein coding genes, only 3381 genes were catalogued with a known variant associated with a disease or syndrome.

In contrast to OMIM, HGMD seeks to be a comprehensive database of all variants with reported disease association.[64,65] The number of new reports of germline mutations in the literature was less than 250 per year through 1990, but throughout the 1990s, reports grew into the thousands.[64] As of 2016, there were 166,768 variants from 6905 genes cataloged in HGMD. The types of variants included 92,974 missense or nonsense; 15,168 splicing; 24,957 small deletions; 10,415 small insertions; and 12,565 gross deletions. Although HGMD is one of the largest databases, there are reports of incorrect annotations arising from database issues or problems with the primary literature.[66] The annotation issue is demonstrated by a report that found that 80% of the HGMD disease-causing variants had an allele frequency of more than 5% in the 1000 Genomes Project dataset; however, rare diseases would be expected to have variant frequencies much less than 5%.[66]

The chief limitation of databases such as OMIM and HGMD is that they rely on published reports. As new variants of known genes are discovered in research or clinical laboratories, they are rarely published. The recognition of the under representation of clinically significant variants resulted in the ClinVar project, which allows for the contribution of annotated variants by clinical laboratories, research laboratories, and the literature into a publicly available database.[67] The dataset that combines submitter, variant, and phenotype is given an accession number with the prefix "SCV" (Submitted Clinical Variant).

INFORMATICS

The modern era of human genome sequencing is underpinned by massively parallel sequencing. As suggested by the name of the technology, both the method as well as the amount of data is massive. Although a single human genome is approximately 3 billion bases, the amount of sequencing needed to accurately determine those bases may exceed 90 billion bases.[68] The data storage requirements are typically more than 0.5 terabytes per human genome. Fortunately, as the scale of sequencing has increased, tools have been developed to manage and analyze the information. There have been many recent reviews and evaluations of existing software tools.[69]

In brief, both publicly available tools and commercial software are assembled into what is referred to as a pipeline. In the pipeline, the information is processed in a serial manner (Fig. 45.5). First, raw sequencing data is saved in a file format such as FASTQ. The sequencing data are composed of data from millions of short sequencing reads. An alignment program uses rules that align the short sequencing reads to the reference genome. Depending on the coverage required, there may be tens to thousands of sequencing reads at a single nucleotide position. After alignment, the bases are "called" or determined by the software algorithm. The base call is dependent on a variety of factors, including the quality of the read (Q-score; Box 45.4) and the percentage of reads at the nucleotide position that are in agreement. At a single nucleotide position, there may be more than one base, which would be expected in the case of a heterozygous

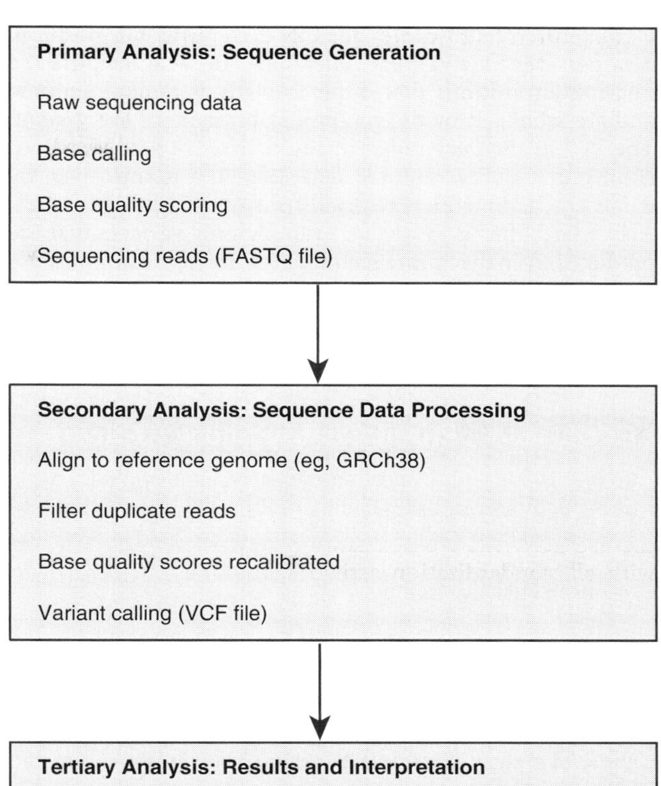

FIGURE 45.5 Bioinformatics pipeline. The analysis of data from massively parallel sequencing can be broadly considered to occur in three phases. *Primary analysis:* The raw output (eg, optical or electronic signals) from the sequencing instrument is transformed into data that describe the individual bases of DNA as well as the quality and confidence of the base call at each position. These reads of DNA are assembled into a FASTQ data file. *Secondary analysis:* The data file is then assembled onto a reference sequence. For human DNA sequencing, this is typically a reference genome such as GRCh38. If the fragments of DNA were prepared by randomly sheared fragments, then the sampling of a wide diversity of fragments improves quality and is ensured by sequencing that is from exact duplicates. When the fragments are assembled against the reference genome, the quality of each of the base calls at specific nucleotide positions can be determined. The variant at each position is then determined and reported in a single variant call file (VCF). *Tertiary analysis:* The variants are then queried against multiple databases that have information on population frequency and clinical significance. Based on these queries, the variants can be prioritized in terms of importance to the given scientific question or clinical scenario. (Modified from Oliver GR, Hart SN, Klee EW. Bioinformatics for clinical next generation sequencing. *Clin Chem* 2015;61:124-135.)

variant. After the bases are called for each nucleotide position, a variant call file (VCF) is generated. The VCF includes the nucleotide positions that differ from the reference genome and are tabulated by the genomic coordinate of the variant. The VCF is then examined by another set of software algorithms that query multiple databases; the examination by databases is sometimes referred to as filtering (Table 45.6). A standard filter is to further examine only variants that are predicted to change protein coding (eg, missense or nonsense variants). Other filters may be based on the frequency of specific variants in various populations. The frequency of the variant in populations is useful for determining if there is a consequence for a variant. For example, if the variant occurs in a gene implicated in a rare disease that occurs in fewer than 1 in 100,000 individuals, then that variant should occur much less frequently than 1% in any population. In addition to population databases, there are databases that catalogue variants with clinical phenotype information or reports in the published literature. Finally, rather than an examination of databases, tools that predict the importance of variants to protein structure or function may be used. These predictive tools are not always accurate, but they may be helpful to prioritize the examination of a long queue of variants from a sequencing study.

BOX 45.4 Phred Quality Score (Q-Score)[73-75]

In the 1990s, Phil Green at the University of Washington developed software to automatically read the fluorescent sequence chromatograms generated from Sanger sequencing. The original software, Phred (**Ph**il's **r**ead **ed**itor), used the following basic parameters:

1. Find the predicted location of peaks.
2. Find the observed location of peaks.
3. Match predicted and observed peaks.
4. Find missing peaks.

A component of Phred was an estimator of the error probability of a base call. A quality value (Q-score) was generated from the formula:

$q = -10 \times \log_{10}(p)$

q = quality value

p = estimated error for a base call

Some representative examples of quality value (q) scores:

Q-score of 30 (Q30): The probability (*p*) is 1/1,000 of being incorrect.

Q-score of 20 (Q20): The probability (*p*) is 1/100 of being incorrect.

Q-score of 10 (Q10): The probability (*p*) is 1/10 of being incorrect.

Although massively parallel sequencing does not generate a Sanger sequencing type chromatogram, the convention of a Phred Q-score is still used to calculate the quality (and accuracy) of a sequenced base. Under ideal conditions, current massively parallel sequencing can achieve more than 90% of bases at Q30.

TABLE 45.6 Tertiary Analysis Databases and Software Tools*

	Annotation Source	Description	Web Address
Population frequency based	1000 Genomes Project	Whole-genome sequencing data on 2577 individuals with ancestry from East Asia, South Asia, Africa, Europe and the Americas	www.1000genomes.org
	NHLBI ESP	NHLBI Exome Sequencing Project, exome variant server. Variant data from ~6500 exomes, including 2203 African Americans and 4300 European Americans	evs.gs.washington.edu/EVS
	HapMap Project	Haplotype Mapping. Multiethnic, international database of common genetic variants	hapmap.ncbi.nlm.nih.gov
	ExAC	Exome Aggregation Consortium. Data from >60,000 individuals as part of various disease-specific and population studies	exac.broadinstitute.org
Evidence based	OMIM	Online Mendelian Inheritance in Man. Curated catalog of genes and genetic disorders. Prototypical or important variants are shown; however, the catalog is not intended to be an exhaustive compendium of all variants	www.omim.org
	LOVD	Leiden Open Variation Database. Open source database of human variation.	www.lovd.nl/3.0/home
	HGMD	Human Gene Mutation Database. Proprietary database of variants correlated with human disease	www.hgmd.cf.ac.uk/ac/index.php
	ClinVar	Clinical Variant. Human variation correlated to phenotype	www.ncbi.nlm.nih.gov/clinvar
	dbVAR	Database of Genomic Structural Variation. Genomic structural variation.	www.ncbi.nlm.nih.gov/dbvar

TABLE 45.6 Tertiary Analysis Databases and Software Tools—cont'd

	Annotation Source	Description	Web Address
Prediction based	Align GVGD	Align Grantham Variation Grantham Difference. Web-based software that combines biophysical properties and protein sequence alignments to generate a score ranging from deleterious to neutral.	http://agvgd.hci.utah.edu/index.php
	ANNOVAR	Annotation of Variants including gene location (eg, exonic, splicing, UTR, intronic).	annovar.openbioinformatics.org/en/lates/
	Mutation Taster	Web-based software that generates a probability of pathogenicity based on multiple data sources.	www.mutationtaster.org/
	SIFT	Sorts Intolerant From Tolerant substitutions. Web or locally available software to predict the consequence of an amino acid change	sift.jcvi.org/
	Polyphen-2	Polymorphism Phenotyping v2. Web or locally available software to predict the consequence of an amino acid change	genetics.bwh.harvard.edu/pph2/

*Many database and software tools are available for tertiary analysis of variants, and only a few are listed here. These tools may either by publicly available or restricted for use by subscription or special permission.
NHLBI, National Heart, Lung, and Blood Institute; *UTR,* untranslated region.
Modified from Oliver GR, Hart SN, Klee EW. Bioinformatics for clinical next generation sequencing. *Clin Chem* 2015;61:124-135.

SELECTED REFERENCES

For a full list of references for this chapter, please refer to ExpertConsult.com.

4. Lander ES, Linton LM, Birren B, et al. Initial sequencing and analysis of the human genome. *Nature* 2001;**409**:860–921.
5. Venter JC, Adams MD, Myers EW, et al. The sequence of the human genome. *Science* 2001;**291**:1304–51.
6. Finishing the euchromatic sequence of the human genome. *Nature* 2004;**431**:931–45.
8. Callaway E. 'Platinum' genome takes on disease. *Nature* 2014;**515**:323.
10. Pendleton M, Sebra R, Pang AW, et al. Assembly and diploid architecture of an individual human genome via single-molecule technologies. *Nat Methods* 2015.
11. Amaral PP, Dinger ME, Mercer TR, et al. The eukaryotic genome as an RNA machine. *Science* 2008;**319**:1787–9.
14. Fleischmann RD, Adams MD, White O, et al. Whole-genome random sequencing and assembly of *Haemophilus influenzae rd*. *Science* 1995;**269**:496–512.
22. Carninci P, Kasukawa T, Katayama S, et al. The transcriptional landscape of the mammalian genome. *Science* 2005;**309**:1559–63.
24. Mendes Soares LM, Valcarcel J. The expanding transcriptome: the genome as the 'book of sand'. *EMBO J* 2006;**25**:923–31.
26. Cech TR, Steitz JA. The noncoding RNA revolution-trashing old rules to forge new ones. *Cell* 2014;**157**:77–94.
31. Abecasis GR, Altshuler D, Auton A, et al. A map of human genome variation from population-scale sequencing. *Nature* 2010;**467**:1061–73.
32. Abecasis GR, Auton A, Brooks LD, et al. An integrated map of genetic variation from 1,092 human genomes. *Nature* 2012;**491**:56–65.
35. Redon R, Ishikawa S, Fitch KR, et al. Global variation in copy number in the human genome. *Nature* 2006;**444**:444–54.
42. Willems T, Gymrek M, Highnam G, et al. The landscape of human STR variation. *Genome Res* 2014;**24**:1894–904.
46. de Koning AP, Gu W, Castoe TA, et al. Repetitive elements may comprise over two-thirds of the human genome. *PLoS Genet* 2011;**7**:e1002384.
52. An integrated encyclopedia of DNA elements in the human genome. *Nature* 2012;**489**:57–74.
61. Sherry ST, Ward MH, Kholodov M, et al. dbSNP: the NCBI database of genetic variation. *Nucleic Acids Res* 2001;**29**:308–11.
67. Landrum MJ, Lee JM, Riley GR, et al. Clinvar: Public archive of relationships among sequence variation and human phenotype. *Nucleic Acids Res* 2014;**42**:D980–5.
69. Pabinger S, Dander A, Fischer M, et al. A survey of tools for variant analysis of next-generation genome sequencing data. *Brief Bioinform* 2014;**15**:256–78.
76. Oliver GR, Hart SN, Klee EW. Bioinformatics for clinical next generation sequencing. *Clin Chem* 2015;**61**:124–35.

46

Nucleic Acid Isolation

Stephanie A. Thatcher

ABSTRACT

Background

Effective isolation of nucleic acids (NAs) is important for clinical molecular methods, including polymerase chain reaction (PCR) and sequencing. Many NA sample preparation techniques (including commercial kits) are available to isolate NA for molecular detection. Solid-phase NA separation and automation are now commonly used in clinical and research laboratories.

Content

Optimal NA isolation includes lysis from diverse sources such as human cells, viruses, bacterial spores or protozoan oocysts, and purification of DNA or RNA. Techniques involve sample exposure to chemicals, enzymes, or binding matrices that reduce sample volume, variability, and complexity to achieve purity goals. The isolated NA should be efficiently separated from inhibitors of a downstream molecular assay. The best preparation method depends on the requirements for a particular application. Goals may include flexibility for multiple sample types, large batch processing, speed, or high-purity NA. Consistent results for today's molecular methods can usually be obtained by the right combination of lysis, concentration, purification, and efficiency for NA isolation.

47

Nucleic Acid Techniques

Carl T. Wittwer and G. Mike Makrigiorgos

ABSTRACT

Background

The expansion and power of molecular diagnostics is enabled by techniques that modify, amplify, detect, discriminate, and sequence nucleic acids (NAs). Molecular diagnostic techniques are getting faster, better, and cheaper. If these trends translate to clinical medicine, we all win.

Content

Nucleic acids are usually first purified and then amplified to provide enough NA to be easily detected and analyzed. However, not all techniques require NA purification or amplification before analysis. Although the polymerase chain reaction (PCR) remains the most common method of amplification for both research and clinical diagnostics, molecular tests that use isothermal amplification methods are now approved by the US Food and Drug Administration, and some are Clinical Laboratory Improvement Amendments waived. Radioactive detection has been replaced by fluorescence and, in some cases, electronic methods. Separation methods, particularly electrophoresis, once dominated NA analysis and are still used today. However, the advantages of closed systems that detect, identify, and quantify without separation, such as real-time PCR and melting analysis, simplify the workflow and reduce the time required. Multiplexed methods enable the physician to go beyond single target queries and can provide diagnostic answers for clinical syndromes. The specificity of NA hybridization is still central to most methods. Microarrays have great merit in research, and copy number arrays have proven clinical utility. Sequencing methods have progressed from labor-intensive base termination ladders visualized on gels, to the current workhorse of massively parallel methods that sequence during synthesis, to the promise of single molecule sequencing.

INTRODUCTION

The structure of DNA was solved in 1953,[1] with semiconservative replication demonstrated in 1958,[2] providing a conceptual background for nucleic acid (NA) replication and analysis. Restriction enzymes,[3] oligonucleotide synthesis,[4] and reverse transcriptase all become known and available around 1970.[5,6] Southern blotting, perhaps the first practical molecular diagnostic technique, appeared in 1975 using restriction enzyme digestion and size separation on agarose gels.[7] Southern blotting typically detects large structural alterations such as deletions, duplications, insertions, and rearrangements but can also detect single nucleotide variants (SNVs) if they disrupt restriction sites. Southern blotting was the first method with adequate sensitivity and specificity for DNA analysis of single-copy genes in complex genomes. Northern blotting is a parallel technique that analyzes RNA instead of DNA to size RNA transcripts and was developed in 1977.[8] However, both Southern and Northern blotting are seldom used today because they require large amounts of NAs and are also very labor intensive and time consuming. They are covered in more detail in the fifth edition of this book.[9]

DNA sequencing with chain-terminating inhibitors (dideoxynucleotides) was developed in 1977 using gels for size separation.[10] Initially sequencing was radioactive with separation on plates, but fluorescent analysis, automation, and a move to capillaries over the next 30 years increased the utility of this "gold standard" method. Originally described in 1985, the polymerase chain reaction (PCR) was greatly improved in 1988 by using heat-stable polymerases.[11] Of all molecular techniques, PCR has become the most popular method in molecular diagnostics, and many variants and improvements exist, particularly real-time PCR for quantification, which was first described in 1992,[12] with commercial instrumentation becoming available in 1997.[13,14]

DNA microarrays appeared in the 1990s with oligonucleotides attached to glass plates.[15] Applications included RNA expression profiling in 1995[16] followed by genomic arrays for SNVs and copy number comparisons. As a counterpoint to the complexity of arrays, fluorescent melting analysis, first used in 1997,[17] was upgraded in 2003 with higher resolution as a simple tool for genetic analysis.[18]

Massively parallel sequencing, first published in 2005,[19,20] continues to develop into a dominant technology because of the massive number of bases sequenced. Also called next-generation sequencing (NGS), we prefer instead the descriptive term massively parallel sequencing (MPS) rather than a temporal reference that will outdate.

Today, molecular diagnostics continues to advance as a rapidly progressing and highly competitive field, both in academics and in industry. This growth is reflected in the number of publications in molecular diagnostics in recent years (Fig. 47.1).[21] In this chapter, our intent is to focus on understanding the mechanisms of NA techniques in use today.

We begin by considering pretreatment methods for NAs and then focus on amplification techniques that are often necessary to observe or quantify NA sequences of interest. Next, the tools used to detect or visualize NAs are discussed, along with methods that allow identification, quantification, and segregation of individual NA species. Finally, we end with the extraordinary power of massively parallel sequencing. Important terms and definitions are listed in Box 47.1.

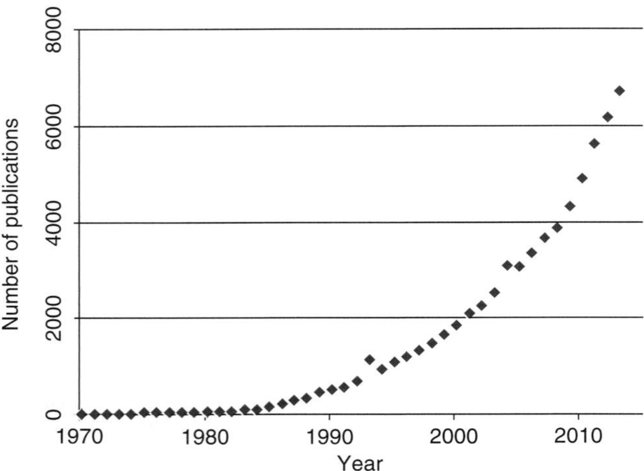

FIGURE 47.1 Molecular diagnostics publications, 1970 to 2013. (Reprinted with permission of the publisher from Chiu RWK, Lo YMD, Wittwer CT. Molecular diagnostics: a revolution in progress. *Clin Chem* 2015;61:1–3. Copyright 2015 AACC.)

NUCLEIC ACID PREPARATION

Conventional NA testing requires (1) NA isolation of DNA, RNA, or both; (2) amplification of the NA; and (3) detection, analysis, or quantification. Sometimes one step can be eliminated or two steps can be combined depending on the sample type and quantity of the target. For example, direct amplification from blood, serum, plasma, cerebrospinal fluid, nasopharyngeal swabs, and other sources may require little or no sample preparation for PCR when high temperatures for denaturation can make sufficient NAs available. However, quantification and sensitivity may suffer with low extraction efficiency and sample dilution. Single-molecule detection and single-molecule sequencing do not always require amplification, although whole-genome amplification is often used in single-cell analysis. Separate amplification and detection are not necessary in real-time PCR, and product melting can be seamlessly added or measured during PCR for additional analysis.[22]

DNA and RNA isolation are covered in Chapter 46. In addition to NA isolation, sometimes it is necessary to prepare samples for amplification or analysis by enzymatic or nonenzymatic means. For example, the enzyme reverse transcriptase may be needed to convert RNA to DNA. Massively parallel sequencing usually requires library preparation that may include enzymatic fragmentation with nonspecific DNAses, end repair of the generated fragments with a polymerase to produce blunt ends, 5′- phosphorylation with a kinase, A-tailing with a polymerase, and adaptor ligation with a ligase.[23] Alternatively, a transpososome complex containing a transposase and double-stranded sequencing adaptors can be used to streamline fragmentation to ligation in one

BOX 47.1 Important Terms and Definitions

Adapter: Oligonucleotides that are ligated to library fragments in order to provide consensus priming sites.

Allele-specific polymerase chain reaction (PCR): A version of PCR in which only one allele at a locus is amplified. Specificity is achieved by designing one or both PCR primers so that they overlap the site of sequence variance between alternative alleles.

Amplicon: The product of an amplification reaction, such as PCR.

Antisense RNA (asRNA): A single-stranded RNA that is complementary to a messenger RNA (mRNA) strand transcribed within a cell.

Asymmetric PCR: A version of PCR that preferentially amplifies one strand of the target DNA.

Branched-chain signal amplification: A molecular probe technique that uses branched DNA (bDNA) as a means to amplify the hybridization signal.

Conformation-sensitive gel electrophoresis (CSGE): A type of electrophoretic mutation scanning in which a segment of DNA is screened for mismatch pairing between normal and variant base pairs.

Copy number variant (CNV): A segment of DNA with copy-number differences between genomes.

Coverage: The percent of target bases that were sequenced at least a given number of times.

Denaturing gradient gel electrophoresis (DGGE): An electrophoretic method for separating DNA fragments according to their mobility under increasingly denaturing conditions (usually increasing formamide or urea concentrations). See also TGGE, SSCP and heteroduplex analysis.

Deoxyribonucleotide triphosphates (dNTPs): Usually dATP, dCTP, dGTP, and dTTP, the building blocks of DNA.

DNA library: A collection of DNA fragments with ligated adapters that will be sequenced.

Dideoxy-termination sequencing (Sanger sequencing): A method of DNA sequencing based on the selective incorporation of chain-terminating dideoxynucleotides by DNA polymerase during in vitro DNA replication.

Digital polymerase chain reaction (digital PCR or dPCR): A modification of PCR with the sample separated into many partitions so that some partitions have no template (0) and others have one or more (1).

Insert: Part of the original DNA that has been fragmented before ligation to adapters.

Fluorescent in situ hybridization (FISH): A genetic mapping technique using fluorescent tags for analysis of chromosomes and genetic abnormalities. FISH can also be referred to as chromosome painting.

gb: One billion bases or 1 gigabase (1,000,000,000 bases).

BOX 47.1 Important Terms and Definitions—cont'd

Heteroduplex: A DNA duplex with internal mismatches or loops.

Heteroduplex analysis (HDA): A type of mutation scanning in which a segment of DNA is screened by gel or capillary electrophoresis for mismatch pairing between normal and variant base pairs.

Homoduplex: A perfectly matched DNA duplex.

Hybridization: The annealing or pairing of two DNA strands.

Insertion: An extra DNA sequence that is present in one sample compared with a reference sequence.

kb: One thousand bases or 1 kilobase (1,000 bases).

Loop-mediated isothermal amplification (LAMP): A single tube technique for the amplification of DNA that uses a single temperature incubation.

Massively parallel sequencing (MPS): Sequencing of many fragments of DNA simultaneously.

Mate-pair sequence: Sequence obtained from both ends of a DNA fragment that is typically 5000 to 10,000 bases long.

mb: One million bases or 1 megabase (1,000,000 bases).

Melting curve: A measurement of the dissociation of double-stranded DNA during heating.

Multiplex ligation-dependent probe amplification (MLPA): A variation of the multiplex polymerase chain reaction that assesses the copy number of several targets by permitting multiple targets to be amplified with only a single primer pair.

Next-generation sequencing (NGS): Massively parallel sequencing. The term *massively parallel sequencing* is preferred.

Northern blot analysis: A technique for identifying specific sequences of RNA in which RNA molecules are (1) separated by electrophoresis, (2) transferred to nitrocellulose, and (3) identified with a suitable probe.

Nucleic acid analogs: Compounds that are analogous (structurally similar) to naturally occurring RNA and DNA. They are used in chemotherapy and molecular biology research.

Oligonucleotide: A short single-stranded polymer of nucleic acid.

Oligonucleotide ligation assay (OLA): A technique for determining the presence or absence of a specific nucleotide pair within a target gene, often indicating whether the gene is wild type (normal) or mutant (defective).

Paired-end sequence: Sequence from both ends of a DNA fragment typically hundreds of bases long.

Peptide nucleic acid (PNA): An artificially synthesized polymer similar to DNA or RNA with peptide instead of phosphodiester bonds. The term is somewhat of a misnomer because PNA is not an acid.

Polony: A microscopic colony of clonal temples used in massively parallel sequencing. A polony may be generated by polymerase chain reaction, bridge amplification, or isothermal amplification.

Polymerase chain reaction (PCR): An in vitro method for exponentially amplifying DNA.

Primer: An oligonucleotide that serves to initiate polymerase-catalyzed addition of nucleotides by annealing to a template strand.

Pyrosequencing: A method of DNA sequencing based on the "sequencing by synthesis" principle that relies on the detection of pyrophosphate release on nucleotide incorporation.

Read: The nucleotide sequence inferred by sequencing of a template.

Read length: Number of bases sequenced.

Real-time PCR: Observation of PCR during amplification at least once each cycle.

Restriction fragment length polymorphism (RFLP): A genetic polymorphism revealed by changes in the sizes of DNA fragments after restriction enzyme digestion and electrophoresis.

Reverse transcriptase: A polymerase that catalyzes synthesis of DNA from an RNA template.

Rolling circle amplification (RCA): A probe amplification method with a linear probe that is ligated to form a circle in the presence of template. The circle is replicated continuously by a polymerase and one or more primers.

Sanger sequencing: See dideoxy-termination sequencing.

Serial invasive signal amplification: A signal enhancing technique that combines two invasive signal amplification reactions in series in a single-tube format. The cleaved 5′-arm from the target-specific primary reaction is used to drive a secondary invasive reaction, resulting in a total signal amplification of more than seven orders of magnitude in about 4 hours.

Single nucleotide variants (SNV) chip: A type of DNA microarray that can detect single nucleotide variants, insertions, and deletions. Also known as a single nucleotide polymorphism (SNP) chip.

Single-stranded conformational polymorphism (SSCP): A gel electrophoresis technique where single-stranded DNA segments are identified by their abnormal migration patterns.

Southern blot: A method for detecting DNA sequence variants after restriction enzyme digestion and size separation by electrophoresis. Hybridization with a labeled probe reveals sequence variants that result in a change in distance between restriction sites, including (1) deletions, (2) duplications, (3) insertions, and (4) rearrangements.

Strand displacement amplification (SDA): An amplification technique that uses two types of primers, DNA polymerase, and a restriction endonuclease to exponentially produce single-stranded amplicons asynchronously.

Temperature-gradient gel electrophoresis (TGGE): A form of electrophoresis that uses temperature to denature the sample as it moves across an acrylamide gel.

Transcription-mediated amplification (TMA): An amplification method that uses RNA polymerase and DNA reverse transcriptase to produce RNA amplicon from a target nucleic acid. TMA is used to amplify both RNA and DNA.

Transcriptome: The set of all RNA molecules, including (1) mRNA, (2) rRNA, (3) tRNA, and other (4) noncoding RNA produced in one or a population of cells.

Virtual karyotyping: A technique used to identify and quantify short sequences of DNA from specific loci all over a genome to obtain information that reflects a karyotype.

Whole-genome amplification (WGA): A nonspecific amplification technique that produces an amplified product representative of the initial starting material (whole genome).

step.[24] Enzymes that act on NAs are covered in Chapter 44. Nonenzymatic methods may also be used to process NAs before amplification or analysis.

Nucleic Acid Fragmentation

Boiling, acid–base treatment, sonication, mechanical shearing, and chemical cleavage can be used to cut DNA or RNA into smaller fragments to make subsequent analysis more efficient or to form libraries. Boiling is a simple way to fragment genomic DNA so that a long initial denaturation period is not necessary in PCR. Although DNA is fragmented by acid and RNA is fragmented by base, these methods are seldom used except in bulk procedures such as blotting. Sonication and acoustic shearing are common methods to fragment NA for library preparation and are used in massively parallel sequencing. Depending on the frequency and geometry of the sample and acoustic generator, fragments averaging from 100 to 20,000 bases can be produced. Hydrodynamic shearing can also be obtained by compressed air to atomize the liquid into a fine mist (nebulization), forcing the solution through a fine-gauge needle, or through a pressure cell. For chemical cleavage, several metal-ion–catalyzed chemistries can cleave single- and double-stranded NAs. Some alkylating compounds can cleave and label NAs at the same time. One example is 5-bromomethyl-fluorescein, which is catalyzed by metal ions to fragment RNA or DNA; then those fragments are simultaneously labeled with fluorescein for microarray analysis.[25] Another example of chemical treatment of DNA is the use of hydroxylamine or osmium tetroxide followed by cleavage of mismatches with piperidine as a way to detect and locate mutations.[26]

Bisulfite Treatment for Methylation Analysis

Bisulfite treatment of DNA is often used to analyze the methylation status of cytosine (C) residues in DNA. Sodium bisulfite ($NaHSO_3$),[27] optionally used together with ammonium bisulfite,[28] converts C into uracil (U), but does not affect 5-methylcytosine. The chemical process of bisulfite treatment is shown in Fig. 47.2. The process works effectively only on single-stranded DNA (ssDNA), so the sample needs to be denatured by heat, alkali, or chaotropic agents such as urea or formamide. Analysis of the bisulfite-treated DNA is usually performed after NA amplification. DNA polymerases used for amplification will recognize 5-methylcytosine as C (no change), but an unmethylated C is converted to U and will be recognized as a T (sequence change of C to T). Many methods can be used to detect and quantify the altered sequences that result from bisulfite treatment of methylated DNA, including allele-specific amplification, detection with probes, melting techniques, and sequencing.[29] One limitation of bisulfite treatment is significant degradation of DNA. Depending on the protocol, as much as 90% of the DNA can be lost. Prior affinity enrichment of methylated DNA may be used before bisulfite treatment. For example, methylated DNA can be enriched by immunoprecipitation with an antibody raised against DNA containing 5-methylcytosine.[30] Up to 90-fold enrichment of methylated DNA can be achieved by immunoprecipitation. Another method is to use a methylated DNA binding protein to capture double-stranded methylated DNA on an affinity column.[31]

AMPLIFICATION TECHNIQUES

Molecular diagnostics requires techniques to detect extremely low concentrations of NAs in a background of complex genomic structure. Achieving sensitive detection limits is a central concern for clinical applications of NA analysis. Techniques that increase the amount of the NA target, the detection signal, or the probe are referred to as *amplification methods.* Examples of amplification methods are listed in Table 47.1. In *target amplification,* a well-defined segment of the NA (the target sequence) is copied many times by in vitro methods. Areas outside the target are not amplified. In *signal amplification,* the amount of target stays the same, but the signal is increased by one of several methods, including sequential hybridization of branching NA structures and continuous enzyme action on substrate that may be recycled. Finally, in *probe amplification,* the probe (or a product of the probe) is amplified only in the presence of the target. Amplification techniques often can achieve more than a million-fold amplification in less than 1 hour.

POINTS TO REMEMBER

Nucleic Acid Amplification Methods

- May amplify the target, the signal, or the probe
- May be isothermal or cycle through different temperatures
- Cycling speed is limited by instrumentation, not biochemistry
- May be analyzed on gels or in real-time
- May be qualitative, quantitative, or digital
- Require positive and negative controls

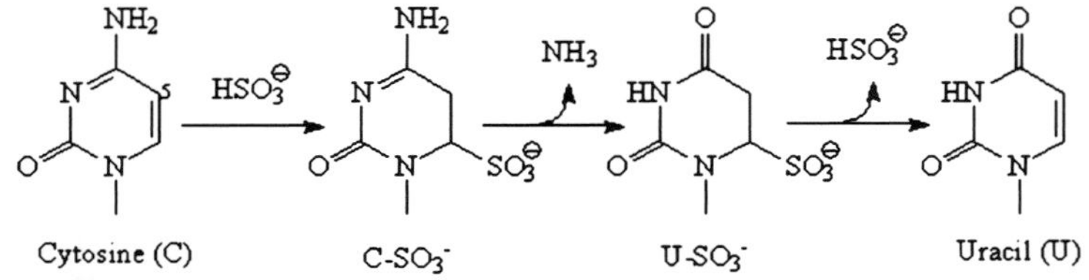

FIGURE 47.2 Bisulfite-mediated conversion of cytosine (C) to uracil (U) occurs in three steps. The first step is the addition of bisulfite to C. This reaction occurs at acid pH. The second step is the deamination of cytidine–bisulfite ($C\text{-}SO_3^-$) to produce uracil–bisulfite ($U\text{-}SO_3^-$), which is optimal at a pH of 5 to 6. Before analysis, $U\text{-}SO_3^-$ is converted to U by adjusting the pH to alkali. The majority of methylation on the C residue in mammalian cells occurs at the carbon 5 position (shown in the structure of C), resulting in 5-methylcytosine, which is resistant to bisulfite-mediated conversion.

TABLE 47.1 Common Amplification Techniques

Techniques	Type	Enzymes Required
Polymerase chain reaction (PCR)	Target	DNA polymerase (thermostable)
Transcription-mediated amplification (TMA)	Target	Reverse transcriptase, RNA polymerase, RNase H
Self-sustained sequence replication (3SR)		
Nucleic acid sequence–based amplification (NASBA)		
Strand displacement amplification (SDA)	Target	*Hinc*II, DNA polymerase I (5′- exo-deficient)
Loop-mediated amplification (LAMP)	Target	DNA polymerase
Helicase dependent amplification (HDA)	Target	Helicase, DNA polymerase
Recombinase polymerase amplification (RPA)	Target	Recombinase, single-strand binding protein, polymerase
Whole-genome amplification (WGA)	Target	Φ29 DNA polymerase
Multiple displacement amplification (MDA)		
Antisense RNA amplification (aRNA)	Target	T4 DNA polymerase, Klenow, S1 nuclease, T7 polymerase
Branched DNA (bDNA)	Signal	Alkaline phosphatase
Serial invasive signal amplification	Signal	Cleavase
Rolling circle amplification (RCA)	Probe	Φ29 DNA polymerase

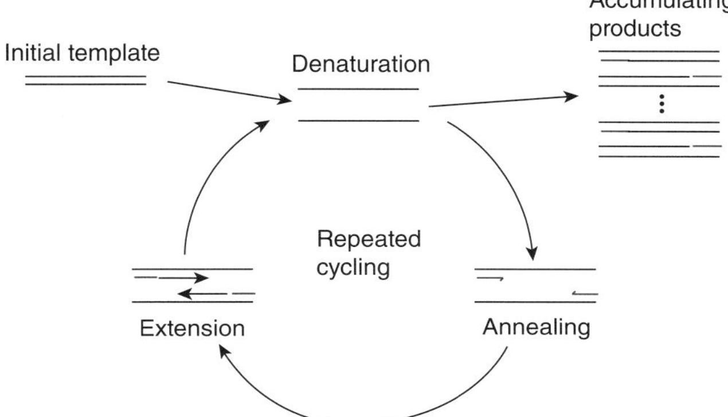

FIGURE 47.3 Simple schematic of the polymerase chain reaction. Amplification of the initial template requires denaturation by heat, allowing primers to anneal at a lower temperature, followed by primer extension at an intermediate temperature. In each cycle, a doubling of the DNA product occurs. After 20 to 40 cycles, the product accumulates more than 1 million-fold.

Polymerase Chain Reaction—Target Amplification

When the amount of target NA is increased by synthetic in vitro methods, target amplification occurs. PCR[11] is the best known and most widely applied of the target amplification methods. Because of the commercial availability of thermostable DNA polymerases, kits, and instrumentation, this method has been widely adopted in research and is routinely used in the clinical laboratory.

Details of the PCR Process

Polymerase chain reaction requires (1) a thermostable DNA polymerase, (2) deoxynucleotides of each base (collectively referred to as *dNTPs*), (3) a DNA strand that includes the sequence to be amplified, and (4) a pair of oligonucleotides (referred to as *primers*) that are complementary to opposite strands that define the target sequence. In the first step, target duplexes are denatured into single strands by heat (Fig. 47.3). When the mixture is cooled, primers provided in great excess (usually over 1 million times the concentration of the initial target) specifically anneal to complementary sequences on the target. After the primers are annealed, the action of the polymerase synthesizes two new DNA strands by extending each of the two primers at their 3′ end. The primers are designed to recognize sequences of the target that are close enough together such that the polymerase extends each strand far enough to include the priming site of the other primer. Usually, the optimal temperature for polymerization (or DNA synthesis) is an intermediate temperature between the annealing temperature (at which primer hybridizes to its target) and the denaturation temperature (at which the newly generated DNA strand dissociates from its template). The second cycle also begins with denaturation, but now twice as many strands (the original genomic DNA and the extension products from the first cycle) are available for primer annealing and subsequent extension. Temperature cycling (typically) uses three temperatures: (1) a high temperature sufficient to denature the target sequence, typically 90° to 97°C but can be lower depending on the melting temperature of the product; (2) a low temperature that allows annealing of the primers to the target, typically 50° to 65°C; and (3) a third temperature optimal for polymerase extension, typically 65° to 75°C. A more complete schematic of PCR is shown in Fig. 47.4, detailing why only products of defined length are generated. The instrument that takes samples through the multiple steps of changing temperature is known as a *thermocycler.*

Repetitive thermocycling results in the exponential accumulation of the short product (consisting of primers and all intervening sequences). If the efficiency of each cycle is perfect, the number of target sequences doubles each cycle (the efficiency is 100% or 1.0). PCR efficiency depends on the primers, the temperature-cycling conditions, and any inhibitors that might limit amplification. Amplified products accumulate exponentially in the beginning cycles of PCR. At some point, however, the efficiency of amplification falls and eventually the amount of product plateaus (Fig. 47.5) as the result of exhaustion of components or competition between primer and product annealing (ie, the single strands of product are at such high concentrations that they anneal to each other rather than to the primers). The S-curve shape is similar to the logistical model for population growth. In a

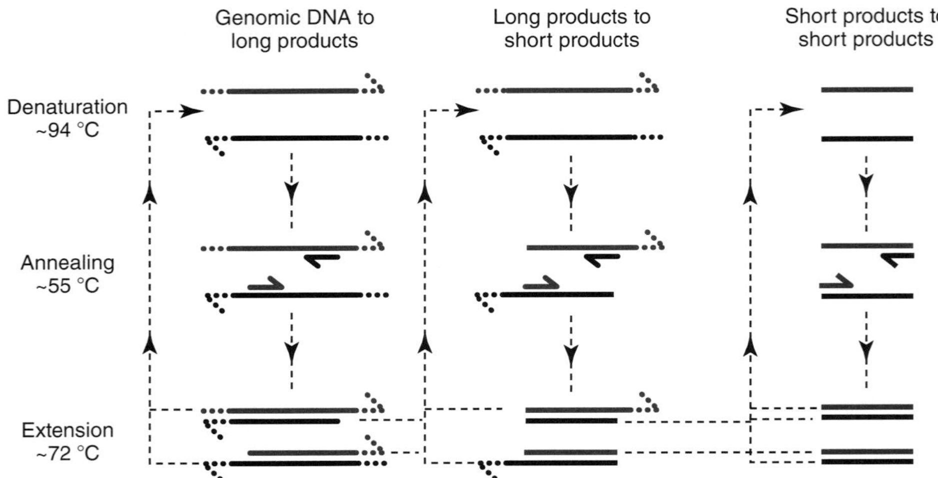

FIGURE 47.4 A more detailed schematic of polymerase chain reaction. Repetitive cycles of denaturation, annealing, and extension are paced by temperature cycling of the reaction. Two primers (indicated as short segments) anneal to opposite template strands *(long red and black lines)* to define the region to be amplified. Extension occurs from the 3′-ends *(indicated with half arrowheads).* In each cycle, genomic DNA is denatured and annealed to primers that extend in opposite directions across the same region, producing long products of undefined length. Long products generated by extension of one of the primers anneal to the other primer during the next cycle, producing short products of defined length. Any short products present produce more short products. After n cycles, 2^n new copies of the amplified region (n long products + [2^n − n] short products) are generated from each original genomic copy. A similar approach can be used to amplify RNA targets by initial reverse transcription of the RNA to produce a DNA template.

typical PCR reaction using 0.5 μmol/L of each primer, the maximum DNA concentration typically achieved is about 100 billion copies/μL.

With the addition of reverse transcriptase, RNA targets can be converted into cDNA and then successfully amplified. Reverse transcription and DNA amplification are most often catalyzed by two different polymerases. In one-step reverse transcriptase polymerase chain reaction (RT-PCR), both enzymes are present in a common buffer, and typically PCR primers are used for both reverse transcription and DNA amplification. Some thermostable enzymes have both DNA polymerase and reverse transcriptase activities so that both steps can be performed in the same tube with the same enzyme. In two-step RT-PCR, the reverse transcription is performed first, usually with random hexamers or a poly-dT oligonucleotide (to prime the poly-A tail of most mRNA). After reverse transcription, the second PCR step is performed on cDNA with specific primers.

After amplification, the products can be detected by various methods. Gel electrophoresis with ethidium bromide staining is a classical method that separates products by size and may suffice for many applications. For fine size discrimination down to a single base, one of the primers can be fluorescently labeled and the post-PCR fragments separated in capillaries on instruments that are typically used for conventional Sanger dideoxy-termination sequencing. Alternatively, some form of hybridization assay can be used to verify or analyze the amplified product. Automated methods are always attractive, and closed-tube methods, in which amplified products are never exposed to the open environment, are particularly advantageous to avoid contamination of future reactions with the products of a prior reaction. Adding a fluorescent dye or probe before amplification allows optical monitoring to follow the reaction as it progresses (real-time PCR) or after the reaction is complete (endpoint melting) without the need to process the sample for a separate analysis step.

Polymerase Chain Reaction Kinetics

It is natural to think about PCR in terms of three events—denaturation of double-stranded target, annealing of primers to their targets, and extension of the DNA strand from the primer—that occur at three different temperatures, each requiring a certain amount of time. Indeed, it is common to perform PCR by holding the reaction mixture at three different temperatures (eg, denaturation at 94°C, annealing at 55°C, and extension at 72°C). Standard thermocyclers that use conical tubes focus on accurate temperature control of the heating block at equilibrium, not on dynamic control of the sample temperature throughout cycling. As a result, sample temperatures are not well defined during transitions, and long cycle times have become standard to ensure that samples reach target temperatures. Reproducibility between instruments and manufacturers is poor, and PCR may require an hour or more to complete 30 cycles of amplification.

The kinetics of denaturation, annealing, and extension suggest that rapid transitions between temperatures with minimal or no pauses (temperature plateaus) provide a better paradigm of PCR amplification (Fig. 47.6). Denaturation, annealing, and extension are very rapid reactions as shown by experiments in capillaries.[32] The use of temperature "spikes" at denaturation and annealing, instead of extended temperature plateaus, allows for rapid cycling with the appropriate instrumentation.[33] The actual time required for PCR depends on the size of the product, but when it is less than 500 base pairs (bp), 30 cycles are easily completed in 15 minutes. Furthermore, rapid amplification improves specificity. Fig. 47.7

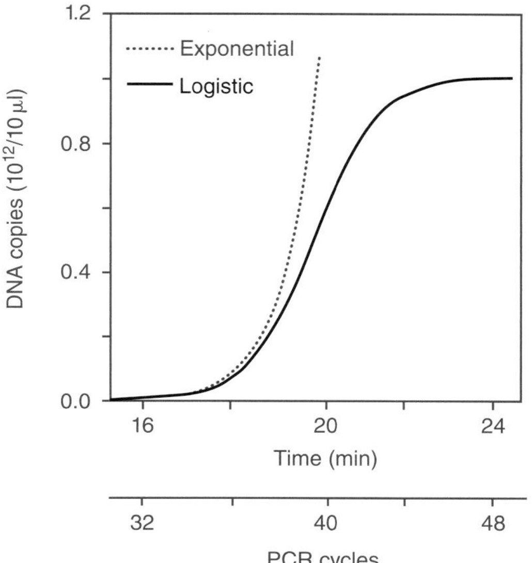

FIGURE 47.5 Exponential and logistic curves for DNA amplified by polymerase chain reaction (PCR). A doubling time of 30 seconds is assumed for PCR, that is, given the equation $N_t = N_0e^{rt}$, in which N_t is the amount of DNA at time t and N_0 is the initial amount of DNA, and r is 1.386 min^{-1} for PCR. A carrying capacity of 100 billion copies of PCR product per µL was used, assuming that the reaction is primer limited at one third the primer concentration (initially at 0.5 µmol/L, or 300 billion primer pairs per µL). Starting with only one target copy, it takes 23 minutes (46 cycles) to amplify the target to saturation when the doubling efficiency is 100%. (Modified with permission of the publisher from Wittwer CT, Kusukawa N. Real-time PCR. In: Persing DH, Tenover FC, Versalovic J, eds. *Molecular microbiology: diagnostic principles and practice.* Washington, DC: ASM Press, 2004:71–84. Copyright 2004 ASM Press.)

shows PCR amplification of the same product amplified at different cycling speeds. With conventional slow cycling, many nonspecific products are generated (see Fig. 47.7, *A*). These products disappear as the cycling time is decreased (see Fig. 47.7, *B* to *D*). In fact, amplification yield and product specificity are optimal when denaturation and annealing times are minimal. However, very rapid cycling may compromise PCR efficiency that is critical for quantitative PCR.

Requirements for denaturation, annealing, and extension in PCR have been reviewed.[34] Initial denaturation of genomic DNA may be required before PCR cycling, depending on how the DNA sample was prepared. Prior boiling of the sample or an initial denaturation step of a few seconds may be necessary to denature very longs strands of genomic DNA. During PCR, however, denaturation of the shorter products occurs very rapidly. Even for long PCR products, denaturation is complete in less than 1 second after the denaturation temperature is reached. Anything greater than a denaturation time of 0 serves only to degrade the polymerase. If longer denaturation times are required, either the sample is not reaching temperature or heat-activated polymerases are being used. Product specificity is optimal when annealing times are less than 1 second. Longer annealing times may be required if the primer concentrations are low. The required extension time for each cycle depends on the length of the PCR product. Extension is not instantaneous, although it is much faster than common practice would suggest. Extension rates of typical polymerases under in vitro conditions are 50 to 100 bases per second. Molecules are fast; people and PCR instruments are slow. Indeed, by increasing the primer and polymerase concentrations 10- to 20-fold, a 60–base pair fragment of genomic DNA was amplified with good efficiency, yield, and specificity in less than 15 seconds.[35] This was achieved with 35 cycles of PCR (each <0.5 seconds) and did not require the use of any hot start method.

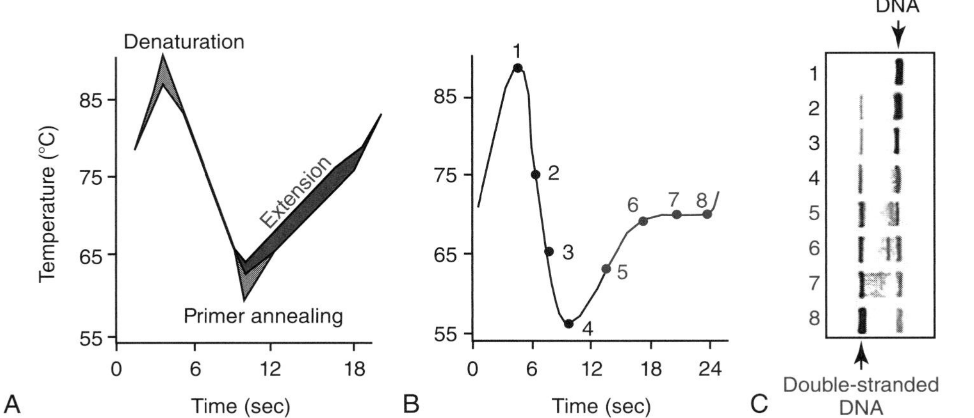

FIGURE 47.6 A visual demonstration of polymerase chain reaction (PCR) kinetics. The three phases of PCR (denaturation, annealing, and extension) occur as the temperature continuously changes **(A)**. Toward the end of temperature cycling, the reaction contains single- and double-stranded PCR products. When different points of the cycle **(B)** are sampled and analyzed, the transition from denatured single-stranded DNA to double-stranded DNA appears as a continuum **(C)**. Sampling is by snap cooling in ice water with analysis on cold agarose gels to best separate single- from double-stranded products. Progression of the extension reaction can be followed by additional bands appearing between the single- and double-stranded DNA (time points *5* to *7*). (Modified with permission from Wittwer CT, Herrmann MG. Rapid thermal cycling and PCR kinetics. In: Innis M, Gelfand D, Sninsky J, eds. *PCR applications*. San Diego: Academic Press, 1999:211–229. Copyright 1999 Academic Press.)

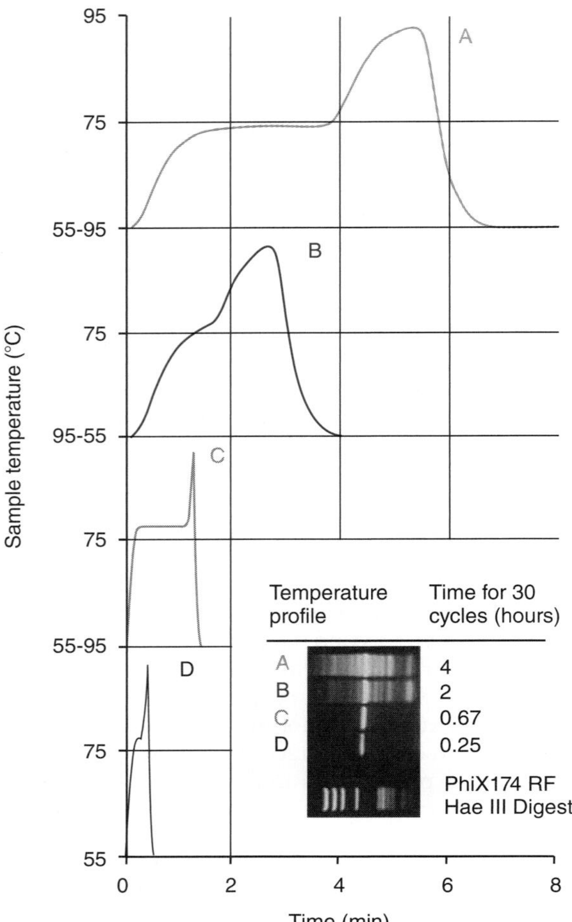

FIGURE 47.7 Rapid polymerase chain reaction improves product specificity. Human genomic DNA samples were cycled 30 times through temperature profiles *A, B, C,* and *D*. Increased specificity of amplification of the 536 bp β-globin fragment of human genomic DNA is seen with faster cycling (*C* and *D*). (Reprinted by permission of the publisher from Wittwer CT, Garling DJ. Rapid cycle DNA amplification: time and temperature optimization. *BioTechniques* 1991;10:76–83. Copyright 1991 Eaton Publishing.)

Polymerase chain reaction products can be as small as 40 bp to about 40 kilobases (kb). To amplify products longer than 2 kb, mixtures of polymerases that include some 3′-exonuclease activity to edit mismatched nucleotides are usually used. Instead of separate annealing and extension temperatures, both processes can be carried out at the same temperature, resulting in two-temperature, instead of three-temperature, cycling. *Taq* DNA polymerase and other polymerases have a terminal transferase activity that may add a single unpaired nucleotide to the 3′-end of PCR product strands. In the presence of all four dNTPs, dATP is preferentially added. This means that many of the double-stranded products generated by PCR will have a protruding A at one or both 3′ ends. Although this does not influence most detection protocols, it can complicate some systems with high size resolution. On the other hand, this feature can be useful in high-efficiency cloning and library construction in massively parallel sequencing.[36]

Polymerase Chain Reaction Optimization

In addition to temperature-cycling conditions, the specificity of PCR depends on the choice of primers and the Mg^{2+} concentration. Mg^{2+} is a polymerase cofactor and also stabilizes the DNA double helix. Low concentrations of Mg^{2+} favor specificity, but high concentrations favor sensitivity. Typical Mg^{2+} concentrations in legacy PCR are rather limited (1.5–2.5 mmol/L), although greater concentrations may be needed to offset chelation of Mg^{2+} by dNTPs, ethylenediaminetetraacetic acid (EDTA), or citrate in the sample.[37] Furthermore, Mg^{2+} concentrations up to 5 mmol/L are required with cycle speeds below 1 seconds.[35] Some common components of PCR buffers, such as K^+, inhibit polymerase extension 75% at 50 mmol/L.[38]

Polymerase chain reaction sensitivity and specificity can be compromised by the formation of unintended low molecular weight artifacts. This process is initiated before PCR, when the primers, template, and polymerase are all together at temperatures below the annealing temperature of the PCR primers. At low temperatures, if a primer momentarily anneals to another primer or to an unintended region, the polymerase may extend the complex. If the extension product, in turn, is primed and extended, then unintended, double-stranded products can be formed (eg, primer-dimers) that serve as amplification templates throughout the reaction. Primer-dimers can be distinguished from the intended target by their molecular weight or melting temperature, but they also influence the efficiency of the intended amplification and decrease assay sensitivity.

The formation of primer-dimers can be minimized in several ways. Almost all limit the activity of polymerase until the temperature is increased (thus the strategy is often collectively called a *hot start*). One method of hot start involves the use of antibody (or an aptamer) to bind and inactivate the polymerase at room temperature. The binding agent is released upon heating, allowing polymerase extension. Another method uses wax or paraffin to create a physical barrier between the essential components in the reaction. Finally, the polymerase, primers, or dNTPs can be chemically blocked so that extension cannot occur until activated by heat, usually requiring an initial denaturation period of 2 to 20 minutes. In an alternative approach, primers are designed to favor a self-annealing, hairpin formation at low temperatures, thus reducing the formation of primer dimers. After the temperature is raised, the primers become linearized and can bind the target DNA, resulting in polymerase extension.

Primer Design

The choice of primers often dictates the quality and success of the amplification reaction. To select primers, the sequence of the target must be known. Some guidelines for primer selection are intuitive and helpful:

1. Make sure the primers anneal to opposite DNA strands of your target with their 3′-ends directed toward each other. The shorter the distance between the primers, the smaller the PCR product and the easier it is to amplify with high efficiency and greater speed. By limiting the extension time, shorter products are amplified with greater efficiency than longer products. With rapid control of temperature cycling, short extension periods selectively amplify shorter products because longer products do not have the time to fully extend.

2. Avoid primers that anneal to themselves or to other primers and particularly avoid complementation at the 3′-end of primers.
3. Choose primers that are specific to the target. Avoid simple sequence repeats and common repeated sequences, such as Alu repeats. If your target has close relatives, design your primers so that they will anneal only to your intended target. Targets that need to be avoided include pseudogenes (for genomic DNA) and related bacterial or viral strains (for microorganisms).
4. Avoid primers that have sequence complementary to internal sequences of the intended product, especially at their 3′-ends.
5. Typically, choose primers between 18 and 25 bases that are matched in melting temperature (Tm) to each other. A primer greater than 17 bases long has a good chance of being unique in the human genome.
6. It is important to avoid sequences similar to your primers that are present in the background DNA likely to be present in your assay. The National Center for Biotechnology Information (NCBI) Basic Local Alignment Search Tool (BLAST) is commonly used to search for similar sequences.[39]
7. Mismatches are better tolerated at the 5′-end rather than the 3′-end of primers. Mismatches at the 3′-end base are most discriminatory and can be used for allele-specific amplification. For efficient amplification, try to completely match at least the first 6 bases at the 3′-end that are important for polymerase binding. Variation at the 5′-end is better tolerated and can be used to introduce restriction sites as long as melting temperature (Tm) differences are considered. Primers can also include 5′-tails that are not homologous to the target for subsequent amplification or detection.

Many primer selection programs are available commercially and others can be freely obtained over the Internet. However, very few of the selection rules have been empirically tested.

Polymerase Chain Reaction Contamination, Inhibition, and Controls

Because PCR typically produces about 1 trillion copies of the target, a small amount of previously amplified product in a new sample reaction will result in false-positive results. Thus, minute aerosol droplets contain enough PCR product for robust amplification. PCR products can contaminate: (1) reagents, (2) pipettes, and (3) glassware. Simple laboratory precautions[40] can minimize contamination by using (1) physically separated areas for pre- and postamplification steps, (2) positive-displacement or barrier filter pipettes to minimize aerosol contamination, and (3) prior preparation and storage of individual or combined ("master mix") reaction components in small aliquots. Chemical methods can prevent contamination from affecting future reactions.[9] These include substituting U for T in PCR with subsequent degradation of the incorporated Us by uracil N-glycosylase or irradiation of DNA product with ultraviolet light. The most effective way of preventing contamination is to contain the product within a closed tube as in real-time PCR. Even with contamination precautions, a negative control or blank reaction (including all reactants except target DNA) is one of the most important controls for PCR.

One advantage of PCR is that it does not require highly purified NA to achieve a successful amplification. In practice, however, clinical samples may contain unpredictable amounts of impurities that can inhibit polymerase activity. Consequently, to ensure reliable amplification in clinical analyses, some form of NA purification is often used (see Chapter 46). The diverse nature of PCR inhibitors within clinical specimens requires demonstration that the sample (or preparation of NA purified from it) will allow amplification. Although such confirmation is automatic with genotyping assays, detection and quantification reactions typically use a control NA sequence different from the target that is added to the sample (or to NA extracted from the sample). Failure to amplify this positive control indicates that further purification of the sample is required to remove inhibitors.

Multiplex Polymerase Chain Reaction and Nested Polymerase Chain Reaction

Multiplex PCR refers to amplifying more than one target simultaneously in the same solution. This can be done by using consensus primers that bind to and amplify more than one bacterial species, for example, ribosomal sequences with high variation internal to the primers, but flanking identical sequence that can be used for consensus primer binding. Usually, however, multiple primer sets are designed for multiple targets and amplified in the same solution at the same time. Although potential primer interactions increase exponentially with multiplex PCR, it works surprising well most of the time as long as the number of PCR cycles is kept low. If lower primer concentrations are used, the annealing time may need to be increased to maintain efficient annealing. Multiplex PCR is often called "preamplification" if it is followed by an additional amplification reaction.

If PCR is performed with a pair of outer primers and then that PCR product is amplified yet again with a set of inner primers, this is referred to as *nested PCR*. Typically, the first round PCR product is diluted 1000 to 1 million times before the inner (nested) primers are added. The advantage of nested PCR is that both sensitivity and specificity increase. The disadvantage is increased potential for contamination, particularly if the first round of PCR products is handled manually for dilution and transfer. Multiplex PCR followed by nested PCR has been used in a closed-tube system for multiplex detection of infectious agents.[41]

Asymmetric Polymerase Chain Reaction

Conventional PCR uses primers that are present in equal amounts, thereby ensuring that most of the DNA products are double stranded. *Asymmetric PCR* uses different concentrations of the two primers to generate more of one strand than of the other. For instance, the use of one primer at 0.5 μmol/L and the other at 0.005 μmol/L produces mostly ssDNA. Yield of the product, however, may be low with this technique. With less extreme ratios (eg, one primer at 0.5 μmol/L and the other at 0.2 μmol/L), the yield is mostly preserved, with one strand produced in enough excess to make it readily available for probe hybridization.

One way to improve the efficiency of asymmetric PCR is to equalize the Tms of the excess and limiting primers. The lower concentration of the limiting primer results in a lower Tm than the excess primer. In "linear after the exponential" (LATE-PCR),[42] the stability of the limiting primer is raised

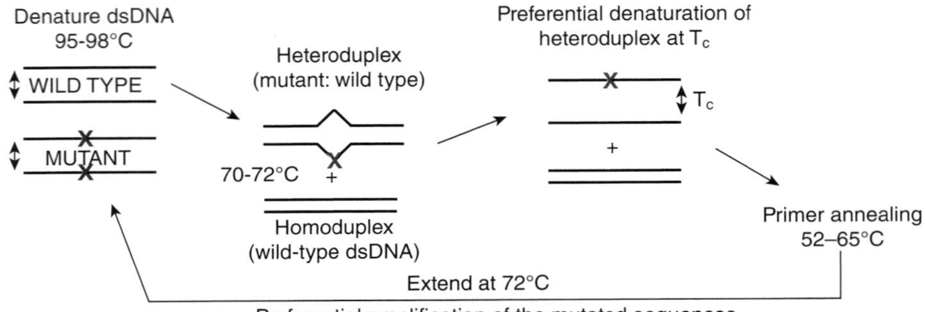

FIGURE 47.8 Schematic of COLD-PCR (co-amplification at lower denaturation temperature polymerase chain reaction). The technique enriches any sequence variant between PCR primers without requiring prior knowledge of variant type or position. Several preliminary rounds of regular PCR from genomic DNA are used to generate an initial amount of PCR product. Then a modified PCR temperature cycle is used for COLD-PCR. After DNA denaturation at 95 to 98°C, the PCR products are incubated at a temperature at which the primers do not bind (eg, 70°C for 2 to 8 minutes) for reannealing and cross-hybridization. Cross-hybridization of mutant and wild-type alleles forms mismatch-containing structures (heteroduplexes) with lower melting temperatures than the fully matched structures (homoduplexes). The temperature is next increased to a critical denaturation temperature (T_c) to preferentially denature the heteroduplex products (a single T_c is used for any mutation along the PCR product; however, different PCR products have different critical denaturation temperatures). The temperature is then reduced for primer annealing (eg, 55°C) and then increased to 72°C for primer extension, thus preferentially amplifying the variant alleles. COLD-PCR is effective for short DNA fragments 50 to 200 bp in length.

sufficiently (typically by making it longer) to counteract the effect of its lower concentration. As a result, the two primers have a comparable ability to bind the template during the initial cycles of PCR. After exponential amplification, linear amplification provides ample template for downstream hybridization assays.

Selective Amplification of Sequence Variants by Polymerase Chain Reaction

Allele-specific PCR enables preferential amplification of one genetic allele over another by placing the 3′-end of one primer at the polymorphic site. The variant that is better matched to the primer extends more readily than the other allele. This strategy can be used to distinguish a gene from its pseudogenes and for genotyping SNVs. Allele-specific PCR can also be used to determine haplotypes.[43]

Polymerase chain reaction can also be modified to enrich for variants internal to the primer binding sites. "Co-amplification at lower denaturation temperature PCR" (COLD-PCR) enriches variants irrespective of their type or position within PCR products smaller than 200 bp.[44] Mismatch-containing sequences have a slightly lower denaturation temperature than fully homologous sequences. During PCR cycling (Fig. 47.8), a product hybridization step after denaturation enables mutation-containing product strands to bind to wild-type strands, forming *heteroduplexes*. The temperature of this step is too high for primers to bind. Next, the temperature of the reaction is raised to a critical denaturation temperature (T_c) that generates preferential denaturation of the mismatch-containing sequences. The temperature is then lowered to allow primers to bind leading to preferential replication of mutation-containing sequences. By repeating this protocol over several PCR cycles, mutation-containing strands are preferentially amplified over wild-type strands. With identification of the correct T_c to within 0.5°C, variant enrichment of 10- to 20-fold for Tm-decreasing (G:C to A:T) or Tm-retaining (eg, T:A to A:T) variants and 5- to 10-fold for Tm-increasing (A:T to G:C) variants is typical. The enrichment increases if a second round of COLD-PCR is applied. Different modifications can enable higher mutation enrichment in a single step[45,46] or restrict enrichment to Tm-decreasing mutations.[47] Because during bisulfite treatment of DNA, unmethylated sequences undergo several C to T changes that decrease Tm, COLD-PCR may also be used for enriching unmethylated sequences.[48] Among various downstream detection methods, high-resolution melting[49-51] or sequencing[52-54] is most often used.

Detection Limits of Polymerase Chain Reaction

When PCR is performed under optimal conditions, a single copy of the target can be detected. In practice, however, the statistical probability of distributing at least a single copy from a dilute template solution into the PCR must be considered. The Poisson distribution indicates that if, on average, one target copy is present per tube, 37% of the tubes will have no target, 37% will have one target, and the remainder will have more than one target. If there is an average of two copies per tube, approximately 14% of the tubes will have no template and will be false negatives. About three copies on average are necessary for 95% of the tubes to include at least one copy. Therefore, the limit of detection (95% probability) of any single PCR cannot be lower than three copies per reaction. About five copies on average are necessary for 99% of the tubes to include at least one copy. This limitation of low copy analysis holds true for any amplification technique. However, digital PCR analyzes many reactions in parallel and can quantify less than one copy (on average) per reaction.

Digital Polymerase Chain Reaction

Conventional PCR averages the amplification results of many individual template molecules. Digital or single-molecule PCR is a technique that uses a dilute solution of template distributed across many reaction compartments or "partitions." Each partition either has or does not have PCR template molecules to amplify. After PCR, the partitions are scored as either positive (one or more initial templates) or negative (no initial template) for a digital readout. Thousands or even millions of partitions are typically scored. The partitions may be aqueous PCR droplets in oil or formed on chips by microfluidics.

Digital PCR can identify and quantify rare sequence variants, precisely determine copy number changes, establish the concentration of PCR standards, and determine the haplotype of variants that are on the same PCR product.[55] When properly performed, digital PCR does not require the standard curves routinely used in quantitative PCR. Digital PCR is less prone to background DNA competition because competing DNA is divided between positive and negative partitions. For example, if only 0.1% of the partitions are positive for a rare variant, 99.9% of the background DNA is in negative wells. The variant-to-background ratio is increased by a factor of 1000 in the positive wells, and better amplification of the variant can be expected. Common PCR inhibitors may not be as apparent in digital PCR because a positive threshold is reached even under conditions of moderate inhibition that would affect bulk quantitative PCR.[56]

Digital PCR results are derived from the average number of initial templates per partition, a value known as λ. Estimates of λ from experimental measurements are determined by Poisson statistics. The precision of the λ estimate increases with the number of partitions. Precision also decreases as λ gets too low (only a few partitions are positive) or too high (nearly all partitions are positive) and is optimal when λ equals 1.59.[57] Consequently, for best precision, a prior estimate of concentration is necessary. Coefficients of variation can be estimated by the Poisson distribution or determined more exactly by the binomial expansion. Single-molecule amplification and digital analysis has also been reported for other amplification methods including loop-mediated isothermal amplification[58] and recombinase polymerase amplification.[59]

Single-molecule PCR is commonly used in massively parallel sequencing methods for clonal amplification. The partitions may be minute aqueous droplets in a water-in-oil emulsion *(emulsion PCR)*,[60] PCR colonies *(polonies)* on a thin film of acrylamide gel,[61] clusters on the surface of a planar flow cell generated by bridge amplification,[62] or beads with clonally amplified template attached to their surface.[19,20,63] When amplification is observed in one of these massively parallel reactions, chances are that clonal amplification occurred from a single template molecule.

Additional Target Amplification Methods

In addition to PCR, many other methods of target amplification have been developed; some have found clinical use and are described in the next sections. These include isothermal amplification methods in which heat denaturation has been replaced by accessory proteins (helicase, recombinase) or strand displacement. These methods still resemble PCR in the products formed. Other methods do not resemble PCR, forming entirely different products based on hairpin extension or the transcription of RNA to DNA.

Transcription-Based Amplification Methods

Transcription-based amplification methods are modeled after the replication of retroviruses. These methods are known by various names, including transcription-mediated

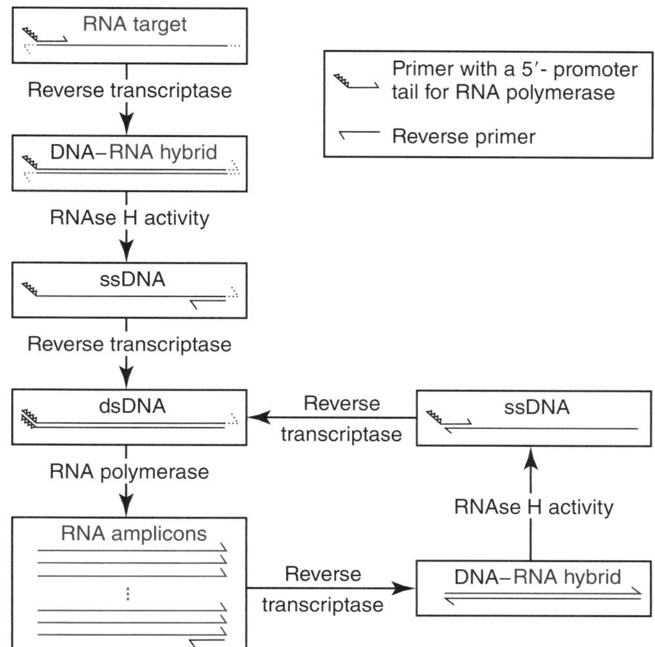

FIGURE 47.9 Schematic diagram of transcription-mediated amplification (TMA). Starting with a single-stranded RNA target, a primer with an RNA polymerase promoter on its 5′-end is extended by reverse transcriptase to form a DNA–RNA hybrid. The reverse transcriptase also has RNAse H activity that subsequently degrades the RNA strand to leave single-stranded DNA (ssDNA). A second primer then binds to the ssDNA, and extension forms double-stranded DNA (dsDNA) with the attached RNA polymerase promoter. RNA polymerase then makes 100 to 1000 copies of RNA, some of which are again primed by the second primer. Repeated cycles of reverse transcription, DNA–RNA hybrid degradation by RNAse H activity, dsDNA formation by reverse transcriptase, and further transcription by RNA polymerase exponentially produce ssRNA amplicons. Single-stranded targets are amplified isothermally, and double-stranded targets are first denatured to single strands.

amplification (TMA),[64,65] NA sequence–based amplification (NASBA),[66] and self-sustained sequence replication (3SR) assays.[67] They amplify their target without temperature cycling (isothermally) and use the collective activities of reverse transcriptase, RNase H, and RNA polymerase. The most widely used is TMA, illustrated in Fig. 47.9. Two primers, a reverse transcriptase, and an RNA polymerase are used. The primer complementary to the RNA target has a 5′-tail that includes a promoter sequence for RNA polymerase. This primer anneals to the target RNA and is extended by the reverse transcriptase, creating an RNA–DNA duplex. The RNA strand is degraded by the RNAse H activity of the reverse transcriptase, allowing the second primer to anneal. The reverse transcriptase then extends the second primer to create double-stranded DNA (dsDNA) that includes the promoter. RNA polymerase recognizes the promoter and initiates transcription, producing 100 to 1000 copies of RNA for each DNA template. Each strand of RNA then binds and extends the second primer, forming an RNA–DNA hybrid; the RNA in the hybrid is degraded, the promoter primer binds and extends to produce dsDNA that can be transcribed, and the cycle repeats. As in PCR, all reagents are included, and amplification is exponential with completion in less than 1 hour. Unlike PCR, these methods do not require temperature cycling (except for an initial heat denaturation if a DNA template is used). They are particularly advantageous when the target is RNA (eg, human immunodeficiency virus [HIV] and hepatitis C virus [HCV] in blood bank NA testing).

Loop-Mediated Amplification Methods

Instead of producing products of a defined length, loop-mediated amplification (LAMP) produces a wide range of different DNA structures with branches and loops. In the basic version, two strand displacement primers and two loop-forming primers recognize six segments in the target.[68] The inner two primers each include a 5′-tail that is complementary to the target sequence. After extension of the inner primers, hairpins or loops can form on each end, one of which will have a free 3′-end that can further extend. This loop formation is similar to self-probing[69] and snapback[70] primers, except that the 3′-end is not blocked. The two outer primers are used for displacement of the inner extension products to produce the starting material for cyclic amplification. The chain reaction includes both extension of the free 3′-ends and additional priming from the inner primers to the exposed single strands in the loops. The amplification results in a mixture of products with ever more loops and branching structures of increasing complexity. In another version of LAMP, allele-specific amplification with five primers and one competitive probe recognizes seven segments in the target.[71] In both versions, a variety of products are formed, and the reactions can be completed in less than 1 hour.

Strand Displacement Amplification

Similar to loop-mediated amplification, strand displacement amplification (SDA)[72] requires initial generation of starting material before the chain reaction. DNA is first heat denatured in the presence of four primers: two outer displacement primers and two inner primers with 5′-tails that includes a restriction site. An exonuclease-negative polymerase with good displacement activity is added in the presence of dCTP, dGTP, dUTP, and a modified deoxynucleotide (dATPαS), incorporating both the restriction site and the modified dATPαS into products that are ready to enter into exponential amplification. Exponential amplification occurs at 37°C by (1) nicking of the restriction enzyme site by the restriction enzyme (double-strand cutting is prevented by dATPαS); (2) extension from the nicked site with strand displacement; (3) priming of the displaced strand with the original inner primer that includes the restriction site; and (4) extension of both the primer and displaced strand, forming a new doubled-stranded product with the restriction site. Steps 1 through 4 are repeated over and over again for exponential amplification.

Variants of Polymerase Chain Reaction That Do Not Require Heat Denaturation

Variants of PCR have been developed that replace the need for heat denaturation with enzymatic separation of the double helix. These methods do not require thermal cycling and better reflect the normal DNA replication process, although the end products are the same as in the PCR. For example, helicase-dependent amplification (HDA)[73] uses the unwinding enzyme, helicase, to separate the double helix into single stands. As originally described, additional proteins were needed to stabilize the process that was performed at 37°C. Later, using a heat-stable helicase and polymerase allowed amplification at 60° to 65°C without the need for any other accessory proteins.[74] Another technique, recombinase polymerase amplification (RPA), uses a recombinase to scan dsDNA for priming sites, causing strand exchange to anneal the primers and single-stranded binding proteins to stabilize the loop structure long enough for strand displacement primer extension.[75] Two opposing primers exponentially replicate a short DNA fragment as in PCR, but the reaction is performed at 37°C without temperature cycling.

Whole-Genome and Whole-Transcriptome Amplification

Instead of specific amplification of one target to improve sensitivity, methods that amplify all genomic DNA or mRNAs are useful when the target is in short supply. For example, *multiple-displacement amplification* uses exonuclease-resistant random hexamers and a highly processive polymerase to amplify DNA nonspecifically.[76] Initial DNA denaturation is not necessary, and the reaction proceeds isothermally. Similarly, messenger RNA can be generically amplified with a poly(T) primer modified with an RNA polymerase promoter.[77] After reverse transcription, second-strand DNA synthesis and transcription, antisense RNA is produced. Both whole genome and antisense RNA amplification are also useful as NA purification methods before amplification or detection.

Signal and Probe Amplification Methods

It is not always necessary to amplify the target DNA or RNA sequence. Instead of target amplification, signal amplification or probe amplification can be used.

Branched-Chain DNA: Signal Amplification

Instead of increasing the concentration of target, signal amplification techniques use NAs to magnify the detection signal. The branched-chain DNA (bDNA) method is one of these techniques in common use. The bDNA approach hybridizes the target NA to multiple capture probes affixed to a microtiter well.[78] This is followed by hybridization to a series of "extender," "preamplifier," and "amplifier" probes. The final, highly branched amplifier probe includes multiple copies of signal-generating enzymes that act on a chemiluminescent substrate to produce light. Nucleotide analogs isoC and isoG (isomers of C and G that are complementary to each other but not to other nucleotides) are often used to increase the specificity of the signaling cascade.

Serial Invasive Amplification: Signal Amplification

When two probes overlap on one target, an "invasive" cleavage reaction can be catalyzed by certain structure-specific nucleases. The cleaved fragment, in turn, can cause invasive cleavage of a secondary probe in the shape of a hairpin. The hairpin probe can be designed as a fluorogenic indicator by using a reporter–quencher pair of dyes that are separated by cleavage. This serial sequence of events (primary invasion and cleavage followed by secondary invasion and cleavage of an indicator probe) is known as the serial invasive signal amplification reaction.[79] After DNA denaturation, cooling, and the addition of enzymes, the reaction is run at a temperature at which both the primary and secondary reactions recycle.

Rolling Circle Amplification: Probe Amplification

If a primer is annealed to a closed circle of DNA in the presence of a processive, displacing polymerase, the complement of the circle will be synthesized over and over again with displacement of the tandem repeats.[80] If two primers are used in opposite orientation, progressively more complex branches will be formed in an exponential reaction. The rolling circle can be formed by ligation of the two ends of a linear probe on template DNA. Ligation may happen directly, after polymerization through a gap, or after annealing of an additional, allele-specific oligonucleotide.

Endpoint Quantification in Amplification Assays

Molecular diagnostic assays may be qualitative (detect the presence or absence of a target or genotype identification) or quantitative (quantify the original concentration of a target sequence in the sample). When amplification is part of the assay, many variables need to be controlled carefully for accurate and precise quantification. Variation in extraction efficiency, the presence of enzyme inhibitors, lot-to-lot variation in enzyme and reagent performance, and day-to-day variation in reaction and detection conditions need to be addressed by quantitative methods. With reverse transcriptase assays, even more variables (reverse transcription efficiency and choice of reference genes) need to be considered.

Quantitative analysis at the endpoint of amplification is usually carried out with the use of calibrators with known amounts of target or a target mimic. Sample NA may be quantified by comparison with an *internal standard* of known amount that is added at the time of sample processing to control for efficiency of NA purification. These internal standards can be DNA fragments, plasmids, or RNA packaged into synthetic phage or virus particles to mimic real viruses.[81]

Real-time (continuous) analysis is simpler and more powerful for quantification than most endpoint analyses. Reactions are monitored at each cycle and initial target concentrations are typically calculated from the change (usually increase) in fluorescence with cycle number. Digital PCR is analyzed at the endpoint of amplification and provides potential advantages in precision, copy number, and rare variant analysis. Guidelines for performing and reporting quantitative real-time PCR (qPCR)[82] and digital PCR (dPCR)[83] experiments are good guides for both novice and experienced users.

DETECTION TECHNIQUES

Molecular diagnostics uses both generic and specific methods of NA detection. NAs can be quantified in bulk by optical techniques of absorbance and fluorescence (these are discussed in Chapter 46). Specific methods of detection and quantification usually use sequence-specific primers or probes with fluorescent or electronic detection.

Nucleic Acid Probes

Ultraviolet absorbance and fluorescent dyes in themselves do not discriminate between different NA sequences (ie, they are not sequence specific). Specificity in NA assays almost always comes from the hybridization of two complementary NA strands. Many reporter molecules can be covalently attached or incorporated into NA probes. Use of these probes can reveal the physical presence or location of sequences complementary to the NA portion of the probe. The first probes used in NA detection were radioactively labeled. Radioactive probes have a short shelf life limited by isotopic decay and radiolysis of the NA. This inherent instability, along with concerns of radioisotope safety and disposal, restricts the use of radioactive probes in the clinical laboratory. Although they are not discussed further here, prior versions of this chapter in earlier editions provide more detail.[9]

Indirect Detection of Hybridized Probes

The first practical example of nonradioactive probes used a biotin-labeled analog of dUTP.[84] Despite the altered steric configuration, this nucleotide is incorporated by most DNA polymerases. Other functional groups, such as digoxigenin, may also be used as affinity labels through chemical linkage to a dUTP and incorporation into polynucleotides. Alternatively, oligonucleotide probes can be labeled during synthesis with biotin or amino linkers for subsequent attachment to indicator molecules. Labels at the 5′- or 3′-end of the molecule are usually preferred because central modifications typically interfere more with hybridization.

Biotin and other affinity labels do not generate detectable signals on their own. However, they can initiate signal amplification mediated by high-affinity binding with antibodies, or in the case of biotin, with streptavidin. These binding molecules can be linked to enzymes—such as alkaline phosphatase, peroxidase, or luciferase—connecting a single target to a single enzyme. Enzyme activity is monitored by detecting catalytic turnover of enzyme substrates that result in colorimetric, fluorescent, or chemiluminescent signals.

Affinity labels can be used to capture and localize targets to an area of a solid support. For example, biotinylated probes can be affixed to a streptavidin-coated surface. After incubation with the target NA, a second probe is added, which may be directly labeled with fluorescence or conjugated through another affinity label to an enzyme. Any background or nonspecific localization of reagents results in amplification of an undesired signal along with the desired signal, and these methods usually require multiple separation and washing steps to decrease the background.

Fluorescent Labels

Advances in oligonucleotide synthesis and fluorescence detection have made fluorescently labeled probes the preferred reporter for NA analysis. Many fluorescent labels are now available, allowing color multiplexing for applications such as DNA sequencing, fragment length analysis, DNA arrays, and real-time PCR as reviewed later in this chapter. Techniques such as fluorescence polarization, fluorescence resonance energy transfer (FRET), and fluorescence quenching can provide additional detection specificity. Fluorescence polarization can be used to distinguish free from bound label, if the molecular rotation of the probe changes upon binding.[85] Molecular rotation primarily depends on the size of the molecule, so binding of a small probe onto a large target results in a polarization increase that can be measured. FRET techniques depend on the distance between two spectrally distinct fluorescent labels. Two labeled probes may be brought closer together by adjacent hybridization. Alternatively, two labels on the same probe may end up farther apart by hydrolysis or hybridization. Fluorescence quenching or augmentation does not always require FRET. For example, fluorescence may change merely by hybridization of a fluorescent oligonucleotide to its target. The effect depends on the dye and on inherent quenching from G residues in the target or probe.[86,87] Alternatively, quenching moieties can be directly incorporated into probes.[87,88]

Electrochemical Detection

Electrochemical detection of NAs is attractive for its simplicity. Hybridization events can be detected by redox indicators that recognize the DNA duplex or by other hybridization-induced changes in electrochemical parameters, such as conductivity or capacitance.[89,90] Usually, PCR amplification is performed before detection, so that many molecules are available and a bulk signal is generated to increase sensitivity. Electronic detection is also used in massively parallel sequencing, in which single nucleotide extension (SNE) from a clonally covered DNA bead produces a change in pH that is detected by complementary metal oxide semiconductor (CMOS) sensors.[63] Direct electronic sequencing of single molecules is also possible by detecting current changes that occur when a single strand of DNA passes through a nanopore.[91]

DISCRIMINATION TECHNIQUES

Nucleic acid discrimination techniques are divided into three categories: (1) electrophoretic methods that physically separate NAs based on molecular size or shape; (2) alternatives to electrophoresis that determine the size, base content, or sequence of NAs without electrophoresis, including high-performance liquid chromatography (HPLC), mass spectrometry, and pyrosequencing; and (3) hybridization assays that identify specific NAs by annealing or melting of complementary NAs. Some techniques use both electrophoresis and hybridization.

Electrophoresis

Both DNA and RNA are negatively charged and migrate toward the positively charged electrode when an electrical field is present within an appropriately buffered solution. Separation of different NAs occurs when mixtures are allowed to travel through a neutral sieving polymer under the electrical field. Separation is based primarily on molecular size, with smaller molecules traveling faster through the polymer than larger ones (Fig. 47.10). When very large molecules (≥50 kb) have to be separated, pulsed electrical fields are used to help move these molecules through the polymer matrix.[92] Separation also occurs based on the physical conformation, or shape, of the molecule. For instance, (1) single-stranded molecules may fold into secondary structures or they may stay as flexible linear structures; (2) linear double-stranded molecules may form heteroduplexes with mismatched bases, or they may stay in their original homoduplex forms; and (3) circular double-stranded NAs may be nicked and take a relaxed open-circular structure, or they can be in a more compact superhelical structure. Under nondenaturing conditions, each of these shapes may influence the way NA molecules travel through the electrophoretic matrix. Separation based on shape can provide useful information, but it can also confuse size-based analysis. Electrophoresis of DNA is performed under nondenaturing or denaturing conditions depending on the application.

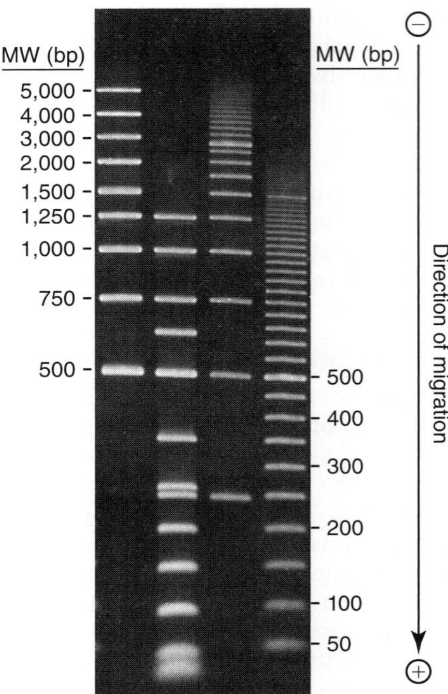

FIGURE 47.10 A photograph of multiple DNA fragments after agarose gel electrophoresis (1% w/v, SeaKem LE agarose gel) showing the separation of double-stranded DNA molecules by size. *MW,* Molecular weight. (Photograph courtesy Lonza Rockland Inc, Rockland, Maine.)

RNA electrophoresis is commonly performed as a quality control check before transcript quantification or microarray expression analysis. RNA can be degraded easily by tissue or environmental RNAses, so it is important to assess the quality of the RNA used in these methods. Because RNA often has secondary structure, electrophoresis is usually performed under denaturing conditions to abolish these structures. Microfluidic chips with integrated microelectrophoresis channels are commercially available to rapidly assess RNA integrity by inspection of ribosomal RNA peaks (Fig. 47.11). Although specific transcripts are not detected by this method, only small amounts of starting RNA are needed.

Agarose and *polyacrylamide* are the two types of polymers commonly used in electrophoresis. Several chemical variants of the polymers are commercially available and are tailored for different separation ranges and applications. The choice of polymer and polymer concentration (usually expressed as % w/v) is dictated by (1) the size of NA to be separated, (2) the resolution that is required, and (3) how the result will be visualized and analyzed. Using various concentrations, an agarose gel can separate NA fragments as small as 20 bp to more than 10 mb (10,000 kb), including chromosomes of yeast, fungi, and parasites. However, the resolution of agarose is limited, usually to a size difference of 2% to 5%. Agarose polymers are cast in trays (sometimes commercially supplied as precast gels) and submerged in buffer. The gels are permeable to fluorescent NA–binding dyes, and results may be recorded as a photographic image of the stained gel under illumination.

Polyacrylamide polymers are suited for high-resolution separation (down to about 0.1% size differences) of short molecules (up to about 2 kb) and are the primary

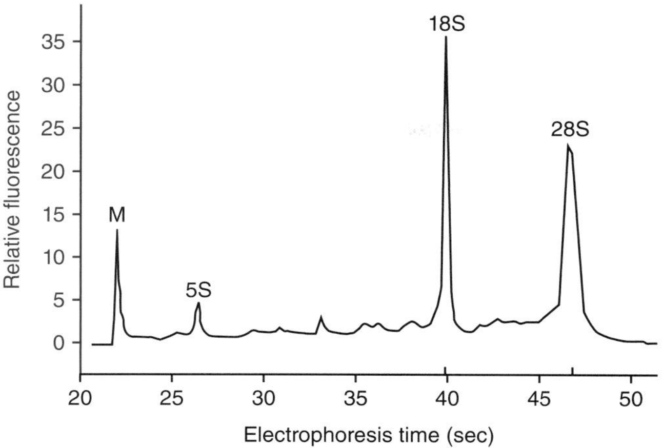

FIGURE 47.11 Microelectrophoresis of human white blood cell (WBC) RNA. After isolation of WBCs and extraction of total RNA, samples were denatured, stained with a fluorescent dye, and applied to a commercial microelectrophoresis platform for assessment of RNA quality. Prominent 18S and 28S bands of ribosomal RNA suggest the RNA is largely intact. Also indicated are a reference marker (M) and the 5S ribosomal band. Note that electrophoresis was performed in less than 1 minute.

polymers for single-stranded NA separation, such as dideoxy-termination sequencing. Polyacrylamide may be used as a linear polymer solution, which is filled in capillaries *(capillary electrophoresis),* or as cross-linked gels, which are cast between two plastic or glass plates *(slab gel electrophoresis).* Polyacrylamide gels are permeable to fluorescent stains, and NAs can also be silver stained. In addition, the optical clarity of polyacrylamide polymers makes them ideal for visualizing emission signals from fluorescently-labeled fragments using laser-induced fluorescence detection. Table 47.2 lists common electrophoresis-based techniques.

TABLE 47.2 Commonly Used Electrophoresis-Based Techniques

Techniques Using Electrophoresis	Abbreviation	Primary Application
Polymerase chain reaction (or reverse transcriptase polymerase chain reaction) length	PCR (or RT-PCR)	Detection
Polymerase chain reaction /restriction fragment length polymorphism	PCR/RFLP	Detection
Southern blotting		Detection
Northern blotting		Detection
Dideoxy-termination sequencing (Sanger)		Sequencing
Single-nucleotide extension assay	SNE	Genotyping
Oligonucleotide ligation assay	OLA	Genotyping
Multiplex ligation-dependent probe amplification	MLPA	Quantification
Heteroduplex migration assay	HDA	Scanning
Conformation-sensitive gel electrophoresis	CSGE	Scanning
Single-strand conformation polymorphism analysis	SSCP, SSCA	Scanning
Denaturing gradient gel electrophoresis	DGGE	Scanning
Temperature gradient electrophoresis	TGGE, TGCE	Scanning
Temperature cycling capillary electrophoresis	TCCE	Scanning

Polymerase Chain Reaction Product Length

Polymerase chain reaction product analysis by electrophoresis is frequently used to query the product size and specificity of PCR. PCR products are visualized by staining the gel with a fluorescent DNA-binding dye, such as ethidium bromide. In some cases, the presence of an amplification product is directly diagnostic (eg, detection of sequences found only in a bacterium, virus, or fungus in a human sample). The specificity of the amplification reaction is verified by the known size of the fragment and the lack of extraneous bands. Internal negative and positive controls are used to control for potential contamination and PCR inhibitors.

Small insertions, deletions, rearrangements, and changes in the number of repeated sequences can also be detected by monitoring PCR product length on gels. Length differences may be large and easily visualized with agarose gel electrophoresis, or they may be small enough to require a denaturing polyacrylamide matrix. Fluorescent primers may be incorporated into the product during PCR to simplify detection of fragment lengths. These techniques are commonly used in the diagnosis of inherited diseases and in identity assessment.

Restriction Fragment Length Polymorphism

DNA extracted from a cell is extremely long and is usually cut into shorter fragments before electrophoresis to enhance mobility. Restriction endonucleases cut dsDNA into fragments of reproducible size; the same enzyme produces the same fragments in different specimens if they contain the same DNA sequence. If an alteration in the DNA abolishes or creates a cleavage site recognized by the enzyme (or changes the spacing between two cleavage sites), different sized fragments will be produced. These changes in fragment lengths (or polymorphisms) that result from restriction digestion are called restriction fragment length polymorphisms (RFLPs). However, restriction digestion of genomic DNA produces thousands of fragments. To be useful, specific fragments need to be visualized with probes such as in Northern and Southern blotting.[9]

Polymerase Chain Reaction/Restriction Fragment Length Polymorphisms

Many sequence alterations (eg, single base changes) do not affect the length of DNA. However, they can be amplified easily by PCR, and many can be detected as RFLPs after treatment with restriction enzymes. After PCR, the products are digested with one or more enzymes and analyzed by electrophoresis. For example, if a sample has a variant that disrupts an enzyme recognition site, it can be distinguished from a sample that does not have the variant. Such an assay

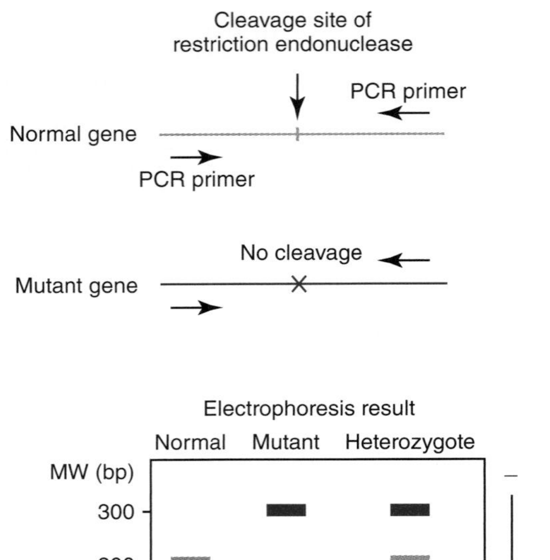

FIGURE 47.12 An example of polymerase chain reaction (PCR) restriction fragment length polymorphism (PCR-RFLP). A DNA fragment amplified by PCR carries a site (a unique sequence of generally four or more bases) that is recognized and cleaved by a restriction endonuclease. If a mutation is present, this site is altered and is no longer recognized by the enzyme. Electrophoresis reveals that the fragment from a normal specimen was indeed cut by the enzyme, generating two fragments shorter than the original length, but the fragment from a homozygous mutant was not cut, and the original length of the PCR product is preserved. In a heterozygous mutant, both the original fragment and the shorter fragments are visible. *MW,* Molecular weight.

will produce one uncut PCR fragment when the variant is present and two shorter fragments with normal DNA (Fig. 47.12). If the variant is present as a heterozygote (one normal and one variant copy of DNA), then one long and two shorter fragments will be observed. Usually it is possible to design the assay so that the fragments can be easily resolved by agarose electrophoresis. One variant of this method uses reverse-transcribed mRNA, which lacks the introns that would be present in the DNA. In this way, multiple exons can be analyzed in a single PCR. To detect rare variants that create a restriction site, this method can be modified by ligating an oligonucleotide to the cut site and using this oligonucleotide as one of the primers in a subsequent PCR amplification. The presence of the variant can be identified with enhanced sensitivity using either electrophoresis or real-time PCR.[93]

Conformation-Sensitive Scanning Techniques

Several electrophoretic methods can be used to scan for sequence variants after PCR amplification. For example, heteroduplex analysis (HDA), also known as conformation-sensitive gel electrophoresis (CSGE),[94] reveals the presence of variants by the altered mobility of dsDNA fragments that contain one or more mismatched bases (a heteroduplex) versus one that is perfectly matched (a homoduplex). Denaturing gradient gel electrophoresis (DGGE)[95] and temperature-gradient gel electrophoresis (TGGE)[96,97] detect heteroduplexes by their lower stability. As the temperature or denaturing gradients are increased, heteroduplexes melt at lower temperatures, and eventually the strands separate, altering the gel migration. Single-strand conformation polymorphism analysis (SSCP or SSCA)[98] monitors the folding of single DNA strands produced by PCR. Electrophoretic mobility is a function of size and shape of the folded single-stranded molecules. Many of these methods, originally developed on slab gels, now have counterparts with separations by capillary electrophoresis. For example, cycling temperature capillary electrophoresis (CTCE)[99] has been proposed for pangenomic scanning for unknown point mutations. Scanning electrophoretic techniques have lost popularity as sequencing costs have decreased. Instead, direct dideoxy sequencing and massively parallel sequencing not only identify that a variant is present but also provide the variant sequence. Another alternative that does not require electrophoretic separation or expensive equipment is high-resolution melting. Additional details of scanning electrophoretic methods can be found in the previous edition of this chapter.[9]

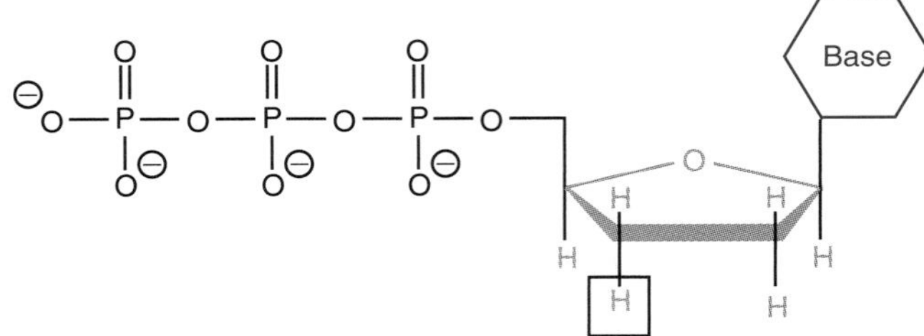

FIGURE 47.13 A dideoxynucleotide. Notice the absence of the 3′-OH that is usually present in standard deoxynucleotides. This lack of a 3′-OH prevents polymerase extension because no phosphodiester bond can form. Incorporation of a dideoxynucleotide forces termination of polymerase extension.

Dideoxy-Termination Sequencing (Sanger Sequencing)

Dideoxy-termination sequencing[100] of DNA is routinely performed in the clinical laboratory. RNA can also be sequenced by first converting RNA to DNA by reverse transcriptase. NA sequence is determined and compared with a reference sequence with an error rate of approximately 0.1% (one misidentified base in 1000). Often the sequence is analyzed on both strands (sense and antisense) for even greater accuracy. Any deviation from the reference sequence is identified by using various available computer software programs to compare the sequences. Base changes, including synonymous changes that do not alter the protein sequence, as well as nonsynonymous changes resulting in altered amino acids, stop codons, and small insertions and deletions, are identified. However, larger deletions and rearrangements spanning the sequencing primer binding sites are not detected.

The most common sequencing strategy uses PCR in the first step to amplify the region of interest followed by a chain-termination reaction developed in the late 1970s.[10] This reaction generates fragments that are terminated at various lengths by incorporation of one of the four dideoxynucleotide base analogs during extension from a sequencing primer. Dideoxynucleotides lack both 3′- and 2′-hydroxyl groups on the pentose ring (Fig. 47.13). Because DNA chain elongation requires the addition of deoxynucleotides to the 3′OH group, incorporation of dideoxynucleotides terminates chain extension. The most common method for generating these terminated fragments is *cycle sequencing,* repeating

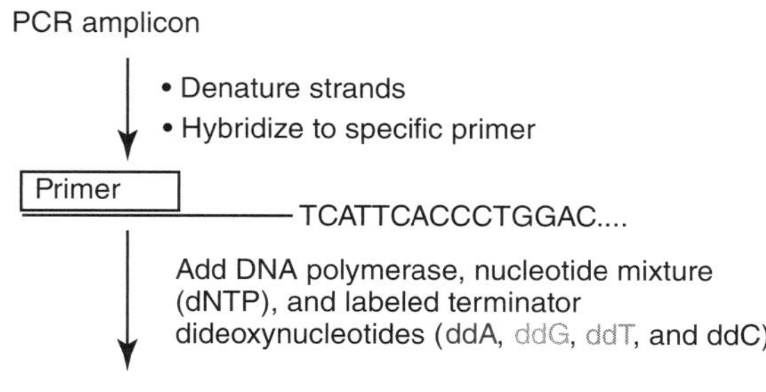

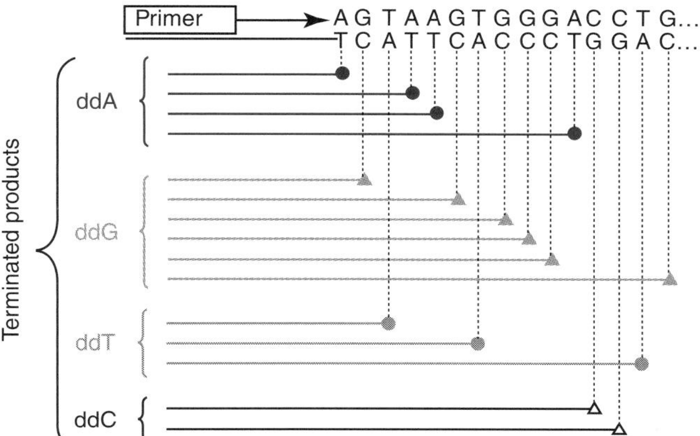

FIGURE 47.14 The dideoxy-termination reaction for sequencing. A polymerase chain reaction (PCR) product is denatured and hybridized to a specific oligonucleotide primer. As the DNA polymerase extends the primer by incorporating bases (deoxynucleotides [dNTPs]) complementary to the template, it occasionally incorporates a terminator dideoxynucleotide base analog (ddA, ddG, ddT, or ddC) that stops further extension. The result is a mixture of extended products of varying lengths. Each terminator base may be labeled with one of four different fluorescent tags (shown as different symbols in the diagram). Alternatively, the primer can carry four different fluorescent tags in individual chain-termination reactions (containing only one dideoxy nucleoside triphosphate [ddNTP]) performed in separate tubes. The original procedure incorporated a radioactive dNTP during extension, allowing monochromatic detection of the truncated fragments in four electrophoresis lanes.

the steps of annealing, chain extension-termination, and denaturation by temperature cycling, similar to PCR (Fig. 47.14). The fragments generated are tagged with a fluorescent dye (with the use of labeled primers or labeled terminator dideoxynucleotides), are separated by electrophoresis, and are detected by fluorescence as the fragments travel past a detector (Fig. 47.15). When fluorescently labeled primers are used, four tubes are needed, each with one of the four dideoxy-terminators. If four colors are used, the termination reactions can be combined before electrophoresis, and only one capillary is necessary. After PCR and cycle sequencing, about 600 to 800 bases can be resolved in less than 2 hours by capillary electrophoresis, and 96 or 384 samples can be run in parallel.

RNA sequencing in the clinical laboratory is commonly used in viral genotyping such as HIV for drug resistance and HCV to establish prognosis and appropriate therapy. Sequencing is also used for bacterial speciation by analysis of ribosomal DNA, to identify mutations in many genetic diseases, and in cancer. Dideoxy sequencing, even of only one gene (including exons and splice sites), in the clinical laboratory for the detection of disease-causing mutations is still an expensive proposition, with the cost of analysis proportional to the size of the gene. This is especially true for population screening (in which most samples will not have a mutation) but also for patients with symptoms of the disease. Massively parallel sequencing vastly reduces these costs and will be discussed later.

Single Nucleotide Extension

Also known as *single-base primer extension* or *minisequencing,* SNE assays[101] involve the annealing of an oligonucleotide primer to a single-stranded PCR product at a location that is immediately adjacent to, but does not include, the site of the single base variant followed by enzymatic extension of the primer in the presence of polymerase and dideoxynucleotide terminators. For example, each of the four terminators can be labeled with a unique fluorescent label so that it is possible to detect which base was incorporated. SNE assays can be multiplexed on capillary electrophoresis instruments by varying the lengths of the primers so that each SNV is resolved by size in one electrophoresis run. Many SNE detection methods are available other than electrophoresis, including (1) photometric detection on microtiter plates, (2) product capture detection systems on DNA microarrays, (3) bead hybridization assays detected by flow cytometry, (4) solution-based fluorescence polarization detection systems, and (5) mass spectrometry. SNE assays are particularly useful when the target of interest contains 5 to 50 disease-causing single base variants. SNE assays do not work well if variants are present in the primer-binding site. Nor are they usually designed to detect variants at a position other than immediately adjacent to the 3′-end of a primer.

Oligonucleotide Ligation

Another assay format frequently used for variant detection is the oligonucleotide ligation assay (OLA).[102] Two oligonucleotide probes are hybridized to adjacent sequences of amplified target DNA, with the variation site positioned at the end of one probe (Fig. 47.16). DNA ligase covalently joins the two probes only if both probes are perfectly hybridized to the target, including the polymorphic base. A probe matching the normal base and another probe matching the variant base are usually prepared. These two can be discriminated through differential electrophoretic mobility by varying the length of their 5′-tails. These tails can be noncomplementary poly A or poly C tails or penta-ethylene oxide (PEO) units. The probe hybridizing to both alleles (the *common probe*) provides the reporter molecule, usually a fluorescent label. Multiplexing is achieved by attaching different fluorescent labels to the common probes and by varying the length of the tails on the allele-specific probes. After ligation, probes for multiple variants are separated by denaturing capillary electrophoresis.

Multiplex Ligation-Dependent Probe Amplification

Multiplex ligation-dependent probe amplification (MLPA)[103] is a convenient method for relative quantification of up to 10

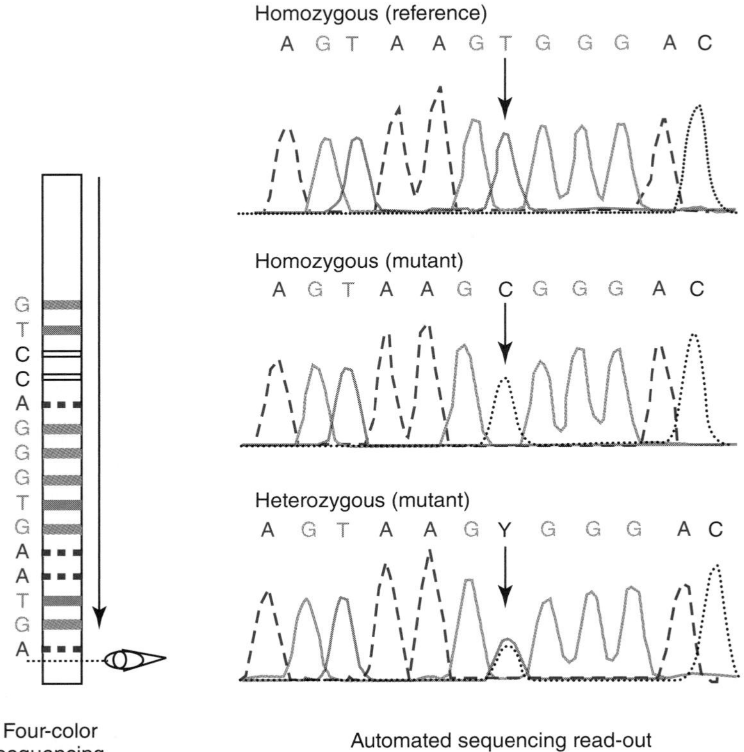

FIGURE 47.15 Schematic of dideoxy-termination DNA sequencing. Extension products (see Fig. 47.13) are labeled with different color dyes for each of the four terminator reactions and are separated by electrophoresis. The four-color strategy allows automated endpoint fluorescence detection *(eye icon)*. The direction of fragment migration is from top to bottom. The sequence is read from left to right in the electropherogram generated by the sequencer. Examples of a reference sample (homozygous T at the polymorphic site), a mutant sample (homozygous C), and a heterozygous mutant sample (T and C, reported as Y) are shown.

to 50 targets. This method is particularly useful in screening for deletions or duplications of exons, multiple exons, or whole genes. For each target, two probes are designed that hybridize adjacent to each other so that they can be ligated. The two probes have unique tails that do not hybridize to the target and that are the same between targets. After hybridization and ligation, the probes are amplified by PCR with a common primer pair (complementary to the tails). One of the primers is fluorescently labeled at its 5′-end. Because probes of different lengths are used, multiple PCR products of different sizes are produced and separated by capillary electrophoresis. Relative peak heights or areas are compared for relative quantification.

Alternatives to Electrophoresis

Electrophoresis is not the only method to determine the size, base content, and/or sequence of NAs. Some of these alternatives to electrophoresis are attractive in the clinical laboratory because of compatibility with automation and capacity for high throughput. Some examples include pyrosequencing, mass spectrometry, and high-pressure liquid chromatography.

Pyrosequencing

Pyrosequencing[104] is a sequencing-by-synthesis method that does not require dideoxy-termination or electrophoresis. A sequencing primer is hybridized to a single-stranded template generated by PCR. Four enzymes, a DNA polymerase, ATP sulfurylase, luciferase, and apyrase, and two substrates—adenosine 5′-phosphosulfate and luciferin—are included in the reaction mixture (Fig. 47.17). One of the four dNTPs is added to the reaction, with dATPαS substituted for dATP because it is incorporated by the polymerase but is not a luciferase substrate. If the base is complementary to the template strand, DNA polymerase catalyzes its incorporation. Each incorporation event is accompanied by release of a pyrophosphate (PPi) so that the quantity of PPi produced is equimolar to the amount of incorporated nucleotide. The release of PPi is monitored by conversion of PPi and adenosine 5′-phosphosulfate into adenosine triphosphate (ATP) by ATP sulfurylase, and ATP in turn drives conversion of luciferin into oxyluciferin, which generates visible light. The light produced is proportional to the number of nucleotides incorporated. Apyrase, which is a nucleotide-degrading enzyme, continuously degrades ATP and unincorporated dNTP. This switches off the light in preparation for the next dNTP addition. As the process is repeated by adding one dNTP at a time, the complementary DNA strand is built, and the nucleotide sequence is determined.

Mass Spectrometry

Matrix-assisted laser-desorption ionization time-of-flight (MALDI-TOF) mass spectrometry can be used to genotype

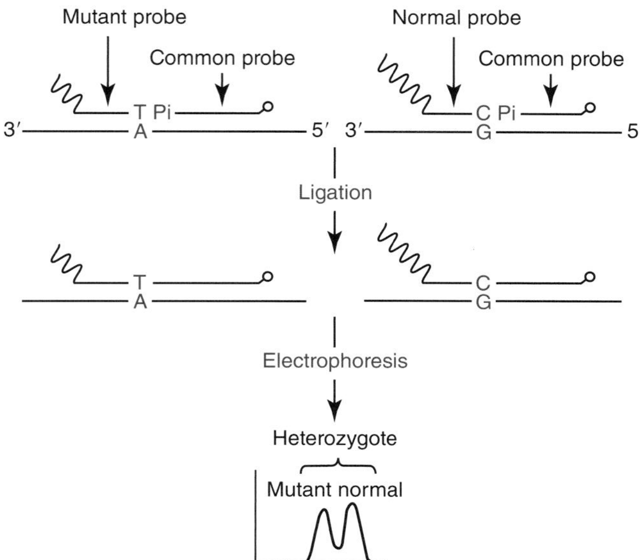

FIGURE 47.16 Oligonucleotide ligation assay of a heterozygous single nucleotide variant (SNV). A mutant probe with a 3′-T *(upper left)* hybridizes to the mutant DNA with an opposing *A,* and a normal probe with a 3′-C *(upper right)* hybridizes to the normal DNA with an opposing *G.* The probes are also attached to mobility modifying tails of different lengths *(wavy lines).* Hybridized next to these probes is the common probe with a 5′-phosphate (Pi) and a 3′-fluorescent tag. In the presence of ligase, adjacent probes are covalently joined to generate longer probes, each with a fluorescent tag and a mobility-modifying tail. Probes that are mismatched to the target at their 3′-ends may hybridize, but they are not ligated. Electrophoresis and endpoint, laser-induced detection of ligated probes reveal the different alleles by their different mobility. Many SNVs can be analyzed in one electrophoresis assay by varying tail lengths or by using multicolor fluorescence tags.

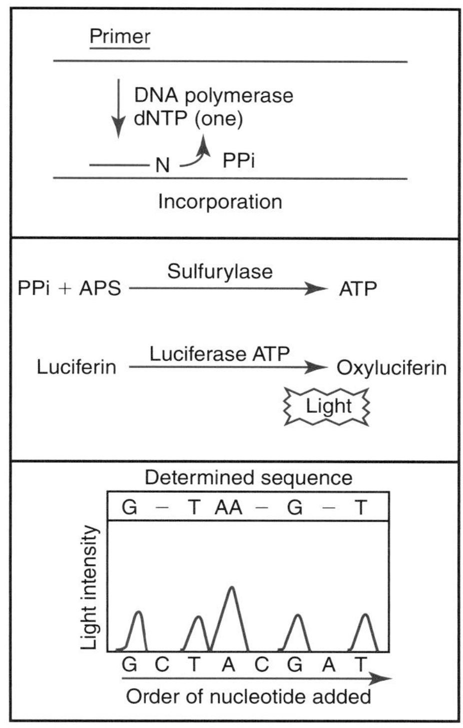

FIGURE 47.17 Schematic of pyrosequencing. Individual deoxynucleotides (dNTPs) are added one by one to the single-stranded template, a primer, and a polymerase. Pyrophosphate is generated if the dNTP is complementary to the next base on the template *(top).* Any pyrophosphate produced reacts with adenosine-5′-phosphosulfate (APS) to produce adenosine triphosphate (ATP), which in turn generates light in the presence of luciferase *(middle).* The sequence can be determined from the order of dTNP addition and from the intensity of light produced *(bottom).*

sequence variants.[105,106] With mass spectrometry, no label is necessary because the alleles differ in mass. After isolation of genomic DNA, a specific DNA fragment, including the variant site, is amplified by PCR. Heat-labile alkaline phosphatase is added to the reaction to dephosphorylate any residual nucleotides, preventing future incorporation and interference with the primer extension assay. Samples are then heated to inactivate the alkaline phosphatase. An extension primer is hybridized directly or closely adjacent to the polymorphic site. Unlabeled deoxynucleotides are incorporated and terminated with a dideoxynucleotide, generating allele-specific diagnostic products of different mass. Salt is removed from the sample, and approximately 10 nL is spotted onto an array coated with 3-hydroxypicolinic acid. This is placed into the MALDI-TOF instrument, which measures the mass of the extension products. After the mass is measured, the genotype is determined (Fig. 47.18). Despite the complexity, automated systems processing 384 to 1536 samples at once are available.

Another use of mass spectroscopy is infectious agent identification. After PCR, electrospray-ionization mass spectrometry determines the exact mass of the PCR product, a process known as PCR/ESI-MS. Because mass rather than sequence is determined, there is some risk of misidentification, but this can be avoided by careful choice of primers and selecting more than one target if necessary. For example, 10 bacterial

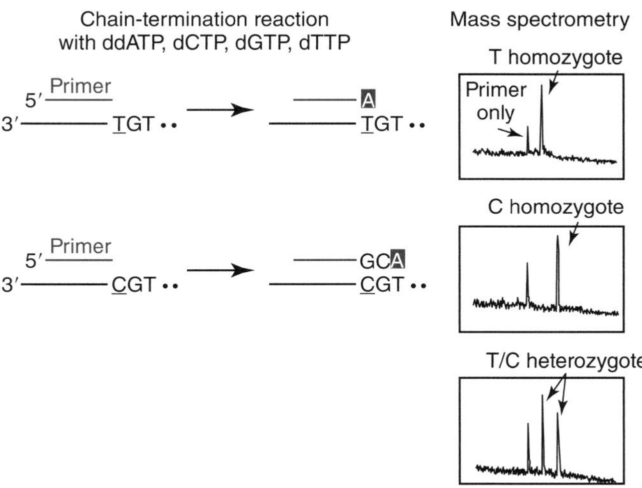

FIGURE 47.18 Sequence polymorphism analysis by mass spectrometry. The underlined base is the polymorphic site in the template (T or C). The single-stranded template is primed and extended in the presence of three deoxynucleotides (dNTPs) and one dideoxy nucleotide triphosphate (ddNTP), producing fragments of different mass depending on the sequence. The boxed "A" in this example indicates the incorporated terminator adenine base. The mass of terminated products is precisely measured by matrix-assisted laser-desorption ionization time-of-flight (MALDI-TOF) mass spectrometry.

and 4 viral biothreat clusters were amplified by PCR using two to four targets each.[107] The pathogenic strains within each cluster were then distinguished from near neighbors by ESI-MS.

High-Performance Liquid Chromatography

High-performance liquid chromatography is commonly used for separating and purifying oligonucleotides. Separation usually is based on ion-pair, reversed-phase chromatography and is particularly useful for purifying fluorescently labeled probes guided by absorbance and fluorescence elution profiles.

A variant of this technology is denaturing HPLC (dHPLC). dHPLC is run at a single elevated temperature to partially denature dsDNA. Similar to gel-based heteroduplex detection, dHPLC reveals the presence of heteroduplexes as additional peaks that are shifted in retention compared with homoduplexes.[108] Retention of dsDNA is governed by electrostatic interactions and an acetonitrile gradient. DNA detection is most often performed by UV absorbance, although fluorescence or mass spectroscopy can also be used. Limitations of dHPLC include sequential (one at a time) analysis and the need to analyze some samples at multiple temperatures when more than one melting domain is present.

Hybridization Assays

All hybridization assays are based on the ability of single-stranded NAs to form specific double-stranded hybrids. The process requires (1) that probe and target NAs are mixed under conditions that allow specific complementary base pairing and (2) that a method is available to detect any resulting double-stranded NAs. A *probe* indicates a NA whose identity is known, and the *target* or *sample* is a NA whose identity or abundance is revealed by hybridization. In some of the methods discussed here, hybridization occurs between a target in solution and a probe that is tethered to a solid surface. In *homogeneous* or *real-time* techniques, both the probes and the targets are in solution, and hybridization and detection occur without washing steps. Some of the homogeneous methods also monitor the dissociation of hybridized duplexes under controlled heating, revealing the identities of the hybridized duplexes by *melting curve* signatures.

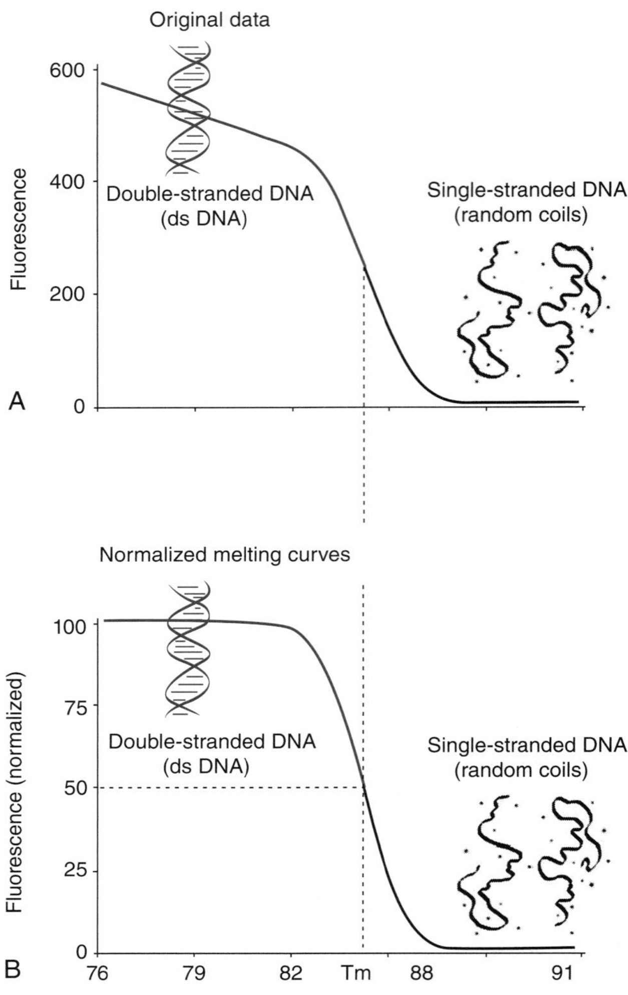

FIGURE 47.19 Fluorescence melting curve of a polymerase chain reaction (PCR) product. PCR-amplified DNA was melted in the presence of the cyanine dye, LCGreen Plus. **A,** Fluorescence gradually decreases as the temperature is increased until a more rapid decrease occurs near the DNA melting temperature (Tm) of the PCR product. **B,** The data are normalized between 0% and 100% after background removal to obtain constant fluorescence outside of the transition. (Modified with permission of the publisher from Wittwer CT, Kusukawa N. Real-time PCR and Melting Analysis. In Persing DH, Tenover FC, Tang YW, et al, eds. *Molecular microbiology: diagnostic principles and practice.* 2nd ed. Washington, DC: ASM Press; 2011:63–82. Copyright 2011 ASM Press.)

Thermodynamics

The favored structure of DNA under physiologic conditions is an ordered double-stranded helix held together by noncovalent interactions. The duplex structure is most stable when all opposing bases are complementary, allowing for maximal hydrogen bonding and base stacking. The noncovalent binding between two DNA strands is both specific (ie, sequence dependent) and reversible. Denaturing agents (eg, high temperature, formamide, or extremes of pH) favor dissociation of the double-stranded molecule into two separate random coils (Fig. 47.19). On removal of the denaturant, single strands attempt to reform duplexes, strongly favoring interactions that maximize complementary base pairing. Because temperature is the denaturant most easily manipulated, double- to single-strand transformation is referred to as *melting,* and the temperature at which half of the DNA is melted is the *melting temperature,* or *Tm,* of the duplex. Duplexes with mismatched base pairs are less stable than those with a perfect sequence match and thus melt at lower temperatures. The reverse process, in which two complementary strands recombine to form a stable duplex molecule, is referred to as *annealing* or *hybridization.* Hybridization can occur between DNA strands, RNA strands, and strands of NA analogs (eg, peptide NAs[109]) in all combinations.

The hybridization environment defines the degree of base pair mismatch that can be tolerated in a duplex structure. Conditions of high *stringency* (low salt concentration, high formamide concentration, and high temperature) require exact base pairing. As the stringency is lowered by increasing the salt concentration, lowering the formamide concentration, or lowering temperature, more base pair mismatches can be tolerated in a duplex structure. The stringency of a hybridization reaction is determined by hybridization conditions and any washing steps designed to remove nonspecific NA. In real-time PCR and melting analysis, the hybridization solution is the buffer in which PCR occurs, and there are no washing steps.

Kinetics

The kinetics of solution-phase hybridizations is second order, being proportional to the concentrations of both hybridizing strands.[110] The rate-limiting step is nucleation, in which a small number of base pairs are formed in the correct orientation followed by rapid "zippering" of complementary sequences. In the case of a probe present in great excess to the target, hybridization proceeds as a pseudo first-order reaction, depending only on the concentration of the target. However, the time required to hybridize the probe to a given fraction of the target remains proportional to the probe concentration. For example, during most of PCR, the concentration of primers is much greater than that of the target, and the reaction rate during each annealing step depends on the concentration of available single-stranded product, but the time required to anneal primers to a certain fraction of the target is proportional to the primer concentration.

The availability of NAs for hybridization can also be an issue. In PCR, primer annealing competes with the formation of double-stranded product. As the concentration of product increases during PCR, some double-stranded product is formed before primer annealing can occur (see Fig. 47.6). Similarly, when double-stranded probes are used at high concentrations, probe self-annealing interferes with probe–target hybridization. Available hybridization sites can also be limited by the intramolecular secondary structure of the probe or target.

In addition to probe concentration and availability, the length of the probe and the NA complexity affect hybridization rates. Rates are directly proportional to the square root of the probe length and inversely proportional to complexity, defined as the total number of base pairs present in nonrepeating sequences. Mismatches up to about 10% have little effect on hybridization rates.

Hybridization rates are also influenced by many factors in the reaction environment, most notably temperature and ionic strength. Above the Tm, no stable hybrids are present, although transient complexes may form. As the temperature is lowered below the Tm, hybridization rates increase until a broad maximum occurs about 20° to 25°C below the Tm. Hybridization rates also increase with ionic strength. Divalent cations such as Mg^{2+} have a much stronger effect than monovalent cations such as Na^+ or K^+.

When the NA target or probe is immobilized on a solid support, hybridization kinetics are even more complex. Many of the preceding observations still hold true, but the rate and extent of solid-phase hybridization are lower than with solution-phase hybridization. Depending on the concentrations of the reactants, solid-phase hybridization can be nucleation limited or diffusion limited. Optimal efficiency of solid-phase hybridization is achieved under conditions that facilitate diffusion of the probe to the support and that favor hybridization over strand reassociation if double-stranded probes are used. This usually means a small volume of hybridization solution and relatively low probe concentrations. In practice, solid-phase hybridization assays are empirically designed. Time of hybridization and probe concentration are the two variables most frequently adjusted. Conditions that tend to maximize the extent of hybridization and minimize the background or nonspecific attachment of the probe are selected.

Probes

Similar to antibodies in immunoassays, probes in NA hybridization assays can be labeled in many ways to detect hybridization. Probes may be cloned (recombinant), generated by PCR, or synthesized (oligonucleotides). They may be DNA, RNA, or NA analogs and single or double stranded. Selection, purification, and labeling of probes are crucial to the success of hybridization assays.

Cloned Probes. Cloned probes consist of a known segment of DNA inserted into a plasmid vector that is propagated by growth in a bacterium. Many different plasmid vectors are available; pBR322 was one of the first in common use.[111] Some plasmids, such as the F plasmid of *Escherichia coli,* can be used to carry insert sizes that are very long (several hundred kilobases) and are called *bacterial artificial chromosomes.* The entire plasmid DNA (insert plus vector sequences) may be used as a probe, or the insert may be purified first from the vector sequences. The latter method is obviously more cumbersome but may result in reduced background. The resulting probe is a dsDNA probe, and it must be denatured before use.

Some vectors contain RNA promoter regions adjacent to the inserted DNA sequence. These regions permit generation of RNA transcripts from the DNA insert. Because only one strand is copied during RNA synthesis, single-stranded RNA probes are generated. Controlling the orientation of the insert in relation to the promoter region allows the production of transcripts in the "sense" direction (ie, same as mRNA) or the "antisense" direction (ie, complementary to mRNA).

Polymerase Chain Reaction–Generated Probes. Polymerase chain reaction–generated probes are simple to prepare.[112] During amplification, the PCR product typically is labeled with nucleotides that are fluorescent or have attached affinity labels. If desired, single-stranded probes can be obtained by amplifying with a biotin-labeled primer followed by solid-phase separation with streptavidin.

Oligonucleotide Probes. Oligonucleotide probes are even easier to obtain than PCR-generated probes. These probes are usually 15 to 45 bases of single-stranded NA that are chemically synthesized as a specified base sequence. Most commonly, they are DNA, but RNA or NA analogs can also be synthesized. Automated, efficient, and accurate methods of synthesis continue to lower the cost of production. Sequence information is now routinely available in public databases,[113] and a similarity check for probe sequence can be performed using public algorithms.[39] Probe sequences must be carefully chosen to minimize cross-hybridization with pseudogenes (eukaryotes) or related species (bacteria and viruses). The melting temperature of the probe should allow both favorable hybrid stability and discrimination against related sequences under the stringency of the assay. Oligonucleotide probes are often prepared with covalent attachment of a reporter molecule (eg, a fluorescent dye) or affinity labels that allow them to be attached to solid supports. Probes used in homogeneous (real-time) PCR are usually oligonucleotides with a fluorescent label.

Estimating Melting Temperature of Oligonucleotide Probes. Probe Tm prediction based on nearest neighbor thermodynamic parameters has improved with compilation of a unified database.[114] Consideration of all possible single-base mismatches and dangling ends further extends the usefulness of these estimates.[115] However, prediction parameters are typically determined using 1-M NaCl, far from typical assay conditions, so it is not surprising that predicted Tms are often at variance from observation. Empirical correction factors[37,116] that may include the concentrations of various cations, dNTPs, the target, and common additives may enhance prediction accuracy and are often used in software programs and websites for in silico Tm estimation. Most fluorescent dyes also stabilize duplexes,[18,117] but this increase in Tm is seldom incorporated into predictions. For these reasons, absolute Tm predictions may not be accurate with common laboratory conditions and PCR buffers. However, relative Tms (ie, the difference in Tm between two related probes, such as a probe that is matched and one that is mismatched to a single base variant) are considerably more accurate.[118]

Purity of Labeled Oligonucleotide Probes. The purity of labeled oligonucleotide probes is important for hybridization assays and critical in real-time PCR. Commercial oligonucleotides with a fluorescent label are of variable quality, and their concentration and purity should be assessed before use. Mass spectroscopy and coelution of absorbance (A_{260}) and fluorescence peaks on reversed-phase HPLC can indicate probe purity. Quantitative estimates of probe purity can also be obtained by simple absorbance measurements as previously described in the prior edition of this textbook.[9]

Examples of Hybridization Assays

Hybridization reactions can be divided into two broad categories: (1) *solid phase,* in which either probe or target is tethered to a solid support while the other is in solution, and (2) *solution phase,* in which both are in solution (Box 47.2). Several classical methods first hybridize in solution and then separate the bound from the unbound labeled probe. Exclusion chromatography and binding by hydroxyapatite, magnetic particles, or other affinity capture methods allow selective measurement of the labeled probe–target hybrid.

BOX 47.2 Hybridization Assays

Solid-Phase Hybridization

Dot blot and line probe assays
Arrays (microarrays and medium-density arrays)
Micro-bead assays
In situ hybridization
Southern and Northern blotting
Massively parallel sequencing on beads or planar flow cells

Solution Phase Hybridization

Real-time (or homogeneous) polymerase chain reaction
Melting analysis
Single-molecule sequencing
Many classical techniques

Solid Phase Hybridization

Solid-phase assays are useful because multiple samples can be processed together, which facilitates (1) control, (2) washing, and (3) separation procedures. Hybridization on a solid support is, however, less efficient than solution-hybridization, and the kinetics are slower and more difficult to predict. Both solid-phase and liquid-phase assays are used routinely in the clinical laboratory. Solid-phase assays include (1) dot blots, (2) line probes, (3) microspheres, (4) microarrays, and (5) in situ hybridization.

Dot Blot and Line Probe Assays. Conventional hybridization assays on membranes are known as dot blot or line probe assays, depending on the geometry of the individual spots. The NAs are applied with suction, forming a shape that is either round (dot) or elongated (line or slot). After immobilization, the membrane is incubated with complementary NA at a constant temperature followed by one or more washes to discriminate matched from mismatched NA. The method allows multiple simultaneous hybridizations under identical conditions.

Two general formats are used for these assays: Either multiple samples are affixed to the solid support and interrogated by a small number of probes ("sample down"), or multiple probes are attached to the support and a small number of samples are used ("probe down"). Results of dot blot and line probe assays are usually qualitative. If hybridization has occurred, a signal is generated at the specified spot, and a simple yes-or-no interpretation is given. Similar assays have been developed substituting microtiter plate wells for filters. This requires chemical modification of the plastic wells to bind short DNA probes at one end, allowing the bound probes to hybridize to sample and is more amenable to automation of washing and detection.

Medium-Density Arrays. Dot blot and line probe assays have largely been replaced by medium-density arrays that typically analyze 20 to 500 spots. Medium-density arrays are used for testing multiple mutations simultaneously in specimens for various applications, including genetic diseases, oncology, and pharmacogenetics.[119,120] These arrays do not need to be attached to a two-dimensional surface as long as their "address" can be decoded. For example, microspheres can be coded by fluorescence intensity in two different channels, and fluorescence in a third channel monitors hybridization. All channels can be read simultaneously using a flow cytometer.[121]

Many different types of medium-density and microarrays are available. The surface of an array may be glass, gold-coated piezoelectric crystals, gel pads with embedded microelectrodes, or microspheres. The bound NAs are often oligonucleotides 20 to 80 bases in length that may be conventionally synthesized and spotted onto the chip or directly synthesized in situ. Arrays can be made of expressed sequence tags (200–500 bases) or bacterial artificial chromosomes (100–200 kb). Instead of an array of probes, sample DNA or cDNA may also be bound to an array surface. After hybridization, detection may be fluorescent, electronic, or by mass spectrometry. Fluorescence is most common, and excitation may use epifluorescence, confocal, laser scanning, or surface plasmon resonance with imaging at various wavelengths, usually with a CCD camera.

Microarrays. Increasing further the density of hybridization assays, microarrays (also called DNA arrays, DNA chips,

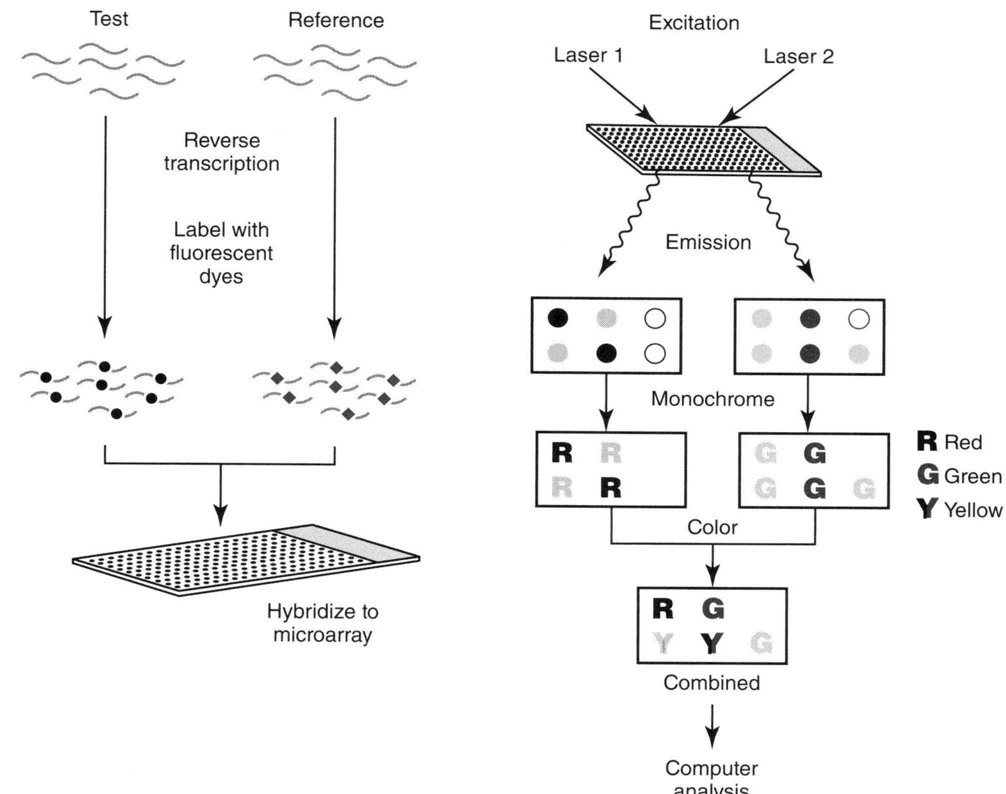

FIGURE 47.20 A two-color microarray experiment. An array of DNA oligonucleotides with sequences of messenger RNA are affixed to a glass slide. Messenger RNAs in the test and reference specimen are converted into differentially labeled cDNA by reverse transcription and incorporation of two different fluorescent dyes. The two samples are hybridized together onto the array. The array is washed, and the image is captured twice, each time with a laser of a wavelength that excites one of the dyes but not the other. The monochromatic images are then converted to two colors (green [G] for the test sample and red [R] for the reference), and the images are combined. If the abundance of cDNA is the same in each of the two samples, then the composite spot will be shown as yellow (Y). If one is in greater abundance, then that color will be preserved. Up- and downregulation of gene expression are then analyzed by software.

or Biochips) were introduced in the mid-1990s.[16] Compared with medium-density arrays, spot sizes in microarrays are decreased (typically to <200 microns in diameter) such that one array contains thousands to millions of spots. This dimensional change requires (1) specialized detection equipment, (2) software, and (3) informatics to analyze the data. Because of their high density, microarrays have attracted intense interest among researchers who wish to monitor the whole genome for (1) SNVs, (2) gene expression, or (3) copy number variation.

Because SNVs represent the most common genetic difference among individuals, much effort has focused on correlating SNV genotypes to phenotype and disease association. SNV microarrays have been used in many genome-wide association studies (GWAS). Microarrays that analyze human SNVs ("SNV chips") provide the technology to genotype most known human SNVs in one experiment. Nearby SNV alleles tend to cluster together as haplotypes, so disease association by haplotype simplifies the analysis. Although some valuable markers have been found by these GWAS,[122] the yield of useful disease markers obtained by these methods has been disappointing, and many difficulties remain, such as identifying adequate control populations.[123] SNV arrays can also be used to genotype SNVs of known association with disease and to assess copy number variation. Cytogenomic arrays, including SNV and comparative genomic hybridization (CGH) arrays, can analyze the entire genome, providing chromosome maps of copy number changes (large insertions and deletions) across each chromosome.

Gene expression microarrays quantify the relative amounts of different messenger RNAs in test and reference samples. An example of a two-color microarray for gene expression is shown in Fig. 47.20. Probes that hybridize to mRNA are usually directly synthesized on microarrays. Modern gene expression arrays have been used to measure the mRNA transcribed from all human genes in one experiment. They have been applied to almost every conceivable human circumstance, including (1) neoplastic, (2) inflammatory, and (3) psychiatric conditions. It is expected that application of this technology will lead to better (1) diagnosis, (2) molecular staging, (3) prognosis, and (4) therapy through understanding of disease pathogenesis. In oncology, gene expression microarrays have led to new diagnostic and prognostic markers in breast cancer,[124] bladder cancer,[125] leukemia,[126] and sarcoma,[127] among others.

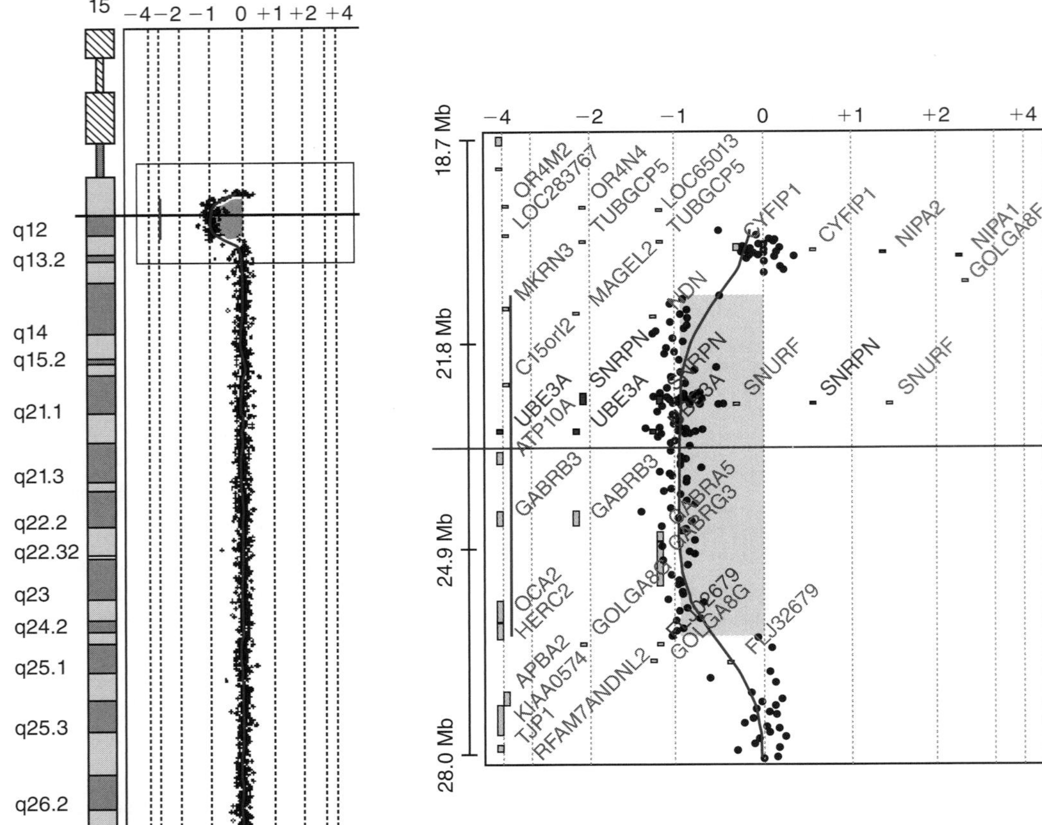

FIGURE 47.21 Copy number variation identified with a comparative genomic hybridization array made from oligonucleotides. DNA from a subject is fragmented, labeled with Cy5, and hybridized onto a microarray, together with Cy3-labeled reference DNA. On the array are nearly 44,000 oligonucleotide probes, each about 60 bases long and tiled across the whole genome at an average spacing of 75 kb. Shown on the *left panel* are results of probes on chromosome 15 (all other chromosomes are analyzed in this assay but are not shown). Each *dot* represents a specific probe to which the subject's DNA hybridizes. Their positions (0, −1, +1, and so on) reflect the dosage of the subject's DNA relative to the reference DNA. A majority of the probes line up on "0," indicating no quantitative difference compared with the reference DNA. Probes in the 15q11 to 15q13 region, however, are on the "−1" line, indicating that the subject has a deletion of that region in one of the chromosomes. A closer view of that region *(right panel)* shows that among the deleted genes are *UBE3A,* which causes Angelman syndrome, and *SNRPN,* which causes Prader-Willi syndrome. Because the method does not distinguish the methylation status of the deleted alleles, this result alone cannot determine which of the two disorders the subject has. (Courtesy Sarah South, PhD, ARUP Laboratories.)

Even with great progress, expression arrays are used directly in only a few clinical diagnostic and prognostic tests. Most arrays are used in marker discovery projects for selection of a smaller panel of expression targets that are then analyzed by other quantitative methods, such as real-time PCR, that provide greater precision and dynamic range.

Another important clinical application of microarrays is the genome-wide analysis of deletions and duplications, referred to as copy number variants (CNVs). CNV analysis using microarrays is replacing traditional cytogenetic chromosome analysis (karyotyping) and fluorescence in situ hybridization (FISH) analysis for detection of genome-wide copy number alterations. Similar to gene expression arrays, many of the CNV arrays use two-color comparative hybridization to determine the gene dosage in a specimen compared with a normal reference genome (array comparative genomic hybridization [aCGH]). Arrays for CGH use oligonucleotide probes for very high resolution and data density. An example of CNV analysis using aCGH is shown in Fig. 47.21. SNV arrays also are used to detect copy number changes by loss of heterozygosity (this method is sometimes referred to as *virtual karyotyping*). Unlike aCGH, SNV arrays have the advantage of analyzing the specimen without the need to mix in a reference genome. SNV arrays also are able to detect copy number neutral changes caused by inversions or uniparental disomy that are not detected by aCGH methods. When a copy number change is found of potential clinical significance, it can be verified by an orthogonal method such as FISH or high-resolution melting.[128]

In Situ Hybridization. In situ hybridization is a specialized type of solid support assay with morphologically intact tissues, cells, or chromosomes affixed to a glass microscope slide to provide the matrix for hybridization. The process is analogous to immunohistochemistry, except that NA probes are used instead of antibodies. The strength of the method lies in linking morphologic evaluation with detection of specific NA sequences. When fluorescent probes are applied to metaphase chromosome spreads or interphase nuclei, the technique is referred to as FISH. Numeric aberrations or translocations of chromosomes can be detected rapidly. FISH can also be combined with immunohistochemistry so that information on both the amount of protein expression and the gene dosage can be found on the same slide. In situ hybridization is appropriate when localization of a target in tissue is important. However, experience in histology is necessary for accurate interpretation. In situ hybridization can provide information on the level of mRNA expression but not on the size or structure of the mRNA. As might be expected, hybridization within a tissue matrix is more variable than in solution or on well-characterized chemical surfaces.

Single-Copy Visualization. If an NA probe is labeled with many fluorescent molecules, it is possible to optically visualize a single copy of the NA target by fluorescent microscopy. One technique uses reporter probes that are labeled with a long string of multicolored fluorescent labels.[129] Several tandem color segments are placed on the reporter probe with each segment consisting of about 100 fluorophores. The combination of different color segments uniquely identifies the target. The target NA is hybridized with the probes each linked to capture probe that are (1) washed, (2) immobilized, (3) stretched, and (4) oriented on the surface of an optical slide. Each captured target is then identified by the color code of the reporter and is counted (see Fig. 50.3). Although the sensitivity of this technique is not as high as that of real-time PCR, up to 150 reporter probes have been multiplexed in one reaction. One application of this technique is direct measurement of mRNA expression in tissue specimens prepared from formalin-fixed paraffin blocks without the need for cDNA preparation or PCR.

Solution Phase Hybridization: Real-Time Polymerase Chain Reaction and Melting Analysis

Several classical hybridization methods use probe-target hybridization in solution. For example, hybrid capture uses an antibody that is specific for RNA–DNA hybrid molecules that are formed during solution-phase hybridization of a DNA sample and an unlabeled RNA probe. The assay also has been adapted to a microtiter plate format for automation of washing and detection. Solution phase hybridization has also been combined with (1) amplification, (2) detection, and (3) quantification steps all in the same tube. Such closed-tube, real-time assays do not require any additions, washing, or separation steps.

Real-time PCR and melting analysis are considered "dynamic" hybridization assays in which the formation or dissociation of the probe–target duplex (or product duplex) is monitored in real time. Data are collected throughout NA amplification rather than just at the endpoint. The technique uses fluorescent reporters and instruments to record hybridization during thermal cycling. The data obtained provide information on the (1) identity, (2) quantity, and (3) melting characteristics of the NA sample. Fluorescent dyes or probes are added to the PCR mixture before amplification. By measuring the fluorescence at each cycle of amplification, the amount of initial template present before PCR can be calculated. During the entire process, the same reaction tube is used for amplification and fluorescence monitoring, and no (1) sample transfers, (2) reagent additions, or (3) gel separation steps are required. This eliminates the risk of product contamination in subsequent reactions. Because the process is simple and fast, real-time PCR has replaced many conventional techniques in the clinical laboratory.

Real-time PCR monitors the accumulation of double-stranded PCR products with the fluorescence signal recorded once each cycle (Fig. 47.22).[12,130] If target DNA is present, fluorescence increases. How early during PCR one begins to see a signal depends on the initial amount of target DNA, and this provides a systematic method of quantification. Furthermore, when fluorescence is continuously monitored as the temperature is raised, a melting curve can be generated. Often the negative derivative of this melting curve is plotted to visually aid a person in estimating the melting temperature as peaks in the plot. Melting analysis can be used to verify the identity of the amplified product and to detect sequence variants.

Dyes and Probes. Many different fluorescence generating systems are used in real-time PCR; some of the more common ones are shown in Fig. 47.23. Many methods use probes with sequences complementary to the target. Others rely on dsDNA binding dyes and the specificity afforded by PCR primers. Some have the additional option of melting analysis to measure the melting temperature of the probe or product.

Certain cyanine dyes increase their fluorescence in the presence of dsDNA that is produced during PCR (see Fig. 47.23, *A*).[22,131] dsDNA binding dyes are commonly used for real-time quantification, particularly in the research setting when the specificity of a probe and its added cost is not needed. They also allow melting analysis of the product at the end of PCR.

Labeled primers can also be used to monitor PCR. In one system, a primer with a 5′-hairpin is labeled with a fluorophore and a quencher so that fluorescence is quenched in the hairpin conformation. When the primer straightens out during PCR, fluorescence increases.[132] If the sequence of the primer is carefully considered, the quencher moiety is not necessary.[86] Nonhairpin primers with a single label can also be used for detection and genotyping because of changes in fluorescence that occur with hybridization.[133]

One advantage of fluorescently labeled primers over dsDNA dyes is that multiplexing is possible. However, with both dsDNA dyes and labeled primers, reaction specificity depends on the primers. Any double-stranded product that is formed will be detected, including primer-dimers. Therefore, hot start techniques to increase specificity and melting curve analysis to confirm the desired product are useful.

The use of fluorescent probes in PCR adds another level of specificity to the process. Fluorescent probes that hybridize to PCR products during amplification change fluorescence by two possible mechanisms: (1) a covalent bond between two dyes is broken by hydrolysis or is made through ligation, or (2) the fluorescence change follows reversible hybridization of the probe to the target. Following this distinction, when an irreversible covalent bond is involved, the probes are called *hydrolysis probes.* When probes reversibly change fluorescence on duplex formation, they are called *hybridization probes.* One difference between the two probe types is

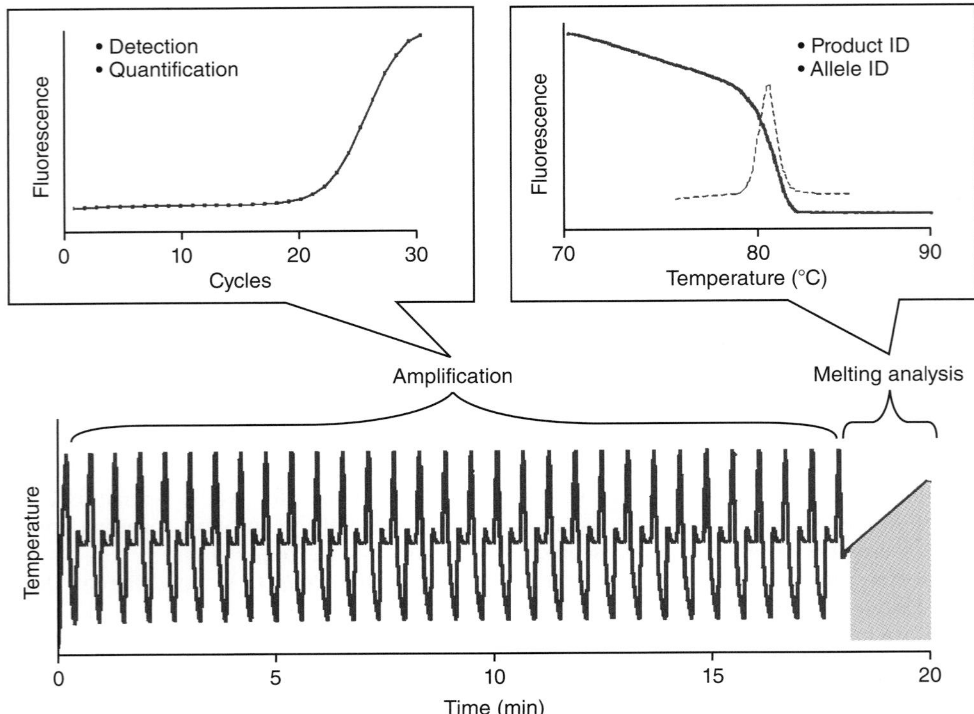

FIGURE 47.22 Real-time monitoring during amplification and melting analysis. The *bottom panel* shows a typical rapid-cycle temperature profile that is followed by a temperature ramp for melting analysis. When fluorescence is monitored once each cycle during amplification, the presence or absence and the quantification of the specific target are obtained. When fluorescence is monitored continuously through the melting phase *(shaded area),* melting analysis can verify target identification and establishes genotype. (Modified with permission of the publisher from Wittwer CT, Kusukawa N. Real-time PCR. In: Persing DH, Tenover FC, Versalovic J, et al, eds. *Molecular microbiology: diagnostic principles and practice.* Washington, DC: ASM Press, 2004:71–84.)

that melting analysis is characteristic of hybridization probes, but hydrolysis probes usually have weak, if any, melting signature.

Hydrolysis probes (exonuclease probes) are synthesized with a quencher molecule positioned to quench the fluorescence of another label. If the probe is hydrolyzed between the fluorophore and the quencher during PCR, fluorescence will increase. The most common implementation uses the 5′-exonuclease activity of some DNA polymerases to hydrolyze the probe and dissociate the labels (see Fig. 47.23, *B*). This method has been simplified by putting the fluorophores on opposite ends of the probe.[134] Dual-labeled probes can also be cleaved using a DNAzyme (a DNA molecule that acts as a catalyst) generated during PCR.[135] Finally, irreversible ligation can be used for homogeneous genotyping with a fluorescent readout.[136] Hydrolysis probes generate fluorescence through changes in covalent bonds. The change in fluorescence signal is irreversible, and melting analysis of the hydrolyzed probe is seldom useful.

Hybridization probes change fluorescence upon hybridization, usually by fluorescence resonance energy transfer (FRET).[22,137] Two interacting fluorophores are typically placed on adjacent probes as dual hybridization probes (see Fig. 47.23, *C*). Only one probe with one fluorophore may be necessary if fluorescence is quenched by deoxyguanosine residues.[138] Another single-labeled probe design uses thiazole orange attached to a peptide NA.[139] In each of these designs, the fluorescence change that occurs with hybridization is reversible upon melting.

Hairpin probes (molecular beacons) typically have a fluorophore and a quencher at the 3′ and 5′-ends of a hairpin stem (see Fig. 47.23, *D*). Fluorescence increases when the distance between the quencher and the reporter increases upon target hybridization.[88] Compared with linear probes, hairpin probes discriminate mismatches with greater temperature changes.[140] Hairpin probes of different colors can be combined with melting curve analysis for highly multiplexed assays.[141]

Self-probing primers are modified at their 5′-end to include a hairpin probe with a fluorophore and quencher on opposite ends of the stem (see Fig. 47.23, *E*).[69] The hairpin loop is complementary to the primer extension product of the same strand that is generated during PCR. Through intramolecular hybridization, the quencher is separated from the fluorophore, and fluorescence increases. A blocker prevents copying the hairpin during PCR.

Highly quenched probes have a very efficient quencher at the 3′-end and a minor groove binder and fluorophore at the 5′-end (see Fig. 47.23, *F*).[142] Background fluorescence is claimed to be very low because of the combined effect of the quencher and minor groove binders. Upon hybridization, fluorescence increases because the fluorophore and quencher are separated, a process that can be reversed by melting. The minor groove binders increase probe stability, allowing the

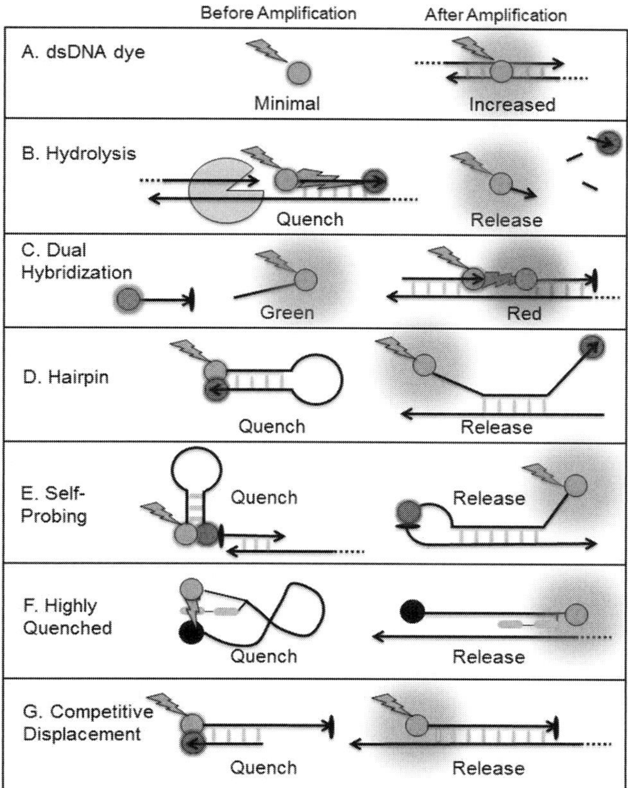

FIGURE 47.23 Common probes and dyes for real-time polymerase chain reaction (PCR). **A,** Double-stranded DNA dyes show a significant increase in fluorescence after DNA amplification. **B,** Hydrolysis probes are cleaved between a fluorescent reporter and a quencher, resulting in increased fluorescence. **C,** Dual hybridization probes. Fluorescence resonance energy transfer (FRET) is illustrated between a donor and acceptor fluorophore. The *thin vertical oval* indicates termination of the 3′-end of the probe to prevent polymerase extension. **D,** Hairpin probes are quenched in the native conformation but increase in fluorescence when hybridized. **E,** Self-probing primers retain their native, quenched conformation until they are incorporated into a double-stranded product. **F,** Highly quenched probes use a combination of minor groove binders and a very efficient quencher to limit background fluorescence. Upon hybridization, fluorescence increases. **G,** Competitive displacement probes have reporters and quenchers on opposite strands. The quenching probe is displaced by the accumulating PCR product and fluorescence increases. There are several forms of this type of probe. (Modified with permission of the publisher from Nolte FS, Wittwer CT. Nucleic acid amplification methods overview. In: Persing DH, Tenover FC, Versalovic J, et al, eds. *Molecular microbiology: diagnostic principles and practice.* 3rd ed. Washington, DC: ASM Press; 2015.)

use of smaller probes when sequence variation of the target is high.

Competitive displacement probes come in several different varieties. In all cases, the fluorophore and quencher are on opposite strands, usually at 3′- and 5′- ends opposing each other. In its most basic form, generation of target strands during PCR displaces one labeled strand by competitive hybridization, separating fluorophore and quencher and generating fluorescence.[143] One design adds a 5′-labeled tail to one primer along with a 3′-quenching anti-primer complementary to the tail.[144] Additional designs for probes and antiprobes have recently been described that include mismatches in the antiprobe to favor displacement.[145] Another design uses partially double-stranded probes with one strand shorter than the other to also favor displacement (see Fig. 47.23, *G*).[146]

POINTS TO REMEMBER

Fluorescent Indicators

- May be dyes or probes
- Dyes are less expensive and less specific
- Melting analysis increases specificity
- May function by hybridization, hydrolysis, ligation, or displacement
- Single base variants can be detected by probes or high-resolution melting
- Enable real-time PCR in a closed system

Detection and Quantification in Real-Time PCR

When fluorescence is monitored once each cycle in the presence of a dye, the data closely follow the expected logistic shape discussed earlier (see Figs. 47.5 and 47.24, *top left*). However, with hydrolysis probes, fluorescence is cumulative and continues to increase even after the amount of product reaches a plateau (Fig. 47.24, *top middle*). In contrast, reactions monitored with hybridization probes may show a decrease in fluorescence at high cycle number[14] (Fig. 47.24, *top right*). Despite differences in the curve shape, all real-time systems follow the amount of product being produced during PCR, and this information is used for detection and quantification.

Detection. A fluorescent signal that increases during PCR and follows one of the expected curve shapes suggests that the specific target is present and was amplified. In contrast, a signal that stays at background even after 40 PCR cycles suggests that the target is absent and that no amplification occurred. Algorithms that analyze the entire curve may be more robust than simple threshold methods.[147] Positive controls (to rule out inhibitory factors) and negative controls (to rule out product contamination and nonspecific signal generation) are necessary. If the fluorescent signal is reversible with hybridization, melting analysis can verify the expected Tm of the probe or product.

Multiplex detection is possible with probes that are labeled with different colors or with probes and/or amplicons that have different melting temperatures. Examples in the clinical laboratory include probe multiplexing to detect the presence of more than one infectious organism, or to discriminate an internal control template from the target.

Quantification. Real-time PCR offers a convenient and systematic approach to quantification by monitoring the amount of product in each cycle. Some of the first clinical uses of quantitative real-time PCR were in the assessment of viral load, particularly for HIV and HCV. The clinical need for quantification is well established, and real-time methods give rapid and precise answers. However, other amplification systems, particularly transcription-based and branched DNA methods, are also used in this high-volume and highly competitive field. Additional quantitative applications of real-time PCR in clinical use are myriad and include quantification of mRNA (after reverse transcription) to monitor minimal residual disease and disease burden in leukemia with disease

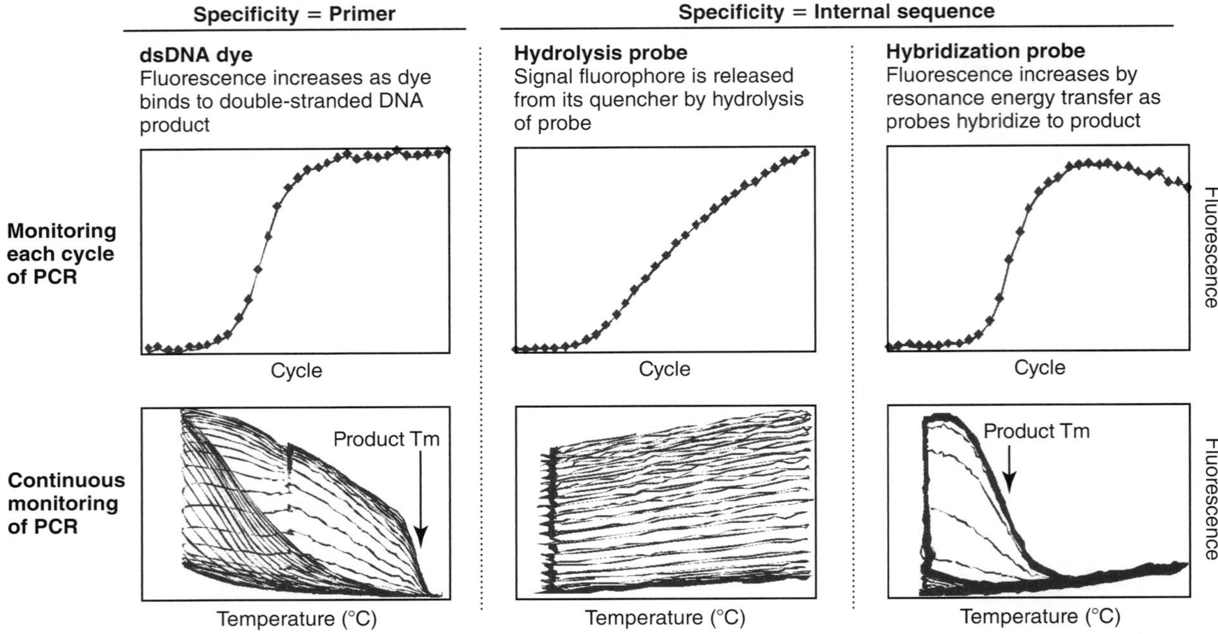

FIGURE 47.24 Monitoring polymerase chain reaction (PCR) in real time. The *top row* shows data collected once each PCR cycle, and the *bottom row* shows data collected continuously (5 times per second) during all PCR cycles. Three different reporter systems are shown. *dsDNA,* Double-stranded DNA; *Tm,* melting temperature. (Modified with permission of the publisher from Wittwer CT, Kusukawa N. Real-time PCR. In: Persing DH, Tenover FC, Versalovic J, et al, eds. *Molecular microbiology: diagnostic principles and practice.* Washington, DC: ASM Press; 2004:71–84.)

specific markers such as *BCR-ABL*, gene expression studies, and assessment of gene dosage in genetics and oncology.

Digital PCR has some advantages over real-time PCR, including precision and rare-allele analysis. However, one of the advantages of real-time PCR is its large dynamic range. Fig. 47.25 shows an extended range of quantification standards in a typical real-time PCR. As the initial template concentration increases, the curves shift to earlier cycles. The extent of this shift depends on the PCR efficiency (Table 47.3). The cycle at which fluorescence rises correlates inversely with the log of the initial template concentration and is the quantification cycle or Cq. This "cycle" is actually a *virtual* cycle that includes a fractional component determined by interpolation, which can be calculated by several methods. One method uses the maximum of the *second derivative* of the curve to determine Cq (Fig. 47.26). The second derivative of the amplification curve is derived from the shape of the curve and is estimated numerically with polynomials[148] without the need to adjust baselines or worry about normalizing the fluorescence values. Alternatively, in *threshold analysis,* a fluorescence level is selected that intersects with the amplification curves, and fractional cycle numbers are found by interpolation. However, when the sample fluorescence does not reach the threshold (as may happen with low copy samples), quantification is not possible.

Accuracy and Precision. The accuracy of real-time PCR quantification depends not only on the method chosen to analyze the curves but also on the quality of the quantification standards used. Purified PCR products quantified by

TABLE 47.3 Correlation Between Polymerase Chain Reaction Efficiency, the Slope of the Standard Curve, and the Percentage of Polymerase Chain Reaction Product After 30 Cycles

Slope of Standard Curve*	PCR Efficiency (%)	PCR Product After 30 Cycles (% Expected)
–3.32	100	100
–3.35	99	86
–3.38	97.5	69
–3.45	95	47
–3.59	90	22
–3.74	85	10
–3.92	80	4
–4.34	70	1
–4.90	60	0.1
–5.68	50	0.02

*Assuming the log (initial template) is plotted on the *x*-axis as the independent variable and the quantification cycle is plotted on the *y*-axis as the dependent variable, the slope of the calibration curve is as follows: Slope = ΔCycle/ΔLog [initial template]. Percent PCR efficiency is calculated as $(10^{-1/\text{Slope}} - 1) \times 100$.
PCR, Polymerase chain reaction.

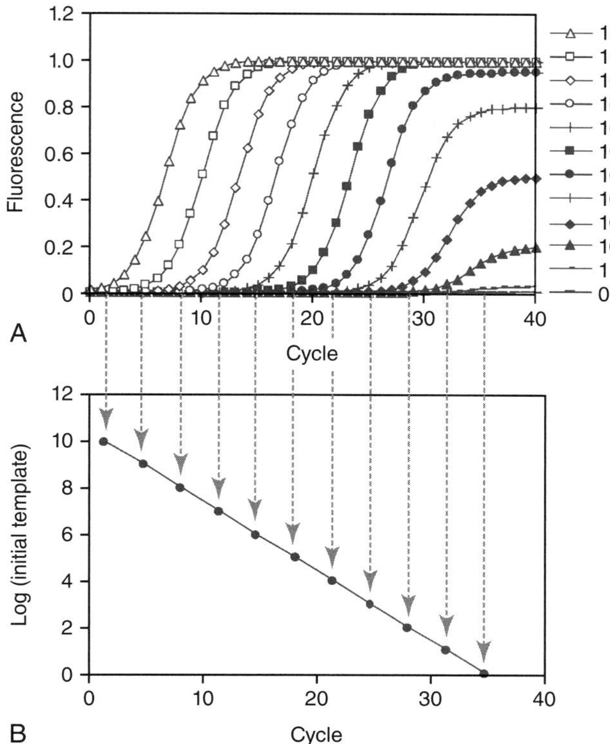

FIGURE 47.25 Quantification by real-time polymerase chain reaction. Shown are typical real-time curves for amplification reactions of varying initial target concentrations **(A)** and the log of the initial concentration plotted against the quantification cycle **(B)** as calculated by the second derivative maximum (see Fig. 47.26). (Modified with permission of the publisher from Wittwer CT, Kusukawa N. Real-time PCR. In: Persing DH, Tenover FC, Versalovic J, et al, eds. *Molecular microbiology: diagnostic principles and practice*. Washington, DC: ASM Press; 2004:71–84.)

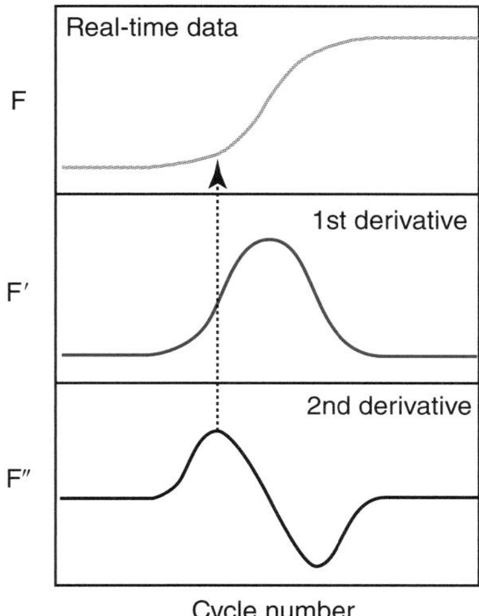

FIGURE 47.26 Estimation of the fractional cycle number for quantification. Real-time fluorescence data *(F)* from the amplification reaction are shown with the first *(F′)* and second *(F″)* derivatives. The maximum of the second derivative provides one way to determine the quantification cycle, Cq. (Modified with permission of the publisher from Wittwer CT, Kusukawa N. Real-time PCR. In: Persing DH, Tenover FC, Versalovic J, et al, eds. Molecular microbiology: diagnostic principles and practice. Washington, DC: ASM Press; 2004:71–84.)

spectrophotometry are easily obtained. When serially diluted, these calibrators can accurately quantify the amount of target in human genomic DNA.[148] Synthesized oligonucleotides, purified plasmids, and genomic DNA can also be used as calibrators. *Limiting dilution* analysis can also determine the amount of "amplifiable" DNA.[149] As previously mentioned, digital PCR is a great method to quantify PCR standards, and absolute reference standards are available for some targets.[150] Sometimes absolute quantification is not needed, and quantification relative to one or more reference genes is performed. In this case, selection of the reference genes and PCR efficiency are critical. The precision of quantitative real-time PCR depends on the initial number of template copies in the reaction. When the initial target concentration is low, imprecision is high. When this is the case, digital PCR may be a better choice.

Melting Analysis

When fluorescence is monitored continuously within each cycle of PCR, the hybridization characteristics of PCR products and probes can be observed.[34] Continuous spirals of fluorescence versus temperature are produced (see Fig. 47.24, *bottom panels*).[22] With dyes, the melting characteristics of the amplified DNA identify the product.[17] Little, if any, hybridization information is revealed with hydrolysis probes, whereas the melting of hybridization probes is readily apparent. Probe melting occurs at a characteristic temperature that can be exploited to confirm target identity and to analyze sequence variants under the probe.

For routine testing in the clinical laboratory, a single melting curve is usually performed at the end of PCR instead of monitoring hybridization throughout the entire PCR process (see Fig. 47.22). Genotyping is best performed in the same tube by monitoring the melting of hybridized duplexes during controlled heating, producing a melting curve signature for the duplex. Such a signature monitors melting over a range of temperatures in contrast to the single-temperature analysis of conventional hybridization techniques, such as dot blots or microarrays. The advantages of complete melting curves also apply when different homogeneous techniques are compared. Real-time amplification and melting analysis make up a powerful combination that requires only temperature control and sampling of fluorescence. When hybridization probes are used, rapid cooling maximizes formation of probe–target duplexes while minimizing formation of the duplex PCR product. Primer asymmetry and use of 5′-exonuclease–deficient polymerases can augment the probe signal.

Homogeneous Single Nucleotide Variant Typing

Many methods are available for SNV genotyping, and the method of choice depends on several factors, including turnaround time, batch size, and throughput requirements. The necessities of high-volume genomic research are different from those of a clinical reference laboratory, a medical clinic, or the STAT laboratories of the future. Many targeted genotyping techniques require complex separation or detection equipment (or both). Real-time PCR with melting curve analysis allows detection, quantification, and genotyping in less than 30 minutes (see Fig. 47.22) in a homogeneous system that does not require ancillary processing or additional equipment.

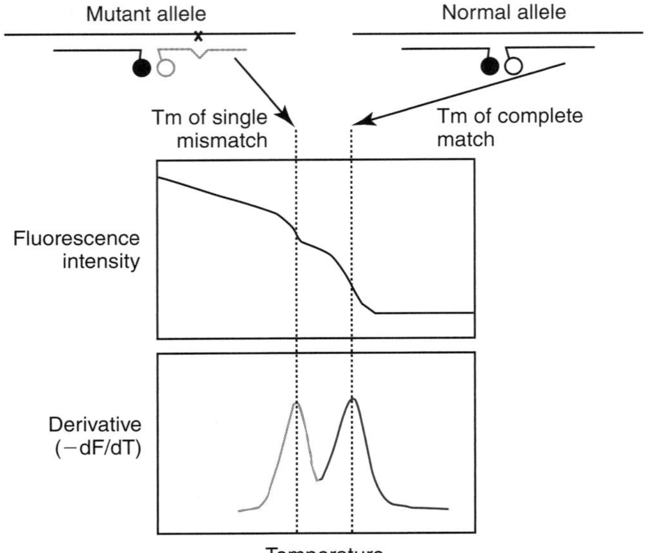

FIGURE 47.27 Melting curve single nucleotide variant (SNV) genotyping. A heterozygous specimen with an SNV under one probe is amplified and melted. Two temperature transitions are visible: one from the mutant allele that is mismatched with the probe and melts at a lower temperature and one from the normal allele that is completely matched with the probe and melts at a higher temperature. The derivative plot shows the melting temperatures (Tms) of both the mutant-probe and the normal-probe duplexes as peaks. (Modified with permission of the publisher from Bernard PS, Pritham GH, Wittwer CT. Color multiplexing hybridization probes using the apolipoprotein E locus as a model system for genotyping. *Anal Biochem* 1999;273:221–228. Copyright 1999 Academic Press.)

For example, a hybridization probe pair with one probe placed over a heterozygous polymorphism is shown in Fig. 47.27. In this example, the reporter probe is complementary to the normal allele. As the temperature is increased, the mismatched mutant hybrid melts first, giving the first transition, followed by the matched normal hybrid. The melting temperatures of both hybrids are easily seen in derivative plots.[148] A well-optimized probe design will provide a Tm difference of 4° to 10°C for a single base mismatch under the probe.

Single nucleotide variant genotyping by melting curve analysis can be achieved with a variety of probe and dye methods. Fig. 47.28, *A*, shows the hybridization probe pair just discussed. Virtually the same result can be achieved by using a single hybridization probe in which the fluorescent signal is quenched on the free probe, but is enhanced as it forms a hybrid with the target (see Fig. 47.28, *B*).[138] Fig. 47.28, *C*, shows genotyping with an *unlabeled probe* and a saturating DNA binding dye.[151] Both probe and amplicon melting transitions are present. Fig. 47.28, *D*, shows similar results using a *snapback primer*,[70] an unlabeled probe attached as a 5′-tail to one of the primers. The advantage of these last two methods is that they do not require fluorescently labeled probes. Finally, SNV genotyping is possible by amplicon melting with a saturating DNA binding dye (see Fig. 47.28, *E*).[152]

The many methods of homogeneous SNV typing differ greatly in their level of complexity (Table 47.4). The number

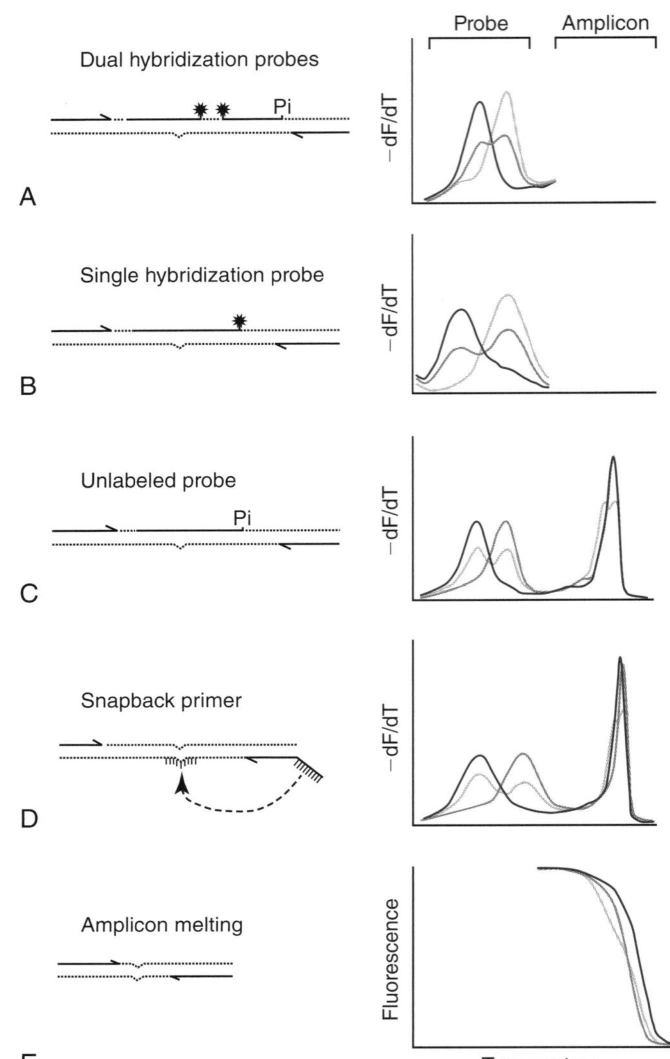

FIGURE 47.28 Five melting designs for single nucleotide variant (SNV) genotyping and corresponding melting curve results. The traditional dual hybridization probe design **(A)** uses a pair of probes: one labeled with an acceptor fluorophore and the other with a donor fluorophore. The single hybridization probe design **(B)** lacks the second probe. The unlabeled probe design **(C)** does not require a covalently attached fluorescent label, using instead a saturating DNA binding dye in solution. Snapback primers **(D)** are similar to unlabeled probes, with the probe attached to one primer as a 5′-tail. Finally, amplicon melting **(E)** uses only two regular polymerase chain reaction primers. Amplicon melting relies on high-resolution melting analysis to distinguish the small differences among genotypes. The two homozygotes are differentiated by melting temperature (Tm), and the heterozygote differs in shape because of the contribution from heteroduplexes. P_i indicates a 3′-phosphate or other blocker that prevents polymerase extension. dF/dT, Rate of fluorescence change.

of oligonucleotides required varies from 2 to 5. The simpler techniques do not require probes at all, although some of the more complex methods require up to three labels or modifications on each probe. All of these methods use fluorescence and solution hybridization. Some that use melting analysis can detect more than two alleles if present; those based on

TABLE 47.4 Comparison of Homogeneous (Closed-Tube) Genotyping Methods (in Order of Increasing Complexity)

Method	Oligonucleotides	Modifications	Comments
Amplicon melting	2	0	Simplest and least expensive
Snapback primers	2	1	Self-complementary 5′-tail
Allele-specific PCR (real time)	3	0	Requires one well for each allele
Unlabeled probes	3	1	3′-phosphate on probe
Allele-specific PCR (melting)	3	1–2	GC* clamps
Single hybridization probe	3	1–2	3′-phosphate if 5′-fluorophore
Dual hybridization probes	4	2–3	3′-phosphate if 5′-fluorophore
Hydrolysis probes	4	4	
Dual-labeled hairpin probes	4	4	
Self-probing amplicon	3–4	6	
Minor groove binder hydrolysis probe	4	6	
Serial invasive signal amplification	5	4	

*Short 5′-oligonucleotide tail of G and C bases used to modify allele melting temperatures.
PCR, Polymerase chain reaction.

allele-specific amplification or endpoint analysis are limited to two.

The five simplest homogeneous SNV typing methods do not use fluorescently labeled probes. Amplicon melting requires only two primers and a heteroduplex-detecting DNA dye (see Fig. 47.28, *E*).[152] The snapback primer system also requires only two primers—one with a self-probing 5′-tail (see Fig. 47.28, *E*).[70] Unlabeled probe genotyping requires two primers and one 3′-blocked probe (see Fig. 47.28, *C*).[151] Allele-specific PCR requires three primers and is based on a preference by the polymerase to extend only a perfectly matched primer. Genotyping can be obtained in two wells by monitoring fluorescence at each cycle[153] or in one well by incorporating GC-clamp(s) so that alleles can be differentiated at the end of PCR by their melting temperatures.[154] Intermediate in complexity are hybridization probe melting assays. Designs with single[138] or dual hybridization[155] probes are shown in Fig. 47.28, *A* and *B*. The more complex closed-tube methods for SNV genotyping are endpoint assays. Allele-specific hydrolysis[87] and hairpin probes[156] are commonly used. Self-probing amplicons[69] and minor groove binder hydrolysis probes[157] both require three modifications on two probes for SNV typing. Finally, serial invasive signal amplification is a method of homogeneous genotyping that does not require PCR but uses the largest number of oligonucleotides for homogeneous genotyping.[79]

High-Resolution Melting Analysis

The temperature difference between genotypes in amplicon melting can be small (see Fig. 47.28, *E*), requiring high-resolution melting for accurate genotyping. High-resolution melting detects heteroduplexes with better sensitivity than gel methods and does not require any processing or separation.[158] Although legacy fluorescent melting analysis can distinguish PCR products that differed by about 1° to 2°C,[17] high-resolution melting instruments now provide precision and resolution improvement of at least 10-fold[18] and require only a few minutes.[159] Typically, melting data are normalized between 0% and 100% fluorescence, and different homozygotes are distinguished by Tm. Heterozygotes are best detected when comparing the melting curve shapes by shifting the curves along the temperature axis until they overlap. An example of heteroduplex detection and SNV genotyping by melting curve analysis is shown in Fig. 47.29 in which a PCR product melts in two domains. Domain prediction can be very useful in melting assay design.[160] Major applications of high-resolution melting include genotyping, mutation scanning, and sequence matching.[161-163] Targeted copy number assessment is a new application that may be even better than copy number determination by digital PCR.[128]

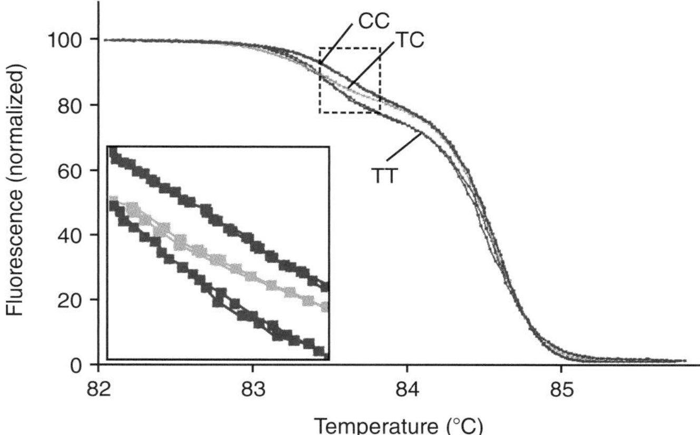

FIGURE 47.29 A single base change in a 544-bp fragment detected by melting analysis. Shown are high-resolution melting curves of polymerase chain reaction products from the gene *HTR2A* carrying a single nucleotide variant (SNV). Results are shown for six individuals, two different individuals for each of the three genotypes: wild-type homozygote (TT), mutant homozygote (CC), and heterozygote (TC). Two melting domains are present because of differing GC content. The SNV was present in the lower melting domain. The *inset* magnifies a portion of the data, showing that all three genotypes can be discriminated. (Modified by permission of the publisher from Wittwer CT, Reed GH, Gundry CN, et al. High-resolution genotyping by amplicon melting analysis using LC Green. *Clin Chem* 2003;49:853–860. Copyright AACC.)

TABLE 47.5 Characteristics of Massively Parallel Sequencing Methods

Method	Principle	Detection	Clonal	Run Time	Output Per Run	Read Length (bp)
Synthesis	Pyrophosphate release	Chemiluminescence	Emulsion PCR	10–23 hours	40–700 mb	400–700
Synthesis	pH change	Electronic CMOS	Emulsion PCR	3–4 hours	1.5–10 gb	125–400
Synthesis	Reversible terminator	Fluorescence	Bridge amplification	2.7–12 days	15–600 gb	200–600*
Ligation	Multiple ligation events	Fluorescence	Emulsion PCR	10 days	300 gb	110
Single molecule	Zero-mode waveguide	Fluorescence	No	2 days	5 gb	10 kb
Single molecule	Conductivity	Electronic	No	Minutes to Days	Depends	5 kb

*Includes both paired end reads (sequencing from both ends).
CMOS, Complementary metal oxide semiconductor; *PCR*, polymerase chain reaction.

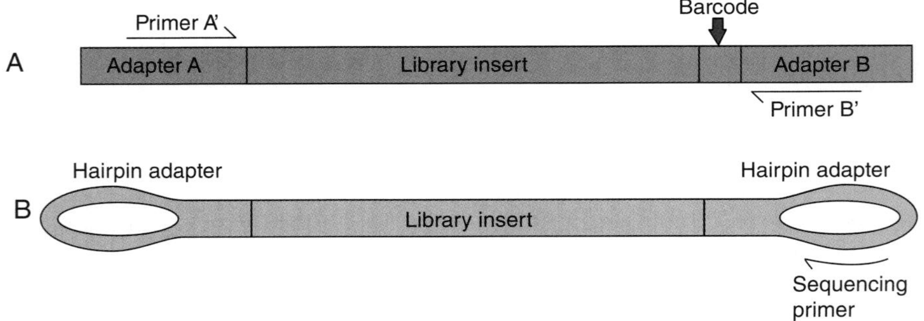

FIGURE 47.30 Diagram of different library formats used in massively parallel sequencing. **A,** Two adapters that include consensus PCR priming sites are ligated onto each end of the library inserts produced by fragmentation. If multiplexing different samples is desired, a barcode is added so that each read can be assigned to a specific sample. **B,** A library insert is bounded by hairpin adapters that allow primer binding to the single-stranded loops on each end for rolling circle amplification.

Massively Parallel Sequencing

The need to understand the full extent of genome-wide human variation has led to the development of new massively parallel sequencing techniques.[164-166] Compared with dideoxy-termination sequencing, these techniques generate up to 1 billion more bases of sequence data in one operation at 10,000 to 100,000 times lower cost per base. These techniques continue to evolve such that throughput and cost continue to improve. Much of the progress that has been made in this technology is dependent on advances in optical data processing, bioinformatics, and overall computer power. As the cost, turnaround time, and convenience of these methods continue to decrease, they increasingly will be used in the clinical laboratory. Indeed, clinical laboratory standards for massively parallel sequencing have already appeared.[167,168] Clonal sequencing methods replicate a single DNA strand to form a clonal template in order to generate sufficient signal for detection. In contrast, single-molecule sequencing methods must be sensitive enough to detect single molecules of DNA. Characteristics of massively parallel sequencing methods are summarized in Table 47.5.

Sequencing From Clones

Clonal sequencing methods start with producing a shotgun (random) library of fragments that are typically 70 to 1000 bases in length, although some methods require 6- to 20-kb fragments. Fragmentation is usually physical or enzymatic.[23] Physical methods include sonication, acoustic shearing, and hydrodynamic shearing. Enzymatic fragmentation can be from restriction endonucleases, nonspecific DNAses, or a tranposase enzyme that simultaneously fragments and adds adapter sequences. In all cases, conditions can be modified to produce different fragment sizes.

Adapter sequences are typically added to each end of the random fragments. The primary role of these adapters is to provide common priming sites for each fragment to initiate massively parallel sequencing reactions. One primer set amplifies a massive array (beads or planer flow cell) of library inserts. Adapters also facilitate initial capture of DNA fragments onto solid surfaces and spatially restrict clonal amplification products generated from the fragments onto beads or spots on an array surface. The fragment ends typically need to be "polished" by filling in any missing bases and optionally adding a single extra A to the 3′-ends to facilitate ligation to the adapters. If multiplexing of different DNA samples is desired, a sequence "barcode" is often added as well to identify which DNA sample the clone arose from. A typical library insert with adapters and a barcode is shown in Fig. 47.30, *A*. The libraries are then partitioned according to size to select a band optimal for the downstream sequencing technology. Clonal amplification is usually performed by either emulsion PCR or bridge amplification.

Emulsion Polymerase Chain Reaction. In emulsion PCR, one strand of a library element is captured on one bead and is

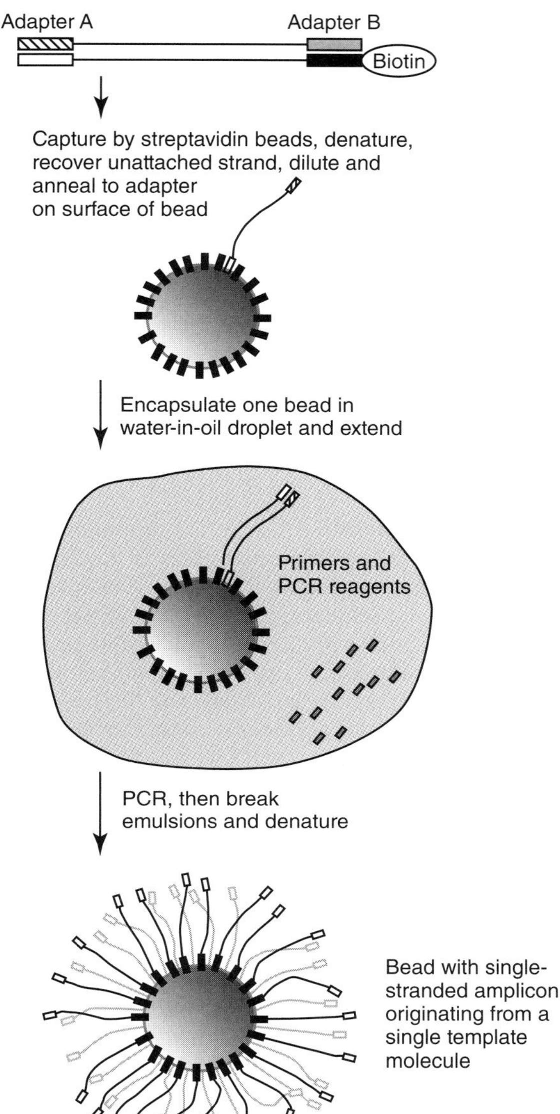

FIGURE 47.31 Emulsion polymerase chain reaction (PCR). Two adapters (*adapters A* and *B*) are randomly ligated to DNA fragments. Adapter B has a biotin on its 5′ end. Fragments with adapter B on one or both ends are captured by streptavidin beads, but fragments with only adapter A are washed away (not shown). Then the fragments are denatured, and the free strand with adapter A and adapter B at each end is collected (fragments with adapter B on both ends will not be released from the streptavidin bead). One molecule of the single-stranded template is then captured on a bead coated with adapter and is encapsulated inside a water-in-oil droplet that contains PCR reagents and primers. After PCR, the emulsion is broken, and the DNA is denatured. This generates a bead with a large number of clonal single strands tethered to it. The bead is then deposited into one of many wells on a fiber optic or onto a glass slide for sequence analysis (not shown).

clonally amplified inside a water-in-oil droplet, generating a bead covered with single-stranded PCR products (Fig. 47.31). The emulsion is formed by mixing beads (each covered with one primer), aqueous PCR components (including the other primer, polymerase, and dNTPs), and a mixture of oils under agitation to ideally form droplets that each contain only one bead and one library insert. The two primers are complementary to the adapters; one coats the bead surface, and one is free in solution. During emulsion PCR, all of the beads are amplified together in aqueous microdroplets dispersed in oil. The emulsion is amplified in a standard PCR thermal cycler. After PCR and denaturation, millions of copies of identical single-stranded PCR products are on each bead with each bead carrying distinct, oriented inserts flanked by the adapters. The emulsion is then broken and, after elimination of empty beads, is ready for sequencing.

Bridge Amplification. Bridge amplification generates clusters of single-stranded PCR products tethered to the surface of a planar flow cell (Fig. 47.32).[62] In contrast to the clonal bead generation of emulsion PCR, the amplification occurs on a flat surface. The primers, complementary to the adapters, are both attached to the surface, either randomly or in a fixed pattern. The library DNA is then denatured to form single strands that hybridize to the primers on the surface. After extension of the surface-bound primers, the original template strands are washed away under denaturing conditions. What follows is called bridge amplification, which is very similar to PCR except that both primers are bound to the surface, so that single strands bound to the surface must bend over to find their opposite primer, resulting in a double-stranded bridge after extension. Instead of denaturing with heat as in PCR, the flow cell is kept at 60°C, and a chemical denaturant is introduced to dissociate the two bridge strands, except now both strands are attached to the planer surface. When the flow cell is flushed with a polymerase and dNTPs under favorable extension conditions, both can find new primers to form additional bridges. The process repeats until about 1000 copies are formed. One of the bound primers can be designed to include a cleavable site (either chemical or enzymatic) so that one strand can be removed after denaturation. After capping the 3′- end of the single strands with ddNTPs (to prevent any undesired extension with the closely packed templates), the surface is ready for sequencing.

Sequencing by Synthesis

Sequencing by synthesis can be detected by (1) pyrophosphate release, (2) a pH decrease, or (3) the fluorescence of reversible terminators. The clonal amplification methods allow parallel observation of thousands to millions of strand extensions, greatly increasing the signal strength. However, the extensions must be controlled at each step because continuous strand extension would not remain synchronous between strands. This is achieved by immobilizing the clones into arrays so that reagents can be applied sequentially (no pun intended).

Pyrosequencing.[19] Pyrosequencing was used in the first massively parallel sequencing platform but has become less popular in recent years because of lower throughput and higher cost. Clonal beads are fit into picoliter reaction chambers formed in etched individual fibers of a fiberoptic cable. Solutions of dATPαS, dCTP, dGTP, or dTTP are passed over chambers one at a time under conditions that favor extension. If there is a base match, the nucleotide will be incorporated, and pyrophosphate will be released. Pyrosequencing signal generation occurs by linked enzymatic reactions, leading to luciferase chemiluminescence, and is covered earlier in this chapter (including the replacement of dATP with dATPαS to prevent interference with the linked enzymatic reactions).

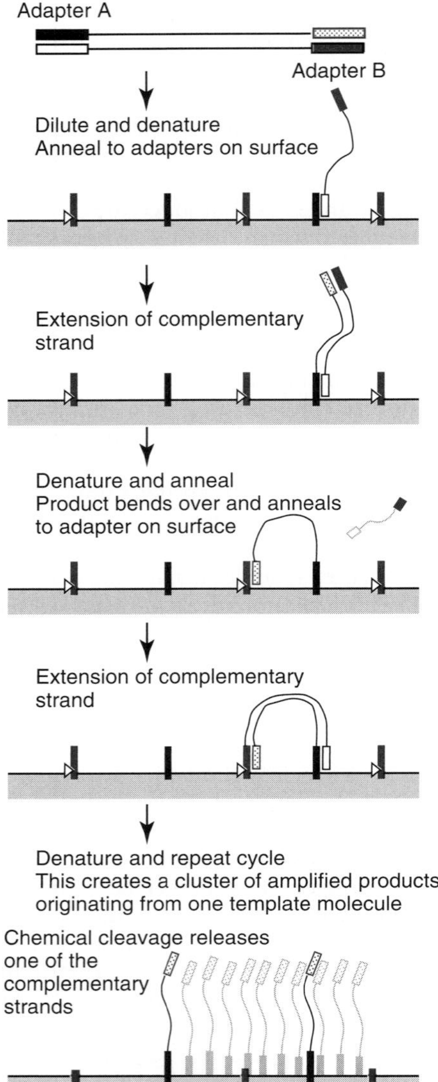
Adapter A
Adapter B
Dilute and denature
Anneal to adapters on surface
Extension of complementary strand
Denature and anneal
Product bends over and anneals to adapter on surface
Extension of complementary strand
Denature and repeat cycle
This creates a cluster of amplified products originating from one template molecule
Chemical cleavage releases one of the complementary strands

FIGURE 47.32 Bridge amplification. Two adapters (*adapters A* and *B*) are ligated to a DNA template. After they are diluted and denatured into single strands, the template is captured onto a flow cell surface by annealing to one of the two surface-bound primers that share sequences with adapter A or B. The polymerase reagent introduced into the flow cell extends the primer and generates the complementary strand of the template. The denaturant (usually sodium hydroxide) is introduced to the flow cell to release the original template strand. The free end of the newly synthesized strand anneals to a nearby primer by bending over, and a second round of reagent addition catalyzes the synthesis of another complementary strand. By repeating many of these cycles, a clonal cluster that consists of about 1000 copies of single-stranded template tethered to the surface is generated. This cluster is still a mixture of both complementary strands. One of the strands is selectively eliminated by treatment with periodic acid that cleaves a diol linkage present in one of the surface-bound primers *(open triangle on red primer)*. The cluster now contains only one of the template strands and is ready for sequence analysis.

The light produced is captured by the individual light fibers and detected on a CCD. If more than one base occurs in a row (a homopolymer stretch), multiple bases of that nucleotide will be incorporated, and the signal will be proportionately higher. As the number of identical bases increases, if becomes harder to determine their exact number.

Semiconductor Sequencing.[63] Similar to pyrosequencing detection, clonal beads are used as template. However, the beads are arrayed on semiconductor sensors modified to detect pH changes.[169] The chip does not detect light but a slight change in pH produced as a consequence of conversion of a dNTP into pyrophosphate by the many clones on the bead. Similar to pyrosequencing, homopolymer stretches can be problematic. By leveraging semiconductor technology development, the chip has rapidly increased in performance by decreasing the size of the beads and sensor wells and increasing the size of the chip. Run times are as short as 3 to 4 hours.

Reversible Terminators. After bridge amplification on a planar flow cell, one of four nucleotides is passed through the flow cell under conditions that favor extension. Unlike pyrosequencing and semiconductor sequencing, the nucleotides are fluorescent terminators so that only one base is incorporated, avoiding the problems with homopolymer stretches. Each nucleotide has a different fluorescent label so that each can be distinguished by color. Furthermore, the fluorescent terminators are reversible, which means that the blocked 3′-end can be regenerated by simple chemical means provided by the flow cell. Each cycle involves (1) adding polymerase and dNTPs as fluorescently labeled terminators under conditions that favor extension, (2) washing the flow cell, (3) imaging the fluorescence, (4) cleaving the fluorescent terminator, and (5) washing the flow cell. Output per run is up to 600 gb in 1 day.

Sequencing by Ligation

Instead of a polymerase and sequencing by synthesis, sequencing by ligation uses a ligase and a mixture of probes about eight bases long (Fig. 47.33). The template is either a clonal bead formed by emulsion PCR (similar to pyrophosphate and semiconductor sequencing) or a colony formed by isothermal amplification directly on a planer surface.[170] First, an anchor oligonucleotide is hybridized to a known portion of the immobilized template. Then a mixture of probes about eight bases long compete for ligation to the anchor. Each of the competing probes has one position with a defined base (A, T, G, or C) indicated by the color of a fluorescent label at the far end of the probe. The remaining bases of the probe may be degenerate (meaning that all four bases are used in the synthesis, creating a combination of 4^m different probes, where m is the number of degenerate base positions), or they may be universal bases (nucleotide analogs that pair with any of the four bases). The terminal fluorescent label blocks further concatenation of probes. At a stringent temperature, only the ligated anchor–probe complex remains hybridized to the template, and the defined base position is decoded by the color of the fluorescent label. The next cycle begins by stripping away the anchor–probe complex from the template and repeating the process but offset by one base by using a different anchor. Eventually, a short string of bases immediately adjacent to the anchoring site is determined. A variant of the technique uses two defined bases on each

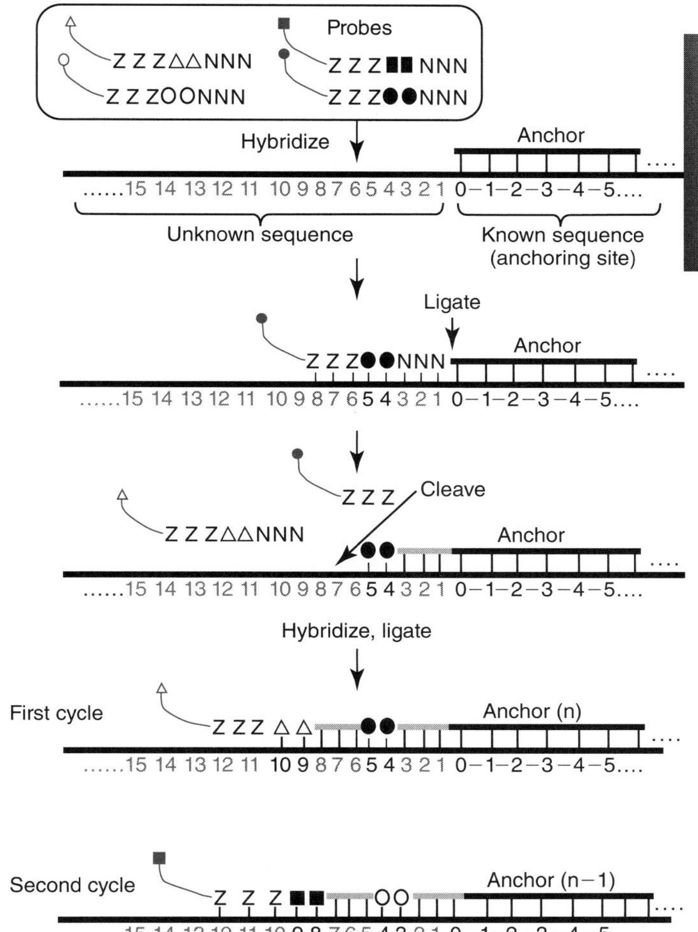

FIGURE 47.33 Sequencing by ligation (two-base encoding method). An anchor oligonucleotide is hybridized to known sequences of the template (anchoring site). Structures of octamer (8-mer) probes are shown. *N* represents a degenerate base (A, T, C, or G), *Z* represents a universal base that pairs with any base, and the defined bases *(closed circle, open circle, closed square, open triangle)* occupy the fourth and fifth base positions. The probes are color coded by one of four labels *(red),* with each color representing a set of four two-base combinations (eg, color 1 is AT, TA, CG, or GC; color 2 is AC, CA, TG, or GT; color 3 is TC, CT, AG, or GA; and color 4 is AA, TT, GG, or CC). When a probe hybridizes to the sequence adjacent to the anchoring site, ligase will connect the probe to the anchor. After the color is recorded, part of the probe is cleaved, and the label is removed together with some of the probe bases. This makes it possible for another probe to ligate to the extending complex. In fact, many rounds of ligation and cleavage can be performed, each time elongating the anchor–probe complex and providing additional two-base possibilities. After a few rounds of probe ligation and cleavage, the anchor–probe complex is stripped, and the next cycle, which is offset by one base, repeats the process. Cycles are repeated until one of the defined bases on the probe pairs with a known base on the anchoring site, allowing decoding of all of the two-base combinations. For example, in the first cycle, two-base possibilities for positions 4, 5, 9, and 10 are determined. In the second cycle, which is offset by one base (n-1), possibilities for positions 3, 4, 8, and 9 are determined. This process is repeated until the defined base on the probe pairs with the first base on the anchoring site (position 0). Because the identity of that base is known, the 0/1 base combination is decoded, which in turn decodes base position 2 and so on, until all of the two-base combinations are decoded.

labeled probe and extends the read length by cleaving part of the probe after recording the label. Although massively parallel, the read length averages less than 75 bases.

Single-Molecule Sequencing

Single-molecule sequencing methods do not require template amplification. Base reads do not require synching with other clonal strands because there are none. Sensitive optical or electronic methods are required to detect base sequence in a single molecule.[171] If long reads and high accuracy are achieved, advantages include efficient sequence assembly, analyses of repetitive sequences, de novo sequencing, mapping of chromosomal rearrangements, and fusions. In contrast, massively parallel sequencing methods usually generate short sequence reads (30–700 bases long) that have to be aligned and analyzed to derive a consensus, then stitched together, and compared with reference genome sequences. Accurate assembly of sequence data relies on sufficient coverage and/or redundancy across the sequenced region.[172]

Real-Time Single Molecule Sequencing With Fluorescent Nucleotides.[171] Library preparation is unique for this method because fragmentation is tuned to provide about 10-kb inserts, and the adapters are designed as hairpins. The result is a double-stranded insert bounded by identical 27 base single-stranded loops on each end (see Fig. 47.30, *B*). Sequencing primers are annealed to the loop region and bound to a single polymerase molecule at the bottom of a zero-mode waveguide to form an active polymerase complex. The zero-mode waveguide allows single molecule detection of transient fluorescent labels that are covalently attached to the terminal phosphate of each dNTP. The four dNTPs are added to the wells with different labels that can be distinguished optically. When a fluorescent dNTP pairs with its complement near to the polymerase active site, it is in a perfect position for fluorescence detection. After being incorporated into the growing strand, the terminal fluorescent label (attached to pyrophosphate) diffuses away from the polymerase. The fluorescent signals are acquired continuously at high speed as the primer proceeds around the loop by rolling circle amplification. The process can be stopped after one loop or continued for multiple reads for error checking. Base reads of up to 40,000 to 50,000 contiguous bases have been reported.

Nanopore Sequencing.[173] Another single-molecule sequencing approach that does not require amplification and uses electronic, rather than optical, detection is nanopore sequencing. Single DNA strands are channeled through nanopores formed by immobilized proteins. Passage of individual DNA bases through the protein nanopore generates characteristic electrical signals that can reveal the identity of the base (or combination of bases) traversing the nanopore. In essence, this is similar to a nano-sized Coulter counter that quantifies base differences on a single strand of DNA rather than cell size. Kilobases of NAs can potentially be sequenced in a single read. The method is nondestructive and can discriminate methylated DNA bases as well as normal bases.[174] A number of nanopores are currently under study (α-hemolysin, *Mycobacterium smegmatis* porin A [MspA], and others), and solid-state nanopores are also being intensively investigated. Shorter and narrower nanopores that interrogate single bases would be ideal, but current material limitations allow about four bases within the nanopore at the same time.

SELECTED REFERENCES

For a full list of references for this chapter, please refer to ExpertConsult.com.

10. Sanger F, Nicklen S, Coulson AR. DNA sequencing with chain-terminating inhibitors. *Proc Natl Acad Sci USA* 1977;**74**:5463–7.
11. Saiki RK, Gelfand DH, Stoffel S, et al. Primer-directed enzymatic amplification of DNA with a thermostable DNA polymerase. *Science* 1988;**239**:487–91.
12. Higuchi R, Dollinger G, Walsh PS, et al. Simultaneous amplification and detection of specific DNA sequences. *Biotechnology (N Y)* 1992;**10**:413–17.
16. Schena M, Shalon D, Davis RW, et al. Quantitative monitoring of gene expression patterns with a complementary DNA microarray. *Science* 1995;**270**:467–70.
22. Wittwer CT, Herrmann MG, Moss AA, et al. Continuous fluorescence monitoring of rapid cycle DNA amplification. *Biotechniques* 1997;**22**:130–1, 4–8.
35. Farrar JS, Wittwer CT. Extreme PCR: efficient and specific DNA amplification in 15-60 seconds. *Clin Chem* 2015;**61**:145–53.
44. Li J, Wang L, Mamon H, et al. Replacing PCR with COLD-PCR enriches variant DNA sequences and redefines the sensitivity of genetic testing. *Nat Med* 2008;**14**:579–84.
56. Dingle TC, Sedlak RH, Cook L, et al. Tolerance of droplet-digital PCR vs real-time quantitative PCR to inhibitory substances. *Clin Chem* 2013;**59**:1670–2.
62. Bentley DR, Balasubramanian S, Swerdlow HP, et al. Accurate whole human genome sequencing using reversible terminator chemistry. *Nature* 2008;**456**:53–9.
82. Bustin SA, Benes V, Garson JA, et al. The MIQE guidelines: minimum information for publication of quantitative real-time PCR experiments. *Clin Chem* 2009;**55**:611–22.
87. Lee LG, Connell CR, Bloch W. Allelic discrimination by nick-translation PCR with fluorogenic probes. *Nucleic Acids Res* 1993;**21**:3761–6.
91. Laszlo AH, Derrington IM, Ross BC, et al. Decoding long nanopore sequencing reads of natural DNA. *Nat Biotechnol* 2014;**32**:829–33.
114. SantaLucia J Jr. A unified view of polymer, dumbbell, and oligonucleotide DNA nearest-neighbor thermodynamics. *Proc Natl Acad Sci USA* 1998;**95**:1460–5.
124. Reis-Filho JS, Pusztai L. Gene expression profiling in breast cancer: classification, prognostication, and prediction. *Lancet* 2011;**378**:1812–23.
152. Liew M, Pryor R, Palais R, et al. Genotyping of single-nucleotide polymorphisms by high-resolution melting of small amplicons. *Clin Chem* 2004;**50**:1156–64.
163. Vossen RH, Aten E, Roos A, et al. High-resolution melting analysis (HRMA): more than just sequence variant screening. *Hum Mutat* 2009;**30**:860–6.
169. Sakurai T, Husimi Y. Real-time monitoring of DNA polymerase reactions by a micro ISFET pH sensor. *Anal Chem* 1992;**64**:1996–7.
170. Ma Z, Lee RW, Li B, et al. Isothermal amplification method for next-generation sequencing. *Proc Natl Acad Sci USA* 2013;**110**:14320–3.
171. Eid J, Fehr A, Gray J, et al. Real-time DNA sequencing from single polymerase molecules. *Science* 2009;**323**:133–8.
173. Steinbock LJ, Radenovic A. The emergence of nanopores in next-generation sequencing. *Nanotechnology* 2015;**26**:074003.

48

Molecular Microbiology

*Frederick S. Nolte**

ABSTRACT

Background

Nucleic acid (NA) amplification techniques are now commonly used to diagnose and manage patients with infectious diseases. The growth in the number of Food and Drug Administration–approved test kits and analyte-specific reagents has facilitated the use of this technology in clinical laboratories. Technological advances in NA amplification techniques, automation, NA sequencing, and multiplex analysis have reinvigorated the field and created new opportunities for growth. Simple, sample-in, answer-out molecular test systems are now widely available that can be deployed in a variety of laboratory and clinical settings. Molecular microbiology remains the leading area in molecular pathology in terms of both the numbers of tests performed and clinical relevance. NA-based tests have reduced the dependency of the clinical microbiology laboratory on more traditional antigen detection and culture methods and created new opportunities for the laboratory to impact patient care.

Content

This chapter reviews NA testing as it applies to specific pathogens or infectious disease syndromes, with a focus on those diseases for which NA testing is now considered the standard of care and highlights the unique challenges and opportunities that these tests present for clinical laboratories.

INTRODUCTION

Since the publication of the fifth edition of this textbook, significant changes have occurred in the practice of diagnostic molecular microbiology. Nucleic acid (NA) amplification techniques are now commonly used to diagnose and manage patients with infectious diseases. The growth in the number of Food and Drug Administration (FDA)–approved test kits and analyte-specific reagents (ASRs) has facilitated the use of this technology in clinical laboratories. Technological advances in NA amplification techniques, automation, NA sequencing, and multiplex analysis have reinvigorated the field and created new opportunities for growth. Simple, sample-in, answer-out molecular test systems are now widely available that can be deployed in a variety of laboratory and clinical settings.

Molecular microbiology remains the leading area in molecular pathology in terms of both the numbers of tests performed and clinical relevance. NA-based tests have reduced the dependency of the clinical microbiology laboratory on more traditional antigen detection and culture methods and created new opportunities for the laboratory to impact patient care. This chapter reviews NA testing as it applies to specific pathogens or infectious disease syndromes, with a focus on diseases for which NA testing is now considered the standard of care and highlights the unique challenges and opportunities that these tests present for clinical laboratories. A complete and current list of all FDA-cleared and FDA-approved microbial NA based tests can be found at http://www.fda.gov/MedicalDevices/ProductsandMedicalProcedures/InVitroDiagnostics/ucm330711.htm. Readers are directed to *Molecular Microbiology: Diagnostic Principles and Practice*, 3rd edition, for a more comprehensive and in depth examination of this dynamic and exciting discipline.[1]

VIRAL SYNDROMES

Human Immunodeficiency Virus 1

Human immunodeficiency virus 1 (HIV-1), the causative agent of the acquired immunodeficiency syndrome (AIDS), is an RNA virus belonging to the genus *Lentivirus* of the family *Retroviridae*. Replication of the virus is complex and involves reverse transcription of the RNA genome into a double-stranded DNA molecule or provirus, which is integrated into the host genome. HIV-1 enters the cell using CD4 as a receptor and CXCR4 or CCR5 as a coreceptor. In general, CCR5 coreceptors are found on macrophages, and CXCR4 coreceptors are found on T cells. Determining the cellular tropism of the virus has become important now that an antiretroviral drug targets the CCR5 coreceptor. The HIV-1 reverse transcriptase (RT) enzyme does not have proofreading capabilities, leading to the significant genetic diversity of HIV-1. Several distinct genetic subtypes or clades have been identified and are categorized into three groups: major (M), outlier (O), and N (nonmajor and nonoutlier). Recently, a new group P has been identified that is closely related to a gorilla simian immunodeficiency virus.[2] The major group is

*The author wishes to acknowledge the contributions of Aaron D. Bossler and Angela M. Caliendo who authored this chapter in the previous edition.

divided into nine clades (A–K) and circulating recombinant forms (CRFs), which are determined on the basis of sequence diversity within the HIV-1 *gag* and *env* genes.[3] Group M virus is found worldwide, with clade B predominating in Europe and North America, clade C in Africa and India, and clade E in much of Southeast Asia. The complex replication cycle and genetic diversity are two important factors that influence the design and interpretation of HIV-1 molecular assays.

The management of patients with HIV-1 infection was transformed by tests performed to measure the concentrations of HIV-1 RNA in blood (viral load testing) and tests for resistance to antiviral drugs. With these tools, it is possible to maximize the effectiveness of antiretroviral therapy (ART) for an individual.

The first HIV-1 viral load test was approved by the FDA in 1996 and rapidly became the standard of care for monitoring response to ART. Early studies found that patients who have higher viral loads progressed more rapidly to AIDS and death than those with low viral loads.[4-6]

Viral load testing is now widely accepted as a marker of response to ART. The guidelines for initiation of therapy based on viral load have changed as our understanding of disease progression at higher CD4 cell counts has improved. With the availability of newer more potent and less toxic drugs, ART is recommended for all HIV-infected individuals regardless of their CD4 cell count or viral load (DHHS Panel on Antiretroviral Guidelines, http://AIDSinfo.nih.gov). After treatment is initiated, viral load testing is crucial for monitoring response to therapy and should be measured in all HIV-infected individuals at the time of entry into care when therapy is initiated and at a regular interval (usually 3–4 months) while on therapy. The standard of care is to treat with a combination of antiretroviral drugs, which are classified based on their viral targets: nucleoside reverse transcriptase inhibitors (NRTIs), non-nucleoside reverse transcriptase inhibitors (NNRTIs), protease inhibitors (PIs), fusion inhibitors, integrase inhibitors (also known as integrase strand transfer inhibitors [INSTIs]), and CCR5 entry inhibitors. Current Department of Health and Human Services Panel on Antiretroviral Guidelines (http://aidsinfo.nih.gov/guidelines) recommend an initial regimen of two NRTIs and an NNRTI, a PI, or an INSTI. The pretreatment viral load values influence the treatment regimen because some regimens are less effective in patients with high viral loads. After initiation of appropriate therapy, there is typically a 2 $\log_{10}$ or greater decrease in viral load within 2 to 3 months. The goal for a patient is to achieve a viral load below the limit of detection of the most sensitive assays (20–50 copies/mL). Data have shown that the lower the absolute viral load, the better the clinical and virologic outcomes.[7,8] Guidelines recommend quantifying plasma HIV-1 RNA immediately before initiating therapy and 2 to 8 weeks later, with the goal to achieve an undetectable viral load level within 16 to 24 weeks of initiating therapy. It is important to determine early in the treatment course if there is suboptimal viral load suppression, so that factors affecting adherence can be assessed and, if needed, the regimen altered. After the initial response has been characterized, the viral load should be monitored every 3 to 4 months to ensure the response to therapy is sustained.

Of note, viral blips (defined as a detectable viral load usually <400 copies/mL) occur in successfully treated individuals and are not predictive of virologic failure.[9] For this reason, *virologic failure* is defined as a sustained viral load of more than 200 copies/mL.

Viral load testing also aids in the diagnosis of acute HIV-1 infection (the window period after infection that occurs before detectable antibody production), although the currently available viral load assays are not FDA approved for diagnostic purposes. During this period of early infection, patients typically have very high viral loads ranging from 10^5 to 10^7 copies/mL.[10] HIV RNA testing is recommended in the 2014 updated HIV diagnostic testing algorithm for patients who are reactive in a fourth-generation immunoassay but test negative in a supplemental HIV-1/HIV-2 antibody differentiation test, primarily to better detect acute HIV-1 infections.[11] However, only one HIV RNA test is FDA approved for diagnosis, the APTIMA HIV-1 qualitative assay (Hologic, San Diego, CA), and it is not widely available in clinical laboratories. Hospital laboratories would benefit from an FDA diagnostic claim for viral load testing that is done reflexively in the above diagnostic algorithm because verifying this claim at a local laboratory level is overly burdensome.

A proviral DNA test, AMPLICOR HIV-1 DNA polymerase chain reaction (PCR) (Roche Diagnostics), is available as a research use only (RUO) test that is helpful in neonates born to HIV-1–infected mothers receiving ART. Both antiretroviral agents and maternal antibody cross the placenta. Antiretroviral agents can suppress the replication of the virus in neonates, and RNA tests can be falsely negative early after birth. Maternal HIV-1 antibody can persist in neonates for up to 2 years after birth and is therefore not a reliable marker of neonatal infection.

Currently there are three commercially available, FDA-approved HIV-1 viral load assays. Two of these assays use real-time PCR, cobas AmpliPrep/cobas TaqMan HIV-1, version 2.0 (Roche Diagnostics), and m2000 RealTime System (Abbott Molecular); the third, Versant HIV-1 RNA 3.0 (Siemens), uses branched DNA signal amplification. The amplification method, gene targets, and dynamic ranges for these assays are given in Table 48.1. Newly emerging NA amplification tests (NAATs) and platforms have the potential for true point-of-care testing for HIV RNA,[12] and several (eg, Alere, BioHelix, Cepheid, and Iquum/Roche) are in commercial development. These tests may have application in detecting acute infections, confirming screening tests, and determining viral loads in resource-poor settings.

Most clinical laboratories are using one of the real-time PCR assays because of their lower limits of detection and quantification and increased dynamic range compared with older-generation PCR assays and the branched DNA assay. Genotype bias was a significant problem in some of the earlier viral load assays because the gene targets chosen were not highly conserved among the different HIV-1 subtypes. However, this problem has been addressed, and the current versions of the Roche and Abbott real-time PCR assays both accurately quantify group M, group O, and CRFs of HIV-1.[13] The intra-assay imprecision of HIV-1 viral load assays is approximately 0.12 to 0.2 $\log_{10}$ copies/mL. The biologic variation of viral load in patients not receiving therapy is approximately 0.3 $\log_{10}$ copies/mL.[14] Consequently, changes in viral load must exceed 0.5 $\log_{10}$ copies/mL (a threefold change) to suggest a meaningful change in viral replication.

TABLE 48.1 Commercially Available Food and Drug Administration–Approved Viral Load Assays

Virus	Assay (Manufacturer)	Method	Gene Target	Dynamic Range
HIV-1	Versant 3.0 (Siemens)	Branched DNA	*pol*	75–500,000 copies/mL
	cobas Ampliprep/cobas TaqMan 2.0 (Roche)	RT-real-time PCR	*gag, LTR*	20–10,000,000 copies/mL
	RealTime (Abbott)	RT-real-time PCR	*int*	40–10,000,000 copies/mL
HCV	Versant 3.0 (Siemens)	Branched DNA	*5′ UTR*	615–7,700,000 IU/mL
	cobas Ampliprep/cobas TaqMan Test 2.0 (Roche)	RT-real-time PCR	*5′ UTR*	43–69,000,000 IU/mL
	RealTime (Abbott)	RT-real-time PCR	*5′ UTR*	12–100,000,00 IU/mL
HBV	cobas Ampliprep/cobas TaqMan Test 2.0 (Roche)	Real-time PCR	*Precore/core*	20–170,000,000 IU/mL
	RealTime (Abbott)	Real-time PCR	*Surface*	10–1,000,000,000 IU/mL
CMV	cobas Ampliprep/cobas TaqMan Test (Roche)	Real-time PCR	*UL54*	137–9,100,000 IU/mL
	artus RGQ MDx (Qiagen)	Real-time PCR	*MIE*	119–79,400,000 IU/mL

CMV, Cytomegalovirus; *HIV,* human immunodeficiency virus; *HBV,* hepatitis C virus; *HCV,* hepatitis B virus; *PCR,* polymerase chain reaction; *RT,* reverse transcriptase.

Viral load testing is routinely performed on plasma specimens, and ethylenediaminetetraacetic acid (EDTA) is the anticoagulant of choice. Acid–citrate–dextrose is also an acceptable anticoagulant, but blood anticoagulated in heparin is unacceptable for most tests. It is critical to handle clinical specimens properly to minimize the risk of RNA degradation during specimen collection and transport. Plasma should be separated within 6 hours of collection and ideally stored at −20°C, although plasma viral RNA is stable at 4°C for several days. For laboratories testing specimens collected at remote sites, sample handling can require careful attention. Special blood collection containers, or tubes, are available that contain a gel that provides a physical barrier between the plasma and cells after centrifugation. The tubes can be shipped without the need to transfer the plasma into a separate tube. Tubes should not be frozen before pouring off of the plasma because this may lead to falsely elevated viral load assays.[15,16]

Six general classes of antiretroviral drugs are used in clinical care: NRTIs, NNRTIs, PIs, fusion inhibitors, INSTIs, and CCR5 entry inhibitors. Viral resistance can occur with each of these drug classes, particularly when viral replication is not maximally suppressed during therapy. The current standard of care is to use regimens that contain a combination of drugs because resistance is less likely to occur on the complex regimens than on monotherapy.

The clinical utility of antiviral resistance testing in HIV-1–infected individuals is well established, and regularly updated guidelines for its use can be found at http://AIDSinfo.nih.gov. Current DHHS Panel on Antiretroviral Guidelines recommend that resistance testing be performed in the following situations: (1) before initiation of ART in treatment-naïve patients, (2) to guide the selection of active drugs when changing antiretroviral regimens, (3) for the management of suboptimal viral load reduction, and (4) in all pregnant women before the initiation of therapy.

HIV-1 resistance testing can be done by genotypic or phenotypic methods. Genotypic assays identify specific mutations or nucleotide changes that are associated with decreased susceptibility to an antiviral drug. Phenotypic assays are performed by the creation of a pseudoviral vector and measuring its replicative capacity in varying concentrations of drug and comparing it with replication of wild-type virus. Both genotypic and phenotypic methods are used clinically for assessing antiviral resistance in patients, with phenotypic testing usually reserved for drug-experienced patients with complicated resistance profiles.

This discussion is limited to automated sequencing methods for genotypic resistance because these are the methods used most often to inform treatment decisions. Currently available FDA-cleared assays will detect mutations in the RT and protease genes; modifications of existing assays are needed to detect resistance mutations associated with other classes of drugs such as integrase and fusion inhibitors.

The first step in genotypic assays is the isolation of HIV-1 RNA from plasma followed by reverse transcriptase polymerase chain reaction (RT-PCR) amplification and sequencing of RT and protease genes. Analysis of the results involves sequence alignment and editing, mutation identification by comparison with wild-type sequence, and interpretation of the clinical significance of the mutations identified. Most clinical laboratories performing genotypic resistance testing rely on commercial assays that provide reagents and software programs to assist with interpretation of the results. Two assays have been cleared by the FDA: the Trugene HIV-1 Genotyping Kit and OpenGene DNA Sequencing System (Siemens Healthcare Diagnostics) and the ViroSeq HIV-1 Genotyping System (Abbott Molecular).

Interpretation of genotypic resistance testing is complex. Interpretation of resistance mutations uses "rules-based" software that takes into account cross-resistance and interactions of mutations. The commercially available systems generate a summary report that lists the various mutations that have been identified in the RT and protease genes, and each drug is reported as resistant, possibly resistant, no evidence of resistance, or insufficient evidence. A comprehensive discussion of the specific mutations associated with each antiretroviral drug and the interactions of mutations is beyond the scope of this chapter but is available from a variety of sources (eg, http://www.iasusa.org, http://hivdb.stanford.edu/).

A limitation of currently used genotypic and phenotypic assays is that they can detect only those mutants that make up at least 20% of the total viral population. Regimens chosen based on resistance testing may not always be effective because the minority populations will quickly predominate in the presence of drug. Drug selection pressure is also needed for some resistance mutations to persist at detectable concentrations in the viral population; when drug therapy is discontinued, the wild-type virus may quickly predominate. For this reason, it is recommended that specimens for resistance testing be obtained while the patient is on ART. The minimum viral load required for reliable resistance testing is approximately 1000 copies/mL. Because genotyping assays are especially sensitive to RNA degradation, care must be taken to properly handle the specimen after collection.

POINTS TO REMEMBER

Human Immunodeficiency Virus

- This RNA virus exhibits significant genetic diversity globally and within individual patients.
- HIV RNA is the earliest marker of infection.
- Viral load testing is a widely accepted marker of response to therapy with the goal of suppression to undetectable amounts.
- Special care should be taken in sample processing to avoid spurious increases in HIV viral load tests.
- HIV resistance genotyping should be performed on all therapy-naïve patients before initiation of ART and in selection of active drugs when changing therapy.

Hepatitis

Hepatitis C Virus

Approximately 3.2 million persons in the United States are living with active hepatitis C virus (HCV) infection, which is a major cause of chronic liver disease. After acute infection, 80% to 85% of individuals develop a chronic infection, and 2% to 4% of these individuals develop cirrhosis and end-stage liver disease, making end-stage liver disease secondary to HCV the most common indication for liver transplantation in the United States. Molecular tests for detection, quantification, and genotyping of HCV are standards of care for the diagnosis and management of patients with hepatitis C.

Hepatitis C virus is an RNA virus with a positive-sense, single-stranded genome of approximately 9500 nt encoding a single polyprotein of about 3000 amino acids. The long open reading frame is flanked at each end by short untranslated regions (UTRs). The genome structure is most similar to viruses of the family *Flaviviridae*, which includes many of the arthropod-borne viruses. As in other flaviviruses, the three N-terminal proteins of HCV (core, envelope 1 [E1]) and envelope 2 [E2]) are probably structural and the four C-terminal proteins (nonstructural 2, 3, 4, and 5) are thought to function in viral replication. HCV is classified within the family *Flaviviridae* in its own genus, *Hepacivirus*.

The 5′ UTR is a highly conserved region of 341 nt and has a complex secondary structure. It contains an internal ribosome entry site and is important in the translation of the long open reading frame. The 3′ UTR contains a short region that varies in sequence and length followed by a polypyrimidine stretch of variable length and finally a highly conserved sequence of 98 nt, which constitutes the terminus of the genome. The function of the 3′ UTR is not known but is thought to be essential for viral replication.

The E1 and E2 regions of HCV are the most variable regions within the genome at both the nucleotide and amino acid levels. Two regions in E2, called hypervariable regions 1 and 2 (HVR1 and HRV2, respectively), show extreme sequence variability, which is thought to result from selective pressure by antiviral antibodies. E2 also contains the binding site for CD81, one of the putative cell receptors or coreceptors for HCV.

The nonstructural regions 2 (NS2) and 3 (NS3) contain a zinc-dependent autoprotease that cleaves the polyprotein at the NS2–NS3 junction. The aminoterminal portion of the NS3 protein also is a serine protease that cleaves the polyprotein at several sites. The carboxyterminal portion of the NS3 protein has helicase activity, which is important for HCV replication. The NS4A protein is a cofactor for NS3 serine protease. The NS5B region encodes the RNA-dependent RNA polymerase, which replicates the viral genome. A region in NS5A has been linked to interferon-α (IFN-α) response and therefore is called the IFN-α–sensitivity determining region.

The first complete HCV genome sequence was reported by Choo et al in 1991.[17] As additional genome sequences from isolates from different parts of the world were determined and compared, it was evident that HCV exists as distinct genotypes with as much as 35% sequence diversity over the whole viral genome.[18] Much of the early literature on genotyping is confusing because investigators developed and used their own classification schemes. However, a consensus nomenclature system was developed in 1994. In this system, the genotypes are numbered using Arabic numerals in order of their discovery, and the more closely related strains within some types are designated as subtypes with lowercase letters. The complex of genetic variants found within an individual isolate is termed the "quasispecies." The quasispecies results from the accumulation of mutations that occur during viral replication in the host.

The genotype and subtype assignments and nomenclature rules for HCV have recently been updated.[19] There are now 7 major genotypes and 67 subtypes of HCV recognized with another 20 provisional subtypes. HCV strains belonging to different genotypes differ at 30% to 35% of nucleotides and those that belong to the same subtype differ at fewer than 15% of nucleotides at the genome level.

Hepatitis C virus genotypes 1, 2, and 3 are found throughout the world, but there are clear differences in their distribution.[20] HCV subtypes 1a, 1b, 2a, 2b, 2c, and 3a are responsible for more than 90% of infections in North and South America, Europe, and Japan. In the United States, type 1 accounts for approximately 70% of the infections with equal distribution between subtypes 1a and 1b. Viral genotype does not correlate with disease progression.[21,22]

Detection of HCV RNA in serum or plasma by NA amplification methods is important for confirming the diagnosis of HCV, distinguishing active from resolved infection, assessing the virologic response to therapy, and screening the blood supply. These tests are incorporated into diagnostic algorithms for hepatitis C proposed by the Centers for Disease Control and Prevention (CDC),[23] American Association for the Study of Liver Diseases,[24] and National Academy of Clinical Biochemistry.[25]

The detection of HCV RNA in the plasma or serum is the earliest marker of infection, appearing 1 to 2 weeks after infection and weeks before elevation of liver enzymes or the appearance of anti-HCV antibodies. Approximately 80% of individuals infected with HCV will be chronically infected with the virus. In antibody-positive individuals, HCV RNA tests can distinguish active from resolved infections. In patients with a high pretest probability of infection, a positive serologic screening test result is usually confirmed with a test for HCV RNA rather than the recombinant immunoblot assay (RIBA). This strategy is cost-effective and more informative than using the RIBA to confirm positive antibody screening tests in a diagnostic setting.[26] However, with the discontinuation of the HCV RIBA by the manufacturer in 2012, all reactive HCV antibody screening tests should be followed by FDA-approved HCV RNA testing.[27]

Hepatitis C virus RNA testing also is helpful for the diagnosis of infection in infants born to HCV-infected mothers because of the persistence of maternal antibody and in immunocompromised or debilitated patients who may have blunted serologic responses. An HCV RNA test also should be used for patients suspected of having an acute infection and in patients with hepatitis of no identifiable cause.

Hepatitis C virus RNA tests are the most reliable means of identifying patients with active HCV infection. A negative HCV RNA test result in a serologically positive individual may indicate that the infection has resolved or that the viremia is intermittent. Up to 15% of chronically infected individuals have intermittent viremia and, as a result, a single negative HCV RNA determination may not be sufficient to exclude active infection when the index of clinical suspicion is high.[28] In these individuals a second specimen should be collected and tested.

The use of anti-HCV antibody tests to screen the blood supply has dramatically reduced the risk of transfusion-associated HCV infection in developed countries. The risk in the United States from blood that is negative for anti- HCV antibodies is less than 1 in 103,000 transfused units.[29] To drive the risk of infection from transfusion even lower, blood donor pools currently are tested for the presence of HCV RNA.[30] The serologic screening tests for HCV have a 70-day window period of seronegativity, and antigen detection tests are not yet available for blood product screening. HCV RNA testing is estimated to reduce the detection window by 25 days and reduce the number of transfused infectious units from 116 to 32 per year.[31]

Assays for the detection and quantification of HCV core antigen in serum have recently been commercially developed but are not yet FDA cleared for diagnostic use.[32-36] These tests significantly shorten the serologically silent window period using seroconversion panels, and their performance correlates closely with RNA detection tests in blood donors. However, the analytical sensitivity is less than most RNA tests, at approximately 10,000 IU/mL. The analytical sensitivity of the core antigen test is too high to be used in the monitoring of late events during and after treatment. Antigen detection may represent a cost-effective alternative to HCV RNA testing to distinguish active from resolved infections in resource-poor settings.

Hepatitis C viral load testing is useful in pretreatment evaluations of patients being considered for therapy because a viral load of less 600,000 IU/mL is one of several predictors of achieving a sustained virologic response.[37,38] Other factors associated with achieving a sustained response to therapy include the absence of cirrhosis, age younger than 40 years, female gender, white race, viral genotype 2 or 3, and presence of two copies of the C allele at position rs12979860 near the gene for IFN lambda 3 (*IFNL3*, *IL28B*).[39,40]

Hepatitis C viral load does not predict disease progression and is not associated with severity of liver disease.[41] This is in sharp contrast to HIV-1, in which the viral load is the principal factor determining the rate of disease progression. Monitoring HCV viral load in untreated patients is not warranted and should be discouraged. Until recently, the standard therapy for patients with chronic HCV infection was pegylated IFN-α in combination with ribavirin administered for either 48 weeks for HCV genotype 1, 4, 5, and 6 infections or for 24 weeks for HCV genotype 2 and 3 infections. Sustained virologic response (SVR) rates were attained in 40% to 50% of patients with genotype 1 and in 80% or more of those with genotype 2 and 3 infections. SVR was defined as the absence of detectable HCV RNA in plasma or serum as determined with a test that has a limit of detection of 50 IU/mL or less and is considered a virologic cure.

The first direct-acting antivirals (DAAs) for treatment of hepatitis C were approved by the FDA in 2011. Both are NS3/4A serine protease inhibitors, boceprevir (BOC) (Merck) and telaprevir (TVR) (Vertex). These DAA agents are used in combination with pegylated IFN-α and ribavirin. Triple therapy for genotype 1 infections has led to approximately a 30% increase in SVR over the previous standard of care therapy in all patient subgroups. TVR also has activity against genotype 2 infections but not against genotype 3 infections. BOC appears to have activity against both genotypes 2 and 3 infections. However, neither drug should be used to treat patients with genotype 2 and 3 infections because SVR rates with pegylated IFN-α and ribavirin alone are much higher.[42]

The important time points for response-guided therapy are at 8, 12, and 24 weeks for BOC and 4, 12, and 24 weeks for TVR. Treatment with all three drugs should be stopped if HCV RNA is greater than 100 IU/mL at week 12 or detectable at week 24 for BOC triple therapy and if HCV RNA is greater than 1000 IU/mL at weeks 4 or 12 or detectable at week 24 with TVR.

The goal of treatment is a SVR, defined as no detectable HCV RNA in serum or plasma by a highly sensitive assay (limit of detection ≤10–15 IU/mL) 6 months after the end of treatment. Patients who achieve a SVR have little or no chance of virologic relapse of their disease.

In 2013, two more potent DAAs were approved by the FDA: sofosbuvir (Gilead), a NS5B polymerase inhibitor,[43] and simeprevir (Johnson & Johnson) a second-generation protease inhibitor.[44] Sofosbuvir was approved in combination with pegylated IFN-α and ribavirin for treatment of genotypes 1 and 4 and in combination with ribavirin alone for genotypes 2 and 3. Simeprevir was approved by the FDA for treatment of genotype 1 infections in combination with pegylated IFN-α and ribavirin but only for patients with genotype 1 who have not failed therapy with first-generation protease inhibitors.

Monitoring of viral load during treatment does not affect management decisions with a sofosbuvir-based regimen because treatment failure is almost exclusively caused by relapse.[43] However, given the expense of the drugs and the potential risk of viral resistance with inappropriate use, viral load testing at week 4 and at the end of treatment (either week 12 or 24 depending on the regimen) seems prudent.

The viral load should be determined at weeks 4, 12, and 24 to assess treatment response and possible cessation of therapy in patients treated with simeprevir, pegylated IFN-α, and ribavirin. Discontinuation is warranted for patients who are unlikely to achieve a SVR based on the virologic response during treatment. If HCV RNA is greater than 25 IU/mL at week 4, the entire regimen should be discontinued. If the HCV RNA is greater than 25 IU/mL at week 12 or 24 after the simeprevir has been completed, the pegylated IFN-α and ribavirin should be discontinued.[44]

Numerous other DAAs have been developed and are currently in clinical trials. These include NS3/4A protease inhibitors, NS5B polymerase inhibitors, and inhibitors of host cell proteins required for HCV replication. The most current recommendations for all aspects of HCV treatment can be found at http://www.hcvguidelines.org.

Currently, three FDA-approved HCV viral load assays are available commercially. Two of these assays use real-time PCR, cobas AmpliPrep/cobas TaqMan, version 2.0 (Roche Diagnostics), and m2000 RealTime System (Abbott Molecular); the third uses branched DNA signal amplification, Versant 3.0 (Siemens). The amplification method, gene targets, and dynamic ranges for these assays are given in Table 48.1. The commercially available assays are calibrated against a World Health Organization (WHO) international calibration standard and report results in IU/mL. The first version of the cobas TaqMan HCV test had a genotype bias particularly against genotype 4 samples. The second version of the assay has been modified to enhance its ability to accurately quantify all of the major HCV genotypes.[45,46]

The development of the WHO first international HCV RNA standard and its acceptance by the manufacturers of HCV RNA assays as a calibrator was a significant advance in HCV RNA quantification.[47] However, despite the implementation of an international standard, HCV RNA measurements are not equivalent between the different assays.[48,49] Therefore, patients should ideally be tested with the same assay during the course of their treatment to minimize the potential for patient management errors.[50]

Although a number of baseline factors are predictive of response to treatment of chronic hepatitis C infection, HCV genotype is a strong and consistent predictor for achieving a SVR to pegylated IFN-α and ribavirin. In the large clinical trials of combination therapy with pegylated IFN-α and ribavirin, only 30% of patients infected with genotype 1 had a SVR compared with 65% of patients infected with genotypes 2 or 3.[37,38]

The determination of HCV subtypes has no clinical relevance in patients treated with IFN-α and ribavirin, but different treatment durations based on viral load kinetics are recommended for patients with different HCV genotypes. However, the emergence of resistant variants and virologic breakthrough were more common in patients infected with HCV subtype 1a than 1b when treated with TVR triple therapy.[51] HCV subtyping may play a role in helping to select treatment regimens and predict the development of resistance to DAA drugs. In addition, triple therapy with a protease inhibitor is not recommended for patients infected with genotypes 2 and 3.

Antiviral-resistance mutations that cluster around the catalytic site of the NS3/4A serine protease emerge during protease inhibitor therapy and are associated with failure and relapse.[42] Similar resistant variants are detected in both BOC- and TVR-treated patients, suggesting that cross-resistance occurs with these protease inhibitors. Also antiviral-resistant variants are found in about 5% of patients before treatment but do not appear to impact response to either protease inhibitor. Currently, there is no role for antiviral resistance genotyping at baseline or during treatment with the protease inhibitors.[52]

Several mutations in the NS3/4A protease are associated with reduced susceptibility to simeprevir. One of the most common and clinically relevant mutations is the substitution Q80K. This mutation may be present at baseline in approximately 30% of patients with genotype 1a and is associated with lower SVR rates. For patients with genotype 1a, Q80K mutation testing is recommended and patients with this variant should be offered other treatment options.[53]

A variety of laboratory-developed and commercial assays are used for HCV genotyping. The methods include NA sequencing, reverse hybridization, subtype-specific PCR, DNA fragment length polymorphism, heteroduplex mobility analysis, melting curve analysis, and serologic genotyping. Currently, there is only one FDA-approved HCV genotyping assay, the Abbott RealTime HCV Genotype II assay.[54] It uses real-time PCR and multiple hydrolysis probes to amplify and differentiate genotypes 1 to 6 and subtype 1a and 1b. The 5′ UTR is the target to identify the genotype and the NS5B is the target for subtyping genotype 1 samples. The results from this test have shown good overall agreement with direct sequencing methods. However, relatively high rates of indeterminate results and inability to distinguish all genotype 1 subtypes are limitations.

A commercially available reverse hybridization line probe assay is the most commonly used method for genotyping HCV among clinical laboratories participating in the HCV proficiency-testing surveys of the College of American Pathologists. This reverse hybridization assay was developed by Innogenetics (Fujirebio Europe) and is now marketed as the Versant HCV Genotype 2.0 Assay by Siemens. In this line probe assay (LiPA), biotinylated PCR products from the 5′ UTR and core regions of the HCV genome are hybridized under stringent conditions with oligonucleotide probes attached to a nitrocellulose strip: 19 type- and subtype-specific probes interrogate the 5′ UTR and an additional three probes interrogate the core region. The core region probes were added to provide better discrimination of subtypes 1a and 1b and genotype 6.[55] Hybridized PCR products are detected with a streptavidin–alkaline phosphatase conjugate. The pattern of reactive lines defines the genotype and in some cases the subtype. The assay discriminates among genotypes 1a, 1b, 2a/c, 2b, 3a, 3b, 3c, 3k, 4a/c/d, 4b, 4e, 4h, 5a, and 6a/b. The Versant HCV Genotype 2.0 Assay correctly identifies genotypes and distinguishes subtypes 1a and 1b when compared with sequencing but may not be able to adequately identify the other subtypes.[56] Mixed genotype infections can be recognized as unusual patterns of hybridization signals. However, the LiPA requires a considerable amount of amplicon for typing, and the assay may regularly fail when the viral load is less than 10^4 copies/mL.

Sequence analysis of amplified subgenomic sequences is the most definitive way to genotype HCV strains. Genotyping schemes based on sequencing variable genes such as E1, Core, and NS5B provide enough resolution to determine types and subtypes.[57,58] The 5′ UTR is too highly conserved to discriminate all subtypes reliably. Genotyping methods targeting highly variable regions have higher failure rates because of primer mismatches and failed amplification reactions. Sequencing reactions can be performed directly on PCR products or on cloned amplicons. Mixed infections with multiple genotypes may be missed by sequence analysis. Definitive detection of mixed infections requires analysis of a large number of clones. Cloning may, however, emphasize artifactual nucleotide substitutions introduced by the DNA polymerase during amplification or by selection during the cloning procedure and is generally not practical for clinical laboratories.

A standardized direct sequencing system for HCV genotyping is commercially available (Siemens). The Trugene HCV 5′NC genotyping kit targets the 5′ UTR (nt 96 to 282) and employs proprietary single-tube chemistry.[59] This method can be used with the 244-base-pair amplicon generated by either the Roche Amplicor HCV or Amplicor HCV Monitor tests as the sequencing template after a column purification step.[60] The sequencing chemistry produces bidirectional sequences. The software acquires the sequence data, and each pair of forward and reverse sequences is combined. A reference sequence library module contains approximately 200 sequences from the six major genotypes and 24 subtypes of HCV. The software automatically aligns the patient HCV sequence with the reference sequences in the library and reports type, subtype, and closest isolate determinations. The Trugene HCV 5′NC genotyping system is a reliable method for determining HCV genotypes, but similar to all approaches targeting the conserved 5′ UTR, cannot reliably distinguish all HCV subtypes.[60,61]

The practice of using sequence analysis of a single subgenomic region for HCV genotyping has been challenged by the description of naturally occurring intergenotypic recombinants of two HCV genotypes.[62-65] The recombinant forms have been detected in patients in Russia (genotypes 2k and 1b), Vietnam (genotypes 2 and 6), and France (genotypes 2 and 5), as well as in experimentally infected chimpanzees (genotypes 1a and 1b).

A novel HCV genotyping method using a solid phase electrochemical array was developed by GenMark Diagnostics. The method uses sequence specific capture of a PCR amplicon from the HCV 5′ UTR by surface-bound oligonucleotide capture probes formed within a preassembled monolayer with electrochemical detection using ferrocene-labeled oligonucleotide signal probes. High genotype concordance between the GenMark and LiPA HCV tests was observed; however, there were minor discrepancies in genotype 1 subtype identifications by the two tests due to differences in the regions of the HCV genome interrogated.[66]

The widespread use of tests not cleared by the FDA for HCV genotyping has placed an increased burden on clinical laboratories to verify the performance characteristics of these tests before clinical use. When validating HCV genotyping tests, laboratories should take advantage of the published evaluations and commercially available genotype panels to streamline the verification process.

The College of American Pathologists has a well-established proficiency testing program for laboratories performing tests for detection, quantification, and characterization of HCV RNA. These surveys have shown a steady improvement in the performance of laboratories over time that probably reflects progress in both the available technologies and laboratory practices.

POINTS TO REMEMBER

Hepatitis C Virus

- There are approximately 3.2 million people living with active HCV infections in the United States. HCV is a common cause of chronic liver disease.
- HCV viral load does not predict progression or severity of liver disease but is important in distinguishing active from resolved infections and as a widely accepted marker of response to therapy.
- Although there are seven major HCV genotypes and numerous subtypes that differ in geographical distribution, genotype 1 infections predominate in much of the developed world and have, historically, been the most difficult to successfully treat using IFN-α and ribavirin.
- Treatment response rates for genotype 1 infections have dramatically improved with the FDA clearance of DAA agents that target HCV proteases and polymerase.
- Currently, there is no role for HCV resistance genotyping in guiding therapy, but that may change as the number of DAA agents increases.

Hepatitis B Virus

Hepatitis B virus (HBV) is a small enveloped DNA virus belonging to the family *Hepadnaviridae* and causes transient or persistent (chronic) infection of the liver. This family is divided into two genera, orthohepadnavirus and avihepadnavirus, which infect mammals or birds as natural hosts, respectively.[67] They possess a narrow host range determined by the initial steps of viral attachment and entry. Approximately 2 billion people have serologic evidence of hepatitis B, and of these, approximately 350 million people have chronic infections.[68] Depending on viral and host factors, the outcomes of infection with HBV range from clearance to mild or severe chronic hepatitis (CHB) to the development of cirrhosis or hepatocellular carcinoma (HCC).[69,70] The evolution of increasingly sensitive methods for HBV DNA detection and its accurate quantification has created an important role for molecular testing in routine patient care. Improved methods for sequencing and single mutation detection have led to tests that document mutational change in the viral genome. Currently, NA testing plays a critical role in the overall care of HBV-infected patients.

The HBV genome is a 3.2-kilobase relaxed circular, partially double-stranded DNA molecule. It has four partially overlapping open reading frames encoding the viral envelope (pre-S and S), nucleocapsid (precore and core), polymerase, and X proteins. After binding to hepatocytes, the virion is taken up into the cell by endocytosis and uncoated. The partially double-stranded DNA genome is converted to a covalently closed circular DNA (cccDNA) in the cell nucleus. The cccDNA is used as a template for transcription of the pregenomic RNA (pgRNA) and messenger RNA in the cell nucleus. The pgRNA moves into the host cell cytoplasm and serves as the template for translation of the HBV RT as well as the core protein by the cellular translational proteins. Concurrently, the HBV RT reverse transcribes the pgRNA to a new circular DNA molecule. Early in the replication cycle, some of the newly synthesized genomes will circulate back to the nucleus to maintain and increase the pool of cccDNA.[71]

Although HBV is a DNA virus, it replicates by an RT that lacks proofreading activity and, as a result, is prone to errors. The overlapping open reading frames of the genome limit the types of mutations that can be tolerated. However, variations in HBV sequences have been detected in almost all regions of the genome. Consequently, HBV exists as quasispecies, and different patients may be infected with different strains and genotypes.

Seven phylogenetic genotypes (A through H) of HBV have been identified, most of which have distinct geographic distribution. Genotypes are defined by intergroup divergence of greater than 8% in the complete genome nucleotide sequence. All known genotypes have been found in the United States with the prevalence of A, B, C, D, and E to G being 35%, 22%, 31%, 10%, and 2%, respectively.[72] Recent data suggest that HBV genotype plays an important role in the progression of HBV-related liver disease as well as response to IFN-α and pegylated IFN-α; however, HBV genotyping is not necessary in routine clinical practice.[73]

Serologic assays with high sensitivity, specificity, and reproducibility have been developed to detect HBV antigens and their respective antibodies. This complicated system of serologic markers is used for diagnosis of HBV infection and to define the phase of infection, degree of infectivity, prognosis, and patient's immune status. The presence of HBV DNA in the serum is a marker of viral replication in the liver and has replaced hepatitis B e antigen (HBeAg) as the most sensitive marker of viral replication. HBeAg is the extracellular form of the hepatitis B core protein. Molecular assays to quantify blood HBV DNA are useful for the initial evaluation of HBV infections, monitoring of patients with chronic infections, and assessing the efficacy of antiviral treatment.[71,73] In addition, U.S. blood donors are routinely screened for HBV DNA by qualitative tests to detect donors in the early stage of infection.[74] Antiviral resistance mutations are detected by molecular methods that identify known mutations associated with drug resistance.

The initial evaluation of patients found to have hepatitis B surface antigen (HBsAg) in serum should include routine liver tests and a variety of virologic tests, including HBV DNA testing.[73] Chronic HBV infection is a disease of variable course, and establishing baseline laboratory values at the time of diagnosis is important clinically for the tracking of disease progression over time and to evaluate candidates for liver biopsy. Monitoring disease activity in chronically HBV-infected patients is best done by measuring aminotransferase (ALT) at regular intervals in HBeAg-positive patients. However, serial HBV DNA testing is recommended in HBeAg-negative patients. The determination of serum HBV DNA (viral load) is important in the pretreatment evaluation and monitoring of therapeutic response in patients with chronic infection.[73] Currently, therapy for chronic HBV infection does not eradicate the virus and has limited long-term efficacy. The decision to treat should be based on ALT elevations; the presence of HBeAg or HBV DNA (or both); viral load of greater than 2000 IU/mL; the presence of moderate disease activity and fibrosis on liver biopsy; and virologic testing to exclude concurrent infections with hepatitis D virus (HDV), HCV, and HIV. The treatment goals for chronic hepatitis B are to achieve sustained suppression of HBV replication and to prevent further progression of liver disease. Parameters used to indicate treatment response include normalization of serum ALT, decrease in serum HBV DNA, and loss of HBeAg with or without detection of anti-HBeAg. Currently, there are eight FDA-approved therapies for chronic HBV infection: IFN-α, pegylated IFN-α2a, four nucleoside analogs (lamivudine, telbivudine, entecavir, and emtricitabine), and two nucleotide analogs (adefovir and tenofovir). Several factors predict a favorable response to IFN treatment with the most important being high ALT and low serum HBV DNA viral load, which are indirect markers of immune clearance.

Therapy usually does not eradicate the virus because the covalently closed circular form of the HBV genome is difficult to eliminate from the liver and the existence of extrahepatic reservoirs of HBV. Endpoints of treatment have traditionally been clearance of HBeAg, development of anti-HBe antibodies, and undetectable serum HBV DNA using insensitive hybridization assays with detection limits of approximately 10^6 genome copies/mL. Achieving these endpoints usually is accompanied by resolution of liver disease as evidenced by normalization of ALT and decreased inflammation on liver biopsy. The response usually is sustained at long-term follow-up. Nevertheless, most responders continue to have detectable HBV DNA when sensitive NA amplification tests are used. Responses to antiviral therapy are categorized as biochemical, virologic, or histologic and as on therapy or sustained off therapy.[73]

Several variations in the nucleotide sequence of HBV have important clinical consequences. An important mutation in the gene encoding HBsAg is a glycine-to-arginine substitution at codon 145 (G145R) in the conserved "a" determinant, which causes decreased affinity of the HBsAg for anti-HBs antibodies.[75] HBV with this mutation has been found in children of HBsAg-positive mothers who develop HBV infection despite vaccination and an adequate anti-HBs antibody response after vaccination, as well as in liver transplant recipients who have recurrent infection despite administration of HBV immune globulin.[76,77] These immune escape mutants have raised concern about vaccine efficacy and serologically silent infections. The G145R mutation has been reported in many countries and is responsible for 2% to 40% of vaccine failures. Although there is diminished binding to anti-HBs antibodies, the vast majority of S mutants can be readily detected with the current generation of HBsAg tests. Thus, an initial concern that widespread use of HBV immune globulin and vaccination would result in HBV mutants that would escape detection in the HBsAg test was unfounded.

Mutations in the basal core promoter and the precore genes affect the synthesis of HBeAg and commonly arise under immune pressure.[78] The most common basal core promoter mutation has a dual change of A to T at nt 1762 (T1762) and G to A at nt 1764 (A1764) that diminishes the amount of mRNA and hence HBeAg secretion.[79] The predominant precore mutation is a G to A change at nt 1896 (A1896), which leads to premature termination of the precore protein at codon 28, thus preventing the production of HBeAg.[80] The A1896 mutation is infrequent in North America and Western Europe but is geographically widespread. This geographic variability in frequency is related to the predominant genotypes in a geographic region because the mutation is found only in genotypes B, C, D, and E.

The A1896 mutation was first reported in patients with chronic active hepatitis or fulminant hepatitis. However, the A1896 mutation also can be present in asymptomatic

TABLE 48.2 Antiviral Agents and the Hepatitis B Virus Polymerase Mutations Associated With Resistance

Antiviral Agent	Drug Class	Resistance Mutations
Lamivudine	Nucleoside analog (cytidine)	(L180M + M204V/I/S), A181V/T, S202G/I
Telbivudine	Nucleoside analog (dTTP)	M204I, A181T/V
Entecavir	Nucleoside analog (2-deoxyguanosine)	T184S/C/G/A/I/L/F/M, S202G/C/I, M250V/I/L
Emtricitabine	Nucleoside analog (cytidine)	M204V/I
Adefovir	Nucleotide analog (dATP)	A181V/T, N236T
Tenofovir	Nucleotide analog (dATP)	A194T, N2263T, A181V/T

dATP, Deoxyadenosine triphosphate; *dTTP*, deoxythymidine triphosphate.

carriers, and viruses with this mutation replicate no more efficiently than wild-type HBV. Thus, the pathophysiologic significance of this mutation is unclear.[81] However, the clinical picture of persistent HBV replication and active liver disease in HBeAg-negative patients appears to be increasingly prevalent, and in some regions, the A1896-mutant virus may be more prevalent than the wild-type virus.

Therapy for chronic hepatitis B requires long courses of treatment with nucleoside or nucleotide analogs. A major concern with long-term therapy is the development of antiviral resistance by mutation in one or more domains of the gene encoding the HBV polymerase. The rate at which resistant mutants are selected is related to pretreatment serum HBV DNA viral load, rapidity of viral suppression, duration of treatment, and prior antiviral exposure. The incidence of genotypic resistance also varies with the sensitivity of the methods used to detect resistance mutations and the patient population tested.

Typically, when a patient experiences a virologic breakthrough, defined as an increase in serum HBV DNA greater than 1 log_{10} above nadir after achieving a virologic response during continued treatment, HBV resistance genotyping should be performed. The standardized nomenclature of HBV antiviral resistance mutations in the polymerase is shown in Table 48.2.[71,82,83] No HBV mutations are associated with resistance to IFN-α or pegylated IFN-α2a.

There are a number of commercially available tests for quantification of HBV DNA in serum and plasma, but only two tests have United States-In Vitro Diagnostics (US-IVD) regulatory status. These tests—the cobas AmpliPrep/cobas TaqMan (Roche) and the Real-time (Abbott) HBV tests—both use real-time PCR (see Table 48.1). The others produced by Cepheid, Qiagen, and Siemens are CE (*Conformité Européenne*, meaning European Conformity) marked and RUO kits or ASRs in the United States.

A WHO international HBV standard was first created in 2001 in response to the recognized need to standardize HBV DNA quantification assays.[84] However, despite the availability of HBV DNA standards, the various quantitative assays usually have different conversion factors for copies to IU/mL, which may reflect their different amplification and detection chemistries. Laboratories should report HBV viral load test results in IU/mL as both log_{10} transformed and arithmetic values. HBV is included in the hepatitis viral load proficiency testing surveys available from the College of American Pathologists.

Two HBV genotyping systems are commercially available as RUO kits. Innogenetics (Fujirebio Europe) offers three different line probe assays for (1) HBV phylogenetic genotyping; (2) detection of precore mutations; and (3) detection of all relevant lamivudine, emtricitabine, telbivudine, adefovir, and entecavir resistance mutations as well as known compensatory mutations.[85,86] All assays use PCR to amplify portions of the relevant genes to produce a biotinylated product. The PCR products are denatured and hybridized to a series of informative probes immobilized on a nitrocellulose strip. The hybrids are visualized on the strip after addition of streptavidin–alkaline phosphatase and a colorimetric substrate. The mutations are identified by the colored patterns of PCR product hybridization to the probes. The line probe assays typically have better sensitivity for detection of sequence variants than direct Sanger sequencing.

The TRUGENE HBV genotyping test (Siemens) uses two fluorescently labeled DNA primers and PCR to amplify a portion of the HBsAg gene and overlapping polymerase gene, with bidirectional sequencing of these amplicons, and a software module that includes a sequence database that identifies the phylogenetic genotype (A to H) as well as mutations associated with resistance to the nucleoside and nucleotide analog drugs.[87] The sequence ladder is resolved on a polyacrylamide slab gel. The total analysis time is approximately 8 hours, including the time required for DNA extraction and purification.

The standardized nomenclature for reporting of HBV antiviral resistance mutations shown Table 48.2 should be used when resistance genotyping is performed. The inability of genotyping assays to detect minor populations of circulating HBV is a significant technical issue. In general, direct sequencing is limited to resolution of populations that are more than 20% of the viral population.

Transplant Recipients

Cytomegalovirus

Cytomegalovirus (CMV), a member of the *Herpesviridae* family, is an enveloped, double-stranded DNA virus. It has a large (240-kb) genome with approximately 95% DNA homology among different strains. CMV usually causes asymptomatic or minor infections in immunocompetent individuals but remains an important pathogen in immunocompromised individuals, including persons with AIDS, transplant recipients, and those on immune-modulating drugs. Primary infection is usually asymptomatic in immunocompetent persons, although a small percentage of individuals with CMV infection may develop a syndrome similar to mononucleosis. After primary infection, a lifelong latent infection is established that does not cause clinical symptoms. However, if an infected individual becomes immunocompromised, the virus can reactivate, leading to a wide variety of clinical syndromes.

The most severe CMV infections are seen in patients who acquire their primary infection while immunocompromised. In persons with AIDS, CMV disease rarely occurs when the CD4+ cell count is above 100 cells/mm^3; the most common clinical presentations are retinitis, esophagitis, and colitis. In transplant recipients, the occurrence and severity of CMV disease are related to the CMV serostatus of the organ donor and recipient, the type of organ transplanted, and the overall degree of immunosuppression. For example, CMV disease tends to be more severe in lung transplant recipients than in renal transplant recipients. For all types of solid organ recipients, the most severe disease occurs when CMV-seronegative recipients receive an organ from a CMV-seropositive donor and the primary CMV infection occurs while the person is immunosuppressed. In contrast, CMV-seropositive recipients of hematopoietic stem cells from CMV-seronegative donors are at highest risk of CMV diseases after hematopoietic stem cell transplant (HSCT). CMV disease can also occur in seropositive individuals, whether they receive an organ from a seropositive or seronegative donor. Clinical findings associated with CMV disease in transplant recipients are diverse and include interstitial pneumonitis; esophagitis and colitis; fever; leukopenia; and, less commonly, retinitis and encephalitis.

The diagnosis of CMV disease represents a challenge because latent infections are common. Immunocompromised individuals can have an asymptomatic, clinically insignificant, low-level, persistent infection that must be distinguished from clinically important active CMV disease. The distinction can be challenging when sensitive molecular assays are used that can detect small amounts of CMV DNA in clinical specimens.

Traditionally, the diagnosis of CMV disease relied on the detection of CMV from clinical specimens by the use of cell culture techniques in human diploid fibroblasts. Although considered the gold standard, these conventional culture methods are labor intensive and have a turnaround time (TAT) of 1 to 3 weeks. In addition, the assays lack adequate sensitivity for detecting CMV in blood specimens. The rapid shell-vial culture method can provide results in 1 to 2 days and is useful for detection of CMV in tissue, respiratory, and urine specimens. However, this method may also fail to detect CMV in blood. For many years, laboratories relied on a CMV antigenemia assay, which detects the matrix protein pp65 in circulating polymorphonuclear white blood cells. This semiquantitative assay is more rapid than culture, and the number of CMV antigen-positive cells correlates with the likelihood of CMV disease, but the assay is labor intensive, subjective, and nonstandardized and, consequently, is no longer done in most clinical laboratories.

Considering the limitations of culture, there is great interest in using NA testing for the detection and quantification of CMV DNA in blood specimens. The clinical uses of CMV molecular assays are diverse and include (1) initiation of preemptive therapy, (2) diagnosis of active CMV disease, and (3) monitoring of response to therapy. Preemptive therapy identifies a group of individuals at higher risk for developing CMV disease. For example, all members of the group would be tested for the presence of CMV DNA in their blood or plasma, and only those testing positive would be treated. Therapy is administered before development of symptoms in an attempt to prevent the onset of active disease. By contrast, with prophylactic therapy, all patients in the group are treated, without further stratification of risk, thus involving treatment of a greater number of patients. Preemptive therapy has become the standard of care for management of HSCT recipients.

Molecular assays are useful to diagnose active CMV disease because CMV DNA concentrations are higher in patients with active CMV disease than in those with asymptomatic infection.[88-91] Quantitative PCR from plasma or whole blood is now commonly used to diagnose CMV disease and monitor response to therapy. Until recently, there have been no FDA-approved CMV viral load tests, and laboratories used a variety of different laboratory-developed tests for detection and quantification of CMV DNA. Therefore, the threshold or viral load cutoff at which a diagnosis is made or preemptive therapy is begun has varied among institutions and transplant populations. Because a universal viral load cutoff for defining CMV disease has not been established, health care providers should rely on the trend of viral load values over time rather a value obtained at a single point in time for diagnosis and patient management.

After active CMV disease has been diagnosed, molecular assays are useful in monitoring response to therapy. Viral load values decrease rapidly after appropriate antiviral therapy is begun, and CMV DNA is cleared from the plasma within several weeks of initiation of therapy.[92-94] Failure of viral loads to decrease promptly should raise concerns of possible treatment failure because persistently elevated concentrations of CMV DNA during therapy indicates therapeutic resistance. Molecular assays can also identify patients at risk for relapsing CMV infection. In solid organ transplant recipients, patients with a detectable viral load after completing 14 days of ganciclovir therapy for CMV infection are at increased risk of relapse. The rate of decline in CMV DNA after initiation of therapy can be also used to predict risk of relapse of CMV infection.[94]

Cytomegalovirus DNA concentrations are also useful in assessing the risk of developing CMV disease in persons with AIDS. Detection of CMV DNA in plasma is associated with increased risk of developing CMV disease and increased risk of death. In addition, each $\log_{10}$ increase in viral load (ie, each 10-fold increase in concentration) has been associated with a threefold increase in the risk of developing CMV disease.[95]

Currently, there are only two FDA-approved CMV viral load assays (see Table 48.1): CAP/CTM CMV test (Roche) and artus CMV RGQ MDx (Qiagen). Both are based on real-time PCR, are calibrated against the WHO CMV standard, and consequently report results in international units per milliliter. The Roche test amplifies a portion of *UL54* gene and the Qiagen test amplifies a portion of the *MIE* gene. Both assays have similar lower limits of quantification, but the Qiagen assay has a 10-fold greater dynamic range. Despite the availability of an international standard and of FDA-approved assays, there is still considerable interlaboratory variability of results in CMV proficiency testing surveys.[96]

Epstein-Barr Virus

Epstein-Barr virus (EBV) is a double-stranded DNA virus belonging to the *Herpesviridae* family. The seroprevalence of EBV is greater than 95% among adults older than the age of 40 years, and primary infection is followed by lifelong latency with reactivation of infection in immunocompromised hosts. In transplant recipients, EBV infection may cause malaise, fever, headache, and sore throat, but it is also associated with posttransplantation lymphoproliferative disease (PTLD), a significant cause of morbidity and mortality. PTLD is a spectrum of lymphocytic proliferation that ranges from benign lymphocytic hyperplasia to potentially fatal malignant lymphoma. The process is often multicentric and may involve the central nervous system (CNS), eyes, gastrointestinal (GI) tract (with bleeding and perforation), liver, spleen, lymph nodes, lungs, allograft, oropharynx, and other organs. Clinical presentations vary and include, but are not limited to, adenopathy, fever (including "fever of unknown origin"), abdominal pain, anorexia, jaundice, bowel perforation, GI bleeding, renal dysfunction, liver dysfunction, pneumothorax, pulmonary infiltrates or nodules, and weight loss.

The pathogenesis of PTLD involves the exponential proliferation of B cells as a result of uncontrolled EBV infection. Risk factors include a donor and recipient serologic mismatch (eg, donor positive/recipient negative), a high degree of immunosuppression (particularly the use of antilymphocyte therapy for rejection), and a high EBV viral load.[97] Most cases of PTLD occur during the first year after transplant, and the cumulative incidence ranges from 1% to 2% in HSCT and liver transplant recipients and up to 11% to 33% in intestinal or multiorgan transplant recipients.[98]

Treatment of EBV-related lymphoproliferative disease is challenging. After lymphoproliferative disease is established, antiviral treatment is not effective, and immunosuppression must be reduced. Murine humanized chimeric anti-CD20 monoclonal antibody (rituximab) has been helpful in some cases; some patients require chemotherapy, radiation therapy, or both. Adoptive immunotherapy using donor-derived cloned EBV-specific cytotoxic T cells may be useful for prophylaxis and treatment of lymphoproliferative disease in allogeneic HSCT and solid organ transplant recipients.

Increases in EBV viral load may be detected in patients before the development of EBV-associated PTLD[99-102]); viral loads typically decrease with effective therapy. Whereas a high EBV DNA viral load is a strong predictor for the development of PTLD, low-level EBV viral load occurs relatively frequently and may resolve without intervention.[103,104] To complicate the matter, some pediatric liver and heart transplant recipients may exhibit chronic high EBV viral loads.[105,106] Available assays lack standardization, and the optimal assay technique, sample type (ie, whole blood, lymphocytes, plasma), and sampling schedule are not defined. Nevertheless, EBV viral load assays are generally sensitive, specific, precise, linear across a wide dynamic range, rapid, reasonably inexpensive, and, overall, useful in patient care.[107] Although there are no defined "trigger points" predictive of PTLD, persistently detectable concentrations of EBV DNA by PCR (cutoffs vary between programs) typically result in a thorough evaluation for PTLD (eg, computed tomography of the chest, abdomen, and pelvis).

Epstein-Barr virus viral load testing is also indicated in transplant recipients who present with lymphadenopathy, fever, or other signs and symptoms suggestive of lymphoproliferative disease. A high EBV load should trigger the search for mass lesions or organ dysfunction pinpointing potential sites of disease, which should be biopsied.

Currently, there are no FDA-approved EBV viral load tests available. A wide variety of commercially available primers and probes for different gene targets are used in the laboratory developed tests (LDTs) deployed in clinical laboratories.[108] There is no consensus on the best target gene or specimen type (whole blood, white blood cells, or plasma); however, the first WHO international standard for EBV DNA was developed to address variation between assay results attributable to calibration (http://www.nibsc.org/documents/ifu/09-260.pdf).

The definitive diagnosis of PTLD requires biopsy. Tissues from patients with EBV-associated lymphoproliferative disease may show monoclonal, oligoclonal, or polyclonal lesions. The diagnosis of EBV-associated lymphoproliferative disease requires demonstration of EBV DNA, RNA, or protein in biopsy tissue. In situ hybridization targeting EBER1, EBER2, or both is the gold standard assay for determining whether a lymphoproliferative process is EBV related. Commercial systems for EBER in situ hybridization are available from Ventana, Leica, Dako, Invitrogen, and Biogenex.[107]

BK Virus

BK virus (BKV) is a member of family *Polyomaviridae*, which also includes JC virus (JCV) and simian virus 40 (SV40). It is an enveloped, double-stranded DNA virus that shares approximately 70% sequence homology with JCV and SV40. Seroprevalence reaches nearly 100% in early childhood, generally after an asymptomatic primary infection (although fever and nonspecific upper respiratory tract symptoms may occur).[109] Seroprevalence declines to 60% to 80% in adulthood. After primary infection, the virus can remain latent in many sites, most notably the epithelium of the urinary tract and lymphoid cells, until an immunosuppressed state allows reactivation and replication of the virus. Replication of BKV in immunocompromised hosts may be asymptomatic or cause organ dysfunction, affecting the kidney, bladder, or ureter. BKV disease in the urinary system manifests as hemorrhagic or nonhemorrhagic cystitis and with ureteric stenosis in bone marrow and solid organ transplant recipients.[110] It also causes polyomavirus-associated nephropathy (PVAN) in renal transplant recipients.[111]

Hemorrhagic cystitis (HC) is a cause of morbidity and occasional mortality in patients undergoing bone marrow transplantation.[112] The manifestations range from microscopic hematuria to severe bladder hemorrhage leading to clot retention and renal failure. Its incidence varies from 7% to 68% of bone marrow transplant recipients. Although mild HC usually resolves with supportive care, severe HC may require bladder irrigation, cystoscopy, and cauterization.[113] BKV was observed in early studies to be associated with the development of HC during bone marrow transplantation; however, later studies using sensitive PCR assays showed that BKV DNA could be detected in the blood and urine of patients with or without HC.[114-116] Recently, quantitative assays for BKV DNA in urine have demonstrated that patients with HC have higher peak BK viruria and larger total amounts of BKV excreted during bone marrow transplantation compared with asymptomatic patients.[117,118]

Although BKV was first isolated from the urine of a renal transplant recipient in 1971,[119] the association between nephropathy and the presence of BKV in renal transplant recipients was not reported until 1995.[120] BKV replication in renal allografts can lead to progressive graft dysfunction and, potentially, graft failure. Although the recognition of PVAN in renal transplant recipients coincided with the use of newer immunosuppressive drugs such as tacrolimus, sirolimus, and mycophenolate mofetil, risk factors for development of PVAN have not been elucidated.[121] The prevalence of PVAN ranges from 1% to 10% in kidney transplant recipients with loss of allograft function in about one third to half of these cases.[121] The disease appears to result from reactivation of BKV infection in the donor allograft.

The signs and symptoms of PVAN are mild and nonspecific, often with only a gradual increase in serum creatinine over weeks as the allograft loses function.[122] A definitive diagnosis of PVAN is obtained through histopathology of the biopsied kidney; the characteristic PVAN pattern includes viral cytopathic changes in epithelial cells and interstitial inflammation and fibrosis. However, these changes are not pathognomonic for PVAN, and most centers use immunohistochemical staining with antibodies specific for polyomavirus proteins or in situ hybridization to confirm the diagnosis.[121] Because of the focal nature of the nephropathy and the possibility of sampling error, a negative biopsy does not rule out PVAN. Biopsy of the kidney is an invasive procedure that is impractical for serial monitoring, early diagnosis, and clinical management of patients with PVAN. Other less invasive diagnostic methods for PVAN have also been assessed. Urine cytology may reveal renal epithelial cells with intranuclear viral inclusion bodies, termed *decoy cells.*[123] The sensitivity and specificity of decoy cells for diagnosing PVAN is 99% and 95%, respectively, but the positive predictive value varies between 27% and 90%. Quantification of BKV DNA or mRNA in urine by NA amplification methods has been proposed as a method to monitor changes in BKV replication.[124-127] However, physiological changes of urine constituents and use of different urine fractions may give rise to considerable variation in viral load values that may complicate the identification of diagnostic thresholds and quantitative cross-sectional and longitudinal studies.[111] PCR methods for detection and quantitation of BK viremia have emerged as clinically useful tools in the diagnosis and management of PVAN because viremia precedes development of nephropathy in almost all cases.[128-131]

In 2005, an expert interdisciplinary panel recommended the use of either urine cytology or NA amplification tests to screen renal transplant recipients for BK viruria every 3 months up to 2 years posttransplant or when allograft dysfunction occurs or biopsy is performed.[121] Patients with positive screening test results should have an adjunct quantitative NA amplification test performed using urine or plasma. Patients with urine DNA loads of more than 10^7 copies/mL or plasma DNA loads of more than 10^4 copies/mL that persist for more than 3 weeks have presumptive PVAN and a renal biopsy should be performed to confirm the diagnosis.

Reducing the intensity of maintenance immunosuppression is the primary intervention in patients with PVAN. No effective antiviral agents for BKV are available, but low-dose cidofovir has been used for treatment of cases not amenable or refractory to decreased maintenance immunosuppression.[121] Viral load in urine or plasma should be monitored every 2 to 4 weeks to gauge the effectiveness of the intervention.

Currently, real-time PCR is the method of choice for BKV DNA quantification because of its simplicity and wide dynamic range of 6 to 7 $\log_{10}$ virus copies/mL. Such high concentrations in plasma are uncommon but can exceed 10^{12} copies/mL. Although BK viral load tests have become a standard of care for diagnosis and monitoring of patients with PVAN, there is neither consensus in the design of PCR assays nor recognized standard reference material. As a consequence, the assays developed by different laboratories may give markedly different results, requiring individual laboratories to establish and verify their own clinical threshold values.

Polymerase chain reaction assay design is complicated by the high degree of homology between the genomes of the different human polyomaviruses. Gene targets for BKV-specific assays include coding sequences for VP1, large T antigen, and agnoprotein because these sequences are sufficiently variable among human polyomaviruses.[130]

BKV is classified into seven subtypes based on phylogenetic analysis of full-genome sequences, subtypes Ia, Ic, II, III, IV, V, and VI.[132] Hoffman et al[133] compared seven *Taq*Man real-time PCR primer–probe sets in conjunction with two different reference standards to quantify BKV DNA in urine samples. They observed substantial disagreement among assays attributable both to features of the primer and probe design and to choice of reference material. The most significant source of error were primer and probe mismatches caused by BKV subtype polymorphisms, primarily among subtype III and IV isolates. However, they found less subtype bias among the seven assays for the more common subtypes Ia, V, and VI. The assay that provided the most reliable measure of all subtypes included a mixture of primers and probes that targeted both the VP1 and large T antigen sequences.

SEXUALLY TRANSMITTED INFECTIONS

Chlamydia trachomatis and *Neisseria gonorrhoeae*

Testing for *Chlamydia trachomatis* (CT) and *Neisseria gonorrhoeae* (NG) is discussed together because several of the available NA amplification tests (NAATs) for these pathogens are multiplex assays. Although both CT and NG can cause a variety of clinical infections, the focus here is on genital infections.

Detection of CT is a challenging and important public health issue. CT is a major cause of sexually transmitted infections (STIs), with an estimated 1 million cases occurring annually among sexually active adolescents and young adults in the United States.[134] More than half of the infections are asymptomatic.[135] Even when symptomatic, the diagnosis can be missed as the manifestations are protean. In men, CT infection may present as urethritis, epididymitis, prostatitis, or proctitis.[136,137] and as cervicitis, endometritis, and urethritis in women, with 10% to 40% of infections in women progressing to pelvic inflammatory disease (PID) if untreated.[138,139] Related complications include chronic pelvic pain, ectopic pregnancy, and infertility. In the United States, CT infection is the likely cause of most secondary infertility in women. In pregnant women, there is the additional risk of transmitting the infection to the newborn during labor and delivery, leading to pneumonia or conjunctivitis in the newborn.

N. gonorrhoeae infection, too, may present in various ways, and the clinical presentations overlap with those of CT. Men may have acute urethritis with discharge, epididymitis, prostatitis, and urethral strictures. In women, NG infection can produce cervicitis, which, if left untreated, can lead to PID, abscesses, or salpingitis.

Traditional methods for the diagnosis of CT infection include cell culture, antigen detection by immunofluorescence, enzyme immunoassay (EIA), and nonamplified NA probes. These traditional methods have been replaced in most laboratories by amplified NA tests, which provide greater sensitivity in detecting CT from genital specimens. For NG, which was traditionally diagnosed based on culture methods that relied on selective culture media, NA testing does not offer significant improvement in sensitivity compared with culture when culture is performed under appropriate conditions. NG is highly susceptible to extreme temperatures and desiccation, which can lead to decreased sensitivity of detection by culture, particularly when specimen transport is required before culture.[140] NA testing for NG offers a sensitive and reliable alternative to culture since it is easier to maintain the integrity of the target NA than it is to maintain the organism's viability.

In addition to high diagnostic and analytical sensitivity and specificity, NA testing offers several advantages over conventional culture and antigen detection methods for the diagnosis of CT and NG. Testing for both pathogens can be done on a single specimen, and for some multiplex assays, testing is performed in a single reaction. Unlike the infectious organism itself, the DNA and RNA of NG and CT are quite stable in commercial transport devices, thus accounting for some of the increased diagnostic sensitivity of these assays compared with culture. The stability of NA avoids the necessity of immediate transport to the laboratory, and specimens may be stored refrigerated or at room temperature before transport. Transport and storage requirements vary among tests, so it is important to refer to the package insert for specific details. An additional advantage of NA testing is the use of urine specimens, which for women allows testing to be done without the need for a pelvic examination. In men, urine offers a convenient and diagnostically sensitive alternative to collection with a urethral swab and increases the likelihood that asymptomatic men will agree to be tested.

NAATs for the detection of CT and NG from clinical specimens use a variety of specimens, including cervical and vaginal swabs, urethral swabs, and urine from both asymptomatic and symptomatic individuals. Not all assays are cleared by the FDA for use in the United States for all conditions and age ranges, and the current assays are not FDA-cleared for oropharyngeal, rectal, or conjunctival specimens. However, many of these tests have been assessed for diagnosing infections in multiple extragenital anatomic sites in men, women, and children. Current CDC guidelines for laboratory-based detection of CT and NG recommend NAATs for oropharyngeal and rectal specimens and for use in evaluating cases of adult and pediatric sexual abuse.[141] However, use of these tests outside of the FDA-approved indications requires that laboratories establish the specifications for performance characteristics according to Clinical Laboratory Improvement Amendments (CLIA) regulations. Performance characteristics vary among assays (details are available in the package inserts), but some general comments can be made. The diagnostic sensitivity of the tests varies according to the specimen type and whether the patient is asymptomatic or symptomatic. Interpretation of the results of NA testing for CT can be challenging because many studies have shown these assays to be more diagnostically sensitive than culture, which was previously used as the gold standard for clinical trials. For men, the diagnostic sensitivity of testing urine specimens is nearly equivalent to that of testing urethral swabs. A limited volume (20–50 mL) of first-passed urine is preferred because larger volumes will lead to a decreased concentration of the organism in the sample and thus reduced diagnostic sensitivity. With proper specimen collection, male urethral swabs and urine specimens have a sensitivity of nearly 100% for the detection of NG or CT infection. For women, vaginal and cervical swab specimens provide the highest sensitivity for the detection of NG and CT infection, with many studies showing a sensitivity of 90% to 95%. Vaginal swabs are preferred because they are easier to collect. Urine specimens can be used, but they generally result in a lower diagnostic sensitivity than cervical swabs (75%–85%). An alternative to urine testing in women is the use of self-collected vaginal swabs, which have been shown in some studies to have a diagnostic sensitivity that is equal to that obtained with cervical swabs; several commercial tests have been cleared for use with vaginal swabs.

Decisions regarding the selection of a specific amplification test for the detection of CT and NG should not be based solely on the cost of reagents. Other key factors to consider include test performance characteristics, such as diagnostic sensitivity and specificity, and applicability for urine and swab specimens in both symptomatic and asymptomatic individuals. Ideally, the test should include an internal control, particularly if a crude lysate is used in the assay. Other factors to consider are degree of automation, ease of use, work flow issues, and space and equipment needs.

Historically, for several of the NG assays, reduced specificity was due to presence of the gene target in nongonococcal *Neisseria* spp.[142,143] Currently, only the ProbeTec tests (Becton-Dickinson) produce false-positive results with commensal species including *Neisseria lactamica*, *Neisseria subflava*, and *Neisseria cinerea* (Table 48.3). None of the NAATs for CT have known biological false-positive results because of presence of the gene target in other organisms. Other sources of false-positive results include carryover contamination of amplified product and cross-contamination during specimen collection, transport, or processing. Concerns over these issues have led to consideration of supplemental testing for all CT- or NG-positive specimens using alternative target tests because false-positive results can have psychosocial and medicolegal ramifications.[144] However current recommendations do not advise confirming all positive NAATs unless otherwise indicated in the package insert or for tests with known cross-reactivity with commensal *Neisseria* spp.[141] False-positive results in a low-prevalence population can significantly reduce the predictive value of a positive result.

Because DNA can persist in urine samples for up to 3 weeks after completion of therapy, test of cure using NA testing is discouraged. If this must be done, then testing should be delayed for at least 3 weeks after therapy is completed to allow time for clearance of the DNA of the pathogen.

False-negative results from inhibition of amplification are a consideration for both NG and CT testing and can occur with both cervical swabs and urine specimens. Inhibition rates may vary considerably depending on the amplification and NA extraction methods used. For tests using a crude lysate (eg, ProbeTec), inhibition rates tend to be higher than those seen with the APTIMA Combo test, which uses a target capture method to purify NA. For assays that test a crude

TABLE 48.3 Amplification Methods and Target Regions for Food and Drug Administration–Cleared Nucleic Acid Amplification Tests for Detection of *Chlamydia trachomatis* and *Neisseria gonorrhoeae*

Assay (Manufacturer)	Method	*C. trachomatis* Target	*N. gonorrhoeae* Target
Abbott RealTime CT/NG (Abbott)	Real-time PCR	Two distinct regions in cryptic plasmid	*Opa* gene region
Aptima COMBO 2 assay (Hologic/Gen-Probe)	Transcription-mediated amplification	23S rRNA region	16S rRNA region
Aptima CT assay		16S rRNA region	
Aptima GC assay			Distinct 16s rRNA region
BD ProbeTec Q^x CT Amplified DNA assay	Strand displacement amplification	One region in the cryptic plasmid	
BD ProbeTec Q^x GC Amplified DNA assay			Chromosomal pilin gene-inverting protein homologue*
Xpert CT/NG test (Cepheid)	Real-time PCR	One distinct chromosomal region	Two distinct chromosomal regions
cobas CT/NG test (Roche)	Real-time PCR	One cryptic plasmid and one chromosomal region	DR-9A and DR-9B regions

*False-positive test results with some commensal *Neisseria* spp. may occur.
CT, Chlamydia trachomatis; *NG, Neisseria gonorrhoeae*; *PCR,* polymerase chain reaction.

lysate, it is useful to amplify another NA sequence as an internal control (or "amplification control") to assess for inhibition of amplification. Results are reported as negative for NG or CT only when amplification of the internal control is documented.

A conserved, cryptic plasmid is found in more than 99% of strains of CT and contains the gene target for several NAATs. However, a new variant (nv) strain of CT emerged in Sweden in 2006 with a 377-base-pair deletion in the cryptic plasmid, which contained the target for several of the CT tests. This deletion led to false-negative results with some but not all of the tests that targeted the cryptic plasmid.[145] The current versions of all the NAATs for CT have been modified to detect the nv strain of CT. Obviously, tests that target the sequences contained on the cryptic plasmid will not detect the rare strain of CT that lacks the plasmid.

Performing CT and NG testing on liquid cytology media is a matter of interest because a single specimen can be used for cervical cancer screening (Papanicolaou [Pap] and human papillomavirus [HPV] tests) and for CT or NG testing.[146] The latter two tests are performed on the liquid specimen that remains after completion of the PAP and HPV testing. However, several drawbacks to this approach must be considered. The instruments used to prepare PAP tests were not designed to control for cross-contamination during processing, and this may lead to false-positive results. CT and NG testing are performed after the PAP smear and HPV testing are complete, delaying diagnosis and treatment of CT or NG infection. Moreover, the remaining specimen may be inadequate to complete CT and NG testing, thus requiring the patient to make a return visit for collection of an additional sample. Removing an aliquot for CT and NG testing before Pap testing is performed ("pre-aliquoting") may be helpful in overcoming some of these issues, provided adequate volume of sample remains for PAP and HPV testing. This approach does not completely remove the risk of cross-contamination, so specimens must be handled in a manner consistent with procedures used in molecular laboratories. In addition, not all NAATs for CT and NG have been FDA approved for use with liquid cytology media, and those that have may not have been cleared for both types of media (Hologic PreservCyt and BD SurePath).

POINTS TO REMEMBER

Chlamydia trachomatis* and *Neisseria gonorrhoeae

- NAATs are the recommended test method for detection of CT and NG genital tract, oropharyngeal, and rectal infections, but they have not been cleared by the FDA for the latter two infections.
- Routine repeat testing of NAAT-positive specimens is not recommended because this practice does not improve the positive predictive value of the test.
- Positive reactions with nongonococcal *Neisseria* spp. have been reported with some NAATs and the use of an alternative target NAAT might be needed to avoid false-positive results for NG.
- CT and NG DNA can persist in samples from successfully treated patients for up to 3 weeks; therefore, tests of cure using NAATs are discouraged.

Trichomonas vaginalis

Trichomoniasis is an STI caused by the protozoan *Trichomonas vaginalis*. Although *T. vaginalis* infection is not a reportable disease in the United States, it is the most prevalent nonviral STI in the United States.[147] *T. vaginalis* infection may present as vaginitis in women and urethritis in men; however, it is frequently asymptomatic. Infection with *T. vaginalis* may also cause additional adverse health outcomes, including PID in women, as well as infertility and increased incidence of HIV transmission in women and men. Current recommendations for *T. vaginalis* diagnosis and treatment can be found at http://www.cdc.gov/std/tg2015/default.htm and available diagnostic tests range from simple microscopy to NAATs.

Microscopic examination of vaginal fluid or urethral discharge for *T. vaginalis* (wet mount) in the clinic is the most commonly used test. It has low sensitivity (51%–65%) but with experienced observers can be highly specific.[148]

Culture has long been considered the gold standard test, but it requires special medium and 5 days to complete. However, recent studies indicate that the sensitivity of culture may be as low as 75% to 96%.[148] Pap tests are not suitable for routine screening or diagnosis because of low sensitivity.[149] There is a single rapid antigen test for *T. vaginalis* (OSOM, Sekisui Diagnostics) that is FDA cleared for use as a point-of-care test for female patients. Test specifications include sensitivity of 82% to 95% and specificity of 97% to 100%.[150]

The Affirm VPIII Microbial Identification test is an FDA-cleared test that uses nonamplified NA probes to detect three organisms associated with vaginitis: *T. vaginalis*, *Gardnerella vaginalis*, and *Candida albicans*. Its sensitivity and specificity for detection of *T. vaginalis* are 63% and 99.9%, respectively.[151] NAATs are the most sensitive tests available for detection of *T. vaginalis*. A variety of LDT NAATs are more sensitive than the previous gold-standard test of culture but with a more rapid analysis time. Currently, there are two FDA-cleared NAATs for detection of *T. vaginalis* from female patients only. The APTIMA *Trichomonas vaginalis* assay (Hologic/Gen-Probe) detects *T. vaginalis* RNA by transcription-mediated amplification, and its sensitivity and specificity are both 95% to 100%.[148,151,152] It also offers the opportunity to test for *T. vaginalis* from the same sample submitted for CT and NG testing with their APTIMA Combo 2 assay because the test runs on the same platform. The BD Probe Tec TV Q^x Amplified DNA assay detects *T. vaginalis* using strand displacement amplification on the Viper system with performance characteristics similar to the APTIMA assay.[153] Tests for CT and NG can also be performed on the Viper system.

The laboratory diagnosis of trichomoniasis remains challenging particularly in men. Considerations for selection of diagnostic methods should include testing location, analysis time, performance characteristics, and the cost to perform the test.

Herpes Simplex Virus

Herpes simplex virus (HSV) is a double-stranded DNA virus surrounded by a lipid glycoprotein envelope. HSV persists as a latent infection in specific target cells despite the host immune response, often resulting in recurrent disease. Genital herpes is a chronic viral infection. Two serotypes of HSV have been identified, HSV-1 and HSV-2. Most cases of recurrent genital herpes in the United States are caused by HSV-2. However, an increasing proportion of anogenital herpetic infections in some populations is now attributed to HSV-1. HSV-1 is usually associated with oral lesions. The CDC estimates that 776,000 new HSV-2 infections occur each year in the United States. Most genital herpes infections are transmitted by persons unaware of their infections. Up to 90% of persons seropositive for HSV-2 antibody have not been diagnosed with genital herpes. However, many have mild or unrecognized disease, and probably most, if not all, shed virus from the genital area intermittently.

Clinical diagnosis of HSV is insensitive and nonspecific; therefore, the clinical diagnosis of genital herpes should be confirmed by laboratory testing. Many infected persons do not experience the multiple vesicular or ulcerative lesions typical of genital herpes. Both virologic and type-specific serologic tests are used to confirm the diagnosis.[154]

Cell culture and NAATs are the preferred virologic tests for persons who seek diagnosis and treatment of genital ulcers or other mucocutaneous lesions. The sensitivity of viral culture is low, especially for recurrent lesions, and declines rapidly as lesions begin to heal. NAATs for HSV DNA are increasingly used in many laboratories, and several tests are now cleared by the FDA for anogenital specimens.[155,156] NAATs are the preferred tests for detecting HSV in spinal fluid for diagnosis of HSV infection of the CNS and are discussed later in this chapter. Both culture and NAATs should determine whether the infection is due to HSV-1 or HSV-2 because recurrences and asymptomatic shedding are much less frequent for HSV-1 than for HSV-2 genital infections.[157] Failure to detect HSV by culture or NAAT does not rule out HSV infection because viral shedding is intermittent. The use of Tzanck preparations or Pap tests to detect cytologic changes produced by HSV are insensitive and nonspecific and should not be used for genital HSV infections.

Serologic tests detect type-specific and nonspecific antibodies to HSV that develop during the first several weeks to few months after infection and persist indefinitely. Type-specific serologic tests based on antigens specific for HSV-1 (gG1) and HSV-2 (gG2) are commercially available. Because almost all HSV-2 infections are sexually acquired, type-specific HSV-2 antibody indicates anogenital infection. However, the presence of HSV-1 antibody does not distinguish anogenital from orolabial infection. Type-specific HSV serologic assays might be useful in the following scenarios: (1) recurrent genital symptoms or atypical symptoms with negative HSV PCR or culture, (2) clinical diagnosis of genital herpes without laboratory confirmation, and (3) a patient whose partner has genital herpes. HSV serologic testing should be considered for persons presenting for an STI evaluation (especially for those persons with multiple sex partners), persons with HIV infection, and men who have sex with men at increased risk for HIV acquisition.[158]

Human Papillomavirus

Human papillomaviruses are small, double-stranded DNA viruses that infect squamous epithelium, subverting normal cell growth and potentially leading to squamous cell carcinoma (SCC). HPV is not a single virus but a family of more than 150 related viral genotypes that are distinguished based on sequence analysis of the L1 region of the viral genome. Anogenital HPV infections are common in both men and women. It is estimated that more than 24 million men and women in the United States are currently infected with HPV. HPV is an STI; it is most common among sexually active young women ages 15 through 25 years. In one study, cervicovaginal HPV was found in up to 43% of sexually active college women during a 3-year period.[159] Infections, however, are usually transient, and progression to cancer requires persistence of viral infection over several years. The types of HPV that are spread through sexual contact are classified as low or high risk for progression to malignancy, and there are multiple types. Infections with low-risk HPV such as types 6 and 11 can lead to benign genital warts or condyloma acuminata and have a low likelihood of progressing to malignancy. In contrast, high-risk types such as types 16, 18, and 45 are associated with development of SCC of the anogenital region and oropharynx. Currently, there are 14 high-risk (HR) HPV types recognized. The cervix is particularly affected, and worldwide, cervical SCC continues to cause significant morbidity and mortality (5% of cancer deaths).

Productive infections usually result in cytologic and histologic changes, including cellular and nuclear enlargement, nuclear hyperchromasia, and perinuclear halos (koilocytosis). These changes can be identified on a stained smear of cells collected from the cervix (the "Pap smear," developed by Dr. George Papanicolaou in the 1940s) or in a biopsy taken during colposcopy or a loop electrosurgical excision procedure. The Pap smear has been used very successfully to identify women with cervical cancer and, more important, for the detection of precursor lesions, so that biopsy or excision can be performed to remove the lesion earlier in the disease process before metastasis can occur. With the introduction of liquid cytology media and automated cytology processors, the procedure is more appropriately called the Pap test because "smears" are no longer used.

The histologic types of squamous precursor lesions are divided into three categories: mild dysplasia, or cervical intraepithelial neoplasia (CIN1); moderate dysplasia, or CIN2; and severe dysplasia, or carcinoma in situ, or CIN3. In the Bethesda System for Cytologic Classification, squamous precursor lesions are divided into low- and high-grade squamous intraepithelial lesions (LSIL and HSIL). LSIL corresponds with CIN1, and HSIL corresponds to CIN2 and CIN3. Frequently, the cytologic evaluation demonstrates mildly atypical cells that do not meet these criteria and are referred to as atypical squamous cells of undetermined significance (ASCUS); these cells may correspond to an early HPV infection. The prevalence of ASCUS on Pap tests is approximately 5% to 10%, with rates as high as 20% reported in sexually active women.

Screening for cervical cancer with cytology testing has been very effective in reducing cervical cancer in the United States. For many years, the approach was an annual Pap test. In 2000 the Hybrid Capture 2 (HC2) test (Qiagen/Digene) for detection of HR HPV types was approved by the FDA for screening women who had ASCUS detected by the Pap test to determine the need for colposcopy. At the time, the Hybrid Capture 2 test was the only FDA-approved test available. In 2003, the FDA approved expanding the use of this test to include screening preformed in conjunction with a Pap test for women over the age of 30 years, referred to as "co-testing." Co-testing allows women to extend the testing interval to 5 years if both test results are negative.[160] In 2014, the FDA approved the use of an HR HPV test (cobas HPV test, Roche) for primary cervical cancer screening for women older than the age of 25 years, without the need for a concomitant Pap test. When using the HR HPV test as the primary screening test, a Pap test is performed only when specific HR HPV types are detected (HPV-16 and -18 are excluded). Colposcopy is performed without an intervening Pap test in women who test positive for HPV-16 and -18. This algorithm was based primarily on the results of a single large FDA registration study for the cobas HPV test.[161] Interim clinical guidance is available for the use of primary HR HPV testing in cervical cancer screening.[162] However, there is still considerable debate about whether co-testing or HR HPV as a primary screening test is the optimal approach for cervical cancer screening.[163]

Four tests for the detection of HR HPV types have been cleared by the FDA for use in the United States: HC2 test, Cervista HPV HR (Hologic/Gen-Probe), cobas HPV test (Roche), and Aptima HPV test (Hologic/Gen-Probe). In addition, two different FDA-cleared tests to specifically identify HPV types 16 and 18 (Cervista) and types 16 and 18/45 (Aptima) are available. The features of these tests are compared in Table 48.4. All of these tests have been cleared by the FDA for use with ThinPrep PreservCyt liquid-based cytology medium (Hologic) but not with the other commonly used SurePath medium (Becton-Dickinson).

TABLE 48.4 **Features of Food and Drug Administration–Cleared High-Risk Human Papillomavirus Tests**

Feature	HC2	Cervista	cobas	Aptima
Technology	Hybrid capture	Cleavase/Invader	Real-time PCR	Transcription-mediated amplification
Target(s)	Multigene	L1, E6, E7	L1	E6, E7 mRNA
LOD and clinical cutoff	5000 copies/reaction	1250–7500 copies/reaction	300–2400 copies/mL	20–240 copies/reaction
Cross reaction with low-risk types	6, 11, 40, 42, 53, 66, 67, 70, 82/82v	67, 70	None reported	26, 67, 70, 82
Internal control	None	Human histone 2 gene	Human β-globin gene	Process
HPV-16/-18 genotyping	No	Yes (separate test)	Yes (integrated)	Yes (separate test also includes type 45)
Automation	Semiautomated and automated	Semiautomated and automated	Automated (cobas 4800)	Automated (Tigris and Panther)
Sample type (volume)	ThinPrep (4 mL), sample transport medium	ThinPrep (2 mL)	ThinPrep (1 mL)	ThinPrep (1 mL)
Prealiquot required	No	No	Yes	Yes
Expanded STI menu	CT/NG	None	CT/NG, HSV 1/2	CT/NG, TV
Primary screening indication	No	No	Yes	No

CT, Chlamydia trachomatis; *HSV*, herpes simplex virus; *LOD*, limit of detection; NG, *Neisseria gonorrhoeae*; *PCR*, polymerase chain reaction; *STI*, sexually transmitted infection; *TV*, *Trichomonas vaginalis*

The HC2 test relies on hybridization of a RNA probe to the HPV DNA followed by use of an antibody for capture of the duplex (RNA-DNA) hybrids and then detection with chemiluminescent signal amplification. The test uses a pool of RNA probes spanning the entire genome that are specific for 13 HR HPV types. The specific type is not identified. The test uses a 96-well microtiter plate format and can be performed manually or with the semiautomated Rapid Capture system (Qiagen) for reagent and plate handling. It is also cleared for use on Digene specimen transport media (STM). The HC2 test has been used in several large studies and reproducibly demonstrates high sensitivity of 93% to 96%, but false-positive results occur as a result of cross-reaction with low-risk HPV types.[164]

The Cervista HPV HR assay also uses a signal amplification method that is based on cleavase/invader technology and detects the same 13 high-risk types as HC2 test plus type 66. A combination of DNA probes and invader oligonucleotides targeting the L1, E6, and E7 sequences and secondary fluorescently labeled probes are divided into three phylogenetically related reactions that are performed on 96-well microtiter plates. Unlike the HC2 assay, this assay includes an internal control with each reaction. Both assays have detection limits of around 3000 to 5000 genome copies per milliliter. The Cervista HPV HR assay has less cross-reactivity with low-risk types. Studies comparing the two assays demonstrate concordance of 82% to 88%.[165] However, the Cervista test may have poor specificity compared with other tests for HR HPV.[166,167] The Cervista HPV-16 and -18 genotyping test uses the same cleavase/invader technology.

The cobas HPV Test is the first real-time PCR method approved by the FDA for cervical cancer screening.[161] It uses a multiplexed primer and hydrolysis probe assay to individually detect both HPV types 16 and 18 simultaneously with the 12 other HR HPV types using different fluorescently labeled probes. The assay includes detection of the human β-globin gene as an internal control for extraction and amplification adequacy. The cobas 4800 system uses automated bead-based NA extraction and PCR assembly. The sensitivity and specificity is similar to the HC2 and Cervista HR HPV assays. Currently, this is the only FDA-cleared test that has an indication for primary screening.

The Aptima HPV assay targets the viral mRNA for the E6/E7 HPV genes for the 14 HR HPV types. The E6 and E7 genes of HR HPV types are known oncogenes. Proteins expressed from E6-E7 polycistronic mRNA alter cellular p53 and retinoblastoma protein functions, leading to disruption of cell-cycle check points and genome instability. Targeting the mRNA of these oncogenic elements may be a more effective approach to detect cervical disease than detection of HPV genomic DNA.[168] The APTIMA HPV Assay involves three main steps, which take place in a single tube: target capture, target amplification by transcription-mediated amplification, and detection of the amplicons by the hybridization protection assay. The assay also incorporates an internal control to monitor NA capture, amplification, and detection, as well as operator or instrument error. Unlike the internal controls used in the Cervista and Roche assays, it does not assess specimen adequacy (cellularity). An adjunctive test to detect and differentiate HPV type 16 and 18/45 based on the same principle described is also available from Hologic/Gen-Probe.

POINTS TO REMEMBER

Human Papillomavirus

- Most HPV infections in women are transient and progression to cervical cancer requires persistent infection with one of the 14 HR oncogenic types of which 16, 18, and 45 are most common.
- HR HPV testing is recommended in conjunction with the Pap test for cervical cancer screening in women older than 30 years of age (co-testing).
- Co-testing allows women to extend the testing interval to 5 years if both test results are negative because HPV DNA is more sensitive than the Pap test for detection of women with significant cervical lesions.
- Currently, there are four FDA-cleared tests for HR HPV types, each based on a different amplification method: hybrid capture, cleavase/invader, real-time PCR, and transcription mediated amplification.

RESPIRATORY TRACT INFECTIONS

Viruses

The viruses that infect the respiratory tract consist of large and diverse groups that cause disease in humans, and new ones continue to be discovered. The more common viruses that infect humans include influenza A and B, parainfluenza virus (PIV) types 1 to 4, respiratory syncytial virus (RSV), metapneumovirus, adenoviruses (>50 different types), rhinoviruses (>100 different types), and coronaviruses (4 types). The disease spectrum ranges from the common cold to severe life-threatening pneumonia. It can be difficult to differentiate the viral origin based on signs and symptoms alone, and treatment options vary depending on the viral etiology. Infection with these viruses has demonstrated the potential for global public health threats of epidemic and pandemic proportions. The 1918 influenza A pandemic, human deaths caused by infection with avian influenza A H5N1 in 1997,[169] the severe acute respiratory syndrome (SARS) coronavirus outbreak in 2003, the 2009 pandemic caused by the novel multiply-reassorted (swinelike) influenza A H1N1, and the emergence of Middle East respiratory syndrome (MERS) coronavirus in 2012 on the Arabian peninsula are all reminders of the potential threats to human health posed by novel respiratory viruses.[170] Detection of emerging respiratory viruses will require multiple modalities, but molecular methods have been crucial to their discovery and characterization and in the development of diagnostic tools.

Acute respiratory viral infection (1) is a leading cause of hospitalization and death in infants and young children; (2) contributes to problems of asthma exacerbation, otitis media, and lower respiratory tract infection; and (3) contributes to acute disease in immunocompromised and elderly patients. Rapid diagnosis aids in effective treatment (eg, with antiviral medications such as oseltamivir for influenza A virus infection) and management (eg, reduction in inappropriately prescribed antibiotics for viral infection and infection control).

Rapid antigen-based EIAs provide short TATs (minutes) but are hampered by poor diagnostic sensitivity compared with culture methods or molecular assays and low positive predictive values, especially when the prevalence is low. Direct

TABLE 48.5 Parameters of Different Food and Drug Administration–Cleared Respiratory Virus Panels

Parameter	Luminex xTAG RVPv1	Luminex xTAG RVP-Fast	FilmArray	eSensor
Amplicon detection method	Fluorescence-labeled bead array	Fluorescence-labeled bead array	Melting curve analysis	Voltammetry
On-board sample processing	No	No	Yes	No
Post-PCR manipulation	Yes	Yes	No	Yes
Hands-on-time (min)	70	45	3	55
Throughput	High	High	Low	Moderate
Analysis time (hr)	7	4	1	6
Total time to results (hr)*	9	6	1.1	8
Complexity	High	High	Low	Moderate
Pathogens detected	ADV INF A (H1, H3) INF B MPV RSV (A, B) RV/EV PIV (1, 2, 3)	ADV INF A (H1, H3) INF B MPV RSV RV/EV	ADV INF A (H1, H3, 09H1) INF B MPV RSV RV/EV PIV (1, 2, 3, 4) COV (HKU1, NL63, 229E, OC43) *Bordetella pertussis* *Chlamydophila pneumoniae* *Mycoplasma pneumoniae*	ADV (B/E, C) INF A (H1, H3, 09H1) INF B MPV RSV (A, B) RV PIV (1, 2, 3,)

*Includes the time required for nucleic acid extraction.
ADV, Adenovirus; *COV,* coronavirus *EV,* enterovirus; *INFA,* influenza A virus; *INFB,* influenza B virus; *MPV,* metapneumovirus; *PCR,* polymerase chain reaction; PIV, parainfluenza virus; *RSV,* respiratory syncytial virus; *RV,* rhinovirus.

fluorescent antibody (DFA) detection assays for viral antigens on centrifuged cellular material from nasopharyngeal swabs, aspirates, or wash specimens demonstrate greater rates of detection than the rapid antigen assays and provide results in a relatively short time frame of 2 to 4 hours. Detection rates, however, are lower for antigen detection methods than for NAATs.

Cell culture methods, although slower than antigen detection methods, have been considered the gold standard for detection of a wide range of viral pathogens. In recent years, culture methods have been optimized for detection by combining multiple cell lines and improving the TAT from weeks to days through the use of shell-vial spin amplification cultures. Here, the patient's specimen is concentrated onto cells grown on a coverslip, and fluorescent antibody detection is performed after 16 to 24 hours of incubation instead of waiting for the development of a cytopathic effect. Although this has hastened the time to detection, 1 to 2 days is still required along with significant technologist labor, and it is not quite as sensitive as molecular methods of detection.

Molecular detection of respiratory viruses offers several advantages over traditional virologic culture or antigen detection. Most important, analytical sensitivity of molecular assays, primarily using PCR or real-time PCR, is consistently better than that of traditional methods.[171-174] Results from molecular testing are more accurate, and thus the patient benefits from the most appropriate treatment decision; also, infection control practitioners can more effectively implement strategies to prevent or reduce nosocomial transmission. Molecular assays can be designed to detect a wide range of viral pathogens, including viruses that are difficult to culture.

Despite the advantages of NAATs for respiratory virus detection, their adoption by clinical laboratories was initially slow because of the limited capacity of real-time PCR assays for multiplexing. There are numerous LDTs and FDA-cleared real-time PCR assays capable of detecting one to three different viruses in single reactions, but to provide comprehensive coverage for respiratory viruses, a panel of such assays needed to be deployed, an approach not practical for most laboratories.

Currently, there are several FDA-cleared multiplexed respiratory virus panels capable of detecting up to 20 different viral targets, thus providing simplified approaches to comprehensive diagnostics for respiratory viruses.[175] See Table 48.5 for an overview of the important parameters of these respiratory virus panels. These tests are truly transformative for the laboratory in that they can replace the combination of limited multiplex NAATs, antigen detection tests, and culture-based methods that were traditionally used in clinical laboratories to detect respiratory viruses and thus dramatically increase diagnostic yield.

The xTAG Respiratory Viral Panel (RVP) v1 assay is a multiplexed RT-PCR–based assay with fluorescently color-coded microsphere (bead) hybridization for simultaneous detection and identification of 12 respiratory viruses and subtypes.[175] The multiplexed RT-PCR primers amplify conserved regions of the viruses, and the products are labeled with biotin-containing deoxynucleotides in a second target-specific primer extension reaction. The extension product has a proprietary tag sequence incorporated for hybridization to the virus-specific probe on the color-coded bead. After hybridization, phycoerythrin-conjugated streptavidin is bound by the biotin-labeled primer extension products, and the fluorescent signal is quantified on the Luminex xMAP instrument. The instrument contains two lasers: one for identification of the microbe by a color-coded bead and the other for detection of the phycoerythrin signal attached to the primer extension product. The data are recorded as mean fluorescent intensities, and the software analyzes the data and reports the positive results. The assay includes a separate lambda phage amplification control and an MS-2 bacteriophage internal control for extraction and amplification. The original version of the assay was modified to reduce the number steps and analysis time (RVP-Fast), but it does not include the parainfluenza viruses, and it is not as sensitive overall as its predecessor. Because there are a number of post-PCR processing steps in both versions of the test, care must be taken to avoid amplicon cross-contamination and false-positive results.

BioFire Diagnostics developed a PCR instrument called the FilmArray and an associated reagent pouch that together are capable of simultaneously detecting multiple organisms in the same sample. The FilmArray pouch contains freeze-dried reagents to perform NA purification; reverse transcription; and nested, multiplex PCR followed by high-resolution melting analysis. The FilmArray Respiratory Panel (RP) was designed for simultaneous detection and identification of 17 viral and 3 bacterial respiratory pathogens (see Table 48.5). The test is initiated by loading water and an unprocessed patient nasopharyngeal swab specimen mixed with lysis buffer into the FilmArray RP pouch. The pouch is then placed into the FilmArray instrument. The software has a simple interface that requires only identification of the specimen and pouch barcode to initiate a run. Multiplexed two-stage RT-PCR followed by high-resolution melting analysis of the target amplicons is used to detect each of the panel analytes.[176] Results are reported in an hour; currently, the instrument is designed to test a single sample per run, though multiple instruments can be linked. Because it is a completely closed system, false-positive results caused by amplicon cross-contamination are not an issue.

The eSensor system (GenMark Dx) uses electrochemical-detection-based DNA microarrays.[177] These microarrays are composed of a printed circuit board consisting of an array of 76 gold-plated electrodes. Each electrode is modified with a multicomponent, self-assembled monolayer that includes presynthesized oligonucleotide capture probes. NA detection is based on a sandwich assay principle. Signal and capture probes are designed with sequences complementary to immediately adjacent regions on the corresponding target DNA sequence. A three-member complex is formed between the capture probe, target sequence, and signal probe based on sequence-specific hybridization. This process brings the 5′ end of the signal probe containing electrochemically active ferrocene labels into close proximity to the electrode surface. The ferrous ion in each ferrocene group undergoes cyclic oxidation and reduction, leading to loss or gain of an electron, which is measured as current at the electrode surface using alternating-current voltammetry. Higher-order harmonic signal analysis also facilitates discrimination of ferrocene-dependent faradic current from background capacitive current.

The eSensor cartridge consists of a printed circuit board, a cover, and a microfluidic component. The microfluidic component includes a diaphragm pump and check valves in line with a serpentine channel that forms the hybridization channel above the array of electrodes. The eSensor instrument consists of a base module and up to three cartridge-processing towers, each with eight slots for cartridges. The cartridge slots operate independently of each other. The throughput of a three-tower system can reach 300 tests in 8 hours. A respiratory pathogen panel for the eSensor system that detects 14 different types and subtypes of respiratory viruses (see Table 48.5) is FDA cleared.[178] Because this test requires post-PCR manipulations of the sample, care must be taken to avoid false-positive tests caused by amplicon cross-contamination.

The Verigene system (Nanosphere) uses PCR amplification and gold nanoparticle-labeled probes to detect target NA hybridized to capture oligonucleotides arrayed on a glass slide. Silver signal amplification is then performed on the gold nanoparticle probes that are hybridized to the captured DNA targets of interest. The Verigene reader optically scans the slide for silver signal, processes the data, and produces a qualitative result. A test for detection of influenza A virus, influenza A virus subtype H3, influenza A virus subtype 2009 H1N1, influenza B, and RSV subtypes A and B is cleared by the FDA for the Verigene system.[179] The system is capable of much higher-order multiplexing and a respiratory panel that detects 13 viral and 3 bacterial targets has been developed and is available in the United States as an RUO product.

Molecular testing for respiratory viruses will likely continue to include tests designed to detect a limited number of viruses of particular importance (eg, influenza A and B viruses and RSV), as well as tests that detect a broad array of viruses because there are clinical needs for both types of tests. The use of comprehensive respiratory virus panels greatly increases diagnostic yield and the ability to detect mixed viral infections. However, the clinical significance of mixed infections is not well documented or understood. In addition, there are test options that range from simple, "sample in answer out" systems to complex tests that require multiple manual steps, meeting different niches for various clinical laboratory settings. In fact, point-of-care molecular testing for respiratory viruses is now possible with the recent development of a CLIA-waived test for influenza A and B viruses (Alere). It delivers results in 15 minutes and can be performed by nonlaboratory personnel, and its performance characteristics are similar to those of NAATs performed in laboratories.[180]

Mycobacterium tuberculosis

Mycobacterium tuberculosis causes a wide range of clinical infections, including pulmonary disease; miliary tuberculosis; meningitis; pleurisy, pericarditis, and peritonitis; GI disease; genitourinary disease, and lymphadenitis. *M. tuberculosis* infection was in steady decline in the United States with an all-time low in the late 1990s, when the number of reported cases began to increase.[181] This resurgence was related to the AIDS epidemic, homelessness, and a decreased focus on tuberculosis control programs. The infection rate continues to rise in foreign-born persons as the result of immigration from countries with a high prevalence of *M. tuberculosis* infection. This increase in *M. tuberculosis* infection has focused considerable attention on the development of assays for its rapid diagnosis; molecular methods are at the center of this effort.

Conventional tests for laboratory confirmation of tuberculosis include acid-fast bacilli (AFB) smear microscopy, which can produce results in 24 hours, and culture, which requires 2 to 6 weeks to produce results.[182,183] Although rapid and inexpensive, AFB smear microscopy is limited by its poor sensitivity (45%–80% with culture-confirmed pulmonary tuberculosis cases) and its poor positive predictive value (50%–80%) for tuberculosis in settings in which nontuberculous mycobacteria are commonly isolated.[183-185]

Compared with AFB smear microscopy, the added value of NAATs include (1) their greater positive predictive value (>95%) than AFB smear-positive specimens when nontuberculous mycobacteria are common and(2) their ability to rapidly confirm the presence of *M. tuberculosis* in 60% to 70% smear-negative, culture-positive specimens.[183-187] Compared with culture, NAATs can detect the presence of *M. tuberculosis* in specimens weeks earlier for 80% to 90% of patients suspected to have pulmonary tuberculosis ultimately confirmed by culture.[184,186,187] These advantages can impact patient care and tuberculosis control efforts, such as by avoiding unnecessary contact investigations or respiratory isolation for patients whose AFB smear-positive specimens do not contain *M. tuberculosis.*

The CDC recommends that NAATs be performed on at least one (preferably the first) respiratory specimen from each patient suspected of pulmonary tuberculosis for whom a diagnosis of tuberculosis is being considered but has not yet been established and for whom the test result would alter case management or tuberculosis control activities.[188] NAATs can also be used to inform the decision to discontinue airborne infection isolation precautions in health care settings.[189,190] NAATs do not replace the need for culture; all patients suspected of tuberculosis should have specimens collected for mycobacterial culture.[188]

Currently, two FDA-approved NAATs are available for direct detection of *M. tuberculosis* in clinical specimens: the Amplified *Mycobacterium tuberculosis* Direct test (MTD test, Hologic/Gen-Probe) and the Xpert MTB/RIF assay (Cepheid). The MTD test is based on transcription-mediated amplification of ribosomal RNA and can be used to test both AFB smear-positive and smear-negative respiratory specimens. The Xpert MTB/RIF assay uses real-time PCR to detect the DNA of *M. tuberculosis* and the mutations in the *rpoB* gene associated with rifampin resistance in sputum specimens. Rifampin resistance most often coexists with isoniazid resistance so detection of rifampin resistance serves as a marker for potentially multidrug-resistant *M. tuberculosis* strains. Similar to the other assays developed by Cepheid, the Xpert MTB/RIF assay uses a disposable cartridge that automates the NA extraction, target amplification, and amplicon detection in conjunction with the GeneXpert Instrument System. Sensitivity and specificity of the Xpert MTB/RIF assay for detection of *M. tuberculosis* appear to be comparable to other FDA-approved NAATs for this use. Sensitivity of detection of rifampin resistance was 95% and specificity 99% in a multicenter study using archived and prospective specimens from subjects suspected of having tuberculosis.[191]

Because the prevalence of rifampin resistance is low in the United States, a positive result indicating a mutation in the *rpoB* gene should be confirmed by rapid DNA sequencing for prompt reassessment of the treatment regimen and followed by growth-based drug susceptibility testing.[190] The CDC offers these services free of charge.

Bordetella pertussis

The genus *Bordetella* is composed of eight species, four of which can cause respiratory disease in humans: *B. bronchiseptica*, *B. holmesii*, *B. parapertussis*, and *B. pertussis*. Whooping cough, or pertussis, is a highly contagious respiratory disease caused by *B. pertussis*. Despite widespread childhood vaccination, more than 28,660 cases were reported in the United States in 2014. (http://www.cdc.gov/pertussis/downloads/pertuss-surv-report-2014.pdf). The reported cases represent only the "tip of the iceberg" with an estimated 800,000 to 3.3 million cases occurring in the United States annually. Although pertussis occurs most often in children younger than 1 year of age, the incidence in older children has increased substantially in recent years. Adolescents and adults, in whom immunity wanes several years after prior infection or vaccination, transmit the organism to susceptible infants. Pertussis in older children and adults is usually characterized by prolonged cough without the inspiratory whoop or post-tussive vomiting that typically is observed in infants.

B. parapertussis may be responsible for up to 20% of pertussis-like disease, more often in young children.[192] Illness is generally milder than that caused by *B. pertussis*. *B. bronchiseptica* is an infrequent cause of disease in humans, usually occurring in immunocompromised individuals. Cases usually have exposure to farm animals or pets, which serve as the natural hosts for *B. bronchiseptica*.[193] *B. holmesii* is the most recently recognized species to be associated with pertussis-like illness in humans.[194] All four species play a significant role in human respiratory disease, and they should be considered in the design of NAATs for patients with pertussis-like disease.[195]

The laboratory diagnosis of pertussis has been fundamentally transformed in the past 2 decades. Culture and DFA staining of nasopharyngeal secretions are now largely replaced by NAATs in clinical laboratories. Although culture is specific for diagnosis, it is relatively insensitive. The fastidious nature and slow growth of the *B. pertussis* make it difficult to isolate. Although DFA staining can provide rapid results, it is neither sensitive nor specific. Serologic testing can be useful late in the disease when the organism may not be detectable by culture or NAAT and in the investigation of outbreaks, but the tests are not standardized, so the results may be difficult to interpret.

NAATs are important tools for the diagnosis of pertussis with enhanced sensitivity and rapid turnaround compared with culture and are now considered standard of care, but they can give both false-positive and false-negative results as discussed later. A variety of LDTs primarily based on real-time PCR with different performance characteristics are deployed in clinical laboratories. Currently, there are only two FDA-approved NAATs for *B. pertussis*, one a stand-alone test based on loop-mediated amplification (Meridian Biosciences) and the other as part of a respiratory panel (BioFire Diagnostics).

A number of different gene targets have been used in NAATs for *Bordetella* spp., some of which are shared among the different species.[195] Most NAATs are based on detection of multicopy insertion sequences (IS), which can increase the sensitivity of the tests. IS*481* is the most validated target for *B. pertussis*, but it can also be found in *B. holmesii* and *B. bronchiseptica*; therefore, tests based on this target alone are of limited value, particularly when used in an outbreak setting. IS*1001* is found in *B. parapertussis* and *B. bronchiseptica* but not in *B. holmesii*. IS*1002* is found in *B. pertussis* and *parapertussis* but not in *B. holmesii* or *bronchiseptica*. Multiplex PCR targeting all three ISs may allow detection and differentiation of the major pathogens that infect humans, *B. pertussis*, *B. parapertussis*, and *B. holmesii*.

A number of assays based on single copy gene targets have also been described.[195] The promoter region of the pertussis toxin operon is often used in diagnostic assays. However, it is also present in *B. parapertussis* and *B. bronchiseptica*, but because of mutations in the promoter region, it is not expressed. It is not found in *B. holmesii*. The mutations in the promoter region found in *B. parapertussis* and *B. bronchiseptica* can be exploited in real-time PCR assays that use post-amplification analysis by melting temperature to distinguish the amplicons from the different species. Pertactin, filamentous hemagglutinin, adenylate cyclase, REC A, flagellin, and BP3385 gene sequences are also shared among the different species. BP283 and BP485 gene targets are reported to be specific for *B. pertussis*.[196] With the exception of the pertussis toxin gene, none of the other single gene targets has been extensively validated in diagnostic assays.

The positive predictive value of NAATs remains their biggest challenge. IS481-based tests will detect *B. holmesii* and *B. bronchiseptica*, which for clinical and epidemiologic purposes are considered biological false-positive results. Environmental contamination with *B. pertussis* DNA in patient clinics has been identified as a source of pseudo-outbreaks of disease.[197] The positive predictive value of NAATs for *B. pertussis* can be increased by amplifying gene targets not shared by other species, using multiplex assays or a two-tiered approach to confirm positives, creating an indeterminate range for assays that target multicopy ISs, segregating "clean" and "dirty" areas in the clinic and the laboratory, and testing only symptomatic patients.[195] Further guidance for health care professionals for the use and interpretation of NAATs for *B. pertussis* can be found on the CDC's website (http://www.cdc.gov/pertussis/clinical/diagnostic-testing/diagnosis-pcr-bestpractices.html).

BLOODSTREAM INFECTIONS

Positive Blood Culture Identification

One of the most important functions of clinical microbiology laboratories is the detection of bloodstream infections. Using conventional grow-based systems, when the blood culture system signals positive, typically within 12 to 72 hours of incubation for most pathogens, the blood culture broth is Gram stained and then subcultured to solid medium. When colonies grow on this medium, identification and antimicrobial susceptibility tests are performed. This typically takes an additional 24 to 48 hours to complete after the blood culture signals positive. Direct inoculation of conventional identification and susceptibility tests using positive blood culture broth can reduce the time required to obtain results by eliminating the subculture to solid medium, but this practice is not FDA approved for automated identification and susceptibility test systems.

A variety of NA-based tests have been developed to expedite identification of organisms in positive blood cultures. FDA-approved tests include peptide NA fluorescent in situ hybridization (PNA FISH) probes, real-time PCR assays for detection of single or limited numbers of pathogens, and high-order multiplex blood culture identification panels based on nested PCR and gold nanoparticle microarrays.[198] Matrix-assisted laser desorption ionization time-of-flight mass spectrometry (MALDI-TOF) uses proteomics rather than genomics to identify pathogens based on the mass spectrum of proteins found in the microorganisms. It has been applied to the direct identification of microorganisms from positive blood culture bottles.[199] The key features of these methods are listed in Table 48.6.

PNA FISH probes are DNA probes in which the negatively charged sugar phosphate backbone is replaced by a noncharged peptide backbone. This results in rapid binding to DNA targets because there is no electrostatic repulsion with the target.[200] PNA FISH probes are available for rapid identification of *Staphylococcus aureus* and coagulase-negative staphylococci; *Enterococcus faecalis* and other enterococci; *Escherichia coli*, *Klebsiella pneumoniae*, and *Pseudomonas aeruginosa*; and *Candida albicans*, and/or *C. parapsilosis*, *C. tropicalis* and *C. glabrata* and/or *C. krusei* (AdvanDx). The most recent protocol involves approximately 5 minutes of hands-on time and 30 minutes for results. Access to a

TABLE 48.6 Key Features of Rapid Blood Culture Identification Methods

Feature	Nested Multiplex PCR FilmArray	Gold Nanoparticle Microarray	PNA FISH	MALDI-TOF MS
Inclusivity*	+++	+++	+	++++
Hands on time	2 min	5 min	5 min	30 min
Time to result	1 hr	2.5 hr	30 min	35 min
Technical complexity	+	++	++	+++
Antibiotic resistance genes (*n*)	Yes (3)	Yes (9)	No	No
Reagent cost	$$$$	$$$	$$	$

*Relative ability to identify common bloodstream pathogens.

MALDI-TOF MS, Matrix-assisted laser desorption ionization time-of-flight mass spectrometry; *PCR,* polymerase chain reaction; *PNA FISH,* peptide nucleic acid fluorescent in situ hybridization.

BOX 48.1 Comparison of Organisms and Antibiotic Resistance Genes Included in the FilmArray and Verigene Blood Culture Identification Panels

FilmArray

Gram Positive
Enterococcus spp.
Listeria monocytogenes
Staphylococcus spp.
 S. aureus
Streptococcus
 S. agalactiae
 S. pneumoniae
 S. pyogenes
Gram Negative
Acinetobacter baumannii
Haemophilus influenzae
Neisseria meningitidis
Pseudomonas aeruginosa
Enterobacteriaceae
 Enterobacter cloacae complex
 Escherichia coli
 Klebsiella pneumoniae
 K. oxytoca
 Proteus spp.
 Serratia marcescens
Yeast
Candida albicans
C. glabrata
C. krusei
C. parapsilosis
C. tropicalis
Antibiotic Resistance Genes
mecA
vanA/B
bla_{KPC}

Verigene

Gram Positive
Staphylococcus spp.
 S. aureus
 S. epidermidis
 S. lugdunensis
Streptococcus spp.
 S. anginosus group
 S. agalactiae
 S. pneumoniae
 S. pyogenes
Enterococcus faecalis
E. faecium
Listeria spp.
Antibiotic Resistance Genes
mecA
vanA
vanB

Gram Negative
E. coli/Shigella
Klebsiella pneumoniae
K. oxytoca
Pseudomonas aeruginosa
Acinetobacter spp.
Proteus spp.
Citrobacter spp.
Enterobacter spp.
Antibiotic Resistance Genes
bla_{KPC}
bla_{NDM}
$bla_{CTx\text{-}M}$
bla_{VIM}
bla_{IMP}
bla_{OxA}

fluorescence microscope with a special filter is required to read the stained slides.

A number of laboratory-developed NAATs for direct identification of single or a limited number of organisms directly from blood cultures have been described, but in general, they have not gained widespread acceptance in clinical laboratories. The number of commercially available assays for this application is also limited. *S. aureus* bacteremia requires prompt microbiologic diagnosis and appropriate antibiotic administration. Vancomycin is the standard treatment for suspected *S. aureus* bacteremia because in most centers, 50% or more of isolates are methicillin-resistant *S. aureus* (MRSA); however, it is less effective than methicillin for treating methicillin-susceptible *S. aureus* (MSSA) strains. Therefore, it is not surprising that many of the methods for rapid identification of bloodstream pathogens focused on the differentiation of MRSA from MSSA. Two FDA-approved real-time PCR assays for detection and differentiation of MRSA and MSSA directly from positive blood cultures are the BD GeneOhm StaphSR (BD Diagnostics) and the Xpert MRSA/SA BC (Cepheid) assays.[201,202] Each assay has limitations in accurately differentiating MRSA from MSSA largely because of assay design and selection of gene targets. See this chapter's section on antibacterial drug resistance for more details.

Two high-order multiplex assays have been approved by the FDA for identification of microorganisms from blood culture bottles, the Verigene Gram-Positive and Gram-Negative Blood Culture Tests (Nanosphere) and the FilmArray Blood Culture Identification (BCID) Panel (BioFire Diagnostics).[203-205] The organisms and antibiotic resistance genes included in each of the panels are listed in Box 48.1.

The FilmArray BCID panel uses the same technology as the respiratory panel described previously to detect 24 genus- or species-specific targets including gram-positive and gram-negative bacteria, *Candida* spp., and thee antibiotic resistance genes in approximately 1 hour.[205] This panel identifies from 80% to 90% of all positive blood cultures and provides important information about resistance to methicillin in staphylococci, vancomycin resistance in enterococci, and carbapenemase production in enteric gram-negative rods.

The Verigene BCID panels use Nanogold microarray technology to identify organisms from positive blood culture bottles without NA amplification. The gram-positive or gram-negative panel (or both) is chosen based on the results of the Gram stain that is performed when the bottle signals positive. The gram-positive panel detects 12 genus- or species-specific targets and 3 antibiotic resistance genes, and the gram-negative panel detects 8 genus- or species-specific targets and 9 antibiotic resistance genes in about 2.5 hours with minimal hands-on time. The gram-positive panel detects *mecA*, *vanA*, and *vanB* genes, and the gram-negative panel detects six different β-lactamase genes. A Verigene yeast blood culture panel is in development that will include *C. albicans, C. dubliniensis, C. glabrata, C. krusei, C. parapsilosis, C. tropicalis, C. gattii,* and *Cryptococcus neoformans.*

The FilmArray and Verigene panels provide comprehensive approaches to rapid identification of the vast majority of blood pathogens and important information about susceptibility of these pathogens to antibiotics. When coupled with active antimicrobial stewardship program interventions, the results of these tests will likely have a positive impact on the clinical outcomes of patients with sepsis.[206]

Direct Pathogen Detection

The methods discussed in the preceding section provide opportunities to expedite the identification of microorganisms when a blood culture signals positive and as such represent significant advances. However, blood cultures require 1 to 5 days of incubation before they are positive, and this timeline is inconsistent with the need to obtain rapid answers to inform treatment decisions in patients with sepsis. Direct detection of pathogens in blood without the need for culture would be ideal but presents a number of challenges. Specimen preparation, enrichment for pathogen DNA, and integration of the front-end specimen preparation with a back-end molecular analysis that identifies virtually all pathogens are major obstacles to success. Also, highly sensitive molecular methods for direct detection of microbial DNA in blood present significant challenges for validation given the known limitations of the sensitivity of culture, the current gold standard.

The Roche SeptiFast system has been available longer than any other method for direct detection of microorganisms in the blood.[207] It uses real-time PCR performed on a LightCycler instrument that targets the ribosomal internal transcribed spacer region. The target DNA is amplified in three parallel, multiplex, real-time PCR assays for detection of 10 gram-positive, 10 gram-negative, and 5 fungal pathogens. Melting curve analysis is used to reliably differentiate the pathogens. The assay is technically complex, requires large amounts of hands-on time, and has an analysis time of about 6 hours. Several evaluations have reported lower sensitivities and specificities in clinical settings when compared with blood cultures.[208-211]

Another molecular approach to direct detection of pathogens in blood and other body fluids has been developed by Ibis Biosciences, a subsidiary of Abbott Molecular. This method combines broad-range PCR with electrospray ionization time-of-flight mass spectrometry (PCR/ESI-MS). The technology has been described in great detail elsewhere,[212] but briefly, it works by coupling conserved-site PCR reactions that are able to amplify shared genes from diverse microorganisms to ESI-MS. Measurement of amplicon mass provides species-specific signatures that can be matched to known signatures in a database. After PCR amplification, ESI-MS analysis is performed on the amplicon mixtures, and the A, G, C, and T base compositions are compared with a database of known base compositions derived from existing sequence data. This technology accurately identifies diverse microbes from blood, other body fluids, and tissues in research settings.[213] The PCR/ESI-MS system was evaluated for the direct detection of bacteria and *Candida* spp. in the blood of 331 patients with suspected bloodstream infections and was found 83% sensitive and 94% specific compared with culture.[214] Replicate testing of the discrepant samples by PCR/ESI-MS resulted in increased sensitivity (91%) and specificity (99%) when confirmed infections were considered true positives. Ibis/Abbott has developed an automated and integrated platform for PCR/ES-MS analysis of clinical samples called IRIDICA. A bloodstream infection assay for this new platform that identifies up to 500 different organisms and four antibiotic resistance genes is currently in clinical trials.

Another novel technology that shows promise for direct detection of pathogens in blood is T2 magnetic resonance (T2MR)–based biosensing.[215] T2 Biosystems has developed an assay to directly identify *Candida* spp. in the blood of patients with suspected candidemia. In this assay, the *Candida* cells are lysed, their DNA is amplified by PCR, and the amplified product is detected directly in the whole-blood matrix by amplicon-induced agglomeration of superparamagnetic nanoparticles. Nanoparticle clustering yields changes in the T2 (spin-spin) relaxation time, making it detectable by magnetic resonance. A small portable T2MR instrument for rapid and precise T2 relaxation measurements has been designed for standard PCR tubes. The T2Dx instrument automates all of the steps in the assay with approximately 5 minutes of hands on time, and results are available within 3 to 5 hours. The T2 *Candida* panel is FDA approved, and the clinical trial data showed an overall sensitivity and specificity of 91.1% and 99.4%, respectively.[216] T2 Biosystems has a panel in development for direct detection of bacteria in blood.

CENTRAL NERVOUS SYSTEM

Herpes Simplex Virus

Herpes simplex virus types 1 and 2 produce various clinical syndromes involving the skin, eye, CNS, and genital tract. Although NA testing has been used to detect HSV DNA in all of these clinical manifestations, this discussion focuses on the use of HSV PCR for the diagnosis of CNS infections because NA amplification testing is widely viewed as the standard of care for diagnosis.

Herpes simplex virus causes both encephalitis and meningitis. In adults, whereas HSV encephalitis is usually attributable to infection with HSV type 1, HSV meningitis is most commonly caused by HSV type 2. HSV encephalitis is a severe infection with high morbidity and mortality; treatment with acyclovir reduces the mortality rate from approximately 70% in those with untreated infection to 19% to 28%. Neurologic impairment is common (≈50%) in those who survive.[217] HSV encephalitis may reflect primary infection or reactivation of latent infection. HSV meningitis is usually a self-limited disease that resolves over the course of several days without therapy. In some patients, the disease may recur as a lymphocytic meningitis over a period of years.[218]

Neonatal HSV infection occurs 1 in 3500 to 1 in 5000 deliveries in the United States. It is most commonly acquired by intrapartum contact with infected maternal genital secretions and is usually HSV type 2. In newborns, three general presentations of the disease are known: skin, eye, and mouth disease, which account for approximately 45%

of infections; encephalitis, which accounts for 35%; and disseminated disease, which accounts for 20%. Because disseminated disease is often associated with neurologic disease, CNS disease occurs in about 50% of newborns with neonatal HSV infection.

Herpes simplex virus encephalitis cannot be distinguished clinically from encephalitis caused by other viruses such as West Nile Virus, St. Louis encephalitis virus, and Eastern equine encephalitis virus. Historically, the gold standard for the diagnosis of HSV encephalitis required brain biopsy with identification of HSV by cell culture or immunohistochemical staining. This approach provided high sensitivity (99%) and specificity (100%), but it required an invasive procedure, and several days elapsed before results were available. Viral culture of cerebrospinal fluid (CSF) has a sensitivity of less than 10% for the diagnosis of HSV encephalitis in adults. Tests that measure HSV antigen or antibody in CSF have diagnostic sensitivities of 75% to 85% and diagnostic specificities of 60% to 90%.[217] Because of the limitations of conventional methods, there was interest in assessing the clinical utility of PCR for the detection of HSV DNA from CSF of patients with encephalitis. The two largest studies compared HSV PCR on CSF specimens versus brain biopsy in patients with suspected HSV encephalitis.[219,220] The sensitivity and specificity of PCR were greater than 95%, and the sensitivity of HSV PCR did not decrease significantly until 5 to 7 days after the start of therapy. PCR is positive early in the course of illness, usually within the first 24 hours of symptoms, and in some individuals, HSV DNA can persist in the CSF for weeks after therapy is initiated.

The clinical utility of HSV PCR has also been established for the diagnosis of neonatal HSV infection. In one study, HSV DNA was detected in the CSF of 76% (26 of 34) of infants with CNS disease; 94% (13 of 14) of those with disseminated infection; and 24% (7 of 29) of infants with skin, eye, or mouth disease.[221] The persistence of HSV DNA in the CSF of newborns for longer than 1 week after therapy initiation is associated with a poor outcome.[222] Based on these findings, detection of HSV DNA in CSF by PCR has become the standard of care for the diagnosis of HSV encephalitis and neonatal HSV infection. In newborns with disseminated disease, HSV DNA may be detected in serum or plasma specimens and is useful diagnostically in newborns if it is not possible to do a lumbar puncture. Although the sensitivity of HSV PCR is high, it is not 100%, so a negative PCR test result may not rule out neurologic disease caused by HSV, particularly if the pretest probability is high. In this situation, it is important to consider repeat testing.

As with HSV encephalitis, HSV meningitis cannot be distinguished clinically from other viral meningitides, although recurrence of viral meningitis is a strong clue that HSV may be the etiologic agent. Unlike HSV encephalitis, HSV meningitis has not been the subject of large studies evaluating the clinical utility of PCR for diagnosis. Nonetheless, because the sensitivity of viral culture of CSF specimens is only 50%, HSV PCR of CSF is commonly used in the evaluation of meningitis and has been described as accurate in anecdotal reports.[223]

Several molecular tests for the detection of HSV DNA from genital specimens have been cleared by the FDA, but only one, the Simplexa HSV 1 and 2 Direct Kit (Focus Diagnostics), has been cleared for use with CSF specimens. Several companies provide primers and probes as ASRs, which can be used as components in LDTs.

Molecular tests are often designed to detect HSV types 1 and 2 with equal sensitivity. Distinguishing between HSV types 1 and 2 may not be necessary because the clinical management of CNS disease is the same for both infections. Primers used for the detection of HSV DNA commonly target the polymerase, glycoprotein B, glycoprotein D, or thymidine kinase genes. It is important that the primers not amplify DNA from other herpesviruses that are associated with neurologic disease; these include cytomegalovirus, varicella zoster virus, human herpes virus type 6, and Epstein-Barr virus.

Herpes simplex virus PCR assays need low detection limits (several hundred copies per milliliter of specimen) to be useful in evaluating neurologic disease. This is particularly true for the diagnosis of meningitis, in which CSF concentrations of DNA tend to be lower than those seen with encephalitis. HSV neurologic disease rarely occurs in individuals without an increased CSF white blood cell count or protein concentration. Caution should be exercised in applying this generalization to immunocompromised individuals because they may not mount a typical inflammatory response to HSV infection. Although HSV PCR of CSF specimens is clearly the gold standard for the diagnosis of neurologic disease, results should be interpreted with caution because neither sensitivity nor specificity is 100%. Test results should always be interpreted within the context of the clinical presentation of the patient. If results do not correlate with the clinical impression, repeat testing should be performed 3 to 7 days later because initial negative PCR results can occur in a small but notable number of patients with confirmed HSV encephalitis.

Enterovirus

The enteroviruses (EVs) are a diverse group of single-stranded RNA viruses belonging to the *Picornaviridae* family. Currently, human EVs are divided into seven species: EV A to D and rhinoviruses A to C. The EV species A to D contain viruses formerly referred as coxsackieviruses, EVs, polioviruses, and echoviruses. The genus Parechovirus (PeV) comprises 16 different serotypes that were originally thought to be echoviruses. Although the genomic organization is similar to EVs, the origin of PeVs is uncertain. Numerous clinical presentations are seen with EV and PeV infections, including acute aseptic meningitis, encephalitis, exanthems, conjunctivitis, acute respiratory disease, GI disease, myopericarditis, and sepsis-like syndrome in neonates. Diagnoses typically are based on clinical presentation and NAATs.

Virus culture methods have several drawbacks, including the requirement to inoculate multiple cell lines because no single cell line is optimal for all EV types, the inability to grow some EV types in cell culture, the limited diagnostic sensitivity of cell culture (65%–75%), and the long TAT of 3 to 8 days for those EVs that do grow in cell culture.[224] The long TAT for culture means that results are rarely available in a time frame to influence clinical management. NAATs offer several important advantages over cell culture, including improved sensitivity and TAT. As a result, NA testing is considered the new gold standard for the diagnosis of aseptic meningitis and neonatal sepsis syndrome caused by EV and PeV infections.

Two methods are used for the detection of enteroviral RNA from clinical specimens: RT-PCR and NA sequence–based amplification. The primers used in clinical testing most commonly target the highly conserved 5′ URT of the genome and detect polioviruses and EVs.[225] These primers do not detect parechoviruses, although these viruses can cause aseptic meningitis. In general, molecular assays have good detection limits ranging from 0.1 to 50 tissue culture infectious doses ($TCID_{50}$) per test. The assays are quite specific, but sequence similarities may allow amplification of some types of rhinoviruses.[226,227] Currently, two tests for the detection of EVs from CSF specimens have been cleared by the FDA: the NucliSENS EasyQ Enterovirus (bioMérieux) and Xpert EV (Cepheid). However, the NucliSENS Easy Q EV assay is no longer commercially available. The Xpert EV test has a sensitivity of 97% and a specificity of 100% for the diagnosis of enteroviral meningitis.[228] The Xpert test has the advantage of being very simple to perform: The specimen and reagents are added to a cartridge, which is inserted into the instrument. NA extraction, amplification, and detection are fully automated, and results are available within about 2.5 hours. The system permits random access, which allows for on-demand testing.

Nucleic acid testing for the diagnosis of enteroviral infection has been evaluated in a variety of clinical studies, with testing showing sensitivities equal to or greater than that of cell culture, a high specificity, and faster TATs than cell culture. Several studies have suggested that the use of molecular methods for the diagnosis of enteroviral infection in infants and pediatric patients can lead to an overall cost savings by reducing the use of antibiotics and imaging studies.[229-231] To maximize the benefits for patient care and cost savings, testing should be available on a daily basis.

As mentioned earlier, many EV molecular assays detect rhinoviruses, and most detect polioviruses. These two factors can lead to unexpected and misleading positive results when respiratory or stool specimens are tested. The diagnosis of EV meningitis should be based on testing of CSF specimens, and sepsis syndrome is best diagnosed in neonates by testing serum, plasma, or CSF samples.

GASTROENTERITIS

Clostridium difficile

Clostridium difficile is a gram-positive spore-forming anaerobic bacillus that is frequently found in the stool flora of healthy infants but is rarely found in the stool flora of healthy adults and children older than 12 months. The organism is acquired by ingesting spores, which survive the gastric acid barrier and germinate in the colon. Alteration of the intestinal flora with the use of antibiotics facilitates colonization of the intestinal tract. After being colonized, patients may develop symptoms of diarrhea or colitis. Most strains of *C. difficile* make two toxins: toxin A and toxin B; the regulatory proteins TcdR and TcdC control expression of the toxin A (*tcdA*) and B (*tcdB*) genes. These toxins are responsible for symptomatic disease; strains that lack these toxin genes do not cause diarrhea or colitis. Toxin B may be more important for production of disease than toxin A.[232] Detection of these toxins or of their activity is essential in diagnostic tests for *C. difficile*–associated disease. An additional toxin, the binary toxin, has been described in some strains of *C. difficile,* and recent reports have suggested that strains encoding the binary toxin (CDT) have a deletion in the *tcdC* gene, leading to overexpression of toxins A and B (ribotype 027), and are causing outbreaks of more severe disease.[233]

C. difficile is a frequent cause of antibiotic-associated diarrhea and colitis both in the hospital and community. In hospitals, the risk of infection increases with the length of hospital stay, and use of antimicrobial therapy greatly increases the likelihood of acquiring *C. difficile* colitis. *C. difficile* causes a spectrum of disease ranging from asymptomatic carrier state to fulminant, relapsing, and fatal colitis. Diarrhea may be mild to severe. Pseudomembranous colitis is a classic presentation of *C. difficile* disease, and toxic megacolon may also be seen. Although clindamycin, penicillins, and cephalosporins have commonly been associated with disease, almost all antibiotics can cause similar disease.

Various non-NA tests are available for the diagnosis of *C. difficile* infection. Culture of the organism alone is not helpful in the diagnosis because there needs to be confirmation that the organism produces toxins. The cell culture cytotoxicity test neutralization assay (CCNA), which detects the cytopathic effect of toxin B, is considered the gold standard for the diagnosis of clinically important *C. difficile* infection. The test is highly sensitive and specific but is labor intensive and technically demanding. The TAT of 1 to 3 days limits its clinical utility.[234] The most commonly used tests are EIAs and lateral flow devices that detect toxin A, toxin B, or both. Overall these tests have lower sensitivities (45%–95%) and specificities (75%–100%) than the cytotoxicity test. In general, EIAs that detect both toxins A and B are preferred because some strains may not produce toxin A. An alternative testing approach is detection of the common antigen glutamate dehydrogenase (GDH). The test does not distinguish between toxigenic and nontoxigenic strains and cannot be used alone for the diagnosis of *C. difficile* disease. A positive result needs to be confirmed with the cytotoxicity test, a toxin EIA, or a NAAT for the detection of toxin B gene. The GDH test is a useful screening test because it has a high negative predictive value. One study evaluated a two-step approach using the GDH test as the initial screen followed by a CCNA for antigen-positive specimens to confirm the presence of toxin. A negative antigen test result was more than 99% predictive of a negative CCNA.[235] A limitation of this approach is the delay in obtaining a result because of the long TAT of the CCNA test. More recently, multistep algorithms using GDH, toxin EIA, and NAATs have been deployed in clinical laboratories.[236]

In view of the limitations of traditional methods, molecular tests are a good alternative for the diagnosis of *C. difficile* infection. The first NAAT for detection of *C. difficile* in stool was approved in 2009. At the time of this writing, 15 different platforms are FDA approved and available for testing using a variety of methods, including real-time PCR, loop-mediated amplification, helicase-dependent amplification, and microarray technology. Some platforms are designed for low-volume laboratories and on-demand testing, and others are more amenable to high-volume, batch mode testing. These assays detect a variety of gene targets, including *tcdA, tcdB, cdt*, and Δ117 deletion in *tcdC,* the latter two as surrogates for identification of the ribotype 027 strain.

Although NAATs have replaced other methods in clinical laboratories for diagnosis of *C. difficile* infection and have very high negative predictive values and analytical and clinical sensitivities, there are concerns about their specificity and positive predictive value because they will detect colonization as well as infection.[236] As mentioned earlier, some laboratories have implemented multistep diagnostic test algorithms using GDH, toxin EIA, and NAAT; however, these algorithms con complicate and delay final results, may not be reimbursed, and may ultimately be less cost effective than NAAT alone. Regardless of how a laboratory chooses to deploy NAAT testing, it should be limited to only patients with diarrhea to increase the pretest probability of disease and thus help mitigate concerns about detecting patients who are asymptomatically colonized with toxigenic strains.

POINTS TO REMEMBER

Clostridium difficile

- *C. difficile*–associated disease spectrum ranges from mild antibiotic-associated diarrhea to life-threatening toxic megacolon and occurs both in hospitals and the community.
- NAATs for detection of the toxin B gene of *C. difficile* have several advantages over traditional methods for diagnosis, including increased analytical and clinical sensitivity, high negative predictive value, and decreased analysis time.
- Concerns about the specificity and positive predictive value of NAATs have led some laboratories to adopt multistep diagnostic algorithms to help mitigate the problem of detecting patients asymptomatically colonized with toxigenic strains of *C. difficile*.

Gastrointestinal Pathogen Panels

Infectious gastroenteritis (IGE) is a leading cause of global morbidity and mortality. Diarrheal disease disproportionally affects developing nations, but IGE remains a significant problem in industrialized countries as well. Each year, approximately 178.8 million cases of IGE occur in the United States, resulting in 474,000 hospitalizations and 5000 deaths.[237] IGE is associated with a diverse array of etiologic agents, including bacteria, viruses, and parasites. Clinical presentation does little to aid with a specific etiologic diagnosis because diarrhea is the predominant symptom regardless of the etiology. Accurate identification of the etiology of IGE provides important information that impacts individual patient management, infection control, and public health interventions.

Common diagnostic practice in the United States requires that providers choose among a variety of tests, including antigen detection tests, culture, ova and parasite microscopic examination, and single-target NAATs, for detection of the responsible organism or toxin. In addition, the selection of tests may be informed by patient's age, severity of disease, immunocompromised state, duration and type of diarrhea, travel history, and time of year.[238] Often the clinician is unsure of what pathogens are included in each test and consequently may miss testing for specific pathogens of interest. In the laboratory, the battery of tests required to detect all possible pathogens is laborious and expensive to maintain, can require special expertise, and may have an unacceptably long TAT. In addition, the conventional microbiologic tests have limited sensitivity for many of the major pathogens.

The application of NA amplification methods could have significant impact on the diagnosis, treatment, and understanding of the epidemiology of IGE.[239] At the time of this writing, there were five FDA-approved enteric pathogen panels. A comparison of their key features is shown in Table 48.7. The systems use a variety of different technologies and differ in the number and types of targets included in the assay and the overall platform design and throughput. The Prodesse ProGrastro SSCS assay (Hologic/Gen-Probe) uses real-time PCR to detect and differentiate among *Salmonella* spp., *Shigella* spp., and *Campylobacter* spp., as well as Shiga toxin 1 *(stx1)* and Shiga toxin 2 *(stx2)* genes as indicators of Shiga-toxin producing *E. coli* in two separate master mixes.[240] Separate NA extraction and manual PCR setup are required. The BD MAX EBP (BD Diagnostics) uses a single real-time PCR master mix to detect essentially the same pathogens and toxins: *Salmonella* spp., *Shigella* spp. or enteroinvasive *E. coli*, *Campylobacter* spp., and *stx1/stx2*. However, the BD MAX automates all of the steps from sample preparation to target amplification and detection.[241]

Other systems have been developed to expand the panel of bacteria detected and include viral and protozoal pathogens.

TABLE 48.7 Comparison of Different Food and Drug Administration–Approved Enteric Pathogen Panel Platforms

Feature	ProGastro SSCS	BD MAX EBP	Verigene EP	xTag GPP	FilmArray GI
Technology	Real-time PCR	Real-time PCR	PCR and gold nanoparticle microarray	PCR and bead array	Nested PCR and melting curve analysis
Automation	Separate extraction, manual PCR setup	Sample to result	Sample to result	Separate extraction, manual PCR setup, post-PCR amplicon transfer	Sample to result
Throughput	Batch (16/thermal cycler)	Batch (24)	1/run	Batch (limited by extractor)	1/run
Analysis time (hr)	3	1.5	2	4	1
Targets	5 (3 bacteria, 2 toxins)	4 (3 bacteria, 1 toxin)	9 (5 bacteria, 2 toxins, 2 viruses)	14 (8 bacteria, 3 viruses, 3 protozoa)	21 (12 bacteria, 5 viruses, 4 protozoa)
Relative cost/test	$$	$	$$$	$$$	$$$

PCR, Polymerase chain reaction.

The Luminex xTAG GPP uses multiplex endpoint PCR and liquid bead array to detect and differentiate eight bacteria, three viruses, and three protozoa, including *Campylobacter* spp., *C. difficile* (toxins A and B), *E. coli* 0157, enterotoxigenic *E. coli*, Shiga-like toxin producing *E. coli*, *Salmonella* spp., *Shigella* spp., *Vibrio cholera*, adenovirus 40/41, norovirus GI/GII, rotavirus A, *Cryptosporidium* spp. *Entamoeba histolytica*, and *Giardia* spp.[242] This system provides for high throughput but requires a separate NA extraction step and post-PCR amplicon manipulation, which can lead to false-positive results caused by amplicon carry-over cross-contamination. It also has the longest analysis time of the available systems.

The Verigene uses multiplex PCR and a gold nanoparticle microarray to detect five bacteria, two toxins, and two viruses, including *Campylobacter* spp., *Salmonella* spp., *Shigella* spp. *Vibrio* spp., *Yersinia enterocolitica*, stx1, stx2, norovirus, and rotavirus.[243] It is a simple to use "sample in, answer out" system, but it has limited throughput because only one sample per instrument can be run at a time.

The FilmArray uses nested multiplex PCR and melting curve analysis to detect 12 bacteria, 5 viruses, and 4 protozoa, including *Campylobacter* spp., *C. difficile* toxin A/B, *Plesiomonas shigelloides*, *Salmonella* spp., *Vibrio* spp., *V. cholerae*, *Y. enterocolitica*, enteroaggregative *E. coli*, enteropathogenic *E. coli*, enterotoxigenic *E. coli*, Shiga-like toxin-producing *E. coli*, *E. coli* 0157, adenovirus F 40/41, astrovirus, norovirus GI/GII, rotavirus A, sapovirus, *Cryptosporidium* spp., *Cyclospora cayetanensis*, *E. histolytica*, and *G. lamblia*.[244] This is the most comprehensive enteric pathogen panel currently available. Similar to all of the FilmArray products, it is simple to use and provides results in about 1 hour. Its chief limitations are low throughput and high cost.

Laboratories can choose from a variety of test platforms based on whether a more focused or broader approach to IGE pathogen detection is desired. Also, the technical complexity and required throughput are important variables that may influence the approach chosen for this application. Current stool test algorithms using conventional methods typically require clinicians to consider which pathogens might be associated with the disease and choose among a variety of tests to ensure that all pathogens are covered. It is not surprising that this piecemeal approach often fails to yield positive results. The use of comprehensive pathogen panels dramatically increases diagnostic yield, but with this comes the unique challenge of interpreting the results from patients with multiple pathogens detected. In the FDA clinical trial of the FilmArray GI Panel, at least one potential pathogen was detected in 53.5% of specimens, and among these, multiple potential pathogens were detected in 32.9%.[244] Asymptomatic infections with *C. difficile*, *Cryptosporidium* spp., and *G. lamblia* are not uncommon, and some of the other IGE pathogens such as *Salmonella* spp. and norovirus can be shed for weeks after resolution of symptoms. Comprehensive panels consolidate testing platforms for agents of IGE and substantially reduce, but not completely eliminate, the need for culture because isolates are needed for epidemiologic surveillance and occasionally for antibiotic susceptibility testing.

ANTIBACTERIAL DRUG RESISTANCE

The detection of antibiotic resistance is one of the most important functions of the clinical microbiology laboratory. This has traditionally been done by phenotypic methods. However, the delays inherent in phenotypic tests can lead to delays in appropriate therapy and adverse clinical outcomes. Molecular methods offer faster alternatives for detection of antibiotic resistance, but the genotypic approach has its own set of challenges because of the complexity of antibiotic resistance. In addition, the detection of a resistance gene may not necessarily imply phenotypic resistance if the gene is expressed at low levels or is not functional. Advances in technology and our understanding of the genetics of antibiotic resistance will likely make the use of molecular detection for antibiotic resistance more widespread in the future. This section focuses on the commonly used resistance targets, currently MRSA, vancomycin-resistant enterococci (VRE), and β-lactamases in gram-negative bacteria.

Because *S. aureus* is among the most common cause of bacterial infections in the industrialized world, particular attention has been focused on assays to rapidly differentiate MRSA from MSSA for diagnosis of infection and surveillance for infection control purposes. Molecular assays that recognize MRSA based on detection of a single target detect the junction between the staphylococcal cassette chromosome *mec* element (SCC*mec*), which carries the *mecA* resistance and other genes, and the flanking *orfX* gene.[245] This assay design has several limitations, including false-negative results caused by SCC*mec* variants and false-positive results caused by MSSA strains that carry SCCmec remnants lacking the *mecA* gene, sometimes referred to as "empty cassettes," or that carry SCCmec with a nonfunctional *mecA* gene.[245-247] An alternative approach to molecular detection of MRSA combines a *mecA* target and a second gene target specific for *S. aureus* such as *sa442, nuc, femA-femB, spa,* or *Idh1*.[248] At the time of this writing, there were five companies with FDA-approved assays for molecular detection of MRSA or MRSA and MSSA (BD Diagnostics, Cepheid, Elitech, Roche, and bioMérieux). In addition to these stand-alone assays, molecular detection of MRSA is incorporated into the blood culture identification panels discussed previously. These assays are intended for use in surveillance testing or to assist in the diagnosis of infections. Depending on the platform, the tests can be run on demand or in batches. Studies indicate that use of molecular methods for rapid identification of patients who are colonized with MRSA may be a cost-effective infection control strategy.[249,250]

Enterococci are commensal residents of the GI tract and female genital tract that account for about 10% of hospital-acquired infections. The vast majority of enterococcal infections are caused by *Enterococcus faecalis* and *E. faecium* and occur primarily in patients requiring long-term care. The emergence of VRE in hospitals is concerning because vancomycin is often used empirically to treat a wide variety of infections. Infection with VRE is associated with increased morbidity and mortality because of the propensity of VRE to infect patients already at high risk for comorbidity.[251]

In the United States, about 30% of enterococci are resistant to vancomycin. High-level vancomycin resistance in enterococci occurs via acquisition of mobile transposable elements carrying the *vanA* or *vanB* genes. *E. faecium* is more frequently resistant to vancomycin than *E. faecalis*, and *vanA* is more commonly found than *vanB* in resistant strains. As with MRSA, the rapid detection of VRE colonization to prevent health care–associated infections is widely recommended.[252]

Molecular assays work well for this application.[253,254] Three FDA-approved molecular assays are marketed for rapid detection of VRE from perianal and rectal swabs. The BD GeneOhm and IMDx assays detect both *vanA* and *vanB*, and the Cepheid assay detects *vanA* alone. All are based on real-time PCR, but only the Cepheid assay is designed for on-demand testing. Aside from rare reports of *vanA* in *S. aureus* and *Streptococcus* spp., detection of *vanA* is highly specific for VRE. However, *vanB* can be found in a wide variety of commensal nonenterococcal bacteria, so detection of *vanB* requires confirmation of VRE by culture. As with *mecA*, assays for detection of *vanA* and *vanB* have also been incorporated in the commercially available blood culture identification panels.

One of the greatest threats to our antibiotic formulary is the emergence of β-lactamases in gram-negative bacteria with the capabilities of hydrolyzing broad-spectrum penicillins, cephalosporins, and carbapenems. These enzymes include extended-spectrum β-lactamases (ESBLs), AmpCs, and carbapenemases. The accurate detection of these enzymes is important for both treatment decisions and infection control purposes. Detection of these organisms harboring these broad-spectrum β-lactamases by phenotypic methods is imperfect.[255,256] A rapid, inexpensive, multiplex molecular assay to detect the genes encoding these enzymes would be clinically useful but presently is an unmet need. One of the biggest challenges to molecular detection is the great diversity of β-lactamases, with more than 200 described ESBLs and numerous classes of carbapenemases, including *K. pneumoniae* carbapenemase (KPC), New Delhi metallo-β-lactamase (NDM), Verona integrin-encoded metallo-β-lactamase (VIM), imipenem metallo-β-lactamase (IMP), and oxacillinase (OXA). An additional challenge is that the detection of the gene(s) does not provide information about copy number and expression, which are important to phenotypic expression of resistance to β-lactam and carbapenem antibiotics.

A number of LDTs and RUO kits have been developed for molecular detection of a variety of broad-spectrum β-lactamase genes that range from single target assays to detect KPC to highly multiplexed assays detecting multiple ESBLs, multiple AMPCs, KPC, NDM, VIM, IMP, and OXA-48.[257-262] Both the Biofire FilmArray and Verigene BCID panels include assays to detect KPC, and the Verigene panel detects genes encoding for five additional broad-spectrum β-lactamases, CTX-M, NDM, VIM, IMP, and OXA.

HUMAN MICROBIOME AND METAGENOMICS

Microbial inhabitants outnumber our own body's cells by about 10 to 1 and at a genomic level have 100-fold greater gene content than the human genome. Interest in elucidating the role of resident organisms in human health and disease has flourished over the past decade with the advent of new technologies for interrogating complex microbial communities. The microbiome is the totality of microbes, their genetic information, and the milieu in which they interact.[263] It includes bacteria, fungi, viruses and phages, and parasites, but most of the emphasis to date has been on the bacterial component of the microbiome. However, progress is being made toward defining the human virome and the role that it plays in complex microbial communities.[264]

Metagenomics refers to the concept that a collection of genes sequenced from the environment could be analyzed in a way analogous to the study of a single genome. It has been facilitated by advances in NA sequencing technology, and this technology has permitted the study of microbial communities directly in their natural environment, thus bypassing the need for isolation and cultivation of individual species. We now know that the majority of microorganisms from the human body cannot be cultured in vitro. Most taxonomic metagenomic studies have used targeted sequencing of the phylogenetically informative regions of the 16s rRNA gene from bacteria because it has long been the gold standard method for bacterial identification, and there are large sequence databases and sophisticated analysis tools available.[265] However, 16s rRNA gene sequencing does not provide enough information for comprehensive microbiome studies. To overcome the limitations of single gene-based amplicon sequencing, researchers have used whole-genome shotgun sequencing on massively parallel sequencing platforms. Whole-genome approaches permit identification and annotation of diverse sets of microbial genes that encode many different biochemical or metabolic functions, thus providing functional metagenomic information.

In 2007, the Human Microbiome Project was launched by the National Institutes of Health with the overarching goal of developing tools and resources for characterization of the human microbiome and to relate it to human health and disease.[266-268] Initial microbiome comparisons across 18 different body sites confirmed high interindividual variation with four phyla of bacteria, *Actinobacteria*, *Bacteroidetes*, *Firmicutes*, and *Proteobacteria* predominating across all body sites.[269] Additionally, the composition of the gut microbiome is most often characterized by smooth abundance gradients of key organisms and does not cluster individuals into discrete microbiome types.[268] However, the microbiome at other body sites such as the vagina can show such clustering.[266] An important point that emerged from these early studies is that although the microbial communities varied among individuals, the metabolic pathways encoded by these organisms were consistently present, forming a functional "core" to the microbiome at all body sites.[268,270,271] Although the pathways and processes of this core were consistent, the specific genes associated with these functions varied.

Alterations of the microbiome in many different disease states have been described.[263] A complete review of this topic is beyond the scope of this chapter, but some specific examples are given in Table 48.8. Establishing a causal link between microbiome changes and a specific disease often is challenging because most studies have been observational, the disease entities themselves may not be well defined, and the pathogenesis may be multifactorial.

However, it seems clear that future approaches in medical microbiology will be shaped in part by developments in metagenomics and human microbiome research. The identification of single agents of infection will be supplemented by techniques that will determine the relative composition of microbiomes in the context of different infections and other disease states. Recent evidence that recurrent *C. difficile* infections can be treated by reconstituting the normal colon microbiota in the patient by transferring feces from a normal donor is a good example of how a better understanding of changes in the microbiome composition can lead to effective

TABLE 48.8 Association of Human Disease With Changes in the Microbiome

Disease	Relevant Change
Psoriasis	Increased ratio of *Firmicutes* to *Actinobacteria*[280]
Reflux esophagitis	Esophageal microbiota dominated by gram-negative anaerobes; gastric microbiota with low or absent *Helicobacter pylori*[281,282]
Obesity	*Reduced ratio of Bacteroidetes to Firmicutes*[283,284]
Childhood-onset asthma	Absent gastric *H. pylori* (especially cytotoxin-associated gene genotype[285,286]
Inflammatory bowel disease (colitis)	Increased *Enterobacteriaceae*[287]
Functional bowel diseases	Increased *Veillonella* spp. and *Lactobacillus* spp.[288]
Colorectal carcinoma	Increased *Fusobacterium* spp.[289,290]
Cardiovascular disease	Gut-dependent metabolism of phosphatidylcholine[291]

Modified from Cho I, Blaser MJ. The human microbiome: at the interface of health and disease. *Nat Rev Genet* 2012;13:260–270.

treatments options.[272] Differences in the composition of the microbiome that may cause or contribute to noninfectious diseases may offer new opportunities for clinical microbiology laboratories to impact other areas of medicine. Finally, metagenomic techniques will facilitate the discovery of previously unrecognized pathogens and increase our understanding of how changes in the microbiome may contribute to infectious diseases.

FUTURE DIRECTIONS

Molecular microbiology will continue to be one of the leading growth areas in laboratory medicine. The number of applications of this technology in clinical microbiology will continue to increase, and the technology will increasingly be deployed in clinical laboratories as it becomes less technically complex and thus more accessible. However, now more than ever, clinical and financial outcomes data will be needed to justify the use of this often expensive technology in an era of declining reimbursement and increased cost consciousness.

The clinical utility of molecular testing for infectious diseases is now well established, and the gap between the availability of FDA-cleared and -approved tests and clinical need is improving. However, the pending enhanced oversight of LDTs and restriction of the use of RUO and IUO reagents and systems by the FDA could limit the ability of laboratories to develop tests to meet clinical needs not met by IVD products (http://www.fda.gov/downloads/medicaldevices/deviceregulationandguidance/guidancedocuments/ucm416684.pdf).

Although considerable progress has been made in recent years, other important needs remain unmet, including the availability of international standards and traceable and commutable calibrators that can be used for assay verification and validation. These materials, when widely available, should improve agreement of the results between or among different tests and aid in the establishment of their clinical utility. Another need is for the continued development of effective proficiency testing programs that will help ensure that the results of molecular tests are reliable and reproducible among laboratories.

Digital PCR is the next advance in the evolution of quantitative PCR methods. Digital PCR has many applications, including detection and quantification of low numbers of pathogen sequences. It can provide a lower limit of detection than real-time PCR methods with better precision at very low concentrations. As opposed to relative quantification, digital PCR provides absolute quantification with no need for reference standards. Currently, digital PCR is used as a research tool, but it may find applications in clinical laboratories to resolve ambiguous results obtained with quantitative real-time PCR assays or for creating accurate viral reference standards as the technology becomes less costly.[273,274]

To a great extent, the future of molecular microbiology depends on automation. Many of the available tests are labor intensive, with much of the labor devoted to tedious sample processing methods. Several fully automated systems for molecular diagnostics have been developed for high- and midvolume laboratories, but most suffer from a limited test menu. To increase access to molecular tests, simple, affordable, fully automated, random access platforms with broad test menus are needed, particularly for laboratories that have a low- and midvolume of testing. NA testing for infectious diseases at the point of care is beginning to enter clinical practice in developed and developing countries, particularly for applications that require short TATs and in settings where a centralized laboratory approach is not feasible.[275]

The use of multiplex NA-based assays to screen at-risk patients for panels of probable pathogens remains a goal for molecular microbiology. Several such tests are currently available, but success to date has been limited by technical complexity of some systems. The development of simple, multiparametric technologies is key to providing molecular tests with the same broad diagnostic range provided by culture and other conventional methods for syndromic diagnosis of infectious diseases.

Metagenomic studies have provided new insights into the human microbiome and alterations in these communities of microorganisms have been linked to a number of disease states. With the continued decrease in the cost of massively parallel NA sequencing and the increasing availability of the necessary bioinformatics tools, it is likely that our understanding of the human microbiome will result in novel microbiome-focused diagnostics and clinical interventions. In addition, the massively parallel sequencing platforms that have enabled metagenomics will be increasingly used in epidemiological investigations[276,277] and new pathogen discovery.[278,279]

SELECTED REFERENCES

For a full list of references for this chapter, please refer to ExpertConsult.com.

11. Centers for Disease Control and Prevention and Association of Public Health Laboratories. Laboratory Testing for the Diagnosis of HIV Infection: Updated Recommendations.

Available at: <http://stacks.cdc.gov/view/cdc/23447>; Published June 27, 2014.

27. Centers for Disease Control and Prevention. Testing for HCV infection: an update of Guidance for Clinicians and Laboratorians. *MMWR Recomm Rep* 2013;**62**:362–5.
71. Horvath R, Tegtmeier GE. Hepatitis B and D Viruses. In: Versalovic J, et al., editors. *Manual of clinical microbiology*. 10th ed. Washington DC: ASM Press; 2011.
93. Caliendo AM, St. George K, Allega J, et al. Distinguishing cytomegalovirus (CMV) infection and disease with CMV nucleic acid assays. *J Clin Microbiol* 2002;**40**:1581–6.
107. Gulley ML, Tang W. Laboratory assays for Epstein-Barr virus-related disease. *J Mol Diagn* 2008;**10**:279–92.
121. Hirsch HH, Brennan DC, Drachenberg CB, et al. Polyomavirus-associated nephropathy in renal transplantation: interdisciplinary analyses and recommendations. *Transplantation* 2005;**79**:1277–86.
141. Centers for Disease Control and Prevention. Recommendations for the Laboratory-Based Detection of Chlamydia trachomatis and Neisseria gonorrhoeae. *MMWR Recomm Rep* 2014;**63**(RR–2):1–19.
152. Schwebke JR, Hobbs MM, Taylor SN, et al. Molecular testing for Trichomonas vaginalis in women: results from a prospective U. S. Clinical trial. *J Clin Microbiol* 2011;**49**:4106–11.
154. Scoular A. Using evidence base on genital herpes: optimizing the use of diagnostic tests and information provision. *Sex Transm Infect* 2002;**78**:160–5.
160. Saslow D, Solomon D, Lawson HW, et al. American Cancer Society, American Society for Colposcopy and Cervical Pathology, and the American Society for Clinical Pathology screening guidelines for the prevention and early detection of cervical cancer. *CA Cancer J Clin* 2012;**62**:147–72.
175. Popowitch EB, O'Neill SS, Miller MB. Comparison of Biofire FilmArray RP, Genmark eSensor RVP, Luminex xTAG RVPv1 and Luminex RVP Fast multiplex assays for detection of respiratory viruses. *J Clin Microbiol* 2013;**51**:1528–33.
188. Centers for Disease Control and Prevention. Updated guidelines for the use of nucleic acid amplification tests in the diagnosis of tuberculosis. *MMWR Recomm Rep* 2009;**58**:7–10.
195. Loeffelholtz M. Towards improved accuracy of Bordetella pertussis nucleic acid amplification tests. *J Clin Microbiol* 2012;**50**:2186–90.
198. Pence MA, TeKippe EM, Burnham C-A. Diagnostic assays for identification of microorganisms and antimicrobial resistance determinants directly from positive blood culture broth. *Clin Lab Med* 2013;**33**:651–84.
208. Josefson P, Strålin K, Ohlin T, et al. Evaluation of a commercial multiplex PCR test (SeptiFast) in the etiological diagnosis of community-onset bloodstream infections. *Eur J Clin Microbiol Infect Dis* 2011;**30**:1127–34.
220. Lakeman F, Whitley RJ. Diagnosis of herpes simplex encephalitis: application of polymerase chain reaction to cerebrospinal fluid from brain-biopsied patients and correlation with disease. National Institute of Allergy and Infectious Diseases Collaborative Antiviral Study Group. *J Infect Dis* 1995;**171**:857.
231. Ramers C, Billman G, Hartin M, et al. Impact of a diagnostic cerebrospinal fluid enterovirus polymerase chain reaction test on patient management. *JAMA* 2000;**283**:2680–5.
236. Wilcox MH, Planche T, Fang FC. What is the role of algorithmic approaches for diagnosis of Clostridium difficile infection? *J Clin Microbiol* 2011;**48**:4347–53.
239. Reddington K, Tuite N, Minogue E, et al. A current overview of commercially available nucleic acid diagnostic approaches to detect and identify human gastroenteritis pathogens. *Biomol Detect Quantif* 2014;**1**:2–7.
248. Carroll KC. Rapid diagnostics for methicillin-resistant Staphylococcus aureus: current status. *Mol Diagn Ther* 2008;**12**:15–24.
263. Cho I, Blaser MJ. The human microbiome: at the interface of health and disease. *Nat Rev Genet* 2012;**13**:260–70.

49

Genetics

Cindy L. Vnencak-Jones and D. Hunter Best

ABSTRACT

Background

The invention of polymerase chain reaction along with the chemistry of fluorescently labeled molecules, high density DNA single nucleotide polymorphism arrays for genome-wide association studies (GWAS), massively parallel sequencing (MPS) technology, the development of chromosomal microarrays, the availability of public databases, and advances in bioinformatics have revolutionized the field of human genetics. The collective use of GWAS and exome- and whole-genome DNA sequencing has facilitated disease discovery and the identification of pathogenic variants for diseases in which the underlying genetic cause was previously unknown. This knowledge has enhanced the efforts for personalized medicine, or a tailored approach to therapy based on an individual's genotype.

Content

This chapter discusses recent advances in the field using some common inherited autosomal recessive, autosomal dominant, and X-linked diseases as examples. In addition, some common mitochondrial, imprinting, and complex disorders and inherited cancers are reviewed. For each disease, information regarding the clinical phenotype, gene, protein function, treatment, and currently used clinical molecular diagnostic techniques are summarized.

DISEASES WITH MENDELIAN INHERITANCE

Autosomal Recessive Disorders

An individual with an autosomal recessive disease has inherited two abnormal alleles at a given locus by receiving one mutant allele from each carrier parent; the disease-causing gene is on one of the autosomes (1–22) and not on a sex chromosome (X or Y). Typically, the carrier parent with one abnormal allele has no clinical features of the disease yet possesses a 50% risk of donating the mutant allele to his or her offspring. Matings in which both partners are carriers of an abnormal allele have a 25% chance of producing a child with both normal alleles, a 50% chance of having a child that has received only one abnormal allele, and a 25% chance of having an affected child. The affected patient may be homozygous for a specific mutation by receiving the same mutation from each parent or may be a compound heterozygote having received a different mutation from each parent. The specific mutations present influence the clinical severity of the disease and account for variability in the expression of the disease between patients, referred to as genotype–phenotype correlation. Modifier genes and environmental factors also play a role in determining the patient's phenotype. Among pedigrees illustrating autosomal recessive disorders, males and females are equally affected, and for rare diseases, consanguinity is likely to be observed. Table 49.1 provides a list of some of the inherited autosomal recessive disorders commonly tested in clinical molecular diagnostic laboratories.

Cystic Fibrosis

Cystic fibrosis (CF) (Online Mendelian Inheritance in Man [OMIM] #219700) is one of the most common autosomal recessive diseases in people of Northern European ancestry with an estimated incidence in the United States of about 1 in 2500 and a carrier frequency of about 1 in 25.[1] Within other ethnic populations, the disease has an estimated incidence of 1 in 2300 Ashkenazi Jews, 1 in 8500 Hispanics, 1 in 17,000 African Americans, and 1 in 35,000 Asian Americans.[2] CF is a multisystem disorder characterized by progressive pulmonary disease, pancreatic insufficiency, elevated sweat electrolytes, male infertility, and a predisposition to sinonasal disease. An abnormal sweat chloride concentration is considered the gold standard for the diagnosis of CF, and a result of 60 mmol/L or greater is considered diagnostic of CF. However, some patients with disease-causing mutations may have indeterminate or borderline values of 30 to 59 mmol/L if they are younger than 6 months of age or 40 to 59 mmol/L if they are older than 6 months of age.[3,4] Although values of less than 30 mmol/L or less than 40 mmol/L, respectively make the diagnosis of CF less likely, normal measurements can be obtained in some patients. By virtue of the intricacies of this test, it is recommended that these tests only be performed at a Cystic Fibrosis Foundation–accredited care center (https://www.cff.org). Interestingly, the phenotypic expression of the disease is heterogeneous, ranging from meconium ileus and severe respiratory disease in infants to mild pulmonary symptoms and no evidence of gastrointestinal problems in adulthood. Atypical CF patients with a nonclassic presentation may have involvement of only one organ, as in congenital bilateral absence of the vas deferens (CBAVD), pancreatitis, rhinosinusitis, or nasal polyps.[3,5,6] Variability in expression is explained by both allelic heterogeneity at the CF gene locus and genetic variation in modifier genes. Loss or decreased amounts of the disease-associated protein cause mucous

TABLE 49.1 Examples of Autosomal Recessive Disorders

Disease	Gene	Location	OMIM Entry #	Incidence
α_1-Antitrypsin	*SERPINA1*	14q32.13	613490	1 in 5000–7000
Canavan disease	*ASPA*	17p13.2	271900	1 in 6400–13,400 Ashkenazi Jews (less common in other populations)
Friedreich ataxia	*FXN*	9q21.11	229300	1 in 25,000–50,000
Gaucher disease type I	*GBA*	1q22	230800	1 in 850 Ashkenazi Jews (less common in other populations)
Glycogen storage disease	*G6PC*	17q21.31	232200	1 in 100,000
Hereditary hemochromatosis	*HFE*	6p22.2	235200	1 in 200–350
Hurler syndrome: mucopolysaccharidosis type 1	*IDUA*	4p16.3	607014	1 in 100,000
Medium-chain acyl-coenzyme A dehydrogenase (MCAD) deficiency	*ACADM*	1p31.1	201450	1 in 4900–17,000
Niemann-Pick type C	*NPC1*	18q11.2	257220	1 in 100,000–150,000
Tay Sachs disease	*HEXA*	15q23	272800	1 in 3500 Ashkenazi Jews (less common in other populations)

OMIM, Online Mendelian Inheritance in Man.

accumulation and airway obstruction; recurrent infection with pathogens, such as *Pseudomonas aeruginosa, Burkholderia cepacia, Staphylococcus aureus,* and *Haemophilus influenzae;* and excessive inflammation with progressive lung damage and ultimately respiratory failure.[7-9] Because morbidity and mortality are most related to severe lung disease, daily management of these patients is to prevent bacterial lung infections through physical therapy of the chest and early or aggressive treatments to eradicate bacterial colonization. Although originally considered a fatal childhood disease, the US Cystic Fibrosis Foundation reported that in 2008, more than 45% of patients were older than 18 years of age. Furthermore, the median survival age among approximately 23,000 patients with CF who received care through one of the nationwide CF care centers was 37.4 years with the life expectancy of patients born now in their 50s. The increase in survival age is due to organ transplantation, improved nutrition, and new therapies.[10-13] The disease is complex with clinical management of most patients at one of more than 110 specialized care centers in the CF Care Center Network.[14-16] This approach provides widespread communication among health care providers who are experts in the care of patients with CF and enables monitoring of a large population of patients with respect to treatment outcome, health care, and disease-specific variables.

The severity and frequency of the disease led to an intensive search for the gene, which was eventually cloned in 1989.[17-19] The CF gene maps to chromosome 7q31.2 with 27 exons encoding a transcript of approximately 6.5 kb. The CF transmembrane conductance regulator protein (CFTR) has 1480 amino acids and is a member of the ATP-binding cassette (ABC) transporter superfamily of membrane transport proteins. CFTR consists of two transmembrane domains (TMDs), each containing six hydrophobic transmembrane sections and one hydrophilic intracellular nucleotide-binding domain (NBD).[18] The TMD/NBD segments are linked by a highly charged regulatory domain containing multiple sites for phosphorylation and activation. The molecule is unique among ABC proteins because it does not actively transport but rather serves as an ATP-gated chloride ion channel pore within the lipid bilayer, predominantly at the apical membrane of secretory epithelial cells. In addition to epithelial chloride conductance as an ion channel, CFTR mediates the passage of bicarbonate and other small ions, including sodium and potassium, from the intracellular compartment to the extracellular surface.[20-23] Whereas opening and closing of the channel requires ATP binding and hydrolysis (ATP-gated channel), channel activity requires phosphorylation of the cytoplasmic regulatory domain by protein kinase A. The wide clinical diversity of CF is based in part on the varying effects conferred on this protein from the more than 2000 mutations reported within this gene.[24]

Because CF is an autosomal recessive disorder, patients with CF must have two mutant *CFTR* alleles to develop the disease. Some mutations are "private" and unique to a family; others may be common among CF patients. Patients may be homozygous with two copies of the same mutation, or they may be compound heterozygotes with one copy of one mutation and one copy of a second mutation. More than half of all mutations are missense or frameshift mutations, with exon 14 containing the largest number of different disease-causing mutations.[24] The types of mutations and frequencies of each differ significantly among populations.[25] Mutations can be divided into six classes based on their effect on the protein[26] (Table 49.2). Class I mutations result in no functional protein production and include nonsense or frameshift mutations that cause premature truncation of the protein, splice site mutations, and exon or gene deletions or rearrangements. Class II mutations are the most common and are associated with defective processing of CFTR and the inability of the protein to reach the apical cell surface. Class II mutations cause misfolding of the fully translated CFTR protein and result from an amino acid alteration such as a deletion or a missense mutation. In the case of class I and II mutations, CFTR is not present on the apical cell membrane, and as predicted, these mutations are typically associated with a severe disease phenotype. Class III and IV mutations are generally due to missense mutations that result in full-length CFTR expression at the cell membrane. Class III mutations are more severe, resulting in defective regulation; class IV mutations generally cause a milder phenotype with reduced conduction of ion flow. Class V mutations are associated with reduced

TABLE 49.2 American College of Obstetricians and Gynecologists/American College of Medical Genetics Recommended Mutation Panel for Cystic Fibrosis Carrier Screening

Mutation Frequency Among Patients With Clinically Diagnosed Cystic Fibrosis (%)						
***CFTR* Mutation**	**Mutation Class**	**Ashkenazi Jewish**	**Non-Hispanic White**	**Hispanic White**	**African American**	**Asian American**
p.Phe508del	II	31.41	72.42	54.38	44.07	38.95
p.Gly542Ter	I	7.55	2.28	5.10	1.45	0.00
p.Trp1282Ter	I	45.92	1.50	0.63	0.24	0.00
p.Gly551Asp	III	0.22	2.25	0.56	1.21	3.15
c.621+1G>T	I	0.00	1.57	0.26	1.11	0.00
p.Asn1303Lys	II	2.78	1.27	1.66	0.35	0.76
p.Arg553Ter	I	0.00	0.87	2.81	2.32	0.76
p.Ile507del	II	0.22	0.88	0.68	1.87	0.00
c.3489+10kbC>T	V	4.77	0.58	1.57	0.17	5.31
c.3120+1G>T	V	0.10	0.08	0.16	9.57	0.00
p.Arg117His	IV	0.00	0.70	0.11	0.06	0.00
c.1717-1G>T	I	0.67	0.48	0.27	0.37	0.00
c.2789+5G>A	V	0.10	0.48	0.16	0.00	0.00
p.Arg347Pro	IV	0.00	0.45	0.16	0.06	0.00
c.711+1G>T	I	0.10	0.43	0.23	0.00	0.00
p.Arg334Trp	IV	0.00	0.14	1.78	0.49	0.00
p.Arg560Thr	II	0.00	0.38	0.00	0.17	0.00
p.Arg1162Ter	I	0.00	0.23	0.58	0.66	0.00
c.3659delC	I	0.00	0.34	0.13	0.06	0.00
p.Ala455Glu	V	0.00	0.34	0.05	0.00	0.00
p.Gly85Glu	II	0.00	0.29	0.23	0.12	0.00
c.2184delA	I	0.10	0.17	0.16	0.05	0.00
c.1898+1G>A	I	0.10	0.16	0.05	0.06	0.00
Total		**94.04**	**88.29**	**71.72**	**64.46**	**48.93**

Modified from Watson MS, Cutting GR, Desnick RJ, et al. Cystic fibrosis population carrier screening: 2004 revision of American College of Medical Genetics mutation panel. *Genet Med* 2004;6:387-391.

amounts of CFTR at the cell membrane and are most often associated with abnormal splicing and decreased amounts of normal *CFTR* messenger RNA (mRNA). These mutations may be associated with a severe phenotype (c.621+1G>T) or a mild phenotype (c.2789+5G>A). Last, class VI mutations cause decreased stability of CFTR in the membrane. In this chapter, the nomenclature for variants follows the Human Genome Variation Society (http://www.hgvs.org/mutnomen), and variants are specified by either the amino acid in the protein (p.) or by the base in the cDNA (c.).

The most common mutation, p.Phe508del (c.1521_1523delCTT), is a class II mutation and is detected in about 70% of CF alleles in whites of Northern European descent. This CFTR protein is misfolded and not properly processed by the endoplasmic reticulum with the majority of the protein rapidly degraded.[27] Whereas common mutations p.Gly542Ter and p.Trp1282Ter are class I mutations and cause premature translation termination and premature truncation of the protein, mutation p.Gly551Asp results in a full-length CFTR that reaches the apical membrane but improperly regulates the chloride channel.[28,29] Infertile males with only the genital form of CF—congenital bilateral absence of the vas deferens (CBAVD)—usually have a mutation associated with a severe phenotype on one allele and a mutation associated with a mild phenotype on the second allele. The most frequently reported *CFTR* genotype in this population is the 5T polymorphism in intron 8, c.1210-12T(5), which corresponds to a sequence of five thymidines.[3] This 5T variant is observed in about 5% of *CFTR* alleles and is less common than the 7T or 9T alleles, c.1210-12T(7) or c.1210-12T(9). The 5T variant affects mRNA splicing and can cause exon 9 to be deleted; without exon 9, the chloride channel is not functional.[30-32] An adjacent polymorphic TG dinucleotide sequence c.1210-34TG(9-13) regulates the efficiency of mRNA splicing, with the higher number of TG repeats c.1210-34TG(13) associated with decreased efficiency of splicing.[33] Thus, the c.1210-12T(5) c.1210-34TG(12) or c.1210-12T(5) c.1210-34TG(13) allele is more commonly associated with an abnormal phenotype than is the c.1210-12T(5) c.1210-34TG(11) allele.

Understanding the effect of each mutation on the CFTR protein is important for choosing the corrective drug therapy required for each patient.[12,13,26,34] Therapy for patients with class I or II mutations is the most challenging because CFTR in most cases is absent or in reduced amounts. Gene therapy to deliver a functional CFTR protein is one effective way to treat these patients and is also applicable to CF patients with mutations in classes other than I or II. Alternatively, for patients in this group with a nonsense stop codon such as p.Gly542Ter, the drug ataluren, an orally administered small molecule that enables readthrough of the transcript, has been attempted. Unfortunately, aminoglycoside antibiotics frequently used by patients with CF can potentially inhibit this molecule, rendering it less effective in a subset of patients. For some class II and for all class III mutations, the potentiator ivacaftor has been administered to increase the effectiveness of chloride transfer through the channel. This drug improves the clinical outcome of patients, especially for those with the common mutation p.Gly551Asp. This drug is also used in patients with mutations in class IV, V, and VI. Ivacaftor has proven more effective in some class II mutations, most notably the common p.Phe508del mutation, in combination with a second small molecule, lumacaftor. Lumacaftor, a CFTR corrector molecule, helps the misfolded p.Phe508del protein reach the cell surface. Most recently, antisense oligonucleotides have been examined as a potential therapy for some class V mutations.[35]

The *CFTR* genotype and clinical phenotype correlations are most closely related for pancreatic involvement rather than for pulmonary manifestations of the disease.[36,37] Most patients with two "severe" mutations, which cause a "severe" CF phenotype, usually classes I to III, have pancreatic insufficiency, but patients with one or two "mild" mutations, which cause a "mild" CF phenotype, generally classes IV to VI, have pancreatic sufficiency (PS) but have an increased risk of developing pancreatitis.[38] Furthermore, CF patients with PS generally have milder disease with longer overall survival, a later age of diagnosis, and lower sweat chloride levels. Although mutations in *CFTR* confer susceptibility to pancreatitis, variants in several other genes inherited in combination with or without *CFTR* variants are seen in patients with chronic pancreatitis.[39] In contrast, lung disease is more dependent on environmental factors and genetic modifiers.[7,38,40] Environmental modulating factors of lung disease include secondhand smoke and varying exposure to pathogens.[41] Genes that modify lung disease among patients with identical genotypes include inflammatory response genes that code for cytokines such as transforming growth factor β1 (TGF-β1) or interleukin-8 (IL8) or pathogen response genes such as mannose binding lectin 2 *(MBL2)*. Other modifying variants may include genes whose proteins are associated with tissue damage or repair, such as glutathione S-transferases *(GSTs)* or nitric oxide synthetases *(NOS1, NOS3)*. Genes that encode proteins for ion transport or cytoskeleton structure such as voltage-gated chloride channel protein or keratin 8 type 2 protein may also modulate the phenotype.[38] More recently, miRNAs have been proposed to explain the observed clinical heterogeneity among patients with the same mutation.[42]

DNA testing for the identification of *CFTR* mutations is performed for a variety of reasons (Box 49.1). It is performed to confirm the diagnosis of disease in patients with equivocal sweat chloride results or when an insufficient amount of sweat is collected and no results are obtained from the test. The presence of two known pathogenic *CFTR* mutations is diagnostic for CF. A diagnosis of CF can be considered in the patient with a *CFTR*-related disorder such as chronic pancreatitis, CBAVD, or sinusitis. In known CF patients, mutation analysis can be requested to help predict the prognosis based on genotype–phenotype correlations and initiate mutation-specific treatment options. At the same time, identifying the *CFTR* gene mutations that are present in the proband and how they segregate in the family enables preimplantation diagnosis or prenatal testing for subsequent pregnancies if desired and allows carrier or diagnostic testing for other at-risk family members. Similarly, state-sponsored newborn screening (NBS) programs have detected infants with CF and at the same time have identified at-risk family members and enabled carrier or diagnostic genetic testing. Most important, NBS allows for early diagnosis and referral to CF care centers for early intervention and management of CF-related clinical symptoms. In the United States, NBS for CF is conducted in all 50 states and the District of Columbia and is based on the measurement of immunoreactive trypsinogen (IRT) from dried blood spots to detect elevated levels of this pancreatic enzyme. However, states vary in their NBS algorithms. In some states, a positive result is followed by IRT retesting; in others, blood from the newborn is submitted for *CFTR* mutation analysis.[43,44] Confirmation of the diagnosis requires a sweat chloride test but may not always be effective in infants younger than 2 weeks.[43] A diagnostic conundrum occurs when sweat chloride testing is normal or intermediate and the phenotypic consequence of one or two of the *CFTR* variants detected is uncertain. In the United States, these children do not meet the diagnostic criteria and are classified as having *CFTR*-related metabolic syndrome.[45] These patients should be monitored closely and may ultimately develop symptoms of CF, albeit with a milder disease course.[46] Other patients with CF-like disease with borderline sweat chloride results and clinical features associate with CF but no *CFTR* gene variants detected may have complex genotypes with variants in one or more genes possibly in a contributory oligogenic fashion.[47] Some couples referred for CF carrier testing or prenatal testing of the fetus have no family history of CF but rather the presentation of hyperechogenic bowel in the fetus on routine ultrasonography.

BOX 49.1 Referrals for *CFTR* Mutation Analysis

- Confirm diagnosis of cystic fibrosis
- Determine prognosis
- Screen patient with pancreatitis
- Family member testing
- Newborn screening
- Preconception couples
- Expectant couples
- Prenatal testing—at-risk fetus
- Prenatal testing—hyperechogenic bowel
- Preimplantation genetic diagnosis
- Infertile male with congenital bilateral absence of the vas deferens
- Semen and oocyte donors

Cystic fibrosis carrier screening may be offered as a single gene-specific test or may be included within high-throughput large carrier screening panels that detect both common *CFTR* gene mutations as well as targeted mutations in other genes.[48,49] Although these more extensive panels provide additional information to patients, they contain genes for inherited conditions for which population-based screening is not recommended in current practice guidelines.[50] CF carrier screening for preconception and expectant couples was first recommended in October 2001 by the American College of Obstetricians and Gynecologists (ACOG) in conjunction with the American College of Medical Genetics (ACMG). A core

TABLE 49.3 Cystic Fibrosis Mutation Carrier Risk

	Ashkenazi Jewish	Non-Hispanic White	Hispanic White	African American	Asian American
Detection rate of ACOG/ACMG 23 mutation panel (%)	94	88	72	64	49
Estimated carrier risk in population	1/24	1/25	1/58	1/61	1/94
Estimated residual carrier risk after no mutation detected on screening panel	1/380	1/200	1/200	1/170	1/180

ACMG, American College of Medical Genetics; *ACOG,* American College of Obstetricians and Gynecologists.
Modified from ACOG committee opinion no. 486: update on carrier screening for cystic fibrosis. *Obstet Gynecol* 2011;117:1028-1031.

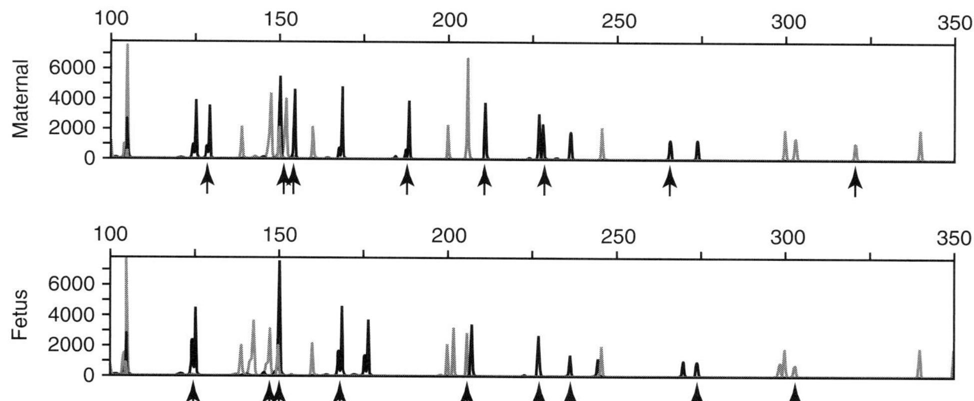

FIGURE 49.1 Electropherograms obtained after polymerase chain reaction (PCR) amplification of maternal *(upper panel)* and fetal *(lower panel)* DNA at nine independently segregating loci and one gender-specific marker. Extracted maternal and fetal DNA were amplified by PCR using a multiplex PCR assay with fluorescent labeled primers (AmpFLSTR Profiler Plus ID PCR Amplification Kit; Applied Biosystems, Foster City, California). Amplicons were detected after capillary electrophoresis on an ABI 3130*xl* Genetic Analyzer and were analyzed using GeneMapper software (Applied Biosystems). Amplicon sizes in bases are noted at the top of the figure and the relative amount of fluorescence detected for each amplicon is measured by the peak height (y-axis). *Arrows* in the *upper panel* denote maternal alleles absent in the fetal DNA specimen. *Arrows* in the *bottom panel* indicate maternal alleles inherited by the fetus.

panel of the most common mutations includes those with an estimated prevalence of at least 0.1% of CF mutant alleles and a carrier detection rate of about 88% for non-Hispanic whites (see Table 49.2).[51] The intent of the screening panel is to identify individuals at risk for classical CF, not isolated CBAVD; thus it is recommended that the 5T/7T/9T status be reviewed and reported only in the presence of variant p.Arg117His, which can be in *cis* with either the 5T or 7T variant. This allows for distinction between p.Arg117His-5T and p.Arg117His-7T individuals and enables genetic counseling and potential prenatal testing options for individuals who are *CFTR* p.Arg117His-5T positive and are at risk of having an offspring with a classic CF phenotype if their reproductive partner is also a carrier of CF. Although CF is more common in the white and Ashkenazi Jewish populations, the standard of care recommended by the ACOG is to make CF testing available to all preconception or expectant couples, especially because it is becoming more difficult to assign a single ethnicity to a patient to best determine the carrier risk.[1] Counseling for CF carrier testing is complex and should include information about CF and CFTR-related disorders and the a priori likelihood of having a child with CF based on personal and family history and ethnicity.[52] Furthermore, it is important for the patient to understand the inability of the screening panel to detect all CF mutations and the residual risk of being a carrier despite a negative test result (Table 49.3).[1] This is especially important for patients in ethnic groups for which the *CFTR* gene mutation detection level is reduced. The genetics professional should discuss the possibility of stigmatization or anxiety associated with being a carrier of a genetic disease and how knowing this information may affect her pregnancy. After DNA testing, it is very important for the genetics professional to know relevant family history when interpreting and reporting the test results to the patient and reproductive partner to accurately assess the risk to the couple of having a child with CF.

In families at risk for a child with CF, prenatal testing of the fetus may be requested. In these prenatal cases and for all DNA testing of fetal DNA, it is the standard of care that the DNA extracted from the fetus be tested for the presence of maternal contamination because the presence of maternal DNA can interfere with interpretation of test results. This is best performed by using polymerase chain reaction (PCR) amplification for highly polymorphic short tandem repeat loci coupled with capillary electrophoresis (Fig. 49.1). In the case of prenatal *CFTR* gene mutation testing with a maternal carrier, if the fetus actually has no mutant *CFTR* allele but the extracted fetal DNA is contaminated with maternal DNA, the mutant maternal *CFTR* allele could be detected, and the fetal DNA test result could be erroneously interpreted as a carrier of a mutant *CFTR* gene. Furthermore, if the fetus inherited a paternal *CFTR* mutation and maternal DNA contaminated the fetal DNA specimen, the fetal DNA test results could show the presence of two *CFTR* gene mutations, and the fetal DNA test result could be erroneously interpreted as a compound heterozygote affected with CF.

CFTR gene mutation testing is performed using a laboratory developed test or one of a variety of commercially available platforms with kits cleared by the US Food and Drug Administration (FDA). The number of mutations detected by each assay is variable, and the median turnaround time is 14 days.[53] Furthermore, because the detection rate of the 23 mutation gene panel is lower in some ethnicities, laboratories serving such populations should consider supplementing this screening panel with additional mutation analysis.[54] Although full gene sequencing by Sanger or massively parallel sequencing (MPS) can be done to detect *CFTR* gene mutations, current practice guidelines do not recommend this methodology for CF carrier screening.[1] Rather, sequencing of the *CFTR* gene should be performed in the context of (1) confirming the diagnosis of CF in a newborn with a positive IRT and a clinical suspicion of CF but no or only one *CFTR* gene mutation was detected with the 23 common mutation panel, (2) identification of *CFTR* mutations in a CF patient in which both *CFTR* mutations were not detected with the 23 *CFTR* gene mutation panel, and (3) confirmation of CF in a patient with a *CFTR*-related disease to rule out CF. In all cases, if *CFTR* gene mutations are identified by sequencing in the proband, targeted analysis to specifically screen for that mutation in at-risk family members may be performed.

Spinal Muscular Atrophy

The spinal muscular atrophies (SMAs) are a heterogeneous group of neurodegenerative disorders characterized by progressive loss of motor neurons in the spinal cord and lower brainstem with muscle weakness and atrophy. A wide clinical spectrum is observed with variability in age of onset, motor function impairment, and inheritance patterns, with 33 contributing genes thus far.[55] SMN-related SMA or SMA5q is an autosomal recessive disorder that accounts for up to 95% of SMAs, has an incidence of 1 in 6000 to 10,000 births, and is a leading cause of death in infants. SMA5q is caused by mutations in the survival motor neuron 1 gene *(SMN1)* and is divided into four types based on clinical presentation and age of onset.[56] Type 1 (OMIM #253300) is the most common (50%); it is associated with age of onset younger than 6 months and has a median survival time of less than 1 year. These children have profound hypotonia, no control of head movement, and are unable to sit. Intercostal muscle weakness leads to respiratory failure and tongue fasciculation, dysphagia, and fatigue, making feeding difficult, worsening the condition, and increasing the risk of aspiration pneumonia. A subdivision of this group into type 1 (0–6 months) and type 0 with prenatal onset and severe disease at birth has been proposed.[56] SMA type II (OMIM #253550), representing about 20% of cases, has an age of onset between 7 and 18 months with median survival into the third decade of life. These children can sit, and some can stand, although none can walk independently. SMA type III (OMIM #253400) is seen in about 30% of patients and has an age of onset after 18 months. These patients have a mild phenotype with gradually progressive disease but a normal life expectancy. SMA type IV (OMIM #271150) is rare and is the mildest of all forms. This type was initially characterized by muscle weakness in the second or third decade of life. These patients are ambulatory and have a normal lifespan.

The gene for SMA, *SMN1*, was mapped to chromosome 5q11.2-13.3 in 1990 and cloned in 1995.[57-59] This gene contains 9 exons (numbered 1, 2a, 2b, and 3–8) spanning about 28,000 bases and encodes a 1.7 kb mRNA transcript producing a 38-kDa protein composed of 294 amino acids that is ubiquitously expressed in the nucleus and cytoplasm.[60] The SMN protein is one of nine core proteins in a multiprotein complex that also contains the proteins Unrip and Gemins2-8.[61] This complex is enriched in the nucleus in size and number to form Gems.[62] The SMN-GEMINs is essential for the cytoplasmic assembly of small ribonucleoproteins (snRNPs) into the spliceosome, critical components for pre-mRNA splicing.[63] SMN is essential during embryogenesis, evidenced by embryonic lethality in *SMN1* knockout mice.[64] In the majority of cases, SMA results from homozygous deletions of *SMN1*. Some SMA cases result from gene conversion of *SMN1*, and in 2% to 5% of cases, patients are compound heterozygotes with an *SMN1* deletion on one allele and a pathogenic loss-of-function or point mutation on the second allele.[65,66] In rare cases, a point mutation in *SMN1* is present on both alleles.

SMN1 is contained within a large inverted repeat sequence that contains the highly homologous *SMN2* gene. *SMN2* differs from *SMN1* by only five bases; it lies in the opposite orientation and is centromeric to *SMN1*.[58,67] Although the five bases that differ between *SMN1* and *SMN2* do not affect the amino acid sequence of the protein, a C-to-T transition in exon 7 of *SMN2* corresponding to codon 280 causes alternative splicing and the deletion of exon 7 in 90% of *SMN2* transcripts.[68] Without exon 7, SMN is unstable and is unable to efficiently oligomerize to form the SMN complex that drives snRNP assembly.[69] Thus, even though most patients with SMA have intact *SMN2* genes, they still have disease because most *SMN2* transcripts do not contain exon 7 (SMAΔ7). Thus the pathogenesis of the disease in most patients results from no *SMN1* transcripts, few full length *SMN2* transcripts, limited functional SMN protein, reduced snRNP assembly, and ultimately aberrant mRNA splicing.

The *SMN2* gene is in part a modifier of the severity of SMA, and its effect is based on the *SMN2* gene copy number.[65,70,71] Some *SMN1* deletion haplotypes also contain an *SMN2* deletion, but other *SMN1* deletion haplotypes may have two or even three copies of *SMN2*. In patients with milder forms of the disease, three or four copies of *SMN2* may be present.[65] Increased *SMN2* copies result in production of more *SMN2* transcripts, some of which translate to functional SMN protein, thereby providing some normal SMN protein for required cellular functions. Prior et al described three unrelated individuals with *SMN1* homozygous deletions and 1 or 2 *SMN2* genes but an unexpected mild phenotype.[72] A point mutation in exon 7 of *SMN2* in these patients created an exonic splicing enhancer element and increased levels of full-length *SMN2* transcript to regain increased cellular levels of SMN protein despite the homozygous loss of *SMN1*. Although *SMN2* copy number or transcripts from *SMN2* are known to influence SMA severity, other uncharacterized factors appear to be contributory. Males with identical biallelic *SMN1* deletions and identical *SMN2* copy numbers appear to be more severely affected than females, and the SMA phenotype is variable even within families whose members share identical genotypes.[73]

Treatment for SMA is supportive for the management of respiratory insufficiency, nutritional deficiency, and orthopedic needs.[74] Because *SMN2* serves to modify the SMA phenotype, it can provide a therapeutic target for treatment by correcting aberrant splicing of *SMN2* using antisense oligonucleotides (ASOs) to allow for full-length transcription of SMN2 and a functional SMN protein. This approach has been successful in mice and more recently in pigs.[75,76] Clinical trials using ASOs are under way. Clinical trials using administration of small molecules to protect motor neuron loss or prevent RNA degradation are also in progress, and emerging therapies using gene or stem cell therapy are planned.[74,77,78]

DNA testing for SMA is performed using a variety of techniques.[79] Diagnostic or carrier testing for SMA can be complicated by (1) the polymorphic nature of the *SMN* locus, with alleles containing varying copy numbers of *SMN1* and/or *SMN2* genes; (2) the degree of homology between *SMN1* and *SMN2*; (3) a small percentage of affected alleles with point mutations rather than deletions within *SMN1*; and (4) a 2% rate of de novo cases, which most frequently occur during paternal meiosis.[65,80] A common diagnostic assay for SMA includes PCR amplification coupled with restriction endonuclease digestion with *DraI* and gel electrophoresis.[81] Only amplicons derived from *SMN2* will contain the restriction site; those generated from *SMN1* do not. Because most SMA-affected patients have *SMN1* deletions involving exon 7, no bands corresponding to *SMN1* are observed. Although this assay is simple and robust, it is not quantitative and cannot determine the *SMN2* copy number, which is required for prognosis, nor can this assay detect other *SMN1* pathogenic mutations. *SMN2* copy number determination requires a quantitative method of analysis such as quantitative PCR or multiplex ligation-dependent probe amplification.

Although population-based carrier screening for SMA has been endorsed by the American College of Medical Genetics and Genomics, the committee on Genetics in the ACOG supports SMA testing in patients with a family history of SMA but does not recommend population-based preconception or prenatal testing at this time.[82,83] With an early age of onset for most SMA patients and the prospects of therapeutic treatment of this disease, NBS for SMA would allow early identification of patients and enable timely treatment intervention, thereby minimizing the severity of the disease. However, no state NBS programs currently include SMA.

Nonsyndromic Hearing Loss and Deafness

More than 100 genetic loci have been linked to nonsyndromic hearing loss and deafness, and most demonstrate an autosomal recessive mode of inheritance.[84] The most common autosomal recessive nonsyndromic hearing loss and deafness locus is DFNB1 (DeaFNess autosomal recessive [B] locus 1), which in most cases is associated with congenital, nonprogressive moderate to profound impairment and no other clinical phenotypic findings.[85] DFNB1 mutations occur in the gene gap junction protein beta-2 *(GJB2)* encoding the protein connexin 26 (OMIM #220290).[86] Also mapped to this region on chromosome 13q12.11 is the gap junction protein beta-6 *(GJB6)* gene encoding the protein connexin 30, which is also associated with DFNB1 autosomal recessive nonsyndromic hearing loss and deafness (OMIM #612645).

The incidence of newborn or prelingual hearing loss is about two to three per 1000 births in the United States, and although the etiology is heterogeneous, including cytomegalovirus infection and other environmental causes, the primary cause is genetic.[87] Because the presentation of deafness at this age is considered relatively common and early intervention in these patients is associated with improved clinical outcomes, newborn hearing screening programs are mandated across the United States. Newborns identified with a sensorineural loss in either ear are referred for audiologic confirmatory testing and, if a sensorineural loss is confirmed, are further referred for genetic evaluation, including a physical examination and pre- and postnatal history. If there is a strong suspicion of a genetic basis for hearing loss, DNA testing is ordered to make or confirm a diagnosis.[88]

The first linkage of a gene to autosomal recessive nonsyndromic hearing loss on chromosome 13q was by Guilford and colleagues in 1994.[89] In 1996, the connexin 26 gene *(GJB2)* was mapped to 13q11-q12, and the following year, mutations in this gene were identified as disease-causing in Pakistani families with profound deafness.[90,91] The *GJB2* gene encodes a member of the other gap junction protein genes with gap junction family of connexin proteins.[92] *GJB2* is flanked by other gap junction proteins with gap junction protein beta-6 *(GJB6)* positioned 5′ to *GJB2* and gap junction protein alpha-3 *(GJA3)* located 3′ to *GJB2*. Common to other connexin genes, although the 5510-bp gene has two exons, only the second exon contains coding sequences for this 26-kDa, 226-amino-acid protein. More than 20 genes encode the connexin proteins, which are expressed throughout the body, most notably in the skin, nervous tissue, heart, muscle, and ear. Each protein has four TMDs connected by two extracellular loops and one intracellular cytoplasmic loop, with the amino and carboxyl termini located in the cytoplasm.[93,94] Connexin proteins oligomerize to form a hexameric connexon or hemichannel of identical (homomeric) or different (heteromeric) connexin proteins dependent on the tissue.[92,95] The connexon formed in the plasma membrane of one cell aligns with the connexon from the plasma membrane of the adjacent cell to form gap junction channels in the extracellular space. These channels allow for the exchange of ions and small molecules between adjacent cells. Connexin 26 and connexin 30 are widely expressed in epithelial cells and interspersed hair cells of the cochlea as well as in the connective tissue, and to a lesser extent, connexins 29, 31, 43, and 45 have also been detected.[87,96,97] In the cochlea, normal hearing requires properly functioning gap junctions for the movement and homeostasis of potassium ions between these cells.

More than 200 *GJB2* gene mutations have been described with most associated with a loss of normal function of the connexin 26 protein.[98] The different *GJB2* mutations result in varying effects on connexin 26 and ultimately on gap function. Mutations can affect the proper formation of the gap junction, a loss of function of the gap junction, or a loss of permeability of selected ions through the gap junction, or mutations can cause a gain of function with abnormal opening and increased gap junction activity.[97] The most common mutation, c.35delG, has a carrier frequency as high as 3% to 4% in some white populations and the highest worldwide carrier rate of 1.5%.[99,100] This is a frameshift mutation resulting in premature termination of the protein, and its relative frequency in multiple populations suggests an ancestral founder mutation. Other common *GJB2* frameshift founder mutations include c.167delT and c.235delC, which are common in the Ashkenazi Jewish and Asian populations, respectively.[101,102] The c.35delG mutation can be homozygous or present with another *GJB2* gene mutation on the second allele. In addition to *GJB2* c.35delG, a less common mutation that is frequently included in a first-tier genetic screening test for nonsyndromic autosomal recessive hearing loss is mutation *GJB6*-D13S1830.[103-105] *GJB6*-D13S1830 is a 342-kb deletion encompassing a portion of the *GJB6* gene and the 5′ regulatory sequences of *GJB2*, thus disrupting normal expression of *GJB2*. This mutation is most commonly associated with *GJB2* c.35delG in compound heterozygous patients with one copy of each mutation, or this mutation can be detected in a homozygous state in which it is present on both alleles of the patient.

Although most *GJB2* gene mutations cause a loss of function and demonstrate autosomal recessive inheritance, some mutations in the first extracellular domain of the protein in a heterozygous state have a dominant-negative effect on connexin 26.[106] In these cases, the production and subsequent incorporation of a mutant protein into the hexameric connexon structure results in abnormal function of the gap junction. These autosomal dominant nonsyndromic hearing loss *GJB2* mutations (OMIM#601544) and similar dominant *GJB6* gene mutations (OMIM#604418) define DFNA3 (DeaFNess autosomal dominant [A] locus 3).[107] Gap junctions are also important in the epidermis for intercellular communication, and connexin 26 as well as connexin proteins 30, 30.3, 31, and 43 are widely expressed here and are important for growth and differentiation of keratinocytes.[94] Some *GJB2* gene mutations demonstrating autosomal dominant inheritance patterns are associated with syndromic hearing loss and characteristic skin diseases such as Bart-Pumphrey syndrome (OMIM#149200), Vohwinkel syndrome (OMIM#124500), and others.[94,108]

Genetic testing to identify the pathogenic variant associated with hearing loss is important to families for diagnosis, determining recurrence risks, enabling subsequent targeted mutation analysis for at-risk family members, and determining the likely degree of hearing impairment for the child (ie, mild, moderate, severe or profound).[85] However, despite the presence of the same mutation within family members, modifier genes and environmental factors influence the phenotype such that the degree of hearing impairment may be different between siblings.[85] After a thorough examination of the newborn by the clinical geneticist and a review of family and patient medical history, nonsyndromic autosomal recessive hearing loss may be suspected. Because up to 50% of these patients have *GJB2* gene mutations including the common 342 kb deletion *GJB6*-D13S1830, full-gene *GJB2* Sanger sequencing and *GJB6*-D13S1830 deletion mutation analysis is often performed (Fig. 49.2).[105] Because the etiology of hearing loss is heterogeneous, if no mutation is detected or if the clinical suspicion of a *GJB2* gene mutation is not high, MPS with targeted panels containing genes known to cause hearing loss is suggested.[86,109,110] Although MPS targeted panels increase the diagnostic yield and the likelihood of finding the pathogenic disease-causing mutation(s), some patients will not have disease variants identified because

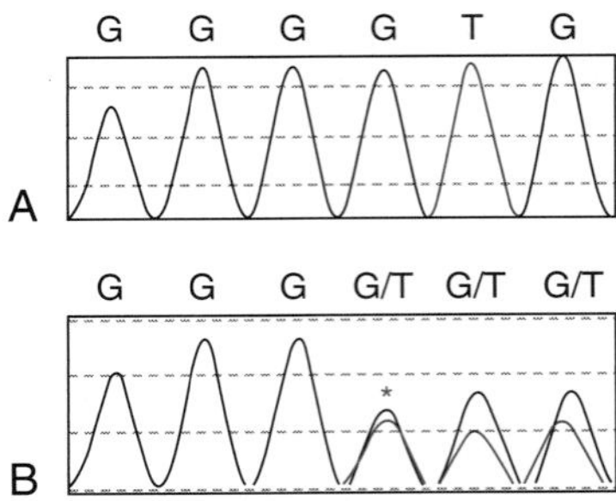

FIGURE 49.2 Sanger sequencing of the *GJB2* gene illustrating a wild-type sequence **(A)** and on a patient with the common c.35delG mutation (**B**, *asterisk*). This mutation results in a frameshift and premature truncation of the protein.

their pathogenic mutation(s) are in genes not included in the panel. In these cases, and if clinically indicated, whole-exome sequencing can be done to identify pathogenic variants in novel candidate genes segregating in the family.[111]

Regardless of the etiology of the hearing loss, these patients and their families require a multidisciplinary team of both health care professionals to manage the clinical needs of the patient and family support services to assist them in adjusting to these new and challenging circumstances.[88] Treatment for patients with hearing loss is dependent on the degree of impairment, including hearing aids or cochlear implantation. Early cochlear implantation surgery results in significant speech perception and language advantages.[112]

Autosomal Dominant Diseases

In autosomal dominant disorders, a single abnormal allele is sufficient to cause disease despite the presence of a normal allele. An individual with an autosomal dominant disease may have inherited an abnormal allele from an affected parent, or the mutant allele may have arisen de novo as a new mutation during gametogenesis in an unaffected parent. The disease-causing gene is on one of the autosomes (1–22) and is not on a sex chromosome (X or Y). An affected individual has a 50% risk of donating the mutant allele to each offspring. Different mutations within the gene may have varying effects on the protein, causing variability in clinical expression between patients who have pathogenic mutations. In some instances, known mutant gene carriers have no clinical symptoms of the disease, a phenomenon referred to as *reduced penetrance*; however, they still possess a 50% risk of donating the mutant allele to each offspring. Differences in phenotypic expression of the disease between patients who share identical gene mutations are commonly explained by the effects of modifier genes or environmental influences (or both). Among pedigrees illustrating autosomal dominant inheritance, both males and females are affected, and male-to-male transmission is observed (unlike X-linked inheritance). Table 49.4 provides a list of some of the inherited autosomal dominant disorders commonly tested in clinical molecular diagnostic laboratories.

Huntington Disease

Huntington disease (HD; OMIM#143100) is an autosomal dominant, late-onset neurodegenerative disorder with an incidence of about 3 to 10 per 100,000 in most populations but may be as high as 10 to 15 in some populations of Western European origin. First described by George Huntington in

TABLE 49.4 Examples of Autosomal Dominant Disorders

Disease	Gene(s)	Location	OMIM Entry #	Incidence
Achondroplasia	*FGFR3*	4p16.3	100800	1 in 26,000–28,000
CHARGE syndrome	*CHD7*	8q12.1-q12.2	214800	1 in 10,000
Familial hypercholesterolemia	*LDLR*	19p13.2	143890	1 in 200–500
Hereditary hemorrhagic telangiectasia	*ACVRL1*	9q34.11	187300	1 in 10,000
	ENG	12q13.13		
	GDF2	10q11.22		
	SMAD4	18q21.2		
Long QT syndrome	Numerous	—	192500	1 in 3000–7000
Myotonic dystrophy type 1	*DMPK*	19q13.32	160900	1 in 20,000
Neurofibromatosis type 1	*NF1*	17q11.2	162200	1 in 3000
Polycystic kidney disease	*PKD1*	16p13.3	173900	1 in 400–1000
	PKD2	4q22.1	613095	
Retinoblastoma	*RB1*	13q14.2	180200	1 in 15,000–20,000
Tuberous sclerosis	*TSC1*	9q34.13	191100	1 in 5,800
	TSC2	16p13.3	613254	

OMIM, Online Mendelian Inheritance in Man.

1872,[113] this progressive disease is characterized by choreic movement, cognitive decline, and ultimately dementia and psychiatric disturbances.[114,115] The mean age of onset is between 35 and 44 years, but subtle changes in personality may be evident before diagnosis. Approximately 25% of patients first display symptoms after the age of 50 years, and about 5% to 10% of patients have juvenile HD with the age of onset before 20 years.[116] The median survival time is 15 to 20 years after the onset of symptoms. Early in the disease, primary symptoms include cognitive deficits; clumsiness; and mood disturbances such as depression, anxiety, irritability, and apathy.[114,116] The next stage of the disease is associated with slurred speech (dysarthria), impairment of voluntary movements, hyperreflexia, chorea, gait abnormalities, and behavioral disturbances such as intermittent explosiveness and aggression. As the disease advances, bradykinesia, rigidity, dementia, dystonia, dysphagia, severe weight loss, sleep disturbances, and incontinence occur. The HD phenotype is initially caused by selective loss of the medium spiny neurons in the striatum, but in later stages of the disease, there are cortical atrophy and widespread degeneration.

In 1983, Gusella and associates reported linkage between DNA marker D4S10, on the short arm of chromosome 4, and HD, based on studies of a large kindred in Venezuela.[117] Through an international collaborative effort, 10 years after its initial localization, the HD gene was cloned.[118] The molecular basis for HD was determined to be an expansion of a glutamine-encoding CAG trinucleotide repeat in exon 1 of the HD gene, *HTT*. This was confirmed in a worldwide study by the identification of expanded CAG-repeat alleles in HD patients from 565 families, representing 43 national or ethnic groups.[119] In this initial international study, the median CAG-repeat length was reported to be 44 in affected patients and 18 in control participants. Normal CAG repeat lengths range from 10 to 26, repeats of 27 to 35 are considered intermediate or "mutable," repeats of 36 to 39 are considered HD alleles associated with reduced penetrance of the disease, and repeats of 40 or greater are diagnostic of HD (Fig. 49.3).

HD is one of many trinucleotide repeat expansion diseases associated with neurologic and neuromuscular

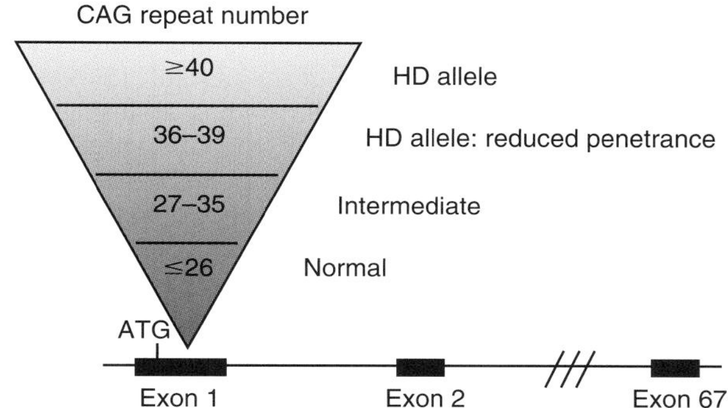

FIGURE 49.3 Schematic representation of the polyglutamine-encoding CAG repeat in exon 1 of the HD gene and associated alleles. A CAG-repeat number of 26 or less is considered normal. CAG-repeat numbers of 27 to 35 are intermediate, and although they are not associated with an abnormal phenotype, these alleles are susceptible to meiotic expansion to an HD allele. CAG repeats of 36 to 39 are considered HD alleles with reduced penetrance, indicating that both unaffected and affected patients have been reported with alleles of this size. CAG repeats of 40 or more are associated with HD with complete penetrance.

dysfunction.[120,121] In HD, the number of CAG repeats is inversely correlated with the age at onset of the disease. Patients with onset as early as 2 years of life have a repeat number approaching 100 or greater, and late-onset-disease patients have repeat numbers of 36 to 39.[122,123] Although the CAG-repeat number accounts for the majority of variance in age of onset for HD (≈70%), the remainder of the variance comes from modifier genes and environmental factors. Analysis of the large Venezuelan HD kindreds encompassing 18,149 individuals spanning 10 generations indicates that 40% of the nongenetic variance is due to heritable modifier genes and 60% to environmental factors.[124] The CAG repeat number and polyglutamine length in the normal huntingtin protein (htt) is not a modifier of age of onset for HD.[125] Genes that encode proteins that interact with htt regulate the expression of *HTT*, dysregulate energy metabolism in the cell, and alter neurotransmitter receptor function have all been considered as modifier genes, but no correlation with age of onset or penetrance has been found.[126]

Pathogenic mutations in *HTT* causing HD in the absence of a family history occur from expansion of a CAG-intermediate allele, which occurs almost exclusively through paternal transmission, although maternal intermediate allele expansion has been reported.[127,128] Intermediate alleles are present in about 1% of the population. The instability of these alleles may be influenced by flanking DNA sequences, which may enhance the formation of hairpin loop structures and cause replication slippage.[129,130] Studies in the HD mouse model have proposed that variations in mismatch repair genes may modify somatic CAG expansion and disease progression.[131,132] Single sperm analysis studies have demonstrated 11% instability (9% expansions and 2.5% contractions) in CAG repeats of 30 compared with 0.6% instability (contractions only) seen in average-sized alleles of 15 to 18 repeats, indicating that CAG instability increases as the repeat number increases.[133] CAG repeats of 36 showed 53% instability, and CAG repeats from 38 to 51 had instability ranging from 92% to 99%. In addition to the CAG repeat number, *cis*-elements may play a role in CAG-repeat instability.[134] In families with HD, the onset of symptoms occurs at a progressively younger age in successive generations, a pattern referred to as *anticipation.* Anticipation is explained by meiotic expansion of the unstable CAG repeat during transmission by the affected parent, resulting in an even higher CAG-repeat number in the offspring and an earlier age of onset. In addition, although 69% of affected father–child pairs show expansion, only 32% of affected mother–child pairs demonstrate expansion. Furthermore, less than 2% of maternal expansions result in a change of more than five repeats, but up to 21% of paternal transmissions increase by more than 7 repeats.[135] For this reason, the affected parent in most cases of juvenile-onset HD is the father. However, the largest reported CAG-repeat number of approximately 130 occurred via maternal expansion of 70 CAG repeats.[136]

The *HTT* gene contains 67 exons and encodes a novel protein, huntingtin (htt), with 3144 amino acids and a molecular mass of approximately 350 kDa.[137] Htt is ubiquitously expressed in both neural and nonneural tissue with highest levels in the brain.[138,139] Htt is required for neuronal development with the complete absence of htt being lethal in mice.[140] Htt is predominantly localized in the cytoplasm, but lesser amounts are also found in the nucleus.[141,142] The structure of htt includes the CAG encoded polyglutamine repeat, a proline-rich domain, and 3 HEAT repeats, which form a rodlike helical scaffold to which other components can attach and are involved in intracellular transport and a nuclear localization domain at the C terminal end. The HEAT acronym is derived from four proteins found to also contain this amino acid sequence and unique structure: **H**untingtin, **E**longation factor 3, regulatory **A** subunit of protein phosphatase 2A and **T**OR1. In neurons, htt is associated with synaptic vesicles and microtubules and is abundant in dendrites and nerve terminals. Huntingtin interacts with more than 200 proteins, including those involved in intracellular trafficking and signaling, cytoskeletal organization, endocytosis, and transcription regulation.[143] Mutant htt with expanded polyglutamine tracks are effectively transcribed and translated, but as a result of the increase in glutamine residues, the protein is misfolded.[144] This abnormal folding conveys a gain of function and an increased amyloid-like ability to form protein aggregates, sequestering other cellular proteins preventing their normal function, thereby disrupting normal protein homeostasis and conferring neurotoxicity. Interestingly, patients with two expanded CAG-repeat alleles do not have more severe disease than heterozygotes.[119]

HD remains an incurable complex disease requiring a multidisciplinary approach and medication to treat the motor, psychiatric, and cognitive symptoms of the disease.[145,146] Current therapeutic strategies include the use of antisense-oligonucleotides specific for HD-associated single nucleotide polymorphisms (SNPs), or RNA interference (RNAi) technology for CAG-expanded allele inhibition.[147-149]

DNA testing for HD is performed using PCR to determine the CAG-repeat number.[150] The most common method includes PCR with fluorescently labeled primers coupled with capillary electrophoresis (Fig. 49.4).[151] Technical standards and guidelines for HD diagnostic testing for clinical laboratories have been developed by the American College of Medical Genetics and Genomics.[150]

Many ethical issues are associated with HD testing, primarily as they relate to presymptomatic testing (Box 49.2). The first policy statement on ethical issues related to predictive genetic testing for HD was adopted in 1989 at a joint meeting with representatives from the International Huntington Association and the World Federation of Neurology.[152] At that time, the gene had not yet been cloned, and predictive testing was performed using linkage studies and the at-risk patient was quoted only the likelihood of inheriting the mutant allele. These tests were less than perfect and provided, at best, results in only 60% to 75% of families. Moreover, the possibility of recombination resulted in an inaccurate carrier assessment.[153] In other families, living affected members were not available, or markers were not informative. After the gene had been cloned and direct mutation analysis was possible, risk assessments were reversed in a small percentage of patients.[154]

However, after the gene was cloned, direct mutation analysis for CAG repeat number was implemented, and guidelines for predictive testing using direct mutation analysis were established.[155,156] The approach used for presymptomatic HD testing has become the model for late-onset single-gene disorders, and similar formats have been applied to other late-onset inherited diseases.[157,158] This model includes a multidisciplinary team involving neurology, psychiatry, and genetics specialists; pretest evaluation and counseling; individual support from family members or close friends; and posttest follow-up sessions.[159] Predictive testing should be performed for patients 18 years of age or older and only with informed consent. Informed consent implies that the patient has been thoroughly counseled and clearly understands both the advantages and the disadvantages of knowing the results. An advantage of having this test is the removal of uncertainty regarding whether patients have or have not inherited the mutant allele and thus a feeling of relief for those who have not inherited a mutant *HTT* allele. This knowledge can help patients plan their career goals and personal affairs involving marriage, children, and long-term care insurance. Disadvantages of knowing this information include, but are not limited to, (1) the feeling of "survivor's guilt" in those who learn that they have not inherited a mutant allele while other family members have, (2) fear from learning that they have inherited a mutant *HTT* allele and will develop this incurable

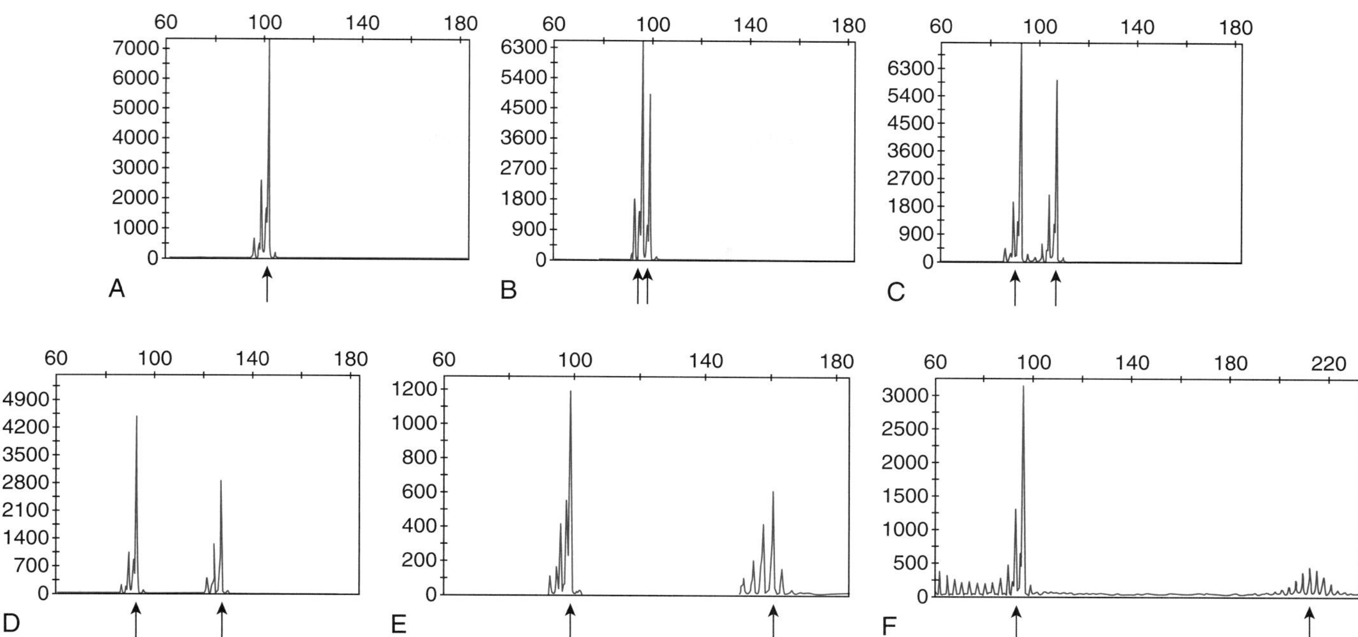

FIGURE 49.4 Electropherograms representing various patterns observed in patients referred for Huntington disease (HD) testing. The polyglutamine-encoding CAG repeat in exon 1 is amplified by polymerase chain reaction (PCR) using flanking oligonucleotide primers, one of which is labeled with a fluorescent dye. Amplicon sizes in bases are noted at the top of the figure, and the relative amount of fluorescence detected for each amplicon is measured by the peak height (y-axis). *Arrows* indicate the predominant amplicons observed for each patient with the size of the amplicons corresponding to the CAG repeat number. Additional smaller peaks not indicated by arrows represent "stutter" peaks and result from strand slippage during PCR of repetitive sequences. **A,** Patient 1 has amplicons 101 bp in length corresponding to 20 CAG repeats on both HD alleles. **B,** Patient 2 has 95- and 98-bp amplicons, corresponding to CAG repeats of 18 and 19. **C,** Patient 3 has 92- and 107-bp amplicons representing CAG repeats of 17 and 22, respectively. The diagnosis of HD can be ruled out in these three patients. **D,** Patient 4 has 92- and 128-bp amplicons corresponding to CAG repeats of 17 and 29. The results would not support a diagnosis of HD. However, a CAG repeat of 29 is considered an intermediate allele and can undergo meiotic expansion to an HD allele during gamete formation. **E,** Patient 5 has CAG repeats of 19 and 39, as depicted by amplicons 98 and 158 bp in length. In a symptomatic patient, these results would support the diagnosis of HD. However, in a presymptomatic patient, the phenotype of an HD allele with reduced penetrance cannot be predicted with certainty. **F,** Patient 6 has CAG repeats corresponding to 18 and 57 with amplicons 95 and 212 bp in length. These results confirm the diagnosis of HD in this patient. Genetic counseling regarding the implications of HD DNA findings is indicated.

BOX 49.2 Ethical Issues Associated With Presymptomatic DNA Testing for Huntington Disease

Patients must be 18 years of age or older.

The decision to proceed with testing must be voluntary and informed.

Genetic counseling regarding the benefits and pitfalls of testing is required.

A support partner is needed for the patient for counseling and the testing process.

Diagnosis of Huntington disease in the family should be confirmed by DNA testing before presymptomatic testing.

Psychiatric assessment of patient is necessary before testing.

Follow-up genetic counseling is recommended after delivery of results.

Prenatal testing of fetuses is controversial; preimplantation diagnosis is available.

disease, (3) potential risk of discrimination in employment, (4) concern for passing this gene on to their offspring, and (5) uncertainty of developing the disease if a mutant *HTT* allele with 36 to 39 CAG repeats is identified.

When at all possible, the patient should be accompanied by a trusted friend or loved one throughout the counseling and testing procedure. This person can provide stability to the patient by being able to intimately speak to the patient about the situation and discuss the information shared at the counseling sessions. Most important, as a part of this process, the partner will be present when the results of testing are revealed and can provide comfort and support as needed both then and in the following days, weeks, or months. Ultimately, however, it is the patient's decision to proceed with this testing and to accept both the benefits and pitfalls of knowing this information. The patient's decision to proceed must be his or hers, without coercion from family members, clinicians, friends, or employers.

For at-risk individuals requesting mutation studies, their mental stability should be considered for the safety of the patient; a psychiatric assessment is often part of the testing protocol because HD test results can precipitate depression. Results of the psychiatric evaluation can influence the timing of the DNA test, postponing it until such time when the patient is considered mentally able to deal with the possibly devastating news. Suicidal tendencies are present in both at-risk patients and those with HD.[160,161]

Because HD is a delayed-onset disease, as the asymptomatic at-risk patient ages, the risk of testing positive with an expanded CAG repeat decreases.[162] Thus if the patient elects not to have predictive testing, the genetic counselor can provide information regarding the probability that an HD mutation exists, which, based on the individual's age, may provide some comfort to the patient. Most individuals who seek presymptomatic testing have a mean age of about 40 years and are more often female.[163] Some individuals may begin the multistep counseling process and then withdraw from the study without receiving test results. If possible, before presymptomatic mutation testing, the diagnosis of HD should be confirmed in an affected member of the family to be certain that the disease segregating in the family is HD. A normal *HTT* CAG repeat number does not rule out a different, dominantly inherited neurodegenerative disease in the family for which the patient likely retains a risk of development.

Counseling in families with no prior family history of HD can be challenging when the expanded CAG repeat appears to be de novo. Multiple factors can explain this phenomenon, including (1) expansion of an intermediate-sized allele (27–35), (2) premature death of an adult asymptomatic yet affected individual with a reduced or full penetrance allele, (3) misdiagnosis of HD in other family members, (4) alternative paternity, and (5) undisclosed adoption. Without understanding the mechanism of a new mutation in the affected individual, a priori risk assessment for HD in at risk family members may be inaccurate. Thus, counseling for the risk of HD is only prudent after accurate DNA testing.

Prenatal testing for HD, another complicated issue associated with this disease, may not be provided in all laboratories that perform routine HD testing for several reasons. Ethical issues include possible pregnancy termination for a late-onset disorder, presymptomatic testing of the child if the parents choose not to terminate, and technical issues that may compromise testing of chorionic villus and amniocentesis samples. As an alternative for prenatal testing, preimplantation genetic diagnosis (PGD) can be performed.[164] In PGD, in vitro fertilization is used to produce embryos that then undergo a single cell biopsy for genetic analysis. After PCR testing has been used to determine the *HTT* CAG-repeat numbers, embryos with normal HD alleles are implanted. This method, which combines direct mutation analysis and PGD, eliminates the necessity for subsequent prenatal testing to determine the HD status of the fetus. Exclusion testing whereby only embryos who have not inherited an affected allele are implanted without disclosing information regarding the *HTT* CAG repeat numbers in all tested embryos is an option for some families that do not wish to know the genotype of the asymptomatic at-risk parent.[165,166]

Marfan Syndrome

Marfan syndrome (MFS; OMIM #154700) is a relatively common autosomal dominant multisystem connective tissue disorder with primary manifestations involving the ocular, musculoskeletal, and cardiovascular systems with an estimated worldwide incidence of about 1 in 5000.[167,168] The most common ocular feature of MFS is myopia, but other associated features include unilateral or bilateral ectopia lentis (60%), or retinal detachment. In addition, patients with MFS are at increased risk for glaucoma and cataracts at a younger age as compared with the general population. Characteristic facial features may include a long narrow face, deep-set and downward-slanting eyes, flat cheek bones, and micrognathia. Skeletal abnormalities arise from bone overgrowth and joint hypermobility. MFS patients are tall with frequent clinical findings including pectus excavatum or pectus carinatum, caused by overgrowth of the ribs, which can interfere with pulmonary function and require surgery. Patients typically have an arm span-to-height ratio greater than 1.05 and a reduced upper body-to-lower extremity ratio. Scoliosis is present in about half of patients; it can be mild to severe and is progressive. Morbidity and early mortality are linked to cardiovascular manifestations of the disorder, which are characterized by progressive dilation of the aortic root, predisposition to aortic dissection, mitral and tricuspid valve prolapse with or without regurgitation, and dilation of the proximal pulmonary artery. Wide phenotypic variability is observed, with some patients presenting as neonates with severe and progressive disease that is sometimes fatal, but others can remain undiagnosed until adulthood. An early diagnosis is associated with an improved long-term outcome.[169,170] Unfortunately, for undiagnosed patients, presentation may be sudden premature death caused by aortic dissection or rupture.[171,172]

The diagnosis of MFS is based on family history of the disease; however, as many as 25% of MFS arise from a new mutation with no family history of disease.[173] In the absence of a documented family history of MFS, currently the clinical diagnosis of MFS is made using the revised Ghent diagnostics nosology with most of the emphasis on the presence of an aortic root aneurysm and ectopia lentis.[168] In the absence of one or both of these, a mutation in the gene associated with MFS or manifestations in other MFS-related organ systems are required. Some MFS features may be isolated findings and not associated with MFS, and some overlap with other genetic syndromes.[167,168] Because most MFS clinical manifestations increase with age, these criteria may make diagnosis in the pediatric patient more difficult, and often these patients may carry a diagnosis of "potential" MFS and require periodic follow-up visits for reevaluation.[167]

MFS is associated with mutations in the fibrillin-1 gene (*FBN1*) mapped to chromosome 15q21.1.[173-175] The gene spans 237,414 bp, is composed of 65 exons, and encodes a 10 kb mRNA, prefibrillin-1.[176] *FBN1* is ubiquitously expressed in connective tissue. The 320-kDa, 2871-amino-acid extracellular glycoprotein, fibrillin-1, self-assembles into macroaggregates to serve as the primary structural component of 10-nm-diameter microfibrils located throughout the basal lamina in both elastic and nonelastic tissue.[176-178] In elastin-expressing tissue, such as blood vessels, lung, and skin, microfibrils make up the scaffold for elastin assembly within the extracellular matrix (ECM). In nonelastic tissue, including the ciliary zonule of the eye and of basement membranes, they have an anchoring function and provide tensile strength.[179] In most cases in which the mutation causes abnormal fibrilin-1 protein, a dominant negative effect occurs when fibrillin-1 is incorporated into the microfibril, resulting in functionally inferior connective tissue. In other cases, disease results from reduced protein production or haploinsufficiency. Fibrillin-1 contains several motifs, including 47 cysteine-rich epidermal growth factor-like (EGF) domains, most of which bind calcium.[180] These domains are interspersed with 7 TGF-β binding protein-like (TB) domains, and there are two hybrid domains with sequences similar to both the EGF and TB motifs.[180] Latent TGF-β binding proteins interact with fibrillin-1 and together bind TGF-β to inactivate and thereby prevent signaling through the SMAD 2/3 pathway.[177,179,181,182] Dysregulation of TGF-β signaling affects the development of vascular smooth muscle and the integrity of the ECM.

Mutations in *FBN1* are heterogeneous with almost 2000 reported throughout the gene.[183] Point mutations represent the largest category at 66%; 20% are small deletions or insertions, 11% are splice site mutations, and the remainder represent large deletions or duplications. In all cases, increased TGF-β signaling is observed. Phenotype–genotype studies have shown that neonatal MFS or early onset and severe MFS is associated with mutations spanning exons 24 to 32.[184,185] These patients also have an increased likelihood of developing ectopia lentis, ascending aortic dilation, mitral valve anomalies, scoliosis, and a reduced life expectancy. This region of the protein contains the longest stretch of EGF-like domains and is thought to be important for microfibril biogenesis. In-frame missense mutations are more often associated with more severe complications of MFS than are mutations predicted to cause premature truncation of the protein, and ectopia lentis is more frequently seen in patients with a missense mutation resulting in cysteine than with other missense mutations.[184] Furthermore, because wide phenotypic variability is observed even for individuals harboring the same recurrent mutation, modifier genes likely play a role in the MFS phenotype.[184] Interestingly, the phenotypic expression of MFS may be related in part to varying degrees of expression between the normal and mutant allele, and these differences may also be tissue specific.[186] The lack of consistent genotype–phenotype correlations provides little prognostic value for individual patient management. Although variability in expression is observed, *FBN1* mutations are considered highly penetrant.

Management of patients with MFS is similar to that of patients with other inherited multisystem disorders, involving a team approach with specialists in many areas of medicine including a cardiologist, ophthalmologist, orthopedist, and geneticist. Because the pathogenesis of MFS is due to dysregulation of TGF-β and increased TGF-β signaling, one pharmacologic treatment for MFS is the drug losartan, an angiotensin II type 1 receptor inhibitor used to inhibit excessive TGF-β signaling and slow aortic growth.[187] More recent studies suggest that this therapy may be more effective in patients with *FBN1* haploinsufficiency as opposed to dominant negative *FBN1* mutations.[188] Other successful treatments for aortic aneurysms associated with MFS include β-blockers and statins or tetracycline to inhibit TGF-β signaling through inhibition of matrix metalloproteinase-2 and -9 and ERK inhibitors to inhibit ERK signaling.[187] Clinical trials investigating the best therapy to treat patients with MFS and other aortopathies are ongoing. Annual ophthalmologic and transthoracic echocardiographic imaging is important for monitoring, and prophylactic surgery for aortic root replacement is recommended when the aortic root reaches a critical diameter of 5.5 cm.[189,190] Lifestyle changes to limit physical activity to low-impact sports in order to prevent physical exhaustion are recommended to prevent high blood pressure and aortic wall stress.

FBN1 is one of the largest human genes, and although it is labor intensive and costly, DNA sequencing is the gold standard for genetic testing for MFS. This may be most effective in patients when the clinical diagnosis of MFS is likely.[191] After a *FBN1* mutation has been identified within a family, predictive targeted *FBN1* mutation specific testing for at-risk family members can be performed and enables early diagnosis and proper management in identified mutation positive family members. However, despite extensive *FBN1* analysis, 7% to 30% of MFS patients will have no mutation detected. These cases could reflect patients with *FBN1* mutations that are contained within regions of the gene that cannot be detected by current screening techniques.[192] Alternatively, these may be patients who have a phenotype suspicious for MFS but who do not meet the strict Ghent diagnostic criteria. MPS with a targeted panel of genes, which includes *FBN1* as well as other candidate genes associated with thoracic aortic aneurysms or aortic dissections, may be an efficient screening method. Associated syndromes and genes may include Loeys-Dietz *(SMAD3, TGFBR1, TGFBR2)* Ehlers-Danlos type IV *(COL3A1)*, or genes associated with thoracic aortic aneurysm and dissections (*ACAT2, MYH11, MYLK, TGFBR1,* and *TGFBR2*).[193] Collectively, these disorders are described as aortopathies. Aortopathies are a common cause of morbidity and mortality in the United States. In fact, it is reported that aneurysm of the aorta is responsible for 1% to 2% of all deaths in the Western world.[194] MPS-based testing using an aortopathy gene panel is rapidly becoming the first-line diagnostic test for individuals who present with a phenotype that could fit any one of multiple disorders (eg, MFS and Loeys-Dietz syndrome).

Multiple Endocrine Neoplasia

Multiple endocrine neoplasia (MEN) is an autosomal dominant disorder characterized by the presence of tumors in two or more endocrine glands. There are two major types of MEN disease: type 1 (MEN1, which is also known as Wermer syndrome) and type 2 (MEN2, which is also known as Sipple syndrome). Both MEN1 and MEN2 are clinically distinct and should be considered as independent disorders with separate genetic causes.

Multiple endocrine neoplasia type 1 (OMIM #131100) is a relatively common disorder with an estimated incidence ranging from 1 in 10,000 to 30,000.[195,196] MEN1 is characterized by the presence of any of many (>20) tumor types, and a clinical diagnosis requires that an individual have at least two endocrine tumors that are parathyroid, pituitary, or gastroenteropancreatic in nature.[196] Parathyroid tumors are the most common tumors observed in MEN1 and occur in approximately 95% of patients.[197] Consequently, hyperparathyroidism resulting from overproduction of hormones by parathyroid tumors is a common early manifestation.[196,198] Parathyroid tumors also often cause hypercalcemia, which ultimately results in a multitude of medical issues (ie, depression, nausea, vomiting, kidney stones, and hypertension, among others).[196] Pancreatic islet cell tumors are the second most common tumors observed in MEN1 with approximately 40% of patients developing a neoplasm of this area.[197,198] Pancreatic tumors are of particular importance in MEN1 because gastrinomas (Zollinger-Ellison syndrome) are the most common cause of morbidity in patients with this disease.[197] Pituitary tumors occur in 30% of patients with MEN1 and represent the third most prevalent tumor type. Of note, a multitude of non–endocrine-associated tumors (carcinoid, adrenocorticoid, facial angiofibromas, lipomas, meningiomas, among others) commonly occur in patients with MEN1.[196-198]

Using a combination of linkage analysis and deletion mapping techniques, investigators in several groups were able to identify a region on chromosome 11 (11q13) likely to contain the gene responsible for MEN1.[199-208] In 1997, the gene causative for MEN1 was identified and named multiple endocrine neoplasia I *(MEN1)*.[209,210] The *MEN1* gene contains ten exons that encode a 610 amino acid protein known as menin.[209] Menin is a ubiquitously expressed protein that can localize to either the nucleus or cytoplasm.[211,212] However, other than clearly defined nuclear localization signals, menin lacks functional domains homologous to those observed in other proteins, making it difficult to predict how it functions.[213] Menin protein interactions suggest that it functions in transcriptional regulation, cell division and proliferation, and genome stability.[213-216] Based on loss of heterozygosity (LOH) patterns observed during gene identification, *MEN1* was considered a likely tumor suppressor gene. Several studies have since shown that overexpression of menin in vitro results in suppression of cellular proliferation.[217-219] Furthermore, the loss of menin results in immortalization of cells.[220] Taken together, these data support a tumor suppressor role for menin, but its specific function is not yet known.

To date, more than 500 unique disease-causing mutations have been described in the *MEN1* gene.[216] Mutations are located in all coding exons of the gene, and there are no significant mutational hot spots. The bulk of mutations reported in *MEN1* are those that lead to truncated forms of the menin protein (eg, frameshift, nonsense, gross deletions).[216] Most known mutations in *MEN1* result in the loss of nuclear localization, and loss of function appears to be the mechanism of disease.[196,216] However, there are no clear genotype–phenotype correlations in patients with MEN1. *MEN1* missense mutations, which are unlikely to be loss of function, have been reported in individuals with familial isolated hyperparathyroidism (FIHP).[221-223] There have also been several truncating mutations reported in FIHP that also occur in classic MEN1 disease.[216] It is therefore not possible to predict the course of disease based on genotype alone.

Molecular diagnosis of MEN1 typically involves Sanger sequencing of the entire coding region of the *MEN1* gene. This method detects disease-causing mutations in 80% to 90% of familial cases and 65% of isolated cases.[196,224,225] Symptomatic individuals with negative Sanger sequencing results should be screened for gross deletions and duplications. Testing for large deletions and duplications (typically performed by multiplex ligation-dependent probe amplification [MLPA]) detects mutations in an additional 1% to 4% of patients.[196,216,226-230] Combining both techniques, a causative mutation is found in approximately 95% of familial MEN1 cases. After a causative germline mutation is identified in a family, other at-risk family members should be offered targeted testing for the identified mutation as soon as possible because the disease may begin to show manifestations as early as 5 years of age.[231] Because MEN1 is autosomal dominant, the risk of MEN1 in the child of an affected individual is 50%. Approximately 10% of mutations identified in *MEN1* are de novo, so recurrence risk is much lower in families where the proband is the child of individuals in which no *MEN1* gene mutation has been identified and correct parentage has been confirmed.[216] However, all children of an individual with a de novo change have a 50% chance of inheriting the causative mutation.

Treatment of MEN1 disease is largely driven by the presentation of disease in the individual patient. Surgical intervention is recommended to remove all functional tumors as well as those that are greater than 4 cm in size or demonstrate rapid growth.[231] In some cases in which pancreatic tumors become metastatic (or are inoperable), chemotherapy may be used.[231] Individuals with hyperparathyroidism may undergo a subtotal or total parathyroidectomy.[231] Thymectomy may be performed prophylactically to prevent the development of carcinoid tumors, but in most cases, it is performed after tumor development.[196,231] Presymptomatic individuals with a known disease-causing mutation in *MEN1* should undergo routine clinical screening for early detection of cancer.

Multiple endocrine neoplasia type 2 is divided into three phenotypically distinct subtypes: MEN2A (OMIM #171400), MEN2B (OMIM #162300), and familial medullary thyroid carcinoma (FMTC, OMIM #155240). Unlike MEN1, tumors associated with MEN2 disease are highly malignant and life threatening. The MEN2A and MEN2B subtypes are both characterized by medullary thyroid carcinoma (MTC) and pheochromocytoma but also have unique distinguishing features. MEN2A is the most common form of MEN2 disease and accounts for approximately 55% of patients. It is characterized by MTC with pheochromocytomas in 50% of patients and parathyroid adenoma in approximately 20% of patients.[197,232] A clinical diagnosis of MEN2A requires the presence of both MTC and pheochromocytoma or a parathyroid adenoma (or parathyroid hyperplasia) in a single individual.[232] MEN2B is much less common, representing only 5% to 10% of MEN2 patients.[197,198] It is characterized by MTC with pheochromocytoma but very little risk for parathyroid adenoma. MEN2B patients also commonly have mucosal neuromas of the lips or tongue, marfanoid habitus, distinctive facies, intestinal autonomic ganglion dysfunction, and medullated corneal fibers.[197,232] A clinical diagnosis of MEN2B typically requires the presence of most of these features in addition to MTC. FMTC accounts for 35% of MEN2 cases and is characterized by MTC in the absence of other malignancies.[197,198] FMTC is clinically diagnosed in families with four or more individuals affected with MTC alone.[232] Interestingly, the onset of disease varies significantly between the subtypes of this disorder. The onset of MTC is typically observed in early adulthood in MEN2A, in early childhood in MEN2B, and often in middle age in FMTC patients.[232]

Using a combination of linkage analysis and gene mapping techniques the gene causative for MEN2A was located in a 480-kilobase region of chromosome 10q11.2.[233-236] The proto-oncogene *RET* was later identified as causative for both MEN2A and FMTC[236,237] and MEN2B.[238,239] *RET* is a proto-oncogene containing 21 exons that encode an 1114-amino-acid protein called RET. RET is a receptor tyrosine kinase for members of the glial cell line–derived neurotrophic factor

TABLE 49.5 Examples of X-Linked Disorders

Disease	Gene	Location	OMIM Entry #	Incidence
Fabry disease	*GLA*	Xq22.1	301500	1 in 50,000 males
Hemophilia A	*HEMA*	Xq28	306700	1 in 4000–5000 males
Hemophilia B	*HEMB*	Xq27.1	306900	1 in 20,000 males
Hunter syndrome: mucopolysaccharidosis type II	*IDS*	Xq28	309900	1 in 100,000 males
Incontinentia pigmenti	*IP*	Xq28	308300	1 in 1,000,000 females
Lesch-Nyhan syndrome	*HRPT1*	Xq26.2-26.3	300322	1 in 380,000 males
Menkes disease	*ATP7A*	Xq21.1	309400	1 in 100,000 males
Ornithine transcarbamylase deficiency	*OTC*	Xp11.4	300461	1 in 14,000 males
Severe combined immunodeficiency	*IL2RG*	Xq13.1	300400	1 in 50,000–100,000 males
Wiskott Aldrich syndrome	*WAS*	Xp11.23	301000	1 in 100,000 males

OMIM, Online Mendelian Inheritance in Man.

family (GDNF) of signaling molecules.[240-243] RET contains three functional domains: an extracellular ligand-binding domain, a TMD, and a cytoplasmic tyrosine kinase domain.[244] It is involved in several signaling pathways during development that control proliferation, differentiation, survival, and migration of enteric nervous system progenitor cells.[244] Not surprisingly, *RET* gene mutations that result in MEN2 disease are activating in nature.[245] Interestingly, mutations that inactivate the *RET* gene result in Hirschsprung disease (OMIM #142623), a disorder characterized by the absence of neuronal ganglion cells in the large intestine.[246,247]

More than 100 variants have been described in the *RET* gene in association with the MEN2 phenotype with several mutation hotspots.[248] In fact, mutations at *RET* codon 634 account for more than 85% of familial MEN2A, and mutations in three cysteine residues located at codons 609, 618, and 620 account for 50% of FMTC.[197,232] Similarly, a single mutation resulting in a change from methionine to threonine at codon 918 (p.Met918Thr) in *RET* exon 16 accounts for 95% of MEN2B patients.[198] Because the bulk of MEN2-associated *RET* gene mutations are limited to exons 10, 11, and 13 to 16, molecular testing is typically limited to Sanger sequencing of these regions. When a diagnosis of MEN2B is suspected, targeted testing for the p.Met918Thr mutation is often performed first. All subtypes of MEN2 are inherited in an autosomal dominant manner, so any individual found to have a disease-causing *RET* mutation has a 50% chance of passing the disease-causing allele to each of his or her offspring. Five percent of MEN2A-related and 50% of MEN2B-related *RET* gene mutations are caused by a de novo change.[232] In these cases, the children of an individual with a de novo mutation also have a 50% chance of inheriting the disease.

Treatment of MEN2 is dependent on the disease presentation. Individuals with MTC typically undergo thyroidectomy and lymph node dissection.[232] Patients with pheochromocytoma have laparoscopic adrenalectomy.[198] Presymptomatic individuals with a disease-causing *RET* mutation should be screened regularly to detect early manifestations of disease. These individuals may also elect to have prophylactic thyroidectomy to prevent MTC.[232]

X-Linked Diseases

In X-linked diseases, the mutant allele resides on the X chromosome. In X-linked recessive diseases, females are heterozygous carriers of the disease with one normal and one mutant allele and are typically not affected. Males receiving the mutant allele from their mothers are considered hemizygous with one mutant allele and no normal allele. All daughters of affected males are carriers of a mutant allele. A carrier female has a 25% chance of transmitting her normal allele to a son, a 25% chance of having an affected son, a 25% chance of having a daughter who carries the mutant allele, and a 25% chance of having a daughter who receives her normal allele. In the absence of a family history, an affected male can have a mutant allele that arose de novo as a new mutation during gametogenesis in the formation of the egg. Roughly one third of all cases of X-linked disorders represent de novo new mutations with the absence of a family history. In these cases, the mother is not a carrier of a mutant allele and is not at risk for having subsequent affected children. In pedigrees associated with X-linked recessive conditions, typically only males are affected, and male-to-male transmission of the disease is not seen. In less frequent, X-linked dominant diseases, one copy of the mutant allele is sufficient to cause disease despite the presence of a normal allele. In these disease processes, females are affected, and in males with only a single mutant allele, these diseases are often lethal. Table 49.5 provides a list of some of the inherited X-linked disorders commonly tested in clinical molecular diagnostic laboratories.

Duchenne Muscular Dystrophy

Duchenne muscular dystrophy (DMD; OMIM #310200) is a fatal X-linked recessive disorder characterized by progressive skeletal muscle wasting. The incidence of DMD is about 1 in 3500 male births, making it the most common severe neuromuscular disease in humans. Classic DMD presents in early childhood, with delayed motor skills or an abnormal gait. This is followed by progressive muscle weakness, calf hypertrophy, and grossly elevated serum creatine kinase (>10× normal) caused by degenerating muscle fibers. A muscle biopsy will show variation in fiber size, necrosis, inflammation, fibrosis, and fiber regeneration and may be required for confirmation of disease in about 5% of patients in whom no DNA mutation is identified. Immunohistochemistry (IHC) staining using antibodies directed against different epitopes of the DMD encoded protein, dystrophin, shows complete or almost complete absence of carboxy-terminal antigens in the majority of DMD patients. Progressive weakness initially affects the lower extremities, causing most DMD patients to require wheelchairs between 10 and 15 years of age. Continual degeneration and regeneration and inflammation of muscle eventually lead to the replacement of muscle tissue by adipose and connective tissue and progressive disease. Scoliosis is common and affects respiratory function. Chronic respiratory insufficiency develops in all patients. Cardiac disease is most commonly dilated cardiomyopathy (DCM) caused by cardiac fibrosis or rhythm and conduction abnormalities. Cardiorespiratory failure is the primary cause of death.[249] In some patients, however, only the heart is affected, causing DMD-associated X-linked DCM (OMIM #302045).[250] Additionally, many patients with DMD exhibit lower IQs and nonprogressive cognitive impairment.[251] Clinical management of patients with DMD is complex, requiring a multidisciplinary team approach.[252,253] Glucocorticoids are used to slow muscle weakness, angiotensin-converting enzyme inhibitors, β-blockers and diuretics for cardiac disease, and noninvasive ventilation for respiratory care. In addition to health care professionals in these respective areas, team members in the areas of psychosocial, gastrointestinal, pain, and speech and language are required. Although elevated serum creatine kinase (CK) levels can be measured from blood spots, NBS for DMD, enabling early identification of affected children and potential better outcomes from early intervention has not been implemented in the United States. This may be in part due to false-positive elevated CK levels as a result of the birthing process and the lack of evidence to support early intervention in DMD patients.[254] A two-tiered pilot program performing both CK and DNA analysis on dried blood spots was successfully implemented in Ohio, screening 37,649 newborn males and identifying 6 affected patients.[254] As novel therapies for DMD continue to develop and the efficacy of targeted treatment for early intervention is validated, NBS for DMD may be adopted.[255]

Because DMD is an X-linked recessive disorder, most carrier females are asymptomatic. Similar to other X-linked diseases, the varying degree of clinical manifestations among carrier females depends on the degree of inactivation of the X chromosome harboring the mutant *DMD* gene in various tissues where the DMD protein is expressed.[256] Up to as many as 20% of carriers can display some symptoms of DMD and Becker muscular dystrophy (BMD). Most frequently observed is muscle weakness with elevated serum CK levels or cardiac involvement, including DCM or left ventricle dilation. Females with severe disease most often result from skewed lyonization in carrier females or an X-autosome translocation involving the *DMD* gene.[257-261]

Cytogenetic abnormalities in DMD patients and DNA linkage studies localized the DMD locus to chromosome Xp21.[258,259,262-264] By mixing DNA enhanced for X-linked genes from a 49, XXXXY cell line with DNA from a patient with DMD and a cytogenetic deletion in Xp21, Kunkel and colleagues cleverly used subtraction hybridization to clone the DNA corresponding to the patient's deletion.[265] During hybridization, Xp21 sequences from the cell line had no complementary sequences with which to anneal in the patient's DNA; thus, they were available for cloning. The *DMD* gene (Xp21.2) is complex and is one of the largest genes in the human genome, spanning 2.4 megabases. DMD contains 79 exons, representing less than 1% of the gene, and encodes a 14 kb mRNA.[266] The gene has multiple tissue-specific promoters that transcribe various full-length dystrophin isoforms differing in their amino terminal sequences. The full-length protein product, dystrophin, contains 3685 amino acids; has a molecular weight of 427 kDa; and contains four distinct domains, including an actin-binding domain, a central rod domain with spectrin-like repeats, a cysteine-rich domain, and a unique COOH-terminal domain. Dystrophin is predominantly expressed in skeletal, cardiac, and smooth muscle. Additional dystrophin isoforms transcribed from four internal promoters and splice variants are found in nonmuscle organs throughout the body.[267] Dystrophin is a rodlike cytoskeletal protein and is a critical component of the dystrophin-associated protein complex (DAPC).[268]

The DAPC interacts with a host of cytoskeletal, transmembrane, extracellular, trafficking, and intracellular signaling proteins. In skeletal muscle, DAPC plays a structural role by connecting the actin cytoskeleton to the ECM, stabilizing the sarcolemma of muscle fibers during repeated cycles of contraction and relaxation, and transmitting force generated in the muscle sarcomeres to the ECM.[269] The DAPC is also important for Ca^{2+} homeostasis. In the absence of normal dystrophin and the DAPC, the sarcolemmal integrity is compromised, allowing an influx of calcium, immune cells, and cytokines to occur, causing the activation of proteases and the breakdown of the ECM. Secondary morphologic findings including autophagy, necrosis, and fibrosis are associated with progressive muscle wasting.[269,270] Dysregulation of matrix metalloproteinases important for normal muscle repair may also contribute to the pathogenesis in muscle tissue. In addition, there is abnormal signaling of nuclear factor-kappa β, mitogen-activated protein kinases (MAPK), and phosphatidylinositol 3 kinase/AKT pathways.[269]

DMD gene mutations are heterogeneous.[271] Intragenic deletions encompassing one or more exons represent 70% of mutations and affect the translational reading frame of the protein leading to a truncated and nonfunctional protein. Duplications of one or more exons are observed in about 5% of patients. Point mutations account for the majority of remaining mutations, but small insertions, deletions, or splice site mutations are also detected.

Becker muscular dystrophy (OMIM #300376) is a milder and less common form of muscular dystrophy with an estimated incidence of 1 in 18,500 births. BMD is an allelic variation of DMD that is caused by different mutations within the *DMD* gene that result in either reduced protein levels or a partially functional protein. As such, BMD is associated with a milder phenotype, with only half of BMD patients displaying symptoms of disease by 10 years of age with the mean age of death in the mid-40s.[271-276] About 85% of BMD patients have deletions of one or more exons; 5% to 10% have duplications involving one or more exons; and 5% to 10% have a small insertion, deletion, or point mutation. The BMD phenotype is variable and is associated with the type of mutation and the resulting effect on the corresponding structural characteristics of dystrophin.[277] Patients with deletions involving the distal rod domain of dystrophin (exons 45 to 60) show the mild BMD phenotype and in some cases remain free of symptoms until their 50s. However, BMD patients with deletions involving the amino-terminal domain of dystrophin (exons 1–9) have a more severe BMD phenotype with an earlier age of onset and more rapid progression of disease.

Patients with DCM may have a mutation at the dystrophin locus, resulting in *DMD*-associated X-linked DCM.[250,278-282]

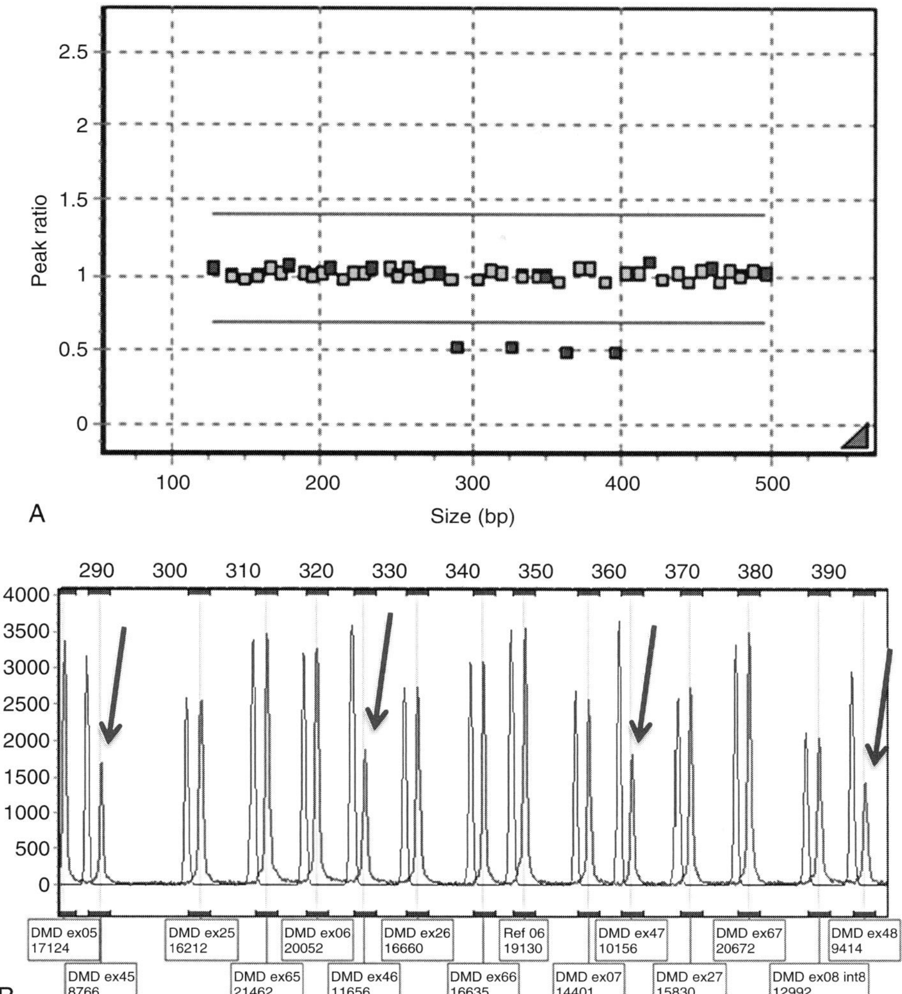

FIGURE 49.5 Deletion/duplication analysis of the *DMD* gene in a female patient by multiplex ligation-dependent probe amplification (MLPA). **A,** Wild-type (normal) alleles demonstrate a peak ratio of about 1. In this example, the patient is positive for a deletion of exons 45 to 48 *(red squares).* Note that the deleted exons show a peak ratio of approximately 0.5. **B,** Electropherogram data showing the reduction in peak height (y-axis, relative fluorescence) for exons 45 to 48 *(arrows)* in one haplotype *(grey peaks)* relative to the other control haplotype *(red).*

DCM is characterized by dilation of the left ventricle and reduced left ventricular systolic function and is a rapidly progressive, fatal disease with an onset of symptoms early in the third decade of life.[283] The lack of the functional dystrophin isoform in the heart results from altered tissue-specific transcription or alternative splicing from mutations involving the promoter region or exon 1, splice sites, or specific exonic duplications and deletions.[283] Although mutations in *DMD* can cause DCM, mutations in other genes are also associated with this phenotype.[284]

Because of the tremendous size and diversity of mutations within the *DMD* gene, DNA testing for DMD presents a challenge for clinical laboratories. DNA testing confirms the diagnosis, identifies the pathogenic mutations segregating in the family, and enables targeted analysis for carrier testing of at-risk females as well as prenatal or preimplantation testing as requested. Deletion and duplication testing for all 79 exons is most frequently performed by multiplex ligation-dependent probe amplification assay (Fig. 49.5).[285] This method determines whether each exon is present, deleted, or doubled compared with control DNA. Alternatively, microarray-based comparative genomic hybridization can be used for deletion and duplication screening.[286] Sanger sequence analysis is typically performed for the remaining 30% of mutations.[286] However more recently, targeted MPS has been used for DMD analysis.[286,287] In about 2% of DMD and BMD patients, the DNA mutation is not identified. Although a muscle biopsy can be used to confirm the diagnosis, in the absence of the pathogenic mutation, targeted mutational analysis is not possible for additional family members, and risk assessment for carrier females can be complex.[288] Particularly difficult are sporadic cases of DMD or BMD in which no other family member with DMD or BMD is known and no mutation in the affected individual is detected. Generally, one third of sporadic cases are thought to represent a new mutation in the mother's gamete from which that individual was derived.

Thus, neither the mother nor female siblings would be carriers, and the risk to the mother for a second affected son would be considered minimal. Alternatively, a female in these families could be a carrier who, although clinically asymptomatic, would be at risk of having an affected child. Furthermore, carrier assessment can be complicated by the phenomenon of germline mosaicism, in which no *DMD* gene mutation is present in lymphocyte DNA but a *DMD* gene mutation is present in germline tissue.[288] These mutations occur during mitosis in germline proliferation and explain the report of multiple affected children of women whose lymphocyte DNA contains no *DMD* mutation. If no mutation within the family is known, linkage analysis using intragenic and DMD flanking polymorphic markers can be used for carrier, prenatal, and preimplantation genetic testing.[262,289]

Although no curative treatment for DMD is available, innovative therapies are emerging.[268,290] Recombinant adeno-associated virus vectors have been used to restore 90% of strength in *mdx* mice by delivery of shortened dystrophin gene constructs. Suppression of nonsense mutations causing premature truncation of the dystrophin protein generated by point mutations in about 10% to 15% of patients can be accomplished with some success using the drug ataluren. Alternatively, for the majority of patients with gene deletions or duplications, exon skipping using antisense oligonucleotide therapy targeting specific exons has been successful for exon 51 using the drugs drisapersen or eteplirsen.[268,291] Clinical trials for these and other drugs are ongoing.[68,290-292] Alternative therapeutic approaches and new targets linked to the pathogenesis of the disease are being evaluated including use of the patient's stem cells, gene editing by homologous recombination, nonhomologous end joining, and increased expression of dystrophin similar proteins.[293-296]

Fragile X Syndrome

Fragile X syndrome (OMIM #300624) is one of the most commonly inherited forms of intellectual disability, with an estimated incidence of approximately 1 in 4000 males and approximately 1 in 5000 to 8000 females.[297] The name of the condition reflects the cytogenetic abnormality of a breakpoint or fragile site in the X chromosome. The clinical syndrome was first described by Martin and Bell in 1943 in a family with sex-linked mental retardation in both males and females yet who had no dysmorphic features.[298] The disease was later redefined by Lubs, who noted the presence of a marker X chromosome in leukocytes of males incubated in cell culture media depleted of folate and thymidine and that segregated with mental retardation within the family.[299]

The chromosomal locus for this fragile site was later localized to Xq27.3.[300] Common clinical features associated with fragile X syndrome are intellectual disability, delayed motor and speech development, macroorchidism, long face, prominent forehead and jaw, large ears, flat feet, and abnormal behavioral characteristics (eg, hyperactivity, hand flapping, temper tantrums, persevering speech patterns, poor eye contact, and autism spectrum disorder [ASD]).[301] Fragile X syndrome represents about 5% of patients with ASD.[301] These features often are less frequent and milder in affected females than in affected males because of random X inactivation of the abnormal fragile X gene in females and the expression of the normal gene in roughly half of their tissues. The primary molecular basis of fragile X syndrome includes expansion of the 5′UTR (untranslated region) CGG repeat sequence that is coupled with hypermethylation and histone deacetylation of this region and the adjacent CpG island in the promoter region of the *FMR1* gene.[302-306] This results in transcriptional silencing of the gene and no production of the associated *FMR1* protein, FMRP. Males with full expansion alleles but incomplete methylation, methylation mosaic males, or males with *FMR1* alleles differing in size within or between tissues may have a more positive clinical outcome.[307]

As a sex-linked disease, fragile X syndrome has a complicated inheritance pattern. Affected females are heterozygous for the mutation, and unaffected males can transmit the mutation through the family. For this reason, Sherman and colleagues proposed that fragile X syndrome was an X-linked dominant disorder with reduced penetrance (79% for males and 35% for females), but the penetrance of the disease appeared to increase in subsequent generations within a family.[308,309] The mechanism of this "Sherman paradox" was resolved when the gene causing fragile X syndrome, *FMR1* (*F*ragile X *m*ental *r*etardation 1), was cloned in 1991.[302,310-313] *FMR1* was the first gene discovered to cause disease through expansion of an unstable trinucleotide repeat sequence. The gene spans 38 kb, with 17 exons, and encodes a 4.4-kb mRNA transcript that contains 190 bp of the 5′UTR.[314] *FMR1* mRNA is expressed in neural and nonneural tissues during embryonic development and throughout life.[315] Interestingly, multiple mRNA splice variants have been identified in humans, mice, and fruit flies, although the roles of their associated FMRP isoforms are not clear.[316] The primary FMR1 protein, FMRP, is a 71-kDa transacting RNA-binding protein with multiple domains including two chromatin-binding domains (Agenet 1 and 2); a nuclear localization signal; a nuclear export signal domain; and three RNA-binding domains, KH1, KH2, and a RGG box.[316] FMRP is most abundant in the testes and the brain, correlating with the two most prominent features of this disease, intellectual disability and macro-orchidism. In the neurons, FMRP shuttles mRNAs from the nucleus to the cytoplasm, but it predominantly resides in postsynaptic spaces of dendritic spines, where it is associated with polyribosomes and plays a role in the regulation of translation of mRNAs important for synaptic plasticity.[316] Several models have been proposed to explain the process by which FMRP inhibits mRNA translation, including (1) blockage of translation initiation, (2) stalling of the polyribosome during translation, and (3) repression of translation via the RNA interference pathway.[316] Thus, loss of function of FMRP in fragile X patients results in abnormal translation profiles and altered synapse structure and signaling. FMRP mRNA targets are large in number yet are specific, with binding occurring only to mRNA transcripts with specific motifs.[317] Most well-characterized is FMRPs normal steady-state repression of translationally upregulated mRNAs in response to stimulation of group 1 metabotrophic glutamate receptors (mGluRs). Upon mGluR activation, FMRP is dephosphorylated, translation inhibition ceases, mRNA translation is enabled, and long-term depression of synaptic transmission occurs. In the absence of FMRP in fragile X patients, there is constitutive translation of these mRNAs in the absence of mGluR activation and excessive and prolonged synaptic long-term depression. However, clinical trials using GluR antagonists for patients with fragile X have been largely unsuccessful.[318] In addition, FMRP associates with mRNAs encoding for

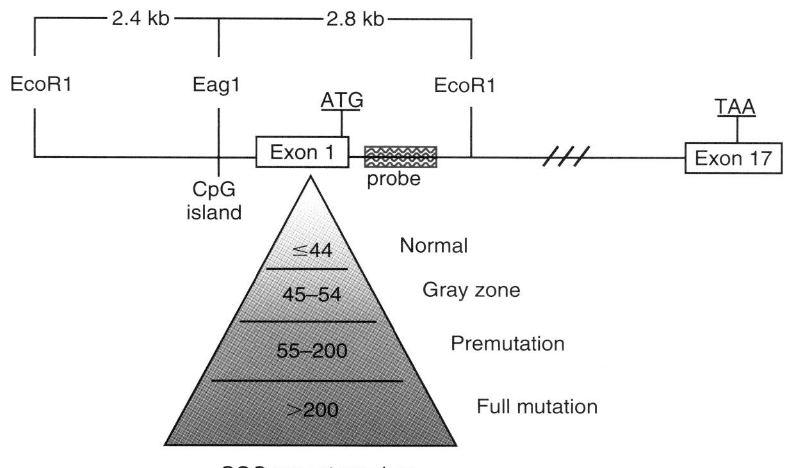

FIGURE 49.6 Schematic representation of the CGG repeat in exon 1 of *FMR1* and associated alleles. A CGG-repeat number less than or equal to 44 is normal. A CGG-repeat number of 45 to 54 is in the gray zone and can expand to a premutation in some families. A CGG-repeat number of 55 to 200 is an unstable premutation allele and is prone to expand to a full mutation allele during female meiosis. A CGG-repeat number in excess of 200 is considered a full mutation and is diagnostic of fragile X syndrome. Restriction endonuclease *EcoRI* and methylation sensitive restriction enzyme *EagI* are used to digest genomic DNA before hybridization with a ^{32}P-labeled probe (see Figure 49.7).

subunits of the neurotransmitter gamma-aminobutyric acid (GABA) receptor.[319,320] *Fmr1* knockout mice display reduced $GABA_A$ receptors, associated altered GABA concentrations, abnormal $GABA_A$ receptor signaling, and overall decreased GABAergic input. Because these aberrations are believed to play a role in the pathogenesis of fragile X syndrome, clinical trials targeting this pathway are underway.

FMR1 alleles contain blocks of CGG repeats usually 7 to 13 repeats in length, which can be interspersed with single AGG repeats.[321,322] Allelic diversity results from the variable numbers and lengths of these CGG-repeat blocks. Normal alleles have 5 to 44 repeats; gray zone, intermediate, or borderline alleles have 45 to 54 repeats; premutation alleles have 55 to 200; and full mutation expansion alleles contain more than 200 repeats (Fig. 49.6).[323] Individuals with a normal number of CGG repeats do not have fragile X syndrome, nor are they at risk of having an affected child. Individuals with 45 to 54 repeats represent alleles in the upper range of normal. These individuals do not have fragile X syndrome, yet some families may have a slightly increased risk of repeat instability and expansion to a *FMR1* premutation allele in their offspring. Premutation alleles are unstable and can expand to a full mutation allele and are associated with a risk of an offspring with fragile X syndrome. However, this expansion is largely confined to maternal transmission. Alternatively, premutation alleles can remain stable or increase to a larger premutation allele. Less commonly, a premutation allele can contract to a smaller premutation allele, a gray zone allele, or even to a normal allele.[324] The risk of CGG expansion from a premutation to a full mutation allele is dependent on both cis- and trans-acting factors, including the number of pure uninterrupted CGG repeats, the number and position of interspersed AGG repeats, maternal age, haplotype background, and less well-characterized heritable factors.[325-330] As the CGG-repeat length increases, the risk of expansion from a premutation to a full mutation in premutation carrier females increases. A carrier woman with a premutation CGG repeat length of 55 to 59 has about a 5% risk of expansion to a full mutation, a woman with a repeat length of 70 to 79 has a 31% risk of expansion, and a woman with a CGG-repeat length greater than 100 has close to a 100% chance of expansion.[331] Although CGG repeat length is the best predictor of maternal premutation expansion, AGG interruptions reduce the risk of transmission for CGG repeat lengths below 100. Nolin et al examined 457 maternal transmissions, including intermediate (45–54) and small premutation alleles (55–69) and reported that 97% of premutation alleles with 0 AGG repeats were unstable, displaying an increase in CGG repeat number compared with only 19% of alleles with 2 interspersed AGG repeats. Only 9 of these 457 transmissions resulted in a full mutation, which originated from a CGG repeat with no interspersed AGG repeats. This study supports the low frequency of full mutation expansion from CGG repeat numbers below 65 and the relevance of AGG repeats for reducing the risk of expansion.[329] Thus, the presence of AGG repeat numbers within CGG repeats can be incorporated into risk assessment for the premutation carrier patient at risk of having a child with fragile X syndrome.[327,329]

Most CGG expansion occurs before zygote formation. CGG expansion that occurs after zygote formation will result in mosaicism with the presence of cells containing either a premutation or full mutation *FMR1* allele. CGG repeat expansion occurs during DNA replication through either the incorporation of looped DNA intermediates on the nascent leading or lagging strand or stalling and restarting of the replication fork.[325,332] Alternatively, trinucleotide repeat expansion may occur at the time of DNA repair of single-strand breaks during the excision of damaged DNA.

Premutation carriers do not have fragile X syndrome. Although *FMR1* is overexpressed in these individuals, FMRP is significantly diminished, indicating reduced translation efficiency.[316] The incidence of a premutation allele in females is estimated to be between 1 in 130 to 250 females.[333] About 20% of premutation carrier females have fragile X associated primary ovarian insufficiency (FXPOI) with cessation of menstrual periods before 40 years of age.[334] Interestingly, women with premutation alleles between 70 and 90 repeats have the highest risk of developing FXPOI. Toxicity from increased expression of premutation *FMR1* mRNA contributes to these clinical symptoms. As expected, full mutation carrier females with no *FMR1* mRNA do not develop ovarian dysfunction, suggesting that decreased or absent FMRP is not contributory to this phenotype. Recently, reports suggest that premutation carrier females are at an increased risk for other medical, reproductive, psychiatric, and cognitive features compared with noncarrier control participants.[335]

Premutation carrier males are less common and are estimated at 1 in 250–810 males.[333] Although premutation carrier males do not have fragile X syndrome, they do have neurodevelopmental problems, including higher rates of attention deficit disorder, shyness, social deficits, and ASDs.[333] As adults, about one third of premutation carrier males older than the age of 50 years exhibit fragile X associated tremor and ataxia syndrome (FXTAS) with 17% of males between the ages of 50 and 59 years and as many as 75% of males older than 80 years of age affected.[336] FXTAS is a neurodegenerative syndrome characterized by progressive intention tremor, cerebellar gait ataxia, parkinsonism, neuropathy, cognitive decline, psychiatric features, and generalized brain atrophy.[337] Although predominantly in premutation carrier males, FXTAS can be seen in up to 16% of premutation carrier females. The lower incidence of FXTAS in females may be explained by the presence of a second X chromosome with a normal *FMR1* gene expressed in approximately half of all cells. The pathogenesis of FXTAS likely results from multiple factors, including (1) increased expression of *FMR1* mRNA, resulting in a gain-of-function through sequestration of specific proteins and a loss of their normal function; (2) translation of unique (CGG) proteins without an AUG start site; or (3) antisense transcription from the *FMR1* locus and decreased production of FMRP.[338]

DNA testing for fragile X syndrome can be performed using Southern blot analysis to detect the 5′UTR CGG repeat expansion as well as hypermethylation of this region, yet PCR analysis is required to accurately determine the precise CGG-repeat number (Fig. 49.7). However, because this is a CG-rich sequence, large premutation and full mutation alleles were at one time difficult to amplify by PCR. These regions can now be successfully amplified using three primers, including the typical forward and reverse primer specific to this unique area within the genome as well as a third oligonucleotide complementary to the CGG repeat itself (Fig. 49.8).[339,340] The methylation status of the CGG repeat in a full mutation allele can also be assessed using PCR.[341] These advances can alleviate the need for Southern blot analysis and reduce both the time required to perform the test and the overall turnaround time.

FMR1 DNA testing for fragile X syndrome is often requested for children with (1) the fragile X phenotype, (2) developmental delay, (3) intellectual disability, (4) ASD, or (5) family members of individuals with a diagnosis of fragile X syndrome. Fragile X DNA testing is performed for carrier testing in at-risk pregnant or preconception female patients with a family history of fragile X or intellectual disability of unknown cause. Prenatal testing can be performed on chorionic villi tissue or cultured amniocytes for at-risk pregnancies. Preimplantation diagnosis for fragile X syndrome has been reported but can be complicated by ovarian dysfunction in premutation carrier females.[342] *FMR1* premutation allele testing is performed on patients with clinical suspicion of FXPOI or FXTAS. NBS for fragile X syndrome, although feasible from blood spots as demonstrated from several pilot

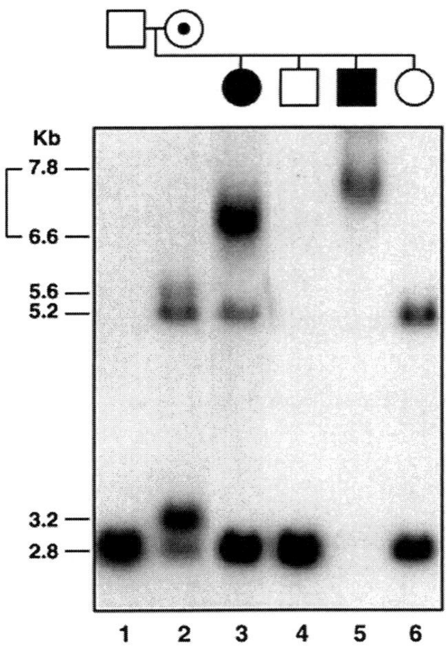

FIGURE 49.7 Southern blot analysis for the diagnosis of fragile X syndrome. Patient DNA is simultaneously digested with restriction endonucleases *EcoR*1 and *Eag*1, blotted to a nylon membrane, and hybridized with a ^{32}P-labeled probe adjacent to exon 1 of *FMR1* (see Figure 49.6). *Eag*1 is a methylation-sensitive restriction endonuclease that will not cleave the recognition sequence if the cytosine in the sequence is methylated. A normal male DNA pattern is seen in the father *(lane 1)* with a CGG-repeat number of 20 on his single X chromosome and in the brother *(lane 4)*, who has a CGG repeat of 22. This generates a band about 2.8 kb in length, corresponding to *Eag*1-*EcoR*1 fragments (see Figure 49.6). A normal female DNA pattern with a CGG-repeat number of 20 on one X chromosome and a CGG-repeat number of 22 on her second X chromosome *(lane 6)* generates two bands: one at about 2.8 kb and a second at 5.2 kb. *EcoR*1-*EcoR*1 fragments 5.2 kb in length result from methylated DNA sequences characteristic of the lyonized chromosome in each cell that is not digested with restriction endonuclease *Eag*1. DNA in *lane 2* is characteristic of a premutation carrier female with one normal allele having a CGG-repeat number of 22 (band at about 2.8 kb) and a second premutation allele with a CGG repeat number of 90 (band at about 3.0 kb). In premutation carrier females, the lyonized (methylated) cells of the X chromosome with the premutation allele is larger than 5.2 kb because of the increased CGG-repeat number and in this case is about 5.4 kb in length. *Lane 3* is diagnostic of a female with fragile X syndrome with one normal allele and one full mutation allele that is completely methylated and transcriptionally silenced. The full mutation allele arose from expansion of the maternal 90 CGG premutation allele *(lane 2)* during meiosis and the normal allele with a CGG repeat number of 20 she inherited from her father *(lane 1)*. The banding pattern observed in *lane 5* is that of an affected male with fragile X syndrome, illustrating the typical expanded allele that is fully methylated in all cells.

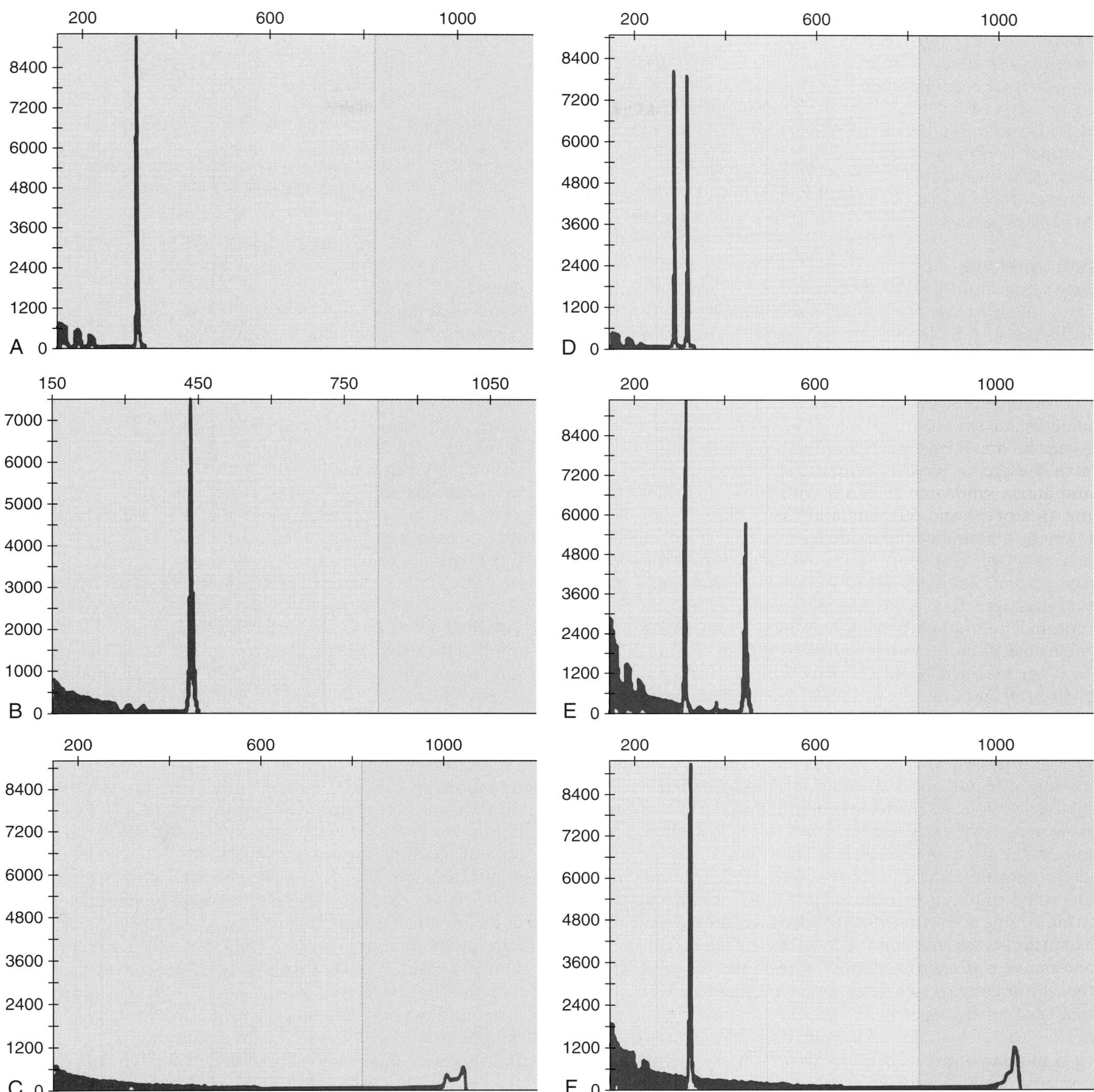

FIGURE 49.8 Electropherograms of polymerase chain reaction (PCR) products of the CGG repeat number in exon 1 of the *FMR1* gene. Amplicon sizes in bases are noted at the top of the figure and the relative amount of fluorescence detected for each amplicon is measured by the peak height (y-axis). Results were generated using the AmplideX kit (Asuragen, Inc). PCR products were amplified by using a primer pair flanking the CGG repeat of the *FMR1* gene and a 15-bp oligonucleotide as a primer within the CGG repeat itself. **A,** Subject 1 is a normal male with a CGG repeat number of 29 corresponding to an amplicon of 316 bp in length. **B,** Subject 2 represents a premutation carrier male with a CGG repeat number of 67 and an amplicon 430 bp in length. **C,** Subject 3 is the characteristic full mutation pattern obtained from a male with fragile X syndrome with more than 200 CGG repeats. **D,** Subject 4 is a pattern from a normal female with CGG repeats of 20 and 30 corresponding to amplicons at 289 bp and 319 bp, respectively. **E,** Subject 5 is a premutation female with CGG repeats of 29 and 74 corresponding to amplicons of 316 bp and 454 bp, respectively. **F,** Subject 6 is characteristic of a female affected with fragile X syndrome with both a normal *FMR1* allele with 31 CGG repeats corresponding to an amplicon of 322 bp, and a second *FMR1* allele with a full mutation with CGG repeats greater than 200 *(pink shaded area).*

studies, remains controversial and currently is not included in NBS panels.[343] NBS enables early detection and intervention for the affected child but also identifies at-risk family members who did not consent to this test and may not wish to know personal health information regarding their own risk for late-onset disorders such as FXPOI and FXTAS. Educational resources and counseling programs regarding the medical implications of the various *FMR1* alleles identified through NBS need to be established before implementation of such programs.

Rett Syndrome

Rett syndrome (OMIM #312750) is an X-linked dominant cause of inherited intellectual disability with an estimated incidence of 1 in 10,000 female births.[344] This disorder was first described in a cohort of patients with identical wringing of their hands by Dr. Andreas Rett in 1966.[345] However, it was not until the 1980s when additional studies described similar patients that the syndrome was given its name. Rett syndrome is characterized by progression in stages with initial normal development up to age 18 months followed by a period of developmental inactivity and overall signs of failure to thrive (eg, microcephaly, weight loss).[346] This stage is quickly followed by a period of rapid developmental regression and the loss of purposeful hand movement. It is during this period that patients exhibit signs of autism and profound intellectual disability. Rett syndrome is also marked by progressive motor deterioration that typically results in patients being wheelchair bound by their teens.[346] Although some patients have unexplained death,[347] many patients survive into the sixth or seventh decade of life. It should be noted that Rett syndrome is almost exclusively observed in females because *MECP2* mutations in males are typically embryonic lethal.

Identification of the genetic cause of Rett syndrome was initially difficult because traditional linkage methods were ineffective because of the sporadic nature of the disease.[346] However, using exclusion mapping methods, it was determined that the causative gene for Rett syndrome was located at chromosome Xq28.[348-352] Systematic analysis of this region identified mutations in the methyl-CpG binding protein 2 (*MECP2*) gene as causative for Rett syndrome in 1999,[353] The *MECP2* gene is composed of four exons that produce two different protein isoforms.[346,354] The protein produced by the *MECP2* gene is a chromosome binding protein expressed in all tissues that specifically targets 5-methyl cytosine residues.[355] MECP2 contains three functional domains: a methyl-CpG binding domain (MBD),[356] a transcriptional repression domain (TRD),[357] and a C-terminal domain (CTD).[358] The MBD specifically binds to methylated cytosine residues and shows a preference for binding to CpG dinucleotide sequences that are adjacent to A/T-rich motifs.[359] Downstream from the MBD is the TRD, which is critical in the interaction of MECP2 with histone deacetylases and other transcription corepressors.[346,353,354,358,360,361] Finally, the CTD enables MECP2 binding to the nucleosome core and allows the protein to bind to naked DNA.[346,354] All of these domains are essential for the MECP2 protein to properly function, and mutations in each of these domains have been found in patients with Rett syndrome.

MECP2 gene mutations are identified in approximately 95% of patients with a classic Rett syndrome phenotype.[346] To date, more than 400 *MECP2* gene mutations have been reported in the literature, and newly identified mutations are regularly added to the RettBASE online mutation database.[362,363] Described pathogenic *MECP2* gene mutations include nonsense, missense, frameshift, and large deletions.[362,363] Interestingly, mutations at eight common residues account for approximately 70% of all cases.[346,354] These common mutations all occur in CpG dinucleotides and include p.Arg106, p.Arg133, p.Thr158, p.Arg168, p.Arg255, p.Arg270, p.Arg294, and p.Arg306 (Fig. 49.9). Because there is a large degree of phenotypic heterogeneity in patients with Rett syndrome, several studies have been performed to correlate genotype with phenotype. Truncating (nonsense or frameshift) mutations cause a more severe phenotype than missense mutations, and mutations that occur in the CTD typically result in milder disease presentation.[346,364] The majority of mutations in *MECP2* are de novo events.[365,366] However, there are cases in which mutations are maternally inherited from an individual who is either unaffected or mildly affected because of skewed X-inactivation. It is therefore important to establish whether a pathogenic mutation is de novo or maternally derived because the recurrence risk in future pregnancies of mutation-positive females with skewed X-inactivation approaches 50%.

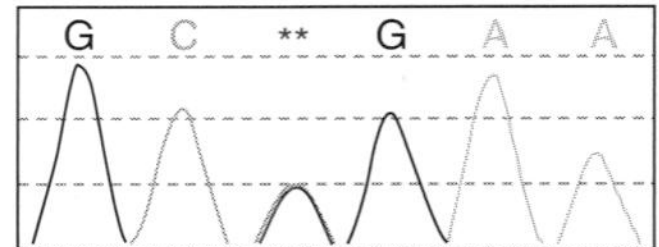

FIGURE 49.9 Sanger sequencing of the *MECP2* gene illustrating a common pathogenic mutation (c.808C>T) at p.Arg270 *(asterisk)*. This C>T transition mutation results in a stop codon (TGA) and premature truncation of the protein.

Because of the heterogeneous nature of disease-causing mutations in *MECP2*, clinical testing for confirmation of a diagnosis of Rett syndrome typically involves DNA sequencing of the entire *MECP2* gene coding region. If mutations are not identified by sequencing analysis, large deletion and duplication analysis (typically MLPA) is performed. This combination detects approximately 95% of causative mutations in patients with a clinical diagnosis of Rett syndrome. Recently, mutations in the *CDKL5* and *FOXG1* genes have been shown to cause variant forms of Rett syndrome and should therefore be considered for follow-up testing in individuals not found to have mutations in *MECP2*.[367-373] Rett syndrome treatment is largely based on the manifestations of disease and therefore should be tailored to each individual patient.

Complex Diseases

A complex or multifactorial inheritance pattern suggests interaction of one or more genes in combination with lifestyles and one or more environmental factors. Multifactorial diseases can be prevalent in some families with several affected family members, but the disease does not follow typical Mendelian inheritance patterns. A disease may present in multiple family members because of the sharing of similar disease-predisposing alleles and often sharing of similar daily habits, routines, and diet. The specific genes, lifestyle habits, and environmental factors and their respective contribution in predisposition to disease vary among diseases and are difficult to elucidate. Twin studies are often used to determine the relative importance of each component. Among twins who were raised together, a greater concordance of disease among monozygotic (MZ) twins (who share all of their genes) than among dizygotic (DZ) twins (who share 50% of their genes) provides strong evidence of a genetic component of the disease. Conversely, disease concordance of less than 100% in MZ twins is strong evidence that nongenetic factors play a role in the disease process. Large genome-wide association studies (GWAS) are used to identify genes and genetic variants that play a role in the pathogenesis of common complex diseases. Examples of complex adult-onset diseases, include type 1 diabetes, rheumatoid arthritis, multiple sclerosis, osteoporosis, Parkinson disease, Alzheimer disease, hypertension, atrial fibrillation, alcoholism, schizophrenia, depression, obesity, and thrombophilia.

Thrombophilia

Thrombophilia is defined as an abnormality of hemostasis with a predisposition to thrombosis. A common complication of venous thromboembolism (VTE) is the development of a deep vein thrombosis (DVT) or a more serious, and potentially fatal, pulmonary embolism. Thrombophilia (OMIM #188050) is a multifactorial disorder resulting from the interaction of genetic, lifestyle, and environmental factors. Risk factors include the use of oral contraceptives, hormone replacement therapy, trauma, obesity, malignancy, surgery, immobility, pregnancy, and advanced age.[374,375]

Protein products of many genes are involved in the anticoagulation and coagulation pathway to regulate hemostasis. Hypercoagulability, or an alteration in the coagulation pathway that predisposes to thrombosis, can be caused by variants in genes encoding proteins involved in the coagulation pathway.[376] Although familial thrombophilia can be attributed to mutations in genes encoding protein C, *PROC* (OMIM #176860); protein S, *PROS1* (OMIM #612336) or antithrombin III, *SERPINC1* (OMIM #107300), 50% to 60% of familial thrombophilia is associated with variants in genes encoding coagulation factor V, *FV* (OMIM #188055) or factor II, *F2* (OMIM #176930). In 1993, Dahlbäck reported that familial thrombophilia caused resistance to activated protein C (APC).[377] In 1994, Bertina and colleagues reported linkage of a common G-to-A base substitution at nucleotide 1691 (c.1691G>A) in exon 10 of the *FV* gene with the APC resistance phenotype.[378] This nucleotide change results in an arginine-to-glutamine substitution in the FV protein at codon 506 (p.Arg506Gln) and is commonly referred to as FV Leiden, named for the Dutch city where it was discovered.[378] The c.1691G>A substitution is common in the white population of Northern European descent with a reported frequency of about 3% to 5%, but it is absent in other populations, including those in Africa and Southeast Asia.

The *FV* gene is localized to chromosome 1q24.2, is about 70 kb, contains 25 exons, and encodes a 330 kDa protein.[379] In the coagulation pathway, FV is converted to an activated form, FVa, by thrombin. FVa is a cofactor for activated factor X, FXa, and is required for the conversion of prothrombin (F2) to thrombin (F2a). Thrombin is essential for the last step of the coagulation cascade by catalyzing the conversion of fibrinogen to fibrin for clot formation. Activated FV is converted to an inactive form by APC. The arginine residue at codon 506 is one of three peptide bonds (Arg306, Arg506, and Arg679) cleaved by APC to inactivate FV and decrease the affinity to FXa, thereby reducing the conversion of prothrombin to thrombin.[380,381] Substitution of a glutamine residue at this site prolongs APC inactivation of FVa by approximately 10-fold, thereby shifting the balance of hemostasis to favor coagulation and increasing thrombin production.[382]

Heterozygous *FV* gene c.1691G>A carriers have a lifelong 7.9-fold increased relative risk of venous thrombosis compared with an increased relative risk for homozygotes as high as 80-fold.[375,383] However, FV Leiden does not confer increased risk for arterial thrombosis.[384] The mean age of onset of symptoms associated with thrombosis is 44 years for heterozygotes and 31 years for homozygotes.[383] *FV* c.1691G>A carriers represent about 25% of patients with idiopathic VTE, 30% to 50% of patients with recurrent VTE, 20% to 60% of oral contraceptive–associated VTE, 20% to 40% of pregnancy-associated VTE, and 8% to 30% of patients with pregnancy loss.[385] Although *FV* gene mutations are considered dominant (heterozygous mutations carriers can be symptomatic), many heterozygous carriers remain asymptomatic because thrombophilia is a complex disease resulting from the interaction of genetic, lifestyle, and environmental factors.[383,386]

Several years later also in Leiden, Poort and coworkers described a genetic variant in the 3′ untranslated region of the *F2* gene present in 18% of patients with a documented family history of venous thrombosis.[387] The *F2* gene maps to chromosome 11p11.2, is 21 kb in length, contains 14 exons, and encodes a 70-kDa protein.[388] The *F2* 3′ variant that segregated with disease, c.*97G>A, results in increased levels of plasma coagulation F2, prothrombin, and a 2.8-fold lifelong increased risk of venous thrombosis.[387] This variant allele is largely confined to white populations at a frequency of 1% to 2% and is rare in other populations. FII requires activation and conversion to thrombin by FXa and FVa to catalyze the conversion of fibrinogen to fibrin, the last step of blood clot formation. The G-to-A substitution does not alter the coding region of the protein; rather, it enhances prothrombin mRNA stability and ultimately results in increased production of both prothrombin and thrombin.[389]

The risk of venous thrombosis is increased 16-fold in *F2* c.*97 G>A carriers using oral contraceptives, and the risk of cerebral vein thrombosis increases 149-fold.[390,391] In the white population, this base substitution is present in 6.2% of patients with venous thrombosis compared with 2.3% of control participants.

Inherited together, *FV* c.1691G>A and *F2* c.*97G>A convey an increased relative risk for a VTE event, an example of additive genetic effects associated with a complex disease.[392-394] Metaanalysis shows a higher risk for severe preeclampsia in women with *FV* or *F2* variants, with odds ratios of 1.9 and 2.01, respectively.[395]

Venous thromboembolism most often is classified as "provoked" with one or more predisposing risk factors; however, in 25% to 50% of cases, it is "unprovoked" with the precipitating cause not determined. The initial treatment of patients with VTE uses both heparin and vitamin K antagonists (eg, warfarin).[396] After several days, the heparin is discontinued, and warfarin therapy is continued. For "provoked" VTE, therapy is discontinued after 3 months for distal DVT and 6 months for proximal DVT or PE. Therapy may be altered based on the type of thrombotic event, the type of precipitating event, or the absence of a triggering cause. The recurrence risk is higher

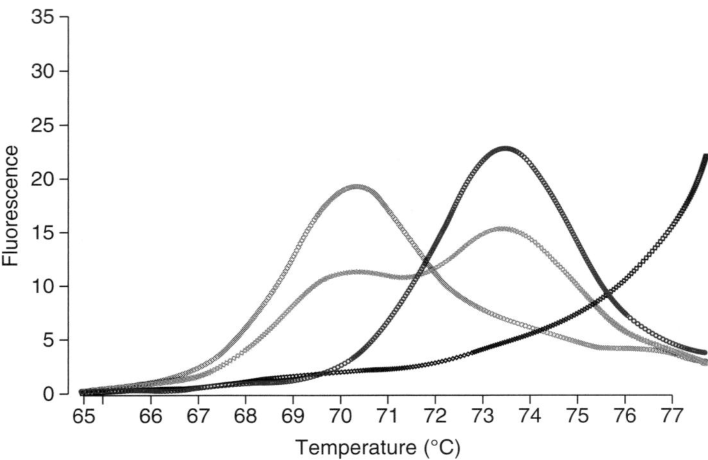

FIGURE 49.10 Interrogation of the common c.*97G>A mutation in the *F2* gene by melting curve analysis. A perfectly matched probe is more tightly bound to the polymerase chain reaction (PCR) product and therefore will melt at a higher temperature than when there is a nucleotide mismatch between the probe and the PCR product. In this example, the probe perfectly matches the wild-type allele *(red)*. When the *F2* c.*97G>A mutation is heterozygous, the probe binds to the mutant allele imperfectly (with a lower melting temperature) and to the wild-type allele perfectly, resulting in the presence of two peaks *(pink)*. When a patient is homozygous for the c.*97G>A mutation, only an imperfect match is possible, resulting a single peak at the lower temperature *(gray)*. A no-template control is always included to rule out potential DNA contamination *(black)*.

in "unprovoked" VTE and in patients with cancer, suggesting prolonged or indefinite anticoagulant therapy.[397] D-dimer levels may identify patients for continued anticoagulation therapy.[398,399] Antithrombic agents may be most advantageous in the management of pregnancy VTE and associated thrombophilia.[400] To avoid the risk of bleeding with sometimes fatal complications, treatment is regularly monitored using prothrombin time reported as the international normalized ratio (INR) ideally achieving an INR of 2.0 to 3.0. Because of the challenges with warfarin therapy, new oral anticoagulants have been developed and effectively used to prevent recurrence of VTE. These include FIIa and FXa inhibitors, and most recently a FIXa inhibitor that does not require regular laboratory monitoring.[401] These drugs carry a lower risk of bleeding complications and appear to provide similar efficacy compared to standard treatment.[401-406]

Another genetic risk factor for predisposition to thrombophilia is a common 1-bp guanine deletion/insertion (4G/5G) polymorphism at c.-817dupG in the promoter region of the *SERPINE1* gene located on chromosome 7q22.1 (OMIM#173360).[407,408] This gene is approximately 12.2 kb in length with 9 exons and encodes a mature 379-amino-acid protein with a molecular weight of about 42.7 kDa.[409-411] This protein, plasminogen activator inhibitor-1 (PAI-1), is a member of the serine protease inhibitor family and is released by endothelial cells to block the degradation of fibrin clots. Increased levels of PAI-1 can be associated with thrombophilia, and the *SERPINE1* 4G allele is associated with higher transcription levels than the 5G allele.[407,412,413] Testing for common variants in the 5,10-methylenetetrahydroflate reductase *(MTHFR)* gene, c.665C>T and c.1286A>C, once thought to convey a slight risk for thrombophilia, are not as frequently used for routine clinical evaluation of this disease.[414]

Many DNA testing platforms have been used for the detection of *FV* c.1691G>A and *F2* c.*97G>A variants, including Invader technology, PCR coupled with restriction-endonuclease digestion and gel electrophoresis, or real-time PCR followed by melting curve analysis with fluorescence resonance energy transfer probes (Fig. 49.10). The most common testing methods for the 4G/5G *SERPINE1* polymorphism involve the use of PCR and melting curve analysis or PCR coupled with capillary electrophoresis and fragment analysis. Any testing platform is acceptable for clinical use as long as the procedure has been properly validated in a CLIA-certified laboratory that follows appropriate regulatory and quality assurance guidelines.

DNA testing for factor V may be requested when a patient tests positive on the functional activated protein C resistance assay to both confirm the diagnosis and distinguish between *FV* c.1691G>A heterozygotes and homozygotes.[415] At many hospitals, screening for FV abnormalities using the functional activated protein C resistance assay is the preferred method because it is both cost effective and can be automated.[416] However, DNA testing should be ordered in place of the functional assay for patients taking FIIa or FVa oral inhibitors (eg, argatroban, dabigatran, bivalirudin, or rivaroxaban) because these can interfere with the functional assay causing a falsely normal result. Similarly, inaccurate results can be obtained in patients with lupus anticoagulants.[415] The clinical utility of knowing the *FV* or *F2* genotype has been debated because it may not affect the clinical management of patients.[417-419] Yet testing for *FV* and *F2* variants is common in clinical practice, and most experts believe that testing is appropriate for targeted patients, including those with (1) venous thrombosis or pulmonary embolism before 50 years of age; (2) venous thrombosis at an unusual site (hepatic, mesenteric, portal, or cerebral veins); (3) recurrent VTE; (4) VTE and a strong family history of thrombotic disease; (5) VTE in pregnancy, postpartum, or associated with contraceptive use or hormone replacement therapy; or (6) unexplained recurrent pregnancy loss.[420-423] However, routine screening before hormone use is not routinely performed, nor is it considered cost-effective. Modifications to patient management after knowledge of this information may involve length of treatment with anticoagulants and management of other procoagulation risk factors. First-degree relatives of *FV* or *F2* variant positive patients are at a higher risk of related thrombotic events if the proband was younger and experienced an "unprovoked" thrombophilic event. DNA testing for *FV* or *F2* variants is not recommended for the general population, prenatal carrier screening or NBS. In addition, variants at two other factor V arginine-cleavage sites have been reported, but these variants are rare and are not part of routine *FV* DNA testing.[424] Although *FV* or *F2* variants are present in 50% to 60% of families with inherited thrombophilia, defects in protein C, protein S, and antithrombin are detected in 10% to 15% of families with inherited venous thrombosis. These less common coagulation deficiencies are typically diagnosed through immunologic or functional assays that do not involve DNA testing. Furthermore, unlike *FV* and *F2* genes, no single common variants in *PROC*, *PROS1*, or *SERPINEC1* have been identified.

Hereditary Pancreatitis

Hereditary pancreatitis (HP; OMIM# 167800) occurs in approximately 1 in 300,000 individuals in the Western world.[425] HP traditionally refers to the occurrence of pancreatitis in two or more individuals in two or more generations of a family.[426] Additionally, HP can refer to individuals with disease-causing germline mutations in any of the genes associated with the disorder.[426] Individuals affected with HP are typically characterized by acute pancreatitis (disease with a duration of a few days to a few weeks) that eventually progresses to chronic pancreatitis (disease with a duration >6 months) over a period of years.[426] The onset of symptoms is difficult to predict, but most individuals with HP are first affected with acute pancreatitis by age 10 years and chronic disease by age 20 years.[427] Given the inflammatory nature of the disease, HP patients are also at higher risk for pancreatic cancer than the general population and should be routinely screened.[428] The complex nature of disease (and variable penetrance) indicates that although genetics is a risk factor for disease, several environmental factors (eg, diet, tobacco use, alcohol consumption) also contribute to disease manifestations.[427] Mutations in the protease, serine, 1 *(PRSS1)* gene (also known as cationic trypsinogen, located at chromosome 7q35) are the most common genetic cause of pancreatitis, accounting for 60% to 100% of HP families.[426,427] Cationic trypsinogen is the main isoform of trypsinogen in human pancreatic juice and is involved in facilitating zymogen activation.[429-431] Mutations in the *PRSS1* gene cause a gain of function and typically result in the constitutive autoactivation of the cationic trypsinogen protein.[432-436] These mutations are inherited in an autosomal dominant manner with variable penetrance.[425] In fact, several studies conducted using large HP patient cohorts have reported that the penetrance of *PRSS1* mutations ranges between 40% and 96%[437-444]; therefore, predicting disease progression in presymptomatic individuals who carry pathogenic *PRSS1* gene mutations is not possible because symptoms and onset are extremely variable even among affected members of the same family.

Several additional genetic risk factors for pancreatitis have been identified.[445-447] In 1998, mutations in the *CFTR* gene (located at chromosome 7q31.2) were reported as a genetic cause of pancreatitis.[447] As discussed in detail earlier, *CFTR* gene mutations are causative for the multisystem autosomal recessive disorder CF. One of the most common features of CF is altered pancreatic function, so the discovery of genetic mutations in the *CFTR* gene in patients with isolated pancreatic disease is not surprising. However, unlike individuals with classic CF disease who carry two severe *CFTR* gene mutations, pancreatitis patients often carry a severe pathogenic *CFTR* gene mutation on one chromosome and a mild mutation on the other (or a mild mutation on both chromosomes).[447] About 30% of patients with pancreatitis remained idiopathic and did not have mutations in *PRSS1* or *CFTR*. In 2000, autosomal recessive mutations in the serine protease inhibitor, Kazal type 1 *(SPINK1)* gene (located at chromosome 5q32), were reported as an additional cause of HP.[446] In this study, 96 patients with chronic pancreatitis were tested for mutations in the *SPINK1* gene, and 23% of the patients tested positive for mutations.[446] Interestingly, a single mutation in codon 34 (p.Asn34Ser) was the most common mutation identified.[446] The *SPINK1* gene produces a protein (SPINK1) that prevents premature trypsinogen activation through the inhibition of trypsin activity in the pancreas.[448] Therefore, *SPINK1* mutations may cause a decrease in the ability of SPINK1 protein to inhibit trypsin.[446] However, functional studies have been inconclusive and the exact mechanism by which *SPINK1* mutations cause pancreatitis remains unknown.

Mutations in the chymotrypsin C *(CTRC)* gene (located at chromosome 1p36.21) are the most recently described genetic cause of HP.[445] An international team of investigators screened a large cohort of German pancreatitis patients (n = 901) for mutations in the *CTRC* gene.[445] *CTRC* mutations were identified in 3.3% of this patient group, and subsequent studies in an Indian population identified *CTRC* variants in 14.1% of affected individuals.[445] Given the overrepresentation of *CTRC* variants in patients with pancreatitis (compared with control populations), the authors were able to conclude that mutations in the *CTRC* gene increase the risk for pancreatitis.[445] The *CTRC* gene produces a digestive enzyme called chymotrypsin C (CTRC) that promotes proteolytic inactivation of trypsinogen and trypsin and is essential for limiting intrapancreatic trypsinogen activation.[449,450] Functional studies indicate that mutations in *CTRC* are loss of function, resulting in diminished secretion ability, impaired catalytic activity, and an inability to degrade trypsin.[450] Similar to *SPINK1*, mutations in the *CTRC* gene are autosomal recessive and require the presence of two pathogenic mutations to cause disease.

DNA testing for pancreatitis is most often performed stepwise with Sanger sequencing of the *PRSS1* gene as the first step. The identification of a single pathogenic *PRSS1* gene mutation confirms a diagnosis of HP in symptomatic patients and indicates a substantial risk for the development of disease in an asymptomatic individual. If *PRSS1* analysis is negative, Sanger sequencing of *CFTR*, *SPINK1*, and *CTRC* can be considered. All three of these genes are inherited in an autosomal recessive manner, and therefore identifying two pathogenic mutations is required to confirm a diagnosis in a symptomatic individual. The identification of a single pathogenic mutation may increase the risk for pancreatitis but, by itself, is not causative for disease. Comprehensive testing of all four HP-associated genes can be performed as the initial test in HP patients. However, this may increase the complexity of the results obtained (eg, variants of uncertain significance), so patients should be counseled carefully before ordering such a panel.

Even with the advances over the past decade in our understanding of the genetics responsible for HP, cases remain that are not explained by mutations in a single gene. These individuals appear to have complex disease that involves a number of pathogenic mutations in several genes (ie, *CFTR* and *SPINK1*) suggesting that gene–gene interactions govern their disease.[426] In fact, as many as one third of pancreatitis cases (acute and chronic) result from complex inheritance patterns.[426,451] In some cases, environmental factors may play a more significant role than genetics in the development of this disease.[451]

Treatment for HP varies between acute and chronic disease. Pain management is the primary focus for patients with acute pancreatitis.[426] Patients with acute disease are also counseled to abstain from activities that will predispose them to future attacks (eg, smoking, alcohol consumption).[426,427] Patients with chronic pancreatitis may be treated with pancreatic enzyme replacement therapy to aid with digestion.[427] In some severe cases, patients may undergo total pancreatectomy with islet autotransplantation.[426] Additional treatment should be based on manifestations of disease such as diabetes mellitus.

Hereditary Breast and Ovarian Cancer

Breast cancer is the most common cancer in women with about 1 in 8 developing invasive cancer during their lifetime.[452] Approximately 10% of breast cancers appear to be familial, exhibiting dominant inheritance. Inherited breast cancer is associated with multiple cases of breast or ovarian cancer within the family, an early age of disease onset, bilateral disease or multiple cancers in the same breast, and an increased prevalence of male breast cancer. Epithelial carcinoma of the ovary is the fifth leading cause of death in women.[453]

Most hereditary breast and ovarian cancer (HBOC) is caused by mutations in *BRCA1* (OMIM #113705) or *BRCA2* (OMIM #600185). In addition to a predisposition to breast and ovarian cancer, germline mutation carriers are at an increased risk for pancreas cancer. and male carriers are at an increased risk for prostate and male breast cancer.[454] The incidence of *BRCA1/BRCA2* mutations in the United States is estimated to be between 1 in 300 to 500.[455] However, the combined frequency of two founder mutations in *BRCA1* (185delAG, 5382insC) and one in *BRCA2* (6174delT) in the Ashkenazi Jewish population is as high as almost 3%.[456]

Although dominantly inherited, *BRCA1/BRCA2* mutation carriers do not possess a 100% certainty of developing cancer. Rather, as tumor suppressor genes, inactivation of both alleles is required for tumorigenesis. In a patient who has inherited a mutant *BRCA1* or *BRCA2* allele, the second normal allele is mutated and most often deleted via somatic mutation in cancer cells. By the age of 70 years, *BRCA1* mutation carriers have a 44% to 75% risk of developing breast cancer, an 83% chance of developing contralateral breast cancer after an initial cancer is found, and a 43% to 76% possibility of developing ovarian cancer.[457] Slightly lower frequencies are observed for *BRCA2* mutation carriers who have a 41% to 70% risk of developing breast cancer, a 62% chance of developing contralateral breast cancer, and a 7.4% to 34% possibility of developing ovarian cancer by 70 years of age. Penetrance of the disease in *BRCA1/BRCA2* mutation carriers is determined by both other genes and lifestyle and environmental factors. Identified susceptibility factors influencing development of disease include parity, body mass index, age at menarche, menopause and first full-term pregnancy, breastfeeding, smoking, and oral contraceptive usage.[458,459] Additional genetic susceptibility factors include variants in multiple genes or genetic regions such as *FGFR2, TOX3, MAP3K1, LSP1, SLC4A7*, 2q35, and 5p12 for *BRCA2* germline mutation carriers and variants in *TOX3* and genetic factors located at 2q35 for *BRCA1* germline mutation carriers.[460] Understanding susceptibility factors, both environmental and genetic, aid in appropriate counseling for patients by either increasing or decreasing their overall risks for the development of cancer and help guide their clinical management decisions for surgical interventions. However, to prevent disease in *BRCA1/BRCA2* mutation carrier women, population-based testing for all women as routine medical care has been proposed.[461] This screening would identify germline mutation carriers and enable appropriate clinical management to reduce their lifetime cancer risks.

In a large study, Mayaddat and colleagues compared the pathologic characteristics between *BRCA1* and *BRCA2* mutation–positive breast and ovarian tumors.[462] *BRCA1*-mutated breast tumors were most frequently invasive ductal carcinomas (80%), grade 3 (77%) with the majority of tumors (69%) triple negative (TN) for the expression of estrogen (ER), progestin (PR) and *HER2*. *BRCA2* mutation positive breast tumors likewise were predominantly invasive ductal carcinomas (83%) but with relatively equal numbers of grade 2 (43%) and grade 3 (50%) observed. However, unlike *BRCA1* mutation–positive tumors, only 16% were TN. Medullary carcinomas were more frequent in *BRCA1* mutation–positive tumors (9.4%) compared with *BRCA2* (2.2%), and invasive lobular was seen more frequently in *BRCA2* mutation positive tumors (8.4%) compared with *BRCA1* mutated tumors (2.2%). Interestingly, *BRCA1*-mutated TN tumors were highest in patients with an earlier age of onset, but TN tumors were more common in tumors from *BRCA2*-positive carriers with an older age of onset. Both *BRCA1* and *BRCA2* mutation–positive ovarian tumors were morphologically similar, with most serous (66% and 70%) and grade 3 (77% and 73%), respectively. Overall, about 15% of ovarian cancers are associated with germline mutations in *BRCA1/BRCA2*, and up to 25% of high-grade serous tumors are positive for germline mutations in one of these two genes.[463] Although the median age for ovarian cancer is close to 60 years, it is about 10 years earlier in patients with a genetic predisposition to this disease.

Using DNA linkage studies, Hall and coworkers mapped the gene for early-onset familial breast cancer to chromosome 17q21.[464] In 1994, *BRCA1* was cloned; it was later confirmed by several other investigators as the susceptibility gene in breast and ovarian cancer kindreds.[465-467] The *BRCA1* gene on chromosome 17q21.31 spans 80 kb and is composed of 24 exons; 22 encode the 7.8-kb mRNA that is translated into a protein of 1863 amino acids. Exon 11, encoding 60% of the protein, is alternatively spliced in a number of tissues. In families not linked to *BRCA1*, a second susceptibility locus at chromosome 13q12-13 was proposed, and in 1995, *BRCA2* was cloned.[468-470] The *BRCA2* gene spans 70 kb, contains 27 exons, encodes an 11.5-kb mRNA, and is translated into a protein of 3418 amino acids.

BRCA1 is a widely expressed multifunctional protein that maintains genomic stability in the repair of double-strand breaks in DNA via the homologous recombination pathway and cell cycle checkpoint control.[471,472] BRCA1 also plays a role in transcription regulation, chromatin architecture, apoptosis, mRNA splicing, and ubiquitination of multiple proteins. Although a distinctly different protein, BRCA2 is also important in the repair of double-strand DNA breaks and in transcription regulation.[473,474] Because BRCA1/ BRCA2-deficient tumors have aberrant DNA repair pathways, they are more sensitive to treatment options causing DNA damage such as platinum-based chemotherapies cisplatin and carboplatin.[473] Clinical trials using PARP (poly ADP ribose polymerase) inhibitors for the treatment of patients with BRCA1/ BRCA2-deficient tumors have been effective.[475] PARP1 is required for base excision repair and repair of DNA single-strand breaks. When PARP1 inhibition occurs in BRCA1/BRCA2 tumors, both double- and single-strand DNA breaks are not repaired, and cell death occurs. However, similar to other targeted therapy, resistant clones develop, and the effectiveness of therapy diminishes.

Variants in *BRCA1* and *BRCA2* are heterogeneous and are located throughout each gene with founder mutations identified in many different ethnic populations.[476] Most variants represent loss-of-function alleles, with more than 75% of the reported variants as deletions, nonsense mutations, or insertions, with deletions representing the majority. Many pathogenic missense mutations occur at critical BRCA1- or BRCA2-protein binding sites that are required for normal function. Although the majority of mutations detected are obviously pathogenic (eg, nonsense or frameshift mutations causing premature truncation of the protein), some detected gene variations may be family specific and may not result in an obvious biologic functional change to the protein based on in silico analysis.[477] These variants of unknown significance (VUS) are most often missense, splice site, or small in-frame insertions or deletions. These may be as common as 7% to 15% of the reported BRCA variants in individuals of European ancestry and can be even higher for patients of other ethnicities for which common variants have not been well characterized.[478] Segregation studies confirming linkage of VUS with disease can be performed if archived tissue or DNA from multiple family members is available.[477] Unfortunately, in many situations, DNA from an adequate number of family members to perform these studies is not possible. The clinical significance for some VUS may become clear by sharing data between laboratories; however, at some testing sites, these databases remain proprietary.[479]

In families in which the clinical history is suggestive of hereditary breast and ovarian cancer, DNA tests for *BRCA1* and *BRCA2* may be requested. Testing should be considered for a woman if (1) there are at least three cases in her family of breast, ovarian, or pancreatic cancer at an early age or aggressive prostate cancer; (2) she has breast or epithelial ovarian cancer and is younger than 45 years; (3) both breast and ovarian cancers are present in her or in a family member; (4) she has breast or ovarian cancer and is of Ashkenazi Jewish descent; (5) she has a male relative with breast cancer; (6) she has a family member with a known *BRCA1* or *BRCA2* mutation; or (7) she has breast cancer and a family history of *BRCA1*- or *BRCA2*-related tumors.[480] In addition, *BRCA1* and *BRCA2* testing should be performed on any man with breast cancer. Nevertheless, *BRCA1* and *BRCA2* mutations can be found in families that do not meet these criteria, and mutations may not be found even when expected.

Before testing, a genetic professional should discuss the likelihood of a *BRCA1* or *BRCA2* mutation, the types of variants that may be identified, and that offspring and other family members may also be at risk for having a mutation.[481] Mathematical models are available to determine the likelihood of *BRCA1* or *BRCA2* mutations, and these models can be used to assist in counseling.[482,483] After a *BRCA* mutation has been detected, targeted mutation analysis can be performed in presymptomatic family members at risk for inheriting the mutation. Counseling for presymptomatic patients may include discussing psychological issues involving the fear of cancer or medical procedures and cancer surveillance and potential risk-reducing surgery options if a mutation is identified. Management of presymptomatic *BRCA1* or *BRCA2* mutation–positive women is complex. The National Comprehensive Cancer Network Clinical Practice Guidelines has established surgical and surveillance guidelines to decrease the risk of disease in these women.[480] The patient may wish to have prophylactic mastectomy, salpingo-oophorectomy, or both. In the United States, it is estimated that these elective procedures are performed at a frequency of 20% to 49% and 37% to 60%, respectively.[478] Alternatively, she may choose to use increased surveillance and prevention strategies for the early detection of breast and ovarian cancer. Surveillance for breast cancer in *BRCA1* or *BRCA2* mutation–positive individuals should include annual mammography and breast magnetic resonance imaging beginning at 25 years of age. Surveillance for ovarian cancer should include transvaginal ultrasonography and CA-125 measurement every 6 months beginning at age 35 or 10 years earlier than the earliest age of onset in the family. Clinical management for patients with a *BRCA1* or *BRCA2* VUS is challenging, and the use of risk-reducing surgeries is appropriately lower.[478] In these cases, because the VUS may ultimately be reclassified as benign, counseling is recommended depending on personal and family medical history rather than solely on *BRCA* mutations.

For presymptomatic patients with a family history but no prior DNA testing for breast or ovarian cancer, the genetic professional should explain before testing the possibility of a VUS result and continued anxiety and uncertainty. In addition, the patient should understand the possibility of false-negative results because (1) not all possible *BRCA1* or *BRCA2* gene mutations are tested or (2) there may be possible mutations in another breast cancer susceptibility gene. Because only 25% of familial breast and/or ovarian cancer is due to *BRCA* mutations, MPS analysis for a panel of breast- and/or ovarian-related cancer predisposing genes may be more appropriate and more cost effective (Table 49.6).[484-489] This strategy reduces the possibility of a false-negative result by increasing the mutation detection rate by a small percentage. Appropriate patient surveillance and management depend on the mutant gene identified.[490] Because founder gene mutations are observed for some susceptibility genes, a specific gene test or cancer panel may be requested based on the ethnicity of the patient and the presence of that gene in a panel. If multiple cancers are reported in the family in

TABLE 49.6 Common Inherited Breast, Gynecologic, and Gastrointestinal Cancer Susceptibility Genes

Gene	Location	Name	Function	Associated Cancer	Disease
APC	5q22.2	Adenomatous polyposis coli	Control of cell proliferation	Colon, small bowel, thyroid, liver, pancreas	Familial adenomatous polyposis
ATM	11q22.3	Ataxia-telangiectasia mutated	Cell cycle control	Breast, ovarian, gastric, hematologic	Ataxia-telangiectasia
AXIN2	17q24.1	Axin 2	Assumed WNT signaling pathway regulator	Colon	Oligodontia-colorectal cancer syndrome
BARD1	2q35	*BRCA1*-associated ring domain 1	DNA repair, apoptosis, cell cycle arrest	Breast, ovarian, brain	Familial breast cancer
BMPR1A	10q23.2	Bone morphogenetic protein receptor, type IA	Cell signaling, proliferation, and differentiation	Colon, stomach, pancreas	Familial juvenile polyposis
BRCA1	17q21.31	Breast cancer 1, early onset	DNA repair	Breast, ovarian, prostate, pancreas	Hereditary breast and ovarian cancer
BRCA2	13q13.1	Breast cancer 2, early onset	DNA repair	Breast, ovarian, prostate, pancreas, brain, kidney, gastric	Hereditary breast and ovarian cancer
BRIP1	17q23.2	*BRCA1*-interacting protein C-terminal helicase 1	DNA helicase, DNA repair	Breast, ovarian, hematologic	Fanconi anemia type J, familial breast cancer
CDH1	16q22.1	E-cadherin	Cell signaling, adhesion, and proliferation	Gastric, breast, ovarian, endometrium, prostate	Hereditary diffuse gastric cancer
CDKN2A	9p21.3	Cyclin-dependent kinase inhibitor 2A	Cell cycle control	Pancreas, skin	Pancreatic cancer/ melanoma syndrome
CHEK2	22q12.1	Checkpoint kinase 2	Cell cycle control	Breast, prostate, colon, bone	Li-Fraumeni syndrome
EPCAM	2p21	Epithelial cell adhesion molecule	Cell adhesion, signaling, proliferation, differentiation, and migration	Colon, endometrium, ovary, stomach, small bowel, hepatobiliary tract, urinary tract, brain, pancreas, sebaceous	Lynch syndrome
GREM1	15q13.3	Gremlin 1	Control of cell proliferation	Colon	Hereditary mixed polyposis syndrome
MLH1	3p22.3	MutL homolog 1	DNA mismatch repair	Colon, endometrium, ovary, stomach, small bowel, hepatobiliary tract, urinary tract, brain, pancreas, sebaceous	Lynch syndrome
MSH2	2p21	MutS homolog 2	DNA mismatch repair	Colon, endometrium, ovary, stomach, small bowel, hepatobiliary tract, urinary tract, brain, pancreas, sebaceous	Lynch syndrome
MSH6	2p16.3	MutS homolog 6	DNA mismatch repair	Colon, endometrium, ovary, stomach, small bowel, hepatobiliary tract, urinary tract, brain, pancreas, sebaceous	Lynch syndrome
MUTYH	1p34.1	Mut Y homolog	DNA repair	Colon	*MUTYH*-associated polyposis
POLD1	19q13.33	Polymerase (DNA-directed), delta 1, catalytic subunit	DNA replication and repair	Colon, endometrium	CRC-polymerase proofreading-associated polyposis syndrome
POLE	12q24.33	Polymerase (DNA-directed), epsilon, catalytic subunit	DNA replication and repair	Colon	CRC-polymerase proofreading-associated polyposis syndrome

TABLE 49.6 Common Inherited Breast, Gynecologic, and Gastrointestinal Cancer Susceptibility Genes—cont'd

Gene	Location	Name	Function	Associated Cancer	Disease
PALB2	16p12.2	Partner and localizer of *BRCA2*	DNA repair	Breast, pancreas	Familial breast cancer; Fanconi anemia type N
PMS2	7p22.1	PMS2 postmeiotic segregation increased 2	DNA mismatch repair	Colon, endometrium, ovary, stomach, small bowel, hepatobiliary tract, urinary tract, brain, pancreas, sebaceous	Lynch syndrome
PTEN	10q23.31	Phosphatase and tension homolog	Cell cycle control	Breast, thyroid, renal, endometrium, colon, skin, CNS	PTEN hamartoma tumor syndrome
RAD51C	17q22	RAD51 paralog C	DNA repair	Breast, ovarian	Familial breast and ovarian cancer
RAD51D	17q12	RAD51 paralog D	DNA repair	Breast, ovarian	Familial breast and ovarian cancer
SMAD4	18q21.2	SMAD family member 4	Cell signaling and control of proliferation	Colon, stomach, pancreas	Familial juvenile polyposis
STK11	19p13.3	Serine/threonine kinase 11	Cell signaling and control of proliferation	Breast, colon, ovary, stomach, lung, pancreas	Peutz-Jeghers syndrome
TP53	17p13	Tumor protein p53	DNA repair; cell cycle control	Breast, brain, renal, adrenal, hematologic	Li-Fraumeni syndrome

CNS, Central nervous system; *CRC*, colorectal cancer; *PTEN*, phosphatase and tensin homolog.

addition to breast or ovarian cancer, a more comprehensive cancer susceptibility panel may be advised as a first-tier testing strategy.[488] The genetic professional must be ever mindful of the insurance coverage for the patient and the financial resources available to the patient for testing to be sure to maximize efficacy of the testing yet minimize unnecessary costs to the patient and carefully determine the appropriate first-tier test to order, whether it is a single gene test, small targeted cancer-specific panel, or a larger comprehensive cancer panel. Regardless of the MPS cancer panel chosen, pathogenic mutations are detected in only about 30% of cases suggestive of familial breast cancer.[486]

One limitation of this personalized medicine approach and increased clinical utilization of MPS panels is the increase in the number of rare missense variants detected, many of which are VUS. These are detected at a rate of about 0.008 variants per 1000 bases of exonic DNA that is sequenced.[491] Thus, while providing more comprehensive testing to patients, the lack of certainty regarding clinical relevance of VUS will remain challenging for health care providers in the care and management of patients and will likely be disconcerting to patients. In addition to the identification of the problematic VUS, expanded genetic testing also reveals variants in cancer susceptibility genes that are less well characterized than *BRCA1* and *BRCA2*. Many of these genes demonstrate reduced penetrance, making it difficult to translate the identification of a variant to a calculable cancer risk, and for many, clinical recommendations and guidelines have not yet been established.[492]

Inherited Colon Cancer

Colorectal cancer (CRC) is the third most common cancer in the United States with close to 150,000 new cases each year and about 50,000 deaths annually. About 3% to 5% of CRC cases are associated with inherited mutations linked to highly penetrant colon cancer syndromes.[493] In as many as one third of cases, familial clustering is observed, thereby suggesting the involvement of less penetrant susceptibility genes and environmental factors. Environmental risk factors include obesity; lack of exercise; moderate to heavy alcohol use; smoking; increased consumption of red or processed meats; and reduced whole-grain fiber, fruits, and vegetables.[453] About 85% of carcinomas arise from transformation of the normal mucosa to adenomas and then to carcinomas, and carcinoma arises through the serrated polyp pathway in 15%.[494] The molecular basis of CRC is a complex multistep process that involves genetic and epigenetic alterations. The various molecular pathways of disease convey different clinical features, prognosis, treatment plans, and pathological findings.

The microsatellite instability (MSI) pathway represents about 15% to 20% of CRC cases and is characterized by inherited, inactivating mutations in genes involved in DNA mismatch repair (MMR) or by acquired epigenetic silencing of these genes. MMR is a ubiquitous DNA repair process that occurs in all dividing cells. Because of a dysfunctional MMR system, DNA replication errors within microsatellite repeats or short tandem repeat sequences of 1 to 6 base pairs in length remain uncorrected and accumulate throughout the genome. Expansion or contraction of the microsatellite-repeat number in noncoding areas of the genome is of little significance; however, the predisposition to CRC results when changes occur within coding microsatellites of the genome and specifically within targeted genes whose protein products are involved in cell growth *(TGFβR2)*, apoptosis *(BAX)*, or DNA repair *(MSH6)*.[495,496]

The chromosomal instability (CIN) pathway is observed in 75% to 80% of CRC cases and was first proposed more than 25 years ago.[497] The CIN pathway is characterized by inherited or somatic mutations causing inactivation of the tumor suppressor gene *APC*, resulting in activation of the Wnt signaling pathway coupled with the acquired loss of chromosomal material as tumorigenesis progresses. These karyotypic changes most frequently involve the chromosomal regions of 5q, 18q and 17p encompassing tumor suppressor genes *APC, DCC, SMAD2,* SMAD4, *TP53,* and adjacent DNA sequences. Activating mutations in codons 12, 13, and 61 of the *KRAS* proto-oncogene on chromosome 12p12.1 is also common.[494] Collectively, this molecular profile results in unrestrained cell growth, proliferation, and loss of apoptosis. The tumors derived from the CIN pathway are microsatellite stable because CIN and MSI pathways are considered mutually exclusive.

The CpG island methylator phenotype (CIMP) is considered a subset of the MSI pathway by which CRC may arise.[498] As a subset of MSI tumors, these tumors are expectedly CIN negative, and CpG island hypermethylation occurs in a characteristic pattern of specific genes. These epigenetic changes cause silencing of the respective genes with no transcription; therefore, ultimately no translation of the associated gene product.[499] CIMP tumors can be further classified based on the degree of methylation and the number of genes in which hypermethylation is observed.[500] CIMP tumors typically display MSI because the MMR gene, *MLH1*, is hypermethylated.

Lynch Syndrome

The most common CRC susceptibility syndrome is Lynch syndrome (LS; OMIM #120435), also referred to as hereditary nonpolyposis colorectal cancer (HNPCC), which represents about 3% to 5% of all CRC cases. This disorder has an incidence of about 1 in 500 and is named after Dr. Henry Lynch's observation of an autosomal dominant predisposition to early-onset CRC with stomach and endometrial tumors in two large Midwestern kindreds.[501] LS is a heterogeneous disorder caused by one of multiple genes, manifests a variable age of onset, demonstrates reduced penetrance with lifetime risks of CRC of 50% to 70%, and confers increased risks for other associated tumors.[502] CRC in LS patients is distinguished by a few polyps that possess an accelerated transformation potential to carcinoma in as little as 2 to 3 years. This predisposing event is linked to germline mutations in MMR genes that are associated with the MSI pathway. Both CRC tumors in LS families and sporadic tumors with MSI, more commonly occur in the proximal part of the colon (right sided). These tumors are typically associated with a better prognosis but, in the absence of MMR proteins, have a poor response to adjuvant 5-FU based chemotherapy.[503] Histologically, these tumors display infiltrating lymphocytes, are mucinous with signet ring cells, and are poorly differentiated.

The first MMR gene was mapped to chromosome 2p15-16 using large LS kindreds.[504] Simultaneously, MSI was noted in a subset of sporadic CRC.[505,506] The MMR genes associated with LS include *MSH2* (2p15-16), *MSH6* (2p15-16), *MLH1* (3p21), and *PMS2* (7p22).[507] The majority of LS mutations are observed in *MSH2* (40%) and *MLH1* (50%).[496] A small percentage of patients with LS (1%–3%) have germline deletions affecting the epithelial cell adhesion molecule *(EPCAM)* gene (2p21), resulting in silencing of the downstream *MSH2* gene and no translation of the associated MSH2 protein.

Lynch syndrome–related *MMR* gene mutations are diverse and are located throughout these genes. Almost all errors made during DNA replication are repaired through the proofreading 3′-to-5′ exonuclease activity of DNA polymerase. Uncorrected errors of mismatched bases between the two strands are repaired before cell division by the MMR proteins, a process that is critical for maintaining genomic stability.[503] In addition to providing the repair of a mismatched base–base pair, the MMR system repairs "loop outs" from small insertions or deletions, unmatched bases that can occur during replication of a microsatellite or small repetitive sequences. The repair process includes three steps: (1) recognition of the mismatch, (2) excision, and (3) resynthesis to restore the correct sequence. In the MMR process, the MLH1 and PMS2 proteins dimerize facilitating the binding of other proteins involved in MMR, and the MSH2 protein forms a heterodimer with the *MSH6* gene product to identify mismatches.[507] When the normal function of MMR proteins is altered through DNA mutations, mismatched bases generated through DNA replication are not fixed, leading to strands of DNA with repeats of different lengths. In LS, a germline mutation in an MMR gene is inherited, causing one allele to be nonfunctional. In the tumor tissue of these patients, the second allele is inactivated through a somatic mutation or is deleted, a phenomena referred to as LOH (Fig. 49.11). Uncorrected somatic replication errors thus accumulate in noncoding and insignificant locations throughout the genome but also in the coding regions of genes involved in cell growth, signaling, and DNA repair. Approximately 15% to 20% of all CRC display MSI. In non-LS cases, MSI is attributed to epigenetic silencing of *MLH1* expression through biallelic methylation.[508]

To assist clinicians in identifying patients in LS kindreds, several criteria have been adopted, including the Amsterdam criteria first developed in 1990 and the more inclusive Bethesda criteria developed in 1998.[509,510] These recommendations have further evolved to maximize the identification of index cases in these families.[511,512] MSI testing should be performed on CRC tumor tissue if one of the following criteria is met: (1) age younger than 50 years; (2) regardless of age, synchronous or metachronous CRC or the presence of other LS-associated tumors, including the endometrium, ovary, stomach, hepatobiliary system, small bowel, ureter, renal, pelvis, and brain; (3) age younger than 60 with histology demonstrating a typical MSI pattern of tumor-infiltrating lymphocytes, Crohn-like lymphocytic reaction, mucinous–signet ring differentiation, or a medullary growth pattern; (4) the patient has one or more first-degree relatives with a LS-related tumor that was diagnosed before age 50 years; or (5) there are two or more first- or second-degree relatives with CRC or LS-related tumors, regardless of their age.[512] Despite these revised guidelines, some index cases are still not identified, so universal screening for all CRC in patients younger than 70 years of age has been recommended.[513] Equally important is screening for LS in patients with endometrial cancer (EC) because approximately 3% of patients with EC have an MMR gene mutation. The lifetime risk of EC in LS women is 25% to 60% with an average age at diagnosis between 48 and 62 years.[514,515] The lifetime risk for developing ovarian cancer is 1% to 3% with 10% to 15% of hereditary ovarian cancer caused by LS.[516] Synchronous tumors of the endometrium and ovary

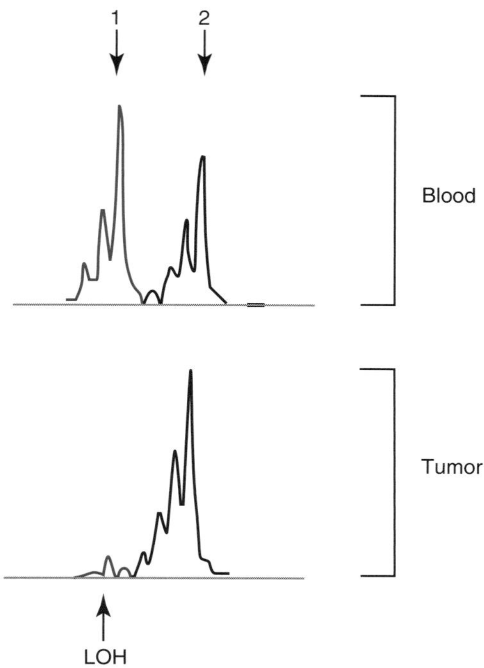

FIGURE 49.11 Electropherograms illustrating loss of heterozygosity (LOH) in tumor DNA. Patient DNA is extracted from peripheral blood and tumor tissue. Polymerase chain reaction of a microsatellite repeat locus contained within the chromosomal region thought to be deleted during tumorigenesis is performed. One of the primers is labeled with a fluorescent dye, and amplicons are subjected to capillary electrophoresis. Relative amplicon size is on the x-axis, and relative fluorescence is on the y-axis. Constitutive DNA from the patient's blood illustrates heterozygosity for this marker as alleles 1 and 2. In DNA from the tumor, a single peak suggesting a homozygous pattern is observed. Thus, LOH is present in the tumor DNA. The absence of one of the amplicons signifies the loss of the second allele and indicates loss of chromosomal material at this particular locus.

may be observed in as many as 20% of women with LS.[517] In many women with LS, EC often precedes CRC as their initial malignancy. Identification of their increased risks of LS-related tumors can be followed by increased surveillance, counseling, and testing for at-risk family members. For these reasons, universal screening for all newly diagnosed EC has been proposed because a significant percentage of LS patients are missed when relying on MMR-associated tumor morphology or patient indices such as age (<50 years) and history.[518-520]

Molecular testing for MSI can identify defects in MMR genes through germline or somatic changes, and IHC testing is performed to detect expression of MMR proteins.[521] MSI testing by PCR may be the preferred method in some facilities. Alternatively, IHC testing may be performed if MSI testing is not readily available or if there is a limited amount of tumor tissue. In some settings, however, both molecular MSI testing and IHC testing are performed concurrently to account for possible false-negative results that may be obtained from either methodology. At many institutions, a multidisciplinary team develops and agrees on a standard protocol for universal screening of suspected LS patients. This practice, however, is not well adopted by many community hospitals.[522] Because mononucleotide microsatellite repeats are more susceptible to MMR errors, MSI testing is most often performed using a multiplex PCR for several mononucleotide loci and requires normal adjacent tissue for comparison (Fig. 49.12). More recently, MSI has been detected with MPS.[523] MSI is characterized by the expansion or contraction of DNA sequences through the insertion or deletion of repeated sequences. If MSI is detected at two or more of five loci, or more than 30% of the loci analyzed, the tumor has a "high" frequency of MSI (MSI-H). If MSI is detected at one locus, or less than 30%, the tumor has a "low" frequency of MSI (MSI-L). If MSI is not detected at any locus, the tumor is considered to be microsatellite stable (MSS). MSI-L or MSS results greatly reduce the likelihood of LS.

If MSI-H is detected, it is necessary to determine whether the MSI results from an inherited inactivating germline MMR gene mutation or from the more frequent somatic CpG methylation of *MLH1* seen commonly in sporadic CRC. Because somatic CpG methylation of *MLH1* is frequently associated with a somatic *BRAF* proto-oncogene p.Val600Glu mutation, this test is often performed as a reflex test on tumor tissue DNA after MSI-H results are obtained (Fig. 49.13).[524] If a somatic *BRAF* p.Val600Glu mutation is detected, LS is unlikely. If, however, no *BRAF* gene mutation is detected, a germline MMR gene mutation is more likely, and the testing algorithm continues with *MLH1* promoter hypermethylation studies of tumor tissue DNA. If epigenetic biallelic *MLH1* gene promoter hypermethylation is detected, a sporadic CRC tumor is the diagnosis. Conversely, the lack of *MLH1* promoter hypermethylation indicates the possibility of LS, and DNA sequence analysis of MMR genes from the patient's peripheral blood lymphocytes to identify a germline MMR gene mutation is performed.[507]

The presence of a germline MMR mutation confirms the diagnosis of LS. If IHC testing has been performed, the IHC pattern obtained may direct which MMR gene to sequence. For example, whereas the loss of MSH2 expression would suggest an inactivating mutation in the *MSH2* gene, the loss of expression of MSH6 would indicate a mutation in the *MSH6* gene. Thus gene-specific, *MSH2* or *MSH6*, Sanger DNA sequencing can be requested to search for an unknown mutation. However, IHC-directed gene testing is not always concordant, and IHC is not always performed. Therefore, germline testing on DNA extracted from a peripheral blood specimen for a MPS LS specific panel with all four MMR genes and *EPCAM* may be considered. After a specific mutation has been identified in a patient with LS, directed Sanger DNA sequencing analysis may be used to screen at-risk family members for the specific mutation that is segregating in the family.

Both pre- and posttest genetic counseling are indicated. Before testing, the genetics professional should review the family history, assess the psychosocial needs of the patient, review risk counseling, and discuss genetic testing and possible outcomes. Prediction models can be used to determine the probability of identifying an MMR gene mutation.[525] Posttest counseling includes disclosing the results and implications to the patient and his or her family members. The genetics professional should provide a management and surveillance plan for the patient based on the MMR gene involved and the identified mutation.[526]

Lynch syndrome–associated gene mutations are heterogeneous; most are nonsense or frameshift mutations expected to result in premature truncation of the protein and loss of

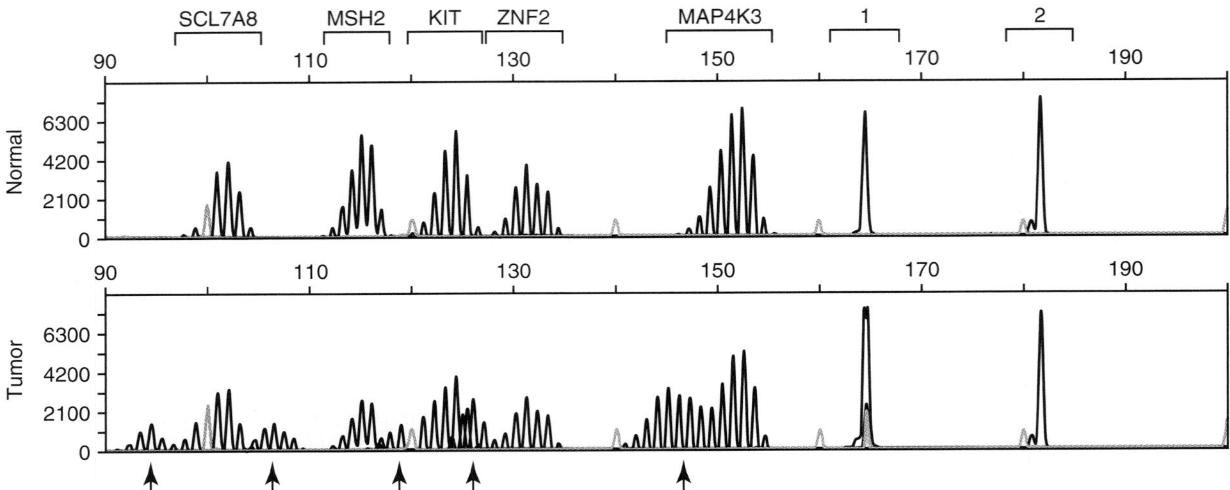

FIGURE 49.12 Electropherograms illustrating microsatellite instability (MSI) in tumor DNA. Patient DNA is extracted from peripheral blood or normal tissue and is compared with DNA extracted from tumor tissue. DNA is amplified in a multiplex polymerase chain reaction (PCR) assay using fluorescent labeled primers corresponding to five mononucleotide loci *(SCL7A8, MSH2, KIT, ZNF2,* and *MAP4K3)* and two pentanucleotide loci (1 and 2) (Promega Corporation, Madison, WI). Amplicon sizes in bases are noted at the top of the figure, and the relative amount of fluorescence detected for each amplicon is measured by the peak height (y-axis). Multiple peaks seen at each locus represent "stutter" peaks and result from strand slippage during PCR of repetitive sequences. *Arrows* denote a shift in product size at five of five mononucleotide loci, indicating microsatellite instability. Identical patterns between normal and tumor DNA at the polymorphic pentanucleotide markers suggest that normal and tumor DNA are derived from the same individual.

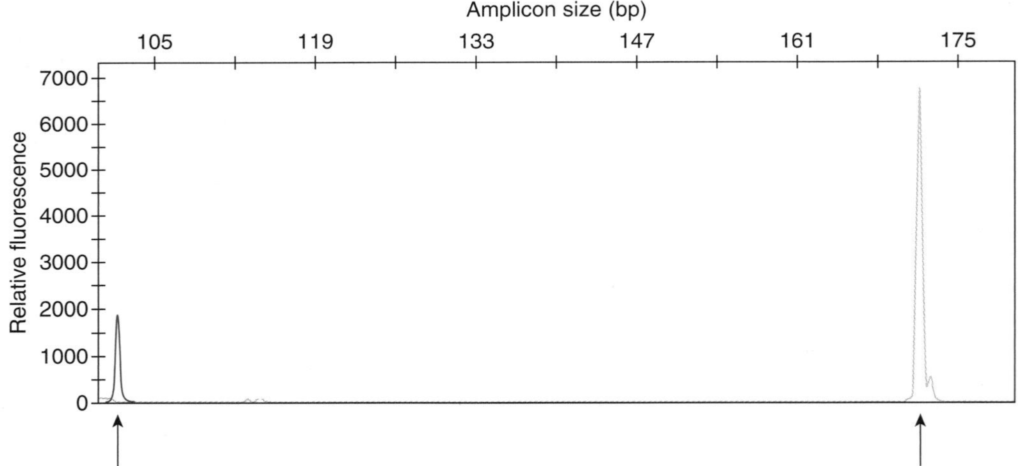

FIGURE 49.13 Detection of *BRAF* mutation c.1799T>A (p.Val600Glu) by allele-specific polymerase chain reaction (PCR). Amplicon sizes in bases are noted at the top of the figure, and the relative amount of fluorescence detected for each amplicon is measured by the peak height (y-axis). *BRAF* mutation c.1799T>A can be rapidly detected using allele-specific PCR coupled with capillary electrophoresis. DNA was extracted from a paraffin-embedded MSI-H (microsatellite instability–high) colon tumor. An internal control 171-bp fragment was amplified using a primer pair flanking exon 15 with the 3′ primer fluorescently labeled. In the same reaction, a 101-bp allele specific amplicon was generated with the same 5′ forward primer and a second 3′-fluorescently labeled primer specific for *BRAF* c.1799T>A.[524] The *right arrow* points to the internal control, and the *left arrow* confirms the presence of mutation *BRAF* c.1799T>A (p.Val600Glu) in the tumor, thereby suggesting that the MSI-H phenotype observed in the colon tumor is associated with sporadic colon cancer and not to mutations in an *MMR* gene associated with Lynch syndrome.

function.[527] The majority of germline mutations occur in *MLH1* and *MSH2* and to a lesser degree in the *MSH6* gene. Mutations in the *PMS2* gene are the least common. Whether Sanger- or MPS-based DNA sequencing analysis is used, an inherent problem is the identification of sequence VUS, which are most often missense or possible splice variants and for which no significant biologic function can be determined. Thus, it is difficult to assign a pathologic role to these variants without functional assays to confirm their relevance in the disease process. Because of this, the International Society for Gastrointestinal Hereditary Tumours (InSiGHT) developed a database with close to 2500 reported constitutional variants identified in LS patients.[527] With a multidisciplinary approach, this group systematically applied a standard classification scheme for the database variants and determined the clinical recommendations for each.[528] This comprehensive approach assists in risk assessments for specific gene mutations and facilitates appropriate care and management for families. Challenging however, are "private" variants segregating within a single family and the associated uncertainty of characterizing those genotype–phenotype correlations and predictive risk assessments for specific mutations based on the clinical findings in just one family.

Overall genotype–phenotype correlations for MMR genes indicate that individuals with *MLH1/MSH2* gene mutations have the earliest age of onset and highest risk for developing CRC by age 70 years.[502,529] *MSH6* gene mutations convey the lowest lifetime risk of CRC to female carriers (10%), yet *MSH6* gene mutation–positive carriers have the highest risk of extracolorectal cancer by age 70 years. *PMS2* gene mutation carriers have a lower penetrance of disease and a lower risk of extracolorectal cancer.

If an MMR gene mutation in a patient is identified, at-risk adult family members can pursue presymptomatic testing with appropriate genetic counseling. Similar to presymptomatic testing for other adult-onset disorders, the counseling session should include verification of the family history and discussion of the clinical course of the disease, including risk of developing the disease and issues associated with disease management. Discussions should be incorporated into the session, including how the patient will act on both positive and negative results, feelings of survivor guilt or stigmatization, and the possibility of discrimination for insurance and employment. If a germline mutation is detected in the presymptomatic patient, a colonoscopy should be performed every 1 or 2 years beginning at age 20 to 25 years or 10 years younger than the youngest age of diagnosis in the family.[530] Surveillance for EC and ovarian cancer for at-risk women with LS should include transvaginal ultrasonography and endometrial biopsy every 1 to 2 years beginning at 30 to 35 years of age.[530] Furthermore, prophylactic hysterectomy and bilateral salpingo-oophorectomy can be considered for women who have completed childbearing. Alternatively, if genetic testing is not pursued, relatives should begin an intensive screening program with colonoscopy every 1 to 2 years, starting between 20 and 30 years of age, and then annually after age 40 years. If no pathogenic MMR germline mutation is detected in the proband despite MSI and IHC testing suggestive of a MMR germline mutation and LS, presymptomatic DNA testing for family members is not possible. These mutation-negative families or Lynch-like families may have (1) a MMR VUS that may eventually be reclassified, (2) a MMR gene mutation in a region of the genome that is not screened, (3) a structural variant not detected by current methodologies, or (4) a germline mutation in other yet to be determined MMR genes or genes that regulate MMR genes.[519] Although detection of a mutation in a family that meets LS criteria is not always possible, heightened surveillance of the proband and at-risk family members should be implemented.

In addition, *MLH1* and *MSH2* mutations have been identified in about 70% of patients with Muir-Torre syndrome (MTS) at frequencies of 10% and 90%, respectively. MTS is characterized by at least one sebaceous gland neoplasia, adenoma or carcinoma, and one or more visceral tumors, which most frequently are colorectal or endometrial, although other LS-associated tumors may be seen. MTS is considered a subtype of LS with a mean age at diagnosis around 50 years.[531] Because sebaceous neoplasms may be sporadic, LS confirmation is recommended. In rare cases, patients with biallelic germline mutations in an MMR gene result in constitutional mismatch repair deficiency syndrome (OMIM #276300) with early-onset CRC and childhood hematologic or brain tumors.

Familial Adenomatous Polyposis

Familial adenomatous polyposis (FAP; OMIM #175100) is an autosomal dominant disorder with an incidence of about 1 in 8000 to 15,000 characterized by hundreds to thousands of adenomatous polyps both in the colon and rectum. This disorder has a high penetrance, conveying a lifetime risk of CRC in untreated mutation carriers of close to 100%. FAP accounts for 1% of CRC cases observed in the United States. Interestingly, in about 20% of cases, no family history exists, and the disease is the result of a new mutation. Polyps appear during the second decade of life in about half of the patients.[532] CRC ultimately develops approximately 10 to 15 years after the onset of polyposis, with the median age of CRC about 40 years of age without surgical intervention.[532,533] It is the sheer number of polyps in these patients that increases the likelihood that one will progress to cancer. For this reason, close surveillance of these patients is indicated, and colectomy is advised when multiple adenomas are observed or if high-grade histologic findings are reported. Furthermore, patients with FAP have an increased risk of developing other malignancies, including carcinoma of the small bowel, most often in the duodenum or periampulla; papillary thyroid carcinoma; hepatoblastoma; pancreatic cancer; and brain tumors.[534] In addition, these patients have a 7% to 20% lifetime risk of developing benign extraintestinal manifestations of the disease, including adrenal or desmoid tumors, osteomas, congenital hypertrophy of the retinal epithelium, and dental abnormalities.[534] Desmoid tumors in vital areas have been reported as a cause of death in as many as 21% of patients with FAP.[535] Thus, close clinical surveillance of FAP patients and at-risk family members is critical to reducing CRC and CRC-associated mortality and APC-associated complications.

Familial adenomatous polyposis is caused by germline mutations in the adenomatous polyposis coli *(APC)* gene, which was cloned in 1991.[536-538] The *APC* gene encodes 8535 base pairs contained within 15 exons and produces a protein of 2843 amino acids and a molecular weight of about 310 kDa. The APC protein is a multidomain, multifunctional protein with multiple binding partners that play key roles in regulating the β-catenin level in the Wnt signaling pathway.[539,540] This protein is also involved in other cellular processes, including cell adhesion and migration, DNA repair, apoptosis, FAK/Src signaling, microtubule assembly, and chromosome segregation.[540,541] However, the main tumor suppressor function of APC appears to be its regulation of the proto-oncoprotein β-catenin and canonical Wnt signaling. In this process, APC together with glycogen synthase kinase-3β and axin regulate the amount of β-catenin through the phosphorylation of cytoplasmic β-catenin for ubiquitin-dependent degradation. In the absence of functional APC, β-catenin is unregulated and accumulates in the nucleus, leading to ligand independent constitutive Wnt signaling and transcription mediated by lymphoid enhancer-binding factor/T-cell factor (LEF/TCF) transcription factors, resulting in the upregulation of genes involved in proliferation.[542] For this reason, APC is commonly referred to as a "gatekeeper" of tumor progression.[540,541,543] Similar to autosomal dominant inherited mutations in other tumor suppressor genes, the normal allele must also be inactivated to manifest the disease phenotype. Therapeutic approaches targeting the multifaceted functions of APC have been reported.[540]

Sanger and MPS DNA sequencing studies have identified well over 1500 germline mutations in *APC,* most of which result in truncated proteins because of small frameshift or nonsense mutations.[528] Gross rearrangements have been identified using MLPA.[544,545] Despite the heterogeneous nature of these mutations, two hot spots occur with 10% and 15% of all mutations found specifically at codons 1061 and 1309, respectively. Additionally, about 33% of mutations occur between these two sites. Genotype–phenotype correlations exist for some *APC* mutations. The AAAAG deletion at codon 1309 is associated with a younger age of onset.[546] Classic FAP is primarily observed from mutations occurring between exon 5 and the 5′ portion of exon 15, the largest of all exons spanning 6.5 kb. Patients with FAP who have mutations between codons 1250 and 1464 or truncating mutations between codons 1403 and 1578 have a severe phenotype and are at increased risk for extracolonic disease.[547,548] Attenuated FAP (AFAP) is seen in about 8% to 10% of patients with FAP and is associated with fewer colonic polyps (10–100) and an older age of onset for both the development of polyps and cancer.[549-552] These patients typically have truncating mutations at the extreme 5′ end of the gene (codons 1–163) or mutations at the carboxyl-terminal end of the gene (codons 1860–1987). Intra- and interfamilial phenotypic variability exists even in the presence of identical mutations and may be explained by a modifier gene or genes.[553,554]

If APC is suspected, full gene sequence analysis is recommended coupled with deletion and duplication analysis.[507,544] If the mutation within the family can be identified, at-risk family members as young as 10 to 12 years of age may be referred for genetic counseling and presymptomatic DNA testing.[555] Although DNA testing on an asymptomatic minor is usually not endorsed by the genetic community, in this scenario, early identification of the mutation in these patients will clearly affect their clinical management because intense screening programs and possible prophylactic colectomy may be initiated as early as the second decade of life. If a mutation is detected in the family, endoscopy should be performed every 2 years and if adenomas are detected, colonoscopy should be performed every year until the colectomy is performed.[556] Annual thyroid and abdominal ultrasonography for detection of thyroid malignancy and desmoid tumors may also be included in the surveillance screening. Family members who test negative for the mutation do not have increased risk of CRC, can avoid these intensive screening programs, and should follow the screening programs for the general population. If the mutation in the family cannot be identified, screening with sigmoidoscopy is recommended every 2 years, starting as early as age 10 to 12 years. Furthermore, when repeatedly negative sigmoidoscopy results are obtained, the frequency of such examinations can be reduced in each subsequent decade of life, and frequent surveillance may be discontinued at age 50 years.[556] Because AFAP is associated with a later age of onset and most adenomas are in the right part of the colon, colonoscopy is the recommended screening method beginning at 18 to 20 years of age.

In 2002, *APC* mutation-negative adenomatous polyposis patients were found to have biallelic mutations in the base excision repair gene *MUTYH*, a disorder known as MYH-associated polyposis (MAP; OMIM #604933).[557,558] This gene contains 16 exons, is located on chromosome 1p34.3-p32.1, and encodes an adenine-specific DNA glycosylase involved in DNA base excision repair (BER). This protein removes adenine when it is inappropriately paired with guanine, cytosine, or oxidatively damaged DNA containing 8-oxo-7,8-dihydroguanine. If not repaired, these mispairings can result in G : C to T : A transversion mutations in the *APC* gene and sometimes the *KRAS* gene as well.[557,559] *MUTYH* gene mutation–positive patients have CRC at a mean age of 51.7 ± 9.5 years.[560] Incomplete penetrance is observed, and the polyp burden is variable with typical patients having between 10 and 100 polyps. Close surveillance of these patients is recommended, similar to that provided for AFAP, with screening beginning as early as 18 to 20 years of age and colonoscopy performed every 2 years. In addition, although this is an autosomal recessive condition, heterozygous carriers with only one *MUTYH* gene mutation are at increased risk for CRC, thus indicating that close clinical surveillance may be indicated in this population as well.[560,561]

Mutations in the *MUTYH* gene are heterogeneous and scattered throughout the gene with more than 300 unique variants reported.[528] Most variants cause amino acid substitutions in the gene, and ethnic-specific common mutations are observed.[562] Patients can be homozygous for the same mutation or compound heterozygotes with two different mutations. DNA testing for *MUTYH* gene mutations can be targeted to common mutations or known mutations segregating in the family. Alternatively, full gene sequencing of the *MUTYH* gene can be requested. If *MUTYH* DNA sequence analysis results are negative, *APC* testing may be offered.[507]

Clinical presentation and personal and family history should be carefully reviewed when determining the most appropriate molecular testing to recommend. In cases of higher disease certainty, gene-specific Sanger DNA sequencing is more cost effective. However, in some families, MPS using a targeted comprehensive panel of susceptibility genes for colon cancer may afford a higher likelihood for identification of the disease gene segregating in the family in a faster and more cost-effective manner (see Table 49.6).[563]

MITOCHONDRIAL DNA DISEASES

Mitochondria are organelles ubiquitous to the cytoplasm of all eukaryotic cells of animals, higher plants, and some

POINTS TO REMEMBER

Inherited Cancer

- Disease can result from the inheritance of a single activating mutation in a proto-oncogene.
- Disease can result from the inheritance of a single loss-of-function mutation in a tumor suppressor or mismatch repair gene followed by somatic inactivation of the second allele.
- Age of onset and type of tumor(s) observed within family members are variable.
- MPS-based disease specific tumor panels are currently most often used to identify the gene mutation segregating in the family.
- Routine clinical surveillance screening is initiated in mutation-positive asymptomatic family members.
- Genetic counseling is an important component of patient care and management.

microorganisms. Mitochondria generate energy for cellular processes by producing ATP through oxidative phosphorylation (OXPHOS); they are important in maintaining both calcium homeostasis and various intracellular signaling cascades, including apoptosis.[564-566] The matrix of the mitochondrion is surrounded by a cardiolipin-rich inner membrane, and both are enclosed by a second outer membrane. Within the matrix are copies of mitochondrial DNA (mtDNA). Each mitochondria contains between about 2 and 10 copies of mtDNA, so with hundreds of mitochondria per cell, an estimated 10^3 to 10^4 copies of mtDNA exist within each cell, with brain, skeletal, and cardiac muscle having particularly high concentrations. Alterations in mtDNA copy number or mutations in mtDNA are associated with both inherited and acquired diseases.[567-569] The mitochondrial genome is composed of a double-stranded, circular DNA molecule containing 16,569 base pairs that encodes 37 genes, including two ribosomal RNAs (rRNA), 22 transfer RNAs (tRNA), and 13 subunits required for the OXPHOS system, with 7 belonging to complex I, 1 to complex III, 3 to complex IV, and 2 to complex V.[570] Most subunits involved in the OXPHOS system are nuclear encoded, as are several nuclear gene products that regulate mitochondrial gene expression. The mitochondrial genetic code is slightly different from the universal code. For example, in mtDNA, TGA codes for tryptophan rather than a termination codon, and all mitochondrial-translated mRNA contains codons requiring only 22 mitochondrial-encoded tRNA molecules for translation rather than the 31 predicted by Crick's wobble hypothesis.[571,572] The high copy number of mtDNA per cell coupled with a small genome and highly polymorphic sequence variations among individuals makes mtDNA sequence analysis an ideal tool for forensic studies.[573,574]

Mitochondria-related diseases have an incidence of 1 in 1000 to 5000 and can result from mutations in nuclear DNA (85%–90%) or, as first reported in 1988, from mutations in the mitochondrial genome (10%–15%).[575-577] Mutations in mtDNA occur at a higher rate than nuclear DNA, probably because of differences in chromatin structure, lack of DNA repair machinery, and the continual generation of reactive oxygen species. Mitochondrial genetics is different from Mendelian genetics in several aspects. First, all mtDNA is maternally inherited, with mature oocytes having the highest mtDNA copy number per cell at 10^5 and with sperm having the lowest mtDNA copy number per cell at 10^2. After fertilization, sperm mtDNA is selectively degraded so that only maternal mtDNA remains. Thus, if a mother is carrying an mtDNA mutation, it will be transmitted to all of her children, but only her daughters can transmit the disease to their offspring. Although this is considered the rule, paternal mtDNA inheritance has been reported and may result from incomplete degradation of sperm mtDNA in early embryogenesis.[578,579] If a mtDNA mutation arises, it will exist among a population of normal mtDNA. This coexistence of normal and mutant mtDNA copies within the same cell is referred to as *heteroplasmy* and is the second unique feature of mitochondrial genetics. Third, during cell division, the proportions of normal and mutant mtDNA can shift as mitochondria, and their accompanying genomes are partitioned into daughter cells. Thus, in development and differentiation, the proportions of normal and mutant mtDNA can vary among cells and tissues within the body. Last, the percentage of mutant mtDNA required within a cell, tissue, or organ system to produce a deleterious phenotype is referred to as the *threshold effect*. The threshold for disease varies among people, energetic requirements for tissue, and the mtDNA mutation. Genetic counseling for families with mtDNA disorders is complicated by an inability to accurately predict phenotype caused by heteroplasmy and the threshold effect.

Two types of mtDNA mutations exist: those that affect mitochondrial protein synthesis (tRNA and rRNA genes) and those within the protein-encoding genes themselves.[580,581] Traditionally, testing for mtDNA mutations was performed by direct Sanger sequencing or by targeted mutation testing for specific disease-related mutations. Over the past several years, most clinical laboratories have moved to MPS-based testing for the detection of mtDNA alterations. Recently, the Mitochondrial Medicine Society released a consensus statement on the diagnosis of mitochondrial diseases.[582] This statement indicates that MPS-based testing of the entire mitochondrial genome is now the preferred method for the diagnosis of a suspected mitochondrial disorder and should be considered the first-line DNA-based test (as opposed to targeted mutation analysis).[582] MPS-based testing for mtDNA mutations usually involves a preliminary long-range PCR to amplify the entire mitochondrial genome.[583-585] After this step is complete, the amplified mtDNA is processed, sequenced, and then analyzed.[584] mtDNA mutations identified by MPS-based methods are usually confirmed by a secondary method (eg, Sanger sequencing). Using MPS-based testing and subsequent mutational confirmation techniques, investigators have been able to reproducibly detect heteroplasmy levels of approximately 10%.[583,584] Because of the limitations in the detection of heteroplasmy using MPS-based methods, some laboratories are continuing to use PCR-based methods capable of detecting lower levels of heteroplasmy to target specific disease-causing mtDNA mutations. Although mtDNA mutations are now associated with a significant number of inherited diseases, acquired mtDNA deletions are associated with the aging process, and mitochondrial dysfunction is associated with neurodegenerative diseases and cancer.[568] Many somatic mtDNA mutations occur via damage by oxygen free radicals produced as byproducts of aerobic metabolism.[586,587]

Clinical treatment of mitochondrial disorders is largely supportive in nature. Several treatment modalities are currently under investigation (eg, antioxidant therapy, gene therapy, stimulation of mitochondrial biosynthesis, among others).[588] However, these potential treatments remain largely experimental.

Leber Hereditary Optic Neuropathy

Leber hereditary optic neuropathy (LHON; OMIN #53500), the most common mitochondrial disease, was the first linked to maternal inheritance through a mutation in the mtDNA.[575] LHON is characterized by acute or subacute bilateral loss of central vision caused by focal degeneration of the retinal ganglion cell (RGC) layer and, in some individuals, impairment of optic nerve function.[589] The specific nature of the disease in terms of RGC degeneration is unknown, but it could be caused by differences in superoxide regulation.[590] Age of onset is typically in the second to fourth decade of life, and after initial symptoms, both eyes are usually affected within 6 months. Approximately 50% of males and only 10% of females who possess an LHON mtDNA mutation will develop disease.[589] In addition, yet to be defined environmental factors, nuclear-encoded modifier genes that affect mtDNA expression, mtDNA products, or mitochondrial metabolism may modify the phenotypic expression of LHON. The explanation for differences in rates between genders has not been determined but could be related to genes on the X chromosome.[591-593] It has also been suggested that sex hormones may provide a protective effect in females. Experiments using LHON cybrid cell lines indicate that the presence of estrogens results in more efficient oxidative phosphorylation suggesting that hormones explain gender differences in LHON.[594] Genetic counseling in LHON is complicated because the amount of mutant mtDNA transmitted by heteroplasmic females is not predictable. Furthermore, genetic testing does not predict which individuals will develop visual symptoms.[595] LHON can be confused with autosomal dominant optic atrophy (OMIN #165500), which shares a similar ocular phenotype but results from mutations in the gene *OPA1* (3q28-29). It is interesting to note that OPA1 is a nuclear-encoded mitochondrial protein required for mitochondrial fusion, maintenance of cristae architecture, and regulation of apoptosis.[566]

Leber hereditary optic neuropathy is a disorder caused by OXPHOS deficiency. Although many mutations have been associated with this disease, mtDNA mutations m.3460G>A, m.11778G>A, and m.14484T>C represent 90% of those identified.[596] Mutation m.11778G>A was the first described, is the most common, and accounts for at least 50% of cases. In most affected individuals, LHON mutations appear to be homoplasmic, with only mutant mtDNA detected, but in 15% of cases, the mutations are heteroplasmic, with a mixture of both normal and mutant mtDNA detected.[597,598] Each of the common mutations affects a subunit of the nicotinamide adenine dinucleotide: ubiquinone oxidoreductase in complex I of the OXPHOS pathway. The mechanism by which these mutations cause the LHON phenotype is not well understood.[599]

Leigh Syndrome

Leigh syndrome (OMIM #256000), or subacute necrotizing encephalopathy, is a progressive neurodegenerative disorder that most often leads to death before the age of 5 years. In contrast to LHON, most patients present within the first year of life with hypotonia, failure to thrive, psychomotor regression, ocular movement abnormalities, ataxia, and brainstem and basal ganglia dysfunction caused by severe dysfunction of mitochondrial energy metabolism. The clinical phenotype for Leigh syndrome is variable in patients with the same pathogenic mtDNA mutation and results from differences in the percentages of mutant mtDNA among organs and tissues within an individual.[600,601] However, it appears that heteroplasmy alone cannot explain the differences in phenotypic presentation because individuals with high levels of the common Leigh syndrome mutation m.8993T>C present with other disease manifestations.[602]

Leigh syndrome exhibits extensive genetic heterogeneity, with disease-causing mutations identified in both nuclear-encoded genes and mtDNA, making both Mendelian and maternal patterns of inheritance possible for this syndrome.[602] Mutations in more than 35 genes have been described to cause Leigh syndrome.[602] The most common mitochondrial-encoded mutation associated with Leigh syndrome is seen in the *MT-ATPase 6* gene (complex V) with a T>G transversion mutation at nucleotide m.8993. The most common nuclear-encoded mutation associated with Leigh syndrome is in the *SURF1* gene (9q34), which encodes a cytochrome oxidase assembly factor. Regardless of which gene is involved, the overall prognosis of these patients is generally poor, and treatment of mitochondrial disease is in its infancy.[588] Because of the lethality of Leigh syndrome, PGD can be considered and has been successfully performed with the implantation of a disease-free embryo.[603]

Mitochondrial Encephalomyopathy, Lactic Acidosis, and Stroke-Like Episodes

Mitochondrial encephalomyopathy, lactic acidosis, and stroke-like episodes (MELAS; OMIM #540000) is a multisystem disorder characterized by generalized tonic-clonic seizures, recurrent headaches and vomiting, hearing loss, exercise intolerance, and proximal limb weakness.[604] Manifestations of MELAS routinely appear in early childhood, and the disease is commonly fatal by young adulthood.[605] As with other mitochondrial disorders, phenotypic presentation in MELAS is widely variable among individuals. In fact, it is not possible to predict the course of disease even among individuals with the same mutation or in the same family.[567,605,606]

The disorder is primarily caused by mutations in the mitochondrial tRNA encoding gene *MT-TL1*.[607] A single *MT-TL1* A>G transition mutation located at nucleotide m.3243 is responsible for disease in approximately 80% of MELAS patients.[604] An additional two *MT-TL1* point mutations (m.3271T>C and m.3252A>G) are responsible for disease in approximately 12% of patients.[604] Mutations in a second mitochondrial gene (*MT-ND5*) that encodes the NADH-ubiquinone oxidoreductase subunit 5 are also a relatively common cause of MELAS.[608] Although several causative mutations have been described in the *MT-ND5* gene, a single point mutation m.13513G>A is by far the most common.[609] There are also rare cases in which causative mutations have been identified in other mitochondrial (and some nuclear) genes.[604]

Myoclonic Epilepsy Associated With Ragged Red Fibers

Myoclonic epilepsy associated with ragged red fibers (MERRF; OMIM #545000) is characterized by myoclonus, epilepsy, ataxia, dementia, muscle weakness, hearing loss, short stature, and optic atrophy.[610] MERRF patients commonly undergo a period of normal development before showing manifestations of disease in childhood.[610] The "ragged red fibers" denote the hallmark finding of frayed muscle fibers observed in muscle biopsies from these patients. Although the clinical presentation of MERRF can vary widely, there are four key characteristics required for diagnosis: myoclonus, ataxia, generalized epilepsy, and ragged red fibers observed in the muscle biopsy.[610]

The disorder is caused by mutations in mitochondrial tRNA genes that result in altered translational efficiency.[568,611] Mutations in several tRNA genes have been described in this disorder, but the most frequently observed alteration (m.8344A>G) occurs in the *MT-TK* gene that encodes the $tRNA^{Lys}$.[612] A single point *MT-TK* point mutation (m.8344A>G) is causative in approximately 80% of MERRF patients. Three additional *MT-TK* gene mutations (m.8356T>C, m.8361G>A, and m.8363G>A) are responsible for disease in an additional 10%.[610] Rare mutations in the *MT-TI*, *MT-TP*, *MT-TF*, and *MT-TL1* genes also result in MERRF. There is much heterogeneity in the presentation of MERRF patients. In fact, a large percentage of patients with the common m.8344A>G mutation do not exhibit all four of the hallmark findings of MERRF,[613] suggesting further refinement of diagnostic criteria in the future.

Kearns-Sayre Syndrome

Kearns-Sayre Syndrome (KSS; OMIM #530000) is a progressive multisystem disorder with onset occurring before age 20 years. KSS is defined by the presence of progressive external ophthalmoplegia and pigmentary retinopathy and at least one additional hallmark finding (cardiac conduction block, cerebrospinal fluid protein concentrations of >100 mg/dL, or cerebellar ataxia).[568,569] Additional clinical findings of KSS may include ptosis, hearing loss, short stature, limb weakness, dementia, hypoparathyroidism, and others.[569] The disease often results in early adulthood death. Unlike most other mitochondrial disorders, KSS usually results from de novo alterations that likely occur in the maternal oocyte during germline development or embryogenesis.[569,614]

In the late 1980s, large deletions in mtDNA were identified as the cause of KSS.[576,615] The size of these deletions varies among individuals, but a common deletion approximately 4.9 kb in size is found in approximately 30% of KSS patients.[615] Studies indicate that regardless of the deletion size, the removal of critical tRNAs needed for protein synthesis results in the disease phenotype.[569] Additionally, the variable presence of deleted mtDNA in specific tissues results in the clinical phenotype of patients.[568] Patients with KSS often have partially deleted mtDNAs in all tissues examined, which is likely to explain the multisystem involvement of this disorder.[568]

Clinical DNA testing for KSS involves the use of deletion and duplication analysis performed by any number of testing modalities (eg, CGH microarray, quantitative PCR, MLPA). Deletion and duplication testing detects disease-causing mutations in 90% of patients affected with KSS.[569] Patients with a KSS phenotype that test negative for deletions may pursue MPS-based mitochondrial genome sequencing because rare point mutations can cause a KSS-like phenotype.

IMPRINTING

Imprinting refers to the differential marking or "imprinting" of specific paternally and maternally inherited alleles during gametogenesis, resulting in differential expression of those genes. Such imprints on the DNA during gametogenesis must be maintained through DNA replication in the somatic cells of the offspring, must be reversible from generation to generation, and must influence transcription. DNA methylation is the primary mechanism for genomic imprinting. The number of imprinted genes in the human genome is estimated to be fewer than 200, and most are clustered around imprinting control centers. Alterations in normal imprinting patterns can result in disease.[616]

Prader-Willi and Angelman Syndromes

Prader-Willi syndrome (PWS; OMIM #176270) is a complex multisystem, neurogenetic disorder with an incidence of 1 in 10,000–30,000. PWS along with Angelman syndrome (AS), were the first reported human disorders resulting from imprinting. Prenatally, fetuses with PWS exhibit diminished movement, peculiar fetal position, and often polyhydramnios.[617] At birth, dysmorphic features, small hands and feet, and hypogonadism are observed, and the child has persistent hypotonia that results in poor feeding and failure to thrive.[618] Development is delayed for both motor skills and language, and this delay continues throughout life, with a mean IQ of 60 to 70. Early in childhood, a unique and characteristic insatiable appetite that is hypothalamic in origin presents; obesity ensues with associated complications and is the major cause of morbidity, mortality, and sleep disorders.[619] In addition, patients have short stature and abnormal body composition characteristic of growth hormone deficiency. This aspect of the disorder can be treated with exogenous growth hormone, although many other aspects of this disease are difficult to manage and require a multidisciplinary approach.[620,621] Children with PWS can develop behavioral disorders, and psychiatric disorders can be present in up to 10% of young adults.

Angelman syndrome (OMIM #105830) is a neurogenetic disorder with a similar incidence in the population as PWS. The AS clinical phenotype includes intellectual disability (IQ <40), inappropriate bouts of laughter, absence of speech, gait ataxia, progressive microcephaly, dysmorphic facial features, and epilepsy.[622] Because these patients demonstrate bursts of laughter and smiling, AS is sometimes referred to as the "happy puppet syndrome." Unique electroencephalographic patterns are seen in most individuals with AS younger than 2 years of age and can be helpful in diagnosing the condition. As many as 6% of patients who display both intellectual disability and epilepsy may have AS. Some of the phenotypic features associated with AS can be nonspecific or can occur separately in other syndromes or nonsyndromic conditions; thus, a constellation of findings with associated laughter, unique smiling, and happy demeanor of people with AS helps in the diagnosis.

Apparent from the characteristic physical findings, PWS and AS are clinically distinct syndromes, yet each results from different genetic alterations involving an imprinted segment within 8 million bases on chromosome 15q11.2-q13. The genes at both ends of this region have biparental expression, but they flank genes that demonstrate exclusively paternal or maternal expression. The expression of either paternal or maternal genes is controlled by an imprinting center (IC) with the imprinting "reset" during gametogenesis between parent and offspring of a different gender.[618] If paternally expressed genes in this region are missing, defective, or epigenetically silenced through DNA methylation and only an inactive, nonexpressed maternal allele remains, PWS is observed. Conversely, if maternally expressed genes in this region are not functional and only the inactive paternal allele remains, the clinical phenotype will be AS.

The most 5′ gene in the paternally expressed region is *MKRN3* that encodes makorin ring finger protein 3, with several zinc finger motifs and no introns.[623] Adjacent to *MKRN3* are the structurally similar and intronless genes *MAGEL2* (alias *NDNL1*) coding melanoma antigen family L2 and *NDN*, a melanoma antigen family member, which is involved in terminal differentiation of neurons.[624,625] This region also contains the locus *SNRPN-SNURF*, small nuclear ribonucleoprotein polypeptide N *(SNRPN)* that is involved in mRNA processing and splicing and *SNURF* (*SNRPN* upstream reading frame), which is found in the nucleus, contains 71 amino acids, may bind RNA, and has a C-terminal motif similar to ubiquitin. Last are multiple C/D box snoRNA genes, which are noncoding RNA molecules that modify both rRNA and snRNA by the methylation of the ribose 2′-hydroxyl group.[626,627] Sahoo et al were the first to link the loss of paternal snoRNA genes to PWS.[628] The mechanism by which the absence of these genes results in the pathogenesis of PWS is not clearly understood.

Loss of normally expressed paternal genes on chromosome 15q11-q13 resulting in PWS can occur by several mechanisms (Table 49.7).[619] Most commonly, PWS (65%–75%) results from a de novo deletion after unequal homologous recombination involving one of two common centromeric breakpoints (BP1 or BP2) and one of multiple telomeric breakpoints (BP3–BP6) on the paternal allele.[629] This renders the zygote monosomic for these genes, and the zygote possesses only the maternal copy of this region. Alternatively, 20% to 30% of cases of PWS are caused by uniparental disomy (UPD). In the case of PWS, although two copies of the genes located in 15q11.2-q13 exist, both are maternal in origin and in most cases arise from meiosis I nondisjunction followed by postzygotic mitotic loss of the third, paternally derived chromosome 15 via a process referred to as *trisomy rescue*. This mechanism rescues the zygote from trisomy 15, a condition that is incompatible with life.[630] Although the fetus is genetically complete with two chromosome 15s (disomy), both chromosomes are received from the mother (uniparental), and no expression of paternally expressed genes occurs in this imprinted region. Not surprisingly, maternal age has been reported to be significantly higher in PWS patients resulting from UPD caused by maternal meiosis I nondisjunction than in PWS patients resulting from a de novo deletion.[631] Some cases of PWS result from microdeletions encompassing the paternal IC or, in 2% of cases, from abnormal methylation at this site.[632] A mutation involving the IC prevents this *cis*-acting control center from resetting the imprint in the germline. These mutations will result in PWS because if they are present on the maternal chromosome of phenotypically normal fathers, they will be transmitted to offspring because now the paternal chromosome will maintain the maternal imprint and will be silenced. Finally, fewer than 1% of PWS cases are caused by chromosomal rearrangements disrupting the genes in the 15q11.2-q13 region.[633] Some genotype–phenotype correlations have been noted. Patients with PWS with UPD are more likely to have psychotic episodes, compulsive behaviors (eg, skin picking), and ASDs than are PWS patients with deletions.[634,635]

The maternally expressed gene *UBE3A* is telomeric to the snoRNA genes and oriented in the opposite orientation on chromosome 15q11.2-q13.[636,637] The *UBE3A* gene encompasses 120 kb; contains 16 exons; and encodes E3 ubiquitin protein ligase, which is involved in the ubiquitin proteasome degradation pathway.[638] Three protein isoforms are produced from this gene by alternative splicing, and they differ at their N-termini.[639] Interestingly, in the brain, only the maternal *UBE3A* allele is expressed; however, both alleles are expressed in other tissues.[640] A second gene, *ATP10A*, is upstream from *UBE3A* and is also preferentially expressed only from the maternal allele.

Similar to PWS, most patients with AS (70%–75%) have a deletion of the critical 15q1.21-q13 region. However, unlike PWS, in AS, the disease-causing deletion occurs on the maternal allele. In 3% to 7% of AS patients, the syndrome is attributed to UPD from the inheritance of two paternally derived chromosome 15s; as a consequence, there is no transcription of *UBE3A*. An IC defect has been described in 2% to 3% of patients with AS ; a chromosome rearrangement has been reported in fewer than1%; and in 10% of cases, a *UBE3A* mutation has been detected.[632,641,642] Most of the *UBE3A* gene mutations are frameshift or nonsense mutations and result in loss of function.[643] Using the AS mouse model, a possible treatment for this disease could be increasing expression of the normal paternal allele and silencing the mutant transcript

TABLE 49.7 Molecular Mechanisms for Prader-Willi and Angelman Syndromes

Molecular Mechanism of Disease	Angelman Syndrome (Frequency)	Prader-Willi Syndrome (Frequency)
Deletion of 15q11-13	Loss of maternal allele (70%–75%)	Loss of paternal allele (65%–75%)
Uniparental disomy	Two paternal chromosomes (3%–7%)	Two maternal chromosomes (20%–30%)
Imprinting center defect epimutations or microdeletions	Maternal allele (2%–3%)	Paternal allele (2%)
UBE3A mutation	10%	Not applicable
Rearrangement involving 15q11-13	Maternal allele (<1%)	Paternal allele (<1%)
Cause not identified	10%	Rare

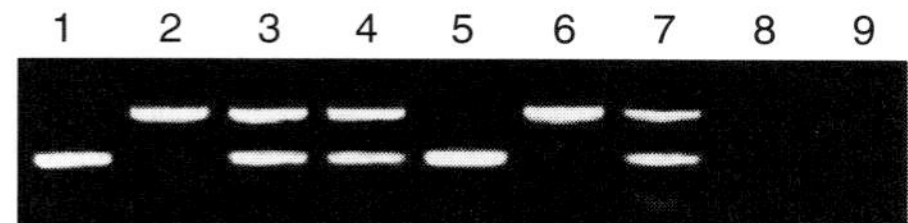

FIGURE 49.14 Methylation-specific polymerase chain reaction (PCR) for the diagnosis of Prader-Willi syndrome (PWS) and Angelman syndrome (AS). Extracted DNA is treated with sodium bisulfate before amplification using multiplex PCR and oligonucleotide primers specific for modified DNA. PCR products are subjected to gel electrophoresis. Normal individuals show two amplicons representing their methylated maternal allele and unmethylated paternal allele. PWS patients show only the maternal allele, and AS patients show only the paternal allele. Patient DNA with patterns diagnostic of AS *(lanes 1* and *5)* and PWS *(lanes 2* and *6)* and patients with normal methylation patterns *(lanes 3* and *4)* are shown. Normal control DNA patterns and a negative control reaction in which no template DNA was added are indicated in *lanes 7 and 8,* respectively. No amplification products are observed in unmodified normal control DNA *(lane 9),* illustrating the specificity of PCR primers prepared specifically for sodium bisulfate–modified DNA. (Courtesy Jack Tarleton, PhD, Director of Genetics Laboratory, Fullerton Genetics Center, Mission Health System, Asheville, North Carolina.)

with antisense oligonucleotides.[644] In about 10% of AS cases, the molecular basis of the disease has not been determined. It is possible that these patients are misdiagnosed with AS and rather are similar to AS but clinically and molecularly separate from those with AS.[645] Genotype–phenotype associations are known, including the fact that patients with AS with deletions are more likely to have hypopigmentation of skin, eye, and hair or microcephaly and are more likely to be severely affected.[646] In contrast, patients with AS arising from UPD have normal head circumference and are more often mildly affected.

Diagnostic testing for individuals suspected of having AS or PWS can involve a variety of laboratory techniques and testing algorithms. Methylation-specific PCR (msPCR) coupled with gel electrophoresis is one cost-effective approach (Fig. 49.14). In methylation-specific PCR, genomic DNA is treated with sodium bisulfite to convert unmethylated cytosine residues to uracil without altering the methylated cytosine residues (those silenced in the 15q11.2-13 region). Subsequent PCR reactions use oligonucleotide primers specific to DNA strands that contain uracil (from unmethylated cytosines) or cytosine (from methylated cytosines).[647,648] Methylation-specific PCR (msPCR) provides a rapid and reliable diagnostic test for PWS or AS. Fewer than 1% of PWS cases and about 20% of AS cases are not detected by this assay. Additionally, msPCR coupled with melting curve analysis or methylation-specific MLPA can be used.[649-651] Although msPCR is frequently the first tier of testing and can be used to diagnose PWS or AS, it cannot determine the molecular basis of disease. If the msPCR result is positive, chromosomal microarray analysis will identify chromosome deletions, and in UPD cases, the parental origin of both chromosomes can be determined.[652-654] Alternatively, if the msPCR result is positive, fluorescent in situ hybridization (FISH) studies will detect deletions, and in UPD cases, molecular testing using polymorphic short tandem repeat sequences coupled with capillary electrophoresis will detect UPD.[655] Patients with PWS and patients with a chromosomal rearrangement disrupting the genes in this area will not be identified by these testing methods nor will AS patients with a *UBE3A* mutation. Rather, in these cases, a routine karyotype or DNA sequence analysis is required for diagnosis. Testing for PWS and AS is critical because knowledge regarding the molecular mechanism of disease is important for accurately determining recurrence risk to the family.[656] For example, although mutations causing AS can arise de novo (eg, UPD with a <1% recurrence risk), other AS-causing mutations can be silently transmitted through several generations. If a *UBE3A* mutation arose de novo on a paternal allele transmitted to a son, the son could transmit the mutation to a son or daughter to produce a normal phenotype. However, although this son could transmit the silenced *UBE3A* mutation to his offspring, his sister could donate her mutated *UBE3A* paternally derived allele to her offspring, and the child would have AS. The recurrence risk for her to have another affected child in this case would be 50%.

POINTS TO REMEMBER

Inherited Diseases

- Mitochondrial and imprinting disorders follow non-Mendelian patterns of inheritance.
- Complex diseases result from the contribution of both genetic and environmental factors and do not follow Mendelian inheritance patterns.
- For most genes, pathogenic mutations are located throughout the gene and are heterogeneous in nature.
- For some disease genes, the type of mutation and effect on the encoded protein can predict the clinical phenotype and identify targeted therapy for patient care.
- Diagnostic DNA testing is complicated by genetic and allelic heterogeneity.
- Genetic counseling is an important component of patient care and management.

EXPANDED CARRIER SCREENING

Carrier screening refers to the use of genetic testing to determine individuals who are at risk of having a child affected with an autosomal recessive disorder. Carrier screening for disorders has long been a mainstay of genetic laboratories and has increased dramatically over the past decade. Carrier screening for some common lethal disorders (eg, CF) is considered the standard of care in prenatal patients regardless of ethnicity.[2] For some ethnic groups, such as Ashkenazi Jews, the carrier frequency for several lethal disorders is relatively high.[657] As a result, screening for many of these disorders (eg, Tay-Sachs, Canavan) has long been recommended to Ashkenazi Jewish couples during preconception and prenatal counseling.[657]

Conventional carrier screening used mutation panels (eg, the ACMG *CFTR* 23 mutation panel) that identify the majority of mutation carriers for a single disorder. Over the past several years, carrier screening (particularly in preconception/prenatal care) has shifted toward new testing platforms that simultaneously screen for hundreds of common disease-associated point mutations. With the advent of these new technologies many laboratories are offering expanded carrier screening (ECS) panels. Initially, ECS panels simply increased the number of mutations or variants that were tested in a single gene (eg, *CFTR*). More recently, ECS panels have broadened to include known mutations or variants for a multitude (>100 in some cases) of inherited disorders in a single test.[658] The clear advantage of ECS panels is that they provide a cost-effective method to screen for multiple genetic disorders. In many cases, the cost of an ECS panel is less than screening for a single gene by traditional means. ECS panels also provide patients with carrier status data on additional disorders not routinely included on traditional carrier screening panels. However, ECS panels have come under criticism because of several drawbacks.

Traditionally, mutations included on carrier screening panels were selected based on confirmed pathogenicity and the carrier frequency of the mutation.[51] With the advent of ECS panels, some laboratories have included variants with reduced penetrance or mild clinical effects.[659,660] Some expanded CF screening panels include variants that are known to have variable clinical impact and in some cases result in no discernible phenotype.[659] The inclusion of such variants in a genetic screening assay can be confusing and lead individuals to make reproductive decisions without a complete understanding of the information provided.[659,661] Some disorders that have been selected for inclusion on commercially available ECS panels do not meet generally accepted criteria for carrier screening.[661,662] For example, some disorders are rare and have a reported incidence of less than 1 per million births.[49,662] Not surprisingly, the targeted mutations in many of these rare disorders only account for a small fraction of the mutations capable of causing disease. A negative screening result in an individual with a family history for a rare disorder may give a false sense of security. Because of this low sensitivity, if a mutation is identified in one partner for a rare disorder, that individual's reproductive partner likely will undergo full gene sequencing for the causative gene, thus increasing the costs of screening dramatically.[662] ECS panels have also been criticized for including mutations (and functional polymorphisms) of variable penetrance that are very common in certain ethnic groups or society at large (eg, factor V Leiden, *HFE*-related hemochromatosis, MTHFR deficiency).[661] Typically, disorders with such high frequency in the population are not recommended for carrier screening because their clinical implications are uncertain. The identification of these mutations or variants in the context of preconception (or prenatal) counseling are especially controversial because fetal testing for some of these disorders (eg, MTHFR deficiency) is not routinely offered in the United States.[661] The clinical validity of some of the variants that are included on prenatal screening panels is unclear.

Another aspect of ECS panels that merits mention is the inclusion of adult onset disorders. Some disorders (eg, familial Mediterranean fever, α_1-antitrypsin deficiency, *GJB2*-related nonsyndromic hearing loss, atypical CF) have variable ages of onset and disease manifestations. Carrier screening for mutations that cause these disorders in individuals of reproductive age can provide an unexpected diagnosis of a disease that they have not yet developed. In one recent study, 78 of 23,453 individuals tested were identified as either compound heterozygous or homozygous for disease-causing mutations.[49] Of the patients identified, only three patients reported a previous diagnosis or history of disease.[49] These data illustrate the complex counseling-related issues that ECS panels have created. Because traditional carrier screening has focused on severe, disease-causing mutations, the likelihood of diagnosing an asymptomatic individual with disease was very low. The newer ECS panels require that all patients undergoing such screening be properly advised as to the potential testing outcomes.

To address the issues associated with ECS testing, the ACMG released a position statement regarding prenatal and preconception ECS that outlined criteria for inclusion of diseases or mutations on a carrier screening panel, including (1) a clearly defined clinical association; (2) most at-risk patients would choose fetal testing to aid in preconception or prenatal decision making; (3) a clearly defined residual risk for individuals that test negative; and (4) for any adult-onset disorder that may affect the individual being tested, pretest counseling and consent should be performed.[663] Recently, several professional societies released a joint statement regarding the use of ECS panels.[50] These statements can guide physicians in offering, consenting, and counseling patients about ECS panels and their results.[50]

The clinical use of ECS panels has only just begun. As with any new technology and the increase in data that it provides, unforeseen ethical issues can arise. As the use of ECS panels becomes widespread and professional organizations (eg, the ACMG) develop formal guidelines, many of the issues outlined here will be resolved. However, preconception and prenatal genetic counseling will continue to be important in helping patients to understand the clinical implications of their screening results.

MASSIVELY PARALLEL SEQUENCING

Massively parallel sequencing (also referred to as next-generation sequencing) is a high-throughput DNA sequencing technology capable of generating data on a genomic scale in a short period of days (see Chapter 47 on nucleic acid techniques). Not since the introduction of PCR in the 1980s has a technology revolutionized the field of molecular diagnostics like MPS has in the past few years. At the most basic level, MPS uses similar concepts to traditional capillary-based Sanger sequencing in that fluorescently labeled dNTPs are used to determine the template sequence. However, the distinct advantage of MPS is its ability to perform simultaneous sequencing reactions on millions of target sequences at a vastly lower cost per base than traditional Sanger sequencing. There are several different MPS methods, but most have similar sample preparation workflows. Typically, DNA fragmentation is followed by insert selection, library formation, and clonal amplification. Then sequencing by synthesis signals is acquired by measuring pyrophosphate release, generation of hydrogen ions, or the fluorescence of reversible terminators. This massively parallel clonal sequencing of library inserts generates gigabases of sequencing data at a cost that is feasible for clinical testing. One drawback to such massive data generation is that bioinformatics filtering processes are required to efficiently interpret the numerous variants identified. Data filtering in MPS typically involves the utilization of publicly available variant databases (eg, dbSNP; Exome Aggregation Consortium [ExAC], National Heart, Lung, and Blood Institute Exome Sequencing Project) to eliminate variants that occur at high frequency in the general population and therefore are likely benign. After the common variants have been filtered, locus-specific mutation databases and in silico prediction programs (eg, SIFT and PolyPhen2) can aid in the

TABLE 49.8 Commonly Ordered Massively Parallel Sequencing–Based Gene Panels

Panel Name	Included Disorders*	Targeted Patient Group
Aortopathy disorders	Ehlers-Danlos syndrome (I, II, and IV), Loeys-Deitz syndrome, Marfan syndrome	Individuals with disease affecting any aortic section
Breast and ovarian hereditary cancer	Hereditary breast and ovarian cancer syndrome	Individuals with a strong family history of breast and ovarian cancer; individuals with early onset of breast or ovarian cancer
Cardiomyopathy disorders	Dilated cardiomyopathy, hypertrophic cardiomyopathy, long QT syndrome	Individuals with a suspected diagnosis of a hereditary cardiomyopathy disorder
Expanded carrier screening	Numerous (>100)	Individuals planning pregnancy or prenatal reproductive partners
Hearing loss	Keratitis–ichthyosis–deafness syndrome, nonsyndromic hearing loss, Usher syndrome	Individuals with a suspected diagnosis of either syndromic or nonsyndromic hearing loss
Hereditary endocrine cancer	Multiple endocrine neoplasia type 1, multiple endocrine neoplasia type 2, Von Hippel-Lindau disease	Individuals with a family history of endocrine cancer; individuals with a personal history of endocrine cancer
Hereditary gastrointestinal cancer	Familial adenomatous polyposis, juvenile polyposis syndrome, Lynch syndrome	Individuals with a personal or family history of gastrointestinal cancer
Noonan spectrum disorders	Cardiofaciocutaneous syndrome, Costello syndrome, Noonan syndrome	Individuals with a suspected diagnosis of Noonan syndrome or a related disorder
Periodic fever syndromes	Familial Mediterranean fever, Majeed syndrome, Muckle-Wells syndrome	Individuals with a suspected diagnosis of a periodic fever syndrome
X-linked intellectual disability	Rett syndrome, Duchenne muscular dystrophy, ornithine transcarbamylase deficiency	Individuals with intellectual disability inherited in an X-linked manner

*This is a selected list of commonly included disorders and is not comprehensive.

interpretation of potential disease-causing variants. Variants are then classified as pathogenic, likely pathogenic, uncertain significance, likely benign, or benign.[664] Data filtering systems are commercially available to help in the interpretation of MPS data, but many laboratories have chosen to develop their own software pipelines internally.

One of the most significant advantages of MPS for diagnostic testing is the ability to target all genes known to be associated with a specific diagnosis (or phenotype) in a single test that is comparable in price and turnaround time to that of Sanger sequencing for a single-gene analysis. These targeted gene panels are the most commonly ordered clinical tests using MPS technology. Before development of MPS, testing patients for causative mutations in multiple genes that cause a single syndrome was a very expensive and time-consuming process. For example, retinitis pigmentosa (RP, OMIM #268000) is a group of inherited degenerative ocular disorders that affects 1 in 3000 to 7000 people.[665] Locus heterogeneity is a hallmark of RP because mutations in more than 60 genes have been reported to cause this disease. Using traditional Sanger sequencing to determine the underlying molecular alteration would be cost prohibitive for most patients with RP, yet an MPS RP gene panel is cost effective and timely. RP is one example of how MPS implementation has advanced our ability to provide a molecular diagnosis for a genetically heterogeneous disorder. Table 49.8 lists some commonly ordered MPS-based gene panels. MPS also enables the sequencing of very large genes at a reasonable cost (eg, the *DMD* gene that causes DMD and BMD). The flexibility of MPS selection and library preparation can provide a comprehensive test of more than 100 genes (eg, an X-Linked Intellectual Disabilities Panel) or a more targeted panel that analyzes a handful of genes associated with a specific phenotype (eg, a hereditary gastrointestinal cancer panel). Over the next few years, it is likely that MPS will be widely implemented in diagnostic laboratories, Sanger sequencing assays will decline in use, and sequencing technology will continue to evolve.

WHOLE-EXOME SEQUENCING

Whole-exome sequencing (WES) refers to an MPS-based DNA sequencing method that specifically targets the coding regions (exons) and directly adjacent intronic regions for the majority of the approximately 20,000 genes known to exist in the human genome. Although the exome only accounts for approximately 1% of the human genome, mutations in gene encoding regions are responsible for the vast majority of human inherited diseases. On average, WES is able to identify an underlying genetic alteration in approximately 25% to 50% of patients (depending on the inclusion criteria).[666-668] This makes WES an effective diagnostic tool for patients with a phenotype that suggests an inherited disorder that does not fit the clinical characteristics of previously described syndromes.[666,669]

Most exome sequencing performed in clinical laboratories currently uses a hybridization based capture method of tagged (biotinylated) probes targeted to specific areas of the fragmented template DNA.[670] These probes are bound to magnetic beads allowing a simple washing process to separate targeted DNA regions from the excess unwanted (intronic) DNA.[670] After this enrichment process, the DNA is ready to be sequenced. Several exome capture kits are commercially available, making WES easily performed in most molecular diagnostic laboratories. Often, the limiting factor in implementing WES is the large amount of data produced; therefore, a well-defined bioinformatics workflow is critical for the timely reporting of WES results. Several data analysis programs are commercially available to aid in the interpretation of WES data, and many publications describe informatics workflows.[671]

Clinical WES sequencing is often performed on both the symptomatic proband and their (typically asymptomatic) parents (often referred to as a trio). Sequencing parents helps with interpretation of sequence variants that are identified in the proband. For example, if a potentially pathogenic variant is identified in the proband but not observed in the parental samples, that variant is likely de novo (assuming confirmed paternity) and potentially causative. Likewise, if a potentially pathogenic variant is identified in a gene that is dominantly inherited but is also identified in an asymptomatic parent, it is less likely to cause the patient's phenotype. Parental samples can also be used to establish phase in the detection of two pathogenic mutations in a gene inherited in an autosomal recessive manner. Use of familial samples to aid interpretation of WES results is a powerful tool capable of dramatically increasing clinical sensitivity of the test and should be pursued in all patients undergoing WES.

WES has been implemented widely in clinical diagnostic laboratories in the United States, and thousands of patients have been tested by this method. WES should be considered in patients with a phenotype suspected to be caused by a mutation in a single gene when known single-gene disorders have been eliminated.[669] Careful consideration should always be given to the patient's presentation before determining whether or not WES is the appropriate test for a given phenotype. Specifically, a detailed family history, a systematic characterization of the patient's phenotype, and a careful literature review is recommended before ordering WES.[669] Obtaining this information can help determine if the patient is actually affected by a previously described, but rare, syndrome with a known genetic cause that should be ruled out before proceeding to WES.[669] In many cases, a single gene test or a targeted MPS-based gene panel with multiple genes may be the appropriate first test to order. To aid clinicians in determining which molecular testing protocol is best for their patients, algorithms have been developed.[672,673] These testing algorithms suggest that individuals with multiple nonspecific clinical findings or with a clinical presentation associated with marked genetic heterogeneity (eg, intellectual disability) are good candidates for WES.[672,673] Individuals with distinctive clinical features, family history of a specific disorder, or indicative findings for specific disorders should be counseled to pursue either single-gene or MPS-based gene panel testing.[672,673] Using these testing guidelines, approximately 50% of patients received a genetic diagnosis using "traditional" methods of diagnosis.[673] Single-gene testing is therefore not obsolete because of WES but continues to be the appropriate diagnostic tool in many clinical cases.

Counseling for WES is highly complex because issues relating to test results must be considered. The risk of identifying a VUS exists in all sequencing-based genetic tests. However, the risk for the identification of a VUS increases dramatically for WES. Patient counseling for WES should always include a discussion of VUSs because these are likely to appear on any WES report even though the clinical implications of these findings are unclear.[672] Patients should be counseled on the possibility that incidental findings may include the identification of pathogenic mutations in clinically actionable genes (eg, *BRCA1*) that are unrelated to the patient's current phenotype. The return of incidental findings (IFs) in WES is a controversial topic and has resulted in the ACMG formalizing recommendations for which IFs should be returned to the patient.[674] The ACMG recommendations provide a list of 56 genes that represent the "minimum" IFs that should be reported to the clinician when a pathogenic variant is identified regardless of the clinical indication for testing.[674] The gene list generated by the ACMG was developed to include genes for conditions that are verifiable by other diagnostic methods and that cause highly penetrant disorders that would likely benefit from medical intervention.[674] The release of the ACMG recommendations was met by criticism because the guidelines were seen by some to violate existing ethical norms in genetic testing and the patient's right to autonomy by suggesting that IFs in the 56-gene list should be returned regardless of patient preference.[674,675] In response to criticism from its members, the ACMG released a statement in April 2014 revising its recommendations to allow patients to opt out of receiving incidental findings. Even after this revision, debate continues among members of the ACMG and clinical geneticists regarding how IFs should be returned to patients.[676] Recommendations on the return of IFs likely will continue to evolve as WES genomic testing becomes more commonplace in clinics.[677]

Over the past several years, WES has proven to be an invaluable research tool in the discovery of the underlying genetic alterations for many Mendelian disorders.[678-680] In some cases, these discoveries identified the first known genetic cause of a disorder (eg, Miller syndrome, Kabuki syndrome), and in others, additional genes were discovered to cause an already well-defined phenotype (eg, RP, nonsyndromic hearing loss, osteogenesis imperfecta, intellectual disability, and many others).[681-687] WES studies also have elucidated alternative phenotypes caused by mutations in genes already known to cause a genetic disorder.[688-690] The benefits of these discoveries in the clinical diagnosis and treatment of patients cannot be overstated. Identification of the underlying molecular alteration (and molecular pathogenesis) that results in a specific disease is the first step in developing treatment modalities. Because of the discoveries made by WES, the next decade will see a vast improvement in the treatment of many inherited disorders. Within the next decade, as WES technology improves and WES costs decline, the underlying cause for the vast majority of inherited genetic disorders may become known.

CYTOGENOMICS

The term *cytogenomics* describes the application of molecular techniques to cytogenetics. In a broad sense, this applies to FISH. In FISH analysis, a fluorescently labeled DNA molecule serves as a "probe" and is hybridized to metaphase chromosomes or interphase nuclei, and the fluorescent probes are visualized using a fluorescent microscope.[691] In a more narrow sense, cytogenomics applies to the use of chromosome microarray (CMA) technology, including array comparative genomic hybridization (aCGH) and SNP arrays.[692] SNP and aCGH arrays have revolutionized the field of cytogenetics as important tools for both clinical diagnosis and disease discovery.[693] However, these technologies do not identify balanced translocations or inversions, both of which require routine karyotyping, FISH analysis, or both.

Instrumentation and associated kits for aCGH and SNP arrays are commercially available. Platforms and methods vary, including the probe size, spacing between the probes on the array, copy number resolutions, and probe sensitivity.[692,694] In aCGH, the patient and control DNA are labeled with two different fluorochromes and co-hybridized to the array, but with a SNP array, no control DNA is used; rather, the fluorescent signals are measured against a reference pattern.[692] Both aCGH and SNP arrays can detect copy number variants (CNVs). In addition, SNP arrays provide the genotype and determine if the patient is homozygous (AA, BB) or heterozygous (AB) for each SNP present on the array. SNP genotype analysis allows long stretches of homologous DNA sequences, also referred to as regions of homology (ROHs) or regions with an absence of heterozygosity (AOHs), to be identified. These segments of DNA are important to identify UPD in the diagnosis of imprinting disorders.[695,696] However, detection of an ROH or AOH could represent an incidental or unexpected finding of parental relatedness or consanguinity. Depending on the degree of homozygosity, these findings could suggest incestral mating. Standards and guidelines for laboratory reporting of incidental findings suggestive of consanguinity have been developed by the ACMG, and care must be taken by clinicians in communicating these results to patients.[697,698]

CMA's clinical utility is in the diagnosis and management of patients referred for multiple congenital anomalies, developmental delay or intellectual disability, and ASDs.[699-701] The ACMG recommends CMA as a first-tier genetic test for patients with these conditions, and practice standards and guidelines for these applications have been established.[702] Interestingly, CMA analysis can identify CNVs of clinical significance in as many as 21% of patients with ASDs.[703] Common ASD CNV hot spots are known, and a database of previously reported CNVs with a documented association with ASDs is available for reference.[703-705] FISH, MLPA, or real-time PCR studies are often used for confirmation of novel aberrant CNV findings to prevent false-positive reporting (Fig. 49.15). Public databases (eg, Database of Genomic Variants,[706] Ensembl,[707] National Center for Biotechnology Information[708]) are used to determine the genes that are contained within the CNV and that may be either lost or gained. Generally, the larger the CNV and the more genes contained within the DNA region of interest, the more the variant is likely to have a clinical consequence and the more likely a deletion is to be pathogenic compared with duplications.[704] After careful review of various databases, peer-reviewed publications, and the clinical findings of the patient, the significance of the CNV is reported using guidelines established by the ACMG.[709] Results may be pathogenic or benign or may be reported as uncertain clinical significance. Furthermore, a variant of uncertain clinical significance can be further classified as likely pathogenic or likely benign.[709] Appropriate literature should be referenced, and the variant should be reported according to standard CNV nomenclature. To ascertain the significance of any variant with uncertain clinical significance, parental specimens should be requested (Fig. 49.16).

Chromosome microarray is also appropriate for prenatal testing when abnormal ultrasound findings are evident or for additional information when a normal karyotype is unexpected.[710,711] CMA testing can be performed on DNA extracted from cultured amniocytes or chorionic villi tissue. However, CMA testing in prenatal cases can be especially challenging if a variant of uncertain clinical significance is identified because it may be difficult to predict the postnatal effect.[710] CMA analysis on DNA extracted from representative tissue of products of conception can be useful in determining the etiology of the pregnancy loss.[712]

In addition to using aCGH and SNP arrays to detect constitutional or germline changes associated with disease, these arrays are also used on hematologic and solid tumors.[713,714] In somatic tissue, the detection of copy number changes can define regions of DNA and specific genes involved in the pathogenesis of neoplastic processes. In addition, the ability of SNP arrays to determine genotype enables the identification of copy neutral LOH. Similar to constitutional UPD seen with imprinting disorders, copy neutral LOH is a somatic event and indicates two copies of the same chromosomal region. This may involve part of the chromosome or the entire chromosome, and most often, the region involved harbors a "driver" mutation in a particular gene that promotes growth and proliferation for the neoplastic process.[713]

POINTS TO REMEMBER

Clinical Utility of Molecular Methods

- Targeted PCR amplification is most useful in the identification of common pathogenic point mutations.
- msPCR is capable of determining the methylation status of DNA and is often used in the diagnosis of imprinting disorders.
- Full-gene Sanger sequencing is typically used to identify pathogenic point mutations and small insertion or deletion mutations in disorders associated with a single disease-causing gene.
- MPS is the ideal technology to use for the identification of a pathogenic point mutation or a small insertion or deletion mutation in disorders caused by mutations in any of a number of genes.
- MLPA is most useful in the detection of large (exon level or bigger) deletions or duplications in three or fewer disease-causing genes.
- Array-based technology is most useful in the simultaneous detection of large deletions or duplications in numerous genes.

REPORTING OF TEST RESULTS

As the preceding pages show, DNA testing for inherited diseases is complex, and thoroughly conveying genetic test results is important. Results must be presented so they can be easily and accurately understood by a professional whose expertise may not be genetics because in many instances, primary care providers communicate test results to the patient. With the increasing clinical demand for genetic testing and the increasing numbers of laboratories performing such tests, uniformity in communicating these complex results to referring clinicians is important, and failure to include pertinent information in these reports constitutes a deficiency in the molecular pathology laboratory inspection checklist of the College of American Pathologists (CAP).[715] A comprehensive

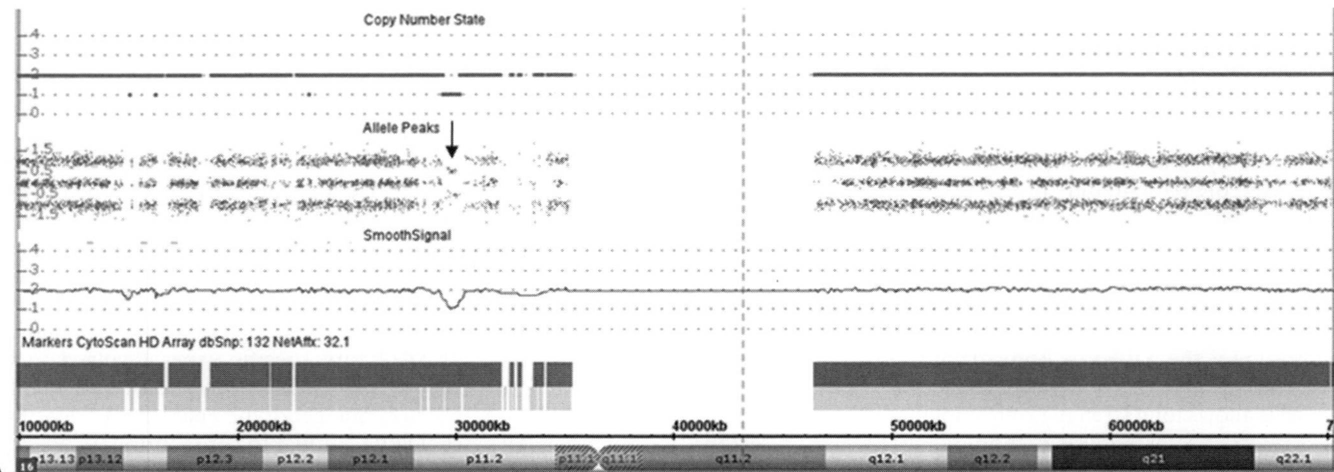

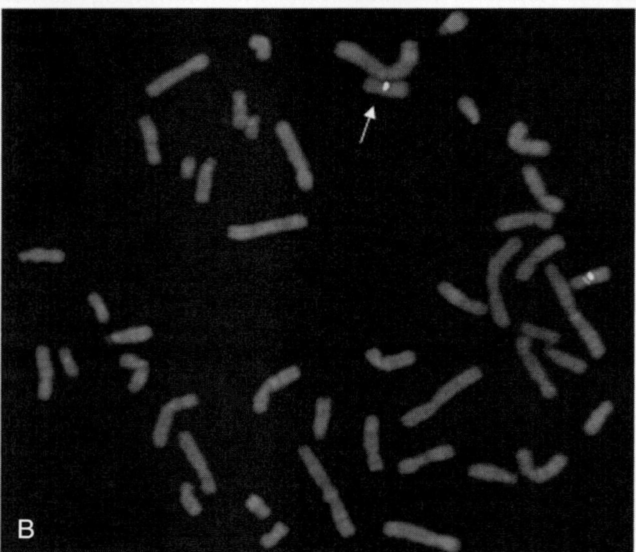

FIGURE 49.15 Loss of 16p11.2 detected by microarray analysis with confirmatory testing performed by fluorescent in situ hybridization (FISH) analysis. **A,** DNA from a patient referred for autism was analyzed using the Affymetrix CytoScan platform. The copy number state *(top)*, allele peaks *(middle)*, and smooth signal pattern of the copy number *(lower rows)* are shown. A partial ideogram of chromosome 16 is shown to localize the data to the corresponding chromosomal bands. A 751-kb loss of nucleotides 29,427,215 to 30,177,916, localized to chromosome band 16p11.2 as denoted by the *arrow,* is shown. Given that only 1 copy of DNA sequence is present at this site, the allele peak single nucleotide polymorphism pattern for this region shows only two lines (AA and BB), and the remaining portions of the chromosome have the characteristic three-line pattern (AA, AB, and BB). The repeat sequences localized to the pericentromeric region of chromosome 16 are excluded from the array (absence of *bars*) because they are not uniquely localized to chromosome 16 and could cross hybridize to other chromosomes. **B,** FISH results obtained using a red probe (PR11-301D18) specific for band 16p11.2 including nucleotides 29,776,142-29,961,746 and an aqua pericentromeric control probe (D16Z3) for chromosome 16 to assess probe hybridization efficiency and identify both chromosomes 16. After hybridization, the metaphase spreads showed a normal pattern for the control probe (one signal on each chromosome 16), but an abnormal pattern for the test probe (one probe signal on a structurally normal chromosome 16, with no signal observed on a structurally abnormal chromosome 16 *[arrow]*). Based on the banding pattern (reverse DAPI and GTG [not shown]) and morphology of the chromosomes, this loss resulted from an interstitial deletion [del(16)(p11.2p11.2)(PR11-301D18-,D16Z3+)] that was not detected by routine karyotype analysis. (Courtesy Dr. Colleen Jackson-Cook, Director Cytogenetics Laboratory, Department of Pathology, Virginia Commonwealth University Health System).

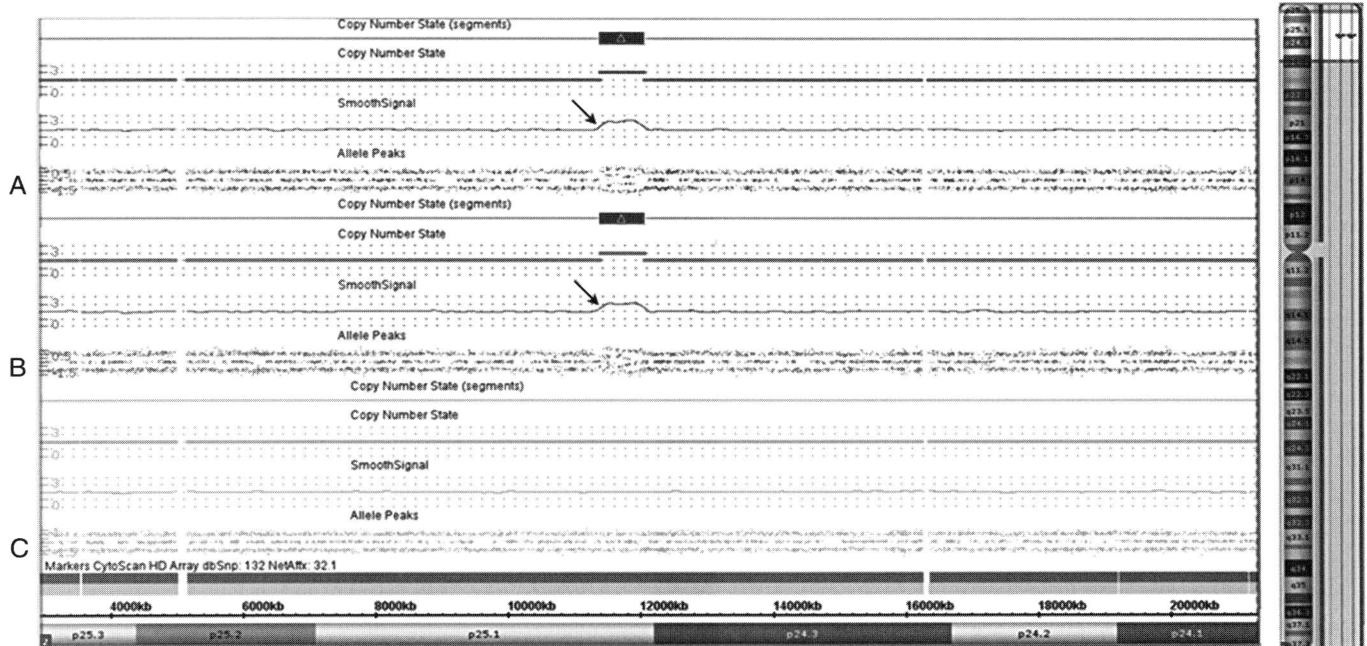

FIGURE 49.16 Detection of inherited copy number gain at chromosome region 2p25.1 by microarray analysis. DNA from a 7-year-old male patient referred for developmental delay was analyzed using an Affymetrix CytoScan platform. A copy number variant (CNV) of uncertain clinical significance representing a 654-kb copy number gain (three copies involving nucleotides 11,410,614–12,064,438) was identified in the patient *(row a)*. The *arrow* denotes the gain of DNA to three copies in the smooth signal and copy number state plots; with four "bands" (AAA, AAB, ABB, and BBB) being observed in the allele peak pattern. A partial ideogram of chromosome 2 is shown horizontally to show the location of the CNV detected in the patient and the location of the CNV relative to the entire chromosome number 2 as seen on the vertical orientation. Maternal *(row b)* and paternal *(row c)* specimens were requested for analysis to determine if the CNV observed in the patient was inherited or represented a de novo event. The results indicate the presence of no CNVs in the paternal DNA but show that the CNV in the patient is of maternal origin. Furthermore, the CNV in the maternal sample is identical to that observed in the patient and demonstrates that the CNV was stably inherited, thereby suggesting that this CNV is benign. The data shown for each family member includes the copy number state *(top rows of each case)*, smooth signal of copy number values *(middle rows of each case)*, and allele peaks *(lower rows of each case)*. (Courtesy Dr. Colleen Jackson-Cook, Director Cytogenetics Laboratory, Department of Pathology, Virginia Commonwealth University Health System).

genetic report should include the patient's name, medical record number or birth date, sex of the patient, ethnicity of the patient (if relevant), type of specimen and date received, specimen's laboratory identification number, laboratory test requested, name and address of laboratory performing the test, name and address of referring health care professional or hospital, date of the report, analytic interpretation of the results using standard nomenclature for all variants identified, detailed description of the method used (citing literature if needed), and sensitivity and specificity of the assay (eg, number of variants analyzed, percentage of variants not detected, possibility of genetic heterogeneity, chance of genetic recombination). All sequence variants are classified as one of the following: pathogenic, likely pathogenic, uncertain significance, likely benign, or benign.[664,716] In silico tools such as PolyPhen2, SIFT, and MutationTaster should be listed if they were used to determine significance of the variant.[716] The DNA and protein change, if applicable, should be listed using guidelines of the Human Genome Variation Society.[717] The laboratory should include the reference sequence and genome build and provide genomic coordinates for the variant. The report must also include a clinical interpretation of the findings as applicable. Although preparation of the clinical interpretation can be labor intensive, this section is vital to most genetic reports and is important for describing the clinical significance of the results as they apply specifically to the patient and his or her family. This section should include a brief clinical history of patient (indicating the reason for testing) and may discuss recurrence risk, genotype–phenotype correlation or penetrance, associated disease or carrier risk calculations for other members of his or her family, and citations of literature as needed. Importantly, a statement that genetic counseling for the patient is indicated must be included.

Furthermore, because many assays performed in clinical DNA laboratories are laboratory-developed tests or procedures that have been developed, designed, or validated by the laboratory and are not approved by the FDA, reports must include a disclaimer to state this fact. Class I analyte-specific reagents may be purchased from a vendor and sold for a specific test, or they may be independently purchased by the laboratory and assembled into a laboratory-designed test.

An example of the disclaimer would state: "This test was developed and its performance characteristics determined by [laboratory name]. It has not been cleared or approved by the U.S. Food and Drug Administration." In addition, the CAP recommends inclusion of these additional statements: "The FDA does not require this test to go through premarket FDA review. This test is used for clinical purposes. It should not be regarded as investigational or for research. This laboratory is certified under the Clinical Laboratory Improvement Amendments (CLIA) as qualified to perform high-complexity clinical laboratory testing."[715] Last, reports should be reviewed and signed by the laboratory director or a qualified designee.

LABORATORY REGULATION

Regulatory oversight of clinical laboratories is essential to maintaining consistency across testing centers. All molecular genetic laboratories offering clinical testing should be CLIA certified and be actively participating in proficiency testing. In most cases, molecular laboratories are accredited by the CAP, which is considered to be the gold standard. CAP accreditation requires that laboratories undergo biannual inspection by an outside team of laboratory scientists using a specified checklist of requirements.[715] Maintaining accreditation requires that any deficiencies identified during a CAP inspection must be corrected. Laboratories are required to perform proficiency testing, which covers the scope of the tests performed in the laboratory. CAP provides proficiency testing samples or packets for a number of commonly ordered tests (eg, HD, fragile X). CAP also provides method-based proficiency testing to verify that a clinical laboratory using a general method (eg, Sanger sequencing) reports results consistent with those of other clinical laboratories. For tests that are offered clinically but are not covered by CAP proficiency testing, other means of confirming test accuracy must be pursued. This can involve sample exchanges with other laboratories that offer a similar clinical test or can simply be internal proficiency testing whereby a sample is randomly selected and is anonymously retested (among other patient samples) to confirm that the same results are obtained. Regardless of the method used, adequate records of proficiency testing results must be kept, and any discrepancies among results must be investigated and addressed. More information on the CAP accreditation and proficiency testing process can be found at http://www.cap.org.

Over the past several years, regulation of molecular genetic testing has become the focus of government agencies. The rise of companies that offer direct-to-consumer (DTC) genetic testing with no involvement of medical professionals or counselors elicited significant concerns regarding the accuracy and clinical validity of some genetic tests. In 2006, the Government Accountability Office (GAO) investigated the activities of multiple DTC genetic testing companies and found that many of the tests being offered were medically unsound or of no practical use. The GAO findings increased the concerns that many agencies had previously voiced regarding DTC genetic testing and complex genetic testing in general. In 2011, the National Institutes of Health started a voluntary registry of genetic tests available in the US. Subsequently, the FDA announced that they would also start reviewing all (non–FDA-approved) laboratory-developed tests. These actions may mark the first steps in what could be an increase in government oversight of genetic testing.

SELECTED REFERENCES

For a full list of references for this chapter, please refer to ExpertConsult.com.

12. Bell SC, De Boeck K, Amaral MD. New pharmacological approaches for cystic fibrosis: promises, progress, pitfalls. *Pharmacol Ther* 2015;**145**:19–34.
55. Farrar MA, Kiernan MC. The genetics of spinal muscular atrophy: progress and challenges. *Neurother* 2014.
79. Nurputra DK, Lai PS, Harahap NI, et al. Spinal muscular atrophy: from gene discovery to clinical trials. *Ann Hum Genet* 2013;**77**:435–63.
88. Alford RL, Arnos KS, Fox M, et al. American College of Medical Genetics and Genomics guideline for the clinical evaluation and etiologic diagnosis of hearing loss. *Genet Med* 2014;**16**:347–55.
147. Kay C, Skotte NH, Southwell AL, et al. Personalized gene silencing therapeutics for Huntington disease. *Clin Genet* 2014;**86**:29–36.
159. MacLeod R, Tibben A, Frontali M, et al. Recommendations for the predictive genetic test in Huntington's disease. *Clin Genet* 2013;**83**:221–31.
188. Franken R, den Hartog AW, Radonic T, et al. Beneficial outcome of losartan therapy depends on type of FBN1 mutation in Marfan syndrome. *Circ Cardiovasc Genet* 2015;**8**:383–8.
190. Radke RM, Baumgartner H. Diagnosis and treatment of Marfan syndrome: an update. *Heart* 2014;**100**:1382–91.
198. Walls GV. Multiple endocrine neoplasia (MEN) syndromes. *Semin Pediatr Surg* 2014;**23**:96–101.
267. Blake DJ, Weir A, Newey SE, et al. Function and genetics of dystrophin and dystrophin-related proteins in muscle. *Physiol Rev* 2002;**82**:291–329.
290. Seto JT, Bengtsson NE, Chamberlain JS. Therapy of genetic disorders-novel therapies for Duchenne muscular dystrophy. *Curr Pediatr Rep* 2014;**2**:102–12.
316. Santoro MR, Bray SM, Warren ST. Molecular mechanisms of fragile X syndrome: a twenty-year perspective. *Annu Rev Pathol* 2012;**7**:219–45.
346. Chahrour M, Zoghbi HY. The story of Rett syndrome: from clinic to neurobiology. *Neuron* 2007;**56**:422–37.
376. Martinelli I, De Stefano V, Mannucci PM. Inherited risk factors for venous thromboembolism. *Nat Rev Cardiol* 2014;**11**:140–56.
425. Rebours V, Levy P, Ruszniewski P. An overview of hereditary pancreatitis. *Dig Liver Dis* 2012;**44**:8–15.
480. Daly MB, Axilbund JE, Buys S, et al. Genetic/familial high-risk assessment: breast and ovarian. *J Natl Compr Canc Netw* 2010;**8**:562–94.
488. Hall MJ, Forman AD, Pilarski R, et al. Gene panel testing for inherited cancer risk. *J Natl Compr Canc Netw* 2014;**12**:1339–46.
489. Hampel H, Bennett RL, Buchanan A, et al. A practice guideline from the American College of Medical Genetics and Genomics and the National Society of Genetic Counselors: referral indications for cancer predisposition assessment. *Genet Med* 2015;**17**:70–87.
567. Davis RL, Sue CM. The genetics of mitochondrial disease. *Semin Neurol* 2011;**31**:519–30.

568. Schon EA, DiMauro S, Hirano M. Human mitochondrial DNA: roles of inherited and somatic mutations. *Nat Rev Genet* 2012;**13**:878–90.
616. Ishida M, Moore GE. The role of imprinted genes in humans. *Mol Aspects Med* 2013;**34**:826–40.
656. Ramsden SC, Clayton-Smith J, Birch R, et al. Practice guidelines for the molecular analysis of Prader-Willi and Angelman syndromes. *BMC Med Genet* 2010;**11**:70.
661. Wienke S, Brown K, Farmer M, et al. Expanded carrier screening panels–does bigger mean better? *J Community Genet* 2014;**5**:191–8.
666. Yang Y, Muzny DM, Reid JG, et al. Clinical whole-exome sequencing for the diagnosis of Mendelian disorders. *N Engl J Med* 2013;**369**:1502–11.
668. Need AC, Shashi V, Hitomi Y, et al. Clinical application of exome sequencing in undiagnosed genetic conditions. *J Med Genet* 2012;**49**:353–61.
716. Bahcall OG. Genetic testing: ACMG guides on the interpretation of sequence variants. *Nat Rev Genet* 2015;**16**:256–7.

50

Solid Tumor Genomics

Elaine R. Mardis

ABSTRACT

Background

Since the initial report of the finished human genome reference sequence in 2004,[1] cancer genetics research has focused on using this reference as a template for characterizing the somatic genomic alterations that underlie cancer's development and the germline genomic alterations that underlie human susceptibility to develop cancer. Because technology has enabled a transition from polymerase chain reaction (PCR)–based mutation discovery, to microarray-based copy number detection, to massively parallel sequencing (MPS) assays that provide a comprehensive somatic landscape of the cancer genome, our understanding of cancer genome alterations has increased in scope while becoming increasingly refined.[2]

Content

Modern day cancer diagnostic assays have been devised based on the cumulative knowledge gained from large-scale cancer genomics discovery efforts. These studies of tens to thousands of cancers across many tissues of origin have catalogued the genomic landscape of human cancers by MPS and often included data from RNA expression and DNA methylation. This chapter outlines aspects of these molecular assays of solid tissue malignancies in the clinical setting that have been enabled by research-based discovery work over the past approximately 20 years.

CONSIDERATIONS FOR SOLID TUMOR GENOMICS

Sampling and Preservation Methods

Solid tumors can be sampled by a variety of procedures that yield different amounts of tumor cells from which DNA, RNA, or both, can be isolated for diagnostic assays. In the ideal setting, the number of assays required for pathological evaluation of the tumor would dictate the amount of sampling done; however, the typical scenario involves a limited amount of a sample that restricts the comprehensiveness of assays that can be performed. This scenario has become even more common with the introduction of nucleic acid–based assays to the diagnostic repertoire because they require tissue that must first satisfy the standard diagnostics of microscopy-based pathology. As will be discussed, the increasing use of MPS in genomic assays of solid tumors has somewhat ameliorated this dilemma.

Briefly, solid tumors can be sampled using either fine needle aspiration or core biopsy procedures.[3] These are often done in advance of surgery or in patients with nonresectable tumors as determined by imaging, to provide a sample for pathology-based examination and diagnosis. Fine needle aspiration (21–25 gauge needle) generates a minimal amount of tissue and can consist of a few tumor cells in the fluid that is co-aspirated into the needle.[4,5] Core biopsies (18–21 gauge needle) can obtain intact and solid cores from the tumor mass. If imaging such as ultrasound or computed tomography scanning is used to guide the biopsy needle to the tumor mass, several passes are made for better sampling. Alternatively, for patients with resectable cancer without plans for neoadjuvant therapy, the tumor mass is removed at surgery and may be preserved either as a bulk resection sample or sampled with core needle biopsies that are preserved for pathology-based assays according to the clinical protocol being followed.

Once the tumor biopsy or resected tumor is obtained, the tissue can be preserved by several methods. Historically, pathology of solid tumors has focused on preservation methods that stabilize proteins and other cellular structural components, preserving tissue structure for microscopic visualization in the presence of specific staining or immunohistochemistry. Hence, tissue fixation by soaking in formalin or formaldehyde was developed to stabilize the cellular proteins. Subsequent embedding in paraffin wax is performed to create an impervious, room temperature stable substrate. Once the paraffinized tissue has solidified into a block, thin sections can be cut for subsequent characterization and diagnosis by staining and microscopic examination. Although this approach is facile and preserves tissues for long-term storage at room temperature, formalin causes crosslinking with cytosine residues in DNA and RNA. Subsequent oxidation results in breaks in the nucleic acid sugar-phosphate backbone, thereby degrading the nucleic acids. The degradation is time-dependent, however, such that preserved tissues that have been formalin-fixed and paraffin-embedded (FFPE) for less than 3 years are, in general, equivalent to fresh frozen tissues in terms of yield and quality of nucleic acids. Because diagnostic assays of solid tumors have begun to include nucleic acids, alternative preservatives and preservation methods are now being used. These methods include flash freezing tissue at −80°C (dry ice acetone bath) or immersion in nucleic acid stabilizers. Stabilizer examples include freezing tissues in optimal cutting temperature (OCT) compound

(Tissue-Plus OCT, Thermo Fisher Scientific), and preserving nucleic acids in tissues by addition of liquid reagents (PAXgene tissue STABILIZER, Qiagen or RNAlater, Thermo Fisher Scientific).[6]

Staining and Selection of Tumor Cells

Several staining methods have been developed to examine the preserved needle biopsy or resection materials obtained in solid tumor sampling. The most basic assay is referred to as an Hematoxylin and Eosin stain (H&E) and readily identifies tumor and normal cells in a tissue section under a light microscope (Fig. 50.1). H&E staining is not only used to diagnose cancer, but also to enumerate cancerous cells in a tissue section to provide an estimate of the percentage of tumor nuclei present. Because solid tumors are a mixture of tumor cells and various normal cells, this estimate of tumor "cellularity" indicates how tumor rich the sample is relative to other needle biopsies or other portions of the bulk tumor. Tumor features such as necrotic areas may be also identified in the microscopic evaluation. In sections with evident necrosis, a process of macro-dissection to cut away the non-necrotic sections for subsequent nucleic acid isolation can be pursued. In tumor types such as prostate and pancreatic adenocarcinomas, there is a low proportion of tumor nuclei present relative to the surrounding normal cells (eg, stroma and immune cells). In these tumor types, a laser capture microdissection (LCM) instrument can be used to isolate tumor cells from surrounding normal cells before nucleic acid isolation (Fig. 50.2). The LCM imaging system produces

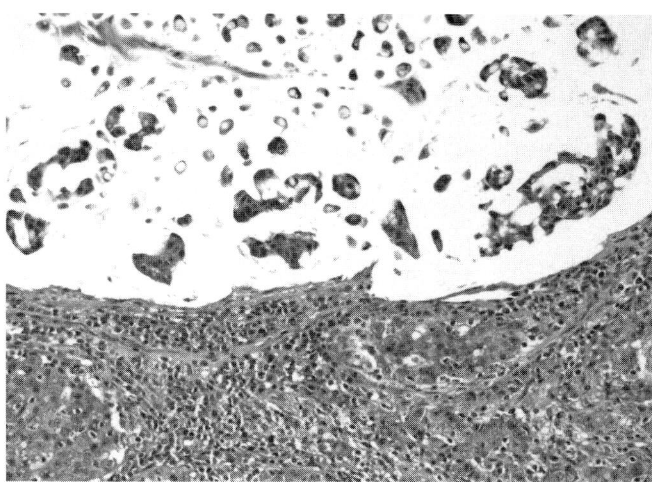

FIGURE 50.1 Illustration of an Hematoxylin and Eosin *(H&E)* Stained Tumor Section (Invasive Colon Adenocarcinoma). This adenocarcinoma has both mucinous *(top)* and medullary *(bottom)* histologic features. In addition, tumor-infiltrating lymphocytes are prominent in the portion with medullary features. These histologic features are frequently found in colon cancers that develop in patients with Lynch syndrome. Lynch syndrome is an autosomal dominant disorder caused by a DNA mismatch repair gene defect (magnification 200×, H&E stain).

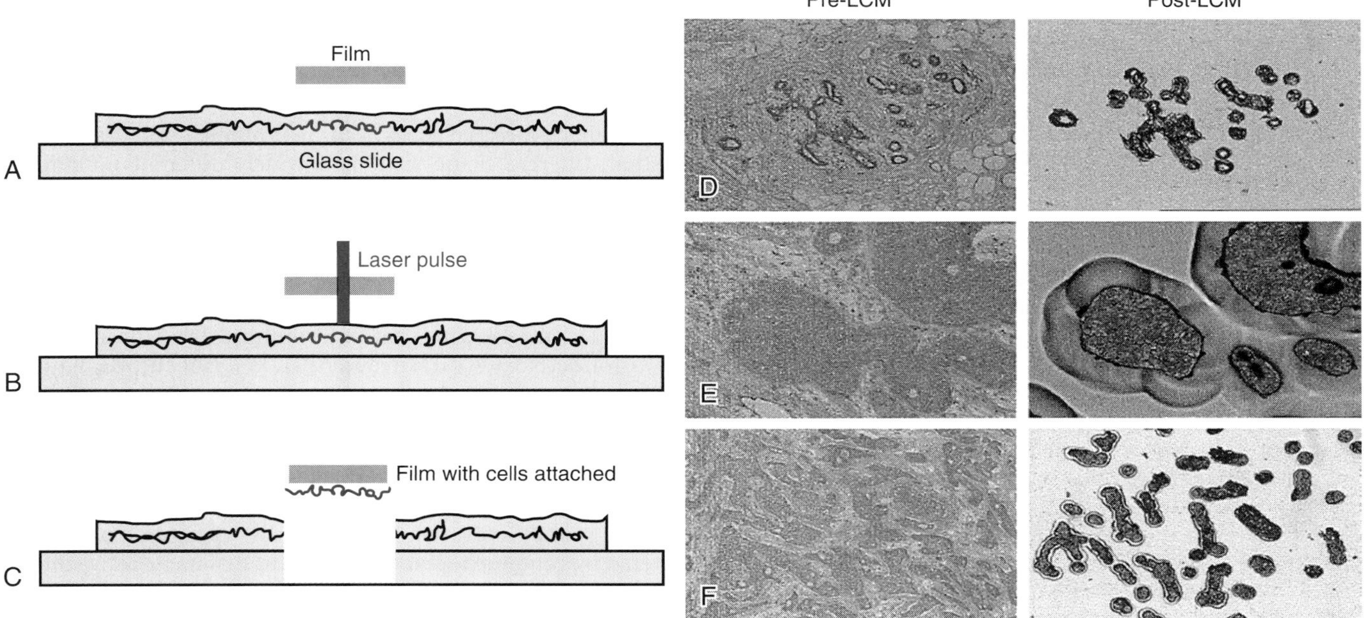

FIGURE 50.2 Laser Capture Microdissection (LCM). **A**, An optically clear film is layered over a tissue section on a glass slide that is viewed through a microscope to locate the cells of interest. **B,** A laser pulse then affixes the film to the tissue of interest *(red)* that can then be removed from the slide for further processing **(C).** LCM can also remove the cells that are not of interest from the slide. For example, selection of residual normal **(D)** breast glands, **(E)** carcinoma in situ, or **(F)** infiltrating ductal carcinoma of the breast is possible. (Photomicrographs reprinted with permission from Palmer-Toy DE, Sarracino DA, Sgroi D, LeVangie R, Leopold PE. Direct acquisition of matrix-assisted laser desorption/ionization time-of-flight mass spectra from laser capture microdissected tissues. *Clin Chem* 2000;46:1513–1516. Copyright AACC Press.)

an image of the tumor section, and an operator uses software to identify the tumor cells for harvest. A membrane is placed adjacent to the tumor section, and the LCM fires an infrared laser pulse at each tumor cell identified for harvest, thereby affixing it to the membrane. Subsequent cutting of tissue and membrane is performed by a ultraviolet laser, completing a laser-induced forward transfer for cellular isolation. Once the desired number of tumor cells is harvested, the membrane goes through a series of processing steps to isolate DNA or RNA (or both) from the captured cells.

Another staining-based method to identify tumor-specific antigens is immunohistochemistry; in this technique, a protein- or protein-epitope–specific antibody is coupled to an enzyme (eg, horseradish peroxidase) to identify tumor cells in a tissue section expressing that protein. Examples of immunohistochemistry stains include those for estrogen and progesterone receptors, and the cellular proliferation marker Ki-67 (MIB-1).

GENOMIC ANALYSIS OF SOLID TUMORS

Background

Although we have known for many decades that cancer's origins lie in changes to the cellular genome, only recently have technologies become available to profile the mutations in genes. Initial gene cloning efforts in the early 1980s identified the chromosomal locations and sequences of many oncogenes and tumor suppressors in the human genome.[7-9] The decoding of the human genome, coupled with technological advances, opened the door to genome-wide studies of cancer. For example, learning the sequences of human genes enabled the construction of microarrays to query RNA expression in tumors (described in Chapter 47). By using advanced bioinformatic analysis approaches (eg, clustering algorithms),[10] similarities and differences in gene expression across tumors from a single tissue site (eg, lung adenocarcinoma) were revealed.[11] Clusters of gene expression, when correlated with other pathology-based categories, revealed subtypes within a given tissue site, such as the intrinsic subtypes of breast cancer.[12] Similarly, single nucleotide polymorphism–based microarrays could be used to identify gross-scale chromosomal aberrations by comparing normalized signal strength between tumor and normal DNA.[13] As explored in the following, conducting research-based inquiries of cancer genomes with these tools provided the means by which the clinical usefulness (diagnosis, prognosis, treatment decision) of the resulting classifications was demonstrated, thereby providing a rationale for the approach to translate them into clinical laboratory assays. More recently, the introduction of MPS platforms and associated methods for exploring cancer genes, genomes, and transcriptomes (expressed RNAs) have supplanted foundational technologies such as capillary sequencing and microarrays. MPS methods have the potential to produce more quantitative data while simultaneously expanding the identification of somatic alterations. The first application of MPS to decode a cancer genome was published in 2008[14] when Ley and colleagues sequenced and compared the whole genome sequence (WGS) data from a patient with FAB M1 (normal karyotype) acute myeloid leukemia (AML) to a matched normal skin sample. The second WGS case published[15] was also on a single patient AML sample, and it revealed an unexpected mutation in the gene *IDH1* (a metabolic enzyme in the glycolytic pathway). This *IDH1* mutation was then characterized as a recurrent mutation in a panel of 188 AML samples and associated with a poor prognosis. From these single patient beginnings, the field of cancer genomics has exploded to characterize tens of thousands of cases by 2015.

> **POINTS TO REMEMBER**
>
> **Cancer Genomics**
> - Gene expression microarrays were initially used to characterize large numbers of human cancers.
> - Cancer gene cloning efforts and the completed Human Genome Sequence enabled the use of PCR and sequencing efforts to catalog cancer mutations.
> - MPS enables the identification of somatic alterations in targeted gene panels, in all known genes, or the whole genome.
> - The scale of massively parallel cancer sequencing has permitted large studies of DNA and RNA from the major solid tissue malignancies.

Large-Scale Discovery Efforts

One consequence of rapid, high-throughput and inexpensive sequencing has been the production of large data sets that explore the mutational, transcriptional, and methylation landscape of thousands of tumors representing major human cancer types. Examples of these large-scale discovery projects include The Cancer Genome Atlas (http://cancergenome.nih.gov), the International Cancer Genome Consortium (https://icgc.org), the Pediatric Cancer Genome Project (http://www.pediatriccancergenomeproject.org/site), and numerous other government and privately funded cancer genomics efforts. The resulting tumor type-specific "omics" catalogues revealed several unexpected discoveries, including the fact that many mutated genes occur in multiple tumor types[16] and that different tissue sites have widely different mutational burdens.[17] These efforts also identified new classes of mutated genes that had previously not been considered as contributing to cancer development. Included in these new classes of genes were proteins involved in the spliceosome complex (U2AF3, SF3B1), proteins involved in cellular metabolism (IDH1, IDH2), and proteins that contribute to DNA packaging in histones (H3.3, ARID1A, and ARID1B). Not surprisingly, the greatly expanded characterization of the cancer mutational landscape afforded by these large-scale projects revealed that most known cancer-associated genes had a multitude of previously unknown mutations, some of which were recurrent. Due to the magnitude of these efforts in a relatively short time span, the overwhelming number of mutations discovered by genomic methods have yet to be functionally studied to determine their effects on the resulting protein.

Once significant progress was made in the individual cancer-specific studies, for example, meta- or "pan can" analyses of these catalogues were pursued, further reinforcing the similarities and differences between tissue sites by virtue of integration across various "omic" data sets. The similarities, in particular, challenge long-held notions about tissue site specificity of therapeutic approaches and introduce the concept that oncogenic "drivers" present in cancers from different tissues could respond to similar targeted therapeutic interventions. These metaanalyses further reinforced the complexity of cancer in that each tumor arises due to a unique and intricate interplay of molecular events. Although some occur more commonly than others, the impact on protein function and amount ultimately manifests in activated or repressed cellular pathways. Hence, cancer is a disease of pathway alterations, rather than a specific gene and/or protein alteration, and therapeutic decision-making should occur using this framework.

Pre-Massively Parallel Sequencing Approaches to "Hotspot" Characterization

The discovery of oncogenes and their activating mutations (also known as "hot spot" or "gain of function" mutations) emerged from gene cloning efforts in the 1980s and 1990s. The description of PCR by Kary Mullis and Fred Faloona[18] tremendously facilitated the selective amplification and sequencing of these genes from DNA isolates of solid tumor blocks. The concomitant development of an automated fluorescent Sanger sequencing instrument by Leroy Hood's group[19] and its commercialization ultimately led to a combined PCR and sequencing assay to detect these hot spot mutations in a few days' time. Automated software to identify variants in capillary electropherograms further facilitated rapid analysis and interpretation of sequencing results (see also the Phred Quality Score, Box 45-5 in Chapter 45). The clinical usefulness of hotspot characterization to identify a drug target in solid tumors was initiated by three studies in lung adenocarcinoma published in 2004.[20-22] These results demonstrated that patients who responded to a new class of targeted therapies called tyrosine kinase inhibitors carried mutations in the tyrosine kinase domain of the epidermal growth factor receptor *(EGFR)* gene. The correlation of these mutations to treatment response initiated a paradigm in which the clinical assay for hotspot mutations became the companion diagnostic for the targeted therapy.

RNA-Based Approaches

The development and use of microarrays to query gene expression and correlate the analyzed data to clinical features has been widely used in the research setting to identify clinically relevant subtypes within specific malignancies. Samples that group into a specific subtype were evaluated in the context of correlative data types such as patient outcome (eg, overall survival, disease-specific survival, or progression-free survival) or treatment, or both. Correlative gene expression analyses can subtype disease and determine treatment as tested in clinical trials. An example of the translation of gene expression assays to clinical tests is the US Food and Drug Administration (FDA)–approved Mammaprint microarray diagnostic from Agendia (www.agendia.com) that originated from a 70-gene breast cancer expression profiling test developed in the Netherlands.[23] Results of this assay indicate whether node negative estrogen receptor positive (ER+) or negative (ER–) patients are at low risk or high risk for disease recurrence. When combined with other clinical risk factors, the Mammaprint score contributes to determining whether a patient will benefit from adjuvant chemotherapy.

The expression of genes previously determined to predict outcomes or characterize subtypes can also be compared with reverse transcriptase quantitative PCR (RT-qPCR). This method is described in Chapter 47, and begins with total RNA isolated from tumor cells, converted to DNA, and subjected to gene-specific amplification by PCR in a specialized instrument that acquires fluorescence at each amplification cycle. Such "real-time" data are then analyzed for each gene to calculate its expression relative to those of previously selected calibrating genes (reference genes). Typically, reference genes are specific to the tissue and/or tumor type of interest and are selected because their expression is constant across multiple samples. By analyzing the qPCR-based gene expression levels of specific subtype-determining genes from banked samples with known outcomes, a classifier algorithm can be derived that returns a risk of recurrence (ROR) score. Oncologists may use the ROR score in combination with other pathology assay results to determine which treatment the patient will receive. An example of such an assay is the Oncotype Dx breast cancer risk of recurrence assay used to classify ROR for women with node-negative ER+ breast cancer.[24]

A third type of RNA quantitation uses a specialized instrument that detects and identifies specific gene transcripts based on combinations of fluorophores ("barcodes") with which they are labeled. In this system, shown in Fig. 50.3, an initial hybridization step permits gene-specific "capture" probes to hybridize to the extracted RNA from the tumor sample. A second "reporter" probe that contains the fluorescent barcode for that gene also hybridizes near the capture probe hybridization site on the transcript. The resulting mixture is placed onto a silicon substrate derivatized with streptavidin, and the biotin-labeled capture probes immobilize each labeled transcript on the substrate. The application of an electric current across the substrate linearizes the RNAs and orders the fluorophores. A scanning step then excites the fluorescent dyes and detects their emission wavelengths across an *x-y* coordinate grid. The scanning step enumerates each barcoded molecule on the silicon substrate, thereby quantitating, and through software-based decoding, identifying each transcript of interest and its absolute expression level. This approach was commercialized by Nanostring, Inc. and currently forms the basis of a clinical assay for breast cancer risk of recurrence (Prosigna).

MASSIVE PARALLEL SEQUENCING OF SOLID TUMOR SAMPLES

Clinical assays of solid tumors using MPS to identify somatic mutations in multiple genes ("gene panels") or in all annotated genes (the "exome") have been developed for several reasons, including: (1) large-scale, MPS-based discovery efforts have identified mutated genes in the major adult and pediatric cancers; (2) specific genes and/or mutations have been studied in clinically annotated sample sets, and their mutational status correlates with outcome (and is therefore prognostic); and (3) novel small molecule- and antibody-based targeted therapies have been developed to address specific somatic alterations, and therefore, the mutational signature of a patient's somatic genome can identify targeted therapies based on predicted gene–drug interactions.

Although testing multiple genes from a single tumor DNA isolate could be accomplished using combinations of individual clinical assays to evaluate individual gene and/or hotspot mutation status, often tumor material is limited due to the size of a biopsy and the need to use the material

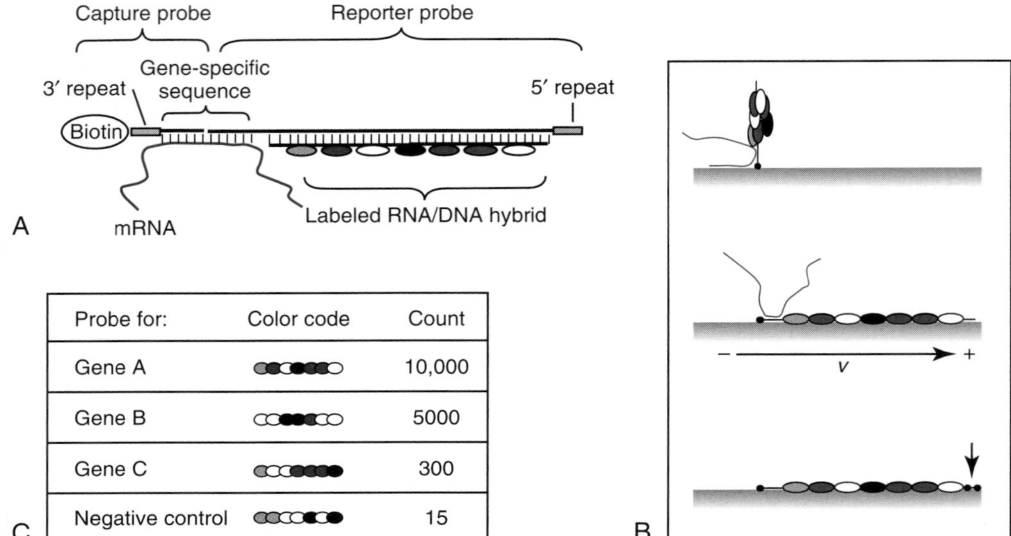

Probe for:	Color code	Count
Gene A		10,000
Gene B		5000
Gene C		300
Negative control		15

FIGURE 50.3 Single Molecule Detection of Messenger RNA (mRNA). **A**, A pair of probes (one capture probe and one reporter probe) hybridizes to the RNA target in solution through gene-specific probe sequences. The reporter probe has seven color segments, each segment is made of approximately 900 RNA bases that are labeled with approximately 100 hundred fluorophores of one type. The labeled portion of the probe is a DNA/RNA hybrid that can be observed as a approximate 3-nm fluorescent spot. **B**, *(top)* The target complex is immobilized on a streptavidin-coated slide through the biotin moieties on the capture probe. *(Middle)* An electrical current is applied, and the complex is stretched. *(Bottom)* The reporter probe is immobilized in extended form by biotin-labeled oligonucleotides complementary to its 5′ repeat sequence. **C**, The color code of the probe fluors is read by an epi-fluorescent microscope, and each unique probe is counted. Normally, a number of negative control probes are present in the hybridization solution to establish nonspecific background counts.

for other more conventional pathology assays such as H&E and immunohistochemistry. Hence, MPS-based assays make more efficient use of precious diagnostic material, especially when so many genes that are potentially mutated can provide important information regarding patient care.

Borrowing from the design of PCR-based hotspot mutation assays, MPS assays often study only the tumor-derived DNA. This is an economic decision because performing the same assay on the matched normal tissue (adjacent nonmalignant or peripheral blood monocytic cell–derived DNA from blood) essentially doubles the cost of the assay. However, there is a fundamental difference between a hotspot assay and an MPS assay; namely, the breadth of genomic territory studied by MPS assays is much larger. As such, variants that lie outside of known hotspots will be identified and may still contribute to the patient's prognostic or therapeutic diagnosis. Further, as shown by focused and large-scale cancer genomics studies, known germline susceptibility loci, such as *BRCA1*, *BRCA2*, *TP53*, and *APC*, are also mutated in the somatic genome. Hence, comparing tumor to normal gene sequences may have important consequences for understanding whether variants that are identified are inherited or acquired.[25] Obviously, determining somatic versus germline origin is important for the patient because the former may help to identify a therapeutic path and the latter will ethically and responsibly involve genetic counseling and enable possible further testing of parents, children, and siblings.

Due to the heterogeneity of solid tumors and the increasing knowledge that certain mutations in genes, if present at low levels in the tumor cell population, can predict early onset of acquired resistance to targeted therapies,[26] MPS-based assays must provide a high depth of tumor sequence data coverage for each gene in the assay. Coverage is defined as the number of sequencing reads that align uniquely at a given gene locus, where each read providing coverage depth must be from a unique DNA fragment. High coverage can be defined as 300- to 1000-fold read depth and can be challenging to obtain when MPS libraries are constructed from low amounts of input DNA because there are fewer unique molecules available for ligation to the adapters in the library construction step.[27] The issue of uniqueness is exacerbated because the use of PCR to amplify the completed library can lead to PCR-based "jackpotting" (preferential amplification of certain sequences). This, in turn, can bias the representation in the completed library. In general, with 500-fold or higher coverage, detecting mutations can be accomplished even from low percentage tumor cellularity samples (10% to 20%), but detecting low prevalence mutations becomes less likely with decreasing tumor cell percentages. High coverage is also important to attain because not all probes capture complementary sequences with the same avidity. When this deficiency is combined with representation bias from MPS processes downstream of capture, lowered coverage at certain sites may result. Hence, higher coverage overall may reduce or eliminate low and/or no coverage sites, thereby reducing the incidence of false negative results or type II errors, wherein a mutation is missed due to lack of coverage in the tumor or the normal gene.

Whole Genome Sequencing

Ideally, the most unbiased characterization of each cancer sample by MPS-based methods should be pursued to optimize the likelihood of identifying all druggable targets in the genome. This is best accomplished using WGS, which can deliver the totality of point mutations, small insertions and deletions, structural variants (including copy number alterations), and other large chromosomal rearrangements in a tumor-to-normal genome comparison. Different technologies for performing WGS are covered in Chapter 47. However, at this time, WGS is rarely performed as a clinical assay that can inform solid tumor therapeutic interventions due to the following limitations. First, the genome is quite large (3 gb), and although new MPS instrumentation can produce the data rapidly (eg, the Illumina HiSeq X produces 30-fold coverage for 16 human genomes in 3 days), the effort to analyze a whole genome comparison of tumor tissue to matched normal tissue and compile a clinical report is in conflict with the time frame needed to inform the oncologist's decision-making process. Second, due to the need for high coverage of the tumor genome, generating the necessary 100-fold or higher WGS coverage needed for confident variant detection remains cost prohibitive. Third, most of the somatic variants will be uninterpretable in terms of their impact on tumor progression because they will lie outside of genes. Fourth, many variants in the coding sequences will not be interpretable in terms of their impact on the protein's function as a potential driver of disease development (ie, gain or loss of function). However, the latter issue is not unique to WGS assays, but reflects on all MPS assay results in terms of the difficulty of interpreting variants. Due to these limitations, among others, it is presently rare (circa 2015) for whole genome comparisons of tumor tissue to normal tissue to be assayed in the clinical diagnostics setting.

Selective Enrichment by Hybridization Capture

Locus-selective or hybridization capture methods have been developed that use synthetic probes designed to hybridize the human loci and/or genes of interest as a means of selectively isolating sequences from a whole human genome library. MPS of the captured sequences is followed by alignment of the reads to the human genome reference sequence, identifying the loci of interest for mutational analysis by applying a Browser Extensible Data format file[28] to delineate the specific genomic regions that should be examined for variants in the tumor tissue compared with normal tissue, and reporting any mutations that are identified. Depending upon the assay, either a select set of genes or hotspots, or the entire annotated gene set of the human (the exome) can be captured. There are several commercially available exome reagents, including "clinical" exome reagents that offer enhanced hybridization times of 2 to 4 hours (compared with approximately 72 hours for research reagents).

As the number of loci assayed by this approach increase, so do both the analysis time and the complexity of the mutational signature. The decision to include drug-targetable genes that carry novel, non-canonical mutations with untested drug interactions is one challenge that can arise in the clinical interpretation of these assays.

Although there is a desire to develop assays with small numbers of genes and/or hotspot loci that will (1) keep cost per assay low, (2) speed the interpretation of data, and (3) decrease the detection of non-canonical mutations, the ability of gene-selective hybridization capture to subset the genome does have a lower limit. In particular, when targeting loci that total less than approximately 300 kb, inefficiencies of selective hybridization capture predominate, requiring increased sequencing coverage to achieve the desired coverage of the targeted genes. In particular, the lower the target space for hybrid capture, the larger the effect of so-called "off target" reads. These spurious hybridization events result in the capture of nontarget sequences by capture probes and effectively decrease the overall coverage achieved from on-target reads.

Multiplex Polymerase Chain Reaction Approach

Because of the lower limit described for hybrid capture, one alternative that has been used in clinical assays of solid tumors is multiplex PCR. In this type of assay, careful design of PCR primer pairs that target the selected loci for mutation detection achieves the coincident amplification of all loci in a single reaction. Multiplex PCR has the distinct advantages of: (1) selectively amplifying smaller target regions of the genome below that which is optimal for selective hybridization capture; (2) requiring only 5 to 10 ng of DNA for the PCR; and (3) focusing mutation detection on a relatively small portion of the genome in an efficient manner. These assays are also relatively inexpensive to perform, and by post-PCR addition of DNA barcoded linkers for MPS, they can be multiplexed with other patients onto a single MPS instrument run. There are obvious limitations to multiplex PCR that include: (1) the ability to design PCR primers with similar T_m, uniqueness, and lack of interprimer complementarity to diminish amplification artifacts (eg, primer dimers, hybrid amplicons); and (2) the presence of pseudogenes and highly conserved regions of gene families may preclude unique amplification of specific gene sequences. PCR primers are often designed with FFPE-associated degradation in mind to produce small products of less than 100 bp; therefore, these require a large number of primers to cover a large gene, which further complicates the design process and/or complicates obtaining complete coverage from the resulting amplicons. Despite the limitations, multiplex PCR assays are widely used in clinical testing of solid tumors. The challenges of overcoming these limitations can be circumvented by purchasing prequalified multiplex PCR primer sets from commercial vendors, many of which frequently include tested medically relevant genes for different types of clinical questions, including cancer mutation hotspots.

RNA Sequencing of Solid Tumor Isolates

RNA isolates from cancer samples can be assayed using MPS technologies (RNA-seq) by simply converting the RNA to DNA via RT before library construction. There are several nuances to this general statement that require further detail, as follows. First, RNA can be reliably amplified if the starting quantities are low, such as isolates from a fine needle aspiration or core biopsy. Second, coding RNAs can be selected from a total RNA population by implementing a polyA selection step. This selection works because messenger RNAs (mRNAs) are polyadenylated at their 3′ ends and thereby can hybridize to superparamagnetic beads with covalently attached polyT sequences. Typically, mRNA represents only 2% of the total RNA population, so the resulting yields will be quite small if one begins with a limited total RNA isolate. In practice, polyA selection is not advised if the starting amount of total RNA is less than 2 μg. Third, because the number of genes transcribed in any given tissue and/or tumor is quite variable in the number and range of expression levels, the notion of coverage as presented for DNA assays does not typically apply to RNA-seq. Rather, a set number of sequencing reads are produced, aligned to the genome, and evaluated. As discussed, FFPE preservation can cause fractionation of the RNA in a tumor sample, so an initial evaluation of the quantity and intactness of the RNA isolate is advised when there are sufficient quantities obtained to permit an initial quality control (QC). This evaluation can be accomplished using a variety of sensitive devices such as the Agilent Bioanalyzer with an RNA Picochip or Agilent TapeStation. As a general rule, RNA that is degraded to an average length of 300 bp or less will not perform well in RNA-seq library construction.

There are valid reasons to assay the transcribed genes in a solid tumor sample in the clinic, including: (1) DNA sequencing assays do not reflect higher order changes in the tumor genome, such as methylation or chromatin packaging that can influence the amount of RNA produced from a gene; (2) in high mutation load tumors such as melanomas and lung squamous or adenocarcinomas, RNA-seq can indicate which of the thousands of mutations identified from DNA sequencing assays are actually being transcribed and could therefore be targeted with a specific therapy; (3) alternatively spliced transcript (isoform) expression can only be detected at the level of RNA and may be important in a diagnostic, prognostic, or therapeutic context; and (4) predicted gene fusions from DNA assays can be verified by the presence of the predicted fusion transcript in the RNA-seq data. Despite these advantages, RNA-seq is rarely pursued in the clinical setting for several reasons. Adding another assay increases the cost of clinical testing and adds time to the delivery of information back to the ordering physician. Furthermore, RNA is an unstable molecule, and preservation techniques such as FFPE degrade RNA more noticeably than DNA, especially if the temperature of the paraffin bath is above 65°C. RNA can be reliably amplified before sequencing when only limited amounts are available from a clinical sample. Alternatively, limited quantities of RNA or degraded RNA from FFPE-preserved tissue can be sequenced by subjecting the MPS library to an intermediate selective hybridization capture step with the same types of reagents used for DNA.[29] Perhaps most daunting is the bioinformatic analysis of RNA-seq data, because there are many different algorithms to evaluate the data once reads are aligned to the human genome reference, depending upon whether straightforward determination of gene expression is the goal, or identifying fusion transcripts, alternative transcript expression, or other types of specialized inquiry are pursued.[30] Despite the challenges, there is increasing recognition that DNA assays alone do not provide a complete picture of the drug-specific vulnerabilities of a solid tumor.

Detection of Cancer Mutations in Body Fluids

Cancer cells are characterized by their rapid growth and proliferation, which infers that they turn over rapidly. In so doing, the cells release DNA into bodily fluids that can be assayed by sequencing and other nucleic acid detection techniques. Chapter 52 describes high-sensitivity, blood-based detection of cancer-specific mutations from circulating tumor cells and circulating tumor DNA. Also referred to as a "liquid biopsy," these sources provide tumor DNA for either diagnosis or therapeutic response monitoring that requires only a blood draw and specific processing steps to obtain the analyte without biopsy. In addition to blood-based tests, several commercially available noninvasive assays use either feces or urine as the analyte and survey a single marker or small number of markers for evidence of cancer-specific DNA or RNA. Hence, these are screening or diagnostic assays and are primarily used for detection of cancer.

One such screening assay is marketed as Cologuard by Exact Sciences and uses stool DNA to detect 11 distinct colorectal cancer biomarkers that are a combination of methylation markers (NDRG4 and BMP3) and mutations (eg, *KRAS*), as well as a hemoglobin immunoassay. This assay was compared in a clinical trial of 9989 participants to a standard fecal immunochemical test (FIT) in which 0.7% of participants had a colon cancer diagnosis and 7.6% had advanced precancerous lesions by colonoscopy.[31] The assay had 92.3% sensitivity to detect colorectal cancer compared with the 73.8% sensitivity of the FIT assay. Sensitivity for advanced precancerous lesions was 42.4% compared with 23.8% for FIT. However, the multitarget stool assay had a lower specificity compared with the FIT test (89.8% compared with 96.4% for FIT) in patients with negative colonoscopy. As a result, Cologuard is an FDA-approved assay in which a positive test result is suggestive of a follow-up colonoscopy to confirm the presence of cancer in the rectum or colon.

There are two available urine-based noninvasive tests that detect prostate cancer, both of which detect specific RNA markers. These tests use urine obtained subsequent to a digital rectal examination of the prostate, which is sufficient mechanical stimulation to release prostate cancer cells into the urine. The Progensa assay from Hologic gained FDA approval in 2012. This quantitative real-time PCR assay evaluates the expression of two genes, prostate specific antigen *(PSA)* and *PCA3*, both of which are overexpressed in prostate cancer. The data analysis compares *PCA3* to *PSA* expression as a ratio that generates a PCA3 score. This score helps determine the need for repeat prostate biopsies in men who have had a previous negative biopsy. In a clinical trial, the Progensa assay had a negative predictive value of 90%. Following a positive assay by Progensa, prostate biopsy is needed for a definitive diagnosis.

The Mi prostate score test is a laboratory-developed test by the University of Michigan that quantifies both *PCA3* and the *TMPRSS2:ERG* fusion transcript (http://www.mlabs.umich.edu/files/pdfs/MiPS_FAQ.pdf). The *TMPRSS2:ERG* gene fusion occurs in 47% of prostate cancers as a known driver event. This test was validated in a cohort of 1225 patients with no history of prostate cancer[32] and was shown to enhance the usefulness of serum PSA for predicting prostate cancer risk and clinically relevant cancer on biopsy.

POINTS TO REMEMBER

Cancer Genomics Assays

- DNA and RNA can be isolated from cancer cells for further study.
- There are multiple technology platforms for directed gene assays of mutations or RNA expression levels.
- MPS assays of DNA permit a broad survey of genetic variation and can detect both germline and somatic alterations.
- Targeted gene assays can detect specific mutations from DNA or quantify both expression and fusion transcripts in RNA.

INTERPRETING SOMATIC ALTERATIONS IN A CLINICAL CONTEXT

The use of MPS-based solid tumor diagnostics is increasing across clinical laboratories, both commercial and academic, largely due to the increasing knowledge of somatic alterations in cancers, to the increasing numbers of targeted therapies designed to interact with known cancer-relevant alterations, and to the demands of patients and oncologists to add this information to the evidence being considered in determining the treatment regimen for the patient. Progress in this area is confounded by the need to relate somatic alterations to other clinical data, such as the diagnosis of a specific tumor type or subtype, the range of possible patient outcomes, and therapeutic response. Additional studies of the functional impact of a somatic alteration, how that functional impact may contribute to the onset or progression of the cancer, or how and/or whether the alteration interacts with a variety of potential therapies based on putative drug–gene interactions are often needed. Drug studies typically involve preclinical testing in cell lines or other disease models, followed by clinical trials that require 1 or more years to compare patient outcomes when patients carrying the gene alteration(s) are treated with a specific therapy in comparison to patients treated with the standard of care. In essence, there is often a significant delay between the research-based discovery of a somatic alteration and when its full clinical implication can be established. The clinical sequencing pipeline and how to determine which of the identified mutations in a cancer biopsy should be evaluated further in terms of their prognostic, diagnostic, or therapeutic value have been described.[33,34] There are also publicly available curated cancer mutation databases that permit a look-up of known cancer genes and mutations that offer prognostic, diagnostic, and therapeutic information, including TARGET (www.broadinstitute.org/cancer/cga/target) and CIViC (www.civicdb.org).

Prognostic Interpretation

Understanding the prognostic or outcome-related value of a specific gene alteration depends upon a number of factors, such as the prevalence of the disease, the time to establish outcome, the specific outcome measure, and the uniformity of patient care in each group. The time to establish outcome can vary widely; for example, patients with lung squamous cell carcinoma or glioblastoma typically present with metastatic disease or progression in 6 to 18 months after a primary diagnosis, whereas ER+ breast cancer may relapse after 15 to 20 years. The defined outcome may be overall survival, disease-specific survival, complete pathologic response, or other responses. Some examples of prognostic mutations and their ability to assort to different disease subtypes are seen in gliomas,[35] colorectal,[36] endometrial,[37] and ovarian[38] cancers.

Diagnostic Interpretation

Multigene capture panels that detect alterations in known cancer susceptibility genes such as *TP53, APC, BRCA1/2*, and others in germline DNA can be used to identify inherited cancer susceptibility. These assays are discussed in Chapter 49. Diagnostic characterization of solid tumor DNA based on somatic alterations is taking on increased significance due to the availability of targeted therapies that correspond to these somatic alterations. Non-small cell lung cancers, especially

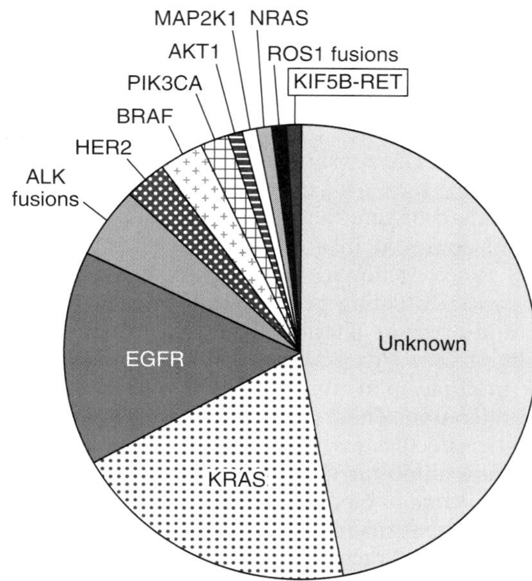

FIGURE 50.4 Molecular Subsets of Lung Adenocarcinoma. The clinically important driver mutations and fusions identified to date from molecular studies of lung adenocarcinoma. The width of the chart wedge for each driver event corresponds to its percentage distribution in the disease. (Reprinted by permission from Macmillan Publishers Ltd. From Pao W, Hutchinson KE. Chipping away at the lung cancer genome. *Nat Med* 2012;18:349–351.)

adenocarcinomas, perhaps provide the richest example of sequencing-based diagnosis and therapeutic option guidance among the solid tumors. In 2012, the spectrum of genomic alterations in genes that drove the development of non-small cell lung adenocarcinomas encompassed approximately 50% of the disease, of which approximately 40% were therapeutically targeted (Fig. 50.4).[39] Increasingly, a gene panel assay is pursued to sequence these genes or gene fusions, and can indicate one or several targeted therapies that represent the first line of therapy. This paradigm shift represents a remarkable transition in medical practice over just a 10-year period from when lung adenocarcinoma mutations that predicted response to tyrosine kinase inhibitors were first described, and is indicative of the directions in diagnostic pathology for other solid cancers. However, there are several challenges to this paradigm that merit further discussion.

Challenges of Variants of Unknown Significance

As somatic gene panel assays expand to generate sequence data across the length of each gene rather than from focused hotspots, more variants are identified. In particular, the resulting breadth of variant discovery permits the detection of variants for which no clear indication of response for a given therapeutic indication might be available. These variants of unknown significance (VUS) raise issues with regard to whether the result should be reported because the therapeutic indication is uncertain. Although basic science experiments may eventually characterize the functional impact of all variants in all cancer-related genes, most molecular pathology groups that are conducting selective hybridization capture panel assays of cancers are instead developing local databases to catalogue VUS in an effort to initially provide a record of whether the variant has been seen in previously completed assays. Over time, data mining of electronic medical records for patients with variants, targeted therapy, and response data recorded may transition VUS to therapeutic indications.

Challenges of Off-Label Indications

The current process for clinical trials of new therapies in cancer toward FDA approval rests on a paradigm in which trials compare each new therapy in a specific tumor type to the standard of care therapy. Hence, cancer therapies are tested and approved in a disease site–specific manner. By contrast, cancer genomics efforts have demonstrated that known cancer-initiating gene alterations occur in multiple disease and/or tissue sites.[16,40] This fact, in turn, raises the possibility that a given targeted therapy might be effective for multiple solid tumor types that all carry the same somatic alteration. There is support for multiple tissue–site therapeutic effectiveness, including the FDA-approved use of the kinase inhibitor Gleevec (imatinib) in both chronic myeloid leukemia (a blood cancer) targeting *ABL* kinase and in gastrointestinal stromal tumors targeting *KIT*.[41] Another example is EGFR-targeting therapies with FDA approval for use in lung adenocarcinomas, head and neck squamous cell carcinomas, and colorectal cancers with somatically altered *EGFR*.[42-44] These approved tissue sites each required a separate series of clinical trials to gain FDA approval. However, in solid tumor assays with gene panels, off-label indications will arise due to the shared nature of cancer-initiating mutations across different tissue sites. This challenge occurs when a gene with a functional mutation is detected that indicates a therapy not yet approved in the specific tissue site of origin. Current changes in clinical trial design are attempting to address this issue by creating either a trial design such as National Cancer Institute's Molecular Analysis for Therapy Choice (MATCH),[45] which assigns patients with a druggable mutation and/or gene to a specific therapy (basket trial) or a design that studies only a single tissue site but permits multiple therapies to be assigned depending upon the mutation identified (umbrella trial).[46]

Importance of Tissue Biology

A further confounder of the shared nature of cancer-initiating mutations that can defeat a seemingly clear therapeutic indication is that the accompanying tissue biology may render the therapy ineffective in a particular tissue. One such example is the presence of point mutations in *BRAF* with corresponding targeted therapies shown by clinical trials to provide therapeutic benefit in melanomas.[47] However, a clinical trial of patients with colorectal adenocarcinomas carrying the same functional *BRAF* V600E mutation was stopped due to a lack of therapeutic benefit. Subsequent research from Bernard's laboratory showed definitively this lack of benefit in colorectal cancer was due to up-regulation of other tyrosine kinases that compensated for the inhibition of mutated *BRAF*.[48] Hence, tissue biology must be considered in the prediction of therapeutic response. Importantly, this study also demonstrated that a combination of BRAF and EGFR inhibitors, which were predicted to alleviate the compensatory mechanism, rendered a therapeutic benefit.[49]

SUMMARY AND CONCLUDING REMARKS

Solid tumor gene-based assays are in a dramatic transition to multigene testing. This trend is driven by (1) the increasing use of selective hybridization capture or other targeting approaches coupled with MPS, (2) the discovery of somatic alterations in the genomes of cancer cells, and (3) the emerging number of targeted therapies that address specific cancer-initiating genes or gene families. The comprehensive nature of multigene assays creates specific challenges, mainly due to the impedance mismatch between cancer mutation discovery and the functional characterization of those alterations that either contribute to the development and progression of cancer or do not contribute to it. The need to accelerate testing of new therapeutics across multiple tissue sites at once is slowly being addressed by new clinical trial designs to identify the most effective therapies for a given gene, alteration, and tissue site. Ultimately, the widespread use of multigene testing for cancer diagnosis, prognosis, and therapeutic decision-making rests in the demonstration of clinical usefulness, which is established for some tissue sites, but as yet, not for all.

SELECTED REFERENCES

For a full list of references for this chapter, please refer to ExpertConsult.com.

1. International Human Genome Sequencing C. Finishing the euchromatic sequence of the human genome. *Nature* 2004;**431**:931–45.
4. de Biase D, Visani M, Baccarini P, et al. Next generation sequencing improves the accuracy of KRAS mutation analysis in endoscopic ultrasound fine needle aspiration pancreatic lesions. *PLoS ONE* 2014;**9**:e87651.
12. Sorlie T, Perou CM, Tibshirani R, et al. Gene expression patterns of breast carcinomas distinguish tumor subclasses with clinical implications. *Proc Natl Acad Sci USA* 2001;**98**: 10869–74.
14. Ley TJ, Mardis ER, Ding L, et al. DNA sequencing of a cytogenetically normal acute myeloid leukaemia genome. *Nature* 2008;**456**:66–72.
16. Kandoth C, McLellan MD, Vandin F, et al. Mutational landscape and significance across 12 major cancer types. *Nature* 2013;**502**:333–9.
20. Paez JG, Janne PA, Lee JC, et al. EGFR mutations in lung cancer: correlation with clinical response to gefitinib therapy. *Science* 2004;**304**:1497–500.
21. Lynch TJ, Bell DW, Sordella R, et al. Activating mutations in the epidermal growth factor receptor underlying responsiveness of non-small-cell lung cancer to gefitinib. *N Engl J Med* 2004;**350**:2129–39.
22. Pao W, Miller V, Zakowski M, et al. EGF receptor gene mutations are common in lung cancers from "never smokers" and are associated with sensitivity of tumors to gefitinib and erlotinib. *Proc Natl Acad Sci USA* 2004;**101**: 13306–11.
25. Jones S, Anagnostou V, Lytle K, et al. Personalized genomic analyses for cancer mutation discovery and interpretation. *Sci Transl Med* 2015;**7**:283ra53.
26. Engelman JA, Zejnullahu K, Mitsudomi T, et al. MET amplification leads to gefitinib resistance in lung cancer by activating ERBB3 signaling. *Science* 2007;**316**: 1039–43.
33. Van Allen EM, Wagle N, Stojanov P, et al. Whole-exome sequencing and clinical interpretation of formalin-fixed,

paraffin-embedded tumor samples to guide precision cancer medicine. *Nat Med* 2014;**20**:682–8.

36. Popovici V, Budinska E, Bosman FT, et al. Context-dependent interpretation of the prognostic value of BRAF and KRAS mutations in colorectal cancer. *BMC Cancer* 2013;**13**:439.
42. Janne PA, Johnson BE. Effect of epidermal growth factor receptor tyrosine kinase domain mutations on the outcome of patients with non-small cell lung cancer treated with epidermal growth factor receptor tyrosine kinase inhibitors. *Clin Cancer Res* 2006;**12**:4416s–20s.
44. Dietel M, Johrens K, Laffert M, et al. Predictive molecular pathology and its role in targeted cancer therapy: a review focusing on clinical relevance. *Cancer Gene Ther* 2013;**20**:211–21.
46. Redig AJ, Janne PA. Basket trials and the evolution of clinical trial design in an era of genomic medicine. *J Clin Oncol* 2015;**33**:975–7.
48. Prahallad A, Sun C, Huang S, et al. Unresponsiveness of colon cancer to BRAF(V600E) inhibition through feedback activation of EGFR. *Nature* 2012;**483**:100–3.

51

Genetic Aspects of Hematopoietic Malignancies

Todd W. Kelley and Jay L. Patel

ABSTRACT

Background

The field of hematology has long been at the forefront of using genetic testing to improve clinical outcomes. There have been many benefits for patients with hematopoietic malignancies, including improved diagnostic accuracy, prognostic stratification, and identification of new therapeutic targets. Molecular methods such as polymerase chain reaction, dideoxy-termination sequencing, and fluorescence in situ hybridization have been a routine part of the practice of hematopathology for many years. However, like other areas of oncology, the last few years have seen further advances in the understanding of the genetic basis of these neoplasms, primarily due to the influence of new sequencing technologies. Massively parallel sequencing has made routine what was just a few years ago unthinkable.

Content

In this chapter we cover the genetic abnormalities common in hematopoietic malignancies, including many of the newest discoveries. We approach hematopoietic malignancies from a laboratory standpoint starting with structural chromosomal abnormalities and translocations and moving to smaller-scale genetic changes found in single genes and finally to epigenetic changes. We compare and contrast the various laboratory methods used to query these abnormalities and highlight the utility of new and advancing technologies and platforms, including array-based methods and massively parallel sequencing. Finally, the chapter ends with a discussion of lymphoid clonality testing, an area of hematology testing that is also benefiting from the influence of modern sequencing technology.

RECURRENT TRANSLOCATIONS AND STRUCTURAL CHROMOSOMAL ABNORMALITIES

Many hematopoietic malignancies harbor underlying chromosomal abnormalities, including balanced and unbalanced translocations and large-scale structural changes such as deletions or duplications. Some of these abnormalities are characteristic of certain disease subtypes and are thus repeatedly, or recurrently, found in different individuals with the same disease. Recurrent genetic abnormalities of all types are found across the spectrum of hematopoietic malignancies. This theme is revisited throughout this chapter.

Chromosomal abnormalities may be detectable by conventional cytogenetics or may require more specialized molecular techniques. The specificity and utility of these findings are variable and highly context-dependent. While there are some genetic lesions that are disease defining, most others have utility in diagnosis, prognosis, and clinical management. Proper diagnosis and classification of acute myelogenous leukemia (AML) and acute lymphoblastic leukemia (ALL), according to the WHO classification, require karyotyping and/or fluorescent in situ hybridization (FISH) studies, in conjunction with morphologic, immunophenotypic, and clinical correlation.[1] The workup of myeloid neoplasms such as myelodysplastic syndromes (MDS) and myeloproliferative neoplasms (MPNs) also often includes these types of ancillary studies. Chromosomal analysis requires bone marrow aspirate samples that are amenable to cytogenetic testing.[2]

A hallmark of certain subtypes of mature B-cell lymphoproliferative disorders is the presence of a balanced translocation involving *IGH* on chromosome 14q32 with a proto-oncogene—for example, *BCL2* in the case of follicular lymphoma. The latter is thereby placed under the influence of *IGH* enhancer elements, resulting in dysregulated expression and lymphomagenesis. The mechanistic details underlying the development of recurrent translocations in hematolymphoid neoplasms continue to be the subject of investigation.

The normal process of lymphocyte antigen receptor gene rearrangement and sequence remodeling, which are necessary for proper B- and T-cell function, is vulnerable to mistakes. Antigen receptor rearrangement occurs in a sequential fashion involving recombination of *IGH*-V, D, and J gene segments mediated by an enzyme complex in which the nucleases RAG1 and RAG2 introduce double-strand DNA breaks adjacent to specific recombination signal sequences (described in more detail in the "Clonality Testing in Hematopoietic Malignancies" section). The presence of recombination signal sequences adjacent to *IGH-BCL2* breakpoints in follicular lymphoma provides evidence for the involvement of failed V(D)J recombination in translocation events involving *IGH*.[3] The precise mechanism of DNA breakage at oncogene loci is less clear but may involve the ability of RAG1 and RAG2 proteins to additionally act as transposases, with the ability to catalyze excision and subsequent integration of a DNA fragment into another molecule via a transesterification reaction.[4] However, aberrant V(D)J recombination–associated events do not account for the entirety of oncogenic translocations leading to lymphoma development. Consider that while the number of B- and T-lymphocytes produced by the human body is roughly equal and both undergo V(D)J recombination, the clear majority of lymphoid neoplasms are of B-cell lineage. This discrepancy is explained in part by the fact that B cells undergo secondary antibody diversification by somatic hypermutation and class switch recombination after migration into the germinal centers of peripheral lymphoid tissue; these processes inherently involve high mutational rates and provide additional opportunities for pathogenic events to manifest during B-cell development. *IGH* breakpoints in most cases of sporadic Burkitt lymphoma, for example, occur 3' to the switch region adjacent to the mu constant segment (C_μ), consistent with a mechanism involving abnormal class switch recombination.[5] T-cell development, in comparison, does not undergo similar mutation-prone events.

Recent studies of mutation events in B cells during somatic hypermutation and class switch recombination have centered on the enzymatic role of activation-induced cytidine deaminase (AID). AID is highly expressed in the germinal center microenvironment, where it normally introduces mutations into variable and class switching regions of immunoglobulin genes to promote increased diversity of the immunoglobulin antigen-binding repertoire. AID is transcription-dependent and acts by deamination of cytidine to uracil in single-stranded DNA targets, which is propagated as a uracil-guanine mismatch and replicated as a cytidine-thymine transition. Alternatively, the uracil residue may be removed by uracil DNA glycolase to create an abasic site, which is recognized by nucleases or proofreading DNA polymerases.[6] Aberrant targeting of AID at the genomic level contributes to genomic instability in B cells and appears to occur preferentially in highly transcribed super-enhancer domains that are also linked to other promoters and enhancers to form a regulatory cluster.[7] Further, AID initiation occurs in association with focal regions of target genes in which sense and antisense transcription converge.[8] These recent discoveries provide a framework for understanding the role of AID in nonimmunoglobulin genes, including *MYC*, *BCL6*, and *PAX5*. Aberrant AID activity confers a predisposition to the development of mutations and chromosomal aberrations found in many B-cell lymphomas.

Lymphoid Disorders

Precursor lymphoid neoplasms are primarily diseases of children and adolescents and are composed of lymphoblasts committed to B or T cell lineage as defined by immunophenotypic features. B-lymphoblastic leukemia (B-ALL) is significantly more common than its T cell–derived counterpart and usually presents with cytopenias accompanying florid peripheral blood and bone marrow disease. T-lymphoblastic leukemia/lymphoma (T-ALL) may manifest as a nodal disease, frequently in association with a mediastinal mass, and shows variable bone marrow involvement. Classification of B lymphoblastic leukemia is based in part on detection of certain recurrent genetic abnormalities that often confer a specific clinicopathologic phenotype and carry prognostic implications (Table 51.1). For detection of chromosomal abnormalities, routine karyotyping along with FISH analysis is the clinical approach used by most laboratories. While T-lymphoblastic leukemia/lymphoma is not currently subclassified according to genetic findings, an abnormal karyotype is found in the majority of cases.

Mature lymphoid neoplasms are diagnosed largely based on morphology and immunophenotypic features. Cytogenetic and/or FISH studies are typically not required in order to appropriately diagnose and subclassify most cases due to the use of surrogate markers. For example, overexpression of cyclin D1 by immunohistochemistry is often used as presumptive evidence of the presence of t(11;14)(q13;q32); *IGH-CCND1* in the case of mantle cell lymphomas if the overall features are otherwise consistent.

B-Lymphoblastic Leukemia/Lymphoma

B-lymphoblastic leukemia with t(v;11q23); *KMT2A* (previously known as *MLL*) rearrangements (see Fig. 51.1 for an explanation of the general format used to represent chromosomal abnormalities) are characterized by a translocation between *KMT2A* on 11q23 and any one of a large number of potential fusion partners, the most common of which is *AFF1* on 4q21. These translocations confer high-risk disease due to aberrant expression of the epigenetic regulator *KMT2A*. *KMT2A* rearrangements represent the most likely recurrent chromosomal abnormality in infantile B-lymphoblastic leukemia and may occur in utero.[9] Patients are typically younger than 2 years of age and characteristically present with marked leukocytosis and central nervous system involvement. *KMT2A* rearrangements in lymphoblastic leukemia are typically detected by FISH studies using a break-apart probe spanning the 11q23 region. This FISH strategy employs locus-specific probes designed to flank a known breakpoint region. When a translocation is present, the probes are separated (they "break apart") and only primary colors are observed (eg, red and green), whereas normal cells demonstrate the secondary color (eg, yellow).

B-lymphoblastic leukemia with t(9;22)(q34;q11.2) is a high-risk disease characterized by production of a fusion protein with constitutively active ABL1 tyrosine kinase activity (*BCR-ABL1*; known as the Philadelphia chromosome). This is the most common recurrent genetic abnormality in

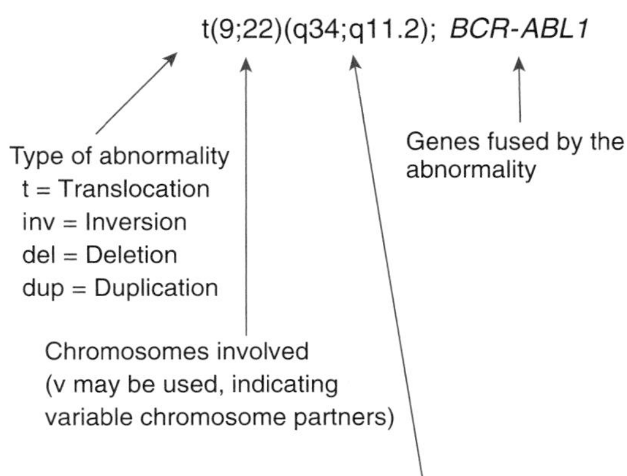

FIGURE 51.1 Format used to represent chromosomal abnormalities.

TABLE 51.1 Select Recurrent Chromosomal Abnormalities in Lymphoid Malignancies

Genetic Abnormality	Disease	Incidence	Prognosis	Clinical Notes
t(v;11q23); *KMT2A* rearranged	B-ALL	5%	Poor	Most common form of infant ALL
t(9;22)(q34;q11.2); *BCR-ABL1*	B-ALL	5% (pediatric) 25% (adult)	Poor	p190 (minor) isoform typical in children, p210 (major) common in adults, quantitative RT-PCR for monitoring
t(12;21)(p13;q22); *ETV6-RUNX1*	B-ALL	25% (pediatric) 3% (adults)	Very good	Balanced cryptic translocation, detection requires FISH
t(5;14)(q31;q32); *IL3-IGH*	B-ALL	1%	Intermediate	Eosinophilia
(1;19)(q23;p13.3); *TCF3-PBX1*	B-ALL	5%	Intermediate	—
Hyperdiploidy (>50 chromosomes)	B-ALL	25%	Very good	"Triple trisomy" of chromosomes 4, 10, and 17 particularly favorable
Hypodiploidy (24–44 chromosomes)	B-ALL	1%	Variable	Prognosis depends on degree of chromosome loss, near haploid patients fare particularly poorly
iAMP21	B-ALL	2%	Poor	Detectable by FISH for *RUNX1* on chromosome 21
t(1;14)(p32;q11); *TRD-TAL1*	T-ALL	3%	Intermediate	Difficult to detect due to cryptic deletion at 1p32
t(1;7)(p32q35); *TRB-TAL1*	T-ALL	1%	Intermediate	—
t(10;14)(q24;q11); *TRD-TLX1*	T-ALL	4%	Good	—
t(8;14)(q24;q32); *IGH-MYC*	BL	75%	Good	Aggressive disease but curable, *IGH-MYC* rare in DLBCL
t(2;8)(p12;q24); *IGK-MYC*	BL	15%	Good	Aggressive disease but curable
t(8;22)(q24;q11); *IGL-MYC*	BL	10%	Good	Aggressive disease but curable
t(14;18)(q32;q21); *IGH-BCL2*	FL, DLBCL	90% (FL) 20%-30% (DLBCL)	Variable	Prognosis in FL depends on grade and clinical stage. Aggressive in combination with *MYC* rearrangement —"double-hit."
t(v;3q27); *BCL6* rearrangement	FL, DLBCL	5%-10% (FL) 30% (DLBCL)	Variable	Aggressive disease when in combination with *MYC* rearrangement —"double-hit"
t(v;8q24); *MYC* rearrangement	DLBCL	10%	Poor	Common in plasmablastic lymphoma
t(11;14)(q13;q32); *IGH-CCND1*	MCL, MM	100%	Poor	FISH preferred for detection, association with lymphoplasmacytic morphology in MM
t(11;18)(q21;q21); *BIRC3-MALT1*	EMZL	40% (lung) 30% (stomach)	Good	Nonresponsive to *H. pylori*–directed antibiotic therapy, low likelihood of DLBCL transformation
del17p13; *TP53* deletion	MM	10% to 15%	Poor	Associated with disease progression
t(2;5)(p23;q35.1); *NPM1-ALK*	ALK+ ALCL	85%	Good	Indirect evidence provided by immunohistochemistry
6p25.3; *DUSP22* rearrangement	ALK- ALCL	30%	Good	Prognosis similar to ALK+ ALCL, FISH for detection
3q27; *TP63* rearrangement	ALK- ALCL	8%	Very poor	FISH for detection

Incidence is estimated with respect to disease category.
B-ALL, B-lymphoblastic leukemia/lymphoma; *T-ALL,* T-lymphoblastic leukemia/lymphoma; *BL,* Burkitt lymphoma; *DLBCL,* diffuse large B cell lymphoma; *FL,* follicular lymphoma; *MCL,* mantle cell lymphoma; *MM,* multiple myeloma; *EMZL,* extranodal marginal zone lymphoma; *ALCL,* anaplastic large cell lymphoma.

adult B-lymphoblastic leukemia patients and confers poor prognosis among all age groups. Patients may benefit from tyrosine kinase inhibitor (TKI) therapy in addition to traditional high-dose chemotherapy. While t(9;22)(q34;q11.2) is reliably detected by FISH, the type of *BCR-ABL1* fusions present should be confirmed by quantitative reverse transcription-PCR for purposes of ongoing monitoring during treatment and minimal residual disease detection. The p190 kDa fusion protein (e1a2 transcript) is seen in pediatric disease, while adults may demonstrate either the p190 kDa form or the larger p210 kDa form (e13a2 [b2a2] or e14a2 [b3a2] transcript). The latter is also seen in almost all cases of chronic myelogenous leukemia (CML). *BCR-ABL1* fusion transcripts are described in more detail later in this section.

The balanced cryptic (not identifiable by routine karyotype analysis) translocation t(12;21)(p13;q22); *ETV6-RUNX1* requires FISH for detection and is the most common recurrent abnormality in childhood B-ALL, accounting for 25% of cases. Its incidence decreases with age, and *ETV6-RUNX1* is only rarely seen in adult B-ALL. The event appears to occur early in leukemogenesis and results in an abnormal fusion of the transcription factor *ETV6* and the DNA-binding domain of *RUNX1*. The fusion protein interferes with the normal function of *RUNX1*, a factor that is critical for hematopoietic cell differentiation. Patients with B-ALL and *ETV6-RUNX1* have an excellent prognosis and achieve cure in greater than 90% of cases.

In contrast to mature B-cell malignancies, B-ALL rarely demonstrates translocations involving immunoglobulin loci. An exception is B-ALL with t(5;14)(q31;q32); *IL3-IGH*. The cytokine interleukin-3 (IL-3) is constitutively overexpressed as a result of being brought under the control of the *IGH* enhancer. One consequence is variable secondary eosinophilia, potentially leading to end-organ damage to sensitive tissues such as cardiac muscle. Otherwise, the clinical characteristics and prognosis associated with this rare disease are similar to B-ALL in general.

B-lymphoblastic leukemia with t(1;19)(q23;p13.3); *TCF3-PBX1* accounts for approximately 6% of cases in children and less than 5% in adults. The genetic abnormality is a translocation between the transcription factors *TCF3* and *PBX1*, resulting in creation of a leukemogenic fusion gene in which the DNA binding domain of *TCF3* is replaced with that of *PBX1*. This results in constitutive transcriptional activity of genes regulated by the PBX protein family. The prognosis of *TCF3-PBX1*–positive B-ALL is similar to other subtypes with comparable risk factors.

Numerical chromosomal abnormalities are relatively common in B-lymphoblastic leukemia and define additional subtypes of the disease. Precise definitions vary, but generally cases with greater than 50 chromosomes are referred to as hyperdiploid, while those with less than 45 chromosomes are designated hypodiploid. Concurrent structural abnormalities may be encountered but are uncommon. B-ALL with hyperdiploidy is seen in 25% of childhood disease and decreases in incidence with age. The prognosis is very good, and achievement of cure is highly likely with standard therapy. The number of chromosomes may be less important than the specific chromosomes involved. Patients with three copies of chromosomes 4, 10, and 17, so-called "triple-trisomy ALL," have an excellent prognosis. Hypodiploid B-ALL is seen in less than 5% of patients overall. Prognosis is generally poor and appears to be correlated to the degree of chromosome loss, with near-diploid (44 chromosomes) and high-hypodiploid (40 to 43 chromosomes) patients faring relatively well. Low-hypodiploid (32 to 39 chromosomes) cases show a high frequency of *TP53* mutations (often germline) along with *IKZF2* and *RB1* abnormalities.[10] Near-haploid (24 to 31 chromosomes) B-ALL is associated with *RAS* mutations and other alterations targeting receptor tyrosine kinase signaling.

Intrachromosomal amplification of chromosome 21 (iAMP21) occurs as a primary genetic event in approximately 2% of childhood B lymphoblastic leukemia and arises from the effect of "gene dosage" due to copy-number alterations of potentially hundreds of linked genes. The iAMP21 abnormality in B-ALL is associated with older age at presentation (median age is 9 years) and with low white blood cell counts. FISH testing with probes to the *RUNX1* locus demonstrates the presence of five or more signals on a single chromosome. Recent data show that B-ALL patients with iAMP21 fare poorly when treated according to standard-risk protocols and benefit from high-risk ALL therapy.[11]

T-Lymphoblastic Leukemia/Lymphoma

The most frequent nonrandom cytogenetic abnormalities seen in T-lymphoblastic leukemia/lymphoma are translocations involving T cell receptor (TCR) loci on chromosomes 7 (*TRA* and *TRD*) and 14 (*TRB* and *TRG*) in association with various partner genes. Many of these rearrangements involve dysregulation of T cell–specific cellular transcription factors, resulting in disruption of normal maturation or uncontrolled cellular proliferation. One frequent genetic target is *TAL1*, which is rearranged in approximately 60% of cases of T-ALL. Other genes implicated in T-ALL–related translocations include *TLX1*, *TLX3*, *MYC*, *LMO1*, *LMO2*, and *LYL1*.[12] The prognostic significance of these rearrangements is generally not well established, but *TLX1* abnormalities appear to correlate with improved clinical outcome, while *LYL1* and *TAL1* rearrangements appear to be less favorable. The Philadelphia chromosome, t(9;22)(q34;q11.2), is rarely detected in T-ALL but confers a poor prognosis.[13] Chromosomal deletions also occur in T-ALL, the most important of which involves the short arm of chromosome 9 and is seen in approximately 30% of cases. This results in loss of the important tumor suppressor gene *CDKN2A* and compromised cell cycle control. Notably, cryptic abnormalities are frequently found in T-ALL. Activating mutations in *NOTCH1*, which encodes a protein critical for early T cell development, have been demonstrated in the majority of T-ALL patients and appear to be associated with a favorable outcome. Increased NOTCH1 signaling can arise from point mutations, insertions, deletions, or, rarely, translocations, and appears to play an important role in leukemogenesis.[14]

Burkitt Lymphoma

Burkitt lymphoma was the first lymphoma shown to harbor a recurrent genetic abnormality, and in many ways it serves as an archetype for the study of mature B cell non-Hodgkin lymphomas.[15] Translocations involving the immunoglobulin locus and the *MYC* oncogene on 8q24 are primary genetic events in most cases of Burkitt lymphoma. The typical finding is t(8;14)(q24;q32), resulting in formation of a derivative chromosome 14 in which *MYC* is brought under control of the *IGH* locus, leading to constitutive *MYC* expression. Variant translocations involving *MYC* and the immunoglobulin light chain loci at 2p12 *(IGK)* and 22q11 *(IGL)* are seen in 5% to 10% of cases. MYC overexpression contributes to genomic instability through various mechanisms, including disruption of DNA double-strand break repair pathways, as well as both activation and repression of transcriptional activity. *IG-MYC* translocations are not specific for Burkitt lymphoma and occur as secondary events in a minor subset of other aggressive B cell non-Hodgkin lymphomas, as well as, rarely, in plasma cell myeloma and B-lymphoblastic leukemia. Burkitt lymphoma is perhaps most reliably defined by gene expression profiling with a molecular signature distinct from diffuse large B cell lymphoma, but such testing remains unavailable in most clinical settings.[16]

Follicular Lymphoma

A translocation involving *IGH* at 14q32 and *BCL2* on 18q21 is present in up to 90% of cases of follicular lymphoma. *BCL2* is thereby placed under the influence of the *IGH* promoter, and the result is overexpression of the antiapoptotic protein bcl-2. *IGH-BCL2* translocations are also found in approximately 20% to 30% of cases of diffuse large B-cell lymphoma (DLBCL). Surprisingly, t(14;18) can sometimes be detected in histologically benign lymph nodes or tonsillar tissue (usually

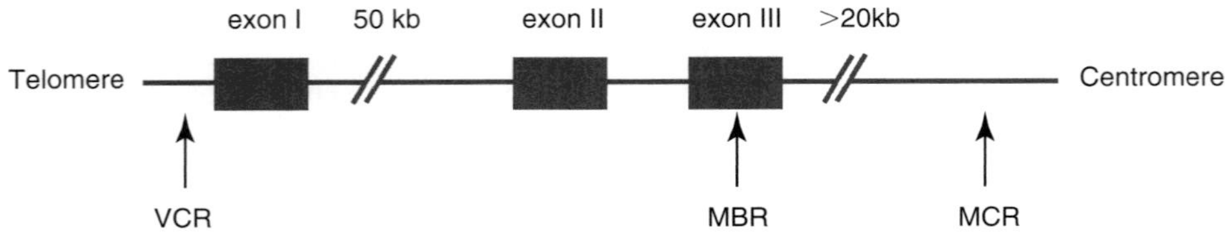

FIGURE 51.2 Schematic depiction of the architecture of *BCL2* on chromosome 18q21 with exons depicted as rectangles. *IGH-BCL2* translocation breakpoints occur most often within the major breakpoint cluster region (MBR, 50% to 60%) or the minor breakpoint cluster region (MCR, 20% to 25%). In approximately 10% of translocations, the *BCL2* breakpoint occurs in the variable cluster region (VCR) found upstream of exon 1 and will not be detected by most PCR assays.

at low levels) in otherwise normal individuals and is therefore not definitively diagnostic of lymphoma in isolation.[17] Additional genetic aberrations are present in most cases of follicular lymphoma, including a variety of chromosomal gains and losses.[18] Notably, 10% to 15% of follicular lymphoma, particularly high-grade cases, lack t(14;18). Approximately 80% to 90% of the breakpoints on 18q21 are located either in the major breakpoint region (MBR) found within the 3' untranslated region of exon 3 of *BCL2* or in the minor cluster region (MCR) found 3' further downstream of exon 3 and are amenable to detection by multiplex PCR using consensus primer sets (Fig. 51.2). Less common breakpoints (10%), many of which are found upstream of exon one of *BCL2*, are not targeted by typical PCR assays.[19] For this reason, FISH is often used to detect t(14;18).

Diffuse Large B-Cell Lymphoma

Diffuse large B-cell lymphoma (DLBCL) is a genetically heterogeneous group of large B cell lymphomas that display a variety of underlying chromosomal abnormalities, including t(14;18)(q32;q21). In addition to *IGH-BCL2* rearrangement, which may signify evolution from preexisting follicular lymphoma, rearrangements of the transcriptional regulator *BCL6* on 3q27 are common. The prevalence of *BCL6* somatic mutations and translocations is explained by the fact that *BCL6* is one of several other genes expressed in the germinal center that are known to normally undergo the process of somatic hypermutation, as does the variable region of *IGH*.[20] *MYC* rearrangements are also present in approximately 10% of patients. A subset of high-grade B cell lymphoma patients with variable histology harbor concurrent rearrangements of *MYC* in combination with *BCL2* or *BCL6*, a phenomenon referred to as "double-hit" lymphoma.[21] Rarely, all three abnormalities may be observed, in which case the designation "triple-hit" B cell lymphoma may be used. In either situation, the clinical phenotype is particularly aggressive. Due to the aggressive nature of the disease and a propensity for involvement of the central nervous system, prompt recognition of these patients is warranted for purposes of therapeutic decision making and prognostic stratification. This requires FISH testing at the time of initial diagnosis.

Mantle Cell Lymphoma

Mantle cell lymphoma is characterized by t(11;14)(q13;q32); *IGH-CCND1* in nearly all cases. The juxtaposition of the *CCND1* gene, encoding cyclin D1, with the *IGH* enhancer is a primary genetic event and results in increased progression through the cell cycle due to cyclin D1 protein overexpression.[22] The latter is detectable by immunohistochemistry, which often renders direct molecular genetic demonstration of *IGH-CCND1* unnecessary for diagnosis in most settings. However, clinical scenarios often arise in which mantle cell lymphoma is in the differential diagnosis but cyclin D1 immunohistochemical evaluation is not feasible, perhaps due to specimen limitations (eg, peripheral blood). In these situations, alternative testing is required. FISH represents the most sensitive testing strategy and is capable of detecting nearly 100% of translocations, assuming that cells harboring the translocation are present above established sensitivity thresholds.[23] Notably, t(11;14)(q13;q32) is also seen in 5% to 10% of plasma cell myeloma patients. Numerous breakpoints involving the *CCND1* locus may be encountered in mantle cell lymphoma and span a 350-kilobase region on 11q13. Approximately 40% of these breakpoints are clustered in a 1-kilobase segment referred to as the major translocation cluster (MTC) found 110 kb downstream of the *CCND1* locus (Fig. 51.3). Most PCR-based assays do not interrogate *CCND1* breakpoints outside the MTC. Translocations with breakpoints outside of this region are therefore not detected, and the sensitivity of these assays is only 40% to 50%.

Extranodal Marginal Zone Lymphoma (MALT Lymphoma)

Several recurrent translocations have been described in extranodal marginal zone lymphoma (MALT lymphoma), and their incidence varies with the anatomic site of disease. The t(11;18)(q21;q21) occurs mostly in gastric and pulmonary MALT lymphoma and results in *BIRC3-MALT1* fusion.[24] Detection is important because patients with t(11;18) are less likely to respond to antibiotic therapy directed at *H. pylori* and only rarely progress to large-cell lymphoma.[25] Three additional translocations—t(14;18)(p14;q32), t(1;14)(p22;q32), and t(3;14)(p22q32)—are seen with relatively low incidence but reinforce the paradigm of proto-oncogenes (*MALT1*, *BCL10*, and *FOXP1*, respectively) under the control of the *IGH* enhancer complex in B cell lymphoproliferative disorders.

Multiple Myeloma

Multiple myeloma is a clinically and genetically heterogeneous clonal disorder of terminally differentiated plasma cells. Incorporation of clinicopathologic and radiographic findings, including bone marrow evaluation, is often necessary for definitive diagnosis. Karyotypic and/or FISH abnormalities are detectable in a large proportion of cases and include a variety of aberrations. The most common abnormalities appear to be early events and include either trisomies of various chromosomes resulting in hyperdiploidy or translocations involving the *IGH* locus at 14q32. *IGH* translocation

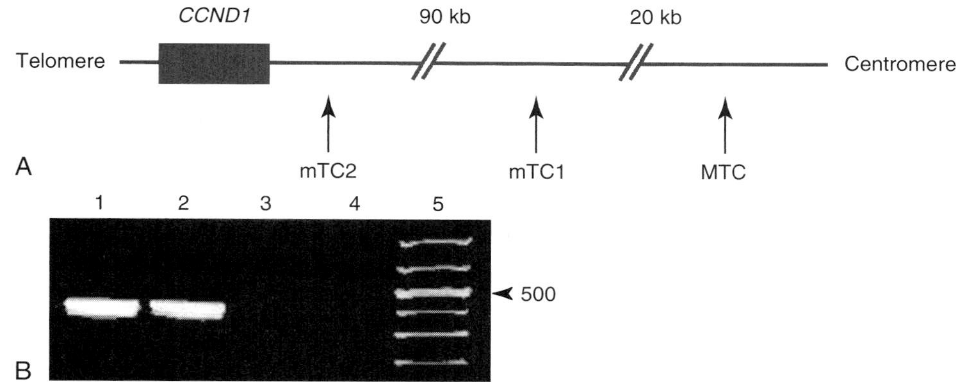

FIGURE 51.3 **A,** Schematic representation of the organization of *CCND1* on 11q13 and the range of breakpoint locations observed in *IGH-CCND1* translocation. The rectangle represents the *CCND1* gene. Various breakpoints may be observed and approximately 40% cluster in the major translocation cluster (MTC), the target of most PCR assays. Most of the remaining breakpoints occur in the minor translocation cluster 1 or 2 regions (mTC1 or mTC2). Note the relatively large distances involved because translocation breakpoints may span a region upward of 350 kb downstream of the *CCND1* locus. **B,** Example of an *IGH-CCND1* PCR assay with primers targeting the MTC followed by agarose gel electrophoresis. Lane 1 is a positive control, lane 2 is the patient sample, lane 3 is a negative control, and lane 4 is a no-template control with lane 5 showing the molecular size marker. The patient sample shows a strong discrete band at approximately 450 bp, comparable to the positive control. Note that the size of the PCR product may vary according to the specific *CCND1* breakpoint involved.

partners include, in decreasing frequency, *CCND1* (11q13), *FGFR3/MMSET* (4p16.3), *C-MAF* (16q23), *CCND3* (6p21), and *MAFB* (20q11). Monosomy 13 or deletion of 13q14 is also observed with regularity in plasma cell myeloma (40%), particularly in its leukemic form (70%). Disease progression is associated with acquisition of various additional genetic abnormalities, perhaps the most important of which is deletion of the tumor suppressor *TP53* at 17p13.[26] *TP53* deletion signals high-risk disease with significantly decreased overall survival and additionally may serve as a marker of extramedullary involvement.[27]

Anaplastic Large Cell Lymphoma

Examples of recurrent chromosomal abnormalities are less common in mature T cell lymphomas. Anaplastic lymphoma kinase (ALK)–positive anaplastic large cell lymphoma (ALCL), the hallmark of which is translocation of the tyrosine kinase receptor *ALK*, is one exception. The most common translocation, t(2;5)(p23;q35.1), accounts for 85% of cases and involves fusion of *ALK* to nucleophosmin *(NPM1)*, resulting in nuclear and cytoplasmic expression of ALK. Numerous, less-frequent variant translocation partners have also been described. *ALK* rearrangements are not disease-specific and are seen in a subset of non–small cell lung cancers. *NPM1-ALK* and variant fusions can be detected by FISH and other means, but this is usually unnecessary because normal postnatal human tissues, except for rare central nervous system constituents, lack ALK expression. Therefore the presence of an *ALK* translocation can be inferred quickly and cost effectively by the immunohistochemical detection of ALK protein expression in the neoplastic cells. Notably, ALK inhibitor therapies are in development, and treatment with these agents may lead to the acquisition of *ALK* kinase domain activating mutations conferring drug resistance.[28]

ALK-negative anaplastic large cell lymphoma is a T cell lymphoma that shares essentially identical morphologic and immunohistochemical features with ALK-positive ALCL, but it occurs in older patients and lacks both *ALK* rearrangements and ALK protein expression. ALK-negative ALCL has a worse prognosis relative to ALK-positive ALCL, possibly justifying a more aggressive therapeutic approach. Recent studies have revealed genetic heterogeneity in these cases. Patients with ALK-negative ALCL and rearrangement of *DUSP22* on 6p25.3 (demonstrated by FISH) fare relatively well, with overall survival resembling ALK-positive disease.[29] Rearrangements of *TP63* on 3q27 appear to be mutually exclusive with regard to *DUSP22* and imply a very poor prognosis.

Myeloid Disorders

Myeloid malignancies are a relatively diverse group of diseases that arise as a consequence of a variety of genetic aberrations. Generally they are classified in the WHO system as myeloproliferative neoplasms (MPN), myelodysplastic syndromes (MDS), myelodysplastic/myeloproliferative overlap neoplasms (MDS/MPN), and acute myeloid leukemia (AML). They are further subclassified through the synthesis of cytologic, morphologic, clinical, and genetic findings (Table 51.2). A variety of laboratory tests are important for genetic evaluation, including cytogenetic karyotyping, FISH, array-based genotyping (eg, single nucleotide polymorphism arrays), and molecular techniques such as PCR and sequencing, including both dideoxy-termination (Sanger) sequencing and massively parallel sequencing. Gene mutations are detectable only by molecular techniques. Such mutations and the techniques used to detect them are the focus of the "Gene Mutations in Hematopoietic Malignancies" section.

Acute Myeloid Leukemias

Core binding factor–associated acute myeloid leukemias (AMLs) are unified by molecular pathophysiology and include t(8;21)(q22;q22); *RUNX1-RUNX1T1* and inv(16)(q13.1;q22); *CBFB-MYH11*. The core binding factor is a

TABLE 51.2 **Selected Recurrent Chromosomal Abnormalities in Myeloid Neoplasms**

Genetic Abnormality	Disease	Incidence	Prognosis	Clinical Notes
t(8;21)(q22;q22); *RUNX1-RUNX1T1*	AML	10%	Good	Core binding factor leukemia, favorable prognosis partly negated by concurrent *KIT* mutation (20%-25%)
inv(16)(q13.1;q22); *CBFB-MYH11*	AML	10%	Good	Core binding factor leukemia, favorable prognosis negated by concurrent *KIT* mutation (30%)
t(15;17)(q24;q12); *PML-RARA*	AML	7%	Good	Hematologic emergency (risk of DIC), FISH is test of choice for diagnostic confirmation, responsive to ATRA, monitor with quantitative RT-PCR
t(9;11)(p22;q23); *MLLT3-KMT2A*	AML	5%	Poor	More common in pediatric AML (12%), monocytic differentiation, gingival hypertrophy, risk of DIC
t(6;9)(p23q34); *DEK-NUP214*	AML, MDS	1%	Very poor	Basophilia, may arise de novo or in the setting of MDS, frequent *FLT3* ITD (70%)
inv3(q21;q26.2); *RPN1-EVI1*	AML, MDS	2%	Very poor	Normal or increased platelet count, may arise de novo or in the setting of MDS, occasional *FLT3* ITD (13%)
t(1;22)(p13;q13); *RBM15-MKL1*	AML	<1%	Good	Pediatric disease associated with Down syndrome, megakaryoblastic differentiation, somatic *GATA1* mutations
del(5q) or monosomy 5	MDS	10%	Good	Excellent response to lenalidomide when del(5q) is sole abnormality, *TP53* mutations confer poor response
del(7q) or monosomy 7	MDS	10%	Intermediate	Poor prognosis with monosomy 7
del(11q)	MDS	3%	Very good	—
del(12p)	MDS	12%	Good	—
del(20q)	MDS	8%	Good	Insufficient to diagnose MDS as a sole abnormality
i(17q) or t(17p); *TP53* deletion	MDS	5%	Intermediate	Acquired (pseudo) Pelger-Huet anomaly
Trisomy 8	MDS	10%	Intermediate	Common but nonspecific, seen in other myeloid neoplasms
Normal	MDS	50%	Good	Somatic mutations by massively parallel sequencing
Complex (>3 unrelated defects)	MDS	7%	Very poor	High risk of evolution to AML
t(9;22)(q34;q11.2); *BCR-ABL1*	CML	100%	Good	Response to TKI therapy monitored by quantitative RT-PCR, myeloid or B lymphoblastic blast phase possible
del(4q12); *FIP1L1-PDGFRA*	CEL	Rare	Unknown	May present as AML or T-LBL, cryptic deletion detectable by FISH for *CHIC2*, responsive to TKI
t(5;12)(q33;p12); *ETV6-PDGFRB*	CMML	Rare	Unknown	Eosinophilia, responsive to TKI
t(v;8p11); *FGFR1* rearranged	Variable	Rare	Very poor	Stem cell disease with lymphomatous presentation common, unresponsive to TKI

Incidence is estimated with respect to disease category.
AML, Acute myeloid leukemia; *MDS,* myelodysplastic syndrome; *CML,* chronic myelogeneous leukemia; *CEL,* chronic eosinophilic leukemia; *CMML,* chronic myelomonocytic leukemia; *T-LBL,* T-lymphoblastic lymphoma; *DIC,* disseminated intravascular coagulation; *ATRA,* all-*trans*-retinoic acid; *ITD,* internal tandem duplication; *TKI,* tyrosine kinase inhibitors.

heterodimeric protein composed of alpha and beta subunits encoded by *RUNX1* and *CBFB*, respectively, which is normally involved in regulation of hematopoiesis. The *RUNX1-RUNX1T1* and *CBFB-MYH11* abnormalities disrupt this function, resulting in the impairment of differentiation leading to the accumulation of immature myeloid blasts. A finding of either t(8;21)(q22;q22); *RUNX1-RUNX1T1* or inv(16)(q13.1;q22); *CBFB-MYH11* is diagnostic of acute leukemia, regardless of blast count. Patients with either of these two AML subtypes respond well to cytarabine-based consolidation chemotherapy.[30] Importantly, prognosis is adversely affected by activating *KIT* gene mutations in exon 8 or 17, which are present in up to 30% of cases.[31] FISH is preferred for detection at diagnosis, while quantitative reverse transcription PCR is highly sensitive and ideally suited for disease monitoring. Minimal residual disease testing has clear prognostic significance in the setting of core binding factor AML.[32] *RUNX1-RUNX1T1* fusion transcripts are readily detectable by reverse transcription-PCR (RT-PCR) utilizing relatively simple primer sets due to the clustering of breakpoints at a limited number of intronic sites.[33] Three dominant *CBFB-MYH11* fusion transcripts (types A, D, and E) corresponding to different breakpoints account for over 95% of inv(16)-positive AML cases and are also amenable to detection by RT-PCR.

The presence of the balanced reciprocal translocation t(15;17)(q24;q12); *PML-RARA* is diagnostic of acute promyelocytic leukemia. The chimeric fusion protein resulting from the translocation mediates an arrest in myeloid differentiation at the promyelocyte stage. Timely recognition is required due to the high risk of disseminated intravascular coagulation (DIC) seen in these patients and the associated clinical ramifications. Prompt DIC prophylaxis may prevent a bleeding diathesis that otherwise could be fatal. Morphologic and flow cytometric studies allow for a presumptive diagnosis in most cases, but genetic confirmation of *PML-RARA* is nevertheless required. FISH is the test of choice at diagnosis due to high sensitivity and typically rapid turnaround time. Rare cryptic *PML-RARA* fusions have been documented, which are not detectable by routine karyotyping.[34] The disease is responsive to therapy with all-*trans*-retinoic acid, which drives the terminal differentiation of the neoplastic cells and is used in combination with anthracyclines or arsenic trioxide to induce durable remission in 80% to 90% of patients.[35] Variant *RARA* fusion partners may be seen on occasion, the most important of which is *ZBTB16* at 11q23. Recognition is important due to the lack of therapeutic response to all-*trans*-retinoic acid.[36] Assessment of response to therapy by a quantitative RT-PCR–based monitoring test has emerged as standard practice and appears to improve clinical outcome.[37] Three *PML-RARA* fusion transcripts (bcr1, bcr2, and bcr3) may be encountered corresponding to breakpoints at different regions of *PML* at 15q24 (Fig. 51.4). *RARA* breakpoints are clustered within intron 2 in a 15 kb region on 17q12. The bcr3 fusion results in a relatively short transcript and may be associated with the presence of *FLT3* mutations.

Translocations involving the *KMT2A* gene and various partner genes occur with some frequency in AML cases, most commonly in children. Over 80 *KMT2A* translocation partners have been described. In AML, the most common is t(9;11)(p22;q23); *MLLT3-KMT2A*, which is routinely detectable by FISH. This disease is often associated with extramedullary manifestations, and patients classically present with gingival hyperplasia or cutaneous lesions due to tissue infiltration by the leukemia cells. Due to the heterogeneity of the translocation breakpoints, a widely applicable quantitative RT-PCR assay for disease monitoring is difficult to design, but testing can be performed on those patients with more common breakpoints.[38]

A subset of cases of acute myeloid leukemia may arise from a preexisting myelodysplastic syndrome (MDS), and therefore some genetic features common to both diseases are observed. Two examples are t(6;9)(p23q34); *DEK-NUP214* and inv(3)(q21;q26.2); *RPN1-EVI1*.[39,40] Both are associated with multilineage dysplasia and occur in 1% to 2% of AML patients overall. As expected, prognosis is generally poor. *FLT3* mutations are frequently detected in AML with *DEK-NUP214*, which has a tendency to affect younger adults and children, and it is unclear whether the negative prognostic implication is independent of *FLT3* status. *FLT3* mutations are relatively uncommon in AML with inv(3) in which *RPN1* acts as an enhancer of the oncogene *EVI1* to drive cellular proliferation possibly in collaboration with *RAS*-pathway mutations.[41]

A particularly rare form of AML occurs in infants and children with Down syndrome and involves fusion of *RBM15* to *MKL1* as a result of t(1;22)(p13;q13). The fusion gene's precise role in leukemogenesis is unclear, but transcriptional activation and modulation of chromatin organization are likely mechanisms.[42] Somatic N-terminal truncating *GATA1*

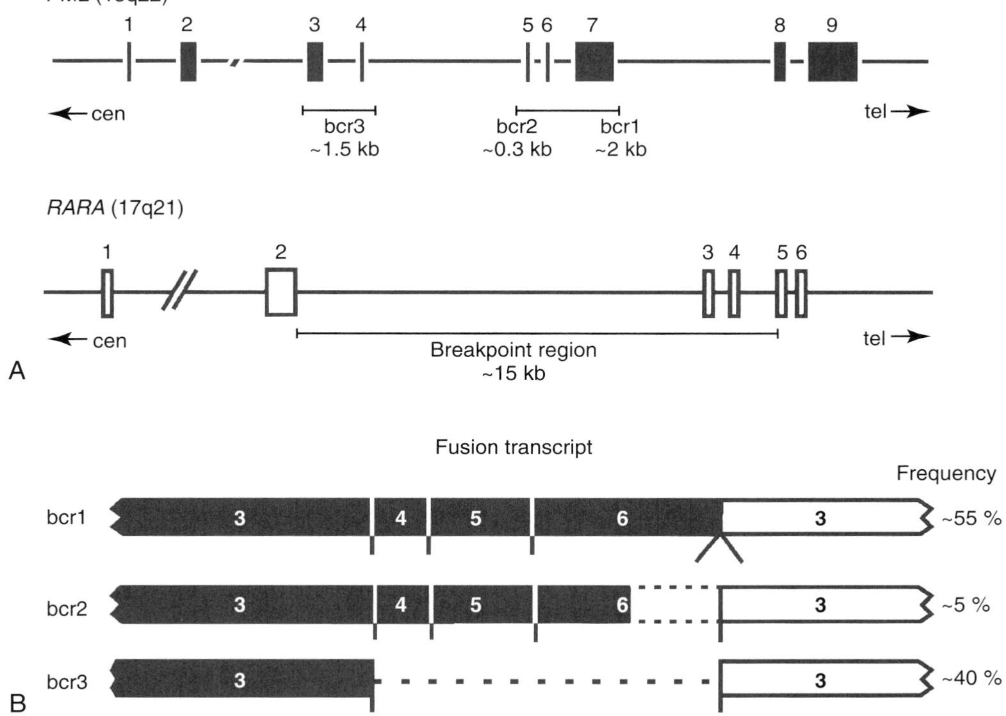

FIGURE 51.4 Schematic representation of the *PML* and *RARA* genes and typical breakpoints involved in the t(15;17)(q24;q12) diagnostic of acute promyelocytic leukemia. **A,** *PML* exons are shown as red rectangles, and *RARA* exons are in white. Translocation breakpoints in *PML* are found in one of three breakpoint cluster regions (bcr1, bcr2, and bcr3), while *RARA* breakpoints are clustered in a single intronic region. **B,** The configuration of the *PML-RARA* fusion transcripts corresponding to different *PML* breakpoint cluster regions along with their relative frequency is shown. *cen,* Centromere; *tel,* telomere.

mutations are common in patients with Down syndrome–associated AML but do not affect prognosis. *GATA1* mutations are also seen in individuals with Down syndrome who develop transient abnormal myelopoiesis (TAM), a disorder which may mimic AML but usually resolves in the first 6 months of life.[43] These two conditions are not readily distinguishable, especially in early infancy, and careful clinical correlation is necessary.

Chronic Myelogeneous Leukemia

The discovery in 1960 of a recurrent chromosomal abnormality in patients with a disease then known as chronic granulocytic leukemia by Peter Nowell and David Hungerford was a landmark observation. This was followed 13 years later by Janet Rowley's demonstration of a consistent reciprocal translocation between 9q34 and 22q11.2, resulting in a der(22q) (now known as the Philadelphia chromosome) found in virtually all cases of chronic myelogenous leukemia (CML).[44,45] Another 10 years would pass before the precise breakpoints were cloned, and it was shown that the translocation results in juxtaposition of the *ABL1* proto-oncogene on 9q34 to *BCR* on 22q11.2 with formation of a novel *BCR-ABL1* fusion gene.[46] This results in constitutive ABL1 protein tyrosine kinase activity and dysregulated cellular proliferation. Documentation of t(9;22)(q34;q11.2); *BCR-ABL1* fusion is necessary for diagnosis and is readily demonstrated by metaphase cytogenetics, FISH and/or RT-PCR.

Distinct *BCR-ABL1* fusion transcripts, which correspond to variably sized fusion proteins, are encountered based on the translocation breakpoints (Fig. 51.5). The *ABL1* breakpoint is largely conserved at a location upstream of exon 2. The bulk of *ABL1* is therefore fused to BCR and preserves the ABL1 kinase domain. The major breakpoint cluster region (M-bcr) is the location of the majority of *BCR* breakpoints in CML, and up to half of the *BCR* breakpoints in Philadelphia chromosome–positive (Ph+) adult B-ALL. MBR breakpoints occur between exons 13 or 15, resulting in a fusion transcript consisting of e13a2 (b2a2) or e14a2 (b3a2), both of which encode the p210 kDa *BCR-ABL1* isoform typical of CML.

Less frequently, BCR breakpoints occur in the minor breakpoint cluster region (m-bcr) between *BCR* exon 1 and exon 2, resulting in a shorter e1a2 fusion transcript encoding the p190 kDa fusion protein seen rarely in CML but commonly in pediatric Ph+ B-ALL. At initial diagnosis, CML patients may harbor low levels of e1a2 transcript detectable by RT-PCR in addition to the M-bcr transcript. This phenomenon is likely due to alternative splicing, and it is important to note that for purposes of disease monitoring, only the M-bcr transcript should be followed by RT-PCR. Occasionally, e1a2 is the exclusive transcript detected in CML and is associated with monocytic proliferation resembling chronic myelomonocytic leukemia. Rare cases of CML harbor *BCR* breakpoints that occur in the mu breakpoint cluster region (μ-BCR) at exon 19 (c3), resulting in an e19a2 (c3a2) fusion. The corresponding *BCR-ABL1* protein is larger (p230 kDa) and is characteristically seen in association with marked neutrophilic maturation that may mimic chronic neutrophilic leukemia. Notably, most RT-PCR assays are not designed to detect the e19a2 fusion transcript, so FISH studies should be recommended if clinical suspicion for CML persists despite a negative RT-PCR result.

Despite dramatic improvement in long-term survival, treatment of CML patients with TKIs does not typically result in cure. This is evidenced by the fact that low levels of *BCR-ABL1* persist even in patients who achieve a major molecular response. Over time, point mutations in the *BCR-ABL*1 kinase domain may develop in a subset of patients and confer resistance to the TKI.[47] This resistance may be overcome by changing therapy to a different TKI. Documentation of a *BCR-ABL1* kinase domain mutation in a patient with suboptimal or failed response to first-line TKI therapy may therefore be indicated and can be accomplished by Sanger sequencing and, increasingly, by massively parallel sequencing. The latter strategy may offer additional testing benefits,[48] as will be discussed in the "Gene mutations in hematopoietic malignancies" section of this chapter.

Myelodysplastic Syndromes

The most common chromosomal abnormalities observed in myelodysplastic syndromes (MDSs) take the form of unbalanced structural chromosomal deletions or gains (Table 51.2). Deletion of the long arm (q arm) or outright loss of chromosome 5 or 7 is seen relatively frequently. Balanced abnormalities are rare in MDS, but they do occur and show some overlap with recurrent translocations found in AML. These findings provide evidence of clonality that is particularly useful when the differential diagnosis in a cytopenic patient includes reactive conditions that must be excluded. Indeed, several chromosomal aberrations can provide presumptive evidence of MDS in the setting of persistent cytopenias, even in the absence of sufficient morphologic evidence of dysplasia.[1] In addition, many of these cytogenetic abnormalities have established prognostic significance and are an integral component of the widely applied International Prognostic Scoring System for MDS.[49] For example, a complex cytogenetic profile (greater than three unrelated defects) is a harbinger of evolution to AML and portends a very poor prognosis. Copy number alterations or copy number neutral loss of heterozygosity (eg, *TP53*) also occur in MDSs and are detectable by array methods.[50,51]

Myeloid and Lymphoid Neoplasms With Eosinophilia and Abnormalities of PDGFRA, PDGFRB, or FGFR1

A rare but distinct group of myeloid and lymphoid neoplasms demonstrate variable clinical presentations but are unified by eosinophilia and gene fusions involving the receptor protein tyrosine kinases *PDGFRA*, *PDGFRB*, or *FGFR1* (see Table 51.2).[52] Patients with *PDGFRA*-associated disease most often present with a myeloproliferative neoplasm resembling chronic eosinophilic syndrome, but a range of presentations, including acute myeloid leukemia and T-lymphoblastic leukemia/lymphoma, are possible. A *FIP1L1-PDGFRA* fusion is formed as a result of a cryptic deletion at chromosome 4q12. FISH is well suited for the detection of this abnormality, and probes targeting *FIP1L1*, *PDGFRA*, and *CHIC2* (also located at chromosome 4q12) are often employed. Fusion of the *FIP1L1* and *PDGFRA* loci results in loss of the *CHIC2* locus and creates a signal pattern detectable by FISH. An *ETV6-PDGRFB* fusion resulting from t(5;12)(q33;p12) is the most commonly observed fusion involving the *PDGFRB* gene and typically occurs in the context of a chronic myelomonocytic leukemia-like disorder, often with eosinophilia. *PDGRFB*-associated translocations are detectable by routine

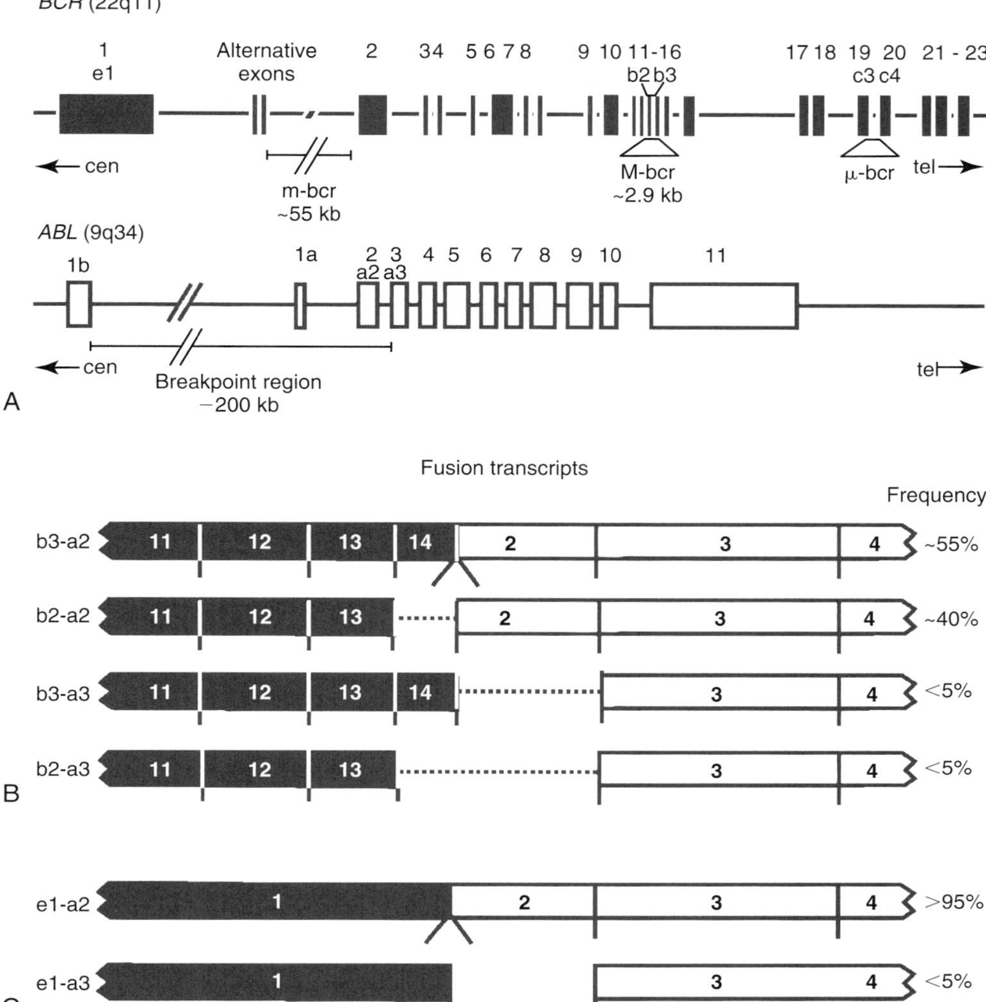

FIGURE 51.5 Schematic representation of the *BCR* and *ABL1* genes and typical breakpoints regions involved in the t(9;22)(q34;q11.2) characteristic of chronic myelogenous leukemia (CML) and a subset of B-lymphoblastic leukemia (B-ALL). **A,** *BCR* exons are shown as red rectangles, and *ABL* exons are in white. *BCR* translocation breakpoints are found in one of three locations: the major breakpoint cluster region (M-bcr), the minor breakpoint cluster region, and the mu breakpoint cluster region (μ-BCR). *ABL* breakpoints are clustered in a single conserved region upstream of exon a2 (or rarely exon a3). **B,** Configuration and relative frequency of *BCR-ABL1* fusion transcripts involving the M-bcr encountered in CML. The e13a2 (b2a2) or e14a2 (b3a2) transcripts encode a p210 kDa protein and are seen in most cases of CML along with a proportion of adult B-ALL. **C,** Configuration and relative frequency of *BCR-ABL1* fusion transcripts involving the m-bcr commonly encountered in B-lymphoblastic leukemia. The e1a2 transcript encodes a p190 kDa protein and is rarely seen in CML but quite frequently in pediatric B-ALL. *cen,* Centromere; *tel,* telomere.

karyotype. Prompt recognition of these diseases is crucial because end-organ damage due to eosinophilia may result in significant morbidity. In addition, most patients with *PDGFRA* and *PDGFRB* abnormalities are highly sensitive to treatment with the TKI imatinib.[53] *FGFR1*-related myeloid and lymphoid neoplasms are characteristically heterogeneous and may manifest as chronic eosinophilic leukemia, acute myeloid leukemia, or T- or B-lymphoblastic leukemia/ lymphoma, among other possibilities. Various fusion partners have been reported, notably including *BCR*, but rearrangement of *FGFR1* at 8p11 is a constant finding. This is readily detectable by karyotyping. Patients with this abnormality have a very poor prognosis disease that is unresponsive to TKI therapy.

Test Applications

Cytogenetics

Conventional cytogenetics refers to visual analysis of a karyotype composed of a complete set of metaphase-arrested chromosomes typically stained by Giemsa (G-banding). G-banding highlights light and dark zones corresponding to A-T-rich and G-C-rich regions of chromosomes. This decades-old technique remains very important for the comprehensive bone marrow evaluation of patients with acute leukemia or a myelodysplastic syndrome. G-banded karyotyping enabled the discovery of many of the recurring translocations characteristic of specific hematologic diseases. Karyotyping provides a genome-scale perspective and is well suited for uncovering large-scale chromosomal aberrations (resolution greater than 5 Mb) including reciprocal translocations, large deletions, and aneuploidy. Cryptic rearrangements and small insertions or deletions are likely to be missed by conventional karyotype and require more sensitive techniques for detection. Karyotyping is a labor-intensive process that requires considerable expertise for performance and interpretation. In addition, because cell growth in culture is required, turnaround times often range from 3 to 7 days, making this technique inappropriate for urgent clinical scenarios such as detection of t(15;17)(q24;q12); *PML-RARA*.

Fluorescence in Situ Hybridization

Fluorescence in situ hybridization (FISH) continues to be a powerful tool in the modern cytogenetics laboratory due to its ability to overcome several of the limitations of conventional G-banded karyotype. This technique utilizes fluorescently labeled DNA probes designed to hybridize to specific sequences on metaphase or interphase chromosomal preparations. Resolution is improved to approximately 2 Mb. FISH allows detection of cryptic chromosomal abnormalities such as translocations or deletions, which may not be identifiable by routine karyotype. The proliferation of FISH testing has been facilitated by the commercial availability of extensive libraries of probes targeting various recurrent abnormalities. A variety of specimen types can be used, importantly including paraffin-embedded formalin fixed samples, because FISH assays do not require viable cells or growth in culture. Break-apart FISH probes allow for identification of gene rearrangements without a priori knowledge of the translocation partner, of which there may be numerous possibilities. For example, an *MLL* break-apart probe (*KMT2A* gene) spanning the appropriate 11q23 region can effectively confirm or exclude the presence of an *MLL* rearrangement without having to query any of the dozens of potential MLL translocation partners. Global assessment of copy number changes is not possible by FISH because only a limited number of probes are utilized.

Single Nucleotide Polymorphism Array

Gene amplification is found in a variety of hematolymphoid neoplasms and may contribute to disease pathogenesis.[54] Array-based strategies offer a method by which to identify potentially important copy number changes that are not detectable by conventional karyotyping or FISH studies. Such arrays are based on genome-wide analysis of common single nucleotide polymorphisms (SNPs) using genomic DNA prepared from both tumor and normal reference samples. Copy number changes and copy neutral loss of heterozygosity are detectable by this method, but balanced translocations are not. Therefore this technique is best utilized as an adjunct tool in combination with conventional cytogenetics and/or FISH testing.

Polymerase Chain Reaction

Conventional polymerase chain reaction (PCR) assays targeting recurrent translocations are occasionally employed in the diagnostic workup of hematopoietic malignancies when evidence of a particular gene fusion (eg, *IGH-BCL2*) is sought. Depending on the context, test sensitivity may be limited due to marked heterogeneity in translocation breakpoints and the fact that abnormal mRNA fusion transcripts may not be produced by a particular abnormality (eg, *IGH-BCL2*). For this reason, FISH is often a preferable alternative for identification of lymphoma-associated translocations involving the *IGH* locus. On the other hand, RT-PCR allows for detection of abnormal mRNA fusion transcripts where applicable, such as in the setting of AML-associated translocations t(8;21)(q22;q22); *RUNX1-RUNX1T1*, t(15;17)(q22;q12); *PML-RARA*, inv(16)(p13.1;q22); *CBFB-MYH11* or in the t(9;22)(q34;q11.2); *BCR-ABL1*–positive leukemias. In RT-PCR assays, mRNA acts as a template for transcription of complementary DNA (cDNA) that is utilized as a template for subsequent PCR reactions. These reactions utilize assay-specific primers spanning the breakpoint of interest and thus will only yield a PCR product in the context of abnormal fusion transcripts.

The advent of technologies allowing real-time detection of PCR products has greatly facilitated the quantitative analysis of pathologic gene fusion transcripts seen in specific diseases. Although several technologies are available (see Chapter 47), oligonucleotide hydrolysis probes are commonly used for quantitative RT-PCR assays. The most important clinical application of quantitative RT-PCR is in minimal residual disease testing or disease monitoring. An important example is in the clinical diagnosis and management of chronic myelogeneous leukemia (Fig. 51.6). Routine molecular monitoring of response to TKI therapy in CML is the standard of care. Testing should be performed at diagnosis and periodically throughout the course of treatment. A three-log or greater reduction in *BCR-ABL1* transcript levels within 18 months of initiation of therapy is designated a major molecular response (MMR) and portends a high likelihood of a favorable long-term outcome.[55] Quantitative PCR assays, therefore, should be designed and validated with clinically important levels of sensitivity in mind.

POINTS TO REMEMBER

Recurrent Translocations and Structural Chromosomal Abnormalities

- Recurrent genetic abnormalities are those that are repeatedly found in different patients with the same or similar diseases.
- Recurrent translocations are common in mature B-cell non-Hodgkin lymphoma and prototypically involve immunoglobulin gene loci.
- Detection of balanced translocations and other abnormalities is crucial in the diagnosis and prognostication of acute leukemia and mature myeloid malignancies.
- Preferred detection methods vary depending on the specific genetic abnormality and clinical context (eg, FISH for diagnosis vs. quantitative RT-PCR for disease monitoring).
- Massively parallel sequencing may allow for more efficient detection of multiple translocations or large-scale genomic alterations, but technical challenges exist.

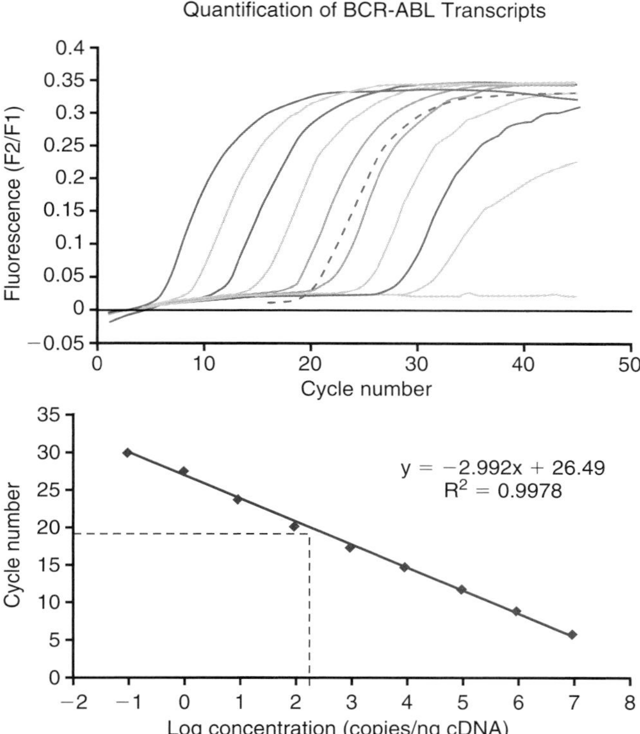

FIGURE 51.6 An example of quantitative reverse transcription PCR (RT-PCR) for enumeration of *BCR-ABL1* transcripts. The upper panel shows amplification curves for standards containing serial log dilutions of *BCR-ABL1* fusion transcripts ranging from 10^0 to 10^9 copies *(solid lines)* and an unknown patient sample *(dotted line)*. The lower panel shows the standard curve for the reaction that plots cycle number versus the log of the template concentration. The cycle threshold is then used to quantitate the *BCR-ABL1* transcript copy number (CN) in the patient sample. For normalization purposes, total *ABL1* transcripts can be analyzed separately in an identical fashion to generate a ratio of *BCR-ABL1* CN to *ABL1* CN referred to as the *normalized copy number* (NCN). The patient NCN can then be converted to the international standard scale (IS).

GENE MUTATIONS IN HEMATOPOIETIC MALIGNANCIES

This chapter is organized by genetic mechanism (translocations, single-gene mutations) and test methodology. For example, cytogenetics and FISH are used for translocations and copy number changes. SNP arrays unveil more cryptic cytogenetic abnormalities, including copy neutral loss of heterozygosity, and molecular studies are employed for targeted detection of abnormal gene fusions and single-gene abnormalities. However, in terms of biology and pathophysiology, such distinctions are artificial. Many different types of genetic abnormalities may be present in a neoplasm, in many cases acting in concert to promote the development and progression of the disease. This section covers gene mutations, including insertions, deletions, and single-nucleotide variants (SNVs), that occur across the spectrum of hematopoietic malignancies and that are not detectable by karyotyping or FISH-based assays but rather by molecular techniques such as PCR and sequencing. In some disorders, such mutations may be the only detectable genetic abnormality and are likely sufficient in and of themselves to promote development of the neoplasm (eg, *BRAF* Val600Glu and hairy cell leukemia). In other cases multiple single-gene mutations are present and may occur along with structural chromosomal abnormalities and/or translocations detectable by classical karyotyping or FISH (eg, myelodysplastic syndromes and acute myeloid leukemia) and with epigenetic changes that must be queried by yet additional testing modalities. In addition, copy number changes may be present and typically require additional, array-based technologies for detection. A comparison of these common testing strategies used to evaluate structural and focal genetic abnormalities in hematopoietic neoplasms is summarized in Table 51.3.

Mechanisms

Mutations can result from exposure to mutagenic agents (ie, ionizing radiation or chemotherapeutic agents) or randomly during the process of DNA replication during cell division. Thus mutation rates at any particular nucleotide position depend on a variety of factors, including nucleotide stability due to genome context (eg, homopolymer tracts or repetitive sequences) or chemical modification (eg, methylation), the error rate of DNA synthesis, and the accuracy and effectiveness of DNA repair mechanisms. Mutations may therefore leave a signature with clues about the original mechanism that resulted in the error.[56]

Mutations that correlate most closely with aging include C to T transition mutations that arise in CpG dinucleotides due to spontaneous deamination of 5-methylcytosine to thymine. Indeed, there is a positive correlation between the number of such mutations and the age of the patient at the time of cancer diagnosis.[56] Chemotherapeutic alkylating agents such as cyclophosphamide also have a characteristic mutation signature involving C to T mutations.[57] Interestingly, and perhaps not unexpectedly, there is also a positive correlation between the number of divisions of normal tissue stem cells and the rate of malignancies among tissue types.[58] This finding suggests that the majority of malignant processes, including those involving the hematopoietic system, are derived from the evolution of chance mutations that occur during the process of DNA replication and not from some environmental or toxic insult. Mutations that arise in a stem cell may be noncontributory to the process of malignant transformation. However, they remain a component of the malignant clone and are detectable if queried in an appropriate manner—for example, by whole genome sequencing. These have come to be known as "passenger" mutations and can sometimes be segregated from true disease "driver" mutations that occur in coding regions, at splice sites, or in RNA genes because they are not recurrent over large disease-specific patient cohorts. As more data are generated, the differentiation between passenger and driver will become easier.

Myeloid Diseases

Two landmark studies with very similar findings published in late 2014 offer important insight into the development of myeloid malignancies.[59,60] Both of these studies described an age-associated rate of mutation in genes known to be involved in myeloid cancers in older individuals who had no evidence of a hematopoietic malignancy. Both studies found that the mutations were primarily in the same three

TABLE 51.3 Testing Strategies Commonly Used to Evaluate Genetic Abnormalities in Hematopoietic Neoplasms

Testing Methodology	Pan-Genomic or Targeted	Sensitivity	Detection of Single Nucleotide Variants (SNVs)	Detection of Small Insertions and Deletions (<10^2 Base Pairs)	Detection of Copy Number Changes	Detection of Balanced Chromosomal Translocations	Detection of CN-LOH	Cost
Karyotyping by metaphase cytogenetics	Pan-genomic	Low	No	No	Yes	Yes	No	Moderate
FISH	Targeted	Low	No	No	Yes	Yes	No	Low
SNP arrays	Pan-genomic	Low	No	No	Yes	No	Yes	Moderate
Quantitative PCR techniques	Targeted	High	Yes	No	No	Yes	No	Low
Sanger sequencing	Targeted	Low	Yes	Yes	No	No	No	Low
Massively parallel sequencing mutation panels	Targeted	High	Yes	Yes	Yes/No*	Yes/No*	Yes/No*	Moderate
Whole genome sequencing	Pan-genomic	Low	Yes	Yes	Yes/No*	Yes/No*	Yes/No*	High

*Some bioinformatics pipelines have the capacity to detect copy number changes and chromosomal rearrangements if designed appropriately.

CN-LOH, Copy neutral loss of heterozygosity.

Modified from Nybakken GE, Bagg A. The genetic basis and expanding role of molecular analysis in the diagnosis, prognosis, and therapeutic design for myelodysplastic syndromes. J Mol Diagn 2014;16:145–58.

genes: *ASXL1, TET2,* and *DNMT3A.* Patients with mutations had an elevated risk for the subsequent development of a hematologic neoplasm.[59] The most common somatic variants were the C to T transition mutations that are typically associated with aging.[59] It has long been known that clonal hematopoiesis is a feature that is detectable in a subset of older individuals, and these studies provide further support for this observation. The implication of these studies is that these mutations are a part of a founding clone and, in and of themselves, are not sufficient to promote the development of an overt hematological malignancy but are predisposing to additional genetic abnormalities that eventually lead to clinical disease.

In myeloid cancers recurrent driver mutations tend to affect discrete cellular pathways and regulatory mechanisms. Although many genes tend to be recurrently mutated in specific myeloid malignancies, there is a large degree of overlap among the various disease entities and there are few, if any, true disease-defining mutations (Table 51.4). Generally the affected pathways may be classified into those involving signal transduction (eg, *JAK2, KIT, CSF3R, MPL, FLT3, CALR, PTPN11, NRAS/KRAS*), epigenetic modifiers (eg, *TET2, IDH1, IDH2, EZH2, DNMT3A*), the RNA splicing complex known as the spliceosome (*SF3B1, SRSF2, ZRSR2*), the cohesion complex involved in sister chromatid separation during meiosis and mitosis (*STAG2, RAD21*), myeloid transcription factors (*CEBPA, RUNX1*), and chromatin modifiers (*ASXL1, EZH2*). Some of these genes are more associated with specific histologically defined myeloid malignancies—for example, *FLT3* mutations and AML or *JAK2* mutations—and myeloproliferative neoplasms such as polycythemia vera, while others are found more widely across the spectrum of myeloid diseases—for example, *TET2* mutations. The order in which mutations arise also appears to have consequences with respect to the overall clinical and pathophysiologic features of a disease process. For example, patients with myeloproliferative neoplasms who acquire *JAK2* mutations prior to acquiring a *TET2* mutation are more likely to have erythrocytosis and have increased sensitivity to *JAK2* inhibitor therapies versus those patients who acquired *JAK2* mutations after a *TET2* mutation.[61]

Signal Transduction Pathways: Disease-Specific Signaling Mutations

Signal transduction pathways define cellular communication networks that allow cells to communicate with other cells and with the extracellular environment via cell surface receptors. These receptors are often linked to tyrosine and serine/threonine kinases that serve to propagate the message, ultimately to the nucleus where modulation of gene expression results in some change in cellular activity. Important pathways in myeloid malignancies include growth factor signaling pathways linked to JAK-STAT signaling and other cell surface receptors linked to the RAS-ERK (mitogen activated

TABLE 51.4 **Recurrently Mutated Genes in Myeloid Malignancies**

Gene	MPN	MDS	MDS/MPN	De novo AML	Secondary AML	Effect*
JAK2	++	−	+	−	−	Gain
MPL	+	−	−	−	−	Gain
CALR	++	−	+	−	−	Gain
FLT3	−	−	−	++	−	Gain
NPM1	−	−	+	++	−	Gain
CEBPA	−	−	−	+	−	Loss
RUNX1	−	+	++	+	−	Loss
KIT	+	−	−	+	−	Gain
CSF3R	+	−	+	−	−	Gain
DNMT3A	+	+	+	++	−	Loss
TET2	+	++	++	++	+	Loss
IDH1/2	+	+	+	++	+	Gain
SF3B1	−	+	+	−	+	Unknown
SRSF2	−	+	++	+	++	Unknown
STAG2	−	+	−	−	++	Loss
ASXL1	++	++	++	+	++	Unknown
EZH2	+	+	+	−	++	Loss
TP53	+	+	+	+	+	Loss

*Gain = gain of function. Loss = loss of function. − = rare (<2% to 3%). + = moderate frequency overall or high frequency in certain small defined subsets (eg, KIT mutations and systemic mastocytosis). ++ = high frequency overall (>~15%).

protein kinase; MAPK) pathway, among others. Thus, the mutations that occur in signaling pathways tend to affect tyrosine kinase mediated signal transduction and often result in constitutively active tyrosine kinases. Activating mutations like these tend to result from recurrent so-called "hot spots" often in regulatory or enzymatic (ie, tyrosine kinase) domains of these important signaling molecules.

JAK2

JAK2 is a protein tyrosine kinase that is mutated in MPNs, including nearly all cases of polycythemia vera and approximately half of cases of essential thrombocythemia and primary myelofibrosis. The most common *JAK2* mutation is c.1849G>T, p.Val617Phe, which occurs in the autoinhibitory pseudokinase (JH2) domain of *JAK2* and imparts dysregulated kinase activity. The JAK2 protein is a prominent component of JAK-STAT dependent growth factor signaling pathways, including those downstream of the erythropoietin (EPO) receptor (EPOR). In MPNs, this abnormality results in *JAK2*-mutated progenitor cells that are abnormally EPO independent. The phenomenon of EPO-independent progenitor cells in patients with polycythemia vera was well recognized many years prior to the discovery of the presence of activating *JAK2* mutations.[62] Frequently, homozygous *JAK2* mutations are present in neoplastic cells in MPNs and may be a result of loss of heterozygosity (LOH) due to mitotic recombination.[63] In fact, LOH had originally been observed at the *JAK2* locus at chromosome 9p prior to the identification of *JAK2* mutations. The observation of recurrent LOH at chromosome 9p prompted the original analysis of the genes located in this region, including *JAK2*.[64] The detection of a *JAK2* p.Val617Phe mutation is important in the workup of a patient suspected of having a myeloproliferative neoplasm and allows neoplasia to be distinguished from benign reactive-type disorders in the differential diagnosis.

When the *JAK2* p.Val617Phe mutation was discovered, there was an initial hope that therapeutic inhibition of JAK2 would produce results similar to those seen with the ABL1 kinase inhibitor imatinib in CML patients. However, the experience with JAK2 inhibitors has not been the panacea that was initially expected. The first JAK2 inhibitor approved in the United State was ruxolitinib, a selective oral inhibitor of JAK1 and JAK2. A series of trials in patients with myelofibrosis, including primary myelofibrosis, postessential thrombocythemia myelofibrosis, and postpolycythemia vera myelofibrosis showed that ruxolitinib reduced patient spleen size and improved the overall burden of symptoms but had uncertain benefits on survival.[65] In a more recent study in patients with polycythemia vera who had an inadequate response to standard treatment with hydroxyurea, ruxolitinib treatment demonstrated clear benefits in terms of disease symptoms and promoted a modest mean reduction in the *JAK2* p.Val617Phe mutant allele burden of −12.2% at 32 weeks of treatment.[66] Overall, it is clear that JAK2 inhibitor therapy markedly improves the quality of life of MPN patients, but, in contrast to the success of imatinib and other TKIs in CML patients, JAK2 inhibition may not improve overall survival rates in patients with MPNs.

KIT

KIT is a receptor protein tyrosine kinase expressed by hematopoietic progenitor cells. *KIT* mutations occur primarily in the tyrosine kinase domain. They are found in most cases of systemic mastocytosis, a MPN that manifests primarily as a mast cell expansion. Patients present with symptoms such as flushing and diarrhea from increased mast cells and their associated secretory products. *KIT* mutations are also found in a subset of cases of core binding factor (CBF) AML, which collectively includes cases with t(8;21)(q22;q22); *RUNX1-RUNX1T1* or inv(16)(p13.1;q22); *CBFB-MYH11* abnormalities, which both involve the same transcription factor complex. The most common *KIT* mutation in both AML and systemic mastocytosis is the *KIT* c. 2447A>T, p.Asp816Val mutation, which results in constitutive protein tyrosine kinase activity. *KIT* mutations may also be present in exon 8, the extracellular domain, and these are commonly in-frame insertions or deletions that also lead to constitutive activation of KIT receptor signaling. Cases of CBF-AML with *KIT* mutations have a higher risk of relapse, and these patients are considered intermediate risk compared to CBF AML cases without *KIT* mutations, which are considered low risk.[31] Because of this, testing for *KIT* mutations is the standard of care in those patients with CBF-AML and inv(16)(p13.1;q22); *CBFB-MYH11* or t(8;21)(q22;q22); *RUNX1-RUNX1T1* abnormalities. *KIT* mutations are also seen in nonhematopoietic malignancies such as melanoma and gastrointestinal stromal tumors (GIST), among others. Certain patients with *KIT*-mutated tumors—for example, GISTs—respond quite well to treatment with the TKI imatinib.[67] The small subset of systemic mastocytosis patients who lack a *KIT p.Asp816Val* mutation may also respond to imatinib, while those with the mutation are resistant.[68]

CSF3R

Activating mutations in the receptor for colony stimulating factor 3 (*CSF3R*) are present in most cases of chronic neutrophilic leukemia, a rare *BCR-ABL1*-negative expansion of mature granulocytes in blood and bone marrow without features of dysplasia.[69,70] *CSF3R* mutations have also been described in patients with atypical chronic myeloid leukemia, an MDS/MPN neoplasm with morphologic features distinct from those of chronic neutrophilic leukemia. However, some degree of controversy exists concerning the presence of *CSF3R* mutations in atypical chronic myeloid leukemia, and if strict criteria from the World Health Organization (WHO) classification system are applied, then *CSF3R* mutations appear much more specific for chronic neutrophilic leukemia.[70] Most mutations occur at codon 618 (p.Thr618Ile; sometimes annotated as p.Thr595Ile) in the membrane proximal extracellular domain and result in hyperactive signaling through the JAK-STAT pathway. Other membrane proximal mutations occur as well, albeit with lower frequencies. However, a significant subset of cases also have frameshift or nonsense mutations in the cytoplasmic domain of *CSF3R* that result in truncation of the CSF3R protein with enhanced signaling through other pathways such as those involving SRC kinases. These are identical to the *CSF3R* truncation mutations that are sometimes observed in patients with severe congenital neutropenia. This syndrome is frequently due to germline mutations in *ELANE*. The subsequent acquisition of somatic *CSF3R* mutations in these patients appears to herald progression to MDS or AML, an outcome for which these individuals are known to be at increased risk. Patients with membrane proximal *CSF3R* mutations and resultant hyperactive JAK-STAT signaling may respond best to treatment with a JAK inhibitor such as ruxolitinib, while those with truncating mutations appear to respond best to treatment with a SRC kinase inhibitor such as dasatinib.[71] In a small subset of cases of chronic neutrophilic leukemia and atypical chronic myeloid leukemia, *CSF3R* mutations may cooperate with mutations in the oncogene *SETBP1* to promote the development of the diseases. Stronger associations exist between *SETBP1* mutations and *ASXL1* mutations, which are very frequently found together in patients with MDS/MPN neoplasms.[72] Recurrent cooperating mutation pairs have been identified across the spectrum of myeloid malignancies and may yield insight into the resultant pathophysiology of the neoplastic cells.

FLT3

FLT3 encodes a receptor protein tyrosine kinase involved in the regulation of hematopoiesis. *FLT3* is one of the most frequently mutated genes in adult de novo AML, along with *NPM1* and *DNMT3A*,[73] and is associated with cytogenetically normal AML (CN-AML). In de novo AML, *FLT3* mutations are present in approximately 25% to 30% of cases.[73] *FLT3* mutations are also found frequently in AML with t(15;17)(q22;q12); *PML-RARA* and in AML with t(6;9)(p23;q34); *DEK-NUP214*.[74] Mutations in *FLT3* are most frequently internal tandem duplication (*FLT3*-ITD) mutations. These are in-frame insertions from three to hundreds of base pairs in length in the juxtamembrane domain (exon 14) that result in constitutive receptor activation. Point mutations also occur in exon 20 in the FLT3 tyrosine kinase domain (FLT3-TKD). These occur most commonly at position D835 (D835Y>D835H/V/E) and also result in constitutive receptor activation.[75] In spite of their apparent biological similarities, *FLT3*-ITD and *FLT3*–TKD mutations do not carry the same clinical significance. *FLT3*-ITD mutations are associated with poor outcome due to a very high likelihood of relapse after first remission. In addition, those patients with the highest *FLT3*-ITD mutant allele burdens (often referred to as a *FLT3*-ITD allelic ratio) do worse than those with lower levels, so testing strategies may be designed to assess mutant allele frequencies as well. Typically *FLT* allelic ratios are derived by capillary electrophoresis of amplicons from a PCR that spans the region. This is accomplished via a comparison of wild-type and mutant product relative fluorescence (Fig. 51.7). *FLT3*-TKD mutations are found in less than 10% of cases and do not appear to affect prognosis.[75] However, *FLT3*-TKD mutations may be a source of TKI resistance because certain point mutations interfere with TKI binding. *FLT3* mutations are known to be unstable. Patients without evidence of *FLT3*-ITD mutation at diagnosis may relapse with a clone carrying *FLT3*-ITD mutation and vice versa. This underscores the fact that leukemia clones present at relapse may differ substantially from the dominant clone that was initially present at diagnosis. The unstable nature of *FLT3* mutations in AML makes them less suitable for use as a minimal residual disease marker.

As monotherapy, FLT3 inhibition has shown only limited success in early phase clinical trials that have been conducted thus far in AML patients. Therefore current strategies are primarily focused on the addition of FLT3 inhibitors to the commonly used chemotherapeutic regimens. Combination therapies are being explored using the FLT3 inhibitors midostaurin, quizartinib, and others with some fairly promising early results.[76] However, to date, the optimum treatment for *FLT3*-ITD mutated AML remains early allogeneic stem cell transplantation during first remission before the almost inevitable relapse occurs.

CALR

In late 2013, two landmark studies were published showing that the majority of patients with essential thrombocythemia

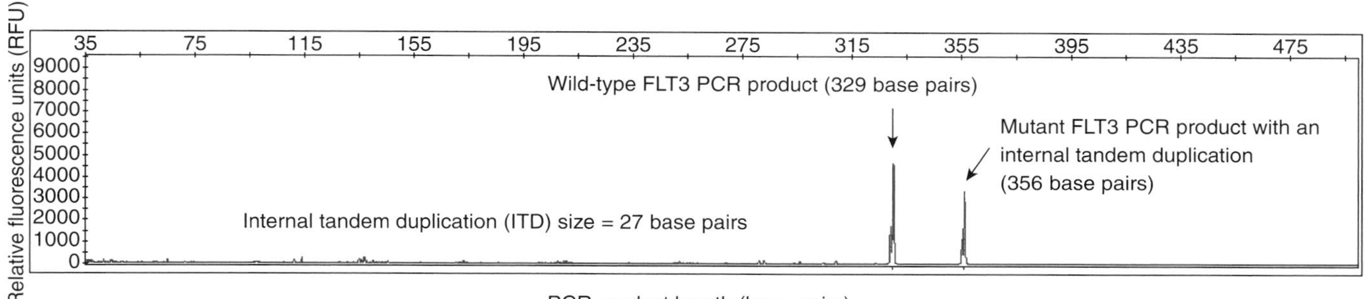

FIGURE 51.7 An example of results from a test for detection of *FLT3* internal tandem duplication (ITD) mutations. In this strategy, a DNA sample is subjected to PCR amplification using primers flanking the region of exon 14 where the insertions occur. The resulting amplicons are resolved by capillary electrophoresis. In this example, the wild-type *FLT3* PCR product is evident (329 base pairs) along with an abnormal *FLT3* amplicon of 356 base pairs representing an in-frame *FLT3* insertion (an internal tandem duplication) of 27 base pairs. A negative test result would demonstrate only the wild-type PCR fragment of 329 base pairs.

or primary myelofibrosis who lack *JAK2 p.Val617Phe* mutations have mutations in *CALR*.[77,78] *CALR* and *JAK2* mutations are mutually exclusive in patients with these diseases, and most of the remaining small subset of patients with essential thrombocythemia or primary myelofibrosis without *JAK2* or *CALR* mutations have mutations in *MPL*, the gene that encodes the receptor for thrombopoietin (TPO). A small subset of individuals lack *JAK2*, *CALR*, and *MPL* mutations and are known as "triple negative." *CALR* mutations are not seen in polycythemia vera patients, making the detection of *CALR* mutations useful for disease subclassification.

CALR encodes a protein, calreticulin, which appears to have multiple functions, including as a calcium-binding endoplasmic reticulum (ER) chaperone. Calreticulin has a C-terminal acidic domain with calcium binding motifs and an ER retention motif (the amino sequence is Lys-Asp-Glu-Leu). The *CALR* gene has 9 exons. *CALR* mutations are recurrent frameshifts in exon 9, most commonly a 52–base pair deletion (known as a type 1 variant) or a 5–base pair insertion (known as a type 2 variant). All *CALR* mutations demonstrate the same abnormal reading frame, shifted by 1 base pair. The mutations result in the production of an abnormal protein with a C-terminus that lacks the ER retention motif and that gains a novel 36 amino acid sequence with a basic, rather than acidic, charge.[77,79] There have been reports of *CALR* mutated myelofibrosis patients responding to treatment with JAK2 inhibitors, suggesting that JAK-STAT signaling is also important in *CALR*-mutated patients.[80] Individuals with primary myelofibrosis with *CALR* mutations appear to have a better prognosis than those with primary myelofibrosis with a *JAK2 p.Val617Phe* mutation or an *MPL* mutation.[81] Interestingly, primary myelofibrosis patients in the "triple negative" subgroup (negative for mutations in *CALR*, *JAK2*, and *MPL*), have the worst outcome.[81]

Mutations in Epigenetic Regulators

Mutations in genes that function in pathways involved in the epigenetic regulation of gene expression are extremely common and important across the spectrum of myeloid malignancies. Mutations result in aberrant function of several related mechanisms of epigenetic regulation. These include DNA methylation, DNA hydroxymethylation, histone modification via methylation and acetylation, metabolic pathways, and others.[82] The end result is abnormal epigenetic regulation and concomitant altered gene expression patterns that result in abnormal cellular differentiation and ultimately lead to the clinical manifestations of disease.

DNA methylation of the C-5 position of cytosine to form 5-methylcytosine in the context of CpG dinucleotides is a fundamentally important mechanism in the regulation of gene expression. Such CpG motifs are clustered in the genome into so-called CpG islands that tend to occur in gene promoter regions. The methylation of CpG islands within promoters results in repression of the expression of the associated downstream genes. In myeloid malignancies, there are recurrent and abnormal methylation patterns that have been observed as a result of aberrant function of genes involved in gene methylation.[83,84] Normally, CpG islands tend to be relatively hypomethylated. Conversely, in the context of many cancers, including myeloid malignancies, CpG islands are frequently found to be hypermethylated, particularly those that are associated with tumor suppressor genes. This mechanism serves to suppress their expression. Mutations in epigenetic regulators are common in AML, MDS, and MDS/MPN neoplasms, but are also occasionally seen in patients with MPNs. Four of the most commonly mutated genes in myeloid malignancies are involved in epigenetic regulatory functions: *DNMT3A*, *TET2*, *IDH1*, and *IDH2*.

DNMT3A

The *DNMT3A* gene encodes a DNA methyltransferase that participates in the de novo methylation of cytosines within CpG dinucleotides. Other closely related genes include *DNMT1*, which stabilizes methylation, and the methyltransferase *DNMT3B*. *DNMT3A* mutations are present in about 10% of cases of MDS and in 20% to 25% of cases of cytogenetically normal AML (CN-AML). The majority of mutations occur in a hotspot at Arg882 (approximately 60%) in the C-terminal methyltransferase domain, while frame-shift, nonsense, and splice-site mutations predicted to inactivate the gene account for most of the remainder of mutations identified.[84] Mutations at R882 result in reduced DNA methylation compared to the wild-type protein,[85] and the most common mutation at this codon, p.Arg882His, binds and inhibits wild-type *DNMT3A* in a dominant negative manner.[86] Thus the majority of mutations found in *DNMT3A* appear to suppress methyltransferase activity either through reduced expression of functional *DNMT3A* or by expression of a dominant negative form that binds and inactivates wild-type *DNMT3A* protein. In terms of prognostic significance, the findings for patients with *DNMT3A* mutations have been mixed. Many, but not all, studies have found a negative impact of mutated *DNMT3A* on outcome in AML patients.[84,87]

TET2

The *TET2* (ten-eleven translocation gene 2) gene encodes an alpha-ketoglutarate dependent 5-methylcytosine dioxygenase with an important role in demethylation of 5-methylcytosine. In myeloid neoplasms, acquired somatic mutations of *TET2* often result in loss of function of the TET2 protein and include frameshift, nonsense, and missense mutations throughout the coding sequence.[88] Somatic *TET2* mutations are found in patients with MPN, AML, and MDS/MPN neoplasms, such as chronic myelomonocytic leukemia.[83] The activity of wild-type TET2 protein results in the conversion of 5-methylcytosine to 5-hydroxymethylcytosine. The latter is subsequently converted to unmodified cytosine. In individuals with *TET2* loss-of-function mutations, there is a measurable loss of 5-hydroxymethylcytosine in genomic DNA from bone marrow cells, supporting a model where TET2 plays a critical role in the overall regulation of gene expression through the formation of 5-hydroxymethylcytosine.[89] Loss of heterozygosity has been frequently reported at the *TET2* locus at chromosome 4q24, including copy number neutral loss of heterozygosity as well as deletions, and this may result in homozygous or hemizygous mutations.[88] There is also evidence of multiple (biallelic) *TET2* mutations in patients with myeloid neoplasms, suggesting there is a selective advantage when both *TET2* alleles are mutated and inactivated in a neoplastic clone.[83] The observations of biallelic *TET2* loss-of-function mutations and loss of heterozygosity at chromosome 4q24 in *TET2*-mutated patients are evidence that *TET2* is a classic tumor suppressor gene.

IDH1 and *IDH2*

Mutations in the *IDH1* (isocitrate dehydrogenase 1) gene were originally detected in a whole genome sequencing study performed on a group of patients with AML.[90] In subsequent studies, mutations in *IDH2* (isocitrate dehydrogenase 2), the mitochondrial homologue of *IDH1*, were also found in other myeloid malignancies.[91] The mutations center on key arginine that resides in the catalytic sites of *IDH1* (Arg132) and *IDH2* (Arg140 and Arg172). In the Krebs cycle, isocitrate dehydrogenase coverts isocitrate to alpha-ketoglutarate. Mutations at Arg132 in *IDH1* or Arg140/Arg172 in *IDH2* confer novel (neomorphic) enzymatic activity that results in the formation of the oncometabolite 2-hydroxyglutarate rather than alpha-ketoglutarate (see Fig. 51.8 for a comparison of the structures of alpha-ketoglutarate and 2-hydroxyglutarate).[92,93] 2-Hydroxyglutarate accumulates and competitively inhibits alpha-ketoglutarate-dependent dioxygenases, including *TET2*, in affected individuals.[94] Thus *IDH1/IDH2* mutations impair TET2 enzymatic function. As such, mutations in *IDH1/IDH2* and *TET2* tend to be mutually exclusive in myeloid malignancies.

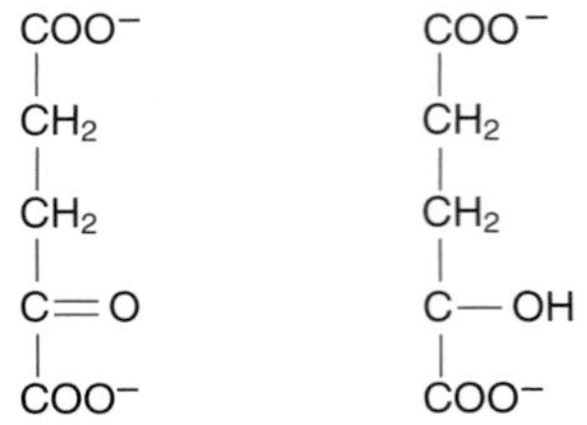

COO^- – CH_2 – CH_2 – C=O – COO^-

alpha-ketoglutarate

COO^- – CH_2 – CH_2 – C–OH – COO^-

2-hydroxyglutarate

FIGURE 51.8 Structures of alpha-ketoglutarate and 2-hydroxyglutarate.

Cases with *TET2* or *IDH1/IDH2* mutations display similar epigenetic abnormalities characterized by histone and DNA hypermethylation.[94] *IDH1/IDH2* mutations are found most frequently in patients with cytogenetically normal AML but are also seen to a lesser degree in cases of MDS and in MDS/MPN neoplasms.[95] Selective inhibitors of mutated *IDH1/IDH2* reverse the abnormal histone and DNA hypermethylation, and thus inhibition of mutant forms of isocitrate dehydrogenase is potentially a promising pharmacotherapeutic strategy.[96] An oral inhibitor of mutant IDH2 appears particularly effective at inducing differentiation and ultimately clearance of leukemic blasts in *IDH2*-mutated AML patients and may obviate the need for highly toxic chemotherapy regimens in these patients.[96] *IDH1* and *IDH2* mutations have also been identified in nonmyeloid hematopoietic malignancies, including T cell lymphoma and in nonhematopoietic tumors, including many gliomas.

Mutations in the RNA Spliceosome

The RNA spliceosome is a large multimeric protein/RNA complex that functions to remove introns and ligate exons from immature precursor messenger RNA (mRNA), resulting in the formation of mature mRNA transcripts. For many genes, multiple possible normal splice variants may be created with sometimes differing functions. Mutations in components of the spliceosome are quite common in myeloid malignancies, particularly in cases of MDS or AML that developed from MDS or MPN (so-called secondary AML). Spliceosome mutations are uncommon in de novo AML and MPNs that have not progressed to AML. Spliceosome mutations have also been identified in lymphoid malignancies, primarily in chronic lymphocytic leukemia and almost always in the gene *SF3B1*. In myeloid cancers, the most commonly mutated spliceosome components include *SF3B1*, *SRSF2*, *U2AF1*, and *ZRSR2*.[97] Mutations in *SF3B1* are found in the majority of cases of MDS with ring sideroblasts.[98,99] Ring sideroblasts are abnormal erythroblasts with iron-containing mitochondria present in a ring pattern that are visible on an iron-stained bone marrow aspirate sample. This observation highlights an important genotype-phenotype association. Although the mechanistic reason for the presence of ring sideroblasts in cases with *SF3B1* mutations is unclear, it correlates to *SF3B1* haploinsufficiency.[100] Cases of MDS with *SF3B1* mutations have a better prognosis with lower risk of AML progression compared to cases of MDS without *SF3B1* mutations.[99] Conversely, MDS patients with mutations in *SRSF2* demonstrate adverse outcome with more rapid progression to AML.[101] Almost half of cases of chronic myelomonocytic leukemia demonstrate mutations in *SRSF2*, and some have mutations in *ZRSR2*.[102,103] Mutations in *SRSF2* most commonly are missense variants affecting codon Pro95 and include p.Pro95His, p.Pro95Leu, and p.Pro95Arg.[102] Mutations in *SF3B1* are most commonly missense variants affecting codon Lys700 (p.Lys700Glu), as well as missense variants affecting codons Glu622, Arg625, His662, and Lys666.[98]

As these patterns suggest, spliceosome mutations do not appear to be simple loss-of-function mutations but rather are hypothesized to change the nature of the splice variants that are generated. Missplicing of pre-mRNA can change the ratio of physiologic splice variants or may lead to the generation of new, abnormal splice variants lacking certain exons, a process known as exon skipping. In the context of *U2AF1* mutations in myeloid neoplasms, distinct patterns of missplicing were observed in functionally related genes, including those involved in regulation of the cell cycle.[104] However, the identity and nature of most splice variants that result from spliceosome mutations are unknown. Spliceosome mutations are not generally seen in pairs but do coexist with nonspliceosomal mutations, commonly with *TET2*.[105]

Mutations in the Cohesin Complex

The cohesin complex is a multimeric protein structure involved in critical genetic regulatory mechanisms, including the segregation of sister chromatids during cell division and the regulation of gene expression. It is composed of four core subunits encoded by the genes: *SMC1*, *SMC3*, *STAG2*, and *RAD21*. Overall, somatic cohesin mutations are seen in approximately 12% of patients with myeloid malignancies and appear most commonly in AML.[106,107] Cohesin mutations are mutually exclusive but may cooccur with other mutations common in AML, including in *NPM1*, *RUNX1*, and *RAS*.[107] Mutations in *STAG2* are often nonsense or frameshift variants that likely result in loss of function, while missense mutations are typical for the other cohesion components.[108] The functional role for cohesin mutations in leukemogenesis is unclear but likely involves alterations in gene expression patterns. MDS patients with cohesin mutations have a worse overall survival compared to MDS patients without cohesin mutations.[107]

Mutations in Myeloid Transcription Factors and Chromatin Modifiers

The transcription factor CCAAT/enhancer binding protein-alpha (*CEBPA*) is critical for expression of myeloid-specific genes and for the repression of proliferation, both of which are necessary for the differentiation of myeloid lineage cells. *CEBPA* expression is highest in differentiated myeloid cells and lowest in hematopoietic progenitor cells.[109] *CEBPA* is an intronless gene approximately 1 kilobase in length with a basic leucine zipper domain (bZIP), which is important for DNA binding at promoter regions, and two N-terminal transactivation (TAD) domains, which are important for protein-protein binding. *CEBPA* can be alternatively transcribed into a long isoform (p42) and a short isoform (p30). The latter lacks the two N-terminal transactivation domains. These two isoforms are translated into proteins with slightly different functions.[110] In AML patients, the mutations are often biallelic in nature. Frequently, individuals with biallelic somatic *CEBPA* mutations demonstrate an N-terminal mutation at one of the TAD domains in one allele and a second bZIP domain mutation in the other allele.[111] *CEBPA* mutations are most commonly seen in normal karyotype AML patients and are associated with good prognosis, but only in those patients with biallelic mutations representing approximately 5% of cases.[112] Germline *CEBPA* mutations are a cause of congenital forms of AML that arise when a second somatic *CEBPA* mutation is acquired in an individual with a single germline mutation.[113]

RUNX1 (runt-related transcription factor -1) is a heterodimeric transcription factor important for hematopoietic cell differentiation and maintenance. Translocations involving the *RUNX1* gene are relatively common in myeloid malignancies and include t(8;21)(q22;q22); *RUNX1-RUNX1T1* and t(3;21)(q26;q22); *EVI1-RUNX1*. In ALL, t(12;21)(p13;q22); *ETV6-RUNX1* is found. *RUNX1* copy number alterations and gene mutations also contribute to the pathogenesis of hematopoietic malignancies. The RUNX1 protein contains an evolutionarily conserved runt-domain, which is important for DNA binding and heterodimerization. Mutations involving *RUNX1* predominantly occur in the runt domain and disrupt *RUNX1* function and include frameshift, nonsense, and missense variants. *RUNX1* mutations are observed in patients with AML, MDS, and chronic myelomonocytic leukemia. Patients with AML with mutated *RUNX1* have shorter survival and tend to display resistance to chemotherapy.[114]

Polycomb group proteins are critical, evolutionarily conserved epigenetic regulators first discovered in *Drosophila melanogaster* (fruit flies). They are involved in histone modification and chromatin remodeling, and their activity results in gene silencing. They function within multiprotein transcriptional-repressive complexes. Two of the major complexes are known as polycomb repressive complex 1 and 2 (PRC1 and PRC2). PRC1 and PRC2 act together but have distinct biochemical roles. *ASXL1* is one polycomb group gene commonly mutated in myeloid malignancies. Mutations in exon 12 of *ASXL1* are found across the spectrum of myeloid malignancies with frequencies from approximately 5% in de novo AML to almost 40% in chronic myelomonocytic leukemia.[115] *ASXL1* mutations are also common in individuals with primary myelofibrosis and are associated with worse outcome in these patients.[116] In fact, *ASXL1* mutations appear to predict worse outcome across all myeloid neoplasms.[115,117,118] The exact biologic functions of *ASXL1* remain unclear, but it may regulate histone H3 lysine 27 (H3K27) methylation status, which influences chromatin structure. It also interacts with a variety of other polycomb complex proteins, including *EZH2* and *SUZ12*. *ASXL1* may be responsible for recruitment and localization of this complex to certain important regions of the genome such as *HOXA* genes.[119] *ASXL1* mutations appear to be primarily localized to the last exon (exon 12) and result in production of an abnormal truncated protein product. It is unclear if these mutations are simple loss-of-function mutations, if they are dominant negative, or if loss of the C-terminus results in a gain-of-function by the truncated protein. The most frequently encountered mutation is a duplication of a nucleotide in a homopolymer track consisting of an 8–base pair guanine repeat (c.1943dupG), resulting in a frameshift initially thought to be a PCR artifact,[120] but that is now accepted as a true somatic variant located in a mutation hot-spot. *ASXL1* mutations are commonly seen together with mutations in *SETBP1* in patients with MDS/MPN.[72]

EZH2 and *SUZ12* are a part of the polycomb repressive complex 2 (PRC2), the activity of which is modified by *ASXL1*. PRC2 is involved in the repression of gene expression via trimethylation of histone H3K27. *EZH2* is a H3K27 histone methyltransferase that is also found mutated in myeloid malignancies. *EZH2* mutations appear to be true loss-of-function variants resulting from deletion, nonsense, and frameshift-type mutations. Such mutations result in enhanced expression of genes epigenetically regulated by *EZH2*.[121] *EZH2* mutations are most common in patients with primary myelofibrosis.[122,123] Patients with primary myelofibrosis with *EZH2* mutations have higher leukocyte counts, higher blast counts, larger spleens, and reduced overall survival.[124] The functional consequence of mutated *EZH2* in myeloid cancers stands in contrast to the observation of *EZH2* mutations in B-cell lymphoma, where they are primarily gain-of-function variants (see below). This contrast highlights the importance of lineage context in the pathophysiology of these complex genetic regulatory pathways.

TP53

The tumor suppressor p53 regulates a variety of critical anticancer functions and is nicknamed the "guardian of the genome." Its functions include regulation of cell cycle entry and exit at various checkpoints, maintenance of cellular senescence, modulation of autophagy, and control of apoptosis.[125] Patients with germline *TP53* mutations (Li-Fraumeni syndrome) have a very high risk for the development of cancers, often sarcoma or breast cancer. In general, dysregulation of p53-dependent signaling networks is a common feature of aggressive malignancies, including those of the hematopoietic system. Genetic abnormalities that result in loss of p53 activity include chromosomal deletions of the *TP53* gene locus on chromosome 17 (17p), loss of function mutations in the *TP53* gene, and epigenetic suppression of *TP53* expression. The presence of del17p or *TP53* mutations is strongly associated with poor prognosis in cancer patients.

In myeloid malignancies, *TP53* mutations are seen most frequently in patients with AML, MDS, and primary myelofibrosis. *TP53* mutations are loss-of-function variants, including insertions, deletions, nonsense mutations, and splice site mutations that result in the production of truncated protein products. In AML, *TP53* mutations are commonly associated with complex (three or more) karyotypic abnormalities.[126] AML patients with both complex karyotypes and *TP53* mutations have an extremely poor prognosis.[126] *TP53* mutations are commonly seen in a subtype of myeloid cancer that develops following exposure to cytotoxic chemotherapy for another malignancy called therapy-related AML (tAML) or therapy-related MDS (tMDS), depending on the blast count at diagnosis, although this distinction has little prognostic significance. The myeloid clones that expand following chemotherapy represent rare hematopoietic stem and progenitor cells (HSPCs) with age-related *TP53* mutations, rather than newly induced *TP53* mutated clones.[127]

NPM1

NPM1 (nucleophosmin) is a multifunctional nucleolar phosphoprotein that continuously shuttles between the nucleus and the cytoplasm. Mutations in the *NPM1* gene are quite common in AML patients and are seen in approximately 50% to 60% of cases of normal karyotype AML, making it one of the most common genetic abnormalities in this disease. Mutations in *NPM1* are found in exon 11 (formerly known as exon 12) and are characteristically tetranucleotide insertions. The most common insertion is a TCTG duplication termed *type A*. The mutation results in abnormal accumulation of mutated *NPM1* protein in the cytoplasm. The finding of abnormal cytoplasmic staining for *NPM1* by immunohistochemistry is a surrogate method that may be used to detect *NPM1* mutations in formalin fixed paraffin embedded tissue.[128] The mutations are almost always heterozygous and appear to act in a dominant negative fashion. They are usually stable at relapse (ie, present at relapse if they were present at diagnosis) and can be used as a marker for the presence of minimal residual disease in posttreatment follow-up samples.[129] *NPM1* mutations are associated with favorable prognosis in acute myeloid leukemia patients who do not have coexisting *FLT3*-internal tandem duplication mutations.[130]

Lymphoid Diseases

Whereas myeloid neoplasms tend to have overlapping mutation profiles with fewer disease-specific mutations, the somatic mutations found in lymphoid disorders are slightly more disease specific, although significant overlap still exists, particularly in T cell lymphoproliferative disorders. Due to this, the discussion of mutations in lymphoid neoplasms is structured by disease rather than by pathway. In addition, the pathophysiology of certain lymphoproliferative disorders is driven much more by the presence of specific translocations rather than single-gene mutations—for example, follicular lymphoma and the t(14;18)(q32;q21); *IGH-BCL2* translocation. The focus in this section is on those disorders where single-gene mutations, rather than balanced translocations, are of central importance with clearcut diagnostic, therapeutic, and/or prognostic significance.

Mature B-Cell Lymphoproliferative Disorders

The spectrum of B-cell lymphoproliferative disorders runs the gamut from those that are relatively indolent and typically incurable, such as chronic lymphocytic leukemia (CLL), to those with a much higher proliferative rate that can be quite aggressive but that may also be cured in certain circumstances, including diffuse large B-cell lymphoma (DLBCL) and Burkitt lymphoma. New therapeutic options are needed for many of these disorders, and the somatic mutations discussed are the targets for much of these efforts. The morphologic and histopathologic subclassification of these diseases are not discussed in detail here.

One theme that is applicable to many types of B cell lymphoproliferative disorders is that they often have dysregulated activation of the B cell receptor (BCR) signaling pathway and thus may be susceptible to inhibitors of BCR signaling, including those targeting Bruton's tyrosine kinase (BTK) or phosphatidylinositide 3-kinase (PI3K). In addition to somatic mutations, other mechanisms may promote inappropriate BCR signaling, including chronic antigenic stimulation by certain microorganisms—for example, *Helicobacter pylori* infection and the development of gastric extranodal marginal zone B cell lymphoma of mucosa-associated lymphoid tissue (MALT lymphoma). Thus both intrinsic and extrinsic activators of the BCR pathway may promote the development of these diseases.

Hairy Cell Leukemia

Hairy cell leukemia is an indolent B cell lymphoproliferative disorder typically diagnosed based on immunophenotypic findings assessed by flow cytometry and/or immunohistochemistry along with characteristic neoplastic cells with "hairy" cytoplasmic projections. Although the diagnosis is typically straightforward based on the clinical and laboratory findings, there are occasional cases that can cause diagnostic difficulty. For these cases, identification of the presence of the *BRAF* p.Val600Glu mutation is diagnostically important. *BRAF* p.Val600Glu mutations are present in nearly all cases of classic hairy cell leukemia and absent in other B cell lymphoproliferative disorders, including those that may cause diagnostic confusion with hairy cell leukemia.[131] The mutation promotes constitutive signaling through the MEK-ERK pathway, downstream of RAS, as demonstrated by high levels of phosphorylated (activated) ERK in the leukemia cells.[132] BRAF inhibitor therapies are available and have been used with some success in other tumors with BRAF-activating mutations such as melanoma. In patients with hairy cell leukemia, combined BRAF and MEK inhibition appears effective at inducing apoptosis in the leukemic cells and thus offers another treatment option for hairy cell leukemia patients who fail or are intolerant to other therapies currently in use.[133]

Lymphoplasmacytic Lymphoma

Lymphoplasmacytic lymphoma is a low-grade B cell lymphoproliferative disorder with plasmacytoid morphology and commonly associated with an immunoglobulin-M (IgM) monoclonal protein and hyperviscosity due to increased serum protein levels. The combination of an IgM monoclonal protein and hyperviscosity constitutes a clinical syndrome known as Waldenstrom macroglobulinemia. Most cases of lymphoplasmacytic lymphoma (approximately 90%) carry an activating mutation (usually, p.Leu265Pro) in *MYD88* (myeloid differentiation factor 88) that encodes an adapter protein in the Toll-like receptor (TLR) signaling pathway that affects the innate immune response to bacterial pathogens.[134] Wild-type MYD88 protein promotes the assembly of a multimeric complex with the serine-threonine kinase interleukin-1 receptor–associated kinase 4 (IRAK-4). The complex activates IRAK-1 and IRAK-2, ultimately leading to activation of nuclear factor-kappa B (NF-κβ). *MYD88* p.Leu265Pro mutations occur in an important domain (Toll-Interleukin 1 receptor; TIR) that functions in oligomerization/homodimerization with other TIR domains. The presence of *MYD88* p.Leu265Pro enhances the formation of MYD88-dependent signaling complexes, resulting in abnormal activation of NF-KB signaling. This appears to require signaling through BTK.[135] In support of a role for BTK in *MYD88* p.Leu265Pro signaling, a therapeutic inhibitor of BTK (ibrutinib) induces killing of lymphoplasmacytic lymphoma cells in vitro.[135] This observation served as the rationale for testing the efficacy of ibrutinib in patients with lymphoplasmacytic lymphoma, and early results have been encouraging.[136]

Diffuse Large B Cell Lymphoma

Diffuse large B cell lymphoma (DLBCL) is an aggressive lymphoma of large B cells that may be classified into various subtypes based on histopathologic and clinical findings. The subtypes include primary DLBCL of the CNS, T cell/histiocyte-rich large B cell lymphoma, Epstein-Barr virus (EBV) positive DLBCL, and DLBCL, not otherwise specified (NOS). DLBCL, NOS may be further segregated into activated B cell–type (ABC) and germinal center B cell (GCB)–type based on gene expression profiling or, more commonly in clinical practice, by expression of surrogate markers by immunohistochemistry.[137] Here again, BCR signaling may be important in the disease, and BCR pathway mutations appear particularly relevant to the pathogenesis of ABC-DLBCL. The B cell receptor comprises surface immunoglobulin (Ig) associated with the signaling molecules CD79a and CD79b, which contain signaling motifs in their intracellular domains called immunoreceptor tyrosine–based activating motifs (ITAMs). ITAMs are paired canonical tyrosine–containing sequences (YXXL/I; where X is any amino acid) separated by six to eight amino acids. Somatic mutations affecting the ITAMs of CD79a and CD79b have been identified in ABC-DLBCL cell lines and patient samples. The mutations increase expression of surface B cell receptors and attenuate negative regulatory mechanisms, thus enhancing BCR signaling.[138] The mutations that occur in the first tyrosine residue of the ITAM result in the maintenance of surface B cell receptor expression, even under chronic active stimulating conditions, that otherwise, in normal cells, leads to downregulation of receptor expression and concomitant decreased cellular activation.[138] *CD79B* mutations, along with mutations in *MYD88*, are more frequent in ABC-type DLBCL, whereas mutations in *EZH2* are more frequent in GCB-type DLBCL.[139] In DLBCL, *EZH2* mutations (primarily at codon Y641 and at codon A677) result in a gain of function, and samples harboring the mutations display increased levels of histone H3K27 trimethylation.[140,141] As pointed out previously, this is in contrast to the loss-of-function variants observed in myeloid malignancies. EZH2 inhibitor drugs are being tested in early-stage clinical trials in patients with *EZH2* mutated B-cell lymphomas.

Chronic Lymphocytic Leukemia

Chronic lymphocytic leukemia (CLL) is a B cell lymphoproliferative disorder of small, mature B cells that have an immunophenotype characterized by expression of pan B cell markers along with CD23, aberrant expression of CD5, and a restricted pattern of immunoglobulin light chain expression. Many prognostic markers have been described, most of which are not discussed in detail here. A few of the more important prognostic markers include *IGH* variable segment somatic hypermutation status (unmutated correlates with poor outcome), ZAP70 protein expression (positivity correlates with poor outcome), and cytogenetic findings (del17p and del11q correlate with poor outcome). Numerous single-gene mutations have recently been identified in CLL, some of which appear to have important prognostic significance. These include mutations in *NOTCH1, MYD88, BIRC3, TP53,* and *SF3B1*. In terms of prognostic significance, mutations in *TP53* and *SF3B1* are independently associated with poor outcome.[142] The poor prognostic outcome observed in *SF3B1*-mutated CLL patients is in contrast to *SF3B1*-mutated MDS patients who appear to have a more favorable outcome. The mechanistic role of *SF3B1* mutations in CLL is unclear but likely involves the production of abnormal mRNA splice variants.

Mature T and NK Cell Lymphoproliferative Disorders

Similar to mature B cell lymphoproliferative disorders, T and NK cell lymphoproliferative disorders include indolent disorders such as T cell large granular lymphocyte (LGL) leukemia, which can be difficult to distinguish from a reactive process, to aggressive disorders such as peripheral T cell lymphoma. It also includes neoplasms in which viral infection plays a significant etiologic role. These include adult T cell leukemia/lymphoma, in which human T cell leukemia virus type-1 (HTLV-1) infection is causative, and extranodal NK/T cell lymphoma, where EBV is universally present in a clonally integrated state in the neoplastic cells. In terms of somatic single-gene mutations and affected pathways, aberrant JAK-STAT pathway signal transduction is very commonly involved in the pathogenesis.

T cell LGL leukemia is a rare clonal disorder of cytotoxic T cells that typically does not progress but that can be associated with severe cytopenias that may themselves be a cause of significant morbidity. A significant subset of these patients (approximately 40%) demonstrate acquired somatic mutations in the signal transducer and activator of transcription 3 *(STAT3)* gene, which encodes a transcription factor important for cytokine and growth factor signaling that is downstream of JAK kinases in various signaling pathways.[143] *STAT3* mutations are located in an important signaling domain called the src homology 2 (SH2) domain that promotes homodimerization by mediating binding to tyrosine phosphorylated STAT3 monomers. *STAT3* mutations lead to inappropriate STAT3 dimerization, phosphorylation, and translocation to the nucleus and increased transcription of STAT3 gene targets in the leukemia cells. Other LGL leukemia patients with wild-type *STAT3* may demonstrate similar SH2 domain mutations in the *STAT5* gene or in genes that influence STAT mediated signaling.[144,145] Dysregulated JAK-STAT signaling is critically important across the spectrum of T-cell lymphoproliferative disorders. Gain-of-function mutations in *JAK2* and *STAT3* have been observed in angioimmunoblastic T cell lymphoma, an aggressive peripheral T cell lymphoma primarily seen in older individuals.[146] Similarly, mutually exclusive gain-of-function mutations in *JAK1*, *JAK3,* and *STAT5B* have been identified in T cell prolymphocytic leukemia (T-PLL), an aggressive T-cell leukemia that frequently demonstrates translocations involving *TCL1* or *MTCP1*.[147] T-PLL may also demonstrate mutations in *IL2RG*, encoding the common gamma chain important for signaling from the IL2 and other cytokine receptors. *IL2RG* mutations in T-PLL also upregulate of JAK-STAT signaling in the leukemia cells.[147] Thus T-PLL appears to arise as a result of the combined effects of the common translocations acting in concert with gene mutations that activate JAK-STAT signaling.

B/T Lymphoblastic Leukemia/Lymphoma

Lymphoblastic leukemia is a neoplasm of immature lymphoid progenitor cells typically displaying evidence of B- or T-lymphoid differentiation. As discussed, B-lymphoblastic leukemias are subclassified on the presence of discrete recurrent cytogenetic abnormalities such as translocations or hypodiploidy or hyperdiploidy. As outlined in the "Recurrent Translocations and Structural Chromosomal Abnormalities" section, the detection of these abnormalities has prognostic significance. Copy number changes and gene mutations not detectable by karyotyping or FISH are also present in cases of lymphoblastic leukemia, and these may provide additional clinically important information. The commonly affected genes are those important for lymphoid differentiation, maturation, and signaling, including *IKZF1*, *NOTCH1*, *PAX5*, and *PTEN1*. However, copy number changes at these loci, rather than gene mutations, appear to be the most common mechanism. *IKZF1* codes for a transcription factor that is important in the development of lymphoid lineage cells and is a tumor suppressor that is frequently deleted in cases of B-lymphoblastic leukemia, including most cases of B-lymphoblastic leukemia with t(9;22)(q34;q11.2); *BCR-ABL1*. *IKZF* deletions include complete loss due to structural abnormalities of chromosome 7 (the gene is located at chromosome 7p), kilobase scale deletions involving *IKZF* (often exons 4-7), and, finally, frameshift, missense, and nonsense mutations.[148] The genetic abnormalities affecting *IKZF* highlight the complexity of testing that is required for analysis. The different types of abnormalities affecting *IKZF* collectively require metaphase cytogenetics, FISH, array-based copy number analysis, and molecular techniques for comprehensive coverage. Detection may be clinically important because *IKZF* abnormalities are associated with poor prognosis of patients with B-lymphoblastic leukemia.

Acquired Drug Resistance Mutations

Patients with either CML or Ph+ lymphoblastic leukemia are treated with ABL1 TKIs. These include the first-generation TKI (imatinib), second-generation TKIs (dasatinib and nilotinib), or third-generation TKIs (bosutinib and ponatinib). A subset of patients may develop acquired mutations in the tyrosine kinase domain of *ABL1* that impede drug binding. When this occurs, patients will manifest signs of resistance typically evident in rising levels of *BCR-ABL1* transcripts detected by a routine quantitative RT-PCR. Many mutations have been identified, and dozens are recurrent across the spectrum of patients treated with TKIs. The identification of one or more mutations is important for clinical treatment because the sensitivity of *BCR-ABL1* to the available TKIs differs depending on which mutation is present. For example, patients who develop imatinib resistance due to the emergence of a clone harboring an *ABL1* p.Tyr253His mutation would also be relatively resistant to treatment with the second-generation TKI nilotinib but sensitive to treatment with the second-generation TKI dasatinib. However, mutations at the so-called gatekeeper residue Thr315, most commonly a p.Thr315Ile mutation, result in resistance to all but one of the currently approved therapies (ponatinib).

In a subset of patients, particularly those who have been treated with multiple sequential TKIs, more than one mutation may arise in the same clone (ie, on the same *BCR-ABL1* allele). These are commonly referred to as compound mutations, and they may impart resistance profiles that differ substantially from those seen when either mutation alone is present. Certain compound mutations, such as p.Glu255Val with p.Thr315Ile, display resistance to ponatinib, whereas either mutation occurring alone does not.[149] The compound mutations that have been identified in patients tend to center around a dozen or so key residues that are frequently found mutated alone.[149] Thus the typical sequence of events in the development of a compound mutation is likely similar in most patients. First, the acquisition and outgrowth of an initial single mutation (X) in a key residue occurs. This is followed by the acquisition of a second mutation (Y) in a clone harboring mutation X, thereby generating a new clone with two mutations (X + Y). At this time, both clone X and clone X + Y coexist in the patient, although clone X + Y may quickly dominate due to enhanced resistance properties. Strategies for analyzing and evaluating the complex clonal architecture in patients with *BCR-ABL1*-positive leukemias who have developed resistance mutations are often imperfect. Sanger sequencing is not typically useful because the data generated consist of a mixture of sequences and clonal relationships are mostly lost. Other techniques, such as massively parallel sequencing, offer more promise because the sequence data comprises single-molecule sequences and not mixtures, and therefore the clonal architecture is retained.[48]

Acquired resistance mutations also occur in patients with CLL who have undergone therapy with the BTK inhibitor, ibrutinib. A *BTK* p.Cys481Ser mutation has been seen in multiple patients. This mutation decreases the affinity of ibrutinib for BTK and reduces its ability to inhibit BTK tyrosine kinase activity. It also renders inhibition reversible instead of the irreversible inhibition seen with wild-type *BTK*.[150] Mutations have also been observed in PLCγ2 *(PLCG2)*, a downstream effector of BTK. These mutations likely circumvent ibrutinib-induced inhibition of BTK by leading to constitutive activation of PLCγ2 through gain of function and BTK-independent activation of B cell receptor signaling pathways.[150] The mutations include *PLCG2* p.Arg665Trp and p.Leu845Phe.

Laboratory Techniques for the Detection of Single-Gene Variants

The clinically important variants outlined in this section include highly recurrent single nucleotide variants such as *JAK2* c.1849G>T, p.Val617Phe or *IDH1* c.394C>T, p. Arg132Cys, and more complex insertions or deletions that may result in a frameshift and lead to loss of function and that are not as recurrent. When deciding which type of testing strategy to use for a particular gene, many factors must be considered (see Table 51.3). These include the nature of the targeted variants (ie, single nucleotide variants vs. insertions and deletions); performance characteristics, including test sensitivity and precision, cost, throughput, and ease of interpretation; and the type of result desired (qualitative vs. quantitative). For example, in the context of a test for a recurrent single nucleotide variant that is used as a marker of response to a targeted therapy, it would be desirable to employ a strategy that is highly sensitive and quantitative with a very narrow focus—for example, allele-specific PCR. This strategy would likely result in the ability to detect specific single nucleotide variants down to an allele frequency of less than 1%. On the other hand, the strategy chosen for detection of loss-of-function mutations that result from various insertions or deletions occurring throughout a single or perhaps in multiple exons of a gene would likely be relatively insensitive but have much broader coverage. An example would be a test such as Sanger sequencing that typically has a comparatively poor sensitivity of approximately 10% to 20% variant allele frequency. Sensitivity is critically important for somatic mutation testing in hematopoietic disorders because there is almost always a variable degree of normal background polyclonal hematopoiesis that serves to dilute signals from the abnormal variant(s). Mutation-specific antibodies have also been developed for certain common, recurrent missense mutations that result in the production of an abnormal protein product. Many are quite specific when used in the appropriate context. For example, antibodies to IDH1 p.Arg132His are available and may be less expensive than molecular methods.[151]

Massively Parallel Sequencing for Somatic Variants in Hematopoietic Malignancies

Massively parallel sequencing (also known as next-generation sequencing or NGS) as a testing strategy is becoming more commonplace in the clinical hematology laboratory and offers numerous advantages to traditional techniques. Currently, panel-based testing, rather than whole exome or whole genome sequencing, is most frequently utilized in the clinical laboratory. Such panels combine a relatively small number of gene targets, at least compared to the breadth of sequence covered by whole genome or whole exome sequencing. Panels are composed of genes that are recurrently mutated in a particular disease or class of disease. For example, a panel comprising a few dozen genes frequently mutated in myeloid malignancies is a strategy currently employed by a variety of clinical laboratories. To enhance the representation of specific gene targets for sequencing, PCR- or hybrid capture–based enrichment is commonly employed. The end result is very high coverage (usually greater than 1000×) of a clinically important set of targets. This degree of coverage depth yields test sensitivities that may be as low as 1% to 2% variant allele frequency, far better than what is possible by Sanger sequencing but not as good as what is achievable by targeted allele-specific PCR assays or digital droplet PCR.

In general, the workflow for massively parallel sequencing panels is similar, regardless of the exact methods or platforms used (see Chapters 45 and 47). In brief, it consists of (1) DNA extraction; (2) sequencing library preparation; (3) target enrichment by PCR or hybrid capture; (4) hybridization of library fragments to a solid surface (ie, flow cell); (5) clonal amplification of library fragments; (6) massively parallel sequencing; (7) data analysis, including variant identification and annotation; and (8) variant interpretation. The variant identification and annotation step is a computationally intensive process requiring a bioinformatics pipeline employing data analysis algorithms to sort and align the generated sequencing data (reads) to a reference sequence and to identify variants (see Chapter 45). A variant is simply a position or positions within the generated sequence that differ from a reference sequence. Typically, the majority of the identified variants represent benign germline polymorphisms unrelated to the disease process. However, a subset may represent true clinically important somatic mutations present only in cancer cells and/or clinically important germline abnormalities associated with a cancer predisposition. Finally, some variants may represent sequencing error and need to be identified as such.

Currently, there is debate about the necessity of comparing the results obtained from massively parallel sequencing of tumor tissue to results obtained from paired "normal" tissues from the same patient obtained at the same time. The rationale is that this allows for the distinction between variants that are truly somatic (pathogenic) and thus not present in normal tissue and those that are germline (likely nonpathogenic) and thus present in both normal and tumor tissue. This comparison may also help in the identification of systematic errors that may be introduced during various stages of the testing process. For example, PCR or sequencing errors tend to occur at highly repetitive sequences that may also be a so-called "hot spots" for somatic variants. In a patient with a solid tumor, a concurrent skin biopsy obtained from normal skin, a buccal swab, or peripheral blood white cells could be used as the paired normal tissue. However, in patients with hematopoietic malignancies, particularly bone marrow–based myeloid or lymphoid disorders, it may be difficult to obtain normal tissue that is not contaminated with granulocytes or lymphocytes that may be derived from the abnormal clone and thus harbor the same somatic variants. It may be necessary to resort to other strategies such as fluorescence activated cell sorting (FACS) to obtain a population of cells that are not part of the malignant clone. Sorted T cell populations have been used as paired normal controls in the context of B cell malignancies such as chronic lymphocytic leukemia.[152] The sequencing of paired normal tissue alongside tumor DNA reduces the rate of false-positive findings in clinically actionable genes that could otherwise result in the use of targeted therapies that are unlikely to be effective.[153] However, sequencing of paired normal tissue essentially doubles the cost and effort involved in testing. Thorough test validation to identify systematic sequencing errors and a careful, measured, and evidence-based approach to variant interpretation, including tiered reporting of variants into separate classes containing those variants of known clinical significance and those variants of unknown clinical significance (so-called "VUSs"), may mitigate the need for sequencing paired normal tissue. This matter remains unsettled, and the arguments for and against will continue to evolve.

POINTS TO REMEMBER

Gene Mutations in Hematopoietic Malignancies

- Massively parallel sequencing is revolutionizing the laboratory-based evaluation of hematopoietic malignancies by allowing for the simultaneous evaluation of dozens to hundreds of genes in the context of testing panels.
- In myeloid malignancies, gene mutations tend to affect a discrete series of cellular pathways involved in cell signaling and genetic regulation.
- In B cell lymphoproliferative disorders, gene mutations tend to affect B cell receptor signaling pathways.
- In T cell lymphoproliferative disorders, gene mutations tend to affect JAK-STAT signaling pathways.

ROLE OF GENETIC REGULATORY MECHANISMS IN HEMATOPOIETIC MALIGNANCIES

The regulation of gene expression involves a host of interacting pathways, a number of which are affected by the genetic abnormalities that occur in hematopoietic malignancies, including those of both lymphoid and myeloid differentiation. As outlined above, these include methylation of cytosine bases in CpG islands by DNA methyltransferases, modulation of the activity of transcriptional enhancers and repressors, chemical modification of histones, and thus chromatin structure by a host of changes, including methylation, acetylation, phosphorylation, and ubiquitination. Abnormal patterns of expression of certain microRNAs, often due to structural chromosomal abnormalities or epigenetic changes, are another mechanism for regulation of gene expression and appear quite important in the pathophysiology of cancer, including various hematopoietic malignancies.[154] The end result of aberrant epigenetics is the development of abnormal gene expression patterns, often leading to a stem cell–like state and a lack of terminal differentiation. The abnormal gene expression pattern can be identified and may itself be of diagnostic or prognostic significance.

Methylation Patterns

Methylation is regulated by DNA methyltransferases, including *DNMT1*, *DNMT3A*, and *DNMT3B*. As outlined above, *DNMT3A* is frequently mutated in myeloid malignancies, but the presence of *DNMT3A* mutations does not necessarily correlate with changes in the global methylation state,[84] although the presence of recurrent *DNMT3A* missense mutations appears to disrupt enzymatic function.[85] It is likely that more focal changes in methylation, and therefore focal changes in gene expression, contribute to the pathophysiology of *DNMT3A*-mutated AML. In fact, hypermethylation of CpG islands is commonly observed in cancer cells. Drugs, such as 5-azacitidine, that reduce methylation by inhibiting methyltransferases, so-called hypomethylating agents, can be effective in certain myeloid malignancies such as MDS. DNA hypermethylation has been associated with poor risk and progression of MDS to AML.[155]

Measurement of DNA methylation status can be performed using chromatographic methods such as high-performance liquid chromatography (HPLC) to very precisely measure overall levels of methylated and unmethylated cytosine. However, this method does not give any information about local CpG methylation. To measure more focal changes, which may be more informative, bisulfite sequencing can be performed. Bisulfite treatment is used to convert unmethylated cytosine to uracil, while methylcytosine remains unconverted. Uracil is then converted to thymine when PCR is amplified and sequenced, usually by pyrosequencing. In this way the methylation status of individual cytosines can be assessed.

Micro RNA Expression Patterns

The discovery of small noncoding regulatory RNA (microRNA; miRNA) represented an entirely new and unappreciated paradigm for the regulation of gene expression. Mature, processed miRNA bind to the 3' untranslated region of target mRNA sequences, where there is sufficient, but usually imperfect, sequence complementarity. The binding of miRNA to target mRNA sequences leads to decreased translation through various pathways mediated by inhibition, inactivation, or degradation of the bound mRNA molecule. Various miRNAs have been associated with the pathophysiology of hematological malignancies and may add prognostic information but are not currently part of the routine clinical workup of patients with hematological malignancies.

Gene Expression Profiling

Gene expression profiling, wherein the expression levels of a series of mRNA transcripts are measured and compared to standards using microarray technology, is becoming more widely employed in the clinical hematology laboratory, although it is still not a common test. One use for gene expression profiling in the clinical laboratory is "cell of origin" testing to determine the differentiation state of cases of diffuse large B cell lymphoma, either activated B cell–type or germinal center B cell–type. Patients with activated B cell–type diffuse large B cell lymphoma appear to have a worse clinical outcome compared to those with germinal center B cell–type lymphoma when treated with standard front-line therapy with rituximab, cyclophosphamide, doxorubicin, vincristine, and prednisone (known as R-CHOP therapy).[156] In the future this distinction is likely to become even more clinically important because the two profiles may be associated with distinct outcomes in the setting of combination therapies incorporating the kinase inhibitor ibrutinib as well as those incorporating the proteasome inhibitor bortezomib.[157,158] Gene expression profiling is considered the gold standard for making this distinction, although in clinical practice most of the testing is done via the surrogate method of immunohistochemistry. However, a significant number of cases are misclassified by immunohistochemistry, potentially leading to inappropriate treatment decisions.[156] The gene expression profiling test is performed using a Bayesian algorithm to assign a profile to either of the two classes, or as unclassifiable, based on statistical probability.[159] Activated B cell–type diffuse large B cell lymphoma tends to display relative overexpression of genes associated with plasmacytic differentiation, while germinal center types demonstrate higher expression of genes seen in normal germinal center B cells.

A number of expression profiles have been published in other hematopoietic malignancies with claimed prognostic implications. However, for the most part none are in widespread use in clinical practice. Multiple myeloma, a systemic disease caused by the expansion of clonal plasma cells and the overproduction of clonal immunoglobulin heavy and/or light chains, is one promising area where gene expression profiling appears to provide clinically useful information. One 70-gene panel has been used in a number of studies and predicts prognosis based on a score derived from the profiling performed on purified bone marrow plasma cells with high analytical reproducibility and low variation.[160]

CLONALITY TESTING IN HEMATOPOIETIC MALIGNANCIES

Lymphoid Clonality Testing

Cancers, including those of hematopoietic origin, are composed of a population of cells derived from a parental cell that has undergone neoplastic transformation. The daughter cells are therefore "monoclonal" by definition and share important biologic characteristics that may be exploited by molecular genetic testing strategies. Putative lymphoproliferative disorders are particularly amenable to clonality testing by molecular methods due to the nature of the role of lymphocytes in immunity and the fact that they express antigen receptors. In the context of adaptive immune function, B-lymphocytes mediate the humoral immune response via the production of immunoglobulins, while T-lymphocytes mediate the cellular immune response. The specificity of these processes requires lymphocytes to be capable of producing an almost unlimited array of antigen receptors. This is accomplished in large part by recombination of germline immunoglobulin (Ig) and T cell receptor (TCR) gene segments in B and T cells, respectively, which results in highly diverse Ig and TCR antigen binding repertoires (Figs. 51.9 and 51.10).[161,162] Clonality has historically been less readily demonstrable in myeloid malignancies but can be shown indirectly in female patients by studying the pattern of inactivation of genes encoded on the X chromosome. However, given the progress of modern genetic testing strategies, it is much easier to demonstrate evidence of a clonal genetic abnormality in myeloid malignancies rather than rely on a surrogate marker of clonality such as X-inactivation patterns.

Although not required in most instances, evidence of monoclonality may aid in the diagnosis of hematologic malignancy in challenging cases such as those presenting with unusual clinical or morphologic features. However, clonality assays are fraught with potential for misinterpretation and should be treated as ancillary diagnostic studies. The recognition of small clonal hematopoietic cell populations, of both myeloid and lymphoid origin, in the peripheral blood of hematologically normal individuals further highlights the need for a comprehensive diagnostic approach.[59,163]

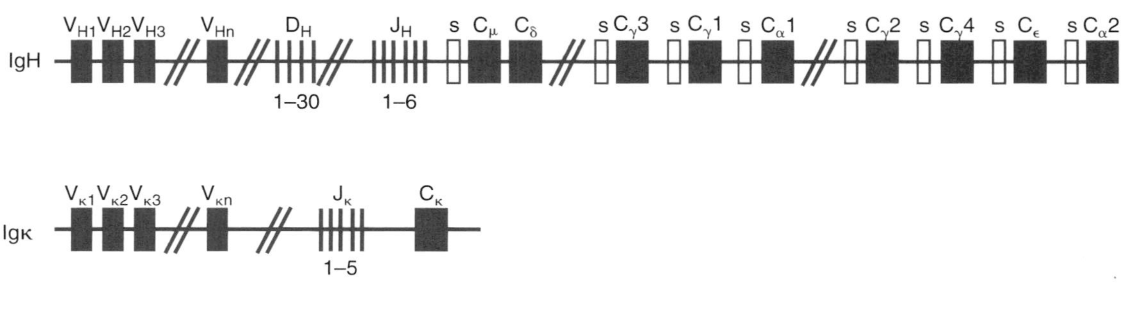

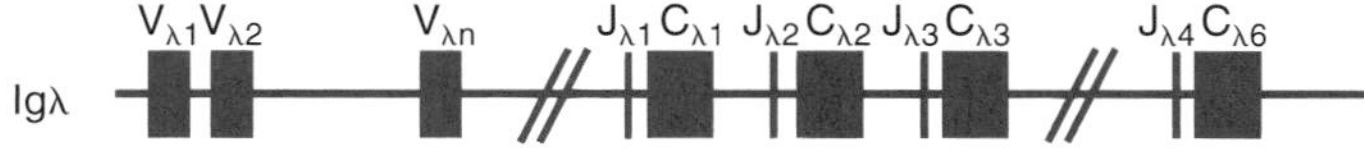

FIGURE 51.9 Schematic representation of immunoglobulin heavy chain *(IGH)*, kappa light chain *(IGK)*, and lambda light chain *(IGL)* genetic loci in germline configuration. *IGH* contains diversity gene segments, whereas *IGK* and *IGL* do not. Switch regions (s) involved in class switch recombination are indicated adjacent to constant (C) gene segments. *V*, Variable; *D*, diversity; *J*, joining.

TABLE 51.5 Chromosomal Location and Number of V, D, and J Segments Potentially Available for Rearrangement of Immunoglobulin and T Cell Receptor Loci

	RECOMBINATION HIERARCHY						
	B Cells →			T Cells →			
Genetic Locus	***IGH***	***IGK***	***IGL***	***TRD***	***TRG***	***TRB***	***TRA***
Chromosomal location	14q32.33	2p11.2	22q11.2	14q11.2	7p14	7q34	14q11.2
V gene segments	123–129	76	73–74	8	12–15	67	54
D gene segments	27	—	—	3	—	2	—
J gene segments	9	5	7–11	4	5	14	61

Data from Lefranc MP, Giudicelli V, Duroux P, Jabado-Michaloud J, Folch G, Aouinti S, et al. IMGT, the international ImMunoGeneTics information system 25 years on. Nucleic Acids Res 2015;43:D413–22.

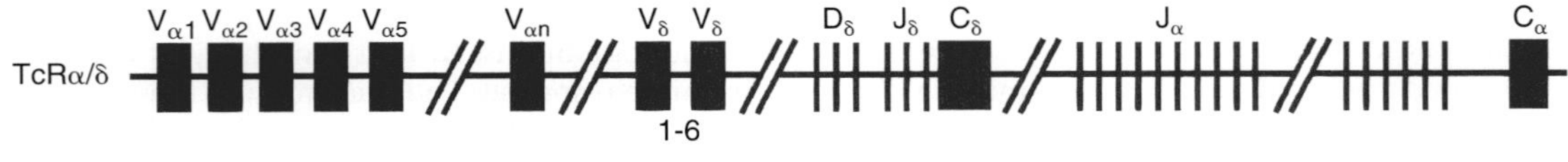

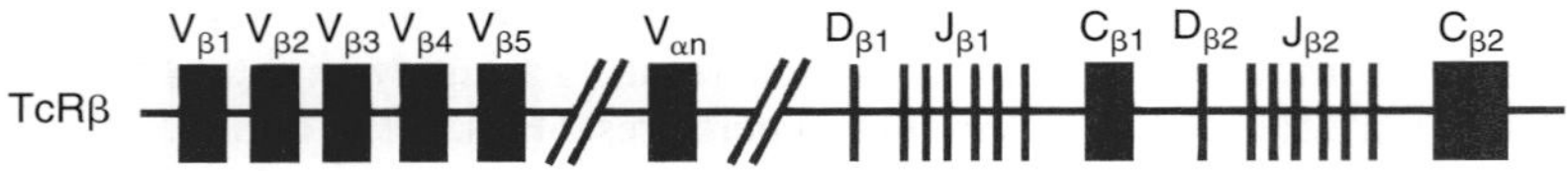

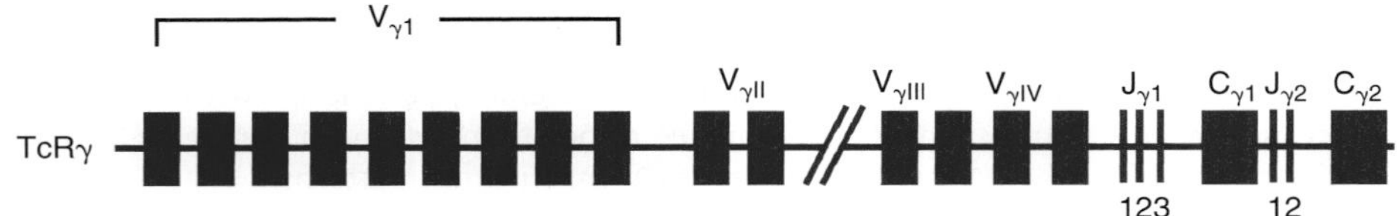

FIGURE 51.10 Schematic representation of T cell antigen receptor genes *TRA*, *TRD*, *TRB*, and *TRG* in germline configuration. *TRB* and *TRD* loci contain diversity gene segments (D), whereas *TRD* and *TRG* do not. Note that *TRD* is located in between the V and J segments of *TRA* and is deleted in the process of productive TRA rearrangement. *V,* Variable; *D,* diversity; *J,* joining; *C,* constant; *TcRα/δ,* TRA/TRD; *TcRβ,* TRB; *TcRγ,* TRG.

V(D)J Recombination in Normal B- and T-Lymphocytes

The genes encoding the immunoglobulin (Ig) and TCR proteins are the targets for DNA-based lymphoid clonality assays. The Ig and TCR gene loci, with some exceptions, are composed of a series of variable (V), diversity (D), joining (J), and constant (C) regions (Table 51.5). The V, D, and J segments recombine during early lymphocyte development in a process known as V(D)J recombination (Fig. 51.11). In B cells, recombination takes place in the bone marrow, whereas T cell maturation occurs primarily in the thymus. The result is that each B or T cell harbors a distinct productive V(D)J rearrangement that is unique in sequence and usually also in length. Monoclonal lymphoid populations, having been derived from a single progenitor cell of origin in most instances, can be expected to demonstrate identical rearrangements, a fact that is exploited for the purposes of clonality testing.

The recombination events are choreographed by an enzyme complex in which the nucleases RAG1 and RAG2 introduce double-strand DNA breaks adjacent to recombination signal sequences.[164] Recombination signal sequences are present downstream of V-gene segments, at each side of D-gene segments, and upstream of J-gene segments. D to J rearrangement is followed by a V to D-J rearrangement. Immunoglobulin

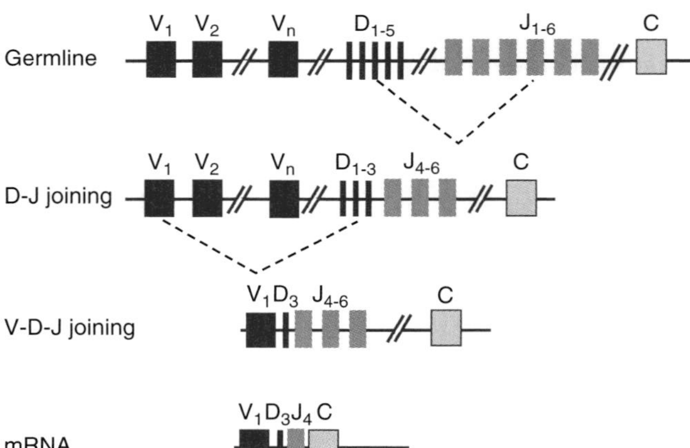

FIGURE 51.11 Schematic depiction of VDJ recombination using the immunoglobulin heavy chain locus *(IGH)* as an example. The process is initiated by D to J segment joining, after which V to D-J rearrangement occurs. Antigen receptor loci that lack diversity segments proceed directly with V to J rearrangement. Following RNA splicing, the *IGH* VDJ transcript is juxtaposed to constant (C) region genes to complete the VDJC transcript. T cell antigen receptor gene loci undergo rearrangement via an analogous process.

light chains kappa *(IGK)* and lambda *(IGL)*, as well as the TCR alpha *(TRA)* and gamma *(TRG)*, lack diversity segments and proceed directly with V to J rearrangement. The imprecise nature of the joining reactions in V(D)J recombination, which are subject to deletion and random insertion of nucleotides, also contributes to the variability of functional rearrangements. Through these mechanisms, phenomenal diversity of Ig and TCR molecules (estimated $>10^{12}$) is achieved. B cells further diversify the repertoire of rearranged antigen receptor molecules by somatic hypermutation, a process that occurs in the germinal center of lymph nodes.

Antigen receptor rearrangements normally occur in a hierarchical sequence. In B cells, *IGH* rearranges, followed by *IGK*. If recombination of *IGK* fails to produce a productive rearrangement, a kappa-deleting element located near the constant region undergoes rearrangement and results in its deletion. *IGL* is the last immunoglobulin gene to participate in recombination and is a less desirable target for clonality investigation. The high frequency of detectable *IGH* and/or *IGK* monoclonal rearrangements in malignant B-cell proliferations (>95%) typically obviates the need for analysis of *IGL*.

T cells begin with rearrangement of the gene encoding TCR delta *(TRD)*, followed by *TRG*, TCR beta *(TRB)*, and finally TCR alpha *(TRA)*. Productive *TRD* rearrangement results in surface expression of the gamma-delta TCR that defines a minor subset of T cells that are preferentially found in mucocutaneous sites. In most T cells, V to J rearrangement of *TRA* results in deletion of *TRD* due to its location between *TRA* V- and J-gene segments. Expression of the common alpha-beta TCR generally follows. The ubiquitous presence of *TRG* rearrangements in T cells, regardless of the type of TCR expressed, lends itself to utilization in clonality studies.

Identification of Clonal Rearrangements in the Workup of Lymphoid Malignancies

The diagnosis of lymphoid malignancies requires a comprehensive approach, including careful consideration of clinical findings, patient history, histopathology, and immunophenotype. The preponderance of lymphoid proliferations can be effectively separated into benign and malignant diagnostic categories based on this strategy. However, a definitive diagnosis may prove difficult in a minor subset of cases (5% to 10%). In such instances, clonality assays may provide additional diagnostic support. Knowledge of the underlying biology and the normal pattern of maturation is essential for interpretation of the clonality results. The finding of a monoclonal immunoglobulin or T cell receptor gene rearrangement may support a diagnosis of lymphoma, particularly in the setting of an atypical lymphoid proliferation showing subtle or otherwise challenging morphologic and immunophenotypic features. Monoclonal immunoglobulin or T cell receptor gene rearrangements are detectable in greater than 95% of cases of mature B cell and T cell neoplasms, respectively.[165]

Monoclonal rearrangements of Ig and TCR genes may also be identified in the context of certain reactive processes. For example, T cell clonality testing is occasionally "positive" in patients with viral infection, immune dysfunction, post-transplantation, or even in certain normal individuals.[166,167] Prominent B cell clones may be found in histologically reactive lymph nodes (particularly with HIV infection or in pediatric patients) and in autoimmune states such as rheumatoid arthritis.[168] A small population of monoclonal B cells, termed *monoclonal B cell lymphocytosis*, is found with surprising frequency in otherwise healthy adults.[169] Evidence of clonality, therefore, does not equate to malignancy. Further, antigen receptor rearrangements are not helpful for lineage determination due to lineage infidelity, a phenomenon particularly well illustrated by precursor lymphoid malignancies.[170] Ig rearrangements may be detectable in up to 15% of cases of T-lymphoblastic leukemia, while up to 40% of cases of B-lymphoblastic leukemia show monoclonal TCR rearrangement. Lineage infidelity is less common, but it can occur in mature T and B cell lymphomas as well. B cell clonality studies cannot distinguish between plasmablastic lymphoma and plasma cell myeloma, a clinically important distinction in which both neoplasms would be expected to harbor monoclonal Ig rearrangements. Coexisting clonal Ig and TCR rearrangements are frequently encountered in patients with angioimmunoblastic T cell lymphoma.[171] Such limitations require that clonality testing always be interpreted within the larger clinical context.

Conversely, lack of evidence of clonality does not necessarily mean benign. For example, a negative TCR gene rearrangement study does not exclude the possibility of an NK cell-derived malignancy in which the neoplastic cells would exhibit germline TCR. The limit of detection of lymphocyte clonality assays, in terms of proportion of clonal cells required in a given sample, varies by testing methodology and ranges from 1% to 10%. Scarcity of malignant cells, often in association with an exuberant cytokine-driven reactive cellular background, is a hallmark of some B cell malignancies, including Hodgkin lymphoma and T cell/histiocyte-rich large B cell lymphoma. Unless specialized techniques are employed to enrich for tumor cells (eg, laser microdissection), attempts at B cell clonality testing in such situations are likely to yield a false-negative result.

Myeloid Clonality Testing

From a historical perspective, clonality investigation of myeloid proliferations was inherently more difficult due to the lack of accessibility of specific genetic markers. To this end, X-chromosome inactivation analysis can provide an indirect method of clonality assessment in most female patients. Females normally have two copies of the X chromosome—one derived maternally and the other paternally. One of these copies is randomly inactivated during embryonic development in a process known as lyonization. When either the maternal or paternal X-chromosome is preferentially inactivated, a nonrandom or skewed pattern of inactivation is usually demonstrable and may serve as evidence of clonality.

The human androgen receptor gene *(AR)* is the most commonly used target of X-chromosome inactivation assays. The *AR* locus contains a hypervariable CAG short tandem repeat that is most often (but not always) heterozygous and in close proximity to cleavage sites of methylation-sensitive restriction enzymes (eg, *HpaII* and *HhaI*).[172] Because X-chromosome inactivation is associated with hypermethylation of cytosine residues, active (unmethylated) alleles are digested by the enzymes and can be distinguished by PCR and subsequent fragment analysis from inactive (methylated) alleles, which are not cut. The ratio of methylated and unmethylated alleles is then assessed and used to determine clonality based on skewing from the theoretically expected normal distribution (50:50). This assay can also determine clonality in NK cell proliferations that, like their myeloid counterparts, lack immunoglobulin or T cell receptor rearrangements.[173]

While capable of providing evidence of clonality in a subset of patients, X-chromosome inactivation studies are seldom performed in today's clinical laboratory. In addition to the obvious limitation with regard to patient gender, the method is subject to other important limitations that may complicate interpretation. One limitation is nonrandom X-chromosome inactivation, which occurs with some frequency in older females and results in skewing of lyonization ratios, potentially mimicking clonality.[174] Diagnosis of myeloid neoplasms is typically accomplished through comprehensive clinical and morphologic evaluation in conjunction with selective use of molecular genetic studies and conventional cytogenetics/FISH. The discovery of mutually exclusive genetic abnormalities involving *JAK2*, *CALR*, and *MPL* in the vast majority of myeloproliferative neoplasms, for example, has rendered X-chromosome inactivation-based clonality studies obsolete with respect to diagnosis of these malignancies. The emergence of massively parallel sequencing allows efficient mutation analysis of gene panels that, in addition to providing prognostic and/or predictive information, may also provide evidence of clonality in patients with morphologically equivocal or otherwise diagnostically challenging myeloid neoplasms.

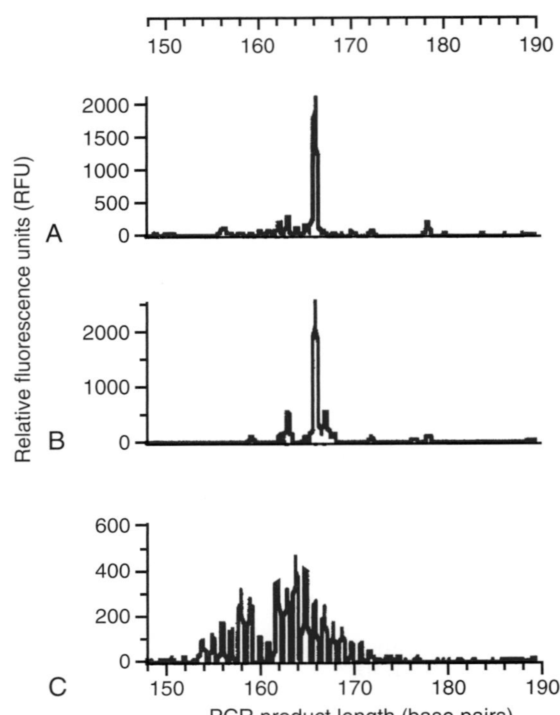

FIGURE 51.12 An example of T cell clonality testing by PCR of the *TRG* locus. The PCR products are resolved by capillary electrophoresis. **A** and **B** each show a dominant peak with amplitude at least five times background, representing monoclonal rearrangements of the same size (166 bp). **C** illustrates a typical polyclonal pattern, with a Gaussian distribution of rearrangements.

Test Applications

Southern Blotting

At one time, Southern blot–based lymphoid clonality assays were recognized as the "gold standard" for specificity. However, this method suffers from a number of practical limitations that have contributed to its decline. Southern blot–based clonality assays utilize multiple restriction endonucleases (eg, *EcoRI*, *BamHI*, and *HindIII*) carefully chosen in order to digest DNA at specific sites within the corresponding antigen receptor genes. The resulting fragments from each enzymatic digestion undergo separation by gel electrophoresis, followed by transfer and immobilization to a membrane. Complementary labeled probes, usually targeted to the *IGH* or *TRG* J-segment, are hybridized to the membrane. The hallmark of a monoclonal rearrangement is the detection of distinct, novel fragments (visualized as distinct bands on the Southern blot) that differ from the pattern seen in the germline, nonrearranged controls indicating the presence of a dominant (clonal) rearrangement in the sample. Polyclonal rearrangements in a normal T or B cell population will yield a smear and no distinct bands, indicating that no dominant rearrangement is present.

The principal shortcomings of clonality assessment by Southern blotting relate to the time-consuming, labor-intensive nature of the method, limited sensitivity, and restrictive specimen requirements. Formalin-fixed paraffin embedded tissue, a common clinical sample type in lymphoma diagnosis, provides DNA of insufficient quality for Southern blot– based testing due to DNA degradation and cross-linking. PCR-based clonality testing has largely overcome these limitations without significant sacrifices in performance.

Polymerase Chain Reaction

PCR-based clonality test methods seek to amplify DNA across the V(D)J junction of rearranged Ig and TCR loci in order to capture the repertoire of unique rearrangements. Upon analysis by capillary electrophoresis, the lengths of the PCR products typically follow a Gaussian distribution due to junction size heterogeneity. A clonal population of B or T cells results in the overabundance of a unique V(D)J junction sequence evidenced by a spike emerging from the Gaussian background of polyclonal fragments (Fig. 51.12). Typically, a peak has to be at least twofold higher than the Gaussian background to be called clonal. To amplify all possible V and J combinations of a locus, multiplexing strategies have been devised to limit the number of required PCR reactions.[19] In addition, V-segment consensus primers are targeted toward framework sequences that define the Ig domain structure and are conserved between V-segments. Despite these efforts, sources of possible false negatives and false positives remain. High levels of somatic hypermutation observed in some B cell lymphoma subtypes such as follicular lymphoma may result in V gene segment alterations that could compromise consensus primer recognition. Multiple V(D)J fragments of different sequences but identical length can lead to false clonal peaks by capillary electrophoresis, especially when studying less complex loci such as *TRG*.[175]

Massively Parallel Sequencing

Massively parallel sequencing strategies allow for sequencing the entire repertoire of junction sequences for an Ig or TCR locus. Typically 100,000 to 400,000 reads are obtained that can be attributed to 15,000 to 30,000 unique rearrangements in a typical clinical sample.[176] The number of sequencing reads obtained for a particular V(D)J rearrangement is proportional to the relative size of the clone harboring that particular rearrangement. Similar to capillary electrophoresis, the analysis is performed on the repertoire of PCR-amplified rearrangements. However, the use of a single-tube multiplexed PCR amplification strategy is highly desirable in order to preserve the relative abundance of the different V and J elements present in the original repertoire.[176] Clonality is determined based on the relative abundance of a particular sequence compared to the background of polyclonal sequences. Using massively parallel sequencing (Fig. 51.13), different rearrangements that result in PCR products of identical length

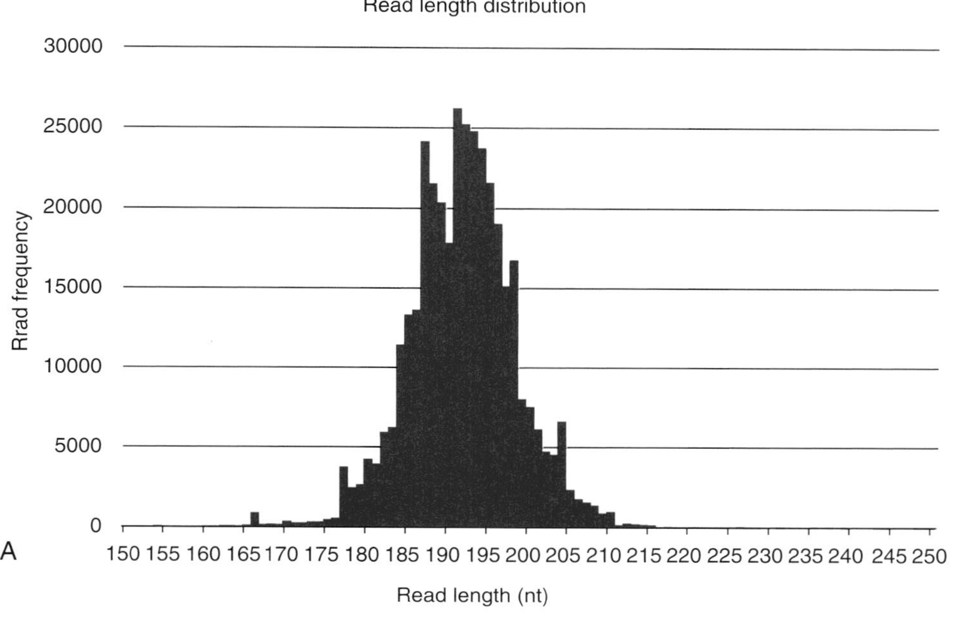

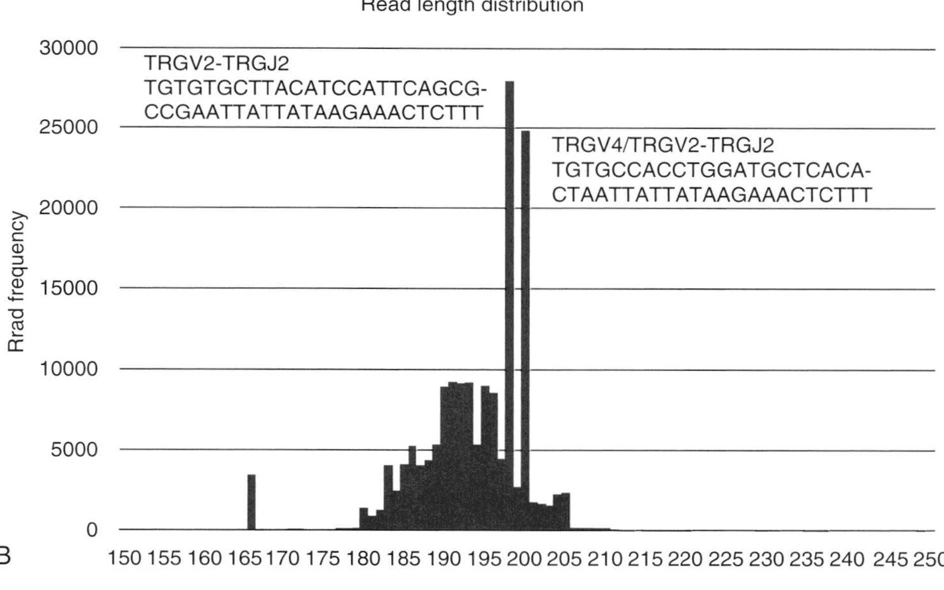

FIGURE 51.13 Examples of T cell clonality analysis by massively parallel sequencing of *TRG* rearrangements. **A,** A polyclonal (normal) pattern. Individual read clusters representing distinct rearrangements each represent 1% or less of total reads, indicating that no dominant clonal rearrangements are present. The histogram shows a Gaussian distribution when read frequencies are graphed according to length (total number of reads: 499,238). **B,** A monoclonal pattern. The top two sequence clusters, with V-J segments and complete TRG junctional sequences shown, represent 12.1% and 10.5% of total reads and show a sixfold difference over the background. The histogram shows a non-Gaussian distribution of read frequencies graphed according to length and illustrates the biallelic nature of the monoclonal rearrangement (total number of reads: 358,674). *nt,* Nucleotides.

can be resolved based on sequence data potentially resulting in a lower false-positive rate. In addition, identification of the junction sequence present in neoplastic cells constitutes a very sensitive marker for subsequent use in minimal residual disease detection at very low levels (0.1% to 0.01% of cells) over the course of treatment, possibly allowing early prediction of relapse.[176]

POINTS TO REMEMBER

Clonality Testing in Hematopoietic Malignancies

- The unique biology of B and T cell antigen receptor gene rearrangement allows for molecular genetic assessment of clonality.
- Failure to interpret clonality assay results within the appropriate clinicopathologic context may lead to diagnostic error.
- Monoclonal T cell receptor and immunoglobulin gene rearrangements may be demonstrable in benign clinical settings.
- Clonality assays employing massively parallel sequencing may be particularly useful for monitoring a previously documented clone.

CONCLUSION

The spectrum of genetic abnormalities present in hematopoietic malignancies requires the use of many complex testing strategies for comprehensive detection. These testing strategies include detection of translocations, copy number changes, gene mutations, and epigenetic abnormalities. As the number and type of clinically actionable genetic variants continue to grow, the laboratory evaluation of these patients will likely become a more multidisciplinary effort. However, traditional clinical, laboratory, and pathologic methods remain central to patient diagnosis and management and are unlikely to be supplanted in the near future by genetic testing.

SELECTED REFERENCES

For a full list of references for this chapter, please refer to ExpertConsult.com.

1. Vardiman JW, Thiele J, Arber DA, et al. The 2008 revision of the World Health Organization (WHO) classification of myeloid neoplasms and acute leukemia: Rationale and important changes. *Blood* 2009;**114**:937–51.
4. Kuppers R, Dalla-Favera R. Mechanisms of chromosomal translocations in B cell lymphomas. *Oncogene* 2001;**20**: 5580–94.
6. Pasqualucci L, Bhagat G, Jankovic M, et al. AID is required for germinal center-derived lymphomagenesis. *Nat Genet* 2008;**40**:108–12.
10. Holmfeldt L, Wei L, Diaz-Flores E, et al. The genomic landscape of hypodiploid acute lymphoblastic leukemia. *Nat Genet* 2013;**45**:242–52.
14. Weng AP, Ferrando AA, Lee W, et al. Activating mutations of NOTCH1 in human t cell acute lymphoblastic leukemia. *Science* 2004;**306**:269–71.
16. Dave SS, Fu K, Wright GW, et al. Molecular diagnosis of Burkitt's lymphoma. *N Engl J Med* 2006;**354**:2431–42.
19. van Dongen JJ, Langerak AW, Bruggemann M, et al. Design and standardization of PCR primers and protocols for detection of clonal immunoglobulin and T-cell receptor gene recombinations in suspect lymphoproliferations: Report of the BIOMED-2 concerted action BMH4-CT98-3936. *Leukemia* 2003;**17**:2257–317.
37. Kayser S, Schlenk RF, Grimwade D, et al. Minimal residual disease-directed therapy in acute myeloid leukemia. *Blood* 2015;**125**:2331–5.
47. Soverini S, Hochhaus A, Nicolini FE, et al. BCR-ABL kinase domain mutation analysis in chronic myeloid leukemia patients treated with tyrosine kinase inhibitors: Recommendations from an expert panel on behalf of European LeukemiaNet. *Blood* 2011;**118**:1208–15.
49. Greenberg PL, Tuechler H, Schanz J, et al. Revised international prognostic scoring system for myelodysplastic syndromes. *Blood* 2012;**120**:2454–65.
56. Alexandrov LB, Nik-Zainal S, Wedge DC, et al. Signatures of mutational processes in human cancer. *Nature* 2013;**500**: 415–21.
58. Tomasetti C, Vogelstein B. Cancer etiology. Variation in cancer risk among tissues can be explained by the number of stem cell divisions. *Science* 2015;**347**:78–81.
59. Jaiswal S, Fontanillas P, Flannick J, et al. Age-related clonal hematopoiesis associated with adverse outcomes. *N Engl J Med* 2014;**371**:2488–98.
60. Genovese G, Kahler AK, Handsaker RE, et al. Clonal hematopoiesis and blood-cancer risk inferred from blood DNA sequence. *N Engl J Med* 2014;**371**:2477–87.
73. Cancer Genome Atlas Research N. Genomic and epigenomic landscapes of adult de novo acute myeloid leukemia. *N Engl J Med* 2013;**368**:2059–74.
90. Mardis ER, Ding L, Dooling DJ, et al. Recurring mutations found by sequencing an acute myeloid leukemia genome. *N Engl J Med* 2009;**361**:1058–66.
93. Dang L, White DW, Gross S, et al. Cancer-associated IDH1 mutations produce 2-hydroxyglutarate. *Nature* 2010; **465**:966.
97. Abdel-Wahab O, Levine R. The spliceosome as an indicted conspirator in myeloid malignancies. *Cancer Cell* 2011;**20**:420–3.
127. Wong TN, Ramsingh G, Young AL, et al. Role of TP53 mutations in the origin and evolution of therapy-related acute myeloid leukaemia. *Nature* 2015;**518**:552–5.
139. Zhang J, Grubor V, Love CL, et al. Genetic heterogeneity of diffuse large B-cell lymphoma. *Proc Natl Acad Sci USA* 2013;**110**:1398–403.
159. Wright G, Tan B, Rosenwald A, et al. A gene expression-based method to diagnose clinically distinct subgroups of diffuse large B cell lymphoma. *Proc Natl Acad Sci USA* 2003;**100**:9991–6.

Circulating Tumor Cells and Circulating Tumor DNA

*Evi Lianidou and Dave Hoon**

ABSTRACT

Background

Classic tissue biopsies or surgical resections are invasive procedures that capture only a single snapshot in the evolution of cancer. In contrast, a blood-based test or "liquid biopsy" has the potential to characterize the evolution of a solid tumor in real time by extracting molecular information from circulating tumor cells (CTCs), circulating tumor DNA (ctDNA), circulating miRNAs, or exosomes. Molecular characterization of CTCs and ctDNA holds considerable promise for the identification of therapeutic targets and resistance mechanisms and for real-time monitoring of the efficacy of systemic therapies. The major potential advantage of CTC and ctDNA analysis is that they are minimally invasive and can be serially repeated.

Content

This overview is focused on the diagnostic, prognostic, and predictive value of CTCs and ctDNA in cancer patients. It includes key studies in different cancers and incorporates the latest advances in genome-wide analysis of ctDNA. Focus includes (1) CTC isolation, enumeration, and detection systems; (2) clinical applications of CTC; (3) different forms of ctDNA; (4) ctDNA isolation and detection systems; (5) clinical applications of ctDNA; (6) quality control and standardization of liquid biopsy assays; (7) the potential of liquid biopsy in the clinical laboratory; and (8) the potential of the molecular characterization of CTCs and ctDNA analysis as a liquid biopsy for individualized therapy. With respect to the clinical laboratory, the development of targeted molecular assays as companion diagnostics, for disease monitoring, and even for early cancer detection are all potential possibilities at various stages of development.

Cancer genomes are not static but change over the course of therapy. The term *liquid biopsy* refers to blood-based cancer testing and often involves detailed molecular analysis of the tumor from circulating genetic material in the peripheral blood. This genetic information is derived mainly from circulating tumor cells (CTCs), circulating tumor DNA (ctDNA), circulating miRNAs, and exosomes (Fig. 52.1). Liquid biopsy offers a simple and noninvasive insight into a patient's cancer. Blood-based targeted molecular assays have potential utility as companion diagnostics, in disease monitoring, and even early cancer detection.[1-3]

Currently the most promising and readily applicable role for liquid biopsy is the profiling of CTCs or ctDNA as a way to monitor patients in the course of therapy—particularly by using novel technologies for a better and earlier indication of either response or emerging resistance to a particular treatment. The next logical step is to couple this ability with analysis of the genomic landscape of CTCs or ctDNA to better understand the mechanisms of evolving resistance and hopefully to guide treatment strategies to overcome resistance. The utility of liquid biopsy is not just limited to being a mirror of tissue biopsy, but it is a potential tool that can detect unique and impactful information about a patient's cancer that tissue testing cannot. Just a few years ago, the liquid biopsy approach was limited to research studies, but it is now entering prospective clinical trials as a companion diagnostic for evaluation. It can be used for patients whose tumors are hard to access or when the site of the primary tumor is unknown. It may in the future enable decisions for activating genomic targeted therapies in patients who have failed treatment on a particular drug regimen (Fig. 52.2).

Potentially, liquid biopsy may aid in the investigation of the evolution of subclonal cancer cell populations. Liquid biopsy may be a minimally invasive method for determining dominant clones to direct targeted therapies against. There is hope that this approach can illuminate strategies to combine drugs that affect the dominant mutated populations and also inhibit other subclonal populations from expanding. This approach may impact the definition of minimal residual disease because it can change the clinician's ability to predict the risk of recurrence in early-stage cancer patients whose tumors have been surgically removed. The most exciting potential clinical application of blood-based cancer testing is early cancer detection.

Liquid biopsy as a diagnostic, prognostic, and theranostic tool is appealing because it is minimally invasive and easily performed in a serial manner. However, there are several

*This work was supported by the CANCER-ID project (E.L.) and by the Dr. Miriam and Sheldon G. Adelson Medical Research Foundation (AMRF; D.H.), Weil Family Foundation, and Gonda Foundation (D.H.). We would also like to thank Ms. Anupam Singh (MSc student) and Mrs. Nousha Javanmardi for their editorial assistance. We would like to thank Ms. Cleo Parisi (PhD student) for her assistance in organizing the references and Mr. Ilias Agelidis (MSc student) for his assistance in designing Figs. 52.1 and 52.6.

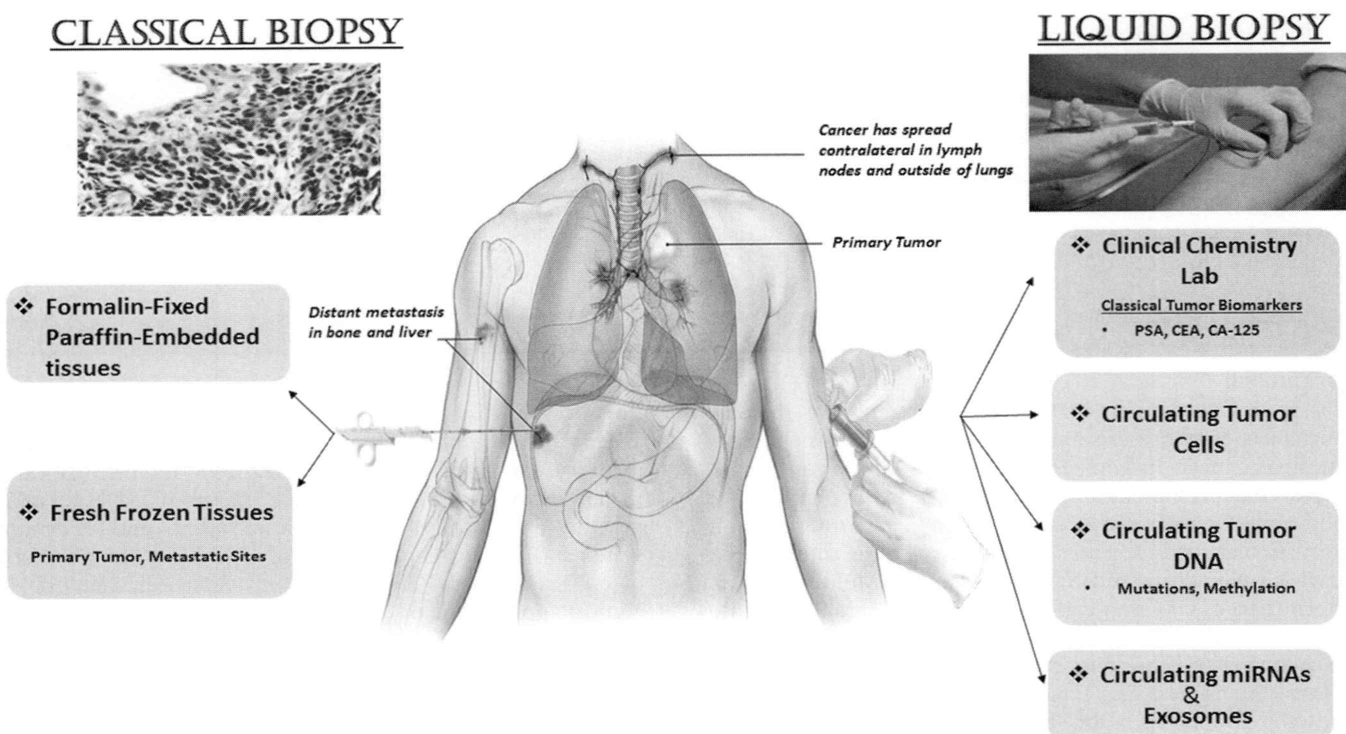

FIGURE 52.1 Classic versus liquid biopsy approaches.

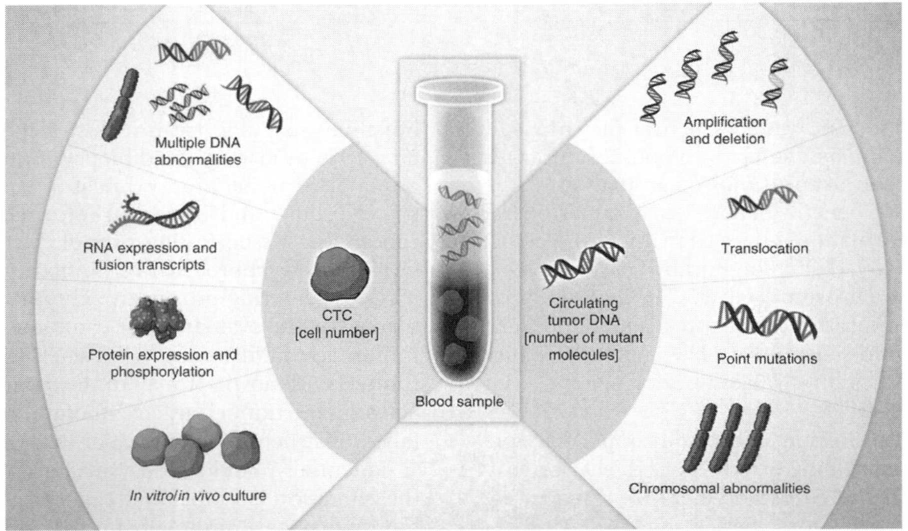

FIGURE 52.2 Circulating tumor cells (CTCs) and circulating tumor DNA (ctDNA). The potential of liquid biopsy for the evaluation and management of cancer patients from CTCs includes nucleic acid analysis, protein expression and phosphorylation, and in vivo and in vitro cultures. Analysis of ctDNA is limited to DNA. (From Haber DA, Velculescu VE. Blood-based analyses of cancer: circulating tumor cells and circulating tumor DNA. *Cancer Discov* 2014;4:650–61. Copyright 2014 American Association for Cancer Research.)

barriers to the routine clinical use of liquid biopsy: (1) numerous technologies are available for the detection of circulating cancer biomarkers, (2) more and more biomarkers for evaluation of CTCs and ctDNA are required, (3) well-designed comparison studies between liquid biopsy (CTCs and/or ctDNA) with conventional biopsy samples are still needed, (4) it is still difficult to control the preanalytical phase to obtain robust and reproducible results, (5) currently available techniques are costly, and (6) the turnaround time is currently too slow for maximal clinical utility.

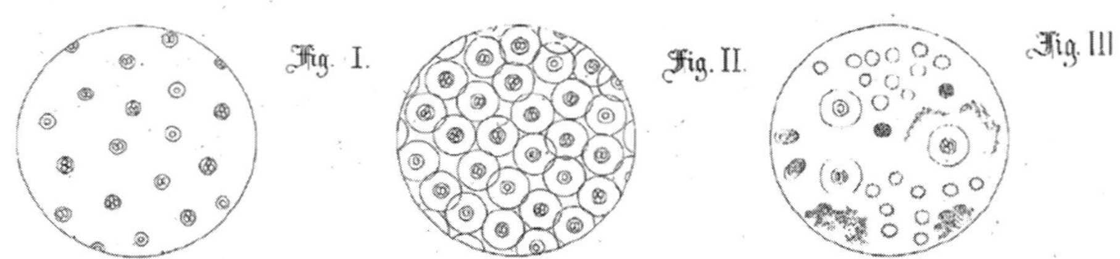

FIGURE 52.3 Historical medical journal article by Thomas Ashworth from 1869 describing circulating tumor cells (I) blood smear from a normal donor, (II) section of tumor from the patient, and (III) blood smear of patient. The larger cells in the blood smear of the patient are circulating tumor cells (From Ashworth TR. A case of cancer in which cells similar to those in the tumours were seen in the blood after death. *Med J Australia* 1869;14:146–47.)

POINTS TO REMEMBER

Liquid Biopsy

- The liquid biopsy approach extracts molecular information from the tumor by detailed analysis of circulating tumor-derived genetic material in the bloodstream. The sources of this material are circulating tumor cells (CTCs), circulating tumor DNA (ctDNA), circulating miRNAs, and exosomes.
- Liquid biopsy can provide detailed information on tumor genome evolution over time through conventional peripheral blood sampling that can be used for serial monitoring of a patient.

CIRCULATING TUMOR CELLS

Circulating Tumor Cells: Historical Background

The presence of circulating tumor cells (CTCs) was first reported in 1869 by Thomas Ashworth (Fig. 52.3).[4] In 2005, the clinical importance of disseminated tumor cells (DTCs) in the bone marrow of breast cancer patients was shown.[5] However, analysis of DTCs in bone marrow is invasive and thus difficult to repeat. CTCs are rare cells that originate from primary and metastatic tumors that have managed to get into the circulation and that may extravasate to different organs. Only a small fraction of CTCs will develop into metastasis.[6] CTCs are a major player in the liquid biopsy approach and may provide real-time information on a patient's disease status. Cancer metastasis is the main cause of cancer-related death, and dissemination of tumor cells through the blood circulation is an important intermediate step that also exemplifies the switch from localized to systemic disease.[7]

Many advances have been made in the detection and molecular characterization of CTCs. The presence of CTCs in peripheral blood has been linked to worse prognosis and early relapse in various types of solid cancers.[8] The FDA has cleared the CellSearch system for breast (2004), colorectal (2008), and prostate (2008) cancer based on the critical role that CTCs play in the metastatic spread of carcinomas.[9] Detection of CTCs is correlated with decreased progression-free survival (PFS) and overall survival (OS) in both operable breast cancer and metastatic breast cancer.

CTCs are targets for understanding tumor biology and tumor cell dissemination in humans. Their molecular characterization offers an exciting approach to understanding resistance to established therapies and elucidating the complex biology of metastasis.[10] Further research on the molecular characterization of CTCs should contribute to a better understanding of the biology of metastatic development in cancer patients and the identification of novel therapeutic targets, especially after elucidating the relationship of CTCs to cancer stem cells. This approach may provide individualized targeted treatments and spare breast cancer patients unnecessary and ineffective therapies.[11]

CTCs are rare, and the amount of available sample is limited, presenting formidable analytical and technical challenges. Recent technical advancements in CTC detection and characterization include multiplex reverse transcription quantitative PCR (RT-qPCR) methods, image-based approaches, and microfilter and microchip devices for their isolation. However, direct comparison of different methods for detecting CTCs in blood from patients with breast cancer has revealed a substantial variation in the detection rates[12,13] There is a lack of standardization in reference material, which hampers the implementation of CTC measurement in clinical routine practice. The potential of CTC analysis is now widely recognized, although many challenges remain(Fig. 52.4).[14]

Circulating Tumor Cells: Analytical Techniques

General Overview

The isolation and further analysis of highly pure CTCs are difficult because these cells are extremely rare in the peripheral blood.[15] Typically, CTCs are coisolated with a background of peripheral blood mononuclear cells. The combination of high-throughput and automated CTC isolation technologies with generally accepted and validated downstream molecular assays is necessary for the routine use of CTC-based diagnostics in the clinical management of cancer patients.

CTC analysis includes isolation/enrichment, detection, enumeration, and molecular characterization. The main analytical systems used are described below, and an outline is presented in Fig. 52.5. Recent advances in this area, as described in recently published reviews, can further supplement this information.[7,16-19]

The main strategies for CTC isolation/enrichment are based on separation by density, size, and/or electrical charge, or by immunomagnetic isolation of specific proteins on their cell surface. A variety of microfluidic and filtration devices has been developed and are currently under evaluation for the isolation and enrichment of CTCs, including in vivo capture and isolation of viable single CTCs. Detection systems for CTC analysis are typically protein- and image-based, although an increasing number of molecular assays are now performed on nucleic acids. Reliable single CTC isolation

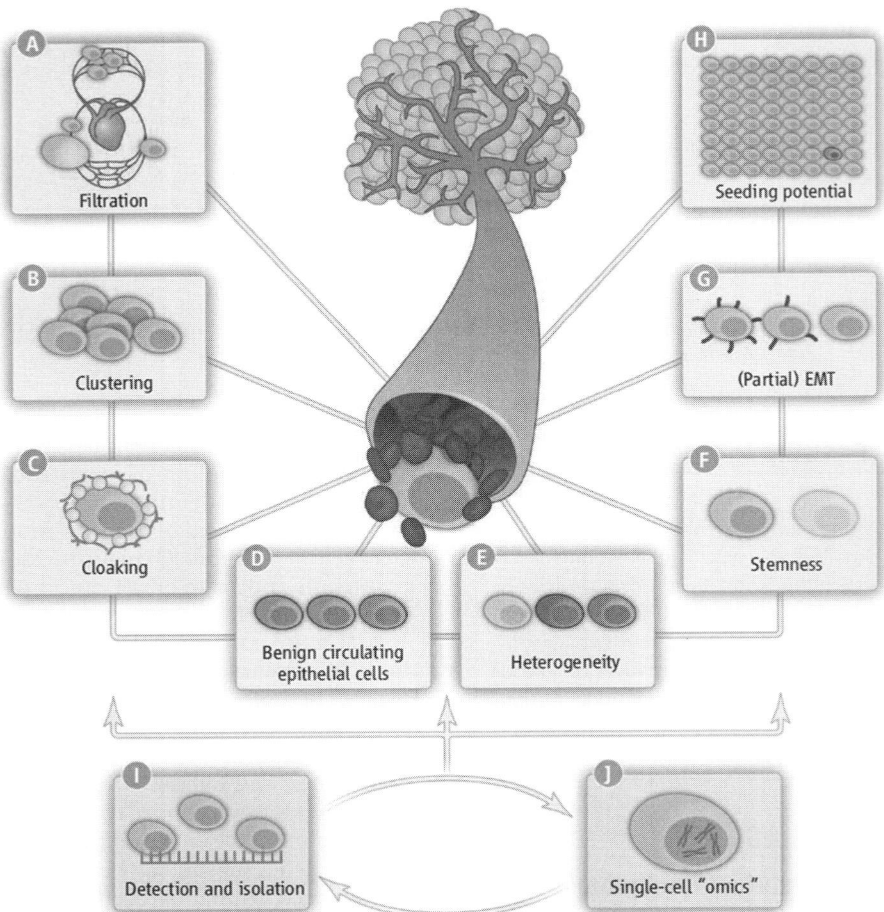

FIGURE 52.4 Challenges in CTC research. Biophysical factors that may diminish the detection of CTCs include (A) filtration of large CTCs in smaller capillaries, (B) clustering of tumor cells that lodge in capillaries, and (C) cloaking of CTCs by platelets or coagulation factors. Biological factors that complicate the detection and isolation of clinically relevant populations of CTCs that rely on epithelial markers include (D) the presence of benign circulating epithelial cells, (E) the large heterogeneity among CTCs, (F) the possible stemness of a subpopulation of CTCs, (G) the (partial) epithelial-mesenchymal transition (EMT) that some CTCs undergo during dissemination, and (H) the unclear seeding potential of detected CTCs. Future research should use technologies focused on (I) improving the detection and isolation of CTCs and (J) single-cell "omics." (From Plaks V, Koopman D, Werb Z. Circulating tumor cells. *Science* 2013;341:1186–88. Copyright 2013 American Association for the Advancement of Science.)

followed by massive parallel sequencing (see Chapters 47 and 50) may open new frontiers for the management of patients.

The CellSearch System

The CellSearch system (Janssen Diagnostics, Raritan, N.J.) is considered the gold standard for detecting CTCs in the clinical setting because it was used in many clinical studies correlating CTC enumeration and prognosis. Epithelial CTCs are detected and enumerated in blood against a backdrop of millions of leukocytes and rely on epithelial cell adhesion molecule (EpCAM)–based immunomagnetic separation. This system has been cleared by the US Food and Drug Administration for prognostication and disease monitoring in patients with metastatic breast (2004), colon (2008), and prostate (2008) cancer and is still the only FDA-cleared system for clinical CTC measurement in metastatic cancer.[20]

In CellSearch, immunofluorescence is used for CTC detection based on specific markers for CTCs such as cytoplasmic epithelial cytokeratins (8, 18, and 19), leukocytes with CD45, and cell viability as indicated by 4',6-diamidino-2-phenylindole (DAPI) staining. This system is based on a combination of positive immunomagnetic enrichment of CTCs and automated digital microscopy. More specifically (Fig. 52.6), the CTC enumeration steps are (1) CTCs are labeled with magnetic beads coated with an antibody against EpCAM, an epithelial marker expressed by the cell membrane of the majority (but not all) of CTCs; (2) CTCs are immunomagnetically captured and concentrated; and (3) CTCs are stained with phycoerythrin (PE)-labeled anti-CK antibodies (CK-PE). Cell nuclei are then fluorescently stained with DAPI. In addition, leukocytes are stained with allophycocyanin (APC)-labeled anti-CD45 antibodies (CD45-APC), and

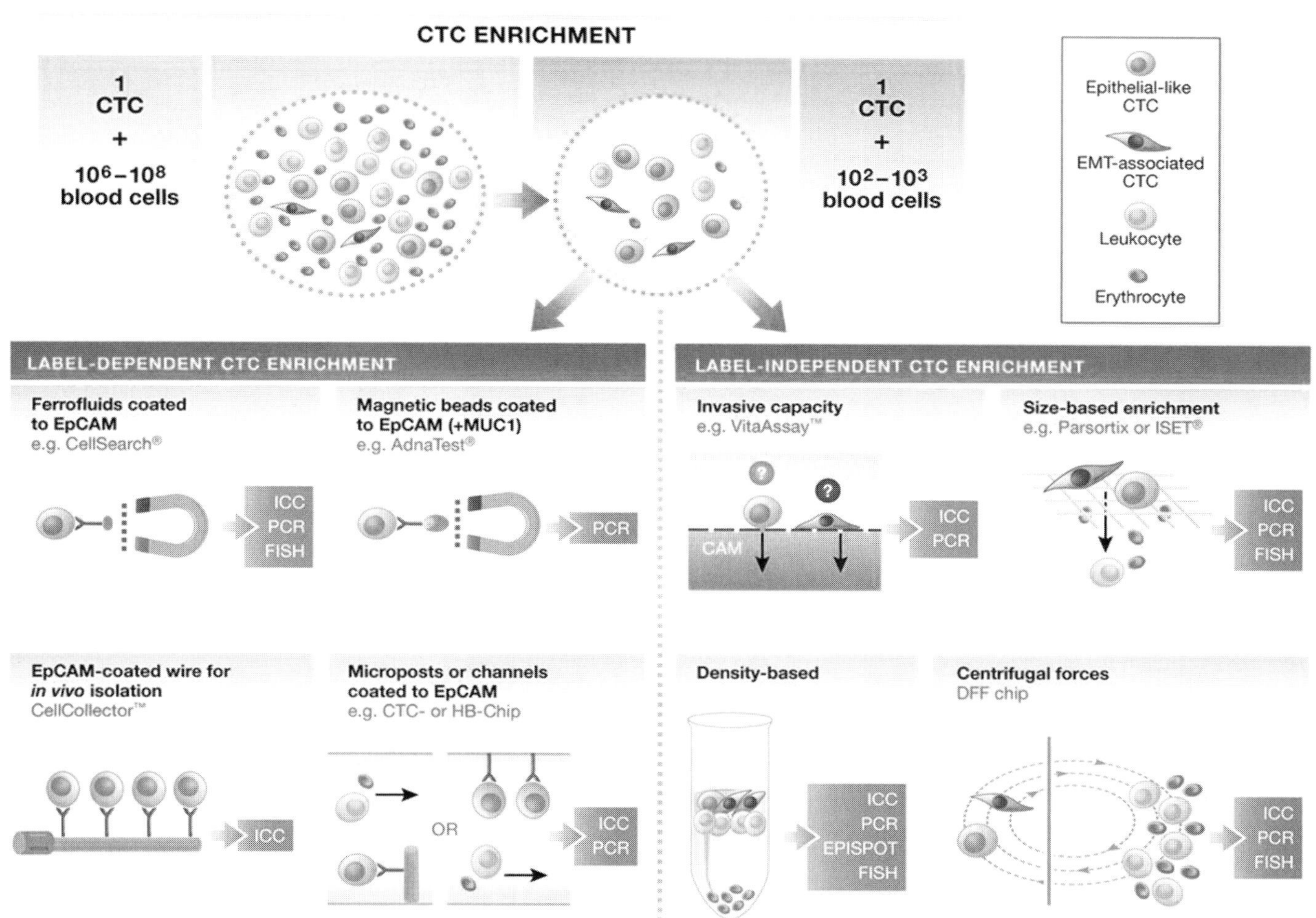

FIGURE 52.5 Overview of CTC enrichment and identification systems. A cartoon of CTC enrichment is shown at the top with depletion of RBCs and leukocytes, leaving mostly epithelial-like CTCs and epithelial mesenchymal transition (EMT)–associated CTCs. Enrichments of 10^4 to 10^5 can be achieved. Enrichment strategies for CTCs can be separated into label-dependent and label-independent techniques. Among label-dependent techniques, immunomagnetic assays targeting EpCAM (epithelial cell adhesion molecule) and sometimes MUC-1 (a cell-surface glycoprotein) are the most common. The antibodies can be attached to ferrofluids (CellSearch, Janssen Diagnostics, Raritan, N.J.), magnetic coated beads (AdnaTest,Qiagen Hanover, Germany), wires (CellCollector, Gilupi GmbH, Potsdam, Germany), microposts (CTC-Chip,[82] or herringbone channels (HB-Chip).[467] Label-independent methods include invasion into a cell adhesion matrix (CAM) (Vita-Assay, Vitatex, Stony Brook, N.Y.), enrichment by size (Parsortix, ANGLE, Guildford, UK) and ISET,[72] enrichment by density (Ficoll gradients), and vortex flows in curvilinear channels known as Dean flow fractionation (DFF).[468] A combination of different enrichment strategies is also practicable. Captured tumor cells are ready for molecular characterization by immunocytochemistry (ICC), using antibodies for tumor-specific markers, or by PCR approaches targeting tumor-specific mRNA or DNA sequences. Additionally, fluorescence in situ hybridization (FISH) can be used for the detection of tumor-specific gene aberrations, or tumor-specific proteins released by CTCs can be detected with labeled antibodies on immobilized membranes by "epithelial immunoSPOT" assays (EPISPOT).[469] (Modified from Joosse SA, Gorges TM, Pantel K. Biology, detection, and clinical implications of circulating tumor cells. *EMBO Mol Med.* 2014;7:1–11. Copyright 2014 Wiley-VCH Verlag.)

cellular fixation is performed; and (4) concentrated, stained tumor cells are examined by fluorescence microscopy to assess labeling by PE, DAPI, and APC, thereby distinguishing tumor cells from leukocytes (Fig. 52.7). By using these fluorescent labels, CD45-APC fluorescence indicates the presence of leukocytes, while CK-PE indicates the presence of epithelial cells. A subcomponent of the CellSearch, the CellSpotter Analyzer, is a semiautomated fluorescence microscope that is used to enumerate the fluorescently labeled cells that are immunomagnetically selected and aligned. This system additionally allows for the detection of a fourth protein biomarker of choice, depending on the type of cancer being investigated—for example, human epidermal growth factor receptor 2 (HER-2) in breast cancer. Moreover, downstream molecular characterization of CTCs is possible because DNA can be isolated from cells captured in the CellSearch

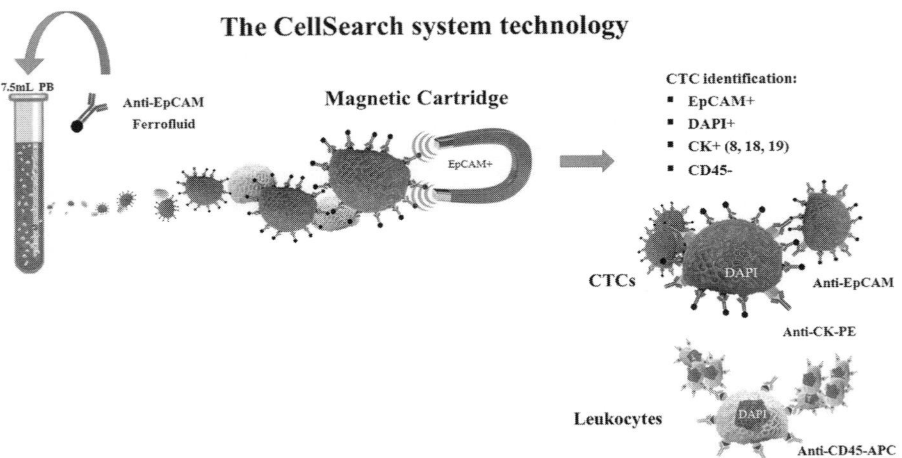

FIGURE 52.6 Positive immunomagnetic isolation and staining of CTC on the CellSearch system. Most nucleated cells in the blood are white blood cells (WBC). CTCs are enriched by a magnetic cartridge and are identified by being EpCAM+, CK+, and CD45–. After isolation, they can be enumerated and/or characterized.

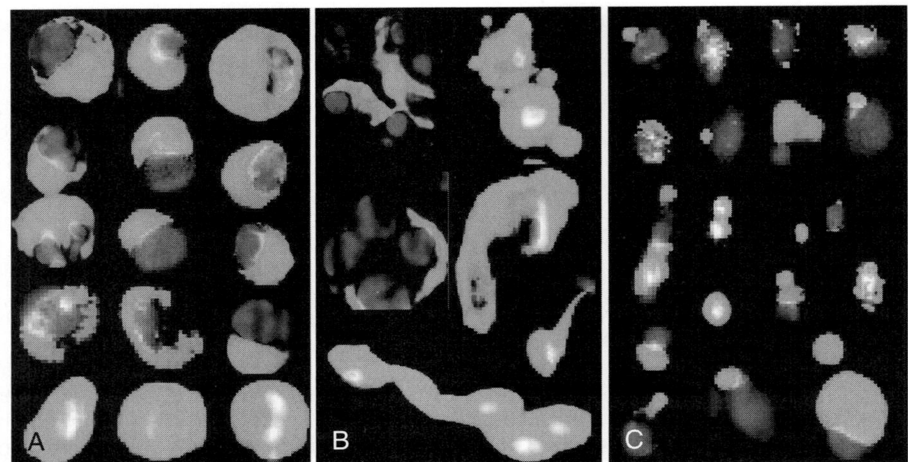

FIGURE 52.7 Gallery of CTC images from the CellSpotter Analyzer of the CellSearch system obtained from 7.5 mL of blood from cancer patients. EpCAM is stained *light gray*, and nuclear DNA is stained *dark gray*. Images that have no nuclear DNA are not viable cells and are not counted. Panel A shows examples of typical intact CTCs, panel B shows examples of intact CTCs present as clusters or with odd shapes that are present less frequently, and panel C provides examples of CTC fragments and apoptotic CTCs. Images presented in panel C are not included in CTC counts but are frequently observed in CTC analysis of carcinoma patients. A full color version of this figure is available online at ExpertConsult.com.

cartridge.[21] However, this application of CellSeach is not FDA-cleared.

The main advantages of the CellSearch system are its ease of use and high reproducibility. The preanalytical phase in this system is controlled by collecting blood in special tubes containing a cell preservative that enables sample transportation and stability. All analytical steps are well controlled and automated, similar to a standardized biochemical analyzer. The blood tubes are placed into an automated sample preparation system that uses ferro-fluids loaded with an antibody against EpCAM to capture CTCs (Fig. 52.8). The CellSearch System can enumerate CTCs in 7.5 mL of peripheral blood and can detect down to one cell. The analytical accuracy, precision, linearity, and diagnostic specificity of this system were first validated in 2004.[21] A prospective multicenter validation study at three independent laboratories showed that CTC counts remained stable for 72 hours after blood sample collection, even at room temperature.[22] Interassay variability was below 5% for 299 analyzed control samples, and the mean recovery rate of tumor cells spiked into normal blood at the 4- to 12-cell level was 82% and 80%, respectively. Within-run precision was evaluated in two different centers

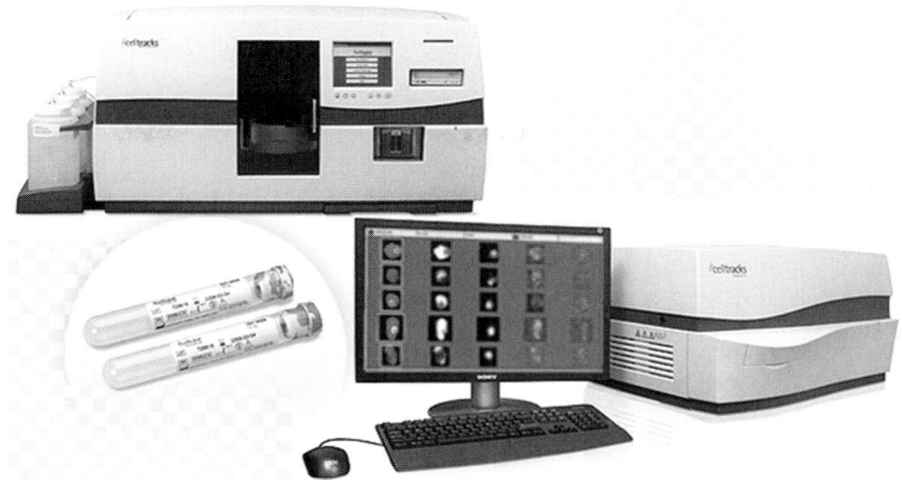

FIGURE 52.8 The CellSearch CTC detection and enumeration system. See text for discussion (Image reproduced by permission of Janssen Diagnostics LLC from *https://www.cellsearchctc.com/product-systems-overview/cellsearch-system-overview*.)

by eight replicates of the same spiked samples, and CVs were 18.4% to 26% for low cell numbers and 2.1% to 11.6% for high numbers of spiked cells.

The majority of evidence supporting the use of CTCs in clinical decision making has been related to epithelial CTC enumeration using the CellSearch system. However, the system has several limitations. The main drawback of CellSearch is that it depends entirely on the expression of the epithelial marker EpCAM on CTCs. This means that CTCs that do not express EpCAM because of epithelial mesenchymal transition (EMT) are not detected, as is the case for a subpopulation of highly aggressive breast cancer stem cells.[23] Another limitation is that gene expression cannot be performed on CTCs isolated with CellSearch because the cell preservative used inhibits downstream RNA analysis.

Leon Terstappen's group, which developed the CellSearch system, evaluated different ways to express changes in CTC counts with respect to overall survival. They clarified that CTC measurements on a patient at successive times may show a decline in CTCs. However, for low CTC numbers, this decline may result from either a true decline in the number of CTCs in the patient's blood, or it may arise from a Poisson sampling error. They propose that a static CTC cutoff is the best method to determine whether a therapy is effective, and they provide a lookup table from which the significance of a change in CTCs can be derived.[24]

An automated CTC counting algorithm to eliminate the variability in manual counting of CTCs has been validated on prostate, breast, and colorectal cancer CTC images. By using this approach, CTCs were identified and morphological features extracted from images stored by the CellSearch system. The automated CTC counts were strongly correlated with clinical outcomes in metastatic breast, colorectal, and prostate cancers.[25] Recent advances in the classification of CTCs captured by the CellSearch system and the implications of their features and numbers have been recently reviewed.[26]

Since its introduction, CellSearch has been widely used in many clinical labs worldwide, and numerous clinical studies have been performed.[27] The enumeration of CTCs continues to hold great promise in guiding treatment decisions in breast cancer patients. However, guidelines on how to use CTC enumeration by CellSearch in clinical decisions in both primary and metastatic breast cancer are still lacking.[28]

Isolation/Enrichment Systems for CTC Analysis

CTCs can be infrequent, depending on the cancer stage. One CTC may be present among 10^6 to 10^8 peripheral blood cells. CTC isolation and enrichment from peripheral blood are thus extremely challenging and very demanding. It is not only that these cells circulate at very low numbers, but they are heterogeneous even within the same patient. Highly standardized and robust isolation protocols are necessary for downstream CTC analysis and molecular characterization. Toward this goal, a lot of effort has focused on developing novel technologies for the isolation and enrichment of CTCs from peripheral blood. These can be categorized into two main systems based on the different properties of CTCs that distinguish them from surrounding normal hematopoietic cells: (1) label-independent systems based on physical properties, such as size, density, electric charge, and deformability that may utilize microfluidics, and (2) label-dependent systems based on biological properties of CTCs, such as expression of specific proteins on their cell surface. These include immunomagnetic bead separation systems with positive and/or negative selection. Approaches using both physical and biologic properties are common. In vivo methods for increasing CTC yield have also been developed.

The most important systems for the isolation/enrichment of CTCs are discussed in the following text. In many cases these technologies are complementary to one another because they target different properties of CTCs and may define unique CTC populations.

Label-Dependent CTC Isolation/Enrichment Systems

Positive Selection. Positive selection is the most widely used CTC isolation/enrichment system. This approach captures CTCs through specific monoclonal antibodies against epithelial cell surface markers that are expressed on CTCs but are absent from normal leukocytes. CTCs can be tagged using antibody-conjugated magnetic microbeads (diameter: 0.5–5 μm) or nanoparticles (diameter: 50–250 nm) that bind to a specific surface antigen. Intracellular antigens like cytokeratins can also be used as targets.[29,30] Immunomagnetic assays require a short incubation (~30 minutes) for antigen/antibody binding that couples the cells to magnetic beads, followed by isolation of the cells using a magnetic field (see Fig. 52.5).

Various antigens have been exploited for the positive immunomagnetic isolation of CTCs. Among these, EpCAM is the most common. This approach is well established in terms of proven clinical significance of the captured cells. However, capture with EpCAM has the disadvantage of missing some cells that are undergoing EMT. We also now know that CTCs are highly heterogeneous, but one approach to partially overcome this issue is to use a "cocktail" of antibodies that targets multiple antigens.[29,31-33] Along these lines, several organ- or tumor-specific markers, such as carcinoembryonic antigen (CEA), epidermal growth factor receptor (EGFR), prostate-specific antigen, HER-2, cell surface–associated mucin 1 (MUC-1), ephrin receptor B4 (EphB4), insulin-like growth factor 1 receptor (IGF-1R), cadherin-11 (CAD11), and tumor-associated glycoprotein 72 (TAG-72), have been used to isolate CTCs.[34,35] Cell surface vimentin on CTCs is a good marker for epithelial cancers undergoing EMT. By using a specific monoclonal antibody against vimentin, EMT-CTCs were detected in patients undergoing postsurgery adjuvant chemotherapy for metastatic colon cancer.[36] These isolated EMT-CTCs were characterized further using EMT-specific markers, fluorescent in situ hybridization, and single-cell mutation analysis. This antibody exhibited high specificity and sensitivity toward different epithelial cancer cells and was used to detect and enumerate EMT-CTCs from patients. The number of EMT-CTCs detected correlated with the therapeutic outcome of the disease. According to these results, cell surface vimentin is a promising marker for the isolation of EMT-CTCs from a wide variety of tumor types.[36]

Another example of positive selection is the MagSweeper, an immunomagnetic cell separator.[37,38] In this device, magnetic beads are coated with an antibody targeting epithelial cell surface markers. These immunomagnetic beads are added into blood samples, and cancer cells are attached to the beads. This device gently enriches target cells and eliminates cells that are not bound to magnetic particles by using centrifugal forces. The isolated cells are easily accessible and can be extracted individually based on their physical characteristics to deplete any cells nonspecifically bound to beads.[37,38] The same group has recently developed the magnetic sifter, a miniature microfluidic chip with a dense array of magnetic pores; tumor cells are labeled with magnetic nanoparticles and are captured from whole blood with high efficiency.[39] The use of isolation technologies that take advantage of magnetic fields may lead the way to routine preparation and characterization of liquid biopsies from cancer patients.

Negative Selection. This isolation approach is completely independent of the phenotype of CTCs and is based on the depletion of noncancerous peripheral blood cells by first lysing red blood cells (RBCs) and further using specific markers for white blood cells (WBCs) like CD45 or CD61 to magnetically remove WBCs from the sample.[40-42] Another variation of CTC enrichment by negative depletion is the commercially available RosetteSep system (StemCell technologies, Canada), which uses a mixture of antibodies that link RBCs to one another and to WBCs. In this way, the majority of the erythrocytes and leukocytes in the peripheral blood sample are depleted, thereby negatively enriching the sample with tumor cells if present. This approach is independent of the expression of EpCAM on CTCs and has better recoveries than the conventional density gradient method for the isolation of CTCs from normal leukocytes in blood.[43]

Flow Cytometry–Based Technologies. Multiparameter flow cytometry was firstly evaluated for the detection of human tumor cells in experimental mouse models of breast cancer.[44] This methodology was later adapted for the analysis of tumor dissemination to bone marrow and lymph nodes, in combination with laser scanning cytometry.[45] It is feasible to isolate CTCs from peripheral blood with high purity through fluorescence-activated cell sorting and profile them downstream via gene expression analysis.[46-48] Recently, cell sorting was used to isolate CTCs from CellSearch isolates and perform downstream high-resolution genomic profiling at the single-cell level.[49]

Label-Independent CTC Isolation/Enrichment Systems

Systems Based on Density. Density gradient centrifugation using commercially available reagents (eg, Ficoll, GE Healthcare Life Sciences, Pittsburgh, Penn.) is one of the most widely used approaches for CTC enrichment.[50,51] It is based on the lower density of mononuclear cells (including CTCs) compared to RBCs and polymorphonuclear leukocytes.[52] The OncoQuick system (Greiner Bio-One, Germany) is an improved version of this approach that uses a porous membrane placed on top of the gradient media to prevent mixing.[53] Experiments performed in cell lines have shown CTC recovery rates of 70% to 90%.[54] Although simple and inexpensive, the OncoQuick system has a relatively low yield and enrichment when compared to the CellSearch system because in the same group of 61 patients, at least one CTC was detected in 23% with OncoQuick and in 54% with CellSearch.[55]

Systems Based on CTC Size. Size-based isolation systems are independent of tumor markers and separate CTCs (that are usually larger) from smaller leukocytes. Several different size–based systems have been developed and include membrane filters, microfluidic chips, and hydrodynamic methods.[56,57] The first CTC filtration device was described by Vona and colleagues in 2000.[58] Since then, filtration devices have been improved, and many downstream applications have been developed. Filters used for CTC isolation/enrichment are often disposable porous membranes (usually polycarbonate) containing numerous randomly distributed 7- to 8-μm-diameter holes that allow blood constituents to cross but capture the larger CTCs.[58,59] Specific microfabrication techniques have been applied to build microfilters with controlled pore distribution, size, and geometry,[60-62] and different materials like polycarbonate,[58,59,63-66] parylene C,[67] nickel,[60] and, most recently, silicon[68] have been tested for fabrication of these membranes. Live CTCs isolated in this way can be further cultured in vitro for downstream studies.

Specifically designed polycarbonate membrane filter kits are usually accompanied by specific syringes or pumps so the pressure on the filter is optimized to keep fragile CTCs intact. Commercially available filtering devices for CTC isolation include ScreenCell (ScreenCell Inc., France), the ISET system (isolation by size of epithelial tumor cells, RareCells, France), and the CellSieve system (CREATV MicroTech, Potomac, Md.). Another filter-based microdevice that is both a capture and analysis platform capable of performing multiplexed imaging and genetic analysis has the potential to enable routine CTC analysis in the clinical setting.[67]

ScreenCell filters allow the isolation of live, spiked cancer cells or paraformaldehyde-fixed CTCs.[59] The performance of this technology for CTC capture was evaluated in 76 patients and has potential as a diagnostic blood test for lung cancer.[69] The ISET filtration system allows for cytomorphological, immunocytological, and genetic characterization of CTCs. This isolation approach is sensitive and can detect one single tumor cell added to 1 mL of blood. It is also simple and fast, consisting of only one filtration step.[58] Furthermore, ISET-isolated tumor cells can be subsequently recovered from the filter and evaluated by immunohistochemistry and/or molecular-genetic analyses.[70] In non–small cell lung cancer, this system can detect CTCs with a hybrid (epithelial/mesenchymal) phenotype, isolate anaplastic lymphoma receptor tyrosine kinase (ALK)–positive CTCs,[71] and isolate ROS-rearranged CTCs.[72] By using the CellSieve filtering system, very large cells (25 to 300 microns), called cancer-associated macrophage-like cells, were recently identified in the peripheral blood of cancer patients.[73]

CTC isolation by size filtration is simple and reliable; filtration and staining are easy to perform, and the method is rapid. CTCs can be identified using classic cytopathologic criteria. No complex instrumentation or specific training is needed. However, false-positive results can be obtained by using filtration devices. This is due to the presence of normal epithelial cells, which are collected by an intradermic needle and can be misinterpreted as CTCs. Moreover, endothelial cells or rare hematologic cells such as megakaryocytes may also be present on the filter. For this reason, downstream cytomorphological, immunocytochemical, and molecular characterization are important to rule out cells that are not CTCs.[74]

Separation Based on the Electric Charge of CTCs. CTCs are different from peripheral blood mononuclear cells with respect to morphology and dielectric properties. Dielectrophoresis (DEP) is a technology for CTC isolation based on electrical properties of cancer cells. Dielectric properties (polarizability) of cells are dependent on cell diameter, membrane area, density, conductivity, and volume. Depending on their phenotype and morphology, different cells have different dielectric properties, which is the principle employed for electro-kinetic isolation of CTCs.[75]

DEP can precisely manipulate and collect single cells. The DEPArray (Silicon Biosystems, Menarini group, IT) is a microfluidic device consisting of 320 × 320 arrayed electrodes generating over 10,000 spherical DEP cages that can guide single CTCs to predetermined spatial coordinates. This lab-on-a-chip platform is completely independent of the expression of antibodies on the cell surface and can be used for quick, arrayed, software-guided binding of individual CTCs. This system has been evaluated in the clinical setting with a goal toward showing superior performance in single-cell CTC analysis (Fig. 52.9).[76] Dielectrophoretic manipulation and isolation of single CTCs at 100% purity has been achieved from preenriched blood samples.[77] The single-use, microfluidic cartridge contains an array of individually controllable electrodes, each with embedded sensors. This circuitry enables the creation of DEP cages around cells. After imaging, individual cells of interest are gently moved to specific locations on the cartridge—for example, for cell–cell interaction studies—or into the holding chamber for isolation and recovery.[77,78] This system can be used in combination with other CTC platforms, such as the CellSearch, for downstream single CTC molecular characterization.[77,79,80]

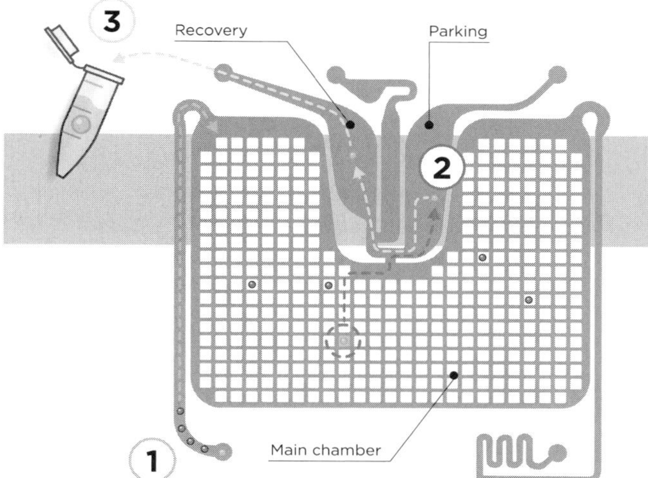

FIGURE 52.9 The DEPArray Cartridge for the isolation of single CTCs (Menarini Silicon Biosystems). The system is based on dielectrophoresis. The sequential steps are (1) inject, trap, and image cells; (2) move the cells of interest into the parking chamber; and (3) move the individual or multiple cells into the recovery chamber. (Image reproduced by permission of Menarini Silicon Biosystems from http://cdn2.hubspot.net/hubfs/304284/Brochures/Silicon_Biosystems_DEPArray_Brochure_2015.pdf?t=1466668511037.)

Microfluidic Systems for CTC Isolation/Enrichment. The main advantages of microfluidic systems for CTC isolation/enrichment are their simplicity and the potential to be fully automated, unlike traditional affinity-based CTC isolation techniques. The main disadvantage up to now is the long time needed to run each sample and the low capacity in terms of the volume of peripheral blood that can be processed. These systems are based on a combination of precisely defined topography of microstructures (traps) with laminar flow in microchannels.[7,81]

The first specific microfluidic device for CTC isolation was described in 2007. This "CTC-Chip" was a silicon chamber etched with 78,000 microposts that were coated with an anti-EpCAM antibody.[82] Captured CTCs attached to microposts were visualized by staining with antibodies against cytokeratin or tissue-specific markers. Using this design, approximately 60% of cancer cells have been recovered from spiked whole blood samples. Due to the high rate of collisions enabled by the dense array of microposts, varying expressions of EpCAM by target cells do not affect the recovery rate. However, in this first device, many false-positive results were detected in a healthy individual's blood.[82] The same group has further developed a simpler device, the "HB-chip," which is characterized by a herringbone structure and reliable coating of the inner surface with antibodies. Moreover, the chambers are made out of transparent materials that enhance high-resolution imaging, including the use of transmitted light microscopy.[83] The latest development of this group is the "CTC-iChip," another microfluidic CTC capture platform that is capable of sorting rare CTCs from

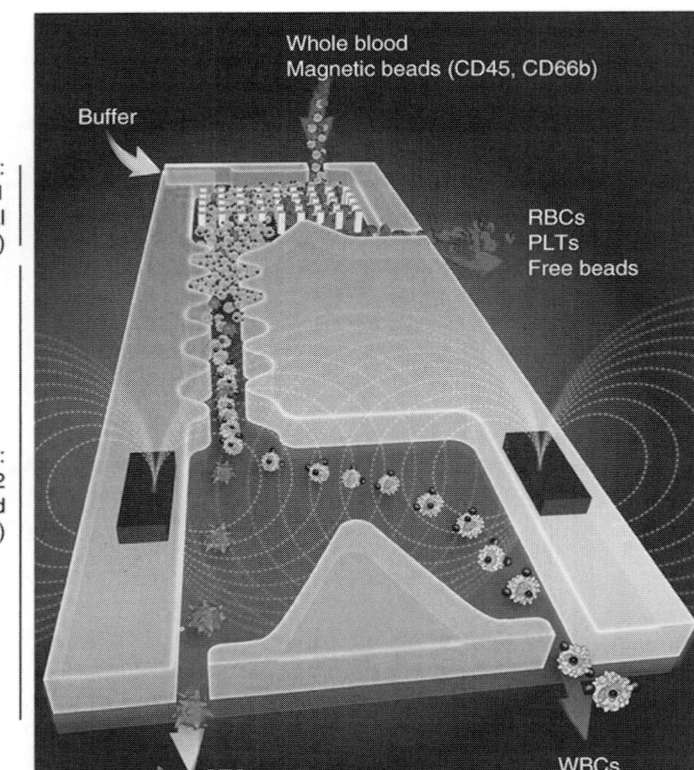

FIGURE 52.10 The CTC-iChip schematic. The CTC-iChip is composed of two separate microfluidic devices that house three different microfluidic components engineered for inline operation: deterministic lateral displacement to remove nucleated cells from whole blood by size-based deflection by using a specially designed array of posts performed in CTC-iChip1, inertial focusing to line up cells to prepare for precise magnetic separation, and magnetophoresis for sensitive separation of bead-labeled WBCs and unlabeled CTCs, which are performed in CTC-iChip2. *PLTs,* Platelets. (From Karabacak NM, Spuhler PS, Fachin F, Lim EJ, Pai V, Ozkumur E, et al. Microfluidic, marker-free isolation of circulating tumor cells from blood samples. *Nat Protoc.* 2014;9:694–710. Copyright 2014 Nature Publishing Group.)

whole blood at 10^7cells/s (Fig. 52.10). This device can isolate CTCs using strategies that are either label-dependent or label-independent and thus is applicable to virtually all cancers. The CTC-iChip was recently evaluated in an expanded set of both epithelial and nonepithelial cancers, including lung, prostate, pancreas, breast, and melanoma. CTC sorting in solution allows high-quality, clinically standardized, morphological and immunohistochemical analyses, as well as RNA-based single-cell molecular characterization.[84]

Most microfluidic devices are reliant on three-dimensional structures that limit the characterization of cells on the chip. Recently, Nagrath's group isolated CTCs from blood samples from patients with pancreatic, breast, and lung cancers by using functionalized graphene oxide nanosheets on a patterned gold surface.[85] This method allows for CTC capture with high sensitivity. A variety of highly sophisticated microfluidic devices have been developed by this group,[86,87] some of which have enabled further culturing of isolated cells on the chip. Recently, this group also developed an in situ capture and culture methodology for ex vivo expansion of CTCs using a three-dimensional co-culture model, simulating a tumor microenvironment to support tumor development. They managed to successfully expand CTCs isolated from early-stage lung cancer patients and characterize them further by both Sanger sequencing and massively parallel sequencing, as summarized in Fig. 52.11.[88]

A multiplexed microfluidic chip was recently developed and clinically validated for the ultra-high-throughput, low-cost, and label-free enrichment of CTCs.[89] Retrieved cells were unlabeled and viable, enabling potential propagation and real-time downstream analysis using massively parallel sequencing or proteomic analysis (Fig. 52.12).[89] In a separate study, HER-2 was used as an alternative to EpCAM in a novel microfluidic device for the isolation of CTCs from peripheral blood of patients with HER-2-expressing solid tumors.[90] In summary, microfluidic devices for CTC isolation have been described, and this number is increasing continuously.[57,91-98]

In Vivo Systems for CTC Isolation/Enrichment. The recent development of in vivo systems for CTC isolation from whole blood adds another dimension to the field of CTC isolation (Fig. 52.13). These systems aim to overcome the limitation of small blood sample volumes inherent to the ex-vivo CTC isolation techniques previously described.

Leukapheresis is a laboratory procedure in which WBCs or peripheral blood stem cells are separated from blood. During leukapheresis, a patient's blood is passed through a machine

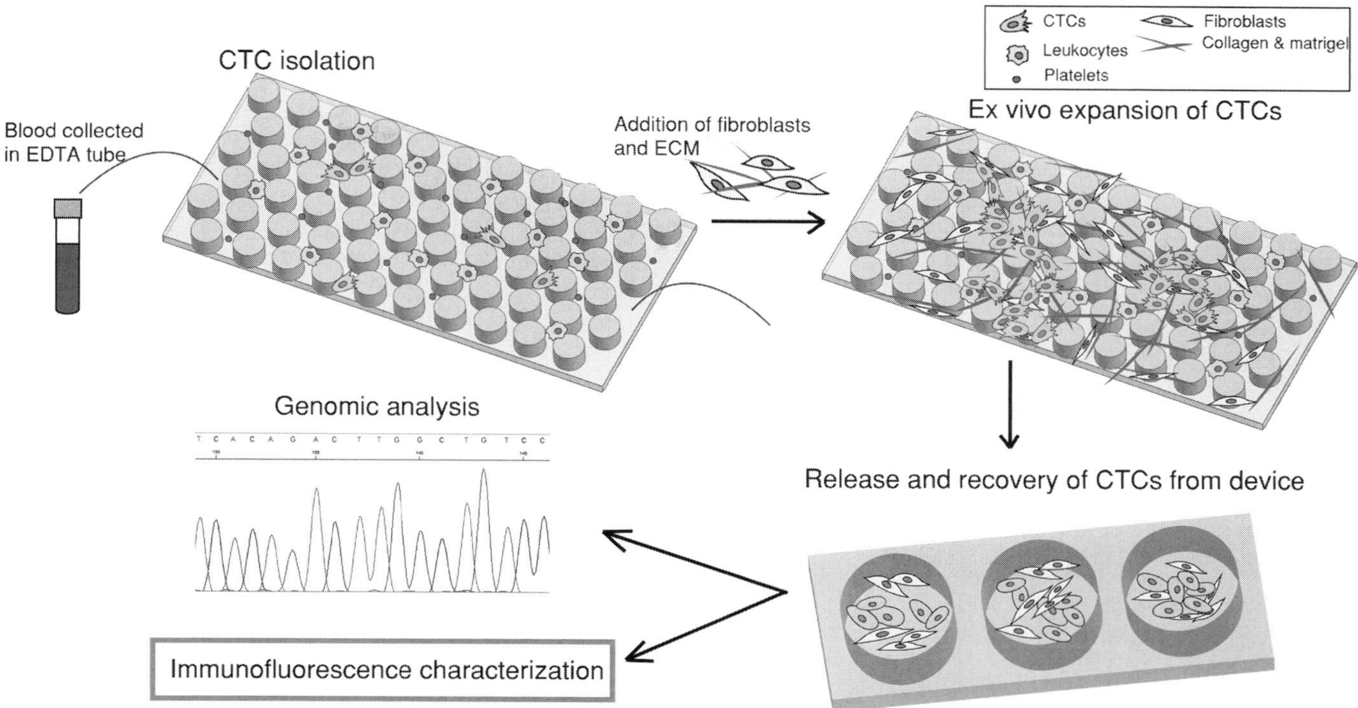

FIGURE 52.11 Expansion of CTCs from early-stage lung cancer patients using microfluidics. The first step is to capture CTCs by flow of a patient blood sample through a CTC-capture chip. The second step is to introduce fibroblasts and extracellular matrix (ECM) to the same chip to establish a co-culture environment for ex vivo expansion of CTCs. The third step is to release and recover CTCs from the device, and the fourth step is downstream characterization. (From Zhang Z, Shiratsuchi H, Lin J, Chen G, Reddy RM, Azizi E, Fouladdel et al. Expansion of CTCs from early stage lung cancer patients using a microfluidic co-culture model. *Oncotarget* 2014;5:12383–97. Copyright 2014 Impact Journals, LLC.)

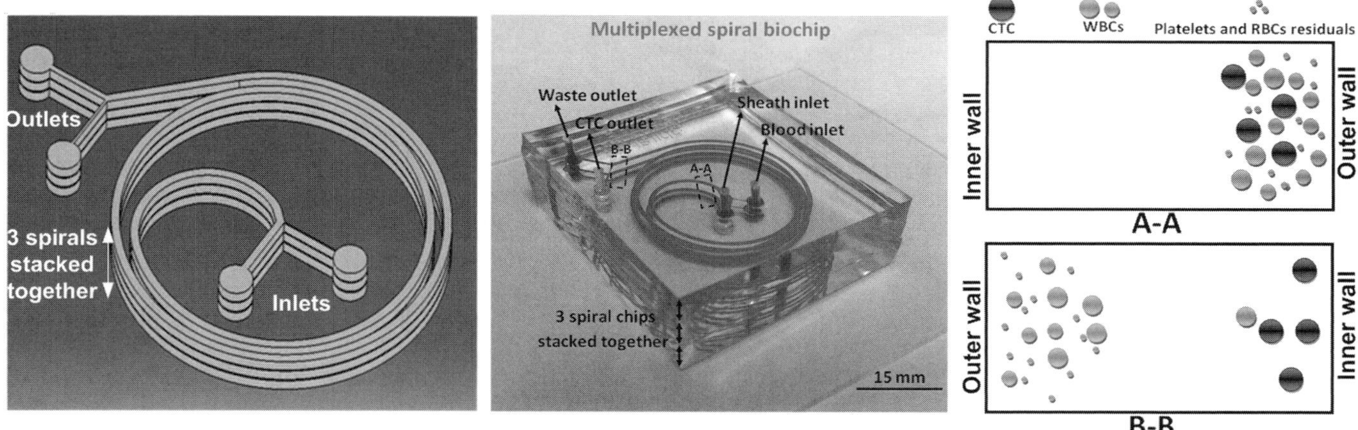

FIGURE 52.12 The design *(left)* and a photograph *(middle)* of a parallel spiral microfluidic device for separating CTCs. Blood sample and sheath fluid are pumped through the device using two separate syringe pumps. Under the influence of inertial lift and Dean drag forces in the fluid flow, CTCs focus near the microchannel inner wall, while WBCs and platelets go through one Dean cycle and migrate toward the outer wall, thus achieving separation. A full color version of this figure is available online at ExpertConsult.com. (Modified from Khoo BL, Warkiani ME, Tan DS, Bhagat AA, Irwin D, Lau DP, et al. Clinical validation of an ultra high-throughput spiral microfluidics for the detection and enrichment of viable circulating tumor cells. *PLoS One*. 2014;9:e99409.)

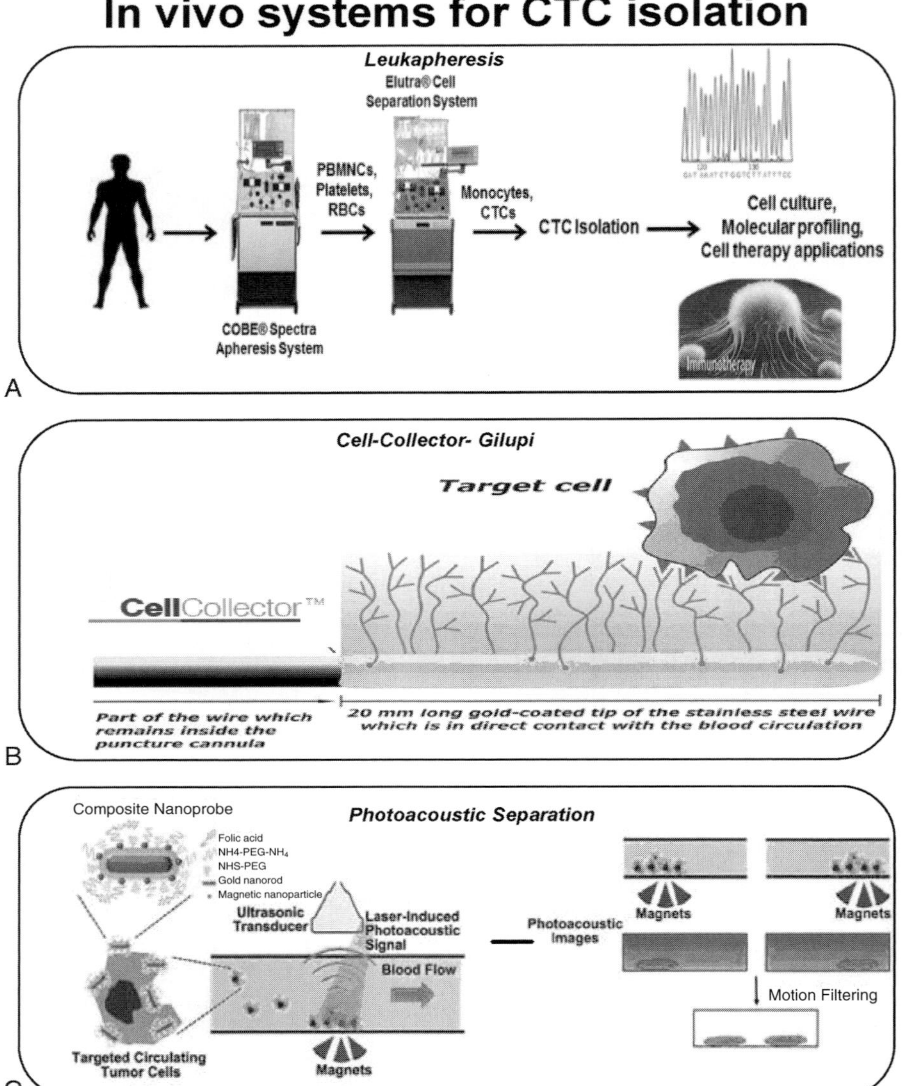

FIGURE 52.13 In vivo systems for CTC isolation and detection. **A,** Blood cells harvested by apheresis can be further processed by leukophoresis to isolate monocytes and CTCs (COBE and Elutara, both from Terumo BCT, Lakewood, Colo.). Additional processing to isolate CTCs allows molecular profiling and potential immunotherapy. **B,** A nanowire coated with EpCAM antibodies can be inserted into a vein for in vivo binding of CTCs (Cell-Collector, Gilupi GmbH, Germany). **C,** Photoacoustic flow cytometry using ultrasound and a pulsed IR laser can count CTCs in blood vessels up to 3 mm deep. Photoacoustic separations of CTCs may be possible with magnetic nanoprobes. (**A,** Modified from Greene BT, Hughes AD, King MR. Circulating tumor cells: the substrate of personalized medicine? *Front Oncol* 2012;2:69. **B,** From GILUPI NanoMedizin. **C,** Modified from Wei CW, Xia JJ, Pelivanov I, et al. Magnetomotive photoacoustic imaging spots circulating tumor cells. *Biophotonics* 2013;20: 34–36.)

that removes the WBCs or peripheral blood stem cells and then returns the balance of the blood back to the patient (Fig. 52.13A). Eifler and colleagues first showed that isolation of CTCs via leukapheresis was feasible.[99] A recent study that screened leukapheresis products generated from up to 25 L of processed blood per patient demonstrated that CTCs can be detected in more than 90% of nonmetastatic breast cancer patients.[100]

Another novel in vivo CTC isolation system is the CellCollector (Gilupi GmbH, Germany) (Fig. 52.13B). CellCollector is a nanowire that is coated at its tip (2 cm of length) with pure gold, to which chimeric antibodies directed to EpCAM are covalently attached. The CellCollector is placed into the antecubital vein of a cancer patient for in vivo binding of rare CTCs from the patient's entire circulating blood pool of several liters.[101] More CTCs to support multiple downstream assays are available as compared to traditional in vitro approaches with samples of 7 to 15 mL of blood. This approach increases the chances of isolating rare tumor cells, especially in the early stages of the disease.

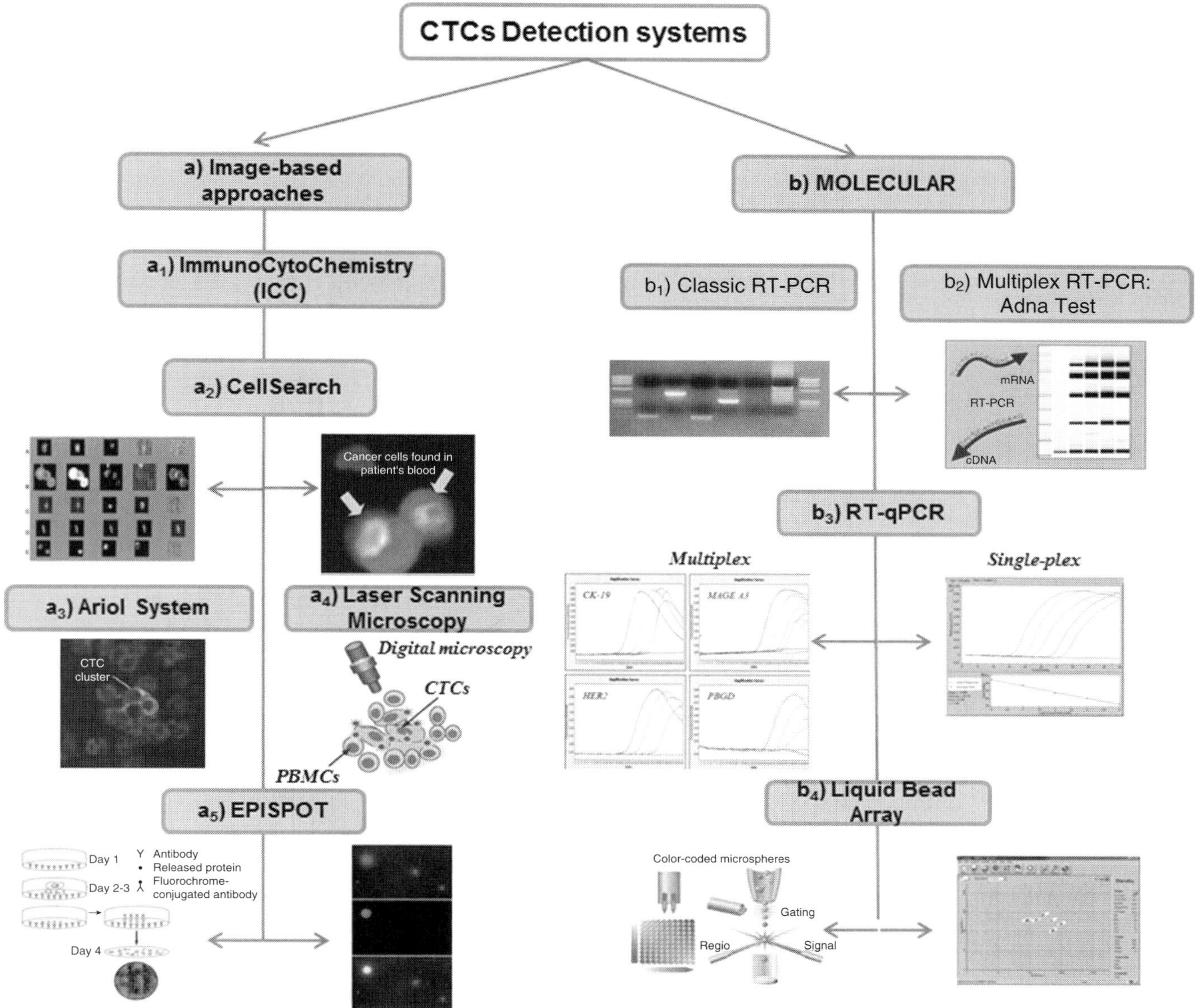

FIGURE 52.14 Main approaches for CTC detection and molecular characterization. **A,** Image-based approaches: (A_1) classic immunocytochemistry (ICC), (A_2) CellSearch system (FDA cleared), (A_3) digital image capture and analysis (Ariol system, Leica Biosystems, Buffalo Grove, Ill.), (A_4) laser-scanning cytometry, and (A_5) EPISPOT assay (detects tumor-specific proteins released by CTCs). **B,** Molecular assays based on nucleic acid analysis: (B_1) classic reverse transcriptase PCR (RT-PCR), (B_2) multiplex RT-PCR—for example, the AdnaTest for breast cancer (Qiagen Hannover, Germany), (B_3) singleplex or multiplex RT-qPCR, and (B_4) liquid bead array. (Modified with permission of the publisher from Lianidou ES, Markou A. Circulating tumor cells in breast cancer: detection systems, molecular characterization, and future challenges. *Clin Chem.* 2011;57:1242–55. Copyright 2011 American Association of Clinical Chemistry.)

Photoacoustic flow cytometry can also detect CTCs in vivo (Fig. 52.13C). A high–pulse repetition rate diode laser shines light through the skin into a vessel that is up to 3 mm deep to detect acoustic vibrations that result from the absorption of laser light by target nanoparticles.[102] By using this technology, circulating melanoma cells were detected in blood.[103] In vivo isolation technologies for CTC detection are now being evaluated in many centers; their future use will depend on the results of these clinical evaluation studies.

CTC Analysis: Detection and Molecular Characterization

CTC detection and molecular characterization are achieved by immunofluorescence; molecular nucleic acid analysis, including RT-qPCR and multiplex RT-qPCR; and detection of tumor-specific proteins released by CTCs. An outline of the main approaches for CTC detection is presented in Fig. 52.14.

Image-Based Approaches. Detection of epithelial CTCs by immunofluorescence using anti-CK antibodies is currently

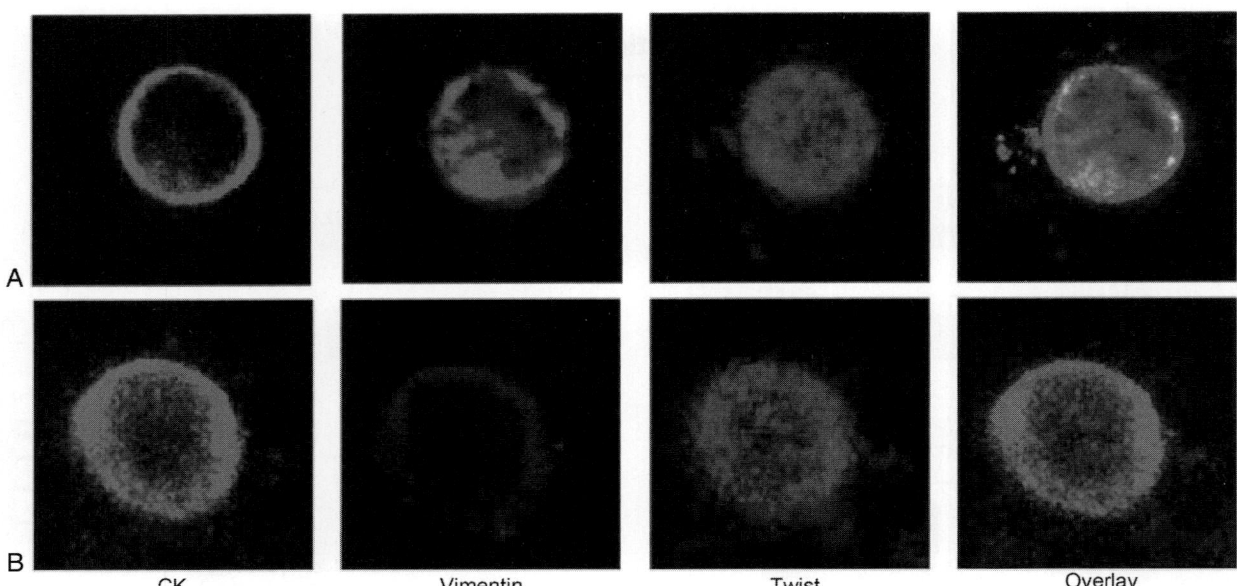

FIGURE 52.15 Digital image capture and analysis of CTCs. Representative confocal laser-scanning photomicrographs of CTC cytospins after negative immunomagnetic separation in a patient with metastatic breast cancer showing coexpression of cytokeratin, Twist and vimentin (Ariol system, Leica Biosystems, Buffalo Grove, Ill.). Cells were triple-stained for cytokeratin (CK), vimentin, and Twist. Original magnification is 600×. **A,** A CTC expressing CK, Twist, and vimentin. **B,** A CTC expressing CK and Twist, but not vimentin. A full color version of this figure is available online at ExpertConsult .com. (From Kallergi G, Papadaki MA, Politaki E, et al. Epithelial to mesenchymal transition markers expressed in circulating tumour cells of early and metastatic breast cancer patients. *Breast Cancer Res.* 2011;13:R59.)

the most validated and standardized approach and also allows for morphological interpretation of positive events. However, detection of CTC by classical immunofluorescence, typically done by trained pathologists through visual observation of stained cytokeratin-positive epithelial CTCs, is time-consuming and may take days if many samples are to be analyzed. Additional image-based modalities include detecting CTCs with multiple antibodies (eg, against cytokeratin, Her-2, and the stem cell antigens ALDH1, CD44, and CD24) labeled with different fluorochromes (DyLight Technology, ThermoFisher) and spectral image analysis to separate the different emissions.[104] Another technology is the laser scanning cytometer, a fast and quantitative automated microscopic procedure for screening with up to 10,000-fold enrichment. However, large numbers of apparent CTCs are detected even in healthy donors, possibly because of nonspecific binding of antibodies.[105] A third example of an image analysis method is the Ariol high-throughout automated image analysis system (Leica Biosystems, Germany) that has been widely used for high-definition imaging of CTCs (Fig. 52.15). The high-definition circulating tumor cell assay is a fluid-phase biopsy approach that identifies CTCs by high-definition imaging without any surface protein-based enrichment at a high enough definition to satisfy diagnostic pathology image quality requirements. This system has been evaluated in various types of cancers, such as lung, colorectal, and prostate.[106-109]

Molecular Assays. Molecular assays for CTC detection and molecular characterization take advantage of the sensitivity and specificity of PCR and the high throughput of massively parallel sequencing (MPS). Molecular assays have been widely applied for CTC detection and characterization and can interrogate CTCs at the single-cell level. CTC molecular assays include RT-qPCR, multiplex RT-qPCR, methylation-specific PCR, allele-specific PCR, fluorescent in situ hybridization, array comparative genomic hybridization (arrayCGH), and MPS technologies.

PCR assays are very sensitive and can analyze both RNA and DNA. PCR assays can be designed in silico, automated, and subjected to internal and external quality control systems.[19,110] In silico design of PCR assays using databases and specific software programs can avoid cross-reactions with nontarget genes. Molecular assays can be quantitative, high throughput, and easy to perform and usually require a very small sample amount for analysis. Especially when multiplex PCR is used, many targets can be evaluated from the same sample, thus enabling a multiparametric approach for the often limited CTC sample. In contrast to imaging approaches, measurements obtained by molecular assays are objective and quantifiable. Molecular assays are relatively low cost, high throughput, and amenable to quantifiable quality control. Another advantage is that many molecular methods can be automated. Fully automated systems for RNA and DNA isolation and downstream PCR analysis are already used in routine molecular in vitro diagnostics labs.

The main disadvantages of molecular assays are preanalytical issues concerning CTC stability during sample shipment and storage, a problem that CellSearch has solved for capture, staining, and image analysis. However, molecular assays currently require immediate handling of blood samples for CTC isolation and downstream analysis, a fact that hinders long-distance shipment of samples. Moreover, PCR assays require specially designed lab areas to avoid end-product contamination. Separate areas are usually needed for RNA/DNA isolation, setting up the reactions, and amplification and analysis. Unless single-cell analysis is performed, molecular assays provide only bulk information on a sample. For example, in mRNA analysis, it is not known whether transcripts are coexpressed in the same cell or derived from different cell populations.

PCR-Based Assays. PCR-based assays can be highly specific and sensitive. RT-qPCR assays targeting specific expression of genes in cancer cells and not in peripheral blood mononuclear cells are especially sensitive, with the ability to detect one cancer cell in the presence of more than 10^6 leukocytes.[111] However, this requires the detection of mRNA markers that are specifically expressed in CTCs and not expressed in leukocytes. In all cases, cutoffs should be estimated based on the expression values of these markers in a significant number of healthy donor samples that should be analyzed in exactly the same way as patient samples. RT-qPCR assays are high throughput and easy to perform because they are based on the isolation of total RNA from viable CTCs and subsequent RT-PCR amplification of tumor- or epithelial-specific targets.

Cytokeratins are not only used as biomarkers in imaging but are also used as biomarkers in RT-PCR as well. *KRT19* (the gene for CK-19) is an especially specific and sensitive marker for CTCs, provided that the primers used are well designed to avoid false-positive results due to the presence of the *CK-19* pseudogene. Using a highly specific EpCAM-independent RT-qPCR assay,[112,113] *KRT19* was a molecular marker of prognostic significance for OS and PFS in early breast cancer before, during, and after chemotherapy.[114-116]

Other targets can also be used for CTC detection. Smirnov and colleagues studied the expression profile of many genes on CTCs and observed that *AGR2, S100A14, S100A16, FABP1*, and other specific genes could be used for the detection of CTCs in the peripheral blood of advanced cancer patients.[117] Since then, many research groups have described the use of RT-PCR to characterize single or multiple targets of CTCs in cancer patients.

Another advantage of RT-qPCR is the flexibility it offers, especially in multiplexing. Multiplexing minimizes time, cost, and conserves available nucleic acid. Only a few transcripts provide adequate sensitivity individually, but combinations of transcripts may produce better sensitivity for CTC detection. AdnaGen (Qiagen, Hamburg) is commercializing a number of molecular diagnostic kits for different types of cancer based on RT-PCR. These kits use positive immunomagnetic isolation of CTC, followed by RT-PCR and electrophoretic detection with a Bioanalyzer (Agilent Technologies) instrument.[118,119] A quantitative gene expression profiling methodology based on RT-qPCR requires only one breast cancer CTC and amplifies a set of genes with no or minor expression by leukocytes.[120] Several mRNA markers may be useful for RT-PCR–based detection of CTCs. Quantification of these mRNAs is essential to distinguish normal expression in blood cells from that due to the presence of CTCs. A technical protocol to measure the expression of thousands of genes in CTCs captured with magnetic beads linked to EpCAM and the carcinoma-associated mucin, MUC-1, was recently reported. The expression profiles were reproducible and the technology suitable for prospective studies to assess the clinical utility of CTCs.[121]

Another approach using multiplex PCR is the liquid bead array (Luminex) that is automated and often present in clinical labs for a variety of applications.[122] A sensitive and specific CTC gene expression assay using multiplexed PCR coupled to a liquid bead array has been developed and validated.[123] Five established CTC genes—the HER-2 gene *ERRB2*, the mammaglobin A gene *SCGB2A2*, the *CK-19* gene *KRT19*, the melanoma antigen family A1 gene *MAGEA1*, the twist basic helix-loop-helix family 1 gene *TWIST1*, and one reference gene *HMBS*—were simultaneously amplified and detected in the same reaction using only 1 μL of cDNA from CTCs. Up to 100 genes in CTCs can be studied.[123]

Fluorescence in Situ Hybridization and RNA in Situ Hybridization. Fluorescence in situ hybridization (FISH) is widely used in the CTC field to verify *HER-2* amplification status and detect the presence of genomic rearrangements, such as *ALK* in lung cancer, and the androgen receptor in prostate cancer. In most cases FISH analysis has followed CellSearch selection and staining. After enumeration of cytokeratin+, CD45–, nucleated cells, the cells are fixed in the cartridge to maintain their original position and hybridized to FISH probes. Next, fluorescence images of the FISH probes are acquired. Heterogeneity of chromosomal abnormalities is observed between CTCs of different patients and among CTCs of the same patient.[124,125]

RNA in situ hybridization is also used for CTC detection; a system called CTCscope detects a multitude of tumor-specific markers from single CTCs. Breast cancer CTC transcripts of eight epithelial markers and three EMT markers have been evaluated.[126] RNA in situ hybridization can also characterize circulating brain tumor cells at the single-cell level isolated with microfluidics from patients with glioblastoma.[127] Both these techniques are mainly used in the research setting.

Array comparative genomic hybridization (arrayCGH) has also been used to detect DNA copy number changes in single CTCs. Multiplex FISH in combination with array CGH revealed that occult disseminated cells are characterized by very complex numerical and structural aberrations. Array CGH in micrometastatic cells allows for high-resolution assessment of copy number changes, pinpointing commonly gained or lost regions to narrow down the regions critically involved in metastasis.[128] Using a combination of whole genome amplification (WGA) technology and high-resolution oligonucleotide arrayCGH, reliable detection of numerical genomic alterations as small as 0.1 Mb in a single cell is possible. Analysis of single cells from well-characterized cell lines and single normal cells confirmed the stringent quantitative nature of the amplification and hybridization protocol (Fig. 52.16).[129] Comprehensive genomic profiling of CTCs can be achieved by combining arrayCGH and MPS technology. An integrated process to isolate, quantify, and sequence whole exomes of CTCs suggests that mapping of greater than 99.9955 of the CTC exome is possible,[130] indicating the clinical potential for CTC genomics in the future.

Protein Analyses on CTCs (EPISPOT Assay). The epithelial immunoSPOT (EPISPOT, a specific type of ELISPOT or enzyme-linked immunoSPOT) assay was developed to detect tumor-specific proteins released by viable CTCs. This assay detects proteins secreted/released/shed from single epithelial cancer cells. Cells are cultured for a short time on a membrane coated with antibodies that capture the secreted/released/shed proteins, with subsequent detection by secondary antibodies

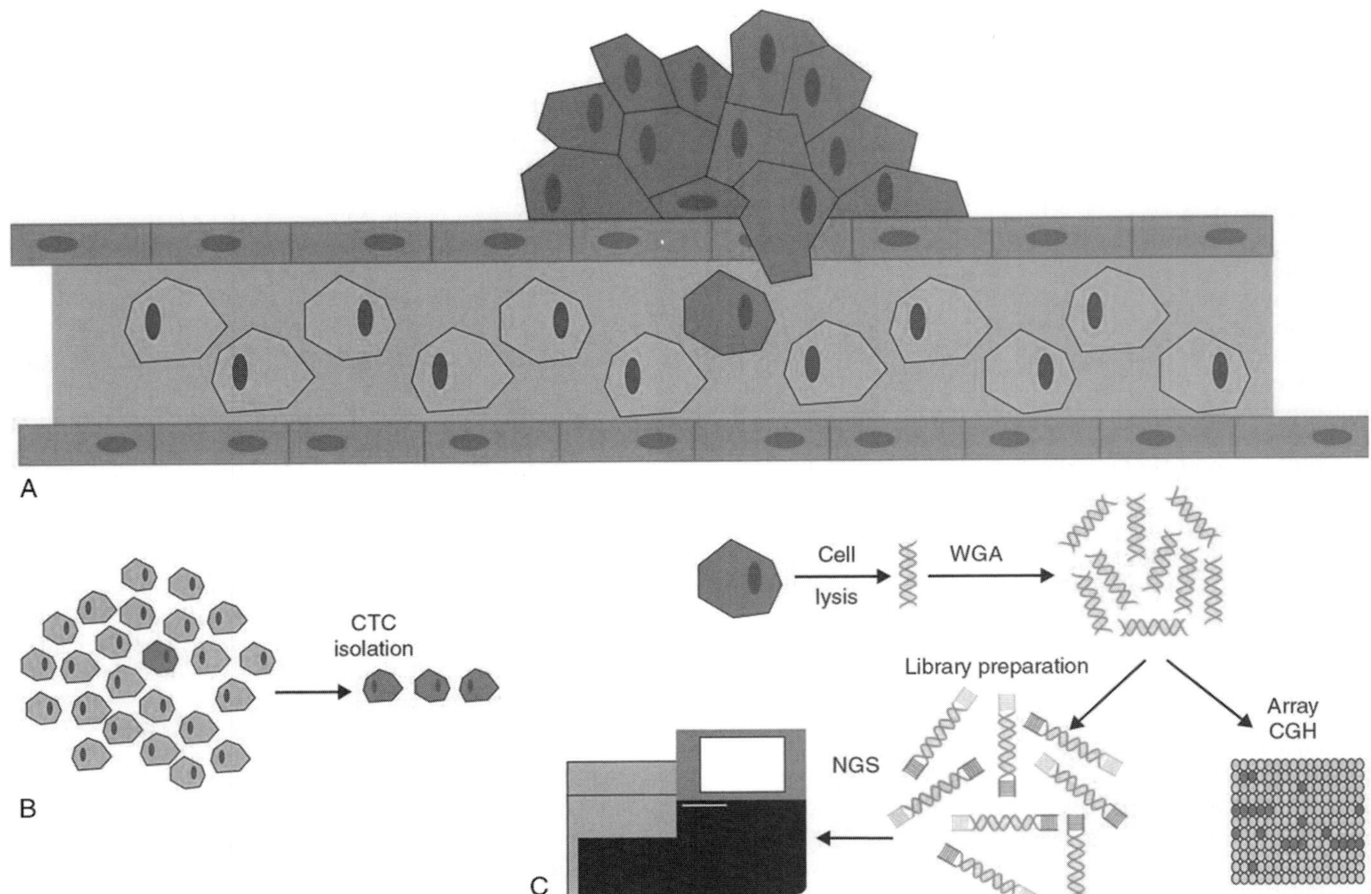

FIGURE 52.16 Workflow of CTC analysis by array comparative genomic hybridization and massively parallel sequencing. **A,** CTCs *(light blue cells)* are rare cells in the circulation; the vast majority of nucleated cells are normal blood cells *(orange)*. **B,** CTCs are isolated by one of many methods. **C,** After cell lysis, DNA is accessible for whole genome amplification (WGA). The WGA products can be analyzed for copy number changes on an array platform by comparative genomic hybridization (arrayCGH). Alternatively, libraries can be prepared and subjected to massively parallel sequencing (also known as next-generation sequencing, or NGS). By NGS, both copy number changes and mutations within genes can be detected. (From Heitzer E, Auer M, Ulz P, Geigl JB, Speicher MR. Circulating tumor cells and DNA as liquid biopsies. *Genome Med.* 2013;5:73. Copyright 2013 BioMed Central.)

labeled with fluorochromes. This assay has been used in many types of solid cancers, such as breast, colorectal, prostate, and others.[75]

Single-Cell Analysis of CTCs. CTCs are highly heterogeneous, even within the same individual.[131] This has been verified by using reliable single-CTC isolation followed by MPS to clearly reveal differences among CTCs. This powerful combination offers a new dimension in CTC molecular characterization. Using the DEPArray system (see Fig. 52.9) for isolation of single CTCs, Peeters and colleagues have obtained reliable gene expression profiles from single cells and groups of up to 10 cells.[77]

MPS technologies reveal that intratumor heterogeneity may reflect tumor evolution and adaptation that hinder personalized medicine strategies developed from results on single-tumor biopsy samples.[132,133] Analysis of CTCs reduces this complexity because CTCs are present in blood in low cell numbers that provide a better picture for individualized treatments because they represent both cells that have disseminated from the primary tumor and cells from secondary metastases. Heitzer and colleagues performed the first comprehensive genomic profiling of CTCs in patients with stage IV colorectal carcinoma using arrayCGH and MPS. Mutations in driver genes of the primary tumor and metastasis were also detected in the corresponding CTCs. Mutations that appeared exclusively in CTCs were later found by additional deep sequencing in metastases from the same patient.[134]

The importance of characterizing single CTCs to investigate their molecular heterogeneity is clear. Polzer and colleagues combined enrichment and isolation of pure CTCs with a WGA method for single cells.[135] Focusing on metastatic breast cancer, both molecular heterogeneity between single CTCs and between CTCs and the primary tumors were identified. Some individual CTCs were resistant to HER2-targeted therapies, suggesting ongoing microevolution at late-stage disease relevant to personalized treatment decisions and acquired drug resistance.[135] Toward this direction, the

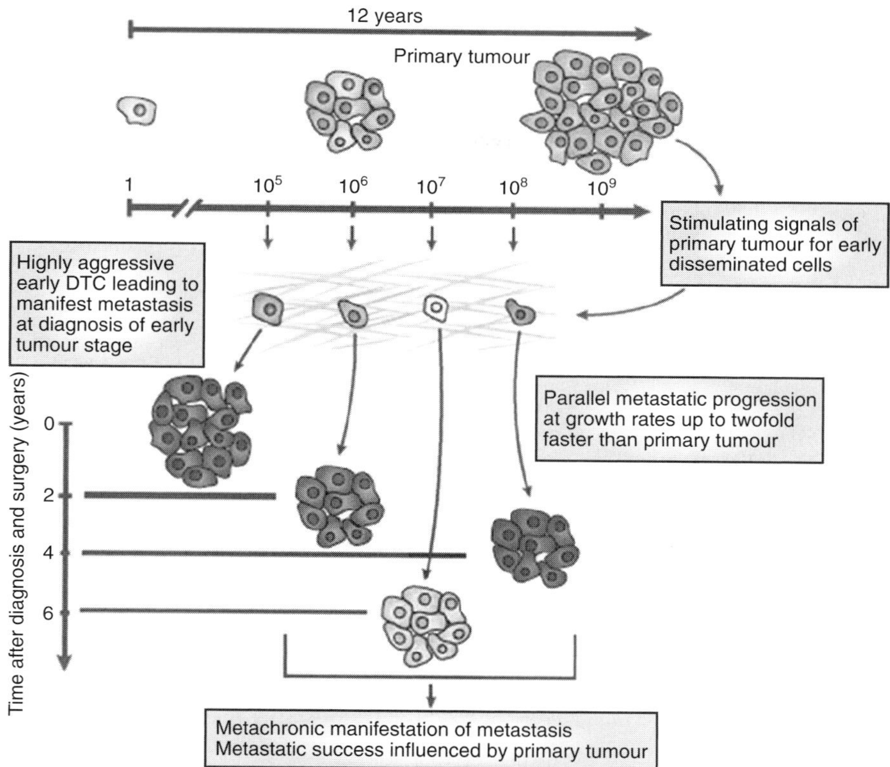

FIGURE 52.17 The parallel progression model of tumor metastasis. In the parallel progression model, several waves of disseminated tumor cells may originate before diagnosis and may progress in parallel at different rates in different organs. (From Klein CA. Parallel progression of primary tumours and metastases. *Nat Rev Cancer.* 2009;9:302–12.)

heterogeneity of *PIK3CA* mutation status within single CTCs isolated from individual metastatic breast cancer patients was recently studied by combining the CellSearch and DEPArray technologies.[80] *TP53* mutations were also found in single CTCs using this method.[79]

CTCs: "A Window to Metastasis"

In 1889, in the very first issue of *Lancet*, Steve Paget described "the seed and soil hypothesis," in which "metastasis depends on the cross talk between selected cancer cells (the seed) and specific organ microenvironments (the soil)," a hypothesis revisited many years later by Fidler.[136] Detailing the mechanism of metastasis remains a very hot topic in cancer research today.[14,137] According to the parallel progression model recently proposed by Klein,[6,138] parallel, independent metastases may arise from early disseminated tumor cells (Fig. 52.17). Analysis of disease course, tumor growth rates, autopsy studies, clinical trials, and molecular genetic analyses of primary and disseminated tumor cells all contribute to our understanding of systemic cancer.[6,138] Molecular characterization of CTCs provides a level of detail not previously possible and may be the key to our further understanding of metastatic progression.

CTC biology can be viewed as a "window to metastasis" because CTCs play a critical role in the metastatic spread of carcinomas (see Figs. 52.17 and 52.18).[7,8] If CTCs are effectively targeted or kept in a dormant state, the cancer may be prevented from progressing to metastatic disease. Molecular characterization of CTCs from patients may be the shortest path to determine which and when patients might relapse and to identify specific mechanisms to target these cells. Dormancy gene signatures that identify individuals with dormant disease have also been explored.[139,140] In contrast, CTCs with stemness and EMT features display enhanced malignant and metastatic potential. The role of CTCs in treatment failure and disease progression is likely explained by their biological processes, such as EMT, stemness features, dormancy, and heterogeneity.[141]

Epithelial and Mesenchymal Transitions of CTCs

Epithelial-mesenchymal transition (EMT) is an essential process in the metastatic cascade.[23,142-144] This biological process is highly associated with an invasive phenotype and enables detachment of tumor cells from the primary site and migration. The reverse process of mesenchymal epithelial transition (MET) might play a crucial role in the further steps of metastasis when CTCs seed distant organs and establish metastasis (Fig. 52.18). The mechanisms and the interplay of EMT and MET have been intensively studied, but only limited data suggest the existence of the EMT process in CTCs. It is now clear that CTCs from metastatic breast cancer patients exhibit heterogeneous epithelial and mesenchymal phenotypes and display higher frequencies of partial or full-blown mesenchymal phenotype than carcinoma cells within primary tumors. Mesenchymal-like CTCs are also elevated in patients who are refractory to therapy.[142]

Currently, most systems that detect CTCs, including the CellSearch system, are based on the expression of the

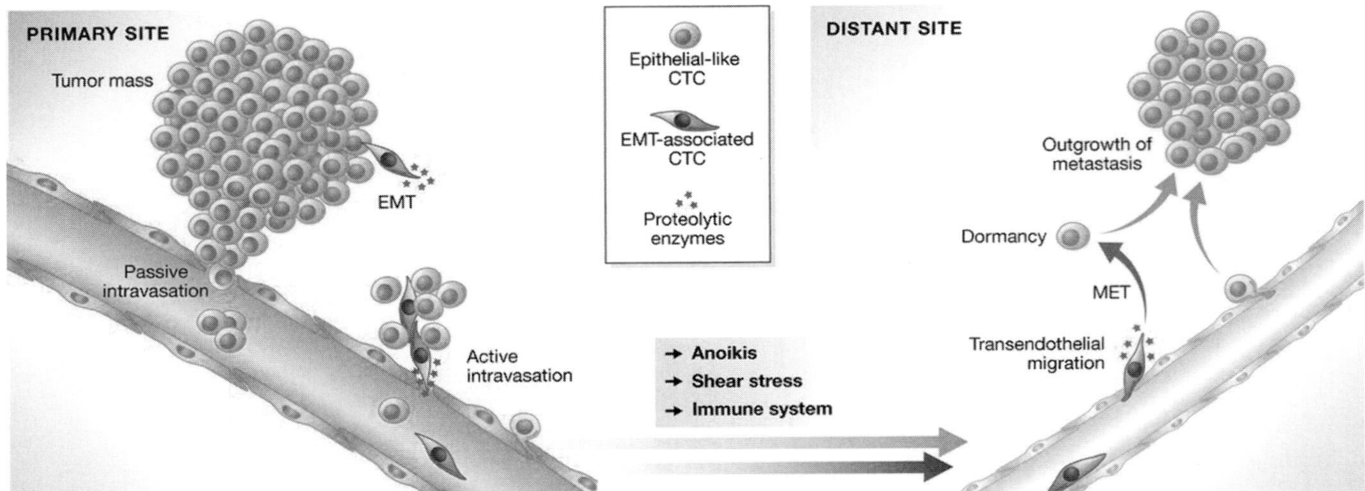

FIGURE 52.18 The metastatic cascade. Tumor cells may enter the bloodstream passively or actively via biological events caused by epithelial mesenchymal transition or centrosome amplification. Disseminating tumor cells must overcome several hurdles, including shear stress in the bloodstream, the immune system both inside and outside of the blood circulation, and anoikis (programmed cell death induced by a cell detaching from the extracellular matrix). Once at a distant site, tumor cells may extravasate, undergo mesenchymal epithelial transition, and grow locally to become a metastasis or remain in dormancy. (From Joosse SA, Gorges TM, Pantel K. Biology, detection, and clinical implications of circulating tumor cells. *EMBO Mol Med.* 2014;7:1–11.)

epithelial marker EpCAM and do not specifically identify CTC subtypes with EMT. Only recently, EMT-related markers have been applied in CTC studies. Three EMT markers (*TWIST1, AKT2,* and *PI3Kα*) and the stem cell marker *ALDH1* were evaluated in CTCs from 502 primary breast cancer patients by a multiplex RT-PCR assay.[145] A subset of CTCs showed EMT and stem cell characteristics. The expression levels of EMT-inducing transcription factors (*TWIST1, SNAIL1, SLUG, ZEB1,* and *FOXC2*) were also determined in CTCs from primary breast cancer patients.[146] In another study, rare primary tumor cells simultaneously expressed mesenchymal and epithelial markers, but mesenchymal cells were highly enriched in CTCs, and serial monitoring suggested an association of mesenchymal CTCs with disease progression.[147] Mesenchymal CTCs occurred as both single cells and multicellular clusters, expressed known EMT regulators, including transforming growth factor (TGF)-β pathway components and the *FOXC1* transcription factor. These data support a role for EMT in the blood-borne dissemination of human breast cancer.[147] When the EMT phenotype of CTCs was studied through the expression of two important EMT-connected genes—namely, *VIM* and *SNAIL*—using cytokeratin-negative CTCs from nonmetastatic breast cancer patients, the simultaneous detection of both EGFR and EMT markers may improve prognostic or predictive information.[148] A new assay based on triple immunofluorescence examines the coexpression of ALDH1 (a stemness marker) and TWIST (an EMT marker) of single CTCs in patients with breast cancer. A differential expression pattern for these markers in CTCs was observed both in early and metastatic disease. CTCs expressing high ALDH1 along with nuclear TWIST were more frequently found in patients with metastatic breast cancer, suggesting that CTCs undergoing EMT may prevail during disease progression.[149]

Gorges and colleagues reported low CTC numbers in patients with late metastatic cancers.[150] These results prompted the search for new markers, including those for mesenchymal-like subpopulations. Plastin-3 is an EMT marker in CTCs in colorectal cancer. Aberrant expression of plastin-3 was associated with increased CTCs and poor prognosis in colorectal cancer and may be involved in the regulation of EMT.[151] Cell-surface vimentin is specifically expressed on the surface of CTCs from epithelial cancers undergoing EMT, and the number of CTCs undergoing EMT correlates with disease outcome.

Cytokeratins are widely used for the identification of CTCs by immunocytochemistry, but even these established markers might be modulated during EMT. Breast cancer cells display a complex pattern of cytokeratin expression with potential biological relevance. Individual cytokeratin antibodies may recognize only certain cytokeratins, and important subsets of biologically relevant CTCs in cancer patients may be missed.[152] EMT and MET transitions are central to the metastatic potential of CTCs; the elucidation of their role in the clinical outcome of cancer patients can be achieved by CTC analysis in single cells.

CTCs and Cancer Stem Cells

Stemness is the ability of cells to self-renew and differentiate into cancer cells.[153] There is substantial evidence that many cancers are driven by a population of cells that display stem cell properties. These cells, called cancer stem cells (CSCs) or tumor initiating cells, not only drive tumor initiation and growth but also mediate tumor metastasis and therapeutic resistance. There is in vitro and clinical evidence that CSCs mediate metastasis and treatment resistance in breast cancer. Novel strategies to isolate CTCs that contain CSCs and the use of patient-derived xenograft models in preclinical breast cancer research have been developed to study the biology of CSCs.[154] Therapeutic resistance, underlying tumor recurrence, and the lack of curative treatments in metastatic disease raise the question as to whether conventional anticancer therapies target the right cells. Indeed, these treatments might miss CSCs that are resistant to many current cancer treatments, including chemotherapy and radiation therapy.[155] Emerging data suggest that the remarkable clinical efficacy of HER-2 targeting agents may be related to their ability to target the breast CSC population. In breast cancers that do not display HER-2 gene amplification, HER-2 is selectively expressed in the CSC population. This expression is regulated by the tumor microenvironment, suggesting that novel and effective adjuvant therapies may need to target the CSC population.[156,157]

EMT induction not only allows for cancer cells to disseminate from the primary tumor but also promotes their self-renewal capability.[158] Breast CSCs have elevated tumorigenicity required for metastatic outgrowth, while EMT may promote CSC character and endows breast cancer cells with enhanced invasive and migratory potential.[159] Emerging evidence indicates that CSCs and EMT cooperate to produce CTCs that are highly competent for metastasis.[160] CTCs with both CSC and EMT characteristics have been identified in the bloodstream of patients with metastatic disease.[118,145] Furthermore, the expression of stemness and EMT markers in CTCs is associated with resistance to conventional anticancer therapies and treatment failure.[158] Some subsets of CTCs have a putative breast cancer stem cell phenotype and express EMT markers. The first evidence of the existence of this putative stemlike phenotype within disseminated breast cancer cells in the bone marrow in early breast cancer patients was shown in 2006.[160] The expression of cancer stem cell markers such as CD44, CD24, or ALDH1, both by molecular assays[118] and imaging,[161] has also been shown in CTCs.[118,161,162]

CTCs: Clinical Significance, Molecular Characterization, and Its Impact on Individualized Treatment of Cancer Patients

Breast Cancer

The clinical significance of CTCs has been extensively evaluated in patients with breast cancer. Many clinical studies have shown that CTC detection is associated with OS and PFS both in early and metastatic breast cancer. A comprehensive metaanalysis of published literature on the prognostic relevance of CTC clearly indicates that the detection of CTCs is a reliable prognostic factor in patients both with early-stage and metastatic breast cancer.[163]

At the moment, many clinical studies are evaluating the potential of CTC testing in the routine management of breast cancer patients.[164] A number of prospective interventional studies are designed to demonstrate that CTC enumeration/characterization may improve the management of breast cancer patients and aim to assess CTC-guided hormone therapy versus chemotherapy decisions in M1 patients, changes in CTC counts during treatment in metastatic patients, and anti–HER-2 treatments in HER-2–negative breast cancer patients selected on the basis of CTCs detection/characterization. The results of these trials will be very important for CTC implementation in the routine management of breast cancer patients.[165]

Clinical Significance of CTCs in Metastatic Breast Cancer. In a seminal paper in 2004, Cristofanilli and colleagues demonstrated that CTCs are an independent prognostic factor for PFS and OS in patients with metastatic breast cancer (MBC).[9] The CellSearch system was used with a cutoff of 5 CTCs/7.5 mL of peripheral blood. This paper led to the FDA clearance of the CellSearch assay in MBC. Many clinical studies have since verified the importance of CTC enumeration in MBC.[162,166-170] It is now clear that MBC patients who present basal counts of 5 CTCs/7.5 mL of blood or greater have a poor prognosis and that enumeration of CTCs during treatment predicts progression of disease earlier than conventional imaging tests.[162] Changing chemotherapy and switching to an alternate cytotoxic therapy was not effective in prolonging OS in patients with persistent increase in CTCs.[171] The independent prognostic effect of CTC count by CellSearch on PFS and OS was further confirmed across 20 studies at 17 European centers that included 1944 eligible patients.[172] CTC analysis may predict the effect of treatment earlier than imaging.[173-175] The prognostic significance of CTC detection is also supported by numerous clinical studies performed on systems other than the CellSearch. RT-PCR assays, especially for the epithelial marker cytokeratin-19 (*CK-19*) alone or in combination with other transcripts, can identify CTCs in MBC.[12] Before the initiation of front-line treatment in patients with MBC, the median PFS and OS were significantly shorter when *CK-19* mRNA-positive CTCs were detected compared with patients who were negative for *CK-19* mRNA.[176] The presence of baseline *CK-19* mRNA-positive CTCs was associated with poor prognosis, and a decrease in mammoglobin mRNA in CTCs may correlate to therapeutic response.[177] The detection of viable CTCs that excrete *CK-19* correlates with OS using the EPISPOT assay.[178]

Clinical Significance of CTCs in Early Breast Cancer. In early breast cancer, CTC numbers are low, and molecular assays are most successful for detection. Nested RT-PCR for *CK-19* expression in the peripheral blood of node-negative breast cancer patients was first shown to be of prognostic value in 2002.[179] Detection of *CK-19* transcripts by using an EpCAM-independent RT-qPCR assay in peripheral blood of early breast cancer patients[112,113] was an independent prognostic factor for disease-free survival (DFS) and OS before,[114] during,[115] and after[116] chemotherapy. Before administration of adjuvant chemotherapy, CTC detection based on *CK-19* positivity by RT-qPCR predicted poor clinical outcome mainly in patients with ER-negative, triple-negative, and HER-2–positive early-stage breast cancer.[180] By using the same EpCAM-independent assay, persistent CTC detection during the first 5 years of follow-up indicated resistance to chemotherapy and hormonal therapy and predicted late relapses in patients with operable breast cancer.[181] Elimination of these *CK-19* mRNA-positive CTCs during adjuvant chemotherapy reflects successful treatment.[182]

CellSearch has also been used in early disease stages, but it requires more than 7.5 mL of blood. By using CellSearch, detection of one or more CTCs in 7.5 mL of blood before neoadjuvant chemotherapy accurately predicted OS.[183] In another CellSearch study, chemonaive patients with nonmetastatic breast cancer at the time of definitive surgery were studied. After a median follow-up of 35 months, the presence of one or more CTCs predicted early recurrence and decreased OS.[184] The REMAGUS02 neoadjuvant study was the first to report the significance of CellSearch CTC detection on distant metastasis-free survival and OS. The detection of CTCs was independently associated with a significantly worse outcome but mainly during the first 3 to 4 years of follow-up.[185] In the German SUCCESS trial, the presence of CTCs was associated with poor DFS, distant DFS, breast cancer–specific survival, and OS, and the prognosis was worse in patients with at least 5 CTCs/30 mL blood. CTCs were confirmed as independent prognostic markers by multivariable analysis for DFS and OS.[186] These findings may change the clinical management of early breast cancer because they clearly indicate the metastatic potential of CTC early in the disease.

Molecular Characterization of CTCs in Breast Cancer and Its Impact on Individualized Treatment. The main goal of adjuvant therapy is to prevent distant recurrences by targeting residual disseminated tumor cells. However, almost 70% of deaths in patients with early breast cancer occur after 5 years, showing that residual disease can be dormant for very long periods. Differences between primary tumors and CTCs could be of crucial importance for therapeutic decisions. In breast cancer, molecular characterization of CTCs may help identify therapeutic targets and resistance mechanisms and to stratify breast cancer patients.[11,187-189] Molecular characterization of CTCs may help to identify new druggable targets in MBC patients.[162] The application of extremely powerful MPS technologies to single CTCs may find a place in the management of patients. However, it is currently a technical challenge for the clinical lab to perform these tests on CTCs on a regular basis, under standardized conditions, with robust and accredited methodologies.

HER-2. In breast cancer, anti–HER-2 therapies are prescribed according to the HER-2 status of the primary tumor, as assessed by immunohistochemistry or FISH. However, a continuously growing body of evidence indicates that CTC HER-2 status can be different from that of the corresponding primary tumor. Moreover, CTC HER-2 status can change over time, particularly during disease recurrence or progression.[110,119,190-194] By using CellSearch and an automated algorithm to evaluate CTC HER-2 expression, heterogeneity even within the same patient, is the rule.[25] Many research groups have shown that HER-2–positive CTCs can be detected in patients with HER-2–negative primary tumors.[190,193-197]

The HER-2 status of CTCs was correlated to the clinical response of HER-2–targeted therapies in the first "liquid biopsy trial" completed in 2012. Georgoulias and colleagues investigated the effect of trastuzumab in a small number of patients who were HER-2 negative in the primary tumor but were positive for CK(+)/HER2(+) CTCs as evaluated by immunofluorescence. These patients were randomized into two groups, and one group received trastuzumab, while the other received a placebo. After trastuzumab administration, 75% of the women became *CK-19* mRNA-negative, the risk of disease recurrence was reduced, and the median DFS was longer.[198] Similarly, a multicenter phase II trial evaluated the activity of lapatinib in MBC patients with HER-2–negative primary tumors and HER-2–positive CTCs using the CellSearch.[199] The TREAT-CTC trial, initiated in 2012, is a randomized phase II trial for patients with HER-2 negative primary breast cancer but HER-2–positive CTCs. This trial is specifically designed to test the efficacy of trastuzumab in HER-2–negative early breast cancer.

Endocrine Treatment. Endocrine treatment is the preferred systemic treatment in MBC patients who have had an estrogen receptor (ER)–positive primary tumor or metastatic lesions. However, 20% of these patients do not benefit from this therapy and demonstrate further metastatic progress. A possible explanation for failure of endocrine therapy might be the heterogeneity of ER expression in CTCs. Similar to the HER-2 story, there is a growing body of evidence that hormone receptor status can change over time, especially during disease recurrence or progression in breast cancer patients.[110,119,190-194] In this context, reevaluation of hormone receptor status by molecular characterization of CTCs is a strategy with potential clinical application. Optimal individualized treatment could be selected by characterizing ER status in CTCs and comparing it to the primary tumor.[200] The commercially available AdnaTest Breast Cancer kit (AdnaGen, Qiagen, Germany) can detect EpCAM, MUC-1, and HER-2 transcripts in CTCs; it was found that a major proportion of CTCs in MBC patients showed EMT and tumor stem cell characteristics.[118] Interestingly, when ER and progesterone receptor (PR) CTC expression was assessed by RT-PCR, CTCs were mostly triple-negative regardless of the ER, PR, and HER-2 status of the primary tumor.[119] CTCs frequently lack ER expression in MBC patients with ER-positive primary tumors and show a considerable intrapatient heterogeneity, which may reflect a mechanism to escape endocrine therapy. Single-cell analysis based on WGA and MPS did not support a role for *ESR1* mutations.[201] In nonmetastatic breast cancer patients, the expression of estrogen, progesterone, and epidermal growth factor receptor (EGFR) by immunofluorescence experiments revealed heterogeneous expression of these hormonal receptors in single CTCs in the same patient.[202]

EMT and Stem Cell Markers on CTCs. EMT and tumor stem cell characteristics were detected in CTCs from metastatic breast cancer patients.[118] CTCs expressing TWIST and vimentin were identified in patients with both metastatic and early breast cancer.[203] Subpopulations of CTCs with putative stem cell progenitor phenotypes in patients with MBC was shown by triple-marker immunofluorescence microscopy.[161] Serial monitoring of CTCs in patients with breast cancer reveals simultaneous expression of mesenchymal and epithelial markers. Mesenchymal cells expressing known EMT regulators, including transforming growth factor (TGF)-β pathway components and the FOXC1 transcription factor, were associated with disease progression.[147]

Apoptosis and Clinical Dormancy on CTCs. CTCs and DTCs can enter a state of dormancy and become resistant to targeted or conventional therapies.[139] Our understanding of the biology of dormant DTCs and CTCs is currently limited. Adjuvant chemotherapy reduced both the number of CTCs per patient and the number of proliferating CTCs.[146] Apoptotic CTCs were detected in patients with breast cancer irrespective of their clinical status, although more were detected in early cancer compared to metastatic cancer.[204] Apoptotic CTCs were more frequently encountered during follow-up in those patients who remained disease-free compared to those with subsequent late relapse.[205] These results indicate that the detection of CTCs that survive despite adjuvant therapy implies that CTC elimination should be attempted using agents targeting their distinctive molecular characteristics.

DNA Methylation in CTCs. Recent studies have shown that DNA methylation silences many key tumor and metastasis suppressor genes in CTCs, including those that suppress growth and proliferation, invasiveness, epithelial differentiation, and stemness like *CST6, BRMS1,* and *SOX17*.[206-208]

Overall, CTC analysis is highly correlative to systemic disease spreading and disease outcome in breast cancer patients. Monitoring of CTCs can predict early subclinical metastasis recurrence and monitor progression during and after treatment. Many clinical studies support the potential utility of CTC detection in breast cancer.

Prostate Cancer. In prostate cancer, CTCs have been extensively studied and validated as a prognostic tool.[209] In advanced prostate cancer, CTC enumeration on the CellSearch system is FDA-cleared as a prognostic test of survival at baseline and posttreatment. Integration into routine clinical practice is ongoing.[211] The main CTC studies in advanced and localized prostate cancer highlight the important gains as well as the challenges posed by various approaches and their implications for advancing prostate cancer management.[210,211]

Clinical Significance of CTCs in Metastatic Prostate Cancer. In 2001, CTC numbers were first quantified in the circulation of patients with metastatic prostate cancer. This change in CTC numbers was of prognostic significance.[212] Later, CTC enumeration before therapy was also related to prognosis. The shedding of CTCs into the circulation was an intrinsic property of the tumor, distinct from the extent of the disease.[213] In 2008, the FDA cleared the CellSearch assay for the enumeration of CTCs in castration-resistant prostate cancer (CRPC) based on data presented by de Bono and colleagues,[214] who showed that CTC enumeration had prognostic value as an independent predictor of OS in CRPC. This study was followed by many others, confirming that CTC enumeration can be used to monitor disease status.[215,216] In patients with metastatic hormone-sensitive prostate cancer, correlation of prostate-specific antigen, Gleason score, and TNM stage with CTC counts showed that CTCs could correctly stage prostate cancer and assess prognosis.[217,218] According to the results of a prospective phase III trial, baseline CTC counts were prognostic and could be used as an early metric to help redirect and optimize therapy.[219]

Clinical Significance of CTCs in Early Prostate Cancer. In early-stage prostate cancer, posttreatment reduction in CTCs may indicate radiation therapy response[220] and can assist in the decision between systemic or local treatment.[221] Recent trials in patients with CRPC are incorporating the detection of CTCs, imaging, and patient-reported outcomes to improve future drug development and patient management.[222]

Molecular Characterization of CTCs in Prostate Cancer and Its Impact on Individualized Treatment. Advances in the understanding of prostate cancer signaling pathways have led to the development and subsequent approval of multiple novel therapies, especially for metastatic castration-resistant prostate cancer. The androgen receptor (AR) is a key target in prostate cancer, and many current therapies for metastatic CRPC target AR signaling. For example, abiraterone and enzalutamide are novel endocrine treatments that abrogate AR signaling in CRPC, but resistance to these therapies is also common. CRPC therapeutic intervention after clinical progression may be achieved through the characterization of AR activity. Biopsies of bone metastases can also assess AR activity but are highly invasive. On the other hand, the molecular characterization of CTCs offers a minimally invasive approach to study late-stage disease. However, patient benefit is variable with these agents, so development of other predictive biomarkers is very important. In addition to CTC enumeration by CellSearch, molecular profiling may better reflect tumor evolution in an individual during the pressure of systemic therapies.[223]

Pretreatment detection of androgen receptor splice variant-7 (AR-V7) in CTCs from CRPC patients is associated with resistance to enzalutamide and abiraterone.[224] Such androgen ablation therapy induces expression of constitutively active AR splice variants that drive disease progression. Recently, the same group confirmed these results by conducting CTC-based AR-V7 analysis at baseline, during therapy, and at progression.[225] Nuclear AR expression in CTCs of CRPC patients treated with enzalutamide and abiraterone was recently evaluated in real-time using the CellSearch system and an automated algorithm to identify CTCs.[226] Large intrapatient heterogeneity of CTC AR expression was observed, including AR-positive CD45-negative CTCs that were CK-negative. The number of these CK-19–negative cells correlated with traditional CTCs and associated with an even worse outcome on univariate analysis. This is important because these events are completely missed by using standard CellSearch detection.[226] A recent study, based on fluorescence-activated cell sorting for CTC isolation and downstream molecular characterization of AR expression, revealed a very high interpatient and intrapatient heterogeneity of the expression and localization of the AR. Increased AR expression and nuclear localization were associated with elevated coexpression of a marker of proliferation, Ki-67, consistent with a continued role for AR expression in castration-resistant disease. However, despite this heterogeneity, it was clear that CTCs from patients with prior exposure to abiraterone had increased AR expression compared to CTCs from patients who were abiraterone naive. Thus the evaluation of AR expression in CTCs is critical for the management of patients with advanced prostate cancer.[227]

Taxanes are a standard of care therapy for CRPC. According to a recent study, two clinically relevant AR splice variants, AR-V567 and AR-V7, differentially associated with microtubules and dynein motor protein, resulting in differential taxane sensitivity in vitro and in vivo. Androgen receptor variants that accumulate in CRPC cells utilize distinct pathways of nuclear import that affect the antitumor efficacy of taxanes, suggesting a mechanistic rationale to customize treatments for patients with CRPC that might improve outcomes.[228]

Clinical trials that evaluate the efficacy of drugs in CRPC need new clinical endpoints that are valid surrogates for survival. In a clinical trial of abiraterone plus prednisone versus prednisone alone for patients with metastatic CRPC, Scher and colleagues evaluated CTC enumeration as a surrogate outcome. They developed a biomarker panel that includes CTC number and LDH concentration as a surrogate for survival at the individual patient level.[229]

Although these findings would require large-scale prospective validation before routine clinical practice, they do show the strong potential of CTC analysis for the management of prostate cancer. Serial CTC AR-V7 expression testing may soon be implemented in clinical practice. This should also provide further insights into tumor evolution.

Overall, CTC analysis is highly correlative to systemic disease spread and disease outcome in prostate cancer patients. Recent clinical studies support the potential utility of CTC molecular characterization, especially in respect to androgen receptor mutations, splice variants, and response to targeted therapies in prostate cancer.

Colorectal Cancer

A metaanalysis of 12 studies revealed prognostic value of CTCs and DTCs in patients with metastatic colorectal cancer.[230] CTC number was an independent predictor of cancer recurrence in six out of nine studies that examined the detection of postoperative CTCs in CRC.[231] The prognostic significance of CTCs in colorectal cancer has been recently reviewed.[232]

Clinical Significance of CTCs in Metastatic Colorectal Cancer. The CellSearch assay was cleared by the FDA for metastatic CRC in 2008.[233] In advanced colorectal cancer, CTC enumeration before and during treatment independently predicts PFS and OS and provides additional information beyond CT imaging,[234-236] while surgical resection of metastases immediately decreases CTC levels.[237] CTC numbers are higher in the mesenteric venous blood compartments of patients with CRC, and viable CTCs are trapped in the liver, a finding that may possibly explain the high rates of liver metastasis in this type of cancer.[238] Six CTC markers (tissue specific and EMT transcripts) used in metastatic CRC patients identified therapy-refractory patients not detected by standard image techniques. Patients with increased CTCs numbers, even when classified as responders by computed tomography, showed significantly shorter survival times.[239] The presence of CTCs in stage III colon cancer patients undergoing curative resection followed by mFOLFOX chemotherapy, as determined by telomerase reverse transcriptase, CK-19, CK-20, and CEA transcripts, was an independent predictor of postchemotherapeutic relapse and strongly correlated with DFS and OS.[240]

Clinical Significance of CTCs in Early Colorectal Cancer. CTC studies in nonmetastatic CRC are more limited compared to metastatic CRC, due to the very low number of CTCs. It was shown that preoperative CTC detection is an independent prognostic marker in nonmetastatic CRC,[241] and the presence of CTCs correlates with reduced DFS in patients with nonmetastatic CRC.[242] CTC detection might help in the selection of high-risk stage II CRC candidates for adjuvant chemotherapy.[243] CEA, CK, and CD133 expression were used to evaluate the clinical significance of CTCs as a prognostic factor for OS and DFS in patients with colorectal cancer after curative surgery. In patients with Duke's stage B and C CRC who required adjuvant chemotherapy, detection of CEA/CK/CD133 mRNA in CTCs predicted risk of recurrence and poor prognosis.[244]

Molecular Characterization of CTCs in Colorectal Cancer and Its Impact on Individualized Treatment. Patients with benign inflammatory diseases of the colon can harbor viable circulating epithelial cells that are detected as "CTCs" on the CellSearch system because they are of epithelial origin and CD45 negative.[245] Hence, further molecular characterization of CTCs is important in colorectal cancer. A considerable portion of viable CTCs are trapped in the liver, as shown by their enumeration in the peripheral and mesenteric blood, using both the CellSearch and EPISPOT assays,[246] potentially explaining the high incidence of liver metastasis in colon cancer. Anti-EGFR therapy in metastatic colorectal cancer may select for *KRAS* and *BRAF* mutations. However, the occurrence of these mutations in metastatic colorectal cancer may vary among primary tumors, CTCs, and metastatic tumors.[247,248] Using the CellSearch system, the expression of *EGFR*, *EGFR* gene amplification, *KRAS*, *BRAF*, and *PIK3CA* mutations were evaluated in single CTCs of patients with metastatic colorectal cancer,[249] and the concordance between *KRAS* mutations in CTCs and primary tumors was 50%.[78] *APC*, *KRAS*, and *PIK3CA* mutations that were found in CTCs were also present at subclonal levels in the primary tumors and metastases from the same patients.[134] When *KRAS* mutations were investigated in CTCs from patients with metastatic CRC throughout the course of the disease and compared to the corresponding primary tumors, CTCs exhibited different *KRAS* mutations during treatment.[250] Plastin-3 is a marker for CTCs undergoing EMT and is associated with colorectal cancer prognosis, particularly in patients with Duke's B and C stage tumors.[251] Patients with CTC positivity at baseline had a shorter median PFS compared to patients with no CTCs, and a significant correlation was also found between CTC detection during treatment and radiographic findings at 6 months.[236] CTCs are promising markers for the evaluation and prediction of treatment responses in rectal cancer patients, superior to CEA. CTC number correlates with treatment outcome, but not serum CEA.[252]

In conclusion, CTC analysis highly correlates to systemic disease spread and disease outcome in colorectal cancer patients. Many clinical studies support the potential utility of CTC detection in colorectal cancer.

Lung Cancer

Lung cancer biopsies are difficult to obtain, while a liquid biopsy of CTCs is relatively easy. However, CTCs in lung cancer are difficult to detect because they seldom have epithelial characteristics. Detection methods that rely on epithelial markers to identify CTCs may not be effective. Even so, there is evidence that in lung cancer CTC numbers are prognostic and that CTCs counted before and after treatment mirror treatment response. In patients with molecularly defined subtypes of non–small cell lung cancer, CTCs demonstrate the same molecular changes as the cancer cells of the tumor.[253] Chronic obstructive pulmonary disease is a risk factor for lung cancer, and monitoring CTCs in these patients may allow for early diagnosis.[254]

Clinical Significance of CTCs in Non–Small Cell Lung Cancer. The presence of EpCAM/MUC-1 mRNA-positive CTCs in non–small cell lung cancer (NSCLC) patients preoperatively and postoperatively revealed shortened DFS and OS.[255] In NSCLC patients undergoing surgery, the presence and the number of CTCs were associated with worse survival.[256] By using the ISET filtration system and immunofluorescence, hybrid CTCs with an EMT phenotype were detected.[257] CTCs are detectable in patients with untreated stage III or IV NSCLC and are prognostic according to another single-center prospective study.[258] Advanced-stage NSCLC patients with elevated CEA had higher numbers of CTCs.[259] Using the ISET filtration system and filter-adapted fluorescence in situ hybridization, genetic alterations of tyrosine kinase oncogenes were examined in CTCs. Specifically, CTCs from four *ROS1*-rearranged NSCLC patients were followed during treatment with the *ROS1*-inhibitor crizotinib.[72]

Clinical Significance of CTCs in Small Cell Lung Cancer. Small cell lung cancer (SCLC) accounts for 15% to 20% of lung cancer cases. It is very aggressive and characterized by early dissemination and dismal prognosis. In most cases, SCLC is not operable, and it is difficult to obtain biopsies to investigate its biology and therapeutic options. In this type of cancer, CTCs circulate in high numbers and are readily accessible through a single blood draw, which can be easily repeated for follow-up over time. A research team that was headed by Dive showed that CTCs in SCLC are tumorigenic in immunocompromised mice; the resultant CTC-derived explants mirror the patient's response to platinum and etoposide chemotherapy and can be used for the selection of appropriate therapies.[260] The same group showed that in patients with SCLC undergoing standard treatment, CTCs and CTC clusters, called circulating tumor microemboli (CTM), can be detected and are independent prognostic factors.[261] Evaluating the presence of CTM also improved diagnostic accuracy in NSCLC patients based on clinical and imaging data.[262] The change in CTC count after the first cycle of chemotherapy, evaluated by using the CellSearch system, provided useful prognostic information in SCLC[263] and was the strongest response predictor for chemotherapy and survival.[261]

Molecular Characterization of CTCs in Lung Cancer and Its Impact on Individualized Treatment. CTCs isolated from early-stage lung cancer patients have been successfully expanded through cell culture. After CTC isolation with an in situ capture and culture methodology, ex vivo expansion of CTCs is performed using a three-dimensional co-culture model. These expanded lung CTCs carried mutations of *TP53* identical to those observed in the matched primary tumors.[264] Mutations were first detected in CTCs of NSCLC patients in 2008.[265] In this study, NSCLC patients with EpCAM-positive CTCs carrying *EGFR* mutations had faster disease progression than CTCs who lacked mutations. In another study, a mutation panel for six genes (*EGFR, KRAS, BRAF, NRAS, AKT1,* and *PIK3CA*) revealed only one *EGFR* mutation (exon 19 deletion) in the 38 patient samples analyzed.[266] In some of these studies, the analytical sensitivity may not be high enough to detect all variants. The CellSearch System coupled with MPS may be the most sensitive and specific diagnostic tool for CTC evaluation.[267] Crizotinib is an effective molecular treatment for *ALK* rearrangement–positive NSCLC. The companion diagnostic test for *ALK* rearrangements in NSCLC for crizotinib treatment is currently done by tumor biopsy or fine-needle aspiration. By using a filtration technique and FISH, Pailler and colleagues successfully managed to detect *ALK* rearrangements in CTCs of NSCLC patients, enabling both diagnostic testing and monitoring of crizotinib treatment.[268] CellSearch technology was recently adapted to identify tumor cells in malignant pleural effusions. The pleural fluid CellSearch assay may complement traditional cytology in the diagnosis of malignant effusions.[269]

Cutaneous Melanoma

Cutaneous melanoma is a cancer of the skin derived from transformation of melanocytes. Melanoma is mainly a disease of developed countries, with the highest incidence in Australia, North America, and Europe.[270] Unfortunately, melanoma is among the fastest-growing cancers in Western societies. A unique characteristic of primary melanoma is that small lesions more than 2.5 mm deep can be highly metastastic with very poor prognosis compared to similar-size tumors of other cancers, so early detection of CTCs is very important. Melanoma often metastasizes to regional lymph nodes and to distant organs.[270,271] Melanoma metastasis may occur to almost any organ, but brain, liver, and lung are the most common, so CTCs are particularly interesting due to their aggressive ability to metastasize systemically. Recently, the approval of targeted therapies such as *BRAF* mutation inhibitors (vemurafenib, dabrafenib), the MEK inhibitor trametinib, and immune checkpoint inhibitors PDL-1 (pembrolizumab), PD1 (nivolumab), and ipilimumab alone and in combinations have improved OS and DFS considerably.[272-274]

Clinical Significance of CTCs in Cutaneous Melanoma. The systemic spread of melanoma as viewed through CTCs is in essence real-time monitoring of metastasis as it occurs.[275,276] The only approved blood biomarker for melanoma is LDH in American Joint Cancer Committee stage III/IV patients. Because melanoma is highly malignant, it is not surprising that studies have found CTC analysis clinically important. CTC analysis of melanoma patients started in the early 1990s and has progressed through the years, along with advancements in molecular assays.[277-279] Circulating melanoma cells have differentiation lineage and tumor-related gene expression patterns that are not found in peripheral blood leukocytes. RT-qPCR can be performed on blood after lysis of RBCs and mononuclear cell preparation. Unlike most other RT-qPCR CTC assays, analysis of melanoma cells does not require antibody capture through cell surface antigens. There are only a few cell-surface melanoma-associated antigens for targeting antibodies.[280-282] Therefore molecular assays that target melanoma transcripts are often used, including *MART-1, MAGE-A3, PAX3,* and ganglioside *GM2/GD2 glycosyltransferase (GalNAc-T)*.[278,283-285]

Melanoma is heterogeneous in genomic aberrations and transcriptome expression. Therefore it is important to use multiple markers to assess CTCs to improve sensitivity.[281,283,286-288] New approaches to detect CTCs include the inertial focusing spiral microfluidics CTChip in the ClearCell FX system (Clearbridge BioMedics, Singapore). It can separate CTCs by size and mass, followed by RT-qPCR or immunohistochemistry. The system is rapid, and the yield of CTCs from peripheral blood leukocytes is higher than with other methods.[98]

Multiple marker RT-qPCR assays allow monitoring both early- and advanced-stage patients during treatment; several well-annotated studies with long-term follow-up have been published.[284,285,287,289,290] CTC monitoring post- and pretreatment also predicts OS in surgically resected disease-free stage III/IV patients. A recent multicenter international phase III trial demonstrated that CTC analysis predicts the outcome of melanoma patients with positive sentinel lymph nodes after their resection with disease-free status.[290] Multimarker RT-qPCR analysis may be helpful in identifying patients who have high risk of systemic disease progression after surgery or therapy.

Molecular Characterization of Isolated CTCs From Melanoma Patients. Melanoma CTCs are unique in their associated antigens, mRNA expression patterns, and genomic aberrations.[280,281,286,291-293] Recently, an in-depth genomic analysis was performed on paired primary tumors and CTCs whereby copy number aberrations and loss of heterozygosity were analyzed. CTCs were captured by several anti-ganglioside cell surface human IgM monoclonal antibodies and then subjected to a genome-wide SNP array (Array 6.0, Affymetrix, Santa Clara, Calif.).[282] IgM provides better capture of CTCs than IgG. Greater than 90% of SNPs were concordant between the primary tumor and isolated CTCs. Several frequent copy number aberrations were identified and validated in a separate cohort of patients with advanced-stage melanoma. These studies indicate the presence of many unexplored key copy number variants in CTCs that can be used to monitor patients' progression. Other groups have reported known genomic mutations in *BRAF* and *KIT,* using isolated melanoma CTCs.[294,295]

Overall CTC analysis is highly correlated to systemic disease spread and disease outcome in melanoma patients. With the availability of new and improved therapeutics in melanoma, the monitoring of CTCs may be important to assess early subclinical recurrence and progression both during and after treatment. Phase II and III clinical trials support the potential utility of melanoma patient CTC detection and analysis.

Ovarian Cancer

Molecular assays are most commonly used for the characterization of CTCs in ovarian cancer. A panel of six genes for the PCR-based detection of CTCs in endometrial, cervical, and ovarian cancers detected CTCs in 44% of cervical, 64% of endometrial, and 19% of ovarian cancers.[296] This same group later identified additional markers for CTCs in patients with epithelial ovarian cancer and evaluated their impact on clinical outcome.[297] Aktas and colleagues investigated CTCs in the blood of 122 ovarian cancer patients at primary diagnosis and after platinum-based chemotherapy by using immunomagnetic enrichment and multiplex RT-PCR (AdnaTest, Qiagen, Germany). They reported that CTCs correlated with shorter OS before surgery and after chemotherapy.[298] When ovarian cancer is studied on the CellSearch system, some studies show that elevated CTCs impart an unfavorable prognosis,[299] while others find no correlation.[300] Even if CTCs are associated with poor outcomes in ovarian cancer, clinical implementation will require uniform methodology and prospective validation.[301] By using a cell adhesion matrix for functional enrichment and identification, the presence of CTCs was correlated with shorter OS and PFS and had a better positive predictive value than CA-125.[302]

Platinum resistance constitutes one of the most recognized clinical challenges for ovarian cancer. Molecular CTC analysis in ovarian cancer correlates with platinum resistance. Although the immunohistochemistry of ERCC1 protein in primary tumors does not predict platinum resistance, ERCC1 (+) CTCs do predict platinum resistance at primary diagnosis of ovarian cancer.[303] A recent metaanalysis of eight studies, including 1184 patients, showed that patients with ERCC1(+) CTCs had significantly shorter OS and DFS than patients with ERCC1(−) CTCs.[304]

Pancreatic Cancer

Pancreatic cancers frequently spread to the liver, lung, and skeletal system, suggesting that pancreatic tumor cells must be able to intravasate and travel through the circulation to distant organs. The presence of CTCs correlates with an unfavorable outcome in pancreatic cancer.[305,306] However, as stated by Gall and colleagues, CTCs are rare in pancreatic cancer, and it is unclear whether CTCs actually contribute toward tumor invasiveness and spread in such an aggressive cancer.[307] A recent metaanalysis including nine studies with a total of 623 pancreatic cancer patients showed that 268 CTC-positive patients had poorer PFS and OS compared to 355 CTC-negative patients.[308] Larger studies, as well as characterization of the CTC population, are required to achieve further insight into the clinical implications of CTC analysis in pancreatic cancer.

Head and Neck Cancer

Head and neck squamous cell carcinoma (HNSCC) is the sixth most common cancer and causes high morbidity due to the lack of early detection. A recent comprehensive review details studies over the past 5 years on the detection of CTCs in HNSCC.[309] When CTCs from locally advanced NHSCC are enriched by the CellSearch system, CTCs are detected in only a low fraction of cases.[310] A metaanalysis of eight studies and 433 patients with HNSCC concluded that the presence of CTCs portends a poor prognosis compared to patients without CTCs.[311] In patients with HNSCC undergoing surgical intervention, patients with no detectable CTCs had a higher probability of longer DFS.[312,313] In both of these studies, CTCs were isolated only by negative enrichment that is not dependent on the expression of surface epithelial markers. Another prospective multicentric study evaluated the role of CTC detection in locally advanced head and neck cancer; a decrease in the CTC number or their absence throughout the treatment was related to nonprogressive disease.[314] Current staging methods for squamous cell carcinomas of the oral cavity need to be improved to predict the risk to individual patients. This can be achieved by counting bone marrow DTCs and peripheral blood CTCs that predict relapse with higher sensitivity than routine staging procedures.[315] The persistence of CTCs after upfront tumor surgery may be useful for the identification of patients who benefit from treatment intensification in locally advanced HNSCC.[316]

Hepatocellular Carcinoma

CTC analysis in hepatocellular carcinoma (HCC) is a new field.[163] A large variation of CTCs with epithelial, mesenchymal, liver-specific, and mixed characteristics, including different size ranges, is observed among patient groups and is associated with therapeutic outcome.[317] Frequent EpCAM+ CTCs in intermediate or advanced HCC are seen.[318] In HCC patients undergoing curative resection, stem cell-like phenotypes have been observed in EpCAM+ CTCs. Preoperative CTC numbers predicted tumor recurrence in HCC patients after surgery, especially in patient subgroups with α-fetoprotein concentrations of up to 400 ng/mL.[319]

Bladder Cancer

CTCs may be used as a noninvasive, real-time tool for the stratification of early-stage bladder cancer patients according to individual risk of progression.[320] The potential prognostic value of CTCs in patients with advanced nonmetastatic urothelial carcinoma of the bladder was shown in a recent clinical study, where CTC-positive patients had significantly higher risks of disease recurrence, as well as cancer-specific and overall mortality.[321] CellSearch was also used to detect and evaluate prospectively the biological significance of CTC in patients with nonmetastatic, advanced bladder cancer; according to this study, the presence of CTCs may be predictive for early systemic disease because CTCs were detected in 30% of patients with nonmetastatic disease.[322] The prognosis of T1G3 bladder cancer is highly variable and unpredictable from clinical and pathological prognostic factors. When survivin-expressing CTCs were evaluated in patients with T1G3 bladder tumors, the presence of CTCs was an independent prognostic factor for DFS.[323] However, in metastatic urothelial carcinoma, CTCs could not predict extravesical disease and were not a clinically useful parameter for directing therapeutic decisions.[324]

POINTS TO REMEMBER

CTCs

- CTC enumeration tests in metastatic breast, colorectal, and prostate cancer are cleared by the FDA.
- A plethora of analytical systems are available for CTC isolation, detection, and molecular characterization that are currently under analytical and clinical evaluation.
- CTC molecular characterization may be translated into individualized targeted treatments.
- Single-cell analysis of CTCs holds considerable promise for the identification of therapeutic targets and resistance mechanisms in CTCs, as well as for real-time monitoring of the efficacy of systemic therapies.
- Quality control and standardization of CTC isolation, detection, and molecular characterization are required for the incorporation of CTC analysis into routine clinical laboratory practice.

CIRCULATING TUMOR DNA

Circulating tumor DNA (ctDNA) isolation, detection, and analysis have significantly improved over the past 2 decades. Several comprehensive reviews have been published.[325-331] Key studies are reviewed in this chapter. Different forms of ctDNA in several cancer types and their roles in clinical oncology also are examined.

Origin and Function of ctDNA

Free circulating DNA can be found in both cancer patients and noncancer patients with various pathologies, including trauma, inflammatory diseases, and autoimmune diseases. This chapter focuses on the circulating DNA in plasma or serum of cancer patients (ctDNA). Most ctDNA is from cancer cells, although some may be from the tumor microenvironment. ctDNA can be actively or passively released by tumor cells and enter different fluid compartments of the body such as lymphatics, urine, blood, semen, saliva, and cerebral spinal fluid.[332,333] ctDNA may also be from CTCs that are disrupted in the bloodstream. ctDNA may have physiological functions that influence normal cells, particularly those adjacent to the tumor. Single- and double-stranded DNA bind to toll-like receptors (TLRs) expressed on the surface of tumor cells and tumor-infiltrating cells.[334] ctDNA can bind to TLRs on leukocytes and activate various specific signal transduction pathways that could alter host-immune responses to tumor cells in the tumor microenvironment. Activation of TLRs can initiate signal transduction pathways that result in cytokine release and other functional changes in the targeted binding cells. The release of ctDNA may have direct effects on tumor microenvironment immune cells, as well as distant organ sites. This may be an important ctDNA physiological influence in the host. ctDNA also may act through horizontal gene transfection into normal cells in the tumor microenvironment.[337] Cellular transformation and tumorigenesis have been implicated with oncogene-containing DNA transfected in vivo.[336-338]

Types of ctDNA

Multiple forms of ctDNA exist in the blood of cancer patients (Figs. 52.19 and 52.20). The most frequent ctDNA results reported are mutations. Tumor mutations in several cancers have drawn more attention because of the availability of respective targeted therapies that are FDA approved in clinical oncology. However, in addition to mutations (single-nucleotide variants, small insertions and small deletions), there are additional types of aberrations in individual cancers with potential utility.[339] These potential targets include methylation of gene promoter regions of coding and noncoding genomic sequences, microsatellite loss of heterozygosity, DNA integrity, gene fusion, copy number variation, and cancer viral DNA.[339]

These different types of ctDNA vary among individual cancer types, although some genomic aberrations can overlap, particularly with cancers of similar embryonic or carcinogenesis origin. The clinical utility of one type of ctDNA in a specific cancer may not be the same for other cancers. For example, *BRAF* mutations are found in several cancers, including melanoma, colorectal, and lung, but they are only partially responsive to therapy with limited long-term response. BRAF inhibitors in melanoma have the highest response overall. Thus ctDNA BRAF mutations may potentially be useful for several types of solid tumor cancers. Several solid tumor cancers have viral etiology, whereby viral specific ctDNA can be used for detection (see the viral section below for more details).

Isolation of ctDNA

The amount and quality of ctDNA are very important for reproducible and accurate assays. Multiple techniques have been used for the isolation of ctDNA, including laboratory developed methods and commercial kits. Unfortunately, there are currently no set standards for isolation or quantification. Isolation of ctDNA is logistically laborious, and there are issues with reproducibility among and within runs.[340] More accurate, robust, and consistent isolation of ctDNA is needed, particularly with small volumes of serum/plasma. Also, these procedures must be standardized to simplify performance across multiple centers and become established laboratory regulations. Both commercial kits and in-house approaches for ctDNA isolation may involve proprietary chemicals and reagents that require centrifugation, bead hybridization, and/or column separations. Yields from different assays can vary considerably.

Quantification of ctDNA

There are many assays for quantification of specific ctDNA fragments. Usually, qPCR assays that incorporate hydrolysis or other types of probes, peptide or locked nucleic acid clamping, and digital PCR are used. However, because only small amounts of ctDNA may be recovered from plasma or serum, reproducible quantification is difficult, accuracy may be low, and false-negative ctDNA results may occur. The issue then becomes how much ctDNA to use in individual assays, and

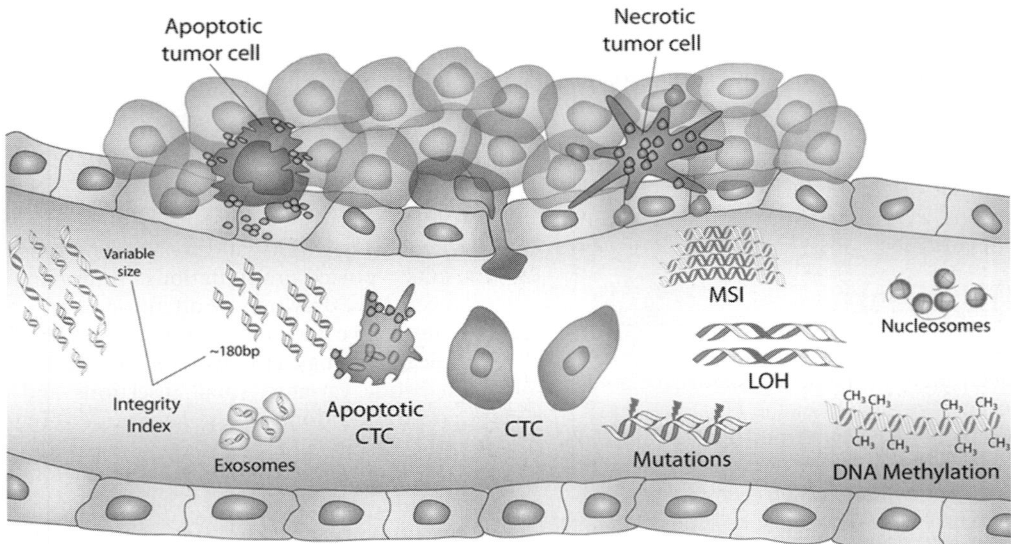

FIGURE 52.19 Schematic representation of circulating tumor DNA (ctDNA) in the systemic circulation. ctDNA arises from apoptosis or necrosis of primary and metastatic solid tumors and from degradation of CTCs. In the circulation, ctDNA is of variable size, can be quantified by an integrity index, and is often enriched with multiples of 180 bp fragments that wind around nucleosomes. In the circulation, ctDNA may be contained within vesicles, attached to nucleosomes or free in solution. Analysis of ctDNA can identify tumor mutations, microsatellite instability (MSI), loss of heterozygosity (LOH), and methylation patterns. Apoptosis of normal cells also results in circulating DNA that dilutes the variant fraction of abnormal DNA.

that requires overall quantification of ctDNA. Quantification methods for purified ctDNA include UV spectrophotometry, electrophoresis, double-stranded (eg, PicoGreen) or single-stranded (eg, OligoGreen) DNA assays (ThermoFisher), qPCR, and digital PCR. Isolated ctDNA can vary in purity and be double-stranded or single-stranded, and it may be complexed to histones, all of which can affect quantification. UV spectrophotometry can assess protein contamination, but it is typically not sensitive enough for ctDNA quantification. Electrophoresis also lacks sensitivity, and quantification is difficult. If enough ctDNA is available, multiple assays can be performed to increase confidence, such as digital PCR, qPCR, and/or PicoGreen assays. ctDNA quantification for downstream assays remains an area that needs improvement.

Massive Parallel Sequencing

Massive parallel sequencing (MPS) can analyze the full sequence of multiple genes at once. MPS provides wider coverage of genes and their aberrations with verification of the ctDNA detection accuracy. MPS analysis of ctDNA continues to improve,[341-345] but it may not be as sensitive as qPCR assays for specific gene targets that have been well optimized for low copy detection. Nevertheless, the development of more sensitive MPS techniques and targeted qPCR with reduced costs will continue to make ctDNA more useful in companion diagnostics.

MPS provides much wider genomic coverage than specific qPCR assays. For example, in an exome analysis of ctDNA, thousands of DNA genes are analyzed for all sequence variants that may be present. The MPS approach allows analysis of many genomic aberrations, including deletions, copy number changes, and mutations, providing a comprehensive profile of ctDNA. Although MPS requires optimization, only one gene panel can cover many tumors, in contrast to multiple qPCR assays that target specific genes and must be optimized for each tumor type. As MPS becomes more cost efficient, targeted gene panels and whole exon sequencing of ctDNA may reveal many specific variants to guide targeted therapies in clinical trials.

The current issues with MPS are the high costs and laborious preparations of libraries from small amounts of extracted DNA from serum or plasma. Bioinformatics also remains a problem, with many different methods for analyzing and reporting results. Reporting needs to be better standardized for easy clinical interpretation. Digital single-molecule sequencing with digital informatics is a new approach that allows for targeted gene sequencing at high sensitivity and specificity for ctDNA analysis.[346-350]

Plasma Versus Serum for ctDNA

ctDNA has been assessed both in plasma and serum of cancer patients. Fetal circulating DNA testing has focused on plasma with CLIA approval using stabilizing DNA blood tubes (cell-free DNA BCT, Streck, Omaha, Neb.) for consistent collection and preservation at room temperature for up to 72 hours before extraction. In general, serum has more ctDNA than plasma and has the advantage of no interference from preservatives. However, plasma is preferred over serum because clotting in serum causes trapped leukocytes to release DNA that can interfere in ctDNA detection. Collection of plasma for ctDNA requires expedient centrifugation and filtration of contaminant cells such as leukocytes and CTCs prior to cryopreservation to prevent cells from breaking up and releasing DNA.

The field of ctDNA analysis takes advantage of well-developed assays designed for tumor tissues. However, the

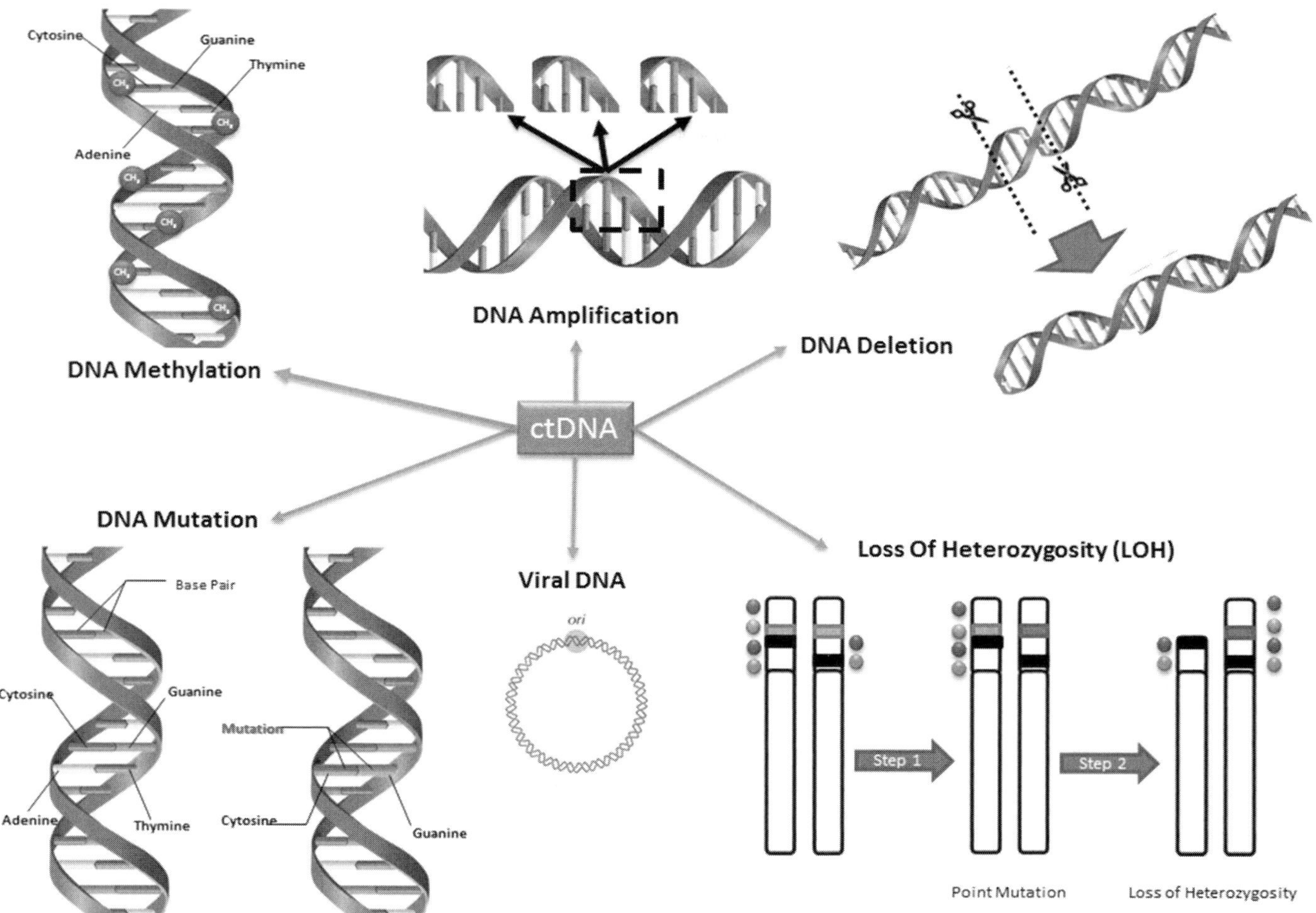

FIGURE 52.20 Examples of genomic variation revealed by analysis of ctDNA in blood. Variants include abnormal DNA methylation patterns, copy number variations (amplifications, deletions, insertions), point mutations, and loss of heterozygosity. Nonhuman DNA, including viral and bacterial DNA, may also be found in the circulation.

extracted amount of ctDNA can be quite low, and, depending on the particular assay, low copy numbers of ctDNA may not be detectable. Uncertain detection limits plague ctDNA analysis. Low copy number ctDNA is particularly problematic in methylation assays when bisulphite treatment is required. On the other hand, ctDNA assays may be easier to interpret than tumor assays because of limited tumor-derived DNA background.

Early assays required large volumes of blood, varying from 0.5 to 10 mL, but improvements in sensitivity and efficiency have lowered the amounts needed. Most current ctDNA assays require less than 2 mL of plasma or serum as the extraction efficiency of methods and laboratories improve. With the demand of various clinical blood tests in cancer patients, lower blood requirements are more practical and also better tolerated by patients.

ctDNA is also present in body fluids other than blood. Urine is an important fluid to detect ctDNA for urogenital cancers.[351-353] However, degradation of DNA in urine is a concern. Cerebrospinal fluid (CSF) is also a potential source for detection of brain tumor ctDNA mutations.[332] CSF in general has less proteins, lipids, and cells compared to blood, which allows for easier extraction of ctDNA. However, the amount of ctDNA in CSF is far less than in blood. ctDNA can also be monitored in pleural and peritoneal fluids for cancer-related progression. These latter fluids can provide a large source of cell-free DNA for very comprehensive analysis of genomic aberrations before and after treatment.

Tumor-Specific ctDNA Mutations

Tumor-specific mutations in ctDNA are most commonly studied in cancer patients. Tumor mutations in ctDNA become increasingly important when the mutations have approved targeted therapies as companion diagnostics and are associated with therapeutic response.[354-376] ctDNA mutations can easily be assessed with high sensitivity and specificity by qPCR or MPS.[346,377] Table 52.1 lists the mutations detected in ctDNA for different cancers. Most mutations can now be detected in ctDNA as well as tumor tissue. Using digital sequencing (Guardent Health, Redwood City, Calif.), complete exomes of genes for ctDNA mutations and amplifications have been reported.[350,366,378]

In NSCLC, mutations in *EGFR* include deletions in exon 19, affecting the amino acid motif ELREA (delE746-A750) and an amino acid substitution (L858R) in exon 21.[379-383]

TABLE 52.1 Detection of Circulating Tumor DNA (ctDNA) Mutations in Various Cancers

Cancer	Gene	Reference
Breast	*PIK3CA, BMI1, SMC4, FANCD2, MED1, ATM, PDGFRA, GAS6, TP53, ESR1, PTEN, AKT1, IDH2 SMAD4*	355, 356, 358, 364, 366, 369, 370, 458
Ovarian	*RB1, ZEB2, MTOR, CES4A, BUB1, PARP8*	458
Non–small cell lung cancer	*KRAS, EGFR, TP53, NFKB1*	359, 364, 366, 368, 376, 379–385, 458
Melanoma	*BRAFV600, TP53, E2H2*	346, 358, 371
Pancreatic	*KRAS, TP53, APC, SMAD4, FBXW7*	349, 357
Hepatocellular carcinoma	*TP53*	459
Colorectal cancer and other gastrointestinal malignancies	*KRAS, WTKRAS, NRAS, BRAF, EGFR, cKIT, PIK3CA*	347, 354, 356, 363, 365, 372–375, 378
Cervical	*KRAS, TP53*	460

These genomic aberrations result in constitutively activated EGFR tyrosine kinase. These EGFR activation changes are responsive to EGFR tyrosine kinase inhibitor (TKI) therapies (gefitnib, erlotinib) in up to 78% of patients, as shown in multiple studies. Recently, detection of *EGFR* mutations in ctDNA has mirrored the *EGFR* mutation status in associated lung tumors.[378,384] In lung cancer patients treated with erlotinib, the presence of *EGFR* L858R ctDNA was associated with a decrease in OS; however, exon 19 deletions detected in ctDNA were associated with increased OS. When serial peripheral blood sampling for ctDNA was assessed, acquired drug resistance correlated with the appearance of *EGFR* T290M.[366] Anti-EGFR drug therapies can be monitored by assessing different ctDNA mutations.[385] Currently, these companion ctDNA diagnostics are being verified in the clinic. Assessment of ctDNA mutations in blood during treatment and follow-up provide information to the clinician about new mutations that were not present in the original tumor. New strategies for initiating targeted therapies based on ctDNA analysis (Fig. 52.21) may replace biopsy of metastases for new gene mutations arising during follow-up.

Gene Amplification in ctDNA

Amplification of *ERBB2*, *BRAF*, and *MET* have been observed in various cancers.[386-389] More types of tumors with these amplifications and more types of amplifications in various tumors will likely be found as techniques to assess gene amplification in ctDNA develop. For example, androgen receptor amplification in prostate cancer can be detected from ctDNA and may be a resistance mechanism for patients on enzalutamide and abiraterone.[389] Table 52.2 lists amplifications detected in different cancers. As MPS becomes more sensitive for the detection of gene amplification, it will be easier to detect amplifications from ctDNA assays.

Copy Number Variation in ctDNA

MPS can measure copy number variants (CNVs) in ctDNA.[344,359,390-392] This new strategy for ctDNA analysis is currently very costly. There are multiple CNVs on specific chromosome arms that are frequent for individual types of cancers. CNVs may cover multiple genes or noncoding sequences and can be valuable biomarkers of tumor progression. For example, 9p1q deletions are found frequently in melanoma and other solid tumors. The main technical issues are, again, low amounts of ctDNA and bioinformatics analysis.

Microsatellite Instability and Loss of Heterozygosity in ctDNA

Microsatellite instability revealed as a loss of heterogeneity (LOH) is common in many cancers and occurs in specific chromosome regions.[393-400] LOH of tumors revealed by ctDNA can correlate with clinical outcome. However, technical issues in assessing LOH of specific chromosome loci can make some assays difficult to interpret and others uninformative. To assess LOH, multiple primer sets to specific loci have to be run to obtain an accurate profile. PCR products are conventionally evaluated by gel electrophoresis with variable sensitivity. Recently, more accurate assays performed by capillary electrophoresis arrays with discrimination down to a few base pairs have appeared. ctDNA LOH analysis now has strong prognostic and diagnostic significance in many different cancer types (Table 52.3). It remains to be seen if ctDNA LOH can be assessed through MPS.

Methylated ctDNA

Methylated ctDNA is detectable in cancer patients and has utility in both early detection and treatment monitoring. Typically, gene promoter regions contain CpG sites that are hypermethylated or hypomethylated to control transcription. In cancer, the promoter regions of tumor suppressor genes may be hypermethylated to limit transcription, and oncogene transcription may be increased by hypomethylation. In the blood of cancer patients, methylated CpG ctDNA can be detected and used for prognosis and as markers of treatment response.[208,285,401-427] Cancer genes that are known to be controlled by methylation are listed in Table 52.4. However, some promoter CpG sites can be nonspecifically hypermethylated and not involved in gene transcription. Therefore, one has to carefully select the regulatory CpG sites in the promoter region for analysis. More than one site can be regulatory, and methylation can vary throughout the gene promoter. This can cause difficulty in interpreting methylated ctDNA results. During tumor progression, promoters typically become hypermethylated. Apparent hypomethylated CpG sites in ctDNA may result from normal cell shedding of hypomethylated DNA. Normal cell regulatory genes can also change in methylation status and be used for methylated ctDNA

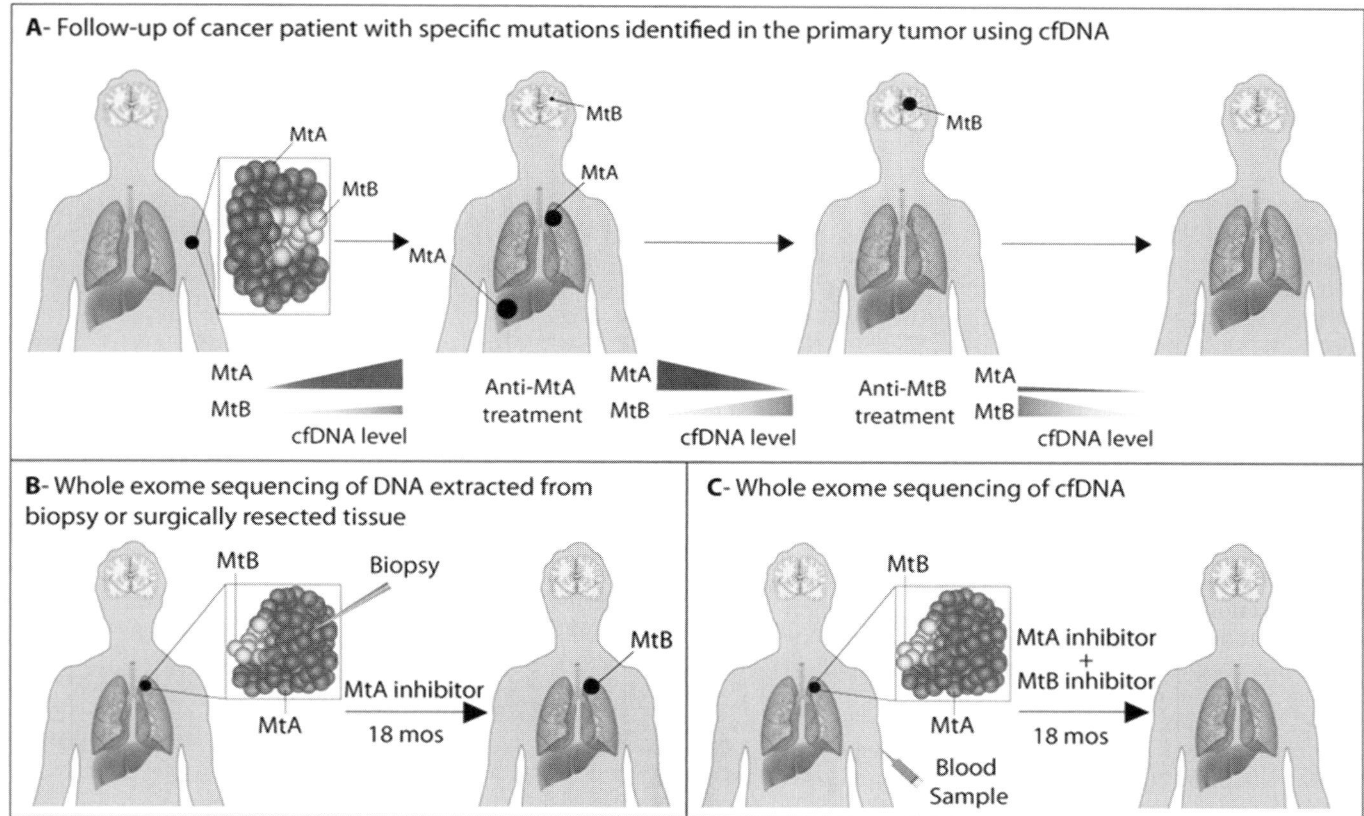

FIGURE 52.21 Examples of ctDNA analysis in cancer patients with multiple mutations. **A,** A melanoma patient presents a heterogeneous primary tumor with both mutation profile A (MtA) and mutation profile B (MtB). Initial circulating free DNA (cfDNA) assessment indicates a higher level of MtA as a consequence of being the predominant tumor subclone. After starting with anti-MtA therapy, MtA clones decrease, while MtB may increase. If the MtB burden increases, anti-mtB treatment can be initiated, potentially clearing both clones by personalized treatment. **B,** A resected tumor of a patient with non–small cell lung carcinoma is analyzed, revealing the targetable mutation L858R in *EGFR* but missing a minor clone harboring *BRAF* V600E. After 1 year of anti-EGFR treatment, the patient relapses with a tumor harboring *BRAF* V600E. **C,** Whole genome sequencing of cfDNA identifies both L858 *EGFR* and an underrepresented subclone with a V600E *BRAF* mutation. In this diagnostic setting, both targetable mutations could be considered for treatment selection and potential cure.

TABLE 52.2 Cell-Free DNA Copy Number Variants (CNVs) and Amplification in Various Cancers

Cancer	CNV	Reference
Prostate	*AR, CYP17A1* CNV	342, 387
Breast	*HER2* amp, *ERBB2, CDK6*	384, 387
Esophageal	*CCND1* amp	386
Liver	Multiple chromosomes	390
Colorectal	*ERBB2, CDK6, EGFR, BRAF, MYC, SMO*	347, 387

TABLE 52.3 Circulating Tumor DNA (ctDNA) Loss of Heterozygosity (LOH) Sites in Various Cancers

Cancer	LOH Site	Reference
Non–small cell lung cancer	D9S286, D9S942, GATA49D12, D13S170	461
Breast	D8S321, D1S228, D14S51, D14S62, D17S855	395, 397, 399, 400
Melanoma	12q22-23	393, 396, 398
Colorectal	D18S59, D18S1140, D18S976	462
Ovarian	D10S1765, D13S218	463
Prostate	D9S171, D10S591, D8S261, D6S286, D8S262, D18S70	408

TABLE 52.4 Circulating Tumor DNA (ctDNA) Methylation in Various Cancers

Cancer	Methylation Gene	Reference
Colorectal	*MGMT, P16, RAR-ß2, RASSFIA, APC, SOX17, SEPT9*	208, 405–407, 416
Breast	*APC, RASSF1, DAPESR1,SOX17,PCDH10, PAX 5 RARβ2, APC, GSTP1*	411, 417, 418, 424, 427
Gastric	*XAF1,CKIT, PDGFRA*	363, 412
Melanoma	*AIM1,LINE1, MGMT, ESR1, RAR-ß2, RASF1*	285, 401–405
Lung	*RAR-ß2,PAX5, MGMT, DCC, BRMS1*	415, 420, 422–424
Prostate	*RASSF1A, GSTP1, RAR-ß2, ARHGAP6*	408, 410, 422, 426
Thyroid (papillary thyroid carcinoma)	*BRAF (V600E)*	369
Liver	*LINE1, RASSF1*	409, 428
Ovary	*KRAS,RASSF1, CALCA, EP300, H1C1, PAX5*	420, 421, 460
Brain	*MGMT*	425

analysis. An example is estrogen receptor (ER) methylation, which increases in advanced melanoma patients and can be detected in ctDNA.[403]

Recently, methylated SEPT9 ctDNA has been detected in early-stage colon cancer, specifically in asymptomatic average-risk individuals undergoing screening.[405-407] These studies included multiple colorectal cancer patients and healthy cohorts and are a good example of the potential for ctDNA analysis to identify early-stage cancer and serve as a cancer screening test. The assay still needs improvement before widespread clinical use because it requires up to 15 mL of blood, and the sensitivity for early-stage colorectal cancer and precancerous adenomas is not optimal. Interestingly, sensitivity of SEPT9 ctDNA detection is not accurate in late-stage CRC.[405,406]

Some methylation ctDNA biomarkers occur in more than one type of cancer. Some common methylated ctDNA markers found in multiple types of cancer include *RASSF1*, *ESR1*, *CDKN2A*, *RARB*, and *MGMT* (see Table 52.4). This limits the specificity of methylation ctDNA biomarkers for early detection in patients without cancer. Nevertheless, methylated ctDNA biomarkers have potential utility in patients with a specific type of cancer. Identification of specific-functional hypermethylated CpG sites in the promoter region of genes may lead to better specificity. One of the drawbacks of methylated ctDNA is that promoter regions of genes can be hypermethylated in both benign and malignant cancers.

There are several types of assays that detect methylated ctDNA. These assays include quantitative methylation-specific PCR, mass spectrometry, pyrosequencing, and array hybridization. Each technique has pros and cons, but all require bisulphite conversion that is laborious and destroys a large fraction of the rare ctDNA during the process. The reliance on bisulphite treatment limits the sensitivity of methylation ctDNA assays until new approaches for methylation detection are developed. Typically, real-time PCR assays are more quantitative and sensitive than the other methods.

Noncoding ctDNA

With whole genome sequencing, repetitive noncoding sequences such as long interspersed nucleotide elements (LINEs) and short interspersed nucleotide elements (SINEs) are also potential biomarkers in multiple cancers.[331,339,402,428,429] There are many variants in the LINE family, such as the *LINE1* subfamily consisting of 6–8 kb CpG-rich DNA elements. Their function is not completely understood, but some act as retrotransposons and, when hypomethylated, increase tumor genomic instability. The human genome contains over 5 million copies of *LINE1*, representing almost 17% of the entire genome and are commonly found in ctDNA. The hypomethylated *LINE1* status in tumor tissues can be assessed as hypomethylated ctDNA. In normal tissue, the *LINE1* subfamily is usually hypermethylated, but in cancers such as melanoma, breast cancer, hepatocellular carcinoma, colorectal cancer, and prostate cancer, *LINE1* elements are hypomethylated and activated. SINEs, mostly *ALU* sequences, are assessed in ctDNA by a DNA integrity index that is described below.

TABLE 52.5 Viral Circulating Tumor DNA (ctDNA) in Various Cancers

Cancer	Virus	Reference
Nasopharyngeal carcinoma	Epstein Barr virus	430–434
Liver	Hepatitis B virus	437, 459
Head and neck	Human papilloma virus	435, 436, 438

Viral ctDNA

Several cancers have an etiology strongly linked to viral DNA integration. In these cancers, ctDNA can be tested for specific cell-free viral DNA (Table 52.5). The advantage of assessing viral ctDNA is the high specificity and detection sensitivity because of the unique viral sequences. The most notable and extensive assessment for clinical utility of viral ctDNA is Epstein Barr virus (EBV) detection in nasopharyngeal cancer (NPC).[430,431] NPC is one of the most common malignancies in southern China and Southeast Asia. Patients with metastatic disease have a poor prognosis. Plasma EBV DNA in NPC patients is a well-established ctDNA biomarker. Studies have shown its utility in assessing clinically concealed residual NPC after curative-intent radiotherapy. Furthermore, EBV ctDNA is associated with treatment outcome prediction.[432] Plasma EBV ctDNA is useful in screening early-stage NPC and is relatively low in cost.[433] Radiotherapy and combination chemoradiotherapy are major treatment modalities for NPC, whereby in the setting of these treatments, plasma EBV ctDNA levels can help assess treatment response and outcome.[434] EBV ctDNA is one of the best examples of the clinical utility of ctDNA biomarkers.

Additional examples of viral ctDNA include human papilloma virus (HPV) for head and neck cancer[435,436] and cervical cancer, and hepatitis virus B for hepatocellular carcinoma.[437] In cervical cancer patients, the specificity of HPV ctDNA detection can be improved by analyzing the cell–viral DNA junction sequences in individual patients.[438] This involves assessing the specific cell genomic locus that the viral DNA integrates into. Although most current viral ctDNA assays are based on quantitative PCR, MPS assays have great potential in the future because they can cover larger DNA or RNA sequences. In the future, as new associations of cancer with virus etiology are found, new ctDNA assays may be developed to improve monitoring these viral-related cancers

ctDNA Integrity

Another approach to evaluating ctDNA is to examine its size, often referred to as "integrity." DNA fragment size can be used to determine the origin of cell-free DNA from either apoptotic or necrotic cells.[439-441] Programmed cell death under normal conditions is accompanied by an organized degradation of the DNA, which results in small and uniform DNA fragments (approximately 140–200 bp). In contrast, cell necrosis, which is a frequent event in solid tumors, generates a wide spectrum of DNA fragment lengths, including those greater than 200 bp as a consequence of digestion. The increased DNA integrity of cell-free DNA in different cancers[442] can be quantified as an integrity index that compares long to short cell-free DNA.

The DNA integrity index may be calculated in different ways. AC electrokinetics can separate cell-free DNA fragments by size (Biological Dynamics, Calif.). However, ctDNA integrity is usually assessed by qPCR of different fragment sizes, often from noncoding repeats such as *ALU*.[331,429,443] *ALU* sequences are approximately 300 bp in length and are found on all human chromosomes, being the most abundant transposable elements of the human genome. Umetani and colleagues developed a method using qPCR to directly measure the integrity of cell-free DNA without DNA purification.[441] The integrity index was calculated as the ratio between a 115-bp (small) amplicon and a 247-bp (large) amplicon of *ALU*. Another DNA integrity index distinguished between lymph node–negative and lymph node–positive breast cancer patients.[444] In this breast cancer study, the integrity index was derived from the quantification cycle of qPCR for two amplicons (one of 400 bp and the other 100 bp). DNA integrity was calculated as the ratio of the 400 bp fragment to total DNA and was clinically useful for detecting breast cancer progression.

The index of integrity has been successfully applied to detect multiple malignancies including breast, colorectal, esophagus, head and neck, kidney, melanoma, nasopharyngeal, periampullary, and prostate cancer (Table 52.6).[444-452] Persistence of a high DNA integrity index after radiotherapy is associated with poor prognosis in nasopharyngeal carcinoma patients.[453] The DNA integrity index is also associated with response to preoperative chemotherapy in rectal carcinoma patients.[454]

DNA integrity analysis is a ctDNA biomarker with applications in many cancers, although the specific calculations and cutoffs may vary between cancer types. Isolation methods may also bias enrichment of different size fragments. As new methods become available for quantification of a larger size range of ctDNA, these assays may increase in utility.

TABLE 52.6 Circulating Tumor DNA (ctDNA) Integrity in Various Cancers

Cancer	Integrity Sites	Reference
Breast	ALU	441, 449
Melanoma	Nonspecific	450
Colorectal	ALU, LINE1	429, 441, 452, 454
Esophageal	Nonspecific	451
Head and neck	Nonspecific	445, 448
Renal	Nonspecific	446
Bladder	Nonspecific	464
Brain	ALU	465
Prostate	Nonspecific	447
Ovarian	Nonspecific	466
Liver	Nonspecific	409

Half-Life of ctDNA

The half-life of ctDNA is important in the assessment of cancer patients. Understanding the rapid clearance and/or degradation from circulation is needed to interpret patient results. Unfortunately, it has been difficult to determine the actual half-life of ctDNA in cancer patients. In fetal cell–free DNA analysis, clearance from maternal blood occurs within 30 minutes.[455] However, in cancer patients, we do not know how long ctDNA survives in the circulation or the kinetics of its clearance. Long-fragment ctDNA (>250 bp) is cleared more rapidly than shorter fragments. Important factors may include degradation by enzymes in blood, binding to blood lipids/proteins, binding to nucleoprotein, uptake by leukocytes in blood and tissues, and clearance by normal physiological mechanisms in the liver and kidney. Tumors located in highly vascular organs or with active angiogenesis will have higher access and release into the systemic circulation. In addition, ctDNA can be taken up by cells in the surrounding microenvironment, as well as be incorporated into vesicles of cancer cells and released as exosomes.[456,457] Although not strictly free ctDNA, exosomes are an additional source of ctDNA. This topic is difficult to address in patients because many physiologic events can control ctDNA half-life in blood. Further studies are needed in patients who are disease free by surgical resection and assessed for ctDNA before and several years after surgery.

ctDNA Detection by Single-Marker Versus Multimarker Approach Assays

The approach of multimarker versus single-marker assays is clearly essential in most cancers. Because of tumor heterogeneity and continual genomic/epigenomic changes during tumor progression, multiple-marker assays are often necessary for diagnosis and monitoring. Furthermore, therapeutics can modify the molecular profile of tumors, particularly when drug resistance develops. Most patients with distant metastasis have molecular heterogeneity between clinical and subclinical metastasis. Multiple molecular markers and platforms may be necessary to study different genomic/epigenomic aberrations and/or multiple targets within an aberration. Combination drug therapy is often required because monotherapy in many advanced-stage cancers is not sufficient to control long-term tumor progression in melanoma, breast cancer, and colorectal cancer. More information is needed on multiple events occurring before, during, and after treatment. Because signal pathways can change during tumor progression and resistance, more complete profiling of specific gene aberrations may be needed (eg, therapies that target tyrosine kinase activation where resistance development frequently occurs). Cancer genomic changes are complex. It is not surprising that multiple markers and assays are needed for adequate study and understanding.[339] Several studies have been conducted whereby multiple markers have shown better utility than single markers, particularly in melanoma. As we know, cancer is quite heterogeneous, so in genomic changes it is more important to have a panel of markers for efficient detection. For example, very few cancers have a single mutation at higher than 50% frequency.

ctDNA in Clinical Oncology Trials

ctDNA testing is now incorporated into many clinical phase II and III trials, particularly for targeted therapeutics to mutations and fusions. To date, the most reported ctDNA companion diagnostics is *EGFR* mutation analysis in ctDNA, particularly in NSCLC.[368] Many clinical cancer trials have shown the potential utility of ctDNA *EGFR* mutations in monitoring treatment response. As more targeted therapies to particular mutations or fusions are developed, more companion ctDNA assays will likely be incorporated into clinical trials. Companion ctDNA diagnostics can either be specific to the targeted gene or to other tumor biomarkers that correlate to patient response. The merit of MPS ctDNA analysis is that tumor heterogeneity with changing mutations can be monitored in real time and associated with emerging drug resistance. This approach identifies new mutations as they arise in the tumor during treatment or follow-up that may provide guidance for decisions to stop treatment and/or initiate new targeted drug(s). Noninvasive ctDNA assays are a welcome replacement for repeated tumor sampling by core biopsies or fine-needle aspirations.

Future Challenges for ctDNA Analysis

The future of ctDNA lies in the hands of investigators in academia and the pharmaceutical and biotechnology industry to validate assays for CLIA and FDA approval for clinical diagnostics. ctDNA assays provide a unique opportunity to better monitor cancer patients with gene-targeted therapies. However, continued validation in well-defined multicenter clinical trials is necessary. Its technical success depends on the robust, consistent, easy, and efficient isolation of ctDNA in small amounts of blood.

In addition to technical improvements, quantification and reporting methods that allow oncologists to make decisions in patient treatment are critical. Standards for ctDNA will be essential to set quality controls, consistent quantification, and reporting among laboratories. Until regulatory groups start implementing these standards, clinical implementation will remain chaotic. The complexity inherent in cancer has resulted in many approaches to ctDNA measurement. MPS will also generate new challenges and opportunities for ctDNA analysis.

POINTS TO REMEMBER

ctDNA

- ctDNA can identify DNA changes in the primary tumor, including mutations, loss of microsatellite heterozygosity, methylation of gene promoter regions, DNA integrity, amplification, copy number variation, and the presence of viral DNA.
- ctDNA assays can be performed on both serum and plasma.
- There are multiple types of detection assays for ctDNA. Some are highly dependent on the form of ctDNA. Most are based on quantitative PCR.
- Massively parallel sequencing (MPS) in recent years has elevated the level of ctDNA analysis to include whole genome analysis of mutations and copy number variations.
- ctDNA mutation analysis can be successful companion diagnostics for targeted therapies (eg, EGFR mutations in NSCLC treatment).

COMBINED DISCUSSION OF CTC AND CTDNA

Comparison Between CTCs and ctDNA

Both CTC and ctDNA technology and applications have greatly advanced in the last decade. Because liquid biopsy of cancer patients can evaluate either CTC or ctDNA, what are the merits of each? Both assays provide some overlapping information as well as unique information for specific cancers. CTC detection provides real-time information on tumor spread. If CTCs are sampled repetitively over days to weeks and are increasing in number, this may indicate that the tumor is progressing and active metastasis is occurring. Assessing the presence of CTCs in blood may be important before, during, and after therapy because their presence suggests potential metastasis and colonization in distant sites. Continued development of better markers for CTCs that predict survival and establishment of metastasis is important. Molecular characterization of CTCs in addition to quantification will provide more guidance for treatment decisions. Markers expressed by CTCs may allow prediction of what organ site is likely to be colonized.

ctDNA detection indicates there is tumor present, but unlike CTCs, it does not indicate if it is spreading through the circulation. Consistent detection or increasing concentrations over time suggest that the tumor is active (progressing or rapidly renewing cell turnover). ctDNA assays require less blood, typically less than 2 mL, whereas most CTC assays require 7 to 10 mL. When the demand for other blood tests is high, the additional volume required by CTC assays can be a concern. Assays that require less blood will have better patient compliance, particularly for repetitive phlebotomy during treatment and follow-up. Table 52.7 compares the relative merits of CTC and ctDNA analyses.

Quality Control and Logistic Issues of CTCs and ctDNA

CTC and ctDNA assays need better quality control and standardization to provide more consistent reporting and comparisons. There are many different ways to detect and procure CTCs, as well as different downstream assays. The CTC field has attracted many new companies in the

TABLE 52.7 Comparison Between Circulating Tumor DNA (ctDNA) and Circulating Tumor Cells (CTCs)

ctDNA	CTCs
Minimal amount of blood (<2 mL)	Larger blood draw (>7 mL)
Logistically easier to assay due to purity of ctDNA	Logistically difficult to assay due to small number of cells and purity
More informative	Less informative for the sample used
Easily quantifiable due to high-sensitivity molecular assays	Difficult to quantify due to heterogeneity and cell recovery
Easier to assess tumor heterogeneity	Tumor heterogeneity is difficult to assess
Identifies presence of tumor	Identifies presence of tumor
Cannot identify metastasis occurring	Can identify metastasis occurring
Highly diagnostic	Diagnosis not dependable clinically
Prognostic	Prognostic
Can identify tumor resistance during therapy	Poor in identifying tumor resistance during therapy

last 5 years. This is important and supportive for continued advancement, but each company tends to brand its specific techniques and reports, resulting in confusion and poor standardization among companies. The development of quality controls and reporting standards is needed to allow comparisons and determine clinical utility. As better isolation methods develop, downstream analysis has improved and become more informative. Blood CTC analysis can be a tremendous advantage over the necessary sampling error of tumor biopsies. However, because CTCs are heterogeneous, all detected CTCs may not be relevant in assessing metastatic potential. Another issue for CTCs is the volume of blood needed (>5 mL) to accurately assess CTCs, particularly in early-stage cancer patients.

Quality control issues in ctDNA must be improved before wider clinical use. Blood tube collection, transport to a reference or hospital laboratory, ctDNA reference standards, isolation, reproducibility, robustness, accuracy, and reporting format are all issues that need to be addressed. There are currently several clinically validated ctDNA assays available to oncologists.

Prenatal plasma cell–free DNA testing has led the field of circulating nucleic acid assessment and has shown how efficient and useful such testing can be (see Chapter 53). ctDNA assays need to model this approach for cross-validated comparisons of different approaches. Similar to currently accepted blood cancer biomarkers, multicenter validation and reporting must be performed for ctDNA assay acceptance and wide use.

Liquid Biopsy Versus Tumor Biopsy

A major objective in the field is to determine if CTC and ctDNA analysis can replace tumor biopsies. Liquid biopsies are

TABLE 52.8 Comparison Between Circulating Tumor (ctDNA) and Solid Tumor Biopsy

ctDNA	Tumor Biopsy
Repetitive analysis	Minimal biopsy material obtainable
Minimally invasive	Highly invasive
More representative genomic information	Variation from biopsy sampling error
Can be repeated as needed	Difficult to repeat
Can be assessed from small blood draw	Not practical in all anatomical sites
Can monitor tumor heterogeneity	Limited assessment of tumor heterogeneity
Better patient compliance	Poor patient compliance
Cost-effective	Expensive

minimally invasive and can be performed repetitively without the complications of tumor biopsy. Tumor biopsies cannot always be performed because of the tumor site location, and repetitive samples may not be sufficient or representative of the tumor. Repeat ctDNA molecular analysis may be more consistent than tumor biopsies because of tumor sampling error. CTC analysis of genomic aberrations can now be performed with the same potential quality as a tumor biopsy such as a fine-needle aspiration. While initial diagnosis is best performed by tumor biopsy and conventional histopathology, liquid biopsies may in the future be used once validated for targeted therapy stratification and monitoring patients. With the advent of MPS, ctDNA and CTC assays have become more informative and offer better homogeneity than a solid tumor for sequencing analysis. As liquid biopsies become better validated, they may replace some tumor biopsies. ctDNA and CTC analysis may enable more rapid decisions for treatment stratification and treatment modifications during therapy (Table 52.8). A newly formed European consortium, CANCER-ID (http://www.cancer-id.eu/), consisting of 33 partners from 13 countries, aims to establish standard procedures for clinical validation of liquid biopsy biomarkers and to evaluate the clinical utility of ctDNA and CTC in several types of carcinomas, including breast and lung. The objective of the CANCER-ID consortium is to have multicenter prospective trials to evaluate techniques for assessing CTC and ctDNA in different laboratories using specimens from different clinical sites.

CTCs and ctDNA Combined as Companion Blood Biomarkers

The combination of both CTCs and ctDNA as a liquid biopsy may augment the accurate assessment of cancer patients. Both can be used together to provide informative patient results.[285] In addition, the use of liquid biopsy (CTC and/or ctDNA) may be combined with imaging and blood protein/analyte tumor biomarkers to give a more comprehensive evaluation of the patient status. The real challenge is to combine all the information into an interpretable result for the clinician to enable decisions on treatment.

CONCLUSIONS

The development of both CTC and ctDNA liquid biopsies provides many new opportunities for implementation over the next 5 years. These assays, upon validation, may provide better clinical management in treatment monitoring and understanding of tumor progression for many different types of cancers. As new biosensors, molecular procedures, and molecular devices develop in both CTC and ctDNA analysis, the sensitivity and specificity, as well as logistics, will improve. With the resource of the cancer gene atlas (TCGA NIH USA:http://cancergenome.nih.gov/), there is a significant amount of sequencing data of multiple cancer types that can be translated into new CTC and ctDNA targets in the future.

SELECTED REFERENCES

For a full list of references for this chapter, please refer to ExpertConsult.com.

1. Alix-Panabières C, Pantel K. Clinical applications of circulating tumor cells and circulating tumor DNA as liquid biopsy. *Cancer Discov* 2016;**6**:479–91.
9. Cristofanilli M, Budd GT, Ellis MJ, et al. Circulating tumor cells, disease progression, and survival in metastatic breast cancer. *N Engl J Med* 2004;**351**:781–91.
20. Miller MC, Doyle GV, Terstappen LW. Significance of circulating tumor cells detected by the CellSearch™ system in patients with metastatic breast colorectal and prostate cancer. *J Oncol* 2010;**2010**:617421.
82. Nagrath S, Sequist LV, Maheswaran S, et al. Isolation of rare circulating tumour cells in cancer patients by microchip technology. *Nature* 2007;**450**:1235–9.
114. Xenidis N, Perraki M, Kafousi M, et al. Predictive and prognostic value of peripheral blood cytokeratin-19 mRNA-positive cells detected by real-time polymerase chain reaction in node-negative breast cancer patients. *J Clin Oncol* 2006;**24**:3756–62.
134. Heitzer E, Auer M, Gasch C, et al. Complex tumor genomes inferred from single circulating tumor cells by array-CGH and next-generation sequencing. *Cancer Res* 2013;**73**:2965–75.
145. Kasimir-Bauer S, Hoffmann O, Wallwiener D, et al. Expression of stem cell and epithelial-mesenchymal transition markers in primary breast cancer patients with circulating tumor cells. *Breast Cancer Res* 2012; **14**:R15.
165. Bidard FC, Fehm T, Ignatiadis M, et al. Clinical application of circulating tumor cells in breast cancer: overview of the current interventional trials. *Cancer Metastasis Rev* 2013;**32**:179–88.
184. Lucci A, Hall CS, Lodhi AK, et al. Circulating tumour cells in non-metastatic breast cancer: a prospective study. *Lancet Oncol* 2012;**13**:688–95.
198. Georgoulias V, Bozionelou V, Agelaki S, et al. Trastuzumab decreases the incidence of clinical relapses in patients with early breast cancer presenting chemotherapy-resistant CK-19mRNA-positive circulating tumor cells: results of a randomized phase II study. *Ann Oncol* 2012;**23**: 1744–50.
214. de Bono JS, Scher HI, Montgomery RB, et al. Circulating tumor cells predict survival benefit from treatment in metastatic castration-resistant prostate cancer. *Clin Cancer Res* 2008;**14**:6302–9.
224. Antonarakis ES, Lu C, Wang H, et al. AR-V7 and resistance to enzalutamide and abiraterone in prostate cancer. *N Engl J Med* 2014;**371**:1028–38.
244. Iinuma H, Watanabe T, Mimori K, et al. Clinical significance of circulating tumor cells, including cancer stem-like cells, in peripheral blood for recurrence and prognosis in patients with Dukes' stage B and C colorectal cancer. *J Clin Oncol* 2011;**29**:1547–55.
260. Hodgkinson CL, Morrow CJ, Li Y, et al. Tumorigenicity and genetic profiling of circulating tumor cells in small-cell lung cancer. *Nat Med* 2014;**20**:897–903.
268. Pailler E, Adam J, Barthelemy A, et al. Detection of circulating tumor cells harboring a unique ALK rearrangement in ALK-positive non-small-cell lung cancer. *J Clin Oncol* 2013;**31**:2273–81.
325. Schwarzenbach H, Hoon DSB, Pantel K. Cell-free nucleic acids as biomarkers in cancer patients. *Nat Rev Cancer* 2011;**11**:426–37.
339. Marzese DM, Hirose H, Hoon DS. Diagnostic and prognostic value of circulating tumor-related DNA in cancer patients. *Expert Rev Mol Diagn* 2013;**13**:827–44.
354. Bettegowda C, Sausen M, Leary RJ, et al. Detection of circulating tumor DNA in early- and late-stage human malignancies. *Sci Transl Med* 2014;**6**:224ra24.
359. Dawson SJ, Tsui DW, Murtaza M, et al. Analysis of circulating tumor DNA to monitor metastatic breast cancer. *N Engl J Med* 2013;**368**:1199–209.
366. Murtaza M, Dawson SJ, Tsui DW, et al. Non-invasive analysis of acquired resistance to cancer therapy by sequencing of plasma DNA. *Nature* 2013;**497**:108–12.

53

Circulating Nucleic Acids for Prenatal Diagnostics

Rossa W.K. Chiu and Y.M. Dennis Lo

ABSTRACT

Background

Prenatal diagnosis is an important part of prenatal care for many patients. Traditional methods of sampling fetal genetic material for a definitive diagnosis, such as chorionic villus sampling and amniocentesis, are invasive and expose the fetus to the risk of spontaneous miscarriage. The discovery of the presence of fetal cell–free DNA in the circulation of pregnant women led to the possibility of noninvasive genetic and chromosomal assessment of the fetus through the sampling of maternal peripheral blood. The clinical introduction of cell-free fetal DNA (cffDNA) tests has led to a substantial reduction in the number of invasive procedures performed worldwide.

Content

This chapter describes the biological properties of circulating cffDNA, the applications that have been developed, and their clinical uses, and it highlights some analytical features that require careful consideration. Circulating cffDNA is derived from cell turnover of the placenta. This DNA is highly fragmented, with the majority of fragments less than 200 bp in length. Circulating cffDNA exists with a substantial background of maternal DNA. Circulating cffDNA can be detected from early pregnancy onward, and it rapidly disappears from maternal circulation following delivery of the newborn. The analysis of cffDNA is now clinically used for the assessment of sex-linked diseases, fetal blood group incompatibility, fetal chromosomal aneuploidies, and some single-gene diseases. Analytical protocols are designed to maximize the yield of fetal DNA by minimizing maternal DNA contamination and by preserving the abundance of short DNA molecules. The inclusion of internal positive controls for the presence of fetal DNA or the measurement of fetal DNA fraction is an important quality control parameter.

BRIEF OVERVIEW OF THE EARLY DEVELOPMENTS OF PRENATAL GENETIC DIAGNOSTICS

Prenatal diagnosis is an important part of prenatal care for many patients. It encompasses both diagnostic and screening tests that detect or exclude morphological, structural, functional, chromosomal, and molecular defects in a fetus.[1] Amniocentesis was first introduced in 1952 for the prenatal assessment of fetal hemolytic disease.[2] This was followed by karyotyping of amniotic fluid cells in 1966,[3] and then ultrasonography for fetal structural abnormalities in the 1970s.[4,5] Later, maternal serum biochemistry testing was shown to be of value in the screening of neural tube defects[6,7] and fetal aneuploidies.[8] In the early 1980s, chorionic villus sampling (CVS) became available as an alternative to amniocentesis for prenatal genetic assessment.[9] For many years, amniocentesis and CVS were the key approaches for providing fetal genetic material used in prenatal testing.

The main disadvantage of amniocentesis and CVS is the procedural-related risk of fetal miscarriage. The fetal loss rate associated with the performance of these invasive procedures is about 0.5%.[10] Consequently, much effort has been devoted to the development of noninvasive approaches to identify high-risk pregnant women.

STRATEGIES TO MITIGATE RISKS OF INVASIVE PRENATAL DIAGNOSIS

The risk for Down syndrome, with an incidence rate of 1 in 800 pregnancies,[11] is one of the predominant reasons for women seeking prenatal diagnosis. Strategies have been devised to identify high-risk pregnancies by the combined assessment of maternal age, serum biochemical markers, and ultrasonographic findings. The purpose of this assessment is to risk stratify pregnancies where the chance of having an affected fetus is higher than the chance of a procedure-related fetal loss. Different combinations of screening strategies have been practiced, with different levels of specificity and sensitivity.[12]

Maternal Age

The probability of giving birth to an infant with Down syndrome increases with advancing maternal age.[13] The risk of giving birth to an affected infant at term is estimated to be less than 1 in 1000 at a maternal age of 29 years and younger, but it increases to 1 in 385 at 35 years of age.[14] Hence, prior to the development of more elaborate prenatal screening strategies, it was customary to offer prenatal diagnosis to women aged 35 years or older. However, because a significant proportion of women become pregnant before 35 years of age, maternal age alone would only identify 51% of Down syndrome–affected pregnancies at a 14% false-positive rate.[15]

Serum Biochemistry Screening

The combination of maternal age assessment with maternal serum screening of various biomarkers between 15 and 22 weeks of gestation was later developed as a second trimester screening protocol to identify high-risk pregnancies. This screening strategy is referred to as the "triple test," and the serum biomarkers include alpha-fetoprotein, human chorionic gonadotropin, and unconjugated estriol. When the analytical cutoff values are set to give a 5% false-positive rate, the detection sensitivity for Down syndrome is 70%.[16] Testing maternal serum inhibin A and the triple test markers during the second trimester, termed the "quadruple test," provided a detection sensitivity of 75% at a false-positive rate of 5%.[15]

First Trimester Screening

The triple test is used during the second trimester; during the first trimester, alternative Down syndrome screening strategies have been developed. Free β-human chorionic gonadotropin and pregnancy-associated plasma protein A are used for Down syndrome screening in the first trimester.[17,18] Down syndrome is associated with an increase in fetal nuchal translucency measured by first trimester ultrasound.[19] Subsequently, the combination of first trimester biochemical markers, fetal nuchal translucency, and maternal age assessments came to be known as the "first trimester combined test." As a false-positive rate of 5%, the test could detect 95% of Down syndrome fetuses.[20]

The approaches described above have been incorporated into many prenatal screening programs. However, the main disadvantage of these tests lies in their high false-positive rates. Most of the test cutoff values used to identify those deemed to be at high risk had false-positive rates of 5%. This meant that 1 in every 20 women would be labeled as high risk and would need to face the decision of whether or not to undergo an invasive diagnostic procedure. Because the average Down syndrome risk is 1 in 800, this meant that a substantial number of women undergoing an invasive diagnostic procedure did not carry an affected fetus. Therefore there was a need to identify new screening methods that had lower false-positive rates and improved detection rates.

NONINVASIVE FETAL DNA ANALYSIS

The above prenatal screening methods are based on the detection of prenatal phenotypic features that tend to be associated with Down syndrome. It had been reasoned that to improve the sensitivity and specificity of prenatal screening, methods directed at the detection of the core pathology of the condition are needed—for example, trisomy 21 for Down syndrome or the fetal mutations for single-gene diseases. To this end, noninvasive methods have been developed to provide access to fetal DNA for analysis.

Fetal Cells in Maternal Blood

Over a century ago, a German pathologist, Schmorl,[21] observed the presence of trophoblasts in the lung tissues of women who died of preeclampsia. The existence of such circulating fetal cells was later confirmed by molecular techniques based on the detection of chromosome Y DNA sequences in the blood of women pregnant with male fetuses.[22] The idea of noninvasive prenatal diagnosis based on maternal blood sampling began to emerge. It was subsequently realized that intact fetal cells are present in maternal circulation rarely, with about just one cell per milliliter of maternal blood.[23] Protocols have since been developed to isolate and enrich for these rare fetal cells, including fluorescence activated cell sorting[24] and magnetic activated cell sorting.[25] To date, the identification and isolation of intact fetal cells in maternal circulation have remained difficult.[26] However, once isolated, they may be amenable to single-cell whole-genome analysis for the potential identification of fetal genetic and genomic abnormalities.[27] Therefore with further improvement in technologies, circulating fetal cell–based noninvasive prenatal diagnostics may be a clinically viable option in the future.

Cell-Free Fetal DNA in Maternal Plasma

Instead of intact cells, Lo and colleagues[28] searched for fetal DNA in the cell-free portion of maternal blood—namely, plasma and serum. Chromosome Y DNA was detected in the plasma and serum of women who were pregnant with male fetuses but not in women with female fetuses. Since this first report in 1997, much research investigated the properties and potential utilities of circulating cell-free fetal DNA (cffDNA). cffDNA analysis is currently used for routine prenatal testing.

THE BIOLOGY OF CIRCULATING CELL-FREE FETAL NUCLEIC ACIDS IN MATERNAL PLASMA

Every milliliter of maternal plasma contains thousands of genome-equivalents of cell-free DNA, with the fetus contributing a minor proportion.[29] In other words, the majority of the cell-free DNA in maternal plasma is derived from the mother. The median amount of cffDNA as a proportion of the total DNA in maternal plasma, termed the "fetal fraction," is around 10% in the first and second trimesters and around 20% during the third trimester.[30] The absolute concentration of cffDNA increases with gestational age, probably as a consequence of the increase in placental tissue mass. Nonetheless, its abundance in the maternal circulation far exceeds that of intact fetal cells.

POINTS TO REMEMBER

Biological Properties of cffDNA

- cffDNA is a by-product of placental cell turnover.
- cffDNA coexists in maternal plasma with a major background of maternal DNA.
- cffDNA is highly fragmented and is generally less than 200 bp long.
- cffDNA has rapid clearance kinetics and an apparent half-life of 1 hour.
- cffDNA is detectable in early pregnancy. It is most reliably detected from the late first trimester onward.

Fetal DNA molecules are detectable in maternal plasma quite early in pregnancy. Depending on the analytical platform used, cffDNA is detected from around the 10th week of gestation.[31] cffDNA is cleared from maternal plasma very rapidly after delivery.[32] Using sensitive methods to measure cffDNA serially after delivery, the half-life of cffDNA in the postpartum maternal serum is about an hour.[33] No cffDNA could be detected in maternal plasma 1 day after delivery. These observations reveal that fetal DNA molecules in maternal plasma have a high turnover rate with efficient clearance mechanisms. Renal clearance studies performed by serial monitoring of cffDNA in maternal plasma and maternal urine after delivery show that renal excretion is only a minor component of fetal DNA clearance.[33]

Despite the rapid clearance kinetics, cffDNA amounts to some 10% to 20% of the total DNA in maternal plasma; this suggests that substantial amounts of fetal DNA may be released by a tissue source at any point in time. Two lines of evidence demonstrate the placenta as the predominant tissue that releases fetal DNA into the maternal circulation: first, epigenetic markers specific to the placenta are detectable in maternal plasma;[34,35] second, chromosomal abnormalities confined to the placenta are detectable in maternal plasma.[36] On the other hand, the main contributors of cell-free DNA from the mother are maternal hematological cells.[35,37]

Cell-free DNA is a metabolic by-product of cell death and is therefore present in the circulation as short fragments in a "cell-free" form. Using paired-end massively parallel sequencing, Lo and colleagues studied the size profile of maternal plasma DNA in a high-resolution manner (Fig. 53.1).[38] By noting the genomic coordinates of the outermost ends of each plasma DNA molecule, the size of the fragments was determined. The cell-free DNA molecules are generally shorter than 200 bp. The most frequently represented size in plasma is 166 bp in length. 166 bp corresponds to the length of DNA that is wound around a histone core with a linker. This characteristic size reflected that cell-free DNA is mainly derived from mononucleosomes. Interestingly, cffDNA molecules are somewhat shorter, and the most frequently represented size is 142 bp in length.[38] This shorter length corresponds to the length of DNA wound around a histone core without a linker. This implies that the fetal DNA molecules may have undergone further steps of degradation compared to maternal DNA in maternal plasma. In addition to these dominant peaks, there are smaller amounts of cell-free DNA that are successively shorter in 10-bp increments. This observation suggests that DNase participates in the degradation of cell-free DNA because DNase cutting sites are located every 10 bases around the nucleosomal DNA.

DIAGNOSTIC APPLICATIONS OF CIRCULATING CFFDNA

Cell-free fetal DNA is a source of fetal genetic material that may be sampled noninvasively by maternal phlebotomy. Its relative high abundance in maternal plasma from early pregnancy, with no postpartum persistence, has facilitated the development of a number of applications for noninvasive prenatal assessment.

Fetal Sex Assessment for Sex-Associated Disorders

The first report of cffDNA was based on the detection of male fetal DNA sequences in the plasma of women pregnant with male fetuses.[28] This noninvasive test for fetal sex assessment was immediately useful for clinical purposes. The accurate

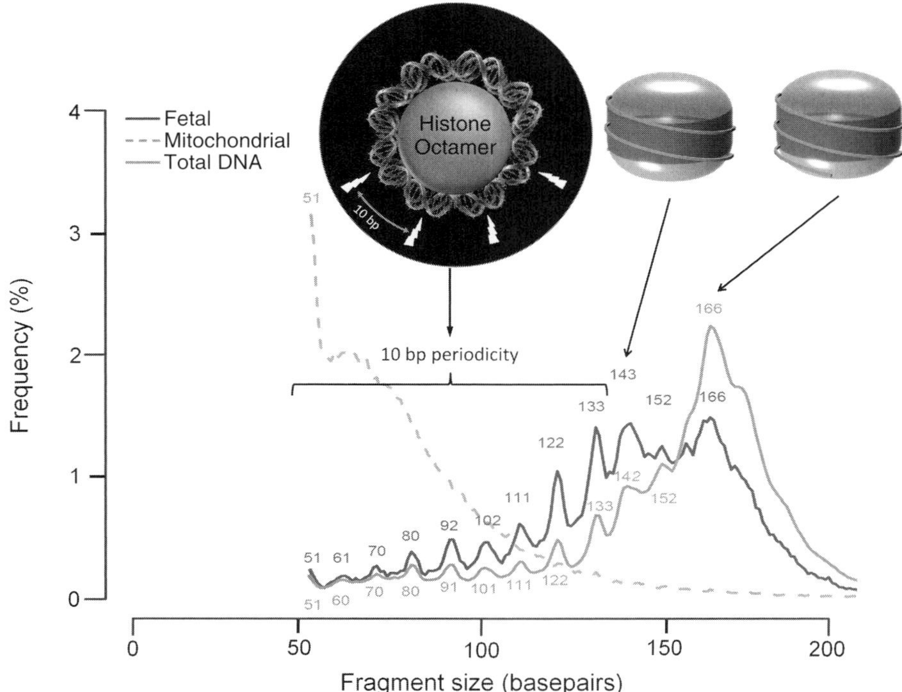

FIGURE 53.1 Size distribution of fetal, mitochondrial, and total DNA. Numbers denote the DNA size in bps at the peaks. Schematic illustrations of the structural organization of a nucleosome are shown above the graph. From left to right, DNA double helix wound around a nucleosomal core unit with the sites for nuclease cleavage shown; a nucleosome core unit (blue) with approximately 146 bp of DNA (red strand) wound around it; and a nucleosomal core unit with an approximately 20-bp linker intact.

POINTS TO REMEMBER

Diagnostic Applications of cffDNA

- Fetal sex assessment for the management of fetal sex–associated diseases.
- Fetal *RHD* genotyping for the management of rhesus D incompatibility.
- Fetal chromosomal aneuploidy screening, especially trisomies 21, 13, and 18.
- Fetal single-gene disease detection, including paternally or maternally transmitted autosomal dominant diseases, autosomal recessive diseases, and sex-linked diseases.

assessment of fetal sex is useful for the prenatal management of diseases with sex-linked patterns of inheritance and conditions such as congenital adrenal hyperplasia, where the disease manifestation differs between male and female offspring. For sex-linked genetic diseases, such as hemophilia and Duchenne muscular dystrophy, invasive prenatal diagnostic procedures could be avoided if the noninvasive fetal sex assessment suggested a female fetus. For congenital adrenal hyperplasia secondary to 21-hydroxylase deficiency, female fetuses are at risk of virilization. Thus steroid therapy and further prenatal genetic assessment may be avoided if the noninvasive fetal sex assessment suggested a male fetus. In general, the specificity for male cffDNA detection approaches 99%.[31] In terms of sensitivity, Devaney and colleagues showed that higher sensitivities could be reached by using later gestational ages, more replicate analyses, and higher-sensitivity analytical approaches.[31] For example, real-time PCR provides higher sensitivity than conventional PCR.

Fetal Rhesus D Status Determination

Rhesus (Rh) D incompatibility occurs when an RhD-negative women is pregnant with a RhD-positive fetus. RhD-negative blood cells lack the RhD antigen. Therefore when the RhD-negative maternal immune cells are presented with the RhD antigen of the RhD-positive fetal blood, alloimmunization occurs. Upon the next pregnancy with an RhD-positive fetus, the sensitized woman and the anti-RhD antibodies may cause destruction of the fetal tissues, causing hemolytical disease of the newborn. However, such risks do not exist if the woman is pregnant with an RhD-negative fetus. Therefore prenatal RhD genotyping of the fetus is useful in the management of RhD-negative pregnant women. The great majority of RhD-negative individuals lack the RhD gene, *RHD*, due to gene deletion. Therefore one could noninvasively assess the fetal RhD status by detecting the presence of *RHD* in the plasma of RhD-negative pregnant women.[39,40] Unlike conventional methods, such as amniocentesis or CVS, noninvasive methods are free from the risk of inducing fetomaternal hemorrhage and further sensitization. In fact, the analysis of cffDNA for noninvasive fetal RhD genotyping has been globally implemented for clinical use. In addition, the test has also been used as the basis for rationalizing the administration of prophylactic anti-D immunoglobulin only to pregnancies involving an RhD-positive fetus.[41] Such an approach may minimize the unnecessary use of the scarce and expensive anti-D immunoglobulin, as well as reduce the need to unnecessarily expose the pregnant woman to the anti-D blood product. Hemolytic disease of the newborn is further discussed in Chapter 69.

Fetal Chromosomal Aneuploidy Screening

Down syndrome is one of the key reasons for couples to consider prenatal diagnosis. Thus there has been a longstanding interest to develop noninvasive tests for Down syndrome assessment based on cffDNA analysis. Down syndrome is typically caused by the presence of an additional dose of chromosome 21—namely, trisomy 21—in the genome of affected individuals. Therefore the key to achieving noninvasive prenatal detection of Down syndrome is to provide evidence that increased copies of chromosome 21 are present in maternal plasma. The majority of the DNA in maternal plasma, including DNA from chromosome 21, originates from the mother who has a normal amount of chromosome 21. If the fetus has trisomy 21, it would contribute additional amounts of chromosome 21 into maternal plasma. Therefore the additional amount of cell-free chromosome 21 DNA molecules in maternal plasma is dependent on the fetal fraction (ie, the percent of fetal DNA in the background of maternal DNA in the plasma). The higher the fetal fraction, the easier the identification of trisomy 21–associated changes in maternal plasma DNA analysis.

Methodological Approaches

To precisely quantify and detect this small additional amount of chromosome 21 DNA, most protocols utilize massively parallel sequencing (see Chapter 47). One approach is based on random or shotgun sequencing of maternal plasma DNA.[42] The rationale is that among the cell-free DNA fragments in maternal plasma, if one sequences a random fraction of all the molecules, the relative amount of DNA obtained from each segment across the genome should reflect the relative DNA contribution of that segment in the genome of the tested individual. To determine the relative amount of DNA from each segment—say, each chromosome—one could determine the number of DNA molecules sequenced from that chromosome as a proportion of all molecules sequenced from the sample. The relative amount, or genomic representation, is then compared with the expected amount for the same chromosome among a control group of samples representing euploid pregnancies (Fig. 53.2). If a sample shows a genomic representation of chromosome 21 that is significantly different (eg, more than 3 standard deviations) from the control group, the amount of chromosome 21 is considered elevated and therefore suggestive of trisomy 21.

Because this approach is based on random whole-genome sequencing, it could in principle be applied to other chromosomal aneuploidies, such as trisomy 18 and trisomy 13, and the sex chromosome aneuploidies, such as Turner syndrome, 45 X0, and Klinefelter syndrome, 47 XXY.[43,44] The protocol could be repurposed for the detection of microdeletion and microduplication syndromes.[45,46] In fact, molecular karyotyping at Mb-level of resolution covering most parts of the genome appears possible.[45,46] Indeed, there is great versatility in the random whole-genome sequencing approach. As described in the section on analytical aspects, the successful implementation of these protocols relies on the precise quantification of the genomic segment of interest. For example, the signal-to-noise ratio for relative quantification of a genomic region is partly governed by the

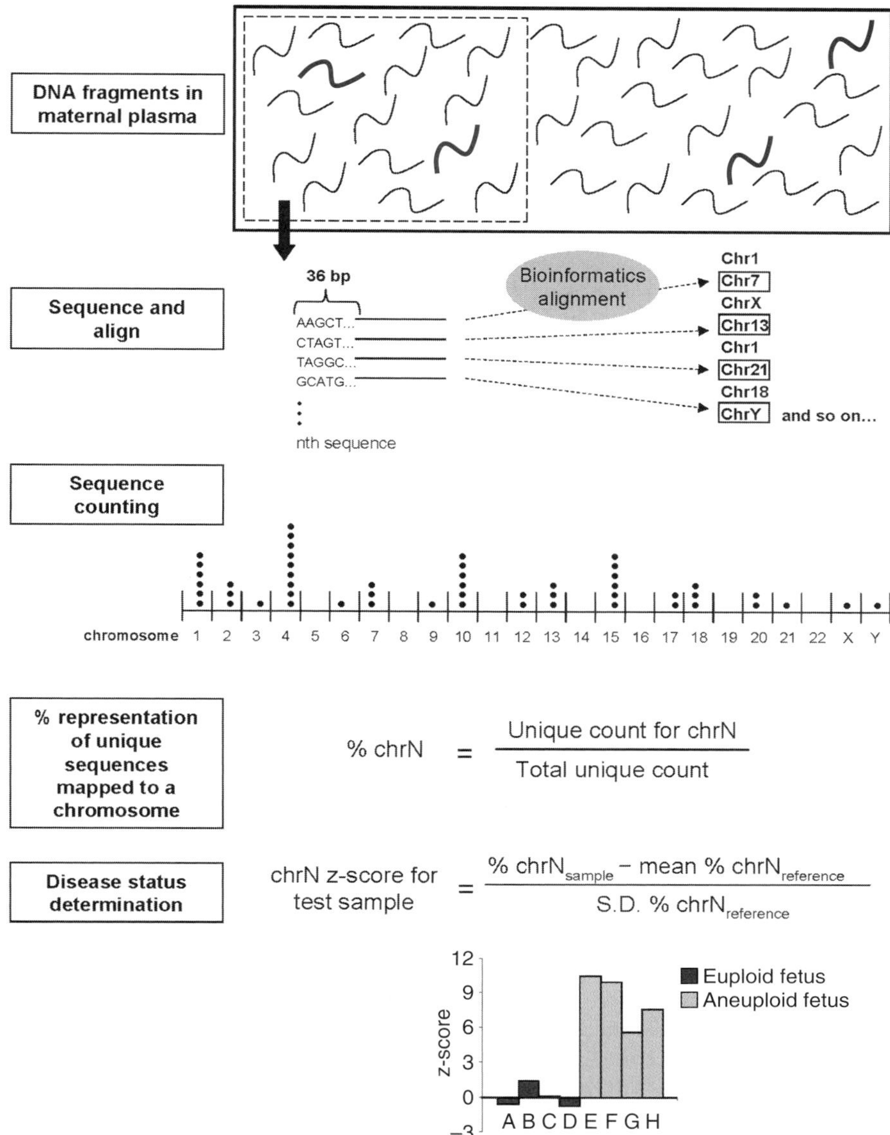

FIGURE 53.2 Schematic illustration of the procedural framework for using massively parallel genomic sequencing for the noninvasive prenatal detection of fetal chromosomal aneuploidy. Fetal DNA (thick red fragments) circulates in maternal plasma as a minor population among a high background of maternal DNA (black fragments). A sample containing representative DNA molecules in maternal plasma is obtained. Plasma DNA molecules are sequenced, and the chromosomal origin of each molecule is identified through mapping to the human reference genome by bioinformatic analysis. The number of sequences mapped to each chromosome is counted and then expressed as a percentage of all unique sequences generated for the sample, termed *%chrN* for chromosome N. Z-scores for each chromosome and each test sample are calculated using the formula shown. The z-score of a potentially aneuploid chromosome is expected to be higher for pregnancies with an aneuploid fetus (cases E to H) than those with a euploid fetus (cases A to D). (From Chiu et al. Noninvasive prenatal diagnosis of fetal chromosomal aneuploidy by massively parallel genomic sequencing of DNA in maternal plasma. *Proc Natl Acad Sci U S A* 2008;105:20458–63.)

sequencing depth.[46,47] Thus the sequencing depth may need to be adjusted if the analysis is intended for the detection of subchromosomal changes instead of whole-chromosome aneuploidies. In addition, target capture of cell-free DNA originating from chromosomal regions of interest followed by targeted analysis could similarly achieve relative genomic representation assessment.[48]

To detect the presence of extra or missing copies of chromosomes, allelic ratio approaches have also been developed. Such approaches take advantage of polymorphic differences between homologous chromosomes between the mother and the fetus.[49] In principle, such polymorphic loci may include loci where the mother is homozygous and the fetus is heterozygous, or when the mother is heterozygous and the fetus is homozygous. The rationale is that when the fetus has aneuploidy, the ratio between alleles on that chromosome will be skewed. However, the extent of skewing between the alleles is dependent on the configuration of the polymorphic markers between the fetus and the mother as well as the fetal fraction. To implement this method, the allelic information of each cell-free DNA fragment needs to be compared to relative amounts of the homologous chromosomes.

Clinical Implementation

cffDNA-based noninvasive prenatal screening for fetal chromosomal aneuploidy became clinically available in 2011.[47] Within 3 years, service availability extended to over 60 countries.[50] In general, cffDNA-based noninvasive prenatal screening achieved detection rates of about 99% for Down syndrome with less than 1% false-positive rates.[51,52] Depending on the specific protocol used, the detection rates for trisomy 18 and trisomy 13 are about or greater than 90% with less than 1% false-positive rates.[51,52] In other words, cffDNA-based prenatal screening achieved better detection sensitivities and specificities than those screening modalities based on maternal serum biochemistry and/or fetal ultrasonography. Consequently, there are now many professional guidelines and recommendations supporting the use of cffDNA-based prenatal assessment for fetal chromosomal aneuploidy screening.[52-55] However, it is noteworthy that there are false-positive cases (see discussion below). Therefore cffDNA assessment is a screening procedure and not a definitive diagnosis. All clinical guidelines recommend that cffDNA tests with positive findings suggestive of chromosomal aneuploidy should be confirmed by tests on fetal genetic material collected by conventional invasive methods such as chorionic villus sampling or amniocentesis.

While the performance profile of the cffDNA-based tests is quite attractive for screening, the direct costs are higher than that of maternal serum biochemistry screening. To balance the overall costs, various modalities for incorporating the cffDNA-based tests into prenatal screening programs have evolved.[51] One option is to recommend cffDNA testing only to pregnant women who are identified as high risk and who would otherwise be recommended for conventional invasive prenatal diagnosis. For example, women who receive a high-risk score upon having undergone the first trimester combined screening test may consider the option of cffDNA testing. In this scenario, the cffDNA assessment is only performed for the 5% of pregnancies with high-risk scores. With their high-specificity profile, the cffDNA tests should be able to further identify 99% of the unaffected pregnancies. As a result, the number of pregnancies recommended for invasive testing would be reduced to only those patients with a positive cffDNA test result. In practice, since the implementation of cffDNA testing in the clinical setting, the reduction in invasive prenatal diagnostic procedures is between 26% and 69%.[56-58]

The two-step screening approach described above has the advantage of reducing the high false-positive rate of the conventional prenatal screening program. However, it does not raise the aneuploidy detection rates that are limited by the detection performance of first-tier screening tests. Consequently, some groups have proposed a "contingent approach" where the threshold to label a pregnancy as "high risk" by the conventional screening tests is relaxed to include a greater proportion of the population (ie, 10% of all pregnancies).[51] Theoretically, this would increase the detection rates for fetal chromosomal aneuploidies without an increase in the overall false-positive rate in the context of a two-tier screening program.

Recently, evidence has emerged that cffDNA tests for chromosomal aneuploidies have similar detection sensitivities and specificities among high- as well as average-risk pregnant women.[59-61] This has led to discussions on applying the cffDNA tests as a primary screening test.[55,62] Bianchi and colleagues[62] reported that the positive predictive values of the cffDNA sequencing tests were substantially higher than that of maternal serum biochemistry–based screening. For trisomy 21 detection, the positive predictive value of cffDNA sequencing was 45.5%, while that of conventional screening was 4.2%. For trisomy 18 detection, the positive predictive value of cffDNA sequencing was 40.0% and 8.3% for conventional screening. In this study, the negative predictive values for trisomy 21 and trisomy 18 detection were 100% for both cffDNA sequencing and conventional screening. If the cost of cffDNA testing could be substantially reduced, cost-benefit studies have identified it as the preferred primary screen for aneuploidies.[63] In this regard, there has been a recent report that single-molecule sequencing may be applied to cffDNA analysis.[64] Such a development may lead to a reduction in costs and the potential for point-of-care noninvasive prenatal testing.

Discordant Results

While cffDNA tests demonstrate high sensitivities and specificities, there are false-negative and false-positive results. Some of the false-negative cases are a result of low fetal DNA fraction.[65] In these cases, the proportion of fetal DNA in the sample is too low to produce a statistically significant change in the genomic representation, even in the presence of chromosome aneuploidy. Other false-negative cases are due to the mosaic nature of some chromosomal abnormalities. Mosaicism refers to the situation when only a proportion of the fetal cells harbor the chromosomal abnormality. Because the proportion of fetal cells that are contributing the DNA from the affected chromosome is reduced, the ability of the analytical protocol to detect the abnormality is also reduced.[65] Interestingly, some of the false-negative cases are a result of the absence of the chromosomal aneuploidy in the placental tissue.[66] In other words, the chromosomal aneuploidy is present in the fetus proper but not in the placenta or is present at an exceedingly low proportion of the placental cells. cffDNA in maternal plasma is mainly placental DNA, and this discrepancy between aneuploidy in the placenta and the fetus may result in false-negative test results.

POINTS TO REMEMBER

Reasons for Discordant cffDNA Results

- False-negative results due to low fetal fraction, mosaicism, and absence of the abnormality in the placenta
- False-positive results due to statistical reasons, confined placental mosaicism, and maternal DNA abnormalities
- Incidental findings could be due to occult maternal malignancy or diseases with plasma DNA abnormalities, such as systemic lupus erythematosus.

False-positivity can be statistical. For example, the chromosome 21 DNA amount is considered elevated when it is 3 S.D. above that of a control population. However, 0.01% of the control population falls beyond 3 S.D. in a one-tailed normal distribution. Therefore the choice of a cutoff value for aneuploidy detection influences the theoretical false-positive rate of the test. A relatively common biological reason for "false-positive" results is confined placental mosaicism.[51] Confined placental mosaicism refers to chromosomal aneuploidy in the placenta but not the fetus proper; one report showed that placental mosaicism occurred in 2% of cases by chorionic villus sampling.[67] Because cffDNA is placental DNA, placental mosaicism may cause false-positive test results reflecting the state of the placenta, not the fetus. In fact, only 13% of mosaic chorionic villus abnormalities are detected in amniocytes.[67] Finally, another reason for "false-positive" fetal aneuploidy detection relates to aneuploidies of the mother. This is especially the case for subclinical mosaic sex chromosome aneuploidies. It has been reported that 8.6% of the sex chromosome aneuploidies detected by cffDNA testing occur when the maternal blood cell DNA showed the same finding.[68] This most commonly occurs with monosomy X (45, X0) and triple X (47, XXX). Consequently, some centers offer reflex confirmatory testing for maternal DNA when the cffDNA test suggests the presence of sex chromosome aneuploidy.[68]

Other non-pregnancy-related diseases may confound the use of cffDNA testing. For example, malignant tumors release cell-free DNA(see Chapter 52).[69] Occult malignancies have been suspected in pregnant women after cffDNA testing.[70] The suspicion arises when multiple chromosomal aneuploidies are detected in the same sample, or the cell-free DNA chromosomal copy number aberration shows a magnitude that is substantially larger than that expected for the measured fetal fraction. Other conditions, such as systemic lupus erythematosus, are also associated with abnormalities in the cell-free DNA profile.[71] If these abnormalities preexist in the plasma of a woman, the cffDNA test interpretation may become more challenging during pregnancy.

In summary, cffDNA results for chromosomal aneuploidy screening may, in rare instances, be inaccurate. Positive results require confirmation by definitive invasive testing. The obstetric history, other obstetric findings, and ultrasound features should be taken into account for the interpretation of the cffDNA tests.

Single-Gene Diseases

Besides fetal chromosomal aneuploidies, many prenatal programs address the screening and diagnosis of single-gene diseases, such as cystic fibrosis, sickle cell anemia, and thalassemias. Noninvasive prenatal diagnosis of autosomal dominant diseases of paternal origin may be achieved in a similar manner to fetal rhesus D genotyping. For example, when a paternal mutation is detected in the plasma of a mother known not to share the same mutation as the father, this may imply that the fetus has inherited the paternal mutation.[72] Maternally inherited mutations, on the other hand, are more challenging to diagnose by cffDNA analysis because cffDNA is surrounded by maternal DNA molecules that harbor the mutation. In view of the maternal DNA interference, the fetal inheritance of the maternal mutation can be assessed by quantifying the ratio between the mutant and the normal alleles in the sample—namely, the relative mutation dosage approach (Fig. 53.3).[73] For example, for a person with a heterozygous mutation, there should be equal amounts of mutant and normal alleles among the cell-free DNA molecules. When the person is pregnant with a heterozygous fetus, the relative amounts between the mutant and normal alleles remain equal. If the fetus has not inherited the maternal mutation and is homozygous for the normal allele, there should be a slight overrepresentation in the normal allele compared with the mutant allele. Finally, if the fetus is homozygous for the mutation (maternal mutation and the same mutation from the father), there would be a slight overrepresentation of the mutant allele when compared with the normal allele. On the other hand, to detect compound heterozygous mutations, a combination approach could be used (ie, direct detection of the paternal mutation combined with the allelic ratio assessment for the maternal mutation in maternal plasma) (see Fig. 53.3).

Protocols that are based on digital PCR[73] or sequencing have been developed for quantifying amounts of the maternal mutant allele and normal allele in maternal plasma. Digital PCR protocols for the noninvasive assessment of beta-thalassemia, hemophilia, and sickle cell disease exist.[73-75] Sequencing-based protocols, such as those for beta-thalassemia[76] and congenital adrenal hyperplasia,[77] use targeted capture of the disease locus. To render the protocols even more cost effective, haplotype-based analyses have been developed, termed *relative haplotype dosage analysis* (RHDO).[38,76,77] In the RHDO method, haplotypes of the mutant and normal alleles are known. During interpretation of the maternal plasma DNA sequencing results, the number of DNA molecules detected that cover SNP alleles belonging to the inheritance block that contains the mutation are counted. The counts from each consecutive informative SNP allele are combined. The same analysis is performed for the homologous allele that does not contain the mutation. The total number of DNA molecules that originate from the haplotype block of the allele containing the mutation are compared with the count for the haplotype block of the allele not containing the mutation. Based on a statistical comparison, an interpretation is made regarding which haplotype block the fetus has likely inherited—namely, the mutant or the normal allele.[38,77] It is envisioned that in the future, targeted sequence analysis covering genomic loci of clinical importance may be the approach of choice to deliver noninvasive prenatal diagnosis of single-gene diseases. To realize this, more convenient methods to generate long-range haplotype information are needed.

NONINVASIVE FETAL 'OMICS

Many advances have occurred in cffDNA analysis. Massively parallel sequencing[38] has enabled an approach to determine the fetal genome noninvasively. Studies have demonstrated that the entire fetal genome is represented in maternal plasma. The fetal genome assembly requires information regarding the paternal genotypes as well as the maternal haplotypes across the genome. Paternal-specific alleles as well as overrepresented maternal haplotype segments that are detected in maternal plasma form the basis for assembling the paternal and maternal portions of the fetal genome. Therefore fetal genotype determination for any disease loci is theoretically possible.

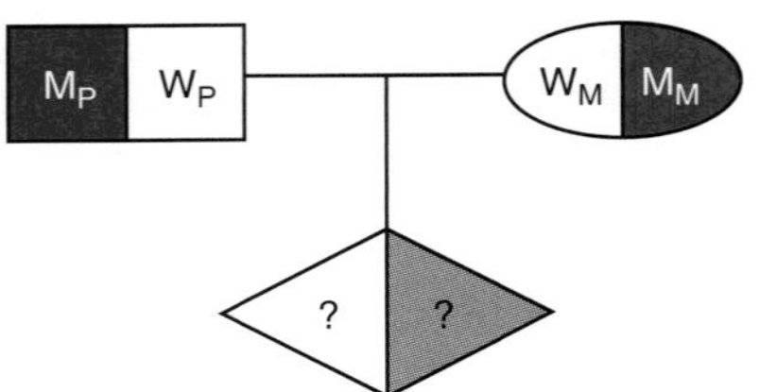

Condition	Approach
Autosomal dominant traits or mutations	
Paternally inherited	Qualitative detection of M_P
Maternally inherited	Quantitative comparison between M_M and W. **If M_M = W, fetus has inherited M_M.** If M_M <W, fetus has not inherited M_M.
Autosomal recessive conditions or diseases	
When M_P and M_M are identical	Quantitative comparison between M and W. If M = W, fetus is heterozygous. If M >W, fetus is homozygous for the mutation. If M <W, fetus has not inherited the mutation.
When M_P and M_M are different	Assess which paternal allele has been transmitted to the fetus by qualitative detection of M_P or W_P by a polymorphism that distinguishes W_P from M_P, M_M, and W_M. Assess which maternal allele has been transmitted to the fetus by quantitative comparison between M_M and W. If M_M = W, fetus has inherited M_M. If M_M <W, fetus has not inherited M_M.

FIGURE 53.3 Approaches to noninvasive prenatal diagnosis of monogenic diseases by maternal plasma DNA analysis. *M,* Mutant allele; *W,* wild-type allele; *M_P,* paternally inherited mutant allele; *W_P,* paternally inherited wild-type allele; *M_M,* maternally inherited mutant allele; *W_M,* maternally inherited wild-type allele.

Besides the fetal genome, the transcriptome[78] and the DNA methylome of the placenta[35] may be determined directly from maternal plasma analysis. These developments are particularly important because they offer the means to monitor placental function. Placental dysfunction occurs or is suspected to occur in some pregnancy-associated diseases, such as preeclampsia, preterm labor, and intrauterine growth retardation. The ability to noninvasively monitor the health of the placenta by molecular means, which was previously not possible, means that the utility of maternal plasma cell-free nucleic acid analysis could be extended beyond the assessment of fetal genetic and chromosomal diseases.

ANALYTICAL ASPECTS

Cell-free nucleic acids exist in plasma in the form of short fragments and are present in low abundance. In addition, the key to successful analysis of cffDNA lies in the preservation and maximization of the fetal fraction in the maternal blood sample. Thus attention to a number of preanalytical and analytical details, as outlined below, is important to ensure the quality of the analysis.

Maternal Blood Sample Collection and Processing

One advantage of cffDNA analysis for prenatal screening is that, unlike maternal serum biochemistry testing, the use of the cffDNA tests is not restricted to a specific gestational period. This is because the cffDNA tests target the detection of the core pathologies of the fetus—for example, inherited mutations or chromosomal aneuploidies. These pathologies exist throughout the pregnancy. However, during the earliest stage of pregnancy, there may not be a sufficient amount of fetal DNA in the maternal circulation. While cffDNA has been detected in maternal plasma in individual pregnant women from as early as 18 days of pregnancy,[79] they become quantitatively sufficient for most testing purposes from about the 11th week of pregnancy. Between 9 to 13 weeks of gestation, 2% of pregnancies show fetal DNA fractions that are below 5% and are prone to potential false-negativity.[47] Therefore some cffDNA testing programs specify the minimum gestational age for samples that are acceptable.[80]

As will be discussed, maximizing the fetal DNA fraction in the maternal sample is a key factor to many cffDNA tests. With such a consideration, maternal plasma is preferred over maternal serum. Clotting of the maternal blood cells results in the release of more maternal DNA into serum as compared to plasma.[29] While the absolute fetal DNA amounts in plasma and serum are similar, the fetal DNA fraction is significantly reduced in serum. Even for plasma, different anticoagulants show varying degrees of efficacy in suppressing the rise in maternal background DNA over time. EDTA is more effective than heparin and citrate in maintaining a relatively stable total plasma DNA concentration and fetal DNA fraction up to about 24 hours after phlebotomy.[81] Some companies now manufacture blood collection tubes containing proprietary cell-stabilizing reagents that are effective in maintaining the plasma DNA concentration and fetal fraction for up to 14 days.[82] The availability of these tubes has helped to facilitate the shipping of maternal blood samples across long distances for cffDNA testing.

After the maternal peripheral blood samples are collected, plasma is harvested via centrifugation. The goal of centrifugation is to minimize the residual maternal blood cells in the sample. Furthermore, it is not recommended to use hemolyzed samples for cffDNA analysis. Reduction in maternal DNA contamination results in maximization of the fetal fraction. Therefore two-step centrifugation protocols are recommended.[83] The plasma supernatant is carefully harvested after the first centrifugation with care not to disturb the underlying maternal blood cell layer. With the second centrifugation, the remaining cells in the form of a cell pellet are separated from the final supernatant. The resultant plasma can be stored frozen until further analysis.

Circulating Cell-Free Fetal DNA Analysis

A significant amount of cffDNA has a length shorter than 100 bp.[38] For plasma DNA extraction, a protocol that is efficient in preserving the small DNA molecules is advantageous.[84] For the same reason, PCR assays intended for cffDNA or placental RNA detection should be designed to amplify shorter products, preferably less than 100 bp.[30,85,86] The fact that circulating fetal DNA molecules are generally shorter than maternal DNA can be used to enhance the detection of fetal DNA. Researchers have used size-selection methods to increase the proportional representation of short DNA within the sample or dataset to improve the detection of fetal DNA.[73,87,88] In addition, the detection of short DNA from maternal plasma can be used to detect fetal disorders.[89] The rationale is that when the fetus has an aneuploidy, such as trisomy 21, there should be an additional dose of short DNA from chromosome 21. Therefore the overall size profile of the chromosome 21 DNA molecules would be shorter than that of other nonaneuploid chromosomes. If the fetus has monosomy X, it is then expected that there would be less short DNA from chromosome X, and thus the overall size profile of chromosome X would be longer than the other nonaneuploid chromosomes.

Besides the need for maximizing the fetal DNA fraction, there are circumstances where it may be advantageous to employ measures to minimize the maternal DNA interference. Unless the fetal DNA sequence of interest is absent in the maternal genome—for example, chromosome Y or *RHD* in rhesus-negative women—the need to minimize the background maternal DNA interference is particularly relevant when one aims to directly detect a fetal-specific sequence in maternal plasma. For example, for the detection of fetal-specific point mutations in maternal plasma, the large background of wild-type DNA often results in nonspecificity of the assay.[90] Researchers have used a number of different approaches to minimize background maternal DNA. Minisequencing or primer extension assays have been designed that only allow the extension of the fetal DNA sequence but not the maternal DNA sequence.[90] Peptide nucleic acid clamping has been used to suppress the maternal DNA from interacting with the detection reagents of the fetal-specific assay.[91] Restriction enzyme cutting has been used to remove the maternal DNA sequence from the sample.[92] Single-molecule or digital PCR is conducted when the average amount of template DNA per reaction well is less than one molecule. Therefore the fetal DNA sequence is separated from the maternal counterpart sequence in the reaction environment and therefore is less prone to nonspecific amplification of the maternal DNA sequence.[73]

Measuring the Fetal DNA Fraction

Analysis of the fetal DNA fraction is an important quality control parameter for cffDNA analysis. For assays that aim to detect the presence of a fetal-specific DNA sequence, such as the presence of chromosome Y sequences for determining male fetal sex and the presence of *RHD* to determine a rhesus D positive fetus, the inclusion of an internal fetal DNA control is preferable. The internal fetal DNA control is particularly useful when the assay reveals that the target sequence is negative. For example, when the chromosome Y assay shows negative results, it may either mean the presence of the female fetus or the lack of fetal DNA in the sample. When the *RHD* assay is negative, it may mean the fetus is rhesus D negative or the sample lacked fetal DNA. The positive detection of an internal fetal DNA control in such situations would exclude the scenario of lack of fetal DNA. Thus the report for the female fetus or rhesus D negative fetus could be issued with confidence.

There are several different methods for detecting the presence of fetal DNA. Some laboratories detect the fetal chromosome Y sequence as the indicator of the presence of fetal DNA, in the case of male fetuses. Some laboratories include the analysis of a panel of polymorphisms with the target sequence analysis. The panel aims to detect alleles that are not present in the maternal DNA or that show a minor contribution as an indicator of the presence of fetal DNA in the sample. Another approach is to detect placental-specific methylation signatures in maternal plasma. These are gene loci where the methylation status is opposite in the placenta as compared to the maternal blood cells. Assays specific for the detection of the placental form of the gene are used for maternal plasma analysis. The assay is designed to only detect the placental and not the maternal form of the DNA sequences. For example, the *RASSF1A* gene was shown to be hypermethylated in the placenta and not the maternal blood cells.[92] The presence of the methylated form of *RASSF1A* in maternal plasma suggests the presence of fetal/placental DNA.

There are a number of cffDNA tests where ensuring the presence of a minimum amount of fetal DNA in the sample—namely, the fetal DNA fraction—is an important quality control parameter.[65] For example, the noninvasive detection of fetal chromosomal aneuploidies by maternal plasma DNA sequencing and the assessment of the fetal inheritance of the maternal allele by relative mutation dosage or relative haplotype dosage all rely on the sample containing a certain minimum amount of fetal DNA.[65,73,77] The statistics developed to determine the presence or absence of a statistically significant difference in chromosome dosage or allelic ratio is dependent on the sample containing at least a certain amount of fetal DNA. Therefore for the tests based on massively parallel sequencing, the proportion of chromosome Y sequences is often used as a fetal fraction measurement for chromosome Y–positive samples.[61] A panel of placenta-specific DNA methylation markers has also been developed to quantify the fetal DNA.[93] Recently, the proportion of short DNA in a sample has also been shown as a reasonable measure of the fetal DNA fraction.[89]

Massively Parallel Maternal Plasma DNA Sequencing

The advantage of massively parallel sequencing–based cffDNA assessment is that many maternal plasma DNA molecules can be analyzed per sample, regardless of whether the DNA fragment is originating from the fetus or the mother. For quantitative sequencing applications, such as for fetal chromosomal aneuploidy detection or relative haplotype dosage analysis, the key to success is to maximize the signal-to-noise ratio of the sequencing data covering the genetic abnormality of interest. Trying to maximize the fetal fraction improves the chance of detecting the fetal abnormality.[65] Increasing the sequencing depth either for random or targeted sequencing improves the precision, and thus reduces the noise, for genomic representation or allelic ratio assessments.[47] The size of the genomic locus of interest also matters. At the same sequencing depth, larger loci, such as whole chromosome aneuploidies, are much easier to detect than subchromosomal aneuploidies.[45,46] Thus protocols for the detection of subchromosomal aneuploidies require higher sequencing depths. The current massively parallel sequencing protocols also suffer from a certain extent of GC bias. To reduce the imprecision surrounding the quantitative measurement of cffDNA by sequencing, GC normalization steps are typically included in the bioinformatics analysis of the data. This is especially important for the detection of aneuploidies in GC-rich chromosomes, such as chromosomes 13 and 18.

On the other hand, current massively parallel sequencing protocols have a sequencing error rate that cannot be ignored. This has an impact on the detection of single-nucleotide variants of the fetus, such as point mutations, polymorphic alleles, and de novo mutations. Because cffDNA is the minor species of DNA in maternal plasma, high-depth sequencing is needed to detect fetal single-nucleotide variants. Yet, the higher the total number of bases sequenced, the higher the chance for sequencing errors.[94] Thus extra care is needed in designing protocols for the detection of fetal single-nucleotide variants by sequencing. For example, targeted capture of loci of interest followed by sequencing is one feasible option. Targeted sequencing allows a high depth to be achieved without sequencing a high total number of bases, thereby reducing the number of sequencing errors detected and improving the signal-to-noise ratio.

CONCLUSION

Cell-free nucleic acids in the maternal circulation are a reliable and noninvasive source of fetal genetic material. Knowledge about their biological properties has translated into useful information for guiding the design of the preanalytical and analytical approaches relevant for cffDNA analysis. cffDNA analysis is useful for the prenatal assessment of fetal chromosomal aneuploidies and genetic diseases. Its effectiveness in some of these areas has led to a major reduction in the number of amniocenteses performed worldwide, causing a paradigm shift in prenatal diagnosis. cffDNA analysis has the potential to detail the entire fetal genome noninvasively before the birth of the child. Nonetheless, the vast amount of information that one may be able to access before the birth of the child has raised some potential concerns and spurred research interests in studying the ethical, legal, and social implications of such technologies.[95] It remains to be seen how noninvasive prenatal diagnostics will continue to develop and how it will contribute to improving and maintaining fetal and maternal health.

POINTS TO REMEMBER

Analytical Factors to Be Mindful of

- EDTA plasma is preferred over serum.
- When delayed blood processing is expected, collection of blood into tubes containing cell-stabilizing agents is recommended.
- Avoid hemolysis.
- Harvest the plasma using protocols to remove as much of the maternal blood cells as possible.
- Use protocols that preserve the short cell-free DNA molecules.
- Design assays to maximize the chance of detecting the short cffDNA molecules.
- Consider approaches to further minimize the effect of the maternal DNA interference.
- Include an internal control to indicate the presence of fetal DNA or measure the fetal DNA fraction.
- Maximize the signal-to-noise ratio of the massively parallel sequencing protocols used for cffDNA analysis.

SELECTED REFERENCES

For a full list of references for this chapter, please refer to ExpertConsult.com.

28. Lo YMD, Corbetta N, Chamberlain PF, et al. Presence of fetal DNA in maternal plasma and serum. *Lancet* 1997;**350**: 485–7.
29. Lo YMD, Tein MS, Lau TK, et al. Quantitative analysis of fetal DNA in maternal plasma and serum: implications for noninvasive prenatal diagnosis. *Am J Hum Genet* 1998;**62**: 768–75.
33. Yu SCY, Lee SW, Jiang P, et al. High-resolution profiling of fetal DNA clearance from maternal plasma by massively parallel sequencing. *Clin Chem* 2013;**59**:1228–37.
36. Masuzaki H, Miura K, Yoshiura KI, et al. Detection of cell free placental DNA in maternal plasma: direct evidence from three cases of confined placental mosaicism. *J Med Genet* 2004;**41**:289–92.
38. Lo YMD, Chan KCA, Sun H, et al. Maternal plasma DNA sequencing reveals the genome-wide genetic and mutational profile of the fetus. *Sci Transl Med* 2010;**2**:61ra91.
39. Lo YMD, Hjelm NM, Fidler C, et al. Prenatal diagnosis of fetal RhD status by molecular analysis of maternal plasma. *N Engl J Med* 1998;**339**:1734–8.
42. Chiu RWK, Chan KCA, Gao Y, et al. Noninvasive prenatal diagnosis of fetal chromosomal aneuploidy by massively parallel genomic sequencing of DNA in maternal plasma. *Proc Natl Acad Sci USA* 2008;**105**:20458–63.

43. Chen EZ, Chiu RWK, Sun H, et al. Noninvasive prenatal diagnosis of fetal trisomy 18 and trisomy 13 by maternal plasma DNA sequencing. *PLoS ONE* 2011;**6**:e21791.
45. Srinivasan A, Bianchi DW, Huang H, et al. Noninvasive detection of fetal subchromosome abnormalities via deep sequencing of maternal plasma. *Am J Hum Genet* 2013;**92**: 167–76.
47. Chiu RWK, Akolekar R, Zheng YW, et al. Non-invasive prenatal assessment of trisomy 21 by multiplexed maternal plasma DNA sequencing: large scale validity study. *BMJ* 2011;**342**:c7401.
48. Sparks AB, Struble CA, Wang ET, et al. Noninvasive prenatal detection and selective analysis of cell-free DNA obtained from maternal blood: evaluation for trisomy 21 and trisomy 18. *Am J Obstet Gynecol* 2012;**206**:319 e1–9.
49. Zimmermann B, Hill M, Gemelos G, et al. Noninvasive prenatal aneuploidy testing of chromosomes 13, 18, 21, x, and y, using targeted sequencing of polymorphic loci. *Prenat Diagn* 2012;**32**:1233–41.
50. Chandrasekharan S, Minear MA, Hung A, et al. Noninvasive prenatal testing goes global. *Sci Transl Med* 2014;**6**:231fs15.
52. Dondorp W, de Wert G, Bombard Y, et al. Non-invasive prenatal testing for aneuploidy and beyond: challenges of responsible innovation in prenatal screening. *Eur J Hum Genet* 2015;doi:10.1038/ejhg.2015.57.
56. Larion S, Warsof SL, Romary L, et al. Association of combined first-trimester screen and noninvasive prenatal testing on diagnostic procedures. *Obstet Gynecol* 2014;**123**: 1303–10.
57. Robson SJ, Hui L. National decline in invasive prenatal diagnostic procedures in association with uptake of combined first trimester and cell-free DNA aneuploidy screening. *Aust N Z J Obstet Gynaecol* 2015;**55**:507–10.
61. Hudecova I, Sahota D, Heung MMS, et al. Maternal plasma fetal DNA fractions in pregnancies with low and high risks for fetal chromosomal aneuploidies. *PLoS ONE* 2014;**9**: e88484.
62. Bianchi DW, Parker RL, Wentworth J, et al. DNA sequencing versus standard prenatal aneuploidy screening. *N Engl J Med* 2014;**370**:799–808.
65. Canick JA, Palomaki GE, Kloza EM, et al. The impact of maternal plasma DNA fetal fraction on next generation sequencing tests for common fetal aneuploidies. *Prenat Diagn* 2013;**33**:667–74.
70. Bianchi DW, Chudova D, Sehnert AJ, et al. Noninvasive prenatal testing and incidental detection of occult maternal malignancies. *JAMA* 2015;**314**:162–9.
77. New MI, Tong YK, Yuen T, et al. Noninvasive prenatal diagnosis of congenital adrenal hyperplasia using cell-free fetal DNA in maternal plasma. *J Clin Endocrinol Metab* 2014;**99**:E1022–30.
83. Chiu RWK, Poon LLM, Lau TK, et al. Effects of blood-processing protocols on fetal and total DNA quantification in maternal plasma. *Clin Chem* 2001;**47**: 1607–13.
95. Greely HT. Get ready for the flood of fetal gene screening. *Nature* 2011;**469**:289–91.

54

Pharmacogenetics

Gwendolyn A. McMillin, Mia Wadelius, and Victoria M. Pratt

ABSTRACT

Background

Pharmacogenetics describes how genes influence drug response. Genes can impact either the pharmacokinetics or pharmacodynamics of a drug to influence the dose required and associated therapeutic or toxic effects. Pharmacogenetic testing performed before drug administration may guide the selection of drugs and drug dosing. Posttherapeutic pharmacogenetic testing can explain an adverse drug reaction, including therapeutic failure.

Content

This chapter reviews pharmacokinetics and pharmacodynamics, the two major processes involved in drug response, and describes how genes that encode for proteins involved in these processes influence drug response. Important nongenetic factors that influence drug response, such as drug formulation differences, drug–drug and food–drug interactions, and clinical status are discussed, along with appropriate specimens and analytical strategies for performing, reporting, and interpreting pharmacogenetic testing results. In addition, specific gene–drug examples are described in detail relative to the nomenclature of genetic variants and allele assignments, genotype-phenotype predictions, clinical applications, and associated guidance for dosing. Specific examples include *ABCB1, CFTR, CYP2C9, CYP2C19, CYP2D6, CYP3A4/5, DPYD, G6PD, HLA-B, NATs, SLCO1B1, TPMT, UGT1A1,* and *VKORC1.*

55

Identity Testing

Victor W. Weedn, Katherine B. Gettings, and Daniele S. Podini

ABSTRACT

Background

DNA has sufficient variation among individuals to discriminate all individuals who have ever lived on the earth or will in the foreseeable future. Furthermore, DNA persists as an identification taggant over the lifetime of the individual and can be obtained from all tissues and fluids—even trace amounts. Accordingly, DNA identity testing has become routine in forensic laboratories around the world. This genetic testing is also useful for parentage and kinship relationship testing as well as certain other clinical applications.

Content

This chapter describes the technologies and methods used in forensic science, parentage, and clinical laboratories for individual identification and genetic relationship testing. Virtually all such testing is based upon capillary electrophoresis (CE) with laser induced fluorescence instrumental analysis following sample collection, DNA extraction, quantification, and polymerase chain reaction (PCR) amplification. Short tandem repeat (STR) testing, using the Federal Bureau of Investigation's (FBI's) combined DNA index system (CODIS) loci, has become routine throughout the United States. An expanded set of 20 STRs will soon replace the original 13 loci. Y-STR analysis, mitochondrial DNA sequencing, and single nucleotide polymorphisms (SNP) tests are important ancillary tests. Massively parallel sequencing and rapid DNA testing will offer new technologic capabilities. Forensic testing must comply with chain-of-custody and other rigorous standards and must be capable of withstanding courtroom scrutiny. The same identity tests are useful for parentage testing, as well as in other clinical applications, such as sample verification, prenatal validation testing, bone marrow transplantation, and loss of heterozygosity (LOH) tumor testing.

SECTION V

Pathophysiology

Exam questions, case studies, and additional resources are available on ExpertConsult.com.
*Full versions of these chapters are available electronically on ExpertConsult.com.

56

Nutrition: Laboratory and Clinical Aspects

William J. Marshall and Ruth M. Ayling

ABSTRACT

Background

Nutrition is relevant to every specialty within overall medical practice. Adequate nutrition, both qualitatively and quantitatively, is essential for normal development, growth, function, and health. Both excessive and insufficient intake of individual nutrients can have adverse consequences. Also, patients with many pathological conditions who have free access to a good diet may benefit from nutritional supplementation or restriction.

Content

This chapter describes all the dietary components that are considered essential to human life, their sources and function, and the consequences of under- or oversupply. It discusses screening methods for malnutrition and the detailed assessment of nutritional status, emphasizing that none of the available techniques for the latter is on its own ideal and that clinical observation remains of paramount importance. The indications for and techniques of nutritional support are described in detail, with particular emphasis on the role of laboratory investigations in assessing its safety and efficacy. The neuroendocrine mechanisms of appetite control are discussed in detail as a preliminary to a discussion of the causes, consequences and management of obesity, arguably the most important nutritional disorder of our age in developed (and increasingly developing) countries. The metabolic consequences of anorexia and bulimia nervosa are described, and reference is made to the many conditions in which nutritional manipulation may benefit conditions not primarily of nutritional origin, ranging from kidney and liver disease to inherited metabolic diseases, many of which are discussed in detail elsewhere in this book.

57

Diabetes Mellitus

David B. Sacks

ABSTRACT

Background

Diabetes mellitus is a common disorder in which patients develop hyperglycemia due to inadequate insulin secretion, defective insulin action, or both. The two major forms of diabetes are type 1 and type 2. The estimated global prevalence of diabetes is approximately 380 million. Many patients with diabetes develop severe debilitating complications, including blindness, renal failure, myocardial infarction peripheral vascular disease, and stroke.

Content

The pathophysiology of the different forms of diabetes is addressed. Hormones that regulate blood glucose concentrations include insulin and the counterregulatory hormones glucagon, epinephrine, and cortisol. Insulin synthesis, mechanism of action, and promotion of glucose uptake into fat and muscle are described. Several analytes that are measured in patients with diabetes are discussed in detail. These include glucose (both in central laboratories and with handheld meters), glycated proteins (such as hemoglobin A1c, fructosamine, and glycated albumin), islet autoantibodies, and urinary albumin. The clinical indications, analytical methods, and sample handling are covered. The vital role played by clinical laboratories in the diagnosis and management of patients with diabetes is emphasized.

Diabetes mellitus is a group of metabolic disorders characterized by hyperglycemia resulting from defects in insulin secretion, insulin action, or both.[1] Some patients may experience acute life-threatening hyperglycemic episodes, such as ketoacidosis or hyperosmolar coma. Acute life-threatening hypoglycemic episodes may occur as a result of therapy. As the disease progresses, patients are at increased risk for the development of specific complications, including *retinopathy* leading to blindness, *nephropathy* leading to renal failure, and *neuropathy* (nerve damage), collectively known as microvascular complications, as well as *atherosclerosis,* which is considered a *macrovascular complication.*[2,3] The last may result in stroke, gangrene, or coronary artery disease.

Diabetes is a common disease, although the exact prevalence is unknown. The number of people with diabetes has increased dramatically worldwide. It was estimated in 2014 that approximately 380 million people have diabetes, and by 2035, this number is predicted to reach 592 million, 80% of whom will live in low- and middle-income countries.[4] In the United States, the prevalence from 1999 to 2002 was 9.3%, 30% of whom were undiagnosed.[5] Analysis of the 2005–2006 National Health and Nutritional Examination Survey (NHANES) using both fasting glucose and oral glucose tolerance testing (OGTT) shows a prevalence of diabetes in the United States in persons 20 years of age and older of 12.9% (equivalent to ≈40 million people).[6] Similarly, the prevalence of diabetes in Asian populations has increased rapidly in recent decades,[7] with China and India ranked first and second, respectively, among countries with the largest diabetic populations. Recent analysis in Chinese adults suggests that in 2010 the estimated prevalence of diabetes and prediabetes was 11.6% and 50.1%, respectively, which is equivalent to 113.9 million persons with diabetes and 493.4 million with prediabetes.[8] The prevalence varies widely among countries, reaching as high as 25% in the Middle East and 35% in the Western Pacific. Information about individual countries—for example, number of patients, prevalence, and deaths—is compiled by the International Diabetes Federation (IDF; http://www.idf.org/sites/default/files/Atlas-poster-2014_EN.pdf). These statistics led to a description of diabetes as "one of the main threats to human health in the twenty-first century."[9] It is estimated that approximately 50% of individuals with diabetes worldwide remain undiagnosed.[4] The prevalence of undiagnosed diabetes in the United States has remained fairly stable; thus the proportion of total diabetes cases that are undiagnosed was reduced to 11% during 2006–2010.[10] The prevalence of diabetes mellitus increases with age, and approximately half of all cases occur in people older than 55 years. In the United States, more than 20% of the population older than 65 years has diabetes.[11] A racial predilection has been noted, and by the age of 65, 33%, 25%, and 17% of Hispanics, blacks, and whites, respectively, in the United States will have diabetes. In 2012, diabetes mellitus was estimated to be responsible for $245 billion in health care expenditures in the United States.[12] The direct costs were $176 billion, with 59% of that total incurred by those 65 years and older. The estimated economic burden of undiagnosed diabetes, prediabetes, and gestational diabetes mellitus in 2012 was $78 billion, producing a total economic burden of over $322 billion.[13] Worldwide diabetes caused at least $612 billion in health expenditures and an estimated 4.9 million deaths in 2014.[4] Acute and chronic complications make diabetes the fourth most common cause of death in the developed world.

CLASSIFICATION

Historical

Diabetes was initially diagnosed by the OGTT. Values greater than two standard deviations above the mean of the value found in a selected population of healthy volunteers without a family history of diabetes mellitus were accepted as diagnostic. This criterion led to the identification of large numbers of asymptomatic people with abnormally high 1- to 2-hour postload glucose values but normal fasting blood glucose. They were presumed to have early or mild diabetes mellitus. In 1975, it was estimated that more than half the population older than 60 years was abnormal. Follow-up of these individuals indicated that most of them with lesser degrees of glucose intolerance did not manifest definite evidence of diabetes mellitus in the next 10 years, and a large percentage returned to normal glucose tolerance.

Most populations have plasma glucose values that exhibit a unimodal, log-normal distribution (a distribution curve that is skewed to the high end but becomes bell shaped on a logarithmic axis). Ethnic groups with a high prevalence of diabetes, such as the Pima Indians and Nauruans, exhibit bimodal blood glucose distributions.[14] Optimal distinction between normal and diabetic individuals in these groups occurs at a fasting glucose around 140 mg/dL (7.8 mmol/L) and glucose concentrations greater than 200 mg/dL (11.1 mmol/L) 2 hours after an oral glucose load. Furthermore, the specific microvascular complications of diabetes were believed to be rare in patients with fasting or 2-hour postprandial plasma glucose concentrations less than 140 or 200 mg/dL (7.8 or 11.1 mmol/L), respectively. These observations formed the basis for the criteria proposed in 1979 by a workgroup of the National Diabetes Data Group[15] and later endorsed by the World Health Organization (WHO) Committee on Diabetes.[16] Lower diagnostic values are used currently.

The 1979 classification scheme recognized two major forms of diabetes: type 1 (insulin-dependent) diabetes mellitus (IDDM) and type 2 (non-insulin-dependent) diabetes mellitus (NIDDM).[15] The terms *juvenile-onset* and *adult-onset diabetes* were abolished. To base the classification on cause rather than on treatment, the American Diabetes Association (ADA) established a workgroup in 1995 to reexamine the classification and diagnosis of diabetes mellitus. The revised classification, published in 1997[1] eliminates the terms *insulin-dependent diabetes mellitus* and *non-insulin-dependent diabetes mellitus,* which now are termed *type 1* and *type 2 diabetes,* respectively (Box 57.1). Furthermore, the categories of previous abnormality of glucose tolerance and potential abnormality of glucose tolerance have been eliminated.

Type 1 Diabetes Mellitus

Approximately 5% to 10% of all cases of diabetes mellitus are included in this category.[17] Patients usually have abrupt onset of symptoms (eg, polyuria, polydipsia, rapid weight loss). They have insulinopenia (a deficiency of insulin) caused by destruction of pancreatic islet β-cells and are dependent on insulin to sustain life and prevent ketosis. Most patients have antibodies that identify an autoimmune process (see later discussion); some have no evidence of autoimmunity and are classified as type 1 idiopathic. The peak incidence occurs in childhood and adolescence. Approximately 75% acquire the disease before the age of 18, but onset in the remainder may occur at any age. Age at presentation is not a criterion for classification.

BOX 57.1 Classification of Diabetes Mellitus

I. Type 1 diabetes
   A. Immune mediated
   B. Idiopathic
II. Type 2 diabetes
III. Other specific types
   A. Genetic defects of β-cell function
   B. Genetic defects in insulin action
   C. Diseases of the exocrine pancreas
   D. Endocrinopathies
   E. Drug or chemical induced
   F. Infections
   G. Uncommon forms of immune-mediated diabetes
   H. Other genetic syndromes sometimes associated with diabetes
IV. Gestational diabetes mellitus

From the American Diabetes Association. Diagnosis and classification of diabetes mellitus. *Diabetes Care* 2014;37(Suppl 1):S81–90.

Type 2 Diabetes Mellitus

This group accounts for approximately 90% of all cases of diabetes.[17] Patients have minimal symptoms, are not prone to ketosis, and are not dependent on insulin to prevent ketonuria. Insulin concentrations may be normal, decreased, or increased, and most people with this form of diabetes have impaired insulin action. Obesity is commonly associated, and weight loss alone usually improves hyperglycemia in these persons. However, many individuals with type 2 diabetes may require dietary intervention, oral antihyperglycemic agents, or insulin to control hyperglycemia. Most patients acquire the disease after age 40, but it may occur in younger people. Type 2 diabetes in children and adolescents is an emerging, significant problem.[9,18,19] Among children in Japan, type 2 diabetes is now more common than type 1.[9]

Specific Types of Diabetes Mellitus Due to Other Causes

This subclass includes uncommon patients in whom hyperglycemia is due to a specific underlying disorder, such as genetic defects of β-cell function; genetic defects in insulin action; diseases of the exocrine pancreas (eg, cystic fibrosis); endocrinopathies (eg, Cushing syndrome, acromegaly, glucagonoma); administration of hormones or drugs known to induce β-cell dysfunction (eg, Dilantin, pentamidine) or to impair insulin action (eg, glucocorticoids, thiazides, β-adrenergics); infection; uncommon forms of immune-mediated diabetes; or other genetic conditions (eg, Down syndrome, Klinefelter syndrome, porphyria; see reference 20 for a detailed list) (see Box 57.1). This was formerly termed *secondary diabetes.* (Additional details can be found in reference 21.)

Gestational Diabetes Mellitus

This is defined as any degree of glucose intolerance (ie, hyperglycemia) with onset or first recognition during pregnancy (ie, diabetic women who become pregnant are not included in this category).[22] Estimates of the frequency of abnormal glucose tolerance during pregnancy range from less than 1% to 28%, depending on the population studied and the diagnostic tests employed.[23] In the United States, gestational diabetes mellitus (GDM) occurs in 6% to 8% of pregnancies (approximately 240,000 cases annually). The prevalence of GDM is increasing, at least in part, due to the considerable increase in obesity. Women with GDM are at significantly greater risk for the subsequent development of type 2 diabetes mellitus, which occurs in 15% to 60%.[24] The risk is particularly high in women who have marked hyperglycemia during or soon after pregnancy, women who are obese, and women whose GDM was diagnosed before 24 weeks' gestation.[25] At 6 to 12 weeks postpartum, all patients who had GDM should be evaluated for diabetes using nonpregnant OGTT criteria. If diabetes is not present, patients should be reevaluated for diabetes at least every 3 years.[26]

Categories of Increased Risk for Diabetes

People who have blood glucose concentrations above normal, but less than those required for a diagnosis of diabetes mellitus, have been recognized for many years. In 1979, this intermediate category was termed *impaired glucose tolerance* (IGT). It was defined as a 2-hour postload plasma glucose following an OGTT of 140 to 199 mg/dL (7.8–11.1 mmol/L).[15] An OGTT is required to assign a patient to this class. To avoid an OGTT, the category of impaired fasting glucose (IFG) was added in 1997 by the ADA[1] and by the WHO in 1999.[27] IFG is diagnosed by a fasting glucose value between those of normal and diabetic individuals—namely, between 100 and 125 mg/dL (5.6 and 6.9 mmol/L). (Note that the WHO and a number of other diabetes organizations define the cutoff for IFG at 110 mg/mL (6.1 mmol/L).[28] In 2009, hemoglobin A1c (HbA_{1c}) was added as a criterion to diagnose diabetes.[29] People with HbA_{1c} values below the cutoff for diabetes—that is, 6.5% (48 mmol/mol)—but above the reference interval are at high risk of developing diabetes.[17] For example, the incidence of diabetes in people with HbA_{1c} between 6.0% and less than 6.5% (42 and 48 mmol/mol) is more than 10 times that of people with lower concentrations. Prospective studies reveal a 5-year cumulative incidence of diabetes ranging from 12% to 25% (three- to eightfold higher than the general population) for people with HbA_{1c} of 5.5% to 6.0% (37–42 mmol/mol).[17]

Individuals with IFG and/or IGT and/or intermediate HbA_{1c} (5.7% to 6.4%; 39–46 mmol/mol) have been referred to as having "prediabetes" because they are at high risk for progressing to diabetes. Moreover, they are at increased risk for the development of cardiovascular disease.[30,31] Nevertheless, there is considerable controversy surrounding prediabetes.[32] For example, IFG, IGT, and HbA_{1c} do not always identify the same individuals.[29] There is also lack of agreement on the cutpoints for IFG and HbA_{1c}. This is due, in large part, to the continuous nature of the risk for the development of diabetes and the concentration of glucose or HbA_{1c}.[29]

HORMONES THAT REGULATE BLOOD GLUCOSE CONCENTRATION

During a brief fast, a precipitous decline in the concentration of blood glucose is prevented by breakdown of glycogen stored in the liver and synthesis of glucose in the liver. Some glucose is derived from gluconeogenesis in the kidneys.[33] These organs contain glucose-6-phosphatase, which is necessary to convert glucose 6-phosphate (derived from gluconeogenesis or glycogenolysis) to glucose. Skeletal muscle lacks this enzyme; muscle glycogen therefore cannot contribute directly to blood glucose. With more prolonged fasting (>42 hours), gluconeogenesis accounts for essentially all glucose production. In contrast, after a meal, the absorbed glucose is converted to glycogen (for storage in the liver and skeletal muscle) or fat (for storage in adipose tissue). Despite large fluctuations in the supply and demand of carbohydrates, the concentration of glucose in the blood is normally maintained within a fairly narrow range by hormones that modulate the movement of glucose into and out of the circulation. These include insulin, which decreases blood glucose, and the counterregulatory hormones (glucagon, epinephrine, cortisol, and growth hormone), which increase blood glucose concentrations (Fig. 57.1).[33] Normal glucose disposal depends on (1) the ability of the pancreas to secrete insulin, (2) the ability of insulin to promote uptake of glucose into peripheral tissue, and (3) the ability of insulin to suppress hepatic glucose production. The major insulin target organs are liver, skeletal muscle, and adipose tissue. These organs exhibit some differences in their responses to insulin. For example, the hormone stimulates glucose uptake through a specific glucose transporter—GLUT4—into muscle and fat cells but not into liver cells.

Insulin

Insulin is a protein hormone produced by the β-cells of the islets of Langerhans in the pancreas. Insulin was the first protein hormone to be sequenced, the first substance to be measured by radioimmunoassay (RIA), and the first compound produced by recombinant DNA technology for clinical use. It is an anabolic hormone that stimulates the uptake of glucose into fat and muscle, promotes the conversion of glucose to glycogen or fat for storage, inhibits glucose production by the liver, stimulates protein synthesis, and inhibits protein breakdown.

Chemistry

Human insulin (molecular weight [MW] 5808 Da) consists of 51 amino acids in two chains (A and B) joined by two disulfide bridges, with a third disulfide bridge within the A chain. The amino acid sequence of human insulin differs slightly from insulin of other species, but the carboxyl terminal region of the B chain (B23 to B26), which appears crucial for the biological actions of insulin, is highly conserved among species. Insulin from most animals is immunologically and biologically similar to human insulin, and in the past, patients were treated with insulin purified from beef or pig pancreas. The most commonly used forms now are recombinant human insulins.

Synthesis

Preproinsulin, a protein of about 100 amino acids (MW 12,000 Da), is formed by ribosomes in the rough endoplasmic reticulum of the pancreatic β-cells (Fig. 57.2). Preproinsulin is not detectable in the circulation under normal conditions because it is rapidly converted by cleaving enzymes to proinsulin (MW 9000 Da), an 86 amino acid polypeptide. This is

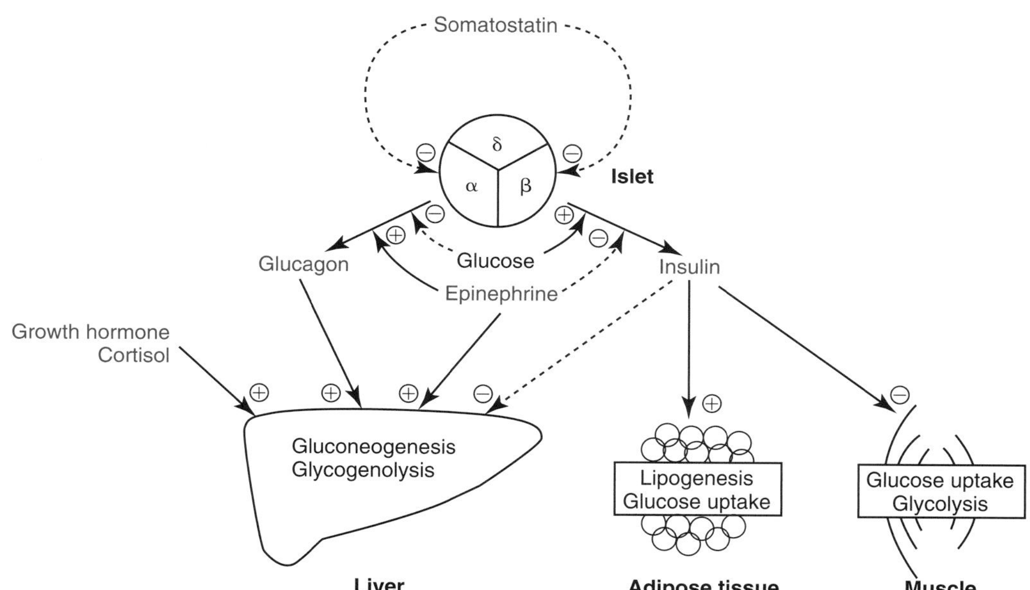

FIGURE 57.1 Hormonal regulation of blood glucose. Cortisol, growth hormone, and epinephrine antagonize the effects of insulin. +, Stimulation; –, inhibition.

stored in secretory granules in the Golgi complex of the β-cells, where proteolytic cleavage to insulin and connecting peptide (C-peptide) occurs.[34] Cleavage of proinsulin is catalyzed by two Ca^{2+}-regulated endopeptidases: prohormone convertases 1 and 2 (PC1 and PC2).[35] PC1 (sometimes designated PC3) hydrolyzes the molecule on the *C*-terminal end of Arg-31 and Arg-32 (at the BC junction) to yield split-32, 33-proinsulin (Fig. 57.3). PC2 cleaves proinsulin on the *C*-terminal side of dibasic residues Lys-64 and Arg-65 (at the AC junction) to generate split-65,66-proinsulin. Each enzymatic hydrolysis reaction is rapidly followed by the removal of two newly exposed *C*-terminal basic amino acids by carboxypeptidase-H to produce insulin and C-peptide.

The split proinsulin intermediates are rarely detected in patient samples because of the relatively high quantity of carboxypeptidase-H. This enzyme produces the more commonly observed proinsulin intermediates, des-31,32-proinsulin and des-64,65-proinsulin (see Fig. 57.3). Most proinsulin processing is sequential. Intact proinsulin is initially hydrolyzed by PC1 or carboxypeptidase-H. The resultant des-31,32-proinsulin is converted by PC2 and carboxypeptidase-H to insulin and C-peptide. Less than 10% of proinsulin is metabolized via des-64-65-proinsulin, which is present in negligible amounts in humans. Des-31,32-proinsulin is the major proinsulin conversion intermediate.[36] Glucose regulates biosynthesis of both proinsulin and PC1, but it has no effect on PC2 or carboxypeptidase-H. At the cell membrane, insulin and C-peptide are released into the portal circulation in equimolar amounts. In addition, small amounts of proinsulin and intermediate cleavage forms enter the circulation.

Release

Glucose is the most important physiological secretagogue for insulin.[37] An increase in blood glucose concentration stimulates insulin secretion within minutes. Insulin release is potentiated by substances such as the incretin hormones glucagon-like peptide 1 (GLP-1) and glucose-dependent insulinotropic polypeptide (GIP), as well as cholecystokinin, peptide YY, and oxyntomodulin, released from the gut in response to food.[37,38] Insulin release is inhibited by hypoglycemia, somatostatin (produced in the pancreatic δ-cells), and various drugs (eg, α-adrenergic agonists, β-adrenergic blockers, diazoxide, phenytoin, phenothiazines, nicotinic acid).[39] In healthy individuals, insulin is secreted in a pulsatile fashion, with glucose and insulin the main signals in the feedback loop. Glucose elicits the release of insulin from the pancreas in two phases. The first phase begins 1 to 2 minutes after intravenous injection of glucose and ends within 10 minutes. This phase, illustrated by the sharp spike in Fig. 57.4A, represents the rapid release of stored insulin. The second phase, beginning at the point where the first phase ends, depends on continuing insulin synthesis and release and lasts until normoglycemia has been restored, usually within 60 to 120 minutes. With progressive failure of β-cell function, the first-phase insulin response to glucose is lost, but other stimuli such as glucagon or amino acids may be able to elicit this response. Although the second-phase insulin response is preserved in most patients with type 2 diabetes mellitus, both the first-phase response (Fig. 57.4B) and normal pulsatile insulin secretion are lost.[15] In contrast, patients with type 1 diabetes mellitus exhibit minimal or no insulin response (Fig. 57.4C).

Degradation

On the first pass through the portal circulation, approximately 50% of the insulin is extracted by the liver, where it is degraded. Because the amount extracted is variable, plasma insulin concentrations may not accurately reflect the rate of insulin secretion. Additional insulin degradation occurs in the kidneys. Insulin is filtered through the glomeruli, reabsorbed, and degraded in the proximal tubules. The basal

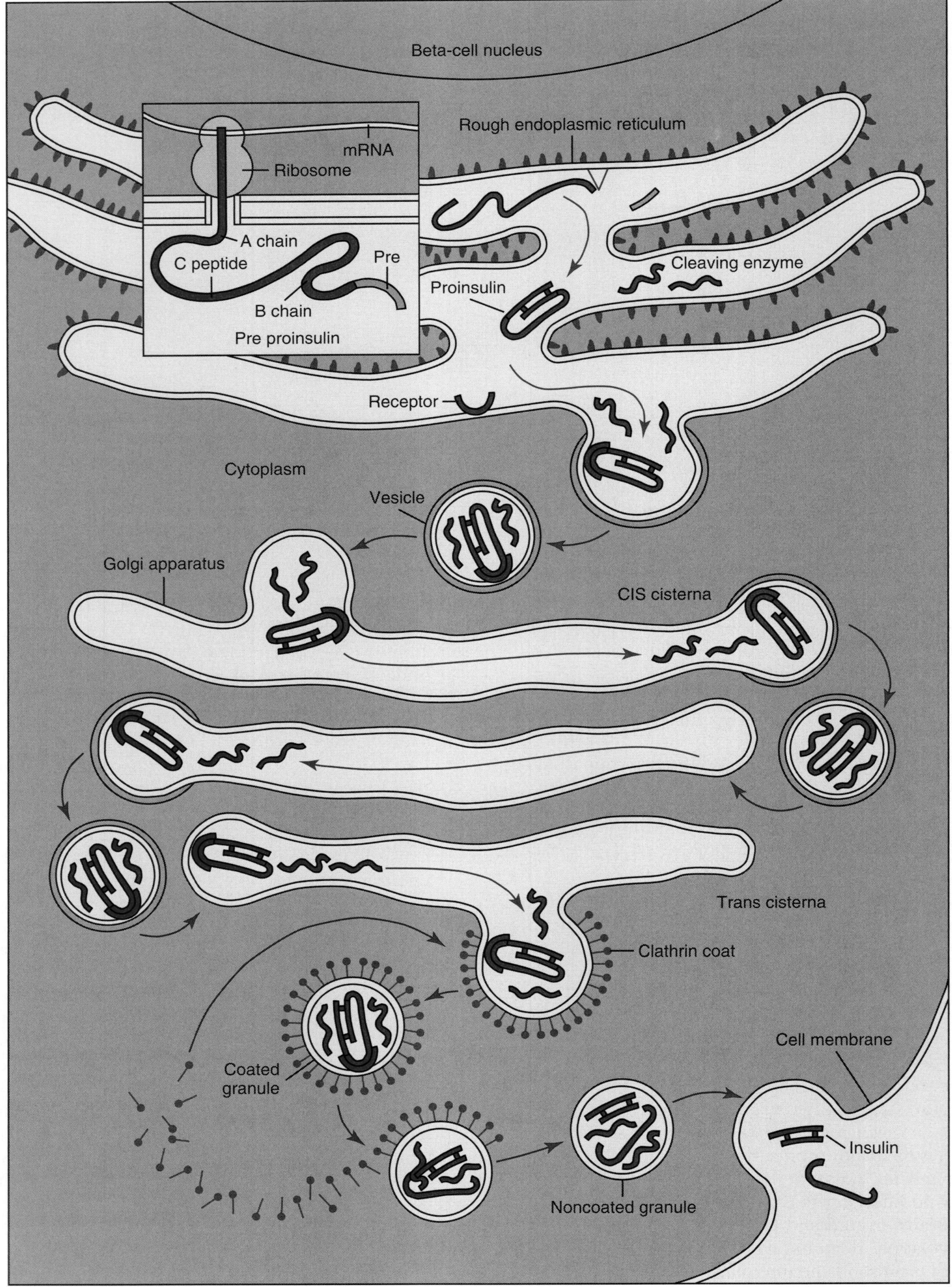

FIGURE 57.2 Insulin synthesis and release from the pancreatic β-cell. (From Orci L, Vassalli J-D, Perrelet A. The insulin factory. *Sci Am* 1988;259:85–94.)

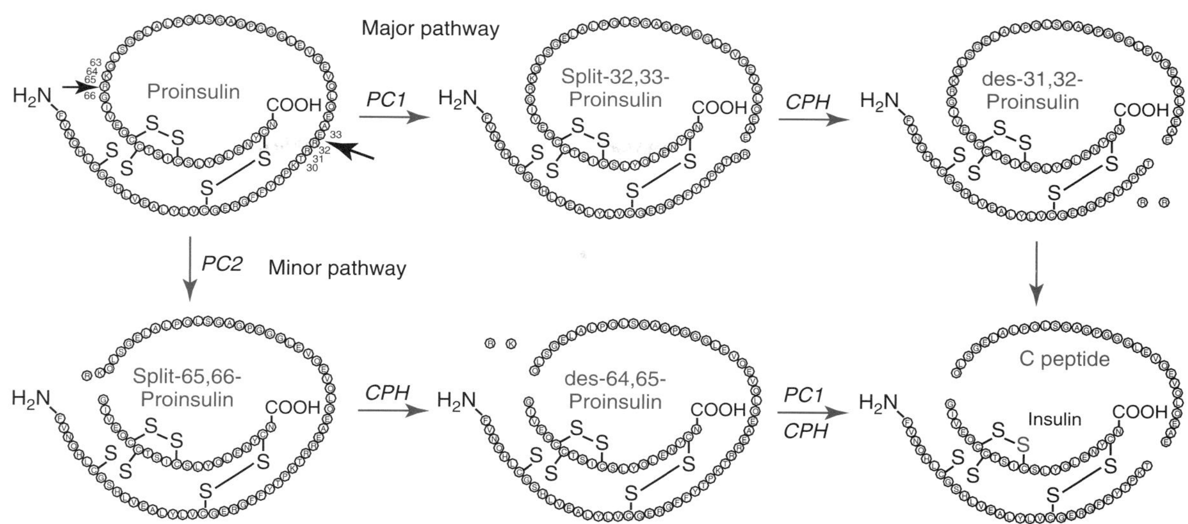

FIGURE 57.3 Processing of proinsulin. The enzymes prohormone convertase 1 and 2 (PC1 and PC2) act on proinsulin to form the appropriate split proinsulins. Carboxypeptidase-H (CPH) removes the two exposed basic amino acid residues *(circles)*.

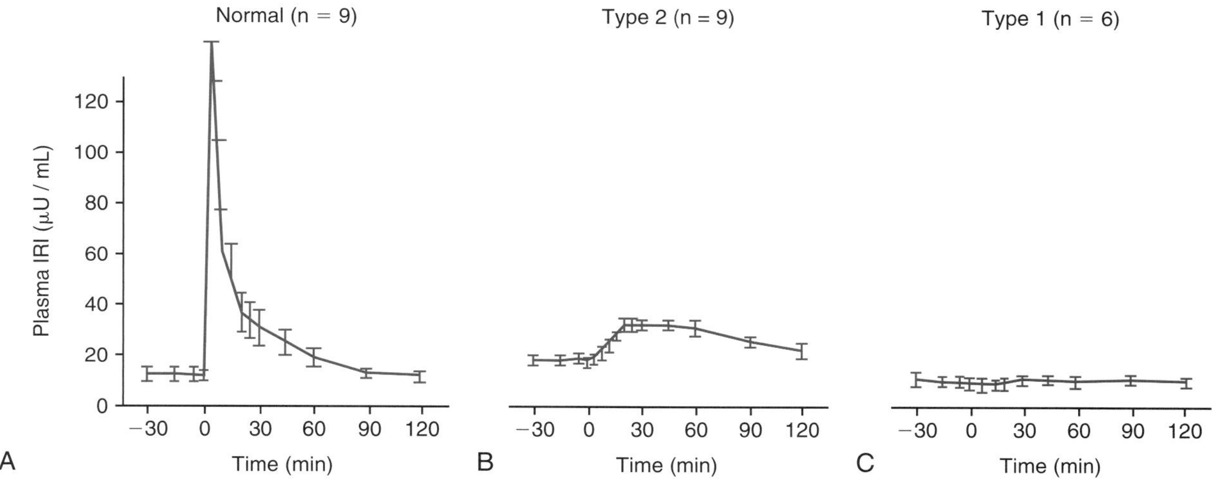

FIGURE 57.4 Response of plasma insulin to glucose stimulation. A 20-g glucose pulse is given intravenously at time 0. **A,** Healthy subjects. **B,** Patients with type 2 diabetes mellitus. **C,** Patients with type 1 diabetes mellitus. Values before time 0 represent baseline. *IRI,* Immunoreactive insulin. (From Pfeifer MA, Halter JB, Porte D Jr. Insulin secretion in diabetes mellitus. *Am J Med* 1981;70:579–88.)

insulin secretory rate is about 1 U (43 μg)/h, with total daily secretion of about 40 U. The half-life of insulin in the circulation is between 4 and 5 minutes.

Proinsulin. Proinsulin, which has relatively low biological activity (approximately 10% of insulin potency), is the major storage form of insulin.[40] Normally, only small amounts (about 3% of the amount of insulin, on a molar basis) of proinsulin enter the circulation. However, the hepatic clearance rate for proinsulin is only 25% of that for insulin, and the half-life of proinsulin is approximately 30 minutes. Therefore, in the fasting state, circulating proinsulin concentrations are approximately 10% to 15% of insulin concentrations.

C-Peptide. Proinsulin is cleaved to a 31 amino acid connecting (C) peptide (MW 3600 Da) and insulin (see Fig. 57.3). C-peptide was initially thought to be devoid of biological activity and was necessary only to ensure the correct structure of insulin.[41] More recent evidence reveals that C-peptide has biological activity, but its possible physiological significance remains controversial.[42] Although insulin and C-peptide are secreted into the portal circulation in equimolar amounts, fasting C-peptide concentrations are 5- to 10-fold higher than those of insulin owing to the longer half-life of C-peptide (approximately 35 minutes). The liver does not extract C-peptide, which is removed from the circulation by the kidneys and degraded, with a fraction excreted unchanged in the urine.

Antibodies to Insulin

Antibodies to insulin develop in almost all patients who are treated with exogenous insulin.[43] These antibodies are usually present at low titer and produce no adverse effects. On rare occasions (usually in insulin-treated patients with

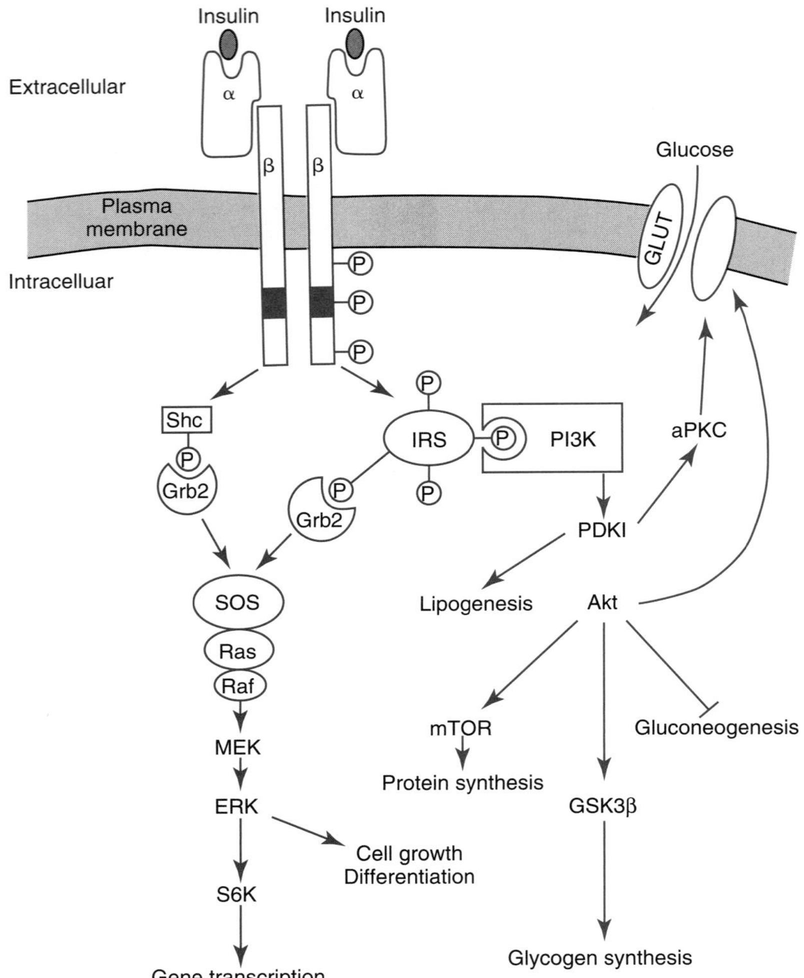

FIGURE 57.5 Mechanism of insulin action. Binding of insulin to the extracellular α-subunit of the insulin receptor induces autophosphorylation of the β-subunit of the receptor and phosphorylation of selected intracellular proteins, such as Shc and the insulin-receptor substrate (IRS) family. These latter phosphoproteins interact with other targets, thereby activating phosphorylation cascades, which result in glucose uptake (into adipose tissue and skeletal muscle), glucose metabolism, synthesis (of glycogen, lipid, and proteins), enhanced gene expression, cell growth, and differentiation. See text for details. *aPKC,* Atypical protein kinase C; *p,* protein phosphorylation.

type 2 diabetes), high titers of insulin antibodies may cause insulin resistance. There are several therapeutic approaches for treating these patients, and a quantitative estimate of the concentration of circulating insulin antibody does not appear to be of significant benefit.[44] Improvement in the purity of animal insulins and the widespread use of human insulin have reduced, but not totally eliminated, antibody production. The use of advanced insulin delivery systems—namely, continuous subcutaneous insulin infusion and inhaled insulin—has resulted in significantly increased concentrations of insulin antibodies.[45] Antibodies to insulin rarely develop in patients who have not received exogenous insulin. There is no evidence to support the use of insulin antibody testing for routine care of patients with diabetes.[44]

Although rare, patients with antibodies to the insulin receptor have been described.[46] On binding the receptor, these antibodies act as antagonists, producing hyperglycemia (eg, in patients with acanthosis nigricans), or agonists, resulting in hypoglycemia.

The Mechanism of Insulin Action

Although the metabolic effects produced by insulin are well known, the molecular mechanism of insulin action remains incompletely understood.[47,48] It is generally accepted that the initial event is the binding of insulin to specific receptors in the plasma membrane (Fig. 57.5). The human insulin receptor, which is well characterized, is a heterotetramer, comprising two α- and two β-subunits. The α-subunit (MW 135,000 Da) is located on the outer surface of the plasma membrane and contains the site where insulin binds. The β-subunit (MW 95,000 Da) extends intracellularly through the plasma membrane and contains an intrinsic tyrosine kinase. Binding of insulin to the α-subunits induces a conformational change in the receptor, resulting in activation of the tyrosine kinase, which catalyzes the phosphorylation of tyrosine residues on several proteins. One of the major substrates for this tyrosine kinase is the receptor itself, which is phosphorylated on multiple tyrosine residues.

TABLE 57.1 Facilitative Human Glucose Transporters

Name	Class	Tissue	Function
GLUT1	I	Erythrocytes, brain, blood–brain barrier, fetal tissues	Basal glucose transport, particularly in erythrocytes, brain and placenta
GLUT2	I	Liver, β-cells of pancreas, small intestine, kidney, brain	Non-rate-limiting glucose transport
GLUT3	I	Brain (neurons), testis	Glucose transport in neurons
GLUT4	I	Skeletal muscle, cardiac muscle, adipose tissue (white and brown)	Insulin-stimulated glucose transport
GLUT5	II	Small intestine, kidney	Transports fructose (not glucose)
GLUT6	III	Brain, spleen, leukocytes	
GLUT7	II	Small intestine, colon, testis, prostate	
GLUT8	III	Testis, brain, adrenal gland, liver, spleen, brown adipose tissue, lung	
GLUT9	II	Kidney, liver, small intestine, placenta, lung, leukocytes	Transports urate
GLUT10	III	Heart, lung, brain, liver, pancreas, placenta, kidney	
GLUT11	II	Heart, skeletal muscle	
GLUT12	III	Heart, prostate, skeletal muscle, placenta	
HMIT (GLUT13)	III	Brain, adipose tissue	Transports *myo*-inositol (not glucose)
GLUT14	I	Testis	

In addition to phosphorylating itself, the insulin receptor catalyzes the tyrosine phosphorylation of various specific intracellular proteins (see Fig. 57.5). These include the four members of the family of insulin-receptor substrate (IRS) proteins (termed IRS-1, IRS-2, IRS-3, and IRS-4), Shc, and Gab-1.[49] The phosphorylated tyrosines on these target proteins act as docking sites for selected intracellular signal transducer proteins.[47] Most of these transducer proteins contain one or more Src homology 2 (SH2) domains. The SH2 domain is a sequence of approximately 100 amino acids that recognizes phosphotyrosine.[50] Sequence differences in the SH2 domain dictate the specificity of binding. SH2-containing proteins depicted in Fig. 57.5 include those labeled phosphatidylinositol 3-kinase (PI3K) and growth factor receptor–bound protein 2 (Grb2), both of which mediate downstream signal transduction events. Similar to other growth factors, insulin stimulates the mitogen-activated protein (MAP) kinase cascade via Ras. In addition, PI3K activates Akt via 3-phosphoinositide dependent protein kinase-1 (PDK1). The effects produced by insulin differ among tissues. In skeletal muscle and adipose tissue, Akt regulates glucose transport by promoting translocation of GLUT4 (the insulin-sensitive glucose transporter) to the plasma membrane. In the liver, Akt phosphorylates and inactivates GSK-3β (glycogen synthase kinase 3β), thereby enhancing glycogen synthesis. Akt also suppresses gluconeogenesis and activates lipogenesis in the liver. Some of these events are listed in Fig. 57.5. The pathways are elaborate with multiple feedback loops. While several components have been identified, there remain considerable gaps in our knowledge and understanding. Investigations have clarified a fundamental concept: that insulin-mediated signaling events are highly degenerate. For example, when two key insulin-signaling molecules, IRS-1 and GLUT4, were knocked out in transgenic mouse experiments, the resulting animals had minor metabolic defects rather than overt diabetes.[51] Similarly, mice with selective knockout of insulin receptors from only skeletal muscle do not develop diabetes.

Glucose Transport

The transport of glucose into cells is modulated by two families of proteins.[52] The sodium-dependent glucose transporters (SGLTs) use the electrochemical sodium gradient to transport glucose against its concentration gradient. SGLTs promote the uptake of glucose and galactose from the lumen of the small bowel and their reabsorption from urine in the kidney. Members of the second family of glucose carriers are called *facilitative glucose transporters* (GLUT), a family of membrane proteins that are encoded by the SLC2 genes (Table 57.1).[53] These transporters are designated GLUT1 to GLUT14, based on the order in which they were identified.[53,54] Eleven have been shown to transport glucose. Many also transport other hexoses, such as galactose, fructose, mannose, and xylose.[53] They can be divided into three classes, based on sequence similarities and characteristics. The best characterized are class I (GLUT1 to GLUT4). Less is known about those in classes II and III. GLUT1 is widely expressed and provides many cells with their basal glucose requirement. GLUT1 in the blood–brain barrier and GLUT3 in neuronal cells provide the constant high concentrations of glucose required by the brain. GLUT1 is responsible for mediating materno-placental transfer of glucose. GLUT2 is expressed in hepatocytes, β-cells of the pancreas, and basolateral membranes of intestinal and renal epithelial cells. It is a low-affinity, high-capacity transport system that allows non-rate-limiting movement of glucose into and out of these cells. GLUT2 is the major glucose transporter of hepatocytes. GLUT3 is the primary mediator of glucose transport into neurons. GLUT4 catalyzes the rate-limiting step for glucose uptake and metabolism in skeletal muscle, the major organ of glucose consumption. GLUT4 is also present in adipose tissue.

When circulating insulin concentrations are low, most of the GLUT4 is localized in intracellular compartments and is inactive. After eating, the pancreas releases insulin, which stimulates the translocation of GLUT4 to the plasma membrane, thereby promoting glucose uptake into skeletal muscle and fat. Insulin-stimulated glucose transport into skeletal muscle is defective in type 2 diabetes mellitus, but the mechanism has not been established.

GLUT9 was initially thought to transport glucose or fructose, but it is established that GLUT9 transports urate. It is required for urate reabsorption in the kidney and appears to be associated with gout. GLUTs 6, 7, 10, 11, 12, and 14 were identified as a result of sequencing the human genome, and their physiological roles remain unclear.[53]

Insulin-Like Growth Factors

Insulin-like growth factors 1 and 2 (IGF-1 and IGF-2) are polypeptides structurally related to insulin.[55] These hormones (previously referred to as *nonsuppressible insulin-like activity* or *somatomedin*) exhibit metabolic and growth-promoting effects similar to those of insulin. Accumulating evidence implicates the IGF axis in the development of several common cancers.[56] IGF-1 (previously known as somatomedin C) is an important mediator of growth hormone action and is one of the major regulators of cell growth and differentiation. The physiological role of IGF-2 is not known. Synthesis of IGF-1 depends on growth hormone and occurs predominantly in the liver. In addition, many other cells produce IGF-1 that does not enter the circulation but acts locally. Circulating IGF concentrations are approximately 1000-fold higher than insulin concentrations, and the hormone is kept inactive by binding to a family of at least six specific binding proteins.[57] These proteins regulate IGF by protecting the ligands in the circulation and delivering them to their target tissue. In contrast to insulin, which is unbound in the circulation, less than 10% of total serum IGF-1 is free. The biological actions of IGF are exerted through specific IGF receptors or the insulin receptor. The IGF-1 receptor is closely related to the insulin receptor in structure and biochemical properties. In contrast, the IGF-2 receptor is quite different; it lacks tyrosine kinase activity, and its physiological relevance is not understood. The IGF-1 receptor has a high affinity for both IGF-1 and IGF-2, but a low affinity for insulin. The IGF-2 receptor has high, low, and no affinity for IGF-2, IGF-1, and insulin, respectively. The insulin receptor binds insulin with high affinity and IGF-1 and IGF-2 with low affinity.

The significance of IGFs in normal carbohydrate metabolism is not known. Exogenous administration produces hypoglycemia, whereas a deficiency of IGF-1 results in dwarfism (pygmies and Laron dwarfs). IGFs, particularly IGF-2, may be produced in excess by extrapancreatic neoplasms, and patients may have fasting hypoglycemia.[58] The high concentrations of both IGF-2 protein in the blood and IGF-2 messenger RNA (mRNA) in tumor extracts have led to the proposal that IGF-2 is the humoral mediator of non–islet cell tumor–induced hypoglycemia.[59] Measurement of plasma IGF-1 concentration may be useful in evaluating growth hormone deficiency and excess (acromegaly), and in monitoring response to nutritional support.

Counterregulatory Hormones

Several hormones have actions opposite to those of insulin. These counterregulatory hormones are catabolic and increase hepatic glucose production initially by enhancing the breakdown of glycogen to glucose (glycogenolysis), and later by stimulating the synthesis of glucose (gluconeogenesis).[33,60] The initial response (within minutes) to low blood glucose is an increase in glucose production, stimulated by glucagon and epinephrine. Over time (3 to 4 hours), growth hormone and cortisol increase glucose mobilization and decrease glucose use (see Fig. 57.1). Evidence also suggests that glucose production by the liver is an inverse function of ambient glucose concentration, independent of hormonal factors *(glucose autoregulation)*. The role of other hormones or neurotransmitters is not clear but appears relatively unimportant. Multiple counterregulatory hormones exhibit both redundancy and hierarchy. Glucagon is the most important, and epinephrine becomes critical when glucagon is deficient. The other factors have lesser roles. These hormones, briefly described here, are discussed further in Chapters 62, 63, 65, and 66.

Glucagon

Glucagon is a 29 amino acid polypeptide secreted by α-cells of the pancreas. It is derived from proglucagon, which is hydrolyzed by prohormone convertase 2 (PC2).[61,62] The major target organ for glucagon is the liver, where it binds to a specific G protein–coupled receptor, which is expressed abundantly in liver and kidney, and to a lesser extent in other tissues, including heart, adipose, pancreas, and brain. Glucagon stimulates the production of glucose in the liver predominantly by glycogenolysis. Gluconeogenesis is also activated, and glycogenesis is inhibited. Glucagon secretion is regulated primarily by plasma glucose concentrations, with low and high plasma glucose being stimulatory and inhibitory, respectively. Long-standing diabetes mellitus impairs the glucagon response to hypoglycemia, resulting in an increased incidence of hypoglycemic episodes. Stress, exercise, and amino acids induce glucagon release. Insulin inhibits glucagon release from the pancreas and decreases glucagon gene expression, thereby attenuating its biosynthesis. Increased glucagon concentrations, secondary to insulin deficiency, are believed to contribute to the hyperglycemia and ketosis of diabetes. In addition to its effects on glycemia, glucagon directly regulates triglyceride, free fatty acid, and bile metabolism. For example, it enhances fatty acid oxidation and ketogenesis in the liver.

Proglucagon is also produced in the distal gut by enteroendocrine L cells and neurons in the nucleus of the solitary tract. In the intestinal L cells, proglucagon is cleaved by prohormone convertase 1/3 (PC1/3) to glucagon-like peptide-1 (GLP-1), GLP-2, oxyntomodulin, glicentin, and intervening peptide 2 (IP2).[62] Food ingestion stimulates secretion of GLP-1, which acts on β-cells of the pancreas to stimulate insulin gene transcription, potentiate glucose-induced insulin secretion, and inhibit glucagon secretion. GLP-1 and GIP (synthesized in and secreted from the duodenum and proximal jejunum) are incretin hormones that are responsible for up to 70% of postprandial insulin secretion.[38,63] GLP-1 receptors are widely expressed, and GLP-1 also regulates glucose concentration through extrapancreatic mechanisms, including inhibiting glucose production and food intake. For these reasons, GLP-1 analogs are generating interest in the treatment of type 2 diabetes,[63] and four (exenatide, liraglutide, albiglutide, and dulaglutide) have received Food and Drug Administration (FDA) approval for use in the United States.

Epinephrine

Epinephrine (also called adrenaline), a catecholamine secreted by the adrenal medulla, stimulates glucose production (glycogenolysis) and decreases glucose use, thereby increasing blood glucose concentrations. It also stimulates glucagon secretion and inhibits insulin secretion by the pancreas (see Fig. 57.1). Epinephrine appears to have a key role in glucose counterregulation when glucagon secretion is impaired (eg, in type 1 diabetes mellitus). Physical or emotional stress increases epinephrine production, releasing glucose for energy. Tumors of the adrenal medulla, known as *pheochromocytomas,* secrete excess epinephrine or norepinephrine and produce moderate hyperglycemia as long as glycogen stores are available in the liver. For more details, see Chapter 63.

Growth Hormone

Growth hormone is a polypeptide secreted by the anterior pituitary gland. It stimulates gluconeogenesis, enhances lipolysis, and antagonizes insulin-stimulated glucose uptake.

Cortisol

Cortisol, secreted by the adrenal cortex in response to adrenocorticotropic hormone (ACTH), stimulates gluconeogenesis and increases the breakdown of protein and fat. Patients with Cushing syndrome have increased cortisol production owing to tumor or hyperplasia of the adrenal cortex and may become hyperglycemic. In contrast, people with Addison disease have adrenocortical insufficiency caused by destruction or atrophy of the adrenal cortex and may exhibit hypoglycemia. For more details, refer to Chapter 66.

Other Hormones Influencing Glucose Metabolism

Thyroxine

Thyroxine, secreted by the thyroid gland, is not directly involved in glucose homeostasis, but it stimulates glycogenolysis and increases the rates of gastric emptying and intestinal glucose absorption. These factors may produce glucose intolerance in thyrotoxic individuals, but patients usually have a fasting plasma glucose concentration in the reference interval.

Somatostatin

Somatostatin, also called growth hormone–inhibiting hormone, is a 14 amino acid peptide found in the gastrointestinal tract, the hypothalamus, and the δ-cells of the pancreatic islets. Although somatostatin does not appear to have a direct effect on carbohydrate metabolism, it inhibits the release of growth hormone from the pituitary. In addition, somatostatin inhibits secretion of glucagon and insulin by the pancreas, thus modulating the reciprocal relationship between these two hormones.

CLINICAL UTILITY OF MEASURING INSULIN, PROINSULIN, C-PEPTIDE, AND GLUCAGON

Box 57.2 lists the clinical conditions in which hormones that regulate glucose—namely, insulin, proinsulin, C-peptide, and glucagon—have been measured. Although there is interest in the possible clinical value of measurement of the concentrations of insulin and its precursors, the assays are useful primarily for research purposes. There is no role for routine testing for insulin, proinsulin, or C-peptide in most patients with diabetes mellitus.[44,64] Measurement of C-peptide is sometimes necessary in the United States for patients to obtain insurance coverage for continuous subcutaneous insulin infusion pumps. Occasionally, C-peptide measurements may help distinguish type 1 from type 2 diabetes in ambiguous cases (eg, patients who have type 2 phenotype, but present with ketoacidosis). It must be emphasized that the diagnostic criteria for diabetes mellitus do not include measurements of hormones, which remain predominantly research tools.

BOX 57.2 Clinical Utility of Insulin, Proinsulin, C-Peptide, and Glucagon Assays

Insulin
Evaluation of fasting hypoglycemia
Evaluation of the polycystic ovary syndrome
Classification of diabetes mellitus
Prediction of diabetes mellitus
Assessment of β-cell activity
Selection of optimal therapy for diabetes
Investigation of insulin resistance
Prediction of the development of coronary artery disease

Proinsulin
Diagnosis of β-cell tumors
Familial hyperproinsulinemia
Cross-reactivity of insulin assays

C-Peptide
Evaluation of fasting hypoglycemia
- β Cell tumors
- Factitious

Classification of diabetes mellitus
Assessment of β-cell activity
Obtaining insurance coverage for insulin pump
Monitoring therapy
- Pancreatectomy
- Transplant (pancreas-islet cell)
- Immunomodulation of type 1 diabetes

Glucagon
Diagnosis of α-cell tumors

Insulin

The primary clinical application of insulin measurement is in the evaluation of patients with fasting hypoglycemia (discussed in more detail in Chapter 33). Measurement of circulating insulin could be helpful in evaluating insulin resistance and insulin secretion. Insulin determination has also been proposed to be of value in selecting the optimal initial therapy for patients with type 2 diabetes mellitus. In theory, the lower the pretreatment insulin concentration, the more appropriate might be insulin or an insulin secretagogue as the treatment of choice. Although intellectually appealing, no evidence suggests that knowledge of the insulin concentration leads to more efficacious treatment. Evidence indicates that increased concentrations of insulin in nondiabetic individuals are an independent predictor of the development of coronary artery disease.[65,66] Nevertheless, it is not clear whether the increased insulin is responsible for the risk of coronary disease, and the clinical value of measuring it in this context is questionable.[44]

In the past, measurement of insulin was advocated by some in the evaluation and management of patients with polycystic ovary syndrome.[44,64] Women with this condition have insulin resistance and abnormal carbohydrate metabolism that may respond to oral antihyperglycemic agents. However, it is not clear whether assessing insulin resistance by measuring insulin concentrations affords any advantage over clinical signs of insulin resistance (body mass index, acanthosis nigricans), and the American College of Obstetrics and Gynecology (ACOG) does not recommend routine measurements of insulin.[67] Although a few investigators have recommended measuring insulin along with glucose during an OGTT as an aid to the early diagnosis of diabetes mellitus, this approach is not recommended.[44,64] Insulin measurements do not add significantly to diabetes risk prediction generated with traditional clinical and laboratory measurements.[68]

Proinsulin

High proinsulin concentrations are usually noted in patients with benign or malignant β-cell tumors of the pancreas. Most patients with β-cell tumors have increased insulin, C-peptide, and proinsulin concentrations, but occasionally only proinsulin is increased[69] because the tumors have defective conversion of proinsulin to insulin. Despite its low biological activity, proinsulin production may be adequate to produce hypoglycemia. In addition, a rare form of familial hyperproinsulinemia, produced by impaired conversion to insulin, has been described. Measurement of proinsulin can be useful to determine the amount of proinsulin-like material that cross-reacts in an insulin assay. Patients with type 2 diabetes have increased proportions of proinsulin and proinsulin conversion intermediates,[70] high concentrations of which are associated with cardiovascular risk factors.[71] Even relatively mild hyperglycemia produces hyperproinsulinemia, with values greater than 40% of insulin concentration in type 2 diabetes.[70] Similarly, women with GDM have higher concentrations of proinsulin and split-32,33-proinsulin than pregnant normoglycemic control subjects. An increased ratio of proinsulin-like molecules to insulin-like molecules at screening has been proposed as a better predictor of GDM than age, obesity, or hyperglycemia.[72] Increased proinsulin concentrations may also be detected in patients with chronic renal failure, cirrhosis, or hyperthyroidism.

Accurate measurement of proinsulin has been difficult for several reasons: the blood concentrations are low; antibody production is difficult; most antisera cross-react with insulin and C-peptide, which are present in much higher concentrations; the assays measure intermediate cleavage forms of proinsulin; and reference preparations of pure proinsulin are not readily available. However, a more sensitive nonequilibrium RIA method for measuring proinsulin was developed by adsorbing the initial antiserum with biosynthetic human C-peptide coupled with agarose to eliminate cross-reactivity with C-peptide.[73,74] An enzyme-linked immunosorbent assay (ELISA) has been described that employs an antibody to C-peptide as the coating antibody and anti-insulin antibody for detection.[75] The detection limit is 0.25 pmol/L.[76]

C-Peptide

Measurement of C-peptide has a number of advantages over insulin measurement. Because hepatic metabolism is negligible, C-peptide concentrations are better indicators of β-cell function than is peripheral insulin concentration.[77] Furthermore, C-peptide assays do not measure exogenous insulin and do not cross-react with insulin antibodies, which interfere with the insulin immunoassay.

Fasting Hypoglycemia

The primary indication for measuring C-peptide is for the evaluation of fasting hypoglycemia. Some patients with insulin-producing β-cell tumors, particularly if hyperinsulinism is intermittent, may exhibit increased C-peptide concentrations with normal insulin concentrations. When hypoglycemia is due to surreptitious insulin injection, insulin concentrations will be high, but C-peptide values will be low;[78] this occurs because C-peptide is not found in commercial insulin preparations and exogenous insulin suppresses β-cell function.

Insulin Secretion

Basal or stimulated (by glucagon or glucose) C-peptide concentrations provide estimates of a patient's insulin secretory capacity and rate. For example, diabetic patients with C-peptide concentrations greater than 1.8 ng/mL (0.60 nmol/L) after stimulation with glucagon behave clinically like patients with type 2 diabetes, and those with low peak C-peptide values (<0.5 ng/mL; <0.16 nmol/L) behave like patients with type 1 diabetes.[79] In rare cases, this strategy may be helpful before discontinuation of insulin treatment (eg, in an obese adolescent). Urinary and fasting serum C-peptide concentrations appear to be of some value in differentiating patients with type 1 diabetes from those with type 2 diabetes.[80] In addition, patients who have type 1 diabetes but who have no C-peptide response are usually more labile than those with some residual β-cell function. Despite these observations, C-peptide measurement has a negligible role in the routine management of patients with diabetes. Medicare patients in the United States must have low C-peptide concentrations to be eligible for insurance coverage of insulin pumps.[44,64]

Monitoring Therapy

Measurement of C-peptide is used to monitor a patient's response to pancreatic surgery. C-peptide should be undetectable after a radical pancreatectomy and should increase after a successful pancreas or islet cell transplant. In addition, C-peptide concentration is used as an endpoint in immunomodulatory trials for the prevention of type 1 diabetes.[81]

Measurements of urine C-peptide are useful when continuous assessment of β-cell function is desired or when frequent blood sampling is not practical. The 24-hour urine C-peptide content (in the absence of renal failure, which produces increased concentrations) correlates well with fasting serum C-peptide concentration or with the sum of C-peptide concentrations in sequential specimens after a glucose load. However, the fraction of secreted C-peptide that is excreted in the urine exhibits high between-subject and within-subject variability, limiting the value of urine C-peptide as a measure of insulin secretion.[82] Some have advocated C-peptide to creatinine ratio in a single urine sample to avoid the problems associated with 24-hour urine collection.[83]

Glucagon

Very high concentrations of glucagon are seen in patients with α-cell tumors of the pancreas called glucagonomas.

Patients with this tumor frequently have weight loss, necrolytic migratory erythema, diabetes mellitus, stomatitis, and diarrhea.[84] Skin lesions often occur first and are frequently overlooked. Most tumors have metastasized when finally diagnosed. Low glucagon concentrations are associated with chronic pancreatitis and long-term sulfonylurea therapy.

METHODS FOR THE MEASUREMENT OF SPECIFIC HORMONES

Insulin

Although insulin has been assayed for over 50 years, no highly accurate, precise, and reliable procedure is available to measure the amount of insulin in a patient sample. Many insulin assays are commercially available.[85-87] The techniques most widely used are immunometric.[86,87] Bioassays, although of greater physiologic relevance because they measure biological activity, are labor intensive and are not widely used. A stable isotope dilution mass spectrometry (IDMS) assay yields lower values than an immunoassay.[88]

Patients treated with exogenous insulin may develop circulating anti-insulin antibodies, which compete with antibodies in the RIA. Endogenous antibodies and their bound insulin can be precipitated from serum with polyethylene glycol (PEG) and free insulin measured by RIA. Total insulin can be determined by eluting antibody-bound insulin with hydrochloric acid (HCl), precipitating the antibody with PEG, and performing RIA. The bound insulin is the difference between total and free insulin. Unless a patient's insulin requirements change dramatically, total insulin concentrations are usually constant in patients with type 1 diabetes, and repeated assays are not necessary.

Principle

In a typical RIA procedure for measuring insulin, ^{125}I-labeled insulin competes with insulin in a patient sample for binding to an insulin-specific antibody immobilized on the walls of a polypropylene tube. The supernatant is decanted, and the bound ^{125}I determined in a gamma counter. The amount of insulin in the sample is established by comparison with a calibration curve obtained by plotting on logit-log scale the percent of total radioactivity bound (B/T%) against the concentration of the calibrators. Various commercial kits for insulin measurement are now available.

Comments

General comments on the measurement of insulin include the following:

1. The term *immunoreactive insulin* is used in reference to assays that may recognize, in addition to insulin, substrates that share antigenic epitopes with insulin. Examples include proinsulin, proinsulin conversion intermediates, and insulin derivatives, produced by glycation or dimerization.
2. Various insulin preparations, including human insulin, are used as insulin calibrators. For ease of comparison of results among laboratories, the insulin calibrator is expressed in terms of international units (IU). One international unit of insulin is equal to approximately 43 µg of the World Health Organization (WHO) First International Reference Preparation (1st IRP) Code 66/304 (National Institute of Biological Standards and Control, South Mimms, Potters Bar, Hertfordshire, United Kingdom), which is 100% human insulin.
3. Antisera raised against insulin show some cross-reactivity with proinsulin but not with C-peptide. Specificity is not a problem in healthy individuals because the low proinsulin concentrations do not appreciably affect the absolute values of insulin. In certain situations (eg, islet cell tumors and diabetic individuals), proinsulin is present at higher concentrations, and direct assay of plasma may falsely overestimate the true insulin concentration. Because proinsulin has very low activity, incorrect conclusions regarding the availability of biologically active insulin may be reached in patients with diabetes. The magnitude of the error depends on the concentration of proinsulin and the extent of cross-reactivity of the antiserum with proinsulin. Monoclonal antibody-based assays that are specific for insulin and do not measure proinsulin,[89] although theoretically advantageous, are not superior to nonspecific assays.[43]
4. A stable (IDMS) assay has been developed to measure insulin, proinsulin, and C-peptide.[88] The difference in mass between the three analytes allows specific measurement of each protein. Comparison of patient samples revealed that most, but not all, results were higher by immunoassay than by mass spectrometry.[88] Thus immunoassays may overestimate insulin, particularly at low concentrations. The high protein concentration in the serum requires extraction of proteins (eg, by immunoaffinity) and purification by high-performance liquid chromatography (HPLC) before quantification by mass spectrometry. This method is not suitable for routine laboratory analysis, but it is the best higher-order measurement procedure available and can be used as a candidate reference measurement procedure.
5. The ADA appointed a task force to standardize the insulin assay.[43] Evaluation of unknown samples by 17 different laboratories revealed a wide range in insulin values, with interlaboratory variation up to threefold.[43] Large differences were observed even among laboratories using the same assays. Use of a common calibrator did not improve agreement among laboratories. Assay coefficients of variation (CVs) ranged from less than 2% to greater than 30%, with ELISAs exhibiting the lowest imprecision. Certain characteristics of some assays, including commercial kits, were unacceptable. The task force judged available proficiency and certification programs for insulin to be inadequate, and recommended the establishment of a central laboratory to provide certification for insulin assays. Complete interlaboratory standardization was deemed to be neither practical nor universally acceptable. ADA recommendations for analysis of insulin[43] are as follows:
   a. Each laboratory should carefully evaluate its insulin assay to ensure acceptable assay performance.
   b. Each laboratory should compare the performance of its assay with others using common calibrators and unknown samples.
   c. Because assay performance may change with time or with new reagents or equipment, performance characteristics must be remeasured periodically.
6. In 2004, the ADA convened an international workgroup to establish guidelines for acceptability of insulin assays and to develop a standardization program that can be used to achieve uniform accuracy-based values.[90] Evaluation of

10 commercial insulin methods from nine manufacturers revealed within-assay CVs ranging from 3.7% to 39%, and seven assays had a CV of 10.6% or less.[90] Interassay CVs ranged from 12% to 66%. Results from six assays agreed within a total error of 32%.[90] Cross-reactivity with proinsulin and split-32,33-proinsulin was less than 2% for nine methods and less than 3% for eight methods, respectively. A common insulin reference preparation failed to improve harmonization of results. The workgroup concluded that not all commercial insulin assays have acceptable performance characteristics. A study in the United Kingdom published at the same time[87] compared 11 commercially available insulin assays and made analogous observations. Insulin values among the different assays varied up to twofold.

The ADA workgroup subsequently compared results of 10 commercial insulin assays against IDMS. Four methods were within 32% of the IDMS concentration.[86] Most methods had bias greater than 15.5%. Bias was reduced by calibration with serum pools, but it remained high for many methods at low insulin concentrations (<60 pmol/L; <10 μIU/mL).

7. Based on biological variability, desirable measurement bias of ±15%, imprecision of 10.6% CV, and total analytical error of 32.0% have been proposed for a single insulin measurement.[90]
8. Patient samples with high values should be diluted with the zero calibrator.
9. The presence of antibodies to insulin produces spuriously increased or decreased (depending on the method used) insulin values.

Reference Intervals

Reference intervals vary among assays, and each laboratory should establish its own reference intervals. After an overnight fast, insulin concentrations in healthy, normal, nonobese people vary from 12 to 150 pmol/L (2–25 μIU/mL). (The conversion factor of 6.0 used to convert μIU/mL [or mIU/L] of insulin to pmol/L is based on an MW of insulin of 5807.58 and specific activity of 30 IU/mg.) More specific assays that have minimal cross-reactivity with proinsulin reveal a fasting plasma insulin concentration of less than 60 pmol/L (10 μIU/mL). Concentrations up to 1200 pmol/L (200 μIU/mL) can be reached during a glucose tolerance test. Representative values for insulin concentrations after glucose are shown in Fig. 57.4. Fasting insulin values are higher in obese, nondiabetic people and lower in trained athletes.

Insulin Antibodies

Assays for insulin antibodies fall into three categories: quantitative radioimmunoelectrophoresis, which measures the binding of immunoglobulin (Ig)G antibody to radiolabeled insulin by rocket immunoelectrophoresis into anti-IgG-containing agarose; RIAs with separation of bound and free insulin by precipitation with PEG or a second antibody; and solid-phase immobilization of insulin to test tubes or Sepharose. These are discussed in greater detail in Reeves.[91]

Proinsulin

Principle

Accurate measurement of proinsulin has been difficult for several reasons: the blood concentrations are low; antibody production is difficult; most antisera cross-react with insulin and C-peptide, which are present in much higher concentrations; the assays measure intermediate cleavage forms of proinsulin; and reference preparations of pure proinsulin were not readily available.[92] Therefore few accurate data are available in the literature on plasma proinsulin. These problems have, to a large extent, been overcome by the availability of biosynthetic proinsulin, which has allowed the production of monoclonal antibodies to proinsulin[36,93] and has provided reliable proinsulin calibrators and reference preparations. An International Reference Preparation for human proinsulin (code 84/611) is available from the National Institute of Biological Standards and Controls (Potters Bar, UK). Earlier assays may have overestimated proinsulin concentrations.[94]

Reference Intervals

Reference intervals for proinsulin are highly dependent on the method of analysis, the degree of cross-reactivity of the antisera, and the purity of proinsulin calibrators. Each laboratory should establish its own reference intervals. Reference intervals in healthy, fasting individuals reported in the literature range from 1.1 to 6.9 pmol/L to 2.1 to 12.6 pmol/L (see reference 95 and the references therein).

C-Peptide

Principle

C-peptide undergoes minimal liver metabolism, and, in contrast to proinsulin assays, assays are not affected by antiinsulin antibodies. However, several methodologic problems produce large between-method variation. These difficulties include variable specificity among different antisera, variable cross-reactivity with proinsulin, and various types of C-peptide preparation used as a calibrator. The CDC formed a committee to harmonize C-peptide measurements. Comparison of 40 serum samples using nine commercial C-peptide assay methods showed within- and between-run CVs ranging from less than 2% to greater than 10% and from less than 2% to greater than 18%, respectively.[96] Some methods had high imprecision, with between-run CVs exceeding 15%. Two IDMS methods for measuring C-peptide have been developed.[97,98] Calibrating C-peptide measurements to a reference method using mass spectrometry increased comparability among laboratories.[96]

Reference Intervals

Each laboratory should establish its own reference interval for C-peptide. Fasting serum concentrations of C-peptide in healthy people range from 0.78 to 1.89 ng/mL (0.25–0.6 nmol/L). After stimulation with glucose or glucagon, values range from 2.73 to 5.64 ng/mL (0.9–1.87 nmol/L), or three to five times the prestimulation value. Urinary C-peptide is usually in the range of 74 ± 26 μg/L (25 ± 8.8 μmol/L). C-peptide is excreted primarily by the kidney, and concentrations in the serum are increased in renal disease.

Glucagon

Principle

A competitive RIA is available for measuring glucagon. ^{125}I-labeled glucagon competes with glucagon in the patient specimen for binding to the polyclonal glucagon antibody. Bound glucagon is separated from free glucagon by the use of PEG and a second antibody. Bound radioactivity for the patient specimen is compared with that of glucagon calibrators. Calibrator values are assigned at the manufacturer using the WHO glucagon international standard (69/194). Immunoassays that do not use radioactivity have been developed. A recent comparison of 10 commercially available assays reveals that some show cross-reactivity with other peptides from proglucagon, and all lack sensitivity at low glucagon concentrations.[99]

Reference Intervals

Fasting plasma concentrations of glucagon vary depending on the method, ranging from 0 to 20 ng/L to up to 135 ng/L (0–5.7 pmol/L to 38.7 pmol/L). Values up to 500 times the upper reference limit may be found in patients with autonomously secreting α-cell neoplasms.

PATHOGENESIS OF TYPE 1 DIABETES MELLITUS

Type 1 diabetes mellitus results from cellular-mediated autoimmune destruction of the insulin-secreting cells of pancreatic β-cells.[100-102] In the vast majority of patients, destruction is mediated by T cells. This is termed *type 1A* or *immune-mediated diabetes* (see Box 57.1). The α-, δ-, and other islet cells are preserved. The islet cells have a chronic mononuclear cell infiltrate, called insulitis. The autoimmune process leading to type 1 diabetes begins months or years before the clinical presentation, and an 80% to 90% reduction in the volume of β-cells is required to induce symptomatic type 1 diabetes. The rate of islet cell destruction is variable and is usually more rapid in children than in adults.

Antibodies

The most practical markers of β-cell autoimmunity are circulating antibodies, which have been detected in the serum years before the onset of hyperglycemia. The best characterized islet autoantibodies are as follows:[44,102,103]

1. *Islet cell cytoplasmic antibodies* (ICAs) react with a sialoglycoconjugate antigen present in the cytoplasm of all endocrine cells of the pancreatic islets. These antibodies are detected in the serum of 0.5% of normal subjects and 75% to 85% of patients with newly diagnosed type 1 diabetes. The antibodies are detected by immunofluorescence microscopy on frozen sections of human pancreatic tails. Results are compared with standard serum of the Immunology of Diabetes Workgroup[104] and are expressed in Juvenile Diabetes Foundation (JDF) units. Although not universal, many laboratories use 10 JDF units on two separate occasions or a single result of greater than or equal to 20 JDF units as a significant titer. The ICA assay is cumbersome, labor intensive, and difficult to standardize. Few clinical laboratories are likely to implement this assay, which has marked interlaboratory variability in sensitivity and specificity.[44]
2. *Insulin autoantibodies* (IAAs) are present in more than 90% of children who develop type 1 diabetes before age 5, but in less than 40% of individuals who develop diabetes after age 12. Their frequency in healthy people is similar to that of ICA. A radioisotopic method that calculates the displaceable insulin radioligand binding after the addition of excess nonradiolabeled insulin is recommended for IAA. Results are positive when concentrations exceed the 99th percentile or the mean +2 (or 3) standard deviations (SDs) in healthy controls. Proficiency evaluation revealed poor concordance for IAA among laboratories.[105] An important caveat is that insulin antibodies develop after insulin therapy, even in those persons who use human insulin.
3. *Antibodies to the 65 kDa isoform of glutamic acid decarboxylase* (GAD65)[106] have been found up to 10 years before the onset of clinical type 1 diabetes and are present in approximately 60% of patients with newly diagnosed type 1 diabetes. GAD65 antibodies may be used to identify patients with apparent type 2 diabetes who will subsequently progress to type 1 diabetes. Several different assay formats have been used for the measurement of anti-GAD65 antibodies, including enzymatic immunoprecipitation assay, radiobinding assay, ELISA, immunofluorescence, and Western blotting.[107] Considerable variability among laboratories has been significantly reduced by the Second International GADAb Workshop.[107] A monoclonal antibody, MICA 3, was suggested as a reference standard. A dual micromethod and RIA performed with ^{3}H-labeled human recombinant GAD65 in a rabbit reticulocyte expression system is used by many laboratories. Methods for measurement of GAD65 are now commercially available.
4. *Insulinoma-associated antigens* (IA-2A and IA-2βA), directed against two tyrosine phosphatases, have been detected in more than 50% of newly diagnosed type 1 diabetes patients. A widely used method to measure IA-2A uses ^{35}S-labeled recombinant IA-2 in a dual micromethod and RIA. Concurrent analysis of IA-2 and GAD65 in a single assay has been reported.[108]
5. *Zinc transporter ZnT8* was identified in 2007 as a major autoantigen in type 1 diabetes.[109] ZnT8 is the least characterized of the autoantibodies in diabetes. Initial analysis identified ZnT8 in 60% to 80% of patients with new-onset type 1 diabetes compared with less than 2% of controls and less than 3% of individuals with type 2 diabetes. More important, antibodies to ZnT8 are detected in approximately 26% of patients with type 1 diabetes who are negative for other islet autoantibodies.[103]

Most islet autoantibodies are measured by quantitative radiobinding assays.[110] Radiolabeled recombinant insulin, GAD65, or IA-2 is incubated with patient's serum, and the amount of radioactivity in the precipitated complex is proportional to the antibody concentration. Nonradioactive ELISA methods have become available for GAD65, IA-2, and ZnT8 (the last was approved by the FDA in 2014 for use in the United States). While RIA remains the most widely used technique for patient samples and clinical studies, new strategies, such as plasmonic chip-based assays,[111,112] are likely to replace the requirement for radiolabel in the future.

The Centers for Disease Control and Prevention (CDC) and the Immunology of Diabetes Society established in 2000 the Diabetes Autoantibody Standardization Program (DASP). The major goals of DASP are to assist laboratories in improving methods, to organize workshops for harmonization of antibody testing for type 1 diabetes, and to provide reference materials.[105,113] DASP provides serum from 50 patients with newly diagnosed type 1 diabetes and from 50 to 100 control individuals. DASP was recently replaced by the Islet Autoantibody Standardization Program (IASP). A WHO standard for GAD65 and IA-2A has been established and allows laboratories to express results in common units.[113] Several workshops have been held. The first assay proficiency evaluation revealed poor performance for IAA among 23 laboratories,[105] and most laboratories continue to have less than acceptable sensitivity and/or specificity.[103] By contrast, good concordance among laboratories was observed for GAD65 and IA-2A,[113] and comparable (although not identical) results have been obtained with subsequent comparisons.[114] Ongoing harmonization is likely to enhance assay performance.

Autoantibody markers of immune destruction are present in 85% to 90% of individuals with immune-mediated diabetes when fasting hyperglycemia is initially detected.[1] Approximately 5% to 10% of white adult patients who have the type 2 diabetes phenotype also have islet cell autoantibodies, particularly to GAD65. This condition has been termed *latent autoimmune diabetes of adulthood* (LADA) (previously termed *type 1.5 diabetes* or *slow-onset diabetes in adults*).[115] Up to 1% to 2% of healthy individuals have a single autoantibody and are at low risk of developing immune-mediated diabetes. Because the prevalence of immune-mediated diabetes is low (~0.3% in the general population in most countries), the positive predictive value of a single autoantibody will be extremely low. A recent study measured IAA, GAD65, and IA-2 in 13,387 children who were at high risk for type 1 diabetes and followed them for 15 years.[116] The number of autoantibodies predicted development of type 1 diabetes, ranging from 10% for one autoantibody to almost 100% if multiple autoantibodies were present. Autoantibodies were not required for diabetes because 0.2% of autoantibody-negative children progressed to type 1 diabetes. The time interval from seroconversion to onset of disease varied from weeks to 18 years.[116] Screening for islet autoantibodies is controversial[44,110] because no acceptable therapy has been documented to reliably prevent or delay the clinical onset of diabetes in islet cell autoantibody-positive individuals.[112]

Although several agents can prevent or reverse type 1 diabetes in mouse models, these approaches have not been successful in humans.[117] Nevertheless, several clinical trials to intervene in the natural history of type 1 are being actively pursued.[81,100,118-120] Therapy is approached at three different stages. Primary prevention is directed at individuals with increased genetic risk who have no signs of autoimmunity or disease. The studies have to be conducted in infancy prior to the development of autoantibodies, and safety is crucial because only a small proportion of participants will develop diabetes. Interventions are predominantly dietary—for example, hydrolyzed casein (avoiding cows' milk), omega-3 fatty acid supplementation, or vitamin D supplementation. Secondary prevention is targeted at individuals with persistent islet autoantibodies. Most strategies focus on immunosuppressive therapy to attenuate the autoimmune response. These can be divided into autoantigen-specific therapies (such as insulin [oral or nasal], alum-formulated recombinant GAD65, or HLA peptides) and nonautoantigen-specific therapies (such as Bacillus Calmette-Guerin [BCG] vaccine, cyclosporine, anti-CD3 monoclonal antibodies, or anti-CD20 monoclonal antibodies). Tertiary prevention or intervention trials recruit patients newly diagnosed with type 1 diabetes where the objective is to preserve residual β-cell function (assessed by measuring C-peptide concentrations in the blood). Strategies include autoantigen-specific therapies, such as proinsulin peptide, and nonautoantigen-specific therapies, such as daclizumab (humanized IgG1 that binds to IL-2 receptor on T cells), rituximab, anakinra (IL-1β receptor antagonist), abatacept (fusion protein of cytotoxic T-lymphocyte protein 4 and immunoglobulin [CTLA4-Ig]), or antithymocyte globulin. Unfortunately, none of the secondary prevention or intervention trials or any of the immunosuppressive agents has preserved β-cell function in the long term. Some experts posit that monotherapy will be insufficient and therapies that combine immunomodulation using an autoantigen with immunosuppressive therapy are necessary.

Genetics

Susceptibility to type 1 diabetes is inherited,[121] but the mode of inheritance is complex and has not been defined. It is a multigenic trait, and the major locus is the major histocompatibility complex on chromosome 6. At least 11 other loci on 9 chromosomes also contribute, with the regulatory region of the insulin gene *INS* on chromosome 11p15 being an important locus. The human leukocyte antigen (HLA)-DQ and -DR genetic factors are by far the most important determinants for risk of type 1 diabetes.[44,122,123] The concordance rate between identical twins is approximately 30%. Approximately 95% of whites with type 1 diabetes express HLA-DR3 or HLA-DR4 histocompatibility antigens. However, up to 40% of the nondiabetic population also express these alleles. In contrast, the HLA-DQB1*0602 allele significantly decreases the risk of type 1 diabetes. HLA typing can indicate absolute risk of diabetes.[44] The risk of a sibling developing diabetes is 1%, 5%, and 10% to 20% if the number of haplotypes shared is none, one, and two, respectively. However, only 10% of patients with type 1 diabetes have an affected first-degree relative. More than 40 non-HLA-susceptibility gene markers have been confirmed, but these have smaller effects than HLA.[122] Non-HLA genetic factors that increase risk include the insulin gene *(INS)*, cytotoxic T-lymphocyte-associated protein 4 *(CTLA4)*, and protein tyrosine phosphatase nonreceptor type 22 (lymphoid) *(PTPN22)*.[44,122,123] The multiplicity of independent chromosomal regions associated with a predisposition to type 1 diabetes suggests that other susceptibility genes will be identified. Routine measurement of genetic markers is not of value at this time for the diagnosis or management of patients with type 1 diabetes.[44]

Environment

Reports describe that environmental factors are involved in initiating diabetes. Viruses, such as rubella, mumps, enterovirus, and Coxsackie virus B, have been implicated.[124] It seems likely that autoimmunity to β-cells is initiated by a viral protein (that shares amino acid sequence with a β-cell protein) or some other environmental insult. Genetic susceptibility and other host factors (eg, HLA type) determine the progression of the β-cell destruction. Epidemiological studies have implicated early exposure to cows' milk as a trigger of type 1 diabetes. This model is contentious and has been debated for decades.[125]

PATHOGENESIS OF TYPE 2 DIABETES MELLITUS

At least two major identifiable pathological defects have been reported in patients with type 2 diabetes.[126,127] One is a decreased ability of insulin to act on peripheral tissue. This is called *insulin resistance* and is thought by many to be the primary underlying pathologic process. The other is *β-cell dysfunction,* which is an inability of the pancreas to produce sufficient insulin to compensate for the insulin resistance. Thus a relative deficiency of insulin occurs early in the disease and absolute insulin deficiency late in the disease. The debate over whether type 2 diabetes is due primarily to a defect in β-cell secretion or to peripheral resistance to insulin, or to both, has been raging for decades. Data are available to support the concept that insulin resistance is the primary defect, preceding the derangement in insulin secretion and clinical diabetes by as much as 20 years.[126,128] Despite the lack of consensus, it is clear that type 2 diabetes mellitus is an extremely heterogeneous disease, and no single cause is adequate to explain the progression from normal glucose tolerance to diabetes. The fundamental molecular defects in insulin resistance and insulin secretion result from a combination of environmental and genetic factors.

Loss of β Cell Function

Increased β-cell demand induced by insulin resistance is ultimately associated with progressive loss of β-cell function that is necessary for the development of fasting hyperglycemia.[129] The major defect is a loss of glucose-induced insulin release (see Fig. 57.4), which is termed *selective glucose unresponsiveness.* Hyperglycemia appears to render the β-cells increasingly unresponsive to glucose (called glucotoxicity), and the degree of dysfunction correlates with both glucose concentration and duration of hyperglycemia. Restoration of euglycemia rapidly resolves the defect. Increased free fatty acids in serum have also been implicated in β-cell failure (lipotoxicity).[130] Other insulin secretory abnormalities in type 2 diabetes include disruption of the normal pulsatile release of insulin and an increased ratio of plasma proinsulin to insulin.[70] The number of β-cells is also reduced in patients with type 2 diabetes.

Insulin Resistance

Insulin resistance is defined as "a decreased biological response to normal concentrations of circulating insulin";[131] it is found in obese, nondiabetic individuals and in patients with type 2 diabetes. The underlying pathophysiologic defect(s) has (have) not been identified, but insulin resistance is usually attributed to a defect in insulin action. Measurement of insulin resistance in a routine clinical setting is difficult, and surrogate measures—namely, fasting insulin concentration or the euglycemic insulin clamp[132]—are used to provide an indirect assessment of insulin function. The euglycemic clamp is performed in the hospital under close supervision. The subject receives a constant intravenous infusion of insulin in one arm with concurrent intravenous infusion of variable amounts of glucose in the other arm to maintain blood glucose at a normal fasting concentration. A broad clinical spectrum of insulin resistance ranges from euglycemia (with marked increase in endogenous insulin) to hyperglycemia (despite large doses of exogenous insulin). Several rare clinical syndromes are also associated with insulin resistance. The prototype is the type A insulin resistance syndrome, which is characterized by hyperinsulinemia, acanthosis nigricans, and ovarian hyperandrogenism.

The insulin resistance syndrome (also known as syndrome X or the metabolic syndrome) is a constellation of associated clinical and laboratory findings, consisting of insulin resistance, hyperinsulinemia, obesity, dyslipidemia (high triglyceride and low high-density lipoprotein [HDL] cholesterol), and hypertension.[133] Individuals with this syndrome are at increased risk for cardiovascular disease. Several different definitions of the metabolic syndrome have been proposed by different organizations. Some consensus was reached in 2009, except for waist circumference. The metabolic syndrome is diagnosed if an individual meets three or more of the following criteria:[134,135]

- Increased waist circumference; population- and country-specific—for example, Europe, Canada, and the United States: greater than 35 inches (>88 cm) (women) or greater than 40 inches (>102 cm) (men)
- Triglycerides greater than 150 mg/dL (>1.7 mmol/L)
- HDL cholesterol less than 51 mg/dL (1.3 mmol/L) (women) or less than 39 mg/dL (1.0 mmol/L) (men)
- Blood pressure greater than or equal to 130/85 mm Hg
- Fasting plasma glucose 100 mg/dL or greater (≥5.6 mmol/L)

The concept of the "metabolic syndrome" has been questioned by several experts, including the person who first described it[136] and major clinical diabetes organizations.[137] A WHO Expert Consultation concluded that while the metabolic syndrome may be useful as an educational concept, it has limited practical utility for diagnosis and management, and further efforts to redefine it are inappropriate.[138]

Environment

Environmental factors, such as diet and exercise, are important determinants in the pathogenesis of type 2 diabetes. Convincing evidence links obesity to the development of type 2 diabetes, but the association is complex. Although 60% to 80% of patients with type 2 diabetes are obese, diabetes develops in less than 15% of obese individuals. In contrast, virtually all obese subjects, even those with normal carbohydrate tolerance, have hyperinsulinemia and are insulin resistant. Other factors, such as family history of type 2 diabetes (genetic predisposition), the duration of obesity, and the distribution of fat are important. Nevertheless, the rising prevalence of diabetes is believed to be a consequence of the increase in obesity (defined as a body mass index ≥30 kg/m^2), which was reported to be 26.7% in US adults in 2009.[139] Evaluation of 84,941 healthy women after 16 years in the Nurses' Health Study revealed that obesity was the most important predictor of type 2 diabetes.[140] Compared with women with body mass indices less than 23, the relative risks of developing diabetes were 38.8 and 20.1 with body mass indices 35 or greater and 30 to 34.9, respectively. It is important to note that intervention can delay or prevent the onset of type 2 diabetes. Two randomized studies documented that lifestyle changes (weight reduction and exercise) in individuals with IGT reduced the incidence of type 2 diabetes.[141,142] Although the weight loss was modest (5% to 7%), the rate of progression to type 2 diabetes was reduced by 58% in both studies. This observation has been validated by several other studies.[143]

An inverse relationship has been noted between the degree of physical activity and the prevalence of type 2 diabetes.

For every 500 kcal increase in daily energy expenditure, a 6% decrease in age-adjusted risk of type 2 diabetes occurs.[144] This effect is independent of both body weight and a parental history of diabetes. The mechanism of the protective effect of exercise is thought to be increased sensitivity to insulin in skeletal muscle and adipose tissue.

Type 2 Diabetes Susceptibility Genes

It is widely acknowledged that genetic factors contribute to the development of type 2 diabetes.[128] For example, the concordance rate for type 2 diabetes in identical twins approaches 100%. Type 2 diabetes is 10 times more likely to occur in an obese person with a diabetic parent than in an equally obese person without a diabetic family history. However, the mode of inheritance is unknown, and type 2 diabetes has been described as a "geneticist's nightmare."[145] Many less common diseases (eg, cystic fibrosis, Duchenne muscular dystrophy) are caused by mutations at a single locus. More common diseases, such as diabetes mellitus, schizophrenia, atherosclerosis, hypertension, and osteoporosis, are not inherited according to simple Mendelian rules. These conditions are genetically more complex, and multiple genetic factors interact with exogenous influences (such as environmental factors) to produce the phenotype.

Numerous mutations of the insulin receptor gene, *INSR*, have been identified.[131] Many patients with these defects have extreme insulin resistance, but the mutations are exceptionally rare and usually are found in only one patient or a single family. A small number of patients have been identified with mutations of substrates for the insulin receptor (eg, IRS-1) that cause diabetes. Few mutations have been described in other potential candidate genes, including those coding for GLUT4 and glycogen synthase.

Multiple factors complicate the search for susceptibility genes in type 2 diabetes.[126] A variety of approaches have produced several genes that are associated with type 2 diabetes. Recent genome-wide association studies (GWAS) have substantially contributed to our understanding of the genetic architecture of type 2 diabetes, with more than 60 genetic loci now identified.[146,147] Most of these genetic loci are associated with the insulin secretion pathway, rather than with insulin resistance. Despite considerable effort to identify the genetic basis of type 2 diabetes mellitus, genetic defects identified to date account for only approximately 5% of patients with type 2 diabetes. Therefore the gene or genes causing common forms of type 2 diabetes remain unknown. Moreover, the risk alleles in these loci all have relatively small effects (odds ratios, 1.1 to 1.3). Combined analysis of 48 different type 2 risk loci did not significantly affect the time from diagnosis to prescription of the first drug.[148]

Maturity-Onset Diabetes of the Young

Initial success in the search for diabetogenes was seen in maturity-onset diabetes of the young (MODY), a rare group of disorders characterized by nonketotic diabetes.[21,149,150] Although some phenotypically resemble type 2 diabetes, MODY usually occurs at a young age (often <25 years) in nonobese patients with diabetes who have a family history of diabetes. The clinical spectrum of MODY is broad, ranging from asymptomatic hyperglycemia to an acute presentation. Thirteen genes are associated with this disorder. MODY2 results from mutations in the gene that encodes glucokinase (an enzyme that phosphorylates glucose in the β-cell), leading to partial deficiency of insulin secretion. Most of the other MODYs are caused by mutations in the genes that encode transcription factors that regulate expression of genes in pancreatic β-cells, resulting in impaired insulin synthesis or secretion or a reduced β-cell mass. MODY mutations have substitution, deletion, or insertion of nucleotides in the coding regions of the genes. These mutations are detected by PCR. OGTT, islet autoantibodies, and C-peptide may be helpful in differentiating MODY from type 1 or type 2 diabetes,[150] but genetic testing is required to establish the diagnosis of MODY.

POINTS TO REMEMBER

Type 2 Diabetes

- Type 2 diabetes is the most common form of diabetes, accounting for approximately 90% of all cases.
- The onset is insidious, and patients have minimal symptoms.
- Many patients have irreversible complications at the time of diagnosis.
- Patients exhibit both insulin resistance and inadequate insulin secretion.
- Insulin resistance is very difficult to measure and at diagnosis patient may have normal, increased, or decreased insulin concentrations.
- The molecular defects are a consequence of both genetic and environmental factors.
- The gene (or genes) that cause the common forms of type 2 diabetes have not been identified.
- Obesity is linked to the development of type 2 diabetes, and lifestyle changes (weight loss and exercise) can delay the onset of the disease,

DIAGNOSIS

For many years the diagnosis of diabetes mellitus was dependent solely on the demonstration of hyperglycemia (Box 57.3). In 2009, an International Expert Committee recommended that diabetes be diagnosed by measurement of hemoglobin A1c (HbA_{1c}), which reflects long-term blood glucose concentrations[29] (for additional information, see "Glycated Hemoglobin" section in this chapter). For type 1 diabetes, the diagnosis is usually easy because hyperglycemia appears abruptly, is severe, and is accompanied by serious metabolic derangements. Diagnosis of type 2 diabetes may be difficult because hyperglycemia often is not severe enough for the patient to notice symptoms of diabetes. Nevertheless, the risk of complications makes it important to identify people with the disease.

The diagnostic criteria recommended in 1979 included the following:

- Classic symptoms of diabetes with unequivocal increase in plasma glucose
- FPG greater than or equal to 140 mg/dL (7.8 mmol/L) on more than one occasion
- A 2-hour and one other postload glucose concentration greater than or equal to 200 mg/dL (11.1 mmol/L) during an OGTT[15]

These criteria were widely adopted but are imperfect. The OGTT is more sensitive for diagnosis than fasting glucose early in the course of type 2 diabetes, resulting in lack of

BOX 57.3 Criteria for the Diagnosis of Diabetes Mellitus

Any one of the following is diagnostic:

1. Hemoglobin A1c (HbA_{1c}) 6.5% (48 mmol/mol)* or greater, OR
2. Fasting plasma glucose (FPG) 126 mg/dL (7.0 mmol/L)† or greater, OR
3. Symptoms of hyperglycemia and casual plasma glucose 200 mg/dL (11.1 mmol/L)‡ or greater, OR
4. Two-hour plasma glucose 200 mg/dL (11.1 mmol/L) or greater during an oral glucose tolerance test (OGTT)§

In the absence of unequivocal hyperglycemia, these criteria should be confirmed by repeating the same test on a different day. Mixing different methods to diagnose diabetes should be avoided.

*The test should be performed in a laboratory using a method that is NGSP-certified and standardized to the DCCT assay. Point-of-care assays should not be used for diagnosis.
†Fasting is defined as no calorie intake for at least 8 hours.
‡Casual is defined as any time of day without regard to time since the last meal. The classic symptoms of hyperglycemia include polyuria, polydipsia, and unexplained weight loss.
§The OGTT should be performed as described by the World Health Organization (WHO), using a glucose load containing the equivalent of 75 g of anhydrous glucose dissolved in water.
Modified from the American Diabetes Association. Standards of medical care in diabetes—2010. *Diabetes Care* 2010;33(Suppl 1): S11–61.

BOX 57.4 Factors Other Than Diabetes That Influence the Oral Glucose Tolerance Test

Patient Preparation
Duration of fast
Prior carbohydrate intake
Medications (eg, thiazides, oral contraceptives, corticosteroids)
Trauma
Intercurrent illness
Age
Activity
Weight

Administration of Glucose
Form of glucose (anhydrous or monohydrate)
Quantity of glucose ingested
Volume in which administered
Rate of ingestion

During the Test
Posture
Anxiety
Caffeine
Smoking
Activity
Time of day
Sample preservation

equivalence between fasting and 2-hour glucose values. Virtually all persons with an FPG concentration of 140 mg/dL (≥7.8 mmol/L) or greater have 2-hour glucose of 200 mg/dL (≥11.1 mmol/L) or greater in an OGTT. In contrast, in persons without previously identified diabetes, fasting glucose of 140 mg/dL (≥7.8 mmol/L) or greater is present in only 25% of those who have 2-hour glucose of 200 mg/dL (≥11.1 mmol/L) or greater. To address these and other discrepancies, the diagnostic criteria were revised in 1997 (see Box 57.3).[1,151] The major modification was lowering the diagnostic threshold for fasting glucose from 140 to 126 mg/dL (7.8 to 7.0 mmol/L) to better identify individuals at risk of retinopathy and nephropathy. The lower cutoff was suggested to provide earlier diagnosis of diabetes, with consequent earlier therapeutic intervention.[151]

Fasting Plasma Glucose Concentrations

FPG concentrations of 126 mg/dL (7.0 mmol/L) or greater on more than one occasion are diagnostic of diabetes mellitus (see Box 57.3). The diagnosis of most cases of diabetes mellitus can be established with this criterion. However, some investigators believe that fasting hyperglycemia may be a relatively late development in the course of type 2 diabetes, delaying the diagnosis and leading to underestimation of the prevalence of diabetes mellitus in the population.[152] Complications of diabetes, such as retinopathy, proteinuria, and neuromuscular disease, are present in approximately 30% of patients at clinical diagnosis of type 2 diabetes, and onset of type 2 diabetes probably occurs at least 4 to 7 years before clinical diagnosis. Screening of high-risk individuals for diabetes is now recommended by the ADA[1,26,153] and a number of other clinical organizations. The ADA recommends that fasting glucose should be measured in all asymptomatic persons at age 45 (or younger in subjects at increased risk), with follow-up testing every 3 years (see discussion later in this chapter). However, no published evidence indicates that treatment based on screening is efficacious.

Oral Glucose Tolerance Test

Serial measurement of plasma glucose before and after a specific amount of glucose given orally should provide a standard method by which to evaluate individuals and establish values for healthy and diseased subjects. Although more sensitive than FPG determinations, glucose tolerance testing is affected by multiple factors that result in *poor reproducibility* (Box 57.4).[154,155] Moreover, approximately 20% of OGTTs fall into the nondiagnostic category (eg, only one blood sample exhibits increased glucose concentration).[155] Unless results are grossly abnormal initially, the OGTT should be performed on two separate occasions to establish the diagnosis of diabetes.

The following conditions should be met before an OGTT is performed: discontinue, when possible, medications known to affect glucose tolerance; perform in the morning after 3 days of unrestricted diet (containing at least 150 g of carbohydrate per day) and activity; and perform the test after a 10- to 16-hour fast only in ambulatory outpatients (bed rest impairs glucose tolerance), who should remain seated during the test without smoking cigarettes. Glucose tolerance testing should not be performed on hospitalized, acutely ill, or inactive patients. The test should begin between 7:00 a.m. and 9:00 a.m. Venous plasma glucose should be measured fasting, and then 2 hours after an oral glucose load. For nonpregnant adults, the recommended load is 75 g, which may not be a maximum stimulus;[15] for children 1.75 g/kg, up to 75 g maximum is given. The glucose should be dissolved in 300 mL of water and ingested over 5 minutes. A commercial, more palatable form of glucose may be ingested, but whether the anhydrous or monohydrate form of glucose should be used is still in question.[156]

An OGTT is not widely used in clinical practice for the diagnosis of diabetes in the United States owing to its lack of reproducibility and inconvenience. The sensitivity of FPG concentrations is lower than the OGTT for diagnosing diabetes, and some authors claim that the OGTT better identifies patients at risk for developing complications of diabetes. An FPG value of less than 100 mg/dL (5.6 mmol/L) or a random glucose concentration of less than 140 mg/dL (7.8 mmol/L) is sufficient to rule out the diagnosis of diabetes mellitus. An OGTT is indicated in the following situations:

- Diagnosis of GDM (discussed later)
- Initial postpartum screening of women with GDM for type 2 diabetes (discussed later)
- Diagnosis of IGT. This remains controversial. Individuals with IGT have increased risk of cardiovascular disease, but many of them do not have IFG by ADA criteria.[64]
- Evaluation of a patient with unexplained nephropathy, neuropathy, or retinopathy, with random glucose concentration less than 140 mg/dL (7.8 mmol/L). Abnormal results in this setting do not necessarily denote a cause-and-effect relationship, and other diseases must be ruled out.
- Population studies for epidemiologic data

As mentioned earlier, current guidelines advocate the use of HbA_{1c} for diagnosis of diabetes in nonpregnant individuals.[157]

AT A GLANCE

Diagnosis of Diabetes

Diabetes is diagnosed if at least one of the following criteria is met:

- Fasting plasma glucose (FPG) 126 mg/dL (7.0 mmol/L) or greater
- Two-hour plasma glucose 200 mg/dL (11.1 mmol/L) or greater during an oral glucose tolerance test
- HbA_{1c} 6.5% (48 mmol/mol) or greater

The same test should be repeated on a different day to confirm the diagnosis.

In individuals with symptoms of hyperglycemia, diabetes can be diagnosed if casual (nonfasting) plasma glucose is 200 mg/dL (11.1 mmol/L) or greater; repeating the assay is unnecessary in symptomatic individuals.

Glucose should be measured in venous plasma.

Glycolysis should be minimized by placing the tube immediately after collection in an ice-water slurry and separating plasma from cells within 30 minutes. If that cannot be achieved, blood should be collected in a tube containing a rapidly effective glycolysis inhibitor such as a citrate buffer.

Plasma glucose and HbA_{1c} should be measured in an accredited laboratory; point-of-care devices are not suitable for screening or diagnosis.

HbA_{1c} analysis should be performed using a method that is NGSP-certified and standardized to the DCCT assay.

Intravenous Glucose Tolerance Test

Poor absorption of orally administered glucose may result in a "flat" tolerance curve. Some patients are unable to tolerate a large oral carbohydrate load or may have altered gastric physiology (eg, after gastric resection). In these patients, an intravenous glucose tolerance test may be performed to eliminate factors related to the rate of glucose absorption. In addition, measurement of the first-phase insulin response can identify the subgroup of individuals with increased concentrations of multiple autoantibodies who are at greatest risk of progression to type 1 diabetes.[158]

Preparation of patients is the same as for the OGTT. The dose of glucose is 0.5 g/kg of body weight (maximum 35 g), given as a 25 g/dL solution. The dose is administered intravenously over 3 minutes ± 15 seconds, and blood is collected every 10 minutes after the midinjection time for 1 hour. A single forearm vein cannula may be used for infusion and sampling, but it should be flushed with saline after the glucose is infused, and dead space should be cleared with several volumes of blood before each sample is drawn. If insulin assays are performed, a specimen is also obtained 5 minutes after the start of the injection. Blood glucose concentrations decrease in an exponential manner, and the rate of glucose disappearance can be calculated from the formula $K = 70/t_{1/2}$, where $t_{1/2}$ is the number of minutes required for the blood glucose value to decrease to one-half of the 10-minute value, and K is the rate of disappearance of blood glucose, expressed as %/min. The glucose values are plotted on a log scale versus time on the abscissa. The best-fitting straight line is drawn through the points, and the time (in minutes) for the glucose concentration to decrease by 50% ($t_{1/2}$) is read. In healthy individuals, K usually exceeds 1.5%; values less than 1.0% are considered diagnostic of diabetes. A poor correlation is found between the results of intravenous and oral glucose tolerance tests.[159] Similar to oral glucose tolerance, intravenous glucose tolerance deteriorates with age.

In the formula $K = 70/t_{1/2}$, the value of 70 is derived from the logarithmic nature of the decrease in glucose concentration over time. The concentration of glucose at 10 minutes will be twice that of the value obtained from the plot $t_{1/2}$. Using natural logarithms, the rate of decrease in glucose concentration, expressed as %/min *(K)*, is given by

$$K = 100\,(\ln 2 - \ln 1)/t_{1/2} = 69.3/t_{1/2} \cong 70/t_{1/2}$$

The main indication for the intravenous glucose tolerance test is in clinical research to evaluate the first-phase insulin response to glucose (see Fig. 57.4).[160] The test is performed as described earlier, but samples are drawn as follows: two baseline samples 5 minutes apart (the latter immediately before infusion) and samples 1, 3, 5, and 10 minutes after the end of the glucose infusion. The first-phase insulin release is usually measured by the sum of the insulin concentrations 1 and 3 minutes after the glucose bolus. Alternatively, the 0- to 10-minute incremental insulin area may be used. Analogous to the OGTT, the intravenous glucose tolerance test has poor reproducibility.

GESTATIONAL DIABETES MELLITUS

Normal pregnancy is associated with increased insulin resistance, especially in the late second and third trimesters. Euglycemia is maintained by increased insulin secretion, with GDM developing in those women who fail to augment insulin sufficiently. Risk factors for GDM include a family history of diabetes in a first-degree relative, obesity, advanced maternal age, glycosuria, and selected adverse outcomes in a previous pregnancy (eg, stillbirth, macrosomia). Recommendations for screening and diagnosis were formulated in 1984 at the Second International Workshop-Conference on Gestational Diabetes Mellitus,[161] and were refined at the Third, Fourth, and Fifth International Workshop-Conferences in 1990, 1998, and 2007,[22] respectively. Despite these workshops, there is considerable disagreement regarding the approaches for screening and diagnosing GDM,[162] with wide variation among countries and often between diabetes and obstetric organizations in a single country.[163] Recommendations for screening range from none (ie, do not screen) to selective (ie, screen only high-risk women) to universal.[162] In addition, screening is performed by measuring glucose fasting, random (regardless of the time of the last meal), or after (usually 1 hour) ingesting oral glucose. An OGTT is usually used to establish the diagnosis. Most criteria for diagnosis of GDM are based on the 1964 O'Sullivan and Mahan recommendations, which were derived from 752 women who had a 3-hour OGTT.[164] If two or more of these values exceeded two SDs above the mean, GDM was diagnosed. The criteria are arbitrary and not related to adverse outcomes of the pregnancy; they predict postpartum development of diabetes. While the cutoffs have been altered in response to modifications in glucose measurements,[162,165] numerous influential clinical organizations continue to promulgate some form of these criteria. However, considerable differences are present among the recommendations. The major items of contention are the amount of the glucose load (75 g or 100 g), the duration of the test (2 hours or 3 hours), the specific cutoffs, and the number of high values necessary (one or two) (see Table 1 in reference 162).

A notable flaw in the GDM diagnostic criteria is that they have been based on the risk of future hyperglycemia, not on clinical sequelae. The Hyperglycemia and Adverse Pregnancy Outcome (HAPO) study was designed to address this deficiency. The objective of the HAPO study was to determine the relationship between maternal blood glucose concentrations and adverse pregnancy outcomes. The prospective, randomized multinational study included 23,316 women who had a 75-g OGTT at 24 to 32 weeks of gestation.[166] Primary outcomes were birth weight over the 90th percentile (macrosomia), primary cesarean section delivery, clinical neonatal hypoglycemia, and cord C-peptide over the 90th percentile (fetal hyperinsulinemia). The findings revealed that the risk of adverse maternal, fetal, and neonatal events increased continuously as a function of maternal glycemia, even within ranges previously considered normal for pregnancy.[166] Similar associations were observed between glycemia and secondary outcomes of the study—namely, preterm birth, shoulder dystocia, preeclampsia, and intensive neonatal care.[166] There were no thresholds at which risk increased (ie, no convenient cutoffs), and each of the three values in the OGTT had an independent contribution to adverse outcome.

To translate the HAPO results into clinical practice, the International Association of Diabetes and Pregnancy Study Groups (IADPSG) sponsored a workshop to develop recommendations for the diagnosis and classification of hyperglycemia in pregnancy.[167] The panel suggested that a 75-g OGTT be performed and a diagnosis of GDM be made if one or more of the following values is equaled or exceeded: FPG (92 mg/dL; 5.1 mmol/L), 1 hour (180 mg/dL; 10.0 mmol/L), and 2 hours (153 mg/dL; 8.5 mmol/L) (Box 57.5, one step). Because only one increased glucose value is required (as opposed to two for prior recommendations), the prevalence of GDM in the United States would rise from approximately 7% to approximately 18% (~250,000 to ~640,000 women per year). Similar increases are anticipated for other countries.

BOX 57.5 Screening for and Diagnosis of Gestational Diabetes Mellitus

One-Step

1. Perform in the morning after an overnight fast of at least 8 hours.
2. Measure fasting venous plasma glucose.
3. Give 75 g of glucose orally.
4. Measure plasma glucose hourly for 2 hours after glucose is given.
5. At least one value must meet or exceed the following:

	Glucose Concentration
Fasting	92 mg/dL (5.1 mmol/L)
1 hour	180 mg/dL (10.0 mmol/L)
2 hours	153 mg/dL (8.5 mmol/L)

Two-Step

Screening (Step 1)

1. Perform at between 24 and 28 weeks' gestation* in all pregnant women not previously diagnosed with diabetes.
2. Give 50 g oral glucose load without regard to time of day or time of last meal.
3. Measure venous plasma glucose at 1 hour.
4. If glucose is 140 mg/dL (7.8 mmol/L) or greater,† proceed to step 2 and perform glucose tolerance test.

Diagnosis (Step 2)

1. Perform in the morning after an overnight fast of at least 8 hours.
2. Measure fasting venous plasma glucose.
3. Give 100 g of glucose orally.
4. Measure plasma glucose hourly for 3 hours after glucose is given.
5. The diagnosis of GDM is made if at least two of the following four plasma glucose concentrations are met or exceeded:

	Carpenter/Coustan	or	NDDG
Fasting	95 mg/dL (5.3 mmol/L)		105 mg/dL (5.8 mmol/L)
1 h	180 mg/dL (10.0 mmol/L)		190 mg/dL (10.6 mmol/L)
2 h	155 mg/dL (8.6 mmol/L)		165 mg/dL (9.2 mmol/L)
3 h	140 mg/dL (7.8 mmol/L)		145 mg/dL (8.0 mmol/L)

*The WHO states that this test can be performed at any time during pregnancy.

†Some experts recommend a cutoff of 135 mg/dL (7.5 mmol/L) in high-risk ethnic minorities with a higher prevalence of GDM.

NDDG, National Diabetes Data Group.

Modified from the American Diabetes Association. Classification and diagnosis of diabetes. *Diabetes Care* 2015;38(Suppl 1):S8–16.

Although they are the first large-scale evidence-based guidelines for GDM that correlate maternal glucose concentrations to outcomes, the IADPSG recommendations are controversial. While adopted in several countries, including Canada, Germany, Italy, Japan, China, and Australia, as well as by the World Health Organization (WHO),[168] in the United States, it has been accepted by the ADA and the Endocrine Society, but not by the ACOG. Moreover, in 2013, an NIH Consensus Development Conference panel supported the continuation of the two-step approach.[169] The main reasons proffered for not switching to the IADPSG criteria are lack of evidence that the additional women identified will have improved outcomes (the HAPO study was observational) and the considerable cost to society incurred by the large increase in the number of individuals with GDM. Universal criteria to diagnose GDM remain elusive.[162]

While GDM is usually asymptomatic and not life-threatening to the mother, it is associated with an increased incidence of neonatal mortality and morbidity, including hypocalcemia, hypoglycemia, and macrosomia.[25,170] Maternal hyperglycemia causes the fetus to secrete more insulin, resulting in stimulation of fetal growth and macrosomia. Recognition is important because therapy can reduce perinatal morbidity and mortality.[171] Maternal complications include a high rate of cesarean delivery and hypertension. In addition, mothers with GDM are at significantly increased risk of subsequent diabetes, predominantly type 2. A metaanalysis and systematic review published in 2009 indicated that women with GDM have a sevenfold increased risk of developing type 2 diabetes compared with those who had a normoglycemic pregnancy.[172] The largest single study observed a 12.6-fold increased risk. The cumulative incidence of type 2 diabetes varies among populations, ranging from about 40% to 70%.[24] It rises markedly in the first 5 years and reaches a plateau after 10 years.

Distinct from GDM is pregnancy in a patient with preexisting diabetes (approximately 19,000 per annum in the United States). This is associated with an increased incidence of congenital malformation, but meticulous glycemic control during the first 8 weeks of pregnancy can significantly decrease the risk of congenital malformation.[173] Tight control results in an increased incidence of maternal hypoglycemia, which is teratogenic in animals but does not cause malformation in humans.[174]

Women with GDM should be screened for diabetes 6 to 12 weeks postpartum using nonpregnant OGTT criteria (see Box 57.3). (HbA_{1c} is not recommended because of the antepartum therapy for hyperglycemia.) If glucose values are normal, glycemia should be reassessed at least every 3 years using either glucose or HbA_{1c}.

CHRONIC COMPLICATIONS OF DIABETES MELLITUS

Pathogenesis

Patients with both type 1 and type 2 diabetes are at high risk for the development of chronic complications.[2,3] Diabetes-specific microvascular pathology in the retinae, renal glomeruli, and peripheral nerves produces retinopathy, nephropathy, and neuropathy. As a result of these microvascular complications, diabetes is the most frequent cause of new cases of blindness in the industrialized world in persons between 25 and 74 years and the leading cause of end-stage renal disease. Diabetes is also associated with a marked increase in atherosclerotic macrovascular disease involving cardiac, cerebral, and peripheral large vessels. The consequence is that patients with diabetes have a high rate of myocardial infarction (the major cause of mortality in diabetes), stroke, and limb amputation. Prospective clinical studies document a strong relationship between hyperglycemia and the development of microvascular complications.[175,176] Both hyperglycemia and insulin resistance appear to be important in the pathogenesis of macrovascular complications.[176-178]

Progress has been made in our understanding of the molecular mechanisms underlying derangements produced by hyperglycemia.[2,177,179] Several hypotheses have been proposed to explain how hyperglycemia causes the neural and vascular pathology. These include increased aldose reductase (or polyol pathway) flux; enhanced formation of advanced glycation end products (AGE); activation of protein kinase C; production of superoxide and other reactive oxygen species (ROS) by the mitochondrial electron transport chain; endoplasmic reticulum stress; increased hexosamine pathway flux; and activation of Src homology-2 domain-containing phosphatase-1 (SHP-1).[177,179] Inhibitors of each of these have been shown to ameliorate diabetes-induced abnormalities in cell culture and animal models.[177] Overproduction of superoxide by the mitochondrial electron transport chain integrates these four apparently disparate mechanisms.[177] Clinical trials are under way using novel therapies specifically directed at the signaling molecules (such as protein kinase C) or employing antioxidants to neutralize the effects of the oxidants.[180]

Effects of Intensive Therapy

Type 1 Diabetes

Although it had been theorized for many years that better glycemic control would decrease rates of long-term complications of diabetes mellitus, it was not until the publication of the Diabetes Control and Complications Trial (DCCT) in 1993[175] that this hypothesis was verified. The DCCT was a multicenter, randomized trial that compared the effects of intensive and conventional insulin therapy on the development and progression of complications in 1441 patients with type 1 diabetes. During the study period, which averaged 6.5 years, intensively managed patients maintained significantly lower mean blood glucose concentrations. Compared with conventional therapy, intensive therapy reduced the risk of retinopathy, nephropathy, and neuropathy by 40% to 75%.[175] Intensive therapy delayed the onset and slowed the progression of these three complications, regardless of age, gender, or duration of diabetes. The absolute risks of retinopathy and nephropathy were proportional to the mean HbA_{1c} (discussed later in the chapter). Although intensive therapy also reduced the development of hypercholesterolemia, major cardiovascular and peripheral vascular diseases were not significantly decreased in the initial assessment. However, analysis after 17 years of follow-up showed that the incidence of cardiovascular disease was 42% lower in the intensively treated group.[181] This landmark study has had a considerable impact on therapeutic goals and comprehension of the pathogenesis of complications of diabetes.

At the conclusion of the DCCT, 95% of participants enrolled in the long-term follow-up study, termed the Epidemiology of Diabetes Interventions and Complications

(EDIC). Five years after the end of the DCCT, no difference in metabolic control (assessed by HbA_{1c} measurements) was noted between the former conventional and intensively treated groups. Nevertheless, further progression of retinopathy, neuropathy, and nephropathy was significantly lower in the former intensive group, demonstrating that the beneficial effects of intensive treatment persisted for at least 19 years beyond the period of strictest intervention.[182-184] The molecular mechanism responsible for this effect, termed *molecular memory*, has not been identified.

Type 2 Diabetes

The role of hyperglycemia in the development of complications in individuals with type 2 diabetes was established in the United Kingdom Prospective Diabetes Study (UKPDS).[176] The UKPDS was a major randomized, multicenter clinical study that included 5102 patients with newly diagnosed type 2 diabetes who were followed for an average of 10 years. Analogous to the findings of the DCCT, the UKPDS demonstrated in patients with type 2 diabetes that intensive treatment diminishes by approximately 10% to 40% the development of microvascular complications.[176] Intensive treatment also decreased the rate of occurrence of macrovascular complications. Although the reduction was not statistically significant initially, follow-up 10 years after the study ended showed a significant reduction in myocardial infarction among patients who had received intensive therapy.[185] Like the EDIC findings, long-term benefits for microvascular complications were observed with follow-up of patients in the UKPDS despite loss of glycemic separation between intensive and standard cohorts after the study ended.[185] An important caveat of both the DCCT and the UKPDS was that intensive therapy produced a threefold increase in the incidence of severe hypoglycemia.[175,176]

ROLE OF THE CLINICAL LABORATORY IN DIABETES MELLITUS

The clinical laboratory has a vital role in both the diagnosis and management of diabetes mellitus.[44] Some of the important variables assayed are outlined in Table 57.2. In 2002, the National Academy of Clinical Biochemistry (referred to as the NACB) published evidence-based guidelines for laboratory analysis in diabetes mellitus.[64] These guidelines were reviewed by the Professional Practice Committee of the ADA and were consistent in those areas where the ADA also published recommendations. Specific recommendations for laboratory testing based on published data or derived from expert consensus are presented.[64] An updated version of these guidelines was published in 2011.[44] The revised guidelines were also published as a Position Statement by the ADA.[186,187] A brief overview is presented here.

Diagnosis

Preclinical (Screening)

Type 1 Diabetes. Evidence from animal studies suggests that immune intervention therapy before the appearance of clinical symptoms can delay or prevent type 1 diabetes. Results from human studies have been disappointing. Notwithstanding the lack of success, a number of large clinical trials are under way to assess a variety of therapeutic strategies designed to delay or prevent the onset of type 1 diabetes.[100,118-120] The Diabetes Prevention Trial-Type 1 (DPT-1) screened 84,228 relatives of patients with diabetes for islet cell antibodies.[188] Half of the 339 individuals deemed to be at high (greater than 50%) risk for disease were randomly assigned to low-dose insulin therapy. Unfortunately, neither insulin injections nor oral insulin delayed the development of type 1 diabetes.[188,189] Despite the negative results, the ADA encourages screening of first-degree relatives of patients with type 1 diabetes by measuring immune-related markers (autoantibodies), provided that individuals who have positive screening results are referred to defined research studies.[190] Until effective intervention therapy becomes available and cost-effective screening strategies are developed for young children, screening for antibodies is not recommended outside of prospective clinical studies.[44]

Some experts have proposed that testing for islet cell autoantibodies may be useful in the following situations: to identify a subset of adults initially thought to have type 2 diabetes but who have islet cell autoantibody markers of type 1 diabetes and progress to insulin dependency; to screen nondiabetic family members who wish to donate a kidney or part of their pancreas for transplantation; to screen women with GDM to identify those at high risk of progression to type 1 diabetes; and to distinguish type 1 from type 2 diabetes in children to institute insulin therapy at the time of diagnosis.[44,64] Wide variability in clinical practice has been noted regarding the use of islet cell autoantibodies. Proponents argue that the results of autoantibody assays are clinically useful, whereas others point to lack of evidence. Although some clinicians, particularly those who treat pediatric patients, use autoantibody assays, clinical studies are necessary to provide outcome data to validate the clinical use of autoantibody assays.

Screening by determining HLA type is not currently warranted, except in research studies.[44] For selected diabetic syndromes—for example, neonatal diabetes—valuable information can now be obtained with definition of disease-associated mutations.[44] A decrease in glucose-stimulated insulin secretion is the first functional abnormality in both type 1 and type 2 diabetes. Nevertheless, tests of insulin secretion are not currently recommended for routine clinical use.

Type 2 Diabetes. Screening of asymptomatic individuals for type 2 diabetes has been the subject of much controversy.[153] The ADA, which previously did not support screening, now advocates screening in all asymptomatic individuals over the age of 45 years.[191,192] Prior screening recommendations were that FPG or the 2-hour OGTT could be used.[26] Current guidelines include the use of HbA_{1c} for screening.[157] If the HbA_{1c} is less than 5.7% (39 mmol/mol) or the FPG is less than 100 mg/dL (5.6 mmol/L), testing should be repeated at 3-year intervals. Testing may be considered at a younger age or may be carried out more frequently in individuals at increased risk of diabetes (eg, family history, members of certain ethnic groups).[191] The rising incidence of type 2 diabetes in adolescents has led to the recommendation for screening overweight youths (BMI >85th percentile) with any two of the following risk factors:

- They have a family history of type 2 diabetes in first- or second-degree relatives.
- They belong to a certain race and/or ethnic group.

TABLE 57.2 **Role of the Laboratory in the Management of Diabetes Mellitus**

Diagnosis	
Preclinical (Screening)	Immunologic markers
	ICA
	IAA
	GAD antibodies
	Protein tyrosine phosphatase antibodies (IA-2)
	Zinc transporter ZnT8 antibodies
	Genetic markers (eg, human leukocyte antigen [HLA])
	Insulin secretion
	Fasting
	Pulses
	In response to a glucose challenge
	Blood glucose
	Oral glucose tolerance test (OGTT)
	Hemoglobin A1c (HbA_{1c})
Clinical	Blood glucose
	Oral glucose tolerance test (OGTT)
	HbA_{1c}
	Ketones (urine and blood)
	Other (eg, insulin, C-peptide, stimulation tests)
Management	
Acute	Glucose
	Blood
	Urine
	Ketones
	Blood
	Urine
	Acid-base status (pH ([H^+]), bicarbonate)
	Lactate
	Other abnormalities related to cellular dehydration or therapy (eg, potassium, sodium, phosphate, osmolality)
Chronic	Glucose
	Blood (fasting, random)
	Urine
	Glycated proteins
	HbA_{1c}
	Fructosamine
	Glycated serum albumin
	1, 5-Anhydroglucitol (1,5-AG)
	Urinary protein
	Albuminuria (previously termed *microalbuminuria*)
	Proteinuria
	Evaluation of complications (eg, creatinine, cholesterol, triglycerides)
	Evaluation of pancreas transplant (C-peptide, insulin)
	Eligibility for insulin pump (C-peptide)

- They have signs of insulin resistance or conditions associated with insulin resistance.
- There is a maternal history of diabetes or GDM during the child's gestation.[64,191,193]

Testing should be done every 3 years starting at 10 years of age. Rationales for screening are that at least 33% of individuals with type 2 diabetes are undiagnosed, complications are often present by the time of diagnosis, and treatment delays the onset of complications.[153] Notwithstanding these recommendations, no published evidence indicates that treatment based on screening has value. However, a recent systematic review identified 16 trials that consistently found that treatment of IFG or IGT was associated with delayed progression to diabetes.[194]

Clinical

The laboratory diagnosis of diabetes is made exclusively by the demonstration of hyperglycemia, by measuring venous plasma glucose or HbA_{1c}. Although other tests (eg, C-peptide, insulin analysis) have been proposed to assist in the diagnosis and classification of the disease, these do not at present have a role outside of research studies.[44]

Management

Acute

In diabetic ketoacidosis,[195] hyperosmolar nonketotic coma,[196] and hypoglycemia, the clinical laboratory has an essential role in both the diagnosis of the condition and monitoring of therapy. Several analytes are frequently measured to guide clinicians in treatment regimens to restore euglycemia and correct other metabolic disturbances. The metabolic abnormalities of these conditions are beyond the scope of this book, and interested readers are referred to recent reviews[195,196] or a standard textbook of medicine. The NACB guidelines[44] also provide information on the tests that are used.

Chronic

The DCCT[175] and UKPDS[176] studies documented a correlation between blood glucose concentrations and the development of long-term complications of diabetes. Measurement of glucose and glycated proteins provides an index of short- and long-term glycemic control, respectively (see section on glycated proteins later in the chapter). Detection and monitoring of complications are achieved by assaying serum creatinine and lipids and assaying urine for albuminuria. The success of newer therapies, such as islet cell or pancreas transplantation, can be monitored by measuring serum C-peptide or insulin concentrations.

SELF-MONITORING OF BLOOD GLUCOSE

Diabetic patients, especially those who need insulin therapy, require careful monitoring to maintain control of blood glucose. This has become particularly important with the results of the DCCT[175] and the recommendation that patients use intensive insulin therapy to achieve nearly normal glycemia. These regimens include multiple daily insulin injections, insulin pumps, and continuous subcutaneous insulin injections. Estimating blood glucose concentrations by monitoring urine glucose concentrations—a simple and convenient method—is undesirable for the following reasons:

1. The renal threshold (the blood glucose concentration above which glucose appears in the urine) averages 160 to 180 mg/dL (8.9–10.0 mmol/L) but varies widely among individuals. It may increase in long-standing diabetes or with age and may be lower in pregnancy or childhood. A decreased threshold (±100 mg/dL; 5.6 mmol/L) is known as *renal glycosuria.*
2. Monitoring of urine glucose concentrations lacks sensitivity and specificity. For example, one study demonstrated that patients with plasma glucose concentrations in the range of 150 to 199 mg/dL (8.3–11.1 mmol/L) exhibited normal urine test results 75% of the time. Furthermore, 9% of patients with plasma glucose concentrations less than 149 mg/dL (8.3 mmol/L) had glycosuria.[197]
3. A negative test result does not distinguish between hypoglycemia, euglycemia, and mild or moderate hyperglycemia.
4. Testing urine using a color chart is not accurate.
5. Other factors (eg, fluid intake, urine concentration, ingestion of salicylates or ascorbic acid, urinary tract infections) may influence test results.

Testing urine for glucose is therefore not adequate for monitoring patients on insulin therapy.[198] Although some evidence suggests that it may be effective for monitoring type 2 diabetes,[199] the ADA states that limitations of urine testing make blood glucose measurements the preferred method of assessing glycemic control.[200]

Glucose Meters

Portable meters for measurement of blood glucose concentrations are used in three major settings: in acute and chronic care facilities (at the patient's bedside and in clinics or hospitals), in physicians' offices, and by patients or their caregivers at home, work, and school. Self-monitoring of blood glucose (SMBG) was performed in the United States in 1993 at least once a day by 40% and 26% of individuals with type 1 and 2 diabetes, respectively.[64] In 2006, the overall rate of daily SMBG had increased to 63.4% among all adults with diabetes in the United States and 86.7% among those treated with insulin.[44,201]

Patients measure their own blood glucose concentration and modify their insulin dose based on this glucose value. It is impractical for patients themselves to perform glucose determinations by the methods used in clinical laboratories, but a large number of simple test strips that are available permit rapid measurements on a drop of whole blood.[198] These use the same methodology as that used for glucose analysis—predominantly glucose oxidase or glucose dehydrogenase. (For more details, see Chapter 33.) In many strips, a dye is colored by the glucose oxidase-peroxidase chromogenic reaction. The reagents are combined in dry form on a small surface area of a test strip, and the colors that develop may be evaluated visually by comparison with a color chart (rarely used anymore) or quantified in a specially designed meter. Visual reading with a color chart is not accurate enough for most clinical circumstances. At the time of this writing (2015), more than 90 different blood glucose meters were commercially available in the United States (numbers differ in other countries). These meters vary in size, weight, calibration method, and other features. They are reviewed annually in the ADA magazine *Diabetes Forecast.*

To perform the measurement, a sample of blood (usually from a finger stick, but anticoagulated whole blood collected in ethylenediaminetetraacetic acid [EDTA] or heparin may also be used) is placed on the test pad, which is attached to a plastic support. The test strip is then inserted into the meter. (In some devices, the strip is inserted into the meter before the sample is applied.) After a fixed period of time, the result appears on a digital display screen. These meters use reflectance photometry or electrochemistry to measure the rate of the reaction or the final concentration of the products. Reflectance photometry measures the amount of light reflected from a test pad containing reagent. In electrochemical systems, the enzymatic reaction in an electrode incorporated on the test strip produces a flow of electrons. The current, which is directly proportional to the concentration of glucose in the sample, is converted to a digital readout. Large variability has been noted among current meters as to the volume of blood required (0.3–1.5 μL), test time (5–45 seconds), and the claimed reading range: 30 to 500 mg/dL (1.7–27.8 mmol/L) to 0 to 600 mg/dL (0–33.3 mmol/L). Calibration is automatic on some devices, whereas others use lot-specific code chips or strips. All manufacturers supply control solutions. Recent advances in technology facilitate data analysis and sharing. Some meters have Bluetooth capabilities (enabling transmission of data to a smart phone or computer), cellular connections that automatically send data to the "cloud," USB ports, and/or communication with an insulin pump. Strict adherence to the instructions is necessary to obtain accurate results. Some meters have a porous membrane that separates erythrocytes, and analysis is performed on the resultant plasma. Whole blood glucose concentrations are approximately 10% to 15% lower than plasma or serum concentrations, but meters can be calibrated to report plasma glucose values, even when the sample is whole blood. An International Federation of Clinical Chemistry and Laboratory Medicine (IFCC) working group recommended that glucose meters be harmonized using a factor of 1.11× to report the concentration of glucose in plasma, irrespective of the sample type or technology.[202]

Analytical Goals

Multiple analytical goals have been proposed for the performance of glucose meters. The rationale for these is not always clear. In 1987, the ADA recommended a goal of total error (in the hands of users) of less than 10% at glucose concentrations of 30 to 400 mg/dL (1.7–22.2 mmol/L) 100% of the time.[203] This recommendation was modified in response to the significant reduction in complications by tight glucose control in the DCCT. The revised performance goal, published in 1996,[198] is for analytical error to be less than 5%. No published studies of glucose meters have achieved this goal. The recommendations promulgated in 2002 by the Clinical and Laboratory Standards Institute (CLSI) (previously called the National Committee for Clinical Laboratory Standards [NCCLS])[204] are that 95% of results should fall within 20% of laboratory-measured glucose concentrations when it is 75 mg/dL (4.2 mmol/L) or greater and within 15 mg/dL (0.83 mmol/L) of a laboratory glucose measurement if the glucose concentration is less than 75 mg/dL (4.2 mmol/L). The 2003 International Organization for Standardization (ISO)[205] recommendations are identical. In both CSLI and ISO guidelines, 5% of these results can be considerably outside these limits. Note that the CLSI guideline is for meter use in acute and chronic care facilities (mainly hospitals), while the ISO guidelines pertain to meters for self-testing (ie, SMBG). Several experts believe these acceptance criteria to be too broad. The CLSI and ISO documents were revised in 2013, with tightening of acceptance criteria. The current CLSI guideline POCT12-A3 indicates that for 95% of the samples, the difference between meter and laboratory measurement must be less than 12.5% when the laboratory glucose value is 100 mg/dL (5.6 mmol/L) or greater and less than 12 mg/dL (0.67 mmol/L) when the glucose concentration is less than 100 mg/dL (5.6 mmol/L). In addition, no more than 2% of results can differ by more than 20% at 75 mg/dL (4.2 mmol/L) or greater and by more than 15 mg/dL (0.83 mmol/L) when the glucose concentration is less than 75 mg/dL (4.2 mmol/L). The revised ISO goals, also issued in 2013, are that for 95% of the samples, the difference between meter and laboratory measurement must be less than 15% when the laboratory glucose value is 100 mg/dL (5.6 mmol/L) or greater and less than 15 mg/dL (0.83 mmol/L) when the glucose concentration is less than 100 mg/dL (5.6 mmol/L). Moreover, 99% of results must be within zones A and B of the consensus error grid (see the next paragraph). In the United States, the FDA issued draft guidance in 2014 for glucose meters. Two separate documents were released: one for home (SMBG) use and one for hospitals. The analytic goals are more stringent than either the CLSI or ISO guidelines. At the time of this writing, the FDA guidance remains in draft form, and the final guidelines are not known.

A different method was proposed by Clarke,[206] who developed an error grid that attempts to define clinically important errors by identifying fairly broad target ranges. The error grid was recently modified to reflect current medical practice.[207]

In addition, a novel approach using simulation modeling reached the conclusion that meters that achieve both a CV and a bias less than 5% rarely lead to major errors in insulin dosing.[208] The lack of consensus on quality goals for glucose meters reflects the absence of agreed-upon objective criteria. When biological variation criteria are used, a goal for total error of 6.9% or less, with an imprecision of 2.9% or less and a bias of 2.2% or less, has been proposed.[44]

Glucose meters are also used to calculate insulin dosage in patients without diabetes on tight glucose control protocols in intensive care units (ICUs). Evidence in 2001[209] showed that intensive insulin therapy significantly reduced mortality and morbidity of critically ill patients in the surgical ICU. A subsequent metaanalysis of multiple randomized control trials failed to identify improved outcomes, but it did detect increased incidence of hypoglycemia.[210] It is important to emphasize that the 2001 study used accurate blood gas analyzers and collected arterial blood samples,[209] whereas subsequent studies often used glucose meters and capillary blood samples. Many factors, such as hypoxia, shock, and low hematocrit, are common in patients in ICUs and can compromise glucose analysis in capillary blood samples.[211] The use of glucose meters in these settings has been questioned by some experts.[212]

Performance of Glucose Meters

The most common errors in SMBG, such as proper application, timing, and removal of excess blood, have been reduced by advances in technology but can still occur. Additional innovations that reduce operator error include systems that abort testing if the sample volume is inadequate, built-in programs that simplify quality control, and increased memory that allows the instrument to store up to several hundred glucose readings that can be downloaded into a computer.

Several factors affect the accuracy and reproducibility of SMBG. These include user variability—up to 50% of values may vary by more than 20% from reference values[198]; hematocrit—the presence of anemia (false increase) or polycythemia (false depression) may result in up to 30% variability; and defective reagent strips or instrument malfunction (rare). Other variables include changes in altitude, environmental temperature, or humidity; hypotension; hypoxia; and high triglyceride concentrations. In addition, these assays are unreliable at very high and very low glucose concentrations (<60 and >500 mg/dL; <3.3 and >27.8 mmol/L). Because dehydration, a common feature of diabetic ketoacidosis, greatly increases blood viscosity, inaccurately low blood glucose results may be obtained. Several drugs interfere, but not with all meters.[213] Another important factor is the lack of correlation among meters, even from a single manufacturer, caused by different assay methods and architecture. Moreover, results from two meters of the same brand have been observed to differ substantially.[214] Patient factors are also important, particularly adequacy of training. Recurrent education at clinic visits and comparison of SMBG with concurrent laboratory glucose analysis improved the accuracy of patients' blood glucose readings.[215] In addition, it is important to evaluate the patient's technique at regular intervals.

The performance of different meters varies widely, but imprecision remains high. Under carefully controlled conditions in which all assays were performed by a single medical technologist, approximately 50% of analyses met the ADA criterion of less than 5% deviation from reference values.[216] Performance of older meters was substantially worse. Note that the performance of glucose meters achieved by medical technologists is better than that achieved by patients. Another study that evaluated meter performance in 226 hospitals by split samples analyzed simultaneously on meters and laboratory glucose analyzers revealed that 45.6%, 25%, and 14% differed from one another by greater than 10%, greater than 15%, and greater than 20%, respectively.[217] Comparison with laboratory values of almost 22,000 measurements of capillary glucose by patients using meters revealed no significant improvement in meter performance between 1989 and 1999.[218] An analysis in 2012 revealed that only 18 of 34 (53%) glucose meters approved for use in Europe fulfilled the minimum accuracy requirements of the 2013 ISO standard.[219] The imprecision of meters precludes their use from the diagnosis of diabetes and limits their usefulness in screening for diabetes.[44]

Indications and Frequency of SMBG

The indications and frequency of self-monitoring vary among patients. SMBG should be performed by all patients treated with insulin. The role of SMBG in patients with type 2 diabetes not treated with insulin has not been defined.[44] A consensus statement by the ADA[198] recommended the following specific indications for SMBG:

- Patients undergoing intensive insulin treatment programs (in this group, glucose should be measured at least four times a day to achieve glycemic control)
- Prevention and detection of hypoglycemia, especially in people who are asymptomatic or unable to recognize the early warning signs
- Avoidance of severe hyperglycemia, particularly in situations of increased risk (eg, medications that alter insulin secretion or action, intercurrent illness, elderly people)
- Adjusted pharmacologic therapy in response to changes in lifestyle, such as exercise or altering food intake
- Determination of the necessity for initiating insulin therapy in GDM.

Glucose meters should not be used to diagnose diabetes mellitus, and their role in screening remains uncertain.[64]

Current ADA recommendations[28] are that patients with type 1 diabetes or on intensive insulin regimens (multiple daily injections or insulin pump therapy) should perform SMBG 6 to 8 times per day—that is, before meals and snacks, occasionally postprandially, at bedtime, before exercise, when they suspect low blood glucose, after treating hypoglycemia, and before critical tasks such as driving. A reduced frequency of SMBG results in deterioration of glycemic control.[220-222] Published studies revealed that self-monitoring is performed by patients much less frequently than recommended.[223] More recent evidence shows a gradual increase, with 63.4% of patients with diabetes now reported to monitor blood glucose at least once daily.[224] Guidelines on the recommended frequency and timing of SMBG vary among international diabetes associations.[225] Recent recommendations suggest that the frequency and timing of SMBG should be dictated by the particular needs and goals of the individual patient.[28,225]

The value of SMBG for patients with type 2 diabetes not on insulin therapy is controversial owing, in part, to the lack of well-designed studies. A metaanalysis of SMBG in non-insulin-treated patients with type 2 diabetes showed that SMBG improved glycemic control.[226] However, many studies in this analysis included patient education, and the contribution of SMBG to glucose control in non-insulin-treated patients remains contentious.[224] Despite controversy in the literature, a survey conducted in 14 countries in 2007 revealed unexpectedly high SMBG use in non-insulin-treated patients, with up to 75% of patients performing SMBG.[227]

MINIMALLY INVASIVE MONITORING OF BLOOD GLUCOSE

A major limitation to performing SMBG is that it is painful and inconvenient. Since the 1960s, attempts have been made to develop a painless method for monitoring blood glucose concentrations. Three general approaches have been used: implanted sensors, minimally invasive monitoring, and noninvasive monitoring.

Implanted Sensors

Several implanted biosensors have been developed and evaluated in both animals and humans. Detection systems are based on enzymes, electrodes, or fluorescence.[228,229] The most widely studied method is an electrochemical sensor that is usually implanted subcutaneously. The first device approved for patient use was the Continuous Glucose Monitoring System (CGMS) (Medtronic, Minneapolis, Minn.); others are now available. All monitoring devices use glucose oxidase to measure glucose every 1 to 5 minutes. The values are sent to a monitor. Results are recorded and, depending on the system, may be downloaded later in the physician's office or are available to the patient in real time. The measurement range is 40 to 400 mg/dL (2.2–22.2 mmol/L) or 20 to 500 mg/dL (1.1–27.8 mmol/L). These devices are subject to some limitations. Implantation of a needle type of sensor into the subcutaneous tissue induces inflammatory responses in the host that alter the sensitivity of the device. Therefore the devices can be worn for only 3 to 7 days. These sensors require calibration by the user every 12 hours with a glucose meter and are subject to the imprecision of the meter. In addition, meters are required for making acute treatment decisions. An important caveat is that changes in glucose concentration in the interstitial fluid occur 4 to 20 minutes later than in the blood.

Another available strategy is the Glucoday (A. Menarini Diagnostics, Florence, Italy), which uses microdialysis and measures glucose outside the body. Fluid is pumped from a storage bag through a microfiber under the skin. The solution carries the glucose sample back to a biosensor, which displays the glucose result every second. This device, which is available in parts of Europe but not in the United States, can be worn for 48 hours.

A randomized study of 322 patients with type 1 diabetes showed that adults aged 25 and older using intensive insulin treatment and real-time continuous glucose monitoring had better long-term glycemic control than patients using intensive insulin therapy and SMBG.[230] Newer features, such as automated suspension of insulin delivery for up to 2 hours when glucose concentrations reach a preset low threshold, have been recently shown to significantly reduce the rate of hypoglycemia[231] and improve HbA_{1c}[232] in patients with type 1 diabetes. CGM may be particularly useful in patients with hypoglycemic unawareness or frequent episodes of hypoglycemia. Automated closed-loop insulin delivery systems (also termed the "artificial pancreas") are a focus of intense research.[233] The system employs a control algorithm that modulates insulin delivery according to real-time interstitial glucose measured by a CGM. Closed-loop systems have been shown to be superior to conventional insulin pump therapy in a controlled research environment, and studies are currently under way to evaluate their performance during home use.

Minimally Invasive Glucose Monitoring

The concept underlying these methods is that the concentration of glucose in the interstitial fluid correlates with the blood glucose concentration. The principle of the FDA-approved Gluco Watch Biographer (Animas Corporation, West Chester, Pennsylvania) involves the application of a low-level electric current to the skin. This induces movement by electro-osmosis of glucose across the skin, where it is measured by a glucose oxidase detector.[234] Glucose concentrations in transdermal fluid and plasma are highly correlated. The clearest application of the Gluco Watch, which is designed to measure glucose three times per hour for up to 12 hours, appears to be in the detection of unsuspected hypoglycemia. Calibration with reference plasma glucose is required. Initial clinical studies reveal reasonable correlation of the Gluco Watch with SMBG.[234] This device has been withdrawn from the market, but it is likely to stimulate enhanced efforts to bring other technologies into clinical use.

Noninvasive Glucose Monitoring

Noninvasive in vivo monitoring of glucose—that is, without implanting a probe or collecting a sample of any type[44]—has been an area of active investigation for many years.[235] The approaches most widely evaluated involve passing a beam of light through a vascular region and analyzing the resulting light. Near-infrared spectroscopic devices measure the absorption or the reflection of light from subcutaneous tissue. Although glucose has a specific absorption at 1035 nm, many substances interfere. A computer, individually calibrated, screens out interfering information to obtain the glucose result. Alternative approaches include Raman scattering spectroscopy and photoacoustic spectroscopy. Notwithstanding the investment of considerable resources, no noninvasive sensing technology is approved for glucose measurement in patients. Major technological hurdles must be overcome before noninvasive sensing technology will be sufficiently reliable to replace existing portable meters, implantable biosensors, or minimally invasive technologies.[44]

POINTS TO REMEMBER

Glucose

- Hyperglycemia results from defects in insulin secretion and/or insulin action.
- Blood glucose homeostasis is regulated by several hormones, including insulin, glucagon, epinephrine, and cortisol.
- Blood glucose concentrations fluctuate widely during the day, depending on food ingestion, exercise, and other factors (eg, stress).
- Self-monitoring of blood glucose using portable meters in patients with diabetes who require insulin has shown to improve patient outcomes.
- Self-monitoring of blood glucose in noninsulin-treated patients is not yet proven to be effective.
- The use of continuous glucose monitoring systems (CGMS), which use subcutaneously implanted glucose sensors, by patients on insulin is increasing.

KETONE BODIES

The development of ketosis requires changes in both adipose tissue and the liver. The primary substrates for ketone body formation are free fatty acids from adipose stores. Normally, long-chain fatty acids are taken up by the liver, reesterified to triglycerides, and stored in the liver or incorporated in very low-density lipoproteins and returned to the plasma. In contrast to other tissue, the brain cannot use free fatty acids for energy. When glucose is unavailable, ketone bodies supply the vast majority of the brain's energy. After a 3-day fast, ketone bodies provide 30% to 40% of the body's energy requirements.[236] In uncontrolled diabetes, the low insulin concentrations result in increased lipolysis and decreased reesterification, thereby increasing plasma free fatty acids. In addition, the higher glucagon/insulin ratio enhances fatty acid oxidation in the liver. Increased counterregulatory hormones also augment lipolysis and ketogenesis in fat and liver, respectively. Thus increased hepatic ketone production and decreased peripheral tissue metabolism lead to acetoacetate accumulation in the blood. A small fraction undergoes spontaneous decarboxylation to form acetone, but most of it is converted to β-hydroxybutyrate. (Strictly speaking, β-hydroxybutyrate is not a ketone body, but it is considered to be equivalent to one as it is reversibly formed from acetoacetate.)

Acetoacetate ⇌ β-Hydroxybutyrate (β-Hydroxybutyrate dehydrogenase (in liver); NADH + $H^{\oplus}$ → $NAD^{\oplus}$)

Acetoacetate + $H^{\oplus}$ → (Spontaneous) Acetone ($H_3C-CO-CH_3$) + CO_2

The relative proportions in which the three ketone bodies are present in blood vary, depending on the redox state of the cell. In healthy people, β-hydroxybutyrate and acetoacetate—which are present at approximately equimolar concentrations[236-238]—constitute virtually all the serum ketones. Acetone is a minor component. In severe diabetes, the ratio of β-hydroxybutyrate to acetoacetate may increase to 6:1 owing to the presence of a large concentration of nicotinamide adenine dinucleotide (NADH), which favors β-hydroxybutyrate production.

None of the commonly used methods for the detection and determination of ketone bodies in serum or urine reacts with all three ketone bodies. Gerhardt's ferric chloride test reacts with acetoacetate only. Tests using nitroprusside are at least 10 times more sensitive to acetoacetate than to acetone, and they give no reaction at all with β-hydroxybutyrate.

Most of the tests for ketosis essentially detect or measure acetoacetate only. This may produce a paradoxical situation. When a patient initially presents in ketoacidosis, the test results for ketones may be only weakly positive. With therapy, β-hydroxybutyrate is converted to acetoacetate, and the ketosis appears to worsen.

Traditional tests for β-hydroxybutyrate are indirect; they require brief boiling of the urine to remove acetone and acetoacetate by evaporation (acetoacetate first breaks down spontaneously to acetone), followed by gentle oxidation of β-hydroxybutyrate to acetoacetate and acetone with peroxide, ferric ions, or dichromate. The acetoacetate thus formed can be detected with Gerhardt's test or by one of the procedures in which nitroprusside is used.

Specific determination of β-hydroxybutyrate in urine is not considered to be a routine procedure. A paper strip for semiquantitative measurement of β-hydroxybutyrate in serum and urine has been described[239] but has not gained general acceptance. Quantitative enzymatic assays for β-hydroxybutyrate that can be performed directly on blood or serum have become commercially available. Originally available as a benchtop analyzer (KetoSite, GDS Diagnostics, Elkhart, Indiana), handheld devices are also available now (Precision Xtra, Abbott Diagnostics, Abbott Park, Illinois; Nova Max Plus, Nova Biomedical, Waltham, Massachusetts, and STAT-Site, Stanbio Laboratory, Boeme, Texas).[240]

Clinical Significance

Excessive formation of ketone bodies results in increased blood concentrations (ketonemia) and increased excretion in the urine (ketonuria). This process is observed in conditions associated with reduced availability of carbohydrates (such as starvation or frequent vomiting) or decreased use of carbohydrates (such as diabetes mellitus, glycogen storage disease type I [von Gierke disease], and alkalosis). The popular high-fat, low-carbohydrate diets are ketogenic and increase ketone bodies in the circulation. Diabetes mellitus and alcohol consumption are the most common causes of ketoacidosis in adults. (Hyperglycemia is not usually present in the latter condition.) Ingestion of isopropyl alcohol and salicylate poisoning can also produce ketoacidosis. Urine ketone test results are positive in approximately 30% of first morning void specimens from pregnant women. Semiquantitative determination of ketone bodies in blood is more accurate than determination of these compounds in urine in the treatment of diabetic ketoacidosis. Although not always excreted in proportion to blood ketone concentrations, because of convenience, urine ketones are widely used for monitoring control in patients with type 1 diabetes. The ADA states that urine ketone testing is an important part of monitoring by patients with diabetes, particularly those with type 1 diabetes, pregnancy with preexisting diabetes, and GDM.[200] Patients with type 1 diabetes should test for ketones during acute illness or stress, with consistent increases in blood glucose (>300 mg/dL; >16.7 mmol/L), during pregnancy, or when symptoms of ketoacidosis are present.[200] Measurement of ketones in urine and blood is widely performed in patients with diabetes for both diagnosis and monitoring of diabetic ketoacidosis.[44]

Determination of Ketone Bodies in Body Fluids

Although quantitative determination of individual ketone bodies is possible, these methods are not used as routine tests. The semiquantitative Acetest or Ketostix (Bayer Health Care, Pine Brook, New Jersey) are frequently used but are insensitive to β-hydroxybutyrate.[241] It is important to bear in mind, therefore, that a negative nitroprusside test result does not rule out ketoacidosis.

Detection of Ketone Bodies by Acetest

Acetest tablets contain a mixture of glycine, sodium nitroprusside, disodium phosphate, and lactose. Acetoacetate or acetone (to a lesser extent) in the presence of glycine forms a lavender-purple complex with nitroprusside. β-Hydroxybutyrate does not react with nitroprusside. The disodium phosphate provides an optimum pH for the reaction, and lactose enhances the color.[242]

False-positive results may occur with urine specimens containing very large quantities of phenylketones, drugs containing sulfhydryls (eg, angiotensin converting enzyme inhibitors), or specimens preserved with 8-hydroxyquinoline. L-Dopa metabolites may produce an atypical reaction that could be interpreted as a positive result. False-negative results have been reported with highly acidic urine specimens (eg, after large intake of vitamin C), when reagents are exposed to air or are out of date.

Detection of Ketone Bodies by Ketostix

Ketostix is a modification of the nitroprusside test in which a reagent strip is used instead of a tablet. The Ketostix test gives a positive reaction within 15 seconds with a specimen containing at least 50 mg of acetoacetate per liter. The accompanying color chart gives readings for ketone concentrations of 50, 150, 400, 800, and 1600 mg/L. Acetone also reacts, but the test is less sensitive to it.

Determination of β-Hydroxybutyrate

A 1995 short report on patients with diabetic ketoacidosis indicated that β-hydroxybutyrate correlated better than acetoacetate with changes in acid-base status.[243] In this test, β-hydroxybutyrate in the presence of nicotinamide adenine dinucleotide (NAD+) is converted by β-hydroxybutyrate dehydrogenase to acetoacetate, producing nicotinamide adenine dinucleotide (NADH). Diaphorase catalyzes the reduction of nitroblue tetrazolium (NBT) by NADH to produce a purple compound, and its absorbance is read in a special meter that provides a digital readout. Some blood glucose meters can measure β-hydroxybutyrate with an appropriate test strip.

$$\beta\text{-Hydroxybutyrate} \xrightleftharpoons[\text{NAD}^{\oplus} \curvearrowright \text{NADH} + \text{H}^{\oplus}]{\beta\text{-Hydroxybutyrate dehydrogenase}} \text{Acetoacetate}$$

$$\text{NADH} + \text{NBT} \xrightarrow{\textit{Diaphorase}} \text{NAD}^{\oplus} + \text{Reduced NBT}$$

Determination of Ketone Bodies in Urine

Acetest, Ketostix, Ketosis Test Strips (LW Scientific, Lawrenceville, Georgia), and Trueplus Ketone Test Strips® (Nipro Diagnostics, Osaka, Japan) are suitable for detecting ketone bodies in urine. The sensitivity and specificity of these tests are the same as outlined for serum.

Reference Interval

Serum β-hydroxybutyrate values vary from 0.21 to 2.81 mg/dL (0.02–0.27 mmol/L) in healthy people after an overnight fast. Ketone bodies in the blood can reach 20 mg/dL (2 mmol/L) with prolonged exercise.[236] Patients with diabetic ketoacidosis usually have β-hydroxybutyrate concentrations greater than 20 mg/dL (2 mmol/L).

GLYCATED PROTEINS

Measurement of glycated proteins, primarily GHb, is effective in monitoring long-term glucose control in people with diabetes mellitus. It provides a retrospective index of integrated plasma glucose values over an extended period of time and is not subject to the wide fluctuations observed when blood glucose concentrations are assayed. GHb concentrations therefore are a valuable and widely used adjunct to blood glucose determinations for monitoring long-term glycemic control. In addition, GHb has recently been recommended for the diagnosis of diabetes and is a measure of risk for the development of microvascular complications of diabetes.

Glycated Hemoglobin

In this chapter, the term *glycated hemoglobin* is used to refer to the set of all glycated hemoglobins, including glycated forms of hemoglobins other than hemoglobin A, such as hemoglobin S and C. The terms *glycated hemoglobin, glycohemoglobin, "glycosylated"* (which should not be used because it refers to proteins in which carbohydrates have been attached enzymatically) *hemoglobin,* HbA_1, and HbA_{1c} have all been used to refer to hemoglobin that has been modified by the nonenzymatic addition of glucose residues. However, these terms are not interchangeable. The set of glycated hemoglobins includes HbA_1 and other nonenzymatically formed hemoglobin-glucose adducts; HbA_1 is made up of HbA_{1a}, HbA_{1b}, and HbA_{1c}. To eliminate this confusing nomenclature and to remove mention of hemoglobin, which is confusing to patients because it has no obvious relation to diabetes or glucose, the term *A1c test* has been suggested. As described in the text, most of the available studies on the effects of metabolic control on complication rates (at least for the DCCT and UKPDS) used assay methods that quantified HbA_{1c} specifically, as do most clinical laboratories.

Glycation is the nonenzymatic addition of a sugar residue to amino groups of proteins. Human adult hemoglobin (Hb) usually consists of HbA (97% of the total), HbA_2 (2.5%),

TABLE 57.3 Nomenclature of Selected Hemoglobins

Name	Component(s)
HbA	Constitutes ≈97% adult hemoglobin
HbA_0	Synonymous with HbA
HbA_{1a1}	HbA with fructose 1,6-diphosphate attached to the *N*-terminal valine of the β-chain
HbA_{1a2}	HbA with glucose 6-phosphate attached to the *N*-terminal valine of the β-chain
HbA_{1a}	Comprises HbA_{1a1} and HbA_{1a2}
HbA_{1b}	HbA with pyruvic acid attached to the *N*-terminal valine of the β-chain
HbA_{1c}	HbA with glucose attached to the *N*-terminal valine of the β-chain
Pre-HbA_{1c}	Unstable Schiff base (aldimine); a labile intermediary component in the formation of HbA_{1c}
HbA_1	Consists of HbA_{1a}, HbA_{1b}, and HbA_{1c}
Total glycated hemoglobin*	Consists of HbA_{1c} and other hemoglobin-carbohydrate adducts

*Also termed *glycated hemoglobin* or *glycohemoglobin.*
Hb, Hemoglobin.

and HbF (0.5%). HbA is made up of four polypeptide chains: two α- and two β-chains. Chromatographic analysis of HbA identifies several minor hemoglobins—namely, HbA_{1a}, HbA_{1b}, and HbA_{1c}—which are collectively referred to as HbA_1, fast hemoglobins (because they migrate more rapidly than HbA in an electrical field), glycohemoglobins, or glycated hemoglobins (Table 57.3). The Joint Commission on Biochemical Nomenclature of the International Union of Pure and Applied Chemistry recommends the term *neoglycoprotein* for such derivatives and the term *glycation* to describe this process. Therefore although *glycosylated* and *glucosylated* have been widely used in the literature, the term *glycated* is preferred. HbA_{1c} is formed by the condensation of glucose with the *N*-terminal valine residue of each β-chain of HbA to form an unstable Schiff base (aldimine, pre-HbA_{1c}; Fig. 57.6). The Schiff base may dissociate or may undergo an Amadori rearrangement to form a stable ketoamine, HbA_{1c}. HbA_{1a1} and HbA_{1a2}, which make up HbA_{1a}, have fructose 1,6-diphosphate and glucose-6-phosphate, respectively, attached to the amino terminal of the β-chain (see Table 57.3). The structure of HbA_{1b}, identified by mass spectrometry, contains pyruvic acid linked to the amino terminal valine of the β-chain, probably by a ketamine or enamine bond. HbA_{1c} is the major fraction, constituting approximately 80% of HbA_1.

Glycation may also occur at sites other than the end of the β-chain, such as lysine residues, or the α-chain. These GHbs, referred to as glycated HbA_0 or total glycated hemoglobin (see Table 57.3), cannot be separated from nonglycated hemoglobin by methods based on charge, but they are measureable by boronate affinity chromatography.

Formation of GHb is essentially irreversible, and the concentration in the blood depends on both the life span of the red blood cell (RBC; average life span is 120 days) and the blood glucose concentration. Because the rate of formation of GHb is directly proportional to the concentration of glucose

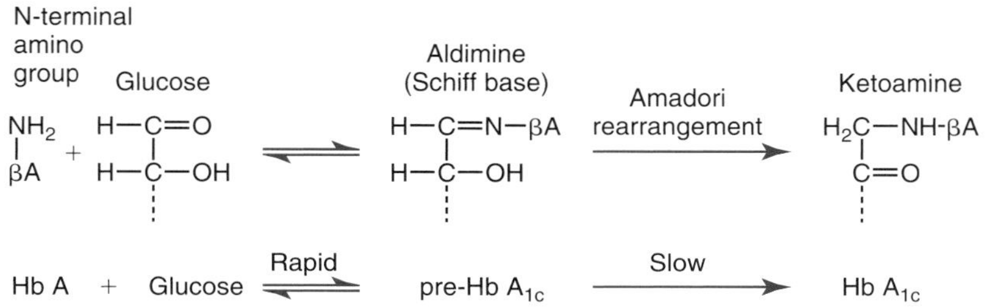

N-terminal amino group + Glucose ⇌ Aldimine (Schiff base) —Amadori rearrangement→ Ketoamine

NH_2–βA + H–C=O / H–C–OH ⇌ H–C=N–βA / H–C–OH → H_2C–NH-βA / C=O

Hb A + Glucose ⇌ (Rapid) pre-Hb A_{1c} → (Slow) Hb A_{1c}

FIGURE 57.6 Formation of hemoglobin A_{1c}.

in the blood, the GHb concentration represents integrated values for glucose over the preceding 8 to 12 weeks. This provides an additional criterion for assessing glucose control because GHb values are free of the influence of day-to-day glucose fluctuations and are unaffected by recent exercise or food ingestion.[155] It is important to realize that the contribution of the plasma glucose concentration to GHb depends on the time interval, with more recent values providing a larger contribution than earlier values. The plasma glucose in the preceding 1 month determines 50% of the HbA_{1c}, whereas days 60 to 120 determine only 25%.[244] After a sudden alteration in blood glucose concentrations, the rate of change of HbA_{1c} is rapid during the initial 2 months, followed by a more gradual change approaching steady state 3 months later.

Interpretation of GHb depends on red blood cells having a normal life span. Patients with hemolytic disease or other conditions with shortened red blood cell survival exhibit a substantial reduction in GHb.[245] Similarly, individuals with recent significant blood loss have falsely low values owing to a higher fraction of young erythrocytes. GHb concentrations can still be used to monitor these patients, but values must be compared with previous values from the same patient—not with published reference intervals. High GHb concentrations have been reported in iron deficiency anemia.[246] The mechanism is unknown, but increased glycation by malondialdehyde has been proposed.[247] The effects of hemoglobin variants (such as HbF, HbS, and HbC) depend on the specific method of analysis used (discussed later).[245] Depending on the particular hemoglobinopathy and assay, results may be spuriously increased or decreased. Most manufacturers of HbA_{1c} assays have modified their assays to eliminate interference from many of the common hemoglobin variants. Therefore accurate measurement of HbA_{1c} is possible by selecting an appropriate instrument, provided the erythrocyte life span is not altered (see www.NGSP.org for additional information). Another source of error in certain methods is carbamylated hemoglobin. This is formed when isocyanic acid, which is derived from urea, is covalently attached to hemoglobin. Renal failure is common in diabetic patients and results in high concentrations of urea in the blood. Carbamylated hemoglobin does not interfere with most modern methods of HbA_{1c} analysis.[246] Most of the interferents produce relatively small effects, and for the vast majority of patients with diabetes, HbA_{1c} can be measured accurately.

Labile intermediates (pre-HbA_{1c}, Schiff base) may be included in measurements of HbA_{1c}, especially in the common ion-exchange methods,[248] and produce misleadingly high results. The labile fraction changes rapidly with acute changes in blood glucose concentration and thus is not an indicator of long-term glycemic control. Pre-HbA_{1c} amounts to 5% to 8% of total HbA_1 in healthy individuals and ranges from 8% to 30% in patients with diabetes, depending on the degree of control of blood glucose concentration at or near the time of blood sampling.[249] If the analytical method measures both fractions, the labile pre-HbA_{1c} should be removed first to prevent falsely increased results. In the absence of glucose, pre-HbA_{1c} reverts to glucose and HbA (see Fig. 57.6). This provides the basis for some procedures to eliminate the labile fraction by incubating washed red blood cells in saline. In some boronate affinity methods, the assay conditions favor rapid dissociation of the Schiff base.

Clinical Utility

Diagnosis of Diabetes. A major change in the diagnosis of diabetes was recommended in 2009.[29,250] An International Expert Committee advised that HbA_{1c} could be used for the diagnosis of diabetes (see Box 57.3). An HbA_{1c} value of 6.5% (48 mmol/mol) or greater was selected as the decision point, based on the prevalence of retinopathy.[29] This recommendation has been endorsed by both the ADA[251] and the WHO. HbA_{1c} concentrations of 5.7% to 6.4% (39–46 mmol/mol) indicate subjects at high risk of developing diabetes. Note that some organizations define high risk as HbA_{1c} concentrations of 5.5% to 6.4% (37–46 mmol/mol).[252] HbA_{1c} was also recommended as an alternative to glucose for screening for diabetes. This last recommendation has also been accepted by the ADA[251] and other clinical organizations.

Monitoring Diabetes. GHb has been firmly established as an index of long-term blood glucose concentrations and as a measure of the risk for development of microvascular complications in patients with diabetes mellitus.[200] Several influential clinical diabetes organizations recommend that HbA_{1c} should be measured routinely in all patients with diabetes to document their degree of glycemic control and to assess response to treatment.[44] GHb was a cornerstone of the DCCT.[175] (To prevent assay variability—see section on assay standardization later in this chapter—all GHb assays in the DCCT were done in a single laboratory that measured HbA_{1c} by HPLC.) The DCCT documented a direct relationship between blood glucose concentrations (assessed by HbA_{1c}) and the risk for development and progression of microvascular complications.[175] The absolute risks of retinopathy and nephropathy were directly proportional to the mean HbA_{1c} concentration. The risk of retinopathy increased continuously with increasing HbA_{1c}, and a single measure of HbA_{1c} predicted the progression of retinopathy 4 years later. Subsequent analysis revealed that the mean HbA_{1c} was the dominant predictor of retinopathy progression, and a 10% lower HbA_{1c} concentration was associated with a 45% lower risk.[253] The risk of microvascular complications varies continuously with HbA_{1c}, and there is no HbA_{1c} concentration below which the risk is eliminated.

Analogous correlations between HbA_{1c} and complications were observed in patients with type 2 diabetes in the UKPDS trial.[176] To ensure that HbA_{1c} results in the UKPDS were comparable with DCCT findings, an ion-exchange HPLC method calibrated to the DCCT was used. Mean HbA_{1c} values for the intensively treated and conventionally treated groups were 7.0% and 7.9% (53 and 63 mmol/mol), respectively.[176] Despite the relatively small difference in HbA_{1c}, microvascular complications were reduced by approximately 25%. Each 1% reduction in HbA_{1c} (eg, from 8% to 7% [equivalent to from 64 to 53 mmol/mol]) was associated with risk reductions of 37% for microvascular disease, 21% for death related to diabetes, and 14% for myocardial infarction.[176] In patients without diabetes, HbA_{1c} is directly related to cardiovascular disease. In the European Prospective Investigation into Cancer and Nutrition (EPIC-Norfolk), an increase of 1% in HbA_{1c} was associated with a 28% increase in the risk of death.[254] Based on the DCCT and the UKPDS, major clinical diabetes organizations recommend that the goal for most patients with diabetes should be HbA_{1c} less than 6.5% to 7% (48 to 53 mmol/mol).[255] The more frequent use of this test in the management of patients is reflected in the increased number of laboratories participating in College of American Pathologists (CAP) GHb surveys. In 1985, 1990, 2003, 2009, and 2014, approximately 300, 700, 2000, 3250 and 3500 laboratories, respectively, were enrolled in the GHb surveys.

POINTS TO REMEMBER

HbA_{1c}

- Glycated hemoglobin is formed by nonenzymatic attachment of glucose to hemoglobin.
- HbA_{1c} has glucose attached to the *N*-terminal Val of the beta chain of hemoglobin.
- The concentration of HbA_{1c} depends on the concentration of glucose in the blood and the erythrocyte life span.
- The average erythrocyte life span is 120 days, and HbA_{1c} therefore reflects the average blood glucose concentration over the preceding 8 to 12 weeks.
- Any condition that substantially changes erythrocyte life span will alter HbA_{1c}.
- HbA_{1c} is used to diagnose diabetes, monitor glycemic control, evaluate the need to change therapy, and predict the development of microvascular complications.

Methods for the Determination of Glycated Hemoglobins

More than 150 different methods have been described for the determination of GHbs. Most methods separate GHb from nonglycated hemoglobin using techniques based on charge differences (ion-exchange chromatography, HPLC, electrophoresis, and isoelectric focusing) or structural differences (affinity chromatography and immunoassay).[256] Chemical analysis (enzymatic, photometry, and spectrophotometry) has also been used. Recently, methods have become commercially available that use capillary electrophoresis or an enzymatic assay that specifically measure HbA_{1c}. Regardless of the method used, the result is expressed as a percentage of total hemoglobin. Analysis by gel electrophoresis, isoelectric focusing, or photometry is rarely used and is not addressed further here. (Interested readers are referred to earlier editions of this book.) The selection of a method by a laboratory is influenced by several factors, including sample volume, patient population, and cost. It is advisable to consult clinicians in this process. The ADA recommends that laboratories use only HbA_{1c} assays that are certified by the NGSP (previously termed the National Glycohemoglobin Standardization Program) as traceable to the DCCT reference.[200] These assays are listed on the NGSP website (www.NGSP.org) and are updated several times a year.

The GHb assays most widely used in the United States are depicted in Table 57.4. These data are based on results from 1947, 2396, and 3225 laboratories participating in quality control surveys conducted by the CAP in 1995, 2009, and 2014, respectively. The results demonstrate that by 2009 virtually all laboratories used immunoassay or ion-exchange chromatography. HbA_{1c} was measured by more than 99% of laboratories (see Table 57.4). Total GHb and HbA_1 measurements had essentially disappeared. These results reflect considerable changes from the methods used in 1995, when affinity chromatography was the most common analytical method (see Table 57.4). Also, only 60% of laboratories reported HbA_{1c} in 1995. In addition, variation among mean values—both between and within methods—and imprecision were substantially lower in 2009 and 2014. Note that the CAP samples are prepared from human whole blood, which allows direct comparison among different methods and instruments. It should be borne in mind that these data refer only to these CAP surveys and are weighted to laboratories that participate (~15% of participants are from outside the United States). All of the methods described in the subsequent text are commercially available.

Ion-Exchange Minicolumns. Ion-exchange chromatography separates hemoglobin variants on the basis of charge. The cation-exchange resin (negatively charged), packed in a disposable minicolumn, has an affinity for hemoglobin, which is positively charged. The patient's sample is hemolyzed, and an aliquot of the hemolysate is applied to the column. A buffer is applied and the eluent is collected. The ionic strength and pH of the eluent buffer are selected so that GHbs are less positively charged than HbA, do not bind as well to the negatively charged resin, and therefore are eluted first. The GHbs—($A_{1a} + A_{1b} + A_{1c}$), expressed collectively as HbA_1—are measured in a spectrophotometer. A second buffer of different ionic strength can be added to the column to elute the more positively charged main hemoglobin fraction. This is read in the spectrophotometer, and GHb is expressed as a percentage of total hemoglobin. Alternatively, only the HbA_1 is eluted, and a separate dilution of the original hemolysate is made, against which the HbA_1 is compared. Numerous commercial modifications have been developed. Simple agitation of resins with hemolysates (batch technique) to adsorb HbA has also been described. In this approach, the supernatant solution containing the HbA_1 fraction is removed by filtration or centrifugation. Methods that separate HbA_{1a+b} from HbA_{1c} by using two different buffers have also been described.[257] Most of the current commercial ion-exchange methods use HPLC.

In all ion-exchange column methods, it is important to control the temperature of the reagents and columns to obtain accurate and reproducible results. This is best done by thermostatting the columns. Alternatively, a temperature correction factor can be applied if the room temperature

TABLE 57.4 Methods of Glycated Hemoglobin Analysis*

Method	Component Reported	YEAR: 1995 (*n* = 1947)[†]				2009 (*n* = 2396)				2014 (*n* = 3225)			
		Number[‡]	% of Total	Mean, %[§]	CV, %[§]	Number[‡]	% of Total	Mean, %[‖]	CV, %[§]	Number[‡]	% of Total	Mean, %[‖]	CV, %[§]
Methods Based on Charge Differences													
Ion exchange			15				35				30		
	HbA_{1c}	279		4.9–5.7	4.4–13.8	832		6.0–6.3	1.3–3	969		6.6–6.8	1.8–2.8
	HbA_1	22		6.5	15.2	—[¶]							
Electrophoresis**			12								<1		
	HbA_{1c}	138		4.9	16.5	0		—	—	15		6.4	2.0
	HbA_1	99		6.4–7.8	9.6–12.7	—							
Methods based on structural differences													
Affinity			66				<1				4		
	HbA_{1c}	642		6.5	8.1	12		5.9	2.3	130		6.5–6.6	1.8–2.7
	Total GHb	638		5.9–7.9	6.9–9.3	0		—	—	—			
Immunoassay			7				65				64		
	HbA_{1c}	129		5.7	3.5	1552		5.7–6.2	2.7–8	2077		6.4–7.1	2.2–5.6
Methods Based on Chemical Reactivity													
Enzymatic											1		
	HbA1c									34		6.5	1.6

*Results are based on 1995 CAP Survey, Set EC-B, Specimen GH-03, 2009 CAP Survey, Set GH2-A, Specimen GH2-02, and 2014 CAP Survey, Set GH2-B, Specimen GH2-04 (© 1995, 2009, and 2014, College of American Pathologists; data used with permission). See text for discussion of methods.

[†] *n* is the number of laboratories that participated in the survey.

[‡] Indicates how many laboratories use the indicated method.

[§] Where more than one value is listed, the data vary among commercial assays. The range is presented.

[‖] The NGSP values in 2009 and 2014 were 6.0% and 6.6%, respectively.

[¶] Number of participants was too low to permit statistical analysis.

**Original methods used agar gel electrophoresis. Current (2014) method uses capillary electrophoresis.

CV, Coefficient of variation; *GHb,* glycated hemoglobin; *Hb,* hemoglobin.

differs from the specified optimum. In addition, rigid control of pH and ionic strength must be maintained. Sample storage conditions are also important.

The labile pre-HbA_1 fractions elute with the stable ketoamine and produce spuriously high values unless destroyed by pretreatment of the red blood cells. Spuriously increased values are also obtained when the charge on hemoglobin is altered by the attachment of noncarbohydrate moieties, which may co-chromatograph with GHbs, as in uremia (carbamylated hemoglobin), alcoholism, lead poisoning, or chronic treatment with large doses of aspirin (acetylated hemoglobin). Hemoglobin variants or chemically modified hemoglobins that elute separately from HbA and HbA_{1c} have little effect on HbA_{1c} measurements. If the modified hemoglobin (or its glycated derivative) cannot be separated from HbA or HbA_{1c}, spuriously increased or reduced results will be obtained.[245] A variant that elutes with HbA_{1c} will yield a gross overestimation of HbA_{1c}, and a variant that coelutes with HbA will underestimate HbA_{1c}. Note that a single variant may falsely increase or decrease HbA_{1c}, depending on the method used.[245]

High-Performance Liquid Chromatography. HbA_{1c} and other hemoglobin fractions can be separated by HPLC, which employs cation-exchange chromatography.[258] Several fully automated systems are commercially available. Assays require only 5 μL of whole blood, and finger stick samples can be collected in a capillary tube for analysis (although venous blood is most commonly used). Anticoagulated blood is diluted with a hemolysis reagent containing borate. Samples are incubated at 37°C for 30 minutes to remove the Schiff base and are inserted into the autosampler. (Some instruments have a shorter preincubation step, and others separate labile A_{1c} chromatographically, eliminating the step to remove the Schiff base.[259]) A step gradient using three phosphate buffers of increasing ionic strength is passed through the column. Detection is performed at both 415 and 690 nm, and results are quantified by integrating the area under the peaks. Analysis time is as short as 3 to 5 minutes. All HPLC methods had CVs less than 3.0% in a 2014 CAP survey (see Table 57.4). HbA_{1c} by HPLC was used for analysis of all patient samples in the DCCT.[258]

Immunoassay. Assays for HbA_{1c} have been developed using antibodies raised against the Amadori product of glucose (ketoamine linkage) plus the first few (four to eight) amino acids at the *N*-terminal end of the β-chain of hemoglobin.[260,261] A widely used assay measures HbA_{1c} in whole blood by inhibition of latex agglutination. The agglutinator, a synthetic polymer containing multiple copies of the immunoreactive portion of HbA_{1c}, binds the anti-HbA_{1c} monoclonal antibody that is attached to latex beads. This agglutination produces light scattering, measured as an increase in absorbance. HbA_{1c} in the patient's sample competes for the antibody on the latex, inhibiting agglutination and thereby decreasing light scattering. Enzyme immunoassays using monoclonal antibodies are commercially available, and most exhibit reasonable imprecision (see Table 57.4). These assays are generally calibrated to give values that match and correlate with HPLC values. The antibodies do not recognize labile intermediates or other GHbs (such as HbA_{1a} or HbA_{1b}) because both ketoamine with glucose and specific amino acid sequences are required for binding. Similarly, several hemoglobin variants, such as HbF, HbA_2, HbS, and carbamylated hemoglobin, are not detected.[245] The procedure has been adapted for capillary blood samples using a benchtop analyzer with reagent cartridges designed for use in physicians' office laboratories.

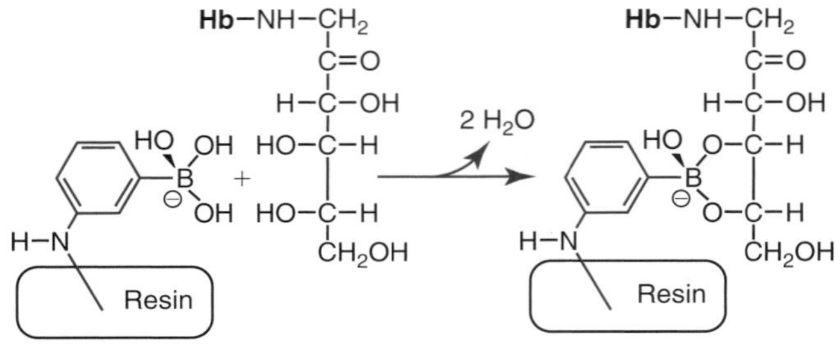

Hb–NH–CH₂ / C=O / H–C–OH / HO–C–H / HO–C–H / CH₂OH + immobilized boronic acid (HO, OH, B⁻, OH; H–N, Resin) → 2 H₂O → Boronic acid-glycated hemoglobin complex

Immobilized boronic acid — Glycated hemoglobin — Boronic acid-glycated hemoglobin complex

FIGURE 57.7 Reaction of glycated hemoglobin (GHb) with immobilized boronic acid.

Affinity Chromatography. Affinity gel columns are used to separate GHb, which binds to the column, from the nonglycated fraction. *m*-Aminophenylboronic acid is immobilized by cross-linking to beaded agarose or another matrix (eg, glass fiber). The boronic acid reacts with the *cis*-diol groups of glucose bound to hemoglobin to form a reversible five-member ring complex, thus selectively holding the GHb on the column (Fig. 57.7). The nonglycated hemoglobin does not bind. Sorbitol is then added to elute the GHb. Absorbance of bound and nonbound fractions, measured at 415 nm, is used to calculate the percentage of GHb.

A commercial assay is performed on an automated analyzer that uses a soluble reagent consisting of dihydroxyboronate coupled with high molecular weight polyacrylic acid.[262] GHb binds to the boronate. The polyanionic-glycated hemoglobin affinity complex attaches by electrostatic interactions to the cationic surface of the solid-phase matrix (ion capture). Nonglycated hemoglobin does not bind and is removed in a wash step. GHb is quantified by measuring quenching by hemoglobin of the fluorescence of an added fluorophore, 4-methyl-umbelliferone. Total hemoglobin is determined by fluorescence quenching of a second sample containing sorbitol. The sorbitol competes for boronate binding sites, and both nonglycated hemoglobin and GHb contribute to inhibition of the quenching. The fluorescence measurements are converted to glycated and total hemoglobin concentrations from separate stored calibration curves.

The major advantages of affinity chromatography are that there is no interference from nonglycated hemoglobins and there is negligible interference from the labile intermediate form of HbA_{1c}. It is unaffected by variations in temperature and has reasonably good precision. Importantly, hemoglobin variants such as HbS, HbC, HbD, or HbE produce little effect. Affinity methods measure total GHb. This includes components other than HbA_{1c} because the assay detects ketoamine structures on lysine and valine residues on both α- and β-chains of hemoglobin.

Although the method detects all GHbs, most commercially available systems are calibrated to report a standardized HbA_{1c} value. The value is derived from an equation obtained from linear regression between total GHb and HbA_{1c} analysis by HPLC.[262] A linear relationship has been demonstrated, and standardized HbA_{1c} values are thus comparable to values obtained by methods specific for HbA_{1c}. Columns and reagents are commercially available.

Capillary Electrophoresis. HbA_{1c} was first identified in 1968 on agar gel electrophoresis at pH 6.2.[263] With development of better alternatives, electrophoretic methods disappeared from use (see Table 57.4). The development of capillary electrophoresis has generated renewed interest in the technique. Advantages of capillary electrophoresis include high resolving ability (due to the high voltage that can be applied) and small sample volume (discussed in more detail in Chapter 15).[264] Briefly, charged molecules are separated by their electrophoretic mobility in an alkaline buffer (pH 9.4), as well as by electrolyte pH and electroosmotic flow. Hemoglobins are detected by absorption spectroscopy at the cathodic end of the capillary. An automated liquid-flow capillary electrophoresis method to measure HbA_{1c} is commercially available and has been approved by the FDA in the United States.

Enzymatic Assays. Enzymatic assays to measure HbA_{1c} have been developed recently based on a method in which fructosyl peptide oxidase catalyzes the oxidative deglycation of *N*-(deoxyfructosyl)-Val-His.[265] Erythrocytes are lysed, and sodium nitrite is added to oxidize total hemoglobin to methemoglobin. Addition of sodium azide produces azidomethemoglobin, which is quantified on a spectrophotometer at 476 nm.[266] Neutral protease is added to release fructosyl dipeptide (ie, *N*-(deoxyfructosyl)-Val-His) from the *N*-terminal of the β-chain of HbA_{1c}. Fructosyl peptide oxidase hydrolyzes the fructosyl dipeptide, releasing hydrogen peroxide, which reacts with a chromogen in the presence of peroxidase, and the color is measured by absorbance at 660 nm. The procedure has been adapted for analysis on a high throughput automated analyzer,[266] and the method has been approved by the FDA for use in the United States. A kit is also commercially available (Diazyme, Poway, California) that can be used on many automated analyzers.

Removal of Labile Glycated Hemoglobin From Red Blood Cells

The concentration of the labile form of HbA_{1c} (Schiff base) fluctuates rapidly in response to acute changes in plasma glucose concentrations and should be removed before analysis by charge-based assays. This may be accomplished by incubating red blood cells in saline[267] or in buffer solutions at pH 5 to 6,[268] or by dialysis or ultrafiltration of hemolysates. Most kits for column assays contain reagents to remove this labile component.

Assay Standardization

Clinical laboratories measure GHb with diverse assays that use multiple methods and quantify different components. The DCCT results accentuated the need for accurate GHb measurement and provided a strong impetus for standardization of GHb assays. At the end of the DCCT, it was noted that absence of both a reference method and a single GHb standard had generated confusion.[269] Interlaboratory comparisons were not possible, and even a single quality control sample analyzed by a single method exhibited interlaboratory CVs as high as 16.5%. Similar large variability among laboratories was observed in Europe.[270] Committees were established under the auspices of the American Association for Clinical Chemistry (AACC) in 1993 and the IFCC in 1995 to standardize GHb assays.[271]

The NGSP was established in 1996 to implement the protocol developed by the AACC to calibrate GHb results to DCCT-equivalent values. Employing a network of reference laboratories, the NGSP interacts with manufacturers of GHb methods to help them calibrate their methods and trace values to the DCCT.[272] Manufacturers apply for certification by performing precision testing according to CLSI EP5-A guidelines and report results in DCCT-equivalent HbA_{1c} values. This calibration effort has markedly improved harmonization of results and has reduced imprecision.[271,272] Results obtained using NGSP-certified assays can be compared directly with results of the DCCT and UKPDS, allowing alignment with clinical outcomes data. The ADA recommends that clinical laboratories use only assays certified by the NGSP and participate in proficiency testing offered by the CAP. The CAP GHb survey uses pooled whole blood specimens at several HbA_{1c} concentrations. Target values are assigned by the NGSP network. Thus individual laboratories can directly compare their HbA_{1c} results with those of the DCCT and UKPDS.

A different approach was adopted by the IFCC. A working group was established to devise a reference system for standardization based on HbA_{1c}. The IFCC group developed a mixture of purified HbA_{1c} and HbA_0 as primary reference material.[273] Two candidate reference methods—electrospray ionization mass spectrometry (ESI-MS) and capillary electrophoresis—were proposed.[273] These specifically measure the glycated *N*-terminal valine of the β-chain of hemoglobin. Analysis is performed by digesting the hemoglobin molecule with endoproteinase Glu-C, which cleaves the β-chain between Glu-6 and Glu-7, releasing the *N*-terminal hexapeptide. Glycated and nonglycated hexapeptides are separated and quantified by HPLC-ESI-MS or by HPLC-capillary electrophoresis.[273] HbA_{1c} is measured as the ratio between glycated and nonglycated *N*-terminal hexapeptides. The IFCC Working Group has established a network of laboratories to implement and maintain the reference system.[274] Comparisons between IFCC and NGSP reference methods (and reference systems from Japan and Sweden) indicate a close and stable relationship and allow manufacturers to calibrate their instruments to a higher-level reference method.[274] However, HbA_{1c} results obtained using IFCC reference methods are 1.5% to 2% absolute HbA_{1c} units lower than those of the NGSP (and lower than other reference systems). The difference is probably due to measurement of glycated components other than HbA_{1c} by HPLC. The IFCC method is a higher-order reference method and is not designed to be used for routine analysis of patient samples.

Reporting HbA_{1c}

HbA_{1c} is reported as a percentage of total hemoglobin in the NGSP system. These values, which are equivalent to those reported in the DCCT and the UKPDS, represent the most widely used reporting system in patient care and the published literature. The IFCC method reports HbA_{1c} as mmol/mol (HbA_{1c}/total Hb).[275] Comparison between the IFCC and NGSP networks produced a master equation that permits conversion between the two reference systems.[276] For example, an HbA_{1c} result of 7% (in NGSP/DCCT/UKPDS units) is equivalent to 53 mmol/mol (in IFCC units). Calculators that convert units are freely available at several websites (eg, http://www.ngsp.org/convert1.asp). Many journals now require that HbA_{1c} values be reported in both NGSP/DCCT and SI units.[277]

A multinational, prospective study (termed A_{1c} Derived Average Glucose [ADAG]) evaluated the relationship between HbA_{1c} concentrations and long-term glucose values.[278] A linear correlation was observed, permitting estimated average glucose (eAG) to be calculated from the HbA_{1c} measurement. The regression equations are as follows (note that in both of these equations, HbA_{1c} is expressed in NGSP % units):

$$\text{eAG mg/dL} = 28.7 \times HbA_{1c} - 46.7$$
$$\text{eAG mmol/L} = 1.59 \times HbA_{1c} - 2.59$$

For example, an HbA_{1c} NGSP value of 7% (53 mmol/mol in IFCC units) translates into an eAG of 154 mg/dL (8.54 mmol/L). Some clinicians and many diabetes educators believe that the eAG will facilitate communication with patients.[279] The ADA and the AACC recommend that laboratories report both HbA_{1c} and eAG. Nevertheless, the concept of expressing HbA_{1c} in terms of average glucose is not accepted by all.[280,281]

Performance Goals

Some expert groups have proposed goals for HbA_{1c} assay accuracy and precision, and these have tightened over the years. Within-subject biological variation of HbA_{1c} is low, with CV_I less than 2%. Recent ADA guidelines recommend an intralaboratory CV of less than 2% and an interlaboratory CV of less than 3.5%.[44] For a single method, the goal should be an interlaboratory CV of less than 3.5%.

Specimen Collection and Storage

Patients do not have to fast. Venous blood should be collected in tubes containing EDTA or oxalate together with fluoride. Sample stability depends on the assay method used.[44] Whole blood may be stored at 4°C for up to 1 week. Above 4°C, HbA_{1a+b} increases in a time- and temperature-dependent manner, but HbA_{1c} is only slightly affected.[282] Storage of samples at −20°C is not recommended for ion-exchange methods.[283] For most methods, whole blood samples stored at −70°C or colder are stable for at least 18 months,[284] with reports of stability up to 14 years.[285] Heparinized samples should be assayed within 2 days and may not be suitable for some methods of analysis (eg, electrophoresis).

Reference Intervals

Values for GHbs are expressed as a percentage of total blood hemoglobin. One of three major GHb species—HbA_1, HbA_{1c}, or total GHb—is usually measured. The United States and many other countries, including Canada, Australia, New Zealand, and the United Kingdom, now report virtually all results as HbA_{1c}. Reference intervals vary, depending on the GHb component measured. The reference interval for HbA_{1c} (using an NGSP-certified method) is 4% to 6% (20 to 42 mmol/mol).

The effects of age on reference intervals are controversial.[44] Some studies show age-related increases (approximately 0.1% per decade after age 30), and other reports show no increase.[286-288] It is not known whether these small but statistically significant increases in HbA_{1c} concentrations with age have any clinical significance. Results are not affected by acute illness. Within-subject biological variation is minimal, as mentioned before.[289] In patients with poorly controlled diabetes mellitus, values may extend to twice the upper limit of the reference interval or more, but they rarely exceed 15% HbA_{1c}. Values greater than 15% (140 mmol/mol) should prompt additional studies to determine the possible presence of variant hemoglobin.[245] Note that target values derived from DCCT and UKPDS and recommended by the ADA and other organizations, not the reference values, are used to evaluate metabolic control in diabetic patients.

There is no specific value of HbA_{1c} below which the risk of diabetic complications is eliminated completely. The ADA states that the goal of treatment in general should be to maintain HbA_{1c} at less than 7% (53 mmol/mol).[26] (Some organizations recommend an HbA_{1c} target of less than 6.5% (48 mmol/mol).) HbA_{1c} goals should be individualized. These goal values are applicable only if the assay method is certified by the NGSP as traceable to the DCCT reference. Each laboratory should establish its own nondiabetic reference interval. Assay precision is important because each 1% change in the NGSP value of HbA_{1c} represents an approximate 30 mg/dL (1.7 mmol/L) change in average blood glucose.

No consensus has been reached on optimum frequency of testing. The ADA recommends that HbA_{1c} should be routinely monitored at least every 6 months in patients meeting treatment goals (and who have stable glycemic control).[26] These recommendations are for patients with type 1 or type 2 diabetes. A recent analysis of more than 79,000 patients revealed that the optimum testing frequency to maximize reduction in HbA_{1c} was every 3 months; testing less frequently was associated with deteriorating control.[290]

Glycated Serum Proteins

In selected patients with diabetes mellitus (eg, GDM, change in therapy), assays may be needed that are more sensitive than GHb to shorter-term alterations in average blood glucose concentrations. Nonenzymatic attachment of glucose to amino groups of proteins other than hemoglobin (eg, serum proteins, membrane proteins, lens crystallins) to form ketoamines also occurs. Because serum proteins turn over more rapidly than erythrocytes (the circulating half-life of albumin is about 14–20 days), the concentration of glycated serum albumin reflects glucose control over a period of 2 to 3 weeks. Therefore both deterioration of control and improvement with therapy are evident earlier than with HbA_{1c}. In addition, glycated serum proteins are not influenced by changes in erythrocyte life span and can be used to monitor glycemia in patients with conditions (eg, hemolysis, blood transfusion) that alter HbA_{1c} independently of glycemia.

Fructosamine

Clinical Significance. Fructosamine is the generic name for plasma protein ketoamines (for reviews, see references 291 and 292). The name refers to the structure of the ketoamine rearrangement product formed by the interaction of glucose with the ε-amino group on lysine residues of albumin. Analogous to GHb, measurement of fructosamine may be used as an index of the average concentration of blood glucose over an extended period of time but one that is about one-fourth as long as the time examined with GHb.

Because all glycated serum proteins are fructosamines and albumin is the most abundant serum protein, measurement of fructosamine is thought to be largely a measure of glycated albumin, but this has been questioned by some investigators.[293] Although the fructosamine assay can be automated and is cheaper and faster than GHb, there is a lack of consensus on its clinical utility. For example, evaluation of 65 studies led the authors to conclude that fructosamine determination is not a reliable test, and it has not been evaluated sufficiently for routine clinical use.[294] In contrast, a review of essentially the same data concluded that fructosamine could provide information useful in the management of diabetes.[291] Early work using the original assay, introduced in 1983,[295,296] indicated that fructosamine concentrations were significantly higher in diabetic individuals than in healthy subjects. Over the succeeding decade, the assay underwent numerous modifications because several artifacts were identified that rendered data from the first-generation fructosamine assay difficult to interpret. These include apparent lack of specificity for glycated proteins (up to 60% of the value was due to non-fructosamine-reducing substances), lack of standardization among laboratories, difficulty in calibrating the assay, and interference by urates and hyperlipidemia.[297] Substantial modifications produced second-generation assays that contain uricase and higher detergent concentrations and are calibrated with glycated lysine.[298] In addition, an industry standard was adopted. These improvements resulted in average fructosamine values in nondiabetic individuals that are approximately 10% of those obtained with the first-generation assay. Some clinical evidence suggests that fructosamine may be useful in the elderly[299] and in those with gestational diabetes.[300] However, there is limited evidence relating it to the complications of diabetes, and there is no agreed target for optimum glycemic control. An important limitation is the lack of long-term prospective studies with clinical outcomes.[301] The potential role of the second-generation fructosamine assay in providing rapid, reliable, inexpensive, and technically easy monitoring of glycemic control requires evaluation. The clinical value of fructosamine has not been firmly established, and further studies are required to determine whether it is useful for routine monitoring of patients' glycemic control.[44]

Because fructosamine determination monitors short-term glycemic changes different from GHb, it may have a role in conjunction with GHb rather than instead of it. In addition, fructosamine may be useful in patients in whom GHb is of limited value—for example, decreased erythrocyte life span. Gross changes in protein concentration and half-life may have large effects on the proportion of protein that is glycated. Thus fructosamine results may be invalid in patients with nephrotic syndrome, cirrhosis of the liver, or dysproteinemias, or after rapid changes in acute-phase reactants. Initial reports indicated that, in the absence of significant alterations in serum protein concentrations, fructosamine results were independent of protein concentrations.[302] However, this observation has been questioned by other investigators, who recommend that fructosamine values be corrected for protein concentrations. This issue remains to be resolved. It is generally accepted that the test should not be performed when serum albumin is less than 30 g/L. Although it was initially postulated that the fructosamine assay would replace the OGTT, there is no role for the fructosamine assay in the diagnosis of diabetes mellitus. A few studies have evaluated fructosamine in identifying women with GDM.[303] Most of these include few patients and use different GDM diagnostic criteria and fructosamine thresholds. Measurement of fructosamine should not be used to screen patients for GDM.[303]

Determination of Fructosamine. Methods for measuring glycated serum proteins include affinity chromatography using immobilized phenylboronic acid (similar to the GHb assay);[304] HPLC of glycated lysine residues after hydrolysis of the glycated proteins;[305] a photometric procedure in which mild acid hydrolysis releases 5-hydroxymethylfurfural (proteins are precipitated with trichloroacetic acid and the supernatant is reacted with 2-thiobarbituric acid);[306] and other procedures using phenylhydrazine and ε-*N*-(2-furoylmethyl)-L-lysine (furosine). None of these assays is popular because they are not suitable for routine clinical laboratories. The development of monoclonal antibodies to glycated albumin,[307] although theoretically advantageous, has not yet resulted in the widespread availability of commercial assays. It should be noted that prolonged storage at ultra-low temperatures (−96°C) prevents in vitro glycation of serum proteins.[308]

An alternative method for the measurement of fructosamine is a modification[298,309] of the original method of Johnson and colleagues.[296] This method is conducted under alkaline conditions and results in fructosamine undergoing an Amadori rearrangement, with the resultant compounds having reducing activity that can be differentiated from other reducing substances. In the presence of carbonate buffer, fructosamine rearranges to the eneaminol form, which reduces NBT to a formazan (Fig. 57.8). Absorbance at 530 nm is measured at two time points, and the absorbance change is proportional to the fructosamine concentration. A 10-minute preincubation is necessary to allow fast-reacting interfering reducing substances to react. It is unnecessary to remove endogenous glucose from patients' samples because a pH greater than 11 is required for glucose to reduce NBT. The assay is easily automated and has excellent between-batch analytical precision. Hemoglobin (>100 mg/dL) and bilirubin (>4 mg/dL) may interfere; therefore moderate to grossly hemolyzed and icteric samples should not be used. Ascorbic acid concentrations greater than 5 mg/dL may cause negative interference. Kits are commercially available (Roche Diagnostics, Indianapolis, Indiana).

Enzymatic methods have also been described.[310] Samples are incubated with proteinase K, which cleaves serum proteins into smaller fragments. The next step is addition of the enzyme fructosaminase, which catalyzes the oxidative degradation of the glycated peptides, resulting in the release of H_2O_2, which is quantified. The assay, which can be run on

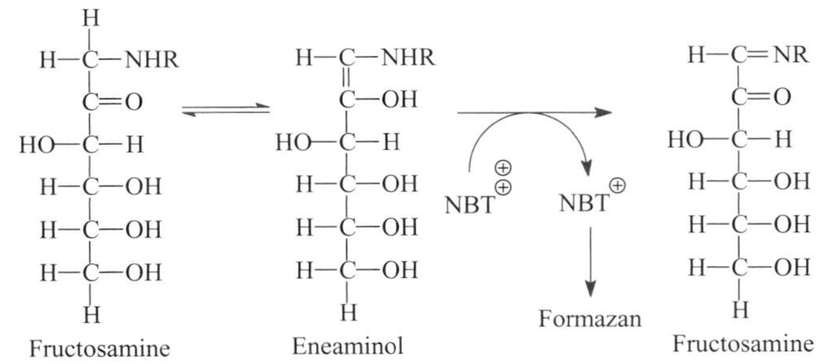

FIGURE 57.8 Reaction of fructosamine with nitroblue tetrazolium (NBT).

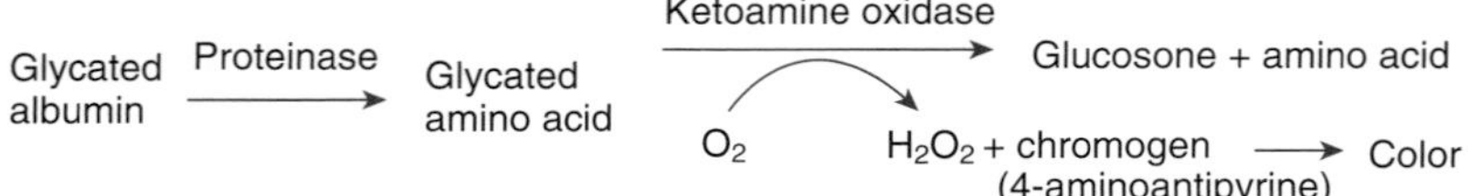

FIGURE 57.9 Hydrolysis of glycated albumin.

an automated analyzer, is commercially available (GlycoGap, Diazyme, Poway, California) and has been approved by the FDA for use in the United States. Unlike the NBT assay, the fructosaminase assay is reported to have no significant interference at up to 7.5 mg/dL (128 umol/L) bilirubin and 200 mg/dL (124 mmol/L) hemoglobin. An assay that measures fructosamine by oxidizing the ketoamine bond using ketoamine oxidase, with release of hydrogen peroxide that is quantified by a photometric reaction, is also commercially available (Randox, Antrim, United Kingdom).

Reference Intervals. Values in a nondiabetic population are 205 to 285 μmol/L using a colorimetric assay. The reference interval corrected for albumin is 191 to 265 μmol/L. The reference interval for the enzymatic assay is reported to be 151 to 300 μmol/L.

Glycated Albumin

Albumin, which comprises approximately 60% of total serum protein, makes up 80% or more of total glycated serum proteins.[311] The *N*-terminus and 59 lysine residues are potential glycation sites, and it is not known how many of these are glycated in vivo. Analysis of human plasma by HPLC tandem mass spectrometry and [$^{13}C_6$]glucose labeling identified 35 different glycation sites on albumin.[312] Assays that measure only glycated albumin, rather than all glycated serum proteins (ie, fructosamine), are commercially available.

The clinical use of glycated albumin is limited by the same caveats that apply to fructosamine—namely, limited evidence relating it to the complications of diabetes and lack of long-term prospective studies with clinical outcomes. Further studies are required to determine whether it is useful for routine monitoring of patients' glycemic control.[44]

Determination of Glycated Albumin. Several different methods have been used to quantify glycated albumin.[311,313,314] These include a colorimetric procedure in which mild acid hydrolysis releases 5-hydroxymethylfurfural (proteins are precipitated with trichloroacetic acid and the supernatant is reacted with 2-thiobarbituric acid);[306] RIA using beads coated with antibody to albumin and ^{125}I-labeled antibody directed against glucitol-lysine epitopes of glycated albumin previously reduced by sodium borohydride ($NaBH_4$) to reduce the Schiff base;[315] ELISA in which glycated albumin binds to a monoclonal antibody coated on a plate, followed by incubation with an enzyme-linked antihuman albumin antibody (Exocell, Philadelphia, Pennsylvania.); enzyme-linked boronate immunoassay where boronic acid-HRP conjugate binds to the cis-diols of glycated albumin, which is immobilized by an antihuman albumin antibody coated onto microtiter plate;[316] affinity chromatography using immobilized phenylboronic acid, followed by elution and measurement of albumin;[304] boronate affinity chromatography; HPLC with anion exchange chromatography to separate albumin, followed by boronate affinity chromatography to separate glycated from nonglycated albumin;[317] enzymatic assay using ketoamine oxidase;[318] and mass spectrometry.[319,320]

Probably the most widely used method globally is enzymatic. The assay has two steps. In the first, endogenous glycated amino acids are eliminated by oxidation with ketoamine oxidase.[318] In the second step, glycated albumin is hydrolyzed by an albumin-specific proteinase to glycated amino acids, which are subsequently oxidized by ketoamine oxidase to glucosone, producing hydrogen peroxide (Fig. 57.9). This is quantified with the chromogen 4-aminoantipyrene by measuring absorbance at 546/700 nm. Total albumin is measured with bromocresol purple, and glycated albumin is expressed as a percentage of total albumin. This assay is commercially available (Lucica GA-L, Asahi Kasei Pharma Corporation, Tokyo, Japan) in several countries and has been used in numerous published studies. At the time of this writing, it is not available in the United States.

Reference Intervals. Reference intervals vary considerably, depending on the method, ranging from 0.8% to 1.4% to 18% to 22%.[311,313] The reference interval for the enzymatic assay, which is expressed as a percentage of total albumin, is 11.9% to 15.8%.

No significant gender differences have been observed, but values in blacks are significantly higher than in whites.[313] Within-subject biological variation is low (CVi 2.1%), but between-subject variation is reported to be 10.6%.[321] In patients with poorly controlled diabetes, values may increase by up to fivefold. Factors that influence albumin metabolism have been reported to alter glycated albumin independently of glycemia. These include the nephrotic syndrome, thyroid disease, cirrhosis of the liver, smoking, hyperuricemia, and hypertriglyceridemia.[322] Samples can be stored as long as 23 years at −70°C.[323]

Advanced Glycation End Products

The molecular mechanism by which hyperglycemia produces toxic effects is unknown, but glycation of tissue proteins may be important. Nonenzymatic attachment of glucose to long-lived proteins, lipids, or nucleic acids produces stable Amadori early-glycated products. These undergo a series of additional rearrangements, dehydration, and fragmentation reactions, resulting in stable advanced glycation end products (AGEs). A series of distinct biochemical reactions produce multiple heterogeneous AGEs,[324,325] with more than 20 identified, including *N*-(carboxymethyl)lysine (CML), pentosidine, pyrraline, and glyoxal lysine dimer.[326] The amounts of these products do not return to normal when hyperglycemia is corrected, and they accumulate continuously over the life span of the protein. Hyperglycemia accelerates the formation of protein-bound AGE, and patients with diabetes mellitus thus have more AGE than healthy subjects. Through effects on the functional properties of protein and extracellular matrix, AGE may contribute to the microvascular and macrovascular complications of diabetes mellitus.[177,327] There is evidence that AGE in the diet contributes to AGE accumulation in tissues.

Measurement of AGEs in the circulation has also been used as a biomarker to monitor the complications of diabetes.[324] However, the diverse structures and composition of AGEs has resulted in assay difficulties. Analysis by ELISA has lacked standardization, yielding variable results.[328] The development of stable isotope dilution analysis liquid chromatography-tandem mass spectrometry, in conjunction with careful preanalytic sample preparation, shows potential to resolve these problems.[325] Some AGE products fluoresce, which forms the basis of noninvasive measurement of skin autofluorescence with a portable reader. Some studies have revealed a positive association of skin autofluorescence with complications of diabetes,[329] but adjustment for HbA_{1c} rendered associations nonsignificant.[330] Limitations of skin autofluorescence measurements include lack of specificity for AGE, while most AGEs are not fluorescent.[325]

Some of the family of heterogeneous AGEs can activate the receptor for AGE (RAGE) to induce intracellular signaling that leads to enhanced oxidative stress and the production of proinflammatory cytokines.[324,327] RAGE is a member of the immunoglobulin superfamily and is expressed on the surface of several cells, including endothelial and kidney. A truncated form of RAGE, termed *soluble RAGE* (sRAGE), is produced mainly by proteolysis of RAGE and is found in serum.[324] An ELISA is commercially available to measure sRAGE. However, the relationship between sRAGE concentrations and adverse outcomes in diabetes is contentious, with some published studies claiming increased sRAGE,[331] while others observe decreased sRAGE.[332] Further studies are required to clarify the association between sRAGE and health outcomes.

Promising findings have been obtained in studies of recombinant sRAGE in animals, suggesting that this may be a therapeutic approach in humans. Similarly, inhibitors of AGE formation, such as aminoguanidine, have been shown to prevent several of the complications of diabetes in experimental animal models. While initial clinical trials in patients failed to show a significant benefit of anti-AGE therapy, this continues to be an area of active research.[324]

1,5-ANHYDROGLUCITOL

Another marker of long-term glycemia is 1,5-anhydroglucitol (1,5-AG), which reflects glucose concentrations over the preceding 2 to 14 days.[333,334] It is a 1-deoxy form of glucose that originates predominantly from the diet, with the vast majority (>99.9%) normally being reabsorbed from the glomerular filtrate by the SGLT4 sodium-dependent glucose transporter. When blood glucose concentrations exceed the renal threshold (usually about 180 mg/dL [10.0 mmol/L]), reabsorption of 1,5-AG decreases, leading to a rapid reduction in serum 1,5-AG concentrations. Therefore low 1,5-AG indicates hyperglycemia, correlating particularly with postprandial blood glucose concentration.[334] An automated assay is commercially available (and FDA-approved for use in the United States) (GlycoMark, Nippon Kayaku, Tokyo, Japan). The two-step colorimetric assay uses glucokinase initially to convert all the glucose in the sample to glucose 6-phosphate to prevent it from interfering in the second step. Then pyranose oxidase oxidizes the C-2 hydroxyl group of 1,5-AG, generating hydrogen peroxide, which is detected by colorimetry using peroxidase. The reference interval is 10.2 to 33.8 µg/mL (males) and 5.9 to 31.8 µg/mL (females). Several factors unrelated to glycemia may alter 1,5-AG values, including diet, medications, renal disease, and liver disease.[334] A recent study found a significant association between low 1,5-AG concentrations and the risk of retinopathy and chronic kidney disease in patients with diabetes.[335] Nevertheless, there is limited evidence linking it to outcomes, and the clinical value of measuring 1,5-AG remains to be established.

ALBUMINURIA

Clinical Significance

Patients with diabetes mellitus are at high risk of developing renal damage. End-stage renal disease requiring dialysis or transplantation develops in approximately one-third of patients with type 1 diabetes,[336] and diabetes is the most common cause of end-stage renal disease in the United States and Europe.[337] Although nephropathy is less common in patients with type 2 diabetes, approximately 60% of all cases of diabetic nephropathy occur in these patients because of the higher incidence of this form of diabetes. Early detection of diabetic nephropathy relies on tests of urinary excretion of albumin. Persistent proteinuria detectable by routine screening tests (equivalent to a urinary albumin excretion rate [AER] >200 µg/min or >300 mg/24 h) indicates overt diabetic nephropathy. This is usually associated with long-standing disease and is unusual less than 5 years after the onset of type 1 diabetes. Once diabetic nephropathy occurs, renal function deteriorates rapidly and renal insufficiency evolves. Treatment at this stage can retard the rate of progression without stopping or reversing the renal damage. Preceding this stage is a period of increased AER not detected by routine dipstick methods. This range of 20 to 200 µg/min (or 30–300 mg/24 h) of increased AER has been called *microalbuminuria*, although current nomenclature has eliminated the terms *microalbuminuria* and *macroalbuminuria*. (Note that it is not defined in terms of urinary albumin concentration, although the ratio of the urinary albumin concentration to the urinary creatinine concentration [albumin-to-creatinine ratio (ACR)] in an untimed urine specimen can be used as a substitute for albumin measurements in a timed collection of urine, as described later.) The term *microalbuminuria*, although widely used, is misleading. It implies a small version of the albumin molecule rather than an excretion rate of albumin greater than normal but less than that detectable by routine methods. Use of the term is discouraged.[338]

The presence of increased AER denotes an increase in the transcapillary escape rate of albumin and therefore is a marker of microvascular disease. Persistent AER greater than 20 µg/min represents a 20-fold greater risk for the development of clinically overt renal disease in patients with type 1 and type 2 diabetes. Prospective studies have demonstrated that increased urinary albumin excretion precedes and is highly predictive of diabetic nephropathy, end-stage renal disease, cardiovascular mortality, and total mortality in patients with diabetes mellitus.[337,339] The DCCT and the UKPDS showed that intensive diabetes therapy can significantly reduce the risk of development of increased AER and overt nephropathy in individuals with diabetes.[175,176] Increased AER also identifies a group of nondiabetic subjects at increased risk for coronary artery disease.[75,340] Interventions, such as control of blood glucose concentrations and blood pressure, particularly with angiotensin-converting enzyme (ACE) inhibitors, slow the rate of decline in renal function.[337]

Methods for Measuring Albuminuria

No consensus has been reached about how a urine sample should be collected for measuring albumin. Variations in urine flow rate in a person may be corrected by expressing albumin as a ratio to creatinine (ie, ACR). AER is increased by physiological and other factors (eg, exercise within 24 hours, posture, diuresis), infection, fever, marked hyperglycemia, and marked hypertension. Samples should not be collected after exertion, in the presence of urinary tract infection, during acute illness, immediately after surgery, or after an acute fluid load. The urine samples that are currently considered acceptable include 24-hour collection; overnight (8 to 12 hours, timed) collection; 1- to 2-hour timed collection (in laboratory or clinic); and first morning sample for simultaneous albumin and creatinine measurement. Only results for timed specimens can be reported as mg albumin excreted per hour, but the AER is more practical and convenient for the patient and is the recommended method.[44] A first morning void sample is best because it has lower within-person variation for the albumin-to-creatinine ratio than a random urine sample.[44,341] At least three separate specimens, collected on different days, should be assayed because of high within-subject biological variation (CVi of 30% to 50%) and diurnal variation (50% to 100% higher during the day). The ACR in the first morning void sample has a within-subject CVi of 31%.[342] Urine should be stored at 4°C after collection. Alternatively, 2 mL of 50 g/L sodium azide can be added per 500 mL of urine, but preservatives are not recommended for some assays. Bacterial contamination and glucose have no effect. Specimens are stable in untreated urine for at least a week at 4°C or −20°C and for at least five months at −80°C. Freezing samples has been reported to decrease albumin,[343] but mixing immediately before assay eliminates this effect. Neither centrifugation nor filtration is necessary before storage at −20°C or −80°C. The albumin concentration decreases by 0.27%/day at −20°C.[44]

Screening tests should be positive in greater than 95% of patients with albuminuria.[44] Patients who screen positive should have quantitative measurement of urine albumin in an accredited laboratory.[44] The analytical CV of methods to measure low concentrations of albuminuria should be greater than 15%.[44] Most quantitative assays achieve this target.[44] An estimated glomerular fitration rate (eGFR) should also be calculated from serum creatinine in patients who have a positive screening test. Serum creatinine and eGFR should be performed at least annually in all adults with diabetes because some patients have decreased GFR without albuminuria.[28]

Semiquantitative Assays

Several semiquantitative assays are available for screening for albuminuria. These test strips, most of which are optimized to read "positive" at a predetermined albumin concentration, have been recommended for screening programs. In view of the wide variability in AER, it must be borne in mind that a "normal" value does not rule out renal disease. Because these assays measure albumin concentration, dilute urine may yield a false-negative test result. Refrigerated urine samples should be allowed to reach at least 10°C before analysis. Chemstrip Micral (Roche Diagnostics Indianapolis, Ind.) uses a monoclonal antialbumin IgG labeled with colloidal gold. The albumin in the urine binds to the antibody-gold conjugate in a zone on the test strip. Excess conjugate is retained in a separation zone containing immobilized human albumin, and only albumin bound to the antibody–enzyme immunocomplex diffuses to the reaction zone. The test strip is dipped into the urine for 5 seconds, and the intensity of the color after 1 minute is proportional to the urinary albumin concentration. Direct visual comparison is made with printed color blocks, with 0, 20, 50, and 100 mg/L. No interference is observed with drugs (except oxytetracycline), glucose, urea, or other proteins. Urine samples with albumin concentrations greater than 100 to 300 mg/L may be diluted and reassayed. The assigned concentration of the color block is multiplied by the dilution factor to obtain the concentration in the sample. These semiquantitative assays have been recommended for screening only.

A number of strips that measured only albumin—for example, Microbumintest, Albu Screen, and Albu Sure—are no longer commercially available; some have been replaced by point-of-care tests that measure both albumin and creatinine and report an ACR. Clinitek Microalbumin (Siemens, Deerfield, Illinois) measures albumin by dye-binding with bromophenol blue and creatinine with an enzyme assay using peroxidase. The strips are read in a reflectance meter. Results are reported as less than 30, 30 to 300, or greater than 300 mg/g (<3.4, 3.4–33.9, or >33.9 mg/mmol). Hemoglobin, myoglobin, contamination of the urine (eg, with soaps, detergents, antiseptics, or skin cleansers), and certain drugs (eg, cimetidine, pyridium, or nitrofurantoin) may interefere. The assay is stated to detect albumin and creatinine at concentrations of 20 to 40 mg/L and 10 mg/dL (0.9 mmol/L), respectively. Aution (Arkray, Kyoto, Japan) also uses a small reflectometer to measure albumin and creatinine on a test strip.[344] Automated readers are more accurate than manual assessment of reagent strips.

Currently available dipstick tests do not have adequate analytical sensitivity to detect low levels of albuminuria.[44] This conclusion was confirmed in a recent systematic review of the diagnostic accuracy of point-of-care tests for detecting albuminuri.[345] The authors observed that results of individual studies vary widely, with sensitivities ranging from 18% to 92.9% and specificities ranging from 60% to 100%. Pooling data yielded a sensitivity of 76% and a specificity of 93% for semiquantitative tests.[345] The negative likelihood ratio was 0.26, indicating that a negative test does not rule out albuminuria.

Quantitative Assays

All sensitive, specific assays for urine albumin use immunochemistry with antibodies to human albumin. Four methods are available: RIA, ELISA, radial immunodiffusion, and immunoturbidimetry.[346] Each method has advantages and disadvantages. The immunoturbidimetric assay is the most reliable and should be considered the standard for comparison.[44] Detection limits range from 16 ug/L for RIA to 2 to 5 mg/L for the other methods.[44] Although dye-binding[347] and protein precipitation[348] assays have been described, these are insensitive and nonspecific and should not be used. The international standard reference material for serum albumin measurement was adopted as the standard reference material for urine albumin measurement.[349] The sensitivity and specificity for detecting albuminuria are 96% and 98%, respectively.[345] The negative likelihood ratio of 0.04 meets performance standards,[44] and quantitative assays can be used to exclude albuminuria.

Radial Immunodiffusion. Radial immunodiffusion has not gained wide acceptance because it requires long incubation and a high level of technical skill and cannot be automated. The antibody is incorporated into an agar gel. Aliquots of samples and calibrators are added to wells and are allowed to diffuse into the agar. The antigen–antibody complexes precipitate at equilibrium, and after staining, the distance of migration is measured.

Radioimmunoassay. Standard RIA methods have been described[350] with ^{125}I-labeled albumin and antialbumin antiserum, but reagents are radioactive and have a short shelf life. Commercial kits are available.

Enzyme-Linked Immunosorbent Assay. Both competitive and "sandwich" ELISAs are available.[351,352] Although the competitive ELISA is faster because it uses only one incubation with an antibody, it is reported to be less sensitive and exhibits large imprecision. ELISA can be performed on a microplate reader, allowing semiautomation. In the sandwich assay, the primary antibody (antialbumin antiserum) is fixed on the plastic plate, which is then washed. Samples, controls, and calibrators are added, and the complexes are detected and quantified by a second antibody conjugated to an enzyme label.

Immunoturbidimetry. Albumin in the urine sample forms an insoluble complex with antibodies to human albumin. PEG accelerates complex formation. The turbidity caused by these complexes is measured by a spectrophotometer at 340 nm or 531 nm and is a measure of albumin concentration. The background absorbance of the initial urine sample is subtracted automatically. This method is simple and less expensive than RIA, and rapid analysis of large numbers of samples is possible. Assays may be performed as kinetic or equilibrium reactions. Kits are commercially available for use with automated analyzers (Roche Diagnostics, Siemens). A point-of-care device that uses a cartridge that measures albumin and creatinine and reports an ACR is commercially available (DCA Vantage, Siemens).

Reference Intervals

	ALBUMINURIA			
	μg/min	**mg/24 h**	**mg/g Creatinine**	**mg/mmol Creatinine**
Normal	<20	<30	<30	<3.5
High albuminuria	20–200	30–300	30–300	3.5–30
Very high albuminuria*	>200	>300	>300	>30

*Also termed overt nephropathy. Previously called clinical albuminuria.

The ADA position statement[28] recommends initial albuminuria measurement in patients with type 1 diabetes who have had diabetes for 5 years or longer, and in all type 2 diabetic patients. Because of the difficulty involved in dating the onset of type 2 diabetes, screening should commence at diagnosis. Analysis should be performed annually in all patients who have a negative screening result. Screening may be performed with a semiquantitative assay. If the screening result is positive, albuminuria should be evaluated by a quantitative assay.[44] Diagnosis requires the demonstration of albuminuria in at least two of three samples measured within a 3- to 6-month period.

If the confirmatory test result is positive, treatment with an ACE inhibitor or an angiotensin-receptor blocker should be initiated. ACE inhibitors delay progression to overt nephropathy, and the National Kidney Foundation recommends their use in both normotensive and hypertensive type 1 and 2 diabetic patients.[353] The role of monitoring albuminuria in patients on ACE inhibitor therapy is less clear, although many experts recommend continued surveillance.[28] Untreated, the albuminuria would increase by 10% to 30% per year, whereas the albumin-to-creatinine ratio in patients on ACE inhibitors should stabilize or decrease by up to 50%.

The mean value for AER (5 to 10 mg/day) in young, healthy adults generally increases with age.[338] Several factors are associated with a higher AER. These include large body size, upright posture, pregnancy, exercise, fever, and activation of the renin-angiotensin system.[338] Diurnal and day-to-day variations are large. Urine ACR in untimed spot urine correlates well with AER in timed specimens.[44,354] An early-morning sample is optimal because it has lower within-subject variation.[44] Clinical laboratories should measure creatinine when urine albumin (or total protein) are requested and express the results as ACR (or protein to creatinine ratio) in addition to total albumin (or protein) concentration.[338]

SELECTED REFERENCES

For a full list of references for this chapter, please refer to ExpertConsult.com.

1. American Diabetes Association. Report of the expert committee on the diagnosis and classification of diabetes mellitus. *Diabetes Care* 1997;**20**:1183–97.
17. American Diabetes A. Diagnosis and classification of diabetes mellitus. *Diabetes Care* 2014;**37**(Suppl. 1):S81–90.
28. Standards of medical care in diabetes—2014. *Diabetes Care* 2014;**37**(Suppl. 1):S14–80.
44. Sacks DB, Arnold M, Bakris GL, et al. Guidelines and recommendations for laboratory analysis in the diagnosis and management of diabetes mellitus. *Clin Chem* 2011;**57**: e1–47.
60. Gerich JE. Lilly lecture 1988. Glucose counterregulation and its impact on diabetes mellitus. *Diabetes* 1988;**37**:1608–17.
102. Atkinson MA, Eisenbarth GS, Michels AW. Type 1 diabetes. *Lancet* 2014;**383**:69–82.
120. Lernmark A, Larsson HE. Immune therapy in type 1 diabetes mellitus. *Nat Rev Endocrinol* 2013;**9**:92–103.
138. Simmons RK, Alberti KG, Gale EA, et al. The metabolic syndrome: useful concept or clinical tool? Report of a WHO expert consultation. *Diabetologia* 2010;**53**:600–5.
143. Schellenberg ES, Dryden DM, Vandermeer B, et al. Lifestyle interventions for patients with and at risk for type 2 diabetes: a systematic review and meta-analysis. *Ann Intern Med* 2013;**159**:543–51.
155. Sacks DB. A1c versus glucose testing: a comparison. *Diabetes Care* 2011;**34**:518–23.

165. Coustan DR. Gestational diabetes mellitus. *Clin Chem* 2013;**59**:1310–21.
166. Metzger BE, Lowe LP, Dyer AR, et al. Hyperglycemia and adverse pregnancy outcomes. *N Engl J Med* 2008;**358**:1991–2002.
195. Kamel KS, Halperin ML. Acid-base problems in diabetic ketoacidosis. *N Engl J Med* 2015;**372**:546–54.
209. van den Berghe G, Wouters P, Weekers F, et al. Intensive insulin therapy in the critically ill patients. *N Engl J Med* 2001;**345**:1359–67.
212. Scott MG, Bruns DE, Boyd JC, et al. Tight glucose control in the intensive care unit: are glucose meters up to the task? *Clin Chem* 2009;**55**:18–20.
236. Laffel L. Ketone bodies: a review of physiology, pathophysiology and application of monitoring to diabetes. *Diabetes Metab Res Rev* 1999;**15**:412–26.
245. Bry L, Chen PC, Sacks DB. Effects of hemoglobin variants and chemically modified derivatives on assays for glycohemoglobin. *Clin Chem* 2001;**47**:153–63.
271. Little RR, Rohlfing CL, Sacks DB. Status of hemoglobin A1c measurement and goals for improvement: from chaos to order for improving diabetes care. *Clin Chem* 2011;**57**:205–14.
311. Cohen MP. Clinical, pathophysiological and structure/function consequences of modification of albumin by Amadori-glucose adducts. *Biochim Biophys Acta* 2013;**1830**:5480–5.
338. Levey AS, Becker C, Inker LA. Glomerular filtration rate and albuminuria for detection and staging of acute and chronic kidney disease in adults: a systematic review. *JAMA* 2015;**313**:837–46.

58

Cardiac Function

Fred S. Apple, Jens Peter Goetze, and Allan S. Jaffe

ABSTRACT

Background

Biomarkers play a powerful role in the detection of myocardial injury, including acute myocardial infarction (AMI), and in the diagnosis and ruling out of heart failure (HF). In the appropriate settings with the available clinical symptoms, imaging and electrocardiogram, cardiac troponin I (cTnI) or T (cTnT) detects MI and natriuretic peptides (NPs) diagnose HF. These biomarkers improve patient management with earlier diagnosis, triage, and the assessment of short- and long-term outcomes while containing medical financial costs.

Content

Concepts and definitions of myocardial anatomy and physiology of the heart are described, along with structural changes that occur during the onset and progression of heart disease. Analytical and biochemical characteristics of cTnI, cTnT, BNP, and NT-proBNP and the assays used to measure them are discussed. The clinical role of cTn is discussed regarding the definition of AMI, appropriate serial measures following a patient's presentation to rule in or out MI, and how high-sensitivity assays will assist in the earlier diagnosis of MI and provide a high negative predictive value to aid in managing outpatients. Outcome studies are reviewed to demonstrate the role of cTn in risk stratification and appropriate therapy management. The clinical role of BNP/NT-proBNP is discussed regarding defining acute and chronic HF, appropriate measurements on a patient's presentation that are necessary to distinguish pulmonary from myocardial dysfunction, and how novel NP assays may assist in earlier outcomes assessment and post-MI dysfunction. Finally, potential novel biomarkers for detecting inflammation, plaque rupture, and ischemia are discussed.

Although the heart is an efficient and durable pump, a variety of pathologic processes are known to diminish cardiac function, possibly leading to a multiplicity of dysfunctional clinical states. Heart failure (HF), cases of which are increasing as we improve the treatment of acute ischemic heart disease, and acute ischemic heart disease are the most common cardiac diseases. Often other processes associated with abnormal biomarkers result in an HF syndrome.[1]

The term acute myocardial infarction (AMI) refers to a situation in which death of myocytes is due to an imbalance between myocardial oxygen supply and demand.[2] When the blood supply to the heart is interrupted, gross necrosis of the myocardium results. In addition, a substantial number of cells die as the result of apoptosis. Such extensive damage is most often associated with a thrombotic occlusion superimposed on coronary atherosclerosis. Initially, it was thought that the population of myocytes was fixed; however, it is now believed that the migration of a variety of precursor stem cells has the potential at least to replace some of the damaged myocytes. It is now thought that the process of plaque rupture or erosion and thrombosis is one of the ways in which coronary atherosclerosis progresses, and that we recognize only more severe events.[3,4] Total loss of coronary blood flow results in a clinical syndrome associated with what is known as ST segment elevation AMI (STE AMI). Partial loss of coronary perfusion, if severe, can lead to necrosis as well, which is generally less severe and is known as non–ST elevation myocardial infarction (NSTEMI). Other events of still lesser severity may be missed entirely or may be called angina, which can range from stable to unstable. With the increasing sensitivity of cardiac troponin (cTn) measurements, the frequency of unstable angina is disappearing and more small NSTEMIs are being diagnosed.[5]

In the United States, there are approximately 1.6 million admissions for acute ischemic heart disease per year. Approximately 525,000 patients will have an initial AMI annually and another 210,000 recurrent AMI.[6] Coronary heart disease causes over 25% of all deaths in the United States. Historically, most deaths caused by ischemic heart disease were acute, but as our therapeutic abilities have increased, the disease is becoming more chronic. Deaths that occur acutely result from ventricular arrhythmias or pump dysfunction and congestive heart failure (CHF) with or without cardiogenic shock. Death rates are sharply age dependent, both during hospitalization and in the year after infarction. The US yearly economic burden of cardiovascular disease is in excess of $315.4 billion (2012) and by 2030 is estimated to be $918 billion.[1]

Before the advent of coronary care units, treatment of AMI was directed toward allowing healing of the infarcted area. The concept that infarctions evolve over time and that their size can be moderated led to rethinking of this passive philosophy.[7] We now know that reestablishment of perfusion reduces the extent of myocardial injury and is an important determinant of prognosis.[8] Today the management of AMI suggested by most guidelines is aggressive and invasively oriented in the hope of reducing the extent of myocardial damage and thus improving prognosis.[9,10] In addition, prevention is finally being recognized as a key element in the long-term treatment of patients with atherosclerosis. Recently, different types of MI have been recognized. Those not related to acute plaque rupture events particularly deserve consideration because they less often require invasive management.[2,11]

BASIC ANATOMY

The average human adult heart weighs approximately 325 g in men and 275 g in women and is 12 cm in length. The heart is a hollow muscular organ, shaped like a blunt cone, and is approximately the size of a human fist. It is located in the mediastinum, between the lower lobes of each lung, and rests on the diaphragm. It is enclosed in a sac called the pericardium. The cardiac wall is composed of three layers: the epicardium, which is the outermost layer; a middle layer; and an inner layer, called the endocardium. The heart has four chambers. The two upper chambers are termed the right and left atria, and the two lower chambers are termed the right and left ventricles (Fig. 58.1). Under normal circumstances, the atria are compliant structures, so that intracavitary pressure is

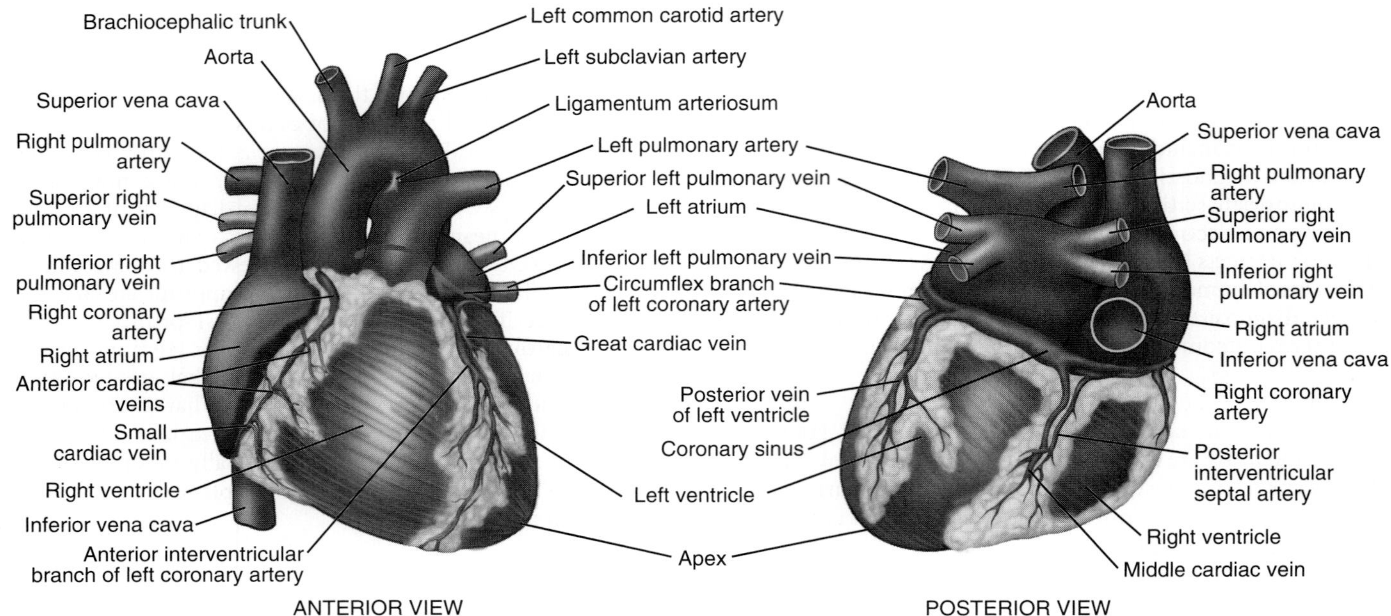

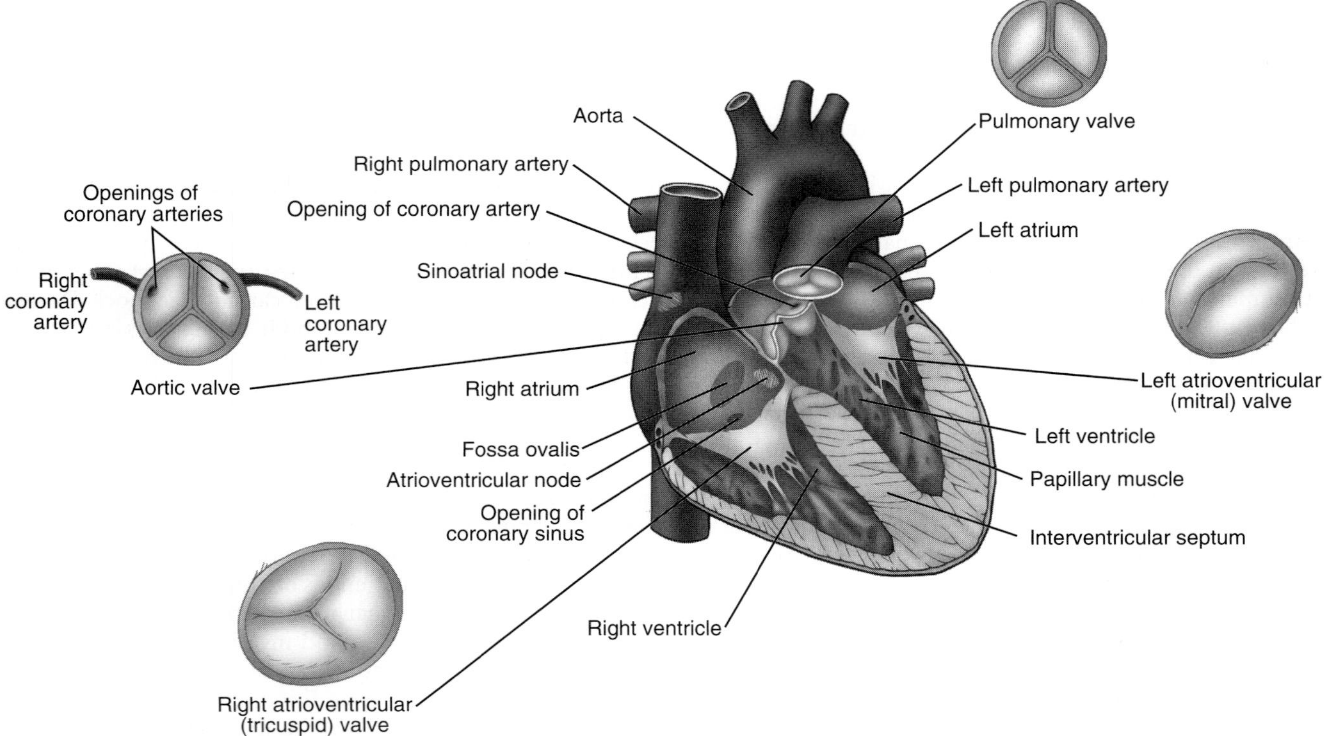

FIGURE 58.1 Anatomy of the heart. (From *Dorland's illustrated medical dictionary.* 32nd ed. Philadelphia: Saunders; 2011, Panel 18.)

low. When anatomy is normal, each atrium is connected to its ventricle through an atrioventricular (AV) valve, which opens and closes (see discussion later in this chapter). The valve on the left side is called the mitral valve and the one on the right side, the tricuspid valve. The right ventricle is banana shaped and pumps blood into the pulmonary artery through a trileaflet pulmonic valve. The left ventricle pumps blood into the aorta through a trileaflet aortic valve. The ventricles, especially the left ventricle, are thicker and less compliant in keeping with the need to generate higher pressures than the right ventricle, and intercavitary pressures are much higher than in the atria. Under normal conditions, the conduction or electrical system of the heart coordinates the sequential contraction of first the atria and then the ventricles. Given that they are connected, each side can affect the other. Under normal circumstances, the sequence of activation optimizes this interaction and thus the efficiency of cardiac function. The right and left coronary arteries originate from two of three cusps of the aortic valve. They provide blood flow and thus nutritive perfusion to the heart. The largest vessels are on the epicardium, and these can be accessed therapeutically fairly easily. Subsequent smaller branches divide to supply the remaining myocardium. The endocardium is the layer most susceptible to ischemia because its perfusion relies on the smallest vessels.

The myocardium contains bundles of striated muscle fibers, each of which is typically 10 to 15 mm in diameter and 30 to 60 mm in length. The work of the heart is generated by the alternating contraction and relaxation of these fibers. The fibers are composed of the cardiac-specific contractile proteins actin and myosin and regulatory proteins called troponins. They also contain a variety of enzymes and proteins that are vital for energy use, such as myoglobin, creatine kinase (CK), and lactate dehydrogenase (LD), some of which can be used as markers of cardiac injury.[2]

PHYSIOLOGY

Cardiac Cycle

A typical cardiac cycle consists of two intervals known as systole and diastole (Fig. 58.2). During diastole, oxygenated blood returns from the lungs to the left atrium via the pulmonary veins and deoxygenated blood returns from other parts of the body to fill the right atrium. During this period, the AV valves are open, allowing passive filling of the ventricle. At the end of diastole, the atria contract, forcing additional blood through the AV valves and into the respective ventricles. During systole, the ventricles contract. This closes the AV valves when ventricular pressure exceeds atrial pressure, and the pulmonary and aortic valves are opened when ventricular pressure exceeds pressure in the pulmonary arteries and/or the aorta, and blood flows into those conduits. During systole, a normal blood pressure in the aorta is typically 120 mm Hg; during diastole, it falls to about 70 mm Hg. At rest, the heart pumps between 60 and 80 times per minute. Stroke volume (ie, the amount of blood expelled with each contraction) is roughly 50 mL, so cardiac output per minute is roughly 3 L. Typically, values are corrected for body surface area and are usually in the range of 2.5 to 3.6 L/min/m^2. Measurements of cardiac output and ventricular filling pressures are the standards for assessing cardiac performance and function. Furthermore, therapeutic intervention in patients with heart disease often includes assessment of cardiac output and ventricular pressures.

Cardiac Conducting System

The cardiac cycle is tightly controlled by the cardiac conducting system, which initiates electrical impulses and carries them via a specialized conducting system to the myocardium. The surface electrocardiogram (ECG) records changes in potential and is a graphic tracing of the variations in electrical potential caused by excitation of the heart muscle and detected at the body surface.[12] Clinically, the ECG is used to identify (1) anatomic, (2) metabolic, (3) ionic, and (4) hemodynamic changes in the heart. The clinical sensitivity and specificity of ECG abnormalities are influenced by a wide spectrum of physiologic and anatomic changes and by the clinical situation.

Under normal circumstances, cardiac cycles are similar and each includes three major components (Fig. 58.3): atrial depolarization (the P wave), ventricular depolarization (the QRS complex), and repolarization (the ST segment and T wave). Atrial depolarization, which is depicted by the P wave, produces atrial contraction. Ventricular depolarization, marked by the QRS complex, produces contraction of the ventricles. It is composed of as many as three deflections: (1) the Q wave, which when present is the first negative deflection; (2) the R wave, which is the first positive deflection; and (3) the S wave, which is a negative deflection after the R wave. On occasion, there is an R′, which is a second positive deflection. Whether each of these occurs depends on the path of depolarization of the ventricles, as does the significance. Thus not every QRS complex will have discrete Q, R, and S waves. The ST segment and the T wave are produced by electrical recovery of the ventricles, and their mean electrical vector is under normal circumstances concordant (ie, in roughly the same direction) with the mean QRS vector.

A routine ECG is composed of 12 leads. Six are called limb leads (I, II, III, aV_R, aV_L, and aV_F) because they are recorded between arm and leg electrodes; six are called precordial or chest leads (V_1, V_2, V_3, V_4, V_5, and V_6) and are recorded across the sternum and left precordium. Each lead records the same electrical impulse but in a different position relative to the heart. Areas of abnormality on the ECG are localized by analyzing differences between the tracing in question and a normal ECG in the 12 different leads.

CARDIAC DISEASE

Cardiac disease occurs in many forms. This chapter briefly covers CHF and acute coronary syndromes (ACSs), such as AMI. The vast number of other cardiac diseases are not discussed in depth here because of the smaller role of clinical laboratory tests in these disorders.

Congestive Heart Failure

CHF is a syndrome characterized by ineffective pumping of the heart, often leading to an accumulation of fluid in the lungs. At least half comes as a result of the loss of the function of the cardiac tissue and is called heart failure with reduced ejection fraction (HFREF). The other half is due to increased stiffness of the cardiac muscle. This type of HF is referred to as heart failure with preserved ejection fraction or HFPEF.[13] Other forms include those related to valvular heart disease and so-called high-output HF. The condition is one in which there is an abnormality of cardiac function such that the heart cannot pump sufficient blood to

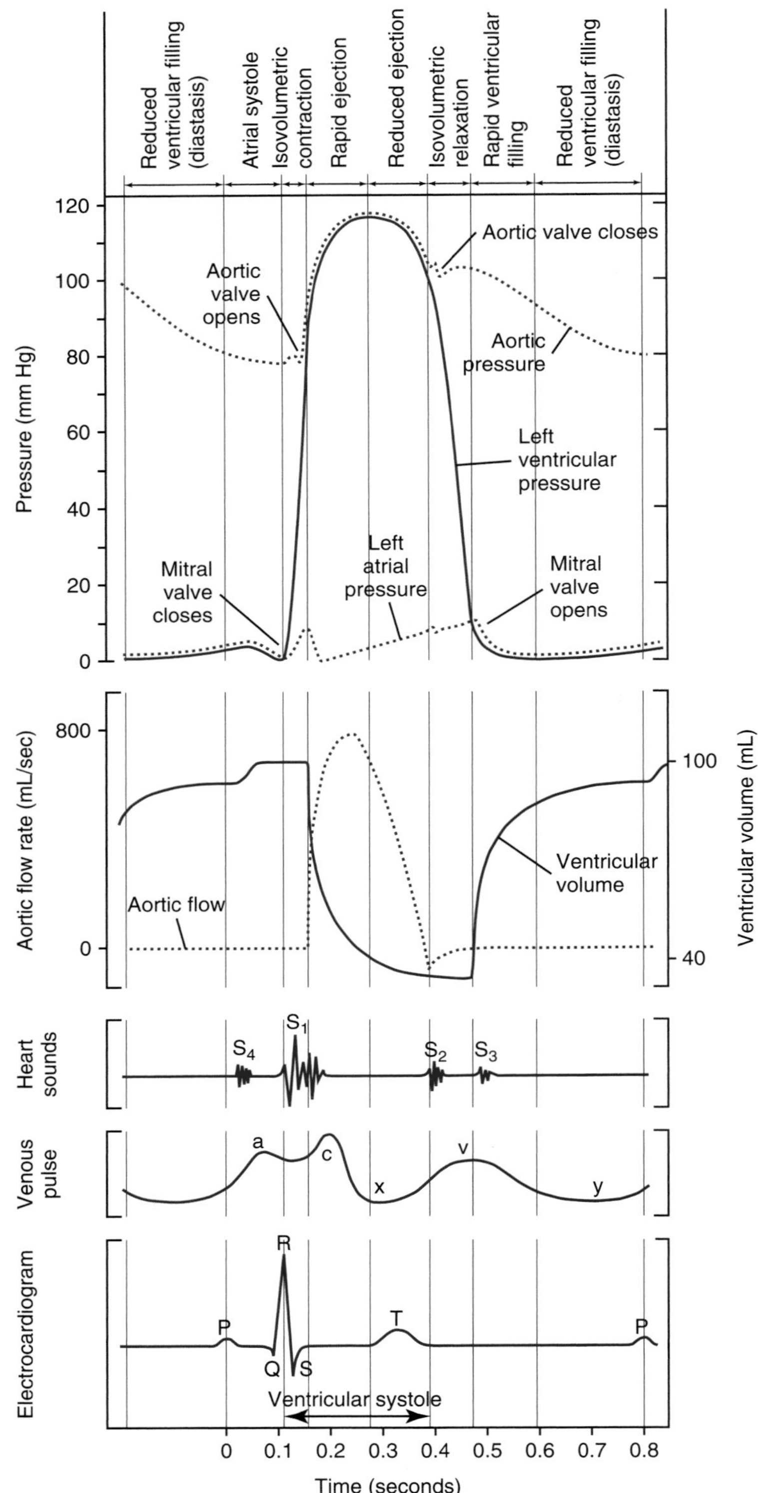

FIGURE 58.2 The cardiac cycle. (From *Dorland's illustrated medical dictionary.* 30th ed. Philadelphia: Saunders, 2003, with permission from the National Kidney Foundation.)

satisfy the requirements of metabolizing tissues, which are abnormally high.

Epidemiology

In the United States, CHF is the only cardiovascular disease with an increasing incidence. The National Heart, Lung, and Blood Institute estimates current prevalence at 4.8 million Americans and 23 million worldwide with CHF.[14] There are approximately 580,000 new cases each year, with approximately 1 million admissions to hospitals for CHF per year.[14] CHF is the leading cause of hospitalization in individuals 65 years of age and older.

Therapeutic options for patients with HFPEF are more limited than for those who have systolic abnormalities.[15] Current prognosis depends on disease severity, but overall it is poor. Mortality at 5 years is approximately 50%, and 10-year mortality is 90%.[14]

These poor outcomes are not without substantial cost, estimated at $24 billion per year in the United States.

Currently, CHF patients are staged with the New York Heart Association (NYHA) functional classifications I to IV. Class I patients are generally considered asymptomatic, with no restrictions on physical activity; class IV patients are often symptomatic at rest, with severe limitations on physical activity. The problem with this classification system is that much of it is based on subjective criteria. Thus patients with comorbidities that reduce their activities are hard to classify. In addition, dyspnea, which is the primary symptom in many of these individuals, has many causes. Finally, many patients with ventricular dysfunction modify their activities to accomplish activities of daily living and thus lack overt symptoms until late in their disease. Therefore patients with CHF often go undiagnosed and untreated early in their disease or are misdiagnosed because of conditions such as pulmonary disease. Initiating treatment in the more advanced disease state (higher degree of irreversible cardiac function and patient deconditioning) is challenging and more expensive (often requiring extended inpatient stay) and leaves patients with considerable morbidity on a daily basis. Obviously, misdiagnoses often lead to patient morbidity. That is the reason why natriuretic peptides have been such an important advance in facilitating the diagnosis of HF.[16,17]

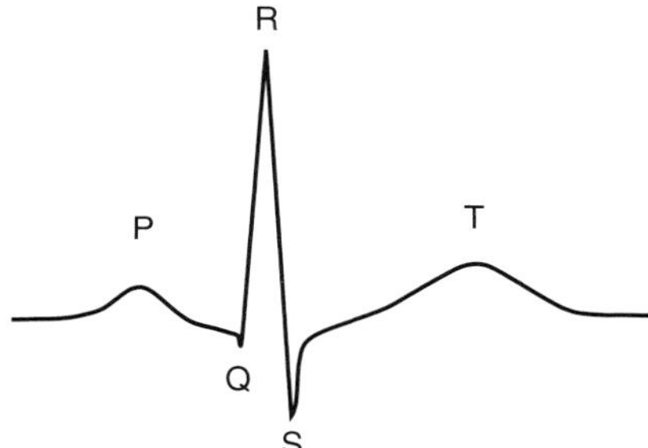

FIGURE 58.3 Electrocardiogram, serial tracing of a normal single heartbeat. Each beat manifests as five major waves: P, Q, R, S, and T. The QRS complex represents the ventricular contraction.

Acute Coronary Syndrome

The term ACS encompasses patients who present with unstable ischemic heart disease.[5] If they have ST segment elevation, their events are called ST elevation myocardial infarctions (STEMI) (Fig. 58.4). Usually, but not always, these individuals develop Q waves on their ECGs, hence the term Q-wave MI. If patients do not have STE but have biochemical criteria for cardiac injury, they are called NSTEMI, and most do not develop ECG Q waves. Those who have unstable ischemia and do not manifest necrosis are designated patients with unstable angina (UA). Most of these syndromes occur in response to an acute event in the coronary artery, when circulation to a region of the heart is obstructed for some reason. If the obstruction is high grade and persists, necrosis usually ensues. Because necrosis is known to take some time to develop, it is apparent that opening the blocked coronary artery in a timely fashion can often prevent some of the death of myocardial tissue. This is clearly the case with STEMI. With non-STEMI (American Heart Association [AHA]/ American College of Cardiology [ACC] guidelines), early but not immediate intervention is advocated, because most often the infarct-related coronary artery is not totally occluded, and thus immediate intervention is less necessary. These syndromes are usually but not always associated with chest discomfort (see discussion later in this chapter).[18,19]

The major cause of ACS is atherosclerosis, which contributes to significant narrowing of the artery lumen and a tendency for plaque disruption and thrombus formation.[3,4,10] Myocardial ischemia and infarction are usually segmental diseases. In up to 90% of patients with these diseases, focal occlusion of only one of the three large coronary vessels or branches occurs. The resulting impaired contractile performance of that segment occurs within seconds and is initially restricted to the affected segment(s). Myocardial ischemia and subsequent infarction usually begin in the endocardium and spread toward the epicardium.[7] The extent of myocardial injury reflects (1) the extent of occlusion, (2) the needs of the area deprived of perfusion, and (3) the duration of the imbalance in coronary supply. Irreversible cardiac injury consistently occurs in animals when the occlusion is complete for at least 15 to 20 minutes. Most damage occurs within the first 2 to 3 hours. Restoration of flow within the first 60 to 90 minutes evokes maximal salvage of tissue, but benefits of

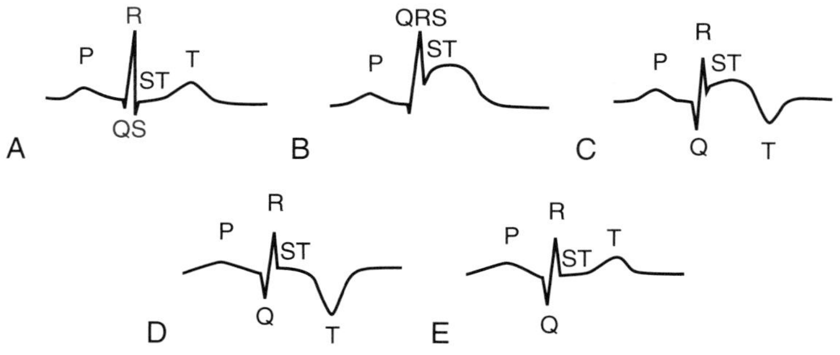

FIGURE 58.4 Electrocardiogram, serial tracing of a patient with an acute myocardial infarction. The sequence is *A*, normal; *B*, hours after infarction, the ST segment becomes elevated; *C*, hours to days later, the T wave inverts and the Q wave becomes larger; *D*, days to weeks later, the ST segment returns to near normal; and *E*, weeks to months later, the T wave becomes upright again, but the large Q wave may remain.

increased survival are possible up to 4 to 6 hours. In some situations, the restoration of coronary perfusion even later is of benefit.[18,19] The percentage of tissue at risk for necrosis (infarct size) depends on the amount of antegrade flow, the existing collateral flow, which is highly variable and difficult to predict, and the metabolic needs of the tissue.[20-22]

In almost all instances, the left ventricle is affected by AMI. However, with right coronary and/or circumflex occlusion, the right ventricle also can be involved, and there is a clinical syndrome in which damage to the right ventricle predominates and is the major determinant of hemodynamics. Coronary thrombi will undergo spontaneous lysis, even if untreated, in approximately 50% of cases within 10 days. However, for patients with STE AMI, opening the vessel earlier with clot-dissolving agents (thrombolysis) and/or percutaneous intervention (PCI) can often save myocardium and lives (Fig. 58.5). At present, immediate PCI with stenting is the preferred therapy for STE AMI. However, many hospitals cannot or do not offer urgent PCI 24 hours per day, 365 days per year. Thus clot-dissolving medications still play a major role in the treatment of these patients. In addition, it is now apparent that urgent but not necessarily immediate invasive revascularization benefits those with NSTEMI.[19] These individuals usually have only partial coronary occlusion and smaller amounts of cardiac damage acutely. However, untreated, repetitive episodes often eventually damage larger amounts of myocardium, leading to increased morbidity and mortality over time. Treatments such as newer anticoagulants and antiplatelet and antiinflammatory agents, in conjunction with coronary revascularization, save lives in this group.

The prognosis for patients with ischemia but without necrosis is far better. Some studies based on biomarkers would suggest that in patients with no troponin elevation, interventional therapies may be harmful.[23] Many of these patients are

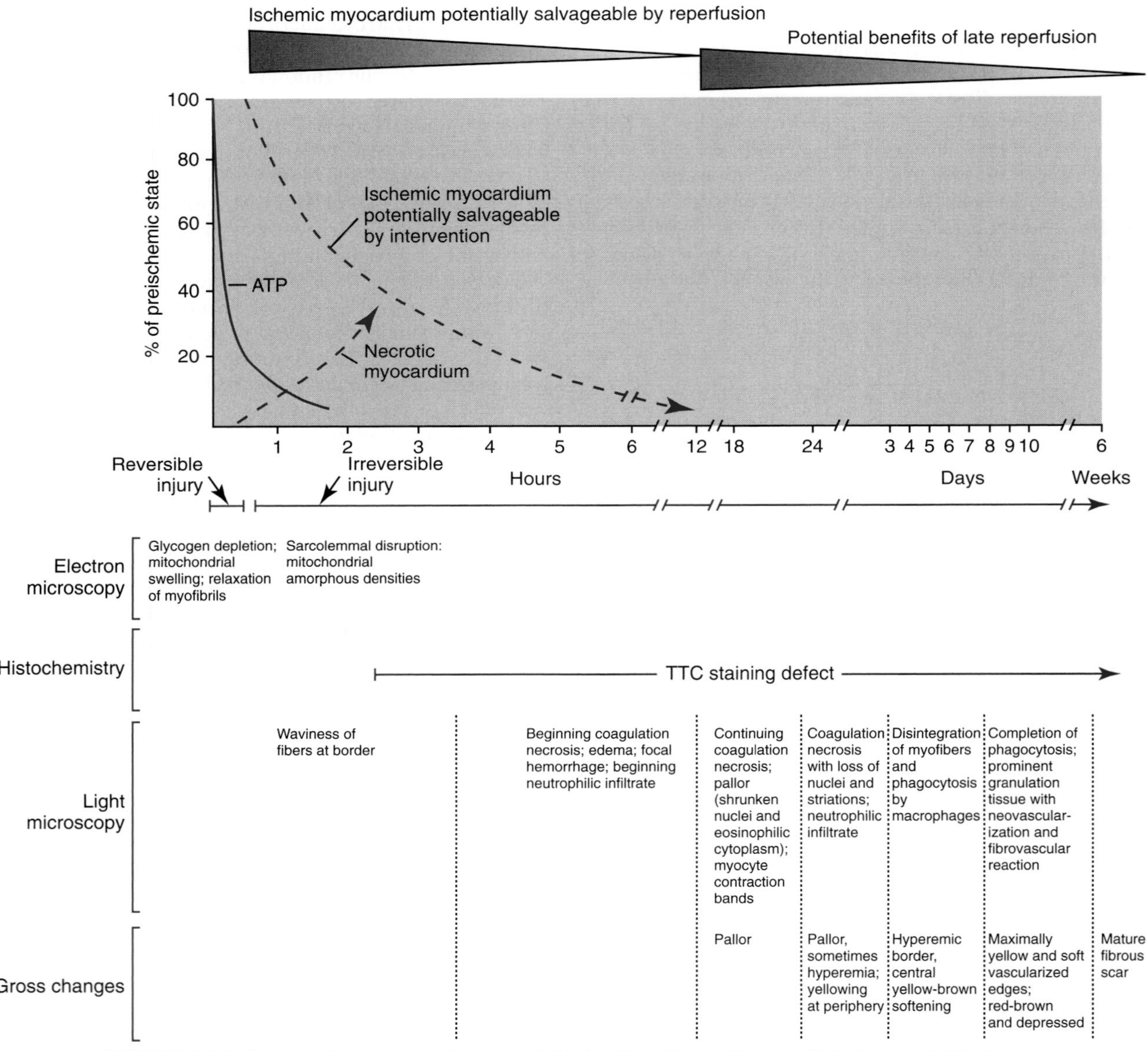

FIGURE 58.5 Temporal sequence of myocardial infarction. (From Antman EM, Braunwald E. Acute myocardial infarction. In: Braunwald E, ed. *Heart disease: a textbook of cardiovascular medicine.* 5th ed. Philadelphia: WB Saunders; 1997:1189.)

women who are known to have lower levels of cTn. With high-sensitivity assays, they will require different cutoff values, but the use of such assays will identify more women who are at risk.[24] A major determinant of mortality and morbidity is the amount of myocardial damage that occurs. With STE AMI, most damage is acute, whereas with NSTEMI, damage may evolve as the result of repetitive events over many months; thus interrupting the process improves survival.

Precipitating Factors

In many patients with AMI, no precipitating factor can be identified. Studies have noted the following patient activities at the onset of AMI: (1) heavy physical exertion, 13%; (2) modest or usual exertion, 18%; (3) surgical procedure, 6%; (4) rest, 51%; and (5) sleep, 8%. Exertion before infarction is somewhat more common among patients without preexisting angina than in those who have a history of angina.[25]

Causes of infarction other than acute atherothrombotic coronary occlusion have been identified. For example, prolonged vasospasm can induce infarction, and spontaneous dissection is becoming more commonly appreciated in women, many of who have fibromuscular dysplasia.[26] In addition, it is now clear that some patients, particularly women, can have acute infarction with normal-appearing angiographic coronary arteries.[27] Other conditions (Box 58.1) can cause the death of cardiomyocytes, leading to a biochemical signal (such as increased circulating concentrations of cTns) of myocyte damage, but these conditions should not be confused with MI.[2] Pulmonary embolism (PE) is another common cause of biochemical elevations that is secondary to right ventricular damage related to acute increases in wall stress and reduced subendocardial perfusion.[28-30]

BOX 58.1 Elevation of Troponins Without Overt Ischemic Heart Disease

- Trauma (including contusion, ablation, pacing, and cardioversion)
- Congestive heart failure—acute and chronic
- Aortic valve disease and hypertrophic cardiomyopathy with significant left ventricular hypertrophy
- Hypertension
- Hypotension, often with arrhythmias
- Postoperative noncardiac surgery patients who seem to do well
- Renal failure
- Critically ill patients, especially those with diabetes, respiratory failure
- Drug toxicity (eg, Adriamycin, 5-fluorouracil, herceptin, snake venoms)
- Hypothyroidism
- Coronary vasospasm, including apical ballooning syndrome
- Inflammatory disease (eg, myocarditis, parvovirus B19, Kawasaki's disease, sarcoid, smallpox vaccination)
- Post–percutaneous intervention patients whose condition appears to be uncomplicated
- Pulmonary embolism, severe pulmonary hypertension
- Sepsis
- Burns, especially if total body surface area is greater than 30%
- Infiltrative disease, including amyloidosis, hemochromatosis, sarcoidosis, and scleroderma
- Acute neurologic disease, including cerebrovascular accident, subarachnoid bleeds
- Rhabdomyolysis with cardiac injury
- Transplant vasculopathy
- Vital exhaustion

Chronobiology

There is a pronounced periodicity for the time of onset of STE AMI.[25,31,32] Often an AMI occurs in the morning hours soon after rising; this is a period of (1) increasing adrenergic activity, (2) increased plasma fibrinogen levels, (3) increased inhibition of fibrinolysis, and (4) increased platelet adhesiveness. Studies have demonstrated that the early morning peak in MI parallels the peak incidence of death from ischemic heart disease, which occurs at approximately 8 AM to 9 AM. A second peak has been noted at approximately 5 PM. Diurnal differences affect many physiologic and biochemical parameters; the early morning hours are associated with rises in plasma catecholamines and cortisol and increases in platelet aggregability. Tissue plasminogen activator activity is low and plasminogen activator inhibitor activity is high during the early morning hours. Thus it is possible that some cyclic aspects of combined vasospastic, prothrombotic, and fibrinolytic factors, in the setting of preexisting atherosclerosis, lead to AMI. NSTEMI does not exhibit this diurnal pattern.

Prognosis

STE and non-STE infarctions have distinctly different short-term prognoses. STE AMI is associated with higher early and in-hospital mortality. It is said that mortality associated with STE AMI can occur up to 6 months after the event, but the vast majority (at least two-thirds) occur during the first 30 or 40 days. It is this risk that coronary recanalization seems to benefit. NSTE AMI is associated with lower acute mortality and complication rates but a longer period of vulnerability to reinfarction and death. As a result, 1- to 2-year survival rates are similar to those for STEMI.[10] This is why intervention has been so effective in this group.

Clinical History

The clinical history remains of substantial value.[8] A prodromal history of angina is elicited in 40% to 50% of patients with AMI. Among patients with AMI who present with prodromal symptoms, approximately one-third have had symptoms from 1 to 4 weeks before hospitalization; in the remaining two-thirds, symptoms predate admission by a week or less, with one-third of patients having had symptoms for 24 hours or less.

In most patients the pain of AMI is severe, but it is rarely intolerable. The pain may be prolonged, lasting up to 30 minutes. The discomfort is described as constricting, crushing, oppressing, or compressing; often the patient complains of something sitting on or squeezing the chest. Although usually described as a squeezing, choking, viselike, or heavy pain, it may be characterized as a stabbing, knifelike, boring, or burning discomfort. The pain is usually retrosternal in location, spreading frequently to both sides of the chest, and favoring the left side. Often the pain radiates down the left arm. Some patients note only a dull ache or numbness in the wrists in association with severe substernal discomfort. In some instances, the pain of AMI may begin in the epigastrium, simulating a variety of abdominal disorders; this often causes MI to be misdiagnosed as indigestion. In other patients, the discomfort of AMI radiates to the shoulders, upper extremities, neck, and jaw, again usually favoring the left side. In patients with preexisting angina, the pain of infarction usually resembles that of the angina pain with respect to features and location. However, it is generally much more severe, lasts longer, and/or is not relieved by rest and nitroglycerin.

Older individuals, patients with diabetes, and women often present atypically. For example, among individuals older than 80 years, less than 50% of those with AMI will have chest discomfort at the time of AMI. Sometimes these patients will present with shortness of breath, fatigue, or even confusion. The pain of AMI may have disappeared by the time a physician first encounters the patient (or the patient reaches the hospital), or it may persist for a few hours.

Myocardial Changes After Acute Myocardial Infarction

Fig. 58.5 shows the temporal sequence of early biochemical, histochemical, and histologic findings after the onset of AMI. On gross pathologic examination, AMI can be divided into subendocardial (nontransmural) infarctions and transmural infarctions.[33] In the former, necrosis involves the endocardium, the intramural myocardium, or both without extending all the way through the ventricular wall to the epicardium. In the latter, myocardial necrosis involves the full thickness of the ventricular wall. The histologic pattern of necrosis may differ: contraction band injury occurs almost twice as often in nontransmural infarctions as in transmural infarctions. Unfortunately, the pathologic changes correlate poorly with clinical, ECG, and biochemical markers of necrosis, which is why those terms are no longer used clinically. Statistically, patients are more apt to have STE MI Q waves on the ECG and larger biochemical signals when the infarction is transmural pathologically.

Ultrastructural (Electron Microscopic) Changes in Myocardium. In experimental infarction, the earliest ultrastructural changes in cardiac muscle after occlusion of a coronary artery, noted within 20 minutes by electron microscopy, consists of reduction in the size and number of glycogen granules, intracellular edema, and swelling and distortion of the transverse tubular system, the sarcoplasmic reticulum, and the mitochondria. These early changes are partially reversible. Changes after 60 minutes of occlusion include myocardial cell swelling; mitochondrial abnormalities, such as swelling and internal disruption; development of amorphous, flocculent aggregation and margination of nuclear chromatin; and relaxation of myofibrils. After 20 minutes to 2 hours of ischemia, changes in some cells become irreversible, and progression of these alterations occurs; additional changes include swollen sacs of the sarcoplasmic reticulum at the level of the A band, greatly enlarged mitochondria with few cristae, thinning and fractionation of myofilaments, disorientation of myofibrils, and clumping of mitochondria. Cells irreversibly damaged by ischemia are usually swollen, with an enlarged sarcoplasmic reticulum. Defects in the plasma membrane may appear, and the mitochondria are fragmented. Many of these changes become more intense when blood flow is restored.

Histologic (Light Microscopic) Changes in Myocardium. Although it was previously believed that no light microscopic changes could be seen in infarcted myocardium until 8 hours after interruption of blood flow, in some infarcts a pattern of wavy myocardial fibers may be seen 1 to 3 hours after onset, especially at the periphery of the infarct.[33] After 8 hours, edema of the interstitium becomes evident, as do increased fatty deposits in the muscle fibers, along with infiltration of neutrophilic polymorphonuclear leukocytes and red blood cells.

By 24 hours, clumping of the cytoplasm and loss of cross-striations are seen, with the appearance of irregular cross-bands in the involved myocardial fibers. The nuclei sometimes even disappear. Myocardial capillaries in the involved region dilate, and polymorphonuclear leukocytes accumulate, first at the periphery and then in the center of the infarct. During the first 3 days, the interstitial tissue becomes edematous. Generally, on approximately day 4 after infarction, removal of necrotic fibers by macrophages begins, again commencing at the periphery. By day 8, the necrotic muscle fibers have become dissolved; by about 10 days, the number of polymorphonuclear leukocytes is reduced, and granulation tissue first appears at the periphery. Removal of necrotic muscle cells continues until the fourth to sixth week after infarction, by which time much of the necrotic myocardium has been removed. This process continues, along with increasing collagenization of the infarcted area. By the sixth week, the infarcted area usually has been converted to a firm connective tissue scar with interspersed intact muscle fibers.

Gross Changes in Myocardium. Gross alterations of the myocardium are difficult to identify until at least 6 to 12 hours after the onset of necrosis.[33] However, several histochemical approaches have been used to identify zones of necrosis that can be observed after only 2 to 3 hours. Initially, the myocardium in the affected region may appear pale and slightly swollen. By 18 to 36 hours after onset of the infarct, the myocardium is tan or reddish purple (because of trapped erythrocytes). These changes persist for approximately 48 hours; the infarct then turns gray, and fine yellow lines, secondary to neutrophilic infiltration, appear at its periphery. This zone gradually widens and during the next few days extends throughout the infarct.

Eight to 10 days after infarction, the thickness of the cardiac wall in the area of the infarct is reduced as necrotic muscle is removed by mononuclear cells. The cut surface of an infarct of this age is yellow and is surrounded by a reddish purple band of granulation tissue that extends through the necrotic tissue by 3 to 4 weeks. Over the next 2 to 3 months, the infarcted area gradually acquires a gelatinous, gray appearance, eventually converting into a shrunken, thin, firm scar that whitens and firms progressively with time. This process begins at the periphery of the infarct and gradually moves centrally. In addition, more hemorrhage is seen in the area of damage because of the use of potent thrombolytic and anticoagulant agents.

Development and Progression of Atherosclerosis

Intrinsic to modern day understanding of ischemic heart disease and to the intense interest in the development of markers of inflammation is the concept that atherosclerosis is a chronic inflammatory disease.[34] The concept is that some event damages the endothelium of blood vessels, which facilitates the egress of lipid into the subendothelial space. Putative injurious stimuli include turbulent flow in a blood vessel, which could occur for example because of hypertension or a noxious metabolite from a lipid fraction. This damage tends to occur at branch points of blood vessels. Regardless of the initial stimulus, once damaged, low-density lipoprotein (LDL) can cross into the vessel wall more easily in a nicotinamide adenine dinucleotide phosphate (NADPH) oxidase–mediated fashion. Whether minimal oxidation facilitates that egress or it occurs once the LDL is within the vessel wall is unclear, but a minimal degree of oxidation once in the vessel wall facilitates the egress of smooth muscle cells from the media of the vessel and macrophages that ingest cholesterol, hence the rationale for the measurement of oxidized lipids in blood. The process of atherosclerosis progresses slowly, with involvement of lymphocytes, monocytes, macrophages, and smooth muscle cells. The dynamic within a given plaque may vary, but there clearly is an inflammatory milieu, in part mediated by substances such as CD40 ligand, which can be measured directly or indirectly as C-reactive protein (CRP). Interleukins (IL)-1, IL-6, IL-8, and IL-18 also participate to various extents as part of this chronic inflammatory process. This process involves adherence of white blood cells to the damaged endothelial surface, with subsequent degranulation and elaboration of myeloperoxidase. A procoagulant component is due predominantly to the presence of tissue factor, which is localized immediately under the cap of the plaque. Intermittent instability is noted because of inflammatory products within the plaque that release chemicals, such as metalloproteinases. Initially the plaque expands by stretching the adventitia through a process of small ruptures with release of procoagulant and proinflammatory materials and then remodeling over time as antiinflammatory and anticoagulant and thrombolytic substances are elaborated. This process of stretching the adventitia preserves the lumen such that by the time luminal encroachment occurs, there is a very large plaque burden.[35]

A categorization of plaques has been proposed to facilitate identification of those at risk for rupture that could lead to an acute event. It is acknowledged that the propensity for a plaque to rupture probably reflects a systemic predilection rather than a local one. Thus, for a given patient at risk, there likely are many plaques that are metabolically at risk for rupture at any given time.[3,4] High-risk plaques have the following:

1. an active inflammatory environment that not only may be intrinsic but may be stimulated additionally by systemic infection;
2. a thin fibrous cap on the endothelial surface with a large lipid core that is filled with procoagulant substances, predominantly tissue factor;
3. endothelial denudation and fissuring caused by the elaboration of metalloproteinases;
4. local high shear stress, usually because they are severe, at branch points in the vessel.

Events likely occur because of superimposed thrombosis. This can be the result of erosions on the surface of the plaque or more often rupture of the plaque at its edges, where the cap is thinnest and most of the metalloproteinases reside. If rupture induces total thrombotic occlusion, the event is usually an STE AMI. If lesser degrees of occlusion occur, an NSTE AMI or UA may ensue. One of the causes that may participate in subtotal occlusive plaque rupture involves platelets and abnormal coronary vasomotion. It is known that diseased coronary arteries respond atypically to many stimuli, often constricting rather than dilating. Because the cross-sectional area of a vessel is related to the square of the radius, even modest amounts of constriction can markedly increase the extent of occlusion. Whether constriction occurs first, leading to changes of coronary flow and platelet aggregation on the plaque, or whether platelets stick and cause the aggregation, is not certain, but these processes reinforce one another. Platelets secrete vasoconstricting substances in response to a denuded area, which expresses cell adhesion molecule (CAM) receptors. This, in addition to stagnant blood flow, will cause platelets and white blood cells to adhere to the surfaces of vessels. It appears likely that platelets adhere and enhance vasoconstriction and then break off, causing small vessel emboli, sometimes in association with plaque debris and sometimes without. These processes, in addition to a reduction in flow, can lead to necrosis or at least recurrent ischemia. It is apparent that the process that eventually leads to acute events involves a systemic propensity to platelet aggregation and inflammation, because effluent flowing from the nonculprit vessel (distant from the putative coronary lesion causing the acute event) elaborates inflammatory mediators (eg, myeloperoxidase) similar to those observed from the affected vessel. Finally, necrosis when present stimulates an acute-phase reaction and inflammation. Given this pathophysiology, many therapies are now oriented toward inhibition of thrombosis, fibrinolysis, platelet aggregation, and inflammation. Many inflammatory markers are used diagnostically and for assessment of therapeutic efficiency.

Diagnosis of Acute Myocardial Infarction

The diagnosis of AMI established by the World Health Organization in 1986 included biomarkers as an integral part of the disorder and required that at least two of the following criteria be met: (1) a history of chest pain, (2) evolutionary changes on the ECG, and/or (3) elevations of serial cardiac markers to a level two times the normal value. However, over time, it became rare for a diagnosis of AMI to be made in the absence of biochemical evidence of myocardial injury. A 2000 European Society of Cardiology/American College of Cardiology (ESC/ACC) consensus conference[36] updated in 2007 and 2012 (Global Task Force)[2,11] codified the role of markers by advocating that the diagnosis should be regarded as evidence of myocardial injury based on markers of cardiac damage in the appropriate clinical situation (Box 58.2).[11] The guidelines thus recognized the reality that neither the clinical presentation nor the ECG had adequate sensitivity and specificity. This guideline does not suggest that all elevations of these biomarkers should elicit a diagnosis of AMI—only those associated with appropriate clinical and ECG findings (see discussion later in this chapter). When elevations that are not caused by acute ischemia occur, the clinician is obligated to search for another cause for the elevation.[37-40] In the 2007 revision of the guidelines, several types of AMI were recognized, including the spontaneous type, which is associated with plaque rupture or erosion, and the type associated with fixed or transient coronary abnormalities but not thrombotic occlusion. These are discussed in greater detail in the following paragraphs. It is also recognized that one can have a classic AMI and succumb before markers are obtained or become elevated, and cardiac injury can occur in association with cardiac procedures.[11] In addition, criteria for different types of MI, including after coronary interventions and bypass surgery were suggested (Box 58.3).

BOX 58.2 Criteria for the Definition of Acute Myocardial Infarction

1. Detection of a rise and/or fall of cardiac biomarker values (preferably cardiac troponin) with at least one value above the 99th percentile upper reference interval and with at least one of the following.
   a. Ischemic symptoms
   b. ECG changes of new ischemia (new ST-T changes or new left bundle branch block)
   c. Development of pathologic Q waves in the electrocardiogram
   d. Imaging evidence of new loss of viable myocardium or new regional wall motion abnormality
   e. Identification of an intracoronary thrombus by angiography or autopsy
2. Pathologic Q waves with or without symptoms in the absence of nonischemic causes
3. Imaging evidence of a region of loss of viable myocardium that is thinned and fails to contract in the absence of a nonischemic cause
4. Pathologic findings of a prior myocardial infarction.

Modified from Thygesen K, Alpert JS, Jaffe AS, Simoons ML, Chaitman BR, White HD, et al. Third universal definition of myocardial infarction. *J Am Coll Cardiol* 2012;60:1581–1598.

Electrocardiography Findings. At one time, the initial ECG was thought to be diagnostic of AMI in approximately 50% of patients.[41] As the frequency of STE AMI has diminished and the diagnosis has been made with increasingly greater sensitivity, this percentage has been greatly reduced. Serial tracings are helpful for STE AMI but not for what is now almost 70% of AMIs that are known as non-STE (NSTE) AMIs. The classic ECG changes of an STE AMI is ST segment elevation, which often evolves to the development of Q waves if intervention is not provided (see Fig. 58.4). Pericarditis, some normal variants, and transient causes that may result in myocardial injury such as myocarditis are well described and on occasion can mimic the changes of AMI. Most NSTE AMIs manifest as ST segment depression, with or without T-wave changes, as T-wave changes alone, or on occasion in the absence of any ECG findings. Those with ST segment change have a substantially worse prognosis.[11]

In some patients, the clinical history and ECG may be definitive. In others, they may not be as clear. Many other clinical aspects might suggest acute ischemia as the origin of a given biomarker elevation. For example, the finding of significant coronary obstructive lesions, especially in a pattern suggestive of recent plaque rupture, is highly suggestive. At times, a positive stress test with or without imaging may be what helps in making the diagnosis. However, if the clinical situation is not suggestive, other sources for cardiac injury should be sought.

BOX 58.3 Clinical Classification of Myocardial Infarction Types

Type 1: Spontaneous myocardial infarction (MI)

Related to atherosclerotic plaque rupture, ulceration, fissuring, erosion, or dissection with resulting intraluminal thrombosis in one or more of the coronary arteries leading to decreased myocardial blood flow or distal platelet emboli with ensuing myocyte necrosis. The patient may have underlying severe coronary artery disease (CAD) but on occasion nonobstructive or no CAD.

Type 2: MI secondary to ischemia imbalance

Myocardial injury with necrosis in which a condition other than CAD contributes to an imbalance between myocardial oxygen supply and/or demand, for example, coronary endothelial dysfunction, coronary artery spasm, coronary embolism, tachyarrhythmia, bradyarrhythmia, anemia, respiratory failure, hypotension, and hypertension with or without left ventriucular hypertrophy.

Type 3: MI resulting in death when biomarker values are unavailable

Cardiac death with symptoms suggestive of myocardial ischemia and presumed new ischemic electrocardiogram (ECG) changes or new left bundle branch block (LBBB), but death occurring before blood samples could be obtained or before cardiac biomarkers could rise; in rare cases cardiac biomarkers were not collected.

Type 4a: MI related to percutaneous coronary innervation (PCI)

MI associated with PCI is arbitrarily defined by elevation of cardiac troponin (cTn) values greater than 5 × 99th percentile upper reference interval in patients with normal baseline values (<99th percentile upper reference interval) or a rise of cTn values above 20% if the baseline values are elevated and are stable or falling. In addition, (1) symptoms suggestive of myocardial ischemia; (2) new ischemic ECG changes or LBBB; (3) angiographic loss of patency of a major coronary artery or a side branch or persistent slow- or no-flow or embolism; or (4) imaging demonstration of new loss of viable myocardium or new regional wall motion abnormality are required.

Type 4b: MI related to stent thrombosis

MI related to stent thrombosis is detected by coronary angiography or autopsy in the setting of myocardial ischemia and with a rise and/or fall of cardiac biomarker values, with at least one value above the 99th percentile upper reference interval.

Type 5: MI related to CABG

MI associated with CABG is arbitrarily defined by elevation of cardiac bimarker values greater than 10 × 99th percentile upper reference interval in patients with normal baseline cTn values (<99th percentile upper reference interval). In addition, (1) new pathologic Q waves or new LBBB, (2) angiographic documented new graft or new native coronary artery occlusion, or (3) imaging evidence of new loss of myocardium or new regional wall motion abnormality.

From Thygesen K, Alpert JS, Jaffe AS, Simoons ML, Chaitman BR, White HD, et al. Third universal definition of myocardial infarction. *J Am Coll Cardiol* 2012;60:1581–1598.

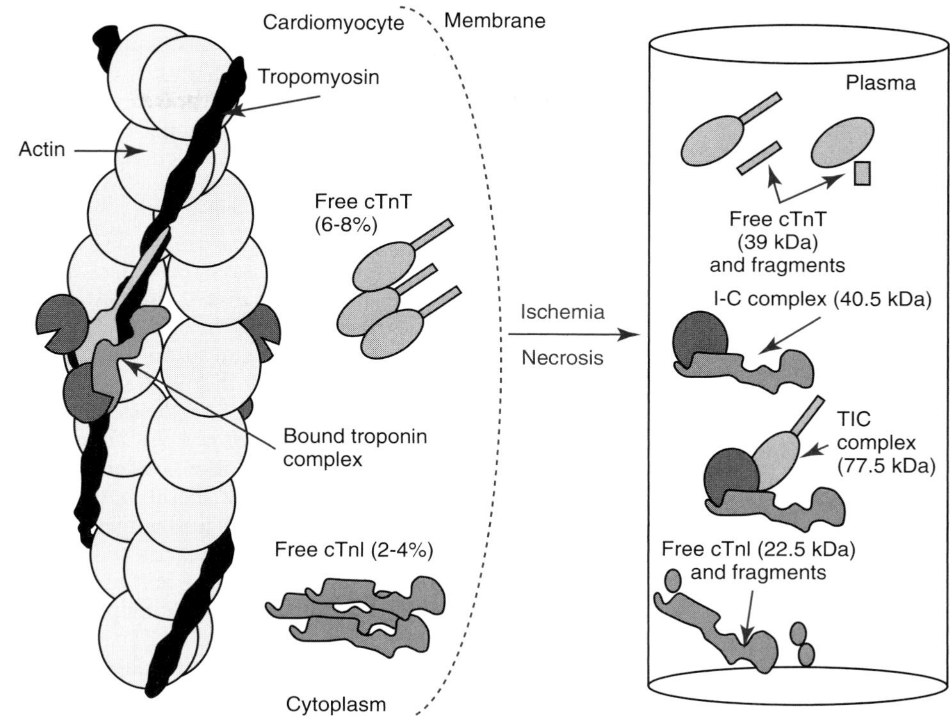

FIGURE 58.6 Structure of cardiac troponin *(cTn)* complex and troponin forms released after myofibril necrosis. *cTn1,* Cardiac troponin I; *cTnT,* cardiac troponin T. (From Gaze DC, Collinson PO. Multiple molecular forms of circulating cardiac troponin: analytical and clinical significance. *Ann Clin Biochem* 2008;45:349–359. Figure courtesy Paul Collinson.)

BIOMARKERS IN ACUTE CORONARY SYNDROME

Analytical Considerations

Myocardial damage detected by increases of cTn is almost invariably associated with adverse clinical outcomes. This statement summarizes more than 25 years of analytical and clinical investigations pertaining to the clinical utility of cTnI and cTnT. This section of the chapter will focus on cTn biochemistry; the analytical aspects of assays used to measure cTn in whole blood, serum, and plasma; preanalytical and analytical specifications that manufacturers of cTn assays need to strive to optimize; 99th percentile (normal) upper reference interval* determinations; central laboratory and point-of-care (POC) testing strategies; recommendations for implementation of high-sensitivity cTn assays; and suggestions for appropriate (cost) utilization recommendations for serial orders in clinical practice to assist in ruling in and ruling out AMI.

Biochemistry

The contractile proteins of the myofibril include the three troponin regulatory proteins (Fig. 58.6).[42-44] The troponins are a complex of three protein subunits: troponin C (the calcium-binding component), troponin I (the inhibitory component), and troponin T (the tropomyosin-binding component). The subunits exist in a number of isoforms. The distribution of these isoforms varies between cardiac muscle and slow- and fast-twitch skeletal muscle. Only two major isoforms of troponin C are found in human heart and skeletal muscle. These are characteristic of slow- and fast-twitch skeletal muscle. The heart isoform is identical to the slow-twitch skeletal muscle isoform, thus the reason why cTnC was never developed as a cardiac-specific biomarker. Isoforms of cardiac-specific troponin T (cTnT) and cardiac-specific troponin I (cTnI) also have been identified and are the products of unique genes.[45-48] Troponin is localized primarily in the myofibrils (94% to 97%), with a smaller cytoplasmic fraction (3% to 6%).[49] Some experts in the field think that 100% of cTn is myofibril bound and that the cytoplasmic fraction represents a more easily mobilizable fraction, rather than representing a different cellular localization.

cTnI and cTnT have different amino acid sequences from the skeletal isoforms and are encoded by unique genes. Human cTnI has an additional 31 amino-acid residue on the amino terminal end compared with skeletal muscle TnI, giving it complete cardiac specificity. Only one isoform of cTnI has been identified. cTnI is not expressed in normal, regenerating, or diseased human or animal skeletal muscle.[45] cTnT is encoded for by a different gene than the one that encodes for skeletal muscle isoforms. An 11 amino acid amino-terminal residue gives this marker unique cardiac specificity. However, during human fetal development, in regenerating rat skeletal muscle, and in diseased human skeletal muscle, small amounts of cTnT are expressed as one of four identified isoforms in skeletal muscle.[46,50,51] In humans, cTnT isoform expression has been demonstrated in skeletal muscle specimens obtained from patients with muscular dystrophy, polymyositis, dermatomyositis, and end-stage

*Laboratories should verify that these ranges are appropriate for use in their own settings.

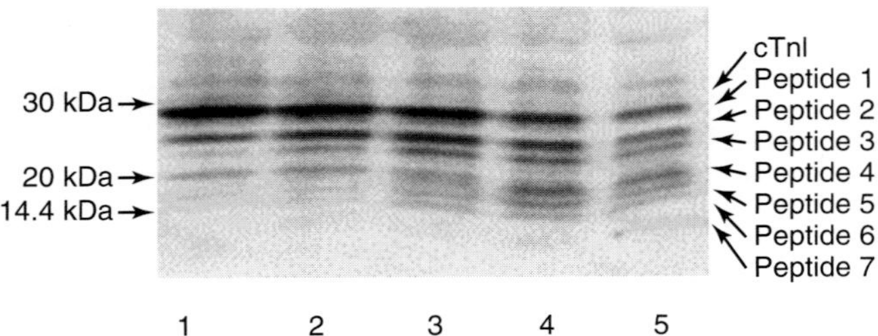

FIGURE 58.7 Western blot analysis of endogenous cardiac troponin I *(cTnI)* proteolysis in human heart tissue visualized with monoclonal anti-cTnI antibody. Protein extracts from tissue samples were incubated at 37°C for 0 h (lane 1), 2 h (lane 2), 5 h (lane 3), 8 h (lane 4), and 20 h (lane 5), separated by 10% to 20% gradient sodium dodecyl sulfate (SDS)-gel electrophoresis, transferred to a nitrocellulose membrane, and visualized by MAb 19C7. The apparent molecular masses and peptides are marked by *arrows.* (From Katrukha AG, Bereznikova AV, Filatov VL, Esakova TV, Kolosova OV, Pettersson K, et al. Degradation of cardiac troponin I: implication for reliable immunodetection. *Clin Chem* 1998;44:2433–2440.)

renal disease.[46,52-57] Thus care is necessary to choose antibody pairs for the cTnT assay that do not detect these reexpressed isoforms or the immunoreactive proteins expressed in neuromuscular skeletal diseases that show cross-reactivity to the commercial cTnT assays because false-positive, noncardiac, cTnT results can occur (as discussed later).[56-59] A substantial body of evidence shows that after myocardial injury or because of genetic disposition, multiple forms of cTn are elaborated both in tissue and in blood (Fig. 58.7).[40,48,60] These include the T-I-C ternary complex, IC binary complex, and free I; multiple modification of these three forms can occur, involving oxidation, reduction, phosphorylation, and dephosphorylation, as well as both C- and N-terminal degradation. Depending on the selection of antibodies used to detect cTnI, different antibody configurations can lead to a substantially different recognition pattern.[42] The conclusions derived from these observations are that assays need to be developed in which the antibodies recognize epitopes in the stable region of cTnI and, ideally, demonstrate an equimolar response to the different cTnI forms that circulate in the blood. At present, standardization of cTnI assays has not been obtained.[61,62]

Immunoassays

Cummins and coworkers[47] were the first to develop a radioimmunoassay (RIA) to measure cTnI, using polyclonal anti-cTnI antibodies.[47] The first monoclonal enzyme-linked immunosorbent assay, an anti-cTnI antibody–based immunoassay, was described by Bodor and colleagues.[63] Numerous manufacturers have now described the development of monoclonal antibody–based diagnostic immunoassays for the measurement of cTnI in serum.[42,64-75] As shown in Table 58.1, contemporary, POC, and high-sensitivity (hs-cTn) assays are marketed worldwide for patient testing. Fig. 58.8 demonstrates the similarities and differences in capture and detection antibodies in the heterogeneous assays used in clinical practice. In addition to these quantitative assays, several qualitative (positive/negative) assays are also marketed. Two hs-cTnI and hs-cTnT assays with improved analytical sensitivity are commercially available worldwide outside the United States: hs-cTnI (Abbott, Chicago, Illinois) and hs-cTnT (Roche, Branford, Connecticut). Neither has been cleared by the US Food and Drug Administration (FDA) for use in the United States.[76]

Two challenges limit the ease of switching from one assay to another in clinical practice or research.[77] First, no primary reference cTnI material is currently available for manufacturers to use in standardizing cTnI assays. Second, measured assay concentrations fail to be consistent because cTnI circulates in its various forms and the different antibodies used in the available assays recognize different epitopes of cTnI even for different assays and instruments marketed by the same manufacturer. The cTnI Standardization Subcommittee of the American Association for Clinical Chemistry (AACC) in collaboration with the National Institute of Standards and Technology (NIST) developed a cTnI reference material (SRM 2921) that is a TnC-cTnI-cTnT complex purified from human heart under nondenaturing conditions.[78] A cTnI value was assigned by a combination of reversed-phase liquid chromatography with ultraviolet detection and amino acid analysis. However, it appears to be of limited value, at best used for the potential of harmonization or possible use for cTnI traceability, but is not helpful as a common calibration material for either cTnI or cTnT. For complete standardization for cTnI assays, manufacturers would need to agree to use the same capture and detection antibodies showing similar specificity for cTnI molecules circulating in the blood. This would also overcome matrix effects that a current International Federation of Clinical Chemistry and Laboratory Medicine (IFCC) working group is investigating based on a serum-based common reference material for calibration.[62] Several adaptations of the Roche cTnT immunoassay have been described over the years.[79,80] The current FDA-cleared assay available in the United States (4th generation) and the assay used worldwide outside the United States (hs-cTnT) involve two monoclonal, anti-cTnT antibodies. Although skeletal muscle TnT is no longer a potential interferent, recent studies in patients with neuromuscular disease have described false-positive cTnT findings in plasma, proposed to be an immunoreactive protein that does cross-react with both cTnT assays.[56,57] Because of calibration differences between the 4th generation, high-sensitivity (hs-TnT), and POC assays, minor differences in measured cTnT concentration have been shown.[81]

Assay Specifications

In 2001 and 2004 the IFCC Committee on Standardization of Markers of Cardiac Damage (C-SMCD) recommended quality specifications for cTn assays.[82,83] These specifications were intended for use by the manufacturers of commercial assays and by clinical laboratories using cTn assays. The overall goal was to attempt to establish uniform criteria so that all assays could be evaluated objectively for their analytical qualities and clinical performance. Both analytical and preanalytical factors were addressed. An adequate description of the analytical principles, method design, and assay components should include (1) antibody specificity and epitope locations identified need to be delineated; (2) epitopes located on the stable part of the cTnI molecule should be a priority; (3) assays need to clarify whether different cTnI forms (eg, binary vs. ternary complex) are recognized in an equimolar fashion by the antibodies used; (4) specific relative responses need to be described for each of the cTnI forms (free cTnI,

TABLE 58.1 Analytical Characteristics of Commercial and Research High-Sensitivity Cardiac Troponin I and T Assays as Stated by Manufacturer

Company/ Platform/Assay	LOD (μg/L)	99th % (μg/L)	%CV at 99th (%)	10% CV (μg/L)	Risk Stratification	Epitopes Recognized by Antibodies	Detection Antibody Tag
Contemporary Assays							
Abbott ARCHITECT	<0.01	0.028	15.0	0.032	No	C: 87-91, 24-40; D: 41-49	Acridinium
Beckman Coulter Access 2	0.01	0.04	14.0	0.06	Yes	C: 41-49; D: 24-40	ALP
Roche E170	0.01	<0.01	18.0	0.03	Yes	C: 125-131; D: 136-147	Ruthenium
Siemens Centaur Ultra	0.006	0.04	10.0	0.03	Yes	C: 41-49, 87-91; D: 27-40	Acridinium
Siemens Dimension RxL	0.04	0.07	20.0	0.14	Yes	C: 27-32; D: 41-56	ALP
Siemens VISTA	0.015	0.045	10.0	0.04	Yes	C: 27-32; D: 41-56	Chemiluminescent
Tosoh AIA II	0.06	<0.06	8.5	0.09	No	C: 41-49; D: 87-91	ALP
Ortho Vitros ECi ES	0.012	0.034	10.0	0.034	Yes	C: 24-40, 41-49; D: 87-91	HRP
Point-of-Care Assays							
Abbott i-STAT	0.02	0.08	16.5	0.10	Yes	C: 41-49, 88-91; D: 28-39,62-78	ALP
Alere Triage	0.05	<0.05	NA	NA	No	C: NA; D: 27-40	Fluorophor
bioMerieux Vidas Ultra	0.01	0.01	27.7	0.11	No	C: 41-49, 22-29; D: 87-91, 7B9	ALP
LSI Medience PATHFAST	0.008	0.029	5.1	0.014	No	C: 41-49; D:71-116, 163-209	ALP
Radiometer AQT90 cTnI	0.0095	0.023	17.7	0.039	NA	C: 41-49, 190-196; D: 137-149	Europium
Radiometer AQT90 cTnT	0.01	0.017	20.0	0.03	NA	C: 125-131; D:136-147	Europium
Response Biomedical RAMP	0.03	<0.1	18.5	0.21	No	C: 85-92; D: 26-38	Flourophor
Roche Cardiac Reader	<0.05	<0.05	NA	NA	No	C: 125-131; D:136-147	Gold particles
Siemens Stratus CS	0.03	0.07	10.0	0.06	Yes	C: 27-32; D: 41-56	ALP
Trinity Meritas	0.019	0.036	17.0	NA	No	C: 24-40, 41-49, D; 88-90, 137-148, 190-196	Fluorophor
High-Sensitivity Assays	**ng/L**	**M/F (ng/L)**		**ng/L**	**% Normals Measurable**		
Abbott ARCHITECT STAT hs-cTnI	1.2	34/16	<6.0	3	96	C: 24-40; D: 41-49	Acridinium
Beckman Coulter Access hs-cTnI	2.1	11/9	<5.0	3.3	80	C: 41-49; D: 24-40	ALP
Ortho Vitros hs-cTnI	1.0	19/16	<5.0	6.5	75	C: 24-40, 41-49; D: 87-91	HRP
Roche E170 hs-cTnT	5	20/13	<8.0	13	25	C: 136-147; D: 125-131	Ruthenium
Siemens Vista hs-cTnI	0.8	55/33	<5.0	3	86	C: 30-35; D: 41-56, 171-8	Gold-nanoparticles
Singulex Erenna hs-cTnI	0.1	27/15	<5.0	0.9	100	C: 41-49; D: 27-41	Capillary flow Fluorescence

hs-cTnI, High-sensitivity cardiac troponin I; *LOD,* limit of detection; Sex-specific 99th percentiles; *F,* female; *M,* male.

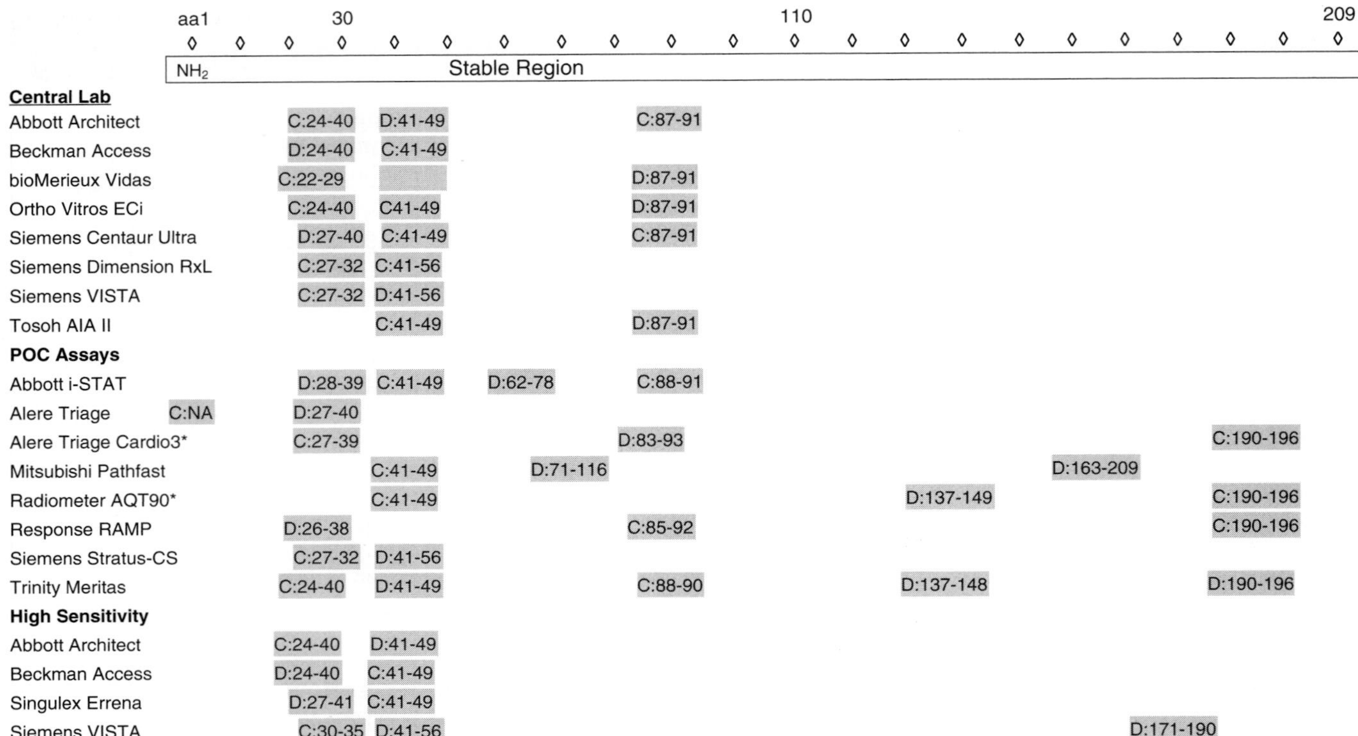

FIGURE 58.8 Amino acid sequence of cardiac troponin I (cTnI) with identification of epitopes used by capture and detection antibodies in contemporary, point of care *(POC)*, and high-sensitivity cTnI assays.

the 1-C binary complex, the T-I-C ternary complex, and oxidized, reduced, and phosphorylated isoforms of the three cTnI forms); (5) the effects of different anticoagulants on binding of cTnI need to be addressed; and (6) the source of material used to calibrate cTn assays, specifically for cTnI, should be reported (Box 58.4).

Regarding hs-cTn assays, recent publications have attempted to provide guidance to regulatory agencies, health care providers, and laboratories.[76,84] First, a meeting between US laboratory medicine, emergency medicine, and cardiology biomarker experts and the FDA resulted in an opinion/perspective article with the objective of providing guidelines for uniform analytical and clinical standards for 510k studies being performed by manufacturers seeking cTnI and cTnT 510k assay clearance. Recommendations provided to the FDA addressed the following points: (1) the number of reference individuals for determination of a 99th percentile upper reference interval, (2) limit of quantification, (3) total imprecision requirements, (4) enrollment of subjects for diagnostic studies, (5) patient adjudication processes, and (6) clinical end points and time limits to assess outcomes. A primary focus was to ensure that the suggested protocols also apply to hs-cTn assays. Unfortunately, the expert recommendations were not endorsed by the FDA. Second, a recent publication from the IFCC Task Force on Clinical Applications of Cardiac Bio-Markers (TF-CB), comprising an international group of laboratory medicine, emergency medicine, and cardiology biomarker experts, endorsed the following analytical recommendations pertaining to the implementation and use of hs-cTnI and hs-cTnT assays: (A) the 99th percentile URL is universally endorsed as the reference cutoff to aid in the diagnosis of AMI; (B) key components to implement hs-cTn assays in practice include: (1) 99th percentile should be determined in a healthy population; (2) 99th percentile from either peer-reviewed literature or from manufacturers' product information are acceptable; (3) 99th percentile for hs-cTn assays should be measured with an analytical imprecision of 10% or less (% coefficient of variation [CV]); (4) hs-assays should measure cTn above the limit of detection in 50% or more of healthy subjects; (C) factors that may influence hs-cTn assay 99th percentile include: (1) age—cTn increases with increasing age, especially older than 60 years; (2) gender—men have higher

BOX 58.4 Quality Specifications: Cardiac Troponin Assays

Analytical Factors

1. Antibody specificity: Recognize epitopes as part of molecule and equimolar for all forms
2. Influence of anticoagulants
3. Calibration against natural form of molecule
4. Defined type of material useful for dilutions
5. Demonstrated recovery and linearity of method
6. Described detection limit and imprecision (10% coefficient of variation)
7. Addressing interferents (ie, rheumatoid factor, heterophile antibodies)

Preanalytical Factors

1. Storage time and temperature conditions
2. Centrifugation effects: Gel separators
3. Serum-plasma: Whole blood correlations

values than women; (3) assay method—the 99th percentile should be determined for each assay, because assays are not standardized; (4) specimen type—the 99th percentile should be determined for serum, plasma, and/or whole blood; (D) 99th percentile values should be established or confirmed: (1) with the appropriate statistical power for each gender (men and women); (2) using a minimum 300 male and 300 female subjects (by gender) if establishing 99th percentiles; (3) using a minimum of 20 subjects if confirming 99th percentiles; and (4) with an appropriate one-tailed nonparametric statistical method.

It has been acknowledged that with imaging, even more comorbidities are detected that lower values for the 99th percentile modestly.[85,86] However, the imposition of imaging in all subjects involved in normal range studies is not logistically or financially feasible. This fact, however, implies that there will likely be a rare patient who will have a rising and/or falling pattern with a substantial change in values whose peak value is just below the 99th percentile upper reference interval. This patient should be recognized and reclassified by those caring for the patient as meeting criteria for cardiac injury and in the proper setting, AMI.

Defining 99th Percentile Normal Reference Intervals for Cardiac Troponin Assays

Advancements in cTn assay technology have created a conundrum for clinicians and laboratory scientists, who must determine which assays are best for optimal patient care. International guidelines have defined an increased cTn above the 99th percentile upper reference interval as an abnormal result, as described in the clinical section.[2,11,65,87,88] Whether a clinical laboratory defines an abnormal result above the 99th percentile as a critical value needs to be assessed and determined by each individual laboratory. What is lacking, unfortunately, is a consensus, uniform approach to define the 99th percentile across the heterogeneity of assays. A recent review article has addressed the vast literature regarding defining normality, on a global basis.[89] In spite of evidence-based literature demonstrating that cTn concentrations tend to increase in individuals older than 60 years, likely because of unrecognized comorbidities, 99th percentiles are often determined across wide age ranges using subjects as old as 80 years (convenience samples).[64,90,91] Further frustrating the problem of selecting relevant reference subjects is the fact that in clinically defined normal individuals without known cardiovascular disease, increased cTn concentrations are indicative of a significantly higher risk for death. Given such problems, most laboratories (1) accept the manufacturer's reference interval from the package insert, (2) perform an underpowered normal study to establish a reference interval or (3) accept a cutoff value published in the literature. Global implementation of the 99th percentile URL has not been accepted by laboratories, most likely because of pressures by clinicians who have been concerned that the imprecision of assays at the 99th percentile does not always meet the Global Task Force Third Universal Definition of MI recommendation of a 10% CV at the 99th percentile; analytical noise around the 99th percentile could result in a false-positive increase of cTn in patients without myocardial injury. However, the Global Task Force Universal Definition does clearly state that assays are clinically usable with up to a 20% CV at the 99th percentile, and necessitates for at least two serial samples to demonstrate a rising or falling cTn pattern.[2]

Guideline-Supported Recommendations

Consensus guidelines from the Global Task Force for the Third Universal Definition of Myocardial Infarction, the National Academy of Clinical Biochemistry (NACB), the ACC/AHA and Epidemiology groups, the ACC Foundation, and the European Clinical and Laboratory groups have recommended that, in patients who present with ischemic symptoms, a rising or falling serial pattern with at least one cTn concentration higher than the 99th percentile upper reference interval during the first 24 hours after onset of symptoms indicates myocardial necrosis. If this elevation occurs in the clinical setting of ischemia consistent with MI, that diagnosis should be made (see Box 58.2). It is recommended that cTn assays with appropriate quality control and optimal total imprecision (CV ≤10%) at the 99th percentile upper reference interval are preferred.[83,85] Better imprecision at low cTn concentrations appears to improve the value of cTn as a diagnostic and risk indicator, as will be discussed in the clinical section. Use of cTn assays with intermediate imprecision (10 to 20% CV) at the 99th percentile, however, is deemed clinically acceptable and does not lead to patient misclassifications when serial cTn results are interpreted.

A challenge that arises as hs-cTn assays with improved analytical sensitivity become incorporated in laboratory practice is determining how these new assays compare with the older contemporary assays. Diagnostic sensitivities using specimens collected at presentation for detection of MI have improved from 15% to 35% for early generations of cTn assays, to 50% to 75% for contemporary assays, and to more than 80% for hs-assays. To exclude an AMI with contemporary assays, the Global Task Force recommended a 6-hour period for assessing the optimal negative predictive value (NPV) for ruling out AMI. With hs-cTn assays, the period for ruling out an AMI with greater than 99% NPV has decreased to less than 2 to 3 hours. The goal is to better define the clinical playing field for assays used to assist in the diagnosis of MI, rule out MI, and better stratify patients for risk for adverse events. Further, several studies have now shown by using hs-assays that in patients presenting with a low clinical likelihood of ACS, a cTnT value below the limit of detection (LOD) or limit of blank (LOB) with a nondiagnostic ECG can be used to rule out AMI in less than 1 to 2 hours, and with a NPV greater than 99% (see clinical section). With more sensitive hs-cTn assays, however, the LOD or LOB will not be useful because everyone will have a measurable value. However, it is likely that a very low value will be determined that will allow for the use of this strategy. As the use of hs-cTn assays grows worldwide, triage of patients in the emergency department (ED) will be significantly improved, allowing for more rapid triage to an appropriate level of care, earlier discharge home, with minimal risk for an adverse event. In addition hs-cTn assays should also allow for more rapid throughput of patients waiting to be triaged in the ED. However, no POC cTn assays currently qualify as hs-assays.

Defining Reference Populations

To solve the conundrum of differences across assays, larger population-based direct comparisons of contemporary assays used in clinical practice with hs-cTn assays that are already in

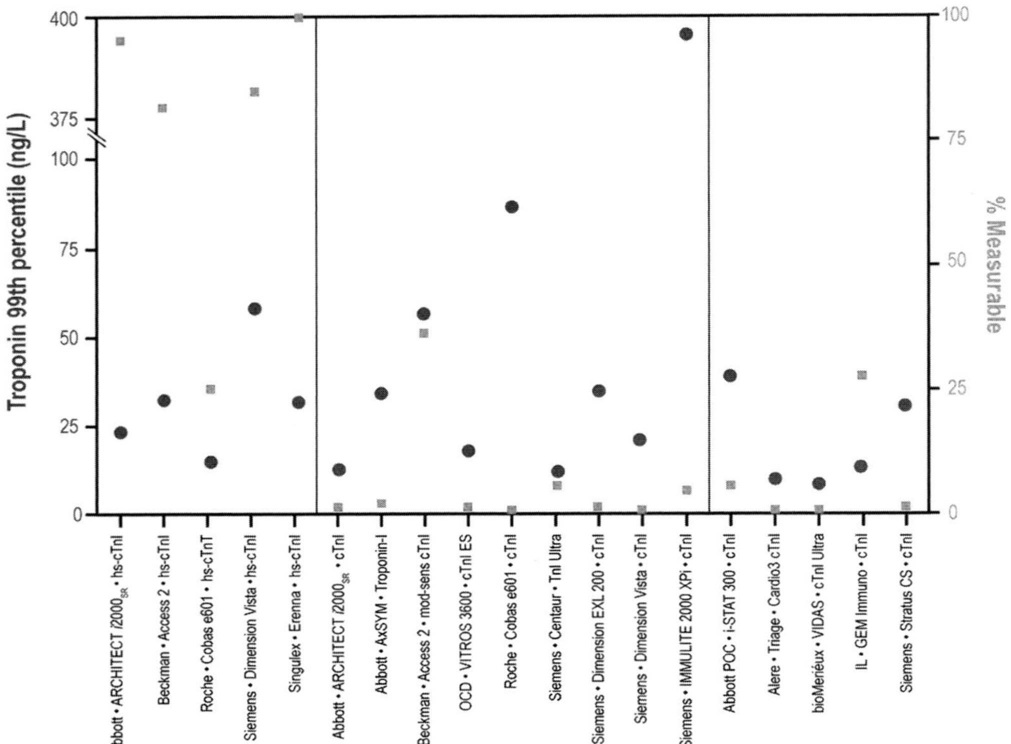

FIGURE 58.9 Comparison of both 99th percentile values *(circles)* and percent measurable concentrations *(boxes)* in a presumably healthy population for 19 cardiac troponin assays designated by hs *(left)*, sensitive-contemporary *(middle)*, and POC *(right)*, *mod-sens,* Modified-sensitive. (From Apple FS, Ler R, Murakami MM. Determination of 19 cardiac troponin I and T assay 99th percentile values from a common presumably healthy population. *Clin Chem* 2012;58:1574–1581.)

the marketplace are needed.[92] One rational approach would be to use a common normal reference population within a focused, healthy, age-defined group to establish 99th percentile upper reference intervals. Multiple studies using first-generation, contemporary, and hs-cTn assays have demonstrated that the cTn 99th percentile strongly depends on selection of individuals to be included in the reference population. Examining multiple contemporary, POC, and hs-assays, the percent of measurable concentrations below the 99th percentile concentration ranged from 1% to 98% across assays (Fig. 58.9). Further, the 99th percentile upper reference interval variability among assays was substantial, further exemplifying the lack of cTnI and cTnT assay standardization. The hs-cTn assays demonstrated near-Gaussian distributions (Fig. 58.10), with sex-derived upper reference interval differences that are not possible with contemporary and POC assays.

Defining Assays Analytical Characteristics

To overcome the barrier for accurate interpretation of cTn values in clinical practice, a two-tiered system of analysis using both 99th percentiles and imprecision values at the 99th percentile, based on a young, healthy reference population that is diversified by sex, race, and ethnicity, has been proposed.[64] This approach has been challenged because (1) it does not provide an age-matched normal cohort matching the ACS patient population that typically presents to rule out an AMI and (2) it is not based on clinical diagnostic or outcomes data at the 99th percentile upper reference interval.[93] The approach was based on a published scorecard concept to capture the essence of which assays are acceptable for use in clinical practice and to facilitate the transition to hs-cTn assays. The proposed assay-dependent scorecard shown in Table 58.2 is based on designations of the total imprecision (% CV) of each assay at the 99th percentile and how many specimens from normal individuals have cTn concentrations that are actually measurable below the 99th percentile.[64] The ultimate goal is to have all assays be level 4 guideline acceptable. A point of controversy does exist regarding the way Roche has commercially designated their cTnT assay as high-sensitivity; the evidence-based literature does not support its designation as an hs-assay because the assay measures less than 50% of normal subjects above the LOD (see Fig. 58.9). The likely clinical effects of using assays rated by the scorecard as "guideline acceptable" or "clinically usable" include: (1) all providers will more accurately detect patients within the normal range as well as with minor myocardial injury, independent of the pathophysiologic mechanism; (2) emergency medicine physicians will achieve improvements in triage through earlier ruling out (improved NPV) and ruling in (improved sensitivity) of patients with MI; (3) cardiology, internal medicine (hospitalists), and family practice physicians will see improved outcomes for both inpatients (hospitalized, short-term risk) and outpatients (posthospitalization, long-term risk) because of the ability to detect injury earlier compared to other diagnostic tools; (4) other medical specialty physicians will be better

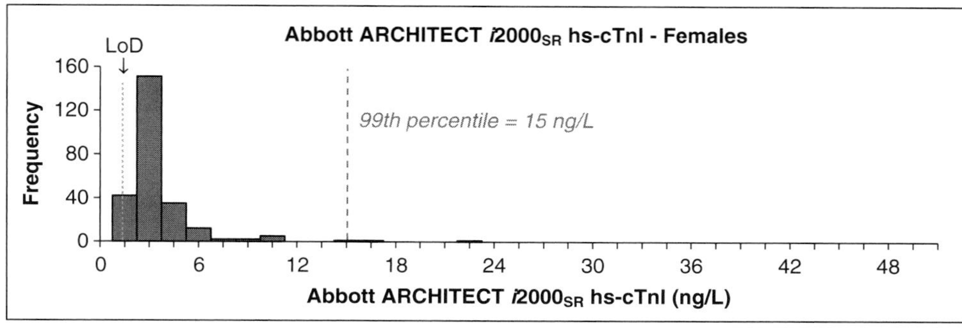

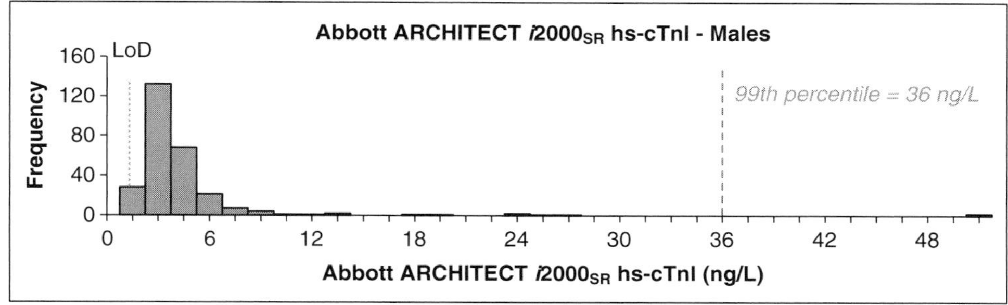

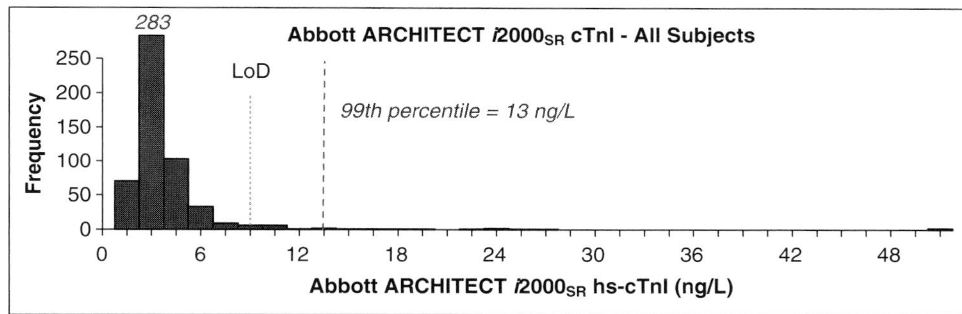

FIGURE 58.10 Histograms of plasma specimens from apparently healthy individuals measured for cTnI by high-sensitivity (by gender) and contemporary assays. *Hs-cTnI,* High-sensitivity cardiac troponin I. (Modified from Apple FS, Ler R, Murakami MM. Determination of 19 cardiac troponin I and T assay 99th percentile values from a common presumably healthy population. *Clin Chem* 2012;58:1574–1581.)

able to identify patients, often without clinical symptoms, who may be at risk of cardiac-related adverse outcomes; and (5) clinical trial investigators will be able to identify appropriate and optimal patient reenrollment and outcome measures.

Optimal discrimination between a small amount of myocardial injury and analytical noise requires assays that have low limits of quantitation (LOQ; lowest concentration at 20% CV) and LOD, and require high imprecision at low cTn concentrations. Efforts to improve the imprecision of cTn assays are always warranted. Irrespective of how the testing is performed, whether in the central laboratory or at the bedside using POC assays, manufacturers need to define the imprecision profile (ie, the scatter graph showing the %CV vs. increasing cTn concentrations obtained using the Clinical and Laboratory Standards Institute [CLSI] EP5-A2 protocol) by assessing pools of human samples containing different cTn concentrations (Fig. 58.11).[83] In particular, at least two cTn concentrations that cover the range between the LOD and the 99th percentile decision limit of the assay are recommended to be included. Imprecision characteristics, including the 10 and 20% CV concentration, the LOD, and

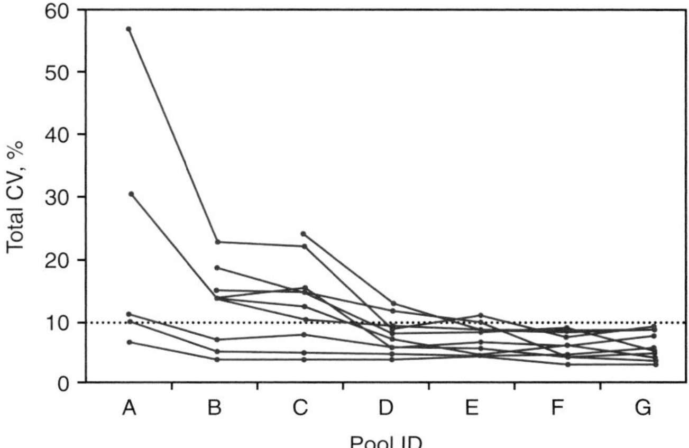

FIGURE 58.11 Cardiac troponin I imprecision profiles for human serum pools using different cardiac troponin I (cTnI) assays, with 10% coefficient of variation *(CV)* concentration indicated by the dashed line. (From Panteghini M, Pagani F, Yeo KT, Apple FS, Christenson RH, Dati F, et al. Evaluation of imprecision for cardiac troponin assays at low-range concentrations. *Clin Chem* 2004;50:327–332.)

TABLE 58.2 Cardiac Troponin Assay Scorecard Designations

Company/ Platform/Assay*	Acceptance Designation	Assay Designation
Contemporary		
Abbott Architect	Clinically usable	Level 1
Beckman Access Accu+3	Clinically usable	Level 2
LSI Medience PATHFAST	Guideline acceptable	Level 1
Ortho Clinical Diag. Vitros ES	Guideline acceptable	Level 1
Roche Elecsys E170	Clinically usable	Level 1
Siemens Centaur Ultra	Guideline acceptable	Level 1
Siemens Dimension RxL	Clinically usable	Level 1
Siemens Stratus CS	Guideline acceptable	Level 1
Siemens VISTA	Guideline acceptable	Level 1
Tosoh AIA II	Clinically usable	Level 1
Point of Care		
Abbott i-STAT	Clinically usable	Level 1
Alere Triage	Not acceptable	Level 1
bioMerieux Vidas Ultra	Not acceptable	Level 1
Radiometer AQT90 cTnI	Clinically usable	Level 1
Radiometer AQT90 cTnT	Clinically usable	Level 1
Response Biomedical RAMP	Clinically usable	Level 1
Trinity cTnI	Clinically usable	Level 1
High-Sensitivity Assays		
Abbott hs-cTnI	Guideline acceptable	Level 4
Beckman hs-cTnI	Guideline acceptable	Level 4
Ortho-Clinical Diagnostics	Guideline acceptable	Level 4
Roche hs-cTnT	Guideline acceptable	Level 2
Singulex hs-cTnI	Guideline acceptable	Level 4

*Per manufacturer's package insert; *NA,* insufficient information to designate.

Assay designation: Measurable normal values below 99th percentile—level 4: ≥95%; level 3: 75 to <95%; level 2: 50 to <75%; level 1: <50%.

Acceptance criteria: %CV at 99th percentile—guideline acceptable ≤10%, clinically usable >10 to 20%, not acceptable >20%.

CV, Coefficient of variation.

Modified from reference Apple FS. A new season for cardiac troponin assays: it's time to keep a scorecard. *Clin Chem* 2009;55:1303–1306.

99th percentile data from currently commercially available assays, are shown in Table 58.1. It is a matter of concern in the context of clinical practice that there still is some variability for an individual patient's cTn concentration when the same sample is measured with the same manufacturer's assay but in different laboratories. Such discrepancies highlight the need for local analytical validation whenever feasible. Laboratories at a minimum should determine total imprecision and should continue to monitor assay performance over time using internal quality control materials that include the lowest concentration corresponding to the 10% and 20% CVs, as well as at the 99th percentile value if different from the 10% CV concentration. Patient specimen comparisons such as regression analysis and bias assessment should be performed according to CLSI guidelines.

Many organizations, including the NACB, IFCC, Global Task Force, and Cardiology and Epidemiology Societies have outlined the following analytical recommendations for cTn (as well as for other biomarkers of ACS). Objectives were to recommend the appropriate implementation and utilization of cardiac biomarkers, specifically cTn, to aid in the diagnosis of MI, complementing the quality specifications for the cTn assay previously published.[11,94]

1. Reference decision intervals should be established for each cardiac biomarker based on a population of normal, healthy individuals without a known history of heart disease (reference population). For cTn I (cTnI) and T (cTnT), as well as for myocardial-bound creatine kinase (CK-MB) mass, the 99th percentile upper reference interval should be the decision limit for myocardial injury.
2. A minimum of 300 men and 300 women per group of healthy individuals is required for appropriate statistical determination of a normal reference URL for both cTn and CK-MB.
3. One decision interval, the 99th percentile, is recommended as the optimum cutoff for cTnI, cTnT, and CK-MB mass. Patients with ACS with cTnI and cTnT results above the decision interval should be labeled as having myocardial injury and at high risk.
4. Monitoring imprecision in clinical practice using quality control materials at the 99th percentile is important to be able to follow the potential of analytical day-to-day drift for assays, especially when new lots of reagents and calibrators are put into practice.
5. Assays for cTn should strive for total imprecision (%CV) of 10% or less at the 99th percentile.
6. Before introduction into clinical practice, cardiac biomarker assays must be characterized with respect to potential interferences, including rheumatoid factors, human antimouse antibodies, and heterophile antibodies. Preanalytical and analytical assay characteristics should include biomarker stability (over time and across temperature ranges) for each acceptable specimen type used in clinical practice and identification of antibody/epitope recognition sites for each biomarker. Analytical and preanalytical specifications developed by professional groups such as the IFCC should be followed.
7. Serum, plasma, and anticoagulated whole blood are acceptable specimens for the analysis of cardiac biomarkers. Choice of specimen must be based on sufficient evidence and the known characteristics of individual biomarker assays.

8. hs-cTn assays should report concentrations using whole number, with the nanogram per liter unit.

Understanding what is truly normal for cTn using high-sensitivity assays in clinical practice will be a major step forward in the cardiac biomarker field. The authors of this chapter continue to advocate for worldwide acceptance of the 99th percentile cTn value as the MI diagnostic upper reference interval.

POINTS TO REMEMBER

High-Sensitivity Cardiac Troponin Assays

Defined by:

- %CV 10% or less at 99th percentile
- cTn above the limit of detection (LOD) in 50% or greater of normal

Values will be reported as whole values, in nanogram per liter, and sex-specific cutoffs

Point-of-Care Testing

The NACB has developed Laboratory Medicine Practice Guidelines for POC testing for the use of cardiac biomarkers in ACS, which will be updated in 2017.[95] These guidelines address administrative issues, cost-effective usage, and clinical and technical performance of cardiac biomarkers in the ED. Eleven proposed elements of the guidelines are as follows:

1. Members of EDs, primary care physicians, cardiologists, hospital administrators, and clinical laboratory staff should work collectively to develop an accelerated protocol for the use of biomarkers in the evaluation of patients with possible ACS.
2. This protocol should be applied to facilitate the diagnosis of MI in the ED or to continue the diagnosis at other locations in the hospital.
3. Quality assurance measures should be used with monitoring to reduce medical errors and improve patient treatment.
4. Blood collection should be referenced to the time of presentation in the ED and, if available, to the reported time of symptom onset.
5. The interdisciplinary team should include personnel who are knowledgeable about local reimbursement.
6. The laboratory should perform biomarker testing with a maximum turnaround time (TAT) of 1 hour and optimally 30 minutes. The TAT is defined as the time from blood collection to reporting of results to the provider.
7. Institutions that cannot consistently provide a 1-hour TAT should consider POC testing assays if clinically necessary.
8. Performance specifications and characteristics for central laboratory and POC testing assays should not differ.
9. Laboratory personnel must be involved in selection of POC assays, training of individuals to perform the analysis (whether laboratory or nonlaboratory personnel), maintenance of POC equipment, oversight of proficiency and competency of operators, and compliance with requirements of regulatory agencies.
10. POC assays should provide quantitative results.
11. Manufacturers are encouraged to work closely with professional organizations to develop structured committees and establish quality performance specifications for new biomarkers.

At present, no hs-cTn assays are available in a POC assay format.[96] For both POC and central laboratory testing, and for practical considerations, anticoagulated whole blood or plasma appears to be the optimal specimen for rapid emergent processing. This eliminates the extra time needed for clotting and additional sample handling. However, differences have been described among plasma, whole blood, and serum specimens for cTnI concentration measurement by an individual assay. Both ethylenediaminetetraacetic acid (EDTA) and heparin are known to interfere with cTnI and cTnT antibody-binding affinity, as well as produce some matrix effect differences.[97] It is not recommended that different sample types are mixed during an individual's work-up when serial, timed samples are being drawn to rule in or out an MI. The interfering effect of blood tube additives has been extensively described in the Chapter 5.

Although clinicians and laboratorians continue to publish guidelines supporting TATs of less than 60 minutes for cTn, most studies demonstrate that TAT expectations are not being met in a large proportion of hospitals. As an example, the College of Pathologists (CAP) Q-Probe Survey study[98] of 7020 cTn and 4368 CK-MB determinations in 159 hospitals demonstrated that median and 90th percentile TATs for troponin and CK-MB were as follows: 74.5 minutes, 129 minutes; and 82 minutes, 131 minutes, respectively.[99] Less than 25% of hospitals were able to meet the less than 60-minute TAT, representing the biomarker order-to-report time. However, data have shown that implementation of POC cTn testing can decrease TATs to less than 30 minutes in cardiology critical care and short-stay units.[95,100-105]

The following example demonstrates how an institution that addressed a poor TAT problem for cTn improved laboratory services through cross-department cooperation.[101,106] Based at a 400-bed county hospital with 120,000 patient presentations per year through the ED, approximately 30,000 cTn orders per year were tested for both outpatients and the 1800 to 2000 patients admitted for short- or long-term care. A 2-month survey of the TAT for cTn showed a 90% TAT of 118 minutes. To better meet the published guideline of 60 minutes 100% of the time, the laboratory medical director, the emergency medicine staff whose primary responsibility involved ACS MI presentations, and the cardiology medical director who was responsible for the 11-bed cardiac 24- to 48-hour observation unit (cardiac short-stay unit [CSSU]), 28-bed telemetry unit, and 8-bed cardiac care unit (CCU) met and designed an ACS triage protocol, outlined in Fig. 58.12. POC cTnI assay systems (using whole blood, Stratus CS) were placed in the small ED laboratory, staffed by the clinical laboratory around the clock, in support of the hospital's level 1 trauma center. Additional POC assays were placed in the CSSU, in which 42 nurses were trained by the laboratories' POC coordinators. The flow of specimens was such that initial presentation cTnI requests ordered through the ED were analyzed in the ED laboratory—approximately 6000 to 8000 per year. TAT from the time of blood draw to the provider result report was less than 18 minutes, 100% of the time. The use of POC testing eliminated the additional time needed to transport and process specimens that would have been needed to analyze specimens in the central laboratory. Patients admitted to the hospital to rule in or rule out MI

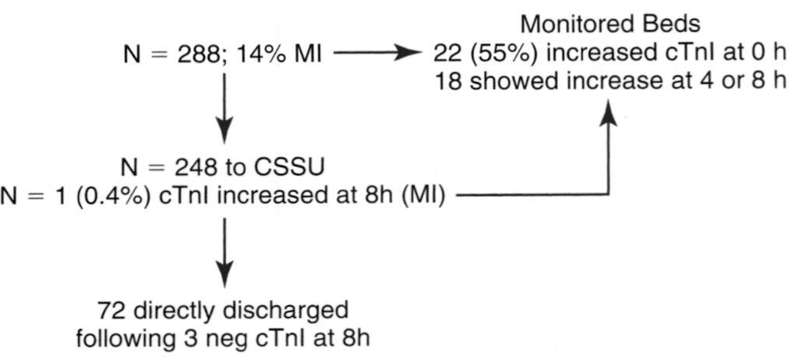

FIGURE 58.12 Role of cardiac troponin testing correlated with patient flow in the triage process from the emergency department *(ED)*, cardiac short stay unit *(CSSU)*, and coronary care unit. *ACS*, Acute coronary syndrome; *cTnI*, cardiac troponin I; *MI*, myocardial infarction; *ROC*, receiver operating characteristic; *TAT*, turnaround time. (From Apple FS, Chung AY, Kogut ME, Bubany S, Murakami MM. Decreased patient charges following implementation of point-of-care cardiac troponin monitoring in acute coronary syndrome patients in a community hospital cardiology unit. *Clin Chim Acta* 2006;370:191–195.)

who were at low risk were admitted to the CSSU, where staff nurses provided less than 20-minute TAT 100% of the time from blood draw to results to provider. In the CSSU, in compliance with the hospital protocol that at least a 6-hour postpresentation sample had to remain normal for cTnI, two blood specimens, in addition to the ED presentation sample, were measured at 4 and 8 hours. The uniform timed ordering protocol for ruling out MI included four timed draws at 0, 4, 8, and 12 hours. In patients admitted to the telemetry unit or the CCU, a dedicated blood draw was tubed to the central laboratory, where specimens were given priority-testing status, and thus met a TAT of less than 60 minutes 98% of the time. During this process, it was recognized that POC testing was not cost-effective for patients in telemetry or CCU units. These were mostly patients at moderate to high risk in whom a clinical diagnosis had already been made; thus urgent cTn values were less necessary. The CSSU was successful in decreasing the length of stay in the unit by 0.8 day through implementation of POC testing, allowing triage to lower levels of care and/or discharge on a 24/7 basis. Although the direct cost per assay reagent increased from $3.83 (central laboratory) to $10.51 (POC testing), the overall cost to the patient decreased by more than $4000 per admission (Fig. 58.13), primarily based on decreased bed charges from a more costly cardiac bed to a less expensive general medicine bed or to discharge. These data highlight the continued need for laboratory services and health care providers to work together to develop better processes to meet a TAT less than 60 minutes, as requested by physicians. It is important to

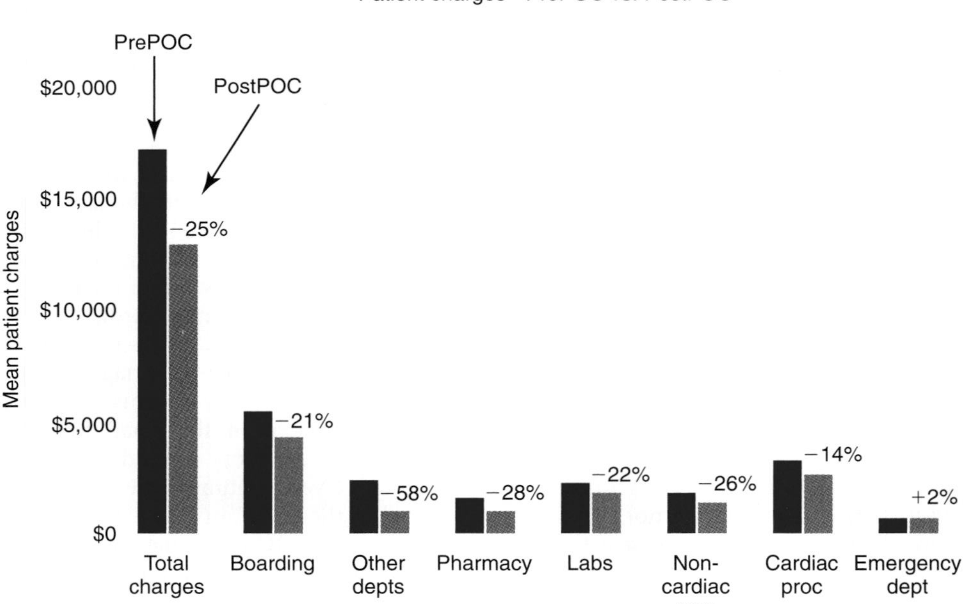

FIGURE 58.13 Financial impact of incorporating point-of-care *(POC)* cardiac troponin I testing into a cardiology service compared with central laboratory cTnI testing. In each pair of bars, the left and right bars indicate the costs before and after introduction of POC testing, respectively. (From Apple FS, Chung AY, Kogut ME, Bubany S, Murakami MM. Decreased patient charges following implementation of point-of-care cardiac troponin monitoring in acute coronary syndrome patients in a community hospital cardiology unit. *Clin Chim Acta* 2006;370:191–195.)

indicate that only two POC testing assays (Siemens Stratus CS and LSI Medience PATHFAST) demonstrate optimal (10% CV at the 99th percentile) analytical sensitivity.

It has been shown that a less sensitive POC assay may miss a positive cTn value that would be detected as increased by a more sensitive contemporary assay, as noted in Fig. 58.14. Further, POC cTnI assays also suffer from the lack of assay standardization. Fig. 58.15 shows that in a representative patient presenting with an evolving AMI, serial cTnI concentrations vary substantially between three POC assays versus a contemporary assay, with substantial variability in clinical sensitivities between assays.[107] Contrary to the poor analytical sensitivity of POC assays, Fig. 58.16 shows that for an hs-cTnI assay, rising values are detected earlier even compared to a contemporary cTnI during the early course of an AMI.

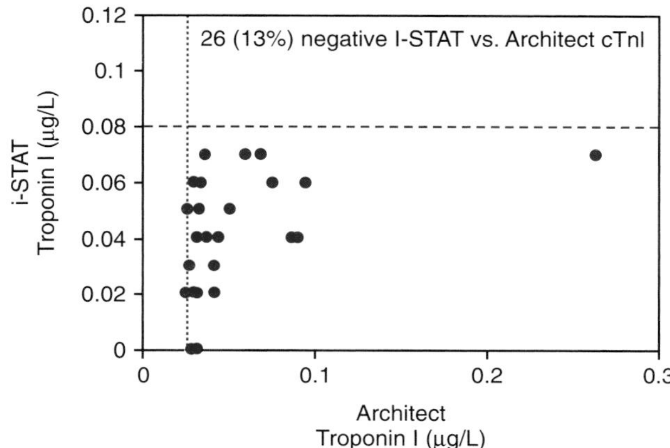

FIGURE 58.14 Scatterplot of i-STAT–negative and Architect-positive samples. The *dotted line* represents the 99th percentile cutoff for each instrument. *cTnI,* Cardiac troponin I. (Courtesy of Jasbir Singh. From Singh J, Akbar MS, Adabag S. Discordance of cardiac troponin I assays on the point-of-care i-STAT and Architect assays from Abbott Diagnostics. *Clin Chim Acta* 2009;403:259–260.)

Appropriate Use of Cardiac Troponin for the Diagnosis of Myocardial Infarction

Although numerous international guidelines have suggested general times that cTn testing should be used to evaluate ruling in or out an AMI after a patient presents to an ED, few studies have actually examined the appropriate use (actual orders placed by providers) of cTn testing in a clinical setting. It is not atypical for the laboratory to receive excessive, unrational cTn test orders well after a patient has been ruled in or ruled out for an MI, at a considerable unnecessary expense to the health care system. There is a substantial diversity across hospitals within the United States and internationally on how cTn testing is ordered, ranging from a hospital-wide serial order-set (such as at presentation, 3, 6, and12 hours) to the ability to order cTn as a single test order at any time without any uniformity across a hospital/medical center. These orders are often complicated within teaching hospitals where both attending physicians and resident physicians may place multiple order sets, with substantial duplication and excessive cTn testing. Two studies have made interesting observations

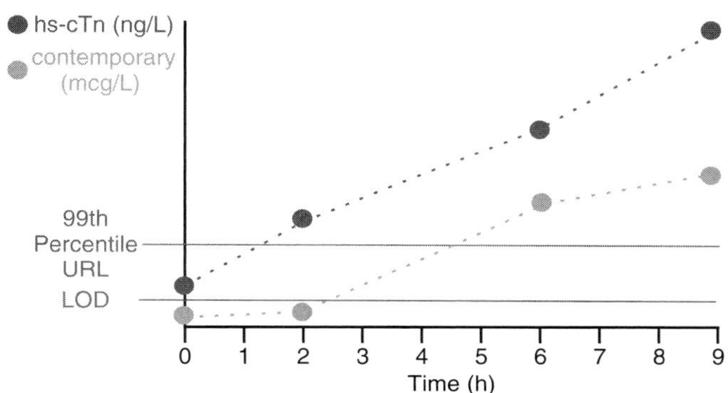

FIGURE 58.16 Cardiac troponin I kinetics comparing high-sensitivity and contemporary assays in a patient presenting with 30 minutes of an acute myocardial infarction. *Hs-cTn,* High-sensitivity cardiac troponin; *LOD,* limit of detection; *URL,* upper reference limit.

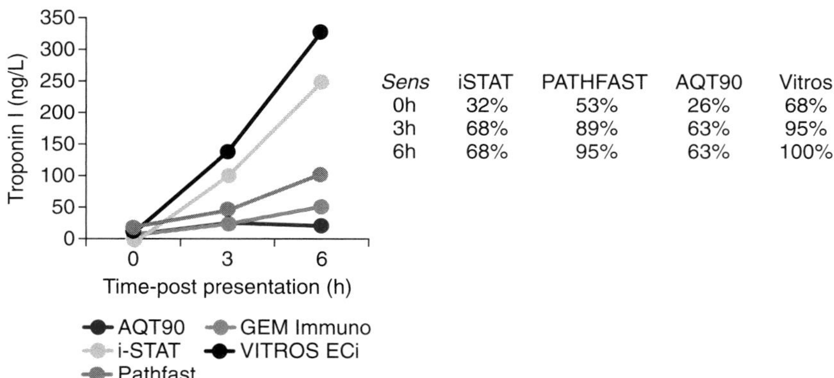

Sens	iSTAT	PATHFAST	AQT90	Vitros
0h	32%	53%	26%	68%
3h	68%	89%	63%	95%
6h	68%	95%	63%	100%

FIGURE 58.15 Serial cTnI findings for a representative myocardial infarction patient plotted as a function of time (hours) vs. cTnI concentration for 5 cTnI assays; respective clinical sensitivities shown at baseline for assays. (From Palamalai V, Murakami MM, Apple FS. Diagnostic performance of four point of care cardiac troponin I assays to rule in and rule out acute myocardial infarction. *Clin Biochem* 2013;46:1631–1635.)

in this regard.[108,109] First, in a monitored telemetry unit staffed by attending and resident physicians, an excessive number of cTnI tests were ordered after the diagnosis of both an MI (48% over testing) and no-MI (39% over testing) already had been established, with an average of approximately 6 to 7 cTn tests per diagnosis. Second, in the course of reviewing approximately 6000 cTn orders over 2 months in a 420-bed primary care hospital, providers (42% of whom were residents) acknowledged and overrode an electronic alert 97% of the time after a second set of serial cTn orders was placed, with 93% in non–ACS-related patients. The overall conclusions from these representative studies were that better education and monitoring of cTnI orders in the diagnosis or exclusion of MI is needed, with the need for electronic ordering review and/or hard stop to be implemented. Proactive test use by laboratory professionals regarding cTn orders, working in concert with their clinical colleagues and information technology counterparts, should become a high priority in clinical laboratory practice to assist in health care savings.

Clinical Use of Cardiac Troponin

History

cTns have been available for clinical use since 1995, when the first cTn T (cTnT) assay was approved. Since that time, it has become clear that enhanced cardiac specificity and particularly improved sensitivity lead to more frequent and more accurate diagnosis of cardiovascular abnormalities especially with the implementation of high-sensitivity cTn assays (Fig. 58.17).[110] Initial use of these assays was influenced in large part by the previous use of markers such as CK-MB. CK-MB is substantially less sensitive and less cardiac specific than cTn, but because of its long use, it had become entrenched in the thinking of clinicians and laboratorians. For this reason, perhaps, the first set of guidelines by the NACB attempted to compromise between the use of these two markers in setting guidelines for clinical use.[94] These guidelines suggested that there should be two cutoffs. One cutoff was selected to be equivalent to values of CK-MB in the clinical identification of patients. This cutoff, known as the receiver operating characteristic (ROC) curve–derived cutoff value, considered CK-MB the gold standard, as it had been for years. However, this cutoff did not take advantage of the increased analytical sensitivity of cTn values.[111] A second cutoff was recommended for use at a lower level (the 97.5th percentile of a normal patient population), which was poorly clinically defined, above which patients were considered to have cardiac injury. But even patients with a classic history of AMI were designated as having "unstable angina with minimal myocardial

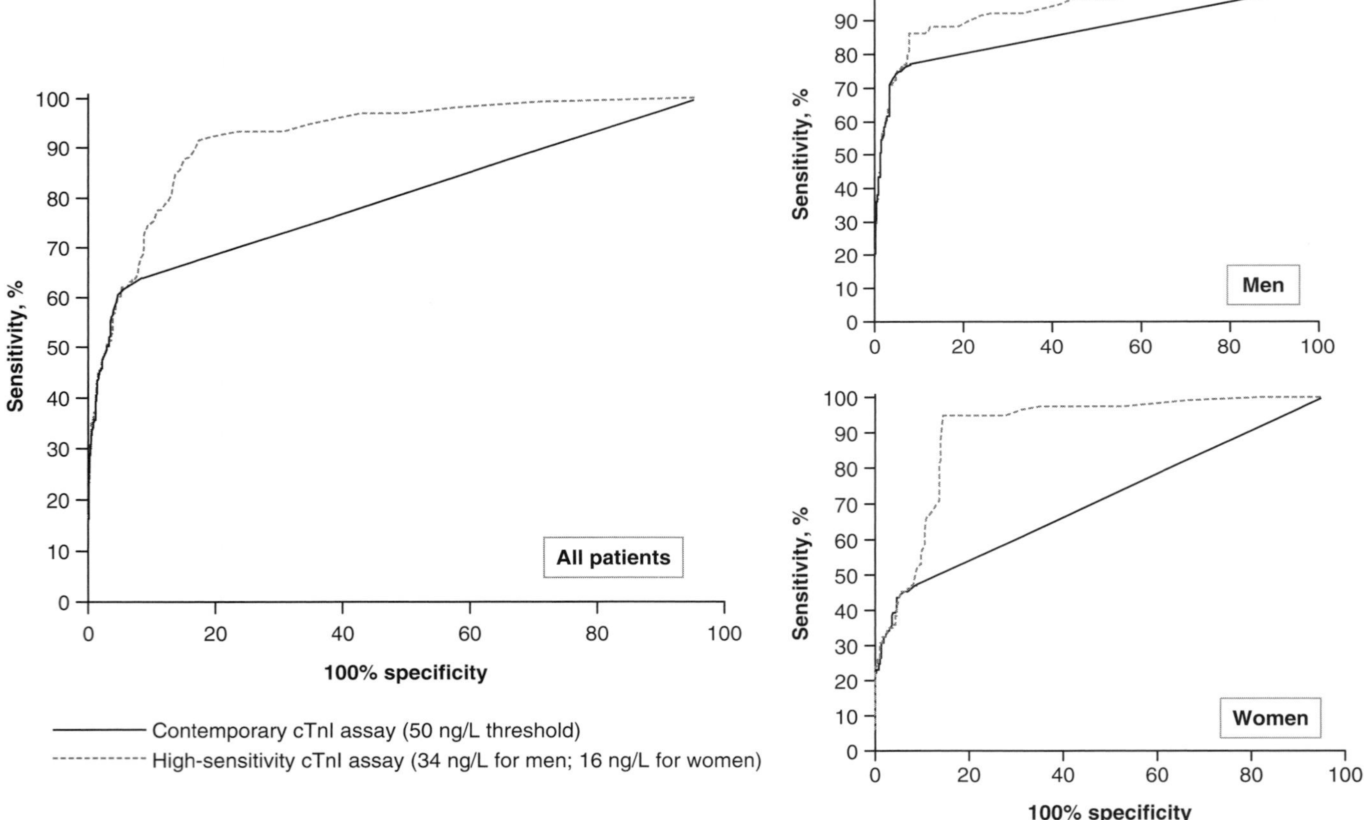

FIGURE 58.17 Receiver operating characteristic (ROC) curve analyses of cardiac troponin I *(cTnI)* comparing high-sensitivity, by gender, and contemporary assays for the diagnosis of acute myocardial infarction. (From Shah AS, Griffiths M, Lee KK, McAllister DA, Hunter AL, Ferry AV, et al. High sensitivity cardiac troponin and the under-diagnosis of myocardial infarction in women: prospective cohort study. *BMJ* 2015;350:g7873.)

necrosis." The guidelines followed extensive research demonstrating large numbers of patients with chest pain (roughly an additional 33%) whose prognoses in terms of subsequent frequency and timing of events were identical, and who had increased cTn values but normal CK-MB values.[111] These findings were documented despite the fact that the initial version of cTn assays was relatively insensitive compared with contemporary assays.

This concept of using prognosis to confirm diagnosis rapidly became the paradigm not only for cTn but for the validation of most other markers as well. It was not until 1999, when a task force empaneled by the ESC/ACC took issue with these guidelines, that the concept of using only one cutoff value was initiated.[112] ESC/ACC guidelines suggested the use, not of the 97.5th percentile of a reference population but the 99th percentile, in recognition of increased sensitivity of cTn that led to many elevations that were difficult to explain. This had the potential benefit of reducing the overlap to 1% between those with disease and normal individuals.[38] It was conceptually important because even by this time, it was clear that enhanced sensitivity of cTn was leading to the identification of a substantial number of patients in whom the cause of cardiac injury (see later sections) could not be determined. This is often the case when one moves from a relatively insensitive measure to one that has substantially greater sensitivity (ie, when one uncovers new diagnostically and prognostically important increases).[113-115] Nonetheless, clinicians had difficulty understanding this because such elevations had not been described previously and the pathophysiology was obscure. This problem continues today as newer cTn assays become increasingly sensitive. The ESC/ACC biochemical group at that time also recommended that the 99th percentile should be measurable with excellent precision and suggested, not mandated, a criterion of 10% CV or less at the 99th percentile. The group did not, however, recommend that if assays did not reach that level of precision, the decision values should be raised above the 99th percentile value. Unfortunately, this was the extrapolation of some, and it led to even greater heterogeneity in how cTn values were interpreted.

Some individuals persisted in using the NACB recommendations, some used the ESC/ACC recommendations, and some because of fear of false-positive results caused by imprecision employed a value higher than the 99th percentile, usually at the level of the 10% CV value. Add to this the fact that local laboratories often felt the need (appropriately) to validate the assays in their own hands and came up with different values, and one can see how the use of cTn values became fragmented and idiosyncratic. This problem also led to tremendous heterogeneity in the published literature and attendant confusion on the part of clinicians.[116-118]

It is now very clear that normal cTn values are substantially lower than concentrations that are being reported for healthy individuals by contemporary assays (see Table 58.1). (The reported concentrations in healthy individuals often represent "noise" (<LOD) in the contemporary assays, see Fig. 58.9). hs-cTn assays are beginning (worldwide outside the United States) to have the ability to measure healthy individuals' low concentrations accurately, but only two (the Roche hs-cTnT assay and the Abbott hs-cTnI assay) have been commercially released for clinical use and, as of this time, they are unavailable in the United States because they have not yet been cleared by the FDA.[119-121] Nonetheless, this documentation and a wealth of clinical information has made it clear that for contemporary assays, the 99th percentile value is the key value to use when measuring cardiac cTn.[70,122-124] Any value above the 99th percentile should be considered abnormal. Concerns about false-positive results induced by such criteria should be minimal because assuming adequate quality assurance of the assays, even reduced imprecision should not lead to false-positive results provided cTn is measured in two serial samples.[125] Usually reduced imprecision simply impairs the sensitivity of the assay. Statistical modeling of this issue suggests that the clinical impact of using even an imprecise assay is negligible with regard to false-positive results.

For this reason, along with the clinical data, the criteria in all guideline papers now include use of the 99th percentile.[2,87] Although some studies have suggested a return to the use of the 97.5th percentile value for high-sensitivity cTn assays, this is unlikely to occur until and unless important clinical reasons for such a change can be demonstrated.[2,84,126] Once one recognizes that the 99th percentile is the criterion for abnormality, one can progress to understanding how to use cTn in a variety of clinical situations. The recent publication of several papers has clearly demonstrated this point, which will be discussed in the following section.

Use of Cardiac Troponin for the Diagnosis of Acute Myocardial Infarction

AMI is a state characterized by abnormalities between nutrient perfusion and myocardial oxygen consumption. It is usually diagnosed when abnormalities in coronary flow at least in part contribute to the pathogenesis of cardiac injury. Because of the high sensitivity and specificity of cTn for the heart, it has become the cornerstone of the diagnosis of MI (see Box 58.2). As shown in Fig. 58.18, high-sensitivity cTn assays eliminate the noise of contemporary (and POC) assays, providing greater reliability of true measurement

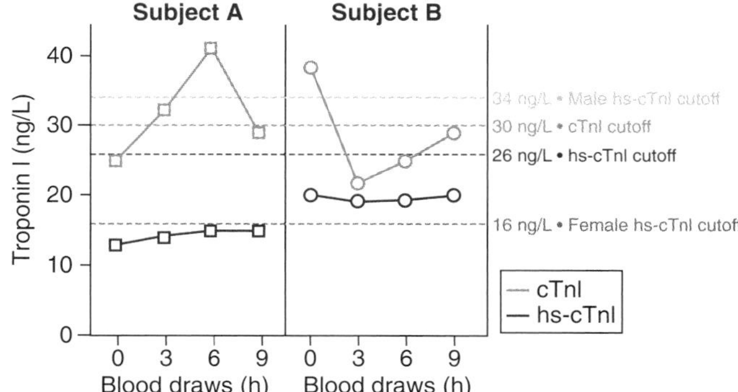

FIGURE 58.18 Representative serial cardiac troponin I *(cTnI)* concentrations in two patients measured by a contemporary and a high-sensitivity cTnI *(hs-cTnI)* (with sex-specific cutoffs) assay demonstrating analytical "noise" of the contemporary assay. (From Sandoval Y, Smith SW, Schulz KM, Murakami MM, Love SA, Nicholson J, Apple FS. Diagnosis of type 1 and type 2 myocardial infarction using a high-sensitivity cardiac troponin I assay with gender-specific 99th percentiles based on the Third Universal Definition of Myocardial Infarction classification system. *Clin Chem* 2015;61:657–663.)

of cTn at the 99th percentile upper reference interval. Accordingly, an increased value of cTn is needed in the appropriate clinical setting with values that manifest a rising or falling pattern for the diagnosis of AMI. Further, with the increased use of high-sensitivity assays, earlier and more accurate diagnoses will be made. Specifics of the MI definition are as follows.

The clinical substrate (usually risk factors for AMI in the patient) is key. An increased cTn value is not synonymous with the diagnosis of MI.[100] First, both the substrate (such as risk factors) and the presentation (most often chest discomfort) must be compatible with the diagnosis. At times, imaging, whether performed at the time of intervention by angiography or thereafter, may provide proof of the substrate.[2,78,87,127] Many clinical situations can mimic AMI, the most common of which is myocarditis. Apical ballooning is another.[128-132] Because of the increased sensitivity of cTn, clinicians need to be astute to the possibility that a given elevation in cTn, even with a rising pattern suggesting that it is acute, may not be due to ischemic heart disease (see Box 58.1).[110] This is conceptually difficult for many clinicians because when CK-MB, which was reasonably insensitive, was used, most substantive elevations were associated with coronary heart disease, albeit not all.

Acute events leading to cardiac injury usually will manifest a changing pattern of values.[2,132-138] The rationale for this is that as assays have become more sensitive, it has become clear that elevations of cTn can exist chronically.[56,139-149] The most overt case of this is seen in patients with renal failure.[139] This is also the pattern manifest when artifactual increases occur as the result of analytical problems caused by interferences from human antimouse antibodies and heterophilic antibodies in the blood of some patients.[150,151] However, hs-cTn assays do not appear prone to as many analytical problems as early generations of assays. Although patients with chronic elevations (not those with artifactual causes) are at long-term high risk, they are not necessarily at high risk over the short term. For this reason, the guidelines groups have advocated the need for a rising pattern of cTn values in patients who present early after the onset of symptoms, because such increases usually are indicative of an acute process. However, the acute process may not be AMI. Whether AMI is present is a clinical decision, when cTn values are not rising, one might seriously question whether acute disease of any kind is present or whether the elevations are of a more chronic nature. Care is necessary to ensure that one does not miss individuals who come in late after the onset of symptoms, whose cTn values may be near peak values, or whose values are on the long persistent tail of the time-concentration curve. They may appear not to have a changing pattern of values because they are near the peak of the time-concentration curve or on the gradual down-slope. This can occur in up to 26% of patients.[152]

With increasingly sensitive assays, there will be more AMIs that are not due to plaque rupture (so called supply-demand type 2 AMI) because these usually elaborate less cTn than plaque rupture events (type 1 AMI).[153-155] However, the criteria for a rising and/or falling pattern do not differ.[156] These will occur more frequently in women than in men. There are good data that the use of sex-specific cutoff values with hs-cTn assays improve the diagnosis of these patients.[124]

The guidelines distinguish five types of MI (see Box 58.3); two will be considered here because they both manifest with chest discomfort and increased biomarkers. One is the so-called spontaneous, or "wild type," in which acute plaque rupture leads to some degree of thrombosis, or an episode in which platelet accretion occurs on a plaque, leading to thrombosis.[2,87] The second type includes coronary abnormalities with possible supply-demand imbalance, vasospasm, or endothelial dysfunction, which provides evidence of myocardial injury. For example, supply-demand imbalance with fixed coronary artery disease (CAD) is thought to be the cause of most perioperative MIs,[157] and these patients do not require the same care as those with a spontaneous AMI.[87]

Individuals with spontaneous AMI can have STEMI or non-STEMI as indicated by the ECG pattern they manifest.[2,28,19] Data indicate that immediate treatment aimed at opening the occluded artery is mandatory for patients with STEMI. This should be done based on the ECG pattern alone, even before biomarker values become available to assist with diagnosis. Opening of the artery is currently done with primary PCI and/or thrombolytic agents. The former is preferred when the two are available in similar time frames. With prompt coronary recanalization, the amount of myocardium lost is minimized and mortality is reduced.[18] It should be noted that coronary recanalization increases the rapidity of biomarker release, and thus the rate of rise of the time-concentration curve is increased and the time to peak values is shortened (Fig. 58.19).[110]

A non-STEMI is less often associated with total coronary occlusion and usually is identified by ECG changes, which show not ST segment elevation but rather ST segment depression or T-wave changes. Given the sensitivity of cTn for this diagnosis, the ECG is even at times totally normal. Patients who present with chest pain as a result of CAD should have risk factors, an appropriate presentation, or imaging evidence

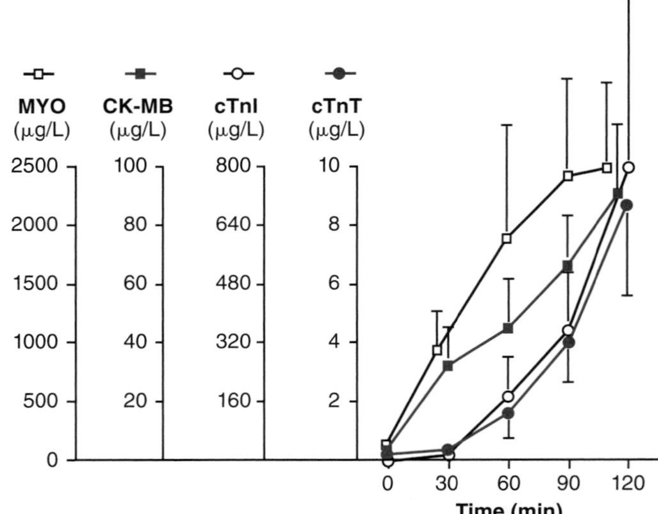

FIGURE 58.19 Time course (mean and standard error) of serum cardiac troponin I *(cTnI)*, cardiac troponin T *(cTnT)*, creatine kinase-2 *(CK-MB)*, and myoglobin *(MYO)* concentrations after initiation of thrombolytic therapy in patients with thrombolysis in myocardial infarction (TIMI) grade 3 reperfusion flow. (From Apple FS, Sharkey SW, Henry TD. Early serum cardiac troponin I and T concentrations following successful thrombolysis for acute myocardial infarction. *Clin Chem* 1995;41:1197–1198.)

of this syndrome. Patients with an increased cTn, using contemporary assays and the recommended 99th percentile upper reference interval are known to have more severe coronary heart disease than individuals without increased cTns. Likely for this reason they also have more procoagulant activity. Multiple intervention studies have shown that these patients benefit from aggressive anticoagulation, including heparin (the data for low molecular weight heparin are much stronger than the data for unfractionated heparin), glycoprotein IIb/IIIa antiplatelet agents, and an early invasive strategy consisting of PCI or coronary artery bypass grafting (CABG). Use of these strategies in patients without increased cTn values has been shown to be of no benefit and, in some trials, has actually proved detrimental.[23] For these patients, expeditious but not necessarily immediate coronary interventions are suggested.[18] Clinical trials have not yet been done to define the prognosis and/or treatment approaches for those with elevated hs-cTn values that are below the level of detection of contemporary assays, but the adverse prognostic significance appears from preliminary studies to be preserved.[152-155] However, given the increased frequency of type 2 MIs, it is unclear that invasive intervention will be necessary in all such patients.

However, not all patients have easily identifiable culprit lesions in which to intervene, and this explains some apparent spontaneous AMIs without severe CAD.[27,128,138,158-160] These patients, often women, may have endothelial dysfunction, coronary vasospasm, coronary dissection, or some other transient process that has resolved before investigation. These patients have type 2 MI according to the guidelines. This group might also include those individuals who have fixed but stable CAD but have some degree of damage as a result of excessive myocardial oxygen consumption, such as that caused by severe tachycardia, hypotension, or hypertension. Coronary arteries that are diseased tend to vasoconstrict rather than dilating in response to stimuli that would normally evoke vasodilation and increases in coronary flow.[159] These patients are probably fundamentally different from individuals who have spontaneous MIs and likely are not a subgroup that has nearly as much procoagulant activity; it is unclear whether they benefit from interventional therapy. This may be one of the reasons why women who tend to have more severe endothelial dysfunction seem to have a different profile.[27,158] Nonetheless, depending on the specific study reviewed, 10% to 30% of patients may not have an identifiable lesion that has caused the event, leading to consideration of this alternative pathophysiology.[159] From the perspective of diagnosis, however, the cTn criteria are identical.

Distinctions among the MI types have to be made on the basis of clinical characteristics and other diagnostic studies. It is now clear that women can have type 2 MI secondary to spontaneous coronary dissection.[26] It used to be thought that this occurred almost exclusively during pregnancy, but that is clearly not the case. This diagnosis can be easily missed angiographically and is associated in at least half of patients with coronary tortuosity[161] and evidence of fibromuscular dysplasia in other vascular beds.[162] Preliminary data suggest that unless these patients are hemodynamically compromised or have total coronary occlusion, a strategy of watchful waiting rather than intervention may be preferred.[163]

Other types of MIs are recognized.[2,11] First, one type does not use biomarkers at all. This includes patients who may present classically with both chest pain and ECG changes but succumb either before blood tests can be obtained or before enough time has elapsed for the circulating concentration of cTn to exceed the 99th percentile. Two other types of MIs have been designated; these are related to PCI and CABG and will be covered later under "Special Situations."

Operationalization of a Changing Pattern of Cardiac Troponin Values

This is a challenging area. Minor changes in values may be due to analytical causes. In general, two values are different if they differ by more than 2.77 standard deviations (SDs) (assuming the variances are comparable at the two concentrations).[120] Ideally, both analytical and biological variation would be included in calculation of the SDs.[77,164] Unfortunately, analysis of biological variation requires studies of stable subjects, and only the hs-cTn assays can provide data on healthy people. Thus, at present, the analysis has focused on the use of data on analytical imprecision alone. At high concentrations of cTns, the CV is 5% to 7%, so a difference of 20% is unlikely to be attributable to measurement imprecision.[2] But as values begin to approach the low concentrations corresponding to the 99th percentile value, analytical %CV increases, making the relative difference between two consecutive values prone to increases by random error alone.[120] Local analysis of imprecision should be used to guide interpretation of differences in results for consecutive samples, with larger percentage changes necessary to suggest real change at very low levels of cTn. Defining a consistent period for analysis is also key to an accurate approach to this analysis. High-sensitivity assays help with this problem; their lower imprecision at low cTn concentrations make it possible to calculate a reference change value (RCV).[77,120,164,165] Studies of several hs-cTn assays show RCV values (biological variation) ranging from 50% to 85% (as shown in Table 58.3).[77,166] Although it is now clear that these values may work well when the baseline value is near the 99th percentile upper reference interval, when the baseline value is elevated, these values are less sensitive. Accordingly, a recommendation has been made for hs-cTnT to use a 50% change near the 99th percentile upper reference interval and a 20% change when the baseline value is elevated.[167] Similar percent change recommendations are not yet available for hs-cTnI assays. Others have advocated for the use of absolute concentration change criteria. In general, these are similar to percentage criteria when baseline values are near the 99th percentile upper reference interval but are much lower when the baseline values are elevated. It appears that these values provide better accuracy, especially when the baseline value is elevated, compared to percent criteria.[121,152,168,169] What is known is that individual assays will need to develop their own change values because there will not be a universal value that will be applicable to all cTnI assays. Clinical studies in this area have generally used convenience cohorts, have often incomplete sample sets, have used insensitive gold standards, and lack early patients, all of which enhance the apparent diagnostic abilities of hs-cTn.[170] Some studies, in an attempt to reduce the time to diagnosis or exclusion of AMI, have divided a validated number from 6 hours and applied it at shorter intervals with the assumption that biomarker release is continuous and constant. This is not a reasonable approach. Furthermore, often the values that need to be documented are outside of the analytical

AT A GLANCE

Strategies for ruling in and ruling out acute MI with contemporary and high-sensitivity cTn assays.

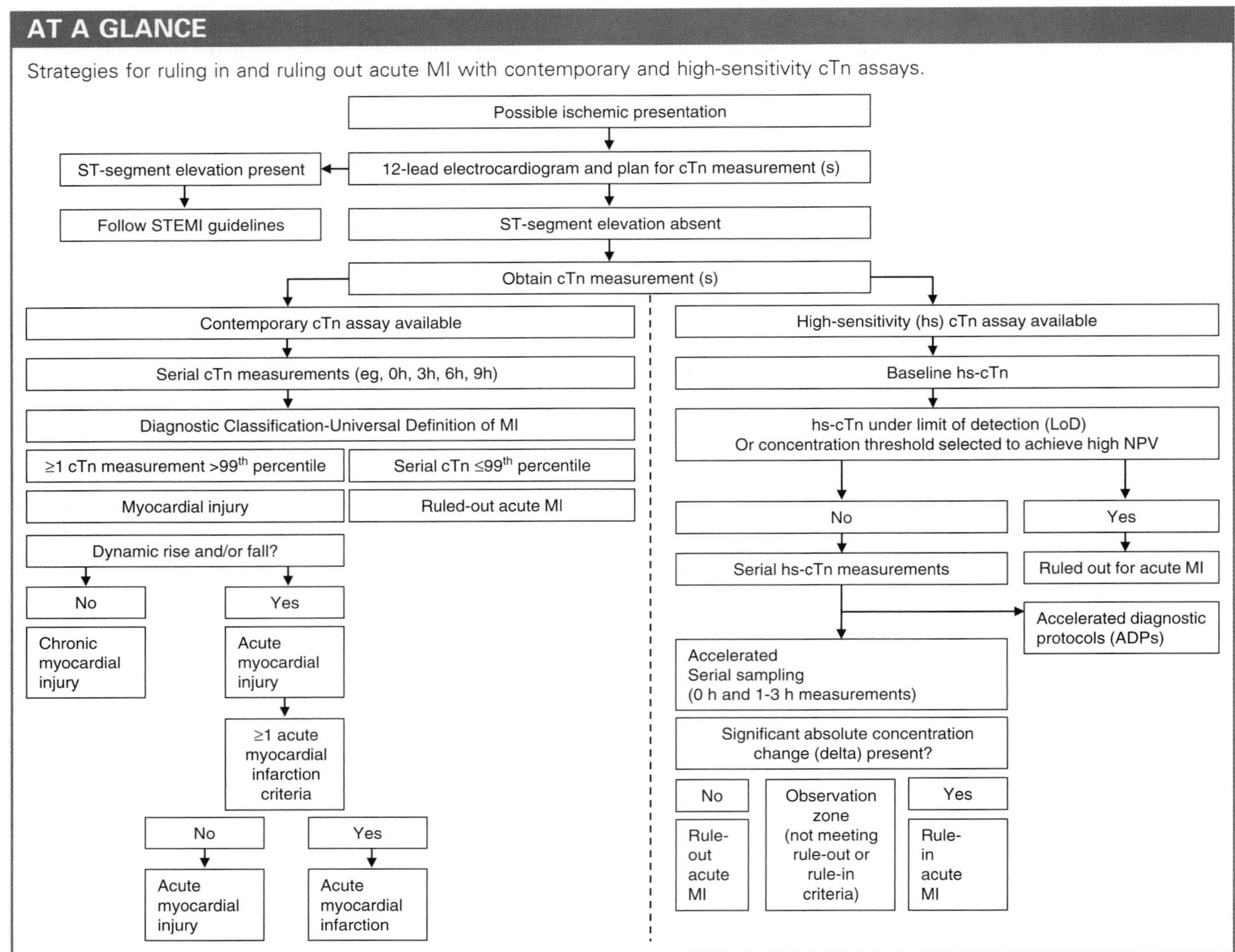

TABLE 58.3 Short-Term Analytical and Biological Variation of High-Sensitivity Cardiac Troponin Assays

	Abbott	Beckman	Roche (E170)	Siemens	Singulex
CV_A (%)	13.8	14.5	7.8	13.0	8.3
CV_I (%)	15.2	6.1	15.0	12.9	9.7
CV_G (%)	70.5	34.8	NA	12.3	57
Index of individuality	0.22	0.46	NA	0.11	0.21
RCV (%)	NA	NA	47.0	NA	NA
RCV increase (%)	69.3	63.8	NA	57.5	46.0
RCV decrease (%)	–40.9	–38.9	NA	–36.5	–32.
Within-subject mean (ng/L)	3.5	4.9	NA	5.5	2.8

CV_A, Analytical variation; *CV_I,* within-subject biological variation; *CV_G,* between-subject biological variation; *NA,* not available; *RCV,* reference change value; *RCV,* percentage applies to the parametric data; *RCV,* increase and decrease percentages refer to nonparametric data and are log-transformed.

From Apple FS, Collinson PO. Analytical characteristics of high-sensitivity cardiac troponin assays. *Clin Chem* 2012;58:54–61.

capabilities of hs-cTn assays.[170] It is likely that shorter time intervals can be achieved with hs-cTn assays to rule in and rule out AMI, but they should be implemented with care and attention to the problems indicated previously and with the concept that there will be some exceptions to the rules (see later discussion).

Special Situations With Acute Myocardial Infarction

After Percutaneous Coronary Intervention

It has long been appreciated that interventions done on the coronary arteries can result in the release from heart muscle of biomarkers indicative of cardiac injury.[171] For this reason, a variety of criteria have been promulgated, starting years ago with CK-MB. It was shown initially that elevations of CK-MB that occurred after the procedure were highly predictive of adverse events over the long term. These findings were difficult to explain because the amount of injury involved often was very minor but was nonetheless easy to document with sophisticated techniques such as cardiac magnetic resonance imaging (cMRI). However, controversy about the mechanisms continued and a large number are being hypothesized. The advent of cTn biomarkers has rendered this issue far less complex. Patients who have elevations of circulating cTn and who present with acute coronary problems have much more severe abnormalities in coronary anatomy than those who do not have cTn elevations.[172] In recent studies, the baseline cTn value has been added to the analysis of these post-PCI elevations.[173-175] This was done for many years, but not with assays that measured cTn concentrations even close to the 99th percentile. Accordingly, it is only recently that the data have confirmed several important conceptual issues.

The first concept is that a vast majority of patients with significant elevations (threefold to fivefold increase in CK-MB or cTn) that in the past were associated with an adverse prognosis are those with increased cTn values at baseline. This usually (although not always) is indicative of an acute presentation and therefore a rising pattern of values. In the setting with a rising pattern of values, it is hard to know whether one should attribute the increases to the PCI or to the initial insult.[175] Nonetheless, when one incorporates the baseline value into the analysis, most of the prognostic significance of the postprocedure cTn values is ablated.[173-175] Data suggest that it is only at an elevation of cTn at baseline that marked postprocedure elevations in cTn are apt to be frequently found, suggesting that in most instances at least a blend of the two processes occurs. These issues have been confounded not only by failure to use appropriate cutoffs for cTn, but by the use of insensitive cTn assays. More recent guidelines clarify this circumstance substantially by indicating that if one has an increased cTn at baseline before PCI, the diagnosis of post-PCI injury is confounded and cannot be made.[2] Thus a normal baseline cTn is required in almost all instances to identify procedure-related myocardial injury. If the baseline cTn is increased, subsequent increases may or may not be able to be attributable to the procedure itself and a diagnosis of post-PCI injury cannot be made with absolute confidence.

Marked elevations, as indicated previously, are uncommon but can occur. When they do occur, they are rarely of cardiovascular importance, in the sense that the more marked elevations are easily presaged by clinical information at the time of the procedure. Thus post-PCI cTn values add very little that is new. In addition, it is unclear whether patients have an adverse cardiovascular prognosis over time. In the most recent analysis done by using the most appropriate cutoff values and contemporary cTn assays, borderline statistical significance was attributed to post-PCI elevations.[174] However, most events that did occur were noted during procedures in patients who had severe underlying noncardiac comorbidities and therefore underwent palliative procedures. The event rate, if patients with non–cardiac-related subsequent complications are excluded, would not have been of statistical importance; even if their inclusion were of only borderline significance. Thus it now appears that collection of this information after PCI is not necessary. Recent data suggest that values even modestly below the 99th percentile upper reference interval have important prognostic significance, presaging in our opinion, the likelihood that with hs-cTn assays, this effect will be strengthened and the prognostic impact of post-PCI values attenuated still further.

Nonetheless, criteria still exist for these occasional patients who may have post-PCI injury. The appropriate cutoff cTn value is unclear, but it is clear that very few patients will reach the marked threefold to fivefold elevation previously advocated if the baseline cTn is not increased.[173] This is likely to change, however, with hs-cTn assays. If cTn is increased post-PCI more than fivefold, with a normal baseline cTn value assumed, the patient can be diagnosed as having had a periprocedural MI if they have had symptoms or have ECG changes and/or had complications of the procedure.[2] No specific therapy is mandated. Regarding biomarker changes that occur after reperfusion of an occluded vessel after PCI or thrombolytic therapy in AMI patients, greater than twofold increases in biomarkers occur within 90 minutes of reperfusion, the rate of increase of biomarkers within the first 4 hours separates reperfused from nonreperfused patients, and after myocardial reperfusion in AMI patients, washouts of all biomarkers parallel each other.[176-180] However, increased washout does not define the level of reperfusion and cannot be used to define a post-PCI AMI.

One unique subset needs to be taken into account, and that is the small group of patients who may have chronic preprocedure elevations in cTn. These individuals will manifest a rising pattern, albeit from an increased baseline, when they have events, including post-PCI events. Accordingly, what has been suggested is that the criteria used for reinfarction of an increased value of 20% or more should be used to define post-PCI infarction in this group.[87]

Post–Coronary Artery Bypass Graft Myocardial Infarction

Abundant data indicate that after cardiac surgery patients have elevations in cardiac cTn. Indeed, in the vast majority of studies, such elevations are of prognostic importance—the higher the elevation, the worse the prognosis.[181-183] However, the underlying propensity for elevation is moderated in part by the details of the procedure. For example, procedures that are done off cardiopulmonary bypass evoke less cTn release,[181] as might be expected, because they cause less direct cardiac injury. In addition, a relationship has been noted between the duration of cross-clamp time and the amount of biomarker elaborated, the temperature of the cardioplegia, and the duration of the procedure. Most of the injury as assessed from cMRI studies is subendocardial and often apical. Higher post-CABG biomarker values are associated with transmural injury.[184,185] Thus procedures that are longer, such as those that include valve replacement, are very likely to evoke more cardiac damage than those that are shorter. Accordingly, finding a single value that separates all of these different subsets is impossible. Accordingly, most recent guidelines have elected not to try to define separate criteria for subsets of these procedures, but instead have preferred to define a single cutoff that can be used for all the situations already described for which ancillary criteria need to be employed. Most recent guidelines support a fivefold increase in cTn after the procedure and add additional criteria such as ECG changes, changes with imaging, and the development of new regional wall-motion abnormalities.

The value of such an approach is that it allows use of a single cTn cutoff. The downside of the approach is that this cutoff lacks some precision when it comes to the types of procedures performed. It might be better to devise specific criteria for each subset of the procedures. This is an extensive task because of multiple variations in the way in which cardiac surgery is done. Nonetheless, the key concept is that the prognostic impact of increased cTn concentrations is related to the magnitude of the increase. Unfortunately, because of the complexity of these considerations, no one has been able to define a value at which increases in cTn can be attributed to a specific coronary-related event such as graft or native vessel occlusion.[186] Thus, although the aggregate amount of marker that is released is prognostic (for both CK-MB and cTn), it does not distinguish the mechanism of injury. The guidelines nonetheless recommend the diagnosis of post-CABG AMI if there is a 10-fold increase in cTn in conjunction with additional imaging or clinical features of AMI.[2] Similar criteria are recommended for other invasive procedures such as transcatheter aortic valve replacement.

Evaluating Possible Acute Myocardial Infarction

Evaluating Possible Acute Myocardial Infarction: The Importance of Clinical Context

Unfortunately, the clinical presentation of patients with possible AMI can be highly variable, as indicated earlier. For that reason, ED physicians often are concerned that they might miss AMI.[187] In addition, when patients have a low pretest likelihood of AMI, even the most predictive symptom or sign will not increase the likelihood of AMI sufficiently for diagnosis. The same can be said for signs and symptoms thought to be atypical for AMI.[188] For these reasons, many patients who are very unlikely to have AMI are often evaluated with cTn measurements, which explains in part why most studies define the frequency of AMI in consecutive ED patients in the single digits in the United States.[188] At some sites in Europe, this is not the case, and this does not receive sufficient attention when evaluating these studies.[189] Thus the interpretation of an elevated cTn value is very different in low-risk patients than in high-risk patients. A variety of shortened protocols have been developed for low-risk patients. Unfortunately, an ideal classification system has not yet been developed. Instead, those used to define risk in patients with possible ACS, such as the thrombolysis in myocardial infarction (TIMI) and Global Registry of Acute Coronary Events (GRACE) risk scores, have been employed.[19] It should be recognized that these schemes, though a good first step, may require modification depending on the specifics of the local situation and for specific patients. Nonetheless, scores of 0 or 1 with the TIMI score and/or less than 140 with the GRACE score have been used to define low-risk groups in whom more rapid rule-out protocols might be used. Several protocols have been proposed with contemporary assays[190,191] and an even larger number with hs-cTn assays.[145,160,192-194] For patients at high risk, the emphasis is on ruling in AMI. There also have been proposals to facilitate these rule-in decisions with hs-cTn assays, which are controversial; based on serial cTn collections at 1, 2, and 3 hours after presentation[170,195,196]; this group probably should not be evaluated with rapid rule-out protocols, and the importance of an elevated cTn value is very different. It is essential for clinicians to take these considerations into account when evaluating patients.

Further, pediatricians are often asked to assist in evaluation of a baby or child with a cTn increase. The first question is what clinical rationale was used to obtain a cTn measurement. Studies have shown that measurements of cTn can be higher during the first 2 weeks of age as well as throughout adolescence, in comparison to established 99th percentile upper reference intervals for adults.[197,198] Whether this reflects evidence of cardiac necrosis is not always clear. However, acute injury should be able to be determined with confidence if rising cTn concentrations are documented with serial draws and the increased cTn concentrations fit the clinical presentation. Further, an isolated single increase or chronic increases that may not show rising or falling values need to be clinically evaluated carefully because results may suggest that in children the 99th percentile may not be a reliable index of silent cardiac disease but rather may be indicating low-grade intercurrent illness. Additional studies are needed in this clinical area as hs-assays become more prevalently used in pediatric practice.

Evaluation of Possible Acute Myocardial Infarction With Cardiac Troponins by Risk Subset

Low-Risk Patients

The major issue with low-risk patients is not inclusion of AMI but its exclusion. It is clear from previous literature that if one can define the time of onset of symptoms accurately, a normal cTn value at 6 hours after the onset of symptoms excludes AMI with a high NPV.[19,113] Precise identification of the time of onset of symptoms is often problematic. Therefore the time clock for cTn measurements should begin at the time of presentation.[19] Several approaches have been advocated both with contemporary cTn assays and hs-cTn assays. With contemporary assays, values that are within the normal range over a 2-hour period exclude AMI in most low-risk patients (TIMI 0 and TIMI 1).[190,191] Caveats important to note include that most of these patients did not present particularly early, almost all were at low risk, and most had very extensive follow-up, with additional testing.[190] Thus care is required in patients who present early, are not at low risk, and may not have adequate follow-up.

The opportunities to detect AMI in low-risk patients using hs-cTn assays are likely to increase. Because values increase with the development of cardiovascular comorbidities, very low values of hs-cTn assays may be indicative of a very low risk.[86,144] In addition to having a low risk profile and a normal ECG, additional information that integrates the presence of sensitive detection of cTn release may allow for facile rule out of AMI. Several manuscripts have probed this strategy using undetectable values (less than LOD or LOB) of hs-cTnT.[145,160,193] The frequency of these findings has varied markedly, many studies have not included sufficient numbers of early patients, and many studies have not provided adequate clinical evaluations. It appears likely, especially for low-risk patients, that an undetectable or very low cTn value with hs-cTn assays will work to help identify the roughly 20% of patients who may benefit from being identified at the time of presentation and who can be immediately discharged as long as good clinical follow-up is available.[193] Additional data based on hs-cTn assays that detect values in almost everyone have developed approaches for a 2-hour rule out in TIMI 0 or TIMI 1 patients, and such a strategy has been shown to work.[194] It is especially likely that a very low cTn level with an hs-cTn assay will be able to be defined, with some patients able to be discharged based on the initial sample. A variety of combined rule-in and rule-out proposals have been made that rely on RCV criteria. They were covered previously and will be discussed later as well.[170] However, a representative study to highlight the role of using only hs-cTn assays to provide an early rule out of AMI was recently published.[199] The study identified a low plasma cTn concentration (<5 ng/L) using an hs-cTnI assay (Abbott) at the time of presentation of a patient thought to have ACS that would exclude MI and demonstrate that these patients would be at very low risk (NPV 99.6%) for cardiac events at 30 days and could be safely discharged from hospital and have further investigation in the outpatient setting if appropriate. The authors do not suggest that all patients with less than 5 ng/L should be discharged from the ED, because there may be other reasons or comorbid conditions that will necessitate hospital admission. At present, no other biomarkers, including copeptin, addressed later in this chapter, provides added clinical value for either diagnostic accuracy or risk outcomes assessment.

Intermediate-Risk and High-Risk Patients

Rule-in algorithms are appropriate in intermediate-risk and high-risk patients. With conventional cTn assays and the use of appropriate 99th percentile upper reference intervals, most AMIs are identified within 3 hours from the time of symptom onset.[200] Patients who are at high risk and have an initial cTn elevation likely can be considered to have an acute presentation per guidelines.[19] Subsequent confirmation is nonetheless imperative. There will be times when a late rule in will occur, for example, in patients in whom there is poor blood flow to the damaged area.[19] It usually requires 6 hours to be sure that an AMI has not occurred (high NPV). With contemporary assays, the possibility of a diagnosis of unstable angina must still be entertained. Hs-cTn assays may facilitate earlier evaluations (NPV >98% within 3 hours), although the number of patients with a new AMI will not be high.[201] The European guidelines suggest that the diagnosis of AMI can be established in most patients within 3 hours with hs-cTn assays. However, they do not define the criteria that should be used or even identify which cTn assays they believe are high sensitivity.[202] This has led to 1-, 2-, and 3-hour rule-out strategies based on finding significant changes in the initial hs-cTn values over time.[194-196] As indicated previously, many of these have design problems (see section "Operationalization of a Changing Pattern of Cardiac Troponin Values"). Their use should be considered speculative at present. It also

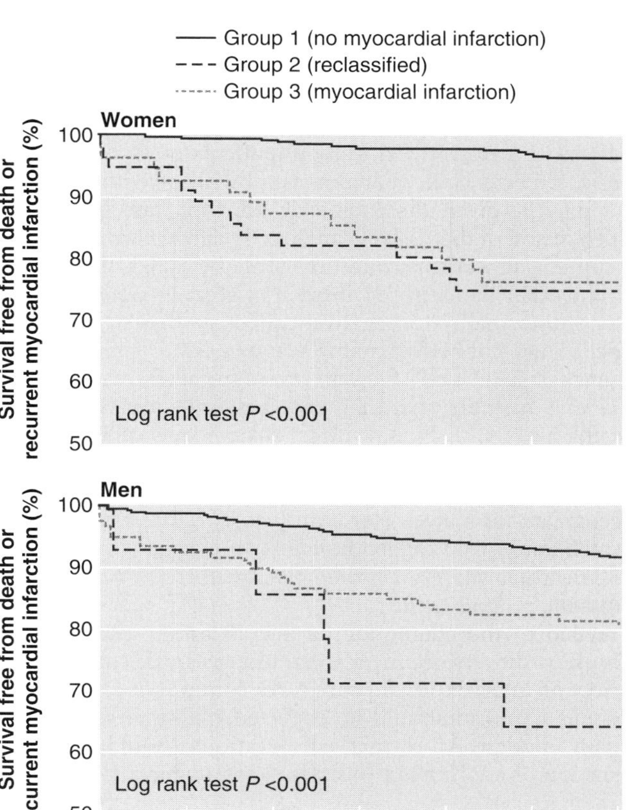

FIGURE 58.20 Survival free from death or recurrent myocardial infarction (MI) in women and men with suspected acute coronary syndrome. Outcomes are shown for women and men with no MI *(solid line)* and with MI *(dashed red line),* in which both assays were concordant, and for those reclassified as having MI using the high-sensitivity assay with sex-specific thresholds *(dashed pink line).* (From Shah AS, Griffiths M, Lee KK, McAllister DA, Hunter AL, Ferry AV, et al. High sensitivity cardiac troponin and the under-diagnosis of myocardial infarction in women: prospective cohort study. *BMJ* 2015;350:g7873.)

should be clear that some patients who present later after the onset of symptoms may not have a changing pattern of values.[152] A recent study by Mills and coworkers demonstrates the power of the implementation of hs-cTn assays, with gender-specific 99th percentile upper reference intervals, for risk stratification.[124] Kaplan–Meier curves showing survival free from death or recurrent MI in women and men with suspected ACS varied depending on the use of a contemporary or hs-cTn assay. Outcomes are shown in Fig. 58.20 for women and men with no MI and with MI, in which both assays were concordant. However, for patients reclassified as having MI using the hs-cTnI assay and sex-specific thresholds, a greater number of at-risk patients were detected.

OTHER CAUSES OF ACUTE CARDIAC TROPONIN ELEVATION IN THE ABSENCE OF ACUTE ISCHEMIC HEART DISEASE

Many acute diseases are associated with elevated cTns (see Box 58.1), and the frequency of such elevations will increase with the advent of hs-cTn assays.[201] This can occur for many reasons,[203-206] including direct trauma to the heart, implantable cardioverter-defibrillator (ICD) firings, biopsies, and cardioversions. Also, some patients may have type 2 MI, as indicated previously. Critically ill patients often have tachycardia, hypertension, or hypotension with or without drugs that may be given therapeutically, such as catecholamines, which in and of themselves can directly damage myocardium. In some instances this condition could be called type 2 AMI. On the other hand, in the absence of at least some coronary artery abnormality to negatively affect perfusion, these episodes would not be designated as type 2 AMI. Patients in the absence of CAD who have very severe supply-demand imbalance may have elevated cTn, and these individuals probably do not have AMI. Finally, direct toxic effects of circulating cytokines and catecholamines can cause severe myocardial toxicity. Such is the case in sepsis. Thus consideration of each mechanism for a given elevation is important. A representative tabulation is provided here.

Trauma

Contusion, slow potential cardiac ablation, pacing, ICD firings, cardioversion, myocardial biopsy, and closure after a variety of interventional procedures commonly cause elevations in cTn and should be expected. These elevations are usually modest. More marked elevations should engender suspicion of additional processes.

Congestive Heart Failure

HF can cause acute elevations,[207] and elevations have been noted during long-term monitoring of patients, as well.[208] In both circumstances, they are markedly adverse prognostic signals and indicate more severe HF and an increased proximate likelihood of mortality. Such patterns can be rising but need not be, especially with more chronic HF. The prognostic significance of cTn is additive to that of the natriuretic peptides. Elevations are usually modest. With hs-cTn assays, these increases will be more frequent but potentially more informative as well. Acutely, increases will be common and preliminary information suggests that the patterns of these elevations may be prognostically important[209]; with hs-cTn assays providing better prognostic information[77] and a better way to monitor treatment.[210-212] Although many patients with HF have CAD, the cTn elevations observed occur in patients both with and without coronary heart disease, so they should not be used to include the diagnosis of AMI absent additional findings to suggest acute ischemic heart disease.[213]

Severe Valvular Heart Disease

Severe valvular heart disease with volume or pressure overload can be associated with elevations in cTn. Elevations may be more apt to occur with cTnI for volume overload via a calpain-mediated mechanism and may be more common with cTnT with left ventricular hypertrophy (LVH).

Hypertension

Hypertension in and of itself can cause LVH or cardiac enlargement, which increases wall stress and reduces nutritive perfusion, causing increases in cTn. LVH is associated with reduced subendocardial perfusion caused by increased wall stress; therefore subendocardial injury may occur in response to severe hypertension.[214] Obviously, because hypertension is a risk factor for CAD, these processes may be exacerbated by each other, but this is not necessary for elevations to be observed. Elevations most often are modest. With hs-cTn assays, it is now appreciated that individuals with LVH (most often a consequence of hypertension) who have elevated hs-cTn values are at very high risk for both HF and mortality.[146]

Hypotension and Tachycardia

Hypotension and tachycardia can be synergistic with underlying coronary abnormalities or may occur independently.[215] Nonetheless, at some point their severity can be sufficient to cause some degree of cTn release, usually modest.

Postoperative Noncardiac Surgery Patients

Data indicate that elevations of cTn postoperatively are negatively prognostic.[157,216] Many of these events are probably due to type 2 MI, but obviously not all of them. Indeed, autopsy studies suggest that half of those events that result in mortality are type 1 MIs.[157] In vascular surgery patients, which is the group best studied, these cTn elevations seem to be related to underlying coronary heart disease in association with an abnormality in acute myocardial oxygen consumption, usually hypertension or hypotension and/or tachycardia, anemia, and the like.[157,217] This is an area of expanding interest because it has become clear that an increasing number of non–cardiac surgery patients suffer events in the hospital, and it is likely that a more diverse group of patients will soon be elucidated. Causes of observed elevations may differ among the groups involved and may include, for example, PE, which is common in postoperative patients. hs-cTn assays will cause this area to explode. Preliminary data suggest that up to 45% of postoperative patients will have cTn elevations.[218] There will be a desire to suggest all of these individuals have ischemic heart disease, but the data for that have not been developed.[219] However, AMI should be considered only if there is a rising and/or falling pattern of hs-cTn. Solitary elevations should evoke a search for possible causes. For that reason, a baseline value is suggested. To emphasize, increases of cTns do not automatically suggest AMI but are associated with myocardial injury. Not only will it help in detection of a rising pattern of values, indicative of an acute event, but it will also identify high-risk patients.[220] Mortality, even in patients undergoing noncardiac surgery, is higher in patients with myocardial injury presenting with postprocedure cTn increases than in patients with a cTn in the normal range.

Patients With Renal Failure

Patients with end-stage renal failure often have elevations in cTn that are highly prognostic.[221] Elevations occur more frequently with cTnT than with cTnI, perhaps because processing of the two proteins is different in the renal failure circumstance. Nonetheless, elevations are highly prognostic in this group, but not necessarily for CAD.[222] A large percentage of renal failure patients die of sudden cardiac death. One should not presume that all cTn elevations occur in such groups, although this group does have an increased prevalence of CAD. The diagnosis of AMI still can be easily made using the presence of a rising and/or falling pattern.[86,221] Almost all patients with end-stage disease will have elevations using the hs-cTnT assay, but only approximately 30% with an hs-cTnI assay.[223] In addition, it is now clear that the distribution of hs-cTn values is increased with even lesser degrees of renal dysfunction.[86]

Critically Ill Patients

These individuals may or may not have underlying coronary heart disease, which is negatively synergistic with their acute illness, but they often have reasons for very substantial increases in myocardial oxygen consumption.[224,225] Elevations in cTn are common and usually modest but nonetheless are highly negative prognostically in the short and long term. In patients with acute respiratory failure, elevations of cTn are strongly related to short- and long-term outcomes.[134] In those with sepsis, the association is less strong short term but very powerful during long-term follow-up.[135] Elevations of hs-cTn seem best related to abnormalities in diastolic function and right ventricular dysfunction.[136] Patients with gastrointestinal bleeding are not at greater risk short term, and there is no signal that invasive evaluation is a problem. However, they are at substantial long-term risk.[137]

Drug Toxicity

Carbon monoxide poisoning is an archetypical example of drug toxicity.[226] Elevations in response to drug toxicity have prognostic significance. Recent data show that detection[227] and early treatment can obviate the effects of some toxic chemotherapies by monitoring cTn and, when elevations occur, by using angiotensin-converting enzyme inhibitors.[228] Snakebite venom can be another cause. It is very likely that over time a far larger number of drug toxicities will be documented.

Inflammatory Heart Disease

Myocarditis, when acute, commonly causes elevations of cTn.[229] Myocarditis also can cause coronary vasospasm and is a common mimicker of ACSs.[230] Elevation in this circumstance can be very high, even higher than that associated with acute infarction, or very modest, depending on whether patients have acute or chronic conditions. Roughly 50% of the patients in whom AMI is suspected but in whom coronary anatomy is deemed to be normal, have myocarditis confirmed by magnetic resonance imaging.[128,138]

Pulmonary Embolism

In general, the degree of cTn elevation is related to the degree of right ventricular dysfunction and therefore to the severity of pulmonary hypertension induced.[28,30] Increased cTn defines a patient who is at high risk; some have advocated that it should be used as an indication for the use of thrombolytic therapy of PE. This recommendation is premature at the present time. Elevations that occur with PE usually resolve within 40 hours. If they do not, recurrent emboli or another cause should be considered, along with or independent of PE.

Sepsis

Severe septicemia with hypotension probably has multifactorial causes for increases in cTn.[224,231,232] Such increases are often related to elaboration of toxic cytokines such as tumor necrosis factor alpha (TNF-α) and heat shock proteins. Initially a relationship was noted between the magnitude of cTn elevation and the extent of myocardial depression associated with cTn elevation that was above that associated with a modest increase in cTn. Some of this may be due to the use of catecholamines, which are directly myocardial toxins, to treat these patients[233] and may contribute to the supply-demand imbalance associated with type 2 AMI. It has reported that hs-cTn elevations seem best related to abnormalities in diastolic function and right ventricular dysfunction.[136]

Burns

Only when they are severe are elevations observed; this probably reflects the marked hemodynamic changes associated with severe burns.[234]

Acute Neurologic Disease

Increases probably represent reflex stimulation from the central nervous system.[235-237] A very substantial literature suggests that such is the case and that such increases seem to be related to insults in the midbrain[238]; they are particularly prominent with subarachnoid bleeds. Such elevations are highly prognostic but not necessarily for coronary heart disease. Seizures can also cause elevations.

Rhabdomyolysis

Rhabdomyolysis can occur systemically with associated cardiac injury.[71]

Transplant Vasculopathy

Monitoring of cTn has not been useful as an early marker, but elevations do occur with both transplant vasculopathy and rejection.

Vital Exhaustion

Severe exercise has been shown to cause release of cTn.[239-242] Whether this implies an element of minor myocardial injury or whether this could be release of cTn from the early releasable pool is a difficult issue. Nonetheless, studies suggest that patients, despite some having cMRI evidence of cardiac injury, do well and do not require emergency hospitalization.[243]

Chronic Elevations of Cardiac Troponin

Any chronic cardiac comorbidity, whether it is CAD, LVH, HF, or diabetes, can be associated with elevations in cTn. In general, these patients are the ones who have the most severe disease and poorest prognosis. Recent data suggest that patients with chronic heart disease at risk for subsequent events can be identified simply by looking at whether a cTn is detectable or not. This ability to predict those at risk is even better with hs-cTn.[147,148] In addition, LVH and HF, both of which can cause increased wall stress and reduced subendocardial myocardial perfusion, are known to be associated with elevations in cTn. With hs-cTn assays, these elevations are substantially prognostic.[146] The prognostic significance of elevations in older individuals is clear. It is also the case that elevations of hs-cTn in patients with putatively stable heart disease define a high-risk group.[56,149,244] How to improve management of this group is unclear.

Hypothyroidism

Hypothyroidism is a rare cause of cTn elevation.[245] Usually, hypothyroidism in the modern era is detected fairly early and treated, and it seems to take fairly severe hypothyroidism for elevations in cTn to occur. This is in contrast to previous literature, which suggested a high frequency of elevated

CK-MB. Given the cTn data, it is likely that CK-MB elevations were due to skeletal muscle abnormalities, rather than cardiac problems, as some might have initially surmised.

Infiltrative Diseases

Amyloid[246,247] and cardiomyopathies such as hemochromatosis are capable of causing increased cTns. In general, elevations are modest but very negatively prognostic.

Potential of Analytical False-Positive Findings

In addition, the possibility that chronic elevations are artifactual always should be considered. Heterophilic antibodies can interfere in cTn assays (though less commonly in contemporary and hs-cTn assays than in the past) by binding to antibodies in the reagent. Some patients have antibodies that bind cTn, creating immunoglobulin-cTn complexes that are poorly cleared from the circulation, leading to increased concentrations of cTn in blood that do not indicate cardiac injury. When clinicians observe an unexpected cTn result, they should notify the laboratory that has protocols to test for known interferents. Usually, when an interferent is present, dilution studies fail to give a linear pattern. Heterophile-blocking reagents can be used to minimize the effects of heterophilic antibodies. On occasion, even more sophisticated methods may be necessary to document false-positive results. Recently, false-positive elevations of cTnT have been reported to result from skeletal muscle injury.[248] Nonetheless, false-positive elevations appear to be relatively uncommon with current cTn assays.

Clinical Use of Myocardial-Bound Creatine Kinase

Considering CK-MB an obsolete test has met with considerable resistance,[10,249-251] in part because of difficulty clinicians have had in understanding how to use cTn measurements. This has been fueled in part by heterogeneity in the cTn assays available, diversity in the cutoffs intermittently advocated, and difficulty in understanding how to respond to elevations in cTn that are seen with cTns but not with CK-MB, because cTn is more diagnostically sensitive (myocardial tissue specific) than CK-MB. Nonetheless, several groups have advocated that CK-MB assays should be eliminated. The major push for this comes from the thought that not only do they add expense while not adding clinical value but because clinicians who continue to rely on CK-MB often do patients a disservice. In addition, these assays retard clinicians' ability to learn how to use cTn measurements properly, which would be more efficacious in almost every situation. Accordingly, serious consideration should be given by laboratories to discontinuing the use of CK-MB. Testing is not essential even for skeletal muscle disease in which total CK is appropriate, but it does eliminate a source of what some would argue is confusion for clinicians. This position has been well articulated,[251] and its use is now discouraged in recent guidelines.[19]

Those who advocate continued use of CK-MB point to a small number of instances that are worthy of consideration. The first includes the most controversial, which is the area of recurrent infarction after an index AMI. When initial guidelines for the use of cTn were developed, how well one would do in diagnosing recurrent injury with cTn was called into question because cTn elevations persist for so long. The data now confirm that cTn values detect acute recurrent injury very well (Fig. 58.21) and that reelevations occur with sufficient robustness that they can be detected promptly.[252] Second, from principles related to sensitivity and specificity (see earlier), some would argue that cTn would be clearly superior in this area. Nonetheless, the diagnosis of reinfarction is common after non–Q-wave MI, and because CK-MB was initially used to unmask this, people have retained some enthusiasm for its use. This occurred in part because in the past, if individuals had chest pain, this did not trigger a rapid evaluation. Thus, because CK-MB was thought to return to normal earlier, its elevation was helpful. However, this is not the case with contemporary and hs-cTn assays. Third, in modern practice, most patients with ACS are seen when chest pain is present and serial values are obtained. Thus, in the series by Apple and Murakami,[252] every patient identified had normal values of CK-MB, which subsequently increased to reach an abnormal threshold (see Fig. 58.21). Accordingly, with serial samples measured for both cTnI and CK-MB, CK-MB possessed no characteristics that would make it superior to cTn.

Fourth, when patients have recurrent chest discomfort, most immediately go back for coronary angiography to evaluate whether the chest pain is indicative of a problem with the area that has undergone intervention (eg, stent thrombosis) or whether severe diminution in flow is present in that vessel. Thus the only patients who are really held for evaluation are those in whom there is uncertainty about the diagnosis, and for this group, one needs to wait for serial samples. Indeed, this is the recommendation of the ACC/AHA committee on the management of patients with unstable angina and non–Q-wave MI and does still problematically include CK-MB.[19] Fifth, the other major indication that some advocate using CK-MB for is in patients who undergo PCI. The problems with this approach are indicated earlier, in the section on post-PCI AMI. Therefore very few to no indications exist to justify the use of CK-MB, except when cTn measurements are unavailable. This is a rare circumstance in the United States and in most of Western Europe but probably does occur elsewhere in the world, perhaps in countries with a much lower incidence of MI or countries that are resource poor and cannot afford the equipment needed to measure cTn. In this circumstance, most countries would rely on total CK, moving back even another step. In addition, immunoassays for cTn and CK-MB are reasonably comparably priced and use similar types of equipment. Nonetheless, if CK-MB is to be used, mass assays are considered far preferable. This is due to the fact that they are more sensitive and less prone to artifactual elevations. Increases in CK-MB from skeletal muscle injury clearly confound this measure and need to be taken into account. Use of the relative index (CK-MB divided by total CK), which used to be advocated by some because the percentage of CK-MB in cardiac muscle is so much higher than that in skeletal muscle, was discredited during the initial evaluation of cTn assays. The specificity of diagnosis is clearly improved when the index is used, but because so much CK is present in skeletal muscle, modest concurrent cardiac injury does not provide an adequate signal, so that sensitivity is lost.

Differences between males and females in reference intervals for CK-MB are likely related to differences in body mass.[253] Thus, if CK-MB is used, gender-specific reference intervals must be used, which improves the sensitivity.[254-256] This will correct in part for the relative lack of sensitivity of CK-MB, particularly in women. When used, the same

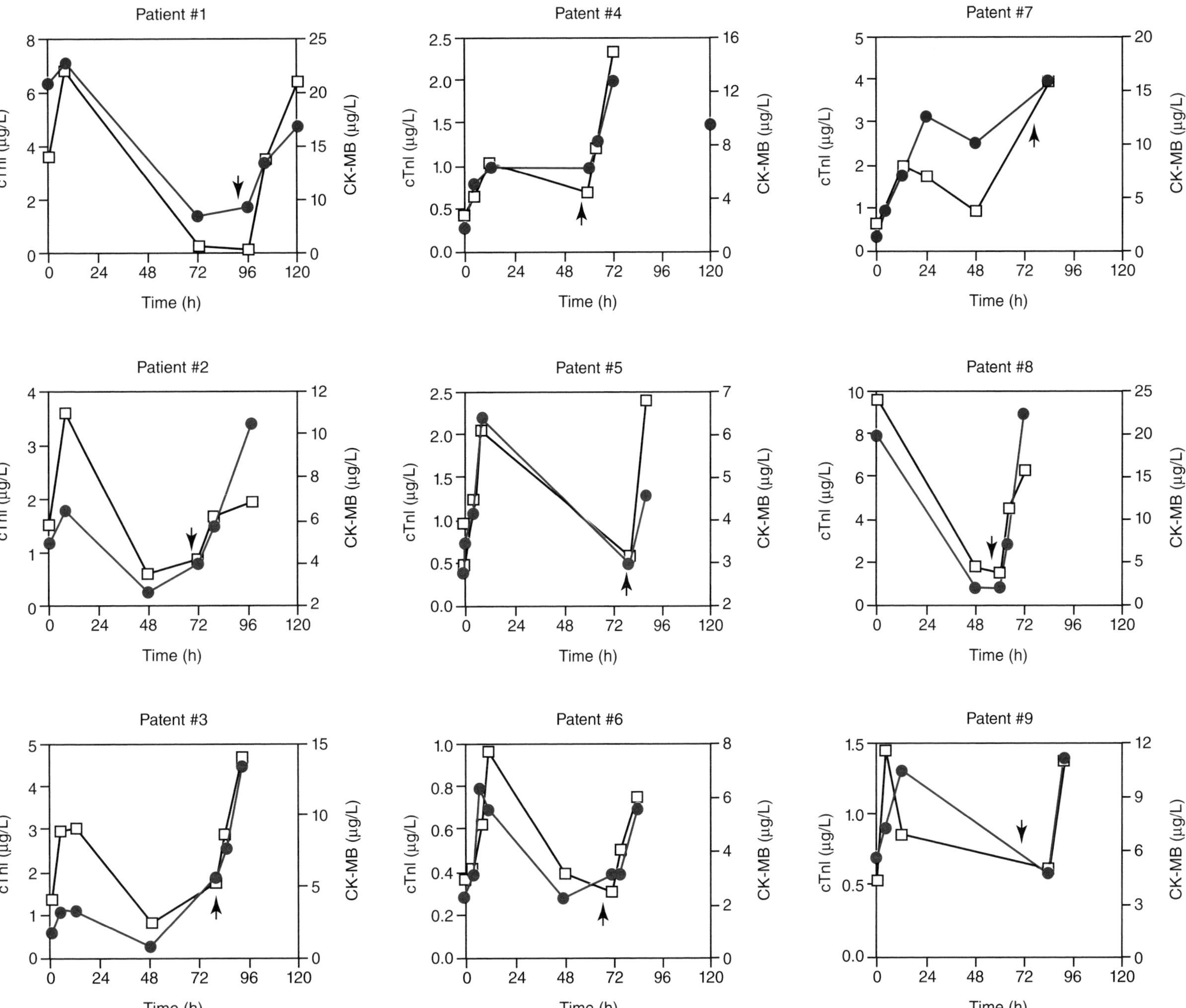

FIGURE 58.21 Time course of changes in biomarker concentrations in nine myocardial infarction patients who experienced reinfarction during hospitalization. *Red closed circles,* CTnI; *black open squares,* CK-MB, myocardial-bound creatine kinase. (From Apple FS, Murakami MM. Cardiac troponin and myocardial-bound creatine kinase monitoring during in-hospital myocardial reinfarction. *Clin Chem* 2005;51:460–463.)

criteria as with cTn should be employed (ie, a rising and/or falling pattern of results with at least one value above the 99th percentile of a normal reference population). However, very clear data indicate that elevations of CK-MB when cTn is normal identify patients who have skeletal muscle injury and not cardiac injury, as suggested strongly by the fact that these individuals do extremely well prognostically and do not appear to have an increased incidence of subsequent cardiovascular events.[257]

Normal skeletal muscle, depending on its location, contains very little CK-MB.[258] Percentages as high as 5% to 7% have been reported, but values less than 2% are much more common. Some differences are related to slow- versus fast-twitch muscle and thus also to race. Severe skeletal muscle injury after trauma or surgery can lead to absolute elevations of CK-MB to above the upper reference interval for CK-MB in serum. However, the percent CK-MB in serum would be low (percentages advocated vary, but in comparisons of activity versus activity, a percentage less than 5% is often used, and when CK activity is compared with CK-MB mass, a percentage less than 2.5% is usually advocated).[258] Increases in serum total CK and CK-MB in several patient groups present a diagnostic challenge to the clinician. Persistent elevations of serum CK-MB resulting from chronic muscle disease occur in patients with muscular dystrophy, end-stage renal disease, or polymyositis and in healthy subjects who undergo extreme exercise or physical activity. The increase in serum CK-MB in runners, for example, may be related to adaptation by skeletal muscle during regular training and after acute exercise, resulting in increased CK-MB tissue concentrations.[259]

The CARdiac MArker Guideline Uptake in Europe (CARMAGUE) study published in 2012 has demonstrated that 60% of laboratories in Europe are still offering total CK in addition to cTn in suspected cases of ACS.[260] As discussed in numerous international guidelines, including the Third Universal Definition of Myocardial Infarction, the only clinical utility of using either CK-MB would be in the absence of cTn testing. Further, the only clinical utility of using CK would be in the absence of both cTn and CK-MB because neither adds any clinical diagnostic or outcomes risk assessment data to cTn for patients presenting to rule in or rule out MI. The study also demonstrated that quite a large proportion of laboratories are still using alanine aminotransferase and aspartate aminotransferase; both are considered dinosaurs in the field of cardiac biomarkers and should not be used.

Biomarker That May Be Helpful: Copeptin

Copeptin is the preform of arginine vasopressin (AVP). It is cleaved from vasopressin and has a longer half-life, making measurement much easier.[261] It correlates well with AVP, which is cleared very rapidly from the blood. Because AVP is a stress hormone, copeptin has been used to define hemodynamic stress in two clinical situations: possible AMI and patients with HF. The assay itself is robust.[262] The first generation had a cutoff value of 14 ng/mL, but a more sensitive iteration is now available with a cutoff value of 10 ng/mL. Copeptin rises very rapidly in response to hemodynamic stress and falls rapidly as well. Its clinical use to rule out AMI has been predicated on its rapid increase. Thus elevations may precede those of cTn even in patients who present very early after the onset of AMI.[263,264] Thus a normal copeptin value has been touted to provide accurate exclusion of AMI.[262,263] The initial studies were done with conventional assays using well-defined cTn cutoff values to make the gold standard diagnosis of AMI.[263,264] However, many of the subsequent clinical trials used local cTn assays with variable cutoff values, leading to questions about the diagnosis of AMI.[265] Nonetheless, excellent discriminative accuracy has been shown for the ruling out of AMI on the initial sample at the time of presentation.[263,264] This would then in theory allow for a substantial number of patients with possible AMI to be discharged based on values from the first sample, an attractive characteristic. However, there have been several concerns about the use of copeptin. One has been that many studies have not been as rigorous as would be ideal in making the diagnosis of AMI. In addition, many studies have not included large numbers of patients presenting early after the onset of AMI. In addition, it is likely that this strategy will work only in patients who present without other major comorbidities that would evoke a stress response.[266] Thus such strategies will need to compete with those that have been developed to exclude AMI with hs-cTn. In those sorts of studies, the relative yield of copeptin has been markedly diminished.[267] Whether the small incremental yield with copeptin justifies the use of another biomarker, with its associated costs, with hs-cTn measurements is much less clear. Finally, it is clear that in some studies, the predictive accuracy of copeptin has been less than ideal but has been rescued by the judgment of the clinicians involved in the study.[268]

In HF patients, AVP is thought to be an important neurohormonal compensation that becomes dysregulated. However, trials of AVP inhibitors have thus far been null. Increasing values of copeptin are prognostic both at baseline and during follow-up, especially in patients with hyponatremia.[269,270] This raises the possibility that the marker may allow for the identification of patients who are in need or AVP inhibition and allow for more focused use of this therapy.

Biomarkers No Longer of Clinical Use

Because of the lack of clinical utility the following biomarkers will not be discussed: CK isoenzymes, CK muscle type (CK-MM) (CK-1), and CK brain type (CK-BB) (CK-3); CK isoforms CK-MM and CK-MB; myoglobin; and LD isoenzymes LD1, LD2, LD3, LD4, and LD5.

CONGESTIVE HEART FAILURE

Natriuretic Peptides: Analytical Considerations

An endocrine phenotype of the heart muscle was suggested by anatomical findings half a century after the principal discovery of endocrine substances by Drs. Starling and Bayliss.[271] In the 1960s, electron microscopy revealed granules in the cytoplasm of atrial myocytes, which structurally resemble secretory granules in known peptide hormone–producing cells.[272,273] In 1981 the Canadian physiologist Adolfo de Bold and colleagues[274] reported that infusion of atrial tissue extracts elicits renal excretion of sodium and water. Moreover, a rapid decrease in blood pressure and increase in blood hematocrit was observed and the substance was named atrial natriuretic factor. This f-factor was then purified and identified as a

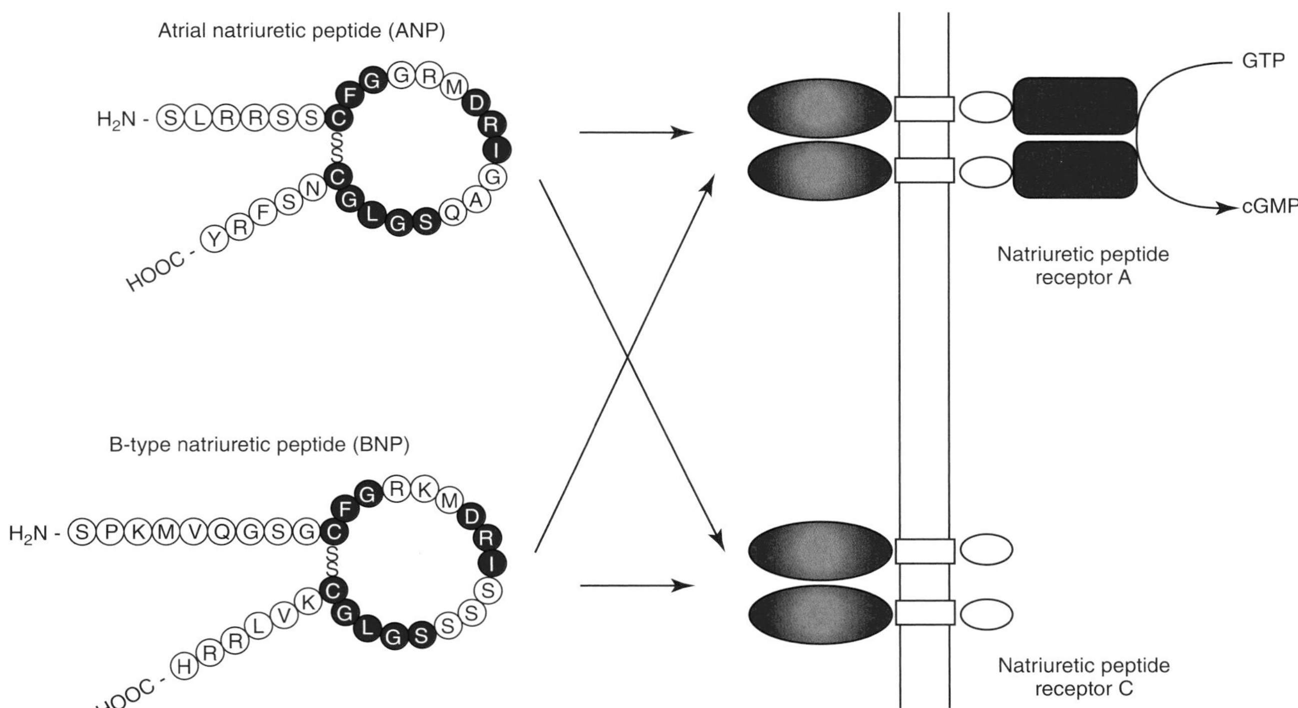

FIGURE 58.22 Schematic presentation of human atrial and B-type natriuretic peptides with their principal receptors. Homolog amino acid residues between the natriuretic peptides are marked in *bold circles*. The natriuretic peptide receptor *(NPR)*-A mediates atrial natriuretic peptide *(ANP)* and brain natriuretic peptide *(BNP)* signal transduction through induction of cyclic guanosine monophosphate *(cGMP)*. The NPR-C receptor lacks the intracellular domain and has been classed primarily as a clearance receptor. *GTP*, Guanosine triphosphate.

peptide comprising 28 amino acid residues and renamed atrial natriuretic peptide (ANP).[275,276] This discovery paved the way for identification of two structurally related peptides in the porcine brain: brain natriuretic peptide (BNP) and C-type natriuretic peptide (CNP).[277-280] However, BNP is mainly expressed in the heart and the name "brain" natriuretic peptide is now replaced with B-type natriuretic peptide (Fig. 58.22).[279,280] CNP is expressed in the invertebrate heart and can be considered the ancestor gene for the natriuretic peptide family.[281] Nevertheless, the CNP gene is not expressed to the same extent in mammalian hearts and should not be considered a cardiac-derived hormone in humans, in which the gene dominantly is expressed in other tissues, including the vasculature and the male reproductive glands.[282,283] Other members of the natriuretic peptide family include Dendroaspis natriuretic peptide (DNP) and urodilatin. In addition, attempts are now being made to develop designer therapeutic peptides that are chimeras between various natriuretic peptides. This chapter will focus on ANP and BNP predominantly because they are the only natriuretic peptides used diagnostically.

The endocrine heart gained clinical interest when it was reported that patients with cardiac disease display increased concentrations of ANP in plasma.[284,285] In parallel, BNP circulates in highly increased concentrations in patients with CHF.[286,287] The concept of a quantitative plasma marker in the HF syndrome was thereby introduced and has been intensely pursued with a dominant focus on clinical applications. In addition to the bioactive end products, N-terminal fragments from the precursor peptides (proANP and proBNP) were also shown to circulate in HF plasma and provided new molecular targets for biochemical detection.[281,284,288-290] As of today, proBNP-derived peptides have become the preferred routine markers in HF diagnostics and prognosis because of the available automated assays, and the clinical relevance of peptide measurement is still being extensively reviewed.[291-298] In contrast to the clinical focus on the diagnostic possibilities, less is known concerning the biosynthesis of proANP and proBNP-derived peptides.[298-300] The posttranslational phase of gene expression and the cellular secretion remain incompletely characterized. The first data on the molecular composition in tissue and plasma suggested a simple cellular maturation with only one endoproteolytic cleavage before secretion. However, cardiac myocytes possess a biosynthetic apparatus, including several enzymes for propeptide processing, and cardiac prohormone maturation has proved much more complex than initially assumed. Clinical studies have revealed that plasma concentrations of the different proBNP-derived peptides vary greatly, which suggests that cardiac myocytes may not always release biosynthetic products on a simple equimolar basis.[301,302]

Peptide Nomenclature and Biosynthesis

Some confusion has arisen because of the incoherent nomenclature of cardiac natriuretic peptides. In some ways, this confusion reflects the underlying lack of knowledge of the biosynthetic products, which has led researchers to apply nonspecific terms for the measured substances. A stringent nomenclature is, however, essential for a uniform understanding of peptide structure and function.[303] If the measured peptide is not readily distinguishable by its name, simple comparisons of reported concentrations may confuse and at worst lead to incorrect decisions. For instance, some of the abbreviations used do not identify the measured peptide(s), which should be the primary goal with the name. A common abbreviation—NT-proBNP—is used for one particular analytical method; it refers to the measurement of nonglycosylated proBNP 1-76, against which the immunoanalysis is calibrated. But the abbreviation does not provide specific information on the primary structure that is actually measured, which includes the intact precursor (proBNP 1-108) and with some cross-reactivity to the glycosylated forms (see later discussion). Other investigators have used broader terms for plasma measurement, such as N-BNP, which refers to measurement of intact proBNP 1-108 as well as its N-terminal fragment(s). However, this abbreviation leaves the less astute user with the impression that it is the N-terminus of BNP that is measured. The use of abbreviations such as BNP 77-108 is simply incorrect (BNP only includes 32 amino acid residues). Thus BNP-32 is synonymous with proBNP 77-108. A rational nomenclature needs to be structurally informative and should see the name in relation to its origin, that is, with insight in and reference to biosynthesis of the precursor. If this information is not available, then that should be stated. In the following section, a nomenclature based on these premises will be attempted.

The Pretranslational Phase of B-Type Natriuretic Peptide Gene Expression

Human atrial (ANP) and B-type (BNP) natriuretic peptide are encoded by genes located on chromosome 1.[304,305] In rodents, the genes are located on chromosome 4 (mouse) or chromosome 5 (rat). The overall gene structure is simple and resembles other peptide hormone genes in size and composition with three exons separated by two introns. For both ANP and BNP, the major part of the coding sequence resides in exon 2. Genetic polymorphisms and mutations have been reported in both genes as well as in the natriuretic peptide receptor genes.[306] Although the impact of genetic variation in the ANP and BNP systems remains to be fully established, it seems reasonable to suspect that it may affect the plasma concentrations in a heritable manner, which in fact has been reported in the general population.[307] However, associations between mutations and risk for disease are more interesting. Genetic variance in cardiac natriuretic peptides may thus be involved in the pathophysiology of a common metabolic disorder.[294] To complicate matters further, diabetes mellitus induces increased risk for development of cardiovascular disease with concomitant changes in cardiac natriuretic peptide expression.[308] In addition to the promoter polymorphism, a frame shift mutation in the ANP gene has been reported in heritable atrial fibrillation. The frame shift introduces a C-terminally extended ANP peptide.[309] Whether the "mutant" ANP exerts stimulatory or inhibitory effects (or no changes) on the natriuretic peptide receptors is still a fascinating question for future experimental studies.

The mature ANP and BNP transcripts consist of approximately 500 to 700 base pairs. Although a review of intracellular regulation of natriuretic gene transcription is extensive and has been reviewed elsewhere,[310-313] both genes seem regulated by the same transcriptional factors including p38 mitogen-activated protein kinase (MAPK). p38 MAPK activates the transcription factor nucleic factor-κB (NF-κB) and subsequently ANP and BNP gene transcription.[314] Vasoactive substances such as catecholamines and angiotensin II increase natriuretic gene transcription in a p38 MAPK–dependent manner. Myocyte stretching increases the intracellular calcium concentration and modulates calcium-binding proteins that regulate downstream modulators, including calcineurin, which stimulates myocyte natriuretic gene expression.[315] Thus cardiac natriuretic gene expression can be modulated by blocking the p38 MAPK and the calcineurin pathways. Finally, the hypoxia inducible transcription factor (HIF) 1-α activates both ANP and BNP transcription, which is of importance in ischemic heart disease.[316,317] One scenario in which the ANP and BNP genes seem not to be coregulated is in inflammation driven by specific cytokines, in which BNP gene expression increases and ANP gene expression is unaffected.[318] This differential gene expression has led to the suggestion that ANP and BNP gene products might be clinically useful when measured in concert during conditions with both hemodynamic changes and a proinflammatory drive on the cardiac myocytes, as seen after cardiac transplantation.[319]

One feature of ANP and BNP mRNA regulation should be recapitulated. Although gene expression is regulated at the transcriptional level, another relevant mechanism is changes in mRNA stability and the half-life of the transcripts. This RNA regulatory mechanism has been demonstrated for BNP mRNA through stimulation of α-adrenergic receptors.[320,321] The BNP mRNA stabilization is thought to be mediated though the elements in the 3′ untranslated region, which is not present in the ANP gene. Consequently, mRNA stabilization seems only to involve BNP and not ANP mRNA.

The Primary Structure of ProBrain Natriuretic Peptide

Human proBNP comprises 108 amino acid residues (Fig. 58.22). The primary structure is slightly shorter in the mouse but with a similar C-terminal region, including the receptor binding motif. Mammalian precursor sequences have been deduced from complementary DNA (cDNA) sequences that encode the entire preprostructure.[322-325] Amino acid homology among species is largely confined to the amino- and carboxy-terminal regions, whereas the remaining prostructure varies considerably among animals. Moreover, the principal motifs for amino acid modifications and enzymatic prohormone processing are not well conserved across species.

In addition to proBNP, human preproBNP contains an N-terminal hydrophobic signal peptide of 26 amino acid residues (Fig. 58.23). As with most regulatory peptides, this sequence is removed during translation before synthesis of the C-terminal part of the precursor is completed. Interestingly, a fragment stemming from the signal peptide has been identified in cardiac tissue and in plasma from patients with cardiac disease.[326] However, preproBNP does not exist as a separate entity but is only a theoretical structure. On the other hand, proBNP is an existing polypeptide, which has been shown by chromatographic profiling and sequence-specific immunoassays.[281,289,290,327,328] The precursor molecule remains to be purified, together with the processing intermediates

cDNA-Deduced proBNP Sequences in Four Mammals

Cat	HPLGGPGPAS--EASAIQELLDGLRDTVSELQEAQMALGPLQQGHSPAESWEAQEEPPAR 58
Dog	HPLGGPGPAS--EASAIQELLDGLRDTVSELQEAQMALGPLQQGHSPAESWEAQEEPPAR 58
Man	HPLGSPGSASDLETSGLQEQRNHLQGKLSELQVEQTSLEPLQESPRPTGVWKSREVATEG 60
Mouse	YPLGSPSQSP--EQFKMQKLLELIREKSEEMAQRQLLKD---QG--------LTKEHPKR 47
Cat	VLAPHDNVLRALRRLGSSKMMRDSRCFGRRLDRIGSLSGLGCNVLRRH 106
Dog	VLAPHDNVLRALRRLGSSKMMRDSRCFGRRLDRIGSLSGLGCNVLRRH 106
Man	IRGHRKMVLYTLRAPRSPKMVQGSGCFGRKMDRISSSSGLGCKVLRRH 108
Mouse	VLRSQGSTLRVQQRPQNSKVTHISSCFGHKIDRIGSVSRLGCNALKLL 95

FIGURE 58.23 The primary structure of proBNP (pro-brain natriuretic peptide) in four mammals. The human proBNP sequence comprises 108 amino acid residues. The precursor sequence is evolutionary and is conserved in the C-terminal region that makes up the bioactive natriuretic peptide. In contrast, the cleavage site corresponding to position 73-76 in the human sequence is not well conserved. Amino acids are indicated by their single-letter codes.

thereof, apart from the C-terminal 32 amino acid cleavage product, that is, BNP-32, and the N-terminal region of the precursor.[329-333] Thus, whenever the primary proBNP structure is mentioned, it should be remembered that it refers to the cDNA-deduced preprosequence combined with antibody-based data from chromatographic elution, Western blotting, or immunoassays.

The Posttranslational Phase of B-Type Natriuretic Peptide Gene Expression

Posttranslational BNP processing has become a subject of increasing interest. One factor contributing to this may relate to the troublesome lack of useful in vitro cellular models. Although neonatal atrial myocytes can be cultured for short periods, they do not anatomically or functionally resemble differentiated atrial, or for that matter ventricular, myocytes. Moreover, only a few immunoassays have been available for characterizing the molecular heterogeneity of the processing intermediates. Recent advances through mass spectrometry combined with the development of sequence-specific antibodies have nevertheless revealed a complex cardiac biosynthesis of cardiac natriuretic peptides.

Disulfide Bond Formation

The proBNP structure appears simple (see Figs. 58.22 and 58.23). In humans, it is divided into two principal regions by a cleavage site in position 73-76 (Arg-Ala-Pro-Arg). The first region is the N-terminal fragment proBNP 1-76, and the second region is the C-terminal BNP-32 (proBNP 77-108). In contrast to other prohormones, proBNP does not contain a C-terminal flanking region. The C-terminal region contains a ring structure formed by a disulfide bond between the cystyl residues in position 86 and 102, respectively (see Fig. 58.22). The ring formation is essential for receptor binding and biological activity.[334] This crucial modification in ANP and BNP synthesis takes place in the endoplasmic reticulum and may be considered the first step in posttranslational processing. The protein disulfide isomerase family and thioldisulfide oxidoreductases are likely candidate enzymes involved in cardiac myocyte disulfide bond formation. Interestingly, cardiac expression of the protein disulfide isomerase transcript was recently reported to be upregulated in cardiac disease.[335] Cellular experiments in vitro further suggest a direct cardioprotective effect of this regulation. It may be that not all cardiac natriuretic peptides are activated through this enzymatic process, which introduces the earliest possible regulatory step in natriuretic peptide biosynthesis and hormone activation. Regulation of protein disulfide isomerase has been classified as endoplasmic reticulum stress, which is a hallmark of several pathologic disorders, including diabetes mellitus, neurodegenerative disorders, and ischemic heart disease.[336]

Glycosylation

Larger forms of BNP than the purified BNP-32 were first suspected from gel filtration studies of cardiac tissue extracts and plasma from patients with severe cardiac disease.[289,290,337,338] Some data even suggested molecular forms larger than the predicted precursor. Independently, several groups observed immunoreactive forms with molecular masses of 25 to 45 kDa in cardiac tissue and plasma (Fig. 58.24). Intact proBNP, however, has an expected mass of approximately 11 kDa based on the primary structure. Whether the peculiar elution patterns were in vitro artifacts or represented peptide binding to other molecules was put aside when it was shown that human proBNP exists as an O-linked glycoprotein.[339] In the precursor structure, the midregion (proBNP 36-71) contains seven seryl and threonyl residues, where O-linked glycosylation occurs either fully or partially (Fig. 58.25). This major modification of a polypeptide apparently does not affect the overall structure of the precursor.[298] On the other hand, the presence of carbohydrate groups clearly affects immunodetection if the epitope recognition resides within this region.[340] No specific immunoassay has yet been developed against the glycosylated forms, and the ratio between glycosylated and nonglycosylated proBNP products can be deduced only from assays that measure the nonglycosylated forms or cross-react with both forms. Whether O-linked glycosylation is an "unlimited" posttranslational modification or is affected by increased BNP gene expression, as in heart disease, will be an important question for future studies. It should also be noted that the ANP precursor also may be subject to glycosylation.[341] In addition, the proBNP sequence varies considerably across species in the midregion (see Fig. 58.23), which probably makes glycosylation a species-specific modification. Finally, it is not known whether atrial and ventricular myocytes possess the same capacity to glycosylate natriuretic precursor peptides.

Glycosylation could perhaps be a biochemical target for diagnostic applications, if the modification is affected by cardiac disease and/or reflects changes in BNP gene

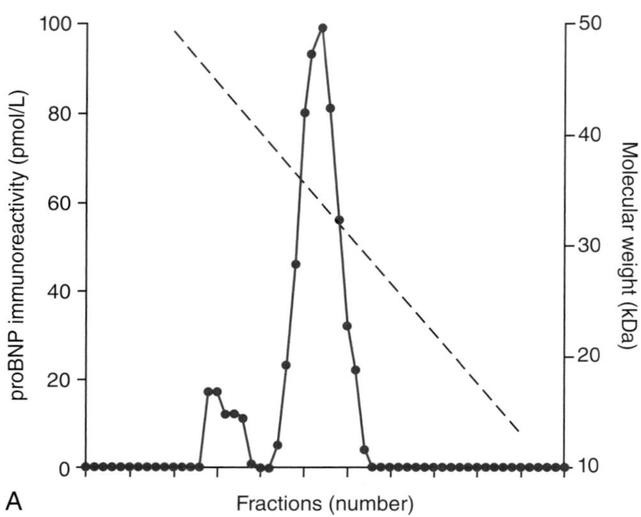

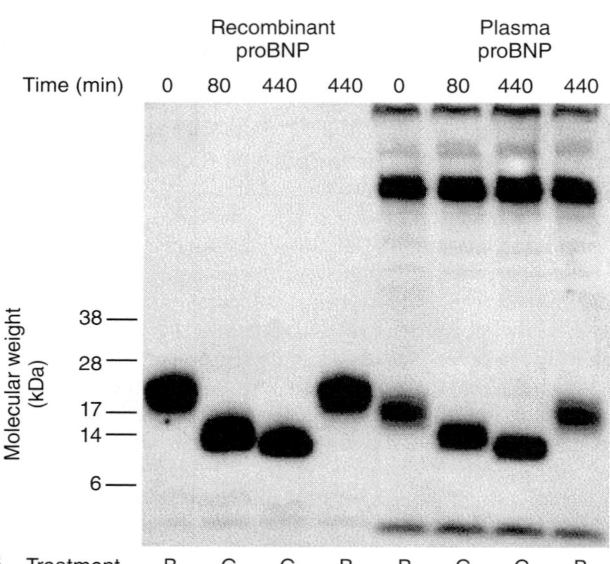

FIGURE 58.24 A, Chromatographic profile of pro-brain natriuretic peptide (proBNP) immunoreactivity in human atrial tissue. Cardiac tissue extract was subjected to size exclusion high-performance liquid chromatography (HPLC). Molecular size calibrators, eluted in a separate run, were used in determining molecular sizes *(dashed line).* The proBNP immunoreactivity eluted in positions approximately three times higher than the theoretical molecular weight of intact proBNP. **B,** Western blotting of recombinant *(left)* and patient *(right)* proBNP in buffer *(B)* or after deglycosylation *(G).* The incubation time is also listed. (Modified from Schellenberger U, O'Rear J, Guzzetta A, Jue RA, Protter AA, Pollitt NS. The precursor to B-type natriuretic peptide is an O-linked glycoprotein. *Arch Biochem Biophys* 2006;451:160–166, with permission.)

expression. Most captivating, however, is the potential impact of early biosynthetic glycosylation on cellular sorting and the subsequent precursor processing. Because O-linked glycosylation can occur close to the principal maturation site in position 74-76 (on the threonyl residue in position 71), the presence of carbohydrate groups can affect processing and

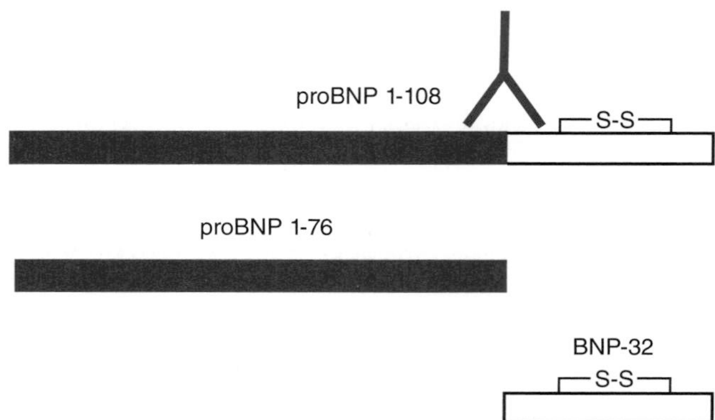

FIGURE 58.25 Immunoassay for detection of unprocessed human pro-brain natriuretic peptide *(proBNP).* The assay uses antibody recognition of an epitope spanning the Arg-Ala-Pro-Arg site (proBNP74-76) thought to be cleaved by corin. *S-S,* Disulfide bond.

hormonal maturation.[342] In turn, this modification could regulate prohormone cleavage by either blocking or guiding endoproteolytic enzymes, which may leave the propeptide with reduced or no biological activity. Such posttranslational regulation has been shown for other regulatory peptides, for example, insulin-like growth factor II.[343] Conceptually, immunoreactive BNP with little or no biological activity has been nicknamed "junk-BNP." This "junk" may nevertheless prove to be the most useful peptide forms for diagnostic measurement.

Endoproteolysis

Human proBNP was first suggested to be cleaved by the ubiquitous endoprotease furin; furin and the BNP gene are coexpressed in cardiac myocytes.[344,345] The Arg-Ala-Pro-Arg motif in position 73-76 in human proBNP has been shown to be a target for furin-mediated cleavage. In fact, endoproteolytic processing can be blocked in vitro by inhibition of furin, and furin has been shown to be essential for maturation of the structurally related CNP. A novel protease named corin has been identified from human heart cDNA.[346,347] Corin is a serine protease that can cleave both proANP and proBNP in vitro, presumably at a similar cleavage site.[348-351] Corin contains a transmembrane domain anchored in the cell membrane and is thought to cleave the precursors on secretion. The enzymatic activity, however, does not require the transmembrane domain because a mutant soluble form also is capable of processing proANP.[352] A role of corin in the processing of cardiac natriuretic peptides in vivo has been further substantiated by genetic coupling of corin mutations to clinical phenotypes that can be explained by reduced ANP and BNP bioactivity in circulation such as hypertension.[353,354] Corin thus seems to be a relevant candidate for cardiac processing of natriuretic peptides generating the N-terminal processing fragments and C-terminal bioactive peptides.[351] Of note, no study has yet demonstrated exactly where corin cleaves the proBNP structure. Moreover, atrial posttranslational processing of proANP and proBNP is likely to differ from ventricular processing because isolated atrial granules have been reported to contain both unprocessed proANP and mature BNP-32.[355] Corin activity alone can therefore not fully explain the endoproteolytic maturation of cardiac natriuretic propeptides. It should be mentioned that the putative corin site in the BNP precursor is not conserved between mammals, and it would accordingly be interesting to examine whether human corin can cleave precursor peptides from other mammalian species.

A well-established family of intracellular processing enzymes deeply involved in prohormone maturation is the proprotein/prohormone convertases (PCs). In addition to the already mentioned furin, the subtilisin-like endoproteases PC1/3 and PC2 are also expressed in the mammalian heart,[356,357] and PC1/3 expression has been demonstrated in both normal and pathologic human cardiac tissue.[358] Atrial myocytes transfected with an adenoviral vector expressing PC1/3 processes proANP to both mature ANP and to a truncated form.[359] Although the precise cleavage site was not established and the processing capacity was somewhat inefficient, this singular report does underscore the possibility that proteases other than furin and corin may be involved in the posttranslational endoproteolysis of proANP and proBNP. PC1/3 is active in secretory granules and could therefore be an important regulator of atrial proBNP processing. Cardiac PC1/3 expression has been reported to be upregulated at the transcriptional level in heart disease.[360] Unfortunately, there are no data on other proBNP-derived fragments stemming from endoproteolytic processing. This may reflect the lack of specific tools for identifying such peptide fragments, which requires antibodies directed at epitopes other than the ones used so far for biochemical identification. Sandwich-based immunoassays are usually not ideal for this type of experiment. The precursor sequence contains several basic amino acid residues that potentially could represent cleavage sites for the PCs, and the molecular characterization may not be complete when it comes to identifying processing intermediates from the natriuretic peptide precursors.

Exoproteolysis

N-terminal trimming of proBNP-derived peptides seems to be a biological feature because both the N-terminus of the biosynthetic precursor and the C-terminal bioactive BNP product contain an amino acid motif for aminopeptidase recognition and cleavage. Both the N-terminus of proBNP and BNP-32 (proBNP 77-108) contain a prolyl residue in position 2 (His-Pro and Ser-Pro, respectively). Although prolyl residues are important for peptide structure and folding, they also can be involved in exoproteolytic trimming when located near the N-terminus.[361] N-terminal trimming has in fact recently been demonstrated for BNP in vitro.[288] Synthetic BNP-32 (proBNP 77-108) incubated in the presence of the dipeptidyl peptidase (DPP) IV removes the N-terminal Ser-Pro residues. DPP-IV is an enzyme located mainly on endothelial cells and in the circulation with a preference for cleaving N-termini with either prolyl or alanyl residues in the second position.[362] Thus this DPP-IV cleavage in BNP-32 cannot per se be considered as a part of the biosynthetic maturation but is rather related to the elimination phase. An N-terminally trimmed form of proBNP lacking the His-Pro residues in position 1-2 also has been reported in HF patients.[363] This report disclosed that a truncated proBNP 3-108 form circulates in increased concentrations in HF patients. In this context, it is noteworthy that the initial report on glycosylated proBNP in a recombinant expression system (CHO cells) also identified a truncated proBNP 3-108 form in cell extracts.[339] Although this finding may be explained by experimental handling of extracts and medium, it could also imply that N-terminal exoproteolysis is a biosynthetic event. N-terminal trimming as part of peptide biosynthesis has been demonstrated, for instance, for melitin, which is a secretory peptide produced in honey bee venom glands.[364,365] In mammalian cells, intracellular aminopeptidase has been reported in compartments different from the lysosomes, suggesting N-terminal trimming as a possible part of the biosynthetic peptide maturation.[366,367] Whether the trimming of BNP and its molecular precursor serves an actual regulatory function in cardiac natriuretic peptide physiology remains an open question for future experimental research. It could be speculated that aminoterminal trimming affects the metabolic fate of the peptides and thus their turnover in circulation. There are, however, no data available on an actual biological relevance of these trimmings.

Cellular Storage and Secretion

BNP gene expression is a feature of both atrial and ventricular myocytes. In the normal heart, the main site of BNP expression is in the atrial regions.[368,369] Ventricular BNP gene expression increases drastically in cardiac disease that affects the ventricles, that is, CHF.[370] The observation of ventricular BNP gene expression in ventricular disease may have given rise to the common statement that BNP is predominantly a ventricular hormone. Atrial and ventricular myocytes, however, differ considerably with respect to their endocrine phenotypes, and it is reasonable to expect major differences in peptide storage and secretion patterns.[371,372] For instance, it is well established that atrial myocytes contain intracellular granules for peptide storage and maturation, which actually contributed to the primary hypothesis of the endocrine heart.[272,273] Atrial granules contain both intact precursors and biosynthetic end products, that is, bioactive ANP-28 and BNP-32. In contrast, normal ventricular myocytes do not seem to express such granules and normal ventricular myocytes do not contain proBNP-derived peptides.[368] A few reports have observed granules and proBNP-derived peptides in ventricular myocytes sampled from pathologic hearts.[373-375] Thus ventricular myocytes not only regulate the BNP gene at the transcriptional and posttranslational level but also seem to be able to differentiate with respect to the biosynthetic apparatus per se. An acidic protein class involved in granule formation is the chromogranins.[376] Chromogranins, or just granins, comprise at least three proteins (A, B, and C) that possess aggregation characteristics suggesting a function in the formation of secretory granules. Cardiac expression of chromogranin A and B has been established.[377-379] The focus on cardiac chromogranins, however, has mainly been on the potential biological activity of chromogranin-derived fragments (the vasostatins) or on plasma measurement for diagnostic purposes.[380] Whether cardiac chromogranins are involved in the biosynthesis of ANP and BNP through formation of granules remains an area for future studies. It should be recapitulated that chromogranin A–deficient mice do not reveal obvious changes in granule formation in, for instance, adrenal chromaffin cells.[381] Cardiac chromogranin B also has been suggested to be directly involved in BNP gene expression through a Ca^{2+}-dependent induction of the BNP promoter.[377] Further in vitro experiments targeted at proANP and proBNP maturation in cardiac cell systems devoid of chromogranin A and B may thus reveal a specific role for the granins in storage and secretion of natriuretic peptides.

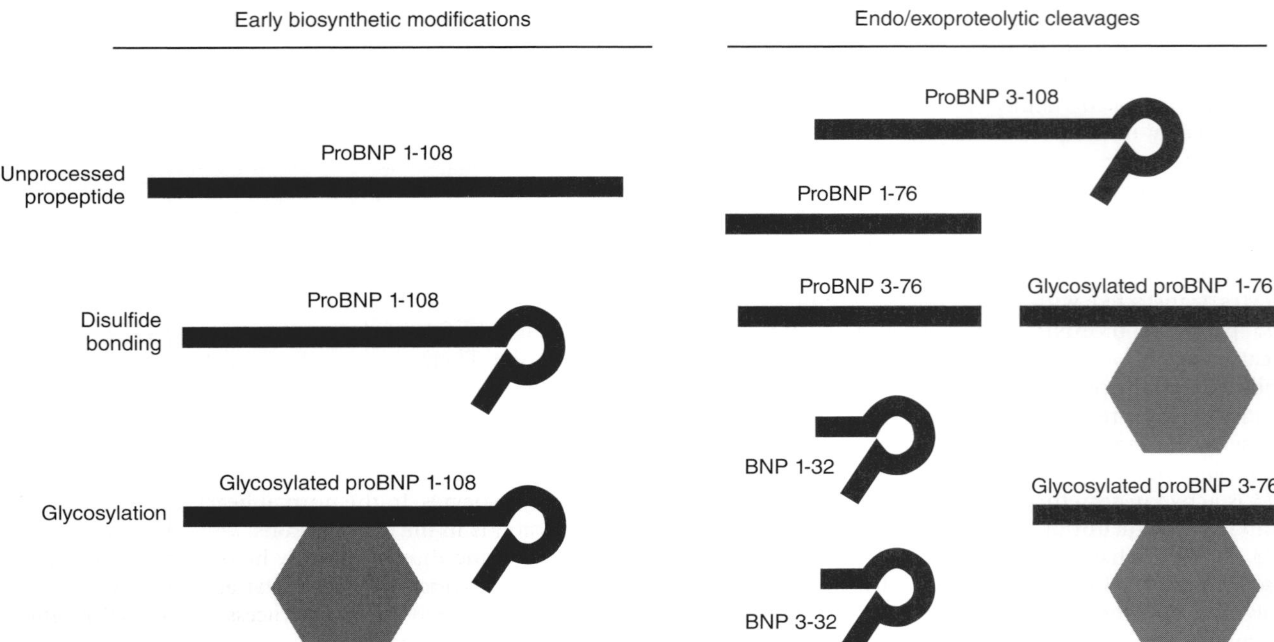

FIGURE 58.26 Schematic presentation of possible pro-brain natriuretic peptide *(proBNP)*-derived peptide products. Note that most peptides are not chemically identified but rather are suggested by biochemical methods that rely on antibody recognition. Carbohydrate is indicated by the *hexagons.*

ProBNP-Derived Peptides in Plasma

ProBNP-derived peptides are secreted by cardiac myocytes and circulate in plasma. Their molecular heterogeneity has primarily been characterized by chromatography in combination with sequence-specific immunoassays. Much of our present conception of the cellular synthesis is in fact derived from the plasma phase, which represents the sum of secretion and metabolism. The picomolar concentrations in plasma limit the possibilities for full biochemical identification and underscore a careful understanding of epitope recognition by the immunoassays. With this in mind, it is established that bioactive BNP is secreted from the heart and circulates without binding to plasma proteins.[382] Synthetic BNP-32 (proBNP 77-108) is trimmed when incubated in whole blood, generating a BNP form lacking the two N-terminal amino acid residues.[338,383] As mentioned earlier, this molecular form can be generated in vitro by enzymatic trimming by DPP-IV and possibly other aminopeptidases.[288] Further processing of plasma BNP seems to involve degradation with a loss of bioactivity though disruption of the ring structure mediated by neutral endopeptidase (NEP 24.11) or by receptor-mediated cellular uptake. Although this has been known for some time, the therapeutic potential of inhibiting neutral endopeptidase with increased plasma concentrations of "beneficial "natriuretic peptides is an appealing strategy.[384] The metabolic fate of BNP-32 has been reported to be 13 to 20 minutes.[385,386] Immunoreactive BNP is also excreted in urine, but the precise contribution of renal excretion to renal metabolism is not yet clarified. A minor degree of hepatic clearance also has been shown, which is not significantly altered in patients with liver failure.[387]

In addition to bioactive BNP, other proBNP-derived fragments circulate in plasma.[388,389] These fragments are commonly referred to as N-terminal proBNP, but the molecular heterogeneity also includes the intact precursor, in particular in HF patients.[290,302,390] Cardiac secretion of proBNP and its N-terminal fragments has been demonstrated by blood sampling from the coronary sinus. The molar ratio of secreted proBNP 1-76 to intact proBNP is not yet fully clarified but is likely to depend on cardiac status, that is, more unprocessed precursor compared to biosynthetic cleavage products in severe HF (Fig. 58.26). In the metabolic phase, there are still major discrepancies in the suggested half-life of N-terminal precursor fragments, which at least partially reflect the epitope recognition in the assays. Theoretically, the half-life of proBNP 1-76 in circulation should be approximately 25 minutes[391] and thus not differ greatly from the established metabolism of BNP-32 (proBNP 77-108). One report, however, suggested a considerably longer half-life (~90 minutes after cardiac pacing), which would fit well with the higher plasma concentrations of N-terminal proBNP fragments compared to bioactive BNP in healthy individuals and in cardiac patients. As our perception of the molecular heterogeneity in plasma has changed radically over the last several years, there is an urgent need for new pharmacokinetic experiments to separate the biosynthetic phase from the peripheral elimination. Ideally, experiments should be performed by classic peptide infusion strategies with measurement across organ beds.

Biosynthesis and Assay Calibration

Elucidation of cardiac natriuretic peptide biosynthesis has disclosed a complex posttranslational maturation that produces a variety of peptides targeted for cellular secretion (Fig. 58.26). The different phases of gene expression are not only region-specific but also depend on changes within the secretory apparatus in cardiac myocytes. The main clinical applications of the peptides today strongly relates to plasma measurement in cardiovascular diagnostics and prognosis. The immunoassays thus need to be designed with insight into the biosynthesis of the peptides. Another defining aspect of immunoassay measurement is the choice of calibrator. This aspect has so far not been scrutinized by researchers apart from the observation of disturbingly large discrepancies across the different assays.[392] On the other hand, it has not been possible to raise meaningful assay calibration issues before now, until the existence of a complex molecular heterogeneity has been established. One way of bypassing this lack of information has been introduced as a "processing-independent assay," which in principle quantifies one in vitro cleavage product that represents all the secreted precursor molecules. This assay then can be calibrated with the specific cleavage product and assay measurement performed on a stoichiometrically correct basis. If one is to choose a proBNP-derived calibrator peptide for plasma measurement, it becomes more blurry. As the ratio of bioactive BNP to intact precursor shifts toward less processed biosynthetic products, the dominant "disease" form might be chosen over the more prevalent forms in healthy individuals. However, large comparative studies still have not revealed major differences between BNP or proBNP measurements in terms of overall clinical performance. One report on assay calibration has shown that assays directed at the C-terminal BNP region do not really cross-react with the larger biosynthetic products.[392] Plasma measurement based on assays directed against the N-terminal proBNP fragment is, however, greatly influenced by the degree of O-linked glycosylation. Clearly, this issue is far from settled and our present perception of "normal" concentrations of the different biosynthetic products may still have to be redefined.

Inefficient Prohormone Maturation in Heart Failure

HF patients display highly increased plasma concentrations of bioactive ANP and BNP. With a dramatic upregulation of the gene expression and concomitant high concentrations of immunoreactive ANP and BNP in plasma, it seems reasonable to expect increased natriuresis. The common presentation of HF, however, is congestion, sodium retention, and edema. Although HF is a complex syndrome with both activation and inhibition of multiple neurohumoral systems, the paradoxical lack of ANP and BNP bioactivity is still compelling. HF patients respond to intravenous administration of chemically synthesized ANP and BNP, which has led to the introduction of a BNP-32 analog, nesiritide.[393] This peptide is a potent drug in HF, which raised serious concerns regarding patient safety by causing unwanted hypotension.[394] Experts have further explored the possibilities of natriuretic peptide drugs by constructing structurally related peptides that possess natriuretic effects but without the undesirable hypotension.[395] Obviously, this research area could prove of major relevance to medical therapy because all the different physiologic effects of natriuretic peptides could have specific roles in modern treatment of HF and other cardiovascular pathologic processes.

The endocrine paradox of sodium and water retention in HF, in which the gold standard biomarkers are the cardiac natriuretic peptides, relates to insufficient post-translational maturation of the biosynthetic precursors.[396] A well-established analogy to this phenomenon is enhanced secretion of proinsulin over mature insulin in patients with type 2 diabetes. In the early stages of the disease, selective proinsulin measurement is therefore a valuable tool in evaluating pancreatic β-cell dysfunction. A shift toward secretion of unprocessed precursors in cardiac disease also may represent early involvement of ventricular expression and secretion because efficient precursor maturation seems to dominantly be an endocrine feature of atrial biosynthesis. In support of this explanation, the intracellular processing enzymes involved in ANP and BNP maturation are dominantly expressed in atrial myocytes. Moreover, the ventricular myocytes do not, at least in the early stages of disease, contain secretory granules for peptide storage and maturation. The posttranslational processing of ventricular precursors may not be efficient in the production of needed natriuretic potency, although immunoassays cross-react to various degrees with the unprocessed biosynthetic products. Though speculative, there may be large individual differences in the heart's ability to process the precursor peptides, which could help explain the highly variable HF phenotypes. The ratio of mature BNP to unprocessed proBNP might be of diagnostic relevance in parallel with the present application of proinsulin to insulin measurement. These considerations are consistent with recent data that suggest that with acute HF, there is less perturbation of the natriuretic peptide system and specifically less glycosylation at theorine 71, which allows for more efficient conversion of proBNP to NTproBNP and bioactive BNP.[13] This might explain why some studies have shown a rapid change in BNP values with diuresis in patients who present acutely.[14] With more chronic HF, glycosylation is more prominent, and thus there is less active BNP and the system likely requires more time and a greater degree of change to manifest clinical significance.

If specific assays for the various forms are applied together, it may be possible to define an early endocrine hallmark of the HF syndrome that could aid clinicians in tailoring diuretic therapy according to the patient-specific ability to ameliorate congestion through secretion of bioactive natriuretic hormones.

ANALYTICAL CONSIDERATIONS OF BIOMARKERS ASSAYS IN HEART FAILURE

In 2005 the IFCC Committee on Standardization of Markers of Cardiac Damage established the first recommended analytical and preanalytical quality specifications for natriuretic peptide (NP) assays.[397] The objectives were intended for use by the manufacturers of commercial assays and by clinical laboratories using NP assays. The overall goal was to attempt to establish uniform criteria so all NP assays could objectively be evaluated for their analytical qualities and clinical performance. As BNP and NT-proBNP become more integrated into clinical practice as diagnostic and prognostic biomarkers, understanding differences among individual assay characteristics is extremely important. The influence of clinical, analytical, and preanalytical factors on the increasing number of BNP and NT-proBNP assays available (as shown in Table 58.4), shows the need for a better understanding by clinicians on how to interpret findings of different studies predicated on BNP or NT-proBNP concentrations monitored by different assays.[398-400] The laboratory community must also

TABLE 58.4 Analytical Characteristics of Commercial Brain Natriuretic Peptide and N-Terminal ProBNP Assays per Manufacturer

Assay	Capture Antibody	Detection Antibody	Standard Material	FDA Claim
BNP				
Inverness (Biosite) Triage	NH_2 terminus and part of the ring structure (Scios), murine monoclonal AB, aa 5-13	BNP (Biosite), murine Omniclonal AB, epitope not characterized	Recombinant BNP	Diagnosis of HF Assess severity of HF Risk for ACS Risk for HF
Beckman Coulter Access, Access 2, DxI	NH_2 terminus and part of the ring structure (Scios), murine monoclonal AB, aa 5-13	BNP (Biosite), murine Omniclonal AB, epitope not characterized	Recombinant BNP	Diagnosis of HF Assess severity of HF Risk for ACS Risk for HF
Abbott Architect, AxSYM, iSTAT	NH_2 terminus and part of the ring structure (Scios), murine monoclonal AB, aa 5-13	COOH terminus, murine monoclonal AB, aa 26-32	Synthetic BNP 32	Assist in diagnosis of HF Assess severity of disease
Siemens (Bayer) ACS 180, Advia Centaur, Advia Centaur CP	COOH terminus (BC-203), murine monoclonal AB, aa 27-32	Ring structure (KY-hBNP-II), murine monoclonal AB, aa 14-21	Synthetic BNP	Aid in diagnosis and assessment of severity of HF Predict survival and likelihood of future HF in ACS patients
Shionogi	Ring structure (KY-hBNP-II), murine monoclonal AB, aa 14-21	COOH terminus (BC-203), murine monoclonal AB, aa 27-32	Synthetic BNP	Not FDA cleared
NT-proBNP				
Roche proBNP I Elecsys, E170	NH_2 terminus polyclonal sheep AB, aa 1-21	Central molecule, polyclonal sheep AB, aa 39-50	Synthetic NT-proBNP 1-76	Diagnosis of HF Assess severity of HF Risk for ACS Risk for HF
Roche proBNP II Elecsys, E170	Murine monoclonal AB, aa 27-31	Sheep monoclonal AB, aa 42-46	Synthetic NT-proBNP 1-76	Treatment monitoring in LVD
Siemens (Dade Behring) Dimension RxL, Stratus CS, Dimension VISTA	NH_2 terminus monoclonal sheep AB, aa 22-28	Central molecule, sheep monoclonal AB, aa 42-46	Synthetic NT-proBNP 1-76	Aid in the diagnosis of CHF and assessment of severity Risk stratification of patients with ACS and HF
Radiometer AQT90	NH_2 terminus polyclonal sheep AB, aa 1-21	Central molecule, polyclonal sheep AB, aa 39-50	Synthetic NT-proBNP 1-76	Aid in the diagnosis of CHF and assessment of severity
Ortho-Clinical Diagnostics Vitros ECi	NH_2 terminus polyclonal sheep AB, aa 1-21	Central molecule, polyclonal sheep AB, aa 39-50	Synthetic NT-proBNP 1-76	Aid diagnosis of CHF Risk stratification of ACS and CHF Risk assessment of CV events and mortality in patients at risk for HF with stable CAD Assess severity of HF
Response Biomedical RAMP	Murine monoclonal AB, aa 27-31	Central molecule, polyclonal sheep AB, aa 39-50	Synthetic NT-proBNP 1-76	Diagnosis of HF Assess severity of HF
bioMérieux VIDAS	NH_2 terminus polyclonal sheep AB, aa 1-21	Central molecule, polyclonal sheep AB, aa 39-50	Synthetic NT-proBNP 1-76	Diagnosis of HF
LSI Medience PATHFAST	NH_2 terminus polyclonal sheep AB, aa 1-21	Central molecule, polyclonal sheep AB, aa 39-50	Synthetic NT-proBNP 1-76	Aid diagnosis of CHF Assess severity of CHF Risk stratification in ACS and stable CAD
Nanogen LifeSign DXpress Reader	Monoclonal (mouse) and polyclonal (goat) ABs	Polyclonal sheep AB	Synthetic NT-proBNP 1-76	Diagnosis of HF

aa, Amino acids; *AB,* antibody; *ACS,* acute coronary syndrome; *BNP,* brain natriuretic peptide; *CAD,* coronary artery disease; *CHF,* congestive heart failure; *CV,* cardiovascular; *FDA,* US Food and Drug Administration; *HF,* heart failure; *LVD,* left ventricular dysfunction; *NA,* not available; *NT-pro BNP,* N-terminal pro-BNP.

work closely with the in vitro diagnostics companies, to assist in defining the numerous assay characteristics.[401] When BNP or NT-proBNP assays are used as biomarkers for diagnosis, therapy decisions, and prognosis, or used in clinical trials or studies, they should be well characterized, as suggested in the list of recommendations that follows. It is further recommended that when designing studies using BNP or NT-proBNP, investigators should review the Standards for Reporting Diagnostic Accuracy[402] initiative for both assay characterization issues as well as for clinical and patient enrollment issues when monitoring BNP or NT-proBNP levels.

A growing diversity of BNP and NT-proBNP assays are used worldwide, emphasizing the need for both analytical and clinical validation of all commercial assays to support definite clinical acceptance of these new biomarkers. At present, four companies have FDA-cleared BNP assays (Alere, Siemens, Abbott including POC, Beckman Coulter using Alere reagents) and several companies have FDA-cleared NT-proBNP assays (Roche, and others that use Roche antibodies and calibrators: Siemens, bioMerieux, Response Biomedical, LSI Medience, Ortho-Clinical Diagnostics, Radiometer, and Nanogen). POC platforms (Response Biomedical, LSI Medience, Radiometer, Alere) are suitable for whole blood use. Preliminary data from research assays for proBNP have been described by BioRad, HyTest, and Alere.[392] Further, Thermo-Fischer-BRAHMS has received FDA clearance for MR-proANP as being substantially equivalent to BNP as a biomarker to rule out and confirm HF. As the number of assays for all four NP biomarkers grows, it is even more essential that appropriate clinical and analytical assay criteria are uniformly adapted. The accurate clinical performance of each BNP or NT-proBNP assay, and likely proBNP in the future, which may serve as the basis for life-and-death medical decisions, sets the stage to establish assay criteria as indispensable. Limited clinical data is available for MR-proANP.[403,404]

BNP and NT-proBNP are determined by a number of different immunoassays using antibodies directed to different epitopes located on the antigen molecules (see Table 58.4). For BNP one antibody binds to the ring structure and the other antibody to either the carboxy- or amino-terminal end. Degradation of BNP (amino acids [a.a.] 77 to 108) is known to occur by proteolytic cleavage of serine and proline residues in vivo and in vitro (see Fig. 58.26).[337,397,405] This degradation may affect antibody affinities and thus be responsible for differences in stabilities of BNP-32 monitored by different commercial BNP assays, as discussed earlier. For NT-proBNP (a.a. 1-76) monitoring, an improved understanding of potential cross-reactivity with split products of the N-terminal portion of NT-proBNP and proBNP itself are needed. For both assays, BNP and NT-proBNP, minimizing interferents from heterophilic antibodies and rheumatoid factor, for example, need to be optimized. The influence, stabilizing or destabilizing, of anticoagulant additives, as well as the type of collection tube, have been well described.[337,406] For BNP, EDTA-anticoagulated whole blood or plasma appears to be the only acceptable specimen choice. For NT-proBNP, serum, heparin plasma, and EDTA plasma (reads 10% lower) appear acceptable. Plastic blood collection tubes are necessary for BNP, while for NT-proBNP, either glass or plastic is acceptable. There also is an assay that is more specific for proBNP using antibodies to amino acids 76-78.

In the clinical setting,[348,407-410] BNP and NT-proBNP assay characteristics need to be better understood or better established for optimal consideration as diagnostic and prognostic biomarkers, as discussed later. Further, recent observations that proBNP, the precursor peptide that splits into BNP and NT-proBNP, appears to have cross-reactivity with both BNP and NT-proBNP assays and may have substantial implications regarding clinical usage.[327] Indeed, some would argue most of what is measured in HF patients is proBNP. The influence of age, gender, ethnicity, and non-HF pathologic processes has been shown to substantially influence what may otherwise be considered a normal reference concentration.[397,411] Renal impairment has been shown to substantially increase NT-proBNP concentrations and BNP to a lesser extent.[397,412-416]

For BNP a single cutoff at 100 pg/mL (ng/L) has been designated, likely driven by the FDA clearance at this value as the ROC curve value optimized for diagnostic accuracy. However, as shown in Fig. 58.27, values in normal subjects older than 75 years appear to be either falsely increased or are not normal, with the 100-pg/mL cutoff detecting occult pathologic processes. For NT-proBNP the FDA-cleared cutoffs are age-based for younger than 75 years at 125 pg/mL and older than 75 years at 450 pg/mL. Again, these cutoffs appear to misclassify many normal subjects, as shown Fig. 58.27. Clinical studies (proBNP Investigation of Dyspnea in the Emergency [PRIDE]) have more appropriately defined age-derived and renal function–derived cutoffs as shown in Fig. 58.28, designated by 50 years of age and estimated glomerular filtration rate (eGFR) at 60 mL/min per 1.73 m^2, with an optimal NPV at less than 300 pg/mL that is age, gender, and eGFR independent. Obesity also has been shown to have an association with BNP and NT-proBNP measurements[417-419]; with an inverse relationship between increased BMI and BNP decrease in CHF patients. HF patients who receive the drug nesiritide (human recombinant BNP) for therapy and management may have confounding BNP results because nesiritide is molecularly identical to endogenous BNP. Thus,

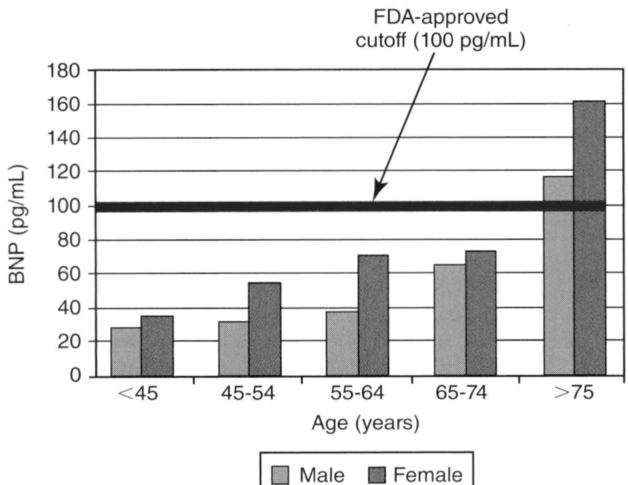

FIGURE 58.27 Representative brain natriuretic peptide *(BNP)* concentration distributions in normal males and females by decade (years) with indication of the US Food and Drug Administration *(FDA)*-cleared 100 pg/mL (ng/L) cutoff value.

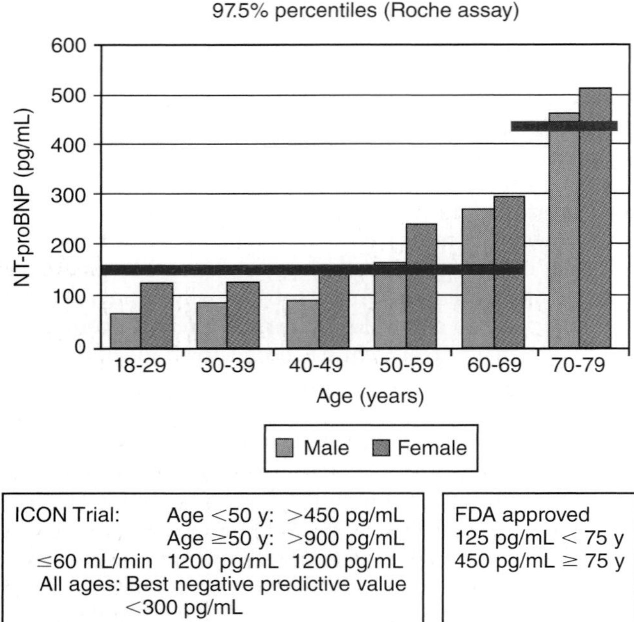

FIGURE 58.28 Representative N-terminal pro-brain natriuretic peptide *(NT-proBNP)* concentration distributions in normal males and females by decade (years) with indication of the US Food and Drug Administration *(FDA)*-cleared age-related cutoff values compared with those recommended by the International Collaborative on NT-proBNP ICON) trial determined by age and renal function.

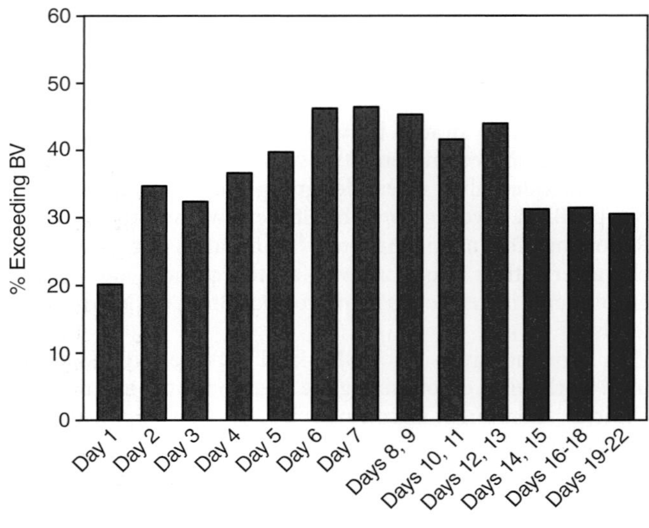

FIGURE 58.29 Variability of brain natriuretic peptide (BNP) concentrations by day from initial admission order, with demonstration that more than 50% exceed biological variability *(BV)* (100% change) over a 2-week period. (From Wu AH, Smith A, Appel FS. Optimum blood collection intervals for B-type natriuretic peptide testing in patients with heart failure. *Am J Cardiol* 2004;93:1562–1563, with permission from Excerpta Medica.)

if BNP were to be monitored for regulation of nesiritide infusion within a time window before an appropriate decrease of the exogenous BNP could occur (half-life ~22 minutes), the potential for falsely increased concentrations could arise. Nesiritide does not directly confound NT-proBNP measurements. Finally, a lack of understanding of the physiologic and biological variability of BNP and NT-proBNP in HF patients may cause clinicians to misinterpret changing (increasing or decreasing) BNP and NT-proBNP concentrations in the context of establishing the success or failure of therapy. It has been shown that both BNP and NT-proBNP exhibit a within-subject biological variability of 35% to 45%.[420] Thus, when considering what is clinically, significantly different between serial BNP or NT-proBNP values, a reference change value of 80% is necessary. This is what has been documented in patients with chronic HF. A small study has demonstrated that in HF patients monitored for BNP over at least two periods during 2 weeks for BNP, that less than 50% of concentrations were found to be outside the expected biological variability (Fig. 58.29). However, it may be that the benefit in outcomes reported reflects the fact that those with reductions will continue to have their values decrease more substantially and thus become for a larger percent of patients beyond the reference change interval. This implies that BNP or NT-proBNP monitoring may be overused and reemphasizes its role as a confirmatory biomarker and not a test that clinicians should solely rely on to manage HF patients.

Presently, no data are available that have established a correlation between BNP and NT-proBNP concentrations using commercially available technology. In addition, the literature is scattered with reports of home-brewed BNP and NT-proBNP assays that may add to the confusion of clinicians when interpreting and comparing data from different studies; whether in diagnosing or ruling out HF, managing HF, screening for asymptomatic left ventricular dysfunction, or for risk stratification and prognostication for patients with HF, ACS, or other pathologic processes. One must consider the assay used, the clinical evidence available based on the individual assay, and the aim of the biomarker-based studies. No peer-reviewed literature has demonstrated that the two assays are analytically equivalent at present. Thus, until large studies are available, which hopefully will include proBNP measurements as well, caution is suggested before the conclusions based on one particular BNP or NT-proBNP assay are translated to another assay.

The following practice guidelines have been recommended by the NACB and IFCC Committee for Standardization of Markers of Cardiac Damage pertaining to analytical issues for biomarkers of HF.

1. Normal reference interval (95th or 97.5th percentile) should be independently established for both BNP and NT-proBNP based on age (by decade) and gender. Each commercial assay should be validated separately. The effect of ethnicity and renal function needs to be evaluated as a possible independent variable.
2. ROC curves should be established to evaluate the clinical effectiveness and to establish optimal medical decision cutoffs for both BNP and NT-proBNP assays for diagnostic usefulness.

3. Assays for BNP and NT-proBNP should have a total imprecision (%CV) of ≤15% at both their age- and gender-defined upper reference intervals, as well as at the NYHA-defined medical decision concentrations.
4. Before introduction into clinical practice, BNP and NT-proBNP assays must be characterized with respect to the following preanalytical and analytical issues:
   Preanalytical:
   a. effect of storage time and temperature
   b. influence of different anticoagulants
   c. influence of gel separator tubes
   d. plastic blood collection tubes are necessary for BNP; for NT-proBNP either glass or plastic are acceptable

   Analytical:
   a. identification of both antibody recognition epitopes
   b. cross-reactivity characteristics with related natriuretic peptides, including NT-proANP, ANP, CNP, BNP, and glycosylated and nonglycosylated NT-proBNP and proBNP
   c. identification of interferences from heterophile antibodies, rheumatoid factors, and human anti-mouse antibodies
   d. description of calibration material used, how the material was defined, and the concentration value assigned
   e. clarification of dilution responses
5. For both BNP and NT-proBNP, until a primary reference material is defined for either assay for appropriate calibration of assays: (a) measurements should be reported in nanogram per liter units, not picomole per milliliter; and (b) patient specimen comparisons and regression analysis should be performed, along CLSI guidelines, to establish the degree of or lack of harmonization across the dynamic range of each assay. Specifically, harmonization around the current presumed optimal diagnostic medical decision cutoff of 100 ng/L for BNP should be validated. Because there is only one source of antibodies and calibrators for NT-proBNP (Roche), harmonization of NT-proBNP assays should not be a problem.
6. For both BNP and NT-proBNP biological variability has been defined as at least 50% and in many studies higher. Therefore caution should be exercised in interpreting less than 50% to 80% concentration changes as reflective of medical therapy. However, consistent trends should be followed as clinically important.

In summary, laboratorians and clinicians must be cognizant of the numerous considerations inherent in the NPs as markers for management of cardiology patients, including the form of the biomarker itself (BNP or NT-proBNP); the lack of standardization of immunoassays; that reference and medical decision limits are dependent on age and gender; that biological variation of NPs in individuals is inherently high; the diagnostic time window (admission or monitoring trends over time); the clinical setting in which NPs are used (eg, general practice, emergency room, and coronary care unit); the patient subset being tested (ie, renal failure, sepsis); and whether application is for diagnostic use, prognostic use, or for a future potential application of therapeutic guidance. All of these aspects must be taken into consideration with the implementation of biomarkers such as NPs to avoid the possibility for misinterpretation of a result for patient care.

Clinical Use of Natriuretic Peptides

BNP, NT-proBNP, and novel NP assays that are being developed have proved of assistance to clinicians in the evaluation of patients with impaired left ventricular function, with or without CHF and those with coronary heart disease.[421-427] On the other hand, the more we have learned about natriuretic peptides, the more complicated the biology of these biomarkers has become (see previous discussion).

Use in the Diagnosis of Congestive Heart Failure

The initial validation of natriuretic peptides was done based on the ability to improve the diagnosis of CHF. The situations chosen to test this hypothesis were not in sophisticated cardiology offices but in the ED and primary care practices.[16,17] The emergency setting is an extremely busy environment in which there is often a severe press for time, making cautious and careful evaluation more difficult. In addition, ED physicians are generalists having to triage problems related to trauma, infectious disease, and a variety of other complaints relating to almost any organ system. Some are very sophisticated in regard to cardiovascular issues and the presenting symptoms and cardiovascular examination associated with HF, and some are not very good at all. Accordingly, some have objected to the use of this as the primary testing ground for the use of natriuretic peptides for the diagnosis of HF. General internists are in a similar position, especially in the outpatient setting where these evaluations are done where they have limited resources and a heterogeneity of expertise related to this particular diagnosis. Thus the relatively marginal improvement in diagnostic yield (74% to 81% in the Breathing Not Properly [BNP] trial and 92% to 96% in the PRIDE trial) is not terribly impressive in one sense. However, in parsing the data, it is clear that the majority of the benefit of the use of natriuretic peptides for diagnosis resides in the triage of patients in whom clinicians are ambivalent, as recently documented.[428] When patients have a very low risk for HF, it is not clear that natriuretic peptides help at all, and, similarly, when they have a classic presentation, they have such a high frequency of HF and such a high pretest probability that natriuretic peptides are unlikely to be helpful. However, there is a group of patients with dyspnea in whom the clinician is ambivalent and it is this group in which natriuretic peptides are helpful. Of importance in the interpretation of natriuretic peptides in this situation is that marginal values often are not helpful. The BNP trial suggested the use of one cutoff value at 100 ng/L to make the diagnosis of HF. This value could have been altered to increase either sensitivity or specificity (Fig. 58.30).[429] However, 26% of the population had values between 100 and 500 ng/L. One-third of this group did not have CHF according to subsequent adjudication, and two-thirds did, but unfortunately, there was no cutoff value that distinguished these groups. For this reason, a group of investigators (ICON) analyzed their data with NT-proBNP looking to generate values that will help to both include and exclude disease.[430] This is an extremely valuable approach. They report that a value for NT-proBNP less than 300 ng/L effectively excludes CHF. Values over 450 ng/L in individuals who are younger than 50 years rules in HF, and values above 900 ng/L diagnose HF in patients who are over the age of 50. As is clear, there are gaps between these values describing the fact that clinical judgment is still importantly necessary

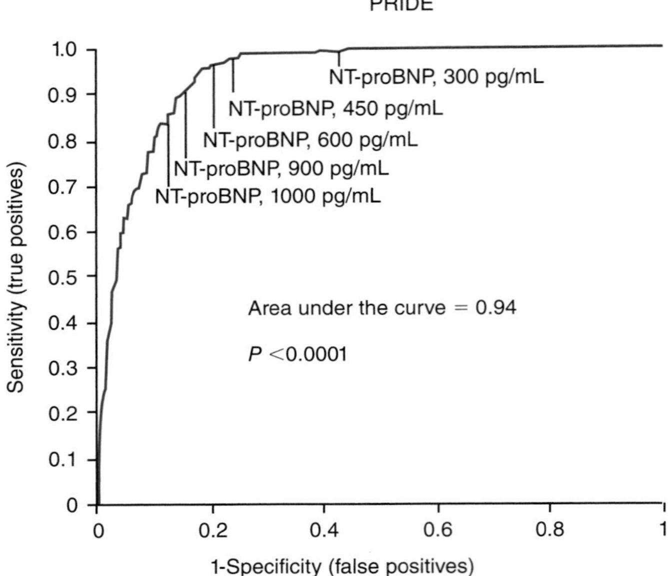

Cut point	Sensitivity	Specificity	Positive predictive value	Negative predictive value	Accuracy
300 pg/mL	99%	68%	62%	99%	79%
450 pg/mL	98%	76%	68%	99%	83%
600 pg/mL	96%	81%	73%	97%	86%
900 pg/mL	90%	85%	76%	94%	87%
1000 pg/mL	87%	86%	78%	91%	87%

Breathing Not Properly

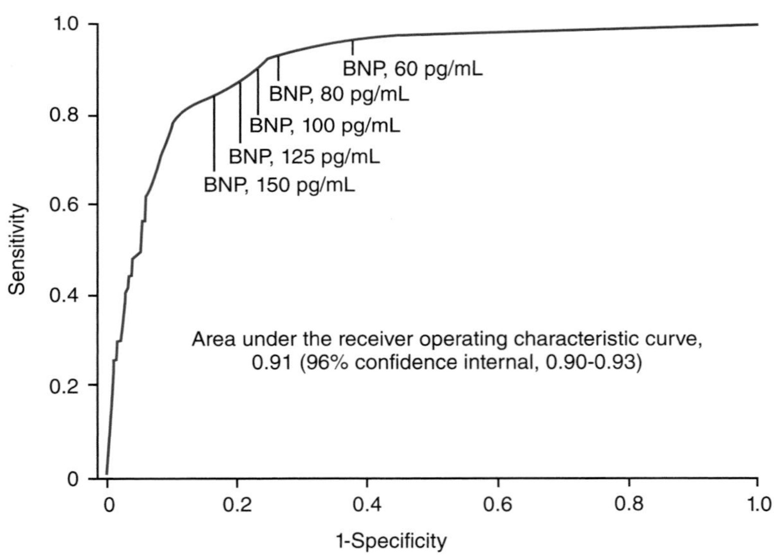

BNP pg/mL	Sensitivity (%)	Specificity (%)	Positive predictive value (%)	Negative predictive value (%)	Accuracy (%)
50	97 (98-98)	62 (60-66)	71 (68-74)	96 (94-97)	79
80	98 (91-96)	74 (70-77)	77 (76-80)	92 (89-94)	83
100	90 (88-92)	76 (73-78)	79 (78-81)	92 (87-91)	83
125	87 (86-90)	79 (78-82)	80 (78-83)	87 (84-89)	83
150	86 (82-88)	83 (80-86)	83 (80-86)	85 (83-88)	84

FIGURE 58.30 Receiver operating characteristic (ROC) analysis for brain natriuretic peptide *(BNP)* and N-terminal pro-brain natriuretic peptide *(NTproBNP)* for the diagnosis of acute heart failure. (From Tang WH, Francis GS, Morrow DA, et al. National Academy of Clinical Biochemistry Laboratory Medicine practice guidelines: clinical utilization of cardiac biomarker testing in heart failure. *Circulation* 2007;116:e99–e109.)

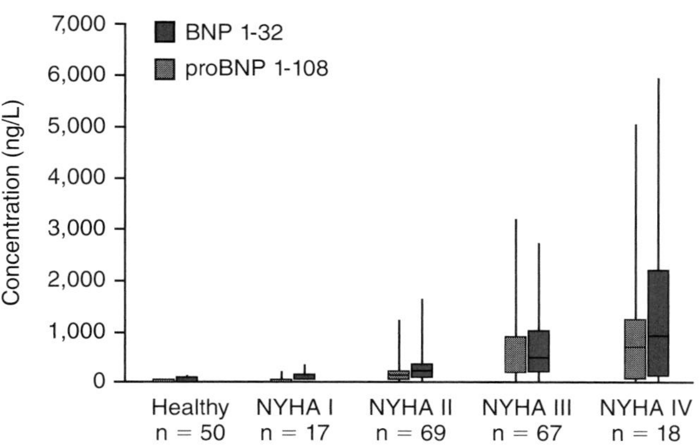

FIGURE 58.31 Relationship between pro-brain natriuretic peptide *(NTproBNP)* 1-108 and New York Heart Association *(NYAC)* classifications. *BNP,* Brain natriuretic peptide. (From Giuliani I, Rieunier F, Larue C, et al. Assay for measurement of intact B-type natriuretic peptide prohormone in blood. *Clin Chem* 2006;52:1054–1061.)

BOX 58.5 Causes of Increased Natriuretic Peptides

1. Acute or chronic systolic or diastolic heart failure
2. Left ventricular hypertrophy
3. Inflammatory cardiac disease
4. Systemic arterial hypertension with left ventricular hypertrophy
5. Pulmonary hypertension
6. Acute or chronic renal failure
7. Ascitic liver cirrhosis
8. Endocrine disorders (eg, hyperaldosteronism, Cushing's syndrome)
9. Sepsis

in the use of natriuretic peptides. It is for this reason why most guidelines groups have not suggested the routine use of natriuretic peptides for diagnosis in every patient who presents with dyspnea.[29,431,432] Instead, they recommend the judicious use in patients in whom the diagnosis is not clear. It is axiomatic to suggest that consideration of gender, age, and weight (see previous discussion) in interpreting such values is advised. In addition, it is clear that the worse the clinical class of the HF, the higher is the natriuretic peptide levels (Fig. 58.31). The diagnosis may be problematic, especially in patients who have other comorbidities.[39,433,434] Chronic obstructive pulmonary disease and cardiovascular disease frequently overlap, and it is in these sorts of patients in whom the optimal use of natriuretic peptides for diagnosis likely resides. Other disease processes (Box 58.5) can cause elevations and must be taken into account by including the clinical situation into interpretation of the natriuretic peptide values. It should be noted that both the proBNP assay indicated above and a novel proANP assay are equivalent to BNP and NTproBNP for the diagnosis of HF in the ED.

Special Situations

Several additional caveats are necessary clinically. There is an increasing epidemic of HF with preserved ventricular function (Box 58.6). Controversy exists concerning the mechanisms for this clinical entity and some even question its existence, but a stiff, noncompliant left ventricle is clearly an important contributor. Unfortunately, the therapeutic modalities used for treatment have been shown to be ineffective.[15] In addition, because natriuretic peptides are predominantly released in response to end systolic wall stress, values are much lower in this disease state. Thus natriuretic peptides provide aid in the inclusion or exclusion of HF secondary to systolic dysfunction, but do not provide similarly robust triage in patients with diastolic dysfunction, heart failure with preserved systolic function (HEFPEF). The presence of primary or secondary valvular abnormalities that increase the pressure of volume overload, and particularly the latter, will cause increases in natriuretic peptide values because they increase wall stress and may be useful diagnostically to define severe disease and/or decompensation. Thus the presence of these abnormalities must be taken into account when interpreting natriuretic peptide values. Additionally, the presence of atrial fibrillation defines a group of patients with underlying cardiovascular disease. Natriuretic peptides both in the presence and absence of HF will be higher in this setting, and this needs to be taken into account in interpreting values for diagnostic purposes. Finally, abnormalities in right ventricular function, even when the result of volume overload that will cause increases in wall stress, are associated with a blunted natriuretic peptide response, likely because of the smaller mass of myocardium involved. The constricted pericardium inhibits increases in wall stress, and thus natriuretic peptide values often are not elevated despite overt HF unless the constrictive process is superimposed on prior cardiac disease.[435]

BOX 58.6 Special Situations of Elevated Natriuretic Peptides

1. Well heart failure patients
2. Heart failure secondary to diastolic dysfunction
3. Acute mitral regurgitation
4. Pulmonary edema less than 1 hour old
5. Constrictive epicarditis
6. Other cases "upstream" from
   a. Left ventricle
   b. Mitral stenosis
   c. Atrial myxoma

Modified from van Kimmenade RR, Januzzi JL, Jr. Emerging biomarkers in heart failure. *Clin Chem* 2012;58:127–138.

Screening for Ventricular Dysfunction

The use of natriuretic peptides for screening to identify patients with impaired ventricular function that has not previously been appreciated has also been proposed. The sensitivity and specificity of such an approach is far less than that of the acute circumstance, and for that reason most groups have not advocated the use of this analyte in that area, but as the criteria for diagnosis improve as more specific assays are developed, this may be an area in which natriuretic peptides will be of value, especially if confined to high-risk groups.[436-439]

Prognostic Use of Natriuretic Peptides

Some have argued for the ubiquitous use of natriuretic peptides in all patients with dyspnea. The logic for such an approach is related to the fact that individuals with higher natriuretic peptide values have a more adverse prognosis (Fig. 58.32) in general than those with lower levels when they present either acutely or chronically.[410,430,440-448] There may be an exception to the idea that higher levels are always more negatively prognostic.[449] There is a report that in the extremely ill end-stage patient lower values are observed, which could reflect exhaustion of the natriuretic peptide system, but these observations remain to be confirmed. Thus one could argue that obtaining a natriuretic peptide value at the time of admission to hospital in a patient who has suspected CHF is valuable from the perspective of determining eventual risk. Indeed, it is well established that values obtained in this circumstance are highly prognostic with very high risk ratios and with higher values by and large being associated with worse disease. Maximal prognostic significance usually is associated with the value at the time of discharge. Thus a reasonable strategy would be to obtain one level at the time of admission and one at the time of discharge. Recent data suggest that if natriuretic peptide values are reduced substantially during hospitalization, patients tend to do better. However, most of the reductions that have been reported are modest compared to the biological variability (see earlier discussion). Thus it is hard to know how to interpret these changes, especially in individual patients. Recent data in the outpatient setting suggest that the changes needed to overcome biologic variability of 80% or greater (see Fig. 58.32) are necessary to see substantive alterations in prognosis.[450,451] Nonetheless, in the clinical perspective, there probably are differences between those individuals with more chronic disease and those with only acute disease. Those with more chronic disease have a chronically induced natriuretic peptide system that probably

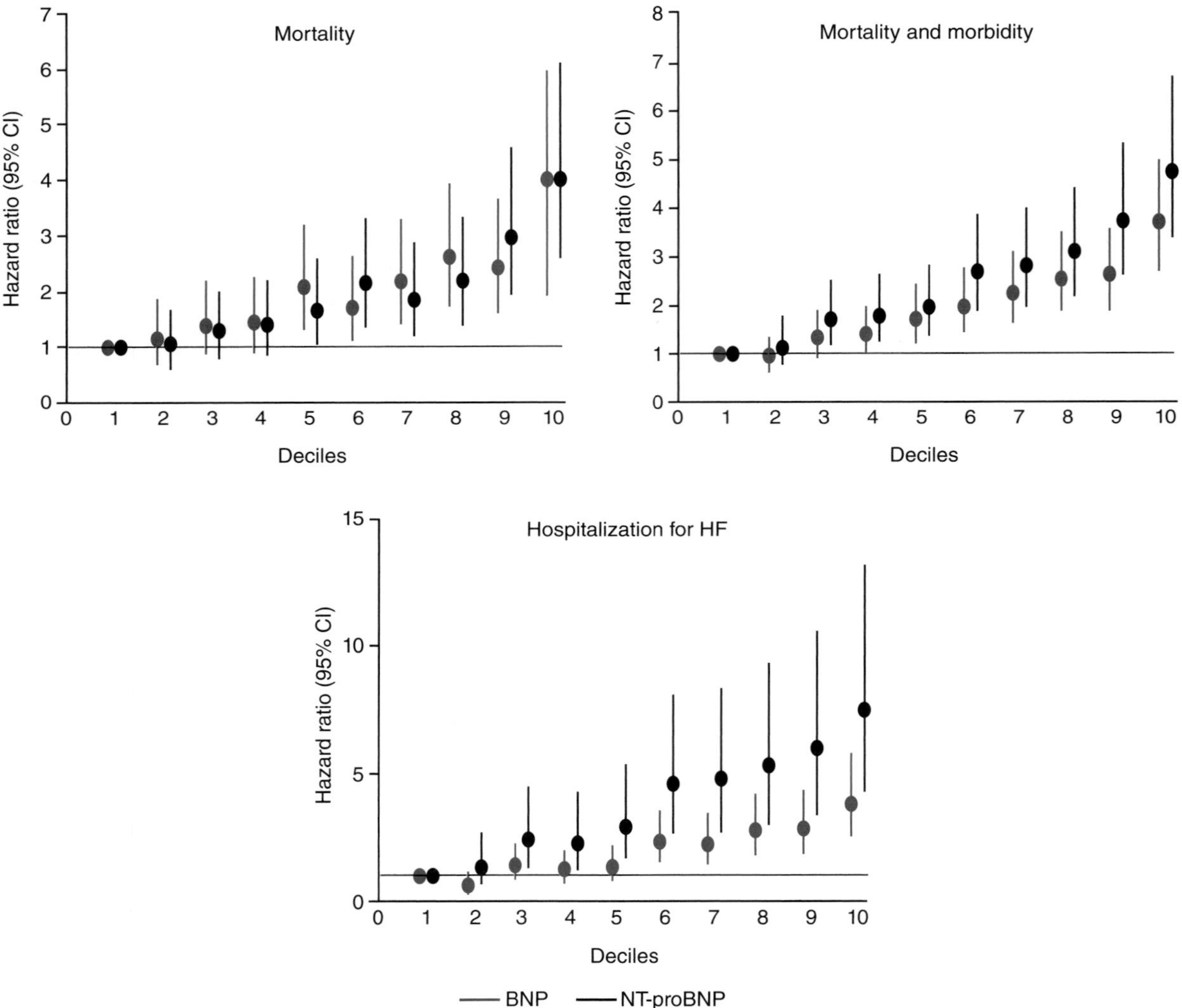
Mortality
Hazard ratio (95% CI)
Deciles
Mortality and morbidity
Hospitalization for HF
BNP
NT-proBNP
Covariates for adjustment: age, gender, NYHA class, ischemic etiology, LVEF, LVIDd, serum creatinine and bilirubin, randomized treatment, prescription of β-blockers, digitalis and diuretics, presence of AF or diabetes at study entry.

FIGURE 58.32 Relationships of brain natriuretic peptide *(BNP)* and N-terminal pro-brain natriuretic peptide *(NT-proBNP)* values and outcomes. *AF,* Atrial fibrillation; *HF,* heart failure; *LVEF,* left ventricular ejection fraction; *LVIDd,* left ventricular internal diameter end diastole; *NYHA,* New York Heart Association. (From Anand IS, Fisher LD, Chiang YT, et al. Changes in brain natriuretic peptide and norepinephrine over time and mortality and morbidity in the Valsartan Heart Failure Trial [Val-HeFT]. *Circulation* 2003;107:1278–1283.)

responds more slowly than individuals who have simply an acute diathesis in whom natriuretic peptide levels may respond somewhat more rapidly. Accordingly, some degree of subclassifying these patients in regard to these parameters is key. Unfortunately, there are no good studies defining what to do if natriuretic peptide levels do not respond rapidly and aggressively to change. It would be important if one could show that keeping patients in the hospital, for example, would mitigate some of these problems, but that information is simply not available at present. Some studies have actually claimed benefit in reducing costs, but at times those studies have included very long hospital stays.[452] Thus management decisions cannot be made based solely on these values. In addition, extreme care is necessary because of the subset of patients who may have low levels if they are quite chronically ill and the heterogeneity of values associated with differences in body physiognomy likely related to the clearance of the natriuretic peptides.

Use of Natriuretic Peptides to Guide Therapy

Perhaps the most interesting use of these markers is in the patient with HF with the hope of finding the ability to titer therapy more efficaciously in these individuals.[453-458] The logic of this approach suggests that many individuals are not as astute as they could be to their symptoms and that having an objective measure may be helpful. This has recently been tested in several randomized controlled trials. The first, Systolic Heart Failure Treatment Supported by BNP (STARS-BNP) suggested benefit to such an approach, but subsequent trials have not confirmed those findings. Two other studies have been presented, but not published at this time. The negative results have been argued to be due in part to the fact that in many of the trials a large percentage of the patients have been elderly (younger than 75 years of age) and the thought is that elderly patients may not tolerate the increased doses of therapeutic agents used in the management protocols predicated on natriuretic peptides. Indeed, if those older than 75 years of age are excluded, there is substantial benefit to this strategy.[459] If this were a finding in only one trial, it might be viewed highly cynically, which is why the reports of the other studies are awaited anxiously. If confirmed, the idea of using natriuretic peptides to adjust therapy so as to reduce values toward normal or a change from baseline of greater than 80% has the possibility of markedly improving prognosis. A large randomized controlled trial is in progress.

New challenges have been posed by the development of neprilysin inhibitors, which in theory inhibit the degradation of bioactive BNP. They have been linked to angiotensin receptor blockers (ARBs) in an agent called LCZ696, which is a combination of valsartan and the inhibitor named sacubitril.[460,461] Sacubitril has been combined with an ARB because neprilysin also degrades bradykinin amongst multiple other proteins and the association of this effect with ARBs exacerbates angioedema. The combination has been shown to markedly improve prognosis in patients with modest (mostly class 2) HF. One possible mechanism suggested has been that the agent works by reducing the degradation of BNP, and in the index randomized controlled trial the agent resulted in increases in BNP values and decreases in NT-proBNP values. It is likely given the complexity of the natriuretic peptide system that this is oversimplistic and that the agent may work by its effects on multiple proteins, including adrenomedullin, bradykinin, substance P, ANP, endothelin 1, and/or angiotensin 2. It is unclear how/if the effects shown in the recent trial will affect the use of natriuretic peptide measurements. A novel assay for neprilysin has been developed, and the values appear to have important prognostic significance.

Other Situations

Several investigations suggest that natriuretic peptides can be used to determine when to intervene in patients with aortic stenosis and mitral regurgitation.[462-465] Unfortunately, usually only one value has been used and those values (corrected for differences in the assays) tend to be quite low. Thus it is unclear how to distinguish these values from those of normal or less severely affected individuals. However, it is possible that using changes in natriuretic peptides over time might provide a better paradigm. In some severe situations, changes in natriuretic peptides can be associated with severe CHF in the absence of elevated levels of natriuretic peptides. These include very acute HF before the stimulus to produce increased levels of natriuretic peptides has had time to occur. In addition, cases in which the abnormality is above the ventricle, such as atrial myxoma or with mitral stenosis, can present with HF and normal natriuretic peptide values. Finally, constrictive pericarditis is associated with low values because increases in wall stress are precluded by the constricting pericardium.

Other situations in which natriuretic peptides are elevated include any disease that increases blood volume and thus wall stress, such as sepsis, anemia, renal dysfunction, Cushing syndrome, and/or hyperaldosteronism, hypertension with LVH, and cirrhosis. Some have suggested that values can be used to assess prognosis in patients with renal failure, albeit using higher cutoff values, and it does appear that the mechanisms for release are still the same.[374] However, mixing values between GFR groups is likely to be fraught with confusion. Using values within groups (eg, those with severe disease on or off chronic dialysis) appears much more productive.[399,466]

Ischemic Heart Disease

Several investigations have suggested that natriuretic peptides can be used to assess prognosis in patients who present with ACS and normal cTn values.[4,467-476] Most of these studies have used relatively insensitive cTn assays or higher cutoff values, but such assays and cutoff values are still in common use. If so, the finding of an elevated natriuretic peptide level may be helpful. In one study, such patients benefited from an invasive strategy.[23] The subgroup involved was mostly female, and it appears that women may have lower cTn levels than men. However, if this strategy is to be used, a relatively low cutoff value has been advocated (80 ng/L with the Alere BNP assay). Whether these low values will allow adequate discrimination in large groups of patients is unclear. However, it is clear that the use of natriuretic peptides may be helpful after the acute episode in predicting the subsequent risk for events. Indeed, over time in some studies they appear to be even more prognostic than troponin.[477] Thus, eventually, it is likely that natriuretic peptides may become part of a long-term risk stratification panel. Natriuretic peptides are also elaborated, albeit to a modest extent in those with positive treadmill stress tests.[478] Some of this release comes directly from the coronary arteries. Elevations also occur in those with diastolic abnormalities.[479] The changes appear too small to be used diagnostically.

Novel Biomarkers Used in Prognosis

ST2

ST2 is a new biomarker that has potential utility in patients with HF and perhaps acute ischemic heart disease as well. It has been known as an inflammatory biomarker for years, but it was the discovery that the soluble form also was released by stretch of cardiomyocytes and macrophages that led to investigations concerning its utility in cardiovascular diseases.[480] ST2 has three isoforms. One is within the cell, and binding by IL33 to that transmembrane receptor results in antihypertrophic and antifibrotic effects. It also works through intracellular nuclear transcription regulatory processes, which evokes inflammatory cytokines and an immune response. Its aggregate effects are thought to be protective. However, in response to stretch and inflammation, the soluble form is secreted and binds to IL33 and by doing so prevents binding to the transmembrane receptor and thus abrogates these protective effects.[481] There have been assays for ST2, but one has been perfected that is more sensitive and is FDA approved.[482] It has good analytic characteristics with an LOD of 1.3 ng/mL and an LOQ of 2.4 ng/mL. However, there likely are multiple requisite forms (those bound to IL33 and others that are free). Normal values ought to be sex specific, but the FDA has suggested a cutoff value of 35 ng/mL and has not required sex-specific values. ST2 has only modest biological variation.[483] Clinically, increased values do not add diagnostically to other markers. Thus, in HF, ST2 is less valuable as a diagnostic marker than BNP. However, it is more prognostic for death and/or HF exacerbations[484] and in most studies it remains prognostic despite other biomarkers and often reduces or eliminates the prognostic impact of those other markers, including BNP.[485,486] This may be because it integrates both inflammatory and stretch-related processes in its prognostic approach. Importantly, ST2 is reduced by therapies known to have a positive impact on clinical outcomes such as β-blockers[487] and mineralocorticoid antagonists.[488] In comparative HF studies, it fares better than other markers thought to look at fibrotic pathways.[489,490]

In patients with acute ischemic heart disease, ST2 levels increase to peak approximately 6 to 18 hours after symptom onset. Levels in the upper quartile independently doubled the risk for cardiovascular death and HF.[491,492] Weaker associations occur with nonSTEMI.[493] ST2 predicts short-term (30-day) and long-term (>1 year) death and HF independent of clinical indicators, but not when NTproBNP and the GRACE score are included in models.

This is a promising marker that has a chance to become important clinically if and when the proper studies are done.

Galectin-3

Galectin-3 is an interesting marker that plays a central role in the fibrotic process. In response to cellular injury, the inflammatory and wound healing responses evoke the egress of macrophages into the injured area. These macrophages release galectin-3, which is a β-galactoside–binding lectin that stimulates myofibroblasts to stimulate collagen formation and thus scar formation.[494] Experimental models are robust in supporting this role in multiple tissues, but particularly the heart and the kidney, and supporting the concept that mineralocorticoid antagonists and modified citrus pectin inhibit the process.[495-497] Galectin-3 also mediates cell-cell and cell–extracellular matrix adhesion, cell growth and differentiation, cell cycle regulation, apoptosis, angiogenesis, tumor genesis, tumor growth, metastasis, and immune reactions. Gene knockout experiments confirm the central role of this protein. Thus it is thought that elevated galectin-3, once stimulated, remains elevated and marks individuals who are prone to develop fibrosis.

The original assay had reasonable analytical characteristics with a normal range from 3.8 ng/mL to 21.0 ng/mL[498] but that rise modestly in the presence of cardiovascular comorbidities.[498] Values do not change markedly over time,[499] but biological variation is substantial. Clinically, elevated galectin-3 is associated with an increased incidence of adverse outcomes after AMI and in community patients as well as even when controlled for other important covariates. Such data have been shown in patients with acute[500] as well as chronic HF[501] and patients with diastolic HF.[502] In the Heart Failure–A Controlled Trial Investigating Outcomes of Exercise (HF ACTION) registry, it was markedly prognostic.[503] It is also prognostic for the development of HF in patients who present with ACS.[504] Several of these studies have also suggested that elevated values in patients hospitalized with HF can predict readmissions.[505] However, the suggestion was made that a 15% change should/could be used as a criterion. This is substantially less than biological variation. Recently, it has been reported that changes in renal function cause systemic increases in galectin-3. This fact could explain part of its prognostic accuracy in patients with HF[506] but also complicate the use of the marker. In head-to-head comparisons with ST2, galectin-3 has been knocked out of the prognostic models.[489,490] Galectin-3 is a promising marker, but much better data and particularly treatment-related information are required before it will be useful as a routine clinical marker.

The Future

The potential future use of natriuretic peptides, as indicated in the analytical sections, is growing as we understand more about the biochemistry and mechanisms of natriuretic peptide release. It appears that CHF is in part a clinical syndrome characterized by abnormalities in how the natriuretic peptide system works. The system synthesizes and releases large amounts of protein, but much of the protein is poorly functional. Whether this is because it is inadequately cleaved or whether it is due to glycosylation or other biochemical processes has yet to be determined. However, what is clear is that very little circulating active BNP is present in patients with HF.[389] Most of what appears to circulate is proBNP that is uncleaved, suggesting probable abnormalities in corin and furin that are indigenous to the pathophysiology of CHF. If

POINTS TO REMEMBER

Measurement of BNP or NT-proBNP

- Most useful in ruling out HF in the ED
- Confirms diagnosis of HF in patients with suggestive clinical symptoms

TABLE 58.5 Biomarkers in Heart Failure

Pathophysiology	Biomarker
Inflammation*,†,‡	C-reactive protein
	Tumor necrosis factor-α
	Fas (APO-1)
	Interleukins-1, -6, and -18
Oxidative stress*,†,§	Oxidized low-density lipoproteins
	Myeloperoxidase
	Urinary biopyrrins
	Urinary and plasma isoprostanes
	Plasma malondialdehyde
Myocyte injury*,†,§	Cardiac-specific troponins I and T
	Myosin light-chain kinase I
	Heart-type fatty acid protein
	Myocardial-bound creatine kinase
Myocyte stress†,§,¶	BNP
	NT-proBNP
	MR-proANP
	ST2
Extracellular matrix remodeling*,†,§	Matrix metalloproteinases
	Tissue inhibitors of metalloproteinases
	Collagen propeptides
New biomarkers†	Chromogranin
	Galectin 3
	Osteoprotegerin
	Adiponectin
	Growth differentiation factor 15
Neurohormones*,†,§	Norepinephrine
	Renin
	Angiotensin II
	Arginine vasopressin
	Endothelin

*Biomarkers in this category aid in elucidating the pathogenesis of heart failure.
†Biomarkers in this category provide prognostic information and enhance risk stratification.
‡Biomarkers in this category can be used to identify subjects at risk for heart failure.
§Biomarkers in this category are potential targets of therapy.
¶Biomarkers in this category are useful in the diagnosis of heart failure and in monitoring therapy.
Modified from Braunwald E. Biomarkers in heart failure. *N Engl J Med* 2008;358:2148–2159.

one could manipulate these systems to facilitate the presence of active BNP or of other fragments that might have biological importance, one might substantially improve CHF. These are some of the approaches currently being pursued in the hope of improving therapy for this very large group of patients.

In addition, novel biomarkers (Table 58.5 and Box 58.7) have the potential to contribute substantially to this work. Recent data suggest that intact proBNP can be measured directly, which may lead to better understanding of underlying pathophysiology. As with other natriuretic peptides, its circulating concentration tracks with the clinical class of HF (see Fig. 58.31).[140] In addition, a new test for ANP has been developed (MR-proANP) that may have some advantages. Preliminary data suggest that it is equivalent to other natriuretic peptides in its ability to diagnose acute HF.[415] Such testing might allow the more rapidly responding atrial peptide and the more slow to respond B-type natriuretic peptide to be used synergistically. Again, additional research is necessary.

Natriuretic peptides may be of additional value in several different intriguing areas that are being explored. One is sudden cardiac death. Several studies have associated elevated natriuretic peptide values with mortality and/or ICD discharges.[507,508] A second area involves the follow-up of patients who received cardiac resynchronization therapy devices. It appears that higher values help define a group apt to benefit, and although it takes some time for natriuretic peptides to fall, their reduction is associated with clinical benefit over time.[418] Finally, several suggestions have indicated that BNP may be useful in helping diagnose PEs when they occur and to determine prognosis. Unfortunately, levels often are not markedly elevated, but with time this indication may be developed more fully.

Another area that needs to be discussed involves multimarker testing. It is clear that for ischemic heart disease, the addition of natriuretic peptides to other markers in a multimarker strategy improves risk stratification, especially over the long term.[485,486] It also appears that benefit may be derived from the prediction of events in older, less acutely ill individuals. Recently, the group from Uppsala reported a rather striking improvement in the prediction of events (changes in the κ coefficient statistic from 0.644 to 0.766) with the use of a multimarker panel that included natriuretic peptides. The panel included cTn, NT-proBNP, cystatin C, and CRP. If confirmed, this approach may become more widely used for risk prediction.

BIOMARKERS OF INTEREST (ALTHOUGH THEY ARE NOT CURRENTLY USED ROUTINELY)

Fig. 58.33 portrays a biochemical profile in coronary vascular disease that correlates staging of biomarker release into the circulation with various pathophysiologic mechanisms of ACS and HF. As shown in Table 58.5 and Box 58.7, numerous biomarkers have been studied and used for different clinical reasons, and other promising novel biomarkers are becoming established alongside cTn and NPs as routine clinical tools. We highlight some characteristics of several of these here. This list is not meant to be all inclusive.

C-Reactive Protein

CRP is an acute-phase reactant that was initially developed to evaluate patients with infection.[127,507-510] It now appears that concentrations below those seen in infection but above healthy values (as measured by high-sensitivity CRP [hsCRP] assays) can be a marker of the atherosclerotic process because both chronic and acute atherosclerotic processes involve an inflammatory component (see Chapter 34). Among the ligands that can stimulate CRP are TNF and IL-1, which are thought to stimulate IL-6, which then causes the elaboration of CRP from the liver (see Chapter 34). It is now clear that CRP itself can enhance the inflammatory and prothrombotic response. A large number of assays for hsCRP are available, as is a standard protocol for their reporting.

For primary prevention, values greater than 3 mg/L are considered high risk. Recent data suggest that using hsCRP

BOX 58.7 Biomarkers in Acute Coronary Syndrome

Serologic Biomarkers of Arterial Vulnerability
Lipid profile
- Apo B
- Lp(a)
- LDL particle number
- CETP
- Lp-PLA_2
- Inflammation

hs-CRP
sICAM-1
IL-6
IL-18
SAA
MPO
sCD40
- Oxidized LDL
- GPX1 activity
- Nitrotyrosine
- Homocysteine
- Cystatin C
- Natriuretic peptides
- ADMA
- MMP-9
- TIMP-1

Structural Markers of Arterial Vulnerability
Carotid IMT
Coronary artery calcium

Functional Markers of Arterial Vulnerability
Blood pressure
Endothelial dysfunction
Arterial stiffness
Ankle-brachial index
Urine albumin excretion

Serologic Markers of Blood Vulnerability
Fibrinogen
D-Dimer

Decreased Fibrinolysis
TPA/PAI-1

Increased Coagulation
von Willebrand factor

Structural Markers of Myocardial Vulnerability
Exercise stress echo
PET

Serologic Markers of Myocardial Injury
Cardiac troponins

ADMA, Asymmetric dimethylarginine; *Apo,* apolipoprotein; *CETP,* cholesterol ester transfer protein; *hs-CRP,* high-sensitivity C-reactive protein; *IL,* interleukin; *IMT,* Intimal-medial thickness; *LDL,* low-density lipoprotein; *Lp(a),* lipoprotein a; *Lp-PLA_2,* phospholipase A2; *MMP,* matrix metalloproteinase; *MPO,* myeloperoxidase; *PET,* positron emission tomography; *SAA,* serum amyloid A; *sCD40,* soluble CD40 ligand; *sICAM,* soluble intracellular adhesion molecule; *TIMP,* tissue inhibitor of metalloproteinase; *TPA/PAI,* tissue plasminogen activator/plasminogen activator inhibitor-1.

data with the calculated LDL is a potent way to predict risk. For risk stratification in primary prevention the use of routine hsCRP is not recommended by the AHA/CDC panel. When used, less than 1 mg/L is considered low risk, 1 to 3 mg/L intermediate risk, and more than 3 mg/L high risk.

In patients who present with ACS, the initial value for hsCRP has prognostic significance. Whether it is short or long term depends on the study. In most studies, the influence of cTn measurements is the predominant short-term prognostic factor, and hsCRP adds to long-term prognosis. However, this is not always the case. Of interest, hsCRP measurements, similar to BNP, seem to predict death, but not recurrent infarction. This could be true because of the effect of mortality, which can confound multivariable models, but it is different from the data related to cTn (see discussion in this chapter).[122] It should be appreciated that once necrosis has occurred, hsCRP values rise and the ability to use them prognostically is attenuated.

Serum Amyloid Protein A

Serum amyloid protein A, an acute-phase protein and an apolipoprotein, has been used with hsCRP in cross-sectional studies. It can be synergistic with hsCRP[511] but is much less commonly used. At present, no standardized assays, reference interval studies, nor consistent assay validations are available.

sCD40 Ligand

CD40 ligand is a transmembrane protein related to TNF. It has multiple prothrombotic and proatherogenic effects. What is usually measured is the soluble form of the receptor, sCD40 ligand, which has been shown to be a predictor of events after acute presentation.[512] At present, standardized assays, reference interval studies, or consistent assay validations are not available. Recent data raise substantial questions about the analytical stability in the samples that have been used to evaluate this particular marker.[513]

Cytokines

A variety of stimulatory and inhibitory interleukins (TNF, IL-1, IL-6, IL-8, IL-12, IL-18) are thought to help mediate the elaboration of CRP and the development of atherosclerosis and acute events.[514] These cytokines may stimulate or inhibit leukocytes, often through T cell–mediated processes and effects on monocytes, which are indigenous to atherogenesis.[515] In some studies, IL-6 is more prognostic than hsCRP. These cytokines often have inhibitors and/or binding proteins that modulate their effects. At present, standardized assays, reference intervals studies, and consistent assay validations are not available.

MYELOPEROXIDASE

Myeloperoxidase (MPO) is released when neutrophils aggregate; this may indicate an active inflammatory response in blood vessels. It has been shown to be elevated chronically when chronic coronary artery disease (CAD) is present.[516] It is increased when patients present with ACS.[517,518] Initial prognostic studies were encouraging but were done without adequate consideration of other analytes and specifically cTn. A multibiomarker study has shown that myeloperoxidase as a prognostic tool depended on the outcomes studied (cardiac

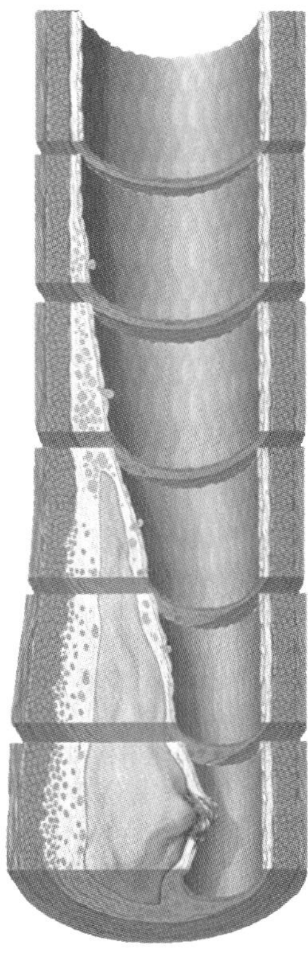

- Proinflammatory Cytokines
  - IL-6, TNFα
- Plaque Destabilization
  - MPO, MMPs, CAMs
- Plaque Rupture
  - sCD40L, PIGF, PAPP-A
- Acute Phase Reactants
  - hs-CRP, serum amyloid
- Ischemia
  - Choline, FFAu, copeptin, GPBB
- Necrosis
  - cTnT, cTnI, CKMB, myoglobin, FABP
- Myocardial Dysfunction/CHF
  - BNP, NT-proBNP, MR-proANP, proBNP, ST2, GDF-15, galactin

FIGURE 58.33 Complete spectrum of acute coronary pathophysiologic process from initiation of atherosclerosis to cell death to myocardial dysfunction. *BNP,* Brain natriuretic peptide; *CAM,* cellular adhesion molecule; *CHF,* congestive heart failure; *CK-MB,* myocardial-bound creatine kinase; *cTnI,* cardiac troponin I; *cTnT,* cardiac troponin T; *FFAu,* unbound free fatty acids; *FABP,* fatty acid binding protein; *GDF-15,* growth differentiation factor-15; *GPBB,* gycogen phosporylase BB; *hs-CRP,* high-sensitivity C-reactive protein; *IL,* interleukin; *MMP,* matrix metalloproteinases; *MPO,* myeloperoxidase; *MR-proBNP,* mid-range pro atrial natriuretic peptide; *NT-proBNP,* N-terminal pro-brain natriuretic peptide; *PAPP-A,* pregnancy-associated plasma protein A; *proBNP,* pro-brain natriuretic peptide; *sCD40L,* soluble CD40 ligand; *TNF-α,* tumor necrosis factor-alpha. (Modified from Apple F. Cardiac ischemia: where no biomarker has gone before. *Clin Lab News* 2009;35:8–10.)

death) and the demographics of the patient population enrolled.[519] Accordingly, additional studies are needed. At present, no standardized assays, reference interval studies, nor consistent assay validations are available. Further, it has been demonstrated that the type of specimen collected is critical for the stability and accurate measurement of myeloperoxidase.[520] For further information on this enzyme, see Chapter 29.

Lipoprotein-Associated Phospholipase A_2

Phospholipase A2 (Lp-PLA_2) is a phospholipase associated with LDL that is thought to be an inflammatory marker. It was previously known as platelet-activating factor acetyl hydrolase. It is synthesized by monocytes and lymphocytes and is thought to cleave oxidized lipids to produce lipid fragments that are more atherogenic and that increase endothelial adhesion. An FDA-approved assay for this analyte includes obligatory reference intervals. It has been shown to be predictive of events in a primary prevention cohort, even when hsCRP is present in the model, suggesting that it measures something different from what is measured by the acute-phase reactants associated with hsCRP.[521,522] The mass assay has significant preanalytical problems. An activity assay has just recently been approved which should help.[523] Unfortunately, recent trials with inhibitors have been null.[524-526]

Pregnancy-Associated Plasma Protein A

Pregnancy-associated plasma protein A (PAPP-A) is a metalloproteinase that is thought to be expressed in plaques that may be prone to rupture. It is most often bound to mature basic protein. The literature in this regard is mixed at present concerning its use.[527-529] At present, standardized assays, reference interval studies, and consistent assay validations are not available. Recent data suggest that heparin administration in MI patients is associated with increased PAPP-A concentrations; this may limit its prognostic role. Recent attempts to develop assays for the IGF fragments that may be more representative of free PAPP-A have been associated with variable results as well.[530,531]

Oxidized Low-Density Lipoprotein

Oxidized LDL has been attributed a key role in the development of atherosclerosis (see Chapter 34). Several methods have been used to measure it, but they yield potentially different data. Some have correlated malondialdehyde LDL with the development of atherosclerosis and short-term events.[532] Direct identification with antibodies suggests that oxidized

LDL may be released from vessels and may colocalize with lipoprotein a [Lp(a)] after acute events.[533]

Placental Growth Factor

Placental growth factor is an angiogenic factor related to vascular endothelial growth factor (VEGF), which stimulates smooth muscle cells and macrophages.[534,535] It also increases TNF and monocyte chemoattractant protein-1 (MCP-1). A novel assay for this analyte is thought to provide additional prognostic information on patients who present with ACS.[536] At present, standardized assays, reference interval studies, and consistent assay validations are not available.

Matrix Metalloproteinases

Matrix metalloproteinases (MMPs) can degrade the collagen matrix in coronary artery or myocardium. They are integral to remodeling of the coronary artery and/or the heart after acute events. Elaboration of MMP-9, a gelatinase, is thought to be important in plaque destabilization; thus some have tried to measure it as a prognostic index.[536] Other MMPs participate in the elaboration of extracellular matrix in the heart. Many MMPs also have inhibitors (tissue inhibitors of metalloproteinase [TIMPs]) that modulate their effects. At present, standardized assays, reference interval studies, and consistent assay validations are not available. Recent data suggest that this marker along with others may be helpful for evaluating patients with HF with preserved ejection fraction.[537]

Monocyte Chemotactic Protein

Monocyte chemotactic protein (MCP-1) is a chemokine that is thought to be responsible for the recruitment of monocytes into atherosclerotic plaque. It has been reported to be elevated in patients with ACS and to have long-term predictive value.[538] However, at present, standardized assays, reference interval studies, and consistent assay validations are not available.

Tissue Plasminogen Activator Antigen and Plasminogen Activator Inhibitor-1

Tissue plasminogen activator (t-PA) is the body's physiologic fibrinolytic activator. Plasminogen activator inhibitor-1 (PAI-1), its endogenous inhibitor, binds to t-PA (see Chapter 59). Inhibition of fibrinolysis has been suggested to be a reason for recurrent infarction; the fact that maximal inhibition usually occurs in the early morning hours provides a potential explanation for the circadian variability of AMI.[539] It may also be the reason why persons with diabetes have such unstable disease; the growth factor properties of insulin stimulate increases in PAI-1.[540] An accurate assessment of this system includes both t-PA and PAI-1, along with some assessment of bound versus free levels.

Soprostanes

Isoprostanes are the end breakdown products of lipid peroxidation, and urinary levels have been used to assess the level of oxidative stress.[541,542] It is thought that oxidation of LDL is essential for the development of atherosclerosis, and that high-density lipoprotein (HDL) and other antioxidants work by antagonizing this oxidative stress. Urinary isoprostanes give some assessment of this critical process. The most commonly measured are F_2-isoprostanes, but a large number of others are available for measurement. It does appear that they will eventually be helpful in assessing oxidative stress.

Urinary Thromboxane

Urinary thromboxane is the end metabolite of thromboxane A2, which is a measure of platelet aggregation. Urinary levels are elevated in patients with unstable coronary disease, in keeping with the known participation of platelets in the pathogenesis of CAD. This level is difficult to ascertain, and collecting urine in the acute situation is at times problematic. Recent data with a mass spectrometry assay that eliminates the measurement of the 2′3′component correlates far less well with ischemic heart disease, leading to questions about the value of this marker.

Adhesion Molecules

Adhesion molecules are a wide variety of molecules that can potentially be measured as a way of assessing the adherence of leukocytes, platelets, or other adhesive proteins to the endothelial matrix.[543] Some are receptors. Examples include platelet-endothelial adhesion molecule 1 (PECAM-1), P-selectin, E-selectin, and VCAM-1 (vascular cell adhesion molecule 1). At times, the receptor itself is measured, but often it is a soluble portion that circulates that is measured. At present, standardized assays, reference interval studies, and consistent assay validations are not available.

Choline

Choline is released after stimulation by phospholipase D and has been touted as a test of prognosis in patients with chest discomfort.[544] At present, standardized assays, reference interval studies, and consistent assay validations are not available.

Unbound Free Fatty Acid

Unbound free fatty acid (uFFA)[536] has been touted as a marker of ischemia. Most fatty acid is bound, and ischemia is thought to increase the small unbound fraction. Initial studies have reported mixed results. At present, standardized assays, reference interval studies, and consistent assay validations are not available.

Nourin

Nourin I is a small protein released rapidly by stressed myocytes. It induces changes in a variety of inflammatory cytokines and attracts neutrophils. Preliminary studies have been done to attempt to validate its use. At present, standardized assays, reference interval studies, and consistent assay validations are not available.

SELECTED REFERENCES

For a full list of references for this chapter, please refer to ExpertConsult.com.

2. Thygesen K, Alpert JS, Jaffe AS, et al. Third universal definition of myocardial infarction. *J Am Coll Cardiol* 2012;**60**:1581–98.
17. Maisel AS, Krishnaswamy P, Nowak RM, et al. Rapid measurement of B-type natriuretic peptide in the emergency diagnosis of heart failure. *N Engl J Med* 2002;**347**:161–7.
21. Roberts R, Henry PD, Sobel BE. An improved basis for enzymatic estimation of infarct size. *Circulation* 1975;**52**:743–54.

60. Katrukha AG, Bereznikova AV, Esakova TV, et al. Troponin I is released in bloodstream of patients with acute myocardial infarction not in free form but as complex. *Clin Chem* 1997;**43**:1379–85.
63. Bodor GS, Porter S, Landt Y, et al. Development of monoclonal antibodies for an assay of cardiac troponin-I and preliminary results in suspected cases of myocardial infarction. *Clin Chem* 1992;**38**:2203–14.
87. Morrow DA, Cannon CP, Jesse RL, et al. National Academy of Clinical Biochemistry Laboratory Medicine Practice Guidelines: clinical characteristics and utilization of biochemical markers in acute coronary syndromes. *Clin Chem* 2007;**53**:552–74.
92. Apple FS, Ler R, Murakami MM. Determination of 19 cardiac troponin I and T assay 99th percentile values from a common presumably healthy population. *Clin Chem* 2012;**58**:1574–81.
124. Shah AS, Griffiths M, Lee KK, et al. High sensitivity cardiac troponin and the under-diagnosis of myocardial infarction in women: prospective cohort study. *BMJ* 2015;**350**:g7873.
156. Sandoval Y, Thordsen SE, Smith SW, et al. Cardiac troponin changes to distinguish type 1 and type 2 myocardial infarction and 180-day mortality risk. *Eur Heart J Acute Cardiovasc Care* 2014;**3**:317–25.
190. Than M, Cullen L, Aldous S, et al. 2-Hour accelerated diagnostic protocol to assess patients with chest pain symptoms using contemporary troponins as the only biomarker: the ADAPT trial. *J Am Coll Cardiol* 2012;**59**:2091–8.
194. Cullen L, Mueller C, Parsonage WA, et al. Validation of high-sensitivity troponin I in a 2-hour diagnostic strategy to assess 30-day outcomes in emergency department patients with possible acute coronary syndrome. *J Am Coll Cardiol* 2013;**62**:1242–9.
199. Shah AS, Anand A, Sandoval Y, et al. High-sensitivity cardiac troponin I at presentation in patients with suspected acute coronary syndrome: a cohort study. *Lancet* 2015;**386**:2481–8.
244. Omland T, de Lemos JA, Sabatine MS, et al. A sensitive cardiac troponin T assay in stable coronary artery disease. *N Engl J Med* 2009;**361**:2538–47.
397. Apple FS, Panteghini M, Ravkilde J, et al. Quality specifications for B-type natriuretic peptide assays. *Clin Chem* 2005;**51**:486–93.
430. Januzzi JL, van Kimmenade R, Lainchbury J, et al. NT-proBNP testing for diagnosis and short-term prognosis in acute destabilized heart failure: an international pooled analysis of 1256 patients: the International Collaborative of NT-proBNP Study. *Eur Heart J* 2006;**27**:330–7.
432. Tang WH, Francis GS, Morrow DA, et al. National Academy of Clinical Biochemistry Laboratory Medicine practice guidelines: clinical utilization of cardiac biomarker testing in heart failure. *Circulation* 2007;**116**:e99–109.
501. Ridker PM. Clinical application of C-reactive protein for cardiovascular disease detection and prevention. *Circulation* 2003;**107**:363–9.

ADDITIONAL READING

Apple FS, Blankenburg S, Morrow D. Impact of clinical markers, proteomics and genomics in cardiovascular disease. *Clin Chem*, Special Issue, January 2012.

59

Kidney Disease

*Michael P. Delaney and Edmund J. Lamb**

ABSTRACT

Background
The kidneys play a central role in homeostasis, and reduced renal function strongly correlates with increasing morbidity and mortality. Laboratory investigations are central to the diagnosis and management of kidney disease, and investigations of kidney function constitute a significant element of the workload of most clinical laboratories.

Content
This chapter describes the basic anatomy and physiology of the kidneys as a foundation for understanding the pathophysiology of disease and the rationale for diagnostic and management strategies in kidney disease. Classification and management of both acute and chronic kidney diseases are described, including detailed examination of the major complications (cardiovascular, mineral and bone, electrolyte, anemia) and causes (genetic, diabetes, hypertension, renovascular, glomerular and tubular diseases, myeloma, nephrolithiasis) of kidney disease. The chapter ends with a detailed description of renal replacement therapy (dialysis and transplantation). Wherever possible, throughout the chapter statements are based on the most current clinical trial evidence or published expert guidelines and national registry data.

The kidneys play a central role in the homeostatic mechanisms of the human body, and reduced renal function strongly correlates with increasing morbidity and mortality. Biochemical investigations, both routine and specialized, are an important part of the clinician's diagnostic armamentarium, and investigations of kidney function constitute a significant element of the workload of most laboratories. The aim of this chapter is to ensure that the clinical chemist/biochemist understands the perspective of the nephrologist when dealing with laboratory investigations for patients with kidney disease. The basic anatomy and physiology of the kidneys are described as a foundation for understanding the pathophysiology of disease and the rationale for diagnostic and management strategies in kidney disease. Key analytical methods employed during the investigation of kidney disease are dealt with in Chapter 32.

ANATOMY

The kidneys form a paired organ system located in the retroperitoneal space. They extend from the level of the lower part of the 11th thoracic vertebra to the upper portion of the 3rd lumbar vertebra, with the right kidney situated slightly lower than the left. The adult kidney is about 12 cm long and weighs about 150 g (Fig. 59.1). The kidneys have both sympathetic and parasympathetic nerve supplies, whose function appears to be predominantly associated with vasomotor activity. The renal lymphatic drainage includes fine lymphatics in the glomerulus, some in close proximity to the juxtaglomerular apparatus (JGA[†]), which are associated with removal of material from the glomerular mesangial cells.

Blood Supply

In most cases, each kidney receives its blood supply from a single renal artery derived from the abdominal aorta. However, multiple renal arteries occur commonly. The renal artery divides into posterior and anterior elements, and ultimately into the afferent arterioles, which expand into the highly specialized capillary beds that form the glomeruli (Fig. 59.2). These capillaries then rejoin to form the efferent arteriole that then forms the capillary plexuses and the elongated vessels (the *vasa recta*) that pass around the remaining parts of the nephron, the proximal and distal tubules, the loop of Henle, and the collecting duct, providing oxygen and nutrients and removing ions, molecules, and water, which have been reabsorbed by the nephron. The efferent arteriole then merges with renal venules to form the renal veins, which merge into the inferior vena cava.

*We are grateful for the data supplied by the United States Renal Data System (USRDS). The interpretation and reporting of these data are the responsibility of the authors and in no way should be seen as an official policy or interpretation of the US government. We are also grateful for data supplied by the United Kingdom Renal Registry. The interpretation and reporting of these data are the responsibility of the authors and in no way should be seen as an official policy or interpretation of the UK Renal Registry. We also acknowledge the input of Professor Christopher Price to previous editions of this chapter.

[†]For a complete list of abbreviations used in this chapter, please refer to ExpertConsult.com.

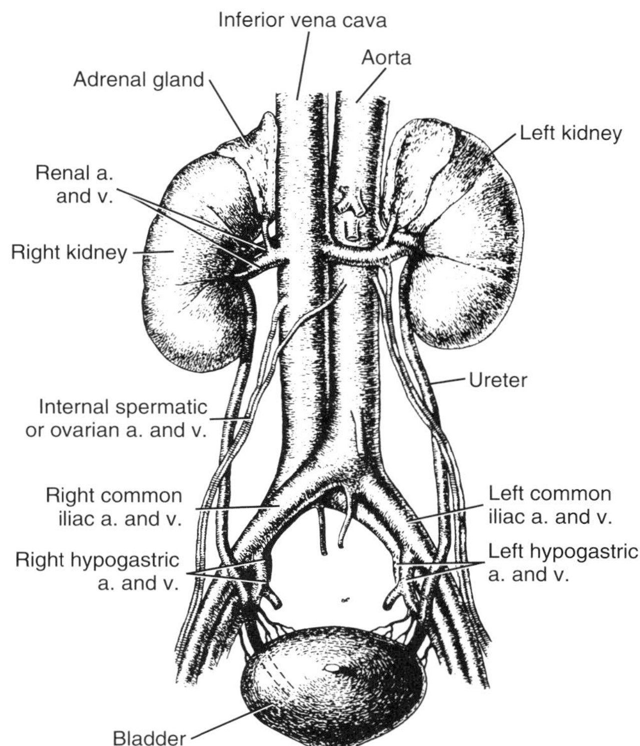

FIGURE 59.1 Vascular and anatomic relationships of the kidneys in man. (From Leaf A, Cotran RS. *Renal pathophysiology*. 3rd ed. Oxford: Oxford University Press, 1985. Reproduced by permission of Oxford University Press.)

In adults, the kidneys receive approximately 25% of the cardiac output, about 90% of which supplies the renal cortex, maintaining the highly active tubular cells. Maintenance of renal blood flow is essential to kidney function, and a complex array of intrarenal regulatory mechanisms ensure that it is maintained across a wide range of systemic blood pressures (see discussion later in this chapter). The renal glomerular perfusion pressure is maintained at a constant 45 mm Hg across systemic pressures between 90 and 200 mm Hg.

Nephron

The functional unit of the kidney is the *nephron*. Each kidney has been reported to contain between 600,000 and 1.5 million nephrons.[1] The number of nephrons that an individual is born with (the "nephron dose") may determine that individual's susceptibility to renal injury. The nephron consists of a glomerulus, proximal tubule, loop of Henle, distal tubule, and collecting duct (see Fig. 59.2). The collecting ducts ultimately combine to develop into the renal calyces, where the urine collects before passing along the ureter and into the bladder. The kidney is divided into several lobes. The outer, darker region of each lobe—the cortex—consists of most of the glomeruli and the proximal and distal tubules. The cortex surrounds a paler inner region—the medulla—which is further divided into a number of conical areas known as the renal pyramids, the apex of which extends toward the renal pelvis, forming papillae. Medullary rays are visible striations in the renal pyramids that connect the kidney cortex with the medulla. They are composed of descending (straight proximal) and ascending (straight distal) thick limbs of Henle and collecting ducts and associated blood vessels (the vasa recta). The central hilus is where blood vessels, lymphatics, and the renal pelvis (containing the ureter) join the kidney.

Glomerulus

The glomerulus is formed from a specialized capillary network. Each capillary develops into approximately 40 glomerular loops around 200 µm in size and consisting of a variety of different cell types supported on a specialized basement membrane (Fig. 59.3A). Some endothelial and epithelial cells act in concert with the specialized glomerular basement membrane (GBM) to form the glomerular filtration barrier, in addition to mesangial cells.

The *capillary endothelial* cells are about 40 nm thick and are in contact with one another. However, in contrast to the continuous endothelial linings seen elsewhere in the body, circular fenestrations (pores) with diameters of approximately 60 nm collectively constitute 20% to 50% of the glomerular endothelial surface.[2] The endothelium permits virtually free access of plasma and small solutes to the basement membrane. However, although the fenestrations are far larger than the diameter of albumin (3.5 nm), it is thought that permselectivity to such larger molecules begins at the level of the endothelium because of the endothelial surface lining—a glycocalyx coating of negatively charged glycoproteins, glycosaminoglycans, proteoglycans, and absorbed plasma proteins, including orosomucoid and albumin. Estimates of the thickness of this layer vary depending on the visualization and preparation techniques used, but it may be between 200 and 400 nm thick.[2]

The *basement membrane* (Fig. 59.3B) of the glomerular capillaries is much thicker (approximately 300 nm) than that of other vascular beds and consists of three distinct electron-dense layers: the *lamina rara interna*, the *lamina densa*, and the *lamina rara externa*. The lamina densa consists of a close feltwork of fine, mainly type IV, collagen fibrils (each 3 to 5 nm thick) embedded in a gel-like matrix of laminin, nidogen/entactin, glycoproteins, and proteoglycans such as agrin and perlecan. The lamina densa forms the main size discriminant barrier to protein passage into the tubular lumen. The other two layers of the basement membrane are rich in negatively charged polyanionic glycoproteins, such as heparan sulfate; these may form a charge discriminant barrier to the passage of proteins, although the importance of the GBM in charge discrimination is still uncertain.[2]

The *epithelial cells* of the glomerulus line the outside of the glomerular capillaries, thus facing Bowman's capsule and the primary urine (see Fig. 59.3A). These cells are called *podocytes* and have an unusual octopus-like structure in that they have a large number of cytoplasmic extensions or foot processes that are embedded in the basement membrane. Foot processes are anchored to the GBM via integrin molecules and dystroglycans and are divided into primary and secondary. The secondary processes between adjacent cells interdigitate to form filtration slits, which are 25 to 60 nm wide.[2] The podocytes are covered by a complex diaphragm ("slit diaphragm"), some of the molecular components of which (eg, nephrin) appear crucial for the maintenance of larger proteins within the circulation. The resulting structure is relatively impermeable to most proteins above 60 kDa, but passage of proteins is modulated by their charge and shape. Podocytes are also covered by a glycocalyx of sulfated molecules, including

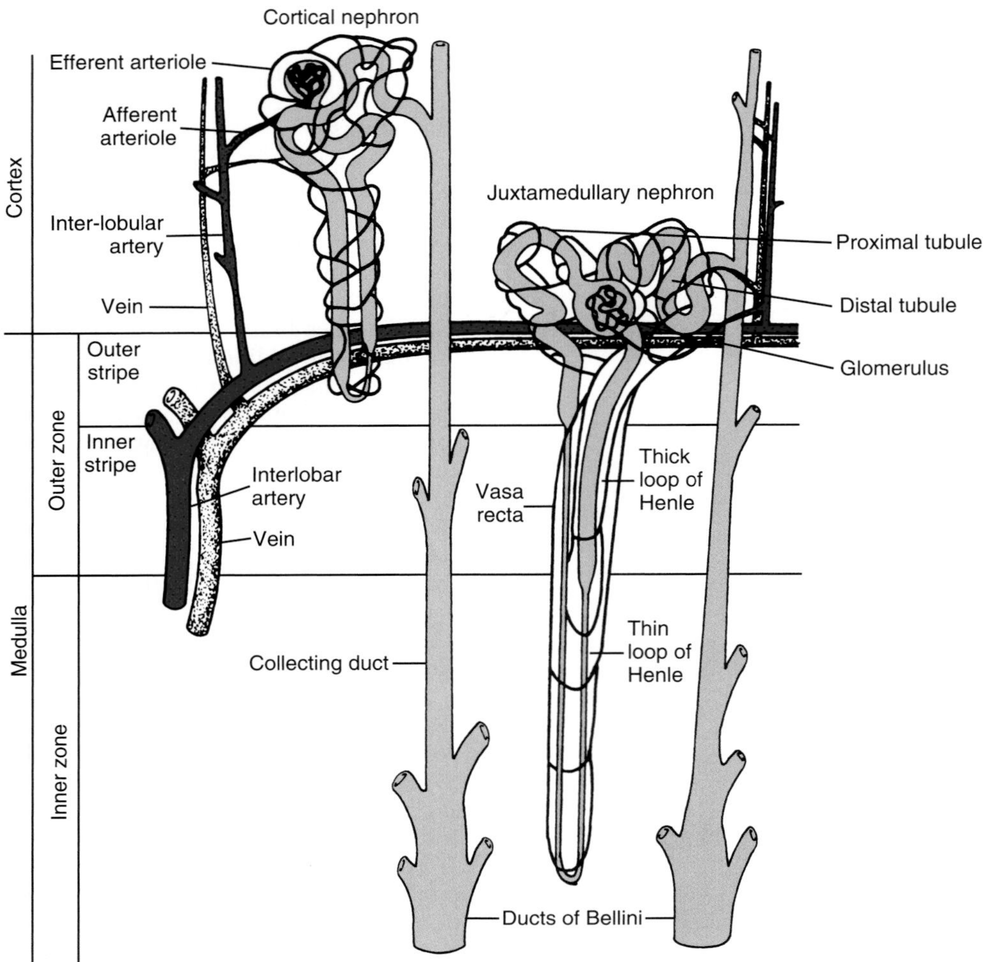

FIGURE 59.2 Diagrammatic representation of the nephron, the functional unit of the kidney, illustrating the anatomic and vascular arrangements. (From Pitts RF: *Physiology of the kidney and body fluids.* 3rd ed. Chicago: Year Book Medical Publishers, 1974:8p.)

FIGURE 59.3 The glomerular cells and the glomerular filtration barrier. **A,** Longitudinal section through a glomerulus and its juxtaglomerular apparatus. The capillary tuft consists of a network of specialized capillaries, which are outlined by a fenestrated endothelium (E). At the vascular pole, the afferent arteriole (AA) enters, branching into capillaries immediately after its entrance; the efferent arteriole (EA) is established inside the tuft and passes through the glomerular stalk before leaving at the vascular pole. The capillary network and the mesangium are enclosed in a common compartment bounded by the glomerular basement membrane (GBM). Note that there is no basement membrane at the interface between the capillary endothelium and the mesangium. The glomerular visceral epithelium consists of highly branched podocytes (POs), which, in a typical interdigitating pattern, cover the outer aspect of the GBM. At the vascular pole, the visceral epithelium and the GBM are reflected into the parietal epithelium (PE) of the Bowman capsule, which passes over into the epithelium of the proximal tubule (PT) at the urinary pole. At the vascular pole, the glomerular mesangium is continuous with the extraglomerular mesangium (EGM), which consists of extraglomerular mesangial cells and an extraglomerular mesangial matrix. The EGM and the granular cells (G) of the afferent arteriole, along with the macula densa (MD), establish the juxtaglomerular apparatus. All cells that are suggested to be of smooth muscle origin are shown in black. **B,** Glomerular capillary wall. In glomerular filtration, filtered fluid is believed to traverse the capillary wall via an extracellular route—that is, through endothelial fenestrae, basement membrane, and slit diaphragms. Circulating polyanions (eg, albumin) are thought to be retarded by the rich distribution in inner barriers of negatively charged sialylated glycoproteins (*shaded area* in schematic diagram) and by the slit diaphragms formed from adjacent interdigitating podocyte cells (see main text). *F,* Foot processes; *M,* messenger cells; *N,* sympathetic nerve terminals; *US,* urinary space. (**A,** from Elger M, Kriz W. The renal glomerulus—the structural basis of ultrafiltration. In: Cameron JS, Davison AM, Grunfeld JP, Kerr D, Ritz E, eds. *Oxford Textbook of Clinical Nephrology (vol. 1).* 2nd ed. Oxford: Oxford University Press, 1998: Chapter 3.1. Reproduced by permission of Oxford University Press. **B,** from Brenner BM, Beeuwkes R, III. The kidney in health and disease: III. The renal circulations. *Hospital Practice* 1978;13:35–46.)

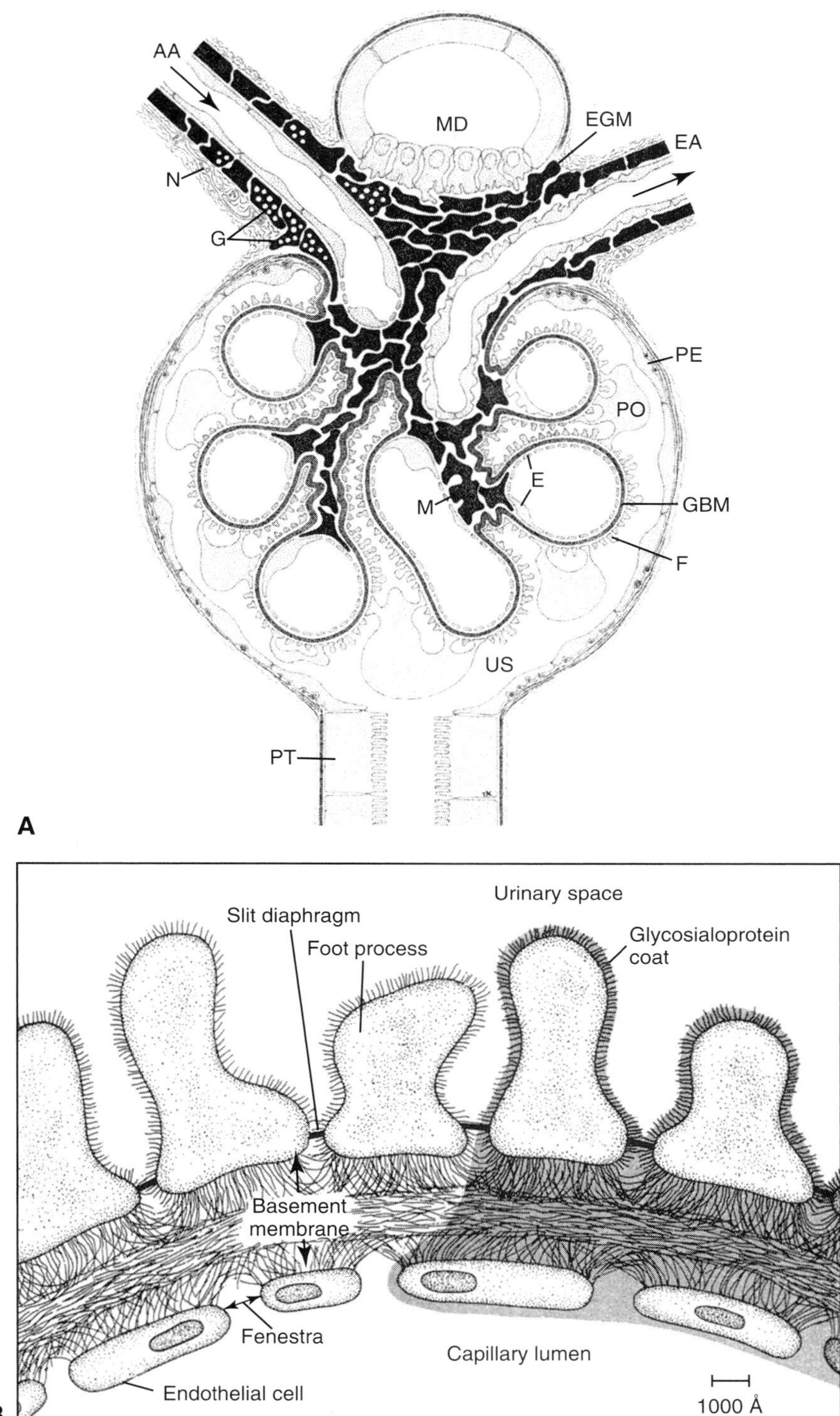

glycosaminoglycans and glycoconjugates (eg, podocalyxin). The surface anionic charge helps to maintain the foot process structure and the distance between the parietal and visceral epithelial cells constituting Bowman's space.

The final cellular components of the glomerulus are the *mesangial cells,* which are found in the central part ("stalk") of the glomerulus between and within the capillary loops suspended in a matrix that they synthesize. They are in direct contact with glomerular endothelial cells and the inner layer of the GBM (lamina rara interna) and also with the extraglomerular mesangium and the JGA (see Fig. 59.3A). Mesangial cells have the characteristics of smooth muscle

TABLE 59.1 Metabolic Functions of the Different Parts of the Nephron

	Proximal		Loop of Henle		Distal Tubule		Collecting Duct	
Molecule	**R**	**S**	**R**	**S**	**R**	**S**	**R**	**S**
Urea	+			(+)			+	
Proteins	+							
Peptides	+							
Phosphate	+							
Sulfate	+							
Organic anions			+					
Urate	+	+						
Sodium	+		+		+		+	
Chloride	+		+		+		+	
Water	+		+				+	
Potassium	+		+	(+)		+	+	
Hydrogen ion		+		+		+	+	+
Bicarbonate	+		+		+		+	+
Ammonium		+	+					+
Calcium	+		+		+		+	

R, Reabsorption; *S,* secretion; + indicates function; (+) indicates partial function.

cells (pericytes), in that they are rich in microfilaments and respond to and produce a variety of stimuli (eg, angiotensin II [AII] and arginine vasopressin [antidiuretic hormone; ADH]).[3] Mesangial matrix is rich in collagens and proteoglycans but is different in composition from the matrix of the GBM. Its composition and volume are tightly regulated in health but can be markedly altered during certain diseases (eg, diabetic nephropathy, immunoglobulin (Ig)A nephropathy). Mesangial cells have both structural and housekeeping functions. They have anchoring filaments to GBM opposite the podocytes, and their contractile properties enable them to alter intraglomerular capillary flow and glomerular ultrafiltration surface area, and thereby single nephron glomerular filtration rate (GFR). The cells appear to respond to capillary stretch by generating soluble factors such as vascular endothelial growth factor and transforming growth factor-β (TGF-β) and by activating intracellular signaling pathways. Mesangial cells also have specific and nonspecific mechanisms for removing macromolecules that reach the mesangial and subendothelial space, preventing their accumulation. These mechanisms include phagocytosis and degradation by the cells and trafficking along the mesangial stalk to the juxtaglomerular region, followed by elimination via the renal lymphatics or by regurgitation into the glomerular capillary.

Proximal Tubule

The Bowman capsule forms the beginning of the tightly coiled, proximal convoluted tubule *(pars convoluta)*, which on its progress toward the renal medulla becomes straightened and is then called the *pars recta.* The proximal tubule is about 15 mm long. The epithelial cells lining the convoluted section are cuboidal/columnar cells with a luminal brush border consisting of millions of microvilli, which expand the surface area for absorption of tubular fluid. The proximal tubule is the most metabolically active part of the nephron (Table 59.1).

Loop of Henle

The pars recta drains into the descending thin loop of Henle, which after passing through a hairpin loop becomes first the thin ascending limb and then the thick ascending limb. The cells of the thin ascending limb are very similar to those in the descending (with little brush border, flattened and interdigitated), but important differences are evident in their permeability to water and in their capability for active transport. The thick ascending limb is lined with cuboidal/columnar cells similar in size to those in the proximal tubule, but they do not possess a brush border. At the end of the thick ascending limb, near where it reenters the cortex and closely associates with the glomerulus and the efferent arteriole, a cluster of cells known as the *macula densa* is present (Fig. 59.4). The main role of the loop of Henle is to assist in generating concentrated urine, hypertonic with respect to plasma; it also has several other functions (see Table 59.1).

Distal Convoluted Tubule

The distal convoluted tubule begins at a variable distance beyond the macula densa and extends to the first fusion with other tubules to form the collecting ducts. The cells of the distal convoluted tubule are tall and cuboidal and contain numerous mitochondria. Na, K-ATPase activity is higher than in any other segment of the nephron, being located in the basolateral membrane and providing the main driving force for ion transport. Reabsorption of sodium and chloride, with passive reabsorption of water, is the main function of the distal convoluted tubule (see later).

Collecting Duct

The collecting ducts are formed from approximately six distal tubules. These are successively joined by other tubules to form the ducts of Bellini, which ultimately drain into a renal calyx. Two main cell types are found in the collecting duct: principal

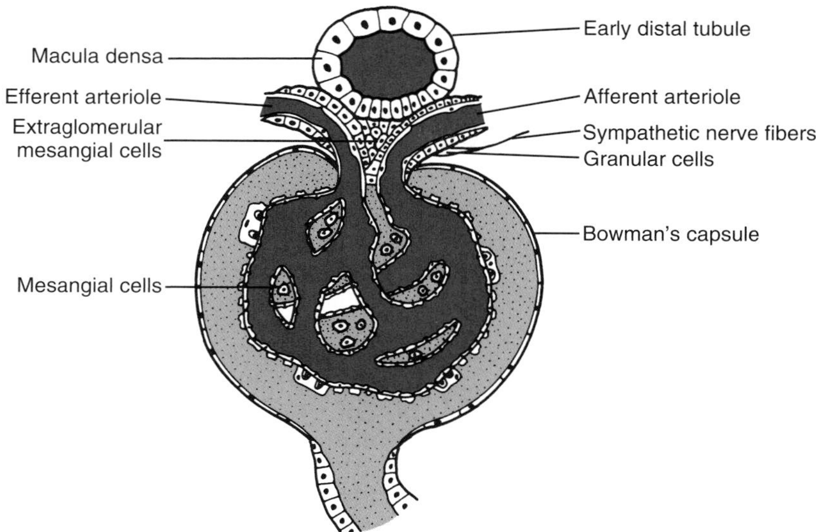

FIGURE 59.4 The juxtaglomerular apparatus. The beginning of the distal tubule (ie, where the loop of Henle reenters the cortex) lies very close to the afferent and efferent arterioles, and the cells of both the afferent arteriole and the tubule show specialization. The cells of the afferent arteriole are thickened, granular (juxtaglomerular) cells that are innervated by sympathetic nerve fibers. The mesangial cells are irregularly shaped and contain filaments of contractile proteins. Identical cells are found just outside the glomerulus and are termed *extraglomerular mesangial cells* or *Goormaghtigh cells*. (From Lote CJ. *Principles of renal physiology*. 4th ed. London: Kluwer Academic Publishers, 2000:Chapter 2.)

(light) cells and intercalated (dark) cells. Intercalated cells have a dark granular cytoplasm with high carbonic anhydrase activity but no Na, K-ATPase activity.

Juxtaglomerular Apparatus

Where the thick ascending limb of the loop of Henle passes very close to the glomerulus of its own nephron, the cells of the tubule and the afferent arteriole show regional specialization (see Fig. 59.4). The tubule forms the macula densa; the arteriolar cells are filled with granules (containing renin or its inactive precursor, prorenin) and are innervated with sympathetic nerve fibers. This area, called the JGA, plays an important part in maintaining systemic blood pressure through regulation of the circulating intravascular blood volume and sodium concentration via the renin-angiotensin-aldosterone system (RAAS). The proteolytic enzyme renin is released primarily in response to decreased afferent arteriolar pressure and decreased intraluminal sodium delivery to the macula densa. Renin is an enzyme of the hydrolase class that catalyzes cleavage of the leucine-leucine bond in angiotensinogen to generate angiotensin I. Renin release from the macula densa is also influenced by nitric oxide, renal cortical prostaglandins (predominantly PGI_2), and the sympathetic nervous system. Angiotensin I is converted in the lungs by angiotensin-converting enzyme (ACE) to the potent vasoconstrictor and stimulator of aldosterone release, AII. Vasoconstriction and aldosterone release (with increased distal tubular sodium retention) act in concert with the other action of AII to increase the release of the nonapeptide vasopressin and to increase proximal tubular sodium reabsorption, intravascular volume and pressure. AII also has an inhibitory effect on renin release as part of a negative feedback loop.

Renal Interstitium

In a normal renal cortex, the interstitium is sparse (7% to 9% by volume) because the tubules lie very close together; however, a large proportion of the reabsorbed tubular fluid has to traverse a true interstitial space before entering the capillaries. The interstitium contains a variety of cell types, including lymphocytes and fibroblast-like cells.[4]

The medullary interstitium contains a further specialized cell—lipid-laden interstitial cells—which are arranged in a characteristic ladder-like pattern across the loop of Henle and the capillaries. The extracellular space is rich in glycosaminoglycans, resulting in a gelatinous matrix that contains various poorly characterized osmolytes, osmotically active molecules that help stabilize the high osmotic gradient essential to the countercurrent mechanism involved in the generation of hyperosmotic urine. The interstitium becomes very important in a variety of kidney diseases, and its expansion, as a consequence or cause of nephron loss, plays an important part in progressive kidney disease. Interstitial expansion includes cellular infiltration and increased interstitial matrix synthesis and interstitial fibrosis.

KIDNEY FUNCTION AND PHYSIOLOGY

The kidneys regulate and maintain the constant optimal chemical composition of the blood and the interstitial and intracellular fluids throughout the body—the internal milieu—through integration of the major renal functions—namely filtration, reabsorption, and excretion. Mechanisms of differential reabsorption and secretion, located in the tubule of a nephron, are the effectors of regulation (Table 59.2).

TABLE 59.2 Important Components of Kidney Function

Function	Examples
Filtration	Preparation of an ultrafiltrate
Reabsorptive	Glucose, amino acids, electrolytes, proteins
Homeostatic	Extracellular volume, acid-base status, blood pressure, electrolytes
Metabolic	Synthetic: glutathione, glyconeogenesis, ammonia
	Catabolic: hormones, cytokines
Endocrine	Erythropoietin synthesis, activation of vitamin D, renin release

Excretory and Reabsorptive Functions

The *excretory function* of the kidneys serves to rid the body of many end products of metabolism and of excessive inorganic substances ingested in the diet. Waste products include the nonprotein nitrogenous compounds urea, creatinine, and uric acid; a number of other organic acids, including amino acids, are excreted in small quantities. Dietary intake contains a variable and usually excessive supply of sodium, potassium, chloride, calcium, phosphate, magnesium, sulfate, and bicarbonate. The efficiency of the homeostatic role of kidney function is illustrated by the way the sodium content of the body is maintained essentially constant, regardless of whether daily sodium intake is 1 or 150 mmol or more. Daily intake of water is also variable and may, on occasion, greatly exceed the requirements of the body. Under such circumstances, water becomes additional waste material requiring excretion. To achieve excretion of metabolic wastes and ingested surpluses without disrupting homeostasis, the kidneys must exercise both their *excretory* and *reabsorptive* functions.

Mechanisms for the regulation of electrolytes, nitrogenous wastes, and organic acids are similar, although not identical. For all except potassium and hydrogen ions and a few organic acids, the maximal excretory rate is limited or established by their plasma concentrations and the rate of their filtration through the glomeruli. Bulk transfer of substances from blood to glomerular filtrate determines the initial mass on which the nephron must operate to produce and excrete urine. Thus the maximal amount of substance excreted in urine does not exceed the amount transferred through the glomeruli by ultrafiltration, except in the case of those substances capable of being secreted by tubular cells. Depending on the activity of the renal tubular epithelial cells and their several reabsorptive capacities, excreted amounts of urinary constituents are in general less than the amounts filtered. Because of this general behavior, for many substances an estimate of the excretory capacity of the kidneys can be obtained by measuring the GFR or some variable that is closely related to it. The primary objective in evaluating renal excretory function is to detect quantitatively the degradation of normal capacities or the improvement of impaired ones.

Definitions

Urine is defined as a fluid excreted by the kidneys, passed through the ureters, stored in the bladder, and discharged through the urethra. In health, it is sterile and clear and has an amber color, a slightly acid pH (approximately 5.0–6.0), and a characteristic odor. In addition to dissolved compounds, it contains a number of cellular fragments and complete cells, derived from normal turnover of tubular cells, casts, and crystals (formed elements). Urinary casts are cylindrical proteinaceous structures formed in the distal convoluted tubule and collecting ducts, which dislodge and pass into the urine, where they can be detected by microscopy.

Urination, also termed *micturition,* is the discharge of urine. In normal adults, adequate homeostasis is maintained with a urine output of 400 to 2000 mL/d. Alterations in urinary output are described as *anuria* (<100 mL/d), *oliguria* (<400 mL/d), or *polyuria* (>3 L/d or 50 mL/kg body weight/d). The most common disorder of micturition is altered frequency, which may be associated with increased urinary volume or with partial urinary tract obstruction (eg, in prostatic hypertrophy).

Formation of Urine—an Overview

The first step in urine formation is filtration of plasma water at the glomeruli. A net filtration pressure of about 17 mm Hg in the capillary bed of the tuft drives the filtrate through the glomerular membrane. The filtrate is called an *ultrafiltrate* because its composition is essentially the same as that of plasma but with a notable reduction in molecules of molecular weight exceeding 15 kDa. Each nephron produces about 100 μL of ultrafiltrate per day. Overall, approximately 170 to 200 L of ultrafiltrate passes through the glomeruli daily. In the passage of ultrafiltrate through the tubules, reabsorption of solutes and water in various regions of the tubules reduces the total urine volume.

Transport of solutes and water occurs both across and between the epithelial cells that line the renal tubules. Transport is both active (energy requiring) and passive, but many of the so-called passive transport processes are dependent on or secondary to active transport processes, particularly those involving sodium transport. All known transport processes involve receptor or mediator molecules, the activity of many of which is regulated by phosphorylation facilitated by protein kinase C or A. Their renal distribution has been shown to correlate with known regional functional activities, but the same transporters, or isoforms of them, can be found in other tissues, particularly the digestive tract. For instance, at least five independent proximal tubular transport processes may be noted for amino acids, including those for basic amino acids plus cystine, glutamic and aspartic acid, neutral amino acids, imino amino acids, and glycine.[5] Inherited disorders of tubular transporters, discussed later in this chapter, may occur, as well as a well-known generalized disorder affecting all of the transport processes, causing Fanconi syndrome and resulting in decreased reabsorption of electrolytes and nutrients (eg, glucose, amino acids).

Direct coupling of adenosine triphosphate (ATP) hydrolysis is an example of an active transport process. The most important enzymatic transporter in the nephron is Na, K-ATPase, which is located on the basolateral membranes of the tubuloepithelial cells. Na, K-ATPase accounts for much of renal oxygen consumption and drives more than 99% of renal sodium reabsorption (Fig. 59.5). Other examples of primary active transport mechanisms include a Ca-ATPase, an H-ATPase, and an H, K-ATPase. These enzymes establish ionic gradients, polarizing cell membranes and thus driving secondary transport processes.

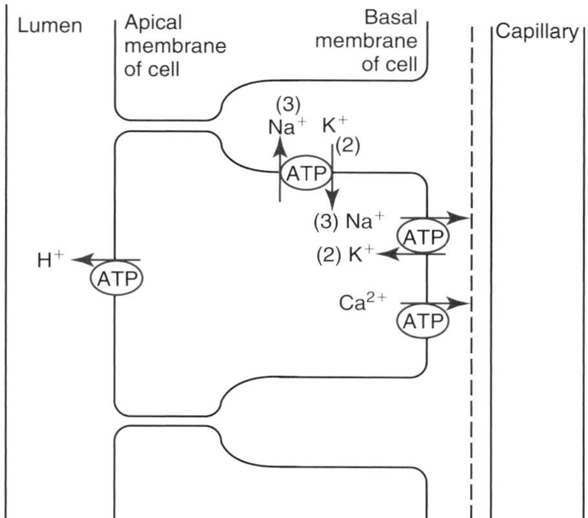

FIGURE 59.5 Tubular reabsorptive mechanisms: the major primary active transport processes in the proximal nephron. The renal tubular epithelium consists of a single layer of cells. At the luminal side, adjacent cells are in contact (the tight junction), whereas toward the basal side of the cells, there are gaps between adjacent cells (lateral intercellular spaces). (From Lote CJ. *Principles of renal physiology*. 4th ed. London: Kluwer Academic Publishers, 2000:Chapter 4.)

Many renal epithelial cell membranes also contain proteins that act as ion channels. For example, there is one for sodium that is closed by amiloride and modulated by hormones such as atrial natriuretic peptide (ANP). Ion channels enable much faster rates of transport than ATPases but are relatively fewer in number—for example, approximately 100 sodium and chloride channels versus 10^7 Na, K-ATPase molecules per cell.

Different regions of the tubule have been shown to specialize in certain functions. The proximal tubule facilitates the reabsorption of 60% to 80% of the glomerular filtrate volume—including 70% of the filtered load of sodium and chloride, and most of the potassium, glucose, bicarbonate, calcium, phosphate, sulfate, and other ions—and secreting 90% of the hydrogen ion excreted by the kidney (see Table 59.1). Glucose is virtually completely reabsorbed, predominantly in the proximal tubule by a passive but sodium-dependent process that is saturated at a blood glucose concentration of about 180 mg/dL (10 mmol/L). Uric acid is also reabsorbed in the proximal tubule by a passive sodium-dependent mechanism, but there is also an active secretory mechanism. Creatinine is secreted but only to a small extent—approximately 2.5 µmol/min.

Certain nonbiological compounds, such as phenolsulfonphthalein and *p*-aminohippurate, are secreted by the proximal tubule and have been used for the evaluation of renal tubular secretory capacity. When blood concentrations of creatinine increase above normal, creatinine is secreted in this region of the nephron. In the loop of Henle, chloride and more sodium without water are reabsorbed, generating dilute urine. Water reabsorption in the more distal tubules and collecting ducts is then regulated by vasopressin. In the distal tubule, secretion is the prominent activity; organic ions, potassium ions, and hydrogen ions are transported from the blood in the efferent arteriole into the tubular fluid.

Tubular epithelial cells synthesize a vast range of growth factors and cytokines in response to a variety of stimuli that can have both autocrine and paracrine effects. All cells secrete a range of cell adhesion molecules that are essential for cellular attachment to the tubular basement membrane.

Regulatory Function

Electrolyte Homeostasis

A complex interplay has been noted between the tubular transport systems regulating individual electrolytes. For simplicity, we have considered each electrolyte individually and have restricted our discussion to the systems of major physiologic, pharmacologic, and pathologic significance.

Sodium. Sodium reabsorption is required for the reabsorption of water and many solutes. The proximal tubule is highly permeable to sodium, and the net flux of reabsorption from the tubular lumen is achieved against a high backflux, particularly from paracellular (transport that occurs between tubular epithelial cells by passive diffusion or solvent drag) movement. Approximately 60% of filtered sodium is reabsorbed in the proximal tubule in an energy-dependent manner, driven by basolateral Na, K-ATPase pumps. Approximately 80% of sodium entering proximal tubular cells does so in exchange for hydrogen ion secretion, facilitated by apical Na-H exchangers. This process in turn permits bicarbonate reabsorption via carbonic anhydrases that are present in both the brush border and the intracellular compartment. A variety of apical sodium cotransporters also allow for reabsorption of other organic and inorganic solutes (eg, chloride, calcium, phosphates, bicarbonate, sulfates,[6] glucose, urea, amino acids). Sodium transport activity is regulated by many factors, including protein kinase–dependent phosphorylation, which can increase both activity and channel numbers.

A further 30% of filtered sodium is reabsorbed in the thick ascending limb of the loop of Henle, where it is achieved by an apical, bumetanide-sensitive, 130 kDa, electroneutral, Na-K-2Cl cotransporter (NKCC2), itself driven by a favorable inward gradient generated by the basolateral Na, K-ATPase pump (Fig. 59.6). NKCC2 is a kidney-specific member of a class of such channels found throughout secretory epithelia. Activation of these cotransporters appears, in part, to be a result of cell shrinkage. The distal tubule reabsorbs 5% to 8% of sodium via the apical thiazide-sensitive Na-Cl cotransporter (NCCT). Final sodium balance is achieved in the collecting duct via selective amiloride-sensitive, apical sodium channels (ENaCs) in exchange for potassium. ENaCs are controlled in part by the effects of aldosterone on the mineralocorticoid receptor (Fig. 59.7).

Potassium. Approximately 90% of daily potassium loss occurs via renal elimination. Potassium is freely filtered across the glomerulus and normally is almost completely reabsorbed in the proximal tubule. However, most regulatory mechanisms affect the loop of Henle, the distal tubule, and the collecting duct. Indeed, urinary losses can exceed filtered load, indicating the importance of distal secretion. Determinants of urinary potassium loss are dietary intake of potassium and plasma potassium concentration, acid-base disturbances (acidosis reduces potassium secretion and vice versa), circulating vasopressin concentration (vasopressin increases potassium loss[7]), tubular flow rate (increased flow rate increases potassium loss[8]), and aldosterone secretion (enhances potassium loss and increases sodium retention).[9]

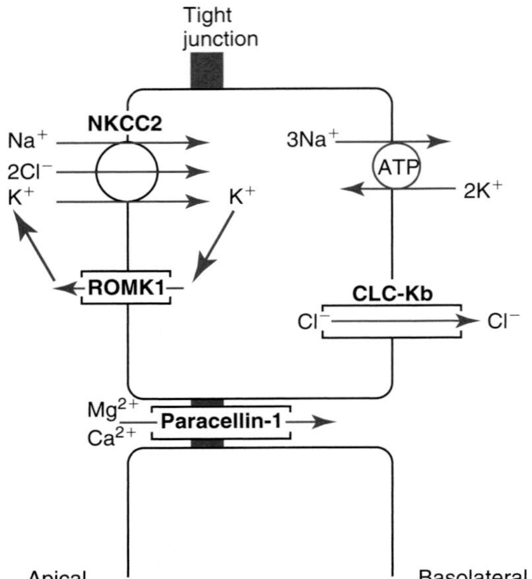

FIGURE 59.6 Schematic diagram showing the major pathways of solute reabsorption in the thick ascending limb of the loop of Henle. Sodium chloride is reabsorbed by the apical NKCC2 transporter. This electroneutral transport is driven by the low intracellular sodium and chloride concentrations generated by the basolateral Na, K-ATPase and the basolateral chloride channel CLC-Kb. The availability of potassium is rate-limiting for NKCC2, so potassium entering the cell is recycled back to the lumen via the ROMKI potassium channel. This potassium movement is electrogenic and drives paracellular resorption of Mg^{2+} and Ca^{2+} via paracellin-1. Mutations in NKCC2, ROMK1, or CLC-Kb cause Bartter syndrome. Mutations in paracellin-1 lead to disruption of this paracellular pathway and the tubular disease known as hypomagnesemic hypercalciuric nephrolithiasis.[11] (From Sayer JA, Pearce SHS. Diagnosis and clinical biochemistry of inherited tubulopathies. *Ann Clin Biochem* 2001;38:459–70.)

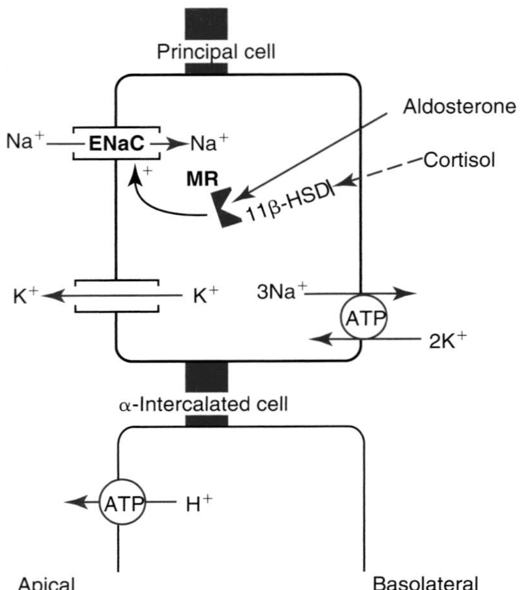

FIGURE 59.7 Schematic diagram showing the major pathways of solute reabsorption in the collecting duct. In principal cells, sodium reabsorption occurs through the amiloride-sensitive epithelial sodium channel (ENaC). Sodium reabsorption is influenced by the actions of aldosterone on the mineralocorticoid receptor (MR), with hyperaldosteronism producing an increase in channel activity. Cortisol, if permitted, will also bind to the MR, but a degree of specificity is maintained by 11β-hydroxysteroid dehydrogenase (11β-HSD), which inactivates cortisol to cortisone. Sodium uptake drives potassium secretion from principal cells and proton secretion from α-intercalated cells. In Liddle syndrome, mutations lead to an increase in ENaC activity, with increased sodium reabsorption and consequent potassium and proton loss. In pseudohypoaldosteronism type Ia, loss-of-function mutations inactivate ENaC, whereas in pseudohypoaldosteronism type Ib, there are MR abnormalities. Both lead to reduced sodium entry via ENaC, causing salt wasting and decreased secretion of potassium and protons. Licorice causes hypertension and a hypokalemic metabolic alkalosis by inactivating 11β-HSD, allowing cortisol to act as a mineralocorticoid. (From Sayer JA, Pearce SHS. Diagnosis and clinical biochemistry of inherited tubulopathies. *Ann Clin Biochem* 2001;38:459–70.)

Potassium ions are actively accumulated within tubular cells as a result of basolateral Na, K-ATPase activity, resulting in increase of intracellular potassium concentration to above its electrochemical equilibrium. Several types of potassium channels with a range of functions exist: (1) maintenance of a negative resting cell membrane potential, (2) regulation of intracellular volume, (3) recycling of potassium across apical and basolateral membranes to supply NKCC2 and enable sodium reabsorption, and (4) potassium secretion in the cortical collecting tubule.[10] As mentioned previously, potassium is reabsorbed with sodium by NKCC2 in the thick ascending limb of the loop of Henle, but it is recycled back into the lumen by renal outer medullary potassium-secreting channel 1 (ROMK1), thus generating an electrical gradient that drives passive paracellular reabsorption of calcium and magnesium down their electrochemical gradient[11] (see Fig. 59.6). ROMK1 is a pH-sensitive, membrane-spanning protein with several serine residues. At least two of these residues require phosphorylation by protein kinase A for the channel to be active.[10]

In the principal cells of the collecting duct, sodium reabsorption via ENaC is accompanied by movement of potassium into the lumen through potassium channels or through a K-Cl symporter (see Fig. 59.7). A *symporter* is an integral membrane protein that is involved in movement of two or more different molecules or ions across a phospholipid membrane such as the plasma membrane in the same direction and is therefore a type of cotransporter.

Chloride. Approximately 60% of chloride is reabsorbed in the proximal tubule. In the early part of the proximal tubule, avid reabsorption of sodium in combination with glucose and amino acids occurs, creating a lumen-negative potential difference. The negative potential difference drives chloride reabsorption by diffusion through the paracellular pathway. Preferential reabsorption of glucose, amino acids, and bicarbonate in association with sodium in the early proximal tubule causes an increase in the luminal chloride concentration. This high chloride composition heralds the second phase of proximal chloride (and sodium) reabsorption: passive diffusion of sodium chloride via the paracellular pathway, and active reabsorption involving several antiporter systems, by which chloride is exchanged for secretion of other anions (eg, bicarbonate, formate, oxalate). An *antiporter* (also called an exchanger or a countertransporter) is an integral membrane protein that is involved in secondary active transport of two or more different molecules or ions (ie, solutes) across a phospholipid membrane such as the plasma membrane in opposite directions. In the thick ascending limb of the loop of Henle, further chloride reabsorption occurs in association with sodium via NKCC2. The concentration gradient is maintained by a basolateral chloride channel (CLC-Kb) (see Fig. 59.6).[12]

Calcium. Approximately 98% of filtered calcium is reabsorbed: 65% to 75% in the proximal tubule (via a paracellular pathway), 20% to 25% in the thick ascending limb of the loop of Henle, 10% in the distal tubule, and, finally, small amounts in the collecting ducts. Calcium reabsorption is predominantly a passive process linked to active sodium reabsorption. For example, in the thick ascending limb of the loop of Henle, paracellular calcium transport is driven by the potential difference created by ROMK1. Active processes, particularly in the distal tubule, tightly regulate the final amount of calcium excreted. Here, calcium reabsorption is transcellular, occurring against the existing electrochemical gradient, and is stimulated by parathyroid hormone (PTH). Following entry into the cell from the lumen via an apical epithelial active transport mechanism (epithelial calcium channel 1, ECaC1), calcium binds to calbindin-D and is delivered to the basolateral membrane. Here it is extruded by a plasma membrane calcium-ATPase 1b (PMCA1b) and a Na-Ca exchanger (NCX1). Transcription of messenger RNA coding for both ECaC1 and calbindin is stimulated by calcitriol (1,25(OH_2)D_3), possibly synthesized locally in the distal nephron and acting in a paracrine and autocrine fashion. A functional vitamin D response element has been identified in the promoter region of the calbindin-D gene, along with a putative site in the ECaC1 gene. ECaC1 is a pH-sensitive, 83-kDa protein with six transmembrane-spanning domains. Activation of the ion channel probably involves protein kinase C phosphorylation. Evidence indicates that stimulation of the renal calcium-sensing receptor by calcium in the tubular lumen can directly affect tubular reabsorption of calcium, independent of the effects of calciotropic hormones.[13]

Phosphate. Reabsorption of phosphate occurs predominantly in the proximal tubule and is mediated by a secondary active transport mechanism. Three families (types I, II, and III) of sodium-dependent, phosphate cotransporters have been identified, of which type IIa (NPT2a, SLC34A1), a 640 amino acid protein located in the apical plasma membrane, is thought to be the most physiologically important. NPT2a sodium-phosphate transporter is electrogenic (ie, involves the inward flux of a positive charge), with three sodium ions and one phosphate ion (preferentially divalent) being transferred. Acute regulation of transport is achieved primarily by an alteration in the amount of NPT2a protein present in the apical membrane, with longer-term changes also involving increased transcription of the protein (eg, in response to 1,25(OH_2)D_3). Tonic levels of NPT2a in the apical membrane are thought to be high, with regulation predominantly involving internalization of the protein. Increased intracellular movement of the channel from the plasma membrane to the lysosomes is believed to follow both protein kinase A and C phosphorylation initiated by PTH receptor binding.[14,15] Fibroblast growth factor 23 (FGF-23), is a 32-kDa phosphate-regulating peptide, largely produced by bone cells. It was discovered during the 1990s following studies of severe hereditary osteomalacia characterized by severe hypophosphatemia and inappropriate phosphaturia.[16] Its major action is the inhibition of sodium-coupled reabsorption of inorganic phosphate in the renal proximal tubule. Autosomal dominant hypophosphatemic rickets is due to a mutation in the FGF-23 gene that results in a hyperstable form of this protein.[17] The current paradigm suggests that phosphate ingestion and/or hyperphosphatemia causes FGF-23 release into the circulation from skeletal osteocytes and osteoblasts. FGF-23 interacts with receptors within the kidney via a transmembrane protein—klotho—thereby inhibiting the sodium-coupled phosphate cotransporter in the proximal tubule (Na-Pi type IIa, or NPt2a) and causing phosphaturia. FGF-23 also inhibits 1α–vitamin D hydroxylase, leading to reduced calcitriol production. These effects will reduce plasma phosphate concentrations. FGF23 may act in concert with PTH by reducing expression of NPT2a at the proximal tubule brush border, hence promoting phosphaturia.[18] Efflux of phosphate across the basolateral membrane may involve an anion-exchange mechanism and/or a phosphate leak.

Normally less than 20% of the filtered load of phosphate is excreted into the urine, but above a plasma phosphate concentration of approximately 3.6 mg/dL (1.2 mmol/L), increments in urinary phosphate excretion increase linearly with the filtered load, suggesting that there is T_m (tubular maximal uptake) for phosphate. The T_m for phosphate is decreased by increases in the circulating PTH concentration and the ratio of T_m for phosphate to GFR (T_mP/GFR). T_mP/GFR has been used as a test in the differential diagnosis of hypercalcemia. Although superseded in this context by modern PTH assays, it may be useful in the investigation of inherited disorders of tubular phosphate handling.[19]

Bicarbonate and Hydrogen Ion. The kidney plays a central role in the maintenance of acid-base homeostasis through reabsorption of filtered bicarbonate and secretion of ammonium and acid. The tubular mechanisms underlying these processes are discussed in Chapter 60.

Water Homeostasis

Approximately 180 L glomerular filtrate is formed each day. The unique physiology of the kidney enables approximately 99% of this to be reabsorbed in the production of urine with variable osmolality (between 50 and 1400 mOsmol/kg H_2O at extremes of water intake). Plasma membranes of all mammalian cells are water permeable but to variable degrees. In the kidney, different segments of the nephron show differing permeability to water, enabling the body to both retain water and produce urine of variable concentration. Water reabsorption occurs both isosmotically, in association with electrolyte reabsorption in the proximal tubule, and differentially, in the loop of Henle, distal tubule, and collecting duct in response to the action of vasopressin. Absorption of water depends on the driving force for water reabsorption (predominantly active sodium transport) and the osmotic equilibration of water across the tubular epithelium. The generation of concentrated urine depends on medullary hyperosmolality. This in turn requires low water permeability in some kidney segments (ascending limb of the loop of Henle), whereas in other kidney segments (eg, proximal tubule), there is a requirement for high water permeability. Differing permeability and facilitation of hormonal control appear to be largely caused by differential expression along the nephron of a family of proteins known as the aquaporins (AQPs), which act as water channels.

At least 11 different mammalian AQPs have been identified, of which 7 (AQP1, -2, -3, -4, -6, -7, and -8) are expressed in the kidney.[20,21] Many of these have extrarenal expression sites as well (eg, AQP1 may be important in fluid removal across the peritoneal membrane). Two asparagine-proline-alanine sequences in the molecule are thought to interact in the membrane to form a pathway for water translocation. AQP1, which is found in the proximal tubule and the descending thin limb of the loop of Henle, constitutes almost 3% of total membrane protein in the kidney. It appears to be constitutively expressed and is present in both the apical and basolateral plasma membranes, representing entry and exit ports for water transport across the cell, respectively. Approximately 70% of water reabsorption occurs at this site, predominantly via a transcellular (eg, AQP1) rather than a paracellular route. Water reabsorption in the proximal tubule passively follows sodium reabsorption, so fluid entering the loop of Henle is still almost isosmotic with plasma.

Urinary concentration is predominantly achieved by countercurrent multiplication in the loop of Henle (Fig. 59.8).[22,23] The descending thin limb is very permeable to water, but the ascending limb and the collecting duct are not (the collecting ducts are also poorly permeable to urea). Fluid entering the loop of Henle is isotonic to plasma but is hypotonic on leaving it. The ascending limb has active sodium reabsorption driven by Na, K-ATPase with electroneutralizing transport of chloride, a combined process that can be inhibited by the so-called loop diuretics (eg, furosemide; see later in this chapter). In this section of the nephron, sodium reabsorption is not accompanied by water, creating a hypertonic medullary interstitium and facilitating water reabsorption from the anatomically adjacent descending limb. The descending limb cells are permeable to sodium chloride, which is cycled from the descending limb back to the ascending limb. Continuous flow along the loop generates an osmotic gradient at the tip of the loop that can reach 1400 mOsmol/kg H_2O. Approximately 5% of water is reabsorbed in the loop of Henle.

A further 10% of water reabsorption occurs in the distal tubule, with the remainder (>20 L/d) reabsorbed in the collecting ducts. Entry of water into the collecting duct cells occurs via apical AQP2 channels, with exit probably occurring via basolateral AQP3 (cortical and outer medullary collecting ducts) and AQP4 (inner medullary collecting ducts). AQP2 appears to be the primary target for vasopressin regulation of water reabsorption. AQP2 is stored in subapical vesicles in the collecting duct cells. In response to vasopressin stimulation, these vesicles are cycled through, and inserted into, the plasma membrane by a cytoskeletal, dynein-mediated transport process. Stimulation occurs following binding of vasopressin to a V_2 receptor in the basolateral plasma membrane of the principal cells of the collecting duct, which promotes a cyclic adenosine monophosphate (cAMP)/protein kinase A cascade, resulting in phosphorylation and activation of AQP2. Vasopressin regulates the acute cellular water-retaining response (AQP2 trafficking) and its

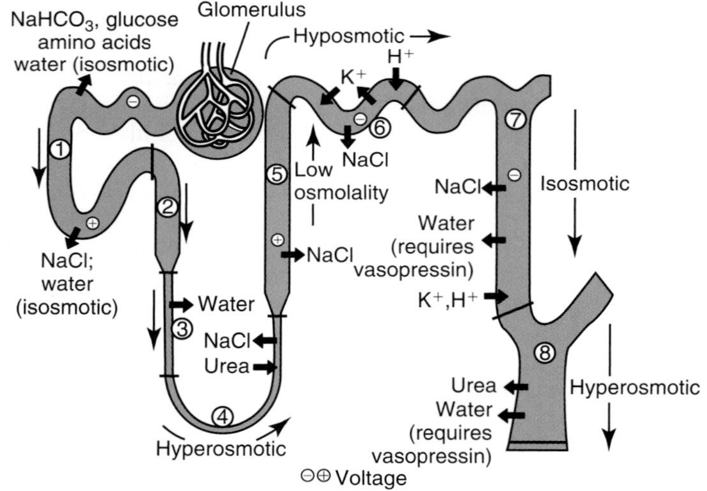

FIGURE 59.8 Countercurrent multiplication mechanism: schematic representation of the principal processes of transport in the nephron. In the convoluted portion of the proximal tubule *(1)*, salts and water are reabsorbed at high rates in isotonic proportions. Bulk reabsorption of most of the filtrate (65% to 70%) and virtually complete reabsorption of glucose, amino acids, and bicarbonate take place in this segment. In the pars recta *(2)*, organic acids are secreted, and continuous reabsorption of sodium chloride takes place. The loop of Henle comprises three segments: the thin descending *(3)* and ascending *(4)* limbs and the thick ascending limb *(5)*. The fluid becomes hyperosmotic because of water abstraction as it flows toward the bend of the loop, and it becomes hyposmotic because of sodium chloride reabsorption as it flows toward the distal convoluted tubule *(6)*. Active sodium reabsorption occurs in the distal convoluted tubule and in the cortical collecting tubule *(7)*. This latter segment is water impermeable in the absence of vasopressin (antidiuretic hormone, ADH), and the reabsorption of sodium in this segment is increased by aldosterone. The collecting duct *(8)* allows equilibration of water with the hyperosmotic interstitium when vasopressin is present. For additional details, see text. (From Burg MB: The nephron in transport of sodium, amino acids, and glucose. *Hospital Practice* 1978;13:100. Modified from a drawing by A. Iselin.)

longer-term regulation via a conditioning effect on AQP2 gene transcription. The AQP2 gene has a cAMP response element that is involved in the long-term upregulation of AQP2 expression by vasopressin. It is likely that there are also vasopressin-independent regulatory pathways of AQP2 expression. Membrane insertion of AQP2 allows water to pass into the collecting duct cells under the influence of medullary hyperosmolality. Maintenance of medullary hyperosmolality depends on efficient fluid removal, which is the function of the ascending *vasa recta*, a specialized medullary vasculature, and the close anatomic relations of all medullary constituents (see Fig. 59.2). AQP2 expression is decreased in a variety of polyuric conditions (eg, diabetes insipidus, lithium treatment, hypokalemia, hypercalcemia, urinary obstruction) and is increased in some water-retaining states (eg, heart failure, cirrhosis, and pregnancy).[21,24] A variety of V_2 receptor antagonists have been designed that block the actions of vasopressin. In contrast to diuretics, these agents promote the excretion of electroyte-free water and have exciting therapeutic potential in water-retaining states.[24]

Vasopressin also increases the permeability of collecting duct cells to urea, which is the major osmotically active component of luminal fluid in the distal tubule. Fluid of high urea concentration therefore enters the deepest layers of the medullary interstitium, passing down its concentration gradient, contributing to medullary hyperosmolality. Regulation of vasopressin excretion is of vital importance to fluid homeostasis. Normal plasma osmolality is maintained very tightly between 280 and 290 mOsmol/kg H_2O and is regulated by means of specific osmoreceptors found in the anterior hypothalamus. These receptors modulate the release of vasopressin and also affect thirst. Vasopressin release may be stimulated by hypotension, hypovolemia, and vomiting independently of osmoregulation.

Endocrine Function

The *endocrine functions* of the kidneys may be regarded as primary because the kidneys are endocrine organs producing hormones or as secondary because the kidneys are a site of action for hormones produced or activated elsewhere. In addition, the kidneys are a site of degradation for hormones such as insulin and aldosterone. In their primary endocrine function, the kidneys produce erythropoietin (EPO), prostaglandins and thromboxanes, $1,25(OH_2)D_3$, and renin. The importance of renin in the maintenance of systemic blood pressure was discussed earlier (see "Juxtaglomerular Apparatus").

Erythropoietin

EPO is a large glycoprotein hormone (Mr 34 kDa) containing 165 amino acids responsible for stimulating erythroid progenitor cells within the bone marrow to produce red blood cells. It is secreted chiefly by renal peritubular capillary endothelial cells in the adult and by the liver in the fetus. Physiologically, the kidneys sense a reduction in oxygen delivery to tissues by blood and release EPO, thereby stimulating erythropoiesis. Conversely, with a surplus of oxygen in blood traversing the kidneys, as in some forms of polycythemia, the release of EPO into blood is diminished. The use of recombinant human erythropoietin (rhEPO, epoetin) in the management of anemia of kidney disease is discussed later.

Prostaglandins and Thromboxanes

Prostaglandins and thromboxanes are synthesized from arachidonic acid by the cyclooxygenase (COX) enzyme system (see Chapter 34). The COX system is present in many parts of the kidney and has an important role in regulating the physiologic action of other hormones on renal vascular tone, mesangial contractility, and tubular processing of salt and water. Prostaglandins have a critical role in renal hemodynamics, control of tubular function, and renin release. The major renal vasodilatory prostaglandin is PGE_2, which is synthesized predominantly in the medulla. The major vasoconstrictor prostaglandin is thromboxane A_2, which is produced primarily within the renal cortex.[25] PGE_2 increases renal blood flow rate, inhibits sodium reabsorption in the distal nephron and collecting duct, and stimulates renin release.[25] These actions promote natriuresis and diuresis. In patients with chronic kidney disease (CKD), renal PGE_2 production is increased, representing a compensatory response to loss of nephron mass.[26] Vasodilatory prostaglandins are synthesized following stimulation with renal sympathetic adrenergic and AII-dependent mechanisms to offset or modulate vasoconstriction.[27] In the tubule, prostaglandins act as autocoids, exerting their effects locally, near the site of synthesis.

In pathophysiologic circumstances, including various forms of acute kidney injury (AKI), thromboxane A_2 and various prostaglandins may have a significant role in inflammation and alteration of vascular tone. The effects of nonsteroidal antiinflammatory drugs (NSAIDs) on renal prostaglandin metabolism are considered later in this chapter. The lipoxygenase pathway, which leads to formation of leukotrienes, is also present within the kidneys, although the major source of leukotrienes in inflammatory disease of the kidneys is infiltrating white cells and macrophages.

$1,25(OH_2)D_3$

The kidneys are primarily responsible for producing $1,25(OH_2)D_3$ from 25-hydroxycholecalciferol as a result of the action of the enzyme 25-hydroxycholecalciferol 1α-hydroxylase found in proximal tubular epithelial cells. Regulation of this system is considered in Chapter 64. The management of renal mineral-bone disorders is considered later in this chapter.

Glomerular Filtration Rate

The GFR is considered to be the most reliable measure of the functional capacity of the kidneys and is often thought of as indicative of the number of functioning nephrons. As a physiologic measurement, it has proved to be the most sensitive and specific marker of changes in overall renal function. Measurement of GFR is discussed in Chapter 32.

The rate of formation of glomerular filtrate depends on the balance between hydrostatic and oncotic forces along the afferent arteriole and across the glomerular filter. The net pressure difference must be sufficient not only to drive filtration across the glomerular filtration barrier but also to drive the ultrafiltrate along the tubules against their inherent resistance to flow. In the absence of sufficient pressure, the lumina of the tubules will collapse. This balance of forces can be expressed as follows:

$$\text{Rate of Filtration} = K_f\left(\left(P_{GCap} + \Pi_{BC}\right) - \left(P_{BG} + \Pi_{GCap}\right)\right)$$

Where:
K_f = (hydraulic permeability × surface area)
P_{GCap} = glomerular-capillary hydrostatic pressure
Π_{BC} = oncotic pressure in Bowman's capsule
P_{BC} = hydrostatic pressure in Bowman's capsule
Π_{GCap} = oncotic pressure in the glomerular capillary

Because the oncotic pressure in Bowman's capsule (Π_{BC}) can be considered negligible (protein concentration is usually 10–100 mg/L), this equation becomes:

$$\text{Rate of Filtration} = K_f\left(P_{GCap} - P_{BC} - \Pi_{GCap}\right)$$

Changes in K_f can be caused by drugs and by glomerular disease, but it is also physiologically regulated. Mesangial cell contraction, which is thought to be the main mechanism, causes a reduction in K_f, tending to reduce GFR. Net P_{GCap} represents a balance between renal arterial pressure and afferent and efferent arteriolar resistance. Although an increase in arterial pressure will tend to increase P_{GCap}, the magnitude of the change is modulated by differential manipulation of afferent and efferent tone, which can result in minimal change to the P_{GCap}. When the renal blood flow is low, oncotic pressure can change as the plasma passes along the renal capillaries. As filtrate is removed, the oncotic pressure rises, and by the end of the capillary, the net filtration rate may become zero; thus GFR falls, and this limits the amount of filtrate that can be obtained from a given volume of plasma. The average ($P_{GCap} - P_{BC} - \Pi_{GCap}$) or net filtration pressure is about 17 mm Hg. This pressure is sufficient to drive the filtration of 180 L of fluid per day because the K_f for glomerular capillaries is several orders of magnitude greater than for nonrenal capillaries.

Regulation of GFR

The factors involved in the regulation of GFR are listed in Table 59.3. Autoregulation of renal blood flow and GFR is widely thought to be explained by the *myogenic theory.* This theory is based on the principle that an increase in wall tension of the afferent arterioles, brought about by an increase in perfusion pressure, causes automatic contraction of arteriolar smooth muscle, thus increasing resistance and keeping the flow constant despite the increase in perfusion pressure.

The *tubuloglomerular feedback mechanism,* involving the *macula densa* and release of the vasodilator adenosine, must also be considered. Although not fully understood, this mechanism appears to regulate GFR, with changes in renal blood flow as a secondary consequence. For individual nephrons, evidence indicates that each single nephron GFR is influenced by the composition of the tubular fluid in the distal tubule, which in turn is influenced by the filtration rate. The *macula densa* is thought to sense the distal tubular sodium chloride content, its osmolality, or the rate at which sodium chloride is transported. The *macula densa* then signals the JGA via an uncertain mechanism to cause the release of adenosine and possibly AII and prostaglandins, which in turn affects vascular resistance. (Vascular resistance is the resistance to flow that must be overcome to push blood through the circulatory system.)

The result of the combination of myogenic mechanisms and tubuloglomerular feedback is that the net filtration pressure or P_{GCap} be kept reasonably constant over a wide range of systemic arterial pressures. It should be noted that renal blood flow and GFR change across this range of systemic pressures but to a significantly smaller extent than would be predicted if these autoregulatory mechanisms were not in place.

Other factors influencing renal blood flow are provided in Table 59.4. The afferent and efferent arterioles are richly supplied with renal sympathetic nerves. Epinephrine acts via α-adrenergic receptors, leading to constriction of both arterioles and causing a decrease in renal blood flow.

Nitric oxide (NO) has been identified as an important vasodilator produced by vascular endothelial cells. NO is synthesized from L-arginine and oxygen by nitric oxide synthase (NOS), of which three isoenzymes are differentially located and regulated. Within the kidney are eNOS (endothelial) and iNOS (inducible) isoenzymes. Activation of NOS has been shown to occur as a result of shear stress (eg, increased arteriolar tone). A variety of physiologic vasoconstrictors are present, including acetylcholine, bradykinin, endothelin, and serotonin; a rise in intracellular ionized calcium is required for the vasoconstrictors. NO synthesis is now known to play an important role in the regulation of human vascular tone and has a crucial role in control of blood pressure and kidney function.[28-30] NOS has also been found in the *macula densa* and has been implicated in the regulation of renin release.

TABLE 59.3 Summary of Factors That Influence the Glomerular Filtration Rate

	Major Influencing Factors	Effect on GFR
K_f	Increased glomerular surface area due to relaxation of mesangial cells	Increase
	Decreased glomerular surface area due to contraction of mesangial cells	Decrease
P_{GCap}	Altered renal arterial pressure	
	Afferent dilation	Increase
	Afferent constriction	Decrease
	Efferent constriction	Increase
	Efferent dilation	Decrease
P_{BC}	Increased intratubular pressure (eg, tubular obstruction)	Decrease
Π_{GCap}	Altered plasma oncotic pressure: increased	Decrease
	Altered renal blood flow: decreased	Decrease

Age and the Kidney

Kidney function varies throughout life. In utero, urine is produced by the developing fetus from about the ninth week of gestation. Nephrogenesis is complete by approximately 35 weeks' gestation, although kidney function remains immature during the first 2 years of life. The kidney of the term infant receives approximately 6% of the cardiac output, compared with 25% in adults. Renal vascular resistance is relatively high, and the low renal blood flow is particularly directed to the medulla and inner cortex. The gradual increase in renal blood flow that occurs with increasing age is directed mainly to the outer cortex and is mediated by local neurohormonal

TABLE 59.4 Factors Altering Renal Artery Tone and Renal Blood Flow

	EFFECT ON		EFFECT ON	
Factor	Afferent Arteriole	Efferent Arteriole	RBF	GFR
Adenosine	Constriction	Dilation	N	N→NE
Angiotensin II	Constriction	Constriction	N	N
Epinephrine/norepinephrine	Constriction	Constriction	N	N→NE
Vasopressin	Constriction	Constriction	NE	N→NE
Endothelin	Constriction	Constriction	NE	N→NE
Leukotrienes	Constriction	Constriction	NE	N→NE
Thromboxane A_2	Constriction	Constriction	NE	N→NE
Prostaglandins (PGE_2, PGI_2)	Dilation	Dilation	NE	NE
Nitric oxide	Dilation	Dilation	N	N
Atrial natriuretic factor	Dilation	Constriction	N	N→P
Dopamine	—	Dilation	N	N

NE, Negligible; *N*, negative; *P*, positive; *RBF*, renal blood flow; *GFR*, glomerular filtration rate.

mechanisms.[31] The GFR at birth is approximately 30 mL/min/1.73 m^2.[32] It increases rapidly during the first weeks of life to reach approximately 70 mL/min/1.73 m^2 by age 16 days.[32] Normal adult values are achieved by age 14 years. Tubular functions, including salt and water conservation, are also immature at birth. Birth is associated with rapid changes in kidney function, with a switch to salt and water conservation mediated by catecholamines, the renin-angiotensin system, vasopressin, glucocorticoids, and thyroid hormone.[32] The immaturity of the neonatal kidney contributes to the relatively common problems of water and electrolyte disturbances in infants. These disturbances are more likely to occur in premature infants, particularly those born before 35 weeks' gestation.

Aging is associated with a range of structural changes in the kidney, which begin in early middle age, including decreasing kidney weight and number of glomeruli, with the cortical glomeruli being particularly affected.[33,34] Changes in the afferent and efferent arteriolar systems are evident, with formation of direct channels (shunts) between afferent and efferent arterioles in the medulla. Aging is also associated with the development of tubulointerstitial fibrosis, loss of tubular mass, and decreasing length of the proximal tubule.

Structural change is accompanied by functional changes, which in many respects are the reverse of those seen in early life. On average, GFR declines with age by approximately 1 mL/min/1.73 m^2/year over the age of 40 years.[35-38] Renal blood flow, particularly to the cortical area, also decreases with age, while the filtration fraction (ie, GFR/renal plasma flow)[35] and renal vascular resistance[39,40] increase. Tubular function, such as the ability to concentrate urine and excrete a water and salt load, is decreased, and nocturnal polyuria is common. Renal salt conservation is impaired,[33] and the prevalence of albuminuria rises over the age of approximately 40 years.[41,42]

It is not known whether these changes are the result of a normal aging process (ie, involutional) or whether they are caused by the interplay of pathology and age. Cumulative exposure to common causes of CKD such as atherosclerosis,[34] hypertension,[43,44] heart failure,[45] diabetes,[46] obstructive nephropathy, infection, immune insult, nephrotoxins such as lead,[47] and dietary protein[48,49] increases with age, and it is difficult to separate these effects from those of "healthy" aging. In the absence of these and other identifiable causes of kidney disease, many individuals have stable GFR as they age.

Loss of kidney function with aging appears to be heterogeneous and is not inevitable.[39,50] Kidney function may be well preserved in healthy older people, and assumptions with respect to GFR based solely on age could be erroneous. Conversely, attention to the common causes of CKD could preserve function in older people.[51] Kidney disease is more common among older people. Studies from England,[52] France,[53] and Iceland[54] have demonstrated a near exponential rise in CKD with age. Data from the United States show the prevalence of GFR between 30 and 60 mL/min/1.73 m^2 to be 4.3% of the total noninstitutionalized population overall, but this rises to 25% among those over 70 years.[55] The prevalence may be even higher among institutionalized older people (eg, 82% of a residential home population were identified as having a GFR <60 mL/min/1.73 m^2).[56] The incidence of AKI also increases with age.[57]

GLOMERULAR AND TUBULAR PROTEIN HANDLING

Glomerular Sieving

Approximately 10 kg/d of protein is presented to the glomerular filtration barrier, with only approximately 1 g passing into the proximal tubule.[58] Glomerular permselectivity to proteins is a function of the integrated actions of endothelial cells, the GBM, and the podocytes, although the exact contribution and importance of each are still a matter of some debate.[58,59] A variety of methods have been used to study the permeability of the glomerular barrier, including urinalysis in vivo, micropuncture of single nephrons, isolated perfused kidneys, isolated glomeruli, isolated GBMs, and artificial membranes. All of these techniques have contributed to knowledge of glomerular permeability characteristics, and all also have advantages and disadvantages. For example, micropuncture techniques may damage the barrier; animal models may differ from human, permselectivity characteristics vary even among different rat species.[60] These issues have been reviewed by Haraldsson and associates.[2] Additionally, a range of different markers, including endogenous and modified proteins, dextran, and Ficoll polymers, have been used to study glomerular permeability.[2] The glomerular permeability of a molecule is expressed in terms of its glomerular sieving coefficient (GSC). Molecules smaller than approximately the molecular weight of inulin (5 kDa) are freely filtered. Therefore inulin, urea, creatinine, glucose, and electrolytes all have a GSC of 1.0. Classic experiments in the 1970s used linear dextran chains of varying molecular weight and charge to study glomerular filtration characteristics. However, linear carbohydrate chains do not necessarily behave in the same manner as a globular protein of equal molecular weight or charge. For example, neutral dextran chains of 15 kDa (diameter 2.4 nm) have a GSC of 1.0, whereas the smaller β2-microglobulin (11.8 kDa; diameter 1.6 nm) has a GSC of 0.7.[61] Linear molecules have a higher GSC than globular proteins, and thus theoretical glomerular pore dimensions based on dextran studies were overestimated. More recently, Ficoll polymers were used. These are neutral, heavily cross-linked, sucrose-epichlorohydrin copolymers that behave as rigid hydrated spheres and are thought to behave more like globular proteins in their sieving behavior.[2]

As a result of such studies, some general conclusions can be drawn with respect to glomerular protein handling. The glomerulus acts as a selective filter of the blood passing through its capillaries, restricting the passage of macromolecules in a size-, charge-, and shape/configuration-dependent manner. Sieving coefficients decrease as molecular size increases, are lower for anionic proteins than for neutral proteins of equivalent size, and are lower for globular rather than elongated proteins. Examples of the GSC for major urinary proteins are listed in Table 32.2.

The protein concentration in the glomerular filtrate has been measured in several animal models by direct glomerular puncture. The concentration of total protein found is in the range of several hundred mg/L (approximately 1% of plasma), with albumin concentrations ranging from less than 40 to a few hundred mg/L. The filtered load of protein depends on the product of the GSC and the free plasma concentration: therefore the albumin load per nephron is much greater than that of the other filtered proteins.[61,62] In general, proteins larger than albumin (66 kDa diameter 3.5 nm, charge −23) are retained by the healthy glomerulus and are termed *high molecular weight proteins*. However, lower molecular weight proteins are also retained to a significant extent.

Tubular Reabsorption

The final urinary concentration of proteins depends on both the filtered load and the efficiency of the proximal tubular reabsorptive process, as well as any contribution of tubular secretion. Proteins are reabsorbed by receptor-mediated, low-affinity, high-capacity processes. Megalin (600 kDa) and cubulin (460 kDa) are endocytic, multiligand receptors that are important in protein reabsorption.[60,63] Megalin belongs to the low-density lipoprotein (LDL) receptor family, whereas cubulin is identical to the intestinal intrinsic factor-vitamin B12 receptor. In the kidney, both are localized in clathrin-coated pits in the apical brush border of renal proximal tubular cells and bind filtered proteins in a calcium-dependent process. This apparatus is found throughout the proximal tubule, although there are notably fewer clathrin-coated pits and vesicles in the S3 segment. Megalin appears capable of both binding and internalizing its ligands, whereas the cubulin-ligand complex requires megalin to be internalized. Some proteins such as albumin will bind to either receptor, whereas others are specific (eg, transferrin binds to cubulin only, retinol-binding protein (RBP) and α_1-microglobulin to megalin only).

Once proteins have been internalized, they are transported by the endocytic vesicle and fuse with lysosomes. Proteolysis occurs, and the resultant amino acids are released into the tubulointerstitial space across the basolateral surface of the tubular epithelial cell. The membrane vesicles are then recycled to the brush border to complete the reabsorption cycle. Some small peptide fragments of proteins may be released back into the urinary space. Recent evidence suggests that interaction with a receptor known as neonatal Fc receptor within the endosomes may also result in transcytosis of albumin—that is, transport of intact reabsorbed albumin across the tubular epithelial cell and back into the circulation.[60] In health, the reabsorptive mechanism removes 99% of the filtered protein, thus retaining most of the essential amino acid constituents for reuse.[61,62,64] Capture of filtered transport proteins is also important in conserving vitamin status (eg, vitamin A associated with RBP).

The tubular reabsorptive process is saturable. Any increase in the filtered load (caused by glomerular damage, increased glomerular vascular permeability [eg, inflammatory response], or increased circulating concentration of low molecular weight proteins) or decrease in reabsorptive capacity (caused by tubular damage) can result in increased urinary protein loss *(proteinuria)*.

Tubular secretion of proteins also contributes to urinary total protein concentration—in particular, in health, Tamm Horsfall glycoprotein (THG) accounts for about 50% of urinary total protein. THG (200 kDa), a highly glycosylated acidic protein, is secreted into the tubular fluid only by the thick ascending limb and the early distal convoluted tubule and is thought to play a role in inhibiting kidney stone formation.[65,66] It is a major constituent of renal tubular casts along with albumin and traces of other proteins. Investigation for proteinuria is mandatory in any patient with suspected kidney disease and is considered in Chapter 32.

Consequences of Proteinuria

It is increasingly accepted that proteinuria is not only a marker of but also contributes directly to progression of kidney disease.[67,68] The accumulation of proteins in abnormal amounts in the tubular lumen may trigger an inflammatory reaction, which in turn may contribute to interstitial structural damage and expansion, and progression of kidney disease.[69] Increasing evidence suggests that megalin may not just be a scavenger receptor for albumin but that it may have signaling functions that regulate cell survival. Excessive quantities of albumin in the tubular lumen may downregulate proximal tubular megalin expression, increasing cell sensitivity to apoptosis.[70] Evidence gathered from in vitro studies suggests that glomerular filtration of abnormal amounts or types of protein induces mesangial cell injury, leading to glomerulosclerosis, and that these same proteins can have adverse effects on proximal tubular cell function.[71] Numerous studies have demonstrated that proteinuria is a potent risk marker for progression of renal disease in both nondiabetic[72-75] and diabetic[76,77] kidney disease. Furthermore, reducing proteinuria slows the rate of progression of proteinuric kidney disease. This effect has been observed in clinical trials in patients treated with ACE inhibitors and angiotensin II receptor blockers (ARBs), given alone or in combination.[78,79] These drugs reduce protein excretion by reducing intraglomerular filtration pressure and possibly by stabilizing the glomerular epithelial cell slit diaphragm proteins.[80,81] Consequently, reduction of proteinuria is an important therapeutic target.[82-84]

PATHOPHYSIOLOGY OF KIDNEY DISEASE

Despite the diverse initial causes of injury to the kidney, progression of kidney disease leading to loss of function and ultimately to kidney failure is a remarkably monotonous process characterized by early inflammation, followed by accumulation and deposition of extracellular matrix, tubulointerstitial fibrosis, tubular atrophy, and glomerulosclerosis. Proteinuria is thought to be one of the most important risk factors for progression of kidney diseases (see earlier). Nephrons are also lost via toxic, anoxic, or immunologic injury that initially may occur in the glomerulus, the tubule, or both together. Glomerular damage can involve endothelial, epithelial, or mesangial cells and/or the basement membrane.

The RAAS plays a pivotal role in many of the pathophysiologic changes that cause kidney injury and is an important therapeutic target (Fig. 59.9).[85] Renal cells are able to produce AII in a concentration that is much higher than in the systemic circulation, and AII generates potentially toxic reactive oxygen species within renal cells affecting signal transduction. In addition, many profibrogenic and proinflammatory mediators are induced within the kidney by AII. Aldosterone has been reported to enhance profibrogenic processes. Inflammatory mediators released include cytokines, chemokines, and growth factors, such as TGF-β, monocyte chemoattractant protein-1 (MCP-1), interleukin-6 (IL-6), interferon-γ, and tissue necrosis factor-α (TNF-α); these inflammatory factors activate resident lymphocytes and macrophages and recruit additional cells from the peripheral circulation. Thus cellular infiltration is a common but not a universal finding in renal biopsy specimens. These activated cells can cause T cell–mediated cell lysis, activation, and proliferation of interstitial fibroblasts. Fibroblast activity results in increased extracellular matrix synthesis and eventually in glomerular and tubular fibrosis. Extracellular matrix expansion causes disruption of local blood flow, exaggerating regional ischemia, and a vicious cycle of inflammation, fibrosis, and cell death is propagated.

Elucidation of this common pathway is incomplete but is the focus of considerable research interest because novel therapies are required to reduce progression and ideally to reverse fibrosis.[86] A strong relationship has been described for proteinuria and MCP-1-mediated interstitial damage in a prospective study of patients undergoing kidney biopsy for CKD.[87] In rodent models, anti-MCP-1 gene therapy reduced interstitial inflammation and fibrosis.[88] Increased production and activity of TGF-β have also been demonstrated in glomerular disease; this acts as a key mediator, along with AII, of fibrogenesis.[86] Data support the hypothesis that during tubulointerstitial fibrosis, α-smooth muscle actin-expressing mesenchymal cells might derive from the tubular epithelium via epithelial-mesenchymal transition (EMT) under the influence of TGF-β.[89] Strategies to block the process of EMT are being explored for future therapeutic targets in CKD. For example, an endogenous antagonist of TGF-β-induced EMT has been identified as bone morphogenic protein-7, a member of the TGF-β superfamily. Systemic administration of bone morphogenic protein-7 repaired severely damaged tubular cells in mice and reversed renal injury.[90]

The kidneys have considerable ability to increase their functional capacity in response to injury. Thus a significant reduction in functioning renal mass (50% to 60%) may occur before the onset of any significant symptoms or even before any major biochemical alterations appear. The most sensitive and specific measure of functional change—the GFR—can be reduced to less than 60 mL/min/1.73 m^2 before signs and symptoms of kidney failure will be observed. This increase in workload per nephron is thought to be an important cause of progressive renal injury.[91] A well-recognized hypothesis suggests that independent of primary renal injury, a point is reached in the decline in nephron number when further loss becomes inevitable and progressive as a consequence of a common pathway leading to interstitial fibrosis.[92]

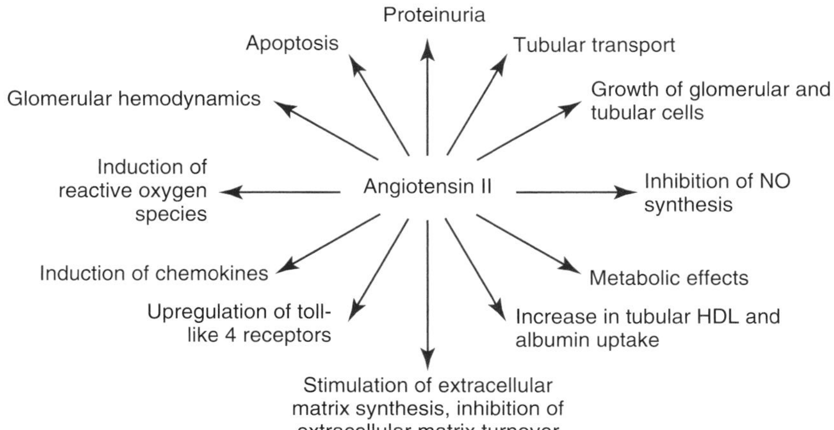

FIGURE 59.9 Role of angiotensin II in renal pathology. Angiotensin II is a cytokine with many effects on the kidney, clearly beyond its classical function as a hemodynamic mediator. (From Ruster C, Wolf G: Renin-angiotensin-aldosterone system and progression of renal disease. *J Am Soc Nephrol* 2006;17:2985–91.)

Overview of Kidney Disease and Its Clinical Manifestations

Most often kidney disease is detected opportunistically by measurement of blood pressure and urine and blood testing in asymptomatic individuals. Such testing can occur in the primary care setting or for health clearance purposes for insurance. Typical findings include isolated hematuria and isolated proteinuria. Kidney disease may also present with macroscopic hematuria, swollen ankles, headaches and visual disturbances due to severe hypertension, or as a manifestation of systemic disease such as in the vasculitides and systemic lupus erythematosus (SLE) (specific kidney diseases are discussed in greater detail later). Symptoms suggestive of advanced kidney disease include fatigue, nausea, vomiting, poor appetite, shortness of breath, fluid retention, poor memory, loss of libido, and itching. Unfortunately, many individuals present very late in their disease and may require urgent dialysis with no previous experience with the specialist nephrology service. These patients have a poor prognosis compared with patients who have been cared for in a multidisciplinary specialist environment for at least 1 year. Therefore early recognition of kidney disease is of paramount importance to outcome.

AT A GLANCE

Who Should Be Tested for Chronic Kidney Disease?

Monitor glomerular filtration rate (GFR) at least annually in people prescribed drugs known to be nephrotoxic, such as calcineurin inhibitors (for example, cyclosporin or tacrolimus), lithium, and NSAIDs.

Offer testing for CKD using estimated GFR and urinary albumin to creatinine ratio (ACR) to people with any of the following risk factors:

- Diabetes
- Hypertension
- Acute kidney injury
- Cardiovascular disease (ischemic heart disease, chronic heart failure, peripheral vascular disease, or cerebral vascular disease)
- Structural renal tract disease, recurrent renal calculi, or prostatic hypertrophy
- Multisystem diseases with potential kidney involvement—for example, systemic lupus erythematosus
- Family history of kidney failure (GFR category G5) or hereditary kidney disease
- Opportunistic detection of hematuria

Do not use age, gender, or ethnicity as risk markers to test people for CKD. In the absence of metabolic syndrome, diabetes, or hypertension, do not use obesity alone as a risk marker to test people for CKD.

Modified from National Institute for Health and Care Excellence. Chronic kidney disease. Early identification and management of chronic kidney disease in adults in primary and secondary care. 2014. http://www.nice.org.uk/nicemedia/live/13712/66658/.pdf.

Detection and diagnosis of kidney disease require a detailed history to include current symptoms, past medical and family history, social history, and a full drug history. A focused examination may identify potential causes of kidney disease, such as obstructive uropathy in which the bladder is easily palpable, or may indicate vascular disease associated with narrowing of the arteries supplying the kidneys (renal artery stenosis), systemic disease, or de novo kidney disease. Blood pressure measurement and urinalysis (see Chapter 32) are crucial baseline assessments. Examination of the skin may reveal evidence of advanced kidney disease with excoriations due to the intense itch that can occur. Signs of fluid overload can be seen in the ankles, or effusions may be noted in the chest. Abdominal examination may detect a palpable bladder, renal bruits, or enlarged kidneys. Fundoscopic examination is performed in hypertensive and diabetic patients to identify microvascular damage to the retina.

Kidney disease may present with heavy blood and protein detected in a sample of the urine—a so-called "active urinary sediment." An acute "nephritic" syndrome may occur as the result of postinfectious glomerulonephritis—for example, following a streptococcal throat or skin infection. The patient presents with poor urine output, edema, hypertension, and brown-colored urine. This pattern of acute nephritis is commonly seen in the developing world and is relatively unusual in developed countries.

Proteinuria may be the only indicator of kidney disease in many people. Proteinuria, particularly if in excess of 1 g/d, is indicative of glomerular disease. Most cases of glomerular disease are chronic, and patients may be followed for many years with monitoring of GFR and quantification of proteinuria.

Kidney disease presenting as nephrotic syndrome is characterized by the triad of heavy proteinuria (typically defined as exceeding an arbitrary threshold of 3 g/d), hypoalbuminemia, and edema. It is almost always caused by glomerular disease as opposed to tubular proteinuria. Several distinct pathological entities that may cause nephrotic syndrome include minimal change nephropathy, focal segmental glomerular sclerosis, and membranous nephropathy (these are discussed later). Nephrotic syndrome can also be a manifestation of diabetic kidney disease (diabetic nephropathy).

Kidney disease often accompanies systemic diseases such as diabetes mellitus, vasculitis, SLE, and plasma cell dyscrasias. The whole spectrum of kidney involvement may be seen, including an active urinary sediment, isolated proteinuria or hematuria, nephrotic syndrome, and rapidly progressive kidney failure.

Imaging of the renal tract to include the kidneys, ureters, bladder, and prostate gland is very important in many kidney diseases and provides useful information. It is mandatory in all cases of new AKI (see later) to identify the size and symmetry of the kidneys and to exclude obstruction to urine flow anywhere within the tract. Renal ultrasound, the imaging technique of choice in most cases, gives reliable data on the size of the kidneys and evidence of obstruction where present. Additionally, underlying structural abnormalities such as polycystic kidneys, renal cysts and tumors, and anatomic and congenital malformations may be demonstrated. Renal ultrasonography is easy, cheap, noninvasive, and without risk. Computed tomography (CT) imaging of the kidney-ureter-bladder has largely superseded intravenous pyelography in identifying kidney stones and structural diseases of the urinary tract. Invasive investigations of the urinary tract, particularly in patients with obstruction and hematuria, include cystoscopic examination of the bladder lining under direct vision, which allows for selective cannulation of each ureteric orifice and imaging with x-rays following injection of radio-contrast medium (retrograde study). The level of the lesion in an obstructed kidney can be ascertained by percutaneous insertion of a catheter into the kidney via a nephrostomy and subsequent injection of contrast via the nephrostomy tube, with x-rays taken as the contrast is drained from the kidney into the ureter and bladder (antegrade study).

Nuclear medicine scintigraphy is used to identify scars or cortical defects within kidneys and to assess the differential function of each kidney relative to the other. In addition, patients with well-preserved kidney function who are suspected of having renal artery stenosis can be challenged with an ACE inhibitor, such as captopril. This investigation assesses whether the flow of the radioisotope alters significantly following captopril administration. Radioisotopes are also utilized in some cases when obstruction is suspected but cannot be reliably demonstrated on ultrasound scanning or when the collecting system with the kidney is dilated to assess whether there is a functional obstruction. Excretion of the radioisotope is tested following the administration of the loop diuretic furosemide.

In patients with suspected renal artery disease, examination of the blood supply is necessary. Noninvasive imaging is preferred for diagnosis, and modalities include contrast enhanced CT angiography and magnetic resonance angiogram following intravenous gadolinium contrast injection. In cases requiring confirmation, or when an intervention to open the artery is proposed, selective renal angiography under x-ray screening can be performed following cannulation of the arterial tree via the femoral artery in the groin or an upper limb artery.

Despite all these investigations, it is occasionally necessary to perform a kidney biopsy. Biopsy typically is indicated in patients with either nephrotic syndrome, moderate proteinuria in the presence of hematuria, rapidly progressive disease, and AKI, and in patients with CKD (see below) that is progressive despite attention to treatments targeted to preserve kidney function. A biopsy is taken from one kidney only following injection of local anesthetic. To minimize the risk of bleeding, the lower pole of the kidney is chosen because the lower pole is away from the hilum, where the major blood vessels are present. The lower pole is identified using ultrasound scanning, and a semiautomatic needle device is placed on the capsule of the kidney and is released into the cortex and medulla. A sample of tissue is obtained, and light microscopy, immunofluorescence, or immunoperoxidase staining is performed, as well as electron microscopy. It should be emphasized that although approximately 13% of the adult population is estimated to have CKD,[93] only a minority of patients undergo a kidney biopsy. A kidney biopsy should be undertaken only for nonmalignant disease in a specialist nephrology setting. Histopathologic examination of the specimen confirms the diagnosis and gives some indication of prognosis and the need for specific treatment.

Terminology of Kidney Disease

The terminology associated with kidney disease has been amended and is clarified here. Previously, renal failure was divided into either *acute renal failure* (ARF) or *chronic renal failure* (CRF). These terms indicate the rate at which damage occurs, rather than the mechanism by which it occurs. The term *renal* has largely been replaced by *kidney* when referring to *chronic* disease because it is more easily understood by patients and nonspecialists. The commonly used term *acute renal failure* (ARF) has been replaced by *acute kidney injury* (AKI). Kidney *failure* is defined as a GFR of less than 15 mL/min/1.73 m^2.[94] Not all patients with kidney failure require renal replacement therapy (RRT, dialysis, or transplantation) to sustain life. *End-stage renal disease* (ESRD) is a US government–defined term that indicates the need for long-term chronic RRT. Each patient with ESRD is registered through the Medical Evidence form (2728) that all dialysis and transplant providers must submit. The term now includes both Medicare and non-Medicare populations.

Classification of Chronic Kidney Disease

Earlier studies to identify the incidence, causes, and complications of CKD largely focused on advanced disease and kidney failure. Because the numbers of patients with ESRD continue to rise, with associated poor prognosis despite modern replacement therapies (eg, 33% 5-year survival on dialysis) and an enormous health care cost (eg, $23 billion total Medicare spending on ESRD in the United States in 2006),[95] it has been recognized that CKD is an important public health problem emphasizing the need for earlier identification and treatment. Historically, data obtained from epidemiologic surveys were compromised by lack of consistent surrogate markers of kidney function to identify established disease. For example, serum creatinine, calculated creatinine clearance, and measured creatinine clearance were variously used. Landmark guidelines developed in the United States by the National Kidney Foundation—Kidney Disease Outcomes Quality Initiative (NKF-K/DOQI)[96] attempted to evaluate, classify, and stratify CKD. These guidelines were published in 2002 and were based upon categories of GFR. They have subsequently been revised and updated by Kidney Disease: Improving Global Outcomes (KDIGO)[94,97] and broadly adopted by other national organizations, such as the National Institute for Health and Care Excellence (NICE) in the United Kingdom[98] (Table 59.5). The KDIGO 2012 guideline added a second dimension to the classification system with three identified levels of albuminuria,[94] acknowledging the powerful additional prognostic information imparted by the presence of proteinuria (see Chapter 32).[99,100]

In the 2012 KDIGO system, CKD is *defined* as abnormalities of kidney structure or function, present for at least three months, with implications for health.[94] Abnormalities in kidney structure (damage) generally precede abnormalities in kidney function (Fig. 59.10). Most commonly, observed abnormalities in function are decreased GFR and/or increased albuminuria, although urinary sediment abnormalities, pathologic/imaging abnormalities, genetic disorders, or a history of renal transplantation must also be considered. CKD is *classified* based on cause, GFR category, and albuminuria category. The KDIGO guideline stratifies GFR from category G1 ($\geq$90 mL/min/1.73 m^2) through to G5 (GFR <15 mL/min/1.73 m^2). A GFR of less than 60 mL/min/1.73 m^2 (G3 to G5) is considered decreased. Category G3 is subdivided into G3A (GFR 45–59 mL/min/1.73 m^2) and G3B (GFR 30–44 mL/min/1.73 m^2), on the basis of the differing epidemiologic and prognostic significances of these GFR levels. Proteinuria is graded in albuminuria

TABLE 59.5 Classification of Chronic Kidney Disease Indicating Prognosis and Secondary/Tertiary Care Referral Decision Making by GFR and Albuminuria Categories

				Persistent Albuminuria Categories: Description and Range		
				A1	**A2**	**A3**
				Normal to mildly increased	Moderately increased	Severely increased
				<30 mg/g (<3 mg/mmol)	30–300 mg/g (3–30 mg/mmol)	>300 mg/g (>30 mg/mmol)
Glomerular filtration rate categories (mL/min/ 1.73 m^2): description and range	G1	Normal or high	>90	55.6	1.9 Monitor	0.4 Refer*
	G2	Mildly decreased	60–89	32.9	2.2 Monitor	0.3 Refer*
	G3a	Mildly to moderately decreased	45–59	3.6 Monitor	0.8 Monitor	0.2 Refer
	G3b	Moderately to severely decreased	30–44	1.0 Monitor	0.4 Monitor	0.2 Refer
	G4	Severely decreased	15–29	0.2 Refer*	0.1 Refer*	0.1 Refer
	G5	Kidney failure	<15	<0.1 Refer	<0.1 Refer	0.1 Refer

DARK RED: very high risk; MIDDLE RED: high risk; RED: moderately increased risk; LIGHT RED: low risk (if no other markers of kidney disease, no CKD).

NOTE: Numbers in the cells show the proportion (in %) of the adult population in the United States.[526]

*Referring clinicians may wish to discuss with their local nephrology service, depending on local arrangements regarding referral and monitoring.

Modified from Kidney Disease Improving Global Outcomes. Clinical practice guideline for the evaluation and management of chronic kidney disease. *Kidney International* 2013;3:1–150.

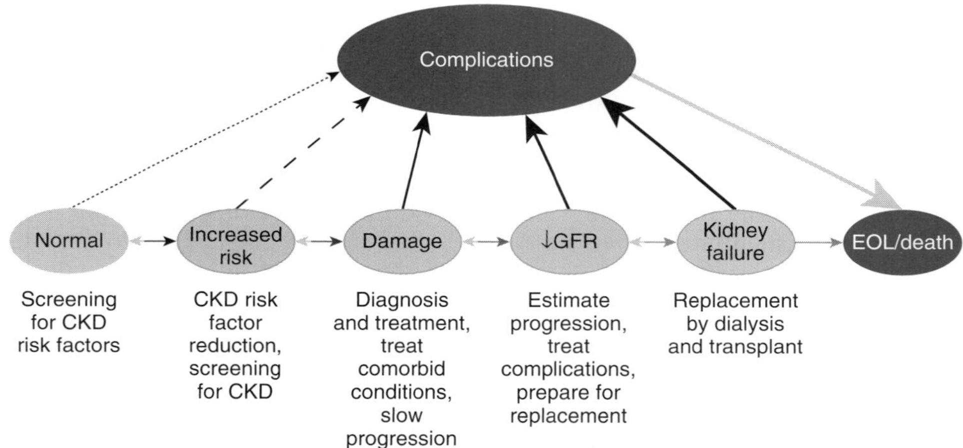

FIGURE 59.10 Conceptual model of CKD. Continuum of development, progression, and complications of CKD and strategies to improve outcomes. Horizontal arrows between circles represent development, progression, and remission of CKD. Left-pointing horizontal arrowheads signify that remission is less frequent than progression. Diagonal arrows represent occurrence of complications of CKD, including drug toxicity, endocrine and metabolic complications, cardiovascular disease, and others, such as infection, cognitive impairment, and frailty. Complications might also arise from adverse effects of interventions to prevent or treat the disease. *CKD,* Chronic kidney disease; *EOL,* end-of-life care and/or conservative management; *GFR,* glomerular filtration rate. (Modified from National Kidney Foundation. K/DOQI clinical practice guidelines for chronic kidney disease: evaluation, classification, and stratification. *Am J Kidney Dis* 2002;39:S1–266.)

categories, from A1 (30 mg/d) through A2 (30–300 mg/d) to A3 (>300 mg/d). For example, a patient with a GFR of 50 mL/min/1.73 m^2 and albumin loss of 200 mg/d would be classified G3a,A2. Although the cutoff levels between stages are somewhat arbitrary, the classification allows for consistency in prevalence reporting for epidemiological studies, facilitates undertaking of comparative studies and analysis, and allows focused treatment schedules for individual patients (see Table 59.5).[101]

Since the introduction of the classification system in 2002, the documented prevalence of CKD has increased, and recognition of the importance of CKD led to the introduction of new diagnostic codes in 2006 (ICD-9-CM diagnosis codes). The importance of early diagnosis of CKD is highlighted by the fact that 40% of the patients who started dialysis—so-called "incident" patients—in the United States in 2006 had not previously seen a nephrologist, and most had not had a serum creatinine measurement within the previous year.[95] One of the concerns regarding classification is the high prevalence of CKD imposed by the classification system itself. In the United States, it is estimated that 27 million individuals have CKD, representing almost 1 in 7 adults.[93] Population samples from elsewhere indicate similar prevalence rates. Most individuals with CKD do not progress to ESRD with prevalence rates of patients in GFR category G3 10 to 20 times higher than the prevalence rates of GFR categories G4 and G5 (see Table 59.5).[102,103] There is some concern that many individuals being identified with G3 CKD are not at increased risk;[102,104] use of cystatin C to delineate risk in this population has been proposed (see Chapter 32).[94,98,105]

The annual acceptance rate for RRT increased worldwide during the latter part of the 20th century but has reached a plateau in both the United States[106] and the United Kingdom[107] in recent years. The annual acceptance rate in the United Kingdom in 2013 was 109 per million population (pmp),[107] and in the United States during 2011, it was 357 pmp, although much higher among African Americans and Native Americans (Fig. 59.11).[106] The age of patients accepted for RRT is increasing: In 2013 in the United Kingdom, the median age of patients starting renal replacement therapy was 64.5 years.[107] It should be noted that the incidence of ESRD increases with age. The prevalence rates of patients with ESRD are also increasing and reached 1901 pmp in 2011 in the United States.[106]

The main causes of CKD leading to kidney failure from 1980 to 2012 in the United States are indicated in Fig. 59.12.

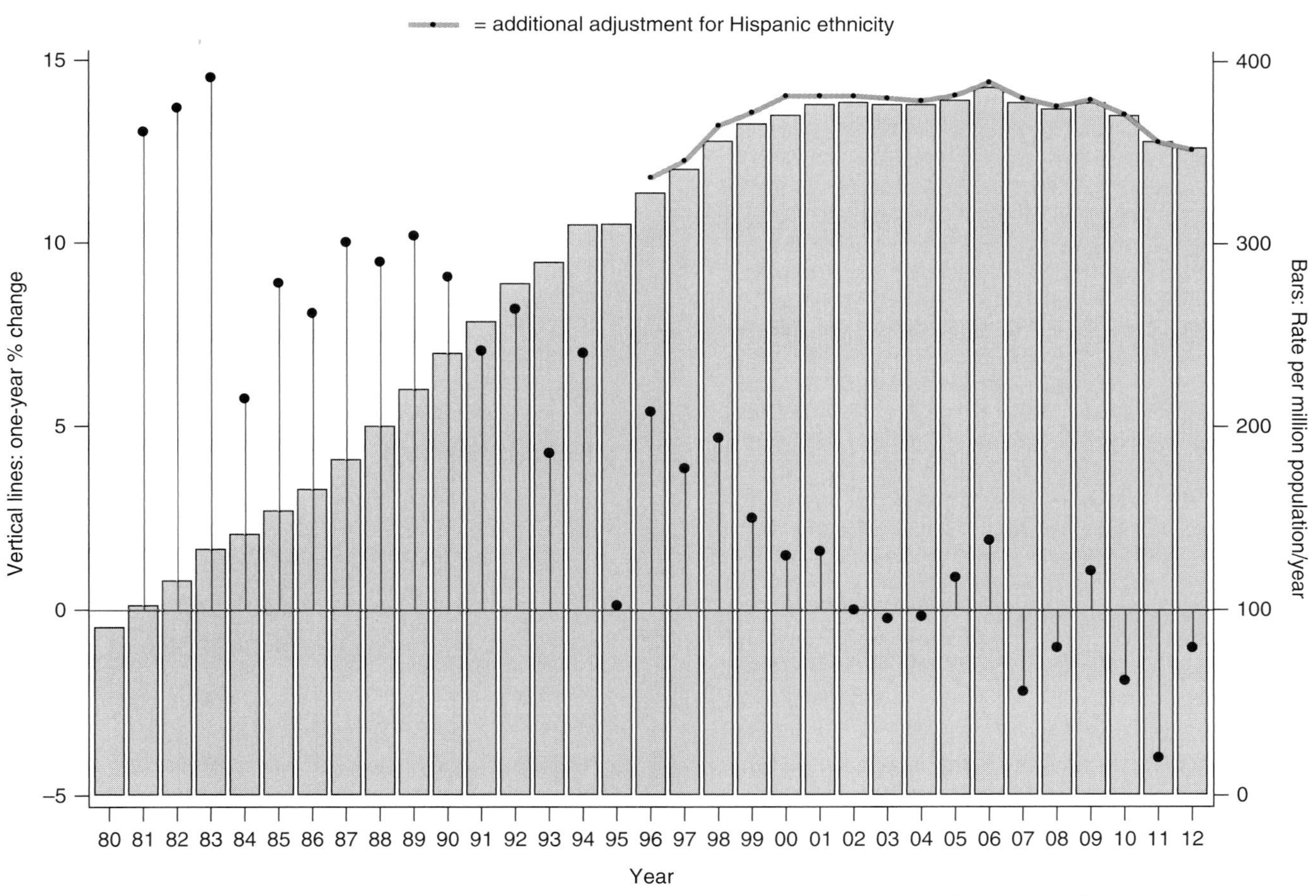

FIGURE 59.11 Trends in the adjusted (for age, sex, and race) incidence rate of ESRD, per million/year (bars; scale on right), and annual percent change in the adjusted (for age, sex, and race) incidence rate of ESRD (lines; scale on left) in the US population, 1980–2012.The number of incident (newly reported) ESRD cases in 2012 was 114,813. After a year-by-year rise in this number over 3 decades from 1980 to 2010, it now appears to have plateaued or declined slightly, with the number of incident ESRD cases lower in both 2011 and 2012 than in 2010. The incidence rate of ESRD per million/year virtually plateaued beginning in 2000 and has declined each year since 2009 to an adjusted incidence rate of 353 per million/year in 2012. This rate was the lowest since 1997. These findings provide further indication that the sustained rise in ESRD incidence through the 1980s and 1990s, both counts and rates, has not continued. Future analyses are needed to assess the causes of these trends. The standard population was the US population in 2011. (From United States Renal Data System, 2013 USRDS annual data report: *An overview of the epidemiology of kidney disease in the United States*. National Institutes of Health, National Institute of Diabetes and Digestive and Kidney Diseases, Bethesda, MD, 2014.[106])

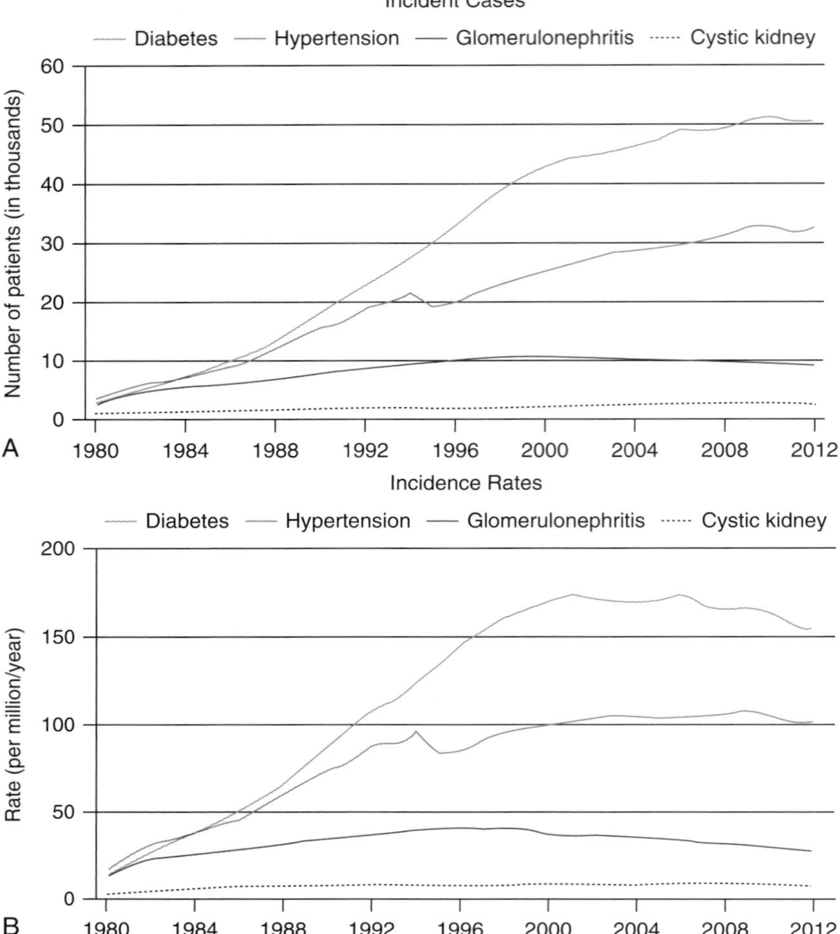

FIGURE 59.12 Trends in (A) end-stage renal disease (ESRD) incident cases, in thousands, and (B) adjusted (for age, sex, and race) ESRD incidence rate, per million/year, by primary cause of ESRD, in the US population, 1980–2012. The data show that diabetes as a cause of ESRD peaked in around 2010 and has fallen thereafter, but it remains the most common diagnosis of new ESRD in the United States. The incidence of ESRD due to glomerulonephritis peaked in the mid-1990s. The lower panel (B) shows some reduction in diabetes as the cause of ESRD in adjusted data. (From United States Renal Data System, 2013 USRDS annual data report: *An overview of the epidemiology of kidney disease in the United States*. National Institutes of Health, National Institute of Diabetes and Digestive and Kidney Diseases, Bethesda, Md., 2014.[106])

As indicated, diabetes mellitus is the largest single cause of advanced CKD and accounts for almost 50% of new dialysis patients in the United States. Hypertension is the underlying diagnosis in around 25% of new dialysis patients and is also particularly prevalent among African Americans. The myriad of kidney diseases, including glomerulonephritis; infective, hereditary, systemic, interstitial, and obstructive conditions; and those of unknown origin, account for the remainder. In the United Kingdom, diabetic nephropathy as a cause of kidney failure is seen in approximately 25% of new patients.[107]

Ethnic origin also modifies risk of kidney disease.[108] The lifetime risk of developing ESRD in 20-year-old black men and women has been estimated to be 7.3% and 7.8%, respectively, compared with 2.5% in white men and 1.8% in white women.[109] Family history of kidney disease is also a risk factor for developing ESRD. For example, a ninefold increased risk for ESRD has been noted in the African American community for those individuals with a first-degree relative with ESRD.[110] Therefore genetic influences may be involved in the development of kidney disease and the rate of progression to ESRD.

In summary, the presence of kidney disease can be easily identified through simple blood and urine testing. Subsequent diagnosis of the cause of kidney disease relies on medical history, examination, and laboratory and radiologic investigations and is discussed in the relevant disease sections later in this chapter.

General Management of CKD

Complications of CKD that develop before the need for RRT are numerous and include cardiovascular disease, metabolic acidosis, bone disease, and anemia. There is a broad, and often causal, relationship between the burden of illness and the level of GFR. Rate of progression of CKD, irrespective of underlying cause, is dependent on both nonmodifiable

AT A GLANCE

Defining and Classifying Chronic Kidney Disease

CKD is defined as abnormalities of kidney structure or function, present for at least 3 months, with implications for health.

Markers of reduced kidney function or damage include:

- Reduced glomerular filtration rate (GFR <60 mL/min/1.73 m^2)
- Albuminuria (≥30 mg/24 h; ACR ≥30 mg/g [≥3 mg/mmol])
- Urine sediment abnormalities
- Electrolyte and other abnormalities due to tubular disorders
- Abnormalities detected by histology
- Structural abnormalities detected by imaging
- History of kidney transplantation

Assign GFR and albuminuria categories as described in Table 59.5.

Modified from Kidney Disease Improving Global Outcomes. Clinical practice guideline for the evaluation and management of chronic kidney disease. *Kidney International* 2013;3:1–150.

factors, such as age, gender, race, and level of kidney function at diagnosis, and modifiable characteristics, including proteinuria, blood pressure control, and smoking. Progression and specific treatment options for diabetic and hypertensive nephropathy are discussed separately later. The current discussion focuses on optimal treatment for nondiabetic CKD.

Lowering blood pressure and reducing proteinuria have been shown to ameliorate the progression of CKD. The Modification of Diet in Renal Disease (MDRD) study compared the rates of decline in GFR in 840 patients with various causes of CKD versus a "usual" or "low" blood pressure goal.[111] Patients with type 1 diabetes were excluded. Outcome data suggest that a low blood pressure goal had some beneficial effect in those patients with higher levels of proteinuria.[111,112] The study supported the concept that proteinuria is an independent risk factor for progression of kidney disease. For patients with proteinuria greater than 1 g/d, the suggested target for mean blood pressure was 92 mm Hg (125/75 mm Hg).[74] The target blood pressure recommended by the seventh report of the Joint National Committee on Prevention, Detection, Evaluation, and Treatment of High Blood Pressure (JNC 7) is 130/80 mm Hg for patients with diabetes or kidney disease.[113] There is concern that lower blood pressures may be associated with worse outcomes in some patients. Hence, target ranges in addition to thresholds are sometimes recommended. In the United Kingdom, a target systolic blood pressure of less than 140 mm Hg (range 120–139 mm Hg) and diastolic blood pressure less than 90 mm Hg is recommended for most patients with CKD.[98] A lower-target systolic blood pressure of less than 130 mm Hg (target range 120–129 mm Hg) and diastolic target of less than 80 mm Hg are recommended in patients with an ACR of greater than 70 mg/mmol (approximately equivalent to >1 g/d proteinuria) and/or diabetes.[98]Data from the Third National Health and Nutrition Examination Survey (NHANES III) (1988–1994) reveal that among hypertensive individuals with an increased serum creatinine concentration, 75% were on antihypertensive treatment, and only 11% had their blood pressure reduced to lower than 130/85 mm Hg.[114]

ACE inhibitors are more effective than other antihypertensive drugs in slowing the rate of progression of proteinuric CKD,[78,115,116] although they do induce a mild decrease in GFR (<10 mL/min/1.73 m^2). It should also be noted that the evidence base for ACE inhibitor use in the setting of CKD may not be generalizable to older (>70 years) nonproteinuric adults, who form the majority of patients with CKD.[117] The development of hypotension, AKI, or hyperkalemia (plasma potassium concentration >5.5 mmol/L) should prompt discontinuation of the drug until other causes have been excluded. Short-term studies show that ARBs have effects on blood pressure and proteinuria that are similar to those of ACE inhibitors.

Low-nitrogen (protein) diets have been advocated from the early years of treatment of severe chronic uremia.[118] The very-low-protein diets tested in the MDRD study were of marginal benefit in these well-supervised patients with very low renal function, but they are not well adhered to in practice, may lead to negative nitrogen balance, and are not recommended. Protein intake is restricted spontaneously to approximately 0.6 to 0.8 g/kg/d by uremic patients not receiving dietary advice.[119] To prevent malnutrition, patients receive professional dietary advice, with diets containing an increased proportion of protein and a total calorie content of up to 35 kcal/kg/d. The NHANES III has confirmed an association with reduced GFR and malnutrition in noninstitutionalized individuals studied in a cross-sectional survey of more than 5000 participants stratified according to GFR.[120]

Recently, a relatively small trial suggested that bicarbonate supplementation can slow the rate of progression of CKD.[121] This hypothesis is undergoing further testing in several clinical trials.[122,123] Although intuitively one might expect correction of renal acidosis to be beneficial, unanticipated secondary effects may impact on patient survival (eg, increased vascular calcification following alkalinization or increased risk of heart failure).[124] General health measures, including cessation of cigarette smoking, should be encouraged.

Cardiovascular Complications of CKD

The spectrum of cardiovascular pathology predominant among patients with CKD (hypertensive cardiomyopathy, arrhythmias, heart failure, valvular disease, and peripheral vascular disease) differs from that predominant in the general population (atheromatous coronary artery disease).[125] The incidence of cardiovascular disease is 7- to 10-fold greater in patients with CKD than in non-CKD age- and gender-matched controls.[126] By the time patients develop the need for RRT, there is an approximately 17 times greater risk of cardiovascular death or nonfatal myocardial infarction among age- and gender-matched individuals without kidney disease.[125,127] Among patients treated by dialysis, the prevalence of coronary artery disease is approximately 40%, and the prevalence of left ventricular hypertrophy (LVH) is approximately 75%.[128,129] Cardiovascular mortality, defined as death caused by arrhythmias, cardiomyopathy, cardiac arrest, myocardial infarction, atherosclerotic heart disease, and pulmonary edema, has been estimated to be approximately 9% per year in dialysis patients, accounting for 50% of deaths of all patients with ESRD. Even after stratification by age, gender, race, and the presence or absence of diabetes, cardiovascular mortality in dialysis patients is 10 to 20 times higher than in the general population (Fig. 59.13).[130,131] Patients with

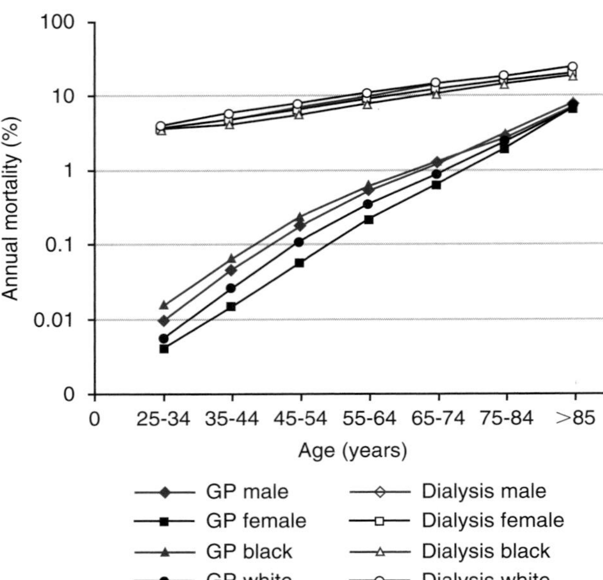

FIGURE 59.13 Cardiovascular disease mortality defined by death caused by arrhythmias, cardiomyopathy, cardiac arrest, myocardial infarction, atherosclerotic heart disease, and pulmonary edema in the general population (GP). Data from NCHS multiple cause of mortality data files compared with end-stage renal disease (ESRD) treated by dialysis. Data are stratified by age, race, and gender. (From Foley RN, Parfrey PS, Sarnak MJ. Clinical epidemiology of cardiovascular disease in chronic renal disease. *Am J Kidney Dis* 1998;32[suppl 3]:S112–19, with permission from the National Kidney Foundation.)

BOX 59.1 Traditional and Chronic Kidney Disease–Related Risk Factors for Cardiovascular Disease in CKD

Traditional Risk Factors for Cardiovascular Disease

Older age
Male gender
White race
Hypertension
Increased LDL cholesterol
Decreased HDL cholesterol
Smoking
Diabetes mellitus
Menopause
Sedentary lifestyle
Family history

CKD-Related Risk Factors for Cardiovascular Disease

Extracellular fluid overload
Left ventricular hypertrophy
Proteinuria
Anemia
Abnormal calcium and phosphate metabolism (vascular calcification)
Dyslipidemia
MIA syndrome
Infection
Thrombogenic factors
Oxidative stress
Increased homocysteine
Uremic toxins

LDL, Low-density lipoprotein; *HDL,* high-density lipoprotein; *MIA,* malnutrition inflammation atherosclerosis.

ESRD should be considered in the highest-risk group for subsequent cardiovascular events.

Risk factors for cardiovascular disease in CKD consist of a mixture of the traditional and CKD-specific factors. Traditional risk factors such as diabetes, hypertension, and dyslipidemia are more likely in CKD patients.[126] In addition, there are a number of CKD-related risk factors (Box 59.1).

Observational studies indicate that cardiovascular disease occurs at an early stage in CKD.[132] Thus, among middle-aged men, increases in serum creatinine concentration (>1.5 mg/dL [>130 μmol/L]) are associated with an age-adjusted relative risk of 1.5 for coronary disease and 3.0 for stroke. Reduction of GFR is associated with increased risk of composite endpoints of cardiovascular death, myocardial infarction, and stroke.[133] Proteinuria has also been shown to be associated with increased risk of cardiovascular disease, cardiovascular mortality, and all-cause mortality.[134-136] These associations may arise because (1) CKD causes an increased level of cardiovascular disease, (2) cardiovascular disease causes CKD, or (3) some other factor, such as diabetes and hypertension, causes both CKD and cardiovascular disease. Significantly, there are many more patients with category G3 than category G5 GFR (see Table 59.5). For example, a longitudinal study of patients with G3/4 GFR in the United States reported an age-adjusted rate for development of ESRD of 0.67 per 100 person-years, compared to the rate for cardiovascular death of 5.25 per 100 person-years.[137]

Two large prospective randomized controlled studies reported significant reductions in cardiovascular morbidity and mortality associated with ACE inhibitor treatment among patients at high risk for future cardiovascular events.[138,139] A secondary analysis of the Prevention of Events with ACE Inhibition (PEACE) trial data revealed a higher risk of death among patients with an estimated GFR of less than 60 mL/min/1.73 m^2 at baseline and a significant reduction in all-cause mortality associated with ACE inhibitor treatment in this subgroup.[140] Whereas none of the studies already mentioned specifically included patients with CKD, and all excluded patients with severe renal impairment, these data do provide support for the notion that ACE inhibitor treatment reduces cardiovascular risk in high-risk patients. Because cardiovascular disease remains the most important cause of death among CKD patients, it seems reasonable to recommend ACE inhibitor or ARB treatment for reduction of cardiovascular risk and for slowing of CKD progression. The use of ACE inhibitors must be tailored to the individual patient. Guidance in the United Kingdom is to use renin-angiotensin system antagonists in people with CKD and (1) diabetes and an ACR of 3 mg/mmol or more; (2) hypertension and an ACR of 30 mg/mmol or more; and (3) an ACR of 70 mg/mmol or more (irrespective of hypertension or cardiovascular disease).[98] There is the risk of a marked deterioration in kidney function in patients with cardiovascular disease and CKD during an acute, intercurrent illness. Recent guidance has recommended temporary discontinuation ("drug holidays") during such illnesses.[94] It is unclear how this message will be transferable to individual patients in practice.

Left Ventricular Hypertrophy

Among dialysis patients, the prevalence of congestive heart failure is approximately 40%. Both coronary artery disease and LVH are risk factors for the development of heart failure. In practice, it is difficult to determine whether cardiac failure reflects left ventricular dysfunction or extracellular fluid volume overload. LVH is demonstrable early in the course of CKD, with the proportion of patients with LVH increasing as kidney function declines. Univariate analysis of a single-center cohort of CKD patients in Canada revealed that age, systolic blood pressure, and hemoglobin were significantly different between the groups with or without LVH.[141] For each 5 mm Hg increase in systolic BP, the risk of LVH increased by 3%. A fall in blood hemoglobin concentration of 1 g/dL increased the risk of LVH by 6%. A large prospective multicenter study confirmed progressive increases in left ventricular mass index (LVMI) over a 12-month period, with the incidence of new LVH at 10% per year.[142] Again, lower hemoglobin concentrations and higher systolic blood pressures were associated with left ventricular growth. Anemia has both direct and indirect effects on left ventricular function and growth. Cardiac output increases because of a combination of increased cardiac preload and a reduction in afterload. Such changes lead to ventricular remodeling, with initial left ventricular dilation followed by subsequent hypertrophy. In ESRD other factors also contribute to LVH, including hypertension, volume expansion, and the metabolic consequences of uremia, to which may be added the effects of diabetes.[143]

Dyslipidemia in CKD

Various dyslipidemias are associated with CKD.[126,144,145] The pattern of dyslipidemia in CKD differs from that seen in non-CKD. It is characterized by an accumulation of partially metabolized triglyceride-rich particles (predominantly very-low-density lipoprotein [VLDL] and intermediate-density lipoprotein [IDL] remnants), mainly due to abnormal lipase function.[146] This causes hypertriglyceridemia and low high-density lipoprotein (HDL) cholesterol. Although total cholesterol concentration may be normal, there is often a highly abnormal lipid subfraction profile with a predominance of atherogenic small, dense LDL particles.[125] In a large cross-sectional analysis of 1047 hemodialysis patients in the Dialysis Morbidity and Mortality Study, only 20% of patients had low-risk lipid concentrations (ie, LDL cholesterol <130 mg/dL [3.36 mmol/L], HDL cholesterol >40 mg/dL [1.03 mmol/L], and triglycerides <150 mg/dL [1.69 mmol/L]).[147] Low cholesterol was found to be associated with increased mortality, but this is probably a reflection of other conditions that lower cholesterol, such as inflammation and malnutrition ("reverse causality"). It is possible that other, nontraditional atherogenic lipoprotein abnormalities (eg, lipoprotein (a) and oxidized LDL) are present in hemodialysis patients.[148,149] Similar profiles are seen in peritoneal dialysis patients.

Lipoprotein (a) concentrations are also increased in CKD. Baseline data from the Chronic Renal Impairment in Birmingham (CRIB) study, confirmed dyslipidemia in early CKD.[126] Patients had lower HDL and LDL cholesterol and higher triglyceride concentrations.

The challenge to the nephrology community is to establish whether interventions to modify the pattern of dyslipidemia with lifestyle changes and drug treatment will preserve kidney function and reduce cardiovascular morbidity and mortality. At present, no large, adequately controlled trials are testing the hypotheses that treatment of dyslipidemia preserves kidney function. There is a shortage of good trial data on which to base recommendations in CKD patients in general and more specifically among dialysis patients. The major trials of intervention with statins (3-hydroxy-3-methylglutaryl-Co-enzyme A [HMG-CoA] reductase inhibitors) in the general population and those with established cardiovascular disease have been limited with reference to CKD because such patients have often been excluded from the trials as perceived to be at too high risk for inclusion.[150,151] The Heart Protection Study randomly allocated 20,536 adults with coronary artery disease, occlusive disease of noncoronary arteries, or diabetes to simvastatin (40 mg) or placebo.[152] In a subgroup analysis of more than 1300 patients with serum creatinine concentration between 1.2 and 2.3 mg/dL (110 and 200 μmol/L), fewer major vascular events were reported in the simvastatin group. The 4D Study investigated the use of atorvastatin in more than 1200 patients with type 2 diabetes mellitus undergoing hemodialysis and followed for a median period of 4 years. The study group concluded that atorvastatin had no statistically significant effect on the composite primary endpoint of cardiovascular death, nonfatal myocardial infarction, and stroke.[153] A more recent study, AURORA, evaluated the use of rosuvastatin in subjects on hemodialysis and failed to demonstrate any beneficial effects of statins on cardiovascular outcomes despite markedly reduced lipid concentrations.[154] Although these studies have limitations, the most likely explanation for the lack of benefit associated with the use of statins is that patients on dialysis have a different type of cardiovascular disease than individuals with earlier stages of CKD. The Study of Heart and Renal Protection (SHARP) evaluated the use of cholesterol lowering with simvastatin and ezetimibe in a broad range of more than 9000 patients with CKD, including 3000 dialysis patients. Benefit in terms of both cardiovascular risk reduction and amelioration of progression of CKD were studied. There were significant reductions in atherosclerotic endpoints, including nonhemorrhagic stroke and arterial revascularization in the treated patients followed for a median of 4.9 years.[155]

Guidelines from the United Kingdom Renal Association[156] recommend that statins should be considered for primary prevention in all patients with CKD and GFR greater than 15 mL/min/1.73 m^2 and also for renal transplant patients if their 10-year risk of cardiovascular disease is calculated as greater than 20% according to the guidelines of the Joint British Societies.[157] The target total cholesterol should be less than 156 mg/dL (<4 mmol/L) or a 25% reduction from baseline, and a fasting LDL cholesterol of less than 78 mg/dL (<2 mmol/L) or a 30% reduction from baseline should be achieved, whichever is the greater reduction in all patients.[156] However, the Joint British Societies risk calculations have not been validated in patients with kidney disease, and lipid-lowering guidance remains controversial,[158] particularly in patients receiving dialysis. The KDIGO Lipid Working Group did not recommend specific lipid targets for patients with CKD due to safety concerns regarding the use of high-dose statins.[159] They recommend that statins, or statins with ezetimibe, be offered to adults over age 50 in the setting of GFR less than 60 mL/min/1.73 m^2 but not treated with renal replacement therapies (dialysis and transplantation).[159] With respect to patients commencing dialysis or changing RRT modality, the United Kingdom Renal Association recommends that statins should not be withdrawn from patients in whom they were previously indicated.[156]

Vascular Calcification

It has been known for many years that patients with kidney failure have vascular calcification. Serial x-ray studies and ultrasound imaging of large arteries confirm increased calcification in patients on dialysis over many years.[160] Studies from France have linked the presence of vascular calcification with reduced survival on dialysis.[161-163] Calcification of the major arteries occurs along the intimal lining of blood vessels in association with atheroma. However, in CKD, medial and adventitial calcification also occurs, reducing the compliance of the vessel. Reductions in vessel compliance can be observed by measuring pulse wave velocities along major arteries such as the aorta. The pulse wave velocity is increased in stiff (less compliant) vessels, causing the rebound pulse wave to return more quickly to the heart during the cardiac cycle. Early rebound of the pulse wave places extra strain on the heart, leading to LVH.[161] Vascular calcification has been studied in both CKD and non-CKD populations using modern sophisticated imaging. Electron beam CT acquires serial sections of the aortic arch, the coronary vessels, and the aorta. Areas of calcification can be identified and allocated a calcium score (Agatston score).[164] This approach cannot distinguish between intimal and medial calcification, but in non-CKD patients, the higher the calcium score, the more predictive it is of stenotic vascular disease.[165,166] Dialysis patients as young as 20 years exhibit vascular calcification, and calcium scores increased rapidly thereafter.[167]

The pathophysiology of vascular calcification in CKD patients is an exciting area of study, with many new developments and hypotheses. Vascular calcification was previously thought to be a passive process caused by precipitation of mineral from the circulation. However, it is increasingly recognized that vascular calcification is a tightly regulated process with true bone marrow, osteo/chondrocytic cells, cytokines, matrix proteins, and matrix vesicles characteristic of mature bone-forming cells (osteoblasts) within calcified vascular lesions.[168-171] Mineralization-regulating proteins are deposited at sites of vascular calcification. The generation of a matrix gamma-carboxyglutamic acid (Gla) protein knockout mouse, which exhibits extensive and lethal calcification and cartilaginous metaplasia of the media of all elastic arteries, has refocused attention on the role of Gla-containing proteins in vascular calcification.[168] A number of proteins, including matrix Gla protein, osteonectin, and osteoprotegerin, are constitutively expressed by vascular smooth muscle cells in normal media but are downregulated in calcified arteries. In calcified plaques, vascular smooth muscle cells express osteoblast-like gene expression profiles, as demonstrated by in situ hybridization,[169] and are able to transdifferentiate into osteo/chondrocytic cells in the arterial wall and to orchestrate bone formation and calcification in response to multiple factors such as hypertension, reactive oxygen species, advanced glycation end products, lipids, and inflammatory proteins. Identification of natural inhibitors of calcification in plasma, such as human fetuin-A (α_2-Heremans Schmid glycoprotein, AHSG) and matrix-Gla protein, suggests that the vascular endothelium may be continually subjected to calcification stresses and that regulatory systems break down in uremia. A cross-sectional study in hemodialysis patients demonstrated that AHSG concentrations were significantly lower in plasma of patients on hemodialysis than in healthy controls.[172]

The use of calcium-containing oral phosphate binders (see later) may be associated with increased risk of calcification.[167] The Treat to Goal study explored the use of a noncalcium, nonaluminum-containing phosphate binder, sevelamer hydrochloride, in 200 hemodialysis patients from Europe and North America.[173] This study demonstrated significant attenuation in the rate of calcification of vessels with sevelamer hydrochloride at 12 months. Patients were less likely to develop hypercalcemia and had lower plasma LDL cholesterol concentrations, but a tendency toward worsening acidosis was noted. Still other studies have identified a potential survival benefit for new ("incident") hemodialysis patients derived from treatment with sevelamer hydrochloride compared with calcium-based oral phosphate binders when treatment was provided for at least 18 months.[174] However, a study comparing sevelamer hydrochloride versus calcium-based binders in more than 2000 prevalent hemodialysis patients failed to show a significant difference between therapies in terms of all-cause mortality and cause-specific mortality.[175]

Disturbances in Calcium and Phosphate Metabolism

CKD is associated with complex metabolic disturbances in divalent ion and phosphate metabolism. Although this is commonly referred to as *renal osteodystrophy,* there has been a paradigm shift in terms of calcium, phosphate, and PTH management in patients receiving dialysis. The impetus for this change in approach has been recognition of the importance of the previously unheralded phosphate moiety in terms of increased risk of death in ESRD and the almost universal development of *cardiovascular calcification* (see earlier) that is seen in dialysis patients. It is likely that treatment of hyperphosphatemia in dialysis patients with calcium-based therapies may be contributing to vascular calcification; therefore these two problems are intricately linked. In an effort to clarify the terminology of renal metabolic bone disease, KDIGO proposed that the term *CKD-mineral and bone disorder* (CKD-MBD) should be used to describe the syndrome of biochemical, bone, and extraskeletal calcification abnormalities that occur in patients with CKD and that the term *renal osteodystrophy* should be used exclusively to define alterations in bone morphology, following bone biopsy, associated with CKD.[176]

As GFR declines, plasma phosphate concentration rises and ionized calcium concentration declines. The consequence of this is increased production of PTH by the parathyroid glands. PTH-producing cells are regulated tightly through complex feedback mechanisms to maintain normocalcemia (see Chapter 64). The calcium-sensing receptor (CaSR) is stimulated by calcium and has an inhibitory effect on PTH production.[177] In addition, phosphate has been reported to directly stimulate the production of PTH in vitro.[178] Elegant early experiments on dogs with varying levels of induced kidney failure confirmed the increase in PTH as GFR falls, with attenuation noted in animals fed a modified diet with very low levels of phosphate (Fig. 59.14).[179] FGF-23 may stimulate PTH production. FGF-23 concentrations increase

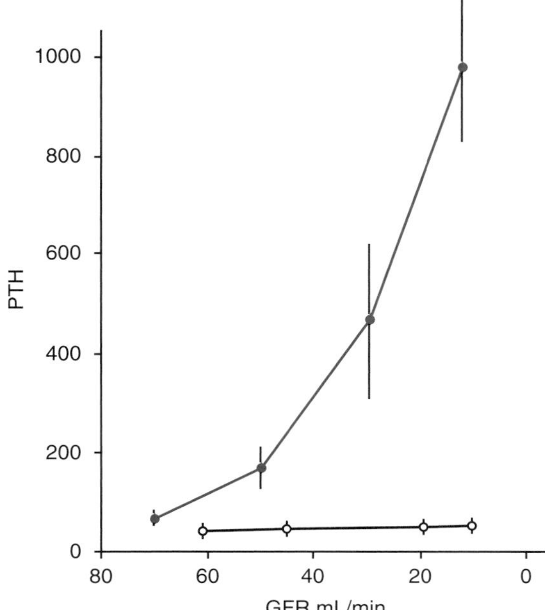

FIGURE 59.14 The relationship between parathyroid hormone (PTH) concentration and glomerular filtration rate (GFR) in two groups of dogs: those maintained on a normal phosphate diet (closed circles) and those maintained on a diet containing less than 100 mg of phosphate per day (open circles). The vertical lines represent ±1 SEM. PTH is expressed in μEq/mL. (From Slatopolsky E, Caglar S, Pennell JP, Taggart DD, Canterbury JM, Reiss E, et al. On the pathogenesis of hyperparathyroidism in chronic experimental renal insufficiency in the dog. *J Clin Invest* 1971;50:492–9.)

markedly in CKD (between 10 and 600 times higher than the normal range) and are correlated with predialysis phosphate concentrations but not with bone mineral density.[180] Ongoing studies are evaluating the importance of this peptide in terms of skeletal resistance to PTH as seen in CKD patients.

In addition to hyperphosphatemia contributing to hypocalcemia, reduced 1α-hydroxylation of 25-hydroxycholecalciferol by the renal proximal tubular cells may lead to reduced production of calcitriol, the active form of vitamin D and a vitamin D receptor activator. Vitamin D is required in health to promote calcium and phosphate absorption from the gut. PTH-producing cells in the parathyroid gland have receptors for vitamin D (VDRs). The VDR is a 427 amino acid peptide that is widely found in tissues, including parathyroid glands, intestine, and osteoblast-like cells. Binding of vitamin D to the VDR inhibits PTH production. The result of these complex metabolic disturbances is secondary hyperparathyroidism. Increased secretion of PTH stimulates resorption of calcium and phosphate from the major calcium reservoir, the bone. Problems can develop early, and patients with a GFR of less than 45 mL/min/1.73 m^2 should be evaluated for these metabolic disturbances.[94] Secondary hyperparathyroidism classically causes bone changes consistent with osteitis fibrosa cystica. Bony erosions and intramedullary cysts are seen because of direct effects of PTH on osteoclasts and osteoblasts. Unchecked, this can lead to bone pain and fracture. Severe secondary hyperparathyroidism is associated with hyperplasia of the glands and ultimately with nodular hyperplasia. These grossly enlarged glands tend to be resistant to medical therapies of secondary hyperparathyroidism (see later) because they have significantly reduced expression of both the CaSR and VDR. Eventually, PTH secretion can become unhinged completely from feedback control; this autonomous production is called *tertiary hyperparathyroidism*. In this setting, medical treatment has failed and parathyroidectomy may be required,[176] although significant morbidity and mortality may be associated with this procedure with no improvement in fracture rate observed at 1 year postsurgery.[181]

A severe and often terminal manifestation of long-standing ESRD is calcemic uremic arteriolopathy *(calciphylaxis)*. Calciphylaxis is characterized by calcium deposition within the arterioles of the microcirculation, leading to destruction of the vessel and in turn causing necrosis of tissues, particularly the skin and adipose tissue on the legs and torso.

Adynamic bone is characterized by low turnover and poor bone formation and is highly prevalent in CKD patients. It is more common in older people and those with diabetes and malnutrition. Adynamic bone is associated with a low PTH concentration and abnormal calcium balance, hyperphosphatemia, and acidosis. Progression of CKD adds to the risk profile for adynamic bone because 1,25-dihydroxyvitamin D becomes markedly reduced in advanced CKD.[182] Diagnosis of adynamic bone is ultimately made on bone biopsy, but patients are reluctant to undertake this procedure. Unfortunately, PTH alone does not correlate with bone biopsy findings. However, serum bone–specific alkaline phosphatase measured using an immunoassay technique has good predictive value in separating high from low bone turnover, particularly in combination with PTH measurements.[183,184] Although adynamic bone has not proved to be associated with increased fracture risk in ESRD patients, dialysis patients with this condition are less able to incorporate calcium into bone and are at increased risk of vascular calcification.[185] Excessive use of vitamin D analogs (eg, alfacalcidol [1α-hydroxyvitamin D3]) is implicated in the high prevalence of adynamic bone in dialysis patients. Bone disease in CKD is also complicated by the relatively high prevalence of hypogonadism in men on dialysis and the high prevalence of osteoporosis in postmenopausal women.

High concentrations of plasma phosphate are associated with increased mortality in hemodialysis patients.[186] In at least 50% of hemodialysis patients, the serum phosphate is greater than 6.0 mg/dL (1.9 mmol/L), and in 25% of patients, it is greater than 7.2 mg/dL (2.3 mmol/L). Higher corrected calcium and PTH concentrations are associated with death in hemodialysis patients. Patients with low phosphate concentrations are also at increased risk of death (relative risk of death increased by approximately 50% with phosphate <3 mg/dL) because low phosphate is associated with intercurrent illness and malnutrition. The UK Renal Association standard for midweek predialysis serum phosphate concentration is 3.3 to 5.3 mg/dL (1.1 to 1.7 mmol/L).[156] KDIGO published detailed international guidance on bone mineral metabolism in CKD in 2009 with the recommendation to maintain serum phosphate within the normal range in CKD and as close to the normal range as possible in patients receiving dialysis (Table 59.6).[176] Achievement of these targets is variable between dialysis providers, with approximately 57% of hemodialysis patients within the phosphate target and 57% within the relatively new and widened PTH target range of

TABLE 59.6 The KDIGO Target Guidelines for Plasma Calcium, Phosphate, and PTH Concentrations in Chronic Kidney Disease Patients

GFR Category	Phosphate	Calcium (Adjusted for Albumin)	Parathyroid Hormone
3–5	Laboratory reference intervals	Laboratory reference intervals	Target level unknown, but if above upper limit of normal for the assay, assess vitamin D status and treat insufficiency and deficiency
5D	Maintain as close to laboratory reference intervals as possible	Laboratory reference intervals	Maintain within 2 to 9 times the upper limit of normal for the assay

5D, Patients receiving dialysis.
Table developed from Kidney Disease Improving Global Outcomes. KDIGO clinical practice guideline for the diagnosis, evaluation, prevention, and treatment of chronic kidney disease—Mineral and bone disorder (CKD-MBD). *Kidney Int Suppl* 2009:S1–130.

TABLE 59.7 Examples of Available Oral Phosphate Binders

Phosphate Binder	Advantages	Disadvantages
Aluminum salts	Calcium free High binder efficiency regardless of pH Cheap Moderate tablet burden	Risk of aluminum toxicity Requires frequent monitoring—extra cost
Calcium carbonate	Aluminum free Moderate binding efficacy Relatively low cost Moderate tablet burden Chewable	Calcium containing—potential risk of hypercalcemia and ectopic calcification Parathyroid hormone oversuppression Gastrointestinal side effects Efficacy pH dependent
Calcium acetate	Aluminum free Higher efficacy than calcichew/sevelamer Moderately cheap Lower calcium load than calcium carbonate Can be combined with magnesium to reduce calcium load	Calcium containing—potential risk of hypercalcemia and ectopic calcification, PTH oversuppresion Gastrointestinal side effects Large tablets, nonchewable formulation
Sevelamer hydrochloride and sevelamer carbonate	Aluminum and calcium free No gastrointestinal absorption Moderate efficacy Reduces total and low-density lipoprotein cholesterol Powder for mixing with water available	Relatively costly High pill burden Large tablets Gastrointestinal side effects Binds fat-soluble vitamins
Lanthanum carbonate	Aluminum and calcium free Minimal gastrointestinal absorption High efficacy across full pH range Chewable formulation Low tablet burden Powder available to disperse on meal	Relatively costly Gastrointestinal side effects

PTH, Parathyroid hormone.

150 to 680 ng/L (16–72 pmol/L).[107] Simultaneous "control" of all three bone disease surrogates in CKD—that is, serum calcium, phosphate, and PTH—was achieved in half of all dialysis patients during 2013.[107]

Strategies to reduce phosphate concentrations are employed routinely in the treatment of patients on dialysis. Inorganic phosphate within the blood accounts for less than 0.1% of total body phosphate. Clearance of phosphate on intermittent hemodialysis is approximately one-third of that seen with urea and is subject to postdialysis rebound because of efflux from the intracellular to the extracellular space. Phosphate is present in many foods and is linearly associated with protein ingestion. The recommended allowance of phosphate is reduced for patients on dialysis to around 800 mg/d. Treatment with vitamin D analogs increases gut absorption of phosphate from approximately 65% to almost 85%. The use of phosphate binders, taken with meals, is almost universal in dialysis patients; treatment may include calcium-containing and non-calcium-containing binders (Table 59.7). Prescribing of phosphate binders should be individualized for each patient because each binder has pros and cons. Interest has focused on the increased propensity to vascular calcification noted in those dialysis patients receiving calcium-containing phosphate binders. These binders reduce phosphate absorption to 30% to 40% and decrease serum phosphate concentrations. However, a systematic review of randomized controlled trials concluded that no evidence suggests that phosphate binders reduce all-cause or cardiovascular mortality compared with placebo.[187] An updated metaanalysis comparing calcium-based with non-calcium-based oral phosphate binders in patients with CKD, the majority of whom were receiving hemodialysis, concluded that there was a 22% risk reduction for all-cause mortality in those patients assigned a non-calcium-containing binder.[188] This suggests that high exposure to calcium-containing phosphate binders is detrimental, contributing to a positive calcium balance, and reflecting physicians' historical practice of trying to compensate for the reduced production of activated vitamin D in these patients. In summary, patients on conventional three times weekly dialysis are in a net positive phosphate balance. Control of hyperphosphatemia can be regained following a kidney transplant. However, what more can be achieved in those patients maintained on hemodialysis? The Frequent Hemodialysis Network (FHN) Trial describes resolution of hyperphosphatemia in patients receiving six times per week hemodialysis.[189]

Medical treatment strategies are designed to limit phosphate intake and normalize calcium. With the advent of vitamin D analogs, it has been possible to supplement vitamin D, resulting in increased plasma calcium concentrations and switching off of PTH production. Unfortunately, the commonly used analogs, such as 1α-hydroxyvitamin D3, also lead to increased absorption of calcium and phosphate from the gut. In the setting of aggressive treatment with vitamin D analogs, hypercalcemia may develop that is associated with low, suppressed concentrations of PTH. Alternative vitamin D receptor activators, such as paricalcitol, are associated with improved survival in US dialysis patients and have a lower incidence of treatment-related hyperphosphatemia and hypercalcemia than calcitriol.[190,191] The vitamin D receptor is ubiquitous and its stimulation has wide-ranging effects on the cardiovascular and immune systems; this may explain the benefits of treatment in CKD patients over and above the effects on reducing PTH.[192]

A further development in the management of CKD-MBD has been the generation of calcimimetic agents such as cinacalcet.[193,194] Calcimimetics can mimic calcium by directly stimulating the CaSR and can affect the molecular configuration of the CaSR to enhance its sensitivity to extracellular calcium.[194] Stimulation of the CaSR switches off PTH production selectively with no risk of increased phosphate absorption. Use of cinacalcet has increased the proportion of patients who reach the biochemical management targets for CKD-MBD[195] and has reduced the need for parathyroidectomy in patients with secondary hyperparathyroidism;[196] a reduction in fracture rate has also been observed.[197] However, a major prospective randomized controlled trial (Evaluation of Cinacalcet HCL Therapy to Lower CardioVascular Events [EVOLVE]) in hemodialysis patients with moderate to severe secondary hyperparathyroidism did not demonstrate significant cardiovascular event or mortality reduction.[195]

Aluminum Toxicity

A causative factor for renal bone disease, historically, has been aluminum intoxication (see Chapter 42). Aluminum concentrations in dialysis fluids were previously high, but with modern dialysis facilities, this is no longer such a problem. However, some dialysis patients are treated intermittently with aluminum-containing phosphate binders; therefore regular monitoring of blood aluminum concentration is recommended in such patients.[156] Aluminum accumulation has been associated with deposition along the mineralization surface of the osteoid and a low-turnover form of bone disease. Aluminum accumulation may be treated by infusions of the chelating agent desferrioxamine. Aluminum intoxication may be associated with neurologic disturbances characterized by dementia (dialysis dementia) and with a hypochromic microcytic anemia.

Anemia

The World Health Organization defines anemia, when the patient is at sea level, as a blood hemoglobin concentration of less than 13 g/dL (130 g/L) in adult men and less than 12 g/dL (120 g/L) in adult, nonpregnant women.[198] It is clearly established that anemia is inevitable as CKD progresses. Therapies are available to correct anemia; therefore it is mandatory that a patient with CKD should be assessed for anemia. The KDIGO 2012 Clinical Practice Guideline for the Evaluation and Management of CKD recommends that an estimated GFR of less than 60 mL/min/1.73 m^2 should be the cutoff value for determining the presence or absence of anemia and that, additionally, CKD should be considered as a possible cause of anemia when the GFR is less than 60 mL/min/1.73 m^2.[94] It is more likely to be the cause if the GFR is less than 30 mL/min/1.73 m^2 (<45 mL/min/1.73 m^2 in patients with diabetes) and no other cause (eg, blood loss, folic acid or vitamin B_{12} deficiency) is identified. The prevalence of anemia increases as GFR declines. In the NHANES III dataset the prevalence of anemia (defined as Hb <12 g/dL in men, Hb <11 g/dL in women) was 33% at a GFR of 15 mL/min/1.73 m^2 and 9% at a GFR of 30 mL/min/1.73 m^2.[55] CKD-related anemia occurs earlier in patients with diabetes and is highly prevalent among such patients.[199] In the United Kingdom, the median hemoglobin of patients starting dialysis is 9.7 g/dL.[107]

Detection is important because if left untreated, anemia causes many of the side effects of CKD, such as fatigue, breathlessness on exertion, intolerance to cold, and decreased exercise capacity. As indicated earlier, it is also a major factor in the high prevalence of cardiovascular disease in patients with CKD and contributes to the development of LVH. In patients on dialysis, large observational studies have clearly shown that anemia is associated with increased mortality rates and increased hospitalization.[200-203] In hemodialysis patients, hematocrit levels of 33% to 36% (corresponding to hemoglobin concentrations of 11 to 12 g/dL) were associated with the lowest risk for all-cause and cardiac mortality,[202] and these patients also had the lowest risk of hospitalization.[203,204]

Etiology of Anemia in CKD. The etiology of anemia in CKD is multifactorial. A major cause, however, is the loss of peritubular fibroblasts within the renal cortex that synthesize EPO. Failure of EPO production in the kidney leads to inappropriately low concentrations within the blood for the concomitant hemoglobin concentration. Other causes of anemia include absolute or functional iron deficiency, folic acid and vitamin B_{12} deficiencies, infections, and chronic inflammation. Red cell survival may also be reduced. Hemodialysis patients tend to have more severe anemia than peritoneal dialysis patients because of greater blood losses and hemolysis.

Several national and international organizations have published algorithms for the treatment of anemia in CKD and dialysis patients.[205-207] Recent concerns regarding the safety of treatment designed to *correct* anemia in CKD has led to revised guidelines, such that zealous attention to correction using the highest dose of erythropoiesis stimulating agents (ESAs) is avoided. The KDIGO recommendations include not intentionally increasing the hemoglobin above 11.5 g/dL.[205] The NICE guideline recommends that treatment should aim to maintain hemoglobin between 10.0 and 12.0 g/dL in adults.[206] Mainstays of treatment are iron supplementation and the use of ESAs. Warnings, indications, precautions, and instructions for dosing and administration of ESAs are available from national regulatory agencies, including the US Food and Drug Administration (FDA), and from product package inserts.

Assessment of Iron and Iron Supplementation. Iron status is assessed by measurement of serum ferritin and transferrin saturation. Transferrin saturation gives an indication of iron "delivery." Ferritin is used to represent iron stores. In patients with CKD, a serum ferritin concentration less than 100 μg/L is considered to suggest iron deficiency, and a serum ferritin of 100 to 200 μg/L in association with transferrin saturation less than 20% represents "functional" iron deficiency. Treatment of anemia in CKD requires adequate iron stores. A very high concentration of ferritin (>800 μg/L) may suggest iron overload (see Chapter 38). However, these indices have limitations (eg, a high ferritin concentration is also generated by an inflammatory process; transferrin varies with nutritional state and is also influenced by inflammation; high biological variation[208]). Clinical hematology laboratories may offer an automated estimate of the percentage of hypochromic red blood cells. A level above 10% is indicative of functional iron deficiency, and the target is less than 2.5%.[207]

Iron deficiency (absolute or functional) was the main cause of ESA resistance in the United Kingdom, but this has been solved by iron replacement strategies. In hemodialysis patient populations, the inverse relationship between ESA dose and iron stores continues to maintain a linear relationship up to a mean ferritin of 500 μg/L. Parenteral iron is the treatment of choice for absolute and functional iron deficiency because oral iron has low efficacy in CKD. Parenteral iron can easily be administered during dialysis in patients receiving hemodialysis. Hemodialysis patients have additional iron losses from gastrointestinal bleeding, blood tests, and losses in dialysis lines that result in iron supplementation requirements that outstrip the capacity of the gut to absorb iron. Maintenance intravenous iron in hemodialysis patients greatly reduces ESA requirements and costs.[209] Maintaining iron stores at steady state in a hemodialysis population requires 50 to 60 mg/week of intravenous iron.

In non-dialysis-treated CKD, a randomized study of intravenous iron versus oral iron in predialysis patients demonstrated a greater improvement in hemoglobin outcome in those on intravenous iron but no difference in the proportion of patients who had to commence ESA after the start of the study.[210]

Nevertheless, oral iron is easy and cheap to prescribe and can be used as first-line iron supplementation in nondialysis patients. It is appropriate to treat patients who have not responded to, or have been intolerant of, oral iron with intravenous iron every 6 to 8 weeks to maintain serum ferritin greater than 100 μg/L.

Use of Erythropoiesis-Stimulating Agents. ESAs are human recombinant erythropoietin (rhEPO or epoetin)—that is, synthetic versions of human EPO that are used to treat anemia. Following replenished iron stores and exclusion of other causes of anemia, the addition of ESAs is indicated for the treatment of CKD-related anemia. Measurement of serum EPO concentration is rarely indicated in the setting of renal anemia. The gene for human EPO was cloned in 1985, and epoetin was introduced into clinical practice shortly afterward.[211,212] ESAs are effective in correcting the anemia of CKD in 90% to 95% of patients. The most common side effect is hypertension; therefore blood pressure should be well controlled before treatment is introduced. Hypertension may develop or worsen in a quarter of patients. Failure to respond to treatment requires thorough investigation for many potential causes (Box 59.2). It is estimated that 3 million patients worldwide have received treatment with ESAs. A rare complication of ESA treatment is the generation of neutralizing antibodies to the ESA. These antibodies stop bone marrow erythroid cells from producing mature red blood cells, so-called pure red cell aplasia.[213] If a case of pure red cell aplasia is proven, then no additional recombinant ESAs are administered.

BOX 59.2 Causes of Failure to Respond to Erythropoiesis-Stimulating Agents

Iron status
Occult blood loss
Vitamin B12 or folate deficiency
Infection and inflammation
Inadequate dialysis
Hyperparathyroidism
Aluminum toxicity
Patient adherence
Hypothyroidism
Primary disease activity
Transplant rejection
Malignancy
Pure red cell aplasia

Many clinical benefits are derived from correcting anemia with ESAs, including improved exercise capacity,[214] improved cognitive function,[215] better quality of life,[216,217] and increased libido. Much of the evidence has been taken from studies in dialysis patients. In patients with advanced CKD not yet on dialysis, small nonrandomized studies have suggested that regression of LVH is possible with partial correction of anemia with epoetin.[218,219] Patients who receive an ESA consistently over the 2 years before commencement of dialysis may have improved survival,[220] although larger prospective randomized trials have not confirmed these observations. Two important studies focused on patients not yet on dialysis. The Correction of Hemoglobin and Outcomes in Renal Insufficiency (CHOIR) study showed no benefit of higher hemoglobin outcome (13.5 g/dL vs. 11.3 g/dL) in CKD patients. Higher outcome target hemoglobin concentrations showed increased risk (using composite endpoints of death, myocardial infarction, and hospitalization for congestive cardiac failure) and no incremental improvement in quality of life.[221] The Cardiovascular Risk Reduction in Early Anaemia Treatment with Epoetin Beta (CREATE) study reported early correction of anemia to normal hemoglobin outcome (13.0

to 15.0 g/dL vs. 10.5 to 11.5 g/dL) but did not reduce the risk of cardiovascular events in patients followed for 3 years.[222] Indeed, the hazard ratio for primary endpoints of death from any cause or death from cardiovascular disease consistently (but not significantly) favored the lower hemoglobin target group. LVH remained stable in both groups, and quality of life was significantly better in the higher hemoglobin outcome group.

A large randomized controlled trial has tested the hypothesis that normalization of anemia would have benefits in terms of morbidity and mortality for hemodialysis patients with New York Heart Association (NYHA) heart failure stage I to III.[223] Patients were randomized to normalization of anemia (618 patients and target hemoglobin concentration of 14 g/dL) or to the control group (615 patients and target hemoglobin concentration of 10 g/dL). The study was terminated early because of a nonsignificant higher risk of death in the normalization group (relative risk 1.3, confidence interval [CI] 0.9–1.9). These studies have been instructive in setting the current hemoglobin target of 10.0 to 12.0 g/dL and in recommending ESA dose adjustments when hemoglobin is less than 10.5 or greater than 11.5 g/dL to balance benefit versus safety to patients. It is not recommended to begin treatment with an ESA in the setting of active malignancy or active stroke. Nondialysis CKD patients with a hemoglobin greater than 10 g/dL should not be commenced on an ESA.[205] In dialysis patients, KDIGO recommends avoiding hemoglobin falling below 9 g/dL and that the maintenance level in most patients should be below full correction. The UK Renal Registry reports that 60% of hemodialysis patients have a reported hemoglobin between the acceptable range of 10 and 12 g/dL.[107]

The Uremic Syndrome

Uremia is defined as the excess within the blood of urea, creatinine, and other nitrogenous end products of amino acid and protein metabolism that are normally excreted in the urine. The *uremic syndrome,* the terminal clinical manifestation of kidney failure, is the group of symptoms, physical signs, and abnormal findings on diagnostic studies that result from failure of the kidneys to maintain adequate excretory, regulatory, and endocrine function.

Classic signs of uremia include progressive weakness and easy fatigue, loss of appetite followed by nausea and vomiting, muscle wasting, tremors, abnormal mental function, frequent but shallow respirations, and metabolic acidosis. In patients with kidney failure (GFR <15 mL/min/1.73 m^2), signs and symptoms of uremia or the need for RRT is generally present. The syndrome evolves to produce stupor, coma, and ultimately death unless RRT is provided. Regulation of body fluids is impaired in patients with uremia because of failure to excrete excess ingested fluid or to cope with fluid losses caused by vomiting or diarrhea. Patients also have difficulty excreting a salt load or retaining sodium when intake is low or vascular volume inadequate. Acid excretion is impaired, as is the ability to excrete nitrogenous metabolites from dietary sources. In addition to the consequences of reduced excretory, regulatory, and endocrine function of the kidneys, the uremic syndrome has several systemic manifestations, among them pericarditis, pleuritis, disordered platelet and granulocyte function, and encephalopathy that have been difficult to explain.

TABLE 59.8 Potential Uremic Toxins

Toxin	Effect
Urea	At very high concentrations (>300 mg/dL; >50 mmol/L) can cause headache, vomiting, and fatigue, carbamylation of proteins
Creatinine	Possibly affects glucose tolerance and erythrocyte survival
Cyanate	Causes drowsiness, hyperglycemia; a breakdown product of urea, it can cause carbamylation of proteins, altering protein function
Polyols (eg, myoinositol)	Can cause peripheral neuropathy
Phenols	Can be highly toxic because they are lipid soluble and therefore can cross cell membranes easily
Middle molecules (eg, atrial natriuretic peptide, cystatin C, delta sleep-inducing protein, IL-6, TNF-α, PTH)	Peritoneal dialysis patients clear middle molecules more efficiently than HD patients and show fewer signs of neuropathy than hemodialysis patients (many candidate molecules but none paramount)
β_2-microglobulin	Causative agent in renal amyloid

IL-6, Interleukin 6; *TNF-α,* tumor necrosis factor alpha; *PTH,* parathyroid hormone.

For over 200 years, scientists have been studying the nature of uremia, but no single retained molecule has yet qualified for the title "uremic toxin," and many now agree that a variety of compounds are potential uremic toxins (Table 59.8). At least 90 organic compounds are known to be retained in uremia.[224,225] Many more still unidentified solutes are possibly retained and might exert systemic toxicity. Although urea was the first metabolite to be identified as increased in uremia, this does not appear to be responsible for the systemic manifestations of uremia. Urea is a 60-Da water-soluble compound that has the highest concentrations of presently known uremic retention solutes in uremic plasma. Although its removal by dialysis is directly related to patient survival, the effects of urea on biological systems are not clear. Urea removal by dialysis is not necessarily representative of other molecules retained in the uremic syndrome, particularly protein-bound solutes such as *p*-cresol, or higher molecular weight molecules such as PTH. Urea may be the source of other, more toxic moieties.[226] However, it is more likely that the syndrome is a result of the cumulative effect of many retained compounds, which may act as toxins and may have an effect on metabolism in general—for example, through enzyme inhibition or derangement in membrane transport. The decreased ability of the kidneys to degrade or eliminate hormones may also have a role.

Acute Kidney Injury

Acute kidney injury (AKI) has largely replaced the older term *acute renal failure* and describes a sudden decline in kidney function over hours and days. AKI is an increasingly common and potentially catastrophic complication of systemic illness.

POINTS TO REMEMBER

Biochemical Characteristics of the Uremic Syndrome

Retained Nitrogenous Metabolites

Urea
Cyanate
Creatinine
Guanidine compounds
"Middle molecules"
Uric acid

Fluid, Acid-Base, and Electrolyte Disturbances

Fixed urine osmolality
Metabolic acidosis (decreased blood pH, bicarbonate)
Hyponatremia or hypernatremia
Hypokalemia or hyperkalemia
Hyperchloremia
Hypocalcemia
Hyperphosphatemia
Hypermagnesemia

Carbohydrate Intolerance

Insulin resistance (hypoglycemia may also occur)
Plasma insulin normal or increased
Delayed response to carbohydrate loading
Hyperglucagonemia

Abnormal Lipid Metabolism

Hypertriglyceridemia
Decreased high-density lipoprotein cholesterol
Hyperlipoproteinemia

Altered Endocrine Function

Secondary hyperparathyroidism
Osteomalacia (secondary to abnormal vitamin D metabolism)
Hyperreninemia and hyperaldosteronism
Hyporeninemia
Hypoaldosteronism
Decreased erythropoietin production
Altered thyroxine metabolism
Gonadal dysfunction (increased prolactin and luteinizing hormone, decreased testosterone)

Identifying the true incidence and prevalence of AKI has been difficult because of wide variation in the accepted definition of AKI. Several studies have reported multicenter experience with AKI in the intensive care unit (ICU) setting and note wide variation in practice and outcomes.[227,228]

In 2003, a new classification of AKI was proposed that was based on the combination of susceptibility, nature and timing of insult, biomarker response, urine output, and end-organ consequences.[229] In recognition of the potential clinical importance of small changes in kidney function and the need to standardize definitions of AKI for clinical and research purposes, the RIFLE criteria were adopted by the Acute Dialysis Quality Initiative (ADQI), providing a graded definition of AKI severity.[230] The acronym RIFLE defines three grades of increasing severity of AKI (risk, injury, and failure) and two outcome variables (loss and ESRD). The grades of severity are established on the basis of change in serum creatinine concentration and the decline in urine output from baseline. The

TABLE 59.9 The AKIN Criteria for AKI

AKIN Stage	Serum Creatinine Criteria*	Urine Output Criteria*
1	↑ ≥0.3 mg/dL (≥26 μmol/L) *or* ↑ ≥150% to 200% from baseline	<0.5 mL/kg/hr for >6 h
2	↑ >200% to 300% from baseline	<0.5 mL/kg/hr for >12 h
3	↑ >300% (>3-fold) from baseline *or* ≥4 mg/dL (≥354 μmol/L) with an acute rise of ≥0.5 mg/dL (≥44 μmol/L) in ≤24 h *or* Initiation of renal replacement therapy (irrespective of stage at time of initiation)	<0.3 mL/kg/hr for >24 h *or* Anuria for 12 h

*Only one criterion needs to be fulfilled to qualify for a stage.

most powerful tool to improve outcome in AKI is prevention, and the advantage of the RIFLE criteria is the definition of "risk," where it is envisaged that intervention may prevent injury and failure. More recently the Acute Kidney Injury Network (AKIN) proposed three stages of increasing disease severity (Table 59.9).[231] This working group has modified the RIFLE criteria slightly to incorporate smaller changes in serum creatinine concentration into the definition of risk because it was appreciated that small changes in kidney function can affect outcome. In essence, the AKIN has provided the following diagnostic criteria for AKI: an abrupt (within 48 hours) reduction in kidney function currently defined as an increase in serum creatinine concentration of either 0.3 mg/dL (26 μmol/L); an increase of 50% or greater (1.5-fold from baseline); or a reduction in urine output (documented oliguria <0.5 mL/kg/h for >6 hours).

A prospective study of the initial hospital management of AKI confirmed that in almost 40% of cases, AKI was iatrogenic or preventable.[232] In addition, a report by the National Confidential Enquiry into Patient Outcome and Death *(NCEPOD: Adding Insult to Injury)*, published in 2009,[233] found that opportunities were missed in the treatment of hospitalized patients that should have been rectified earlier and that deaths of people with AKI were easily preventable. The report has driven the focus of care onto AKI risk, identification, treatment, and referral for specialist services, recently summarized in guidance from NICE.[234] Early identification of intravascular volume depletion, cessation of nephrotoxic drugs, and early diagnosis of causative conditions can prevent AKI. Therefore prompt administration of intravenous crystalloid solutions such as 0.9% sodium chloride and balanced salt solutions may prevent further deterioration of AKI in many cases. Patients at risk for AKI include older persons; those with preexisting CKD, sepsis, diabetes, and heart disease; and those taking nephrotoxic drugs, particularly in the setting of hypovolemia. Fluid replacement requirements need careful monitoring and review of the patient, with emphasis on restoring an optimal circulatory volume without developing signs of fluid overload such as pulmonary edema. Additional monitoring may include use of a central venous

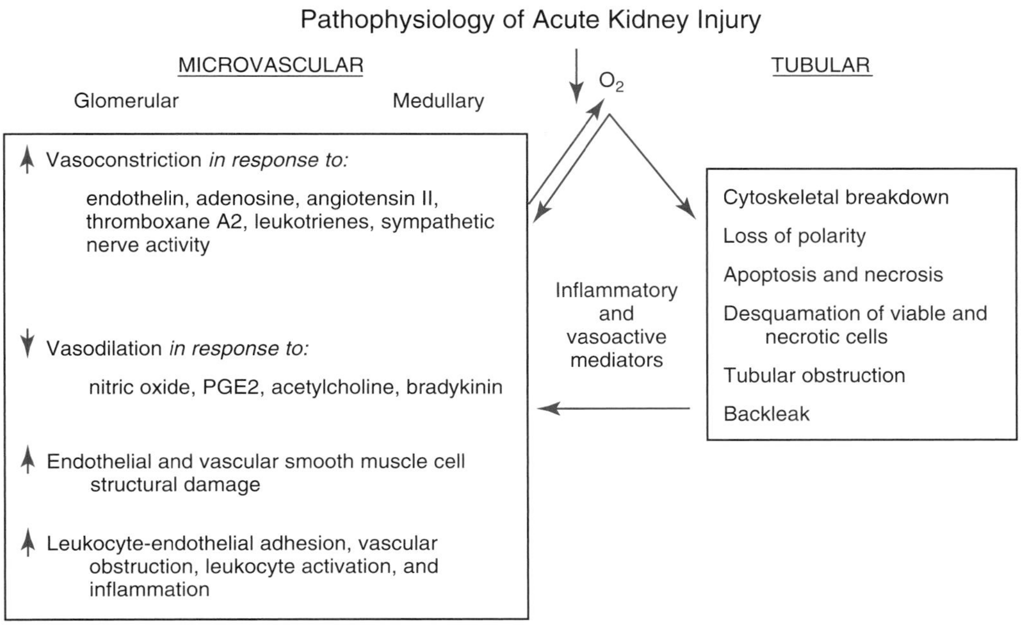

Pathophysiology of Acute Kidney Injury

MICROVASCULAR

Glomerular — Medullary

↑ Vasoconstriction *in response to:*
endothelin, adenosine, angiotensin II, thromboxane A2, leukotrienes, sympathetic nerve activity

↓ Vasodilation *in response to:*
nitric oxide, PGE2, acetylcholine, bradykinin

↑ Endothelial and vascular smooth muscle cell structural damage

↑ Leukocyte-endothelial adhesion, vascular obstruction, leukocyte activation, and inflammation

↓ O_2

Inflammatory and vasoactive mediators

TUBULAR

Cytoskeletal breakdown
Loss of polarity
Apoptosis and necrosis
Desquamation of viable and necrotic cells
Tubular obstruction
Backleak

FIGURE 59.15 Pathogenesis of ischemic acute kidney injury. Hypoxic insults cause vascular responses and tubular damage. (From Bonventre JV, Weinberg JM. Recent advances in the pathophysiology of ischemic acute renal failure. *J Am Soc Nephrol* 2003;14:2199–210.)

pressure (CVP) line. Insertion of a CVP line is a specialist skill that requires cannulation of the internal jugular vein, ideally utilizing ultrasonic guidance facilities. However, where hypovolemia is clinically apparent, the priority is to resuscitate the patient with fluid, rather than delay treatment by establishing invasive monitoring. The target CVP is 8 to 12 cm H_2O. A series of CVP measurements are useful to check response to fluids.

Clinical assessment of AKI should consider whether the precipitant is prerenal, intrarenal (intrinsic), or postrenal. Most commonly, AKI is caused by ischemia, which initiates a complex sequence of hemodynamic changes, endothelial injury, epithelial cell injury, and immunological mechanisms that underpin its initiation and extension.[235] Intrinsic AKI can be caused by primary vascular, glomerular, or interstitial disorders. It is therefore important that all patients presenting with AKI undergo urinalysis to test for infection, hematuria, and proteinuria. In most cases the kidney lesion seen on histology is referred to as acute tubular necrosis (ATN). ATN is caused by ischemic or nephrotoxic injury to the kidney. In 50% of cases of hospital-acquired AKI, the cause is multifactorial. (The term *ATN* is somewhat misleading, insofar as necrosis per se is seldom seen, but rather tubular *damage* occurs.) Although the pathogenesis is uncertain, a well-recognized clinical pattern is associated with the development of ATN, with anuria or oliguria and abnormalities indicating tubular dysfunction (Fig. 59.15).[236] Necrosis of tubular cells need not be extensive, but obstruction by tubular casts, back-leak of glomerular filtrate through gaps in the tubular epithelium caused by cellular denudation, and primary reductions in GFR caused by altered intrarenal hemodynamics, known as tubuloglomerular feedback, may occur.[237] Direct vasoconstriction of glomerular capillaries in response to ischemic insults can also occur and may be mediated by AII, endothelin,[238,239] and serotonin.[240]

Laboratory tests and imaging are crucial in the management of AKI. Tests assist in establishing the underlying diagnosis and excluding obstruction as a cause. Specific investigations are requested if kidney function has not improved following volume correction (Table 59.10). Kidney biopsy is generally reserved for cases of AKI where an ultrasound scan has excluded obstructed kidneys, kidney sizes are maintained, and the cause of AKI is otherwise unexplained and an intrinsic pathology is suspected. Urinary electrolyte measurements are often undertaken in the investigation of AKI. However, in practice, because the treatment of prerenal AKI and ATN requires prompt and continued correction of hypovolemia, the urinary findings are generally unhelpful.

Metabolic acidosis is the most common acid-base disorder in patients with AKI. Reduced renal excretion of potassium and the effects of acidosis on the generation of extracellular potassium may lead to a very high plasma potassium concentration. Severe hyperkalemia (plasma potassium concentration >6.5 mmol/L) is associated with life-threatening cardiac arrhythmias. Emergency treatment of hyperkalemia should be instituted as necessary. Patients who have an abnormal electrocardiogram in the setting of high plasma potassium concentration, or a potassium concentration of 6.5 mmol/L or greater, should receive 10% calcium gluconate intravenously over 2 to 3 minutes through a large-bore peripheral venous cannula or a central line. This treatment stabilizes myocardial cells. However, calcium gluconate will not lower the potassium concentration. Infusion of high concentrations of glucose stimulates insulin secretion from the pancreas and uptake of potassium into the intracellular space. A fall in potassium concentration should be expected within 60 minutes. In addition, low-dose rapid-acting insulin can be administered with the glucose bolus. Blood potassium concentration should be monitored hourly until the risk of a life-threatening cardiac event has passed and no evidence

TABLE 59.10 Investigation of AKI

Test	Indication/Comments
Urine Testing	
Urine reagent strip ("dipstick")	Hematuria and proteinuria may indicate glomerular origin
Red cell casts on microscopy	(Not available universally; may need bedside microscope)
Urine microscopy and culture	Identify urinary tract infection
Urine protein electrophoresis and immunofixation	
Blood Tests	
Baseline Studies	
Urea, electrolytes, and creatinine	Check previous laboratory reports: AKI or AKI with preexisting CKD
Calcium, phosphate, albumin	
Liver function tests	Suspected multiorgan involvement or abnormal coagulation
Acid-base studies	Arterial blood gas or venous plasma bicarbonate concentration
Full blood count	Anemia, hemolysis, thrombocytopenia
Coagulation studies	Evidence of intravascular coagulation; need to normalize if considering kidney biopsy and central line insertion
Selected Additional Investigations	
Blood culture	Any infection, but especially endocarditis, severe pneumonia, or urinary tract sepsis
Creatine kinase	Very high in cases of muscle inflammation and necrosis (rhabdomyolysis)
Lactate dehydrogenase	If high, suspect renal infarction and consider hemolysis
Antineutrophil cytoplasmic antibodies	Vasculitides
Antiglomerular basement membrane antibody	Antiglomerular basement membrane disease
Antinuclear antibodies	SLE
Anti-dsDNA antibodies, extractable nuclear antigens	SLE
Low C3 complement	SLE, MPGN, C3 glomerulopathies
Low C4 complement	Systemic lupus erythematosus, atheroembolism, cryoglobulinemia, MPGN (immune complex positive)
Cryoglobulin	Cryoglobulinemia
Urate	Urate nephropathy
Serum protein electrophoresis	Myeloma
Virology studies	Hepatitis serology, human immunodeficiency virus
Other serology	Antistreptolysin O titer
Imaging	
Chest x-ray	Pulmonary edema, pneumonia, effusions, malignancy, and granulomas
Abdominal x-ray (kidney, ureter, and bladder)	Renal stones
Renal tract ultrasound scan	Identify size and symmetry of kidneys Evidence of an obstructed system Small, shrunken kidneys in advanced CKD
Computed tomography scan	Anatomy and perfusion
Magnetic resonance imaging	Angiography to identify renovascular lesions
Formal angiography	Critical renal artery stenosis
Kidney Biopsy	Reserved for patients with unexplained AKI in whom acute tubular necrosis is not suspected. It is anticipated that additional therapy such as steroids, cytotoxic drugs, and plasma exchange may be required.

CKD, Chronic kidney disease; *dsDNA,* double-stranded DNA; *MPGN,* membranoproliferative glomerulonephritis; *SLE,* systemic lupus erythematosus.

of potassium rebound is found. Blood glucose concentration should be monitored because hypoglycemia may occur following exogenous insulin. Again, care should be taken with 50% glucose infusions that good venous access is established because extravasation can cause severe tissue necrosis.

When hyperkalemia persists despite appropriate medical measures, then RRT should be considered. Options for RRT include intermittent hemodialysis, peritoneal dialysis, and continuous renal replacement therapies (hemofiltration and hemodiafiltration) (see later). The continuous modalities are particularly appropriate for the intensive care unit (ICU) setting in cases of multiple-organ failure. Continuous therapies are useful in the treatment of septic shock, cardiac failure, pancreatitis, and acute respiratory distress syndrome.

They also allow the use of supplementary feeding, which is important in the oliguric patient with established AKI, in whom fluid is restricted to avoid overload.

If the patient survives, recovery usually will occur within days or weeks following removal of the initiating event and requires ongoing careful monitoring. There is an initial polyuric phase because glomerular function recovers before tubular function recovers. This polyuric phase recedes after a few days to weeks. Uncomplicated AKI has a mortality rate of 5% to 10%,[241] although AKI complicating nonrenal organ system failure in the ICU setting is associated with mortality rates approaching 50% to 70%, despite advances in dialysis treatment.[229]

Serum creatinine is the most widely used parameter for everyday assessment of GFR, but it has poor sensitivity and specificity in AKI because it lags behind both kidney injury and recovery. Several urinary and serum biomarkers of early tubular injury are being studied to assess whether injury can be detected before GFR is decreased. These include urinary kidney injury molecule-1 (KIM-1), plasma and urinary neutrophil gelatinase-associated lipocalin (NGAL), and urinary IL-18 (see Chapter 32).

Contrast-Induced Acute Kidney Injury

Many procedures and tests that are undertaken within the hospital environment may contribute to the burden of AKI. In particular, intravascular administration of radiocontrast media during enhanced CT scanning and angiographic procedures accounts for many cases of AKI.[241] This is an important point: Contrast media are commonly administered worldwide,[242] and preventive strategies should be employed in patients with preexisting CKD, particularly in those with GFR of less than 40 mL/min/1.73 m^2, in patients with diabetes mellitus, and those who are dehydrated and at increased risk of developing AKI when undergoing imaging.

Radiocontrast media are iodinated and may be ionic or nonionic. At concentrations required for angiography or CT scanning, the various agents used have differing osmolality. First-generation agents were ionic monomers with a very high osmolality with respect to plasma (eg, 1500–1800 mOsmol/kg). Second-generation agents, such as iohexol, are nonionic monomers with a lower osmolality, although still higher than that of plasma (eg, 600–850 mOsmol/kg). An iso-osmolal agent, iodixanol, is also available (osmolality 290 mOsmol/kg). The use of low- and iso-osmolar agents is associated with a lower incidence of adverse events, including AKI, compared to the older high-osmolar compounds.[243,244] Nevertheless, efforts to prevent AKI should be considered before a radiocontrast load is administered, regardless of the agent used. If possible, alternative investigations should be performed. However, when radiocontrast is required, the patient should be adequately hydrated with crystalloid solutions such as normal saline, isotonic sodium bicarbonate, or balanced salt solutions. More recently, the efficacy of the antioxidant, *N*-acetylcysteine (NAC), commonly administered as part of a strategy to prevent AKI, has been questioned, and although tolerated and safe, it is no longer recommended.[243] The focus of management is identifying the risk, optimizing fluid management, and avoiding use of nephrotoxic drugs. NSAIDs should be avoided because they interfere with vasodilator prostaglandins, causing increased renal vasoconstriction.

POINTS TO REMEMBER

Causes of Acute Kidney Injury (AKI)

- Prerenal AKI:
  - Hemorrhage
  - Diarrhea
  - Postoperative fluid and blood losses
  - Sepsis
  - Acute cardiac failure
- Renal (intrinsic renal disease) AKI:
  - Tubular
    - Any of the 'prerenal' causes that are severe or that are not corrected promptly leading to ATN. Other causes of ATN
    - Drug nephrotoxicity
      - NSAIDs, ACE inhibitors
      - Aminoglycoside antibiotics
      - Amphotericin
    - Contrast nephropathy
    - Poisoning
    - TIN
      - Allergic TIN associated with antibiotics and NSAIDs
      - Sarcoidosis
      - Pyelonephritis
  - Glomerular
    - RPGN (ANCA-associated vasculitides, Goodpasture's disease, SLE, other crescentic glomerulonephritides)
    - Thrombotic microangiopathies
    - Cryoglobulinemia
    - Atheroembolism
  - Vascular
    - Aortic dissection
    - Renal vein thrombosis
  - Miscellaneous
    - Rhabdomyolysis
    - Urate nephropathy
    - Hepatorenal syndrome
- Postrenal AKI:
  - Bladder outflow obstruction
  - Benign and malignant prostate disease
  - Invasive bladder carcinoma
  - Bilateral renal calculi or calculi within a single kidney
  - Retroperitoneal fibrosis

ACE, Angiotensin converting enzyme; *AKI*, acute kidney injury; *ANCA*, antineutrophil cytoplasmic antibody; *ATN*, acute tubular necrosis; *NSAIDs*, nonsteroidal antiinflammatory drugs; *RPGN*, rapidly progressive glomerulonephritis; *SLE*, systemic lupus erythematosus; *TIN*, tubulointerstitial nephritis.

Consideration should be given to withholding the drug metformin at the time of the exposure to contrast in patients with diabetes and CKD.[243] It is imperative that at-risk patients receiving intravenous iodinated contrast agents have a further serum creatinine measurement 48 to 96 hours after the procedure.[94] Gadolinium-based contrast agents are used in enhanced magnetic resonance scanning. These agents are non-nephrotoxic, but can rarely be associated with a serious side effect, nephrogenic systemic fibrosis, in patients with advanced kidney disease including dialysis patients. Where there is no reasonable alternative to contrast-enhanced MRI, the lowest dose of the lowest risk compounds can be administered even to patients with advanced CKD.[243]

DISEASES OF THE KIDNEY

Diabetic Nephropathy

Diabetes mellitus is a state of chronic hyperglycemia sufficient to cause long-term damage to specific tissues, notably the kidney, retina, nerves, and arteries (see Chapter 57). Type 1 diabetes is due to autoimmune destruction of pancreatic islet β-cells, causing loss of insulin secretion. Type 2 diabetes is due to the combination of cellular resistance to insulin and β-cell failure. Tissue lesions are common to both types of diabetes, and chronic hyperglycemia (or a closely related metabolic abnormality) is responsible for diabetic complications, including diabetic nephropathy. The World Health Organization (WHO) and national diabetes agencies have approved diagnostic criteria for diabetes based on venous plasma glucose concentrations, with subsequent guidance in 2011 confirming the acceptability of glycated hemoglobin for this purpose in certain situations (see Chapter 57). In 2012, the WHO estimated that 9% of adults aged over 18 years worldwide were affected by diabetes.[245]

Background

Diabetic nephropathy is a clinical diagnosis based on the finding of proteinuria in a patient with diabetes and in whom there is no evidence of urinary tract infection. Overt nephropathy is characterized by protein loss greater than 0.5 g/d, approximately equivalent to albumin loss of greater than 300 mg/d or category A3 albuminuria. For a variety of reasons, it is preferable to assess proteinuria as albuminuria (see Chapter 32), and albumin has long been uniformly adopted as the "criterion standard" in evaluating diabetes-related kidney damage.[96,246] Category A2 albuminuria, equivalent to urinary albumin loss of between 30 and 300 mg/d, was previously termed *microalbuminuria*, although this terminology is no longer recommended.[94] Diabetic nephropathy is the most common cause of ESRD in the United States. The number of incident patients with diabetes as the cause of ESRD exceeded 50,000 during 2010, but it has fallen slightly since (see Fig. 59.12).[106] Almost 250,000 people receiving RRT in the United States have diabetes as the cause of their ESRD, and this continues to rise steadily at around 2.5% per year.[106] Among patients who require dialysis, those with diabetes have a 22% higher mortality at 1 year and a 15% higher mortality at 5 years than patients without diabetes. Diabetic nephropathy as a cause of ESRD in the United Kingdom is seen in approximately 25% of new patients—a lower percentage than that of the United States and Europe.[107] In the United States, a number of objectives were developed for reducing threats to the health of the nation as part of the Healthy People Initiative. One of the objectives of the Healthy People Initiative (HP 2010 Objective 4.7) was to reduce the incidence rate of ESRD caused by diabetes from 145 per million population in 2003 to 78 per million people by 2010.[247] However, the overall rate for new cases of ESRD caused by diabetes missed this target and was 157 pmp in 2011.[106] The Healthy People Initiative is ongoing, and Healthy People 2020 is active, having been established in 2010. There are several important targets and aspirations related to CKD and ESRD within this program.[106] It is interesting to note that the HP2020 CKD 9.1 objective is to reduce kidney failure due to diabetes to the target of 152 pmp. The prevalence of diabetes as a cause of ESRD is variable among ethnic groups within the United States, with whites having rates approximately 25% of those observed among African Americans.[106]

Diabetic nephropathy is clinically a very slowly developing condition, but ultrastructural evidence of glomerular damage has been found in renal biopsies taken from type 1 diabetic patients within a few years of their diagnosis.[46,248,249] In type 1 diabetes, early macroscopic changes include kidney enlargement and pallor. With disease progression, the kidneys become smaller. Type 2 diabetes is typified by variable kidney contraction caused by associated ischemia. On histologic examination, glomerular changes include diffuse mesangial sclerosis with accentuation of matrix and irregularly thickened basement membranes; sclerotic, acellular mesangial nodules (so-called Kimmelstiel-Wilson lesions); hyaline fibrin cap lesions around peripheral capillary loops; capsular drop lesions located within Bowman capsule; and hyalinosis of arterioles.

Clinical progression is defined in terms of changes in rate of urinary albumin loss and decline in GFR and blood pressure changes (Table 59.11). In type 1 diabetes, it is unusual to develop albuminuria within the first 5 years of diagnosis, but it can occur anytime thereafter, and even after 40 years. Patients with type 1 diabetes and category A2 albuminuria will progress to overt nephropathy at an average rate of 20% over 5 years.[250] Long-term follow-up data on albuminuric patients confirm that 30% regress to normoalbuminuria and the rest remain albuminuric at 10 years.[251] The United Kingdom Prospective Diabetes Study (UKPDS) has described the incidence of albuminuria (equivalent to A2 albuminuria) as 6.5% and overt nephropathy (equivalent to A3 albuminuria) as 0.7% at diagnosis of type 2 diabetes in a large cohort of patients.[252] As albuminuria worsens and blood pressure increases, a relentless decline in GFR occurs.

Family studies of patients with type 1 diabetes have shown that diabetic siblings of patients with nephropathy have a fourfold risk of nephropathy compared with siblings without nephropathy. A family history of hypertension and cardiovascular disease may increase nephropathy rates.[253] Considerable work has been undertaken to look for genetic linkages with the development of nephropathy in diabetes.[254] However, the best available predictor for development of nephropathy is albuminuria.

Pathophysiology

Observational studies have shown that sustained poor glycemic control is associated with a greater risk for development of nephropathy in both type 1 and type 2 diabetes.[145,255-257] The exact mechanism for hyperglycemic tissue damage probably includes (1) glycation of proteins leading to the formation of advanced glycation end products (AGEs), (2) overactivity of the polyol pathway, and (3) generation of reactive oxygen species.[258] Polyols are sugar alcohols formed from their respective sugars under the action of aldose reductase. Glucose is preferentially shunted through the polyol pathway under hyperglycemic conditions, generating sorbitol that accumulates within cells. A key step linking glucotoxicity to cell dysfunction in diabetic nephropathy is the excess of extracellular matrix within the glomerulus and interstitium. A

TABLE 59.11 **Development of Diabetic Nephropathy**

Stage	Designation	Characteristics	Structural Changes	Glomerular Filtration Rate (mL/min/1.73 m²)	Blood Pressure (mm Hg)
I	Hyperfunction	Hyperfiltration	Glomerular hypertrophy	>150	Normal
II	Normoalbuminuria	Normal albumin loss (<30 mg/d)	Basement membrane thickening	150	Normal
III	Incipient diabetic nephropathy	Increased albumin loss (30–300 mg/d)	Albumin loss correlates with structural damage and hypertrophy of remaining glomeruli	125	Increased
IV	Overt diabetic nephropathy	Clinical proteinuria (>300 mg/d)	Advanced structural damage	<100	Hypertension
V	Uremia	Kidney failure	Glomerular closure	0–10	High

number of genes encoding matrix proteins in hyperglycemic conditions have been identified.[259] For example, transcription of the gene for TGF-β is stimulated by hyperglycemia, AGE, AII, and reactive oxygen species.[260-262]

One important consequence of glucose-stimulated TGF-β transcription is upregulation of the insulin-independent GLUT-1 transporter in mesangial cells. Glucose is transported to the cells through GLUT-1 and is metabolized mainly by the glycolytic pathway. Increased de novo synthesis of diacylglycerol results in the activation of protein kinase C and mitogen-activated kinases. Activation of these enzymes can lead to stimulation of certain genes, including TGF-β. Activation of TGF-β can induce the expression of GLUT-1, and these signaling pathways induce the expression of extracellular matrix proteins. The formation of AGE also generates reactive oxygen species, which can activate latent TGF-β.[259] Studies employing neutralizing anti–TGF-β antibodies have provided evidence that the prosclerotic and hypertrophic effects of high ambient glucose in cultured renal cells are largely mediated by autocrine production and activation of TGF-β.[263,264] These antibodies can reverse established nephropathy in animal models.[265,266] Furthermore, glomerular TGF-β mRNA is markedly increased in kidney biopsy specimens from patients with proven diabetic kidney disease, and blood and urine sampling across the renal vascular bed confirms net renal production of TGF-β in diabetic patients.[267] Treatment with the ACE inhibitor captopril lowers circulating TGF-β concentrations in patients with diabetic nephropathy.[268] The receptor for AGE (RAGE) has been identified.[269] RAGE is selectively expressed in the glomerular epithelial cells (podocytes) and not in the mesangial cell or the glomerular endothelium.[270] Increased accumulation of AGE in diabetes engages podocyte RAGE and may lead to increased glomerular permeability.[271] Vascular hyperpermeability, a hallmark feature of diabetes, can be suppressed by inhibiting RAGE in the animal model of diabetes, the streptozotocin-treated rat.[272]

Studies of experimental diabetes in the rat suggest that hyperfiltration alone could cause glomerular changes; conflicting reports have described the effects in humans. Increased GFR could be a predictor of progression to albuminuria, but it is also a reflection of poor metabolic control. In the Diabetes Control and Complications Trial (DCCT),[255] no association was noted between hyperfiltration and subsequent development of albuminuria.[273] Systemic blood pressure is higher in patients with diabetes who subsequently develop albuminuria, although it is not clear which comes first. Tubulointerstitial fibrosis occurs in diabetic nephropathy, in addition to glomerulosclerosis. Decreased GFR correlates with interstitial and glomerular expansion.[274]

Treatment Strategies

The cornerstones of treatment for diabetic nephropathy consist of glycemic control; blood pressure control, particularly with drugs that block the RAAS; and management of cardiovascular risk.[255,257,275,276] Guidelines published by NICE recommend targeting glycated hemoglobin (HbA_{1c}) concentrations to 48 mmol/mol (6.5%) or lower, while acknowledging the need for individualized target setting in certain cases.[277-279] High blood pressure accelerates the progressive increase in albuminuria in patients with initially normal urinary albumin loss and accelerates loss of kidney function in those with overt nephropathy in type 2 diabetes.[280,281] The NKF Task Force on Cardiovascular Disease has recommended a target blood pressure of less than 125/75 mm Hg in diabetic kidney disease.[282] In the United Kingdom, a target blood pressure of less than 130/80 mm Hg is recommended for people with diabetes and CKD (see earlier).[98] ACE inhibitors and ARBs slow the progression of diabetic kidney disease.[79,283-285] A trial reported in 2000 confirmed that even normoalbuminuric patients with type 2 diabetes should be managed with ACE inhibitors or ARBs to prevent cardiovascular events.[138] In addition to lowered systemic blood pressure, such patients have lowered glomerular capillary blood pressure and protein filtration.[286,287] ACE inhibitors and ARBs also reduce AII-mediated effects on glomerular permeability and cell proliferation and fibrosis[81,288] and should be incorporated into the treatment schedules of all patients with type 2 diabetes and those with type 1 diabetes and albuminuria. ACE inhibitors may exacerbate hyperkalemia in patients with advanced kidney disease and/or hyporeninemic hypoaldosteronism. In older patients with renal artery stenosis, they may cause a rapid decline in kidney function. A low-sodium diet potentiates the antihypertensive effect and antiproteinuric effect of AII blockade in type 2 diabetes.[289] Patients should be encouraged to stop smoking because smoking increases the risk of albuminuria.[290] Dyslipidemias should be managed as outlined for nondiabetic proteinuric CKD. For many years, the Steno Diabetes Center in Copenhagen, Denmark, has advocated multifactorial interventions in the management of type 2 diabetes. For example, intensified interventions, including tight glucose regulation; use of RAAS blockers, aspirin, and lipid-lowering agents; and lifestyle changes, were shown to reduce nonfatal cardiovascular disease among patients with type 2 diabetes[291] and subsequently provide beneficial effects with respect to vascular complications and all-cause mortality.[292]

Hypertensive Nephropathy

Hypertension is second only to diabetes as a primary diagnosis of ESRD for incident patients commencing dialysis in the United States (see Fig. 59.12). The incidence is higher in older people and especially among the black population in the United States. Hypertension often develops as a consequence of CKD because of alterations in salt and water metabolism and activation of the sympathetic nervous and renin-angiotensin systems.[293,294] Hypertension can act as an accelerating force in the development of ESRD. As described earlier, treatment of hypertension to predefined target blood pressure values is critical in preventing progression to ESRD.[74,111,295] Various national and international guidelines on the treatment of hypertension have been published, although variability is evident among these recommendations. The JNC 7 report suggests that the risk of cardiovascular disease doubles for each increment in BP of 20/10 mm Hg beginning at 115/75 mm Hg. The report identifies 120/80 mm Hg as normotension. All patients with hypertension (>140/90 mm Hg) should receive lifestyle change advice and antihypertensive medication if necessary.[113]

Large vessel *renovascular disease* can cause hypertension. Primary diseases of the renal arteries usually involve the origin of the renal arteries at the aorta (ostial lesions). Secondary diseases with hypertension and CKD with small vessel and intrarenal disease are referred to as *ischemic nephropathy*. A complex interplay occurs between renal artery stenosis and ischemic nephropathy. Atherosclerosis accounts for more than 90% of renal artery stenosis. The disease is progressive and may cause renal artery occlusion.[296] Prevalence increases with age and is associated with refractory hypertension, low body mass index, smoking, diabetes, and established vascular disease elsewhere. In general, as a marker of established cardiovascular disease, atheromatous renal artery stenosis is associated with a poor prognosis.[297] Diagnosis requires a high index of suspicion and is guided by radiologic examination of the renal arterial anatomy. Patients who receive ACE inhibitors and ARBs may develop AKI in the setting of severe bilateral renovascular disease or severe disease to a single functioning kidney. Kidney function should be carefully monitored following the introduction of these drugs, and a fall of GFR in excess of 15% to 20% should raise the suspicion of renovascular disease. The diagnosis is important to make because radiological placement of intraluminal stents[298] is possible, and surgical repair can be performed to prolong vessel patency.[299] Patients are at risk, however, of atheroembolism following intervention.[300] A correctable atherosclerotic renal artery stenosis (ARAS) lesion is found in less than 1% of all hypertensive patients, so investigation has to be targeted to high-risk groups. However, a note of caution: Two large studies (ASTRAL and STAR) failed to confirm any benefit from radiological interventions in patients with atheromatous renal artery stenosis.[301,302] The implication of these studies is that the disease should be managed medically with attention to traditional cardiovascular risk factor reduction strategies.

Renal artery stenosis in younger patients is characteristically due to fibromuscular dysplasia. The medial part of the artery is most commonly affected and presents radiologically as alternate bands of narrowing and dilatation, giving rise to a "string of beads" appearance. If the diagnosis is made, then hypertension can be cured following balloon angioplasty to the artery in at least 50% of cases.

Noninvasive imaging is readily available and includes CT angiogram and MRI angiography with gadolinium-based contrast media. A rare but potentially fatal disease—nephrogenic systemic fibrosis—has been described in patients with advanced kidney disease receiving gadolinium-based contrast media during MRI. Because many patients who are investigated for ARAS will have CKD, the approach to investigation has changed. Nephrogenic systemic fibrosis was first described in 2000 as a cutaneous scleromyxedema-like disorder in patients with ESRD.[303] Gadolinium-based contrast media are not recommended for patients with advanced renal impairment, particularly those on dialysis.[304] The Royal College of Radiologists in the United Kingdom published updated guidelines in 2015. These acknowledge that on certain occasions, it is necessary for contrast-enhanced MRI to be used in patients with advanced CKD, including those patients on dialysis (see earlier section on contrast-induced AKI).[243]

Glomerular Disease

Glomerular disease is suggested clinically by the finding of blood and protein in the urine on urine reagent strip testing. Proteinuria of greater than 1 g/day (0.88 g/g creatinine; 100 mg/mmol creatinine) in the absence of an overflow-type proteinuria, such as myoglobinuria or light chain–related disease, is invariably glomerular in origin. Although a detailed discussion of each glomerular disease is beyond the scope of this book, the most important diseases are discussed to illustrate the spectrum of disease. For further information regarding clinical guidelines, the reader is directed to the KDIGO *Clinical Practice Guideline for Glomerulonephritis*.[305] Whereas the incidence of kidney failure in the Western world has increased dramatically over recent years, in the United States the incidence rate due to glomerulonephritis has fallen (see Fig. 59.12).[106] In the United Kingdom, glomerulonephritis accounts for 14% of new cases of established renal failure.[306]

Primary Glomerular Disease

Glomerulonephritis can be primary (affecting only the kidneys) or secondary (in which the kidneys are involved as part of a systemic process). Histopathologic classification of glomerulonephritis may appear slightly cumbersome, but it is readily simplified by consideration of the glomerular structures and cells that may be involved and the presence or absence of immune complexes (Table 59.12). In essence, only three cell types are involved—endothelial, epithelial, and mesangial—plus the acellular GBM. The glomerular cells and the GBM have a limited range of response to injury—namely, proliferation, scarring (sclerosis), and GBM thickening. The term *focal* is used if fewer than half of the glomeruli are involved in the disease process as seen on light microscopy, whereas *diffuse glomerulonephritis* refers to cases in which all glomeruli are involved. Immune deposits identified following

TABLE 59.12 Overview of Some Primary Glomerular Diseases

Disease	Histological Findings	Clinical Spectrum	Treatment	Prognosis
IgA nephropathy	Focal mesangial cell proliferation on LM. IgA deposited within mesangial cells on IM.	Variable: incidental finding; episodes of macroscopic hematuria; proteinuria and declining GFR. There is a male preponderance, and the peak incidence occurs in the second and third decades of life. May be associated with systemic vasculitis in HSP.	Generic treatment targeting blood pressure and RAAS blockade. Selected cases receive corticosteroids and cytotoxic drugs.	Variable, but 30% to 40% progress to kidney failure over 20 years.
Minimal change disease (MCD)	Little evidence of cellular involvement on LM. Podocyte foot process effacement demonstrated on EM. No immune deposits.	Most common cause of nephrotic syndrome in children. Usually idiopathic. Relapsing and remitting course.	Oral corticosteroids and cytotoxic drugs.	Does not cause kidney failure. Significant side effects of immunosuppressant drugs.
Focal segmental glomerulosclerosis (FSGS)	Glomerular scarring and nonspecific trapping of immune complexes in scarred areas.	Common cause of nephrotic syndrome in adults. Congenital forms described. Secondary causes include collapsing variety seen in HIVAN.	Idiopathic disease requires corticosteroids and cytotoxic drugs in selected cases.	Nephrotic syndrome commonly refractory to treatment. 30% to 40% develop kidney failure at 10 years.
Membranous nephropathy	Thickened GBM with immune deposits in subepithelial GBM. Classically, "spikes" are seen along the GBM and represent new GBM squeezed between deposits.	Common cause of nephrotic syndrome. Secondary causes in 20% of cases. Idiopathic or primary cause supported by PLA_2R antibody positivity.	Treat underlying condition. Treat idiopathic membranous nephropathy generically, and if progressive, add immunosuppressive drugs,	Variable outcome: "rule of thirds" (see text).

EM, Electron microscopy; *ESRD,* end-stage renal disease; *FSGS,* focal segmental glomerulosclerosis; *GBM,* glomerular basement membrane; *GFR,* glomerular filtration rate; *HIVAN,* human immunodeficiency virus-associated nephropathy; *HSP,* Henoch-Schönlein purpura; *IM,* immunofluorescence or imunoperoxidase microscopy; *LM,* light microscopy; *PLA_2R,* phospholipase A_2 receptor antibody; *RAAS,* renin-angiotensin-aldosterone system.

immunofluorescence or immunoperoxidase staining do not define whether a disease is focal or diffuse.

IgA Nephropathy. IgA nephropathy is an example of a focal glomerulonephritis with focal mesangial cell proliferation demonstrated by light microscopy. However, diffuse and global deposition of the immunoglobulin, IgA, can be demonstrated following immunostaining. It is the most common type of glomerulonephritis worldwide and has a particularly high prevalence around the Pacific rim, where it is commonly reported as an incidental finding in kidney biopsy specimens from potential kidney donors.[307] The disease tends to be slowly progressive (in terms of loss of kidney function), depending, as with most kidney diseases, on the degree of proteinuria, kidney function at time of diagnosis, and degree of interstitial fibrosis on kidney biopsy. Up to 50% of patients exhibit increased concentrations of serum IgA, although diagnosis depends on kidney biopsy findings. Clinical presentation varies considerably from asymptomatic microscopic hematuria to macroscopic hematuria; proteinuria including nephrotic syndrome; and crescentic glomerulonephritis with kidney failure. Episodic macroscopic hematuria is seen in some patients at the same time as an upper respiratory tract infection. IgA nephropathy may also present with established proteinuria, renal impairment, and hypertension. Variation in clinical and histologic features leads to difficulty in reaching conclusions regarding treatment protocols that have been tested in clinical trials.

No treatment is available that specifically modifies mesangial deposition of IgA, and available options are limited to downstream immune and inflammatory events that may lead to scarring. Treatment options range from tonsillectomy in patients with macroscopic hematuria associated with respiratory infection to no treatment in those with isolated microscopic hematuria or those with proteinuria of less than 1 g/d. In progressive disease, all patients are treated in a similar generic fashion as for most kidney diseases, including targeting blood pressure to less than 125/75 mm Hg and using comprehensive RAAS blockade to minimize proteinuria. Assessment of the impact of immunosuppressive therapy is compromised by the heterogeneity of the disease and the duration of a randomized controlled study with sufficient numbers to allow a conclusion. Nevertheless, a large Italian study with more than 10 years of follow-up data demonstrated benefit from oral corticosteroids in high doses for 6

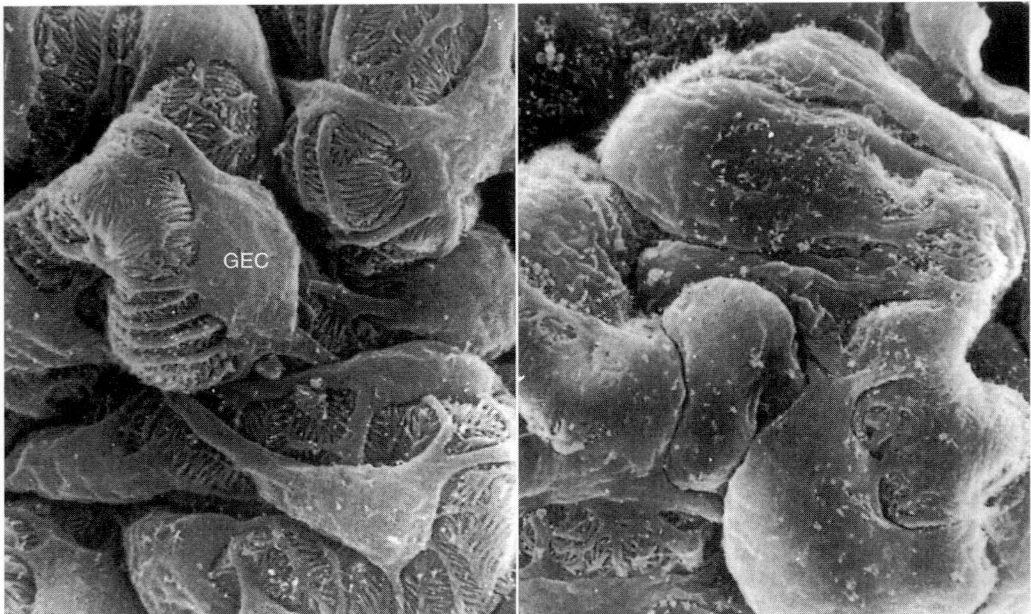

FIGURE 59.16 Graphic example of glomerular changes in nephrotic syndrome. Scanning electron microscopic view of glomerular epithelial podocytes from a vehicle-treated rat *(left)* and a puromycin aminonucleoside (PAN)–treated (180 mg/kg body weight) rat *(right)*. Note the extensive loss of podocyte foot processes, which occurs in response to PAN-induced nephrotic syndrome and illustrates the major cellular changes that can occur in nephrotic syndrome. *GEC,* Glomerular epithelial cell. (From Ricardo SD, Bertram JF, Ryan GB: Antioxidants protect podocyte foot processes in puromycin aminonucleoside–treated rats. *J Am Soc Nephrol* 1994;4:1974–86.)

months.[308,309] In addition, a retrospective study has recently reported benefit from corticosteroids.[310] Cytotoxic therapy can be considered for rapidly progressing or vasculitic IgA.[311]

Nephrotic Syndrome. Nephrotic syndrome is defined as heavy proteinuria (>3 g/d), reduced serum albumin concentration, and edema. In comparison with nephritic syndrome, nephrotic patients may exhibit an otherwise bland urinary sediment with little hematuria. Nephrotic syndrome can occur at any age from neonate to elderly. Although the underlying kidney disease tends to vary with age, in all cases the lesion is within the glomerulus and is associated with damage to the specialized visceral epithelial cells, the podocytes (see earlier). Proteinuria is a consequence of a reduction in the charge-selective properties of the filtration barrier, particularly the GBM, and of alterations in the slit diaphragms of interdigitating foot processes of adjacent podocytes (Fig. 59.16).[312,313] Following the discovery of numerous genes and podocyte proteins that make up the slit diaphragm, the pathophysiology of glomerular proteinuria is beginning to be elucidated. The primary glomerular diseases that cause nephrotic syndrome have recently been termed *podocytopathies,* and a new classification scheme has been proposed that will identify diseases based on both morphology and etiology.[314]

The most common causes of nephrotic syndrome are minimal change disease (MCD), focal segmental glomerulosclerosis (FSGS), and membranous nephropathy (see later). Secondary causes are discussed separately and include diabetic nephropathy, amyloidosis, and SLE. A kidney biopsy is generally undertaken in all adult patients who present with nephrotic syndrome. Nephrotic syndrome is associated with significant morbidity regardless of cause, and patients with the disease have increased cardiovascular disease as a result of marked hyperlipidemia and increased risk of infection and thromboembolic disease. Between 10% and 40% of patients with nephrotic syndrome develop evidence of arterial and venous thromboemboli, particularly deep vein and renal vein thrombosis. Renal vein thrombosis may be unilateral or bilateral and may extend into the inferior vena cava. However, most cases of renal vein thrombosis have an insidious onset and produce no symptoms. Infrequently, patients develop acute renal vein thrombosis and present with signs of renal infarction, including flank pain, and microscopic or gross hematuria. In addition, AKI may supervene in cases of nephrotic syndrome (Box 59.3), and prolonged proteinuria with a poor response to treatment may lead to kidney failure.

BOX 59.3 Causes of AKI in Nephrotic Syndrome

- Acute tubular necrosis usually in MCD and patients older than 50 years of age
- Minimal change disease with acute interstitial nephritis induced by NSAIDs
- Tubular injury in collapsing FSGS, either idiopathic or associated with HIV infection
- Crescentic glomerulonephritis superimposed upon membranous nephropathy

FSGS, Focal segmental glomerulosclerosis; *HIV,* human immunodeficiency virus; *MCD,* minimal change disease; *NSAIDs,* nonsteroidal antiinflammatory drugs.

BOX 59.4 Management of Nephrotic Syndrome

Low-sodium diet
Protein intake of 1.0 g/kg/day
Fluid management: usually includes loop diuretics
Thromboembolism prophylaxis: may include formal anticoagulation in high-risk patients (serum albumin <20 g/L or in nephrotic syndrome due to membranous nephropathy or membranoproliferative glomerulonephritis)
Vigilance for infections
Treatment of hyperlipidemia with 3-hydroxy-3-methylglutaryl-Co-enzyme A (HMG)-CoA-reductase inhibitors (statins)
Treatment of hypertension, primarily with RAAS blockade
Supportive treatment of AKI
Education and psychological support for patients and relatives

AKI, Acute kidney injury; *RAAS,* renin-angiotensin-aldosterone system.

The management of nephrotic syndrome depends on the underlying glomerular lesion, although general principles apply in all cases (Box 59.4). In addition to general measures, specific treatment targeted at inducing remission from proteinuria usually requires a combination of immunosuppressive drugs, including corticosteroids and cytotoxic drugs.

MCD is the most common cause of nephrotic syndrome in children and young adults.[315] The incidence of MCD is estimated at 1 to 5 cases per 100,000 children per year. It typically presents with severe edema and hypoalbuminemia, and urine testing confirms heavy proteinuria. Kidney function is normal, with little evidence of a reduced GFR. MCD does not progress to kidney failure except in some cases of severe refractory disease that may be complicated by glomerular scarring lesions. Nephrotic syndrome in a noninfant child is assumed to be caused by MCD, and a kidney biopsy generally is not performed because the condition typically is responsive to a trial of corticosteroids, with remission within 2 weeks. Following the disappearance of proteinuria, or 1 week after remission is induced, the corticosteroid dose can be reduced and tapered slowly. An attempt to stop treatment may be indicated after 8 weeks. Longer duration of corticosteroid therapy significantly reduces the risk of relapse, and many centers will treat for a minimum of 12 weeks, particularly with a first episode of steroid-responsive nephrotic syndrome. Around 60% of steroid-responsive patients experience multiple relapses. Some of these patients can be managed with low-dose corticosteroids given daily or on alternate days, but relapses do occur, especially if intercurrent infection is present. In addition to the comorbidity associated with nephrotic syndrome, the burden of long-term exposure to corticosteroids and cytotoxic drugs has to be considered. Cyclophosphamide, azathioprine, tacrolimus, and cyclosporin are reserved for refractory cases and can be used as corticosteroid-sparing agents with the aim of reducing relapse rates. Treatment with cyclophosphamide is limited to 8 to 12 weeks to reduce the risk of gonadal toxicity.

The histologic lesion is by definition "minimal" when viewed on light microscopy. However, electron microscopy confirms disruption to the epithelial surface of the glomerular capillary. Podocyte foot processes are detached (effaced) from the GBM, conferring absence of the slit diaphragm, and therefore the final barrier to filtration fails (see Fig. 59.16). The glomerular architecture is restored following prompt treatment with high-dose corticosteroids. In MCD, the onset of nephrotic syndrome is often preceded by an infection or allergic reaction, and it has been proposed that nephrotic syndrome may be the result of an exaggerated response to normal physiologic and immune mechanisms that increase proteinuria during infection. MCD does occur in adults who present with nephrotic syndrome. MCD occasionally complicates NSAID ingestion, and secondary MCD has been described in patients with malignancy (particularly Hodgkin lymphoma).

BOX 59.5 Causes of Secondary Focal Segmental Glomerulosclerosis

Glomerular hypertrophy/hyperfiltration
- Unilateral renal agenesis
- Massive obesity

Scarring due to previous injury
- Focal proliferative glomerulonephritis
- Vasculitis
- Lupus

Toxins (pamidronate)
Human immunodeficiency virus-associated nephropathy (HIVAN)
Heroin nephropathy

Focal segmental glomerulosclerosis (FSGS) is the most important cause of the nephrotic syndrome in adults and remains a frequent cause in children and adolescents, particularly in the United States, Brazil, and many other countries.[316] Genetic studies in children with familial nephrotic syndrome have identified mutations in genes that encode important podocyte proteins.[317,318] Nephrin was the first slit diaphragm protein identified, and mutations in this transmembrane protein cause congenital (Finnish-type) nephrotic syndrome that occurs with a frequency of 1 out of 8200 live births in Finland. Among children with inherited nephrotic syndrome, other podocyte proteins (podocin, α-actinin 4, CD2-AP) have been described; all proteins are crucial to the interaction of the slit diaphragm with the podocyte cytoskeleton. Compelling evidence advocating a soluble permeability factor has been proposed as causing nephrotic syndrome in FSGS. Evidence includes experience in kidney transplantation, whereby FSGS may recur within hours of transplantation of a normal kidney into a recipient with FSGS.[319] The nature of the permeability factor remains unknown, but it can be removed by immunoabsorption to protein A and plasma exchange prior to transplantation.

Several disease processes lead to the description of FSGS on kidney biopsy and are shown in Box 59.5. Proteinuria in secondary FSGS, as in primary FSGS, reflects epithelial injury, although the mechanism is different. Following nephron loss, the remaining glomeruli undergo hypertrophy. Because podocytes are usually in a state of terminal differentiation and unable to replicate, the density of available foot processes to cover the enlarged glomerular surface is decreased. Focal areas of denudation from the GBM ensue, leading to proteinuria. Corticosteroids and other immunosuppressant drugs are not recommended for secondary forms of FSGS or for congenital forms. The treatment of primary disease causing nephrotic syndrome is typically a course of high-dose corticosteroids given for at least 6 months as tolerated. Remission of nephrotic syndrome is characterized by absence of proteinuria, loss of edema, and normalization of serum albumin concentration.

Membranous Nephropathy. The term *membranous nephropathy* reflects the primary histologic change noted on light microscopy: basement membrane thickening with little or no cellular proliferation or infiltration. Immunostaining is typically positive to immunoglobulins and complement components. Electron microscopy (EM) reveals electron-dense deposits within the GBM. Idiopathic membranous nephropathy is a common cause of nephrotic syndrome, accounting for approximately 30% of adult cases. The clinical features are variable and are classically described as ("rule of thirds") (1) a third of cases undergo spontaneous remission of proteinuria and recovery of kidney function; (2) a third of cases have nonprogressive disease but evidence of ongoing proteinuria; and (3) a third of cases continue to exhibit nephrotic syndrome and are at high risk of progressive kidney failure.

The clinical course therefore is difficult to predict at the onset of the disease, although 40% of patients in the control arm of an immunosuppressive treatment trial developed kidney failure after 10 years.[320] Patients generally are observed for 6 months to assess the likely natural history of the condition and are treated generically. In progressive cases and in those who have evidence of nephrotic syndrome for at least 6 months, a course of immunosuppressive drugs is indicated. Typical immunosuppressive schedules include high-dose corticosteroids, calcineurin inhibitors such as cyclosporin, and cytotoxic drugs (chlorambucil and cyclophosphamide).[320,321] The immunosuppressive schedules are targeted at primary membranous nephropathy. A seminal paper from Debiec and colleagues in 2002 described the discovery of an antibody to neutral endopeptidase (a human podocyte antigen) in antenatal cases of membranous nephropathy.[322] Target antigens for nephritogenic antibodies have since been further described. The M-type phospholipase A_2 receptor (PLA_2R) is the first podocyte antigen involved in membranous nephropathy in adults.[323] Detection of autoantibodies directed to PLA_2R (anti-PLA_2R antibody) indicates primary disease rather than a secondary process and guides therapy. Biological agents directed at antibody formation—that is, against, for example, CD20 molecules—include rituximab and are being used in the treatment of the disease.[324]

Secondary causes of membranous nephropathy are associated with a wide spectrum of diseases, including SLE, hepatitis B, falciparum malariae, malignancy, and drugs (eg, gold, penicillamine, captopril). In comparison with idiopathic disease, the clinical outcome depends on the underlying disease process. Underlying malignancy has been thought to be responsible for up to 5% to 10% of cases of membranous nephropathy in adults; the risk is highest in patients older than 60 years of age. A solid tumor (such as carcinoma of the lung, colon, or prostate) is most often involved and usually is clinically obvious.[325]

Rapidly Progressive Glomerulonephritis

Rapidly progressive glomerulonephritis (RPGN) is a heterogeneous group of disorders characterized by a fulminant clinical course that leads to kidney failure in only weeks or months. The clinical picture of RPGN is often preceded by a systemic illness for several months associated with general malaise, weight loss, breathlessness, upper respiratory tract abnormalities, and skin changes. Clinical examination may reveal nailfold infarcts affecting the fingernails and toenails and palpable purple lesions on the skin of the legs. In severe cases, a renal-pulmonary syndrome supervenes with kidney failure and alveolitis with associated pulmonary hemorrhage. In some cases, the condition may be limited to the kidneys (renal-limited vasculitis).

These syndromes are often characterized by focal glomerulonephritis with glomerular ischemia, infarction, and tissue death (necrosis). Following release of inflammatory cytokines and chemokines from the necrotic capillaries, there is proliferation of the epithelial cells of the Bowman capsule. The proliferated cells lie on top of adjacent cells and form a partial circle around the inner rim of the Bowman capsule that is referred to as a *crescent*. Proliferating epithelial cells and macrophages eventually compress the glomeruli and obstruct the proximal convoluted tubules, thus severely compromising nephron function.

RPGN may be classified as idiopathic kidney disease or as a disease secondary to other conditions, such as infectious disease, multisystem disease, and occasionally an adverse reaction to medication. Anti-GBM antibodies may be present along the GBM in anti-GBM disease. Most commonly, however, there is no, or little, immunoglobulin deposition within the glomerulus (so-called "pauci-immune"). Approximately 80% of patients with active pauci-immune necrotizing and crescentic glomerulonephritis have been shown to possess antineutrophil cytoplasmic antibodies (ANCAs), irrespective of the presence or absence of a concomitant systemic vasculitis. This strong association has allowed serologic discrimination of this type of glomerulonephritis from other types of RPGN. Wegener granulomatosis, microscopic polyangiitis, and Churg-Strauss syndrome are small-vessel vasculitides characterized by an association with ANCAs.

ANCA were first reported in 1982 in patients with pauci-immune serologic glomerulonephritis.[326] Three years later, ANCAs were detected by indirect immunofluorescence on human neutrophils in patients with active Wegener granulomatosis.[327] Since 1989, two subtypes of ANCA have been described—cytoplasmic (C-ANCA) and perinuclear (P-ANCA)—reflecting the patterns observed by indirect immunofluorescence microscopy using alcohol-fixed neutrophils as a substrate.[328] C-ANCAs are directed toward a plasma proteinase (PR3) in neutrophil primary granules and are associated with Wegener granulomatosis, whereas the P-ANCA target antigen is usually myeloperoxidase (MPO) and is associated with microscopic polyangiitis.[329,330] Immunoassays have been used to measure anti-PR3 and anti-MPO antibody titers. Vasculitis or angiitis is an inflammatory reaction in the wall of any blood vessel that can have diverse clinical presentations. The exact sequence of events that triggers perivascular inflammation leading to injury is unclear, but ANCAs have been identified that have at least diagnostic and prognostic usefulness. ANCAs appear in the plasma of almost all patients with active and generalized disease and are useful in diagnosis of the disease. However, false positives and false negatives may occur, necessitating histological diagnosis where possible. The use of ANCA to predict relapse of disease is limited, and a response to treatment cannot rely on falling titers but must be assessed utilizing clinical parameters of inflammation.[331] Autoantibodies of other specificities in rheumatoid arthritis, SLE, and inflammatory bowel disease may mimic the P-ANCA pattern, and in isolation, the finding of P-ANCA has a low specificity for vasculitis. The "International Consensus Statement on Testing and Reporting of Antineutrophil Cytoplasmic Antibodies (ANCA)" was developed to optimize ANCA testing.[332] It requires that all sera be tested by indirect immunofluorescence examination of peripheral blood neutrophils and, where there is positive fluorescence, by immunoassays for antibodies against PR3 and MPO. Following this protocol, false-positive rates of less than 1% can be achieved. Testing will be further improved by standardization and use of common immunoassay methods.

Rapidly progressive glomerulonephritis accounts for 15% of patients presenting to specialist nephrology units for renal replacement therapy and therefore is an important disease category to be aware of because if treatment is initiated early, independent kidney function can be restored, particularly if active lesions are seen on biopsy.[333] In addition to measurement of ANCA, C-reactive protein (CRP) is extremely helpful in assessment of the acute-phase reaction in active disease processes and is critical in helping to define disease remission. In patients in whom the CRP has returned to normal, disease remission is indicated; this prompts the clinician to reduce immunosuppressant treatment doses.[334]

Highly intensive immunosuppressive schedules are commenced in patients who present with RPGN. This *induction* phase of treatment is continued until the disease has remitted. Once remission is attained, a longer maintenance phase of treatment with less intensive schedules is commenced. In cases with a high index of suspicion on clinical grounds, treatment should begin empirically. Usually the diagnosis is made following a kidney biopsy and the result of an ANCA or anti-GBM antibody test. High-dose oral prednisolone and oral or intravenous cyclophosphamide are given as standard baseline treatment. Adjunctive treatments that may be used routinely in severe cases include pulses of intravenous methylprednisolone (1 g/d for 3 days) or a series of plasma exchanges.[335] The rationale for these approaches is to switch off production of the antibody and attenuate the proinflammatory response to tissue damage. Patients are closely followed for many months for evidence of disease activity and signs of treatment-related toxicity. This involves monitoring of kidney function, full blood count, ANCA serology, and anti-MPO/PR3 titer, as well as CRP. Following remission of active disease, drug doses are tapered, and cyclophosphamide may be exchanged for azathioprine. Serologic testing for ANCA and measurement of CRP are performed prior to immunosuppressant dose reduction to ensure that the disease activity has abated. Plans for long-term follow-up are made, and treatment is expected to be ongoing for at least 3 to 5 years. Relapses may occur as immunosuppression is reduced or withdrawn. The untreated mortality of ANCA-associated vasculitis is 90% at 1 year.[336] With current management strategies, the mortality rate has fallen to 20% to 30%.[337] The elderly are most susceptible both to the disease and to treatment-related morbidities, particularly infection. Patients who require dialysis or ventilatory support for pulmonary involvement have a higher mortality rate.

Anti-GBM disease (Goodpasture disease) affects 0.5 to 1 per million population per year in the United Kingdom.[338] Serologic detection of anti-GBM antibodies is helpful for assisting diagnosis in cases of RPGN. In this process, the antigens are well characterized and the antibody is directed at the $\alpha 3$ chain of type IV collagen. The disease is characterized by a relative lack of prodromal illness, a very rapid deterioration in kidney function, and a poor prognosis, with 0% renal survival at 12 months if oliguria or anuria develops.[339] The kidney biopsy typically demonstrates crescents in all the glomeruli ("100% crescents"), and each crescent is at a similar stage of development. The GBM stains positively in a linear pattern with anti-GBM antibodies. In addition to renal involvement, lung basement membrane can be affected, leading to pulmonary hemorrhage (Goodpasture syndrome). The environment plays a critical role in determining whether anti-GBM antibodies cause lung injury because pulmonary hemorrhage occurs only in current cigarette smokers.

Systemic Lupus Erythematosus

Systemic lupus erythematosus (SLE) is a chronic inflammatory disease of unknown cause that can affect the skin, joints, kidneys, lungs, nervous system, serous membranes, and/or other organs of the body. The clinical course of SLE is variable and may be characterized by periods of remissions and chronic or acute relapses. Women, especially in their 20s and 30s, are affected more frequently than men. Renal involvement, termed *lupus nephritis*, occurs in up to 60% of adults with SLE. Lupus nephritis is especially common in black and Hispanic patients in the United States.[340] Lupus nephritis may present variably from incidental hematuria and proteinuria, nephrotic syndrome, or a fulminating RPGN. Most (75%) patients with SLE develop an abnormal urinalysis or impaired kidney function during the course of the disease. A pathologic description is required to stage the disease process in lupus nephritis. The classification of lupus nephritis has been revised, and treatment is targeted depending on the stage of disease.[341] In general terms, pathologic findings include a spectrum from focal mesangial proliferation to diffuse global necrotizing glomerulonephritis. Membranous nephropathy may also be present. Detection of lupus nephritis involves urine testing for blood and protein and tests of kidney function. In addition, serologic testing for autoantibodies to nuclear antigens and measurement of complement components C3 and C4 are undertaken (Table 59.13). Significant hypocomplementemia and increased anti–double stranded DNA (anti-dsDNA) titers suggest active disease. Combined use of corticosteroids and intravenous or oral cyclophosphamide has been the conventional treatment for diffuse proliferative lupus nephritis since the 1970s.[342] Treatment duration with cyclophosphamide is limited because of severe toxicity, including gonadal toxicity, hemorrhagic cystitis, bone marrow suppression, and carcinogenicity. Recent data suggest that mycophenolate mofetil and corticosteroids can be as effective, but not superior to, intravenous cyclophosphamide for induction treatment for lupus nephritis.[343]

Acute Nephritic Syndrome

This disorder is characterized by rapid onset of hematuria, proteinuria, reduced GFR, and sodium and water retention, with resulting hypertension and localized peripheral edema.

TABLE 59.13 Laboratory Investigation of Vasculitic Syndromes

Disease	Serological Test	Antigens	Associated Laboratory Features
SLE	ANA including antibodies to dsDNA and ENA (including SM, Ro [SSA], La [SSB], and RNP)	Nuclear antigens	Leukopenia, thrombocytopenia, Coombs test Complement activation: low serum concentrations of C3 and C4 Positive immunofluorescence using *Crithidia luciliae* as substrate Antiphospholipid antibodies—ie, anticardiolipin, lupus anticoagulant, false-positive VDRL
Goodpasture disease	AntiGBM antibody	Epitope on noncollagen domain of type IV collagen	
Small Vessel Vasculitis			
Microscopic polyangiitis	P-ANCA	MPO	↑ CRP
Wegener granulomatosis	C-ANCA	Proteinase 3 (PR3)	↑ CRP
Churg-Strauss syndrome	P-ANCA in some cases	MPO	↑ CRP and eosinophilia
Henoch-Schönlein purpura	None		
Cryoglobulinemia			Cryoglobulins, rheumatoid factor, complement components, hepatitis C
Medium Vessel Vasculitis			
Classical PAN	None		↑ CRP and eosinophilia

ANA, Antinuclear antibodies; *ANCA,* antineutrophil cytoplasmic antibody; *C-ANCA,* cytoplasmic ANCA; *CRP,* C-reactive protein; *dsDNA,* double-stranded DNA; *ENA,* extractable nuclear antigens; *GBM,* glomerular basement membrane; *MPO,* myeloperoxidase; *P-ANCA,* perinuclear ANCA; *PAN,* polyarteritis nodosa; *RNP,* ribonucleoproteins; *SLE,* systemic lupus erythematosus; *VDRL,* Venereal Disease Research Laboratory.

Congestive heart failure and oliguria may also develop. In a number of patients with the acute nephritic syndrome, the pathologic process is related to recent group A β-hemolytic streptococcal infection of the pharynx or, less commonly, the skin. Only certain strains of streptococci are capable of inducing acute nephritis. A latent period averaging about 2 weeks exists between the time of streptococcal infection and clinical evidence of nephritis. In patients suspected of having acute poststreptococcal glomerulonephritis, evidence of recent infection may be found in increased titers of antibodies to streptococcal extracellular products: antistreptolysin O, antihyaluronidase, and antideoxyribonuclease-B. Serial measurements that document rising antibody titers against streptococcal antigens provide stronger evidence of recent infection than is provided by a single determination. Most patients have moderate reductions in total hemolytic complement activity (CH_{50}) and in the C3 component of the complement cascade. Typical poststreptococcal glomerulonephritis is now rare in developed countries, and a kidney biopsy may be performed in adult cases to establish the diagnosis pending serologic test results. A kidney biopsy of patients with poststreptococcal glomerulonephritis reveals diffuse involvement with enlarged hypercellular glomeruli infiltrated by polymorphonuclear leukocytes and monocytes. Electron microscopy reveals deposits, presumably immune complexes, on the epithelial side of the glomerular basement membrane. Abnormal laboratory results are usually present early in the course of acute nephritis. Hematuria, which may be gross ("cola-colored" urine) or microscopic, and proteinuria, usually less than 3 g/d, are almost always present. Red blood cell casts are highly suggestive of glomerulonephritis. These casts are commonly present in urine but are observed only if the specimen is fresh and acidic, centrifugation is light, and sediment (after decantation) is resuspended gently. Large numbers of hyaline and granular casts are common; waxy casts suggest a chronic process and should raise the possibility of acute exacerbation of a preexisting disease. Persistent and severe depression of C3 concentration should suggest membranoproliferative glomerulonephritis (MPGN, also known as mesangiocapillary glomerulonephritis [MCGN]), SLE, endocarditis, or other forms of sepsis. Although depressed levels of complement imply disease activity, they are not useful for grading the severity or determining the prognosis of the illness.

Other causes of acute nephritis include reactions to drugs, acute infection of the kidneys, systemic disease with immune complexes such as SLE, bacterial endocarditis, and finally disease in which the antigen is unknown but is possibly related to antecedent viral infection. These may manifest histologically as MPGN. The finding of immune complexes in these cases in kidney biopsy specimens subjected to immunofluorescence or immunoperoxidase staining should provoke a search for an underlying disease, typically either autoimmune (SLE, Sjogren syndrome), infection (hepatitis B and C), or a monoclonal gammopathy. In some cases complement reactants are present in the absence of immune complexes (immune complex negative MPGN), indicating an underlying C3 glomerulopathy,[344] and provoking a search for alternate pathway complement factor gene mutations and autoantibodies to C3 convertase.

Interstitial Nephritis

A variety of chemical, bacterial, and immunologic injuries to the kidney may cause generalized or localized changes that primarily affect the tubulointerstitium rather than the glomeruli. This group of disorders is characterized by alterations in tubular function that, in advanced cases, may cause secondary vascular and glomerular damage. Interstitial nephritis, including chronic pyelonephritis, is the primary diagnosis, accounting for 3.8% of patients admitted onto dialysis programs in the United States.[247] *Pyelonephritis* is the term associated with a bacterial infection that causes this kind of damage, and it is the most common of the interstitial nephritides.[345] Both acute and chronic types of pyelonephritis may occur; the acute type is most commonly associated with urinary tract infection (UTI). Acute pyelonephritis may develop into chronic pyelonephritis, usually as a result of a renal tract abnormality such as abnormal urethral valves. Interstitial nephritis is also associated with proteinuria that is less severe than in glomerular disease. In addition to conventional pyelonephritis, interstitial nephritis may present in acute and chronic forms and has many causes. Acute allergic interstitial nephritis presents with AKI and marked inflammation of the interstitium. Lymphocytes, polymorphonuclear cells, and eosinophils are prominent. The incidence is variable and depends on kidney biopsy practice. It may account for up to 7% of cases of AKI when an intrinsic kidney disease is diagnosed as opposed to purely toxic and/or ischemic acute tubular damage.[346] Higher values are likely in older people because of the increased incidence of drug reactions. A drug hypersensitivity reaction is the most common form of acute interstitial nephritis. Urinary findings may be normal, or low-level proteinuria and eosinophils may be seen on light microscopy. More than 100 different drugs have been implicated, but NSAIDs and β-lactam antibiotics are the drugs most commonly identified.[347] Nephrotic syndrome may accompany an acute interstitial nephritis associated with NSAIDs. Treatment is directed at removing any causative agent. Steroids are used to promote early resolution of the clinical course, although patients can develop chronic interstitial fibrosis.[348]

Sarcoidosis is a multisystem disorder associated with chronic granulomatous interstitial nephritis. Biochemical abnormalities include hypercalcemia, hypercalciuria, and increased serum ACE activity.[349] The condition may be effectively treated with steroids.

Prostaglandins and NSAIDs in Kidney Disease

NSAIDs block synthesis of prostaglandins by COX. Two isoforms of COX synthesize prostaglandins. COX-1 is a resident or constitutive form, and COX-2 is an inducible form that increases with disorders of inflammation.[350] NSAIDs are nonspecific inhibitors of both COX isoforms. Analgesic nephropathy is a common cause of incident kidney failure in many countries. In Australia, for example, it contributes around 10% of incident ESRD cases, despite awareness of the risk of kidney damage from chronic analgesic ingestion.[351] However, it is essentially a preventable condition for which monitoring of kidney function has proved useful. The incidence of this disease has decreased over the past decade as awareness has improved, and phenacetin was withdrawn from over-the-counter analgesic mixtures. In the United States, 1 in 5 citizens (50 million) report that they use an NSAID for an acute complaint.[352] Although most healthy individuals tolerate NSAIDs well, a study of the older people (mean age, 88 years) demonstrated significant reduction of GFR within 1 week of ingestion of NSAIDs.[353] Renal blood flow, particularly within the medulla, is dependent on systemic and local production of vasodilatory prostaglandins, and analgesic-related kidney damage is seen mostly within the medulla, with late changes causing papillary necrosis and interstitial fibrosis. Hyperkalemia can develop as a consequence of reduced GFR or secondary to hyporeninemic hypoaldosteronism. In addition, NSAIDs can rarely cause nephrotic syndrome and drug-related acute allergic interstitial nephritis.

Plasma Cell Disorders and Kidney Disease

Immunoglobulin (Ig) molecules are formed in secretory B cells (plasma cells) and consist of heavy chains, which denominate the antibody isotype, and either kappa (κ) or lambda (λ) light chains (see Chapter 28). The proportion of Ig containing κ versus λ is 3 : 2 in humans. The molecular weight of light chains is approximately 23 kDa. Excess production of light over heavy chains appears to be required for efficient Ig synthesis, resulting in the release of free light chains into the circulation. In normal individuals, the small quantity of circulating polyclonal light chains is filtered by the glomerulus, and 90% is reabsorbed in the proximal tubule and degraded by proteases. Increased concentrations of filtered light chains lead to alteration in the proximal tubule cells, including prominent cytoplasmic vacuolation, loss of the microvillous border, and epithelial cell exfoliation.[354]

Myeloma or multiple myeloma is a neoplastic proliferation of a clone of plasma cells that produce excessive amounts of a monoclonal (M) protein and free light chains. In multiple myeloma, complete monoclonal Igs (usually IgG or IgA) are accompanied in the plasma by variable concentrations of free light chains that appear in the urine as Bence Jones proteins (named after Henry Bence Jones, who first described these in 1848). M-proteins and free light chains can be identified in the blood and/or the urine in 98% of patients with myeloma using protein electrophoresis and immunofixation. Immunoparesis, with reduction in non-M-protein Ig, is characteristic of myeloma. The free light chain (FLC) immunoassay is now also used to detect monoclonal immunoglobulin.[355] The kidneys are often affected in myeloma, with diverse clinical and pathological presentations. The three most common forms of monoclonal Ig-mediated kidney disease are cast nephropathy, monoclonal Ig deposition disease (MIDD), and AL amyloidosis. Evidence suggests that light chains are directly pathogenic.[356] The pattern of human renal injury associated with monoclonal light chains can be reproduced in mice injected intraperitoneally with large quantities of light chains isolated from patients with myeloma or light chain–associated amyloid (AL-amyloid).[357]

Impairment of kidney function at presentation occurs in almost 50% of patients with myeloma.[358,359] Although most recover following treatment for other factors contributing to renal impairment (eg, dehydration, hypercalcemia, infection, nephrotoxic drugs), about 10% have severe renal involvement caused by the effects of monoclonal free light chains on the kidney. Severe kidney failure may occur in myeloma following deposition of light chains within tubules—so-called "cast nephropathy" ("myeloma kidney"). Cast nephropathy can present acutely, again precipitated by dehydration, hypercalcemia, or NSAIDs, or de novo in the absence of these factors. It occurs when the reabsorptive capacity of proximal tubular cells is exceeded by overproduction of light chains. In myeloma, light chain excretion can exceed 20 g/d. Casts are large and numerous and are found predominantly in the distal convoluted tubule and collecting ducts, causing obstruction to urine flow. They have a hard and fractured appearance, with lamination visible on histologic examination of kidney biopsy specimens. Immunofluorescence confirms that casts are composed of monoclonal free light chains and THG. Casts usually stain exclusively with either anti-κ or anti-λ antibodies, demonstrating so-called "light chain restriction," which is indicative of a malignant process. At biopsy, there is often an interstitial inflammatory infiltrate, and fibrosis and tubular atrophy can be extensive. Not all light chains induce cast formation. The ability of light chains to form casts is based on binding to THG.[66] Light chains interfere with proximal tubule cell function, and this promotes delivery to the distal tubule. A specific binding site for light chains has been identified on THG, and light chains with high affinity appear to be more likely to produce obstructing intratubular casts.[360] Physicochemical determinants of binding of light chains to THG include the isoelectric point (pI) of the light chain. Those molecules with a pI above 5.1 (above the tubular fluid pH in the distal nephron) will have a net positive charge that may promote binding via charge interaction to anionic THG (pI, 3.2). Urinary alkalinization reduces binding of light chains to THG in animal models.[361] Nephrotoxicity may be determined by the ability of light chains to self-associate, leading to the formation of high molecular weight aggregates that are more likely to deposit in tissues, particularly in the setting of volume depletion. However, not all patients with excessive production of monoclonal Ig develop disease. Ig-independent mechanisms include dehydration, hypercalcemia, contrast medium, and NSAIDs.

The clinical features of myeloma include a normochromic normocytic anemia, bone pain with pathologic fractures (back or chest rather than extremities), and hypercalcemia in 20% of patients. Severe kidney failure may dominate the clinical picture, and 84% of patients studied retrospectively with severe renal impairment required dialysis.[362] Only 15% of these patients regained independent kidney function. Treatment has two main objectives: to reverse Ig-independent causes of AKI and to reduce the load of monoclonal immunoglobulin and free lights chains. In addition to chemotherapy protocols, plasma exchange was considered a useful adjunctive treatment to remove excess free light chains and reduce renal injury. However, a study from Canada of 104 patients presenting with myeloma and AKI, randomized to five to seven plasma exchange treatments, in addition to conventional treatment, showed no significant difference in the composite outcome of death, dialysis dependence, and GFR less than 30 mL/min/1.73 m^2 at 6 months.[363] Nevertheless, interest in direct removal of light chain has not abated, and other filtration technologies have been explored, notably extended hours dialysis with large pore membranes. This approach is currently being evaluated in clinical trials (for example, European Trial of Free Light Chain Removal [EULITE][364]).

Excess production of monoclonal light chains (or rarely heavy chains) can cause disorders in which *fragments* are deposited in the kidney and other tissues. Amyloidosis is a condition characterized by extracellular deposition of fibrils in an antiparallel-pleated sheet arrangement. The type of amyloid is defined by the abnormal protein deposited. For example, in "primary amyloid" or "AL-amyloid," fibrils derived from the variable region of light chains are deposited in the tissue. Seventy-five percent are derived from the λ-light chain. Because it is the variable region that is deposited, it is often difficult to assess with immune reactants. Only 50% of AL-amyloid cases are stainable with commercially available antisera to κ and λ. The deposits are fibrillar in nature and bind to Congo red. Amyloid fibrils also bind to the serum amyloid P component, allowing noninvasive evaluation by radiolabeled serum amyloid P scanning.[365] The diagnosis of AL-amyloid can be suspected from the clinical findings of nephrotic range (>3.5 g/d) proteinuria and serum or urinary paraprotein. Amyloidosis is a relatively common cause of nephrotic syndrome in older people. However, 10% to 15% of patients with primary amyloid do not have a detectable serum or urinary paraprotein. Demonstration of a clonal excess of plasma cells on bone marrow biopsy may help with the diagnosis in those without detectable paraprotein. AL-amyloid has a poor prognosis, and mean survival is 18 months, with 50% of patients dying from cardiac failure. Treatment options are unsatisfactory, although prednisolone and melphalan may be tried.[366-368] Circulating free light chains can be detected by the nephelometric immunoassay in most patients with AL-amyloid, and patient outcome following treatment is improved if the concentration of free light chains can be reduced by 50%.[369]

The French Myeloma Group has published results of bone marrow or stem cell transplantation in AL-amyloid.[370] In a retrospective analysis of 21 patients treated with melphalan and stem cell transplantation, 43% died within 1 month, and the remainder had a favorable outcome.

Polycystic Kidney Disease

Autosomal dominant polycystic kidney disease (ADPKD) is the second most common inherited monogenic disease (after familial hypercholesterolemia), with an estimated incidence of 1:1000. It is by far the most common inherited kidney disease; 12.5 million people worldwide are affected.[371] In the United Kingdom, ADPKD is responsible for 11% of new ESRD in patients aged younger than 65 years and 4% of incident patients over age 65 years.[306] The prevalence of the disease ranges from 1 in 200 to 1 in 1000 of the population, but many cases, possibly up to 50%, remain clinically undiagnosed during life. Approximately 50% of ADPKD patients develop kidney failure by age 55 years.[372] It is therefore important to make the diagnosis in affected families and to monitor kidney function regularly. The intervals between estimations of GFR will depend on the stage of CKD, as with other progressive kidney diseases. An important clinical observation is the highly variable phenotype within families. The disease causes the development of multiple kidney cysts and extrarenal cysts occurring in the liver and pancreas. About 10% of ADPKD families have a strong family history of intracranial arterial aneurysm rupture. Hypertension is an early and frequent manifestation, and gross hematuria is a common presenting symptom. On the basis of effectiveness, cost, and safety, ultrasound is the imaging modality most commonly used to make the diagnosis. Screening for polycystic kidney disease is controversial, and age-dependent ultrasound diagnostic criteria for ADPKD have been developed. According to recent criteria, the presence of fewer than two renal cysts has a negative predictive value of 100% and is enough to exclude the disease in at-risk individuals who are 40 years of age and older.[373]

ADPKD is caused by mutations in the genes (*PKD1* and *PKD2*) that encode polycystin 1 and 2, which are located in primary cilia.[374-376] Mutations affecting *PKD1* are more prevalent than those of *PKD2* and tend to have a worse prognosis, with larger kidneys and earlier development of kidney failure. Genetic testing is not used routinely as a screening tool because current techniques identify only 70% of the hundreds of different *PKD1* and *PKD2* mutations.[377] The function of primary cilia is to act as flow sensors in the tubules, with flow-induced deformation resulting in calcium influx that leads to a proliferative cellular response mediated by intracellular cAMP. Animal model studies have demonstrated abnormalities in vasopressin and vasopressin receptors in ADPKD, and these receptors have become therapeutic targets. Other mutations include the *PDK2* mutation on chromosome 4 (110 kDa) and *APKD3*, for which the gene product and the chromosomal location remain unknown.[378] *PKD2* appears to be a more slowly progressive form of the disease.[379] The median age of onset of ESRD with *PKD2* is 15 years later than with *PKD1*. Also, a rare (incidence 1 out of 20,000) autosomal recessive form of the disease may present in childhood.

Specific treatments for ADPKD in clinical practice are currently lacking. Generic treatment should include treatment of hypertension with ACE inhibitors and/or ARBs and maintaining a fluid intake of 2 to 3 L/d to reduce the risk of kidney stone disease. Specific therapies, in development, are targeted at reducing cyst development and enlargement. Estimates of cyst volume can be determined using MRI techniques and changes documented over a relatively short period of time.[380] This has allowed the performance of clinical trials of novel drugs such as the vasopressin V_2-receptor antagonists, Tolvaptan, and antiproliferative drugs such as sirolimus.[381] Tolvaptan has been shown in the 3-year clinical study (TEMPO3:4) to slow the increase in size of the cysts, reduce pain associated with cysts, and slow the rate of change in kidney function.[382] Adverse events, primarily thirst and polyuria, due to anticipated increase in salt-free water excretion, led to discontinuation of the study drug in almost a quarter of the patients. In addition, abnormalities in liver function tests were reported, and the drug is subject to an FDA review. Tolvaptan, under the trade name Jinarc, received its license (marketing authorization) in 2015 in the United Kingdom to slow the progression of cyst development and renal insufficiency in ADPKD in adults with CKD and a GFR of 30 mL/min/1.73 m^2 or higher at initiation of treatment with evidence of rapidly progressing disease. It is also approved for treatment of ADPKD in Japan.[383]

Obstructive Uropathy

Benign prostatic hyperplasia (BPH) is one of the most common types of obstructive uropathy and is an almost universal finding in aging men.[384] For example, for men aged 50 years, the reported prevalence of BPH is 40%, and for men aged over 70 years, it is at least 75%.[385] No close relationship between the degree of enlargement and the symptoms experienced has been observed.[386] Among the most common symptoms are disorders of micturition, in particular increased frequency, and in many cases this can progress to bladder outflow obstruction. Between 10% and 40% of men with bladder outflow obstruction caused by BPH present in acute retention.[384] Approximately 5% of this group have high-pressure chronic retention of urine, which can result in upper urinary tract obstruction and consequently CKD as a result of glomerular and tubular damage. Although medical treatments are available to decrease the rate of enlargement of the prostate, resection of the enlarged gland remains the most common surgical procedure performed on men. Urinary retention can be a chronic disorder, with acute exacerbations requiring bladder decompression by catheterization. If the obstruction is not removed by surgery, progressive kidney injury can occur as a result of backpressure along the urinary tract. It is important to identify those patients at risk of developing CKD because failure to remove their enlarged gland can cause kidney failure. Obstruction can also occur because of kidney stones, which can cause bilateral or unilateral damage. In children, severe kidney damage can be caused by vesicoureteric reflux. One of the main complications of reflux, whether caused by obstruction or an inherited defect, is the increased incidence of urinary tract infection. When the obstruction is relieved, the kidney often regains some independent function. A tendency toward slower progression to kidney failure has been noted in obstructive uropathy compared with other kidney diseases.

Tubular Disease

Types of tubular disease discussed in this section include renal tubular acidoses (RTAs) and inherited tubulopathies.

Renal Tubular Acidoses

The RTAs constitute a diverse group of inherited and acquired disorders affecting the proximal or distal tubule. They are characterized by a hyperchloremic, normal anion gap; metabolic acidosis; and urinary bicarbonate or hydrogen ion excretion inappropriate for the plasma pH. They may result from failure to retain bicarbonate or from the inability of the renal tubules to secrete hydrogen ion. Typically, the GFRs in RTAs are normal or slightly reduced, and there is no retention of anions, such as phosphate and sulfate (as opposed to the acidosis of kidney failure). Before attempting to understand the pathology of these conditions, the reader should ensure a good comprehension of normal renal acid-base (and ammonia) regulation (see Chapter 60).

Classification of RTAs is based on the biochemical expression and region of the defect, rather than on an understanding of the exact molecular defect. The three categories of RTA are distal (dRTA, type I); proximal (pRTA, type II); and type IV, which occurs secondary to aldosterone deficiency or resistance. The term *type III RTA* (mixed proximal/distal defect) has been abandoned by some authors because it is not considered a separate entity.[387] It may arise as the result of a mutation in the gene coding for carbonic anhydrase type 2.[388])

Distal RTA (Type I). Type I dRTA occurs most often in infants (sometimes transiently) and young children, but it may also be encountered in adults, in whom it is more common than pRTA. Clinical features generally include metabolic acidosis, muscle weakness, nephrocalcinosis (ie, diffuse, fine, renal parenchymal calcification), and urolithiasis (ie, the formation of calculi in the urinary tract). Biochemical features typically include hypokalemia, hypocitraturia, and low urinary ammonium ion. Several subtypes may be seen, and urinary pH greater than 5.5 is a common feature.[387,389]

Classic Hypokalemic dRTA (Proton Secretion Defect). Both inherited and acquired forms exist. There is increasing understanding of the genetic causes of dRTA.[390] Inherited forms are associated with mutations in proteins involved in hydrogen ion secretion, including defects of H+, ATPase and anion exchanger 1, or to mutations in carbonic anhydrase. Loss of function mutations affecting H+, ATPase are usually responsible for autosomal recessive forms of dRTA often associated with early or late sensorineural deafness. Medullary sponge kidney is also a primary cause of dRTA, related to the malformation of the distal tubules. Acquired impairment of the hydrogen ion secretion mechanism leading to dRTA may occur in association with a wide range of conditions, in particular a range of autoimmune disorders (eg, SLE, Sjögren syndrome, primary biliary cirrhosis, thyroiditis).[389] Some medications, such as topiramate and acetazolamide, can also inhibit carbonic anhydrase, leading to dRTA. The pathogenesis of nephrocalcinosis and urolithiasis may be the result of decreased urinary citrate excretion secondary to cellular acidosis.

Back-Leak dRTA (Proton Gradient Defect). Although the kidney tubule retains the ability to secrete hydrogen ions, the gradient is not maintained because of back-diffusion, Typically, this occurs in association with specific drug treatments (eg, amphotericin B) that increase the permeability for protons of the apical membrane in the collecting duct, causing back-diffusion of secreted protons.

Voltage-Dependent (Hyperkalemic) dRTA. This is due to failure to maintain an intraluminal negative potential and thus to promote hydrogen (and potassium) ion secretion, primarily due to reduced ENaC activity. Both genetic and acquired forms of reduced ENaC activity occur, with the latter being more common—for example, in association with chronic urinary tract obstruction, CKD, and treatment with amiloride, cyclosporin, lithium, or triamterene. Voltage-dependent (hyperkalemic) dRTA has many features in common with type IV RTA (see discussion later in this chapter).

Incomplete dRTA. This is a less severe, normokalemic form, which may represent an early stage of overt dRTA. Some patients acidify urine at a submaximal rate but at a rate that is generally sufficient to maintain acid-base balance. Potassium wasting, hypokalemia, and hyperchloremia are generally not present. However, when patients are stressed or are given an acid load test, their ability to excrete acid and to lower urine pH is suboptimal, and urinary pH may exceed 5.5.

Proximal RTA (Type II). In pRTA, the primary defect is failure of proximal tubular bicarbonate reabsorption.[391] Proximal RTA may occur as an isolated defect (primary or sporadic type II pRTA) that occurs chiefly in infant males and is commonly associated with growth retardation or that produces a generalized proximal tubular disorder (Fanconi syndrome). Proximal tubular bicarbonate reabsorption is still incompletely understood at the molecular level, but some candidate transporters associated with hereditary forms of pRTA are discussed by Ring and colleagues.[388] Most cases of pRTA are secondary to genetic disorders that affect the proximal tubule (eg, cystinosis, fructose intolerance) or to acquired diseases, including multiple myeloma, Sjögren syndrome, and amyloidosis; heavy metal poisoning (lead, mercury, cadmium); drugs (eg, ifosfamide, valproic acid, tenofovir); and renal transplant rejection. Drugs that act as carbonic anhydrase inhibitors (eg, acetazolamide, topiramate) have also produced a pRTA condition. (Note that several of these disorders and agents also cause dRTA.) In pRTA, the threshold for bicarbonate reabsorption is lowered (from a plasma concentration of 22 mmol/L to 15 mmol/L).[387] Once plasma bicarbonate falls below this threshold, filtered bicarbonate is reclaimed, and urinary pH generally will be less than 5.5. In pRTA, contrary to dRTA, nephrocalcinosis and nephrolithiasis are rarely observed, but metabolic bone disease is common. Other features of the Fanconi syndrome (eg, glycosuria, aminoaciduria, hypophosphatemia, hypouricemia) are commonly present.

Selective Aldosterone Deficiency (Type IV RTA). In type IV RTA, there is failure of distal potassium, and hydrogen ion secretion results from aldosterone deficiency or resistance due to a range of steroid or steroid receptor synthetic defects or from hyporeninemic hypoaldosteronism (eg, due to diabetic nephropathy, tubulointerstitial disease, urinary obstruction, renal transplantation, or SLE). Hyperkalemia, although mild, is a usual manifestation. Type IV RTA associated with pseudohypoaldosteronism type 2 is thought to be due to a mutation in the *WNK* gene, which encodes a protein that interacts with several renal electrolyte transport systems (Table 59.14).[388]

Diagnosis of RTA. The finding of a hyperchloremic metabolic acidosis in a patient without obvious gastrointestinal bicarbonate losses (eg, due to excessive diarrhea or small intestinal fistulas) and with no obvious pharmacologic cause should prompt suspicion of an RTA. The presence of suggestive clinical (eg, nephrocalcinosis in dRTA) or biochemical (eg, hypophosphatemia and hypouricemia as a result of proximal tubular wasting in pRTA) features should also be considered.

In addition to plasma electrolyte (including potassium) measurement, preliminary investigation should include measurement of urinary pH in a fresh, early-morning urine sample. The finding of urine pH greater than 5.5 in the presence of systemic acidosis supports the diagnosis of dRTA, although it is not specific and will also be seen in types II and IV RTAs. If appropriate urinary acidification cannot be demonstrated, further investigation may involve assessing the ability of the kidneys to excrete an acid load (ammonium chloride load test) and to reabsorb filtered bicarbonate (fractional bicarbonate excretion). Additional details on the conduct and interpretation of these tests may be found in a review article.[387]

Treatment of RTA. Treatment of the RTAs is aimed at (1) correcting the biochemical disturbance and, where possible, underlying disorder; (2) improving growth in children; and (3) avoiding the development and progression of CKD. In both type I and II RTAs, bicarbonate is administered to correct the metabolic acidosis. Fludrocortisone and loop diuretics (see "Diuretics" section later) may be used to treat type IV RTA.

Inherited Tubulopathies

The inherited tubulopathies make up a heterogeneous set of disorders often characterized by electrolyte disturbances (see Table 59.14). Many are eponymous and have been described

TABLE 59.14 Characteristics of Some Inherited Tubulopathies

Disorder [OMIM Number]	Protein Defect	Chromosome Localization	Inheritance	Clinical Features/Notes	Biochemical Features
Proximal Tubule					
Lowe syndrome (oculocerebral dystrophy) [309000]	OCRL1	Xq26.1	XR	Hydrophthalmia, cataract, mental retardation, hyporeflexia, hypotonia, and progressive kidney failure: normotensive	Plasma: ↓K, ↓CO_2 Urine: ↑LMWP, ↑AA, ↑PO_4, ↑K
Wilson disease [277900]	ATP7B	13q14.3-q21.1	AR	Liver disease ± neurological symptoms, or both, Kayser-Fleischer rings, normotensive	Plasma: ↑free copper, abnormal LFTs Urine: ↑copper excretion, ↑LMWP, ↑AA, ↑ PO_4,↑Glycosuria
Dent disease (X-linked recessive hypophosphatemic rickets) [300009]	CLCN5	Xp11.22	XR	Nephrocalcinosis, nephrolithiasis, rachitic and osteomalacic bone disease, progressive kidney failure, normotensive	Plasma: ↓PO_4, N/↓K Urine: ↑LMWP, ↑AA, ↑K, ↑Ca, ↑PO_4, ↑Glycosuria
X-linked dominant hypophosphatemic rickets [307800]	PHEX	Xp22.2-p22.1	XD	Growth retardation, rachitic and osteomalacic bone disease, hypophosphatemia, and renal defects in phosphate reabsorption and vitamin D metabolism	Plasma: ↓PO_4, ↑ALP Urine: ↑PO_4
Loop of Henle					
Bartter syndrome					
[601678]	NKCC2 (type I)	15q15-q21.1	AR	Polyuria, polydipsia, muscle weakness, hypovolemia, normotensive or hypotensive (all types). Maternal polyhydramnios, premature birth, perinatal salt wasting, nephrocalcinosis and kidney stones (types I and II), milder phenotype with normocalciuria (type III), sensorineural deafness, motor retardation, renal failure (type IV),	Plasma: ↑renin, ↓K, ↑CO_2, mild ↓Mg in some patients Urine: ↑Ca
[241200]	ROMK (type II)	11q24	AR		
[607364]	ClC-Kb (type III, "classic")	1p36	AR		
[602522]	Barttin (type IV)	1p31	AR		
Hypomagnesemic Hypercalciuric Nephrocalcinosis (magnesium-losing kidney) [248250]	PCLN1	3q27	AR	Nephrocalcinosis, renal failure, ocular/hearing defects, polyuria, polydipsia, recurrent urinary tract infections, recurrent renal colic, normotensive	Plasma: ↓Mg, ↑PTH Urine: ↑Ca, ↑Mg

Continued

TABLE 59.14 Characteristics of Some Inherited Tubulopathies—cont'd

Disorder [OMIM Number]	Protein Defect	Chromosome Localization	Inheritance	Clinical Features/Notes	Biochemical Features
Distal Tubule/Collecting Duct					
Liddle syndrome [177200]*	ENaC (activating)	16p13-p12	AD	Early, and frequently severe, hypertension, stroke	Plasma: ↓renin, ↓K, ↓Mg, ↑CO_2, Urine: ↑K
Pseudohypoaldosteronism type Ia [264350]*	ENaC (inactivating)	12p13, 16p13-p12	AR	Presents in infancy with salt wasting and hypotension; cough, respiratory infections	Plasma: ↑renin, ↓Na, ↑K, ↓CO_2 Urine: ↑K
Pseudohypoaldosteronism type Ib [177735]*	Mineralocorticoid receptor	4q31.1	AD	Presents in infancy with salt wasting and hypotension; milder than type 1a and remits with age	Plasma: ↑renin, ↓Na, ↑K, ↓CO_2, Urine: ↑K
Pseudohypoaldosteronism type II (Gordon syndrome) [145260]	Unknown (?WNK)	1q31-q42 12p13 17q21-q22	AD	Hypertension (± muscle weakness, short stature, intellectual impairment). Correction of physiological abnormalities by thiazide diuretics.	Plasma: ↓renin, ↑K, ↓CO_2, ↑Cl Urine: ↓K
Gitelman syndrome [263800]	NCCT	16q13	AR	Hypotension, weakness, parasthesias, tetany, fatigue, and salt craving. Presentation generally much later in life than in Bartter, and hypocalciuria is typical.	Plasma: ↑renin, ↓K, ↓Mg, ↑CO_2, Urine: ↓calcium : creatinine excretion ratio (useful in distinguishing Gitelman and Bartter). (Note: Biochemically can mimic thiazide use.)
X-linked nephrogenic diabetes insipidus type I [304800]	V2 receptor	Xq28	XR	Hyperthermia, polyuria, polydipsia, dehydration, inability to form concentrated urine, mental retardation if diagnosis delayed. Symptoms in infancy.	Hyperosmolar plasma, dilute urine
Autosomal dominant nephrogenic diabetes insipidus type II [192340]	AQP2	12q13	AD and AR	Polyuria, polydipsia, dehydration, inability to form concentrated urine. Symptoms after first year of life.	Hyperosmolar plasma, dilute urine

Note: This list is not exhaustive. Some of the material in this table has been adapted from Sayer JA, Pearce SHS.[393] A useful resource for further information is the Online Mendelian Inheritance in Man (OMIM) website, which may be searched using the OMIM numbers given in the table (http://www.ncbi.nlm.nih.gov/entrez/query.fcgi?db=OMIM).
*See Fig. 59.7.
AA, Aminoaciduria; *AD,* autosomal dominant; *AR,* autosomal recessive; *LMWP,* low molecular weight proteinuria; *XD,* X-linked dominant; *XR,* X-linked recessive.

clinically for many years. However, enhanced understanding of the molecular biology of the tubular ion channel and transport pumps has delineated the mechanism of disease in many of these disorders. In addition to electrolyte disturbances (particularly of potassium), general reasons to suspect a tubulopathy include a familial disease pattern, renal impairment, nephrocalcinosis, and stone formation, especially if these should present at an early age. In cases in which a diuretic-sensitive channel is affected, these disorders will clearly mimic the effects of diuretic use (see discussion later in this chapter), and exclusion of covert use of diuretics is important. Although they are individually uncommon or rare, an awareness of these disorders is critical for the clinical biochemist when considering the potential differential diagnoses in patients presenting with electrolyte imbalances. A brief description of these disorders follows; for more detailed information, the reader is referred to comprehensive reviews on this subject.[392-395] This section should be considered in conjunction with the description of tubular electrolyte handling (see earlier "Electrolyte Homeostasis").

Bartter Syndrome. This group of autosomal recessive disorders is characterized by renal salt wasting, polyuria, polydipsia, impaired urinary concentrating ability, a hyperreninemic, hypokalemic metabolic alkalosis, low blood pressure, and a mild hypomagnesemia in some patients. Biochemically, the effects resemble those of loop diuretic use, but clinically the phenotype is highly variable. This variability arises because the syndrome encompasses defects of three different transporters/channels in the loop of Henle. The biochemical effects are predictable from knowledge of the function of these transporters and channels (see Fig. 59.6).

Mutations in the genes encoding for NKCC2 (type I) or ROMK1 (type II) are associated with the more severe phenotype, including polyhydramnios, premature birth, life-threatening salt wasting in the perinatal period, and hypercalciuria. Patients with ROMK1 defects tend to have less severe hypokalemia.

The milder ("classic," type III) Bartter syndrome is due to defects in the basolateral pump, CLC-Kb. Although the phenotype is extremely variable (neonatal, life-threatening presentations do occur), patients typically present in the first year of life with weakness and hypovolemia and normal urinary calcium excretion. Nephrocalcinosis and kidney stone formation usually are not features.

A fourth variant of Bartter syndrome (type IV) is due to a mutation in the gene coding for Barttin. Barttin is an essential subunit of CLC-Kb that influences its function and expression in the cell membrane. Bartter syndrome type IV is characterized by severe, early-onset salt wasting, leading to polydramnios, premature birth, and inner-ear deafness.[12]

Gitelman Syndrome. This autosomal recessive disorder is characterized by a hypokalemic, hyperreninemic, hypomagnesemic, metabolic alkalosis. Presentation is generally much later in life than with Bartter syndrome, and hypocalciuria is typical. Clinical features include reduced blood pressure, weakness, paresthesia, tetany, fatigue, and salt craving.[396] The molar urinary calcium/creatinine excretion ratio can be useful in distinguishing between Gitelman ($\leq$0.20) and Bartter (>0.20) syndromes.[397] The molecular defect is in the thiazide-sensitive NCCT transporter (see Fig. 59.6), and the biochemistry can therefore mimic the effects of thiazide use (see "Diuretics" section later).

Liddle Syndrome. This autosomal dominant disorder is characterized by a hypokalemic, hypomagnesemic metabolic alkalosis, but, in contrast to Bartter and Gitelman syndromes, hypertension and hyperreninism also occur. The disease is due to mutations that prevent ENaC from being targeted for internalization. Thus mutant channels remain at the cell surface, resulting in enhanced sodium transport through the channel and consequent enhanced kaliuresis (see Fig. 59.7).

Pseudohypoaldosteronism Type I. This condition presents in infancy with salt wasting, hypotension, hyperkalemia, and significant hyperreninism and aldosteronism. Two different molecular mechanisms are causative. Type Ia (autosomal recessive) is caused by inactivating mutations of the *ENaC* gene, and type Ib (autosomal dominant) is caused by mutations in the mineralocorticoid gene. In both cases, sodium loss in the collecting duct is increased, with consequent retention of potassium.

Dent Disease. Dent disease is an X-linked condition characterized by hypercalciuria and kidney stone formation, low molecular weight proteinuria, aminoaciduria, hypophosphatemia, rickets, and progression to kidney failure.[398] The disease is most commonly (60% of cases) due to single-base change mutations in the gene coding for the tubular endosomal chloride channel CLC-5. CLC-5 has an important role in proximal tubular endocytosis, accounting for the low molecular weight proteinuria that is seen in Dent disease.[395,399] Reduced uptake of PTH by proximal tubular endocytosis results in increased activation of apical PTH receptors in later segments of the nephron, resulting in reduced phosphate reabsorption and phosphaturia. Increased concentrations of PTH also increase 1,25 dihydroxyvitamin D production, enhancing intestinal calcium absorption and ultimately leading to hypercalciuria, which, together with phosphaturia, promotes stone formation.[395] Although X-linked, a mild form of the disease can be seen in females because of lyonization. The related syndromes, X-linked recessive nephrolithiasis, X-linked recessive hypophosphatemic rickets, and Japanese idiopathic low molecular weight proteinuria, are also all related to defects in CLC-5.[400]

Phosphate Disorders. Several disorders of tubular phosphate handling have been described, including X-linked dominant hypophosphatemic rickets (XLH; previously known as vitamin D resistant rickets), autosomal dominant hypophosphatemic rickets, and acquired oncogenic hypophosphatemic osteomalacia. Our understanding of the molecular biology of these and other renal phosphate transport disorders has advanced greatly in recent years.[15] Many other tubulopathies are beyond the scope of this textbook.[392-395] Features of some of these are described in Table 59.14.

Diuretics

Diuretics are among the most widely prescribed drugs. They are used predominantly to treat hypertension and/or disorders associated with fluid overload. All diuretics act by interfering with tubular reabsorption of sodium and/or chloride, thereby promoting water loss from the peripheral circulation. Diuretics are taken up by tubular cells across the basolateral membrane by specific anion- (eg, furosemide, thiazides) or cation- (eg, amiloride, triamterene) exchangers and then are secreted into the lumen through a process that has not been fully elucidated.[394] Different classes of diuretics act at different sites along the nephron. A basic understanding of these processes is helpful in understanding both the potency of different diuretic classes and their importance in the investigation of electrolyte disorders, in particular hypokalemia. Many diuretics will cause hypokalemia to some degree, depending on potency, dose, duration of treatment, and the patient's underlying potassium balance.

Loop Diuretics. Loop diuretics act largely by blocking sodium and chloride reabsorption in the ascending limb of the loop of Henle. Because this is a site at which 30% of sodium reabsorption normally occurs, these are considered potent diuretics. Loop diuretics specifically inhibit NKCC2; therefore they also have an effect on potassium handling in the ascending limb. Consequent changes in transepithelial potential result in a direct kaliuretic effect in this region,[9] causing hypercalciuria (see Fig. 59.6). Loop diuretics also paralyze the macula densa segment, stimulating renin secretion and subsequent aldosterone release, promoting sodium reabsorption and potassium loss in the distal tubule, and thus further exacerbating the kaliuresis. Most significantly, blockage of loop sodium reabsorption results in enhanced delivery of sodium ions to the distal tubule, where sodium is reabsorbed in exchange for potassium secretion.[9] The affinity of loop diuretics for NKCC2 is bumetanide > torasemide > piretanide > furosemide > azosemide.[401] The net effect of loop diuretics is that increased sodium chloride with associated water is lost from the body. Potassium loss as a result of the various mechanisms described here means that hypokalemia is a common side effect.

Thiazide Diuretics. The benzothiadiazine group of compounds inhibits NCCT in the distal tubule. Because only 5% to 10% of sodium reabsorption occurs at this site, these agents are less potent than the loop diuretics, but hypokalemia is still common as a result of increased sodium delivery to the collecting duct. Thiazide diuretics also have secondary effects, resulting in increased calcium reabsorption, which may lead to hypercalcemia.[401]

"Potassium-Sparing" Diuretics. These diuretics act by reducing sodium reabsorption in the collecting duct, thus increasing potassium retention. Spironolactone acts as a competitive antagonist of aldosterone, blocking its stimulatory effects on sodium reabsorption via the mineralocorticoid receptor. Both amiloride and triamterene inhibit ENaC. The danger associated with this group of diuretics is that they can induce hyperkalemia; this is particularly likely to occur in patients with kidney disease.

Diabetes Insipidus

Primary functions of the kidney include conservation of water and production of concentrated urine. A range of conditions are associated with disturbances of the renal concentrating mechanism, resulting in polyuria and an inability to produce hypertonic urine. General conditions giving rise to this picture include hypercalcemia, hypokalemia, and CKD. Specifically, diabetes insipidus is due to the absence of a vasopressin effect, caused by impaired or failed secretion (cranial or central diabetes insipidus) or lack of end-organ response to vasopressin (nephrogenic diabetes insipidus). A further disorder, psychogenic polydipsia, or compulsive water drinking, can also present as diabetes insipidus. Polyuria is common to both diabetes insipidus and diabetes mellitus, but in diabetes insipidus, no hyperglycemia and no glycosuria is present. These individuals may fail to concentrate urine even in response to fluid restriction or synthetic vasopressin as a result of medullary "washout"; sustained fluid ingestion destroys the hyperosmolality of the medulla, which may take some time to recover. Differentiation and the pathology of these three conditions are discussed in Chapter 65. It should be noted that a vast diuresis can be induced by consumption of excessive fluid volumes (eg, among heavy beer drinkers).

Congenital nephrogenic diabetes insipidus is associated with defects that have been characterized at the molecular level (see Table 59.14).[402] Most (>90%) congenital nephrogenic diabetes insipidus patients have mutations in the *AVPR2* gene, which codes for the ADH V2 receptor. This results in an X-linked form of diabetes insipidus, with an estimated prevalence of 4 per 1 million males.[402] In less than10% of cases, an autosomal recessive inheritance pattern is caused by mutations in the *AQP2* gene. Downregulation of *AQP2* has been observed in a variety of acquired forms of diabetes insipidus, including lithium treatment, hypokalemia, hypercalcemia, ureteric obstruction, and, in animal models, chronic kidney failure.[21] Acquired forms of diabetes insipidus are more common than congenital forms.

Assessment of Renal Concentrating Ability: Urinary Osmolality

Urinary concentration can be quantified by measuring specific gravity (see Chapter 32) or by measuring urinary osmolality. For most clinical purposes, measuring specific gravity is probably sufficient,[403] but urinary osmolality measurement is critical in the diagnosis of diabetes insipidus using the water deprivation test (see Chapter 65). Specific gravity may be misleading in certain situations (eg, in the presence of proteinuria or radiocontrast dyes).

Urinary osmolality may vary widely, depending on the state of hydration. After excessive intake of fluids, for example, the osmotic concentration may fall to as low as 50 mOsm/kg H_2O, whereas in individuals with severely restricted fluid intake, concentrations of up to 1400 mOsm/kg H_2O can be observed. In individuals on an average fluid intake, values of 300 to 900 mOsm/kg H_2O are typically seen. If a random urine specimen has an osmolality of greater than 600 mOsm/kg H_2O (after 12 hours of fluid restriction), it generally can be assumed that the renal concentrating ability is normal.

In chronic progressive kidney disease, the concentrating ability of the tubules is diminished, and in ATN, the urinary osmolality, if there is urine output at all, approaches that of plasma. For a discussion on measurement of urinary and plasma osmolality, readers are referred to Chapter 35.

Renal Calculi

Nephrolithiasis is the disease condition associated with the presence of renal calculi. Renal calculi, commonly termed *kidney stones*, occur in the renal pelvis, the ureter, or the bladder. In developed countries, bladder stones are now uncommon because the causative factors of malnutrition and infection have been eliminated.[404] Calcification can also occur scattered throughout the parenchyma (nephrocalcinosis). Kidney stone formation is often considered to be a nutritional or environmental disease, linked to affluence, but genetic or anatomic abnormalities are significant. Approximately 5% to 10% of the population of the Western world are thought to have formed at least one kidney stone by the age of 70 years,[404,405] and the prevalence of kidney stones is increasing.[406] For most stone types, there is a male preponderance. The passage of a stone is associated with severe pain called *renal colic*, which may last for 15 minutes to several hours and is commonly associated with nausea and vomiting.[407] Kidney stone formation contributes to the development of CKD[408,409] and has been associated with vascular calcification, a risk factor for cardiovascular disease, and reduced bone mineral density.[410]

Background

Chemically, urine contains many mineral salts that are present in concentrations that approach their solubility

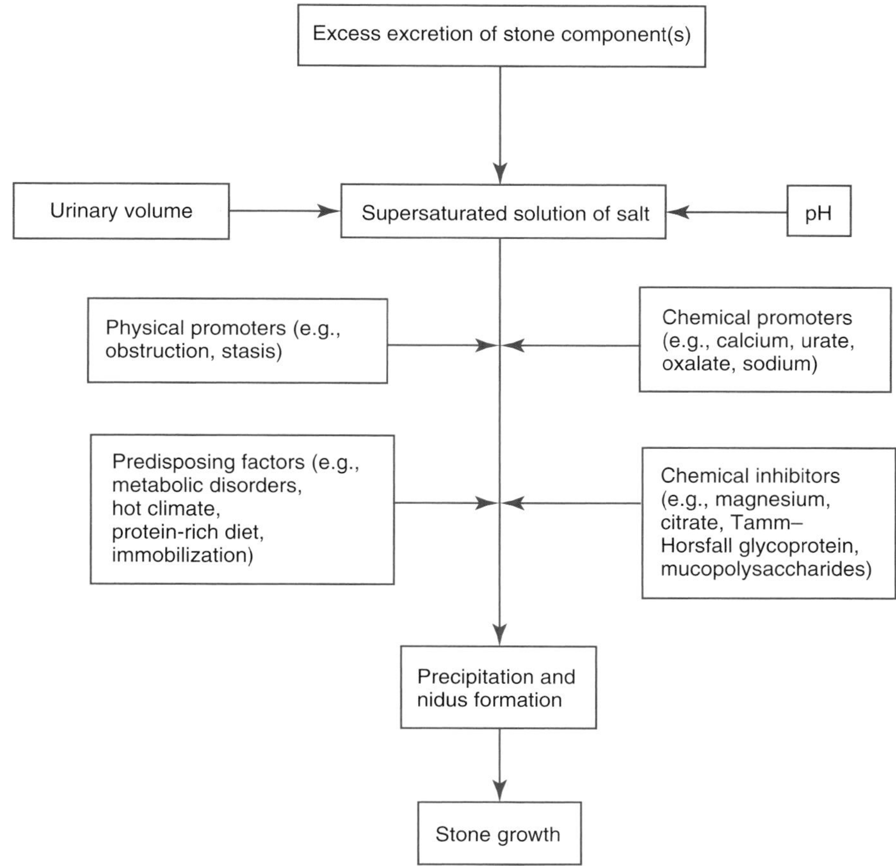

FIGURE 59.17 Diagrammatic representation of the interplay of factors involved in kidney stone formation. High or low pH may act as a promoter or inhibitor of stone formation, depending on the stone type in question (eg, calcium stone formation is favored by inadequate acidification, while urate is less soluble in acidic urine). Controversy exists as to whether formed stones become trapped as they pass through the nephron ("free particle theory") or whether stone formation occurs at damaged sites on the tubule wall ("fixed particle theory").

products at body temperature. Anyone who has seen a urine sample before and after refrigeration has witnessed the consequences of this in the massive crystal deposits that can form on cooling. Crystals can form spontaneously if the salt concentrations are high enough or, alternatively, may bind to organic material, acting as a "seed"; hyaluronic acid, a large glycosaminoglycan, has been suggested as one such promoter of crystal formation.[411] Human urine contains a number of promoters of stone formation and a variety of inhibitors, the concentrations of which can be influenced by dietary and metabolic factors (Fig. 59.17).

Initial diagnosis and examination of stones require radiologic investigation to explore the degree of intrarenal calcification and papillary damage. Plain x-rays are undertaken at initial presentation, although it should be noted that urate and other purine stones and some cystine stones are radiolucent. An intravenous urogram or spiral CT scan may be performed to establish the presence and extent of urinary tract obstruction, intrarenal reflux, and ureteric dilation. Further investigation of the patient with kidney stones or suspected of being a stone former involves analysis of blood, urine, and the stone itself, should one be obtained.[412]

Small stones (<5 mm in diameter) pass spontaneously in the urine as "gravel."[407] Although surgical treatment to remove large staghorn calculi may still be necessary, the most common form of treatment is ultrasonic extracorporeal shock wave lithotripsy (ESWL),[413] which can be applied to stones between 5 mm and 2 cm in diameter. Although this allows noninvasive destruction of stones, the long-term sequelae of exposing the kidney to high-intensity sound waves have not been fully established.[408] Additionally, evidence is mounting that ESWL may be associated with higher recurrence rates than invasive treatment.[414] Percutaneous nephrolithotomy (PCNL) may be required if ESWL fails. PCNL is the preferred approach for removal of struvite stones[415] and may be required for the treatment of cystine stones, which are more resistant to ESWL than other stone types.[416]

After treatment and successful removal of a stone, follow-up monitoring is required; recurrence rates of 30%[417] to 50%[418] are reported. The mechanisms responsible for multiple recurrences of kidney stones in only certain individuals are not completely understood. Factors involved include urine flow (fluid intake), excretion of excess quantities of stone components, the relative absence of a substance or substances in the urine that inhibit stone formation, and urinary pH (see Fig. 59.17). The predominant risk factor is poor hydration, with concentrated urine further increasing the concentrations of the mineral salts, predisposing to crystallization. Urinary concentration at least partially explains the increased incidence of kidney stone disease in hot climates—for example, in the Gulf States.

Kidney Stone Analysis

A majority of kidney stones found in the Western world are composed of calcium oxalate with or without phosphate (frequency 67%), magnesium ammonium phosphate (12%), calcium phosphate (8%), urate (8%), cystine (1% to 2%), or complex mixtures of these substances (2% to 3%).[404] These poorly soluble substances crystallize within an organic matrix, the nature of which is not well understood.

When available, analysis of the chemical constituents of stones may be useful in establishing the cause and in planning rational therapy. Stone analysis complements and guides metabolic investigation of the patients and may be particularly useful in identifying rare stone types (eg, xanthine, dihydroxyadenine), artifacts (eg, Munchausen syndrome), or drugs precipitating in the urinary tract, such as triamterene[419] and indinavir.[420] Conversely, it has been argued that stone analysis is not useful clinically[421] because the stone material that is passed often does not represent the initial metabolic derangement. This is a result of the phenomenon known as *epitaxy*, whereby nonspecific stone material, typically arising as a result of urinary tract infection (eg, struvite), may accumulate on a preexisting "metabolic" nidus, the latter of which may not be detected during stone analysis. Clearly, for stone analysis to be useful, it must be accurate. A variety of techniques have been used over the years. Traditionally, stones were crushed and solubilized, and the resulting solution was analyzed (at several dilutions when appropriate) with the use of conventional qualitative or semiquantitative chemical methods. Such techniques require relatively large amounts of stone, may miss rare and artefactual material, and analytically often perform poorly.[404] More sophisticated approaches, including thermogravimetric analysis,[422] x-ray diffraction crystallography, and especially infrared spectroscopy are preferred, a detailed description of which is beyond the scope of this chapter.[423-425]

Metabolic Investigation of Kidney Stone Formers

Ensuring adequate fluid intake remains the cornerstone of management of stone disease. Specific management of disease depending on the metabolic abnormality present is commonly undertaken, and a treatment rationale is emerging. However, with the exception of urate, there is little evidence to suggest that baseline biochemical evaluation predicts treatment efficacy.[426] Several misconceptions have arisen about the role of diet in stone formation, and optimal treatment at first may appear counterintuitive; some of these paradoxes are discussed here.

Further investigation of stone formers may be guided by knowledge of the type of stone formed. However, increasing use of lithotripsy means that often no stone material is available for analysis. Consequently, a management strategy that focuses on the cause of stone formation and is based on knowledge of blood and urinary composition is useful. Although historically metabolic investigations have often been targeted at recurrent stone formers only, the increasing availability of simple assays for chemical risk factors and the health economic burden of renal colic suggest that they are likely to become more widespread.[421,427,428] However, in some instances, it is not possible to demonstrate a biochemical abnormality in stone-forming individuals beyond a persistently small urine volume.

A variety of metabolic screening strategies have been proposed in stone-forming patients.[404,412,429,430] The chosen strategy should balance convenience for the patient and the laboratory against the ability to intervene therapeutically. For example, although THG is known to inhibit stone formation, in the absence of a specific treatment, there is little merit in measuring it. A reasonable approach should probably include measurement of plasma sodium, potassium, chloride, bicarbonate, creatinine, calcium, phosphate, and urate, together with 24-hour urinary volume, calcium, magnesium, phosphate, oxalate, urate, creatinine, sodium, citrate, and microbiology (to exclude infection). Additionally, urinary pH and cystine should be measured on a fresh, early-morning urine sample. Some investigators have proposed complex "supersaturation indices" that combine the information obtained from these studies in a numeric index.[431-433] Metabolic evaluation should be undertaken at least 6 weeks after the episode of renal colic and ideally should be done on several occasions.[429] Evaluation is most informative when undertaken on an outpatient basis with patients pursuing their normal diet and lifestyle. A brief description of the role of these risk factors is given here, with focus predominantly on the investigation of calcium stone formers. Methodologic approaches to the measurement of urinary oxalate, citrate, and cystine are discussed in Chapter 32.

Calcium. Most of the stones formed in the Western world are composed of calcium, often in association with oxalate, although calcium phosphate and urate may also be present, alone or in combination with calcium oxalate. As a consequence, urinary calcium measurement has been a central investigation. However, the significant role of oxalate is increasingly appreciated, and this has resulted in changes to the optimal management of hypercalciuria. As a rough guide, calcium oxalate stones tend to suggest hyperoxaluria as the main cause, while calcium phosphate stones implicate hypercalciuria and/or failure to adequately acidify urine.[404] A strict definition of hypercalciuria is difficult because of significant overlap between stone-forming and non-stone-forming individuals, but a cutoff of 4 mg/kg body weight (0.1 mmol/kg) is useful.[434,435] Excretion in excess of this, the most common metabolic abnormality seen in calcium stone formers, is observed in up to 50% of patients. The risk of crystal formation is clearly dependent on the concentration of calcium as opposed to its excretion rate.

Traditionally, some investigation strategies focused on whether patients demonstrated hypercalciuria while fasting (*renal hypercalciuria*) or in response to a calcium load (absorptive hypercalciuria).[407] This classification was the basis of an investigative and treatment strategy in patients with absorptive hypercalciuria who have abnormally high intestinal calcium absorption compared with non–stone formers (possibly because of a relative increase in $1{,}25(OH)_2D_3$ concentration and/or changes in intestinal vitamin D receptor activity). Treatment in these patients focused on dietary modification of calcium intake. Patients with renal hypercalciuria are now thought not to have a renal transport defect but to have an increased turnover of skeletal calcium, although management of such patients may involve pharmacologic modification of renal calcium handling (eg, thiazide diuretics).[407]

However, convincing evidence questions the usefulness of this classification and these therapeutic approaches. Dietary restriction of calcium now is generally regarded as ineffective and counterproductive because it results in an increase in intestinal oxalate absorption and increased risk of stone formation.[436,437] Further, patients with hypercalciuria are known to have reduced bone mineral density, and dietary calcium restriction may exacerbate a tendency toward osteopenia and/or osteoporosis.[438,439]

A more useful approach is to classify hypercalciuric patients into hypercalcemic or nonhypercalcemic causes. The former is most commonly due to primary hyperparathyroidism, which is seen in approximately 5% of stone formers. Treatment involves neck exploration and removal of the adenoma, although the risk of a stone recurring remains high for several years after parathyroidectomy.[440]

Nonhypercalcemic causes of hypercalciuria account for the majority of patients and, generally are classified as idiopathic (although causes such as RTA, high sodium intake, and prolonged immobilization should be excluded). Most patients with idiopathic hypercalciuria appear to have a generalized acceleration of calcium transport with increased absorption from the gut, increased mobilization from bone, and abnormal renal calcium conservation, all contributing to hypercalciuria.[435,441] In addition to increasing fluid consumption, idiopathic hypercalciuric patients appear to benefit from a diet that is low in animal protein and sodium.[442,443] Animal protein consumption increases the production of metabolic acids, increasing urinary calcium and uric acid excretion and decreasing urinary citrate (see discussion later in this chapter).[434] High sodium excretion as a result of high consumption inhibits tubular reabsorption of calcium, with a consequent increase in the risk of calcium stone formation. Sodium is easily measured in urine and represents a modifiable risk factor. Other therapeutic maneuvers that may be useful include the use of thiazide diuretics or alkaline citrate, reducing oxalate, and increasing fiber intake.[430] Some of these factors are discussed in greater detail in the following sections. A recent systematic review of randomized controlled trial evidence concluded that there were grounds for recommending increased fluid intake for the prevention of recurrence in people who have formed a single calcium stone. For recurrent calcium stone formers, the use of citrate, allopurinol, and thiazide diuretics further reduced recurrence risk.[426]

Magnesium. With calcium stone disease, magnesium is an inhibitor of stone growth. Magnesium forms complexes with oxalate that are more soluble than calcium oxalate. Increased urinary magnesium therefore inhibits stone formation.[444] Administration of magnesium has been shown to reduce enteral calcium absorption and has been proposed as a treatment for idiopathic hypercalciuric stone formers.[445] However, oral magnesium supplementation may have unpleasant side effects, and a positive benefit in terms of reducing stone recurrence has not been demonstrated.[430]

Urate. Some investigators believe that urate may potentiate calcium stone formation, although this has been questioned.[446] However, hyperuricosuria is common in calcium stone–forming patients, and treatment with allopurinol, by decreasing urate synthesis, reduces the rate of stone recurrence. Allopurinol treatment is therefore recommended for hyperuricosuric patients with calcium stone disease.[430] The formation and management of pure urate stones are discussed in Chapter 32.

Oxalate. Hyperoxaluria is a powerful promoter of calcium oxalate stone formation; indeed, it is more significant in this respect than calcium itself.[404] Oxalate is an end product of metabolism, predominantly derived from the breakdown of glyoxylate and glycine. The plasma concentration of oxalate is 1.0 to 2.4 mg/L (11–27 μmol/L), and it is excreted in the urine at a rate of 17.5 to 35.1 mg/d (200–400 μmol/d).[447] Day-to-day within-individual variability in oxalate excretion has been reported to be approximately 16%.[448] Daily excretion is independently and positively associated with increased weight, BMI, vitamin C intake, and the presence of diabetes.[448]

Hyperoxaluria may occur as a result of excessive dietary intake because of malabsorption and/or steatorrhea (enteric hyperoxaluria), or because of an inborn error of metabolism (primary hyperoxaluria). Enteric hyperoxaluria commonly occurs in association with inflammatory bowel disease and may contribute to an increased incidence of stone formation in such patients.[447] Fat malabsorption contributes to the formation of calcium fatty acid complexes ("soaps") in the intestine, increasing the enteric concentration of unbound oxalate that is absorbed through the damaged bowel wall. Primary hyperoxaluria may be type 1 (glycolic aciduria) or type 2 (L-glyceric aciduria). Patients with type 1 disease present in the first decade of life with recurrent calcium oxalate nephrolithiasis. Inheritance is autosomal recessive and survival is poor. Type 2 disease is rarer and has been claimed to run a milder course, despite the passage of similarly high concentrations of urinary oxalate. The urinary excretion of oxalate may increase to approximately 60 mg/d (700 μmol/d) when a diet containing an excess of oxalate-rich foods is taken and to as much as 260 mg/d (3 mmol/d) in patients with primary hyperoxaluria.

A dietary history may be useful in the evaluation of calcium oxalate stone formers. Patients who are excreting large amounts of oxalate are often offered dietary advice to modify their risk of future stone formation. Foods rich in oxalate include spinach, beets, tea, sorrel, wheat bran, strawberries, rhubarb, black currants, peanuts, and chocolate.[404,407,430] However, only 10% to 15% of urinary oxalate is derived directly from dietary sources,[430] and the relationships between oxalate intake and both risk of nephrolithiasis[449] and urinary oxalate excretion[448] are weak. Paradoxically, epidemiologic evidence has actually demonstrated a protective effect of high tea consumption.[437] This has been attributed to the low bioavailability of oxalate in tea and the inhibition of tubular vasopressin action by caffeine. Patients may be treated with calcium carbonate, which binds oxalate in the gut, rendering it unavailable for absorption. Alternatively, pyridoxine (vitamin B_6) may be used; this increases the catabolism of oxalate to more soluble products.[407] It should be remembered that the use of calcium-lowering diets, once favored in the treatment of calcium stone formers, increases intestinal absorption of oxalate. Measurement of urinary oxalate is discussed in Chapter 32.

Citrate. Urinary citrate inhibits stone formation by forming soluble complexes with calcium. It is present in the diet in many fruits. Excretion (typically between 120 and 930 mg/d (0.6 and 4.8 mmol/d) for adult males and between 250 and 1160 mg/d (1.3 and 6.0 mmol/d) for adult females)[404] is reduced in the calcium stone–forming population, with

50% of stone formers demonstrating hypocitraturia in one study.[417] Urinary citrate measurement may be of value in the assessment of stone-forming risk, particularly in the setting of distal RTA, where the reduction in filtered bicarbonate appears to increase tubular reabsorption of citrate with consequent hypocitraturia.[450] Inadequate urinary acidification compounds the increased risk of calcium stone formation. Treatment with carbonic anhydrase inhibitors (eg, acetazolamide,[451] topiramate)[452,453] mimics distal RTA, with a consequent increase in stone risk. Hypocitraturia may also be seen in malabsorption and urinary tract infection. Administration of oral alkaline citrate increases urinary citrate concentration by increasing the pH of tubular cells. It has been shown to be effective in the treatment of nephrolithiasis,[426] although side effects are reported and compliance is poor. Measurement of urinary citrate is discussed in Chapter 32.

Struvite Stones. Struvite stones (also called *triple phosphate* or *infection stones*) are composed of magnesium ammonium phosphate hexahydrate. Struvite stones may form in the kidney or bladder. The formation of struvite stones requires urinary tract infection with urease-producing organisms, including both gram-negative and gram-positive species from the genera *Proteus, Staphylococcus, Pseudomonas, Providencia,* and *Klebsiella*.[415] When urease is present, water and urea are hydrolyzed to form carbon dioxide and ammonia, which then hydrolyze further to form ammonium and bicarbonate. If urinary pH is greater than 7.2, struvite will form from the product of ammonium and naturally occurring cations in urine such as magnesium and phosphate (carbonate apatite will form if the pH is 6.8 to 7.2).[415]

Struvite stones are more common in females and in certain patient populations (eg, paraplegic individuals, people with congenital urinary tract malformation or stasis due to urinary tract obstruction).[415] The risk of progression to CKD appears higher in patients who develop infection stones than in those with other forms of stone disease.[408]

Cystinuria

Cystinuria is an inherited condition in which excessive urinary excretion of cystine results from a defect in proximal renal tubular reabsorption. (Cystinuria should not be confused with cystinosis, which is a condition associated with intracellular accumulation of cystine but not with excess urinary excretion of cystine.) In the most common form of the disease, there is also excess excretion of the dibasic amino acids (lysine, ornithine, and arginine). These share the same renal tubular transporter, although their presence in excess in urine appears benign. More rarely, isolated cystinuria is seen. This phenotypic classification has been superseded by increased understanding of the genetic basis of the disease. Mutations in either of the genes coding for two components of the dibasic amino acid transport system (*SLC3A1* [type A cystinuria] and *SLC7A9* [type B cystinuria]) cause cystinuria. More than 200 mutations have been reported. Type A is generally a recessive condition, so affected individuals will have genotype AA, but some heterozygotes may develop cystinuria. Type B is usually a dominant condition, but with variable penetrance; both B and BB genotypes may develop cystinuria. Some patients have mutations in both genes (type AB cystinuria). Occasionally there are more than two mutated alleles present (eg, AAB or ABB).[454] A small percentage of patients with cystinuria do not have mutations in either of these genes.[416] There does not appear to be a clear genotype-phenotype association.[454]

The normal urinary excretion of cystine has been reported to be 5 to 48 mg/d (40–400 μmol/d).[404] Its relatively low limit of solubility, 18 mg/dL (1500 μmol/L),[407] is exceeded in many patients with cystinuria,[404] resulting in the formation of hexagonal crystals and, ultimately, cystine stones. Cystinuria may present at any age from infancy to old age, although presentation is most common in the second and third decades.[416,454] Cystinuria is often recurrent and is associated with large kidney stones, including staghorn calculi, and renal impairment.[454]

The finding of a cystine stone should prompt confirmation of cystinuria by urinary analysis.[404] It could be argued, however, that all stone formers should be screened for cystinuria; at least 10% of cystinuric individuals form stones in which cystine cannot be detected, presumably because of epitaxy.[455] The index of suspicion should be increased in patients who are relatively young (<30 years old) stone formers and in those with recurrent or bilateral stones or a positive family history.[416] Once a cystinuric patient is diagnosed, it is important to screen all members of the family, particularly to detect affected siblings.

Treatment of cystinuria is aimed at keeping cystine below its saturation point by maintaining high fluid intake (>3 L/d), particularly at night. Other treatments include reducing cystine (found in animal protein) and salt intake, urinary alkalinization (eg, with potassium citrate; cystine is more soluble in alkaline urine) and chelation with thiol-binding drugs (eg, D-penicillamine or –mercaptopropionylglycine [tiopronin]).[416] Quantitative analysis is an important adjunct for monitoring penicillamine therapy, which can be optimized on the basis of free cystine versus cystine/penicillamine disulfide. Penicillamine itself may cause glomerular damage; thus regular monitoring of urinary protein excretion is recommended. Measurement of urinary cystine is discussed in Chapter 32.

Toxic Nephropathy

A wide variety of nephrotoxins exist in the environment, in some cases associated with particular occupations (eg, heavy metals, such as cadmium and lead; see Chapter 42). Both glomerular and tubulointerstitial damage may result from exposure to toxins; detection of both requires biochemical monitoring of GFR/serum creatinine concentration and tubular and glomerular proteinuria. Anatomic physiologic and biochemical features make the kidney susceptible to insult from a variety of medicinal and environmental agents. Factors contributing to the sensitivity of the kidney include its large blood flow, the concentration of filtered solutes during urine production, and the presence of a variety of xenobiotic transporters and metabolizing enzymes. Toxic nephropathy commonly occurs as a result of decreased renal perfusion because of precipitation within the tubule or because of direct toxic effects at the proximal tubule level. In some cases the conjugation of environmental chemicals (eg, mercury, cadmium) to glutathione and/or cysteine targets these chemicals to the kidney, where inhibition of renal function occurs through a variety of mechanisms that are not completely understood. Although some drugs can cause kidney damage in the presence of normal renal function, a far greater variety of drugs can cause problems in patients with kidney disease, predominantly because of accumulation resulting from decreased renal elimination. A list of drugs and environmental toxins commonly known to cause kidney damage is given in Table 59.15.

RENAL REPLACEMENT THERAPY

Renal replacement therapy (RRT) includes dialysis procedures such as hemodialysis (HD), peritoneal dialysis (PD), continuous hemofiltration (HF), and continuous hemodiafiltration (HDF). These techniques are used to temporarily or permanently remove toxic substances from the blood when the kidneys cannot satisfactorily remove them from the circulation. In addition, kidney transplantation has become an effective form of RRT. Extensive laboratory support is required by an RRT program (Table 59.16).

Background

In 1861, Thomas Graham Bell in Glasgow, Scotland, carried out the first dialysis experiments (and coined the term *dialysis*), separating crystalloids and colloids in a solution. Bell predicted that this technique could have medical application, but this was not realized until nearly 100 years later in the work of Willem Kolff and then Belding Scribner, who made HD a feasible treatment in the early 1960s. Since that time, HD and, more recently, PD have extended the lives of many people, sometimes for up to 20 or 30 years.

Dialysis

Dialysis is the process of separating macromolecules from ions and low molecular weight compounds in solution based on the difference in their rates of diffusion through a semipermeable membrane, through which crystalloids can pass

TABLE 59.15 Toxic Nephropathy: Causes, Patterns, and Markers

Compound Category	Drug/Toxin	Type of Renal Injury/Pathology	Biomarkers/Notes
Antibacterial agents	Aminoglycosides (eg, neomycin, gentamicin, tobramycin, amikacin)	Acute tubular necrosis and interstitial nephritis. Nonoliguric AKI.	Plasma: ↓K, ↓Mg, ↓Ca Urine: ↑LMWP, ↑Glycosuria Nephrotoxicity major and common side effect
	Amphotericin	Initially distal tubular injury followed by medullary injury	Plasma: ↓K, ↑creatinine dRTA
Antiviral/antiprotozoal agents	Acyclovir	Nonoliguric AKI due to tubular obstruction and interstitial inflammation	Crystalluria and hematuria
	Pentamidine	Tubular toxicity	Plasma: ↓Mg, ↓Ca Urine: ↑Mg, ↑Ca
	Indinivar	Nephrolithiasis, irreversible kidney failure in some patients	Crystalluria and hematuria
Radiocontrast agents	Eg, iothalamate, iodixanol	Oliguric or nonoliguric AKI, generally reversible. Proximal tubular damage.	↑Plasma creatinine after contrast administration
Antitumor drugs	Cisplatin	Irreversible dose-related and cumulative kidney failure. TIN with heavy proteinuria. Often AKI.	Urine: ↑Mg, ↑PO4, tubular casts and ↑LMWP in early stages.
	Methotrexate	Nonoliguric AKI. Tubular atrophy and interstitial fibrosis.	Only seen in association with high-dose therapy
	Interleukin-2	Reversible AKI due to ↓RBF	Observed in up to 90% of cases of high-dose therapy
Other drugs	ACE inhibitors	Dramatic ↓GFR due to ↓ efferent arteriolar tone	Especially in the setting of bilateral renal artery stenosis. ↑Plasma creatinine and K.
	5-aminosalicylic acid (eg, mesalazine, olsalazine)	Occasional ATN and irreversible kidney damage	Tubular proteinuria
	Cyclooxygenase (COX)-2 inhibitors	Probably a similar pattern of renal injury to NSAIDs (see below)	
	Lithium	Distal tubular damage with nephrogenic diabetes insipidus ± dRTA	
	Penicillamine	Membranous glomerulopathy with NS, occasionally AKI	Proteinuria
	NSAIDs	Several forms of nephropathy identified, including (1) hemodynamically mediated AKI, (2) TIN ± NS, (3) salt and/or water retention, (4) hyperkalemia, and (5) CKD/ESRD ("analgesic nephropathy")	Depends on type of effect

Continued

TABLE 59.15 Toxic Nephropathy: Causes, Patterns, and Markers—cont'd

Compound Category	Drug/Toxin	Type of Renal Injury/Pathology	Biomarkers/Notes
Heavy metals	Cadmium	Subtle but irreversible TIN	Fanconi syndrome with RTA. ↑Urinary metallothionein.
	Gold	Membranous glomerulopathy but normal GFR maintained	Proteinuria <3.5 g/24 h
	Lead	Proximal tubular atrophy with interstitial fibrosis	Reversible Fanconi syndrome in children with acute poisoning. In lead workers, urinary proteinuria <2 g/24 h in association with ↑plasma urate, hypertension ± gouty arthritis.
	Mercury	Proximal tubular damage with ATN	Urine: ↑LMWP
Other environmental agents	Hydrocarbons (eg paints, dry cleaning solvents)	ATN, chronic TIN, glomerulonephritis. Caused by renal cytochrome P450 metabolism of chloroform to toxic metabolites.	Tubular proteinuria ± ↑plasma creatinine
	Paraquat, diquat	ATN secondary to ↓RBF due to shock and direct toxic effects of paraquat. Intrinsic kidney damage due to production of reactive oxygen species.	↑Plasma creatinine
Drugs used in transplantation	See Table 59.18.		

The list of agents shown is not exclusive but illustrates the range of compounds that may affect the kidney. For further information, readers should consult: Palmer BF, Henrich WL. Toxic nephropathy. In: Brenner BM (ed.) *Brenner and Rector's the Kidney*, 7th ed. Philadelphia: Saunders; 2004 [chapter 34].

ACE, Angiotensin converting enzyme; *AKI,* acute kidney injury; *ATN,* acute tubular necrosis; *CKD,* chronic kidney disease; *dRTA,* distal renal tubular acidosis; *ESRD,* end-stage renal disease; *LMWP,* low molecular weight proteinuria; *NS,* nephrotic syndrome; *NSAIDs,* nonsteroidal antiinflammatory drugs; *TIN,* tubulointerstitial nephropathy.

TABLE 59.16 Laboratory Support for Dialysis Programs

Clinical Condition	Laboratory Tests
Acute Dialysis	
Dialysis disequilibrium	Urea and electrolyes, bicarbonate, calcium
Pyrexia	C-reactive protein, white cell count, blood cultures
Bleeding	Clotting screen, platelets
Chronic Dialysis	
Anemia	Ferritin, transferrin saturation, B12, folate Blood film, PTH, C-reactive protein
Sepsis	C-reactive protein, blood, urine specimens for microscopy, culture, and sensitivity
Nutrition	Albumin, phosphate
Cardiovascular disease risk	Lipid profile
Dialysis-related amyloid	β_2-microglobulin (not routinely measured)
CKD-MBD	Predialysis plasma calcium, phosphate (monthly in hemodialysis patients; every 3 months in peritoneal dialysis patients) Alkaline phosphatase PTH (at least every 3 months) Aluminum in patients receiving aluminum-based phosphate binders (every 3 months)
Adequacy of hemodialysis as assessed by urea clearance	Predialysis and postdialysis urea
Sepsis, abdominal pain in peritoneal dialysis	Microscopy and culture of peritoneal dialysate
Adequacy of peritoneal dialysis as assessed by weekly small solute clearance	Dialysate creatinine, urea
Peritoneal membrane characteristics assessed by peritoneal equilibration test (PET)	Plasma and dialysate glucose and creatinine

CKD, Chronic kidney disease; *MBD,* mineral.

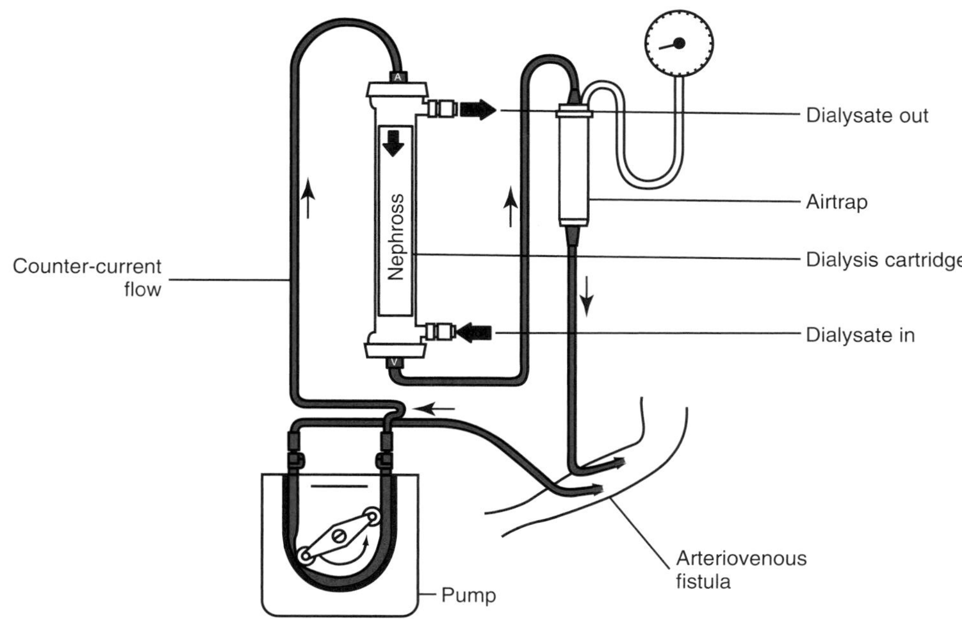

FIGURE 59.18 A hemodialyzer setup.

readily but colloids pass very slowly or not at all. Two distinct physical processes are involved: diffusion and ultrafiltration.

The timing of initiation of dialysis treatment is controversial and requires judgment, taking into account the treatment of metabolic consequences of advanced CKD, the comorbidities of the patient, and the accepted impact of dialysis treatment on quality of life. No absolute recommendation of commencement of dialysis based on GFR alone can be made. KDIGO suggest that dialysis be initiated when one or more of the following are present: symptoms or signs attributable to kidney failure (serositis, acid-base or electrolyte abnormalities, pruritus); inability to control volume status or blood pressure; a progressive deterioration in nutritional status refractory to dietary intervention; or cognitive impairment. This often but not invariably occurs in the GFR range between 5 and 10 mL/min/1.73 m^2.[94] Not all individuals will be suitable for RRT, and in this setting, it is important that the multidisciplinary team facilitates care for people on the "conservative management" pathway.[94] The US Renal Data System reports that 13% of incident patients starting dialysis in 2012 had an estimated GFR below 5 mL/min/1.73 m^2.[456]

Hemodialysis and Hemofiltration

HD is the method most commonly used to treat advanced and permanent kidney failure. Clinically, it is considered the default therapy that is utilized in patients unsuitable for the alternate modalities of PD and kidney transplantation. Operationally, it involves connecting the patient to a circuit into which his or her blood flows to and from a semipermeable large surface area membrane, the hemodialyzer. After filtration to remove wastes and extra fluid, the cleansed blood is returned to the patient. This is a complicated and inconvenient therapy requiring a coordinated effort from a health care team that includes the patient, nephrologist, dialysis nurse, dialysis technician, dietitian, and others.

Description. HD utilizes diffusive and convective mass transfer across a semipermeable membrane. The driving force for diffusion is the concentration gradient between blood and dialysate. Smaller solutes with larger concentration gradients give increased diffusion. The concentration gradient is maintained by using countercurrent flows and high flow rates. Anticoagulated blood is pumped in one direction across the membrane, and the recipient fluid, the dialysate, flows at a rate of 500 to 800 mL/min in the opposite direction, as shown in Fig. 59.18. Water molecules and small molecular weight molecules can cross the membrane, while larger proteins and cellular elements are retained in the vascular space. Convection is the bulk movement of solvent and dissolved solute across the membrane, down a transmembrane hydrostatic pressure gradient. The most important functional part is the dialyzer membrane. Biocompatibility of the dialyzer membrane is an essential requirement because of high surface areas and long contact times. Patients are dialyzed in home-based or hospital-based units, with dialysis usually performed three times a week for sessions lasting between 3 and 5 hours. This dialysis schedule is largely empirical, insofar as it reconciles adequate treatment with breaks between treatments to provide the patient with a reasonable quality of life. Approaches to increase the dose of dialysis have been explored. These include short daily HD that entails a 2- to 3-hour dialysis 6 days per week.[457] Alternatively, slow overnight dialysis for 5 to 7 nights has been employed. These regimens have been reported to improve outcome.[457-459] The Frequent Hemodialysis Network (FHN) Trial, in which patients received six hemodialysis sessions per week, demonstrated improved mortality, biochemical parameters, and LV mass.[189]

HD relies on good vascular access to the circulation of the patient to enable blood to be pumped around the extracorporeal circuit at a rate in excess of 300 mL/min. Suitable vascular access was not achieved until the 1960s. Although Kolff at Groningen Hospital in the Netherlands performed the first dialysis experiments in humans in 1943, the problem of dialysis support with long-term vascular access was not solved until Scribner developed the arteriovenous cannula in 1960. This advance was followed by the development of the surgically created arteriovenous fistula (AVF), introduced by Brescia and colleagues in 1966, which provided permanent vascular access. The Dialysis Outcomes Practice Patterns Study (DOPPS) confirmed a wide variation in how dialysis is achieved throughout the world. For example, most patients in Germany have an AVF as their main access, whereas in the United States, a fistula was used for access in only 13% of patients for their first dialysis in 2006,[95] reflecting suboptimal pre-ESRD care. AVF survival is longer in Europe than in the United States. However, recent coalition initiatives exemplified by the "Fistula First" campaign and the K/DOQI Work Group have delivered service improvements, with national AVF rates reported at 63% as of March 2015 (see Fistula First-Catheter Last dashboard: http://esrdncc.org/ffcl/for-ffcl-professionals/). When used as a patient's first access, AVF survival is considered superior to arteriovenous grafts regarding time to first failure.

Conventional HD uses low-flux dialyzers, allowing diffusive but little convective solute removal. Middle molecule clearance is poor. HF is a convective treatment. Although middle molecule clearances are improved, small molecule clearance is poor. HF is used for continuous treatment in ICUs in the management of AKI. In addition, acute HD and continuous filtration in ICU are utilized in acute poisoning with, for example, ethylene glycol and lithium (see Chapter 41). High-flux HD using biocompatible membranes allows convective and diffusive solute removal. The use of very pure water is crucial in high-flux modes, because dialysis fluid is infused directly into the bloodstream by back-filtration. The Hemodialysis (HEMO) Study, a randomized clinical trial designed to determine whether increasing the dose of dialysis or using a high-flux dialyzer membrane alters major outcomes, concluded that patients undergoing HD thrice weekly derived no major benefit from a higher dialysis dose than that recommended by current US guidelines or from the use of a high-flux membrane.[460] However, subgroup analysis suggested a benefit in patients maintained on dialysis for longer than 3.7 years and in those with diabetes.[461] The Membrane Permeability Outcome study group reported similar results,[462] and the KDOQI recommends the use of high-flux membranes.[463]

HDF is HD in which fluid removal exceeds the desired weight loss, and fluid balance is maintained by the infusion of a sterile pyrogen-free solution. HDF offers the advantages of both HD and HF in a single therapy. The replacement fluid is generated "online" from concentrated bicarbonate, and 20 to 30 L of water is used per session.[464] The result is that HDF provides a 10% to 15% increase in urea clearance compared with HD, along with increased middle molecule clearances. Water for online preparation of substitution solution should meet common standards for dialysis water regarding chemical contaminants, but it should be of higher quality regarding microbiological contaminants. Online HDF has been used extensively in continental Europe over the past 20 years or so.

After several years of HD, patients may develop carpal tunnel syndrome and evidence of amyloid deposition. The main constituent of dialysis-related amyloid is β_2-microglobulin. Circulating concentrations of β_2-microglobulin can be as high as 300 to 400 mg/L. Although no correlation is noted between circulating β_2-microglobulin concentration and the risk of amyloidosis, evidence from the HEMO study indicates that concentrations are correlated with survival.[465] Retrospective data from Lombardy in Italy indicate that there is a 5% risk that carpal tunnel decompression surgery will be required after 8 years of extracorporeal therapy and that a reduction in risk of 42% is seen in those patients treated by HDF and HF compared with conventional HD.[466] It is suggested that patients on PD are less prone to developing amyloidosis.

Fluid management on HD is crucial for patient well-being and survival. Because conventional dialysis is based on a thrice weekly schedule, fluid is accumulated by the patient between dialysis sessions. Many patients are anuric or at least oliguric; therefore unrestricted fluid intake would result in fluid overload and complications of pulmonary edema and hypertension. Patients receiving HD are advised to restrict fluid intake to 1 L/d or so. This allowance is recommended to the individual patient by the dialysis nursing staff and the dietitian to ensure that adequate nutrition is maintained. Nevertheless, many patients find the fluid restriction very difficult to maintain; therefore large weight gains between dialysis sessions are a common occurrence. During the dialysis session, the patient's "dry" or "target" weight is achieved. At dry weight, the fluid compartments are normal; this value is determined by gradually reducing weight until the patient is edema-free and reaches the point below which hypotension occurs on further fluid removal. The dry weight is difficult to reach in patients with abnormal cardiovascular responses, who may become hypotensive despite being relatively fluid replete.

When HD is begun, most patients have a small amount of residual renal function (RRF). This level of RRF may persist for many months and years. The volume of urine produced each day allows greater fluid intake and provides the benefit of reducing large fluctuations in body fluid volumes. RRF should be taken into consideration when dialysis prescriptions are adjusted. The K/DOQI Work Group 2006 updates include recommendations, as opposed to guidelines (opinion-based rather than evidence-based), for preserving RRF in patients receiving HD.[463]

Assessment of Adequacy of Hemodialysis. Assessment of adequacy of dialysis treatment for individual patients in the clinical setting includes consideration of the patient's well-being, cardiovascular risk, nutritional status, and degree of achievable ultrafiltration. It also includes estimates of a number of laboratory parameters such as hemoglobin, phosphate, and albumin, and clearance of the small solutes, urea and creatinine. Although a full description of adequacy is beyond the scope of this text, a brief outline is provided. Urea removal is typically defined by the "Kt/V_{urea}." This ratio is a measure of the amount of plasma cleared of urea ($K \times t$, where t = time in hours) divided by the urea distribution volume (V). The urea distribution volume is considered equivalent to the total body water.[467] Kt/V during a dialysis session is calculated following determination of predialysis and postdialysis plasma urea concentrations, the time of the dialysis session, RRF, total clearance predicted from the dialyzer, and blood and dialysate flow rates. These variables are processed using computerized mathematical formulas. The Kt/V effectively describes the *power* of the dialysis session and continues to be valued as the most precise and accurate measure of dialysis.[463] A retrospective analysis of the National Cooperative Dialysis Study (NCDS) was the first study to identify a threshold in the level of Kt/V and survival in HD.[468] In practice, a simple calculation may be performed to obtain an estimate of dialysis adequacy: the urea reduction ratio (URR). The URR is the percentage fall in plasma urea attained during a dialysis session and is measured as follows:

$$[(\text{Predialysis }\{\text{urea}\} - \text{Postdialysis }\{\text{urea}\})/(\text{predialysis }\{\text{urea}\})] \times 100\%$$

Observational studies in populations of dialysis patients have shown that variations in URR are associated with major differences in mortality.[469]

Following publication of the HEMO study,[460] the KDOQI Work Group 2006 update recommended that the target dose of delivered dialysis as calculated by Kt/V urea kinetic modeling was 1.4 per dialysis session. This dose is consistent with the target single pool Kt/V of approximately 1.4 set by the European Standards Group[470] and is roughly equivalent to a urea reduction ratio of 70% per dialysis for a patient receiving thrice weekly hemodialysis.

Peritoneal Dialysis

Peritoneal dialysis (PD) is a type of dialysis in which dialysate is passed into the patient's peritoneal cavity, with the peritoneum then employed as the dialysis membrane. It was first explored by Ganter in 1923 and initially showed poor results. The modern era of PD started in 1953 with intermittent irrigation of the peritoneal cavity with commercially prepared solutions and access achieved through a single disposable catheter (Fig. 59.19). In 1976, Popovich and colleagues introduced the concept of portable equipment; this approach led to the use of continuous ambulatory peritoneal dialysis (CAPD),[471] a type of PD performed in ambulatory patients during normal activities. Peritoneal dialysis now accounts for 6.2% and 7.4% of the incident and prevalent dialysis populations in the United States, respectively, proportions that have continued to decline over the past decade from peaks of 13% and 11% primarily as the result of an increase in HD capacity.[95] Use of PD varies among countries, depending on access to HD. For example, in the United Kingdom in 2013, at Day 90, 20% of incident patients were receiving PD (compared to 66% receiving hemodialysis and 10% with a functioning transplant),[107] whereas in Mexico, 90% of patients received PD.[472]

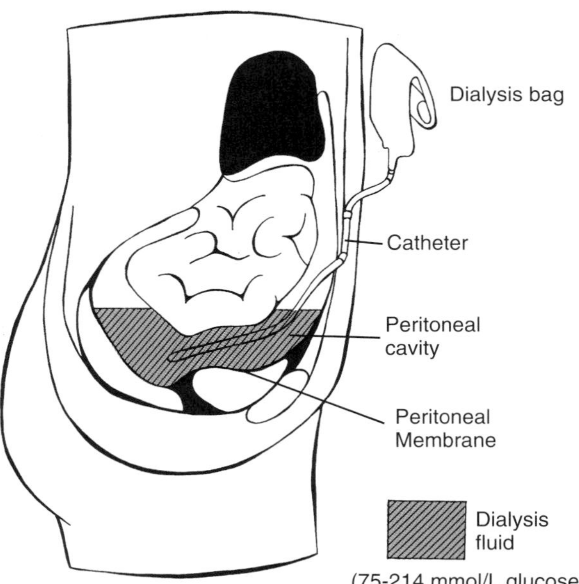

FIGURE 59.19 Diagrammatic sketch of peritoneal dialysis. To convert glucose concentration in mmol/L to mg/dL, multiply by 18. (Redrawn from Nolph KD. Peritoneal anatomy and transport physiology. In: Maher JF, ed. *Replacement of Renal Function by Dialysis*. 3rd ed. Kluwer Academic Publishers/Springer: Dordrecht, The Netherlands 1989: Chapter 23.)

Description. Operationally, PD uses the patient's own peritoneal membrane (surface area approximately 2 m^2), across which fluids and solutes are exchanged between the peritoneal capillary blood and the dialysis solution placed in the peritoneal cavity. Fluid removal (ultrafiltration) is achieved by using dialysis fluids containing high concentrations of dextrose acting as an osmotic agent; as dextrose passes across the peritoneal membrane, the concentration gradient diminishes and the rate of fluid removal decreases. Conventional therapies use four daily exchanges of approximately 2 L of fluid, with approximately 10 L of spent dialysate generated (including ultrafiltration). RRF is critical to the success of PD because only a few milliliters per minute can contribute substantially to urea clearance and creatinine clearance (C_{Cr}), with each additional milliliter resulting in an extra 10 L of clearance per week. Practical reasons for opting for PD include preservation of RRF and vascular access sites, a home treatment facilitating increased patient autonomy, flexibility as to where the treatment can be administered, and ease of self-treatment, with lower capital costs involved. Blood pressure control and extremes of fluid shifts are not as problematic as those that occur on conventional HD.

Automated PD is now widely available. It requires a programmable machine to regulate flow, dwell time, and drainage, and it may be performed at night. Solute clearance can be increased by leaving fluid in the peritoneum during the day and by performing an additional daytime exchange.

The main disadvantage of PD is the risk of infection causing peritonitis. Incidence rates of peritonitis have decreased over the years with the introduction of disconnect PD systems, improved training of patients with regard to meticulous hygiene, and microbiological surveillance protocols. The current standard from the Renal Association in the United Kingdom is that the peritonitis rate should be less than one episode per 18 patient months.[156]

Peritonitis typically presents with a cloudy dialysate effluent and abdominal pain. Additional features such as vomiting and a high temperature suggest serious infection. Blood and dialysate samples should be taken for urgent microbiological analysis and antibiotics administered via the dialysis catheter directly into the peritoneum. If antibiotic treatment fails, then the catheter is removed and the patient is converted to HD. In the majority of cases, the episode of peritonitis responds to treatment, and PD can continue, although it is likely that repeated episodes will cause scarring and fibrosis of the peritoneal membrane, with permanent loss of ultrafiltration. Long-term serious complications may occur, such as sclerosing encapsulating peritonitis caused by adhesions and peritoneal thickening encasing the peritoneal contents and causing bowel obstruction. This unusual condition is associated with increased frequency of peritonitis episodes and longer duration of PD.[473]

Assessment of Adequacy in PD. A series of clinical outcome reports have demonstrated that measures of PD solute removal (urea and creatinine) correlate with patient status and outcome.[474-476] In particular, a multicenter prospective cohort study of 680 incident CAPD patients (Canada–United States [CANUSA] Study) showed that a decrease of 0.1 in weekly urea clearance ratio (defined by Kt/V_{urea}) was associated with a 5% increase in the relative risk of death.[477] Similarly, a decrease of 5 L/wk/1.73 m^2 of total C_{Cr} was associated with a 7% increase in the RR of death. As a consequence of these studies, national guidelines from the United Kingdom,[478] and the United States[479] have set standards of dialysis adequacy in terms of small solute removal. An estimate of adequacy is performed in all patients within 6 to 8 weeks of commencement of dialysis. Additional studies should be performed at least every 6 months.[478]

Obtaining the weekly Kt/V_{urea} requires measurement of the volume of spent dialysate and urine for a complete 24-hour period. The concentration of urea in dialysate (D) compared with plasma (P) is calculated (the D/P ratio), and this value is then multiplied by the volume of the drained effluent to obtain an estimate of Kt. The calculation of "V," or the volume of distribution of urea, is derived from an estimate of total body water.[480,481] An estimate of weekly Kt/V_{urea} is simply the daily clearance multiplied by a factor of 7. These equations are used for both peritoneal and renal clearance, and the total weekly clearance is obtained by addition. Calculation of C_{Cr} is based on the following clearance (C) formula:

$$C = \frac{U\,(\text{or } D) \times V}{P}$$

where U is the concentration of creatinine in urine or dialysate, V is the mean daily drain volume or urine volume (measured in liters), and P is the concentration of creatinine in the plasma. The daily clearances obtained for both urine and dialysate are added together and multiplied by 7 for the total weekly C_{Cr}. Current recommendations from the UK Renal Association include a combined urinary and peritoneal Kt/V_{urea} greater than 1.7/week or a creatinine clearance greater than 50 L/week/1.73 m^2, which should be considered as reflecting minimal treatment doses. The dose should be increased in patients experiencing uremic symptoms.[156]

Compliance with complete collections is mandatory. To reduce sampling errors in patients who void infrequently, urine is collected over a 48-hour period. Dialysate sampling requires that all effluent bags obtained over a 24-hour period should be brought to the center renal unit; this can be difficult because the bags are heavy and bulky. Glucose concentrations in peritoneal dialysis bags may reach 3852 mg/dL (214 mmol/L); it is important that glucose interference in the dialysate creatinine measurement is corrected for when Jaffe assays are used[482] or minimized by the use of an enzymatic creatinine method.[483] An adjunct to assessment of adequacy in PD patients is the peritoneal equilibration test (PET),[484] which assesses peritoneal membrane transport characteristics in terms of creatinine clearance, glucose absorption, and ultrafiltration. The results are used to select dialysis schedules appropriate to the transport characteristics of the patient.

Measurement of adequacy is burdensome, labor intensive, and prone to multiple measurement errors, particularly from volume measurements of urine and dialysate samples; laboratory errors in measurements of urea and creatinine in blood, urine, and dialysate; and finally adjustment of results to predict weekly clearance. Although dialysis center nursing staff and patients may collect the samples required for adequacy testing with the utmost diligence, the very complexity and number of measurements taken will lead to an accumulation of measurement errors. In the opinion of the authors of the NKF-K/DOQI Clinical Practice Guidelines for PD Adequacy, when properly performed, these measures are reproducible enough to be useful in routine clinical practice.[479] However, an alternative, simpler method for defining dialysis adequacy would be very useful in practice.

Malnutrition in Dialysis Patients

Dialysis patients with ESRD tend to have a poor appetite. Protein metabolism is altered in the setting of chronic acidosis and low-grade inflammation. These factors in combination place patients at risk of protein and energy malnourishment. Nutritional screening is recommended in dialysis patients. Such screening may involve measurement of weight, a recent history of edema-free weight loss, the body mass index, and subjective global assessment.[156] Serum albumin is often used as a marker of malnutrition, even though it is a relatively poor nutritional marker.[485] However, good evidence indicates that the lower the albumin concentration, the worse the long-term prognosis.[469,486,487] An albumin concentration of less than 3.5 g/dL (measured by a bromocresol green method) or less than 3.0 g/dL (bromocresol purple method) is indicative of undernutrition. Hypoalbuminemia is associated with increased markers of the acute-phase response, such as CRP.[488,489] Persistent increase of CRP is common in dialysis patients and may occur in the absence of detectable infection. Episodes of peritonitis in PD patients cause significant albumin losses as the result of membrane leakage.

Kidney Transplantation

Kidney transplantation is the most effective form of renal replacement therapy in terms of long-term survival and quality of life.[490] Data provided by the Organ Procurement and Transplantation Network reveal that, as of May 10, 2015, 101,660 patients were on the waiting list for a kidney transplant, and almost 17,000 kidney transplants were performed in the United States in 2012 (http://optn.transplant.hrsa.gov/data/). Median waiting time for a listed patient depends on his or her age. For example, for patients listed between 2003 and 2004, the median waiting time for a child aged 1 to 5 years was approximately 1 year, and for an adult aged 35 to 49 years, it was approximately 5 years. The median time to transplant for a white adult increased from 2.7 years in 1998 to 4.2 years in 2008 (http://srtr.transplant.hrsa.gov/annual_reports/2012/pdf/01_kidney_13.pdf). Although patients with kidney failure should have equitable access to kidney transplantation, currently only 23% of adult patients on dialysis in the United Kingdom are on the active renal transplant waiting list. Patients in transplanting centers are more likely to be listed than those in nontransplanting centers.[107] Waiting time spent on dialysis has been shown to be an important factor in determining mortality. In England and Wales, 45% of patients younger than 65 years were activated on the transplant list within 1 year of starting dialysis, and 66% were activated within 5 years. Evidence suggests that the very best outcomes are achieved following preemptive (ie, before dialysis has become necessary) live donor transplants.[491] This has led to increased emphasis on preemptive transplantation, particularly in the United Kingdom, following the National Service Framework for Renal Services, published in 2004.[492]

Since Joseph Murray in Boston performed the first successful transplant in 1954 from one twin to the other, progressive developments have occurred in this field of medicine. In 1959, Dameshek and Schwartz used 6-mercaptopurine (6-MP) in place of irradiation to precondition patients for bone marrow transplantation. Calne developed this work with the introduction of a safer derivative of 6-MP called azathioprine (AZA). By 1963, maintenance AZA and corticosteroids had become the standard regimen for kidney transplantation. Kidney transplant or "allograft" survival with these treatment protocols was approximately 40% at 12 months. In the late 1970s to early 1980s, cyclosporin was introduced and has since been the mainstay immunosuppressive regimen in combination with AZA and corticosteroids. Cyclosporin-based protocols led to fewer episodes of acute rejection and improved graft survival at 12 months to 80% to 90%. Tacrolimus, mycophenolate mofetil (MMF), sirolimus (Rapamycin), and everolimus (Ever) were developed for use in kidney transplantation in the mid- to late 1990s. Also, there has been progress on the development and use of biological agents (monoclonal or polyclonal antibodies directed against immune response cellular targets) to suppress the immune response to a graft in human transplant recipients. All these advancements have led to increases in graft and patient survival, with 1-year graft survival of approximately 90% being the norm.[493,494] By contrast, long-term graft survival remains a major problem, with half of transplants failing within 14 years, usually as a result of chronic allograft injury or death with a functioning graft. Transplantation medicine provides a constant challenge to balance the immunologic risk of damage to the allograft (rejection) versus the well-being of the recipient, while avoiding excess immunosuppression that increases the likelihood of opportunistic infection and malignancy. In addition, many of the powerful immunosuppressive drugs have idiosyncratic side effect profiles.

Preoperative Assessment

The criteria for acceptance into a transplant program differ slightly from center to center, and it is easier to consider reasons for exclusion (Box 59.6). Two important psychological issues remain to be considered: the concept of organ receipt and potential difficulty in complying with immunosuppressive therapies. Age is no longer a primary issue in an otherwise healthy individual. The median age of incident and prevalent renal transplant patients in the United Kingdom has increased every year, and in 2013, it was 50.3 and 52.8 years, respectively.[107]

Laboratory assessment includes indicators of general operative health (eg, electrolytes, acid-base status, clotting profile, full blood cell count, cross-matching; Boxes 59.7 and 59.8). In addition, a full screen for infectious diseases, particularly cytomegalovirus (CMV), Epstein-Barr virus, hepatitis B and C, varicella-zoster virus, and human immunodeficiency virus (HIV) status, is undertaken; these infections can be activated by immunosuppressive therapy.

BOX 59.6 Exclusion Criteria for Consideration for a Kidney Transplant

- Serious concomitant illness (particularly if likely to shorten life expectancy or to be exacerbated by immunosuppressive treatment)
  - Active malignancy*
  - Inoperable ischemic heart disease
  - Severe chronic lung disease
  - Active systemic infection (eg, tuberculosis)
  - Active immunological disease
  - Severe irreversible hepatic disease
  - Severe peripheral vascular disease
- Severe obesity (body mass index [BMI] >40 kg/m^2)
- Lower urinary tract dysfunction not amenable to surgical repair
- Substance abuse
- Significant psychiatric disturbance

*Malignancy that has been treated with no evidence of recurrence is not an exclusion provided the predefined remission period has elapsed.

The Operation

The donor kidney is usually placed extraperitoneally in the right or left iliac fossa. Anastomoses are constructed joining the transplant renal artery and vein to the recipient's respective iliac vessels. The ureter is joined to the bladder. The recipient native kidneys are left in situ in most cases. Living donor kidneys can be retrieved through open surgery or with the aid of laparoscopic techniques. The workup for a live donor transplant is beyond the scope of this chapter.

Postoperative Assessment

During the initial postoperative phase of 1 to 2 weeks, careful monitoring of serum creatinine and urine output is required to monitor graft function. Most grafts produce measurable amounts of urine within a matter of hours, and this is a clear sign of a functioning graft; however, in a certain proportion, perhaps 5% to 10% of cases, primary nonfunction is apparent. In this subgroup, continuing dialysis support is necessary. In some patients the condition resolves without treatment, but in others a percutaneous kidney biopsy may be necessary to establish whether the graft is still viable and what form of therapy should be initiated. In otherwise uncomplicated cases, the serum creatinine concentration falls rapidly postoperatively (Fig. 59.20). Early allograft rejection episodes are suspected if the creatinine does not fall to the expected level or if there is a creatinine concentration indicating allograft dysfunction. The differential diagnoses of graft dysfunction and complications that may ensue following transplant are summarized in Table 59.17. In the very early postoperative phase, in addition to rejection, graft dysfunction may be a consequence of delayed graft function, immunosuppressive drug toxicity, and acute tubular damage. Relative hypotension and dehydration may also contribute. Renal artery and venous thromboses are rare complications, and ureteric obstruction can be readily diagnosed using ultrasonography. Histologic examination of a transplant biopsy is necessary to aid diagnosis and treatment adjustment. Regular monitoring of kidney function, drug concentrations, and viral polymerase chain reaction (PCR) (particularly for CMV viremia

BOX 59.7 Immunological Aspects of Transplantation

Although a detailed description of the immunological aspects of transplantation is beyond the scope of this chapter, a brief discussion follows to highlight the close collaboration between clinicians and the tissue typing laboratory and to explore some of the recent advances in transplantation. The tissue type identifies an individual based on human leukocyte antigens (HLA) expressed on cells. These antigens are coded by genes of the major (and minor) histo- (tissue) compatibility complex (MHC). Individuals who have received blood transfusions or previous transplants of nonidentical tissue, and females who have had pregnancies develop antibodies to nonself HLA. These antibodies can be detected by analyzing the recipient serum against a panel of cells containing various HLA types or, more recently, the introduction of antigen-specific beads and flow cytometry. If a reaction is noted between donor cells/antigen beads and recipient serum in vitro, then this is indicative of a potential positive crossmatch between the donor organ and the recipient at the time of transplantation. All recipients are tested regularly by the tissue typing service. Highly sensititized individuals form around 30% of those on the transplant waiting list in the United States and have a number of antibodies or an antibody to a common HLA type, resulting in a longer waiting time for a suitable donor kidney in the majority of cases.[524]

ABO blood group incompatibility and HLA crossmatch reactivity between donor organs and recipients result in an accelerated or "hyperacute" rejection of the nonself organ (allograft) and have been traditional barriers to transplantation. Recent developments have led to desensitization protocols to remove the preformed antibodies from the plasma of potential recipients and have permitted transplantation across ABO and HLA barriers. This has permitted previously unsuitable potential live donors to donate. The outcome for recipients of desensitization programs is very encouraging, with 89% of allografts surviving at 22 months follow-up in a single center.[525] Following transplantation, clinicians and the tissue typing laboratory must remain vigilant for the persistence or reappearance of antibodies that may mediate rejection of the allograft.

BOX 59.8 Laboratory Assessment of Potential Kidney Transplant Recipient*

Electrolytes, liver function tests, glucose, C-reactive protein
Acid-base status
Full blood cell count
Clotting profile
Cytomegalovirus (CMV)
Hepatitis B and C
Varicella-zoster virus (VZV)
Epstein-Barr virus (EBV)
Human immunodeficiency virus (HIV) 1 and 2
Toxoplasma
Syphilis serology
Blood group: ABO compatibility
Tissue typing: human leukocyte antigen (HLA)
Index of sensitivity to alloantigens—for example, panel reactive antibodies (PRA) or cumulative frequency (CF) scores

*Tests of cardiac disease, vascular disease, and bladder function are also required in most cases.

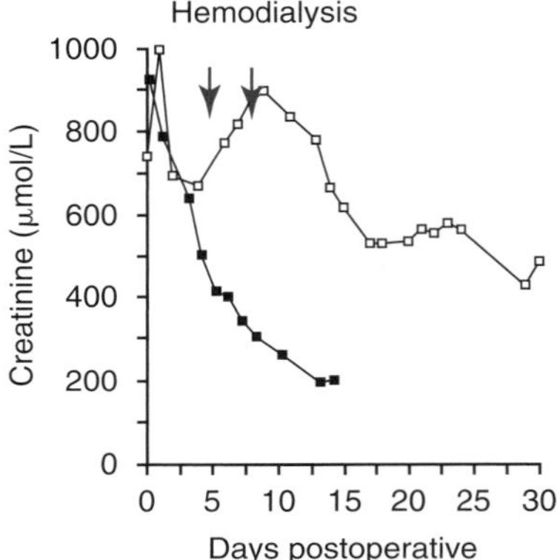

FIGURE 59.20 Posttransplantation biochemical profile. Open squares represent the course of a patient who experienced an early rejection episode (confirmed by biopsy, ↓) and requires initial hemodialysis support. Solid squares represent the typical profile of an uncomplicated transplant recipient. To convert creatinine concentration in μmol/L to mg/dL, multiply by 0.011.

and polyoma viruses such as BK virus) is mandated following kidney transplantation in many centers.

Primary glomerular disease may recur following kidney transplantation, resulting in loss of the graft. An Australian study has confirmed the 10-year incidence of graft loss caused by recurrent glomerulonephritis as 8.4%.[495] Recurrence was the third most frequent cause of graft loss (chronic allograft nephropathy and death with a functioning graft were most common). Compared with the average for all recipients with a primary diagnosis of glomerulonephritis, FSGS (11.8%) and membranoproliferative glomerulonephritis (MPGN), also known as mesangiocapillary glomerulonephritis (MCGN) type 1 (10.2%), were most likely to recur, causing graft loss. In contrast, graft loss due to recurrent IgA and pauci-immune crescentic glomerulonephritis occurred in only 2% of patients at 10-year follow-up.

Allograft Rejection. The immune response to the foreign graft (allograft) is very brisk, and allograft rejection may occur in response to nonidentical HLA molecules. The majority of rejection episodes are asymptomatic, manifested by a rise in creatinine concentration above the baseline for the patient. However, biopsy of the kidney transplant is necessary to confirm the cause of graft dysfunction and to identify the type of rejection that is occurring. A systematic classification system is employed ("Banff classification") to report transplant biopsy specimens.[496] The latest updates from the Banff report have increasingly recognized the importance of humoral (antibody-mediated) rejection as a cause of allograft failure during the whole life of the transplant. Rejection has classically been divided into cellular and vascular types and typically has been qualified by the speed of onset of graft dysfunction and the time since transplant. The recent classification builds on this but incorporates antibody-mediated rejection (acute or chronic) and T cell–mediated rejection (again, acute or chronic). Advances in the diagnoses of humoral rejection have included identification of

TABLE 59.17 Complications Following Kidney Transplantation

	Immediate Posttransplant	Early Posttransplant Period Until 3 Months	3 to 12 Months	After 1 Year	Comments
Surgical complications	Renal venous thrombosis, arterial thrombosis Pelvic lymphocele adjacent to the transplanted kidney Ureteric obstruction			Ureteric obstruction, renal artery stenosis	Increased incidence of lymphocele reported with sirolimus
Kidney	Acute tubular necrosis with delayed graft function				Dialysis treatment may need to be continued. Transplant usually recovers following adjustment of CNI doses. Electrolytes and creatinine should be measured daily.
(a) Immunological	Hyperacute rejection: occurs as a consequence of preformed antibodies in recipient serum to donor blood group or HLA antigens resulting in graft failure. Plasma exchange may be initiated but transplant nephrectomy likely.	Acute rejection in 20% to 60% of patients. Associated with rise in serum creatinine concentration. Confirmed on biopsy. Pathological description includes vascular and cellular infiltration by immune reactive cells. Requires urgent treatment with high-dose corticosteroids.	(a) Chronic allograft injury. Heralded by rising serum creatinine, proteinuria, and hypertension. Common cause of graft failure in the long term. Complex pathogenesis with a combination of donor-specific and recipient influences. Humoral (antibody-mediated) rejection increasingly recognized as contributing to immunological injury. Transplant biopsy may show peritubular capillary stain for complement degradation product C4d. (b) Subclinical rejection not suspected from serum creatinine concentration. This is a pathological diagnosis from transplant biopsy and is treated with high-dose corticosteroids.		Transplant centers may perform biopsy protocols at 3, 6, and 12 months to guide therapy. Clinical episode of rejection considered if serum creatinine concentration increases from baseline. Monitor recipient serum for anti-HLA antibodies, particularly donor-specific antibodies. Reduction in immunosuppression during maintenance phase of stable transplants.
(b) Recurrent disease	Glomerular disease such as FSGS and MPGN may occur early and lead to graft failure.		Risk of antiGBM disease in patients with Alport syndrome Familial hemolytic-uremic syndrome		Low risk of recurrent disease causing graft failure in diabetes and IgA nephropathy.
Infection	Chest infection Urinary tract infection Septicemia	Opportunistic infections: PCP, CMV infection, and reactivation. High-risk cases include donor-positive and recipient-negative for prior exposure to CMV (D+/D−). Prophylactic antiviral drugs recommended in high-risk patients. Varicella-zoster virus, polyoma virus (BK virus nephropathy), candidiasis.	CMV viremia in high-risk cases following discontinuation of prophylactic antiviral medication		Increased risk of infection in all patients receiving immunosuppression. Patients advised to receive influenza vaccine annually and vaccination against pneumococcus. Regular screening for viremia by PCR methodology. Routine staining of transplant biopsy specimens for SV40 to identify BK virus nephropathy. C-reactive protein, urine microscopy, cultures performed. Blood cultures, chest x-ray.

Continued

TABLE 59.17 Complications Following Kidney Transplantation—cont'd

	Immediate Posttransplant	Early Posttransplant Period Until 3 Months	3 to 12 Months	After 1 Year	Comments
Drug-related toxicity	See Table 59.18.				
Lymphoproliferative		PTLD. Typically associated with EBV expression in patients exposed to highly potent immunosuppressive protocols.	PTLD. Includes non-EBV-related lymphoma.	PTLD. Includes non-EBV-related lymphoma.	EBV-PCR. CT/MRI scans of chest, abdomen, and pelvis. Tissue diagnosis mandatory from lymph node and bone marrow. Serum lactate dehydrogenase activity increased.
Malignancy	Increased risk of nonmelanotic skin malignancy and solid organ malignancy in all patients				
Cardiovascular disease	Increased incidence of cardiovascular disease following transplantation. Death with a functioning graft is a common cause of "graft failure." The majority of transplant patients require treatment for hypertension and dyslipidipemias.				

CMV, Cytomegalovirus; *CNI,* calcineurin inhibitor; *EBV,* Epstein-Barr virus; *FSGS,* focal segmental glomerulosclerosis; *GBM,* glomerular basement membrane; *MPGN,* membranoproliferative glomerulonephritis; *PCP, Pneumocystis carinii* pneumonia; *PCR,* polymerase chain reaction; *PTLD,* posttransplant lymphoproliferative diseases; *SV40,* simian virus 40 (cross-reacts with BK virus).

complement-fixing alloantibody along capillary walls within the transplant following the development of a stain for C4d product.[497] In addition, donor-specific anti-HLA antibodies can often be detected in the serum of the recipient during the course of the transplant and may predict graft dysfunction in some cases.[498,499] It is accepted that antibody and T cell–mediated rejection may coexist as causes of immunologic damage to the allograft. Allograft rejection typically is treated by escalating immunosuppression schedules, and treatment may include antithymocyte globulin and/or high-dose corticosteroids. Subclinical rejection is also described whereby there is no apparent rise in creatinine concentration, but rejection is diagnosed following a protocol biopsy.

Immunosuppression and Therapeutic Drug Monitoring. As mentioned earlier, the introduction of immunosuppressive drugs in the 1970s led to vast improvement in the success rate of kidney transplantation. However, currently used drugs have potentially numerous and serious side effects that are summarized in Table 59.18.

Following the introduction of cyclosporin in the 1980s, a dramatic increase in 1-year graft survival resulted from the reduction in the number of acute rejection episodes.[500] However, a number of important side effects have been observed. Nephrotoxicity was soon apparent in early clinical trials[501] and remains a major clinical problem. During the 1990s, tacrolimus was introduced, and 1-year graft and patient survival rates were equivalent to those achieved with cyclosporin therapy, although rates of acute rejection episodes were lower.[502-505] Five-year follow-up data suggest improved graft survival with tacrolimus compared with cyclosporin.[506]

Sirolimus, in contrast to cyclosporin, does not cause nephrotoxicity, gingival hyperplasia, or tremor. However, patients treated with sirolimus have a higher incidence of thrombocytopenia, hyperlipidemia, and lymphocele formation.[507] Sirolimus and mycophenolate mofetil (MMF), both introduced during the late 1990s, have been studied in the setting of cyclosporin withdrawal and cyclosporine-free strategies in kidney transplantation,[493,508-512] the hypothesis being that withdrawal or avoidance of cyclosporin would improve long-term outcomes because there is no nephrotoxic stimulus. It has been shown in a multinational study that withdrawal of cyclosporin within 3 months of transplantation is feasible.[509] Studies have also shown that sirolimus in combination with MMF is safe and is associated with low rates of acute transplant rejection at 12 months.[493] Patients also received basiliximab, a monoclonal antibody to a specific target (CD 25) of T-cell activation that occurred in response to a nonidentical graft. However, Ekberg and colleagues found that the use of MMF, corticosteroids, and daclizumab induction was associated with increased risk of rejection if cyclosporin was withdrawn by month 6 following the transplant, compared with continuation of low-dose cyclosporin.[511]

Cyclosporin is insoluble and is presented for clinical use as a microemulsion. It has a narrow therapeutic window, and in clinical transplantation, it is important to monitor the blood concentration frequently. The most widely accepted practice is to monitor the "trough" concentration (C-0) just before the next dose. Accepted trough concentrations range from 100 to 300 µg/L (see Table 59.18 and Chapter 40). The highest concentrations are targeted during the induction phase of treatment for 2 to 3 months; subsequently, lower maintenance concentrations are desirable. The trough concentration within the blood may not provide a truly accurate guide to total drug exposure because wide variation in absorption is seen over the first 2 to 4 hours following dosing.[513] This is important in that most of the pharmacodynamic effects of cyclosporin occur within 2 hours.[514] Studies from Canada suggest that trough concentrations do not reflect clinical outcomes in terms of acute rejection rates,[515] although high trough concentrations were associated with increased nephrotoxicity. A 2-hour drug (C-2) concentration correlated well with a formal area under the curve measurements and

TABLE 59.18 **Noninfectious Complications of Immunosuppressant Drugs**

Drug	Drug Dose	Target Therapeutic Range*	Toxicity Profile
Corticosteroids—eg, prednisone	Dose depends on weight of patient and time since transplant. Typically, 40 mg daily during first week and tapering to 5 mg at 6 months and withdrawal at 12 months.	Not appropriate	Increased risk of developing diabetes mellitus Deterioration in diabetes control Osteopenia Osteoporosis Psychosis Fat redistribution Hypertension Dyslipidemia Cataracts Weight gain
Calcineurin Inhibitors			
Cyclosporin	Variable Depends on weight, time since transplant and achieved drug concentration. Dose given in 2 divided doses and predose trough concentration measured in morning blood sample	200–300 µg/L for first 3–12 months. Thereafter, aim for 100 µg/L.	Nephrotoxicity Hypertension Neurotoxicity Hemolytic-uremic syndrome Tubular electrolyte abnormalities (hypophosphatemia, hypomagnesemia, hyperkalemia) Hirsutism Gingival hyperplasia Bone pains Dyslipidemia
Tacrolimus			As for cyclosporin, except no hirsutism or gingival hyperplasia Increased risk of diabetes mellitus Cardiomyopathy (children) Alopecia
Mycophenolate mofetil	Initially 2 g daily in divided doses	Not routinely measured	Abdominal pain Diarrhea Myelosuppression
Sirolimus	Dose depends on weight and achieved drug concentration. The drug is administered once daily.	Level depends on time since transplant. Typical early (less than 3 months) targets are 8–12 µg/L and thereafter 4–8 µg/L.	Lymphocele (a fluid-filled collection near to transplanted kidney) Thrombocytopenia Hyperlipidemia
Azathioprine	Usual starting dose of 2 mg/kg body weight in a single daily dose	Levels not measured. Because the enzyme thiopurine methyltransferase (TPMT) metabolizes azathioprine, the risk of myelosuppression is increased in patients with low activity of the enzyme. Enzyme activity may be determined prior to commencing treatment, and full blood counts are performed for several weeks following commencement of drug.	Myelosuppression Severe interaction if used with allopurinol (treatment for gout)
Selected biological agents			
AntiCD25 monoclonal antibodies: basiliximab and daclizumab	Given at time of transplant and once thereafter		Very well tolerated
Polyclonal antithymocyte globulin (ATG) and antilymphocyte globulin (ALG), and monoclonal OKT3	Given in response to refractory rejection episodes in selected patients		Increased risk of malignancy, posttransplant lymphoproliferative disease Hypersensitivity reactions

*These are not recommendations but are illustrative and will vary among centers.

is predictive of nephrotoxicity and acute rejection episodes. Among kidney transplant patients, the trough level of tacrolimus is correlated with acute rejection episodes and nephrotoxicity.[516] Trough concentrations also guide sirolimus therapy (see Table 59.18).[517]

MMF is morpholinoethyl ester of mycophenolic acid (MPA), a potent and reversible inhibitor of inosine monophosphate dehydrogenase isoform 2 (IMPDH), and it has become the single most used immunosuppressant in solid organ transplantation. Excellent results have been obtained with a fixed-dose regimen. IMPDH is a target for immunosuppression because lymphocytes depend on the de novo guanosine nucleotide synthesis pathway for DNA synthesis and cell division.[518] MMF, because it is a prodrug of MPA, is rapidly absorbed following an oral dose and is deesterified to MPA, which is highly protein bound. Free MPA concentrations determine the level of immunosuppressive activity, and this can be affected by hypoalbuminemia and renal insufficiency. Adverse events related to mycophenolate formulations include gastrointestinal disturbances, hematologic disorders (leucopenia and anemia), and infections.

Therapeutic drug monitoring of MPA is possible using HPLC and immunoassay techniques (see Chapter 40). However, it has not been universally accepted in kidney transplantation programs because prospective studies have given conflicting information of its value.[519] For example, in the *Adaption de Posologie du Mycophénolate en Greffe Renale* (APOMYGRE) study, a concentration-controlled regimen based on MPA area-under-the-curve measurements was associated with fewer rejection episodes than the use of a standard fixed dose of mycophenolate mofetil.[520] The Fixed Dose–Concentration Controlled (FDCC) study compared a fixed-dose regimen of 2 g of MMF with a concentration-controlled regimen based on abbreviated MPA area-under-the-curve measurements (target concentrations of 30 to 60 mg × h/L) in 901 patients who were treated with cyclosporin or tacrolimus.[521] An overall benefit could not be demonstrated in this large cohort over 12 months, despite an association with low MPA area-under-the-curve measurements and biopsy-proven acute rejection. In APOMYGRE and FDCC, no correlation between MPA predose trough concentrations or area-under-the-curve measurements and MMF-related adverse events was observed in the first year after transplantation, despite differences in MPA exposure. A consensus report highlights that the use of imprecise definitions for adverse events, multicausality of adverse effects, including concomitant drugs, time elapsed between MPA measurement and event, assay used for MPA quantification, and associated toxicity profiles of concomitant immunosuppressive medications undermine the ability to demonstrate a relationship between drug exposure and toxicity.[519]

In summary, long-term graft failure is a major problem, and graft loss accounts for the return of increasing numbers of patients to dialysis. The most common cause of graft loss is death with a functioning graft. Kidney failure carries a considerable burden of cardiovascular morbidity. Although some risk factors, such as volume overload and anemia, are improved following transplantation, others, including dyslipidemia and hypertension, persist. The drugs used to prevent rejection can exacerbate these. Challenges to the nephrology community are complex and include improving access to transplantation, reducing side effects of the powerful drugs used to prevent rejection, and reducing in cardiovascular risk profiles for individual patients.

Simultaneous Pancreas-Kidney Transplantation

Patients with kidney failure and diabetes, predominantly type 1, but increasingly certain patients with type 2, and limited secondary complications of diabetes may be considered for simultaneous pancreas and kidney (SPK) transplantation. Patients tend to be younger than kidney-only recipients (eg, aged between 20 and 40 years). A 2011 analysis of 25,000 recipients of a pancreas transplant reported to the International Pancreas Transplant Registry (IPTR) in the United States since 1966 shows that the majority of recipients receive a simultaneous kidney and pancreas (75%), with 18% receiving a pancreas after kidney (PAK) and 7% pancreas only.[522] Patient survival now reaches over 95% at 1 year posttransplant and over 83% after 5 years. The data also show increasing age of the typical recipient and utilization of pancreas transplantation in C-peptide positive type 2 diabetic patients (from 2% in 1995 to 7% in 2010). These results compare favorably with those of cadaveric kidney-only transplantation in diabetes. The main reason for the survival advantage of SPK over kidney only is the fact that younger donors and recipients are selected and the waiting time for the dual transplant is much shorter than for kidney-only transplants. In effect, the kidney-only "waiting-list" is a pool of patients with kidneys allocated primarily by tissue matching and age, whereas the SPK-listed patients are on a list rather than in the pool. A separate prospective observational study examined the impact of SPK transplant in terms of quality of life.[523] At 3 years, SPK patients report greater improvements than kidney-only recipients in physical functioning, bodily pain, general health, and perception of improvements to secondary complications of diabetes.

The surgical technique for SPK involves whole-organ pancreas transplantation with the duodenal segment draining either into the urinary bladder through a duodenocystostomy or, more commonly today, enterically via an anastomosis between the graft duodenal segment and the recipient small bowel. The kidney is attached as usual to the iliac vessels, and the donor ureter is inserted into the bladder separately. Postoperatively, blood glucose concentrations are monitored closely, and intravenous insulin is given as necessary. Exocrine pancreatic secretion can be measured in the urine for bladder-drained pancreas allografts. The major fear is rejection, and a number of parameters are monitored, including plasma glucose, amylase, lipase, and 12- or 24-hour urinary amylase (again for bladder-drained allografts). For patients with bladder drainage, enteric conversion may be required for refractory problems, such as dehydration, metabolic acidosis, chronic urethritis caused by trypsinogen activation, urinary tract infection, and recurrent reflux pancreatitis. Because of high fluid, bicarbonate, and electrolyte losses into the urine in these patients, the need for supplementation is increased in SPK recipients. There is a long-term need for high-dose oral sodium bicarbonate supplementation in bladder-drained pancreatic transplantation because of exocrine secretory losses. Hyperamylasemia is common postoperatively and may or may not signify allograft rejection. Immunosuppressive schedules vary among centers and include induction therapy with monoclonal or polyclonal anti–T cell agents and a combination of the drugs outlined previously. Diagnosis of pancreatic rejection in the absence of a simultaneous kidney transplant is very difficult. Signs of rejection include fever, pain, hematuria, reduction of urinary amylase, and unexplained hyperglycemia. Organ scanning and biopsy are also used. However, the function of the kidney in SPK mirrors the pancreas; therefore immunosuppression can be tailored to the requirements of the kidney.

SELECTED REFERENCES

For a full list of references for this chapter, please refer to ExpertConsult.com.

2. Haraldsson B, Nystrom J, Deen WM. Properties of the glomerular barrier and mechanisms of proteinuria. *Physiol Rev* 2008;**88**:451–87.
36. Davies DF, Shock NW. Age changes in glomerular filtration rate, effective renal plasma flow, and tubular excretory capacity in adult males. *J Clin Invest* 1950;**29**:496–507.
78. Ruggenenti P, Perna A, Gherardi G, et al. Renal function and requirement for dialysis in chronic nephropathy patients on long-term ramipril: rEIN follow-up trial. Gruppo Italiano di Studi Epidemiologici in Nefrologia (GISEN). Ramipril Efficacy in Nephropathy. *Lancet* 1998;**352**:1252–6.
93. Coresh J, Selvin E, Stevens LA, et al. Prevalence of chronic kidney disease in the United States. *JAMA* 2007;**298**: 2038–47.
94. Kidney Disease Improving Global Outcomes. Clinical practice guideline for the evaluation and management of chronic kidney disease. *Kidney Int* 2013;**3**:1–150.
100. Matsushita K, van der Velde M, Astor BC, et al. Association of estimated glomerular filtration rate and albuminuria with all-cause and cardiovascular mortality in general population cohorts: a collaborative meta-analysis. *Lancet* 2010;**375**:2073–81.
105. Lamb EJ, Stevens PE, Deeks JJ. What is the best glomerular filtration marker to identify people with chronic kidney disease most likely to have poor outcomes? *BMJ* 2015;**350**:g7667.
106. Collins AJ, Foley RN, Chavers B, et al. US Renal Data System 2013 Annual Data Report. *Am J Kidney Dis* 2014;**63**:A7.
159. Wanner C, Tonelli M. KDIGO clinical practice guideline for lipid management in CKD: summary of recommendation statements and clinical approach to the patient. *Kidney Int* 2014;**85**:1303–9.
176. Kidney Disease Improving Global Outcomes. KDIGO clinical practice guideline for the diagnosis, evaluation, prevention, and treatment of chronic kidney disease-mineral and bone disorder (CKD-MBD). *Kidney Int Suppl* 2009;S1–130.
179. Slatopolsky E, Caglar S, Pennell JP, et al. On the pathogenesis of hyperparathyroidism in chronic experimental renal insufficiency in the dog. *J Clin Invest* 1971;**50**:492–9.
205. Kidney Disease Improving Global Outcomes. KDIGO clinical practice guideline for anemia in chronic kidney disease. *Kidney Int* 2012;**2**:279–335.
234. National Institute for Health and Care Excellence. Acute kidney injury: prevention, detection and management of acute kidney injury up to the point of renal replacement therapy (CG169). <http://wwwniceorguk/guidance/cg169> 2013.
255. Diabetes Control and Complications Trial Research Group. The effect of intensive treatment of diabetes on the development and progression of long-term complications in insulin-dependent diabetes mellitus. The Diabetes Control and Complications Trial Research Group. *N Engl J Med* 1993;**329**:977–86.
257. United Kingdom Prospective Diabetes Study (UKPDS) Group. Intensive blood-glucose control with sulphonylureas or insulin compared with conventional treatment and risk of complications in patients with type 2 diabetes (UKPDS 33). *Lancet* 1998;**352**:837–53.
305. Kidney Disease Improving Global Outcomes (KDIGO). KDIGO clinical practice guideline for glomerulonephritis. *Kidney Int* 2012;(Suppl. 2):139–274.
383. Chapman AB, Devuyst O, Eckardt KU, et al. Autosomal-dominant polycystic kidney disease (ADPKD): executive summary from a Kidney Disease: improving Global Outcomes (KDIGO) Controversies Conference. *Kidney Int* 2015;**88**:17–27.
395. Loudon KW, Fry AC. The renal channelopathies. *Ann Clin Biochem* 2014;**51**:441–58.
463. National Kidney Foundation. Clinical practice guidelines for hemodialysis adequacy, update 2006. *Am J Kidney Dis* 2006;**48**(Suppl. 1):S2–90.
479. National Kidney Foundation. II. NKF-K/DOQI clinical practice guidelines for peritoneal dialysis adequacy: update 2000. *Am J Kidney Dis* 2001;**37**:S65–136.

60

Disorders of Water, Electrolytes, and Acid–Base Metabolism

Steven Cheng, Emily I. Schindler, and Mitchell G. Scott

ABSTRACT

Background

A complex yet elegant system of chemical buffers together with highly specialized mechanisms of the lungs and kidneys continuously work in tandem to ensure a precise balance of water, electrolytes, and pH in both the intracellular and extracellular compartments of the human body. Although these systems display impressive resilience and responsiveness to perturbation by illness or injury, they do have limits, at which point medical evaluation and treatment are required.

Content

This chapter describes the various fluid compartments in the body and reasons for differences in composition between these compartments. Laboratory testing algorithms are used to investigate and treat perturbations of water and electrolytes in pathologic settings, including the role of such simple tests as urine electrolytes. Similarly, testing algorithms and mnemonic tools are presented to diagnose and manage disturbances in acid-base homeostasis. The clinical laboratorian needs to understand the nuances and pitfalls associated with these algorithms and associated tests to provide accurate and meaningful results to the clinician.

Adaptation to terrestrial life led to the evolution of physiologic systems to maintain the composition of the internal milieu of animals, including humans. These systems require the interaction of multiple organ systems such as the kidneys, lungs, heart, liver, brain, and lymphatics. In particular, a variety of chemical buffers and highly specialized mechanisms of the lungs and kidneys work together to regulate water, electrolytes, and pH between and within intracellular and extracellular compartments. Perturbations in the dynamic equilibria that exist for water, electrolytes, and pH may arise from external (eg, trauma, changes in altitude, ingestion of toxic substances) or internal (eg, normal metabolism, disease state) sources. Endogenous correction of these imbalances may not always be adequate; at these times, the clinical laboratory can provide valuable information for guiding therapy.*

TOTAL BODY WATER: VOLUME AND DISTRIBUTION

During gestation, ≈90% of fetal body weight is water.[1] Water is 70% of body weight for full-term infants. Water gradually decreases as percent of body weight, so that it accounts for 60% of body weight in adolescents and adult males,[1] and ≈55% for adult females. As depicted in Fig. 60.1, approximately two-thirds of total body water (TBW) is distributed into the intracellular fluid (ICF) compartment, and one-third exists in the extracellular fluid (ECF) compartment. The ECF may be further subdivided into interstitial (≈75% of ECF) and intravascular (≈25% of ECF) compartments, which are separated by the capillary endothelium. The average adult has ≈5 L of blood volume (intravascular compartment) and a plasma volume of ≈3.0 L when the hematocrit is 40%. Although fluid from other clinically relevant ECF compartments (eg, cerebrospinal fluid [CSF],[2] urine) may be analyzed in the clinical laboratory, most laboratory tests used to determine hydration, electrolyte, and acid-base status are performed on samples from the intravascular compartment.

The minimum daily requirement for water can be estimated from renal (1200 to 1500 mL in urine) and "insensible" losses (≈400 to 700 mL as a result of evaporation from the skin and respiratory tract). Activity, environmental conditions, and disease all have dramatic effects on daily water (and electrolyte) requirements. On average, an adult must take in ≈1.5 to 2.0 L of water daily to maintain fluid balance. Because primary regulatory mechanisms are designed to first maintain *intracellular* hydration status, imbalances in TBW are initially reflected in the ECF compartment. Table 60.1 lists common causes and clinical manifestations of expansion and contraction of the ECF compartment.

WATER AND ELECTROLYTES: COMPOSITION OF BODY FLUIDS

The primary cationic (positively charged) electrolytes are sodium (Na^+), potassium (K^+), calcium (Ca^{2+}), and magnesium (Mg^{2+}), whereas the anions (negatively charged) include

*Laboratories should verify that these ranges are appropriate for use in their own settings.

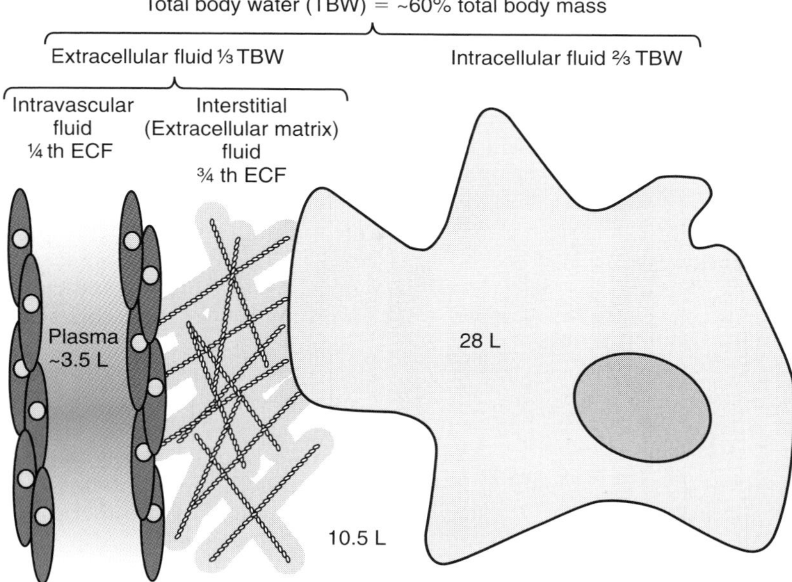

FIGURE 60.1 Volume and distribution of total body water. Note that the intracellular and extracellular fluid compartments (ICF and ECF, respectively) are separated by cellular plasma membranes, and within the ECF, interstitial and intravascular fluids are separated by the capillary endothelium (red cells). The volumes indicated represent water and not total volume. Endothelial cells = red; interstitial cell = gray; collagen matrix fibers = black cables.

TABLE 60.1 Causes and Clinical Manifestations of Changes in Extracellular Fluid Volume

	Clinical Manifestations	Causes
ECF loss	Thirst, anorexia, nausea, lightheadedness, orthostatic hypotension, syncope, tachycardia, oliguria, decreased skin turgor and "sunken eyes," shock, coma, death	Trauma (and other causes of acute blood loss), "third-spacing" of fluid (eg, burns, pancreatitis, peritonitis), vomiting, diarrhea, diuretics, renal or adrenal (ie, sodium wasting) disease
ECF gain	Weight gain, edema, dyspnea (secondary to pulmonary edema), tachycardia, jugular venous distention, portal hypertension (ascites), esophageal varices	Heart failure, cirrhosis, nephrotic syndrome, iatrogenic (intravenous fluid overload)

ECF, Extracellular fluid.

TABLE 60.2 Electrolyte and Water Composition of Body Fluid Compartments*

Component	Plasma	Interstitial Fluid	Intracellular Fluid[†]
Volume, H_2O (TBW = 42 L)	3.5 L	10.5 L	28 L
Na^+	142	145	12
K^+	4	4	156
Ca^{2+}	4.8	4-6	0.6
Mg^{2+}	2	1-2	26
Trace elements	1	—	—
Total cations	155	—	—
Cl^-	103	114	4
HCO_3^-	27	31	12
$Protein^-$	16	—	55
Organic $acids^-$	5	—	—
HPO_4^{2-}	2	—	—
SO_4^{2-}	1	—	—

*All electrolyte values are expressed in millimoles per liter of *fluid.* Because the H_2O content of plasma is ≈93% by volume, the corresponding electrolyte concentrations in plasma water are ≈10% higher. Note that the *molar concentration* of divalent ions is half the depicted value.

[†]These values are derived from skeletal muscle.

TBW, Total body water.

chloride (Cl^-), bicarbonate (HCO_3^-), phosphate (HPO_4^{2-}, $H_2PO_4^-$), sulfate (SO_4^{2-}), organic ions such as lactate, and negatively charged proteins. Electrolyte concentrations of the body fluid compartments are shown in Table 60.2. Na^+, K^+, Cl^-, and HCO_3^- in the plasma or serum are commonly analyzed in an *electrolyte profile* because their concentrations provide the most relevant information about the osmotic, hydration, and acid-base status of the body. Although hydrogen (H^+) is a cation, its concentration is approximately 1 million–fold lower in plasma than the major electrolytes listed in Table 60.2 (10^{-9} mol/L vs. 10^{-3} mol/L) and is negligible in terms of osmotic activity.

Any increase in the concentration of one anion is accompanied by a corresponding decrease in other anions, or by an increase in one or more cations or both because total electrical neutrality must be maintained. Similarly, any decrease in the concentration of anions involves a corresponding increase in other anions, a decrease in cations, or both. In the case of polyvalent ions (eg, Ca^{2+}, Mg^{2+}), it is important to distinguish between the substance concentration of the ion itself and the concentration of the ion charge. Thus, although the concentration of total calcium ions in normal plasma is ≈2.5 mmol/L, the concentration of the total calcium ion *charge* is 5.0 mmol/L (also called 5 milliequivalents per liter [mEq/L]).

Extracellular and Intracellular Compartments

The extracellular compartment is composed of plasma and interstitial fluid.

Plasma

Plasma generally has a volume of 1300 to 1800 mL/m^2 of body surface and constitutes approximately 5% of the body volume (≈3.5 L for a 66-kg subject). Total body volume is derived from body mass by using an estimated body density of 1.06 kg/L. Table 60.2 describes the electrolyte composition of plasma. The mass concentration of water in normal plasma is approximately 0.933 kg/L, depending on the protein and lipid content (see "Electrolyte Exclusion Effect" in Chapter 35). Thus a concentration of sodium in the plasma of 140 mmol/L would correspond to a molality of sodium in plasma water of 150 mmol/kg H_2O (140 mmol/L divided by 0.933 kg/L). The concentration of net protein ions in plasma is ≈12 mmol/L.[3]

Interstitial Fluid

Interstitial fluid is essentially an ultrafiltrate of blood plasma (see Fig. 60.1). When all extracellular spaces except plasma are included, the volume accounts for about 26% (10.5 L) of the total body volume. Plasma is separated from the interstitial fluid by the endothelial lining of the capillaries, which acts as a semipermeable membrane and allows passage of water and diffusible solutes but not compounds of high molecular mass proteins. The exchange of water between the interstitial and intravascular compartments is governed by Starling forces, which demonstrates that the net movement of fluid across a capillary membrane is a function of membrane permeability and differences in hydrostatic and oncotic pressures on the two sides of the membrane.[1] The "impermeability" to proteins is not absolute, and in some pathologic conditions causing shock, such as bacterial sepsis, the permeability of the vascular endothelium increases dramatically, resulting in leakage of albumin, a reduction in the effective circulating volume, and hypotension. If not aggressively treated with intravenous fluids and/or vasopressors, this condition can result in death as the result of decreased cerebral perfusion.

Intracellular Fluid

The exact composition of ICF is difficult to measure. Data for ICF (see Table 60.2), therefore, are considered only approximations. The ICF constitutes ≈66% of the total body volume (see Fig. 60.1).

Reasons for Composition Differences of Body Fluids

The composition of ICF can differ markedly from that of ECF because of separation of these compartments by the cell membrane. The composition differences are a consequence of both the Gibbs-Donnan equilibrium and active and passive transport of ions, as well as active transport of larger molecules.

Gibbs-Donnan Equilibrium

Two solutions separated by a semipermeable membrane will establish an equilibrium, so that all ions are equally distributed in both compartments, provided the solutes can move freely through the membrane. At the state of equilibrium, the total ion concentration and therefore the total concentration of osmotically active particles are equal on both sides of the membrane.

If solutions on two sides of a membrane contain different concentrations of ions that cannot freely move through the membrane (eg, proteins), distribution of diffusible ions (eg, electrolytes) at the steady state will be unequal, but the sum of the concentrations of ions in one compartment is equal to the sum of ions in the other compartment. This is referred to as Gibbs-Donnan law.[4] Also, the law of electrical neutrality is obeyed for both compartments. An example of the uneven distribution of an ion in two compartments with different protein content (nondiffusible ions) is the concentration of chloride ions in plasma and CSF. As a result of increased selectivity of the blood-brain barrier against proteins, Cl^- ions are ≈15% higher in CSF to establish electrical and osmotic equilibrium.[2] Cells, most notably those of the CNS, that contain nondiffusible protein anions can withstand only a limited and temporary difference in osmotic pressure across the cell membrane. Osmotic pressure is normally identical inside and outside the cells because the cell membrane can correct concentration differences by excluding some small ions through active, energy-requiring transport processes. If these processes cease, the cells will swell and eventually will burst (osmotic lysis).

Distribution of Ions by Active and Passive Transport

Examination of Table 60.2 reveals that the electrolyte compositions of blood plasma and interstitial fluid are similar and differ markedly from that of ICF. The major ECF ions are Na^+, Cl^-, and HCO_3^-, but in ICF, the main ions are K^+, Mg^{2+}, organic phosphates, and protein. This unequal distribution of ions is due to active transport of Na^+ from inside to outside the cell against an electrochemical gradient. An active sodium pump deriving its energy from glycolysis-generated adenosine triphosphate (ATP) is present in most cell membranes and frequently is coupled with transport of K^+ into the cell.

In addition to the Na^+/K^+-ATPase, a ubiquitous Na^+-H^+ exchanger (often referred to as an *antiporter*) actively pumps H^+ out of the ICF in exchange for Na^+.[5] This exchanger is critical for maintaining intracellular pH homeostasis. At least six different isoforms of this transmembrane protein have been identified.[5] Of particular importance is the role of this exchanger for acid-base regulation in renal tubular cells, as discussed later in this chapter.

Electrolytes

Disorders of Na^+, K^+, Cl^-, and HCO_3^- will now be separately considered, even though disorders of electrolyte and water homeostasis need a systematic evaluation rather than an individual review of each ion.[6]

Sodium

Disorders of Na^+ homeostasis can occur because of excessive loss, gain, or retention of Na^+, or as the result of excessive loss, gain, or retention of H_2O. It is difficult to separate disorders of Na^+ and H_2O balance because of their close relationship in establishing normal osmolality in all body water compartments.[7] As described in detail in Chapter 59, the primary organ for regulating body water and extracellular Na^+ is the kidney. As a brief introduction to this section, it is important to remind the reader of the functions of healthy kidneys.

The human body is in a dynamic state of flux as fluids and electrolytes are constantly being gained through mechanisms such as thirst and hunger and lost through processes such as sweating and urination. Homeostasis within a narrow window is necessary for life, and the body must defend against excessive gains or losses. Although certain behavioral adaptations are undoubtedly important (eg, drinking when thirsty to prevent water and volume loss) others may be more debatable (as in the case of dietary sodium restriction).[8] The kidney is responsible not only for clearing uremic toxins from the circulation but also in maintaining balance and defending electrolyte homeostasis across a wide range of these gains and losses. In the proximal tubules, 70% to 80% of filtered Na^+ is actively reabsorbed, with H_2O and Cl^- following passively to maintain electrical neutrality and osmotic equivalence. In the descending loop of Henle, H_2O, but not electrolytes, is passively reabsorbed because of the high osmotic strength of interstitial fluid in the renal medulla. In the ascending loop of Henle, Cl^- is reabsorbed actively, with Na^+ following. At the level of the distal tubule, the first of the two primary Na^+/H_2O regulating processes occurs. Here, aldosterone stimulates the cortical collecting ducts to reabsorb Na^+ (with water following passively) and secrete K^+ (and to a lesser extent, H^+) to maintain electrical neutrality. Aldosterone is produced by the adrenal cortex in response to angiotensin II derived by the action of renin. The secretion of renin by renal juxtaglomerular cells is stimulated by low chloride, β-adrenergic activity, and low arteriolar pressure.[9] Thus, when the kidneys are hypoperfused (as occurs when blood volume decreases, or when the renal arteries are obstructed), the distal tubules, under the influence of aldosterone, reclaim Na^+.

Further water regulation in the kidney occurs from the distal tubule through the collecting duct, where tubular permeability to H_2O is under the influence of vasopressin (also called antidiuretic hormone [ADH]) (see Chapters 59 and 65). Vasopressin is released by the posterior pituitary under the influence of baroreceptors in the aortic arch and hypothalamic chemoreceptors that are responsive to circulating osmolality, which is primarily a reflection of Na^+ concentration. When ECF volume is decreased, or when plasma osmolality is increased, vasopressin is secreted, tubular permeability to H_2O increases via aquaporins, and H_2O is reabsorbed in an attempt to restore blood volume or to decrease osmolality. In contrast, when ECF volume is increased or osmolality decreased, vasopressin secretion is inhibited, and more H_2O is excreted in the urine (diuresis).

Besides the kidney, the body's only other mechanism for restoring Na^+/H_2O homeostasis is ingestion of H_2O. Thirst is stimulated by decreased blood volume or hyperosmolality. It is important to remember that baroreceptors that influence renal handling of Na^+ and H_2O, and thirst, sense changes only in the intravascular blood volume and not the total ECF, whereas osmoreceptors in the brain, such as the organum vasculosum lamina terminalis (OVLT) neurons sense the osmolality of the ECF surrounding the cells. Laboratory assessment of water and electrolyte disorders is made primarily from the blood volume (plasma); the clinician must assess the status of TBW and blood volume before interpreting laboratory values. The physical findings of these disorders are as important as the laboratory values in management of water and electrolyte disorders (see Table 60.1).

Hyponatremia

Hyponatremia is defined as a decreased plasma Na^+ concentration (defined as <130 to 135 mmol/L without consensus agreement of the definition).[10] Hyponatremia typically manifests clinically as nausea, generalized weakness, and mental confusion at values below 120 mmol/L, and severe mental confusion plus seizures at less than 105 mmol/L.[11] The rapidity of development of hyponatremia influences the Na^+ concentrations at which symptoms develop (ie, clinically apparent symptoms may manifest at higher Na^+ concentrations [≈125 mmol/L] when hyponatremia develops rapidly).[11] It is important to note that symptoms are due to changes in osmolality rather than to the Na^+ concentration per se. Central nervous system (CNS) symptoms are due to movement of H_2O into cells to maintain osmotic balance and subsequent swelling of CNS cells. These symptoms can occur more rapidly in children, so there is a need to be particularly vigilant in the pediatric population.

Hyponatremia can be hypo-osmotic, hyperosmotic, or iso-osmotic. Thus measurement of plasma osmolality is an important initial step in the assessment of hyponatremia. Of these, the most common form is hypo-osmotic hyponatremia. Fig. 60.2 describes an algorithm for laboratory measurements and physical examination findings in the differential diagnosis of plasma Na^+ less than 135 mmol/L.

Hypo-Osmotic Hyponatremia. Typically, when plasma Na^+ concentration is low, calculated or measured osmolality also will be low. This type of hyponatremia can be due to excess loss of Na^+ *(depletional hyponatremia)* or increased ECF volume *(dilutional hyponatremia)*. Differentiating these initially requires clinical assessment of TBW and ECF volume by history and physical examination.

Depletional hyponatremia results from a loss of Na^+ from the ECF space that exceeds the concomitant loss of water. The net loss of Na^+ from the ECF space also stimulates thirst and production of vasopressin, both of which contribute to the maintenance of hyponatremia. Hypovolemia is apparent in the physical examination (orthostatic hypotension, tachycardia, decreased skin turgor). If urine Na^+ is low (<10 mmol/L), the kidneys are properly retaining filtered Na^+ and the loss is extrarenal, most commonly from the gastrointestinal tract or skin (see Fig. 60.2). Preventing ongoing loss and restoring ECF volume with isotonic fluid is sufficient to correct hyponatremia in these situations. Alternatively, if urine Na^+ is increased in this setting (generally >20 mmol/L), renal loss of Na^+ is likely. Renal loss of Na^+ occurs with (1) osmotic diuresis, (2) use of diuretics (which inhibit reabsorption of Cl^- and Na^+ in the ascending loop), (3) adrenal insufficiency (no aldosterone or cortisone prevents distal tubule reabsorption of Na^+), or (4) salt-wasting nephropathies, as can occur with

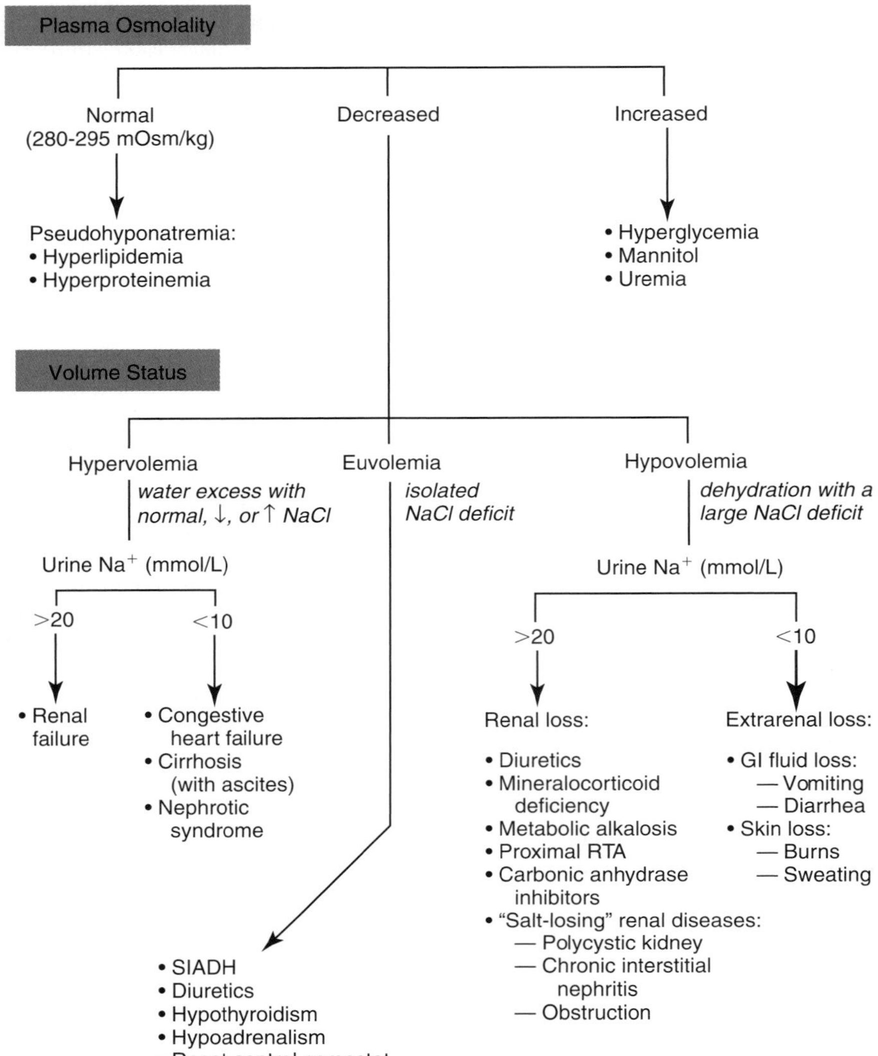

FIGURE 60.2 Algorithm for the differential diagnosis of hyponatremia. *GI,* Gastrointestinal; *RTA,* renal tubular acidosis; *SIADH,* syndrome of inappropriate secretion of antidiuretic hormone. (Modified from Kirkpatrick W, Kreisberg R. Acid-base and electrolyte disorders. In: Liu P, editor. *Blue book of diagnostic tests.* Philadelphia: WB Saunders; 1986:239–254.)

interstitial nephritis and tubular recovery after acute tubular necrosis or obstructive nephropathy. Renal loss of Na^+ in excess of H_2O can also occur in metabolic alkalosis from prolonged vomiting, because increased renal HCO_3^- excretion is accompanied by Na^+ ions. In this case, urine sodium is increased (>20 mmol/L), but urine chloride remains low. In proximal renal tubular acidosis (RTA) type 2, bicarbonate is lost because of a defect in HCO_3^- reabsorption, and Na^+ is coexcreted to maintain electrical neutrality. As with extrarenal Na^+ loss, management of hyponatremia attributable to renal Na^+ loss is centered around the reversal of underlying cause and restoration of ECF volume.

Dilutional hyponatremia is a result of excess H_2O retention and often can be detected during the physical examination as edema. In advanced renal failure, water is retained because of decreased filtration and H_2O excretion. When ECF is increased but the circulating blood volume is decreased, as occurs in hepatic cirrhosis and nephrotic syndrome, a vicious cycle is established. The decreased blood volume is sensed by baroreceptors and results in increased aldosterone and vasopressin, even though ECF volume is excessive. The kidneys reabsorb Na^+ and H_2O in response to increased aldosterone and vasopressin in an attempt to restore the blood volume, resulting in further increases in ECF and further dilution of Na^+. In dilutional hyponatremia, the low serum sodium concentrations reflect the severity of the underlying disease process. Management should be focused on the treatment of the underlying disease, as correction of Na^+ concentrations alone have no effect on overall morbidity or mortality.[11]

In hypo-osmotic hyponatremia with a normal or euvolemic volume status, the most common causes are the syndrome of inappropriate antidiuretic hormone (ADH) (vasopressin) (SIADH), primary polydipsia, and endocrine disorders such as adrenal insufficiency and hypothyroidism (see Fig. 60.2). Adrenal insufficiency causes hyponatremia through increased cortisol-releasing hormone, which stimulates vasopressin release,[12] while hypothyroidism impairs free H_2O excretion. SIADH describes hyponatremia attributable to "inappropriate" vasopressin release, as from a malignancy, which stimulates excessive H_2O retention and increased urine osmolality.[13] Free water restriction is the mainstay of therapy in SIADH. However, in severe or symptomatic hyponatremia from any cause, the use of hypertonic saline solutions may be required to correct serum Na^+ concentrations.[11] In such cases, the hyponatremia must be corrected cautiously because too rapid correction can lead to brain demyelination. The pons is particularly sensitive to this, and rapid correction can lead to central pontine myelinolysis. Current recommendations are to increase Na^+ by 0.5 to 2.0 mmol/L per hour and not to exceed a total increase in Na^+ greater than 18 to 25 mmol/L over 48 hours.[14]

Finally, euvolemic hyponatremia also can be found in primary polydipsia when water intake is greater than the renal capacity to excrete excess H_2O. This can be the result of psychiatric illness, but diseases that cause hypothalamic disorders, such as sarcoidosis, also may cause polydipsia by altering the thirst reflex (see Fig. 60.2).

Hyperosmotic Hyponatremia. Hyponatremia in the presence of increased quantities of other solutes in the ECF is the result of an extracellular shift of water or an intracellular shift of Na^+ to maintain osmotic balance between ECF and ICF compartments. The most common cause of this type of hyponatremia is severe hyperglycemia (see Fig. 60.2). As a general rule, Na^+ is decreased by ≈1.6 to 2.0 mmol/L for every 100 mg/dL (5.6 mmol/L) increase in glucose above 100 mg/dL (5.6 mmol/L).[14] Correction of hyperglycemia will restore normal blood Na^+. It also may occur when mannitol and glycine, used for irrigation during certain surgical procedures, enter the intravascular fluid compartment.

Isosmotic Hyponatremia. If the measured Na^+ concentration in plasma is decreased, but measured plasma osmolality, glucose, and urea are normal, the most likely explanation is pseudohyponatremia caused by the electrolyte exclusion effect (see Chapter 35). This occurs when Na^+ is measured by an indirect ion-selective electrode in patients with severe hyperlipidemia or hyperproteinemia.

Hypernatremia

Hypernatremia (plasma Na^+ >150 mmol/L) is always hyperosmolar. Symptoms of hypernatremia are primarily neurologic (because of neuronal cell loss of H_2O to the ECF) and include tremors, irritability, ataxia, confusion, and coma.[7,11] As with hyponatremia, the rapidity of development of hypernatremia will determine the plasma Na^+ concentration at which symptoms occur. Acute development may cause symptoms at 160 mmol/L, although in chronic hypernatremia, symptoms may not occur until Na^+ exceeds 175 mmol/L. In chronic hypernatremia, the intracellular osmolality of CNS cells will increase to protect against intracellular dehydration. Because of this, rapid correction of hypernatremia can cause dangerous cerebral edema because CNS cells will take up too much water if the ICF is hyperosmotic when normonatremia is achieved.[11]

In many cases, the symptoms of hypernatremia may be masked by underlying conditions. Hypernatremia rarely occurs in an alert patient with a normal thirst response and access to water. Most cases are observed in patients with altered mental status or infants, both of whom may not be capable of rehydrating themselves.

Hypernatremia arises in the setting of (1) hypovolemia (excessive water loss or failure to replace normal water losses), (2) hypervolemia (a net Na^+ gain in excess of water gain), or (3) normovolemia. Again, assessment of TBW status by physical examination and measurement of urine Na^+ and osmolality are important steps in establishing a diagnosis (Fig. 60.3).

Hypovolemic Hypernatremia. Hypernatremia in the setting of decreased ECF is caused by renal or extrarenal loss of hypo-osmotic fluid, leading to dehydration. Thus, once hypovolemia is established by physical examination, measurement of urine Na^+ and osmolality is used to determine the source of fluid loss. Patients who have large extrarenal losses will have concentrated urine (often >800 mOsmol/L) with low urine Na^+ (<20 mmol/L), reflecting a proper renal response to conserve Na^+ and water to restore ECF volume. Extrarenal causes include diarrhea, skin losses (burns, fever, or excessive sweating), and respiratory losses coupled with failure to replace the water. When gastrointestinal loss is excluded, and the patient has normal mental status and access to H_2O, a hypothalamic disorder (tumor or granuloma) inducing diabetes insipidus (DI) should be suspected.[11]

In patients with poorly controlled diabetes with glucose values greater than 600 mg/dL (33.3 mmol/L), an osmotic diuresis can occur that results in extreme dehydration and hypernatremia. This condition is referred to as hyperosmolar hyperglycemic nonketotic syndrome and occurs most commonly in elderly individuals with type 1 diabetes.

Normovolemic Hypernatremia. Hypernatremia in the presence of normal ECF volume is often a prelude to hypovolemic hypernatremia. Insensible losses through the lung or skin must be suspected and are characterized by concentrated urine as the kidneys conserve water. Another cause of normovolemic hypernatremia is water diuresis, which is manifested by polyuria (see Fig. 60.3). The differential for polyuria (generally defined as >3 L urine output/d) is a water or solute diuresis. Solute diuresis is exemplified by the osmotic diuresis of diabetes mellitus and generally is characterized by urine osmolality greater than 300 mOsmol/L and hyponatremia (see previous discussion in this chapter). Water diuresis, a manifestation of DI, is characterized by dilute urine (osmolality <250 mOsmol/L) and hypernatremia.[11] DI can be central or nephrogenic.[15] Central DI is due to decreased or absent vasopressin secretion resulting from head trauma, hypophysectomy, pituitary tumor, or granulomatous disease. Nephrogenic DI is due to renal resistance to vasopressin as a result of drugs (eg, lithium, demeclocycline, amphotericin, propoxyphene); electrolyte disorders (eg, hypercalcemia, hypokalemia); sickle cell anemia or Sjögren syndrome, which affect collecting duct responsiveness to vasopressin; or, more rarely, mutant vasopressin receptors.[16] When thirst and access to water are uncompromised, many patients with DI will remain normonatremic because their free water losses are offset by intake. Such patients display symptoms of only polyuria and polydipsia. However, overt hypernatremia can become manifest with progression of underlying causes, impaired thirst, or restricted access to water. Administration of vasopressin can be used to treat central DI, although patients with nephrogenic DI may be resistant to it. Correction of underlying disorders or discontinuation of offending drugs may be required to normalize Na^+ concentrations in nephrogenic DI.[11]

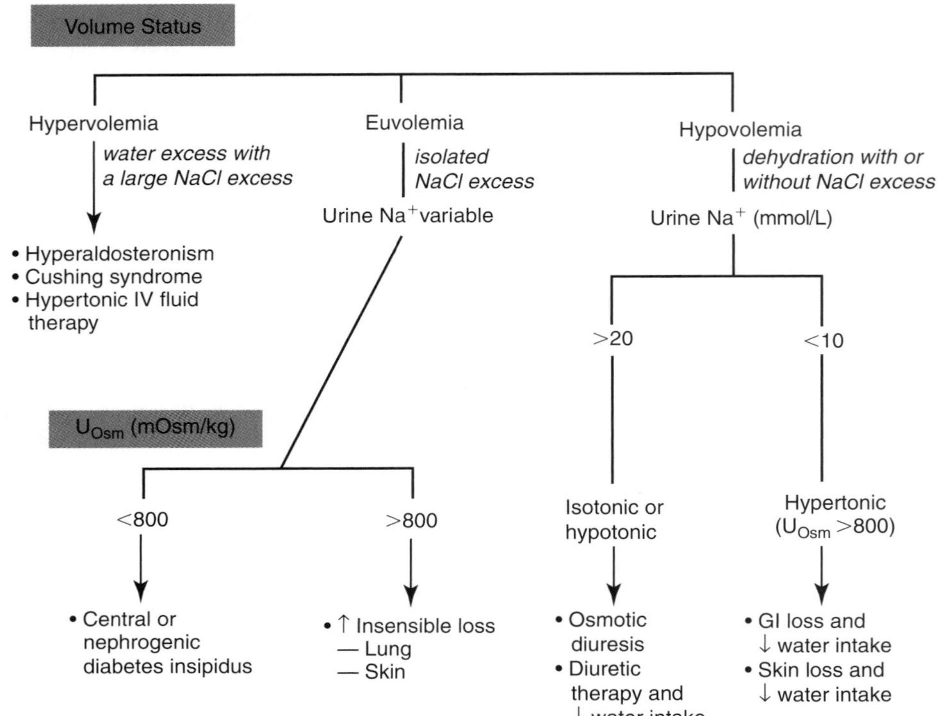

FIGURE 60.3 Algorithm for the differential diagnosis of hypernatremia. (Modified from Kirkpatrick W, Kreisberg R. Acid-base and electrolyte disorders. In: Liu P, editor. *Blue book of diagnostic tests.* Philadelphia: WB Saunders; 1986:239–254.)

Hypervolemic Hypernatremia. The presence of excess TBW and hypernatremia indicates a net gain of water and Na^+, with Na^+ gain in excess of water (see Fig. 60.3). This rare condition is observed most commonly in hospitalized patients receiving hypertonic saline or sodium bicarbonate.

Potassium

The total body potassium of a 70-kg subject is ≈3.5 mol (40 to 59 mmol/kg), of which only 1.5 to 2% is present in the ECF. Nevertheless, plasma K^+ is often a good indicator of total K^+ stores. Disturbance of K^+ homeostasis has serious consequences. For example, a decrease in extracellular K^+ (hypokalemia) is characterized by muscle weakness, irritability, and paralysis. Plasma K^+ concentrations less than 3.0 mmol/L are often associated with marked neuromuscular symptoms and indicate a critical degree of intracellular depletion. At lower concentrations, tachycardia and cardiac conduction defects are apparent on electrocardiogram (ECG) (flattened T waves) and can lead to cardiac arrest.[11]

High extracellular K^+ (hyperkalemia) concentrations may produce symptoms of mental confusion, weakness, tingling, flaccid paralysis of the extremities, and weakness of the respiratory muscles.[11] Cardiac effects of hyperkalemia include bradycardia and conduction defects evident on the electrocardiogram as prolonged PR and QRS intervals and "peaked" T waves. Prolonged, severe hyperkalemia greater than 7.0 mmol/L can lead to peripheral vascular collapse and cardiac arrest. Symptoms or ECG abnormalities are almost always present at K^+ concentrations above 6.5 mmol/L. Concentrations greater than 10.0 mmol/L in most cases are fatal, although fatalities can occur at significantly lower values.

Hypokalemia

Causes of hypokalemia (plasma K^+ <3.5 mmol/L) are classified as redistribution of extracellular K^+ into ICF, or true K^+ deficits, caused by decreased intake or loss of potassium-rich body fluids (Fig. 60.4).

Redistribution. Intracellular redistribution of K^+ is illustrated by the fall in plasma K^+ that occurs after insulin therapy for diabetic hyperglycemia. Insulin plays a crucial role in maintaining the intracellular distribution of K^+ through active cellular transport as well as glucose control. Redistribution hypokalemia, in which K^+ moves from ECF into cells as increased H^+ alters the activity of the Na^+/K^+-ATPase, is also a feature of alkalosis.[17] In addition, renal conservation of H^+ in the distal tubule occurs at the expense of K^+. Hypokalemia is highly prevalent in patients with cancer. Pseudohypokalemia can occur in settings of very high white blood cell or platelet counts. For instance, in some patients in leukemic blast crisis there can be time-dependent transport of K^+ into the leukemic cells after a blood sample is drawn. Additionally, use of myelopoietic growth factors after chemotherapy can lead to rapid K^+ uptake by new cells.[18] In these settings it is important to process the samples as quickly as possible. Other causes of intracellular redistribution are listed in Fig. 60.4. Clinically, redistributive hypokalemia is generally a transient phenomenon that is reversed once underlying conditions are corrected.

True Potassium Deficit. Hypokalemia reflecting true total body deficits of K^+ as a consequence of potassium loss can be classified into renal and nonrenal losses, based on daily excretion of K^+ in the urine (see Fig. 60.4). If urine excretion of K^+ is less than 30 mmol/d, it can be concluded that the kidneys

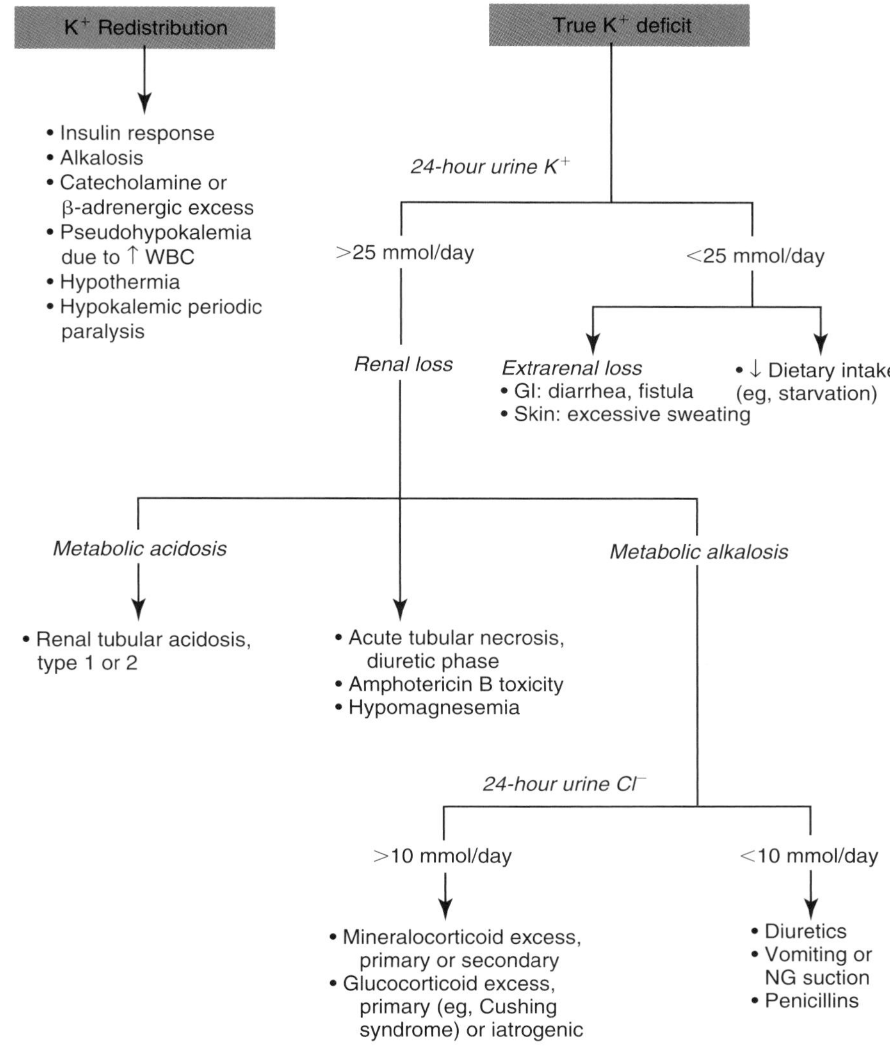

FIGURE 60.4 Algorithm for the differential diagnosis of hypokalemia. *GI,* Gastrointestinal; *NG,* nasogastric; *WBC,* white blood cell. (Modified from Kirkpatrick W, Kreisberg R. Acid-base and electrolyte disorders. In: Liu P, editor. *Blue book of diagnostic tests.* Philadelphia: WB Saunders; 1986:239–254.)

are functioning properly and are attempting to reabsorb K^+. The cause may be decreased K^+ intake or extrarenal loss of K^+-rich fluid. Causes of decreased intake include chronic starvation and postoperative intravenous fluid therapy with K^+-poor solutions. Gastrointestinal loss of K^+ occurs most commonly with diarrhea and loss of gastric fluid through vomiting.

Urine excretion exceeding 25 to 30 mmol/d in a hypokalemic setting is inappropriate and indicates that the kidneys are the primary source of K^+ loss. Renal losses of K^+ may occur during the diuretic (recovery) phase of acute tubular necrosis and during states of excess mineralocorticoid (primary or secondary aldosteronism) or glucocorticoid (Cushing's syndrome) when the distal tubules increase Na^+ reabsorption and K^+ excretion. Renal loss of K^+ is also caused by thiazide and loop diuretics.[19] In addition to redistribution of K^+ into cells in an alkalotic setting, K^+ can be lost from the kidneys in exchange for reclaimed H^+ ions. This cause of true hypokalemia will be evident in low urine Cl^- and an alkaline urine. In patients with cancer, increased renal K^+ loss may be due to chemotherapy (eg, cisplatin)-induced nephron and tubular damage.[18] Magnesium deficiency also can lead to increased renal loss of K^+, which is attributable to a reduction in the inhibitory effect of magnesium on luminal potassium channels.[20]

True potassium deficit requires replacement of potassium. Although there are dietary sources of potassium, such as potatoes and tomatoes, significant K^+ losses may require oral or intravenous supplementation with potassium chloride. The oral route is generally preferred, although intravenous correction should be pursued in patients with severe or symptomatic hypokalemia and those who are unable to take oral medication.[11] In individuals with ongoing sources of potassium losses, such as patients on diuretics, chronic supplementation with a daily regimen of oral potassium chloride is often used.

Hyperkalemia

Hyperkalemia (plasma K^+ >5.0 mmol/L) is a result of (singly or in combination) (1) redistribution, (2) increased intake, or (3) increased retention. In addition, preanalytical conditions—such as hemolysis, thrombocytosis ($>10^6/\mu L$), and leukocytosis ($>10^5/\mu L$ together with delayed sample analysis)—have been known to cause marked pseudohyperkalemia, as described in detail in Chapter 35 (Fig. 60.5).

Redistribution. The transfer of intracellular K^+ into ECF invariably occurs in acidemia as K^+ shifts outward as the result of pH-induced changes in Na^+/K^+-ATPase activity. As a general rule, K^+ concentrations can be expected to rise 0.2 to 0.5 mmol/L for every 0.1-unit drop in pH. When acidemia is corrected, normokalemia will be restored rapidly. Extracellular redistribution of K^+ also may occur in (1) tissue hypoxia; (2) insulin deficiency (eg, diabetic ketoacidosis); (3) massive intravascular hemolysis; (4) severe burns; (5) violent muscular activity, as in status epilepticus; (6) rhabdomyolysis; and (7) tumor lysis syndrome. Finally, important iatrogenic causes of redistribution hyperkalemia include digoxin toxicity and β-adrenergic blockade, especially in patients with diabetes or on dialysis.[11] Redistributive hyperkalemia can be corrected by reversing the aberrations that cause K^+ to shift out of cells. Insulin and sodium bicarbonate are commonly used and have a quick onset of action, particularly in the diabetic or acidemic setting. Drug-induced causes require cessation or dose reduction of the offending agent. Patients with digoxin toxicity should be given antibodies to digoxin as well, because of the high risk for mortality associated with hyperkalemia and supratherapeutic administration of digoxin.

Potassium Retention. When glomerular filtration or renal tubular function is decreased, hyperkalemia will often occur. In the absence of severe renal failure, hyperkalemia is seldom prolonged and may not even occur in some cases. Decreased excretion of K^+ in moderate and acute renal disease and end-stage renal failure (with oliguria or anuria) are the most common causes of prolonged hyperkalemia (see Fig. 60.5). Hyperkalemia occurs along with Na^+ depletion in adrenocortical insufficiency (eg, Addison disease) because diminished Na^+ reabsorption results in decreased tubular K^+ secretion. Drugs that block the production of aldosterone, such as inhibitors of angiotensin-converting enzyme (ACE inhibitors; eg, lisinopril), nonsteroidal anti-inflammatory drugs, and angiotensin II–receptor blockers, may also cause hyperkalemia. Excess administration of potassium-sparing diuretics that block distal tubular K^+ secretion (eg, triamterene, spironolactone) may also cause hyperkalemia.[19] In patients with cancer, hyperkalemia can be caused by adrenal insufficiency secondary to metastases to the adrenal glands, nephrotoxic chemotherapy agents (eg, mitomycin-C, methotrexate, platinum compounds), postrenal obstruction, or tumor lysis syndrome.[18] Treatment of hyperkalemia includes agents that increase cellular uptake of K^+, such as glucose and insulin, sodium bicarbonate, and β_2-adrenergic agonists. The rapid onset of these agents provides a quick reduction in ECF potassium concentrations, thus reducing the risk for immediate life-threatening cardiac effects of hyperkalemia. However, these redistributive effects are only temporizing measures when there is a true excess of potassium, and they need to be coupled with interventions that remove potassium from the circulation. To reduce the total body content of potassium, patients can be given K^+-losing diuretics, cation-exchange

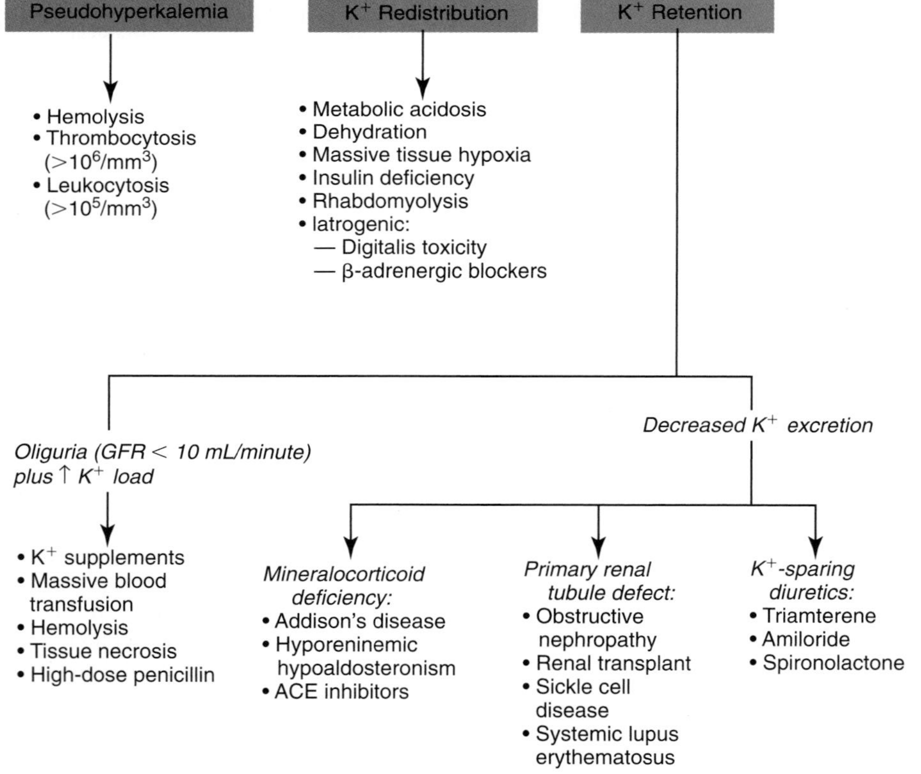

FIGURE 60.5 Algorithm for the differential diagnosis of hyperkalemia. *ACE,* Angiotensin-converting enzyme. (Modified from Kirkpatrick W, Kreisberg R. Acid-base and electrolyte disorders. In: Liu P, editor. *Blue book of diagnostic tests.* Philadelphia: WB Saunders; 1986:239–254.)

resins, and, finally, hemodialysis.[18] Stimulation of renal potassium excretion is preferred, because the use of cation-exchange resins can be associated with bowel necrosis, particularly when given per rectum. Hemodialysis is an option of last resort, removing potassium through an extracorporeal circuit, which stimulates diffusion of potassium out of the circulating blood and into the discarded dialysate.

Chloride

In the absence of acid-base disturbances, Cl^- concentrations in plasma generally will follow those of Na^+. However, determination of plasma Cl^- concentration is useful in the differential diagnosis of acid-base disturbances and is essential for calculating the anion gap. Fluctuations in serum or plasma Cl^- have little clinical consequence, but do serve as signs of an underlying disturbance in fluid or acid-base homeostasis. The specific replacement of chloride is rarely targeted at chloride deficit independently, but it is a corner stone of management for metabolic alkalosis.

Hypochloremia

In general, causes of hypochloremia parallel causes of hyponatremia. Persistent gastric secretion and prolonged vomiting result in significant loss of Cl^- and ultimately in hypochloremic alkalosis and depletion of total body Cl^- with retention of HCO_3^-. Respiratory acidosis, which is accompanied by increased HCO_3^-, is another common cause of decreased Cl^- with normal Na^+.

Hyperchloremia

Increased plasma Cl^- concentration, similar to increased Na^+ concentration, occurs with dehydration, prolonged diarrhea with loss of sodium bicarbonate, DI, and overtreatment with normal saline solutions, which have a Cl^- content of 150 mmol/L. In fact, mounting evidence suggests that use of saline (NaCl) solution for maintenance, intraoperative, and resuscitative therapy can result in a host of hyperchloremia-induced side effects.[21] For these reasons, there is a movement among the surgical community toward more physiologic solutions such as lactated Ringer's solution.[21] A rise in Cl^- concentration also may be seen in respiratory alkalosis because of renal compensation for excreting HCO_3^-.

POINTS TO REMEMBER

- Physical examination is important in assessing TBW status and hyponatremic or hypernatremic disorders
- Urine electrolytes are important to determine if the kidneys are functioning properly in disorders of electrolyte and water balance.
- Patient history can be important in assessing electrolyte disorders. Examples include vomiting, diarrhea, water deprivation, excess perspiration, anuria, diabetes, etc.

ACID-BASE PHYSIOLOGY

Normal metabolic processes result in the production of large amounts of carbonic acid and lesser amounts of sulfuric, phosphoric, and other acids. For example, during a 24-hour period, a person weighing 70 kg disposes of approximately 20 moles of carbon dioxide ([CO_2] the volatile form of carbonic acid) through the lungs, and about 70 to 100 mmol (or ≈1 mmol/kg) of nonvolatile acids (mainly sulfuric and phosphoric acids) through the kidneys. These products of metabolism are transported to the lungs and kidneys via the ECF and blood with no appreciable change in the ECF pH, and with only a minimal difference between arterial (pH 7.35 to 7.45) and venous (pH 7.32 to 7.38) blood. This is accomplished by the buffering capacity of blood and by respiratory and renal regulatory mechanisms.

Acid-Base Balance and Acid-Base Status

A description of acid-base balance involves an accounting of the carbonic (H_2CO_3, HCO_3^-, CO_3^{2-}, and CO_2) and noncarbonic acids and conjugate bases in terms of input (intake plus metabolic production) and output (excretion plus metabolic conversion) over a given time interval. The acid-base status of body fluids is typically assessed by measurements of total CO_2, plasma pH, and PCO_2, because the bicarbonate/carbonic acid system is the most important mammalian buffering system.

The following clinical terms are used to describe acid-base status. *Acidemia* is defined as an arterial blood pH less than 7.35 and *alkalemia* indicates an arterial blood pH greater than 7.45. *Acidosis* and *alkalosis* refer to pathologic states that often lead to acidemia or alkalemia. For example, in common acid-base disorders such as lactic acidosis and diabetic ketoacidosis, intermediate organic acids (lactic acid and β-hydroxybutyric acid, respectively), which normally are metabolized to CO_2 and water, may accumulate to a significant extent, resulting in acidemia. Additionally, more than one type of pathologic process can occur simultaneously, giving rise to a mixed acid-base disturbance, in which the blood pH may be low, high, or within the reference interval.

Acid-Base Parameters: Definitions and Abbreviations

Acids are chemical substances that can donate protons (H^+ ions) in solution and *bases* are substances that accept protons. Strong acids readily give up H^+, whereas strong bases readily accept H^+. Thus the conjugate base of a strong acid is a weak base and vice versa.

pH and pK. The pH of a solution is defined as the negative logarithm of the hydrogen ion activity ($pH = -\log aH^+$). Thus *pH is a dimensionless quantity,* such that a decrease in one pH unit represents a tenfold increase in H^+ activity. The average pH of blood (7.40) corresponds to a hydrogen ion concentration of 40 nmol/L, assuming an activity coefficient of 1. The relationship between hydrogen ion activity and pH is illustrated in Fig. 60.6. This relationship is inverse and nonlinear.

The pK (also, pK' and pK_a) represents the negative logarithm of the ionization constant of a weak acid *(K_a)*; that is, the pK is the pH at which an acid is half dissociated, existing as equal proportions of acid and conjugate base. Acids have pK values less than 7.0, whereas bases have pK values greater than 7.0. The lower the pK, the stronger is the acid, and the higher the pK, the stronger is the conjugate base. For example, the pK of lactic acid is 3.86, and that of ammonium ion NH_4^+ is 9.5. The high pK for the ammonium ion indicates that this species prefers to hold onto its proton, rather than dissociating into NH_3 and H^+.

The pH of plasma may be considered to be a function of two independent variables: (1) the PCO_2, which is regulated

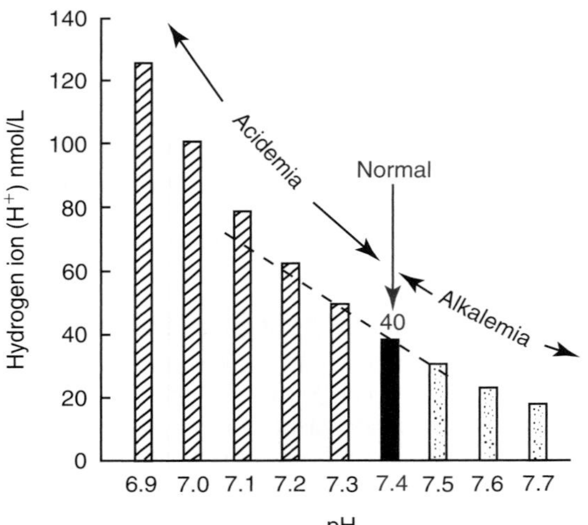

FIGURE 60.6 Relationship of pH to hydrogen ion concentration. A *broken line* is drawn to emphasize the (approximate) linear relationship between hydrogen ion concentration and pH over the pH range of 7.2 to 7.5. (From Narins RG, Emmett M. Simple and mixed acid-base disorders: a practical approach. *Medicine* 1980;59:161–187.)

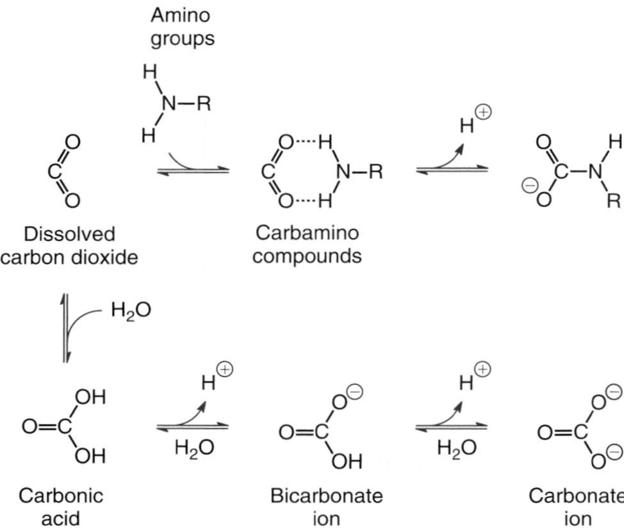

FIGURE 60.7 Reactions of carbon dioxide with water and amino groups. Hydrogen bonding is indicated by a *dotted line.* The carbamino acid is fairly strong (—R—NH—COOH → H^+ + R—NH—COO^-).

by the lungs and represents the acid component of the carbonic acid/bicarbonate buffer system, and (2) the concentration of titratable base (base excess or deficit, which is defined later), which is regulated by the kidneys. The plasma total CO_2 concentration generally is taken as a measure of the base excess or deficit in plasma and ECF.

Bicarbonate and Dissolved Carbon Dioxide. Bicarbonate is the second largest fraction (behind Cl^-) of plasma anions. Conventionally, it is defined to include (1) plasma bicarbonate ion (HCO_3^-), (2) carbonate ion (CO_3^{2-}), and (3) CO_2 bound in plasma carbamino compounds (RCNHCOOH) (Fig. 60.7). Actual bicarbonate ion concentration is not measured in clinical laboratories. The analyte usually measured in plasma is total CO_2, which includes bicarbonate and dissolved CO_2 (dCO_2) but is often referred to as "serum bicarb." At the pH of the blood, the amount of dissolved CO_2 is 700 to 1000 times greater than the amount of carbonic acid (H_2CO_3); therefore $cdCO_2$ is the term used to express their combined concentration. It is calculated from the solubility coefficient of CO_2 in blood at 37°C (α = 0.0306 mmol/L per mm Hg) multiplied by the measured PCO_2 in mm Hg. Thus at a PCO_2 of 40 mm Hg, $cdCO_2$ is 1.224 mmol/L (0.0306 mmol/L × 40 mm Hg). This $cdCO_2$ value can then be used, in the Henderson-Hasselbalch equation, to calculate the total bicarbonate concentration.

Henderson-Hasselbalch Equation. The Henderson-Hasselbalch equation is described in detail in Chapter 35. However, it is important to review here because it enhances understanding of pH regulation of body fluids as it relates to compensatory mechanisms in acid-base disturbances. The equation derived in Chapter 35 can also be written as follows:

$$pH = 6.1 + \log \frac{cHCO_3^-}{cdCO_2}$$

where $cdCO_2$ is equal to α (0.0306 mmol/L per mm Hg) PCO_2 and 6.1 is the pK' for the carbonic acid/bicarbonate system. An alternative expression useful for approximating cH^+ in blood is as follows:

$$cH^+ = K \times \frac{PCO_2}{cHCO_3^-}$$

where $K = 24$ (nmol/L) (mmol/L) (mm Hg^{-1}).

The average normal ratio of the concentrations of bicarbonate and dissolved CO_2 in plasma is 25 (mmol/L)/1.25 (mmol/L) = 20/1. It follows then that any change in the concentration of bicarbonate or dissolved CO_2 relative to each other must be accompanied by a change in pH. Such changes in this important ratio can occur through a change in $cHCO_3^-$ (the renal component) or PCO_2 (the respiratory component). Clinical conditions characterized as *metabolic* disturbances of acid-base balance are classified as primary disturbances in $cHCO_3^-$. Those characterized as *respiratory* disturbances are classified as primary disturbances in $cdCO_2$ (PCO_2). Various compensatory mechanisms attempting to reestablish the normal ratio of $cHCO_3^-/cdCO_2$ may result in changes in bicarbonate concentration, dissolved CO_2 concentration, or both. Application of the Henderson-Hasselbalch equation to human acid-base physiology can be illustrated by a lever-fulcrum (teeter-totter) diagram (Fig. 60.8).

Buffer Systems and Their Role in Regulating the pH of Body Fluids

A buffer is a mixture of a weak acid and a salt of its conjugate base that resists changes in pH when a strong acid or base is added to the solution. If concentrations of the acid and base components of a buffer are equal, the pH will equal the pK. Generally, buffers work best at resisting pH changes in the interval ± 1 pH unit of its pK and are more effective at higher molar concentrations. The action of buffers in the regulation of body pH can be demonstrated by using the bicarbonate

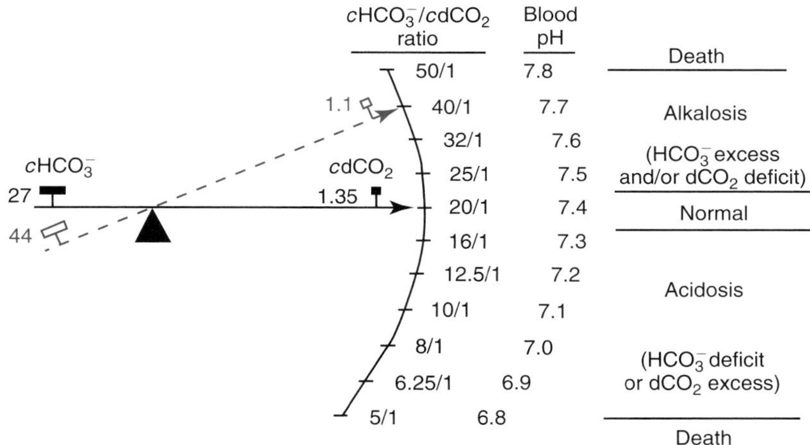

FIGURE 60.8 Scheme demonstrating the relation between pH and the ratio of bicarbonate concentration to the concentration of dissolved CO_2. If the ratio in blood is 20:1 ($cHCO_3^-$ = 27 mmol/$cdCO_2$ = 1.35 mmol/L), the resultant pH will be 7.4, as demonstrated by the *solid beam*. The *dotted line* shows a case of uncompensated alkalosis (bicarbonate excess) with a bicarbonate concentration of 44 mmol/L and a $cdCO_2$ of 1.1 mmol/L. The ratio therefore is 40:1, and the resultant pH is 7.7. In a case of uncompensated acidosis, the pointer of the balance would point to a pH between 6.8 and 7.35, depending on the $cHCO_3^-/cdCO_2$ ratio. (From Weisberg HF. A better understanding of anion-cation ["acid-base"] balance. *Surg Clin North Am* 1959;39:93–120.)

buffer system as an example. If a strong acid is added to a solution containing HCO_3^- and H_2CO_3, the H^+ will react with HCO_3^- to form more H_2CO_3 and subsequently CO_2 and H_2O. The hydrogen ions are thereby bound, and the increase in the H^+ concentration will be minimal.

$$H^+ + HCO_3^- \rightleftharpoons H_2CO_3 \rightleftharpoons CO_2 + H_2O$$

Bicarbonate and Carbonic Acid Buffer System

The most important buffer of plasma is the bicarbonate/carbonic acid pair even though its p*K* is 6.1, and normal plasma pH is 7.4. The normal bicarbonate/dCO_2 ratio is 20:1, which is outside the 10:1 or 1:10 ratio at which buffers work best. However, the effectiveness of the bicarbonate buffer is based on the fact that the lungs can readily dispose of or retain CO_2, and that other than hemoglobin (Hb) and other serum proteins, it is present at higher concentrations than other buffers, with the exception of Hb. In addition, the renal tubules can increase or decrease the rate of reclamation of bicarbonate from the glomerular filtrate (see Chapter 59). The importance of the relatively high concentration of bicarbonate (relative to H^+) becomes apparent when considering that at normal plasma pH, 5 mmol/L of lactate (p*K* ≈3.86) generates ≈5 mmol/L of H^+ ion, which is remarkable given that a normal H^+ ion concentration is only 40 nmol/L. The buffer value (β) is defined as the amount of base required to cause a change in pH of 1 unit. The buffer value of the bicarbonate buffer in plasma is 55.6 mmol/L.[22]

Phosphate Buffer System

At a plasma pH of 7.4, the ratio $cHPO_4^{2-}/cH_2PO_4^-$ is 4:1 (pK′ = 6.8). The total concentration of this buffer in both erythrocytes and plasma accounts for approximately 5% of the nonbicarbonate buffer value of plasma. Organic phosphate, however, in the form of 2,3-diphosphoglycerate (present in erythrocytes in a concentration of about 4.5 mmol/L), accounts for about 16% of the nonbicarbonate buffer value of erythrocytes.

The phosphate buffer reacts with acids and with bases as follows:

$$HPO_4^{\oplus\oplus} + H^{\oplus} \rightarrow H_2PO_4^{\oplus}$$

$$H_2PO_4^{\oplus} + OH^{\ominus} \rightarrow HPO_4^{\oplus\oplus} + H_2O$$

This system is most important in the titration and excretion of acids in urine.

Plasma Protein Buffer System

The buffer value (β) of the nonbicarbonate buffers of plasma totals approximately 7.7 mmol/L at pH 7.40 and a normal plasma protein concentration of 72 g/L. Proteins, especially albumin, account for the greatest portion (>90%) of the nonbicarbonate buffer value of plasma.

The significance of nonbicarbonate buffers of plasma can be illustrated by the chemical reactions during CO_2 equilibration:

$$CO_2 + H_2O \rightarrow H_2CO_3 \rightarrow HCO_3^{\ominus} + H^{\oplus}$$

$$HPr \rightarrow H^{\oplus} + Pr^{\ominus}$$

where the HPr/Pr^- system represents all nonbicarbonate buffers. Because the purpose of this buffer system is to maintain cH^+ constant, for each molecule of HCO_3^- generated, one molecule of nonbicarbonate buffer base disappears. Thus, in alkalosis, the cH^+ from CO_2 equilibration falls and an excess of nonbicarbonate buffer base is the result. As follows, there is a consumption or negative excess of this buffer base in acidosis.

Hemoglobin Buffer System and Whole Blood Base Excess

The buffer value (β) of the nonbicarbonate buffers of erythrocyte fluid is approximately 63 mmol/L at pH 7.20, for an erythrocyte Hb concentration of 21 mmol/L (33.8 g/dL). Hb accounts for the major part (53 mmol/L), with the remainder attributable to 2,3-diphosphoglycerate (2,3-DPG). The imidazole groups of Hb are quantitatively the most important buffer groups with a pK = 7.3.

As in plasma, CO_2 equilibration of whole blood depends on the buffer value of nonbicarbonate buffers. Thus CO_2 equilibration in whole blood depends on Hb concentration and also on pH and oxygenation status. It is possible to derive an approximate equation for whole-blood CO_2 equilibration and calculation of *whole-blood base excess* as follows:

$$\Delta cHCO_3^-(P) = -\beta \times \Delta pH(P) + \frac{\Delta cB'(B)}{\zeta}$$

where

$\Delta cHCO_3^-$ = measured plasma $cHCO_3^-$ (P) − 24.5 mmol/L HCO_3^-

ΔpH = measured pH − the standard pH of 7.40

$\Delta cB'(B)$ = the *whole-blood base excess* (ie, the concentration of titratable base when the blood is titrated with strong acid or base to pH = 7.40 at PCO_2 (Std) and 37°C]

$\beta = \beta_m Hb \times cHb(B) + \beta Pr$, where $\beta_m Hb$ is the molar buffer value of Hb (2.3 mol/mol), $cHb(B)$ is the substance concentration of Hb (Fe) in the blood (unit, mmol/L), and βPr is the buffer value of the plasma proteins (7.7 mmol/L): $\zeta = 1 - cHb(B)/c_{ref}$, where c_{ref} is an empirical parameter (43 mmol/L).

This equation for whole-blood base excess (known as the Van Slyke equation,[23,24]) together with the Henderson-Hasselbalch equation, provides the simplest algorithm for calculation of various acid-base variables, and its clinical use is owed to Ole Siggaard-Andersen, an author of this chapter in the first two editions of this textbook.[23,24]

Isohydric and Chloride Shift

Because of continuous production of CO_2 within tissue cells, there is a concentration gradient for CO_2 from cells to plasma and thus to erythrocytes. Despite this, all buffer systems discussed previously interact through a phenomenon known as the isohydric Cl^- shift, which keeps the $cdCO_2$ and cH^+ (pH) essentially constant between arterial and venous blood. A small portion of the CO_2 entering the plasma stays as dissolved CO_2, thus the slightly higher PCO_2 of venous blood. Most reacts with H_2O to form carbonic acid that dissociates into H^+ and HCO_3^-. The increased amount of H^+ is buffered by plasma buffers (Fig. 60.9, reaction 1). Another small portion combines with the amino groups of proteins and forms carbamino compounds (see Fig. 60.9, reaction 2). The normal concentration of carbamino compounds in the plasma is approximately 0.2 mmol/L. Most of the CO_2 enters erythrocytes and reacts with water to form carbonic acid. This reaction is catalyzed by the enzyme carbonic anhydrase and proceeds at a relatively high rate (see Fig. 60.9, reaction 3). Some CO_2 remains as dissolved CO_2, and some combines with Hb to form $HbCO_2$ (see Fig. 60.9, reaction 4).

The carbonic acid formed in Fig. 60.9, reaction 3 initially increases the H^+ concentration. The pH change, however, is fully or partially compensated by the release of oxygen from O_2Hb, which involves the conversion of stronger acid (O_2Hb) into weaker acid (HHb) that then readily accepts the H^+. Furthermore, the HHb binds significantly more CO_2 in the form of carbamino-CO_2 than does oxyHb. The oxygen released from O_2Hb moves from the erythrocytes through the plasma into the peripheral tissue cells.

Remaining H^+ formed in reaction 3 are buffered by the nonbicarbonate buffers of the erythrocyte fluid, whereas the concentration of HCO_3^- increases to the same extent that the concentration of Hb anion falls. The transformations described so far (see Fig. 60.9, reactions 1 through 5) are referred to as the isohydric shift (ie, a shift in which the H^+ concentration remains unchanged).

However, the equilibrium between plasma and red cells has been disturbed by this isohydric shift. The concentration of HCO_3^- has increased relatively more in the erythrocytes than in the plasma; the pH of plasma has fallen relatively more than the pH of erythrocytes; and the nondiffusible ion concentration in the erythrocytes has fallen because of the increase in protonation of Hb. The membrane potential of the erythrocytes therefore becomes less negative, and the distribution of all diffusible ions must change with the new membrane potential. The ion shifts that occur rapidly include movement of HCO_3^- out of the erythrocytes and movement of Cl^- into

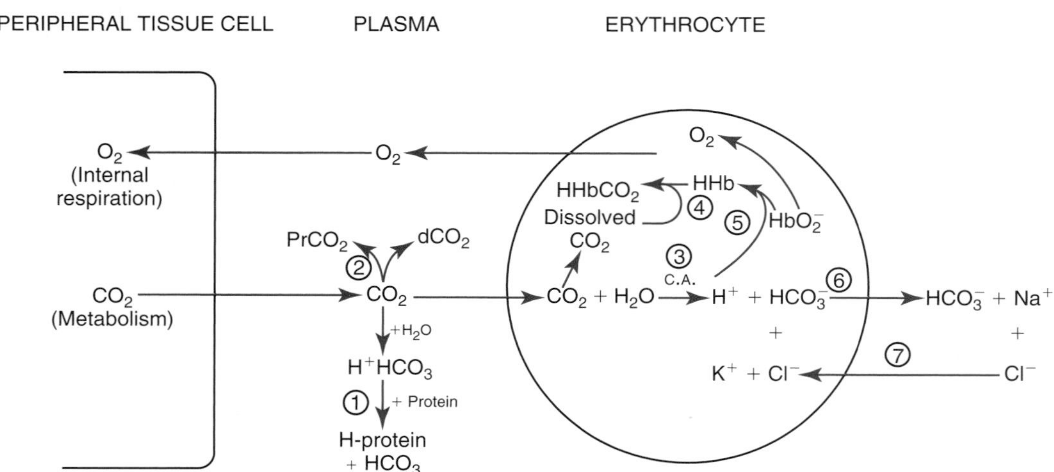

FIGURE 60.9 Scheme demonstrating the isohydric and chloride shift. The *encircled numbers* refer to the reactions described in the text. For details, see text discussion.

the erythrocytes to provide electrochemical balance. This shift of chloride ions is referred to as the chloride shift (see Fig. 60.9, reactions 6 and 7). In the alveoli, low PCO_2 and high PO_2 cause a reversal of reactions 1 through 7, as shown in Fig. 60.9.

Respiratory Mechanism in the Regulation of Acid-Base Balance

In addition to supplying O_2 to tissue cells for normal metabolism, the respiratory mechanism contributes to maintenance of normal body pH through elimination or retention of CO_2 in metabolic acidosis and alkalosis, respectively.

Respiration

Exchange of O_2 and CO_2 in the lungs between alveolar air and blood is called external respiration, in contrast to internal respiration, which occurs at the cellular level. During inspiration, muscular contraction expands intrathoracic volume, decreasing intrapulmonary pressure. Atmospheric air is drawn into the bronchial tree, which terminates at the alveoli, where the exchange of gases between alveolar air and pulmonary blood occurs. Expiration occurs passively as the elastic tissues of the lungs and chest wall rebound and the intrathoracic volume is decreased.

Peripheral venous blood reaches the pulmonary circulation from the right ventricle of the heart and is arterialized in the capillaries of the alveoli by uptake of O_2 and loss of CO_2. Pulmonary venous blood then returns to the left ventricle by way of the left atrium and is pumped to the peripheral tissues. In the capillaries of peripheral tissues, the arterial blood releases O_2 to the tissue cells and takes up CO_2.

In a resting state, the respiration rate is normally 12 to 15 breaths/min. For an average-sized adult with a tidal volume of approximately 0.5 L, 6 to 8 L of air is moved per minute in either direction. Involuntary increases in rate and depth of respiration are regulated by the medullary respiratory center in the brainstem, which is stimulated by central chemoreceptors located on the anterior surface of the medulla oblongata and by peripheral chemoreceptors located in the carotid arteries and aorta. Peripheral chemoreceptors are stimulated by a fall in pH caused by accumulation of CO_2 or a decrease in PO_2. Central chemoreceptors are stimulated only by a decrease in pH of the CSF.

Exchange of Gases in the Lungs and Peripheral Tissues

Diffusion of O_2 and CO_2 across alveolar and cell membranes is governed by gradients in the partial pressure of each gas (Fig. 60.10). Dry air inspired at a pressure of 1 atm (760 mm Hg) consists of 21% O_2 (PO_2 ≈160 mm Hg), 0.03% CO_2 (PCO_2 ≈0.25 mm Hg), 78% nitrogen, and ≈0.1% other inert gases. As inspired air passes over the mucous membranes of the upper respiratory tract, it is warmed to 37°C, becomes saturated with water vapor, and mixes with air in the respiratory tree, resulting in partial pressures of ≈150 mm Hg for O_2, ≈0.3 mm Hg for CO_2, ≈47 mm Hg for H_2O, and ≈563 mm Hg for nitrogen. Further mixing with alveolar air results in partial pressures at the alveolar membrane of ≈105 mm Hg for O_2, ≈40 mm Hg for CO_2, and ≈47 mm Hg for H_2O. Venous blood on the opposite side of the alveolar membrane has PO_2 ≈40 mm Hg and PCO_2 ≈46 mm Hg. Thus the gradient for O_2 is inward, toward the blood, and for CO_2, it is outward, toward the alveoli. CO_2 removal is so efficient that the PCO_2 in expired air is more than 100 times the PCO_2 in inspired air (see Fig. 60.10). In arterial blood, the PO_2 is slightly lower than in alveolar air (90 to 100 vs. 105 mm Hg) as the result of shunting of about 5% of blood that does not equilibrate.

At the arterial end of capillaries of peripheral tissues, the PO_2 at 95 mm Hg is substantially higher than the average PO_2 at the surface of tissue cells (20 mm Hg), and the PCO_2 at 40 mm Hg is substantially lower than that in the cells (50 to 70 mm Hg). Thus, in the tissue capillary, the gradient for O_2 is inward to the cell; for CO_2, it is outward to the capillary blood. The arteriovenous difference in partial pressures is approximately 60 mm Hg for O_2 and 6 mm Hg or less for CO_2.

Respiratory Response to Acid-Base Perturbations

Most metabolic acid-base disorders develop slowly, within hours in diabetic ketoacidosis and months in chronic renal disease. The respiratory system responds immediately to a change in acid-base status, but several hours may be required for the response to become maximal. The maximum response is not attained until both central and peripheral chemoreceptors are fully stimulated. For example, in the early stages of metabolic acidosis, plasma pH decreases, but because H^+ ions equilibrate rather slowly across the blood-brain barrier, the pH in CSF remains nearly normal. However, because peripheral chemoreceptors are stimulated by decreased plasma pH, hyperventilation occurs, and plasma PCO_2 is decreased. When this occurs, the PCO_2 of the CSF decreases immediately because CO_2 equilibrates rapidly across the blood-brain barrier, leading to a rise in pH of the CSF that inhibits the central chemoreceptors. As plasma bicarbonate gradually falls because of acidosis, bicarbonate concentration, and pH in the CSF will also eventually fall. At this point, stimulation of respiration becomes maximal from both central and peripheral chemoreceptors.

Renal Mechanisms in the Regulation of Acid-Base Balance

The average pH of plasma and the glomerular filtrate is ≈ 7.4, whereas the average urinary pH is ≈6.0, reflecting renal excretion of nonvolatile acids. Various functions of the kidneys respond to different alterations in acid-base status. In the case of acidosis, excretion of acids is increased and that of base is conserved; in alkalosis, the opposite occurs. The pH of the urine changes correspondingly and may vary in random specimens from pH 4.5 to 8.0. The ability to excrete variable amounts of acid or base makes the kidney the final defense mechanism against changes in body pH.

The various acids produced during metabolic processes are buffered in the ECF at the expense of HCO_3^-. Renal excretion of acid and conservation of HCO_3^- occur through several mechanisms, including (1) Na^+-H^+ exchange, (2) production of ammonia and excretion of NH_4^+, and (3) reclamation of HCO_3^-.

Na^+-H^+ Exchange

Nearly all mammalian cells contain a plasma membrane ATP-hydrolyzing protein capable of exchanging sodium ions for protons—the so-called Na^+-H^+ exchanger, of which there are six isoforms (Fig. 60.11).[5] In the renal tubules, two isoforms, NHE-1 and NHE-3, appear predominant. These isoforms extrude H^+ ions into the tubular fluid in exchange for Na^+ ions.

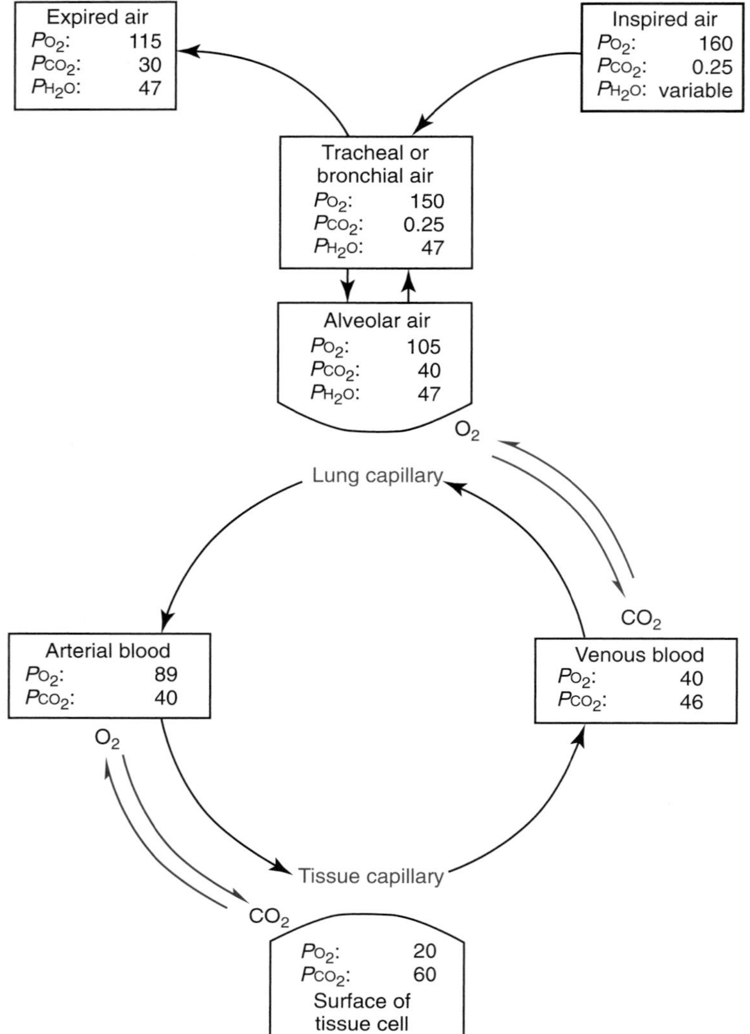

FIGURE 60.10 Partial pressures of oxygen and carbon dioxide in air, blood, and tissue. Values shown are approximations in mm Hg and are calculated assuming a 5% shunt. *Red arrows* show directions of gradients. (Modified from Tietz NW. *Fundamentals of clinical chemistry,* 3rd ed. Philadelphia: WB Saunders; 1987.)

Na^+-H^+ exchange is enhanced in states of acidosis and inhibited in alkalosis. Both NHE-1 and NHE-3 are transcriptionally upregulated in response to acidotic states.[5] The proximal tubules, however, cannot maintain an H^+ gradient of more than ≈1 pH unit, whereas the distal tubules cannot maintain more than ≈3 pH units. Thus maximum urine acidity is reached at ≈pH 4.4. In types 1 and 4 RTA, this exchange process is defective and may lead to a decrease in blood pH. In RTA type 1, an increase in urinary pH is often noted.

Potassium ions compete with H^+ in the renal tubular Na^+-H^+ exchanger. If the intracellular K^+ concentration of renal tubular cells is high, more K^+ and less H^+ are exchanged for Na^+. As a result, the urine becomes less acidic, thereby increasing the acidity of body fluids. If K^+ is depleted, more H^+ ions are exchanged for Na^+; the urine becomes more acidic and the body fluids more alkaline. Thus hyperkalemia contributes to acidosis and hypokalemia to alkalosis.

Renal Production of Ammonia and Excretion of Ammonium Ions

Renal tubular cells are able to generate ammonia from glutamine and other amino acids derived from muscle and liver cells according to the reaction in Fig. 60.12.

The ammonium ion produced dissociates into ammonia and hydrogen ions to a degree dependent on the pH (see Fig. 60.11). At normal blood pH, the ratio of NH_4^+/NH_3 is approximately 100 to 1. Ammonia is a gas that diffuses readily across the cell membrane into the tubular lumen, where it combines with hydrogen ions to form ammonium ions (see Fig. 60.11). At the acid pH of urine, the equilibrium between NH_4^+ and NH_3 shifts markedly to the left (≈10,000 to 1), strongly favoring formation of NH_4^+. The NH_4^+ formed in the tubular lumen cannot easily cross cell membranes and thus is trapped in the tubular urine and excreted with anions such as phosphate, chloride, or sulfate. In normal individuals, NH_4^+ production in the tubular lumen accounts for the

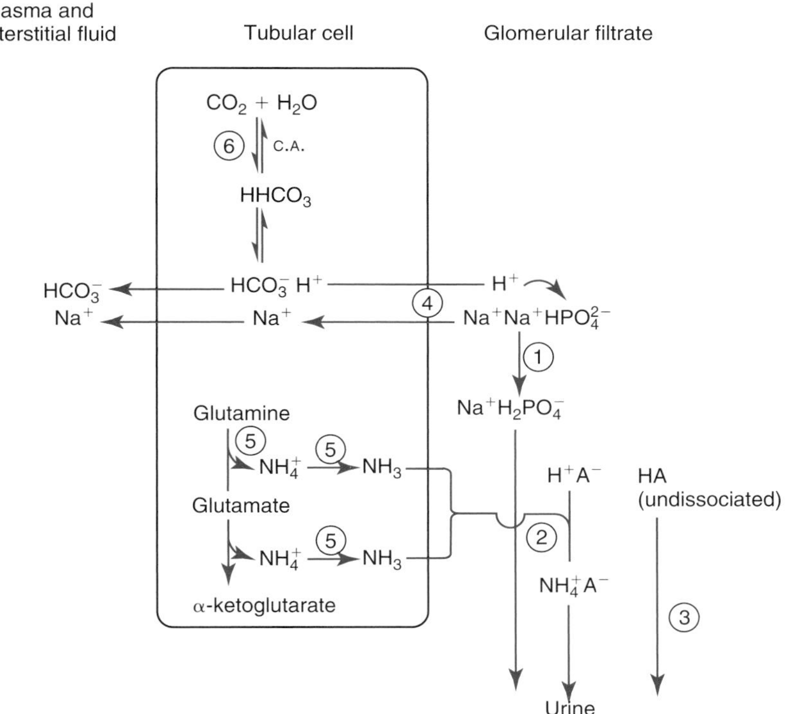

FIGURE 60.11 Hydrogen ion excretion, sodium hydrogen ion exchange, and ammonia production in the renal tubules. *1,* Conversion of HPO_4^{2-} to $H_2PO_4^-$; *2,* reaction of hydrogen ions with NH_3; *3,* excretion of undissociated acids; *4,* Na^+-H^+ exchange; *5,* NH_3 production; and *6,* synthesis of carbonic acid from CO_2.

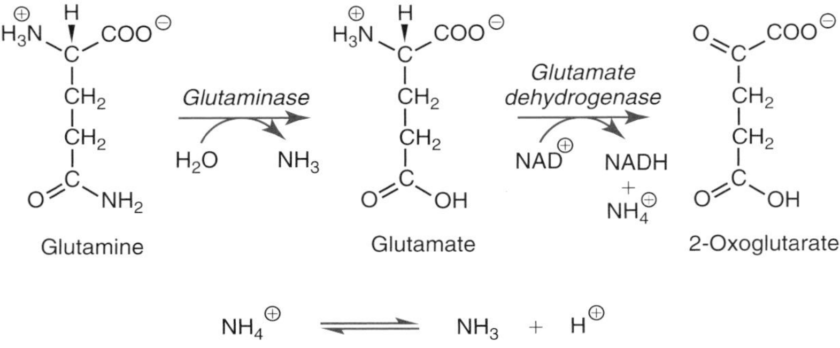

FIGURE 60.12 Generation of ammonia from glutamine by renal tubular cells.

excretion of ≈60% (30 to 60 mmol) of the hydrogen ions. Finally, the α-oxoglutarate produced in this reaction is converted to bicarbonate (up to 270 mmol/d) that helps replenish bicarbonate neutralized by metabolic acid production. The amount of H^+ excreted bound to NH_3 can be measured as NH_4^+. The H^+ required for NH_4^+ formation may be present in the glomerular filtrate or may be generated within tubular cells by carbonic anhydrase synthesis of carbonic acid from CO_2 (see Figs. 60-11 and 60-12). These H^+ ions are secreted into the tubular lumen through the Na^+-H^+ exchangers (see Fig. 60.11).

Excretion of Hydrogen as Dihydrogen Phosphate

H^+ secreted into the tubular lumen by the Na^+-H^+ exchanger also may react with hydrogen phosphate (HPO_4^-) to form dihydrogen phosphate ($H_2PO_4^{2-}$) (see Fig. 60.11). Under normal physiologic conditions, ≈30 mmol of H^+ is excreted per day as $H_2PO_4^-$. Acidemia increases phosphate excretion and thus provides additional buffer for reaction with H^+. A decrease in the glomerular filtration rate (GFR) results in a decrease in $H_2PO_4^-$ excretion.

Reclamation of Filtered Bicarbonate

The unmodified glomerular filtrate has the same concentration of HCO_3^- as plasma does; however, with increasing acidification of proximal tubular urine, the HCO_3^- concentration is decreased. Excreted H^+ reacts with HCO_3^- (catalyzed by carbonic anhydrase, in the brush border of the proximal tubular cells) to form H_2CO_3 and subsequently CO_2 and H_2O (Fig. 60.13).

This increase in urinary CO_2 causes CO_2 to diffuse across the tubular cell membrane into the tubular cell, where it

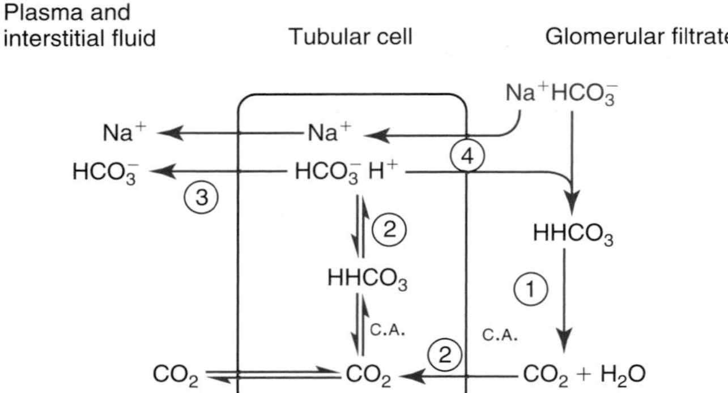

FIGURE 60.13 Reclamation of bicarbonate by tubular cells. *1,* Formation of CO_2 from bicarbonate in the tubular fluid; *2,* formation of H^+ and HCO_3^- from CO_2 in the tubular cell; *3,* new generation of HCO_3^-; and *4,* Na^+-H^+ exchange.

reacts with H_2O in the presence of cytoplasmic carbonic anhydrase to form H_2CO_3 and subsequently H^+ and HCO_3^- (see Fig. 60.13). Thus reclamation of bicarbonate consists of diffusion of CO_2 into tubular cells and its subsequent conversion to HCO_3^-. The increase in HCO_3^- helps maintain or restore a normal pH in the circulation. Normally, ≈90% of filtered HCO_3^- (or ~4500 mmol/d) is reclaimed in the proximal tubule, which parallels Na^+ reabsorption. Thus, for each mmol H^+ secreted into the tubular fluid, 1 mmol Na^+ and 1 mmol HCO_3^- enter the tubular cell and return to the general circulation. When plasma HCO_3^- concentration increases above ≈28 mmol/L, the capacity of the proximal and distal tubules to reclaim HCO_3^- is exceeded and HCO_3^- is excreted in the urine. RTA type 2 is caused by a decreased ability to reabsorb HCO_3^- in the proximal tubules, leading to a decrease in blood pH.

CONDITIONS ASSOCIATED WITH ABNORMAL ACID-BASE STATUS AND ABNORMAL ELECTROLYTE COMPOSITION OF THE BLOOD

Abnormalities in acid-base status of the blood are always accompanied by characteristic changes in electrolyte concentrations in the plasma. H^+ ions cannot accumulate without concomitant accumulation of anions, such as Cl^- or lactate, or without exchange for cations, such as K^+ or Na^+. Consequently, the electrolyte composition of blood serum or plasma is often determined along with measurements of blood gases and pH to assess acid-base disturbances.

Acid-base disturbances are traditionally classified as (1) metabolic acidosis, (2) metabolic alkalosis, (3) respiratory acidosis, or (4) respiratory alkalosis. In simple, straightforward acid-base disorders, the laboratory parameters observed for these groups are shown in Table 60.3. However, interpretation of laboratory values to classify these disorders is rarely straightforward because of compensatory responses by the respiratory and renal systems.

A logical approach to the classification of acid-base disorders is to consider that an acidosis can occur only as the result of one (or a combination) of three mechanisms: (1) increased addition of acid, (2) decreased elimination of acid, and (3) increased loss of base. Similarly, alkalosis occurs only by (1) increased addition of base, (2) decreased elimination of base, and (3) increased loss of acid. Dufour[25] illustrated this simple concept by depicting the body as a two-tank vat, one of acid and one of base, with inputs and outputs for each vat (Fig. 60.14).

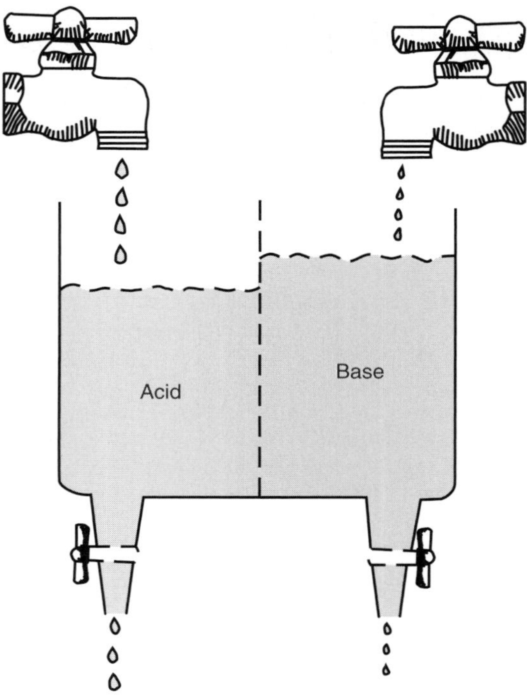

FIGURE 60.14 Simple depiction of the body as a two-vat system of acid and base. At equilibrium, input and output from each vat are equal. (From Dufour DR. Acid-base disorders. In: Dufour DR, Christenson RH, editors: *Professional practice in clinical chemistry: a review.* Washington, DC: AACC Press; 1995:604–635.)

Metabolic Acidosis (Primary Bicarbonate Deficit)

Metabolic acidosis is readily detected by decreased plasma bicarbonate (or a negative extracellular base excess)—the primary perturbation in this acid-base disorder.[26] Causes include the following:

1. Increased production of organic acids that exceeds the rate of elimination (eg, production of acetoacetic acid and β-hydroxybutyric acid in diabetic ketoacidosis). Bicarbonate is "lost" in the buffering of excess acid.
2. Reduced excretion of acids (H^+) as occurs in renal failure and some RTAs, resulting in an accumulation of acid that consumes bicarbonate.
3. Excessive loss of bicarbonate secondary to increased renal excretion (decreased tubular reclamation) or excessive loss of duodenal fluid (as in diarrhea). Plasma $cHCO_3^-$ falls; the fall is associated with a rise in the concentration of inorganic anions (mostly chloride) or, rarely, a concomitant fall in the sodium concentration.

When any of these conditions exists, the ratio of $cHCO_3^-/cCO_2$ is decreased because of the primary decrease in bicarbonate. The resulting drop in pH stimulates respiratory compensation via hyperventilation, which lowers PCO_2 in order to raise the pH.

TABLE 60.3 Classification and Characteristics of Simple Acid-Base Disorders

	Primary Change	Compensatory Response	Expected Compensation
Metabolic			
Acidosis	↓$cHCO_3^-$	↓ PCO_2	$PCO_2 = 1.5\,(cHCO_3^-) + 8 \pm 2$ PCO_2 falls by 1 to 1.3 mm Hg for each mmol/L fall in $cHCO_3^-$ Last two digits of pH = PCO_2 (eg, if PCO_2 = 28, pH = 7.28) $cHCO_3^-$ + 15 = last two digits of pH ($cHCO_3^-$ = 15, pH = 7.30)
Alkalosis	↑$cHCO_3^-$	↑ PCO_2	PCO_2 increases 6 mm Hg for each 10-mmol/L rise in $cHCO_3^-$ $cHCO_3^-$ + 15 = last 2 digits of pH ($cHCO_3^-$ = 35, pH = 7.50)
Respiratory			
Acidosis			
Acute	↑ PCO_2	↑$cHCO_3^-$	$cHCO_3^-$ increases by 1 mmol/L for each 10-mm Hg rise in PCO_2
Chronic	↑ PCO_2	↑$cHCO_3^-$	$cHCO_3^-$ increases by 3.5 mmol/L for each 10-mm Hg rise in PCO_2
Alkalosis			
Acute	↓ PCO_2	↓$cHCO_3^-$	$cHCO_3^-$ falls by 2 mmol/L for each 10-mm Hg fall in PCO_2
Chronic	↓ PCO_2	↓$cHCO_3^-$	$cHCO_3^-$ falls by 5 mmol/L for each 10-mm Hg fall in PCO_2

From Narins RG, Gardner LB. Simple acid-base disturbances. *Med Clin North Am* 1981;65:321–346.

TABLE 60.4 Conditions of Metabolic Acidoses With High and Normal Anion Gaps

Cause	Retained Acid(s)	Other Laboratory Findings
High Anion Gap (MUD PILES)		
Methanol	Formate	↑ Osmolal gap (>15 mOsmol/kg)
Uremia	Sulfuric, phosphoric, organic	↑ Urea and serum creatinine
Diabetes mellitus	Acetoacetate and β-hydroxybutyrate	↑ Plasma and urine glucose, hydroxybutyrate
Paraldehyde toxicity/ Paracetamol (acetaminophen)	Acetate, chloracetate/pyroglutamate (5-oxoproline)	
Isoniazid or Iron	Organic, mainly lactate	
Lactic acidosis	Lactate	
Ethylene glycol	Hippurate, glycolate, oxalate	↑ Osmolal gap (>15 mOsmol/kg), urine oxalate crystals
Salicylate	Salicylate	Respiratory alkalosis
Normal Anion Gap		
Gastrointestinal fluid loss/diarrhea	Primary loss of bicarbonate	Hypokalemia
Acetazolamide	Bicarbonate wasting	
Renal tubular acidosis		
Type 1	Decreased H^+ secretion	Hypokalemia
Type 2	Bicarbonate wasting	Hypokalemia
Type 4	Aldosterone deficiency or resistance	Hyperkalemia
Pancreatitis		
Pancreatic fistula	Bicarbonate wasting	

Increased Anion Gap Acidosis (Organic Acidosis)

Metabolic acidoses are classified as those associated with an increased anion gap or a normal anion gap (Table 60.4). The concept of the anion gap was originally devised as a quality control rule when it was noted that if the sum of Cl^- and HCO_3^- values was subtracted from the Na^+ values ($Na^+ - [Cl^- + HCO_3^-]$), the difference, or "gap," averaged 12 mmol/L in healthy subjects.[27] This apparent gap is due to unmeasured anions (eg, proteins, SO_4^{2-}, $H_2PO_4^{2-}$) that are present in plasma. In reality, unmeasured cations (calcium, magnesium, organic cations) should be included in the equation with sodium and potassium, but their concentration in the blood is relatively small compared with circulating sodium concentrations. The anion gap is increased in most patients with a metabolic acidosis. The presence of an increased anion gap is often the first indication of a metabolic acidosis and should be assessed in the electrolyte profiles of all patients.[27] The gap is also slightly increased in the absence of acidosis by very low calcium, magnesium, or potassium concentrations, because lower concentrations of these "unmeasured" cations will result in lower values of anions (Fig. 60.15).

All anion gap metabolic acidoses, besides inborn errors of metabolism, can be explained by one (or a combination) of

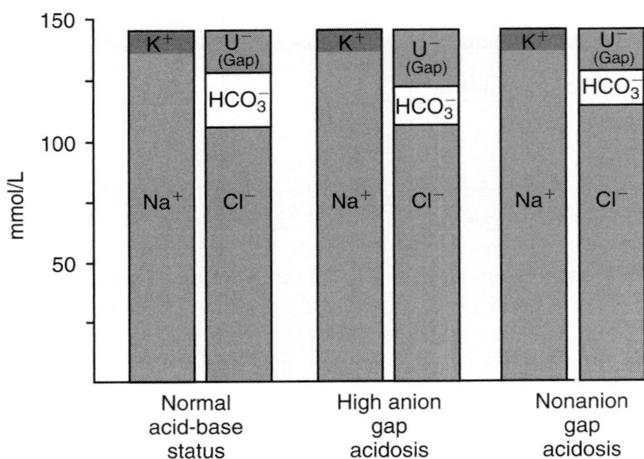

FIGURE 60.15 Simple "Gambelgram" depiction of normal gap, anion gap acidosis, and nonanion gap acidosis. Cations, Na^+ and K^+, are in *left bar* for each condition, whereas measured (Cl^- and HCO_2^-) and unmeasured (U^-) anions are in *right bar* for each condition.

BOX 60.1 A New Mnemonic for High Anion Gap Acidosis (GOLD MARK)

G	Glycols (ethylene and propylene)
O	Oxoproline
L	L-Lactate
D	D-Lactate (short-bowel syndrome)
M	Methanol
A	Aspirin
R	Renal failure
K	Ketoacids

eight underlying mechanisms listed here according to the common mnemonic device MUDPILES (see Table 60.4).[28] The physiologic basis for the anion gap in these conditions is the consumption of bicarbonate in buffering excess acid. Cl^- values remain normal when the excess acid is any other than HCl, because lost bicarbonate is replaced by unmeasured anions. It should be mentioned that a new mnemonic for increased anion gap acidosis has been suggested: GOLD MARK[28] (Box 60.1).

Methanol. Although nontoxic itself, methanol is metabolized by the liver to formaldehyde and formic acid. Accumulation of this acid leads to metabolic acidosis with a high anion gap and to clinical symptoms of optic papillitis ("snowfield" blindness), retinal edema, and ultimately blindness caused by optic nerve atrophy, as well as neurologic defects that may lead to coma. Methanol and other ingested alcohols such as ethylene glycol, ethanol, and isopropanol will increase the osmolality of plasma. Thus, in the presence of a high anion gap acidosis, determination of the osmolal gap (see Chapter 35) will help determine the source of the unmeasured anion and may suggest specific toxicologic analyses.[29] Toxic alcohol ingestions are often treated with fomepizole, which competitively inhibits alcohol dehydrogenase and reduces the generation of toxic metabolites. Hemodialysis also may be required to remove high concentrations of accumulated alcohols directly from the bloodstream.

Uremia of Renal Failure. Loss of functional renal tubular mass results in decreased ammonia formation, decreased Na^+-H^+ exchange, and decreased GFR. All lead to decreased acid excretion (see Chapter 59). Acidosis usually develops if GFR falls below 20 mL/min. Serum creatinine and urea concentrations usually are increased and are used as an estimate of the degree of renal damage or, more appropriately, as an estimate of remaining functional renal capacity. Although the presence of mild acidosis alone can be managed conservatively in chronic kidney disease, the presence of other uremic symptoms, including intractable nausea, vomiting, and fatigue, are indications for the initiation of dialysis.

Diabetes or Ketoacidosis. The pathogenesis of ketoacidosis is discussed in detail in Chapter 57. Ketoacids such as β-hydroxybutyrate and 2-oxoglutarate accumulate and represent the unmeasured anions. Accumulation of these ketone bodies causes a decrease in HCO_3^-, a normal serum chloride, and a high anion gap. Ketoacids also accumulate in states of starvation and alcoholic malnutrition. Treatment is directed at the process that is generating the ketoacids, most commonly insulin deficiency or starvation.

Paraldehyde or Paracetamol (Pyroglutamic Acid). Historically used as a treatment for alcohol withdrawal, paraldehyde is not common today. Paraldehyde toxicity may develop after chronic paraldehyde ingestion. The pathogenesis is poorly defined, but the acidosis may actually be a ketosis (nitroprusside negative) with β-hydroxybutyric acid as the main acidic product as well as acetic and chloracetic acid.[27] Patients with paraldehyde toxicity have a pungent, apple-like odor to their breath.

Chronic paracetamol (acetaminophen in the United States) use by patients with decreased glutathione stores can lead to an accumulation of pyroglutamic acid (5-oxoproline) that results in an anion gap.[30] Pyroglutamic acid is an intracellular intermediate in the γ-glutamyl cycle that is glutathione dependent. An anion gap acidosis usually develops only in chronic paracetamol users that have other co-morbidities such as malnutrition, chronic renal failure, or liver disease. Cessation of the drug is mandatory.

Isoniazid, Iron, or Ischemia. These seemingly unrelated causes of high anion gap acidosis share a common feature: the accumulation of organic acids, with a predominance of lactic acid. Thus the "three Is" actually represent special cases in the general category of lactic acidosis, which is described next. Both isoniazid, an antimycobacterial agent commonly used in the treatment or prophylaxis of tuberculosis, and iron toxicity involve the production of toxic peroxides that act as mitochondrial poisons and interfere with normal cellular respiration. In addition, isoniazid may be hepatotoxic, leading to significant liver damage and impairment of lactate clearance.[27]

Tissue ischemia may result from many causes; in general, hypoperfusion leads to hypoxia of cells, resulting in anaerobic metabolism with accumulation of organic (mainly lactic) acids.

Lactic Acidosis. Lactic acid, present in blood as the lactate ion ($pK = 3.86$), is an intermediate of carbohydrate metabolism that is derived mainly from muscle cells and erythrocytes (see Chapter 33). It represents the end product of anaerobic metabolism and is normally metabolized by the liver. Therefore, blood lactate concentration is affected by the rate of production and the rate of metabolism, both of which depend on adequate tissue perfusion. An increase in the concentration of lactate to greater than 3 mmol/L with the associated increase in H^+ is considered lactic acidosis.[11]

Lactic acidosis caused by severe tissue hypoxia is seen in severe anemia, shock, cardiac arrest, and pulmonary insufficiency. Severe oxygen deprivation of tissue blocks aerobic oxidation of pyruvic acid in the tricarboxylic acid cycle, resulting in the reduction of pyruvate to form lactate. Extreme deterioration of the cellular oxidative process is associated with marked tachypnea, weakness, fatigue, stupor, and finally coma. Conditions at these later stages are frequently irreversible, even if treatment is instituted. If the source of lactate can be rectified, lactate is rapidly metabolized to CO_2, which then is eliminated by an intact respiratory system.

Lactic acidosis may be caused by (1) drugs and toxins such as ethanol, methanol, isoniazid, metformin, and excess iron; (2) acquired and hereditary defects in enzymes involved in gluconeogenesis; (3) disorders such as uremia, liver failure, tumors, and seizures; (4) anesthesia; and (5) abnormal intestinal bacteria producing D-lactate. Most common methods for lactate do not detect D-lactate acidosis; this form of lactic acidosis should be considered only in patients with short-bowel syndromes or after other gastrointestinal surgeries resulting in "blind loops."[31] Treatment is directed toward the underlying cause of lactic acid accumulation. Extracorporeal removal of lactate through dialysis has not been shown to be effective.

During vigorous, anaerobic exercise, lactate concentrations may increase significantly from an average normal concentration of ≈0.9 mmol/L to ≈12 mmol/L. However, under healthy conditions, the lactate is rapidly metabolized to CO_2, so the "acidosis" is transient only as hyperventilation eliminates the CO_2.

Lactate in spinal fluid normally parallels blood values. In cases of biochemical alterations in the CNS system, however, CSF lactate values change independently of blood values. Increased CSF lactate concentrations may be seen in intracranial hemorrhage, bacterial meningitis, epilepsy, and other CNS disorders.[2]

Ethylene Glycol. Ingested ethylene glycol is metabolized primarily to glycolic and oxalic acids. Its metabolism leads to an acidosis with high anion and osmolal gaps. Accumulation of toxic metabolites also may contribute to lactic acid production that further contributes to the acidosis. Precipitation of calcium oxalate and hippurate crystals in the urinary tract may lead to acute renal failure. Clinically, patients develop a variety of neurologic symptoms that may lead to coma. Treatment of alcohol toxicities has been described previously (see "Methanol")

Salicylate Intoxication. Acidosis generally occurs with blood salicylate concentrations above 30 mg/dL (2.1 mmol/L). Salicylate, itself an unmeasured anion, alters peripheral metabolism, leading to the production of various organic acids. Management of salicylate toxicity can be complex, with a number of superimposed acid-base disturbances occurring simultaneously. Early consultative input from critical care or toxicology is recommended, along with possible nephrology assessment for hemodialysis.

Normal Anion Gap Acidosis (Inorganic Acidosis)

In contrast to high anion gap acidoses, in which bicarbonate is consumed from buffering excess H^+, the cause of acidosis in the presence of a normal anion gap is the loss of bicarbonate-rich fluid from the kidney or the gastrointestinal tract (see Table 60.4). As bicarbonate is lost, more Cl^- ions are reabsorbed with Na^+ or K^+ to maintain electrical neutrality, so that hyperchloremia ensues (see Fig. 60.15). Normal anion gap acidosis can be divided into *hypokalemic, normokalemic,* and *hyperkalemic* acidoses, which can be helpful in the differential diagnosis of this type of disorder (see subsequent section on RTA type 4).

Gastrointestinal Losses. Diarrhea may cause acidosis as a result of loss of Na^+, K^+, and HCO_3^-. One of the primary exocrine functions of the pancreas is production of HCO_3^- to neutralize gastric contents on entry into the duodenum. If the water, K^+, and HCO_3^- in the intestine are not reabsorbed, a hypokalemic, normal anion gap metabolic acidosis will develop. The resulting hyperchloremia is due to replacement of lost bicarbonate with Cl^- to maintain electrical balance.

Renal Tubular Acidoses. These syndromes are characterized by loss of bicarbonate secondary to decreased tubular secretion of H^+ (distal or type 1 RTA) or decreased reabsorption of HCO_3^- (proximal or type 2 RTA).[32] Because the major urine-acidifying power of the kidneys rests in the distal tubules, proximal and distal RTAs may be differentiated by measurement of urine pH after administration of acid. In proximal RTA, urine pH becomes less than 5.5, whereas in distal RTA, the distal tubules are compromised and urine pH is greater than 5.5.[32] RTA type 4 is due to decreased aldosterone or aldosterone resistance leading to decreased Na^+ reabsorption and thus decreased H^+ and K^+ secretion. It can be differentiated from type 1 by the increased K^+.[32]

Carbonic Anhydrase Inhibitors. Acetazolamide is the most commonly used drug in this class of therapeutic agents. It is used for urine alkalinization and in patients with open-angle glaucoma or acute mountain (altitude) sickness.[19] Inhibition of carbonic anhydrase causes wasting of Na^+, K^+, and HCO_3^- in the proximal tubules and represents a pharmacologically induced proximal RTA similar to type 2 RTA.

Compensatory Mechanisms in Metabolic Acidosis

The buffer systems of the blood (mainly the bicarbonate/carbonic acid buffer) minimize changes in pH. In acidoses, the bicarbonate concentration decreases to yield a ratio of $cHCO_3^-/cdCO_2$ or less than 20:1. The respiratory compensatory mechanism responds to correct the ratio with increased rate and depth of respiration to eliminate CO_2. Table 60.3 depicts expected compensation in various cases of acidoses and alkaloses and corresponding laboratory intervals.

Respiratory Compensatory Mechanism. The decrease in pH in metabolic acidosis stimulates hyperventilation (Kussmaul respiration), which results in the elimination of carbonic acid as CO_2, a decrease in PCO_2 (hypocapnia), and thus a decrease in $cdCO_2$. There is also a decrease in $cHCO_3^-$ that is smaller than that in $cdCO_2$. For example, the ratio of $cHCO_3^-/cdCO_2$ might be 16:1.28 (12.5:1) for a pH of 7.2 before compensation, and 14.5:0.9 (16:1) for a pH of 7.30 after compensation (see Fig. 60.8).

Renal Compensatory Mechanism. If possible, the kidneys respond to restore the normal pH through increased excretion of acid and preservation of base (increased rate of Na^+-H^+ exchange, increased ammonia formation, and increased reabsorption of bicarbonate). When the renal compensating mechanisms are functioning, urine acidity and ammonia are increased. The total amount of H^+ excreted may be as great as 500 mmol/d. As a result, $cHCO_3^-/cdCO_2$ will increase, for example, to 22:1.1 (20:1) for a pH of 7.40. This is a fully compensated metabolic acidosis, because the pH has returned to normal; however, acidosis still exists because a process that consumes HCO_3^- persists.

Metabolic Alkalosis (Primary Bicarbonate Excess)

Alkalosis occurs when excess base is added to the system, base elimination is decreased, or acid-rich fluids are lost[25,33] (see At a Glance: Conditions Leading to Metabolic Alkalosis). Any of these can lead to a primary bicarbonate excess, such that the ratio of $cHCO_3^-/cdCO_2$ becomes greater than 20:1. For instance, a primary increase in bicarbonate to 48 mmol/L will alter the $cHCO_3^-/cdCO_2$ to 48:1.5 (32:1) for a pH of 7.6 (see Fig. 60.8). The patient will hypoventilate to raise PCO_2, thereby lowering the pH toward normal. However, hypoxia usually prevents the patient from achieving a PCO_2 greater than 55 mm Hg. Above pH 7.55, tetany may develop, even in the presence of a normal serum total calcium concentration. The cause of the tetany is a decreased concentration of ionized calcium resulting from increased binding of calcium ions by albumin. Measurement of urine Cl^- can be helpful because causes of metabolic alkalosis fall into Cl^- responsive, Cl^- resistant, and exogenous base categories (see Fig. 60.4).

AT A GLANCE

Conditions Leading to Metabolic Alkalosis

Chloride Responsive (Urine Chloride Less Than 10 mmol/L)

- Contraction alkaloses
  - Prolonged vomiting or nasogastric suction
  - Pyloric or upper duodenal obstruction
  - Prolonged or abusive diuretic therapy (loop diuretics)
  - Dehydration
- Posthypercapnic state
- Cystic fibrosis (systemic ineffective reabsorption of Cl^-)

Chloride-Resistant (Urine Cl^- Greater Than 20 mmol/L)

- Mineralocorticoid excess
  - Primary hyperaldosteronism (adrenal adenoma or, rarely, carcinoma)
  - Bilateral adrenal hyperplasia
  - Secondary hyperaldosteronism
  - Congenital adrenal hyperplasia (resulting from adrenal enzyme deficiencies in cortisol production (11β- or 17α-hydroxylase)]
- Glucocorticoid excess
  - Primary adrenal adenoma (Cushing'syndrome)
  - Pituitary adenoma secreting adrenocorticotropic hormone (Cushing' disease)
  - Exogenous cortisol therapy
  - Excessive licorice ingestion
- Bartter syndrome (defective renal Cl^- reabsorption)

Exogenous Base

- Iatrogenic
  - Bicarbonate-containing intravenous fluid therapy
  - Massive blood transfusion (sodium citrate overload)
  - Antacids and cation-exchange resins in dialysis patients
  - High-dose carbenicillin or penicillin (associated with hypokalemia)
- Milk-alkali syndrome

Chloride-Responsive Metabolic Alkalosis

Most cases of Cl^--responsive metabolic alkalosis occur as a result of hypovolemia. When the ECF is severely depleted, the resulting acid-base disorder is often referred to as contraction alkalosis. Hypovolemia will result in increased reabsorption of Na^+, along with increased absorption and excretion of K^+ and H^+. Urine Cl^- will be less than 10 mmol/L because both the available Cl^- and HCO_3^- are reabsorbed with Na^+. Urine Na^+ is not useful for classifying metabolic alkalosis, because an obligatory loss of Na^+ will occur when filtered HCO_3^- exceeds reclamation. Common causes of contraction alkalosis include prolonged vomiting or nasogastric suction, pyloric or upper duodenal obstruction, and the use of certain diuretics. After prolonged vomiting or gastric suction, excessive loss of hydrochloric acid from the stomach and hypovolemia occur. In this hypochloremic, hypovolemic setting, the kidneys preferentially reabsorb Na^+ to restore volume, and excess bicarbonate is reabsorbed in the absence of sufficient Cl^- to maintain electrical neutrality. In addition, H^+ and K^+ are secreted in exchange for Na^+. Urine Cl^- will be less than 10 mmol/L in this setting (see Fig. 60.4). Treatment consists of replacing TBW with water and NaCl tablets or saline infusion.

Diuretic Therapy. Prolonged administration of certain diuretics has been known to cause an alkalosis similar to that observed in a hypovolemic setting. Most common are those acting on the ascending limb of the loop of Henle (eg, furosemide [Lasix]) that block sodium, potassium, and chloride reabsorption.[19] The resulting increase in Na^+ concentration reaching the distal convoluted tubule, particularly when combined with activation of the renin-angiotensin-aldosterone axis, leads to increased urinary excretion of K^+ and H^+. Loss of K^+ with furosemide is much greater than with thiazides. Continued abuse or unmonitored use of loop diuretics can lead to volume contraction and a contraction alkalosis. This is commonly seen among those using diuretics for the purpose of weight loss.

Chloride-Resistant Metabolic Alkalosis

This condition is far less common than Cl^--responsive metabolic alkalosis and is almost always associated with an underlying disease (primary hyperaldosteronism, Cushing's syndrome, or Bartter's syndrome) or with excess addition of exogenous base. In these conditions, urine Cl^- will usually be greater than 20 mmol/L.

In states of adrenocortical excess (endogenous or pharmacologic, primary or secondary), K^+ and H^+ are "wasted" by the kidneys as a consequence of increased Na^+ reabsorption stimulated by increased aldosterone or cortisol. The attendant hypokalemia often further contributes to the alkalosis and should be treated with K^+ replacement therapy. The decreased tubular K^+ concentration stimulates NH_3 production and thus renal H^+ excretion as NH_4^+. This is accompanied by enhanced HCO_3^- reabsorption (see Figs. 60-3 and 60-12). Diseases in which endogenous mineralocorticoids, glucocorticoids, or both are increased include primary and secondary hyperaldosteronism, bilateral adrenal hyperplasia, pituitary ACTH-producing adenoma (Cushing's disease), and primary adrenal adenomas producing glucocorticoids (Cushing's syndrome) or aldosterone.

Excessive licorice ingestion may cause a form of Cl^--resistant alkalosis. Black licorice contains glycyrrhizic acid, which inhibits the enzyme 11-β hydroxysteroid dehydrogenase, which catalyzes the conversion of cortisol to cortisone.[34] The excess cortisol exerts a mineralocorticoid effect on the distal tubule aldosterone receptors.

Finally, a rare cause of Cl^--resistant metabolic alkalosis are several genetic (autosomal recessive) defects in Cl^- reabsorption within the thick ascending limb of the loop of Henle—conditions known collectively as Bartter's syndrome.[35]

Exogenous Base

Examples in this category include citrate toxicity after massive blood transfusion, aggressive intravenous therapy with bicarbonate solutions, and ingestion of large quantities of antacids in the treatment of gastritis or peptic ulcer (milk-alkali syndrome).[36] The latter is far less commonly seen since the introduction and now widespread use of H_2-receptor antagonists and proton pump inhibitors.

Compensatory Mechanisms in Metabolic Alkalosis

The compensatory mechanisms for metabolic alkalosis include both respiratory compensation and, if physiologically possible, renal compensation. The increase in pH depresses the respiratory center, causing retention of CO_2 (hypercapnia), which in turn causes an increase in cH_2CO_3 and $cdCO_2$. Thus the ratio of $cHCO_3^-/cdCO_2$, which was originally increased, approaches its normal value, although the actual concentrations of both $cHCO_3^-$ and $cdCO_2$ remain increased. The kidneys respond to the state of alkalosis by decreased Na^+-H^+ exchange, decreased formation of ammonia, and decreased reclamation of bicarbonate. This response is blunted, however, in conditions of hypokalemia and hypovolemia.

Laboratory Findings in Metabolic Alkalosis

Plasma values for $cHCO_3^-$, $cdCO_2$, and PCO_2, and therefore the plasma total CO_2 concentration, are increased, and the ratio of $cHCO_3^-/cdCO_2$ is high. In uncomplicated metabolic alkalosis, the PCO_2 is increased by ≈6 mm Hg for each 10 mmol/L rise in $cHCO_3^-$. A higher than expected PCO_2 may indicate superimposed respiratory acidosis. The extent of increase in pH in uncompensated metabolic alkalosis can be estimated by adding 15 to the $cHCO_3^-$ to give the last two digits of the pH. If the $cHCO_3^-$ is 35 mmol/L, the estimated pH would be 7.50 (35 + 15 = 50). In cases of prolonged vomiting, Cl^- (and sometimes K^+) concentrations are low because of loss of these ions through the vomitus. Protein values may be increased owing to dehydration, and if food intake is inadequate, formation of ketoacids may increase the organic acid fraction. In cases of excessive administration of $NaHCO_3$, Na^+ concentrations are increased.

In patients with adequate renal function, urinary pH values are usually increased as the result of decreased excretion of acid and increased excretion of bicarbonate. Urinary ammonium values are decreased because of decreased formation of ammonium in the tubules.

Respiratory Acidosis

Any condition that decreases elimination of CO_2 through the lungs results in an increase in PCO_2 (hypercapnia) and dCO_2 (respiratory acidosis). Thus respiratory acidosis occurs only through decreased elimination of CO_2. Causes of decreased CO_2 elimination (See At a Glance: Conditions Leading to Respiratory Acidosis) are classified as acute or chronic.

POINTS TO REMEMBER

- In determining the differential for an anion gap acidosis, two mnemonic devices MUDPILES and GOLDMARK can be helpful (see Table 60.1 and Box 60.1).
- Volume depletion is very often accompanied by a hypochloremic metabolic alkalosis.
- Normal anion gap acidosis is due to loss of bicarbonate-rich fluid via the gastrointestinal tract (diarrhea) (pancreatic fistula) or the renal tubular acidoses.

Alternatively, these conditions may be separated into those caused by factors that directly depress the respiratory center (such as centrally acting drugs, CNS trauma, or infection) and those that affect the respiratory apparatus or cause mechanical obstruction of the airways. Chronic obstructive pulmonary disease (COPD) is the most common cause. An increase in PCO_2 results in an increase in $cdCO_2$ (and thus H_2CO_3, which dissociates to H^+ and HCO_3^-), which in turn causes a decrease in the $cHCO_3^-/cdCO_2$ ratio (eg, the ratio may be 28 : 1.7 [16 : 1] for a pH of ≈7.30; see Fig. 60.8). Doubling of PCO_2 will cause a fall in pH of approximately 0.23 when other factors remain constant.

AT A GLANCE

Conditions Leading to Respiratory Acidosis

Factors That Directly Depress the Respiratory Center
- Narcotics and barbiturates
- CNS trauma, tumors, and degenerative disorders
- Infections of the CNS such as encephalitis and meningitis
- Comatose states such as cerebrovascular accident secondary to intracranial hemorrhage
- Primary central hypoventilation

Conditions That Affect the Respiratory Apparatus
- COPD (most common cause)
- Severe pulmonary fibrosis
- Status asthmaticus (severe)
- Disease of the upper airways such as laryngospasm or tumor
- Pulmonary infection (severe)
- Impaired lung motion secondary to pleural effusion or pneumothorax
- Acute respiratory distress syndrome
- Chest wall disease and chest wall deformity
- Neurologic disorders affecting the muscles of respiration
- Opioids

Others
- Abdominal distention, as in peritonitis and ascites
- Extreme obesity (pickwickian syndrome)
- Sleep disorders such as sleep apnea

Compensatory Mechanisms in Respiratory Acidosis

Compensation for respiratory acidosis occurs immediately via buffers, and over time via the kidneys and, if possible, the lungs. Excess carbonic acid present in blood is buffered to a great extent by the Hb and protein buffer systems[3] (see Fig. 60.9). Buffering of CO_2 causes a slight rise in $cHCO_3^-$.

Thus, in the immediate posthypercapnic state, this compensation may appear as a metabolic alkalosis. The kidneys respond to respiratory acidosis similarly to the way they respond to metabolic acidosis, namely, with (1) increased Na^+-H^+ exchange, (2) increased ammonia formation, and (3) increased reclamation of bicarbonate. In a partially compensated chronic respiratory acidosis at steady state, the plasma pH is returned approximately halfway toward normal compared with the acute (uncompensated) situation. Renal compensation is not effective before 6 to 12 hours and is not optimal until 2 to 3 days. In chronic respiratory acidosis, such as occurs in patients with COPD, full renal compensation may be seen even in patients with very high PCO_2 (>50 mm Hg). However, patients with severe COPD often present with a superimposed metabolic alkalosis arising from a variety of causes, such as prolonged administration of diuretics.

The increase in PCO_2 stimulates the respiratory center, resulting in an increased pulmonary rate and depth of respiration, provided that the primary defect is not in the respiratory center. Elimination of CO_2 through the lungs results in a decrease in $cdCO_2$; thus the ratio of $cHCO_3^-/cdCO_2$ and pH approach normal.

Laboratory Findings in Respiratory Acidosis

Plasma $cdCO_2$, PCO_2, $cHCO_3^-$, and therefore $ctCO_2$ are increased in respiratory acidoses. Because of an increase in $cdCO_2$, the ratio of $cHCO_3^-/cdCO_2$ is decreased, resulting in a decreased pH. In the acute phase, $cHCO_3^-$ will increase by ≈1 mmol/L for each 10 mm Hg rise in PCO_2. If respiratory acidosis persists, the change will be ≈3.5 mmol/L, mainly as a result of renal compensation. For every increase in PCO_2 of 25 mm Hg, pH decreases in the acute phase by ≈0.10 pH unit and in chronic conditions by slightly less than 0.05 pH unit. For example, if the PCO_2 increases acutely by 30 mm Hg, the pH drops to ≈7.20. The same PCO_2 increase in a chronic condition results in a pH of ≈7.31. The plasma chloride decreases as plasma bicarbonate increases. Hyperkalemia may occur but is not as predictable as in some forms of metabolic acidosis. For every 0.1-unit decrease in pH, there is generally an inverse change of 0.6 mmol/L in K^+. Urinary acidity and ammonium content are increased as the kidney attempts to compensate.

Respiratory Alkalosis

A decrease in PCO_2 (hypocapnia) and the resulting primary deficit in $cdCO_2$ (respiratory alkalosis) are caused by an increased rate and/or depth of respiration. Therefore the basic cause of respiratory alkalosis is excess elimination of acid by the respiratory route. Excessive elimination of CO_2 reduces the PCO_2 and causes an increase in the $cHCO_3^-/cdCO_2$ ratio. The latter shifts the normal equilibrium of the bicarbonate/carbonic acid buffer system, reducing the hydrogen ion concentration and increasing the pH. This shift also results in a decrease in $cHCO_3^-$, which somewhat ameliorates the change in pH. Analogous to causes of respiratory acidosis, causes of respiratory alkalosis can be classified as those with a direct stimulatory effect on the respiratory center and those resulting from effects on the pulmonary system. These and some additional conditions underlying respiratory alkaloses are listed in At a Glance: Factors Causing Respiratory Alkalosis.

POINTS TO REMEMBER

- Respiratory acidosis results in an increased PCO_2 secondary to the inability of the lungs to eliminate CO_2.
- Respiratory alkalosis is result of excess elimination of CO_2 via hyperventilation.
- Respiratory compensatory mechanisms in primary metabolic acidosis or alkalosis settings should not be interpreted as respiratory disorders.

AT A GLANCE

Factors Causing Respiratory Alkalosis

Nonpulmonary Stimulation of Respiratory Center

- Anxiety, hysteria
- Febrile state
- Gram-negative septicemia
- Metabolic encephalopathy (eg, secondary to liver disease)
- CNS infection such as meningitis and encephalitis
- Cerebrovascular accident
- Intracranial surgery
- Hypoxia (eg, severe anemia, high altitudes [acute condition])
- Drugs and agents such as salicylates, catecholamines, and progesterone
- Pregnancy, mainly third trimester (increased progesterone?)
- Hyperthyroidism

Pulmonary Disorders*

- Pneumonia
- Pulmonary emboli
- Interstitial lung disease
- Large right-to-left shunt (PCO_2 <50 mm Hg)
- Congestive heart failure
- Respiratory compensation after correction of metabolic acidosis

Others

- Ventilator-induced hyperventilation

*The severe stages of some of these disorders may be associated with respiratory acidosis if elimination of CO_2 is severely impaired.

Compensatory Mechanisms in Respiratory Alkalosis

The compensatory mechanisms respond to respiratory alkalosis in two stages. In the first stage, erythrocyte and tissue buffers provide H^+ ions that consume a small amount of HCO_3^-. The second stage becomes operational in prolonged respiratory alkalosis and depends on renal compensation as described for metabolic alkalosis (decreased reclamation of bicarbonate).

Laboratory Findings in Respiratory Alkalosis

In this condition, $cdCO_2$, PCO_2, $cHCO_3^-$, and thus total CO_2 concentration, all decrease. The ratio of $cHCO_3^-/cdCO_2$ is increased, causing an increase in pH. During the acute phase, $cHCO_3^-$ falls by 2 mmol/L for each decrease of 10 mm Hg in PCO_2 (ie, if the PCO_2 falls by 20 mm Hg, $cHCO_3^-$ is decreased by 4 mmol/L). For the same decrease of 20 mm Hg in PCO_2, the (H^+) will decrease by 16 nmol/L. The resulting alkalosis (lower H^+) will result in a greater binding of Ca^{2+} by albumin and a lower free Ca^{2+}, which can lead to hypocalcemic symptoms of tetany such as Chvostek's and Trousseu's signs (see Chapter 64).

If the original cH^+ was 40 nmol/L, it would now be 24 nmol/L (40 − 16 = 24), which corresponds to a pH of 7.61 (see Fig. 60.6). Finally, individuals living at high altitudes chronically hyperventilate because of hypoxia and have PCO_2 values lower than those seen at sea level.

REFERENCES

1. Ruth JL, Wassner SJ. Body composition: salt and water. *Pediatr Rev* 2006;**27**:181–7, quiz 8.
2. Watson MA, Scott MG. Clinical utility of biochemical analysis of cerebrospinal fluid. *Clin Chem* 1995;**41**:343–60.
3. Figge J, Rossing TH, Fencl V. The role of serum proteins in acid-base equilibria. *J Lab Clin Med* 1991;**117**:453–67.
4. Nguyen MK, Kurtz I. Quantitative interrelationship between Gibbs-Donnan equilibrium, osmolality of body fluid compartments, and plasma water sodium concentration. *J Appl Physiol* 2006;**100**:1293–300.
5. Putney LK, Denker SP, Barber DL. The changing face of the Na^+/H^+ exchanger, NHE1: structure, regulation, and cellular actions. *Annu Rev Pharmacol Toxicol* 2002;**42**:527–52.
6. Palmer BF. Approach to fluid and electrolyte disorders and acid-base problems. *Prim Care* 2008;**35**:195–213, v.
7. Adrogue HJ, Madias NE. Hypernatremia. *N Engl J Med* 2000;**342**:1493–9.
8. Oparil S. Low sodium intake: cardiovascular health benefit or risk? *N Engl J Med* 2014;**371**:677–9.
9. Skott O. Renin. *Am J Physiol Regul Integr Comp Physiol* 2002;**282**:R937–9.
10. Verbalis JG, Goldsmith SR, Greenberg A, et al. Hyponatremia treatment guidelines 2007: expert panel recommendations. *Am J Med* 2007;**120**:S1–21.
11. Jang J, Cheng S. Fluid and electrolyte management. In: Godara H, Hirbe A, Nassif M, et al., editors. *The Washington manual of medical therapeutics*. 34th ed. Philadelphia, PA: Lippincott Williams & Wilkins; 2014.
12. van der Hoek J, Hoorn EJ, de Jong GM, et al. Severe hyponatremia with high urine sodium and osmolality. *Clin Chem* 2009;**55**:1905–8.
13. Ellison DH, Berl T. Clinical practice: the syndrome of inappropriate antidiuresis. *N Engl J Med* 2007;**356**:2064–72.
14. Verbalis JG. Hyponatremia and hypoosmolar disorders. In: Greenberg A, Cheung AK, editors. *Primer on kidney diseases*. Philadelphia, PA: Saunders; 2005. p. 55–65.
15. Robertson GL. Diabetes insipidus. *Endocrinol Metab Clin North Am* 1995;**24**:549–72.
16. Birnbaumer M. The V2 vasopressin receptor mutations and fluid homeostasis. *Cardiovasc Res* 2001;**51**:409–15.
17. Kaplan JH. Biochemistry of Na,K-ATPase. *Annu Rev Biochem* 2002;**71**:511–35.
18. Miltiadous G, Christidis D, Kalogirou M, et al. Causes and mechanisms of acid-base and electrolyte abnormalities in cancer patients. *Eur J Intern Med* 2008;**19**:1–7.
19. Jackson E. Diuretics. In: Hardman JG, Linbird LE, editors. *Goodman and Gilman's the pharmacological basis of therapeutics*. 10th ed. New York: McGraw-Hill; 2001. p. 763–7.
20. Huang CL, Kuo E. Mechanism of hypokalemia in magnesium deficiency. *J Am Soc Nephrol* 2007;**18**:2649–52.
21. Handy JM, Soni N. Physiological effects of hyperchloraemia and acidosis. *Br J Anaesth* 2008;**101**:141–50.
22. Siggaard-Andersen O, Fogh-Andersen N. Base excess or buffer base (strong ion difference) as measure of a non-respiratory acid-base disturbance. *Acta Anaesthesiol Scand Suppl* 1995;**107**:123–8.
23. Siggaard-Andersen O. An acid-base chart for arterial blood with normal and pathophysiological reference areas. *Scand J Clin Lab Invest* 1971;**27**:239–45.
24. Siggaard-Andersen O. The Van Slyke equation. *Scand J Clin Lab Invest Suppl* 1977;**146**:15–20.
25. Dufour DR. Acid-base disorders. In: Dufour R, Christenson RH, editors. *Professional practice in clinical chemistry: a review*. Washington, DC: AACC Press; 1995. p. 604–35.
26. Adrogue HJ, Madias NE. Management of life-threatening acid-base disorders: first of two parts. *N Engl J Med* 1998;**338**:26–34.
27. Rice M, Ismail B, Pillow MT. Approach to metabolic acidosis in the emergency department. *Emerg Med Clin North Am* 2014;**32**:403–20.
28. Mehta AN, Emmett JB, Emmett M. Gold mark: an anion gap mnemonic for the 21st century. *Lancet* 2008;**372**:892.
29. Dorwart WV, Chalmers L. Comparison of methods for calculating serum osmolality from chemical concentrations, and the prognostic value of such calculations. *Clin Chem* 1975;**21**:190–4.
30. Fenves AZ, Kirkpatrick HM 3rd, Patel VV, et al. Increased anion gap metabolic acidosis as a result of 5-oxoproline (pyroglutamic acid): a role for acetaminophen. *Clin J Am Soc Nephrol* 2006;**1**:441–7.
31. Kadakia SC. D-lactic acidosis in a patient with jejunoileal bypass. *J Clin Gastroenterol* 1995;**20**:154–6.
32. Lash JP, Arruda JA. Laboratory evaluation of renal tubular acidosis. *Clin Lab Med* 1993;**13**:117–29.
33. Adrogue HJ, Madias NE. Management of life-threatening acid-base disorders. II. *N Engl J Med* 1998;**338**:107–11.
34. Farese RV Jr, Biglieri EG, Shackleton CH, et al. Licorice-induced hypermineralocorticoidism. *N Engl J Med* 1991;**325**:1223–7.
35. Chesney R. Specific renal tubular disorders. In: Goldman L, Bennett J, editors. *Cecil textbook of medicine*. 21st ed. Philadelphia, PA: WB Saunders; 2000. p. 605–10.
36. Gabriely I, Leu JP, Barzel US. Clinical problem-solving: back to basics. *N Engl J Med* 2008;**358**:1952–6.

61

Liver Disease

*William Rosenberg, Tony Badrick, and Sudeep Tanwar**

ABSTRACT

Background

The liver is the largest and most complex organ in the body. The anatomy of the liver is intricate, and its function is dependent on the close interaction of resident cell lineages; the arterial, venous, and portal vasculature; and the biliary system. The liver plays a central role in numerous biochemical processes, executing metabolic and catabolic functions that are vital for homeostasis and health. Biochemical tests can be used to determine both the cause and prognosis of liver diseases.

Content

This chapter reviews the anatomy and physiology of the liver, the major causes of acute and chronic liver diseases, and the patterns of biochemical test results associated with these disorders.

The chapter describes how the functions of the liver can be investigated through the measurement of the enzymes and proteins it produces and the processes that it regulates. The chapter also explains how clinical chemistry can provide powerful insights into the health of the liver and the likely etiology of disease.

In chronic liver disease, inflammation initiates liver fibrosis, which leads to cirrhosis. This chapter describes how biochemical markers of liver fibrosis can be used to determine both the severity and prognosis of liver disease.

This chapter covers the use of biochemical tests to help determine the etiology, chronicity, severity, and prognosis of a wide range of liver pathologies. Diagnostic strategies that can be used to determine the most likely pathology and probable etiology of the major acute and chronic liver disorders are outlined.

The liver has a central and critical biochemical role in the metabolism, digestion, detoxification, and elimination of substances from the body. All blood from the intestinal tract initially passes through the liver, where products derived from digestion of food are processed, transformed, and (in some cases) stored. These include amino acids, carbohydrates, fatty acids, cholesterol, lipids, vitamins, and minerals (see Chapters 28, 33, 34, and 37, respectively). Most major plasma proteins (with the exception of immunoglobulins [Igs] and the von Willebrand factor) are mainly or exclusively synthesized in the liver. The liver responds to multiple hormonal and neural stimuli to regulate blood glucose concentrations. Not only does it extract glucose from blood for use in generating energy, it also stores dietary glucose as glycogen for later use. The liver is also the major site for gluconeogenesis, which is critical for maintaining blood glucose concentration in the fasting state. The liver is central in lipid metabolism; it extracts and processes dietary lipids, and it is the principal site of cholesterol, triglyceride, and lipoprotein synthesis. Another major liver function is the synthesis of bile acids from cholesterol, with secretion of these compounds into the bile, which facilitates the absorption of dietary fat and fat-soluble vitamins. The liver is also the primary site of metabolism of both endogenous substances and exogenous compounds (eg, drugs and toxins). This process, known as biotransformation, converts lipophilic substances to hydrophilic ones for subsequent elimination. The liver is a major site of catabolism of hormones, and thus participates in regulation of plasma hormone concentrations. The liver is also involved in hormone synthesis, producing such hormones as insulin-like growth factor 1, angiotensinogen, hepcidin, thrombopoietin, erythropoietin, and the prohormone 25-OH vitamin D. Many of these hepatic functions can be assessed by laboratory procedures to gain insight into the integrity of the liver.

As a large organ, the liver shares with many other organs the ability to perform its functions with extensive reserve capacity. In many cases, individuals with liver disease maintain normal function despite extensive liver damage. In such cases, liver disease may be recognized only by using tests that detect injury. Most commonly, this is accomplished by measuring plasma activities of enzymes found within liver cells, which are released in somewhat specific patterns with different forms of injury. Chronic liver injury often involves fibrosis in the liver; markers of the fibrotic process might be indicators of the degree of injury. Chronic damage is often due to chronic inflammation; cytokines alter the pattern of liver protein production, which allows detection of inflammation (although not necessarily that involving the liver). Some proteins are produced in increased amounts with liver regeneration and neoplasia; such markers may be useful in detecting liver cell proliferation.

*The authors gratefully acknowledge the original contributions by Drs. D. Robert Dufour, Keith G. Tolman, and Robert Rej, upon which portions of this chapter are based.

The chapter begins with a discussion of the anatomy and biochemical functions of the liver. Various disease states that involve the liver are then discussed. The chapter concludes with a discussion of the use of laboratory test results in recognizing and characterizing patterns of liver injury.

ANATOMY OF THE LIVER

The adult liver weighs approximately 1.2 to 1.5 kg. It is located beneath the diaphragm in the right upper quadrant of the abdomen and is protected by the ribs and held in place by ligamentous attachments.

Gross Anatomy

The liver is divided into left and right anatomic lobes by the falciform ligament, an anterior extension of the peritoneal folds that connects the liver to the diaphragm and the anterior abdominal wall (Fig. 61.1). Two smaller lobes are found on the posterior surface (caudate lobe) and the inferior surface (quadrate lobe) of the right lobe. Riedel's lobe, an anatomic extension of the right lobe of the liver, consists of a projection that may feel like a mobile tumor in the right abdomen.

The liver has a dual blood supply. The portal vein, which carries blood from the spleen and nutrient-enriched blood from the gastrointestinal (GI) tract, supplies approximately 70% of the blood supply; the hepatic artery, a branch of the celiac axis, provides oxygen-enriched arterial blood. Each supplies approximately half of the oxygen reaching the liver, making it highly resistant to infarction. Ultimately, these two blood supplies merge and flow into the sinusoids that course between individual hepatocytes. Venous drainage from the liver ultimately converges into the right and left hepatic veins, which exit on the posterior surface of the liver and join the inferior vena cava near its entry into the right atrium.

The liver is covered by an anterior reflection of the peritoneum known as Glisson's capsule. Other extensions of

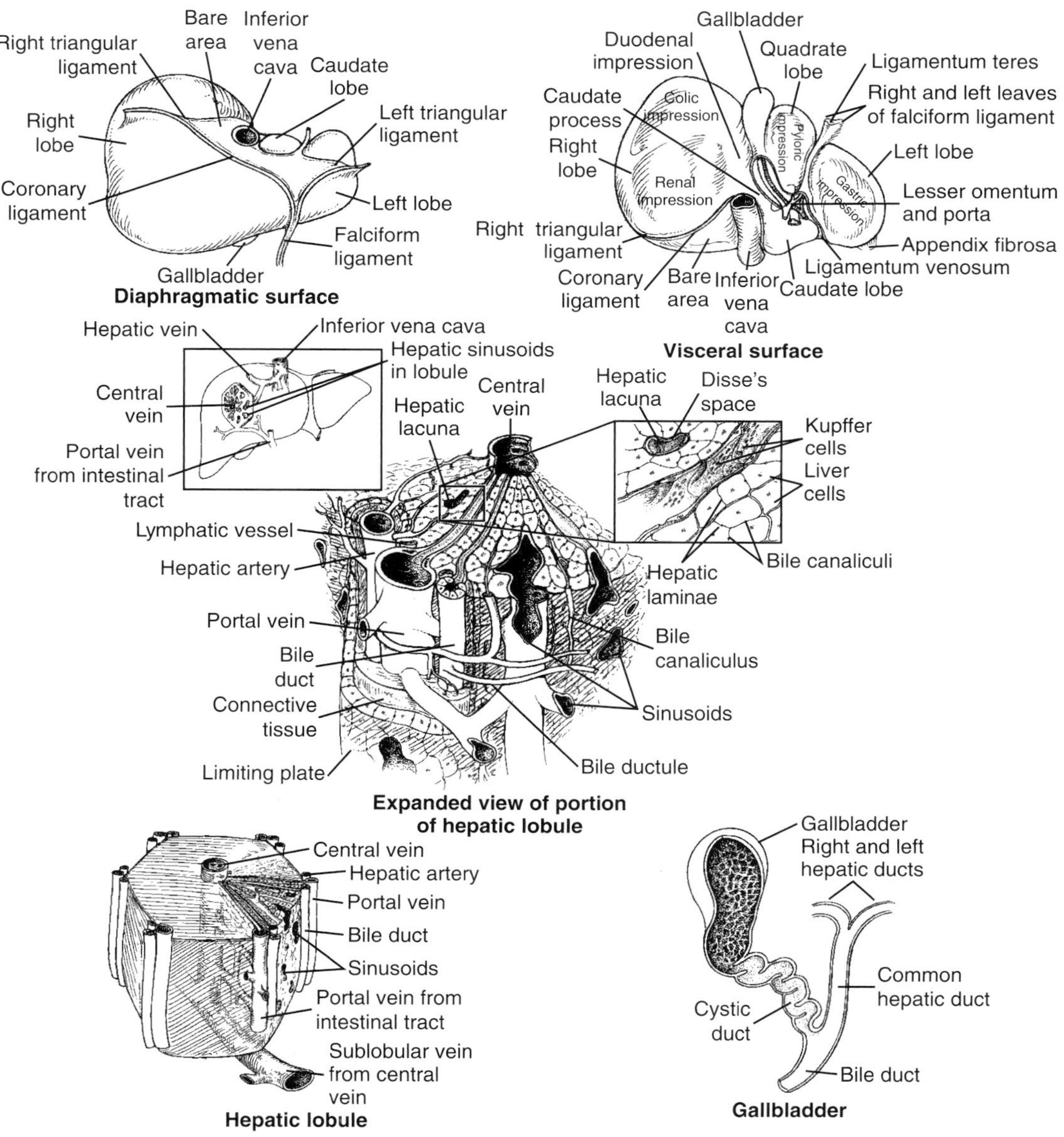

FIGURE 61.1 Structure of the liver. (From *Dorland's Illustrated Medical Dictionary*. 30th ed. Philadelphia: Saunders; 2003, plate 26.)

the peritoneum form ligaments that hold the liver in place. Internal extensions of the capsule provide an internal supporting framework that divides the liver into lobules and ultimately surrounds blood vessels and nerves. One of the ligaments, the ligamentum teres, is the vestigial remnant of the umbilical vein; it connects the umbilicus to the inferior border of the liver. When portal hypertension occurs, the umbilical veins may reopen, leading to venous dilatation around the umbilicus (termed caput medusae).

The nerve supply to the liver comes from the vagus and phrenic nerves, and the sympathetic ganglia originating from cell bodies in the spinal cord that are located between the seventh and tenth thoracic vertebrae. These merge to accompany the hepatic arteries and bile ducts throughout the liver.

Biliary drainage originates at the bile canaliculi; these grooves between adjacent hepatocytes form ductules that merge to create the intrahepatic bile ducts, which ultimately join to form the right and left hepatic bile ducts, which exit from the liver at the porta hepatis and combine to form the common hepatic duct. The hepatic duct is joined by the cystic duct that drains the gallbladder to form the common bile duct (see Fig. 61.1). The common bile duct then enters the duodenum (usually with the pancreatic duct) at the ampulla of Vater. The duodenal portion of the common bile duct is surrounded by longitudinal and circular muscle fibers that form the sphincter of Oddi. This musculature relaxes when the gallbladder contracts, allowing bile to enter the duodenum; in its normally contracted state, the sphincter prevents reflux of acidic duodenal contents into the bile duct. The gallbladder, which is located on the undersurface of the right lobe of the liver, is the site for storage and concentration of bile, a complex mixture of bile salts and waste products. In the adult, it averages approximately 10 cm in length and has a capacity of 30 to 50 mL of bile. Hormonal stimuli initiated by food ingestion cause contraction of the muscular wall of the gallbladder, releasing bile salts into the intestine to facilitate digestion of fat.

Microscopic Anatomy

The functional anatomical unit of the liver is the acinus, which is adjacent to the portal triad (which consists of a branch of each of the portal vein, hepatic artery, and bile duct). Each acinus is a diamond-shaped mass of liver parenchyma that is supplied by a terminal branch of the portal vein and of the hepatic artery, and is drained by a terminal branch of the bile duct. The blood vessels radiate toward the periphery, forming sinusoids, which perfuse the liver and ultimately drain into the central (terminal) hepatic vein (Fig. 61.2). The sinusoids are lined by fenestrated endothelial cells (which allows free filtration of blood) and phagocytic Kupffer cells (see Fig. 61.1). The Kupffer cells are derived from blood monocytes. They contain lysosomes with hydrolytic enzymes that break down phagocytized foreign particles (eg, bacteria). They also have Ig and complement receptors, and are the main site for clearance of antigen–antibody complexes from blood. Kupffer cells secrete interleukins (ILs), tumor necrosis factor (TNF), collagenase, prostaglandins, and other factors involved in inflammatory responses.

Hepatocytes are the major functioning cells in the liver and are responsible for approximately 70% of liver mass. They perform most of the metabolic and synthetic functions of the liver. Two other cell types are found in small numbers within the liver. The stellate cells (sometimes referred to as Ito cells) are located between the endothelial lining of

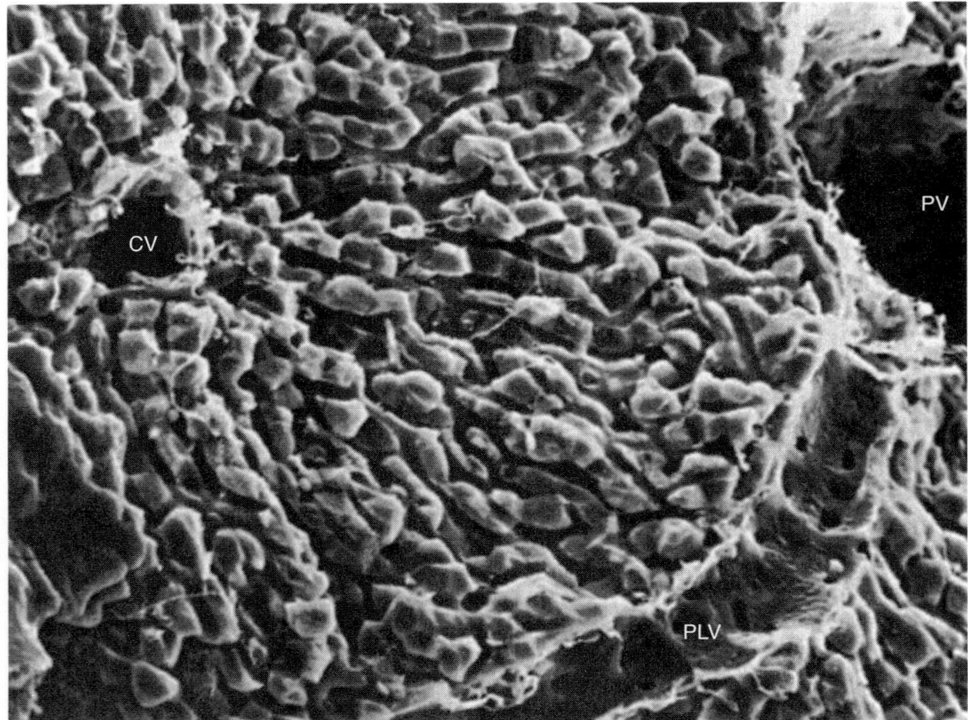

FIGURE 61.2 A low-magnification scanning electron micrograph depicting a portion of a liver lobule from a rat liver. *CV*, Central vein; *PLV*, perilobular venules; *PV*, portal vein. (From Zakim O, Boyer TD. *Hepatology: A Textbook of Liver Disease*. 3rd ed. Philadelphia: WB Saunders; 1996. p. 9.)

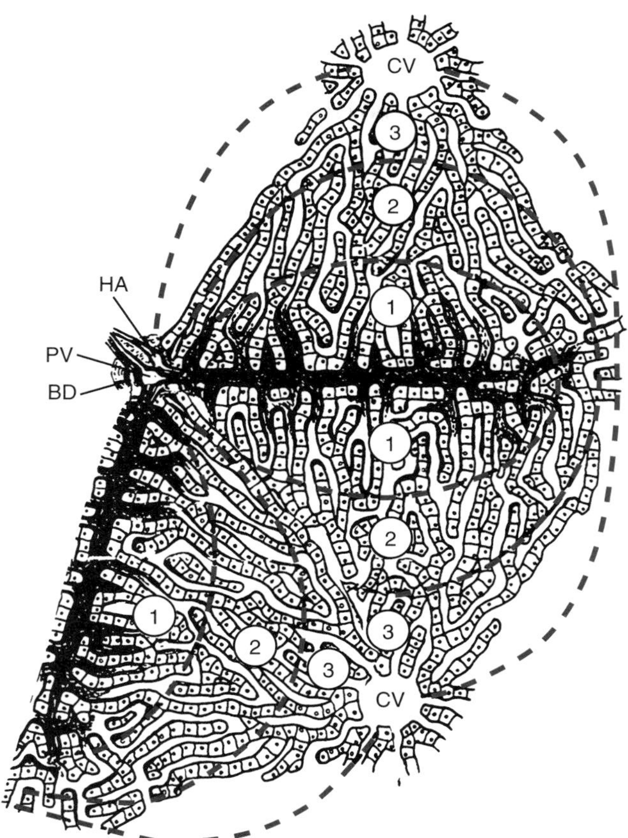

FIGURE 61.3 Blood supply of the simple liver acinus. Zones 1, 2, and 3 indicate corresponding volumes in a portion of an adjacent acinar unit. Oxygen tension and the nutrient level in the blood in sinusoids decrease from zone 1 through zone 3. *BD*, Bile duct; *CV*, central vein; *HA*, hepatic artery; *PV*, portal vein. (From Zakim O, Boyer TD. *Hepatology: A Textbook of Liver Disease.* 3rd ed. Philadelphia: WB Saunders; 1996. p. 10.)

the sinusoids, and the hepatocytes are within a small cleft referred to as the space of Disse. In their normal, quiescent state, stellate cells serve as a site of storage for fat-soluble vitamins, particularly vitamin A. When stimulated, stellate cells are morphologically and functionally transformed. They synthesize collagen and are the cells responsible for fibrosis, and eventually, cirrhosis. They also synthesize nitric oxide, which helps to regulate intrahepatic blood flow. Oval cells, found near the portal areas around small bile passages, are believed to be liver stem cells involved in regeneration of hepatocytes and bile ducts after liver injury.[1]

The blood supply to each acinus consists of three zones (Fig. 61.3). Zone 1, the area immediately adjacent to the portal tract, is enriched with lysosomes and mitochondria. Zone 1 appears to be involved in protecting the liver from external injury and providing a base for hepatic regeneration. Zone 2 predominantly contains hepatocytes that perform the major metabolic functions of the liver. The periphery of the acinus, zone 3, is enriched with endoplasmic reticulum, is active metabolically, and has relatively low oxygen tension. This area is most susceptible to injury.

Ultrastructure of the Hepatocyte

Hepatocytes contain a well-developed organelle substructure (Fig. 61.4). Mitochondria, which constitute approximately 18% of hepatocyte volume, are the sites of oxidative phosphorylation and energy production. They contain enzymes involved in the citric acid cycle and in β-oxidation of fatty acids. The rough endoplasmic reticulum is the site of synthesis of many proteins, including albumin, coagulation factors, enzymes (eg, glucose 6-phosphatase), and triglycerides. The smooth endoplasmic reticulum contains microsomes that are involved in bilirubin conjugation, detoxification (cytochrome P_{450}–dependent isoenzymes), steroid synthesis, cholesterol synthesis, and bile acid synthesis. Several microsomal enzymes, including γ-glutamyltransferase, are induced by many drugs and inhibited by others. This is the site of most drug metabolism and many important drug interactions.

Peroxisomes are found near the smooth endoplasmic reticulum and contain oxidases that use molecular oxygen to modify a variety of substrates, leading to the production of hydrogen peroxide. They also contain catalase, which decomposes hydrogen peroxide. Peroxisomes catalyze the β-oxidation of fatty acids that have 7 to 18 chain lengths. Approximately 5% to 20% of the metabolism of ethanol also occurs in the peroxisomes. Lysosomes are dense organelles that contain hydrolytic enzymes that act as scavengers. Deposition of iron, lipofucsin, bile pigments, and copper occurs in the lysosomes. The Golgi apparatus lies near the canaliculus and is involved in the secretion of various substances, including bile acids and albumin.

BIOCHEMICAL FUNCTIONS OF THE LIVER

The liver is involved in various excretory, synthetic, and metabolic functions. Clinical laboratories perform numerous tests that are useful in the biochemical assessment of these functions.

Hepatic Excretory Function

Organic compounds of both endogenous and exogenous origin are extracted from the sinusoidal blood, biotransformed, and excreted into the bile or urine. Assessment of this excretory function provides valuable clinical information. The most frequently used tests involve the measurement of plasma concentrations of endogenously produced compounds, such as bilirubin and bile acids. In specialist centers, these tests may be augmented by determination of the rate of clearance of exogenous compounds, such as aminopyrine, lidocaine, and caffeine.

Bilirubin

Bilirubin is the orange-yellow pigment derived from heme, which is mainly a product of red blood cell turnover. It is extracted and biotransformed in the liver and excreted in bile and urine. The chemistry, biochemistry, and analytical methodology for bilirubin and related compounds are discussed in Chapter 38; a brief overview of factors relevant to an understanding of liver disease is included here.

Bilirubin is transported from sites of production (mainly the spleen) and is loosely bound to albumin in its native, unconjugated form. Bilirubin is transported across the hepatocyte membrane and is rapidly conjugated with glucuronic acid to produce bilirubin glucuronides, which are then excreted into bile by an energy-dependent process. This process is highly efficient, and bilirubin conjugates are detectable in normal plasma only with the use of highly sensitive

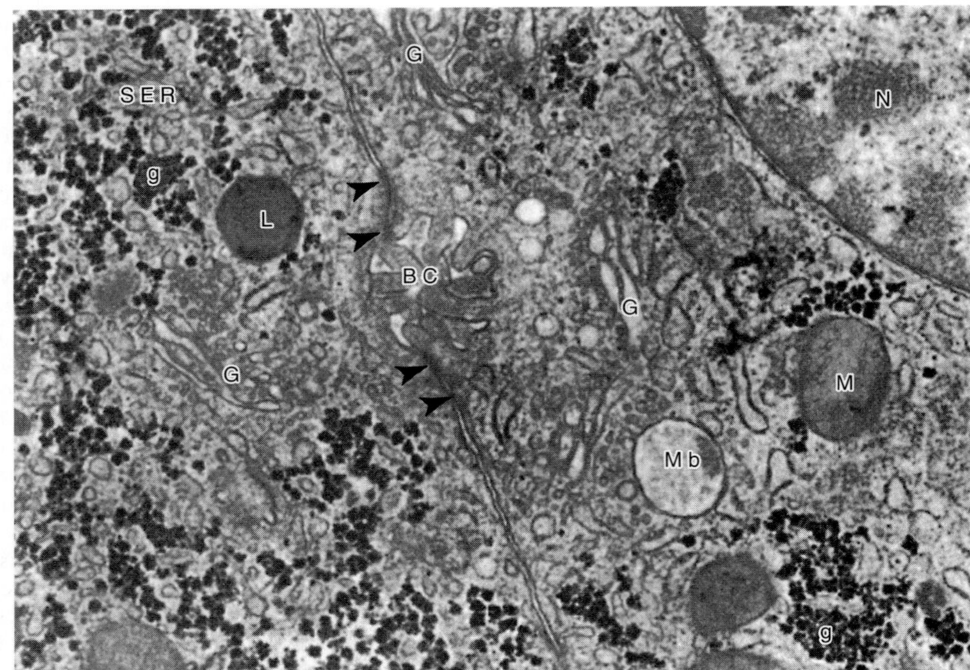

FIGURE 61.4 Portions of two human liver cells showing the relationship of the organelles and a typical bile canaliculus (BC). *Arrowheads* indicate light junctions. *G*, Golgi; *g*, glycogen; *L*, lysosome; *M*, mitochondria; *Mb*, microbody; *N*, nucleus; *SER*, smooth endoplasmic reticulum. (From Zakim O, Boyer TD. *Hepatology: A Textbook of Liver Disease*. 3rd ed. Philadelphia: WB Saunders; 1996. p. 20.)

techniques. In the presence of bilirubin monoglucuronide, albumin (and other proteins) can be postsynthetically modified by covalent attachment to lysine residues. In the case of albumin, this produces a protein-bound form termed biliprotein or δ-bilirubin. Increases in conjugated bilirubin or δ-bilirubin are highly specific markers of hepatic dysfunction (except in the presence of rare inherited disorders that impair excretion of conjugated bilirubin, such as Dubin-Johnson syndrome). In the intestinal tract, bilirubin glucuronides are hydrolyzed and reduced by bacteria to form colorless urobilinogens, which undergo an enterohepatic circulation. A small fraction (2 to 5%) escapes the liver and is excreted in urine. In the colon, urobilinogens spontaneously oxidize to stool pigments stercobilin, mesobilin, and urobilin.

Increased plasma bilirubin typically is classified as primarily indirect (an approximation of unconjugated bilirubin) or direct (an approximation of the sum of conjugated bilirubin and biliprotein). Increased indirect bilirubin indicates overproduction of bilirubin, which is usually caused by hemolysis, or decreased metabolism by the liver, which is primarily caused by congenital defects involving uridine 5′-phosphate-glucuronyl transferase. With severe liver injury, which occurs with fulminant hepatic failure and end-stage cirrhosis, liver disease may cause primarily unconjugated hyperbilirubinemia. Increased urine urobilinogen occurs when bilirubin delivery to the intestinal tract is increased (as with hemolysis, or after recovery from hepatitis or obstruction) or when liver clearance is decreased, which occurs in portal hypertension.

Increased direct bilirubin generally results from functional or mechanical impairment in bilirubin excretion from the hepatocyte. Increased conjugated bilirubin is found in most cases of acute hepatitis and cholestasis (stoppage or suppression of the flow of bile); the percentage of direct bilirubin is similar in both types of liver disease.[2] Urine bilirubin reflects increased plasma concentrations of conjugated bilirubin. With resolution of liver disease, conjugated bilirubin is rapidly cleared, and biliprotein may become the only form present; urine bilirubin is typically absent in such circumstances. Increased conjugated bilirubin is rarely seen with congenital defects in bilirubin excretion, such as Dubin-Johnson syndrome, and with impaired bilirubin excretion, which occurs in sepsis or other acute illness.

Bile Acids

Regulation of bile acid metabolism is a major function of the liver. Alterations in bile acid metabolism are usually a reflection of liver dysfunction. Cholesterol homeostasis is in large part maintained by the conversion of cholesterol to bile acids and subsequent regulation of bile acid metabolism. Bile acids themselves provide surface-active detergent molecules that facilitate both hepatic excretion of cholesterol and solubilization of lipids for intestinal absorption. Bile acid homeostasis requires normal terminal ileum function to absorb bile acids for recirculation (enterohepatic circulation). Alterations in hepatic bile acid synthesis, intracellular metabolism, excretion, intestinal absorption, or plasma extraction are reflected in derangements of bile acid metabolism.

Chemistry. Four major bile acids are known. Cholic acid and chenodeoxycholic acid, the primary bile acids, are synthesized in the liver. The sequence of reactions involved in the synthesis of cholic acid from cholesterol is shown in Fig. 61.5. To date, nine inborn errors of bile acid synthesis have

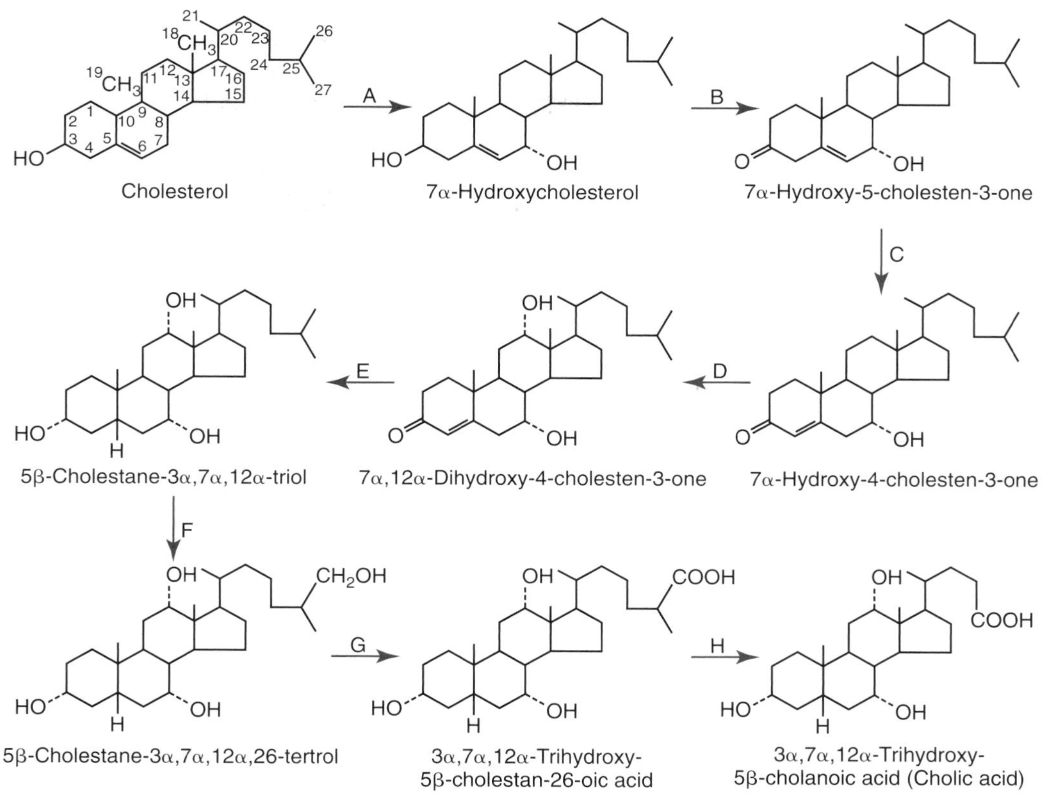

FIGURE 61.5 The biosynthetic pathways of cholesterol conversion to cholic acid. **A**, 7-α-Hydroxylation of cholesterol (addition of –OH group at position 7-α-configuration), the rate-limiting step in the biosynthetic pathway. **B**, Oxidation of the 3-β-hydroxyl group (to form 3-oxo compound). **C**, Isomerization of the 5-ene structure. **D**, 12-α-Hydroxylation (for cholic acid only). **E**, Saturation of the double bond and reduction of the 3-one group. **F**, Hydroxylation of the side chain at C-26 position. **G**, Side chain oxidation to cholestanoic acid. **H**, Hydroxylation at C-24 and β-oxidation to reduce the length of the side chain. (From Balistreri WF, Setchel KDR. Clinical implications of bile acid metabolism. In: Silverberg M, Daum F, editors. *Textbook of Pediatric Gastroenterology*. 2nd ed. Chicago: Year Book Medical Publishers; 1988. p. 72–89. By permission of Mosby, Inc.)

been identified; these can present with neonatal hepatitis, fat malabsorption, or neurologic defects that can progress to chronic liver disease or liver failure and death.[3] The primary bile acids are metabolized (by bacterial 7α-dehydroxylase) in the intestinal lumen to the secondary bile acids—deoxycholic acid and lithocholic acid. Bile acids (through their carboxylate groups) are conjugated in the liver with the amino acid glycine or taurine. This decreases passive absorption in the biliary tree and proximal small intestine, but permits conservation through active transport in the terminal ileum. Approximately 0.1 to 0.6 g of bile acids is lost in the feces daily.

Because they possess both polar and nonpolar regions, molecules of bile acids are able to solubilize biliary lipids. Such molecules align at water–lipid interfaces and reduce surface tension, acting as detergents. In an aqueous solution, bile acids aggregate to form small polymolecular aggregates approximately 5 nm in diameter called micelles, which are capable of incorporating cholesterol and phospholipids to form mixed micelles. Micellar solubilization of these water-insoluble constituents maintains cholesterol in solution. In the intestinal lumen, dietary cholesterol and the products of triglyceride digestion (predominantly free fatty acids and monoglycerides) are incorporated into mixed micelles. Micelles deliver lipolytic products to the mucosal surface. To carry out these functions, a critical micellar bile acid concentration of approximately 2 mmol/L is necessary. Bile acids are thus important for ensuring the solubility of cholesterol (a major component of most gallstones) in bile and dietary lipids (including fat-soluble vitamins) in the intestinal lumen.

Clinical Significance of Bile Acids. In view of the multiple processes involved in bile acid synthesis, conjugation, and excretion, and in its hepatic and intestinal uptake, several potential sites for primary or secondary disturbances have been identified (Box 61.1). With hepatocyte dysfunction (which occurs in many liver disorders), decreased bile acid synthesis results in low primary bile acid concentrations and a decreased ratio of primary to secondary bile acids in plasma; in addition, decreased extraction from plasma often leads to increased concentrations of bile acids, particularly in the nonfasting state. With cholestatic disorders, decreased delivery of primary bile acids to the intestine with resulting decreased secondary bile acid production causes an increased ratio of primary to secondary bile acids, as well as increased total bile acid concentrations. With intestinal disease (including bypass operations that may be performed to treat obesity), increased fecal loss of bile acids leads to decreased concentrations of both primary and secondary bile acids and often a

BOX 61.1 Disturbances in Bile Acid Metabolism

Defective bile acid synthesis
Inherited defects in bile acid synthesis
Acquired defects in bile acid synthesis secondary to liver disease
Extrahepatic bile duct obstruction
Bile acid malabsorption
Effective uptake or altered intracellular metabolism

decrease in plasma cholesterol concentration caused by an increased need for bile acid synthesis. Although plasma bile acid concentrations are abnormal in many situations, their measurement adds little to standard tests of liver function, and they are rarely used in clinical medicine except in the investigation of unexplained pruritus.

Analytical Methods. Analytical techniques used to quantify total or individual bile acids in biological fluids include gas-liquid chromatography, high-performance liquid chromatography (HPLC), enzymatic assay, radioimmunoassay, enzyme-linked immunosorbent assay (ELISA), and tandem mass spectrometry.

Hepatic Synthetic Function

The liver has extensive synthetic capacity and plays a major role in the regulation of protein, carbohydrate, and lipid metabolism (see Chapters 28, 33, and 34). A bidirectional flux of precursors and products, such as glucose, amino acids, free fatty acids, and other nutrients, occurs across the hepatocyte membrane. Normal blood glucose concentrations are maintained during short fasts by the breakdown of hepatic glycogen and during prolonged fasts by hepatic gluconeogenesis. The primary sources of carbon atoms for gluconeogenesis are amino acids derived from muscle proteins. To a lesser extent, lactate (produced in skeletal muscle and erythrocytes) and glycerol (obtained from hydrolysis of triglycerides) also serve as substrates for gluconeogenesis. In humans, the oxidation of odd-numbered fatty acids yields propionyl-coenzyme A (CoA), which can be converted to glucose. However, the formation of glucose in this manner is not quantitatively significant. Protein, triglyceride, fatty acid, cholesterol, and bile acid synthesis also occur within the liver.

Protein Synthesis

The liver is the primary site of the synthesis of most plasma proteins (see Chapter 28). Synthesis occurs in the rough endoplasmic reticulum of hepatocytes, followed by release into the hepatic sinusoids. Although disturbances of protein synthesis occur as a consequence of impaired hepatic function, a variety of other factors may affect plasma protein concentrations. These include decreased availability of amino acids (malnutrition, maldigestion, and malabsorption), catabolic states (hyperthyroidism, Cushing syndrome, burns, postsurgery recovery), protein-losing states (nephrotic syndrome and protein-losing enteropathy), actions of cytokines (decrease in transport proteins, such as albumin, transferrin, and lipoproteins, but an increase in inflammatory response modifiers such as α_1-antitrypsin [AAT], ceruloplasmin, and α_2-macroglobulin), action of hormones (such as growth hormone [GH], cortisol, estrogen, androgens, and thyroid hormones) to increase or decrease production of specific proteins, and congenital deficiency states (Wilson disease and AAT deficiency). In addition, the liver has a significant reserve capacity that prevents protein concentrations from decreasing unless liver damage is extensive. In addition, many liver proteins have relatively long half-lives, such as albumin, which lasts approximately 3 weeks. For this reason, the sensitivity and specificity of protein concentrations for diagnosis of liver disease are far from ideal.

The patterns of plasma protein alterations seen in liver disease depend on the type, severity, and duration of liver injury. For example, in acute hepatic dysfunction, there is usually little change in the plasma protein profile or the total plasma protein concentration; with fulminant hepatic failure or severe liver injury, concentrations of short-lived hepatic proteins (such as transthyretin and prothrombin) fall quickly and become abnormal, whereas those of proteins with longer half-lives are normal or minimally changed. In cirrhosis, concentrations of liver-synthesized plasma proteins and Igs decrease and increase, respectively. Serial determination of plasma proteins provides prognostic information; for example, worsening of prothrombin time (PT) during acute hepatitis suggests a poor prognosis.

Plasma Proteins

Albumin. Albumin, the most commonly measured plasma protein, is synthesized exclusively by the liver. The rate of synthesis varies, depending on the hormonal environment, nutritional status, age, and other local factors. In inflammatory conditions, IL-6 inhibits albumin synthesis but induces synthesis of acute-phase response proteins. With liver disease, hypoalbuminemia is noted primarily in cirrhosis, autoimmune hepatitis (AIH), and alcoholic hepatitis. The mechanism is multifactorial. In cirrhosis, hepatic synthesis of albumin may be decreased, normal, or increased. Loss of albumin into ascitic fluid seems to be responsible for the decrease in albumin in many cases. One important consideration in measurement of albumin is the inaccuracy of dye-binding methods in patients with liver disease. Although bromocresol green measurements tend to overestimate albumin concentration at low concentrations,[4] bromocresol purple methods give falsely low values in patients with jaundice because of the interference of bilirubin at the site of binding.[5]

Transthyretin. This protein has a short half-life of 24 to 48 hours, making it a sensitive indicator of current synthetic ability. Transthyretin is typically decreased in cirrhosis (among other conditions) as a result of decreased synthesis. It is more commonly used as a measurement of nutritional status.

Immunoglobulins. Plasma Ig concentrations are commonly increased in cirrhosis, AIH, and primary biliary cirrhosis (PBC), but they are normal in most other types of liver disease. IgG is increased in AIH and cirrhosis; IgM is increased in PBC. IgA tends to be increased in all types of cirrhosis. None of these findings are specific, and they are seldom used in the diagnosis of liver disease.

Ceruloplasmin. The concentration of this protein is decreased in Wilson disease, cirrhosis, and many causes of chronic hepatitis, but it may be increased by inflammation, cholestasis, hemochromatosis, pregnancy, and estrogen therapy. It is discussed in greater detail in the section on Wilson Disease.

TABLE 61.1 Blood Coagulation Factors

Number or Abbreviation	Name
I	Fibrinogen*
II	Prothrombin*†
III	Tissue factor
IV	Calcium (Ca2+)
V	Proaccelerin*
VI	—
VII	Proconvertin*†
VIII	Antihemophilic factor
IX	Christmas factor*†
X	Stuart-Prower factor†
XI	Plasma thromboplastin antecedent*
XII	Hageman factor*
XIII	Fibrin-stabilizing factor* (Laki-Lorand factor)
PK	Prekallikrein (Fletcher factor)*
HMWK	High-molecular-weight kininogen*

*Protein synthesized in liver.
†Synthesis requires vitamin K.

Alpha$_1$-Antitrypsin. Concentrations of this protein, which is the major serine protease inhibitor (serpin) in plasma, is decreased in homozygous deficiency and cirrhosis, and is increased by acute inflammation. It is discussed in greater detail later in the section on Alpha$_1$-Antitrypsin Deficiency.

Alpha-Fetoprotein. The concentration of this protein, a normal component of fetal blood, falls to adult values by 1 year of age. Mild increases are seen in patients with acute and chronic hepatitis, and indicate hepatocellular regeneration. It is present at higher concentrations in hepatocellular carcinoma (HCC), and is discussed in greater detail later and in Chapter 31.

Coagulation Proteins. The coagulation proteins that are synthesized in the liver are listed in Table 61.1. These proteins interact to produce a fibrin clot (see Chapter 71). Inhibitors of the coagulation system, including antithrombin, protein C, and protein S, are also synthesized in the liver. Some of the coagulation factors (II, VII, IX, and X) require vitamin K for posttranslational carboxylation within the hepatocyte. Proteins C and S are also carboxylated by a vitamin K–dependent enzyme. Activated protein C in plasma inhibits coagulation by inactivating factors V and VIII. Parenchymal liver disease of sufficient severity to impair protein synthesis or obstructive liver disease sufficient to impair intestinal absorption of vitamin K is therefore a potential cause of bleeding disorders. Because of the great functional reserve of the liver, failure of hemostasis usually does not occur except in severe or longstanding liver disease.

PT depends on the activity of fibrinogen (factor I), prothrombin (factor II), and factors V, VII, and X. Because all of these factors are made in the liver, and several are vitamin K–dependent, a prolonged PT often indicates the presence of significant liver disease. In cholestasis, vitamin K deficiency may cause an increase in PT. In this case, the coagulation abnormality is corrected in 1 to 2 days by parenteral injection of 10 mg of vitamin K. In contrast, if PT is prolonged because of hepatocellular disease, factor synthesis is decreased, and administration of vitamin K does not typically correct the problem. PT is also prolonged in some patients with liver disease because of the presence of dysfibrinogenemia, an abnormal form of fibrinogen that does not clot normally, which may predispose patients to thrombosis.[6]

The method for reporting PT in liver disease remains controversial. PT measures the time for plasma to clot after exposure to tissue factor. Reagents differ in the amount of tissue factor present; in patients on warfarin, clotting times are more greatly prolonged when lower amounts of tissue factor and other reagents that stimulate clotting are in the reagents. This makes a reagent more sensitive to clotting factor abnormalities, but makes standardization of results among laboratories difficult. The international normalized ratio (INR) was developed by the World Health Organization (WHO) and the International Committee on Thrombosis and Hemostasis for reporting the results of blood coagulation (clotting) tests. All results are standardized using the international sensitivity index (ISI) for the particular thromboplastin reagent and instrument combination used to perform the test. In practice, it requires determination of the ISI based on the slope of the relationship between PT using the reagent and that using a reference method in patients on warfarin. The INR is then calculated as follows:

$$INR = \left[\frac{\text{PT (patient)}}{\text{PT (geometric mean of normal)}}\right]^{ISI}$$

INR has been found to standardize interpretation of PT measurements among laboratories for those taking warfarin. Unfortunately, INR does not have the same relationship with impairment of clotting in individuals with liver disease.[7] The apparent explanation lies in the mechanism of clotting factor deficiency in liver disease and warfarin administration. Although liver disease inhibits synthesis of clotting factors, warfarin impairs vitamin K–dependent carboxylation, which impairs the ability of the factors to bind calcium. These noncarboxylated clotting factors (termed proteins induced by vitamin K absence [PIVKAs]) appear to act as inhibitors of coagulation; thus, when lower amounts of tissue factor are present, clotting times are more prolonged.[8] In contrast, in liver disease, factor deficiency is due to impaired factor synthesis, and no PIVKAs are present (except in HCC, as discussed later in this chapter). This leads to lesser increases in PT in individuals with liver disease and an underestimation of the degree of clotting impairment when reagents with a low ISI are used. Studies have shown that calculation of a different ISI using plasma samples from patients with liver disease can standardize PT results with different reagents,[9,10] but to date, such liver ISI information is not readily available to laboratories.

Lipid and Lipoprotein Synthesis. The liver plays a key role in the metabolism of lipids and lipoproteins (see Chapter 34). On a daily basis, approximately 33% of the fatty acids originating from adipose tissue enter the liver, where they undergo esterification into triglycerides or are oxidized. Oxidation is favored in the fasting state and esterification is favored in the nonfasting state. Excessive esterification results in fatty liver, a disorder in which excess triglycerides are deposited in large vacuoles that displace other cellular components. Most cholesterol is synthesized endogenously, in the liver. It and cholesterol of dietary origin enter the hepatic pool, where they are converted to bile acids, incorporated into lipoproteins, or used in the synthesis of liver cell membranes. The relative rates of secretion of bile acids, cholesterol, and lecithin are important factors in the pathogenesis of cholesterol gallstones.

Urea Synthesis. Patients with end-stage liver disease may have low concentrations of urea in plasma (see Chapters 32 and 59). The rate of urea excretion in urine is lower in these patients than that in healthy individuals. In addition, plasma concentrations of urea precursors—ammonia and amino acids—are elevated. Lower specific activities of enzymes involved in urea synthesis are also seen. These findings suggest that patients with liver disease have an impaired ability to metabolize protein nitrogen and to synthesize urea. The rate of hepatic urea synthesis also depends on exogenous intake of nitrogen and on endogenous protein catabolism.

Hepatic Metabolic Function

A recurring theme is the central importance of the liver in metabolic and regulatory pathways. The functional expression of the complex, integrated organelle structure includes the metabolism of drugs (activation and detoxification) and the disposal of exogenous and endogenous substances, such as galactose and ammonia. In addition, metabolic abnormalities due to specific inherited enzyme deficiencies can affect the liver. A classic example is galactosemia. In this condition, congenital absence of galactose 1-phosphate uridyltransferase allows accumulation of the toxic metabolite galactose 1-phosphate, which causes injury to the liver, brain, and kidneys.

Ammonia Metabolism

Biochemistry and Physiology. The major source of circulating ammonia is the GI tract. Plasma ammonia concentration in the hepatic portal vein is typically fivefold to tenfold higher than that in the systemic circulation. It is derived from the action of bacterial proteases, ureases, and amine oxidases on the contents of the colon and from the hydrolysis of glutamine in both the small and large intestines. Under normal circumstances, most of the portal vein ammonia load is metabolized to urea in hepatocytes through the Krebs-Henseleit (urea) cycle during the first pass through the liver; this process includes intramitochondrial and cytosolic enzyme-catalyzed steps (Fig. 61.6).

Ammonia enters the tissue of the central nervous system by passive diffusion. The rate of entry increases in proportion to the plasma concentration and is dependent on pH. Ammonia crosses the blood–brain barrier more readily than

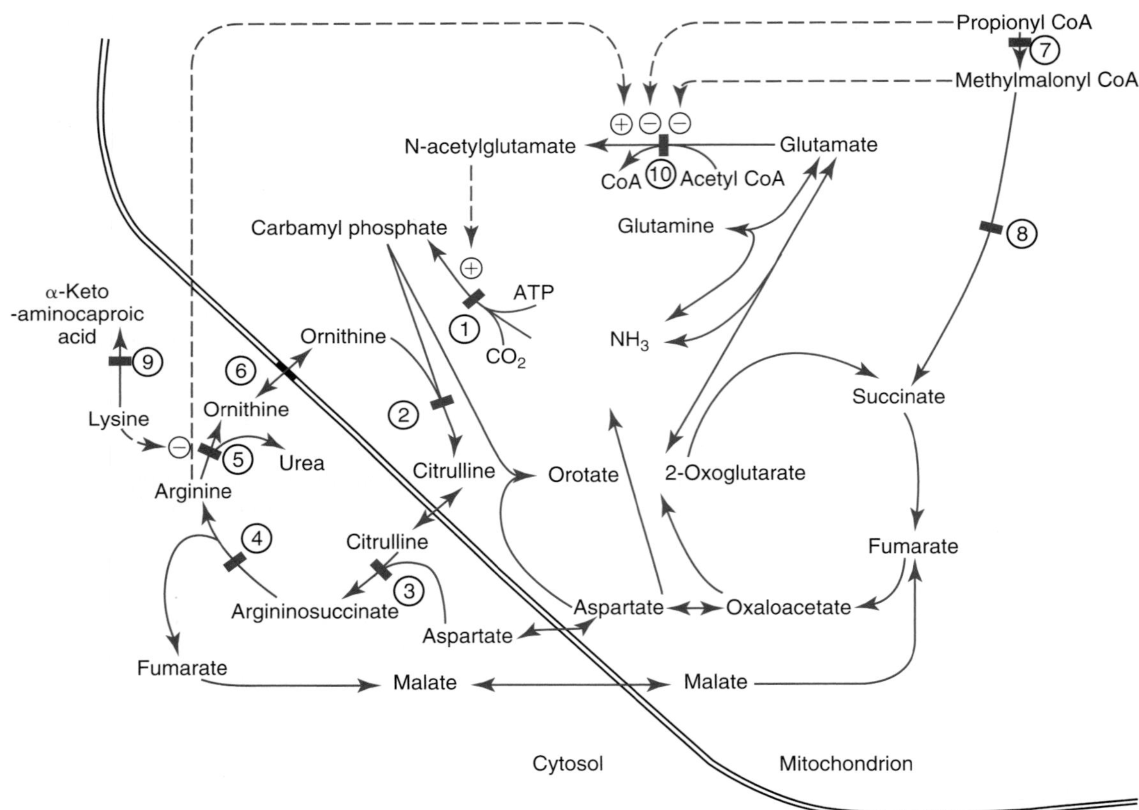

FIGURE 61.6 Major metabolic pathways for the use of ammonia by the hepatocyte. *Solid bars* indicate the sites of primary enzyme defects in various metabolic disorders associated with hyperammonemia: (1) carbamyl phosphate synthetase 1, (2) ornithine transcarbamylase, (3) argininosuccinate synthetase, (4) argininosuccinate lyase, (5) arginase, (6) mitochondrial ornithine transport, (7) propionyl coenzyme-A (CoA) carboxylase, (8) methylmalonyl CoA mutase, (9) L-lysine dehydrogenase, and (10) N-acetyl glutamine synthetase. *Dotted lines* indicate the site of pathway activation (+) or inhibition (–). (From Flannery OB, Hsia YE, Wolf B. Current status of hyperammonemia syndromes. *Hepatology* 1982;2:495–506.)

the ammonium ion. As pH increases, the rate of entry of ammonia into the central nervous system tissue increases as the result of an increase in ammonia relative to ammonium. Because the acid dissociation constant (pK_a) of ammonia is 9.1 at 37°C, approximately 3% of total blood ammonia is ammonia at the normal physiological pH of 7.4. An increase in pH to 7.6 produces an increase in ammonia to approximately 5% of total blood ammonia, which is a 67% increase in concentration.

Clinical Significance. Animal and human studies have shown that an elevated concentration of ammonia (hyperammonemia) exerts toxic effects on the central nervous system. Several causes, both inherited and acquired, of hyperammonemia are known. Inherited deficiencies of urea cycle enzymes are the major cause of hyperammonemia in infants.[11] The two major inherited disorders are those that involve the metabolism of the dibasic amino acids lysine and ornithine and those that involve the metabolism of organic acids, such as propionic acid, methylmalonic acid, isovaleric acid, and others (see Chapter 70).

The main acquired causes of hyperammonemia are advanced liver disease and renal failure. Severe or chronic liver failure (which occurs in fulminant hepatitis or cirrhosis, respectively) leads to significant impairment of normal ammonia metabolism. Reye syndrome, which is primarily a central nervous system disorder with minor hepatic dysfunction, is also associated with hyperammonemia. Hepatic encephalopathy in the cirrhotic patient is often precipitated by GI bleeding, which enhances ammonia production through bacterial metabolism of protein found in blood. Other precipitating causes of encephalopathy include excess dietary protein, constipation, infection, drugs (particularly central nervous system depressants and those that alter blood biochemistry such as diuretics), and electrolyte and acid-base imbalance. Because cirrhosis is accompanied by portosystemic shunting, ammonia clearance is impaired, leading to increased concentrations of blood ammonia. Impaired renal function also causes hyperammonemia. As blood urea concentration increases, more diffuses into the GI tract, where it is converted to ammonia.

The fasting venous plasma ammonia concentration is useful in the differential diagnosis of encephalopathy, when it is unclear whether encephalopathy is of hepatic origin.[12] It is especially helpful in diagnosing Reye syndrome and the inherited disorders of urea metabolism, as well as increased ammonia concentrations due to drugs such as salicylates or valproate. In acute liver injury, ammonia concentrations more than 200 μmol/L are associated with cerebral edema and a poor prognosis,[13] and it has been suggested that ammonia concentrations should be used as part of the evaluation of prognosis in acute liver failure.[14] However, plasma ammonia is not useful in patients with known chronic liver disease.[15] Although ammonia concentrations are higher as the degree of encephalopathy worsens, significant overlap between concentrations is seen in different stages of encephalopathy, and approximately 70% of those with cirrhosis without encephalopathy have elevated ammonia concentrations.[16] Ammonia concentrations may actually better reflect the presence of shunting blood around the portal veins than the degree of liver dysfunction.[17]

Analytical Methodology. Both enzymatic and chemical methods are used to measure ammonia in body fluids. An enzymatic assay with glutamate dehydrogenase is the most frequently used method. Plasma ammonia measurement is particularly susceptible to contamination, leading to falsely elevated concentrations. Common preanalytical problems are discussed in Chapter 4 on Sample Handling and Processing.

Reference Intervals. For the enzymatic method, the reference interval is 15 to 45 μg/dL (11–32 μmol/L). For more details on age-dependent values, see the Appendix on Reference Intervals. Laboratories should verify that these ranges are appropriate for use in their own settings.

Carbohydrate Metabolism

Because the liver is a major processor of dietary and endogenous carbohydrates, liver disease affects carbohydrate metabolism in a variety of ways (see Chapter 33). However, none of the conventional modes of evaluating carbohydrate metabolism have value in the diagnosis of liver disease. Because the liver is the major site of both glycogen storage and gluconeogenesis, hypoglycemia is a common complication in certain liver diseases, particularly Reye syndrome, fulminant hepatic failure, advanced cirrhosis, and HCC.

Xenobiotic Metabolism and Excretion

Xenobiotics are chemical substances that are foreign to the biological system. Biochemically, they are cleared and/or metabolized by the liver; some have been used as the basis of tests of liver function. Rates of metabolism of these compounds are sometimes referred to as quantitative liver function tests, to distinguish them from the more commonly used term, liver function tests, which is often used to refer to measurements of liver-associated enzymes. As liver disease progresses, quantitative liver function test results gradually worsen, but their measurement adds little to that obtained by widely used tests such as bilirubin, albumin, and INR measurement.[18] Even when these tests are used, significant overlap of values is noted in persons with cirrhosis and less severe degrees of liver scarring, which limits their usefulness.

Dye Excretion Tests. Dye excretion tests, such as bromsulphthalein (BSP) and indocyanine green clearance, were formerly used as indicators of liver disease. With the development of more sensitive and specific indicators of liver disease, dye excretion tests have become obsolete, although until the 1970s, BSP was the most frequently used dye excretion test. Because of reports of fatalities resulting from hypersensitivity and other adverse effects, BSP use has been discontinued. Indocyanine green clearance is still occasionally used[19] for investigating hepatic blood flow and for predicting clearance rates of drugs that undergo first-pass clearance by the liver, such as lignocaine. Typical indocyanine green clearance values in healthy subjects range from 6.5 to 14 mL/min/kg body weight.

Drug Clearance Tests. A variety of drugs that are metabolized by the liver have been used to study the action of various P_{450} (mixed-function oxidase) enzymes. Aminopyrine is demethylated to form carbon dioxide and aminoantipyrine. With the use of ^{13}C- or ^{14}C-labeled aminopyrine, the resulting isotopically labeled carbon dioxide is measured in breath as a reflection of functioning liver mass. Decreases in metabolism are common in persons with cirrhosis,[20] but metabolism is also affected by other factors such as cigarette smoking and use of drugs such as oral contraceptives; significant intraindividual variation in results has been noted.[21] Overall diagnostic sensitivity is similar to that of other more routine laboratory tests.[22]

Caffeine clearance is altered during hepatic injury; it is prolonged in both chronic hepatitis and cirrhosis.[23] Caffeine is rapidly and nearly completely absorbed from the GI tract and then undergoes N-demethylation by the hepatic mixed-function oxidase system. A single dose of caffeine (3.5 mg/kg to a maximum dose of 200 mg, dissolved in water, fruit juice, or milk for oral administration) is administered. This caffeine dose is equivalent to that found in one cup of brewed coffee or in one can of a commercial soft drink.

Blood (or salivary samples) obtained before and at timed intervals after caffeine ingestion can be analyzed by reversed-phase HPLC or immunoassay. A close correlation is found between plasma and salivary caffeine concentrations. Caffeine half-life is approximately 5.5 hours in healthy adults and 3 hours in healthy children, with clearance of approximately 2 mL/min/kg in healthy adults and 10 mL/min/kg in healthy children. Caffeine clearance correlates with the aminopyrine breath test and has similar limitations, although it is less subject to effects of variables, such as smoking and oral contraceptive use.[21] Lidocaine undergoes N-deethylation in the liver by cytochrome P_{450} to form monoethylglycinexylidide (MEGX); the rate of appearance of MEGX in plasma reflects hepatic lidocaine clearance. Because lidocaine is highly extracted, its clearance is flow dependent. Thus, alterations in hepatic blood flow also influence lidocaine elimination.[24] Lidocaine (1 mg/kg) is given by intravenous bolus; plasma is obtained at baseline and at 15 minutes for MEGX concentration (time of plateau concentration in healthy individuals). MEGX is most commonly measured using an immunoassay. Lidocaine clearance has been used to assess liver transplantation function, but its use is limited by the effect of hypoperfusion (which occurs in sepsis or volume depletion).[25]

Hepatic Storage Function

Because individual cells are unable to store a sufficient supply of energy-rich carbohydrate substrates, the liver serves as the major site for their storage. For example, hepatic storage of glycogen allows the release of glucose to other tissue when the need exists (eg, when plasma concentrations of glucose decrease). Other tissues, such as muscle and adipose tissue, store proteins and triglycerides, respectively, and are capable of adaptation. Depending on the availability of oxidizable fuels, these tissues also switch from the storage mode to the synthesis or release mode during periods of decreased carbohydrate intake.

CLINICAL MANIFESTATIONS OF LIVER DISEASE

Various characteristics indicate the presence of liver disease, including fibrosis, jaundice, portal hypertension, abnormal renal function, altered drug metabolism, nutritional and metabolic abnormalities, disordered hemostasis, and release of enzymes into various body fluids.

Liver Fibrosis

Pathogenesis of Liver Fibrosis

As the first solid organ beyond the gut to process ingested antigens, the liver is constantly exposed to antigen-rich blood; therefore, it is a major line of defense against such antigens, especially microorganisms. Both the adaptive and innate immune systems of the liver are highly evolved to serve this function. Fibrosis should be considered as a normal component of the innate immune response to tissue injury, and as such, is controlled by the cells and products of the immune system.[26] Both the innate and adaptive immune systems play an important role in hepatic fibrosis modulation. For example, in the liver, type I collagen (which predominates in fibrotic scar) protects hepatocytes against toxic stimuli. In the liver this inflammation can be due to acute viral hepatitis, AIH, alcohol or bile salt exposure, or fatty liver disease. Hepatic dysfunction is caused by degeneration and necrosis of epithelial cells (hepatocytes and/or cholangiocytes), replacement of liver parenchyma by fibrotic tissues and regenerative nodules, and loss of liver function. In the liver, when the inflammatory insult becomes chronic, fibrosis can then lead to apoptosis and loss of the architectural integrity of the liver and cirrhosis. Regeneration of these epithelial cells is essential for architectural and functional recovery of the organ.[27]

The process of hepatic fibrosis involves the activation of hepatic stellate cells (HSCs) (or portal fibroblasts in biliary disease), Kupffer cells, and an array of other cells, proteins, and signaling pathways. The complexities of these interactions are becoming better understood, and the currently known roles of the many players are summarized in the following.

Hepatic Stellate Cells. HSCs reside in the space of Disse, interposed between the endothelium and hepatocytes,[28] where they encircle the liver sinusoids. After liver injury, HSCs become activated by the products of apoptotic mesenchymal cells, which leads to the conversion of a resting vitamin A–rich cell (a quiescent HSC) to one that has lost vitamin A droplets by autophagy, which leads to increased proliferation and contraction, and the release of proinflammatory, profibrogenic, and promitogenic cytokines. The activated HSCs become contractile myofibroblasts that generate a scar that forms around the injury site.

HSC activation can be divided into two phases: initiation and perpetuation.[29] Initiation, which is also known as the preinflammatory stage, refers to early changes in gene expression and phenotype. It is the result of primarily paracrine stimulation from damaged parenchymal cells. Maintenance of these stimuli leads to a perpetuation phase that is regulated by autocrine and paracrine stimuli. Perpetuation involves at least six distinct changes in HSC behavior, including proliferation, chemotaxis, fibrogenesis, contractility, matrix degradation, and retinoid loss.[30]

Myofibroblasts. The profibrotic myofibroblasts are the master regulators of the fibrotic response because of their scar-producing, proliferative, migratory, contractile, immunomodulatory, and phagocytic properties. Myofibroblasts are the prototypical mesenchymal cell type that regulates repair after an injury in a range of tissues, including liver, kidneys, skin, lungs, and bone marrow, as well as the central nervous system.[31] Myofibroblasts, once activated, are capable of enhanced migration and deposition of extracellular matrix (ECM) components.[30,32] Although HSCs are the primary source of this fibrogenic population in the liver,[30] other cells such as bone marrow–derived cells, portal fibroblasts, and epithelial-to-mesenchymal transition from hepatocytes and cholangiocytes also contribute to fibrogenesis, although their exact role in disease is not completely understood.

Role of the Extracellular Matrix. In the normal liver, the ECM provides structural and biochemical support to the surrounding cells and is composed mainly of a number of structural proteins collagens IV and VI), as well as a range of growth factors and matrix metalloproteinases (MMPs) that are specifically bound and preserved in latent forms.[33] The ECM can modulate the activation and proliferation of HSCs, angiogenesis, and the availability and activity of growth factors and MMPs. The ECM also provides cells with signals for polarization, adhesion, migration, proliferation, survival, and differentiation. ECM–cell interactions are determined largely by specific membrane adhesion receptors. The ECM may prevent apoptosis in the damaged liver and also prevent growth factor proteolysis.[33] Interactions between ECM and its surrounding cells are bidirectional. After injury, the fibrillary collagens I and III predominate together with fibronectin.[27] Liver fibrosis as a consequence of liver injury entails both qualitative and quantitative changes in ECM composition as a result of an imbalance between the rates of matrix synthesis and degradation. The ECM becomes progressively insoluble and resistant to protease digestion because of the thickening of fibrotic septae and increased cross-linking.[34,35]

Matrix Metalloproteinases. MMPs, also known as matrixins, are the major family of calcium-dependent enzymes that degrade collagenous and noncollagenous ECM substrates. There are 25 members of this tightly regulated family, which are classified on the basis of their substrate specificity: interstitial collagenases, gelatinases, stromelysins, membrane types, and metalloelastases. MMPs are secreted as inactive proenzymes, have complex transcriptional control, and their action is inhibited by a family of endogenous proteinase inhibitors known as tissue inhibitors of metalloproteinases (TIMPs).[34,36,37] Four TIMP members bind reversibly to the active site of all MMPs and have different affinities for specific MMPs. Thus, TIMPs play an important role in preventing degradation of the accumulating matrix during liver injury by antagonizing the activity of MMPs. TIMP-1 has also an antiapoptotic effect on HSCs; it prevents clearance of activated HSCs during injury and promotes their survival through induction of B-cell lymphoma 2.[38] HSCs are a key source of MMPs, especially MMP-2, -3, -9, and -13. In chronic human liver disease and animal models of fibrosis, concentrations of MMP-1 and/or -13 do not change, but there is a progressive increase in TIMP-1 and -2 as fibrosis advances. TIMP expression can be detected soon (6 hours) after liver injury and may precede the induction of procollagen I.[39]

Cytokines. Fibrosis usually follows an inflammatory insult; therefore, certain cytokines secreted by a range of cells, including Kupffer cells, HSCs, hepatocytes, natural killer cells, lymphocytes, and dendritic cells play a key role in the response. These include the chemokines (monocyte chemotactic protein-1, RANTES [Regulated on Activation, Normal T Expressed and Secreted; also known as CCL5 or C-C motif chemokine ligand 5], IL-8), interferons (IFN-α, IFN-γ), ILs (IL-1, IL-6, IL-10), growth factors, adipokines, and soluble neurohumoral ligands (endocannabinoids). Adipokines (adipose tissue cytokines) are polypeptides secreted mainly by adipocytes, and to a lesser extent, by stromal cells, including macrophages, fibroblasts, and infiltrating monocytes. Leptin and adiponectin are the main adipokines implicated in liver injury.[40,41]

Hepatocytes. The hepatocytes are the major cell type in the liver and are also involved in the process of fibrosis and cirrhosis. Normally, hepatocytes can regenerate removed liver tissue rapidly, but in chronic disease states, they appear to become senescent with respect to this function, but the HSCs become activated and are sufficient to regenerate the biliary and hepatocellular epithelium.[42]

Kupffer Cells. Kupffer cells are specialized, self-renewing, long-lived macrophages located in the liver that line the walls of the sinusoids that form part of the reticuloendothelial system. Their role is to regulate the local immune system in response to bacteria, bacterial toxins, and debris that are derived from the GI tract. Kupffer cell activation is responsible for early ethanol-induced liver injury, which is common in chronic alcoholics. Chronic alcoholism and liver injury involve a two-hit system. If the toxic effect of alcohol is considered to be the first "hit," the second hit is characterized by activation of the Toll-like receptor 4 and CD14, which are receptors on the Kupffer cells that internalize endotoxin (lipopolysaccharide). This activates the transcription of proinflammatory cytokines (TNF-α) and production of prooxidant superoxides. TNF then activates the HSCs, which leads to collagen synthesis and fibrosis. In response to hepatic injury, the liver macrophage populations change. During hepatic inflammation and fibrosis, the number of Kupffer cells decrease, and they are gradually replaced by monocyte-derived macrophages. The Kupffer cells have a key role in early response to injury and are replenished as the inflammation and fibrosis subsides. The macrophages secrete cytokines TNF-α and IL-1 β, which stimulates the activation of HSCs and ECM synthesis. Hepatic macrophages are also involved in matrix remodeling and play an important role in matrix degradation through increased MMP-13 production during resolution of liver fibrosis.[42,43]

Lymphocytes. The relative balance of T-helper 1 (TH1) and T-helper 2 (TH2) cells has an impact on the outcome of fibrosis. TH1 cells are antifibrotic, whereas TH2 are strongly profibrotic. IL-13, which is associated with TH2, stimulates transforming growth factor (TGF)-β1 synthesis and upregulates MMP-9. TH1 cells are associated with IFN-γ, and IL-12 suppresses collagen deposition by regulating the balance of MMP and TIMPs. There are other T-cell subsets that may also play a role, including TH17, which stimulates Kupffer cells, HSCs, and choliangiocytes, and the secretion of proinflammatory cytokines, such as IL-1β, IL-6, TNF, and TGF-β. The influence of these different T-cell populations on the fibrosis process is probably dependent on the underlying cause of the injury. Innate natural killer T cells are proinflammatory and may have a role in initiating and perpetuating fibrosis, whereas γδ T cells may be antifibrotic by promoting HSC apoptosis.[27]

Liver Sinusoidal Endothelial Cells. The highly fenestrated liver sinusoidal endothelial cells (LSECs) constitute the sinusoidal wall or endothelium of the liver, where they act as a dynamic filter that facilitates the exchange of metabolites and fluids between the blood and the hepatocytes. Defenestration and capillarization of the LSECs can lead to impaired substrate exchange and hepatic dysfunction. However, differentiated LSECs promote reversion of activated HSCs to quiescence and thereby accelerate regression and prevent progression of fibrosis.[27]

Platelets. Platelets have the features of inflammatory cells and release factors, such as platelet-derived growth factor (PDGF), vascular endothelial growth factor (VEGF), TGF-α, which induce angiogenesis, wound healing, liver regeneration, and metastasis.[44] In chronic hepatitis, blood platelet numbers gradually fall, which is reflected in liver fibrosis. The thrombocytopenia seen in chronic hepatitis has many causes, including increased splenic breakdown of platelets and pooling, and decreased marrow production. However, there may be a role for platelets in the pathogenesis of liver fibrosis and hepatic cell carcinoma. Platelets accumulate in noncancerous liver tissues of patients with cirrhosis and chronic hepatitis as blood platelet numbers drop. In chronic hepatitis C infection, platelets accumulate in the sinusoidal space mediated by the activated reticuloendothelial system (RES) involving Kupffer cells. HSCs express the PDGF receptor, which is the most basic mediator involved with platelet granules and is involved with fibrosis and malignancy. When HSCs express this receptor, they are susceptible to PDGF contained in platelets, and this may be why platelets accumulate in patients with chronic hepatitis.[44] Platelets also accumulate in cancerous tissue in the blood space through a mechanism that involves Kupffer cells.

Reversibility of Fibrosis

Hepatic fibrosis is reversed or stabilized in up to 80% of patients who are treated with conventional regimens.[45-47] In humans, successful treatment of the underlying disease may reverse liver fibrosis. Regression of liver fibrosis has been observed in patients with iron and copper overload; alcohol-induced liver injury; chronic hepatitis B, C, and D; hemochromatosis; secondary biliary cirrhosis; nonalcoholic steatohepatitis (NASH); and AIH.

Two key events in fibrosis resolution are the degradation of the fibrillar ECM and reduction in myofibroblast survival. TIMPs play an important role in preventing degradation of the accumulating matrix during liver injury by antagonizing the activity of MMPs and promoting survival of activated HSCs. In contrast, several mediators have been implicated in inducing apoptosis and clearance of HSCs. Similarly, p21 and p16 proteins can limit the fibrogenic response by promoting senescence of HSCs.

Jaundice

Jaundice (or icterus) is a physical sign characterized by a yellow appearance of the skin, mucous membranes, and sclera caused by bilirubin deposition. It is the most specific clinical manifestation of hepatobiliary dysfunction, but is not present in many individuals with liver disease (especially chronic liver disease) and may occur in states of bilirubin overproduction (such as hemolysis). Jaundice is seen most easily in the sclera of the eyes, where yellow contrasts sharply with the usual bright white color. Jaundice is usually apparent clinically when the plasma bilirubin concentration reaches 2 to 3 mg/dL (34–51 μmol/L), although higher concentrations may be required when fluorescent lighting is used. When bilirubin clearance from the liver to the intestinal tract is impaired (as in acute hepatitis and bile duct obstruction), acholic (gray colored) stools may be noted. Bilirubin is the source of stercobilin, which produces the brown color of normal stools. Increases in plasma-conjugated bilirubin lead to orange-brown colored urine, because conjugated bilirubin is water soluble. Jaundice may also be due to disorders of bilirubin metabolism. Bilirubin metabolism and classification of jaundice are discussed in more detail in Chapter 38.

Portal Hypertension

The portal circulation handles all venous outflow of the GI tract, the spleen, the pancreas, and the gallbladder (Fig. 61.7). The portal vein is formed by the union of the splenic vein and the superior mesenteric vein. Portal flow is normally 1000 to 1200 mL/min, with pressure of 5 to 7 mm Hg. Portal hypertension occurs when portal flow is obstructed anywhere along its course. Causes of obstruction leading to portal hypertension are classified by site: presinusoidal, sinusoidal, and postsinusoidal. Presinusoidal portal hypertension is most commonly caused by portal vein thrombosis or schistosomiasis, but may also occur with increased portal flow, such as occurs with Felty syndrome (a combination of chronic rheumatoid arthritis, splenomegaly, leukopenia, vasculitis that may be manifest by pigmented spots on the lower extremities, and sometimes other evidence of hypersplenism, such as anemia and thrombocytopenia). Sinusoidal hypertension is most commonly caused by cirrhosis, but may occur transiently with acute and chronic hepatitis or acute fatty liver. The most important cause of postsinusoidal hypertension is hepatic vein occlusion or Budd-Chiari syndrome,[48] in which sudden obstruction or occlusion of the hepatic veins (associated with myeloproliferative disorders in one-half of cases) causes hepatomegaly, abdominal pain, severe ascites, mild jaundice, with acute portal hypertension, and may progress to long-standing portal hypertension and liver failure.[49] The most common cause of postsinusoidal hypertension is cardiac disease, most commonly congestive heart failure. Chronic congestive heart failure is usually associated with portal hypertension and ascites, and may even lead to increased activities of aminotransferases.[50] Other causes include abscesses, membranous obstruction of the vena cava, and venoocclusive disease (as may be seen in patients after bone marrow transplantation). The causes of increased resistance to blood flow through the liver include the previously described static factors and may be compounded by the dynamic alterations in vascular and sinusoidal tone due to contraction of hepatic myofibroblasts and vasoactive compounds. These dynamic factors may cause acute rises in portal pressure, resulting in complications such as variceal hemorrhage. Although increased portal resistance is the major factor that causes portal hypertension, it is often accompanied by decreased resistance to blood flow through other blood vessels, which enhances blood flow through the portal veins.

When portal pressure increases, the portal venous system becomes dilated and forms collateral connections to the systemic venous flow (Fig. 61.8), leading to portosystemic shunting. Initially, this is clinically silent, but as portal hypertension worsens, it compromises many of the metabolic functions of the liver. One such abnormality is altered estrogen metabolism, which increases the ratio of plasma estrogen to testosterone concentrations. Clinical consequences include spider telangiectasias and palmar erythema, gynecomastia in men, and abnormal vaginal bleeding and irregular menstrual periods in women. Impaired protein metabolic functions cause the accumulation of ammonia and abnormal neurotransmitters,

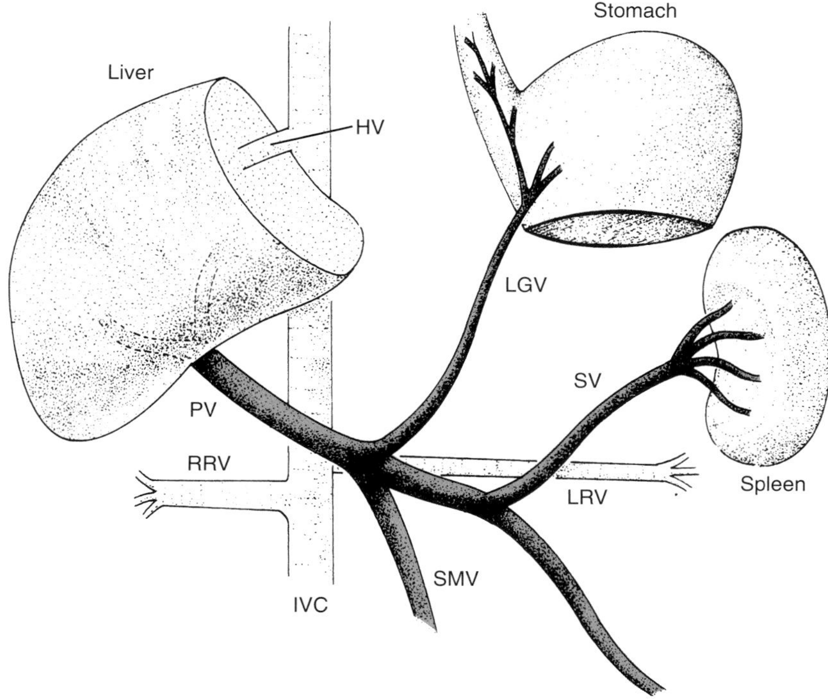

FIGURE 61.7 The portal-venous system. *HV*, Hepatic vein; *IMV*, inferior mesenteric vein; *IVC*, inferior vena cava; *LGV*, left gastric vein; *LRV*, left renal vein; *PV*, portal vein; *RRV*, right renal vein; *SMV*, superior mesenteric vein; *SV*, splenic vein. (From Zakim O, Boyer TD. *Hepatology: A Textbook of Liver Disease.* 3rd ed. Philadelphia: WB Saunders; 1996. p. 721.)

ultimately leading to hepatic encephalopathy.[51] Because most nutrients arrive through the portal vein, synthetic functions are also impaired, leading to hypoalbuminemia (contributing to ascites), decreased clotting factors (predisposing to bleeding), and reduced thrombolytic factors, such as antithrombin (predisposing to venous thrombosis).

Bleeding Esophageal Varices

The most life-threatening consequence of portosystemic shunting is the development of varices (enlarged and tortuous veins), which can occur throughout the GI tract but are most common in the esophagus, stomach, and rectum, at sites of portosystemic anastamosis. Bleeding from varices is one of the leading causes of morbidity and mortality in patients with cirrhosis. Varices are present at the time of diagnosis of cirrhosis in approximately 40% of patients and occur in an additional 6% per year.[52] Normal portal pressure ranges between 1 and 5 mm Hg. When the portal pressure exceeds 10 mm Hg, collateral portosystemic shunts may open, with an increased risk of bleeding once the portal pressure exceeds 12 mm Hg. The major consequences of varices are rupture and bleeding, usually presenting as hematemesis. Treatment of portal hypertension and varices is directed at obliterating the dilated blood vessels or reducing portal pressure. Pressure can be reduced by pharmacological agents, such as nonselective β-adrenergic blockers, but if this is not effective, invasive procedures can be used, most commonly by putting rubber bands around large varices (banding), or if this is not successful, by placing a stent through the jugular and hepatic veins to connect to the portal vein (transjugular intrahepatic portosystemic shunting).[53] Because portal flow is already significantly reduced before shunting, minimal change in liver function is usually seen, but the incidence of hepatic encephalopathy after the placement of shunts is markedly increased.

Ascites

Ascites is the effusion and accumulation of fluid in the abdominal cavity. Ascites is the most common clinical finding in patients with portal hypertension. Ascites itself is not life threatening, but it is uncomfortable and may compromise respiration (from upward displacement of the diaphragm and compression of the lungs). It predisposes individuals to spontaneous bacterial peritonitis, which is life threatening (see the following).

The pathogenesis of ascites is complex because of a number of simultaneously operating factors. Of these, the most important are increased hydrostatic portal venous pressure, with increased resistance to flow, decreased colloid osmotic (oncotic) pressure due to hypoalbuminemia, and leakage of protein-enriched fluid from the surface of the liver, which increases intraperitoneal colloid pressure. The primary event is probably peripheral vasodilation due to an imbalance of vasoactive factors, including endothelins. The net effect of these forces is shrinkage of the central blood volume, which decreases renal perfusion and leads to sodium retention through activation of the renin–angiotensin system. Sodium retention leads to water retention, but because of increased portal hydrostatic pressure and decreased intravascular colloid pressure, the fluid leaks into the so-called third space, causing ascites and edema.

Ascites has many causes, and it is important to differentiate ascites secondary to portal hypertension from ascites due to other causes. This is done by analyzing ascitic fluid.

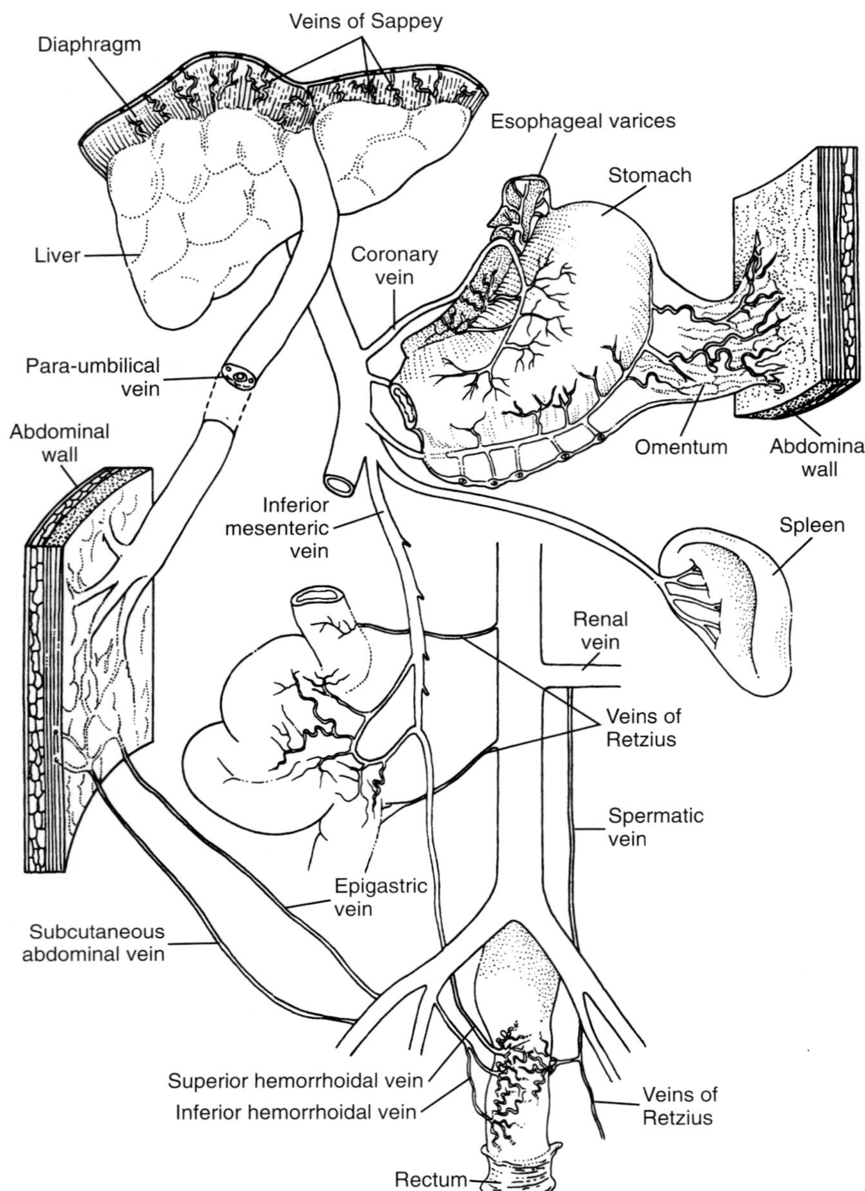

FIGURE 61.8 Sites of portosystemic collateral circulation in cirrhosis of the liver. (From Sherlock S, Dooley J, editors. *Diseases of the Liver and Biliary System.* 9th ed. London: Blackwell Scientific Publications; 1993. p. 134.)

The feature that best distinguishes portal hypertension is an increase in the serum/ascites albumin gradient. A gradient greater than 1.1 g/dL (11 g/L) is characteristic of ascites caused by portal hypertension,[54] but a high serum/ascites albumin gradient can also be seen in congestive heart failure or nephrotic syndrome. For more details on the biochemical tests in peritoneal fluid, refer to Chapter 43 on Body Fluids.

Ascites due to portal hypertension is managed by creating a negative sodium balance or by relieving portal hypertension. A negative sodium balance can be obtained by reducing sodium intake and enhancing sodium excretion using diuretics. In cirrhosis, activation of the renin-aldosterone axis (caused by a variety of factors) necessitates use of agents that act at the distal nephron as the primary diuretic used, but these can be combined with other diuretics that act more proximally. In patients who require more urgent treatment for relief of symptoms, or who do not respond adequately to diuretics, ascitic fluid may be removed with a catheter placed percutaneously through the abdominal wall (paracentesis). More than 10 L of fluid may be drained to relieve patient discomfort or respiratory compromise. Removal of more than 4 L of ascites requires concomitant plasma volume expansion to prevent renal failure; albumin is effective as an expander.[55]

Spontaneous Bacterial Peritonitis

Ascites predisposes to spontaneous bacterial peritonitis, defined as peritoneal infection (typically Gram negative), in the absence of mechanical disruption of the bowel.[56] The condition usually presents in an individual with known cirrhosis and manifests by the development of abdominal pain, fever, or leukocytosis. The diagnosis is established by examination of the ascitic fluid; more than 250 neutrophils/mL (or >500 neutrophils/mL in the absence of a positive blood culture) is considered diagnostic. In contrast, secondary peritonitis is usually associated with higher neutrophil counts, along with high protein and low glucose in ascitic fluid. Several studies have suggested that dipsticks that detect the presence of leukocyte esterase could be used to identify increased leukocytes and to diagnose spontaneous bacterial peritonitis; however, a recent review found poor sensitivity and frequent false-negative results in asymptomatic patients.[57,58] Unless cell counts are not available (eg, in an office setting or in a remote site), use of dipsticks for leukocyte esterase is not recommended. Culture of ascites may be negative in up to 60% of cases, but infection should be treated empirically if symptoms and signs are indicative of spontaneous bacterial peritonitis (SBP).

Hepatic (Portosystemic) Encephalopathy

Hepatic encephalopathy is a metabolic disorder characterized by a wide spectrum of neuropsychiatric dysfunction.[51,59] It may occur as an acute syndrome in patients with acute hepatic failure, or as a chronic, relapsing syndrome associated with cirrhosis. As implied by the synonym, chronic hepatic encephalopathy occurs in the setting of portosystemic shunting, usually as a result of cirrhosis. It may occur as the result of a range of metabolic disturbances, including dehydration, electrolyte imbalances, ingestion of excess protein, bleeding, sepsis, renal dysfunction, hypoxia, portosystemic shunting, increased demands on hepatic function (eg, surgery), and commonly due to drugs, particularly those that act on the central nervous system (eg, benzodiazepines).

The clinical syndrome is variable but follows a reasonably predictable course. Disturbed consciousness always occurs. It usually starts as hypersomnia and progresses to sleep reversal, in which the patient tends to sleep through the day and be awake at night. This is followed by decreased spontaneous movement, apathy, and gradually increasing levels of coma. Personality changes may be conspicuous, especially in patients with chronic disease. Irritability and disturbed social behavior may follow. Intellectual deterioration occurs and generally progresses to overt confusion. Neurologic abnormalities include slurred speech, a characteristic flapping tremor called asterixis, increased muscle tone, and abnormal reflexes. Disturbed gait may ensue. In chronic encephalopathy, these changes typically fluctuate over time and follow a waxing and waning course. Acute encephalopathy progresses rapidly, often within hours, and is characterized by cerebral edema, which may result in brainstem herniation and death.

The pathophysiology of hepatic encephalopathy is not completely understood but includes an increased sensitivity to dietary proteins. Ammonia concentrations are typically increased with acute encephalopathy[60] and are often but not invariably increased with chronic encephalopathy. A reduction in plasma ammonia concentration is often associated with symptomatic improvement. However, because plasma ammonia concentrations do not correlate with the severity of the encephalopathy, it has been suggested that other factors are involved.[61] It is recognized that a variety of neurotransmitter systems are dysfunctional in hepatic encephalopathy, but the exact cause of the changes is not known. One important contributor is the endogenous benzodiazepine agonist system.

The diagnosis of chronic hepatic encephalopathy is usually made on clinical grounds. Plasma ammonia concentrations are rarely helpful for diagnosis or for monitoring the patient's disorder; normal ammonia concentrations are helpful in excluding hepatic encephalopathy as a cause of cerebral dysfunction when the clinical picture is not clear. As alluded to earlier, ammonia is more helpful in acute encephalopathy in proving a hepatic cause, and is of some prognostic importance in acute liver failure.[14] Elevated ammonia concentrations in this situation suggest acute hepatic failure or Reye syndrome. The most reliable diagnostic assessment is the electroencephalogram, which is usually abnormal in patients with symptomatic hepatic encephalopathy, with triphasic waves over the frontal lobes that oscillate at 5 Hz and δ-wave activity in the most advanced stages of the condition.[51]

Treatment is largely empirical, based on observations that intestinal bacteria and protein loads in the intestinal tract are important in the symptoms of hepatic encephalopathy. Lactulose has long been known to reduce symptoms in chronic hepatic encephalopathy. Antibiotic treatment with a nonabsorbable antibiotic (eg, rifaxamin) reduces the number of bacteria and is especially helpful in patients with GI bleeding. Patients with acute encephalopathy may require measures to reduce intracranial pressure, such as osmotic diuretics.

Hepatorenal Syndrome

Hepatorenal syndrome (HRS) refers to decreased renal function secondary to hepatic disease. Portal hypertension is a common factor in all cases of HRS that develop in chronic liver disease, but HRS may also occur in acute liver failure. Although formerly believed to be a rapidly progressing, terminal event in a person with end-stage liver disease, it is now recognized that HRS falls into two major varieties.[62] Type 2 HRS is more common; it represents a slowly progressive or stable decline in renal function that is due to peripheral vasodilation and renal vasoconstriction. Type 1, or classic HRS, represents rapidly declining renal function, which is usually seen in a person with preexisting type 2 HRS. Type 1 HRS usually develops in the setting of an acute decrease in blood pressure, which is often due to spontaneous bacterial peritonitis or variceal bleeding.

A common feature in both forms of HRS is activation of the renin–angiotensin–aldosterone axis, which is caused by intravascular volume depletion.[15] As with other forms of prerenal azotemia (elevated concentrations of urea, creatinine, and other compounds rich in nitrogen), HRS in the untreated patient is generally associated with increased antidiuretic hormone and with profound thirst. This leads to the development of hyponatremia, hypokalemia, metabolic alkalosis, low urine sodium, high urine potassium excretion, and high urine osmolality. Plasma urea and creatinine concentrations, and creatinine clearance are not reliable indicators of renal function in HRS.[63] Urea production by the liver is often decreased in advanced liver disease; it is also increased after upper GI bleeding, which is a common cause of worsening renal function in HRS. Creatinine production by muscle is reduced in cirrhosis, causing a misleadingly low plasma creatinine concentration and creatinine clearance. Although plasma cystatin-C concentration has better correlation with the measured glomerular filtration rate (GFR),[64,65] it has not been widely adopted for monitoring persons with cirrhosis, and one study has suggested that it may be misleading after liver transplantation.[66]

Despite its limitations, the most widely accepted criterion for diagnosis of HRS is an increase in plasma creatinine concentration or a reduction in estimated GFR. Because no specific clinical or laboratory features of HRS have been identified, diagnosis depends on the presence of severe liver disease, a rise in creatinine to more than 1.5 mg/dL (133 μmol/L), no evidence of other renal disease by urinalysis and clinical history, and lack of improvement in renal function with treatments that increase intravascular volume (such as stopping diuretics, or administration of fluids and/or albumin).[62] The latter two criteria are important because laboratory findings are similar to those of volume depletion, with low urine output, low urine sodium concentration, and increased urine osmolality.

Treatment of HRS is best accomplished by increasing systemic vascular resistance, using the vasopressin analog terlipressin, octreotide, and midadrine, in conjunction with intravascular volume expansion. The choice of agents remains controversial, but albumin infusion has been shown to reduce both the incidence of HRS and mortality. Measures that reduce portal venous pressure, such as a transjugular intrahepatic portosystemic shunt, may also be effective but may be contraindicated due to hepatic encephalopathy. Both approaches have shown promise in improving renal function in HRS.[67]

Altered Drug Metabolism

Because of the central role of the liver in drug metabolism and disposition, alterations in drug metabolism may occur in patients with liver disease. In general, this is reflected in delayed metabolism. Only patients with evidence of liver failure, such as encephalopathy, coagulopathy, or ascites, need alterations in dosing. In general, patients with liver disease are not more susceptible to drug-induced hepatotoxicity. However, those with alcoholic liver disease who continue to consume alcohol are susceptible to liver injury from acetaminophen, even at therapeutic doses.[68]

Nutritional and Metabolic Abnormalities

The intake and disposition of nutrients in patients with chronic liver disease are altered, which subjects them to nutritional imbalance. Severe metabolic and nutritional derangements have been observed in cirrhotic patients, including alterations in glucose metabolism caused by insulin resistance, and hypokalemia caused by secondary hyperaldosteronism. In addition, hypoalbuminemia is frequently present because of decreased production and sinusoidal leakage of albumin in patients with portal hypertension. Also, in patients with chronic cholestasis, impaired delivery of bile salts to the duodenum may result in malabsorption of lipids and fat-soluble vitamins, leading to deficiencies in vitamins A, D, E, and K (see Chapters 37 and 56). Vitamin A deficiency in association with liver disease may cause night blindness, but rarely progresses to serious visual impairment. Vitamin D deficiency causes osteopenia, and in severe cases, osteomalacia. Osteopenic bone disease may be one of the most crippling results of chronic cholestatic liver disease, such as PBC.[69] Vitamin E deficiency is of little clinical significance. Vitamin K deficiency leads to hypoprothrombinemia, with easy bruising and bleeding.

Disordered Hemostasis in Liver Disease

As discussed earlier and in Chapter 71, the liver manufactures most of the soluble clotting factors (the major exceptions being factor VIII and von Willebrand factor) and a number of inhibitors of clotting (proteins C and S, antithrombin III). The liver also clears activated clotting factors from the circulation. Bile acids are necessary for vitamin K absorption and are needed to produce the active forms of several clotting factors, as well as proteins C and S. Disorders of fibrinogen also occur in liver disease. For example, dysfibrinogenemia may be seen in both acute and chronic liver disease, and leads to prolongation of the partial thromboplastin time.[70] Patients with AIH may have anticardiolipin antibodies and antibodies to platelets. The liver is the major source of thrombopoietin, which is needed to produce platelets. Portal hypertension results in splenomegaly, which often leads to thrombocytopenia. In addition, persons with liver disease often have evidence of platelet-associated antibodies,[71] although their contribution to low platelet counts in liver disease is questionable.[72]

Although these facts suggest that hemostatic problems are common in patients with liver disease, discordance is often noted between the degree of abnormality of laboratory tests of coagulation and clinical evidence of bleeding.[73-75] Even in patients bleeding from esophageal varices and who have prolonged clotting times, administration of blood components (including activated factor VII) has not been associated with any clinical difference in degree of bleeding or need for blood transfusions.[75]

Enzymes Released From Diseased Liver Tissue

Because hepatic function is often normal in many patients with liver disease, the plasma activities of several cytosolic, mitochondrial, and membrane-associated enzymes are measured because they are increased in many forms of liver disease. Because plasma enzyme measurements are discussed in greater detail in Chapter 29, only those factors relevant to an understanding of liver disease will be summarized here.

Reference Intervals for Alanine Aminotransferase

One area of significant concern is the reference intervals for liver-associated enzymes, particularly for alanine aminotransferase (ALT; EC 2.6.1.2). In most laboratories, reference intervals are based on samples of the apparently healthy population. For ALT, that upper reference interval is often approximately 40 to 45 U/L in men, but many laboratories have upper reference intervals of 65 to 70 U/L, depending upon the methods used.[76] These differences are greater than can be explained by analytical differences among methods.[76] Although ALT values are approximately 40% lower in females (a difference found even in children[77]), not all laboratories have different reference intervals for the two sexes. For more information, refer to the Appendix on Reference Intervals and to the CALIPER database on pediatric reference intervals: http://www.sickkids.ca/Caliperproject/intervals/index.html.

However, population-based reference intervals may not be adequate for identifying persons with liver disease or for recognizing persons who may be at risk for metabolic syndrome or cardiovascular disease. Because many chronic liver disorders (eg, hepatitis C, alcoholic liver disease, nonalcoholic fatty liver disease [NAFLD]) are prevalent in the population, such reference intervals may include many persons with liver disease. A widely cited Italian study, which excluded persons with known or likely liver disease, suggested lowering reference intervals for ALT to approximately 30 U/L in males and 19 U/L in females.[78] However, racial and ethnic variations should be considered.

A study among dialysis patients (who had 25% lower aspartate aminotransferase [AST] and ALT compared with healthy controls) in Taiwan found that the optimal cutoff value for detecting viral hepatitis was 17 U/L.[79] In Korea, risk of development of liver steatosis increased with increasing serum ALT activity, even among those within its usual reference intervals,[80] which was also true with risk of death from cardiovascular disease.[81] A study using the Framingham study offspring in the United States found that risk of metabolic syndrome and cardiovascular disease increased significantly with ALT, which was above the lowest quartile of the normal reference intervals.[82] The National Academy of Clinical Biochemistry and the American Association for the Study of Liver Diseases (AASLD) guidelines on liver-related tests recommend that health-related reference intervals should be developed for ALT.[83] These data provide some preliminary information toward that end.

ALT levels are affected by many factors, including lifestyle; reference interval determinations using apparently healthy individuals may contain individuals with undetected liver disease, such as hepatitis C or NAFLD. Different methods for determining ALT activity also produce different results with the same population. Therefore, the physician must be aware of the reference interval for a particular laboratory's method but also should be cautious in interpreting a normal ALT in a particular patient. The debate about the upper cutoff for ALT activity is ongoing and will require a reevaluation of the risk–benefit and cost-effectiveness of any change to the conventional model of using a population-derived upper reference interval.[84-86]

Factors Affecting Plasma Enzyme Quantities

Because the pattern and degree of elevation of enzyme activity vary with the type of liver disease, their measurement is extremely helpful in the recognition and differential diagnosis of liver damage. Several factors govern the ability of liver enzymes to assist in diagnosis, including their tissue specificity, subcellular distribution, relative activity of enzyme activity in liver and plasma, patterns of release, and clearance from plasma.

Tissue Specificity

Four enzymes, ALT, AST (EC 2.6.1.1), alkaline phosphatase (ALP; 3.1.3.1), and γ-glutamyltransferase (GGT; EC 2.3.2.2) are commonly used to detect liver injury. ALT and GGT are present in several tissues, but increased plasma activities primarily reflect liver injury. AST is found in the liver and muscle (cardiac and skeletal), and to a limited extent in red cells. ALP is found in a number of tissues, but in normal individuals, it primarily reflects bone and liver sources. Thus, based on tissue distribution, ALT and GGT would seem to be the most specific markers for liver injury.

Subcellular Distribution

Enzymes are found at different locations within cells. AST and ALT are cytosolic enzymes. As such, they can be released with cell injury and appear in plasma relatively rapidly. AST and ALT have both mitochondrial and cytosolic isoenzymes in hepatocytes and other cells containing these enzymes. In the case of ALT, the relative amount of mitochondrial isoenzyme is small, and its plasma half-life is extremely short, making it of no diagnostic significance. In the case of AST, the mitochondrial isoenzyme represents a significant fraction of total AST within hepatocytes. In contrast, ALP and GGT are membrane-bound glycoprotein enzymes. The most important location of both enzymes is on the canalicular membrane of hepatocytes.

Relative Activity in Liver and Plasma

For cytoplasmic enzymes, the relative amount of enzyme in the liver relative to plasma is an important determinant of diagnostic sensitivity. The activity of AST within hepatocytes is approximately twice that of ALT, although plasma activities are similar. The relative amount of enzyme in tissue is not necessarily the same in disease; in cirrhosis and malnutrition, and with alcohol abuse, greater decreases are seen in cytoplasmic ALT than in cytoplasmic AST.[87] In addition, other mechanisms may be responsible for this difference in enzyme activity. The development of immunoassays for measuring ALT has led to the observation of discordance between enzymatic activity and mass in several types of liver disease.[88] In chronic hepatitis and in healthy individuals, ALT activity and mass change in parallel. In acute hepatitis, activity is increased to a much greater degree than mass; the opposite pattern is seen in cirrhosis and HCC. Additional studies are necessary to confirm these findings, but these results suggest that poorly understood factors still affect enzyme activity.

Mechanisms of Release

Several mechanisms appear to be involved in the release of enzymes from hepatocytes. Cell injury, the simplest mechanism, appears to allow leakage of cytoplasmic enzymes from cells, but minimal release of other types of enzymes. Thus, necroinflammatory disease leads to release of AST and ALT, but not of a mitochondrial isoenzyme of AST nor ALP or GGT. Alcohol appears to induce expression of mitochondrial AST on the surface of hepatocytes.[89]

The mechanism of release of membrane-bound enzymes such as GGT and ALP into the circulation is less well understood. Synthesis of GGT and ALP appears to be increased in the diseased human liver.[90] How this enhanced synthesis of tissue-bound enzymes translates into increased activity in plasma is not clear. However, fragments of hepatocyte membrane rich in GGT and ALP activity have been detected in the plasma of patients with cholestasis; this process may be a result of membrane fragmentation by bile acids. Furthermore, bile acids, which are detergents, could solubilize and release GGT and ALP from plasma membranes. In vitro studies of membranes treated with bile acids have shown that this possibility exists.[91]

Rate of Clearance of Enzyme From Plasma

Clearance of liver enzymes from plasma occurs at variable rates. The half-life of ALT is 47 hours and that of cytosolic AST is 17 hours; thus although more AST is released from the liver, the much longer half-life of ALT leads to higher activities of ALT than AST in most forms of hepatocellular injury. The half-life of the liver isoenzyme of ALP has been variously reported as from 1 to 10 days; the former figure

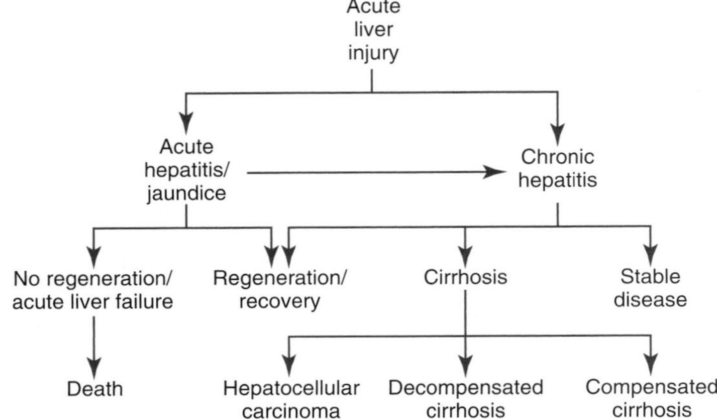

FIGURE 61.9 Natural history of liver disease. With acute injury to the liver, several outcomes are possible. In many individuals, damage is clinically inapparent and recovery occurs with clearance of the causative agent. In some, clinical acute hepatitis occurs. In most of these, clearance of the causative agent results in complete recovery; in a small minority, damage is so severe that acute liver failure (fulminant hepatitis) develops, which is usually fatal without liver transplantation. A variable percentage of persons with acute liver injury (dependent on the cause) progress to chronic hepatitis. In some, recovery eventually occurs naturally or following treatment of the underlying cause. Among those in whom chronic hepatitis persists, many will never progress to cirrhosis. Most of those who do will remain well for many years, but approximately 3% per year develop decompensated cirrhosis (bleeding varices, ascites, hepatic encephalopathy) or hepatocellular carcinoma. These are the most common causes of death from liver disease.

appears to correspond better to changes seen with removal of gallstones. The half-life of GGT has been reported as 4.1 days. The mechanism by which enzymes are removed from the circulation is not completely known, although receptor-mediated endocytosis by liver macrophages is likely involved.

DISEASES OF THE LIVER

The liver has a limited number of ways of responding to injury.[92] Acute injury to the liver may be asymptomatic, but often presents as jaundice. The major acute liver disorders are acute hepatitis and cholestasis. Chronic liver injury generally takes the clinical form of chronic hepatitis; its long-term complications include cirrhosis and HCC. The discussion of liver disease will focus mainly on these patterns and on a few diseases that differ from this general pattern.

Mechanisms and Patterns of Injury

Cell death occurs by necrosis (death of cell) or apoptosis (programmed cell death) or both. The target cell determines the pattern of injury, with hepatocyte injury leading to hepatocellular disease and biliary cell injury leading to cholestasis. All cellular injury induces fibrosis as an adaptive or healing response, with the duration of injury and genetic factors determining whether cirrhosis and ultimately carcinoma occur (Fig. 61.9).

Cellular necrosis occurs as the result of an injurious environment and has been referred to as "murder." It is characterized by cellular swelling with loss of membrane integrity. Toxic injury from compounds such as carbon tetrachloride, aspirin, and acetaminophen (Fig. 61.10) occurs for the most part by necrosis. Apoptosis occurs as the result of accelerated programmed death in which the cell participates in its own demise and thus commits "suicide." It is characterized by cell shrinkage, with nuclear chromatin condensation and fragmentation forming apoptotic bodies. Regardless of the cause, cell death typically leads to leakage of cytoplasmic enzymes. Most forms of hepatitis are associated with apoptosis.

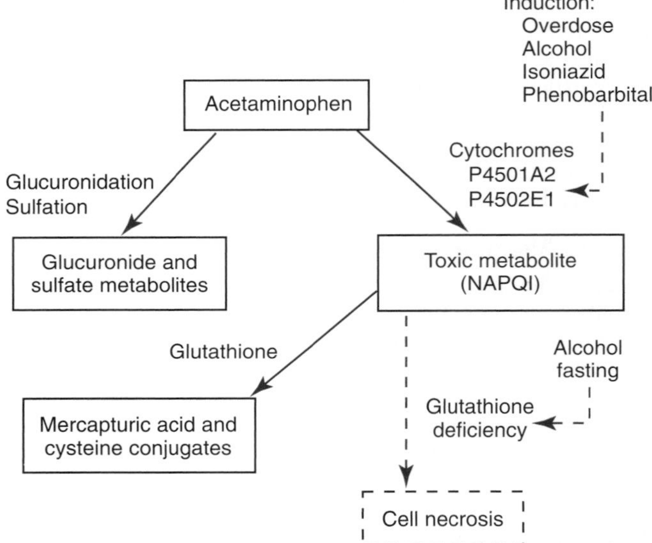

FIGURE 61.10 Metabolism of acetaminophen by the liver.

Laboratory tests are helpful in distinguishing between the pattern of injury (hepatocellular vs cholestatic), the chronicity of injury (acute vs chronic), and the severity of injury (mild vs severe). In general, the aminotransferase enzymes and ALP are used to distinguish the pattern, the plasma albumin determines the chronicity, and the PT or factor V concentration determines the severity. Classically, liver fibrosis has been assessed using liver biopsy, but in recent years

TABLE 61.2 Types of Viral Hepatitis

	A	B	C	D	E	G
Type	RNA	DNA	RNA	Partial	RNA	RNA
Incubation period, days	45–50	30–150	15–160	30–150	20–40	Unknown
Transmission						
Fecal–oral	Yes	No	Minimal	No	Yes	No
Household	Yes	Min	Min	Yes	Yes	No
Vertical	No	Yes	Min	Yes	No	Yes
Blood	Rare	Yes	Yes	Yes	Unknown	Yes
Sexual	No	Yes	Min	Yes	Unknown	Yes
Diagnosis	Anti-HAV IgM	HBsAg, PCR, anti-HBc IgM	Anti-HCV, PCR	Anti-HDV	Anti-HEV	Anti-HGV
Carrier state	No	Yes	Yes	Yes	Yes	Yes
Risk of chronic hepatitis	No	Depends on age, immune status	50–70%	Yes	Rare†	No
Risk of liver cancer	No	Yes	Yes	No	No	No
Prevention						
Vaccine	Yes	Yes	No	Yes*	No	No
Immunoglobulin	Yes	Yes	No	Yes*	No	No
Response to interferon	Not used	30%	40–80%	Yes	Not used	Yes

*Vaccination and passive immunization against HBV protects against HDV infection.
†Only with severe immunosuppression.
HAV, Hepatitis A virus; *HBc*, hepatitis B core antigen; *HBsAg*, hepatitis B surface antigen; *HCV*, hepatitis C virus; *HDV*, hepatitis D virus; *HEV*, hepatitis E virus; *HGV*, hepatitis G virus; *IgM*, immunoglobulin M; *PCR*, polymerase chain reaction.

several noninvasive methods of assessment of liver fibrosis have been described and evaluated. Although liver biopsy yields incomparable information about the nature, severity, and chronicity of liver disease, noninvasive tests may provide more accurate assessment of liver fibrosis, and in particular, disease severity and prognosis.

Disorders of Bilirubin Metabolism

Defects in bilirubin metabolism resulting in jaundice are known to occur at each step in the metabolic pathway (see Chapter 38). Disorders related to these defects are discussed in Chapter 38.

Hepatic Viral Infection

Five viruses (hepatitis A, B, C, D, and E) have been identified as causes of infections that primarily target the liver. In addition, certain other viruses may infect the liver as part of a more generalized infection, of which the more important causes include cytomegalovirus (CMV), Epstein-Barr virus (EBV), and herpes simplex virus (HSV). Several other viruses have been proposed as causes of liver injury; these include hepatitis G virus[93] (HGV; discussed later), transfusion-transmitted virus,[94] and the closely related SEN virus.[95] Although all three are blood-borne chronic viral infections, and in the case of transfusion-transmitted virus and SEN, have been known to replicate in the liver, none of these viruses appear to cause acute or chronic liver injury.[96-98] The various hepatitis viruses are outlined in Table 61.2.

Hepatitis A Virus

Hepatitis A virus (HAV) has historically accounted for approximately one-fourth to one-third of cases of clinical acute hepatitis in the United States and 20% to 25% worldwide. Since the mid-1980s, a vaccine has been available for HAV, and incidence has declined to its lowest ever in the United States.[99] Current recommendations are that all children should be immunized for HAV, along with adults at high risk for HAV,[100] as well as persons planning international travel and individuals exposed to HAV.[101] Although most commonly an infection in children and adolescents before the introduction of widespread immunization, the disease has now become more common in developed countries in adults than children; it is most common in young adult men, particularly in people exposed to sewage, those who eat raw seafood, people who inject drugs, and in men who have sex with men.[102] It tends to be most virulent in middle-aged and older people. Epidemics have been associated with waterborne and foodborne contamination. Ingestion of raw shellfish from contaminated waters has caused both sporadic and epidemic cases. Although not as common a cause of liver infection as hepatitis B, it is more frequently associated with jaundice when it occurs in adults than hepatitis B or C; an estimated 50% to 70% of infected adults develop jaundice, and mortality is almost 2% with infection in those older than 60 years of age.[99] In contrast, hepatitis A infection in children is rarely associated with jaundice, and thus is usually not detected clinically. Hepatitis A may cause severe hepatitis and death in those who have chronic hepatitis, particularly hepatitis B or C.[103]

Hepatitis A is caused by a 27-nm RNA picornavirus. It has four capsid proteins (VP1–4), but only one serotype has been identified. The virus is not cytopathic to hepatocytes, but causes liver injury by stimulating both cellular and humoral immune responses. Hepatitis A occurs in sporadic and epidemic forms, with an incubation period of 15 to 50 days. The clinical course of acute hepatitis A is usually that of a mild flu-like illness that lasts for a few days to a few weeks. There is no chronic form of hepatitis A, but cholestasis (manifested by several weeks of jaundice and pruritus) may occur in some adults. Although a rare occurrence, relapse has been known to happen 1 to 3 months after the acute illness in up to 5% of patients. It resembles the acute illness and is associated with viremia, but recovery always ensues.

Although tests for HAV RNA are available for research purposes, diagnosis of HAV is based primarily on serologic tests for antibodies to HAV. Total anti-HAV is believed to be protective and occurs with natural exposure to HAV and to HAV vaccine. With natural exposure, HAV antibodies appear to persist for life.[104] IgM antibodies to HAV are always present at the time of diagnosis of acute hepatitis A and generally remain present for 3 to 6 months, although they may persist for longer in approximately 14% of individuals.[105] With the falling prevalence of HAV, the number of cases of acute HAV reported to the Centers for Disease Control and Prevention (CDC) that are due to false-positive results exceeds the frequency of actual cases of HAV.[106] For this reason, IgM anti-HAV should be used only in the clinical setting of acute hepatitis.

Three types of effective vaccines are available. A monovalent vaccine against HAV, a combined HAV and hepatitis B virus (HBV) vaccine, and a combined HAV and typhoid vaccine. Vaccination followed by a booster at 12 months will provide immunity for up to 20 years.

Hepatitis B Virus

HBV is the most common cause of acute hepatitis, and the most common chronic viral infection worldwide. An estimated 350 million individuals are chronically infected with HBV, and several times as many individuals have been exposed to HBV. The frequency of chronic HBV infection varies worldwide, and it is highest in most of central and southeast Asia, central Africa, and southern Europe (prevalence >8% of the population) and intermediate (2% to 8%) in most of the rest of Asia, Africa, and South America. It occurs rarely among those born in North America and Europe[107]; one study found that 86% of US residents with chronic HBV were actually born outside the United States.[108] In endemic areas, the incidence of new infection has decreased markedly in those places where HBV vaccine has been introduced. HBV is transmitted through body fluids, primarily by parenteral or sexual contact; it can be transmitted from mother to child, usually at or after delivery (termed vertical transmission). In parts of the world with high rates of chronic infection, much of the transmission is vertical. The residual risk from transfusion is estimated to be 1 in 600,000.[109]

Hepatitis B is caused by a 42-nm DNA virus that is a member of the hepadnavirus family. The DNA is partially double stranded and contains 3200 nucleotides with overlapping coding regions, leading to several major open reading frames. The S gene codes for several different length variants of surface protein; the smallest form, hepatitis B surface antigen (HBsAg), is produced independently of and in excess of the amount needed for viral replication; the largest form (S1) makes up the surface coat of circulating viral particles. The C gene encodes the hepatitis B core antigen (HBcAg), which is part of the infectious core of the virus. The X gene codes for a transactivating factor that may be involved with viral replication and the development of malignancy. The precore and basal core promoter regions code for production of hepatitis B e antigen (HBeAg), which is a protein found only in those with (but separate from) circulating viral particles. The final major viral protein is a polymerase, which has several different enzymatically active sites. Hepadnaviruses are unusual among DNA viruses because they produce the first strand of DNA from a form of viral messenger RNA (mRNA), using the reverse transcriptase activity of HBV polymerase. This error-prone reproductive strategy, along with an extremely high rate of viral replication in chronically infected individuals, leads to a high rate of mutation in HBV. The significance of several mutants is described later.

Hepatitis B was first described in the 1960s by Blumberg and colleagues after discovery of a protein, termed the Australia antigen, which was initially believed to be a tumor marker for leukemia.[110] Subsequent studies confirmed it to be a marker for a form of hepatitis initially termed serum hepatitis. Later work established that this was HBsAg. The complete HBV virion (Dane particle) consists of a core containing DNA attached to DNA polymerase and HBcAg, surrounded by the S1 form of surface protein. HBsAg and other forms of surface protein contain a common determinant, a, and four subdeterminants designated d, y, w, and r. These determinants are responsible for determining HBV genotypes; the eight major genotypes, termed A through H, have less than 92% homology with other types.[111] Geographic differences in genotype distribution have been noted; genotype A predominates among those infected in North America, whereas genotype C is the dominant form in those infected in Asia. Although not routinely determined at present, evidence indicates that genotype is an important predictor of the natural course of HBV and response to certain forms of treatment.[112] For example, genotypes A1 and F1 are associated with HCC in young adults and (in Alaska with genotype F1) children.[113] Genotype C has a higher risk of development of cirrhosis and HCC than is the case with most other genotypes. Genotype C has a low likelihood of response to INF treatment.

Several mutants of HBV may have clinical importance (see the following).

Pathogenesis of Hepatitis B. The HBV virus is not directly cytopathic. The liver damage associated with HBV infection is mediated by the immune response to HBV with innate and adaptive inflammatory immune responses causing hepatocyte necrosis and apoptosis that is accompanied by wound healing response, which results in liver fibrosis. This results in the typical histological picture of viral hepatitis characterized by hepatic inflammation with interface hepatitis and fibrosis. Recognition of the importance of the immune response to HBV has led to the classification of stages of chronic hepatitis based on the host immune response. In the early "immune-tolerant" phase of chronic infection,[114] the host mounts little in the way of an immune response to high levels of viral replication. This is characterized by high levels of viremia, normal ALT levels, and eAg positive eAb negative serology. Once host immunity is activated, hepatitis ensues, characterized by falling levels of viremia, elevated transaminases, and fluctuating serology. This phase is termed the immune-reactive phase. In most cases, this phase gives way to a prolonged period of immune control with inactive disease characterized by eAg negativity, eAb positivity, low or undetectable HBV viremia, and normal transaminases. In a minority of eAg negative patients, the emergence of replicative mutants results in rising HBV DNA titers that may be accompanied by immune activation and an HBVeAg negative hepatitis. In some cases, this pattern of disease may fluctuate with periods of activity and periods of inactive hepatitis, making diagnosis difficult and dependent on frequent blood tests. Both chronic eAg negative hepatitis and fluctuating eAg negative hepatitis are associated with progressive fibrosis and hepatocellular cancer, and should be looked for in patients with eAg negative disease. Normal blood tests for HBV DNA and ALT every 2 to 3 months over 12 months should exclude active hepatitis in more than 90% of cases.

Hepatitis B e Antigen and Hepatitis B e Antigen Mutants. Hepatitis B e antigen is a protein of uncertain function produced by viral mRNA. It is released into the circulation by infected hepatocytes and may be involved as a "decoy" that prevents the immune system from attacking HBV viral particles. The most common HBV mutations involve the regions that code for production of HBeAg. The highest frequency is for a mutation at nucleotide 1896 that inserts a stop codon in the mRNA, preventing production of HBeAg. Mutations in the precore promoter region, particularly at nucleotides 1762 and 1764, are associated with reduced production of normal HBeAg. Such mutants are associated with undetectable HBeAg and are usually found in patients with detectable levels of anti-HBe. Precore and core promoter mutants are found in most individuals chronically infected with HBV in areas with high rates of infection, such as Asia and Southern Europe. In North America, it is estimated that 10% to 20% of individuals with chronic HBV infection have such precore mutants.[115] Such mutants may be present at the time of infection or may develop during the course of disease. Although initially it was believed that individuals infected with such mutants were much more likely to have severe acute infection, the high prevalence of such mutants suggests that this is not the case. Infection with these mutant strains is associated with a higher risk of development of HCC, and risk is stronger for the basal core promoter mutations.[116]

Polymerase Mutants. Treatment with antiviral agents that inhibit the reverse transcriptase domain of HBV polymerase is now the most widely used therapy for chronic HBV.[117] As with HIV, specific amino acid substitutions have been linked to resistance with several of the commonly used agents, particularly lamivudine and adefovir. The longer these agents are used, the greater is the likelihood that resistant mutants will emerge. Testing to detect resistant mutants is becoming more widely performed, particularly in individuals who have been exposed to more than one reverse transcriptase inhibitor (such as those who also are infected with HIV). Nucleotide and nucleoside polymerase inhibitors that are highly potent and present a higher barrier to resistance (eg, tenofovir and entecavir) are much less likely to select resistance and can be used long-term to suppress viremia. However, it is mandatory that patients prescribed these drugs are checked regularly for adherence to treatment, therapeutic effectiveness, and for the emergence of mutants.

Hepatitis B Surface Antigen Mutants. Mutations in the "a" determinant of HBsAg are the most important HBsAg mutants. Antibody to HBsAg, which is developed by natural exposure or by the HBV vaccine, is primarily directed against the "a" determinant. Exposure to strains that have mutations in this domain can result in infection despite the presence of protective titers of anti-HBs. In areas where HBV is endemic, up to 25% of cases of HBV in immunized infants are due to infection by such mutants.[118,119] In addition, the reagents used to detect HBsAg are antibodies to anti-HBs; therefore, mutant strains can be missed by HBsAg assays.[120-122] The ability of reagents to identify these mutant strains differs, mainly because of the specific epitopes recognized by the antibody (or antibodies) used in the assay.[123] Use of assays with antibodies to multiple epitopes improves detection of such mutant strains.[124] At present, the importance of such mutant strains is unknown. Data suggest that most individuals infected with mutant strains have such viral particles at low titers, usually in the presence of larger amounts of wild-type virus. Thus, most infected persons will be detected by the current assays for HBV. However, some infected individuals (perhaps more commonly those immunized for HBV) will be missed by some current assays.

Immunization. Hepatitis B may be prevented by passive (hepatitis B immune globulin [HBIG]) or active (hepatitis B recombinant vaccine) immunization. In the United States, current data suggest that more than 90% of children have been immunized against HBV infection, leading to a historically low incidence of acute HBV infection. Because infants born to HBsAg mothers have a high risk of developing chronic HBV infection, routine prenatal testing for HBsAg is needed to identify infants at risk. Infection occurs in only approximately 2% of infants before birth[125]; postexposure prophylaxis (typically used in infants of HBsAg positive mothers), which consists of passive immunization with 0.06 mL/kg of HBIG and the first dose of hepatitis B vaccine within 24 hours of birth is more than 95% effective in preventing infection.[126] A universal immunization program in Taiwan, where vertical transmission of HBV was endemic, has greatly reduced the death rate from HCC in young individuals.[127]

Diagnostic Tests for Hepatitis B. More diagnostic tests exist to measure hepatitis B than any of the hepatitis viruses; consequently, interpretation of results is complicated. Testing currently primarily involves ELISA or related techniques to measure viral antigens or antibodies, but nucleic acid–based tests are becoming more widely used.

HBsAg, the most widely used marker for detecting current hepatitis B infection, is detected by kits using antibody to HBsAg. Occasionally, false-positive results occur in testing, particularly during pregnancy; a neutralization assay is available. Low-level reactivity (as evaluated by the ratio of the signal from the sample to that of the cutoff for distinguishing positive and negative, termed the signal/cutoff [S/C] ratio) is highly predictive of samples that fail to confirm neutralization.[128] False-negative results can occur with mutants in the surface antigen (as previously described), and they occur more commonly in early HBV infection. Most assays are qualitative; quantitative HBsAg assays have been available in Europe for more than a decade. Some studies have shown a direct relationship (in untreated individuals) between quantitative HBV DNA and viral load[129]; others have not.[130] Declines in quantitative HBsAg during treatment have been found to be predictive of response to treatment for chronic HBV,[131,132] and lower levels of HBsAg may identify patients with HBeAg negative disease who do not require long-term treatment to maintain viral suppression.

Antibody to the hepatitis B core antigen (anti-HBc) is the most commonly detected antibody against HBV. Two assays are usually used: IgM and total anti-HBc. IgM anti-HBc assays typically use a large dilution of plasma (1:100) before analysis to reduce the likelihood of positivity in individuals with chronic HBV. The total antibody assay measures both IgM and IgG antibodies. Anti-HBc appears to last longer than anti-HBs in natural infection, and is still present in 97% of previously infected individuals more than 30 years after exposure.[133] Isolated anti-HBc is a relatively common finding, particularly in the setting of hepatitis C virus (HCV) coinfection,[134] but is also found in immunosuppressed individuals. Although this may represent a false-positive result, particularly as a transient phenomenon after influenza vaccination, current guidelines on hepatitis B recommend consideration of individuals with isolated anti-HBc as having been exposed to HBV.[135]

Antibody to the HBsAg (anti-HBs) is considered evidence of immunity to hepatitis B and is the only marker found in those have received the hepatitis B vaccine. The WHO has developed reference material that contains 10 IU/mL of anti-HBs. Current guidelines suggest that immunocompetent individuals who achieve an anti-HBs of ≥10 IU/mL have lifelong immunity to hepatitis B.

The HBeAg and antibody to the e antigen (anti-HBe) are typically used only in the setting of chronic HBV infection. Although HBeAg typically appears at about the same time as HBsAg in acute hepatitis, it is rarely used as a marker for acute infection. In chronic infection, HBeAg has historically been used as a marker of persistence of infectious virus; its clearance and the appearance of anti-HBe have been used as indicators of conversion to the nonreplicating state and as goals of antiviral treatment. With widespread availability of HBV DNA assays with low detection limits, the discordance between HBeAg and the presence of infectious viral particles has become apparent. Although most untreated patients with HBV who are HBeAg positive have high viral loads (usually >10^6 IU/mL), detectable HBV DNA is also found (usually with lower viral load) in approximately 70% of those who are HBeAg negative. When HBeAg positive individuals are treated with polymerase inhibitors, loss of HBV DNA occurs in the majority, and HBeAg usually remains detectable. Loss of HBeAg during treatment, with development of anti-HBe, indicates a high likelihood that viral suppression will be maintained after discontinuation of treatment.[117] In contrast, in those with HBV viremia who were HBeAg negative (and anti-HBe positive) before treatment, discontinuation of treatment usually leads to recurrence of viremia. Thus, HBeAg remains an important marker for monitoring therapy, but has largely been replaced by HBV DNA for detection of those who harbor the infectious virus.

Hepatitis B viral DNA is now routinely measured using amplification techniques. The WHO has established an international reference material for HBV DNA, and results are typically reported in international units per milliliter[136]; conversion from copies per milliliter differs on the basis of viral load and is different for various assays. Because much older literature and some currently published papers still report HBV DNA in copies per milliliter, a rough conversion factor is 5 copies/mL = 1 IU/mL. Currently, assays that use amplification, particularly polymerase chain reaction (PCR) methods, have detection limits of 100 IU/mL, although nonamplified assays are still available. It is unclear what amount of HBV DNA represents clinically important viremia; however, data (primarily from Taiwan) have shown that risk of progression to cirrhosis or HCC increases at viral loads at more than 10,000 copies/mL (2000 IU/mL).[137] Current treatment guidelines suggest that this number should be used as one criterion in treatment decision-making.[138]

Hepatitis B mutants and genotypes are usually determined by direct sequencing or with the use of line probes.

Hepatitis C Virus. The HCV is the cause of most cases previously known as non-A, non-B hepatitis. It was recognized in 1989[139] and fully characterized 2 years later.[140] It is the most common cause of chronic viral hepatitis in North America, Europe, and Japan, and is estimated to infect approximately 170 million individuals worldwide. Although HBV infection appears to have been present for a long time, evidence suggests that HCV is a more recently developing viral infection, because rates of HCV-related liver disease have been increasing in many parts of the world. Predictions are that HCV-related end-stage chronic liver disease will increase twofold to threefold over the next 20 to 30 years.[141] HCV infection primarily occurs through plasma; major risk factors are injection drug use and transfusion. For example, before the recognition of and availability of tests for HCV, the frequency of posttransfusion hepatitis (mainly due to HCV) was 3.5%[142]; the risk of HCV transmission by transfusion is currently estimated at 1:2,000,000.[109] Because of its mode of spread, HCV infection is rare in children; the only common causes of pediatric infections are vertical transmission from an infected mother (estimated to occur in ≈5% of infected women[143]) and previously transfusion of infected blood products. In countries where standards of hygiene are suboptimal, unsterile medical and ritual practices continue to account for new infections.

HCV is a single-stranded enveloped RNA virus of the flavivirus family, which includes other hepatitis viruses (yellow fever virus) and viruses that cause unrelated disease (such as West Nile virus). HCV RNA contains one reading frame (Fig. 61.11). The resulting polypeptide is cleaved to core and envelope antigens, and a number of nonstructural proteins, including a polymerase, a protease, and an INF response element. As an RNA virus, HCV is subject to a high rate of spontaneous mutation, giving rise to large numbers of variants. This results in six major genotypes (<70% nucleotide homology), along with a number of subtypes (77% to 80% homology).[144,145] According to various global reviews, genotype 1 (G1) is the most common (46%; affecting ≈83 million cases, one-third of which are in East Asia), followed by G3 (22% to 31%; ≈54 million), G2 (13%; ≈22 million), and G4 (13%; ≈22 million).[146,147] In a chronically infected individual, numerous quasispecies (>90% homology) develop over time. These quasispecies seem to be important in establishing

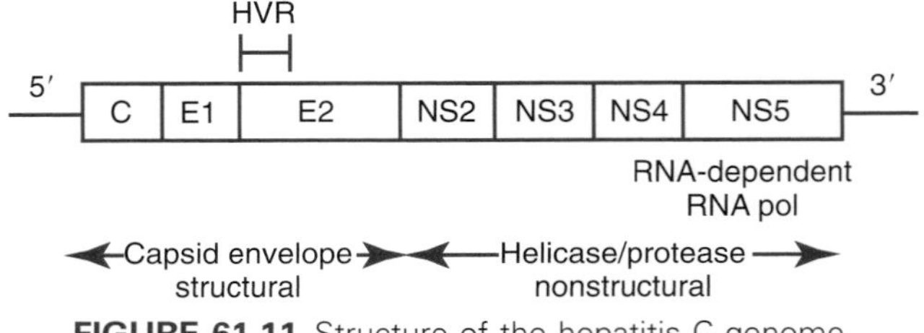

FIGURE 61.11 Structure of the hepatitis C genome.

chronic infection[148] and appear to be related to the fluctuating nature of chronic inflammation in chronic HCV infection.[149] Quasispecies are unique to the individual infected; those infected from a common source show different patterns of mutation.[150]

Chronic HCV infection is associated with evidence of chronic liver injury in most cases. Elevations in liver-associated enzymes, particularly ALT, are usually mild and fluctuate between normal and abnormal in most infected individuals. In an estimated 15% to 20% of cases, cirrhosis becomes evident an average of 20 to 30 years after exposure. HCC may develop once cirrhosis is present, at an average rate of 1.5 to 3 cases per year. In North America, Europe, and Japan, HCV is the most common risk factor in the development of HCC. Various extrahepatic manifestations of chronic HCV infection may be noted; the most common are cryoglobulinemia and porphyria cutanea tarda (see Chapter 39 on Porphyrias). Epidemiologic evidence has linked HCV to increased risk of lymphoma and type 2 diabetes mellitus.

Prevention. Prevention of hepatitis C has proved more difficult than that of HAV and HBV. However, an 80% decrease in the incidence of acute HCV has occurred,[99] which is similar to what occurred with HAV and HBV; this is believed to be due to testing of blood donors for HCV and to safe injection practices that have been instituted to reduce the risk of HIV infection. Vaccine development has been difficult because of the many subspecies of virus and the presence of many quasispecies with different antigenic determinants. The dramatic evolution in treatments for HCV over the last two decades has culminated in the development of drugs capable of eradicating infection in more than 90% of cases of most genotypes of HCV.[151]

Diagnostic Tests for Hepatitis C. Measurement of the antibody to HCV (anti-HCV) is the principal screening test for HCV exposure. These tests, which use ELISAs and related microparticle chemiluminescence formats, detect the presence of antibodies to one or more HCV antigens (derived by recombinant technology from yeast cultures or through production of synthetic peptides). Although the initial assay detected only antibody to a single antigen, subsequent tests have used antigens from four different regions of the HCV genome. Second-generation assays become positive an average of 12 weeks after exposure, and third-generation assays become positive an average of 9 weeks after exposure. After comparison with a cutoff value, results are interpreted as positive or negative. As is true for HBsAg, samples with a low S/C ratio are often false positive, whereas false-positive results are rare in samples with a high S/C ratio.[152,153] Current CDC recommendations suggest use of an S/C ratio of less than 3.8 for both second- and third-generation ELISA assays, and an S/C ratio less than 8.0 for the chemiluminescence assay, to define low-positive results.[135] Samples with a low S/C ratio are recommended to be confirmed, ideally with the use of a recombinant immunoblot assay (RIBA).

RIBA is a technique similar in principle to Western blotting. HCV antigens used in anti-HCV assays are typically blotted onto a membrane as dots, and reactivity is detected after incubation with serum. Results are interpreted as negative if there is less than 1+ reactivity with any of the four antigens, indeterminate if there is 1+ or greater reactivity to only a single antigen (or to more than one antigen along with the nonspecific yeast marker superoxide dismutase), and positive with 1+ or greater reactivity to multiple antigens. Third-generation RIBAs have considerably fewer indeterminate results than second-generation RIBAs.

HCV RNA measurement has become the most widely used test to detect current HCV infection. Typical of RNA in general, HCV RNA is labile in whole blood because of the action of RNAses primarily found in blood cells. Rapid separation of serum from a clot is critical for accurate measurement of HCV RNA. If serum is separated from the clot by centrifugation within 1 hour, HCV RNA does not show an appreciable decline until 6 hours after collection. If serum is physically separated from cells within 1 hour, samples are stable at room temperature for 3 days, at refrigerator temperatures for 1 week, and indefinitely if frozen.[154] Samples collected in ethylenediaminetetraacetic acid, which inhibits enzyme activity, are stable for 24 hours, even if plasma is not separated from red cells.[155]

Assays for HCV RNA historically were divided into qualitative and quantitative variants. An international reference material for quantification of HCV RNA has been developed,[156] and quantitative HCV RNA assay results are calibrated using this material and are reported in international units per milliliter. The relationship between international units per milliliter and copies per milliliter differs significantly for different assays. Results expressed in international units per milliliter agree within 1 log in approximately 90% of samples, but discrepant results do occur.[157] Until recently, qualitative assays had significantly lower detection limits than quantitative assays, but quantitative assays using real-time PCR have equivalent or lower detection limits compared with qualitative assays. If assays with detection limits of 10 to 20 IU/mL are used (as is the case in many settings), qualitative assays are no longer needed.[158] One of the currently available real-time PCR assays tends to underreport viral load among 15% of individuals infected with genotype 2[159] and may cause falsely negative results with genotype 4.[160]

Hepatitis C core antigen (HCV Ag) is produced by the most constant part of the HCV genome. HCV Ag is one of the major targets of antibody formation, and most HCV Ag circulates bound to antibody. HCV Ag has a similar time course to that of HCV RNA in both acute and chronic HCV infection[161]; the currently available assay for HCV Ag becomes reliably positive when HCV RNA is 20,000 IU/mL or greater.[162] In one laboratory, experience with several thousand HCV RNA samples suggested that less than 5% of untreated HCV RNA–positive individuals had a viral load of less than 20,000 IU/mL. In contrast to HCV RNA, HCV Ag is stable in storage. Currently, no commercial HCV Ag assays are available in North America.

Hepatitis C genotype shows regional diversity and is an important parameter in the development of vaccines and for determining the length and intensity of antiviral therapy.[145-147] Several methods are currently used to determine the infecting genotype. Although serologic assays to detect antibodies to specific genotypes of HCV are available, their correlation with direct tests is approximately 90%,[163] and a significant minority of infected individuals have antibodies to more than one genotype.[164] However, detection of viral RNA of more than one genotype is exceptionally rare. The most reliable method involves direct sequencing of regions of the genome that show characteristic patterns with specific genotypes and subtypes. Commercial assays using the 5′-untranslated region are the most widely used,[165] although assays using the NS5b region are now available. All currently available assays show good agreement on genotype, although they differ in their detection limits.[166] Sequencing methods have the advantage that they can be used to identify treatment resistance–associated variants that may develop under selection pressure from the new directly acting antiviral agents. Line probe assays are also widely used and show good agreement with direct sequencing assays.[167]

Hepatitis D Virus (Delta Agent)

Hepatitis D virus (HDV) is an incomplete, 36-nm RNA particle that cannot replicate on its own.[168] It is coated with HBsAg and is dependent on HBV for its activation. It is thus a satellite virus similar to that seen in plants. The D virus is a single-stranded antisense RNA virus. It is very infectious and strongly associated with intravenous drug use; approximately 10 million individuals have been infected worldwide, although the incidence is declining with the fall in incidence of HBV infection.[169] It occurs as simultaneous infection with hepatitis B (coinfection) or as a superimposed infection in someone with chronic hepatitis B (superinfection). Coinfection usually runs the same time course as acute hepatitis B, and HDV is spontaneously cleared as the hepatitis B resolves, but the risk of fulminant hepatitis is higher than in HBV infection alone, and mortality is higher. Superinfection typically results in chronic HDV infection, suppression of HBV DNA replication, and more rapid progression to cirrhosis (estimated 4%/year) and HCC (estimated 3%/year).[170] It should be assessed in all patients with HBV infection due to the seriousness of coinfection and suspected in patients with HBV infection whose condition worsens.[171] Although it is traditionally diagnosed serologically by detection of anti-HDV (total or IgM) and/or HDV Ag,[172] HDV RNA measurements are often used as evidence of current infection.[173]

Hepatitis E Virus

Hepatitis E virus (HEV) is a 34-nm, single-stranded, unenveloped RNA virus. It accounts for sporadic and epidemic hepatitis in tropical and semitropical countries and in people returning from these areas.[174] Although considered to be rare in Europe and nontropical areas of North America, HEV RNA is frequently isolated from city sewage treatment plants in such nonendemic areas.[175] A number of small outbreaks have occurred in Europe over the past several years[176]; in one institution in England, HEV was responsible for approximately 10% of otherwise undiagnosed cases of acute hepatitis.[177] It is enterically transmitted, as is HAV, and viral RNA has been detected in plasma and in stools.[178] There is probably only one species, although four genotypes are known. Tests to detect an antibody to HEV have been developed; specificity for HEV is high only for assays that detect an antibody to the open reading frame 2 antigen.[179] The prevalence of antibodies to HEV is high in the United States, with 21% of randomly selected individuals having anti-HEV from 1988 to 1994.[180] HEV has been isolated from a number of animals, notably rats[181] and pigs[182]; the significance of this is unclear, although it has been speculated that HEV is a zoonotic disease.[183,184] In several countries, HEV has been linked to ingestion of pork,[176] and in the United States, to ingestion of liver (from unclassified species).[180]

As with HAV, IgM anti-HEV detection of antibodies has been considered diagnostic of acute infection by HEV, but false-positive results have been reported with hepatitis due to CMV and EBV.[185] The clinical course is similar to that of HAV infection, in that HEV typically infects young people, has a self-limited course, and has not been associated with chronicity. Recently, however, chronic infection with HEV has been documented in organ transplantation recipients.[186,187] A peculiar feature of this disease is its virulent course in late pregnancy in India, with mortality generally in the range of 20% to 25%, but rates as high as 50% have been reported.[188] Mortality during pregnancy is not increased in other parts of the world.[189] Mortality is increased among the elderly and in those with chronic liver disease.[177] The interested reader is referred to more recent reviews for further information on the epidemiology, diagnosis, and treatment of HEV infection.[190,191]

Hepatitis G Virus

HGV, also known as GBV-C, is an RNA virus of the flavivirus family and is closely related to HCV.[93] It is most commonly transmitted by plasma[192]; vertical transmission has also been reported.[193] Although it has a very high infection rate in recipients of contaminated blood (>90%), HGV infection appears to have no adverse consequences.[194] Although it has been called a hepatitis virus, viral RNA cannot be isolated from the liver in chronic infection.[195] Coinfection with HCV and HGV is common, but coinfection has no effect on prognosis in HCV.[196,197] HGV and HIV coinfection is common; individuals coinfected with HGV and HIV have lower HIV viral loads and a better prognosis than those infected with HIV alone.[198-200] The pathogenesis of this presumed viral interaction is still unknown,[201] although stimulation of innate immunity may be involved.[202]

Acute Hepatitis

Acute hepatitis refers to an acute injury directed against the hepatocytes. The injury may be mediated directly, which occurs with certain drugs, such as acetaminophen or with ischemia, or indirectly, which occurs with immunologically mediated injury from most of the hepatitis viruses and most drugs, including ethanol. In direct injury, a typical rapid rise in cytosolic enzymes, such as AST, ALT, and lactate dehydrogenase (LDH), is followed by a rapid fall, with rates of decline similar to known half-lives of the enzymes. With immunologic injury, a gradual rise in cytosolic enzymes occurs, followed by a plateau phase and gradual resolution of enzyme elevation. Although jaundice is a key clinical finding in acute hepatitis, it is often absent (as discussed later under the various forms of viral infection). An increase in AST activity to greater than 200 U/L or in ALT activity to greater than 300 U/L has sensitivity and specificity greater than 90% for acute hepatitis.[203]

ALP usually is mildly elevated and typically is less than three times the upper reference limit in 90% of cases of acute hepatitis.[203] Increased plasma concentration of bilirubin, when present, typically is predominantly due to direct reacting bilirubin; indirect bilirubin is higher than direct bilirubin in approximately 15% of cases.[2] The distribution of direct bilirubin percentage is identical in acute hepatitis and bile duct obstruction, making the relative amount of direct bilirubin inconsequential in the differential between hepatitis and obstruction.[2] Liver synthetic function usually

TABLE 61.3 Laboratory Features of Different Forms of Acute Hepatitis

Type	AST/ALT	ALP	Bilirubin	PT (s)	Serology	Other
Viral	8–50× URL	<3× URL	5–15 mg/dL (86–256 μmol/L)	<15	Positive	
HAV					IgM anti-HAV	
HBV					HBsAg, IgM anti-HBc	
HCV					HCV RNA ± anti-HCV	
Alcoholic	<8× URL	>3× URL in 25%	5–15 mg/dL (85–256 μmol/L)	<15	Negative	AST > ALT
Toxic	>50× URL	Normal	<5 mg/dL <85 μmol/L)	>15	Negative	Toxin usually detectable; acute renal failure common
Ischemic	>50× URL	Normal	<5 mg/dL (<85 μmol/L)	>15	Negative	Acute renal failure common
Drug induced	8–50× URL	>3× URL in 50%	5–15 mg/dL (85–256 μmol/L)	<15	Negative	Eosinophilia, skin rash common
Autoimmune	8–50× URL	<3× URL	5–15 mg/dL (85–256 μmol/L)	<15	Positive ANA or ASMA	Low albumin, high globulins
Wilson	8–50× URL	Low normal or decreased	5–15 mg/dL (85–256 μmol/L)	<15	Negative	Hemolytic anemia, renal failure, low ALP common; low ceruloplasmin often absent

ALP, Alkaline phosphatase; *ALT*, alanine aminotransferase; *ANA*, antinuclear antibody; *ASMA*, anti–smooth muscle (or antiactin) antibody; *AST*, aspartate aminotransferase; *HAV*, hepatitis A virus; *HBc*, hepatitis B core antigen; *HBsAg*, hepatitis B surface antigen; *HBV*, hepatitis B virus; *HCV*, hepatitis C virus; *IgM*, immunoglobulin M; *URL*, upper reference limit.

is well preserved in most forms of acute hepatitis. These and other features that are helpful in the differential diagnosis of acute hepatitis are summarized in Table 61.3.

The outcome of acute hepatitis is variable. In most cases, complete recovery occurs, and liver regeneration leads to normal structure and function. With some viruses, failure to clear infection leads to development of chronic hepatitis. In a small percentage of cases, massive destruction of the liver leads to acute (fulminant) hepatic failure, which is associated with high mortality unless liver transplantation is performed.[204,205]

Acute Viral Hepatitis

All forms of acute viral hepatitis have similar pathology and a similar clinical course. They are all diagnosed on the basis of marked elevations in serum aminotransferase activities, usually to between 8 and 50 times the upper reference intervals, with only slight elevations in ALP and little or no effect on hepatic synthetic function. ALT is typically higher than AST because of slower clearance. Enzyme elevations typically peak before peak bilirubin occurs, and remain increased for an average of 4 to 5 weeks (longer for ALT than AST because of its longer half-life). Bilirubin elevation is variable, as is discussed later. The incidence of acute viral hepatitis due to HAV, HBV, and HCV reached historically low levels by 2007. However, the incidence of these infections reported in the most recent report from the CDC in 2013 described an increase in acute cases of all three infections. This has been attributed in part to changes in methodology in 2011, but also to a large outbreak of HAV, inward migration of people carrying HBV, and better diagnoses of cases of HCV infection.[99] For more detailed information on acute viral hepatitis, the reader is referred to the practice guideline of the World Gastroenterology Organisation.[206]

Acute Hepatitis A. In adults, approximately 70% of those with acute HAV infection develop jaundice much more commonly than those with HBV or HCV. In children, acute HAV infection typically goes unrecognized and is often considered to be a viral gastroenteritis or other viral disease, because only 10% of children become jaundiced. The disease is more prolonged and serious in individuals older than age 60 years, can cause liver failure in persons with chronic HCV[103] or cirrhosis,[207] and has high mortality. The specific etiologic diagnosis is made with serologic tests. An IgM antibody (anti-HAV IgM) appears early in the course of the illness and persists for an average of 2 to 6 months; rarely, IgM antibodies may remain positive for a year or longer. The presence of IgM anti-HAV has therefore been considered diagnostic of a recent HAV infection. No antigen tests are available for detection of hepatitis A in serum. Incubation of stool samples with labeled antibodies to hepatitis A and examination with an electron microscope have been used in the past to detect infectious viral particles. Amplification techniques (usually with reverse transcriptase PCR [rt-PCR]) have been used to detect virus in epidemiologic studies, but are not routinely used to diagnose infection.

Acute Hepatitis B. In most of the world, HBV is the most common cause of acute viral hepatitis. As with HAV, most infections in children are clinically silent. An estimated one-third of adolescents and adults with acute HBV infection develop jaundice. The outcome in acute HBV infection is strongly influenced by age and immune status. In healthy adolescents and adults, an estimated 1% to 3% of cases will progress to chronic infection. In a person with immunosuppression, the likelihood of chronic infection increases to 10%. Neonates infected with HBV have a 90% likelihood of chronic infection, and the risk falls gradually during the first 5 years of life.[208]

The serologic course of acute hepatitis B infection is illustrated in Fig. 61.12. HBsAg is the first serologic marker to appear, although HBV DNA may be detectable slightly earlier. HBsAg usually appears 1 to 2 months after infection

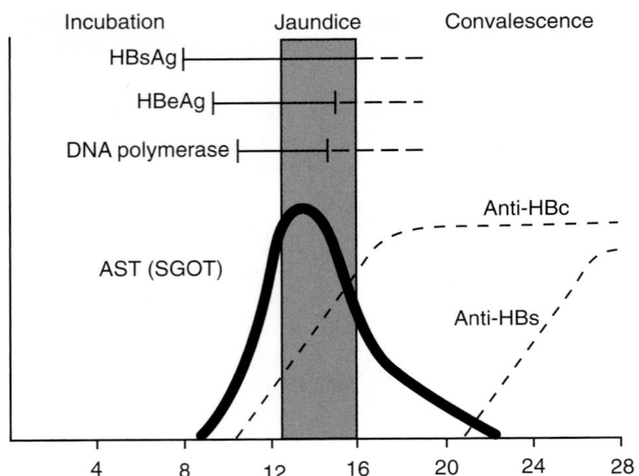

FIGURE 61.12 Course of acute type B hepatitis with recovery. *1,* Onset of hepatitis with jaundice 3 months after exposure; *2,* detection of hepatitis B surface antigen *(HBsAg)* 2 to 8 weeks after exposure, followed by appearance of its antibody *(anti-HBs)* 2 to 4 weeks after HBsAg is no longer detectable; *3,* detection of hepatitis B e antigen *(HBeAg)* shortly after HBsAg disappears (this is usually followed by the appearance of antibody to HbeAg *[anti-HBe],* which persists); *4,* detection of hepatitis B core antibody *(anti-HBc)* at the time of onset of disease 2 to 3 months after exposure. Anti-HBc immunoglobulin M will be detectable in high levels for approximately 5 months. (From Balistreri WF. Viral hepatitis: unique aspects of infection during childhood. *Consultant* 1984;24:131–153.)

and before the onset of clinical illness, and is the last protein marker to disappear. HBV DNA replication is slower than that of HCV; doubling time averages 2 to 3 days.[209] Persistence of HBsAg for longer than 6 months beyond the onset of acute hepatitis indicates chronic infection. HBeAg appears at about the same time as HBsAg; however, because it is not usually measured except in the setting of chronic HBV infection, it usually is not helpful as a marker to document acute infection. The first antibody to appear, which usually coincides with the onset of clinical evidence of hepatitis 3 to 6 months after infection, is the anti-HBc. As with hepatitis A, an IgM antibody is the first to appear and usually persists for 3 to 6 months; it is usually considered diagnostic of acute hepatitis B infection. However, in chronic infection, the IgM antibody may become detectable with flares of severity of disease; thus, it is not completely reliable in recognizing a recent infection.[210] The typical pattern at clinical presentation is positive serology for anti-HBc (both total and IgM), HBsAg, HBeAg (when measured), and negative anti-HBs. A small percentage of individuals have negative HBsAg and anti-HBs at the time of initial presentation, leaving IgM anti-HBc as the only commonly measured marker that is positive; this finding has been termed the core window. With current sensitive assays for HBsAg, it is rare to encounter individuals in the core window. Clearance of HBeAg with development of anti-HBe is the first sign of viral clearance and usually predates loss of HBsAg. Clinically, HBsAg clearance from serum is associated with recovery from acute hepatitis and has been believed to confer life-long immunity to HBV.

Accumulating evidence indicates that HBV remains dormant in the body and HBV DNA circulates in many to most individuals who have recovered from acute hepatitis as evidenced by clearance of HBsAg and acquisition of HBsAb. This has been termed occult HBV infection.[211] Several studies have demonstrated that HBV DNA is still present in low amounts, in both plasma and liver, in most individuals who have had past acute HBV infection and who were HBsAg negative and anti-HBc positive.[134,212,213] Viral loads typically consist of ≤100 copies/mL, and it has been estimated that the number of liver cells infected may be as low as 1%. Such individuals have been shown to transmit HBV infection if their organs are used for transplantation (if treatment to prevent this is not given). The significance of circulating HBV DNA for the individual infected or for others (in the absence of transplantation) seems to be minimal, however, in that liver enzymes are usually normal, and circulating HBV DNA is found mainly in immune complexes.

In recent years, the problem of reactivation of HBV has been increasingly recognized. Reactivation refers to return of viral replication, which is often accompanied by acute liver injury (and in a high percentage of cases, liver failure) in a person with HBsAg but who has inactive viral replication (sometimes also called seroreversion) or less often in patients with occult HBV. Typically, agents that suppress the immune system (chemotherapeutic agents, glucocorticosteroids, antilymphoid treatments) allow return of viral replication that was kept in check by the immune system.[214-217] Withdrawal of immune suppression (including immune restoration in persons with HIV[218]) leads to liver injury. Treatment with lamivudine (or other agents that suppress HBV replication) before immune suppression is highly effective in preventing such reactivation, and guidelines have recommended testing all patients who receive immune suppression for HBV, including testing for HBcAb, before such agents are used.[219,220]

Acute Hepatitis C. Acute HCV infection is responsible for 10% to 15% of cases of acute hepatitis in the United States; an estimated 10% to 30% of those with acute infection develop jaundice. Increased aminotransferases usually develop approximately 6 to 8 weeks after infection. In those cases in which clinical acute hepatitis develops, jaundice typically begins approximately 2 to 3 months after exposure. HCV RNA and HCV Ag are detectable in plasma 2 to 4 weeks after initial exposure. Viremia increases rapidly (average doubling time, 17 hours) and plateaus at high viral loads (often >10^7 IU/mL). In acute hepatitis C infection, anti-HCV is present in a little more than one-half of cases at the time of presentation.[221,222] IgM anti-HCV assays are not commercially available, but in contrast to HAV and HBV, IgM antibodies are encountered in both acute and chronic HCV infection, making the test useless diagnostically.[223] HCV RNA and HCV Ag usually are both present at the time of diagnosis, and viral load is often significantly elevated compared with values seen in chronic hepatitis. Diagnosis of acute HCV is likely if anti-HCV is absent but HCV RNA is positive. Diagnosis of acute HCV is also likely if the HCV RNA viral load is high and the anti-HCV titer is low or increases with time.[223,224] Viral load falls with development of antibodies to one or more HCV proteins, and may become transiently negative. HCV antibodies never appear or disappear in 30% to 50% of those who recover from acute HCV.[225,226] The importance of recognizing acute hepatitis C is that, if virus does not clear spontaneously, treatment is highly effective when given in the first 6 months after diagnosis.[227]

Other Types of Acute Viral Hepatitis. Numerous other viruses can affect the liver, causing acute hepatitis. The most common are EBV and CMV. Features are otherwise typical of viral hepatitis, although signs of systemic infection are often seen as well. Herpes simplex virus occasionally may cause severe hepatitis in adults.[227a] Infection with each of these agents is more commonly associated with hepatitis in the neonatal period, during which it is part of the disseminated infection. Diagnosis of infection with these viruses involves serologic and nucleic acid tests; none are specific to the liver.

Sudden flares of activity in individuals with chronic hepatitis B may mimic acute hepatitis. An acute rise in cytoplasmic enzymes commonly occurs, often in association with jaundice and other clinical features, suggesting an acute liver disease. For example, development of an immune response that leads to clearance of HBeAg or HBsAg is often associated with clinical and enzymatic features of acute hepatitis.[112] Recognition of this cause of the clinical picture of acute hepatitis in a person with chronic hepatitis relies on demonstration of antigen loss and antibody development, along with absence of other causes of acute hepatitis.

Toxic Hepatitis

Toxic hepatitis refers to direct damage of hepatocytes by a toxin or toxic metabolite. Toxic reactions are usually predictable and are directly related to the dose of the agent ingested. In North America and Europe, the most common cause of toxic hepatitis (and the most common cause of acute liver failure) is acetaminophen, a widely used nonprescription pain reliever.[228] The metabolism of acetaminophen is affected by dose, induction of metabolic enzymes, and concentrations of glutathione (see Fig. 61.10). When a large dose of acetaminophen is ingested (the average lethal dose as a single ingestion is 15 g), the metabolic pathways are overwhelmed, glutathione is depleted, and toxic intermediates accumulate, causing liver damage. When metabolic enzymes are induced (such as by ethanol) or glutathione is depleted (which occurs in alcoholism and with starvation), toxicity can occur with relatively small doses of acetaminophen (total doses of 2–4 g).[68] Toxicity can also occur with excessive cumulative doses of acetaminophen; such accidental overdoses appear to be responsible for approximately one-half of cases of toxicity.[229] Diagnosis is often based on history and increased acetaminophen concentrations; in patients who present later, and for whom a history cannot be obtained, measurement of acetaminophen-protein adducts allows diagnosis.[230] The first laboratory abnormality to appear is an increase in PT, followed by increased activity of cytosolic enzymes, with AST tending to be higher than ALT.[231] Peak activities (typically >100 times the upper reference intervals) usually occur by 24 to 48 hours, followed by rapid clearance at rates approximating the known half-lives of the enzymes.[232] PT elevations are typical and are more than 4 seconds above the control value in most cases. Prognosis is related most closely to the prolonged increase in PT[233]; persistent elevation of PT 4 days after ingestion is associated with a poor prognosis.[234] Other markers of risk include development of acute renal failure and the presence of lactic acidosis, particularly if the pH is less than 7.30 ([H^+] >50 nmol/L).

Ischemic Hepatitis (Shock Liver)

Hepatic hypoperfusion (ischemic hepatitis) is one of the most common causes of elevated cytosolic enzymes; in hospital patients, it is the cause of most cases of acute hepatitis.[235,236] Ischemic hepatitis may follow any cause of shock; the most common causes are septic and cardiogenic shock (sometimes termed cardiac hepatopathy[50]). Not all patients with shock develop ischemic hepatitis; in one recent study, only 13.8% of those with septic shock did, but mortality was significantly higher in such patients.[237] Another study found that cardiac dysfunction, especially right heart failure, appeared necessary to cause the clinical picture of ischemic hepatitis.[238] Bilirubin elevations typically are minimal, and they usually peak several days after enzyme activity reaches its greatest point.[239] Laboratory findings are similar to those seen in toxic hepatitis, and acute renal failure is a common complicating factor. Prognosis is primarily related to the underlying cause of hypotension[239]; individuals with prolonged elevation of bilirubin appear to have a poor prognosis.[240]

Reye Syndrome

Acute encephalopathy in combination with fatty degeneration of the viscera was initially described by Reye and associates in Australia in 1963,[241] with nearly simultaneous case descriptions by Johnson and colleagues in the United States.[242] In most of these early cases, the disease was fatal. It most frequently strikes children aged 6 to 11 years and infants, although it may affect individuals of other ages. The syndrome is characterized by a prodromal, febrile viral illness (usually influenza B or varicella), followed by approximately a week of protracted vomiting associated with lethargy and confusion, which may deteriorate rapidly into stupor and coma.[243] At the same time, the liver enlarges, increased aminotransferases and PT develop, and ammonia increases. A prolonged PT more than 3 seconds above normal and a plasma ammonia concentration more than 100 µmol/L usually indicate a poor prognosis. Serum bilirubin concentration is typically normal or only mildly increased. Other laboratory features include hypoglycemia and hyperuricemia.

Only sporadic case descriptions of Reye syndrome were published until 1974, when 379 cases in the United States were reported to the CDC. The mortality rate in this series was 41%. The number of cases peaked in 1980 at 555.[244] At about the same time, articles began to appear linking Reye syndrome with aspirin treatment of viral illness[245]; these were followed by a case control study that strongly implicated salicylate in the pathogenesis of Reye syndrome.[246] Although CDC guidelines recommending avoidance of aspirin in children with febrile illness were not published until 1985,[247] a decline in salicylate use began before this time, and Reye syndrome has again become a rare disease. A 2008 review suggested that children who present with a clinical picture similar to Reye syndrome are actually much more likely to have inborn metabolic errors, particularly those involving the urea cycle or mitochondrial enzymes, and should be evaluated for those before a diagnosis of Reye syndrome is considered.[248]

Other Causes of Acute Hepatitis

Alcoholic hepatitis is discussed more fully in the Alcoholic Liver Disease section later in this chapter. Alcoholic hepatitis is often suspected by the combination of mild elevations in enzymes (peak AST typically <300 U/L), AST/ALT ratio >2, and leukocytosis.[249] Drugs can cause liver injury through a number of mechanisms, but the most common is idiosyncratic, immune-mediated injury to hepatocytes. The most common pattern is similar to that of other types of acute hepatitis; cholestatic hepatitis, with increased aminotransferases and ALP, is more common in drug-induced hepatitis than with other causes of acute hepatitis, but it is present only in a minority of cases (40% in a 2008 US study).[250] Criteria used to recognize drug-induced liver injury include a temporal relationship between drug exposure and onset of hepatitis, exclusion of other known causes of hepatitis, the presence of extrahepatic hypersensitivity (especially skin rash, arthralgia, renal injury, and eosinophilia), the development of liver injury on rechallenge, and ideally, previously published reports of similar reactions.[251] Several standardized approaches for evaluation of possible drug-induced liver disease have been developed.[252-254] Hepatic drug reactions were reported to represent approximately 6% of all adverse drug reactions[255] in a Danish study and approximately 1% of cases of acute hepatitis in an Indian survey.[256] Although usually associated with prescription drugs, complementary and alternative products are becoming increasingly recognized as causes of acute hepatitis,[257,258] and in a US study, these products were responsible for 9% of all cases.[250] Although drug reactions typically develop soon after that start of treatment, several months may elapse between the time of initial exposure and development of acute hepatitis. Approximately 60% of cases cause severe acute hepatitis with jaundice; fatalities can occur,[259] although often death is not due to liver disease.[250] Serious reactions are more common in individuals who are continued on the medication.[260] In 15% to 30% of cases, liver injury persists and becomes chronic after cessation of the drug.[250]

Some of the disorders that usually produce chronic hepatitis (and are discussed more fully later) may occasionally present in an acute fashion. AIH has an acute component in up to 40% of cases. Clinically, it differs from other forms of acute hepatitis because it is characterized by decreased albumin, increased globulins, and a more protracted increase in aminotransferases.[261-263] Acute AIH is diagnosed by the absence of other causes of acute hepatitis and the presence of autoimmune markers (discussed in detail in the section on Chronic Hepatitis). Wilson disease is the result of deficiency of an intracellular adenosine triphosphastase[264-266] and typically presents in childhood with neuropsychiatric findings, which are almost always associated with chronic liver injury. Wilson disease may also present as acute hepatitis that is often associated with fulminant hepatic failure[267]; in one study, 8 of 14 patients who had hepatic injury due to Wilson disease had an acute presentation.[268] The classic biochemical findings of Wilson disease are often absent (low plasma ceruloplasmin, low plasma copper) or misleading (high urine copper is common to all forms of acute hepatitis) in the setting of acute Wilson disease.[267,269] However, in advanced liver disease or acute hepatitis, ceruloplasmin concentrations may be misleading and be in the normal range because of an acute inflammatory response. Additional features often suggest the diagnosis, including nonimmune hemolytic anemia, acute tubular necrosis, and a low ratio of serum ALP (in units per liter) to bilirubin (in milligrams per deciliter). One recent study found that if this ratio was less than 4, sensitivity was 94% and specificity was 96%, which is far superior to tests such as ceruloplasmin and plasma copper.[270]

Other Disorders With Laboratory Findings Similar to Acute Hepatitis

Several conditions mimic the laboratory picture of acute hepatitis. Hemolytic anemia can cause jaundice, increased plasma LDH activity, and slight increases in AST and ALT. In contrast to hepatitis, the increase in bilirubin is predominantly (often >80%) indirect reacting. LDH activity is elevated to several times that of AST, and AST activity usually is several times that of ALT. Acute injury to skeletal or cardiac muscle may cause significant increases in AST, and to a lesser extent, ALT, but the ratio of AST/ALT activity is generally more than 3 at presentation (although, as with liver injury, the shorter half-life of AST will cause the ratio to become less than 1 with time, usually after 3 days).[271] Plasma bilirubin concentration is not usually elevated, but mild increases in unconjugated bilirubin from metabolism of myoglobin may be seen in severe skeletal muscle injury. Acute bile duct obstruction, particularly when caused by gallstones, can resemble acute hepatitis. In the early stages of obstruction, transient increases in AST and ALT are common,[272] and their activities may rarely exceed 2000 U/L.[273,274] Increases in ALP develop more slowly than those of the aminotransferases, masking the presence of cholestasis early in the course. Increases in bilirubin are typically predominantly directly reacting, creating a presentation similar to that seen in acute hepatitis. Even if obstruction persists, aminotransferase activity falls rapidly, with AST typically returning to normal within 8 days[275] and ALP activity gradually increasing. ALP activities more than 300 U/L in this setting strongly suggest the presence of obstructive jaundice.[276] Acute biliary obstruction by gallstones is often accompanied by acute pancreatitis; increased plasma amylase and lipase activities should suggest biliary tract obstruction as the cause of any noted liver abnormalities.

Approach to the Patient With Acute Hepatitis

Once a diagnosis of acute hepatitis has been established, additional laboratory testing is usually required to determine the cause. Although the incidence of acute viral hepatitis has decreased, serologic studies should be performed to rule out infectious causes. A typical panel of tests should include IgM anti-HAV, HBsAg, IgM anti-HBc, anti-HCV, and HCV RNA (or HCV core antigen, if available). Marked elevations (>100 times the upper reference intervals) in AST or ALT, particularly if AST is higher than ALT, should suggest the possibility of toxic or ischemic liver injury. Minimal increases (<8 times the reference interval) in AST, with AST greater than ALT, in a patient with jaundice and leukocytosis indicate likely alcoholic hepatitis. Imaging studies of the biliary tract are appropriate to rule out obstruction in those who present with sudden onset of symptoms, especially if accompanied by right upper quadrant pain and tenderness, laboratory evidence of pancreatitis, or a history of gallstones. The presence of increased plasma globulin and decreased albumin concentrations, or the presence of hemolytic anemia and acute renal failure, should suggest the possibility of AIH or Wilson disease, respectively.

Follow-Up of Acute Hepatitis

Important uses of laboratory tests in acute hepatitis are to identify individuals with fulminant hepatic failure, to document recovery, and to determine clearance of any infectious agents. The most important tests in determining the extent of injury are not plasma activities of cytosolic enzymes, but evidence of impaired liver function. The most important indicator of prognosis in acute viral hepatitis is impairment in synthetic function, with PT a widely accepted indicator. In acute viral or alcoholic hepatitis, a PT of more than 3 seconds above normal is associated with a poor prognosis,[233] whereas in toxic hepatitis, persistent elevation more than 4 days after ingestion has prognostic importance.[234] Low concentrations of other markers of synthetic function, such as transthyretin or actin-free Gc globulin,[277] or of markers of hepatocyte regeneration, such as α-fetoprotein,[278] have been found to predict poor prognosis. In alcoholic hepatitis, bilirubin and INR are the most reliable predictors of prognosis; several indexes, discussed later in the section on Alcoholic Liver Disease, have been used to predict risk of death and need for treatment.[249] Plasma activities of cytosolic enzyme decrease rapidly in ischemic and toxic hepatitis or obstruction, regardless of outcome, and fall more gradually in viral and alcoholic hepatitis, but are not helpful in evaluating outcome. With hepatitis B and C, cytosolic enzyme activities may return to normal even if viral replication persists[279,280]; serologic tests are the only reliable means to evaluate resolution of infection.

Chronic Hepatitis

Chronic hepatitis is defined as chronic inflammation of the liver that persists for at least 6 months, or signs and symptoms of chronic liver disease in the presence of elevated cytosolic enzymes.[281] It is characterized by ongoing inflammatory

POINTS TO REMEMBER

Assessment of Viral Hepatitis

- In all cases of viral hepatitis, it is prudent to test patients for each of the major blood born viruses: HBV, HCV, and HIV.
- In viremic patients, testing should include measurement of viral nucleic acid (HBV DNA and HCV RNA).
- Hepatic inflammation is indicated by the extent of elevation of aminotransferases, but these are neither sensitive nor specific.
- The staging of severity of chronic viral hepatitis is determined by the severity of liver fibrosis. Liver fibrosis can be assessed using noninvasive blood tests, fibroelastography, imaging or liver biopsy, or any combination of these tests.

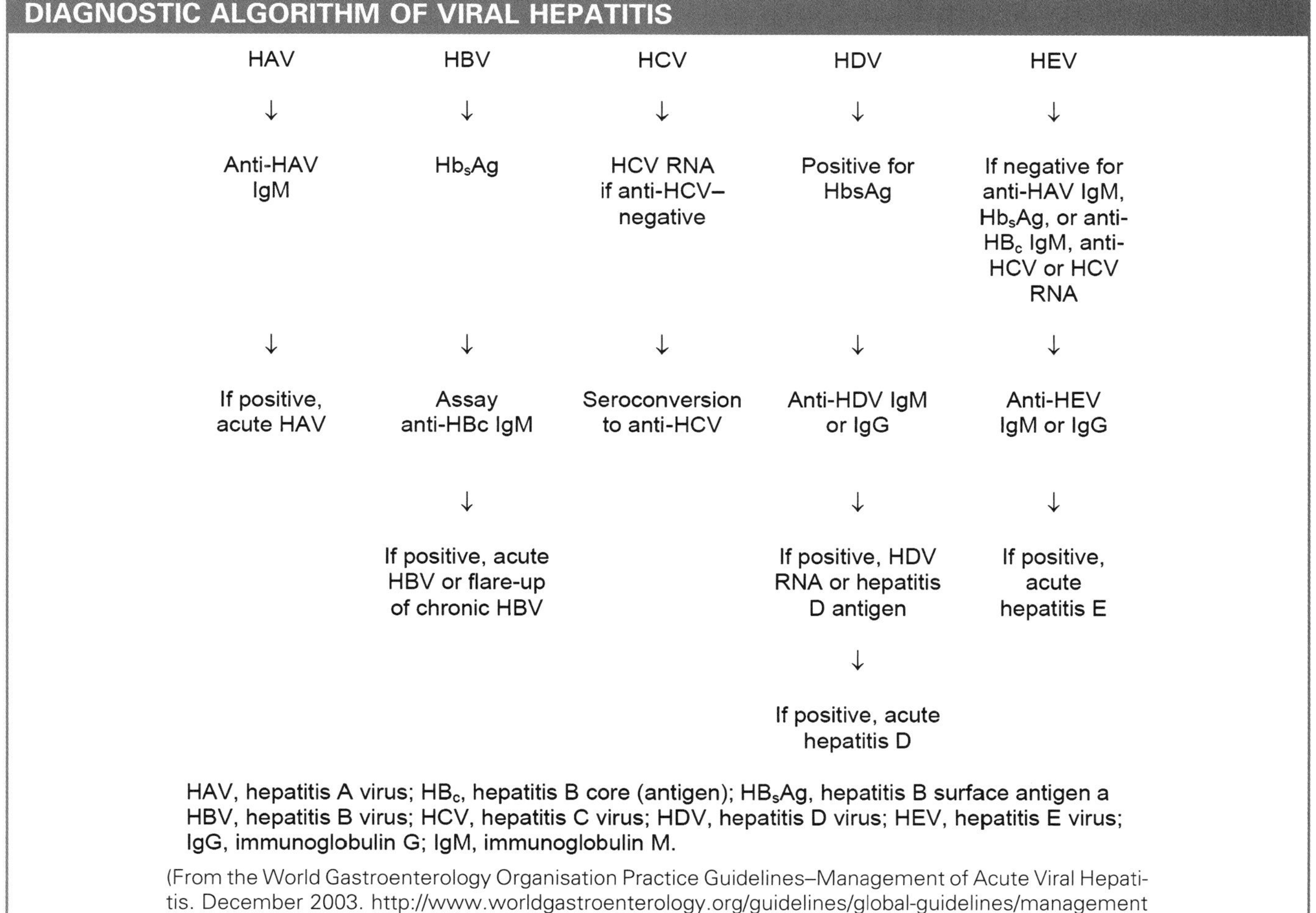

HAV, hepatitis A virus; HB_c, hepatitis B core (antigen); HB_sAg, hepatitis B surface antigen a HBV, hepatitis B virus; HCV, hepatitis C virus; HDV, hepatitis D virus; HEV, hepatitis E virus; IgG, immunoglobulin G; IgM, immunoglobulin M.

(From the World Gastroenterology Organisation Practice Guidelines–Management of Acute Viral Hepatitis. December 2003. http://www.worldgastroenterology.org/guidelines/global-guidelines/management-of-acute-viral-hepatitis/acute-viral-hepatitis-english.)

TABLE 61.4 Causes of Chronic Hepatitis and Diagnostic Strategies

Cause	Diagnosis
Hepatitis B	History, HBsAg, anti-HBs, anti-HBc, HBV DNA
Hepatitis C	Anti-HCV, HCV RNA by PCR
Autoimmune type 1	ANA, anti–smooth muscle antibody
Autoimmune type 2	SLA, anti-LKM1
Wilson disease	Ceruloplasmin
Drugs	History
AAT deficiency	AAT phenotype
Nonalcoholic fatty liver disease	Metabolic syndrome, liver ultrasound, liver biopsy
Idiopathic	Liver biopsy, absence of markers

ANA, Antinuclear antibody; *AAT*, α1-Antitrypsin; *HBc*, hepatitis B core antigen; *HBsAg*, hepatitis B surface antigen; *HBV*, hepatitis B virus; *HCV*, hepatitis C virus; *LKM1*, liver-kidney microsomal antigen type 1; *PCR*, polymerase chain reaction; *SLA*, soluble liver antigen.

damage to hepatocytes, which are often accompanied by hepatocyte regeneration and scarring. Formerly, chronic hepatitis was subdivided into three forms (chronic persistent, chronic lobular, and chronic active) based on histologic characteristics. It was recognized that individuals often had each of these diseases at different points in time, and often in different areas of the liver in the same biopsy. Current classifications describe the cause and evaluate the severity of inflammatory injury (termed grade) and the extent of fibrosis (termed stage). The importance of these findings will be discussed in detail later. Common causes of chronic hepatitis and tests used to make a specific etiologic diagnosis are listed in Table 61.4.

The clinical features of chronic hepatitis are highly variable. Most patients are asymptomatic, but nonspecific features, such as fatigue, lack of concentration, and weakness may be present. Most patients are diagnosed because of an unexplained abnormality in aminotransferase activities or detection of positive results on a screening test for a cause of chronic hepatitis. Moderate elevations in plasma aminotransferase activities (an average of approximately twofold, and in most cases, less than fivefold) are characteristic, whereas results of most other tests are normal. Normal aminotransferase activities do not rule out histologic evidence of chronic hepatitis, especially in the presence of chronic viral hepatitis or NASH.[158,282,283] Characteristically, ALT is elevated to a greater degree than AST,[284] although elevations in both are common; reversal of the AST/ALT activity ratio to more than 1 suggests coexisting alcohol abuse or development of cirrhosis in patients with a variety of causes of chronic liver disease[285-288] (as discussed in greater detail later in this chapter). One study found that the AST/ALT ratio was significantly higher in women than in men[289]; however, in most studies in which the AST/ALT ratio was used, separate analyses were not done by sex. Although ALT is relatively specific for the liver, skeletal muscle sources for AST and ALT should always be considered, especially in physically active young individuals.[271,290,291] A finding of persistent elevation of aminotransferase activity should lead to an evaluation for chronic hepatitis using the tests outlined in Table 61.4. A liver biopsy may be helpful in determining the cause, assessing severity, and following treatment. A specific etiologic diagnosis is essential because it dictates the treatment. The most common causes of chronic hepatitis are chronic HBV, HCV, and NASH, but a variety of other disease processes may cause chronic hepatitis.

Chronic Hepatitis B

Worldwide, HBV infection is the most important cause of chronic hepatitis.[292] According to the WHO, approximately 350 million individuals worldwide have chronic HBV infection; most cases are found in Asia, Africa, and southern Europe.

In most circumstances, HBV is not cytopathic because the injury results from an immune-mediated inflammatory attack against hepatocytes. Chronic hepatitis results when the immune response is incomplete and the virus is not eliminated from infected cells. This leads to a continuing cycle of viral replication, reinfection of regenerating hepatocytes, and immune damage to newly infected cells that is inadequate to clear infection. The details are not completely understood, but it appears that in normal circumstances, hepatocytes express surface markers (in this case, HBcAg and human leukocyte antigen [HLA] class 1 proteins).[293] Primed lymphocytes then attack the infected hepatocytes.[294] It appears that many chronic hepatitis B patients are deficient in or have an inadequate response to INF, and by inference, are unable to express HLA antigens that would attract an appropriate lymphocyte response.[295] The discovery of INF deficiency led to the successful use of IFN-α therapy in chronic HBV.

The clinical presentation may be complicated by various extrahepatic complications (which occur in 1% to 10% of those with HBV[208]), including polyarteritis, glomerulonephritis, polymyalgia rheumatica, cryoglobulinemia, myocarditis, and Guillain-Barré syndrome. These conditions are associated with circulating immune complexes containing HBsAg.[296] Immunocompromised persons, such as HBV/HIV coinfected individuals, typically have higher replication markers, less hepatic inflammation, and poorer survival than those with HIV alone.[297,298]

The natural history of chronic hepatitis B (defined by the persistence of HBsAg) varies.[112] Features of the different stages of chronic HBV are given in Table 61.5. It is convenient to divide chronic hepatitis B infection into two basic types—replicative and nonreplicative—although transitions between these stages are common. In the chronic replicative form, viral DNA is found in the cytoplasm of infected hepatocytes, and complete viral particles are produced and released into the circulation. In the replicating form of infection, viral loads in plasma are usually high (>10^5 copies/mL, often >10^8 copies/mL, or >20,000 IU/mL, often >2× 10^7 IU/mL; 1 IU/mL = 5.6 copies/mL). In those infected later in life who develop chronic hepatitis, evidence of hepatocyte injury (elevated aminotransferase activity and inflammation in liver biopsy sections) is found in most cases (termed immune active[112] or chronic active phase). However, in those infected early in life, evidence of hepatocyte injury is often minimal; this has been referred to as the immunotolerant phase of chronic HBV. Those in the immune tolerant phase may transition to the immune active phase, but do not always

TABLE 61.5 Patterns of Chronic Hepatitis B Virus Infection

Type	AST/ALT	HBsAg	HBeAg	Anti-HBc	HBV DNA
Occult	Normal	Negative	Negative	Positive	Negative*
Immune control	Normal	Positive	Negative	Positive	Negative*
Immune tolerant	Normal	Positive	Negative/Positive	Positive	Positive
Immune active	Increased	Positive	Positive	Positive	Positive, viral load usually >106 IU/mL
HBeAg-negative chronic hepatitis	Increased	Positive	Negative	Positive	Positive, viral load usually <106 IU/mL

*May have very low level (usually <102 IU/mL) in serum.
ALT, Alanine aminotransferase; *AST,* aspartate aminotransferase; *HBc,* hepatitis B core antigen; *HBeAg,* hepatitis B e antigen; *HBsAg,* hepatitis B surface antigen; *HBV,* hepatitis B virus.

do so. In the nonreplicating form, circulating viral load is low or undetectable, and evidence of hepatocyte injury is usually absent. This variant has been termed the HBV carrier state, although current terminology describes this phase as the immune control phase. Traditionally, HBeAg had been used to differentiate replicative and nonreplicative types of chronic hepatitis, with negative HBeAg and positive anti-HBe believed to indicate the nonreplicating stage of infection. As discussed earlier, however, this distinction is inaccurate, and classification is based on HBV DNA concentrations, along with ALT activities and histology.[112] All of the three phases of chronic HBV are associated with the presence of HBsAg in serum. As mentioned earlier, occult HBV infection is present in many individuals previously exposed to HBV, but it is not associated with inflammation in the liver or elevated aminotransferases.

In general, chronic HBV passes through stages in untreated persons. For those infected early in life, the immune tolerant phase is usually followed by an immune active phase that may vary in duration and may cause significant liver damage. This phase usually gives way to a protracted period of immune control, with HBsAg positivity or occult infection if HBsAg is cleared. For those infected individuals who go on to have chronic infection as older children or adults, the immune tolerant phase may be a short period or absent, leading straight into the immune active phase. Approximately 8% to 10% of persons per year will transition from the immune active to the immune control phase of chronic HBV.[117] A variable, but low, proportion of those in the immune control phase will revert to the immune active phase (mainly dependent on genotype).[112] Approximately 0.5% to 1% of persons per year will convert from HBsAg positive to HBsAg negative, entering the occult phase of infection (or, in a minority, resolved HBV). Each of these transitions can be associated with an acute rise in aminotransferase activities in a clinical picture that mimicks acute viral hepatitis, as discussed earlier.

For individuals who have chronic replicating infection, the major risk is development of cirrhosis and HCC. An estimated 20% to 30% of individuals with chronic hepatitis B will develop cirrhosis over a 20-year follow-up period; the risk is directly related to the amount of HBV DNA, with risk progressively increasing at viral loads of more than 2000 IU/mL (10,000 copies/mL).[299] Once cirrhosis has developed, a 1.5% to 5% annual risk of development of HCC is noted. Although the risk of HCC is lower in individuals with HBV infection who do not have cirrhosis, risk is directly related to viral load and rises at quantities above 2000 IU/mL.[300] Even a person in the nonreplicating stage of infection has a 10-fold higher risk of HCC.[137] On a worldwide basis, hepatitis B infection is the most common cause of liver cancer.

Efficacy of treatment is typically measured by response of ALT and/or AST and HBV DNA; goals of treatment include normalization of ALT and suppression of HBV DNA below the limits of detection of assays, ideally with detection limits of approximately 20 to 50 IU/mL. With polymerase inhibitors, approximately 70% to 80% of patients will achieve these goals within 1 year of treatment. Duration of treatment is largely dependent on HBeAg status before the start of therapy, and for those who are HBeAg positive before treatment, the duration depends on the response of HBeAg on therapy. For those who are HBeAg negative, treatment typically is continued indefinitely, as long as treatment is effective. For those who are HBeAg positive before treatment, loss of HBeAg and development of anti-HBe indicate a high likelihood of maintenance of HBV DNA control and normalization of ALT once treatment is stopped (after 6–12 months of further treatment once anti-HBe appears). With INF therapy, response rates to 1 year of treatment are somewhat lower than with polymerase inhibitors, but treatment requires only 6 to 12 months. Loss of HBsAg is uncommon; with most agents, the likelihood of loss of HBsAg usually is not higher than that in untreated persons, although it may be higher with INF and tenofovir.[117]

Chronic Hepatitis C

Approximately 170 million individuals worldwide have been diagnosed with chronic HCV infection; most cases are found in North America, Northern Europe, and Japan.[301] In contrast to HBV, the risk of chronic hepatitis does not appear related to age at exposure (although perinatal infection is uncommon with HCV), and the likelihood of chronic infection is much higher overall. Many studies state an approximate 80% to 85% likelihood of chronic infection by HCV; this interpretation is based on the frequency of finding HCV RNA on a chronic basis among those who are anti-HCV positive. However, as mentioned earlier, many individuals who clear HCV with acute exposure never develop or lose anti-HCV. Among persons followed prospectively after an acute HCV infection, chronic HCV infection actually developed in only about 50% to 70%.[226,302,303] Once viremia becomes established beyond 6 months after initial exposure, it essentially never resolves spontaneously; in one study of 320 patients followed serially for more than 3 years, only 6 patients with end-stage liver disease lost detectable HCV RNA.[304] HCV viral load fluctuates little over time; in most individuals, viral load differs by less than 0.5 log,[305,306] and gradually increases by an average of 0.2 to 0.3 log/year.[305,307] It is estimated that approximately 20% to 30% of patients with hepatitis C will progress to cirrhosis over a period of 20 years.[308] The frequency of progression appears to be increased by age older than 40 years at the time of infection, male sex, alcohol abuse,[309] and immunosuppression, but it is less than 5% after 20 years of infection in those infected during the first 20 to 30 years of life.[226,302,303,310] In those who develop recurrent HCV after liver transplantation, the response rate is lower, and the rate of progression to cirrhosis is faster than in primary infection. As with HBV, the likelihood of progression to HCC is between 1.5% and 5% per year in those with cirrhosis.[311]

The clinical picture of chronic HCV is similar to that of HBV in producing chronic hepatitis. Infection with HCV is characterized by fluctuating ALT activities over time. Only about one-third of those with chronic HCV have continually increased ALT, and many of these individuals show variation in ALT activity.[312] It is common for individuals with fluctuating values to have multiple normal ALT activity values interspersed with elevated values.[280,313] Individuals with normal ALT tend to have milder fibrosis and less severe disease on liver biopsy, but a minority have advanced fibrosis.[158] In contrast to HBV, individuals with continually normal ALT activity have a similar rate of response to antiviral treatment.[158]

Dramatic advances in the treatment of chronic hepatitis C have revolutionized outcomes for patients and changed the requirements for laboratory testing in the management of patients on treatment. Directly acting antiviral agents that target critical HCV proteins have been shown to cure infection in most patients. Tests for evaluating chronic HCV infection and its treatment are shown in Table 61.6. Although this remains a rapidly evolving field, it is highly likely that it will be possible to cure infection within the next decade[314] in any patient capable of adhering to a full course of treatment. HCV susceptibility to these drugs is determined by HCV genotype; therefore, genotyping before treatment remains mandatory. This permits the treating clinician to select the most appropriate combination of drugs and the correct duration of therapy. Tests are used to monitor response to treatment by measuring serum HCV RNA concentrations during and 4 and 12 weeks after the end of treatment. Patients who have undetectable HCV RNA 12 weeks after the end of treatment are considered cured. The extent to which liver fibrosis reverses in patients who attain clearance of HCV still needs to be established, but studies of patients who have been cured using INF-based therapies suggest that the long-term risks of liver cancer and bleeding varices are reduced even in cirrhotic patients who attain clearance of HCV.[315]

Hepatitis B and C Coinfection. Approximately 2% to 10% of individuals infected with HCV are coinfected with HBV; of those with chronic HBV, 15% to 20% are also HCV positive.[316,317] Clinical and laboratory features of coinfected patients are somewhat contradictory and differ from those in individuals infected with a single hepatitis virus. Coinfected patients have lower viral loads than do those with single infection.[318] In patients with chronic HBV who develop acute HCV infection, the likelihood of progressing to chronic HCV infection is low,[319] and acute infection with HBV can lead to clearance of HCV.[320] These features would suggest a beneficial effect of coinfection. In contrast, patients with chronic HBV/HCV coinfection have more rapid progression to cirrhosis.[321] Patients with acute coinfection have severe acute hepatitis more frequently.[317,322] Some studies suggest a high frequency of HBV DNA viral replication in the liver even in the absence of circulating HBsAg; such subclinically coinfected patients have more severe liver injury and a higher frequency of cirrhosis.[323,324] Despite some favorable findings, the outcome of hepatitis in coinfected patients seems to be worse than for those infected with only a single agent.

Nonalcoholic Fatty Liver Disease and Nonalcoholic Steatohepatitis

Nonalcoholic fatty liver disease is now a major cause of chronic liver disease and is increasing in prevalence.[325] Ludwig and colleagues first described patients who had histologic features identical to those of alcoholic hepatitis (including hepatocyte ballooning, presence of Mallory hyaline, and neutrophil infiltration), but who had no history of heavy alcohol intake and did not have AST values higher than ALT values.[326] They introduced the term NASH to describe this entity, which was more common in women than in men, and was usually associated with diabetes and/or obesity. (Because alcohol ingestion is common in the population, and alcoholic liver disease does not occur with daily ingestion of less than 20 g

TABLE 61.6 Tests for Evaluating Chronic Hepatitis C Virus (HCV) Infection and Its Treatment

Time of Testing	Test	Condition	Use/Interpretation
Pretreatment	HCV viral load	Detectable	Baseline (to compare with 12-wk value)
	Genotype	2 or 3 vs other	Length of treatment (24-wk genotype if 2 or 3, 48 wk if other genotype)
4 wks on treatment	HCV viral load	Undetectable	Rapid virologic response—high likelihood of treatment success
12 wks on treatment	HCV viral load	<2 log drop	Stop treatment (nonresponder)*
		>2 log drop	Continue treatment (on treatment responder)
End of treatment†	Sensitive HCV RNA‡	Detectable	Nonresponder or breakthrough (if was previously undetectable)
24 wks after completion	Sensitive HCV RNA§	Not detectable	Treatment responder
		Detectable	Relapser
		Not detectable	Sustained virologic responder

*Less than 3% chance of sustained virologic response; some continue treatment to 24 weeks and reevaluate.
†Done at 24 weeks if genotype 2 or 3, done at 48 weeks if other genotypes; not all recommend evaluating end of treatment response.
‡Lower detection limit less than 50 IU/mL.
§Done only if genotype not 2 or 3.

ethanol, this threshold has been suggested as the maximum alcohol intake compatible with a diagnosis of NAFLD).[327,328] It is now recognized that NAFLD is associated strongly with the presence of the metabolic syndrome; almost half of individuals who meet the criteria for metabolic syndrome have NAFLD, and as many as 20% to 30% of the population in North America and Europe has NAFLD,[329] making it far and away the most common form of liver disease and an extremely common condition in the population in the developed world.[330] Approximately 10% of those with NAFLD have the more severe form, NASH. The frequency in obese or diabetic individuals is much higher, with NAFLD in 60% to 75% and NASH in 20% to 25%.[328,331] Prospective studies of patients with liver disease have confirmed that NASH is a common cause of elevated liver enzymes in an unselected population of patients referred to gastroenterologists or seen in primary care settings.[332-334] The frequency of cirrhosis in NASH is not well established, but it has been suggested that NASH may be a major cause of cryptogenic cirrhosis, that is, cirrhosis for which no underlying cause can be determined. Because weight loss develops with chronic illness, fat may disappear from the liver, leaving only fibrosis.

Current evidence suggests that accumulation of fat in NAFLD is a consequence of insulin resistance. A variety of mechanisms may lead to insulin resistance, including genetic predisposition, increased concentrations of free fatty acids, and the presence of cytokines such as TNF-α. Because TNF-α is produced at a rate that correlates with body fat mass, and is critical to development of insulin resistance in obesity, it may be a key factor in the development of NAFLD. However, the pathogenesis is likely to be more complicated because a variety of other factors lead to increased fat accumulation in the liver, including increased carbohydrate intake, certain drugs, and mutations in lipid synthesis, but they have not been associated with the development of NASH.

A clinical approach to the identification of patients with NASH typically involves a compatible clinical history and the presence of steatosis on imaging studies, exclusion of other causes of liver injury, and may include liver biopsy to confirm the diagnosis and determine the extent of injury (but not if patients improve clinically with weight loss and exercise). Although increased activities of liver enzymes are often used to distinguish NASH from other forms of NAFLD, the degree of necroinflammatory damage is not related to elevations in AST or ALT activity, and the likelihood of significant liver damage is similar in those with normal or elevated ALT.[283] The search for laboratory tests capable of identifying the minority of patients with NASH among the large numbers of individuals with NAFLD have highlighted CK18[335,336] and PIIINP[337] as potential serum markers of NASH.

Greater progress has been made in the identification and validation of blood tests for liver fibrosis in NAFLD with a variety of indirect and direct tests being validated for this purpose, including the NAFLD Fibrosis Score, BARD (calculated from body mass index, AST/ALT ratio and diabetes), and the Enhanced Liver Fibrosis (ELF) test.[273,337a–339]

Of these, both the NASH Fibrosis Score and ELF tests have been shown to predict long-term outcomes in NAFLD. It remains to be seen if these tests either alone or in conjunction with other tests will be capable of accurately stratifying patients with NAFLD into those with NASH and those with fibrosis.

To date, major treatments for NAFLD have been aimed at lowering body weight and fat content. Loss of weight is often associated with decreased ALT values; in one study, a 1% decrease in weight was associated with an 8% decrease in ALT activity.[340] The association of NAFLD with insulin resistance has suggested treatment with antidiabetic medications, particularly those that increase insulin responsiveness (such as peroxisome proliferator-activated receptor-γ agonists and metformin); studies have not been conclusive as to the benefits of such treatment.[341]

Autoimmune Hepatitis

AIH represents a rapidly progressive form of chronic hepatitis, with up to 40% 6-month mortality in untreated individuals[342]; it is associated with the presence of autoimmune markers. It is relatively uncommon, with an annual incidence of 1.9 cases per 100,000 population in the United States,[343] but it is responsible for 3% to 6% of all liver transplantations[344]; the disease recurs in approximately 30% of patients after transplantation.[345] As with most autoimmune diseases, there is a strong female predominance. Forms of AIH have been found in individuals of all ages, with no racial or ethnic predilection. It has been associated with specific HLA haplotypes, notably DR3 and DR4, as is true for many other autoimmune diseases. Practice guidelines on autoimmune chronic hepatitis have been developed by the AASLD.[346]

AIH is associated with the presence of liver and nonliver autoantibodies in plasma. These are helpful in diagnosis but are not likely to be the cause of liver injury. The most important antibodies for diagnosis include antinuclear antibody (ANA), anti–smooth muscle (or anti-actin) antibody (ASMA), anti-liver–kidney microsomal antigen type 1, and antisoluble liver antigen (SLA), which is insensitive but highly specific. A variety of other autoantibodies are found frequently in AIH, some of which are found in other disorders. A summary of the most common autoantibodies, their associations, and their molecular targets (when known) is given in Table 61.7. Tests for these autoimmune markers initially used cell or tissue preparations studied by indirect immunofluorescence, but these have largely been replaced by assays that detect antibodies to purified proteins. Individuals who are negative for common autoantibodies, but who otherwise meet criteria for diagnosis, have a similar prognosis and response to treatment.[347]

Criteria for the diagnosis of AIH were developed by an international group[348] and subsequently revised[349]; a simplified scoring system has also been developed.[350] The simplified criteria include exclusion of viral hepatitis, increased plasma IgG concentration, positive autoantibodies, and compatible histologic features.

It is controversial whether AIH should be further divided into subtypes; the international group that codified diagnostic criteria does not recommend use of subtypes,[349] but many authorities recognize three different forms (types 1, 2, and 3). Although differences in epidemiology may be evident among the different forms, there do not seem to be differences in clinical course or response to treatment. Type 1, which is the most common form and the only one seen frequently in North America, is predominantly a disease of middle-aged women. It is characterized by ASMA or anti-actin (found in 87% of cases) and/or ANA (found in 67% of cases); one or the other is present in nearly 100% of cases. Because of the

TABLE 61.7 Serologic Markers of Autoimmune Liver Disease

Antibody Name	Antigen Target	Associations
Antiactin	Actin	AIH type 1; more specific than ASMA, poor response to corticosteroids, early age of onset
Anti-asialoglycoprotein receptor	Transmembrane antigen binding protein	AIH, correlate with activity, disappear with successful treatment
Anti–LKM1	Cytochrome P450 2D6	AIH type 2; seen in only 4% of US cases; usually in children
Anti–liver-specific cytosol	Enzyme (possibly formiminotransferase cyclodeaminase or argininosuccinate lyase)	AIH in younger patients, often with anti-LKM1, primary sclerosing cholangitis; vary with activity of disease
Antimitochondrial antibody	Dihydrolipoamide acyltransferase	Primary biliary cirrhosis
Antineutrophil cytoplasmic antibodies	Bactericidal/permeability protein, cathepsin G, lactoferrin	PSC (50–70%), ulcerative colitis (50–70%), AIH; nonspecific
Antinuclear antibody	Multiple targets (centromere, ribonucleoproteins); may not be detected by ELISA	AIH type 1, some PSC cases
ASMA	Actin, tubulin, vimentin, desmin, skelitin	AIH type 1, seen in other autoimmune diseases in lower titers
Antisoluble liver antigen/ liver pancreas	UGA tRNA suppressor–associated transfer protein	AIH type 3; specific for AIH, correlate with relapse after corticosteroid withdrawal

AIH, Autoimmune hepatitis; *ASMA*, anti–smooth muscle antigen; *ELISA*, enzyme-linked immunosorbent assay; LKM1, liver-kidney microsome; *PSC*, primary sclerosing cholangitis.

nonspecific nature of these antibodies, the strength of the antibody reaction (titer or immunoassay signal) is important in determining the likelihood of AIH. In children, the strength of the reaction is typically lower than in adults. Type 2 AIH, which characteristically occurs in children (although 20% occurs in adults), represents up to 20% of cases in Europe. It is associated with antibodies to liver–kidney microsomal antigen 1 or cytochrome P_{450} 2D6 (CYP2D6).[351] Some cross-reactivity has been noted between this antibody and certain HCV antigens, leading to positive anti-CYP2D6 in individuals with HCV infection. The epitopes recognized by anti-HCV antibodies are different from those in persons with type 2 AIH.[352] Type 3 often lacks other autoimmune markers but is positive for antibodies to soluble liver antigen liver–pancreas. This antibody is directed against the UGA tRNA suppressor-associated antigenic protein.[353]

Immunosuppressive treatment using prednisone, alone or in combination with azathioprine, is effective in inducing clinical remission of disease in approximately 80% of cases; other immunosuppressants are now being used to reduce dependence on corticosteroids.[354] Because inherited differences in the activity of thiopurine methyltransferase affect approximately 10% of the population,[355] it has been recommended that pretreatment determination of enzyme activity should be used to reduce the likelihood of toxicity. Remission typically begins with improvement in symptoms, followed by normalization in laboratory abnormalities, and finally, histologic resolution. Laboratory remission generally does not occur until after at least 12 months of treatment, but it almost always occurs within 24 months in responders. Histologic remission is less common and usually requires at least 3 to 6 months longer than laboratory evidence of remission.[342] Sustained remission can persist off-treatment in 80% of those with normal histology after therapy, but relapse occurs in 50% within 6 months if inflammation persists in the liver biopsy.[356] Liver biochemistry and serum IgG concentrations can be used to identify patients in whom immunosuppression can be safely withdrawn.[357]

Inherited Liver Disease Presenting as Chronic Hepatitis

Inherited liver diseases that present as chronic hepatitis include hemochromatosis, Wilson disease, and AAT deficiency.

Hemochromatosis. Hereditary hemochromatosis (HH) is an autosomal recessive disorder of iron metabolism that results in excessive iron absorption and accumulation in tissues, specifically in the parenchymal cells of the liver, heart, pancreas, and other organs (see also Chapters 38 and 42). HH is caused by mutations that affect any of the proteins that control the entry of iron into the circulation. These proteins include hepcidin, HFE, transferrin receptor 2 (Tfr2), hemojuvelin (HJV) (these proteins all sense iron accumulation that hepcidin acts to correct) and the protein ferroportin (Fpn), which is a cellular transporter of iron down-regulated by hepcidin. Hepcidin is believed to be the major regulator of dietary iron absorption and cellular iron release. It exerts its regulatory function by counteracting the function of Fpn, the major cellular iron exporter in the membrane of macrophages, hepatocytes, and the basolateral site of enterocytes. Hepcidin induces the internalization and degradation of Fpn, which results in increased intracellular iron stores, decreased dietary iron absorption, and decreased circulating iron concentrations. Patients with most forms of HH are unable to appropriately upregulate hepcidin synthesis in response to increased iron stores. This dysregulation is caused by defects in certain genes encoding for positive regulators of hepcidin (*HFE*, *tfr2*, *hjv;* see the following).[358]

HH is primarily a disease in men and postmenopausal women with common clinical features, including lethargy and weakness, arthralgia, loss of libido, upper abdominal discomfort, hepatomegaly, grey/bronze skin pigmentation, testicular atrophy, and joint swelling and/or tenderness. Untreated, HH can lead to serious complications, including liver fibrosis and cirrhosis with HCC in approximately 30% of patients with cirrhosis, diabetes mellitus, and cardiomyopathy, and arrhythmias. Cardiac and endocrine cells are more susceptible to rapid iron loading because they have more mitochondria and less antioxidants.[359]

The gene for HH has long been linked to chromosome 6, close to the genes for the HLA system; it has been definitively identified and termed the *HFE* gene, which codes for a transmembrane protein similar to the class I major histocompatibility complex (MHC) molecule.[360,361] The protein product of the *HFE* gene is a 343-residue type I transmembrane glycoprotein that resembles the MHC class I proteins in sequence and three-dimensional structure (CC). Both the HFE and MHC class I proteins contain a membrane-bound heavy chain with three extracellular domains. HFE protein regulates iron uptake by binding to the transferrin receptor (TfR) on cell membranes and acts as an iron sensor that controls the release of hepcidin. Most cases of hemochromatosis are caused by alterations in the genes that regulate hepcidin synthesis, including *HFE*, *Tjr2*, and *Hjv*. Deficiency of hepcidin activity in macrophages and enterocytes leads to unrestricted Fpn-mediated iron export into the circulation. Hepcidin secretion is part of the innate immune response induced by inflammation and infection that serves to restrict available iron for use by invading pathogens.[359,362] In North America and Europe, more than 90% of individuals with HH are homozygous for a single point mutation that inserts a tyrosine instead of cysteine at residue 282 (termed the C282Y mutation).[362] Although it is a frequent genetic trait (estimated 1 in 8 persons of northern European ancestry are carriers, with approximately 1 in 250 being homozygous), most individuals who are homozygous for this mutation do not develop evidence of iron overload. A large population-based study showed that only 28% of males and approximately 1% of females homozygous for the C282Y mutation develop HH.[363]

Up to approximately 60% to 70% of C282Y homozygotes will develop iron overload during their life. Approximately 2% of people with HH have a C282Y gene mutation in one of their copies of the HFE gene and the H63D mutation from the other parent. Clearly, the family members of individuals with HH, unaffected C282Y, compound heterozygotes, and C282Y heterozygotes will be at increased risk of having HH and should be advised to have the gene test and iron studies performed.[364,365]

Liver disease due to hemochromatosis is rare in younger individuals, but becomes more common after the age of 30 years. Liver function tests are frequently normal in asymptomatic patients but may be abnormal in symptomatic patients. The most useful tests are fasting transferrin saturation and serum ferritin. The transferrin saturation reflects increased iron absorption, and a value more than 45% is the most sensitive marker of early iron overload, but neither a raised fasting transferrin saturation nor ferritin concentration is diagnostic of HH. Ferritin is also an acute-phase reactant and can be raised nonspecifically in the presence of alcohol consumption, inflammation, and other liver disease. Serum ferritin is considered to be abnormal when it is more than 250 μg/L in premenopausal women and more than 300 μg/L in men and postmenopausal women. If the fasting transferrin saturation or serum ferritin is elevated on more than one occasion, HH should be suspected, even if there are no clinical symptoms or abnormal liver function tests. In this situation, the *HFE* gene test should be requested. Iron studies may be normal in individuals with a genetic predisposition to HH who have not developed iron overload. Up to 40% of homozygotes have normal results in iron studies, which may be due to overt (blood donation) or covert (gynecological or GI) blood loss. The likelihood of liver disease is related to serum ferritin concentrations. Follow-up of all patients with iron overload should occur regardless of the HFE gene test. It is suggested that if the patient is C282Y homozygous without iron overload, then iron studies should be repeated every 2 to 5 years. If the patient is C282Y homozygotic and has iron overload, then lifelong venesection is necessary, usually every 2 to 3 months after the results of iron studies have become normal. The patient should also reduce their red meat and alcohol intake. Non-cirrhotic patients who are treated early have a normal life expectancy. Cirrhosis is unlikely if the ferritin is less than 1000 μg/L, plasma AST activities are normal, and there is no hepatomegaly. Cirrhotic patients rarely regress to normal and have a lifelong risk of HCC.[364,365]

Wilson Disease. Wilson disease is an autosomal recessive disorder of copper metabolism.[265] It has a gene frequency of 1 in 200 and a disease frequency of 1 in 30,000. It is due to 1 of more than 200 mutations in a gene on chromosome 13 that codes for a copper-transporting adenosine triphosphatase (ATP7B).[264,266] This enzyme, found mainly in the liver, is involved in movement of copper into bile; deficiency leads to accumulation of copper in the liver and eventually in other tissues. Guidelines on diagnosis and treatment of Wilson disease have been updated.[366]

Wilson disease usually manifests at age younger than 30 years,[367] and for reasons that are unknown, patients usually present either with the hepatic or the neuropsychiatric form of the disease. In children, hepatic involvement tends to predominate, whereas in adolescents and adults, the neuropsychiatric form becomes more common. Patients presenting with neuropsychiatric manifestations commonly have advanced liver disease at the time of presentation, whereas those presenting with liver disease may have little in the way of neurologic damage. Hepatic manifestations include fulminant hepatitis (as discussed earlier), but more commonly chronic hepatitis, with or without cirrhosis, is the presenting finding.[368,369] Occasionally, the features mimic those of AIH, with increased plasma globulins and positive ANAs.[370]

The classic clinical finding of increased copper deposition in the eye is the Kayser-Fleischer ring, caused by deposition of copper at the edge of the cornea. Although found in approximately 95% of patients with neurologic or psychiatric manifestations, it is present in only approximately one-half of patients with hepatic forms of Wilson disease[269] and is rarely present in children.[371] As mentioned earlier, hemolytic anemia and renal failure commonly accompany acute forms of Wilson disease; hemolytic anemia may be episodic even in chronic forms of Wilson disease.[366]

Several laboratory tests are available for the diagnosis of Wilson disease; ceruloplasmin measurement is discussed in detail in Chapter 28 and copper measurement in Chapters 37 and 42. Test results are often affected by other conditions, sometimes making diagnosis difficult. Classic findings of Wilson disease include decreased plasma ceruloplasmin, decreased total plasma copper, increased plasma-free (or non-ceruloplasmin) copper, increased urine copper excretion, and increased hepatic copper content. Ceruloplasmin is a ferroxidase that typically is measured by enzymatic activity or by immunoassay. Controversy is ongoing over which assay format is preferable, and guidelines have not specified one type.[281,366] Plasma ceruloplasmin concentrations are low in infants, gradually rise to higher concentrations than adult concentrations in early childhood, then gradually decline to adult concentrations. Use of age-appropriate reference intervals is critical for diagnosis in children. Ceruloplasmin is an acute-phase protein, and its synthesis is induced by estrogen; concentrations may be falsely normal with acute illness or with high estrogen states. Low concentrations of ceruloplasmin are seen with malnutrition, in protein-losing states, and in cirrhosis of any cause. These preanalytical variables cause ceruloplasmin to have a low predictive value as a single test for Wilson disease; in one study of patients with chronic hepatitis, the positive predictive value was only 6%.[372] Ceruloplasmin is also decreased in approximately 20% of heterozygous carriers of the Wilson disease gene.[373] Because most plasma copper is bound to ceruloplasmin, total plasma copper is affected by factors that affect ceruloplasmin. Some experts recommend estimation of free (non-ceruloplasmin) copper as the difference between total copper (micrograms per deciliter) and ceruloplasmin (3× mg/dL); values more than 25 μg/dL (3.9 μmol/L) suggest Wilson disease.[374] Measurement of urine copper excretion is the most specific noninvasive test for Wilson disease; 24-hour urine copper excretion is typically more than 100 μg/24 hours (15.7 μmol/24 hours) in Wilson disease. Unfortunately, the clinical sensitivity of copper excretion appears to be only 75% to 85%.[269,371]

Treatment of active, symptomatic Wilson disease is aimed at increasing urine copper excretion to eliminate excess copper from tissue. The primary therapy for Wilson disease usually involves chelating agents such as D-penicillamine and trientine, which is now more widely used because of its lower rate of side effects. Zinc (particularly zinc acetate) inhibits copper absorption from the intestinal tract; it is usually used for maintenance treatment after copper chelation, but it can also be used as initial therapy. Monitoring treatment (particularly with zinc) by annual measurement of urine copper excretion can be helpful in ensuring that excess copper is no longer being excreted.[366]

Alpha$_1$-Antitrypsin Deficiency. Alpha$_1$-antitrypsin is the most important of the serine protease inhibitors (collectively termed serpins; see also Chapter 28). As its name implies, AAT inhibits trypsin, but it also inhibits other proteolytic enzymes, including neutrophil-derived elastase, cathepsin G, and proteinase 3. The gene for AAT (originally called *PI*, but now called SERPINA1) is located on chromosome 14. Several genetic variants of AAT (differing by a single amino acid) have been classified on the basis of their electrophoretic mobility; the slowest migrating of these was termed the Z variant. Some variants, particularly S and Z, form loop sheet polymers,[375] causing impaired release from the endoplasmic reticulum, hepatocytic inclusions of AAT, and reduced plasma concentrations. The most severe forms of disease have been associated with homozygosity for the Z variant, which is found in 1 in 1000 to 2000 individuals in Europe and North America.[376] However, it is estimated that only approximately 10% of those with AAT deficiency develop clinical disease.[377]

The effects of AAT deficiency on the liver are controversial. In neonates, AAT deficiency is often associated with hepatitis; in one study, almost one-third of infants with prolonged jaundice were found to be AAT deficient.[378] Approximately 20% of AAT-deficient infants develop hepatitis,[379] with up to 25% 1-year mortality.[380] However, in those who survive the first year, evidence of liver injury diminishes and usually resolves by age 12 years.[381,382] At age 18 years, none of 183 individuals with AAT deficiency had clinical evidence of liver disease, none had elevated plasma procollagen III peptide concentrations, and less than 20% had increased concentrations of liver-associated enzymes.[383]

Data on the association of AAT deficiency with liver disease in adults are somewhat contradictory.[384] In several studies, cirrhosis was present in one-third to one-half of those with AAT deficiency, and HCC was present in approximately one-third of those with cirrhosis.[385,386] The frequency was similar in those with heterozygous and homozygous presence of the PiZ variant.[386] In two studies of patients with cryptogenic liver disease, the frequency of the PiZ heterozygotes was significantly higher than that found in the general population.[387,388] However, two other studies found a similar frequency of liver disease in those with AAT deficiency and controls.[389,390] Some evidence suggests that AAT deficiency may increase risk of liver damage from other factors. In one study, most individuals with AAT deficiency and liver injury were also positive for anti-HCV; only 11% had no other liver risk factors.[391] In those with AAT deficiency and no evidence of liver disease (usually viral-related), life expectancy was no different from that of healthy controls. A 2007 research conference found evidence that defects in degradation of AAT underlie differences in protein accumulation, which is necessary for the development of liver disease.[392] It is likely that, as with hemochromatosis, the abnormal form of AAT is necessary, but perhaps not sufficient, to cause liver disease.

AAT is estimated by protein electrophoresis, in which it constitutes most of the α_1-globulin band; this was the original means by which AAT deficiency was recognized.[385] It can also be quantified by a variety of other techniques (see Chapter 21). AAT is an acute-phase response protein; misleadingly normal concentrations have been reported in approximately 40% of PiZ heterozygotes,[393] although rarely in PiZZ homozygotes. This is due to the acute-phase response elevating AAT concentrations into the reference range, a consequence that may affect other proteins produced by the liver, including ferritin and ceruloplasmin. Determination of phenotype was typically accomplished by isoelectric focusing and had been recommended as the diagnostic test of choice in one guideline,[281] but phenotyping cannot distinguish true homozygotes from heterozygotes who have a null genotype on the other *AAT* gene. Molecular tests are now available to determine *AAT* genotype.[394] Because the prognosis may vary between those who are actually homozygous for the Z variant and those with null phenotype, molecular testing of the SERPINA1 gene is considered preferable.[377]

Drug-Induced Liver Injury

As discussed earlier, most cases of drug-induced liver injury present as acute hepatitis. Less commonly, drugs have produced chronic liver injury in a pattern that mimicks chronic hepatitis or other chronic liver injury (chronic cholestasis and hepatic granulomas).[395] The drugs most commonly linked to chronic hepatitis are nitrofurantoin, methyldopa, and hydroxy-3-methylglutaryl-CoA reductase inhibitors; however, a large number of drugs have been associated with liver injury,[396] and herbal medications have been linked to chronic hepatitis.[397,398] In individuals with increased activities of aminotransferases and no obvious cause, prescription drug use was significantly more likely to be present than in those with a known cause for elevated enzyme activities.[399] As with acute drug reactions, establishing drugs as the cause of chronic hepatitis is difficult; temporal relationships to drug ingestion are not as clear as with acute hepatitis, and reactions can be seen first in those who have been taking the medication for many months.[400,401] Most chronic drug reactions resolve when administration of the drug is discontinued.[402,403]

Significance of Chronic Hepatitis

In many cases, chronic hepatitis is a disease with minimal consequences. As mentioned earlier, an average of 20% to 30% of individuals with chronic HBV or HCV progress to cirrhosis over a 20-year period. However, cirrhosis was the sixth leading cause of death in the United States in 35 to 44 year olds and the fourth leading cause of death in 45 to 54 year olds in 2012 (the most recent year for which full data are available).[404] The frequency of cirrhosis and HCC has been increasing in much of the Western world,[405] mostly caused by the increase in cases related to HCV. The proportions of individuals with HCV with cirrhosis and HCC are expected to double by 2020, and the number of deaths caused by liver disease is expected to almost triple.[141] The ability to predict which patients are at increased risk for such late complications of chronic hepatitis would allow more appropriate treatment. Even with the advent of highly effective and well-tolerated treatments for HCV, it is likely to be decades before the burden of infection is brought under control sufficiently to reduce the incidence of complications of disease and the necessity for liver transplantation,[314] making the search for a prophylactic vaccine an imperative.

Fibrosis and necroinflammatory activity are the two major components of chronic hepatitis. The extent of fibrosis (stage) is strongly related to the risk of progression,[406-408] whereas necroinflammatory activity (grade) is correlated with progression in some,[408-410] but not all,[411,412] studies. Because ALT activity is strongly correlated with necroinflammatory activity,[413] it is also associated with risk of progression to cirrhosis in some, but not all, studies. Clinical variables are associated with risk of progression as well; these include age at infection, male sex, alcohol intake, and the presence of immunosuppression.[411,414-416]

The process of scar formation in the liver involves numerous factors and differs in some important ways from that in other sites in the body.[417,418] Increasing evidence suggests that the process of fibrosis is reversible, even when cirrhosis is histologically present.[47] For example, two studies found that successful treatment of HBV[419] and HCV[420] was associated with reversal of cirrhosis in 50% to 75% of cases. Although the principal component of hepatic scars is type III collagen, other components include type I and type IV collagen, laminin, elastin, and fibronectin. Proteoglycans, especially hyaluronate, are also involved in scar formation. Production of scar in the liver is affected by the rate of enzymatic degradation; a variety of MMPs are found in areas of scar formation, along with several TIMPs. MMPs are involved in degradation of the normal connective tissue of the liver (a necessary prequel to fibrosis), but they are also involved in breakdown and remodeling of collagen. HSCs are critical in this process; they produce both MMP and TIMP, as well as collagen and other matrix materials.[29,421] Recruitment and activation of stellate cells involve the action of a number of cytokines, particularly TGF-β, PDGF, and IL-6.[29] Evidence indicates that a variety of other cells also contribute to development of scar tissue within the liver.[422]

As discussed earlier in the chapter, the gold standard for evaluation of the extent of liver damage has been liver biopsy. Because the degree of injury is not uniform throughout the liver, the sample taken may not be representative of the extent of damage.[423] This has led to interest in the use of laboratory tests to predict the extent of fibrosis in the liver as described previously. Increasingly, these tests are being used to stratify and monitor patients with chronic liver disease.

Alcoholic Liver Disease

Alcoholic liver disease differs clinically and biochemically from other forms of hepatitis and liver disease.[424] It is a common cause of liver disease in the developed world, but the incidence of acute alcoholic hepatitis and death from alcoholic cirrhosis is declining in North America and Europe.[425,426] Risk factors for developing alcoholic liver disease include the following.

1. *Duration and magnitude of alcohol ingestion.* As discussed later in the chapter, alcoholic liver disease does not occur in all individuals with chronic ethanol intake; although there appears to be a threshold intake of 40 g/day in men and 10 g/day in women,[427] meta-analysis of published studies shows that risk increases even at intakes of less than 25 g/day.[428] Most individuals with alcoholic liver disease ingest more than 80 g of alcohol per day.[429] Daily drinking appears to be riskier than intermittent drinking.
2. *Sex.* There is a greater likelihood of progression to cirrhosis in women.[430] Although some studies have suggested that this is due to lower activities of gastric mucosal alcohol dehydrogenase in women, 2002 data show that this is true only in younger women, and that older women actually have higher activities than older men.[431]
3. *Hepatitis B or C infection.* Both may increase the severity of liver damage in persons who drink heavily, and both correlate with degree of liver damage. For example, antibodies to HCV are several times more common in individuals with alcoholic hepatitis than in alcoholic individuals without hepatitis or in age- and sex-matched controls, suggesting a synergistic role for HCV.[432]
4. *Genetic factors.* As discussed later, an inherited predisposition to alcoholism has been clearly established. *HFE* gene mutations are more common in alcoholic individuals with liver disease than in those with no evidence of liver disease.[433]
5. *Nutritional status.* Protein-calorie malnutrition is extremely common among alcoholic individuals. Malnutrition may be due not only to poor intake but also to abnormal nutrient metabolism. Although poor nutrition may contribute to the evolution of alcoholic liver disease, adequate nutrition does not prevent its development. Studies suggest that obesity may be a risk factor (perhaps because of the presence of coexisting NAFLD).

Alcohol is metabolized to acetaldehyde by cytosolic alcohol dehydrogenase and microsomal enzymes (primarily CYP2E1). Acetaldehyde is subsequently metabolized to acetyl-CoA by aldehyde dehydrogenase. This is further broken down to acetate, which may be converted to carbon dioxide and water through the citric acid cycle to be converted to fatty acids. The latter is a major mechanism for induction of fatty liver by alcohol, but acetaldehyde is probably the primary toxin. It causes most of the injury to liver cells, as well as the induction of collagen synthesis leading to fibrosis, and ultimately, cirrhosis.

The mechanism for liver injury in alcohol abuse is still unclear. Only a minority of patients (less than one-third) who abuse alcohol develop alcoholic liver disease,[434] and only 5% of the heaviest drinkers develop cirrhosis.[249] Acetylation of a variety of liver proteins occurs with alcohol abuse, leading to loss of function of affected proteins in many cases.[435] Antibodies to acetylated liver proteins have been detected in patients with alcoholic liver disease.[436,437] Alcohol causes damage to intestinal epithelial cells, leading to release of lipopolysaccharide, which can also damage liver cells.[438] Activation of innate immunity, through either or both of these mechanisms, appears to be central to damage in alcoholic liver disease.[439] A variety of other metabolic changes have been observed in alcoholic liver disease, including changes in methionine metabolism and oxidative stress.[440]

Genetic factors seem to play a role in both alcohol abuse[441,442] and alcoholic liver disease.[443] As much as 40% to 60% of alcohol abuse is due to inherited factors.[441] Much effort has been expended in finding specific genetic markers; some of the more commonly implicated specific genes are those coding for alcohol dehydrogenase and several brain receptors, including those for γ-aminobutyric acid and acetylcholine. Genetic variants in alcohol-metabolizing enzymes (including alcohol dehydrogenase, aldehyde dehydrogenase, and microsomal enzymes such as CYP2E1) are linked to alcohol abuse. However, most believe that multiple genes are involved in alcohol abuse. Genetic factors may also be important in determining which persons with alcohol abuse develop liver disease; as with alcohol abuse itself, as much as half of the risk of cirrhosis is due to genetic factors.[444] Similar genes may be involved; a 2009 study showed that alcoholic individuals with cirrhosis were much more likely to have mutations in CPP2E1 and γ-aminobutyric acid receptors than alcoholics without cirrhosis.[445]

Acute alcoholic hepatitis clinically is an acute febrile illness[249] that is characteristically associated with leukocytosis[446] and increased plasma concentrations of acute-phase response proteins.[447] It causes mild increases in cytosolic enzymes; AST activity is typically more than two times greater than that of ALT,[447a] and it is rare for AST to be more than eight times the upper reference interval.[446] Among the factors involved in causing the higher AST/ALT ratio in alcoholic hepatitis are damage to mitochondria, causing release of mitochondrial AST,[448,449] deficiency of pyridoxal 5′-phosphate,[450] and a reduction in ALT content within the liver.[450] A cholestatic form of the disease, with increases in ALP activity to greater than three times the upper reference interval, is seen in up to 20% of cases; it is associated with higher mortality.[451] Increases in bilirubin are common, and reduced liver-synthesized protein concentrations are commonly present. Increased bilirubin, decreased albumin, and prolonged PT are poor prognostic markers in alcoholic hepatitis.[452] The Maddrey discriminant function (4.6 × (PT – Control PT)) + Plasma bilirubin (milligrams per deciliter)) value of more than 32 identifies individuals with a high mortality rate,[427] and a Model for End-Stage Liver Disease (MELD) score more than 11 has been found to have similar sensitivity and better specificity.[453]

A large number of biochemical markers have been proposed for the detection of excessive alcohol consumption.[454-456] Among routine laboratory tests, the most widely used are GGT and mean corpuscular volume (MCV). Serum GGT activity is commonly used as a screening test for alcohol abuse. However, GGT is an inducible enzyme that is elevated by many drugs and a variety of other factors such as cigarette smoking and other forms of liver disease.[83] The threshold for positivity is approximately 2 drinks/day, and elevation is more common in those who drink regularly than in binge drinkers. Although the clinical sensitivity of GGT for alcohol abuse is in the range of 70%, specificity is poor.[457] GGT remains elevated for an average of 25 days after alcohol abstention.[458] MCV has similar clinical sensitivity, and specificity is low.[457]

Alcohol leads to production of isoforms of transferrin with low sialic acid content, termed carbohydrate-deficient transferrin (CDT; also called hyposialyl- and asialyltransferrin). The use of CDT for detecting problem drinkers has been reviewed.[459] CDT returns to a normal concentration in a mean of 10 days with abstention from alcohol.[458] In a pilot study, CDT was found to be the only test to reliably distinguish alcoholic hepatitis from NALFD.[460] It has been suggested that combining markers such as CDT and GGT will enhance accuracy in identifying problem drinkers.[457] CDT is frequently elevated in persons with end-stage liver disease, regardless of cause.[461]

Other markers of alcohol abuse have been studied, but with fewer data than for the markers mentioned earlier. Fatty acid ethyl esters are formed with acute and long-term alcohol intake.[462] Similarly, alcohol metabolites combine with glucuronic acid, forming ethylglucuronides in patients who abuse alcohol.[463] Acetaldehyde adducts with serum proteins[464] and sialic acid[465] have also been evaluated as markers of alcohol abuse. Proteomic techniques have been used to try to identify additional markers,[466] with the suggestion that these will perform better than the currently used markers (eg, GGT and CDT).

POINTS TO REMEMBER

Most Common Causes of Chronic Liver Disease

- Alcohol
- Fatty liver disease
- Chronic viral hepatitis B or hepatitis C

Cirrhosis

Cirrhosis, which is defined anatomically as diffuse fibrosis with nodular regeneration, represents the end stage of scar formation and regeneration in chronic liver injury. This response to injury occurs independently of the etiology and thus it is not possible, in most circumstances, to determine the cause of cirrhosis based on histology. Classically, cirrhosis has been classified as micronodular, macronodular, or mixed, based on the histology and gross appearance of

AT A GLANCE

Causes of Chronic Liver Disease

Often the cause of chronic liver disease is not immediately obvious. In this situation, a systematic approach to differential diagnosis should be taken, gathering history, and the findings of clinical examination, blood and urine tests, as well as imaging and biopsy.

The following categories of causes of chronic liver disease should be considered:

- Toxins: alcohol, drugs
- Viruses: HBV, HCV
- Metabolic liver diseases: fatty liver disease, hemochromatosis, AAT deficiency, Wilson disease
- Immune-mediated liver diseases: AIH, primary biliary cirrhosis, primary sclerosing cholangitis
- Infiltration of the liver
- Tumors: benign and malignant (primary, secondary)

the liver. However, this is considered inadequate for etiologic or prognostic purposes. Consequently, it is more common to classify cirrhosis on the basis of its presumed or known etiology. Common causes of cirrhosis and their therapies are listed in Table 61.8. Virtually all chronic liver diseases are known to lead to cirrhosis (see Fig. 61.9), but most cases of cirrhosis occur as a result of chronic hepatitis.

In the early stages of transition from chronic hepatitis to cirrhosis, termed compensated cirrhosis, no signs or symptoms of liver damage may be present. Laboratory abnormalities usually appear before clinical findings, such as ascites, gynecomastia, palmar erythema, and portal hypertension, begin to develop. The earliest laboratory abnormalities to develop in cirrhosis are a fall in platelet count, an increase in PT, a decrease in the plasma albumin-to-globulin concentration ratio to less than 1, and an increase in the AST/ALT activity ratio to more than 1.[467,468] Generally, in those with documented cirrhosis, decompensation occurs slowly, at a rate of approximately 3% per year; 10-year survival with compensated cirrhosis is 90%.[469] However, once decompensation occurs, 10-year survival is only approximately 20%.[469] However, prognosis varies with etiology and may be influenced dramatically by response to treatment (as is the case in viral hepatitis B and C) or by abstinence from alcohol in alcoholic liver disease. Jaundice is a late finding in decompensated cirrhosis. A variety of staging systems have been used to predict prognosis in cirrhosis. For many years, the most common classification system was the Child-Pugh class system, summarized in Table 61.9. Currently, the MELD score is used to identify patients with advanced cirrhosis who may be candidates for liver transplantation; it appears superior to the Child-Pugh scoring system in predicting short-term survival.[470-472] The MELD score is calculated as:

$$\begin{aligned}\text{MELD Score} = {} & (0.957 \times \ln(\text{serum creatinine}) \\ & + 0.378 \times \ln(\text{serum bilirubin}) \\ & + 1.120 \times \ln(\text{INR}) + 0.643) \\ & \times 10\ (\text{if hemodialysis, value for} \\ & \text{creatinine is automatically set to 4.0})\end{aligned}$$

or in SI units as:

$$\begin{aligned}\text{MELD Score} = {} & 10 \times ((0.957 \times \ln(\text{creatinine}/88.4)) \\ & + (0.378 \times \ln(\text{bilirubin}/17.1)) \\ & + (1.12 \times \ln(\text{INR}))) + 6.43\end{aligned}$$

Risk of death over 3 months is low in those with MELD scores less than10, intermediate in those with scores of 10 to 20, and high in those with scores of more than 20.[473] Various modifications of the MELD score have been developed.

TABLE 61.8 Causes and Treatment of Cirrhosis

Cause	Treatment
Viral	
Hepatitis B	Administration of nucleoside or nucleotide HBV DNA polymerase inhibitors or pegylated α-interferon
Hepatitis C	Directly acting antiviral inhibitors of HCV and/or pegylated α-interferon with or without ribavirin
Toxic	
Alcohol	Abstinence, liver transplantation
Metabolic	
Hemochromatosis	Phlebotomy
Wilson disease	Penicillamine, zinc trientine
α1-Antitrypsin deficiency	Gene therapy, protein administration
Nonalcoholic fatty liver disease	Diet, exercise, insulin sensitizers
Biliary	
Primary biliary cirrhosis	Ursodeoxycholic acid
Primary sclerosing cholangitis	Liver transplantation
Autoimmune hepatitis	Corticosteroids, azathioprine, other immunosuppressants
Idiopathic	Consider immunosuppression
Advanced cirrhosis, irrespective of cause	Liver transplantation

HBV, Hepatitis B virus; *HCV*, hepatitis C virus.

TABLE 61.9 Child-Pugh System for Classifying Severity of Cirrhosis

Feature	1 Point	2 Points	3 Points
Encephalopathy	None	Grade 1–2	Grade 3–4
Ascites	None	Slight	Moderate-severe
Albumin, g/dL	>3.5	2.8–3.5	<2.8
Prothrombin time, seconds prolonged	<4	4–6	>6
Bilirubin, mg/dL (μmol/L)	<4 (<68)	4–10 (68–170	>10 (>170)

Scoring: <7 points: class A; 7 to 9 points: class B; >9 points: class C.

Children younger than age 12 years should be assessed by the Pediatric End-Stage Liver Disease (PELD) Score. If a patient has had two or more hemodialysis treatments or 24 hours of continuous venovenous hemodialysis in the week before the time of the scoring, creatinine will be set to 4 mg/dL (353.6 μmol/L), the maximum creatinine level allowed in the model. For patients with HCC, the PELD/MELD score is increased according to an algorithm established by the United Network for Organ Sharing. Additional information about the MELD and PELD scores and web-based calculators can be found at http://optn.transplant.hrsa.gov/resources/by-organ/liver-intestine.

Laboratory findings in cirrhosis reflect ongoing liver injury and decreased hepatic function. Plasma activities of aminotransferases are variable in cirrhosis and reflect underlying necroinflammatory activity. If the cause of cirrhosis has been eliminated (as by abstinence from ethanol or successful treatment of viral hepatitis), aminotransferase activity is often within the reference interval. If aminotransferases remain increased, risk of development of HCC is increased.[474] As described earlier, the ratio of AST/ALT activity is often more than 1 in cirrhosis; this is usually a result of a fall in ALT and minimal change in AST activities. The mechanism for these changes is not clear, but there appears to be a decrease in the production of enzymatically active ALT in cirrhotic individuals,[475] along with a high ratio of immunoreactive to enzymatically active ALT in plasma.[88] Increases in AFP are common in cirrhotic patients, even in the absence of HCC.[476]

Acute on Chronic Liver Failure

Patients with compensated liver cirrhosis may experience decompensation due to a wide variety of precipitating factors, including infection, metabolic disturbance, bleeding, and protein overload. An international consortium of hepatologists has collected data on cirrhotic patients to identify markers of acute decompensation of cirrhosis that they have termed "Acute on Chronic Liver Failure" (ACLF).[477] This syndrome is characterized by acute decompensation (ascites, encephalopathy, GI hemorrhage, and/or bacterial infections), organ failure (liver, kidney, brain, coagulation, respiration, circulation), and high short-term mortality (ie, 28-day mortality rate ≥15%).[15] The European Association for the Study of the Liver Chronic Liver Failure "CLIF Consortium" has derived the Chronic Liver Failure-Sequential Organ Failure Assessment score, which combines biochemical markers, including bilirubin, INR and platelet count, with assessment of organ failure to derive a prognostic score that can be used to predict outcomes in patients with liver failure.[478] The use of the term ACLF in place of "decompensated cirrhosis" has been suggested as a means of highlighting the onset of acute liver dysfunction, which is often accompanied by other organ dysfunction due to an acute insult, in the context of cirrhosis, and to differentiate ACLF from decompensation due to gradual and progressive loss of liver function. The emphasis on determining other organ dysfunction may be clinically important, but the value of differentiating ACLF from decompensated cirrhosis remains controversial.

Hepatic Glycogenoses

The glycogenoses are a group of disorders that are characterized by excessive and/or aberrant glycogen storage in various tissues.[479] Most of these have deficient glucose production by the liver, leading to hypoglycemia. All are inherited by autosomal recessive transmission, except for type IV, which is sex linked. The hepatic glycogen storage diseases and their enzyme defects are listed in Table 61.10 and discussed in more detail in Chapter 33 on Carbohydrates. Most of these disorders are associated with growth retardation and hepatosplenomegaly. Mental development is usually normal. Hypoglycemia is a prominent feature in types I, III, and VI, and needs to be treated with continuous glucose feeding of uncooked cornstarch, which results in slow release of glucose. The diagnosis is based on the demonstration of excess glycogen in the liver biopsy and in vitro identification of the abnormal enzyme or aberrant glycogen. Prognosis and treatment vary with each entity (for more details, see Chapter 33).

Cholestatic Liver Disease

Cholestasis (stoppage or suppression of the flow of bile) is characterized by retention of bile within the excretory system. The term obstruction is often used inappropriately, because cholestasis has been known to occur without mechanical obstruction to the biliary tract. Although intrahepatic cholestasis may be due to functional or mechanical problems, extrahepatic cholestasis is always due to physical obstruction of the bile ducts by gallstones, biliary strictures, and tumors. The major cholestatic diseases include mechanical obstruction of the bile ducts, PBC, and primary sclerosing cholangitis (PSC). Other cholestatic disorders include post–bone marrow transplantation cholangiopathy, post–liver

TABLE 61.10 Hepatic Glycogen Storage Diseases

Type	Eponym	Enzyme Defect	Involved Tissues
0		Glycogen synthetase	Liver
I	von Gierke	Ia glucose 6-phosphatase Ib translocase for glucose 6-phosphatase Ic phosphate/pyrophosphate translocase	Liver, kidney, intestines
II	Pompe	Lysosomal acid α-1,4 glucosidase	Most tissues
III	Cori	Amylo-1,6 glucosidase debranching enzyme	Liver, muscle, WBCs
IV	Anderson	Amylo-1,4–1,6 trans-glucosidase (branching enzyme)	Most tissue
VI	Hers	Liver phosphorylase	Liver, WBCs
VII		Phosphorylase activation	Liver
IXa		Phosphorylase kinase	Liver, WBCs, RBCs

RBCs, Red blood cells; *WBCs*, white blood cells.

transplantation cholangiopathy, drug-induced cholestasis, AIDS cholangiopathy, parenteral nutrition (see Chapter 56 on Nutrition), and bilirubinostasis of acute illness. Cholestatic hepatitis, which was discussed previously, may also cause cholestasis, but generally presents in a fashion similar to hepatitis. There are specific types of cholestasis that can occur in pregnancy; these are discussed in Chapter 69 on pregnancy related disorders.

The clinical consequences of prolonged cholestasis are related to impaired biliary drainage. Deficiency of bile acids in the intestinal tract leads to malabsorption of fat and the fat-soluble vitamins A, D, E, and K (see Chapters 37, 56, and 64, and the Bile Acids section of this chapter). Vitamin A malabsorption results in night blindness. Vitamin D malabsorption leads to calcium and phosphate malabsorption, causing rickets in children and osteomalacia in adults. Vitamin K malabsorption results in deficiency of coagulation factors II, VII, IX, and X, leading to prolonged clotting times, and sometimes, bleeding. Lack of excretion of normal bile contents results in their accumulation in plasma. Bile acid retention leads to increased bile acid concentrations in plasma. Bilirubin retention leads to jaundice, dark urine, and pale stools. Increased bilirubin generally occurs only with complete obstruction, and thus, is more commonly seen with extrahepatic rather than intrahepatic cholestasis.

Laboratory features of cholestasis vary, depending on whether the process causes complete or partial impairment of biliary drainage. A common feature of all cholestatic disorders is an increase in plasma activities of canalicular enzymes, such as ALP and GGT. Because this process involves both increased synthesis of enzyme and release of enzyme from its membrane-bound forms, a short lag period is generally seen between the onset of cholestasis and the increase in plasma activities. In the early stages of an acute mechanical obstruction (especially from gallstones), transient increases may be noted in plasma activities of liver cytosolic enzymes, such as AST and ALT. Activities of plasma AST and ALT may exceed 400 U/L, and in 1% to 2% of cases are greater than 2000 U/L. Even in the presence of continued obstruction, AST and ALT activity gradually decreases, and AST is typically within the reference interval within 8 to 10 days. Increases in total bilirubin typically occur only with complete extrahepatic obstruction, although they may be seen with extensive intrahepatic cholestasis. Increases in direct bilirubin are more commonly seen, and direct bilirubin has been reported to be the most sensitive functional test for the presence of cholestasis. Prolonged PT is the most commonly detected coagulation abnormality. It usually is corrected by administration of parenteral vitamin K. Accumulation of cholesterol is associated with the development of an abnormal lipoprotein, termed lipoprotein-X,[480,481] which contains phospholipids, cholesterol, fragments of cell membrane (along with ALP),[482] and albumin; the lipid may deposit in connective tissue, producing xanthomas.[483] Although it is often measured as low-density lipoprotein cholesterol,[484] lipoprotein-X is actually antiatherogenic.[483,485]

Mechanical Bile Duct Obstruction

The most common cause of cholestasis is biliary tract obstruction by space-occupying lesions.[486] Extrahepatic bile duct obstruction occurs most commonly as the result of gallstones in the common bile duct or because of tumors in the head of the pancreas or duodenum. Other causes of extrahepatic obstruction include (1) bile duct strictures, (2) extrinsic compression of the bile ducts by enlarged lymph nodes, (3) congenital biliary atresia, and (4) PSC. Extrahepatic obstruction is commonly associated with jaundice, especially when obstruction is complete. Elevation in canalicular enzymes is common, but is not present in all cases[487]; marked increases (>3× the upper reference limit) are more common with gallstones as a cause of obstruction.[276] Transient increases in aminotransferases are more common with choledocholithiasis than with other causes of extrahepatic obstruction.[488] Transient increases in CA 19-9 occur with bile duct obstruction[489]; this is an important consideration, because CA 19-9 is often used as a diagnostic test for pancreatic and bile duct carcinoma (for more details see Chapter 31 on Tumor Markers). A key feature of extrahepatic obstruction is dilation of more proximal and intrahepatic bile ducts, which can be visualized by imaging studies.

Intrahepatic cholestasis caused by mechanical obstruction is also common, but is rarely associated with jaundice or with visibly dilated ducts on imaging studies, although it may be associated with increased direct bilirubin. Jaundice typically occurs only with lesions that are large, or are located near the porta hepatis, where they may obstruct both hepatic ducts. Common causes of intrahepatic obstruction include tumors (particularly metastases), granulomatous diseases (such as sarcoidosis and tuberculosis), and infiltrative processes (such as lymphoma, leukemia, and extramedullary hematopoiesis).

Primary Biliary Cirrhosis

PBC, or non-suppurative destructive cholangitis, is an uncommon autoimmune disorder that targets intrahepatic bile ducts.[490,491] Its prevalence is approximately 2 to 8 per 100,000 population in the developed world, but is much lower in developing areas. The median age at onset is 50 years, and the female-to-male ratio is approximately 6:1. An association with HLA class II antigen DR8 has been noted in some populations. A family history of PBC is seen in 1% to 4% of cases. In up to 80% of cases, the condition is associated with other autoimmune processes, most commonly Sjögren syndrome and hypothyroidism (which often develops before the onset of PBC).[492]

The pathogenesis of PBC is not well understood. However, it is known that destruction of the bile duct is mediated by T cells in the presence of upregulation of HLA class I antigens on hepatocytes and HLA class II antigens on biliary epithelial cells.[493] Although the target antigens of the T cells have not been identified, at least 95% of patients have antimitochondrial antibodies that react against the dihydrolipoamide acyltransferase component of the pyruvate decarboxylase complex.[494] Part of this complex is found on the apical surface of biliary epithelial cells, suggesting a role for this antigen as an immune target.[495] In individuals with coexisting Sjögren syndrome, the antigen is also expressed on the surface of salivary gland cells.[496]

PBC typically presents as an asymptomatic elevation of ALP, but may present with features of cholestasis, particularly pruritus or with fatigue.[497] Metabolic bone disease and xanthomas are common complications of PBC.[498] Occasionally, autoantibodies are detected (usually because of the presence of another autoimmune disease or because of a family history of PBC) before elevation of ALP.[499] Aminotransferase activities are increased in 50% of cases, but are more than twice the upper reference limit appears in only 20% of cases.[500] Increased bilirubin is a late finding and is important in predicting decompensation.[501] Antibodies to mitochondria or to the recombinant pyruvate decarboxylase complex appear similar in sensitivity, although the latter are more specific.[502] A liver biopsy is not required for diagnosis in most cases, but may be helpful in those with low titer antibodies or with a greater than twofold increase in aminotransferase activity.

The natural history of PBC is one of slow progression to portal hypertension, often without development of cirrhosis; the average time from diagnosis to death in untreated patients is 22 years.[497] Development of jaundice is the most important indicator of advanced disease and serves as the most important prognostic test.[498] Medical management of PBC consists of ursodeoxycholic acid therapy; most evidence suggests that survival is improved in treated patients.[498] Although a rare complication, the relative risk of developing HCC is significantly increased in individuals with PBC.[503] Liver transplantation is the only definitive treatment, but even when it is performed, PBC may recur in the transplanted organ.[504]

Biochemical tests and direct markers of liver fibrosis have been studied as surrogate markers of disease severity and prognostic markers of survival in PBC. Of these, the ELF test (see section of this chapter on Direct Biomarkers of Liver Fibrosis) has been shown to be the most accurate in determining prognosis.[505]

Primary Sclerosing Cholangitis

PSC is a chronic inflammatory disease of the biliary tree that most commonly affects the extrahepatic bile ducts; involvement of intrahepatic ducts, with extrahepatic involvement or as an isolated finding, is also possible.[506,507] In contrast to PBC, PSC has a male predominance (60% to 70%) and a younger median age at onset (30 years). In 70% to 90% of patients, PSC is associated with ulcerative colitis, which usually (but not always) precedes onset of PSC; conversely, only approximately 2% to 4% of patients with ulcerative colitis develop PSC.[506] This has led to speculation that bacterial antigens in portal blood might be involved in the pathogenesis of PSC.[508] An autoimmune component is likely because 97% of patients with PSC have one or more autoantibodies present in their plasma.[509] The prevalence of PSC is similar to that of PBC, but geographic differences in prevalence have been observed; it is most common in Northern Europe, where PSC is the most common indication for liver transplantation.[510,511] A markedly increased prevalence of HLA antigens B8 and DR3 has been noted.[512]

The clinical presentation of PSC, similar to that of PBC, is typically an asymptomatic patient with elevated ALP activities found during routine laboratory screening. Symptoms are ultimately present in most patients with PSC; the most common are pruritus and intermittent abdominal pain, but fever may also be present.[507] Treatment, whether medical or surgical, may improve both the results of laboratory tests and symptoms, but does not improve long-term survival.[513,514] Transplantation, the major treatment available for end-stage PSC, results in a high rate of long-term survival. Although PSC recurs after transplantation in approximately 20% to 35% of cases, it does not appear to affect survival.[515] Transplantation also appears to increase the severity of underlying ulcerative colitis, when present.[516] The major cause of death in individuals with PSC is cholangiocarcinoma, which ultimately develops in up to 40% of patients.[506,507] Transplantation in the presence of cholangiocarcinoma is associated with rapid development of metastatic disease and poor survival.[511,517] PSC also increases the likelihood of colon carcinoma in individuals with coexisting ulcerative colitis, although the risk is not affected by liver transplantation.[518]

At the time of diagnosis, most patients with PSC have elevated ALP activities and other canalicular enzymes; bilirubin concentration is typically normal, although it may increase with acute exacerbations. The diagnosis of PSC is based on the typical radiographic appearance of beading and irregularity of the bile ducts. Antineutrophil cytoplasmic antibodies are present in approximately 80% of patients[519] but are not specific for PSC; they are also present in PBC and AIH. Typically, the antibodies have an atypical perinuclear pattern because they are located around the nucleus in formalin- and methanol-fixed preparations. Antigens include lactoferrin, bactericidal and/or permeability increasing protein, and cathepsin G.[509]

Because of the discontinuous nature of the histological lesion in PSC, liver biopsy is of limited value in staging disease severity, but magnetic resonance cholangiopancreatography provides a view of the entire biliary tree. Similar to PBC, the enhanced liver fibrosis test, which is a combination of direct markers of liver fibrosis, has been demonstrated as the best prognostic biochemical marker for PSC.[520]

Drug-Induced Liver Injury

Drugs are a common cause of cholestasis, causing approximately 15% of cases.[521,522] Drug reactions are especially common in older individuals, among whom up to 50% of individuals have increased enzymes because of medications.[521] Nonmedicinal drugs are also increasingly recognized as a cause of cholestasis.[523] Drugs can cause a cholestatic picture by two major mechanisms.[524] In some cases, only conjugated bilirubin is increased, whereas canalicular enzymes are not elevated. This picture, which is often seen with estrogen and anabolic steroids, appears to be due to inhibition of production of the multidrug resistance protein-2[525] an ABC transporter that transports drug-conjugates and divalent bile salt conjugates into bile. More commonly, drugs induce a cholestatic hepatitis, as discussed earlier. The National Institutes of Health website, http://livertox.nih.gov, and recent reviews provide further information and excellent support in the investigation of suspected drug-induced liver toxicity.[402,526,527]

Gallstones

Gallstones are solid formations in the gallbladder that are composed of cholesterol and bile salts. Although they vary in chemical composition, they generally contain a mixture of cholesterol, bilirubin, calcium, and mucoproteins. In the United States, 70% to 85% of all gallstones are predominantly cholesterol, and more than 10% of the adult population is affected.

Three major types of gallstones are cholesterol, pigmented, and the most common, mixed. These stones form whenever bile is supersaturated with cholesterol or unconjugated bilirubin. For these stones or cholesterol gallstones to form, bile must be supersaturated with cholesterol. Whenever an increase in cholesterol or a decrease in bile acids or lecithin occurs, bile becomes lithogenic and cholesterol may precipitate. Factors that predispose to cholesterol hypersecretion include obesity, aging, certain drugs such as clofibrate and nicotine, and certain hormones such as estrogen. Factors that decrease bile acid secretion include terminal ileal disease and cholestatic diseases, such as PBC, PSC, and cystic fibrosis. Genetic factors also appear to be involved. Within racial groups, women are more frequently affected than men. Diet may play a role because it appears that people who ingest diets high in polyunsaturated fats have a higher incidence, whereas those with a diet high in fiber have a decreased incidence.

Pigmented gallstones are associated with conditions in which the bilirubin concentration is increased, such as hemolytic anemia, or when bilirubin becomes insoluble (ie, deconjugated), such as occurs in cholestasis or chronic biliary infection.

Rare Causes of Cholestasis

Several other disorders are associated with cholestasis. Because they occur in specific settings, they are often suggested by the clinical picture. Laboratory tests are of little help in establishing the correct diagnosis.

Cholestasis may develop following bone marrow transplantation because of a variety of factors. Acute graft versus host disease (GVHD) is a consequence of the infusion of allogeneic immunocompetent T-lymphoid cells into an immunocompromised host that cannot reject these cells.[528] Periductular epithelial cells are the primary targets of injury in both acute and chronic GVHD.[529] Clinical features of GVHD include skin rash, intestinal symptoms (nausea, vomiting, diarrhea, and abdominal pain), and cholestasis. The histologic appearance is characteristic, but a liver biopsy is somewhat hazardous in these patients; thus most cases are diagnosed on clinical grounds.

Although acute liver transplantation rejection is associated with necroinflammatory changes and increased aminotransferases, chronic rejection is often associated with cholestasis. The primary targets of immunologic injury are bile ductules and blood vessels.[530] Because of cholestasis, plasma bile acids are often increased early in the process of rejection. Increased numbers of canalicular membranes are often the first evidence of rejection.[530] Although eosinophilia is common in rejection,[531] it is also a common finding in drug-induced cholestasis and thus is not helpful in the differential diagnosis.

AIDS cholangiopathies are caused by organisms not previously known to infect the biliary tree; they have become less common with reduction in the frequency of immunosuppression because of combination antiretroviral treatment. Cryptosporidium is the most common organism. Microsporidium, CMV, *Mycobacterium avium* complex, and cyclospora have also been identified. The clinical presentation usually includes abdominal pain, diarrhea, and cholestasis manifested by threefold to tenfold elevations in plasma ALP, mild elevations in aminotransferases, and rarely, jaundice. Papillary stenosis at the ampulla of Vater is present in patients with pain, and the bile ducts have features of PSC. Cholangiography is needed for the diagnosis, but is indicated only in patients with pain. Brushings and biopsies at the time of cholangiography will establish the diagnosis. Treatment is primarily endoscopic. Sphincterotomy will give pain relief in approximately 70% of patients.

TABLE 61.11 Classification of Hepatic Tumors

Type	Benign	Malignant
Epithelial	Adenoma Bile duct adenoma Cystadenoma Carcinoid Focal nodular hyperplasia Diffuse nodular hyperplasia	Hepatocellular carcinoma Cholangiocarcinoma Cystadenocarcinoma Squamous carcinoma
Mesenchymal tumors	Cavernous hemangioma Fibroma Leiomyoma Hematoma	Hemangiosarcoma Fibrosarcoma Leiomyosarcoma Hepatoblastoma
Metastatic tumors (most common sources)	Colon Pancreas Stomach Breast Lung Unknown primary	

Hepatic Tumors

The liver is host to a wide variety of benign and malignant primary tumors. It is the second most common site of metastases; metastatic tumors account for 90% to 95% of all hepatic malignancies. Primary tumors may arise from many cell lines in the liver, but they arise most commonly from parenchymal and biliary epithelial cells and from mesenchymal cells (Table 61.11). The two most important primary liver tumors are HCC and cholangiocarcinoma.

Hepatocellular Carcinoma

HCC is the fifth most common cancer worldwide and a leading cause of cancer death; more than 500,000 cases occur annually, with a similar number of deaths.[532] Wide geographic and ethnic variations are noted in the incidence, suggesting that both host and environmental factors are involved in its origin. For example, approximately 75% of HCC cases occur in Asia, with an annual incidence of HCC in China of approximately 30 cases per 100,000 males. Worldwide, the incidence is twofold to threefold higher among men than among women. The incidence of HCC has been increasing in the United States[533,534] and much of Europe because of the increasing frequency of cirrhosis caused by HCV; however, incidence has declined in many parts of the world because of the success in prevention of infection by HBV.[535,536] Although cirrhosis is present in most patients with HCC, it is absent in approximately 25% to 30% of cases, often in association with HBV.[537,538] More importantly, the presence of cirrhosis had been recognized before diagnosis of HCC in approximately one-third of cases.[538,539] Wide variations in the incidence of HCC are associated with different causes of cirrhosis. For example, HCC commonly occurs in cirrhosis caused by alcohol abuse, hemochromatosis, AAT deficiency, HBV, and

HCV, but it is rare that it is caused by AIH and Wilson disease.

In most parts of the world, the major risk factors for development of HCC are infection with HBV or HCV. In Asia, Africa, and Alaska, the major risk factor is HBV infection. The presence of HBsAg and HBeAg is associated with a relative risk of HCC of 60, whereas the presence of HBsAg with negative HBeAg is associated with a relative risk of 10.[540] This is probably due to the lower viral loads in HBeAg negative chronic HBV; in all forms of chronic HBV, risk of HCC is directly related to viral load.[300] Once cirrhosis has developed, the rate of development of HCC is approximately 1.5% to 5% per year in both HBV and HCV[292,541]; the relative risk of HCC doubles in those coinfected with these viruses.[542] The risk of HCC is higher in those with cirrhosis who have elevated aminotransferase activities than in those with normal ALT activity.[474,543] The mechanism of increased risk in HBV is believed to be related to integration of HBV DNA into the host genome, possibly caused by the action of the HBV X gene, which may block the activity of p53.[544,545] The mechanism of increased risk of HCC in HCV has not been identified, but may be related to ongoing injury.

Aflatoxin, a product of *Aspergillus flavus* contamination of grain, has been linked to risk of HCC; although it is harmless, it is metabolized to aflatoxin 8,9-epoxide. This reactive intermediate binds to guanosine bases in DNA, leading to mutagenesis. If the formed adduct is not repaired, G-to-T transversion occurs in codon 249 of the *TP53* gene (p53), causing an inactivating mutation.[546] Under normal circumstances, the mutagenic aflatoxin 8,9-epoxide is rendered harmless by glutathione S-transferase, which converts it to a glutathione conjugate, which in turn is metabolized to 1,2-dihydrodiol by epoxide hydrolase.[547] However, both detoxifying enzymes are polymorphic in humans, and the mutant forms are less active. Patients with HCC are more likely to have the mutant forms of epoxide hydrolase and glutathione-S-transferase; this allows accumulation of the epoxide.[548]

The clinical presentation of HCC is variable and usually does not occur until late in the course of disease, when the tumor is large and resection is impossible. In some cases, acute decompensation occurs in a patient with cirrhosis, but clinical presentation may include detection of a right upper quadrant mass, shock due to hemorrhage into the peritoneal cavity, or right upper quadrant pain. Nonspecific signs and symptoms, such as fever, malaise, anorexia, and anemia, are common, and jaundice may occur with central tumors that obstruct biliary drainage. In a small number of cases, paraneoplastic features, such as hypoglycemia, hypercalcemia (due to parathyroid hormone–related peptide production), or erythrocytosis (due to erythropoietin production), may be the initial presenting findings; such paraneoplastic findings occur in up to 20% of cases, usually in association with poor prognosis.[549,550] Laboratory findings include those of cirrhosis and cholestasis, and (except for tumor markers discussed later) are nonspecific.

Because treatment usually is not possible in individuals with clinically diagnosed HCC, much interest has focused on screening high-risk individuals. Most professional societies have not advocated screening for HCC in Europe or North America, although the AASLD has endorsed screening of high-risk patients every 6 to 12 months.[551] Although some data have suggested that screening is effective in detecting small, treatable tumors, other data have not been as supportive.

The most common screening programs have used plasma tumor marker concentrations or tumor markers plus imaging studies; the AASLD recommends imaging as the primary screening modality and recommends against using only tumor markers (although tumor markers were noted to be useful as an addition to imaging).[551] Ultrasound is typically used as the imaging modality for screening because of its low cost. The tumor marker most widely used for screening purposes is AFP; it is typically quantified using assays that measure its total concentration. Although it appears to be relatively sensitive,[552] elevation of AFP is common in individuals with chronic hepatitis and cirrhosis, which is the group at highest risk for HCC. In our experience, AFP above the upper reference limit has a positive predictive value of only 16% for HCC. Use of higher cutoff values than the upper reference limit improves clinical specificity of total AFP, at the expense of clinical sensitivity; for example, at a cutoff of 20 ng/mL, approximately three times the upper reference limit, sensitivity is only 60%.[551] As discussed in Chapter 31 on Tumor Markers, modified forms of AFP are more specific for tumors, particularly the L3 isoform recognized by lens culinaris (lentil) lectin. The L3 isoform by itself has low sensitivity for HCC,[553] and it is the only positive tumor marker in only a small number of cases. In contrast, specificity and positive predictive value are significantly improved when the L3 isoform is combined with the AFP total.[553] An L3 isoform more than 15% of total AFP may be associated with more aggressive and less well-differentiated tumors.[554]

Des-γ-carboxy prothrombin (DCP)—also called PIVKA-2 (factor II PIVKA)—is the inactive form of prothrombin found in individuals taking warfarin or other vitamin K antagonists. Its plasma concentration was first found to be increased in HCC in 1984,[555] but its measurement was not widely used until the early 1990s. Initial studies found that DCP was increased in some patients who did not have elevated AFP, but was insensitive to small HCC that might be curable. DCP immunoassays with lowered detection limits have been developed and have shown increased sensitivity for small HCC, and DCP seems directly related to tumor size[556] and prognosis.[553] Pretreatment with vitamin K, to eliminate other causes of increased DCP, further improves specificity.[557] DCP is best used as an adjunct to AFP, because tumors often produce one or the other tumor marker.[558]

Treatment of HCC is dependent on the extent of the tumor. Small tumors are often treated by transplantation, after which there is a low rate of recurrence. Local techniques, such as ethanol injection, chemoembolization, and use of radiofrequency ablation, are increasingly used before transplantation or instead of transplantation. Larger tumors generally are not resectable, but may be treated by chemoembolization if a single feeding vessel is identified. A novel approach to identifying micrometastases has been described using rt-PCR to amplify mRNA for AFP to detect recurrence or metastasis.[559]

Tumors of the Gallbladder and Bile Ducts

Benign lesions such as papillomas or adenomas may be seen as an incidental finding at cholecystectomy; malignant disease of the gallbladder is uncommon. Cholelithiasis may be an etiologic factor, because 85% of gallbladder carcinomas occur in patients with gallstones. However, less than 1% of patients with gallstones develop carcinoma. It has been suggested that a calcified gallbladder is especially prone to malignant transformation. Various pathologic forms exist, including papillary adenocarcinoma, squamous cell carcinoma, and anaplastic tumors. These tumors usually arise in the neck of the gallbladder and spread rapidly, causing obstruction and cholestasis. Physical examination reveals a hard, tender mass in the gallbladder fossa. These lesions are particularly difficult to treat, and most cases are inoperable at the time of diagnosis.

Cholangiocarcinoma, or primary carcinoma of the bile ducts, can arise at any point in the biliary tree, including the small intrahepatic bile duct radicals. This lesion is typically associated with underlying liver disease, such as PSC, congenital cystic lesions, or chronic infestation with *Clonorchis sinensis*. The clinical presentation is that of cholestasis, including jaundice, dark urine, tan-colored stool, and pruritus. This condition is differentiated from other cholestatic diseases by visualizing the biliary tree.

DIAGNOSTIC STRATEGY

Liver function tests are useful in detecting and diagnosing liver disease and dysfunction, as well as in evaluating severity, monitoring therapy, and assessing prognosis. They are also useful in directing further diagnostic workup. The array of tests useful for these purposes (Table 61.12) includes measurement in plasma of total and direct bilirubin, protein, and albumin concentrations, and the activity of enzymes such as the aminotransferases (AST and ALT), ALP, and GGT. By using a combination of these tests, it is possible to categorize broad types of liver disease, which can then be more accurately diagnosed through disease-specific tests. An algorithm for this process is presented in Fig. 61.13. It should be born in mind that all diagnostic tests should be applied after determining the pretest probability of disease and in the full knowledge of the test performance to derive a posttest probability of disease.[560]

TABLE 61.12 Tests of Hepatic Function and Injury

Test	Utility
Bilirubin	Diagnosing jaundice, modest correlation with severity
Alkaline phosphatase	Diagnosing disorders of metabolism and disorders of the newborn
Bilirubin fractionation	Diagnosing cholestasis and space-occupying lesions
AST	Sensitive test of hepatocellular disease; AST > ALT in alcoholic disease
ALT	Sensitive and more specific test of hepatocellular disease
Gamma-glutamyltransferase	Prognostic indicator for increased cardiovascular and all-cause mortality
Albumin	Indicator of chronicity and severity
Prothrombin time	Indicator of severity of cholestasis

ALT, Alanine aminotransferase; *AST*, Aspartate aminotransferase.

Plasma Enzymes

In practice, plasma aminotransferases and ALP are the most useful tests, because they allow differentiation of hepatocellular disease from cholestatic disease in most cases. The importance of this distinction cannot be overstated: failure to recognize cholestatic disease caused by extrahepatic biliary obstruction will result in liver failure if the obstruction is not quickly corrected. It is also important to recognize that there may be a grey zone of mixed hepatocellular and cholestatic disease wherein the tests do not distinguish one disease from the other. In this case, it is wise to assume that the problem is cholestatic and rule out biliary obstruction. In all cases, the use of imaging to look for evidence and causes of biliary obstruction must be a high priority, with ultrasound being the cheapest and mostly widely available imaging modality.

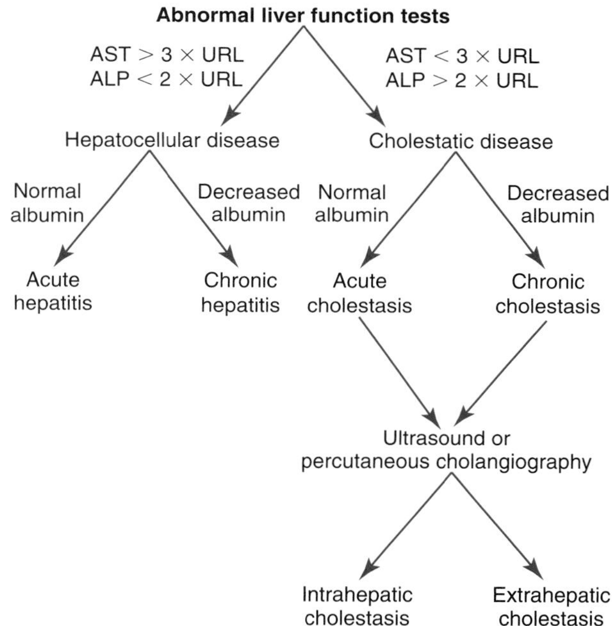

FIGURE 61.13 Algorithm for using abnormal liver function tests to classify and diagnose various types of liver disease. Initial evaluation is best accomplished by examining the pattern of liver-associated enzymes. If elevation primarily affects one of the aminotransferases, then hepatocellular disease is likely; an increase primarily in alkaline phosphatase *(ALP)* suggests a cholestatic disorder. If only ALP is elevated, then it is appropriate to consider nonhepatic sources before further investigation (using measurement of other canalicular enzymes such as γ-glutamyltransferase *[GGT]* or ALP isoenzymes). If the liver is the source of elevated ALP, then an imaging study to evaluate the ducts is the next test performed; dilated ducts establish a mechanical cause of obstruction, and normal ducts indicate intrahepatic cholestasis requiring further evaluation, as discussed in the text. Predominant increases in aminotransferases suggest hepatocellular injury; values more than 10× upper reference limit *(URL)* usually indicate acute hepatitis, and lower values are typical of chronic hepatitis. If aspartate aminotransferase *(AST)* is higher than alanine aminotransferase *(ALT)*, common causes include early hepatic injury, nonhepatic injury (such as muscle injury), and with mildly increased values, cirrhosis.

Patients are occasionally seen with isolated elevations in ALP or aminotransferase enzyme activities. In practice, an isolated increase in ALP activity is difficult to interpret. In children, benign transient hyperphosphatasemia should always be considered. In adults, it is necessary to first confirm that the ALP is of hepatobiliary origin. This can be done by isoenzyme fractionation (see Chapter 29 on Serum Enzymes) or GGT, which tends to parallel the activity of ALP in cholestasis. The most important aspect of the workup is to rule out space-occupying lesions by visualizing the liver with computed tomography, and biliary tract disease by visualizing the biliary tree with ultrasound or magnetic resonance cholangiography.

Elevated plasma activities of AST and ALT are common in many disorders. To determine whether this elevation is liver related, administration of all drugs and alcohol intake (especially if AST is higher than ALT) should be discontinued. If the elevation persists, ultrasound (looking for a nonalcoholic fatty liver) and hepatitis B and C serology should be performed. More than 50% of isolated enzyme elevations of liver origin will be caused by these disorders. A liver biopsy is often needed to allow a more specific diagnosis. No reliable test other than liver biopsy can be used to detect fibrosis. The investigation of the patient with isolated elevations of liver enzymes in the absence of overt liver disease represents the investigation and differential diagnosis of all chronic liver disease. The common causes are described elsewhere in this chapter, but include alcohol, drugs, fatty liver disease, and viral, metabolic, and immune causes of liver disease; the investigation involves taking a thorough history, physical examination, and imaging.

Evidence is accumulating that GGT, as a marker of oxidative stress, is associated with increased cardiovascular and all-cause mortality.[561,562] It has shown prognostic value in assessing adverse outcomes after acute coronary syndrome and/or acute myocardial infarction and chronic cardiac disorders. Increasing GGT over time is associated with type 2 diabetes and the metabolic syndrome. These associations are weaker than that of cholesterol and smoking, and current evidence is limited that measuring GGT improves cardiovascular disease risk prediction beyond conventional risk factors.[561,562]

Albumin

Serum albumin measurements are useful in assessing the chronicity and severity of liver disease. For example, the plasma albumin concentration is decreased in advanced chronic liver disease. However, its usefulness for this purpose is somewhat limited because the plasma albumin concentration may also be decreased in severe acute liver disease and is lowered by many other disorders, and nonspecifically in acute illness. Serial measurements of plasma albumin can be used in chronic liver disease to assess deterioration in the patient's condition.

Prothrombin Time

PT measurements can be used to differentiate between cholestasis and severe hepatocellular disease. In practice, PT should be measured again after vitamin K injection, because cholestasis may cause a decrease in PT as the result of malabsorption of vitamin K. The patient has cholestasis if the PT corrects after vitamin K replacement (10 mg subcutaneously or intramuscularly, followed by PT measurement 24 hours later). Over time, if the PT does not return to normal, the patient has severe hepatocellular disease.

Bilirubin

Serial measurement of serum bilirubin concentration is helpful in assessing the severity of liver damage in several types of liver disease (eg, alcoholic hepatitis, cirrhosis). In acute hepatitis, bilirubin peaks later than enzyme activities, and bilirubin remains elevated for longer than urine bilirubin because of the presence of biliprotein (δ-bilirubin). Increases in bilirubin in most liver diseases are primarily due to an increase in conjugated bilirubin, which is usually detected as direct reacting bilirubin. An increase in unconjugated bilirubin usually is not due to liver disease, although severe acute hepatitis and cirrhosis are often associated with elevations primarily of unconjugated bilirubin, and autoantibody negative hemolytic anemia is a feature of Wilson disease.

Patients are frequently seen with isolated elevations in bilirubin concentration and normal levels of liver-associated enzymes. Increased unconjugated (indirect reacting) bilirubin in such situations is usually due to increased production of bilirubin (hemolysis, rhabdomyolysis, large hematomas), which is prehepatic or due to impaired conjugation (inherited decrease in activity of conjugation in Gilbert syndrome or Crigler-Najjar syndrome, drug-induced inhibition of enzyme activity by atazanavir, immaturity of liver in physiologic jaundice of the newborn). Gilbert syndrome is the most common cause of isolated unconjugated hyperbilirubinemia, and concentrations of bilirubin characteristically increase with fasting or intercurrent illness. Increases in conjugated (direct reacting) bilirubin are common in seriously ill individuals (bilirubinostasis of sepsis) and are less common with inherited defects in excretion of conjugated bilirubin (Dubin-Johnson syndrome, Rotor syndrome). An algorithm for differentiating the familial causes of hyperbilirubinemia is presented in Fig. 61.14. For more information, refer to the Bilirubin section of Chapter 38.

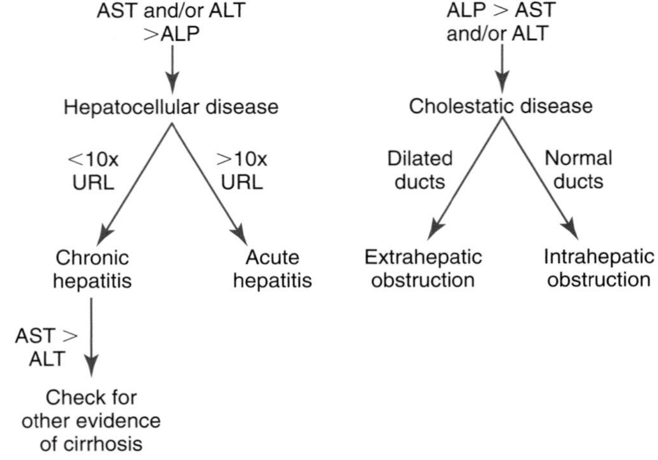

FIGURE 61.14 Algorithm for differentiating familial causes of hyperbilirubinemia.

POINTS TO REMEMBER

Liver Function Test Abnormalities

- Patterns of liver test abnormalities denote the predominant type of liver injury.
- Predominant elevation of aminotransferases (ALT and AST) suggests parenchymal liver injury or hepatitis.
- Predominant elevation of biliary enzymes (ALP and GGT) suggest bile duct injury, cholestasis, or cholangitis.
- Elevation of bilirubin suggests cholestasis. Obstruction of the biliary tree should be excluded as a cause of hyperbilirubinemia.
- Hepatic synthetic function is assessed by measuring albumin and clotting (PT or INR).

Liver Fibrosis Assessment

Chronic liver disease is characterized by progressive hepatic fibrosis, which over time culminates in the development of cirrhosis and its complications of portal hypertension, HCC, and liver failure.[563] The reference standard for staging liver disease is the histological staging of a liver biopsy specimen. Liver biopsy is invasive and resource-intensive even under optimal conditions, and it is far from a perfect reference standard. Even in experienced centers, biopsy is associated with complications such as pain (20%), serious morbidity (0.6%) (including bleeding that requires intervention), and even death (0.01%).[564] Aside from the hazards associated with the procedure itself, sampling variability may under or over stage fibrosis in as many of 20% of liver biopsies.[564] Moreover, the accuracy and reliability of liver biopsy is compromised by sampling error[565] as well as inter- and intra-observer variability.[566] For a confident histopathologic fibrosis stage to be assigned to a biopsy, the liver biopsy specimen must be of adequate size (eg, 15 mm or five portal tracts). Nevertheless, at this size, a liver biopsy specimen represents only 1/50,000th of the liver, and it is well documented that liver histologic changes can vary within a particular liver segment or lobe. Accordingly, it has been argued that the maximum diagnostic accuracy of liver biopsy under optimal circumstances could be no more than 90%.[567] Because of the associated morbidity, the use of liver biopsy to perform longitudinal monitoring of liver disease raises ethical considerations and has contributed to the quest for noninvasive tests that can replace biopsy. The high reproducibility and low coefficients of variation associated with automated blood and biochemical tests have resulted in considerable interest in the use of blood tests to assess fibrosis. However, it should be recognized that liver histology generates more information than just assessment of liver fibrosis; therefore, the place and importance of liver biopsy should not be underestimated. It should be recognized that even if it were possible to develop perfect blood tests, they would not replace histology.

Biomarkers of Fibrosis

Due to the limitations of liver biopsy, several noninvasive methods have been developed to detect progressive liver fibrosis and stage liver disease. Over the past two decades, numerous serum markers or biomarkers have been identified and described. In contrast to a liver biopsy, biomarkers are less invasive, with minimal associated procedural morbidity. Serum biomarkers of fibrosis can be categorized into direct serum markers (measuring parameters directly related to both the fibrolytic and fibrogenic processes involved in liver matrix turnover) and indirect serum markers (combinations of serum parameters that are related to liver function, including AST and ALT).[563]

Candidate Biomarker Derivation. Typically in biomarker derivation studies, a "training set" of patients with defined severity of chronic liver disease is used, and putative candidate biomarkers are measured. The diagnostic performance of the biomarkers is then determined by measuring their ability to detect the stage of liver fibrosis determined by liver biopsy. Fibrosis stages are usually dichotomized into diagnostic targets, such as those with and without mild (eg, meta-analysis of histological data in viral hepatitis [METAVIR] F0-1), moderate (eg, METAVIR F2-4), advanced (eg, METAVIR F3-4) liver fibrosis, and cirrhosis (eg, METAVIR F4). Thereafter, logistic regression modeling is used to derive a predictive algorithm that includes an individual biomarker or a combination of biomarkers. The diagnostic accuracy of a biomarker algorithm to correctly identify a particular stage of fibrosis can be examined by a receiver-operator characteristic curve, which plots sensitivity against 1-specificity for all values of the biomarker as a continuous variable. The area under the receiver-operator characteristic curve (AUC) ranges between 0 (a test with 0% sensitivity and 0% specificity) and 1 (a test with 100% sensitivity and 100% specificity). Typically, good diagnostic test performance is defined as an AUC of more than 0.8 by convention. However, it should be noted that if sampling error and inter- and intra-observer variability limit the sensitivity and specificity of the liver biopsy itself to 90%, then a truly perfect biomarker of fibrosis could obtain a maximum AUC of no more than 0.9.[568] Thereafter, biomarker algorithms derived from a training set are validated in an independent cohort of patients ("validation set"), and their AUCs calculated. For more information on how new biomarkers are developed and evaluated, refer to Chapter 2 on Statistical Methodologies in Laboratory Medicine and Chapter 9 on Evidence-Based Laboratory Medicine.

Direct Biomarkers. Direct biomarkers exhibit biological plausibility because they represent alterations of ECM composition that occur during hepatic fibrosis. The most widely studied direct biomarker is hyaluronic acid (HA), a glycosaminoglycan that is synthesized by HSCs and degraded by liver sinusoidal cells.[569] Other direct biomarkers include terminal peptide of procollagen III,[440] TIMP-1,[570] type IV collagen,[571] and TGF-β.[572] As derived by logistic regression, panels of direct biomarkers have been also described. Combinations of direct biomarkers can result in superior diagnostic performance for the detection of fibrosis compared with their constituent components. The ELF[573] test is a combination of HA, TIMP-1, and procollagen III that has been validated for the detection of fibrosis in a variety of liver diseases, including viral hepatitis B[574] and C,[575] NAFLD in children[576] and adults,[339] and PBC[505] and PSC.[520] FIBROSpect (Prometheus, Mayo Medical Laboratories, Rochester, Minnesota) is a combination of the direct biomarkers HA, TIMP-1, and α_2-macroglobulin.[577]

Indirect Biomarkers. By contrast, indirect biomarkers reflect parameters that are altered because of changes in hepatic function that arise in the context of a particular stage of liver fibrosis. Indirect biomarkers include biochemical or hematological variables that are synthesized or regulated by the liver (for example, clotting factors, cholesterol, and bilirubin), or indicate inflammation (for example, aminotransferases). Hitherto, the AST-to-platelet ratio has been one of the most studied indirect biomarkers of liver fibrosis.[578] The AST-to-platelet ratio is calculated by dividing AST by the upper limit of normal of AST (for the sex of the patient) and the platelet count, and multiplying by 100. Another indirect biomarker is Fib-4, which is a combination of AST, ALT, age, and platelet count.[579] The Forns index is an indirect biomarker panel that consists of age, GGT, cholesterol and platelet count.[580]

Hybrid Biomarkers. Indirect biomarkers can also be combined with direct biomarkers to form combination or hybrid biomarkers. Fibrometer is a hybrid biomarker that uses age, platelets, prothrombin index, AST, α_2-macroglobulin, HA, and urea.[581] Hepascore is a combination of bilirubin, GGT, HA, α_2-macroglobulin, age, and sex.[582] Fibrotest is a combination of GGT, bilirubin, haptoglobin, α_2-macroglobulin, apolipoprotein A1, age, and sex.[583]

Imaging Modalities. Conventional imaging techniques including ultrasonography, computed tomography, and magnetic resonance imaging can detect liver cirrhosis by identifying and detecting characteristic morphologic changes that occur in the cirrhotic state, including liver surface nodularity and the presence of portal hypertension. These conventional imaging findings have an intermediate specificity but a low sensitivity for a diagnosis of compensated cirrhosis. Moreover, conventional imaging modalities perform poorly for the detection of lesser degrees of fibrosis. These failings of conventional imaging modalities to quantify liver fibrosis have driven the development of novel imaging technologies. Nevertheless, in contrast to serum markers, imaging modalities for fibrosis are time consuming and are more suited for use in a secondary care setting.

The most widely studied imaging modality for the detection of liver fibrosis is Transient Elastography (Fibroscan, Echosens, France). In this modality, a specialized transducer emits painless mild amplitude, low-frequency vibrations into the liver, which propagates a shear wave. Assessment of the velocity of this shear wave allows interpretation of liver stiffness, and by inference, the degree of liver fibrosis. The results are available instantaneously, and the volume of liver assessed equates to a 1- by 4-cm cylinder, far exceeding the tissue volume reviewed by liver biopsy. Although its usefulness in obese patients has increased with the advent of new probes (XL probe), a failure rate of 1% with the XL probe and 15% with the standard M probe is still associated with the procedure.[584]

An alternative form of ultrasound elastography is the acoustic radiation force impulse (ARFI) imaging.[585] ARFI technology can be integrated into standard ultrasound units; it interrogates the mechanical properties of the liver tissue by evaluating the attenuation of propagated acoustic waves. In addition, because it is used in standard ultrasound apparatus, ARFI can localize areas of abnormality and perform a simultaneous abdominal and liver ultrasound.

Advances in magnetic resonance imaging technology have precipitated interest in magnetic resonance elastography.[586] Magnetic resonance elastography provides a uniform assessment of the overall liver, but is expensive, time-consuming, and limited in those with metallic implants and those who experience claustrophobia.

Prognosis and Monitoring. Noninvasive tests have been shown to be better than liver biopsy at determining prognosis in chronic liver diseases,[587] and therefore, may be a useful adjunct to liver biopsy when assessing a patient. A further advantage of noninvasive testing compared with liver biopsy is the readiness with which blood tests or imaging can be repeated to track changes in disease severity over time and in response to interventions. This use is proving particularly valuable in determining the impact of treatments for specific chronic liver diseases such as viral hepatitis and in monitoring responses to new antifibrotic therapies in clinical trials as part of drug discovery. For these reasons, noninvasive tests of liver fibrosis are gaining increasing acceptance as valuable additions to the repertoire of tests in the assessment and monitoring of patients with chronic liver disease.

LIVER TRANSPLANTATION

Clinical biochemistry plays an important role in the management of patients before and after transplantation. As described previously in this chapter, algorithms incorporating biochemical and other clinical parameters have been developed for the assessment of the need for transplantation in patients with acute and chronic liver disease. These include the formerly described Child-Pugh-Turcotte, MELD, and United Kingdom Endstage Liver Disease Score classifications. Posttransplantation, the main focus of management is on detecting graft failure, organ rejection, and monitoring the efficacy of immunosuppression. Laboratories are closely involved in monitoring the levels of liver enzymes, tests of hepatic synthetic function, therapeutic drug monitoring, and monitoring for viruses, including recurrence of HBV or HCV and CMV, which may complicate the course of recovery in immune-suppressed patients.

A detailed description of the interpretation of the results of these tests in the context of liver transplantation is beyond the scope of this text. The goal of the transplantation physician is to be alert for evidence of cellular rejection as indicated by elevations of liver enzymes while monitoring the concentrations of immunosuppressive drugs and potential evidence of their toxicity, which is primarily indicated by renal impairment or leukopenia. Unfortunately, the current assays for cellular rejection are not sufficiently specific, and elevations in liver enzymes may be the result of many other causes in patients who receive transplants. Furthermore, the assays of the major immunosuppressive agents are inaccurate and do not permit precise prediction of therapeutic doses. Thus, the monitoring and treatment of patients after transplantation remain the domain of expert and experienced clinicians working in close partnership with clinical chemists and other members of the multidisciplinary transplantation team.

SELECTED REFERENCES

For a full list of references for this chapter, please refer to ExpertConsult.com.

15. Arroyo V, Fernandez J, Ginès P. Pathogenesis and treatment of hepatorenal syndrome. *Semin Liver Dis* 2008;**28**:81–95.
30. Friedman SL. Evolving challenges in hepatic fibrosis. *Nat Rev Gastroenterol Hepatol* 2010;**7**:425–36.
47. Friedman S, Bansa LM. Reversal of hepatic fibrosis—fact or fantasy? *Hepatology* 2006;**43**:S82–8.

83. Dufour D, Lott J, Nolte F, et al. Diagnosis and monitoring of hepatic injury. I. Performance characteristics of laboratory tests. *Clin Chem* 2000;**46**:2027–49.
112. McMahon B. The natural history of chronic hepatitis B virus infection. *Hepatology* 2009;**49**:S45–55.
139. Choo QL, Kuo G, Weiner A, et al. Isolation of a cDNA clone derived from a blood-borne non-A, non-B viral hepatitis genome. *Science* 1989;**244**:359–62.
151. Lam BP, Jeffers T, Younoszai Z, et al. The changing landscape of hepatitis C virus therapy: focus on interferon-free treatment. *Therap Adv Gastroenterol* 2015;**8**:298–312.
214. *EASL. Clinical Practice Guidelines. Management of chronic hepatitis B.* 2012; <http://www.easl.eu/research/our-contributions/clinical-practice-guidelines/detail/management-of-chronic-hepatitis-b-virus-infection>.
228. Lee W. Acetaminophen-related acute liver failure in the United States. *Hepatol Res* 2008;**38**:S3–8.
249. Lucey M, Marthurin P, Morgan T. Alcoholic hepatitis. *N Engl J Med* 2009;**360**:2758–69.
268. Gow P, Smallwood R, Angus P, et al. Diagnosis of Wilson's disease: an experience over three decades. *Gut* 2000;**46**:415–19.
286. Fontana R, Lok A. Noninvasive monitoring of patients with chronic hepatitis C. *Hepatology* 2002;**36**:S57–64.
325. Day CP. Non-alcoholic fatty liver disease: a massive problem. *Clin Med* 2011;**11**:176–8.
339. Guha IN, Parkes J, Roderick P, et al. Non-invasive markers of fibrosis in nonalcoholic fatty liver disease: validating the European Liver Fibrosis panel and exploring simple markers. *Hepatology* 2008;**47**:455–60.
350. Hennes E, Zeniya M, Czaja A, et al. Simplified criteria for the diagnosis of autoimmune hepatitis. *Hepatology* 2008;**48**:169–76.
359. Pietrangelo A. Hereditary hemochromatosis: pathogenesis, diagnosis and treatment. *Gastroenterology* 2010;**139**:393–408.
473. Kamath P, Wiesner R, Malinchoc M, et al. A model to predict survival in patients with end-stage liver disease. *Hepatology* 2001;**33**:464–70.
498. Lindor K, Gershwin M, Poupon R, et al. Primary biliary cirrhosis. *Hepatology* 2009;**50**:291–308.
521. Zimmerman H. Drug-induced liver disease. *Clin Liver Dis* 2000;**4**:73–96.
573. Rosenberg WM, Voelker M, Thiel R, et al. Serum markers detect the presence of liver fibrosis: a cohort study. *Gastroenterology* 2004;**127**:1704–13.

62

Gastric, Pancreatic, and Intestinal Function

Roy A. Sherwood, Natalie E. Walsham, and Ingvar Bjarnason

ABSTRACT

Background
The stomach, intestinal tract, and pancreas are closely related, both anatomically and functionally, and clinical manifestations, such as diarrhea or malabsorption, may be associated with disease or disorders of any of these organs. It is therefore appropriate to discuss them together. Advances in imaging techniques and improvements in endoscopic procedures has led to many traditional laboratory tests of gastrointestinal (GI) and pancreatic function becoming obsolete. However, in recent years, there has been a resurgence in the role of the laboratory in the investigation of the GI tract, particularly with the development of noninvasive biomarkers of GI tract inflammation and in the detection of pancreatic insufficiency.

Content
In this chapter, the anatomy and physiology of the GI tract and the normal processes of digestion and absorption are reviewed. Disorders of the stomach, pancreas, and intestine in which the laboratory plays a role in diagnosis and monitoring are discussed. The chapter concludes with an overview of GI regulatory hormones and neuroendocrine tumors in which GI symptoms are prominent and sections on strategies for the investigation of malabsorption and diarrhea.

INTRODUCTION TO THE ANATOMY AND PHYSIOLOGY OF THE GASTROINTESTINAL TRACT

The major organs of the gastrointestinal (GI) tract include the stomach, small and large intestines, pancreas, and gallbladder, all of which are involved in the digestive processes that commence with the ingestion of food and water and culminate with the excretion of waste products as feces.

Anatomy

The GI tract is a hollow tube, approximately 8 m in length, beginning with the mouth and ending with the anus. The esophagus, which is approximately 25 cm in length, is a muscular tube connecting the pharynx to the stomach. The laboratory has little role in the investigation of disorders of the esophagus, so this chapter will focus on the stomach, intestines, and pancreas.

Stomach

The stomach consists of three major zones: the cardiac zone, the body, and the pyloric zone (Fig. 62.1). The upper cardiac zone includes the fundus and contains mucus and pepsinogen II–secreting surface epithelial cells and endocrine secreting cells. The body of the stomach contains cells or cell groups of many different types: surface epithelial cells that secrete mucus; parietal cells that secrete hydrochloric acid and intrinsic factor; chief cells that secrete groups I and II pepsinogens; enterochromaffin cells that secrete serotonin, and other endocrine cells. The pyloric zone is subdivided into the antrum (approximately the distal third of the stomach), the pyloric canal, and the sphincter. The cells of the pyloric zone secrete mucus, group II pepsinogens, serotonin, and gastrin, but not hydrochloric acid. In the stomach, food is converted into a semifluid, homogeneous material (chyme) that passes through the pyloric sphincter into the small intestine. The digestion of proteins begins with the action of pepsin produced in the stomach.

Small Intestine

The small intestine consists of three parts: the duodenum, jejunum, and ileum. In the adult, the small intestine is approximately 6 m in length and its cross-section decreases as it proceeds distally. The duodenum is approximately 25 cm long and is the shortest part of the small intestine. The jejunum and ileum make up the remainder of the small intestine, with the ileum constituting the distal 3.5 m.

The wall of the small intestine consists of four layers: mucous, submucous, muscular, and serous. The internal surface of the upper part of the small intestine contains valve-like circular folds (valvulae conniventes or plicae circulares) that project 3 to 10 mm into the lumen. Covering the entire mucous surface are small (1 mm) finger-like projections (villi) that increase the absorptive surface area. The luminal surface of each epithelial cell consists of some 1700 microvilli projecting approximately 1 μm from the cell. The folds, villi, and microvilli increase the absorptive surface area 600-fold to approximately 250 m^2, which is comparable to the area of a doubles lawn tennis court.

Large Intestine

The large intestine is approximately 1.5 m in length, extending from the ileum to the anus and includes the cecum, appendix, colon, rectum, and anal canal. The cecum is a blind pouch

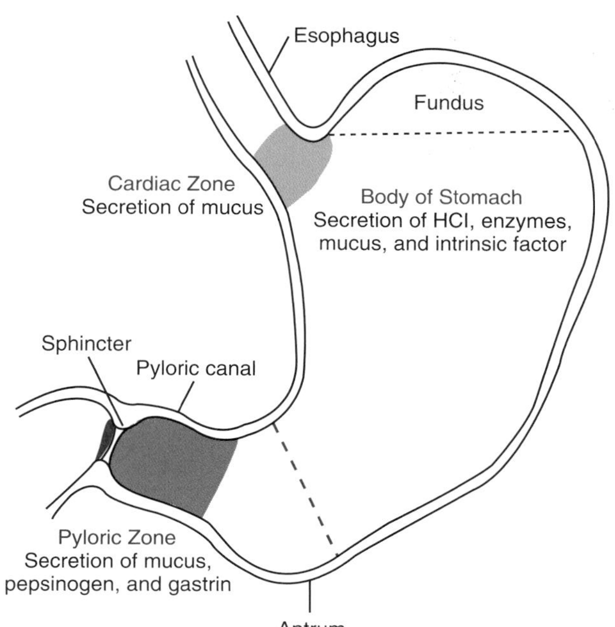

FIGURE 62.1 Schematic drawing of the stomach with major zones. *GI,* Gastrointestinal; *IBD,* inflammatory bowel disease; *IBS,* inflammatory bowel syndrome; *NSAID,* nonsteroidal antiinflammatory drug.

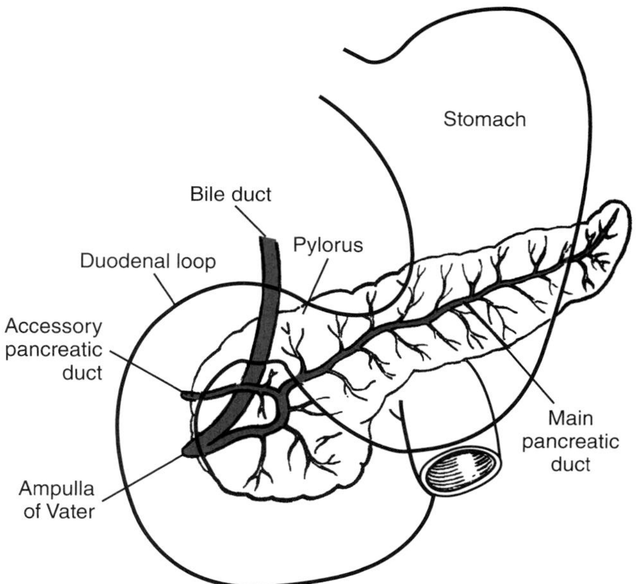

FIGURE 62.2 Cross-section through the pancreas.

that begins the large intestine; it is connected to the terminal ileum via the ileocecal sphincter (or valve). The appendix is connected to the blind end of the cecum. The colon is approximately 1 m long and is divided into the ascending, transverse, descending, and sigmoid sections. The sigmoid colon connects to the rectum, which is approximately 15 cm long and connects to the anal canal.

Pancreas

The pancreas is 12 to 15 cm long and lies across the posterior wall of the abdominal cavity. The head is located in the duodenal curve, with the body and tail extending to the left to the spleen (Fig. 62.2). The pancreas secretes a juice containing digestive enzymes and bicarbonate that enters the duodenum through the ampulla of Vater and the sphincter of Oddi to mix with the bolus of food coming from the stomach.

PHASES OF DIGESTION

The processes of digestion can be divided into neurogenic, gastric, and intestinal phases.

Neurogenic Phase

The neurogenic, or cephalic, phase is initiated by the intake of food into the mouth; the sight, smell, and taste of food stimulates the cerebral cortex and subsequently the vagal nuclei.

Gastric Phase

When food enters the stomach the resulting distention initiates the gastric phase of digestion mediated by local and vagal reflexes. Hydrochloric acid release is caused by direct vagal stimulation of the parietal cells, local distention of the antrum, and vagal stimulation of antral cells to secrete gastrin, which in turn stimulates the release of hydrochloric acid from parietal cells, and release of gastrin stimulated by the near neutralization (pH 5.0 to 7.0) of the stomach contents entering the pyloric zone. Gastrin also stimulates antral motility, secretion of pepsinogens and of pancreatic fluid rich in enzymes, and release of hormones such as secretin, insulin, acetylcholine, somatostatin, and pancreatic polypeptide (for details refer to section on GI regulatory peptides). As a result of the acid environment pepsinogen is rapidly converted to the active proteolytic enzyme pepsin. Food is mixed by contractions of the stomach and is partially degraded into chyme by the chemical secretions of the stomach. The pylorus plays a role in emptying chyme into the duodenum by virtue of its strong musculature.

Intestinal Phase

The intestinal phase of digestion begins when the weakly acidic digestive products of proteins enter the duodenum. Many hormones and other regulatory peptides are released by both neural and local stimulation and act within the GI tract to regulate digestion and absorption. Digestion, absorption, and storage functions are stimulated or inhibited by different hormones, creating a control system that regulates the action of intestinal hormones and provides for secretion of bile acids, bicarbonate, and numerous enzymes involved in the digestion of food.

During the intestinal phase, carbohydrates, proteins, and fats are broken down and absorbed. Most nutrients, including vitamins and minerals, have been absorbed by the time the food passes from the jejunum and ileum into the large intestine. In the large intestine, water is actively absorbed, electrolyte balance is regulated, and bacterial actions take place. These processes result in the formation of feces.

Processes of Digestion and Absorption

The total quantity of fluid absorbed each day by the gut is estimated to be approximately 9 L, which is composed of 2 L oral intake, 1.5 L saliva, 2.5 L gastric juice, 0.5 L bile, 1.5 L

TABLE 62.1 Brush Border Oligosaccharidases

Enzyme	Principal Substrate	Products
Lactase (EC 3.2.1.23)	Lactose	Glucose + galactose
Sucrase (EC 3.2.1.48)	Maltose/sucrose	Glucose or fructose + glucose
Isomaltase (EC 3.2.1.10)	1,6-α-linkages in Isomaltose and α-dextrins	Glucose
	Maltose	Glucose
Trehalase (EC 3.2.1.28)	Trehalose	Glucose
Glucoamylase complex (EC 3.2.1.20)		
Glucoamylase-(maltase)-1 and glucoamylase-(maltase)-2 (have similar substrate specificities)	1,4-α-linkages at nonreducing ends of amylose, amylopectin, glycogen and straight-chain 1,4-α-glucopyranosyl oligomers, including maltose	Glucose

From Semenza G, Auricchio S, Mantei N. Small-intestinal disaccharidases. In: Scriver CR, Beaudet AL, Sly WS, Valle D, editors. *The Metabolic and Molecular Bases of Inherited Disease*. 8th ed. New York: McGraw-Hill; 2001:1623–1650.

pancreatic juice, and 1 L intestinal secretions. More than 90% of this fluid is absorbed in the small intestine. The maximal absorptive capacity for fluid is probably at least 20 L. Several hundred grams of carbohydrates, 100 g of fat, and 50 to 100 g of amino acids are absorbed daily in the small gut, but the maximal absorptive capacity is believed to be at least 10 times higher. This considerable reserve capacity may explain the lack of symptoms from mild disease processes, at least in the early stages. The efficiency of absorption is due to the unique features of the absorptive surface of the bowel and the relationship of the epithelial cells to the underlying rich vascular plexus and the lymphatic vessels.

Digestion of food starts in the mouth through the action of salivary amylase and lingual lipase, but principally takes place both within the lumen of the small intestine and at the mucosal (brush border) surface. Defects of digestion may occur at one or more stages of this process. The terms *maldigestion* and *malabsorption* refer to different functional abnormalities. *Maldigestion* is a dysfunction of the digestive process that may occur at various sites in the GI tract. For example, a reduction in the acidity in the stomach will reduce peptic digestion of protein, whereas hyperacidity of the duodenum (eg, due to overproduction of gastrin by tumor in the Zollinger-Ellison syndrome) can inactivate pancreatic enzymes; loss of brush border enzymes in the small intestine as a result of a variety of conditions can prevent oligosaccharides and disaccharides from being further hydrolyzed; pancreatic insufficiency will reduce intraluminal enzyme activity in the small gut, causing maldigestion of fats and proteins. Inherited disorders of the exocrine pancreas can cause maldigestion by causing pancreatic insufficiency secondary to chronic pancreatic inflammation. In contrast, malabsorption is strictly a dysfunction of the absorptive process in the small gut resulting from reduction in the size of the absorptive surface caused by responses to factors including gluten, inflammation, infection, surgical resection, and infiltration. Various transport defects also lead to malabsorption of specific substances (eg, glucose-galactose malabsorption, zinc deficiency in the congenital disorder acrodermatitis enteropathica). In clinical practice, however, the term *malabsorption* is often used to encompass all aspects of impaired digestion and absorption.

In the following three sections, the digestion and absorption of carbohydrates, fats, and proteins will be discussed separately. It must be remembered, however, that a complex interplay takes place among nutrients, regulatory peptides, enzymes, gallbladder and pancreatic function, and bowel motility, leading to an integrated absorptive process that commences with the ingestion of food and culminates in the excretion of feces.

Digestion and Absorption of Carbohydrates

After the action of salivary and pancreatic α-amylases on dietary starch and glycogen, the carbohydrate content of the small intestine consists of newly formed maltose; ingested monosaccharides; dietary disaccharides such as lactose, sucrose, maltose, and trehalose; oligosaccharides such as dextrins and maltotriose, and indigestible oligosaccharides and polysaccharides such as cellulose, agar, and other dietary fibers.

The brush border enzymes with disaccharidase and oligosaccharidase activity are listed in Table 62.1. The sucrase-isomaltase complex comprises most (80%) of the sucrase, isomaltase, and maltase activity of the small intestine. It hydrolyzes sucrose to its constituent monosaccharides, cleaves glucose from α-limit dextrins with 1,6 bonds, and hydrolyzes maltose. The activity of the complex is fourfold to fivefold greater in the jejunum than in the ileum. Changes in diet have a marked effect on the expression of the complex; starvation leads to a rapid decline in activity that is rapidly restored on refeeding. Secretion of all small intestinal saccharidases may decrease with infection or inflammation of the small bowel to the extent that carbohydrate malabsorption occurs, leading to diarrhea, flatulence, and weight loss. Paradoxically, diabetes mellitus causes a striking increase in sucrase-isomaltase activity; an increase is also observed in monosaccharide and amino acid transport.

The lactase–phlorizin hydrolase complex is the only brush border enzyme able to hydrolyze lactose and is therefore essential for the survival of mammals early in life. This complex also has glycosylceraminidase, β-glycosidase, and phlorizin hydrolase activities. Infectious and inflammatory diseases greatly reduce lactase–phlorizin hydrolase activity, leading to symptomatic intolerance to milk (bloating, abdominal pain, diarrhea, and flatulence). Recovery of enzyme activity after intestinal disease may be slow. The activity of the complex is resistant to starvation. The developmental regulation of lactase is discussed later in the section on disaccharidase deficiencies. Also present in the brush border is the α-glucosidase maltase-glucoamylase, which removes individual glucose molecules from the nonreducing end of α(1,4) oligosaccharides and disaccharides. This enzyme accounts for approximately 20% of the total maltase activity of the small intestine. Trehalase is also found in the brush border of the small intestine and hydrolyzes trehalose, an α(1,1) disaccharide of glucose found in yeast and mushrooms. The developmental pattern of trehalase appears to follow that of sucrase-isomaltase.

In addition to their actions on disaccharides, the brush border enzymes further hydrolyze the products of amylase action, including maltose, maltotriose, and α-limit dextrins. The brush border enzymes appear to act in an integrated manner in that a flow of substrate occurs from glucoamylase and isomaltase to sucrose, producing the monosaccharides glucose, galactose, and fructose. These monosaccharides are transported into enterocytes by facilitative transport systems such as the sodium-dependent glucose (and galactose) transporter (SGLT1) and the GLUT5 transporter, which transports fructose across the apical membrane of the enterocyte. Subsequently absorbed glucose and fructose are transported across the basolateral membrane, out of the enterocyte, and into the portal system by the GLUT2 transporter.

It is increasingly being recognized that the limiting factor in carbohydrate digestion and absorption may be diffusion from the intestinal lumen to the membrane surface where the enzymes are localized.[1] Normally, little disaccharidase activity is seen in the luminal contents. For most oligosaccharides (with the exception of lactose), hydrolysis is rapid and transport is the rate-limiting step in reducing the concentration of monosaccharides and the osmotic load in the gut. When the transport system is operating at its maximum rate but monosaccharide concentration is still high, inhibition of hydrolases by their monosaccharide products (ie, product inhibition) slows hydrolytic activity, keeping monosaccharide concentrations relatively constant, thereby controlling osmotic load and water concentration in the gut.[1] The importance of this control is evident from the consequences of intestinal disorders in which ingested disaccharide is not split and absorbed, leading to osmotic fluid retention within the lumen, increased fluid secretion into the gut, and increased intestinal motility. Enteric bacteria ferment the unabsorbed sugars producing hydrogen, carbon dioxide, and organic acids, causing abdominal discomfort such as bloating, abdominal distention, cramping, and looseness of bowel motions. Absorption of fermentation products may lead to metabolic acidosis. In the large bowel, the presence of carbon dioxide and organic acids decreases pH and keeps the osmolality high, so that water reabsorption is decreased. The result is an acidic, liquid stool. Normally, however, accumulation of monosaccharide products does not occur, because the transport system is sufficiently fast to remove them. Mucosal lactase activity is the lowest of all the disaccharidases; for lactose, the rate-limiting step in absorption is thought to be hydrolysis. Lactase activity is not increased by feeding large amounts of lactose, as is the case for maltase and sucrase with maltose and sucrose feeding, respectively. Lactase, maltase, and sucrase all show circadian rhythms in their activities; minimum and maximum rates of secretion may vary by a factor of two.[2]

Carbohydrate digestion is not always complete in the small intestine. It is likely that some starch and sucrose, as much as 10% of that ingested, normally pass undigested and unabsorbed into the colon. It has been estimated that colonic bacteria require 70 g of carbohydrate per day. Much of this is derived from endogenous sources, such as glycoproteins from GI secretions, with the remainder coming from unabsorbed dietary carbohydrate and dietary fiber. Up to 15% of the carbohydrate from white bread reaches the colon, and the effects of indigestible oligosaccharides on reaching the large bowel are well known. Bacterial action creates short-chain fatty acids that are rapidly absorbed by the colonic mucosa and are thought to provide fuel for the colonocytes. Starch and oligosaccharides are osmotically active and draw water into the gut and retain luminal fluidity. The colon, however, can absorb up to four times the normal colonic water load; for this reason, diarrhea is not always present in oligosaccharide malabsorption.

Digestion and Absorption of Lipids

The recommended daily fat intake in Europe and North America is 70 to 85 g. Less than 5 g/24 h is recoverable in feces, indicating the overall efficiency of the normal processes of fat digestion and absorption. Most dietary fat is in the form of long-chain triacylglycerols (triglycerides). Pancreatic lipase is quantitatively the most important hydrolytic enzyme, but the contribution of gastric lipase to overall hydrolysis should not be underestimated. Gastric lipase is secreted by the gastric mucosa and normally accounts for up to 17.5% of fatty acids released from triglycerides following a meal.[2] The enzyme has a wide pH optimum and is active in both the stomach and duodenum. This nonpancreatic lipase may have a significant role in lipid digestion when pancreatic function is impaired and in the neonatal period before pancreatic lipase activity is fully developed. A lingual lipase is also produced, but is thought to be of little significance in humans.

Fats are first emulsified in the stomach by its churning action and are stabilized by interaction with luminal lecithin and protein fragments. The lingual and gastric lipases do not require bile salts or cofactors for their action; they have a pH optimum of 3 to 6, and their action produces 1,2-diacylglycerols and fatty acids. These products further stabilize the surface of the triglyceride emulsion and in the duodenum promote the binding of pancreatic colipase. In addition, the liberated fatty acids stimulate release of cholecystokinin (CCK) from the duodenal mucosa.

Pancreatic lipase, in the presence of bile salts and colipase, acts at the oil-water interface of the triglyceride emulsion to produce fatty acids and 2-monoacylglycerols. Colipase is secreted by the pancreas as an inactive proenzyme, which is then converted to the active form by trypsin. Other significant enzymes involved in the breakdown of fats are cholesterol ester hydrolase, phospholipase A2, and a nonspecific bile salt-activated lipase.

Only a small proportion of ingested triacylglycerol is completely hydrolyzed to glycerol and fatty acids. These products form micelles with bile salts and lysophosphoglycerides; the micelles convey the nonpolar lipid molecules from the lumen to the epithelial cell surface and dissociate there to produce a high concentration of monoglycerols, lysophosphoglycerides, and fatty acids, which partition into the mucosal cell. Absorption involves both passive and active transport processes and is facilitated by a fatty acid–binding protein in the cytosol of the cell that has a high affinity for fatty acids.[3] Within the cell, triacylglycerols are resynthesized from the absorbed 2-monoacylglycerols and fatty acids. The triacylglycerols, together with phospholipids, cholesterol and

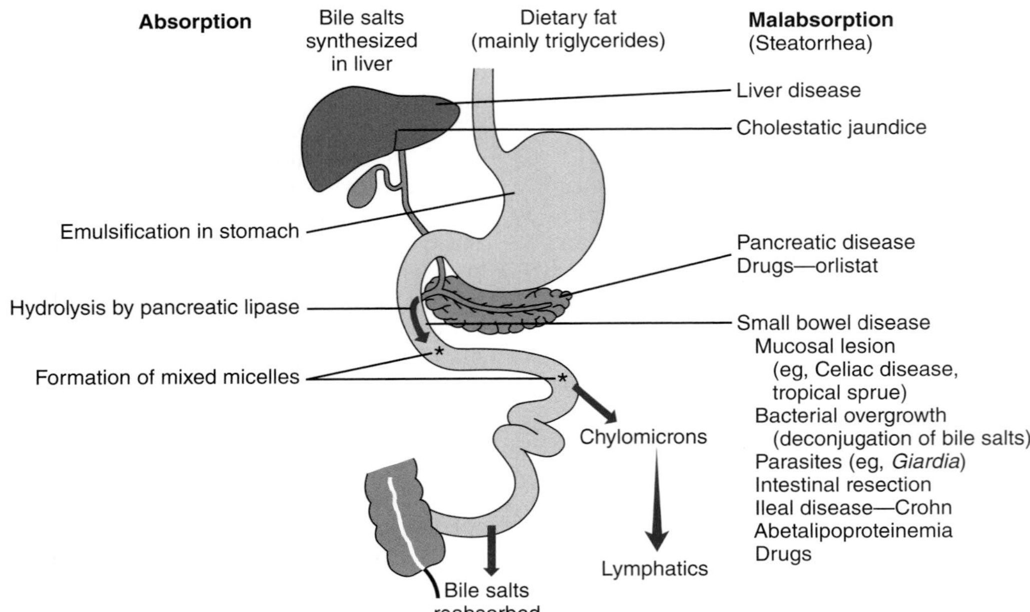

FIGURE 62.3 Summary of the processes involved in fat absorption and malabsorption. (From Clark ML, Silk DB. Gastrointestinal disease. In: Kumar P, Clark M, editors. *Clinical Medicine.* 6th ed. Edinburgh: Saunders; 2005:265–345.)

its ester, fat-soluble vitamins, and apolipoprotein B-48, are formed into chylomicrons that are then released by exocytosis into the lymphatic system of the small bowel. The absorption of long-chain fatty acids is facilitated by transmembrane fatty acid transport proteins.

From the lymphatic system, chylomicrons enter the bloodstream via the thoracic duct and are distributed to the liver, adipose tissue, and other organs. Medium- and short-chain fatty acids (chain length <12 carbon atoms) in mixed triglycerides are preferentially split by lipases and pass into the aqueous phase, from which they are rapidly absorbed. Medium-chain triglycerides can be absorbed without complete lipolysis and in the absence of bile. They do not require micellar solubilization and are transported from the intestinal epithelial cells predominantly via the hepatic portal vein. Fig. 62.3 summarizes the processes involved in fat absorption and conditions that compromise the efficiency of one or more stages in these process that can result in fat malabsorption.[2]

Digestion and Absorption of Proteins

The average daily intake of protein in developed countries is approximately 100 g compared with an estimated requirement for adults of 50 to 70 g. Another 50 to 60 g of protein enters the intestinal tract daily in GI secretions and from desquamated mucosal cells. Normal daily fecal loss of protein is about 10 g.

Protein digestion is initiated in the stomach by the action of pepsin in a highly acidic medium. The acidity also helps denature dietary proteins, unfolding the polypeptide chains for better access by the gastric, pancreatic, and intestinal proteolytic enzymes. The polypeptides and amino acids produced in the stomach by the action of pepsin are potent secretagogues for hormones that stimulate the pancreas and intestine. Stimulated pancreatic secretion contains proenzyme forms of the proteolytic enzymes trypsin, chymotrypsin, elastase, exopeptidases, and carboxypeptidases. Proteolytic enzymes may be endopeptidases (eg, pepsin, trypsin, chymotrypsin, elastase), which hydrolyze peptide bonds within the polypeptide chain, or exopeptidases, which hydrolyze peptide bonds of the terminal amino acids (eg, carboxypeptidase, aminopeptidase). Stimulation of the intestine by GI hormones liberates several proteolytic enzymes from the brush border. One of them, enterokinase, selectively cleaves a hexapeptide from the N-terminus of trypsinogen to form trypsin. Trypsin then activates more trypsin (autocatalysis) and also converts other pancreatic proenzymes into their active forms. The action of the pancreatic enzymes on partially digested proteins within the lumen produces peptides that are 2 to 6 amino acid residues in length, as well as single amino acids. The peptides are largely hydrolyzed to single amino acids by the aminopeptidases and dipeptidases of the brush border before absorption, although some dipeptides and tripeptides are absorbed and hydrolyzed to amino acids by cytosolic peptidases within the enterocytes. Multiple carrier systems with overlapping specificities for the 20 essential amino acids are involved in the transport of amino acids into cells. Absorption of amino acids by these transport systems is faster in the jejunum than the ileum. The amino acids pass across the enterocyte basolateral membrane by passive diffusion and by active transport systems, which are distinct from those at the brush border membrane. The underlying rich vascular plexus is drained by the portal circulation, and it is by this route that absorbed amino acids reach the liver and then the systemic circulation.

Individuals with achlorhydria or total gastrectomy have normal protein digestion and absorption because small intestinal function compensates for the lack of pepsin activity. Pancreatic and small intestinal diseases are the major causes of protein maldigestion and malabsorption. However, fecal loss of protein rarely becomes significant in pancreatic insufficiency until trypsin secretion falls to less than 10% of normal. Two rare disorders, trypsin deficiency and enterokinase deficiency, have far-reaching effects on the efficiency of protein digestion, as would be expected from their roles in the activation of proteolytic proenzymes.

Mucosal diseases may affect protein assimilation through a number of mechanisms. Reduction in the number of mucosal cells decreases peptidase activity in the intestine and the absorptive capacity for amino acids. Disease may increase the turnover of intestinal cells and their rate of desquamation. This cell loss, together with increased losses of plasma proteins from the damaged intestinal surface, can cause a negative nitrogen balance. Surgical resection of the intestine not only reduces the total absorptive surface area but also may remove a segment of the gut that is specialized for absorption of certain nutrients (eg, resection of the distal ileum removes the active transport system for vitamin B_{12}–intrinsic factor complex). Resection also may alter intestinal motility leading to stasis and bacterial overgrowth that can intensify a negative nitrogen balance. Also, rare hereditary defects in amino acid transporters (eg, Hartnup disease) may produce distinct syndromes.

STOMACH: DISEASES AND LABORATORY INVESTIGATIONS

Growth in endoscopic procedures, with direct visualization of the interior of the stomach, has largely removed the need for the laboratory to carry out investigation of gastric contents. Situations remain, however, in which the laboratory continues to play a role in diagnosing gastric diseases and in monitoring the effectiveness of treatment. This section describes peptic ulcer disease and tests for *Helicobacter pylori*.

Helicobacter pylori

In 1985, an association was made between the presence of a spiral-shaped bacterium, *H. pylori*, and peptic ulcer diseases.[4-7] *H. pylori* is now accepted to be the predominant cause of gastric and duodenal ulcers, the remainder being associated with the long-term use of nonsteroidal antiinflammatory drugs (NSAIDS) and, rarely, gastrinomas. Most estimates suggest that *H. pylori* is present in the mucus layer of the stomach in half of the world's population. In Europe 30% to 50% of adults and in the United States at least 20% of the adult population are infected with the bacterium. Chronic infection produces an inflammatory response (gastritis) and carries an increased risk for developing a peptic ulcer (3- to 10-fold) and/or adenocarcinoma (2- to 10-fold).[8] Up to 90% of gastric cancer patients are infected with *H. pylori* compared to 40% to 60% of age-matched controls.[9,10] In a European study comparing the prevalence of *H. pylori* versus gastric cancer rates in 13 countries, a significant correlation was found between the infection rate and gastric cancer incidence and mortality.[11] *H. pylori* may cause dyspepsia in the absence of an ulcer, and current recommendations suggest a low threshold for testing for *H. pylori* and some advocate treatment without testing.

The mode of transmission of *H. pylori* is unclear. In many cases the infection appears to originate in childhood, presumably by the fecal-oral route, because the prevalence is higher in developing countries and is inversely related to food hygiene. Almost all individuals infected with *H. pylori* develop chronic gastritis, but only 10% of cases manifest as peptic ulcers. *H. pylori* infection predominantly affects the gastric mucosa, with the antrum usually the most densely colonized area. At least 95% of patients with duodenal ulcers have *H. pylori* infection, and eradication of the organism results in healing of the ulcer and a reduction in relapse rates.[12] There is considerable variation in whether an individual infected with *H. pylori* will develop clinically significant disease. This variation is governed by a number of factors including the site of infection, virulence factors (eg, vacuolating cytotoxins [VAC], CagA protein), mucus secretion and extent of pepsinogen secretion.[13] Infection of the mid-body of the stomach is the commonest form, occurs in people with a strong immune system and involves a type of *H. pylori* with low expression of CagA and VAC. However, if the infection is in the antrum, the inflammation causes the G cells to become hyperactive with a resulting disproportionate secretion of gastrin in response to food and gastric distention and consequent increases in acid output.[13] Basal acid output has been shown to be higher in *H. pylori*–infected subjects, and this resolves after eradication of the organism.[14] Hypergastrinemia is believed to be only one of the mechanisms leading to increased acid output. Studies using the neuropeptide gastrin-releasing peptide (GRP) suggest that impairment of inhibiting control mechanisms regulating acid production may be responsible for the increase in acid output in *H. pylori* infection.[14]

H. pylori produces urease, and hydrolysis of this endogenously produced urea to bicarbonate and ammonia may create a more hospitable environment for the survival of the organism in the stomach. This ability of *H. pylori* to hydrolyze urea forms the basis of urea breath tests and direct urease tests on gastric biopsy samples.

Diagnostic Tests for *Helicobacter pylori*

In theory it would be possible to carry out endoscopy on all patients who have symptoms that could be associated with *H. pylori* infection, but in the real world this is not practical nor would it be acceptable to the patient population. Numerous invasive and noninvasive diagnostic tests for *H. pylori* have been described (Box 62.1) and many have been reviewed.[15]

At gastroduodenoscopy, biopsies can be taken from the gastric mucosa from which the organism can be visually detected or cultured. The antrum is the preferred site, but multiple biopsies from the anterior and posterior walls of

BOX 62.1 Diagnostic Tests for *Helicobacter pylori*

- Invasive tests: Using gastric mucosal biopsy samples
- Histology: Microscopy after Giemsa or silver staining
- Histology: Microscopy after immunohistochemical staining
- Direct urease test: Biopsy included in urea/indicator solution—visual end point
- Culture: Incubation in suitable media for 4 to 10 days
- Polymerase chain reaction: Amplification of specific DNA sequences
- Noninvasive tests: Using breath, blood, saliva, or feces
- Breath tests: Rise in $^{14}CO_2$ or $^{13}CO_2$ after ingestion of ^{14}C- or ^{13}C-labeled urea
- Serum, saliva, or feces tests: Detection of IgG antibody

the antrum and the body of the stomach are recommended to avoid false-negative results in cases in which colonization is patchy. False-negative results may also occur when biopsies are taken during treatment with proton pump inhibitors (PPIs) or within 2 weeks of stopping PPI therapy, because these drugs alter the intragastric distribution of *H. pylori* and suppress its activity.[16] PPIs also can lead to false-negative urea breath test results. If PPIs cannot be withheld for at least 2 weeks before a breath test, negative results should be interpreted with caution. Histamine (H_2)-receptor antagonists should be stopped at least 24 hours before a breath test. Antacids do not affect the test results. Commercially available kits can be used to identify *H. pylori* in gastric biopsy samples. These are based on a gel that incorporates urea and an indicator that changes color at an alkaline pH. The action of urease present in *H. pylori* cleaves the urea to bicarbonate and ammonia, raising the pH and inducing a color change in the indicator.

Tests for *H. pylori* are required for the diagnosis of infection and in some situations to ascertain whether eradication therapy has been successful. High sensitivity is required to ensure that positive findings are not missed; similarly, high specificity is essential to prevent inappropriate use of eradication therapy. The Maastricht III Consensus Guidelines[17] recommend a "test and treat" strategy in adults with appropriate dyspeptic symptoms who are younger than 45 years of age using a breath test or stool antigen test. The age limit may vary depending on local prevalence and the age distribution of gastric cancer (eg, in the United Kingdom, testing and treatment are now an option in any patients with uncomplicated dyspepsia, although for those aged 55 years and older with unexplained and persistent recent-onset dyspepsia alone, consideration should be given for endoscopy).[18] Successful eradication of *H. pylori* should be confirmed with the urea breath test or by a monoclonal antibody–based stool antigen test if urea breath tests are not available. Other national guidelines confirm the urea breath test as the preferred procedure, both for initial diagnosis and for confirmation of eradication.[18-20] Testing to confirm eradication should be done at least 4 weeks after completion of the course of treatment.

The urea breath test for *H. pylori* is currently the most widely used method for the noninvasive diagnosis of infection. Urea labeled with carbon-13 is given orally as a drink or a capsule. *H. pylori* rapidly hydrolyzes the urea to produce labeled bicarbonate that is absorbed into the bloodstream and broken down to be exhaled as $^{13}CO_2$. In the absence of urease the urea is absorbed intact and renally excreted. Breath samples are collected before and 45 to 60 minutes after drinking the labeled urea. The detection of labeled carbon, which is not radioactive, is usually carried out by mass spectrometry. The breath test has sensitivity and specificity for *H. pylori* in excess of 95% and can be used both for diagnosis and to assess the success of eradication therapy.

Serologic methods are available to detect *H. pylori*–specific antibodies (immunoglobulin G [IgG] or IgA), but have some drawbacks compared to the urea breath test. The systemic antibody response is variable, with equivocal results often occurring in subjects older than 50 years. The sensitivity (92%) and specificity (83%) are also lower than those for the breath test.[17] Serologic tests cannot be used to confirm eradication of the bacterium because of the persistence of the antibodies for variable periods after completion of treatment. Point-of-care devices exist to detect *H. pylori* antibodies, but current evidence is these perform poorly in terms of both sensitivity and specificity and cannot be recommended.[17] These tests may be useful in specific situations, such as when PPI therapy cannot be withheld because of ulcers that are bleeding.[17]

H. pylori is shed in feces, and several tests have been described that can detect the organism. Polyclonal or monoclonal antibodies to *H. pylori* can be configured into various immunoassay formats, although sensitivity and specificity are lower than for breath tests. Commercial kits are available that use polymerase chain reaction to amplify nuclear sequences specific for *H. pylori* in feces (or saliva) and have a sensitivity and specificity of 95% and 94%, respectively. In time, stool tests for *H. pylori* may replace the urea breath test, particularly in assessing whether eradication has been successful.

POINTS TO REMEMBER

Helicobacter pylori

- *H. pylori* is the predominant cause of gastric and duodenal ulcers.
- There is an increased risk for gastric cancer with *H. pylori* infection.
- The urea breath test is useful in the diagnosis of *H. pylori* infection.
- Tests based on serologic/molecular techniques are available to detect antibodies to *H. pylori* in blood or feces.

Gastric Acid Secretion and Gastrinomas

Before the discovery of the role of *H. pylori,* patients with gastric or duodenal ulcers were often tested for hyperacidity of the stomach, either in the basal state or after stimulation. Patients with duodenal ulcers are typically hypersecretors of acid, whereas those with peptic ulcers are more often normal or low secretors, but there was significant overlap between the two groups of patients. Collection of gastric juice and analysis of acid output was at one time extensively carried out in the investigation of possible gastrinomas. This invasive technique has now been replaced by the greater availability of plasma gastrin measurements, endoscopy, and imaging modalities, including computed tomography (CT), magnetic resonance imaging (MRI), positron emission tomography (PET), and octreotide scanning.

Gastrin

Three molecular forms of gastrin occur in blood and tissues: G-34, G-17, and G-14; they are linear polypeptides of 34, 17, and 14 amino acids, respectively.[21,22] In addition to these forms, G-71, G-52, and G-6 are present in small amounts. Gastrins originate from the cleavage of a single precursor, preprogastrin, a peptide consisting of 101 amino acids. The smallest peptide sequence of gastrin possessing biological activity is the carboxy-terminal tetrapeptide (G-4), but on a molar basis is only 10% to 20% as potent as G-17. A synthetic pentapeptide (pentagastrin) was used in the past to stimulate acid secretion for collection and analysis but is rarely used now.

Gastrin is produced and stored mainly by endocrine cells (G cells) of the antral mucosa and to a lesser extent by G cells of the proximal duodenum and Δ cells of the pancreatic islets. After secretion, gastrin is transported by the blood through the liver to the parietal cells of the fundus of the stomach, where it stimulates the secretion of gastric acid. Gastrin also stimulates secretion of gastric pepsinogens and intrinsic factor by the gastric mucosa, release of secretin from the small intestinal mucosa and secretion of pancreatic bicarbonate and enzymes and hepatic bile; it increases gastric and intestinal motility, mucosal growth, and blood flow to the stomach. It is secreted in response to antral distention from food and by the presence of amino acids, peptides, and polypeptides in the stomach from partially digested proteins. Other stimuli of gastrin include alcohol, caffeine, insulin-induced hypoglycemia, and calcium.

Maximal secretion of gastrin occurs at an antral pH of 5 to 7. At pH 2.5, secretion of gastrin is reduced by approximately 80%, with maximal suppression occurring at pH 1. Secretion is inhibited by the direct action of acid on the G cells. This negative feedback prevents excess acid production regardless of the stimulant.

The principal circulating form of gastrin is in healthy individuals and in patients with hypergastrinemia is G-34. Trypsin cleaves G-34 into two fragments, one of which has the amino acid sequence of G-17. On a molar basis, G-17 is 6 to 8 times more potent than G-34 as a stimulant of gastric acid secretion. In the fasting state, the ratio of G-34 to G-17 is approximately 2 : 1. After meals, the concentration of G-34 doubles but that of G-17 increases fourfold so the ratio approaches 1 : 1. The half-lives of endogenous G-17 and G-34 in the circulation are approximately 6 and 36 minutes, respectively; this difference probably accounts for the higher concentration of G-34 in the fasting state.

Gastrinoma and the Zollinger-Ellison Syndrome

In 1955, Zollinger and Ellison described a syndrome consisting of multiple peptic ulcers, gastric hypersecretion, and non–β islet cell tumors of the pancreas secreting gastrin.[23-25] Gastrinomas are a rare cause (<0.5%) of gastroduodenal ulcers. The persistently high circulating gastrin concentrations lead to hypersecretion of gastric acid and increased parietal cell mass as the hormone is trophic to parietal cells. Most cases occur between the ages of 30 and 50 years, although the condition has been reported in patients as young as 7 and as old as 90 years of age. It is more common in men (60% of cases) than in women.

Symptoms may be those of *H. pylori* peptic ulcer disease but also can include diarrhea (secondary to inactivation of pancreatic enzymes in the acidic environment). Duodenal ulceration and ulcers resistant to standard therapies must be considered suspicious. Gastrinomas are most often sporadic, but also may be associated with multiple endocrine neoplasia type 1 (MEN1, Wermer's syndrome), a syndrome characterized by the presence of two or more tumors sited in the pituitary, parathyroid glands, or pancreas. MEN1 is also associated with an increased prevalence of adrenal, thyroid, and carcinoid tumors (see Chapter 63).

Gastrinomas are commonly located in the pancreas, but can arise from the stomach, duodenum, or other tissues. They are more often (60%) malignant than benign, with metastases frequently present at the time of diagnosis. Measurement of plasma gastrin in a fasting sample is the initial step in aiding the differential diagnosis. A mildly elevated plasma gastrin concentration may be observed in long-term PPI therapy, hypochlorhydria, pernicious anemia, and G-cell hyperplasia. *H. pylori* infection also can lead to increased plasma gastrin and in some cases atrophic gastritis.[26] Increases in plasma gastrin in chronic renal failure appear to be related to the severity of renal impairment.[25]

Fasting plasma gastrin concentrations in the Zollinger-Ellison syndrome are usually markedly increased, and a concentration more than 10 times the upper limit of the reference range in the presence of gastric acid hypersecretion is virtually diagnostic of a gastrinoma. No correlation has been observed between the severity of symptoms and the extent of plasma gastrin elevation. However, the fasting plasma gastrin concentration at presentation in sporadic gastrinomas is related to the extent of tumor burden and the presence of hepatic metastases and is therefore of prognostic value.[27]

Measurement of Plasma Gastrin

In plasma from healthy subjects, the predominant forms of gastrin are amidated G-34 and G-17. In patients with gastrinomas, the gastrins found in the circulation display unpredictable heterogeneity with a shift toward larger peptides. For the detection of gastrinomas, the assay should be able to detect all secreted forms of gastrin to prevent false-negative findings.[28] Gastrin is unstable in serum or plasma, and samples may lose up to 50% of their immunoreactivity over 48 hours at 2° to 8°C because of the action of proteolytic enzymes. Blood samples should be collected into tubes containing an anticoagulant (eg, heparin) and a protease inhibitor (eg, aprotinin) to prevent degradation. Samples should be processed rapidly and the plasma stored at −20°C until assayed.

INTESTINAL DISORDERS AND THEIR LABORATORY INVESTIGATION

This section includes discussion of celiac disease, disaccharidase deficiency, bacterial overgrowth, bile salt malabsorption, inflammatory bowel disease (IBD), and protein-losing enteropathy and the main laboratory investigations associated with the diagnosis and monitoring of these disorders.

Celiac Disease

Pathophysiology of Celiac Disease

Celiac disease occurs in genetically predisposed subjects as a consequence of an inappropriate T cell–mediated immune response to ingestion of gluten from wheat and to similar proteins in barley and rye.[29-33] The role of genetic factors in celiac disease has been recognized for many years; a 70% concordance for celiac disease has been reported in identical twins and typically 10% of first-degree relatives of an affected individual will be found to have the disease, with a further 20% to 25% having nonspecific small bowel changes. The major genetic component has been localized to the human leukocyte antigen (HLA) region of chromosome 6. Approximately 95% of subjects with celiac disease express a specific HLA heterodimer (HLA DQ2 α/β). Most white populations have a high frequency (20% to 30%) of DQ2, but only a small minority will develop celiac disease.

The external trigger to the development of celiac disease in genetically susceptible individuals is found in gluten, which is the complex group of proteins found in wheat and other grains. The major toxic proteins of wheat are the gliadins that account for 50% of the wheat protein, with homologous proteins (the hordeins and secalins) occurring in barley and rye, respectively. All proteins (and peptides) that are toxic to the small bowel mucosa in subjects with celiac disease contain large amounts of glutamine.

The identification in 1997 of small bowel tissue transglutaminase as the autoantigen of celiac disease has led to a greater understanding of the pathogenesis of the condition.[34] The tissue transglutaminases are a family of calcium-dependent enzymes that are released from cells during wound healing. They catalyze the cross-linking or deamidation of proteins leading to stabilization of the wound area. Expression of the enzyme is increased during apoptosis and in active celiac disease. Deamidation of gliadin peptides enhances their binding to HLA DQ2/DQ8 and increases recognition of these peptides by gut-derived T cells from subjects with celiac disease.[35] The characteristic enteropathy is then induced by the release of interferon-γ and other proinflammatory cytokines.

A 33–amino acid peptide of gluten appears to be the primary initiator of the inflammatory response.[36] It is resistant to breakdown by all gastric, pancreatic, and brush border membrane proteases, thus allowing it to reach the small intestine intact. Homologs of the peptide are found in food grains that are toxic to patients with celiac disease but are absent from nontoxic food grains. The peptide can be detoxified by exposure to a bacterial prolyl endopeptidase, suggesting a therapeutic strategy for celiac disease.[36]

Increased intestinal permeability in untreated celiac disease that is reversible on withdrawal of gluten from the diet has been recognized since the early 1980s.[37] Evidence suggests that this increase in paracellular permeability may be mediated by increased expression of zonulin,[38] a protein that opens small intestinal tight junctions, or by decreased expression of intercellular epithelial cell adhesion molecules such as Z0-1, catenin, and cadherin,[39] The zonulin pathway is now thought to play a significant role in the entry of allergens into cells and hence in the autoimmune response.[40]

Clinical Considerations

Celiac disease is a common disorder in white populations with a prevalence of approximately 1%.[41,42] It also occurs in northern Indian and North African populations. It is rare among people of Chinese, Japanese, and African Caribbean origin. The prevalence in North America has been found to be similar to that in Europe.[43,44]

A wide spectrum of clinical manifestations of celiac disease is seen, with most diagnoses being made in adult life.[45,46] Classic celiac disease, manifesting in infancy with failure to thrive, abdominal distention, and diarrhea, is now uncommon in developed countries. Most adults present with nonspecific symptoms; the condition may be picked up during the investigation of patients suspected of having irritable bowel syndrome (IBS). Mild iron deficiency is common. The initial presentation may be seen by a wide range of clinical specialties, as shown in Table 62.2. A strong association with other autoimmune diseases, especially type 1 diabetes and autoimmune thyroid disease, has been reported. In type 1 diabetes, the prevalence of celiac disease is approximately 5% and serologic screening to detect these cases has been advocated.[47]

Tests for Celiac Disease

Serologic tests have played a significant role in raising awareness of the high prevalence of this disorder and appropriately standardized tests have high clinical sensitivity and specificity for diagnosis and monitoring of compliance with a gluten-free diet. Table 62.3 compares the sensitivity and specificity of the serologic tests commonly used for the diagnosis of celiac disease.

Historically, serologic testing for celiac disease involved testing for antigliadin antibodies and antiendomysial antibodies by indirect immunofluorescence. The sensitivity and specificity of these tests was poor, and they have largely been superseded by measurement of antibodies against tissue transglutaminase (TGA) and deaminated gliadin peptide (DGP) antibodies.[48] Both IgG and IgA tests are available for these antibodies in the form of quantitative enzyme-linked immunosorbent assays (ELISAs). The diagnostic accuracy of DGP-IgA is similar to that of TGA-IgA, with sensitivities in the range of 85% to 90% and a specificity of approximately 95%. Sensitivity for DGP-IgG is not as good as that for

TABLE 62.2 Sample of Clinical Specialties to Which a Child or Adult With Celiac Disease May Present

Clinical specialty	Symptoms/manifestations
General medicine	Tired all the time
Gastroenterology	Diarrrhea, flatulence, weight loss
Hematology	Anemia
Obstetrics/gynecology	Infertility
Orthopedics	Fracture, osteopenia
Dermatology	Dermatitis herpetiformis, hyperkeratosis
Neurology	Peripheral neuropathy
Rheumatology	Arthropathy
Endocrinology	Short stature, thyroid disease
Diabetes	Diarrhea, anemia

TABLE 62.3 Comparison of Serologic Tests for Celiac Disease

Antibody	Method	Sensitivity(%)	Specificity(%)
IgA-endomysial antibody	Immunofluorescence on monkey esophagus or human umbilical cord	80-100	>99
IgA-antigliadin antibody	Quantitative ELISA	75-95%	95
IgA-antitissue transglutaminase antibody	Quantitative ELISA	>90	>99
IgA-deamidated gliadin peptide antibody	Quantitative ELISA	90	90

DGP-IgA but has a specificity approaching 99%. Subjects with selective IgA deficiency (plasma IgA concentration <0.05 g/L, incidence ~1 in 600) are at greater risk for celiac disease. The tests directed at the IgA antibodies to TGA and DGP may produce false-negative results in these patients, so total IgA always should be measured when requesting serologic tests for celiac disease. When IgA deficiency is identified, the IgG-based tests should be used to confirm or exclude a diagnosis of celiac disease. No current recommendations suggest that DGP-based tests should replace tests based on TGA antibodies, but support has been increasing for their use in both adult and pediatric populations.[49,50] The response to gluten withdrawal can be assessed clinically, by serologic tests or by endoscopic or wireless capsule techniques. The latter are invasive and expensive and are now less frequently used for this purpose.

Strict adherence to a gluten-free diet leads to mucosal healing in celiac disease and reduces the risk for bowel malignancy (small bowel lymphoma). TGA can be used as a marker for monitoring dietary adherence in addition to its diagnostic role. Failure of symptoms to respond to a prescribed gluten-free diet may indicate nonadherence to the diet, other coexisting conditions such as small bowel overgrowth, lactose intolerance, microscopic colitis, or the presence of refractory celiac disease. The latter is characterized by persistent villous atrophy with an increase in intraepithelial lymphocytes in the small bowel while the patient is on a strict long-term gluten-free diet.[51] In both responsive and refractory celiac disease, antibody titers are typically decreased with dietary therapy and remain within reference intervals unless individuals are reexposed to gluten.

Two types of refractory celiac disease may occur and are differentiated by the types of T-cell populations found in the intestinal mucosa—polyclonal in type 1 disease and clonal in type 2 disease. Differentiation of the two types is accomplished by immunohistochemical, flow cytometric, or T-cell–receptor γ-gene rearrangement analysis of intestinal mucosal T cells. Type 2 celiac disease has an unfavorable prognosis and typically is viewed as a precursor to enteropathy-associated T-cell lymphoma (EATL).

Disaccharidase Deficiencies

The presence of the brush border disaccharidases is essential for carbohydrate absorption, and a reduction in their activity leads to carbohydrate malabsorption and intolerance.[52,53] Carbohydrate malabsorption can result in osmotic diarrhea with abdominal pain and distention and flatulence resembling the symptoms of IBS. Inherited disorders of sucrase-isomaltase and of transport proteins causing glucose-galactose malabsorption and fructose malabsorption have been described but are rare (see later discussion). Adult lactase deficiency is common in humans and in certain ethnic groups is the normal state.

Lactase Deficiency

Lactase activity has its highest prevalence in the earliest months of life and declines after weaning. The prevalence of lactase deficiency varies widely with ethnic origin; although only 5% to 15% of northern Europeans are lactase deficient, hypolactasia or alactasia can be found in more than 70% of those of African and Asian origin (Table 62.4) and approaches 19% in the Inuit. Congenital lactase deficiency is a very rare

TABLE 62.4 Prevalence of Hypolactasia in Adults

Racial Group	Prevalence (%)
Chinese	>90
African-Americans	54-81
Asians	60-90
Greeks	60-78
North Europeans	5-30

BOX 62.2 Methods for Detecting Lactase Deficiency

- Lactase in mucosal biopsy
- Oral lactose tolerance
  - Measure increase in plasma glucose or galactose
  - Measure increase in breath H_2 or $^{13}CO_2$
  - Measure urinary excretion of lactose after oral load

disorder that becomes apparent once the infant has been exposed to milk feeds. Stools have a low pH and contain large amounts of lactose and glucose, the latter being produced by bacterial degradation of undigested lactose. Secondary lactase deficiency is common in celiac disease owing to villous atrophy but also may occur in tropical sprue, small bowel Crohn disease, radiation enteritis, giardiasis and other bowel infections, chronic alcoholism with malnutrition, and the enteropathy associated with acquired immunodeficiency syndrome (AIDS).[52]

Tests for Lactase Deficiency

Many methods have been proposed for the diagnosis of lactase deficiency (Box 62.2). Disaccharidase activities can be measured in jejunal biopsies, although this is rarely done in routine practice.[53] The xylose absorption test was first introduced as a test for carbohydrate malabsorption in the 1930s. In humans, D-xylose, a pentose sugar of plant origin, is absorbed by a passive mechanism in the jejunum. After an oral dose of D-xylose it can be measured in blood or urine samples. It is now accepted that the amount of xylose excreted is affected not just by reduced absorption in the gut but also by renal, hepatic, and cardiac disease, and the test is no longer widely available. Oral lactose tolerance tests, measuring the increase in plasma glucose after ingestion of lactose have been used to diagnose lactase deficiency. The usual dose of lactose is 50 g, but lower doses should be used in children (2 g/kg up to a maximum of 50 g). Blood samples are taken over a 2-hour period and the peak increment in glucose recorded; a rise greater than 1.1 mmol/L (20 mg/dL) for capillary samples or greater than 1.4 mmol/L (>25 mg/dL) for venous plasma excludes lactase deficiency.[54,55] The xylose absorption test has largely been superseded by the hydrogen breath test (Box 62.3).

Hydrogen Breath Tests

Hydrogen is not a normal end product of mammalian metabolism, and hydrogen in breath is derived from bacterial metabolism in the intestinal tract.[56] After lactose ingestion, the disaccharide is normally broken down into its constituent

BOX 62.3 Protocol for Lactose Tolerance Test With Measurement of Breath Hydrogen

- Meal before 07:00 hours (restriction on wheat and fiber), then fasting until test completed
- Brush teeth (night and morning) or use mouthwash
- Measure end-expiratory fasting breath H_2
- Give lactose solution (50 g in 180 mL water for adults)
- Rinse mouth with further 20 mL water and swallow
- Measure breath H_2 at 15, 30, 60, 90, and 120 minutes
- Test can be stopped if earlier rise of more than 20 ppm above fasting level

monosaccharides, which are absorbed. In the presence of lactase deficiency, unabsorbed disaccharide passes into the large bowel, where bacteria act on it to produce hydrogen that is absorbed into the systemic circulation and subsequently exhaled. Breath hydrogen can be measured by a variety of techniques based on the electrochemical detection of hydrogen; both laboratory and hand-held point-of-care devices are available.[55] Fasting breath hydrogen is normally less than 5 ppm (5 μL/L), and concentrations greater than 20 ppm (20 μL/L) at 2 hours after oral administration of 50 g lactose in adults (2 g/kg up to a maximum of 50 g in children) are suggestive of malabsorption or bacterial overgrowth.[55,57,58] A lower cutoff of 10 ppm (10 μL/L) has been suggested that can improve diagnostic sensitivity without altering specificity.[59] Occasionally, higher than normal concentrations may occur within the first 30 minutes after lactose ingestion; this may indicate very rapid transit of lactose to the cecum or bacterial overgrowth. In some individuals (estimated at 2% to 13%), the large bowel bacteria do not produce hydrogen[57,60,61] and fasting breath hydrogen will be low; in such individuals a normal result cannot exclude lactase deficiency. A positive breath hydrogen result after ingestion of lactose also may occur in glucose-galactose malabsorption; this can be confirmed or excluded by repeating the test substituting 25 g each of glucose and galactose for the lactose. An increase in breath hydrogen confirms the diagnosis. Lactose intolerance or malabsorption has become a very topical issue with clinicians as well as dieticians and nutritionists. Many of these have abandoned any measurements to confirm malabsorption-maldigestion and simply rely on exacerbation of symptoms with the ingestion of a pint of milk. Alternatively, they may make the diagnosis based on symptomatic improvement when patients are placed on a dairy-free diet.

Sucrase-Isomaltase and Trehalose Deficiencies and Monosaccharide Malabsorption

Sucrase-isomaltase deficiency usually manifests clinically in infancy when sucrose and fruits are first introduced into the diet[62] but can present in adulthood.[63,64] The deficiency is rare in whites and is more common in Inuits. Secondary deficiency can occur in other GI tract disorders, such as transiently after gastroenteritis. Trehalase deficiency is a rare disorder[65,66] except in Greenland, where it occurs in 8% of the population.[67] It is manifested by diarrhea after the ingestion of mushrooms.

BOX 62.4 Abnormalities of the Small Intestine Associated With Bacterial Overgrowth

- Jejunal diverticuli
- Crohn disease
- Autonomic neuropathy
- Scleroderma (systemic sclerosis)
- Pseudo-obstruction
- Postgastrectomy

Malabsorption of monosaccharides also can cause intestinal symptoms more commonly attributed to maldigestion of disaccharides. Glucose-galactose malabsorption is also inherited as an autosomal recessive trait. Symptoms occur in the affected neonate as soon as milk is introduced but also can follow ingestion of glucose- or galactose-containing foods. Symptoms caused by fructose malabsorption occur after ingestion of fruit. This dietary disorder is different from hereditary fructose intolerance, in which the hepatic enzyme aldolase is absent.

The breath hydrogen test described previously can be used to diagnose sucrase-isomaltase deficiency, with 50 g sucrose replacing lactose. An increase in breath hydrogen greater than 20 ppm (20 μL/L) within 2 hours is diagnostic. It is rarely necessary to test for trehalase deficiency, although a breath test using 25 g trehalose has been described.[68]

Bacterial Overgrowth

The proximal small intestine (duodenum and jejunum) normally contains few bacteria. Most ingested bacteria do not survive the acidic environment of the stomach; therefore few live organisms enter the small bowel. The motility of the jejunum prevents fecal-type organisms from progressing up into the jejunum from the cecum. The ileum normally contains some fecal-type bacteria. Colonization of the upper small bowel is described as bacterial overgrowth and usually occurs as a consequence of other abnormalities (structural or motility disorders) of the small intestine (Box 62.4). Gastric hypochlorhydria (associated with the use of PPIs) may contribute to bacterial overgrowth. Abnormalities in the systemic immune system (eg, isolated IgA deficiency, hypogammaglobulinemia, combined immunodeficiency, infection with the human immunodeficiency virus [HIV]) can result in bacterial overgrowth. Impaired motility, pancreatic insufficiency, intrinsic small bowel disease, or surgically induced blind loops are often associated with bacterial overgrowth.

Small bowel bacterial overgrowth can be asymptomatic or associated with nonspecific symptoms that include abdominal distention, flatulence, and diarrhea resembling IBS.[69] Bacteria colonizing the small bowel (eg, *Escherichia coli* and *Bacteroides* species) deconjugate and dehydroxylate bile salts, resulting in conjugated bile salt deficiency and mild fat malabsorption. Bacterial metabolism of vitamin B_{12} can occur, leading to deficiency, whereas plasma folate concentration may be increased owing to production by the bacteria.

The gold standard diagnostic procedure is microbiologic examination of small bowel contents, but this is seldom practical.[69] Noninvasive procedures based on oral administration of substances metabolized by bacteria to yield products that can be detected in breath are now the most common tests for bacterial overgrowth, but there is controversy as to which test to use and their sensitivity/specificity.[70]

The ^{14}C-glycocholate breath test was one of the first tests to be used for noninvasive diagnosis of bacterial overgrowth but have been superseded by tests that avoid the use of radioactive isotopes. Small bowel bacterial breath tests in routine use involve test substances labeled with ^{13}C and the breath hydrogen tests.[71] Lactulose is not normally absorbed from the small bowel and is therefore available for metabolism by bacteria throughout the gut; alternatively, labeled glucose can be used. In a normal subject, breath hydrogen does not increase until the substrate reaches the large intestine and the time from ingestion to a rise in breath hydrogen is an indicator of small bowel transit time. In bacterial overgrowth an early rise in breath hydrogen of at least 20 ppm (20 μl/L) is observed within 30 minutes of ingestion. The early increase is diagnostic when it can be distinguished clearly from the later colonic phase. Frequent measurements are essential (eg, at 5-minute intervals) for the first 30 minutes.[72] The finding of an increased breath hydrogen output has high specificity for bacterial overgrowth but poor sensitivity.[72] Variations in gastric emptying rate and small bowel transit times limit the diagnostic accuracy of the breath tests.

Bile Acid Malabsorption

Bile acids are synthesized in the liver and pass into the lumen of the small bowel via the gallbladder. Bile acids are present in bile as taurine or glycine conjugates; because the pH of bile is slightly alkaline and contains significant amounts of sodium and potassium, most of the bile acids and their conjugates exist as salts (ie, bile salts). In practice, the terms *bile acids* and *bile salts* are frequently used synonymously. Their major function is to act as surface-active agents, forming micelles and facilitating the digestion of triglycerides and the absorption of cholesterol and fat-soluble vitamins. Little reabsorption of bile acids occurs in the proximal small bowel, but normally more than 90% is reabsorbed in the terminal ileum. The bile acids return to the liver via the portal circulation and can be resecreted into bile (enterohepatic circulation). Less than 10% of secreted bile acid is lost in the feces (~0.2 to 0.6 g/24 h).

Bile acid malabsorption leading to chronic diarrhea occurs when ileal disease is present, or after resection of the terminal ileum; it also may occur after cholecystectomy and is present in some patients with IBS.[73] Malabsorption of bile salts produces diarrhea by two different mechanisms. When significant bile salt depletion occurs, the deficiency of intraluminal bile salts leads to fat malabsorption and steatorrhea. More commonly, malabsorption of bile salts in the ileum leads to increased concentrations of bile salts in the colon, where they alter water and electrolyte absorption. This leads to net secretion of water into the lumen and diarrhea. Bile salt malabsorption is probably an underdiagnosed condition and should be suspected in patients with unexplained chronic diarrhea.[74-76]

The most widely used test for bile acid malabsorption involves oral administration of the synthetic radiolabeled bile acid[75] selenohomocholyltaurine (SeHCAT). Whole-body gamma counting is used to determine the basal level at 1 hour and then repeated at 7 days when in normal subjects more than 15% of the dose is retained. Retention of less than 10% of SeHCAT at 7 days can predict a good response to bile acid sequestrants.

Two blood tests have been proposed as alternatives to SeHCAT to avoid administration of a radioactive substance; fibroblast growth factor-19 (FGF-19) and 7α-hydroxy-4-cholesten-3-one (C4). C4 is the intermediary step between cholesterol and taurocholic acid and reflects the activity of hepatic cholesterol 7α-hydroxylase and therefore, because this is the rate-limiting enzyme, the rate of bile acid synthesis. Bile acid malabsorption is associated with increased plasma concentrations of C4 as hepatic synthesis is up-regulated to maintain the pool of circulating bile acids.[77] The presence of bile acids in the ileum has been shown to stimulate the production of FGF-19.[78] Good correlation has been demonstrated between both serum C4 and FGF-19 and SeHCAT.[79] Several publications have demonstrated good sensitivity for identifying bile acid–induced diarrhea.[80,81]

With growing awareness of the role of bile salt malabsorption in chronic diarrhea in a proportion of patients with IBS or inflammatory bowel disease (IBD), and the therapeutic effectiveness of cholestyramine, measurement of C4 and/or FGF-19 may become routine.[82]

POINTS TO REMEMBER

Malabsorption

- Carbohydrate malabsorption can occur in disaccharidase deficiency.
- Celiac disease causes malabsorption by reduction in the villous surface area.
- Fat malabsorption is associated with exocrine pancreatic insufficiency.
- Fecal elastase is a useful test for exocrine pancreatic insufficiency.

Inflammatory Bowel Disease and Irritable Bowel Syndrome

Intestinal symptoms including abdominal pain or discomfort with diarrhea or constipation are common to both IBD and IBS. IBD includes ulcerative colitis (UC) and Crohn disease (CD), as well as a number of microscopic inflammatory bowel conditions. IBS is a functional bowel disorder for which there is no identifiable pathologic process or known cause. Although IBS may produce symptoms that are sufficient to interfere with daily life, it is seldom associated with serious morbidity. IBS may affect up to 10% to 20% of the adult population in the developed world, with a typical age at presentation of 20 to 30 years and a female preponderance.[83] The prevalence of UC is approximately 100 to 200 per 100,000 people and of CD approximately 50 to 100 per 100,000 people, with no significant difference between genders.[83] There is, however, a difference in prevalence with ethnic origin, with IBD being more common among whites than individuals of Asian or African origin. Up to 20% of cases of IBD manifest in childhood, although the most common age at presentation is between 15 and 30 years of age. Both UC and CD are chronic conditions that tend to follow a remitting and relapsing course. The prognosis of patients with CD tends to be worse than that of UC, although in the latter it is estimated that up to 10% of patients will require surgical intervention within 10 years of diagnosis.

The cause of IBD is not fully understood, but both genetic and environmental factors have been implicated.[84] Genome-wide association studies have identified over 160 susceptibility loci/genes that are significantly associated with IBD.[85,86] Studies in monozygotic twins, however, have shown a lower than expected concordance rate (15% to 19% for UC, 27% to 50% for CD) if IBD were simply an inherited disorder. It is thought that individuals with a genetic predisposition to IBD need to be exposed to a range of environmental triggers that affect the host's immunity. The enteric GI microbiota are now accepted as a central etiologic factor in the pathogenesis of IBD, although the mechanistic details are lacking.[86,87] Tissue damage is a consequence of neutrophil activation and the production of proinflammatory cytokines and chemokines. The success of treatments based on immunosuppressive agents or tumor necrosis factor-alpha (TNF-α) inhibitors appears to support an immune basis for the development of IBD.[84] Environmental factors implicated in triggering the development of active disease include a protective effect of breastfeeding and an increased risk in patients who have recurrent GI infections or exposure to drug therapy (antibiotics, oral contraceptives, NSAIDs) along with socioeconomic factors, stress, smoking, and diet.[84]

The conventional diagnostic pathway includes a full blood count to detect/exclude anemia, markers of generalized inflammation (erythrocyte sedimentation rate [ESR] and C-reactive protein [CRP]) and serologic testing for celiac disease (see earlier section on tests for celiac disease). In the past 20 years, there have been significant advances in biomarkers that can aid in differentiating IBD from IBS and in monitoring disease activity or response to treatment. Most of these are fecal markers.[88]

Calprotectin

Calprotectin is a member of the S100 family of zinc- and calcium-binding proteins and is a heterodimer of S100A8/9. First discovered in 1980, it accounts for approximately 60% of cytosolic protein in neutrophils.[89] It is also present in monocytes and macrophages at lower concentrations than in neutrophils and may have antimicrobial properties.[90] Any disruption to the mucosal architecture of the GI tract allows neutrophils that accumulate at sites of active inflammation to be released into the lumen and subsequently shed in feces.[91] The fecal concentration of calprotectin has been shown to correlate well with the gold standard indium-111–labeled granulocyte test and is directly related to the extent of inflammation.[92] Calprotectin appears to be evenly distributed in fecal samples and has reasonable stability at room temperature.[93]

The initial studies of fecal calprotectin were on its ability to differentiate between IBS and IBD. In a study of 602 consecutive referrals from primary care to a gastroenterology clinic at King's College Hospital (London, United Kingdom) patients had fecal calprotectin measured and were assessed for IBS using the Rome questionnaire.[94] The sensitivity and specificity for calprotectin for the detection of organic disease were 89% and 79%, respectively. Combining calprotectin with the Rome questionnaire had a predictive value approaching 100%.

In the past decade, there have been many studies of the value of fecal calprotectin for distinguishing IBD from IBS and these have been the subject of several meta-analyses.[95-99] The studies included in these meta-analyses included only patients already in secondary or tertiary care and may have been biased by preselection of patients in primary care before referral. A retrospective analysis of data from 946 patients from 48 primary care practices found a sensitivity of 82% and a specificity of 77%.[100] Nevertheless, the (UK) National Institute for Health and Care Excellence (NICE) has recommended the widespread use of calprotectin in general practice to select patients at high risk for having IBD for referral to gastroenterologists, with the vast majority of the rest with IBS (normal calprotectin) remaining in primary care and treated appropriately. The cost savings of this approach are substantial.

Calprotectin has been found to differentiate between active and inactive IBD.[101] The aim of treatment of IBD is currently to secure and maintain remission, with the ultimate aim of achieving mucosal healing.[102] Assessment of treatment efficacy until recently has been based on clinical scores, including the Crohn Disease Activity Index (CDAI) and the Ulcerative Colitis Disease Activity Index (UCDAI), and by changes in ESR and CRP. However, many patients in clinical remission have increased fecal calprotectin concentrations and it is perhaps these who would benefit from escalation of treatment to achieve mucosal healing. Several studies have demonstrated that a fall in the fecal calprotectin concentration indicates a good response to treatment and that this can precede any clinical response.[103-106] It has been recommended that fecal calprotectin should be included in the range of tests before consideration of initiating or changing IBD therapy.[107] Various studies have provided data on the use of fecal calprotectin in predicting relapse or recurrence of IBD and these have been reviewed.[108] Treating the inflammatory component of IBD, regardless of symptoms, promises to alter the natural history of the disease in a way similar to that seen in rheumatoid arthritis.

Fecal calprotectin is not, however, specific to IBD and has been shown to be increased in patients with colorectal carcinoma,[109] the chronic use of NSAIDs,[110] bacterial infections,[111] and diverticular disease.[112]

Other Fecal Markers

M2-PK. The glycolytic enzyme pyruvate kinase is present in normal cells as tissue-specific isoenzymes (L-PK in liver, M1-PK in muscle and brain, and R-PK in erythrocytes). These isoenzymes exist as tetramers, but in rapidly dividing cells a dimeric form has been described (M2-PK). Serum M2-PK was originally proposed as a marker of renal cell carcinoma but was found to be increased in fecal samples from patients with colorectal carcinoma.[113] It is essentially a marker of increased cellular turnover and was shown to be high in patients with IBD, exhibiting a good correlation with calprotectin.[114] In a study of 105 gastroenterology outpatients and 94 controls, fecal M2-PK had a sensitivity of 93% and a specificity of 92% compared to 67% and 88%, respectively, for calprotectin.[115]

Lactoferrin. Lactoferrin, a major whey protein, is a red, iron-binding protein present in polymorphonuclear neutrophils and secretions, including breast milk that possibly has bacteriostatic properties.[116] Lactoferrin, like calprotectin, is present in neutrophils in higher concentrations than in any other cells. A number of studies have been carried out with lactoferrin alone or in combination with other markers.[117]

ALGORITHM FOR THE USE OF FECAL CALPROTECTIN IN DIFFERENTIATING INFLAMMATORY BOWEL SYNDROME AND INFLAMMATORY BOWEL DISEASE

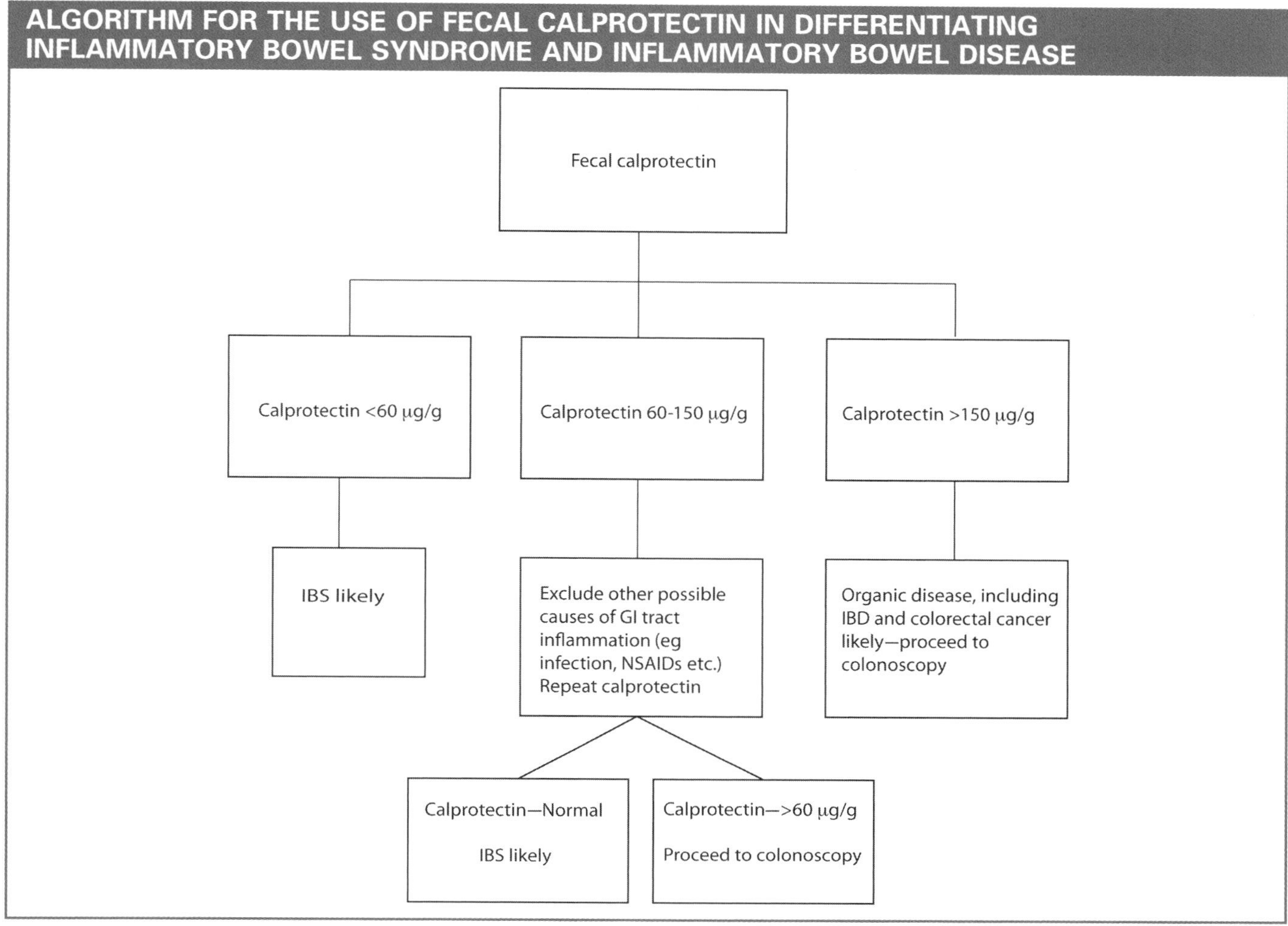

Combining fecal lactoferrin and calprotectin did not confer additional benefit in any of the studies in which both were measured.

S10012. Like calprotectin, S100A12 is a member of the S100 family of calcium-binding proteins. It is present in neutrophils and may have proinflammatory properties. The number of studies of fecal S100A12 in patients with GI symptoms is limited, and the majority are in children.[88] Further studies are required before the potential value of this marker can be fully assessed.

Therapeutic Drug Monitoring in Patients With Inflammatory Bowel Disease

The increasing use of thiopurine analogs (azathioprine [AZA] and mercaptopurine [MP]) and the introduction of the anti–tissue necrosis factor (anti-TNF) drugs infliximab (IFX) and adalimumab (ADA) have led to the introduction of the concept of therapeutic drug monitoring to gastroenterology.[118] The metabolism of AZA (a prodrug) is complex involving a number of enzymatic pathways that result in active, inactive, and potentially toxic metabolites.[119] The key enzyme in the pathway is thiopurine methyltransferase (TPMT), which converts MP into the potentially hepatotoxic metabolite 6-methylmercaptopurine (MMP). The therapeutically active metabolite 6-thioguanine (6-TG) is formed via an alternative pathway involving the enzyme thioinosine monophosphate. Although 6-TG is a favorable metabolite, high concentrations cause myelosuppression with the potential result of life-threatening infection. TPMT has a polymorphism that results in a homozygous state with very low enzyme activity (1 in 300 of the population), a heterozygous state with intermediate activity (10% of the population), and the normal wild type (89%).[120] Measurement of red cell TPMT activity has become a prerequisite before starting patients on AZA therapy because the presence of the low metabolic activity phenotype is a relative contraindication to the use of thiopurine analogs, and those who are heterozygous will require a reduced dose. Similarly, measurement of the plasma concentration of 6-TG can be used to assess adherence or the adequacy of dosage.

The anti-TNF drugs, particularly IFX and ADA, have proved effective in inducing and maintaining remission in patients with IBD. However, because these drugs are themselves humanized antibodies against TNF, many patients develop antibodies against them. Simultaneous measurement of the plasma drug concentrations and the antibodies against them has meant that a failure to sustain a beneficial response to anti-TNF therapy can be correctly ascribed to either subtherapeutic drug concentrations or the presence of antidrug antibodies and alternative therapies can be devised and initiated.[118] ELISA methods are commercially available for the measurement of both IFX and ADA and their corresponding antibodies. For further information see the thiopurines section of Chapter 40.

Assessment of Functional Small Bowel Length

The amino acid citrulline, which is involved in the urea cycle, is predominantly synthesized in the enterocytes of the small intestine. The short bowel syndrome can be present after major surgical resection of the gut in the treatment of Crohn disease or necrosis. The remaining small bowel length can be estimated at surgery, but this is unreliable at lengths over 50 to 80 cm. Plasma citrulline concentrations have been shown to correlate well with small bowel length and absorption of xylose ($P < .001$), but not with CRP, CDAI, or ESR.[121] Plasma citrulline measurements therefore appear to be a noninvasive means of assessing small bowel absorptive capacity that is not influenced by intestinal inflammation.

Protein-Losing Enteropathy

Loss of significant quantities of plasma proteins into the bowel lumen and their subsequent excretion in feces is associated with a range of GI disorders. These include IBD, diseases in which the intestinal lymphatics are obstructed (eg, lymphoma, Whipple disease), and disorders of immune status such as systemic lupus erythematosus and some food allergies.

In the healthy bowel, fecal protein is largely derived from enterocytes shed from the mucosal surface and from intestinal secretions. The normal GI loss of albumin is less than 10% of albumin catabolism, representing a daily loss of less than 1% to 2% of the circulating protein pool.[122] In protein-losing enteropathy, this may increase to 40%, resulting in hypoalbuminemia and edema.

The diagnosis of protein-losing enteropathy should be considered in the investigation of patients with hypoalbuminemia in whom renal loss, liver disease, and malnutrition have been excluded. Methods using the administration of radioactive albumin or dextran are the gold standards but are seldom used now.

Fecal excretion of α_1-antiprotease inhibitor (AAT) can be used as a marker of GI protein loss. AAT is a 54-kDa glycoprotein (formerly called α_1-antitrypsin) present in plasma at a concentration of approximately 1.0 to 2.0 g/L that is resistant to degradation in the GI tract. Increased AAT excretion can be found in both small and large bowel disease and is applicable to both adults and children.[123,124] Interpretation must be made with knowledge of the plasma AAT concentration because the test is invalid in the presence of low plasma AAT concentrations (eg, in AAT deficiency or impaired hepatic synthesis).

POINTS TO REMEMBER

Inflammatory Bowel Disease

- Crohn disease and ulcerative colitis are the most common IBDs.
- Fecal calprotectin can help distinguish IBD from IBS.
- Fecal calprotectin is related to disease activity and can predict relapse in IBD.
- Therapeutic drug monitoring is valuable when treating IBD with anti–TNF-α agents

PANCREAS: DISEASE AND ASSESSMENT OF EXOCRINE PANCREATIC FUNCTION

The pancreas plays a central role in the absorptive process for carbohydrates, fats, and proteins. Disorders of the exocrine pancreas therefore are frequently associated with symptoms of malabsorption such as diarrhea or steatorrhea. In this section, pediatric and adult exocrine pancreatic disorders are briefly discussed and tests that can be used to assess exocrine pancreatic function are described. Information on neuroendocrine tumors of the pancreas is also provided. Textbooks on gastroenterology or medicine provide much greater detail on the clinical aspects of exocrine pancreatic disorder.[125,126]

Pediatric Disorders of the Exocrine Pancreas

Pancreatic disorders of childhood have been reviewed[127] and are summarized in Box 62.5.

Cystic fibrosis (CF) is the most common severe autosomal recessive disease, with an estimated gene frequency in Western Europe and the United States of between 1 : 25 and 1 : 35 and a disease incidence of approximately 1 in 2500 to 1 in 3200. The pathogenesis and diagnosis of CF are described in Chapter 35. Pancreatic insufficiency is present in the neonatal period in 65% of infants with CF, and a further 15% develop it during infancy and early childhood. The 20% who do not develop pancreatic insufficiency have a better prognosis and develop fewer complications.

Measurement of pancreatic elastase-1 in feces (see section on noninvasive tests of exocrine function) is considered to be a reliable test for pancreatic insufficiency in infants over the age of 2 weeks with CF and in older children at the time of diagnosis.[128-130] This test also can be used to detect the onset of pancreatic insufficiency in those previously sufficient.

Recurrent bouts of acute pancreatitis in childhood should arouse a suspicion of a hereditary cause. Two gene defects have been shown to be associated with pancreatitis that manifests

BOX 62.5 Spectrum of Pancreatic Disease in Childhood

Disorders of Morphogenesis

- Annular pancreas, pancreas divisum, pancreatic hypoplasia and agenesis, heterotopic pancreas

Inherited Syndromes Affecting the Pancreas

- Cystic fibrosis
- Scwachman-Diamond syndrome, Johnson-Blizzard syndrome, Pearson bone marrow pancreas syndrome

Gene Mutations Leading to Pancreatic Disease

- Hereditary pancreatitis, cationic trypsinogen gene mutations, trypsin inhibitor gene mutations

Pancreatic Insufficiency Syndrome

- Isolated enzyme deficiencies: Lipase, colipase, enterokinase
- Pancreatic insufficiency secondary to other disorders
- Celiac disease

Acquired Pancreatitis in Childhood

- Idiopathic, traumatic, drugs, viral, metabolic, collagen vascular disease, autoimmune, fibrosing, nutritional (trophic) in childhood: the cationic trypsinogen gene *(PRSS1)* and the serine protease inhibitor Kazal type 1 *(SPINK1)* gene.[131] The majority of patients with *PRSS1*-related hereditary pancreatitis have a pathogenic mutation in exons 2 or 3 of the *PRSS1* gene. Duplication or triplication of the *PRSS1* gene has been reported to cause hereditary pancreatitis. The mechanism is assumed to be inappropriate activation of trypsin with consequent proteolytic action causing cell damage. Approximately 22% of patients with idiopathic pancreatitis have been reported to have at least one copy of the c.101A>G (p.Asn34Ser) mutation in the *SPINK1* gene compared to approximately 2.5% of the general population. This protease inhibitor is believed to be the principal inhibitor of trypsin and chymotrypsin within the pancreas, and the mutation results in a loss of its inhibitory capacity.

Adult Disorders of the Exocrine Pancreas

The major exocrine pancreatic disorders manifesting in adult life are acute pancreatitis, chronic pancreatitis, and carcinoma of the pancreas. The use of enzyme tests in diagnosis of acute pancreatitis is discussed in Chapter 29. The causes of pancreatitis are given in Box 62.6.

Chronic pancreatitis is defined by irreversible pancreatic damage with histologic evidence of inflammation and fibrosis leading to destruction of cells and loss of endocrine and exocrine function. In developed nations, the most common cause is alcohol (60% to 90% of all cases of chronic pancreatitis), although because only 5% to 15% of heavy drinkers develop the disease, other predisposing factors must be present (eg, smoking, diet high in fat and protein). The role of invasive and noninvasive pancreatic exocrine tests in chronic pancreatitis has been reviewed.[132]

BOX 62.6 Causes of Pancreatitis in Adults

Acute

- Gallstones
- Alcohol
- Infection (eg, mumps, Coxsackie B)
- Pancreatic tumors
- Drugs (eg, azathioprine, estrogens, corticosteroids, didanosine)
- Iatrogenic (eg, postsurgical, endoscopic retrograde cholangiopancreatography)
- Hyperlipidemias
- Miscellaneous (eg, trauma, scorpion bite, cardiac surgery)
- Idiopathic

Chronic

- Alcohol
- Tropical (nutritional)
- Hereditary (trypsinogen and inhibitory gene defects, cystic fibrosis)
- Idiopathic
- Trauma
- Hypercalcemia

From Burroughs AK, Westaby D. Liver, biliary tract disease and pancreatic disease. In: Kumar P, Clark M, editors. *Clinical Medicine.* 7th ed. Edinburgh: Saunders; 2009:319–385.

Tests of Exocrine Function of the Pancreas

The predominant exocrine function of the pancreas is the production and secretion of pancreatic juice, which is rich in enzymes and bicarbonate. Normal pancreatic juice is colorless and odorless; it has a pH of 8.0 to 8.3 and a specific gravity of 1.007 to 1.042. The total 24-hour volume secreted may be as high as 3000 mL.[133]

Laboratory tests used to assess exocrine pancreatic function can be divided into invasive and noninvasive categories. Invasive tests require GI tract intubation to allow the collection of pancreatic secretions. Noninvasive tests were developed to avoid the need for intubation, which is uncomfortable for the patient, time-consuming, and therefore expensive. Noninvasive tests ("tubeless") are simpler to perform but in general lack the sensitivity and specificity of invasive tests, particularly for the diagnosis of mild pancreatic insufficiency. In recent years, there have been significant advances in imaging techniques for the pancreas; these have grown in importance and are described in Box 62.7.

BOX 62.7 Pancreatic Imaging Procedures

- Plain abdominal radiography
  - May show pancreatic calcification, particularly when alcohol is the cause.
- Ultrasound
  - Useful screening investigation for inflammation and neoplasia. Views may be limited by overlying bowel gas.
- Spiral computed tomography (CT)
  - With contrast enhancement and following a specific pancreatic protocol remains the gold standard imaging technique for the investigation of pancreatic disease.
- Magnetic resonance imaging (MRI)
  - An alternative to CT. Magnetic resonance cholangiopancreatography (MRCP) gives clear definition of the pancreatic duct and the biliary tree. Gallstones (including microcalculi) also may be identified in the biliary tree using MRI/MRCP.
- Endoscopic ultrasound
  - Very useful for identifying distal common bile duct stones, which may be the cause of an episode of acute pancreatitis
  - Can identify early changes of chronic pancreatitis before those evident on other imaging methods.
  - Has an increasing role for staging the operability of pancreatic adenocarcinoma, particularly with respect to vascular invasion.
  - Considered to be the imaging technique of choice for investigating cystic lesions of the pancreas
  - Is a sensitive means of detecting small tumors, particularly those of neuroendocrine origin.
- Endoscopic retrograde cholangiopancreatography (ERCP)
  - This has been considered the gold standard for diagnosing pancreatic disease. However, with MRCP and endoscopic ultrasound, ERCP is restricted to therapeutic intervention.

From Burroughs AK, Westaby D. Liver, biliary tract disease and pancreatic disease. In: Kumar P, Clark M, editors. *Clinical Medicine.* 7th ed. Edinburgh: Saunders; 2009: 319–385.

FIGURE 62.4 Comparison of the amino acid sequences of cholecystokinin (CCK)-8 and ceruletide.

Invasive Tests of Exocrine Pancreatic Function

Total volume of pancreatic juice, the amount of concentration of bicarbonate, and activities of the pancreatic enzymes, amylase, lipase, and trypsin, are measured in duodenal fluid. The Lundh test consists of administering a standardized meal consisting of 6% fat, 15% carbohydrate, and 74% nonnutrient fiber that provides a physiologic stimulus to the pancreas. It is, however, no longer in routine use and is largely of historical interest only.

The secretin-cholecystokinin test is based on the principle that secretion of pancreatic juice and bicarbonate output are related to the functional mass of the pancreas. After an overnight fast a tube is sited in the duodenum to permit the collection of pancreatic juices. Secretin (1 unit/kg body weight) is given intravenously, and the duodenal fluid collected at 15-minute intervals for at least 1 hour. Secretin stimulates the secretion of pancreatic juice and bicarbonate. CCK (or the synthetic equivalent, ceruletide, the C-terminal octapeptide sequence of the intact hormone, where the functional activity resides, Fig. 62.4) then can be given to stimulate the secretion of pancreatic enzymes, allowing a more complete assessment of pancreatic reserve than can be obtained with secretin alone. The secretin-cholecystokinin or secretin-ceruletide tests are considered the gold standard test for assessing pancreatic exocrine function. Although seldom used in adults, this test is still used in infants with pancreatic insufficiency to distinguish between CF and Schwachman-Diamond syndrome (pancreatic α-cell aplasia). In the former, mucous plugs reduce pancreatic secretion but the enzyme concentrations increase in a normal physiologic response to cholescystokinin, whereas in the latter enzyme secretion is absent or minimal.

Noninvasive Tests of Exocrine Pancreatic Function

A range of tubeless tests have been proposed, but none has adequate sensitivity for reliably detecting early pancreatic disease. When malabsorption is present, such tests are of value in confirming or excluding pancreatic disease. Considerable overlap often occurs between results observed in normal individuals and those found in patients with pancreatic disease; this is due mainly to the large functional reserve of the pancreas. It has been estimated that pancreatic insufficiency cannot clearly be demonstrated until at least 50% of the acinar cells have been destroyed. Clinical signs of pancreatic insufficiency often do not appear until 90% of acinar tissue has been destroyed.

The noninvasive tests are based on the reduction in secretion of pancreatic enzymes with measurement of the enzymes in feces (chymotrypsin or elastase) or detection of products of their catalytic reactions, after oral administration of synthetic substrates, in urine (N-benzoyl-L-tyrosine-*p*-aminobenzoic acid (NBT-PABA) or pancreolauryl test), or in breath (^{13}C mixed-chain triglyceride breath test). The NBT-PABA and pancreolauryl substrates are no longer commercially available, and measurement of fecal elastase is currently the noninvasive method of choice for assessing pancreatic insufficiency.

Pancreatic chymotrypsin is almost completely digested in its passage through the gut in adults, but the residual activity of the enzyme in feces is stable for several days at room temperature. Its output in stool correlates poorly with chymotrypsin secretion in duodenal contents when both are measured after stimulation with secretin-CCK. In patients without pancreatic disease, the incidence of falsely low results is approximately 10 to 15% and may be due to voluminous stools (>300 g/24 h) and thus less enzyme per gram of feces; inadequate food intake; partial gastrectomy or mucosal disease (eg, celiac disease), which causes inadequate stimulation of pancreatic secretion; or obstruction of the common bile duct. Falsely normal results in patients with mild pancreatic insufficiency may be as high as 50%.[134] In a collaborative study in children, both fecal chymotrypsin and elastase showed 100% sensitivity for detecting pancreatic insufficiency in CF; but the specificity of chymotrypsin was lower than that of elastase in a control group of children with small intestinal disease.[135]

Pancreatic elastase-1 is a pancreas-specific protease present in pancreatic juice. It is not degraded during passage through the gut, and concentrations in feces are fivefold to sixfold greater than those in pancreatic juice.[136] The enzyme can be measured by ELISA with two monoclonal antibodies specific to the human enzyme. Treatment of patients with pancreatic enzyme supplements therefore does not interfere with the test. Fecal elastase-1 has been evaluated extensively in both CF and adult pancreatic insufficiency, and its use is recommended in both groups.[76,137] Fecal elastase is often undetectable (<15 μg/g) in children with CF, and values below 200 μg/g after 4 weeks of age are indicative of pancreatic insufficiency.

The test has been evaluated in adults against the secretin-CCK test[138-140] and in patients whose diagnosis of chronic pancreatitis has been made on the basis of anatomic and morphologic changes detected by ultrasound and endoscopic retrograde pancreatography or CT.[134,141,142] The test is routinely carried out on a small random fecal sample; thus it might be expected to give inferior diagnostic accuracy compared to evaluations carried out on portions of 24- or 72-hour fecal collections. However, with random fecal samples, specificities of 98% and 100% have been reported in healthy controls and specificities of 90% to 97% in patients with nonpancreatic GI disease. Positive results (ie, <200 μg/g) have been reported in patients with clinical or laboratory evidence of malnutrition who also have IBD or chronic diarrhea (nonpancreatic). These conditions may actually be due to impaired pancreatic

TABLE 62.5 **Characteristics of Prominent Forms of Principal Gut Regulatory Peptides**

Hormone/ Peptide	Molecular Weight (Da)	No. of Amino Acids	Main Gut Localization	Principal Physiologic Action
Gastrin Family				
Cholecystokinin	3918	33	Duodenum and jejunum	Stimulates gallbladder contraction and intestinal motility; stimulates secretion of pancreatic enzymes, insulin, glucagon, and pancreatic polypeptides; has a role in indicating satiety; the C-terminal 8–amino acid peptide (CCK-8) retains full activity
Gastrin-17	2098	17	Gastric antrum and duodenum	Stimulates the secretion of gastric acid pepsinogen, intrinsic factor, and secretin; stimulates intestinal mucosal growth; increase gastric and intestinal motility
Gastrin	3839	34		
Secretin-Glucagon Family				
Secretin	3056	27	Duodenum	Stimulates pancreatic and jejunum secretion of bicarbonate, enzymes and insulin; reduces gastric and intestinal motility, inhibits gastrin release and gastric acid secretion
VIP	3326	28	Enteric nerves	Relaxes smooth muscle of gut, blood, and genitourinary system; increases water and electrolyte secretion from the pancreas and gut; releases hormones from pancreas, gut and hypothalamus
GIP	4976	42	Duodenum and jejunum	Stimulates insulin release; reduces gastric and intestinal motility; increases fluid and electrolyte secretion from the small intestine

GIP, Glucose-dependent insulinotropic peptide; *VIP*, vasoactive intestinal polypeptide.

secretion as a consequence of malnutrition.[142] The authors also suggest that increased bacterial degradation of the enzyme might be the cause of false-positive findings in some patients with bacterial overgrowth. Similar results have been reported in children with nonpancreatic disease; the finding of low fecal elastase in a child with steatorrhea probably indicates coexisting pancreatic insufficiency.[135]

Measurement of pancreatic elastase-1 in feces has high sensitivity for the detection of severe and moderate chronic pancreatitis in adults. It has better sensitivity than other tests for detecting mild chronic pancreatitis and high sensitivity and high negative predictive value for discriminating between diarrhea of pancreatic and nonpancreatic origin. The test is not specific for pancreatitis and detects moderate to severe impairment of pancreatic exocrine secretion from any cause. It is considered to be the most suitable test to confirm pancreatic insufficiency in CF infants older than 2 weeks.[129] A negative test does not exclude mild disease and false-positive results in some nonpancreatic diseases and in very watery samples limit its diagnostic accuracy.

Gastrointestinal Regulatory Peptides

The gut is the largest endocrine organ in the body[23] but is also a major target for many hormones released locally or from other organs. GI regulatory peptides are released from the pancreatic islets (eg, somatostatin) or from endocrine cells spread throughout the gut mucosa and collectively known as the diffuse endocrine system. Many of these peptides (such as vasoactive inhibitory peptide [VIP] and somatostatin) are present in the enteric nerves. They are also found in the central nervous system (CNS) and have important roles in the neuroendocrine control of the gut. Although many of them (eg, secretin and gastrin) fulfil the classic criteria for a hormone by acting on distant cells, others function as neurotransmitters or have local (paracrine) effects on adjacent cells. Collectively, they influence the motility, secretion, digestion, and absorption in the gut. They regulate bile flow and secretion of pancreatic hormones and affect the tonicity of the vascular walls, blood pressure, and cardiac output.

Table 62.5 summarizes the basic chemical characteristics of four of the major GI regulatory peptides and indicates their site of origin and main functions. More detailed descriptions of these peptides are given in the following paragraphs. A list of other regulatory peptides of the GI tract is presented in Table 62.6.

Cholecystokinin

CCK is a linear polypeptide that exists in multiple molecular forms.[22,23] The first form to be isolated was the 33–amino acid peptide CCK-33. Other major forms are CCK-8, CCK-39, and CCK-58. In all forms, the five terminal amino acids are identical to those of gastrin and are necessary, together with a sulfated tyrosyl residue, for physiologic activity. All forms of CCK are produced by enzymatic cleavage of a single 115–amino acid precursor, preprocholecystokinin.

CCK is found in the I-cells of the upper small intestinal mucosa. Mixtures of polypeptides and amino acids (especially tryptophan and phenylalanine) stimulate CCK secretion, whereas pure undigested protein does not elicit a response. Secretion is also stimulated by gastric acid entering the duodenum and by fatty acids with chains of nine or more carbons, especially in the form of micelles. Circulating concentrations of CCK are therefore increased following ingestion of a mixed meal. CCK is rapidly cleared from plasma ($t_{1/2}$

TABLE 62.6 Brief Description of Other Gastrointestinal Regulatory Peptides

Hormone/Peptide	Major Tissue Location	Principal Known Actions
Bombesin	Throughout the gut and pancreas	Stimulates release of CCK and gastrin
Calcitonin gene-related peptide	Enteric nerves	Unclear
Chromogranin A	Neuroendocrine cells	Secretory protein
Enkephalins	Stomach, duodenum	Opiate-like actions
Enteroglucagon	Small intestine, pancreas	Inhibits insulin secretion
Ghrelin	Stomach	Stimulates appetite, increases gastric emptying
GLP-1	Pancreas, ileum	Increases insulin secretion
GLP-2	Ileum, colon	Enterocyte-specific growth hormone
Leptin	Stomach	Appetite control
Motilin	Throughout the gut	Increases gastric emptying and small bowel motility
Neuropeptide Y	Enteric nerves	Regulation of intestinal blood flow
Neurotensin	Ileum	Affects gut motility; increases jejunal and ileal fluid secretion
Pancreastatin	Pancreas	Inhibits pancreatic endocrine and exocrine secretion
Pancreatic polypeptide	Pancreas	Inhibits pancreatic and biliary secretion
PYY	Colon	Inhibits food intake
Somatostatin	Stomach, pancreas	Inhibits secretion and action of many hormones

GLP, Glucagon-like peptide; *PYY,* peptide tyrosine tyrosine.

<3 min), predominantly by the kidneys. Secretion of CCK is completely inhibited after somatostatin infusion.

CCK regulates gallbladder contraction and increases small intestinal motility. It possesses the same terminal pentapeptide as gastrin and therefore has a mild stimulatory effect on gastric acid and pepsinogen secretion, antral motility, and pancreatic bicarbonate secretion. Secretion of the less potent CCK results in decreased output of acid because CCK competes with gastrin for receptor sites on the acid-secreting cells. Conversely, gastrin and CCK are additive in their stimulation of the pancreas and both increase the effects of secretin on pancreatic function. CCK also stimulates pancreatic growth, relaxes the sphincter of Oddi, and stimulates secretion from Brunner (duodenal) glands.

CCK is also present in the brain, with highest concentrations in the cerebral cortex, and the peripheral nervous system; its function in the CNS is unclear. It is released from the GI tract and acts as a short-term, meal-related satiety signal, thus contributing to the regulation of appetite.

Secretin

Secretin, a linear polypeptide containing 27 amino acids, has structural similarities to those of glucagon, VIP, gastric inhibitory polypeptide (GIP) and growth hormone–releasing hormone GHRH. The amino acid residues at 14 positions within the molecule are identical to those found in glucagon; 8 are the same as in GIP, and 9 are the same as in VIP. The intact secretin molecule is required for biological activity.

Secretin is secreted by mucosal S cells located in greatest concentration in the duodenum but present throughout the small intestine. It is released primarily on contact of the S cells with gastric hydrochloric acid; however, as pancreatic juice flows into the duodenum, it neutralizes gastric acid and thereby removes one stimulus for its own secretion. Secretin is not released until the pH is lowered to at least 4.5. Below this pH, secretin release is proportional to the amount of acid entering the duodenum. A pH less than 4.5 normally occurs only in the first few centimeters of the duodenum, with the result that there is little increase in secretin release after a normal meal. Thus secretin release after exposure of S cells to acid may not be an important physiologic stimulus. However, plasma secretin concentrations that are too low to be measured by current methods may stimulate the pancreas in the presence of physiologic concentration of CCK, which is known to strongly potentiate the action of secretin. Undigested fat does not stimulate secretin release, but fatty acids with chains of 10 or more carbons are weak stimulants. Alcohol increases secretin release through stimulation of gastric acid secretion with subsequent lowering of duodenal pH rather than by a direct stimulatory effect. The half-life of secretin is approximately 4 minutes. The kidney is the major site of its degradation. The only known physiologic inhibitor of secretin release is somatostatin.

The primary physiologic role of secretin is stimulation of the pancreas to secrete an increased volume of juice with high bicarbonate content. Other actions include stimulation of bicarbonate and water secretion from the liver and Brunner glands; augmentation of gallbladder contraction and increased hepatic blood flow; weak stimulation of insulin secretion; stimulation of parathyroid hormone secretion; release of pancreatic enzymes and pepsinogen by the chief cells of the stomach; reduction of gastric and duodenal motility; reduction of lower esophageal sphincter pressure; and promotion of pancreatic growth. Secretin inhibits normal gastric secretion (but does not decrease plasma gastrin in the Zollinger-Ellison syndrome) and therefore gastric acid secretion.

Vasoactive Intestinal Polypeptide

VIP is a linear polypeptide consisting of 28 amino acids with structural similarities to those of secretin, GIP, and glucagon. VIP is a neurotransmitter, present throughout the body, and is found in highest concentrations in the nervous system and gut. Unlike secretin and other GI hormones, VIP is not found in the mucosal endocrine cells of the GI tract. VIP-containing nerve fibers are found throughout the GI tract from the esophagus to the colon and in all tissue layers of the gut.

Little is known about the conditions that cause VIP to be released into the circulation. No evidence suggests that VIP is released during digestion, but its secretion is increased by vagal stimulation. It has a plasma half-life of approximately 1 minute, and most of the hormone is inactivated by a single passage through the liver.

VIP has a large number of ill-defined physiologic actions, some of which are shared with other similar polypeptide hormones (secretin and GIP). It acts as a neurotransmitter in the central and autonomic nervous systems and causes vasodilatation and relaxation of the circulatory and genitourinary systems and the gut. Other actions of VIP include an increase of water and electrolyte secretion from the pancreas and gut; release of hormones from the pancreas, gut, and hypothalamus; stimulation of lipolysis, glycolysis, and bile flow; and inhibition of gastrin and gastric acid secretion. Most of the actions of VIP tend to be of short duration because of its rapid degradation.

Gastric Inhibitory Polypeptide

GIP is a linear polypeptide consisting of 42 amino acids. Its N-terminal end has a close resemblance to those of glucagon and secretin, but the C-terminal amino acid sequence of 17 residues is not common to any other known intestinal hormone.

GIP is synthesized and released by K cells located in the duodenal and jejunal mucosa. Plasma GIP is increased by oral administration of glucose or triacylglycerols or intraduodenal infusion of solutions containing a mixture of amino acids; none of these however, increases GIP concentrations when given intravenously. Protein ingestion does not significantly increase GIP. For food components to stimulate GIP they must be absorbed by the intestinal mucosa.

The biological actions of GIP include stimulation of insulin secretion in the presence of hyperglycemia, reduction of intestinal motility with stimulation of small intestine fluid and electrolyte secretion, and (in supraphysiologic concentrations) inhibition of gastric acid, pepsin, and gastrin secretion. The insulinotrophic action of GIP appears to be the most important of its biological actions; as a result, this hormone has been called glucose-dependent insulinotrophic peptide as a more accurate description of its physiologic action.

Gastrointestinal Neuroendocrine Tumors and Tumor Markers

GI neuroendocrine tumors may be endocrine pancreatic tumors or carcinoid tumors arising from enterochromaffin cells that occur throughout the GI tract. Carcinoid tumors are described in Chapter 63. Approximately two-thirds of patients with tumors arising from pancreatic islet cells present with excessive hormone production. This group of tumors includes insulinomas, gastrinomas, VIPomas, glucagonomas, and somatostatinomas. Insulinomas and glucagonomas are not usually associated with GI symptoms. Gastrinomas were discussed earlier. The somatostatinoma syndrome is associated with steatorrhea, gallstones, and hyperglycemia.[143]

The watery diarrhea hypokalemic achlorhydria syndrome (Werner-Morrison syndrome, WDHA syndrome) is a consequence of a tumor producing excessive amounts of VIP. The WDHA syndrome may be suspected in a patient who produces large volumes (>1 L/24 h) of secretory diarrhea with dehydration and hypokalemia. The diagnosis is confirmed by the finding of a high plasma VIP concentration and demonstration of somatostatin-receptor uptake on imaging.

The remaining one-third of patients with neuroendocrine tumors have no specific clinical symptoms associated with the tumors, which are described as nonfunctional.

The pattern of hormonal and precursor production by neuroendocrine tumors is complex. Most secrete several tumor markers. Chromogranin A, a member of a family of secretory proteins, has a diagnostic sensitivity of more than 90% for neuroendocrine tumors. Plasma chromogranin A concentration is elevated in most tumors and is an alternative to more specific markers in monitoring the effectiveness of therapy. Although chromogranin A has high sensitivity, false-positive findings have been observed in several nonendocrine tumors, including prostate cancer.[144]

Chromogranin A has been reported to be slightly increased in IBD and also in other malignancies, including lung, prostate, breast, and uterine. It is increased by the use of PPIs and hydrogen receptor blockers, which can be problematic because many patients suspected of having a neuroendocrine tumor may have started on these in primary care. Chromogranin A is renally excreted so significant renal dysfunction increases the concentration. For these reasons, chromogranin A is usually considered to be a marker of prognosis and for monitoring response to therapy rather than a diagnostic tool.

Investigation of Maldigestion and Malabsorption

This section summarizes causes of malabsorption and suggests a general laboratory approach to these disorders. Table 62.7 summarizes the main causes of malabsorption under the three categories of intraluminal disorders and malabsorption secondary to disorders of either transport into the mucosal cells or transport out of the mucosal cells.

TABLE 62.7 Summary of Disorders Leading to Malabsorption

Disorders of Intraluminal Digestion	
a. Altered gastric function	Postgastrectomy syndrome, Zollinger-Ellison syndrome
b. Pancreatic insufficiency	Chronic pancreatitis, cystic fibrosis, pancreatic cancer
c. Bile acid deficiency	Disease/resection of terminal ileum, small bowel overgrowth
Disorders of Transport Into the Mucosal Cell	
a. Generalized disorders due to reduction in absorptive surface area	Celiac disease, tropical sprue
b. Specific disorders	Hypolactasia, vitamin B_{12} in pernicious anemia, zinc in acrodermatitis enteropathica
Disorders of Transport Out of the Mucosal Cell	
a. Blockage of the lymphatics	Primary lymphangiectasia Abdominal lymphoma
b. Inherited disorders	Abetalipoproteinemia

The clinical presentation of a patient with malabsorption or maldigestion classically includes the following features:

Evidence of general ill health. Anorexia, weight loss, fatigue after minor effort, and dyspnea may be seen. Edema (due to hypoalbuminemia), tetany (low plasma calcium concentration) and dehydration secondary to electrolyte imbalance and water loss may be present. In exocrine pancreatic insufficiency, however, hyperphagia is the rule: patients may often report a very high (5000 kcal/d, 21,000 kJoules/day) food intake without weight gain.

Isolated nutrient deficiencies. Iron, folate, or vitamin B_{12} deficiency may manifest as anemia, which may be mild; vitamin K deficiency as a bleeding tendency; and vitamin D deficiency as bone disease. They are reflected by a variety of signs and symptoms (glossitis, pallor, dermatitis, petechiae, bruising, hematuria, muscle or bone pain, or neurologic abnormalities).

Abdominal symptoms. These include discomfort, distention, flatulence, and borborygmi (rumbling and gurgling sounds resulting from movement of gas in the intestine).

Watery diarrhea and possible steatorrhea. In severe cases of steatorrhea the stool is typically loose, bulky, offensive, greasy, light-colored, and difficult to flush away. Alternatively, the stools may appear normal but may be more bulky or be passed more frequently.

Early manifestation of malabsorption will, however, be more subtle than this list might indicate. The alteration in volume or consistency of the stool may be slight, and only mild symptoms may be attributable to the GI tract. The patient may report only anorexia, fatigue, and lack of interest in daily activities. It is in these cases that the astute physician who suspects malabsorption on clinical grounds will rely on the laboratory to assist in the diagnosis. Initial laboratory investigations consist of routine tests, with abnormalities that may indicate the possibility of malabsorption (eg, blood hemoglobin concentration, mean red cell volume, serum concentrations of folate, ferritin, calcium, albumin, liver enzyme activities, and tests for antibodies in celiac disease).

Evaluation of Fat Absorption

The evaluation of fat absorption or malabsorption is required in only a small minority of patients undergoing investigation for GI disorders, because a firm diagnosis often can be made on clinical grounds alone. The guidelines of the British Society of Gastroenterology state that gastroenterologists should have access to such tests to "assess patients with malabsorption who are proving difficult to diagnose".[145]

Historically the assessment of fat malabsorption was carried out by measurement of fecal fat excretion in a timed (2 to 3 days) fecal collection. This had many limitations and is seldom performed today. Box 62.8 indicates a range of alternative tests that were proposed. Most of these have limitations similar to those for fecal fat measurement, in either their sensitivity and specificity or analytical constraints. Currently, investigation of fat malabsorption is limited to measurement of fecal elastase (see earlier discussion) to identify exocrine pancreatic insufficiency with consequent reduction in secretion of lipase. The ^{13}C mixed-chain triglyceride breath test uses ^{13}C-labeled medium- and long-chain fatty acids as a means of assessing intraluminal pancreatic lipase activity. The labeled substrate is administered orally with a standard meal of toast and butter. Breath samples are collected over a 5-hour period and exhaled $^{13}CO_2$ is expressed as a percentage of the administered dose, with normal excretion in the range of 25% to 40%. The sensitivity and specificity of the test for identifying pancreatic insufficiency has been reported as 89% and 81%, respectively.[146] Similar results have been reported for the ^{14}C-triolein test using a variety of fat loads and procedures.[147] The disadvantage of this test is the need to measure the ^{14}C-labeled CO_2 immediately, which requires the availability of a scintillation counter and facilities for the administration of radioisotopes.

BOX 62.8 Tests for Assessing Fat Absorption and Malabsorption

Measurement of Fecal Fat
- Problems of poor recovery during sample collection (requires use of markers) inadequate dietary fat (minimum of 70 g/d), inaccurate analysis and uncertain interpretation

Butter Fat Test
- Unreliable, poor discrimination

$^{13/14}C$-glyceryl trioleate
- Sensitivity 85%, specificity 93%

Mixed-Chain Triglyceride Breath Test
- Valid test for pancreatic steatorrhea

Fat Globules (Fecal Microscopy)
- Need for standardized procedure

Investigation of Chronic Diarrhea

Although diarrhea is a common problem, no clear definition has existed to distinguish it from the range of stool weight, frequency, consistency, or volume that occurs in the normal population. A 2003 proposal that sought to encompass these different elements suggests that for a Western diet, diarrhea may be defined as "the abnormal passage of loose or liquid stools more than three times daily and/or a volume of stool greater than 200 g/day."[76] Guidelines suggest that diarrhea may be defined as chronic when it has continued for 4 weeks or more; such persistence indicates the likelihood of a non-infectious cause requiring further investigation.

Several quite different mechanisms can lead to diarrhea. In carbohydrate malabsorption, the presence of unabsorbed solutes in the bowel causes osmotic diarrhea as water enters the bowel from tissue. By contrast, the diarrhea of most cases of laxative abuse or VIPomas is due to active secretion of water and electrolytes into the bowel, which is described as secondary diarrhea. IBD causes diarrhea as a consequence of the inflammatory process.

Many diseases more commonly thought to cause "diarrhea" in fact lead to more frequent passage of stools but not usually to an increased stool weight (or volume). Such disorders (eg, IBS) generally fall outside the scope of the definition of chronic diarrhea. Guidelines for the management of IBS are available, and the best results are achieved with an integrated approach to the problem involving clinicians with a special interest, dietitians, a psychiatric-psychologic approach, etc.[148,149]

Box 62.9 describes the many causes of chronic diarrhea; most are due to disease of the colon, in which laboratory

BOX 62.9 Causes of Chronic Diarrhea

Colonic
- Ulcerative colitis
- Crohn disease
- Microscopic colitis

Small Bowel
- Celiac disease
- Small bowel enteropathies (eg, Crohn disease, Whipple disease, tropical sprue, amyloidosis, intestinal lymphangectasia)
- Bile salt malabsorption
- Disaccharidase deficiency
- Small bowel bacterial overgrowth
- Lymphoma
- Giardiasis (and other chronic infections)
- Irritable bowel syndrome

Endocrine
- Hyperthyroidism
- Diabetes
- Hypoparathyroidism
- Addison disease
- Neuroendocrine tumors (eg, VIPoma, carcinoid tumors)

Other
- Chronic laxative abuse (eg, bulemia nervosa)
- Surgical causes (eg, small bowel resection, internal fistulas)
- Drugs and alcohol
- Autonomic neuropathy

Modified from Thomas PD, Forbes A, Green J, Howdle P, Long R, Playford R et al. Guidelines for the investigation of chronic diarrhoea. 2nd edition. *Gut* 2003;52(suppl V):1–15.

diagnostic tests are of little value with the exception of fecal calprotectin for the differentiation of IBS from IBD.

Laxative Abuse

Surreptitious laxative abuse is an important cause of diarrhea that is often overlooked. It may be as common as 20% of cases in secondary or tertiary referral centers.[150,151] In Munchausen syndrome by proxy, adults have administered laxatives surreptitiously to young children. A clinical diagnosis rarely can be made; no single clinical feature reliably predicts a positive test making laboratory support essential. When there is a high index of clinical suspicion urine screens for laxatives may be beneficial.

The pattern of laxative abuse has changed following legislation in several countries banning over-the-counter sales of laxatives containing phenolphthalein, traditionally the most widely abused laxative. Other laxatives encountered by clinical laboratories include colonic stimulants containing bisacodyl or anthraquinones (eg, senna, aloin, cascara). Their absorption, metabolism, and excretion have been reviewed.[152] Magnesium salts are the active ingredients in some over-the-counter laxatives; these may also be abused. Most screens for laxatives are still carried out using thin layer chromatography (TLC), but their interpretation is subjective, requiring experienced staff, and they are slowly being replaced by methods based on gas chromatography–mass spectrometry.[152]

BOX 62.10 Causes of the Acute Abdomen

Common Causes
- Acute appendicitis
- Acute cholecystitis, ascending cholangitis
- Small and large bowel obstruction
- Intussusception, volvulus and strangulated hernias
- Renal/ureteric colic
- Perforated peptic/duodenal ulcer
- Acute pancreatitis
- Acute diverticulitis
- Gynecological conditions (eg, ectopic pregnancy, salpingitis)
- Ruptured aortic aneurysm
- Mesenteric lymphadenitis

Less Common Causes
- Gastroenteritis including *Salmonella, Shigella, Yersinia,* measles virus, etc.
- Crohn disease
- Pyelonephritis
- Meckel diverticulitis
- Acute intermittent porphyria

Conditions That May Simulate the Acute Abdomen
- Myocardial infarction or myocarditis

The Acute Abdomen

The acute abdomen is defined as undiagnosed intense abdominal pain lasting less than 1 week. Many of the diseases that present in this way have a high mortality if not treated surgically, but others may have high morbidity and mortality if surgical intervention is carried out. The clinical diagnosis is based primarily on the nature of the pain. Common causes of the acute abdomen are detailed in Box 62.10. Nonabdominal conditions may simulate an acute abdomen. History and examination often yield a likely diagnosis, but laboratory investigations may help in establishing the diagnosis (eg, pregnancy test in suspected ectopic pregnancy, serum amylase, or lipase in acute pancreatitis). A full blood count may reveal a raised neutrophil count suggestive of infection or anemia secondary to blood loss from the GI tract. Knowledge of renal function and acid-base status is important if surgery is being considered.

Acute Pancreatitis

Acute pancreatitis is an acute inflammatory condition of the pancreas that may have a self-limiting short course but can be fatal. Almost all patients with acute pancreatitis have severe epigastric pain, usually of sudden onset and often radiating to the back. In more severe cases, there is nausea and vomiting, fever, hypotension, shock, and multiorgan failure that may lead to death. Biochemical features of acute pancreatitis include uremia, hypoalbuminemia, hypokalemia, hyperglycemia, metabolic acidosis, hypoxemia, and abnormal liver tests. None of these are invariably present or diagnostic for pancreatitis. In acute necrotizing pancreatitis, methemalbuminemia may be detectable. The use of enzyme measurements in the diagnosis of acute pancreatitis is explained in Chapter 29.

AT A GLANCE

Causes of Acute Pancreatitis

- Gallstones
- Alcohol excess
- Drugs
- Hypertriglyceridemia
- Hypercalcemia
- Trauma
- Infections
- Rare causes, including tumors

SELECTED REFERENCES

For a full list of references for this chapter, please refer to ExpertConsult.com.

3. Lindsay J, Langmead L, Preston S. Gastrointestinal disease. In: Kumar P, Clark M, editors. *Clinical medicine*. 8th ed. Edinburgh: Saunders; 2012.
17. Malfertheiner P, Megraud F, O'Morain C, et al. Current concepts in the management of *Helicobacter pylori* infection: the Maastricht III Consensus Report. *Gut* 2007;**56**:772–81.
23. Barakat MT, Meeran K, Bloom SR. Neuroendocrine tumours. *Endocr Relat Cancer* 2004;**11**:1–18.
33. van Heel DA, West J. Recent advances in celiac disease. *Gut* 2006;1037–46.
48. Armstrong D, Don-Wauchope AC, Verdu EF. Testing for gluten-related disorders in clinical practice: the role of serology in managing the spectrum of gluten sensitivity. *Can J Gastroenterol* 2011;**5**:193–7.
69. Kumar PJ, Clark ML. Malabsorption and weight loss. In: Bloom S, editor. *Practical gastroenterology*. London: Martin Dunitz; 2002. p. 371–82.
74. Smith MJ, Cherian P, Raju GS, et al. Bile acid malabsorption in persistent diarrhoea. *J R Coll Physicians Lond* 2000;**34**:448–51.
75. Thomas PD, Forbes A, Green J, et al. Guidelines for the investigation of chronic diarrhoea. *Gut* 2003;**52**(Suppl. V): v1–15.
84. Ponder A, Long MD. A clinical review of recent findings in the epidemiology of inflammatory bowel disease. *Clin Epidemiol* 2013;**5**:237–47.
88. Sherwood RA. Faecal markers. *J Clin Path* 2012;**65**: 981–5.
95. Gisbert JP, McNicholl AG. Questions and answers on the role of faecal calprotectin as a biological marker in inflammatory bowel disease. *Dig Liver Dis* 2009;**41**:56–66.
108. Walsham NE, Sherwood RA. Fecal calprotectin in inflammatory bowel disease. *Clin Exp Gastroenterol* 2016;**9**:1–9.
118. Yarur AJ, Abreu MT, Deshpande AR, et al. Therapeutic drug monitoring in patients with inflammatory bowel disease. *World J Gastroenterol* 2014;**20**:3475–84.
121. Papadia C, Sherwood RA, Kalantzis C, et al. Plasma citrulline concentration: a reliable marker of small bowel absorptive capacity independent of intestinal inflammation. *Am J Gastroenterol* 2007;**102**:1–9.
129. Leus J, Van Biervliet S, Robberecht E. Detection and follow up of exocrine pancreatic insufficiency in cystic fibrosis: a review. *Eur J Pediatr* 2000;**159**:563–8.
131. Masamune A. Genetics of pancreatitis: the 2014 update. *Tohoku J Exp Med* 2014;**232**:69–77.
142. Masoero G, Zaffino C, Laudi C, et al. Fecal pancreatic elastase 1 in the work up of patients with chronic diarrhea. *Int J Pancreatol* 2000;**28**:175–9.
143. Ardill JES. Circulating markers for endocrine tumors of the gastrointestinal tract. *Ann Clin Biochem* 2008;**45**: 539–59.
145. Thomas PD, Forbes A, Green J, et al. Guidelines for the investigation of chronic diarrhoea. *Gut* 2003;**52**(Suppl. V): v1–15.
152. Duncan A. Screening for surreptitious laxative abuse. *Ann Clin Biochem* 2000;**37**:1–8.

63

Monoamine-Producing Tumors

Graeme Eisenhofer, Stefan Grebe, and Nai-Kong V. Cheung

ABSTRACT

Background

Monoamine-producing tumors include neuroblastomas, pheochromocytomas, paragangliomas, and gastroentero-pancreatic neuroendocrine tumors (GEP-NETs). Synthesis, storage, and secretion of biogenic amines, polypeptide hormones, and proteins are key features of these tumors that both underlie their clinical manifestations and provide a means for laboratory diagnosis. The clinical characteristics and related patterns and types of hormones produced by the tumors are highly heterogeneous. Consequently, no single biomarker can reliably diagnose any tumor group. The heterogeneity not only reflects a host of underlying genetic mutations and downstream tumorigenic pathways but also progenitor cell susceptibility to specific mutations and from which the tumors develop.

Content

This chapter describes the structure, function, and developmental biology of peripheral monoamine systems and provides a comprehensive overview of the laboratory and clinical aspects of various monoamine-producing tumors. Neuroblastomas present in early childhood and develop from neural crest cells halted in their differentiation at the neuroblast stage, from which they can either spontaneously regress or follow an aggressive clinical course. Biochemical diagnosis depends mainly on measurements of urinary homovanillic acid and vanillylmandelic acid, biomarkers that often fail to detect the aggressive forms of disease. Pheochromocytomas and paragangliomas, which also develop from neural crest–derived chromaffin progenitors, are more readily detected by plasma or urinary normetanephrine, metanephrine, or methoxytyramine. Production of these metabolites varies depending on the underlying mutations. GEP-NETs secrete more variable products, requiring careful considerations and interpretation according to clinical manifestations. Choice, interpretation, and development of laboratory tests can be facilitated by an understanding of the underlying biology of monoamine-producing tumors.

64

Bone and Mineral Metabolism

*William D. Fraser**

ABSTRACT

Background

The skeletal system is one of the largest organs in the body and is one of the hallmarks that distinguishes vertebrates from invertebrates. It is the storehouse for 98% to 99% of the body's 1 kg of calcium. Bones are mineralized connective tissue in which type I collagen forms a network of flexible fibers. Mineralization of this network, or matrix, with calcium salts is required to produce the rigid skeleton. Bone is a living tissue that is constantly being remodeled by degradation of old tissue and replacement with new bone matrix. Osteoclasts and osteoblasts are the bone cells mainly responsible for remodeling. Osteocytes are important regulators of bone cell activity that can be estimated by laboratory methods.

Calcium is required for mineralization of bone and is a key regulator of many body processes. Calcium ions play critical roles in intracellular signaling, in regulation of events at the plasma membrane, and in the function of extracellular proteins such as those involved in blood coagulation. The circulating concentration of calcium ions is kept constant under the control of parathyroid hormone (PTH) and metabolites of vitamin D. Deviations of the concentration of free (unbound) calcium outside its very narrow reference interval can cause morbidity and mortality. The importance of the tight regulation of free calcium is underscored by the recognition that skeletal health is allowed to suffer markedly to allow physiologic processes in other organs to be maintained.

Phosphate is also important in bone mineralization and is a component of high-energy molecules. Fibroblast growth factor 23 (FGF23) is involved in regulation of phosphate in combination with PTH and vitamin D metabolites. Bone is increasingly recognized as having endocrine functions playing an important role in regulating metabolic processes.

Content

This chapter provides an overview of skeletal metabolism and then details the clinical chemistry of calcium and other ions, including phosphate and magnesium. Key molecules regulating these minerals in health and disease are described. Measurement of markers of bone metabolism, and the role of molecules involved in major disorders of bone and mineral metabolism are discussed.

OVERVIEW OF SKELETAL METABOLISM

Bone is composed primarily of an extracellular mineralized matrix with a smaller cellular fraction. Bone is a dynamic tissue that is under continuous turnover or *remodeling,* which enables bone to repair damage and adjust strength. *Osteoclasts* and *osteoblasts* are two main types of bone cells located on bone surfaces and are responsible for bone resorption and formation, respectively. *Osteocytes,* the most abundant cells in mature bone, are located in lacunae within the bone matrix. Osteoclasts resorb bone, osteoblasts lay down new bone at a site of previous bone resorption, and osteocytes nourish the skeleton and regulate bone cell activity (Fig. 64.1). Bone remodeling does not occur at random, but occurs instead in discrete packets known as *bone remodeling units.* Bone resorption and bone formation normally are coupled, with synthesis of new bone following the resorption of old. During perimenopause, the remodeling rate is often increased, but with excess resorption (a negative bone balance). The remodeling cycle can be divided into activation, resorption, reversal, formation, and termination/resting phases.

Circulating mononuclear osteoclast precursors are recruited, proliferate, and fuse to form giant multinucleate osteoclasts that resorb bone by producing hydrogen ions to mobilize minerals and lysosomal enzymes to digest the organic matrix. Deep folds of the plasma membrane (ruffled border) are in contact with the bone surface, forming the osteoclastic bone-resorbing compartment (Fig. 64.2). The resorption lacuna contains degradative enzymes such as collagenases, cathepsin K, and several matrix metalloproteinases (MMPs). After resorption ceases, a cement line is deposited in the resorption cavity. Stromal lining cells differentiate to osteoblasts. Osteoblasts form bone by synthesizing the organic matrix, including type I collagen, and participating in the mineralization of newly synthesized matrix. The development of the osteoblast phenotype has been divided into three consecutive phases, each with its typical gene-expression patterns (Fig. 64.3).[1] Osteoblasts/osteoprogenitor cells that are trapped within the bone matrix can develop into osteocytes with mechanosensory properties that can communicate with other bone cells via a network of dendritic processes within canaliculi.

The organic matrix of bone is primarily type I collagen (90%) combined with lesser amounts of a large number of

*The author gratefully acknowledges the contributions to previous editions by Drs. David B. Endres, Michael Kleerekoper, Juha Risteli, Leila Risteli, and Robert K. Rude, upon which portions of this chapter are based.

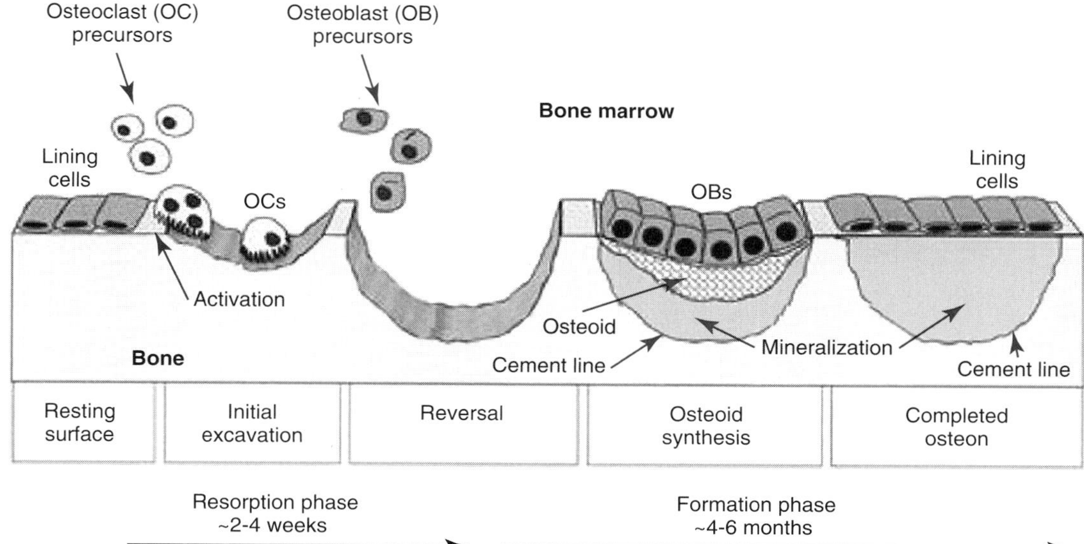

FIGURE 64.1 **Bone Remodeling Sequence.** A cartoon depiction of the sequential action of osteoclasts and osteoblasts in removing old bone and replacing it with new bone. For simplicity of illustration, the cartoon shows remodeling in only two dimensions, whereas in vivo, it occurs in three dimensions, with osteoclasts continuing to enlarge the cavity at one end and osteoblasts beginning to fill it in at the other end. (From Riggs BL, Parfitt AM. Drugs used to treat osteoporosis: the critical need for a uniform nomenclature based on their action on bone remodeling. *J Bone Miner Res* 2005;20:177–84.)

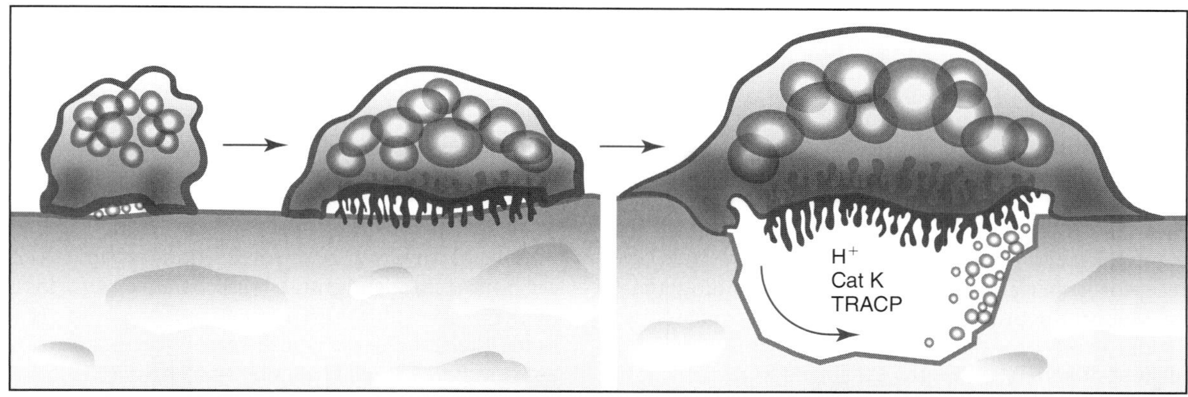

FIGURE 64.2 **Activation of Bone Resorption.** Multinucleated cells are recruited by the action of colony-stimulating factor 1 (CSF-1) and receptor activator for nuclear factor–κB ligand (RANKL) and adhere to bone, undergoing differentiation into mature osteoclasts. RANKL stimulates osteoclast activation by inducing secretion of protons and lytic enzymes into a sealed resorption vacuole formed between the basal surface of the osteoclast and the bone surface. Acidification of the vacuole leads to activation of tartrate-resistant acid phosphatase (TRACP) and cathepsin K (Cat K). (Modified from Boyle WJ, Simonet WS, Lacey DL. Osteoclast differentiation and activation. *Nature* 2003;423:337–42.)

non-collagenous proteins, some of which are found only in bone. Type I collagen is a product of two genes—*COL1A1* on chromosome 17 and *COL1A2* on chromosome 7—that encode two chains of the collagen molecule, called α_1(I) and α_2(I) chains. The organic matrix is mineralized by the deposition of inorganic calcium and phosphate in small crystals with lesser amounts of carbonate, magnesium, sodium, potassium, and various other ions.

The skeleton is not only a storehouse for ions but is essential for locomotion, protection of vital organs, and production and maturation of major components of the hematopoietic system. Bone contains nearly all of the calcium (≈99%), most of the phosphate (85%), and much of the magnesium (55%) of the body. The structural component of bone required for locomotion and protection of organs is the outer cortical shell, which accounts for 80% of skeletal mass. The less robust inner cancellous (trabecular) bone also has a role in the mechanical stability and flexibility of the skeleton, in that disruption of its microarchitecture is the dominant contributor to minimal-trauma fractures.

Cell Signaling in Bone

Control of the bone remodeling cycle is achieved via important signaling pathways. Knowledge and understanding of

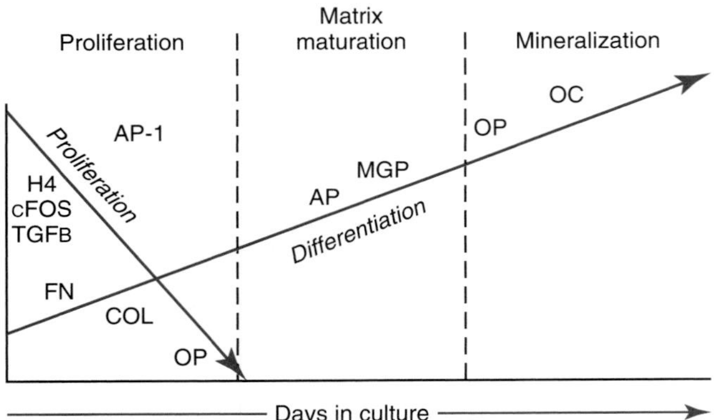

FIGURE 64.3 Schematic Representation of the Development of the Osteoblast Phenotype. The reciprocal relationship between cell growth and differentiation is shown, with *arrows* depicting expression of cell cycle and cell growth–related genes *(proliferation arrow)* and that of genes related to maturation of the osteoblast phenotype and production of the extracellular matrix *(differentiation arrow)*. The three principal periods in the developmental sequence are designated by *vertical broken lines*. *AP,* Alkaline phosphate; *COL,* type I collagen; *MGP,* matrix Gla protein; *OC,* osteocalcin; *OP,* osteopontin. (Modified from Lian JB, Stein GS. Development of the osteoblast phenotype: molecular mechanisms mediating osteoblast growth and differentiation. *Iowa Orthop J* 1995;15;118–40.)

these pathways has resulted in the development of new therapies for metabolic bone disease.[2] Two key signaling pathways are known as *RANK/RANKL/OPG* and *Wnt.*

RANK (receptor activator of nuclear factor–κB) is a membrane protein expressed on the surface of osteoclasts. Its ligand (RANK ligand, or RANKL) is found on the surface of osteoblasts (also on stromal and T cells). Binding of RANK to RANKL activates osteoclasts (see Fig. 64.2). Osteoprotegerin (OPG) is a cytokine (a member of the tumor necrosis factor [TNF] receptor superfamily) and a RANK homolog that can inhibit the production and maturation of osteoclasts by acting as a decoy receptor blocking the interaction of RANK with its ligand RANKL. OPG production is stimulated by estrogens, and the marked decrease in estrogen at menopause diminishes OPG production, resulting in increased activation of osteoclasts and the accelerated bone loss that accompanies the menopause. Antibodies to OPG can be produced by humans that bind OPG resulting in increased RANKL activity that leads to significant increased osteoclast activity and marked bone loss.[3]

The Wnt signaling pathway is complex and is involved in many physiologic systems beyond the skeleton. Key components with respect to skeletal physiology include the frizzled family of G protein–coupled receptor proteins; low-density lipoprotein receptor–related protein 5 encoded by the *LRP5* gene and associated with high bone mass in affected families; cathepsin K; Dickkopf-related protein 1 (DKK1); and sclerostin.[4]

Bone Remodeling

An estimated 10% to 30% of the skeleton is remodeled each year, with wide variation among individuals. Bone growth and turnover are influenced by the metabolism of calcium, phosphate, and magnesium, and several hormones, primarily PTH and 1,25-dihydroxyvitamin D [1,25$(OH)_2$D, calcitriol]. A number of other hormones and factors affect bone formation and resorption, including thyroid hormones, estrogens, androgens, cortisol, insulin, growth hormone, insulin-like growth factors (IGF-I and IGF-II), transforming growth factor-β (TGF-β), fibroblast growth factor 23 (FGF23), and platelet-derived growth factor (PDGF). Numerous cytokines alter bone remodeling, primarily by stimulating resorption; these factors include interleukins (IL)-1, -4, -6, and -11; macrophage and granulocyte/macrophage colony-stimulating factors (GCSF, MCSF), and tumor necrosis factor-α (TNF-α). Findings suggest that leptin, which is secreted by adipocytes, may influence bone formation through leptin receptors on osteoblasts.[5,6]

Exercise, via loading of bone, is a major factor in maintaining bone mass, and immobilization leads to rapid bone loss. Lack of gravity, as occurs during space flight, results in dramatic bone loss.[7]

During childhood and adolescence, bone formation markedly exceeds bone resorption (bone modeling)—a process that ends with epiphyseal closure at the end of puberty and is followed, in women, by a period of consolidation for the next 5 to 10 years, during which time the bone becomes fully mineralized. In healthy individuals, resorption and formation remain in balance for several decades. After menopause, the decline in estrogen triggers an increase in bone resorption that exceeds the capacity of the formation process and results in a rapid decrease in bone mass. This imbalance continues at an accelerated rate for approximately 5 years before slowing down to a slower rate of bone loss, termed *age-related bone loss.* Men do not normally experience the phase of rapid bone loss unless they develop altered physiology such as male hypogonadism, but they do experience longer-term age-related loss at a rate similar to that seen in women. One disease resulting from remodeling imbalance, with loss of bone, is osteoporosis.

Several diseases and medications have adverse effects on bone remodeling and bone balance with loss of bone; in these cases the term *secondary osteoporosis* is used. Systemic skeletal disease is also seen in primary and secondary abnormalities in PTH regulation. This latter group includes osteomalacia caused by deficiency of active metabolites or disruption of the vitamin D endocrine system as seen in patients with chronic kidney disease (CKD). Non-systemic skeletal disease also occurs as in skeletal metastases and Paget disease of bone.

BIOCHEMICAL MEASUREMENTS IN METABOLIC BONE DISEASE

There are several analytes that can be measured in biologic fluids that give important information on bone and calcium metabolism enabling diagnosis of abnormalities and disease. In many cases, these analytes have been the subject of attempts to harmonize measurements[8] and reference intervals so that interpretation of results are consistent across different laboratories. There are some analytes that are difficult to harmonize especially when measured by immunoassays, and it is important to interpret these results in comparison to method and local population–established reference intervals.

Calcium

Calcium is the fifth most common element in the body and the most prevalent cation. An average human body (70 kg) contains about 1 kg, or approximately 25 mol, of calcium (Table 64.1). The skeleton contains approximately 99% of the body's calcium, predominantly as extracellular crystals of an unknown structure and a composition approaching that of hydroxyapatite [$Ca_{10}(PO_4)_6(OH)_2$]. Soft tissues and extracellular fluid contain about 1% of the body's calcium.

Biochemistry and Physiology

In blood, virtually all of the calcium is found in the plasma, which has a mean calcium concentration of 9.5 mg/dL (2.38 mmol/L). Calcium exists in three physicochemical states in plasma (Table 64.2): 50% is free (ionized), 40% is bound to plasma proteins, and 10% is complexed with small diffusible inorganic and organic anions, including bicarbonate, lactate, phosphate, and citrate.[9]

The free calcium fraction is the biologically active form. Its concentration in plasma is tightly regulated by the calcium-regulating molecules PTH and $1,25(OH)_2D$. Synthesis and secretion of PTH by the parathyroid glands is controlled via a calcium-sensing receptor (CaSR), which is a transmembrane receptor on the surface of parathyroid gland cells. A decrease in circulating free calcium is detected at the CaSR, resulting in the chief cells releasing PTH to act via the kidneys (calcium reabsorption), the gut (calcium absorption), and skeleton (bone resorption releasing calcium) to increase free calcium (Fig. 64.4). When calcium increases sufficiently, a classic feedback loop is in place whereby the increase in free calcium interacts with the CaSR, switching off PTH synthesis and release from the parathyroid glands.

About 80% of protein-bound calcium is associated with albumin,[10,11] with the remaining 20% associated with globulins. Because calcium binds to negatively charged sites on proteins, its binding is pH dependent. Alkalosis leads to an increase in the negative charge of proteins increasing binding, resulting in a decrease in free calcium; conversely, acidosis leads to a decrease in negative charge, decreasing binding and resulting in an increase in free calcium. In vitro, for each 0.1-unit change in pH, approximately 0.2 mg/dL (0.05 mmol/L) of inverse change occurs in the serum free calcium concentration.

Calcium can be redistributed among the three plasma pools, acutely or chronically, by alterations in the concentrations of protein and small anions, changes in pH, or changes in the quantities of free calcium and total calcium in the plasma (Fig. 64.5).

Physiologically, calcium may be classified as intracellular or extracellular. Intracellular calcium has key roles in many important physiologic functions, including muscle contraction, hormone secretion, glycogen metabolism, and cell

TABLE 64.1 Distribution of Calcium, Phosphate, and Magnesium in the Body

Tissue	Calcium	Phosphate	Magnesium
Skeleton	99%	85%	55%
Soft tissues	1%	15%	45%
Extracellular fluid	<0.2%	<0.1%	1%
Total	1000 g (25 mol)	600 g (19.4 mol)	25 g (1 mol)

Modified from Aurbach GD, Marx SJ, Speigel AM. Parathyroid hormone, calcitonin, and the calciferols. In: Wilson JD, Foster DW, eds. *Williams Textbook of Endocrinology*. 8th ed. Philadelphia: Saunders; 1992:1397–476.

TABLE 64.2 Physicochemical States of Calcium, Phosphate, and Magnesium in Human Plasma

	APPROXIMATE PERCENT OF TOTAL		
State	Calcium	Phosphate	Magnesium
Free (ionized)	50	55	55
Protein-bound	40	10	30
Complexed	10	35	15
Total, mg/dL	8.6–10.3	2.5–4.5	1.7–2.4
Total mmol/L	2.15–2.57	0.81–1.45	0.70–0.99

Modified from Marshall RW. Plasma fractions. In: Nordin BEC, ed. *Calcium, Phosphate and Magnesium Metabolism*. London: Churchill Livingstone; 1976:162–85.

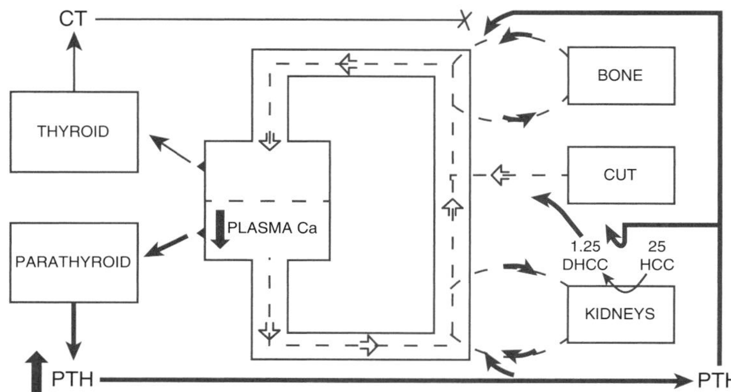

FIGURE 64.4 The regulation of calcium via PTH secretion and its direct and indirect action at the kidneys, intestine, and bone. (Modified from Fraser WD. Hyperparathyroidism. *Lancet* 2009;374:145–58.)

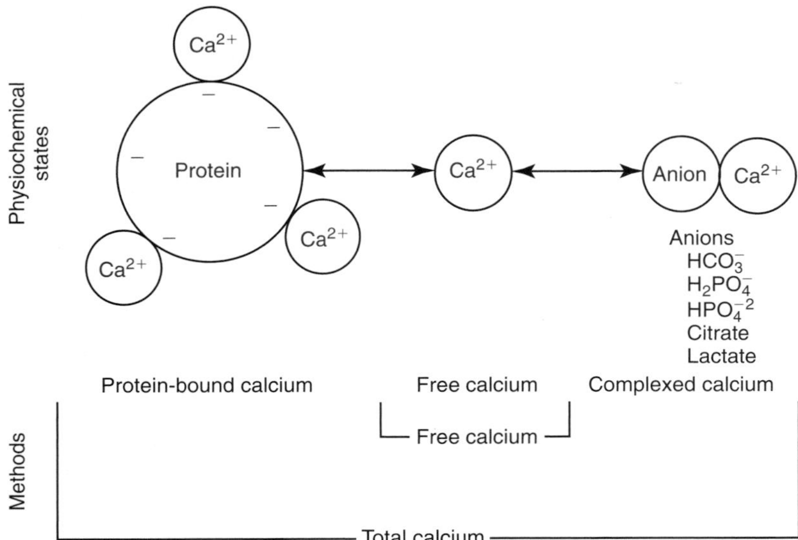

FIGURE 64.5 Equilibria and Determinations of Calcium in Serum. Calcium can move between three physiochemical pools: (1) free calcium, (2) protein-bound calcium, and (3) calcium complexed with inorganic and organic anions. Methods for determining total calcium measure all three pools, whereas methods for determining free calcium measure only that pool.

division.[12] The intracellular concentration of calcium in the cytosol of unstimulated cells is around 0.1 μmol/L, which is less than 1/20,000 of that in extracellular fluid.

Extracellular calcium provides calcium ions for the maintenance of intracellular calcium, bone mineralization, blood coagulation, and plasma membrane potential. Calcium stabilizes the plasma membranes and influences permeability and excitability. A decrease in the plasma free calcium concentration causes increased neuromuscular excitability and can lead to tetany; an increased concentration reduces neuromuscular excitability.

Clinical Significance

Hypocalcemia. Low total plasma calcium (hypocalcemia) may be due to a reduction in albumin-bound calcium, the free fraction of calcium, or both (Box 64.1).[13] Hypoalbuminemia is the most common cause of apparent hypocalcemia on a standard biochemical profile, particularly in hospitalized patients, because 1 g/dL (1 g/L) of albumin binds approximately 0.8 mg/dL (0.02 mmol/L) of calcium. Common clinical conditions associated with low plasma albumin include chronic liver disease, nephrotic syndrome, congestive heart failure, malignancy, malnutrition, and postsurgical volume replacement with saline or colloidal solutions. In these conditions, the concentration of free calcium typically is maintained within its physiologic reference interval. Causes of hypocalcemia are listed in Box 64.1. The most common causes of hypocalcemia are chronic renal failure, hypoparathyroidism, and hypomagnesemia. In CKD, hypoproteinemia, hyperphosphatemia, low plasma 1,25(OH)$_2$D (caused by reduced renal synthesis), and skeletal resistance to PTH can all contribute to hypocalcemia. Magnesium deficiency can also lead to hypocalcemia through several mechanisms, including impairment of PTH secretion by interfering with the fusion of intracellular vesicles containing PTH with the chief cell membrane, and decreased responsiveness of target organs to PTH action (end-organ resistance). Less common causes of hypocalcemia include pseudohypoparathyroidism and activating mutations of the CaSR. Hypoparathyroidism is caused most commonly by parathyroid gland destruction or removal during neck surgery (90%), less commonly by autoimmune endocrine disorders, and rarely by genetic causes. In pseudohypoparathyroidism, patients have an inherited resistance to PTH and, as a result, increased circulating concentrations of PTH.[14] The molecular basis for the most common form, pseudohypoparathyroidism type 1 (Albright's hereditary osteodystrophy [AHO]), is an inactivating mutation in the gene coding for the stimulatory guanine nucleotide-binding protein in the adenylate cyclase complex, resulting in an inability to produce the second-messenger cyclic adenosine monophosphate (cAMP).

Box 64.2 describes the signs and symptoms of hypocalcemia. The severity of symptoms is related to the rate of decrease in plasma free calcium concentration. When symptomatic hypocalcemia is observed, the initial laboratory evaluation may require measurement of ionized calcium and should include assessment of renal function and measurement of blood pH, serum albumin, magnesium, and PTH concentrations. Plasma intact PTH concentrations are low or rarely inappropriately normal in hypoparathyroidism and increased in pseudohypoparathyroidism. Vitamin D deficiency is an uncommon cause of symptomatic hypocalcemia and is characterized by low plasma 25 hydroxyvitamin D (25[OH]D), high PTH (secondary hyperparathyroidism), and high plasma total alkaline phosphatase (ALP). Treatment of symptomatic hypocalcemia may require calcium to be given intravenously, and biochemical response to therapy can be monitored by measurement of serum adjusted calcium. If hypocalcemia is secondary to hypoparathyroidism or pseudohypoparathyroidism, vitamin D or vitamin D analogs plus oral calcium supplements are administered. PTH therapy by injection is available to treat hypoparathyroidism. In hypomagnesemic hypoparathyroidism, intravenous magnesium will be required to return magnesium to within the reference

BOX 64.1 Causes of Hypocalcemia

Artefact/Interference
- Hypoalbuminemia
- EDTA plasma
- Citrated plasma
- Gadolinium salts
- Excessive/rapid infusion of intravenous fluids

Chronic Kidney Disease
- Hyperphosphatemia
- PTH resistance
- Decreased $1,25(OH)_2D$

Hypoparathyroidism
- Postsurgical
- Autoimmune
- Genetic
- Magnesium deficiency
- Postradiation
- Infiltrative process (iron overload, Wilson disease, metastatic tumor, aluminum toxicity)

Pseudohypoparathyroidism

Vitamin D Deficiency or Resistance
- Lack of sunlight exposure
- Nutritional deficiency
- Malabsorption
- Gastric bypass surgery
- End-stage liver disease
- Chronic kidney disease
- Vitamin D–dependent rickets types 1 and 2

Calcium Deposition in Damaged Tissue (Binding with Phosphate/Sulfate)
- Crush injury
- Rhabdomyolysis
- Hemorrhagic and edematous pancreatitis
- Tumor lysis syndrome

Drugs
- Bisphosphonates
- Denosumab
- Imatinib
- Proton pump inhibitors
- Phosphate enemas
- Foscarnet

Malignancy
- Osteoblastic metastases
- Treatment (see drugs)

Healing Phase of Bone Disease (Hungry Bone Syndrome)
- Postparathyroidectomy
- Postthyroidectomy
- Treatment of hematologic malignancies

interval to restore normal control over PTH synthesis and secretion and allow restoration of normocalcemia with calcium supplementation.

Activating mutations of the CaSR as a cause of hypocalcemia have been described. Intervention to correct the hypocalcemia may not be needed long term, but in affected neonates, calcium replacement must be provided until genetic confirmation of CaSR status is obtained. Autoimmune destruction of the parathyroid glands may occur in isolation or in combination with other endocrine abnormalities. Postsurgical hypoparathyroidism is uncommon in patients

BOX 64.2 Signs and Symptoms of Hypocalcemia

Paraesthesia
- Circumoral
- Peripheral (fingers, toes)
- Perianal

Increased Neuromuscular Irritability
- Muscle weakness
- Twitching
- Muscle cramp
- Tetany

Laryngospasm

Bronchospasm

Central Nervous System Abnormalities
- Depression
- Altered mental status
- Seizures
  - Grand mal
  - Petit mal
  - Focal
- Coma

Cardiac
- Hypotension
- Arrythmias
- ECG abnormalities
- Congestive heart failure

Fatigue

Cataracts

undergoing thyroidectomy, surgery for primary hyperparathyroidism (PHPT), or surgery for secondary hyperparathyroidism (SHPT), but is common in patients undergoing radical neck surgery for treatment of head and neck malignancies. Hypocalcemia in the presence of functional parathyroid glands is a very late manifestation of disease because the interaction of PTH and $1,25(OH)_2D$ will maintain normocalcemia until body stores of 25(OH)D are severely depleted (25[OH]D <6 ng/mL, <15 nmol/L) or, in the later stages of CKD when $1,25(OH)_2D$ production is inadequate.

Symptoms of hypocalcemia (see Box 64.2) include tingling/paresthesia around the mouth and in the fingers and toes (regions of relative ischemia/hypoxia). In more severe cases, intense, painful spasm of the fingers and toes develops (tetany) and may be sustained for several minutes. In the most severe cases, life-threatening laryngospasm may occur. These symptoms reflect decreases in the plasma free calcium and may occur despite a normal total calcium concentration when the complexed or protein-bound calcium fraction is increased. This can occur, for example, during massive transfusion (or pheresis), when large quantities of citrated blood are infused rapidly; citrate complexes calcium, leading to lower free calcium concentration without decreasing the total calcium concentration. It is also commonly observed in hysterical overbreathing (anxiety related), where a marked increase in respiratory rate results in respiratory alkalosis with the increased pH (lowered hydrogen ion concentration) causing protein binding of free calcium. An important exception to symptomatic hypocalcemia occurs in CKD when marked acidosis is present. Hypocalcemia triggers muscle contraction, but acidosis impairs muscle contraction. Rapid

BOX 64.3 Causes of Hypercalcemia

Primary Hyperparathyroidism
- Adenoma, hyperplasia, carcinoma
- Familial
  - Familial benign hypercalcemic hypocalciuria (FBHH, FHH)
  - Neonatal severe PHPT
  - Multiple endocrine neoplasia type 1 with pituitary and pancreatic tumors
  - Multiple endocrine neoplasia type 2A with medullary thyroid carcinoma and pheochromocytoma
  - Hyperparathyroidism jaw tumor syndrome
  - Familial isolated PHPT

Malignancy
- With direct skeletal involvement (local osyeolytic hypercalcemia)
  - Direct tumor erosion of the bone
  - Local tumor production of bone-resorbing agents
- No direct skeletal involvement (humoral hypercalcemia of malignancy)
  - Parathyroid hormone–related protein
  - Growth factor(s) (tumor growth factor, epidermal growth factor, platelet-derived growth factor)
- Hematologic malignancy
  - Cytokines (interleukin-1, tumor necrosis factor, lymphotoxin)
  - 1,25-Dihydroxyvitamin D (lymphoma)
  - Coexistent primary hyperparathyroidism
  - Ectopic PTH secretion

Other Endocrine Disorders
- Hyperthyroidism
- Hypothyroidism
- Acromegaly
- Acute adrenal insufficiency
- Pheochromocytoma

Idiopathic Hypercalcemia of Infancy

Loss-of-Function Mutations in *CYP24A1* (25-Hydroxyvitamin D 24-Hydroxylase)
- Absent/low 24,25$(OH)_2$ D

Vitamin Overdose
- Vitamin D
- Vitamin A

Granulomatous Disease
- Sarcoidosis
- Tuberculosis
- Berylliosis
- Coccidioidomycosis

Renal Failure
- Chronic kidney disease
- Acute kidney injury—diuretic phase
- Post–renal transplantation

Drugs
- Calcium ± vitamin D
- Vitamin D and vitamin D analogs
- PTH therapy
- Estrogen/selective estrogen receptor modulators (SERMS)
- Chlorothiazide diuretics
- Lithium
- Growth hormone
- Aminophylline/theophylline

Milk-Alkali Syndrome

Artificial Nutrition (TPN)

Immobilization

End-Stage Liver Disease

Increased Serum Proteins/Abnormal Protein Binding
- Hemoconcentration
- Hyperglobulinemia due to multiple myeloma

Manganese Intoxication

correction of low serum bicarbonate in patients with CKD without confirming that plasma free calcium concentration is maintained may trigger muscle spasm.

Hypercalcemia. Box 64.3 describes the causes of hypercalcemia commonly encountered in clinical practice. Hypercalcemia often results when the influx of calcium into the extracellular fluid compartment from the skeleton, intestine, or kidney is greater than the efflux as, for example, when excessive resorption of bone mineral occurs in malignancy. Hypercalciuria often develops in such situations. When the capacity of the kidney to excrete filtered calcium is exceeded, hypercalcemia develops; where renal failure is present and calcium excretion is decreased, hypocalciuria may paradoxically be present. Hypercalcemia can be caused by increased intestinal absorption (eg, vitamin D intoxication [rare]), increased renal retention (eg, thiazide diuretics), increased skeletal resorption (eg, immobilization), or a combination of mechanisms (eg, PHPT).

PHPT is the most common pathologic cause in outpatients, whereas malignancy is more common in hospitalized patients. Vitamin D (cholecalciferol or ergocalciferol) or vitamin D analog therapy has become one of the most common causes of hypercalcemia detected in laboratory practice. Together, these causes account for 90% to 95% of all cases of hypercalcemia. Algorithms for investigation of hypercalcemia are shown in Figs. 64.6A and B.

PHPT is often characterized by increased secretion of PTH that results in hypercalcemia.[15] It is most often due to a solitary adenoma (80% to 85% of cases), less frequently to hyperplasia involving all glands (~15%), and infrequently to parathyroid carcinoma (<1%).[16]

More than 80% of hyperparathyroid patients in developed countries are free of overt symptoms on presentation because of early detection of this disorder through the widespread use of chemistry panels that include calcium.[15] The most common signs and symptoms of hypercalcemia are nonspecific and are related to the neuromuscular system (Box 64.4). They include fatigue, malaise, and weakness with mild hypercalcemia (calcium <12 mg/dL or <3 mmol/L); depression, apathy, and inability to concentrate may be present at higher calcium concentrations. Hypercalcemia at 12 mg/dL (3 mmol/L) (urine calcium >40 mg/dL [10 mmol/L]) may induce mild nephrogenic diabetes insipidus with polydipsia and polyuria. Renal colic caused by kidney stones can result from chronic hypercalcemia and hypercalciuria. Nephrocalcinosis can lead to slowly developing renal failure.

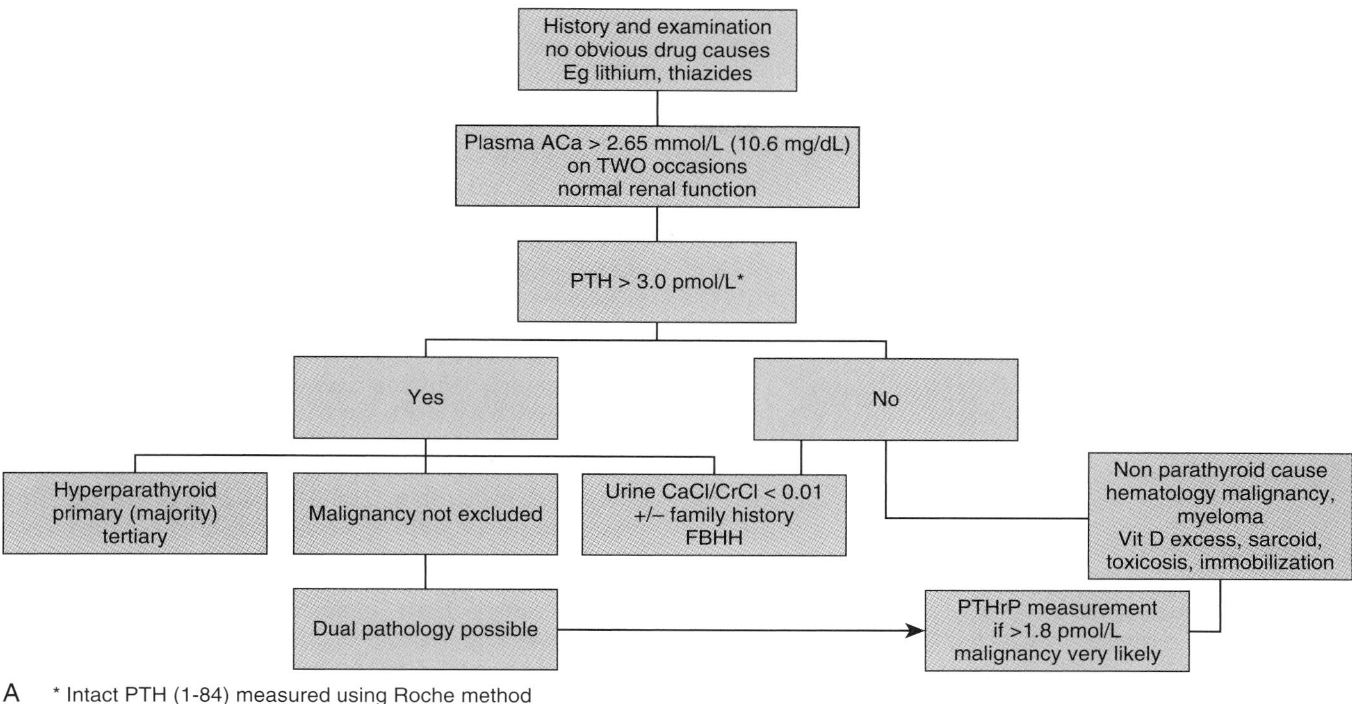

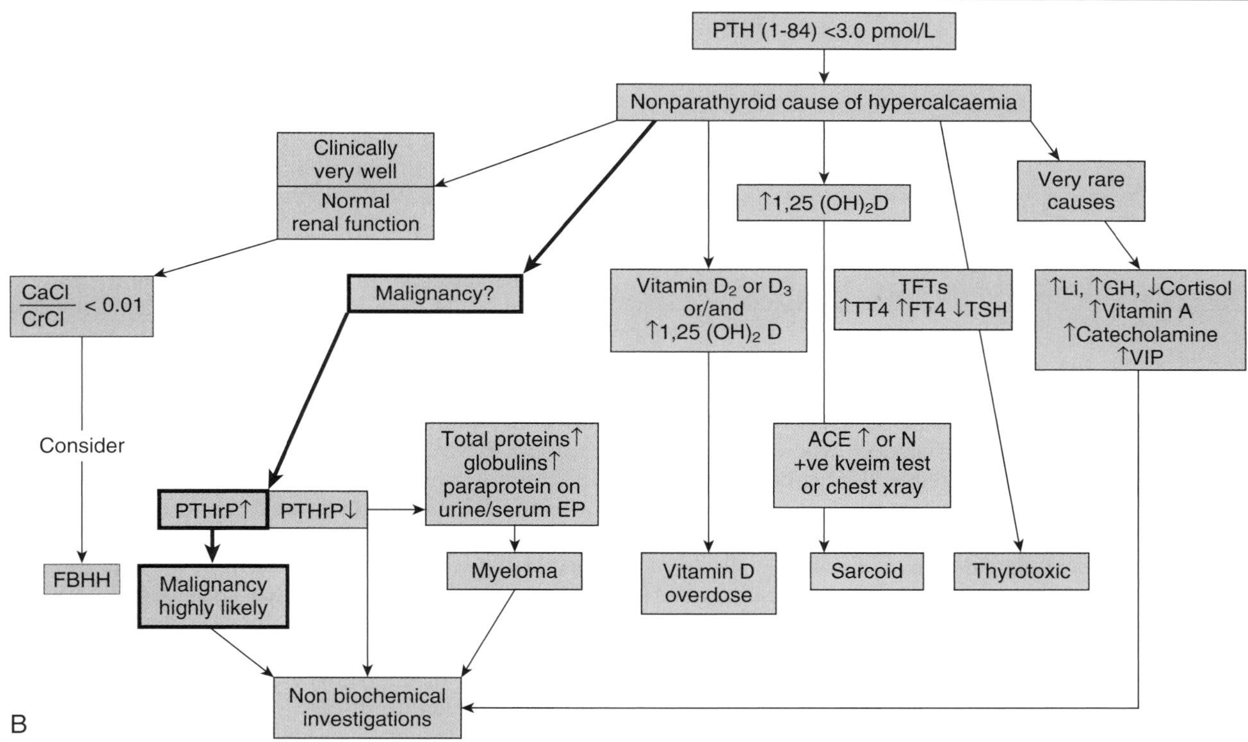

FIGURE 64.6 A, Investigation algorithm for hypercalcemia. **B,** Investigation of non-parathyroid hypercalcemia. *1,25 (OH)2D,* 1,25 Dihydroxyvitamin D; *ACa,* adjusted calcium; *ACE,* angiotensin converting enzyme; *CaCl,* calcium clearance; *CrCl,* creatinine clearance; *EP,* electrophoresis; *FBHH,* familial benign hypocalciuric hypercalcaemia; *FT4,* free tetraidothyronine; *GH,* growth hormone; *Li,* lithium; *PTH,* parathyroid hormone; *PTHrP,* parathyroid hormone related protein; *TFTs,* thyroid function tests; *TSH,* thyroid stimulating hormone; *TTF,* total tetraidothyronine; *VIP,* vasoactive intestinal peptide.

Most patients with PHPT (>60%) are postmenopausal women.

PHPT is diagnosed by laboratory studies. Hypercalcemia should be documented by measuring total calcium and serum albumin and then calculating adjusted calcium, or by measuring free calcium, on more than one occasion. Measurement of intact PTH (with concomitant measurement of calcium) is the most sensitive and specific test for parathyroid function and is central to the differential diagnosis of hypercalcemia. Plasma PTH may not be increased in some patients;

BOX 64.4 Signs and Symptoms of Hypercalcemia

Gastrointestinal
- Nausea
- Vomiting
- Abdominal pain
- Hyperacidity/reflux
- Peptic ulcers
- Constipation
- Pancreatitis

Neurologic
- Weakness
- Tiredness
- Fatigue
- Decreased muscle contraction
- Depression
- Flushing
- Obtundation
- Coma

Renal
- Polyuria (polydipsia)
- Dehydration/prerenal uremia
- Stone formation

Tissue Calcification
- Nephrocalcinosis
- Vascular
- Cardiac
- Cornea (band keratopathy)
- Gastric mucosa

Cardiac
- Decreased muscle contraction
- ECG (prolonged Q-T interval)

however, if within the upper half of the reference interval, it is inappropriate for the prevailing calcium concentration. This should not detract from the diagnosis because, with rare exceptions, non-parathyroid causes of hypercalcemia are associated with very low or suppressed PTH concentrations. Serum $1,25(OH)_2D$ is often in the upper half of the reference interval or is increased in PHPT, as PTH stimulates its production from 25(OH)D. By contrast, $1,25(OH)_2D$ (similarly to PTH) is low-normal or suppressed in non-parathyroid hypercalcemia, except in sarcoidosis or other granulomatous diseases and certain lymphomas, in which pathologic tissues contain the 25-hydroxyvitamin D-1α-hydroxylase required to produce $1,25(OH)_2D$.

PTH increases the renal clearance of bicarbonate and phosphate such that in PHPT a mild hyperchloremic metabolic acidosis may be observed, whereas in non-parathyroid hypercalcemia a mild hypochloremic metabolic alkalosis may be observed. Although hypophosphatemia is often seen in PHPT, measurement of serum phosphate is of limited diagnostic value because hypophosphatemia is also found in hypercalcemic cancer patients.

Symptomatic patients with PHPT should undergo parathyroid surgery. If the patient is asymptomatic, guidelines (Table 64.3) have been established recommending surgery over monitoring depending on serum calcium concentration, creatinine clearance, bone mineral density, and age.[15] In the "Guidelines for Management of Asymptomatic Primary Hyperparathyroidism" from the Fourth International Workshop on the topic,[17] a serum calcium concentration >1 mg/dL (>0.25 mmol/L) above the reference interval was considered an indication for surgical intervention, as was an eGFR <60 mL/min/1.73 m^2. For patients who were to be managed without surgery, annual measurements of serum calcium and creatinine were recommended. The changes in the recommendations over a 23-year period are highlighted in Table 64.3.

Hypercalcemia occurs in 5% to 30% of individuals with cancer.[18] Solid-tissue malignancies, particularly squamous cell carcinomas, commonly produce parathyroid hormone–related peptide (PTHrP), which is secreted into the circulation and stimulates bone resorption. PTHrP binds to the PTH receptor and is the principal mediator of humoral hypercalcemia of malignancy (HHM).[19] Skeletal metastases from cancer can also produce hypercalcemia, but this is often a late manifestation, reflecting a large metastatic burden, and less often presents a diagnostic problem. Cytokines such as lymphotoxin, interleukin-1, tumor necrosis factor, and PTHrP appear to be important mediators of hypercalcemia in multiple myeloma and other hematologic malignancies. Some lymphomas associated with acquired immunodeficiency syndrome or human T-lymphotropic virus type 1 (HTLV-1) infection cause hypercalcemia by producing $1,25(OH)_2D$. Between 5% and 15% of patients with hypercalcemia caused by malignancy have coexisting PHPT.[18,20]

Signs and symptoms of hypercalcemia are more evident in patients with HHM because the plasma calcium increases rapidly and often reaches concentrations higher than those usually seen in PHPT. Lethargy, obtundation, nausea, and vomiting are common symptoms (see Box 64.4).

Samples must be obtained prior to initiating treatment for hypercalcemia as lowering the calcium in HHM will stimulate PTH secretion and can cause diagnostic confusion when hypercalcemia is still present with detectable PTH. Laboratory test selection in non-parathyroid hypercalcemia is outlined in an investigation algorithm (see Fig. 64.6B), with the addition of PTHrP, as required, in some individuals with HHM. PTHrP is less likely to be informative if the PTH is not suppressed.[21] In specific instances (eg, lymphoma, sarcoidosis), measurement of $1,25(OH)_2D$ may be useful.

Therapies are directed toward treating the malignancy, decreasing the plasma calcium concentration by saline diuresis, and decreasing osteoclastic resorption (eg, with bisphosphonates, denosumab, or calcitonin). Corticosteroids can be useful in reducing intestinal absorption of calcium in $1,25(OH)_2D$-mediated hypercalcemia, particularly in sarcoid and granulomatous disease.

Familial benign hypocalciuric hypercalcemia (FBHH) (also called *benign familial hypercalcemia*) is characterized, as its name implies, by the presence of hypercalcemia and hypocalciuria (low fractional calcium excretion). It is due to a loss-of-function mutation in the CaSR in the parathyroid glands and the kidney tubules. Biochemical tests that may help differentiate PHPT from FBHH are listed Box 64.5. Ultimately, genetic testing may be required to confirm the type of CaSR defect that may be present.

Studies of four families and sporadic individual patients with idiopathic hypercalcemia of infancy (see Box 64.3) have identified a genetic basis for this condition.[22] Sequence

TABLE 64.3 Guidelines for Recommending Parathyroidectomy*

	1990	2002	2008	2013
Measurement†				
Serum calcium above upper reference limit	>1–1.6 mg/dL (>0.25–0.4 mmol/L)	>1 mg/dL (>0.25 mmol/L)	>1 mg/dL (>0.25 mmol/L)	>1 mg/dL (0.25 mmol/L)
Skeletal	BMD by DXA: Z-score <–2 (site unspecified)	BMD by DXA: T-score <–2.5 at any site†	BMD by DXA: T-score <–2.5 at any site† Previous fragility fracture‡	A. BMD by DXA: T-score <–2.5 at lumbar spine, total hip, femoral neck, or distal 1/3 radius† B. Vertebral fracture by radiograph, CT, MRI, or VFA‡
Renal	A. eGFR reduced by >30% from expected B. 24-h urine for calcium >400 mg/24 h (>10 mmol/24 h)	A. eGFR reduced by >30% from expected B. 24-h urine for calcium >400 mg/24 h (>10 mmol/24 h)	A. eGFR <60 mL/min B. 24 h urine for calcium not recommended	A. Creatinine clearance <60 mL/min B. 24-h urine for calcium >400 mg/24 h (>10 mmol/24 h) and increased stone risk by biochemical stone risk analysis§ C. Presence of nephrolithiasis or nephrocalcinosis by radiograph, ultrasound, or CT
Age, y	<50	<50	<50	<50

Patients need to meet only one of these criteria to be advised to have parathyroid surgery. They do not have to meet more than one.
*Surgery is also indicated in patients for whom medical surveillance is neither desired nor possible and in patients opting for surgery, in the absence of meeting any guidelines, as long as there are no medical contraindications.
†Consistent with the position established by the ISCD, the use of Z-scores instead of T-scores is recommended in evaluating bone mineral density (BMD) by dual-energy x-ray absorptiometry (DXA) in premenopausal women and men younger than 50 y.
‡The history of a fragility fracture at any site would define someone as having a complication of PHPT, and thus the individual would be automatically considered to be a surgical candidate.
§Most clinicians will first obtain a 24-hour urine for calcium excretion. If marked hypercalciuria is present (>400 mg/d [>10 mmol/d]), further evidence of calcium-containing stone risk should be sought by a urinary biochemical stone risk profile, available through most commercial laboratories. In the presence of abnormal findings indicating increased calcium-containing stone risk and marked hypercalciuria, a guideline for surgery is met.
CT, Computed tomography; *eGFR,* estimated glomerular filtration rate; *h,* hour; *MRI,* magnetic resonance imaging; *VFA,* vertebral fracture assessment; *y,* year.

BOX 64.5 Comparison of Clinical and Biochemical Findings in Familial Benign Hypercalcemic Hypocalciuria (FBHH) and Primary Hyperparathyroidism (1°HPT)

Sign/Symptom/Measurement	FBHH	1°HPT
Age (years)/gender	<40/equal	>50/majority female
Symptoms	Unrelated to calcium	Calcium related
Plasma adjusted calcium	2.55–3.5 mmol/L (10.2–14.0 mg/dL)	2.55–4.5 mmol/L (10.2–18.0 mg/dL)
Intact PTH	Majority within reference interval	Majority above reference interval
pmol/L	(0.9–11.0, median 3)	(2.5–84.5, median 8.2)
Plasma magnesium	Trend higher	Trend lower
mmol/L	(0.78–1.18, median 0.94)	(0.34–1.03, median 0.84)
mg/dL	1.90–2.88, median 2.29	0.83–2.51, median 2.05
Plasma 1,25(OH)$_2$ vitamin D	Within reference interval	Often elevated
pmol/L	(54–134, median 87)	(62–212, median 105)
Ca_{Cl}/Cr_{Cl}	Majority <0.01 (0.001–0.018, median 0.005)	Majority >0.015 (0.001–0.060, median 0.019)

Ca_{Cl}/Cr_{Cl}, Renal calcium clearance/creatinine clearance ratio.

analysis of *CYP24A1,* which encodes 25-hydroxyvitamin D 24-hydroxylase, the key enzyme for degrading the active metabolite of vitamin D_3, revealed recessive mutations in the affected children. In addition, *CYP24A1* mutations were identified in a group of infants in whom severe hypercalcemia developed after bolus prophylaxis with vitamin D. Functional characterization revealed a complete loss of function in all *CYP24A1* mutations.[23] Cases have been reported in adults. The decreased ability to prevent vitamin D actions appears to explain the hypercalcemia seen in some patients.[24]

Measurement of Calcium

The methods used for quantifying calcium in blood can measure the free Ca^{2+} ion or the total concentration of calcium and the subsequent calculation of albumin-adjusted calcium. The term *ionized calcium,* although widely used, is a misnomer because all calcium in plasma or serum is ionized, irrespective of whether or not it is free or is associated with protein or small anions by ionic binding.

Free calcium is the biologically active fraction of blood calcium; it is tightly regulated by PTH and 1,25(OH)$_2$D, and thus is the best indicator of calcium status. Methods for both total, albumin-adjusted, and free calcium are currently in use and have their own sources of error. Adjustment of total calcium for the prevailing albumin concentration is often performed in an attempt to correlate the total calcium concentration to the free calcium. Free calcium measurements and adjusted calcium calculations have been recommended because of the consequences of delayed treatment and the cost of working up patients with misleading total calcium results.[25]

Measurement of Total Calcium

Several methods have been described for total calcium measurement. At present, only photometric, ion-selective electrode (ISE), and occasionally atomic absorption spectrophotometry methods are used in clinical laboratories for measuring serum and urine total calcium.[13]

ISEs for the measurement of total calcium were introduced more recently than photometric methods. The specimen is acidified to convert protein-bound and complexed calcium to free calcium before calcium is measured by ISE.

Photometric Methods. Total calcium is most frequently measured by spectrophotometry using metallochromic indicators or dyes. Of the metallochromic indicators that change color on selectively binding calcium (Fig. 64.7), *o*-cresolphthalein complexone (CPC) (o-Cresolphthalein-3′,3″-bis-methyleneiminodiacetic acid) and arsenazo III are most widely used. These methods, although less accurate and reproducible than atomic absorption spectrometry, have been readily automated on chemistry analyzers.

o-Cresolphthalein Complexone Method. In alkaline solution, the metal-complexing dye CPC forms a red chromophore with calcium; the color is usually measured at a wavelength between 570 and 580 nm. The sample is diluted with acid to release protein-bound and complexed calcium. Organic base, most often diethylamine, 2-amino-2-methyl-1-propanol, or 2-ethylaminoethanol, is added to buffer the reaction and to produce an alkaline pH. Interference by magnesium is reduced: by adding 8-hydroxyquinoline (see Fig. 64.7), by buffering the reaction mixture to near pH 12, and by measuring the absorbance near 580 nm. Urea may be added to reduce the turbidity of lipemic specimens and to enhance complex formation. Blank absorbance may be reduced by adding ethanol or other organic solvents. Calcium forms both 1 : 1 and 2 : 1 complexes with CPC, with the former predominating at lower concentrations.[26] Because the 1 : 1 complex has lower molar absorptivity, the calibration curves are nonlinear at low calcium concentrations. Multipoint calibration of CPC methods has been recommended. Linearity may be improved by adding sodium acetate.[27] The temperature must be carefully controlled because the reaction is temperature sensitive.

Arsenazo III Method. Arsenazo III [1,8-dihydroxynaphthalene-3,6-disulfonic acid-2,7-bis(azo-2)-phenylarsonic acid] (see Fig. 64.7), at mildly acidic pH, has much higher affinity for calcium than magnesium and binds it to produce an intense purple complex. A reaction pH of about 6 is commonly used; imidazole has been used to buffer the reaction. The solution must be thoroughly buffered because the spectral properties of arsenazo III are dependent on pH. Binding of calcium to arsenazo III can be influenced by buffer and sodium concentration. Interference from most biologic pigments is reduced by measuring the calcium–dye complex near 650 nm. Citrate has been reported to cause negative interference, particularly with dry-slide techniques; in these, the only source of fluid is the sample, and the effective concentration of citrate is much higher than in wet-chemistry methods.[28,29] Clinically significant interference may be noted in patients receiving citrated blood or blood products. Unlike CPC, which has limited stability when used as a single reagent, the arsenazo III reagent is stable.[30]

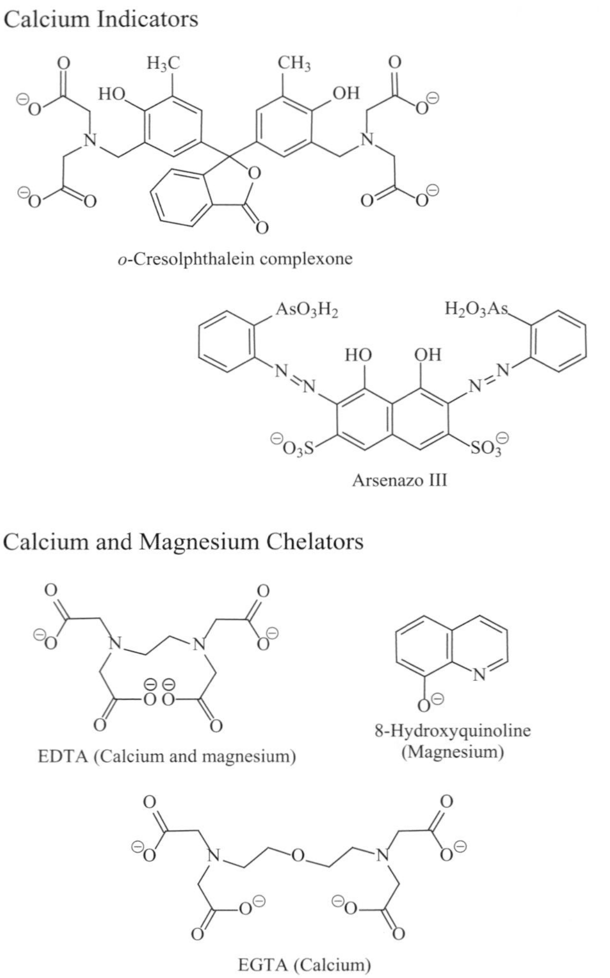

Calcium Indicators

o-Cresolphthalein complexone

Arsenazo III

Calcium and Magnesium Chelators

EDTA (Calcium and magnesium)

8-Hydroxyquinoline (Magnesium)

EGTA (Calcium)

FIGURE 64.7 Metallochromic indicators for calcium and chelators for calcium and magnesium.

Some photometric methods should not be used within 24 hours after a magnetic resonance imaging (MRI) examination of the patient in which gadolinium has been used as contrast medium, particularly if the patient has impaired renal function.[31] A predictive model has been described to calculate, in patients who have received gadodiamide, the minimum length of time to wait before blood collection to avoid pseudohypocalcemia when the Roche *o*-cresolphthalein method is used.[32]

Atomic Absorption Spectrometry Methods. The Clinical Laboratory and Standards Institute (CLSI; formerly known as the National Committee for Clinical Laboratory Standards [NCCLS]) has approved a method by which atomic absorption spectrophotometry (AAS) is used as a reference method in measuring total serum calcium.[33,34] This method has been compared with isotope dilution–mass spectrometry (ID-MS), the definitive method for total serum calcium developed by the National Institute of Standards and Technology. The reference method is reported to have an accuracy of 100 ± 2%, compared with 100 ± 0.2% for ID-MS.[33] Although AAS provides better accuracy and precision for total serum calcium than the widely used photometric methods, it is used by only a few laboratories. It should continue to be used for validating new total calcium methods. For further information, see the following references.[13,25,33-36]

Total Calcium Adjusted for Albumin (Adjusted or Corrected Calcium). Wide variation in the concentrations of compounds that bind calcium in blood may be noted; this variation will affect the measured total calcium concentration without changing the free calcium fraction. Several types of calculation have been suggested to "adjust" the measured calcium concentration. The goal is to produce an adjusted result that would have been found if the concentrations of all compounds that bind calcium had been within their respective reference intervals. In practice, only adjustments based on albumin are commonly used. The term *adjusted calcium* is preferable to *corrected calcium,* because "corrected" may suggest that the result has been corrected because of an error.[37-39]

Adjusted calcium is calculated from total calcium and albumin by first calculating a correction factor by multiplying the deviation of plasma albumin from the mean of its reference interval by the slope of the regression of total calcium against albumin. The following two equations are frequently used for results expressed as mg/dL and mmol/L, respectively:

$$\text{Adjusted total calcium (mg/dL)} = \text{Total calcium (mg/dL)} + 0.8\,[4 - \text{Albumin (g/dL)}]$$

$$\text{Adjusted total calcium (mmol/L)} = \text{Total calcium (mmol/L)} + 0.02\,[40 - \text{Albumin (g/L)}]$$

These are rather simplistic calculations, and in practice it is recommended that laboratories establish equations for their particular reference populations that incorporate linear regression for the different methods used to measure the total calcium and albumin concentrations. Many factors affect the distribution of calcium among free, complexed, and protein-bound fractions (Box 64.6). The reliability of adjustment for serum albumin deteriorates in patients with very low or high serum albumin concentrations[37] and in patients with severe disease and multiple organ failure such as is often seen in intensive care units. Equations that are derived for specific reference patient groups, such as hemodialysis patients[38] or patients with liver disease, may be better than no adjustment in that group of patients. Direct determination of free calcium by ISE is preferable to adjusted calcium, but it should be remembered that ISE methods are also subject to effects due to prevailing albumin concentrations.

Specimen Requirements. Serum and heparinized plasma are the preferred specimens. Citrate, oxalate, and ethylenediaminetetraacetic acid (EDTA) anticoagulants should not be used for the spectrophotometric methods, because they interfere by forming complexes with calcium. Total calcium measurements are little affected by storage, provided that loss of water associated with prolonged refrigerator or freezer storage is prevented (by the use of tightly capped containers designed for such storage), although co-precipitation of calcium with fibrin (eg, in heparinized plasma) or lipids has been reported with storage or freezing. Plastic and glass may also adsorb calcium from dilute solutions during storage.

BOX 64.6 Factors Altering the Distribution Between Protein-Bound, Complexed, and Free Calcium and Compounding the Interpretation of Total Calcium

Factors Altering Protein Binding of Calcium
Altered concentration of albumin or globulins
Abnormal proteins
Heparin
pH
Free fatty acids
Bilirubin
Drugs
Temperature

Factors Altering Complex Formation
Citrate
Bicarbonate
Lactate
Phosphate
Pyruvate and β-hydroxybutyrate
Sulfate
Anion gap

Acidification of urine is recommended to ensure complete dissociation of calcium from complexes that can be formed at high pH seen in some urine samples. The routine necessity of this procedure has been debated.[40]

Interferences. Hemolysis, icterus, lipemia, paraproteins, and magnesium have been reported to interfere positively or negatively with photometric methods. Many methods use bichromatic analysis, multiwavelength corrections, or blanking to reduce interference. Lipemic specimens should be ultracentrifuged before analysis or treated to remove the lipid fraction.

Although hemolysis can cause a negative error because red blood cells contain lower concentrations of calcium than does plasma, more significant errors may be caused by the spectral interference of hemoglobin. Depending on the method used, hemoglobin has been reported to produce negative or positive interference. In photometric methods, if hemolyzed specimens must be analyzed, blanking with ethylene glycol-*O,O′*-bis(2-aminoethyl)-*N,N,N′,N′*-tetraacetic acid (EGTA)-treated serum is suggested.

Individual instruments and methods should be evaluated for their susceptibility to interference from magnesium, hemoglobin, bilirubin, proteins, turbidity, and other interferents. Care should be taken in handling specimens, calibrators, and solutions to prevent contamination with calcium. Any glassware or plastic ware that is reused should be washed with dilute hydrochloric acid, followed by distilled water, to eliminate calcium contamination. Corks/bungs should not be used because they can contaminate specimens with calcium. How the patient is prepared and how the specimen is obtained can have a significant effect on both free and total calcium measurements. For information on these preanalytical effects, see *Patient Preparation and Sources of Preanalytical*

BOX 64.7 Preanalytical Factors Affecting Measurement of Serum Total or Free Calcium

In Vivo

Tourniquet use and venous occlusion
Changes in posture: 10% to 12% increase in total calcium and 5% to 6% increase in free calcium on standing
Exercise
Hyperventilation
Fist clenching
Alimentary status
Alterations in protein binding (see Box 64.6)
Alterations in complex formation (see Box 64.6)

In Vitro

Inappropriate anticoagulants
Dilution with liquid heparin
Interfering levels of heparin
Contamination with calcium
  Bungs, glassware, tubes
Specimen handling
  Alterations in pH (free calcium)
  Adsorption or precipitation of calcium
Spectrophotometric interference
  Hemolysis, icterus, lipemia

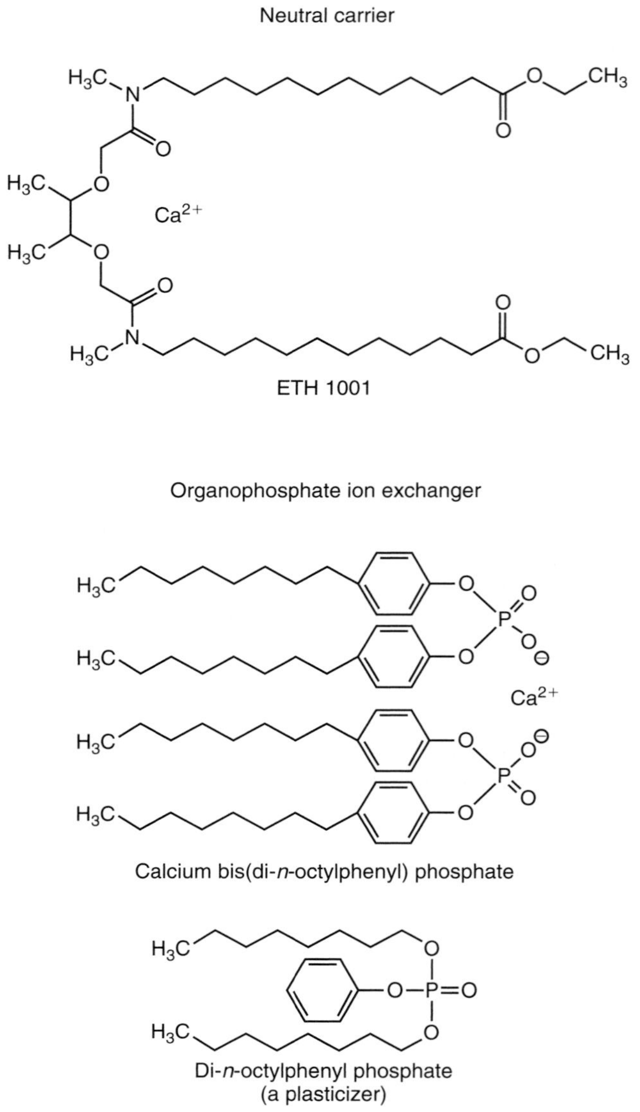

Error for Total and Free Calcium Measurements later in this chapter, Chapter 5, and Box 64.7.

Measurement of Free (Ionized) Calcium

(See also Chapters 14 and 35.)

Many blood gas analyzers, using ISEs, provide rapid whole-blood determinations of plasma free calcium and electrolytes, as well as determinations of blood gases.[13,25,41-43] The free calcium analyzer consists of a system of pumps under microprocessor control that transport calibration solutions, samples, and wash solutions through a measuring cell containing calcium ion–selective, reference, and pH electrodes. Sensitive potentiometers measure the voltage difference between the calcium or pH and reference electrodes for calibrating solutions or samples. A microprocessor calibrates the system and calculates calcium concentration and pH. Most instruments simultaneously measure the actual free calcium and pH at 37°C.

Calcium ISEs contain a calcium-selective membrane that encloses an inner reference solution of calcium chloride often containing saturated silver chloride (AgCl) and physiologic concentrations of sodium chloride and potassium chloride and an internal reference electrode.[13,25,41,44,45] The reference electrode, usually of Ag/AgCl, is immersed in this inner reference solution. Modern calcium ISEs use liquid membranes containing the ion-selective calcium sensor dissolved in an organic liquid trapped in a polymeric matrix. The Ca^{2+} ionophores may be based on a polyvinyl chloride matrix and contain ETH1001 or ETH129 as a carrier. Instead of these two neutral carriers, ion exchangers, such as organophosphate sensors (Fig. 64.8), have been used.[25] Neutral carrier membranes contain an uncharged calcium-selective organic molecule, such as ETH1001, dissolved in a plasticizer and

FIGURE 64.8 Free calcium sensors.

trapped in a polyvinyl chloride membrane. These molecules have a favorable steric and electrostatic pocket or site for selectively binding calcium. Ion exchangers or negatively charged carrier membranes are calcium salts, such as calcium bis(di-*n*-octylphenyl) phosphate, dissolved in di-*n*-octylphenyl phosphonate and trapped in a polyvinyl chloride membrane.

The electrochemical cell is completed by the external reference electrode, an Ag/AgCl or calomel electrode, which is in contact with the specimen through a liquid/liquid junction or a salt bridge of potassium chloride or sodium formate. The potential difference across the cell is logarithmically related to the activity of free calcium ions in the sample by the Nernst equation. By convention, free calcium is converted from activity to concentration with its activity coefficient, which is itself dependent on ionic strength.

Temperature affects electrode response and the extent of calcium binding by protein and small anions. Most free calcium analyzers adjust and maintain samples at 37°C, thereby ensuring that results are physiologically relevant for most patients.

Carryover has been minimized by various techniques, including using flush solutions containing 5 mg/dL (1.25 mmol/L) of free calcium; using the leading edge of the specimen to clean the fluid path, or purging with air.[41] Significant carryover is noted only at extremely low or high concentrations of free calcium.

The International Federation of Clinical Chemistry and Laboratory Medicine (IFCC) has recommended a reference method for free calcium.[46]

Interferences. Because ISEs measure ion activity, they are affected by the ionic strength of a specimen (see Chapter 35).[13,42] Free calcium analyzers (and the associated calibrators) are optimized for specimens of serum, plasma, or whole blood. Because the ionic strength of these fluids is primarily a result of the concentrations of Na^+ and Cl^- ions, calibrators usually are prepared in buffer and sodium chloride with a final ionic strength of 160 mmol/kg.[41-43] Although the range of Na^+ and Cl^+ concentrations usually observed in serum or plasma does not cause a clinically significant error in the measurement of free calcium, significant errors can occur with other specimens unless the matrices and the ionic strength of the calibrators and samples are matched closely.

Modern electrodes have high selectivity for calcium over Na^+, K^+, Mg^{2+}, H^+, and Li^+ ions.[41,42] At normal concentrations, these cations have little effect on the accuracy of free calcium measurements. Wide variations in the concentration of Na^+ and high concentrations of Mg^{2+} and Li^+ may influence the apparent concentration of free calcium. Electrodes are quite insensitive to H^+, with insignificant interference noted between pH 5 and 9.

Many physiologic anions including protein, phosphate, citrate, lactate, sulfate, and oxalate form complexes with calcium ions. Although these anions reduce the concentration of free calcium by complex formation, they do not directly interfere with measurement of the calcium that is free. Protein deposits on the electrode may act as a divalent cation exchanger, resulting in positive interference with high concentrations of Mg^{2+} ions. Older electrodes were sensitive to the concentration of protein in the sample. Newer electrodes use a dialysis membrane or a neutral carrier to reduce or eliminate this protein effect,[41,45,47,48] which typically is less than +0.02 mmol/L (0.08 mg/dL) for 1 g/dL (10 g/L) of protein. Regular instrument maintenance and protein removal are reported to minimize this interference. The type of dialysis technology or protein exclusion technology can result in different effects of protein concentration on free calcium measurement, especially at extremes of albumin concentration.[49]

Chemicals may interfere with the measurement of free calcium. Anionic surfactants and ethanol have been reported to affect the calcium-selective membrane.

Effect of pH. The binding of calcium by protein and small anions is influenced by pH in vitro and in vivo.[41,42] Albumin, with up to 30 binding sites for calcium,[10,11] accounts for approximately 80% of the protein-bound calcium. Increasing the pH of a specimen in vitro increases the ionization and negative charge on albumin and other proteins, leading to an increase in protein-bound calcium and a decrease in free calcium. Decreasing pH in vitro decreases ionization and negative charge, thereby decreasing protein-bound calcium

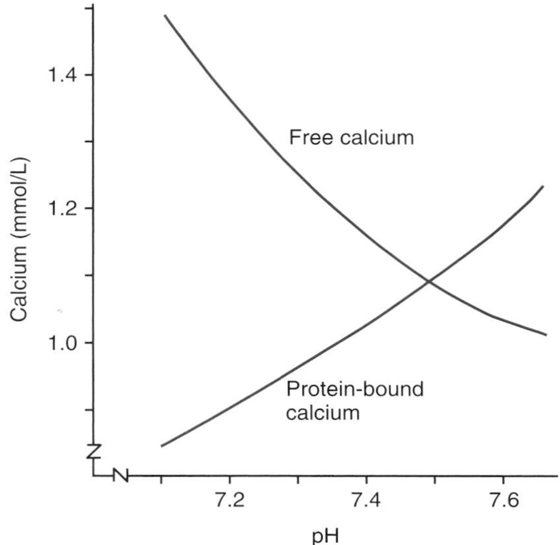

FIGURE 64.9 Effect of pH on free and protein-bound calcium.

and increasing free calcium. Free calcium changes by about 5% for each 0.1-unit change in pH (Fig. 64.9).

Because of this inverse relationship between free calcium and pH, specimens must be analyzed at the patient's in vivo pH. Usually, this requires that specimens are handled to prevent alterations in pH.

Specimen Requirements. Preanalytical considerations, including specimen collection and handling, are particularly important for free calcium. Specimens for free calcium must be collected and handled to minimize alterations in pH and free calcium caused by both loss of CO_2 and metabolism by blood cells. Free calcium may be measured in heparinized whole blood, heparinized plasma, or serum. For most laboratories in which specimens are analyzed rapidly (within minutes of sampling) by the use of blood gas analyzers, heparinized whole blood is preferable because it reduces processing time and the required specimen volume and avoids the alteration in pH associated with centrifugation. All syringes and evacuated tubes should be filled completely, kept tightly sealed, and handled anaerobically to prevent the loss of CO_2 and the increase in pH that may occur when specimens are exposed to air. If other tests are ordered that are not available on the blood gas analyzer, it is best that the sample for free calcium is collected in a separate container to minimize the likelihood that the specimen may be analyzed aerobically. Specimens should also be handled to prevent the decrease in pH caused by the production of lactic acid by glycolysis, by erythrocytes, and by white blood cells. IFCC has published recommendations on sampling, transport, and storage of the samples,[50] and CLSI has published guidelines (C-31A2) for free calcium specimen collection and handling.[51]

Ideally, whole-blood specimens should be analyzed within 15 to 30 minutes of sampling,[50,52,53] although free calcium is reported to be stable in whole-blood specimens for at least 1 hour at room temperature and for 4 hours at 4°C.[41,50,52,53] It has been reported that free calcium was stable for at least 7 hours at room temperature in an evacuated blood collection tube.[54] If specimens cannot be analyzed promptly, they can be collected in an ice-water slurry to minimize metabolism. If measurements of plasma potassium are needed on the sample, cooling will not be appropriate; potassium concentrations will be increased because of the inhibition of ATPase activity at low temperature.[55]

For delayed analysis, serum may be the optimal sample type because of elimination of the anticoagulant and reduction in the occurrence of microclots. Serum specimens can be collected in evacuated gel tubes. These tubes should be filled completely and centrifuged to form an effective barrier between the serum and the clot with its cellular elements. Once centrifuged, specimens are stable for hours at 25°C and for days at 4°C, provided the tube remains sealed. Free calcium has been reported to be less stable in specimens from both acidotic and non-acidotic patients with uremia.[56]

The practice of using aerobic specimens for the measurement of free calcium with correction of the free calcium to pH 7.4[41,57] has been criticized [41,58-60] and is not recommended. The free calcium value at pH 7.4 may be misleading in patients with respiratory and metabolic alkalosis or acidosis.[56] Furthermore, aerobic handling of specimens may lead to irreversible precipitation of calcium-phosphate complexes and a decrease in free calcium in some specimens that have a high total calcium and phosphate content or a high pH (pH >7.9).

Effects of Anticoagulants. Because citrate, oxalate, and EDTA bind calcium and significantly reduce free calcium, heparin is the only acceptable anticoagulant for free calcium determinations. However, heparin, a polyanion, significantly lowers free calcium at the concentrations (≥30–100 U/mL) found in many conventional blood gas syringes (Table 64.4).[42,61] In addition, the use of liquid heparin should be avoided; it can result in errors in free calcium caused by dilution, as well as high and variable concentrations of heparin. Underfilling of heparin sample tubes can result in lower free calcium concentrations.

Several commercially available syringes containing lyophilized heparin are suitable for free calcium determinations: electrolyte-balanced or calcium-titrated heparin syringes (final concentration of 40–50 U/mL); very low heparin syringes with heparin in an inert filler, providing a final heparin concentration of 2 to 3 U/mL; and lithium-zinc heparin syringes.[62] With electrolyte-balanced or calcium-titrated heparin syringes, the heparin is titrated with calcium so that the free calcium is not significantly altered over most observed concentrations (3.6–6.4 mg/dL or 0.9–1.6 mmol/L); however, some bias may be apparent at very low and high free calcium concentrations. Electrolyte-balanced heparin may also produce a bias in specimens with pathologically low protein concentrations.[63] In very low heparin syringes that contain 2 to 3 U/mL of heparin dispersed in a puff of inert proprietary material, the puff allows the heparin to be accurately dispensed during manufacturing and to rapidly dissolve with proper mixing, providing effective anticoagulation. A blend of lithium and zinc heparins has been reported to eliminate the heparin interference in free calcium measurements.[64-66] In addition, lithium-zinc heparin did not alter total calcium, unlike electrolyte-balanced or calcium-titrated heparin. Three-milliliter syringes containing a total of 50 U of a 1 : 1 blend of lithium and zinc heparins did not alter results of any general chemistry tests except total magnesium, which was increased by 0.19 mg/dL (0.08 mmol/L). In practice, individuals obtaining the blood specimen should not place additional liquid heparin in heparinized syringes.

Most evacuated collection tubes, when filled completely, contain concentrations of heparin (15 U/mL) that only slightly decrease free calcium.[67] Specific brands of syringes, evacuated tubes, and heparin should be carefully evaluated. It is important that all syringes and tubes be filled completely to minimize dilution and/or heparin effects.

Calibrators and Quality Controls. Various calibration solutions are used by manufacturers for free calcium analyzers. The buffers in which these calibrators are prepared may have an effect on the liquid junction potential and on calcium binding; however, this is usually corrected for by the instrument software.[41] Until reference solutions are available, it is best to use the calibrators provided by the instrument manufacturer.

Aqueous quality control materials are commercially available for free calcium. Because simple aqueous controls may not reliably detect changes in performance with patient specimens, use of serum-based quality control materials has been recommended.[68] Serum-based controls may be prepared by acidifying serum with 10 μL of 1 mol/L hydrochloric acid and leaving it exposed in the refrigerator for 1 week to remove carbon dioxide. The pH is then adjusted to 7.4, and the serum is aliquoted and frozen. Alternatively, serum-based controls can be equilibrated with carbon dioxide before undergoing analysis.

Patient Preparation and Sources of Preanalytical Error for Total and Free Calcium Measurements

Patient preparation and the manner of specimen collection can significantly affect the results of total and free calcium determinations (see Box 64.7).[41,69]

A common and important source of preanalytical error in the measurement of calcium is the increase in total, but not free, calcium concentration associated with tourniquet use and venous occlusion during sampling.[70] Errors of 0.5 to 1 mg/dL (0.12–0.25 mmol/L) in total calcium may result from the increase in protein-bound calcium caused by the efflux of water from the vascular compartment during stasis. Only small and clinically insignificant increases in free calcium have been reported with venous stasis. If a tourniquet is required, it should be applied just before sampling and released as soon as possible.

Fist clenching or other forearm exercise should be avoided before phlebotomy[70] because forearm exercise causes a

TABLE 64.4 Effects of Heparin on Free Calcium

		FREE CALCIUM	
Specimen	**Heparin, U/mL**	**mg/dL**	**mmol/L**
Serum	0	5.00	1.25
Plasma	44 (Ca-heparin)	4.96	1.24
Plasma	29 (Na-heparin)	4.84	1.21
Plasma	100 (Na-heparin)	3.76	0.94
Whole blood	44 (Ca-heparin)	5.08	1.27
Whole blood	29 (Na-heparin)	5.04	1.26
Whole blood	100 (Na-heparin)	3.88	0.97

Modified from Toffaletti J. Ionized calcium. In: Pesce AJ, Kaplan LA, eds. *Methods in Clinical Chemistry*. St Louis: Mosby; 1987:1010–20.

decrease in pH (owing to lactic acid production) and an increase in free calcium. CLSI and IFCC have published recommendations on blood collection.[51,61]

Changes in posture cause fluid shifts within 10 minutes and thus alter the concentrations of cells and large molecules, including albumin and total calcium (as part of it is protein bound), in the vascular compartment. Standing decreases intravascular water and increases the total calcium concentration by 0.2 to 0.8 mg/dL (0.05–0.2 mmol/L), while recumbency has the opposite effect, whereas a much smaller effect has been reported for free calcium.[41,69,70] One partial explanation (along with hypoalbuminemia) for the mild hypocalcemia observed in many hospitalized patients may be the hemodilution associated with recumbency. This effect can be observed during 24-hour sampling of normal individuals.

Prolonged immobilization and bed rest[71,72] increase bone resorption, which increases total and free calcium. Hyperventilation and exercise decrease and increase the concentration of free calcium, respectively, because of changes in plasma pH.[41,70] Both plasma free calcium concentration and calcium excretion are decreased during the night.[73] Food ingestion has been reported to have various effects but usually causes a mild increase in plasma calcium. Ingestion of calcium salts may increase plasma calcium. Hemolysis can alter free calcium because of dilution and alterations in pH and binding (see the *Interferences* section earlier in this chapter). Sodium perchlorate (Irenat), used in the treatment of hyperthyroidism, may falsely lower the results of free calcium measurement.[74,75]

Reference Intervals for Total and Free Calcium in Serum and Plasma

Total Calcium

The reference interval for serum and plasma calcium is usually defined by an upper limit of 10.1 to 10.5 mg/dL (2.52–2.62 mmol/L) and a lower limit of 8.5 to 8.8 mg/dL (2.12–2.20 mmol/L). The reference interval depends on the method and the reference population chosen. Detailed pediatric reference intervals have been established as part of the CALIPER study and are available in the Appendix.

An analytical goal, or quality specification, for between-day imprecision, expressed as the coefficient of variation (CV), is 0.9% or less based on within-person biologic variation.[76] Current methods achieve between-day CVs of 1.5% or less within laboratories.

Free Calcium

The reference interval of free calcium (in adults) has been reported as 4.6 to 5.3 mg/dL (1.15–1.33 mmol/L). Because of the dependence of free calcium on pH, it is recommended that pH be measured and reported with all free calcium determinations. This will assist the laboratory and the physician in identifying specimens in which inappropriate preanalytical handling has led to an in vitro change in pH. Some laboratories report the free calcium corrected to pH 7.4.

Whole-blood specimens develop a liquid junction potential different from that of serum or plasma because of the presence of erythrocytes.[41,42,45] A positive bias that is directly proportional to the hematocrit has been reported. In addition, free calcium values have been reported to differ among capillary blood, venous blood, and serum samples because of differences in pH. Therefore, reference intervals should be determined by each laboratory using the local instrument, specimen type, and collection protocol, and reference subjects representative of the patient population served.

Physiologic Variation in Calcium

Plasma calcium concentration has been reported to vary with age, gender, and season and during pregnancy and during a 24-hour period.[13,77,78] Total and free calcium have been reported to decline modestly and to remain unchanged in the elderly.[79] In a healthy ambulatory group of men and women residing in the southwest United States, no age-related decline or gender-related difference could be found in total or free calcium values.[80] During pregnancy, total calcium and adjusted calcium decline in parallel with plasma albumin, whereas free calcium is unchanged.[77,78] The fetal circulation is relatively hypercalcemic,[81,82] as evidenced by higher total and free calcium in cord blood than in maternal plasma. Calcium concentrations decline after birth in healthy term neonates during the first few days, but soon increase to concentrations slightly greater than those observed in adults.[82,83]

Interpretation of Total and Free Calcium Results

Calcium status is more accurately determined by measuring free calcium, the tightly regulated, biologically active species.[25,84] Interpretation of total serum calcium value is complicated by its association with protein and inorganic and organic ions. Interpretation of free calcium concentration is less complicated, provided the specimen has been properly obtained, handled, and analyzed. Disagreement between free and total calcium (abnormal total calcium and normal free calcium, or vice versa) values occurs in a high percentage of specimens. One study of 1213 patients suspected of having calcium disorders found disagreement between free calcium and total calcium or adjusted calcium values in 18% and 31% of patients, respectively.[85]

Free calcium is reportedly more useful than total calcium determination in hospitalized patients, especially those undergoing major surgery (Fig. 64.10) who have received citrated blood or platelets, heparin, bicarbonate, intravenous solutions, or calcium.[41] Alterations in blood pH and temperature further reduce the usefulness of a total calcium assay in these patients. Rapid measurement of free calcium, blood gases, and potassium permits maintenance of good cardiac function during liver transplant operations and other major operations such as those in which cardiopulmonary bypass is used. Free calcium is more useful than total calcium determination in patients in intensive care because of abnormal protein concentrations and putative circulating factors that alter calcium binding to albumin. Abnormally low free calcium is frequently found in critically ill patients.[86-88] A study at one hospital where free calcium has replaced total calcium determinations found that 41% of free calcium concentrations were abnormal among inpatients.[25] Of these cases, 31% were below and 10% were above the reference interval. The recovery room, surgical intensive care unit, renal transplantation ward, medical intensive care unit, and medical oncology unit had the highest percentages of abnormal values.

Another study has questioned the value of frequent measurements of free calcium in hospitalized patients.[89] In a large academic hospital setting, serial and daily testing was responsible for a large fraction of free calcium analyses. Half of all patients tested had free calcium concentrations

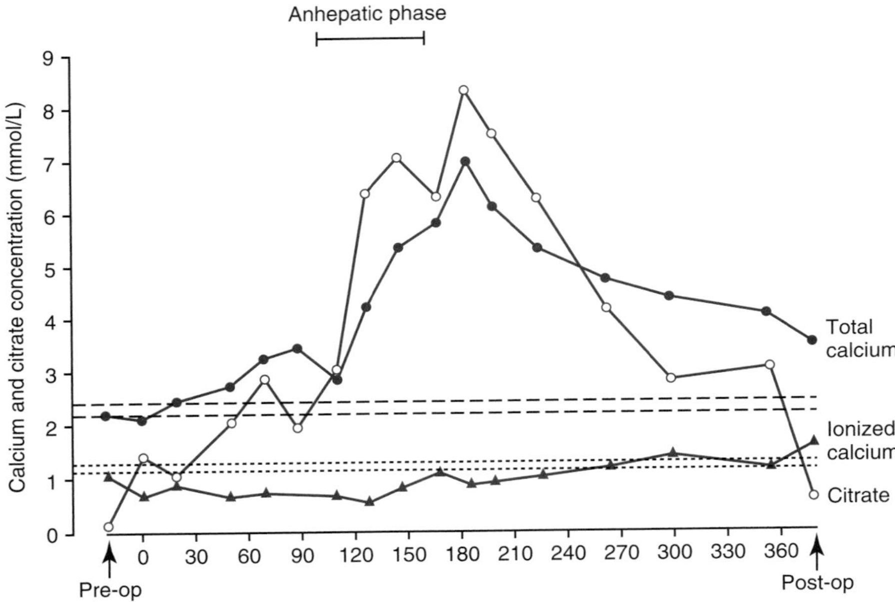

FIGURE 64.10 Free calcium (μ), total calcium (δ), and citrate (σ) concentrations in a patient undergoing liver transplantation. Reference intervals are indicated by the *upper* (total calcium) and *lower* (free calcium) sets of *dashed horizontal lines*. The reference interval for citrate is 0.03 to 0.15 mmol/L. (From Gray TA, Paterson CR. The clinical value of ionized calcium assays. *Ann Clin Biochem* 1988;25:210–9.)

below the reference interval. Free calcium was increased by intravenous administration of calcium, but the increase attributable to administered calcium was small compared with the increase that occurred in patients given no calcium. Retrospective analysis suggested that a total calcium <8 mg/dL (<2 mmol/L) identified most patients with low free calcium <4 mg/dL (<1 mmol/L). Introduction of a reflexive strategy, in different locations, where free calcium was measured only when total calcium was below that limit reduced free calcium testing by 72% to 76% and reduced intravenous calcium gluconate therapy by 45% to 81%. An outcomes study showed no evidence of an increase in adverse events.

Bone and mineral disorders are common in patients with renal disease. The calcium metabolism of these patients is best evaluated by the determination of free calcium because of alterations in protein, pH, protein binding of calcium, and calcium complexes with organic and inorganic anions.

Free calcium may be useful in the diagnosis of hypercalcemia. Patients with subsequently surgically proven PHPT more often have increases in free calcium than in total calcium (Fig. 64.11). Free calcium is more sensitive than total calcium in detecting hypercalcemia associated with malignancy, as may be expected in patients who frequently have decreased plasma albumin concentrations. Less commonly, paraproteins produced in myeloma may bind calcium, complicating the interpretation of total or adjusted calcium measurements.

In neonates, assay of free calcium rather than total calcium is recommended because of its speed and the ability to use small skin-puncture specimens, and because of its greater validity in the presence of hyperphosphatemia, with alterations in pH, and with the persistence of α-fetoprotein after birth.[82]

Urinary Calcium

The rate of urinary calcium excretion reflects calcium intake, intestinal absorption, skeletal resorption, and renal tubular filtration and reabsorption.[9] Healthy men and women excrete up to 300 mg (7.5 mmol) of calcium per day on a diet with unrestricted calcium content, and up to 200 mg (≈5 mmol) per day on a calcium-restricted diet (500 mg or 12.5 mmol dietary calcium per day or less for several days). The reference data for urinary calcium are not well established, and it may be preferable to use a value of 4 mg/kg body weight (0.1 mmol/kg) as the upper reference limit in an individual patient.

The reference interval for urinary calcium (UCa) for spot fasting or timed specimens collected after an overnight fast is <0.16 mg/100 mL (<0.04 mmol/L) of glomerular filtrate (GF), as calculated by the following equation:

$$\text{UCa (mg/100 mL GF)} = \frac{[\text{UCa (mg/dL)}] \times [\text{Serum creatinine (mg/dL)}]}{\text{Urinary creatinine (mg/dL)}}$$

Alternatively, the ratio of urine calcium to urine creatinine can be calculated; reference intervals for the ratio depend on age and sex.

An important but underrecognized contributor to urine calcium excretion is urinary sodium excretion. Patients with hypercalciuria and normal sodium excretion have so-called *renal leak hypercalciuria,* which can result in increased secretion of PTH and can be corrected with the use of a thiazide diuretic. This condition should not be confused with normocalcemic hyperparathyroidism but should be regarded as a form of secondary hyperparathyroidism. Hypercalciuria with increased urinary sodium excretion responds rapidly to a reduced dietary sodium intake.

Under fasting conditions, the intestinal and renal components are relatively fixed, and calcium excretion (mg/100 mL [mmol/L] of GF) in the fasting state is used to assess the skeletal component. A value >0.16 mg/100 mL (>0.04 mmol/L) of GF usually implies an increase in osteoclastic bone

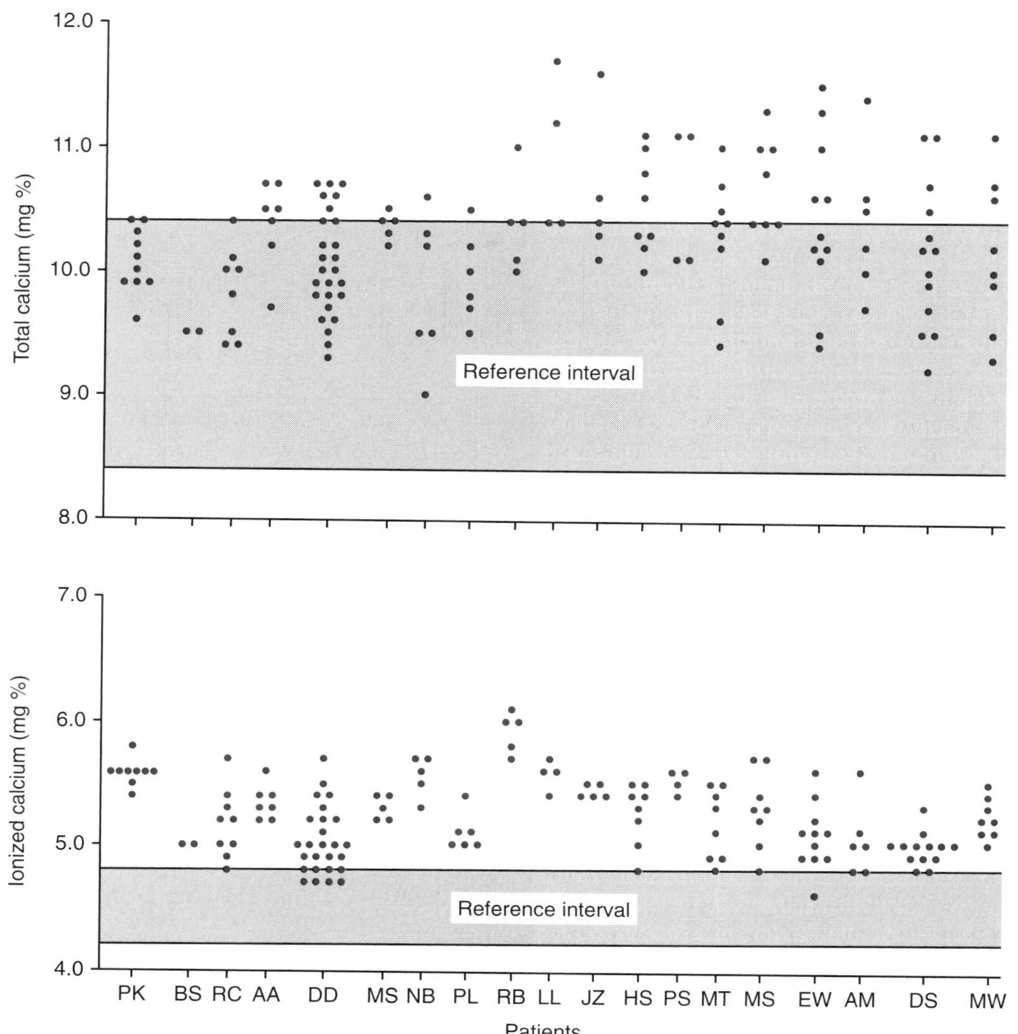

FIGURE 64.11 Concurrent total and free calcium in patients with primary hyperparathyroidism and intermittent total hypercalcemia. *Shaded areas* represent the reference intervals. (From McLeod MK, Monchik JM, Martin HF. The role of ionized calcium in the diagnosis of subtle hypercalcemia in symptomatic primary hyperparathyroidism. *Surgery* 1984;95:667–73.)

resorption. This test is used in assessing renal stone disease and high-turnover osteoporosis.

Calcium salts, such as calcium oxalate, precipitate in urine specimens during and after collection. Specimens may be collected in a container containing acid to prevent calcium salt precipitation. A commonly used acid is HCl, 6 mol/L, with 20 to 30 mL added to the container for a 24-hour collection (1–2 mL for a random specimen). The safety of the patient and the patient's family in handling such a container may be a concern. The measured urinary calcium concentration must be corrected for dilution by the acid solution when the urinary volume is low. The specimen should be kept well-mixed during collection. Specimens collected without acid should be acidified and allowed to stand for 1 hour before thorough remixing and aliquoting. Some have questioned the ability of postcollection acidification to redissolve all of the calcium salts with or without heating.[69]

POINTS TO REMEMBER

Calcium

- The skeleton is the major store of calcium.
- The free calcium is the physiologically important ion and is tightly regulated.
- PTH and vitamin D metabolites combine to regulate calcium via the kidney, intestine, and bone.
- Calcium adjusted for albumin can supply important information regarding an individual's calcium status.
- A calcium sensing receptor is present on the chief cells of the parathyroid gland that is responsive to changes in circulating free calcium.

PHOSPHATE

An adult has about 600 g or approximately 20 mol of phosphorus in inorganic and organic phosphates, of which about 85% is in the skeleton, and the rest is principally in soft tissue (see Table 64.1).[9,90]

Biochemistry and Physiology

Plasma contains both inorganic and organic phosphate, but only inorganic phosphate is measured. Inorganic phosphate exists as both monovalent ($H_2PO_4^-$) and divalent (HPO_4^{2-}) phosphate anions. The ratio of $H_2PO_4^-$ to HPO_4^{2-} is pH dependent and varies from approximately 1:1 in acidosis to 1:4 at pH 7.4 and 1:9 in alkalosis. Approximately 10% of the phosphate in serum is protein-bound; 35% is complexed with sodium, calcium, and magnesium; and the remainder, or 55%, is free (see Table 64.1). The organic phosphate esters are located primarily within the cellular elements of blood.

Inorganic phosphate is a major component of hydroxyapatite in bone; thus it plays an important role in the structural support of the body and provides phosphate for the extracellular and intracellular pool.

In the soft tissue, most phosphate is intracellular. Although both inorganic and organic phosphate is present in cells, most is organic and is incorporated into nucleic acids, phospholipids, phosphoproteins, and high-energy compounds involved in metabolism. ATP and other phosphates, such as creatine phosphate, are involved in many energy-intensive physiologic functions, such as muscle contractility, neurologic function, and electrolyte transport. Phosphate is also an essential element of cyclic nucleotides (such as cAMP) and cofactors such as nicotinamide-adenine dinucleotide phosphate (NADP). It is important for the activity of several enzymes, including adenylate cyclase, 25-hydroxyvitamin D-1α-hydroxylase, and those involved in the production of 2,3-diphosphoglycerate, the key compound regulating the oxygen affinity of hemoglobin. Intracellular phosphate therefore is involved in the regulation of intermediary metabolism of proteins, fats, and carbohydrates, and in gene transcription and cell growth.

Regulation of phosphate is a complex process involving the kidneys, intestine, and skeleton. Plasma phosphate in adults is maintained in the range of 0.7 to 1.4 mmol/L. Throughout 24 hours, plasma phosphate concentration demonstrates a diurnal variation (Fig. 64.12), with a significant increase after the evening meal, a peak in the early hours of the morning, and a decrease to nadir in the early morning.[91] This circadian rhythm is almost completely removed by fasting, demonstrating the importance of dietary intake on the daily changes in phosphate.[92] 1,25(OH)$_2$D can promote phosphate and calcium absorption via the intestine and can increase phosphate mobilization from the bone by stimulating osteoclastic resorption of bone mineral containing hydroxyapatite as the storage form of phosphate.[91] PTH can have effects on phosphate via the kidneys by increasing the expression of the type IIa sodium-phosphate cotransporter (NPT2a) in the proximal tubules and downregulating NPT2a by decreasing the time the transporter remains in the apical membrane of the tubules.[93] PTH action at the tubules promotes phosphaturia and will lower circulating phosphate indirectly. PTH can stimulate both bone resorption and bone formation depending on the fluctuation in PTH and so can either release or deposit phosphate in bone.[92,94] It is clear that the variations observed in PTH and 1,25(OH)$_2$D in health and disease do not fully explain the changes in phosphate homeostasis, and so the existence of "phosphatonin(s)" such as fibroblast growth factor (FGF)23 had been suspected for some time.

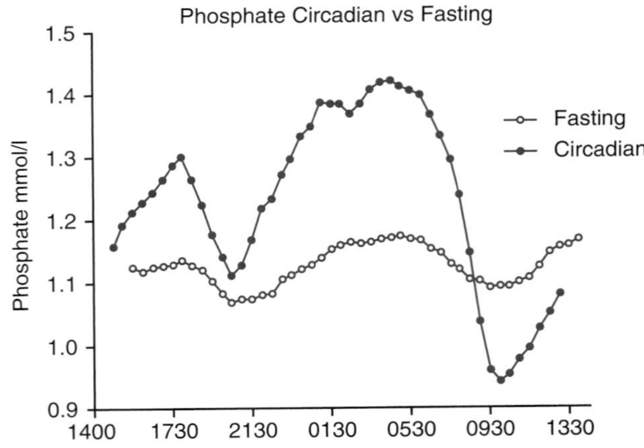

FIGURE 64.12 Normal diurnal rhythm and rhythm after a 96 hour fast. The normal subjects ate meals at 0800, 1200, 1800, and 2230, and they were recumbent from 2300 until 0800. (Modified from Fraser WD, Logue FC, Christie JP, et al. Alteration of the circadian rhythm of intact parathyroid hormone following a 96-hour fast. *Clin Endocrinol [Oxf]* 1994;40:523–8.)

FGF23 is a mid- to long-term modulator of phosphate homeostasis.[95] FGF23 increases fractional excretion of phosphate by the kidneys. It also decreases production of the active form of vitamin D, 1,25(OH)$_2$D, by decreasing the activity of the enzyme responsible for its formation (25-hydroxyvitamin D 1-alpha-hydroxylase). Both of these key activities lead to decreased plasma phosphate concentrations. FGF23 is secreted by bone cells (osteocytes, osteoblasts, and osteoclasts) in response to sustained increased plasma phosphate or increased plasma 1,25(OH)$_2$D. In CKD, FGF23 increases in a compensatory mechanism to counter increasing plasma phosphate. As kidney failure deteriorates further, responsiveness to FGF23 declines (in association with loss of Klotho, the coreceptor for FGF23) reducing FGF23's ability to lower plasma phosphate. The C-terminal fragment of Klotho increases in plasma and further inhibits FGF23 action.[96]

Other phosphatonins that play a role in phosphate metabolism in health and disease are matrix extracellular phosphoglycoprotein (MEPE), frizzled related protein, acidic serine aspartate-rich MEPE-associated motif (ASARM), and FGF7. These molecules can have their effects through bone, kidneys, and the intestine.

Clinical Significance

Disorders of phosphate metabolism can be separated into those causing hypophosphatemia and those causing hyperphosphatemia.

Hypophosphatemia

Hypophosphatemia, defined as the concentration of inorganic phosphate in the serum below the reference interval

BOX 64.8 Causes of Hypophosphatemia and Phosphate Depletion

Intracellular Shift
- Refeeding syndrome
- Glucose/fructose
  - Oral or intravenous
  - Artificial nutrition
- Insulin
- Diabetic ketoacidosis
- Respiratory alkalosis
- Alcoholism
- Severe burns
- Hungry bone syndrome

Lowered Renal Phosphate Threshold
- Primary or secondary hyperparathyroidism
- Oncogenic osteomalacia
- Renal tubular defects
  - Familial hypophosphatemia
  - Fanconi syndrome

Decreased Net Intestinal Phosphate Absorption
- Increased loss
  - Vomiting
  - Diarrhea
  - Phosphate-binding antacids
- Decreased absorption
  - Malabsorption syndrome
  - Vitamin D deficiency

Intracellular Phosphate Loss
- Acidosis
  - Ketoacidosis
  - Lactic acidosis
- Genetic
  - X-linked hypophosphatemic rickets
  - Autosomal dominant hypophosphatemic rickets
  - Autosomal recessive hypophosphatemic rickets
  - Dent disease
  - Hereditary hypophosphatemic rickets with hypercalciuria
  - Vitamin D–resistant rickets types 1 and 2

Drugs
- Acetazolamide
- Anticonvulsants
- Anti–epidermal growth factor (EGF) treatment
- Antiviral drugs (HIV therapy)
- Azacitidine
- Bisphosphonates
- Catecholamines
- Cefottan
- Diuretics
- Estrogens
- Ifosfamide
- Iron polymaltose
- Niacin
- Paracetamol
- Phosphate binding antacids
- Rapamycin
- Salicylate
- Suramin
- Tyrosine kinase inhibitors

(usually <2.5 mg/dL [<0.81 mmol/L]), is relatively common in hospitalized patients (≈2%). Hypophosphatemia is not necessarily associated with intracellular phosphate depletion. Hypophosphatemia may be present when cellular concentrations are normal, and cellular phosphate depletion may exist when plasma concentrations are normal or even high.

Hypophosphatemia or phosphate depletion in blood may be caused by a shift of phosphate from extracellular to intracellular spaces; renal phosphate wasting; decreased intestinal absorption; and loss of intracellular phosphate.[9,90,97] Box 64.8 lists the commonly encountered causes of hypophosphatemia and phosphate depletion.

A shift of phosphate from extracellular to intracellular fluid is a common cause of hypophosphatemia. A major cause of low plasma phosphate is carbohydrate-induced stimulation of insulin secretion, which promotes the transport of glucose and phosphate into insulin-sensitive cells, where phosphate is incorporated into sugar phosphates and ATP. Oral or intravenous carbohydrate and injected insulin decrease plasma phosphate concentration. Refeeding of malnourished individuals creates an anabolic state, causing an intracellular shift of phosphate. In severe cases of nutritional deficiency and the refeeding syndrome, rhabdomyolysis may occur, resulting in normalization of plasma phosphate as phosphate is released from damaged muscle cells. Respiratory alkalosis leads to an increase in intracellular pH, which activates phosphofructokinase and accelerates glycolysis, causing a shift of phosphate into the cell. Low plasma phosphate in these conditions does not indicate a deficiency of phosphate, and hypophosphatemia is self-correcting with stabilization of the patient's condition.

Renal phosphate wasting may also cause hypophosphatemia. Any cause of excessive PTH secretion (primary and secondary hyperparathyroidism) lowers the renal phosphate threshold and may result in hypophosphatemia and phosphate depletion. However, this may not occur if renal failure is the cause of secondary hyperparathyroidism when hyperphosphatemia is more common. The renal phosphate threshold is also lowered in Fanconi syndrome, X-linked hypophosphatemic rickets (XLH), and tumor-induced osteomalacia (TIO).

Hypophosphatemia and phosphate depletion may result from inadequate intestinal phosphate absorption. Patients taking aluminum- or magnesium-containing antacids may develop hypophosphatemia because these antacids bind phosphate in the intestine, rendering it nonabsorbable. The hypophosphatemia observed in patients with malabsorption may be more closely related to their secondary hyperparathyroidism than to malabsorption of phosphate. Because phosphate is abundant in most foods, dietary deprivation is not usually a cause of phosphate depletion in patients with normal intestinal function and an adequate diet.

Intracellular phosphate may be lost in acidosis as a result of catabolism of organic compounds within cells. Diabetic ketoacidosis is associated initially with high-normal to increased plasma phosphate. Treatment of ketosis, hyperglycemia, and acidosis with insulin and intravenous fluids results in intracellular movement of phosphate, urinary loss of phosphate, and a rapid reduction in the plasma phosphate concentration. Consequently, patients being treated for diabetic ketoacidosis may have both intracellular phosphate depletion and hypophosphatemia.

The clinical manifestations of plasma phosphate depletion depend on the length and the degree of deficiency. Moderate hypophosphatemia of 1.5 to 2.4 mg/dL (0.48–0.77 mmol/L) is usually not associated with clinical signs and symptoms (unless chronic, when osteomalacia or rickets develops). Plasma concentrations <1.5 mg/dL (0.48 mmol/L) may produce clinical manifestations. Because phosphate is necessary for the formation of ATP, glycolysis and cellular function are impaired by low intracellular phosphate concentrations. Muscle weakness, acute respiratory failure, cardiac arrhythmia, and decreased cardiac output may occur in phosphate depletion. At very low plasma phosphate concentrations (<1 mg/dL [<0.32 mmol/L]), rhabdomyolysis may be seen. Phosphate depletion in erythrocytes decreases erythrocyte 2,3-diphosphoglycerate, which causes tissue hypoxia as the result of increased affinity of hemoglobin for oxygen. Severe hypophosphatemia (plasma phosphate concentration <0.5 mg/dL [<0.16 mmol/L]) may result in hemolysis of the red blood cells. Mental confusion and frank coma may be secondary to low ATP and tissue hypoxia. If hypophosphatemia is chronic, impaired mineralization of bone produces rickets in children and osteomalacia in adults.

Treatment of hypophosphatemia depends on the degree of hypophosphatemia and on the presence of symptoms. Patients with moderate hypophosphatemia often require only treatment of the underlying disorder and, possibly, oral phosphate supplementation. In patients with marked symptoms of hypophosphatemia, particularly if respiratory muscle weakness is present, parenteral administration of phosphate may be indicated.

Hyperphosphatemia

Common causes of hyperphosphatemia are listed in Box 64.9. The most common cause of hyperphosphatemia is inability of the kidneys to excrete phosphate.[90,97] Hyperphosphatemia is a major clinical problem in CKD (see Chapter 59). In acute kidney injury and CKD, a decrease in glomerular filtration rate reduces the renal excretion of phosphate, resulting in hyperphosphatemia. Moderate increases in plasma phosphate occur in individuals with low PTH (hypoparathyroidism), PTH resistance (pseudohypoparathyroidism), or acromegaly (increased growth hormone) caused by an increased renal phosphate threshold. Growth hormone contributes to the increased renal phosphate threshold and the higher phosphate concentrations observed in children. EDTA therapy has also been associated with hyperphosphatemia.

Increased intake and a shift of phosphate from the tissues into the extracellular fluid are also causes of hyperphosphatemia. Excessive oral, rectal, or intravenous phosphate administration for the treatment of phosphate depletion is a common cause of hyperphosphatemia. Release of phosphate as the result of cell breakdown in cases of rhabdomyolysis, intravascular hemolysis, or chemotherapy of certain malignancies may cause hyperphosphatemia. Hyperphosphatemia may also be associated with acidosis, a consequence of the hydrolysis of intracellular organic phosphate–containing compounds, with the release of phosphate into the plasma.

The clinical manifestations of hyperphosphatemia depend on its rate of onset. A rapid increase in plasma phosphate may be associated with hypocalcemia. Therefore, symptoms may include tetany, seizures, and hypotension (see Box 64.4). Long-term hyperphosphatemia may be associated with secondary hyperparathyroidism, osteitis fibrosa, and soft-tissue calcification of the kidneys, blood vessels, cornea, skin, and periarticular tissue.

Therapy for hyperphosphatemia is directed toward correcting the cause. In renal failure and in hypoparathyroidism, dietary restriction of phosphate and agents that bind phosphate in the intestine (calcium carbonate and others) are useful in lowering the plasma phosphate concentration but are mostly not sufficient to fully reverse hyperphosphatemia.[90,97]

BOX 64.9 Causes of Hyperphosphatemia

Decreased Renal Phosphate Excretion

- Decreased glomerular filtration rate
  - Renal failure, chronic and acute
- Increased tubular reabsorption
  - Hypoparathyroidism
  - Pseudohypoparathyroidism
  - Acromegaly
  - Disodium etidronate (bisphosphonate)

Increased Phosphate Intake/Absorption

- Oral or intravenous administration
- Phosphate-containing laxatives or enemas
- Vitamin D/vitamin D analogs intoxication

Increased Extracellular Phosphate Load

- Transcellular shift
  - Lactic acidosis
  - Respiratory acidosis
  - Untreated diabetic ketoacidosis
  - Malignant hyperpyrexia

Cell Lysis

- Rhabdomyolysis
- Intravascular hemolysis
- Cytotoxic therapy
- Tumor lysis syndrome
- Leukemia
- Lymphoma

Genetic

- Tumoral calcinosis
- Pseudohypoparathyroidism types 1A and 1B
- Autosomal dominant hypoparathyroidism
- Familial isolated hypoparathyroidism
- Blomstrand disease
- Epidermal naevus syndrome
- Osteoglophonic dysplasia

Measurement of Phosphate

Most methods used to measure serum inorganic phosphate are based on the reaction of phosphate ions with ammonium molybdate to form a phosphomolybdate complex that is then measured by a spectrophotometer[13]:

$$7H_3PO_4 + 12(NH_4)_6Mo_7O_{24} \bullet 4H_2O \rightarrow 7(NH_4)_3[PO_4(MoO_3)_{12}] + 51NH^{+4} + 51OH^- + 33H_2O$$

The colorless phosphomolybdate complex may be measured directly by ultraviolet absorption (340 nm) or reduced to molybdenum blue and measured at 600 to 700 nm. An acidic pH is necessary for the formation of complexes, but it must be controlled because both complex formation and reduction of molybdate are dependent on pH. A less acidic pH can result in spontaneous reduction of molybdate. The rate of complex formation is also influenced by protein concentration. Solubilizing agents such as Tween 80 are used to prevent protein precipitation.

Measurement of unreduced complexes has several advantages, including simplicity, speed, and reagent stability, and it is the assay that is used in most laboratory analyzers. Disadvantages of the method include greater interference by hemolysis, icterus, and lipemia when measurements are made at 340 nm.

Many reducing agents have been used in producing the blue phosphomolybdate complex, including aminonaphtholsulfonic acid, stannous chloride, methyl-*p*-aminophenol sulfate, ferrous ammonium sulfate, ascorbic acid, and *N*-phenyl-*p*-phenyldiamine (semidine) HCl. Each of these reagents appears to have some individual advantage, such as increased stability, increased color stability, lower detection limit, or reduced hydrolysis of organic esters. Ferrous sulfate and especially ascorbic acid have often been used for biologic specimens containing organic esters, because they cause fewer breakdowns of labile phosphate esters. Aminonaphtholsulfonic acid has been widely used but is unstable, tends to precipitate, and requires careful timing because color continues to increase for several hours. With this reagent, color formation is increased with heating. Stannous chloride provides greater color intensity. Hydrazine has been added to stannous chloride to stabilize the reagent and improve the linearity. Methyl-*p*-aminophenol sulfate is acid tolerant, allowing for a one-component acid-molybdate reagent. A method using semidine hydrochloride has been published as a "Selected Method" by the American Association for Clinical Chemistry.[98]

Phosphate concentrations can also be determined by several other procedures, including the vanadate-molybdate and enzymatic methods. Vanadate and molybdate form a yellow complex with phosphate at acid pH, but the method tends to overestimate inorganic phosphate because of hydrolysis of organic esters. Enzymatic methods are rarely used.[13]

Specimen Requirements

Serum and heparinized plasma are preferred specimens for the measurement of phosphate. Concentrations of inorganic phosphate are about 0.2 to 0.3 mg/dL (0.06–0.1 mmol/L) lower in heparinized plasma than in serum. Other anticoagulants such as citrate, oxalate, and EDTA may interfere with formation of the phosphomolybdate complex and thus are not suitable.[13]

The apparent concentration of inorganic phosphate in whole-blood specimens may decrease or increase with time, depending on the type of specimen, the storage temperature, and the duration of storage. Phosphate concentrations in plasma or serum are increased by prolonged storage with cells at room temperature or 37°C. Hemolyzed specimens are unacceptable because erythrocytes contain high concentrations of organic phosphate esters, which can be hydrolyzed to inorganic phosphate during storage. Inorganic phosphate increases by 4 to 5 mg/dL (1.29–1.61 mmol/L) per 24 hours in hemolyzed specimens stored at 4°C, and more rapidly at room temperature or 37°C. Glucose phosphates, creatine phosphate, and other organic phosphates may also be hydrolyzed by assay conditions, resulting in overestimation of inorganic phosphate concentrations.

Phosphate is considered to be stable in separated serum for days at 4°C and for months when frozen, provided evaporation and lyophilization are prevented.

Interferences

Depending on the method used, positive or negative interference has been noted with hemolyzed, icteric, and lipemic specimens.[13] Mannitol,[99] fluoride, and monoclonal immunoglobulins[100,101] have also been reported to interfere. Glassware should be properly cleaned and rinsed because phosphate is a common component of many detergents.

Reference Intervals

Phosphate is often referred to as *phosphorus,* a practice that is inaccurate and misleading because only phosphate, not elemental phosphorus, circulates in blood and is measured. When results are reported in molar units (as in SI), the numeric results and the reference intervals are the same for phosphorus and phosphate, but confusion occurs when results are reported in mg/dL.

In adults, the reference interval for serum phosphate is 2.5 to 4.5 mg phosphorus/dL (0.81–1.45 mmol/L). In children, it is 4 to 7 mg phosphorus/dL (1.29–2.26 mmol/L). Adult plasma reference intervals are about 0.2 mg/dL (0.06 mmol/L) lower than for serum (2.3–4.3 mg/dL [0.75–1.39 mmol/L]).

Serum phosphate concentrations are about 50% higher in infants than in adults and decline throughout childhood as a consequence of the ability of growth hormone to increase the renal phosphate threshold.[102] Detailed pediatric reference intervals have been established as part of the CALIPER study and are available in the Appendix. The reference interval for serum phosphate in elderly women is similar to that in younger adult women, whereas in elderly men it is lower than that in younger adult men.[79,80]

Because a significant diurnal variation in plasma phosphate has been reported, fasting morning specimens are recommended (see Fig. 64.12).[13] Concentrations are higher in the afternoon and evening. Plasma phosphate concentrations are influenced by dietary intake and meals and are increased by exercise.

Urinary phosphate excretion varies with age, muscle mass, renal function, PTH, time of day, and other factors. Urinary excretion of phosphate varies widely with diet and is essentially equivalent to dietary intake.[9] On a nonrestricted diet, the reference interval for urinary phosphate is 0.4 to 1.3 g/24 hours (12.9–42 mmol/24 hours).

Urine should be collected in 6 mol/L HCl (20 to 30 mL for a 24-hour specimen) to avoid precipitation of phosphate complexes. Simultaneous measurement of phosphate and creatinine in serum and urine with fasting morning spot or 1- to 2-hour timed collections permits calculation of the renal phosphate threshold ($TmPO_4$/GFR); this calculation is considered the best method for assessing renal tubular reabsorption of phosphate.[13] The clearance of phosphate divided by creatinine clearance can be plotted on a nomogram,[103] and the $TmPO_4$/GFR determined. This index expresses phosphate reabsorption as a function of both serum phosphate concentration and GFR and is more useful than urinary phosphate excretion.

POINTS TO REMEMBER

Phosphate

- Phosphate can be stored in bone combined with calcium as hydroxyapatite.
- Abnormalities of phosphate metabolism can lead to significant bone disorders including rickets.
- Phosphate metabolism is under the regulation of PTH, vitamin D metabolites, and FGF23.
- Phosphate in serum is subject to significant fluctuation throughout the day influenced by nutritional intake.
- Chronic kidney disease results in significant increases in serum phosphate.

MAGNESIUM

Magnesium is the fourth most abundant cation in the body and the second most prevalent intracellular cation.[104,105] The total body magnesium content is about 25 g (~1 mol), of which about 55% resides in the skeleton (see Table 64.1). One-third of skeletal magnesium is exchangeable and is thought to serve as a reservoir for maintaining the extracellular magnesium concentration. About 45% of magnesium is intracellular.

Biochemistry and Physiology

The concentration of magnesium in cells varies from 2.4 to 7.3 mg/dL (1–3 mmol/L). In general, the higher the metabolic activity of a cell, the greater is its magnesium content. Within cells, most of the magnesium is bound to proteins and negatively charged molecules; 80% to 90% of cytosolic magnesium is bound to ATP, and MgATP is the substrate for numerous enzymes. The nucleus, mitochondria, and endoplasmic reticulum contain significant amounts of magnesium. Approximately 0.5% to 5% of the total cellular magnesium is free. Transport of magnesium across the cellular membrane is regulated by a specific magnesium transport system.

Extracellular magnesium accounts for about 1% of the total body magnesium content. About 55% of the magnesium in plasma is free, 30% is associated with proteins (primarily albumin), and 15% is complexed with phosphate, citrate, and other anions (see Table 64.2).

Magnesium is a cofactor for more than 300 enzymes in the body.[90,106] It is required for formation of substrates of enzymes (eg, MgATP is a substrate for numerous enzymes that require ATP). In addition, magnesium is an allosteric activator of many enzyme systems. Examples of enzymes that require magnesium for action include adenylate cyclase, Na^+,K^+-adenosine triphosphatase (ATPase), alkaline phosphatase, Ca^{2+}-ATPase, phosphofructokinase, and creatine kinase. The guanine nucleotide containing regulatory proteins Gs and Gi require magnesium for activity. Magnesium is important in oxidative phosphorylation, glycolysis, cell replication, nucleotide metabolism, and protein biosynthesis. A decrease in the plasma magnesium concentration lowers the threshold of axonal stimulation and increases nerve conduction velocity. Magnesium also influences neurotransmitter release at neuromuscular junctions by competitively inhibiting the entry of calcium into presynaptic nerve terminals. Reducing the plasma magnesium concentration results in increased neuromuscular excitability. Magnesium deficiency can thus result in a variety of metabolic abnormalities and clinical consequences.[90]

The Institute of Medicine recommends a daily magnesium intake of 310 to 420 mg; 20% to 80% of dietary magnesium is absorbed via the small bowel, with absorption being proportional to the amount present in the diet. Both passive and active pathways control absorption. Vitamin D status has minimal effect on magnesium absorption. Passive absorption occurs paracellularly through a favorable electrochemical gradient and solvent-driven cellular uptake. Active absorption is via two magnesium transporters in the large intestine: transient receptor potential melastatin 6 (TRPM6) and TRPM7. It has been suggested that TRPM6 plays an important role in epithelial magnesium uptake. This receptor is expressed along the whole length of the large intestine, whereas TRPM7 is more ubiquitous in its expression and is thought to be involved in cellular magnesium homeostasis.

The kidneys play a major role in regulating magnesium balance. Seventy to 80% of magnesium is ultrafilterable, with 15% to 25% then being reabsorbed passively in the proximal tubules. Sixty-five to 75% is then absorbed paracellularly in the thick ascending limb of the loop of Henle facilitated by the tight junctional protein claudin-16 (also known as *paracellin-1*) and claudin-19. Five to 10% of filtered magnesium is reabsorbed transcellularly via TMRP6 located in the distal convoluted tubules (Fig. 64.13).

Clinical Significance

Disorders of magnesium metabolism can be separated into those causing hypomagnesemia with or without magnesium deficiency and hypermagnesemia.

Hypomagnesemia/Magnesium Deficiency

Hypomagnesemia is common in hospitalized patients.[90,106,107] Box 64.10 outlines the causes of hypomagnesemia. Ten percent of patients admitted to city hospitals and as many as 65% of patients in intensive care units may be hypomagnesemic.[6,90] Moderate or severe magnesium deficiency is usually due to loss of magnesium from the gastrointestinal tract or kidneys.

Vomiting and nasogastric suction may deplete body stores of magnesium in that upper gastrointestinal fluids contain approximately 1.2 mg/dL (~0.5 mmol/L) of magnesium. More commonly, magnesium deficiency is associated with losses from the lower intestine. Diarrhea may result in marked losses of magnesium; therefore, acute diarrheal states, regional enteritis, and ulcerative colitis are frequently complicated by magnesium deficiency. Excessive urinary losses of magnesium from the kidneys are important causes

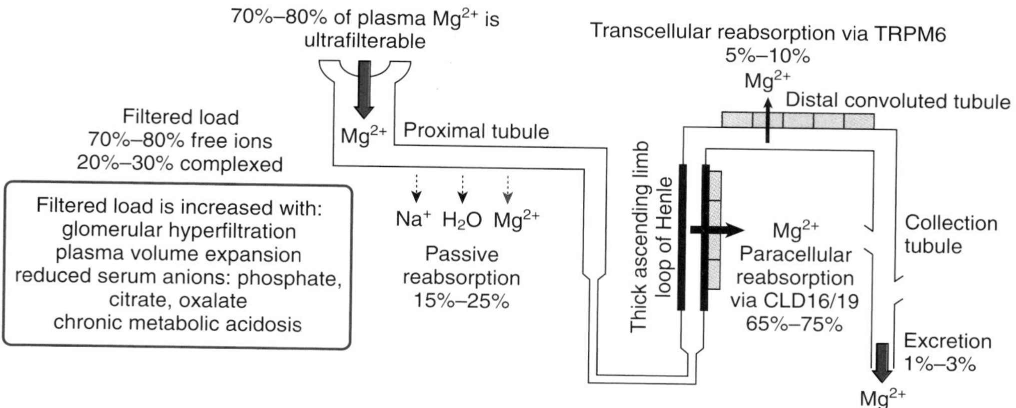

FIGURE 64.13 The regulation of magnesium secretion by the kidney tubule. (From Pham PC, Pham PA, Pham SV, Pham PT, Pham PM, Pham PT. Hypomagnesemia: a clinical perspective. *Int J Nephrol Renovasc Dis* 2014;7:219–30.)

BOX 64.10 Causes of Hypomagnesemia

Gastrointestinal Disorders
- Prolonged nasogastric suction
- Malabsorption syndromes
- Extensive bowel resection
- Acute and chronic diarrhea
- Intestinal and biliary fistulas
- Protein-calorie malnutrition
- Acute hemorrhagic pancreatitis
- Primary hypomagnesemia (neonatal)
- Celiac disease

Renal Loss
- Chronic parenteral fluid therapy
- Osmotic diuresis
  - Glucose (diabetes mellitus)
  - Mannitol
  - Urea

Hypercalcemia

Drugs
- Alcohol
- Diuretics (furosemide, ethacrynic acid)
- Proton pump inhibitors
- Aminoglycosides
- Cisplatin
- Cyclosporine
- Amphotericin B
- Cardiac glycosides
- Pentamidine
- Metabolic acidosis (starvation, ketoacidosis, alcoholism)

Renal Disease
- Chronic pyelonephritis, interstitial nephritis, and glomerulonephritis
- Diuretic phase of acute tubular necrosis
- Postobstructive nephropathy
- Renal tubular acidosis
- Post–renal transplantation

Primary Hypomagnesemia

Phosphate Depletion

Genetic (Affected Molecule in Brackets)
- Hypomagnesemia with secondary hypocalciuria (TRPM6)
- Familial hypomagnesemia with hypercalciuria and nephrocalcinosis (Claudin 16)
- Familial hypomagnesemia with hypercalciuria, nephrocalcinosis, and ocular manifestations (Claudin 19)
- Antenatal Bartter syndrome type I (NKCC2)
- Antenatal Bartter syndrome type II (ROMK)
- Classic Bartter syndrome type III (ClC-Kb)
- Bartter syndrome type V (CaSR)
- Gittelman syndrome (NCCT)
- Isolated recessive hypomagnesemia with normocalcemia (EGF)
- Autosomal dominant hypomagnesemia (CNNM2)

of magnesium deficiency. Clinically important causes include alcohol, diabetes mellitus (osmotic diuresis), loop diuretics (eg, furosemide), aminoglycoside antibiotics, and proton pump inhibitors (eg, omeprazole, lansoprazole). Increased sodium excretion (parenteral fluid therapy) and increased calcium excretion (hypercalcemic states) also result in renal magnesium wasting. Familial hypomagnesemia has been reported in patients with a loss-of-function mutation in TRPM6 and missense mutations in claudin genes.

Because magnesium deficiency is usually secondary to another disease process or to a therapeutic agent, features of the primary disease process may complicate or mask magnesium deficiency. Neuromuscular hyperexcitability with tetany and seizures may be present. These symptoms and signs may also be due to hypocalcemia, and magnesium deficiency is a common cause of hypocalcemia. Hypomagnesemia impairs PTH secretion and causes resistance to PTH in the kidneys and bone; it has been linked to osteoporosis in epidemiologic studies[106] and in animal experiments.[108]

One of the more serious complications of magnesium deficiency is cardiac arrhythmia. Premature atrial complexes, atrial tachycardia and fibrillation, premature ventricular complexes, ventricular tachycardia, torsades de pointes, and ventricular fibrillation may occur with magnesium deficiency.

These effects may be caused in part by the hypokalemia, renal wasting, and intracellular depletion of potassium caused by hypomagnesemia. In hospital practice, it is very common to see a triad of deficiencies involving magnesium, calcium, and potassium.

Although extracellular magnesium accounts for only about 1% of total body magnesium, and plasma magnesium concentrations correlate poorly with total body magnesium, determination of serum magnesium is the most widely used test to assess magnesium deficiency. Hypomagnesemia is often transient and is not an indication of magnesium deficiency. Conversely, intracellular magnesium depletion and magnesium deficiency may exist despite a normal plasma magnesium concentration. Consequently, hypocalcemia, hypokalemia, neuromuscular hyperirritability, and cardiac arrhythmias should be an alert to the possible presence of magnesium deficiency. Other tests less commonly used include the magnesium loading test (also known as the *magnesium tolerance test*)[106] and measurements of intracellular magnesium (eg, in red blood cells, lymphocytes, or skeletal muscle).

Acute symptomatic magnesium deficiency usually is treated with parenteral magnesium; mild depletion may be treated with oral magnesium.[90]

Hypermagnesemia

Magnesium intoxication is not a frequently encountered clinical problem, although a mild to moderate increase in the serum magnesium concentration may be noted in as many as 12% of hospitalized patients.[104] Symptomatic hypermagnesemia is almost always caused by excessive intake, resulting from administration of antacids, enemas, and parenteral fluids containing magnesium (Box 64.11). Many of these patients have concomitant renal failure, thereby limiting the ability of the kidneys to excrete excess magnesium. Magnesium used to treat preeclampsia and eclampsia may cause magnesium intoxication in mothers and their neonates.

BOX 64.11 Causes of Hypermagnesemia

Excessive Intake
- Orally (usually in the presence of chronic renal failure)
  - Antacids
  - Catharsis
- Rectally
  - Purgation
- Parenterally
  - Treatment of pregnancy-induced hypertension
  - Post–cardiac bypass surgery
  - Treatment of magnesium deficiency

Renal Failure
- Chronic (usually with administration of magnesium)
  - Antacid
  - Catharsis
  - Enema
  - Infusion
  - Dialysis
- Acute
  - Rhabdomyolysis

Familial Benign Hypocalciuric Hypercalcemia (FBHH, FHH)

Lithium Ingestion

Depression of the neuromuscular system is the most common manifestation of magnesium intoxication. Deep tendon reflexes disappear at a plasma magnesium concentration above 5 to 9 mg/dL (2.06–3.7 mmol/L), whereas depressed respiration and apnea, caused by voluntary muscle paralysis, may occur at concentrations >10 to 12 mg/dL (4.11–4.94 mmol/L). Higher concentrations may result in cardiac arrest. Somnolence, hypotension, nausea, vomiting, and cutaneous flushing may also be seen. Hypermagnesemia induces a decrease in the plasma concentration of calcium, presumably because of the inhibition of both PTH secretion and end-organ action of PTH by magnesium.

The possibility of magnesium intoxication should be anticipated in patients receiving magnesium, especially those with renal failure. Replacement therapy should be discontinued in patients with mildly to moderately increased serum magnesium. Higher serum concentrations than "normal" are aimed for in the treatment of preeclampsia and eclampsia (4.4–7.3 mg/dL, 1.8–3 mmol/L). Because calcium acutely antagonizes the toxic effects of magnesium and can promote magnesium excretion through the kidneys, patients with severe magnesium intoxication may be treated with intravenous calcium. If necessary, peritoneal dialysis or hemodialysis against a low-magnesium dialysis bath effectively lowers the serum magnesium concentration.[90,104]

Measurement of Total Magnesium

Serum magnesium has been measured by various techniques including photometry, fluorometry, flame emission spectroscopy, and atomic absorption spectrometry (AAS).[13,109,110] Photometric methods are most commonly used by clinical laboratories; although AAS[13,111] is considered the reference method, it is rarely used.

Photometric Methods

Several metallochromic indicators or dyes change color on selectively binding magnesium and have been used to measure it in biologic samples.[13,109,110,112] Calmagite [1-(1-hydroxy-4-methyl-2-phenylazo)-2-naphthol-4-sulfonic acid] (Fig. 64.14), a metallochromic indicator, forms a colored complex with magnesium in alkaline solution, which is measured at 530 to 550 nm.[109,113-115] A calcium-chelating agent, EGTA (see Fig. 64.7), is added to reduce interference by calcium. Reagents may include potassium cyanide (to prevent formation of heavy metal complexes) and polyvinylpyrrolidone and surfactants to reduce interference from protein and lipemia. Methylthymol blue (see Fig. 64.14) forms a blue complex with magnesium, which is measured at around 600 nm.[110,112] EGTA is added to reduce interference by calcium. A formazan dye [1,5-bis(3,5-dichloro-2-hydroxyphenyl)-3-formazan carbonitrile] forms a complex with magnesium at alkaline pH, which has been measured at 630 nm by thin-film reflectance photometry.[116] *N,N′*-[1,2-ethanediylbis(oxy-2,1-phenylene)bis(N-carboxymethyl)] glycine is used to chelate calcium. This thin-film reflectance method shows relatively little interference from icteric, lipemic, and hemolyzed specimens. Increased calcium concentrations cause a measurable but small overestimation. Magon, or xylidyl blue [1-azo-2-hydroxy-3-(2,4-di-methylcarboxanilido)-naphthalene-1′-(2-hydroxybenzene)] (see Fig. 64.14), binds magnesium in alkaline solution, causing a spectral shift and forming a red complex.[117,118] Absorbance most often has been measured

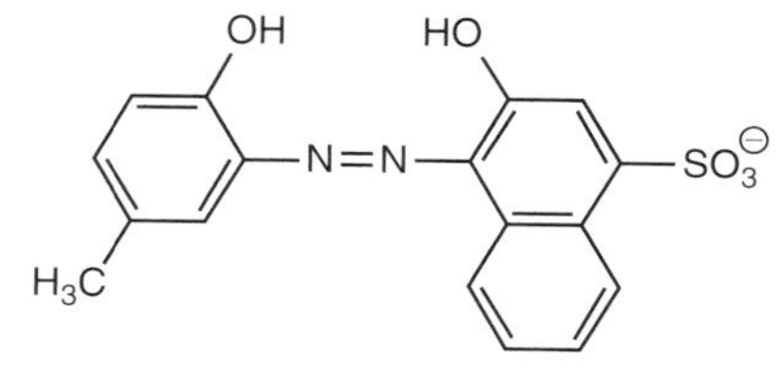

FIGURE 64.14 Metallochromic Indicators for Magnesium.

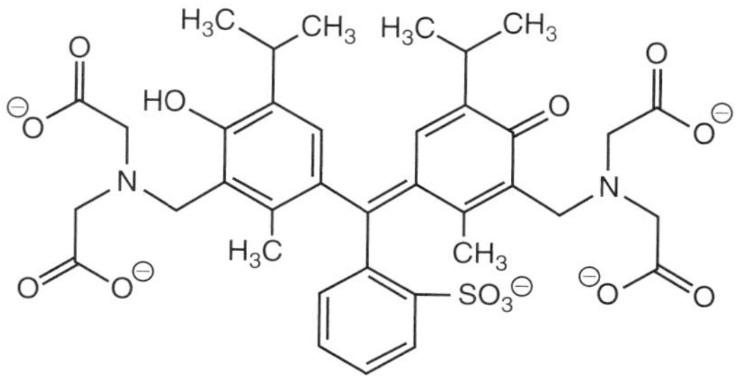

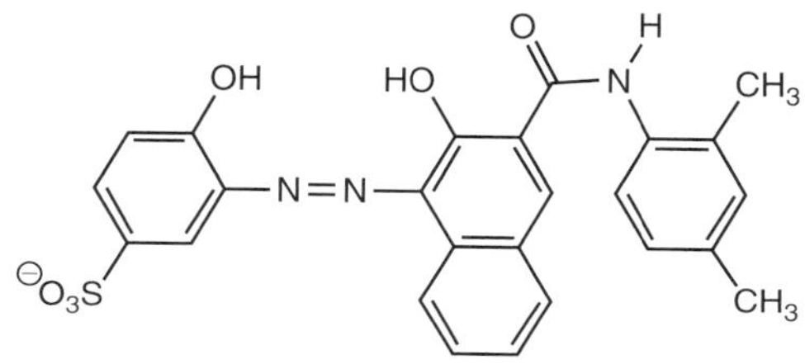

around 600 nm. Calcium and protein interferences are reduced by EGTA and dimethyl sulfoxide, respectively. All of these methods have been applied to automated analyzers.

Atomic Absorption Spectrometry

As with calcium, AAS methods provide greater accuracy and precision for magnesium measurements than do photometric methods.[13] For further information, see the following references.[110,111]

Enzymatic Methods

Enzymatic methods have been developed with hexokinase or another enzyme that uses Mg^{2+}-ATP as a substrate. The rate of the enzyme-catalyzed reaction is dependent on the concentration of magnesium. When hexokinase is used with glucose 6-phosphate dehydrogenase, the rate of the dehydrogenase reaction is monitored by measuring the formation of NADPH by measurement of absorption at 340 nm.[119] A simple one-step reaction using stabilized isocitrate dehydrogenase has been reported.[120,121] This enzyme is activated by magnesium and produces NADPH.

Measurement of Free (Ionized) Magnesium

Instruments for the measurement of free magnesium in whole blood, plasma, or serum were developed in the 1990s.[42,122,123] These instruments use ISEs with neutral carrier ionophores, including ETH5220, ETH7025, or a proprietary ionophore. Current ionophores or electrodes have insufficient selectivity for magnesium over calcium. Thus it is necessary to determine the two ions simultaneously in each sample and to correct the result for Ca^{2+} interference. Also, pH should be measured simultaneously, as the binding of magnesium in plasma is pH dependent.[124]

Comparisons of instruments for free magnesium determinations have been reported.[35,125-128] Differences in measured free magnesium were apparent among analyzers, mainly because of interference from free calcium.

Decreased total serum magnesium is a common finding in hospitalized patients. Magnesium salts are frequently administered to patients for their antiarrhythmic, vasomotor, and neuronal actions, and to patients with preeclampsia, myocardial infarction, and ischemic heart disease. Monitoring of free magnesium concentrations has been suggested because both low and high concentrations can be life-threatening.[90,104,106,129]

Discordance between total and free magnesium measurements has been reported in selected patient populations, including those with cardiovascular disorders, diabetes mellitus, alcoholism, migraine headaches, asthma, renal transplant, and head trauma, and in pregnant women. Interferences in measurements of total magnesium (such as that from thiocyanate in smokers[42]) may explain some of these discrepancies. Free magnesium determinations may be helpful in some of these disorders, in critically ill patients, and during cardiopulmonary bypass, preeclampsia, neonatal distress, and therapy with a number of drugs.[104,105,130]

Specimen Requirements for Total and Free Magnesium

Serum and heparinized plasma are the preferred specimens for measuring free and total magnesium.[122,123] Zinc heparin, lithium-zinc heparin, and some of the newer heparins developed for free calcium determination should be avoided because they significantly increase the apparent free magnesium concentration.[66,123,131] Other anticoagulants, such as citrate, oxalate, and EDTA, are not acceptable because they form complexes with magnesium. Storage of serum for days at 4°C and for months frozen does not affect measured concentrations of total magnesium, provided evaporation of the specimen is prevented.

Serum or plasma must be separated from the clot or red blood cells as soon as possible to prevent an increase in serum/plasma magnesium due to cell leakage. Because erythrocytes contain higher concentrations of magnesium than serum or plasma, hemolyzed specimens are unacceptable. Interference by icterus or lipemia depends on the method and can be decreased by the use of bichromatic analysis or blanking with EDTA. Lipemic specimens should be ultracentrifuged.

Factors that alter free calcium concentration by altering the distribution of calcium between free, protein-bound, and complexed pools can also alter free magnesium concentration. Therefore, specimens should be handled anaerobically to prevent loss of carbon dioxide and analyzed without delay to prevent changes in pH caused by metabolism. As with free calcium, high concentrations of heparin should be avoided. Certain silicones or other tube additives as well as thiocyanate (smokers and diet) interfere with free magnesium determinations.

Magnesium is primarily an intracellular ion. Thus magnesium depletion is not necessarily reflected in decreased concentrations of the metal in plasma. The magnesium status of an individual can be estimated by a parenteral magnesium load test,[132] also known as a *magnesium tolerance test.*[106] In this test, the percentage of magnesium retention is assessed after an intravenous magnesium load. After baseline collection of 24-hour urine, 0.1 mmol/kg body weight of magnesium is administered intravenously in 5% dextrose, and another 24-hour urine collection is carried out. In individuals with adequate magnesium stores, 60% to 80% of the magnesium load is excreted within 24 hours.[106,132]

Urine specimens should be collected in acid (eg, HCl, 6 mol/L, with 20–30 mL added to the container for a 24-hour collection) to prevent precipitation of magnesium complexes. As with calcium, if acid must be added after collection, the entire specimen must be acidified, warmed, and mixed thoroughly before a sample is removed for analysis.

Reference Intervals for Total and Free (Ionized) Magnesium

For adults, reference intervals for total serum magnesium of 1.7 to 2.4 mg/dL (0.66–1.07 mmol/L) have been reported. However, the adequate reference interval is somewhat a matter of debate, as concentrations from the lower end may be associated with cardiovascular risk.[13] Magnesium concentrations in erythrocytes are approximately three times those of plasma. Conversion factors for the units used to express magnesium concentration are given as follows:

$$\text{mmol/L} = \text{mEq/L} \times 0.5 = \text{mg/dL} \times 0.41$$

$$\text{mEq/L} = \text{mmol/L} \times 2 = \text{mg/dL} \times 0.82$$

$$\text{mg/dL} = \text{mEq/L} \times 1.22 = \text{mmol/L} \times 2.43$$

The reference interval for free magnesium is instrument dependent;[13,42] a reference interval for the Nova Biomedical instrument (Nova Biomedical Corp., Waltham, Massachusetts) is 0.45 to 0.60 mmol/L.

Reference intervals for total magnesium in infants, children, and adolescents have been published; they do not differ significantly from those of adults.[13] Detailed pediatric reference intervals have been established as part of the CALIPER study and are available in the Appendix.

HORMONES REGULATING BONE AND MINERAL METABOLISM

PTH and 1,25(OH)$_2$D are the primary hormones regulating bone and mineral metabolism. FGF23 is recognized as an important molecule controlling phosphate homeostasis. Calcitonin has pharmacologic actions, but a physiologic role has not been established in adults. Parathyroid hormone–related peptide (PTHrP) is the principal mediator of HHM, but it also has physiologic functions in fetuses and in women during pregnancy and lactation. Sclerostin inhibits the Wnt signaling pathway that plays a major role in osteoblast development and function and so results in decreased bone formation and turnover.

Parathyroid Hormone

PTH is synthesized and secreted by the parathyroid glands, usually two superior and two inferior, located bilaterally on or near the thyroid gland capsule. The chief cells are responsible for synthesizing, storing, and secreting PTH. The chromosomal location of the gene for PTH is 11p15.3-p15.1.

Biochemistry and Physiology

The concentration of PTH in blood is determined by the rates of its synthesis and secretion by the parathyroid glands and of its metabolism and clearance by the liver and kidneys. The primary regulators of PTH secretion are free calcium, 1,25(OH)2D, and phosphate. PTH acts directly on bone and the kidneys, and indirectly on intestine via 1,25(OH)2D, to increase the plasma concentration of free calcium and ultimately decrease the plasma concentration of phosphate.

Synthesis and Secretion. Parathyroid cells have relatively few secretory granules for the storage of PTH. Thus PTH must be synthesized as needed for secretion. Control of PTH synthesis by calcium and phosphate occurs largely at the post-transcriptional level. Specific proteins bind to a sequence in the 3′-untranslated region of the PTH mRNA with resultant alteration of the stability of the mRNA.[133]

The primary translation product leading to PTH is the 115–amino acid–long pre-pro-PTH (Fig. 64.15).[134,135] The amino-terminal hydrophobic “pre” or leader sequence is involved in transporting PTH across the endoplasmic reticulum membrane into the cisternae. Both the pre sequence and the six–amino acid–long N-terminal “pro” sequence are enzymatically cleaved during intracellular processing and before packaging in the Golgi apparatus. After processing, intact PTH (84 amino acids, molecular mass 9425 Da) is secreted, stored, or degraded intracellularly. Intracellular degradation is increased when plasma calcium concentration is high and secretion of PTH is low. When PTH secretion is high (eg, with low plasma calcium), intracellular degradation of PTH is low. Unlike proinsulin, pro-PTH does not appear to be secreted or to circulate in measurable concentrations. However, together with intact PTH, several C-terminal fragments of the molecule are secreted from the parathyroid glands.[136]

The classic biologic activity of PTH resides in the N-terminal third of the molecule.[136,137] Synthetic PTH(1–34) is at least as potent as intact PTH(1–84) in interacting with the PTH/PTHrP receptor (PTH1R, type 1 PTH receptor) and stimulating calcemic, phosphaturic, and other biologic responses in kidneys and bone. Oxidation of the methionine residues at position 8 or 18 results in loss of biologic activity.

The PTH molecule contains a large number of basic amino acids. The middle portion of the molecule is quite immunogenic because of its hydrophobicity and species specificity. The C-terminal metabolite of PTH, PTH(7–84), has some effects that antagonize those of PTH(1–84)[138] and is involved in some functions of the hormone, having its own receptors in kidneys and bone, that are distinct from those mediated by PTH1R.[136]

The concentration of free calcium in blood or extracellular fluid is the primary acute physiologic regulator of PTH synthesis, metabolism, and secretion.[134,135,139] Free calcium is sensed by a G-protein–coupled CaSR in the plasma membrane of parathyroid cells; intracellular signal transduction pathways following activation of the receptor involve release of free calcium from intracellular stores and opening of plasma membrane calcium channels.[140] The 1078–amino acid CaSR (gene symbol *CASR,* gene location chromosome 3q13.3–q21) is a member of subfamily C of the G-protein–coupled receptors. Other subfamily members include γ-aminobutyric acid type B (GABAB) receptors, metabotropic glutamate receptors (mGluR), and pheromone receptors. The CaSR has a large extracellular domain for the detection of ionized calcium, seven transmembrane domains, and an intracellular domain

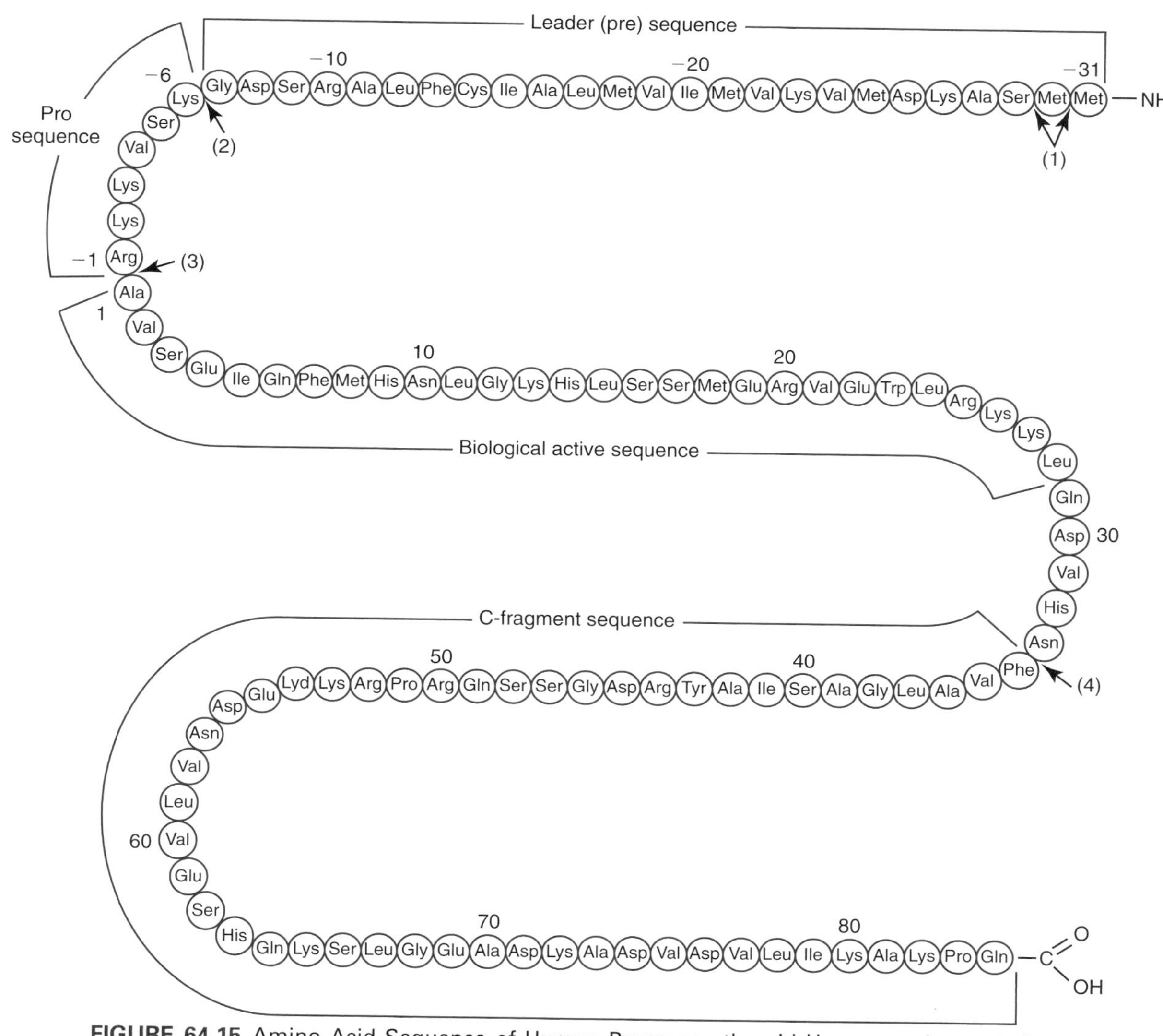

FIGURE 64.15 Amino Acid Sequence of Human Preproparathyroid Hormone. *Arrows* indicate the sites of cleavage by proteases to remove the N-terminal methionine and isoleucine *(1)*, the leader (pre) sequence *(2)*, and the pro sequence *(3)*, producing intact PTH(1–84). Cleavage at position 4 produces inactive carboxyl (C)-terminal fragments. (From Habener JF, Rosenblatt M, Potts JT Jr. Parathyroid hormone: biochemical aspects of biosynthesis, secretion, action, and metabolism. *Physiol Rev* 1984;64:985–1053.)

that couples the receptor to G proteins. An increase in extracellular free calcium concentration inhibits PTH synthesis and secretion and increases PTH metabolism, whereas a decrease has the opposite effect. An inverse sigmoid relationship exists between PTH secretion and free extracellular calcium (Fig. 64.16).[135] Several effectors/diseases can modify this relationship including growth hormone and CKD. Maximal secretion and suppression are attained with mild hypocalcemia and mild hypercalcemia, respectively. The midpoint of this relationship (or set point) is the calcium concentration at which PTH secretion is half maximal. Set points can vary from individual to individual and may be altered by physiologic or pathologic processes.

1,25$(OH)_2$D, phosphate, and magnesium also influence the synthesis and secretion of PTH.[84,134,135] 1,25$(OH)_2$D interacts with vitamin D receptors in the parathyroid glands to chronically decrease PTH secretion by suppressing PTH gene transcription and subsequent secretion. Hyperphosphatemia and hypophosphatemia increase and decrease PTH synthesis and secretion,[141] respectively, and the hyperphosphatemia of CKD leads to parathyroid hyperplasia and hyperparathyroidism. Magnesium probably does not play an important role in PTH secretion except at the extremes of magnesium concentration.[84] Chronic severe hypomagnesemia, such as that occurring in alcoholism, has been associated with impaired PTH secretion, whereas acute hypomagnesemia may stimulate secretion. Chronic hypomagnesemia can cause resistance to the effects of PTH.[142] Hypermagnesemia suppresses PTH secretion via the CaSR, although not as effectively as does calcium.

Circulating PTH demonstrates a circadian rhythm and an appropriate variation in end-organ function throughout 24 hours.[143] Acute fasting abolishes the PTH circadian rhythm,[92] which may reflect the importance of variation in phosphate in controlling the circadian secretion of PTH. The presence of the circadian rhythm has particular importance when taking

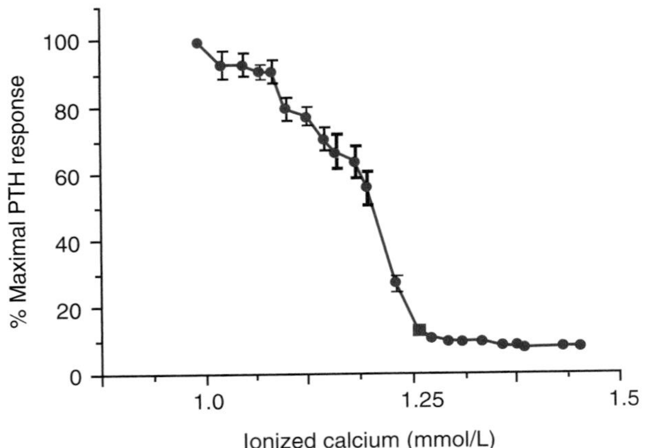

FIGURE 64.16 Regulation of secretion of intact parathyroid hormone (PTH) by calcium in healthy humans. Calcium and ethylenediaminetetraacetic acid (EDTA) were infused to demonstrate the sigmoidal relationship between PTH secretion and free calcium. **Bold** error bars demonstrate areas of the curve where a significant difference in effect on PTH release between increasing free calcium or lowering free calcium exists. (Greater differences are seen in patients with Chronic Kidney Disease.) (From Brown EM. Extracellular Ca^{2+} sensing, regulation of parathyroid cell function, and role of Ca^{2+} and other ions as extracellular [first] messengers. *Physiol Rev* 1991;71:371–411.)

samples for diagnostic purposes. In women, the circadian rhythm is blunted with an earlier and greater increase in PTH at night than in men. This blunted nocturnal rise in PTH in women may explain the poor nocturnal adaptation to fasting found in women who, despite lower calcium intake, do not reduce urinary calcium loss at night as effectively as men. In postmenopausal women with osteoporosis, there is loss of the circadian rhythm for PTH, and there is blunting of the rhythm in normal postmenopausal women when compared with normal premenopausal women.[144] Patients with PHPT lose the circadian rhythm for PTH,[145] and following removal of an adenoma the circadian rhythm is restored.

Biologic Actions. PTH influences calcium and phosphate homeostasis directly through its actions on both bone and kidneys and indirectly through its actions on the intestine through 1,25$(OH)_2$D (see Fig. 64.4).[134,135] The hormone exerts its actions by interacting with type 1 PTH receptors (PTH/PTHrP receptors) located in the plasma membranes of target cells. The PTH 1 receptor (PTH1R) is a G protein coupled receptor (GPCR). Following receptor binding of PTH both adenylate cyclase and phospholipase C are activated resulting in protein phosphorylation, activation of intracellular enzymes, and transport systems resulting in secretion of lysosomal enzymes.[134,146] Two active domains have been identified in the receptor-binding region of PTH that activate two separate second-messenger pathways upon binding to the receptor[147] in its classic target cells; PTH normally activates both pathways.

In the kidneys, PTH has several functions. It induces 25-hydroxyvitamin D-1α-hydroxylase, increasing the production of 1,25$(OH)_2$D, which, in turn, stimulates intestinal absorption of both calcium and phosphate; it increases calcium reabsorption in the distal convoluted tubules; it decreases reabsorption of phosphate by the proximal tubules; and it inhibits Na^+,H^+ antiporter activity, which favors mild hyperchloremic metabolic acidosis in hyperparathyroid states.

The effects of PTH on bone are complex, as evidenced by its stimulation of bone resorption or bone formation, depending on the concentration of PTH, the duration of exposure, and the PTH signaling profile.[134,137] Chronic exposure to high concentrations of PTH leads to increased bone resorption that is a prompt effect important for the maintenance of calcium homeostasis. Intermittent increase and decrease of PTH results in an anabolic effect on bone, and the delayed skeletal effects of PTH are important for extreme systemic needs and skeletal homeostasis. The anabolic effects of intermittent PTH secretion or injection may be mediated by inhibition of sclerostin expression in osteocytes.[148] PTH increases the number of osteoblasts and enhances their differentiation from stromal cells. Different PTH fragments and the intact hormone may have varying effects on osteoblast gene expression.[149] Because of their anabolic effects on bone, PTH(1–34) and PTH(1–84) are used as therapeutic agents for osteoporosis (see *Biochemical Markers of Bone Turnover*).[137]

Despite the extent and rapidity of catabolic effects in bone, it has not been possible to definitively find PTH receptors on osteoclasts, whereas they are found on osteoblasts and adjacent bone marrow stromal cells. These cell types mediate PTH action to osteoclasts via several cytokines and in particular RANKL.[136] Actions include enhanced differentiation of osteoclast precursors and stimulation of resorbing activity in mature osteoclasts. Osteoblasts, via macrophage–colony-stimulating factor (M-CSF), stimulate osteoclast precursor formation from macrophages. Osteoclasts are ultimately derived from the bone marrow and from hematopoietic stem cells located in the bone marrow.

Integration of the direct effects of PTH on bone and kidneys, and of the indirect effects on intestine through 1,25$(OH)_2$D, results in alterations in calcium and phosphate concentrations in blood and urine. In blood, total and free calcium concentrations are increased, whereas the concentration of phosphate is decreased. In urine, inorganic phosphate and cAMP concentrations are increased. Urinary calcium excretion usually is increased because the larger filtered load of calcium, derived from bone resorption and intestinal calcium absorption, overrides the increased tubular reabsorption of calcium. In the absence of disease, the increase in blood free calcium reduces PTH secretion through a negative feedback loop, maintaining homeostasis.

Heterogeneity of Circulating Parathyroid Hormone. PTH circulates partially as the biologically active hormone and partially as a series of N-terminally truncated fragments containing the midregion and C-terminal amino acids. Many of these fragments have been identified[150,151] (Fig. 64.17). The heterogeneity is due to the secretion of both intact hormone and C-terminal fragments by the parathyroid glands, peripheral metabolism of intact hormone by liver and kidneys to C-terminal fragments, and renal clearance of intact hormone and C-terminal fragments (Fig. 64.18). In the parathyroid glands, secretion of intact PTH is increased by hypocalcemia and is greatly reduced or absent in hypercalcemia, whereas some secretion of C-terminal fragments persists in hypercalcemia. Biologically active intact PTH (amino acids 1–84) is rapidly cleared from plasma in normal subjects (half-life <5 minutes) by Kupffer cells of the liver (60% to 70%) and

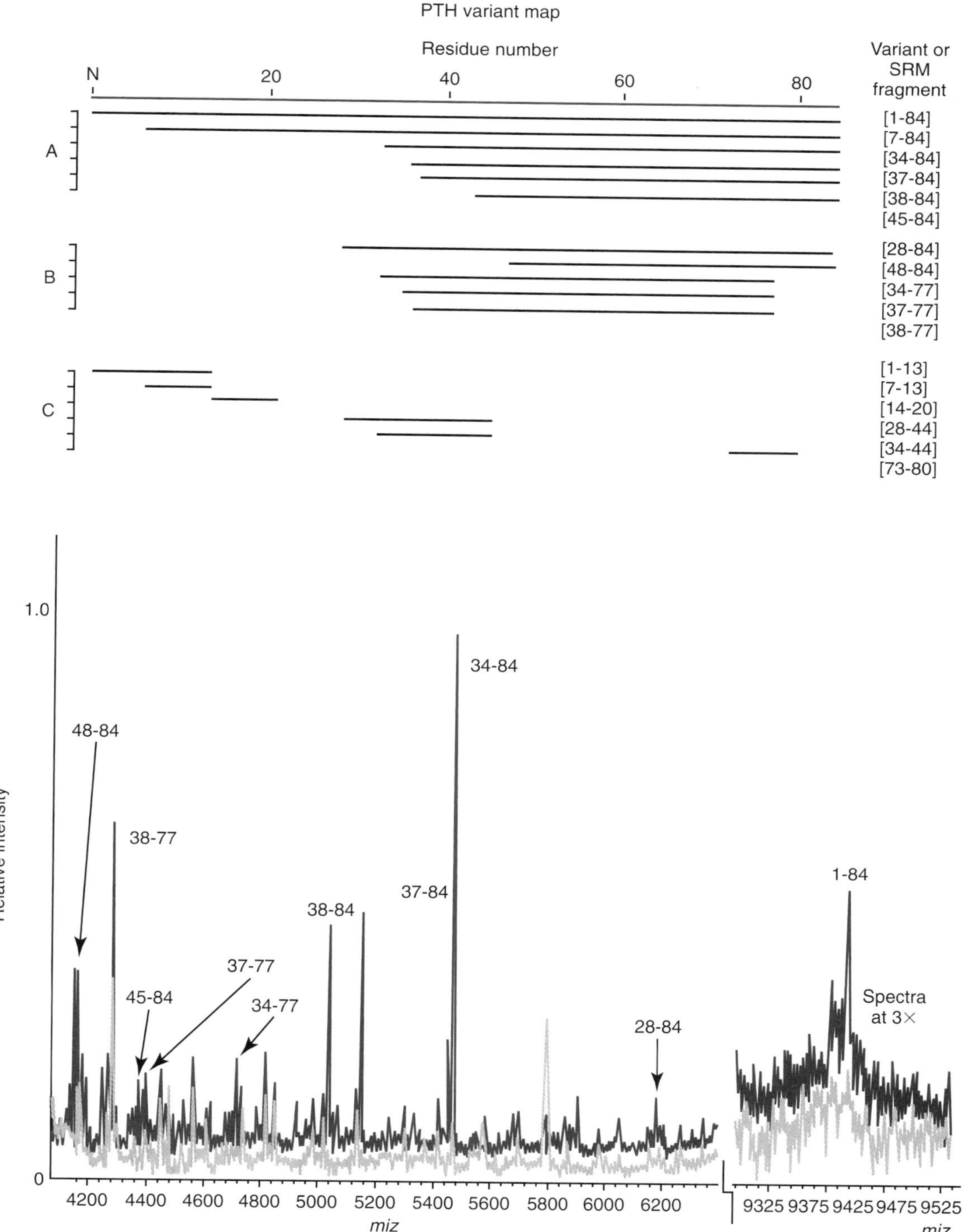

FIGURE 64.17 Parathyroid hormone (PTH) fragments in plasma. *Upper panel: (A)* N-terminally truncated PTH variants identified before 2010. *(B)* Variants added to map from study by Lopez and associates. *(C)* Conserved and truncated tryptic fragments chosen for study reported in *bottom panel. Bottom panel:* Spectra representative of 12 samples from patients with renal failure *(red/upper tracing)* and 12 from healthy controls *(light red/lower tracing)*. The marked species were consistently found at higher relative abundance in the renal failure cohort. (From Lopez MF, Rezai T, Sarracino DA, Prakash A, Krastins B, Athanas M, et al. Selected reaction monitoring—mass spectrometric immunoassay responsive to parathyroid hormone and related variants. *Clin Chem* 2010;56:281–90.)

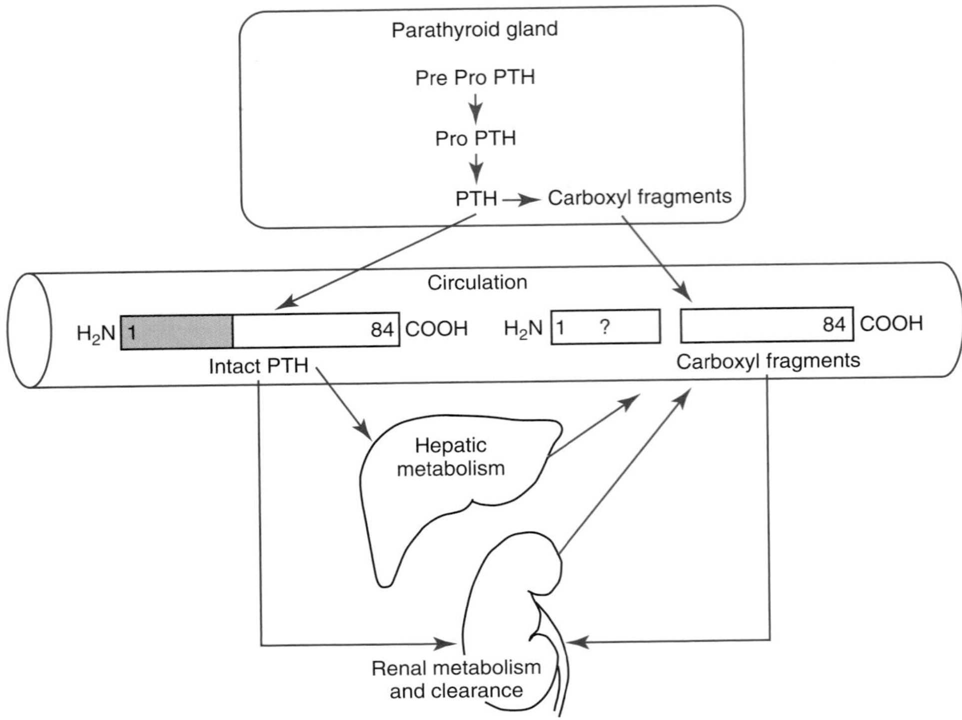

FIGURE 64.18 Secretion, metabolism, clearance, and circulating forms of parathyroid hormone (PTH). Both intact PTH and inactive fragments containing the middle and carboxyl (C)-terminal amino acids are secreted by the parathyroid glands. These inactive fragments are produced by peripheral metabolism of intact PTH by the liver and kidneys. Carboxy-terminal fragments are cleared by the kidneys by glomerular filtration. The half-life and concentration of intact hormone are small compared with those of inactive fragments. (From Endres DB, Villanueva R, Sharp CF Jr, Singer FR. Measurement of parathyroid hormone. *Endocrinol Metab Clin North Am* 1989;18:611–29.)

by glomerular filtration in the kidneys (20% to 30%).[134] Peripheral metabolism appears to inactivate intact hormone without releasing measurable concentrations of biologically active N-terminal fragments that are rapidly removed by the liver.[136,150]

Circulating PTH measured by most immunoassays is composed of both "inactive" fragments and intact hormone. Fragments consisting of the middle and carboxyl regions of the molecule (eg, amino acids 34–84, 36–84) are devoid of the N-terminal region and classic PTH biologic activity and were earlier considered to be inactive degradation products. However, reports have identified separate receptors for C-terminal PTH in bone cells and have suggested that such fragments may affect the maturation and biologic activity of these cells. C-terminal fragments are cleared by glomerular filtration and normally have a half-life of less than 1 hour. Their half-life and circulating concentration are significantly increased in individuals with impaired renal function, in most current assays. In individuals with normal renal function, 5% to 25% of the total circulating PTH is intact hormone, and 75% to 95% consists of C-terminal fragments.[134]

Clinical Significance

Determination of PTH is useful in the differential diagnosis of both hypercalcemia and hypocalcemia, for assessing parathyroid function in renal failure, and for evaluating parathyroid function in bone and mineral disorders.

Measurement of Parathyroid Hormone

Radioimmunoassay (RIA) for PTH was among the first modern immunoassays to be put to clinical use in the 1960s, adding a new dimension to diagnosis and treatment of hypocalcemic and hypercalcemic states. It soon became clear that not all immunoreactive substances measured in blood by the assay were active PTH—a finding that led to the identification of C-terminal fragments of PTH. Subsequent immunoassays were developed to overcome this problem. PTH assays have yielded different measurements as the result of the presence of a series of immunologic determinants along the molecule and the physiologic heterogeneity of circulating PTH-related antigens (Fig. 64.19).[150,152-155] Noncompetitive (sandwich) immunoassays are commonly used for the measurement of intact PTH (Fig. 64.20). RIAs for PTH have been largely discontinued because of their limited specificity and/or sensitivity (see Chapter 23 for further discussion on immunoassays). The midregion and C-terminal methods, which measured primarily C-terminal fragments, often provided poor identification of parathyroid function, as the measured concentration was affected by peripheral metabolism and glomerular filtration of the fragments.[154,156]

PTH assays were developed to measure the intact molecule of PTH(1–84) only and were called *intact assays.* These assays incorporated the use of a noncompetitive (sandwich) immunometric assay (IMA) format using two antibodies:[150,155] (1) a solid-phase capture antibody directed against

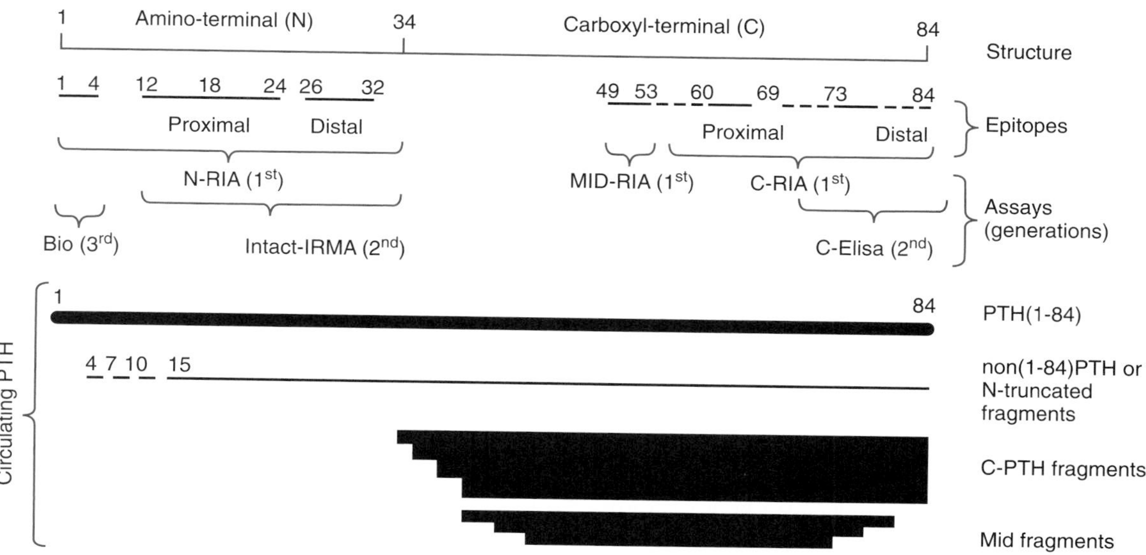

FIGURE 64.19 Relationship between parathyroid hormone (PTH) assays, PTH assay epitopes, and PTH molecular forms detected in circulation. The *upper panel* depicts the structure of human PTH and epitopes detected by various PTH assays. First-generation PTH assays detect full-length PTH(1–84), in addition to PTH fragments. These assays include radioimmunoassays (RIAs) that use antisera specific for the amino-terminal (N-RIA), middle (MID-RIA), or carboxy-terminal (C-RIA) region of PTH. Second-generation "intact PTH" assays detect full-length PTH(1–84) and non–PTH(1–84) fragments. Third-generation PTH assays (Bio) detect the full-length PTH(1–84). The *bottom panel* depicts the PTH molecular forms present in the circulation. (Modified from Henrich LM, Rogol AD, D'Amour P, Levine MA, Hanks JB, Bruns DE. Persistent hypercalcemia after parathyroidectomy in an adolescent and effect of treatment with cinacalcet HCl. *Clin Chem* 2006;52:2286–93.)

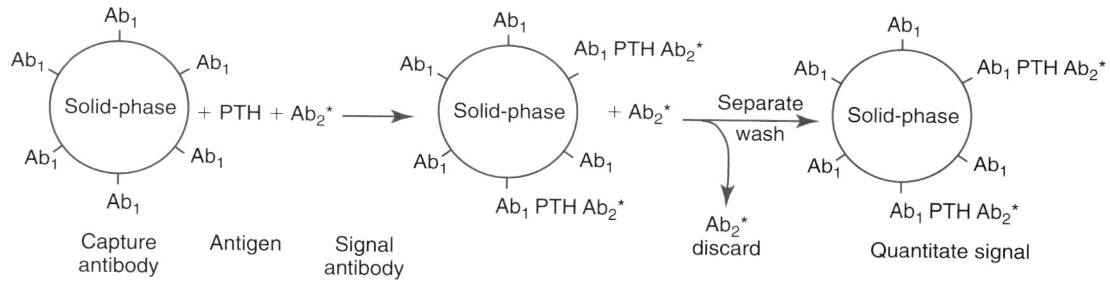

FIGURE 64.20 Principle of a noncompetitive immunoassay for parathyroid hormone (PTH). PTH is reacted with immobilized capture antibody (Ab_1) against one antigenic determinant and with a labeled signal antibody (Ab_2*) against a second antigenic determinant. PTH forms a bridge between the two antibodies, producing a "sandwich" or ternary complex. Both antibodies are added in excess, ensuring that all PTH reacts and is measured. Free signal antibody is separated, and the solid-phase antibody-PTH-labeled antibody complexes are quantified with an appropriate detection system. The signal increases with increasing concentrations of PTH. (Modified from Endres DB, Villanueva R, Sharp CF Jr, Singer FR. Measurement of parathyroid hormone. *Endocrinol Metab Clin North Am* 1989;18:611–29.)

the C-terminus and (2) a labeled detection antibody raised against the N-terminus (amino acids 1–34), or vice versa. The clinical utility of intact PTH assays in diagnosing PHPT and in monitoring secondary hyperparathyroidism is well established.[150,155] It has become clear that they can overestimate the severity of PTH-related bone disease because they can detect several molecular species of PTH, which can be separated when a serum sample is fractionated using high-performance liquid chromatography (HPLC). If PTH concentration in the serum of a patient with end-stage renal disease (ESRD) were decreased to "normal" as measured by these assays, adynamic bone disease was a possible outcome.[150,155] Blood was found to contain N-terminally truncated PTH fragments that are long enough to react in the intact PTH assays but do not bind to the PTH receptor. Therefore, the term *intact* as applied to these immunometric intact PTH assays is somewhat of a misnomer because PTH fragments (eg, PTH[7–84]) are detected along with PTH(1–84).

In the newest PTH assays, the epitope of the N-terminally binding antibody consists of the first four to six amino acids of the PTH molecule.[154,157] Such assays have been variously termed *true intact* PTH assays, *whole* PTH assays, or *cyclase-activating* PTH assays. Despite the theoretical improvement, in clinical practice they have not shown clear advantages over earlier IMMAs.[150,158] In addition to intact PTH, these assays have been reported to detect another molecular species in blood, called *amino PTH* by D'Amour and colleagues,[159] which possibly has its amino-terminal serine residue in a phosphorylated form.

For measuring intact PTH, the capture antibody is most often directed against the carboxyl or middle region of the molecule (eg, amino acid sequences 39–84, 44–84) and the signal antibody against the N-terminal amino acid sequence (1–34).[150] A few methods have reversed this, using capture antibodies against the N-terminal amino acid sequence (eg, amino acids 26–32) and signal antibodies against the middle or C-terminal amino acid sequence (eg, 55–64).[157] With the latter arrangement, a higher concentration of signal antibody is needed because of the high concentration of inactive fragments relative to intact hormone, especially in CKD, potentially adversely impacting sensitivity by increasing the blank (signal in the absence of intact PTH). This can be overcome by adopting a two-step incubation in which non-bound C-terminal fragments can be washed off before incubation with the signal antibody. The specificity of these noncompetitive methods depends on the sequence specificity of the antibodies used; they do not measure classic C-terminal fragments that lack the N-terminal amino acid sequence (1–34).

Antibodies used in IMAs may be monoclonal or polyclonal antibodies purified by affinity chromatography to produce sequence-specific antibodies. Affinity-purified polyclonal antibodies have been widely used, particularly for the signal antibody, because of the difficulty of producing high-affinity monoclonal antibodies against PTH. Capture antibodies are noncovalently bound or are covalently attached to one of a variety of solid phases, including polystyrene beads, plastic tubes, paramagnetic particles, microparticulate cellulose, and sepharose.[160] Signal antibodies most often have been radiolabeled (for immunoradiometric assays [IRMAs]) with ^{125}I, or labeled (for immunochemiluminometric assays [ICMAs]) with a chemiluminescent compound, such as acridinium ester or isoluminol, or an enzyme (enzyme-linked immunosorbent assay [ELISA] or enzyme immunoassay [EIA]), such as alkaline phosphatase (ALP).[157,160] Other assay formats used on fully automated immunoassay analyzers include electrochemiluminescence detection (see Chapter 13). Intact PTH assays available commercially have been listed and compared.[157,161]

N-Terminal–Truncated Parathyroid Hormone and Intact Parathyroid Hormone Methods. The N-terminal–truncated fragment(s) (also called non-[1–84] PTH and PTH[7–84]), which contain all but a few of the N-terminal amino acids of PTH,[162,163] account, on average, for 20% to 50% of intact PTH concentrations measured by early intact PTH assays in healthy subjects and patients with chronic renal failure, respectively. Furthermore, the relative concentration of N-terminal–truncated PTH increases with hypercalcemia and decreases with hypocalcemia. Similar to classic C-terminal fragments, N-terminal–truncated PTH originates from both secretion by the parathyroid glands and peripheral metabolism of intact hormone.[164]

The first noncompetitive methods used for intact PTH cross-reacted with N-terminal–truncated fragment(s), thus overestimating the concentration of biologically active, intact PTH. Synthetic PTH(7–84) has shown cross-reactivities of 40% to 60% in these methods.[163,165] These findings stimulated the development of a new intact PTH, using antibodies against the very N-terminal region of PTH that do not cross-react with synthetic PTH(7–84) (see Fig. 64.20). The newest intact PTH assay utilizes antibodies against PTH(1–4) and even requires the presence of the most N-terminal amino acid, as evidenced by its failure to recognize PTH(2–34).[157,165]

Studies have suggested that N-terminal–truncated PTH (eg, PTH[7–84]) may be biologically active and antagonistic to the action of PTH. Synthetic PTH(7–84), used as the available representative of N-terminal–truncated PTH, decreased serum calcium; antagonized the calcemic, phosphatemic, and phosphaturic effects of intact PTH in thyroparathyroidectomized animals; and was bound by a C-terminal PTH receptor distinct from the PTH/PTHrP receptor.[166]

Because early intact PTH assays measured N-terminal–truncated PTH, they overestimated the concentration of biologically intact hormone. The degree of overestimation is method dependent, but intact PTH is 50% higher on average than PTH(1–84) in patients with PHPT or ESRD.[165]

The inability of some intact PTH methods to accurately measure biologically active intact hormone may explain why such intact PTH assays are not a reliable indicator of bone turnover in dialysis patients and often fail to distinguish patients with low-, normal-, and high-turnover bone disease.[167] Furthermore, treatment of patients to suppress their intact PTH value to normal or near-normal can result in adynamic bone disease. The PTH(1–84)/N-terminal–truncated fragment ratio has been proposed for evaluating bone turnover in renal osteodystrophy on the basis of the ability of PTH(7–84) to antagonize the biologic activity of intact PTH and preliminary experimental evidence for the predictive value of this ratio.[168] The ratio is calculated after intact PTH and PTH(1–84) are measured and N-terminal–truncated fragments are calculated by subtracting PTH(1–84) from intact PTH. This issue is still unclear, however, because subsequent studies were unable to substantiate the greater clinical utility of measuring both PTH(1–84) and intact PTH and calculating this ratio to assess bone turnover in ESRD.[167,169]

The newest intact PTH assays (whole PTH) are not absolutely specific for intact PTH, as evidenced by demonstration of an amino-terminal form of PTH distinct from both the intact hormone and the N-truncated fragment. This form represented approximately 20% of the intact PTH measured with a second-generation intact PTH method.[159] The clinical implications of this form have not yet been established, but it has been reported in patients with hyperparathyroidism and parathyroid carcinoma.

Several studies have highlighted the lack of comparability of current commercial PTH assays, especially when measuring samples from patients with CKD or receiving hemodialysis.[161] This has raised concerns regarding standardization of PTH assays and recognized that the production and implementation of a commutable international standard material is required. An IFCC committee is addressing the question of future standardization of PTH assays using a new standard material, IS 95/646.

Mass spectrometry has been used to characterize PTH fragments and to measure intact PTH.[151,170,171] In the mass-spectrometric method Kumar and colleagues used for measurement of PTH in serum,[171] PTH was captured on antibody-coated beads and was digested by trypsin. The N-terminal 13 amino acids were then quantified by selected reaction monitoring in a liquid chromatography–tandem mass-spectrometry system. The assay showed no detectable cross-reactivity with PTH fragments, including PTH(7–84), which was captured on the antibody-coated beads. Using this method, PTH(7–84) was not detected in the serum of CKD patients, although other large C-terminal fragments have been detected. The sensitivity of the method (60 pg/dL, 6 pmol/L) is not as low as immunoassays.

Specimen Requirements. Specimen requirements may depend on the specific assay method. EDTA plasma is often preferred, but some assays require serum, and results may vary with sample type. In some immunoanalyzers, EDTA interferes with assay signal when in excess by chelating divalent cations needed for enzymatic action of the alkaline phosphatase label.[172] After separation, if EDTA plasma is used in an assay, it should be analyzed within 72 hours if stored at 4°C. Lower concentrations of PTH are observed in serum incubated at room temperature for longer than a few hours, or after one to several days at 4°C. PTH has been reported to be more stable in EDTA plasma;[173] this is a probable consequence of reduced proteolytic activity. There is no consensus on the effects of storing samples in a freezer (–20°C or –80°C) before analysis. PTH can stick to some plastic tubes and result in a decrease in values obtained with sample storage.

Reference Intervals

Reference intervals for PTH vary greatly with the method used[155,157] and can be affected by the vitamin D status of the population sampled.

Typical reference intervals are as follows:

Intact PTH: 10 to 65 pg/mL or 1.1 to 6.8 pmol/L

PTH (1–84): 6 to 40 pg/mL or 0.6 to 42 pmol/L

Interpretation of PTH concentrations must take into account the patient's circulating calcium concentration at the time of sampling.

The upper limit of the reference interval for PTH may be inappropriately high because of the prevalence of vitamin D insufficiency and mild secondary hyperparathyroidism in the reference group. Significantly lower intervals have been established for these methods by excluding individuals with vitamin D insufficiency (see *Vitamin D and Its Metabolites*, subsection *Reference Intervals* later in this chapter).[157]

Intact PTH concentrations vary with age and are low or normal during pregnancy,[78] lower in fetuses and umbilical cord blood,[81] and increased during the first few days of life, in response to neonatal hypocalcemia. Concentrations in children and adolescents are reportedly similar, if not identical, to those in adults.[174] In healthy adults, circulating concentrations of intact PTH increase with age.[80]

Intact PTH is secreted in a pulsatile fashion with an overall circadian rhythm characterized by a nocturnal rise. Measurement of PTH on more than one occasion should assist in preventing misinterpretation of parathyroid status as the result of episodic secretion.

Interpretation of Parathyroid Hormone Results

PTH is the most important test for the differential diagnosis of hypercalcemia. The plasma concentration of intact PTH is increased in most patients with PHPT (Fig. 64.21) and is below normal or close to the lower limit of the reference interval in most patients with non-parathyroid hypercalcemia, including hypercalcemia of malignancy (HCM). In patients with stable hypercalcemia, a PTH value in the upper half of the reference interval is inappropriately high and is suggestive of PHPT. Whenever possible, PTH specimens should be obtained before therapy is provided for hypercalcemia, because PTH secretion may be stimulated by declining serum calcium. Increased or inappropriately detectable PTH in patients with hypercalcemia and malignancy suggests coexisting hyperparathyroidism and malignancy, in that ectopic PTH production appears to be extremely rare. HCM is usually associated with bone metastases (eg, local osteolytic hypercalcemia) and/or production of PTHrP (eg, HHM). PTHrP does not cross-react in any of the PTH immunoassays that have been evaluated. According to one study, whole PTH(1–84) is more sensitive in diagnosing PHPT than intact PTH.[175] In this study, whole PTH(1–84) and intact PTH were increased in 96% and 73% of 56 patients with PHPT, respectively. However if the correct interpretation of inappropriate intact PTH for the prevalent hypercalcemia had been included, then the diagnostic sensitivities were not significantly different.

Measurements of urinary calcium excretion are necessary to confirm hypocalciuria in cases of suspected FBHH (see Box 64.5). Such patients do not usually display hypercalcemia >12 mg/dL (>3 mmol/L). Because having this disorder in the heterozygous state leads to no ill effects, parathyroidectomy is not indicated. However, infants with homozygous FBHH can present with life-threatening hypercalcemia, even requiring emergency parathyroidectomy.

Because of the short half-life of PTH (≤5 minutes), intraoperative determination of intact PTH can be used to assess the completeness of parathyroidectomy and to facilitate minimally invasive parathyroid surgery, thereby improving cost-effectiveness and cosmetic outcomes.[176] PTH is measured just before the incision and again at 20 minutes after resection of the hyperfunctioning parathyroid tissue. The surgeon should not massage the patient's neck at baseline (this can increase PTH) or following parathyroidectomy (when PTH can be released from injured parathyroid glands). A decline of 50% or more is usually considered indicative of the removal of all hyperfunctioning tissue. This is method-dependent, relating to cross-reactivity with various PTH fragments, and method-specific rates of decline in measured PTH need to be established. In contrast to patients with solitary parathyroid adenomas, interpretation of results in patients with multiglandular disease is complicated. Preoperative or intraoperative PTH may be useful for localizing hyperfunctioning parathyroid tissue by sampling multiple veins from the cervical and mediastinal regions. PTH(1–84) may be decreased more rapidly and completely than intact PTH after removal of hyperfunctioning tissue.[177] Postoperative PTH concentrations after thyroidectomy may be predictive of development of hypocalcemia due to a large influx of calcium into bone (hungry bone syndrome).[178]

Subnormal or low-normal PTH is observed in most patients with hypoparathyroidism (see Fig. 64.21); such concentrations are inappropriately low for patients with hypocalcemia. The apparently detectable concentrations observed in many patients with hypoparathyroidism or non-parathyroid hypercalcemia may be a result of the imprecision of methods used at low concentrations, a nonspecific serum (ligand-free

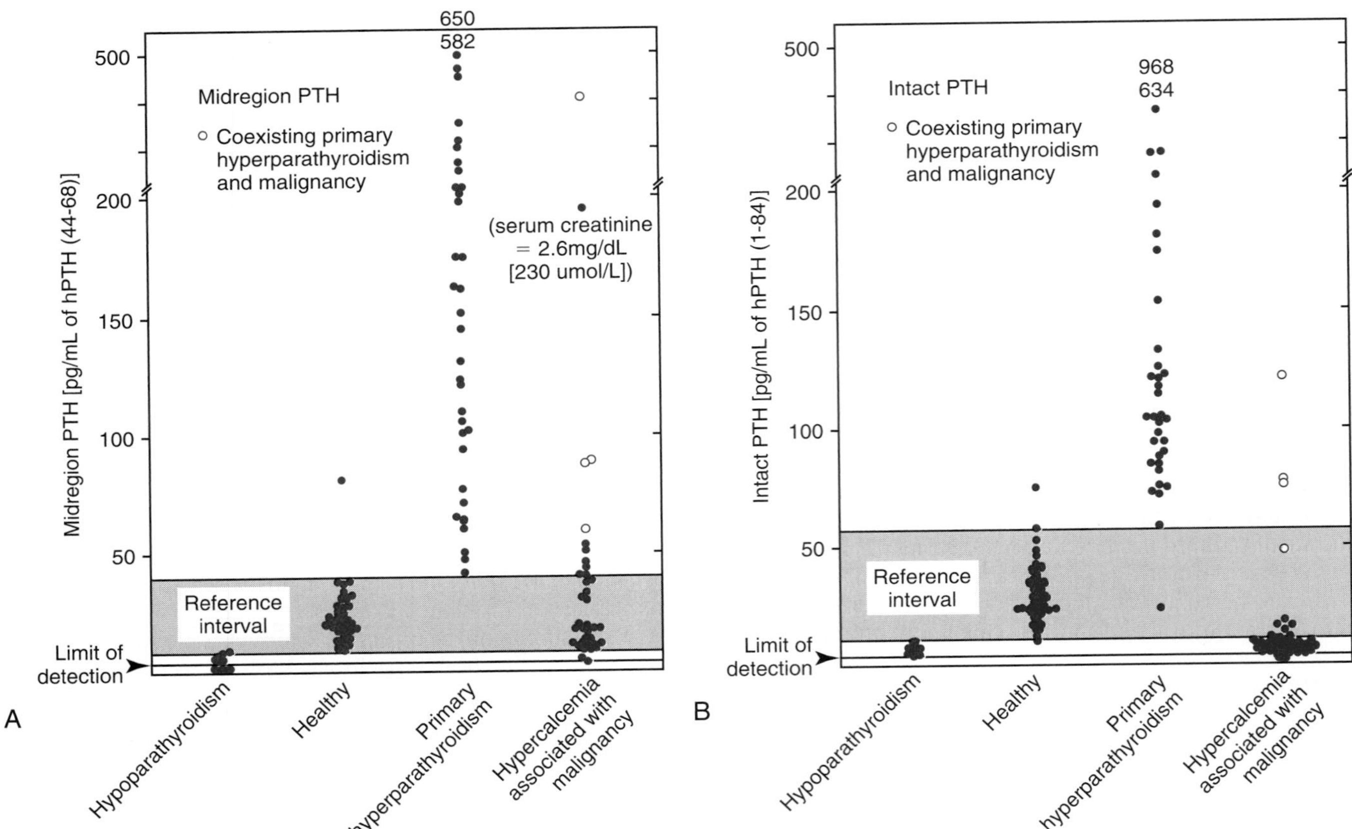

FIGURE 64.21 Parathyroid hormone (PTH) in healthy individuals and patients with primary hyperparathyroidism, hypercalcemia associated with malignancy, and hypoparathyroidism. PTH was measured with immunoassay for its midregion **(A)** and for intact PTH **(B)**. (Modified from Endres DB, Villanueva R, Sharp CF Jr, Singer FR. Measurement of parathyroid hormone. *Endocrinol Metab Clin North Am* 1989;18:611–29.)

matrix) effect, and/or measurement of N-terminal–truncated PTH. More rigorous assessment of the limit of detection of PTH immunoassays and use of the newest intact PTH(1–84) methods may show that concentrations are undetectable in these patients.

In secondary hyperparathyroidism, PTH is increased before total or free calcium becomes abnormally low—a consequence of homeostatic mechanisms for maintenance of serum calcium. Consequently, PTH is more sensitive than calcium in identifying secondary hyperparathyroidism.

In patients with chronic kidney disease (CKD), measurement of PTH is helpful in assessing parathyroid function, in estimating bone turnover, and in improving management. Patients with high-turnover bone disease caused by secondary hyperparathyroidism (advanced osteitis fibrosa) have the highest concentrations of PTH, whereas those with low-turnover, adynamic bone disease, including osteomalacia, have the lowest concentrations whether measured by whole or intact PTH assays (Fig. 64.22). Considerable overlap in whole/intact PTH concentrations is apparent among the various forms of renal osteodystrophy. In dialysis patients, cut points ("decision levels") of <100 or 150 pg/mL (10 or 15 pmol/L) and >250 to 300 pg/mL (25 to 30 pmol/L) have been suggested for distinguishing patients with low-turnover and high-turnover bone disease, respectively. The Kidney Disease Improving Global Outcomes (KDIGO) organization produced guidelines for evaluation and management of mineral and bone disorders and defined therapeutic goals for intact PTH concentrations in patients with CKD stages 3 to 5. In patients with CKD5 the recommendation is made that intact PTH is maintained within two to nine times the upper reference limit.[179] Some nephrologists feel that this recommendation should be reviewed and that this range is too wide.[180]

Parathyroid status is usually determined by measuring PTH on predialysis specimens because various factors, including changes in plasma calcium and the type of dialysis membrane, affect PTH secretion and clearance. Comparison of predialysis and postdialysis specimens has been suggested for determining acute parathyroid responsiveness to alterations in plasma calcium concentrations.

The whole PTH(1–84) assay theoretically should more accurately assess parathyroid status and bone turnover and thus better guide therapy in patients with ESRD compared with the intact PTH assay (see Measurement of Parathyroid Hormone).[167,168]

However, the benefits of the new generation of PTH assays have not been as expected,[181] and it has not been easy to define the therapeutic targets for PTH(1–84).[182] Significant variability and lack of comparability of PTH assays has

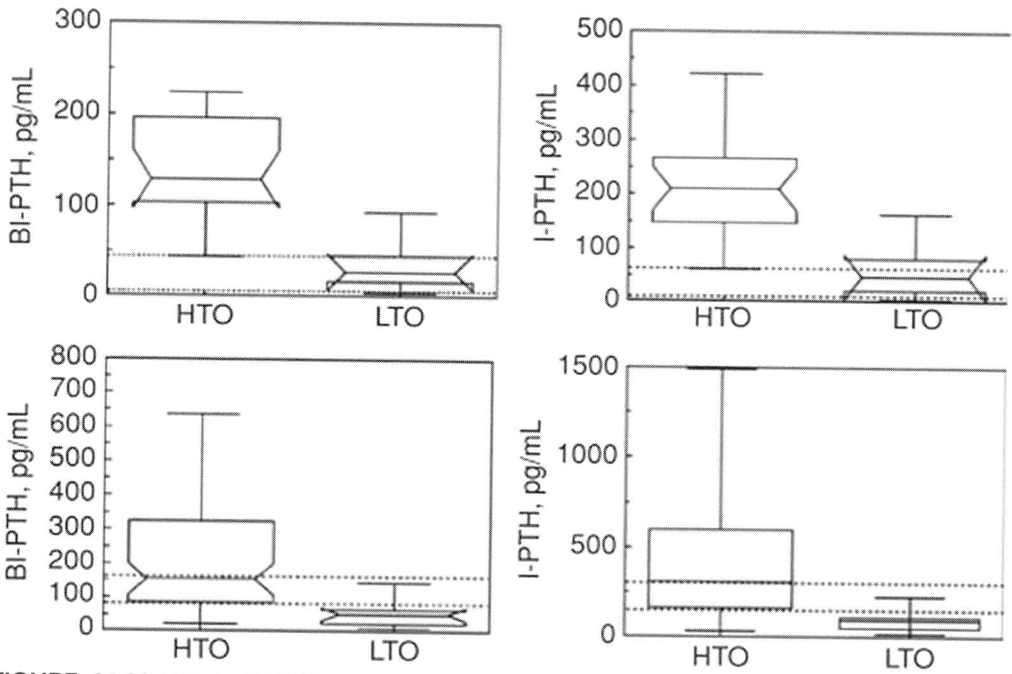

FIGURE 64.22 Whole (BI-PTH) or Intact PTH (I-PTH) concentrations in patients with high bone turnover (HTO) or low bone turnover (LTO) skeletal lesions of renal osteodystrophy. Upper panels CKD 3/4 and lower panels CKD5. The *dashed lines* indicate depict the ranges recommended by the KDOQI guidelines of the National kidney Foundation for patients with CKD5.

been demonstrated, particularly in CKD patients, which is a function of the variation in cross-reactivity of antibodies employed in the assays with C-terminal fragments and a lack of a commutable standard material that can be used to harmonize the assays. Noncompetitive immunoassays for intact PTH or whole PTH(1–84) must have high concentrations of the C-terminal antibody to avoid underestimation of PTH in dialysis patients with secondary hyperparathyroidism who have very high concentrations of C-terminal fragments. Absence of interference can be assessed by confirming that specimens from dialysis patients with the highest concentrations of PTH dilute in a parallel fashion. Alternatively, recovery can be determined by adding a known amount of intact PTH to these specimens.

PTH concentrations may be altered in hyperthyroidism, in hypothyroidism, and with lithium carbonate treatment. PTH is decreased and is inversely correlated with tri-iodothyronine (T3) concentrations in hyperthyroid patients. Plasma PTH is increased in patients who become hypothyroid after radioactive iodine treatment, and is decreased with replacement therapy; these changes apparently are mediated by plasma calcium concentration. Long-term lithium carbonate therapy has been reported to increase parathyroid gland size and circulating intact PTH. Lithium may produce a state of relative resistance to calcium negative feedback, raising PTH concentrations.

An uncommon use for PTH methods measuring C-terminal fragments involves analysis of fluid from suspected parathyroid cysts. Parathyroid cyst fluid appears to contain primarily inactive fragments of PTH, not the intact hormone.[183]

With the development of teriparatide to treat osteoporosis, the use of PTH(1–34) in treatment of hypoparathyroidism and in Ellsworth Howard tests (PTH infusion test) for pseudohypoparathyroidism, it is sometimes necessary to estimate the circulating concentration of PTH(1–34). Automated and plate-based IMAs have been developed that can measure PTH(1–34) and have demonstrated the profile of circulating PTH(1–34) when administered by injection or orally. PTH(1–34) is undetectable in normal subjects.

POINTS TO REMEMBER

Parathyroid Hormone

- Several assays exist for the measurement of parathyroid hormone (PTH). Cross-reactivity with PTH metabolites and standardization remains a current problem resulting in significant variation in values obtained, particularly in chronic kidney disease.
- Measurement of intact PTH is pivotal in the differential diagnosis of calcium disorders.
- Surgical removal of the parathyroid glands is the most common cause of hypoparathyroidism.
- Hypomagnesemia can result in failure of the chief cells to release PTH resulting in hypoparathyroidism. In such cases, patients will not normalize their circulating calcium until there is adequate magnesium replacement.
- PTH by daily injection is a treatment for osteoporosis.

Vitamin D and Its Metabolites

Vitamin D_3 (cholecalciferol) is produced endogenously through exposure of skin to sunlight and is absorbed from foods containing or supplemented with vitamin D_3 or D_2 (ergocalciferol). The vitamin is metabolized to its biologically active form, $1{,}25(OH)_2\,D_3/D_2$, promoted by hormones that

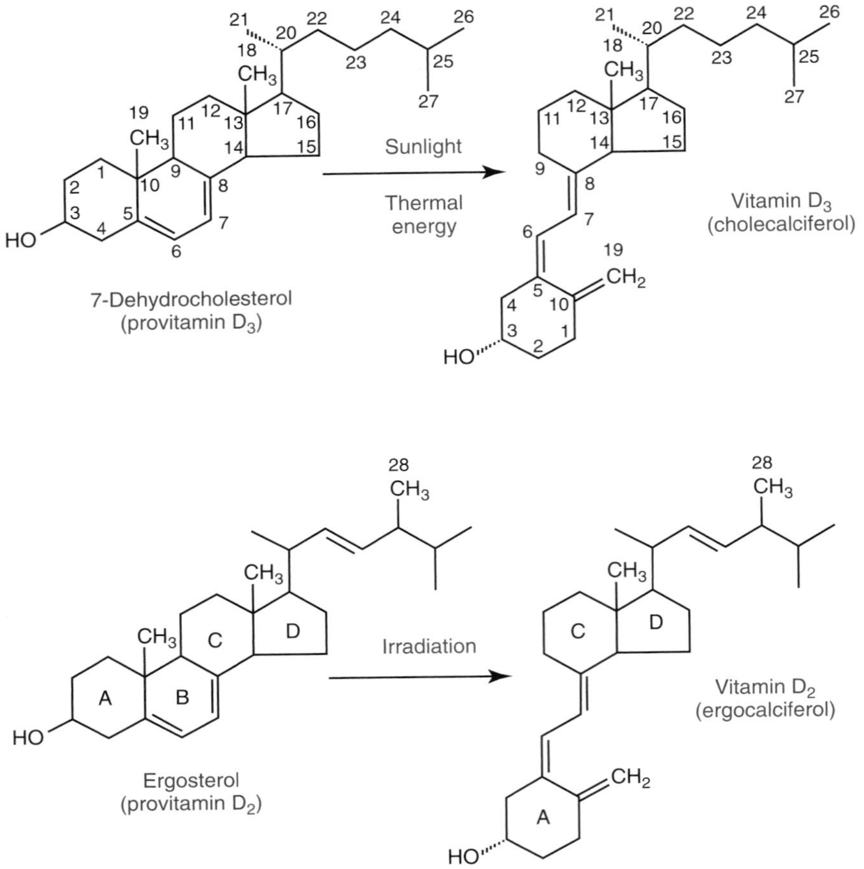

FIGURE 64.23 Structures of vitamin D_3 (cholecalciferol) and vitamin D_2 (ergocalciferol) and their precursors. 7-Cholecalciferol is produced in the skin from 7-dehydrocholesterol on exposure to sunlight. Ergocalciferol is produced commercially by irradiation of ergosterol. (Modified from Holick MF, Adams JS. Vitamin D metabolism and biological function. In: Avioli LV, Krane SM, eds. *Metabolic Bone Disease*. 2nd ed. Philadelphia: Saunders; 1990:155–95.)

regulate calcium and phosphate metabolism. Deficiency of vitamin D results in impaired formation of bone, producing rickets in children and osteomalacia in adults.

Biochemistry and Physiology

Vitamin D and its metabolites may be categorized as cholecalciferols or ergocalciferols (Fig. 64.23). Cholecalciferol (vitamin D_3) is the parent compound of the naturally occurring family and is produced in the skin from 7-dehydrocholesterol on exposure to the ultraviolet B portion of sunlight.[184,185] Latitude, season, aging, sunscreen use, and skin pigmentation influence production of vitamin D_3 by the skin. Vitamin D_2 (ergocalciferol), the parent compound of the other family, is manufactured by irradiation of ergosterol produced by yeasts. Vitamin D_2 differs from vitamin D_3 by the double bond between carbon 22 and carbon 23 and a methyl group on carbon 24. When vitamin D or its metabolites are written without a subscript, the term includes both families (total vitamin D).

Only a few foods, primarily fish liver oils, oily fish, egg yolks, and liver, naturally contain significant amounts of vitamin D. Consequently, before foods were supplemented with vitamin D_2 or vitamin D_3, most vitamin D in the body (90%) was that produced by synthesis in the skin. In North America, a considerable fraction of vitamin D is acquired by ingestion of fortified foods (some cereals, bread products, and milk) or vitamin D supplements. The recommended daily allowance is 400 IU (10 μg). In some European countries, the recommendation for people older than 60 years of age is 800 IU (20 μg). However, some clinicians in the United States are prescribing up to 2000 IU of vitamin D daily in an attempt to treat or prevent osteoporosis and to ensure optimal dietary calcium absorption.[186] There is much debate about the doses of vitamin D that are considered optimal for bone health and can improve vitamin D status sufficiently to result in increases in bone mineral density (BMD) and reduction in risk for fracture. Prospective randomized trials of high-dose vitamin D supplementation have not shown an increase in BMD and muscle function in women,[187] and in some cases a detrimental effect has been observed resulting in increased falls and fractures. There is evidence that increasing the dose of vitamin D supplementation results in a greater proportional production of $24,25(OH)_2D$ and that this may act to block the action of $1,25(OH)_2D$.[188]

Metabolism, Regulation, and Transport

Vitamin D_2 and vitamin D_3 are metabolized to 25-hydroxyvitamin $D_{2/3}$ ($25[OH]D_{2/3}$) in the liver by vitamin D 25-hydroxylase, a cytochrome P450 enzyme (Fig. 64.24).[185,189] The concentration of 25(OH)D in plasma is approximately

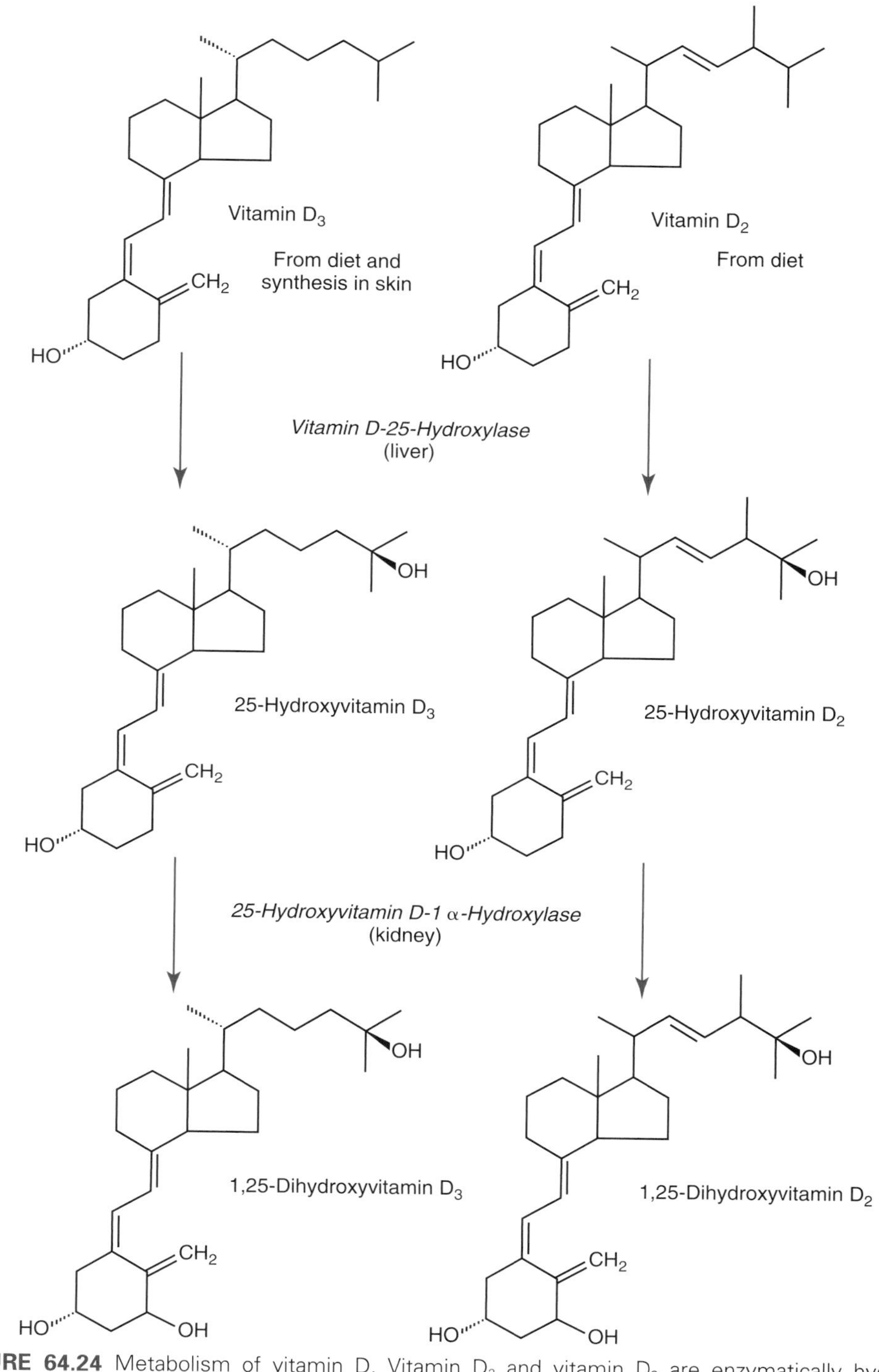

Vitamin D_3

From diet and synthesis in skin

Vitamin D_2

From diet

Vitamin D-25-Hydroxylase
(liver)

25-Hydroxyvitamin D_3

25-Hydroxyvitamin D_2

25-Hydroxyvitamin D-1 α-Hydroxylase
(kidney)

1,25-Dihydroxyvitamin D_3

1,25-Dihydroxyvitamin D_2

FIGURE 64.24 Metabolism of vitamin D. Vitamin D_2 and vitamin D_3 are enzymatically hydroxylated to 25-hydroxyvitamin D in the liver and further to 1,25-dihydroxyvitamin D by the kidneys. 1,25-Dihydroxyvitamin D_2 and 1,25-dihydroxyvitamin D_3 are the biologically active forms of vitamin D.

10 to 65 ng/mL or 25 to 162 nmol/L (Table 64.5). The half-life of circulating 25(OH)D is 2 to 3 weeks. At 25(OH)D concentrations near 30 ng/mL (75 nmol/L), dietary calcium absorption is maximal. Therefore, any reference interval for 25(OH)D should not be confused with the "optimal" or "healthy" range for 25(OH)D. At physiologic concentrations, 25(OH)D is biologically inactive in affecting dietary calcium absorption.

25(OH)D_2 and 25(OH)D_3 are metabolized to 1,25-dihydroxyvitamin D_2 or D_3 (1,25[OH]$_2$D), the biologically active hormone, by 25(OH)D 1α-hydroxylase, a cytochrome P450 enzyme, in the kidneys and placenta (see Fig. 64.24). Normal circulating concentrations are approximately 15 to 60 pg/mL (36–144 pmol/L), about 1/1000 of 25(OH)D (see Table 64.5). The plasma half-life of 1,25(OH)$_2$D is 4 to 6 hours.

TABLE 64.5 Vitamin D and Its Metabolites in Plasma

Compound	Concentration	Free, %	Half-Life
Vitamin D	<0.2–20 ng/mL <0.5–52 nmol/L	—	1–2 days
25-Hydroxyvitamin D	10–65 ng/mL 25–162 nmol/L	0.03	2–3 weeks
1,25-Dihydroxyvitamin D	15–60 pg/mL 36–144 pmol/L	0.4	4–6 hours
24,25-Dihydroxyvitamin D	0.8–2.8 ng/mL 2–7.2 nmol/L	Not established	NA

Circulating concentrations of 1,25(OH)$_2$D are tightly regulated, primarily by PTH, phosphate, calcium, FGF23, and 1,25(OH)$_2$D.[189-191] PTH and hypophosphatemia increase the synthesis of 1,25(OH)$_2$D by increasing 25(OH) D-1α-hydroxylase activity, whereas hypocalcemia acts indirectly by stimulating the secretion of PTH. Hypercalcemia, hyperphosphatemia, FGF23, and 1,25(OH)$_2$D reduce 25(OH)D 1α-hydroxylase and 1,25(OH)$_2$D. 1,25(OH)$_2$D also induces 25(OH)D 24-hydroxylase, an enzyme producing 24,25-dihydroxyvitamin D (24,25[OH]$_2$D), the most prevalent dihydroxylated vitamin D form in plasma. This enzyme is also responsible for inactivating 1,25(OH)$_2$D through the 24-oxidation pathway, leading to formation of 1,23,24,25,26,27 tetranorvitamin D (calcitroic acid).[23] Normal circulating concentrations of 24,25(OH)$_2$D are 0.8 to 2.8 ng/mL (2–7 nmol/ L) with a half-life of 1 to 2 weeks. 24,25(OH)$_2$D can occupy the vitamin D receptor and block the action of 1,25(OH)$_2$D.

In the circulation, vitamin D, 25(OH)D, and 1,25(OH)$_2$D are bound to vitamin D–binding protein (DBP), a specific, high-affinity transport protein also known as *group-specific component of serum* or *Gc-globulin*.[184,190,192] DBP belongs to the albumin and α-fetoprotein gene family. In humans, DBP contains 458 amino acid residues and has a molecular mass of 51,335 Da. DBP is constitutively synthesized by the liver and circulates in great excess (at about 400 mg/L), with <5% of the vitamin D binding sites normally occupied. DBP binds vitamin D and its metabolites, particularly the 25-hydroxylated metabolites 25(OH)D, 24,25(OH)$_2$D, and 1,25(OH)$_2$D.[184,192] Only 0.03% of 25(OH)D and 0.4% of 1,25(OH)$_2$D are normally free in plasma (see Table 64.5). DBP concentrations are increased in pregnancy and with estrogen therapy and are decreased in nephrotic syndrome.

Biologic Actions of 1,25-Dihydroxyvitamin D

1,25(OH)$_2$D helps to maintain calcium and phosphate concentrations in blood through its actions on intestine, bone, kidney, and the parathyroid glands. In the small intestine, 1,25(OH)$_2$D stimulates calcium absorption, primarily in the duodenum, and phosphate absorption by the jejunum and ileum.[184,189,190] Three events serve to absorb calcium from the diet: (1) calcium entry into the brush border cytoplasm, mediated by an epithelial Ca^{2+} transporter or channel (CaT1; gene name *ECAC2;* chromosome 7q34); (2) diffusion of calcium within the cell fostered by calbindin-D9k, which is a cytosolic calcium-binding protein (gene symbol *S100G,* located on the X chromosome, and distinct from calbindin-D28K, located on chromosome 8 [gene symbol *CALB1*]), and (3) exit of calcium from the cell across its basolateral membrane by the action of a CaATPase (eg, a Na^+/Ca^{2+} exchanger). CaT1 synthesis is approximately 90% vitamin D dependent, and calbindin D synthesis is completely dependent on vitamin D. Because knockout mice lacking calbindin D_{9k} expression do not display deficient calcium absorption and can increase calcium absorption in response to vitamin D, the necessity of calbindin-D9k for calcium absorption has been questioned.[193,194] A diet high in calcium downregulates CaT1 and calbindin D expression by downregulating production of 1,25(OH)$_2$D.

At high concentrations, 1,25(OH)$_2$D increases bone resorption by inducing monocytic stem cells in bone marrow to differentiate into osteoclasts and by stimulating osteoblasts to produce cytokines and other factors that influence osteoclast activity. By stimulating osteoblasts, 1,25(OH)$_2$D also increases the circulating concentrations of ALP and osteocalcin. In the kidneys, 1,25(OH)$_2$D inhibits its own synthesis in an ultra-short negative feedback loop and stimulates its own metabolism. 1,25(OH)$_2$D also acts directly on the parathyroid glands to inhibit the synthesis and secretion of PTH. In addition to a direct transcriptional mechanism, 1,25(OH)$_2$D increases the concentrations of the CaSR in the parathyroid gland, thus sensitizing the gland to calcium inhibition.[184]

In target tissues such as bone, 1,25(OH)$_2$D exerts its actions by associating with a specific nuclear vitamin D receptor (VDR), analogous to the steroid receptors for androgens, estrogens, and corticosteroids (see Chapters 68 and 69).[190] This receptor is expressed widely in tissues, and most cells respond to 1,25(OH)$_2$D.[195] The vitamin D receptor can form heterodimers with members of the retinoid X receptor. The vitamin D receptor is a member of the NR1I family, whose other members include the pregnane X receptor (PXR) and the constitutive androstane receptor (CAR). The gene for the vitamin D receptor is located on chromosome 12q1. The vitamin D_3 receptor is 427 amino acids long and binds to DNA through amino acids 21 to 96 with NR C4-type zinc fingers at positions 24 to 44 and 60 to 84. A hinge region encompasses amino acids 97 to 191. The ligand-binding region spans amino acids 192 to 427 with vitamin D–binding regions at amino acids 227 to 237 and 271 to 278. The receptor has many natural variations. At least one natural variant (position 274: R → L) decreases ligand affinity by a factor of 1000.

In addition to the classical vitamin D effects on calcium metabolism, increasing evidence suggests the role of 1,25(OH)$_2$D in regulation of the immune response and in epithelial differentiation. Inverse relationships have been documented between vitamin D metabolite concentration in blood and the incidence of certain cancers[196] and various other disorders. These findings have led to increased demand for vitamin D testing and have prompted calls for increases in the recommended daily intake of vitamin D. Nevertheless, substantial reductions in the rate of development of various cancers through the use of vitamin D have been difficult to demonstrate in clinical trials.[196] There is much debate regarding the optimal replacement concentration of 25(OH)D that should be targeted for optimal bone health and the amount of vitamin D supplement that should be recommended. Recent studies have suggested that "high-dose" therapy is not beneficial.[197]

Clinical Significance

Determination of 25(OH)D may be useful in the differential diagnosis of hypocalcemia, hypercalcemia, or hypercalciuria and for evaluating vitamin D status in health and in bone and mineral disorders. Measurements of 25(OH)D, 1,25$(OH)_2$D, and 24,25$(OH)_2$D have clinical value; however, 1,25$(OH)_2$D and 24,25$(OH)_2$D measurements are rarely needed in routine clinical practice.[198,199] The (UK) National Kidney Foundation guidelines have emphasized that vitamin D nutrition is assessed by measurements of 25(OH)D, *not* measurements of 1,25$(OH)_2$D (eg, see http://www.kidney.org/professionals/kdoqi/guidelines_pedbone/index.htm).

Vitamin D nutritional status is best determined through the measurement of 25(OH)D (Box 64.12), rather than vitamin D, because 25(OH)D is the main circulating form of vitamin D (see Table 64.5); it has a longer half-life [as a result of this, plasma 25(OH)D concentration is less affected by day-to-day variation, exposure to sunlight, or food intake], and because measurement of 25(OH)D is relatively easy compared with the more technically complicated methods used to measure vitamin D.[185,200,201] Groups at higher risk for developing nutritional vitamin D deficiency include breastfed infants, strict vegetarians who abstain from eggs and milk, strict vegans, individuals with darker skin pigmentation, and the elderly.

Measurement of circulating 25(OH)D is useful in selected patients in evaluating hypocalcemia or hypercalcemia, vitamin D status, bone disease, and other disorders of mineral metabolism. Circulating concentrations of 25(OH)D may be decreased by reduced availability of vitamin D; inadequate conversion of vitamin D to 25(OH)D; accelerated metabolism of 25(OH)D; and urinary loss of 25(OH)D with its transport protein DBP. Reduced availability of vitamin D may occur with inadequate exposure to sunlight, dietary deficiency, malabsorption syndromes, and following gastric or small bowel resection. Severe hepatocellular disease has been associated with inadequate conversion of vitamin D to 25(OH)D. Drugs such as phenytoin, phenobarbital, and rifampin induce drug-metabolizing enzymes that accelerate the metabolism of vitamin D and its metabolites. Plasma 25(OH)D concentrations may be reduced in patients with nephrotic syndrome because of the urinary loss of DBP and 25(OH)D.

BOX 64.12 Abnormal Circulating Concentrations of 25(OH)D

Decreased 25(OH)D

- Inadequate exposure to sunlight
- Inadequate dietary vitamin D
- Vitamin D malabsorption
- Severe hepatocellular disease
- Loss of 25-hydroxylase activity
- Increased catabolism (eg, drugs, such as anticonvulsants)
- Increased loss (nephrotic syndrome)

Increased 25(OH)D (hypercalcemia)

- Vitamin D or 25(OH)D intoxication

Serum 25(OH)D concentration is generally accepted as the functional indicator of an individual's vitamin D status.[202] Studies of serum concentrations of 25(OH)D have suggested that a significant proportion of adults in Europe or North America have poor vitamin D status.[203-206] It has been notoriously difficult to harmonize the reference intervals for 25(OH)D used in various laboratories; this may be related in part to differences of opinion regarding the definition of subclinical vitamin D insufficiency in apparently healthy populations.[185,207] The Institute of Medicine has produced pragmatic recommendations based on analysis of existing published studies (See the *Reference Intervals* section later in this chapter).

In patients with hypercalcemia, measurement of 25(OH)D has limited value. Its most common use in this situation is in confirming intoxication after ingestion of large amounts of vitamin D or 25(OH)D; in such patients, the 25(OH)D concentration is typically >100 ng/mL (>250 nmol/L).

A guideline from the Endocrine Society[208] and the UK National Osteoporosis Society recommends that routine screening for vitamin D deficiency is not warranted on a population basis, but is warranted in those at risk for deficiency. Candidates for screening are listed as patients with rickets, osteomalacia, osteoporosis, CKD, hepatic failure, malabsorption syndromes (eg, in cystic fibrosis, inflammatory bowel disease, Crohn disease, bariatric surgery, radiation enteritis), hyperparathyroidism, granuloma-forming disorders (sarcoidosis, tuberculosis, histoplasmosis, coccidiomycosis, berylliosis, Wegener granulomatosis), and some lymphomas; patients on medications, particularly antiseizure medications, glucocorticoids, AIDS medications, and antifungals (eg, ketoconazole, cholestyramine); and African-American and Hispanic children and adults, pregnant and lactating women, older adults with history of falls, older adults with history of nontraumatic fractures, and obese children and adults with BMI >30 kg/m^2).

Measurement of 1,25$(OH)_2$D is diagnostic in vitamin D–dependent rickets types 1 and 2, and helpful in disease states associated with overproduction of 1,25$(OH)_2$D such as granuloma-forming disorders, fungal infection, Hodgkin disease, and other lymphomas. In the last of these, activated macrophages convert 25(OH)D to 1,25$(OH)_2$D. In other situations, the test result gives confirmatory information in the evaluation of hypercalcemia, hypercalciuria, hypocalcemia, and bone and mineral disorders[209] (Box 64.13). Plasma concentrations of 1,25$(OH)_2$D are increased in vitamin D–dependent rickets type 2 (as the result of nonfunctioning VDR) and in 1,25$(OH)_2$D intoxication, and may be increased in PHPT, although the diagnosis of PHPT does not require measurement of 1,25$(OH)_2$D. Patients with PHPT and high concentrations of 1,25$(OH)_2$D do appear to be more prone

BOX 64.13 Abnormal Circulating Concentrations of 1,25(OH)$_2$D

Decreased 1,25(OH)$_2$D
- Renal failure
- Hyperphosphatemia
- Hypomagnesemia
- Hypoparathyroidism
- Pseudohypoparathyroidism
- Vitamin D–dependent rickets, type 1
- Hypercalcemia of malignancy
- Oncogenic osteomalacia

Increased 1,25(OH)$_2$D
- Granulomatous disease
- Primary hyperparathyroidism
- Lymphoma
- 1,25(OH)$_2$D intoxication
- Vitamin D–dependent rickets, type 2
- 24,25 hydroxylase deficiency

to developing hypercalciuria and renal stones. Reduced concentrations of 1,25(OH)$_2$D can be observed in patients with renal failure, HCM, hyperphosphatemia, hypoparathyroidism, pseudohypoparathyroidism type 1, vitamin D–dependent rickets, hypomagnesemia, nephrotic syndrome, and severe hepatocellular disease. Other than in cases of suspected vitamin D–resistant rickets, measurement of 1,25(OH)$_2$D in such circumstances is not required for diagnostic purposes.

Diagnosis of vitamin D deficiency is not based on measurement of 1,25(OH)$_2$D because the circulating concentration of this metabolite is often normal due to compensatory hyperparathyroidism.[209] Nor is the assay useful in confirming intoxication with vitamin D or 25(OH)D, because in this situation, 1,25(OH)$_2$D concentrations may be low, normal, or increased.

24,25(OH)$_2$D measurements are becoming increasingly valuable. The absence of this metabolite allows 1,25(OH)$_2$D to interact with the VDR unopposed and was shown to result in cases of childhood hypercalcemia and stone formation, then was reported in adults and also as the cause of a case of hypercalcemia in pregnancy. It is possible that in patients who lack 24,25(OH)$_2$D (due to a defect in the *CYP24A1* gene), hypercalcemia or other calcium abnormalities will only be observed during periods when an increase in 25(OH)D metabolism to 1,25(OH)$_2$D exists such as during vitamin D supplementation.[24] Higher 25(OH)D concentrations have a strong positive correlation with 24,25(OH)$_2$D, and increasing vitamin D supplementation, particularly high-dose therapy, results in proportionally greater increases in 24,25(OH)$_2$D than 1,25(OH)$_2$D.[188]

Measurement of Vitamin D Metabolites

Specific and sensitive assays have been developed for measuring vitamin D, 25(OH)D, 1,25(OH)$_2$D,[185,200,201] and 24,25(OH)$_2$D.[210,211] All assays should measure D$_2$ and D$_3$ metabolites equally (with equimolar reactivity), because both D$_2$ and D$_3$ are metabolized to produce biologically active 1,25(OH)$_2$D. Separate measurement of the D$_2$ and D$_3$ forms does not necessarily distinguish between dietary and endogenous sources of vitamin D, as food can be supplemented with D$_3$ or D$_2$.

The hydrophobic natures and small circulating concentrations of vitamin D metabolites, together with the possibility of matrix effects, have presented enormous challenges for the development of assays that would be both specific and suitable for high-throughput clinical analysis needs.[200,201] In general, two or three of the following steps are needed in any assay for 25(OH)D, 1,25(OH)$_2$D, or 24,25(OH)$_2$D: deproteinization or extraction, purification, and quantification. The first step frees the metabolites from DBP and may partially purify them. Purification steps, most often using column chromatography, separate the various forms of vitamin D, lipids, and interfering substances. The method of quantification depends on the metabolite that is being measured.

Extraction and Deproteinization. Before the advent of commercially available methods, it was common to use two-phase, liquid-liquid partitions with organic solvents and solvent mixtures, including methylene chloride, hexane, diethyl ether, ethanol/chloroform/water, methylene chloride/methanol, hexane/isopropanol, and cyclohexane/ethyl acetate. Ethanol and methanol have also been used to free 25(OH)D from DBP when 25(OH)D is measured.

Protein precipitation using zinc sulfate is a common step in sample preparation. The most widely used commercially available methods use acetonitrile to deproteinize the specimen and to denature DBP, thereby freeing the vitamin D metabolites.[185,200,201]

There is an assay that uses immunoextraction for 1,25(OH)$_2$D,[212] and this process has been incorporated into an automated method.

Column Chromatography. Differences in their polarities, related to their numbers of hydroxyl groups, have been used to separate vitamin D and its metabolites. With three hydroxyl groups, 1,25(OH)$_2$D and 24,25(OH)$_2$D are more polar than 25(OH)D, with its two hydroxyls, which is in turn more polar than vitamin D, with only one hydroxyl group.

Extracts have been purified by chromatography on, for example, minicolumns of silica, silicic acid, Sephadex LH-20, hydroxyalkoxypropyl Sephadex LH-20 (Lipidex 5000), celite, and alumina. Solid-phase extraction using octadecyl (C$_{18}$)-silica was widely used for measuring 1,25(OH)$_2$D. The most popular method used both a reversed-phase C$_{18}$-silica minicolumn and a normal-phase silica minicolumn to separate vitamin D metabolites. This method was modified by eliminating the silica cartridge and using "phase switching" with a single non–end-capped C$_{18}$OH cartridge.

Measurement of 25-Hydroxyvitamin D. Acceptance of serum 25(OH)D as an indicator of an individual's vitamin D status has resulted in the development of several commercial assays over the past 20 years.[185] The metabolite is measured by competitive protein binding assay (CPBA), competitive or noncompetitive immunoassay (RIA, EIA, ICMA), ultraviolet (UV) absorption after separation by HPLC, or by mass spectrometry after separation by chromatography (see Chapters 16 and 23). Determination by HPLC with UV absorption or mass spectrometry requires appropriate HPLC equipment (see Chapters 16 and 17), specialized training, and a larger sample. Most clinical laboratories that measure 25(OH)D have chosen the more familiar competitive immunoassays. These assays are relatively easy to perform, use widely available reagent sets on multichannel analyzers, and require only a small volume of plasma. Most large commercial manufacturers have incorporated 25(OH)D assays on their platforms. In the Vitamin D External Quality Assessment Scheme (DEQAS) during 2015, the various formats of the Diasorin immunoassay were the commonest methods returned.

External quality assurance surveys and proficiency testing programs have identified some differences of results among the different 25(OH)D assays—RIA, chemiluminescence immunoassay (CLIA), and the newer liquid chromatography–mass spectrometry (LC–MS/MS) methods.[213] The differences in results reflect, in part, firstly differences in calibration of the assays, secondly nonequimolar responses of some assays to 25(OH)D_2 and 25(OH)D_3, and thirdly noncommutable materials used in surveys. Nonequimolar responses are common among the automated methods, but not in LC–MS/MS and HPLC assays.

Care must be taken in interpreting results from external quality assurance surveys and proficiency testing programs. Survey materials that have been processed extensively can be noncommutable and lead to overestimation of between-assay variability. Moreover, survey materials that lack 25(OH)D_2 will give no indication of assays that underrecover that form. DEQAS and the College of American Pathologists have used pooled samples to investigate this problem. These surveys showed that some assays underestimated the total 25(OH)D in the samples with increased 25(OH)D_2, but the gross errors of 100% or more seen in previous surveys were absent. The differences laboratories using LC–MS/MS assays demonstrated were comparable to differences among laboratories using single commercial assays.

Vitamin D–binding protein concentrations have an effect on 25(OH)D estimation using immunoassays probably due to the inability of the displacing reagent employed in the assays to completely dissociate 25(OH)D from VDBP.[214] 24,25$(OH)_2$D has also been demonstrated to cross-react in some immunoassays for 25(OH)D, contributing to overestimation of the 25(OH)D concentration.[215,216] It is hoped that efforts at the NIST, IFCC, and elsewhere will lead to improvements of accuracy and harmonization of these assays.

Radioimmunoassay and Chemiluminescence Immunoassay. Development of a useful antiserum permitted the development of a competitive immunoassay (RIA) for 25(OH)D.[200,201] The antiserum was raised against a bovine serum albumin (BSA) conjugate of a vitamin D analog lacking the side chain [23,24,25,26,27-pentanor vitamin D-C(22)carboxylic acid]. A radioiodinated vitamin D analog [3-aminopropyl derivative of vitamin D-C(22)-amide] was used as the tracer. Samples and calibrators are deproteinized with acetonitrile and analyzed directly without chromatography. Although the antiserum also recognizes 24,25$(OH)_2$D, 25,26$(OH)_2$D, and 25(OH)D-26,23-lactone, the 25(OH)D results obtained are comparable with those obtained by HPLC because of the much lower concentrations of the other metabolites. The RIA has been reported to be less sensitive to interfering substances in serum extracts than is a CPBA that uses DBP.[217] This assay is commercially available as an RIA and as an automated immunoassay based on chemiluminescence (CLIA) detection.[200] The manufacturer replaced the original RIA antiserum in the late 1990s.

Immunoassays for 25(OH)D have appeared from several manufacturers. Some of these assays have underestimated the total concentration of 25(OH)D when 25(OH)D_2 is present.[218] This is a particular concern in the United States, Japan, and the United Kingdom, where the available high-dose supplements are often vitamin D_2.

Competitive Protein-Binding Assays with Vitamin D–Binding Protein. Before the development of immunoassays, 25(OH)D was measured primarily with CPBA with DBP as the specific binder, and with tritiated 25(OH)D_3 (>100 Ci/mmol) as the tracer. Assays based on DBP measure both 25(OH)D_2 and 25(OH)D_3, but it is important to verify that they respond equally to 25(OH)D_2 and 25(OH)D_3. If the assay procedure does not involve a chromatographic step for isolating 25(OH)D, other metabolites are also measured, including 25(OH)D_3-23,26-lactone, 24,25$(OH)_2$D, 25,26$(OH)_2$D, and, to a lesser extent, vitamin D itself, thus overestimating the 25(OH)D concentration by about 10% in healthy subjects. 25(OH)D concentrations are reported to be significantly higher when measured by CPBA than when measured by RIA or HPLC.[205,209]

HPLC and Ultraviolet Absorption. HPLC methods for 25(OH)D have used normal-phase chromatography on silica, reversed-phase chromatography on C_{18}-silica, or a combination of the two followed by quantification by UV absorption at 254 or 265 nm. Most methods have required both extraction and preparative chromatography before HPLC. Methods without preparative chromatography also have been developed using gradient or isocratic reversed-phase HPLC with photodiode-array UV detection.[219,220] A specimen of 0.5 to 1 mL is required because of the limited sensitivity of UV detection. HPLC methods allow 25(OH)D_2 and 25(OH)D_3 to be separated. HPLC is useful for validating the accuracy of immunoassays and CPBAs.[200,201]

LC–MS/MS Assays. Liquid chromatography coupled with tandem mass spectrometry (LC–MS/MS) is commonly used in the measurement of 25(OH)D.[201,221-224] The LC–MS/MS methods are capable of relatively high throughput, with some laboratories producing over 1000 results per day. LC–MS/MS has become more attractive for 25(OH)D measurement as the instrumentation has become widely available in clinical laboratories.

Despite the high selectivity of mass spectrometry, the C-3 epimer of 25(OH)D is not differentiated from 25(OH)D as it has the same mass. Thus, unless the epimer is separated chromatographically before the mass-spectrometric quantification, results of LC–MS/MS assays are increased by the C-3 epimer. This is rarely a problem in adults as the epimer is normally present in only low concentrations, but it is more of a problem in pediatric patients.[223] Some immunoassays also cross-react with the epimer.

In LC–MS/MS assays, samples typically are denatured by the addition of alcohol (such as a methanol-propanol mixture) containing a stable-isotope–labeled internal standard such as $(^2H_6)$25(OH) D_3 (26,26,26,27,27,27-hexadeutero-25-hydroxycholecalciferol). Following extraction, drying, and reconstituting in solvent, the 25(OH)D is chromatographed and analyzed by multiple reaction monitoring. Between-day (total) CVs of 5% to 10% have been reported within individual laboratories, but between-laboratory variability has been a problem, although no worse than for commercially available competitive binding assays.

The 25(OH) metabolites related to D_2 and D_3 can be quantified separately by LC–MS/MS. This may have limited clinical value in some settings,[200] but it is important to report the sum of the two concentrations [25(OH)D_2 + 25(OH)D_3] because vitamin D status depends on the total concentration, not on the individual concentrations. One approach to reporting is to provide the concentrations of both forms, but to provide a reference interval only for the sum of the two.

Measurement of 1,25-Dihydroxyvitamin D. 1,25$(OH)_2$D circulates at approximately 1/1000 of the concentration of 25(OH)D and at significantly lower concentrations than other dihydroxylated metabolites (see Table 64.5)—facts that together with the extreme hydrophobicity and instability of the compound greatly complicate its determination in serum.[185,200] The most widely used methods require extraction, chromatography, and quantification by radioreceptor assay (RRA) or RIA.

Radioreceptor Assay. Assays using vitamin D receptors from calf thymus or chick intestine have been reported but are rarely used in clinical laboratories.

Radioimmunoassay. The first radioimmunoassay for 1,25$(OH)_2$D was introduced in 1978 and required a cumbersome purification.[200] After several assays of similar characteristics had been developed, in 1996 another RIA was introduced, with an iodinated reporter and use of an equivalent serum matrix. For this method, sample purification is not needed.[200,225]

The RIA is more convenient than the RRA for 1,25$(OH)_2$D because a radioiodinated tracer eliminates the need for liquid scintillation counting, and the antiserum eliminates the need to prepare VDR from calf thymus. The RIA uses an antiserum with 1% to 2% cross-reactivity with the more abundant, non–1-hydroxylated vitamin D metabolites and a ^{125}I-labeled tracer prepared from 1,25$(OH)_2$-24,25,26,27,tetranor-C(23)-carboxylic acid and radiolabeled Bolton-Hunter reagent. Before analysis, specimens are deproteinized with acetonitrile, oxidized with sodium metaperiodate, and purified using C_{18}-OH and silica cartridges. Sodium metaperiodate is necessary to eliminate interference by 24,25$(OH)_2$D and 25,26$(OH)_2$D by oxidizing them to their aldehyde and ketone forms, which are easily removed by chromatography. A silica column was added to the single C_{18}-OH cartridge used with the radioreceptor assay, to reduce interference in the RIA. As measured by this RIA, 1,25$(OH)_2$ D_2 has about 70% of the potency of 1,25$(OH)_2D_3$. Recovery of individual samples is not determined, although calibrators are prepared in a stripped serum base and are treated identically to samples. The method does cross-react (13% to 25%) with numerous 1-hydroxylated metabolites, including 1,24,25$(OH)_3$D, 1,25,26$(OH)_3$D, and 1,25$(OH)_2$D-26,23-lactone. 1,25$(OH)_2$D-26,23-lactone is a significant metabolite with a concentration of 0% to 30% of that of 1,25$(OH)_2D_3$. A modification of this method using a single C_{18}-OH "extra-clean" cartridge is commercially available.

Another commercially available RIA has been developed that uses selective immunoextraction of 1,25$(OH)_2$D.[226] This method is reported to have greater cross-reactivity with the 1-hydroxylated metabolites, including 1,25-dihydroxyvitamin D_3-26,23-lactone[227] and calcipotriol,[228] which is used for treating psoriasis. Apparent concentrations of 1,25$(OH)_2$D are significantly higher with this method than with RRA in patients with hypoparathyroidism receiving vitamin D treatment, patients with biliary atresia, vitamin D–intoxicated subjects, and some normal specimens. This assay has been fully automated.

High-Performance Liquid Chromatography, Tandem Mass Spectrometry, and Gas Chromatography–Mass Spectrometry. Measurement of 1,25$(OH)_2$D by direct-detection UV methods is not possible due to its low concentration in blood (in the pg/mL [pmol/L] range). 1,25$(OH)_2$D has few ionizable polar groups, and so techniques to increase the ionization efficiency (derivitization) have been incorporated in all of the published methods.

1,25$(OH)_2D_3$ measurement in serum was achieved by LC–MS/MS after extraction and purification using both reverse phase and normal phase on a C18 cartridge followed by generation of an ammonium adduct prior to positive electrospray ionization. The lowest limit of quantification (LLOQ) was 20 pg/mL (52 pmol/L) using 1 mL of sample. Derivitization using 4-phenyl-1,2,4-triazoline-3,5-dione (PTAD), a Cookson-type reagent, of a solid-phase extracted (SPE) sample and measurement using ultra-performance liquid chromatography (UPLC) electrospray tandem MS allowed simultaneous quantification of a profile of vitamin D metabolites [1,25$(OH)_2D_2$, 1,25$(OH)_2D_3$, 24,25$(OH)_2D_3$, 25(OH)D_2, and 25(OH)D_3] with an LLOQ of 25 pg/mL (65 pmol/L) and a CV of 5% to 16% for 1,25$(OH)_2D_3$.[229] PTAD, also used in a method, was able to quantitate the same four metabolites with significantly improved sensitivity, 5 ng/L (13 pmol/L) for 1,25$(OH)_2D_3$, that employed selective SPE and microflow LC–MS/MS.[230] The SPE procedure enabled high sample loading on the UPLC column. Column sample focusing prevented band-broadening allowing excellent separation, eliminating endogenous interferences while minimizing ion suppression, but with a run time of 27 minutes. Lithium acetate has been used to produce ionizable adducts in a method that uses a complex online sample-processing procedure with the use of a perfusion column followed by a chain of two monolithic columns to clean and enrich the sample prior to quantification on a highly sensitive LC–MS/MS.[229] Both 1,25$(OH)_2D_2$ and 1,25$(OH)_2D_3$ can be measured on 30 μL of sample with an LLOQ for 1,25$(OH)_2D_3$ of 15 pg/mL (39 pmol/L), a CV of 5% to 15% across physiologic concentrations, and a total run time per sample of 30 minutes. An immunoaffinity column and reagents were incorporated into a sample preparation procedure following protein precipitation and SPE. Lithium acetate was used to produce adducts prior to LC–MS/MS analysis. This method removed isobaric interferences and matrix effects resulting in significantly reduced ion suppression, with the resultant LLOQs of 3.9 pg/mL (10.1 pmol/L) for 1,25$(OH)_2D_2$ and 3.4 ng/L (8.8 pmol/L) for 1,25$(OH)_2D_3$ with interassay CVs of 2.5% to 7%. A very similar approach using the ImmunoDiagnosticS (IDS, Boldon Tyne & Wear, United Kingdom) columns for immunoextraction but derivitizing using PTAD prior to UPLC–MS/MS resulted in improved sensitivity with LLOQs of 0.65 pg/mL (1.7 pmol/L) for 1,25$(OH)_2D_2$ and 1.25 ng/L (3 pmol/L) for 1,25$(OH)_2D_3$ with interassay CVs of 8% to 13%. All of the LC–MS/MS methods described earlier are fairly labor-intensive with manual workflows and limited throughput. Future developments will incorporate more online processing, automated sample preparation, and possibly mass tagging to increase throughput.

A report from DEQAS (2015) lists seven categories of methods and 123 users performing 1,25$(OH)_2$D measurement of quality assurance samples. Immunoassay methods dominate the scheme with 96% of users; 68% are performing

TABLE 64.6 **Reported Associations of Serum 25-Hydroxyvitamin D Concentrations With Serum PTH and Bone Histology**

25(OH)D	$1,25(OH)_2D$	PTH Increase	Bone Histology
<5 ng/mL or <12.5 nmol/L	Normal or low	>30%	Incipient or overt osteomalacia
5–10 ng/mL or 12.5–25 nmol/L	Normal	15–30%	High turnover
10–20 ng/mL or 25–50 nmol/L	Normal	5–15%	Normal or high turnover
>20 ng/mL or >50 nmol/L	Normal	—	Normal

From Lips P, van Schoor NM, Bravenboer N. Vitamin D-related disorders. In: Rosen CJ, Compston JE, Lian JB, eds. *Primer on the Metabolic Bone Diseases and Disorders of Mineral Metabolism*. Washington, DC: American Society for Bone and Mineral Research; 2008:329–35.

an IDS method, and 4% report results by LC–MS/MS. The CVs reported are wide for all the methods at around 20% for most samples circulated, and this reflects the difficulty of measurement and a lack of availability of an international standard material.

Measurement of 24,25 Dihydroxyvitamin D. There are no immunoassays with sufficient antibody specificity that enable measurement of $24,25(OH)_2D$. Competitive protein binding assays have been described, but the most common methods currently in use are LC-MS/MS assays. Protein precipitation, displacement from proteins, and purification from samples has adopted previously described methods as for 25(OH) D, and derivitization with PTAD is utilized to achieve the required specificity and sensitivity.

Standardization. There is no international standard material available, so most methods utilize "in-house" standards, produced as previously discussed for 25(OH)D using solvent dissolution, spectrophotometric analysis at 264 nm, and a molar extinction coefficient of 19,400 to calculate the concentration. Human serum stripped of $1,25(OH)_2D_3$ by activated charcoal can then be used to make calibrators of varying concentrations by adding dissolved $1,25(OH)_2D_3$. Some authors report using a substrate addition approach to calculate concentrations, and a commercial standard material, with a consensus mean concentration assigned, is also available.

Troubleshooting Vitamin D Assays. Methods requiring extraction and chromatography should be monitored for recovery of the vitamin D metabolites of interest and for solvent or column blanks. Care must be taken to ensure that D_2 and D_3 metabolites are recovered equally, providing a total measurement of 25(OH)D or $1,25(OH)_2D$. Solvents, chromatographic materials, and cartridges may contain substances that interfere with quantification of vitamin D metabolites by CPBA, RIA, and RRA or UV absorption after HPLC, resulting in an overestimation of vitamin D metabolites. Any interference can be monitored by treating a water blank identically to the specimens. Undetectable concentrations of vitamin D in this blank verify the absence of positive interference.

Calibrators for vitamin D assays should be prepared from stock solutions whose concentration and purity are checked by UV spectrophotometry. Stock solutions are suitable if the ratio of absorbance at 264 nm to that at 228 nm is greater than or equal to 1.5. Stock solutions are adjusted using a molar extinction coefficient of 18,200 L/mol/cm for vitamin D_3 metabolites at 264 nm. Tracers used for recovery must be pure to determine recovery accurately. Both calibrators and tracers can be purified by HPLC.

Specimen Requirements. Serum is typically used for measuring vitamin D metabolites, although plasma is generally acceptable for assays using extraction and chromatography. Once separated from the clot, serum is relatively stable at both room temperature and 4°C; specimens should be frozen if the analysis is delayed. Vitamin D metabolites in serum or plasma do not appear to be sensitive to light and do not require special handling in the laboratory.[201]

Reference Intervals

Reference intervals for vitamin D metabolites are method-dependent. A representative range for $1,25(OH)_2D$ is: 15 to 60 pg/mL (36–144 pmol/L). Lower limits of the reference interval for 25(OH)D of 10 or 15 ng/mL (25–37 nmol/L) have been increasingly criticized as inappropriately low, as even above this limit the vitamin D status of the individual can be insufficient (Table 64.6).[231] Concentrations of <20 to 30 ng/mL (<50–75 nmol/L) can be associated with increased plasma PTH concentrations and reduced calcium absorption. The US Institute of Medicine published a recommendation that the lower limit for vitamin D sufficiency be lowered from 30 to 20 ng/mL (75 to 50 nmol/L) and that concentrations >50 ng/mL (>125 nmol/L) be considered as cause for concern. A reverse *J*–shaped curve has been reported describing the relation between the serum concentration of 25(OH) D and all-cause mortality. Concentrations of 20 to 24 ng/mL (50–60 nmol/L) were associated with the lowest mortality risk, and very low (<4 ng/mL [<10 nmol/L]) or high (>56 nmol/L [>140 nmol/L]) concentrations were associated with increased morbidity and mortality.[232]

The National Health and Nutrition Examination Survey (NHANES) III study reported an unexpectedly high prevalence of vitamin D insufficiency in adults and adolescents in North America.[233,234] For example, vitamin D insufficiency [25(OH) D <20 ng/mL (50 nmol/L)] was exceedingly common during the winter in adult (≥30 years of age) Caucasian men (15%) and women (30%) living in the southern United States. Similar findings have been reported from Europe.[204]

The concentrations of 25(OH)D in African Americans are lower than in non-Hispanic whites, but the clinical significance of this is uncertain. Compared with non-Hispanic whites, African Americans have higher bone mineral density, higher plasma concentrations of PTH and $1,25(OH)_2D$, lower concentrations of biochemical markers of bone remodeling, and lower rates of osteoporosis.

Circulating concentrations of 25(OH)D are increased by exposure to sunlight and show seasonal variation, with the highest concentrations in summer or fall and the lowest concentrations in winter or spring.[79] This has led to the recommendation that testing be done at the end of winter; if results are above the chosen cutoff, the patient is likely to have adequate concentrations throughout the year on his or her usual regimen of sun exposure and oral intake of the vitamin. The concentrations are influenced by latitude, sunscreen use, and skin pigmentation. Plasma 25(OH)D concentrations of 100 ng/mL (250 nmol/L) can be detected in individuals with extensive sun exposure, such as lifeguards.

Concentrations of vitamin D metabolites vary with age and are increased in pregnancy.[77,78] Concentrations of $1,25(OH)_2D$ are higher in children than in adults, with the highest concentrations occurring during periods of greatest growth.[235] Although 25(OH)D and $1,25(OH)_2D$ concentrations have been reported to decrease with age, this decline may be a consequence of poor nutrition, reduced exposure to sunlight, and declining health. Concentrations of these metabolites were unchanged with age in studies limited to healthy and active subjects.

$24,25(OH)_2D$ concentrations are method-dependent, but a reference interval of 2 to 7 nmol/L has been defined in a young, healthy population. Ethnic differences have been reported, with black Americans having lower concentrations than Caucasians. Increasing supplementation with vitamin D results in increasing $24,25(OH)_2D$ concentrations and defects in the *CYP24A1* gene, resulting in reduced 24-hydroxylase activity and decreased $24,25(OH)_2D$ concentrations.

POINTS TO REMEMBER

Vitamin D

- Measurement of 25 hydroxyvitamin D [25(OH)D] is accepted as the best reflection of vitamin D status.
- Tandem mass-spectrometric methods are considered the best way of measuring 25(OH)D.
- A high percentage of the world's population is vitamin D deficient.
- Prolonged deficiency of vitamin D results in rickets in children and osteomalacia in adults.
- Care is required with high-dose vitamin D treatment, as it can result in significant morbidity, increasing falls and fractures in elderly women.

FIBROBLAST GROWTH FACTOR 23

Biochemistry and Physiology

Fibroblast growth factor 23 (FGF23) is a phosphaturic peptide promoting phosphate excretion in urine, also termed a *phosphatonin* (a class of factors regulating phosphate homeostasis).[236,237] FGF23 is a member of the FGF family of growth factors. The *FGF23* gene is located on chromosome 12p3.3. Most FGFs share an internal core region of similarity with 28 highly conserved, and six identical amino acid residues (FGF homology domain).[238,239] Regions thought to be involved in receptor binding are distinct from regions that bind heparin. FGF23 is 26 kDa in weight uncleaved and consists of 251 amino acids. FGF23 is cleaved at the 176-RXXR-179 motif generating inactive amino-terminal and carboxy-terminal fragments.[240]

FGF23 has been found in both embryonic as well as adult tissues.[241] Peptide and mRNA has been detected in heart, liver, lymph nodes, thymus tissue, and brain ventrolateral thalamus. FGF23 has also been shown to have high expression in osteoblasts and osteocytes in mouse and human bone.[242-244]

In contrast to most FGFs, FGF23 is not membrane bound. This results in it acting like a hormone rather than an adhesion molecule/cell surface receptor.

Biologic Actions

FGF23 is involved in the medium- to long-term regulation of circulating phosphate. It acts directly on the kidney via Klotho–FGF receptor complexes to decrease renal phosphate reabsorption through reduction in the sodium proximal tubule transporter 2a protein (NPT2a transporter). Klotho is essential for the action of FGF23 and ensures that the FGF receptors become specific for FGF23. Because of its soluble nature, in contrast to most FGFs, FGF23 needs Klotho to generate a transmembrane signal through FGFR1. Alteration in alpha-Klotho concentrations can result in hypophosphatemic rickets and hyperparathyroidism.[245] Direct administration of FGF23 suppresses renal vitamin D 1α-hydroxylase mRNA and stimulates vitamin D 24-hydroxylase, resulting in low circulating $1,25(OH)_2D$ concentrations[239,246,247] and increased $24,25(OH)_2D$ concentrations. Plasma phosphate and $1,25(OH)_2D$ are increased in the FGF23 knockout mouse, suggesting that FGF23 plays an important role in vitamin D and phosphate homeostasis.[248,249]

Synthesis, Secretion, and Metabolism

The *FGF23* gene has three exons and spans approximately 10 kb of genomic DNA on chromosome 12p3.3. It is highly expressed in osteocytes and osteoblasts, and FGF23 synthesis is positively stimulated by phosphate, $1,25(OH)_2D$, PTH, and the proteolytic cleavage product of the transmembrane protein, Klotho. Iron deficiency stimulates FGF23 production possibly through hypoxia-inducible factor 1α but also results in abnormal metabolism with generation of increased C-terminal fragments. Calcium deficiency suppresses FGF23 production and local bone-derived factors such as dentin matrix protein-1 (DMP-1), and the phosphate-regulating gene with homologies to the endopeptidases on the X chromosome (PHEX) have negative effects on transcription.

FGF23 is synthesized as a 251–amino acid precursor with a 24–amino acid signal peptide, an N-terminal FGF-like homology domain (25-179), and a unique C-terminal (180–251) that mediates high-affinity binding to the Klotho-FGFR complex. Following removal of the 24–amino acid signal peptide, the remaining molecule undergoes both disulfide bond formation and *O*-glycosylation:polypeptide by uridine diphosphate-*N*-acetyl-α-D-galalactosamine:polypeptide *N*-acetylgalactosaminyltransferase 3 (GALNT3). The *O*-glycosylation is important in protecting cleavage of the molecule by serine endopeptidase pro-protein convertases (PC), especially at the consensus sequence R176XXR 179, which results in generation of N-terminal and C-terminal fragments and abolishes FGF23 activity. Metabolism of FGF23 in bone is thought to be mediated by proteolysis by furin, PC5, and PC2 combined with an essential binding co-factor 7B2. There are little data on further metabolism of FGF23 and how or where it is cleared from the circulation, although renal failure results in a significant increase in C-terminal fragments, but hemodialysis only transiently reduces immunologic FGF23 fragments in the circulation. Studies in animals suggest full-length intact FGF23 is cleared almost twice as fast as C-terminal fragments with half-lives of 6 minutes and 12 minutes, respectively.

BOX 64.14 FGF23-Related Diseases

High FGF23

- Chronic kidney disease
- X-linked hypophosphatemia (XLH)
- Autosomal dominant hypophosphatemic rickets (ADHR)
- Tumor-induced or osteogenic osteomalacia (TIO)
- Autosomal recessive hypophosphatemic rickets (ARHR)
- Autosomal recessive hypophosphatemia (ARHP)
- Fibrous dysplasia (FD), McCune-Albright syndrome (MAS)

Low FGF23

- Tumoral calcinosis (TC)
- Hyperglycemic hyperosmolar state
- Inactivating mutations of FGF23

Clinical Significance

FGF23 is increased in plasma in a number of disease states, and its measurement can help point toward several important clinical diagnoses in patients with abnormalities of phosphate metabolism (Box 64.14). There is some evidence that FGF23 may be the best measurement at predicting deterioration in CKD. Several clinical trials are in place looking at treating CKD patients with particular types of phosphate binders such as sevalamer and titrating this therapy using FGF23 concentrations to help prevent the development of CKD-associated complications.

Disease Associated with Abnormal FGF23 Concentrations

Abnormalities in FGF23 production and secretion can be divided into hypophosphatemic and hyperphosphatemic conditions.

X-Linked Hypophosphatemic Rickets. XLH is an X-linked dominant disorder that is fully penetrant with variability in clinical severity. It is classically associated with hypophosphatemia, phosphaturia, normocalcemia, and low plasma $1,25(OH)_2D$. It is the most common form of inheritable rickets, and the bone problems include lower-extremity deformity (usually bowing of the femora and tibiae), bone pain, joint pain, fracture, abnormal calcification of tendons and ligaments, and dental abcess.[250,251]

XLH is caused by inactivating mutations in the phosphate-regulating gene with homologies to endopeptidases on the X chromosome (PHEX).[252-254] PHEX encodes an M13 membrane metalloprotease whose precise substrate has not been identified. An initial study proposed that PHEX cleaved normal FGF23 but not FGF23 produced in autosomal dominant hypophosphatemic rickets or ADHR,[255] but subsequent researchers have not supported these data,[256] and some have suggested protease contamination as a cause for FGF23 metabolism in early experiments.[242]

The Hyp mouse is a valuable model of XLH because it has a 3′ deletion in the *PHEX* gene[257] and displays hypophosphatemia and has an abnormally low circulating $1,25\text{-}(OH)_2D_3$ with growth retardation and bone mineral defects.[258] Experiments on Hyp mice indicate that it is possible to transfer humoral factors between Hyp and wild-type mice, resulting in the XLH phenotype in the wild type.[259] FGF23 expression is increased in Hyp mice as is circulating FGF23. The suggestion has been made that in XLH there is overproduction of FGF23 rather than increased metabolism and that the true PHEX substrate is another regulatory peptide or enzyme involved in sensing phosphate variations.[236]

Animal studies using neutralizing antibodies of FGF23 given to Hyp mice show normalization of plasma phosphate and partial improvement of the bone pathology allowing a rise in the sodium proximal tubules transporter 2 protein (NPT2A protein) and vitamin D 1α-hydroxylase in the renal tubules. It has also been possible to partially correct mineralization defects in these animals by osteoblast-targeted PHEX expression.[260] Antibodies to FGF23 are being assessed in studies of patients with hypophosphatemic rickets.[261]

Autosomal Dominant Hypophosphatemic Rickets. Patients with autosomal dominant hypophosphatemic rickets (ADHR) have a very similar biochemical and clinical presentation to those with XLH. They are hypophosphatemic, phosphaturic, and normocalcemic with inappropriately normal $1,25(OH)_2D$ concentrations. They can present in later life than XLH patients, and so they do not necessarily have florid rickets but do have evidence of osteomalacia. FGF23 elevations in ADHR are due to missense mutations of FGF23 that block its metabolism. Metabolism of FGF23 by serine proteases at amino acids 179 and 180, a subtilisin-like proprotein convertase cleavage site (RXXR motif), is prevented by missense mutations (R176Q, R179W, and R179Q) preventing proteolytic cleavage.[240,247,262,263] FGF23 molecules produced as a result of these mutations are reported to be biologically active[264,265] as they are intact. It is believed, although not proven in humans, that this FGF23 will be stable in the circulation and have a prolonged half-life.

Tumor-Induced Oncogenic Osteomalacia. Tumor-induced oncogenic osteomalacia (TIO), also known as oncogenic osteomalacia (OOM), is an acquired hypophosphatemic syndrome in which FGF23 is produced as a paraneoplastic phenomenon. Patients have predominantly benign mesenchymal tumors, mainly in bone and soft tissues, that present with hypophosphatemia and inappropriately suppressed $1,25(OH)_2D_3$ concentrations. Plasma bone-specific alkaline phosphatase activities may also be increased. Where patients describe muscle weakness, bone biopsy may reveal osteomalacia.[266-269]

FGF23-producing tumors are commonly slow growing and can be hemangiopericytomas, fibromas, or angiosarcomas.[268,270] Malignant tumors causing TIO tend to be more aggressive,[271] and FGF23 concentrations in patients with malignant tumors tend to be higher in the more malignant and advanced cases. Removal of the neoplasm responsible for the FGF23 production restores normal circulating phosphate, resolves the phosphaturia, and results in marked clinical improvement and resolution of the metabolic bone disease.[272-278]

Although FGF23 has been clearly implicated as the causative factor for many of the abnormalities observed in TIO, other tumor-related factors are emerging that may have a role in the pathogenesis of this condition. Factors having discrete effects inhibiting mineralization of bone may be produced: these are called *minhibins*. In addition to FGF23, matrix extracellular phosphoglycoprotein (MEPE) and secreted frizzled-related protein 4 (sFRP4) are purported to be important phosphatonins/minhibins that can be produced by TIO tumors.[279-281] MEPE expression has been detected in almost all TIO tumors screened to date and is absent from

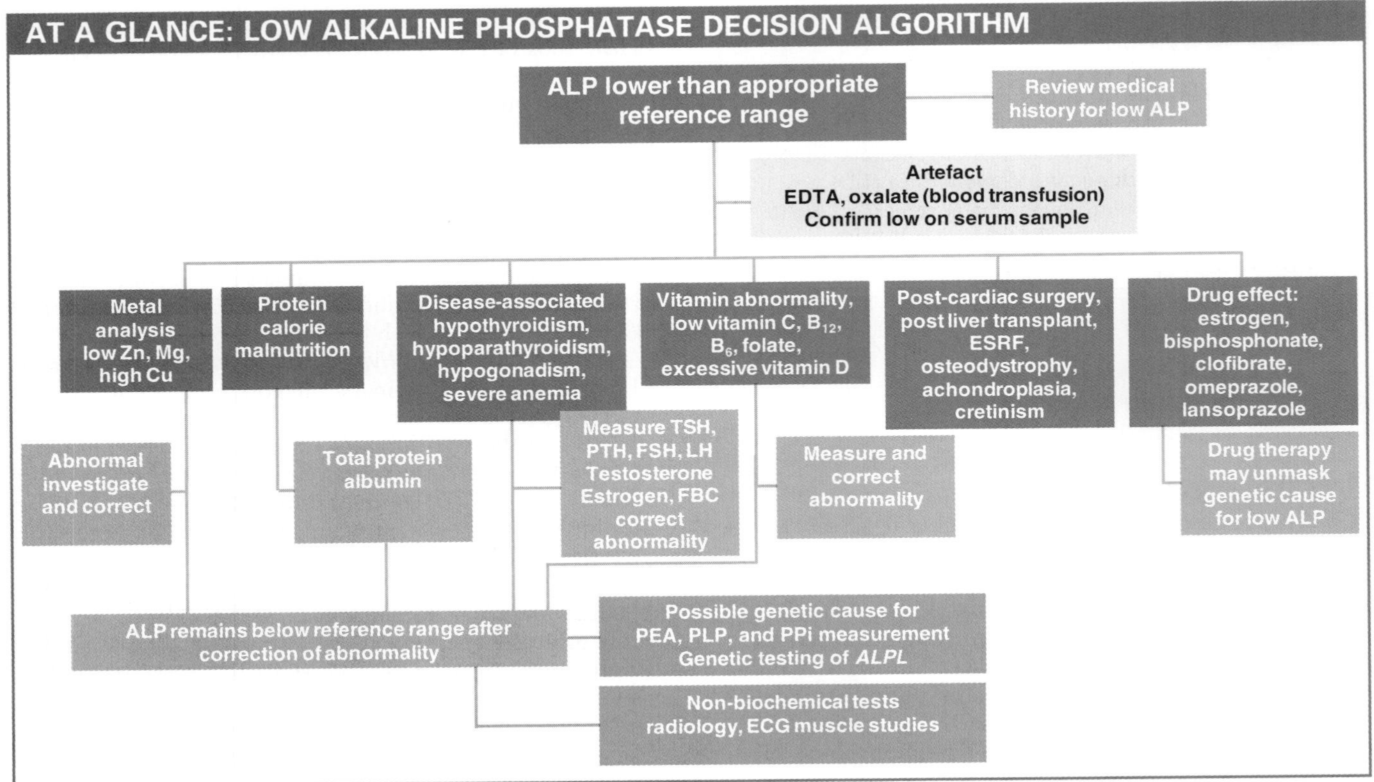

ALP, Total alkaline phosphatase; *ALPL,* tissue nonspecific ALP gene; *Cu,* copper; *ECG,* electrocardiogram; *EDTA,* ethylene diamine tetra acetic acid; *ESRF,* end stage renal failure; *FBC,* full blood count; *FSH,* follicle stimulating hormone; *HPP,* hypophosphatasia; *LH,* lutenising hormone; *Mg,* magnesium; *PEA,* phospho ethanol amine; *PLP,* pyridoxaL phosphate; *PPi,* pyrophosphate; *PTH,* parathyroid hormone; *TSH,* thyroid stimulating hormone; *Zn,* zinc.

non-phosphaturic tumors.[239,279,280,282] Carboxy-terminal cleavage of MEPE by cathepsin B produces a protease-resistant peptide termed *MEPE-ASARM peptide* (acidic serine–aspartate-rich MEPE-associated motif), which can inhibit mineralization and may also affect phosphate metabolism.[281]

Fibrous Dysplasia of Bone. Fibrous dysplasia (FD) is a skeletal disorder in which normal bone is replaced by benign fibro-osseous tissue. It can be polyostotic or monostotic with isolated skeletal lesions, supporting the view that there are different patterns of somatic mosaicism in FD.[283]

McCune-Albright syndrome (MAS) is characterized by skin pigmentation, endocrine disorders including precocious puberty, and FD. These conditions result from postzygotic somatic activating mutations of the *GNAS-1* gene. Mutations of this gene produce disturbances in intracellular signaling (via G-protein Gsα and cAMP activation).[284,285]

Renal phosphate wasting is observed in 50% of FD/MAS patients,[286] mineralization defects are common in FD,[287,288] and rickets/osteomalacia is a rare complication of FD/MAS.[289-291] Bone cell production of calcium- and phosphate-regulating hormones/factors is abnormal with increased osteoblastic PTHrP production[292] and increased interleukin-6 (IL-6) expression.[293-298]

FGF23 is produced by both normal and FD osteoprogenitors and mature bone-forming cells in vivo and in vitro.[242-244] Circulating FGF23 concentrations are increased in FD/MAS patients compared with normal age-matched controls and are negatively correlated with serum phosphate and positively correlated with disease burden and bone turnover.[244,299] Expression of FGF23 within FD lesions in bone is higher when hypophosphatemic osteomalacia is observed.[117] Thus production of FGF23 by FD tissue may play a role in the renal phosphate-wasting syndrome associated with FD/MAS.

Hyperphosphatemic Conditions

Chronic Kidney Disease. CKD is associated with significant increases in plasma phosphate concentrations, and this plays a major role in maintaining the hyperparathyroidism and causing subsequent bone disease in CKD. FGF23 decreases plasma phosphate concentrations by decreasing renal phosphate reabsorption and by suppressing $1,25(OH)_2D$ formation through the inhibition of 1α-hydroxylase activity.[300] It is unknown whether FGF23 is directly responsible for the decreased concentrations of $1,25(OH)_2D$ seen in CKD, or whether this or any other phosphatonins are induced in an attempt to correct the hyperphosphatemia of ESRD.

Measurement of circulating FGF23 in CKD has detected markedly increased concentrations.[276,301,302] The precise mechanism regulating FGF23 production in CKD remains unclear. Phosphate retention is a possible factor, as positive correlations with FGF23 have been observed in CKD.[303] Significantly higher FGF23 concentrations are seen in CKD patients with lower creatinine clearance (CrCl).[303] Positive correlations between PTH and FGF23 concentrations are observed in dialysis patients,[304-306] and total parathyroidectomy results in decreased PTH, decreased plasma phosphate, decreased calcium–phosphate product, and a significant decrease in FGF23.[307]

Of major clinical interest is the finding that FGF23 appears to be a better predictor of refractory hyperparathyroidism (those patients resistant to medical therapy) than current standard measurements (PTH, calcium, and phosphate), with higher FGF23 more likely to be refractory.[306] In a cohort of dialysis patients with PTH greater than 300 pg/mL (>30 pmol/L), analyses using receiver-operated characteristic curves revealed that FGF23 was the best screening test to predict if patients will be refractory to calcitriol therapy.[305]

Familial Tumoral Calcinosis. Patients with familial tumoral calcinosis (FTC) are hyperphosphatemic with increased or inappropriately normal plasma 1,25$(OH)_2D$ concentrations. They present with ectopic calcified masses and vascular calcification.[308-311] The genotype of FTC patients is similar to that of FGF23-null mice, and circulating FGF23 concentrations are low. When a serine residue is substituted for a glycine residue at position 71 (the S71G mutation), this appears to stabilize the full-length FGF23 molecule. As a result, C-terminal fragments of FGF23 are secreted by HEK293 cells in vitro, while the intact protein is retained intracellularly.[256] S129F substitutions occur when a serine residue is changed to a phenylalanine residue at position 129. These substitutions have also been found to result in increased FGF23 breakdown resulting from conformational changes in the FGF23 molecule, producing high concentrations of C-terminal fragments.[312] Biallelic mutations in the *N*-acetylgalactosaminyltransferase 3 *(GALNT3)* gene have been identified in some families as a cause of FTC. The enzyme product of the gene is responsible for posttranslational *O*-glycosylation of proteins at serine or threonine residues, and so abnormalities in this process may result in loss of FGF23 function.[313,314] An M96T mutation of FGF23 at a highly conserved methionine residue has been found to be associated with very severe calcification of cutaneous and extracutaneous tissues.[315]

Measurement of FGF23

FGF23 concentrations have been measured using a number of different immunoassays in several populations. A single-step IMA incorporates an antibody to the C-terminal peptide fragments of FGF23 (cFGF23) that also reacts with the intact molecule (Immutopics, San Clemente, California). The capture antibody initially recognized amino acids 206–222 (first-generation assay), then subsequently amino acids 186–206 (second-generation assay), with a detection antibody directed to amino acids 225–244. This assay therefore provides a combined estimate of both cFGF23 and iFGF23 present in a sample. Immutopics produced an intact-molecule–specific assay, also single-step, with the capture antibody recognizing amino acids 186–206 and detection antibody 51–69. An intact two-step assay for iFGF23 is also available from Kainos Laboratories (Kainos Laboratories Inc., Tokyo, Japan), but the precise epitopes recognized by the antibodies have not been revealed. The format utilizes N-terminal capture and C-terminal detection, and this has been developed into an automated chemiluminescent assay. A single-step cFGF23 assay is available from Biomedica (Biomedica, Vienna, Austria). An iFGF23 assay is also available from Millipore (Millipore, Billerica, Massachusetts). It is becoming clear that these assays can give different results in the same populations, and so great care is required when interpreting the results obtained. All of the assays are calibrated using recombinant human FGF23, but there is no recognized international reference preparation available, and the reporting units vary widely, with the result that reference intervals are considerably different for each assay.

Preanalytical factors are of importance, and the sample type differs among assays. EDTA is the preferred sample for Immutopics' assays, whereas the Kainos assay specifies serum. Experiments have confirmed increased stability of FGF23 in plasma (lithium-heparin or K-EDTA) when measured using Immutopics' methods. Inclusion of protease inhibitors can further reduce the instability of the intact molecule when using the Immutopics iFGF23 assay. Instability seems to be less of an issue with the Kainos and Millipore assays, which might reflect the epitopes detected by the antibodies or the inclusion of protease inhibitors to the buffers used in some assays.

One study compared the ability of the two assays to detect increasing FGF23 with dietary phosphate manipulation. The intact-molecule assay (Kainos) was found to have a better correlation between iFGF23 and phosphate indices. With phosphate loading over 4 days, the intact-molecule assay demonstrated earlier and greater increases in iFGF23 compared to the cFGF23 of the Immutopics assay. There was a weak correlation between the two assays ($r = 0.26$).[316]

An estimation of the half-life of intact FGF23 in the circulation has been made in a patient with normal renal function who had TIO. After removal of a hemangiopericytoma from this 37-year-old man, and sampling over 1 hour, the half-life of FGF23 was calculated to be 21.5 minutes. This short half-life of FGF23 allowed the same investigators to perform localization studies of the tumor causing TIO, using selective venous catheterization and sampling.[278] The half-life may be influenced by production of an abnormal FGF23 molecule by the tumor.

Where direct comparisons in the same patient populations have been performed, a greater percentage of patients were found to have FGF23 above the reference interval in both TIO and XLH when samples were measured using the intact assay (Kainos) compared to the C-terminal assay (Immutopics) (100% vs. 77% in TIO and 83% vs. 45% in XLH).[275]

Low serum iFGF23 has been associated with the hyperphosphatemia of FTC, but increases in cFGF23 of up to 40-fold were found when the condition was assessed with the cFGF23 assay.[107,317] This clearly reflects the differential processing of the molecule that was demonstrated in vitro when the FGF23 missense mutations are present.

Reference Intervals

What is clear is that there is significant variability in the reference intervals quoted and a lack of a standardized approach to development of FGF23 reference intervals. As usually happens once a reference interval has been published by one group, this is often applied by others, and in some cases misquoted, without their establishing a reference interval in their own population.

The reference intervals in healthy adults are as follows:
iFGF 23: 11.7–48.6 pg/mL (Kainos)
cFGF23: 21.6–91 RU/mL (Immutopics)

Interpretation

With the increasing availability of commercial assays for FGF23, there are several reports appearing in which FGF23 has been measured and found to be significantly different in disease from normal. Very high FGF23 concentrations can be obtained by both assays in XLH, TIO, and CKD, indicating that this measurement is not clearly discriminatory between the diseases and that careful use of the FGF23 values in light of the patient's history and examination is required. An FGF23 concentration in the upper quartile of the reference interval may be inappropriate for a prevailing low plasma phosphate concentration and may require further investigation. Increasing severity of CKD results in significant increases in FGF23, and so it is essential to take account of renal function when interpreting FGF23 values. The discrepant values obtained in FTC by the two assays highlight the additional knowledge gained by performing both measurements in certain diseases and the current level of knowledge we have on FGF23 metabolism and function. It is also obvious that a value within the currently quoted reference intervals does not exclude the presence of disease: one of the other proposed phosphotonins/minhibins such as MEPE, MEPE-ASARM, or sFRP4 may be responsible for the biochemical abnormalities observed in such patients.

POINTS TO REMEMBER

FGF23

- Osteocytes are major producers of FGF23.
- Several metabolic bone diseases result from abnormalities of FGF23 secretion and metabolism.
- FGF23 acts at the kidneys to promote phosphate excretion. Klotho is required to allow specific changes in FGF receptors in the kidney permitting FGF23 selective activity.
- Metabolism of FGF23 results in the generation of inactive C-terminal fragments that are measured in some assays.
- FGF23 inhibits alpha hydroxylase in the kidney resulting in a decrease in the circulating concentration of 1,25 dihydroxy vitamin D.

CALCITONIN

Release of calcitonin from the parafollicular or C cells of the thyroid gland is stimulated by circulating calcium. The hormone has been used pharmacologically as an inhibitor of bone resorption, but the physiologic role of endogenous calcitonin is less certain. No apparent alterations in bone or mineral metabolism are evident in humans with calcitonin deficiency or excess. However, calcitonin measurements have a role in the diagnosis and follow-up of medullary thyroid carcinoma, a malignant tumor of the C cells, in particular in its familial form.

The C cells of the thyroid gland arise from the neural crest and are distributed throughout the gland. These are amine precursor uptake and decarboxylation (APUD) cells, which explains the association of thyroid medullary carcinoma with other tumors such as multiple endocrine neoplasia types 2A and 2B (MEN2A and MEN2B).

Biochemistry and Physiology

Calcitonin is a 32–amino acid peptide, with a molecular mass of 3418 Da, an N-terminal disulfide bond linking the cysteine residues 1 and 7, and a C-terminal proline-amide (Fig. 64.25). The hormone interacts with a specific G-protein–coupled receptor that is found on fully differentiated osteoclasts.[293] The structures necessary for biologic function are the C-terminal portion of the molecule, with its proline-amide

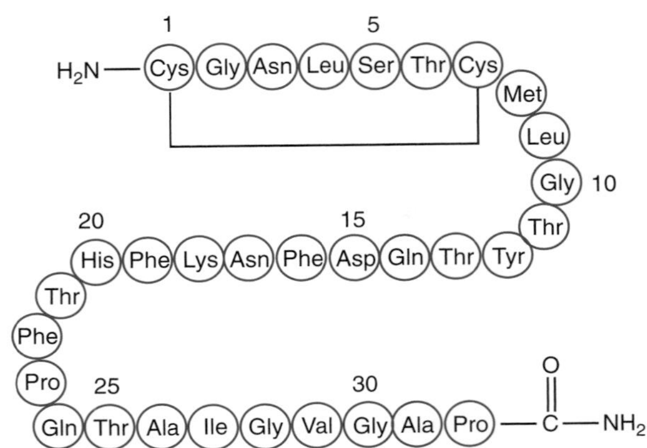

FIGURE 64.25 Amino Acid Sequence of Human Calcitonin.

residue, the disulfide bond between residues 1 and 7, and the methionine residue at position 8. The amino-terminal amino acids are highly conserved. In humans, salmon calcitonin is 10 times as potent as the human hormone and has been used pharmacologically, sometimes in the form of a nasal spray.[293]

The physiologic regulation of calcitonin secretion is incompletely understood, but the best known secretagogue is free calcium in blood. At least in animals, several other peptide hormones (gastrin, cholecystokinin, glucagon, secretin) can stimulate calcitonin secretion, but their physiologic role in humans is uncertain.

Pharmacologic doses of calcitonin reduce plasma calcium and phosphate concentrations primarily by inhibiting osteoclastic bone resorption. Salmon calcitonin has been used to treat Paget disease of bone, osteoporosis, and hypercalcemia caused by increased bone resorption. Pharmacologic doses of calcitonin also decrease the renal tubular reabsorption of calcium and phosphate. Calcitonin seems to exert an analgesic effect, which is not necessarily solely explained by its effects on bone.[293]

Higher concentrations of circulating calcitonin can be observed in young children[318] and during pregnancy and lactation,[77,78] suggesting that the hormone may be important in protecting the skeleton during periods of calcium stress. Evidence in favor of such a hypothesis has been gained from knockout mice that lack calcitonin.[319]

In plasma, multiple forms of calcitonin can be observed both in healthy individuals and in patients with medullary thyroid carcinoma (MTC) or nonthyroidal malignancies. Much of the immunoreactive calcitonin in the circulation is larger than the monomeric hormone.[320] Several reasons for this heterogeneity have been put forward: sulfoxide modification of the monomer, dimerization, glycosylation, the presence of biosynthetic precursors of the monomer, and binding to plasma proteins.

During the biosynthesis of calcitonin, the original product is a larger precursor form known as *procalcitonin*. Procalcitonin (Chapter 28) has attracted attention as a potential infection marker, in relation to the acute-phase response.[321]

Clinical Significance

MTC occurs as a sporadic disease and as part of the multiple endocrine syndromes MEN2A, MEN2B, and familial medullary thyroid carcinoma (FMTC). Together, these account for 5% to 10% of thyroid malignancies, with the sporadic MTC

BOX 64.15 Increased Circulating Concentrations of Calcitonin

C-cell hyperplasia
Medullary thyroid carcinoma
Nonthyroidal cancers
- Oat cell carcinoma, small-cell carcinoma
- Other malignancies

Acute kidney injury, chronic kidney disease
Hypercalcemia
Hypergastrinemia and other gastrointestinal disorders
Pulmonary disease

accounting for about 80% of all MTCs. It has been suggested that routine measurement of serum calcitonin in nodular thyroid disease could assist in detecting unsuspected sporadic MTC. After thyroidectomy of MTC patients, calcitonin serves as a tumor marker in the monitoring of treatment response. For more detailed information on the use of calcitonin measurements in oncology, see Chapter 31.

Calcitonin concentrations are increased occasionally in various nonthyroidal cancers (Box 64.15), both in those arising from the neural crest and in others. Increased concentrations or enhanced response to calcitonin secretagogues (calcium, pentagastrin, or both) has been reported in cases of nonmalignant disease such as acute and chronic renal failure, hypercalcemia, hypergastrinemia and other gastrointestinal disorders, pulmonary disease, and severe illness.

Assays have been reported also for salmon calcitonin, but it has not been possible to predict the treatment response to this drug by monitoring its circulating concentration. Thus it is advisable to follow the treatment by determining clinical parameters and measuring calcium.

Measurement of Calcitonin

Calcitonin is measured by immunoassay, and interpretation of results in principle can be complicated both by the heterogeneity of the circulating antigen and by the varying characteristics of the different assays.

Historically, the first methods described were RIAs; the different assays showed widely differing reference intervals, sensitivities, and specificities, and they suffered differently from matrix effects. More recently, noncompetitive immunoassays (IRMA, ELISA, EIA, ICMA) have been developed and are available from several diagnostic companies;[322] their results still differ markedly.[323] Some assays may give results that are erroneously low at high concentrations (hook effect); samples with concentrations of 344 ng/L or less (≤100 pmol/L) appear to be unaffected.[323,324]

Reference Intervals

The reference intervals for calcitonin are dependent on the method used. They should be determined for healthy and athyroidal individuals, by gender, in each laboratory for basal and stimulated (calcium and pentagastrin provocation tests) conditions. It is a common finding that men show higher basal and stimulated concentrations than women, but this is not necessarily true for every method.

A typical upper limit for the reference interval for basal calcitonin concentration in adults is about 10 pg/mL (2.9 pmol/L); the mean concentrations are lower in women (5.8 pg/mL [1.7 pmol/L]) and higher in men (8.8 pg/mL [2.6 pmol/L]).[318,325] In addition to gender, age, growth, pregnancy, and lactation have been reported to influence[318,326] circulating calcitonin concentrations in healthy individuals, but reference intervals generally are not given by the assay manufacturers for groups other than healthy adults.

Parathyroid Hormone–Related Protein

Parathyroid hormone–related protein (PTHrP) was discovered as an agent responsible for causing the state known as *humoral hypercalcemia of malignancy (HHM)* in certain cancers.[327,328] It later proved to be an autocrine/paracrine factor with a multitude of functions in several organ systems.[329,330] Among these are its effects on chondrocyte biology and endochondral bone formation,[290] as well as on calcium metabolism in the fetus[331,332] and during pregnancy and lactation.[328]

Biochemistry and Physiology

PTHrP is derived from a gene on chromosome 12 that is distinct from the *PTH* gene on chromosome 11. Three isoforms of 139, 141, and 173 amino acids are predicted by alternative messenger RNA (mRNA) splicing (Fig. 64.26).[83] The N-terminal end of the molecule shows close homology to PTH, with 8 of the first 13 amino acids being identical and 3 of the next 21 amino acids being identical. The remainder of the PTHrP molecule shows little homology with PTH. The PTH-like activity of PTHrP is contained within the N-terminal amino acids [PTHrP(1-36)].

The primary transcript can undergo a series of posttranslational modification reactions, resulting in a series of partially overlapping peptides with different biologic activities.[83,328,331]

The common N-terminus explains the ability of PTHrP to interact with the PTH/PTHrP receptor, mimicking the biologic actions of PTH in classic target tissues, including bone and kidneys.[331] Like PTH, PTHrP causes hypercalcemia and hypophosphatemia, and increases urinary cyclic AMP. However, when compared with patients with PHPT, those with PTHrP-induced hypercalcemia have lower concentrations of 1,25$(OH)_2D$ and more typically have metabolic alkalosis (instead of hyperchloremic metabolic acidosis), reduced distal tubular calcium reabsorption, and reduced and uncoupled bone formation.

The presence of several basic amino acid residues in PTHrP suggests that it may undergo extensive posttranslational processing. Forms of PTHrP containing the following amino acids have been detected in serum:[329] PTHrP(1–36) measured by N-terminal assays; PTHrP containing N-terminal and midregion amino acids measured with noncompetitive immunoassays against PTHrP(1–74 or 1–86); midregion fragments, beginning at position 38 and extending 70 to 80 amino acids, measured with midregion assays; carboxyl fragments, beginning at position 107 or 109, measured with antiserum directed against PTHrP(109–138).[328] Midregion and carboxyl forms exert biologic actions distinct from the PTH-like actions associated with the N-terminal region.

Besides its endocrine role in the pathophysiology of HHM, PTHrP participates in normal physiology by acting locally on cells or tissues as an autocrine or paracrine factor.[83,328,330] PTHrP is widely expressed in most normal tissues of fetuses and adults. Although it is unlikely that low circulating concentrations of PTHrP have a significant effect on calcium homeostasis in normal adults, PTHrP exerts endocrine

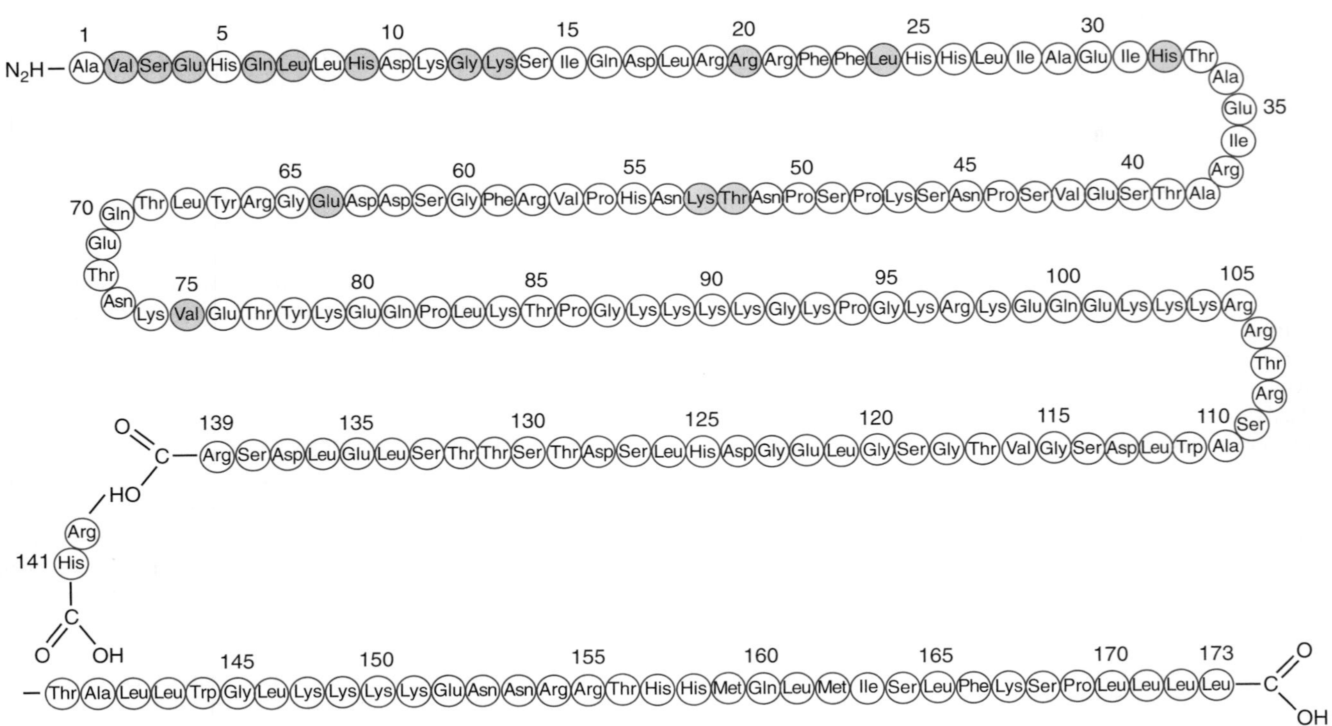

FIGURE 64.26 Amino Acid Sequence of Human Parathyroid Hormone–Related Peptide (PTHrP). Although the exact length of circulating PTHrP is unknown, proteins of 139, 141, and 173 amino acids have been predicted from alternative splicing events. The *shaded circles* show amino acids that are identical in parathyroid hormone (PTH) and PTHrP. (Modified from Hendy GN, Goltzman D. Parathyroid hormone-like peptide. In: *Endocrinology and Metabolism Inservice*. vol. 9. Washington, DC: American Association for Clinical Chemistry; 1991:9–24.)

effects on skeletal development and calcium homeostasis during fetal life[77,81] and lactation.[78] Breast milk contains extremely high concentrations of PTHrP[328] as does amniotic fluid. Examination of the physiologic effects of PTHrP has identified several themes: PTHrP regulates transepithelial calcium transport; it is a potent smooth muscle relaxant; and it regulates growth, differentiation, and development. However, the role of PTHrP in many tissues is unknown.[330]

Clinical Significance

Hypercalcemia associated with malignancy (HCM) is the third most frequent cause of hypercalcemia in hospitalized patients. This common paraneoplastic syndrome is believed to occur primarily through two mechanisms: HHM and local osteolysis. HHM is present in approximately 75% to 80% of patients with hypercalcemia associated with malignancy.[333] HHM is common in patients with squamous (lung, head and neck, esophagus, cervix, vulva, and skin), renal, bladder, and ovarian carcinomas. Hypercalcemia due to skeletal metastases and local osteolysis are common in breast cancer and multiple myeloma, lymphoma, and other hematologic malignancies. The hypercalcemia of a subset of lymphomas (human T-cell leukemia virus-1) appears to be caused by HHM. Breast carcinomas may cause hypercalcemia by HHM and/or skeletal metastases with local osteolysis. It is now well established that PTHrP is the principal mediator of HHM, and by stimulating production of RANKL, causes dramatic uncoupling of bone resorption from bone formation. After it is secreted by tumors, PTHrP circulates and acts on its target tissues (skeleton and kidney) as an endocrine hormone causing hypercalcemia. PTHrP can also be secreted locally by tumors having a paracrine action.

PTHrP determinations are rarely required for diagnosis because HHM nearly always occurs in advanced disease when the diagnosis is clear. The need for PTHrP determination is greater when it becomes important in prognosis,[334] selection of therapy, or monitoring.

Measurement of PTHrP

Several competitive immunoassays have been used to measure PTHrP in sera from patients with HHM. For example, N-terminal [PTHrP(1–34)], midregion [PTHrP(37–67, 37–74)], and C-terminal [PTHrP(109–138)] competitive RIAs have been developed.[327] Of the competitive immunoassays, the N-terminal assays have been used most widely. Affinity chromatography with immobilized antisera against PTHrP, reversed-phase chromatography, and other purification techniques have been used to improve the sensitivity and specificity of these competitive RIAs. C-terminal assays give increased results in patients with renal insufficiency.[327]

More sensitive and noncompetitive immunoassays (IRMAs) have also been developed.[20,327,335,336] Currently available assays use antibodies against PTHrP (sequences 37–74, 1–40, 1–34) as capture antibodies. Their radiolabeled signal antibodies are against PTHrP (sequences 1–36, 60–72, 57–80, 37–67, 50–83), respectively; the idea is to measure molecular species of PTHrP that contain large N-terminal regions. The limit of detection for these assays is reported to be from 0.1 to 1 pmol/L.

Specimen Requirements

PTHrP is unstable in serum and plasma at 4°C and at room temperature unless collected in the presence of protease inhibitors. A combination of aprotinin, leupeptin, pepstatin, and EDTA provides the greatest protection. In general, specimens should be collected with protease inhibitors and kept on ice. Serum or plasma should be promptly separated from the clot and/or cells and frozen, as red cell enzymes are involved in PTHrP degradation.

Reference Intervals

PTHrP concentrations in healthy individuals are dependent on both the assay and the specimen collection, varying from undetectable to up to 5 pmol/L. With sensitive noncompetitive immunoassays, concentrations of between 1 and 2 pmol/L have been reported in some normal subjects. Care in interpretation of values within this concentration range is required as in certain individuals PTHrP may be produced mainly by tumors, producing a measured value between 1 and 2 pmol/L and resulting in hypercalcemia. In these patients, repeat sampling may reveal increasing concentrations of PTHrP with the passage of time confirming PTHrP by a tumor. PTHrP is reported to be detectable in approximately 50% to 80% of healthy individuals with the most sensitive and specific methods such as LC-MS/MS.

Interpretation

PTHrP is increased in 50% to 90% of patients with hypercalcemia associated with malignancy (Fig. 64.27). In addition to squamous cell carcinoma of the lung, head and neck, esophagus, cervix, skin, and other sites, increased concentrations have been found in a wide variety of other malignancies, irrespective of their source or histology. Increased concentrations of PTHrP have been found in breast, renal, bladder, and ovarian carcinomas and in endocrine malignancies with hypercalcemia, including pheochromocytoma and islet carcinomas. PTHrP is increased in hypercalcemic patients with adult T-cell lymphoma/leukemia and B-cell lymphoma. Circulating PTHrP is increased less frequently in patients with hypercalcemia and other hematologic malignancies (eg, multiple myeloma), but local production of PTHrP may play a role in the generation of the hypercalcemia observed.

PTHrP is undetectable or normal in the plasma of most but not all patients with malignancy not associated with hypercalcemia. Increased concentrations of PTHrP have been reported to precede hypercalcemia in some patients with malignancy. Concentrations are normal in patients with PHPT hypoparathyroidism, miscellaneous noncancer causes of hypercalcemia, and chronic renal failure.

Survival is limited in patients with increased PTHrP and hypercalcemia, so the presence of PTHrP is a poor prognostic indicator. Very few patients have a benign cause for an increase in PTHrP, so the test has a high specificity for diagnosing the presence of a cancer in a patient who is hypercalcemic. PTHrP production by tumors is also associated with a poorer response to bisphosphonate therapy, with fewer patients normalizing calcium following standard doses of bisphosphonates and increased requirement for repeated dosing with bisphosphonate.

SCLEROSTIN

Sclerostin is a 190-residue secreted protein member of the Cerberus/Dan protein family. Sclerostin was discovered as a

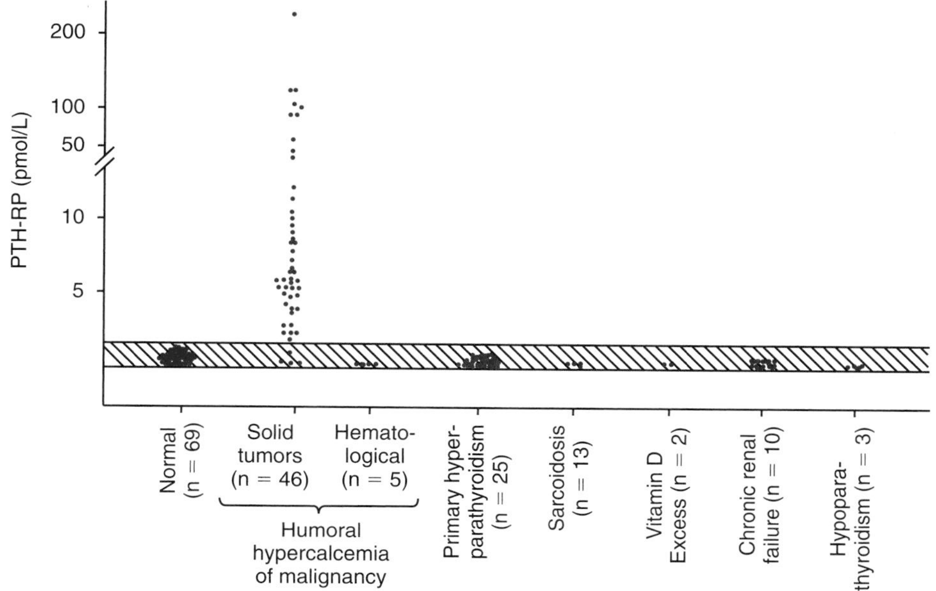

FIGURE 64.27 Parathyroid hormone–related peptide (PTHrP) in healthy patients and patients with malignancies and other disorders. The *hatched area* indicates the reference interval. (Modified from Pandian MR, Morgan CH, Carlton E, Segre GV. Modified immunoradiometric assay of parathyroid hormone-related protein: clinical application in the differential diagnosis of hypercalcemia. *Clin Chem* 1992;38:282–88.)

product of the *SOST* gene localized on chromosome region 17q12–q21 causing sclerosteosis[337,338] and van Buchem syndrome,[339,340] and it was later confirmed in mice in which the *SOST* gene had been deleted[341] or overexpressed.[342] Sclerostin is secreted by osteocytes[343] and articular chondrocytes, and its absence favors bone formation by lack of inhibition of the canonical Wnt/β-catenin signaling,[344,345] leading to osteoblast differentiation, proliferation, and activity.[346,347]

Biochemistry and Physiology

Sclerostin expression by osteocytes is regulated by mechanical forces with immobilization increasing sclerostin positive osteocytes and circulating sclerostin.[348,349] Calcitonin and glucocorticoids are both stimulatory; PTH and estrogen are inhibitory. In the bone microenvironment, prostaglandin E2, oncostatin M, cardiotrophin-1, osteryx, and leukemia inhibitory factor regulate osteocyte sclerostin expression.[350] During osteoblast differentiation, variable sclerostin expression has been noted in response to ephrin signaling and tumor necrosis factor.[351]

Gender, age, and seasonal variability has been reported in circulating sclerostin. There is a significant circadian rhythm in normal men with a nocturnal/early-morning peak (01.00–02.00 hours) following recumbency and a nadir in the early morning after rising from bed (09.00–10.00 hours).[352]

Clinical Significance

Circulating sclerostin concentrations are altered in metabolic bone diseases. They are increased in disorders such as hypoparathyroidism,[353] type II diabetes,[354,355] cancer-induced bone disease,[356] and Paget disease.[357] Sclerostin is decreased in PHPT[358-360] and ankylosing spondylitis,[361] although recently increased disease activity in ankylosing spondylitis has been shown to be associated with higher sclerostin concentrations.[362] Sclerostin is being suggested as a "predictor" and "biomarker" for diseases such as CKD,[363] aortic valve calcification,[364] osteoporotic fracture,[365] and spinal cord injury–induced osteoporosis.[366] Measurement may be invaluable in helping explain how osteocytes regulate bone turnover and in the assessment of therapeutic effectiveness in skeletal disorders.

Measurement of Sclerostin

Several assays are available for measurement of sclerostin using human blood. It has been suggested that heparin as an anticoagulant could interfere with the binding of sclerostin to proteins such as LRP5/6 and the antibodies used in some assays.[367] EDTA plasma and serum are the recommended sample types. Measurements using EDTA plasma are more comparable among assays (lower differences in values and better correlations between kits) than serum.

A number of commercial immunoassays are available to measure sclerostin. Biomedica (Vienna, Austria), R&D Systems (Abingdon, United Kingdom), TECO*medical* (Sissach, Switzerland), and Meso Scale Diagnostics (Rockville, Maryland) all manufacture assays using different antibody types and assay formats. Significant variations exist among the assays[368] reflecting differences in epitopes recognized, detection of intact molecule or fragments, and possible cross-reactivity with sclerostin domain-containing protein 1.

Reference Intervals

Using the Biomedica assay in normal adults, the mean concentrations are as follows: serum 0.8 pmol/L; plasma (EDTA) 1.3 pmol/L; plasma (heparin) 1.2 pmol/L; and plasma (citrate) 1.4 pmol/L.

SUMMARY OF INTEGRATED CONTROL OF MINERAL METABOLISM

The metabolism of calcium is linked intimately with that of phosphate (Fig. 64.28).[9,12,84] The homeostatic mechanisms are directed principally toward the maintenance of normal extracellular calcium and phosphate concentrations, which sustain extracellular and intracellular processes and provide substrate for skeletal mineralization. The parathyroid glands respond to a decrease in free calcium concentration within seconds. During a time of calcium deprivation, the increase in plasma PTH rapidly alters both renal and skeletal metabolism.

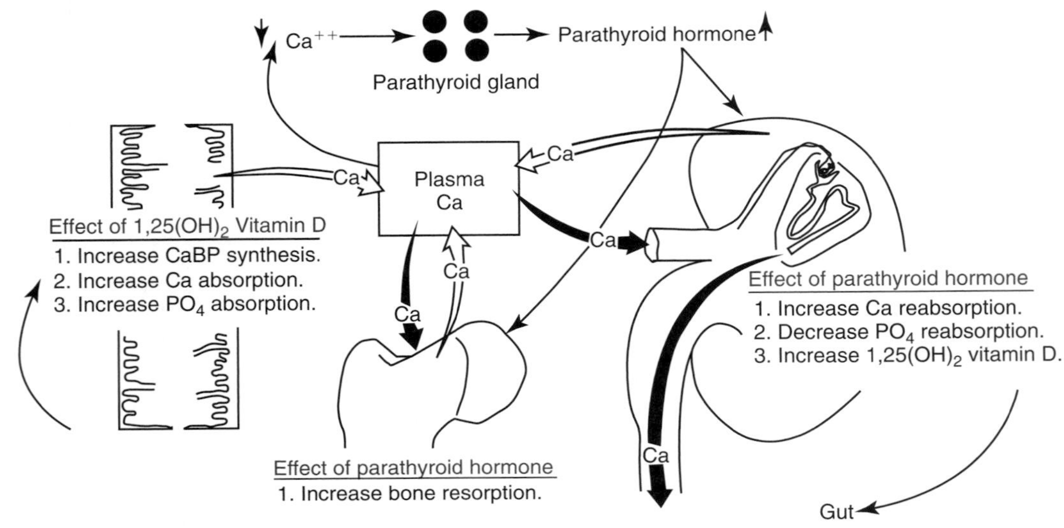

FIGURE 64.28 Integrated control of mineral metabolism. *CaBP,* Calcium-binding protein.

Renal Handling of Calcium and Phosphate

Of the 10 g (~250 mmol) of calcium filtered by the kidneys each day, 65% is reabsorbed in the proximal tubules. Calcium reabsorption there is closely linked to sodium and is independent of PTH. Approximately 10% to 20% of calcium is reclaimed in the thick ascending loops of Henle, and 5% to 10% in the distal convoluted tubules (see Chapter 59). PTH enhances calcium reabsorption at the two latter locations[84] by binding to the PTH receptor.

In contrast to the calcium-conserving effect of PTH on the kidneys, PTH increases renal phosphate excretion by the proximal tubules by directly lowering the renal phosphate threshold. Approximately 6.5 g (~210 mmol) of phosphate is filtered by the kidneys each day. Normally, 85% to 90% is reabsorbed by the renal tubules (proximal and distal). FGF23 has recently been recognized as a key hormone that lowers plasma phosphate concentration.

Intestinal Absorption of Calcium and Phosphate

PTH increases intestinal calcium absorption by increasing $1,25(OH)_2D$, whereas FGF23 decreases $1,25(OH)_2D$. The effects of PTH and FGF23 are mediated by opposite effects on renal 25(OH)D 1α-hydroxylase, which increases the conversion of 25(OH)D to the active vitamin D metabolite, $1,25(OH)_2D$. About 30% to 40% of a daily calcium intake of 1 g (25 mmol) is absorbed. Approximately 100 to 200 mg (2.5–5 mmol) of calcium is secreted into the gut lumen by intestinal secretion; therefore, net calcium absorption is 200 mg/24 hours (5 mmol/24 hours). Calcium is absorbed by both passive diffusion and an active transport system. It is estimated that passive diffusion accounts for absorption of about 10% of ingested calcium per day. Active calcium absorption in the duodenum is under the control of $1,25(OH)_2D$.

Dietary phosphate intake is usually 1.2 to 1.4 g/24 hours (39–45 mmol/24 hours, nearly twice the recommended intake, of which approximately 60% to 70% is absorbed, principally in the jejunum. As with calcium, both passive and active transport systems exist; $1,25(OH)_2D$ is the principal regulator of the active transport of phosphate. PTH-stimulated synthesis of $1,25(OH)_2D$ thus offsets the phosphaturic effect of PTH. High plasma phosphate concentration stimulates secretion of FGF23 by bone cells, thus leading to increased phosphate excretion and also decreased $1,25(OH)_2D$. Phosphate depletion or hypophosphatemia stimulates formation of $1,25(OH)_2D$ by the kidneys. At pharmacologic concentrations, calcitonin has the opposite effect to that of PTH. It is unclear, however, whether calcitonin has any physiologic role in mineral homeostasis in adult humans.

Bone Metabolism

PTH also has an acute effect on the skeleton. Acutely, high PTH decreases collagen synthesis in osteoblasts, but osteoclastic bone resorption is increased, with a net increase in mineral (calcium and phosphate) release from bone into the extracellular fluid. PTH is able to act directly on osteoblasts by interacting with their PTH receptors. The effect of PTH on osteoclasts appears to be indirect, through local mediators produced by the osteoblast [eg, RANK ligand and osteoprotegerin (OPG)] or released from the bone matrix (eg, transforming growth factor-β or TGF-β). Prolonged calcium deprivation results in enhanced recruitment of osteoclasts and an increased number of mature osteoclasts, which continue to resorb bone, releasing calcium, phosphate, and degradation products of the organic matrix. Prolonged exposure to intermittent high PTH eventually also increases osteoblast activity. This anabolic effect has been the rationale for designing PTH analogs that specifically increase bone formation.[137,369] PTH decreases SOST mRNA production and decreases circulating sclerostin, which may contribute to the anabolic action of intermittent PTH treatment.[148]

BIOCHEMICAL MARKERS OF BONE TURNOVER

In recent years, a large number of specific markers have been developed for measuring both bone formation and degradation. Markers of bone formation are products of the osteoblast: the amino-terminal or carboxy-terminal propeptides of type I collagen, PINP, and PICP, respectively, bone-specific alkaline phosphatase (BAP/BSAP/BALP are all used as abbreviations), and osteocalcin. Markers of bone resorption are breakdown products of type I collagen in bone and include the amino-terminal (N-terminal) and carboxy-terminal (C-terminal) cross-linked telopeptide parts of collagen (N-telopeptide [NTX], C-telopeptide [CTX], and C-telopeptide of type I collagen [ICTP]) and the pyridinium cross-links (pyridinoline [PYD] and deoxypyridinoline [DPD]). TRAP5b is an enzyme released from resorbing osteoclasts and measurable in blood. Several reviews on biochemical markers of bone metabolism are available.[370-374] More recently, methods have been developed for the measurement of OPG and RANK ligand—proteins synthesized by the osteoblast that can influence osteoclast formation, activation, and bone resorption. Additional studies are required to determine the roles of RANK ligand and OPG as markers of bone turnover.

Markers of Bone Formation

Bone formation markers, listed in Box 64.16, can be divided into three families, each of them roughly reflecting a specific phase in development of the osteoblast phenotype. During each remodeling cycle, osteoblasts are formed from undifferentiated mesenchymal cells and pass through the phases of proliferation, matrix maturation, and mineralization (see Fig. 64.3).[1] In a steady-state situation without specific disturbances in the production of any of the osteoblast products, the protein products of all three phases should in principle correlate with each other, and their measurements should give the same clinical information on the rate of bone formation. However, marker families can give discordant results if bone formation is affected by a disease state that specifically targets a particular developmental phase of the osteoblast.

Propeptides of Type I Procollagen

Type I collagen accounts for approximately 90% of the organic matrix of bone and provides it with tensile strength.

BOX 64.16 Biochemical Markers of Bone Formation

Propeptides of type I procollagen	PINP and PICP
Bone alkaline phosphatase	BALP
Osteocalcin (bone gla protein [BGP])	OC

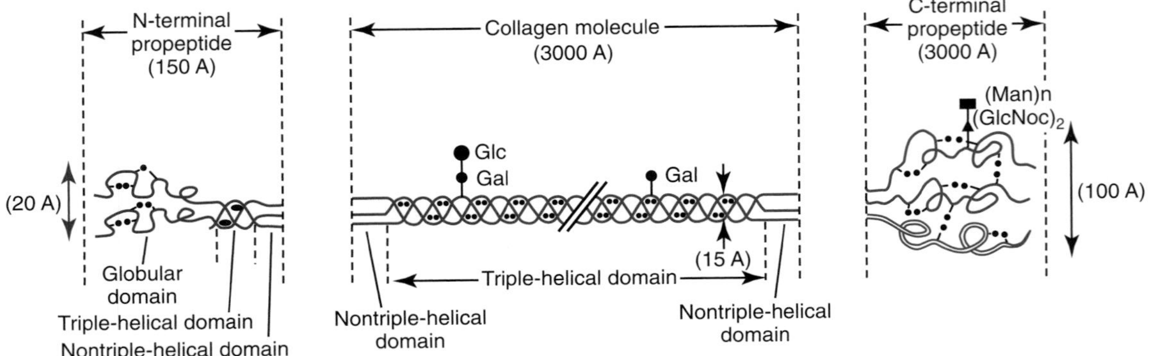

FIGURE 64.29 Schematic Representation of a Type I Procollagen Molecule. The non–triple-helical domains at both ends of the collagen molecule are the telopeptides. The N-terminal propeptide consists of an N-terminal globular domain, a triple-helical domain, and a C-terminal non–triple-helical domain. (From Prockop DJ, Kivirikko KI, Tuderman L, Guzman NA. The biosynthesis of collagen and its disorders. *N Engl J Med* 1979;301:13–23, 77–85.)

TABLE 64.7 Molecular Properties of Propeptides of Type I Procollagen and Corresponding Circulating Antigens

	PINP	PICP
Location	Amino-terminal	Carboxy-terminal
Molecular mass	35,000 Da	100,000 Da
Shape	Elongated	Globular
Chemical nature	Phosphorylated, partially collagenous	Glycoprotein, oligosaccharides of the high-mannose type
Related Serum Antigen		
Homogeneity	One major (trimeric) and one minor (monomeric) form	One form
Size	Same as intact PINP (major) or smaller	Same as PICP
Clearance from blood	Scavenger receptor of liver endothelial cells	Mannose receptor of liver endothelial cells

The type I collagen molecule, a triple helix of two identical α_1(I) chains and a slightly different α_2(I) chain, is synthesized as a precursor type I procollagen that contains large additional domains at both ends of the rodlike collagen molecule (Fig. 64.29). These extensions, known as *propeptides,* are enzymatically cleaved from procollagen in the extracellular space by two different enzymes. Cleavage of the bulky, globular C-terminal propeptide (PICP) is necessary before collagen molecules can be assembled into collagen fibers, whereas the N-terminal propeptide (PINP) may remain longer as a portion of the molecules that are deposited on the surfaces of fibers. In bones, PINP is released before mineralization, but in soft tissues, type I collagen may still contain the N-terminal propeptide (type I pN-collagen). In principle, the concentrations of procollagen propeptides reflect the rate of collagen synthesis in a manner analogous to the way that the C-peptide of insulin serves as an indicator of endogenous insulin production.[372]

Properties of the two propeptides of type I procollagen and the corresponding circulating antigens are summarized in Table 64.7. The plasma PICP antigen is homogenous and corresponds in size to the complete propeptide.[375] Also, plasma PINP antigen in healthy individuals is present mainly in intact, trimeric form.[376] However, in certain situations (eg, ESRD with hemodialysis, bedridden geriatric patients),[182] smaller forms of PINP antigen can be detected in plasma. Their exact origin is not known, but in ascitic fluid the molecular mass of a similar antigen (~10,000 Da) is clearly less than that of an individual monomeric chain of PINP (15,000 Da), suggesting a truncated form of such a chain.[377] In principle, this could represent a degradation fragment of tissue type I pN-collagen, an idea strengthened by the finding that the concentration of this smaller antigen correlates with that of the serum marker of type I collagen degradation, ICTP.[182,377] PINP assays differ with respect to whether they only measure the trimeric form (intact PINP[376]) or both forms (total PINP[378]) of the antigens.

Clearance of Propeptides. For each molecule of type I collagen deposited in the tissues, one molecule of each propeptide is released. For a kilogram of type I collagen synthesized, which is an estimated yearly production rate for adults, about 450 g of propeptide is produced. An efficient recycling mechanism has been noted for this material, which has no known further function once cleaved from procollagen. The intact propeptides are taken up from the circulation via two specific receptor-mediated pathways and are degraded by the endothelial cells of the liver (see Table 64.7).[296,379] PICP and PINP behave differently after exogenous thyroxine treatment, which increases the PINP concentration while PICP is decreased.[380] There are also families with a genetic defect in the uptake mechanism for PICP, which results in an increased concentration of this antigen with no

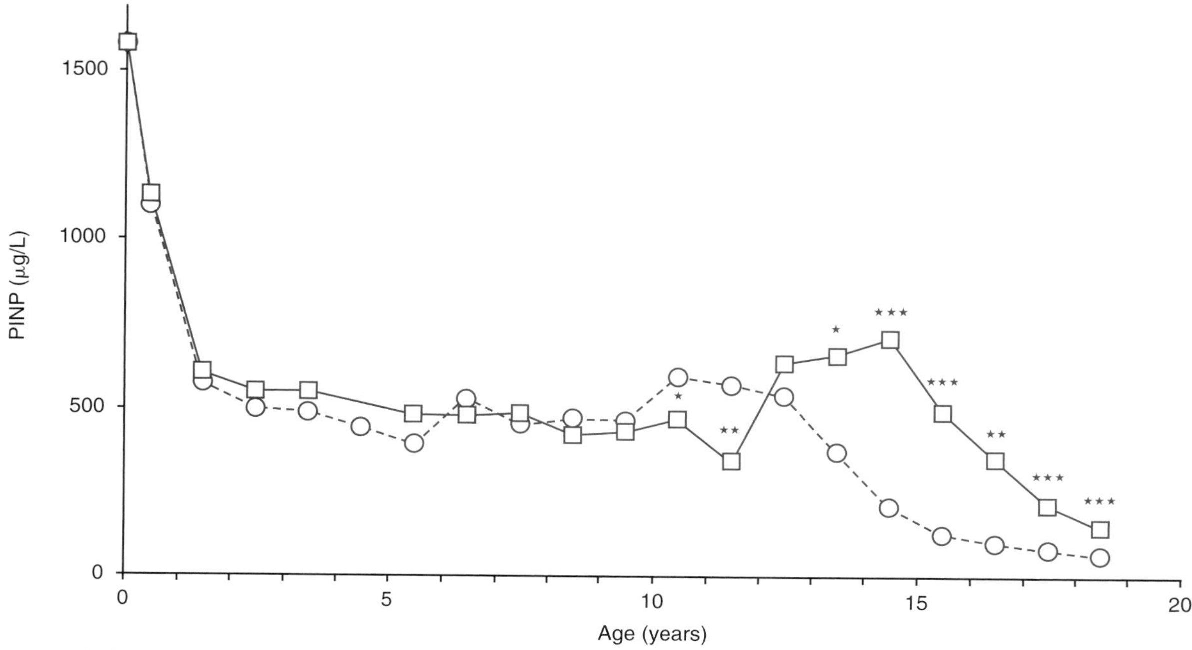

FIGURE 64.30 Serum concentrations of the amino-terminal propeptide of type I procollagen (PINP) in infants, children, and adolescents in relation to age and gender. Geometric means are shown, defined as the arithmetic mean of log-transformed PINP concentrations, raised to the power of 10. η, boys; σ, girls. Geometric means for each age band are plotted at the midpoint of that age band. Unpaired *t*-tests between age-matched boys and girls: *P *<0.05;* **P *<0.01;* ***P *<0.001*. (From Crofton PM, Evans N, Taylor MRH, Holland CV. Procollagen type I amino-terminal propeptide: pediatric reference data and relationship with procollagen type I carboxyl-terminal propeptide. *Clin Chem* 2004;50:2173–6.)

other abnormalities in type I collagen metabolites or other biochemical markers of bone metabolism.[381] When clearance of PINP was studied using an assay that detects both forms of antigens, it was found that renal clearance also occurs for the smaller circulating propeptides.[382]

Clinical Significance. After they are set free from procollagen, the two propeptides behave as two individual proteins, and their fates and metabolism are dependent on their structures. In principle, measurement of either propeptide should give the same information. This is the case when PICP and PINP concentrations are compared *in situ* (eg, during the fibroproliferative response in a healing wound, where the concentrations of both propeptides increase up to 1000-fold in 1 week).[376] In children, circulating propeptides closely reflect the somatic growth rate, and the peak of PICP and PINP concentrations occurs earlier in girls than in boys (Fig. 64.30).[383] During puberty, the increase is greater in boys than in girls.

Various drug therapies affect PINP and PICP concentrations. For example, during the first 2 days of teriparatide [PTH(1–34)] treatment, PINP and PICP increase rapidly and continue to increase until the end of 1 month of treatment to a net increase of 110% (Fig. 64.31).[384] By contrast, large doses of intravenous methylprednisolone decrease PICP rapidly, reflecting the inhibition of bone formation by glucocorticoids.[385] Significant decreases in circulating P1NP and P1CP are observed with antiresorptive therapy such as bisphosphonates and denosumab. Measurement of response to treatment for osteoporosis therapies is the major use of bone formation markers in clinical practice.

Several studies suggest that the serum concentration of PINP is increased more during active bone growth than is the concentration of PICP.[384,386] The ratio of PICP/PINP in serum is expected to be about 3 when the concentrations are expressed as μg/L. In adults, this ratio is indeed about 3, but in children it is less than1.[387] In Paget disease of bone, a similar discrepancy is seen between circulating concentrations of the two propeptides.[388] A low PICP/PINP ratio is associated with aggressive breast cancer.[389]

Specimen Requirements. The preferred sample for measuring either of the procollagen propeptides is serum. The antigens are very stable in serum or plasma. Storage of a serum sample at room temperature for 1 week does not decrease measurable concentrations.[173,375]

Assays for C-Terminal Propeptide and N-Terminal Propeptide. The PICP antigen has been purified from the cell culture medium of human fibroblasts and used for establishing a radioimmunoassay.[375] A similar EIA is commercially available (called *CICP*). Assays for PINP can be divided into two families: intact PINP[200] and total PINP.[378,390,391] So far, only an RIA for intact PINP has been approved by the US Food and Drug Administration (FDA). This assay has been used in several clinical studies, for example, for monitoring the effects of alendronate, denosumab, teriparatide, rososuzomab, and odanacatinib on bone.[384,392-395]

Reference Intervals. The reported reference intervals for PICP are 38 to 202 μg/L in men and 50 to 170 μg/L in women.[375] For intact PINP, the original reference intervals reported in men are 20 to 78 μg/L and 19 to 84 μg/L in women.[376] The reference interval for total PINP in young,

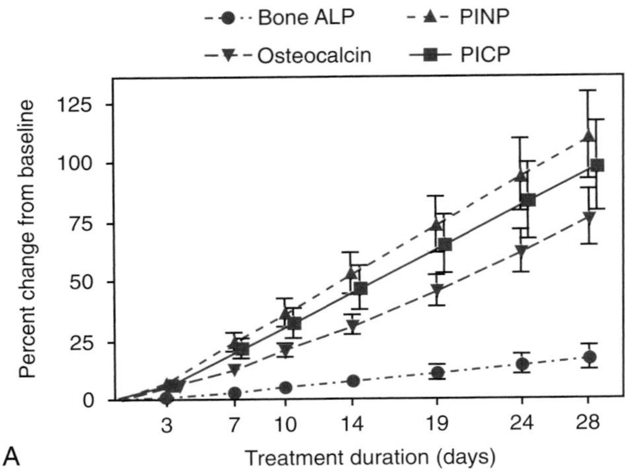

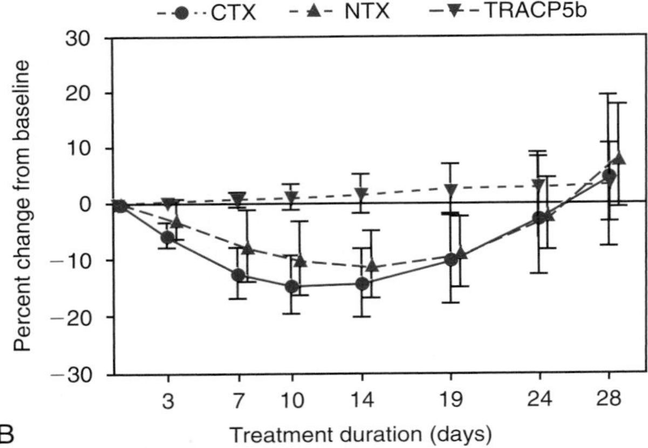

FIGURE 64.31 Changes in biochemical markers of bone metabolism during 28 days of teriparatide [PTH(1–34)] treatment of osteoporosis. *Line plots* show estimated mean and 90% confidence intervals for percentage change from baseline in **(A)** markers of bone formation and **(B)** markers of bone resorption. *Bullet points* at some time points have been slightly shifted horizontally to increase readability. For bone ALP, osteocalcin, PINP, and PICP, all changes from baseline are statistically significant ($P < 0.0001$). For CTX, all changes from baseline until day 19 are statistically significant ($P < 0.0004$). For NTX, all changes from baseline to days 7 to 10 are statistically significant ($P < 0.03$). For TRACP5b, no changes are statistically significant. (From Glover SJ, Eastell R, McCloskey EV, Rogers A, Garnero P, Lowery J, et al. Rapid and robust response of biochemical markers of bone formation to teriparatide therapy. *Bone* 2009;45:1053–8.)

healthy premenopausal women ($n = 637$; 30–39 years of age) is 16.3 to 72.2 μg/L in France, Belgium, the United States, and the United Kingdom.[396] Significant differences have been noted among countries, with significantly higher values in France and Belgium than in the United Kingdom and the United States. The reference interval for total PINP in men is 13.9 to 85.5 μg/L.[397] Children have higher concentrations immediately after birth and later during growth spurts (see Fig. 64.30); reference intervals for children have been reported.[383] In neonates (younger than 1 month of age), the reference interval of intact PINP concentration is very high at 770 to 3202 μg/L. Detailed pediatric reference intervals have been established as part of the CALIPER study and are available in the Appendix.

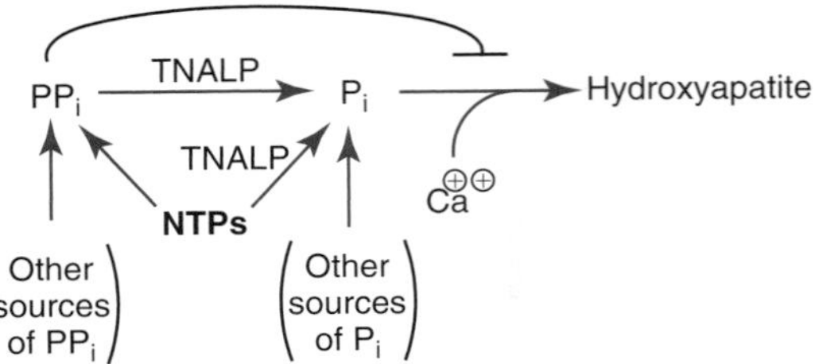

FIGURE 64.32 Schematic representation of the role of bone alkaline phosphatase in hydroxyapatite formation. Alkaline phosphatase catalyzes the hydrolysis of pyrophosphate (PP_i) produced by the activity of nucleoside triphosphate pyrophosphohydrolase from nucleoside triphosphates (NTPs). Alkaline phosphatase has a positive effect on mineralization primarily by controlling the size of the inhibitory pool of PP_i. The enzyme also generates P_i by using NTPs and PP_i as substrates, but other major sources of P_i (eg, intestinal absorption) are likely to contribute to the bulk of the P_i needed for hydroxyapatite deposition. (Modified from Hessle L, Johnson KA, Anderson HC, Narisawa S, Sali A, Goding JW, et al. Tissue-nonspecific alkaline phosphatase and plasma cell membrane glycoprotein-1 are central antagonistic regulators of bone mineralization. *Proc Natl Acad Sci U S A* 2002;99:9445–9.)

Bone Alkaline Phosphatase

Alkaline phosphatases (ALPs; EC 3.1.3.1) are membrane-bound ectoenzymes that catalyze the hydrolysis of monophosphates from ester linkage under alkaline conditions (pH 8–10). Four different gene codes are known for the tissue-nonspecific, intestinal, placental, and germ cell (placental-like) isoenzymes. The alkaline phosphates of liver, bone, and kidney are isoforms of the same gene product, the tissue-nonspecific gene located in chromosome 1 *(TNALP)*. These isoforms are N-glycosylated, and only the liver ALP does not contain O-linked glycans.[398] ALP is attached to the outer surface of cell membranes by a glycosylphosphatidylinositol (GPI) anchor. Plasma ALP is a homodimer in which the anchor has been removed by the action of endogenous or exogenous (eg, plasma) GPI-specific phospholipase D.[399] Bone ALP can be further separated by anion-exchange HPLC or isoelectric focusing into four isoforms—B/I, B1x, B1, and B2, which differ in their sialic acid content.[400,401] Using the same procedure, liver ALP can be divided into three isoforms.[401] As glycoproteins, ALPs are cleared by the liver.

During mineralization of bone, the main function of bone ALP is to hydrolyze inorganic pyrophosphate (PPi) to generate phosphate (Pi) (Fig. 64.32).[402-404] Matrix vesicles are markedly enriched in tissue-nonspecific ALP.[404] The balance between Pi and PPi is thought to be critical for mineralization because PPi inhibits the formation of hydroxyapatite. Studies on TNALP knockout mice, whose condition resembled the human disease hypophosphatasemia (or hypophosphatasia), have suggested that skeletal ALP is necessary for the propagation step but not for the initiation of mineralization.[399,405,406]

Bone ALP is produced by osteoblasts during the matrix maturation phase (see Fig. 64.3),[1] when the newly formed collagenous matrix is prepared for the deposition of mineral. However, because ALP is firmly bound to cell membranes, its release to plasma can be delayed, and the increase in plasma activity takes time.

Clinical Significance. Total ALP or bone ALP provides the highest clinical sensitivity and specificity in the diagnosis and monitoring of Paget disease of bone. Although total ALP is

AT A GLANCE

FGF 23 In Disease States

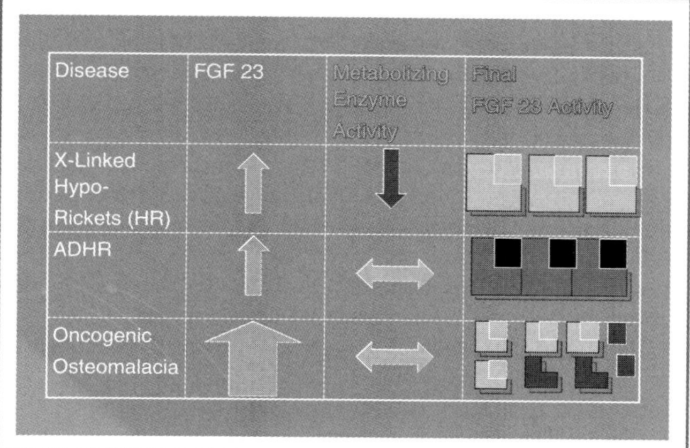

In X-linked hypophosphataemic rickets decreased metabolizing enzyme activity results in increased intact FGF23 *(light colored boxes)*. In autosomal dominant hypophosphataemic rickets (ADHR) an abnormal intact FGF23 *(dark colored boxes)* that is not metabolized by normal enzyme activity circulates resulting in increased intact FGF23. In oncogenic osteomalacia a large amount of intact FGF23 is produced *(light colored boxes)*. This exceeds the metabolizing enzyme capacity, which is producing the dark separate fragments that are composed of inactive N *(larger L-shaped fragment)* and C-terminal *(small squares)* fragments.

used most often, bone ALP is more sensitive than total ALP in mild (often monostotic) disease. ALP is increased in Paget disease and reflects generally increased bone formation in this condition. In recent years, there has been a change in the presentation of Paget disease to a milder phenotype than has been previously reported. As a result, the concentration of ALP at diagnosis is often only 2 to 4 times the upper limit of normal (ULN) rather than 10 times the ULN seen in the past.

In severe osteomalacia, bone ALP may be markedly increased without an increase in bone mineralization because of a mineralizing defect.

Bone ALP is increased in metabolic bone diseases including osteoporosis, osteomalacia and rickets, hyperparathyroidism, renal osteodystrophy, and thyrotoxicosis, and in individuals with acromegaly, bone metastases, and other disorders with increased bone formation.

Because the half-life of ALP is relatively long (≈40 hours), it is less sensitive than procollagen propeptides or osteocalcin to acute treatment effects, such as the effects of large doses of intravenous methylprednisolone.[385] During teriparatide treatment, ALP is not increased as early or as much as procollagen propeptides or osteocalcin (see Fig. 64.31).[384]

ALP and bone ALP are stable in serum in vitro and do not require special specimen handling. ALP has a long half-life in plasma and is relatively unaffected by diurnal variation. Bone ALP is more useful than osteocalcin (as discussed earlier in this chapter) in individuals with impaired renal function because it is not cleared by glomerular filtration.

Because $1,25(OH)_2D$ regulates the synthesis of bone ALP and osteocalcin, both of these markers may be misleading in patients treated with calcitriol and in those with abnormal concentrations of this hormone.

Low total ALP is important to identify as an increasing number of patients are being recognized with hypophosphatasia, for which effective treatment is now available. This calls for evidence-based lower reference intervals for ALP based in the IFCC reference method.[407] Childhood hypophosphatasia can be categorized into three forms, and the severity of the disease is correlated with the concentration of total ALP. Skeletal abnormalities are common in severe hypophosphatasia, and bone ALP is often low. Advances in therapeutics have resulted in the development and registration of a genetically engineered treatment, Asfotase Alfa, which can replace the deficiency of ALP resulting in significant improvement in the condition in affected children.

Measurement of Bone Alkaline Phosphatase. Measurement of the enzymatic activities of total and bone ALP was described in Chapter 29. Although internal standards for ALP isoenzymes have been used to increase assay precision in assays of bone ALP activity,[408] they tend to be technically complicated and labor-intensive, imprecise, insensitive, and inaccurate. Heat denaturation has been criticized because of its irreproducibility or variability. A method using wheat germ agglutinin (WGA) to precipitate bone ALP has been criticized because WGA does not precipitate all bone ALP from serum from Paget disease patients and fails to completely separate bone and liver activity.[409] Lot-to-lot variability of the lectin is also evident.[410]

Several immunoassays have been reported for bone ALP. However, none of the monoclonal antibodies used is completely specific for bone or liver ALP.[411] Two commercially available immunoassays use monoclonal antibodies against bone ALP from SaOS-2 cells. One immunoassay is an IRMA using two monoclonal antibodies—a capture antibody and a radioiodinated signal antibody—preferentially reacting with bone ALP. This two-site immunoassay measures the mass of bone ALP in μg/L. Subsequently, an immunoenzymatic method was developed by replacing the signal antibody with direct measurement of the activity of immobilized bone ALP.[412] A modification of this method is available on an automated immunoassay analyzer using chemiluminescence detection. The other assay uses a single monoclonal antibody against bone ALP. Microtiter plates are coated with this antibody and are used to separate bone ALP from other isoforms and isoenzymes. After immunoseparation, the activity (U/L) of bone ALP is determined with a *p*-nitrophenyl phosphate substrate.

The analytical and clinical performances of these bone ALP immunoassays have been characterized in a series of articles. Unfortunately, current immunoassays are not completely specific for bone ALP and exhibit 7% to 17% cross-reactivity with ALP from liver.[412,413] It has been difficult to exactly determine cross-reactivity with the liver isoform because of limitations of existing preparations and incomplete understanding of the exact nature of circulating isoforms and bone ALP may be misleading in liver disease because of this cross-reactivity of current methods with liver ALP.

Reference Intervals. Plasma concentrations of bone ALP are influenced by age and gender. Concentrations are higher in men and increase with age in both men and women, consistent with the age-related increase in bone turnover. The reference interval of bone ALP with the IRMA is 5 to 20 μg/L. With the immunoabsorption assay, it is 15 to 41.3 U/L for men and 11.6 to 29.6 U/L for premenopausal women. For the automated chemiluminescent immunoenzymatic method, the 95th percentile limit is reported to be 14.3 μg/L for men

Osteocalcin [Bone Gla Protein (BGP)]

1				5					10
Tyr	Leu	Tyr	Gln	Trp	Leu	Gly	Ala	Pro	Val
11				15					20
Pro	Tyr	Pro	Asp	Pro	Leu	**Gla**	Pro	Arg	Arg
21				25					30
Gla	Val	Cys	**Gla**	Leu	Asn	Pro	Asp	Cys	Asp
31				35					40
Glu	Leu	Ala	Asp	His	Ile	Gly	Phe	Gln	Glu
41				45				49	
Ala	Tyr	Arg	Arg	Phe	Tyr	Gly	Pro	Val	

FIGURE 64.33 **Structure of Human Osteocalcin.** Three glutamyl residues at positions 17, 21, and 24 can be carboxylated in a posttranslational, vitamin K–dependent, enzymatic step producing γ-carboxyglutamyl (Gla) residues. A disulfide bond formed between cysteines in positions 23 and 29 stabilizes two antiparallel α-helical structures representing 40% of the overall structure.

and 20.1 μg/L for premenopausal women. Children have much higher concentrations, especially at puberty.[414,415]

Osteocalcin

Osteocalcin (OC), also known as bone gla protein (BGP), is the most abundant noncollagenous protein of human bone. It is a small protein of 49 amino acids with a molecular mass of 5669 Da; its gene, symbol *BGLAP,* is located in chromosome 1. 1,25$(OH)_2$D upregulates OC synthesis. OC contains three glutamyl residues at amino acid positions 17, 21, and 24 (Fig. 64.33), which can be converted to γ-carboxyglutamyl residues by a posttranslational, vitamin K–dependent enzymatic carboxylation. These unique carboxylated amino acids bind calcium ions and are found in various proteins involved in blood coagulation and in calcium transport, deposition, and homeostasis. OC binds calcium and hydroxyapatite, suggesting a physiologic role in bone mineralization.[416]

Osteocalcin knockout mice have increased bone formation compared with wild-type mice.[417] They develop a phenotype marked by higher bone mass and bones of improved functional quality by 6 to 9 months. This could indicate an inhibitory function of OC on osteoblast activity, but further study has demonstrated that osteocalcin has a small role in bone and dentine mineralization, in contrast to another γ-carboxylated protein of bone, matrix gla protein.[418]

Instead of bone formation defects, these knockout mice show decreased insulin and adiponectin secretion, insulin resistance, higher serum glucose concentrations, and increased adiposity.[198] Osteocalcin in fact may be an osteoblast-secreted hormone regulating insulin secretion and sensitivity.[126,419] Leptin formed in adipose tissues, on the other hand, regulates synthesis of osteocalcin in osteoblasts. Adipose cells can also produce osteocalcin.[420]

Both in mice and in men, osteocalcin can be present in the plasma in carboxylated and undercarboxylated forms; it is the undercarboxylated form of osteocalcin that acts as a hormone. The undercarboxylated fraction represents 16% to 21% of the total OC.[421]

Plasma OC is cleared by the kidneys and has a half-life of approximately 5 minutes. OC concentrations are increased in individuals with renal failure. OC exhibits a diurnal variation with a nocturnal peak, dropping by as much as 50% to a morning nadir. Circulating OC is heterogenous; in addition to the intact molecule, several fragments are the result of proteolysis at arginine residues in positions 19, 20, 43, and 44 (see Fig. 64.33). Intact OC has been estimated to account for about 35% of total OC, N-terminal/midregion for about 30%, and other fragments for much less in the circulation.[422] These proportions are different in some conditions (eg, osteoporosis).

In animal models, osteocalcin has been shown to influence glucose homeostasis expanding the role of bone as an endocrine organ.[423] In humans, low osteocalcin was associated with impaired glucose metabolism in men and premenopausal women. In postmenopausal women with increased bone turnover, this relationship was not present.[424]

Clinical Significance. The concentration of OC changes rapidly in situations that affect bone turnover. During teriparatide treatment, OC increases rapidly, but this is less pronounced than with PINP and continues to increase until the end of the first month of treatment (see Fig. 64.31).[384] OC rapidly decreases in patients given large doses of methylprednisolone intravenously.[385] Plasma OC concentration is increased in metabolic bone disease with increased bone formation, including osteoporosis, hyperparathyroidism, renal osteodystrophy, and thyrotoxicosis, and in individuals with fractures, acromegaly, and bone metastases. It is decreased in hypoparathyroidism, hypothyroidism, and growth hormone deficiency, and during estrogen therapy and treatment with glucocorticoids, bisphosphonates, and calcitonin.

OC concentrations may be misleading in several situations. They increase in patients with impaired renal function without a similar increase in bone formation, because OC is cleared by the kidneys. OC may be increased during bed rest without an increase in bone formation. Serum OC may not reflect bone formation in patients treated with 1,25$(OH)_2$D or those with abnormalities in this hormone, because OC is regulated by 1,25$(OH)_2$D.

About 10% to 30% of OC synthesized by the osteoblast is released into the circulation. OC is not a pure marker of bone formation: freshly synthesized OC is secreted in part into the bloodstream and is incorporated in part into the bone matrix.[425] Osteocalcin is also released from the bone matrix during bone resorption; these fragments of OC may contribute to circulating concentrations of osteocalcin. Thus, serum osteocalcin may be considered a marker of bone turnover rather than bone formation.[426] Measurements of OC are used more in research than in clinical practice.

Measurement of Osteocalcin. Many immunoassay methods have been developed for OC since the first assay was reported in 1980.[425] Early OC assays were competitive immunoassays, but noncompetitive methods have been developed.[427] Noncompetitive methods measuring intact OC, especially those measuring both intact OC plus the N-terminal/midregion (1–43) fragment, are of particular interest. These assays do not measure smaller fragments of OC that can be produced during bone resorption. OC concentrations are more stable when measured with assays that recognize both intact hormone (1–49) and the N-terminal/midregion (1–43), because this fragment is produced in vitro by hydrolysis of intact OC.[428]

For most assays, specificities with respect to carboxylated and undercarboxylated forms of OC are not known. An ELISA assay for N-terminal midfragment is independent of the degree of γ-carboxylation of human OC.[428] If the serum sample is precipitated with hydroxyapatite[429] or barium sulfate,[430] the supernatant contains undercarboxylated OC.

The circulating concentration of OC measured in healthy subjects varies widely between methods and laboratories. One study reported that mean values for healthy individuals ranged from 3 to 27 ng/mL.[431] Such variability may be a consequence of differences in specificities and sensitivities of antisera and/or antibodies used in the assays, and in the purity, potency, and immunoreactivity of OC calibrators. Another important source of variation between methods may be their dependence on, or independence of, calcium concentration in the assay. Calcium binding to γ-carboxyglutamyl residues induces a conformational change in OC. Although EDTA is added to some assays to eliminate this effect, other assays require the addition of calcium.

An immunoassay for the undercarboxylated form of osteocalcin has also been developed. This assay uses recombinant human undercarboxylated OC for calibration and two monoclonal antibodies;[421] one of these specifically recognizes the 14–30 sequence, in which the three glutamic acid residues are not carboxylated.

Specimen Requirements. Osteocalcin is rapidly degraded in blood samples at room temperature or at 4°C.[422,432,433] Serum OC concentrations are more stable when assessed with methods measuring both intact OC and the N-terminal/midregion fragment (1–43): concentrations were unchanged after 3 hours at room temperature and after 24 hours at 4°C.[422,433]

Reference Intervals. OC concentrations are influenced by age, gender, and diurnal variation. Men have somewhat higher concentrations of OC than women. OC concentrations have been reported to increase, decrease, or remain unchanged with advancing age as a probable consequence of the heterogeneity of circulating OC and differences in immunoassay specificity. OC concentrations generally are increased during menopause. In a commercially available OC ELISA, the reference interval is 9.6 to 40.8 μg/L in men, 8.4 to 33.9 μg/L in premenopausal women, and 12.8 to 55 μg/L in postmenopausal women. Concentrations are higher in children; the highest concentrations are observed during periods of rapid growth.[414,415]

Biochemical Markers of Bone Resorption

Most markers of bone resorption reflect aspects of the degradation of type I collagen. These markers were initially measured in urine, but serum-based methods have been developed. An osteoclast-derived enzyme, serum tartrate-resistant acid phosphatase (TRAP5b), has also been used to assess bone resorption. Bone resorption markers are listed in Box 64.17.

BOX 64.17 Biochemical Markers of Bone Resorption

Type I Collagen Telopeptides
- N-telopeptide (NTX)
- C-telopeptide (CTX)
- ICTP

Pyridinium Cross-Links
- Free deoxypyridinoline (DPD) and pyridinoline (PYD)
- Total deoxypyridinoline (DPD) and pyridinoline (PYD)

Tartrate-Resistant Acid Phosphatase 5b (TRAP5b)

Collagen Cross-Links

Procollagen undergoes extensive intracellular posttranslational processing, including hydroxylation of proline and lysine residues, glycosylation of hydroxylysine residues, and formation of the collagenous triple helix.[372] After it is secreted, procollagen is converted to collagen during extracellular processing, with enzymatic removal of PINP and PICP (see Fig. 64.29).

Extracellularly, type I collagen molecules are assembled into immature fibrils with limited tensile strength, which then are modified by formation of intramolecular and intermolecular covalent bonds or cross-links.[434] Intermolecular cross-linking sites have been located in short non–triple-helical domains at each end of the type I collagen molecule, called *telopeptides* (see Fig. 64.29). Two hydroxylysine and/or lysine residues in the telopeptide at the amino-terminal end (N-telopeptide) can be linked to a helical site at amino acid 930, and two C-telopeptides can be linked to a helical site at amino acid 87. The activities of two enzymes—intracellular lysyl hydroxylase 2b and extracellular lysyl oxidase—regulate which variant structures of cross-links are formed (Fig. 64.34).[435] Lysyl hydroxylase 2b forms hydroxylysine in telopeptide sequences, and lysyl oxidase deaminates the ε-amino group of lysine or hydroxylysine to produce allysine or hydroxyallysine. After this enzymatic processing of telopeptides, the other reactions are spontaneous, leading to a series of divalent and later trivalent cross-links. Of the latter, pyridinoline and deoxypyridinoline are stable even to acid hydrolysis, whereas the pyrrole variants are quite unstable (see Fig. 64.34). Trivalent cross-links are found in soft tissues and in collagen types other than type I (type II, III etc.).

In soft tissues, only mature, trivalent cross-links are found, but bone contains immature, divalent cross-links because mineralization occurs at the same locations as telopeptide cross-links. C-terminal telopeptide isolated from human bone contains non–cross-linked as well as divalently and trivalently cross-linked telopeptides.[436] Pyridinolines were the first mature cross-links to be identified, but their quantity in bone is relatively low—approximately 1 per 3 to 5 collagen molecules—compared with the quantity of their divalent precursors—1 per collagen molecule.[100,209] The pyrrole cross-links are concentrated at the N-terminal end of human bone collagen.[209] More pyrrole is produced if the activity of lysyl hydroxylase 2b is low in the osteoblast.[100]

Both telopeptides have a sequence including an aspartic acid residue, which as the result of a nonenzymatic reaction, can undergo racemization and β-isomerization.[437,438] Immunoassays detect only one form of these structures, thus decreasing the amount or concentration of antigen detected and creating the possibility that changes in concentration (eg, with treatment) are due in part to changes in the fine structure of the antigen, rather than to changes in total concentration.

Degradation of Bone Collagen. Cathepsin K is the main enzyme that degrades bone collagen within the lacunae of osteoclasts. Its activity alone is sufficient to completely dissolve insoluble collagen of adult human cortical bone.[439] Osteoclasts also produce other proteases, notably several matrix metalloproteinase (MMP) enzymes (eg, MMP-9, MMP-10, MMP-12, MMP-14).[440] Cross-linked telopeptides

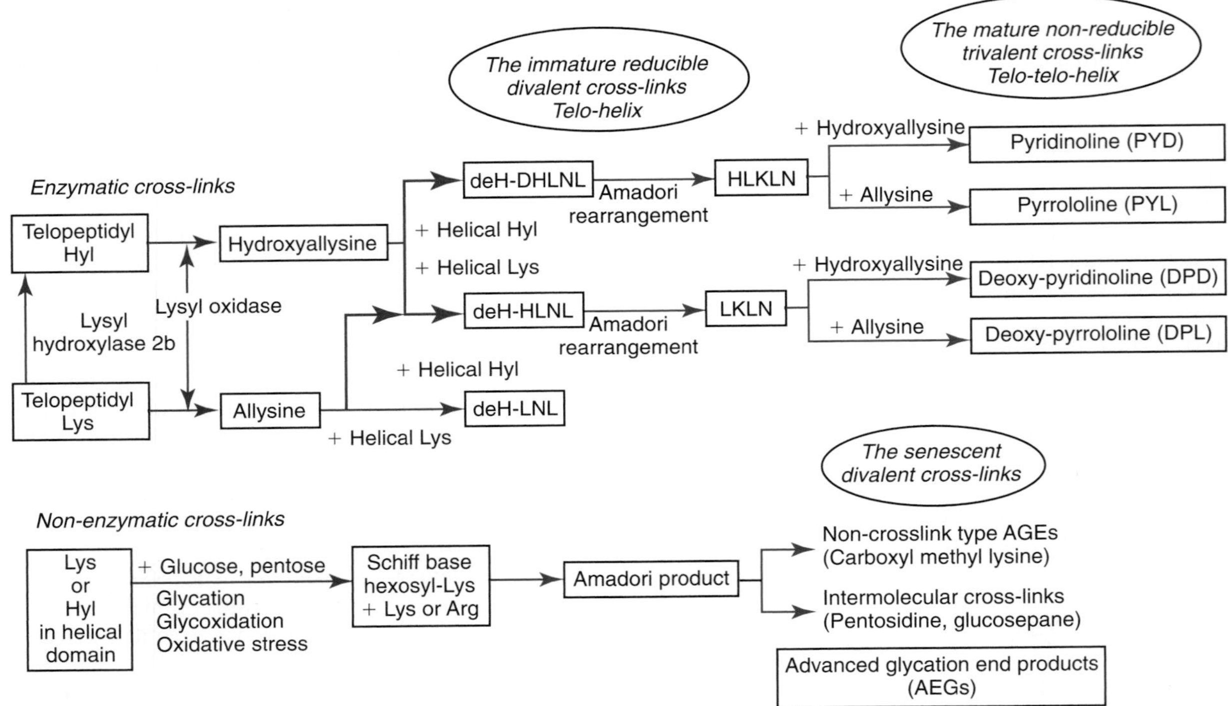

FIGURE 64.34 Pathways of Enzymatic and Nonenzymatic Cross-Link Formation in Bone Collagen. Lysyl hydroxylase 2b- and lysyl oxidase-controlled reactions are the first steps for enzymatic cross-linking within collagen fibers. *deH-DHLNL,* Dehydrodihydroxylysinonorleucine; *deH-HLNL,* dehydrohydroxylysinonorleucine; *deH-LNL,* dehydrolysinonorleucine; *HLKNL,* hydroxylysino-5-ketonorleucine; *LKNL,* lysino-5-ketonorleucine. (Modified from Saito M, Marumo K. Collagen cross-links as a determinant of bone quality: a possible explanation for bone fragility in aging, osteoporosis, and diabetes mellitus. *Osteoporosis Int* 2010;21:195–214.)

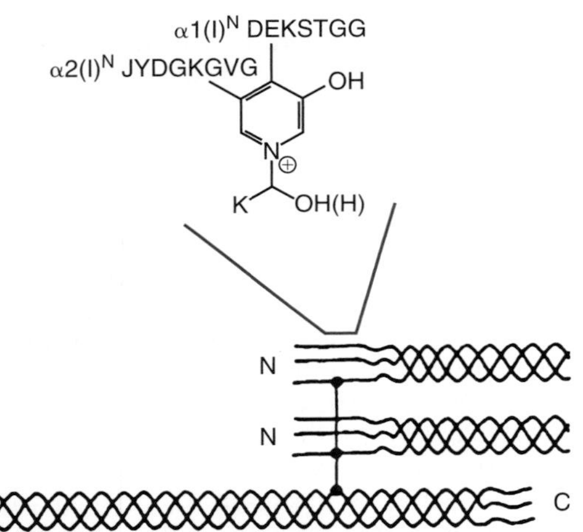

FIGURE 64.35 Structure and Molecular Origin of the N-Telopeptide (NTX) Epitope in Type I Collagen Fibrils. The peptides excreted in urine consist of two telopeptide fragments still linked to the cross-linking residue, which can have a deoxypyridinoline *(as shown here),* a pyridinoline, or a pyrrole structure. (Modified from Atley LM, Mort JS, Lalumiere M, Eyre DR. Proteolysis of human bone collagen by cathepsin K: characterization of the cleavage sites generating the cross-linked N-telopeptide neoepitope. *Bone* 2000;26:241–7.)

are released from type I collagen during bone resorption because cross-links resist proteolysis of adjacent polypeptide chains. This may lead to generation of a neoepitope such as NTX that can be detected by an immunoassay (Fig. 64.35).[441]

For C-terminal telopeptides, two distinct immunoassays—ICTP and CTX—reflect different enzymatic pathways of bone breakdown.[442] Cathepsin K releases CTX antigen but destroys reactivity in the ICTP assay (Fig. 64.36). ICTP antigen is stable after MMP-1, MMP-9, and MMP-13 digestion.[443] It has been suggested that the ICTP assay could be called the *CTX-MMP assay.*[444] The importance of MMPs is demonstrated by pycnodysostosis, a lysosomal disease caused by cathepsin K deficiency.[445] In this disease, ICTP is the major fragment released during bone resorption.[446]

NTX and CTX reflect normal osteoclastic function,[447] whereas ICTP detects pathologic degradation of bone and soft connective tissue as seen in multiple myeloma, bone metastasis, and rheumatoid arthritis.[372] Thus, in rheumatoid arthritis, CTX is generally within the reference interval, whereas ICTP is increased, correlating with markers of inflammation (C-reactive protein and erythrocyte sedimentation rate).[448] It seems that MMPs are important in this condition because lack of cathepsin K activity does not abolish erosion.[449]

Measurement of urinary excretion of hydroxyproline has been used in the past to assess bone turnover or bone resorption, but it is rarely used today. Hydroxyproline is found mainly in collagens, where it accounts for about 13% of total amino acids (note that, strictly, hydroxyproline, like proline is an imino acid). It is needed to stabilize the triple-helical structure at body temperature. When the helical collagenous

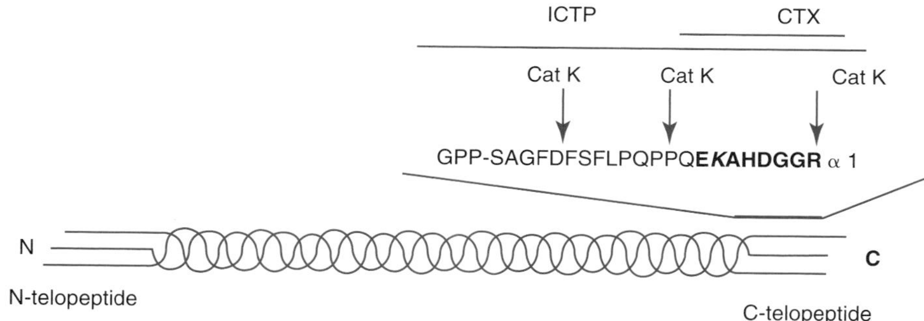

FIGURE 64.36 Schematic representation of the CTX and ICTP epitopes and cathepsin K (Cat K) cleavage sites in the carboxy-terminal telopeptide of type I collagen. The CTX epitope corresponds to an 8–amino acid sequence in the telopeptide part of an α_1(I) chain, whereas the ICTP epitope is a larger conformational epitope, requiring telopeptide parts of two α_1(I) chains, both of which contain the phenylalanine-rich region. As shown in the figure, cathepsin K degrades the ICTP phenotype, while generating CTX. The hydroxylysine residue (K) participates in intramolecular and intermolecular covalent cross-links. (From Garnero P, Ferreras M, Karsdal MA, et al. The type I collagen fragments ICTP and CTX revel distinct enzymatic pathways of bone collagen degradation. *J Bone Miner Res* 2003;18:859–867. Modified from Garnero P, Borel O, Byrjalsen O, et al. The collagenolytic activity of cathepsin K is unique among mammalian proteinases. *J Biol Chem* 2003;273:32347–32352. Modified from Sassi ML, Eriksen H, Risteli L, et al. Immunochemical characterization of assay for carboxyterminal telopeptide of human type I collagen: loss of antigenicity by treatment with cathepsin K. *Bone* 2000;26:367–373.)

sequence is degraded, this amino acid is released and about 90% of it is catabolized in the liver to urea and carbon dioxide. About 10% is excreted in urine, where it can be analyzed by any one of several methods. However, hydroxyproline is not specific for collagen in that other proteins also contain it (eg, complement C1q). In addition, the amino-terminal propeptides of type I and III procollagens, markers of collagen synthesis, include in their structure a triple-helical part, which contains hydroxyproline (see Fig. 64.29). Also, ingestion of meat or gelatin increases hydroxyproline excretion.

Comparison of Urine and Serum Analyses. Urine used to be the sample of choice for measuring bone collagen degradation. Urinary hydroxyproline analysis was replaced by the more sensitive and specific cross-link (DPD, PYD) and telopeptide (CTX, NTX) assays. Urinary measurements need to be corrected for creatinine excretion to adjust for effects of urinary concentration or dilution. This includes a second analyte, which has its own analytical variation that adds to the uncertainty of the result.

Serum and urine telopeptide assays have been compared in several studies; correlation coefficients have varied from 0.6 to 0.9.[450] Kidneys are involved in further degradation of cross-linked peptides; as a result, approximately 40% of total cross-links in the urine are free (ie, not peptide bound).[451] The mean fractional excretion of NTX (0.22) is lower than that of CTX (0.44), indicating that renal degradation is greater for the former analyte.[452]

During antiresorptive treatment, urinary telopeptide assessment may overestimate the decrease in bone resorption because the renal metabolism of these peptides can change. The response to antiresorptive therapy is generally greatest when measured with telopeptide assays, intermediate with the total DPD assay, and lowest with the free DPD assay.[390,453] Fractional excretion of conjugated cross-links is less than 1, whereas that of the free fraction is greater than 1.[454] Serum or plasma assays have replaced urine assays in many countries.

Clinical Significance of Telopeptides and Cross-Links. Increased urinary CTX, NTX, and DPD have been reported in osteoporosis, Paget disease of bone, primary and secondary hyperparathyroidism, hyperthyroidism, and other diseases such as carcinoma metastases, multiple myeloma, and with increased bone resorption or osteolysis.

Inhibition of bone resorption with pharmacologic agents (bisphosphonates, Denosumab) leads to a decrease in serum or plasma or urinary CTX, NTX, and DPD. Markers of bone formation are also decreased because of the coupling of resorption and formation; their reductions are delayed and are not as great as those observed for markers of bone resorption. The most common use in clinical practice is the assessment of response to treatments decreasing bone resorption.

Measurement of Telopeptides and Pyridinium Cross-Links. Several methods are commercially available; the most commonly used are serum and urine assays for NTX and CTX, serum assay for ICTP, and a urine assay for deoxypyridinoline.

N-Telopeptide. NTX in urine is measured with a commercially available ELISA, which uses a monoclonal antibody against the NTX fraction isolated from the urine of healthy adolescents.[455] The antibody recognizes a conformational epitope of the cross-linked α_2(I)N-telopeptide containing the sequence QYDGKGVG, which is a product of osteoclastic proteolysis (see Fig. 64.35). It does not recognize a precursor that is not cross-linked, but it does measure both pyridinolines and pyrroles.[456] Because the assay does not measure precursors of cross-links, only degradation of mature collagen is measured, just as with the pyridinolines. Measurement of NTX provides specificity for bone because DPD cross-links primarily involve the α_2(I) chain of collagen. By contrast, α_1(I) predominates in other tissues. Two-thirds of DPD cross-links in bone collagen are at the NTX site, whereas one-third are at the CTX site. On the other hand, about 85% of the pyrroles are located in the N-telopeptide.[457] The lability and reactivity of pyrroles and their potential for oxidation and hydrolytic ring opening explain the difficulties encountered in isolating and characterizing these structures from NTX antigen.[456] When urine is treated with UV light for 3 days, the apparent concentration of urinary NTX unexpectedly increases by approximately 30%, which probably indicates dissolution of aggregated N-telopeptides.[458]

The commercially available urinary NTX ELISA assay measures only nonisomerized α_2(I) N-telopeptide.[437] However, in adult urine, the amount of β-isomerized NTX-peptide is about 10-fold that of nonisomerized forms.

The NTX method has been adapted for the measurement of N-telopeptides in serum.[149] The use of serum eliminates the need to measure urine creatinine to correct for urine concentration and can significantly reduce within-subject day-to-day variation in NTX measurements. Experimental and clinical data have demonstrated this serum assay to provide a useful index of bone resorption.[450]

C-Telopeptide CTX Assay. Sample type is important for CTX assays. EDTA plasma is the preferred sample, although serum can be used if rapidly separated prior to storing frozen at a minimum of −20°C. The first CTX immunoassays were based on a polyclonal antibody produced in rabbits against a synthetic peptide corresponding to residues 15C to 22C (EKAHDGGR) of the α_1(I) chain of type I collagen.[459] This region includes the cross-linking hydroxylysine at residue 16C. Subsequently, several other methods were developed for measuring CTX in urine and serum or plasma. The most widely used methods recognize the β-isomer, formed during aging of bone by transfer of the peptide backbone from the α-carboxyl group of aspartic acid to the β-carboxyl group of the same amino acid. In healthy human bone, approximately 70% to 80% of C-telopeptides have this β-isomerization, but in Paget disease, it accounts for only about 50% to 60%.[460] This fact introduces additional uncertainly in that β-isomerization and racemization may vary between individuals.[77] All CTX methods require the C-terminal amino acid to be a free arginine.

Serum or plasma CTX is measured using two monoclonal antibodies.[461] With two α_1(I) chain telopeptides in each collagen molecule, the use of two antibodies directed against the β-isomer ensures that only the β-forms are measured. A modification of this method is now available on an automated immunoassay analyzer using electrochemiluminescence detection.[462]

C-Telopeptide ICTP Assay. A radioimmunoassay for the C-terminal telopeptide of type I collagen (ICTP) detects collagen degradation fragments in serum.[463] Rabbit antibodies were raised against a cross-linked C-telopeptide of type I collagen produced by collagenase digestion of human bone. The epitope measured is vulnerable to digestion by cathepsin K (see Fig. 64.33); this method is relatively insensitive to changes in bone resorption caused by normal bone turnover.[442] However, the method is suitable for detecting the osteolytic processes taking place in multiple myeloma[464] and metastatic bone disease, as well as the erosion process in rheumatoid arthritis.

Deoxypyridinoline and Pyridinoline. DPD and PYD were originally measured by HPLC. Today, DPD is measured primarily by immunoassay using automated analyzers or manual ELISA. Unlike most HPLC methods, which measure total DPD and total PYD, the immunoassays for DPD or DPD/PYD measure primarily free, but not peptide-bound, forms. In urine, approximately 40% of PYD and DPD fraction is free and 60% is protein bound.

Comparisons of free and total DPD and PYD suggest that the ratio of free to total pyridinolines varies with physiology, pathophysiology, and treatment.[390,453] Total DPD has been reported to be increased more than free DPD in individuals with disorders involving increased bone resorption (eg, postmenopausal women, women with osteoporosis, Paget disease, hyperthyroidism). Furthermore, short-term bisphosphonate treatment of patients with Paget disease or osteoporosis reduces the total but not the free DPD.

One commercially available ELISA measures both PYD and DPD with equimolar cross-reactivity.[465] Of greater interest for monitoring bone resorption is the commercially available ELISA that measures DPD but not PYD.[466] This method, a competitive ELISA, uses a streptavidin-coated microtiter plate and biotinylated deoxypyridinoline as the solid phase. Sample or calibrator and the monoclonal antibody against DPD are added and incubated. After washing, a second antibody, goat antimouse immunoglobulin (Ig)G conjugated to ALP, is added. The formed immunocomplex is measured after addition of *p*-nitrophenyl phosphate.

More recently, automated immunoanalyzer methods for DPD have become commercially available. The most widely used is a solid-phase, competitive EIA with chemiluminescence detection. The solid-phase antibody is incubated with serum or calibrator and ALP conjugated to DPD. After washing, the immunocomplexes are determined after the addition of substrate.

DPD and PYD can also be measured by HPLC with fluorescence detection.[442] Because approximately 60% of the pyridinolines in urine are contained in peptides, most methods use acid hydrolysis to generate free amino acids. The hydrolysate is fractionated by column chromatography before resolution of the pyridinolines by reverse-phase chromatography. Because the pyridinolines are highly polar at acid pH, ion-pairing agents have been used to increase their retention by reverse-phase columns. Although most methods have used gradient elution, simpler isocratic methods have been described.[467] Fluorometric detection is used to quantify these naturally occurring fluorescent pyridinium compounds. Lack of synthetic calibrators, controversy over the molar fluorescence yield of pyridinolines, and variability of acid hydrolysis have been suggested as factors contributing to differences observed between laboratories.[468]

A tandem MS method has been described with increased sensitivity that can measure both DPD and PYD simultaneously with significant improvement in precision and accuracy for the cross-link molecules.

Specimen Requirements. Serum or plasma is best collected after overnight fasting. Although early studies used 24-hour urine samples, timed or early-morning voided urine has also been used. A second morning void, collected by 10.00 hours, is most commonly recommended.[370] For treatment monitoring, the specimens should be collected at the same time as the baseline specimen. Peak urinary excretion of pyridinolines occurs at about 05.00–08.00 hours, reflecting the nocturnal peak in bone turnover. Urinary pyridinolines reach a nadir between 14.00 and 23.00 hours.

Pyridinolines and telopeptides are relatively stable in urine. Exposure to UV light, but not laboratory lighting, decreases DPD and PYD.[458] Free pyridinolines are especially vulnerable to UV lighting. It is recommended that prolonged exposure to light and exposure to direct sunlight should be avoided.

Reference Intervals. Concentrations of collagen cross-links are influenced by age and gender. Reference intervals

TABLE 64.8 Reference Intervals of Type I Collagen Telopeptides and Deoxypyridinoline Cross-Links

Test	Premenopausal Women	Men
N-Telopeptide		
Serum, nmol BCE/L	8.7–19.8	10.7–22.9
Urine, μmol BCE/mol creatinine	10–110	11–103
C-Telopeptide		
Serum,* ng/L	≤573	≤584
Urine, mg/mol creatinine	220 (128)†	249 (128)†
ICTP		
Serum, μg/L	1.5–5	1.5–5.0
Deoxypyridinoline, Pyridinoline		
Urine Free DPD (μmol/mol creatinine)	3.0–7.4	2.3–5.4
Urine Free PYD (umol/mol creatinine)	9.1–21.4	7.2–18.7

*CTX by automated immunoassay with electrochemiluminescence detection.
†Mean (SD).
BCE, Bone collagen equivalent;[452] ICTP, C-telopeptide of type I collagen.

for NTX, CTX, ICTP, DPD, and PYD are listed in Table 64.8. Concentrations are markedly higher in children, with highest concentrations observed during early infancy and adolescence—periods of rapid bone growth. In adults, concentrations of collagen cross-links are relatively constant between 30 and 45 years of age, but they increase significantly after menopause in women. Age-related increases have also been reported in men.

Tartrate-Resistant Acid Phosphatase (TRACP5b)

Osteoclasts produce and secrete a tartrate-resistant acid phosphatase (see Fig. 64.2) during bone resorption (EC 3.1.3.2).[469] In cell culture, its activity is used to detect and enumerate osteoclasts.[447] Osteoclast number can be increased in bone disorders and is decreased by antiresorptive treatment (such as bisphosphonates and selective estrogen receptor modulators).[470] The activity of this acid phosphatase in serum has been measured by a number of methods, but most previous methods failed to distinguish between two isoforms: TRACP5b produced by the osteoclasts, and TRACP5a produced by inflammatory macrophages and dendritic cells. These isoforms differ in their carbohydrate content: 5a contains a sialic acid and mannose, but 5b only mannose. In addition, isoform 5b is a dimer, whereas 5a is a monomer. Only about 10% of TRACP circulates in an enzymatically active form, the remaining 90% being present as inactive fragments.[471]

Several approaches may be used to measure only TRACP5b activity. In a kinetic method, TRACP5b activity is estimated by subtracting tartrate-resistant fluoride-resistant acid phosphatase activity from total activity.[472] Two commercial immunoassays are also available for TRACP5b. In one of them, monoclonal antibody (O1A) binds both isoforms but no inactive fragments; the activity of bound enzymes is then detected with *p*-nitrophenyl phosphate as a substrate at pH 6.1, which is selective for TRACP5b activity.[473,474] In another assay, two monoclonal antibodies are used. One antibody binds the active 5b isoforms of 5b; the other binds inactive fragments, and the activity of bound enzyme is then detected with the TRACP 5b-selective substrate, 2-chloro-4-nitrophenyl phosphate.[475] The two assays have similar TRACP5b specificity and clinical performance in monitoring antiresorptive treatment.[470]

Specimen Requirements. The preferred sample for measuring TRACP5b is serum. Diurnal variation is minor, probably indicating that the half-life of TRACP5b is longer than those of the other markers of bone resorption.[476] TRACP5b may be relatively unstable on storage, although it has been shown that TRACP5b can be stored for up to 8 hours at room temperature and up to 3 days at 4°C. For long-term storage, it is essential that samples be stored at −80°C.[474] Storage at −20°C for 6 months reduces activity by at least 40%.[474]

Clinical Significance. In response to alendronate, TRACP5b decreased by a mean (SE) of 39% (4%), compared with 49% (4%) to 69% (5%) for urinary telopeptides (CTX and NTX), and 75% (8%) for serum/plasma CTX.[476] TRACP5b activity changes in children; boys 13 to 17 years of age have higher concentrations than girls in the same age group.[48]

Reference Interval. An immunoassay for TRACP5b has upper limits of reference intervals of 4.2 U/L for women and 4.8 U/L for men.

Preanalytical and Analytical Variables of Bone Turnover Marker

Controllable sources of preanalytical variability include sampling time, sample preservation procedures, and food intake. Bone marker concentrations in urine and serum vary with the time of day because of the diurnal variation of bone resorption and formation. Because of the nocturnal peak in bone turnover, most bone markers peak in the early morning hours (04.00–08.00 hours) and reach their nadir in the afternoon (13.00–23.00 hours). The amplitude of this variation is greatest for resorption markers, with nadir values averaging 70% of peak values. Consequently, specimens should be collected at a standardized time of day to minimize the impact of diurnal variability. For urinary markers, collection of the second morning void is often recommended.

Concentrations of urinary resorption markers are usually normalized by dividing by the urinary creatinine concentration. Variability (within- and between-method) in creatinine measurements, within-subject variability in urinary creatinine, and its dependence on muscle mass contribute to the overall variability of urinary resorption markers.

Long-term, within-individual variability of urine markers is generally higher (15% to 60%) than that of plasma markers (5% to 10%). Compared with other bone markers, bone ALP and TRACP5b do not demonstrate much diurnal variation because of their long plasma half-lives.

Food intake has an effect on plasma CTX concentration.[477] The diurnal variation of plasma CTX has a magnitude of about ±40% around the 24-hour mean; fasting reduces circadian variation to about one-fourth.[478] Exercise can also acutely increase the circulating concentrations of plasma CTX. With other bone markers, the clinical impact of feeding versus fasting is small. However, in clinical practice, collection of samples in the fasting and resting state is standard practice.

METABOLIC BONE DISEASES

Metabolic bone disease results from a partial uncoupling or imbalance between bone resorption and formation. Decreased bone mass, or *osteopenia*, is more common than abnormal increases in bone mass. The most prevalent metabolic bone diseases are osteoporosis, osteomalacia and rickets, and renal osteodystrophy. Osteoporosis, the most prevalent metabolic bone disease in developed countries, is characterized by loss of bone mass, microarchitectural deterioration of bone tissue, and increased risk for fracture. Rickets and osteomalacia, which are more common in developing countries, are characterized by defective mineralization of bone matrix. Renal osteodystrophy is a complex condition that develops in response to abnormalities of the endocrine and excretory functions of the kidneys. In addition to these three diseases that affect the skeleton in general, two diseases characterized by localized bone involvement are discussed here: Paget disease of bone and bone metastases as well as one disease with a major genetic component, osteogenesis imperfecta.

Osteoporosis

Osteoporosis, the most prevalent metabolic bone disease in the United States, results in 1.5 million fractures each year.[479] Osteoporosis is associated with increased risk for vertebral, hip, and distal forearm fractures. At 50 years of age, women have a lifetime fracture risk (at any of these three sites) of about 40%. Men have a lifetime fracture risk of approximately one-third that of women. Because trabecular bone turns over at five to seven times the rate of cortical bone, fractures of bones that are predominantly trabecular (vertebrae and distal forearm) occur earlier in life. One-third of women who are older than 65 years of age suffer vertebral crush fractures. Vertebral crush fractures can occur acutely and result in disabling pain and discomfort. Long-term complications include immobility and loss of height. Secondary problems include protuberant abdomen, hiatus hernia, chronic constipation, urinary incontinence, and loss of self-esteem. Many mild vertebral fractures (up to 50%) may be clinically silent when they occur, only to manifest much later as an incidental finding on radiograph.

Fractures of bone with more cortical bone (proximal femur or hip) occur later in life. For women, the lifetime risk for hip fracture is 15%, and for men it is 3%. The mortality rate accompanying hip fracture may be as high as 20% in the 6 months following fracture. Hip fracture mortality is higher in men than in women, increases with age, and is higher for those with coexisting illness and poor prefracture functional status.[479] Twenty-five percent of survivors are confined to long-term care in nursing homes. The annual cost of medical care for osteoporosis in the United States is estimated to be close to $20 billion.

Peak bone mass normally is attained by 30 years of age and begins to decrease slowly after 40 years of age in both men and women. The amount of bone attained during growth is an important determinant of whether clinical osteoporosis develops later in life. Exercise and adequate nutrition play important roles in attaining and maintaining skeletal mass. During early adult life, bone formation is coupled with bone resorption so that bone mass remains stable. Aging is a major risk factor for bone loss because after 40 years of age, bone resorption slightly exceeds bone formation, so that approximately 0.5% of the skeletal mass is lost per year. In women, the decrease in sex steroids at menopause accelerates bone loss (postmenopausal osteoporosis) to about 2% to 3% per year. Osteoporosis is usually due to inadequate bone formation during growth or a pathophysiologic process that impairs osteoblastic bone formation or increases bone resorption. Clinically, osteoporosis is most commonly encountered in postmenopausal women. Advanced age, female gender, and sex steroid deficiency are prominent risk factors. Other risk factors include a family history of osteoporosis, alcohol abuse, smoking, and chronic disease.[480]

After decreased bone mass is documented by bone mass measurements, the diagnostic workup is directed at determining the cause (Box 64.18). Most often, the cause is attributed to age ("senile" osteoporosis), postmenopausal osteoporosis, or both, but it may be secondary to chronic disease, drug therapy, or other causes. If osteoporosis is inconsistent with age or gender (such as in a middle-aged man or a premenopausal woman), laboratory testing should be performed to exclude other secondary causes of osteoporosis, including hyperthyroidism, Cushing syndrome, hypogonadism, PHPT, systemic mastocytosis, and multiple myeloma. Chronic excess of thyroid hormone, cortisol, or PTH may cause osteoporosis. Long-standing hyperthyroidism or excessive thyroid hormone replacement increases bone resorption to a greater extent than formation, leading to osteoporosis. Cortisol markedly decreases bone formation and causes an increase in bone resorption. Patients with Cushing syndrome may have severe osteoporosis. More commonly, patients receiving glucocorticoid therapy for diseases like asthma and rheumatoid arthritis may develop disabling osteoporosis. Hyperparathyroidism occurs most commonly in postmenopausal women and may lead to osteoporosis. Multiple myeloma commonly presents with vertebral crush fracture, and osteoporosis must be considered in these patients.

Bone markers can be used to assess bone turnover in patients with osteoporosis, because the rate of bone turnover (spontaneous or modified by the therapy) is considered an important determinant of bone fragility in postmenopausal and older women.[481] Increased markers of bone turnover indicate increased bone turnover but are not diagnostic for osteoporosis. Markers for both bone resorption and bone formation can, because of coupling of bone formation and resorption, be useful in monitoring the effects of antiresorptive therapy.[481,482] Teriparatide treatment is best monitored by PINP or osteocalcin, but resorption markers may change later during therapy (see Fig. 64.28). The International Osteoporosis Foundation and IFCC recommend one bone formation marker (serum PINP) and one bone resorption marker (plasma CTX) to be used as reference markers.[483]

Prevention of osteoporosis is an important goal. Adequate nutrition and exercise during growth allow achievement of optimal bone mass. High calcium intake (1000–1500 mg/day), adequate vitamin D (at least 400–800 IU/day), sufficient protein intake, and a regular exercise program are helpful in maintaining bone mass and preventing osteoporosis.

The treatment of osteoporosis depends on the cause. In secondary osteoporosis, treatment is directed at the underlying

BOX 64.18 Causes of Osteoporosis

Failure to develop normal skeletal mass during growth and development because of poor nutrition or inadequate exercise

Endocrine deficiency or excess
- Estrogen or testosterone deficiency
- Cushing syndrome
- Hyperthyroidism
- Hyperparathyroidism
- Diabetes

Immobilization or weightlessness/decreased weight bearing
- Long-term bed stay/hospitalization (especially intensive care treatment)
- Poliomyelitis
- Cerebral palsy
- Paraplegia

Bone marrow disorders
- Multiple myeloma
- Leukemia
- Mastocytosis

Defects of collagen synthesis
- Osteogenesis imperfecta
- Marfan syndrome
- Homocystinuria

Inflammatory disorders
- Rheumatoid arthritis
- Inflammatory bowel disease

Malabsorption
- Celiac disease
- Postgastrectomy
- Post–gastric bypass
- Long-term parenteral feeding
- Chronic liver disease

Combination of pathology
- Cystic fibrosis

Drugs
- Alcohol
- Aromatase inhibitors
- Androgen deprivation treatment
- Anticonvulsants
- Caffeine
- Cannabis
- Cyclosporin
- Depot progesterone
- Glucocorticoids
- Heparin
- Methotrexate
- Proton pump inhibitors
- Selective serotonin reuptake inhibitors
- Thiazoladinediones

Idiopathic juvenile osteoporosis

Anorexia nervosa

HIV infection

Autoimmune (anti-osteoprotegerin antibodies)

condition. Most therapies for the treatment of postmenopausal osteoporosis are directed at decreasing osteoclastic bone resorption. Antiresorptive therapies approved by the US FDA include bisphosphonates (alendronate, risedronate, ibandronate, and zoledronate), denosumab (humanized antibody to RANKL), and selective estrogen receptor modulators (raloxifene). Estrogen is approved for management of menopausal symptoms and has an effect on slowing down early postmenopausal bone loss that appears as robust as that of the bisphosphonates. Recombinant hPTH(1–34), also known as *teriparatide,* is the only FDA-approved therapy for stimulating bone formation, but recombinant hPTH(1–84) and strontium ranelate have been approved for this purpose in Europe and in several other countries.

A number of therapies are in phase III studies and are showing promise as future treatments for osteoporosis. Humanized sclerostin antibodies romosozumab and blosozumab have significantly increased bone formation markers (P1NP and ALP) while decreasing the bone resorption marker CTX, and this translated into a significantly increased BMD at all sites measured. Cathepsin K inhibition has been explored as a possible treatment for osteoporosis,[484] and one therapy, Odanacatib, has shown excellent clinical effectiveness resulting in a significant decrease in bone resorption (CTX, NTX, DPD) and a transient decrease in bone formation (Bone ALP, P1NP).

Osteomalacia and Rickets

Osteomalacia and rickets are caused by a mineralization defect that occurs during bone formation, resulting in an increase in osteoid, the unmineralized organic matrix of bone.[231] Defective mineralization produces rickets in children and osteomalacia in adults. Osteomalacia or rickets is usually due to either vitamin D deficiency or phosphate depletion.

The causes of decreased 25(OH)D and $1,25(OH)_2D$ are listed in Boxes 64.12 and 64.13, respectively. Vitamin D deficiency may be secondary to dietary deprivation and/or inadequate exposure to sunlight, vitamin D malabsorption, disorders of vitamin D metabolism, or end-organ resistance to the action of vitamin D. In spite of supplementation in some countries of milk, bread, and some cereals with vitamin D, vitamin D insufficiency may be more common than was previously thought, in both North America and Europe.[233,234] Breast-fed infants, the elderly, strict vegetarians, and individuals with darker skin pigmentation are at increased risk. Although clinical osteomalacia caused by vitamin D deficiency appears to be uncommon, the prevalence of subclinical or mild osteomalacia in the overall population is unknown. Subclinical osteomalacia may coexist with osteoporosis in elderly patients with poor diets and little exposure to sunlight. It has also been shown that mild to moderate vitamin D deficiency may be associated with reduced muscle strength, impaired physical performance, and falls—all factors contributing to osteoporotic fracture.[231] Vitamin D deficiency may develop in patients with malabsorption caused by postgastrectomy syndrome, small bowel disease (eg, celiac disease, tropical sprue), hepatobiliary disease, or pancreatic insufficiency.

Vitamin D resistance is rare. Vitamin D–dependent rickets type 1 is an inherited defect in 25(OH)D-1α-hydroxylase that causes impaired formation of $1,25(OH)_2D$.[231] The disease is manifested in infancy and can be treated with physiologic doses of $1,25(OH)_2D$. Vitamin D–dependent rickets type 2 is an inherited disorder that is characterized by very high plasma concentrations of $1,25(OH)_2D$.[231] This syndrome is caused by resistance to $1,25(OH)_2D$, secondary to defects in the $1,25(OH)_2D$ receptor.

Osteomalacia and rickets may also occur as the result of phosphate depletion. The most common cause of rickets in the United States is hypophosphatemic osteomalacia (also known as *hypophosphatemic vitamin D–resistant rickets* and *vitamin D–resistant rickets*).[97] This disorder is an X-linked dominant inherited trait characterized by renal phosphate wasting. Tubular phosphate wasting can also occur sporadically in adults and as part of Fanconi syndrome. Certain rare mesenchymal tumors may produce a phosphaturic factor (phosphatonin or FGF23, discussed earlier in this chapter), resulting in renal phosphate wasting and osteomalacia.

In developing countries, dietary calcium deprivation may lead to the clinical picture of rickets, without clear vitamin D or phosphate deficiency.[485]

Drugs have also been associated with osteomalacia. Anticonvulsants increase the hepatic catabolism of vitamin D metabolites and also produce end-organ resistance. Phosphate-binding antacids used for treatment of peptic ulcer disease cause osteomalacia by preventing the intestinal absorption of phosphate. Etidronate treatment (eg, of Paget disease, osteoporosis, HCM) can cause a mineralization defect, resulting in osteomalacia.

Clinical manifestations of rickets and osteomalacia are a consequence of the defect in mineralization. Rachitic manifestations include bowing of the extremities, short stature, costochondral junction swelling, indentation of the lower ribs, and flattening of the skull. In adults, bone pain is the most common symptom, and stress fractures and frank skeletal fractures may occur. Radiographs show classic findings in rickets, such as cupping and fraying of the epiphyseal and diaphyseal ends of the long bone. Pseudofractures ("looser zones") are common in adults.

Vitamin D deficiency is diagnosed by measuring serum 25(OH)D (see Table 64.5). Other laboratory findings in rickets and osteomalacia include increased plasma ALP activity, with other alterations in bone and mineral metabolism dependent on the cause and severity of the disorder. ALP is usually increased because of increased osteoblastic activity associated with producing unmineralized osteoid. Plasma calcium may be low-normal or low in vitamin D deficiency, depending on the severity of the disease. Phosphate may be normal or low but falls with the development of secondary hyperparathyroidism. Plasma calcium and PTH concentrations are usually normal in renal tubular defects of phosphate transport. Renal phosphate defects can be best assessed through determination of the renal phosphate threshold.

Treatment of rickets and osteomalacia is dictated by the cause of the disorder. Nutritional rickets and osteomalacia are healed by treatment with physiologic doses of vitamin D, whereas higher doses may be required in malabsorption. Adequate dietary intakes of calcium and phosphorus are critical during therapy. Renal phosphate-wasting syndromes require frequent pharmacologic administration of oral phosphate.

Disorders of Bone and Mineral in Chronic Kidney Disease (Renal Osteodystrophy)

Chronic kidney disease (CKD) is associated with a multitude of disorders of bone and mineral metabolism.[486,487] Renal bone diseases include both high-turnover bone disease (osteitis fibrosa or secondary hyperparathyroidism) and low-turnover bone disease (osteomalacia and adynamic bone disease). Quantitative histomorphometric analysis of bone biopsies, measurement of bone formation by double tetracycline labeling, and special stains are often necessary for correct diagnosis of patients with osteitis fibrosa, osteomalacia, adynamic bone disease, and mixed bone disease of renal osteodystrophy.

Osteitis fibrosa (hyperparathyroid bone disease) is the most common high-turnover bone disease. This disorder is caused by high concentrations of serum PTH in secondary hyperparathyroidism. Secondary hyperparathyroidism is a consequence of the hypocalcemia associated with hyperphosphatemia and $1,25(OH)_2D$ deficiency. Hyperphosphatemia is a result of the inability of the kidneys to excrete phosphate. $1,25(OH)_2D$ deficiency results from the inability of the kidneys to synthesize $1,25(OH)_2D$ because of decreased renal mass and suppression of 25(OH)D-1α-hydroxylase activity by high concentrations of phosphate. Deficiency of $1,25(OH)_2D$ leads to reduced intestinal absorption of calcium, and the inhibition of PTH secretion by $1,25(OH)_2D$ is reduced. Skeletal resistance to PTH also contributes to hypocalcemia and secondary hyperparathyroidism.

Low-turnover bone diseases include osteomalacia and adynamic (also known as *aplastic*) bone disease. Osteomalacia and adynamic bone disease are distinguished by the extent of unmineralized bone matrix or osteoid: osteoid is increased in osteomalacia and normal or low in adynamic bone disease. Osteomalacia in chronic renal failure may reflect vitamin D deficiency caused by decreased renal synthesis of $1,25(OH)_2D$ (see the "Osteomalacia and Rickets" section earlier in this chapter) or aluminum-related disease. In the 1970s and 1980s, aluminum intoxication (commonly caused by aluminum contamination of dialysis water and by therapeutic use of oral aluminum-containing antacids to reduce plasma phosphate by binding phosphate and preventing its intestinal absorption) was a significant contributing factor to the development of osteomalacia and adynamic bone disease. The inability of patients with renal failure to excrete aluminum leads to high concentrations in plasma (see section on aluminum toxicity in Chapter 42) and deposition in bone, inhibiting bone cell function and bone mineralization. Aluminum-related disease is less common today because of reduced use of aluminum-containing antacids and the use of effective means to decrease the concentrations of aluminum in dialysis water. Other causes of adynamic renal bone disease include calcium supplementation, excessive vitamin D administration, treatment of hyperparathyroidism, advanced age and osteoporosis, diabetes, corticosteroid therapy, and immobilization. Today, oversuppression of parathyroid function (brought about by the use of oral calcium carbonate to control hyperphosphatemia and treatment with vitamin D and dialysate solutions containing high calcium to control hyperparathyroidism) is believed to be the main cause of adynamic renal bone disease.

Amyloid deposition may be noted in bone and in other tissues. It is thought to result from reduced degradation of α_2-microglobulin by the kidneys. The amyloid in renal failure is primarily composed of α_2-microglobulin. The fraction of patients with amyloidosis increases with the duration of dialysis therapy; 70% to 80% of patients have clinical features of amyloidosis after 10 or more years of hemodialysis.

Amyloidosis may coexist with high-turnover or low-turnover bone disease.

Bone pain is the most common complaint of patients with renal osteodystrophy. The weight-bearing bones are the site of greatest discomfort, with leg and hip pain and back pain being common. If the patient is a growing child, skeletal deformities may result, with bowing of the extremities, kyphoscoliosis, and slipped femoral epiphyses. Extracellular calcification is also commonly found in periarticular areas, in the medial layer of arteries, and in internal organs (lungs, heart muscle, and other tissue).

The central role of plasma PTH in guiding therapy requires that the PTH assay used can be relied on to measure only the active hormone. This is not true for any of the assay generations (see *Parathyroid Hormone*, subsection *Measurement of Parathyroid Hormone* earlier in this chapter), and kidney disease leads to accumulation of inactive PTH fragments well above the concentrations seen in healthy individuals. Treatment guidelines take this problem into account, but inconsistencies among assays can still lead to situations in which opposite therapeutic decisions could be made for a single patient, depending on the assay used.[157] Studies are clearly needed to test whether modern biomarkers of bone turnover, when used with measurements of circulating PTH concentrations, could more adequately define the type of osteodystrophy.[487]

Biochemical findings in CKD include hyperphosphatemia and hypocalcemia (see Chapter 59). The measured concentration of immunoreactive PTH is generally increased, often dramatically, and $1,25(OH)_2D$ is decreased. Plasma ALP is increased in patients with hyperparathyroidism or osteomalacia. Because magnesium is cleared by the kidney, modest increases in plasma concentration (2–4 mg/dL [0.08–0.16 mmol/L]) are common, especially in those taking magnesium-containing antacids.

Early management of CKD calls for dietary restriction of phosphate and administration of phosphate-binding agents. Calcium supplements added to the diet to prevent secondary hyperparathyroidism may also serve as phosphate binders. Administration of $1,25(OH)_2D$ or other active forms of vitamin D enhances intestinal calcium absorption and may act directly on the parathyroid glands to reduce PTH secretion. Ultimately, dialysis or renal transplantation may be necessary.

Paget Disease of Bone

Paget disease is a localized disease of bone characterized by osteoclastic bone resorption, followed by replacement of bone in a chaotic fashion.[488,489] This disease has a restricted geographic distribution. It is most common in Northern Europe, North America, Australia, and New Zealand in individuals of Anglo-Saxon descent (the prevalence may be up to 5% among people older than 40 years of age), whereas it is extremely uncommon in Asia, Africa, and Scandinavia. Its origin has been linked to genetics, as a family history of Paget disease is reported by 20% to 50% of patients, but also to environmental factors, in particular to a possible paramyxovirus infection (measles, canine distemper, respiratory syncytial). The most important genetic factor identified is a loss-of-function mutation affecting the ubiquitin-binding domain of the sequestosome gene *(SQSTM1)*. Penetrance is high (95% 60 years of age) for *SQSTM1* mutation, and the severity of Paget disease is greatest in patients with *SQSTM1* mutation. The disease typically has late onset, patchy bone involvement, and inclusions that originally were reported to resemble viral nucleocapsids but have been shown to be abnormal protein molecules in the nuclei of osteoclasts. An apparent decline in the frequency and severity of the disease has been reported; this change is believed to be too rapid to be explained by genetics alone.[489,490]

Paget disease may affect one bone (monostotic) or several bones (polyostotic). Signs and symptoms depend on which skeletal site is affected; the skull, femur, pelvis, and vertebrae are most commonly affected. In most affected individuals, the disease is diagnosed from radiographs or laboratory tests (total ALP) performed for another reason. With more extensive disease, localized bone pain and increased warmth may be noted in or over the affected bone. Advanced disease can produce deformities such as skull enlargement and anterior bowing of the weight-bearing bones (femur and tibia). Complications of deformed bone include arthritic symptoms, nerve compression, deafness, spinal nerve compression, and, in rare cases, osteogenic sarcoma.

Laboratory and other findings include increased markers of bone turnover[491] and abnormal radiographs and Technetium bone scans. Radiologic examination demonstrates the characteristic findings of Paget disease: lytic areas in sites of active osteoclastic bone resorption and thickened, expanded, and sclerotic areas in sites where osteoblasts have formed woven bone. The radioisotopic bone scan is the most sensitive test for detecting small, early lesions. The most common finding leading to the diagnosis of Paget disease is increased serum total ALP.

Other biochemical markers of bone formation and degradation give information about the pathologic process taking place. Discrepancies have been noted between the formation markers that reflect different phases of the normal osteoblast phenotype: PINP and total and bone ALP all perform similarly,[491] whereas osteocalcin is less consistently increased. Paget disease leads to a disproportionate increase in serum PINP compared with that of PICP.[388]

Increases in biochemical markers of bone resorption reflect the osteoclastic nature of the disease. In untreated Paget disease, the αCTX derived from relatively newly formed collagen, is raised more (16-fold) than the βCTX (3-fold), which dominates in diseases with generally increased resorption of normal bone such as hyperparathyroidism or hyperthyroidism.[491]

Bone markers are used in diagnosis and therapeutic monitoring. Total ALP (TALP) is usually sufficient, but in patients with hepatocellular injury, a measurement of bone ALP (BALP) or PINP may be helpful.[489]

Therapy is directed at decreasing osteoclastic bone resorption. Intravenous zoledronate is the treatment of choice, resulting in sustained biochemical and clinical response. Other bisphosphonates, such as oral risedronate, are also effective in decreasing bone pain, serum ALP, and other biochemical markers of bone turnover. Calcitonin is now rarely used owing to the transient nature of its therapeutic effect; there are a number of reports of the effectiveness of denosumab, a nonapproved therapy, in Paget disease. Patients occasionally may require surgery for skeletal deformity that limits mobility or for arthritic changes, fractures, or nerve compression.

Osteogenesis Imperfecta

Osteogenesis imperfecta (OI), often termed *brittle bone disease,* is a heterogeneous group of inherited connective tissue disorders that share similar skeletal abnormalities resulting in low bone mass, minimal trauma fractures, and subsequent bone deformity. In its most severe form, it can be lethal in fetal life and in neonates. Several protein defects have been identified, but there is mainly a defect in collagen that predominates resulting in the pathophysiology. There is abnormal production, posttranslational modification, and metabolism of collagen, particularly type I collagen. OI was originally thought to be an autosomal dominant bone dysplasia caused by defects in type I collagen, but discoveries of novel (mainly recessive) genes have demonstrated defects in proteins with very different functions, ranging from structural to enzymatic and from intracellular transport to chaperones. These genes, and corresponding products, include cartilage-associated protein *(CRTAP),* cyclophilin B *(PPIB),* heat shock protein 47 *(SERPINH1),* pigment epithelial-derived factor *(SERPINF1),* FK506-binding protein *(FKBP10),* prolyl 3 hydroxylase *(LEPRE1),* and the transmembrane protein Bril *(IFITM5).*[193,492-497]

Biochemical and molecular studies have identified that milder forms of OI are caused by quantitative defects in type I collagen and that more severe types are caused by structural defects in either of the two chains that form the heterotrimer. When OI is suspected clinically, there is usually a spectrum of signs and symptoms including frontal bossing of the skull, bluish sclera, yellowish teeth, barrel chest/pectus excavatum, joint laxity, vertebral compression, and growth retardation. Recurrent fractures with minimal trauma may lead to suspicion of child abuse. When a diagnosis is in doubt, biochemical studies of collagen expressed by cultured cells, DNA sequencing of type I collagen, and genetic expression plus gene sequencing studies may be of value in confirming the diagnosis.

Most bone biochemistry is within normal limits. Acid phosphatase is increased in type VIII, ALP can be increased postfracture, and there are some reports of increased CTX and PINP in some types of OI (Type III) and in some patients with lower BMD and increased risk for fracture.[498] The profile of urine pyridinoline cross-links and their ratios is reported to be abnormal in different types of OI, and this may help point the way toward a specific diagnosis.[499]

Bisphosphonate therapy is often prescribed in patients with a high risk for fractures, and risedronate has been shown to increase BMD and significantly reduce fracture incidence.[500] Measurement of markers of bone formation and resorption can provide evidence of the therapeutic effect of bisphosphonate treatment.

Involvement of Bone in Malignancy

Bone metastases are the most common skeletal complication of malignancy, occurring in up 70% of patients with advanced breast or prostate cancer, and in 15% to 30% of patients with carcinoma of the lung, colon, stomach, bladder, uterus, rectum, thyroid gland, or kidney.[501] Metastases can have a markedly osteolytic or osteoblastic character, but often they are mixed.[502] Most patients with breast cancer have predominantly osteolytic lesions,[503] but about 15% to 20% of metastases have a predominantly osteoblastic nature. Metastases of prostate cancer are generally regarded as osteoblastic.[502] In most carcinoma metastases, however, both bone degradation and formation take place to some extent, and so both biochemical markers of bone formation and resorption can be of value in assessing the presence of bone metastasis.[504] The lesions of multiple myeloma are purely osteolytic; the tumor cells secrete factors that suppress bone formation; generalized osteoporosis is also a feature of the disease (see Box 64.14).[505,506]

Many biochemical bone markers, reflecting bone formation or bone resorption, have been investigated for their potential for early detection or treatment monitoring of both bone metastases and myeloma.[374] In addition to localized malignant lesions, generalized osteoporosis can complicate the interpretation of most resorption markers, with the possible exception of ICTP. In multiple myeloma, serum ICTP and urinary NTX are the most sensitive tools for estimating increased bone breakdown and may be clinically useful for identifying patients with increased risk for progression of bone disease.[464,507] Resorption markers (eg, deoxypyridinoline [DPD]) respond promptly to antiresorptive therapy (eg, with bisphosphonates) for multiple myeloma,[374] whereas serum ICTP has been reported to predict the overall clinical outcome.[464] TRACP5b activity is increased in various carcinomas with bone involvement,[473,508] but evidence for its clinical value is still quite limited.

In carcinomas with predominantly or partially osteoblastic metastases, bone formation markers such as PINP can help in early detection of skeletal involvement.[4,509]

SELECTED REFERENCES

For a full list of references for this chapter, please refer to www.expertconsult.com.

2. Kearns AE, Khosla S, Kostenuik PJ. Receptor activator of nuclear factor kappaB ligand and osteoprotegerin regulation of bone remodeling in health and disease. *Endocr Rev* 2008;**29**:155–92.
21. Fritchie K, Zedek D, Grenache DG. The clinical utility of parathyroid hormone-related peptide in the assessment of hypercalcemia. *Clin Chim Acta* 2009;**402**:146–9.
23. Schlingmann KP, Kaufmann M, Weber S, et al. Mutations in *CYP24A1* and idiopathic infantile hypercalcemia. *N Engl J Med* 2011;**365**:410–21.
85. Thode J, Juul-Jorgensen B, Bhatia HM, et al. Comparison of serum total calcium, albumin-corrected total calcium, and ionized calcium in 1213 patients with suspected calcium disorders. *Scand J Clin Lab Invest* 1989;**49**:217–23.
139. Brown EM. Calcium receptor and regulation of parathyroid hormone secretion. *Rev Endocr Metab Disord* 2000;**1**: 307–15.
144. Fraser WD, Logue FC, Christie JP, et al. Alteration of the circadian rhythm of intact parathyroid hormone and serum phosphate in women with established postmenopausal osteoporosis. *Osteoporos Int* 1998;**8**:121–6.
163. Lepage R, Roy L, Brossard JH, et al. A non-(1-84) circulating parathyroid hormone (PTH) fragment interferes significantly with intact PTH commercial assay measurements in uremic samples. *Clin Chem* 1998;**44**:805–9.

165. Gao P, Scheibel S, D'Amour P, et al. Development of a novel immunoradiometric assay exclusively for biologically active whole parathyroid hormone 1-84: implications for improvement of accurate assessment of parathyroid function. *J Bone Miner Res* 2001;**16**:605–14.
175. Silverberg SJ, Gao P, Brown I, et al. Clinical utility of an immunoradiometric assay for parathyroid hormone (1-84) in primary hyperparathyroidism. *J Clin Endocrinol Metab* 2003;**88**:4725–30.
179. Kidney Disease: Improving Global Outcomes (KDIGO) CKD-MBD Work Group. KDIGO clinical practice guideline for the diagnosis, evaluation, prevention, and treatment of Chronic Kidney Disease-Mineral and Bone Disorder (CKD-MBD). *Kidney Int Suppl* 2009 Aug;**113**:S1–130.
207. Carter GD, Carter CR, Gunter E, et al. Measurement of vitamin D metabolites: an international perspective on methodology and clinical interpretation. *J Steroid Biochem Mol Biol* 2004;**89-90**:467–71.
236. Quarles LD. FGF23, PHEX, and MEPE regulation of phosphate homeostasis and skeletal mineralization. *Am J Physiol Endocrinol Metab* 2003;**285**:E1–9.
239. Shimada T, Mizutani S, Muto T, et al. Cloning and characterization of FGF23 as a causative factor of tumor-induced osteomalacia. *Proc Natl Acad Sci USA* 2001;**98**:6500–5.
264. Saito H, Kusano K, Kinosaki M, et al. Human fibroblast growth factor-23 mutants suppress Na+-dependent phosphate co-transport activity and 1alpha,25-dihydroxyvitamin D3 production. *J Biol Chem* 2003;**278**:2206–11.
335. Pandian MR, Morgan CH, Carlton E, et al. Modified immunoradiometric assay of parathyroid hormone-related protein: clinical application in the differential diagnosis of hypercalcemia. *Clin Chem* 1992;**38**:282–8.
346. Baron R, Rawadi G. Minireview: Targeting the Wnt/β-catenin pathway to regulate bone formation in the adult skeleton. *Endocrinology* 2007;**48**:2635–43.
350. Compton JT, Lee FY. A review of osteocyte function and the emerging importance of sclerostin. *J Bone Joint Surg Am* 2014;**96**:1659–68.
369. Neer RM, Arnaud CD, Zanchetta JR, et al. Effect of parathyroid hormone (1-34) on fractures and bone mineral density in postmenopausal women with osteoporosis. *N Engl J Med* 2001;**344**:1434–41.
463. Risteli J, Elomaa I, Niemi S, et al. Radioimmunoassay for the pyridinoline cross-linked carboxy-terminal telopeptide of type I collagen: a new serum marker of bone collagen degradation. *Clin Chem* 1993;**39**:635–40.
477. Clowes JA, Hannon RA, Yap TS, et al. Effect of feeding on bone turnover markers and its impact on biological variability of measurements. *Bone* 2002;**30**:886–90.

ADDITIONAL READING

Bilezikian JP, Marcus R, Levine MA. *The parathyroids: basic and clinical concepts*. 2nd ed. San Diego: Academic Press; 2001.

Rosen C, Bouillon R, Compston J, et al., editors. *Primer on the metabolic bone diseases and disorders of mineral metabolism*. 8th ed. Washington, DC: American Society for Bone and Mineral Research; 2013.

Seibel MJ, Robins SP, Bilezikian JP, editors. *Dynamics of bone and cartilage metabolism: principles and clinical applications*. 2nd ed. San Diego: Academic Press; 2006.

65

Pituitary Function and Pathophysiology

*William E. Winter, Ann McCormack, and Roger L. Bertholf**

ABSTRACT

Background

The anterior and posterior lobes of the pituitary gland control processes vital for survival of the individual and survival of the species. Although growth in infancy and childhood depend on nutrition, genetics, and environment, thyroid hormone and growth hormone (GH) are essential contributors to growth. Thyroid hormone is a master regulator of the metabolic rate and neurologic development in utero, in infancy, and in childhood. The stress response requires the participation of cortisol. Together, cortisol and GH help maintain normal plasma glucose levels. Although prolactin is also a stress hormone, its role in lactation is evolutionarily required for the nutrition, hydration, and survival of the newborn and infant. The survival of the species is dependent upon reproduction and the gonadotropins, which regulate spermatogenesis and ovulation beginning during puberty. The posterior pituitary is no less important than the anterior pituitary. Antidiuretic hormone (ADH) is a key regulator of water balance. Because humans are 60% water (and infants and children have proportionately more total body water than adults), maintenance of intracellular and extracellular volumes is necessary for health and survival. Lastly, oxytocin is involved in breast feeding and parturition. Collectively, the most complex endocrine systems involve the cerebral cortex, hypothalamus, anterior and posterior lobes of the pituitary, pituitary hormones, and target organs and tissues.

Content

This chapter focuses on disorders of the anterior and posterior pituitary that produce deficient or excess hormone activity. In some instances, more specific details are provided in other chapters that concern specific hormone systems.

The pituitary gland (also called the hypophysis) regulates the endocrine system by integrating chemical signals from the brain with feedback from the concentration of circulating hormones to stimulate intermittent hormone release from target endocrine glands.[1,2] The pituitary serves as the master gland in maintaining homeostasis by orchestrating the many processes necessary for survival of the individual and the species. There are also many important endocrine systems that operate independently of the pituitary gland, such as the renin-angiotensin-aldosterone system (RAAS),[3] the calcium-parathyroid axis,[4] and the glucose-insulin axis.[5] Each of these systems and/or axes is far more complex than their simple names. For example, maintenance of normal plasma glucose concentrations involves multiple cells, tissues and organs (eg, the islets of Langerhans [β, α, and δ cells], liver, adipose tissue, muscle, and intestine), hormones (eg, insulin, glucagon, GH, cortisol, somatostatin, and the incretins), and various physiological and biochemical events (eg, nutrient absorption, glycolysis, glycogen synthesis, gluconeogenesis, glycogenolysis, lipid, and protein metabolism).

The hypophysis is composed of the adenohypophysis (the anterior lobe of the pituitary; ≈75% of the mass of the pituitary) and the neurohypophysis (the posterior lobe of the pituitary, ≈25% of the mass of the pituitary; also called the pars nervosa) (Fig. 65.1).[6] In turn, the adenohypophysis has three parts: (1) the pars distalis, where most hormone-producing cells are located; (2) the pars tuberalis, which is part of the hypophyseal stalk; and (3) the pars intermedia. The pars intermedia may be referred to as the intermediate lobe of the pituitary, although it is actually part of the adenohypophysis.

The biology of the adenohypophysis is distinctly different from that of the neurohypophysis; the adenohypophysis is controlled by the hypothalamus via releasing or inhibiting hormones, whereas the cell bodies of the neurohypophysis are anatomically located in hypothalamic nuclei, with oxytocin or ADH reaching the neurohypophysis through neurohypophyseal nerve axons.[7] Thus, the neurohypophysis is not a discrete endocrine organ, but rather functions as a reservoir for these two hormones.

The roles of the various hormones secreted by the pituitary are exceedingly diverse and include regulation of (1) the body's response to stress (adrenocorticotropic hormone [ACTH, or corticotropin] and GH), (2) the metabolic rate (thyroid-stimulating hormone [TSH, or thyrotropin]), (3) growth (TSH and GH), (4) reproduction (luteinizing hormone [LH] and follicle-stimulating hormone [FSH]), (5) nourishment for the newborn and infant (prolactin), (6) parturition and milk letdown during breast feeding (oxytocin), and (7) fluid balance and blood pressure regulation in states of stress (ADH, or vasopressin, and cortisol).[8] Some of

*The authors gratefully acknowledge the contributions of Ishwarlal Jialal, Mary Lee Vance, Ronald J. Whitley, A. Wayne Meikle, Nelson B. Watts, and Laurence M. Demers, on which portions of this chapter are based.

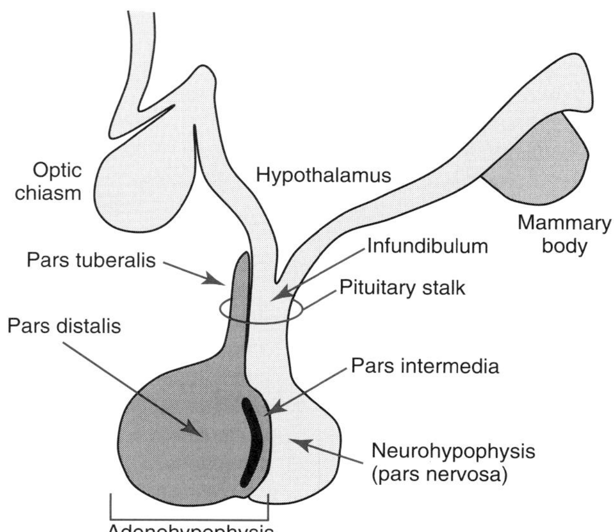

FIGURE 65.1 The Hypophysis (Pituitary Gland) Is Composed of the Adenohypophysis (the Anterior Lobe of the Pituitary) and the Neurohypophysis (the Posterior Lobe of the Pituitary; Pars Nervosa). The adenohypophysis has three parts: the pars distalis, where most of the hormone-producing cells are located; the pars tuberalis, which is part of the pituitary stalk; and the pars intermedia.

the pituitary hormones have specific targets (eg, ACTH, TSH, LH, or FSH), whereas other hormones have multiple targets (eg, GH, prolactin, oxytocin, and ADH). The action of the various hormones is dependent upon the expression of the pertinent receptor in the target cell and associated second messenger systems.

A newly recognized product of the pituitary gland detected in some peri- and postmenopausal women is human chorionic gonadotropin (hCG).[9] Usually, hCG is associated with pregnancy or gestational trophoblastic disease. In early pregnancy, hCG doubles approximately every 48 hours, whereas the concentration of hCG from pituitary or gestational trophoblastic disease origin is relatively stable and does not increase in concentration in the pattern seen in pregnancy. If an elevated hCG of 5 to 14 IU/L is detected in a postmenopausal woman, it is likely to be of pituitary origin if (1) the FSH is elevated (>45 IU/L), (2) the hCG is suppressed after 2 weeks of estrogen replacement, and (3) gestational trophoblastic disease has been excluded.

The placenta produces several hormones that are similar to pituitary hormones: hCG has functional and structural similarity to LH; human placental lactogen (hPL, or somatomammotropin) has actions similar to prolactin and GH; placental GH becomes the predominant maternal GH during gestation; and placental corticotropin-releasing hormone (CRH) concentration rises in the fetus throughout gestation.[10] Placental GH (GH-V) differs from pituitary GH in 13 of 191 amino acids. Furthermore, GH-V exists in glycosylated and nonglycosylated forms, whereas pituitary GH is not glycosylated.

ANATOMY

The pituitary is located at the base of the brain and is protected anteriorly, inferiorly, and posteriorly by the bony sella turcica. Inferior and anterior to the sella is the air-containing sphenoid sinus, which communicates with the nasopharynx. Neurosurgeons take advantage of the proximity of the sphenoid sinus to the pituitary; the preferred surgical route to the pituitary is transsphenoidal (either via a sublabial or endonasal approach).

The pituitary weighs only 0.5 to 0.6 g. The gland is larger in women than in men; its size increases during pregnancy, and it is larger in multiparous women. At the completion of pregnancy, when the pituitary is largest, it is susceptible to infarction if hypovolemic shock develops from hemorrhage after delivery, producing a state of postpartum hypopituitarism called Sheehan syndrome.[11]

If the pituitary is greatly reduced in size or is apparently absent on magnetic resonance imaging (MRI) studies, the sella is said to be "empty."[12] In the empty sella syndrome, the sella may be normal in size or enlarged. An incompetent diaphragma sella with compression of the pituitary gland by a herniating arachnoid can cause an empty sella, or the pituitary may be reduced in size as the result of previous apoplexy into a tumor, radiotherapy, or surgery.

Arterial blood is supplied to the pituitary via the superior and inferior hypophyseal arteries, both of which are branches of the carotid arteries. The superior hypophyseal arteries supply the anterior pituitary and hypophyseal stalk, whereas the inferior hypophyseal arteries supply the posterior pituitary.

Direct delivery of hypothalamic regulatory hormones to the adenohypophysis occurs through the hypothalamic-pituitary portal system, which surrounds the adenohypophysis (pars distalis). A portal system is a vascular apparatus in which blood that initially passes through one capillary network (eg, the hypothalamus) is collected into vessels that subsequently supply a second capillary network (eg, the anterior pituitary). Anatomically, this is similar to the nephron where blood from glomerular capillaries is collected into the efferent arteriole to be distributed again to the peritubular capillaries or vasa recta. In this way, the hypothalamus controls the secretion of adenohypophyseal hormones via delivery of hypothalamic venous blood to the anterior pituitary gland. There is also retrograde flow from the pituitary to the hypothalamus via the portal system.

Pituitary venous drainage is moved to the cavernous and intercavernous sinuses via the lateral hypophyseal veins. The cavernous sinus drains to the superior and inferior petrosal sinuses, which join the transverse sinus to form the jugular vein. This anatomic relationship is clinically important because access to pituitary secretions can be afforded by cannulation of the inferior petrosal venous sinuses.[13] Usually, the neuroradiologist places a catheter into a femoral vein that traverses an iliac vein, inferior vena cava, or superior vena cava to the jugular vein to enter the inferior petrosal venous sinus. Inferior petrosal venous sinus sampling can be helpful in the evaluation of patients with Cushing syndrome to differentiate between Cushing disease (an anterior pituitary corticotropinoma) and ectopic ACTH syndrome.

The internal carotid arteries are located laterally to the pituitary. Above the pituitary is the diaphragma sellae, which comprises circular (intercavernous) sinuses containing venous blood. Anterior and superior to the pituitary is the optic chiasm. These relations are clinically important because pituitary neoplasms can invade or compress these structures, as well as the bony sella turcica. For example, superiorly expanding anterior pituitary adenomas can compress the optic chiasm, typically producing bilateral hemianopsia.[14] In this condition, both lateral visual fields are lost, and patients experience loss of peripheral vision.

PITUITARY EMBRYOLOGY

The adenohypophysis develops in utero from a dorsal evagination of the roof of the stomodeum, which becomes the Rathke pouch.[15] The superior portion of the Rathke pouch constitutes the pars tuberalis (see earlier), whereas the posterior portion of the Rathke pouch develops into the pars intermedia (or intermediate lobe). Transcription factors that regulate the development of the anterior pituitary gland include HESX, FGFR1, LHX3, LHX4, SOX3, Pit-1, PROP1, RIEG, and GLI2.[16-18] Mutations in these transcription factors can cause various types of hypopituitarism, along with other conditions such as septo-optic dysplasia.[18,19] The pars intermedia, which is active only late in pregnancy and in utero, secretes α-, β-, and γ-melanocyte stimulating hormone (MSH), corticotropin-like intermediate lobe peptide, γ-lipotropin, and β-endorphin. MSH is believed to promote melanin synthesis. Lipotropins mobilize fat from adipose tissue, and endorphins are endogenous opioids.[20] The clinical significance of these intermediate lobe products as causes of disease is questionable and is not well understood.

Regulation of Function of the Adenohypophysis

The synthesis and release of the following anterior pituitary hormones are stimulated by hypothalamic-releasing hormones: ACTH, TSH, GH, LH, and FSH.[7] Prolactin is the sole anterior pituitary hormone whose release is predominantly regulated through suppression. Corticotrophs secrete ACTH, thyrotrophs secrete TSH, somatotrophs secrete GH, gonadotrophs secrete both LH and FSH, and lactotrophs (or mammotrophs) secrete prolactin. Except for LH and FSH, each hormone is normally produced by a unique cell type. However, in pathologic circumstances, both GH and prolactin may be secreted by an anterior pituitary adenoma termed a mammosomatotrophinoma. The molecular composition of the anterior pituitary hormones is summarized in Table 65.1.

Multiple levels of control of the hypothalamic-pituitary-end organ-hormone axis are known (Fig. 65.2).[21] Except for prolactin and LH at the midpoint of the menstrual cycle, negative feedback controls secretion of the adenohypophyseal hormones. The long feedback loop involves suppression of the hypothalamic-releasing hormone and the anterior

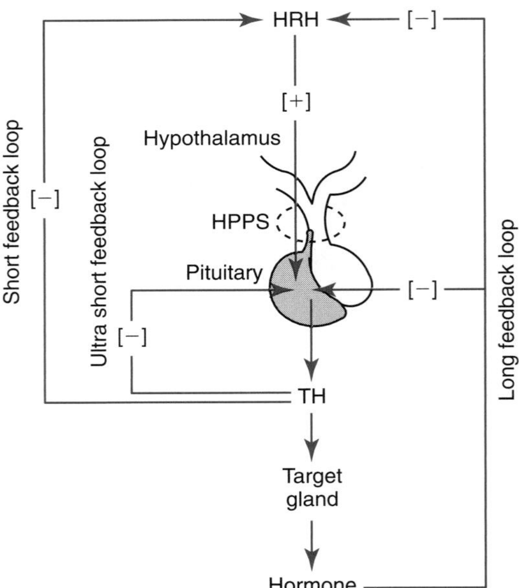

FIGURE 65.2 Many Anterior Pituitary Trophic Hormones (eg, Adrenocorticotropic Hormone *[ACTH]*, Thyroid-Stimulating Hormone *[TSH]*, Growth Hormone *[GH]*, Luteinizing Hormone *[LH]*, Follicle-Stimulating Hormone *[FSH]*) Are Regulated by Hypothalamic Releasing Hormones *(HRHs)*. Releasing hormones secreted by the hypothalamus reach the pituitary via the hypothalamic-pituitary portal system *(HPPS)*. Long feedback loops involve negative feedback of the target cell hormone at the pituitary gland and hypothalamus. The short feedback loop involves the anterior pituitary trophic hormone feeding back at the hypothalamus, whereas the ultra-short feedback loop involves the anterior pituitary hormone feeding back at the anterior pituitary. *[+]*, Stimulation; *[–]*, suppression; *TH*, trophic hormone.

TABLE 65.1 Hypothalamic-Releasing or -Inhibiting Hormones, Their Target Cells, and the Hormone That Is Regulated

Hypothalamic Hormone/Abbreviation	Amino Acids	Anterior Pituitary Target Cell	Hormone Regulated	Amino Acids	MW (kDa)
Corticotropin-releasing hormone (CRH)	41	Corticotroph	ACTH	39	4.5
Thyrotropin-releasing hormone (TRH)	3	Thyrotroph	TSH*	α: 92	28
				β: 118	
Growth hormone–releasing hormone (GHRH)	44	Somatotroph	GH	191	22
				176	20
Somatotropin release–inhibiting hormone† (SRIH)	14	Somatotroph	GH	176	20
Gonadotropin-releasing hormone (GnRH)	10	Gonadotroph	LH*	α: 92	32
				β: 121	
			FSH*	α: 92	30
				β: 111	
Prolactin release-inhibiting hormone (PRIH)	1	Lactotroph	Prolactin	199	22

ACTH, adrenocorticotropic hormone; *FSH*, follicle-stimulating hormone; *GH*, growth hormone; *LH*, luteinizing hormone; *MW*, molecular weight.
*All α-glycoprotein chains are identical, including the α-chain of human chorionic gonadotropin.
†Also known as somatostatin.

pituitary trophic hormone by the hormonal product of the target tissue. The major site of negative feedback for cortisol (regulated by ACTH), insulin-like growth factor-I (IGF-I; regulated by GH), and sex steroids and inhibins (regulated by LH and FSH) is the hypothalamus. In contrast, for thyroid hormone (regulated by TSH), the major site of negative feedback is the anterior pituitary. Retrograde flow from the pituitary to the hypothalamus via the portal system permits the existence of short negative feedback loops in which pituitary hormones suppress the secretion of hypothalamic-releasing hormones. Ultra-short feedback loops also exist in which pituitary hormones inhibit their own secretion. This later event certainly occurs in other endocrine systems. For example, 1,25-dihydroxyvitamin D suppresses its own synthesis by inhibiting the activity of renal 1-α hydroxylase.

POINTS TO REMEMBER

- Most anterior pituitary hormones are predominantly regulated by stimulatory hypothalamic hormones. The exception is prolactin, which is regulated by suppression.
- The pulsatility of release of hypothalamic-releasing hormones can regulate the release of anterior pituitary hormones such as LH and FSH.
- Either hypo- or hyperfunction can develop from pathologic processes involving the hypothalamus, the hypothalamic-pituitary portal system, or the anterior pituitary.
- Reference intervals may depend upon the time of the day that a measurement is obtained, the sex of the subject, their age, and for gonadotropin and sex steroid concentrations in women of reproductive age, their menstrual cycle.

HYPOTHALAMIC REGULATION

The hypothalamus is an area of the brain that produces hormones that control a number of bodily functions, including the release of hormones from the anterior pituitary gland. The hypothalamus is located in the middle of the base of the brain and encapsulates the ventral portion of the third ventricle.

Hormones released by the hypothalamus that regulate the anterior pituitary hormones are listed in Table 65.1. With the exception of ACTH, hypothalamic hormones are structurally smaller than all of the anterior pituitary hormones.

CRH has wide distribution throughout the brain and brainstem.[22] In the hypothalamus, it is released by the paraventricular nucleus (PVN). CRH secretion is stimulated by systemic physiologic stress via (1) neurons of subfornical origin, (2) neurons of the nucleus tractus solitarius, (3) hypothalamic glutamatergic neurons, and (4) 5-hydroxytryptamine–secreting neurons of the raphe nucleus. Neurogenic stress to release CRH also acts via hypothalamic glutamatergic neurons. Stress inhibits hypothalamic GABAergic neurons of the PVN that otherwise would suppress CRH release. Gamma-aminobutyric acid (GABA) serves as an inhibitory neurotransmitter. GABAergic neurons that innervate CRH-secreting neurons also originate from the lateral septum and the bed nucleus of the stria terminalis. ACTH release is stimulated by serotonin, endorphins, and acetylcholine, whereas it is suppressed by GABA. Physiologically, stress, inflammation, and hypoglycemia stimulate ACTH release.

Thyrotropin-releasing hormone (TRH) is a tripeptide product of the PVN of the hypothalamus.[23] TRH-secreting neurons in the PVN are innervated by axons that release (1) norepinephrine, (2) leptin, (3) neuropeptide Y, (4) agouti-related protein, (5) MSH, (6) CRH, or (7) somatostatin. Leptin is produced by adipose tissue and acts to reduce appetite and raise energy expenditure as body fat stores rise. Leptin receptors are expressed in the ventromedial nucleus of the hypothalamus. Leptin (*LPE* gene) deficiency and leptin receptor (*LEPR* gene) deficiency are rare causes of severe, early-onset genetic obesity.[24] Neuropeptide Y and agouti-related protein promote food intake.

The energy state and temperature of the organism influence TRH secretion. In addition to TRH regulation of TSH, TSH secretion is suppressed by (1) thyroid hormones, (2) glucocorticoids, (3) estrogens, and possibly (4) GH. Acute inflammatory cytokines such as interleukin (IL)-1β, IL-6, and tumor necrosis factor (TNF)-α stimulate ACTH release but suppress TRH and TSH. Norepinephrine stimulates TSH release, whereas endorphins, serotonin, and dopamine suppress TSH.

GH–releasing hormone (GHRH) is produced by neurons in the arcuate nucleus of the medial basal hypothalamus. Stimulators of GHRH release include dopamine- and galanin-secreting neurons, and brain stem neurons with catecholaminergic inputs.[25] Galanin is a neuropeptide that is widely expressed in the endocrine, central nervous, and peripheral nervous systems. There are three unique galanin receptors.[26] Hypothalamic somatostatin release–inhibiting hormone (SRIH) suppresses both GHRH release and anterior pituitary GH release. Leptin from adipose tissue and ghrelin from the stomach overall have the effect of increasing GHRH secretion and directly increasing GH concentrations. However, the clinical relevance of these influences and of other GH-releasing peptides (eg, GHRP-6) is not well understood. Ghrelin binds to GH secretagogue receptors, which increases food intake. Ghrelin and obestatin are derived from the ghrelin-obestatin preproprotein. The actions of obestatin may involve reducing anxiety and thirst, enhancing recall, sleep regulation, cell division, and augmented pancreatic enzyme secretion.[27] Hormones that affect GH secretion include estrogen, testosterone, and glucocorticoids. Physiologically, amino acids and hypoglycemia stimulate GH release. Glucagon also stimulates GH release. In turn, the secretion of IGF-I in response to GH is influenced by nutrition, sex steroids, thyroid hormone, and the presence of chronic disease. Malnutrition, sex hormone deficiency in adolescents and adults, hypothyroidism and chronic disease all produce GH resistance to varying extents. Dopamine, endorphins, serotonin, and norepinephrine stimulate GH secretion.

Gonadotropin-releasing hormone (GnRH) regulation is complicated by the fact that GnRH must differentially control LH and FSH secretion, which vary greatly during the menstrual cycle in women.[28] GnRH-secreting neurons are not located in a discrete nucleus, but instead are diffusely distributed in the hypothalamus. Embryologically, these neurons are unusual because they originate outside the central nervous system (CNS). GnRH secretion is stimulated by neurons that secrete (1) galanin-like peptide, (2) kisspeptin, (3) glutamate, (4) neuropeptide Y, and (5) norepinephrine. Kisspeptin, derived from *Kiss* 1 gene expression, is a neuropeptide that regulates puberty and reproduction. Hyperprolactinemia

TABLE 65.2 Hypothalamic-Pituitary-End Organ Physiology

Hypothalamic Hormone	Anterior Pituitary Hormone	Target Organ/Tissue	Target Hormone
CRH	ACTH	Adrenal cortex: zona fasciculata and zona reticularis	Cortisol
TRH	TSH	Thyroid follicular cell	Thyroxine (T_4) and 3,5,3′-triiodothyronine (T_3)
GHRH and SRIH	GH	Liver and many tissues of the body	IGF-I, IGFBP-3, and ALS
GnRH	LH, FSH	Gonad	Sex steroids and inhibins
PRIH	Prolactin	Breast	Not applicable

ACTH, Adrenocorticotropic hormone; *ALS*, acid-labile subunit; CRH, corticotropin-releasing hormone; *FSH*, follicle-stimulating hormone; *GH*, growth hormone; *GHRH*, growth hormone–releasing hormone; *GnRH*, gonadotropin-releasing hormone; *IGFBP-3*, IGF binding protein-3; *IGF-I*, insulin-like growth factor-I; *LH*, luteinizing hormone; *MW*, molecular weight; *PRIH*, prolactin release-inhibiting hormone; *SRIH*, somatotropin release–inhibiting hormone; *TRH*, thyrotropin-releasing hormone.

inhibits *Kiss* 1 gene expression and leads to diminution of GnRH and gonadotropin secretion. Neurons secreting GABA, β-endorphins, and CRH inhibit GnRH. Gonadotropin release is stimulated by norepinephrine, GABA, and acetylcholine, and is suppressed by endorphins, dopamine, and serotonin.

GnRH pulsatility is essential to gonadotroph responsiveness. Tonic release of GnRH will downregulate GnRH receptors on gonadotrophs, which leads to hypogonadism. Therapeutically, downregulation is accomplished with a long-acting GnRH agonist, such as leuprolide acetate (Lupron Depot, AbbVie Inc. North Chicago, Illinois) in the treatment of central precocious puberty in children or the induction of hypogonadism in men with prostate cancer. Conversely, pulsatile GnRH administration is used to initiate puberty and to induce ovulation or spermatogenesis in states of GnRH deficiency. The rate of pulsatility may influence the relative secretion of LH and FSH. In primate studies, GnRH at one pulse per hour preferentially released LH, whereas one pulse every 3 hours caused a decline in LH and a mild rise in FSH.

Anterior Pituitary

In the anterior pituitary, (1) CRH receptors are expressed on corticotrophs, (2) TRH receptors are expressed on thyrotrophs, (3) GHRH receptors are expressed on somatotrophs, (4) GnRH receptors are expressed on gonadotrophs, and (5) prolactin-inhibiting hormone (PRIH) receptors are expressed on lactotrophs. There are two CRH receptors (CRHR1 and CRHR2) that are G-protein–coupled receptors.[29] The gene for CRHR1 is located on chromosome 17q21.31. The gene for CRHR2 is located on chromosome 7p14.3. The TRH receptor is also G-protein coupled. The gene for the TRH receptor is located on chromosome 8q23.1. Chromosome 7p14.3 is the location of the GHRH receptor gene. The gene for the G-protein–coupled GnRH receptor is chromosome 4q. In pathologically high concentrations, TRH stimulates the release of LH and prolactin. Otherwise, TRH does not appear to play a major role in regulating LH or prolactin secretion.

Corticotrophs are stimulated by high concentrations of proinflammatory cytokines, such as IL-1, IL-6, and TNF-α.[30] This emphasizes the interrelationship of the endocrine and immune systems in a hypothalamic-pituitary-adrenal-immune system axis. Through vasopressin type 3 receptors (also known as the arginine vasopressin receptor 1B, V1b receptors, gene location: chromosome 1q32), high concentrations of ADH stimulate corticotrophs to release ACTH.

The hormonal products of each anterior pituitary target cell (if applicable) are listed in Table 65.2 together with a summary of each system. Many of these hormones display circadian (daily), ultradian (more than daily), or infradian (less than daily) variation that reflects changes in hypothalamic control. Deficiency of an individual pituitary hormone is typically called hypopituitarism,[31-33] whereas deficiency of all anterior pituitary hormones is termed panhypopituitarism.

Growth Hormone and Insulin-Like Growth Factors

Linear growth is the consequence of (1) genetic potential, (2) nutrition, (3) the presence or absence of disease, and (4) hormonal effects.[34] Many hormones influence growth, but the most important are GH, thyroid hormone, and sex steroids. Excess glucocorticoids can impair growth in children. GH deficiency produces morbidity in adults, thus GH is essential for health throughout life.

Growth Hormone–Releasing Hormone

The *GHRH* gene is located on chromosome 20q11.2. Prepro-GHRH is a polypeptide chain of 108 amino acids (12.4 kDa). Removal of the 20 amino acid signal (leader) sequence yields the 88 amino acid pro-GHRH. Cleavage of the 11 amino acid N-terminal pro-sequence and the 31 amino acid C-terminal pro-sequence, with release of 2 free amino acids (positions 76–77 with reference to prepro-GHRH), produces the 44 amino acid mature GHRH. The terminal leucine of GHRH is amidated. Alternative splicing of the mRNA (isoform 2) produces a prepro-GHRH protein of 107 amino acids, which is missing amino acid 103.

Somatotropin Release–Inhibiting Hormone

Somatotropin release–inhibiting hormone (SRIH) is also known as somatostatin.[35] It is widely distributed throughout the body (CNS, gut, and δ-cells of the islets of Langerhans) and produces multiple physiologic effects. Somatostatin receptors are widely distributed (see Table 65.3). Somatostatin that functions as SRIH is produced by the paraventricular nucleus of the hypothalamus. In the islets, somatostatin suppresses glucagon and insulin secretion, whereas somatostatin release is stimulated by both of these hormones. In this way, δ-cell somatostatin modulates islet function by smoothing out extremes in the secretion of glucagon and insulin to maintain a stable blood glucose concentration. Somatostatin

TABLE 65.3 Biology of the Somatostatin Receptors

SSTR	Gene Location	Amino Acids/Molecular Weight	SST Binding	Distribution
SSTR1	14q1	391 aa 42.7 kDa	SST-14 >SST-28	Fetal kidney, fetal liver, adult pancreas, brain, lung, jejunum, stomach
SSTR2	17q2	369 aa 41.3 kDa	SST14 and SST-28	Cerebrum, kidney
SSTR3	22q13.1	418 aa 45.8 kDa	SST-14 and SST-28	Brain, pituitary, pancreas
SSTR4	20p11.2	388 aa 42 kDa	SST-14	Fetal and adult brain, lung, stomach, less in kidney, pituitary, adrenals
SSTR5	16p13.3	364 aa 39.2 kDa	SST-28 >SST-14	Adult pituitary, heart, small intestine, adrenal, cerebellum, fetal hypothalamus

aa, Amino acid.

in the gut is found in highest concentration in the duodenum and jejunum.

The somatostatin gene is located on chromosome 3q2. Expression of the somatostatin gene produces the 116 amino acid polypeptide prepro-somatostatin. Cleavage of the signal sequence (24 amino acids) produces pro-somatostatin (92 amino acids), and subsequent cleavage of the N-terminal pro-sequence (64 amino acids) yields a 28 amino acid form of somatostatin (SST-28). SST-28 has an intrachain disulfide bond between amino acids 17 and 28. In many tissues, SST-28 undergoes cleavage to a 14 amino acid form (SST-14) through removal of the N-terminal 14 amino acid sequence by the enzymes prohormone convertase 1/prohormone convertase 2 (PC1/PC2) and carboxypeptidase E (CPE). SST-14 is the major form of somatostatin in the CNS and δ-cells, whereas SST-28 is the major form in the gastrointestinal tract. SST-28 is also the major circulating form of somatostatin. Therefore, somatostatin measurements in peripheral blood do not reflect SRIH secretion. Somatostatin is highly conserved in nature; all vertebrates have the identical sequence for SST-14.[35]

In addition to GH suppression, somatostatin also suppresses TRH, TSH, CRH, and ACTH. However, the effect of somatostatin on the regulation of the adrenal cortical and thyroid axes is usually minor. In the gastrointestinal tract, somatostatin reduces the secretion of multiple hormones, including (1) gastrin, (2) secretin, (3) cholecystokinin, (4) vasoactive intestinal polypeptide, (5) motilin, (6) neurotensin, and (7) pepsin, and reduces gastric pH, intestinal motility, ion and nutrient absorption, and proliferation of the mucosa (see Chapter 62). Calcitonin, catecholamines, renin, and pancreatic exocrine function are suppressed by somatostatin. Somatostatin analogs (eg, octreotide) are used pharmacologically to suppress a variety of hormone overproduction conditions.[36] Indium-111 and gallium-68 labeled octreotide have been used for imaging, and lutetium-177 labeled octreotide has been used in radiotherapy of tumors expressing somatostatin receptors (eg, neuroendocrine tumors).[37] For more information on neuroendocrine tumors, refer to Chapter 63.

Growth Hormone–Releasing Hormone Receptor

The anterior pituitary somatotroph GHRH receptor (GHRHR) is a member of family B-III of the G-coupled receptor superfamily (the "secretin" family).[7] Receptors for (1) secretin, (2) vasoactive intestinal polypeptide, (3) parathyroid hormone (PTH), and (4) calcitonin share partial sequence identity with GHRHR.

Pre-GHRHR is a 423 amino acid polypeptide that is converted to the mature 401 amino acid form of GHRHR by removal of the 22 amino acid signal peptide. The N-terminal extracellular domain is 110 amino acids. GHRHR has 7 transmembrane domains and a 42 amino acid cytoplasmic domain. Amino acid 50 may be glycosylated.

Somatostatin Release–Inhibiting Hormone Receptor

Throughout the body, there are five receptors for somatostatin (SSTR1 through SSTR5; Table 65.3). Each receptor is encoded by a gene located on a separate chromosome. SSTR2 has two alternatively spliced isoforms. All of the SSTR receptors have seven transmembrane domains, and are coupled with a pertussis toxin–sensitive G-protein. SSTR2, SSTR3, SSTR4, and SSTR5 are expressed in the pituitary.

Growth Hormone

Growth hormone has two disulfide bridges (amino acids 54 and 165, and amino acids 182 and 189).[38] Structurally, GH has four main α-helices, and within the connecting loops, it has three mini-helices. Two circulating forms of GH are present: a 22-kDa form that is a 191 amino acid chain (full-length GH) that represents 85% to 90% of circulating GH, and a 20-kDa GH that lacks amino acids 32 through 46.[39] The 20-kDa form of GH results from alternative splicing of the GH mRNA transcript. In addition to the 22- and 20-kDa forms, circulating GH exists as aggregates and oligomers. "Big GH" is a dimer of GH monomers, and "big, big GH" is GH associated with its binding protein (GHBP). GHBP is the external domain of the GH receptor (GHR), which binds GH with high affinity and is produced by cleavage of the GHR. Approximately 55% of all circulating GH forms are monomeric; big GH and big, big GH represent approximately 27% and approximately 18% of circulating GH, respectively. Approximately 50% of GH is not bound to GHBP; approximately 45% is bound to GHBP, and the remaining 5% of GH is bound to low-affinity binding proteins. Considering the multiple forms of GH, it is not surprising that significant analytical biases are observed between different immunoassays for GH.

The gene for GH (chromosome 17q24.2) is a member of the GH subfamily that includes (−5′ to 3′ direction) (1) GH (the GH1 gene), (2) a chorionic somatomammotropin

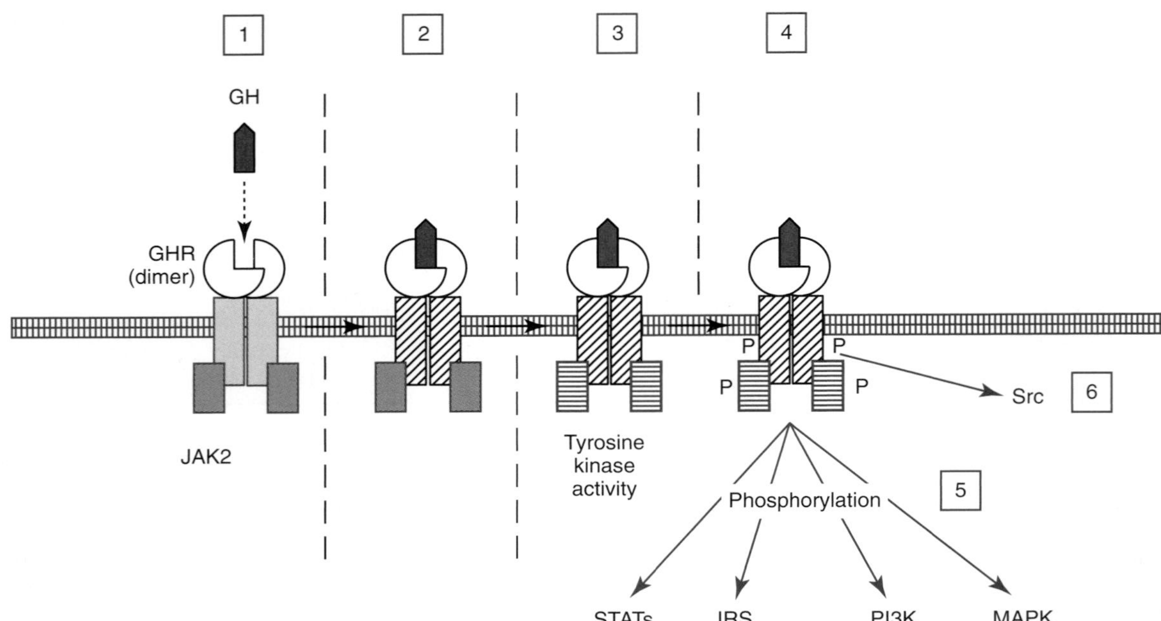

FIGURE 65.3 The Growth Hormone Receptor *(GHR)* Exists as a Cell Surface Dimer in Its Inactive State. With growth hormone *(GH)* binding to the GHR *(1)*, the GHR recruits or activates Janus-associated kinase enzyme *(JAK2) (2)*. JAK2 then achieves tyrosine kinase activity *(3)*, and JAK2 and the GHR are phosphorylated *(4)*. Activated JAK2 triggers several intracellular pathways involving signal transducers and activators of transcription *(STATs)*, the insulin receptor substrate *(IRS)*, phosphatidylinositol 3′-kinase *(PI3K)*, and a mitogen-activated protein kinase *(MAPK) (5)*. Independent of JAK2, GHR signaling can proceed via Src *(6)*.

(hPL) pseudogene designated CSHP, (3) a chorionic somatomammotropin-A designated CSH1, (4) the placentally produced 22-kDa GH variant (GH-V; gene designation GH2), and (5) chorionic somatomammotropin-B (gene designation CSH2).[40] Somatomammotropin (hPL) is a placental hormone with growth-promoting properties. Prolactin (199 amino acids) shares a homologous amino acid sequence with GH, but prolactin, encoded on chromosome 6p22, is not part of the GH complex on 17q24.2.

GH has both direct and indirect activity. Its direct actions will be described in the following sections.[41] The indirect activity of GH is mediated by IGF-I. To initiate its direct and indirect activity, GH binds to receptors (GHR) that appear to be expressed by all tissues.

Growth Hormone Receptor

The GHR is a member of the class 1 hematopoietic cytokine family.[42] Other members of this family include receptors for erythropoietin, granulocyte-macrophage colony-stimulating factor, and various interferons. Structurally, the GHR is a single-chain, 620 amino acid protein (130 kDa). Pre-GHR includes an 18 amino acid leader sequence. The GHR structure includes an extracellular domain (246 amino acids), a transmembrane domain (24 amino acids), and a cytoplasmic domain (350 amino acids).[43] When the extracellular portion of the GHR is shed, the 55-kDa GHBP moiety is released into the circulation.

Four isoforms of the GHR are expressed by alternative splicing of the nascent mRNA. Isoform 1 is the full-length receptor. Isoform 2 differs in the sequence of amino acids 292 to 297 (with reference to pre-GHR) and lacks amino acids 298 to 638. Isoform 3 differs in the sequence of amino acids 292 to 294 and lacks amino acids 295 to 638. An alanine at position four is replaced by aspartic acid, and amino acids 25 to 46 are missing in isoform 4.

The GHR exists as a cell surface dimer in its inactive state (Fig. 65.3). When GH binds to the GHR, the receptor recruits or activates 120-kDa Janus-associated kinase enzymes (JAK2; a type of adapter tyrosine kinase). JAK2 then exerts tyrosine kinase activity by phosphorylating itself and the GHR.[44,45] Phosphorylation activates JAK2, which triggers several intracellular pathways involving (1) signal transducers and activators of transcription (STATs), (2) the insulin receptor substrate, (3) phosphatidylinositol 3′-kinase (PI3K), and (4) a mitogen-activated protein kinase (MAPK). Via receptor-associated kinases, members of the STAT family are phosphorylated to permit the formation of homodimers or heterodimers that act as transcriptional activators once they translocate to the cell nucleus.[46] STAT5b is involved, but it is unclear whether STAT5a is also involved.[47] In its role as a transcription factor, phosphorylated, dimerized STAT5b enters the nucleus to promote gene transcription. Independent of JAK2, GHR signaling can be effected via *Src*, which is a tyrosine kinase. (Note: *Src* is the Rous sarcoma virus protooncogene.)

Insulin-Like Growth Factors

IGF-I is a member of the insulin-related peptide family whose other members include IGF-II, insulin, and relaxin. Stimulated by hCG during pregnancy, relaxin is produced by the corpus luteum verum (the corpus luteum of pregnancy), the decidua (the uterine lining during pregnancy), and the placenta. Relaxin increases collagenase activity to soften and lengthen the cervix and pubic symphysis, and facilitate parturition. Relaxin also reduces uterine contractility by inhibiting myosin kinase activity. In humans, there are three nonallelic relaxin genes: *RLN1, RLN2,* and *RLN3.*

Proinsulin, IGF-I, IGF-II, and relaxin are all composed of two domains (A and B) joined by a connecting domain. The connecting domains vary in sequence and length much more than the A and B domains. The connecting domain of proinsulin is cleaved to release C-peptide (connecting peptide), producing insulin A and B chains. Insulin, IGF-I, IGF-II, and relaxin have two disulfide bridges. IGF-I and IGF-II share 62% homology, and they each share 50% homology with insulin.

The 110 amino acid sequence of preproinsulin includes a signal peptide (amino acids 1–24), the insulin B chain (amino acids 25–54), C-peptide (amino acids 57–87), and the insulin A chain (amino acids 90–110). The two interchain disulfide bonds are between amino acids 31 and 96, and 43 and 109. The single intrachain disulfide bond is between amino acids 95 and 100.

Two forms of prepro–IGF-I are expressed as a consequence of alternative mRNA splicing: IGF-IA and IGF-IB. The IGF-IA preprohormone is 153 amino acids, including a signal peptide (amino acids 1–21), an N-terminal propeptide (amino acids 22–48), IGF-I (70 amino acids), and a C-terminal propeptide (the E domain, amino acids 119–153). The IGF-I polypeptide includes the B domain (amino acids 49–77), the C (connecting) domain (amino acids 78–89), the A domain (amino acids 90–110), and the D domain (amino acids 111–118). Three disulfide bonds are present between amino acids 54 and 96, 66, and 109, and 95 and 100. IGF-I is not glycosylated.

The 195 amino acid IGF-IB preprohormone is composed of a signal peptide (amino acids 1–21), a propeptide (amino acids 22–48), IGF-I (70 amino acids), and another propeptide region (the E domain, amino acids 119–195). Differences in the D domain of the prepro–IGF-I distinguish IGF-IA from IGF-IB; the tertiary structure of the IGF-I proteins and the placement of disulfide bonds are identical between IGF-IA and IGF-IB.

The IGF-II preprohormone comprises 180 amino acids. The first 24 residues constitute the signal (or leader) peptide. After their removal, IGF-II is derived from pro–IGF-II after cleavage of the C-terminal E peptide (amino acids 92–180). Therefore, amino acids 25 to 91 include the B region (amino acids 25–52), the C region (amino acids 53–64), the A region (amino acids 65–85), and the D region (amino acids 86–91) of IGF-II. Isoform I is the full-length prepro–IGF-II (180 amino acids). Formed by alternative splicing, isoform II lacks amino acid 25 (alanine) and is therefore 179 amino acids in length. IGF-II is glycosylated at amino acid 99 and has three intrachain disulfide bonds between amino acids 33 and 71, 45 and 84, and 70 and 75. A potential glycosylation site is amino acid 163.

Prorelaxin is a 185 amino acid protein that contains a signal sequence (amino acids 1–22), a B chain (amino acids 23–53), a connecting propeptide (amino acids 56–158), and an A chain (amino acids 163–185). A–B interchain disulfide bonds can occur between amino acids 35 and 172, and 47 and 185. An additional disulfide bridge may occur between amino acids 171 and 176.

IGF-I and IGF-II circulate together with an IGF binding protein (IGFBP) (specifically IGFBP-3), and the acid-labile subunit (ALS) to form a 150-kDa trimeric protein complex. Approximately 75% to 80% of IGF-I/IGFBP-3 complexes are trimeric; the remaining IGF-I/IGFBP-3 complexes are dimeric and may include other IGFBPs. Less than 1% of the total IGF-I is free (the biologically active form). The binding affinity of IGF-I for the insulin receptor is low (≈7% of insulin affinity), but circulating IGF-I concentrations exceed insulin by three orders of magnitude. Without binding proteins, therefore, IGF-I could cause potentially devastating hypoglycemia.

The trimeric IGF-I-IGFBP-3-ALS complexes do not normally cross capillary membranes because of their size. However, the 50-kDa binary complex and free IGF-I are able to enter the interstitium, where binding to type I IGF receptors can occur.

Most of the circulating IGF-I is produced by hepatocytes.[48] However, IGF-I is also produced locally throughout the body and thus acts as a paracrine and an autocrine hormone. The possible endocrine (systemic) influence of IGF-I on growth is discussed later.

Similar to IGF-I, IGF-II does not normally produce hypoglycemia. However, tumors that secrete a larger than normal form of IGF-II have been described. These usually more than 0.5 kg in size, nonislet cell tumors are most often of mesenchymal or hepatic origin.[49] Big IGF-II does not bind normally to IGFBP-3, and therefore the free IGF-II concentration is greatly elevated, and the molar IGF-II to IGF-I ratio is greater than 10. As a result of IGF-II binding to the insulin receptor, the clinical syndrome is similar to hypoglycemia caused by hyperinsulinism (ie, absence of ketonemia with no elevation of free fatty acids, lactate, or alanine), and insulin itself is suppressed because β-cells are normal. Physiologically, hypoglycemia stimulates the release of counter-regulatory hormones, such as GH, but in this scenario IGF-II suppresses the GH axis. Removal of the tumor leads to the resolution of hypoglycemia.[50,51]

Insulin-Like Growth Factor Binding Proteins

Because of their high affinity (K_d 10^{-10} to 10^{-11} M) for IGFs, IGFBPs are regarded as inhibitors of IGF action.[52a] IGFBPs have higher affinity for IGFs than the IGF receptors. IGFBP-3 has biological actions independent of the IGF/IGF-I receptor axis.[52b] Receptors for IGFBPs have been described. Proteolysis of IGFBPs releases IGF-I; therefore, IGFBP proteases can influence free IGF-I concentrations. Table 65.4 summarizes the features of the seven known IGFBPs.

Receptors for Insulin-Like Growth Factors

Two types of receptors for IGFs have been identified: the type I IGF receptor and the type II IGF receptor (Fig. 65.4).[53] Structurally, the type I IGF receptor is similar to the insulin receptor. Because this receptor does not exclusively bind IGF-I, the terminology "IGF-I receptor" is not recommended. The type I receptor is derived from a single precursor protein of 1367 amino acids that include the 30 amino acid signal peptide. The 706 amino acid (130 kDa) α-chain is extracellular and is bound by a disulfide bond to the transmembrane 90-kDa (627 amino acids) β- chain. Cleavage of the α- and β-chains releases a tetrapeptide (707–710: arginine-lysine-arginine-arginine). Beta-chain amino acids 906 to 929 form a transmembrane domain. The receptor exists as a homodimer (β-α-α-β) with the two α-chains bound to each other by two disulfide bonds. Similar to the type I IGF receptor, the insulin

TABLE 65.4 Characteristics of Insulin-Like Growth Factor Binding Proteins

IGFBP	Chromosome Gene Location	Amino Acids	Affinity for IGF-I vs. IGF-II	Specific Features
1	7p13	234	1 = 2	RGD sequence*
2	2q3	289	1 < 2	RGD sequence*
3	7p13	264	1 = 2	N-glycosylation
4	17q	237	1 = 2	Extra cysteines
5	2q3	252	1 < 2	Ternary complex with ALS
6	12q13	216	1 < 2	O-glycosylation
7	4q12	282	†	Stimulates prostacyclin production

*RGD sequence = Arginine-glycine-aspartic acid.
†Binds IGF-I and IGF-II with low affinity.
ALS, Acid-labile subunit; *IGF*, insulin-like growth factor; *IGFBP*, insulin-like growth factor protein.

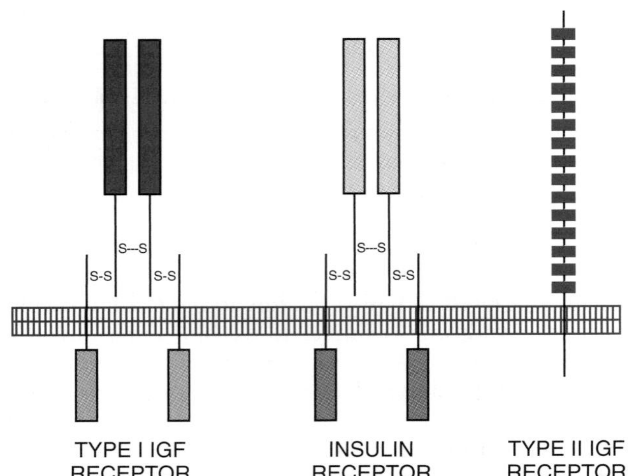

FIGURE 65.4 The Type I Insulin-Like Growth Factor *(IGF)* Receptor Is Structurally Similar to the Insulin Receptor. The structure of the type II IGF receptor is similar to that of the epidermal growth factor receptor.

receptor is a homodimer of two 135-kDa α-chains and two 95-kDa β-chains.

Tyrosine kinase activity in the cytoplasmic portion of the type I IGF receptor β-chain results from binding of an IGF molecule to the cysteine-rich portion of the α-chains (amino acids 148–302), which causes conformational changes in both α- and β-chains. Intracellular signaling involves autophosphorylation and phosphorylation of the 185-kDa insulin receptor substrate 1, which is the predominant target of the active type I IGF receptor. The type I IGF receptor binds IGF-I with higher affinity than IGF-II, and affinity for insulin is lower than the affinity of the receptor for IGF-I or IGF-II. The affinities of the insulin receptor are the opposite: insulin ≫IGF-II >IGF-I.

The type II IGF receptor is structurally dissimilar from the type I IGF receptor and the insulin receptor. The 270-kDa, 2451 amino acid, type II IGF receptor is a monomeric protein that is similar to the epidermal growth factor (EGF) receptor. (Note: The leader sequence is 40 amino acids.) The EGF receptor itself is also known as ErbB1 or HER1. The external portion of the receptor is 2264 amino acids, the transmembrane domain is 23 amino acids, and the cytoplasmic domain is 164 amino acids. Beginning at the N-terminus, thirteen approximately 150 amino acid repeats and a 47 amino acid fibronectin type II domain are followed by 2 more repeats. Evidence indicates at least five glycosylation sites: amino acids 112 (with preference for the pre-type II IGF receptor), 581, 626, 747, and 1246. Two disulfide bonds are found between amino acids 1903 and 1927, and between amino acids 1917 and 1942.

Ligand binding to EGF receptors results in dimerization and tyrosine kinase activation. The external ligand-binding domain of EGFs is composed of numerous short amino acid repeats. The type II IGF receptor removes IGF-II from the circulation. The type II IGF receptor binds mannose-6-phosphate, in addition to IGFs, permitting the uptake and intracellular movement of mannose-6-phosphate–containing lysosomal enzymes. The binding sites for IGFs and mannose-6-phosphate are found on different parts of the receptor. The affinities of the type II IGF receptor are as follows: IGF-II ≫IGF-I >insulin. Because this receptor does not exclusively bind IGF-II, the terminology "IGF-II receptor" is not recommended.

A hybrid receptor consisting of the α–β-chain of the insulin receptor and the α–β-chain of the type I IGF receptor has been described. It has been suggested that these hybrid receptors may allow cancers to respond to insulin.[54] In cancers, insulin is also thought to act through the insulin signaling pathway via insulin receptors and also probably acts through receptors that bind IGF-I. Thus IGF-I also plays a role in cancer biology. Increasing evidence suggests that IGF-I may enhance the growth of many tumors. Thus, the casual use of IGF-I injections in children to enhance growth in short but otherwise normal children is problematic and potentially carcinogenic.

Regulation of Growth Hormone Secretion

Growth hormone ultimately stimulates release of IGF-I, which negatively feeds back to regulate GH release via two hypothalamic hormones: SRIH (or somatostatin; from the hypothalamic paraventricular nucleus) and GHRH (from the hypothalamic infundibular nucleus) (Fig. 65.5). These hypothalamic GH-regulating hormones are carried to the anterior pituitary via the specialized hypothalamic-pituitary portal vascular system. Somatotrophs of the anterior pituitary gland have receptors for both hormones. Somatostatin inhibits GH release, whereas GHRH promotes the release of GH. However, GH release is the predominant hypothalamic

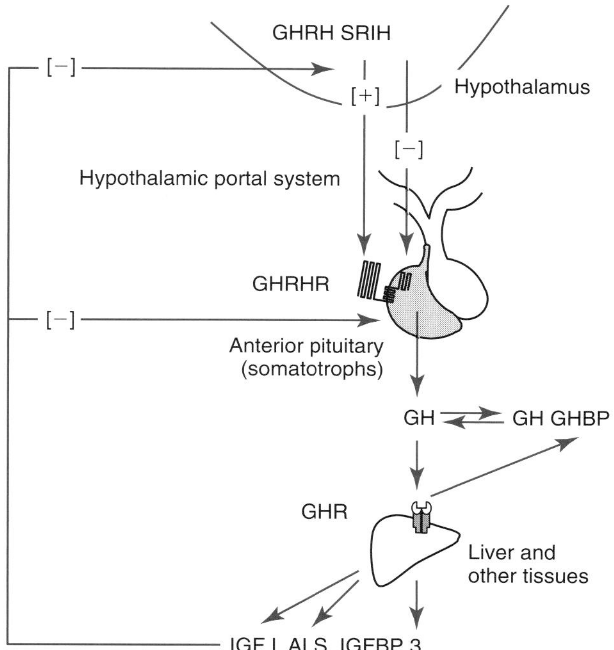

FIGURE 65.5 The Hypothalamus Secretes Growth Hormone–Releasing Hormone *(GHRH)* and Somatotropin Release–Inhibiting Hormone (*SRIH*; Somatostatin), Which Regulate Growth Hormone *(GH)* Release. The receptor for GHRH *(GHRHR)* is illustrated because mutations in this receptor can cause some forms of inherited GH deficiency. GH circulates unbound and bound to its binding protein *(GHBP)*. GHBP is the extracellular domain of the GHR, which is cleaved from the GHR and circulates in the plasma. GH releases IGF-I, IGF binding protein 3 *(IGFBP-3)*, and the acid-labile subunit *(ALS)*. IGF-I negatively feeds back at the anterior pituitary somatotrophs and at the hypothalamus. Because transection of the pituitary stalk leads to GH deficiency, the predominant hypothalamic control of GH is stimulatory via GHRH.

POINTS TO REMEMBER

- GGH deficiency in children should be considered only when other causes of low growth-velocity short stature have been excluded.
- The diagnosis of GH deficiency usually requires repeated stimulation tests, although some endocrinologists will diagnose GH deficiency based solely on the measurement of IGF-I.
- Defects in IGF-I generation and response are rare compared with cases in which GH is deficient.
- GH deficiency does occur in adults, and such adults may benefit from GH replacement.
- GH excess produces the clinical syndrome of gigantism in children and acromegaly in adults.
- GH excess is diagnosed by the failure of GH suppression after an oral glucose load and elevated IGF-I levels.
- Reference intervals for IGF-I are influenced by age, sex, and pubertal stage.

BOX 65.1 Protocol for Glucose Suppression of Growth Hormone Test

Rationale

Normal subjects show suppression of serum growth hormone (GH) concentrations after oral administration of glucose. Subjects with acromegaly fail to exhibit appropriate GH suppression.

Procedure

The test should be performed after an overnight fast with the patient maintained at bed rest. After a baseline blood specimen is collected for GH and glucose measurement, a solution of 75 g of glucose is given orally (in children, 1.75 g/kg to a maximum dose of 75 g). Glucose and serum GH are measured again on specimens collected 30, 60, 90, and 120 minutes later.

Interpretation

Serum GH concentrations in normal individuals fall to less than 1 to 2 µg/L (ie, below the lower limit of detection of the GH assay used). Subjects with acromegaly fail to show this suppression and sometimes show a paradoxical increase in GH concentration. Patients with liver disease, uremia, or heroin addiction may have false-positive results with this test (failure to suppress serum GH concentrations after oral glucose load).

effect, because surgical interruption of the pituitary stalk with destruction of the hypothalamic-pituitary portal system leads to GH deficiency, not excess. In addition to its hypothalamic negative feedback effects, IGF-I directly suppresses pituitary release of GH.

Physiologically, GH secretion is episodic and pulsatile.[55] Consequently, random measurements cannot exclude GH deficiency nor confirm GH excess; between pulses, GH concentrations can be quite low and do not distinguish GH insufficiency from normal production of the hormone. During daytime hours, the plasma concentration of GH in healthy adults remains stable and relatively low (<2 ng/mL; <2 µg/L), with several secretory spikes occurring approximately 3 hours after meals (particularly meals high in protein and arginine) and after exercise. In contrast, during the evening hours, adults and children show a marked rise in GH secretory activity approximately 90 minutes after the onset of sleep; GH concentrations reach a peak value during the period of deepest sleep. This pattern of GH secretion may be important for anabolic and repair processes, and for proper skeletal growth. GH is also increased by psychologic or physical stress and hypoglycemia. Normal GH secretion requires thyroxine and age-appropriate concentrations of testosterone or estrogen.

GH is suppressed by elevations in blood glucose. One of the tests for GH excess measures GH after an oral glucose load (eg, 75 g in adults and 1.75 g/kg in children); the normal response is a GH concentration of less than 1 to 2 ng/mL (1–2 µg/L), depending on the lower limit of detection of the GH immunoassay (Box 65.1). GH also declines with increases in free fatty acid concentrations, rapid eye movement sleep, and aging. In the presence of abnormally high concentrations of glucocorticoids, GH secretion is suppressed. In addition, circulating GH is thought to influence the release of hypothalamic hormones through the short feedback loop. Other hypothalamic hormones, such as TRH and GnRH, do not affect GH release in normal subjects but may provoke GH release in patients with acromegaly.

Age-associated decline in GH production has spawned an industry of dietary supplements purported to "support" GH secretion.[56] These supplements are amino acid preparations that theoretically stimulate release of the subject's own GH. Such dietary supplements have no proven medical value. Use of GH by athletes to enhance strength or promote recovery from injury is prohibited in most sports.

The role of non-GHRH GH secretogogues (eg, ghrelin, various synthetic hexapeptides) in the physiologic control of GH and growth is highly debated.[57] One such secretogogue is ghrelin (28 amino acids, 3.4 kDa; gene name: GHRL; chromosome 3p2). Although ghrelin is produced in the hypothalamus, its highest concentration is found in stomach tissue. In addition, ghrelin is widely distributed in the gastrointestinal tract, heart, lung, and adipose tissue. Ghrelin appears to stimulate food intake and obesity.[58]

Ghrelin binds to the somatotroph GH-secretogogue receptor (gene name: GHSR; isoform 1A: 366 amino acids, 41 kDa; isoform 1B: 289 amino acids, 32 kDa; chromosome 3q26.31), which is distinct from the GHRHR. GHRL, the gene that encodes ghrelin, also encodes the 23 amino acid peptide obestatin. As noted previously, obestatin may decrease food intake and increase satiety, but this has been debated. Obestatin is a ligand for the orphan GPR39 receptor (453 amino acids, 51 kDa; chromosome 2q21). However, despite obestatin binding to the GPR39 receptor, receptor activation may not follow.[59]

Physiologic Actions

Growth hormone effects can be classified as indirect or direct.[60] GH directly raises blood glucose by stimulating gluconeogenesis and reducing insulin sensitivity. Also, it causes adipose tissue lipolysis, and the resulting GH-induced elevations in free fatty acids provide an alternative energy source that serves to spare glucose for CNS use. Therefore when glucose and free fatty acid concentrations are raised at times of stress, in partnership with epinephrine, glucagon, and cortisol, fuels for the fight-or-flight response are provided. GH has other effects on intermediary metabolism: GH stimulates the uptake of nonesterified fatty acids by muscle, and accelerates the mobilization and metabolism of fat from adipose tissue to the liver.

At the epiphysis of growing bone, GH promotes epiphyseal prechondrocyte differentiation. GH directly stimulates the production of the ternary complex of IGF-I, IGFBP-3, and the ALS. In turn, after entering the interstitium, unbound IGF-I binds to type I IGF receptors.

Indirect effects of GH are mediated through IGF-I production, which (together with GH) is necessary for linear growth in childhood. IGF-I is mitogenic and antiapoptotic. Epiphyseal prechondrocyte differentiation stimulated by GH, along with the local effects of IGF-I (also under the control of GH), stimulates the clonal expansion of differentiating chondrocytes.

Thus the overall effect of GH is to promote growth in soft tissue, cartilage, and bone. This action results from stimulation of protein synthesis that is induced in part by an increase in amino acid transport through cell membranes. The effects of GH on bone and muscle are exerted both directly and through the effects of IGF-I under the influence of GH. Increased growth of soft tissue and the skeleton is accompanied by changes in electrolyte metabolism, including positive nitrogen and phosphorous balance, a rise in plasma phosphorous concentration, and a fall in blood urea and amino acid concentrations. Additional responses to GH include increased intestinal absorption of calcium and decreased urinary excretion of sodium and potassium. The metabolic changes most likely are caused by increased uptake of these ions by growing tissue.

IGF-I increases glucose oxidation in adipose tissue and stimulates glucose and amino acid transport into diaphragmatic muscle and heart muscle. Synthesis of collagen and proteoglycans is enhanced by IGF-I, which also has positive effects on calcium, magnesium, and potassium homeostasis. The insulin-like effects of this growth factor have been ascribed in part to its structural similarity to insulin.

Evidence indicates that the local effects of IGF-I (autocrine or paracrine) are predominant in stimulating growth when compared with the systemic effects of IGF-I produced by the liver. When the hepatic IGF-I gene was knocked out in mice (although nonhepatic tissues expressed IGF-I), growth was normal, and IGFBP-3 and ALS concentrations were low. IGF-II may function as a growth factor in utero; however, its secretion in utero is not under the control of GH.

In the absence of GH, IGF-I is not as effective a growth stimulant as it is when GH and IGF-I both are present. IGF-I treatment alone is not recommended as therapy for GH deficiency; IGF-I therapy is reserved for cases of GH resistance due to GHR deficiency (eg, Laron syndrome).[45,61]

GH (through IGF-I) and insulin induce growth in a similar manner because both have protein anabolic effects and stimulate the transport of amino acids into peripheral cells. Their respective effects on glucose homeostasis, however, oppose each other. Most growth-promoting GH effects are delayed rather than immediate and are exerted primarily through IGF-I.

IGF-I concentrations vary widely with age and gender.[62] IGF-I rises during childhood, and during puberty, IGF-I concentrations can be two to three times the adult concentration. After adolescence, IGF-I concentrations show a gradual decline, reaching a steady state in the third decade of life.

GH is not the only determinant of IGF-I concentration in the circulation. Transformation of the GH stimulus to IGF-I production and secretion is modulated by (1) nutrition, (2) the presence or absence of chronic inflammation, (3) thyroid function, (4) glucocorticoids, and (5) sex steroids. IGF-I secretion is reduced by (1) malnutrition, (2) malabsorption (eg, inflammatory bowel disease), (3) celiac disease, (4) cystic fibrosis, (5) chronic disease, (6) hypothyroidism (eg, Hashimoto thyroiditis), and (7) sex hormone deficiency during adolescence. Therefore, a decreased IGF-I concentration is not necessarily synonymous with GH deficiency.

In cases of acquired GH resistance and genetic GH resistance (GHR mutation or signaling disorder), GH concentrations will rise, and high concentrations of GH produce hyperlipidemia and hyperglycemia.[63] Cases of acquired GH resistance are not treated with GH or IGF-I, but instead are treated through resolution of the underlying disorder.

The actions and regulation of IGF-II have been debated.[64] IGF-II is believed to be important for intrauterine growth.

Mice display intrauterine growth retardation when the IGF-II gene is knocked out. Although IGF-II–producing tumors are rare, such tumors can produce hypoglycemia.[46,51] Both IGF-I and IGF-II are of great interest to cancer researchers; the reader is referred to the literature for a detailed discussion of this topic.

Clinical Significance

Clinically important states of GH excess or deficiency are uncommon and are often difficult to diagnose.[65] GH concentrations vary widely under normal circumstances; therefore random measurements of GH, in general, are not diagnostically useful. A single GH measurement cannot distinguish between normal fluctuations and the low or high concentrations that are typical of various diseases. GH measurements are best determined as part of dynamic testing: physiologic or pharmacologic provocative stimuli are used to help diagnose GH deficiency, whereas GH suppression (or lack thereof) following glucose administration is useful in evaluating GH excess.[66] IGF-I concentrations often correlate better with the clinical severity of acromegaly than with glucose-suppressed or basal GH concentrations.[67]

In contrast to GH, a single measurement of IGF-I is considered to be an accurate reflection of GH-IGF-I production, irrespective of the time of the day or meals. IGF-I has a much longer half-life than GH, so its concentration is more stable. The half-life of GH is slightly longer than 15 minutes, whereas the half-life of the trimeric IGF-I-IGFBP-3-ALS complex is 17 to 22 hours. The half-life of unbound IGF-I is only 10 to 20 minutes, but the unbound form of the hormone accounts for less than 1% of the total concentration. Serum concentrations of IGF-I are influenced by (1) age, (2) sex, (3) degree of sexual maturity, (4) thyroid status, and (5) nutritional status. As mentioned previously, IGF-I concentrations are low in GH deficiency and in patients with acute or chronic protein or caloric deprivation. In pediatric endocrinology, measurements of IGFBP-3 have been used in addition to IGF-I measurements to assess GH; however, the value of this approach has not been established. The diagnostic use of GH to stimulate IGF-I production is controversial and is not currently included in standard medical practice.[68]

Growth Hormone Excess

Acromegaly is the rare clinical syndrome in adults that results from GH excess.[69,70] Even less common is gigantism, which results from GH excess in childhood. The clinical features of acromegaly involve overgrowth of the skeleton and soft tissue, producing (1) acral enlargement (enlargement of the extremities), (2) organomegaly (enlarged heart and/or liver), (3) facial coarsening, (4) intestinal polyposis, (5) premature cardiovascular disease, (6) hyperhidrosis (increased sweating), (7) skin tags, (8) joint disease, (9) myopathy with weakness, (10) insulin resistance, and often (11) diabetes mellitus. Premature cardiovascular disease is the most common cause of death in individuals with acromegaly. Gigantism is characterized by extreme tall stature, in addition to the clinical features of acromegaly, as pathologic GH excess occurs before epiphyseal fusion is complete (eg, in children or adolescents).

Most cases of acromegaly (≈95%) result from anterior pituitary GH-secreting tumors (somatotropinomas).[71] Somatotropinomas are usually large macroadenomas (>10 mm in diameter) by the time they come to clinical attention; the vast majority of these tumors are visualized by computed tomography (CT) or magnetic resonance imaging (MRI), which is the preferred method for pituitary imaging. Some anterior pituitary tumors secrete both GH and prolactin (somatomammotropinomas). GH-secreting anterior pituitary adenocarcinomas are exceedingly rare. Approximately 5% of GH-secreting tumors are familial and caused by disorders such as multiple endocrine neoplasia type 1 syndrome, familial acromegaly, Carney syndrome, McCune-Albright syndrome, and familial isolated pituitary adenoma.[72] Approximately 5% of acromegaly cases result from GHRH-secreting hypothalamic tumors, and less than 1% of cases result from extrapituitary somatotropinomas, GHRH-secreting islet cells, or lung or breast tumors.

In severe or advanced cases of GH excess, the diagnosis may be nearly certain on the basis of physical appearance alone. However, in less severe or early cases, the physical changes may be subtle and gradual, so a high degree of clinical suspicion is needed to make an early diagnosis. The reversibility of tissue changes depends largely on the duration of the disease. In addition to soft tissue changes, acromegaly may cause severe disability or death from cardiac, pulmonary, and/or neurologic sequelae. The most important requirement for the diagnosis of acromegaly is the demonstration of inappropriate and excessive GH secretion.[73]

As many as 10% of patients with active acromegaly have random serum GH concentrations that fall within normal reference intervals. Essentially all patients with acromegaly have an abnormal GH response to oral glucose (see Box 65.1). Patients with acromegaly typically show no change in their basal concentration of GH or demonstrate a paradoxical increase in GH[74]; in contrast, normal individuals show suppression of GH concentrations to less than 1.0 ng/mL (<1 μg/L) after a 75-g oral glucose load. Serum IGF-I concentrations are also elevated in active acromegaly, and often correlate better with the clinical severity of acromegaly than do glucose-suppressed or basal GH concentrations.[75] IGF-I measurements are considered to be the most important diagnostic tests in the diagnosis of acromegaly.[76,77]

Growth Hormone Deficiency and Growth Retardation

In children, short stature with a normal growth velocity (≥4–5 cm/years) results from (1) familial short stature, (2) primordial growth failure (prenatal-onset growth failure), or (3) constitutional delay in growth and adolescence (delayed maturation).[78] Short stature with a low growth velocity (<4–5 cm/years) results from genetic short stature, chronic illness, malnutrition, deprivation (nutritional or psychological), Turner syndrome in girls, or endocrine disorders (eg, hypothyroidism, disorders of the GHRH-GH-IGF-I axis, extremely poorly controlled diabetes, rickets, pseudohypoparathyroidism, pseudopseudohypoparathyroidism, and Cushing syndrome).[79]

Idiopathic short stature is the term that is used when children with short stature and a low growth velocity lack evidence of pathology. It has been increasingly recognized that 5% to 15% of these children have a mutation in the *SHOX* (short stature homeobox) gene located on chromosome Xp22.33. Forearm anomalies are common in such children, and they become more evident during puberty.[80]

GH deficiency is not a common cause of growth retardation. Approximately one-half of children evaluated for growth retardation have no specific organic cause; approximately 15% have an endocrine disorder, of which approximately half (approximately 8% of all children with short stature) have GH deficiency. Children with significantly reduced height and low growth velocities with no clear explanation should be screened for GH deficiency once other endocrine disorders have been excluded.

GH deficiency in children is characterized by (1) short stature, (2) low growth velocity, (3) immature facial appearance, (4) retarded bone age on radiologic examination, and (5) increased adiposity. In cases of congenital GH deficiency, size at birth is usually normal because in utero IGF-I does not appear to be under GH control. Micropenis (an abnormally short penis) is evident in some boys with congenital GH deficiency and will resolve with GH replacement in childhood. Micropenis suggests hypopituitarism, although there are other causes for micropenis.[81] Adults with GH deficiency experience (1) reduced muscle mass, (2) increased central adiposity, (3) osteoporosis with decreased bone density, (4) an increase in fracture risk, (5) decreased quality of life, (6) dyslipidemia, and (7) an increased risk for cardiovascular disease.[82] GH deficiency is probably the most common endocrine abnormality in adults with large pituitary adenomas[83] and in patients who have undergone pituitary irradiation. Recovery of hormonal production after surgery for pituitary adenomas occurs uncommonly. GH replacement therapy forms an important part of the clinical care of GH-deficient children. Whether GH therapy is required in GH-deficient adults is somewhat controversial.

GH insufficiency can be a consequence of (1) hypothalamic disease, (2) disruption of the portal system between hypothalamic nuclei and the anterior pituitary, (3) GHRHR loss-of-function mutations, or (4) somatotroph disease. GH deficiency can occur in isolation (isolated GH deficiency) or together with other pituitary deficiencies (multiple pituitary hormone deficiencies [MPHDs] or combined pituitary hormone deficiencies [CPHD]). Patients with isolated GH deficiency should be followed clinically for the development of other pituitary hormone deficiencies because MPHD can evolve over time. Biochemical stimulation testing is necessary to establish the diagnosis of GH deficiency, GH resistance, or MPHD. In most affected children, the cause of GH deficiency is unknown (idiopathic GH deficiency).[84] Approximately one in four children with proven GH deficiency has an organic origin for their GH deficiency; half of these children will be diagnosed with a CNS tumor.[85]

Any type of hypothalamic disease or dysfunction can lead to or be associated with GHRH deficiency, including (1) tumors, (2) inflammation, (3) previous infection, (4) trauma (including previous surgery),[86] (5) bleeding, (6) irradiation, and (7) malformations (eg, septo-optic dysplasia [SOD]).[19] Low-dose irradiation of the hypothalamus and/or pituitary can cause idiopathic GH deficiency, whereas higher doses of irradiation can cause MPHD. SOD is defined by the triad of (1) midline brain defects, such as agenesis of the septum pellucidum and/or corpus callosum, (2) hypoplasia of the optic nerve, and (3) anterior and/or posterior pituitary hormone abnormalities. A small number of cases of SOD are explained by mutations in HESX1, SOX2, and SOX3, all of which are transcription factors. HEXS1 (chromosome 3p14.3) is a paired-like homeobox gene, SOX2 (chromosome 3q26.3) is the SRY (sex-determining region on the Y chromosome) box 2 gene, and SOX3 (chromosome Xq27.1) is the SRY box 3 gene. Midline brain tumors, such as meningiomas, gliomas, germinomas, third ventricle colloid cysts, ependymomas, and optic nerve gliomas, also affect the hypothalamus. Disruptions in the hypothalamic-pituitary portal system can result from tumors, inflammation, previous infection, trauma (including previous surgery), and irradiation.

Congenital GH deficiency from pituitary disease has many causes, including GHRHR gene mutations (idiopathic GH deficiency type IB), GH1 mutations (idiopathic GH deficiency types IA, IB, II, and III, and bioinactive GH), and transcription factor mutations (which usually cause MPHD: LHX3, LHX4, PROP1, Pit-1, RIEG) and malformations (anencephaly and holoprosencephaly) (Table 65.5).[79] Homozygous LHX3 mutations have caused panhypopituitarism, with the exception that ACTH was not affected.[87] Heterozygous LHX4 mutations have caused deficiencies of GH, TSH, and ACTH. PROP1 (name derived from PROphet of Pit-1; POU1F1; Pit-1 stands for "paired-like homeodomain transcription factor")[88] mutations cause deficiencies of GH, prolactin, TSH, and gonadotropins. ACTH deficiency has also occurred in some families. PROP1 gene mutations are inherited as autosomal recessive traits. Pit-1 gene mutations cause GH, prolactin, and variable degrees of TSH deficiencies. These transcription factor mutations may be inherited as autosomal recessive or dominant traits. Heterozygous RIEG gene mutations (PITX2, a paired-like homeobox gene) are the cause of Rieger syndrome, which may include GH deficiency. Features of Rieger syndrome encompass developmental abnormalities of the teeth, the anterior chamber of the eye, and the umbilicus. Mutations in GLI1, GLI2, Shh, ZIC2, SIX3, tgif, PATCHED1, DGF1, and FAST1 have variously been cited as causes of holoprosencephaly.[89] Children with midline facial clefts (cleft lip, cleft palate, or combined)

TABLE 65.5 Growth Hormone Deficiency of Genetic Etiology

Gene/Classification/Inheritance	Mutation	Phenotype
GH1; IA; AR	Deletion, FS, NS	Absent GH expression; immune resistance to GH treatment is common
GH1; IB; AR	Splicing?	Reduced GH; responds to GH treatment*
GHRHR; IB; AR	Possible MS	Reduced GH; responds to GH treatment*
GH1; II; AD	DN	Reduced GH; responds to GH treatment; MPHD is possible
Unknown; III; XLR	—	Reduced GH; responds to GH treatment; agammaglobulinemia is possible

*One third of heterozygotes may be short.

AD, Autosomal dominant inheritance; *AR,* autosomal recessive inheritance; *DN,* dominant negative; *FS,* frameshift; *GH,* growth hormone; *MS,* missense mutation; *NS,* nonsense mutation (stop codon); *XLR,* X-linked recessive; *?,* otherwise not defined.

or a single central incisor can exhibit GH deficiency. Two GH1 gene mutations have been identified to cause bioinactive GH.[90] In these mutations, GH does not have full biological activity but retains normal immunoreactivity. Therefore, in contrast to other forms of pituitary or hypothalamic disease, the GH concentration is not deficient. At least one reference laboratory provides GHRHR, GH1, and GHR gene sequencing services (Athena Diagnostics, Worcester, Massachusetts).[91-93]

Acquired causes of pituitary disease include (1) tumors (anterior pituitary adenoma, craniopharyngioma), (2) congenital cysts (Rathke cleft cyst, arachnoid cyst), (3) infiltrative disease (amyloidosis or histiocytosis), (4) inflammation (autoimmune, granulomatous or IgG4-related hypophysitis), (5) infection, (6) trauma (including surgery), (7) bleeding, (8) irradiation, (9) infarction (pituitary apoplexy from Sheehan syndrome), and (10) metabolic derangement (hemochromatosis, iron overload from long-term transfusion therapy, or certain anemias, such as sideroblastic anemia).[94] Hemochromatosis does not cause hypopituitarism until many decades have passed.[95] Some investigators believe that all patients with “idiopathic” hypopituitarism should be screened for hemochromatosis.[96]

Investigation of Growth Hormone Deficiency. A staged approach for the evaluation of GH secretion is advised.[97] Initial screening can involve one of the following tests: (1) measurement of IGF-I (with or without IGFBP-3), or (2) GH measurement after exercise. A definitive diagnosis of GH deficiency in children requires the performance of a GH stimulation test. All forms of GH testing should be performed after the subject has fasted overnight. If a GH screening test is abnormal, definitive testing should be pursued.[98] If GH adequacy is demonstrated by GH screening tests, definitive GH testing need not be performed unless there is a very high index of suspicion for GH deficiency. In peripubertal children, the likelihood of a falsely abnormal GH screening test can be reduced by pretreatment of both boys and girls with a short course of sex steroids (ethinyl estradiol [40 μg/m^2 daily] for 2 days before testing).[99] The mechanism of sex-steroid priming is unclear; however, sex steroids appear to play a major role in increasing the response of IGF-I to GH at the time of puberty. From clinical experience, GH deficiency is overdiagnosed in some peripubertal children who are tested without the benefit of sex hormone priming.

Exercise physiologically enhances GH release.[100] Typically, in the fasting state, the child exercises vigorously for approximately 20 minutes (eg, running up and down stairs, running on a treadmill). At the completion of the exercise, when the child is tachycardic and sweating, a venous sample is collected for GH measurement (Box 65.2). A baseline GH measurement is not required. A GH concentration may also be obtained 40 minutes after exercise, in case of a delayed GH release.

Finally, screening for GH deficiency can be performed by measuring GH 60 to 90 minutes following clonidine, glucagon, or L-dopa administration. (Note: L-dopa is not currently available in the United States.) Doses of clonidine, glucagon, and L-dopa are identical to doses used in formal GH testing scenarios (see the subsequent text).

It has been argued that measuring GH during sleep is a physiologic assessment of the hypothalamic-somatotroph-GH axis. Some authorities suggest electroencephalographic monitoring with GH measured during deep sleep (eg, stage III, stage IV). More simply, GH could be measured 1 hour after the onset of sleep. However, in reality, these types of sleep studies are cumbersome because they require hospitalization or overnight boarding in a sleep laboratory. In practice, this is rarely done. Furthermore, the high cost of hospitalization or the sleep laboratory suggests that an exercise tolerance test or a simple pharmacologic stimulus would be a more cost-effective approach to initial GH testing.

Reference intervals for IGF-I and IGFBP-3 are age- and sex-dependent.[101] If IGF-I is within its reference interval for age and sex in children, GH deficiency is excluded. If IGF-I is low, definitive GH testing is required. Because IGF-I concentrations can be depressed in states of (1) malnutrition, (2) malabsorption, (3) chronic disease, (4) hypothyroidism, and (5) sex hormone deficiency, a low IGF-I concentration does not confirm GH deficiency. IGFBP-3 is less dependent on good nutrition to achieve normal concentrations, so it may be a superior marker of GH deficiency compared with IGF-I. However, one study failed to demonstrate that measuring IGFBP-3 alone or together with free IGF-I was superior to measuring IGF-I alone as a screening test for GH deficiency.[102] In another study, only approximately 50% of GH-deficient children had a low IGFBP-3 concentration; this finding calls into question its value as a sensitive screening test.[103]

Analytical advantages of IGFBP-3 measurements over IGF-I measurements include the following: (1) IGF-I must be separated from its binding proteins to be measured, but IGFBP-3 does not require a dissociation step; (2) IGFBP-3 is present in higher concentrations than IGF-I; and (3) less age dependency is seen for IGFBP-3 compared with IGF-I.[104] Because of their stability over the course of a day, IGF-I and IGFBP-3 measurements may be obtained randomly. However, some researchers have concluded that IGFBP-3 measurements are too nonspecific to be used for the evaluation of GH deficiency.[105] Furthermore, reports indicate that IGF-I

BOX 65.2 Protocol for the Exercise Stimulation Test for Growth Hormone

Rationale

Brisk exercise normally causes an increase in serum growth hormone (GH) concentrations.

Procedure

The test is best performed in the morning after an overnight fast, but may be done at any time. Vigorous physical exercise (running or calisthenics) is performed for 20 minutes. A venous blood specimen for determination of GH is drawn immediately after termination of exercise.

Interpretation

If the serum GH concentration is 7 to 10 μg/L or greater (depending on the specific GH immunoassay used), GH deficiency is unlikely in children. A normal response in adults is a GH concentration of ≥5 μg/L. In children, a single subnormal response is not diagnostic for GH deficiency and should be confirmed with a second provocative test.

BOX 65.3 Protocol for the Insulin-Induced Hypoglycemia Stimulation Test (Insulin Tolerance Test)

Rationale

The stress of insulin-induced hypoglycemia triggers the release of growth hormone (GH) and adrenocorticotropin hormone (ACTH) from the pituitary gland in normal subjects. The GH response is measured directly. Cortisol is measured as the indication of the ACTH response.

Procedure

The test is done after an overnight fast with the patient at bed rest. An indwelling intravenous (IV) line is inserted. Sampling begins after a 30-minute rest period. Baseline samples are drawn for determination of glucose, GH, and cortisol. Regular insulin, 0.1 to 0.15 U/kg body weight, is injected intravenously. Samples are then obtained at +10, +20, +40, and +60 minutes for glucose, GH, and cortisol determinations. Optional time points are +30, +75, +90, and +120 minutes. To be confident that adequate stress has been applied, the patient must become symptomatic (exhibit sweating or tremor), or the glucose concentration must fall to less than 40 to 45 mg/dL (2.2–2.5 mmol/L). Additional IV insulin may be given if this has not occurred by 30 minutes, in which case sampling should be prolonged by 30 minutes. The physician should be in attendance throughout the test, and 50% dextrose for IV administration should be kept on hand to be used in the event of severe hypoglycemic reaction and after adequate hypoglycemia has been documented. Glucagon (1 mg) should be available for parenteral administration in case IV access is lost. The test is contraindicated in older adult patients and those with a seizure disorder, ischemic heart disease, or cardiovascular insufficiency.

Interpretation

The serum cortisol concentration should increase to a peak value of 18 to 20 μg/dL (497–552 nmol/L) or greater. The serum GH concentration should rise to a peak value of 7 to 10 ng/mL (7–10 μg/L) or greater. No response or inadequate response may be due to pituitary hormone deficiency or a hypothalamic lesion.

BOX 65.4 Protocol for the Arginine Stimulation Test for Growth Hormone

Rationale

In normal subjects, intravenous (IV) administration of arginine hydrochloride stimulates growth hormone (GH) release.

Procedure

The test should be done after an overnight fast with the patient maintained at bed rest. A 10% solution of arginine hydrochloride, 0.5 g/kg body weight (maximum dose = 30 g), is infused intravenously over 30 minutes. Blood samples are drawn for determination of GH before the infusion is started, and 30, 60, and 90 minutes after the infusion is begun. Optional time points are +15 and +120 minutes.

Interpretation

The serum GH concentration should rise to a peak value of 7 to 10 ng/mL (7–10 μg/L) or greater. A subnormal response is seen in GH-deficient subjects, but a single subnormal GH response is not diagnostic for GH deficiency and should be confirmed with a second provocative test.

and IGFBP-3 exhibit imperfect sensitivity and specificity for the diagnosis of GH deficiency.[106]

IGF-I measurements in adults often are not diagnostically helpful.[107] For reasons that are unclear, IGF-I concentrations can be normal in GH-deficient adults. Therefore, a normal IGF-I does not rule out adult GH deficiency. If the IGF-I concentration is low and suspicion for GH deficiency is high (MPHD or childhood-onset severe GH deficiency), some experts would diagnose GH deficiency in the absence of GH testing.[108]

GH responses to insulin-induced hypoglycemia (insulin tolerance test [ITT]) (Box 65.3) and GH responses to centrally acting pharmacologic or biological agents (Box 65.4) are considered definitive tests. The stimuli can be sequential or administered on different days. The classical diagnosis of pediatric GH deficiency requires that GH responses to two different stimuli (Table 65.6) be deficient. In research settings, GHRH and GHRP-6 have been used to stimulate GH release. However, because these agents are not available for clinical use, they are not included in Table 65.6. Note that many variations of these protocols are available because endocrinologists often customize these tests. Diazepam and pentagastrin have been studied as GH secretogogues; however, experience with these agents is limited, and they are not included in Table 65.6.

Of children with appropriate stature for age, approximately 80% will have normal GH responses to one stimulus, and at least 95% will have normal GH responses to at least one of two stimuli. This is why two GH stimuli are generally recommended—to avoid overdiagnosis of GH deficiency. However, the GH Research Society advises that a single definitive abnormal test is adequate to diagnose GH deficiency if the child has (1) confirmed CNS pathology, (2) a history of CNS irradiation, (3) multiple pituitary hormone deficiencies, or (4) a genetic defect.[109]

A history of childhood GH deficiency, CNS disease, trauma, or irradiation is an indication to test adults for GH deficiency.[110,111] Retesting of adults with the diagnosis of childhood GH deficiency is necessary because not all adults with childhood GH deficiency remain GH deficient as adults. In adults, a single abnormal GH response to a stimulus is diagnostic of GH deficiency if the deficiency is congenital or genetic, or if multiple pituitary hormone deficiencies are due to organic disease. Guidelines published in 2009 recommended that a low IGF-I concentration in a patient with three or more pituitary hormone deficiencies is sufficient to diagnose GH deficiency.[112] Unfortunately, GH testing is not very reproducible.[113]

Insulin-induced hypoglycemia (ITT) is often considered to be the gold standard stimulus when hypoglycemia is achieved (glucose <40–45 mg/dL) (<2.2–2.5 mmol/L).[114] The risk associated with this type of test is that untreated severe hypoglycemia can be life threatening. Venous access for infusion of glucose is important during the ITT. If vascular

TABLE 65.6 Growth Hormone Stimuli

GH Stimulus	Dose	GH Sampling* (min)
Glucagon	0.03–0.1 mg/kg, IM, max 1 mg	0, 30, 60, 90, 120, 150, 180, ±240 (maximum response ≈2–3 hours)
L-Dopa	500 mg/M^2 (15 mg/kg) max 500 mg (or) <15 kg: 125 mg 15–30 kg: 250 mg >30 kg: 500 mg	0, 40, 60, 90, 120
Clonidine	0.15 mg/M^2 <13.6 kg: 0.05 mg >13.6 kg: 0.1 mg (0.1 mg/tab)	0, 30, 60, 90
Arginine HCl	0.5 g/kg, max 30 g (10% solution IV over 30 min)	0, ±15, 30, 60, 90, ±120
Insulin tolerance test	0.1 U/kg (0.05–0.15) IV push insulin	0, 10, 20, ±30, 40, 60, ±75, ±90, ±120
Arginine-insulin tolerance test	Arginine: begin at time zero, give insulin at +60 min	0, 30, 60, 70, 80, 100, 120

*Experts may differ on the best interval of GH measurements; ± indicates an optional time point.

GH, Growth hormone; *HCl*, hydrogen chloride; *IM*, intramuscular; *IV*, intravenous.

access is lost during the ITT, glucagon should be readily available for an intramuscular injection (the dose of glucagon is 1 mg). If intravenous access cannot be ensured, stimuli other than insulin should be considered. In general, GH stimulation tests are not conducted by laboratory personnel because of the risks and complexities of testing. Arginine infusion presents the danger of acidosis and even death.[115]

Stimulated GH concentration less than 7 to 10 ng/mL (7–10 μg/L) defines GH deficiency in children.[116] The cutoff defining GH deficiency is method-dependent and subject to interpretation by clinicians and may vary between countries. The definition of GH deficiency also differs between adults and children. In adults, GH deficiency is present when stimulated GH is less than 5 ng/mL (5 μg/L). GH deficiency in adults can be parsed according to the stimulus. For ITTs, a deficient peak GH response is less than 3 ng/mL (3 μg/L). For GHRH plus arginine, a deficient peak GH response is less than 11 ng/mL (<11 μg/L) when the body mass index (BMI) is less than 25 kg/m^2. However if the BMI is 25 to 30 kg/m^2, deficiency is defined as less than 8 ng/mL (<8 μg/L), and for BMI greater than 30 kg/m^2, deficiency is identified as less than 4 ng/mL (<4 μg/L). Because GHRH is not commercially available, and clonidine and arginine alone are not helpful in defining GH deficiency in adults, the ITT remains the best test of GH secretion in adults.

Controversy continues as to what constitutes a normal GH response to stimuli because insulin-induced hypoglycemia is considered by some to be a nonphysiologic stimulus. Discordance between normal stimulated GH concentration and a deficient spontaneous rise in GH concentration has been described as neurosecretory GH deficiency.[117] Neurosecretory GH deficiency can result from CNS or hypothalamic disease. The diagnosis of neurosecretory GH deficiency requires overnight blood sampling with GH measurements every 20 minutes, which is a protocol that ordinarily requires hospitalization. The combined costs of GH assays, physician fees, and inpatient services would exceed several thousand dollars.

The definition of partial GH deficiency is especially problematic because the definition of GH deficiency is itself controversial.[118,119] Eliminating GH stimulation testing has been proposed, with the diagnosis of GH deficiency based on growth parameters, IGF-I, and IGFBP-3 measurements, neuroradiologic investigation, and genetic considerations.[120-122] There is increased pressure to diagnose GH deficiency because the clinical indications for GH therapy are expanding. Non-GH deficient conditions are also sometimes treated with GH (eg, Prader-Willi syndrome, Turner syndrome, and chronic renal failure). There is concern about the long-term risks of GH therapy.[123]

Growth Hormone Resistance

In children with short stature and low growth velocity, if IGF-I is (1) below the reference interval for the child's bone age and gender, (2) if the GH concentration is normal or elevated, and (3) if non–GH-dependent causes of IGF-I deficiency (malnutrition, malabsorption, chronic disease, hypothyroidism, and sex hormone deficiency compared with the patient's bone age) have been excluded, GH resistance should be considered.[124] As uncommon as GH deficiency is in the general pediatric population (1 in 10,000 children), GH resistance as a primary problem is far less frequent.

GH resistance can be congenital, resulting from loss-of-function GHR mutations or GHR signaling defects (STAT5b mutations),[125,126] or from defects in the production of IGF-I itself. Most GHR mutations involve the extracellular domain that involves GH binding to the GHR. Some GHR mutations affect homodimerization. Loss of the intracellular GHR domain can result from splice-site mutations. GHR is not expressed on the cell surface if the transmembrane domain is defective. Recall that circulating GHBP is derived from the extracellular domain of the GHR. Most cases of GHR deficiency display low or absent concentrations of GHBP. STAT5b is necessary for normal GH-GHR signaling to the cell nucleus. These are autosomal recessive disorders. Size at birth is normal because in utero IGF-I production is independent of GH.

IGF-I gene–inactivating mutations or deletions are rare, and only two such mutations have been described. In contrast to GHR and signaling defects, when IGF-I itself cannot be produced because of intrinsic IGF-I gene mutations, intrauterine growth retardation will result, in addition to extrauterine growth failure. Other consequences of IGF-I gene mutations include severe mental retardation, deafness, and micrognathia (mandibular hypoplasia).[127,128]

IGF-I and IGFBP-3 concentrations are low in rare cases of ALS deficiency, whereas baseline and poststimulation GH concentrations are normal.[129] Although adolescence was delayed, adult stature was nearly normal in persons with ALS deficiency.

Acquired GH resistance is far more common than congenital GH resistance. In cases of acquired GH resistance, the IGF-I is low (despite sufficient GH secretion) because of malnutrition, malabsorption, chronic disease, hypothyroidism, or sex hormone deficiency. An acquired form of GH resistance has also been observed in patients with idiopathic GH deficiency type I; they develop GH-inhibitory antibodies when treated with exogenous GH. Because GH is absent in this form of congenital GH deficiency, exogenous GH is seen by the immune system as foreign. Apparently, the resulting antibodies directed against exogenous GH bind to, and inactivate, the GH. This is reminiscent of the development of factor VIII antibodies in some boys with severe hemophilia A, who are treated with exogenous factor VIII.

A number of criteria for GH resistance have been proposed, including (1) height more than 3 SDs below the mean for age; (2) basal GH greater than 2.5 ng/mL (>2.5 μg/L); (3) basal IGF-I less than 50 ng/mL; (4) basal IGFBP-3 more than 2 SDs below the mean for age; (5) an increase in IGF-I of less than 15 ng/mL after 4 days of GH treatment (0.05 mg/kg/day); and (6) increase in IGFBP-3 of less than 0.4 μg/mL after GH treatment. The largest concentrations of subjects with GH resistance are found in Israel and southern Ecuador.[130]

Insulin-Like Growth Factor-I Resistance

Even less common than GH resistance as a cause of growth failure is IGF-I resistance.[131,132] IGF-I resistance is characterized by growth failure despite elevations in GH and IGF-I. In contrast to GH deficiency and GH resistance states, and in common with IGF-I gene mutations, IGF-I resistance causes intrauterine growth retardation and growth failure in childhood. IGF-I resistance can result from mutations in the type I IGF receptor (IGFR) or from downstream signaling mutations.

Rare cases of familial short stature have been ascribed to hemizygosity for the type I IGF receptor gene.[133] Approximately 1 in 50 children with intrauterine growth retardation, short stature, and normal IGF-I concentrations have heterozygous type I IGF receptor mutations.

Measurement of Growth Hormone in Blood

A variety of isotopic and nonisotopic assays for GH are commercially available; most of the modern GH assays use mouse monoclonal antibodies and recombinant-derived GH as the competing (labeled) antigens, or as calibrators. Gravimetrically prepared international reference preparations (IRPs), such as the World Health Organization (WHO) international standard of IRP 80/505 human GH recombinant (hGHr), which has a potency of 3.3 IU/mg of r-hGH, or other reference preparations, such as WHO IRP 66/217 or 88/624, have been developed. International collaborative groups have recommended use of the WHO IRP 98/574 to harmonize GH assays,[134,135] and some commercially available two-site noncompetitive immunoassays have been harmonized to this IRP.[136,137]

Noncompetitive two-site immunoassays for GH are widely available; most include monoclonal antibodies coupled to an enzyme, chemiluminescent, or fluorescent label. Sensitivity as low as 0.05 ng/mL (0.05 μg/L) has been reported for an electrochemiluminescent immunoassay.[137] Mass spectrometric methods for GH measurement have also been described.[138,139] Many of these mass spectrometric methods were developed for detecting GH doping by athletes but are in clinical use as well.

Although GH is filtered in the glomerulus and excreted in the urine, measurement of urinary GH concentration is not clinically useful.

Analytical Challenges

GH is not a single molecular species, but instead exists in the circulation as a heterogeneous mixture of structural isoforms, including monomeric, dimeric, and oligomeric forms, as well as posttranslationally modified monomers with molecular weights ranging from 20 to 22 kDa.[140]

Two genes on chromosome 17q code human GH: the product of one is designated GH-N (or GH1) and is expressed primarily in the pituitary; the other is designated GH-V (or GH2) and is derived from the placenta (see the earlier discussion in this chapter). Both products are 22-kDa proteins, but they differ at 13 residues, and the GH-N isoform is susceptible to deletion of an internal 15 amino acid sequence, producing a 20-kDa GH isoform that accounts for 5% to 10% of the total GH; it has a propensity to dimerize. Normally, the human gene for GH that directs the synthesis of a monomeric 22-kDa protein accounts for most of the GH found in the circulation. The 20-kDa variant has less biological activity and does not react with some GH assays, but antibodies that specifically recognize the 20-kDa variant are available.[141] No clinical indications are known for measuring the 20-kDa form of GH, but it has been suggested that it can be used to detect GH doping in sports (see the following). Because recombinant GH is the 22-kDa isoform, and exogenous GH suppresses endogenous secretion of the hormone, administration of the recombinant hormone should suppress production of the 20-kDa variant; this effect has been demonstrated.[142] The immunoreactivity of the oligomeric (up to pentameric) isoforms of GH has not been well characterized, although it is known that they have reduced bioactivity and clearance.

Approximately one-half of circulating GH is bound to GHBP derived from the extracellular domain of the GH receptor,[143,144] and a small amount (5%–8%) is bound to a low-affinity protein.[145] Generally, anti-GH antibodies have sufficiently higher affinity for GH to compete with GH-binding proteins when enough time is allowed for the GH-protein complexes to dissociate. Therefore, immunoassays provide a good approximation of total hormone concentration. Assays for measuring unbound (free) GH have also been developed.[146] Free GH concentrations are proportional to total GH and are inversely proportional to GHBP, but the clinical usefulness of free GH measurements has not been established. Significant challenges remain in the harmonization of methods for GH measurements.[147,148]

Detecting Growth Hormone Doping in Athletes

Because GH promotes anabolic and lipolytic activities, it has been used by athletes to enhance their physical size, strength, and endurance. In response, the World Anti-Doping Agency has banned the use of GH by athletes competing in sanctioned events. Detecting GH use is challenging, however, because recombinant forms of the hormone are available that are identical to endogenous GH, and normal GH concentrations vary significantly because of the pulsatile nature of hormone release from the pituitary.[149] Although suppression of the

20-kDa GH isoform has showed some promise as a marker of GH doping, most current strategies focus on secondary markers, including IGF and IGFBP.[150-152]

Specimen Collection and Storage

The preferred specimen is serum; plasma with ethylenediaminetetraacetic acid (EDTA) or heparin added to prevent coagulation may also be used, but values are method dependent. Serum specimens should be stored at 2 to 8°C if they are not to be tested within 8 hours. If specimens must be stored for longer periods, they should be frozen at −20°C or colder.

Comments

A single basal or random concentration of GH provides limited diagnostic information. As discussed earlier in this chapter, secretion of GH by the pituitary gland is both episodic and pulsatile, and transient concentrations of up to 40 ng/mL (40 μg/L) have been observed in normal healthy subjects. Serum concentrations are low between pulses in healthy individuals, and some immunoassays are not sensitive enough to distinguish patients with abnormally low concentrations from healthy individuals who have concentrations that happen to fall in the low to normal reference interval. In some individuals, spontaneous low GH secretion is better monitored by using a continuous withdrawal pump or by drawing specimens for GH assay every 20 to 30 minutes over a 12- to 24-hour period (eg, during evaluation of neurogenic GH deficiency). Several stimulation tests have been developed to assess the adequacy of GH secretion (as discussed previously), including the ITT, arginine and GHRH, GHRH and GHRP, and glucagon stimulation tests. Consensus guidelines have been published for diagnosis of GH deficiency; the commonly accepted ITT cutoff for GH deficiency in adults is less than 3 ng/mL (<3 μg/L) after insulin suppression of glucose concentrations to less than 40 mg/dL (<2.2 mmol/L).[153]

Measurement of Insulin-Like Growth Factors

The liver is the primary source of circulating IGF-I (somatomedin C), but autocrine and paracrine production of IGF-I (as controlled by GH) is responsible for growth; IGF-I is the principal mediator of somatotropic GH activity.[154]

IGF-I has a longer biological half-life than GH, so its measurement provides an integrated estimate of GH secretion; it is also a more sensitive measure of GH excess in acromegaly. IGF-II is a fetal GH, and the clinical usefulness of measuring IGF-II is limited to patients being investigated for a possible IGF-II–secreting tumor causing insulin-independent hypoglycemia.[51]

Current IGF-I methods should use a reference material that is traceable to the International Reference Preparation IGF-I 87/518, or the newer WHO First International Standard 02/254.[155] To avoid interference from IGF-binding proteins, many assays isolate IGF using a variety of extraction methods, including (1) gel filtration, (2) acid-ethanol precipitation, (3) cryoprecipitation, (4) C-18 column extraction, or (5) reversed-phase chromatography.[156] Direct (no extraction) procedures are also available, but extraction methods prevent the formation of complexes with carrier proteins and serum proteases. Moreover, extraction procedures are better able to discriminate between GH-deficient patients and age-matched controls. Commercial assays that include chemiluminescent labels are available for measuring IGF-I, usually with minimal cross-reactivity to IGF-II (0%–3%). It is important to establish age- and sex-related reference intervals for IGF-I because of marked differences in hormone concentrations between adults and children and between males and females. Mass spectrometric methods for IGF-I have been described.[157] As with GH methods, harmonization of IGF-I assays remains a challenge.[158-160]IGFBP-3 is the major protein carrier of circulating IGF-I and is an indirect measure of GH activity. IGFBP-3 measurements, therefore, provide additional evidence in cases of suspected GH deficiency. Immunoassays for measuring IGFBP-3 have been reviewed.[161] Measurement of IGF-I has become a staple in the evaluation of GH abnormalities, but problems with interassay agreement remain, mostly related to binding proteins.[158] The availability of reliable reference materials against which immunoassays for IGF-I may be calibrated has been problematic.

Specimen Collection and Storage

Serum or plasma (with heparin or EDTA added to prevent coagulation) is used, depending on the assay method. Samples should be centrifuged within 1 hour of collection and stored frozen at −20°C or colder for up to 30 days. Some procedures use dried whole blood or serum collected on filter paper.[162]

POINTS TO REMEMBER

- Compared with the measurement of other anterior pituitary hormones, prolactin can be measured in the absence of stimulation or suppression.
- There are many causes of hyperprolactinemia that should be considered in the evaluation of hyperprolactinemia.
- The first line of treatment for prolactinomas is medical therapy, with the administration of drugs with dopamine-like action.

Prolactin

Prolactin is secreted by lactotrophs of the adenohypophysis.[163] Prolactin stimulates and sustains lactation in postpartum mammals after the mammary glands have been prepared by other hormones, including estrogens, progesterone, GH, corticosteroids, and insulin.

Biochemistry

Hypothalamic prolactin release inhibitory hormone (PRIH) is dopamine, which is a product of the tuberoinfundibular cells and the hypothalamic tuberohypophyseal dopaminergic system. In lactotrophs, dopamine binds to the type 2 dopamine (D2) receptor, one of five dopamine receptors. Dopamine receptors are located in the caudate putamen, nucleus accumbens, and olfactory tubercle, affecting (1) locomotion, (2) learning, (3) memory, (4) reward, and (5) reinforcement.

The gene for the D2 receptor is located on chromosome 11q2, contains 443 amino acids, and has a mass of 50.6 kDa. The extracellular domain is 37 amino acids, and 7 transmembrane domains are present, along with a 14 amino acid cytoplasmic domain. A large extracellular loop is evident between amino acids 211 and 373. Three potential sites of N-glycosylation have been noted: amino acids 5, 17, and 23. A disulfide bridge may occur between amino acids 107 and 182. Three isoforms of the D2 receptor have been identified: the full-length isoform is referred to as D2 (long); isoform 2 is D2 (short) and lacks amino acids 242 to 270; isoform 3,

D2 (longer), contains a val → trp-glu substitution at position 270. Mutations in the D2 receptor cause dystonia type 11 (myoclonus dystonia, or alcohol-responsive dystonia).

The gene that encodes prolactin was described in the section concerning the GH1 gene. Initially, preprolactin is synthesized (227 amino acids), and after cleavage of the leader sequence, the 199 amino acid prolactin hormone is liberated. Amino acid 59 is the site of putative N-glycosylation. Intrachain disulfide bonds are located between amino acids 32 and 39, 86 and 202, and 219 and 227.

Circulating prolactin exists in several forms: monomeric prolactin (23 kDa, "little" prolactin), dimeric prolactin (48–56 kDa, "big" prolactin), and polymeric prolactin (>100 kDa, "big, big" prolactin). Occasionally, and independent of the presence or absence of disease, IgG autoantibodies against prolactin can bind to prolactin, forming macroprolactin. The presence of macroprolactin elevates the total prolactin concentration, as the result of lower clearance, in the absence of excess prolactin secretion by the anterior pituitary lactotrophs. Failure to recognize macroprolactin can lead to the inappropriate diagnosis of hyperprolactinemia. In nature, many examples of macroproteins resulting from the complex of an antibody and a protein can be found, including macro-creatine kinase, macro-amylase, macro–lactate dehydrogenase, and macro-aspartate aminotransferase.[164]

The gene for the prolactin receptor (PRLR) is located at chromosome 5p13.2. Pre-PRLR is 622 amino acids (69.5 kDa). Upon removal of the signal peptide, the full-length PRLR is released (598 amino acids). The first 210 amino acids of the receptor are extracellular, 24 amino acids are present in the transmembrane domain, and the cytoplasmic domain consists of 364 amino acids. Amino acids 27 to 121 (with reference to preprolactin) represent a fibronectin type III-1 domain, whereas amino acids 127 to 227 represent a fibronectin type III-2 domain. Amino acids 215 to 219 display a WSXWS motif, and amino acids 267 to 275 display a box 1 motif. The WSXWS motif is the tryptophan-serine-wild card-tryptophan-serine sequence located near the lipid bilayer. Box 1 motifs are expressed in the cytoplasmic domain of receptors that engage in JAK2 receptor signaling. Glycosylation may occur at amino acids 59, 104, and 233, and intrachain disulfide bonds occur between amino acids 36 and 46, and 75 and 86. The PRLR forms a homodimer upon binding prolactin.

Eight isoforms of the PRLR have been described. Isoform 1 is the full-length PRLR. In isoform 2, amino acids 24 to 124 are missing. In isoform 3, amino acids 229 (aspartate) and 230 (phenylalanine) are replaced, respectively, by alanine and tryptophan (amino acids 231–622 are missing; therefore, this protein lacks a transmembrane domain, and the protein is soluble). This isoform has been reported as the product of a breast cancer cell line. Isoform 4 has changes in the amino acid sequence of amino acids 338 to 376, with the remaining amino acids deleted, and is nonfunctional. Because of a deletion of part of exon 10, and a frameshift mutation, the sequence of isoform 5 is altered among amino acids 337 to 349; thereafter the remaining amino acids are absent. In isoform 6, amino acids 286 to 288 (lysine-glycine-lysine) are replaced, respectively, by valine, tyrosine, and proline, and the amino acids distal to 288 are absent; this receptor is nonfunctional. Isoform 7 is secreted with changes in amino acids 229 to 268, and amino acids 269 to 622 are absent. Last, isoform 8 begins at amino acid 72, and amino acids 286 to 288 are replaced, respectively, by valine, tyrosine, and proline; the amino acids distal to 288 are absent, as in isoform 6.

Physiology

In women, prolactin is necessary for lactation after delivery of the newborn. Recent work in animal models provides some evidence that the different prolactin isoforms may have independent biological functions. In addition, the discovery of extrapituitary sites of prolactin secretion has also provided insights into a wider function of this hormone.[165] Prolactin is stimulated by breast-feeding, chest wall disease, and stress. Although prolactin is higher during the day than at night, and a night-to-day prolactin ratio greater than 1:2 is considered normal, the ratio has no diagnostic value. Prolactin is measured in its basal state without stimulatory or suppressive manipulation. As with other adenohypophyseal hormones, the release of prolactin is episodic and varies predictably during the day, with lowest concentrations found at midday and highest values found shortly after the onset of deep sleep.

Receptors for prolactin are located in the hypothalamus, breast, and ovaries. Breast development during puberty can occur in the absence of prolactin, but estrogen is required, along with GH and GH-stimulated IGF-I. Fetal breast development is stimulated by parathyroid hormone–related peptide, which shares the N-terminal active domain of parathyroid hormone but has extraparathyroidal origins.

Prolactin secretion by lactotrophs is controlled predominantly through suppression by PRIH.[166] In addition, prolactin may provide feedback centrally to stimulate PRIH in a short negative feedback loop, but this has been difficult to confirm. An ultra-short feedback loop is present where prolactin suppresses its own release. In addition to high concentrations of TRH, other factors that may stimulate prolactin secretion include oxytocin, vasoactive intestinal polypeptide, basic fibroblast growth factor, EGF, hypothalamic prolactin-releasing peptide, galanin, and neurotensin. Identified in the hypothalamus, amygdala, basal ganglia, and dorsal gray matter of the spinal cord, neurotensin is a 13 amino acid peptide neurotransmitter. Neurotensin affects gastrointestinal function and has a role in pain perception.[167]

Estrogen increases prolactin gene transcription and secretion; this explains why prolactin concentrations are higher in women than in men. The upper limit of the prolactin reference interval for women is approximately 20 ng/mL (≈420 mIU/L), whereas in men it is approximately 10 ng/mL (≈210 mIU/L). Prolactin rises during pregnancy because of elevated concentrations of sex steroids (predominantly estradiol). The average serum prolactin during pregnancy is approximately 200 ng/mL (≈4200 mIU/L). Because of increased lactotrophs, the pituitary approximately doubles in size during pregnancy.

The breast is prepared for lactation during pregnancy through the actions of (1) estrogen, (2) progesterone, (3) prolactin, (4) GH-V, (5) hPL, and possibly (6) IGF-I.[168] As the visible size of the breast increases during pregnancy, many microscopic changes also occur in breast tissue. Typically, lactation is not active until after delivery, when estrogen and progesterone concentrations have declined. Prolactin increases amino acid and glucose uptake by breast tissue, and synthesis of α-lactalbumin and β-casein, lactose, and milk fats is increased.

Postpartum, a positive feedback loop is seen between suckling and milk production. Transmitted via nerve fibers from the nipple to the CNS, suckling reduces PRIH, which increases prolactin release. With suckling, prolactin can rise by more than eightfold over baseline. The positive feedback loop of suckling, prolactin secretion, and milk production is a "stimulus-secretion" reflex. However, with continued breast-feeding, prolactin concentrations decline. One report observed mean prolactin concentrations of 162 ng/mL (≈3400 mIU/L) 2 to 4 weeks postpartum, 130 ng/mL (≈2730 mIU/L) 5 to 14 weeks postpartum, and 77 ng/mL (≈1620 mIU/L) 15 to 24 weeks postpartum. Suckling also stimulates oxytocin release, which is discussed in the section of this chapter concerning the posterior pituitary.

Because elevated prolactin concentrations reduce LH and FSH by inhibiting GnRH release (a short feedback loop between prolactin and the hypothalamus), breast-feeding delays the onset of menses after delivery.[169] Lactation amenorrhea is beneficial because it temporarily ensures that the mother can adequately breast-feed her newborn before she becomes pregnant again. It is understood that oligomenorrhea, amenorrhea, and infertility in hyperprolactinemic women, and impotence and oligospermia in hyperprolactinemic men, result from prolactin suppression of GnRH secretion. Prolactin has direct effects on prolactin receptors in the ovaries.

The role of prolactin in the immune system is controversial. At this time, it is difficult to ascribe any major, specific immune function to prolactin.

Hyperprolactinemia

Hyperprolactinemia is the most common hypothalamic-pituitary disorder encountered in clinical endocrinology.[170] Prolactin concentrations may be elevated in women who have only subtle alterations in fertility, such as (1) anovulation with or without menstrual irregularity, (2) amenorrhea and galactorrhea, or (3) galactorrhea alone. In men, prolactin excess usually manifests as a result of low serum testosterone, with reduced libido and central weight gain. Hyperprolactinemia can also cause galactorrhea in men. In addition, men with prolactin-secreting anterior pituitary adenomas more often than women present with macroadenomas and visual field disturbances resulting from a large tumor pressing on the optic chiasm.

An irregular menstrual period frequently reveals a microadenoma (≤10 mm in diameter) in women. Elevated prolactin concentrations are observed in as many as 30% of women with polycystic ovarian syndrome and patients with clinically silent pituitary adenoma. If a borderline elevation of prolactin is found, it is advisable to repeat the measurement on at least two other occasions, taking care to obtain a morning specimen under conditions of minimal excitement or stress to the patient (ie, no trauma and no breast stimulation). Ideally, the patient should not be on any medication that could stimulate prolactin release (discussed in more detail later in this section). The differential diagnosis of hyperprolactinemia is extensive (Table 65.7).

An extremely important cause of hyperprolactinemia is a prolactinoma.[171,172] The higher the prolactin concentration, the greater is the likelihood that hyperprolactinemia is the result of a prolactinoma. As a general rule, prolactin levels more than five times the upper limit of normal almost always indicate a prolactinoma. Hyperprolactinemia due to a macroprolactinoma (>10 mm in diameter) can produce prolactin concentrations into the tens of thousands (ng/mL). Prolactin concentrations greater than 200 ng/mL (approximately 4000 mIU/L) usually indicate a macroprolactinoma. Prolactinomas are diagnostically challenging. Because any degree of hyperprolactinemia can be seen in cases of prolactinoma, if hyperprolactinemia is otherwise not explained, a thorough search for a prolactinoma, including MRI imaging, should be undertaken. Idiopathic hyperprolactinemia does exist but is a diagnosis of exclusion. Mass displacement effects from an anterior pituitary tumor include destruction of the sella turcica, invasion of other structures, compression of the stalk, or optic nerve compression with bitemporal hemianopsia.

TABLE 65.7 Differential Diagnosis of Hyperprolactinemia

PRIH (dopamine) deficiency	Hypothalamic disease
	Interruption in the hypothalamic-pituitary portal system
Drugs	Dopamine antagonists
	Cholinergic antagonists
	Serotonergic antagonists
	Antipsychotic medication
Hormones	Estrogen, pregnancy
Neurogenic	Nursing (nipple stimulation)
	Chest wall disease
	Spinal cord injury
Other diseases	Hypothyroidism (pathologically elevated TRH can release prolactin)
	Chronic renal disease
	Cirrhosis

PRIH, Prolactin release-inhibiting hormone; *TRH*, thyrotropin-releasing hormone.

Early diagnosis of a prolactinoma is critical because therapy with dopamine agonists, such as bromocriptine, can reduce tumor size and control tumor progression.[173] Surgical excision of a prolactinoma usually is considered if there is tumor growth or failure to lower prolactin levels with dopamine agonist therapy (the "dopamine-resistant prolactinoma"), or where there is failure to quickly reverse any associated visual loss or in a patient intolerant of dopamine agonists.

Macroprolactinemia is a common cause of an elevated plasma prolactin concentration; this benign condition should be ruled out before additional diagnostic studies are performed.[174] Macroprolactinemia can result from elevated circulating concentrations of the polymeric forms of prolactin and/or from prolactin-immunoglobulin complexes with molecular masses in excess of 100 kDa.

Polymeric forms of prolactin lack biological activity; thus, none of the sequelae associated with an elevated prolactin concentration (sexual dysfunction and galactorrhea) are present. In addition, macroprolactinemia is not associated with negative or positive feedback effects at the hypothalamus. Because macroprolactin is formed outside of lactotrophs, it is not found in pituitary tissue, and its size prevents entry into the cerebrospinal fluid. Therefore, macroprolactin appears to be confined to the vascular compartment.

Macroprolactinemia, although asymptomatic, is troublesome for clinicians and the laboratory because it is detected by most prolactin immunoassays. In one report, almost 20% of patients who presented for a clinical workup for prolactinoma had hyperprolactinemia attributable to the presence of macroprolactin. Although the prevalence of macroprolactinemia was approximately 1.5% in the population studied, the report suggested that macroprolactinemia is more common than was previously realized. Thus, clinical laboratories must be able to rule out the presence of a macroprolactin.[175] Macroprolactin can be precipitated by the addition of polyethylene glycol (PEG) to serum; this is the most common laboratory approach to detecting macroprolactin (see details in the section *Measurement of Prolactin*.[176]

Another diagnostic challenge in the investigation of hyperprolactinemia is the presence of a pituitary incidentaloma in a patient with elevated prolactin that could potentially lead to inappropriate medical or surgical treatment.[177-179] A lesion identified by MRI cannot unequivocally be associated with hyperprolactinemia because of the possibility of an incidentaloma. Incidental pituitary adenomas are common, occurring in 10% to 20% of the population.[180] Compression of the optic chiasm, or destruction of bone, argues against an incidentaloma, but mild to modest elevations in prolactin concentrations (50–200 ng/mL) are possible when other anterior pituitary tumors compress the hypothalamic-pituitary portal system, impairing the delivery of PRIH to the lactotrophs; the so-called "stalk" effect or pseudoprolactinoma. Treatment with a dopamine agonist should lower prolactin concentrations in cases of a true prolactinoma, but will not reduce prolactin concentration with pseudoprolactinoma. Prolactin measurements are also susceptible to a high-dose hook effect that may lead to a missed diagnosis of a macroprolactinoma.[181] If a macroadenoma is identified by MRI, but the prolactin is only modestly elevated, clinicians may request that the prolactin be remeasured at 1 to 10 and 1 to 100 dilution. If a hook effect is present, the concentration of the diluted sample will be significantly greater than that of the undiluted sample (see Chapter 23 for more detail).

MRI of the pituitary gland is performed as part of the clinical assessment when a prolactinoma is suspected. Unless a pituitary tumor can be demonstrated by MRI, prolactin-secreting microadenoma (≤10 mm in diameter) is diagnosed by exclusion. Because half of all prolactin-secreting microadenomas are too small to be detected by imaging methods, differentiating between a small pituitary tumor, prolactin-cell hyperplasia, and idiopathic hyperprolactinemia may not be possible.

Medications that stimulate prolactin release (through PRIH suppression) are the most common cause of hyperprolactinemia in otherwise healthy individuals.[182,183] When significant elevation of prolactin is confirmed, a careful history should rule out the possibility that medications are the cause. In addition to estrogens, dopamine receptor blockers (such as the phenothiazines) and dopamine antagonists (such as metoclopramide and domperidone used to treat gastrointestinal diseases as an antiemetic) cause significant increases in prolactin. Certain psychiatric drugs, including haloperidol and risperidone and selective serotonin reuptake inhibitors, monoamine oxidase inhibitors and some tricyclics may cause elevated prolactin. Antihypertensive agents (such as β-blockers and calcium channel blockers) and antihistamines (such as cimetidine and ranitidine) are associated with modest elevations in prolactin. Thyrotropin (TSH) measurements should be considered in patients suspected of a prolactinoma, to rule out primary hypothyroidism; in rare cases of severe primary hypothyroidism, TRH will promote release of prolactin. A pregnancy test should be performed in women of reproductive age because pregnancy is a cause of hyperprolactinemia (see Table 65.7).

Prolactin Deficiency

Prolactin is of great clinical importance in the postpartum period, because prolactin is required for lactation.[184] Without the availability of infant formulas or wet nurses, failure of maternal lactation can be fatal to the newborn. However, other than the necessity of breast-feeding, prolactin deficiency in humans may not have adverse consequences.

Measurement of Prolactin

Prolactin assays typically involve noncompetitive, heterogeneous "sandwich" techniques that use two antibodies that recognize different epitopes on the prolactin polypeptide.[185]

Structural variations in circulating prolactin result in biases between immunoassays for this hormone. Monomeric prolactin accounts for more than 85% of the total circulating hormone, but glycosylated and inactive complexed forms ("big" and "big-big" prolactin, respectively) constitute a significant fraction, and immunoreactivity of these prolactin complexes is variable. IgG-bound prolactin, now referred to as macroprolactin, is a relatively common finding in healthy patients, and according to one study, may account for up to 10% of misdiagnoses in hyperprolactinemic patients[175] because renal clearance of the Ig-bound hormone is reduced.[186] IgG-bound prolactin can be separated by gel chromatography, or more conveniently by precipitation of Ig complexes with the addition of PEG. PEG precipitation removes a small fraction of monomeric prolactin as well, but remains a useful method for distinguishing between clinical hyperprolactinemia and prolactin elevations due to prolactin-IgG complexes.[187,188] If the ratio of the precipitated prolactin to the total prolactin is 0.50 or greater, macroprolactinemia is said to be present.[189,190]

Prolactin methods should be calibrated against reference materials with known international unit potency, such as the WHO first IRP 75/504, the second international standard (IS) 83/562, or the third IS 84/500, to allow assay-to-assay comparison. Despite the heterogeneity of prolactin, immunoassays correlate well with bioassay-validated prolactin standards. A method for measuring prolactin by liquid chromatography/multiple reaction monitoring mass spectrometry has been described.[191]

Specimen Collection and Storage

Prolactin is measured in serum or plasma, although individual assays may recommend serum only. Special handling procedures are not necessary; specimens can be stored at 4°C for at least 24 hours, but should be frozen if analysis is delayed for longer than 24 hours. Emotional stress, exercise, ambulation, and a protein-rich diet all stimulate prolactin secretion; thus specimens collected after an overnight fast when the patient is resting provide the most reliable prolactin concentrations.

Adrenocorticotropic Hormone and Related Peptides

Adrenocorticotropic hormone (ACTH; corticotropin) is secreted by adenohypophysis as a derivative of

POINTS TO REMEMBER

- Cushing syndrome can be endogenous or exogenous from the excess administration of glucocorticoids.
- Endogenous Cushing syndrome can result from an anterior pituitary adenoma (ie, Cushing disease), ectopic ACTH or CRH secretion, or a cortisol-secreting adrenocortical tumor.
- ACTH deficiency produces cortisol deficiency, although aldosterone secretion remains intact.

pro-opiomelanocortin (POMC).[192,193] ACTH acts primarily on the adrenal cortex, stimulating its growth and the secretion of corticosteroids (specifically cortisol). ACTH production is increased during physiologic or psychologic stress.

Biochemistry

The biochemistry of ACTH, with its origin from POMC and POMC-derived peptides, is described in detail in Chapter 66.

Regulation of Adrenocorticotropic Hormone Secretion

Many variables affect the secretion of ACTH, which is both pulsatile and circadian in nature. Thus, regulation of pituitary secretion of ACTH by the hypothalamus is complex. The control of ACTH release by the pituitary is an integral part of the neuroendocrine regulation of stress homeostasis.

Cortisol is the major negative feedback hormone for the tonic inhibition of hypothalamic CRH and pituitary ACTH secretion. However, endogenous opioids such as met-enkephalin and β-endorphin, which are produced by the adrenal glands, have a downregulatory effect on the hypothalamic-pituitary-ACTH axis as well. Regulation of ACTH is discussed at length in Chapter 66.

Clinical Significance

Because ACTH synthesis originates from the POMC precursor peptide, its production by the pituitary is closely linked with the secretion of endogenous opioid peptides, such as β-endorphin.[194] The physiologic effects of endogenous opiates include (1) sedation, (2) an increased threshold of pain, and (3) autonomic regulation of respiration, blood pressure, and heart rate. These peptides are also involved in modifying endocrine responses to stress and water balance, and may play a role in the regulation of reproduction and the immune system.

Gonadotropin secretion by the pituitary is under inhibitory control by opioid peptides, as is evident by the effects of β-endorphin analogs on the pulse frequency and amplitude of pituitary LH release. In contrast, β-endorphin antagonists (such as naloxone) can elicit an increase in the amount and pattern of gonadotropin secretion. ACTH secretion is similarly downregulated by endogenous opioid peptides; therefore, naloxone causes an increase in plasma ACTH concentrations.

No diseases have been clearly associated with disordered metabolism of opioid peptides, but changes in their plasma concentrations may accompany other disorders, such as Cushing disease and depression (increased β-endorphin concentrations)[195] or pheochromocytoma (increased enkephalin concentrations; see Chapter 63). Altered concentrations of opioids in cerebrospinal fluid may reflect disorders such as chronic pain syndrome, schizophrenia, and depression.

In summary, the only POMC derivative that is measured in the diagnosis of certain human disease states is ACTH. Further discussion of adrenal disorders, including disorders of ACTH secretion, is found in Chapter 66.

Measurement of Adrenocorticotropic Hormone

Bioassays and receptor assays for ACTH are currently mostly of historical interest. Immunoassays that measure the concentration of ACTH are more common than bioassays or receptor assays. Competitive binding radioimmunoassays (RIAs) have been developed for ACTH; they differ in (1) the choice of radioactive label (125 iodine is the most common), (2) separation system (charcoal adsorption, PEG, or second-antibody precipitation), (3) antibody (N-terminal or C-terminal specificity), and (4) whether preextraction of ACTH is required. Most polyclonal antibodies recognize a segment of the biologically active N-terminal portion of the molecule and react with intact ACTH (amino acids 1–39), N-terminal ACTH fragments (amino acids 1–24), and ACTH precursors (eg, POMC and pro-ACTH).

Immunoradiometric ACTH assays that use labeled monoclonal antibodies in noncompetitive formats have also been developed.[196] In these assays, two monoclonal antibodies (or a polyclonal/monoclonal combination) are directed toward different sites on the ACTH molecule (eg, the N-terminal and C-terminal domains). These double antibody (sandwich) immunoassays can detect ACTH concentrations of 1 to 4 pg/mL (0.22–0.88 pmol/L). Monoclonal immunoassays have improved analytical specificity for intact ACTH, but may not recognize biologically active precursors and fragments.[197] Less specific ACTH immunoassays are sometimes used to detect the presence of these peptide fragments in patients with cancer-related syndromes (eg, ectopic ACTH Cushing syndrome); a two-site immunoradiometric assay has been developed for measuring ACTH precursors in plasma.[198] A direct (unextracted) immunoradiometric test kit for ACTH is commercially available that uses a polyclonal antibody–monoclonal antibody sandwich to detect ACTH; the monoclonal antibody is radiolabeled with 125 iodine. A nonisotopic time-resolved immunofluorometric method has also been reported.[199] ACTH assays have been developed for automated immunoassay platforms using chemiluminescent labels.[200] These methods are more precise than manual methods (coefficients of variation <8%), and analytically, they are sensitive enough to distinguish between low-normal and suppressed hormone secretion.

Quantitative results from different ACTH immunoassays may demonstrate bias as the result of calibration. Currently, manufacturers of commercial ACTH immunoassays usually calibrate their assays with ACTH preparations obtained from research centers, such as human purified ACTH 1-39 (MRC 74/555, 6.2 IU/25 μg), supplied by the National Institute for Biological Standards and Control (United Kingdom), or synthetic ACTH 1-39 (4.71 IU/50 μg), supplied by the US National Hormone and Pituitary Program, which was formerly known as the National Pituitary Agency. For comparison between assays, the calibrators used in a particular assay system must be clearly specified.

Specimen Collection and Storage

Some precautions are necessary in the collection, transportation, and storage of specimens. ACTH is easily oxidized, adsorbs to glass surfaces, and is rapidly degraded by plasma proteases into nonreactive fragments during freezing and thawing of the specimen. Factors that influence plasma ACTH, such as previous administration of corticosteroids, the time of day at which the specimen is collected (diurnal variation), and stress from the venipuncture procedure, should be taken into account. To minimize these problems, it is recommended that blood specimens are collected into prechilled polystyrene (plastic) tubes containing EDTA, immediately placed on ice, and centrifuged at 4°C. Some laboratories recommend the use of protease inhibitors, such as aprotinin (Trasylol). The plasma should be transferred to another plastic tube and frozen at −20°C or colder if analysis is delayed. In chilled samples with the addition of EDTA and aprotinin, the plasma proteases that would otherwise degrade ACTH are inhibited, permitting freezing and thawing without substantial subsequent degradation. Antioxidants, such as mercaptoethanol, may be used to stabilize ACTH. Immediately before the ACTH assay is set up, frozen specimens should be thawed and centrifuged to remove any fibrin clots that can interfere with the assay.

Measurement of Endogenous Opioid Peptides

β-Endorphin is a cleavage product of POMC, which is also the precursor to ACTH and β-lipotropin. Both RIAs and immunoradiometric assays have been developed for measurement of β-endorphin. Commercial assays are widely available, and most reference laboratories offer β-endorphin assays. The concentration of β-endorphin is usually very low or undetectable in healthy subjects, and some analytical methods require extraction procedures to detect meaningful concentrations in plasma. The specificity of commercial antibodies for β-endorphin (relative to β-lipotropin) can be variable, and some assays cross-react as much as 50% with β-lipotropin. Assays based on polyclonal antibodies may produce spuriously high results as the consequence of cross-reactivity with serum IgG (eg, in patients with an IgG myeloma).[201]

Met-enkephalin shares a 5 amino acid N-terminal sequence with β-endorphin but is thought to be derived from pro-enkephalin, rather than POMC. Measurement of met-enkephalin in plasma is difficult because of its very short half-life (2.5 minutes at 37°C). Even if blood is immediately chilled on ice and centrifuged under refrigeration, approximately 50% of met-enkephalin is lost unless the specimen is collected in 23 mmol/L of citric acid. Commercial assays for met-enkephalin have been developed, and anti-enkephalin antibodies are available. Assays for endogenous opioid peptides maybe useful for research purposes but are not currently applicable for solving clinical endocrine problems.

POINTS TO REMEMBER

- Reproduction is likely the most complex endocrine system.
- The secretion of LH and FSH is pulsatile.
- To establish LH and FSH deficiency, GnRH testing may be required.

Gonadotropins (Follicle-Stimulating Hormone, Luteinizing Hormone)

Luteinizing hormone and follicle-stimulating hormone are synthesized by gonadotrophs in the adenohypophysis. The actions of FSH are to (1) stimulate the growth and maturation of ovarian follicles, (2) stimulate estrogen secretion (estradiol), (3) promote, via estrogen, the endometrial changes characteristic of the first phase (proliferative or follicular) of the menstrual cycle, and (4) stimulate spermatogenesis in males. FSH is also called follitropin.

LH and FSH act synergistically to promote ovulation and secretion of androgens (androstenedione) and progesterone. The actions of LH are to (1) promote and maintain the second phase (secretory or luteal) of the menstrual cycle; (2) in females, to assist in the formation of the corpus luteum; and (3) in males, to stimulate the development and functional activity of testicular Leydig cells that produce testosterone. LH is also called interstitial cell–stimulating hormone, or lutropin.

Biochemistry

Under the generic term gonadotropins, LH and FSH control the functional activity of gonads. In males and females, gonadotropin secretion is regulated via GnRH.[202] Pituitary gonadotropin secretion is controlled by feedback from the gonadotropic hormones. In females, estrogen and inhibin regulate LH and FSH secretion, respectively, and in males, testosterone and inhibin regulate LH and FSH release.

Two GnRH genes are present: GnRH1, located at chromosome 8p21, and GnRH2, located at chromosome 20p13. Prepro-GnRH1 is a 92 amino acid, 10.4-kDa polypeptide with a 23 amino acid leader sequence. Removal of the leader sequence produces pro-GnRH1, which comprises 69 amino acids. Release of the C-terminal GnRH-associated peptide-1 yields GnRH1 (amino acids 24–33). Amino acid 24 is modified as a pyrrolidone carboxylic acid, and amino acid 33 is modified as a glycine amide.

GnRH2 is expressed in higher concentrations outside the CNS than within the CNS. *GnRH2* is principally produced in the prostate, bone marrow, and kidneys. PreproGnRH2 is a 120 amino acid (12.9 kDa) polypeptide. Cleavage of the 23 amino acid leader sequence generates proGnRH2, which is 97 amino acids in length. Release of the C-terminal GnRH-associated peptide 2 yields *GnRH2* (amino acids 24–33). Similar to *GnRH1*, amino acid 24 is modified as a pyrrolidone carboxylic acid, and amino acid 33 is modified as a glycine amide. *GnRH2* has three isoforms: isoform 1 is the full-length protein; isoform 2 lacks amino acids 52 to 59; and isoform 3 is missing amino acids 52 to 58.

The receptor for GnRH (GnRHR) is expressed on anterior pituitary gonadotropic cells. The gene for GnRHR is located at chromosome 4q. GnRHR is a 328 amino acid protein; the first 38 amino acids are extracellular, and seven transmembrane domains are present. Only two amino acids are cytoplasmic. The GnRHR is possibly glycosylated at amino acids 18 and 102, and a disulfide bond is probably present between amino acids 114 and 196. Two isoforms of GnRHR are expressed: the full-length protein (isoform 1), and isoform 2, which differs in the amino acid sequence between residues 176 and 328. A putative second GnRHR (GnRH2R) exists, comprising 178 amino acids. However, the gene for GnRH2R (located on chromosome 1) may be a pseudogene.

Both LH and FSH are secreted by gonadotrophs. Similar to TSH and hCG, LH and FSH are glycoprotein α-/β- heterodimers.[203] The α-chain is shared among all four hormones. The glycoprotein α-chain gene is located on chromosome 6q1. The α-chain includes 116 amino acids and weighs 13.1 kDa, including a leader sequence of 24 amino acids; the secreted chain is 92 amino acids. Amino acids 76 and 102 in the α chain are glycosylated. Five disulfide bonds are present at amino acids 31 to 55, 34 to 84, 52 to 106, 56 to 108, and 83 to 111.

The gene for the LH β-chain is located at chromosome 19q13.3. The leader sequence (amino acids 1–20) is followed by the 121 amino acid β-chain, which is the secreted form. The β-chain is glycosylated at amino acid 50, and six disulfide bonds are present at amino acids 29 to 77, 43 to 92, 46 to 130, 54 to 108, 58 to 110, and 113 to 120.

The gene for the FSH β-chain is located at chromosome 11p1. The 129 amino acid pre-FSH β-chain is 14.7 kDa, including an 18 amino acid leader sequence; the secreted FSH β-chain is 111 amino acids. FSH-β is glycosylated at amino acids 25 and 42 and contains six disulfide bonds at amino acids 21 to 69, 35 to 84, 38 to 122, 46 to 100, 50 to 102, and 105 to 112. Isolated α-subunits are devoid of biological activity; the β-subunit of FSH may have slight intrinsic biological activity, but full activity is attained when α- and β-subunits are recombined. This suggests that the presence of both α- and β-subunits is important for specific receptor recognition, and that the β-subunit is responsible for eliciting the specific biological response.

In men, the LH receptor (LHR) is expressed by Leydig cells, whereas in women, the LHR is expressed on theca cells and is induced by FSH on granulosa cells during the follicular phase of the menstrual cycle. The gene for the LHR is located at chromosome 2p21. The pre-LHR protein is 699 amino acids (78.6 kDa). After removal of the leader sequence, LHR comprises 673 amino acids. The extracellular domain is 337 amino acids, followed by 7 transmembrane domains and a cytoplasmic domain of 72 amino acids. Seven leucine-rich repeats are present at amino acids 48 to 71, 97 to 121, 122 to 147, 149 to 171, 172 to 196, 197 to 220, and 221 to 244. Cysteines at positions 643 and 644 are lipidated to S-palmitoyl cysteine. Potential glycosylation sites exist at amino acids 99, 174, 195, 291, 299, and 313. A disulfide bond is likely between amino acids 439 and 514. Two isoforms of LHR are expressed: the long isoform is the full-length LHR, and the short isoform lacks amino acids 227 to 289.

The FSH receptor (FSHR) is expressed on Sertoli cells in men and on granulosa cells in women. Following the 17 amino acid leader sequence is the 678 amino acid FSHR. The extracellular domain is 349 amino acids, with 7 transmembrane domains. The cytoplasmic domain is 65 amino acids. Ten leucine-rich repeats are present at amino acids 18 to 48, 49 to 72, 73 to 97, 98 to 118, 119 to 143, 144 to 169, 170 to 192, 193 to 216, 217 to 240, and 241 to 259. The FSHR has four proven or suspected sites of glycosylation at amino acids 191, 199, 293, and 318; two definitive disulfide bonds (amino acids 18–25 and 23–32); and one possible disulfide bond (amino acids 442–517). Two isoforms of the FSHR are expressed: isoform 1 is the full-length FSHR, and isoform 2 lacks amino acids 224 to 285.

Physiologic Activity

In men, LH stimulates testosterone synthesis and secretion by Leydig cells. In response to FSH, Sertoli cells nourish developing sperm during spermatogenesis.

Based on the two-cell model of estradiol and progesterone production by the adult ovary, androstenedione is produced by theca cells in response to LH stimulation (Fig. 65.6). Granulosa cells do not have direct access to the circulation; therefore, low-density lipoprotein cholesterol is not readily available to granulosa cells in the follicular phase of the menstrual cycle. Consequently, granulosa cell synthesis of sex steroids is dependent on theca cell androstenedione. Granulosa cells initially respond to FSH, and later to FSH plus LH.

FSH has several effects on the ovary during the follicular phase of the menstrual cycle (see Chapter 68). When bound to granulosa cell FSHRs, FSH stimulates granulosa cell proliferation. As a result, a dominant follicle develops containing the ovum that will be expelled midcycle (ovulation) to be captured by the fibria of the fallopian tube. When this event is being stimulated by FSH, granulosa cells use theca cell androstenedione as the precursor for estradiol synthesis. FSH also stimulates the expression of LHRs on the granulosa cells. Estradiol and inhibins from the ovary provide negative feedback for hypothalamic release of GnRH.

At midcycle, as a consequence of the LH surge, the follicle ruptures with release of the ovum (ovulation). The corpus luteum of the ovary (Fig. 65.7) is formed from the remaining theca and granulosa cells. The theca cells (responsive to LH) become the theca lutein cells, and the granulosa cells (now responsive to LH and FSH) are converted to the granulosa lutein cells, which now are vascularized and gain access to low-density lipoprotein (LDL) cholesterol from the circulation. With an adequate supply of cholesterol from LDL, the granulosa lutein cells generate progesterone and estradiol. Estradiol and progesterone convert the proliferative endometrium of the first half of the menstrual cycle to the secretory endometrium of the second (luteal) half of the menstrual cycle.

In the absence of pregnancy (ie, in the absence of hCG), progesterone concentrations decline, and menstruation occurs because the corpus luteum atrophies to become the corpus albicans. However, if a fertilized ovum implants in the uterine wall, the syncytiotrophoblast, via hCG, will maintain the corpus luteum, and menstruation is avoided because of continued secretion of estradiol and progesterone. The corpus luteum (supported by hCG) then becomes the corpus luteum of pregnancy.

Regulation and Clinical Significance

In hypogonadal patients, if gonadotropin concentrations are greatly elevated, hypergonadotropic hypogonadism is diagnosed, indicating that gonadal (end-organ) failure has occurred.[204] Alternatively, if gonadotropin concentrations are consistently low in hypogonadal patients, the diagnosis of hypogonadotropic hypogonadism is likely. To ensure that the pituitary is unable to respond to GnRH, a GnRH stimulation test can be performed.[205,206] GnRH testing should be performed in children (especially boys) in whom hypogonadotropic hypogonadism versus constitutional delay in growth and adolescence (delayed puberty) is a diagnostic dilemma; basal LH and FSH may also be low. If basal LH

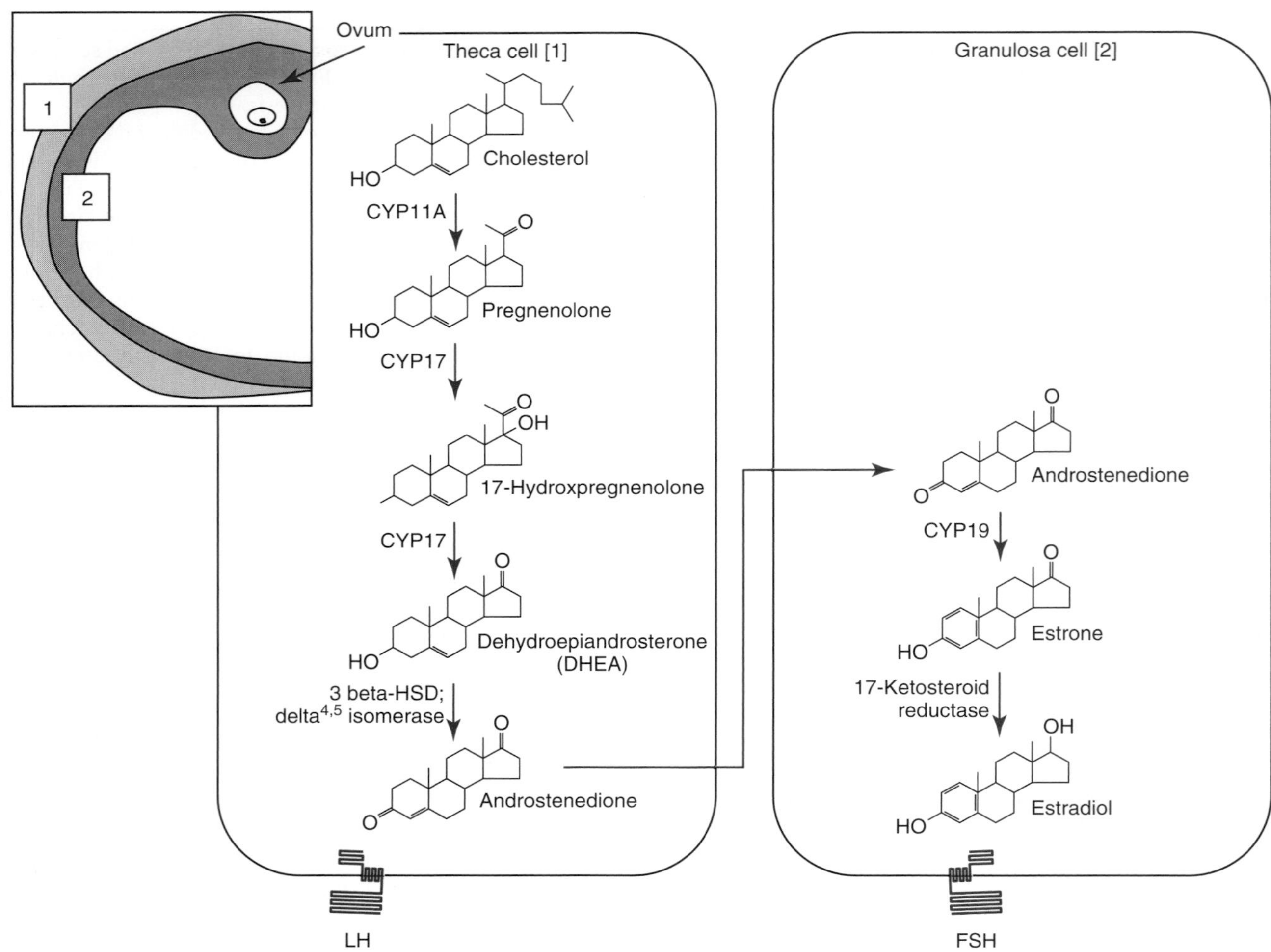

FIGURE 65.6 In the Follicular (Proliferative) Phase of the Menstrual Cycle, Under the Influence of Luteinizing Hormone *(LH)*, Theca Cells *(1)* Produce Androstenedione From Cholesterol (the Intermediary Steps Are Illustrated). Under the influence of follicle-stimulating hormone *(FSH)*, granulosa cells use the androstenedione produced by the theca cells to synthesize estradiol (the intermediary steps are illustrated) *(2)*. *3 Beta-HSD,* 3 Beta-hydroxysteroid dehydrogenase; *CYP11A,* 20,22 desmolase; *CYP17,* 17-hydroxylase activity; *CYP19,* aromatase.

and FSH concentrations are low, but LH and FSH rise substantially after GnRH stimulation, constitutional delay in growth and adolescence is likely, and hypogonadotropic hypogonadism can be excluded. The therapeutic approach to these two conditions is different. Children with constitutional delay in growth and adolescence eventually will enter puberty (although later than their peers), whereas hypogonadotropic hypogonadism will require sex hormone replacement therapy for initiation of puberty. If hypogonadotropic hypogonadism is diagnosed, a thorough search for its cause (eg, a CNS tumor) is essential. Induction of fertility in patients with hypogonadotropic hypogonadism requires gonadotropin replacement. A protocol for performance of the GnRH test is discussed in the following section.

Hypogonadotropic hypogonadism has also been found to result from loss-of-function mutations in the GnRHR gene.[207] Isolated FSH deficiency can result from mutations in the FSH β chain. However, isolated FSH deficiency is a rare cause of infertility in men or women. Men with FSH deficiency (but LH sufficiency) will have normal testosterone concentrations because LH and responding Leydig cells are normal.

Gain-of-function mutations in the LHR cause a hypogonadotropic, familial, male precocious puberty, in which the testes autonomously and prematurely produce testosterone (testotoxicosis).[208] Leydig cell adenomas with LHR mutations can cause precocious puberty.

LHR loss-of-function mutations cause Leydig cell hypoplasia and inadequate virilization of males in utero, leading to ambiguous genitalia.[209] In females, LHR loss-of-function mutations cause oligomenorrhea, amenorrhea, or infertility. FSHR loss-of-function mutations in females result in ovarian dysgenesis.

Central precocious puberty occurs with early activation of the hypothalamic-pituitary-gonadal axis, leading to gonadotropin-driven early puberty (onset of breast development or pubic hair before age 8 years or menses before age 9.5 years in girls, and puberty onset in boys before age 9 years).[210] In most girls (≈95%), no specific cause is identified (idiopathic precocious puberty). Central precocious puberty

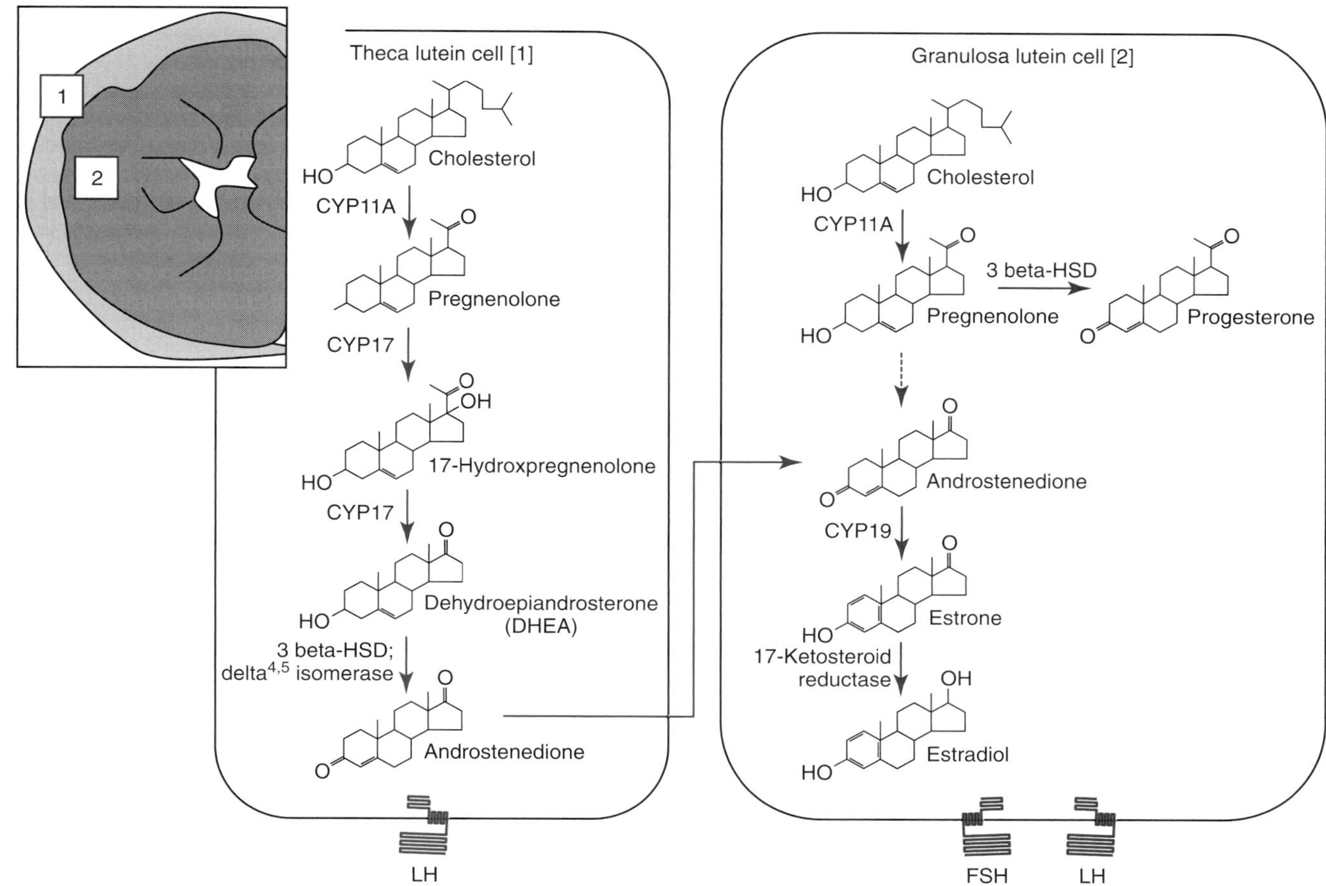

FIGURE 65.7 In the Luteal (Secretory) Phase of the Menstrual Cycle After Ovulation, Under the Influence of Luteinizing Hormone *(LH)*, Theca Lutein Cells *(1)* Produce Androstenedione From Cholesterol (the Intermediary Steps Are Illustrated). Under the influence of follicle-stimulating hormone *(FSH)* and LH, granulosa lutein cells use androstenedione produced by the theca cells to synthesize estradiol, and use cholesterol available from low-density lipoprotein *(LDL)* to synthesize progesterone (the intermediary steps are illustrated) *(2)*. *3 Beta-HSD,* 3 Beta-hydroxysteroid dehydrogenase; *CYP11A,* 20,22 desmolase; *CYP17,* 17-hydroxylase activity; *CYP19,* aromatase.

is uncommon in boys. However, when central precocious puberty occurs in boys, the likelihood of CNS pathology is greater than that in girls.

Other details concerning the regulation and clinical significance of LH and FSH are discussed in Chapter 68.

Measurement of Luteinizing Hormone and Follicle-Stimulating Hormone

The α subunit of LH and FSH is a member of the "cystine knot" superfamily of polypeptides that also includes GH, chorionic gonadotropin (hCG), and thyrotropin (TSH). Therefore, analytical methods for measuring LH and FSH must recognize the unique β subunits of these hormones because the α subunit is shared among several homologous pituitary products as well as hCG.

Two-site (double antibody) heterogeneous immunoassays are currently the most common methods for measuring gonadotropins, and a wide variety of assays have been adapted to automated platforms. Some commercially available methods attach a capture antibody to the surface of test tubes or plastic beads, whereas others use a paramagnetic label or a microparticle to capture the antibody–antigen complexes. Numerous labels have been used for the second antibody, including radioisotopes, enzymes,[211] fluorophores,[212] and chemiluminescent molecules. Immunometric methods for measuring LH and FSH have recently been reviewed.[185,213] The analytical sensitivity of LH assays is especially important in the evaluation of prepubertal children and patients with hypothalamic disorders because LH concentrations are very low.

Calibration of gonadotropin assays is difficult because LH and FSH undergo posttranslational modifications that produce a mixture of closely related compounds.[214] The earliest reference material used for calibration of LH and FSH assays was the second IRP for human menopausal gonadotropins, isolated from the urine of postmenopausal women. However, alterations during metabolism and excretion limited the comparability of this preparation with circulating forms of the hormones, and subsequent calibrators were prepared from extracts derived from the human pituitary gland. Purified pituitary extracts, such as the first and second IRPs for FSH and LH, were available for many years but have been replaced by highly purified extracts that have minimal contamination with cross-reacting glycoproteins.

Manufacturers of older immunoassays for LH and FSH used one or more pituitary-derived reference materials for their working calibrators, but recombinant gonadotropin calibrators are now available.

Biases in analytical results still exist between different immunoassay systems (most notably in LH assays), and results can differ by more than 50%, even when calibrated with the same reference preparation.[215,216] The most likely explanation for the bias is the specificity of the antibodies used in each method. Gonadotropic hormones are glycosylated, and this affects their antigenicity.[217] For example, LH immunoassays using monoclonal antibodies generate considerably lower LH concentrations than RIAs using polyclonal antibodies, presumably because of the greater specificity of monoclonal antibodies, which may recognize only a subset of LH isoforms and epitopes. Other factors that contribute to method-dependent biases include differences in calibration procedures and the assay matrix itself.

Specimen Collection and Storage

Serum is the preferred specimen for gonadotropin measurements. Hemolyzed, lipemic, and/or icteric specimens should not be used. Both hormones are stable for 8 days at room temperature, and for 2 weeks at 4°C; for longer periods, the serum specimen should be frozen at or below −20°C. Because of episodic, circadian, and cyclic variations in the secretion of gonadotropins, meaningful clinical evaluation of these hormones may require determinations in pooled blood specimens, multiple serial blood specimens, or timed urine specimens. Urine specimens should not contain preservatives; storage at or below −20°C is recommended.

Measurement of Urinary Follicle-Stimulating Hormone and Luteinizing Hormone

Clinically, the pulsatile and episodic release of gonadotropins makes a single blood measurement of FSH or LH difficult to interpret. In adults, concentrations of gonadotropins in blood, particularly LH, may differ as much as threefold between blood specimens collected from the same individual 20 minutes apart. In addition, the lower detection limit of many FSH and LH immunoassays may be within the reference interval for these hormones in normal adults. In prepubertal children, most blood assays are not capable of measuring normal concentrations because they are so low. To optimize detection limits for gonadotropin assays in children, urinary FSH or LH assays have been used.[218]

Thyroid-Stimulating Hormone

TSH (thyrotropin), which is synthesized in thyrotrophs of the adenohypophysis, promotes the growth of thyroid follicular cells and sustains and stimulates the hormonal secretion of thyroid gland hormones 3,5,3′,5′ tetraiodothyronine (thyroxine; T4) and 3,5,3′-triiodothyronine (T3).[219]

Biochemistry and Physiology

TSH binds to TSH receptors (TSHRs) located on the surfaces of thyroid follicular cells.[220] TSH (1) stimulates growth and vascularity of the thyroid gland, (2) stimulates growth of thyroid follicular cells, (3) promotes thyroid hormone synthesis by increasing the uptake of iodine (via the sodium-iodide transporter), (4) promotes the organification (reduction) of iodine, (5) promotes the coupling of tyrosines, and (6) promotes the proteolytic release of stored thyroid hormone from thyroglobulin. TSH release is stimulated by TRH and is suppressed by thyroid hormone (principally, circulating T4).

TRH is a modified tripeptide produced by the hypothalamus. The thyroid-releasing hormone receptor (TRHR) is expressed on anterior pituitary thyrotrophs. TRHR is a 398 amino acid protein, and 28 of its amino acids constitute an extracellular domain. Seven transmembrane domains are present, along with a 79 amino acid cytoplasmic domain. Two possible glycosylation sites exist at amino acids 3 and 10, and a disulfide bridge is present between amino acids 98 and 179. Details of TRH and TRHR production are discussed in Chapter 67.

The glycoprotein α chain, shared with FSH, LH, and hCG, was described earlier in this chapter. The β-chain of TSH is encoded on chromosome 1p13. After removal of the 20 amino acid leader sequence, the pro-TSH β-chain consists of 118 amino acids. Cleavage of the six C-terminal residues released from the propeptide yields the TSH β-chain (112 amino acids). TSH is glycosylated at residue 43, and disulfide bonds are likely at amino acids 22 to 72, 36 to 87, 39 to 125, 47 to 103, 51 to 105, and 108 to 115.

Regulation, Clinical Significance, and Analytical Methods

Details concerning the regulation, clinical significance, and measurement of TSH are discussed in detail in Chapter 67.

Assessment of Anterior Pituitary Lobe Reserve

Evaluation of endocrine function is an important part of the management of patients with pituitary disease.[221,222] Detection of hormone deficiencies before and after treatment and recognition of hormone-producing tumors are the two objectives of testing of pituitary function in patients with pituitary disease.[223]

Assessment of anterior and posterior pituitary function in patients with a pituitary tumor is important in the identification of clinically significant hormone deficiency states caused by the tumor, and in the re-evaluation of patients after pituitary surgery or irradiation to detect hormone deficiencies that occur as a result of invasive treatment. Testing of pituitary function usually is performed under basal conditions, but it can be performed under provocative conditions to expose subtle or mild deficiencies observed in disorders of the adrenal gland or gonads. The primary relevance of prolactin deficiency relates to Sheehan syndrome, in which postpartum hemorrhage results in pituitary infarction and panhypopituitarism; this is still an important problem in developing countries. However, Sheehan syndrome can develop years after delivery.[224]

The lower detection limits of the newer two-site immunoassays for the measurement of pituitary hormones make it possible to distinguish an abnormally low value from the lower end of the normal reference interval. Although assessment of a particular aspect of pituitary function should include clinical signs and symptoms of hormone deficiency and measurement of hormones secreted by the pertinent endocrine gland (eg, T4, cortisol, testosterone), newer ultrasensitive assays for TSH, FSH, LH, and ACTH may allow accurate distinction between a pathologically low result and a low-normal result. A scheme for testing of pituitary reserve is proposed in Box 65.5.

BOX 65.5 Assessment of Pituitary Reserve in Surgical Patients

Before Pituitary Surgery

Adrenal function: measurement of morning serum cortisol concentration or cosyntropin stimulation test:

- Thyroid function: free T_4
- Gonadal function: sex hormone determinations (estradiol in women and testosterone in men) and gonadotropins (luteinizing hormone and follicle-stimulating hormone) if sex steroids are low

Shortly After Pituitary Surgery (2 to 4 Days After Surgery)

- Adrenal function: morning serum cortisol concentration
- Thyroid function: deferred
- Gonadal function: deferred

Six Weeks After Pituitary Surgery

- Adrenal function: cosyntropin stimulation test or insulin tolerance test
- Thyroid function: free T_4
- Gonadal function: sex hormone determinations (estradiol in women and testosterone in men)

Hypothalamic-Pituitary-Adrenal Axis

A morning serum cortisol concentration in excess of 18 to 20 µg/dL (497–552 nmol/L) usually provides adequate evidence that the hypothalamic-pituitary-adrenal (HPA) axis is intact and is functioning properly. A typical reference interval for morning cortisol is 5 to 23 µg/dL (138–635 nmol/L). A morning cortisol result can fall within the reference interval, yet may not prove that the patient has a normal HPA axis.

If the morning cortisol is frankly low (<5 µg/dL; <138 nmol/L) or equivocal (5 to <18 µg/dL; 138 to <497), or if a strong clinical suspicion of adrenal insufficiency is present, the cosyntropin (or Synacthen) stimulation test is helpful. Cosyntropin provocation of cortisol release is performed by obtaining a baseline blood specimen for cortisol followed by intravenous (IV) or intramuscular (IM) administration of 250 µg of cosyntropin (an active ACTH analog). Blood specimens are collected 30 and 60 minutes after administration of cosyntropin (see Box 66.1 and Chapter 66 for more detail). A lower dose cosyntropin test (1.0 µg IV) has been proposed as a more sensitive test of impaired pituitary reserve, but its usefulness is still unclear and controversial.[225,226] The use of such testing in the setting of critical illness to assess adrenal function or direct steroid therapy is controversial.[227]

Tests of the entire HPA axis, such as the insulin tolerance test (also called the insulin-induced hypoglycemia stimulation test; see Box 65.3), occasionally are abnormal in patients who have (1) a normal morning cortisol result, (2) a normal response to cosyntropin, and (3) no signs of adrenal insufficiency. Although an abnormality in these sensitive tests suggests some diminution of ACTH reserve, the clinical significance is most relevant when the patient encounters a major stress, such as gastroenteritis. These tests should be reserved for patients who are strongly suspected of having adrenal insufficiency, or whose morning cortisol concentration or response to ACTH has been found to be abnormal. Standard protocols for the performance and interpretation of these tests have been published. These tests involve some patient risk and discomfort and should be performed only under the direct supervision of an experienced physician. Certainly good vascular access should be available for ITTs.

Measurement of ACTH in blood collected at baseline or after stimulation with insulin adds little to the usefulness of the tests discussed previously and generally is not recommended. In patients who have undergone pituitary surgery, the cortisol negative feedback loop to ACTH secretion may take time to normalize. ACTH and cortisol measurements after administration of CRH potentially are a direct test of pituitary ACTH reserve. The insulin-induced hypoglycemia test is currently the definitive test of ACTH and/or cortisol reserve; however, this test is contraindicated in patients aged older than 70 years, those with a history of coronary heart disease, seizure disorder, or general debility. Metyrapone testing, as another test of pituitary ACTH reserve, is discussed in Chapter 66; for details and interpretation, see Box 66.4.

Hypothalamic-Pituitary-Thyroid Axis

Because the current generation of TSH assays provide limits of detection extending to ≤0.01 mIU/L, which is sufficient to distinguish between low-normal and pathologically suppressed TSH secretion, TRH testing usually is not required for assessment of thyroid function.[228] Pharmaceutical TRH currently is not available in the United States.

The sole value of the TRH test is in the diagnosis of a TSH-secreting tumor in a patient presenting with increased free T4 and an inappropriately elevated TSH.[229] In these patients, the TSH response to TRH is impaired. Such patients may also have elevated concentrations of free α subunits.

TRH testing involves the bolus IV administration of TRH (100 µg/m2, or 500 µg total in adults), along with the measurement of TSH at baseline and at 30 minutes. (Note: Some protocols extend TSH measurements to 45 and 60 minutes.) The expected (normal) response is an increase in TSH concentration over the baseline of 5 to 30 mIU/L. Some sources report that a normal response to TRH is a fivefold to tenfold increase in serum TSH concentration within 60 minutes after TRH administration. A TSH change of less than 5 mIU/L indicates TSH suppression (primary hyperthyroidism) or the inability of the pituitary to respond (secondary hypothyroidism). TSH responses greater than 30 mIU/L are consistent with primary hypothyroidism. In tertiary hypothyroidism, TSH will rise slowly in a delayed response pattern.

Hypothalamic-Pituitary-Gonadal Axis

History and physical examination are extremely helpful in evaluating the status of the hypothalamic-pituitary-gonadal axis, particularly in women during their reproductive years.[230,231] Normal menstrual cycles usually indicate an intact hypothalamic-pituitary-gonadal axis in women of reproductive age. A serum progesterone concentration greater than 10 ng/mL (31.8 nmol/L) during the luteal phase of the menstrual cycle supports the diagnosis of ovulation.

Baseline laboratory assessment for hypothalamic-pituitary-gonadal dysregulation should include measurement of serum gonadotropins (LH and FSH) and sex steroids (estradiol in females and testosterone in males). Provocative testing of this axis with GnRH administration and measurements of FSH and LH (Box 65.6) are useful in selected patients. However,

BOX 65.6 Protocol for the Gonadotropin-Releasing Hormone Stimulation Test for Luteinizing Hormone and Follicle-Stimulating Hormone Reserve

Rationale

The hypothalamic releasing hormone gonadotropin-releasing hormone (GnRH) stimulates the pituitary release of both luteinizing hormone (LH) and follicle-stimulating hormone (FSH) in normal individuals. Subnormal responses are seen in some patients with pituitary or hypothalamic disorders. However, the magnitude of LH and FSH responses to GnRH is usually predictable from basal LH and FSH concentrations. This test may be useful in patients in whom the clinical picture and basal gonadotropin measurements are inconclusive.

Procedure

The test may be performed without regard to previous feeding or time of day. After baseline specimens are obtained for LH and FSH measurement, 100 μg or 2.5 μg/kg (to a maximum of 100 μg) GnRH is given intravenously. Samples for LH and FSH determination should be drawn every 15 to 20 minutes for 1 to 2 hours.

Interpretation

LH response should increase by threefold to tenfold. The FSH response is of lesser magnitude (usually a 1.5- to 3-fold increase). Peak responses for both LH and FSH occur between 15 and 30 minutes.

the definition of an appropriate response to GnRH is controversial and depends on the stage of sexual maturation of the subject. After GnRH injection, LH normally rises more than FSH. Two shortened variations of the GnRH test are available: in one variation, leuprolide (a GnRH agonist; 20 μg/kg) is injected subcutaneously, and LH and FSH are measured 3 hours later; in the other variant, 100 μg of GnRH is injected subcutaneously, and LH and FSH are measured 40 minutes later. However, these tests can be unreliable in differentiating pituitary disorders from hypothalamic dysfunction; the physician usually is dependent on an accurate determination of gonadotropins and sex steroids, along with clinical judgment, in differentiating hypothalamic from pituitary disease.

AT A GLANCE

The pituitary is a master gland for many vital endocrine functions regulating growth (GH), thyroid function (thyrotropin), reproduction (LH, FSH, and prolactin), stress responses (corticotropin), parturition (oxytocin), and water balance (antidiuretic hormone).The most common pituitary disorders encompass over or under production of pituitary hormones, and pituitary tumors.

The hypothalamus regulates pituitary hormone release or is the site of synthesis of the posterior pituitary hormones. Like the pituitary, hypothalamic disease can involve over or under production of hypothalamic hormones.

Pituitary Assessment in Surgical Patients

Initial Assessment

Preoperative testing is indicated in patients with large pituitary tumors or specific clinical indications such as suspected ACTH deficiency, when glucocorticoids may be required preoperatively (see Box 65.5), but the gonadal axis may be compromised in patients with microadenomas as well. In addition to the history and physical examination, patients at risk for pituitary insufficiency should be evaluated for endocrine function before surgery is performed, including laboratory measurements of serum prolactin, free T4, LH, FSH, sex steroids (testosterone in males and estradiol in females), IGF-I, GH, serum sodium, and urine specific gravity (or serum and urine osmolality), and a morning serum cortisol or cosyntropin stimulation test.

Perioperative Assessment

The optimum time for retesting endocrine function after pituitary surgery is not known. Many protocols (often based on sparse data) explain how potential cortisol deficiency is managed in the perioperative period. Some neurosurgeons provide "stress" doses (high doses) of glucocorticoids immediately before, during, and after surgery. If the patient had ACTH deficiency preoperatively, IV glucocorticoids can be replaced with oral replacement doses (eg, the equivalent of 12 mg/m^2 per day of hydrocortisone in children, or 20 to 30 mg in adults in divided doses) after 2 to 3 days. If the patient had normal adrenal function preoperatively, exogenous glucocorticoids can be discontinued on the second or third postoperative day. Morning cortisol should be measured 24 hours later; if the result is less than 5 μg/dL (138 nmol/L), ACTH deficiency is likely, and glucocorticoid replacement is indicated. If the 24-hour postoperative cortisol is 10 μg/dL (276 nmol/L) or greater, the HPA axis is normal and glucocorticoid replacement is not required. If cortisol is between 5 and 10 μg/dL (138–276 nmol/L), the patient should be treated with glucocorticoids until provocative testing can be performed (ITT or glucagon stimulation test) safely; the ITT can be used concurrently to assess GH deficiency. Many clinicians prefer to perform a cosyntropin test at least 6 weeks postoperatively as an alternative to elevate the HPA axis.

Some neurosurgeons do not treat with glucocorticoids if preoperative adrenal function is normal,[232] preferring instead to assess postoperative morning cortisol concentration in the patient. If cortisol concentration is less than 3.6 μg/dL (99 nmol/L), ACTH deficiency is present and glucocorticoid treatment is necessary. If cortisol is greater than 16 μg/dL (442 nmol/L), ACTH deficiency is not present, and glucocorticoid treatment is not required. Definitive testing is indicated only for patients with a morning cortisol of 3.6 to 16 μg/dL (99–442 nmol/L); pituitary function in these patients can be evaluated with an ITT or glucagon stimulation test (or cosyntropin test at least 6 weeks postoperatively). Patients with a morning cortisol between 3.6 and 9 μg/dL (99–248 nmol/L) usually receive daily glucocorticoid treatment, whereas those with an morning cortisol between 9 and 16 μg/dL (248–442 nmol/L) are treated only at times of stress.

In the first 6 weeks after pituitary surgery, the cosyntropin test may not be a reliable indicator of HPA axis integrity. During this period, the adrenal response to cosyntropin may be normal, yet endogenous ACTH may be insufficient in the basal state or at times of stress to avoid glucocorticoid insufficiency. Once the adrenal gland atrophies from a deficiency of endogenous ACTH (which may take ≈6 weeks), the cosyntropin challenge becomes abnormal, reflecting endogenous ACTH deficiency.

Postoperative Assessment

It is advisable to wait until 1 month or longer after surgery to evaluate thyroid function (TSH and free T4) and gonadal function (testosterone in males and estradiol in females; see Box 65.5). Early treatment of thyroid and gonadal deficiencies is not critical, and misleading test results might be observed in the early postoperative period. Adrenal function should be reassessed with a 250-μg cosyntropin stimulation test 6 weeks after surgery even if immediate results are subnormal, because ACTH deficiency after pituitary surgery may be transient. Periodic clinical follow-up and laboratory assessment should be tailored to individual circumstances.

Stimulation tests for the secretion of ACTH, GH, and GnRH can be combined. For example, the ITT can be combined with the GnRH stimulation test. The ITT assesses GH and ACTH secretion, whereas the GnRH stimulation test assesses the ability of the anterior pituitary to secrete gonadotropins in response to GnRH.

After pituitary irradiation, patients should be evaluated yearly with measurement of free T4, sex steroids, cortisol and IGF-I.

POINTS TO REMEMBER

- ADH and oxytocin synthesizing cells are located in the hypothalamus.
- ADH and oxytocin are released from axons in the posterior pituitary.
- There are no known diseases of oxytocin deficiency or excess.
- ADH deficiency or resistance causes DI with excess free water loss.
- ADH excess causes SIADH, which results in excess free water retention.

Neurohypophysis

The neurohypophysis (posterior pituitary) is derived from the brain neuroectodermis. Embryologically, ventral evagination of the floor of the third ventricle forms the neurohypophysis.[233] Antidiuretic hormone (ADH; vasopressin) and oxytocin are secreted from the neurohypophysis, the cell bodies of which are located in hypothalamic supraoptic and paraventricular nuclei. These neurons are located in and travel through the median eminence and pituitary stalk, with nerve endings projecting to the posterior lobe of the pituitary gland.

Antidiuretic Hormone

Disorders of ADH involve excess hormone (syndrome of inappropriate ADH [SIADH]) or deficient ADH action (diabetes insipidus [DI]). DI can result from ADH deficiency, ADH resistance, or renal tubular disease; the latter two conditions are termed nephrogenic DI. Disorders of oxytocin secretion have not been described. However, the discovery that receptors for oxytocin are expressed on osteoblasts and osteoclasts opens the door for a role of oxytocin in bone physiology and bone disease.[234]

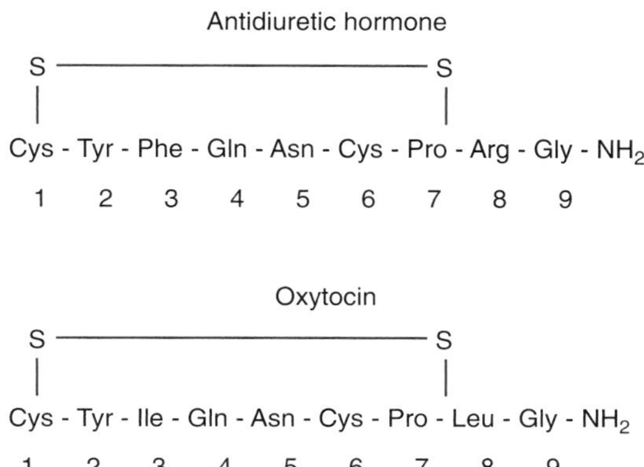

FIGURE 65.8 The Amino Acid Sequences of Antidiuretic Hormone *(ADH)* and Oxytocin Are Compared.

Biochemistry

Both ADH and oxytocin are nonapeptides consisting of a cyclic hexapeptide and a three amino acid side chain (Fig. 65.8). At the physiologic pH of plasma, ADH and oxytocin circulate mainly as unbound (free) hormones.

The *AVP* gene for ADH is located at chromosome 20p13. Prepro-ADH consists of 164 amino acids (17.3 kDa). The gene also encodes neurophysin 2 and copeptin. The first 19 amino acids of prepro-ADH are the leader sequence. Amino acids 20 to 28 constitute the ADH nonapeptide hormone; amino acids 32 to 124 represent neurophysin 2, and amino acids 126 to 164 represent copeptin (C-terminal provasopressin). The glycine residue at position 28 is amidated, and amino acid 131 is glycosylated. Disulfide bonds are definitive or possible at amino acids 20 to 25, 41 to 85, 44 to 58, 52 to 75, 59 to 65, 92 to 104, 98 to 116, and 105 to 110. The disulfide bridge at residues 20 to 25 is within ADH.

The ADH receptor in the renal tubules (specifically, the collecting ducts) is termed the arginine vasopressin receptor 2 (V2 receptor). The V2 receptor is a member of the seven-transmembrane domain G-protein–coupled receptor superfamily, whose other members include the V1a and V1b vasopressin receptors and the oxytocin receptor.

The gene for the V2 receptor is located on chromosome Xq28. The receptor has 371 amino acids (40.3 kDa), including a 38 amino acid extracellular domain, 7 transmembrane domains, and a 43 amino acid cytoplasmic domain. Amino acid 22 may be glycosylated, and amino acids 341 and 342 are lipidated as S-palmitoyl cysteines. Two isoforms of the V2 receptor are known: isoform 1 is the full-length receptor, whereas isoform 2 varies in the sequence of amino acids 305 to 309, and amino acids 310 to 371 are absent.

The V1a receptor (V1 receptor) gene is located at chromosome 12q14. The protein has 418 amino acids and weighs 46.8 kDa. A 52 amino acid extracellular domain is present, along with 7 transmembrane domains and a 67 amino acid cytoplasmic domain. Glycosylation is possible at amino acids 27 and 196. Amino acids 365 and 366 may be lipidated as S-palmitoyl cysteines. A serine residue at position 404 may be phosphorylated to phosphoserine, and a disulfide bond is likely between amino acids 124 and 203.

The V1b receptor (V3 receptor) is encoded by a gene located on chromosome 1q32. The V3 receptor has 424 amino acids (47.0 kDa). A 35 amino acid extracellular domain is present, along with 7 transmembrane domains and an 83 amino acid cytoplasmic domain. The receptor is possibly glycosylated at amino acid 21, and a disulfide bond is likely between amino acids 107 and 186.

The action of ADH is to simulate the movement of aquaporin-2 from the cytoplasm to the basal plasma membrane. In this way, ADH allows the reabsorption of water from the collecting duct. Aquaporin-2 is a 271 amino acid protein (28.8 kDa).[235] The gene encoding aquaporin-2 is located on chromosome 12q1. The external domain contains 16 amino acids, along with 7 transmembrane domains and a 47 amino acid cytoplasmic domain. Phosphoserines are possible or definitive at amino acids 256, 261, and 264, and amino acid 123 is a possible site of glycosylation. Amino acids 68 to 70 and 184 to 186 are NPA (asparagine-proline-alanine) motifs.

Regulation of Antidiuretic Hormone Secretion

Antidiuretic hormone secretion is controlled predominantly by plasma osmolality (tonicity).[236] Plasma osmolality is sensed by osmoreceptors located in cell bodies in or near the magnocellular nuclei of the hypothalamus. Increased osmolality results in ADH release; even relatively small changes in osmolality affect ADH secretion. A 2% increase in extracellular fluid osmolality can stimulate the osmoreceptor to release ADH. Plasma osmolality above 280 mOsm/kg (mmol/kg) is thought to be the osmotic threshold for triggering ADH release.

In addition to the osmoreceptor mechanism of vasopressin release, physiologic regulation of ADH secretion involves a pressure–volume mechanism that is distinct from the osmotic sensor. High-pressure arterial baroreceptors of the aortic arch and carotid sinus, and low-pressure volume receptors in the pulmonary venous system and atria, also regulate ADH release. Therefore, ADH is secreted in response to decreased circulating blood volume, or decreased blood pressure. Other nonosmotic stimuli for ADH release include pain, stress, nausea and vomiting, sleep, exercise, and chemical agents, such as catecholamines, angiotensin II, opiates, prostaglandins, anesthetics, nicotine, and barbiturates.

The thirst center is regulated by many of the same factors that determine ADH release. This center has a higher set point than the osmoreceptors and responds to osmolalities above 290 mOsm/kg. Responses involving ADH, thirst, and renal reabsorption of sodium and water are coordinated in a complex scheme that maintains plasma osmolality in healthy individuals within a narrow interval (~285 to ~295 mOsm/kg [mmol/kg]).

Physiologic Activity

Both ADH and neurophysin 2 are present in secretory vesicles that reach the terminal portion of the axon 12 to 14 hours after they are synthesized (this is also true for oxytocin and neurophysin 1). Upon nerve stimulation, release of neurohypophyseal hormones into the portal circulation occurs via calcium-dependent exocytosis. When a stimulus for secretion of ADH or oxytocin occurs, the stimulus acts on the appropriate magnocellular cell body in the hypothalamus, sending an action potential down the long axon to the posterior pituitary, causing an influx of calcium and the release of hormone from neurosecretory granules.

The exact role of the neurophysins is unclear, but their proper synthesis is necessary for ADH secretion. The biological role of copeptin is unknown. Copeptin is being investigated as a marker of myocardial infarction.[237] Because of analytical difficulties in measuring ADH, some investigators have suggested measuring copeptin as a surrogate for ADH, because copeptin is secreted in amounts stoichiometrically equivalent to ADH, and copeptin is stable in plasma.

The actions of ADH are to conserve free water (via V2 receptors) and stimulate vasoconstriction (via V1a receptors).[238] These effects combine to maintain proper osmolality of the extracellular space (the major action of ADH) and blood pressure through maintenance of circulating blood volume and prevention of dehydration and excessive loss of water.

ADH increases the permeability of renal collecting ducts to water, thereby increasing water reabsorption and concentrating the urine to a higher specific gravity (Fig. 65.9).

An alternative name for ADH is vasopressin (or arginine vasopressin), which emphasizes the vasoconstrictive effects of high concentrations of ADH.[239] These vasoconstrictive effects are manifested when ADH binds to V1a receptors on arterial smooth muscle cells. Note that the major endocrine system regulating blood pressure is the renin-angiotensin-aldosterone system. However, ADH is believed to play an important role in the maintenance of arterial blood pressure during blood loss. Release of ADH into the pituitary portal system also augments the release of ACTH from the adenohypophysis, but does not appear to affect the release of other anterior pituitary hormones.

ADH binding to the V1a receptor stimulates the secretion of vascular endothelial growth factor. The V1a receptor may also affect platelet aggregation, coagulation factor release, and glycogenolysis by its expression on platelets and hepatocytes.

The V1b receptor (V3 receptor) is expressed in the CNS. In this way, ADH can release ACTH to aid in the response to stress. The V1b receptor also has been reported to be expressed in islet cells, influencing insulin secretion.

Clinical Significance

Disorders of ADH activity have been divided into hypofunction (DI) and hyperfunction (SIADH) (Fig. 65.10).[240,241]

Polyuric States and Diabetes Insipidus. Polyuric states are divided into two main categories: (1) deficient ADH action, producing DI (sometimes called "water diabetes"), and (2) excessive oral water intake (psychogenic polydipsia).[242] Inadequate ADH activity can result from ADH deficiency or ADH resistance. Osmotic diuresis may also produce polyuria and polydipsia. Uncontrolled diabetes mellitus with a high glucose load to the kidney is a common cause of osmotic diuresis.

In DI, polyuria results from excessive loss of water into the urine.[243] Under normal circumstances, urine output is predominantly dependent on fluid intake; thus an arbitrary upper limit for normal urine output cannot be defined. When urine output is greater than 2.5 L/day, investigation is usually indicated. In the absence of ADH, urine output may approach 1 L/h. Increased osmolality normally stimulates thirst. Therefore, if a patient with DI has an intact thirst mechanism and free access to water, excessive urinary loss of water should be matched by excessive intake of fluids. This is why DI patients report polydipsia in addition to polyuria. The major laboratory finding in DI is urine of low osmolality and serum sodium within the upper half of the

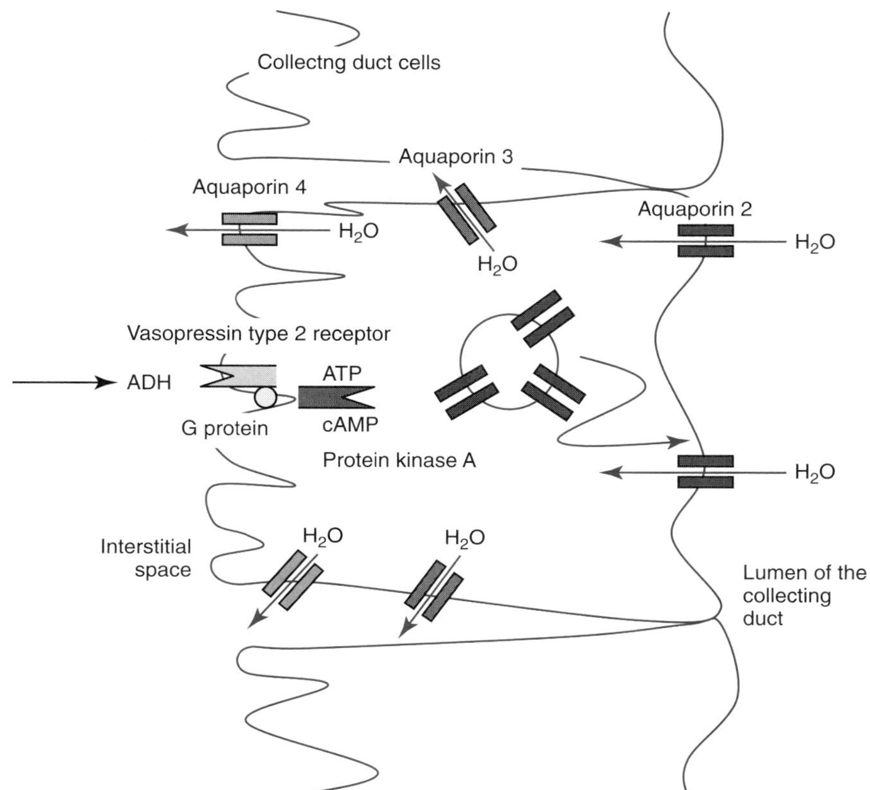

FIGURE 65.9 Vasopressin Type 2 Receptors on Collecting Duct Cells Bind Antidiuretic Hormone *(ADH)*. Via a G-protein system, adenosine triphosphate *(ATP)* is converted to cyclic adenosine 3′,5′-monophosphate (cAMP) via adenylate cyclase with protein kinase A activation. This leads to translocation of aquaporin-2 water channels from an intracellular pool to the apical plasma membrane, allowing free water uptake by cells of the collecting duct. Via the basolateral plasma membrane aquaporin-3 and aquaporin-4 water channels, free water then leaves these cells.

reference interval, with a corresponding high-normal serum osmolality. If water is not available, or the individual with DI is physically impaired or lacks a normal thirst mechanism, serum osmolality rises, serum sodium rises (producing hypernatremia), urine osmolality remains low, and polyuria continues. With dehydration, weight loss is acute (because of fluid loss) and blood pressure falls, inducing tachycardia.

Central DI can result from any destructive hypothalamic lesion or infundibular lesion (Table 65.8). DI resulting from such lesions can equally be termed hypothalamic, neurogenic, central, or cranial DI. Central DI is caused by failure of the posterior pituitary gland to secrete appropriate amounts of ADH in response to rising plasma osmolality. Increased fluid intake promoted by thirst mechanisms usually prevents dehydration in DI. When the thirst center is also abnormal, severe dehydration can occur. Destruction of 80% of ADH-secreting neurons is required to produce central DI. Surgical or traumatic injury to the neurohypophysis may cause transient or permanent DI.

The incidence of central DI is approximately 1 in 25,000 people. In 30% of patients, central DI occurs without apparent cause. The remaining cases are associated with (1) neoplastic disease, (2) neurologic surgery, (3) head trauma, (4) ischemic or hypoxic disorder, (5) granulomatous disease, (6) infection, or (7) autoimmune disorder. A hereditary form of the disorder is transmitted as an autosomal recessive or autosomal dominant trait.[244] Inborn errors in the ADH gene cause deficiency of the hormone. Individuals with familial neurohypophyseal diabetes insipidus (FNHDI) are typically recognized before the age of 6 years and display worsening polyuria and compensatory polydipsia.[245] More than 50 mutations have been identified as causes of FNHDI. Although rare, DI can develop during pregnancy as a result of high circulating concentrations of the enzyme cysteine aminopeptidase (vasopressinase), which inactivates ADH.[246] The vasopressinase may be of placental origin.

DI can result from tubular diseases that affect the responsiveness of renal tubules to ADH (nephrogenic DI). In X-linked congenital DI, an inactivating mutation of the V2 receptor is noted.[247] Loss-of-function mutations in aquaporin-2 cause autosomal recessive and autosomal dominant forms of congenital nephrogenic DI.[248] Chronic hypokalemia and hypercalcemia produce a form of nephrogenic DI that results from downregulation of aquaporin-2 expression.[249]

In the broadest sense, any form of tubular injury with impaired water reabsorption, including (1) polycystic kidney disease, (2) medullary cystic kidney, (3) chronic pyelonephritis, (4) acute tubular necrosis, (5) obstructive uropathy, (6) sickle cell nephropathy, and (7) renal amyloidosis can cause nephrogenic DI. A large number of drugs can cause nephrogenic DI, including (1) lithium,[250,251] (2) various antimicrobials (amphotericin B, rifampin, methicillin, demeclocycline, and foscarnet), and (3) several antineoplastic drugs (cisplatin and ifosfamide). In psychogenic polydipsia

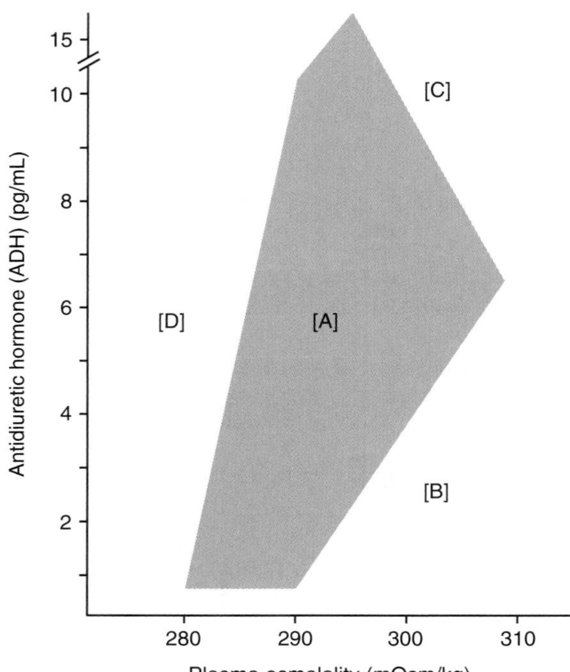

FIGURE 65.10 The Relationship of Plasma Antidiuretic Hormone *(ADH)* to Plasma Osmolality. Region *(A)* is the reference interval and the results observed in subjects with psychogenic polydipsia and excessive water intake. Region *(B)* represents findings in central diabetes insipidus, whereas region *(C)* represents findings in nephrogenic diabetes insipidus. Region *(D)* represents findings in the syndrome of inappropriate ADH *(SIADH)* secretion. (Modified from Zerbe RL, Robertson GL. A comparison of plasma vasopressin measurements with a standard indirect test in the differential diagnosis of polyuria. *N Engl J Med* 1981;305:1539–1546.)

(primary polydipsia), excessive water intake eventually begins to impair the concentrating ability of the kidney.

Investigation of Polyuria. Assuming that diabetes mellitus is excluded, a differential diagnosis of polyuric states can be made using measurements of plasma and urine osmolality and plasma ADH concentrations (if the findings are equivocal).[250,252] A recommended strategy is shown in Box 65.7. A screening test for ADH sufficiency is the measurement of the urine specific gravity in the first morning-voided urine sample. The specific gravity should be 1.010 or greater in patients with adequate ADH secretion. Failure to demonstrate an appropriate urine specific gravity and response in a subject with a history of polyuria and polydipsia should trigger assessment of a basic metabolic panel, urinalysis, serum osmolality, and urine osmolality. Hyperglycemia or glycosuria with an elevated urine specific gravity would suggest diabetes mellitus (see Chapter 57).

Urine osmolality less than 300 mOsm/kg (mmol/kg) combined with serum osmolality more than 300 mOsm/kg (mmol/kg) (or with hypernatremia) is diagnostic for DI. If urine osmolality is above 600 mOsm/kg (mmol/kg), and serum osmolality is below 270 mOsm/kg (mmol/kg), DI is unlikely.

If the diagnosis of DI is unclear, a water deprivation test should be performed, although this is rarely needed.[251,253] Before a water deprivation test, uncontrolled diabetes mellitus should be corrected, and thyroid and adrenal function should be normal (or treated if deficient). Water deprivation testing should not be carried out if the subject is dehydrated at baseline or has renal insufficiency. The overnight water deprivation test is usually conducted in a hospital setting because

TABLE 65.8 Causes of Central Diabetes Insipidus

Congenital	Midline malformations: septo-optic dysplasia, holoprosencephaly, single central incisor, and cleft lip and/or palate
	Malformation of the pituitary (ectopia or hypogenesis)
	Diabetes insipidus-diabetes mellitus-optic atrophy syndrome (Wolfram syndrome)
	Familial diabetes insipidus (autosomal dominant and recessive forms)
Acquired	Tumors (craniopharyngioma, germinoma, pinealoma, optic glioma, pituitary adenoma, metastatic tumor, leukemia)
	Trauma (eg, stalk section)
	Infarction (eg, septic shock, Sheehan syndrome, hypoxic injury)
	Infiltrative disease (sarcoidosis, hypophysitis, histiocytosis)
	Cysts and aneurysms
	Drugs (opiates, alcohol, phenytoin, alpha-adrenergic agents, etc.)
	Infection
	Increased metabolism of ADH (vasopressinase in pregnancy)

ADH, Antidiuretic hormone.

BOX 65.7 Diagnosis of Diabetes Insipidus

Document polyuria (urine volume >2.5 L/day in adults) and exclude glycosuria. If desired, creatinine excretion can be measured as an estimate of the completeness of the urine collection. Substances that influence antidiuretic hormone (ADH) secretion should be avoided (eg, nicotine, alcohol, caffeine). If plasma osmolality is more than 295 mOsm/kg (millimoles per kilogram), or if the serum sodium concentration is more than 145 mEq/L (millimoles per liter), primary polydipsia is unlikely. If the diagnosis of diabetes insipidus is unclear, proceed with the overnight water deprivation test (see text for a description of this test).

Overnight water deprivation test: if the ratio of urine to plasma osmolality is less than 1.5 at the end of the test, primary polydipsia is unlikely. Measure plasma and urine osmolalities, and plasma ADH concentrations at the end of the test; use these relationships to differentiate normal, nephrogenic, and hypothalamic diabetes insipidus, as well as psychogenic polydipsia. If urine osmolality is more than 400 mOsm/kg (millimoles per kilogram) at the end of the test, give 5 U of aqueous vasopressin subcutaneously (minimum, 1 U/m^2). If urine osmolality increases by more than 10%, central diabetes insipidus is probable; if urine osmolality does not increase, nephrogenic diabetes insipidus is highly probable.

of the immediate concerns of profound hypotension and possible mortality.[252-255] Hypertonic saline infusion testing is dangerous and is not used clinically.

The water deprivation test is usually begun on the morning after an overnight fast, unless the history describes large volumes of water ingested and urine produced, in which case the test should begin after breakfast. The subject remains fasting throughout the entire test. A heparin lock is inserted intravenously, so that serial blood samples are obtained easily. Baseline laboratory tests include (1) sodium, (2) potassium, (3) chloride, (4) serum carbon dioxide (CO_2), (5) urea (blood urea nitrogen [BUN]), (6) creatinine, (7) glucose, (8) calcium, and (9) serum osmolality. Potassium and calcium are measured to exclude hypokalemia and hypercalcemia as causes of nephrogenic DI (see later).

Measurements of serum or plasma sodium, chloride, CO_2, and urine pH provide an assessment of the patient's renal tubular acid-base function.[254,256] Renal function and hydration status are evaluated with creatinine and urea (BUN) measurements. A urine specimen is obtained for measurement of urine sodium, urine osmolality, and urine specific gravity. Body weight and vital signs at baseline are recorded. Thereafter, each hour, serum and urine tests are repeated with measurement of hourly urine output, body weight, and urine volume. If ADH measurements are requested, they can be performed at the beginning, middle, and completion of the test; however, ADH measurements are not required for making the diagnosis of DI. The test is continued for 8 to 10 hours unless the diagnosis of DI is confirmed before the full time has elapsed.

One approach that reduces laboratory charges is to perform serum and urine measurements every 4 hours until plasma osmolality reaches 280 mOsm/kg (mmol/kg), when the frequency is increased to every 2 hours. When plasma osmolality reaches 290 mOsm/kg (mmol/kg) or serum sodium exceeds 140 mEq/L (mmol/L), or weight loss nears 3%, the tests are performed hourly. During the water deprivation test, if urine osmolality exceeds 600 mOsm/kg (mmol/kg) on two samples 1 hour apart, or a single urine sample exceeds 1000 mOsm/kg (mmol/kg), DI is effectively ruled out, and the test can be concluded. If urine osmolality is less than 600 mOsm/kg (mmol/kg), and serum osmolality is more than 300 mOsm/kg (mmol/kg), DI is diagnosed, and the test can be concluded. If serum osmolality does not exceed 300 mOsm/kg (mmol/kg), the test should be continued. If mental status changes or hypotension occurs, or weight loss exceeds 3%, the test should be terminated.

If DI is diagnosed during a water deprivation test, aqueous vasopressin is injected subcutaneously (1 U/m^2), or desamino-D-arginine vasopressin (desmopressin) is given IV or IM (2 μg). A decline in urine volume with doubling of urine osmolality over the next 1 to 2 hours identifies the DI as central in origin with the patient being ADH deficient. After exogenous ADH administration, some references define an increase in urine osmolality of 10% or greater over 60 minutes as evidence of ADH deficiency. Failure to respond to exogenous ADH defines nephrogenic DI. Most patients with psychogenic polydipsia have normal urine osmolality after water deprivation, but some fail to produce concentrated urine unless the water deprivation is prolonged. When psychogenic polydipsia is suspected, the patient should be given a minimum of 1 L of normal saline IV to re-establish the renal medullary concentrating gradient, so that the patient can respond appropriately to ADH.

The diagnosis of "partial" DI, in which test results fall between normal and frank DI, is difficult, because no clear-cut boundaries are evident between normal and partial DI, or between partial DI and complete DI.[255,257] In some cases, measurement of ADH in plasma or urine may be required to reach the correct diagnosis. After water deprivation, patients with central DI have low or inappropriately normal plasma ADH concentrations relative to high plasma osmolality or low urine osmolality, whereas patients with nephrogenic DI have high plasma concentrations of ADH when plasma osmolality exceeds 300 mOsm/kg (mmol/kg), and urine osmolality is low. Patients with primary polydipsia have normal concentrations of ADH relative to their plasma osmolality. Because ADH concentrations are most discriminatory when plasma osmolality is high, in the past, ADH was measured after hypertonic saline was administered to the patient. However, this saline infusion test is potentially dangerous and currently is not used by clinical endocrinologists.

Syndrome of Inappropriate Antidiuretic Hormone Secretion. The autonomous, sustained production of ADH in the absence of recognized and appropriate stimuli (such as hyperosmolality) is termed SIADH.[256,258] In this syndrome, plasma ADH concentrations are "inappropriately" elevated relative to decreased plasma osmolality, and relative to normal or increased plasma volume.

SIADH may be the result of one of several factors (Table 65.9), including (1) production of ADH by a malignancy (such as small cell carcinoma of the lung), (2) the presence of acute or chronic disease of the CNS, (3) pulmonary disorders, or it may occur as (4) a side effect of certain drug therapies. In addition, as many as 10% of patients who undergo pituitary surgery have transient SIADH (for 2–3 days) approximately 8 to 9 days after surgery (typically when the patient is at home) that responds to water restriction and resolves spontaneously. This may represent the release of ADH from the posterior

TABLE 65.9 Causes of the Syndrome of Inappropriate Antidiuretic Hormone

CNS disease	Brain tumor Infection (eg, meningitis, encephalitis, abscess) Prolonged seizure Psychiatric disease Stress (eg, prolonged nausea)
Non-CNS tumor (eg, leukemia)	
Pulmonary disease	Hypoxia (eg, neonatal) Infection (eg, pneumonia, emphysema)
Nonpulmonary infection (eg, AIDS)	
Drugs	Drugs with CNS effects (anticonvulsants, antiparkinsonian drugs, antipsychotics, antipyretics, antidepressants) Angiotensin-converting enzyme inhibitors Antineoplastic drugs First-generation sulfonylureas

CNS, Central nervous system.

pituitary or hypothalamus after surgical trauma. A rare form of nephrogenic SIADH results from a gain-of-function mutation in the V2 receptor.[248,259,260]

In SIADH, primary excess of ADH, coupled with unrestricted fluid intake, promotes increased reabsorption of water by the kidney. The consequences are decreased urine volume and increased urine osmolality. The increase in intravascular volume causes hemodilution accompanied by dilutional hyponatremia and low plasma osmolality. Physiologically, hypo-osmolality in blood should result in dilute urine, but in SIADH urine osmolality is inappropriately high for the plasma osmolality. It is important to know that although osmoregulation is tightly controlled, volume regulation always takes precedence over osmoregulation, when the intravascular volume changes by more than 10% (eg, as is the case in SIADH due to fluid overload). Via suppression of the renin-angiotensin-aldosterone axis, volume expansion also decreases renal sodium reabsorption, thus the urine sodium concentration is typically 20 to 40 mEq/L (mmol/L) despite dilutional hyponatremia in blood. This hypervolemia-induced urinary sodium excretion, coupled with water loss, explains why patients with SIADH are euvolemic.

SIADH is a common cause of hyponatremia in hospitalized patients.[257,261] However, other disorders can cause dilutional hyponatremia and must be differentiated from SIADH. These conditions include (1) congestive heart failure, (2) renal insufficiency, (3) nephrotic syndrome, (4) liver cirrhosis, and (5) hypothyroidism. The mechanism of hyponatremia in congestive heart failure, and in nephrotic syndrome and liver cirrhosis is partly due to the compensatory secretion of ADH in response to decreased cardiac output and volume depletion.[258,262] These nonosmotic stimuli for ADH release, mediated through high (aortic arch and carotid sinus) and low (left atrial) pressure baroreceptors, increase the secretion of ADH at any plasma osmolality. Excessive administration of hypotonic fluids and treatment with drugs that stimulate ADH (chlorpropamide, vincristine, carbamazepine, nicotine, phenothiazines, and cyclophosphamide) can also cause dilutional hyponatremia. In addition, hyponatremia may occur from renal or extrarenal sodium loss (depletional hyponatremia) as a result of vomiting, diarrhea, excessive sweating, diuretic abuse, salt-losing nephropathy, or mineralocorticoid deficiency. In these latter conditions, plasma urea is generally increased. Hyponatremia is recognized as a marker of disease severity.[259,263] However, selectively increasing the patient's plasma sodium through fluid manipulation will not improve the outcome; it is the underlying disorder that most likely is responsible for the hyponatremia, as well as the poor clinical outcome.

Clinical manifestations of hyponatremia are nonspecific and include nausea, weakness, and apathy in mild cases, and CNS changes such as lethargy, coma, and seizures in more severe cases.[260,264] No signs or symptoms are specific for SIADH. History, physical examination, and routine laboratory test results often suggest that hyponatremia is dilutional (decreased urea, hemoglobin, or albumin) or depletional (increased urea, hemoglobin, or albumin).

Measurements of sodium and osmolality in blood and urine, combined with clinical assessment of volume status, usually permit the appropriate differential diagnosis of hyponatremic conditions (Box 65.8). The diagnosis of SIADH usually is explored solely on the basis of the clinical scenario and the routine laboratory studies discussed previously.[261,265] SIADH is diagnosed when hyponatremia (<135 mEq/L [mmol/L]) and reduced serum osmolality (<270 to 280 mOsm/kg [mmol/kg]) are present, together with an inappropriately concentrated urine (urine osmolality >100 mOsm/kg [mmol/kg]). Maximally dilute urine normally is 50 to 80 mOsm/kg, and this is expected in the setting of hyponatremia and hypo-osmolality. However, in SIADH, despite serum hypo-osmolality, urine osmolality is typically 250 to 1400 mOsm/kg (mmol/kg). It is important to point out that the urine osmolality does not need to exceed the serum osmolality for the diagnosis of SIADH to be made: the urine need only be inappropriately concentrated with respect to the serum. Urine sodium in SIADH is usually 40 to 60 mEq/L (mmol/L) or greater.

BOX 65.8 Diagnosis of the Syndrome of Inappropriate Antidiuretic Hormone

Document plasma hypo-osmolality (≤275 mOsm/kg [millimoles per kilogram]) and hyponatremia (sodium concentration ≤130 mEq/L [millimoles per liter]). Use the history, physical examination, and appropriate laboratory tests to exclude cardiac, hepatic, renal, thyroid, or adrenal failure, along with the effects of pituitary surgery, diuretic therapy, or medications known to stimulate antidiuretic hormone [ADH[release. (Syndrome of inappropriate ADH [SIADH] cannot be diagnosed unless these factors are corrected.) Measure the urine sodium concentration and osmolality. Urine osmolality greater than plasma osmolality and without correspondingly low urine sodium concentration (usually >40 to 60 mEq/L [millimoles per liter]) indicates that SIADH is probable (see the text for details). If the cause of SIADH is unclear, consider measuring plasma ADH and plasma renin concentrations. SIADH is characterized by high ADH concentration and low renin concentration. If both plasma ADH and renin concentrations are low, a primary defect in renal water excretion is present.

Patients with dilutional hyponatremia resulting from excess water intake (psychogenic polydipsia) have hypotonic plasma, an unremarkable urine sodium concentration (<20 mEq/L [mmol/L]), and a dilute urine (urine osmolality less than that of plasma).[262,266] Patients with depletional hyponatremia caused by extrarenal sodium loss have hypotonic plasma, a low urine sodium concentration (usually <10 to 20 mEq/L [mmol/L]), and urine osmolality greater than that of plasma. Patients with depletional hyponatremia caused by impaired renal sodium conservation have similar results, except that their urine sodium concentrations are inappropriately elevated in the setting of volume depletion. Urinary sodium wasting is evident in an elevated fractional excretion of sodium.

Water load testing is not recommended in cases of suspected SIADH because it may cause acute hyponatremia with significant adverse consequences. Acute oral water loading to excess can produce fatal hyponatremia and cerebral edema.[263,267]

Diagnostic Studies

ADH usually is not measured for diagnostic purposes because ADH excess and deficiency are evident in changes in serum and urine osmolality, serum sodium, and urine volume.[268] Less precise measures of fluid balance include clinical evaluation for dehydration, blood pressure (supine and upright), heart rate, and body weight. Hormone concentration is not measured in some endocrine disorders because the consequent metabolic abnormality is more important. The best example is diabetes mellitus. The diagnosis and management of diabetes mellitus center on measurement of glucose (and now glycosylated hemoglobin) and not on measurement of insulin or C-peptide.

Serum osmolality can be estimated from serum sodium, glucose, and urea (BUN), but is more reliably measured directly by freezing point depression. Vapor pressure osmometry is not as robust an analytical method as freezing point depression (see also Chapter 35). Various formulas are available for estimating serum osmolality; all are based on the fact that sodium represents approximately half of all the ions in serum (each sodium is balanced by an anion, and sodium accounts for almost 95% of all cations); among all nonionic solutes, only glucose and urea have high enough concentrations to substantially affect (alone) osmolality. Hence, osmolality can be estimated by adding together twice the sodium, the glucose, and the urea concentrations (in the United States, glucose and urea (BUN), measured in mg/dL, must be converted to mmol/L by dividing their concentrations by 18 and 2.8, respectively).

Several variations may be seen in the calculation of serum osmolality. The equation

$$\frac{\text{mOsmol}}{\text{kg}} = (2 \times [\text{Na}^+]) + \frac{\left[\text{Glucose}\left(\frac{\text{mg}}{\text{dL}}\right)\right]}{18} + \frac{\left[\text{Urea}\left(\frac{\text{mg}}{\text{dL}}\right)\right]}{2.8}$$

underestimates the true osmolality by 5 to 10 mOsm/kg (mmol/kg) because of the remaining constituents in serum that do not, individually, have significant concentrations, but when combined, they contribute approximately that amount. Some laboratories provide a reference interval that accounts for the difference, whereas others add an average factor (often 8 or 9 mOsm/kg [mmol/kg]) (and use a different reference interval) to make the calculated osmolality a closer estimate of measured osmolality. The equation assumes that the activity coefficient for sodium (Na+) is 1.0, and this is not really the case. Regression analysis of sodium versus measured osmolality produces a slope that corresponds to a factor of approximately 1.86, so some calculations of osmolality (particularly automated calculations) use that factor instead of 2, which results in a bias of approximately 5% between the two equations. As discussed in Chapter 35, the following equations are often recommended:

$$\frac{\text{mOsmol}}{\text{kg}} = (1.86 \times [\text{Na}^+]) + \text{Glucose}\left(\frac{\text{mmol}}{\text{L}}\right) + \text{Urea}\left(\frac{\text{mmol}}{\text{L}}\right) + 9$$

or

$$\frac{\text{mOsmol}}{\text{kg}} = (1.86 \times [\text{Na}^+]) + \text{Glucose}\left(\frac{\text{mg}}{\text{dL}}\right)\Big/18 + \text{Urea}\left(\frac{\text{mg}}{\text{dL}}\right)\Big/2.8 + 9$$

In the absence of proteinuria, hematuria, glycosuria, and other osmotically active substances (such as radiocontrast dyes), urine specific gravity generally reflects urine osmolality.

Measurement of Antidiuretic Hormone

Measurement of ADH typically requires extracting and concentrating the hormone from biological fluids because of its low (pmol/L) concentration and the presence of potentially interfering compounds. ADH can be extracted into acetone, petroleum ether, or ethanol,[269] or it can be chromatographically isolated using octadecyl silica (C-18) columns.[270-272] Although nonisotopic (enzyme) immunoassays have been described,[273,274] most laboratories measure ADH by RIA. Most ADH RIA methods are noncompetitive, and separation of bound and free ligand is commonly achieved using second-antibody precipitation techniques.

An ADH method described by Kluge and colleagues[271] extracts the hormone from 0.5 mL of acidified plasma onto a C-18 column preconditioned with methanol and water. After washing with 0.67 mol/L acetic acid, ADH is eluted from the column with 1.0 g/L trifluoracetic acid in methanol. The extract is dried and reconstituted in 0.25 mL of phosphate buffer containing 2.5 g/L bovine serum albumin, 0.01 mol/L EDTA, and 1 g/L neomycin sulfate. A 100-μL aliquot of reconstituted extract is mixed with 25 μL of polyclonal ADH antisera, and after incubation for 24 hours at 4°C, 125I-labeled ADH is added, followed by incubation for 16 hours. Antigen–antibody complexes are adsorbed on activated charcoal, and after centrifugation, radioactivity is measured in the pellet. This method had an average coefficient of variation of 3.4% over an analytical range of 0.25 to 5.1 ng/L and a minimum detectable concentration of 0.06 ng/L, determined by 3 SD above the mean result for an ADH-free calibrator. Methods for measuring ADH have been recently reviewed.[275]

Vasopressin (ADH) use is banned by the World Anti-Doping Agency, and liquid chromatography and tandem mass spectrometry has been used to detect vasopressin in urine.

Specimen Collection and Storage

Blood specimens for ADH should be collected into prechilled tubes containing EDTA as an anticoagulant. Most procedures recommend that specimens be delivered to the laboratory on ice and centrifuged at 4°C within 30 minutes of collection. The plasma is then removed and stored or shipped frozen at −20°C until analysis is performed. Random urine specimens may be collected without preservatives; alternatively, complete 24-hour urine specimens may be collected in 10 mL of 6 mol/L hydrochloric acid.[276] Significant deterioration of ADH occurs after prolonged storage.

Oxytocin

Oxytocin is a nonapeptide secreted by the magnocellular neurons of the hypothalamus and stored in the neurohypophysis along with ADH. It promotes uterine contractions and milk ejection and contributes to the second stage of labor.[277]

Biochemistry

The structure of oxytocin is similar to that of ADH (see Fig. 65.8), but with a phenylalanine → isoleucine substitution at residue 3, and an arginine → leucine substitution at residue 8.

The gene for oxytocin is located on chromosome 20p13. Prepro-oxytocin is 125 amino acids (12.7 kDa). Similar to the ADH gene, the oxytocin gene encodes two proteins: oxytocin and neurophysin 1. In contrast to prepro-ADH, prepro-oxytocin lacks a sequence analogous to copeptin in ADH. Following the leader sequence of 19 amino acids, the nonapeptide oxytocin is encoded, followed by the 94 amino acid C-terminal propeptide neurophysin 1. The glycine residue at position 28 is amidated. Suspected or definitive disulfide bonds are at amino acids 20 to 25 (within oxytocin), 41 to 85, 44 to 58, 52 to 75, 59 to 65, 92 to 104, and 105 to 110. ADH and oxytocin are highly conserved throughout a variety of species, suggesting that mutations in the genes that encode these proteins are likely to produce serious consequences.

Oxytocin receptors are expressed in the uterine myometrium and myoepithelial cells of the breast. More myometrial receptors are expressed toward the end of pregnancy. The gene for the oxytocin receptor is encoded on chromosome 3p25. Of its 389 amino acids (42.8 kDa), the first 38 amino acids are extracellular, followed by 7 transmembrane domains and a 57 amino acid cytoplasmic domain. Three potential sites of glycosylation are known: amino acids 8, 15, and 26. A disulfide bond may be found between amino acids 112 and 187. Oxytocin receptors occur throughout the CNS, and it is thought that these receptors affect behaviors related to stress, socialization, and maternity.

Regulation of Oxytocin Secretion and Physiologic Activity

Oxytocin is present in both males and females, but its physiologic effects are known only for females.[278] Afferent nerve fibers from the uterus and cervix (and possibly the vagina) communicate with the paraventricular (PVN) and supraoptic nuclei (SON) in the hypothalamus; these are the sites of cell bodies that synthesize oxytocin. Near the conclusion of pregnancy, mechanical stimulation of the cervix by the growing fetus stimulates stretch mechanoreceptors that, in turn, promote oxytocin release from the hypothalamus. Next, uterine contractions during labor trigger additional release of oxytocin. The effect of oxytocin is to increase the strength of uterine contractions, providing positive feedback to oxytocin release until the time of delivery of the fetus. For the myometrium to respond to oxytocin, it must be estrogen primed. Thus, increasing responsiveness of the myometrium to oxytocin is noted near term. Increased sensitivity to oxytocin in the myometrium may reflect changes in oxytocin receptor number and/or responsiveness. Centrally, estrogens enhance the response of oxytocin to these stimuli. The influence of oxytocin on other parts of the brain has been reported. For example, emotional stress inhibits lactation.

With delivery of the newborn and placenta, declining concentrations of sex steroids allow prolactin to trigger active lactation. The role of oxytocin is to stimulate the smooth muscle cells of the breast to propel the milk toward the nipple. These smooth muscle cells (myoepithelial cells) surround the milk-producing cells. With suckling, afferent fibers that travel to the PVN and SON trigger oxytocin release. Contraction of the myoepithelial cells causes "milk let-down" (milk ejection), and milk can leak from the nipple if suckling is not continued.

In summary, oxytocin stimulates uterine smooth muscle contraction during labor and milk duct constriction during suckling that propels milk toward the nipple. Therefore, oxytocin is critical for delivery of the newborn. Likewise, oxytocin is exceedingly important for nourishment and hydration of the newborn and infant.

Clinical disorders involving oxytocin have not been reported. However, oxytocin and its derivatives (pitocin) are used as pharmaceuticals to increase the intensity of uterine contractions during labor (eg, as treatment for prolonged or failed labor) and to prevent or treat postdelivery uterine hemorrhage.

Measurement of Oxytocin

Immunoassays for measuring oxytocin in plasma or urine have been developed but are mostly of research interest, because no clinical indications for measuring oxytocin are known. With most plasma oxytocin assays, a preliminary extraction procedure is required to concentrate the hormone and remove interfering substances.

SUMMARY OF PITUITARY-RELATED DISORDERS

Disorders that result from over- or underproduction of pituitary hormones are tremendously diverse (Table 65.10). Pituitary adenomas may be secretory or nonsecretory.[279] Corticotropinomas secrete ACTH, somatotropinomas secrete GH, and prolactinomas secrete prolactin. Gonadotropinomas usually do not secrete intact LH and/or FSH but may secrete free α subunits.[280] Pituitary adenomas, whether functional or not, can lead to deficiencies of other pituitary hormones through compression and destruction of the adjacent pituitary cells. These topics are reviewed in depth in many chapters in this textbook. Understanding pituitary function and the various diseases that result from pituitary dysfunction is a fundamental and essential aspect of clinical and laboratory medicine practice.

TABLE 65.10 Disorders of Overproduction and Underproduction of Pituitary Hormones

Pituitary Hormone	Consequences of Hormone Excess	Consequences of Hormone Deficiency
ACTH	Cushing disease	Cortisol deficiency
TSH	Central hyperthyroidism	Central hypothyroidism
GH	Children: gigantism Adults: acromegaly	Children: short stature Adults: adult GHD
LH, FSH	Alpha-chain overproduction	Hypogonadism
Prolactin	Galactorrhea, hypogonadism	Inadequate lactation or lactation failure in mothers after delivery
ADH	SIADH	DI

ACTH, Adrenocorticotropic hormone; *ADH*, antidiuretic hormone; *FSH*, follicle-stimulating hormone; *GH*, growth hormone; *LH*, luteinizing hormone; *SIADH*, syndrome of inappropriate ADH; *TSH*, thyroid-stimulating hormone.

SELECTED REFERENCES

For a full list of references for this chapter, please refer to ExpertConsult.com.

4. Cooper MS. Disorders of calcium metabolism and parathyroid disease. *Best Pract Res Clin Endocrinol Metab* 2011;**25**:975–83.
31. Ascoli P, Cavagnini F. Hypopituitarism. *Pituitary* 2006;**9**: 335–42.
34. Winter WE, Hardt NS. Laboratory evaluation of short stature in children. In: Winter WE, Sokoll L, Jialal I, editors. *Handbook of diagnostic endocrinology*. Washington DC: AACC Press; 2008. p. 139–74.
48. LeRoith D. Clinical relevance of systemic and local IGF-I: lessons from animal models. *Pediatr Endocrinol Rev* 2008;**5**(Suppl. 2):739–43.
68. Obara-Moszynska M, Kedzia A, Korman E, et al. Usefulness of growth hormone (GH) stimulation tests and IGF-I concentration measurement in GH deficiency diagnosis. *J Pediatr Endocrinol Metab* 2008;**21**:569–79.
78. Rogol AD, Hayden GF. Etiologies and early diagnosis of short stature and growth failure in children and adolescents. *J Pediatr* 2014;**164**:S1–14.
88. Mullis PE. Genetics of growth hormone deficiency. *Endocrinol Metab Clin North Am* 2007;**36**:17–36.
97. Richmond EJ, Rogol AD. Growth hormone deficiency in children. *Pituitary* 2008;**11**:115–20.
106. Rosenbloom AL, Connor EL. Hypopituitarism and other disorders of the growth hormone-insulin-like growth factor-I axis. In: Lifshitz F, editor. *Pediatric endocrinology*. New York: Informa Healthcare; 2007. p. 65–99.
124. Rosenfeld RG, Hwa V. New molecular mechanisms of GH resistance. *Eur J Endocrinol* 2004;**151**(Suppl. 1):S11–15.
130. Rosenbloom AL, Guevara AJ, Rosenfeld RG, et al. The little women of Loja–growth hormone-receptor deficiency in an inbred population of southern Ecuador. *N Engl J Med* 1990;**323**:1367–74.
135. Clemmons DR. Consensus statement on the standardization and evaluation of growth hormone and insulin-like growth factor assays. *Clin Chem* 2011;**57**:555–9.
153. Ho KK. Consensus guidelines for the diagnosis and treatment of adults with GH deficiency II: a statement of the GH Research Society in association with the European Society for Pediatric Endocrinology, Lawson Wilkins Society, European Society of Endocrinology, Japan Endocrine Society, and Endocrine Society of Australia. *Eur J Endocrinol* 2007;**157**:695–700.
163. Goffin V, Binart N, Touraine P, et al. Prolactin: the new biology of an old hormone. *Annu Rev Physiol* 2002;**64**: 47–67.
165. Bernard V, Young J, Chanson P, et al. New insights in prolactin: pathological implications. *Nat Rev Endocrinol* 2015;**11**:265–75.
177. Molitch ME. Pituitary tumours: pituitary incidentalomas. *Best Pract Res Clin Endocrinol Metab* 2009;**23**:667–75.
181. Agarwal M, Das A, Singh AS. High-dose hook effect in prolactin macroadenomas: a diagnostic concern. *J Hum Reprod Sci* 2010;**3**:160–1.
185. Wheeler MJ. The measurement of LH, FSH, and prolactin. *Methods Mol Biol* 2013;**1065**:105–16.
193. Winter WE, Harris NS. Laboratory approaches to diseases of the adrenal cortex and adrenal medulla. In: Winter WE, Sokoll L, Jialal I, editors. *Diagnostic endocrinology*. Washington, DC: AACC Press; 2008. p. 75–138.
204. Ciccone NA, Kaiser UB. The biology of gonadotroph regulation. *Curr Opin Endocrinol Diabetes Obes* 2009;**16**:321–7.
225. Fleseriu M, Gassner M, Yedinak C, et al. Normal hypothalamic-pituitary-adrenal axis by high-dose cosyntropin testing in patients with abnormal response to low-dose cosyntropin stimulation: a retrospective review. *Endocr Pract* 2010;**16**:64–70.
226. Cemeroglu AP, Kleis L, Postellon DC, et al. Comparison of low-dose and high-dose cosyntropin stimulation testing in children. *Pediatr Int* 2011;**53**:175–80.
236. Ball SG. Vasopressin and disorders of water balance: the physiology and pathophysiology of vasopressin. *Ann Clin Biochem* 2007;**44**:417–31.
238. Boone M, Deen PM. Physiology and pathophysiology of the vasopressin-regulated renal water reabsorption. *Pflugers Arch* 2008;**456**:1005–24.
252. Ghirardello S, Garre ML, Rossi A, et al. The diagnosis of children with central diabetes insipidus. *J Pediatr Endocrinol Metab* 2007;**20**:359–75.
264. Douglas I. Hyponatremia: why it matters, how it presents, how we can manage it. *Cleve Clin J Med* 2006;**73**(Suppl. 3):S4–12.
278. Macdonald K, Macdonald TM. The peptide that binds: a systematic review of oxytocin and its prosocial effects in humans. *Harv Rev Psychiatry* 2010;**18**:1–21.

66

Adrenal Cortex

*Roger L. Bertholf, Mark Cooper, and William E. Winter**

ABSTRACT

Background
The adrenal cortex produces steroid hormones that regulate salt and water balance (mineralocorticoids); metabolism of fat, proteins, and carbohydrates (glucocorticoids); and sexual development (androgens).

Content
Secretion of adrenocortical hormones is influenced by multiple physiological signals originating in the kidney, liver, lungs, pituitary, hypothalamus, and elsewhere. Disease can result from overproduction, as well as deficiency, of adrenocortical hormones. Moreover, excess or deficiency of these hormones can be primary (ie, resulting from adrenal gland dysfunction) or secondary (ie, resulting from dysregulation of stimulating hormones). Mineralocorticoid excess causes hypertension and hypokalemia (called Conn syndrome), whereas deficiency causes salt wasting, sometimes in the form of Addison disease (primary adrenal insufficiency). Glucocorticoid excess causes Cushing syndrome, characterized by hypertension, abdominal obesity, weakness, and abnormal fat distribution. Glucocorticoid deficiency, as in Addison disease, causes weakness, hypotension, and hyperpigmentation of the skin, among other symptoms. Because regulation of adrenocortical hormones is multifactorial, laboratory investigation of adrenal disorders often requires measuring the response to various stimulating factors, both chemical and physiological. Analytical methods are available to measure most adrenocortical hormones.

ANATOMY

The adrenal (or suprarenal) glands are pyramidal shaped, 2 to 3 cm wide, 4 to 6 cm long, and about 1 cm thick. Arterial blood is supplied to the adrenal gland by (1) the superior adrenal (or suprarenal) artery from the inferior phrenic artery (a branch of the aorta); (2) the middle adrenal artery, which is directly from the aorta; and (3) the inferior adrenal artery, a branch of the renal artery. Venous access to the adrenal gland, which is important for diagnostic studies, is obtained through the right adrenal vein that enters into the vena cava at an acute angle or the left adrenal vein that enters into the left renal vein.

The adrenal cortex and the gonads share several metabolic pathways for synthesis of steroid hormones because both are derived from mesodermal anlagen.[1] Two important transcription factors control the development of the adrenal cortex: steroidogenic factor-1 (SF-1) and the dosage-sensitive sex reversal adrenal hypoplasia congenita (AHC) on the X-chromosome gene 1 *(DAX-1)*.[2] SF-1 regulates *DAX-1.*

The postnatal adrenal cortex is composed of three layers: the glomerulosa (10% to 15% of the cortex), the fasciculata (up to 75% of the cortex), and the reticularis (5% to 10% of the cortex). The fetal adrenal cortex, which wanes by 18 months of age, is proportionately larger than adrenal glands observed later in life. The fetal adrenal layer is situated between the definitive cortex and the medulla and contains large steroid-secreting cells arranged in a reticular pattern. At birth, the adrenal gland is nearly equal in weight to that of an adult (8 to 12 grams). The large size of the fetal adrenal gland (≈250 mg/100 g body weight) may explain its propensity to occasionally be traumatized during delivery. Between 3 and 18 months of age, the adrenal glands involute to approximately half their size at birth. Later in life, the adrenal glands are less susceptible to trauma and represent less than 50 mg/100 g of body weight. Adult adrenal glands weigh 4 to 6 g each. Table 66.1 lists the location and action of hormones produced by the adrenal gland.

STEROID BIOCHEMISTRY

Steroids are characterized by a cyclopentanoperhydrophenanthrene nucleus of four aliphatic rings biosynthesized by cyclization of squalene, produced by the mevalonate (also called the HMG-CoA reductase, or isoprenoid) pathway. The steroid backbone consists of three hexacyclic and one pentacyclic carbon rings, designated A, B, C, and D. Sterols are steroids hydroxylated at position 3 on the A ring; cholesterol is a sterol. Cholesterol has a double bond between carbons 5 and 6 and an eight-carbon aliphatic side group at position 17, and it is the precursor for all human steroid hormones (Fig. 66.1). In humans, cholesterol is derived from both dietary sources and de novo synthesis, and it is transported in blood principally in low-density lipoprotein (LDL). An increase in cellular cholesterol concentration inhibits expression of the LDL receptor. Hormones produced by the adrenal cortex include mineralocorticoids, glucocorticoids, and adrenal androgens.

*The authors gratefully acknowledge the contribution of Professor Laurence M. Demers to the fourth edition of this textbook, on which portions of this chapter are based.

Mineralocorticoids (Aldosterone)

Mineralocorticoids bind to the mineralocorticoid receptor (MR) in the distal convoluted tubule (DCT) and collecting duct of the nephron, the colon, and the salivary glands to promote sodium reabsorption and potassium and hydrogen ion excretion.[3] Similar to other steroid and thyroid hormone receptors, the MR functions as a transcription factor. When mineralocorticoid binds to cytoplasmic receptors, the mineralocorticoid-MR complex migrates to the nucleus, where it influences gene transcription. The principal mineralocorticoid is aldosterone, but other compounds with mineralocorticoid activity include 11-deoxycorticosterone (DOC), 18-hydroxycorticosterone, corticosterone, and cortisol.

The *MR* gene encodes the 107-kDa nuclear receptor protein, subfamily 3, group C, member 2 (NR3C2), located on chromosome 4q31.1-31.2. Alternative splicing yields alpha and beta MR mRNA. Aldosterone stimulates epithelial sodium channel (ENaC) activity via serum and glucocorticoid-induced kinase and K-ras, increases expression of mitochondrial ATP-producing genes, and stimulates the basolateral Na^+/K^+-ATPase pump. ENaC, a highly selective ENaC that is amiloride sensitive (amiloride is a K^+-sparing diuretic), has three subunits: the alpha subunit (most important of the three subunits; the sodium channel, non–voltage gated protein 1, alpha coded by *SCNN1A*, chromosome 12p13), the beta subunit (sodium channel, non–voltage gated 1, beta *SCNN1B*, chromosome 16p13-p12), and the gamma subunit (sodium channel, non–voltage gated 1, gamma *SCNN1G*, chromosome 16p13-p12).[4] All ENaC subunits are similar and contain a large N-terminal extracellular domain, two transmembrane spanning domains (M1 and M2), and a short C-terminal intracellular domain.[5] Although aldosterone binds to the MR in the cytoplasm, with subsequent transit of the complex to the nucleus, some free MR is present in the nucleus. The MR binds cortisol and DOC with affinity equal to that of aldosterone. However, the MR is protected from cortisol and DOC by 11 beta-hydroxysteroid dehydrogenase-2 (HSD11B2), which converts cortisol to cortisone (Fig. 66.2). Cortisone does not bind to the MR. Mutations in HSD11B2 may be involved in some cases of essential hypertension.[6] Chronic elevations in angiotensin, which controls aldosterone synthesis and release, produces myocardial fibrosis and inflammatory changes in the renal vasculature.[7] The actions of mineralocorticoids are summarized in Table 66.2.

TABLE 66.1 Anatomy and Products of the Adrenal Gland

Adrenal Layer	Major Product(s)	Action
Cortex		
Zona glomerulosa	Aldosterone	Mineralocorticoid
Zona fasciculata	Cortisol	Glucocorticoid
Zona reticularis	Dehydroepiandrosterone Androstenedione	Adrenal androgen
Medulla	Epinephrine	Catecholamine

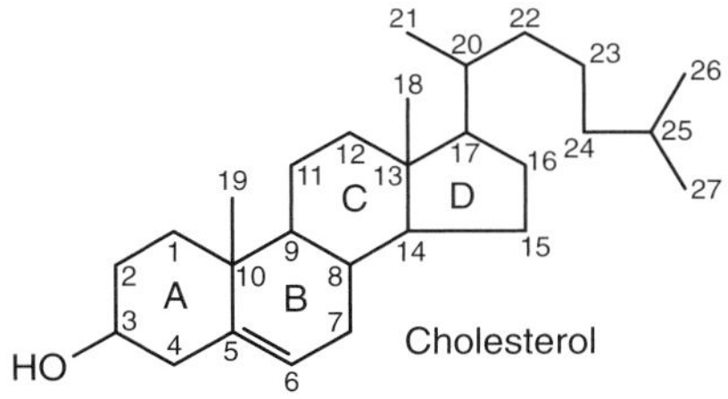

FIGURE 66.1 Steroids are a class of compounds structurally characterized by four interconnected rings labeled *A* to *D*. The carbons are numbered in a standard fashion as illustrated. A sterol is a type of steroid wherein a hydroxyl group is attached to the ring (eg, cholesterol where the hydroxyl group is attached to carbon 3). Cholesterol has a double bond between carbons 5 and 6 and contains an eight-carbon R group.

Glucocorticoids (Cortisol)

Glucocorticoids bind to the glucocorticoid receptor (GR) expressed in a variety of tissues, including lymphocytes, hepatocytes, and bone.[8] The *GR* gene contains 10 exons (exons 1 through 8 plus 9 alpha and 9 beta). Alternative splicing yields GR alpha and beta transcripts. Because of the wide distribution of the GR, glucocorticoid effects are diverse, including changes in intermediary metabolism and

TABLE 66.2 Major Actions of Mineralocorticoids

Action	Adverse Outcome/ Excessive Action	Deficient Action
Sodium retention*	Hypertension	Hypotension
Urinary potassium wasting	Hypokalemia	Hyperkalemia
Urinary hydrogen ion wasting	Alkalosis	

*With consequent H_2O retention.

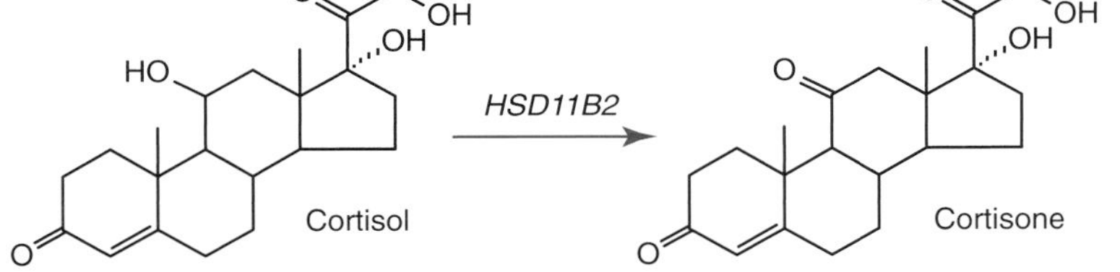

FIGURE 66.2 The mineralocorticoid receptor (MR) is protected from cortisol by 11 beta-hydroxysteroid dehydrogenase-2 (HSD11B2), which converts cortisol to inactive cortisone. Cortisone does not bind to the MR.

TABLE 66.3 Relative Potencies of Corticosteroids

Corticosteroid	Glucocorticoid Activity	Mineralocorticoid Activity
Aldosterone	0.1	400
Corticosterone	0.2	2
Cortisol	1	1
Cortisone	0.7	0.7
Dexamethasone*	50–150	2
11-Deoxycorticosterone	0	20
Fludrocortisone*	10	400
6α-Methylprednisolone*	5	0.5
Prednisolone*	4	0.7
Prednisone*	4	0.7
Triamcinolone*	3	0

*Synthetic.

immunoregulation. Glucocorticoids raise blood glucose concentrations by enhancing the synthesis of gluconeogenic enzymes (eg, glucose-6-phosphatase and phosphoenol pyruvate carboxykinase), increase liver glycogen content by activation of glycogen synthase, and inhibit glycogen phosphorylase, producing insulin resistance in both muscle and adipose tissue and further raising blood glucose concentrations. Excessive catabolism of skeletal muscle causes myopathy, resulting in weakness. Protein catabolism causes thinning of the skin and loss of strength in connective tissues. Excess glucocorticoids may result in bone loss from collagen catabolism and loss of osteoid, leading to fractures and compressed vertebrae.

Glucocorticoids promote redistribution of adipose tissue centrally to the trunk, neck, and face; increased adipocyte differentiation; and lipogenesis in these tissues. Insulin resistance raises very low-density lipoprotein (VLDL) and triglyceride concentrations and lowers high-density lipoprotein concentrations. Insulin resistance decreases the activity of adipose tissue hormone-sensitive lipase, allowing triglyceride hydrolysis to free fatty acids. In the liver, those free fatty acids provide substrate for hepatic triglyceride synthesis and subsequent VLDL production and export. Glucocorticoids increase appetite, thereby increasing caloric intake and weight gain.

When glucocorticoids bind to the cytoplasmic GR, heat shock proteins HSP70 and HSP90 are released.[9] Glucocorticoids are powerful antiinflammatory hormones that inhibit nuclear factor kappaB (NFkappaB) through the induction of IkappaB synthesis.[10] IkappaB binds to cytoplasmic NFkappaB, impairing its entry into the nucleus. Within the nucleus, the GR-cortisol complex binds NFkappaB, preventing it from binding to DNA. Subsequently, GR-cortisol and NFkappaB compete for cofactors that are present in limited supply. Although IkappaB synthesis is enhanced, many proinflammatory genes are repressed, such as cyclo-oxygenase 2, inducible nitric oxide synthase, various interleukins (IL-1, IL-2, and IL-6), tumor necrosis factor-alpha, interferon-gamma, and E-selectin. Adrenocorticotropic hormone (ACTH) also stimulates the release of IL-1, IL-6, and tumor necrosis factor-alpha.[11]

Glucocorticoids help maintain vascular tone and cardiac output and stabilize lysosomal membranes.[12] Glucocorticoids suppress immune hypersensitivity by inhibiting the production of histamine by basophils and mast cells. Modest doses of glucocorticoids can improve mood, but at therapeutic doses, they can cause psychosis. The glucocorticoid and mineralocorticoid activities of various corticosteroids are compared in Table 66.3, and the physiological actions of glucocorticoids are summarized in Table 66.4.

TABLE 66.4 Major Targets of Glucocorticoid Action and Adverse Consequences of Excesses and Deficiencies

	ADVERSE OUTCOME	
Target Tissue	**Excessive Action**	**Deficient Action**
Central Nervous System	Polyphagia	Anorexia
	Depression or psychosis	Depression
Endocrine System		
Carbohydrate metabolism	Hyperglycemia	Hypoglycemia
Glycogen synthesis, gluconeogenesis, insulin resistance	Increased	Decreased
Free fatty acids, triglycerides	Increased	NSE
Body weight	Increased	Decreased
Fat distribution	Centripetal	NSE
Pituitary	Decreased TSH	NSE
Musculoskeletal and Connective Tissue		
Muscle	Atrophy (catabolism)	NSE
Skin	Thinning (catabolism)	NSE
Bone	Osteoporosis	NSE
Immune System	Immunosuppression	NSE

NSE, No specific effect.

Adrenal Androgens (DHEA and Androstenedione)

The adrenal androgens dehydroepiandrosterone (DHEA), dehydroepiandrosterone sulfate (DHEA-S), and androstenedione are peripherally converted to testosterone, which binds to the androgen receptor (described in Chapter 68).[13] Between ages 7 and 8 years, urinary excretion of 17-ketosteroids (breakdown products of adrenal androgens) increases, signaling that puberty will begin within 3 to 5 years.[14]

In males, adrenal androgens such as DHEA and androstenedione are mostly unimportant because testosterone, produced in the testes, is a much more potent androgen. In pubertal and adult women, however, the adrenal androgens produce axillary and pubic hair. Women with Turner syndrome (ie, XO sex chromosome genotype) illustrate the effects of adrenal androgens in women. Because of streak gonads (hypoplastic and dysfunctioning gonads mainly composed of fibrous tissue) and all of their ovarian follicles being atretic before birth, adolescents with Turner syndrome do not experience gonadarche (the period during which the gonads begin to secrete sex hormones). Estrogen deficiency during adolescence is manifest in lack of breast development, primary amenorrhea, and failure of fat redistribution to the hips and buttocks. However, because adrenarche (the increase in activity of the adrenal glands preceding puberty) is normal in adolescents with Turner syndrome, they will develop axillary and pubic hair despite their lack of estrogen.

DHEA is highly sulfated; circulating concentrations of DHEA-S exceed those of DHEA by at least 100-fold. DHEA-S decreases slightly in women following menopause. For detailed age- and sex-dependent reference intervals see Appendix on Reference Intervals. Please note that throughout this chapter, reference intervals are given as a guide only. Laboratories need to verify the transferability of published reference intervals to their local population and analytical methods based on the CLSI C28-A3 guidelines (for details of verification, see Chapter 8 on Reference Intervals).

PHYSIOLOGY AND REGULATION OF ADRENOCORTICAL HORMONES

Steroid hormones are not stored and therefore must be produced as needed. Steroids are lipophilic and pass through cell membranes to exit the hormone-producing cells, enter the circulation to be distributed throughout the body, and enter target cells by passing through the membrane into the cytoplasm, where they bind to receptors. Translocation of the cytosolic hormone-receptor complex into the nucleus results in hormonal activity. Evidence suggests that steroid hormones may affect more than DNA transcription alone. In the circulation, steroids exist as free and protein-bound species.

Aldosterone

Aldosterone production and secretion are regulated by the renin-angiotensin system (Fig. 66.3).[15,16] The rate-limiting component in this system is renin, the release of which is

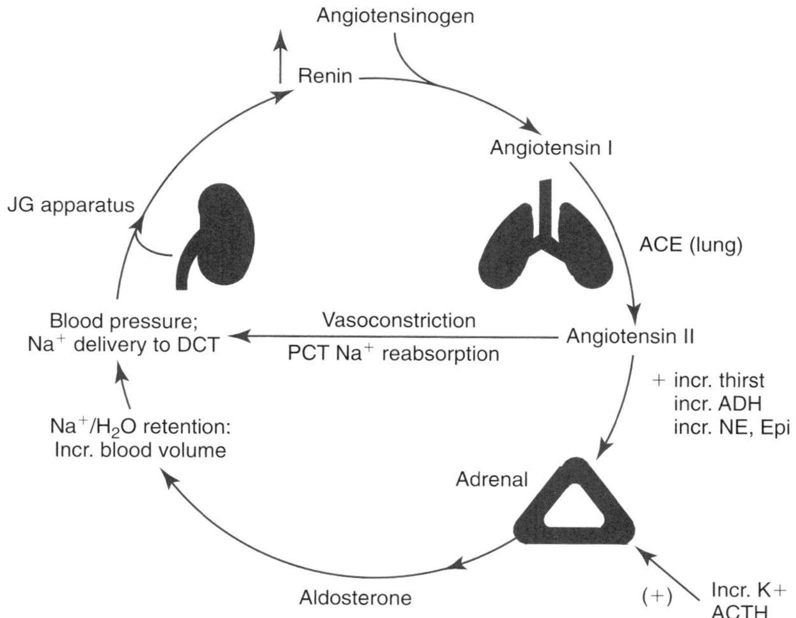

FIGURE 66.3 The juxtaglomerular *(JG)* apparatus monitors hydrostatic pressure in the glomerulus and the sodium concentration in the distal convoluted tubule *(DCT)*. Renin is released in cases of decreased renal perfusion or decreased sodium concentration in the DCT. Renin cleaves angiotensinogen to angiotensin I. Angiotensin-converting enzyme *(ACE)*, predominantly in the lung, converts angiotensin I to angiotensin II. Angiotensin II has powerful vasoconstrictive effects, promotes sodium reabsorption by the proximal convoluted tubule *(PCT)*, and stimulates thirst, antidiuretic hormone *(ADH)* release, catecholamine release, and aldosterone synthesis and secretion. Aldosterone stimulates sodium and water reabsorption, increasing blood volume and blood pressure. Overall these effects enhance renal perfusion. Adrenocorticotropic hormone *(ACTH)* and increased potassium have minor effects in stimulating aldosterone synthesis and secretion. *Epi,* Epinephrine; *NE,* norepinephrine.

regulated by the juxtaglomerular apparatus. The juxtaglomerular apparatus is composed of the juxtaglomerular cells of the afferent arteriole that immediately leads to the glomerulus, lacis cells (extraglomerular mesangial cells located at the vascular pole of the renal corpuscle), and the macula densa.

Juxtaglomerular cells are modified smooth muscle cells that synthesize and secrete renin. Preprorenin is a 406 amino acid protein; removal of a 20 amino acid presequence yields prorenin (386 amino acids). Cleavage of the 46 amino acid prosegment produces the active hormone (340 amino acids, 37 kDa). Both prorenin and renin are released by the juxtaglomerular cells, which have baroreceptors that detect arterial wall stretch produced by renal perfusion pressure; decreased renal perfusion is the primary trigger of renin release. The macula densa contains specialized cells that line the DCT. Anatomically, the DCT passes between the afferent and efferent arterioles of the nephron, which supply blood to and drain blood from the glomerular capillaries, respectively. Compared with other tubular cells, DCT cells are unique in that their nuclei are near the apical (luminal) pole of the cell, whereas the Golgi apparatus is near the basolateral pole of the cell. The macula densa monitors the sodium concentration in the DCT. If a decline in sodium concentration is detected, the macula densa signals the juxtaglomerular cells via prostacyclin to release renin.

Sodium delivery to the DCT is decreased when renal perfusion declines. Sodium delivery to the DCT can decline due to hyponatremia or decreased glomerular filtration rate, both of which stimulate renin release. Sympathetic innervation of the juxtaglomerular cells also influences renin secretion via beta$_1$-adrenoreceptors. For this reason, norepinephrine and dopamine stimulate renin release. Upright posture and catecholamine release thereby stimulate renin release. Potassium also directly stimulates renin release. Overall, renin release is physiologically stimulated by hypovolemia, reduced cardiac output, systemic vasodilatation, selectively reduced renal perfusion, hyponatremia, and stress (mediated by catecholamines).

Angiotensinogen is an approximately 60-kDa alpha$_2$-globulin synthesized by hepatocytes.[17] Renin acts as an aspartyl proteolytic enzyme cleaving 10 N-terminal residues from angiotensinogen to form the decapeptide angiotensin I. Angiotensin I is a prohormone that has no innate activity. Angiotensin-converting enzyme (ACE), a zinc metallopeptidase, removes the two C-terminal residues from angiotensin I to generate the octapeptide angiotensin II.[18] High concentrations of ACE are expressed in the lung, and the enzyme is pathologically expressed in conditions involving macrophage activation such as sarcoidosis. Further degradation of angiotensin II by aminopeptidase A (a glutamyl aminopeptidase) yields the heptapeptide angiotensin III. The ratio of angiotensin II to angiotensin III is usually 4 to 1. An arginyl aminopeptidase generates angiotensin IV from angiotensin III. Angiotensin III and IV are active but overall have less potency than angiotensin II. These steps are summarized in Table 66.5.

Angiotensin II preserves circulating blood volume and maintains blood pressure through several mechanisms: (1) stimulation of aldosterone synthase (CYP11B2) to produce aldosterone; (2) direct vasoconstriction; (3) increased release of epinephrine and norepinephrine from the adrenal medulla, which also act as vasoconstrictors; (4) stimulation of sodium reabsorption in the proximal convoluted tubule (PCT); (5) stimulation of thirst; and (6) stimulated release of antidiuretic hormone (ADH). Angiotensin III has equivalent potency to angiotensin II in stimulating aldosterone secretion.

TABLE 66.5 Angiotensinogen and Derived Peptides

Molecule	Size (Amino Acids; Abbreviation)
Angiotensinogen	485
↓ Renin	
Angiotensin I	10 (A1-10)
↓ Angiotensin-converting enzyme	
Angiotensin II	8 (A1-8)
↓ Amino peptidase A	
Angiotensin III	7 (A2-8)
↓ Arginyl aminopeptidase	
Angiotensin IV	6 (A3-8)

The best-characterized angiotensin receptors are AT1 and AT2, which involve multiple second messenger systems.[19] Most functions of angiotensin II are mediated via the AT1 receptor. Some actions of the stimulated AT2 receptor oppose those of the AT1 receptor (eg, AT2 receptor engagement causes vasodilatation).

Cortisol

Cortisol is regulated through a traditional hypothalamic-pituitary-end organ negative feedback system (Fig. 66.4). Corticotropin-releasing hormone (CRH) is released from the hypothalamus by stress, exercise, and hypoglycemia. Examples of physiological stress include pain, trauma, surgery, and hemorrhage. Examples of psychological stress include severe anxiety and major depression. Prolonged administration of high doses of glucocorticoids either orally or parenterally suppresses the hypothalamic-pituitary-adrenal axis, leading to adrenal atrophy. As a consequence, abrupt termination of exogenous corticosteroids may induce an acute and possibly life-threatening glucocorticoid insufficiency, sometimes called Addisonian crisis.

CRH is produced by the paraventricular nucleus of the hypothalamus. Prohormone convertase-1 (PC1) and PC2 liberate a C-terminal, 43 amino acid CRH precursor from the 196 amino acid preprohormone. Peptidylglycine alpha-amidating mono-oxygenase removes the two C-terminal residues and adds an amine group, producing the 41 amino acid CRH.

Secreted CRH reaches the anterior pituitary gland via the hypothalamic pituitary portal system.[20] Corticotrophs express CRH receptors and comprise about 20% of functional anterior pituitary cells that synthesize, store, and release corticotropin (ACTH; 4.5 kDa).[21] ACTH is also released in response to stimulation by ADH, but to a lesser degree than CRH. The proinflammatory cytokines IL-1, IL-6, and tumor necrosis factor-alpha also stimulate ACTH release. There are two CRH receptors (CRH-R1 and CRH-R2) and three splice variants of CRH-2 (CRH-2alpha, CRH-2beta, and CRH-2gamma). CRH mediates its effects on corticotrophs exclusively through

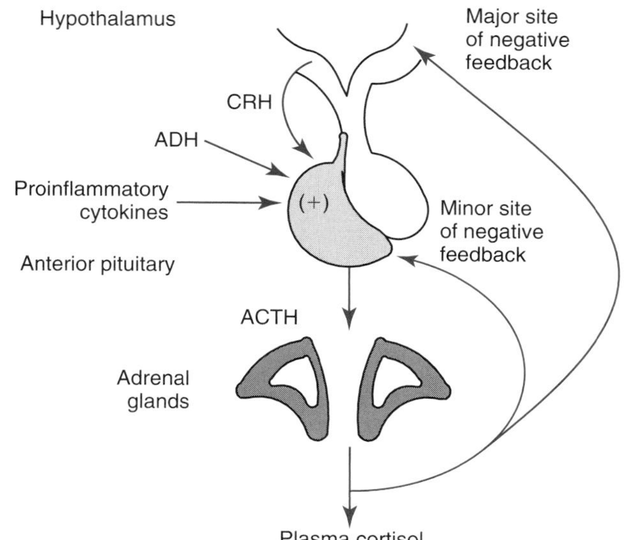

FIGURE 66.4 Cortisol synthesis and release are controlled through a traditional hypothalamic–pituitary–end organ negative feedback loop. Corticotropin-releasing hormone *(CRH)* released from the hypothalamus is delivered to the anterior pituitary via the hypothalamic-pituitary portal system. CRH releases adrenocorticotropic hormone *(ACTH)* from anterior pituitary corticotrophs. Increased concentrations of antidiuretic hormone *(ADH)* and proinflammatory cytokines (eg, IL-1, IL-6, and tumor necrosis factor-alpha) also stimulate ACTH release. ACTH stimulates the synthesis and release of cortisol from the adrenal cortex. Cortisol feeds back negatively at the pituitary, but the major site of negative feedback is the hypothalamus.

CRH-R1. CRH and its receptors are widely distributed throughout the central nervous system (CNS).

ACTH is proteolytically released from its 32-kDa precursor protein, 266 amino acid pro-opiomelanocortin (POMC; gene: 8 kb; chromosome 2p23).[22,23] In the corticotrophs, subtilisin-like proprotein convertase (PC1/3) cleaves POMC into two fragments: the 22-kDa pro-ACTH fragment and beta-lipotropin (amino acids 42–134), whose functions remain poorly understood. PC1/3 releases ACTH (amino acids 1–39) from pro-ACTH. The resulting N-terminal fragment is further cleaved to release pro-gamma-melanocyte-stimulating hormone (MSH) and a joining peptide. ACTH is not further modified in corticotrophs (Fig. 66.5).

The action of PC2 in the hypothalamus, skin, and intermediate lobe melanotrophs is to release gamma-MSH from pro-opiocortin; alpha-melanocyte-stimulating hormone (alpha-MSH; amino acids 1–13) and corticotropin-like intermediate lobe peptide (amino acids 18–39) from ACTH; and gamma-lipotropin (amino acids 42–101) and beta-endorphin (amino acids 104–134) from beta-lipotropin. Finally, beta-MSH (amino acids 84–101) is derived from gamma-lipotropin via PC2 (see Fig. 66.5).

Hyperpigmentation that occurs with ACTH excess appears to be a direct consequence of the MSH-like activity of ACTH and not ACTH cleavage into alpha-MSH.[24] Although gamma and alpha MSH sequences are contained within ACTH and the beta-MSH is contained within gamma-lipotropin (a fragment of beta-lipotropin), MSH is not released by the human anterior pituitary gland.

ACTH circulates systemically and binds to ACTH receptors located on adrenocortical cells. The ACTH receptor is the G-protein–coupled melanocortin-2 receptor (gene location: chromosome 18p11.2).[25] A second messenger system involves adenyl cyclase and cyclic AMP production. ACTH activity is triggered via protein kinase A and protein kinase C, leading to steroidogenesis, increased size and number of adrenocortical cells, and increased size and functional complexity of cellular organelles, resulting in cortisol synthesis and release. Cortisol inhibits hypothalamic and pituitary release of CRH and ACTH, respectively.[26] Other negative feedback loops include ACTH suppression of hypothalamic CRH and an ultra-short feedback loop whereby ACTH suppresses its own release. There is diurnal variation in the secretion of cortisol; highest concentrations occur approximately 2 hours before awakening, and lowest concentrations shortly after falling asleep.

Adrenal Androgens

Regulation of adrenal androgen synthesis and secretion is not well understood. The existence of a pituitary adrenal androgen–stimulating hormone or an adrenocortical androgen–stimulating hormone remains doubtful despite many years of research that sought its existence.[27] The best-characterized regulator of androstenedione and DHEA secretion is ACTH, which may be expected because ACTH regulates CYP17. Diurnal rhythm in adrenal androgen concentrations parallels cortisol variations. Nevertheless, ACTH regulation of adrenal androgens does not explain the normal prepubertal and pubertal increases in adrenal androgen synthesis that occurs in both boys and girls: ACTH does not increase prior to puberty. Evidence indicates that there is posttranslational regulation of 17 to 20 lyase activity of CYP17 through changes in the expression and activity of factors that enhance electron transfer.[28]

BIOSYNTHESIS OF ADRENOCORTICAL HORMONES

An overview of steroid biosynthesis is illustrated in Fig. 66.6, and the major steroidogenic enzymes are listed in Table 66.6.[29]

Aldosterone

Within the cytoplasm of steroid-producing cells, cholesteryl esters are hydrolyzed by the ACTH-responsive steroidogenesis activator protein that functionally is a cholesteryl esterase. Freed cholesterol is transported across the outer mitochondrial membrane by a sterol transfer protein into the mitochondrial intermembranous space. The 30-kDa steroidogenic acute regulatory protein (StAR) then transports cholesterol into the mitochondria.[30,31] StAR-mediated cholesterol transport is a rate-limiting step in steroid hormone synthesis. StAR transcription is enhanced by rising concentrations of cyclic AMP stimulated by receptor-bound ACTH. In the mitochondria, cholesterol is converted to pregnenolone by the action of CYP11A, the cytochrome P450 sidechain cleavage enzyme (P450ssc; gene location: chromosome 15q23-24) that is functionally a 20,22-desmolase that releases isocaproaldehyde from cholesterol. CYP11A thereby converts the C_{27} steroid cholesterol to corresponding C_{21} steroids.

Pregnenolone moves from the mitochondrion to the lumen of the endoplasmic reticulum. In the zona glomerulosa,

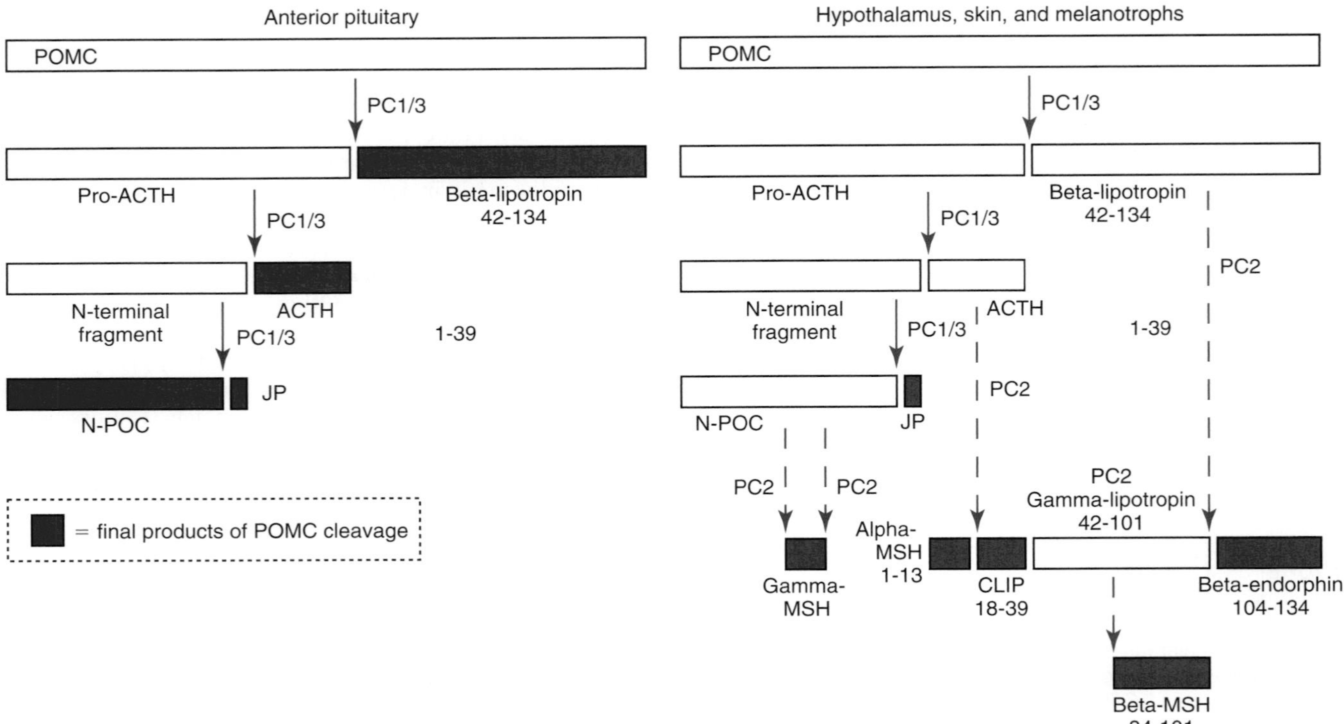

FIGURE 66.5 Adrenocorticotropic hormone *(ACTH)* is derived from pro-opiomelanocortin *(POMC)* by proteolysis. In the corticotrophs through the action of subtilisin-like proprotein convertase PC1/3, POMC is first cleaved into two fragments: the 22 kDa pro-ACTH fragment and beta-lipotropin (amino acids 42–134), the function of which remains poorly understood. Next, PC1/3 releases ACTH (amino acids 1–39) from pro-ACTH. The resulting N-terminal fragment is further cleaved to pro-gamma-MSH *(aka N-POC)* and a joining peptide *(JP)*. ACTH is not further cleaved in corticotrophs. In the hypothalamus, skin, and melanotrophs, further processing of N-POC, ACTH, and beta-lipotropin occurs. The action of PC2 in the hypothalamus, skin, and melanotrophs of the intermediate lobe of the pituitary is to release gamma-MSH from N-POC; alpha-melanocyte stimulating hormone (alpha-MSH; amino acids 1–13) and corticotropin-like intermediate lobe peptide (CLIP, amino acids 18–39) from ACTH and gamma-lipotropin (amino acids 42–101); and beta-endorphin (amino acids 104–134) from beta-lipotropin. Last, beta-MSH (amino acids 84–101) is derived from gamma-lipotropin via PC2.

CYP17 (P450c17) activity is not expressed; therefore pregnenolone is converted to progesterone via the non-P450 enzyme, 3-beta-hydroxysteroid dehydrogenase type 2 (3 beta-HSD; gene location: chromosome 1p13.1). The conversion of pregnenolone to progesterone also requires delta(5)-ketosteroid isomerase, which translocates the double bond from position 5 to position 4 on the steroid backbone. Pregnenolone, 17-hydroxypregnenolone, and DHEA are delta(5) steroids, whereas progesterone, 17-hydroxyprogesterone, and androstenedione are delta(4) steroids based on the location of their double bond.

CYP21, a P450 21 alpha-hydroxylase (P450c21; gene location: chromosome 6p21.3), also expressed in the zona fasciculata, converts progesterone to DOC. DOC migrates back into the mitochondrion, where CYP11B2 (P450 aldo; gene location: 8q24.3) catalyzes its conversion DOC to aldosterone. Normally, little CYP11B1 (P450c11; gene location: 8q24.3) activity occurs in the zona glomerulosa.

CYP11B2 (aldosterone synthase) encompasses three enzymatic activities: an 11-hydroxylase (DOC → corticosterone), an 18-hydroxylase (corticosterone methyl oxidase I; corticosterone → 18-hydroxycorticosterone), and an 18-hydroxydehydrogenase (corticosterone methyl oxidase II; 18-hydroxycorticosterone → aldosterone; see Fig. 66.6).[32] Aldosterone diffuses out of the mitochondrion into the cytoplasm, across the cell membrane, entering the interstitium and then the circulation. Aldosterone secretion varies inversely with urinary sodium and is estimated to be 1 to 80 μg (2.8–222 nmol/L). Aldosterone secretion is approximately one-tenth the rate of cortisol secretion on a weight basis. The half-life of circulating aldosterone is less than 15 minutes.

Whereas CYP11A, CYP17, and CYP11B1 are under ACTH control, CYP11B2 is regulated predominantly by angiotensin II. Thus control of aldosterone synthesis is mostly independent of the anterior pituitary. Cortisol and adrenal androgens are not formed in the zona glomerulosa because the zona glomerulosa does not express CYP17.

Cortisol

Cortisol production follows within minutes of an increase in circulating ACTH concentrations. In the zona fasciculata, where CYP17 (P450c17; gene location: chromosome

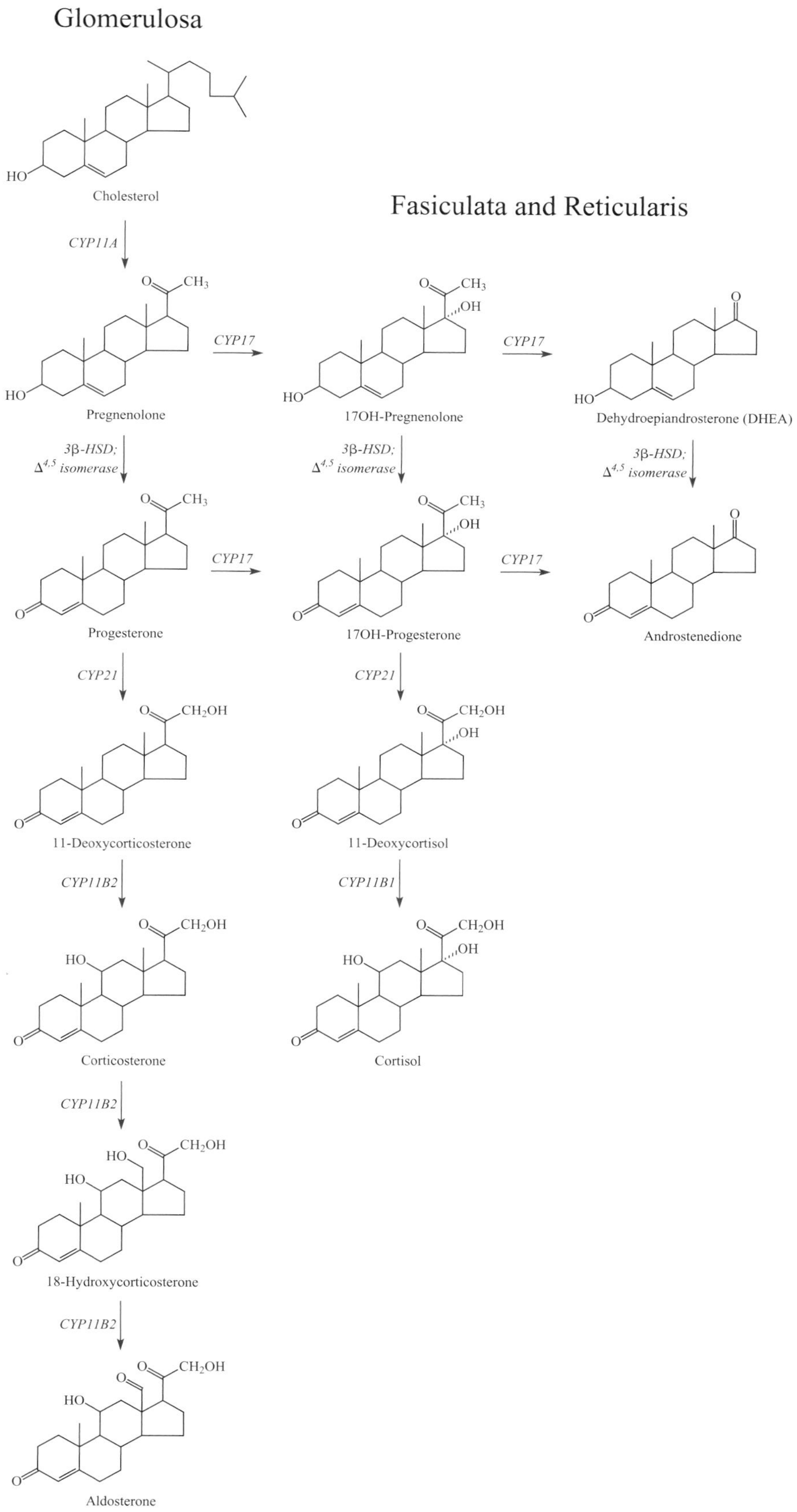

Glomerulosa

Cholesterol

CYP11A

Pregnenolone

3β-HSD; $\Delta^{4,5}$ isomerase

Progesterone

CYP21

11-Deoxycorticosterone

CYP11B2

Corticosterone

CYP11B2

18-Hydroxycorticosterone

CYP11B2

Aldosterone

Fasiculata and Reticularis

CYP17

17OH-Pregnenolone

CYP17

Dehydroepiandrosterone (DHEA)

3β-HSD; $\Delta^{4,5}$ isomerase

CYP17

17OH-Progesterone

CYP17

Androstenedione

CYP21

11-Deoxycortisol

CYP11B1

Cortisol

FIGURE 66.6 The zona glomerulosa is the site of aldosterone synthesis. CYP11B2 is predominantly controlled by angiotensin II, regulating aldosterone synthesis and secretion. In the fasciculata and reticularis layers, cortisol and the adrenal androgens DHEA and androstenedione are produced. CYP11A, 3 beta-HSD, CYP17, CYP21, and CYP11B1 activities are controlled by ACTH.

TABLE 66.6 Major Steroidogenic Enzymes Expressed in Adrenal Cortex

Protein*	P450 Abbreviation	Enzyme Activity(ies)
Major Enzymes Expressed in Zona Glomerulosa		
CYP11A	P450ssc	20,22-Desmolase (20,22-Lyase)
3-Beta HSD (type 2) (gene name: *HSD3B2*)	—	3-Beta hydroxysteroid dehydrogenase
Delta^5-ketosteroid isomerase	—	Delta^5-ketosteroid isomerase
CYP21	P450c21	21-Alpha hydroxylase
CYP11B2	P450 aldo	11-Beta hydroxylase 18-Hydroxylase 18-Oxidase
Major Enzymes Expressed in Zona Fasciculata and Reticularis		
CYP11A	P450ssc	20,22-Desmolase (20,22-Lyase)
3-Beta HSD (type 2) (gene name: *HSD3B2*)	—	3-Beta hydroxysteroid dehydrogenase
Delta^5-ketosteroid isomerase	—	Delta^5-ketosteroid isomerase
CYP17	P450c17	17-Hydroxylase 17,20-Lyase (ZR > ZF)
CYP21	P450c21	21-Alpha hydroxylase
CYP11B1	P450c11	11-Beta hydroxylase

*Usually these terms when italicized refer to the gene name. However, because different sources refer to these enzymes in a variety of ways (gene name vs. enzyme activity), the gene name in roman is used for the protein name.
ZF, Zona fasciculata; *ZR*, zona reticularis.

10q24.3) is expressed, the enzyme hydroxylates pregnenolone to 17-hydroxypregnenolone.[33] CYP17 also has P450 17,20-lyase activity, which is important for adrenal androgen synthesis. 3-Beta-HSD and delta(5)-4-isomerase convert 17-hydroxypregnenolone to 17-hydroxyprogesterone. In the final step outside of the mitochondrion, CYP21 hydroxylates 17-hydroxyprogesterone to 11-deoxycortisol. 11-Deoxycortisol migrates into the mitochondrion, where CYP11B1 (P450c11) converts 11-deoxycortisol to cortisol. The zona fasciculata expresses little CYP11B2 activity. Similar to aldosterone, cortisol diffuses out of the cell and enters the circulation. Normal cortisol secretion is 6 to 14 mg/m^2 per 24 hours. In adults, this is approximately 10 to 20 mg/d (28–55 μmol/d), with some estimates as high as 25 mg/d (60 μmol/d).

Adrenal Androgens

There is debate over the principal site of adrenal androgen synthesis.[34] Traditionally, it has been taught that adrenal androgens are synthesized exclusively in the zona reticularis. However, the activity of 17,20-lyase (17,20-desmolase) that converts 17-hydroxypregnenolone to DHEA (a delta[5] steroid) and 17-hydroxyprogesterone to androstenedione (a delta[4] steroid) is included in the CYP17 protein, described previously. Therefore synthesis of adrenal androgens theoretically could occur within both the zona fasciculata and the zona reticularis. However, adrenal androgen synthesis in the zona reticularis may result from high cytochrome 5b expression, which increases the 17,20-lyase activity of CYP17. CYP17 converts C_{21} steroids into C_{19} steroids. Likewise, cortisol synthesis in the zona reticularis is possible. The conversion of DHEA to DHEA-S is catalyzed by DHEA sulfotransferase (SULT2A1; gene location: chromosome 19q13.3). Based on this model of enzymes partitioned between the mitochondrion and the endoplasmic reticulum, adrenal androgen synthesis is completed within the endoplasmic reticulum because this pathway does not require CYP21, CYP11B1, or CYP11B2, which are located in the mitochondrion.

A small amount of testosterone is produced by the adrenal cortex. DHEA is converted to androstenediol by 17-ketosteroid reductase (17 beta-hydroxysteroid dehydrogenase, 17 beta-OHSD); this is followed by conversion of androstenediol to testosterone by 3-beta HSD and delta(4)-5-isomerase. Peripheral conversion of adrenal androgens to testosterone requires conversion of DHEA to androstenedione and androstenedione to testosterone by 17-ketosteroid reductase. Finally, testosterone is activated to DHT by 5-alpha reductase in target tissues (penis, scrotum, and androgen-dependent hair follicles). Peripheral aromatization of androstenedione yields estrone, whereas peripheral aromatization of testosterone yields estradiol. For testosterone metabolic pathways, refer to Figs. 68.1 and 68.2 in Chapter 68.

Adrenal androgens are the major product of the adrenal cortex, whose total synthesis exceeds 20 to 25 mg/d. The adult adrenal secretes approximately 6 to 8 mg/d of DHEA, 8 to 16 mg/d of DHEA-S, 1.5 mg/d of androstenedione, and 0.05 mg/d of testosterone. Only small amounts of estradiol and estrone and insignificant amounts of progesterone and other precursor steroids are produced by the adrenal cortex.

Adrenal Steroid Synthesis in the Fetus

The fetal adrenal gland lacks adult expression of 3-beta-HSD, resulting in elevated production of DHEA, DHEA-S, and 16-hydroxy DHEA-S (from hydroxylation of DHEA-S in the fetal liver). In utero, adrenal pregnenolone and 17-hydroxypregnenolone enter the fetal circulation and are converted in the placenta into progesterone and 17-hydroxyprogesterone, respectively, via placental 3-beta-HSD. Progesterone and 17-hydroxyprogesterone then return via fetal circulation to the fetal adrenal gland, where they serve as substrates for aldosterone and cortisol, respectively.[35]

Summary of ACTH Activity

The biochemical actions of ACTH on the adrenal cortex include ACTH effects via steroidogenesis activator protein and StAR, increased cholesterol esterase activity, decreased cholesterol ester synthesis, increased cholesterol transport into the mitochondrion, increased CYP11A binding of cholesterol, and increased synthesis of pregnenolone. Mediated by transcription factors (SF-1), expression of CYP11A, CYP17, CYP11B1 (but not CYP11B2), and the LDL receptor is increased. CYP11B2 is regulated by angiotensin II, separating control of the zona glomerulosa from the zona fasciculata. In addition, ACTH and other factors not yet discovered control adrenal androgen synthesis.

ADRENOCORTICAL HORMONES IN THE CIRCULATION

Steroid hormones are 90% to 98% bound to specific carrier proteins or albumin. Steroids that are sulfated or glucuronidated circulate unbound in the plasma. Aldosterone is carried primarily by albumin because cortisol, corticosterone, and 17-hydroxyprogesterone occupy most of the binding sites on corticosteroid-binding globulin (CBG; transcortin), a 58-kDa, 383 amino acid alpha-1 globulin.[36,37] Total cortisol concentration normally exceeds the aldosterone concentration by about 1000-fold, which explains why little aldosterone is carried on CBG. CBG is a serine protease inhibitor (specifically, SERPINA6, clade A—alpha-1 antiprotease, antitrypsin—member 6; gene location: chromosome 14q3) in a superfamily of such protease inhibitors.[38]

In the blood, 80% to 90% of cortisol is bound to CBG, 7% is loosely bound to albumin, and 2% to 3% is unbound (free). When total cortisol rises in Cushing syndrome, the increased fraction of free cortisol is excreted in the urine, increasing the urinary free cortisol (UFC) concentration.[39] At normal concentrations in the blood, only 0.25% to 0.5% of total cortisol is excreted in the urine.

Because more cortisol than aldosterone is bound to CBG, the half-life of cortisol is longer (60–80 minutes) than the half-life of aldosterone (20–30 minutes).[40] In addition to cortisol, progestins are carried by CBG. *Progestin* is a generic term for any substance that produces some or all of the biological effects of progesterone.

CBG concentrations rise in response to increasing estrogen. In pregnancy, CBG concentration may rise two- to threefold. CBG concentrations are also increased in some patients with chronic active hepatitis. CBG concentrations are reduced in nephrosis (as a result of CBG loss in the urine), cirrhosis (because of decreased production), and hyperthyroidism (due to increased metabolism), as well as with glucocorticoid treatment (probably as a result of catabolism). Even with changes in total cortisol due to variations in CBG, the concentration of free cortisol remains stable if the hypothalamic-pituitary-adrenal axis is functioning normally.

DHEA and its sulfated form, DHEA-S, and estradiol are mostly bound to albumin. In contrast, testosterone and dihydrotestosterone (DHT) are carried by sex hormone–binding globulin (SHBG), an approximately 100-kDa homodimer (each monomer is about 50 kDa; 373 amino acids; gene location: chromosome 17p1).[41] Estrogens and thyroid hormone increase SHBG production, whereas insulin, growth hormone, glucocorticoids, androgens, and progestins inhibit SHBG synthesis. SHBG concentrations are higher in children than in adults.

METABOLISM OF ADRENAL STEROIDS

Steroid metabolism occurs primarily in the liver via P450 enzymes; the kidney plays a lesser role in steroid metabolism but an important excretory role.[42] Clearance of steroid hormones involves hydroxylation, dehydrogenation, reduction of double bonds, and conjugation to sulfates or glucuronic acid. Chemical reduction of steroids increases their water solubility and exposes functional sites (such as hydroxyl groups) that can be conjugated to sulfate or glucuronic acid, which increases their solubility in urine, thereby promoting their excretion. Approximately 90% of conjugated steroids are excreted by the kidney.

Aldosterone

Aldosterone is reduced to tetrahydroaldosterone.[43] Glucuronidation produces tetrahydroaldosterone 3-glucuronide, which can be excreted in the urine. Aldosterone is 3 alpha- and 5 alpha-reduced, or 3 alpha- and 5 beta-reduced (Fig. 66.7). Only about 0.5% of unreduced aldosterone is excreted in the urine. Aldosterone is glucuronidated at the carbon 18 position. Cirrhosis, severe congestive heart failure, and ascites impair hepatic metabolism of aldosterone.

Cortisol

Cortisone is formed from cortisol via 11 beta-hydroxysteroid dehydrogenase type 2 (see Fig. 66.7).[44] The 11-hydroxyl group is converted to an 11-oxo group by removal of two hydrogens. Cortisone lacks glucocorticoid activity. (Note: When cortisone is used as a drug, it is activated by hepatic conversion to cortisol via 11-beta hydroxysteroid dehydrogenase type 1, a nicotinamide adenine dinucleotide phosphate-dependent oxo-reductase.) Reduction of the double bonds at carbons 4-5 via delta(4)-5-beta reductase or delta(4)-5-alpha reductase yields dihydrocortisol and dihydrocortisone. Reduction of the ketone groups at carbon 3 produce tetrahydrocortisol (THF) and tetrahydrocortisone (THE), which account for the major portion of cortisol clearance (~50%). The only difference in the outcome of delta(4)-5-beta reductase versus delta(4)-5-alpha reductase activity is the alpha or beta orientation of the hydrogen (5 beta-THF or 5-alpha-THF). Normally, the beta metabolite predominates (5-beta THF:5-alpha-THF ratio = 2:1).

Further metabolism of THF and THE via 20-alpha-hydroxysteroid dehydrogenase or 20-beta-hydroxysteroid dehydrogenase produces alpha and beta cortol and cortolone (the cortoic acids), which account for approximately 30% of cortisol excretion. Opening the carbon 17-20 bond creates a ketone and gives rise to 11 beta-hydroxyetiocholanolone and 11-ketoetiocholanolone, representing about 10% of cortisol excretion. Only about 1% of cortisol is normally excreted as free cortisol or cortisone. Minor cortisol metabolites include 20 alpha-hydroxycortisol and 20 beta-hydroxycortisol, which result from reduction of the carbon 20 ketone, and 6 beta-hydroxycortisol, which results from hydroxylation of carbon 6. Oxidation of carbon 17 in THF and THE yields oxo or hydroxy metabolites (Fig. 66.8).

Of the many cortisol metabolites, more than 95% are conjugated at carbon 3 to glucuronic acid or sulfated at the

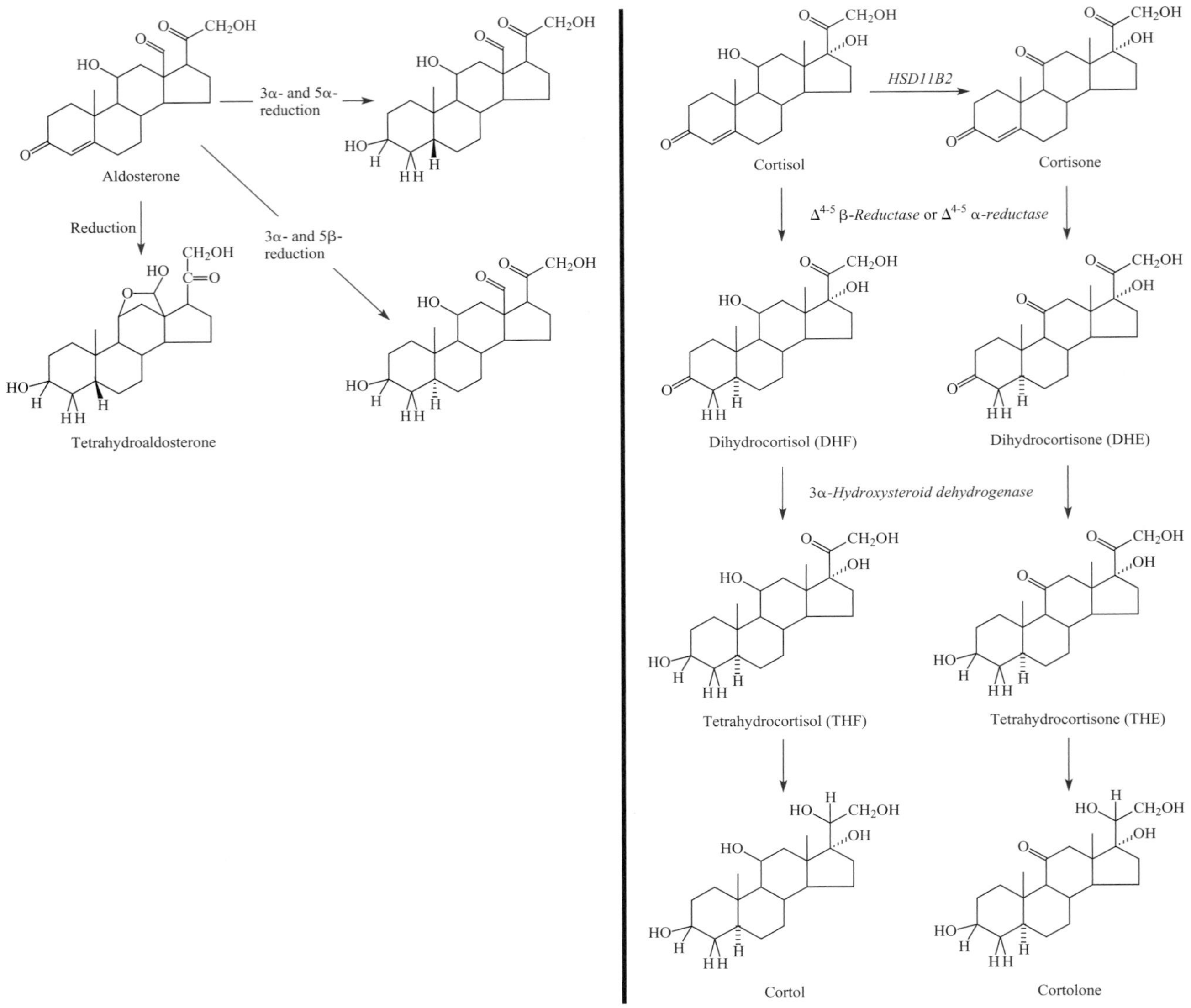

FIGURE 66.7 *Left panel:* Aldosterone metabolism. Aldosterone is reduced to tetrahydroaldosterone. Aldosterone can be 3 alpha- and 5 alpha-reduced or 3 alpha- and 5 beta-reduced. *Right panel:* Cortisol metabolism. Cortisone is formed from cortisol via 11-beta hydroxysteroid dehydrogenase-2 *(HSD11B2)*. Reduction of the double bonds at carbons 4-5 via delta(4)-5 beta reductase or delta(4)-5 alpha reductase yields dihydrocortisol *(DHF)* and dihydrocortisone *(DHE)*. Metabolism with reduction of the ketone groups at carbon 3 results in tetrahydrocortisol *(THF)* and tetrahydrocortisone *(THE)*, which account for approximately 50% of cortisol clearance. Further metabolism of THF and THE via 20-alpha hydroxysteroid dehydrogenase or 20-beta hydroxysteroid dehydrogenase produces alpha and beta cortol and cortolone (the cortoic acids), which account for approximately 30% of cortisol excretion.

C-21 position. Proportionately, the glucuronide metabolites predominate over sulfated metabolites.

Adrenal Androgens

DHEA is sulfated to DHEA-S.[29] These compounds are 7 alpha-hydroxylated or 16-alpha-hydroxylated. Alternatively, 17-ketosteroid reductase reduces the ketone at carbon 17 to a hydroxyl group, yielding androstenediol from DHEA and androstenediol sulfate from DHEA-S. Androstenedione is converted to androsterone via 3-alpha- and 5-alpha-reduction, whereas 3-alpha- and 5-beta-reduction yields etiocholanolone (Fig. 66.9). Similar to cortisol metabolites, adrenal androgen metabolites are glucuronidated or sulfated for urinary excretion.

Urinary Metabolites

Whereas measurement of biliary adrenal steroids is not clinically useful, measurement of the urinary excretion of these compounds is common in the laboratory assessment of adrenal disease. Immunoassays for the major circulating steroid hormones are widely available.

17-Hydroxyprogesterone is metabolically reduced to pregnanetriol, which can be measured in urine. The reduction converts keto groups at the 3-position and the 20-position to

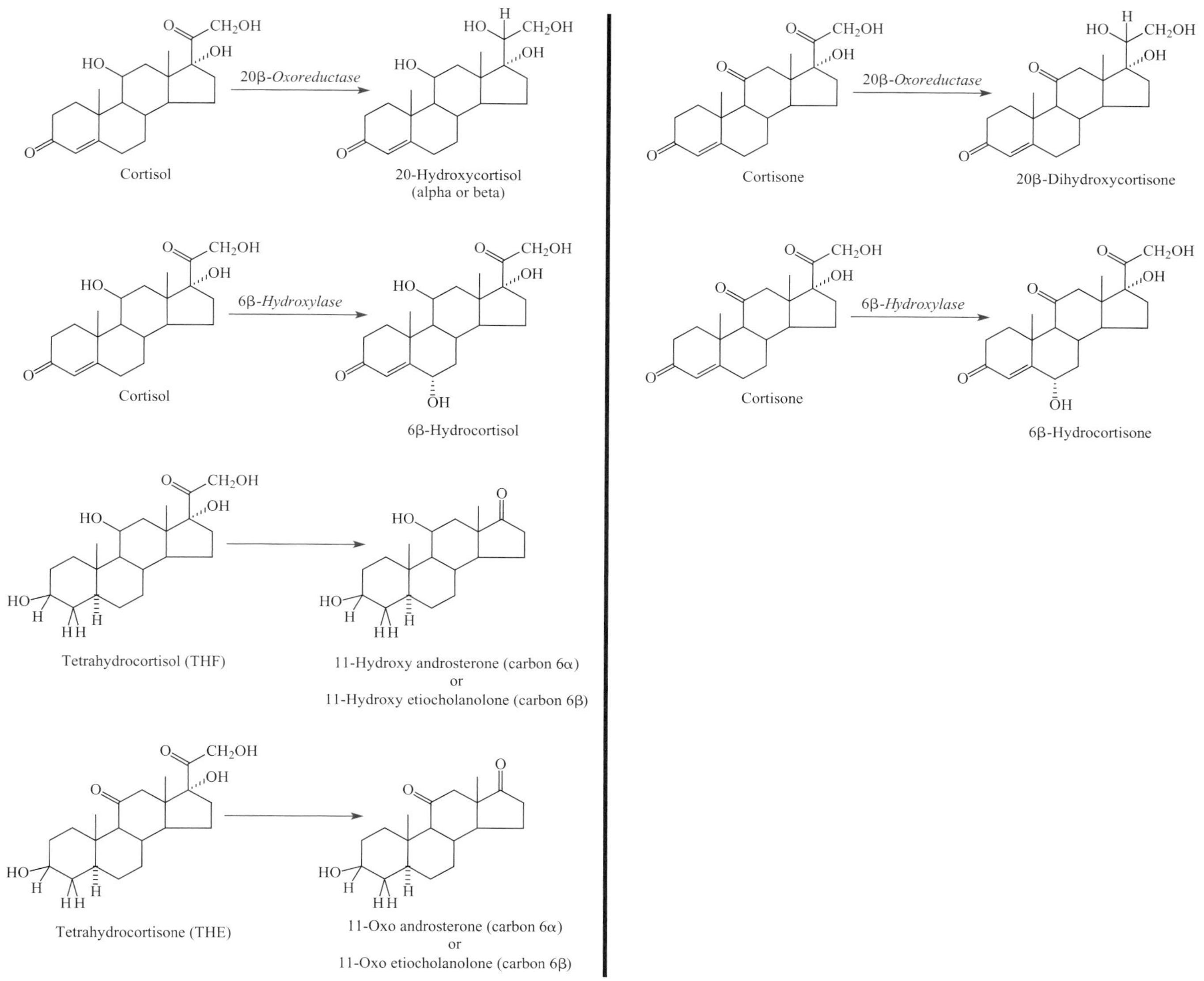

FIGURE 66.8 *Left panel,* Minor cortisol metabolites include 20-alpha-hydroxycortisol and 20-beta-hydroxycortisol, which result from reduction of the carbon 20 ketone, and 6-beta-hydroxycortisol, which results from hydroxylation of carbon 6. Oxidation of carbon 17 in THF and THE yields oxo- or hydroxyl-metabolites. *Right panel,* Minor cortisone metabolites include 20-beta-dihydrocortisone and 6-beta-hydrocortisone.

hydroxyl groups, giving the molecule three hydroxyl groups (hence the term *triol*). Hydroxylation helps solubilize the compound for renal excretion. Before the development of immunoassays for 17-hydroxyprogesterone, a 24-hour urine was collected for measurement of pregnanetriol excretion in cases of congenital adrenal hyperplasia (CAH) due to CYP21 or CYP11B1 deficiency. If these forms of CAH were managed appropriately, ideally the pregnanetriol excretion would return to its reference interval.

The urinary metabolites of 11-deoxycortisol and cortisol are classified as 17-hydroxycorticosteroids (17-OHCS). Analytically, 17-OHCS can be photometrically measured by the reaction of 17,21-dihydroxy-20-oxosteroids with a phenylhydrazine-ethanol-sulfuric acid reagent, producing yellow phenylhydrazones termed *Porter-Silber chromogens.* Measurement of 17-OHCS has been used to differentiate CYP21 deficiency from CYP11B1 deficiency. In CYP21 deficiency, 17-OHCS would not be elevated because both 11-deoxycortisol and cortisol are low. However, because CYP11B1 deficiency increases 11-deoxycortisol (the metabolic block is between 11-deoxycortisol and cortisol), 17-OHCS would be elevated in untreated or undertreated CYP11B1 deficiency. Also, CYP11B1 deficiency and CYP21 deficiency are differentiated by elevated plasma 11-deoxycortisol concentrations in the former.

Urinary metabolites of 17-hydroxyprogesterone, 11-deoxycortisol, and cortisol are 17-ketogenic steroids (17-KGS) because oxidation of these compounds yields a keto group at the 17 position. Ketogenic steroids have been measured using the Zimmermann reaction, in which an alkaline solution of meta-dinitrobenzene reacts with methylene groups at carbon-16 of the 17-ketosteroids. In CYP17

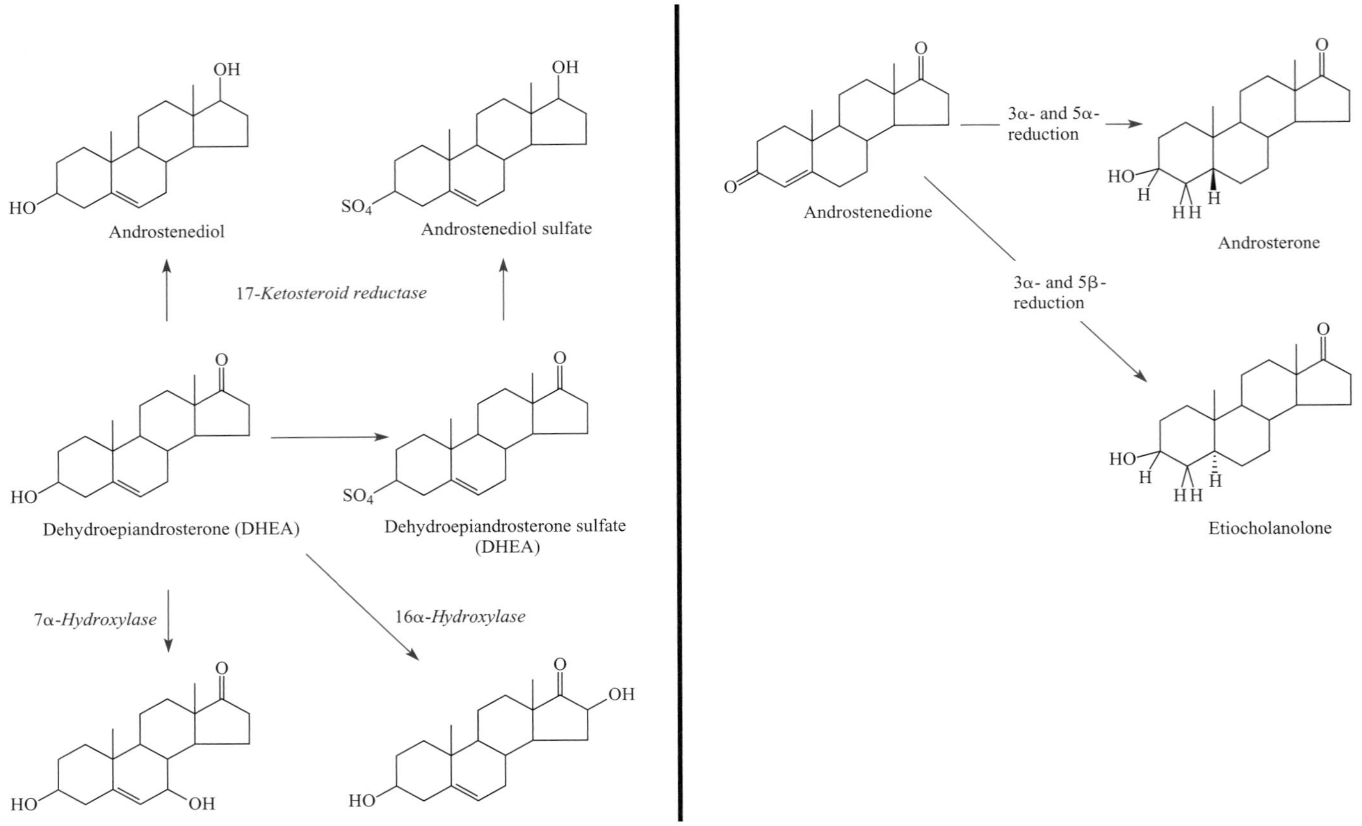

FIGURE 66.9 *Left panel,* DHEA metabolism. DHEA can be 7-alpha-hydroxylated or 16-alpha-hydroxylated. Alternatively, conversion of the carbon 17 ketone group of DHEA and DHEA-S to a hydroxyl can be accomplished by 17-ketosteroid reductase, yielding androstenediol from DHEA and androstenediol sulfate from DHEA-S. *Right panel,* Androstenedione metabolism. Androstenedione is converted to androsterone via 3-alpha- and 5-alpha-reduction, whereas 3-alpha- and 5-beta-reduction yield etiocholanolone.

deficiency, 17-KGS is not elevated. However, in both CYP21 and CYP11B1 deficiencies, when untreated or undertreated, 17-KGS are elevated.

DHEA and androstenedione metabolites are measured in the same way as 17-ketosteroids because both have keto groups in the C-17 position. Testosterone has a hydroxyl group at the C-17 position, and therefore is not a 17-ketosteroid. DHEA and androstenedione are elevated in untreated and undertreated CYP21 and CYP11B1 deficiencies. Fig. 66.10 summarizes these urinary steroid metabolites.

Factors Affecting Adrenal Steroid Metabolism

Cortisol metabolism and clearance affect plasma cortisol concentrations. If the clearance of cortisol is reduced, plasma cortisol increases, whereas enhanced clearance of cortisol decreases its plasma concentration. Rifampin-induced Addisonian crisis from increased cortisol metabolism has been reported. However, in most cases, cortisol, free cortisol, and ACTH are normal, presumably because alterations in the free cortisol concentration will be sensed by the hypothalamus, which will respond by secreting CRH to ultimately return the free cortisol concentration to its reference interval. Table 66.7 lists a number of conditions that affect plasma cortisol concentrations.

DYNAMIC TESTS OF ADRENAL FUNCTION

Several strategies are used to assess adrenal function. These tests are typically designed to differentiate between primary and secondary causes of disease or to detect abnormalities that may not be apparent in the results of static, baseline laboratory measurements. For example, provocative stimulation tests are useful in documenting reduced secretory capacity of adrenocortical hormones.[45] A specific stimulus is applied, and the release of a given hormone is measured during a specified time interval. Also, suppression tests are used to document hypersecretion of the adrenocortical hormones.[46]

ACTH Stimulation (Cosyntropin) Test

ACTH stimulation tests, sometimes referred to as the *cosyntropin test,* assess the functional capacity of the adrenal glands to synthesize cortisol (Boxes 66.1 and 66.2). Cosyntropin (Cortrosyn) is the N-terminal 24 amino acid sequence of ACTH, which includes the biologically active domain. Another name for cosyntropin is *tetracosactrin* (Synacthen). Cosyntropin is a potent stimulator of cortisol secretion and has a very brief half-life and minimal antigenicity. The protocols for the 1-hour (also known as the "Short Synacthen Test") and multiple-day ACTH stimulation test (or "Long or

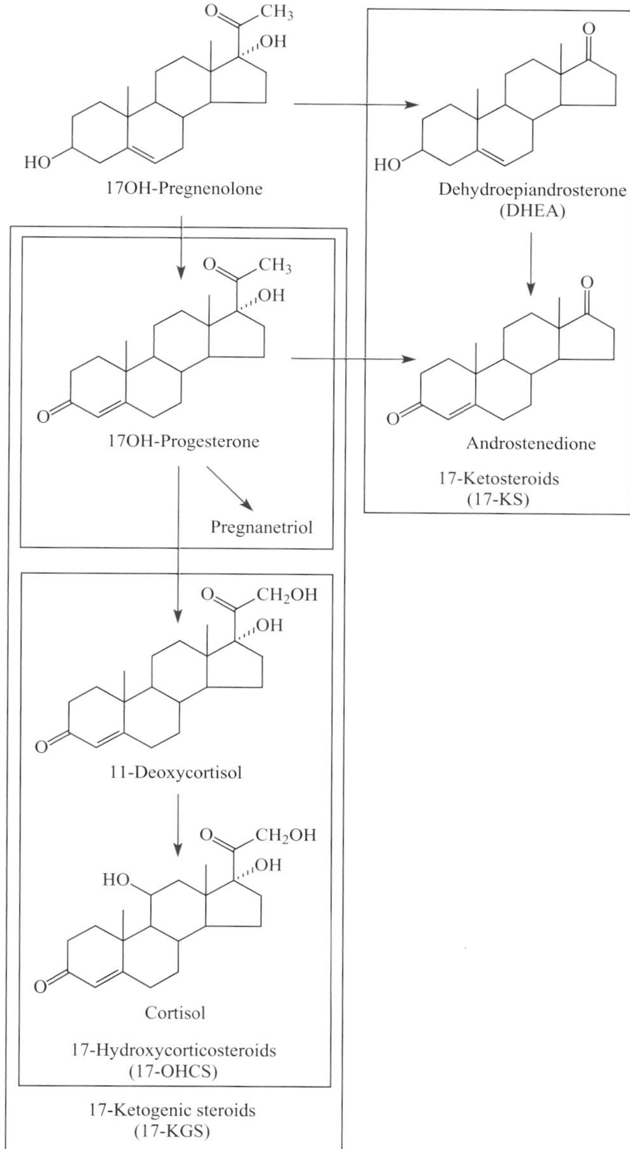

FIGURE 66.10 Urinary metabolites generated from steroids involved in cortisol and adrenal androgen synthesis.

Prolonged Synacthen Test") are shown in Box 66.1 and Box 66.2, respectively.

There is debate over the best dose of cosyntropin (1 μg vs. 250 μg) in the 1-hour stimulation test for the detection of adrenal insufficiency from ACTH deficiency or primary adrenal failure.[47] Some patients have normal responses to 250 μg of ACTH, yet inadequate responses to 1 μg of ACTH. This remains a point of controversy, and the 1-μg ACTH dose has not been universally accepted as superior to the 250-μg dose in detecting glucocorticoid deficiency.[48-50] There is also debate about the most appropriate diagnostic thresholds, especially in view of cortisol assay heterogeneity and variable cross-reactivity of immunoassays with steroid metabolites,[51-53] as well as the time points at which the test is interpreted.[54,55] It is currently debated whether the Short Synacthen Test should be performed at all in acute or intensive care because the rate of false positivity is high and may lead to inappropriate patient management.[56]

CRH Stimulation Test

A direct and selective test of pituitary function is the CRH stimulation test (Box 66.3).[57,58] Administration of ovine CRH stimulates ACTH secretion in normal subjects within 60 to 180 minutes; glucocorticoids inhibit this effect (as in cases of Cushing syndrome [adrenal tumor] or ectopic ACTH secretion by a nonadrenal tumor). In pituitary-dependent Cushing disease, however, the corticotropinoma may respond to exogenous CRH with a normal or exaggerated response. This test may be used to assess adrenocortical hyperfunction or hypofunction. CRH stimulation is also used to diagnose endogenous Cushing syndrome and to distinguish secondary from tertiary ACTH deficiency.

To differentiate pituitary-dependent Cushing disease from ectopic ACTH syndrome, a variation of the CRH stimulation test can be performed that measures ACTH in blood collected from the two inferior petrosal sinuses (IPSs).[59,60] Blood specimens are collected from both right and left IPSs and from a peripheral vein (eg, the inferior vena cava) at −30, 0, +2, +5, +10, and +30 minutes after intravenous administration of ovine CRH (1 μg/kg body weight) over 20 to 60 seconds. The ratio of the IPS concentration to the peripheral venous concentration of plasma ACTH is used to predict the location of excess ACTH secretion. An IPS-to-peripheral vein ratio greater than 2.0 is consistent with a pituitary lesion (Cushing disease), whereas a ratio less than 1.4 to 1.7 supports the diagnosis of an ectopic ACTH syndrome. ACTH release is suppressed in patients with primary adrenal tumors, compared to patients with Cushing disease or the ectopic ACTH syndrome.[61,62] Imaging studies are insufficient to replace laboratory testing for Cushing disease.[63] Even when ectopic ACTH syndrome is diagnosed, radiographic localization of the source tumor can be very difficult.[64,65]

Insulin-Induced Hypoglycemia Stimulation Test

In the insulin-induced hypoglycemia stimulation test, insulin is administered to stimulate CRH release by hypoglycemia; plasma ACTH or cortisol concentrations are measured.[66] This test involves a risk of hypoglycemia (obtundation, seizure, coma, and death) and should be performed only in highly monitored settings. The test should not be performed in patients with a seizure disorder or coronary artery disease. Venous access must be maintained for immediate administration of intravenous glucose if hypoglycemic complications occur.

Metyrapone Stimulation Test

An alternative, although less commonly used, indirect test of hypothalamic-pituitary-adrenal axis function involves the administration of metyrapone, an inhibitor of the 11-beta-hydroxylase enzyme that converts 11-deoxycortisol to cortisol.[67] Several protocols have been designed for metyrapone stimulation testing: a simple and relatively safe protocol for outpatient testing is described in Box 66.4.

Dexamethasone Suppression Test

Elevated cortisol normally inhibits ACTH release from the pituitary gland, resulting in decreased production of cortisol

TABLE 66.7 Conditions That Affect Cortisol Clearance

Endocrinopathy	Cortisol Clearance	Mechanism
Hyperthyroidism	Incr	Inhibition of hepatic 11-beta HSDI and stimulation of 5-alpha reductase and 5-beta reductase
Hypothyroidism	Decr	Stimulation of hepatic 11-beta HSDI and inhibition of 5-alpha reductase and 5-beta reductase
Acromegaly	Incr	Inhibition of hepatic 11-beta HSDI
Cushing syndrome	Incr	Induction of 6 beta-hydroxylase
Solid Organ Dysfunction		
Chronic liver disease (disease including alcoholic cirrhosis)	Decr	Decreased cortisol metabolism
Renal disease	Decr	Reduced renal conversion: cortisol → cortisone
Drugs/Toxins		
Acute alcohol ingestion	Decr	—
Rifampin	Incr	Induction of 6 beta-hydroxylase
Phenytoin	Incr	Induction of 6 beta-hydroxylase
Phenobarbital	Incr	Induction of hepatic mixed-function oxidases
Other		
Aging	Decr	*Note:* Decreased clearance is balanced by decreased synthesis; therefore cortisol concentrations and responses to ACTH are normal.
Starvation	Decr	Balanced by decreased production
Anorexia nervosa	Decr	—

—, Not defined; *decr,* decreased; *incr,* increased.

BOX 66.1 Protocol for the 1-Hour (Rapid) Cosyntropin Stimulation Test

Rationale

Administration of ACTH to normal subjects causes a rapid rise in the serum cortisol concentration. Patients with adrenal destruction (eg, Addison disease) show no change or an inadequate change in serum cortisol concentration after ACTH stimulation. Patients with atrophy of the adrenal cortex caused by exogenous glucocorticoid treatment or dysfunction of the pituitary gland or hypothalamus may show a slight rise in serum cortisol concentration, but not one of normal magnitude.

Procedure

A morning (baseline) blood specimen is collected for determination of serum cortisol concentration; then 250 µg of cosyntropin is administered intramuscularly or intravenously. Blood specimens for serum cortisol determination are collected 30 and 60 minutes after injection.

Interpretation

A peak serum cortisol concentration of 18 to 20 µg/dL (500–550 nmol/L) or greater is a normal response. The expected change (delta) in cortisol concentration is 7 to 10 µg/dL (193–276 nmol/L). The peak cortisol value is more important than the incremental change. The incremental change may not be seen in patients who are tested at times of stress, when their adrenal output of cortisol is already maximally stimulated by endogenous ACTH. Also, it should be noted that clinical thresholds depend on the specific quantitative method used and may vary based on the reference material with which the analytical method is standardized.[51-53]

and other ACTH-dependent steroids by the adrenal cortex. The integrity of this feedback mechanism is tested by administering a potent glucocorticoid, such as dexamethasone and assessing ACTH secretion by measuring serum or urine cortisol concentrations. Several dexamethasone suppression tests are available for clinical use (Boxes 66.5 through 66.7). Dexamethasone does not significantly cross-react with cortisol immunoassays, so the secreted endogenous glucocorticoid—cortisol—can be distinguished from the exogenous glucocorticoid, dexamethasone.

A low dose of dexamethasone (1 mg in adults; 0.3 mg/m^2 in children) administered at 22:00 hours is used to detect true hypersecretion of cortisol (see Box 66.5).[68] Patients with endogenous Cushing syndrome normally fail to suppress their morning cortisol concentration to less than 5 µg/dL (138 nmol/L) with a low dose of dexamethasone.[69] This is a screening test, and confirmation of Cushing syndrome requires measurement of urinary cortisol on at least two separate days or some other combination of tests (eg, midnight cortisol <5 µg/dL [<138 nmol/L], salivary cortisol <0.112 µg/dL [<3.09 nmol/L]).[70,71] A 0.5-mg dose variant of the overnight dexamethasone suppression test has been described and validated.[72] Also, a 2-mg dexamethasone dose has been used to exclude Cushing syndrome in obese patients.[73]

Higher doses of dexamethasone administered over 48 hours can help resolve the differential diagnosis of an

BOX 66.2 Protocol for the Multiple-Day Adrenocorticotropic Hormone Stimulation Test

Rationale

Multiple-day adrenocorticotropic hormone (ACTH) stimulation testing for assessment of adrenal cortex function is required occasionally to evaluate adrenal cortisol responsiveness. A common situation is adrenal insufficiency treated with glucocorticosteroids before the cause has been established. Prolonged ACTH stimulation is used to distinguish primary from secondary and/or tertiary (central) causes of adrenal insufficiency.

Procedure

A total of 250 μg of cosyntropin is injected daily for 3 days. This is followed by an 8-hour infusion of 250 μg of cosyntropin. Urinary free cortisol and serum cortisol are measured daily.

Interpretation

Serum cortisol values of 18 to 20 μg/dL (500–550 nmol/L) or greater exclude primary adrenal insufficiency. Glucocorticoid withdrawal would be required before secondary or tertiary adrenal insufficiency can be assessed. Little or no increase in cortisol secretion, even over successive days, is seen in primary adrenal failure. A progressive (staircase) rise in cortisol is seen over 2 to 3 days in adrenal insufficiency caused by pituitary or hypothalamic disease or corticosteroid suppression. Little or no response is seen in congenital adrenal hyperplasia caused by 21- and 17-hydroxylase deficiencies. Two- and 5-day variations of this test have been used in clinical practice. Also, it should be noted that clinical thresholds depend on the specific quantitative method used and may vary based on the reference material with which the analytical method is standardized.[51-53]

BOX 66.3 Protocol for the Corticotropin-Releasing Hormone Stimulation Test

Rationale

Exogenous corticotropin-releasing hormone (CRH) stimulates the secretion of adrenocorticotropic hormone (ACTH) from the anterior pituitary gland in normal subjects. The subsequent cortisol concentration is an indicator of the ACTH response.

Procedure

Synthetic ovine CRH (corticorelin ovine triflutate), 1 μg/kg body weight, is administered intravenously in bolus form at 09:00 or 20:00 hours. Blood specimens for cortisol and ACTH measurements are collected 15 minutes and immediately before, and 5, 15, 30, 60, 120, and 180 minutes after, CRH injection.

Interpretation

In normal subjects, plasma ACTH concentrations peak 30 minutes after CRH injection (80 ± 7 pg/mL [18 ± 1.5 pmol/L]) at 09:30 h and 29 ± 2.6 pg/mL (6.4 ± 0.6 pmol/L) at 20:30 h; serum cortisol peaks at 60 minutes (13 ± 1 μg/dL [359 ± 28 nmol/L]) at 10:00 h and 17 ± 0.7 μg/dL (469 ± 19 nmol/L) at 21:00 h. Patients with pituitary ACTH deficiency (secondary adrenal insufficiency) have decreased ACTH and cortisol responses. Patients with hypothalamic disease have prolonged ACTH responses and subnormal cortisol responses. Most patients with Cushing syndrome caused by adrenal tumors or nonendocrine ACTH-producing tumors do not respond to CRH injection. Patients with Cushing disease usually respond with a normal or increased ACTH. Responses usually are normal in patients with depression.

BOX 66.4 Protocol for the Overnight Single-Dose Metyrapone Stimulation Test

Rationale

Metyrapone inhibits 11-beta-hydroxylase (CYP11B1), the enzyme that catalyzes the step immediately preceding cortisol synthesis. As the blood concentration of cortisol falls, the negative feedback effect is diminished, causing the release of adrenocorticotropic hormone (ACTH) from the pituitary gland. The stimulatory effect of ACTH on the adrenal cortex leads to a rise in 11-deoxycortisol, the compound immediately preceding cortisol in the biosynthetic pathway.

Procedure

Metyrapone (30 mg/kg body weight) is given orally at midnight with milk or a snack (to delay absorption). At 08:00 hours the following morning, blood is collected for measurement of 11-deoxycortisol, cortisol, and ACTH concentrations.

Interpretation

In normal subjects, 11-deoxycortisol increases from less than 1 μg/dL (29 nmol/L) to greater than 7 μg/dL (200 nmol/L) after metyrapone stimulation, and ACTH values exceed 150 pg/mL (33 pmol/L). No response or an impaired response may be observed in pituitary or hypothalamic disease combined with inadequate enzyme blockade (plasma cortisol >3 μg/dL [>83 nmol/L]) or with Cushing syndrome caused by adrenal tumors or nonendocrine ACTH-secreting tumors. Exaggerated responses may be seen in pituitary Cushing syndrome.

Note: This test is not recommended in cases of suspected Addison disease for fear that suppression of cortisol production might precipitate an Addisonian crisis. However, patients with Addison disease have an inadequate rise in 11-deoxycortisol in response to metyrapone.

BOX 66.5 Protocol for the Overnight Low-Dose Dexamethasone Suppression Test

Rationale

In low doses, dexamethasone, a synthetic glucocorticoid and cortisol analog, suppresses adrenocorticotropic hormone (ACTH) and cortisol production in normal subjects, but not in patients with Cushing syndrome.

Procedure

One milligram of dexamethasone is given orally between 22:00 and 24:00. Blood is collected for measurement of serum cortisol at 08:00 hours the next morning.

Interpretation

In normal subjects, the serum cortisol concentration is suppressed to 2 µg/dL (55 nmol/L) or less after administration of 1 mg of dexamethasone. A postdexamethasone 08:00 hours' cortisol cutoff of less than 5 µg/dL (138 nmol/L) is more sensitive for the detection of Cushing syndrome but is less specific. Most patients with Cushing syndrome do not show adequate suppression, and 08:00 hours' cortisol concentrations are usually 10 µg/dL (276 nmol/L) or greater. Serum cortisol greater than 2 µg/dL (55 nmol/L) may be seen in cases of stress, obesity, infection, acute or chronic illness, alcohol abuse, severe depression, oral contraceptive use, pregnancy, estrogen therapy, failure to take dexamethasone, or treatment with phenytoin or phenobarbital (which can enhance dexamethasone metabolism).

ACTH-secreting pituitary adenoma versus an ectopic ACTH source. Suppression of the basal urinary cortisol excretion by less than 50% is consistent with Cushing disease but not ectopic ACTH syndrome or primary adrenal pathology for hypercortisolism, in which ACTH is not suppressed by high doses of dexamethasone.

On high-dose dexamethasone, suppression will occur in about 60% of patients with Cushing disease. However, failure of suppression on high-dose dexamethasone does not distinguish Cushing disease from the other causes of Cushing syndrome, and other diagnostic approaches must be pursued, such as IPS sampling.

Failure of cortisol suppression by dexamethasone has been observed in patients with depression, severe stress, uncontrolled diabetes mellitus, anorexia nervosa with estrogen administration, who are receiving medications (such as phenytoin) that induce the hepatic cytochrome P450 enzymes that metabolize dexamethasone, and who abuse alcohol.[74,75]

Mineralocorticoid Stimulation Tests

The renin-angiotensin-aldosterone system responds to electrolyte imbalance.[76] Sodium excretion and extracellular fluid volume are inversely correlated with plasma renin and aldosterone concentrations. The fractional excretion of sodium (FENa) reflects the sodium status and is calculated as follows:

$$FENa = \frac{[U_{Na^+}][S_{Cr}]}{[S_{Na^+}][U_{Cr}]} \times 100$$

BOX 66.6 Protocol for the Classic Low-Dose/High-Dose Dexamethasone Suppression Test

Rationale

Normal subjects show a decline in urinary free cortisol (UFC) concentrations in response to low-dose dexamethasone. However, cortisol in patients with excess cortisol production, regardless of the cause, is not suppressed by low-dose dexamethasone. Patients with Cushing syndrome caused by an adrenocorticotropic hormone (ACTH)-producing pituitary adenoma (eg, Cushing disease from a corticotropinoma) may show suppression of cortisol with high-dose dexamethasone. Patients with Cushing syndrome from other causes (adrenocortical adenoma or carcinoma, or ectopic production of ACTH or corticotropin-releasing hormone [CRH]) usually do not demonstrate cortisol suppression with high-dose dexamethasone treatment.

Procedure

Twenty-four-hour urine samples are collected daily for 6 consecutive days. Free cortisol and creatinine are measured in each 24-hour urine sample. UFC is regarded as a more specific measure of cortisol secretion than 17-hydroxycorticosteroids. The first 2 days provide baseline measurements of the excretion of cortisol. Dexamethasone 0.5 mg ("low-dose dexamethasone") is given orally every 6 hours starting at 08:00 hours on day 3 (for a total of eight doses: days 3 and 4). Dexamethasone 2.0 mg ("high-dose dexamethasone") is then given orally every 6 hours starting at 08:00 hours on day 5 (for a total of eight doses: days 5 and 6).

Interpretation

On the first 2 days, urinary excretion of cortisol (ie, the baseline measurements) should be elevated in cases of Cushing syndrome. In cases of true endogenous Cushing syndrome, baseline UFC is usually at least two to three times higher than the upper limit of the reference interval. In normal individuals, baseline UFC excretion should be within the reference interval. Should a normal individual be stressed, psychologically or physiologically, and the baseline UFC is elevated, UFC on days 3 and 4 should be suppressed to less than 50% of the baseline level—that is, UFC suppression was achieved. All subjects with true endogenous hypercortisolism should not suppress on day 3 or 4. If suppression of UFC excretion occurs on days 5 and 6 (or on day 6), Cushing disease is diagnosed. However, not all cases of Cushing disease suppress on high-dose dexamethasone. Therefore failure to suppress on high-dose dexamethasone leaves three diagnostic possibilities: Cushing disease, adrenal adenoma (or, less commonly, adrenal carcinoma), and ectopic ACTH or CRH syndrome. Patients taking phenytoin or phenobarbital (or both) may metabolize dexamethasone more rapidly than normal subjects and may not show appropriate suppression.

FENa is typically less than 1%. The FENa exceeds 1% in tubular disease or injury with sodium wasting. FENa is not valid in patients treated with diuretics.

Mineralocorticoid Suppression Tests

Mineralocorticoid suppression tests are based on salt loading, such as saline infusion or oral salt loading. Mineralocorticoid

BOX 66.7 Protocol for the High-Dose Overnight Dexamethasone Suppression Test

Rationale

The rationale for this test is similar to the rationale for the multiple high-dose dexamethasone suppression test.

Procedure

Four milligrams of dexamethasone is given orally at 23:00 and 24:00 hours. Blood is collected for measurement of plasma cortisol at 07:00 hours or 08:00 hours the next morning, or 8 to 9 hours after dexamethasone is given.

Interpretation

Most patients with Cushing syndrome show at least 50% suppression of the baseline cortisol concentration. If suppression is not greater than 50%, the test should be repeated with 8 to 24 mg of dexamethasone.

BOX 66.8 Protocol for the Saline Suppression Test

Rationale

Rapid volume expansion with intravenous saline should suppress plasma aldosterone in normal subjects, but not in patients with primary hyperaldosteronism.

Procedure

Care must be taken to ensure that the subject is not hypokalemic before beginning the test. The subject is awakened at 06:00 hours and is kept in an upright posture for 2 hours. Blood is collected for measurement of plasma aldosterone at 08:00 hours. The subject then assumes a supine position, and 2 L of isotonic saline 0.9 % (g/dL) is infused over a 4-hour period. Blood is collected at noon for plasma aldosterone measurement.

Interpretation

Normal subjects show a plasma aldosterone concentration of 5 ng/dL (140 pmol/L) or less after saline infusion. Concentrations greater than 10 ng/dL (280 pmol/L) are usually seen in patients with autonomously functioning aldosterone-secreting tumors.

administration has also been used to suppress aldosterone secretion by the adrenal gland. In healthy individuals, acute expansion of plasma volume with salt increases renal perfusion, suppresses renin release, and decreases aldosterone secretion.

The protocol for the saline suppression test is shown in Box 66.8. This test should not be performed in patients with severe hypertension or heart failure. Administration of fludrocortisone, a synthetic mineralocorticoid, normally produces comparable suppression of aldosterone secretion (see fludrocortisone suppression test; Box 66.9). Fludrocortisone should be administered with caution in patients with hypokalemia and heart or renal failure. An alternate suppression test uses the ACE inhibitor captopril.[77] This test is recommended when risks from volume overload (eg, the development of pulmonary edema or hypertension) preclude the use of other procedures. Captopril inhibits the conversion of angiotensin I to angiotensin II, removing the angiotensin II stimulus for aldosterone secretion.

BOX 66.9 Protocol for the Fludrocortisone Suppression Test

Rationale

Fludrocortisone is a potent mineralocorticoid that suppresses aldosterone production in normal subjects, but not in subjects with primary hyperaldosteronism.

Procedure

Hypokalemia must be corrected before starting this test, and serum potassium must be monitored during the test. Fludrocortisone, 0.1 mg every 6 hours, is administered for 3 days. Plasma is collected for aldosterone measurement after a standing position has been maintained for 2 hours (for baseline measurement) and at the end of fludrocortisone administration. Twenty-four-hour urine collections for measurement of aldosterone are obtained 1 day before fludrocortisone administration is started and on day 3 of the test.

Interpretation

Normal subjects show suppression of plasma aldosterone to less than 4 ng/dL (111 pmol/L); urinary aldosterone secretion in normal subjects is 20 μg/d (550 nmol/d) or less on day 3.

Adrenal Androgen Stimulation Tests

The response of adrenal androgen secretion to ACTH stimulation is variable. Plasma DHEA and androstenedione are increased three- to fourfold after 90 minutes of stimulation with ACTH (10 $\mu g/m^2$). DHEA-S, on the other hand, is increased by 30% to 50% with ACTH administration. ACTH stimulation studies are not considered useful in evaluating hypoandrogenic disorders.[78]

Adrenal Androgen Suppression Tests

Overnight suppression using dexamethasone produces small changes in adrenal androgen concentration compared with those of cortisol. Dexamethasone, 0.75 mg, administered at midnight for several days, reliably suppresses adrenal androgen concentrations measured in blood. Tissue stores of these androgens may account in part for the delay in response.[79]

DISORDERS OF THE ADRENAL CORTEX

Thomas Addison first reported hypofunction of the adrenal cortex in 1855.[80] During the past 65 years, many of the diseases associated with abnormal adrenal function have been described.[81] Diseases of the adrenal cortex are classified as resulting from hypofunction or hyperfunction.[82]

Although circulating concentrations of adrenal androgens decline with age, it is unclear whether this simply reflects physiologic changes associated with aging or if it is a pathologic condition that should be treated.[83] Most experts believe the former and do not prescribe adrenal androgens as "treatment" for aging.[84] Adrenal androgen deficiency accompanies primary adrenal failure, but it has no clear pathologic consequences.[85] Excess prenatal adrenal androgens may produce ambiguous genitalia in females. Excess postnatal adrenal androgens can lead to precocious pseudopuberty in boys and hirsutism or virilization in girls. *Pseudopuberty* involves pubertal changes that result from autonomous gonadal or adrenal hypersecretion of sex steroids, independent of the CNS. In central precocious puberty, gonadotropins drive early sexual development.

Adrenal Insufficiency (Addison Disease)

Adrenal insufficiency causing combined mineralocorticoid and glucocorticoid deficiency is a rare disorder with a prevalence of only 4 to 11 cases per 100,000.[86,87] Untreated adrenal insufficiency can be fatal.[88] Cortisol deficiency is classified as primary, secondary, or tertiary.[89]

Primary adrenal insufficiency, also known as Addison disease, results from progressive destruction or dysfunction of the adrenal glands by a systemic disorder, an inborn error of metabolism (endogenous causes), or an exogenous cause such as infection (Table 66.8).[90] Worldwide, infectious disease is the most common cause of primary adrenal insufficiency and includes tuberculosis, fungal infection (histoplasmosis, cryptococcosis, North and South American blastomycosis, sporotrichosis, and coccidiomycosis), and cytomegalovirus infection. Syphilis can produce a syphilitic gumma (a fibrotic and granulomatous lesion) that destroys the adrenal gland. Human immunodeficiency virus (HIV) infection increases the risk of adrenalitis.[91] Autoimmune adrenalitis accounts for more than 70% of cases reported in the Western world, with adrenal autoantibodies measurable in more than 75% of cases.[92] In adrenalitis, the adrenal glands are atrophic, with loss of cortical cells but an intact medulla. Patients with autoimmune adrenalitis can also have pluriglandular autoimmune deficiency syndromes, as described in detail later.

The most common inborn steroidogenic defects involve synthesis of cortisol with or without concurrent aldosterone deficiency, producing CAH.[93] Because such disorders commonly lead to adrenal androgen overproduction, they are discussed in a later section concerning hyperfunction of the adrenal cortex, although such patients present a mixed picture of cortisol deficiency and possible aldosterone deficiency plus adrenal androgen overproduction.

Because the entire adrenal cortex is affected in primary adrenal insufficiency, all classes of adrenal steroids are deficient. The onset of clinical manifestations is usually gradual, and the degree and severity of symptoms depend on the extent of adrenal failure.[94] In early or mild primary adrenal insufficiency, hypofunction may not be evident unless the patient is under stress (eg, following trauma or surgery). Complete glucocorticoid deficiency can manifest in a variety of ways, including fatigue, weakness, weight loss, gastrointestinal disturbance, and fasting hypoglycemia. Mineralocorticoid deficiency leads to dehydration with hypotension, acidosis, hyponatremia, and hyperkalemia. Excessive pituitary release of ACTH, unchecked by the negative feedback system, may cause hyperpigmentation of the skin and mucous membranes.[95]

Measurement of basal ACTH and cortisol concentrations along with ACTH stimulation testing is recommended if primary adrenal insufficiency is indicated by clinical history and symptoms.[96] Basal plasma ACTH concentrations greater than 150 pg/mL (33 pmol/L), along with serum cortisol concentrations less than 5 µg/dL (138 nmol/L), are diagnostic of adrenal insufficiency. A subnormal cortisol response in the cosyntropin (also called synacthen) stimulation test supports the diagnosis of primary adrenal insufficiency. A normal cortisol response to cosyntropin stimulation establishes that the adrenal cortex is capable of releasing cortisol and excludes primary adrenal failure. A subnormal response to cosyntropin stimulation suggests the diagnosis of primary, secondary, or tertiary adrenal failure. The clinical presentation usually assists in the differentiation of primary (hyperpigmentation and hypotension) from secondary or tertiary hypoadrenalism (other trophic hormone deficiencies may be present, such as growth hormone or thyroid-stimulating hormone, but hyperpigmentation and hyperkalemia are absent). If needed, a plasma ACTH concentration can help differentiate primary from secondary and tertiary hypoadrenalism.

Mineralocorticoid and glucocorticoid deficiency may occur in cases of primary adrenal insufficiency. In contrast, when ACTH deficiency (secondary or tertiary) is the cause of adrenal insufficiency, mineralocorticoid secretion is typically normal.[97] A rare cause of isolated glucocorticoid deficiency of adrenal origin is familial glucocorticoid deficiency. In this autosomal recessive disorder, resistance to the effects of ACTH is caused by mutations in *MCR2* or melanocortin 2 receptor accessory protein, although some cases are currently unexplained.[98]

In secondary and tertiary adrenal insufficiency, inadequate cortisol production may be due to destructive processes in the hypothalamus and/or pituitary that result in a decreased ability to secrete CRH (tertiary) or ACTH (secondary).[99] However, the most common cause of tertiary insufficiency is long-term pharmacologic administration of glucocorticoids that suppress CRH, leading to a decrease in both ACTH release and cortisol secretion. Clinical features of secondary and tertiary adrenal insufficiency are similar to those of primary insufficiency, except hyperpigmentation is not present and hypotension is less severe. Mineralocorticoid deficiency, hyperkalemia, and ACTH excess are not seen in secondary or tertiary adrenal insufficiency.

The cosyntropin stimulation test may be used to demonstrate adrenal insufficiency in patients with secondary and tertiary adrenal insufficiency. When results of this test are abnormal, however, it does not identify the cause of adrenal failure. Mild to moderate dysfunction of ACTH secretion may go undetected. Some patients with partial ACTH deficiency maintain sufficient ACTH to prevent adrenal atrophy but are unable to augment ACTH secretion in response to stress or hypoglycemia. In these cases, pituitary ACTH reserve can be investigated with a metyrapone test or an insulin-induced hypoglycemia test. Because of the danger of precipitating Addisonian crisis, neither test should be performed if primary adrenal insufficiency is suspected. Subnormal responses to these tests suggest that pituitary ACTH release is inadequate, thus supporting a diagnosis of secondary or tertiary adrenal insufficiency.

ACTH and cortisol concentrations often are not useful for establishing the diagnosis of secondary adrenal insufficiency. Episodic secretion and circadian variation result in ACTH and cortisol concentrations that overlap between normal subjects and individuals with secondary or tertiary adrenal insufficiency. Elevated basal plasma ACTH in a patient with an abnormal response to acute ACTH stimulation suggests

TABLE 66.8 Causes of Primary Adrenal Insufficiency or Failure of Aldosterone Production

Endogenous Causes	
Autoimmune disease	Sporadic
	Autoimmune polyglandular syndrome type 1 (Addison disease, candidiasis, hypoparathyroidism, and primary gonadal failure)
	Autoimmune polyglandular syndrome type 2 (Addison disease, primary hypothyroidism, primary hypogonadism, diabetes, and pernicious anemia)
Inborn errors	Congenital adrenal hyperplasia
	Congenital adrenal hypoplasia (*DAX-1* mutation)
	Demyelinating disorders: adrenoleukodystrophies
	Childhood X-linked recessive adrenoleukodystrophy (ALD; Brown-Schilder disease)
	Neonatal autosomal recessive ALD
	X-linked recessive adrenomyeloneuropathy (sudanophilic leukodystrophy)
	Familial (isolated) glucocorticoid deficiency (degeneration of fasciculata-reticularis layers)
	Wolman disease (lysosomal acid lipase deficiency)
	Steroidogenic factor-1 mutations
	Mitochondrial forms of Addison disease (Kearns-Sayre syndrome)
	Smith-Lemli-Opitz syndrome (sterol delta-7-reductase mutations)
	Adrenocorticotropic hormone resistance syndromes
Vascular disorders	Intraadrenal hemorrhage (Waterhouse-Friderichsen syndrome): infection (caused by *Neisseria meningitidis, Pseudomonas aeruginosa, Haemophilus influenzae, Streptococcus pyogenes, Streptococcus pneumoniae*) or anticoagulants
Glandular infiltration	Neoplastic
	Leukemia, lymphoma, carcinoma of the lung, carcinoma of the breast
	Nonneoplastic
	Amyloid
	Hemochromatosis
Exogenous Causes	
Infection	Granulomatous disease
	Tuberculosis, sarcoidosis, histoplasmosis, cryptococcosis, blastomycosis (North and South American), sporotrichosis, and coccidiomycosis
	Other infections
	Cytomegalovirus, human immunodeficiency virus
Drugs	Blockers of steroid synthesis: mitotane, aminoglutethimide, trilostane, ketoconazole, metyrapone
	Glucocorticoid receptor blockers: RU-486
Abdominal Irradiation	
Bilateral adrenalectomy	Intraadrenal thrombosis: renal vein thrombosis in neonates, heparin-induced thrombocytopenia, the antiphospholipid syndrome
Causes of Deficient Mineralocorticoid Activity	
Failure of Aldosterone Production (Decreased Aldosterone)	
Hyperreninemia hypoaldosteronism (synthetic deficiency)	Primary adrenal insufficiency
	Selective aldosterone deficiency
	Inborn errors (eg, *CYP11B2* mutations)
	Drug-induced aldosterone suppression
	Heparin (direct inhibition of aldosterone secretion)
	Angiotensin-converting enzyme inhibitors
	Angiotensin receptor blockers
	Hypoaldosteronism in critical illness/hypotension (eg, selective zona glomerulosa injury)
Hyporeninemia hypoaldosteronism (deficient aldosterone stimulation)	Renin deficiency (eg, diabetes, renal failure)
Deficient Aldosterone Action (Resistance to Aldosterone; Elevated Aldosterone)	
Pseudohypoaldosteronism, type 1	Renal
	Multiple-target organ defects
	Early childhood hyperkalemia

primary adrenal failure, whereas low ACTH and subnormal response to the cosyntropin stimulation test suggest a hypothalamic or pituitary disorder.

The multiple-day cosyntropin stimulation test is particularly useful when patients have been receiving glucocorticoid therapy. In primary adrenal insufficiency, the damaged adrenal glands are unresponsive to any course of exogenous cosyntropin administration. Patients with secondary or tertiary adrenal insufficiency usually have an inadequate or absent initial cortisol response because the adrenal glands have been unstimulated for a prolonged time, and steroidogenesis requires the trophic priming of ACTH. Eventually, a delayed or staircase response is observed, indicating reactivation of the normal steroidogenic pathways as the adrenal gland benefits from the trophic actions of ACTH. This test, however, is not used as frequently in this situation because of the availability of better and sensitive ACTH immunoassays that more accurately determine ACTH concentrations at baseline. In primary adrenal insufficiency, the ACTH concentration is disproportionately elevated compared with the decreased plasma cortisol concentration.

The CRH stimulation test (see Box 66.3) is used to differentiate tertiary from secondary adrenal insufficiency.[59] Individuals with tertiary disease produce elevations in ACTH following CRH administration, whereas individuals with secondary disease demonstrate only minimal changes in ACTH concentration.

Although low basal plasma concentrations of DHEA-S occur in primary, secondary, and tertiary forms of adrenal insufficiency, DHEA-S measurements are of little value in the diagnosis of adrenal insufficiency; low concentrations of adrenal androgens are normally observed in young children (before ages 7 to 9) and in the elderly. Patients with HIV infection may have reduced concentrations of DHEA-S.[100] DHEA-S concentrations are helpful in women with hirsutism or patients suspected of having adrenal tumors, or sometimes in the adrenogenital syndrome (eg, CAH).[101]

Measurement of adrenal autoantibodies can be useful in evaluating patients with suspected adrenal insufficiency.[102] Antibodies against the 21 alpha-hydroxylase enzyme or other intracellular antigens have been used to diagnose autoimmune adrenal insufficiency.[103]

The first assay for adrenal autoantibodies utilized indirect immunofluorescence with human adrenal gland as the substrate. Fluorescence of the cortex indicates the presence of adrenal cytoplasmic autoantibodies (ACAs) in the serum.[104] Usually all layers of the adrenal cortex fluoresce, whereas the medulla rarely fluoresces because the adrenal cortical cytoplasmic autoantigens are localized to the microsomes of adrenal cortical cells.[105,106]

Among new-onset patients with Addison disease, 60% to 70% will express ACA. Studies in the 1990s established that target adrenal autoantigens were enzymes whose expression was limited to steroid-producing endocrine glands: 17-hydroxylase and 21-alpha-hydroxylase.[107-110] Autoantibodies to 21-alpha-hydroxylase (P450c21, CYP21) and 17-hydroxylase (P450c17, CYP17) have been detected by immunoprecipitation or enzyme-linked immunosorbent assay (ELISA) techniques. In many comparison studies, ACA and 21-alpha-hydroxylase autoantibody immunoassays performed similarly in identifying humoral adrenal autoimmunity in patients with Addison disease. Once the diagnosis of Addison disease has been established, testing for adrenal antibodies can resolve the underlying cause. In the absence of adrenal autoantibodies, testing for the presence of very long-chain free fatty acids (VLCFAs) is now performed to detect adrenoleukodystrophy. In the absence of abnormalities of VLCFA, other diagnoses must be considered.[111]

In otherwise asymptomatic individuals, detection of ACAs or 21-alpha-hydroxylase autoantibodies predicts the development of Addison disease.[112] The evolution of Addison disease passes through sequential stages: (1) normal to low aldosterone and elevated renin concentrations, (2) a deficient cortisol response to ACTH injection, (3) increased basal ACTH concentrations, and (4) deficient basal cortisol and aldosterone secretion.[113] Autoantibodies against the adrenal cortical cytoplasmic antigens or steroidogenic enzymes precede the clinical appearance of Addison disease;[114,115] however, their predictive power is more evident in children than in adults.[116,117] High-titer autoantibodies are also more predictive of progression to clinical disease.[118,119] Approaches to the diagnosis of Addison disease are provided in the At a Glance: Investigation of Clinically Suspected Addison Disease and At a Glance: Investigation of Suspected ACTH Deficiency features.

Hypoaldosteronism

Deficient aldosterone production occurs in conditions other than Addison disease (see Table 66.8).[120] Isolated aldosterone deficiency accompanied by normal cortisol production is seen in patients with (1) inadequate production of renin by the kidney, which leads to secondary aldosterone deficiency (hyporeninemic hypoaldosteronism); (2) inherited enzyme defects in aldosterone biosynthesis (eg, CYP11B2 deficiency; CYP11B2 = P450 aldo); and (3) acquired forms of primary aldosterone deficiency (heparin therapy and after surgery).[121] The resulting metabolic changes are hyperkalemia and hyponatremia, often with hypochloremic acidosis. Mild or moderate volume depletion, often with postural or unprovoked hypotension, may also occur. Hyporeninemic hypoaldosteronism can be established by demonstrating failure of both plasma renin and aldosterone to increase in response to furosemide stimulation or upright posture. This disorder is more common in older patients and in individuals with diabetes mellitus and nephropathy, who may have a hyperkalemic acidosis with low renin and aldosterone production, and hypertension.

Patients with primary adrenal insufficiency almost always suffer from aldosterone deficiency, in addition to cortisol deficiency.[122] Tests to confirm aldosterone deficiency in such patients are not usually necessary because hyperkalemia and hypotension support the diagnosis of primary adrenal insufficiency in patients with cortisol deficiency, elevated ACTH, and hyperpigmentation.

Glucocorticoid Excess (Cushing Syndrome)

Endogenous Cushing syndrome is the result of autonomous excessive production of cortisol, leading to the classic symptoms that are characteristic of this disorder (Table 66.9).[123] The clinical picture includes truncal obesity, moon face, a "buffalo" hump on the upper back below the neck, supraclavicular fat pads, purple striae, myopathy, hypertension, hirsutism, hypokalemic alkalosis, carbohydrate intolerance, disturbed reproductive function, and neuropsychiatric

AT A GLANCE

Investigation of Clinically Suspected Addison Disease

In cases of clinically suspected Addison disease, at the time of an Addisonian crisis with compatible hyponatremia, hyperkalemia, and acidosis, cortisol concentrations less than 5 µg/dL (<138 nmol/L) are diagnostic for Addison disease. Otherwise, further testing guided by the cortisol concentration is required (either the "stress" cortisol concentration or the average of two 08:00 a.m. cortisol levels). Further testing can include the 1-hour cosyntropin stimulation test or an insulin tolerance test (ITT). If the "stress" or average a.m. cortisol is 18 to 20 µg/dL (500–550 nmol/L) or greater, and the index of suspicion for Addison disease is low, no further testing is required. However, if the index of suspicion for Addison disease is high despite a "stress" or average a.m. cortisol of 18 to 20 µg/dL (500–550 nmol/L) or greater, further testing should be considered. As depicted, results of the 1-hour cosyntropin stimulation test or the ITT determine whether cortisol deficiency is excluded or, alternatively, a multiple-day cosyntropin stimulation test is indicated. Failure to demonstrate increased cortisol production in response to multiple-day cosyntropin stimulation supports the diagnosis of Addison disease (primary adrenal insufficiency). Not shown, but still important: an elevated adrenocorticotropic hormone (ACTH) in the setting of proven cortisol deficiency also supports the diagnosis of Addison disease. If cortisol rises in response to prolonged cosyntropin stimulation, ACTH deficiency is evident (eg, central ACTH deficiency). Note that cortisol assay results will exhibit bias based on calibration materials and other assay characteristics, so decision thresholds may vary and should be established by the laboratory.

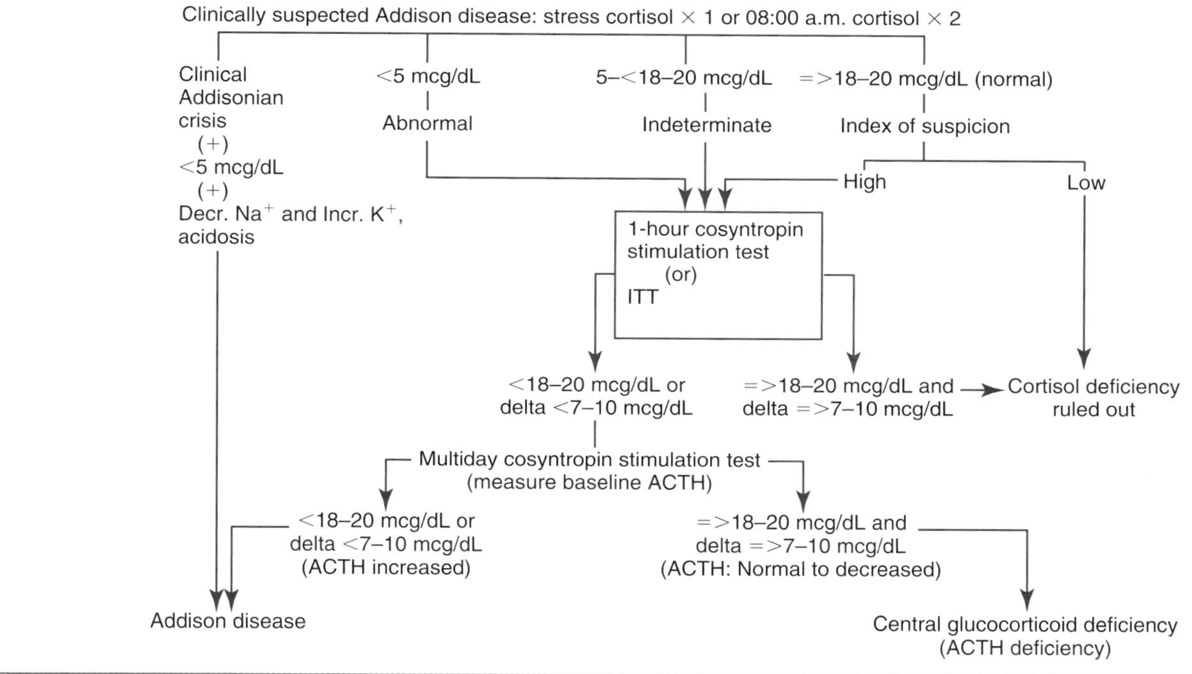

symptoms.[124] Exogenous Cushing syndrome is caused by excessive glucocorticoid therapy.

Endogenous disorders that cause hypersecretion of cortisol and Cushing syndrome may be classified as ACTH dependent or ACTH independent (Fig. 66.11).[125] Cushing disease is the pituitary-dependent form of Cushing syndrome.[126] In Cushing disease, hypersecretion of ACTH by a pituitary microadenoma is the primary defect that leads to bilateral adrenal hyperplasia and cortisol overproduction.[127] In ectopic ACTH syndrome, nonendocrine tumors develop the ability to secrete ACTH or modified ACTH, resulting in bilateral adrenal hyperplasia, unregulated cortisol secretion, and suppression of pituitary ACTH release.[128] Rarely, ectopic secretion of CRH occurs. In ectopic ACTH syndrome, the clinical presentation is usually dominated by the presence of cancer, and the patient may not display classic clinical findings of Cushing syndrome such as centripetal obesity.

Multiple endocrine neoplasia type 1 can cause Cushing syndrome through hypersecretion of ACTH from a pituitary microadenoma, an ectopic ACTH-secreting tumor of the pancreas, or medullary thyroid carcinoma.[129] Cushing syndrome caused by primary adrenal disease suppresses both CRH and ACTH, resulting in atrophy of the nontumorous adrenal zona fasciculata and zona reticularis.[130]

Glucocorticoid-producing adrenal adenomas are usually unilateral, circumscribed, brown-yellow in color, homogeneous in consistency, and weigh less than 30 g.[131] Histologically, the cells appear normal. Glucocorticoid-producing carcinomas are usually irregular in shape and histologically display hemorrhage, necrosis, nuclear pleomorphism, mitotic figures, and capsular and blood vessel invasion. The clinical history is more acute (4–6 months) than in cases of functional adenoma. Adrenal carcinomas have been known to exceed 100 g and may be palpable, and hepatic metastases can

AT A GLANCE

Investigation of Suspected Adrenocorticotropic Hormone Deficiency

When adrenocorticotropic hormone (ACTH) deficiency is suspected (eg, central glucocorticoid deficiency), unless the 08:00 a.m. cortisol is 18 to 20 μg/dL (500–550 nmol/L) or greater and the index of suspicion for ACTH deficiency is low, the 1-hour cosyntropin stimulation test, an insulin tolerance test (ITT), or an overnight metyrapone test is performed. (Note: Metyrapone is not currently available in the United States.) Normal responses to such tests rule out cortisol deficiency. An abnormal response to such testing triggers testing via the multiple-day cosyntropin stimulation test. If cortisol rises in response to prolonged cosyntropin stimulation, ACTH deficiency is evident. Failure to respond to prolonged cosyntropin stimulation indicates primary adrenal failure, and concurrent mineralocorticoid deficiency should be investigated. Note that cortisol assay results will exhibit bias based on calibration materials and other assay characteristics, so decision thresholds may vary and should be established by the laboratory.

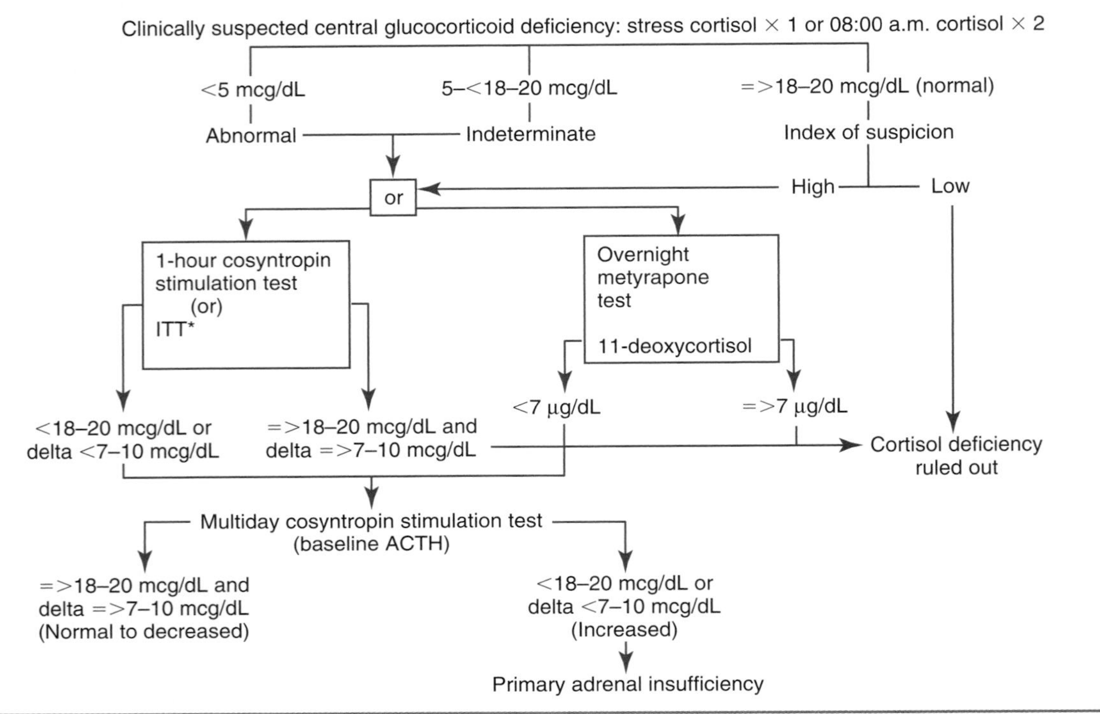

TABLE 66.9 Incidence of Clinical Manifestations in Cushing Syndrome

Clinical Manifestation	Incidence, %
Obesity	90
Hypertension	85
Hyperglycemia and decreased glucose tolerance	80
Menstrual and sexual dysfunction	76
Hirsutism, acne, plethora	72
Striae, atrophic skin	67
Weakness, proximal myopathy	65
Osteoporosis	55
Easy bruisability	55
Psychiatric disturbances	50
Edema	46
Polyuria, polyphagia	16
Ocular changes and exophthalmos	8

produce hepatomegaly. Adrenal carcinomas also occur in the Li-Fraumeni syndrome (*p53* loss-of-function mutations),[132] along with sarcoma, brain tumors, leukemia, lymphoma, and early-onset breast cancer.

Less common than adenomas, adrenal hyperplasia can cause cortisol excess.[133] In bilateral micronodular hyperplasia (also called *primary nodular hyperplasia* or *adrenocortical dysplasia*), nodules of 0.1 to 0.3 cm in diameter are observed that may be pigmented. The clinical outcome is similar to that of adrenal adenoma. Bilateral micronodular hyperplasia can be observed in the Carney complex, which includes growth hormone–producing anterior pituitary adenoma, Sertoli cell tumor, atrial or ventricular myxoma, mammary fibroadenoma, and cutaneous myxoma.[134,135] Affected patients can display a spotty skin pigmentation pattern. In bilateral macronodular hyperplasia (also called *massive macronodular hyperplasia* or *macronodular adrenal dysplasia*), large nodules of 0.2 to larger than 4 cm diameter are evident. Adrenal weight can exceed 100 g. Aberrant expression of a receptor for gastric-inhibitory polypeptide on the surface of tumor

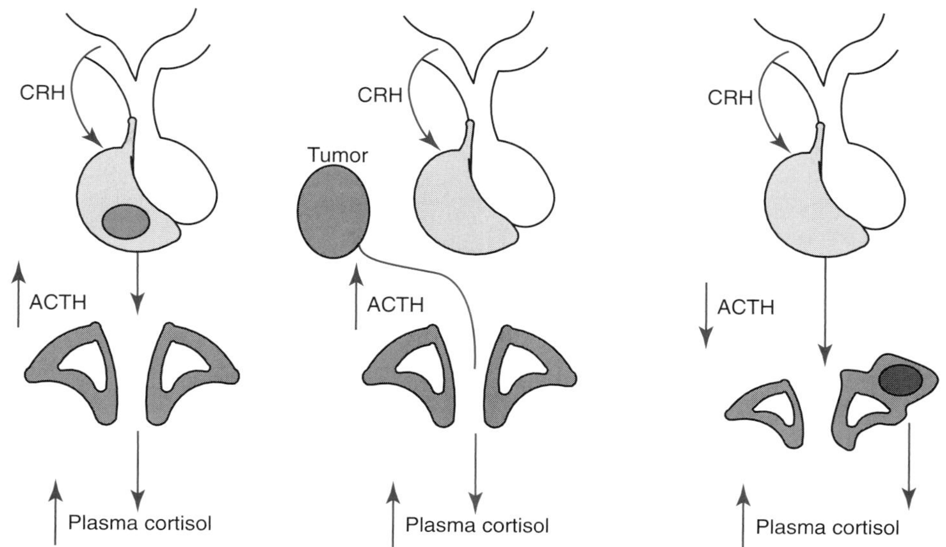

FIGURE 66.11 Endogenous Cushing syndrome can be classified as Cushing disease *(left)*, ectopic adrenocorticotropic hormone *(ACTH)* syndrome *(center)*, or adrenal Cushing syndrome *(right)*. ACTH is elevated in cases of Cushing disease and ectopic ACTH syndrome. ACTH is suppressed in cases of adrenal Cushing syndrome.

cells may result in postprandial hypercortisolism. This condition has been linked to mutations in the *ARMC5* gene.[136]

Screening Tests for Cushing Syndrome

Cushing syndrome is an uncommon disorder, but many of the usual signs and symptoms of this syndrome are seen in patients with normal adrenal function.[137] The initial diagnosis of Cushing syndrome, particularly in mild or early disease, rests on laboratory evidence of excessive and autonomous cortisol production.[138,139] Three simple screening tests are available for detecting Cushing syndrome—namely, 24-hour urine free cortisol, the 1 mg overnight dexamethasone suppression test (for protocol, see Box 66.5), and salivary cortisol. One test is the measurement of 24-hour UFC.[140,141] Under normal circumstances, less than 2% of secreted cortisol appears in urine as free cortisol. A 24-hour UFC excretion of less than 50 μg/d (1380 nmol/day) excludes the diagnosis of Cushing syndrome. Diagnostic accuracy is greater than 90%.[142] However, improper timing of the urine specimen (eg, collection over more than 24 hours), concomitant use of a diuretic, high salt intake, depression, and stress can all cause false-positive results. Any single test that exhibits cortisol excess should not, in itself, be used to prompt highly invasive therapy (eg, transsphenoidal neurosurgery for a suspected pituitary adenoma) without additional evaluation.[143]

The overnight low-dose dexamethasone suppression test, wherein 1 mg of dexamethasone is taken orally between 22:00 and 24:00, is a reliable and convenient screening test for Cushing syndrome. Cortisol concentrations at 08:00 a.m. below 5 μg/dL (1380 nmol/L) are normal and render the diagnosis of Cushing syndrome unlikely. A cortisol concentration of less than 2 μg/dL (55.2 nmol/L) essentially rules out Cushing syndrome. Cortisol values greater than 10 μg/dL (276 nmol/L) after dexamethasone suppression significantly favor the diagnosis of hypercortisolism and require further evaluation.

A multiple low-dose suppression test may also be used. Following low-dose dexamethasone (0.5 mg every 6 hours for 48 hours), plasma cortisol is usually suppressed to less than 2.2 μg/dL (60.7 nmol/L), and UFC is suppressed to less than 25 μg/d (690 nmol/d) in normal subjects. A diagnostic accuracy of 90% has been achieved with simultaneous measurements of cortisol and dexamethasone (to ensure dexamethasone was taken in the proper dose), although this approach is rarely used.

The 2008 Endocrine Society guidelines recommend that two out of the three screening tests—namely, 24-hour urine free cortisol, the 1 mg overnight dexamethasone suppression test, and salivary cortisol—should be abnormal before proceeding to more definitive evaluation.[141,144]

The circadian rhythm of cortisol secretion has been used to screen for Cushing syndrome, although it is considerably less useful than measurement of urinary cortisol, measurement of the morning plasma cortisol concentration following dexamethasone suppression, or plasma or salivary cortisol measurements taken at midnight. A midnight, plasma cortisol greater than 9 μg/dL (248 nmol/L) suggests loss of diurnal variation. The later in the night that cortisol can be measured, the more helpful the test will be. Some patients with Cushing syndrome do not exhibit loss of diurnal variation even with elevations in both morning and night cortisol concentrations; loss of diurnal variation is not a consistent finding in Cushing syndrome. Measuring cortisol at 08:00 a.m. as a screening test for Cushing syndrome is not recommended. If a single cortisol measurement is to be used, plasma or saliva should be collected near midnight.[144] Because of the ease of obtaining saliva, this approach has become widely used. However, analysis in a reference laboratory is usually required because salivary cortisol concentration is much lower than plasma cortisol concentration. Typical salivary cortisol concentrations in healthy individuals are 0.14 to 1.0 μg/dL (4–28 nmol/L) at 07:00 a.m. and 0.07 to 0.22 μg/L (2–6 nmol/L) at 22:00.

TABLE 66.10 Differentiating the Causes of Endogenous Cushing Syndrome

	Cushing Disease Corticotropinoma	Ectopic ACTH Syndrome	Cushing Syndrome Adrenal Tumor
Biochemical Evaluation			
ACTH	Norm, Incr	Norm, Incr	Decr
UFC response to high-dose dexamethasone	Usually declines by >50%	Does not decline by >50%	Does not decline by 50%
Basal and post-CRH ACTH levels	IPS > peripheral	IPS = peripheral	Not performed
Radiologic Evaluation			
CT or MRI			
Pituitary	Abn	Norm	Norm
Adrenal	Norm	Norm	Abn
Other location	Norm	Abn	Norm

Abn, Abnormal; *ACTH,* adrenocorticotropic hormone; *CRH,* corticotropin-releasing hormone; *CT,* computed tomography; *decr,* decreased; *incr,* increased; *IPS,* inferior petrosal sinus; *MRI,* magnetic resonance imaging; *Norm,* normal; *UFC,* urinary free cortisol.

Differential Diagnosis of Cushing Syndrome

Hypercortisolism supports the diagnosis of endogenous Cushing syndrome. More definitive testing should be performed to determine the source of the excess cortisol (Table 66.10 and the At a Glance: Investigation of the Causes of Hypercortisolism and At a Glance: Differentiation of Endogenous Cushing Syndromes features). Plasma ACTH concentrations are low in patients with an adrenal tumor (<10 pg/mL; <2.2 pmol/L) and are normal or moderately elevated in patients with Cushing disease (generally >50 pg/mL; >11 pmol/L). Plasma ACTH is often markedly elevated in patients with nonendocrine ACTH-secreting tumors (ectopic ACTH syndrome) because the tumor source of the ACTH does not respond to negative feedback from cortisol. On the other hand, the ACTH-secreting pituitary adenoma of Cushing disease has an elevated set point for negative feedback; if the cortisol (or other glucocorticoid) concentration is elevated high enough, some measure of negative feedback will occur (eg, 60% of patients with Cushing disease achieve ACTH and UFC suppression when treated with high-dose dexamethasone). Plasma ACTH concentrations greater than 300 pg/mL (66 pmol/L) usually suggest a nonendocrine ACTH-secreting tumor (ectopic ACTH syndrome).

High-dose dexamethasone suppression testing (overnight high dose or multiple-day high dose) is useful in differentiating Cushing syndrome caused by an adrenal tumor or nonendocrine ACTH-secreting tumor from pituitary Cushing disease (see earlier section on Dexamethasone Suppression Test and Box 66.7).

Some patients with Cushing disease may fail to suppress cortisol (plasma or urinary) after high-dose dexamethasone. Such test results can be followed up by administering 1.0 mg (low dose) or 8 mg (high dose) of dexamethasone at midnight (overnight dexamethasone suppression test). Serum is collected at 08:00 a.m. for the measurement of cortisol. In the overnight dexamethasone suppression test, 1 mg of dexamethasone should not suppress cortisol in any form of Cushing syndrome. In patients with adrenal tumor and, with a few exceptions, in those patients with nonendocrine ACTH-secreting tumor, suppression does not occur after the high-dose 8-mg dexamethasone administration. Furthermore, with high-dose dexamethasone testing, less than 10% of patients with Cushing disease fail to show some degree of suppression, although most patients show only 50% to 60% suppression. Failure to suppress cortisol in response to high-dose dexamethasone has occurred in patients with accelerated clearance of dexamethasone due to hepatic cytochrome P450–inducing drugs, such as phenytoin and rifampin. In these patients, measurements of plasma dexamethasone can be useful in gauging the effective concentration.

The CRH stimulation test (see earlier section on CRH Stimulation Test and Box 66.3) produces an exaggerated ACTH or cortisol response, or both, in about 90% of patients with Cushing disease. Usually plasma cortisol increases by 20%, and plasma ACTH increases by 50% following CRH (1.0 μg/kg) administration. Poor responses occur in patients with adrenal tumors and in most patients with nonendocrine ACTH-secreting tumors (usually those having elevated basal concentrations of plasma ACTH). Patients with depression and anorexia nervosa may not exhibit an exaggerated ACTH response to CRH injection.

If the cause of Cushing syndrome is uncertain, measurement of ACTH from inferior petrosal sinus specimens before and after CRH stimulation can be helpful.[59] When ACTH concentrations in inferior petrosal sinus specimens are similar to those of simultaneously obtained peripheral vein specimens (eg, from the inferior vena cava), a nonpituitary source of ACTH is evident. In virtually all patients with ectopic production of ACTH, the ratio of ACTH concentrations between the inferior petrosal sinus and a peripheral venous specimen is less than 1.4 : 1. In contrast, patients with Cushing disease have a ratio greater than 2.0 and an average ratio near 15.[145] Inferior petrosal sinus sampling is not useful for locating the lesion because venous drainage can cross over.[60,146]

Adrenal androgens and plasma DHEA-S are measured to diagnose hirsutism without Cushing syndrome.[147] In patients with Cushing syndrome, plasma DHEA-S is usually normal or moderately elevated (plasma DHEA-S ~500 μg/dL; 13.5 μmol/L). Patients with an adrenal adenoma usually have low (age-adjusted) plasma DHEA-S levels. Plasma DHEA-S in patients with nonendocrine ACTH-secreting tumors are normal to elevated. In patients with congenital adrenal hyperplasia, adrenal androgens are usually suppressed after administration of 0.75 mg per day of dexamethasone for 2 to 3 weeks, but suppression does not occur in patients with adrenal tumors and nonendocrine ACTH-secreting tumors.

CRH stimulation of ACTH after dexamethasone suppression has been used to investigate hypercortisolism. The concept is that a normal individual exposed to dexamethasone would secrete reduced amounts of ACTH in response to CRH compared to a patient with Cushing syndrome. It has been reported that a post-CRH ACTH concentration of 28 pg/mL or greater yielded clinical sensitivity of 95% and specificity of 97% for the recognition of Cushing syndrome, and a 15-minute cortisol of 2.6 μg/dL (71.8 nmol/L) or greater was 90% sensitive and 90% specific.[148] Combined testing by dexamethasone suppression and post-CRH ACTH measurements is being used in psychiatric evaluations.[149]

In addition to suppression and stimulation testing, methods of tumor localization should be used to document the cause of Cushing syndrome. Computed tomography (CT) of the adrenal glands has been helpful in localizing adrenal tumors, macronodular hyperplasia, and bilateral hyperplasia of the adrenal glands.[150] CT in combination with magnetic resonance imaging (MRI) of the pituitary gland can help to detect pituitary microadenomas.[151] However, anatomic abnormalities are not always related to functional abnormalities. For this reason, when an adrenal source of excess cortisol is suggested by CT scanning or MRI, it is prudent that the patient undergo venography with measurement of cortisol in each adrenal vein. In the case of a cortisol-secreting adrenal adenoma, the cortisol should be significantly higher (eg, 50% higher) in one adrenal vein compared with the other. In the case of bilateral hyperplasia causing hypercortisolism, no significant difference (<50%) between sides should be observed. The search for ectopic sources of ACTH can involve conventional radiography, ultrasonography, and CT scanning or MRI for the detection of suspected neoplasms.

Especially challenging are cases of episodic Cushing syndrome, wherein hypercortisolism is not always present. Rare cortisol-secreting adrenal tumors that express incretin receptors have been reported.[152] In these cases, hypercortisolism occurs only with meals.

AT A GLANCE

Investigation of the Causes of Hypercortisolism

When hypercortisolism is established, low-dose/high-dose dexamethasone suppression testing (see Box 66.6 for protocol) can clarify the cause. Suppression of urinary free cortisol (UFC) on low-dose dexamethasone excludes cortisol excess. Suppression on high-dose dexamethasone establishes the diagnosis of Cushing disease, but not all patients with Cushing disease are suppressed on high-dose dexamethasone. Lack of cortisol suppression on high-dose dexamethasone triggers the measurement of adrenocorticotropic hormone (ACTH). Elevated ACTH (>50 pg/mL or >10 pmol/L) favors a central or ectopic source, whereas a suppressed ACTH (<10 pg/mL or <2.2 pmol/L) favors an adrenal lesion.

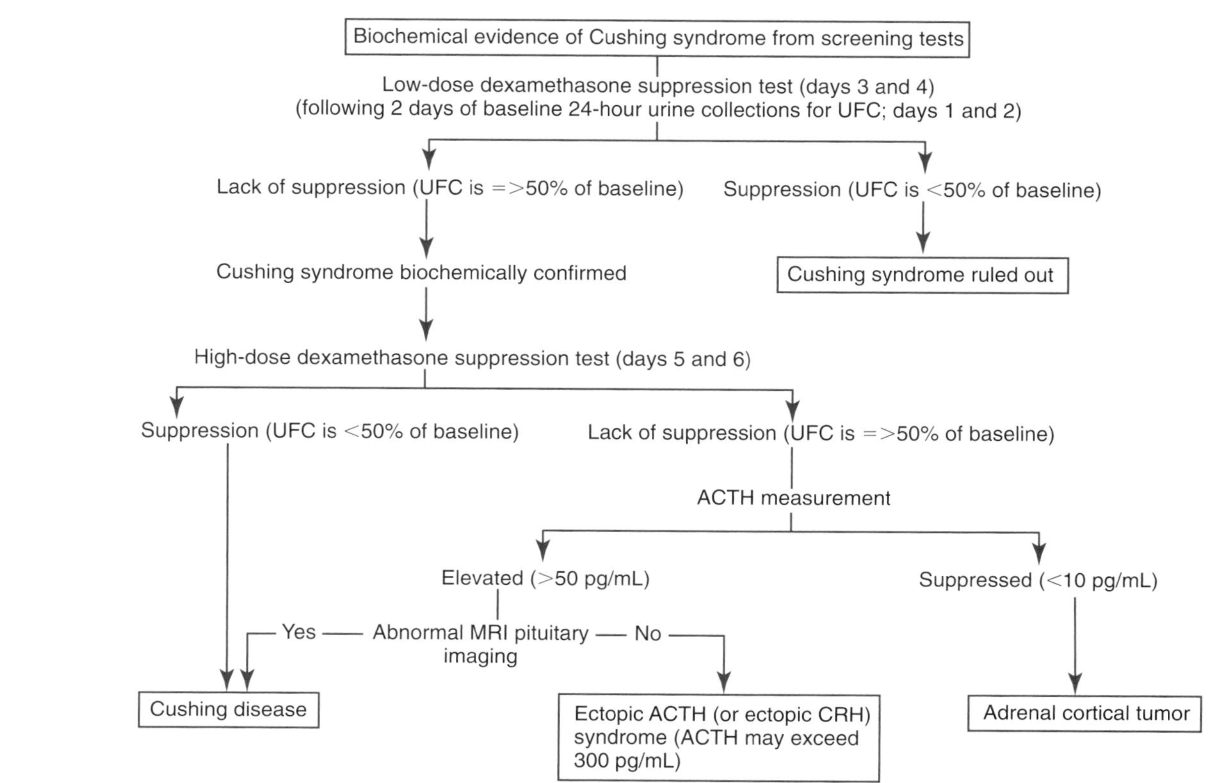

AT A GLANCE

Differentiation of Endogenous Cushing Syndromes

A suppressed adrenocorticotropic hormone (ACTH) establishes the diagnosis of adrenal Cushing syndrome (ie, a cortisol-secreting adrenal cortical tumor). If ACTH is elevated, the pituitary is examined via inferior petrosal sinus sampling (and magnetic resonance imaging scanning) to resolve Cushing disease versus ectopic ACTH syndrome. Elevated ACTH (>50 pg/mL or >10 pmol/L) is an indication for inferior petrosal sinus sampling (IPSS), whereas a suppressed ACTH (<10 pg/mL or <2.2 pmol/L) favors an adrenal lesion.

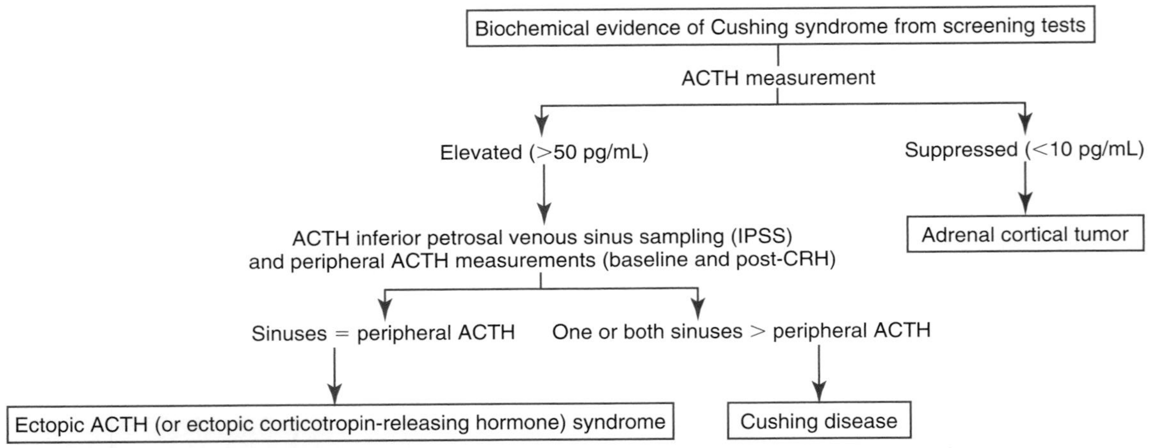

Conditions That Mimic Cushing Syndrome

Alcohol abuse can induce a "pseudo-Cushing syndrome" that mimics the clinical and biochemical features of the disease. The abnormalities are reversible when alcohol consumption stops. HIV infection, anorexia nervosa, and depression are associated with elevated serum cortisol concentrations, and patients with these disorders may have abnormal low-dose, overnight dexamethasone suppression tests (morning cortisol ≥5 μg/dL; ≥138 nmol/L). Cortisol measurements at 24:00 may help exclude Cushing syndrome in these circumstances.[20] However, the clinical features of patients with HIV and anorexia nervosa are not typical in Cushing syndrome. Measurement of UFC and plasma cortisol with the dexamethasone suppression test improves the predictive value in the diagnosis of both Cushing syndrome and depression.[153] In patients with depression, it is best to repeat testing after the depression has been treated.

Obese patients also may display clinical features that mimic Cushing syndrome.[154] Truncal obesity, striae, and enhanced excretion of 17-OHCS are features of Cushing syndrome that occur in normal, obese subjects. UFC, however, is normal in obese individuals and can effectively differentiate normal subjects from those with true Cushing syndrome.[155] Likewise, 48 hours of low-dose dexamethasone (0.5 mg orally every 6 hours) should suppress urinary free cortisol excretion by more than 50% in obese patients.

Congenital Adrenal Hyperplasia

CAH is the most common cause of adrenocortical insufficiency in newborns.[156] However, CAH is discussed under adrenal hormone overproduction syndromes because CAH commonly leads to overproduction of adrenal androgens. CAH presents a mixed picture of cortisol deficiency (hypofunction) and adrenal androgen overproduction (hyperfunction). Rarely, traumatic adrenal hemorrhage or adrenal hemorrhage from sepsis causes adrenal failure in newborns, but CAH is the most common cause of adrenal failure in newborns.

CAH results from loss-of-function mutations in adrenocortical enzymes responsible for cortisol synthesis.[157] These disorders are inherited as autosomal recessive traits. Six enzymes are necessary to convert cholesterol into cortisol: CYP11A (a 20,22-desmolase; sometimes called a 20 alpha-hydroxylase), CYP17 (a 17-hydroxylase), 3 beta-hydroxysteroid dehydrogenase, delta(4)-5-isomerase, CYP21 (a 21-alpha-hydroxylase), and CYP11B1 (an 11-beta-hydroxylase).

With insufficient cortisol production, ACTH concentrations increase and stimulate fetal adrenal hyperplasia in utero.[158-160] 21-Alpha-hydroxylase deficiency (CYP21 deficiency; Fig. 66.12) and 11-beta-hydroxylase deficiency (CYP11B1 deficiency) are the two most common causes of CAH. About 95% of CAH cases result from 21-alpha-hydroxylase deficiency, and 11-beta-hydroxylase deficiency accounts for most of the remaining CAH cases. Other causes of CAH are very rare. The incidence of 21-alpha-hydroxylase CAH in Western societies varies from 1 in 5000 to 15,000 live births.[161]

Newborn screening for 21-alpha-hydroxylase and 11-beta-hydroxylase deficiency by measuring 17-alpha-hydroxyprogesterone (17-OHP) is standard practice in the United States and many other countries.[162-165] Methods based on tandem mass spectrometry can essentially eliminate the risk of false-positive 17-OHP screens.[166,167]

The metabolic block in cortisol biosynthesis leads to an accumulation of precursors, which can then be shunted into production of adrenal androgens.[168] Measurements of the precursor steroids in blood help identify the specific enzyme defect and monitor the response to cortisol replacement therapy. A partial block may cause marked or subtle clinical manifestations, whereas a complete enzyme block can be

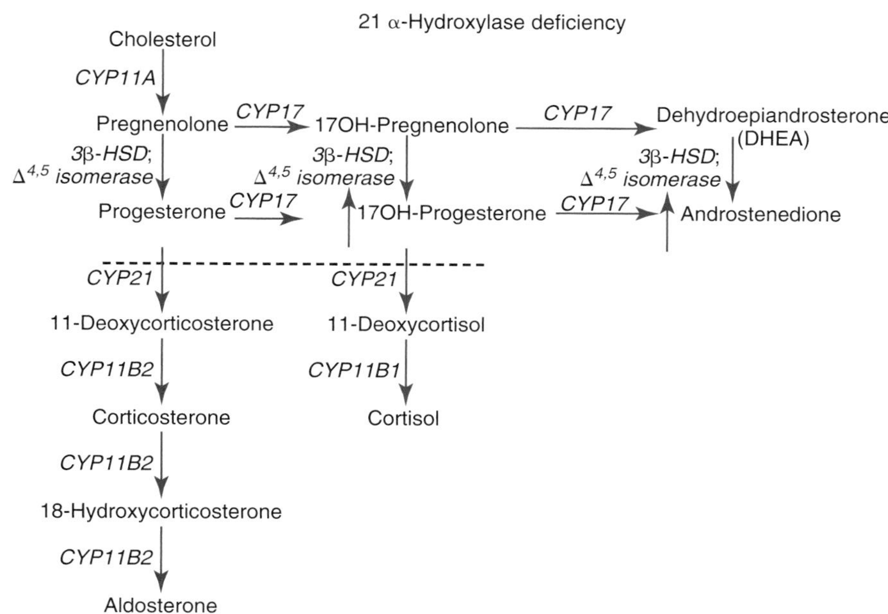

FIGURE 66.12 In 21-alpha-hydroxylase deficiency (CYP21; *dashed line*), cortisol deficiency and possibly aldosterone deficiency are present. Elevations in 17-hydroxyprogesterone and androstenedione are observed.

fatal without treatment. The closer the enzyme block is to the final cortisol product, the less life-threatening are the symptoms.

Because CAH produces elevations of adrenal androgens (DHEA and androstenedione) in utero, virilization of the external genitalia of a female fetus occurs, producing sexual ambiguity (ambiguous genitalia). Only rarely does CAH lead to inadequate male sexual development.

Cortisol deficiency in affected individuals leads to malaise, failure to thrive, hypoglycemia, and vascular instability. In approximately one-half of infants afflicted with 21-alpha-hydroxylase deficiency, insufficient aldosterone production can cause hyponatremia, hyperkalemia, acidosis, dehydration, and hypotension. In its most severe form, this type of "salt-losing" 21-alpha-hydroxylase deficiency clinically presents at 10 to 14 days of age with Addisonian crisis. Untreated, mortality is very high in salt-losing 21-alpha-hydroxylase deficiency. The non–salt-losing form of this disease is customarily referred to as *simple virilizing* 21 alpha-hydroxylase deficiency.

Before newborn screening for CAH with 17-alpha-hydroxyprogesterone measurements was available, the diagnosis of CAH was more common in females than in males.[169] The lower number of males diagnosed with CAH appears to be the result of deaths of undiagnosed males afflicted with salt-losing CAH. The cause of death could have been erroneously ascribed to sepsis or idiopathic dehydration and not to Addisonian crisis. Presently, with newborn CAH screening, the male and female incidences of CAH are approximately equal, which is typical of an autosomal recessive condition.

In 21-alpha-hydroxylase and 11-beta-hydroxylase deficiencies, excess ACTH and the metabolic block in cortisol biosynthesis result in overproduction of adrenal androgens DHEA, DHEA-S, and androstenedione.[170] At birth, females with 21-alpha-hydroxylase deficiency CAH can present with ambiguous genitalia and postnatal virilization (intersex or a disorder of sexual development) and are at risk for neonatal salt-losing Addisonian crisis. Virilization in females varies from mild fusion of the labia, to marked labial fusion with clitoromegaly, to complete masculinization with apparent male external genitalia. Newborn genetic females with CAH can be incorrectly categorized as males with bilaterally undescended testes. Untreated, postnatal females who survive will continue to develop masculine characteristics. Because salt-losing 21-alpha-hydroxylase deficiency is a more severe expression of the inborn error than non–salt-losing 21-alpha-hydroxylase deficiency, salt-losing CAH is associated with more severe virilization in females.

In males, adrenal androgen overproduction in 21-alpha-hydroxylase deficiency produces precocious pseudopuberty and some degree of hyperpigmentation of the male external genitalia during infancy or childhood, or in the neonatal period they present with salt-losing crisis. Untreated, postnatal males will experience early-onset puberty with advanced secondary sex characteristics, and despite an early acceleration in their growth rate and tall stature, they may ultimately suffer from short stature because of premature closure of their epiphyses.[171] The more profound the defect in cortisol biosynthesis, the greater the degree of precocious pseudopuberty in males. True precocious puberty is driven by the pituitary gonadotropins luteinizing hormone and follicle-stimulating hormone and testicular enlargement. In contrast, CAH-induced pseudopuberty does not produce testicular enlargement until true puberty. If adrenal rests are adherent to the testes, they can enlarge with untreated or undertreated CAH (a *rest* is a group of cells that has become displaced and lies embedded in another tissue).

In 11-beta-hydroxylase deficiency (ie, CAH from *CYP11B1* mutations), mineralocorticoid deficiency does not occur.[172] Because the conversion of DOC to corticosterone in the zona glomerulosa is predominantly catalyzed by CYP11B2 (aldosterone synthase, P450 aldo), mineralocorticoid levels are not affected in 11-beta-hydroxylase (CYP11B1) deficiency. Also, elevated ACTH may have some effect in stimulating DOC production, and DOC may be elevated in CYP11B1 11-beta-hydroxylase deficiency.[173] 11-Beta-hydroxylase activity of CYP11B2 is normal in CYP11B1 11-beta-hydroxylase deficiency; therefore DOC may be elevated by the residual 11-beta-hydroxylase activity of CYP11B1 normally present in the zona glomerulosa.

Whereas females with CYP11B1 11-beta-hydroxylase deficiency have ambiguous genitalia and males undergo precocious pseudopuberty, salt loss does not occur in CYP11B1 11-beta-hydroxylase deficiency. Thus electrolyte disturbances and acidosis do not occur, nor does Addisonian crisis develop, in the newborn period or later. However, later in childhood, hypertension, with or without hypokalemia, can develop. The incidence of CYP11B1 11-beta hydroxylase deficiency is approximately 1 in 100,000.

Diagnosis of 21-alpha-hydroxylase deficiency and CYP-11B1 11-beta-hydroxylase deficiency depends on finding elevated concentrations of 17-OHP in plasma or serum. Patients with CYP11B1 11-beta-hydroxylase deficiency are not hypotensive and may develop hypokalemic hypertension during childhood. Biochemically, 17-OHCS are elevated in CYP11B1 11-beta-hydroxylase deficiency (ie, 11-deoxycortisol is elevated and contributes to 17-OHCS), whereas 17-OHCS are low in 21-hydroxylase deficiency (both 11-deoxycortisol and cortisol are low). 11-Deoxycortisol and its urinary metabolite tetrahydrodeoxycortisol (THS) will be elevated in CYP-11B1 11-beta-hydroxylase deficiency, as will the ratio of plasma 11-deoxycortisol to plasma cortisol and the ratio of their urinary metabolites, THS to THF. In 21-alpha-hydroxylase deficiency, the synthesis of both 11-deoxyocortisol and cortisol is impaired, and the ratio of urinary THS to THF is not elevated.

Once a child is diagnosed with CAH, fetal DNA testing in subsequent pregnancies allows prenatal diagnosis of CAH.[169] Prenatal diagnosis of CAH can prompt maternal treatment with high-dose dexamethasone to suppress excess fetal adrenal androgen production. This treatment prevents ambiguous genitalia in females and the androgenic effects of excess fetal adrenal androgens on the fetal brain.[174,175]

A late-onset or attenuated (nonclassical) form of 21-alpha-hydroxylase deficiency can occur in female adolescents, presenting as hirsutism or virilization associated with menstrual irregularities, oligomenorrhea, amenorrhea, and a polycystic ovary–like syndrome.[176,177] Late-onset 21-alpha-hydroxylase deficiency CAH is much milder than the classical prenatal virilizing form of 21-alpha-hydroxylase deficiency. Baseline and post-ACTH 17-OHP concentrations in attenuated 21-alpha-hydroxylase–deficient CAH are higher than in controls, but the values are not as high as those seen in classical 21-alpha-hydroxylase deficiency CAH. Gene carriers (individuals heterozygous for a wild-type allele and a mutant allele) usually have normal basal concentrations of 17-OHP but amplified 17-OHP responses to a cosyntropin challenge.

Early-morning 17-OHP or random androstenedione measurements are used to assess the response to glucocorticoid replacement in CAH patients.[157] With adequate glucocorticoid replacement, 17-OHP or androstenedione should not exceed the upper limit of the reference interval for age and sex. Insufficient glucocorticoid replacement permits excess adrenal production of androgens. Alternatively, overtreatment with glucocorticoids can suppress growth by induction of a mild iatrogenic Cushing syndrome. In patients with 21-alpha-hydroxylase deficiency, aldosterone is replaced with oral fludrocortisone (Fluorinef). Mineralocorticoid replacement is monitored by measuring blood pressure and renin. Inadequate replacement may result in hypertension from elevated renin that increases angiotensin II, causing vasoconstriction despite possible volume depletion. However, mineralocorticoid overdosage can also induce hypertension through excess sodium retention. Hypokalemia and alkalosis are potential consequences of overreplacement with fludrocortisone. The effectiveness of fludrocortisone therapy depends on the presence or absence of normal linear growth, normal sexual development, and 17-OHP and/or adrenal androgen concentrations in the normal range.

17-Alpha-hydroxylase deficiency (CYP17, P450c17) is a rare cause of CAH.[178] Normally, 17-alpha-hydroxylase converts pregnenolone to 17-hydroxypregnenelone and progesterone to 17-OHP in the zona glomerulosa and the zona reticularis. Absence of 17-alpha-hydroxylase activity impedes cortisol biosynthesis. *CYP17* mutations influence sex steroid production in males in utero and in females at the time of puberty because this gene provides zona reticularis and gonadal 17,20-desmolase (lyase) activity. 17,20-Desmolase converts 17-hydroxypregnenelone to DHEA and 17-hydroxyprogesterone to androstenedione. In the gonad, DHEA is the precursor of androstenediol, which is the immediate precursor of testosterone. Thus, in addition to interference in cortisol biosynthesis, *CYP17* mutations preclude sex steroid production of both androgens and estrogens. In contrast, the aldosterone pathway remains intact and salt-wasting does not occur with elevated DOC, causing hypertension in later childhood. Because both *CYP17* and *CYP11B1* mutations can cause hypertension, these conditions are compared in Table 66.11.

Similar to 21-alpha-hydroxylase deficiency and CYP11B1 11-beta-hydroxylase deficiency, ACTH concentrations increase because of cortisol deficiency in 17-alpha-hydroxylase deficiency. Elevated ACTH stimulates mineralocorticoid overproduction in the zona glomerulosa. Salt and water retention suppress aldosterone release. Salt-wasting is not present in 17-alpha-hydroxylase deficiency; in fact, excessive salt and water retention from excessive mineralocorticoid activity frequently produces hypertension in childhood. When sex steroids are not produced, genetic males will appear as sexually ambiguous or phenotypic females with delayed puberty. The uterus, fallopian tubes, and upper one-third of the vagina are absent because of Müllerian inhibiting hormone (or anti-Müllerian hormone) secreted by the Sertoli cells of the testes. Virilization of the external genitalia is reduced or absent in males in utero because of the block in testosterone biosynthesis. In genetic females, genitalia are not ambiguous; however, puberty and menses will not occur spontaneously because estrogens will not be produced.

Another rare form of CAH is 3-beta-hydroxysteroid dehydrogenase deficiency.[179] This enzyme converts ^{5}delta to ^{4}delta steroids (eg, pregnenolone to progesterone, 17-hydroxypregnenolone to 17-OHP, and DHEA to androstenedione). Because the gonads share these pathways with the adrenal glands, males are undervirilized when testosterone production is deficient, and females are overvirilized due to excessive adrenal androgen production. In

TABLE 66.11 **Comparisons of 21-Hydroxylase Deficiency, 11 Beta-Hydroxylase Deficiency, and 17 Alpha-Hydroxylase Deficiency Congenital Adrenal Hyperplasia**

	Enzyme Deficiency 21-Hydroxylase	11β-Hydroxylase	17α-Hydroxylase
Gene	*CYP21*	*CYP11B1*	*CYP17*
Concentrations			
17-OHP	Elevated	Elevated	Depressed
DOC	Depressed	Elevated	Elevated
11-Deoxy-cortisol	Depressed	Elevated	Depressed
Cortisol*	Depressed	Depressed	Depressed
17-KGS	Elevated	Elevated	Depressed
17-OHCS	Depressed	Elevated	Depressed
17-KS	Elevated	Elevated	Depressed
Ambiguous genitalia	In females	In females	In males
Precocious puberty	In boys	In boys	None
Salt loss	Present in approximately 75% of patients	None	None
Hypertension	None	Late childhood/adolescence	Late childhood/adolescence

*In mild forms of congenital adrenal hyperplasia, cortisol may be low-normal from a compensatory elevation in adrenocorticotropic hormone.
17-KGS, 17-Ketogenic steroids; *17-KS,* 17-ketosteroids; *17-OHCS,* 17-hydroxycorticosteroids.

3-beta-hydroxysteroid dehydrogenase deficiency, the ratios of pregnenolone to progesterone, 17-hydroxypregnenolone to 17-OHP, and DHEA to androstenedione are elevated. A late-onset form of this disease has been described in patients with premature pubarche, hirsutism, acne, and menstrual irregularities.

Biochemically, 17-ketosteroid reductase deficiency affects sex steroid synthesis in the gonads, but it does not affect aldosterone or cortisol biosynthesis.[180] 17-Ketosteroid reductase deficiency causes testosterone deficiency in utero with sexual ambiguity in males and primary amenorrhea and failure to enter puberty in females.

The least common, but most severe, form of CAH is not an enzyme deficiency but a disorder involving StAR.[181] StAR mediates the transport of cholesterol across the mitochondrial membrane. A deficiency of StAR is potentially lethal and causes congenital lipoid adrenal hyperplasia when the adrenal glands are saturated with cholesterol and cholesterol esters that are not further metabolized. In this disorder, deficiencies of all steroid hormones are present. Failure of androgen production in males results in ambiguous genitalia.

Functioning Adrenocortical Tumors

Plasma DHEA-S, DHEA, androstenedione, and testosterone concentrations are elevated in patients with virilizing adrenal adenomas and Cushing syndrome.[182] The plasma concentrations of DHEA may also be elevated in women with virilizing ovarian tumors. CT scans along with MRI are useful in differentiating the sites of the tumors.[183] Aldosterone-producing adenomas, referred to as *Conn syndrome,* are typically small microadenomas found in the zona glomerulosa that hypersecrete aldosterone, producing a syndrome characterized by low renin hypertension.[184]

Adrenal carcinomas are rare, with an incidence of only 1 per million; they usually are larger than 4 cm and may cause only virilization, without the typical features of Cushing syndrome.[185] Adrenal carcinomas are more common in women than in men by a 2.5:1 ratio. Most adrenal carcinomas are functional, producing glucocorticoids alone or glucocorticoids and androgens. Plasma DHEA-S, DHEA, and androstenedione concentrations are markedly elevated in patients with functional adrenal carcinomas. Peripheral conversion of adrenal androgens to testosterone results in hirsutism and virilization. DHEA-S concentrations can exceed 1000 μg/dL (27 μmol/L) in patients with adrenal carcinoma and usually are diagnostic for this malignancy. High-dose glucocorticoids do not suppress elevated androgen production.

Feminizing adrenocortical carcinomas are rare.[186,187] These tumors result in elevated plasma DHEA-S, DHEA, androstenedione, estrone, and estradiol concentrations. Gynecomastia and sexual dysfunction occur in males; precocious pseudopuberty occurs in females. Dexamethasone does not suppress cortisol production in these cases.

Nonfunctioning Adrenocortical Tumors

Approximately 2% of the population have an adrenal tumor; most of these tumors are nonfunctioning and benign and are called *incidentalomas* (or *incidentomas*) when found by accident.[188,189] The tumors usually are found when CT or MRI scans of the abdomen are performed that easily detect tumors 1 cm in diameter or 5 g in weight. No virilizing tumor smaller than 1 cm in diameter has been reported. Carcinomas usually weigh more than 30 g.

The challenge occurs when CT or MRI of the abdomen reveals an adrenal mass in a patient lacking clinical evidence of adrenal hyperfunction.[190] The CT or MRI might have been ordered for evaluation of undiagnosed "chronic abdominal pain," for example. An unexpected adrenal mass may prompt screening for Cushing syndrome, hypermineralocorticoidism, and pheochromocytoma. Diagnostically challenging cases with possibly mild hypercortisolism may be revealed.[191] Screening for hypermineralocorticoidism may be as simple as measuring the patient's blood pressure and serum potassium (assuming that the patient has not previously been diagnosed with hypertension and the patient is not on potassium-wasting diuretics). Because adrenal androgen- or estrogen-secreting tumors are very rare, these may be detected solely by taking a history and performing a physical examination with attention to evidence of androgen or estrogen excess.

Screening for pheochromocytoma involves measuring plasma free metanephrine or 24-hour urinary metanephrines and/or catecholamines.

Mineralocorticoid Excess (Hyperaldosteronism)

Primary hyperaldosteronism, also known as *Conn syndrome*, is a syndrome caused by aldosterone excess.[192] In primary hyperaldosteronism, excessive aldosterone production originates within the adrenal gland, whereas in secondary hyperaldosteronism, a stimulus outside the adrenal gland activates the renin-angiotensin system. (Note: The term *aldosteronism* is often used synonymously with *hyperaldosteronism*.) The interaction of renin, angiotensin, and aldosterone is important in the regulation of extracellular fluid volume and blood pressure, the balance of sodium and potassium ions, and acid-base balance.

Renin release from the kidney is regulated by (1) the distal tubule, where chemoreceptor macula densa cells monitor the sodium concentration; (2) the pressure-transducer juxtaglomerular cells, which monitor renal perfusion pressure; (3) the sympathetic nervous system, which controls catecholamine release; and (4) humoral factors such as potassium, atrial natriuretic peptides, and angiotensin II. Secondary events that disrupt normal renin release are much more common than primary abnormalities of renin secretion (Table 66.12).

TABLE 66.12 Causes of Functional Hypermineralocorticoidism

Hyperaldosteronism	Primary (hyporeninemic) • Aldosterone-producing adenoma • Aldosterone-producing carcinoma • Idiopathic adrenal hyperplasia • Unilateral adrenocortical hyperplasia • Glucocorticoid remediable hypertension Secondary (hyperreninemic) • Renin-secreting tumors • Renovascular hypertension • Compensatory (nephrosis, cirrhosis, CHF) • Bartter syndrome • Gitelman syndrome
Deoxycorticosterone (DOC) excess	DOC-secreting adrenal adenoma 11 Beta-hydroxylase (CYP11B1) deficiency 17-Hydroxylase (CYP17) deficiency
Glucocorticoid excess	Cushing syndrome Cortisol resistance
Increased mineralocorticoid action without circulating mineralocorticoid excess	Apparent mineralocorticoid excess (HSD11B2 deficiency) Acquired HSD11B2 inhibition (glycyrrhizic acid induced) • Liddle syndrome (type 1 pseudohyperaldosteronism) • MR gain-of-function mutation (type 2 pseudohyperaldosteronism)

CHF, Congestive heart failure; *MR*, mineralocorticoid receptor.

For example, a decrease in effective plasma volume or mean arterial pressure from sudden blood loss leads to release of renin from the juxtaglomerular cells of the kidneys; more angiotensin I and angiotensin II are formed, and production of aldosterone by the adrenal glands is increased. Angiotensin II promotes sodium reabsorption in the PCT, increases thirst, and increases release of ADH and catecholamines. Overall, angiotensin II promotes retention of sodium and water, an increase in extracellular volume, hydrogen ion wasting, and a decrease in the serum potassium due to enhanced renal potassium excretion. Secondary hyperaldosteronism is common in patients with congestive heart failure, nephrotic syndrome, cirrhosis of the liver, other hypoproteinemic states, or conditions that chronically deplete plasma volume.

Secondary hyperaldosteronism is characterized by volume depletion, edema, and hypokalemic alkalosis. Whereas hypertension is present in primary hyperaldosteronism, it is usually absent in secondary hyperaldosteronism unless the patient has a reninoma or renal artery stenosis. Plasma renin and aldosterone measurements are seldom needed in secondary hyperaldosteronism because factors that contribute to the patient's hypokalemia and alkalosis (eg, secondary hyperaldosteronism in congestive heart failure) are usually apparent. Renin and aldosterone measurements are invaluable, however, in the investigation of primary disturbances in the renin-angiotensin-aldosterone system, assessment of renal artery stenosis, and in arterial hypertension.

Primary Hyperaldosteronism

Primary hyperaldosteronism, first described by Conn in 1955, is characterized by elevated plasma aldosterone and suppressed renin release, along with hypertension and hypokalemic alkalosis. Historically, it was believed that no more than 1% of hypertensive patients have primary hyperaldosteronism. However, results from a 2007 study identified primary hyperaldosteronism in 10% or more of cases otherwise defined as "essential" hypertension.[193]

Clinical indications for a formal evaluation of hyperaldosteronism (measurement of the aldosterone-to-renin ratio)[268] include hypokalemia that is unprovoked by diuretics and lack of response to conventional antihypertensive treatment.[194]

Overproduction of aldosterone may be due to autonomous and inappropriate secretion of aldosterone by (1) an adenoma of one adrenal gland (aldosterone-producing adrenal adenoma [APA], or Conn syndrome), (2) hyperplasia of aldosterone-producing cells in both glands (bilateral idiopathic adrenal hyperplasia [IAH]), (3) an aldosterone-producing adrenal carcinoma, or (4) a rare familial condition known as *glucocorticoid-suppressible hyperaldosteronism* (familial hyperaldosteronism type 1).[195,196] Familial hyperaldosteronism type 2 is the rare occurrence of familial APA, familial hyperaldosteronism from IAH, or combined familial APA and hyperplasia. Another rare cause of hyperaldosteronism is unilateral adrenocortical zona glomerulosa hyperplasia, which can be micronodular or macronodular. Even more rarely, primary hyperaldosteronism results from ectopic aldosterone secretion from the ovary or kidney.

Clinical features of primary hyperaldosteronism generally are related to the consequences of aldosterone overproduction.

Increased retention of sodium, expansion of extracellular fluid volume, and increased tubular secretion of potassium and hydrogen ions are the cardinal manifestations of primary hyperaldosteronism. Hypokalemic alkalosis results from excessive renal excretion of potassium and hydrogen ions. Sodium retention causes a modest expansion of extracellular fluid volume along with an increase in arterial blood pressure.

Diagnosis and Treatment of Primary Hyperaldosteronism

Hypokalemia is the principal sign that primary hyperaldosteronism may be present in a patient with diastolic hypertension. To confirm the diagnosis, it is necessary to demonstrate hyposecretion of renin, which is not appropriately elevated during volume depletion, and hypersecretion of aldosterone, which is not suppressed appropriately during volume expansion.[197] The At a Glance: An Approach to the Differential Diagnosis of Hypokalemic, Alkalotic Hypertension feature shows a suggested scheme for evaluating patients with suspected excessive mineralocorticoid action causing hypertension.

Most patients with autonomous aldosterone overproduction are hypokalemic, but hypokalemia itself does not predict primary hyperaldosteronism. Because some patients with primary hyperaldosteronism are not hypokalemic, primary hyperaldosteronism as a cause of hypertension may be underrecognized. In hyperaldosteronism, urinary potassium excretion is inappropriately high, and a random urine potassium greater than 30 mmol/L is usually indicative of primary hyperaldosteronism or some form of mineralocorticoid excess. If hypokalemia can be shown to be due to nonrenal potassium loss, the diagnosis of hyperaldosteronism does not need to be explored.

Elevated aldosterone and low renin activity are key diagnostic features in primary hyperaldosteronism.[198,199] Other factors influence the secretion of renin and aldosterone, however, and these factors must be considered before further laboratory evaluation.[200] Drugs such as ACE inhibitors, beta blockers, and spironolactone alter renin release, and patients should be withdrawn from these medications for several weeks before the plasma aldosterone-to-renin ratio is determined. When patients with suspected primary hyperaldosteronism are evaluated, it is helpful to compare ambulatory plasma renin activity (PRA) activity to the patient's urinary sodium excretion or stimulate renin production with a potent diuretic such as furosemide (Box 66.10). Elevated PRA can be due to secondary hyperaldosteronism (eg, renovascular hypertension, pheochromocytoma). Low renin activity, on the other hand, suggests primary hyperaldosteronism or low-renin hypertension. The latter may be caused by exogenous or endogenous mineralocorticoids that mimic the action of aldosterone, producing expanded plasma volume, hypertension, and hypokalemia.

The ACE inhibitor captopril has been used for the diagnosis of primary hyperaldosteronism.[201] In individuals who are normotensive or have essential hypertension, acute inhibition of ACE decreases angiotensin-mediated aldosterone production to less than 15 ng/dL, whereas autonomous aldosterone production from an aldosterone-producing adenoma is unaffected by the ACE inhibitor. Determination of plasma renin responsiveness, however, is not sufficient to diagnose primary aldosteronism because renin activity is suppressed in about 25% of patients with essential hypertension. Recently, losartan (an angiotensin II receptor antagonist drug marketed under the name Cozaar) suppression of aldosterone was found to be superior to captopril suppression in the diagnosis of primary hyperaldosteronism.[202]

Primary hyperaldosteronism is differentiated from other hypermineralocorticoid states based on the inappropriate secretion of aldosterone.[203] An elevated plasma or urine aldosterone in a patient with an unequivocally suppressed renin concentration (a plasma aldosterone-to-renin ratio >25–30) is presumptive evidence of primary hyperaldosteronism,[199,204] although the ratio employed will depend on the assays used and, in particular, mass versus activity assays for renin. The aldosterone-to-renin ratio is a screening test, and the chosen cutoff is designed to maximize sensitivity. Because hypokalemia suppresses aldosterone secretion, the potassium deficit should be resolved before aldosterone measurements are performed. To establish aldosterone autonomy, aldosterone production may be suppressed with rapid volume expansion using the saline suppression test (see Box 66.8)[205] with a potent mineralocorticoid such as fludrocortisone (see Box 66.9)[206] or pharmacologically with captopril. Failure of aldosterone to be suppressed by these maneuvers confirms the diagnosis of primary hyperaldosteronism.

Once the diagnosis of primary hyperaldosteronism is established, it is necessary to distinguish between APA and bilateral IAH. This differentiation is vital because most patients with adrenal adenoma respond favorably to surgical removal of the tumor, whereas those with adrenal hyperplasia are managed medically.[207] Localization using imaging techniques[208]—spiral CT scans,[183,209] ultrasonography, and adrenal scanning with NP-59 (^{125}I-6-iodomethyl-19-norcholesterol)—can be helpful, and adrenal venography with or

BOX 66.10 Protocol for the Furosemide Stimulation Test

Rationale

Plasma renin activity (PRA) varies with hydration status and sodium intake. Furosemide, a potent diuretic, stimulates renin secretion.

Procedure

Furosemide (40 to 80 mg) is given orally after an overnight fast. The subject is maintained in an upright posture (sitting, standing, or walking) throughout the test. Blood is collected for measurement of PRA before and 4 hours after furosemide administration.

Interpretation

Responses must be defined for the assay technique used. Patients with renin-dependent forms of hypertension (eg, renovascular hypertension) respond with renin activity approximately five times normal. Increased PRA following furosemide is seen in patients with high-renin essential hypertension, pheochromocytoma, and Bartter syndrome. Patients with hypertension from mineralocorticoid excess (eg, primary hyperaldosteronism) usually have PRA below the lower limit of detection for the PRA assay.

without selective adrenal venous sampling for aldosterone measurements is used to determine whether the right or left adrenal is hypersecreting aldosterone. This is valuable when tumors are too small to be detected by imaging techniques. However, when CT or MRI findings are equated with a functional APA, mistakes can be made (eg, the visualized mass was an incidentaloma and was not the APA).[210] Therefore it has been argued that venography with aldosterone measurements should always be completed before adrenal surgery for a suspected APA to confirm the laterality suggested by CT or MRI. In addition to aldosterone assessment, when performing venography, it is prudent to measure cortisol in the adrenal veins and inferior vena cava to confirm identification of the vein in case one of the adrenal veins is not appropriately cannulated. The usual ratio of cortisol in the adrenal veins to the inferior vena cava is 10 : 1. Adrenal carcinomas are rare causes of primary hyperaldosteronism.[211]

Numerous biochemical clues help in the differential diagnosis of APA versus bilateral IAH. Aldosterone hypersecretion and plasma renin suppression are usually greater with adrenal adenomas. After sodium depletion, or after 2 to 4 hours of upright posture, patients with APA usually show no change or a paradoxical fall in plasma aldosterone, whereas patients with IAH typically show a rise in plasma aldosterone (presumably because the hyperplastic glands are sensitive to increases in renin, and adenomas are insensitive to renin).[212] Plasma concentrations of 18-hydroxycorticosterone are elevated in most patients with APA, but this test is not considered clinically useful.

Adrenal vein catheterization is considered the gold standard for differentiation of an aldosteronoma versus IAH. To correct for variations in cortisol and aldosterone concentrations induced by the stress of venography, a cosyntropin intravenous infusion of 50 μg/h can be provided during the procedure. When the aldosterone-to-cortisol ratios on both sides are compared, aldosteronomas display a mean side-to-side ratio of 18, whereas the ratio in patients with IAH averages 1.8. The consensus is that side-to-side aldosterone-to-cortisol ratios of 4 or greater are consistent with aldosteronoma, whereas side-to-side ratios of 3 or less are consistent with IAH. Ratios greater than 3 and less than 4 fall into a gray zone, and other techniques must be relied upon to differentiate aldosteronoma and IAH.

A small percentage of patients with hypermineralocorticoidism respond to dexamethasone treatment (eg, rare glucocorticoid-remediable hyperaldosteronism, also called *dexamethasone-suppressible hypertension*) with normalization of their blood pressure and correction of their biochemical abnormalities.[213-215] Dexamethasone treatment should be attempted before surgery, particularly in young patients, or when the normal fall in plasma aldosterone concentration after salt depletion and standing does not occur and no unilateral lesion is seen on CT/MRI. Also, a trial treatment of spironolactone, an aldosterone antagonist, usually normalizes blood pressure in patients who are likely to have a good response to surgery. In glucocorticoid-remediable hyperaldosteronism, concentrations of 18-oxocortisol and 18-hydroxycortisol are increased as a result of the gene fusion between CYP11B1, the 11-beta-hydroxylase (P450c11) of the zona fasciculata/reticularis, and CYP11B2 (aldosterone synthase, P450 aldo).

Adrenocortical carcinomas may produce excess mineralocorticoid and cause hypertension with hypokalemia.[216] Aldosterone or DOC, or both, may be produced in excess.[217-219] Mineralocorticoid concentrations do not respond to glucocorticoid therapy or alterations in salt status. CT scans are helpful; adrenal carcinomas are usually large tumors that weigh more than 30 g, whereas aldosterone-producing adenomas are usually much smaller. Carcinomas are similar to adenomas in that furosemide stimulation or upright posture should not elevate renin or aldosterone concentrations.

Other Causes of Excessive Mineralocorticoid Action

Unusual conditions that suggest aldosterone excess but do not involve disorders of renin, angiotensin II, or aldosterone[220] include apparent mineralocorticoid excess (AME), type 1 pseudohyperaldosteronism (Liddle syndrome), type 2 pseudohyperaldosteronism, and cortisol resistance.[221]

AME results from HSD11B2 deficiency or inhibition.[222] Normally, HSD11B2 protects the MR from cortisol by converting cortisol to cortisone in tissues expressing the MR. Cortisone does not bind to the MR. Impaired conversion of cortisol to cortisone allows cortisol to bind to the MR, producing a hypermineralocorticoid effect in the absence of excess aldosterone or DOC. Therefore HSD11B2 deficiency produces an AME because patients can manifest hypertension, hypokalemia, and alkalosis without elevation of aldosterone nor DOC.

AME is inherited as an autosomal recessive trait and presents in childhood. Spironolactone blocks the MR and is used to treat hypertension. Dexamethasone inhibits ACTH and suppresses cortisol production; however, this treatment does not consistently lower the patient's blood pressure.[223] Glycyrrhetinic acid, a component of black licorice, inhibits HSD11B2, causing an acquired form of AME.[224] AME is diagnosed by an increased ratio of cortisol to cortisone and an increased ratio of urinary THF to urinary tetrahydrocorticosterone.[225]

Liddle syndrome (type 1 pseudohyperaldosteronism) results from gain-of-function mutations in the beta or gamma subunit of the amiloride-sensitive ENaC.[226-228] Consequences include excessive sodium reabsorption, expanded blood volume, hypertension, hypokalemia, and alkalosis. Because ENaC activity is autonomous, both renin and aldosterone are suppressed. This disorder responds to triamterene but not to spironolactone (which blocks the MR). Triamterene is believed to inhibit ENaC through a mechanism similar to the action of amiloride. Type 2 pseudohyperaldosteronism is a gain-of-function mutation in the MR associated with early-onset hypertension, with severe exacerbation in pregnancy. An important gene associated with pseudohyperaldosteronism type 2 is NR3C2 (nuclear receptor subfamily 3, group C, member 2), which encodes the MR.

Loss-of-function mutations in the GR cause cortisol resistance.[229] In response to decreased cortisol action, CRH and ACTH concentrations rise, increasing circulating cortisol to a sufficient concentration so functional cortisol deficiency is not present. However, the protective action of HSD11B2 in converting cortisol to cortisone is overwhelmed, resulting in increased binding of cortisol to the MR and excessive mineralocorticoid effects. Treatment with a MR blocker such as spironolactone or dexamethasone, which suppresses ACTH, is effective.

AT A GLANCE

An Approach to the Differential Diagnosis of Hypokalemic, Alkalotic Hypertension

If the concentration of renin is elevated, diagnostic considerations include a juxtaglomerular renin-secreting tumor (reninoma) and renovascular hypertension (assuming that intrinsic renal disease has been ruled out, which can cause elevated renin and aldosterone, leading to hypertension). If renin is suppressed and aldosterone is elevated (an aldosterone-to-renin ratio >20 to 25), imaging and venography can help differentiate between unilateral disease without a discrete mass (rare unilateral adrenal hyperplasia), unilateral disease with a discrete mass (aldosteronoma), bilateral idiopathic adrenal hyperplasia (IAH), or the rare condition of glucocorticoid-remediable hyperaldosteronism (GRH), with no masses or hyperplasia. If aldosterone is not elevated, 11-deoxycorticosterone (DOC) and cortisol should be measured to discriminate between Cushing syndrome (CS) or cortisol resistance (normal DOC and elevated cortisol), DOComa (DOC-secreting adrenal adenoma) or CYP11B2 (aldosterone synthase) deficiency (increased DOC and normal cortisol), deficiency of CYP17 (17-hydroxylase deficiency; increased DOC and decreased cortisol), and end-organ disorders (normal DOC and cortisol). In familial hyperaldosteronism type 2, aldosterone-producing adrenal adenoma (APA), IAH, or combined disease can occur. Plasma aldosterone greater than 100 ng/dL (277 pmol/L) in the presence of a discrete mass in this algorithm favors an aldosterone-producing adenoma, whereas a lower value in the absence of a discrete mass favors IAH.

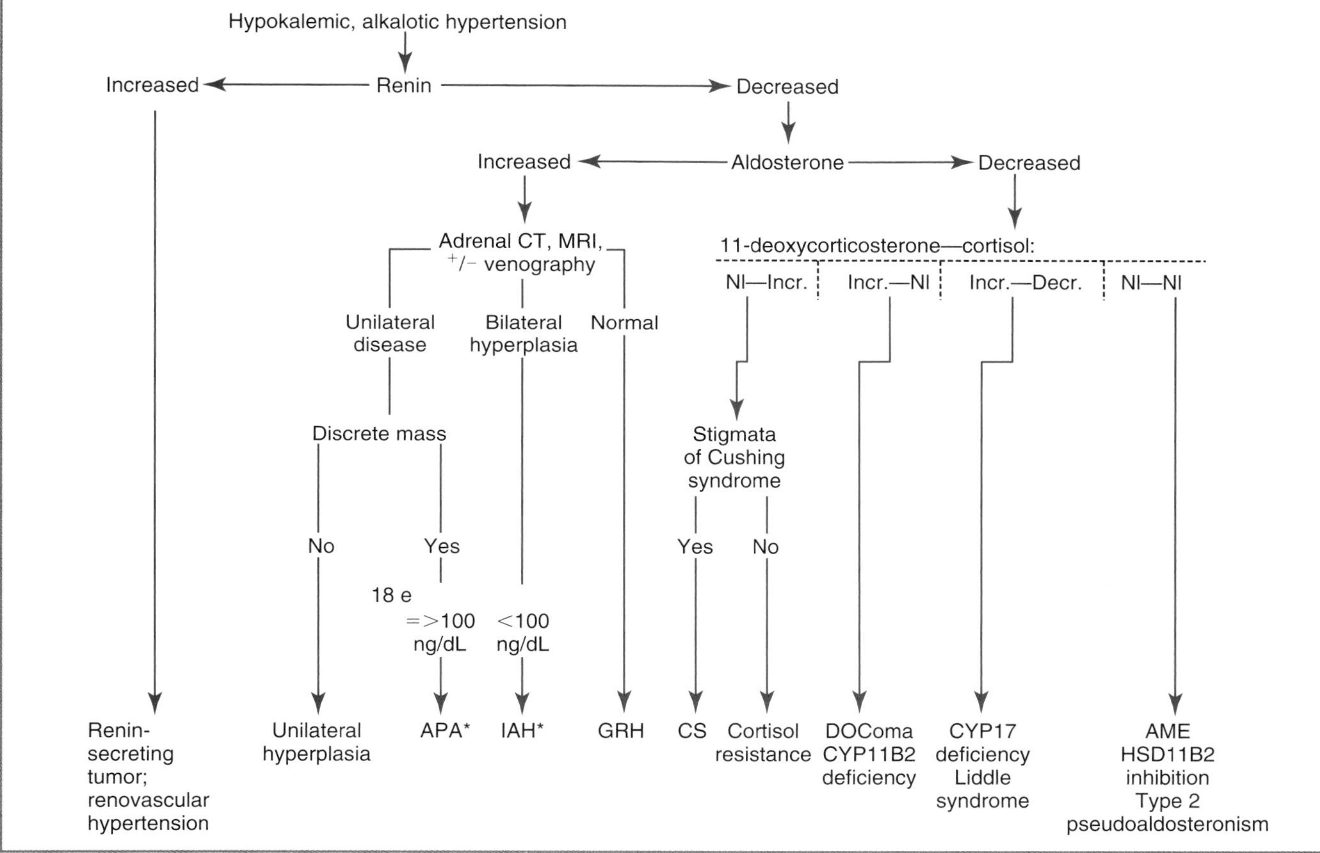

AME, Apparent mineralocorticoid excess; *decr*, decrease; *incr*, increase; *Nl*, normal.

Nonmineralocorticoid-Deficient Causes of Urinary Sodium Loss

Bartter syndrome is a consequence of sodium loss from dysfunction of the ascending, thick loop of Henle or the DCT.[230] Sodium loss evokes a compensatory hyperaldosteronism with increased renin and aldosterone, producing hypokalemia and alkalosis. Bartter syndrome in adults may be asymptomatic, but infants can display failure to thrive, salt craving, polyuria, and polydipsia. Potassium depletion elicits prostaglandin-induced vasodilatation that can exacerbate the compensatory aldosterone release, possibly accounting for the absence of hypertension in Bartter syndrome. A variety of genetic mutations cause urinary sodium loss that leads to secondary hyperaldosteronism with hypokalemia and alkalosis (Table 66.13).

In pseudohypoaldosteronism (PHA; aldosterone resistance), hypoaldosteronism (acidosis, hyperkalemia, possible hypotension) is concurrent with elevated concentrations of aldosterone. PHA may be classified as renal type 1, multiple target organ defects type 1, early childhood hyperkalemia type 1, Spitzer-Weinstein syndrome (adolescent hyperkalemic syndrome), subtype 3 RTA (renal tubular acidosis, IV type 2

TABLE 66.13 **Renal Tubule Disorders Characterized by Loss of Sodium Chloride That Lead to Secondary Hyperaldosteronism***

Subtype	Channel/Transporter	Site of Expression	Gene	Gene Location
Bartter syndrome, classic, 3	Renal chloride channel	ALH	*CLCNKB*	1p36
Bartter syndrome, neonatal, 1	Na^+-K^+-$2Cl^-$ cotransporter	ALH	*NKCC2*	15q15-q21.1
Bartter syndrome, neonatal, 2	Potassium channel (ROMK)	ALH	*KCNJ1*	11q24-q25
Gitelman	Thiazide-sensitive sodium-chloride cotransporter (TSC; a.k.a. NCCT)	DCT	*SLC12A3*	16q13

*Pseudohypoaldosteronism type 1 is not included in this table.
ALH, Ascending loop of Henle; *DCT,* distal convoluted tubule.

PHA), and Gordon syndrome (mineralocorticoid-resistant hyperkalemia, chloride shunt syndrome type 2 PHA).

Renal type 1 PHA results from reduced numbers or function of the renal MR. This occurs as an autosomal dominant or sporadic disorder, and usually the child is asymptomatic by age 2. In multiple-target organ defects type 1 PHA (autosomal recessive), a loss-of-function mutation in ENaC affects the sweat glands, salivary glands, and colon, in addition to the kidney, throughout the patient's life. Early childhood hyperkalemia type 1 PHA is milder than renal type 1 PHA, and its cause is unknown. The child usually outgrows this disorder by age 5.

Whereas renin and aldosterone are elevated in PHA type 1, in PHA type 2, renin and aldosterone are normal or low. Type 2 PHA results from a defect in the distal tubules due to absent WNK1 or WNK4 kinase activity. Gordon syndrome is also most likely due to defects in the WNK kinase activity that increase the activity of the thiazide-sensitive sodium channel cotransporter.[231]

Plasma Renin in Renovascular Hypertension

When used as a screening test, elevated plasma renin after furosemide stimulation, or when correlated with urinary sodium excretion, suggests renal artery stenosis as the cause of hypertension.[232,233] If arteriographic evidence indicates the presence of renal artery stenosis, measurement of plasma renin in specimens obtained from renal vein catheterization is helpful in predicting the response to surgical correction of the renal vascular lesion or nephrectomy.[234] Lateralization of renin in the renal vein to the radiographically involved side, especially after sodium depletion, is predictive of a good response to surgery in 90% of cases (Box 66.11).[235] Comparison of renin activity in the renal artery with that in the renal vein can allow a further distinction.[236]

BOX 66.11 **Protocol for the Differential Renal Vein Renin Test**

Rationale
In renovascular hypertension, plasma renin activity (PRA) is significantly higher in the renal vein on the involved side.

Procedure
The patient should be on a low-sodium, high-potassium diet and receiving a diuretic for 3 days before the procedure. Under fluoroscopic guidance, percutaneous catheterization is performed, and blood samples are obtained from both renal veins and the inferior vena cava for determination of PRA.

Interpretation
Various criteria have been suggested for interpretation. A ratio of PRA (affected side to unaffected side) that is greater than 1.5 suggests functionally significant renovascular disease.

LABORATORY EVALUATION OF ADRENOCORTICAL FUNCTION

Laboratory evaluation of adrenal cortex function centers on measurement of cortisol, the primary corticosteroid; aldosterone, the primary mineralocorticoid; and the sex hormones, of which the adrenal cortex is a secondary source. Chromaffin cells in the adrenal medulla are a source of catecholamines, which are discussed in Chapter 63. Underproduction or overproduction of cortisol and aldosterone produces characteristic clinical syndromes, and genetic defects in steroid hormone biosynthesis produce abnormalities in sex hormone concentrations that are associated with clinical symptoms as well. Therefore measurement of steroid hormones produced in the adrenal cortex is essential to the clinical diagnosis of a variety of endocrine disorders.

Steroid hormones such as those produced in the adrenal cortex share considerable structural similarity based on their terpenoid sterane core, which is modified by functional groups at various locations on the tetracyclic backbone. In general, steroids are lipophilic compounds, but they require additional modification—esterification to fatty acids—to facilitate their transport across cellular membranes. Transport in the bloodstream typically involves carrier proteins (eg, transcortin, SHBG). These properties influence the choice of analytical methods for measuring steroid hormone concentrations; most procedures begin with enzymatic or chemical hydrolysis of steroid esters and displacement of the steroid from carrier proteins through addition of a protein-binding agent such as 8-anilino-1-naphthalene-sulfonic acid (ANS) or salicylate. Photometric and fluorometric measurements of steroids lack specificity unless extraction and purification procedures are used. Immunoassays are practical for the measurement of steroid hormones and are widely available on a variety of automated chemistry platforms, but cross-reactivity with structurally similar hormones often results in bias between various immunochemical methods. Endogenous interferences also occur, for example, near the time of birth, when placental steroid concentrations are very high. Steroids can be extracted into organic solvents and analyzed by chromatographic methods coupled with mass spectrometric detection, which provides sensitive and specific quantitative results for these compounds. In contrast to peptide hormones, most of which exhibit considerable heterogeneity as the result of posttranslational modifications, steroid hormones constitute a relatively homogenous group of compounds that are calibrated against gravimetrically validated synthetic calibrators.

Episodic secretion and circadian variation limit the diagnostic accuracy of basal serum cortisol concentrations.[237] Serum cortisol concentrations are highest in the early-morning hours and vary between 7 and 25 μg/dL (193 and 690 nmol/L) between 04:00 and 12:00 hours. Late afternoon concentrations are about half the morning concentrations and frequently are less than 5 μg/dL (138 nmol/L) between 22:00 and 02:00 hours. A midnight cortisol less than 5 μg/dL (138 nmol/L) is considered normal. Serum cortisol combined with plasma ACTH improves the diagnostic accuracy of basal values, although ACTH concentrations display even greater variation throughout the day than cortisol concentrations.

Choice of Specimen

Steroid hormones have been measured in urine, blood, saliva, and, recently, hair.[238] The choice of specimen depends on the application. For clinical assessment of adrenal function, blood (plasma) measurements are convenient, but conditions that cause the binding protein concentration to increase can produce clinically irrelevant elevations in the total cortisol concentration. Urinary concentrations are helpful in determining time-integrated hormone production and provide useful estimates of free hormone concentrations in blood if an appropriately timed urine specimen collection is available. Measurement of steroid hormones in saliva has been proposed as an alternative to urinary hormone assays to estimate free hormone concentrations in blood, the principal advantage being ease of collection. Hair analysis, while not widely used, may be useful for assessing adrenal hormone production over an extended time.[239]

Urine

Urinary concentrations of a hormone, or its metabolites, provide an approximation of the amount secreted over the time the urine is collected, typically 24 hours. Thus urinary hormone or metabolite measurements are useful when the hormone has a very short biological half-life and/or its secretion is pulsatile or varies in predictable cycles. Timed urine collections suffer variability associated with factors such as completeness of collection and impaired renal function. Urinary metabolites may reflect only a fraction of the active steroid hormones; these metabolites, in turn, may be affected by metabolic disease, as well as diet and medications. Despite these limitations, UFC and measurement of urinary free estradiol, estrone, and testosterone are most useful for estimating the rates at which these steroids are produced and are not affected by variations in the concentrations of proteins that bind hormones, such as CBG and albumin.

UFC obtained from a 24-hour urine collection, an integrated measure of plasma free cortisol, eliminates the circadian influence on cortisol secretion.[240] With increases in total cortisol and stable concentrations of CBG, the serum free cortisol fraction rises substantially and is cleared into the urine. UFC measurements therefore are considered a superior screening test for cortisol excess. In Cushing syndrome, UFC is two to three times the upper limit of the reference interval. The UFC excretion rate in normal subjects is less than 50 μg/d (138 nmol/d) when assayed by high-performance liquid chromatography (HPLC).

Blood

Circulating concentrations of steroids in the blood provide the most direct measure of endocrine activity mediated by these hormones. Immunoassays and chromatographic methods have been developed for measuring most of the clinically relevant steroids in blood; mass spectrometric methods for steroid profiling have recently been reviewed.[241,242] Provocative testing (stimulation and suppression tests, discussed earlier) may require blood samples because of the rapid changes that occur in hormone activity after stimulus or suppression. Many steroid hormones are released in a pulsatile or rhythmic fashion, so their concentrations in isolated blood specimens should take into account these variables.

Mineralocorticoid and adrenal androgen secretion is circadian and episodic in nature, but the dynamic swings in concentration are not as pronounced as with cortisol. It is usually recommended, however, that blood samples for adrenal steroids should be collected in the 07:00 to 10:00–hour time frame for consistency in interpreting the results.

Steroid hormone concentrations in serum and plasma are nearly the same. It has been suggested that steroid hormone concentrations may change in unseparated blood specimens as the result of 17β-hydroxysteroid dehydrogenase activity in red blood cells and macrophages, but stability studies of estradiol, cortisol, testosterone, progesterone, 17α- hydroxyprogesterone, androstenedione, and DHEA-S have failed to reveal clinically significant changes in these hormones in whole blood specimens stored at room temperature for up to 1 week.[243,244]

Saliva

Most steroids of clinical interest have been measured in saliva, and for some steroids, such as cortisol, estriol, testosterone, and progesterone, salivary concentrations appear to correlate with the free hormone concentration in plasma.[245,246] For other steroids (eg, 17α-hydroxyprogesterone, estradiol, aldosterone), the clinical usefulness of salivary measurements has not been established.

Measurement of steroids in saliva is attractive because specimens are simple to collect; this consideration is particularly important in pediatric patients. Several saliva collection devices using absorbent materials have been designed to collect a sufficient volume of saliva for steroid analysis. However, recovery of cortisol from these devices has been questioned. Using cotton swabs, cotton ropes, and hydrocellulose microsponges, Harmon and colleagues demonstrated that recovery of both the volume of saliva specimen and the cortisol concentration were variable, relative to a directly collected ("passive drool") saliva specimen.[247] For further details of saliva collection, please refer to Chapter 43.

Hair

Hair grows at an average rate of 1 cm per month; therefore it can reveal historical blood concentrations of substances that are deposited in the forming hair matrix. Hair has been used as an alternative to urine specimens for the detection of illicit drug use because a number of drugs are detectable in urine for only a few days following exposure.[248] Several reports describe methods for measuring steroid hormones in hair.[238,249-251] These methods have shown potential as diagnostic tools but will require additional validation studies before they can be applied generally.

Basal Peptide and Steroid Hormone Concentrations

Concentrations of adrenal mineralocorticoids and elements of the renin-angiotensin system are routinely measured in body fluids by various immunoassay and mass spectrometric methods.[252,253] As with cortisol, aldosterone is secreted episodically, with the highest circulating concentrations near the time of awakening and the lowest concentrations shortly after sleep onset. Aldosterone concentrations, however, are only modestly stimulated by ACTH secretion. In healthy subjects, consuming a low-sodium diet, maintaining an upright posture, and using diuretics all increase plasma aldosterone concentrations, whereas consuming a high-sodium diet and lying in the supine position decrease aldosterone secretion. Standardized procedures for obtaining blood and urine specimens are required for proper interpretation of test results. It is useful to interpret aldosterone concentrations together with urinary sodium excretion because salt intake can profoundly influence the aldosterone concentration. Normally, the aldosterone concentration is inversely proportional to the urinary sodium concentration.

Because it has enzymatic activity, renin can be measured either by its activity or its mass, and both methods are available; a MALDI-TOF method for measuring renin activity was recently described.[254] PRA is measured by its stimulation of angiotensin I release, which is measured using immunoassay techniques.[255]

Renin release is controlled by many physiologic factors. Consuming low-sodium diets, maintaining an upright posture, and using diuretic medications increase renin release (causing a rise in aldosterone) and should be controlled or eliminated before testing of the renin-angiotensin-aldosterone axis is begun. Because plasma renin varies with sodium balance, it is helpful to interpret ambulatory renin measurements together with urinary sodium excretion. An inverse relationship exists (similar to aldosterone), allowing the identification of low-, normal-, and high-plasma renin groups from a nomogram.[256]

Age, estrogen therapy, and diabetes mellitus without renal failure affect plasma renin results.[161] Patients older than 55 years and those with diabetes have PRA results that are about 50% of normal. Estrogen causes an increase in hepatic synthesis of angiotensinogen, thereby increasing the endogenous substrate concentration for the renin enzyme. This causes inappropriately elevated renin activity for the urinary sodium concentration. Several medications may affect plasma renin activities. ACE inhibitors and spironolactone raise renin concentrations, whereas beta blockers and nonsteroidal antiinflammatory agents block renin release.

Even when time of sampling, posture, drug intake, and diet are controlled, it is often difficult to identify disorders of mineralocorticoid secretion on the basis of basal hormone concentrations alone.[257] A variety of dynamic tests have been developed to assess hypersecretion or hyposecretion of aldosterone and renin.

The diagnosis of adrenal insufficiency in critically ill patients is controversial.[258-262] On one hand, if the diagnosis of cortisol and/or aldosterone deficiency is missed and replacement therapy is not initiated, the patient can die from Addisonian crisis, as might occur in Waterhouse-Friderichsen syndrome (bilateral adrenal hemorrhage). However, inappropriate administration of cortisol in a septic patient can produce immunosuppression that may be fatal. Some investigators believe that free cortisol measurements are diagnostically helpful because CBG concentrations frequently decline from liver disease or acute malnutrition, which could lead to misdiagnosis of cortisol deficiency. In equivocal cases of adrenal insufficiency, some authors caution that a single low cortisol concentration should not be used to make the diagnosis of cortisol deficiency.[262] Just as free testosterone can be estimated from total testosterone and SHBG concentrations, a free cortisol index has been described as the simple ratio of total cortisol to CBG.[263]

Free Versus Bound Steroids

Many hormones circulate in the blood bound to carrier proteins. Hormone-binding proteins serve two functions: They solubilize lipophilic compounds such as steroid hormones to facilitate their transport in the primarily aqueous circulatory environment, and they buffer the concentration of free, active hormone in tissue. Protein-bound hormones are inactive, but the protein-bound reservoir provides a relatively constant, buffered concentration of the free hormone for activity at tissue receptors. However, for hormones that are highly protein bound, the concentration of the binding protein is the principal determinant of the total concentration of hormone. Therefore total hormone concentrations vary significantly, while the free, active hormone concentration remains within physiologically appropriate limits. Measurement of free (unbound) hormone concentrations provides the best indicator of hormone activity, but analytical methods that isolate free hormone concentrations without disrupting the free/bound equilibrium are difficult to design. Antibodies that recognize steroid hormones may have binding affinities that compete with binding proteins and detect significant portions of the bound fraction. Preanalytical methods to separate bound and free fractions often disrupt the physiologic equilibrium between bound and free hormone. Urinary and salivary steroid hormone measurements have been widely used to estimate free hormone concentrations.

Analytical Methods

In contrast to peptide hormones, which may exhibit considerable structural heterogeneity, steroids present less of a challenge in the design of specific analytical methods because these compounds, for the most part, are homogeneous. Sensitive immunometric methods for measuring steroid hormones have been available for decades, and methodological approaches include most, if not all, of the common labels (radioisotope, enzyme, fluorescent, chemiluminescent) and immunoassay designs (heterogeneous, homogeneous, competitive, noncompetitive). A participant survey from a 2009 College of American Pathologists proficiency challenge revealed that, among participating clinical laboratories reporting cortisol results, a vast majority use heterogeneous chemiluminescent or electrochemiluminescent immunoassays. However, analytical methods involving liquid chromatography coupled with tandem mass spectrometry are becoming more common.[264-267]

Measurement of Cortisol

Approximately 90% of circulating cortisol is bound to plasma proteins, primarily to CBG. Cortisol also binds weakly to albumin. The concentration of CBG in the plasma rises in hyperestrogenic states, including pregnancy and oral contraceptive use; therefore total cortisol in serum is increased in these conditions, although free cortisol remains normal. Analytical methods involving extraction or protein precipitation estimate the free and protein-bound cortisol in the circulation, but immunoassays for direct measurement of cortisol have mostly replaced extraction/chromatographic methods for routine cortisol determinations. Methods for measuring cortisol in clinical laboratories have been reviewed.[268,269]

Chromatographic Methods. Gas chromatography (GC),[270,271] thin-layer chromatography (TLC),[272] and HPLC[39,273-276] have been used to measure cortisol. GC and HPLC coupled to mass spectrophotometric detectors (GC/MS, LC/MS, and LC/MS-MS) provide the most specific methods for measuring corticosteroids.[277,278] Cortisol methods based on capillary electrophoresis are also available.[279,280] All of these methods demonstrate high specificity for cortisol but have relatively low throughput and require sample preparation steps before analysis. For example, most HPLC methods require preanalytical extraction of cortisol with solid-phase extraction columns[281] or liquid-liquid extraction[282] prior to separation and detection by reversed- or normal-phase HPLC and a fluorescence or ultraviolet absorption detector.[283] A reference method for serum cortisol using isotope dilution GC/MS has been proposed.[270] GC/MS methods for cortisol typically require extraction of the hormone from plasma and conversion to the methoxime-trimethylsilyl derivative prior to analysis. Deuterated cortisol is available for use as the internal standard.

Although GC/MS has long been considered the reference method for measuring organic compounds, liquid chromatography-tandem mass spectrometry (LC/MS-MS) methods are becoming increasingly common. Liquid chromatography has the advantage of not requiring volatile derivatives, so specimen preparation can be vastly simplified. LC/MS-MS methods have been developed to measure cortisol,[284,285] cortisol and corticosterone,[286] and other corticosteroids.[287-290] LC/MS-MS appears poised to become the method of choice for corticosteroid profiling due to its greater analytical specificity.[267,291,292] However, use of more specific methods may require revising reference limits and decision thresholds for some of these analytes (for further discussion, the reader is referred to the "ACTH Stimulation Test" section earlier).

Immunoassay. In routine laboratory practice, automated immunoassays are the most common methods used for measuring cortisol in serum and urine, and they are widely available on various automated immunoassay platforms. Most cortisol immunoassays in routine use are heterogeneous, competitive-binding assays that do not require extraction of steroids prior to analysis. Cortisol is displaced from CBG and other endogenous binding proteins by protein-binding agents such as ANS or salicylate, low pH, or heat treatment. The efficiency of cortisol displacement from proteins by agents such as ANS may be influenced by the concentration of binding proteins in the specimen. For example, the amount of ANS that is adequate for plasma obtained from healthy men and nonpregnant women may be insufficient to displace cortisol from CBG in pregnancy when CBG concentrations are elevated.

Although economical and widely used, immunoassays designed to measure steroid hormones are limited by cross-reactivity among the many structurally similar compounds in this class.[293] Analytical methods based on chromatography and mass spectrometry have greater specificity for individual steroids, but they are more complex and require expensive instrumentation and skilled technicians. The relative advantages and disadvantages of immunoassays versus chromatography/mass spectrometric methods for measuring steroid hormones were recently reviewed,[291] with the conclusion that mass spectrometric methods, despite their superior analytical performance, are not yet poised to displace immunoassay as the principal method for measuring steroid hormones but will likely surpass immunoassay at some point in the future.

Nonisotopic Immunoassay Methods. Most contemporary automated cortisol immunoassays use nonisotopic labels. Enzyme labels used in these immunoassays include horseradish peroxidase, alkaline phosphatase, or β-galactosidase, and enzyme activity has been measured using photometric,[294-296] fluorescent,[297] or chemiluminescent substrates.[298] Nonenzymatic approaches typically involve fluorescent and chemiluminescent[299] labels, and these are the most common methods currently in use.[300] Both heterogeneous and homogeneous designs have been developed. Most current heterogeneous immunoassays for cortisol involve chemiluminescent labels and magnetic separation. Homogeneous immunoassays for cortisol include the enzyme-multiplied immunoassay technique[299] and the cloned enzyme donor immunoassay.[301] These assays do not require separation of bound and free fractions. Most immunoassay methods for cortisol are available on fully automated immunochemistry platforms.[300]

Other Methods. A highly sensitive method for measuring salivary cortisol using a biosensor based on nanolinking and surface plasmon resonance detection has been described.[33] This method had a detection limit of 49 pg/mL (135 pmol/L) in human saliva, and the technology eventually may give rise to point-of-care instruments that measure salivary cortisol.

Specimen Collection and Storage. Cortisol can be measured in serum, heparinized plasma, or ethylenediaminetetraacetic acid (EDTA) plasma, although some methods recommend against using EDTA plasma because of assay interference. In serum or plasma specimens, cortisol is stable for 7 days at room temperature or refrigerated and is stable for 3 months frozen at −20°C.[244]

Comments. Blood cortisol concentrations parallel ACTH concentrations, with episodic and diurnal minima and maxima observed throughout the day. The cortisol concentration in the evening is normally less than 50% of the morning cortisol concentration. Increased cortisol is associated with stress, glucocorticoid therapy, pregnancy, depression, hypoglycemia, and hyperthyroidism. No significant difference in cortisol concentrations has been observed between men and women, and reference intervals for cortisol are not age dependent. The half-life of cortisol in the circulation is approximately 60 minutes,[244] so concentrations of this hormone in blood can change rapidly. In newborns, a transient rise in cortisol occurs immediately after delivery, but after 12 to 48 hours, cortisol declines to concentrations below umbilical cord blood concentrations; it then increases to a stable reference interval by about 1 week of age. Renal failure does not directly affect serum cortisol, but metabolites that are not cleared in the urine have the potential to cross-react with immunoassays, causing overestimation of blood cortisol concentrations. Extraction of cortisol into an organic solvent may eliminate interference from hydrophilic metabolites. Celite chromatography has been used to "clear" the sample of possible interference before immunoassay measurements are carried out in patients with renal failure.

Measurement of Free Cortisol

Free or unbound cortisol is the biologically active form of the circulating hormone; its concentration is buffered by the large reservoir bound to its transport proteins: CBG and albumin. Various methods have been developed to measure the free fraction of cortisol in serum, including ultrafiltration, equilibrium dialysis, and gel filtration, but these assays are technically demanding and expensive, and they are not in general use.[269] Algorithms have been suggested for estimating the free cortisol concentration on the basis of CBG and albumin concentrations.[302-305] Calculation of the free cortisol "index" based on the CBG concentration may be helpful in interpreting cortisol results.[305]

Measurement of urinary cortisol provides an estimate of the free hormone concentration and for many years has been considered the gold standard screening test for Cushing disease,[124] although salivary cortisol has been recommended as the first-line diagnostic test.[144] Approximately 2% of total cortisol is excreted into the urine, and urinary cortisol may be used as a screening test for cortisol hypersecretion. However, β-hydroxycortisol also appears in the urine and may interfere with some immunoassays used to measure cortisol in urine.[306]

Measurement salivary cortisol (or oral fluid) is a practical and convenient way to assess the free hormone.[307,308] Salivary cortisol reflects the concentration of free cortisol in blood because CBG and albumin, the primary cortisol-binding proteins, do not appear in saliva. Most immunoassay kits for total serum cortisol can be used for the measurement of cortisol in saliva;[309] extraction is not required because saliva contains virtually no cortisol-binding proteins or other cortisol metabolites. The glycoproteins in saliva can be precipitated by freezing and thawing, followed by centrifugation, producing a clear fluid that is free of protein interference. At this point, the challenge in measuring salivary cortisol involves achieving an adequate lower limit of detection because the concentration of cortisol in saliva is less than in serum or plasma.

Unextracted urine may be assayed for cortisol if the antibody has sufficient selectivity, although reference values may differ from those seen in methods that include an extraction step.[310] Even with solvent extraction, most commercial assays for cortisol in urine are subject to interference and imprecision. Chromatographic procedures (such as HPLC) are more specific than immunoassays for measuring urinary cortisol; LC/MS-MS is emerging as the preferred method.[285-287]

Specimen Collection and Storage. A 24-hour urine specimen for cortisol measurement should be collected with 10 g of boric acid to maintain the urine pH below 7.5, and the urine should be refrigerated. After the total volume is measured, a thoroughly mixed aliquot may be stored at −20°C prior to analysis. Care should be taken to ensure an appropriately timed, complete 24-hour collection because an incorrectly timed sample is the largest source of error with this method. Cortisol measurements on randomly collected urines are not useful. A 2009 report described falsely elevated urinary cortisol results attributed to interference from carbamazepine.[311] The drug interfered with the liquid chromatography method used for measuring urinary cortisol. CYP3A4 induction by carbamazepine may also affect the results of the low-dose dexamethasone suppression test through enhanced metabolism of dexamethasone.

Cortisol is stable in saliva for 1 week at 4°C and for 4 months when stored frozen. Freezing of specimens is recommended because it leads to precipitation of salivary glycoproteins and produces a nonviscous liquid supernatant that makes volumetric transfer by pipette more reliable.[310]

Measurement of urinary creatinine sometimes is used to assess the completeness of the collection or to adjust concentrations of urinary constituents in spot urine collections for changes in urine specific gravity related to water intake. Diurnal variations in cortisol production, however, place greater importance on the integrity of the 24-hour urine specimen, in that daily cortisol excretion correlates with the functional adrenal status of the patient. Salivary cortisol measurements serve as a practical and convenient method to assess cortisol secretion in many patients. Morning salivary cortisol concentration is decreased in adrenal insufficiency; evening values are increased in Cushing syndrome.

Measurement of Aldosterone

Measurement of aldosterone is technically challenging because the concentration of this hormone in blood is very low, nearly one-thousandth that of the cortisol concentration. Immunoassays for measuring aldosterone in blood and urine are available.

The cross-reactivity of aldosterone antibodies with other adrenal steroids (eg, DOC, corticosterone) is relatively low (<0.01%). Nevertheless, the concentration of potentially cross-reacting steroids sometimes is very high, requiring some purification of aldosterone before measurement. Unconjugated plasma aldosterone will extract into an organic solvent and can be isolated by chromatography. The addition of tritiated aldosterone as an internal standard corrects for incomplete extraction in radioimmunoassay methods for aldosterone. In urine, unconjugated steroids first are extracted into an organic solvent such as ethyl acetate or methylene chloride after acid hydrolysis of the conjugates. The solvent is evaporated, and the dried extract is reconstituted in a buffer before analysis. Whether the specimen requires purification depends on the diagnostic kit being used and the type of patient being evaluated. For example, specificity is not a significant concern in hypertensive adults without adrenal disease, whereas greater specificity may be needed for newborns and young infants, patients with adrenal disease, and pregnant women, in whom high concentrations of potentially interfering steroids are likely.

An automated heterogeneous immunoassay for aldosterone involving a monoclonal aldosterone antibody and a chemiluminescent tracer has been validated against three RIA methods.[312] This method displays minimal

(<0.05) cross-reactivity with corticosterone, cortisol, DOC, 18-hydroxycorticosterone, and dexamethasone, and a linear range of 15 to 1200 ng/L. A time-resolved fluorescence immunoassay for measuring aldosterone in saliva was described in 2010.[313] LC/MS-MS has also been applied to aldosterone measurements;[314] these results were in close agreement with RIA measurements. The LC/MS-MS method has a detection limit of 2.5 ng/dL (0.069 nmol/L) and a linearity up to 198 ng/dL (5.5 nmol/L).

Specimen Collection and Storage. If possible, the patient should be in an upright position (standing or seated) for at least 2 hours before collection. Plasma (heparin or EDTA) or serum is suitable for aldosterone measurement, although EDTA plasma is preferred. The aldosterone concentration in specimens stored at room temperature begins to decline after 24 hours, although the aldosterone concentration in unseparated blood specimens stored at 32°C for 24 hours is relatively unchanged. The aldosterone concentration in refrigerated or frozen specimens is stable for at least 4 days. For urine assays, a 24-hour urine specimen should be collected with boric acid as a preservative.[244,315]

Measurement of 17-Hydroxyprogesterone

The most common cause of CAH is a deficiency in the 21α-hydroxylase enzyme (CYP21). Measurement of serum or plasma 17-OHP can be used to diagnose almost all cases of CAH. In 21α-hydroxylase deficiency, 17-OHP concentrations may reach several hundred times the upper limit of normal.

Radioimmunoassays for 17-OHP that use antibodies against 17-hydroxyprogesterone-3-carboxymethyloxime-BSA are available; these methods can be used with serum, plasma, saliva, and amniotic fluid. Monoclonal antibody–based methods have also been described.[316] In addition to radioiodinated tracers,[162,317,318] nonisotopic labels used in 17-OHP immunoassays include enzymes with photometric, fluorescent, or chemiluminescent substrates,[316,319-321] and fluorescence-based immunoassays using fluorescein or streptavidin-europium labels,[322] and chemiluminescent labels.[323] Despite the use of highly specific antisera, most immunoassays are susceptible to interference by other corticosteroids that may be present in neonatal and infant plasma specimens.[324,325]

Methods for measuring 17-OHP in serum by GC/MS[326] and LC/MS-MS[264,266,327-329] have been described. For chromatographic analysis, 17-OHP is typically extracted using a liquid-liquid (diethylether/diethylacetate,[329] methyl-tert-butyl-ether[330]), solid-phase,[327] or online[288,328] extraction procedure; these methods have detection limits below 1 nmol/L. LC/MS-MS methods for measuring 17-OHP in dried blood spots obtained from neonates[331,332] and in urine[287] are also available.

Specimen Collection and Storage. Most reports of analytical methods for measuring 17-OHP use serum, although plasma has also been used. Specimens have been stored at 4°C for up to 4 days or at −20°C for up to 1 month. 17-OHP was stable in unseparated blood at room temperature for 1 week.[243]

Screening newborns for 21α-hydroxylase deficiency has been possible since the introduction of 17-OHP immunoassays in 1977.[333] Neonatal specimens can be obtained by heel puncture and collected in capillary tubes or on filter paper. Dried blood specimens are stable and easily transported and are widely used to screen newborns for metabolic defects. It has been reported that the presence of EDTA in dried blood specimens may interfere with 17-OHP results measured by immunometric methods based on lanthanide fluorescence.[334] The utility of salivary 17-OHP measurements has been reviewed,[335] and the principal advantage is ease of collection.[336]

Measurement of 11-Deoxycortisol

Serum or plasma 11-deoxycortisol (compound S) measurements are used to detect 11β-hydroxylase (or C-11 hydroxylase) deficiency or as part of the metyrapone stimulation test. Metyrapone inhibits the 11β-hydroxylase enzyme, and a 40- to 80-fold increase in plasma 11-deoxycortisol is observed after metyrapone stimulation in patients with normal pituitary-adrenal reserve. As a consequence, analytical methods for 11-deoxycortisol in metyrapone stimulation tests do not require particularly high sensitivity.

Nonisotopic methods for measuring 11-deoxycortisol in serum have been described, including enzyme immunoassays,[337,338] fluorometric methods,[339,340] and fluorescence polarization.[341] One method[342] for measurement of 11-deoxycortisol involves the "open-sandwich enzyme immunoassay" technique, which is based on the reassociation of two cloned antibody variable regions by a bridging antigen.

Liquid chromatography/tandem mass spectrometry methods for measuring 11-deoxycortisol have been described, mostly as part of corticosteroid profiles.[287-290,330] These methods typically involve liquid-liquid extraction into an organic solvent, although solid-phase extraction has been used as well.[264,287]

Specimen Collection and Storage. Most of the methods used for measuring 11-deoxycortisol have used serum, although plasma and urine are also used. Data in the literature on the stability of 11-deoxycortisol in stored specimens are lacking.

Measurement of Renin

Methods for measuring renin have been the subject of two reviews,[343,344] upon which most of this discussion is based.

Circulating concentrations of prorenin may be as many as 100-fold greater than the concentration of renin (although a 10:1 ratio of prorenin to renin is more common); therefore even minimal cross-reactivity of prorenin with renin antibodies used in immunoassays to measure renin can be problematic. Assays exist to measure PRA (by monitoring the production of angiotensin I) or the mass of renin by immunoassay. Each approach has advantages and disadvantages.

Measuring Renin Activity. Measuring renin activity (traditionally called PRA) provides an indication of the biologically active fraction of renin in the specimen because it measures the primary function of the enzyme, which is the conversion of angiotensinogen to angiotensin I. Renin activity measurements, however, are difficult to standardize, and two general approaches are used to measure renin activity. In the classic PRA method, first described in 1975,[345] inhibitors of angiotensinase and ACE are added to prevent the conversion of angiotensin I to angiotensin II (some methods "trap" angiotensin I with an antibody to prevent its conversion to angiotensin II), the specimen is incubated at 37°C, and production of angiotensin I is measured. The rate of the reaction is influenced by pH, incubation time, and, most important, the endogenous angiotensinogen concentration in the specimen (which can be increased in pregnancy, glucocorticoid excess, and estrogen administration). Because the angiotensinogen concentration in blood does not ordinarily exceed the K_m for the renin-angiotensinogen complex, its concentration is rate limiting. Therefore the classic PRA method produces results that vary significantly, depending on the endogenous concentration of angiotensinogen. An ELISA method has been described to measure angiotensinogen.[346] PRA procedures are also susceptible to variability associated with storage conditions.[347]

Although several variations of the classic PRA method exist, a typical approach involves the preparation of two aliquots of plasma. One of the aliquots is incubated at 37°C for 3 hours, and the other is kept at 4°C (renin is not active at cold temperature). Following the incubation period, angiotensin I is measured by RIA in both aliquots, and the difference between the two reflects the renin activity, expressed as pg of angiotensin I per mL of plasma. The specificity of the PRA assay can be validated using plasma from anephric patients or deangiotensinized plasma.[348]

A second approach to measuring renin activity uses exogenous angiotensinogen as substrate and thereby avoids the variability associated with endogenous angiotensinogen concentrations. This approach is sometimes called *plasma renin concentration assay*,[343,344] which is a confusing term in that the assay still involves the measurement of activity, rather than concentration. Furthermore, the term is not consistently applied; *plasma renin concentration* has been used in reference to immunoassays that measure the renin concentration, rather than activity.[347,349]

These renin activity methods use angiotensinogen derived from plasma collected from nephrectomized sheep; it is added at a concentration that is several times the K_m for the renin-angiotensinogen complex, ensuring that the reaction rate is limited by renin activity alone. The advantage of using a consistent source of angiotensinogen is that the activity assays can be calibrated against renin reference materials; an International Reference Preparation of human renin (68 out of 356), validated by bioassay, has been available since 1975.[350]

Prorenin exists in two forms, depending on whether the 46 amino acid "pro" segment is in an "open" or "closed" conformation. The open conformation of prorenin has the active site of the enzyme exposed, so this form is enzymatically active. In the blood, approximately 2% of prorenin is in the open conformation, but assay conditions such as cooling and low pH can cause the closed conformation of prorenin to open, which results in an overestimate of physiologic renin activity. Incubation of plasma at 22°C for 24 hours reversibly activates (unfolds) approximately 5% of prorenin,[351] although incubation at 37°C promotes refolding of the "pro" segment to its closed form.[352] In some assays, the closed prorenin is deliberately opened by acidification (pH 3.3) or incubation with trypsin, which removes the "pro" segment from prorenin altogether. These assays measure total renin and prorenin by activating all of the prorenin and following with a standard renin activity assay.[353]

Care must be taken when measuring and interpreting renin activity in patients who are taking renin inhibitors, a relatively new class of drugs used to treat essential hypertension. Aliskiren was the first member of this class of drugs to be approved by the US Food and Drug Administration. Renin activity will be suppressed in these patients, although renin and prorenin concentrations will be high.[343,344]

Measuring Angiotensin I and II. All renin activity assays rely on angiotensin I as a direct measure of renin activity and a surrogate marker for angiotensin II, which is the active form of the hormone. Angiotensin II has a very short half-life (1 to 2 minutes) and is difficult to measure.[354] Monoclonal antibodies with high affinity and specificity have been produced against angiotensin II, and these have been used to develop a direct radioimmunoassay; as little as 0.8 fmol of angiotensin II in 2 mL of plasma has been detected without interference from angiotensin I.[355] When angiotensinogen and ACE are in sufficient supply, however, the concentration of the prohormone angiotensin I is a reliable estimate of renin activity and angiotensin II concentration in blood.[343] Most angiotensin I methods involve radioimmunoassay, but enzyme immunoassays,[356,357] HPLC,[358] and fluorescence polarization methods[359] have also been described. A 2009 report described a homogeneous immunoassay for angiotensin I that is based on luminescent oxygen channeling, a technology involving chemiluminescence stimulated by photoexcited singlet oxygen.[360]

Angiotensin I and angiotensin II have poor immunogenicity because of their small molecular size. They must be conjugated to proteins such as albumin, hemocyanin, or succinylated polylysine to be sufficiently immunogenic to elicit antibodies. Polyclonal antisera usually lack sufficient specificity to distinguish between the decapeptide, heptapeptide, and hexapeptide angiotensins. Problems associated with immunoassay of angiotensins have been reviewed.[353] Angiotensins are labile oligopeptides in plasma and can be generated in vitro, even in frozen plasma. Therefore great care must be taken in the collection and storage of specimens for angiotensin assays.[361]

With continued improvement and availability of nonisotopic immunometric assays for direct measurement of the concentration of renin, activity assays may soon be replaced by direct mass assays for routine assessment of plasma renin. However, because physicians are so familiar with PRA testing results, renin mass assays will require realignment of physician practices.

Measuring Renin Concentration. As an alternative to the PRA assay, the concentration of renin can be measured by immunoassay or mass spectrometry. Immunoassays for renin cross-react with prorenin in both closed and open conformations; assays based on monoclonal antibodies are likely to have the highest specificity for renin. A variety of monoclonal immunoradiometric assays (IRMAs) for renin have been developed, some of which measure renin and prorenin in the open configuration, and others that measure all forms of renin and prorenin.[343] An example of a two-site IRMA was described by Simon and colleagues.[362] This assay uses two monoclonal antibodies, and the specificity of the assay was verified by immunoprecipitation of prorenin with a monoclonal antibody directed to the "pro" sequence. Immunochemiluminometric (ICL) methods for renin are also available, and the results of these assays have been correlated with IRMA results. One such assay[363] involves a biotinylated capture antibody (which recognizes both renin and prorenin)

POINTS TO REMEMBER

- The adrenal gland is the exclusive source of cortisol and aldosterone, and it is a minor source of sex hormones.
- Cortisol is synthesized and released by the adrenal gland in response to adrenocorticotropic hormone (ACTH) secreted by the anterior pituitary gland, which in turn is stimulated by corticotropin-releasing hormone (CRH) secreted by the hypothalamus.
- Aldosterone is synthesized and released by the adrenal gland in response to several factors, including angiotensin II and III, ACTH, and increased plasma potassium concentration.
- Overproduction of cortisol results in various symptoms collectively termed *Cushing syndrome*.
- Adrenal insufficiency can precipitate a life-threatening condition known as Addisonian crisis, due to inadequate secretion of cortisol and aldosterone.
- Cushing syndrome is most often caused by corticosteroid therapy, but it also may be caused by cortisol-, ACTH-, or CRH-secreting tumors.
- Chronic adrenal insufficiency (Addison disease) can be caused by autoimmune, infectious, and metastatic diseases.
- Provocative tests are often required to determine whether adrenal disease is primary (dysfunction of the adrenal gland) or secondary (dysregulation of adrenocortical stimulating hormones).

immobilized to streptavidin-coated magnetic particles, and an acridinium ester–labeled signal antibody that recognizes only renin.[364] The chemiluminescent assay had a limit of detection of less than 0.1 mU/L and a functional sensitivity (CV <20%) of 2.6 mU/L.

Direct renin immunoassays (both IRMA and ICL) have been compared with renin activity assays.[365] With direct renin results expressed in mIU/L and PRA results expressed in ng • mL^{-1} • h^{-1}, the overall correlation coefficient was 0.98, and the standard error of the residuals was 11.8 mU/L. Better interlaboratory agreement with direct renin assay results compared with PRA has been reported.[366]

The aldosterone-to-renin ratio (ARR), based on aldosterone concentration and PRA, was proposed[367] in 1981 as a sensitive screening test for primary hyperaldosteronism in normokalemic patients. The screening thresholds for ARR have been reestablished using measurements of renin concentration, rather than activity.[368]

Specimen Collection and Storage. EDTA plasma is typically used for PRA assays. After centrifugation, plasma should be removed and frozen at −20°C or lower, although the renin concentration is stable in unseparated blood at room temperature for up to 6 hours. Plasma for PRA can be stored frozen up to 1 month before assay, but freeze-thaw cycles should be avoided because of the possible activation of prorenin. At the time of collection, blood should not be chilled or placed on ice because irreversible cryoactivation of prorenin can occur, leading to falsely high estimates of PRA. Serum or plasma collected in another anticoagulant can also be used as long as EDTA is added (3 mmol/L) before incubation because it inhibits ACE. Cryoactivation of prorenin, however, is more likely in serum than in plasma. Hemolyzed specimens should not be used because red blood cells contain angiotensinases.

The patient should be ambulatory for 2 hours before blood collection. A 24-hour urine specimen for sodium is often collected on the day before the renin test to reference the result to salt intake. Specimens with high renin activity can generate considerable amounts of angiotensin I before and during storage, even at −20°C. This will not affect results, however, because angiotensin I is determined with and without the incubation step.

SELECTED REFERENCES

For a full list of references for this chapter, please refer to ExpertConsult.com.

1. Kempna P, Fluck CE. Adrenal gland development and defects. *Best Pract Res Clin Endocrinol Metab* 2008;**22**:77–93.
9. De BK, Haegeman G. Minireview: latest perspectives on antiinflammatory actions of glucocorticoids. *Mol Endocrinol* 2009;**23**:281–91.
20. Papadimitriou A, Priftis KN. Regulation of the hypothalamic-pituitary-adrenal axis. *Neuroimmunomodulation* 2009;**16**:265–71.
29. Ghayee HK, Auchus RJ. Basic concepts and recent developments in human steroid hormone biosynthesis. *Rev Endocr Metab Disord* 2007;**8**:289–300.
30. Miller WL. Steroidogenic enzymes. *Endocr Dev* 2008;**13**: 1–18.
44. Tomlinson JW, Stewart PM. Cortisol metabolism and the role of 11beta-hydroxysteroid dehydrogenase. *Best Pract Res Clin Endocrinol Metab* 2001;**15**:61–78.
45. Nieman LK. Dynamic evaluation of adrenal hypofunction. *J Endocrinol Invest* 2003;**26**:74–82.
82. Vaughan ED Jr. Diseases of the adrenal gland. *Med Clin North Am* 2004;**88**:443–66.
90. Husebye E, Lovas K. Pathogenesis of primary adrenal insufficiency. *Best Pract Res Clin Endocrinol Metab* 2009;**23**: 147–57.
111. Winter WE, Harris NS. Laboratory approaches to diseases of the adrenal cortex and adrenal medulla. In: Winter WE, Sokoll L, Jialal I, editors. *Diagnostic endocrinology*. Washington, DC: AACC Press; 2008. p. 75–138.
125. Schuff KG. Issues in the diagnosis of Cushing's syndrome for the primary care physician. *Prim Care* 2003;**30**:791–9.
141. Nieman LK. Cushing's syndrome: update on signs, symptoms and biochemical screening. *Eur J Endocrinol* 2015;**173**: M33–8.
144. Nieman LK, Biller BM, Findling JW, et al. The diagnosis of Cushing's syndrome: an Endocrine Society Clinical Practice Guideline. *J Clin Endocrinol Metab* 2008;**93**:1526–40.
157. Antal Z, Zhou P. Congenital adrenal hyperplasia: diagnosis, evaluation, and management. *Pediatr Rev* 2009;**30**:e49–57.

67

Thyroid Disorders

Danielle B. Freedman, David Halsall, William J. Marshall, and Christina Ellervik

ABSTRACT

Background

The ability to accurately diagnose thyroid disease using a blood test is arguably one of the greatest triumphs of modern clinical chemistry. Thyroid function tests are now among the most widely requested laboratory investigations. This is because of the relatively high incidence of thyroid disease, the symptoms of the disease often being nonspecific, and effective treatment options for the most common forms of thyroid disease being readily available. However, despite the success of diagnostic and therapeutic interventions, both clinical chemists and clinicians need to be aware of the limitations of these strategies.

Content

This chapter describes the physiology of the normal and abnormal thyroid and the role of the thyroid hormones. This includes the importance of iodine in the correct functioning of the thyroid gland and the effect of common medications and nonthyroidal illness on thyroid function. Laboratory methods for thyroid function tests are critically reviewed. The clinical presentation of thyroid disease is described along with treatment options; this chapter includes sections on thyroid disease in pregnancy, subclinical thyroid disease, and the genetic basis of inherited thyroid diseases.

HISTORICAL LANDMARKS

A total of 179,870 publications on the entry word "thyroid" are registered in PubMed (at the end of 2015), with the first registered from 1842. Up until 1945, the annual number of publications ranged from 1 to 35. After World War II, the number of publications has steadily increased every year, now being approximately 6500 per year. In Box 67.1, historical landmarks are listed in chronological order.

ANATOMY

The thyroid consists of two lobes connected by an isthmus and is similar to a butterfly in shape with the right lobe being slightly larger than the left.[38] It is located in the front of the neck just above the trachea. The gland synthesizes thyroid hormones and calcitonin through two distinct cell types: the epithelial or follicular cells and the parafollicular (or C) cells, respectively.[39] The gland's name derives from its topographic relationship to the laryngeal thyroid cartilage, whose shape resembles a Greek shield or *thureos*.[38] The normal adult thyroid gland weighs 15 to 25 g, but in specific disease states, it can attain a weight of several hundred grams.[38] The thyroid gland receives its blood supply from the carotid arteries, branches of the common carotid artery, and subclavian arteries; blood supply increases in hyperthyroidism.[38]

The thyroid gland is composed of follicles or acini (Fig. 67.1). The height of the follicular cells reflects their biochemical activity (ie, the greater the height, the more thyroid hormone synthetic activity is occurring). In the center of the follicle is the lacuna, which contains colloid composed predominantly of thyroglobulin (Tg). The parafollicular (or C) cells are usually located below the basement membrane but not adjacent to the lacuna of the follicle. Parafollicular cells are very difficult to identify without immunohistochemical staining for calcitonin.

THYROID MORPHOGENESIS AND DYSMORPHOGENESIS

Embryologically, the thyroid gland is formed by fusion of three anlagen that develop from the anterior foregut.[39] During the fourth week of gestation, the foramen cecum develops as an endodermal thickening in the floor of the primitive pharynx at the junction between the first and second pharyngeal pouches, the base of the prospective tongue.[38,39] The medial thyroid primordium derives as a ventral diverticulum at the foramen cecum. The primitive thyroid tissue detaches and descends to a pretracheal position (fourth to seventh weeks).[38] The primitive thyroid tissue differentiates into a hormone-producing gland (the thyroid hormone producing follicular cells) by the end of the third month and is able to concentrate radioiodine and synthesize iodothyronines.[38,40] During its descent, the thyroid is remodeled into a bilobed organ.[39] A pair of lateral primordia from the caudal-most pharyngeal pouch integrates with the rest of the gland and differentiates into calcitonin-producing C-cells.[38,39] It is currently believed that these cells arise from neural crest cells.[38,39] The thyroglossal duct retracts, forms a solid fibrous stalk, and ultimately atrophies; the distal portion of this duct may give rise to a pyramidal lobe in some individuals.[38]

The understanding of this complex morphogenesis has mainly come from animal models,[39] but in the genetic era, understanding of the genetic basis of thyroid dysgenesis has further elucidated stages of normal human thyroid

BOX 67.1 Historical Landmarks in Chronological Order

Circa 3600 bc, early Chinese medical writings described decreases in goiter size upon ingestion of seaweed and burnt sea sponge.[1]

Early 13th century, endemic cretinism was noted in alpine Europe.[2]

16th century, Paracelsus, physician and alchemist, was the first to mention coexistence of endemic goiter and cretinism in the Duchy of Salzburg.[1-3]

1786, Caleb Hillier Parry, a practitioner at Bath, England, was the first person to describe the features of hyperthyroidism (later known as Graves disease).[1,4]

1811, a French chemist, Bernard Courtois, described the chemical properties of an unknown substance, later known as iodine.[5] Joseph Louis Gay-Lussac, Andre Ampere, and Sir Humphry Davy continued his work but with some controversy on whom to credit for the discovery.[6]

1813, Gay-Lussac published the first paper presenting the new element iodine, termed after the Greek word *ioeides*, meaning violet colored.[6]

1819, Jean-Francois Coindet, a physician in Switzerland, published his observations that administration of iodine decreased goiter size.[1,7]

1833, the French chemist Boussingault was the first to hypothesize that salt fortification with iodine would prevent goiter.[8,9]

1835, Robert James Graves (Ireland), published a description of exophthalmic goiter.[10]

1840, Adolph von Basedow (Germany), described toxic goiter.[1,2,11]

1851, 10 iodine pharmaceutical companies showed iodine compounds publicly for the first time at an exhibition in London.[6]

1852, Adolphe Chatin, a French chemist, published the hypothesis that population iodine deficiency was associated with endemic goiter.[9,12]

1880, Ludwig Rehn (Germany) performed the first thyroidectomy on a patient with Graves disease.[13]

1888, on the basis of the work by Gull,[14] Ord,[15] Kocher,[16,17] and Reverdin,[18] the Clinical Society of London linked cretinism, myxedema, and the "cretinism-like" state after thyroidectomy to the same disease, later known as hypothyroidism.[19] Furthermore, they also described delusions and hallucinations linked to the disease.

1891, treatment for hypothyroidism with sheep thyroid extract was first described by Murray.[20]

1896, Eugen Baumann reported the discovery of iodine within the thyroid gland.[21]

1909, Theodor Kocher was awarded the Nobel Prize in Physiology and Medicine for his work on the physiology, pathology, and surgery of the thyroid gland.[17]

1912, Hakaru Hashimoto, a Japanese medical doctor, first described Hashimoto thyroiditis.[22]

1915, Kendall described the crystallization of a compound, which he called thyroxin.[23]

1922, iodine fortification of table salt began in Switzerland.[9]

1927, Harington and Barger described the synthesis of thyroxin.[24]

1938 Hertz, Evans, and Roberts made the short-lived labeled I^{128} for the first use of uptake of a labeled substance in animals.[25,26]

1939 Hamilton and Soley described two other labeled radioiodines, I^{130} and I^{131}, with longer half-lives, to study iodine physiology in humans.[27]

1943, Astwood described thiouracil to treat hyperthyroidism.[28]

1949, Asher revisited the psychiatric symptoms in myxedema and introduced the terminology "myxedema madness."[29]

1952, Carbimazole was introduced.[28]

1952, Triiodothyronine was discovered by Gross and Pitt-Rivers.[30]

1956, Roitt and colleagues reported the presence of circulating thyroid autoantibodies in Hashimoto thyroiditis.[31]

1963, Condliffe purified thyrotropin (thyroid-stimulating hormone).[32] Later the same year, Condliffe together with Odell and Utiger reported the first immunoassay for human thyrotropin.[33]

1970, Braverman, Ingbar, and Sterling described that endogenous triiodothyronine was generated from thyroxine.[34]

1971, Mayberry[35,36] and Hershman[37] independently described use of thyrotropin immunoassays for diagnosis of hypothyroidism.

1980, The World Health Organization published for the first time the global estimate on the prevalence of iodine deficiency or goiter to affect 20% to 60% of the world's population, mostly in developing countries.[9]

Courtesy Christina Ellervik.

morphogenesis.[39] The molecular bases for many of the morphogenetic stages are still uncovered. Understanding how the thyroid reaches a position far from its origin will likely provide further detail on thyroid ectopia.[39]

Thyroid dysgenesis is a collective designation for thyroid agenesis (or athyreosis, ie, the complete lack of thyroid tissue), hypoplasia, hemiagenesis (lacking one lobe), and thyroid ectopia (complete or coexisting with normal positioned tissue, ie, the aberrant location of thyroid tissue along its embryological descent).[38,39,41] The developmental defects have considerable phenotypic variations.[39] Ectopic tissue may coexist with a normally positioned gland.[38] It is important to localize ectopic thyroid tissue before thyroidectomy.[38]

THYROID HORMONES IN FETAL GROWTH

Fetuses are dependent on thyroid hormones for normal growth and organ development,[40] especially brain development and maturation.[42]

Fetal thyroid hormone availability is dependent on placental permeability to maternal thyroid hormones in the first half of gestation and the bioavailability of the fetus' own production during the second half of gestation.[40] Availability and concentrations of the thyroid hormones depend on development of the fetal hypothalamic–pituitary–thyroid (HPT) axis, the thyroid hormone transporters, the deiodinases, gestational age, nutrition, and other intrauterine

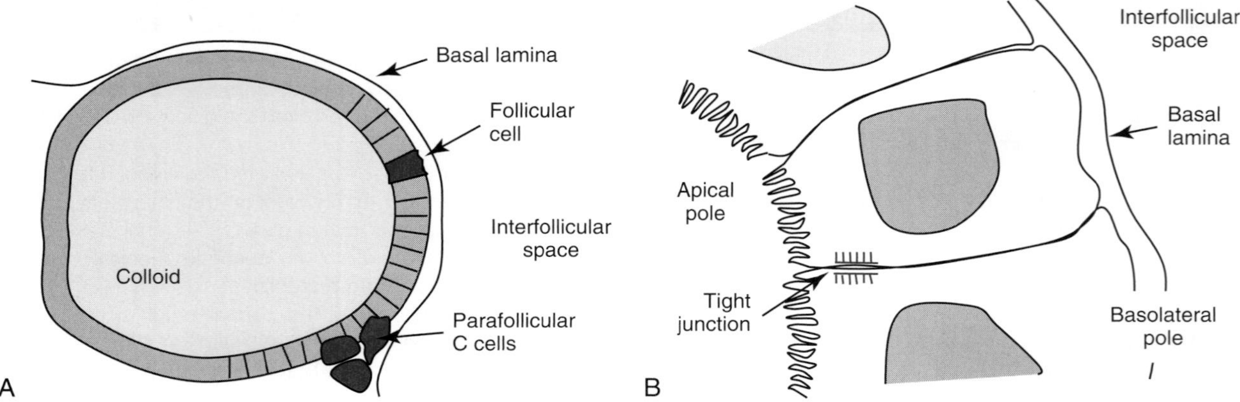

FIGURE 67.1 A, Basic unit of the thyroid gland. The follicle is the basic unit of the thyroid gland. It is composed of thyroid follicular cells surrounding the colloid. Outside the follicular cells is a basal lamina. **B,** Apical and basolateral poles of the follicular cells and tight junctions between the follicular cells. Parafollicular (C cells) that secrete calcitonin can be found beneath or outside the basal lamina. Not pictured between the follicles are capillaries and fibroblasts.

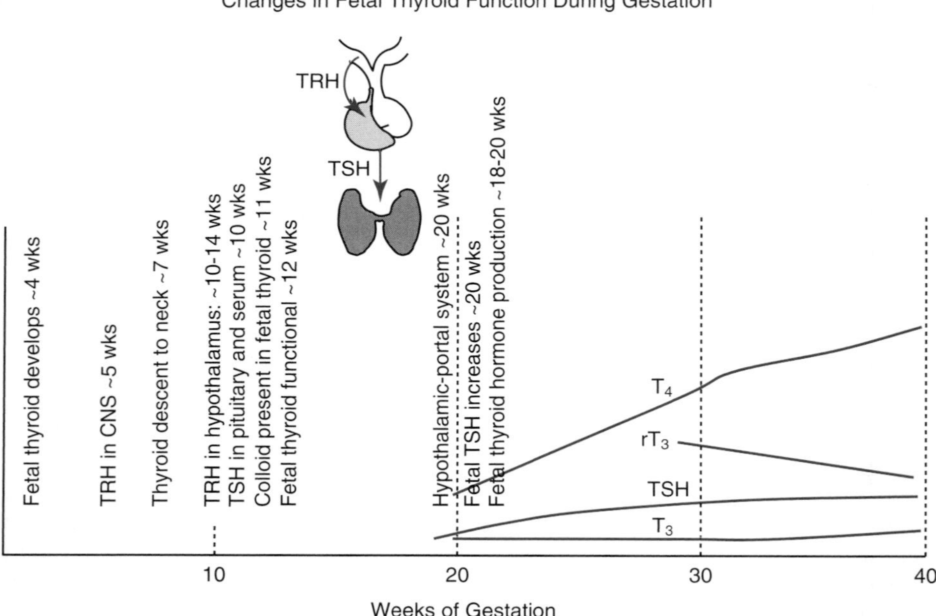

FIGURE 67.2 Changes in fetal thyroid function during gestation. During the first half of gestation, the fetus is dependent on transplacental passage of thyroid hormone. After midgestation, the fetus produces its own thyroid hormone.

endocrine conditions.[40] Maturation of the HPT axis occurs by the middle of the second trimester, enabling the fetus to become responsible for its own production of thyroid hormones by 20 weeks gestation[40]; the axis becomes fully mature and functional around the time of birth. In fetal as well as in adult life, hypothalamic thyrotropin-releasing hormone (TRH) stimulates thyrotropin (thyroid-stimulating hormone [TSH]), which in turn stimulates thyroid hormone synthesis, and the thyroid hormones control their production by negative feedback on the hypothalamus and pituitary.[40] The synthesis of thyroid hormones is dependent on active iodine transport across the placenta.[40] By 10 weeks of gestation, fetal thyroid follicles and thyroxine synthesis are demonstrable (Fig. 67.2). Thyroxine-binding globulin (TBG) and thyroxine (T_4) are first detectable in fetal serum at 8 to 10 weeks of gestation and increase thereafter until they plateau at 35 to 37 weeks.[40] Deiodinases (see later) are responsible for the in utero conversion of T_4 to the bioactive triiodothyronine (T_3) or the relatively bioinactive reverse T_3 (rT3).[40] During most of the fetal life, T_4 is primarily metabolized to rT_3, and clearance of T_3 is high because of the relative concentrations of different deiodinases in fetus and placenta.[40] Toward term, these ratios change, resulting in a rise in fetal plasma T_3, which is important for a range of maturational effects before birth such as pulmonary gas exchange, thermogenesis, hepatic gluconeogenesis, and cardiac adaptions.[40]

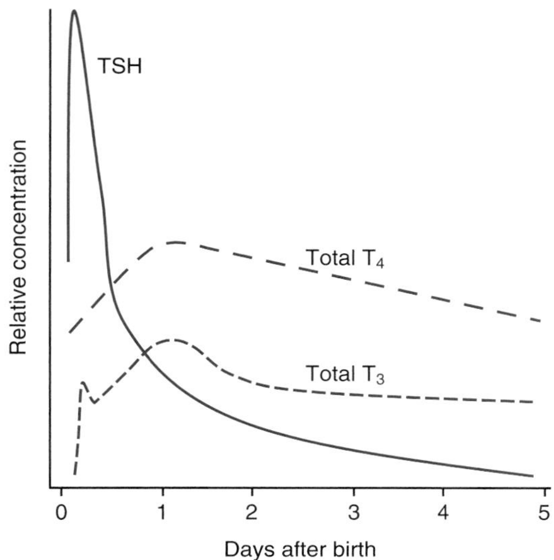

FIGURE 67.3 Concentrations of thyroid hormones for 5 days after birth. After birth, an immediate thyroid-stimulating hormone (TSH) surge peaks at about 30 minutes. Triiodothyronine (T_3) and thyroxine (T_4) rise rapidly, peaking at about 24 hours after delivery. The greater initial rise in T_3 compared with T_4 in the first 24 hours of life likely represents acutely increased conversion of T_4 to T_3. After their peak concentrations, T_4 and T_3 decline to stable concentrations.

Within hours of birth, plasma TSH, T_4, and T_3 concentrations rise rapidly[43] (Fig. 67.3). It is believed that cold stress is responsible for the massive TSH surge. By 2 to 3 days, TSH concentrations fall. Total T_4 falls to adult concentrations by 1 to 2 months of age.[44] The postbirth rise in T_3 results from increased thyroid gland release in response to the rising TSH concentration and also increased conversion of T_4 to T_3 because of the maturation of type I deiodinase enzyme.

BIOCHEMISTRY AND PHYSIOLOGY

Introduction

The major thyroid hormone secreted by the thyroid is T_4 (Table 67.1 shows a list of abbreviations used in the chapter). T_3 is largely produced by peripheral deiodination of T_4, but a small amount of T_3 is also directly secreted by the thyroid.[45] Thyroxine is derived from the amino acid tyrosine and, almost uniquely in physiologically relevant biomolecules, iodine. Two tyrosine molecules are first iodinated then coupled to form the iodothyronine moiety. The nomenclature of iodothyronines is based on the position of iodine on the four possible iodination sites at the meta position on the two tyrosine-derived phenyl rings (Fig. 67.4). The 3 and 5 positions are on the inner or α ring and the 3′ and 5′ positions on the outer or β ring. T_3 is 3,5,3-triiodothyronine; T_4 is tetraiodothyronine. Because T_3 has a higher affinity for the thyroid hormone receptor, it has classically been considered to be the active hormone, with T_4 being a prohormone; however, recent evidence suggests that T_4 may function directly as a hormone as well.[46]

Total T_4 and T_3 are present in plasma at nanomolar concentrations (~100 and 2 nmol/L [7.8 μg/dL and 120 ng/dL], respectively). They are extensively protein bound in

T_4 Tetraiodo-thyronine (Thyroxine) T_3 3,5,3′ Triiodo-thyronine rT_3 3,3′,5′ Triiodo-thyronine

FIGURE 67.4 Chemical structures of iodine-containing thyroid hormones.

TABLE 67.1 Nomenclature and Abbreviations for Thyroid Tests

Name	Abbreviation
Hormones	
Total thyroxine	T_4
Total triiodothyronine (3,5,3′-triiodothyronine)	T_3
Free thyroxine	fT_4
Free triiodothyronine	fT_3
Thyrotropin (thyroid-stimulating hormone)	TSH
Reverse T3 (3,3′,5′-triiodothyronine)	rT_3
Serum-Binding Proteins	
Thyroxine-binding globulin	TBG
Transthyretin (thyroxine-binding prealbumin)	TTR
Albumin	Alb
Tests for Autoimmune Thyroid Disease	
Autoimmune thyroid disease	AITD
Thyroglobulin autoantibodies	Anti-Tg
Thyroperoxidase autoantibodies	Anti-TPO
TSH receptor autoantibodies	Anti-TSHR
Anti-TSHR binding assay	TRAb
TSHR blocking antibodies	Anti-TSHRB
TSHR stimulating antibodies	Anti-TSHRS
Other Hormones, Thyroid-Related Proteins, and Conditions	
Thyroid peroxidase	TPO
Thyrotropin-releasing hormone	TRH
Thyroglobulin	Tg
Thyroid hormone receptor	THR
Deiodinase 1,2,3	D1, D2, D3
Iodotyrosine dehalogenase 1	DEHAL
Sodium/iodide symporter	NIS
TSH receptor	TSHR
Dual oxidase 1 and 2	DUOX1 and DUOX2
Thyroid hormone receptor-α	THRα
Thyroid hormone receptor-β	THRβ

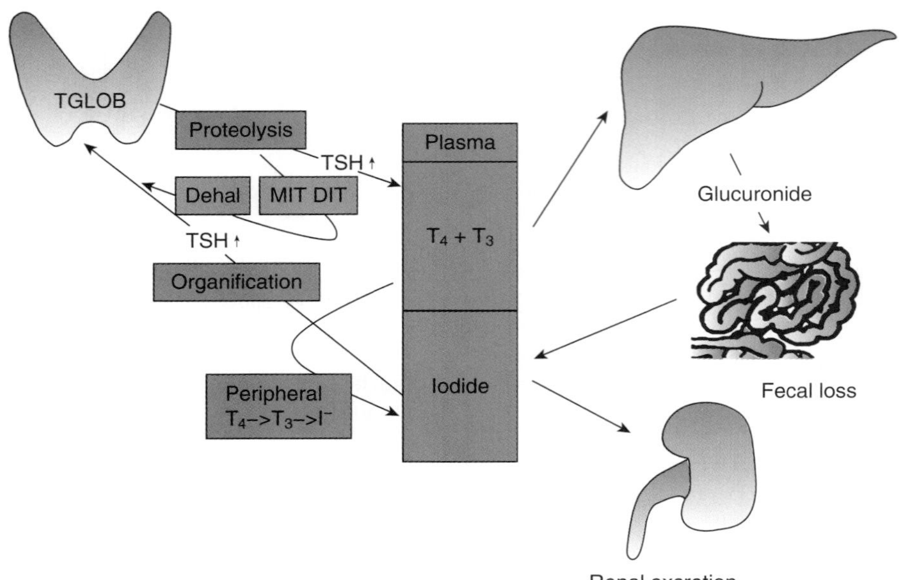

FIGURE 67.5 Synthesis and metabolism of thyroid hormones. Dietary iodine is trapped by the thyroid as iodotyrosine moieties on thyroglobulin (TGLOB) by a process known as organification. Proteolysis releases triiodothyronine (T_3) and thyroxine (T_4) into the plasma, and other iodine derivatives are recycled via dehalogenase. T_4 is metabolized to T_3 in the liver and other tissues by deiodinases. The liver also generates glucuronides that are excreted into the gut and form part of an enterohepatic cycle. Excess iodine is excreted by the kidney. *TSH,* Thyroid stimulating hormone. (Courtesy David Halsall.)

plasma such that the free hormone concentrations are in the picomolar range (~15 and 5 pmol/L [1 ng/dL and 0.3 ng/dL], respectively). As unbound thyroid hormones are transported into cells, the concentration of free hormones better reflects hormone activity.[47] The major plasma thyroid-hormone binding proteins are TBG, transthyretin (TTR), and albumin.[48]

Thyroid hormones are imported into the cell via several relatively recently described carrier proteins. In the cell, T_4 can be further activated to T_3 by iodothyronine deiodinase action, and this can then bind to one of the two nuclear hormone receptors (THRα and THRβ) to exert its physiological function.[49]

Activation and inactivation of T_4 and T_3 are carried out by three iodothyronine deiodinases, which have different tissue distributions and physiological roles.[50-52] Alternate pathways are also involved (see later).[53] Excess iodine produced as a byproduct of thyroid hormone synthesis is effectively scavenged by the thyroidal enzyme iodotyrosine deiodinase 1 (DEHAL)[54] (Fig. 67.5).

The pituitary glycoprotein hormone TSH is the major regulator of thyroid activity, acting through a classic endocrine feedback loop (Fig. 67.6).[55,56] However the action of the deiodinase enzymes on thyroid hormone at the tissue level provides a second regulatory mechanism for hormone action, independent of the concentration of circulating thyroid hormone.[50-52]

Thyroid Hormone Synthesis and Secretion

The adult human thyroid secretes on average 94 to 110 μg of T_4 and 10 to 22 μg of T_3 daily.[57] The major regulator of this process is TSH, which regulates the production of several enzymes in the synthetic pathway.[55,56] The first step

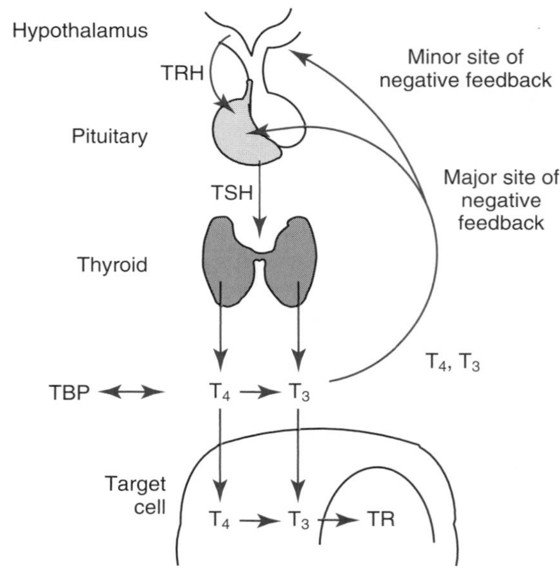

FIGURE 67.6 Metabolic control of thyroid hormones. Thyrotropin-releasing hormone (TRH) from the hypothalamus enters the hypothalamic–pituitary portal system to release thyroid-stimulating hormone (TSH; thyrotropin) from anterior pituitary thyrotrophs. TSH stimulates the release of triiodothyronine (T_3) and thyroxine (T_4) from the thyroid gland, although most T_3 comes from peripheral monodeiodination of T_4 to T_3. More than 99% of T_4 and T_3 is bound to various thyroid hormone–binding proteins (TBP). T_4 and T_3 negatively feedback on the hypothalamus and, more powerfully, the pituitary. T_4 and T_3 enter target tissues, where T_4 is converted to T_3 with T_3 and then binds to the thyroid hormone receptor (TR).

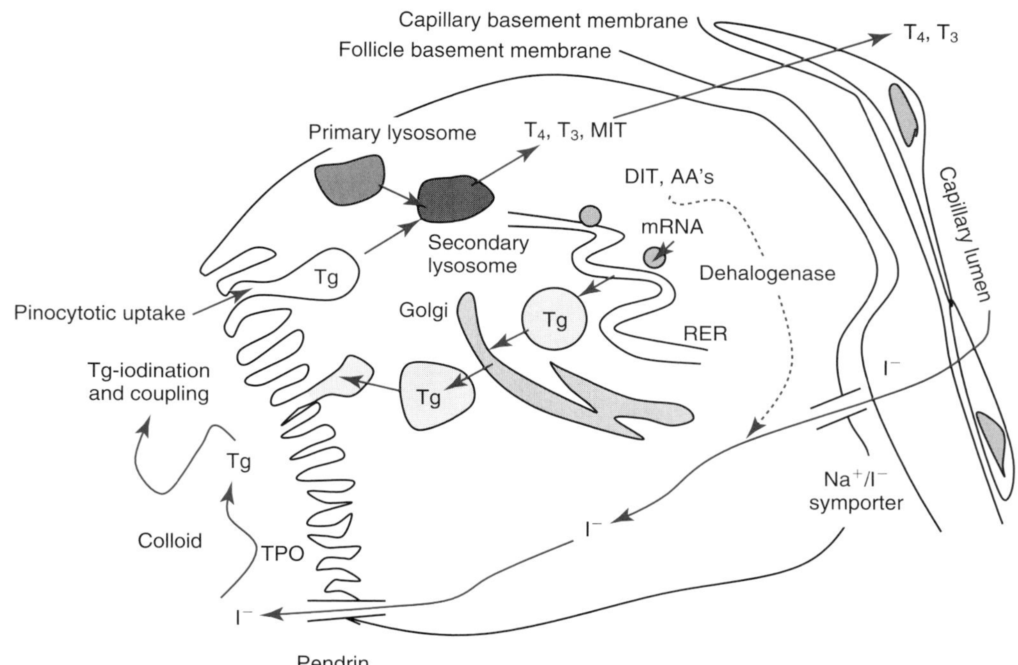

FIGURE 67.7 Synthesis of thyroid hormones begins with absorption of iodine by the thyroid follicular cell and the Na^+/I^- symporter (NIS). From the cytoplasm, iodide moves into the lacunae via pendrin. Within the lacunae, thyroperoxidase (TPO) and the dual oxidases DUOX (not depicted) convert iodide to iodine, leading to iodination of tyrosine residues on thyroglobulin (Tg). Tg is synthesized in the cell and exported to the lacunae. TPO is responsible for the coupling of monoiodotyrosine (MIT) and di-iodotyrosine (DIT) to form triiodothyronine (T_3) and di-iodotyrosine and di-iodotyrosine to form thyroxine (T_4). Upon uptake of iodinated Tg (containing T_4 and T_3) and fusion of this phagosome-like vesicle with a primary lysosome, Tg is degraded in a secondary lysosome, releasing T_4 and T_3 into the circulation, and MIT and DIT undergo deiodination via a dehalogenase to recycle the iodine for new thyroid hormone synthesis.

in thyroid hormone synthesis is the sequestration of iodide into the thyroid gland (Fig. 67.7). Iodine is relatively scarce in unsupplemented diets, and lack of dietary iodine is the major cause of hypothyroidism worldwide.[58] Consequently, a highly efficient system for the sequestration of iodide to the thyroid has evolved. The first step in this process is the active transport of iodide into the thyroid follicular cell against an approximate 30-fold concentration gradient. This is performed by the sodium-iodide (Na^+/I^-) symporter, NIS, which uses the sodium gradient generated by the Na^+/K^+-ATPase.[59] NIS is encoded by the *SLC5A5* gene, a member of the SLC5 solute carrier family. NIS is a 618-amino-acid membrane glycoprotein with 12 predicted transmembrane segments, which resides in the basolateral surface of the thyroid follicular cell. TSH is the primary regulator of NIS function[60,61]; it is likely to be responsible for both the transcription of NIS mRNA as well as translation and targeting of the protein to the plasma membrane. NIS is also expressed in the salivary gland, the gastric mucosa, and the lactating mammary gland but not regulated by TSH. Perchlorate and thiocyanate ions compete with iodide for NIS transport. This forms the basis of the perchlorate discharge test to diagnose T_4 synthetic defects as radiolabeled iodide, which is effectively trapped by the healthy thyroid, will be released if NIS is blocked[62] (see section called Imaging the Thyroid).

After active transport into thyroid follicular cells, iodide is passively transported to the follicular lumen. Although the exact nature of this process is unclear, a further solute carrier (SLC) molecule, pendrin (encoded by *SLC26A*), as well as other as yet unidentified ion channels are involved.[63,64] Pendred syndrome, caused by the loss of function of pendrin, and which causes hearing loss, has only a modest effect on thyroid function; patients typically have a goiter but are euthyroid.[64] An abnormal perchlorate discharge test result is a feature of this syndrome, which suggests that other ion channels as well as pendrin are required for iodide efflux to the follicular lumen. Within the thyroid lumen, iodide is incorporated into the thyroid specific protein Tg by a complex and coordinated process known as "iodine organification." In essence, iodide is oxidized to iodine and is captured and stored as iodotyrosyl residues on Tg within the thyroid lumen. This process requires locally generated hydrogen peroxide and is catalyzed by the enzyme thyroid peroxidase (TPO). TPO catalyses both iodination of tyrosyl residues and the coupling of iodotyrosines to form the T3- and T_4-iodothyronine Tg complexes (Fig. 67.8). The commonly used thionamide class of antithyroid drugs acts at this stage, probably by competing with tyrosyl residues for free iodine.

Thyroglobulin

Thyroglobulin (Tg) is a large thyroid-specific dimeric glycoprotein.[65] It is the major constituent of thyroid lumen, where its concentration is approximately 300 g/L. The mature protein has 2749 amino acid residues, including 66 tyrosines. Although 10 to 15 of these tyrosyl residues can be iodinated, T_4 production occurs only at sites 5, 1291, and 2554.[65] T_3 is

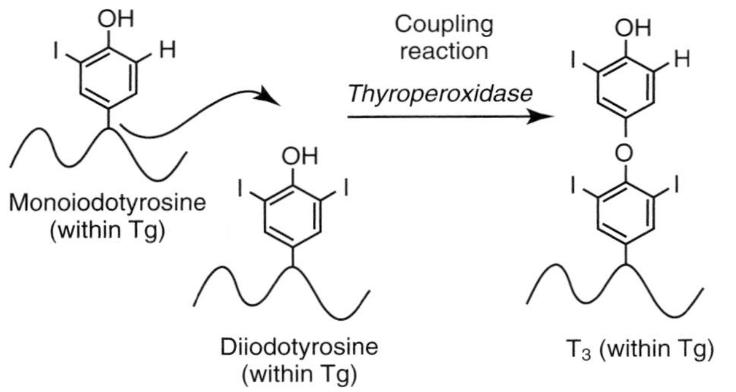

FIGURE 67.8 Chemical coupling of one molecule of monoiodotyrosine and one molecule of di-iodotyrosine to produce one molecule of triiodothyronine (T_3). The reaction is catalyzed by thyroperoxidase.

formed at 2747. The protein is extensively glycosylated, being 10% by weight carbohydrate.

The 48-exon gene encoding Tg contains several thyroid-specific promoters (TTF-1, TTF-2, and PAX8) in common with the *TPO* gene, with which it shares considerable homology.[65] TSH is the major regulator of protein synthesis. Tg acts as both the scaffold and a storage depot for thyroid hormone.[65] Mutations in the gene encoding Tg can cause a spectrum of hypothyroidism from subclinical to overt.[65] Many of these mutations cause the retention of mutated Tg in the endoplasmic reticulum, so these are a form of endoplasmic reticulum storage disease.[65]

Tg is packaged extremely efficiently into the follicular lumen at high concentration.[65] After organification, Tg must be returned to the follicular cell for further processing before secretion. This occurs by a complex but well-characterized process of vesicle-mediated endocytosis, which is regulated by TSH action.[65] Tg is proteolyzed, and thyroid hormone is generated in lysosomes. How the mature prohormone leaves the lysosomes is unclear, but the process is now thought to involve transporter proteins such as monocarboxylate transporter MCT8, which is expressed at the basolateral membrane of follicular cells.

Thyroid Peroxidase

Thyroid peroxidase is a 933-residue heme-containing glycoprotein. It is located at the apical membrane of the follicular cell with the active site accessible to the follicular lumen.[66] The enzyme catalyses the oxidation of iodide by hydrogen peroxide, and in the presence of Tg, iodinates and couples tyrosine residues. Similar to Tg, the synthesis of TPO is regulated by TSH. The mechanism of iodination and iodo-thyronine coupling is not fully elucidated; it is likely to involve oxidation of TPO by hydrogen peroxidase and the generation of an iodine radical from iodine that can then react with the tyrosine to form mono-iodotyrosine and, subsequently, di-iodotyrosine. Further action of TPO generates iodotyrosyl radicals that can combine to form the iodothyronines T_4 and T_3. Mutations in TPO have been described in patients with hypothyroidism caused by defective thyroid hormone synthesis.

Hydrogen peroxide is generated in situ at the apical membrane by two homologous heme-containing NADPH-dependent oxidases, dual oxidases 1 and 2 (DUOX1 and DUOX2).[67] Both are membrane bound. Two maturation factors (DUOXA1 and DUOXA2) are co-transported to the cell membrane and are required for maximum peroxide generation. Peroxide generation by DUOX1 is regulated by TSH via cyclic AMP and DUOX2 via protein kinase C. Mutations in DUOX2 and DUOXA2 have been identified in patients with hypothyroidism caused by defective hormone production. Hydrogen peroxide generation is inhibited by excess iodide, possibly to protect the thyroid from exposure to excess iodine, which would otherwise cause over-production of thyroid hormones. This is the basis of the Wolff–Chaikoff effect, in which excess iodine administration can be used in the treatment of acute hyperthyroidism or "thyroid storm."

TABLE 67.2 Thyroid Hormone Transport in Plasma

Thyroid Binding Protein	TBG	TTR	Albumin
Concentration in plasma (mean normal, mg/L)	16	250	40,000
T_4 capacity (μg/dL)	22	120	1000
Distribution			
T_4	75%	20%	5%
T_3	75%	<5%	20%
Approximate molecular mass (kDa)	54	55	66
Structure	Monomer	Tetramer	Monomer
Number of binding sites for T_4 and T_3	1	2	Several
Association Constant (M^{-1})			
For T_4	1×10^{10}	2×10^{8}*	1.5×10^{6}*
For T_3	1×10^{9}	1×10^{6}	2×10^{5}

*Value given is for the high affinity binding site only.

T_3, Triiodothyronine; *T_4*, thyroxine; *TBG*, thyroxine-binding globulin; *TTR*, transthyretin.

Modified from Feldt-Rasmussen U, Rasmussen ÅK. Thyroid hormone transport and actions. In: Krassas GE, Rivkees SA, Kiess W (eds). *Diseases of the thyroid in childhood and adolescence.* Basel: Karger; 2007:80–103.

Circulating Thyroid Hormone–Binding Proteins

Thyroid hormones are extensively protein bound in plasma, with only 0.03% of total T_4 (tT_4) and 0.3% of total T_3 (tT3) in plasma being circulating free or unbound.[48,68] The three major hormone binding proteins are TBG, TTR, and albumin (Table 67.2).[48,68] TBG has the highest affinity for T_4 and binds 75% of plasma T_4.[68] TTR binds 20% and albumin 5%.[68] Small amounts of T_4 are also bound by lipoproteins, immunoglobulins, and some plasma serpin protease inhibitors. As thyroid hormone enters target cells unbound, the free fraction of hormone in the plasma best represents the biologic activity of the thyroid hormones, the total amount being largely determined by the concentrations of binding proteins. The function of thyroid-binding proteins is somewhat enigmatic because both naturally occurring mutations and knockout animal models do not have an obvious phenotype. Thyroid-binding proteins may be involved in the following processes[48,68]:

- Limiting urinary loss of thyroid hormone
- Buffering fluctuations in thyroid output of hormones

TABLE 67.3 **Characteristics of the Deiodinases**

	D1	D2	D3
Source	Liver, kidneys, thyroid	Brain, pituitary, skeletal muscle	Brain, placenta, fetal tissues
Substrates	$rT_3 \gg T_4 > T_3$	$T_4 > rT_3$	$T_3 > T_4$
Role	Plasma T_3 production, rT_3 clearance, clearance of hormone	Local T_3 production, ? plasma T_3 production	T_3 degradation, prevents exposure of fetus to T_3
Effect of hypothyroidism	Decrease	Increase	Decrease
Effect of hyperthyroidism	Increase	Decrease	Increase
Inhibition by propylthiouracil	Yes	No	No

D1, D2, D3, Deiodinase 1, 2, and 3, respectively; *rT_3,* reverse triiodothyronine; *T_3,* triiodothyronine; *T_4,* thyroxine.

- Acting as a reservoir of thyroid hormone, so the amount of free hormone can be kept constant

It is widely accepted as proof of the "free hormone" hypothesis that changes in plasma concentrations of thyroid-binding proteins affect total thyroid hormone measurements but free hormone concentrations are maintained. This is consistent with the lack of a specific phenotype associated with demonstrable binding protein abnormalities. However, many immunoassays for free thyroid hormones are affected by alterations in binding protein concentrations and return incorrect values, largely because of limitations in assay design rather than to a genuine change in free hormone concentration. Consequently, the clinical chemist needs to be aware that alterations in thyroid-binding protein concentrations are still a cause of abnormal thyroid function test results. Increased concentration or reduced concentration or affinity of TBG for thyroid hormones have been described as causes of raised or lowered total thyroid hormone concentrations. TBG concentration is most commonly increased in conditions of estrogen excess.[68] TBG is reduced by androgens and can be dramatically reduced in terminal illness.[68] Thyroid status also directly affects TBG concentration, most likely owing to the effect of thyroid hormone on protein clearance. Genetic conditions also affect TBG concentration: A variety of mutations have been described that reduce protein concentration or hormone binding affinity as well as TBG excess caused by gene duplication events.[68]

Reduced concentration of TTE or albumin have little effect on total T_4 concentration owing to the relatively small amount of T_4 bound, but increases in either the affinity or concentration of TTE or the affinity of albumin for T_4 have been described as causes of raised total T_4. Familial dysalbuminemic hyperthyroxinemia is the most prevalent (0.01%–1.8%) and best characterized such condition; it causes a dramatic rise in total T_4 (tT_4) and affects many immunoassays for free T_4 to varying degrees.[69]

Thyroid Hormone Uptake and Metabolism

Uptake

Thyroid hormones are imported into cells through several transporter proteins. OATP1C1, MCT8, and MCT10 are likely to be the most important channels because they are most specific for thyroid hormones.[70] OATP1C1 is expressed in brain capillaries; a mouse knockout model has features of central nervous system hypothyroidism. A likely role is for the transport of T_4 across the blood–brain barrier. MCT8 is widely expressed; a mutation in the human *MCT8* gene causes Allan–Heardon–Dudley syndrome, an X-linked condition that presents with severe psychomotor retardation and is associated with elevated plasma T_3 concentrations.[70] MCT10 is highly homologous to MCT8 but has broader substrate specificity, including aromatic amino acids.[70] It is also widely expressed in tissues, including skeletal muscle, the kidneys, the liver, and the intestine. Mutations in the *MCT10* gene have yet to be described.

Metabolism

T_4 is converted to the active thyroid hormone T_3 by two deiodinases, D1 and D2, by outer-ring deiodination[50,51] (see Fig. 67.8). Both T_4 and T_3 are also inactivated by inner-ring deiodination by D1[50] but also more significantly by a third de-iodinase, D3.[52] T_4 is metabolized to 3,3′5′-tri-iodothyronine (reverse T_3, rT_3) and T_3 to 3,3′-di-iodothyronine (3,3′T2). Reverse T_3 is present at low concentrations in the plasma of healthy individuals but is not thought to have any function. Originally, the role of the deiodinases was thought to be to preserve plasma T_3 concentrations despite fluctuations in iodine availability; however, recent evidence suggests that the deiodinases provide a second level of regulation of thyroid hormone signaling at the cellular level by activating or suppressing local T_3 production.[50-52]

The deiodinase enzymes (Table 67.3) are homologous homodimeric membrane selenoproteins of around 30 kDa.[50-52] The modified amino acid selenocysteine is critical for deiodinase function, and defects in the incorporation of selenocysteine into the enzymes are a cause of abnormal thyroid function tests.[50-52]

T_3 and T_4 are mainly metabolized by two deiodinases (D1 and D3) to generate further iodothyronines, which are decarboxylated to generate thyronamines.[50,52] Iodothyronines and thyronamines, also called nonclassical thyroid hormones, are present in plasma at much lower concentrations and have previously been considered inactive breakdown products, but recent research has shown that they may have relevant biologic effects.[71]

Alternate pathways of thyroid hormone metabolism include conjugation (sulfation or sulfonation and glucuronidation) and oxidative deamination of the alanine side chain, leading to the formation of the corresponding iodothyroacetates and ether link cleavage.[53] Excess iodine produced as a byproduct of thyroid hormone synthesis is effectively scavenged by the thyroidal enzyme iodotyrosine dehalogenase 1 (DEHAL)[54] (Fig. 67.5).

T_3 Production. Both D1 and D2 catalyze the outer-ring deiodination (activation) of T_4 to T_3.[50,51] However, the exact role of these two enzymes in human T_3 production remains unclear. The major role of D1 is likely to be scavenging iodine from thyroid hormone metabolites because it has high affinity for conjugated iodothyronines. D2 has a clear role in the production of T_3 in tissues that express this enzyme (brain, anterior pituitary gland, thyroid, and skeletal muscle). Thus, tissues with or without D2 respond differently to T_4 because T_4 is activated intracellularly by D2. D2 may also contribute significantly to the production of circulating T_3.

Thyroid Hormone Inactivation. Inner-ring deiodination by D3 leads to inactivation of T_3 to 3,3′-di-iodothyronine and of T_4 to rT3.[52] As such, D3 expression is also responsible for the plasma T_3 concentration. Knock-out models of D3 have a much more severe phenotype than D1 or D2; this includes increased mortality and growth retardation. Taken together with the up-regulation of this enzyme during fetal development, D3 appears to have a role in protecting developing tissues from potentially deleterious effects of T_3 exposure. These effects may also be carried on into adulthood during regenerative or pathological processes such as heart failure. D3 can also be expressed by tumors, and thus it falls into the category of oncofetal proteins.[52] The uncontrolled expression of D3, by inactivating T_4 and T_3 in tumors such as infantile hemangiomas, can induce a paraneoplastic syndrome called *consumptive hypothyroidism*, a rare but severe condition mostly affecting patients in the first years of life.[52]

Iodothyronines are also metabolized by conjugation with sulfate or glucuronic acid, which renders them more water soluble. Sulfate conjugates are usually kept at low concentrations because of the effects of D1. Glucuronides are detectable in bile and enter the enterohepatic cycle; that is, they are delivered to the intestine, where these metabolites get deconjugated and thyroxine is reabsorbed, and the cycle is repeated. Typically 20% of T_4 produced is excreted in the feces, most likely via glucuronide production (see Fig. 67.5).

Mechanisms of Thyroid Hormone Action

The molecular mechanisms of thyroid hormone action are *genomic* and *nongenomic.*[47] Whereas thyroid hormones exert genomic actions via nuclear receptors, the nongenomic actions are exerted on the plasma membrane, in the cytoplasm, or on organelles such as the mitochondria.[47] Genomic and nongenomic actions may overlap, such that hormonal actions outside the nucleus often result in nuclear transcriptional events regulated by intranuclear receptors as well as other nuclear transcription factors,[47] and nongenomic actions may involve support of trafficking of transcriptional regulators from the cytoplasm to the nucleus.[72] Nongenomic actions are more rapid compared with the genomic actions.[47,73] Nongenomic actions of thyroid hormones T_4 and T_3 begin at the hormone receptor the heterodimeric integrin αvβ3.[47] T_4 has a higher affinity for integrin αvβ3, but T_3 has a higher affinity for the nuclear thyroid hormone receptors, THRα and THRβ.[47]

Nongenomic Actions

Some tissues, particularly muscle, can respond to thyroid hormones more quickly than can be explained by genomic actions.[74] These effects are transcription independent.[75] They may be coordinated by cytosolic THRs via interaction with the PI3 or cAMP kinase pathways or via alternative receptors such as the recently described plasma membrane integrin αvβ3 T_4 receptor.[47]

Genomic Actions

The receptors bind to specific thyroid response elements that are located in the promoter region of thyroid responsive genes. The mechanism of gene regulation by thyroid hormone receptors is complex but well elucidated (Fig. 67.9).[49] In the unliganded state, THRs bind co-repressors such as CoR as well as the retinoic acid receptor and the thyroid response element.[49] In this state, basal transcription of thyroid responsive genes is repressed. T_3 binding displaces the co-repressors and recruits co-activators, causing transcriptional activation via a mechanism likely to involve local chromatin remodeling.[49] Some genes are negatively regulated by thyroid hormone; the mechanism is less well understood, but co-repressors and co-activators are likely to perform reciprocal functions in this situation.[47,49]

The widely expressed THRα and THRβ are tissue dependent and developmentally regulated.[75] The THRα1 form predominates in the brain, heart, gastrointestinal (GI) tract, and skeletal muscle; the THRβ1 form in liver and kidneys; and the THRβ2 form in the pituitary and inner ear.[49] THRα1 is constitutively expressed during embryonic development, but THRβ is expressed during later embryonic development.[75] Mutations have been described for both THRα and THRβ receptors, and the phenotype presented reflect the respective tissue distribution of the receptors.[49]

Biologic Function

Thyroid hormones enhance many intracellular events and promote differentiation and growth. At the molecular level, thyroid hormones[40,42,74,76,77]:

- Increase oxygen consumption in tissues via increased membrane transport (cycling of sodium/potassium ATPase with increased synthesis and consumption of adenosine triphosphate).
- Enhance mitochondrial metabolism (stimulation of mitochondrial respiration and oxidative phosphorylation).
- Regulate calorigenesis and metabolic rate.
- Increase sensitivity to catecholamines with increased heart rate and myocardial contractility, (however, mechanisms responsible for many interactions between thyroid hormones and the sympathetic nervous system have not been identified).
- Stimulate synthesis and carbohydrate metabolism.
- Increase synthesis and degradation of cholesterol and triglycerides (eg, regulation of low-density lipoprotein receptor expression by the liver).
- Increase vitamin requirements.
- Regulate calcium and phosphorous metabolism, stimulating bone turnover (resorption more so than mineralization).
- Regulate and promote normal growth and development in fetuses, neonates, children, and adolescents.
- Regulate and promote neurologic function.

The actions of thyroid hormones increase demand for coenzymes and vitamins.

All the actions above are typically magnified in patients with hyperthyroidism and suppressed in patients with hypothyroidism. It is also noteworthy that hyperthyroidism

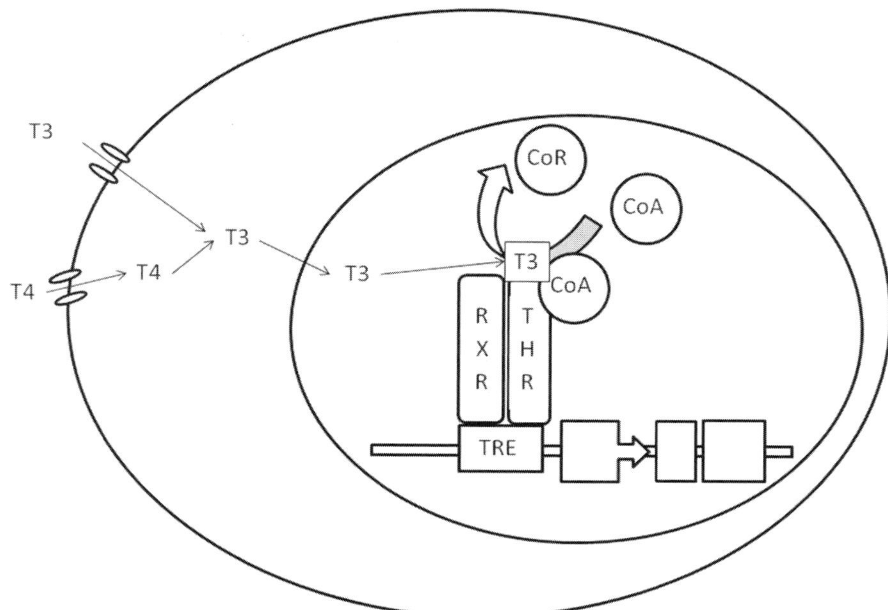

FIGURE 67.9 Mechanism of thyroid hormone receptor action. The thyroid hormone receptor (THR) and retinoid X receptor (RXR) form heterodimers that bind specifically to thyroid hormone response elements (TRE) in the promoter regions of target genes. In the absence of hormone, THR binds co-repressor (CoR) proteins that silence gene expression. (Courtesy David Halsall.)

accelerates the clearance of many drugs, and hypothyroidism decreases their excretion.

Physiological Control of Thyroid Hormone Synthesis and Secretion

Thyroid-stimulating hormone (thyrotropin) is the principal regulator of thyroid hormone synthesis and secretion. Human TSH is secreted by the pituitary thyrotrophs; it is a 28-kDa asymmetric dimeric glycoprotein that consists of a 92-amino-acid α subunit (which is common to the other pituitary glycohormones, including human chorionic gonadotropin, follicle-stimulating hormone, and luteinizing hormone) and a unique 118-amino-acid β chain.[78,79]

The pituitary–thyroid axis is a classic endocrine negative feedback loop because the pituitary TSH secretion is inhibited by thyroid hormones[55,56] (see Fig. 67.6). This effect is mediated by the pituitary thyroid hormone receptor THRβ-2, as discussed earlier, which suppresses transcription of the both the TSH α and β subunit. Thyroid hormone also feeds back at the level of the hypothalamus to inhibit the secretion of the hypothalamic tripeptide hormone TRH (Fig. 67.10) via the THRβ-2 receptor, although this effect is minor compared with the suppression of TSH by the pituitary. TRH is processed from a prohormone containing six copies of the TRH sequence flanked by basic amino acid pairs that are cleaved by the prohormone convertases PC1, PC2, and carboxypeptidase E.[56] The tripeptide is further processed by cyclisation of the N-terminal glutamate and amidation of the C-terminus. TRH is a major positive regulator of TSH transcription, acting via the phospholipase C pathway. TRH also reduces the sensitivity of thyrotrophs to thyroid hormone inhibition, probably by reducing the expression of the thyroid hormone receptor. Mutations in the human TRH receptor cause central hypothyroidism[80]; however, the phenotype is not as severe as in patients with genetic absence of the TSHβ subunit.[81] (Knockout mice models of TRH support this as the mice are not hypothyroid at birth but become so postnatally).

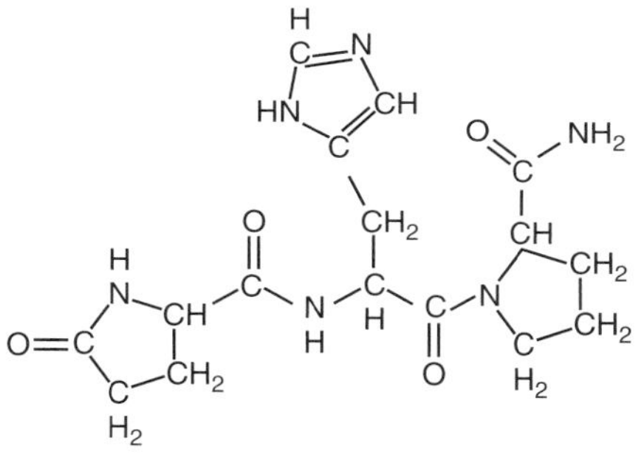

(pyro)Glu-His-Pro(NH_2)

FIGURE 67.10 Chemical structure of the tripeptide thyrotropin-releasing hormone (TRH), L-pyroglutamyl-L-histidyl-L-prolinamide.

Thyroid-stimulating hormone is posttranslationally modified by glycosylation of both the α and β subunits.[79] Glycosylation of TSH affects both its biologic activity and clearance. The variable biologic activity of different glycoforms is not necessarily reflected in the reactivity of the molecule to immunoassay; the intrinsic heterogeneity of the molecule also confounds attempts to standardize immunoassay methods. Glycosylation status is affected by TRH, which tends to increase biological activity. This increased specific activity is also seen in patients with TSH-secreting pituitary tumors and those with thyroid hormone resistance. In contrast, patients with central hypothyroidism secrete less active TSH. TSH clearance is slower in hypothyroid patients and enhanced in toxic patients, also because of differential glycosylation.

The thyroid-stimulating hormone receptor (TSHR) is a member of the G protein–coupled receptor family, with the conserved seven transmembrane domain motif.[82] Human chorionic gonadotropin (hCG) can also activate the TSHR; this is commonly seen in the early weeks of pregnancy when TSH is often suppressed.[82]

IODINE AND THYROID DISORDERS

Iodine (or iodide [I^-] in its ionized form) is a trace element and an essential nutrient. Iodine is an indispensable component of the thyroid hormones T_3 and T_4, respectively. These hormones, together with the thyronamines, are the only iodine-containing hormones in vertebrates. Without iodine, there is no biosynthesis of thyroid hormones. Thus, thyroid function requires an adequate supply of iodine to the thyroid gland.

Geography

Iodide ions in seawater and coastal seaweed beds are oxidized to elemental iodine, which then volatilizes into the atmosphere and is returned to the soil by rain. This process (the iodine cycle) is slow and incomplete in many regions, thus leaving soils and drinking water iodine depleted. Crops grown in these soils are low in iodine, and animals consuming food grown in these soils become iodine deficient. The common iodine-deficient soils are found in mountainous areas such as the Alps, Andes, and Himalayas and areas of frequent flooding such as the Ganges River plain of north eastern India. Central Asia and Africa, Central and Eastern Europe, and the littoral of the Great Lakes of the United States and Canada are other areas of iodine deficiency.[83]

Nutrition

Various foods contain iodine.[84,85] Most iodine is found in the oceans; the concentration of iodine in seawater is approximately 50 μg/L. Foods of marine origin, such as kelp and kombu seaweed, have the highest iodine content. Brown seaweeds contain a particularly high concentration of iodine and have been used as raw material for iodine production since the early 1800s.[86] Other sources include bread, soup, nonorganic milk, and fortified salt. Some vitamin preparations may also be fortified with iodine. The major source of iodine in industrialized countries is iodized salt, and if that is not available, then dairy products.[83] Natural (organic) milk contain very little iodine, but iodine supplements are often given to livestock and increase the iodine content of dairy products.[87] Also, many countries use iodized salt for cooking and seasoning of foods. Potassium iodate (KIO_3) is the recommended form of iodine in salt because it has increased stability in the presence of salt impurities, humidity, and porous packaging compared with potassium iodide (KI).[58,88]

The recommended dietary allowances by the World Health Organization (WHO) are shown in Table 67.4.[58,88] Pregnant and lactating women have higher demands for iodine because of an increase in maternal T_4 production to maintain maternal euthyroidism and also transfer of thyroid hormone to the fetus early in the first trimester.[89]

TABLE 67.4 World Health Organization Recommendations for Iodine Intake by Age or Population Group

Group	Iodine Intake (μg/day)
Children 0–5 yr	90
Children 6–12 yr	120
Adults >12 yr	150
Pregnant women	250
Lactating women	250

Reproduced with permission from Zimmermann MB, Boelaert K. Iodine-deficiency disorders. *Lancet Diabetes Endocrinol* 2015;3:286–295.

Cruciferous vegetables, such as cabbage, kale, cauliflower, and broccoli, contain glucosinolates, and their metabolites compete with iodine for thyroidal uptake.[90] Cassava, linseed, and sweet potato contain cyanogenic glucosides, which can be metabolized to thiocyanates and compete with iodine for thyroidal uptake.

Deficiencies of selenium, iron, or vitamin A exacerbate the effects of iodine deficiency.[91] Pregnant women, who are often iron deficient, and poor maternal iron status can predict both higher TSH and lower T_4 concentrations during pregnancy in areas of borderline iron deficiency.[89]

Iodine-Containing Products and Goitrogens

Exposure to iodine can also occur from iodine and iodophor-derived iodine used as disinfectants; they have a wide range of antimicrobial actions against gram-positive and gram-negative bacteria, fungi, and viruses. Iodophor-derived iodine may be retained in materials used in the construction of milking machines and subsequently released into the milk.[92] Other products containing iodine are certain drugs such as amiodarone, radiology contrast agents such as iopanoic acid and ipodate sodium, and topical antiseptics such as the surgical scrub povidone–iodine (a stable complex between povidone and iodine). Iodine present in medications, supplements, and iodinated contrast agents has concentrations up to several thousand-fold higher than iodine appearing in naturally occurring foods.[93]

Iodine deficiency is the major cause of endemic goiter, but naturally occurring compounds and environmental pollutants may also be goitrogenic.[94,95] Goitrogens can be either agents acting directly on the thyroid gland or cause a goiter by indirect action. Interestingly, cigarette smoking is associated with high plasma concentrations of thiocyanate, which can compete with iodine for uptake into the thyroid.

Public Health Programs

There are two kinds of public health programs for securing optimal thyroid function. One is newborn screening for thyroid function (see section on congenital hypothyroidism); the other is iodization of salt.

It is estimated that 2 billion people worldwide have insufficient iodine intake.[96] In regions that are affected by iodine deficiency, the most effective way to control this is through salt iodization. In the 1910s and 1920s, studies by Swiss and American physicians demonstrated the efficacy of

TABLE 67.5 Iodine Deficiency Disorders by Age Group

Age Groups	Health Consequences of Iodine Deficiency
All ages	Goiter Increased susceptibility of the thyroid gland to nuclear radiation In severe iodine deficiency, hypothyroidism
Fetus	Abortion Stillbirth Congenital anomalies Perinatal mortality
Neonate	Infant mortality Endemic cretinism
Children and adolescents	Impaired mental function Delayed physical development
Adults	Impaired mental function Reduced work productivity Toxic nodular goiter, hyperthyroidism

Reproduced with permission from Zimmerman MB, Boelaert K. Iodine-deficiency disorders. *Lancet Diabetes Endocrinol* 2015;3:286–295.

iodine prophylaxis in the prevention of goiter and cretinism. The Swiss surgeon Hans Eggenberger was the first person to promote a general public health measure by using salt iodization because it is effective, inexpensive, and safe.[97]

During the period from 1970 to 1990, controlled studies in iodine-deficient regions showed that iodine supplementation eliminated new cases of cretinism reduced infant mortality rates, and improved cognitive function in the rest of the population. The new term *iodine-deficiency disorders* (IDDs) has gained recognition as a spectrum of related disorders affecting billions of people[58,98] (Table 67.5). Since 1990, elimination of the IDDs has been an important part of many national nutrition strategies.[58] The WHO and the United Nations Children's Fund (UNICEF) are working closely with the International Council for Control of Iodine Deficiency Disorders (ICCIDD) and the salt industry.

The WHO, UNICEF, and ICCIDD recommend that iodine status of populations should be assessed by median urinary iodine concentration (UIC); however, they have also recently recognized Tg as a sensitive marker.[99] Surveys of iodine intake have been performed in 152 countries, representing 98% of the world's population. People of 74% of the countries have sufficient iodine intake, 19% have insufficient intakes, and 7% have excessive intake.[58] However, only a few countries have done national UIC surveys in pregnant women to detect iodine deficiency.[100,101] Iodine deficiency is not only a problem in developing countries but also a problem in transitioning countries (eg, Russia) and high-income countries (eg, Denmark). Data from 128 member states in UNICEF have shown that overall, 70% of all households worldwide have access to adequately iodized salt[102,103]; about 30% of the member states have attained universal salt iodization, with at least 90% of households consuming adequately iodized salt; about 40% of the member states have coverage in 50% to 89% of households; and about 30% of the countries still have coverage in fewer than 50% of households. However, in Australia, the United Kingdom, and the United States, iodine intakes are falling. The current global push to reduce salt consumption to prevent chronic disease and the policy of salt iodization to control iodine deficiency do not necessarily conflict. Iodization methods can fortify salt to provide adequate iodine even if the intake of salt is reduced, providing that all salt produced is iodized.[104]

In systematic reviews, iodine supplementation has been shown to improve maternal thyroid indices and cognitive function in school-age children.[105] Global meta-analyses investigating the effects of salt iodization particularly are lacking on thyroid and iodine-deficiency endpoints,[106] but median UICs have improved.[107] Universal salt iodization reduced the prevalence of goiter in a period after the intervention, but the fact that the prevalence of goiter and toxic nodular goiter had increased recently suggests that both insufficient and excess iodine may be associated with goiter.[108]

Biochemistry

Dietary iodine controls its own absorption through post-transcriptional regulation of the intestinal Na^+/I^- symporter (NIS).[109] The thyroid gland has autoregulatory mechanisms to handle excess iodine intake involving the sodium iodide symporter.[59] Excess iodine has an inhibitory effect on thyroxine synthesis in intact thyroids.[110] In conditions of adequate dietary iodine supply, the healthy thyroid usually takes up less than 20% of absorbed iodine. However, in chronic iodine deficiency, this fraction can be more than 80%. The thyroid is thus able to adapt to low intakes of dietary iodine by marked modification of its activity. In most adults, if iodine intake falls below 100 µg/day, TSH secretion is augmented. Iodine in plasma has a half-life of approximately 10 hours, but this can be less in iodine deficiency or hyperthyroidism. A healthy adult has up to 20 mg of iodine of which up to 80% is actually in the thyroid. The metabolism of circulating thyroid hormones in peripheral tissues releases iodine that enters the plasma iodine pool, which in turn can be taken up by the thyroid or excreted by the kidney. Approximately 90% of ingested iodine is excreted in the urine and approximately 10% in feces[111] (see Fig. 67.5).

Iodine Deficiency

Both deficient and excessive intakes of iodine can impair thyroid function.[58] The clinical presentations of iodine deficiency are largely age dependent[58] (see Table 67.5). In fetuses, deficiency may cause abortion, stillbirth, and congenital anomalies, and in neonates, deficiency may cause infant mortality and endemic cretinism. In children and adolescents, deficiency may cause impaired mental function, delayed physical development, and low IQ. In adults, deficiency may cause impaired cognitive function, reduced work productivity, thyroid autoimmunity, toxic nodular goiter, and hyperthyroidism. In all ages, goiter is the most visible sign of iodine deficiency but is not specific to it.

In mild iodine deficiency, many people develop simple diffuse goiter, and some develop nodules, but TSH is usually stable.[58,112]

In mild to moderate iodine deficiency, plasma Tg concentrations rise, and the thyroid is enlarged, producing a diffuse goiter. There is increased thyroid activity as a compensation for low iodine intake, but this chronic stimulation increases thyroid nodularity, and multinodular toxic goiter develops in these populations.[58] Thus, TSH is lowered, and there is usually a higher prevalence of hyperthyroidism compared with populations with a sufficient excessive intake. The prevalence of hyperthyroidism transiently increases further when iodized salt is introduced, but with iodine sufficiency, the thyroid activity returns to normal, thus reducing the prevalence of nodular autonomy over the years.[58] Furthermore, in populations with moderate iodine deficiency, there is an increased incidence of solitary toxic adenoma and amiodarone-associated hyperthyroidism.[113]

In moderate to severe iodine deficiency, TSH often increases slightly, T_4 remains normal, and subclinical hypothyroidism (SCH) may develop.[58] In severe, chronic iodine deficiency, iodine concentrations are too low for the production of thyroid hormones, and overt hypothyroidism develops with increased TSH and decreased T_4 and T_3.[58] Most affected individuals develop goiter.[58,114]

A meta-analysis of results from randomized controlled trials of iodine intake or iodine supplements showed that doubling of dietary iodine intake increased UIC by 14% in children and adolescents, by 57% in adults and older adults, and by 81% in pregnant women.[115] Also, daily iodine supplementation in form of potassium iodine decreased TSH by 12% and Tg by 31% decrease in pregnant women.[115]

Correction of iodine deficiency in adult populations, irrespective of severity, reduces thyroid size and the prevalence of diffuse goiter at all ages.[58,116,117] Correction of iodine deficiency in a population with a high prevalence of nodular autonomy usually results in a further increase in the prevalence of hyperthyroidism. However, corrections in adults older than 50 years do not reduce the prevalence of thyroid nodularity because of irreversible fibrotic changes in nodules.[118] Increased iodine intake in an iodine-deficient population leads to a small increase in mild SCH, especially in individuals positive for thyroid antibodies. Individuals with autoimmune thyroiditis are at increased risk of hypothyroidism when exposed to excess iodine. There is no evidence that iodine intake increases the risk of thyroid cancer,[119] but correction of iodine deficiency reduces goiter, a major risk factor for thyroid cancer.[120] Furthermore, correction of iodine deficiency may shift subtypes toward less malignant types of thyroid cancer.[121-123]

Iodine Excess

Thyroid dysfunction may occur in vulnerable patients if exposed to excess iodine. These patients include those with preexisting thyroid disease, older adults, pregnant and lactating women, fetuses, and neonates.[93] Because iodine is present in medications, supplements, and iodinated contrast agents in much higher concentrations than are found in naturally occurring foods,[93] iodine excess can result in adverse thyroidal effects after only a single exposure to these substances.[93] Excess dietary iodine intake in pregnant and lactating women in iodine-replete areas may lead to an increase in plasma TSH concentrations and thus to SCH.[124,125] Amiodarone-induced thyrotoxicosis (AIT) is discussed in another section of this chapter.

POINTS TO REMEMBER

Iodine

- Without iodine, there is no biosynthesis of thyroid hormones.
- Iodine deficiency is a major cause of endemic goiter.
- Most iodine is found in oceans and thus marine life.
- Common iodine deficiency soils are found in mountainous areas, such as the Alps, Andes, and Himalayas.
- IDDs are a spectrum of related disorders affecting billions of people worldwide.
- Switzerland, some parts of Scandinavia, Australia, the United States, and Canada were the only countries that were completely iodine sufficient before 1990.

EXTRATHYROIDAL FACTORS THAT AFFECT THYROID FUNCTION

Epidemiologic Factors

Concentrations of thyrotropin, thyroid hormones, thyroid antibodies, and thyroid-binding proteins are to varying degrees determined genetically[126-130] and by epidemiologic factors such as age,[44,131-137] gender,[131-134] ethnicity,[44,131-134] body mass index,[136] smoking,[138] pregnancy,[139] nutritional iodine,[58] season,[140] nonthyroidal disease,[141] radiation,[142] and medication.[143] Some of these factors are discussed in this section; others have their designated sections in this chapter.

In children, concentrations of plasma tT_3, fT_3, tT_4, free T_4 (fT_4), and TSH decrease with age,[44,135] but tT_4 seem to increase again in girls during puberty.[44,136] Overall, modest gender differences are seen in fT_3, tT_3, and tT_4,[44] and fT_4, tT_3, tT_4 show some ethnic differences.[44] The concentrations of antithyroid antibodies do not seem to affect reference intervals in children.[136] However, TBG concentration increases until 5 years and then decreases with age and is also gender dependent.[135] The most marked changes in concentrations occur after the neonatal period.[135] Seasonal variations in TSH occur, leading to an increased false-positive rate of congenital hypothyroidism in screening programs in the winter (0.9%) compared with the summer (0.6%).[140]

In adults, concentrations of TSH increase with age[131-133] and are higher in whites than in blacks or Hispanics.[144] Antithyroid antibody concentrations increase with age, are higher in women than men, and higher in whites than in blacks.[131,132] Smoking is associated with lower plasma concentrations of TSH and thyroid antibodies and lower risk of hypothyroidism.[138] Concentrations of thyroid antibodies are genetically determined, but environmental triggers, such as radiation exposure, nuclear or medical, or environmental contaminants, increase the risk of autoimmune thyroid disease.[142] T_4 secretion and degradation decrease with age,[145] but plasma fT_4 concentrations remain largely unchanged with increasing age.[131]

In older adults (age older than ~60 years), plasma TSH concentrations increase; the upper limit especially increases markedly.[133] Age-specific TSH reference intervals must be used; if not, the incidence of SCH may be overestimated.[133] tT_3 but not fT_3 concentrations decrease with age.[146] Other factors that should be considered in the interpretation of thyroid function tests in older adults are medications interfering with thyroid function tests[143] and acute or chronic nonthyroidal illness leading to decreased plasma fT_3, low or normal TSH, high rT_3, and relatively normal fT_4 concentrations.[141] As a result, the diagnoses of both subclinical and overt hypothyroidism and hyperthyroidism may pose challenges to clinicians.[146] Higher TSH concentrations with age are associated with increased longevity.[147,148]

Drugs

Many drugs, other than those used for treatment of thyroid disorders, interfere with thyroid hormone homeostasis (Table 67.6) through actions on thyroid hormone synthesis, secretion, transport, metabolism, and absorption.[143,149]

Thyroid hormone homeostasis may be affected at different levels. In the gut, drugs may cause reduced thyroid hormone absorption. In the thyroid, the synthesis or secretion of thyroid hormones may be altered, leading to changes in the plasma concentrations of thyroid hormones. Drugs may also influence the binding of thyroid hormones by competing for hormone-binding sites. Some drugs may modify cellular uptake and metabolism of thyroid hormones or interfere with hormone action at the target tissue level. Some drugs may interfere simultaneously through many actions.

Drugs That May Affect Plasma Thyroid-Stimulating Hormone Concentration

At the pituitary or hypothalamic level, drugs may affect TSH secretion.[149] Dopamine and dopamine agonists, such as bromocriptine and cabergoline used in patients with hyperprolactinemia, may suppress TSH through action on the dopamine D2 receptor. Somatostatin and its analogues may inhibit TSH secretion; these agents can be used clinically in patients with TSH-secreting pituitary adenomas. Other drugs that can suppress TSH secretion include glucocorticoids, metformin, and antiepileptics such as carbamazepine, valproic acid, and phenytoin.[150]

Drugs Affecting the Synthesis and Secretion of Thyroid Hormones

Lithium. Lithium, which is still a widely used drug for the treatment of bipolar disorder, is associated with subclinical and overt hypothyroidism in up to 34% and 15% of patients, respectively.[143,150,151] These may develop even after many years of treatment. Patients should have regular thyroid function tests, at least once or twice per annum. Lithium primarily inhibits thyroid hormone secretion, although it appears also to have effects on iodine trapping, release, and coupling.

Drugs Influencing the Metabolism of Thyroid Hormones

The cytochrome p450 complex consists of more than 100 isoenzymes. Some of these enzymes (CYP3A) can be induced by antiepileptic agents such as phenytoin, phenobarbital, and carbamazepine as well as the antituberculosis drug rifampicin.[143,149,150] Plasma thyroid hormone concentrations can decrease markedly in patients taking these drugs. The effect on TSH are, however, minor. Phenytoin has been shown to displace T_4 and T_3 from the binding site on TBG in vivo. Although this effect is compensated for in vivo by a reduction in tT_4, it is compounded by a possible in vitro effect on fT_4 immunoassays because this displacement effect can be reversed if the serum is diluted during analysis.[152] As the metabolic clearance rate and hepatic metabolism of T_4 increases in patients taking phenytoin, it is likely that in normal subjects, thyroid secretion increases to compensate for the increased metabolism; hypothyroid subjects taking phenytoin need increased doses of levothyroxine.[153]

TABLE 67.6 Effects of Some Drugs on Tests of Thyroid Function

Cause	Drug	Effect
Inhibit TSH secretion	Dopamine L-dopa Glucocorticoids Somatostatin	↓ T_4; ↓ T_3; ↓ TSH
Inhibit thyroid hormone synthesis or release	Iodine Lithium	↓ T_4; ↓ T_3; ↑ TSH
Inhibit conversion of T_4 to T_3	Amiodarone Glucocorticoids Propranolol Propylthiouracil Radiographic contrast agents	↓ T_3; ↑ rT_3; ↓, ⇌, ↑ T_4 and FT_4; ⇌, ↑ TSH
Inhibit binding of T_4/T_3 to serum proteins	Salicylates Phenytoin Carbamazepine Furosemide NSAIDs Heparin (in vitro effect)	↓ T_4; ↓ T_3; ⇌, ↑ FT_4; ⇌TSH
Stimulate metabolism of iodothyronines	Phenobarbital Phenytoin Carbamazepine Rifampicin	↓ T_4; ↓ FT_4; ⇌TSH
Inhibit absorption of ingested T_4	Aluminum hydroxide Ferrous sulfate Cholestyramine Colestipol Iron sucralfate Soybean preparations Kayexalate	↓ T_4; ↓ FT_4; ↑ TSH
Increase in concentration of T_4-binding proteins	Estrogen Clofibrate Opiates (heroin, methadone) 5-Fluorouracil Perphenazine	↑ T_4; ↑ T_3; ⇌FT4; ⇌TSH
Decrease in concentration of T_4-binding proteins	Androgens Glucocorticoids	↓ T_4; ↓ T_3; =FT_4; ⇌TSH

↓, Reduced serum concentration; ↑, increased serum concentration; ⇌ no change; *FT4,* free thyroxine; *NSAID,* nonsteroidal antiinflammatory drug; *rT_3,* reverse triiodothyronine; *T_3,* triiodothyronine; *T_4,* thyroxine.
Data obtained from Smallridge RD. Thyroid function tests. In: Becker KL, editor. *Principles and Practice of Endocrinology and Metabolism.* 7th ed. Philadelphia: JB Lippincott; 1995:299–306.

Rifampicin acts on intracellular thyroid hormone metabolism.[154-156] T_4 kinetic data show that rifampicin increases the plasma clearance rate of T_4; it has little effect on T_3 metabolism. Thus, drugs that enhance the activity of the hepatic p450 enzyme system result in a decrease in plasma tT_4 concentrations because of an acceleration of hepatic metabolism of T_4. As a result, the plasma half-life of T_4 decreases, and its metabolic clearance rate increases. Euthyroid subjects have a slight increase in T_4 production; thus, T_3 concentrations do not change, and plasma TSH may increase slightly but not significantly. Importantly, patients on levothyroxine replacement therapy started on treatment with any of these drugs are likely to require an increase in their dosage.

A number of environmental pollutants, such as organochlorine, pesticides, dioxins, and furans, can induce hepatic uridine diphosphonate glucuronyl transferase (UDPGT), resulting in a lower plasma T_4 concentration.[157]

Drugs Inhibiting Monodeiodination of Thyroxine

5′-Monodeiodinase type 1 is inhibited by several drugs, including propylthiouracil (PTU).[50] Dexamethasone and propranolol can also inhibit this enzyme.[158]

The β-receptor antagonist propranolol is used in the treatment of thyrotoxicosis to alleviate the manifestations of increased sympathetic activity, such as tremor. It is particularly useful in the treatment of thyrotoxic crisis. It can induce a modest reduction in plasma fT_3 concentration and a small increase in rT_3 concentration owing to the inhibition of hepatic monodeiodination, but the clinical benefit far exceeds what might be expected from the modest reduction in plasma T_3 concentrations. This effect is unique to propranolol and is not shared with other β-receptor antagonists or mixed β- and α-receptor antagonists such as labetalol.[159]

Drugs Affecting the Transport and Action of Thyroid Hormones

Many drugs inhibit the binding of T_4 and T_3 to the binding sites on the plasma transport proteins in vitro. These effects often require high concentrations of such drugs.

Nonsteroidal antiinflammatory drugs, including salicylate, inhibit T_4 and T_3 binding to both TBG and TTR.[160] Other nonsteroidals, such as fenclofenac, can displace T_4 from its binding site.[161] Enoxaparin and heparin affect the distribution of T_4 between plasma and its rapidly exchangeable tissue pools. This has been shown to be an in vitro effect caused by nonesterified fatty acid production by lipoprotein lipase released in vivo by heparin.[162]

Drugs Acting at More Than One Site

Some drugs interfere with the thyroid hormone homeostasis at various sites.

Amiodarone. Amiodarone is a class III antiarrhythmic drug that comprises 37% iodine by weight and has structural similarities with thyroid hormones. The drug has a long half-life, large distribution volume, and wide tissue distribution.[163] The mechanisms of amiodarone injury are multifactorial and involve accumulation of iodine, formation of free radicals, and immunologic injury.[163] The effects of amiodarone can be divided into effects occurring in everyone treated with amiodarone, resulting in changes in thyroid function tests ("obligatory effects"),[163] and effects only occurring in some people treated with amiodarone ("facultative effects"),[163] resulting in clinically overt thyrotoxicosis or hypothyroidism.[143,163]

During metabolism of amiodarone, large amounts of iodine are released into the plasma, but renal iodine clearance does not change, resulting in urinary iodine excretion 100 times higher than for the recommended daily iodine intake.[163] The iodine excess causes the thyroid to initially inhibit iodine organification (the Wolff-Chaikoff effect), thereby decreasing T_4 and T_3 production with a resulting TSH increase.[163] This effect can be interpreted as an autoregulatory response of the thyroid gland to avoid excessive production of thyroid hormone when exposed to high doses of exogenous iodine. Later, the thyroid escapes the Wolff-Chaikoff effect, resulting in TSH returning to baseline values after 3 months.[163] Amiodarone also inhibits type 1 deiodinase, resulting in decreased T_3 production and increased rT_3, and inhibits T_4 transport into the liver, resulting in decreased T_4 metabolism and consequently increased plasma T_4.[163] The changes in T_3 and T_4 are observed early during the amiodarone treatment and are sustained during the treatment; therefore, specific reference intervals should be used. In clinical practice, patients who are on long-term amiodarone should have TSH and thyroid antibodies measured at the beginning of therapy and fT_4 and TSH at 6-month intervals. It may take several months for normalization of thyroid function tests after discontinuation of amiodarone treatment.[163]

Amiodarone-induced thyrotoxicosis (AIT) is particularly prevalent (10%) in iodine-deficient regions, in men, and in patients with underlying thyroid disease (eg, nodular goiter or Graves disease).[163] AIT may occur at any time during treatment.[163] There are two types of AIT: type 1 is similar to classic iodine-induced excess of hormone synthesis in patients with preexisting thyroid abnormalities; type 2 resembles a subacute destructive thyroiditis with excess hormone release in patients with no previous thyroid disease, possibly owing to a direct cytotoxic effect of amiodarone. Color-flow Doppler sonography may be able to distinguish between the two types.[163] High-dose thionamides should be initiated in type 1 AIT.[143] Corticosteroids are effective in type 2 AIT.[143]

Amiodarone induced hypothyroidism occurs primarily in iodine-sufficient regions and in women with preexisting anti-TPO antibodies.[163] Amiodarone-induced hypothyroidism develops early after starting treatment.[163] It is thought this may be due to a direct inhibitory effect of the excess iodine supply leading to defective organification and subsequent hormone synthesis. If the patient has underlying disease (eg, Hashimoto thyroiditis, Graves disease), escape from the Wolff-Chaikoff effect is less likely, and permanent hypothyroidism can develop.[163] In addition, amiodarone and its main metabolite desethylamiodarone are weak antagonists of thyroid hormone actions.[163] Treatment of amiodarone-induced hypothyroidism is often challenging because the drug has a long and varying half-life because of mobilization of the drug from lipophilic stores.[163,164] The terminal half-life after cessation of therapy is approximately 40 ± 10 days for amiodarone and 57 ± 27 days for the main metabolite, desethylamiodarone.[163,164] Patients should be managed jointly by a cardiologist and an endocrinologist. In patients with amiodarone-induced hypothyroidism, there is no need to stop the amiodarone, but the patient should be prescribed levothyroxine.

Other Drugs Acting at More Than One Site. Dexamethasone also has multiple effects on the thyroid: It can suppress TSH secretion, reduce plasma T_3 concentration (owing to an inhibitory action on 5′-monodeiodination), and increase rT_3 production.[149,165] In Graves disease, it can reduce T_4

secretion, either by a direct thyroidal effect or by increasing thyroid-stimulating immunoglobulin production. It can also markedly decrease plasma T_3 concentrations.

Cytokines alter thyroid hormone secretion and metabolism. Administration of interferons and interleukins may cause drug-induced thyroiditis.[166,167]

Tyrosine kinase inhibitors are promising new agents used in advanced papillary and medullary thyroid cancer (MTC) when there is resistance to conventional chemotherapy.[168,169] In addition to the effect on cancer growth, they also have an effect on the thyroid gland, and patients treated with levothyroxine may need to increase their dosage. The potential mechanisms seem to be either impairment of enteral absorption, reduction of enterohepatic reabsorption, or increased deiodination and clearance of thyroxine.

Nonthyroidal Illness

Abnormal thyroid function test results are common in patients with both acute and chronic illness and in starvation.[141,170] They are features of a wider neuroendocrine response to illness and stress. The biochemical pattern is typically a low plasma fT_3 concentration with raised rT_3, so this condition is also known as the low fT_3 syndrome. However, with more severe or longstanding illness, plasma fT_4 can also be low with TSH concentrations that can be inappropriately normal or low, but generally are not reduced to the extent seen in hyperthyroidism. Whether fT_4 is genuinely low in nonthyroidal illness (NTI) or is a consequence of assay interference caused by compounds released during illness that can affect the binding of T_4 to its binding proteins remains controversial. Total T_4 is typically low, but reduction in T_4 binding protein concentrations and the possible cleavage of TBG by inflammatory proteases is a dominant contributor to this effect.

Reduced activity of hepatic D1 deiodinase is a major contributory factor to the low plasma fT_3 concentration seen in NTI.[141,170] Hepatic D1 expression is regulated by cytokines and possibly leptin, which may contribute to the starvation response.

The changes in TSH and possible changes in fT_4 are evidence of diminished hypothalamic function, which is well described in severe illness.[141,170] This is also likely to be mediated by cytokine effects, although the nature of these effects is currently poorly defined; a reduction in TRH secretion is a likely mechanism.

Whether the NTI syndrome confers any evolutionary benefit remains a topic of debate. This is more likely to be the case in acute illness or starvation, in which a reduction of energy expenditure may be beneficial but less plausible for the chronically ill patient and unlikely in critically ill patients. The magnitude of the change in thyroid function in NTI has prognostic value.[171] However, the use of thyroid hormone replacement in severely ill patients with NTI remains controversial.[141]

EVALUATION OF THYROID FUNCTION

Serum or Plasma Measurements

The widespread availability of high-sensitivity serum TSH assays is arguably one of the most impressive achievements of modern clinical chemistry. Serum TSH can be accurately measured at picomolar concentration, with minimal cross-reactivity with other highly homologous pituitary hormones present in serum. Given the classic endocrine feedback loop (see Fig. 67.6), TSH concentrations change logarithmically when the thyroid axis is perturbed. Consequently, in the majority of cases, a serum TSH measurement within the reference interval effectively excludes primary thyroid disease. Given the prevalence of thyroid disease and the often nonspecific symptoms, it has become one of the most popular clinical chemistry investigations. Historically, there has been considerable debate concerning the utility of TSH assay alone as a "first-line" test to exclude thyroid disease because measurement of thyroid hormone is also often required to establish a secure diagnosis.[172,173] Robust automated fT_4 assays, which estimate the biologically active fraction of circulating T_4, are also widely available, and a combination of these two assays is a very powerful tool for minimally invasive investigation of the pituitary–thyroid axis. The performance of fT_4 assays is equally impressive; these work in the picomolar (ng/dL) range and against a vast excess of bound thyroid hormone. However, the free hormone assay designs are complex and are based on theoretical and empirical assumptions. Clinical chemists and clinicians need to be aware of the limitations of these assays when interpreting thyroid function tests because overreliance on the numbers generated by these assays can be to the detriment of patient care, albeit in the minority of cases.

Historical nomenclature for both TSH and fT_4 assays is confusing and reflects serial improvements in assay design and performance. TSH assays have a "generational" nomenclature that describes improvement in assay sensitivity, which was required to establish the utility of the assay in hyperthyroid as well as hypothyroid patients. fT_4 assays have an array of terms to describe assay architecture. At this stage in assay development, it is unlikely that any further increase in TSH assay sensitivity will yield a proportionate gain in clinical utility but that there is scope to better harmonize the current TSH assays in clinical use. It also seems unlikely that the "perfect" fT_4 assay, which is truly independent of T_4 binding proteins, can be designed.[174]

Thyroid-Stimulating Hormone Reference Intervals

Because TSH is used as the primary marker of thyroid function, serum TSH concentrations must be interpreted against relevant reference intervals. Within individuals, TSH concentrations are remarkably constant with an intraindividual variation of approximately of 0.5 mIU/L. This is small given the population reference intervals quoted for TSH (eg, 0.35–5.0 mIU/L), so the "reference range" concept may need to be used with caution for TSH and comparison with previous results is likely to be more helpful.

Age, Gender, and Circadian Rhythm. There is little effect of age or gender[175] on TSH concentrations apart from at the extremes of age. The TSH surge during the neonatal period is well described. TSH concentrations can reach in excess of 80 mIU/L but typically drop to below 20 U/L in the first day of life, falling into the adult reference limits during the first month. The effect of old age on the TSH reference interval is a topic of active debate because these ranges are used to define the prevalence of hypo- and hyperthyroidism in this group. Current consensus is that the TSH reference limits increase with age and that the use of age-specific reference intervals is appropriate.[176]

Thyroid-stimulating hormone has a circadian rhythm with peak levels at around midnight and nadir in the morning through noon.[177] Sleep deprivation causes a rise in TSH. The circadian rhythm of TSH is lost during illness.

Thyroid-Stimulating Hormone Population Distribution. The distribution of plasma TSH concentrations in a healthy population is positively skewed. This may be due to "contamination" of the reference population with patients with autoimmune thyroid disease (AITD), which is evidenced by studies of autoimmune markers of thyroid disease in these participants. However, recent evidence suggests that physiological heterogeneity as well as the presence of subclinical disease is also likely to contribute to this asymmetry.[178,179]

What can be concluded from both the relatively wide interindividual variation and the non-Gaussian nature of the reference interval is that a "binomial" approach to TSH reference intervals is too simplistic and that borderline TSH concentrations need to be interpreted in context with clinical findings. Clinically specific cut points for TSH concentration have been proposed, above which intervention for primary hypothyroidism is likely to be beneficial.[180] However, providing a useful sensitive cut point to exclude evolving hypothyroidism is more challenging. One attempt is to define the TSH concentration below which the incidence of thyroid autoantibodies no longer increases. However, using this threshold, a large number of false diagnoses would be made in patients with no clinical evidence of AITD. Given indeterminate results, most authorities recommend periodic measurement of TSH.[180,181]

Measurement of TSH. The majority of clinical laboratories use immunometric assays to measure TSH in serum, typically with chemiluminescent probes and solid phase capture antibodies, and this format gives the required analytical sensitivity. Sensitivity of TSH assays is a major issue because it is necessary to measure well below the population reference interval to differentiate primary hyperthyroidism from other causes of low serum TSH concentration. The previously used "generational" concept for TSH assays is now largely redundant because clinical guidelines now specify the appropriate sensitivity required for TSH assays. In short, first-generation assays were sensitive enough only to discriminate normal from hypothyroid subjects; second-generation assays could detect TSH below the reference interval but not well enough to reliably discriminate primary hyperthyroidism from other causes of low TSH. This can be achieved with third-generation assays.[182] All assays in clinical practice should be "third generation," that is, they should have a coefficient of variation (CV) of less than 20% (functional sensitivity) at a concentration of 0.01 mIU/L.[183,184] It is beholden to the clinical chemist to be aware of and to monitor this aspect of the assay.

The specificity of TSH assays is largely of historical concern because modern assays show little cross-reactivity with the other highly homologous pituitary glycoprotein hormones despite sharing a common α-subunit.

Although the clinical performance of TSH assays is impressive, further challenges for the clinical chemist remain. This is because of the heterogeneity of the TSH molecule. The protein is 25% by mass glycosylated and the pituitary secretes a range of glycoforms that differ with thyroid status. This makes TSH assays difficult to standardize because a homogenous reference preparation will not accurately reflect all isoforms. Harmonization initiatives aiming at equivalence of thyroid function tests are ongoing by the International Federation of Clinical Chemistry and Laboratory Medicine (IFCC) to establish calibration traceability for thyroid hormones.[185-189] Currently, an international reference preparation is not available,[185,190] so it becomes difficult to establish true analytical sensitivity goals for TSH assays. Glycosylation status also affects the relation between TSH immunoreactivity and biologic activity. The utility of TSH immunoassay in secondary (pituitary) thyroid disease is greatly reduced because the pituitary can produce immunoreactive but biologically inactive TSH. This is often quoted as the reason that TSH alone cannot be used as a front-line screening strategy for thyroid disease. Bioassays for serum TSH concentration are available, but these are complex and difficult to standardize and are rarely used in clinical practice.[191]

Both serum and plasma are acceptable substrates for TSH immunoassay. TSH is stable in serum for at least five days at 4°C,[192] and at least 29 years at −25°C.[193]

Free Thyroid Hormones

Most authorities now subscribe to the "free hormone hypothesis," that is, that the measurement of non–protein-bound T_4 in circulation (fT_4) is a more accurate reflection of thyroid status than the total amount of T_4 (free plus bound T_4 or tT_4). This is because tT_4 concentrations are clearly influenced by changes in thyroid-binding proteins as well as HPT axis regulation. However, the measurement of fT_4 presents both theoretical and practical challenges, which limit the utility of this assay.[162,186,194,195] Unbound fT_4 is present in picomolar concentration in plasma and represents only about 0.03% of the total. fT_4 must be measured in spite of this vast excess of bound hormone and in the presence of other iodothyronines such as T_3. All current methods represent varying degrees of compromise because it is difficult to separate bound from free hormone without perturbing the equilibrium between the two species. Several assay designs have been established that have been given confusing and often nonstandard nomenclature.[174] Pragmatically, immunoassays for fT_4 have gained widespread popularity and clinical use, but an awareness of the limitations of these assays is required to prevent misdiagnosis.[162,186]

The first level of assay hierarchy is between "direct" methods, which use a physical separation of bound from free T_4, such as equilibrium dialysis or ultrafiltration, and indirect methods that estimate fT_4 in the presence of T_4 binding proteins. Of the indirect methods, immunoassay methods (see Chapter 23) are almost universally used in clinical chemistry laboratories. Immunoassays are further divided into one- and two-step methods depending on whether a wash step is included to remove serum constituents before the addition of the T_4 immunoassay tracer. Modern immunoassay methods are also "analog" because chemically modified T_4 probes are used rather than historic radiolabeled hormones.

Direct methods are conceptually easier to understand; fT_4 is separated from protein-bound T_4 using a physical method such as dialysis or ultrafiltration. Competitive immunoassay methods were originally used to measure T_4 in the protein-depleted fraction, but these methods are now being replaced with mass spectrometric methods. Although direct methods have been proposed for routine clinical use, the complexity and expense of these methods compared with the easily automatable indirect immunoassay methods has prevented wide-scale implementation of direct fT_4 assays. Dialysis has been proposed as a potential "gold standard" method for fT_4 analysis,[196] but these methods are not infallible and need to be used with caution. The conditions that determine the equilibrium between free and bound T_4 in vivo must be carefully maintained during dialysis. Serum components that have the ability to displace T_4 from its binding proteins represent a particular challenge because the relative concentration of these agents changes during the inevitable serum dilution that occurs after dialysis. Nonesterified fatty acids are the best described displacing agent; these are particularly challenging because they can be generated ex vivo because of the action of lipoprotein lipase.[162]

Indirect immunoassay methods make the assumption that the fT_4:tT_4 equilibrium is maintained during immunoassay to an extent sufficient to return a clinically relevant estimation of fT_4. One-step methods incubate the assay antibody and tracer in the presence of all serum constituents. Two-step or "back-titration" methods allow T_4 to equilibrate with the assay antibody in the presence of all serum components but wash away uncaptured components before back titrating with tracer. Although both methods sequester a significant amount of T_4 from the serum pool during assay, the fT_4:tT_4 equilibrium is maintained sufficiently to provide a reliable estimate of fT_4 under most conditions. Both methods will fail when the nature or concentration of T_4 binding proteins is significantly different in the analytical sample compared with the serum-based calibrator used. This is apparent in samples from patients with genetic abnormalities of thyroid-hormone binding proteins such as familial dysalbuminemic hyperthyroxinemia[69,197] and TBG or TTE deficiency or excess. These effects are assay dependent, with some assay designs more susceptible than others. Patients with autoantibodies generated against T_4 are well described; these antibodies are particularly problematic for one-step assays because they can sequester the immunoassay tracer, giving false-positive results.[197,198] Two-step assays are more resistant to this class of interference because the autoantibody is removed before the immunoassay tracer is added. Both labeled tracer and labeled antibody methods are currently used in clinical practice. Although labeled antibody methods have theoretical advantages in terms of assay sensitivity, susceptibility to anti T_4 antibodies and binding protein abnormalities remain an issue. Harmonization initiatives by the IFCC aim to establish calibration traceability, particularly for free hormones.[185-189]

Total Thyroxine and Triiodothyronine

Total thyroid hormone measurements are now largely used to confirm the results of fT_4 measurements when they are in doubt. Because total thyroid hormone is present in the serum in nanomolar concentrations, it is less of an analytical challenge than the measurement of free hormone. Mass spectrometric measurements are now the method of choice for total thyroid hormone analysis because this technique is relatively straightforward given the sensitivity and selectivity of modern mass spectrometers.[199-201] However competitive immunoassay is still in widespread use. These methods include a displacing agent such as 8-anilino-1-napthalene-sulfonic acid to release thyroid hormone from high-affinity serum binding sites; this is less of an issue for tT_3 methods owing to the weaker binding of T_4 to serum thyroid hormone–binding proteins. The efficiency of this process for tT_4 methods may contribute to relatively poor method comparisons both between immunoassay methods and between immunoassay and mass spectrometry.[187]

Thyroglobulin

Thyroglobulin is detectable in the plasma and as such acts as a marker for the presence of active thyroid tissue. Tg concentrations are determined by thyroid mass; TSH stimulation; and thyroid manipulation, including surgery, fine-needle aspiration (FNA), or thyroid injury.[202] The primary use of serum Tg measurement is as a tumor marker in patients with differentiated thyroid cancer (DTC) who have undergone thyroidectomy.[202] It is also used in the diagnosis of congenital hypothyroidism and may be of use in the differential diagnosis of factitious hyperthyroidism. It is notoriously difficult to measure Tg owing to the heterogeneity of the molecule, largely because of different glycoforms and because of the prevalence of endogenous anti-Tg or antireagent antibodies that interfere with the immunoassay. Current practice for thyroidectomized thyroid cancer patients is to withdraw thyroxine replacement to stimulate endogenous TSH secretion or to use recombinant human TSH to stimulate any residual or neoplastic thyroid tissue.[203] This can be inconvenient, unpleasant, and expensive. Consequently, a Tg assay with the sensitivity to detect Tg in the absence of TSH stimulation (ie, suppressed) is desirable.[204] Three methods are in current use, each with its own advantages and limitations.

- **Competitive immunoassay:** These methods are labor intensive and have lower sensitivity than immunometric assays (~5 ng/mL). However, they may be more robust to antibody interference than the immunometric assays.[205]
- **Immunometric assay:** These methods are now very sensitive (≤0.1 ng/mL) and amenable to automation[206,207] but are still subject to antibody interference. Different methods remain poorly standardized despite the availability of an international reference preparation.[208,209] Immunometric Tg assays should be reported together with anti-Tg results, and Tg should not be used as a tumor marker in the presence of anti-Tg antibodies owing to measurement interference.[210]
- **Peptide mass spectrometric assay**[211,212]: These assays are limited by the relatively poor analytical sensitivity and low available mass range of mass spectrometric methods. However, they offer the promise of robustness to antibody interference. Proteolytic digestion is required to generate specific peptides small enough for analysis. Some form of immunoconcentration step, either of the parent protein[213] or the specific proteolytic peptide,[214] is required to provide the desired analytical sensitivity. Sensitivities of 0.4 ng/mL are now achievable, which, although not as sensitive as immunometric assays, are sufficient for clinical use. The gain in robustness to antibody interference may outweigh the lower sensitivity; however, these methods are complex and are not widely available at the time of writing.

Antithyroid Peroxidase

Anti-TPO assays are in widespread use as a marker of AIDH because their presence is widely accepted as a risk factor for developing hypothyroidism.[215] Historically, TPO autoantibodies (anti-TPO) were detected as thyroid microsomal antibodies using agglutination or immunofluorescence methods. The principle autoantigen was found to be the membrane protein TPO as described earlier (see section on TPO), which led to the development of specific immunometric methods that are more easily automated. Immunometric methods are in widespread use, but despite the availability of an international reference preparation, methods do not agree well. Consequently, results from different assays cannot be compared.[216] Anti-TPO assay is a very sensitive marker for Hashimoto thyroiditis, and it has been implicated in the disease process.[217] The specificity of the assay is less well understood because it is dependent both on the assay and the population studied, being affected by age, gender, ethnicity, and iodine status. Serial measurement of anti-TPO is of little value because the treatment is aimed at the thyroid dysfunction rather than the autoimmune process.[218]

Anti–Thyroid-Stimulating Hormone Receptor Antibodies

The TSHR is a target for both blocking (anti-TSHRB) and stimulating autoantibodies (anti-TSHRS). Graves disease, which is the most common cause of hyperthyroidism in adults, is caused by anti-TSHRS. Competitive assays based on the ability of anti-TSHRB or anti-TSHRS to displace ligand from the TSHR (thyroid receptor binding or TRAb assays) cannot distinguish between these two classes of autoantibody. However, these assays have found clinical use because they have high sensitivity and specificity for the diagnosis of Graves disease.[219] Typically, these assays use a cloned TSHR with either labeled TSH or a labeled monoclonal anti-TSHR as the competitive ligand. TRAb assays are also in widespread use for the management of pregnant women with a history of Graves disease who are at risk of passing anti-TSHRB or anti-TSHRS transplacentally.

Patients who switch between having anti-TSHRB and anti-TSHRS, typically during treatment for thyroid disease, are well described.[220] In this context, the ability to distinguish between autoantibody classes could be useful because it helps decide to withdraw thyroid-blocking agents in a timelier manner. Bioassays based on the downstream effect of the activated TSHR to generate cyclic AMP have been devised that are specific for anti-TSHRB and anti-TSHRS.[221] Current assays use the cloned TSHR constructs linked to luciferase reporters.[222] Because these assays are more complex than the TRAb assays, they are largely confined to research rather than to clinical laboratories.

More recently, a genetically modified TSHR has been designed to be more specific for anti-TSHRS, and this has formed the basis of an anti-TSHRS immunoassay that could be run in a general clinical chemistry laboratory. Although losing the ability to detect anti-TSHRB, initial studies suggest an even greater diagnostic efficacy than for TRAb assays.[223]

Assay Interference

Despite improvement in assay design, the potential for assay interference remains an ongoing challenge for the clinical chemist. Antibody interference is an inherent risk for all immunoassays. Two antibody categories are responsible for interferences in thyroid hormone immunoassays. Autoantibodies particularly interfere with T_4, fT_4, T_3, and fT_3.[224] Heterophilic antibodies interfere particularly with TSH in immunometric assays and fT_4 in competitive assays.[224]

Antibody interference has been greatly reduced by attention to assay architecture and the use of blocking agents or modified antibodies.[224] The incidence of antibody interference is difficult to define and is likely to be method dependent. When suspected, there are several techniques that the clinical chemist can use to demonstrate the presence of this type of interference. However, identifying samples a priori at risk of this type of interference is a formidable challenge given the vast number of thyroid function tests performed. The incidence of assay interference in thyroid function tests is difficult to define, but it is estimated to be as high as 0.5%.[225]

Thyroid-Stimulating Hormone Assay Interference. Antibody interference can affect TSH immunometric assays in two ways. Heterophile or antianimal antibodies can bind to reagent antibodies, causing blocking (negative) or cross-linking (positive) interference.[226,227] Heterophilic antibodies can also be directed against TSH itself. These so-called "macro-TSH" complexes[228] are likely to be immunoreactive but biologically inactive. Method comparison, linearity and recovery studies, immunosubtraction, and gel filtration chromatography methods have all been used to identify this type of interference, but it can be difficult to return an accurate value for biologically active TSH in this situation.

Free Thyroxine Assay Interference. As discussed earlier, fT_4 immunoassays are more prone to assay interference than TSH assays owing to the more complex assay design. As with TSH, assays for fT_4 can be affected by heterophile or anti-animal interference that blocks T_4 binding to the assay reagents (given a false-positive result owing to the competitive assay design) or by antianalyte antibodies (endogenous anti- T_4 antibodies) sequestering the T_4 tracer, again giving a false-positive result.[197,198] The fT_4 assay is also susceptible to factors that perturb the binding of T_4 to its binding proteins during assay conditions. These can be inherited or acquired changes in binding proteins, such as familial dysalbuminemic hyperthyroxinemia (FDH),[69] or the presence of agents that can displace T_4 from its binding proteins. The effect on non-esterified fatty acid (NEFA) generation of heparin and drugs such as phenytoin, which can displace T_4 from albumin, is well described.[162,229] Careful method comparison studies can expose these shortcomings, providing the methods use different assay designs. Physical separation methods such as equilibrium dialysis or ultrafiltration are often cited as gold standard methods, but these too can be affected by displacing agents. The use of total T_4 assay along with TBG estimation can also be useful in this situation.[162]

Algorithm for Laboratory Evaluation of Thyroid Function

The majority of thyroid function tests are easy to interpret and will confirm a clinical suspicion of hyper- or hypothyroidism or rule out thyroid disease with good accuracy. The relationship between TSH and fT_4 has traditionally been described as log-linear (Fig. 67.11); however, the dogma is now being challenged and debated using large epidemiologic studies to describe other mathematical models for the relationship.[230-232] However, given the widespread use of these tests a significant number of results appear confusing, either because they are at odds with clinical findings or the TSH and fT_4 results are discordant. Such results need careful consideration to prevent misdiagnosis[233-235] (Fig. 67.12). Medications (see Table 67.6), intercurrent illness, and physiological changes such as pregnancy can affect thyroid function tests. Assay interference should also be considered as a possible cause

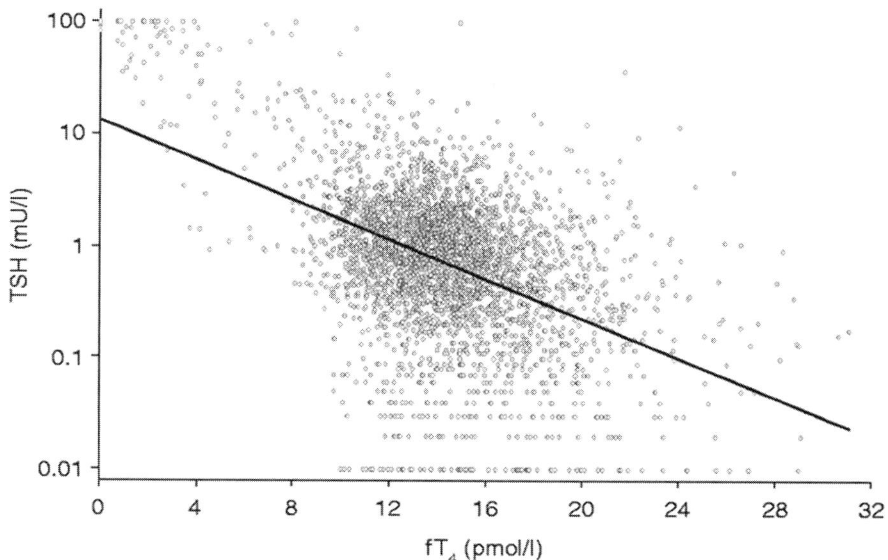

FIGURE 67.11 The log-linear relationship between thyroid-stimulating hormone (TSH) and free thyroxine (fT_4) concentrations in plasma. The *lines* represent the linear regression fitted to the data points. (Modified from Hoermann R, Eckl W, Hoermann C, Larisch R. Complex relationship between free thyroxine and TSH in the regulation of thyroid function. *Eur J Endocrinol* 2010;162:1123–1129.)

of incorrect results. If these are excluded, the possibility of rare genetic and acquired disorders of the HPT axis such as resistance to thyroid hormone or thyrotropinoma (TSHoma) should be considered.

Some general principles are outlined:

1. A plasma TSH concentration within the reference interval excludes primary thyroid disease with good accuracy in most cases. However, TSH will not return an accurate assessment of the HPT axis in the following situations and should not be used alone without a reasonable degree of confidence that these conditions do not exist:
   - Recent treatment for thyrotoxicosis (TSH may remain suppressed even when thyroid hormone concentrations have normalized.)
   - Nonthyroidal illness
   - Medications such as glucocorticoids will transiently depress TSH
   - Central hypothyroidism (eg, hypothalamic and pituitary disorders)
   - TSH-secreting pituitary adenoma (TSHoma)
   - Resistance to thyroid hormone
   - Disorders of thyroid hormone transport or metabolism.

   It is worth considering the relatively wide between-subject variation in TSH and the effects of extremes of age when considering a reference interval with which to compare TSH result, as discussed earlier.
2. TSH and fT_4 concentrations in plasma have an approximately log-linear relation (see Fig. 67.11); paired and consecutive results should be interpreted accordingly. Again, because of the wide interindividual variation of fT_4, comparison with previous results is likely to be more valuable than the use of generic reference intervals. In primary thyroid disease, TSH is likely to change before fT_4 as the axis attempts to restore homeostasis; this leads to the diagnosis of subclinical disease in which TSH is out of the reference interval, but fT_4 is not.[180]
3. Consider the use of additional tests. If TSH is undetectable in patients not on treatment, fT_3 aids the diagnosis of T_3 toxicosis. TRAb has a high sensitivity and specificity for Graves disease. In subclinical disease, consider the use of antithyroid antibody measurement if TSH is elevated because this has prognostic information and can be used to determine retesting intervals.
4. If TSH and fT_4 are discordant, take into account or reassess clinical findings and the a priori odds of these conditions.
5. Patients treated with T_4. To abolish symptoms and normalize TSH concentrations, some individuals return borderline elevated fT_4 concentrations. This may be due to less efficient deiodination of T_4 to T_3. In this situation, fT_3 is typically within the reference interval, which provides reassurance.

The combination of a normal plasma TSH concentration with a slightly elevated fT_4 is most commonly seen in patients on thyroid hormone replacement. Aside from this, the differential diagnosis includes the genetic conditions FDH and THR, and also TSH-secreting pituitary tumours.[233,234]

Familial dysalbuminemic hyperthyroxinemia results in an assay artefact, to which most current fT_4 assays are susceptible to a variable degree.[69,197] In the most common form of FDH (R218H), fT_3 is typically within the reference interval. (Two other forms, L66P and R218P, are associated with elevated T_3 and both elevated T_3 and T_4, respectively.)

Measurement of Urinary Iodine Concentration

The population status of iodine intake is best determined by measurements of UIC.[88,236] Because most of the body's iodine is excreted in urine, UIC is considered a reliable and valid

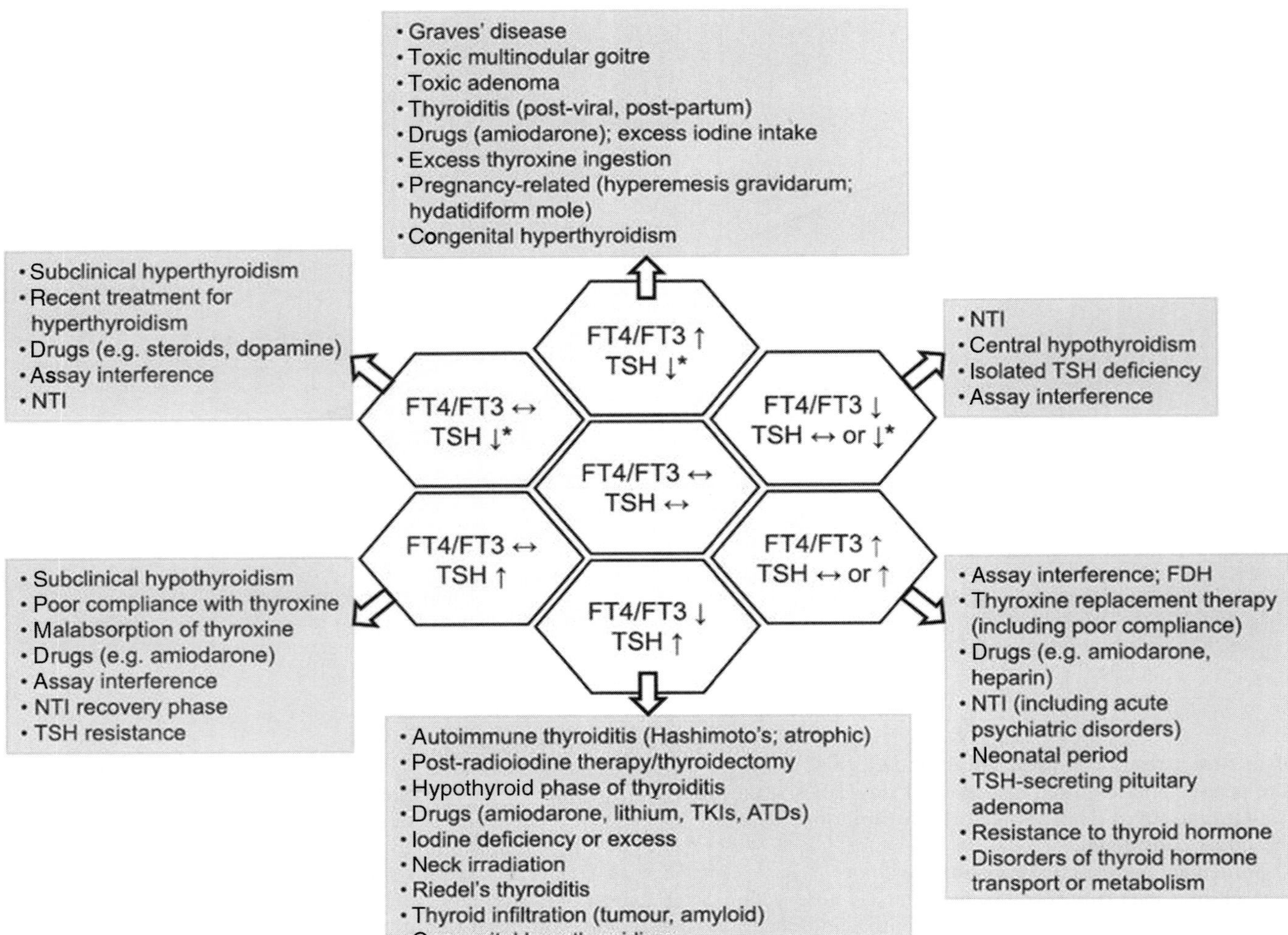

FIGURE 67.12 An algorithm to guide interpretation of thyroid function tests. Different patterns of thyroid function tests and their causes. The *asterisk* signifies that thyroid-stimulating hormone (TSH; thyrotropin) may be either fully suppressed (eg, as seen in classic primary hyperthyroidism) or partially suppressed (ie, measurable but below the lower limit of the reference interval). *ATD,* Antithyroid drug; *FDH,* familial dysalbuminemic hyperthyroxinemia; *FT_4,* free thyroxine; *FT_3,* free triiodothyronine; *NTI,* nonthyroidal illness; TKI, tyrosine kinase inhibitor. (Reproduced from Koulouri O, Gurnell M. How to interpret thyroid function tests. *Clin Med 2013*;13:282–286. Copyright Royal College of Physicians.)

biomarker of the iodine intake and iodine deficiency of the population. Secondary measurements for estimating iodine deficiency are thyroid size, TSH concentration, and thyroid hormones.[88]

The gold standard is 24-hour urine collection. However, in large-scale epidemiologic studies, a random spot urinary measurement is preferred.[237] This is considered to provide a reliable and valid estimate considering the costs, feasibility, and patient convenience.[237] The iodine concentration can be expressed in relation to urinary creatinine excretion or as UIC per liter. Even though the UIC/Cr measurement corrects for the day-to-day variability in iodine intake, water consumption, and the equilibration time for iodine,[236,238] the UIC per liter is the most widely used and internationally accepted form of expression of results.[88] UIC show circadian rhythmicity independent of age, gender, and season[239] with the lowest values in the morning between 8:00 and 11:00 AM increasing progressively between noon and midnight before falling and with intermediate peaks 4 to 5 hours after main meals.[239] The circadian rhythmicity of UIC is important to take into consideration in multinational population studies because morning measurements may not be directly comparable to measurements at other times of the day.[237]

The laboratory tests are collectively called urinary iodine tests, although technically is an assessment of urinary iodide anion concentration. There are several urinary iodine methods with overall good intermethod agreement and acceptable performance characteristics,[240] which are important in multinational comparison studies of iodine intake. Most methods are based on the sensitive colorimetric method of the Sandell–Kolthoff reaction[241] in which urine is first acid digested under mild conditions and iodine is then determined by a catalytic reduction of ceric ammonium sulfate (yellow) to the colorless cerous form in the presence of arsenious acid.[237] The inductively coupled plasma mass spectrometry method has a lower limit of detection.[240]

Imaging the Thyroid

Radionuclide imaging and uptake studies of the thyroid gland were once frequently used in the investigation of thyroid disease, but owing to the availability of ultrasound imaging and FNA and biopsy, they are now of less importance. However, there has been a considerable growth in the use of photon emission computed tomography (PECT) imaging to improve the detection and follow-up of thyroid cancers of a variety of types, especially PECT/computed tomography (CT) imaging with fluro-2-deoxy-D-glucose.

With the proliferation of imaging tests such as CT, magnetic resonance imaging (MRI), and carotid ultrasonography as well as great availability of diagnostic ultrasound devices in primary care and endocrinology doctors' offices, there has been an increase in the detection of incidental nonpalpable thyroid nodules. A small but significant fraction of these nodules is malignant. There is much debate that some of these smaller cancers may not be clinically relevant.[242] Thyroid cancer incidence rates have increased nearly threefold in the past 20 years with very much (but not all) of the increase being cancers smaller than 1 cm in diameter.

Thyroid ultrasonography can demonstrate the type of thyroid enlargement (diffuse or localized) and nature, solid or cystic, single or multiple, thyroid nodules (Table 67.7). Benign nodules (thyroid adenomas, hyperplastic nodules) are hypoechoic relative to normal thyroid tissue, but so are thyroid carcinomas, and the two cannot be distinguished reliably on the basis of size; degree of echogenicity; or presence of a sonographic halo, calcification or vascularization. To do this requires FNA or biopsy of the nodule under ultrasound guidance. Table 67.7 summarizes low- versus high-risk features on ultrasonography. The coexistence of two or more suspicious criteria on ultrasonography greatly increases the risk of thyroid cancer.[243]

TABLE 67.7 Ultrasonography Criteria Assessing Risk of Thyroid Nodule

Features	Low Risk	High Risk
Margins	Well defined*	Poorly defined
Shape	Regular	Irregular
Taller than wide	No	Yes
Microcalcifications	Absent	Present
Echogenicity	Isoechoic or hyperechoic Inhomogenous	Hypoechoic
Structure	Cystic, spongiform, or mixed	Solid
Color-flow Doppler	Peripheral	Intranodular, chaotic
Elastography†	"Low score" (high elasticity)	"High score" (low elasticity)
Pathogenic lymph nodes	Absent	Present

*Eventually with the presence of a peripheral halo. Size is not a reliable predictor of malignancy.

†Elastography requires further evaluation

Modified from Hegedus L. Non isotope techniques of thyroid imaging. In: Braverman LE, Cooper DS, editors. *Werner & Ingbar's The Thyroid.* 10th ed. Philadelphia: Lippincott, Williams & Wilkins; 2012:313. Copyright Lippincott, Williams & Wilkins.

The American Thyroid Association (ATA) in its 2009 Clinical Practice Guidelines recommends that "thyroid sonography should be performed in all patients with known or suspected thyroid nodules." The summary of their recommendations[210] suggests that thyroid ultrasonography should be performed on all patients with known or suspected nodular thyroid disease and should also be used as a screening tool on high-risk patients (eg, history of childhood neck radiation, family history of MTC and multiple endocrine neoplasia [MEN] II).[244]

Real-time ultrasound elastography is a newly developed technique to study the hardness and elasticity of nodules in an effort to differentiate malignant nodules from benign. The majority of thyroid cancers (90%) are solid rather than cystic. Color-flow Doppler sonography is also increasingly being use to distinguish between type I (increased uptake) and type II (decreased or absent uptake) AIT.

The major nuclide imaging agents for thyroid disease have typically been radioactive iodine radioisotopes (^{131}I, ^{123}I, and more recently ^{124}I [PET tracer]).^{99m} Tc pertechnetate (TcO_4^-) is now used extensively. ^{99m}Tc is given intravenously as pertechnetate and is initially concentrated within the gland but is not organified into thyroid hormones and therefore diffuses out of the gland. This fact along with the short half-life of the isotope mean that large doses can be administered without delivery of a high radiation dose to the thyroid. The disadvantages of using ^{99m}Tc are that it cannot reliably be used to identify retrosternal glands, and it does not give information regarding iodine organification.

The use of radioisotopes of iodine (eg, ^{123}I) bypasses this latter problem. ^{123}I delivers a much lower total radiation dose to the gland than the other iodine isotopes and is used when imaging the thyroid tissue in its normal site. The isotope ^{131}I has higher energy and a longer half-life and is useful when deep thyroid tissue is sought or when there is a need to detect functionally active metastatic thyroid carcinoma and treat it by irradiation.

Although quantitative radioactive iodine uptake (RAIU) studies have been superseded by biochemical tests of thyroid function, they may still be useful in identifying patients with hyperthyroidism and negligible uptake (painless thyroiditis) and hyperthyroid patients after treatment with amiodarone for whom ^{131}I therapy would be inappropriate.

Perchlorate Discharge Test

Very rarely, hypothyroidism or goiter results from enzyme defects responsible for the incorporation of iodine into thyroid hormone. In such cases, iodine will be trapped within the thyrocytes but not organified. The perchlorate discharge test[62] can be used to detect defects in iodine oxidation or the iodination of Tg.

Under normal circumstances, iodide ions are rapidly transported into the thyroid gland via NIS. The NIS also concentrates other anions within the thyroid gland, such as thiocyanate (SCN^-), pertechnetate (TcO_4^-), and perchlorate (ClO_4^-). After a dose of labeled perchlorate, if there is an enzyme defect, a supranormal amount of radioiodine is released from the thyroid gland, and the perchlorate discharge of radioiodine is increased. If there is a defect in the NIS (eg, a loss of function mutation), the release of radioiodine is not increased after perchlorate because radioiodine was not initially taken up by the thyroid gland.

POINTS TO REMEMBER

Questions to Ask When Interpreting Thyroid Function Test Results

- Are the results consistent with clinical findings?
- Are the results typical for a particular thyroid disease?
- Any medications that may explain discordant results?
- Any physiological or pathological confounders?
- Consider the use of additional tests (eg, fT_3, TPOAb, TRAb).
- Consider assay interference or rare acquired or genetic pituitary or thyroid syndromes.

THYROID DISEASE

Thyroiditis

Thyroiditis means inflammation of the thyroid. Thyroiditis encompasses many thyroid disorders, some of which have an autoimmune etiology, including Hashimoto thyroiditis, painless sporadic thyroiditis, and painless postpartum thyroiditis[166] (Table 67.8). The prevalence of individuals with high serum concentrations of thyroid antibodies varies with gender, age, and ethnicity[132]; the prevalence is higher in women, in people older than 60 years of age, and in whites. It has been suggested that dietary iodine deficiency may be protective against certain types of thyroiditis because of the geographical variations in incidence seen in Hashimoto thyroiditis, painless postpartum thyroiditis, and painless sporadic thyroiditis.[245,246]

TABLE 67.8 Types of Autoimmune Thyroiditis

	Course	Features
Goitrous (Hashimoto) thyroiditis	Chronic	Goiter, lymphocytic infiltration, fibrosis, thyroid cell hyperplasia
Atrophic thyroiditis (primary myxedema)	Chronic	Atrophy, fibrosis
Juvenile thyroiditis	Chronic (may disappear)	Usually lymphocytic infiltration
Postpartum thyroiditis	Transient: may progress to chronic thyroiditis	Small goiter; some lymphocytic infiltration
Silent (painless) thyroiditis	Transient	Small goiter; some lymphocytic infiltration
Focal thyroiditis	Progressive in some patients	Present in the thyroid glands of 20% of people at autopsy

Reproduced from Weetman AP. Chronic autoimmune thyroiditis. In: Braverman LE, Cooper DS, editors. *Werner & Ingbar's The Thyroid.* 10th ed. Philadelphia: Lippincott, Williams & Wilkins; 2012:56. Copyright Lippincott, Williams & Wilkins.

The different types of thyroiditis may cause thyrotoxicosis, hypothyroidism, or both.[166] All types of thyroiditis may eventually progress to permanent hypothyroidism, and the risk is higher in patients with high serum thyroid antibody concentrations.[247-249] As thyroid function declines, TSH secretion increases, resulting in SCH (elevated TSH, normal T_4 and T_3), and later in overt hypothyroidism with clearly elevated TSH and a preferential expression of T3 but low T_4, and finally, in thyroid failure also low T_3.[166]

Painless Sporadic Thyroiditis, Painless Postpartum Thyroiditis, and Painful Subacute Thyroiditis

Painless sporadic thyroiditis (synonyms: silent sporadic thyroiditis, subacute lymphocytic thyroiditis), painless postpartum thyroiditis (synonyms: postpartum thyroiditis, subacute lymphocytic thyroiditis), and painful subacute thyroiditis (synonym: De Quervain thyroiditis) are pathologically characterized by lymphocytic infiltration in the first two and giant cells and granulomas in the third.[166,250] The inflammatory destruction of the thyroid in these conditions leads to release of preformed thyroid hormones from the damaged gland, leading to a transient thyrotoxicosis. Subsequently, patients become euthyroid, but hypothyroidism develops as the thyroid hormone stores are depleted. An increased plasma concentration of Tg is an early biomarker of inflammatory thyroiditis.[251] The thyrotoxicosis is characterized by decreased TSH and a preferential increase in T_4 in comparison with T_3, reflecting the release of the stored thyroid hormone. The signs and symptoms of thyrotoxicosis in thyroiditis are usually mild. Painless sporadic thyroiditis and painless postpartum thyroiditis are similar except that the latter occurs following pregnancy.[166]

Painless Postpartum Thyroiditis. The term *postpartum thyroiditis* refers to destructive thyroiditis occurring the first 12 months postpartum and *not* to Graves disease, although the two conditions may occur together. The immunologic damage to the thyroid is mediated by complement- and lymphocyte-associated mechanisms.[166] Approximately 4% to 9% of unselected postpartum women develop postpartum thyroiditis,[252,253] although the incidence varies with geographical location. Of women who are euthyroid in the first trimester of pregnancy but test positive for thyroid autoantibodies, 50% will develop postpartum thyroiditis.[252,253] Furthermore, postpartum thyroiditis has been associated with specific human leukocyte antigen (HLA) haplotypes.[254]

Approximately 20% of women develop a triphasic pattern, 50% of women develop isolated hypothyroidism, and 30% develop isolated thyrotoxicosis.[166,252] There is an increased incidence of postpartum thyroiditis in women with Graves disease, type 1 diabetes, chronic viral hepatitis, and systemic lupus erythematosus.[166] The severity of symptoms varies. The thyrotoxic phase is relatively asymptomatic, and the patient may have palpitations and tachycardia. The hypothyroid phase may be more clinically apparent. Postpartum thyroiditis thyrotoxicosis is more common than Graves disease thyrotoxicosis postpartum.[253] The presence of TRAb points toward thyrotoxicosis caused by Graves disease and helps in differentiating it from postpartum thyroiditis thyrotoxicosis.[255] Because there is no excess thyroid hormone production in painless postpartum thyroiditis, antithyroid drugs are contraindicated, but if thyrotoxicosis is severe, it is treated with beta-blockers. Levothyroxine is indicated if plasma TSH is greater than 10.0 mIU/L.[256]

Although the thyrotoxicosis in postpartum thyroiditis always resolves, several long-term studies of the hypothyroid phase show persistence of hypothyroidism in up to 30% of cases.[252] It has been estimated that 50% of women who develop postpartum thyroiditis remained hypothyroid at 1 year after delivery.[257] Women with a previous history of postpartum thyroiditis should have TSH concentration measured annually owing to the increased risk of developing permanent hypothyroidism.[258] Women who are known to be TPO antibody positive should have TSH measured at 6 to 12 weeks of gestation and again at 6 months postpartum if not otherwise clinically indicated.[258]

Painful Subacute Thyroiditis. Painful subacute thyroiditis (De Quervain thyroiditis) usually occurs (2–8 weeks) after a viral upper respiratory tract infection (Coxsackie virus, mumps, measles, adenovirus, and other viral infections).[259] Treatment is symptomatic. Clinical features may include neck pain, swelling, and fever, usually preceded by a prodromal phase with myalgias, pharyngitis, mildly elevated temperature, and fatigue.[166] Approximately half of affected patients have thyrotoxicosis, followed after several weeks by hypothyroidism; the majority recover to normal thyroid function after 3 to 6 months, but late relapses sometimes occur.

Suppurative Thyroiditis

Suppurative thyroiditis is rare and caused by bacterial infection, fungal, or parasitic infections.[166] TPO antibodies are absent, and patients are usually euthyroid. Treatment is with appropriate antibiotics.

Hashimoto Thyroiditis

Hashimoto thyroiditis was first described in 1912 by Hakaru Hashimoto, a Japanese physician.[22,260] Also known as chronic lymphocytic thyroiditis, Hashimoto thyroiditis is the most common type of thyroiditis and in iodine-sufficient areas also the most frequent cause of hypothyroidism and goiter. It leads to the destruction of thyroid follicular cells through a T-cell–mediated autoimmune process.[166,261] Histologically, the gland is infiltrated with lymphocytes and plasma cells, which can lead to the development of secondary lymphoid follicles within the gland which are similar to the secondary follicles observed in normal lymph nodes. The initial finding is usually a firm, symmetric goiter, but over time, the gland can atrophy, reflecting destruction of the gland. The gland may often be lobulated, which sometimes makes it difficult to distinguish from multinodular goiter. Although atrophy may occur in Hashimoto thyroiditis, atrophic thyroiditis may also occur when autoantibodies against the TSHR bind to the receptor and block the action of endogenous TSH. TSHR-blocking autoantibodies can cross the placenta during pregnancy, causing transient hyperthyrotropinemia in infants (elevated TSH with a normal T_4) or even transient congenital hypothyroidism. Therefore, atrophic thyroiditis falls into the spectrum of AITDs.

The diagnosis of Hashimoto thyroiditis is supported by recognition of autoantibodies against TPO (anti-TPO) or Tg (anti-Tg).[66] Ninety percent of patients with chronic lymphocytic thyroiditis (the histologic description of Hashimoto thyroiditis) have anti-TPO at presentation, and 20% to 50% have anti-Tg autoantibodies, making these autoantibodies excellent markers for the condition.[166,262] The thyroid is hypoechogenic on ultrasound examination.

If overt hypothyroidism is present or SCH with high serum thyroid antibody concentrations, patients should be treated with levothyroxine with the goal of normalizing TSH. TSH-suppressing doses can be used short term to reduce goiter size.[166] TSH should be used for monitoring. Serum thyroid antibody concentrations do not decrease with treatment.

There is a strong association between Hashimoto thyroiditis and primary B-cell lymphoma of the thyroid, although this is a rare condition.[263] It is thought that prolonged stimulation of the intrathyroid B cells results in the emergence of a malignant clone. In addition, the frequency of papillary carcinoma may be increased in chronic autoimmune thyroiditis, particularly in women.[264] Pain may indicate the presence of lymphoma. FNA biopsy or surgical biopsy may be required to distinguish between these conditions.

Riedel's Thyroiditis

In this rare condition (also known as Riedel disease or chronic fibrous thyroiditis), the thyroid gland can become fibrotic with possible attachment to adjacent structures that can produce, for example, tracheal compression. Riedel thyroiditis occurs in 0.05% of people with thyroid disease.[166] Painful subacute thyroiditis can also lead to Riedel thyroiditis.[265] It is now believed that Riedel thyroiditis is part of the IgG4-related systemic sclerosing disease spectrum associated with multisystem fibrosis which is also related to Hashimoto thyroiditis.[266-268] The etiology of Riedel thyroiditis is uncertain, although an autoimmune basis has been suggested because of the presence of thyroid antibodies as well as histologic finding of lymphocytes and plasma cells.[267,269] At presentation, most patients are euthyroid, but they become hypothyroid as fibrosis replaces thyroid tissue. The diagnosis is by open biopsy. Treatment is surgical, but immunosuppressants may be effective in the early stages of disease.[166,267]

Autoimmune Thyroid Disease

Autoimmune thyroid disease comprises two main diseases, Hashimoto thyroiditis and Graves disease.[261] The prevalence is estimated to be 5%, but the prevalence of thyroid antibodies in the general population is 10% to 20%.[248,270] AITD is a T cell–mediated disorder leading to an immune attack of the thyroid in an individual with genetic susceptibility accompanied by environmental factors.[261] Examples of factors that increase the risk of AITD include ethnicity, pollutants (smoking, radioiodine), dietary (iodine excess, selenium deficiency), endocrine (female gender, parity, postpartum, oral contraceptives), infections, drugs, and trauma.[271,272]

Pathologically, AITD is characterized by lymphocyte infiltrates within the thyroid. AITD is associated with other autoimmune diseases, either organ specific (autoimmune polyglandular syndromes) or systemic (type 1 diabetes, rheumatoid arthritis, systemic lupus erythematosus, Sjögren syndrome, systemic sclerosis, cryoglobulinemia, sarcoidosis, psoriatic arthritis)[261]; these associations reflect common genetic susceptibilities and common pathogenic mechanisms.[261] Autoimmune disease is also associated with papillary thyroid cancer.[273,274]

Polyglandular Autoimmune Syndromes

Polyglandular autoimmune syndromes (PAS) are rare polyendocrinopathies. PAS is characterized by the failure of at least two endocrine glands (but often several) caused by an immune-mediated destruction of endocrine tissues (eg, thyroid), but failure of nonendocrine organs may also occur.[275,276] Based on age at onset, gender, genetics, autoimmune endocrinopathies, and nonendocrine autoimmune disorders, the syndromes can be divided into two major subtypes: type I (with childhood onset) and type II (with adult onset). Incidence of type I is less than 1 in 100,000 per year. Type II is more common with an incidence of 1 or 2 per 100,000 per year. The order in which the endocrinopathies occur in PAS II vary, but typically type 1 diabetes mellitus is diagnosed first (50% of patients).[275] The most common combination of the endocrinopathies in PAS II is type 1 diabetes and AITD (40% of patients).[275] Schmidt syndrome refers to the combination of autoimmune adrenal insufficiency (Addison disease) with autoimmune hypothyroidism or type 1 diabetes mellitus.[275]

Hypothyroidism

Hypothyroidism is defined as a deficiency in thyroid hormone production or secretion producing a variety of clinical signs and symptoms of hypometabolism. The term *myxoedema* is used in severe or complicated cases but strictly refers only to the appearance of the skin as it becomes infiltrated with glycosaminoglycans.[277]

Hypothyroidism is a common endocrine disorder that is often overlooked but often may present with serious signs and symptoms. The disorder is treatable with a good prognosis.

Hypothyroidism (Boxes 67.2 and 67.3) can be classified according to:

- Age of onset (congenital or acquired)
- HPT level (primary (defect in the thyroid),or secondary (defect in the hypothalamus or pituitary gland, also called central hypothyroidism)
- Severity (overt [clinical], mild [subclinical])
- And duration (permanent or transient)[277]

BOX 67.2 Causes of Hypothyroidism

Primary Hypothyroidism
Thyroid dysgenesis
Destruction of thyroid tissue
Chronic autoimmune thyroiditis: atrophic and goitrous forms
Radiation: ^{131}I therapy for thyrotoxicosis, external radiotherapy to the head and neck for nonthyroid malignant disease
Subtotal and total thyroidectomy
Infiltrative diseases of the thyroid (amyloidosis, sarcoid, lymphoma, hemochromatosis, scleroderma)
Defective thyroid hormone biosynthesis
Congenital defects in thyroid hormonal biosynthesis
Iodine deficiency
Drugs with antithyroid actions: lithium, iodine and iodine-containing drugs, radiographic contrast agents

Central Hypothyroidism (Secondary Hypothyroidism)
Pituitary disease
Hypothalamic disease

Transient Hypothyroidism
Silent (painless) thyroiditis including postpartum thyroiditis
Subacute thyroiditis (De Quervain syndrome)

Epidemiology

A metaanalysis of European studies showed that the prevalence of undiagnosed hypothyroidism was about 5%, the prevalence of previously diagnosed hypothyroidism was about 3%, and the incidence rate of hypothyroidism was about 226 per 100,000 per year.[278] Worldwide, the most common cause of hypothyroidism is still iodine deficiency.[58,103] However, in developed countries where iodine fortification is widespread, the most common cause of primary hypothyroidism is Hashimoto thyroiditis. Hypothyroidism is more common in women than men, increases with age, and is higher in whites than in blacks or Hispanics.[132,249,279]

Etiology

Hypothyroidism has many etiologies[277] (some of which are described in other sections of this chapter), including thyroiditis and in particular autoimmune thyroiditis, postpartum phase, drugs, previous thyroid injury, hypothalamic or pituitary disorders in central hypothyroidism, and iodine deficiency. Congenital hypothyroidism is discussed in a separate section.

BOX 67.3 Primary Hypothyroidism From Other Causes

Thyroid ablation
Radioactive iodine therapy or surgery for
- Graves disease
- Thyrotoxicosis
- Toxic nodular goiter

External radiotherapy for
- Hodgkin and non-Hodgkin lymphoma
- Solid cancers of the head and neck
- Aplastic anemia
- Leukemia

Pharmacologic agents
- Lithium carbonate
- Cytokines (interferon-α, interleukin-2)
- Tyrosine kinase inhibitors
- Amiodarone
- Other drugs: aminoglutethimide, ethionamide, sulfonamides

Infiltrative disorders
- Riedel (invasive fibrous) thyroiditis
- Amyloidosis
- Sarcoidosis
- Hemochromatosis
- Scleroderma
- Cystinosis
- AIDS (including *Pneumocystis* infection)
- Primary thyroid lymphoma

Toxic substances
- Cigarettes
- Industrial and environmental agents

Embryological variants
- Lingual thyroid

Reproduced from Singer PA. Primary hypothyroidism due to other causes. In: Braverman LE, Cooper DS, editors. *Werner & Ingbar's The Thyroid.* 10th ed. Philadelphia: Lippincott, Williams & Wilkins; 2013:552. Copyright Lippincott, Williams & Wilkins.

POINTS TO REMEMBER

Hypothyroidism
- Hypothyroidism is the commonest disorder of thyroid function.
- It is more common in women, and the risk of developing hypothyroidism increases with age.
- Hypothyroidism is a known risk factor for cardiovascular disease.
- Excluding the newborn period and iodine deficiency, AITD is the most common cause of primary hypothyroidism.
- Central hypothyroidism (TSH deficiency) is a rare cause of hypothyroidism.

Previous Thyroid Injury. Acquired primary hypothyroidism may be caused by previous thyroid injury as a result of surgery (thyroidectomy for thyroid cancer) or irradiation (for head and neck malignancy), radioactive iodine therapy for thyrotoxicosis (Graves disease or toxic nodular goiter), or environmental exposure to radioiodine.

Central Hypothyroidism. Central hypothyroidism is caused by an insufficient stimulation by TSH of an otherwise normal thyroid gland.[280] The prevalence is estimated to be 1 in 20,000 to 1 in 80,000 in the general population, accounting for 1 in 1000 hypothyroid patients.[280,281] Neonatal screening programs have shown a prevalence of congenital hypothyroidism of central origin of 1 in 160,000.[282] In the Netherlands, the neonatal screening program using a combined TBG, TSH, and T_4 strategy has shown that central hypothyroidism is diagnosed earlier with milder forms with an incidence of 1 in 16,000.[283]

Central hypothyroidism may arise from pituitary disorders (secondary) or hypothalamic (tertiary) disorders including the pituitary stalk (Box 67.4). Tertiary hypothyroidism is a result of insufficient TSH stimulation by TRH. Anti-POU1F1 (anti-PIT-1) is a unique autoantibody against pituitary transcription factor PIT-1. It is detectable in patients with an acquired combined pituitary hormone deficiency characterized by specific defect in growth hormone (GH), prolactin, and TSH.[284]

Central hypothyroidism can be classified into invasive or compressive lesions, iatrogenic factors (eg, cranial surgery or irradiation), injuries (eg, head traumas), vascular accidents (eg, pituitary apoplexia, postpartum pituitary [Sheehan] syndrome), autoimmune disease (eg, polyglandular autoimmune diseases), infiltrative lesions (eg, iron overload, sarcoidosis), inherited diseases, and infectious diseases (eg, tuberculosis).[277,280] Invasive or compressive lesions include pituitary macroadenomas, craniopharyngiomas, meningiomas or gliomas, Rathke cleft cysts, metastases, empty sella syndrome, and carotid aneurysms.[280] The inherited forms are rare and may include TSHβ mutations[285] or TRH receptor mutations[80] or pituitary transcription factor defects (mutations in *POU1F1, PROP1, HESX1, LHX3, LHX4,* or *LEPR*) with combined pituitary hormone deficiencies including TSH deficiency.[286,287]

Transient or reversible forms of central hypothyroidism can be observed with drugs affecting the neuroendocrine TSH regulation, such as somatostatin analogs, glucocorticoids, or dopaminergic compounds acutely inhibiting TSH secretion; however, the thyroid stimulation may be inadequate to maintain a euthyroid status because the reduction in TSH and thyroid hormone concentrations activates the feedback mechanism.[280] Transient or reversible forms may also occur during recovery from prolonged thyrotoxicosis or severe chronic diseases.[280] Transplacental passage to the fetus of TSH receptor-stimulating antibodies or thyroid hormones from a thyrotoxic mother or corticosteroids or dopamine given to mothers during complicated delivery may also transiently affect neonates' suppression of TSH secretion and central hypothyroidism.[280]

The clinical manifestations of central hypothyroidism (caused by either pituitary or hypothalamic disease) are similar to those of primary hypothyroidism but tend to be less severe (unless diagnosed in infancy). If a mass is taking up space in the cranium, headache, visual field disturbances, and hypopituitarism may develop. Nonthyroidal illness may have a similar picture as central hypothyroidism because of suppression of the hypothalamic–pituitary axis.[141] Undiagnosed central hypothyroidism in infancy leads to cretinism.

The laboratory diagnosis is based on demonstration of low, normal, or slightly elevated TSH concentrations combined with low tT_4 or fT_4 concentrations.[280] In neonatal screening programs, central hypothyroidism can only be identified if TSH and T_4 are both measured.[280,288]

The treatment of central hypothyroidism is the same as that of primary hypothyroidism (ie, with levothyroxine).[289] For optimal levothyroxine replacement therapy in patients with central hypothyroidism, the following conditions must be fulfilled:

- Exclude adrenal insufficiency.
- Follow up for fT_4 measurement should be obtained *before* ingestion of daily levothyroxine tablets.
- Final dose should be based on age and sex (≈1.4–1.7 µg/kg body weight).
- Maintain concentration of circulating fT_4 in the middle of the laboratory reference value.

BOX 67.4 Possible Causes of Central Hypothyroidism

Invasive lesion: pituitary macroadenomas, craniopharyngiomas, meningiomas, gliomas, Rathke cleft cysts, metastases, carotid aneurysms
Iatrogenic: cranial surgery or irradiation, drugs
Injury: head traumas, traumatic delivery
Infarction: postpartum necrosis (Sheehan syndrome), pituitary apoplexy, ictus
Immunologic disease: lymphocytic hypophysitis, circulating anti-POU1F1 antibodies
Infiltrative lesion: sarcoidosis, hemochromatosis, histiocytosis X
Infectious disease: tuberculosis, syphilis, mycoses
Inherited: pituitary transcription factor defects (occasionally with childhood onset), *TSHβ* and *TRHR* mutations
Idiopathic: Other unknown causes
Empty sella syndrome

TSHR, Thyroid releasing hormone receptor gene; *TRHβ,* TSHβ subunit gene.
Reproduced from Persani L, Beck-Peccoz P. Central hypothyroidism. In: Braverman LE, Cooper DS, editors. *Werner & Ingbar's The Thyroid.* 10th ed. Philadelphia: Lippincott, Williams & Wilkins; 2013:561. Copyright Lippincott, Williams & Wilkins.

BOX 67.5 Clinical Manifestations of Hypothyroidism

Symptoms
Fatigue
Lethargy
Sleepiness
Mental impairment
Depression
Cold intolerance
Hoarseness
Dry skin
Hair loss
Decreased perspiration
Weight gain
Decreased appetite
Constipation
Menstrual disturbances (typically menorrhagia) and infertility
Arthralgia
Paraesthesia

Signs
Goiter (may be present)
Slow movements
Slow speech
Hoarseness
Bradycardia
Dry skin
Loss of outer lateral eyebrow
Nonpitting edema (myxedema) (caused by accumulation of glycosaminoglycans in subcutaneous and other interstitial tissue)
Carpal tunnel syndrome
Psychosis
Galactorrhea
Hyporeflexia
Delayed relaxation of reflexes
Myopathy
Congestive cardiac failure (severe hypothyroidism)
Coma (severe hypothyroidism)
Growth failure and mental retardation (undetected congenital hypothyroidism)
Prolonged jaundice (neonatal hypothyroidism) (as a result of immaturity of uridine diphosphonate glucuronyltransferase

- Reassess dose of L-T_4 if additional replacement of pituitary hormone is necessary; it has been shown that undertreatment is possible if TSH concentrations are greater than 0.5 mIU/L.

Symptoms and Signs

Thyroid hormones affect the function of most of the organs and tissues of the body (Box 67.5). The clinical features of thyroid hormone deficiency are therefore quite diverse and may involve multiple systems. The thyroid gland itself may be enlarged as a goiter; either firm or granular in texture; tender or nontender, or normal, small, or impalpable, depending on the etiology of the hypothyroidism.

Cardiovascular System. Hypothyroidism is a known risk factor for cardiovascular disease.[277] Atherosclerosis is most likely a result of the dyslipidemia and the hypertension that can occur with thyroid hormone deficiency. There is an increase of 50% to 60% in peripheral vascular resistance in hypothyroid patients and a 30% to 50% decrease in resting cardiac output. A total of 20% to 40% of patients with hypothyroidism have hypertension, with the diastolic pressure being increased more than the systolic. This is primarily attributable to the increase in systemic vascular resistance. Importantly, all the changes in the cardiovascular function, as well as in lipid metabolism, in patients with hypothyroidism improve in response to treatment with levothyroxine or liothyronine.

Myocardial dysfunction, both systolic and diastolic, occurs with hypothyroidism. Hypothyroidism is also associated with congestive cardiac failure, particularly in individuals with severe thyroid hormone deficiency. Up to 50% of studied patients with thyroid gland failure have pericardial effusions; pericardial tamponade is rare but has been reported.[290]

Gastrointestinal System, Liver, and Pancreas. Despite reduced appetite, most individuals with hypothyroidism show moderate weight gain. This is primarily owing to fluid retention. Hypothyroidism reduces GI tract motility, often causing constipation. Thyroid hormone deficiency can lead to decreased bile flow because of gallbladder hypotonia and also alterations in bile composition. This is probably the underlying reason for the propensity for hypothyroid patients to have bile duct stone formation.[291] Importantly, hypothyroidism caused by Hashimoto thyroiditis is associated with an increase in autoimmune disorders of the GI tract such as pernicious anemia, gluten sensitivity, celiac disease, primary biliary cirrhosis, and autoimmune hepatitis. Primary hypothyroidism is also associated with types 1 and 2 diabetes. The relationship to type 1 may be shared autoimmune predisposition; the relationship to type 2 diabetes is more complex.[292]

Central and Peripheral Nervous Systems. Mental retardation and cretinism are well-recognized complications of endemic iodine deficiency and untreated congenital hypothyroidism. Adults with acquired hypothyroidism are more likely to develop entrapment neuropathies, such as carpal tunnel syndrome, metabolic polyneuropathies and, rarely, cerebellar ataxia. Psychiatric disturbances, particularly depression, are well-known features of hypothyroidism. Thyroid hormone deficiency has also been linked to other neuropsychiatric abnormalities, including poor concentration, impaired memory, cognitive dysfunction, paranoia, hallucinations, and schizophrenia.[293]

Musculoskeletal System. Arthralgia, myalgia, proximal muscle myopathy, and acute exertional rhabdomyolysis have been reported in patients with hypothyroidism.[294]

Skeletal muscles can show abnormal structure on microscopy with loss of striations, edema, swelling of fibers, and relative deficiency of type II fibers. Plasma creatine kinase activity is often increased.

Respiratory System. Abnormal respiratory muscle function may occur in patients with preexisting lung disease leading to exacerbation of any carbon dioxide retention. Upper airway obstruction can also occur from soft tissue enlargement or goiter leading to sleep apnea. They may also develop pleural effusions.

Skin and Connective Tissue. Hypothyroidism can have a marked effect on the epidermis, dermis, sweat glands, hair, and nails. *Myxedema* is the term describing the edema-like skin that results from deposition of glycosaminoglycans (eg, hyaluronic acid) within the dermis. This appears as nonpitting cutaneous edema with firm texture and a pale waxy appearance. Facial puffiness, periorbital edema, and enlargement of the tongue can also occur. There may be associated anemia and hypercarotenemia through impaired conversion of beta carotene into retinol. This can make the skin look pale yellow. The hair becomes coarse, dry, and brittle with alopecia, and there may be thinning of the eyebrows, especially the lateral portion. Vitiligo can occur in patients with autoimmune pathogenesis.

Kidneys and Electrolyte Metabolism. Renal blood flow and glomerular filtration rates (GFRs) are both decreased, but total-body water has been shown to increase in patients with hypothyroidism owing to impaired renal excretion of water. Although exchangeable body sodium is increased, the dilutional effect leads to a mild hyponatremia. Plasma vasopressin concentrations have been reported to be inappropriately increased in some patients.[295]

Reproductive System. Hypothyroidism leads to a reduction in libido and subfertility in men and women.

The frequency of menstrual disturbances, both oligo- and polymenorrhea, in hypothyroidism is approximately three times greater than in the normal population.[296]

Oligospermia can occur; it is thought to be owing to impaired luteinizing hormone secretion. Hypothyroidism leads to a reduction in plasma sex hormone–binding globulin concentration and subsequent reduction in total testosterone. Free testosterone is also reduced in around 60% of hypothyroid men. In hypothyroid men, the prevalence of hypoactive sexual desire, delayed ejaculation, and erectile dysfunction has been estimated to be 64% and of premature ejaculation 7%.[297]

Pituitary and Adrenal Disorders. Lack of thyroid hormone significantly reduces spontaneous nocturnal GH secretion and GH response to stimuli such as insulin-induced hypoglycemia and GH-releasing hormone.[298] In addition, hypothyroidism may inhibit the response of cartilage to insulin like growth factor 1. These abnormalities lead to significant growth failure and short stature in children with hypothyroidism.

With increased TRH release, patients with hypothyroidism sometimes exhibit hyperprolactinemia. Women may thus develop galactorrhea and amenorrhea, and it is imperative that these patients are identified as having primary hypothyroidism to avoid inappropriate treatment for hyperprolactinemia.

In hypothyroid patients, cortisol production rate and metabolic clearance are diminished. However, because both are decreased, the plasma cortisol concentrations remain relatively normal.

Hematology and Hemostasis. Hypothyroid patients frequently have a mild normochromic, normocytic, or slightly macrocytic anaemia. This is due to decreased erythropoiesis as a result of low plasma erythropoietin concentrations and possibly hypocellular bone marrow. Iron deficiency can occur as a result of either impaired intestinal iron absorption or associated achlorhydria or from menorrhagia. Megaloblastic anemia from vitamin B_{12} deficiency is seen in patients with associated pernicious anemia. Low plasma coagulation factor VIII concentrations and prolonged partial thromboplastin time[299] may lead to easy bruising and to excessive bleeding after minor injuries or procedures or during menstruation. Factor IX concentrations and platelet adherence may also be reduced.

Severity of Hypothyroidism

Importantly, hypothyroidism may be overt or subclinical. Overt hypothyroidism is defined by a high serum TSH concentration and low serum fT_4; subclinical hypothyroidism is defined by a high serum TSH (but usually <10 mIU/L) and a normal serum fT_4 concentration.

Subclinical Hypothyroidism

Subclinical hypothyroidism can be classified as mild (TSH between 4 and 9.9 mIU/L) or severe (TSH ≥10 mIU/L)[180,181]; trimester and age-dependent cut-offs differ and should be applied as appropriate. The elevation in TSH should have persisted for 6 to 12 weeks or longer in the setting of fT_4 concentrations that are repeatedly found within the reference interval.[300] The prevalence increases with age and is higher in women than in men. Population prevalence differs; in the United States, it is estimated to be 4% to 9%[132,279] in individuals without known thyroid disease.

The biochemical features of SCH may also be present in patients with overt hypothyroidism, who are inadequately treated, have poor compliance or because of drug-interactions.[301] SCH is more common in iodine-sufficient regions, and iodine supplementation may increase the incidence in mild to moderate iodine-deficient regions.[58,301]

There has been controversy on what should be the upper reference limit for TSH.[300] One of the arguments in favor for a lower limit is that individuals with TSH between 3 and 5 mIU/L more often are positive for TPO antibodies and have a higher rate of progression to overt hypothyroidism.[300,302] Also, plasma TSH concentrations are not normally distributed, and if TSH is transformed to fit a Gaussian distribution, the upper reference limit would be 2.5 mIU/L. The strongest argument against reducing the upper limit is the increased number of individuals that would be given a diagnosis of hypothyroidism without any clinical or therapeutic benefit from this diagnosis.[300,303] Furthermore, there has also been debate on whether and when to treat in SCH (see later discussion of treatment); however, if patients with a laboratory diagnosis of SCH have clinical signs and symptoms, treatment should be instituted.

Evidence from metaanalyses of observational studies have shown that SCH is not associated with increased fracture risk[304,305] or cognitive impairment[306] but is associated with risk of heart failure with TSH of 10 mIU/Lor greater.[307] Meta-analyses and nationwide studies disagree on whether risk is increased for coronary heart disease, fatal coronary heart disease, and all-cause mortality.[308-311]

The results from metaanalyses of randomized clinical trials have not shown consistently beneficial effects of levothyroxine treatment on serum lipid concentrations, myocardial infarction, or all-cause mortality in patients with SCH.[308,312]

Myxedematous Coma. Patients with severe hypothyroidism may present with myxedematous (hypothyroid) coma, a syndrome of decreased consciousness, hypothermia, and other features of hypothyroidism.[313] This condition has a high mortality and requires aggressive treatment in a critical care facility with facilities for mechanical ventilation if required. Treatment includes slow rewarming, fluid replacement, treatment of any precipitating factors (eg, infection), and intravenous hydrocortisone until concurrent adrenal insufficiency has been excluded. There is no consensus as to the optimum regimen for hormone replacement. Levothyroxine should be given intravenously (the dose dependent on the factors discussed later) until the patient can take it orally; triiodothyronine can be added if there is no improvement within 24 to 48 hours.

Laboratory Diagnosis of Hypothyroidism

Serum TSH is the first-line measurement with age-dependent reference interval usually between 0.4 and 4.2 mIU/L (for reference intervals see Appendix). *Overt hypothyroidism* is defined as increased TSH and low fT_4. Autoantibodies should also be measured, indicating an autoimmune etiology.

Patients diagnosed with SCH (defined as increased TSH but fT_4 within the reference interval) should be followed up with repeat measurements together with measurement of TPO antibodies preferably after a 2- to 3-month interval.[181] The presence of antibodies indicates increased risk of progression to overt hypothyroidism. Other conditions in which TSH is elevated but fT_4 is normal encompass recent institution of thyroid hormone replacement therapy (fT_4 returns to normal before TSH declines), poor compliance with treatment in primary hypothyroidism, recovery from nonthyroidal illness, positively interfering heterophilic antibodies, (eg, human antimouse antibodies) in double-antibody immunoassays, and thyroid hormone resistance.

In central hypothyroidism, the laboratory diagnosis is based on low, normal, or slightly elevated TSH combined with low tT_4 or fT_4 concentrations.[280]

Treatment

Levothyroxine sodium (thyroxine) is the treatment of choice for hypothyroidism with few adverse events if used appropriately.[314] It is chemically stable with relatively modest product deterioration during storage. The ATA recommends against the routine use of combination treatment with levothyroxine and liothyronine replacement therapy in patients with primary hypothyroidism because evidence of superiority of combination therapy over monotherapy with levothyroxine is not consistently strong.[289]

Levothyroxine is absorbed in the proximal small bowel; it has a 7-day half-life in plasma because of protein binding and is metabolized to triiodothyronine in the tissues by deiodination. The bioavailability is 60% to 80% in healthy volunteers under fasting, with time to maximum concentration of about 2 hours. Absorption is delayed by food. In hypothyroidism, the time to maximum concentration may be prolonged (≈3 hours), and the bioavailability may be higher.[315]

Optimal treatment is typically about 1.8 µg/kg/day but higher in infants and young children and lower in older adults (0.5 µg/kg/day), in patients with ischemic heart disease, and in patients with SCH.[277] Patients who are thyroidectomized tend to need higher doses than those who have autoimmune thyroiditis.[277] It is essential to appreciate that patients with central hypothyroidism may have concomitant central adrenal insufficiency; this must be always excluded before starting levothyroxine therapy because of the risk of precipitating adrenal crisis.

The European Thyroid Association and ATA are generally in agreement with their recommendations for treatment in SCH.[181,316] Levothyroxine is recommended for younger patients (<65–70 years) with serum TSH levels greater than 10 mIU/L. In younger SCH patients (serum TSH <10 mIU/L) with symptoms suggestive of hypothyroidism, levothyroxine replacement therapy should be considered. If symptoms fail to improve with treatment, levothyroxine should usually be stopped. In those 80 to 85 years or older with elevated serum TSH of 10 mIU/L or les, a wait-and-see strategy is recommended.

Initiation of treatment should start with a dose in the lower end of what is anticipated to be the optimal dosage. It is usually not recommended to start at a low dose with upward titration because this prolongs recovery,[277] but it is essential to do so in patients with longstanding disease or evidence of ischemic heart disease. Steady-state concentrations of the drug are reached by approximately 6 weeks after starting treatment or changing the dose. Patients are customarily advised to take levothyroxine sodium 0 to 60 minutes before breakfast because food and caffeine interfere with its absorption, but bedtime administration is equally effective and may be better suited to patients who take a number of other medications.

In primary hypothyroidism, the treatment goal is to have TSH within the reference interval. In the initial phase of titrating the appropriate dose, changes in TSH lag behind serum thyroid hormone levels; therefore, TSH should be measured no earlier than 4 to 6 weeks after adjustment of thyroxine dosage. According to the ATA guidelines, TSH monitoring is then repeated after 4 to 6 months and then yearly when the patient has reached the optimal dose to maintain euthyroidism.[289] In central hypothyroidism, fT_4 should be monitored, and the treatment goal is to maintain fT_4 concentration toward the upper end of the reference interval to ensure adequate replacement and euthyroidism.[277]

Reasons for an elevated TSH in treated patients include suboptimal dosing (inadequate prescribed dosage, noncompliance), a decrease in endogenous thyroid production (autoimmune thyroiditis), reduced absorption (because of interactions with drugs, eg, iron, calcium carbonate, cholestyramine, sucralfate), comorbid conditions (malabsorption, small bowel surgery), pregnancy (caused by increased TBG, increased clearance, increased body mass), diet (dietary fibers, grapes, soybeans, papaya, and coffee), and increased clearance (drug interactions [phenytoin, carbamazepine, phenobarbital, rifampicin], comorbid conditions [kidney disease])[277,314,315]; in all of these conditions, an increased dose is required. A decreased dose may be required in older adults and with increasing age.[314]

The metabolism of other drugs can also be affected in hypothyroidism. Because of a smaller distribution volume, plasma concentrations of drugs may be higher than is typical, and because of decreased metabolism, the doses of certain drugs may need to be lower. However, dosage adjustment will usually be needed when euthyroidism is restored.[277]

Adverse reactions include clinical or subclinical thyrotoxicosis with increased risk of bone loss and atrial arrhythmias. In patients with ischemic heart disease, thyroxine treatment may worsen myocardial ischemia.[277]

Factors to consider when initiating levothyroxine therapy are patient age, concurrent comorbidities and medication, and lean body mass.[289] In older adults, the TSH reference interval is higher than in younger individuals; therefore, the TSH treatment target should also be higher compared with younger individuals. Older adults often have less lean body mass than younger individuals and thus decreased T_4 turnover; therefore, the dose needed to normalize the TSH is generally lower. The general recommendation by ATA for treatment with levothyroxine in older adults is that, regardless of known heart disease or risk factors for heart disease, levothyroxine should be initiated with low doses and the dose titrated slowly based on TSH.[289]

Thyrotoxicosis

The term *thyrotoxicosis* refers to a condition with excess thyroid hormone. The term *hyperthyroidism* refers to a sustained increase in thyroid hormone biosynthesis and secretion by the thyroid gland.[317] The term *thyrotoxicosis* relates to its clinical manifestations: a syndrome of hypermetabolism and hyperactivity resulting from an elevation of plasma T_4 or T_3 concentration (most usually both). The terms *thyrotoxicosis* and *hyperthyroidism* are not entirely synonymous. For example, thyrotoxicosis can occur as a result of excessive hormone release from the thyroid in the absence of increased synthesis, as may occur in thyroiditis. Excessive intake of thyroid hormones can also cause thyrotoxicosis but not hyperthyroidism. Box 67.6 summarizes the clinical manifestations of thyrotoxicosis.

Epidemiology

A metaanalysis of European studies showed that the prevalence of undiagnosed hyperthyroidism was 1.72%, the prevalence of previously undiagnosed and diagnosed hyperthyroidism combined was 0.75%, and the incidence rate of hyperthyroidism was about 51 per 100,000 per year.[278] The risk increases with age and is higher in women,[249] in iodine-deficient areas,[58,245] and in whites.[318]

The population prevalence of subclinical hyperthyroidism is 0.6% to 2% depending on the cut-off used for TSH concentration[132,301,319]; the prevalence is higher in women and increases with age, with prevalence reported to be 2% in people older than 65 years of age.[132,319,320] In the National Health and Nutrition Examination Survey, 1.8% had TSH less than 0.4 mIU/L (4% in blacks and 1.4% in whites), and 0.7% had TSH less than 0.1 mIU/L.[132] The prevalence is higher in iodine-deficient populations.[245]

The incidence of thyroid storm has been estimated in Japan to be 0.2 persons per 100,000 per year (ie, 0.22% of all thyrotoxic patients and 5.4% of thyrotoxic patients admitted to hospitals).[321]

Graves disease, the commonest cause of hyperthyroidism, affects approximately 0.4% of the US population and occurs more often in women than in men (5:1). Graves disease frequently is associated with other autoimmune disorders.[322] There is a genetic susceptibility to Graves disease, as shown by a sibling occurrence risk of 11.6%[323] and a heritability of 75% in twin studies[324,325]; the rest is environmental with smoking being a significant risk factor.[326-328]

Thyroid-stimulating hormone–secreting anterior pituitary adenomas are very rare and account for about 1% of all pituitary adenomas.[329,330] TSH-secreting tumors may occur at any age and occur with equal frequency in men and women.[330-332]

Causes of Thyrotoxicosis

The causes of thyrotoxicosis are listed in Box 67.7. Thyrotoxicosis is usually associated with hyperthyroidism but not always.[317] Among common causes for thyrotoxicosis associated with hyperthyroidism are (1) *production of abnormal thyroid stimulator* (TSHR-stimulating antibody) in Graves disease and (2) *thyroidal autonomy*, including toxic multinodular

BOX 67.6 Clinical Manifestations of Thyrotoxicosis

Symptoms
Nervousness, stroke, agitation or irritability
Fatigue, lethargy
Weakness
Increased perspiration
Heat intolerance
Tremor
Hyperactivity
Palpitation
Appetite change (usually increase)
Weight change (usually weight loss)
Increased bowel movement
Menstrual disturbances

Signs
Hyperactivity
Tachycardia or atrial arrhythmia
Systolic hypertension
Warm, moist, smooth skin
Stare and eyelid retraction
Tremor
Hyperreflexia
Muscle weakness
Goiter
Thyroid bruits (with Graves disease, exophthalmos, pretibial myxedema, onycholysis, thyroid acropachy)
Digital clubbing, swelling of digits and toes
Periosteal reaction at extremities of bones

BOX 67.7 Causes of Hyperthyroidism

Endogenous Thyroid Disorders
Autoimmune thyroid disease
Graves disease
Hashitoxicosis
Postpartum thyroiditis
Toxic multinodular goiter
Toxic adenoma
Struma ovarii
hCG-induced hyperthyroidism
  Gestational hyperthyroidism
  hCG-secreting tumors (trophoblastic tumor)
Atopic thyroid tissue
Secondary hyperthyroidism (pituitary tumor secreting TSH)

Exogenous Disorders
Thyroid destruction from viral or bacterial thyroiditis, eg, de Quervain
Iodine-induced hyperthyroidism, eg, amiodarone
Thyroid hormone ingestion (thyrotoxicosis factitia)

hCG, Human chorionic gonadotropin; *TSH*, thyroid-stimulating hormone.

goiter and solitary toxic adenoma.[317] Less common causes include (A) *conditions with production of thyroid stimulating hormones* (TSH-secreting pituitary adenoma, pituitary resistance to thyroid hormone, neonatal Graves disease [thyroid-stimulating immunoglobulins], choriocarcinoma [hCG secretion], and hyperemesis gravidarum [hCG secretion]), (B) *conditions with thyroidal autonomy* (eg, congenital hyperthyroidism [activating mutations in the TSHR], struma ovarii), and (C) *drug-induced hyperthyroidism* (iodine, iodine-containing drugs [eg, amiodarone], and radiographic contrast agents).[317]

Common causes for thyrotoxicosis *not* associated with hyperthyroidism include (1) *thyroiditis* (silent painless thyroiditis, postpartum thyroiditis, subacute thyroiditis) and (2) *excess exogenous thyroid hormone* (iatrogenic or factitious).[317] Less common causes include (A) *drug-induced thyroiditis* (eg, amiodarone, interferon alfa, lithium), (B) *acute infectious thyroiditis*, (C) *radiation thyroiditis*, (D) *infarction of thyroid adenoma*, and (E) *"hamburger" thyrotoxicosis* (caused by ingestion of thyroid-contaminated food from animal sources).[317]

The prevalence of the causes varies with iodine intake, such that in iodine-sufficient areas, Graves disease is the most common cause of thyrotoxicosis, accounting for 60% to 90% of cases. But in iodine-deficient areas, thyroidal autonomy is more common.[333] Thyroiditis accounts for about 10% of all causes of thyrotoxicosis.[317] Iodine fortification induces a temporary, modest increase in the incidence of hyperthyroidism in mild to moderate iodine-deficient regions.[334]

POINTS TO REMEMBER

Thyrotoxicosis

- Central hyperthyroidism (TSH-secreting tumors) is a very rare cause of thyrotoxicosis.
- Graves disease is the most common cause of thyrotoxicosis and most of the remaining causes are toxic nodular goiter and toxic adenoma.
- Of all clinical manifestations of thyrotoxicosis, cardiovascular complications represent the highest potential for morbidity and mortality.
- Antithyroid drugs (eg, methimazole) remain mainstay of treatment in Graves disease.
- ^{131}I may be treatment of choice for multinodular goiter and toxic adenoma.
- ^{131}I treatment is absolutely contraindicated in pregnancy or the possibility of pregnancy.

Signs and Symptoms of Thyrotoxicosis and Hyperthyroidism

Thyrotoxicosis can affect any physiological system in the body (see Box 67.6) with the frequency and severity of signs and symptoms varying considerably among patients. Some of the causes produce characteristic clinical signs, for example, orbital and cutaneous manifestations in Graves disease. The age of the patient and presence of concomitant disturbances may have an impact on the clinical features of hyperthyroidism, either exaggerating or diminishing them. For example, older patients may have less marked evidence of sympathetic activation such as anxiety, hyperactivity, or tremor and less weight loss but marked features of cardiovascular dysfunction such as congestive cardiac failure and atrial fibrillation.

Cardiovascular System. Cardiovascular symptoms and signs often predominate.[317] Of the many clinical manifestations of hyperthyroidism, cardiovascular complications represent the highest potential for morbidity and mortality; the rate of cardiovascular death is higher in patients with hyperthyroidism than in euthyroid subjects.[335,336] Typical symptoms in thyrotoxicosis include palpitations, exercise intolerance, exertional dyspnea, angina, chest pain, and tachycardia.[337] Typical signs include systolic hypertension, atrial fibrillation, cardiac hypertrophy, peripheral edema, pulmonary hypertension, and ultimately heart failure.[337]

High circulating concentrations of thyroid hormone have a direct stimulatory effect on cardiac muscle.[337] Heart rate and volume are increased at rest, and peripheral vascular resistance is reduced, which leads to a marked rise in cardiac output in patients who have no preexisting cardiac disease. This results in increased cardiac oxygen demand and risk of ischemia, increasing the risk of atrial arrhythmia (particularly atrial fibrillation) and promoting the development of congestive cardiac failure in susceptible individuals. In patients with preexisting ischemic heart disease, thyrotoxicosis may precipitate angina. Many of these symptoms and signs mimic those that occur in states of increased β-adrenergic activity. However, catecholamine metabolism is usually normal, and urinary excretion of catecholamine metabolites is also normal. Despite this, the adrenergic antagonists (eg, propranolol) do mitigate or even prevent some of the ionotropic and chronotropic responses, particularly to T_3.

Thyroid hormone increases the synthesis and secretion of renin and aldosterone. This contributes to the increase in renal sodium absorption and blood volume that occurs in thyrotoxicosis. Thyrotoxicosis can cause primarily systolic hypertension as a result of the tachycardia.

Metabolic and ischemic cerebrovascular events have both been described in patients with overt hyperthyroidism; embolic events resulting from atrial fibrillation is more common.

Gastrointestinal System and Liver. Increased bowel motility leading to hyperdefecation is a frequent finding in patients with overt hyperthyroidism.[338] There is a shortened small bowel transit time, although true diarrhea does not usually result. Nausea and vomiting are not common but can precede the onset of a thyrotoxic crisis. Weight loss is a common feature of hyperthyroidism owing to increased basal metabolic rate.

Hepatic changes occur with thyroid hormone excess, typically with mild elevations of plasma aminotransferase activities,[339] which may be a result of increased oxygen demand in the face of normal or diminished hepatic blood flow.[340] In severe hyperthyroid states, liver function can be markedly deranged with hypoalbuminemia; marked elevation of plasma aminotransferase and alkaline phosphatase activities can occur. The latter can be of mixed bone and liver origin.

Central and Peripheral Nervous Systems. Tremor associated with thyrotoxicosis is usually most evident in the hands but can occur elsewhere (eg, the lower extremities, trunk, and tongue). It is thought to be caused by β-adrenergic stimulation and responds well to β-adrenergic blocking agents such as propranolol.[341]

Myasthenia gravis can occur rarely (<1%, though more frequently in the general population) in patients with Graves disease, but AITD occurs frequently in patients with myasthenia gravis.[341,342] Seizures are a well-recognized component of thyroid storm but occur only in a minority (<1%) of patients with moderate hyperthyroidism.[341] The exact mechanism is unknown, but seizures and electroencephalogram abnormalities resolve with correction of thyroid hormone concentrations.

Mental and Psychiatric Disorders. Thyrotoxicosis may be associated with a number of neuropsychiatric symptoms, including restlessness; irritability; agitation; emotional lability; anxiety; depression; and, rarely, encephalopathy, psychosis, and coma.[341]

Musculoskeletal System. Some degree of myopathy occurs in the majority of patients with overt hyperthyroidism. It is usually proximal and involves the pelvic girdle and shoulder muscles. Advanced hyperthyroidism can lead to muscle wasting owing to its catabolic effect.

Thyrotoxic periodic paralysis occurs as a result of intracellular shift of potassium in genetically and clinically susceptible patients.[341] It occurs most frequently in Asian men[341]; the disorder typically presents after an episode of carbohydrate ingestion or intense physical exercise. Total-body stores of potassium are normal, but plasma potassium during an episode of paralysis may fall to below 1.5 mmol/L. Treatment is with intravenous potassium, but care has to be taken to avoid rebound hyperkalemia. The addition of β-adrenergic blocking agents can reduce the frequency of repeat attacks while the patients are being returned to a euthyroid state by treatment.

Skeletal involvement includes loss of bone mineral density with increased bone turnover markers, including hydroxyproline, hypercalciuria and, occasionally, hypercalcemia. There have been many studies demonstrating an increased risk of fracture in patients with a history of thyrotoxicosis.[343-345] Indeed, it has been shown there is an increased standardized mortality ratio because of hip fracture among a follow-up population register of patients treated with radioiodine for hyperthyroidism.[346]

Eye Involvement. Hyperthyroidism itself can cause a characteristic "staring" expression (eyelid retraction with sclera being seen above and below the iris). In addition, there is a tendency for the eyelid movement to lag behind that of the globe as patients look forward from a position of maximum upward gaze (eyelid lag).

In addition, specific orbital signs and symptoms occur in patients with Graves disease (Graves ophthalmopathy). This condition is characterized by periorbital and conjunctival edema and erythema (caused by compression of orbital veins, resulting in venous stasis), retraction of the upper eyelid (caused by sympathetic hyperactivity), and proptosis caused by the increased volume of orbital contents.[341] The last two can lead to corneal ulceration because of incomplete eye closure. The complaints include grittiness in the eyes, excess watering, photophobia, retro-orbital pain, gaze-provoked pain, and diplopia.[341] Features of a myopathy in Graves ophthalmopathy include failure of relaxation of involved muscles, most commonly the levator palpebrae superioris and the inferior and medial recti. Risk factors for Graves ophthalmopathy include smoking and radioiodine therapy for hyperthyroidism (especially among smokers).[328,347,348] The onset of eye disease in Graves disease usually coincides with that of thyrotoxicosis, but it is not uncommon for the ophthalmopathy to precede or follow thyrotoxicosis by months or even years. It is usually bilateral but can be asymmetrical in up to 15% of cases.[349]

Respiratory System. Exertional dyspnea is a common manifestation of thyrotoxicosis. It is a result of respiratory muscle weakness, enhanced ventilatory drive, diminished lung compliance, and concurrent cardiovascular complications (eg, congestive cardiac failure).[337,350]

Skin and Hair. Diffuse hair loss is common with prolonged elevation of thyroid hormones.[351] The nails are brittle and may become elevated from the nail bed (onycholysis). The skin is warm, soft, and smooth,[351] and there may be palmar erythema.

Graves disease is associated with unique extrathyroidal manifestations, including ophthalmopathy (see earlier discussion), thyroid dermopathy, and, rarely, acropachy.[352] Thyroid acropachy in patients consists of a triad of digital clubbing of fingers and toes, soft tissue swelling of the hands and feet, and a characteristic periosteal reaction of the distal metatarsals.[351] Thyroid dermopathy presents with indurated purple skin lesions over the anterior tibia (pretibial myxedema); these contain large amounts of glycosaminoglycans.

Renal Function and Electrolytes Metabolism. The GFR is increased owing to the increased renal blood flow that results from increased cardiac output and vasodilatation.[353] Thyrotoxic individuals often complain of increased thirst and mild polyuria even in the absence of an obvious cause such as hyperglycemia. Plasma sodium and potassium concentrations are usually normal, but there may be an increase in urinary magnesium excretion, leading to a low plasma magnesium concentration.

Reproductive System. Hyperthyroidism is associated with impaired reproductive function in both men and women. Menstrual abnormalities are common with either a scanty menstrual loss, an irregular cycle, or both. Although cycles usually remain ovulatory, fertility is reduced.[296,354]

In one study in men with hyperthyroidism, the prevalence of hypoactive sexual desire was 17.6%, erectile dysfunction was 2.9%, premature ejaculation was 50%, and delayed ejaculation was 14.7%.[297] Plasma sex hormone–binding globulin concentration is increased, leading to increased total testosterone and estradiol concentrations. Preferential metabolism of androgen to estrogens may be the reason for gynecomastia seen in a small proportion of men with hyperthyroidism.

Hematology. Anemia not attributable to other causes, such as iron deficiency or vitamin B_{12} deficiency, is a frequent finding in patients with Graves disease.[355] Relative neutropenia and lymphocytosis have also been described in patients with untreated Graves disease.[356] There is also some evidence to suggest that thyrotoxicosis is associated with a hypercoagulable state, but patients requiring anticoagulation appear to have a decreased warfarin dose requirement owing mainly to an increased rate of clotting factor degradation.[357]

Thyroid (Thyrotoxic) Storm. Thyroid storm (also known as thyrotoxic crisis) is a rare, severe, exaggerated, and life-threatening condition of thyrotoxicosis and is triggered by precipitating factors.[313,358] Thyroid storm is most often seen in the context of underlying Graves hyperthyroidism but can complicate thyrotoxicosis of any etiology.[313,358] It is much less common today than in the past owing to earlier diagnosis and treatment of thyrotoxicosis. The results of laboratory tests are indistinguishable from those seen in patients with uncomplicated thyrotoxicosis; the diagnosis of thyroid storm remains a clinical diagnosis. The condition has a potentially high mortality rate, and it is thus often necessary to begin treatment without waiting for biochemical confirmation of the diagnosis.

The key manifestations of thyroid storm may be present in variable degrees. The clinical manifestations depend on severity and include[358,359]:

- Thermoregulatory dysfunction: fever with temperature usually >41°C
- Cardiovascular dysfunction: tachycardia, atrial fibrillation, congestive heart failure (pedal edema [mild]; bibasal rales or crackles [moderate]; pulmonary edema [severe])
- Central nervous system dysfunction: agitation (mild); delirium, psychosis, and extreme lethargy (moderate); seizures, coma (severe)
- GI dysfunction: nausea, vomiting, and diarrhea in mild to moderate forms and jaundice in severe forms with patients being hypotensive because of volume depletion caused by vomiting and diarrhea

Older individuals often present atypically (a variant termed *apathetic thyroid storm)* with apathy, stupor, cardiac failure, coma, and minimal signs of thyrotoxicosis.[358] In this disorder, biochemical evidence of thyroid hormone excess is observed in the absence of any clinical evidence of hyperthyroidism. Alternatively, only a single organ system may be affected. Mortality rates are high, and death occurs because of multiorgan failure in 25% of patients.[321]

Two types of events have been associated with precipitation of thyroid storm, namely an intercurrent illness, surgery, or injury that exacerbates the effects of thyrotoxicosis either systemically or on one or more organ systems or more rarely an acute event that suddenly increases thyroid hormone secretion.[313,358] The best example of the latter is occurrence of thyroid storm soon after thyroidectomy, which was relatively common before the need for preoperative antithyroid therapy was recognized. This is now a rare occurrence.

There are four components to the treatment of patients with thyroid storm[358]:

- Acute resuscitative intervention: airway, breathing, and circulation
- General supportive care: cooling, electrolyte replacement, correction of volume depletion, nutritional support, ventilator support, and organ-specific treatment
- Thyroid-specific therapy (the five Bs): block synthesis with antithyroid medication; block release with iodine; block T_4 into T_3 conversion with propylthiouracil, propranolol, and corticosteroid (rarely amiodarone); beta-blocker; and block enterohepatic circulation with cholestyramine.
- Treatment of precipitating illness
- Maintenance therapy: Antithyroid treatment should be continued until euthyroidism is achieved.

Diagnosis and Differential Diagnosis of Thyrotoxicosis

The laboratory diagnosis of thyrotoxicosis is based on a suppressed or low TSH and increased fT_4 or increased fT_3 or total T_3. TSH is the most sensitive biomarker. A total of 2% to 4% of patients with hyperthyroidism have increased concentration of fT_3 or tT3 but normal concentration of fT_4 (T_3 thyrotoxicosis).[360] However, low TSH can also be caused by other conditions relevant for the diagnosis. Subclinical hyperthyroidism is defined as low TSH with normal circulating concentrations of T_4 and T_3.[317] Low TSH may also be drug induced (glucocorticoids and dopamine)[317] or caused by nonthyroidal illness.

In pituitary adenoma (secondary hyperthyroidism), TSH can be inappropriately normal or high for an elevated concentration of peripheral thyroid hormones.

If the etiology of thyrotoxicosis is uncertain, a RAIU test should be performed; iodine uptake of the thyroid gland is low in thyroiditis and high in Graves disease and autonomous nodules (single or multiple).[359] A thyroid scan should be added in the presence of nodularity[359]; technetium scintigraphy (TcO4) and ^{123}I scintiscan are both useful. Technetium scintigraphy uses pertechnetate that is trapped by the thyroid and not organified, resulting in a low range of normal uptake and high background activity, but total-body radiation exposure is less than for ^{123}I scintiscan.[359] Ultrasonography is only indicated in the differential diagnosis of thyrotoxicosis when radioactive iodine is contraindicated (eg, pregnancy or breastfeeding) or not useful (eg, following recent iodine exposure).[359]

The presence of TRAb (TSHR-stimulating antibodies) effectively confirms a diagnosis of Graves disease.[361] The likelihood of Graves disease is 1000- to 3000-fold greater if TRAb are present.[362] Sensitivity and specificity for third-generation TRAb assays are high.[362] A total of 75% of patients with Graves disease have TPO antibodies, an observation that may help differentiate Graves disease from toxic nodular hyperthyroidism if necessary.[317]

Patients with Graves disease should have a baseline complete blood count, including white blood cell (WBC) count with differential, and a liver profile, including bilirubin and transaminases, before initiating antithyroid drug therapy for Graves disease.[359]

Graves Disease

Graves disease results from an autoantibody that binds to and activates the TSHR, producing excessive release of thyroid hormone and clinical hyperthyroidism.[317,363] In patients with Graves disease, the thyroid gland is no longer under the control of pituitary TSH but is constantly stimulated by the circulating antibodies with TSH-like activity.

Both B and T lymphocytes are known to be directed at three well-characterized thyroid autoantigens, namely Tg, TPO, and TSHR. The majority of the evidence, however, suggests that TSHR is the primary autoantigen of Graves disease and that the immune response to the other two thyroid antigens is reflective of the resulting thyroiditis.

Graves ophthalmopathy has an autoimmune pathogenesis, with important genetic and environmental influences, particularly smoking.[326,328] Orbital muscle, connective tissue, and adipose tissue are infiltrated by lymphocytes and macrophages. The extracellular compartment of extraocular muscles and orbital fibroadipose tissue becomes edematous secondary to deposition of hydrophilic glycosaminoglycans. Acute inflammation can also cause erythema and swelling of the conjunctiva and eyelids, compounded by venous and lymphatic congestion. Muscle inflammation gives way to fatty degeneration and scarring and sometimes tethering and restricted eye movement.

The diagnosis of Graves disease is based on laboratory demonstration of thyrotoxicosis, clinical features (particularly

Graves disease–specific extrathyroidal manifestations, including ophthalmopathy, dermopathy, and [rarely] acropachy), and the presence of a goiter moderate, diffuse and soft goiter over which a vascular bruit may be detectable.[317,360] Ophthalmopathy, thyroid dermopathy, and acropachy occur in 25%, 1.5%, and 0.3 % of patients with Graves disease, respectively.[352] Patients with ophthalmopathy who are smokers have a higher risk of developing or worsening of the condition (6% in nonsmokers vs. 23% in smokers).[328]

Management of Graves Disease. The natural history of the thyrotoxicosis of Graves disease in the majority of patients is of successive relapse and remission over many years. In about 30% of patients, there is a single episode of hyperthyroidism lasting several months followed by prolonged remission and even the eventual development of hypothyroidism up to 20 years thereafter. The development of the guidelines outlined below was commissioned by the American Thyroid Association in association with the American Association of Clinical Endocrinologists (AACE).[359] The choice of treatment varies globally but includes three treatment modalities: antithyroid drugs, surgery, and radioactive iodine (^{131}I).[317,359]

Some important points regarding thyrotoxicosis are as follows (Fig. 67.13):

- Common causes include Graves disease, multinodular goiter, and toxic adenoma.
- Therapy is directed at inhibiting T_4 and T_3 synthesis and release or destroying thyroid tissue.
- Effective control of thyrotoxicosis may require treating the effects of T_4 and T_3 on peripheral tissues.

To elucidate the cause:

- History and physical examination are crucial.
- Anti-TPO abs and TRAb may play a role.
- The use of thyroid ultrasonography, thyroid radioiodine, and thyroid nuclide uptake imaging may be helpful.
- Regular measurements of white blood cell count, especially in the start-up phase because risk of agranulocytosis is highest here. If fever rises rapidly, immediate transfer to emergency department with measurement of blood cell counts. Risk of agranulocytosis is highest in the beginning of treatment. Agranulocytosis can be fatal.

Antithyroid drugs (thionamides): Carbimazole (and its active metabolite, methimazole) and PTU have been used for many years for the treatment of hyperthyroidism. They act principally by inhibiting the action of TPO and therefore thyroid hormone synthesis. Propylthiouracil, unlike carbimazole and methimazole, also decreases the conversion

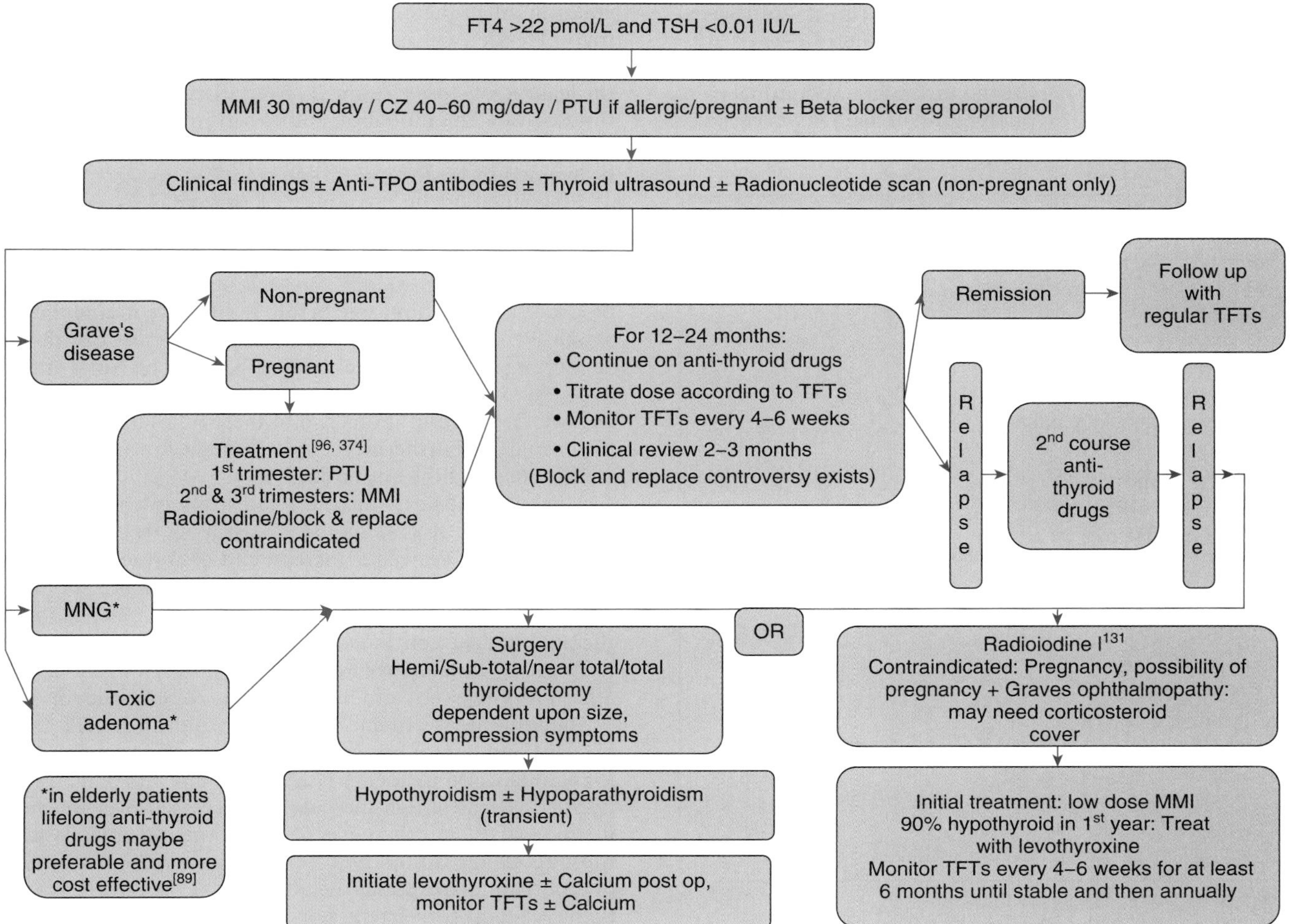

FIGURE 67.13 Guidelines for the treatment of thyrotoxicosis. *CZ,* Carbimazole; *fT₄,* free thyroxine; *MMI,* methimazole; *MNG,* multinodular goiter; *PTU,* propylthiouracil; *TFT,* thyroid function test; *TPO,* thyroid peroxidase; *TSH,* thyroid-stimulating hormone. (Courtesy Danielle Freedman.)

of T_4 to T_3 in peripheral tissues, inhibiting the activity of iodothyronine deiodinase 1 (D1). They are almost completely absorbed, and metabolism is hardly affected by liver or kidney disease.[364]

Before antithyroid drug treatment, patients should have a baseline complete blood cell count, including WBC count with differential, and a liver profile, including bilirubin and transaminases.[359]

Methimazole is the drug of choice for Graves disease, except during the first trimester of pregnancy when PTU is preferred, in thyroid storm, and in patients who experience minor adverse effects with methimazole.[359] Treatment with methimazole is typically given for 12 to 18 months, but the subsequent relapse rate is high.[317] TRAb titers should be measured before stopping antithyroid drug therapy because normal concentrations indicate a greater chance of remission.[359] If hyperthyroidism persists after methimazole treatment, radioactive iodine or thyroidectomy should be considered as alternatives.[359]

Both methimazole and PTU are very (at least 90%) effective in controlling thyrotoxicosis caused by Graves disease. There have recently been concerns about PTU-related hepatotoxicity, and these have led the ATA and the US Food and Drug Administration to recommend that methimazole should be used instead of PTU as first-line therapy unless the patient has an adverse reaction.[359] Adverse effects of antithyroid drugs are listed in Box 67.8. Patients should be advised to consult a physician if they experience pruritic rash, jaundice, light-colored stools or dark urine, arthralgia, abdominal pain, nausea, fatigue, fever, or pharyngitis. If patients experience symptoms suggestive of agranulocytosis or hepatic injury, they should stop medication immediately and call their physicians because these are potential life-threatening conditions.[359] If agranulocytosis is suspected (eg, because of a febrile illness or pharyngitis), a WBC count should be performed. Liver function tests should be performed if the patient develops a pruritic rash, jaundice, light-colored stools or dark urine, joint pain, abdominal pain or bloating, anorexia, nausea, or fatigue.[359] Antihistamine therapy may be used for minor cutaneous reactions without stopping the antithyroid drug.[359] If minor side effects of antithyroid medication persist, the drug should be stopped and treatment changed to another antithyroid medication, radioactive iodine, or surgery. If patients experience serious allergic reactions, prescribing an alternative drug is not recommended.[359]

Methimazole is the recommended first-line therapy in children.[317,359]

Radioiodine therapy: Radioiodine therapy has been widely used for adults with thyrotoxicosis caused both by Graves disease and other common causes such as multinodular goiter. ^{131}I is the isotope of choice. It is effective, safe, and relatively inexpensive. It is administered orally as a single dose in a capsule or in water. It is rapidly and completely absorbed and is then concentrated, oxidized, and organified by thyroid follicular cells. It causes cellular necrosis, which in turn provokes an inflammatory response; patients may develop a mild thyroid tenderness in the few days after treatment. Others may develop transient worsening of their thyrotoxicosis caused by the leakage of stored T_4 and T_3 from disrupted follicles. Over time, chronic inflammation and fibrosis result in a substantial decrease in the size of the thyroid gland. ^{131}I therapy should be avoided in very young children.[317,359]

Pregnancy or the possibility of pregnancy is an absolute contraindication for radioiodine therapy. A negative pregnancy test result 48 hours before administration of radioiodine should be ensured.[359] Pretreatment with β-adrenergic blockade and methimazole before radioactive iodine therapy should be instituted in patients with Graves disease who are at increased risk of complications because of worsening of hyperthyroidism (ie, those who are extremely symptomatic or have fT_4 concentrations two to three times the upper limit of normal).[359] Furthermore, pretreatment for any comorbid conditions should be optimized.[359]

Hypothyroidism is an inevitable consequence of radioiodine therapy. It develops in as many as 90% of patients within the first year after therapy and continues at a rate of 2% to 3% per year.[365] Measurement of fT_4 and tT3 should be done within the first 1 to 2 months after radioactive iodine therapy and be continued at 4- to 6-week intervals while the patient remains thyrotoxic.[359] If hyperthyroidism persists after 6 months, retreatment with ^{131}I is recommended.[359]

Radioiodine treatment for hyperthyroidism is a risk factor for development of cancer of the small bowel and thyroid, but the standardized incidence risk is low (4.81 and 3.25, respectively).[366] Even though the risk has decreased over the years, it still persists, and there is a need for long-term vigilance in those receiving radioiodine.[366,367] Development or worsening of ophthalmopathy may be preventable by glucocorticoid therapy begun concurrently or immediately after radioactive iodine therapy.[359]

Thyroidectomy: Surgery may be the treatment of choice in adolescents and pregnant women who are allergic to or

BOX 67.8 Side Effects of Antithyroid Drugs

Minor

Common (1%–5%)
- Urticaria or other rash
- Arthralgia
- Fever
- Transient granulocytopenia

Uncommon (<1%)
- Gastrointestinal upset
- Abnormalities of taste and smell
- Arthritis

Major

Rare (0.2%–0.5%)
- Agranulocytosis

Very rare (<0.1%)
- Aplastic anemia
- Thrombocytopenia

Toxic hepatitis (PTU)
- Cholestatic hepatitis (MMI)
- Vasculitis, systemic lupus-like syndrome
- Hypoprothrombinemia (PTU)
- Hypoglycemia (caused by anti-insulin antibodies) (MMI)

MMI, Methimazole; *PTU* propylthiouracil.

Reproduced from Cooper DS. Treatment of thyrotoxicosis. In: Braverman LE, Cooper DS, editors. *Werner & Ingbar's The Thyroid.* 10th ed. Philadelphia: Lippincott, Williams & Wilkins; 2013:p497 noncompliant with antithyroid drugs, patients with large goiters or severe ophthalmopathy, and when patients prefer destructive therapy but are apprehensive about radioiodine therapy.[359] Thyroidectomy is highly effective for treating patients with Graves disease, but the patients must be rendered euthyroid before surgery, usually by using methimazole.[359] Antithyroid drugs should be stopped at the time of thyroidectomy and patients weaned from β-adrenergic blockers after surgery.[359] Potassium iodide should be given in the immediate preoperative period.[359] In Graves disease, to avoid the risk of relapse and the requirement for repeat surgery, near-total or total thyroidectomy is undertaken rather than subtotal thyroidectomy.[359] All patients are thus rendered hypothyroid postoperatively and have to be initiated on thyroid hormone replacement immediately postsurgery. Thyroidectomy in children should be chosen when definitive therapy is required and the child is too young for ^{131}I treatment.[317,359] After thyroidectomy, serum calcium or intact parathyroid hormone concentrations should be measured, and oral calcium and calcitriol supplementation should be administered if required based on laboratory results.[359]

Other medications: β-Adrenergic blockade should be considered in all patients with symptomatic thyrotoxicosis.[359] Concurrent corticosteroids should be used in patients with Graves disease and mild active ophthalmopathy who are also smokers or have other risk factors for Graves ophthalmopathy and who are to undergo radioactive iodine therapy.[359]

Toxic Adenomas and Toxic Multinodular Goiter

Toxic adenomas and toxic multinodular goiter are conditions in which thyrocytes function and produce thyroid hormones independently of thyrotropin (TSH) and there is an absence of the TSHR-stimulating antibody. This autonomous secretion of thyroid hormones leads to TSH suppression and ultimately results in thyrotoxicosis. Such thyroid autonomy is a common finding in iodine-deficient areas, where it accounts for up to 60% of cases of thyrotoxicosis. However, thyroid autonomy is rare in regions with sufficient iodine supply (3%–10% of cases with thyrotoxicosis).[58,368]

The cause of toxic adenoma and toxic multinodular goiter is not well understood. Although the picture is far from complete, the most prominent epidemiologic factor for their development is iodine deficiency.[58] There is also a strong correlation with age because older patients have a much higher percentage of nodular transformation in iodine-deficient as well as iodine-sufficient areas.[58] In addition, smoking is considered a risk factor for multinodular goiter in women.[369,370]

One theory is that these disorders arise from colloid goiters.[371] A colloid goiter itself is a disorder of unknown origin in which the thyroid gland enlarges because of increased size of the follicular lacunae.[372] Microscopically, the enlarged lacunae display wide variation in size. However, colloid goiters do not display the follicular cell hyperplasia typical of Graves disease. Patients with colloid goiter lack thyroid autoantibodies, and there is no evidence suggestive of a defect in thyroid hormone synthesis. Over many years, some regions of colloid goiters undergo further hypertrophy, and other areas of atrophy, producing nodules that may become palpable.

Thyroid receptor antibodies are negative in toxic multinodular goiter.[373] The diagnosis of thyroid autonomy is based on three characteristics:

- Confirmation of clinically suspected thyrotoxicosis by thyroid function tests
- Presence of palpable or sonographically demonstrable nodule(s)
- Increased radionuclide (eg, 99mTc) uptake in the nodule(s) combined with a decreased uptake in the surrounding extranodular thyroid tissue

The treatment of toxic multinodular goiter and toxic adenoma is with radioiodine or thyroidectomy.[359] In patients with short-term life expectancy, low-dose carbimazole or methimazole may be an alternative.[317] A decision about radioiodine or thyroidectomy should be based on clinical and demographic factors and patient preference.[359] The treatment goal is a rapid and long-lasting elimination of the hyperthyroid state.[359] If goiter size is large with compressive symptoms, thyroidectomy is usually the better choice. Radioiodine treatment may be preferred with advanced age, small goiter size, or multimorbidity.[317]

Gain-of-Function Mutations of the Thyroid-Stimulating Hormone Receptor

A familial autosomal dominant form of hyperthyroidism has been described that is caused by gain-of-function mutations in the TSH receptor.[374] The gain-of-function mutation places the TSHR in the "on" position in the absence of ligand (TSH) binding. In infants homozygous for such mutations, neonatal thyrotoxicosis, so severe as to require emergency thyroidectomy, has been observed. Certain heterozygous mutations have been reported to cause infantile hyperthyroidism.[375]

Central Hyperthyroidism

Thyroid-stimulating hormone–secreting pituitary adenomas are nearly always benign. A total of 75% of the tumors are macroadenomas, having a diameter larger than 10 mm at the time of diagnosis, but microadenomas (diameter <10 mm) are increasingly recognized owing both to early diagnosis and improvements in imaging techniques.[331,376,377]

Thyroid-stimulating hormone adenomas may show concomitant hypersecretion of other pituitary hormones (GH, prolactin, and less frequently follicle-stimulating hormone and luteinizing hormone) together with the hypersecretion of TSH.[331,377]

Patients with TSH-secreting tumors present with signs and symptoms of thyrotoxicosis, but extrathyroidal manifestations (ie, ophthalmopathy, pretibial myxedema, and acropachy) are absent.[331,377] Goiter is a common finding as a consequence of chronic TSH hyperstimulation. Patients may also have symptoms related to the mass effect of the pituitary adenoma such as visual field defects, headache, or loss of other anterior pituitary function (menstrual disorders, galactorrhea acromegaly).[331,377] Many patients have a long history of thyroid dysfunction often diagnosed as Graves disease, and in one series, about one third had inappropriate thyroidectomy or radioiodine ablation.[330,332,376]

The laboratory diagnosis is based on a nonsuppressed TSH in the presence of high levels of free thyroid hormones (fT_3 and fT_4).[331,377] Other diagnostic criteria include evidence of a pituitary mass on CT or MRI.[331] There are both clinical situations (in particular) and possible laboratory artefacts that may cause a biochemical profile similar to that characteristic of patients with TSH-secreting tumors; these include thyroid hormone resistance, binding protein abnormalities, falsely high fT_4 results, and falsely high (given the high T_4) TSH concentrations. The molar ratio of α-subunit to TSH may serve as a useful tumor marker in the differential diagnosis of a TSH-secreting pituitary adenoma, in which the ratio of α-subunit to TSH concentrations is typically larger than 1 ng/mL, from thyroid hormone resistance syndrome, in which the ratio is less than or equal to 1 ng/mL.[330-332,378] Additional tests that may help with the diagnosis include T_3 suppression and TRH tests. Preoperative petrosal venous sampling can be used for the lateralization of TSH-secreting microadenoma, similar to the diagnosis of ACTH-secreting microadenomas.[379]

Commonly, patients may have a previous history of misdiagnosed primary hyperthyroidism and inappropriate attempts at thyroid ablation.[233] Interestingly, in patients previously treated with thyroid ablation who still present with thyrotoxicosis, plasma TSH concentrations are even higher than in untreated patients. This suggests that tumoral thyrotroph cells may increase their TSH secretion in response to even a small reduction in thyroid hormone concentrations. This is important with regard to treatment of such patients. Furthermore, the distinction between hyperthyroidism caused by a TSH-secreting adenoma and resistance to thyroid hormone is difficult because the clinical presentations overlap.

Transsphenoidal resection is the recommended therapy for TSH-secreting tumors.[331,377] Pharmacologic reduction of TSH secretion can be used as an adjunct to surgery or may be used postsurgery if some tumor still remains. Long-acting somatostatin analogues (eg, octreotide, lanreotide) have been shown to reduce TSH secretion and tumor size in individual cases.[380-382] Dopaminergic agonists, such as bromocriptine and cabergoline, may also be effective in residual or recurrent tumors.[331] If surgery is contraindicated or declined, or in the case of surgical failure, pituitary radiotherapy may be considered. Ablative antithyroid therapy (eg, with antithyroid agents) leads to control of the hyperthyroidism but does not deal with the primary problem and is thus generally not indicated.[331]

Early diagnosis and treatment are essential for a good prognosis. The main prognostic factors are size and invasiveness of the tumor, duration of symptoms, and intensity of hyperthyroidism.[383]

Resistance to Thyroid Hormone

Resistance to thyroid hormone (RTHβ) is usually caused by mutations in the thyroid hormone receptor β (THRβ) gene.[49] The HPT axis is affected with impairment of the central T_3 feedback loop.[49]

A laboratory picture with raised plasma concentrations of thyroid hormones with nonsuppressed TSH (normal or elevated) in the presence of thyrotoxic features and goiter should lead to the suspicion of a TSH-secreting tumor.[49] The differential diagnosis is a TSH-secreting adenoma[233] and the molar ratio of α-subunit:TSH may serve as a useful tumor marker in the differential diagnosis of a TSH-secreting pituitary adenoma from thyroid hormone resistance syndrome (see earlier). In TSH-secreting pituitary adenoma, the ratio of α-subunit:TSH serum concentrations is larger than 1 ng/mL; in thyroid hormone resistance, the ratio is less than or equal to 1 ng/mL.[330-332,378] Further diagnosis is based on imaging and genetic testing with *THRβ* gene sequencing.[49] Dynamic function tests such as the TRH test or T_3 suppression tests are also often required and give the best discrimination.[235]

The typical clinical phenotype is of sinus tachycardia, attention deficit hyperactivity disorder, and goiter.[384] The phenotype is a reflection of tissues expressing thyroid hormone receptor α-isoform being overstimulated and tissues expressing the thyroid hormone receptor β-isoforms 1 and 2 being resistant.[384] The clinical phenotypes can be highly variable, and the pathogenic basis for this may be based on the degree of tissue responsiveness to elevated thyroid hormone levels in a given individual.[49]

Only a few patients have been described with mutations in the thyroid hormone receptor α gene *(THRα)*. The HPT axis is minimally affected, and the central T_3 feedback loop is not impaired.[49] Laboratory results in patients with RTHα show plasma TSH concentration within the normal range, slightly lowered concentrations of fT_4, slightly elevated tT3, and an abnormally low free T_4:T_3 ratio.[49] The clinical phenotype is different from RTHβ, and symptoms and signs have been described as a variable degree of mental retardation, short stature, chronic constipation, and bradycardia.[384]

Hyperthyroidism Caused by Human Chorionic Gonadotropin

Human chorionic gonadotropin–induced hyperthyroidism is observed in gestational transient thyrotoxicosis, resulting from TSHR sensitivity to (appropriately) high hCG concentrations during pregnancy (see later section on thyroid disorders in pregnancy and the hyperemesis gravidarum section of Chapter 69) and to hCG-secreting tumours.[385]

Tumors that secrete hCG, such as choriocarcinoma, hydatidiform mole, and metastatic embryonal carcinoma, can cause hyperthyroidism through hCG stimulation of the TSH receptor.[385,386] Hydatiform mole occurs in between 0.5 and 2.5 per 1000 pregnancies.[387] Choriocarcinoma occurs in 2.5 and 5.0 per 100,000 pregnancies.[388] For more details on these hCG-secreting entities, refer to Chapter 69.

Subclinical Hyperthyroidism

The laboratory diagnosis of subclinical hyperthyroidism is defined by a low plasma TSH with normal concentrations of T_4 and T_3.[317] The condition is classified as mild if TSH is in the range 0.1 to 0.4 mIU/L.[301]

Persistent subclinical hyperthyroidism may be caused by exogenous iatrogenic overdose of levothyroxine or by endogenous causes as in primary hyperthyroidism such as Graves disease, toxic multinodular goiter, or solitary autonomous nodule.[301] Exogenous subclinical hyperthyroidism is the most common and is reversible by reduction of levothyroxine dose.

Transitory subclinical hyperthyroidism may be caused by treatment with radioiodine or antithyroid drugs in patients previously with overt hyperthyroidism or as part of thyroiditis.

Plasma TSH concentrations are lower in blacks, in older adults, in cigarette smokers, during the first trimester of pregnancy, in nonthyroidal illness, and in patients treated with certain drugs (glucocorticoids, dopamine).[301] Therefore, appropriate reference intervals should be used (pregnancy, age, and gender related), and if they are not available, caution must be taken in using population reference limits. In nonthyroidal illness, fT_4 and fT_3 concentrations may also be low.

Low TSH values may also be transitory,[389,390] but some patients may develop overt hyperthyroidism over time, particularly if TSH is suppressed.[391-393] The TSH progression over time also depends on the underlying disease; in patients with solitary autonomous nodules or multinodular goiter, the TSH is more likely to persist or progress, but in patients with Graves disease, TSH more often tends to revert to normal values.[301,394]

Patients with subclinical hyperthyroidism have increased risk of ectopic beats,[395,396] carotid artery plaques and stroke,[397,398] atrial fibrillation,[399-402] heart failure,[307] osteoporosis, and fractures.[304,305,403] For cardiovascular and all-cause mortality, three meta-analyses have shown no increased risk,[309,404,405] but one has shown risk to be increased.[406]

The treatment of patients with asymptomatic hyperthyroidism is much more controversial than the treatment of those with asymptomatic hypothyroidism. In the absence of a clinically compatible cardiac arrhythmia or significantly reduced bone mineral density, there is little justification for treating a patient with subclinical hyperthyroidism with thionamide.[301] Current ATA and AACE guidelines state that when a TSH is persistently below 0.10 mIU/L, treatment of subclinical thyrotoxicosis should be strongly considered for patients older than the age of 65 years, in postmenopausal women who are not taking estrogens or bisphosphonates, and in patients with osteoporosis or cardiac risk factors.[359]

Thyroid Disorders in Pregnancy and Postpartum

It is estimated that approximately 4% of pregnant women have a history of thyroid disease, develop thyroid disease during the pregnancy, or are for the first time diagnosed with thyroid disease 5 years after a pregnancy.[407] Postpartum thyroiditis is discussed earlier in the section on thyroiditis.

Physiological Changes

Plasma tT_3 and tT_4 concentrations increase during pregnancy owing to an increase in TBG concentration. This increase is caused by enhanced hepatic synthesis and reduced metabolism (a result of increased estrogen levels) early in pregnancy, resulting in a 1.5-fold increase in TBG by 6 to 8 weeks of gestation. TBG remains elevated throughout pregnancy.[252,408]

Placental hCG shares the same α subunit with TSH but has a unique β subunit and acts in early pregnancy as a TSH agonist by binding to TSH receptors on the thyroid gland.[252,385,408] The physiological consequences of the mild hCG stimulation of the thyroid in early pregnancy leads to a physiological rise in T_4 and T_3, which, by the HPT axis feedback mechanism, inhibits TSH secretion, causing TSH to fall. The decrease in serum TSH in the first trimester is followed by a rise during the second and third trimesters when the hCG concentrations fall but do not exceed prepregnancy values.[252,385,408] There is transient rise in fT_4 during the first trimester owing to the relative high circulating concentration of hCG and a gradual fall of fT_4 in the second and third trimesters.[409] Changes in fT_3 concentrations are broadly parallel with those of fT_4. TSH is higher in singleton pregnancies than in twin pregnancies.[410]

Hypothyroidism in Pregnancy

A total of 2% to 3% of all iodine-sufficient pregnant women have undiagnosed hypothyroidism,[252,411] mostly SCH. Overt hypothyroidism is estimated to occur in 0.5% of all pregnant women.[252] Worldwide, the most common cause is endemic iodine deficiency. The main cause of hypothyroidism in iodine-sufficient populations is chronic autoimmune thyroiditis.[412] Two percent have isolated hypothyroxinemia (eg, elevated thyroid hormone without plasma TSH elevation and without the presence of autoantibodies).[408] About 10% to 20% of women in the childbearing years have detectable autoantibodies (TPO or Tg autoantibodies).[413]

The diagnosis of hypothyroidism in pregnancy is based, as in nonpregnant subjects, on the finding of an elevated serum TSH concentration with low concentrations of fT_4, using trimester-specific reference intervals (see Appendix). Untreated overt maternal hypothyroidism is associated with adverse maternal and fetal outcomes.[252,414,415] There is an increased risk of miscarriage, preterm delivery, and preeclampsia in the mother. In the newborn, there is an increased risk of neonatal mortality caused by preterm delivery, risk of low for gestational age birth weight, and decreased IQ (see section called "Neonatal Thyroid Function" in Chapter 69). The complications are similar in SCH, but occur at a lower frequency.[301] Also, in euthyroid women positive for autoantibodies, there are increased risks of miscarriage, preterm delivery, and postpartum thyroiditis.[252,416]

Treatment and Monitoring. The ATA recommends levothyroxine treatment for all pregnant women with a TSH concentration above the trimester-specific reference interval with a decreased fT_4, and those with a TSH concentration above 10.0 mIU/L irrespective of fT_4 concentration or with TPO autoantibodies[252,256] (Fig. 67.14). The treatment goal is TSH within trimester-specific reference intervals. In women with SCH who test positive for TPO autoantibodies, the ATA recommends levothyroxine treatment, but for those who test negative for TPO autoantibodies, evidence for treatment is insufficient.[252,256]

In women with SCH in pregnancy who are not initially treated, the ATA recommends monitoring with TSH and fT_4 every 4 weeks or so until 16 to 20 weeks of gestation and at least once between 26 and 32 weeks of gestation.

In euthyroid women not receiving levothyroxine who are TPO autoantibody positive, the ATA recommends monitoring for hypothyroidism during pregnancy. Serum TSH should be evaluated every 4 weeks during the first half of pregnancy and at least once between 26 and 32 weeks of gestation.

In women treated with levothyroxine, lower preconception TSH values within the nonpregnant reference interval reduce the risk of TSH elevation during the first trimester. When pregnant, TSH should be measured every 4 weeks until 20 weeks of gestation and at least once in the second half of pregnancy. The required dose of levothyroxine is typically higher in pregnancy and should be returned to the prepregnancy amount immediately postpartum. Six weeks postpartum, thyroid function tests should be performed again. At that that time, TSH and thyroid hormones are no longer affected by the pregnancy.[252,256]

Isolated hypothyroxinemia should not be treated in pregnancy.[256]

Thyrotoxicosis in Pregnancy

Graves disease occurs in 0.1% to 1% of all pregnancies.[252] Transient gestational hyperthyroidism usually occurs in the first trimester with a prevalence of 2% to 3% in Europeans.[417]

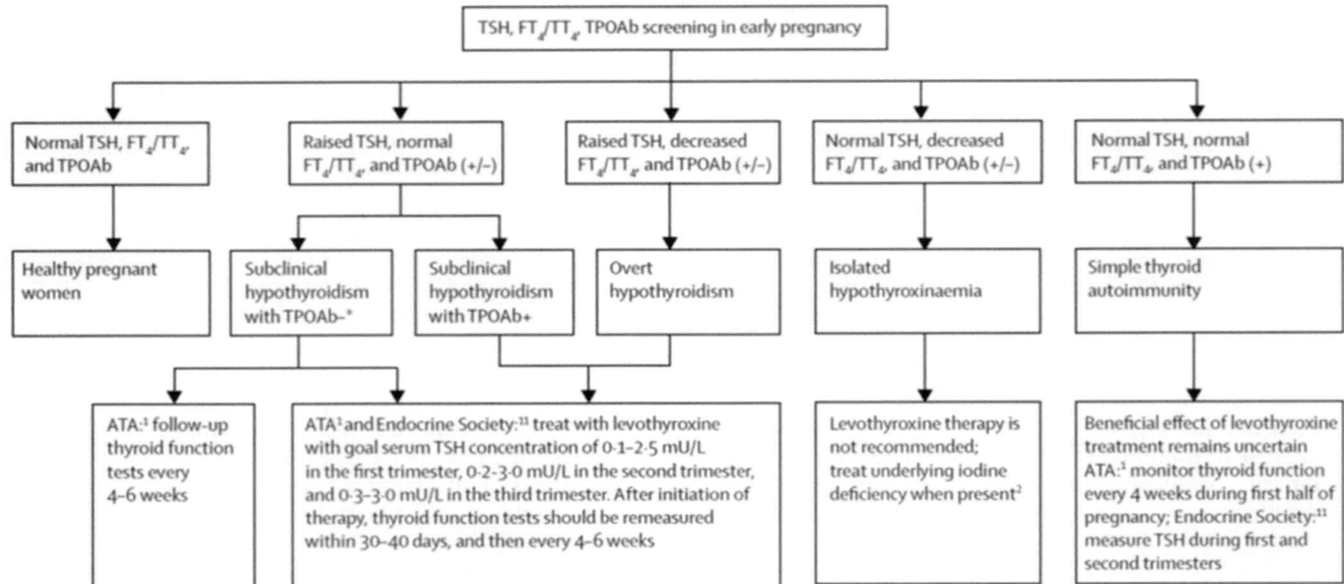

FIGURE 67.14 Screening, diagnosis, and management of hypothyroidism in pregnancy. (Reproduced with permission from Teng W, Shan Z, Patil-Sisodia K, Cooper DS. Hypothyroidism in pregnancy. *Lancet Diabetes Endocrinol* 2013;1:228–237. Based on recommendations from American Thyroid Association [ATA][256] and The Endocrine Society.[258])

The causes of thyrotoxicosis in pregnancy are the same as for thyrotoxicosis generally; however, transient gestational hyperthyroidism is pregnancy specific.[252,417] Thyrotoxicosis may be present before pregnancy or be diagnosed in pregnancy or postpartum.

Diagnosis of Thyrotoxicosis in Pregnancy. The diagnosis of thyrotoxicosis in pregnancy, as at other times, is made by finding a low plasma TSH concentration and elevated concentrations of fT_3, fT_4, or both using trimester-specific reference intervals. Subclinical hyperthyroidism in pregnancy is defined as a low plasma TSH concentration with normal concentrations of fT_4 or fT_3.[252] In patients with Graves disease, TSH and thyroid hormones should be measured every 4 to 6 weeks during pregnancy.[317]

Measurement of TRAb should be reserved for patients with Graves disease who become pregnant or if Graves disease is suspected during pregnancy. In the former, TRAb should be measured at diagnosis and at 24 to 28 weeks gestation because these antibodies can cross the placenta, starting in late second trimester.[252] This to identify high titers that indicate a need for fetal and neonatal monitoring of thyroid size and function[359] even in euthyroid mothers because maternal TRAb antibodies can cross the placenta. Testing for other thyroid autoantibodies is not required, although these are typically present in high titers.

Graves Disease in Pregnancy. Uncontrolled, untreated Graves disease is associated with adverse pregnancy outcomes[418] and risk of maternal heart failure.[419] Risks for the mother include fetal loss, preeclampsia, miscarriage, premature labor, thyroid storm, and congestive heart failure.[252,256,317] Risk for the fetus and neonate include hyperthyroidism caused by TSHR antibodies crossing the placenta (fetal tachycardia, accelerated bone maturation, fetal goiter, intrauterine growth restriction and signs of congestive heart failure, low birthweight for gestational age, poor Apgar scores, and respiratory distress syndrome), risk of hypothyroidism caused by treatment with antithyroid drugs, and congenital abnormalities caused by hyperthyroidism and the teratogenic effects of antithyroid drugs.[252,256,317] Neonatal hyperthyroidism is infrequent and occurs in fewer than 1% of infants born to mothers with Graves disease (effectively 1 in 50,000 neonates). However, if it is not recognized and treated properly, the mortality rate can be as high at 30%.

If Graves disease is diagnosed before pregnancy, the aim should be to achieve a euthyroid state before conception.[252] In patients with a diagnosis of Graves thyrotoxicosis for the first time in pregnancy, the symptoms often will have preceded conception by several months. Many signs and symptoms are commonly seen as normal features of pregnancy, such as mild palpitation, heat intolerance, and shortness of breath on exercise. Features such as a family history of thyroid disease or other autoimmune conditions, the presence of goiter, ophthalmopathy, vitiligo, tachycardia (pulse >100 beats/min), weight loss, or inability to gain weight should help make the diagnosis.[252,317] Anti-TPO antibodies are elevated in most patients with Graves disease, and TRAbs are frequently present.[252,317]

In many pregnant women, Graves disease tends to become exacerbated in the first trimester, improves during later pregnancy, but relapses postpartum.[252,317] As a result of the improvement during pregnancy, the dose of antithyroid drugs may be lowered or even treatment be withdrawn.[252]

In pregnant women with thyrotoxicosis, antithyroid drugs are the treatment of choice. Because of the risk of hepatotoxicity, current guidelines recommend that PTU be used in the first trimester only and should be avoided in the second and third trimesters.[359] The risk of embryopathy with PTU has previously been considered to be low in the first trimester. In the second and third trimesters, methimazole or carbimazole should be used, but these should be avoided during the first trimester (the period of fetal organogenesis) owing to risk of malformation. However, two metaanalyses have shown increased risk of congenital anomalies using PTU, methimazole, or carbimazole, either alone or in switching regimens.[420,421] Combined antithyroid drug and T_4 therapy (block and replacement) is not recommended in pregnancy because it does not prevent neonatal hypothyroidism and usually requires the administration of higher doses of the antithyroid drugs than would otherwise be necessary. Pregnant patients with thyrotoxicosis require careful monitoring to keep the dose of the antithyroid drug to a minimum, especially during the last trimester, because these compounds cross the placenta and may render the fetus hypothyroid.[359] The goal of therapy is to keep fT_4 within or slightly above the trimester-specific reference interval.[317]

Fetal thyroid gland suppression by thionamides is a concern when any pregnant woman with hyperthyroidism is treated. The size of the fetal thyroid gland can be monitored by ultrasonography.[252] TSH and T_4 can be measured in fetal blood obtained by cordocentesis (a high-risk procedure) or in the amniotic fluid.[422] Besides the analytical challenge of measuring the very low concentrations of these hormones in nonplasma body fluids, the choice of an appropriate reference interval can be difficult. Also, it is unlikely that many laboratories have validated measurements of thyroid hormone or TSH in amniotic fluid.

According to the recent ATA and AACE guidelines, breastfeeding is permitted if the daily dose of PTU is less than 300 mg or if methimazole is less than 20 to 30 mg/day.[256]

Thyroidectomy is rarely needed unless a larger goiter compresses the trachea. Subtotal thyroidectomy is an effective management and is usually performed in the second trimester, but there are very few indications.

Therapy with ^{131}I is contraindicated because it can produce fetal hypothyroidism.[256] Subclinical hyperthyroidism does not require treatment in pregnancy.[252]

Transient Gestational Hyperthyroidism and Hyperemesis Gravidarum. Transient gestational thyrotoxicosis is a nonautoimmune hyperthyroidism occurring in pregnant women with a spectrum ranging from no emesis, to emesis, to hyperemesis gravidarum (when dehydration could be so severe that intravenous fluid replacement may be required).[423] Gestational transient thyrotoxicosis occurs in 2% to 3% of all pregnancies and results from activation of TSH receptors by hCG. It is important to distinguish between Graves disease and transient gestational thyrotoxicosis. In both conditions, palpitations, anxiety, hand tremor, and heat intolerance are common clinical manifestations.[256] In transient gestational thyrotoxicosis, thyroid autoantibodies are negative; in Graves disease, diffuse goiter and ophthalmopathy may be present, and thyroid autoantibodies are positive.[256]

Transient gestational thyrotoxicosis may occur in women with hyperemesis gravidarum, in twin or higher-order pregnancies, and in association with hydatiform mole,[252] all conditions in which hCG concentrations are high.[252] Hyperemesis gravidarum occurs in 0.3% to 1% of pregnancies and is characterized by severe nausea and vomiting in the first trimester, leading to more than 5% weight loss, ketonuria, dehydration, and liver and electrolyte abnormalities (particularly hypokalemia).[424] Serum hCG concentrations are positively correlated with the severity of nausea and vomiting.[425] The thyrotoxicosis of hyperemesis gravidarum usually resolves spontaneously within several weeks as the vomiting disappears. The degree of hyperthyroidism is typically mild.[252]

Most patients with hyperemesis gravidarum and transient gestational hyperthyroidism do not require antithyroid medication.[252] Supportive treatment includes rehydration, replacement of electrolytes, and antiemetics.[252,256] Antithyroid drugs are not indicated.[252] However, it is important to exclude concomitant Graves disease because it needs specific treatment.

Thyroid Autoantibodies in Euthyroid Women

Thyroid peroxidase antibodies and Tg antibodies can be detected in 10% to 20% of pregnant women, but most of the women are euthyroid.[413] The presence of the autoantibodies reflects an autoimmune process in the thyroid gland. A meta-analysis has shown that maternal thyroid autoantibodies are strongly associated with miscarriage and preterm delivery.[413] A randomized trial has also shown that treatment with levothyroxine reduces the risks[426] but is currently not recommended by any obstetric, thyroid, or endocrine society.[256,258,316,427]

Postpartum Thyroiditis

Postpartum thyroiditis may be difficult to differentiate from Graves disease. The differences between the two include the presence of goiter, ophthalmopathy, and thyroid receptor (TRAb) antibodies in Graves disease with high iodine or technetium uptake; these are usually not present in thyroiditis. Approximately 4% to 9% of unselected postpartum women develop postpartum thyroiditis,[252,253] although the incidence varies with geographical location. Postpartum thyroiditis often recurs in subsequent pregnancies, and 50% of women eventually develop hypothyroidism. Postpartum thyroiditis only requires beta-blockers for treatment.

Thyroid Function Testing in Pregnancy

Trimester-specific reference intervals for TSH and thyroid hormones should be applied (see Appendix). International guidelines recommend that trimester- and assay-specific reference intervals should be established or verified in each laboratory. If that is not possible, then reference intervals from the ATA should be applied.[256] TSH is a reliable indicator of thyroid function during pregnancy in most cases, with these reference intervals:

- First trimester: 0.1 to 2.5 mIU/L
- Second trimester: 0.2 to 3.0 mIU/L
- Third trimester: 0.3 to 3.0 mIU/L.

Serum fT_4 and fT_3 are in the picomolar range, and to be valid, they are technically difficult to measure because they must be free from interference by the much higher total hormone concentrations (in the nanomolar range).[409] The reliability of immunoassays for the measurement of fT_3 and fT_4 is decreased in pregnancy owing to higher TBG but lower albumin concentrations.[252,428-430] Liquid chromatography–tandem mass spectrometry combined with equilibrium dialysis or ultrafiltration methods are more reliable for both total and free hormone concentrations during pregnancy.[252,409,431,432]

Thyroid Screening in Pregnancy

Thyroid dysfunction during pregnancy may affect maternal health, fetal health, and obstetric outcome. Recommendations for screening for thyroid disorders in pregnancy vary among different clinical associations.[256,258,316,427] The controversies can be narrowed down to whether to screen universally or to use a targeted approach and what criteria should be used for targeted screening, such as age, previous pregnancy-related adverse outcomes, comorbid disease (especially autoimmune disease), presence of thyroid antibodies, obesity, family history of thyroid disease, goiter, medication, iodine availability in the area of living, and previous thyroid disease. The consequence of the different guidelines is different practices among physicians nationally as well as internationally.[433-437]

POINTS TO REMEMBER

Pregnancy

- Use trimester-specific thyroid reference intervals.
- TSH may be misleading in the first trimester and fT_4 values will give a more accurate estimate of clinical status.
- Late in gestation, TSH concentrations are more reliable, but T_4 may fall, especially during the third trimester.
- In some cases, anti-TPO antibodies can provide further information; this can predict risk of hypothyroidism.
- Measurement of TRAb is indicated in all women with active Graves disease or a history of this condition because transplacental transfer of this antibody can cause fetal hyperthyroidism.

SCREENING FOR THYROID DYSFUNCTION

Apart from newborn screening for congenital hypothyroidism, so far no compelling data shows that universal screening of asymptomatic individuals, including pregnant women or older adults, improves the clinical outcome of the patients.[427,438]

In a review on behalf of the US Preventative Services Task Force (USPSTF) from 2015, the conclusion was that more research is needed to determine the clinical benefits associated with universal thyroid screening.[438] The review focused on the benefits and harms of screening and treatment of subclinical and undiagnosed overt hypothyroidism and hyperthyroidism in adults without goiter or thyroid nodules.

However, the USPSTF recommended targeted screening in high-risk groups; also, the ATA recommends targeted screening in pregnant women.[252] The recommended groups for targeted screening are overlapping, including, among others, patients with a personal history of previous thyroid disease or neck irradiation; patients with a family history of thyroid disease, newly diagnosed atrial fibrillation, or a history of goiter; patients with type 1 diabetes or other autoimmune or endocrine disorders; women with infertility or previous preterm delivery or miscarriage; and patients taking drugs known to interfere with thyroid function.

THYROID NEOPLASIA

The prevalence of palpable thyroid nodules in adults is about 5%, the prevalence of nodules found on ultrasonography is 13% to 30%, and the prevalence of nodules found on autopsy is 49% to 57%.[439] The prevalence of cancer in single nodules has been estimated to be 5% and may be less frequent in multinodular goiter.[440] Cancer risk depends on age, sex, radiation exposure, history, family history, and other factors.[210] A recent metaanalysis of observational studies showed that vegetables overall may have a protective effect on thyroid cancer incidence and likewise fish and shellfish in iodine-deficient areas, but no effects were observed in iodine-rich areas.[441]

Thyroid cancer is a rare cause of cancer death (<0.4% in the United States) because the incidence is low (~2%).[442] The female-to-male ratio is 3 to 1.[443] The incidence is increasing,[443] but mortality rates from thyroid cancer have remained stable. Therefore, it is debated whether this increase in cases is due to overdiagnosis, as a consequence of high-resolution imaging,[444] or a true increase caused by environmental factors such as radiation exposure.[443,445]

There are four main types of thyroid cancer (listed from the most common to the least common): differentiated thyroid cancer (DCT), including (1) papillary and (2) follicular thyroid cancer, accounting for more than 90% of thyroid cancers in United States[210]; (3) medullary (<5%)[446,447]; and (4) anaplastic thyroid cancer, accounting for about 2%.[443] Follicular cells give rise to well-differentiated papillary and follicular carcinomas[210] but also the poorly differentiated anaplastic carcinomas, which have a worse prognosis.[448] Parafollicular or C cells secrete calcitonin and give rise to MTC, with an intermediate prognosis.[447] MTC may be sporadic or hereditary, but most cases (80%) are sporadic (ie, not genetically inherited and occur randomly).

The main role for the clinical biochemist is the monitoring of TSH suppression therapy, determination of cancer ablation, the detection of recurrence in patients given definitive treatment such as thyroidectomy, and prognosis.[202]

Diagnosis

Although the diagnosis of thyroid neoplasia is largely reliant on clinical, radiologic, and histologic investigations, serum TSH measurement is a key investigation in a patient presenting with a thyroid nodule. Suppressed TSH is in keeping with an autonomous nodule; these have a low risk of being malignant, but patients may need treatment for thyrotoxicosis. A normal or high TSH should prompt ultrasound investigations with FNA biopsy dependent on results.

Differentiated Thyroid Cancer

These have a favorable prognosis.[442] Evaluation and treatments for DTC are multimodal. Evaluation involves ultrasound, FNA biopsy, imaging, and blood tests. The goals of therapy are to remove the primary tumor and clinically significant lymph node metastases with thyroidectomy and local nodal dissection[210] and to minimize the risk of disease recurrence and metastatic spread with adjuvant therapy radioactive iodine and TSH suppression.[210] Routine TSH suppression therapy for benign thyroid nodules in iodine-sufficient populations is not recommended.[210]

Biochemically, TSH and Tg are useful markers.[210] Serum TSH should be measured during the initial evaluation of a patient with a thyroid nodule.[210] A higher TSH is suspicious for cancer even if TSH is on the higher end of the reference interval.[210] Because TSH is a major trophic factor for thyroid carcinoma, suppression of TSH using exogenous thyroid hormone administration after surgery reduces the risk of recurrence and prevents hypothyroidism.[210] Consequently, the routine measurement of serum TSH, fT_4, and fT_3 is required for patient follow-up. Free T_3 analysis can provide reassurance that these patients have not been rendered overly hyperthyroid. A low or low within the reference interval TSH concentration is suggestive of the presence of some autonomous nodules in patients with multiple nodules.[210]

Serum Tg concentration can be elevated in many thyroid diseases and is not sensitive or specific for thyroid cancer; thus, it is not recommended to measure serum Tg for initial evaluation of thyroid nodules or preoperatively.[210] However, it is a useful marker for disease recurrence in thyroidectomized patients because it should be undetectable. Tg should not be used as a tumor marker in the presence of anti-Tg antibodies owing to measurement interference[210] (see also Chapter 31). TSH stimulation by either temporarily ceasing thyroid hormone replacement or by the administration of recombinant TSH greatly increases the sensitivity of Tg measurement, but this may not be necessary using more sensitive Tg assays.[210] The optimal cut-off for Tg for predicting recurrence is not known. There is a general agreement that a stimulated Tg less than 1 ng/mL with no other radiologic or clinical evidence of disease and in the absence of autoantibodies suggests no evidence of disease, although recurrence has been described below this cut point.[210] Tg should be measured 6 weeks to 3 months after surgery and then every 6 to 12 months,[202,210] but there is no agreement on the ideal timing and frequency of testing.[202,210] Persistently elevated Tg concentrations may indicate either recurrence or a thyroid remnant.[210] Newer Tg assays have a functional sensitivity of 0.1 ng/mL or less (compared to older assays with 1 ng/mL); this allows for earlier identification of recurrence and also avoidance of the use of TSH stimulation.[210]

About 20% to 30% of patients with DTC have Tg antibodies (TgAbs).[209] If Tg cannot be measured on a mass spectrometric method in the presence of Tg antibodies, then TgAbs themselves may be used as surrogate tumor marker instead of Tg.[202,209,449] Both the actual concentrations and values over time may be used.[209,449,450] TgAbs should not be used within the first weeks after thyroidectomy because a transient rise may be caused by TgAbs reacting to released Tg.[209,449,450] However, TgAbs have a role in long-term follow-up after thyroidectomy.[450] Whereas a sustained high level or persistent rise suggests recurrence, a persistent fall suggests low risk of recurrence.[209,449,450]

Immunometric assays used to measure Tg and TgAbs are prone to interferences. The hook effect can cause falsely low values for Tg and TgAbs.[210] Thus, an apparent absence of TgAbs may be a result of antibodies not being detected, and in such instances, low Tg concentrations may be misleading. Furthermore, both Tg and TgAb immunometric assays may be affected by heterophilic antibodies, causing falsely elevated results.[210] If TgAbs are absent on immunometric assays, but pathology shows Hashimoto thyroiditis, then the presence of TgAbs should be suspected.[210] Serially measured Tg and TgAbs should be done on the same analyzer using the same assay.[210]

Medullary Thyroid Cancer

The diagnosis of MTC is based on FNA biopsy, imaging, blood tumor markers, and genetic testing. The standard treatment for patients with sporadic or hereditary MTC is total thyroidectomy and dissection of cervical lymph node compartments depending on serum calcitonin concentrations and ultrasound findings and subsequent replacement with levothyroxine.[447] Radiation or chemotherapy maybe used as palliative measures but not as a cure.[447] The prognosis depends on the spread of the cancer, with localized cancers having a good 10-year prognosis but cancers with peripheral metastases having a poor prognosis.[447] Serum TSH and serum calcium should be measured postoperatively. The goal is to render patients euthyroid and to prevent hypocalcemia.[447]

Calcitonin, produced by C cells, is a valuable blood tumor marker for MTC. Calcitonin is a 32-amino-acid monomeric peptide that is the result of cleavage and posttranslational processing of procalcitonin, which is itself a product of pre-procalcitonin.[447] Serum calcitonin can be used as a screening test in patients with a family history of MTC447, who are at risk of developing the disease. The use of calcitonin as a screening marker in patients with nodular goiter and with no family history is debatable.[447] Calcitonin is also used diagnostically as an immunohistochemical marker.[447] Basal serum calcitonin and carcinoembryonic antigen (CEA) should be measured concurrently.[447] CEA is not a specific biomarker for MTC and is not useful in the early diagnosis of MTC.[447] However, CEA is useful for evaluating disease progression in patients with clinically evident MTC and for monitoring patients after thyroidectomy.[447] All patients diagnosed with MTC should be tested for the genetic mutations associated with hereditary forms of the disease.[447] A small number of patients with sporadic MTC can have RET gene mutations. To predict outcome and plan long-term follow-up in patients treated by thyroidectomy for MTC, TNM (tumor, node, metastasis) classification, the number of lymph node metastases, and postoperative serum calcitonin and CEA should be used.[447] Genetic status also determines prognosis in patients with hereditary MTC.[447]

Measurements of calcitonin may also be used to monitor for persistent or recurrent disease after surgery because the concentrations correlate with tumor burden. The MTC growth rate can be determined by measuring serum levels of calcitonin or CEA over multiple time points to determine the rate at which each marker's value doubles.[447] Furthermore, serum TSH and serum calcium should be measured postoperatively. The goals are to get patients euthyroid and to prevent hypocalcemia.[447]

Measurement of Serum Calcitonin

Blood samples should be drawn in the fasting state. Calcitonin has a low stability in serum at room temperature, so the sample must be immediately spun after coagulation and then frozen and transported on ice to the laboratory. Measurement of calcitonin is by immunoassay. Historically, radioimmunoassay were used, but more recently, automated noncompetitive immunoassays (eg, immunochemiluminometric assays [ICMA]) have largely taken over owing to their high sensitivity and specificity for monomeric calcitonin[446] and comparable analytical performances.[446] With ICMAs, cross-reactivity with procalcitonin and other calcitonin-related peptides is largely eliminated. Measured concentrations of calcitonin may be falsely high (because of heterophilic antibodies) or falsely low (because of a hook effect, as can be seen in patients with a large tumor burden and very high concentrations), causing interpretation problems. Normal reference intervals are higher in men than in women, likely because of a higher C-cell mass.[446,447] Because of intermethod differences pre- and postthyroidectomy and during treatment, concentrations should be measured using the same assay and instrument in the same laboratory. Because reference intervals depend on the method used as well as gender and whether basal or stimulated (calcium and pentagastrin provocation)[446] calcitonin is measured, each laboratory should determine its own reference intervals based on these criteria.

Alternatively, manufacturers' recommendations or reference intervals from relevant literature may be used.[446] Basal serum calcitonin concentrations greater than 100 pg/mL measured by ICMA are suggestive of MTC.[446] The predictive value for MTC of an elevated basal calcitonin is increased by a positive stimulation test result.[446] Simultaneous elevations of serum CEA and calcitonin concentrations in serial measurements indicate disease progression.[447] Misdiagnosis or advanced dedifferentiation of the MTC indicating a poor prognosis should be suspected if patients with advanced MTC have normal or low serum concentrations of calcitonin and CEA.

Other than MTC, calcitonin may also be increased in nonthyroidal cancer, inflammation and sepsis, acute and chronic renal failure, hypercalcemia, pulmonary disease, and hypergastrinemia.[447] Calcitonin may also be high during the first week of life and in low-birthweight children and premature infants.[447] Besides gender and age, growth in children and during pregnancy, and lactation may also influence circulating concentrations of calcitonin.[451] The relevance of calcitonin to bone and mineral metabolism is discussed in Chapter 64.

Anaplastic Thyroid Cancer

Anaplastic thyroid cancer (ATC) is the most infrequent but also the most lethal of the thyroid cancers.[448,452] There is no particular specific circulating biomarker for ATC.

THYROID DISEASE IN CHILDREN

Thyroid disease as described in this chapter can occur at any age; however, some characteristics in newborns, children, and adolescents are worth mentioning. The consequences of a hypofunctioning thyroid (see later) in developing and maturing children may be long lasting if not diagnosed and treated early.[453] Neonatal hyperthyroidism may be caused by transplacental passage of thyroid-stimulating maternal immunoglobulins (due to active maternal Graves' disease[454]) or by activating TSH receptor mutations (see subsequent text).[455] In older children and adolescents, the most common cause of hyperthyroidism is Graves disease,[456] and the most common cause of hypothyroidism in iodine-replete areas is Hashimoto thyroiditis.[457]

Iodine Deficiency in Children

Iodine deficiency leads to reduced thyroid hormone synthesis, increased TSH secretion, which stimulates proliferation of thyroid cells, and consequently thyroid enlargement and goiter.[458] If the iodine deficiency is severe, thyroid hormone production will continue to fall, leading to hypothyroidism. Thyroid hormone plays a vital role in growth and neurodevelopment,[458] and metaanalyses have shown that children living in iodine-deficient areas have IQs that are 6 to 12 points lower than children living in iodine-replete areas.[459,460]

Congenital Hypothyroidism

Before the introduction of newborn screening programs, the incidence of congenital hypothyroidism was estimated to be 1 in 7000 newborns.[453] However, recent surveys estimate the incidence to be 1 in 2000 to 1 in 4000 newborns[461-463]; the incidence is higher in Asians and Hispanics than whites and blacks.[462] The incidence is higher in older compared with younger mothers and in preterm infants versus term infants.[462] Incidence rates are dependent on TSH screening cut-offs. "Cretinism refers to the syndrome of mental retardation, deafness, short stature, and characteristic facial deformities occurring with untreated congenital hypothyroidism."[277]

Congenital hypothyroidism can be categorized into *permanent* and *transient* forms, which again can be divided into *primary* (thyroid disorder), *secondary* (ie, central hypothyroidism; see earlier discussion), and *peripheral*.[461] Permanent congenital hypothyroidism (75%–86%) needs lifelong replacement treatment, but transient forms resolve within weeks to months after birth.[464] Permanent primary congenital hypothyroidism may be caused by defects in thyroid development, thyroid dysgenesis (85%), or dyshormonogenesis (15%), a biosynthesis defect of thyroid hormone production in a structurally normal gland.[39,465] Thyroid dysgenesis may consist of either thyroid agenesis, failure of the gland to descend normally during embryologic development with or without ectopy, or hypoplasia of a normal localized gland.[466] Central hypothyroidism occurs in 1 in 25,000 to 1 in 50,000 newborns.[453]

Transient congenital hypothyroidism is most commonly caused by inadequate maternal iodine intake in areas of endemic iodine deficiency.[461] Transient congenital hypothyroidism may also be caused by maternal antithyroid medication during pregnancy,[453] transfer of maternal blocking antibodies, maternal iodine exposure (eg, amiodarone), liver hemangiomas causing increased production of deiodinase 3, and genetic defects.[461]

Unless born with thyroid agenesis, most newborns with congenital hypothyroidism have some thyroid function.[453] Many newborns, even those with thyroid agenesis, do not present with classic symptoms and signs of hypothyroidism owing to transplacental passage of maternal thyroid hormones.[453] Early symptoms and signs of congenital hypothyroidism include a lethargic infant with increased sleep, prolonged jaundice, myxedematous facies, large fontanels, macroglossia, distended abdomen, hypothermia, and hypotonia.[288,453] Later symptoms and signs include poor sucking effort leading to feeding difficulties, constipation, developmental delay with cognitive and growth retardation, myxedema, umbilical hernia, and decreased activity.[288,453,461] Ten percent of children born with congenital hypothyroidism have other congenital birth defects, and 50% of them have congenital heart defects.[288]

Levothyroxine is the treatment of choice with treatment goals to raise serum T_4 and normalize serum TSH.[467] Levothyroxine treatment can prevent mental retardation in the majority of children (>90%) if commenced within the first 2 weeks of life.[288]

Laboratory Diagnosis of Congenital Hypothyroidism

Newborn screening for congenital hypothyroidism is a successful public health program for secondary prevention of mental retardation.[288] Worldwide it is estimated that 25% of the newborn population undergoes a screening for congenital hypothyroidism.[453,461]

Screening strategies differ between countries with some countries measuring TSH initially with a reflex T_4 if TSH is abnormal. Others measure T_4 as a first-line test and if T_4 is below a certain cut-off reflex test for TSH or measure a combination of TSH, T_4, and Tg to differentiate between primary and secondary causes.[288] The disadvantage of screening programs only measuring TSH with a reflex T_4, is the inability to detect central hypothyroidism.[453] The initial screening occurs on the second to fifth day of life[453]; children discharged from the hospital on the first day of life may have a sample taken at this time. Some programs routinely obtain a second specimen at 2 to 6 weeks of age.[461] Some programs use cord blood at birth, and others use heel prick on filter paper after birth.[461] Many programs now use initial TSH measurement from heel prick blood on filter cards.[461] Filter cards are mailed to a central laboratory. Each program has its own cut-offs for test results. Thyroid hormone levels and TSH are higher in the first days of life but have usually fallen to concentrations typically seen in infancy within the 2 to 4 weeks[461](see Appendix for reference intervals).

An abnormal result on screening should lead to a confirmatory test in a serum sample, but this should not delay treatment.[288,461] Confirmatory testing includes TSH and free or total T_4[461] and should be compared with appropriate age-dependent reference intervals[461] (see Appendix for reference intervals). Further diagnostic tests may include radionuclide thyroid uptake and scanning, thyroid sonography, and serum Tg to determine the subtype of congenital hypothyroidism but should not delay the initiation of treatment.[288,461]

False-positive elevations in TSH may be seen within the 2 first days of life but revealed after repeated testing on a confirmatory test. Transplacental transfer of TSH heterophile antibodies is well described as a false-positive interference in blood spot TSH and maternal thyroid function tests need to be checked in this context.[468] Preterm infants with immature HPT axis and acutely ill term infants may have a late rise in TSH and may not show elevated TSH on the first screening test; many programs have a second screening test for these babies.[288,461] Dopamine used in the treatment of ill premature neonates can also attenuate TSH release.[288] Seasonal variations in TSH occur with an increased false-positive rate of congenital hypothyroidism in the winter (0.9%) compared with the summer (0.6%)[140]; this is in accordance with globally conducted previous studies that have identified an increased prevalence of suspected and confirmed cases of congenital hypothyroidism in the winter months.[140]

GENETICS

Evidence from twin studies has shown that about 65% of baseline TSH and thyroid hormone concentrations are genetically determined,[128,469,470] with about 20% of the variability coming from common genetic variation at the population level.[127] This suggests a genetic basis for narrow intraindividual variation in these hormone concentrations.[471] Several loci have been identified in genome-wide association studies (GWAS) for the circulating concentrations of TSH, thyroid hormones, thyroid autoantibodies,[127,129] and deiodinases.[128,471] Also, GWAS studies have identified common polygenic variations in DTC[472] and papillary thyroid cancer.[473] GWAS may identify pathways, but large cohort studies and experimental cell and animal models are needed to understand the biologic effects and translate the genetic information to human health and disease.[128]

Genetics in Autoimmune Thyroid Disease

Autoimmune susceptibility against the thyroid gland is estimated to affect 5% of the general population, and 80% of this susceptibility is estimated to be explained by genetic factors. The rest is explained by environmental triggers, including dietary iodine, stress, smoking, and infection.[129] Autoimmune susceptibility genes include thyroid-specific genes (Tg and TSHR) and immune-regulatory genes, which are shared with other autoimmune diseases.[272,474] AITD immune-regulatory genes encompasses *FOXP3* and *CD25* involved in establishment of immune self-tolerance, and CD40, CTLA-4, and HLA involved in T-lymphocyte activation and antigen presentation.[272] HLADR3 carries the highest risk.[272] Concordance for AITD is higher among monozygotic twins than among dizygotic twins.[324,475] Twin studies have estimated that 75% of Graves disease is heritable.[324,325]

Genetics in Congenital Hypothyroidism

Thyroid dyshormonogenesis is inherited in an autosomal recessive pattern.[464] Thyroid dysgenesis, on the other hand, is inherited in only approximately 2% of cases; the rest are considered to be sporadic.[464] Monogenetic thyroid dysgenesis can be classified into syndromic and nonsyndromic forms.[464] The sporadic cases of thyroid dysgenesis may also have a genetic component but not a classic Mendelian inheritance; rather, they have a polygenic or epigenetic inheritance.[464]

Genes associated with *thyroid dyshormonogenesis* include genes involved in the steps of thyroid hormone synthesis,[288] including (1) iodine transport into the thyroid follicle through the sodium-iodine symporter NIS[476] and the sodium-independent chloride/iodide transporter pendrin,[64] and (2) iodine incorporation into the nascent thyroid hormone, that is, the enzyme TPO,[477] dual oxidases (DUOX),[478] and the matrix protein Tg.[479]

Nonsyndromic thyroid dysgenesis genes include inactivating mutations in the TSH receptor,[480] and the *syndromic thyroid dysgenesis* include genes for $G_s\alpha$ and for the transcription factors TITF-1, TITF-2, and PAX-8.[465]

Resistance to TSH that results from mutations in *TSHR* causes overt or subclinical congenital hypothyroidism.[480] It has been shown that heterozygous individuals experience stable thyroid hormone concentrations and only mild SCH not amenable to treatment, but homozygous individuals experience low fT_4 over time. requiring treatment with levothyroxine.[481]

Thyroid-Stimulating Receptor Mutations and Resistance to Thyroid-Stimulating Hormone

Cases of familial thyrotoxicosis with absence of evidence of autoimmunity and children with persistent isolated neonatal hyperthyroidism should be evaluated for familial nonautoimmune autosomal dominant hyperthyroidism (FNAH) and persistent sporadic congenital nonautoimmune hyperthyroidism (PSNAH) caused by rare germline mutations in the *TSHR* gene.[482] The mutation changes an amino acid in the transcript and results in a TSHR that is continuously activated with consequent overproduction of thyroid hormones. As a result, the thyroid gland enlarges (goiter) with symptoms of hyperthyroidism. The laboratory diagnosis shows hyperthyroidism confirmed by high serum concentration of fT_4 and low TSH or subclinical hyperthyroidism with only suppressed TSH.[482] Somatic mutations in autonomous adenomas reveal a similar phenotype.[455] Qualitatively, the activating mutations are similar in FNAH, PSNAH, and autonomous adenomas; however, the onset is different.[455]

Thyroid Hormone Receptor Mutations and Resistance to Thyroid Hormone

Two different thyroid hormone receptors are known, thyroid hormone receptor α (THRα) and thyroid hormone receptor β (THRβ), encoded by the *THRA* and *THRB* genes, respectively.[49,384] THRα has three isoforms, the main form being THRα1, and THRβ has two main isoforms, THRβ1 and THRβ2, for mediating thyroid hormone action. The clinical phenotypes in patients with resistance to thyroid hormone α (RTHα) and resistance to thyroid hormone β (RTHβ) are different.[49,384]

Patients with mutations in *THRB* present with resistance to thyroid hormone β (RTHβ) characterized by raised levels of thyroid hormone, normal or elevated levels of TSH, and goiter, suggesting a critical role for *THRB* in negative-feedback regulation.[49,384]

Only a few patients with resistance to thyroid hormone α (RTHα) have been described.[49,483] Patients show features of hypothyroidism, typically growth and developmental retardation, skeletal dysplasia, and constipation caused by effects on the GI tract, skeletal muscle, and skeleton.[49,483] However, these patients have near-normal concentrations of thyroid hormones and TSH, suggesting that the central T_3 feedback loop is not impaired and that the HPT axis is only minimally affected.[49,384] This is in contrast to the clinical phenotype in patients with RTHβ.[49]

SELECTED REFERENCES

For a full list of references for this chapter, please refer to ExpertConsult.com.

44. Bailey D, Colantonio D, Kyriakopoulou L, et al. Marked biological variance in endocrine and biochemical markers in childhood: establishment of pediatric reference intervals using healthy community children from the CALIPER cohort. *Clin Chem* 2013;**59**:1393–405.
58. Zimmermann MB, Boelaert K. Iodine deficiency and thyroid disorders. *Lancet Diabetes Endocrinol* 2015;**3**:286–95.
127. Taylor PN, Porcu E, Chew S, et al. Whole-genome sequence-based analysis of thyroid function. *Nat Commun* 2015;**6**: 5681.
135. Elmlinger MW, Kuhnel W, Lambrecht HG, et al. Reference intervals from birth to adulthood for serum thyroxine (T4), triiodothyronine (T3), free T3, free T4, thyroxine binding globulin (TBG) and thyrotropin (TSH). *Clin Chem Lab Med* 2001;**39**:973–9.
166. Pearce EN, Farwell AP, Braverman LE. Thyroiditis. *N Engl J Med* 2003;**348**:2646–55.
174. Midgley JE. Direct and indirect free thyroxine assay methods: theory and practice. *Clin Chem* 2001;**47**:1353–63.
185. Thienpont LM, Van Uytfanghe K, Beastall G, et al. Report of the IFCC Working Group for Standardization of Thyroid Function Tests; part 1: thyroid-stimulating hormone. *Clin Chem* 2010;**56**:902–11.
187. Thienpont LM, Van Uytfanghe K, Beastall G, et al. Report of the IFCC Working Group for Standardization of Thyroid Function Tests; part 3: total thyroxine and total triiodothyronine. *Clin Chem* 2010;**56**:921–9.
188. Thienpont LM, Van Uytfanghe K, Van Houcke S, et al. A Progress Report of the IFCC Committee for Standardization of Thyroid Function Tests. *Eur Thyroid J* 2014;**3**:109–16.
189. Thienpont LM, Van Uytfanghe K, Van Houcke S. Tests IWGfSoTF. Standardization activities in the field of thyroid function tests: a status report. *Clin Chem Lab Med* 2010;**48**:1577–83.
214. Hoofnagle AN, Becker JO, Wener MH, et al. Quantification of thyroglobulin, a low-abundance serum protein, by immunoaffinity peptide enrichment and tandem mass spectrometry. *Clin Chem* 2008;**54**:1796–804.
252. Stagnaro-Green A, Pearce E. Thyroid disorders in pregnancy. *Nat Rev Endocrinol* 2012;**8**:650–8.
277. Roberts CG, Ladenson PW. Hypothyroidism. *Lancet* 2004;**363**:793–803.
288. Gruters A, Krude H. Detection and treatment of congenital hypothyroidism. *Nat Rev Endocrinol* 2012;**8**:104–13.
301. Cooper DS, Biondi B. Subclinical thyroid disease. *Lancet* 2012;**379**:1142–54.
317. Franklyn JA, Boelaert K. Thyrotoxicosis. *Lancet* 2012;**379**:1155–66.
369. Vestergaard P, Rejnmark L, Weeke J, et al. Smoking as a risk factor for Graves' disease, toxic nodular goiter, and autoimmune hypothyroidism. *Thyroid* 2002;**12**: 69–75.
454. Cooper DS, Laurberg P. Hyperthyroidism in pregnancy. *Lancet Diabetes Endocrinol* 2013;**1**:238–49.

68

Reproductive Endocrinology and Related Disorders

*Robert D. Nerenz, Emily Jungheim, and Ann M. Gronowski**

ABSTRACT

Background

The field of reproductive endocrinology encompasses the hormones of the hypothalamic-pituitary-gonadal axis and the adrenal glands that are crucial for reproductive function. Hypothalamic gonadotropin-releasing hormone (GnRH) directs the pituitary to synthesize and release follicle-stimulating hormone (FSH) and luteinizing hormone (LH), which in turn stimulate gonadal synthesis of the sex steroids that govern the development and maintenance of secondary sex characteristics. In states of reproductive health, serum concentrations of these hormones rise and fall in a tightly regulated and well-characterized pattern. In states of reproductive dysfunction, measurement of these hormones in the clinical laboratory often provides the necessary information to identify the underlying abnormality and guide appropriate treatment.

Content

This chapter discusses the role of reproductive hormones in typical developmental and reproductive processes and describes disease states caused by hormonal dysregulation. The first section covers male reproductive biology, with an emphasis on testosterone synthesis, activity, and transport and explains alterations in hormonal signaling that lead to common reproductive abnormalities. Similarly, the second section discusses female reproductive biology and focuses on the activities of estrogens and progesterone in states of reproductive health and disease. The third section describes the clinical approach to evaluating both male and female infertility. Finally, the fourth section summarizes analytical methods used to measure reproductive hormones in the clinical laboratory, with particular attention given to the strengths, limitations, and ideal clinical applications of immunoassay- and mass spectrometry–based methods.

Reproductive endocrinology encompasses the hormones of the hypothalamic-pituitary-gonadal axis, as well as the adrenal glands (see Chapters 65 and 66). These hormones are crucial for reproductive function and include gonadotropin-releasing hormone (GnRH), luteinizing hormone (LH), follicle-stimulating hormone (FSH), and a multitude of sex steroids. The sex steroids are synthesized by the ovaries, testes, and adrenal glands and are responsible for the manifestation of primary and secondary sex characteristics. This chapter discusses the actions of these hormones in typical developmental and reproductive processes, disease states caused by hormone dysregulation, and current techniques used to measure these hormones in the clinical laboratory. This chapter is divided into four sections: Male Reproductive Biology, Female Reproductive Biology, Infertility, and Methods.

MALE REPRODUCTIVE BIOLOGY

The mature testes synthesize both sperm and androgens. The testes contain a structured network of tightly packed seminiferous tubules. The lumina of the seminiferous tubules are lined by maturing germ cells and Sertoli cells. Sertoli cells play a crucial role in sperm maturation and secrete *inhibin*, a 32-kDa glycoprotein that inhibits the pituitary secretion of FSH. Surrounding the seminiferous tubules are the interstitial Leydig cells, the primary site of androgen production. The principal androgen in man is testosterone, which serves a central role in reproductive physiology. Testosterone is required for sexual differentiation, spermatogenesis, and promotion and maintenance of sexual maturity at puberty. At the cellular level, these effects are mediated by binding of testosterone or its more potent metabolite dihydrotestosterone (DHT) to the androgen receptor or via aromatization to estradiol and subsequent binding to the estrogen receptor. Testicular function is under the control of the hypothalamic-pituitary-gonadal axis.

Hypothalamic-Pituitary-Gonadal Axis

Gonadotropin-releasing hormone (GnRH) is a decapeptide synthesized in the hypothalamus and transported to the anterior pituitary gland, where it stimulates the release of both FSH and LH (see also Chapter 65).

In adult men, GnRH and thus LH and FSH are secreted in pulsatile patterns. A circadian rhythm is present, with higher concentrations found in the early-morning hours and lower concentrations in the late evening.[1] LH acts on Leydig cells to stimulate the conversion of cholesterol to pregnenolone. FSH acts on Sertoli cells and spermatocytes and is central to the initiation (in puberty) and maintenance (in adulthood) of spermatogenesis.[2] Sex steroids and inhibin provide negative

*The authors gratefully acknowledge the original contribution of R.J. Whitley, A.W. Meikle, and N.B. Watts, on which portions of this chapter are based.

feedback control of LH and FSH secretion, respectively. LH secretion is inhibited by testosterone and by its metabolites: estradiol and DHT. FSH may be elevated in disorders in which Sertoli cell numbers (and thus inhibin concentrations) are reduced. Likewise, a reduction in the number of Leydig cells (and thus testosterone secretion) leads to increased LH concentrations.

Androgens

Androgens are a group of C-19 steroids (Fig. 68.1) responsible for masculinization of the genital tract and development and maintenance of male secondary sex characteristics. Testosterone is the principal androgen secreted in men.

Biosynthesis of Testosterone

Testosterone is synthesized primarily by the Leydig cells of the testes (95%) and, to a lesser extent (≈5%) via peripheral conversion from the precursors dehydroepiandrosterone (DHEA) and androstenedione, which are synthesized in the zona reticularis of the adrenal glands (for more information on adrenal androgen synthesis and regulation, refer to Chapter 66). Synthesis of androgens begins with mobilization of cholesterol derived from lipoprotein cholesterol or by de novo synthesis.[3,4] Cholesterol released from the lipid droplets migrates to the inner mitochondrial membrane, where pregnenolone formation is catalyzed by the cholesterol sidechain cleavage enzyme, CYP11A1. Conversion of cholesterol to pregnenolone is the rate-limiting step in testosterone synthesis;[5,6] however, it is thought that the rate of steroidogenesis is determined not by the activity of CYP11A1, but rather by delivery of cholesterol to the enzyme in the inner mitochondrial membrane by the steroidogenic regulatory protein (StAR)—a process thought to be regulated by LH.[7] Following the formation of pregnenolone, four additional enzymatic steps are required to convert cholesterol to testosterone. The pathway for testosterone formation is shown in Fig. 68.1, with the preferred pathway defined by heavy red arrows.

Androgen Transport in Blood

Testosterone and DHT circulate in plasma freely (≈2% to 3%) or bound to plasma proteins. Binding proteins include the specific sex hormone–binding globulin (SHBG) and nonspecific proteins such as albumin. SHBG is an α-globulin that has low capacity for steroids but binds with very high affinity ($K_a = 1 \times 10^8$ to 1×10^9), whereas albumin has high capacity but low affinity ($K_a = 1 \times 10^4$ to 1×10^6).[6] SHBG has the highest affinity for DHT and the lowest for estradiol. In men, testosterone circulates bound 44% to 65% to SHBG and 33% to 50% to albumin, whereas in women testosterone is bound 66% to 78% to SHBG and 20% to 30% to albumin.[8,9]

The biologically active fraction includes free testosterone; some have suggested that albumin-bound testosterone may also be available for tissue uptake.[10,11] Therefore the bioavailable testosterone is equal to approximately 35% of the total quantity (free + albumin-bound). Whether albumin-bound testosterone dissociates sufficiently fast to enter tissues is controversial.[12,13] However, concentrations of bioavailable testosterone correlate with those of free testosterone.[14,15]

Testosterone and SHBG exhibit rhythmic variation in their circulating concentrations. Testosterone concentrations peak at approximately 0400 to 0800 hours, and nadir concentrations occur at between 1600 and 2000 hours.[16,17] Daily variations in SHBG concentrations are similar to those of other proteins and albumin in serum, with major changes related to posture.[17] Concentrations of SHBG are elevated with hyperthyroidism and in hypogonadal men.

Metabolism of Testosterone

Circulating testosterone serves as a precursor for the formation of two additional active metabolites: DHT and estradiol. In one pathway, 5α-reductase converts 6% to 8% of testosterone to DHT. Both testosterone and DHT bind the androgen receptor, but DHT binds with higher affinity. In an alternative pathway, testosterone and androstenedione are converted to estrogens (≈0.3%) through aromatase (CYP19). DHT is formed in androgen target tissues such as the skin and prostate, whereas aromatization occurs in many tissues, especially the liver and adipose tissue. Peripheral aromatization occurs primarily in adipose tissue (of both men and women) because of the high concentration of aromatase in this tissue. The rate of extraglandular aromatization therefore increases with body fat.[18]

Dihydrotestosterone is metabolized to 3α-androstanediol (see Fig. 68.1) and then is conjugated to form 3α-androstanediol glucuronide. These metabolites have been used as markers of DHT production in peripheral tissues. Serum concentrations of 3α-androstanediol glucuronide or 3α-androstanediol reflect the production of DHT in peripheral tissues such as skin.[19,20] However, DHT may also arise from precursors other than testosterone. The reduction in serum 3α-androstanediol glucuronide concentrations noted in patients treated with glucocorticoids that suppress adrenal glucocorticoid and androgen production supports this conclusion.[21]

The main excretory metabolites of androstenedione, testosterone, and DHEA are shown in Fig. 68.2. Except for epitestosterone, these catabolites constitute a group of steroids known as *17-ketosteroids* (17-KS); they are excreted primarily in the urine.

Testosterone Concentrations

Testosterone is required for proper sexual development and function throughout all stages of life: fetal, pubertal, and adult (Fig. 68.3). Fetal testes produce testosterone around the seventh week of gestation, with peak serum concentrations of approximately 250 ng/dL (8.7 nmol/L) observed at the beginning of the second trimester, and with concentrations gradually returning to baseline by birth. Shortly after birth, the concentration of testosterone begins to increase, peaking again at approximately 250 ng/dL (8.7 nmol/L) at 2 to 3 months of age, and then falls to baseline again by 6 to 12 months. The function of this neonatal testosterone surge is not entirely clear, but it is thought to be important for bone growth and remodeling[22] and development of external male genitalia.[23] The concentration of testosterone remains low (<50 ng/dL, 1.7 nmol/L) until puberty, when the concentration of testosterone rises to 500 to 700 ng/dL (17.3–24.3 nmol/L). Testosterone remains elevated through adulthood until around the third to fourth decade.[18]

Men beyond 30 to 40 years of age experience an age-dependent decrease in circulating testosterone concentration. This has been demonstrated consistently in both cross-sectional and longitudinal analyses. Collectively these studies have shown a 0.5% to 2% decrease per year in total serum testosterone from about the fourth decade onward.[24-27] This

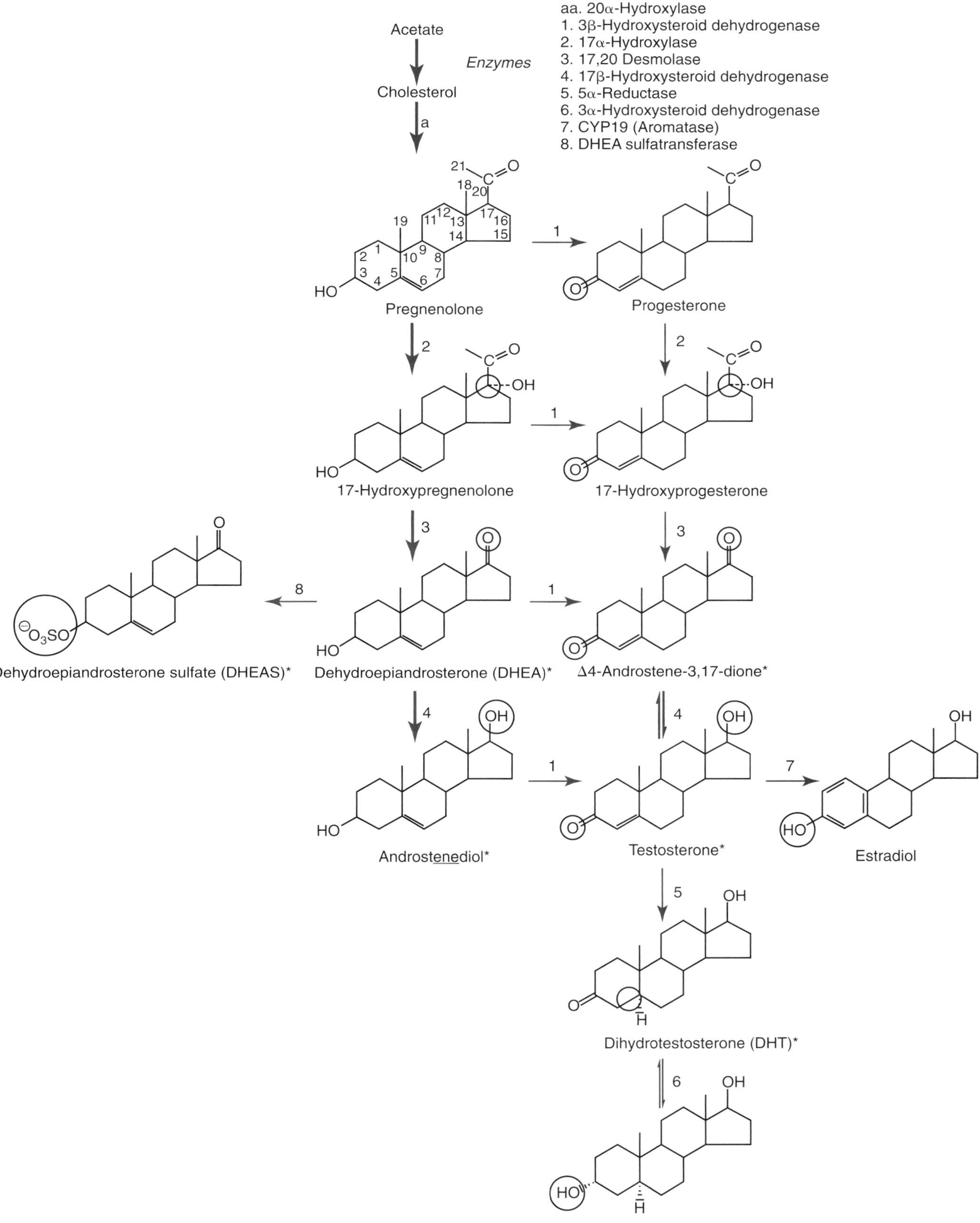

FIGURE 68.1 Biosynthesis of androgens (adrenal glands and testis). The heavy arrows indicate the preferred pathway. The enclosed area represents the site of chemical change. *Denotes androgens.

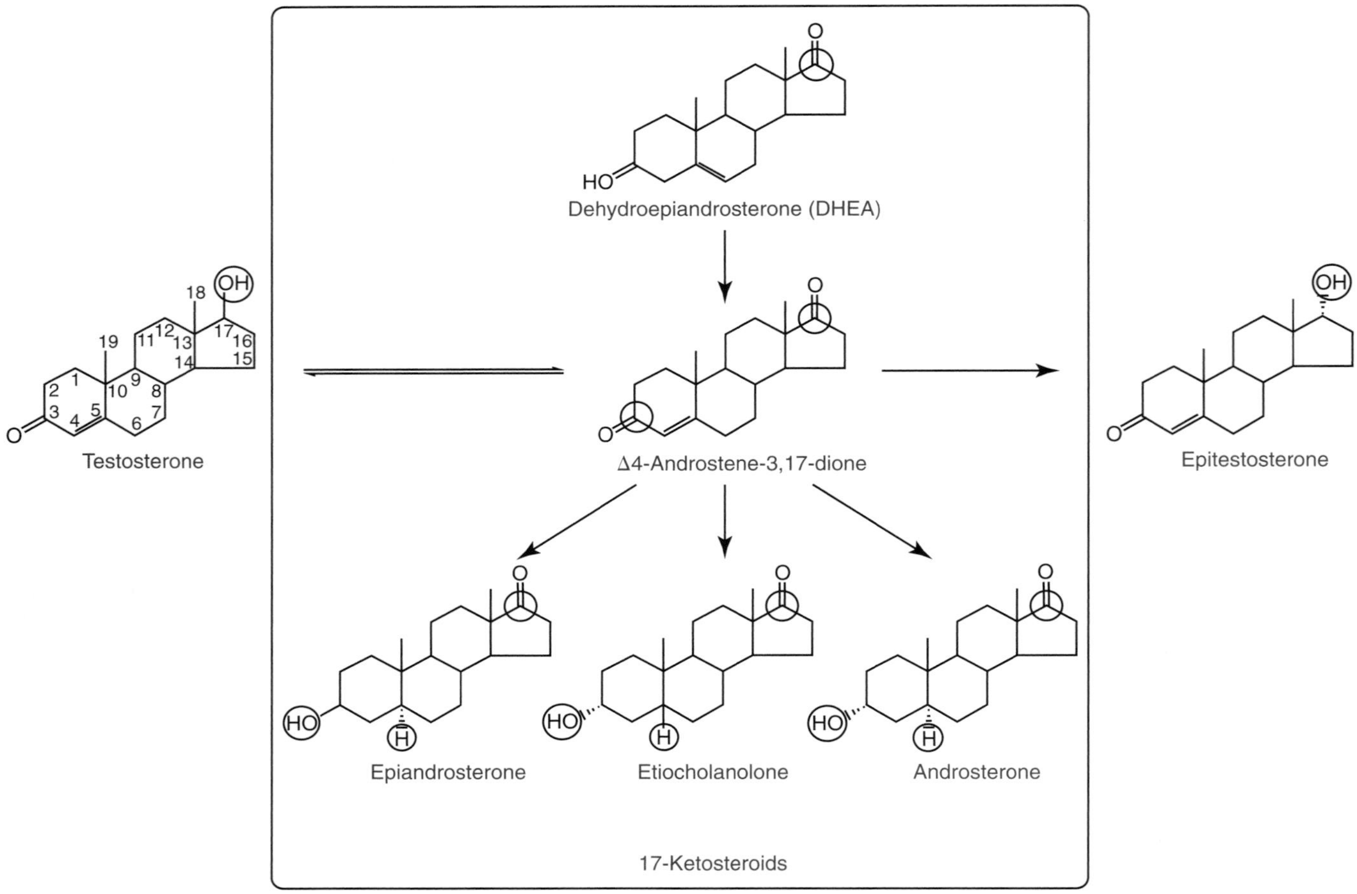

Dehydroepiandrosterone (DHEA)

Testosterone

Δ4-Androstene-3,17-dione

Epitestosterone

Epiandrosterone

Etiocholanolone

Androsterone

17-Ketosteroids

FIGURE 68.2 Catabolism of C19O2 androgens. The circled area represents the site of chemical change.

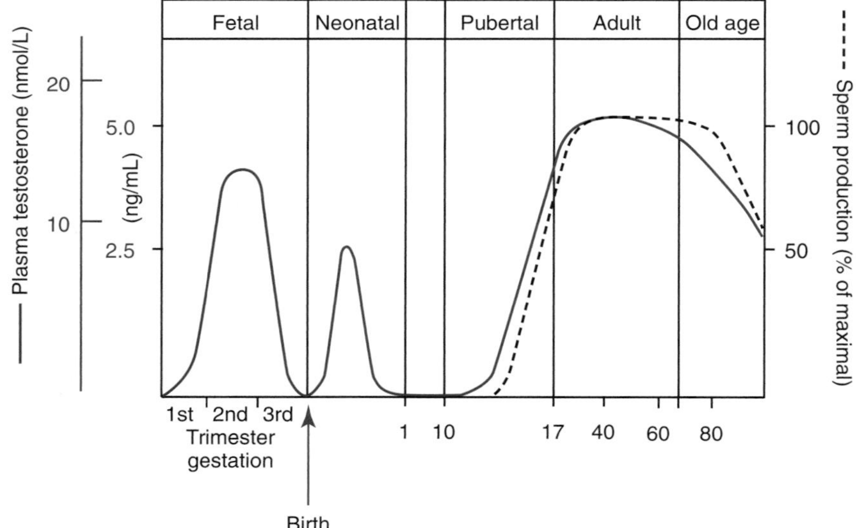

FIGURE 68.3 Schematic diagram of different phases of male sexual function during life as indicated by mean plasma testosterone concentration and sperm production at different ages. (From Griffin JE, Wilson JD. The testis. In: Bondy PK, Rosenberg LE, eds. *Metabolic Control and Disease*. 8th ed. Philadelphia: WB Saunders; 1980:1535–78.)

decline in testosterone is thought to be due to (1) a decrease in Leydig cell numbers, (2) decreased GnRH pulse amplitude, and (3) increases in SHBG.[26] In the past, these decreases in circulating concentrations of testosterone were viewed as a normal part of the aging process. Now, however, these decreases, when accompanied by symptoms of decreased libido, sexual dysfunction, decreased energy levels, and decreased muscle mass, are regarded as a syndrome with a variety of names, such as androgen deficiency in the aging male (ADAM), partial androgen deficiency of the aging male (PADAM), late-onset hypogonadism (LOH), and, erroneously, andropause. The name *andropause* is inaccurate and misleading, given that in contrast to menopause in women, concentrations of sex steroids in men do not decrease sharply with secondary cessation of reproductive function. A name put forward more recently is *testosterone deficiency syndrome (TDS),* highlighting a specific deficit in testosterone as part of the clinical picture.[28,29]

Diagnosis of LOH (TDS) should be based on both clinical and laboratory assessment.[30] Clinically, patients should exhibit symptoms suggestive of testosterone deficiency, such as decreased libido, erectile dysfunction, decreased muscle mass and strength, decreased bone mineral density, and changes in mood. Patients should exhibit one to three of these symptoms with a concomitant low concentration of serum testosterone to fit various diagnostic criteria. Total serum testosterone is the most widely used biochemical parameter for assessment of hypogonadism; although there is no agreed-upon lower limit of normal, recently published consensus recommendations drafted by five professional andrology/urology societies concur that total testosterone above 350 ng/dL (12 nmol/L) does not require testosterone supplementation, whereas patients whose concentrations fall below 230 ng/dL (8 nmol/L) may benefit from testosterone replacement. This value is similar to the 200-ng/dL (6.9-nmol/L) intent-to-treat cutoff published in the 2002 practice guidelines of the American Association of Clinical Endocrinology.[31] The joint societies further recommend, for those patients falling in the gray zone between 230 ng/dL and 350 ng/dL (8–12 nmol/L), repeat measurement of serum total testosterone with measurement of SHBG to calculate free testosterone, or direct measurement of free testosterone by equilibrium dialysis (if available). Measurement of free or bioavailable testosterone should be considered when total testosterone is not diagnostic despite the clinical presentation of hypogonadism.[32]

This is particularly true in the setting of advanced age, where concentrations of SHBG have been shown to be elevated. High concentrations of SHBG may result in normal total testosterone but low free testosterone. Transient decreases in testosterone secondary to acute illness should be excluded during this assessment. Moreover, underlying chronic disease that lowers concentrations of testosterone should be taken into consideration and treated appropriately. To assess whether hypogonadism is primary or secondary, serum LH should be measured; a serum prolactin measurement is indicated when serum testosterone concentrations are lower than 150 ng/dL (5.2 nmol/L) or when secondary hypogonadism is suspected.[33-35] In sum, no absolute cutoffs or specific tests (total vs. bioavailable vs. free testosterone) are recommended for the laboratory diagnosis of hypogonadism in the aging male. Each patient's laboratory results should be interpreted on an individual basis, with particular attention given to those parameters of the biochemistry of testosterone (eg, obesity, age, comorbidities, medications) that may affect the findings.

Some patients may be candidates for treatment with testosterone replacement therapy (TRT). Considerable controversy surrounds TRT, primarily regarding potential adverse effects on prostate and cardiovascular health.[33-35] TRT in younger patients diagnosed with hypogonadism has been proven both safe and effective, but data from prospective randomized controlled trials regarding the efficacy and safety of TRT in the aged population are lacking. Despite this lack of evidence, TRT prescriptions are on the rise[36]; thus a sustained role for the laboratory in the diagnosis of LOH becomes evident, particularly given a growing aging population of males older than 65 years, projected to number some 31.3 million in the United States by the year 2030.[37]

The Endocrine Society's 2010 guidelines[38] recommend TRT only in men with consistent symptoms (fatigue, decreased muscle mass, osteopenia, diminished sexual function), unequivocally low serum testosterone, no personal or family history of prostate cancer, and the absence of poorly controlled heart failure. However, recent work has questioned the utility of TRT in adults, arguing that underlying poor health rather than low testosterone is the true cause of symptoms for the majority of patients evaluated for LOH.[39-41] This is supported by the observation that many symptomatic men do not have low testosterone and many men with low testosterone do not have symptoms.[42] Furthermore, lifestyle changes that result in improved metabolic profiles are often associated with increases in serum testosterone concentrations in individuals with previously low testosterone.[43] Additional evidence suggests an increased risk of cardiovascular events in frail, elderly men or men with underlying cardiovascular disease who receive TRT.[44] In summary, despite the increasing number of patients receiving TRT, it has yet to be conclusively demonstrated that its benefits outweigh the potential risks for the majority of patients.

Male Reproductive Abnormalities

A wide variety of abnormalities affect the male reproductive system before birth, in childhood, or in adulthood. For the purposes of this chapter, they have been divided into categories of (1) hypogonadotropic hypogonadism, (2) hypergonadotropic hypogonadism, (3) defects in androgen action (Box 68.1), (4) erectile dysfunction, and (5) gynecomastia. The effects of these abnormalities on infertility are discussed later in this chapter.

Hypogonadotropic Hypogonadism. Male hypogonadism is a condition caused by decreased function of the testes, which can lead to abnormalities in sexual development if manifested prepubertally. Hypogonadism is classified as *hypo*gonadotropic or *hyper*gonadotropic.

Hypogonadotropic hypogonadism occurs when defects in the hypothalamus or pituitary prevent normal gonadal stimulation. Causative factors include congenital or acquired panhypopituitarism, hypothalamic syndromes, GnRH deficiency, hyperprolactinemia, malnutrition or anorexia, and iatrogenic causes. All of these abnormalities are associated with decreased testosterone and gonadotropin concentrations.

Kallmann syndrome, the most common form of hypogonadotropic hypogonadism, results from a deficiency of GnRH

BOX 68.1 Male Reproductive Abnormalities

Hypogonadotropic Hypogonadism

Panhypopituitarism (congenital or acquired)

Hypothalamic syndrome (acquired or congenital)

- Structural defects (neoplastic, inflammatory, and infiltrative)
- Prader-Willi syndrome
- Laurence-Moon-Biedl syndrome
- GnRH deficiency (Kallmann syndrome)
- Hyperprolactinemia (prolactinoma or drugs)
- Malnutrition and anorexia nervosa
- Drug-induced suppression of luteinizing hormone (androgens, estrogens, tranquilizers, antidepressants, antihypertensives, barbiturates, cimetidine, GnRH analogs, and opiates)

Hypergonadotropic Hypogonadism

Acquired (irradiation, mumps orchitis, castration, and cytotoxic drugs)

Chromosome defects

- Klinefelter syndrome (47,XXY) and mosaics
- Autosomal and sex chromosomes, polyploidies
- True hermaphroditism

Defective androgen biosynthesis

- 20α-Hydroxylase (cholesterol 20,22-desmolase) deficiency
- 17,20-Lyase deficiency
- 3β-Hydroxysteroid dehydrogenase deficiency
- 17α-Hydroxylase deficiency
- 17β-Hydroxysteroid dehydrogenase deficiency

Testicular agenesis

Selective seminiferous tubular disease

Miscellaneous

- Noonan syndrome (short stature, pulmonary valve stenosis, hypertelorism, and ptosis)
- Streak gonads
- Myotonia dystrophica

Acute and chronic disease

Defects in Androgen Action

Complete androgen insensitivity *(testicular feminization)*

Partial androgen sensitivity

- 5α-Reductase deficiency

GnRH, Gonadotropin-releasing hormone.

in the hypothalamus during embryonic development.[45] It is characterized by hypogonadism and anosmia (loss of the sense of smell) in male or female patients and is inherited as an autosomal dominant trait with variable penetrance.[16,46] This syndrome arises from a defect in the migration of GnRH neurons to the hypothalamus. The pituitary disorders are characterized by isolated gonadotropin deficiency with or without growth hormone deficiency. Patients with isolated gonadotropin deficiency display sexual infantilism and long arms and legs; those with combined deficiency do not have long arms and legs. These patients must be distinguished from those with growth delay. In all of these patients, LH, FSH, and testosterone concentrations are lower than normal. However, heterogeneity exists in the degree of gonadotropin deficiency; hence concentrations of LH, FSH, and testosterone have been shown to differ among affected patients.

Hypergonadotropic Hypogonadism

Hypergonadotropic hypogonadism results from a primary gonadal disorder. Patients with primary testicular failure have increased concentrations of LH and FSH and decreased concentrations of testosterone. Causes for primary hypogonadism are categorized as (1) acquired causes (irradiation, castration, mumps orchitis, or cytotoxic drugs), (2) chromosome defects (Klinefelter syndrome), (3) defective androgen synthesis (20α-hydroxylase deficiency), (4) testicular agenesis, (5) seminiferous tubular disease, and (6) other miscellaneous causes. Aging is associated with gonadal failure, specifically, decreased Leydig cell mass and reserve capacity with reduction in pulsatile secretion of GnRH by the hypothalamus, leading to decreased testosterone secretion.[47]

Defects in Androgen Action

The most common and severe defect in androgen action is *androgen insensitivity syndrome* (AIS), a disorder arising from mutations in the androgen receptor gene (AR). AIS may be classified as complete (CAIS) or partial (PAIS), depending on the amount of residual receptor function. Individuals with complete AIS (formerly known as testicular feminization) have a male karyotype (46,XY) with female external genitalia (labia, clitoris, and vaginal opening). The testes are present intraabdominally, and because they produce anti-Müllerian hormone (AMH) (also known as Müllerian inhibitory substance), no uterus, fallopian tubules, or proximal vagina is present. The circulating concentration of testosterone in these patients is greater than or equal to that of a healthy male.[48] Concentrations of LH are increased, presumably because of resistance of the hypothalamic-pituitary system to androgen inhibition.

Males with *5α-reductase deficiency* (5-ARD) do not convert testosterone to the more potent DHT. Because DHT leads to masculinization of external genitalia in utero, males are born with ambiguous genitalia.[49] High ratios of the circulating concentrations of testosterone to DHT are indicative of 5-ARD. Moreover, evidence indicates that DHT formation is deficient in the tissues of the urogenital tract in these patients.[48]

In patients with cryptorchidism or ambiguous genitalia, identification of abdominal gonads is essential for proper diagnosis and treatment. The presence of testicular tissue has traditionally been detected by measurement of Leydig cell testosterone production after stimulation with hCG.[50] A growing appreciation of assessment of Sertoli cell function has been noted. Inhibin and AMH reflect Sertoli cell function and may offer a noninvasive evaluation of seminiferous tubular integrity.[51-54] In one study, the mean plasma AMH concentration in anorchid patients was 0.8 ng/mL (5.7 pmol/L), compared with 48.2 ng/mL (344.1 pmol/L) in patients with normal testes.[52] AMH concentrations are also elevated in boys with delayed puberty and partial androgen insensitivity. Inhibin B may be used as a basal serum marker for the presence and function of testicular tissue in boys with nonpalpable testicles.[55-57]

Studies have shown that boys with anorchia have undetectable serum inhibin B concentrations.[57] Boys with severe testicular damage or gonadal dysgenesis also have undetectable or very low concentrations of inhibin B, whereas normal serum inhibin B concentrations are observed among boys with abdominal "normal" testes.[57]

Erectile Dysfunction

Erectile dysfunction (formerly referred to as *impotence*) is the persistent inability to develop or maintain a penile erection that is sufficient for intercourse and ejaculation in 50% or more of attempts.[16,58] A wide variety of organic and psychologic abnormalities may cause changes in sexual drive and in the ability to have an erection or to ejaculate. Psychogenic erectile dysfunction is the most common diagnosis. Other causes include vascular disease, diabetes mellitus, hypertension, uremia, neurologic disease, hypogonadism, hyperthyroidism and hypothyroidism, neoplasms, and drugs. The physician must pursue a careful evaluation of possible psychologic factors, neuropathy, or vascular abnormalities that may be interfering with proper sexual function. If no obvious explanation for erectile dysfunction can be found, measurement of morning serum testosterone, LH, and thyroid-stimulating hormone (TSH) concentrations has been suggested.[16,59] Elevated gonadotropin concentrations indicate primary hypogonadism. Total and even free testosterone concentrations may be within normal reference intervals, yet still may be subnormal for a given patient if found in the presence of elevated LH or FSH. Hyperprolactinemia is an infrequent cause of erectile dysfunction but should be considered in unusual situations.

Sildenafil (sold under the trade names Viagra, Revatio, and others) was approved by the US Food and Drug Administration (FDA) in April 1998 for use as an oral therapeutic agent for male erectile dysfunction.[60-64] This agent and the drugs tadalafil (Cialis) and vardenafil (Levitra) are selective inhibitors of phosphodiesterase 5 (PDE5).[61] By inhibiting PDE5 in the corpus cavernosum of the penis, these drugs block degradation of cyclic guanosine monophosphate (cGMP), which is increased during sexual arousal. Increased cGMP results in relaxation of vascular smooth muscle and increased inflow of blood. A high-performance liquid chromatography (HPLC) method for sildenafil has been developed.[65]

Gynecomastia

Gynecomastia, the benign growth of glandular breast tissue in men, is a common finding among males of varied ages.[66-68] Gynecomastia, which is associated with an increase in the estrogen/androgen ratio, is commonly associated with three distinct periods of life. First, transient gynecomastia can be found in 60% to 90% of all newborns because of high estrogen concentrations that cross the placenta. The second peak occurs during puberty in 50% to 70% of normal boys. It is usually self-limited and may be due to low serum testosterone, low DHT, or a high estrogen/androgen ratio. The last peak is found in the adult population, most frequently among men aged 50 to 80 years. Gynecomastia may be due to testicular failure, resulting in an increased estrogen/androgen ratio, or to increased body fat, resulting in increased peripheral aromatization of testosterone to estradiol.[66-68]

Gynecomastia may also develop as the result of iatrogenic causes, hyperthyroidism, or liver disease. Liver disease impairs estrogen clearance and SHBG production, leading to increased bioavailable estrogen and subsequent gynecomastia. Finally, germinal cell or nonendocrine tumors that produce human chorionic gonadotropin (hCG), as well as estrogen-producing tumors of the adrenal glands, the testes, or the liver, will cause gynecomastia. hCG stimulates testicular aromatase activity and estrogen production, resulting in gynecomastia.[67] In cases of striking gynecomastia in which history and physical examination point to no specific disorder, measurements of hCG, plasma estradiol, testosterone, and LH concentrations are appropriate.[66] It is important to note that prolactin plays an important role in *galactorrhea* (milk production), but only an indirect role in gynecomastia.

POINTS TO REMEMBER

- GnRH stimulates LH and FSH release, which increase testosterone and sperm production, respectively.
- LH secretion is inhibited by testosterone, and FSH secretion is inhibited by inhibin.
- Testosterone is transported in blood tightly bound to SHBG and loosely bound to albumin.
- Free testosterone is biologically active and represents 2% to 3% of total testosterone.
- Pituitary defects result in hypogonadotropic hypogonadism.
- Primary gonadal defects result in hypergonadotropic hypogonadism.

FEMALE REPRODUCTIVE BIOLOGY

The ovaries produce ova and secrete the sex hormones progesterone and estrogen. Every healthy female neonate possesses approximately 400,000 primordial follicles, each containing an immature ovum. During the reproductive life span of an adult woman, 300 to 400 follicles will reach maturity.[69,70] A single mature follicle is produced during each normal menstrual cycle at approximately day 14. Surrounding the oocyte of the mature follicle are three distinct cell layers: *theca externa, theca interna,* and *granulosa cells.* The theca interna cells are the primary source of androgens, which are transported to adjacent granulosa cells, where they are aromatized to estrogens.[46]

The mature follicle undergoes ovulation by the process of rupture, thereby releasing the oocyte into the proximity of the fallopian tubes. The follicle then fills with blood to form the corpus hemorrhagicum. The granulosa and theca cells of the follicle lining quickly proliferate to form lipid-rich luteal cells, replacing the clotted blood and forming the *corpus luteum* (yellow body). The luteal cells produce estrogen and progesterone. If fertilization and pregnancy occur, the corpus luteum persists and continues to produce estrogen and progesterone. If no pregnancy occurs, the corpus luteum regresses, and the next menstrual cycle begins.

The uterine cavity is lined by the endometrium. The endometrium undergoes cyclic changes in preparation for implantation and pregnancy in response to cyclic changes in estrogen and progesterone. During the follicular phase, the endometrial lining increases in thickness and vascularity in response to increasing circulating concentrations of estrogen; after regression of the corpus luteum, menstruation begins, and the endometrium is shed in response to the withdrawal of progesterone.

Hypothalamic-Pituitary-Gonadal Axis

In adult women, a tightly coordinated feedback system exists among the hypothalamus, anterior pituitary, and ovaries to orchestrate menstruation. FSH serves to stimulate follicular growth, and LH stimulates ovulation and progesterone secretion from the developing corpus luteum. These actions are discussed in greater depth later in this chapter.

Estrogens

Estrogens are responsible for the development and maintenance of female sex organs and female secondary sex characteristics. In conjunction with progesterone, they participate in regulation of the menstrual cycle and of breast and uterine growth, and in the maintenance of pregnancy.

Estrogens affect calcium homeostasis and have a beneficial effect on bone mass. They decrease bone resorption, and in prepubertal girls, estrogen accelerates linear bone growth, resulting in epiphyseal closure. Long-term estrogen depletion is associated with loss of bone mineral content, an increase in stress fractures, and postmenopausal osteoporosis.

Estrogens also have well-established effects on plasma proteins that influence endocrine testing. They increase concentrations of SHBG, corticosteroid-binding globulin, and thyroxine-binding globulin. Hence, boys and girls have comparable concentrations of SHBG, but adult men have SHBG concentrations that are about one-half those of adult women. Concentrations of plasma proteins that bind copper and iron are also elevated in response to estrogen, as are those of high-density and very high-density lipoproteins. In addition, estrogens are believed to play a preventive role in coronary heart disease.[71]

Chemistry

The three most biologically active estrogens in order of potency are estradiol (E_2), estrone (E_1), and estriol (E_3) (Fig. 68.4). Structurally, estrogens are derivatives of the parent hydrocarbon *estrane,* which is an 18-carbon molecule with an aromatic ring A and a methyl group at C-13.[46,72] All estrogens possess a phenolic hydroxyl group at C-3, which gives the compounds acidic properties, and lack a methyl group at C-10. In addition, estrogens may possess a ketone (estrone) or hydroxyl group (estradiol) at position C-17. The phenolic ring A and the hydroxyl group at C-17 are essential for biological activity.

Biosynthesis

The biochemical pathway illustrating aromatization of testosterone to estradiol and androstenedione to estrone is shown in Fig. 68.5. The role of estrogens in normal and abnormal menstrual cycles is described later in this chapter.

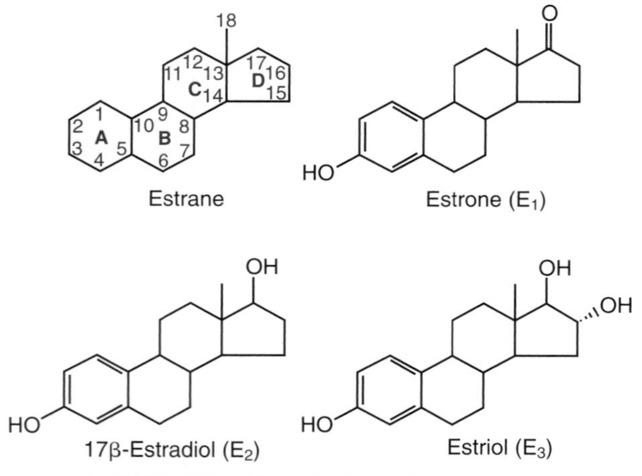

Estrane

Estrone (E_1)

17β-Estradiol (E_2)

Estriol (E_3)

FIGURE 68.4 Biologically active estrogens.

Estrogens are secreted primarily in healthy women by the ovarian follicles and the corpus luteum and during pregnancy by the placenta. The adrenal glands and testes (in men) are also believed to secrete minute quantities of estrogens. The ovary synthesizes estrogens via aromatization of androgens. Synthesis of estrogens begins in the theca interna cells with the enzymatic synthesis of androstenedione from cholesterol. Androstenedione is then transported to the granulosa cells, where it is further metabolized directly to estrone (androstenedione → estrone), or first to testosterone and then to estradiol (androstenedione → testosterone → estradiol). These conversions are catalyzed by the enzyme aromatase. The healthy human ovary produces all three classes of sex steroids: estrogens, progestagens, and androgens; however, estradiol and progesterone are its primary secretory products. Because the ovary lacks both the 21-hydroxylase and 11β–hydroxylase enzymes, glucocorticoids and mineralocorticoids are not produced in the ovary.[46,72] More than 20 estrogens have been identified, but only 17β-estradiol (E_2) and estriol (E_3) are routinely measured clinically. The most potent estrogen secreted by the ovary is 17β-estradiol. Because it is derived almost exclusively from the ovaries, its measurement is often considered sufficient for evaluation of ovarian function.

Estrogens are also produced by peripheral aromatization of androgens, primarily androstenedione. In healthy men and women, approximately 1% of secreted androstenedione is converted to estrone.[46,72] Although the ovaries of postmenopausal women do not secrete estrogens, these women have significant blood concentrations of estrone originating from the peripheral conversion of adrenal androstenedione. Because a major site of this conversion is adipose tissue, estrone is increased in obese postmenopausal women, sometimes yielding enough estrogen to produce bleeding.[46,72,73]

Biosynthesis During Pregnancy

Research has shown that biosynthesis of estrogens differs qualitatively and quantitatively in pregnant women compared with nonpregnant ones. In pregnant women, the major source of estrogens is the placenta, whereas in nonpregnant women, the ovaries are the main site of synthesis.[46,72,74] In contrast to the microgram quantities secreted by nonpregnant women, the quantity of estrogens secreted during pregnancy increases to milligram amounts. The major estrogen secreted by the ovary is estradiol (E_2), whereas the major product secreted by the placenta is estriol (E_3). E_3 is formed in the placenta by sequential desulfation and aromatization of plasma dehydroepiandrosterone sulfate (DHEA-S). Except during pregnancy, measurements of E_3 have little clinical value because in nonpregnant women, E_3 is derived almost exclusively from E_2 (see also Chapter 69).

E_3 is the predominant hormone of late pregnancy. Maternal E_3 is almost entirely (≈90%) derived from fetal and placental sources. It is first detected during the ninth gestational week and gradually increases during the first and second trimesters. Plasma and salivary E_3 concentrations peak approximately 3 to 5 weeks before labor and delivery.[75] This characteristic surge in E_3 has been observed in term, preterm, and postterm pregnancies. Some reports have suggested utility in the measurement of salivary E_3 in the prediction of risk for spontaneous preterm birth.[76-81] This test has a

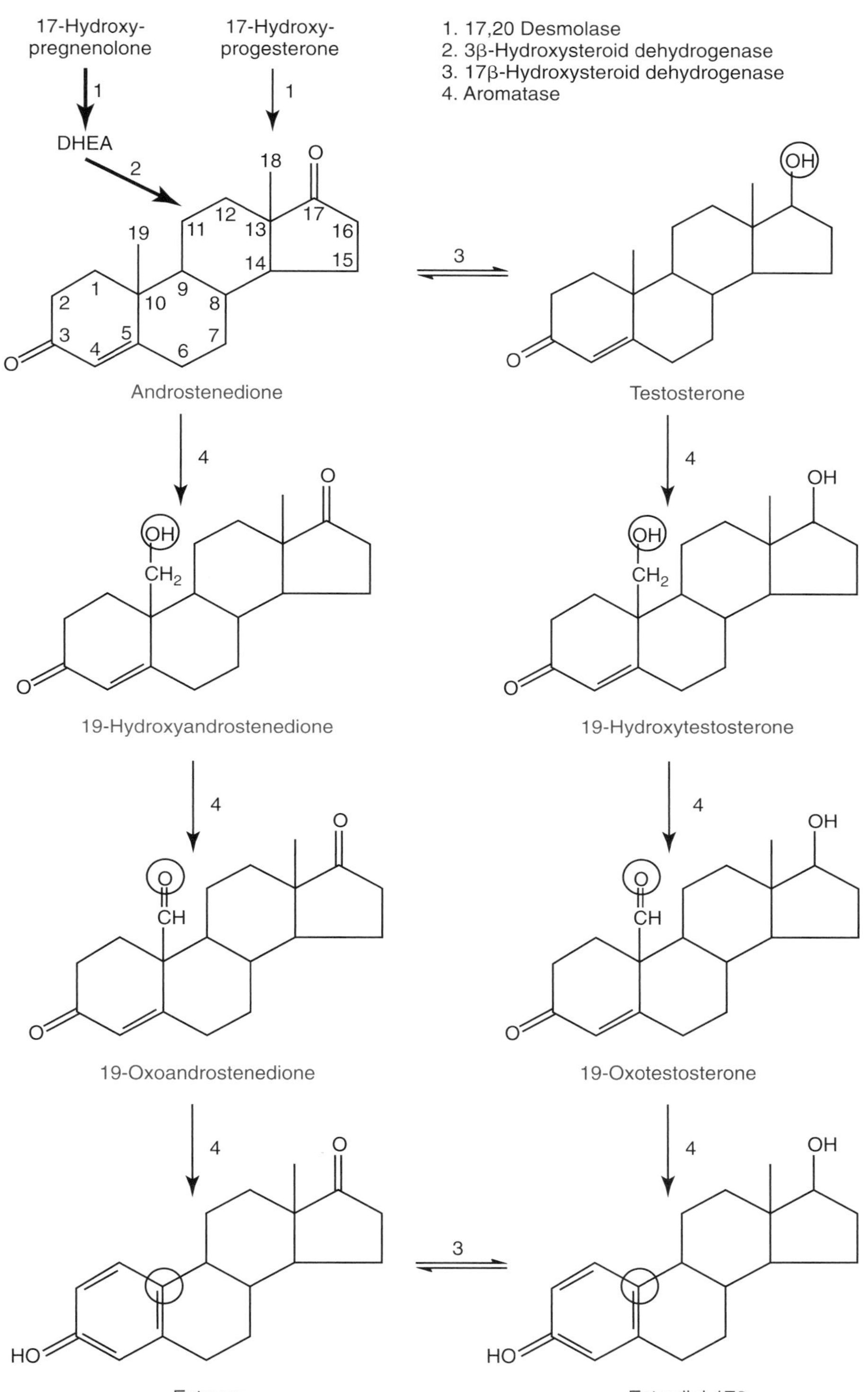

FIGURE 68.5 Biosynthesis of estrogens. Heavy arrows indicate the Δ5-3β-hydroxy pathway. The circled area represents the site of chemical change. See Fig. 68.1 for early synthetic steps.

high negative predictive value but a low positive predictive value. Consequently, the American College of Obstetricians and Gynecologists does not now suggest measuring salivary E_3 concentrations, except for research purposes.[82] Details regarding techniques used to determine serum and salivary E_3 concentrations are discussed later in the section on analytical methods. For further discussion of saliva formation, see Chapter 43.

Serum unconjugated E_3 measurements, along with alpha fetoprotein, hCG, and inhibin A, are commonly used as part of the "quad" maternal screens for Down syndrome–affected fetuses. On average, unconjugated E_3 is 0.72 times less than normal (median value at 16 weeks: 0.30–1.50 μg/L) when fetal Down syndrome is present.[83-86] For more on maternal serum screening, see Chapter 69.

Transport in Blood

More than 97% of circulating E_2 is bound to plasma proteins. It is bound specifically and with high affinity to SHBG and nonspecifically to albumin.[6,8] SHBG concentrations are increased by estrogens and therefore are higher in women than in men. They are also increased during pregnancy, oral contraceptive use, hyperthyroidism, and administration of certain antiepileptic drugs such as phenytoin (Dilantin). SHBG concentrations may decrease in hypothyroidism, obesity, or androgen excess. In women, E_2 circulates bound 40% to 60% to SHBG and 40 to 60% to albumin. SHBG has a higher affinity for testosterone than E_2; therefore in men, E_2 circulates 20% to 30% bound to SHBG and 70% to 80% bound to albumin.[8,9] Only 2% to 3% of total E_2 circulates in free form. In contrast, estrone and estrone sulfate circulate bound almost exclusively to albumin. As with testosterone, both free and albumin-bound fractions of E_2 are thought to be biologically available,[12] but measurement of this fraction has not been shown to be clinically important.

Diurnal variation in blood estrone concentrations occurs in postmenopausal women, presumably reflecting the variation in the androstenedione precursor that originates in the adrenal glands. However, no such diurnal rhythms have been demonstrated for E_2.

Metabolism

The metabolism of E_2 is chiefly an oxidative process dominated by three pathways, of which the fastest is oxidation of the β-hydroxy group at C-17 to a ketone (estradiol → estrone). This process is reversible; however, equilibrium favors the estrone species. Estrone is further oxidized along two pathways: the *2-hydroxylation pathway,* leading to formation of catechol estrogens (2-hydroxyestrone, 2-hydroxyestradiol, and 2-hydroxyestriol and their corresponding methoxy derivatives), and the *16α-hydroxylation pathway,* leading predominantly to formation of E_3(Fig. 68.6).[46,72]

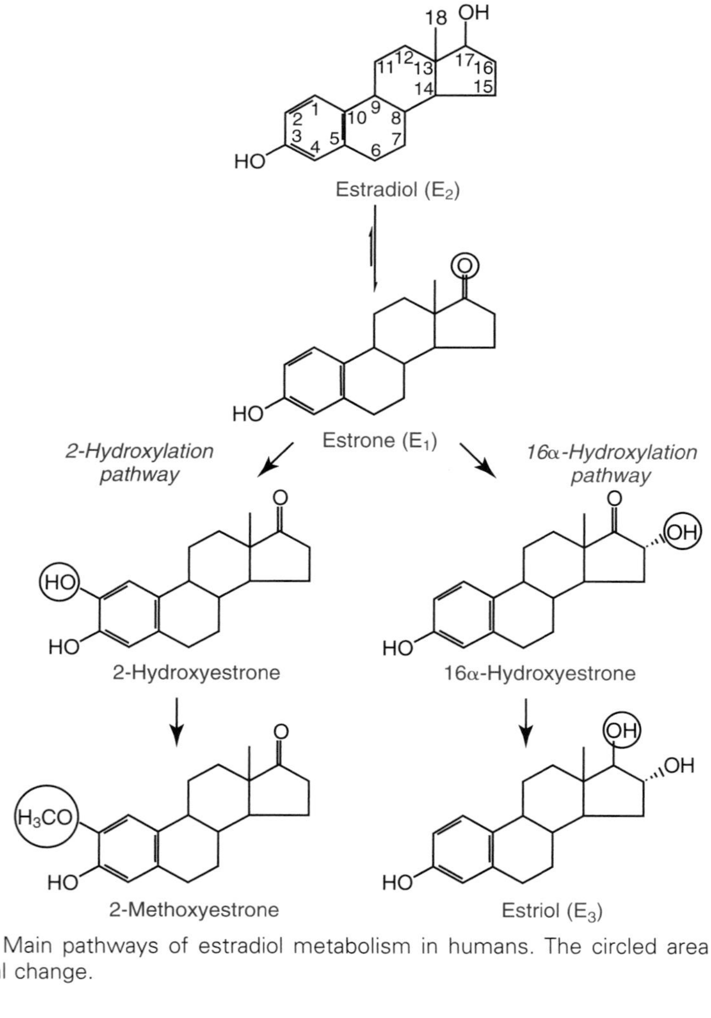

FIGURE 68.6 Main pathways of estradiol metabolism in humans. The circled area represents the site of chemical change.

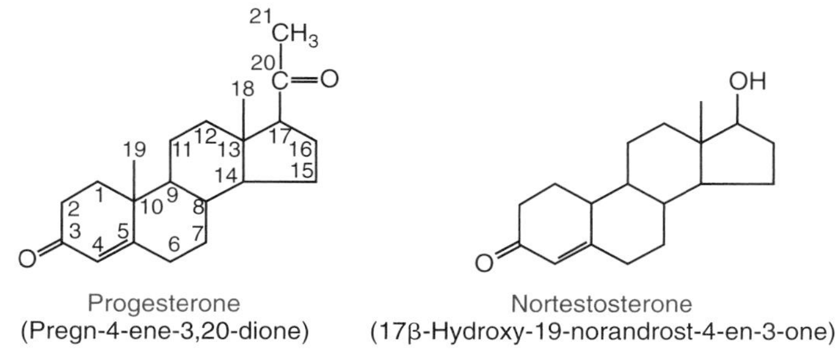

Progesterone
(Pregn-4-ene-3,20-dione)

Nortestosterone
(17β-Hydroxy-19-norandrost-4-en-3-one)

FIGURE 68.7 Structural formulas of progesterone and 19-nortestosterone.

Normally, blood estrone concentrations parallel E_2 concentrations throughout the menstrual cycle, but at one-third to one-half their magnitude. Estrone metabolism is influenced by the metabolic state. For example, obesity and hypothyroidism are associated with an increase in E_3 formation, whereas low body weight and hyperthyroidism are associated with formation of catechol estrogens.[46] Although assays for catechol estrogen measurement are available,[87,88] they have no known current clinical value.

In addition to the oxidative pathways already described, formation of estrogen conjugates has been reported as a major route of estrogen metabolism. The most abundant circulating estrogen conjugates are the sulfates, followed by the glucuronides, with estrone sulfate circulating at concentrations 10-fold higher than unconjugated estrone.[89] Initially, it was thought that sulfate conjugation would lead to an increase in polarity, making the compound more readily excretable; however, estrogen sulfates actually exhibit a longer half-life than do parent estrogens.[89] These observations have led to the idea that estrone sulfate may serve as a precursor for the bioactive estrogens via desulfation and conversion to E_2 by 17β-hydroxysteroid dehydrogenase. In contrast to estrogen sulfates, glucuronidation of estrogens generally is accepted to serve a classic excretory role. Estrogen glucuronides are detectable in both urine and bile.

Progesterone

Progesterone, similar to the estrogens, is a female sex hormone. In conjunction with estrogens, it helps to regulate the accessory organs during the menstrual cycle.[72,73] This hormone is especially important in preparing the uterus for implantation of the blastocyst and in maintaining pregnancy. In nonpregnant women, progesterone is secreted mainly by the corpus luteum. During pregnancy, the placenta becomes the major source of this hormone. Minor sources are the adrenal cortex in both sexes and the testes in men.

Chemistry

The structural formula of progesterone, a C_{21} compound, is shown in Fig. 68.7. Similar to the corticosteroids and testosterone, progesterone (pregn-4-ene-3,20-dione) contains a keto group (at C-3) and a double bond between C-4 and C-5 (Δ^4); both structural characteristics are essential for progestational activity. The two-carbon sidechain (CH_3CO) on C-17 does not seem to be very important for its physiologic action. Indeed, the synthetic compound 19-nortestosterone (Fig. 68.8) and its derivatives, which are widely used as oral contraceptives, are more potent progestational agents than progesterone itself.

Biosynthesis

Biosynthesis of progesterone in ovarian tissues follows the same path from acetate to cholesterol through pregnenolone as it does in the adrenal cortex (see Fig. 68.1).[46,72,90] In luteal tissue, however, low-density lipoprotein cholesterol is thought to serve as the preferred precursor despite the potential of the corpus luteum to synthesize progesterone de novo from acetate.[91] Initiation and control of luteal secretion of progesterone are regulated by LH and FSH.[46,72,92]

Transport in Blood

Progesterone does not have a specific plasma-binding protein but is primarily bound to albumin with a smaller fraction bound to corticosteroid-binding globulin. Reported concentrations for plasma free progesterone vary from 2% to 10% of total concentration, and the percentage of unbound progesterone remains constant throughout the normal menstrual cycle. The production rate of progesterone during the luteal phase reaches as high as 30 mg/d (95 μmol/d), whereas the production rate of progesterone by the placenta during the third trimester of pregnancy is approximately 300 mg/d (950 μmol/d).

Metabolism

The important metabolic events leading to inactivation of progesterone are reduction and conjugation. The main metabolic pathway for the metabolism of progesterone is outlined in Fig. 68.8.

Metabolites of progesterone are classified into three groups based on the degree of reduction:

1. *Pregnanediones.* The C4-5 double bond is reduced, producing two compounds: pregnanedione (hydrogen atom at C-5 is in β-orientation) and allopregnanedione (hydrogen atom at C-5 is in α-orientation).
2. *Pregnanolones.* The keto group at C-3 is reduced, producing hydroxyl groups in α- or β-orientation. However, most urinary pregnanolones exist in the α-configuration.
3. *Pregnanediols.* The keto group at C-20 is also reduced. As in the previous case, metabolites containing the 20-hydroxyl group in α-orientation are quantitatively more important. In fact, urinary measurement of pregnanediol (5β-pregnane-3α,20α-diol) can be used as an index of endogenous production of progesterone because this metabolite is quantitatively very significant, and its concentration correlates with most clinical conditions.

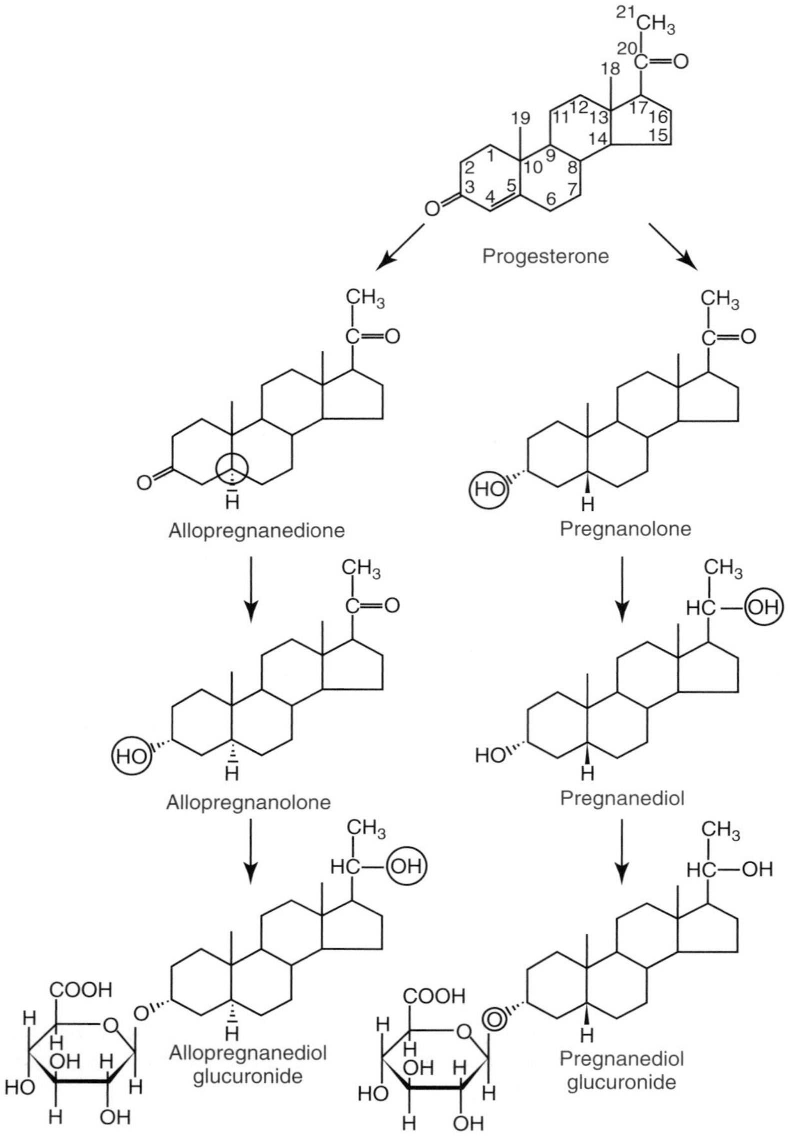

FIGURE 68.8 Metabolism of progesterone. The circled area represents the site of chemical change.

Reduced metabolites are eventually conjugated with glucuronic acid and excreted as water-soluble glucuronides.

Female Reproductive Development

Reproductive development begins with anatomy during the fetal period, a postnatal period of adaptation to reduced maternal sex steroids, and finishes with sexual maturation during puberty. Normal females remain fertile and menstruating until menopause.

Fetal

In the genotypic female, lack of testosterone and AMH causes regression of the wolffian ducts and maintenance of the Müllerian ducts, thus forming the female reproductive tract. Gonadotropin activity in utero is suppressed because of high concentrations of circulating estrogens derived from the mother.[46,72]

Postnatal

When the placenta separates, concentrations of fetal sex steroids drop abruptly. Serum E_2 in neonates is decreased to basal concentrations within 5 to 7 days after birth and persists at this concentration until puberty. The negative feedback action of steroids is now removed, and gonadotropins are released. Postnatal peaks of LH and FSH are measurable for a few months after birth, peaking at 2 to 5 months and then dropping to basal concentrations. During childhood, circulating concentrations of sex steroids and gonadotropins are low and are similar for both sexes. However, in patients with hypogonadism (Turner syndrome), LH and FSH concentrations are higher than in healthy children.[46,72]

Puberty

The transition from sexual immaturity appears to begin with diminished sensitivity of the pituitary gland or hypothalamus, or both, to the negative feedback effect of sex steroids. The mechanism for this change is unclear. As puberty approaches, nocturnal secretion of gonadotropins occurs. Concentrations for LH, FSH, and gonadal steroids rise gradually over several years before stabilizing at adult concentrations when full sexual maturity is reached. In girls, puberty is considered precocious if onset of pubertal development (secondary sex characteristics) occurs before the age of 8 years (see later section on precocious puberty) and is considered delayed if no development has occurred by the age of 13 years or if menarche has not occurred by age 16.5 years.[93,94] It was reported in 2003 that the median age of menarche in the United States is 12.43 years, which is 0.34 year earlier than that reported in 1973.[95,96] This study also found that the median age at menarche of non-Hispanic black (12.06 years) girls is significantly earlier than that of non-Hispanic white (12.55 years) and Mexican American (12.25 years) girls.[95]

Adrenarche precedes puberty by a few years. In girls, the rise in adrenal androgen concentrations (DHEA, DHEA-S, and androstenedione) begins at age 6 to 7 years.[97] This rise in adrenal androgen concentrations lasts until late puberty. A cortical androgen-stimulating hormone may contribute to the rise in adrenal androgens at puberty in both sexes.[98] In girls, puberty is associated with elevations in estrogen secretion by the ovary in response to gonadotropin concentrations that increase in response to GnRH. Estrogen secretion by the ovary increases, causing enlargement of the uterus and breasts. In the breast, estrogen enhances growth of ducts; progesterone augments this effect. As the breast develops, estrogen increases adipose tissue around the lactiferous duct system, contributing to the further enlargement of breast tissue.[46,72] These physiologic and physical processes associated with puberty in girls culminate in *menarche*—the beginning of menstrual function and the first menstrual period.

Normal Menstrual Cycle

During a normal menstrual cycle, a closely coordinated interplay of feedback effects occurs between the hypothalamus, the anterior lobe of the pituitary gland, and the ovaries. In addition, cyclic hormone changes lead to functional and structural changes in the ovaries (follicle maturation, ovulation, and corpus luteum development), uterus (preparation of the endometrium for possible implantation of the fertilized ovum), cervix (to permit transport of sperm), and vagina (Fig. 68.9).

Phases. The menstrual cycle is measured beginning on day 1 as the first day of menstrual bleeding. Each cycle consists of a follicular phase followed by ovulation and then a luteal phase.

Follicular Phase. The *follicular phase*—that is, the selection and growth of the dominant follicle—actually begins during the last few days of the previous luteal phase and terminates at ovulation (see Fig. 68.9). During the early part of the follicular phase, concentrations of FSH rise and then decline up until ovulation (see Fig. 68.9). LH secretion begins to increase around the middle of the follicular phase. Just

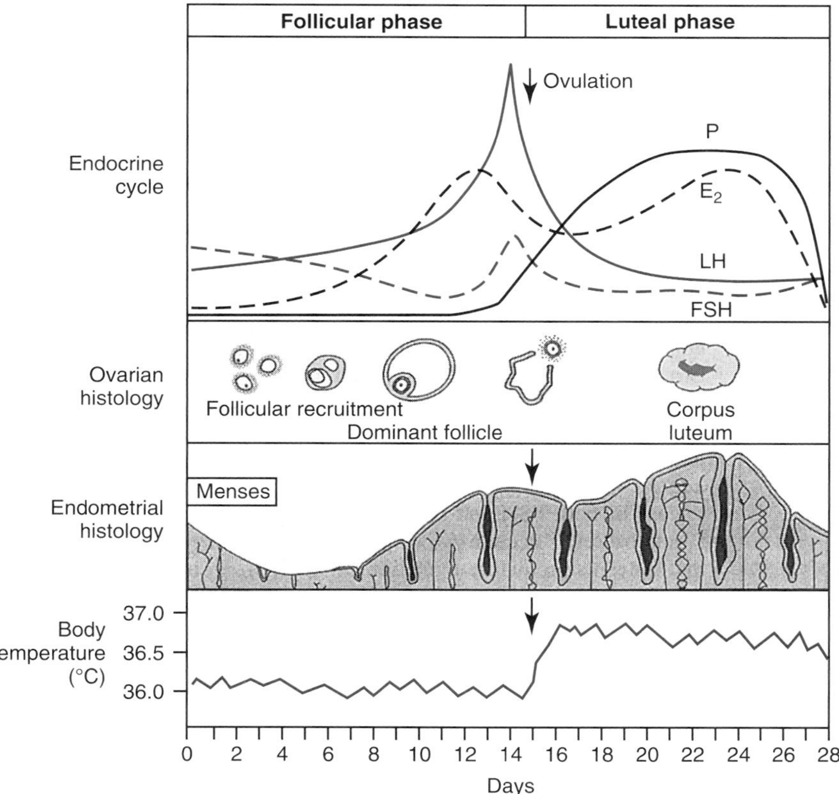

FIGURE 68.9 Hormonal, ovarian, endometrial, and basal body temperature changes throughout the normal menstrual cycle. (From Carr BR, Bradshaw KD. Disorders of the ovary and female reproductive tract. In: Braunwald E, Fauci A, Kasper D, Hauser SL, Longo DL, Jameson JL, eds. *Harrison's Principles of Internal Medicine.* 15th ed. New York: McGraw-Hill, 2001:2158; used with permission.)

before ovulation, estrogen secretion by the follicle increases dramatically; this positively stimulates the hypothalamus and triggers the LH surge. The LH surge is a reliable predictor of ovulation, with onset of the surge for 90% of women occurring 16 to 58 hours before, and the peak occurring 3 to 36 hours before, ovulation.[46] Ovulation occurs around day 14 in a 28-day menstrual cycle.

Luteal Phase. The *luteal phase,* the last half of the cycle, is characterized by increasing production of progesterone and estrogen from the corpus luteum with consequent gradual lowering of LH and FSH concentrations. The concentration of progesterone reaches a peak at about 8 days post ovulation. If ovulation does not occur, the corpus luteum fails to form, and a cyclic rise in progesterone is subnormal. If ovulation and pregnancy occur, hCG maintains the corpus luteum, and progesterone continues to rise. In the absence of conception, the corpus luteum resolves, resulting in a decrease in estrogen and progesterone concentrations and a breakdown of the endometrium. The average duration of menstrual flow is 4 to 6 days, and average menstrual blood loss is 30 mL.[99]

Cycle Variation. Healthy women display considerable variation in cycle length ranging from 26 to 34 days (28 days on average).[46] Much of the cycle variation can be attributed to variation in the length of the follicular phase while the length of the luteal phase remains relatively constant.[100]

Role of Individual Hormones. To explain further the intricacies of the normal menstrual cycle, fluctuations in each major hormone are discussed separately in the following sections with regard to control and effects (see Fig. 68.9).

Gonadotropin-Releasing Hormone. Gonadotropin-releasing hormone triggers the surge of LH that precedes ovulation.[72,73,99] There appear to be two separate feedback centers in the hypothalamus: a tonic negative feedback center in the basal medial hypothalamus and a cyclic positive feedback center in the anterior regions of the hypothalamus. Low concentrations of E_2, such as those that are present during the follicular phase, affect the negative feedback center, whereas high concentrations of E_2, such as those seen just before the midcycle LH peak, trigger the positive feedback center. Progesterone, in combination with estrogen, affects the negative feedback center in the luteal phase. GnRH is released in a pulsatile fashion and has a self-priming effect; the first dose potentiates the effects of subsequent doses. The magnitude of the LH response to GnRH increases steadily through the follicular phase and is greatest at the time of the preovulatory surge of LH, after which it declines again.

Follicle-Stimulating Hormone. A few days before day 1 of the cycle, FSH begins to rise (see Fig. 68.9), probably triggered by a fall in E_2 concentration that briefly eliminates the negative feedback effect.[46,72,74] This rise in FSH initiates the growth of a cohort of ovarian follicles. LH and FSH release is pulsatile throughout the cycle; therefore the values shown in Fig. 68.9 represent integrated concentrations. As estrogen is released from the growing follicles, FSH concentrations fall again and remain low through the follicular phase. By days 5 to 7, a single, dominant follicle is selected for further growth and maturation. The effect of FSH on the maturing follicle is increased through estradiol-induced changes in FSH receptors. FSH, aided by E_2, acts on the cells of the follicle to increase the responsiveness of LH receptors by the time of the midcycle surge. FSH and LH receptors respond with an increase in their number or in their affinity for corresponding gonadotropin. A rise in FSH at midcycle is triggered by progesterone. The function of this peak is not entirely known, but it is thought to stimulate plasminogen activator and increase granulosa cell LH receptors.[46] During the luteal phase, FSH is suppressed by negative feedback from E_2 until a lesser FSH peak, occurring near the end of the cycle, starts off the follicular recruitment for the next cycle.

Luteinizing Hormone. Luteinizing hormone secretion is suppressed in the follicular phase by negative feedback from E_2.[46,72,73] As E_2 production by the developing follicle increases, the effect of E_2 on the positive feedback center becomes important. Increasing release of GnRH from the hypothalamus and increasing the sensitivity of the anterior lobe of the pituitary gland to GnRH lead to the midcycle surge of LH. Ovarian follicle receptors for LH, sensitized by FSH and E_2, transmit the stimulus to enhance differentiation of the theca cell and production of progesterone by the developing corpus luteum. LH production is suppressed during the luteal phase by negative feedback from progesterone combined with E_2, but a low concentration of LH is probably necessary to prolong corpus luteum function.

Estradiol. E_2 production by the ovary decreases near the end of a cycle but begins to increase again under the influence of FSH (see Fig. 68.9).[46,72,73] E_2 enhances the FSH effect on a maturing follicle through changes in FSH receptors of the follicular cells, but it suppresses pituitary FSH and LH release during the follicular phase through negative feedback. Before the mid–follicular phase, estrogen concentrations are less than 50 pg/mL (183.5 pmol/L), but they increase rapidly as the follicle matures. E_2 production increases, reaching a midcycle peak at between 250 and 500 pg/mL (917.5–1835 pmol/L).[6] E_2 concentrations decrease abruptly after ovulation but increase again as the corpus luteum is formed, reaching concentrations of approximately 125 pg/mL (458.8 pmol/L) during the luteal phase.[6] Progesterone produced by the corpus luteum, combined with E_2, exerts a negative effect on the hypothalamus and anterior lobe of the pituitary gland. As a result, LH and FSH secretion is suppressed again during the luteal phase. E_2 is essential for the development of proliferative endometrium and is synergistic with progesterone for the development of changes in the endometrium that initiate shedding; the decrease in negative feedback from E_2 on the anterior lobe of the pituitary gland triggers the FSH surge that begins the development of an ovarian follicle for the next cycle.

E_2 is not the only estrogen produced; estrone secretion, mainly from peripheral sources, also is increased throughout the cycle. Estrogen and progesterone have visible effects on vaginal cytology and cervical mucus, and progesterone elevates body temperature (as discussed later). Changes in androgen production also occur during the menstrual cycle, with a peak at midcycle.

Progesterone. Progesterone is not produced in significant amounts until the midcycle LH surge and ovulation. LH enhances theca cell differentiation and progesterone production, which increase by a factor of 10 to 20 to a maximum about 8 days after the midcycle peak of LH. Progesterone is thought to stimulate the ovulatory peak of FSH and to promote the growth of secretory endometrium, which is necessary for implantation of the fertilized ovum.[46]

Ovulation. An intricate interplay of endocrine events contributes to follicular maturation. Growth of ovarian follicles appears to be continuous. How an individual follicle is singled out for each menstrual cycle is not known; however, the late-cycle peak in FSH concentration is likely important in this process. Once a follicle has been stimulated, E_2 production causes that specific follicle to be more receptive to effects of FSH. The high concentration of E_2 just before midcycle is responsible for triggering positive feedback in the hypothalamus that leads to the midcycle LH surge. After ovulation, LH is suppressed by progesterone and E_2, but the effect of LH on the corpus luteum is increased.[46,72,73,92] In the event of successful fertilization and implantation, corpus luteum function is sustained by hCG produced by trophoblastic cells of the developing embryo with high molecular homology to LH and is capable of binding and stimulating LH receptors. Otherwise, the declining concentration of E_2 leads to regression of the corpus luteum and to the late-cycle FSH peak that starts the process again.

Menopause

Menopause is defined as the permanent cessation of menstruation resulting from loss of ovarian follicular activity. It begins with the ovaries failing to produce adequate amounts of estrogen and inhibin; as a result, gonadotropin production is increased in a continued attempt to stimulate the ovary (Fig. 68.10). The mean age of menopause in the United States is 51 years but varies considerably.[46,101-103] Ovarian failure may occur at any age, but menopause before age 40 years is considered premature.[104]

Hormonal changes begin about 5 years before the actual menopause, as the response of the ovary to gonadotropins begins to decrease and menstrual cycles become increasingly irregular.[102,103,105] The term *perimenopausal* refers to the time interval from onset of these menstrual irregularities to menopause itself. This transition phase will last from 2 to 8 years.[102,105] At this time, FSH concentrations increase and E_2 concentrations decrease, whereas LH and progesterone concentrations remain unchanged, indicating that menstrual cycles remain ovulatory. As estrogen continues to decline, an associated decrease in prolactin concentrations is noted. The decrease in estrogen concentrations gives rise to vasomotor instability and so-called "hot flashes."

After menopause, the ovary continues to produce androgens, particularly testosterone and androstenedione, as a result of increased LH concentrations. In addition, the adrenal gland continues to secrete androgens. The resulting decrease in the estrogen/androgen ratio is the cause of the hirsutism seen in some postmenopausal women.[103] In general, menopause may be diagnosed in women over the age of 45 on the basis of menstrual history and age without relying on laboratory test results, although serum FSH values may be helpful.[106,107] In women younger than 40 with menopausal symptoms and irregular menses, other causes of menstrual irregularities should be ruled out prior to making the diagnosis of primary ovarian insufficiency (POI) or premature ovarian failure (POF). The etiology of POI or POF warrants further investigation.

The issue of hormone replacement therapy (HRT) for vasomotor symptoms, osteoporosis, various cardiac problems, and other disorders has received a great deal of attention, and data concerning the benefits and risks have changed ideas about indications and contraindications. Current guidelines and consensus statements emphasize that each woman's individual medical history, symptoms, and goals for treatment should guide decisions regarding the type of HRT chosen, when treatment is initiated, how treatment is administered, and what dose is used.[108,109] In general, the benefits of HRT before age 60 or within 10 years of menopause are considered to outweigh the risks associated with treatment. Relief of vasomotor symptoms remains the primary indication, but HRT also decreases the risk of osteoporosis-related fractures and modestly decreases the risk of coronary heart disease in women under 60 or within 10 years of menopause. HRT consisting of estrogen alone (ET) is associated with an increased risk of endometrial cancer and is contraindicated in women with an intact uterus or endometriosis. Because of the increased risk of uterine cancer associated with ET, HRT

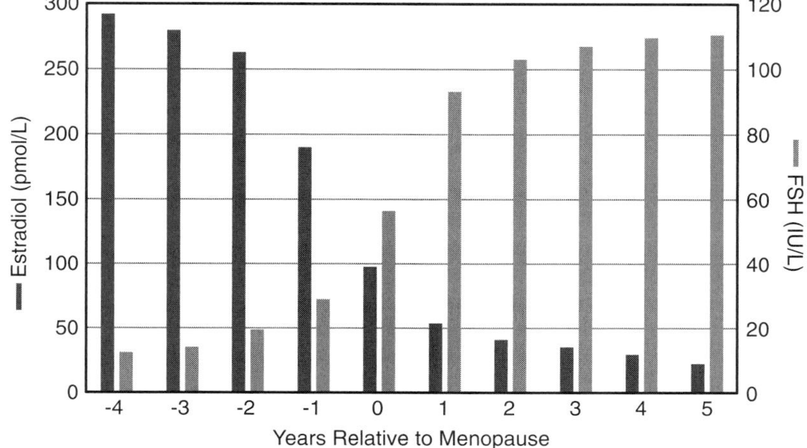

FIGURE 68.10 Geometric means for follicle-stimulating hormone (FSH) and estradiol in relation to the final menstrual period (FMP). The horizontal axis represents time (y) with respect to the FMP (0); negative (positive) numbers represent time before (after) the FMP. (Modified from Burger HG, Dudley EC, Hopper JL, Groome N, Guthrie JR, Green A, et al. Prospectively measured levels of serum follicle-stimulating hormone, estradiol, and the dimeric inhibins during the menopausal transition in a population-based cohort of women. *J Clin Endocrinol Metab* 1999;84:4025–30.)

consisting of estrogen and a progestogen (EPT) is indicated in women with an intact uterus, but it is recommended that these women limit their duration of therapy because the risk of breast cancer increases after 3 to 5 years of EPT treatment. HRT is contraindicated in women with a history of either breast or endometrial cancer. For further details, the reader is directed to recent guidelines and position statements.[108-110]

It is important to note that perimenopausal and postmenopausal women secrete pituitary hCG.[111-114] Serum concentrations generally are low (<13 IU/L), but positive hCG results often cause confusion and can delay important diagnostic tests or treatments. Pituitary versus placental hCG can be confirmed by measuring serum FSH (concentrations of FSH >45 IU/L are consistent with menopause and make pregnancy unlikely) or by 2 weeks of hormone replacement therapy (hormone replacement therapy should decrease LH, FSH, and hCG concentrations).[115,116]

Female Reproductive Abnormalities

A wide variety of abnormalities affect the female reproductive system and have been classified in a variety of ways. For the purposes of this chapter, they have been divided into categories of (1) pseudohermaphroditism, (2) precocious puberty, (3) irregular menses, and (4) menopause. Infertility from the male and female perspective is discussed in a separate section.

Female Pseudohermaphroditism

In pseudohermaphroditism, the gonadal sex varies from the genital sex. The female pseudohermaphrodite is an individual who is genetically female but whose phenotypic characteristics are, to varying degrees, male. In neonates with a 46,XX karyotype and ambiguous genitalia, *congenital adrenal hyperplasia* (CAH) should be considered. CAH is a family of autosomal recessive disorders of adrenal steroidogenesis (see Chapter 66). Each disorder has a specific pattern of hormonal abnormalities, resulting in deficiency or excess of androgens. The molecular genetics of CAH is discussed in detail in several reviews.[117-121] In female fetuses, exposure to androgens before the 12th week of gestation causes ambiguous genitalia; after 13 weeks, it results in clitoral enlargement.[16,46] Because androgen excess occurs before the 12th week of gestation in those with CAH, ambiguous genitalia are almost always present. Only deficiencies of 21-hydroxylase and 11β-hydroxylase are predominantly virilizing disorders. Deficiency of 3β-hydroxysteroid dehydrogenase is rare, but when it occurs, affected girls may exhibit virilization.

Diagnosis of *21-hydroxylase deficiency* is made in infants and children with excess excretion of urinary 17-KS and pregnanetriol (a metabolite of 17-hydroxyprogesterone; see Chapter 66) and elevated concentrations of plasma 17-hydroxyprogesterone and androstenedione.[45,119,122] However, sick and premature infants may have elevated concentrations of 17-hydroxyprogesterone and androstenedione.[45,119] Elevation of 17-hydroxyprogesterone concentrations in early infancy (>3000 ng/dL; 90.9 nmol/L) confirms the diagnosis of this disorder.[45,123] Additionally, molecular diagnostic testing is now available for detection of the mutations that account for most cases (80% to 90%) of 21-hydroxylase deficiency.[124]

An *11β-hydroxylase deficiency* is confirmed by finding elevated plasma concentrations of 11-deoxycortisol and deoxycorticosterone, increased concentrations of their metabolites in urine, and their suppression by glucocorticoid therapy (see Chapter 66). Plasma renin activity and aldosterone concentrations are low in this deficiency.[45,120,125]

Elevated plasma concentrations of 17-hydroxypregnenolone, DHEA, and DHEA-S are found in patients with *3β-hydroxysteroid dehydrogenase deficiency* (see Chapter 66). Plasma concentrations of 17-hydroxyprogesterone may be elevated as a result of peripheral conversion of 17-hydroxypregnenolone. The ratio of 17-hydroxypregnenolone to 17-hydroxyprogesterone is strikingly elevated in these patients.[45,120,126]

Precocious Puberty

Precocious puberty is the development of secondary sexual characteristics in girls younger than 8 years old and boys younger than 9 years old.[127] In 1999, the Lawson Wilkins Pediatric Society issued new recommendations to lower the age standards at which puberty should be considered precocious from 8 to 7 in white girls and to 6 in black girls.[128] These recommendations have been met with criticism because they are based solely on a single epidemiologic study performed by Herman-Giddens and collaborators in 1997.[129] Many argue that the decreased age standards will result in underdiagnosis of this condition.[130-132]

Despite the debate over the age of onset, pediatric endocrinologists agree that it is important to distinguish between benign advanced pubertal conditions and true precocious puberty.[133-138] Early puberty is manifested by the appearance of secondary sexual characteristics such as premature thelarche (premature breast development) for girls, or premature testicular enlargement for boys. When presented as isolated cases, these secondary sexual characteristics are not necessarily considered to be pathologic. However, if a child demonstrates progressive development of the characteristics and/or increased rates of bone growth and maturation, causes of true precocious puberty must be considered.[138]

Precocious puberty has been classified as GnRH dependent or independent.[133-135,138] GnRH-dependent precocious puberty (also called *central precocious puberty*) is due to precocious activation of the hypothalamic-pituitary-gonadal axis. In girls, the cause is most commonly idiopathic (90%); however, idiopathic cases account for less than 10% of central precocious puberty in boys. Central nervous system tumors also have been known to cause central precocious puberty, the most common being hypothalamic hamartoma. Neurofibromatosis has been documented to lead to GnRH-dependent precocious puberty.

GnRH-independent precocious puberty (also called *pseudoprecocious puberty*) refers to precocious sex steroid secretion that is independent of pituitary gonadotropin release. Congenital adrenal hyperplasias (CAH) are a common cause of pseudoprecocious puberty. Classic forms of CAH present with virilization, growth acceleration, and accelerated bone maturation. Nonclassic or late-onset forms usually present in childhood or adolescence with premature adrenarche and acne. In fact, 5% to 10% of children who present with premature adrenarche have late-onset adrenal hyperplasia. Tumors of the adrenal gland, ovaries, and testes that secrete androgens or estrogens may result in GnRH-independent precocious puberty. Signs of puberty exhibited in males around 2 years of age are characteristic of testotoxicosis, a familial male-limited form of precocious puberty. This autosomal dominant disorder is due to activating mutations affecting

LH receptors.[139] The McCune-Albright syndrome is due to mutation of the *GNAS1* gene, which is involved in the signaling of G-proteins associated with gonadotropin receptors.[140] The mutation causes the gonads to function as if both FSH and LH receptors are constitutively activated. Although this mutation results in GnRH-independent precocious puberty in both sexes, it is most common in girls. Precocious puberty, polyostotic fibrous dysplasia, and café au lait pigmentation are hallmarks for McCune-Albright syndrome. Severe hypothyroidism is also associated with GnRH-independent precocious puberty, likely caused by intrinsic FSH activity of high circulating concentrations of TSH. Unlike the other causes, hypothyroid-induced precocious puberty is associated with skeletal and growth delays.

Diagnosis of precocious puberty is based on clinical presentation, a thorough pubertal history, bone age determinations, and laboratory tests performed to assess gonadotropin concentrations and response to exogenous GnRH.[133-138] The GnRH stimulation test is the gold standard for diagnosis of GnRH-dependent precocious puberty. Pubertal responses of LH and FSH to GnRH stimulation are considered diagnostic of precocious puberty when chronological age is inappropriate for the hormone response. A diagnosis of GnRH-dependent precocious puberty can also be made without proceeding to the GnRH stimulation test if baseline plasma LH concentrations are greater than 5 IU/L. The GnRH stimulation test is also used to monitor the effectiveness of GnRH agonist therapy used to treat central precocious puberty.[141-143] Typically, an IV bolus of exogenous GnRH is administered (100 µg or 2.5 µg/kg, maximal dose 100 µg), followed by a single measurement (at 40 to 45 minutes) or serial measurements of LH and FSH concentrations.[134,144-149] A predominant LH response correlates with a pubertal pattern, and cutoffs vary depending on the assay, with sex differences noted. A typical pubertal response is characterized by a rise in LH to 8 IU/L or greater after IV administration of 100 µg GnRH.[94] In girls, peak LH/FSH ratios (>0.66 to 1.0) have been proposed to be diagnostic of central precocious puberty.[150,151] Highly sensitive fluorometric[152] and chemiluminetric[149] immunoassays are now available for use in measuring basal LH concentrations. Basal LH concentrations have been used instead of the GnRH stimulation test for diagnosis of central precocious puberty. A fluorometric assay resulting in a basal concentration of LH greater than 0.6 IU/L in either sex indicates a pubertal pattern and is consistent with precocious puberty. Values less than 0.6 IU/L have been seen with all forms of precocious puberty and require follow-up with a GnRH stimulation test.[152] A similar pattern is observed for immunochemiluminometric assays using a cutoff of 0.3 IU/L.[148,149]

Response to exogenous GnRH is suppressed, and LH and FSH concentrations are low in individuals with GnRH-independent precocious puberty. The diagnosis of GnRH-independent precocious puberty must exclude nonclassic adrenal hyperplasia (NCAH). Basal 17-hydroxyprogesterone concentrations of early-morning samples have been used to screen for 21-hydroxylase–deficient NCAH. A basal 17-hydroxyprogesterone concentration less than 200 ng/dL (6.0 nmol/L) almost always rules out 21-hydroxylase–deficient NCAH. Morning basal 17-hydroxyprogesterone concentrations as low as 82 ng/dL (2.5 nmol/L) have been documented in children with NCAH, but use of this lower threshold value resulted in suboptimal specificity and is not practical for routine clinical use.[153,154] Patients with intermediate (200–500 ng/dL; 6–15 nmol/L) basal 17-hydroxyprogesterone concentrations should undergo an ACTH stimulation test to confirm the presence of 21-hydroxylase–deficient NCAH. This is achieved by measuring the 17-hydroxyprogesterone response to ACTH stimulation. An exaggerated response is expected in cases of NCAH. The Endocrine Society Clinical Guidelines (2010) recommend a 17-hydroxyprogesterone diagnostic cutoff of greater than 1000 ng/dL (30 nmol/L).[155] However, some argue that the cutoff should be raised to greater than 1500 ng/dL (45 nmol/L) or 2000 ng/dL (60 nmol/L) because the value of 1000 ng/dL (30 nmol/L) was set before molecular genotyping became available, and studies have indicated that several nonaffected carriers exhibit 17-hydroxyprogesterone concentrations above 1000 ng/dL (30 nmol/L).[156-158]

Therapy for precocious puberty is dependent on the presenting symptoms and underlying causes.[135-138,159] Isolated premature thelarche or adrenarche does not require therapy. Patients with premature thelarche should be followed for 3 to 6 months and require further evaluation for precocious puberty. Cases of premature adrenarche should be evaluated for NCAH and/or polycystic ovary syndrome in girls with determined insulin resistance. GnRH-dependent precocious puberty is treated with GnRH agonists to inhibit normal gonadotropin release, thereby slowing pubertal progression. Therapy for GnRH-independent precocious puberty is determined by the underlying cause.

Estrogens and Breast Cancer

Suspicions of estrogen-based causes in the development of human breast cancer stem from epidemiological and experimental observations.[160,161] Early menarche and later natural menopause are associated with increased risk of breast cancer. A two-stage mechanism has been postulated: initiation of a precancerous state by ovarian activity during the early reproductive years and continuation of ovarian activity in later years as a promoting influence on already initiated tumor cells. Ovarian estrogen has been assumed to be the causative factor because administration of estrogen negates the protective effects of early oophorectomy. According to the theory, relative concentrations of individual estrogen fractions (E_1, E_2, and E_3) produced in the first decade or so after puberty are important determinants of a woman's lifetime risk of breast cancer.[162] In particular, pregnancy at a young age is associated with both favorable estrogen fraction ratios and decreased risk. Further discussion of the role of estrogen in the genesis of breast cancer can be found in monographs and review articles[163-169] and the previous version of this chapter.[170]

Irregular Menses

Amenorrhea, the absence of menstrual bleeding, is traditionally categorized as primary (women who have never menstruated) or secondary (women in whom menstruation is present for a variable time and then ceases). Amenorrhea is a relatively common disorder, with an estimated prevalence of 5% in the general population and as high as 8.5% in an unselected adolescent postpubescent population.[171]

Primary Amenorrhea. Primary amenorrhea is defined as failure to establish spontaneous periodic menstruation by the age of 16 years regardless of whether secondary sex characteristics have developed.[93,172,173] About 40% of phenotypic females who have primary amenorrhea (nearly always associated with absence of development of secondary sex characteristics) have *Turner syndrome* (45,X karyotype) or *pure gonadal dysgenesis* (46,XX or XY karyotype).[46,90] *Müllerian duct agenesis* or *dysgenesis* with absence of the vagina or uterus is the second most common manifestation, and the third most common is *androgen insensitivity syndrome* (androgen receptor deficiency and normal or elevated plasma testosterone concentrations if the patient is past puberty and is karyotype XY but has female sex characteristics).

A *17α-hydroxylase deficiency* is a rare form of CAH that is associated with delayed puberty, primary amenorrhea, and hypertension. Patients have a 46,XX karyotype with elevated gonadotropins, low sex steroids, hypertension, and hypokalemia.[93,120]

Another rare cause of amenorrhea is the so-called *resistant ovary syndrome.* This primary hypogonadal condition is associated with increased concentrations of plasma FSH and LH and ovaries that contain predominantly primordial follicles. It is thought to arise from a defect in FSH receptors.[46] This disorder can be diagnosed only by examination of an ovarian biopsy specimen, which will exhibit functioning ovarian follicles despite the presence of amenorrhea. Ovulation sometimes is induced in these patients with administration of high doses of gonadotropins.

As discussed earlier, *Kallmann syndrome* involves hypogonadotropic hypogonadism associated with anosmia or hyposmia and is caused by a defect in the formation and migration of GnRH neurons. Sexual infantilism is the prominent manifestation, and primary amenorrhea is common.[46,90] Finally, delayed pubertal development should be considered.

Evaluation of Primary Amenorrhea. When puberty is delayed in a girl, serum gonadotropins should be measured. Low concentrations may indicate pituitary failure, whereas concentrations elevated into the postmenopausal interval indicate definite gonadal failure.[46,90,174] In the latter case, chromosome studies are indicated. In the former case, pituitary function testing and radiography may be helpful. Patients with short stature without Turner syndrome but with primary amenorrhea may have multiple deficiencies of pituitary hormone secretion. In these patients, a craniopharyngioma or pituitary tumor should be suspected. In patients with normal development of secondary sex characteristics and a normal karyotype who experience primary amenorrhea, a structural abnormality blocking the outflow of blood should be suspected.

The diagnosis of *17α-hydroxylase deficiency* is made when the concentration of (1) serum progesterone is greater than 300 ng/dL (9.54 nmol/L); (2) 17α-hydroxyprogesterone is less than 20 ng/dL (0.6 nmol/L); (3) aldosterone is low; and (4) 11-deoxycorticosterone is elevated. Plasma concentrations of 11-deoxycortisol, testosterone, E_2, and DHEA-S are also low. The diagnosis is confirmed with an *ACTH stimulation test* in which baseline concentrations of progesterone and 17α-hydroxyprogesterone are measured first, followed by administration of 0.25 mg ACTH. Diagnosis is made if serum concentrations of progesterone are significantly elevated and 17α-hydroxyprogesterone concentrations are unchanged at 60 minutes after ACTH administration.[93,175]

Secondary Amenorrhea. Secondary amenorrhea is defined as absence of periodic menstruation for at least 6 months in women who have previously experienced menses.[104,172,173,176,177] *Oligomenorrhea* is infrequent menstruation that occurs fewer than eight times per year.[178] With few exceptions, the causes of primary and secondary amenorrhea overlap (Box 68.2). Pregnancy, the most common cause of secondary amenorrhea, must be considered first and ruled out.[172,173,177] Elevated concentrations of prolactin—iatrogenic or induced by a prolactin-secreting tumor—have been found to result in oligomenorrhea or amenorrhea.[172,173,177] About one-third of women with no obvious cause of amenorrhea have elevated prolactin concentrations.[172] It is thought that hyperprolactinemia interferes with GnRH pulsatility, resulting in impaired release of LH and FSH.[179] If hyperprolactinemia is identified, hypothyroidism should be ruled out because correction of hypothyroidism may lead to normalization of plasma prolactin concentrations. Additionally, both hyperthyroidism and hypothyroidism are associated with a variety of menstrual disorders because of their effects on metabolism and interconversion of androgens and estrogens.[172,173,180] In practice, it is helpful to separate patients with secondary amenorrhea into those with and without signs of estrogen production. Many other factors or conditions have been observed to cause secondary amenorrhea, including disorders of the ovary, uterus, pituitary, and hypothalamus and the use of drugs.

Disorders of the ovary, such as *primary ovarian insufficiency (POI)* (also referred to as premature ovarian failure [POF]) and loss of ovarian function, have been known to cause amenorrhea. POI has been defined as failure of ovarian estrogen production that occurs in a hypergonadotropic state at any age between menarche and 40 years.[46,104,172,177] If the patient is younger than 25 years or shorter than 5 feet tall, karyotyping or chromosomal microarray should be performed to rule out the presence of a variety of chromosomal abnormalities involving duplications or absence of the X chromosome or the presence of a Y chromosome.[214] Screening for the fragile X premutation *(FMR1)* should also be performed.[184] Patients with POI may present with symptoms of hypoestrogenism, including hot flashes and high gonadotropin concentrations. Autoimmune disorders have been associated with 20% to 40% of cases of POI that result in destruction of the ovary and in amenorrhea.[46,104,172,177] Patients also may have antibodies to other endocrine and nonendocrine tissues. Other causes for ovarian failure include oophorectomy, cystic degeneration, trauma, infection, galactosemia, interference with blood supply, radiotherapy treatment, and treatment with cytotoxic chemotherapeutic agents. In rare patients, ovarian resistance to gonadotropins may be evident.[46,177]

Secondary amenorrhea may also result from an issue with the outflow tract. The patient with a uterine problem is normal hormonally but does not menstruate. *Asherman syndrome*, or intrauterine adhesions, is the most common outflow tract abnormality that causes amenorrhea. Endometrial damage may occur in response to a dilatation and curettage and to infection of the endometrium.[104,172] Pituitary dysfunction will also cause secondary amenorrhea. This is most often due to intrinsic pituitary tumors. However, Sheehan syndrome and pituitary apoplexy can result in panhypopituitarism. Empty sella syndrome has been reported in 4% to 16% of patients with amenorrhea and galactorrhea.[172]

Evaluation of Secondary Amenorrhea. Evaluation of women with secondary amenorrhea should begin with a careful history that includes a complete description of menstrual patterns. In addition, the patient should be evaluated

BOX 68.2 Causes of Amenorrhea

Primary Amenorrhea

Lower tract defects
- Vaginal aplasia
- Imperforate hymen
- Congenital vaginal atresia

Uterine disorders
- Congenital absence of the uterus
- Endometritis
- Müllerian agenesis (Mayer-Rokitansky-Kuster-Hauser syndrome)

Ovarian disorders
- XO gonadal and X dysgenesis and variants
- XX gonadal dysgenesis
- Turner syndrome
- 17-Hydroxylase deficiency of the ovaries and adrenal glands
- Autoimmune oophoritis
- Resistant ovary syndrome
- Polycystic ovary syndrome

Adrenal disorders (congenital adrenal hyperplasia)

Thyroid disorders (hypothyroidism)

Pituitary-hypothalamic disorders
- Hypopituitarism
- Constitutional delay in the onset of menses (physiologic)
- Nutritional disorders
- Kallmann syndrome

Secondary Amenorrhea

Pregnancy/lactation

Uterine disorders
- Posttraumatic uterine synechiae (Asherman syndrome)
- Progestational agents

Ovarian disorders
- Polycystic ovary syndrome (hypothalamic)
- Ovarian tumor
- Primary ovarian insufficiency (idiopathic, autoimmune, chemotherapy, radiation, injury)
- Antimetabolite therapy

Adrenal disorders
- Late-onset adrenal hyperplasia
- Cushing syndrome
- Virilizing adrenal tumors
- Adrenocorticoid insufficiency

Thyroid disorders
- Hypothyroidism
- Hyperthyroidism

Pituitary disorders
- Acquired hypopituitarism (trauma, tumor, Sheehan syndrome, lymphocytic hypophysitis)
- Physiologic or pathologic hyperprolactinemia

Hypothalamic disorders
- Tumor and infiltrative disease
- Nutritional disorders
- Hypophysitis
- Excessive exercise
- Stress

Iatrogenic
- Antipsychotics (phenothiazines, haloperidol, clozapine, pimozide)
- Antidepressants (tricyclics, monoamine oxidase inhibitors)
- Antihypertensives (calcium channel blockers, methyldopa, reserpine)
- Drugs with estrogenic activity (digitalis, flavonoids, marijuana, oral contraceptives)
- Drugs with ovarian toxicity (busulfan, chlorambucil, cisplatin, cyclophosphamide, fluorouracil)

for galactorrhea, hot flashes, symptoms of hypothyroidism, hirsutism, prior abdominal surgery, pelvis or uterus trauma, medications prescribed, nutritional history, patterns of exercise, previous contraceptive use, weight changes, stress, and chronic disease. The physical examination should determine the visual fields, thyroid size and function, cushingoid appearance, galactorrhea, hirsutism, abdominal masses, pelvic masses, clitoral enlargement, and evidence of malnutrition. Serum or urine β-hCG should be measured to rule out pregnancy. Because both hypothyroidism and hyperprolactinemia have been known to cause amenorrhea, they are easily excluded by measuring concentrations of serum thyroid-stimulating hormone and prolactin.

A 24-hour urine sample for cortisol measurement or an overnight dexamethasone suppression test is performed in those patients suspected of having Cushing syndrome (see Chapter 66). On the basis of the preliminary assessment, MRI of the sella turcica should be performed in patients with evidence of pituitary or hypothalamic disease, or clinical hypoestrogenism. A GnRH stimulation test with measurement of LH and FSH concentrations in those patients with gonadotropin deficiency assists in differentiating hypothalamic disease from pituitary disease. For diagnosis of polycystic ovary disease (PCOS), see the section "Laboratory Evaluation of Hirsutism/Virilization" later in this chapter.

Progesterone Challenge for Evaluating Amenorrhea. When the cause of amenorrhea is unclear after the initial assessment, relative estrogen status should be determined. Serum E_2 can be measured, but results must be interpreted with caution because serum E_2 fluctuates throughout the menstrual cycle. A *progesterone challenge* may be performed as a functional assessment of relative estrogen status.[46,90] Women with an estrogen-primed uterus have withdrawal vaginal bleeding after treatment with oral progestin (medroxyprogesterone acetate; Provera), 30 mg daily for 3 days, 10 mg daily for 5 to 10 days, or 100 to 200 mg of progesterone in oil given intramuscularly. If estrogen concentrations are adequate and the outflow tract is intact, menstrual bleeding should occur within a week of treatment. In patients with withdrawal bleeding, the plasma E_2 concentration is usually greater than 40 pg/mL (146.8 pmol/L).[46,104] However, the progesterone challenge test is subject to false positives because up to 20% of normoestrogenic women with oligomenorrhea do not experience withdrawal bleeding, as well as false negatives because up to 40% of women with oligomenorrhea and reduced plasma E_2 experience withdrawal bleeding.[181] A pelvic ultrasound to evaluate the thickness of the uterine cavity may also be helpful.

If the patient demonstrates withdrawal bleeding after the progestin challenge test, this indicates that the ovaries are producing sufficient estrogen to cause endometrial proliferation and no anatomic obstruction is present. Most of these women have a history of progestin-containing contraceptive use (the progestin-dominant state can thin the endometrium), stress, weight loss, or excessive exercise.

If bleeding fails to occur after progestin challenge, then additional laboratory tests are indicated, including measurement of FSH to localize the problem to the follicle, pituitary, or hypothalamus. High FSH concentrations indicate that the ovarian follicle is not responding to gonadotropin stimulation. A single measurement of FSH greater than 50 IU/L is suggestive of ovarian failure or primary ovarian insufficiency in women younger than 40 years of age

Because of the association of *primary ovarian insufficiency* (POI) with thyroid, parathyroid, or adrenal insufficiency secondary to autoimmune disease, it has been suggested that patients younger than 40 years should be screened for thyroid antibodies.[104] Increasing evidence indicates that young women with spontaneous premature ovarian failure are at increased risk of developing autoimmune adrenal insufficiency.[74,182-184] It has been suggested that adrenal antibodies (21-hydroxylase antibodies or adrenal cortex autoantibodies) should be measured during the initial evaluation of women with spontaneous POI. Periodic monitoring for the development of antiadrenal antibodies should also be performed in women with idiopathic POI. Patients in whom antiadrenal antibodies have been detected and patients with signs and symptoms of adrenal insufficiency should be tested using a standard ACTH stimulation test. The differential diagnosis for evaluation of amenorrhea is listed in Table 68.1. As indicated by the clinical presentation, special additional testing may be required.

Androgen Excess. Amenorrhea due to androgen excess can be due to adult-onset CAH, corticotropin-dependent Cushing syndrome, or polycystic ovary syndrome (PCOS). Patients with androgen excess often will present with acne, obesity, and variable degrees of excess hair on the face, chest, abdomen, and thighs. Some individuals with 21-hydroxylase deficiency do not manifest any developmental abnormalities or salt wasting, but they present with signs of androgen excess. This clinical syndrome, referred to as *nonclassic, adult-onset,* or *late-onset CAH,* may be clinically indistinguishable from PCOS.[156,185,186]

PCOS is characterized by infertility, hirsutism, obesity (in approximately half of those affected), and various menstrual disturbances ranging from amenorrhea to irregular vaginal bleeding (Table 68.2). Women with PCOS have an increased prevalence of diabetes, along with increased risk for coronary heart disease and endometrial cancer. PCOS patients have substantial estrogen production because of the peripheral conversion of androgens to estrogens. Abnormal bleeding patterns seen in PCOS are due to chronic anovulation and lack of progesterone stimulation and withdrawal. Chronic estrogen exposure without progesterone may predispose patients to endometrial cancer. Although this syndrome is associated with polycystic ovaries, they often are not present in women with this syndrome. The name is actually a misnomer in that the ovaries are covered with follicles, not cysts.

PCOS occurs in 4% to 10% of premenopausal women, and the prevalence varies depending on the diagnostic criteria used. The Rotterdam Consensus Criteria define hyperandrogenism, oligomenorrhea or amenorrhea, and polycystic ovaries by ultrasound as the characteristic signs and symptoms and require the presence of two of the three for diagnosis of PCOS.[187] This definition has been criticized by the Androgen Excess Society, which requires the presence of hyperandrogenism in conjunction with either oligomenorrhea/amenorrhea or polycystic ovaries.[188,189] Despite these concerns, current Endocrine Society guidelines recommend the use of the Rotterdam Consensus Criteria.[190]

Because the pathophysiological mechanism is unknown, PCOS remains a diagnosis of exclusion clinically defined by hyperandrogenism with chronic anovulation in women with no other cause.[191] Relatively low FSH and disproportionately high LH concentrations are common in PCOS, although this ratio should not be used in a routine PCOS workup. Some attempt has been made to link PCOS to *leptin,* a hormone that is secreted by adipocytes and is thought to play a role in regulating food intake and metabolism.[192] While animal studies provide suggestive evidence,[193,194] clinical studies have yet to conclusively demonstrate that leptin plays a role in PCOS, and it remains a subject of research interest only.[195,196] Other studies have reported higher serum AMH concentrations in women with PCOS relative to healthy women,[197,198] and ongoing work is evaluating the potential utility of including AMH measurement in PCOS diagnostic criteria.[199]

Recent evidence has demonstrated that biochemical androgen excess in women with PCOS is associated with an increased risk of insulin resistance and other metabolic dysfunction[200,201] and that metabolic disease severity increases with increasing androgen excess.[202] Many women with PCOS have normal serum testosterone concentrations but demonstrate clinically apparent hyperandrogenism. In the presence of oligomenorrhea and/or polycystic-appearing ovaries on ultrasound, this is enough to make the diagnosis of PCOS. On the other hand, measurement of serum androstenedione has been advocated on the grounds that peripheral conversion of androstenedione to testosterone may explain clinical symptoms of hyperandrogenism in women with normal serum testosterone.[203] In a recent study, serum androstenedione detected androgen excess (as defined by either serum testosterone or androstenedione concentrations above the appropriate reference interval) in PCOS patients, fulfilling the Rotterdam consensus criteria with a sensitivity of 88.3% and specificity of 97.7% compared to 65.1% and 88.3% for testosterone.[202] As will be discussed below, routine measurement of androstenedione and testosterone will require widespread use of liquid chromatography-tandem mass spectrometry (LC-MS/MS) due to the limitations of immunoassays in the measurement of androgens in women. For women with clinically apparent virilization, DHEA-S should also be measured along with serum testosterone to rule out an androgen-secreting tumor (see below).

For PCOS patients who are not interested in conceiving, the mainstay of therapy is oral contraceptive pills for regulation of menstrual periods. In many cases, hirsutism is the primary focus of treatment and may be addressed by androgen receptor antagonists, androgen suppressing agents, or 5 alpha-reductase inhibitors. For those who are overweight or obese, weight loss and exercise are advocated. For women

TABLE 68.1 Differential Diagnosis of Secondary Amenorrhea

Causes	FSH	LH	Estrogen (E_2)	Uterine Bleeding After Progesterone
Hypothalamic				
CNS—hypothalamic dysfunction				
Idiopathic	↓ or N	↓ or N	↓ or N	±
Secondary to medications	↓ or N	↓ or N	↓ or N	±
Secondary to stress	↓ or N	↓ or N	↓ or N	±
CNS—hypothalamic dysfunction or failure due to exercise	↓ or N	↓ or N	↓ or N	±
CNS—hypothalamic dysfunction or failure due to weight loss				
Simple weight loss	↓ or N	↓ or N	↓ or N	±
Anorexia nervosa	↓	↓	↓	—
CNS—hypothalamic failure				
Lesions	↓	↓	↓	—
Idiopathic	↓	↓	↓	—
CNS—hypothalamic–adreno-ovarian dysfunction (polycystic ovary syndrome) or hyperandrogenic chronic anovulation	N	↑*	N	+
Pituitary				
Destructive lesions (Sheehan syndrome)	↓	↓	↓	—
Tumor	↓	↓	↓	—
Ovarian				
Premature ovarian failure	↑	↑	↓	—
Loss of ovarian function (oophorectomy, infection, cystic degeneration, chemotherapy, radiation)	↑	↑	↓	—
Uterine				
Uterine synechiae (Asherman syndrome)	N	N	N	—

CNS, Central nervous system; *FSH,* follicle-stimulating hormone; *LH,* luteinizing hormone; *N,* value within normal reference interval; ↓, value below normal reference interval; ↑, value above normal reference interval; ↑*, >25 IU/L, less than menopausal concentration; ±, positive or negative bleeding response to progesterone.

From Davajan V, Kletzky OA. Amenorrhea. In: Mishell DR, Davajan V, Lobo RA, eds. *Infertility, Contraception and Reproductive Endocrinology.* 3rd ed. Boston: Blackwell Scientific Publications, 1991:373.

TABLE 68.2 Clinical Features of the Polycystic Ovary Syndrome*

Clinical Feature	Frequency, %
Hirsutism	65
Acne	25
Obesity	35
Infertility	50
Amenorrhea	35
Oligomenorrhea	40
Regular menstrual cycle	20

*Data were compiled from three studies. Two used ultrasonography as the primary method of diagnosis, one used ovarian histology. Total $n = 1935$.

Modified from Franks S. Polycystic ovary syndrome. *N Engl J Med* 1995;333:853.

with PCOS who wish to conceive, treatment is aimed at ovulation induction. Weight reduction helps to promote ovulation. Medications such as aromatase inhibitors and clomiphene citrate are useful.[191] Metformin may be a helpful adjuvant in women with documented glucose intolerance as measured by a 2-hour oral glucose tolerance test.

Ovarian hyperthecosis, a nonneoplastic lesion of the ovary characterized by the presence of islands of luteinized thecal cells in the ovarian stroma, is sometimes confused with PCOS. Features that distinguish it from PCOS include higher concentrations of testosterone, androstenedione, and DHT derived from ovarian secretion. Thus androgenization is greater than is usually observed in patients with PCOS. Both LH and FSH concentrations are low or low-normal. Insulin resistance and hyperinsulinism are present to a greater degree than in PCOS. Finally, patients with ovarian hyperthecosis fail to ovulate when treated with an antiestrogen such as clomiphene citrate.[204]

Hirsutism and Virilization. Hirsutism is defined as excessive growth of terminal hair in women and children in a distribution similar to that occurring in postpubertal men.[205-207] True hirsutism, which is androgen responsive, has to be distinguished from hypertrichosis, which consists of excessive growth of vellus or non-androgen-responsive hair. Women with androgen-dependent hirsutism may have exposure to excess androgens or may have heightened sensitivity to normal circulating concentrations of androgen.

The causes of hirsutism are listed in Box 68.3. The estimated prevalence for idiopathic hirsutism ranges from 6% to 50% of women evaluated for hirsutism, depending on the definition.[207-210] Typically, idiopathic hirsutism is defined by

BOX 68.3 Causes of Hirsutism

Ovarian
- Severe insulin resistance
- Hyperthecosis, hilus cell or stromal cell hyperplasia
- Androgen-producing ovarian tumor
- Menopause

Adrenal
- Classic congenital hyperplasia
- 21-Hydroxylase deficiency
- 11-Hydroxylase deficiency
- 3β-Hydroxysteroid dehydrogenase deficiency
- Adult or attenuated adrenal hyperplasia
- Androgen-producing adrenal tumor

Familial Hirsutism

Endocrine Disorders
- Polycystic ovary syndrome
- Hyperprolactinemia
- Acromegaly
- Cushing syndrome

Idiopathic Hirsutism (includes increased skin sensitivity to androgens)

Iatrogenic
- Androgens
- Phenytoin
- Diazoxide
- Minoxidil
- Streptomycin
- Cyclosporine
- Danazol
- Metyrapone
- Phenothiazides
- Progestagens (19-nonsteroid derivatives)

normal physical and laboratory findings in hirsute women. Nonneoplastic forms of hirsutism are slow to progress and usually manifest at the time of puberty, when circulating concentrations of androgens increase, after a period of weight gain, or when oral contraceptives have been stopped.[206] Rapid onset of hirsutism suggests an iatrogenic cause or, if associated with virilization, a neoplastic source of androgens. The most common cause of androgen hypersecretion in women is PCOS; 70% to 80% of hirsute women are reportedly afflicted with this disorder.[210] Late-onset CAH (see Chapter 66), acromegaly, hyperprolactinemia, menopause (see earlier section "Menopause"), and ACTH-dependent Cushing syndrome have been observed to cause hirsutism.

Virilization is characterized by clitoral hypertrophy, deepening of the voice, temporal hair recession, baldness, increased libido, decreased body fat, and menstrual irregularities or amenorrhea. Hirsutism is usually associated with normal or slightly elevated serum androgens, whereas virilization is associated with marked increases in ovarian or adrenal androgen production and is an indication for more intensive investigation.[46]

Laboratory Evaluation of Hirsutism/Virilization. The two most important screening tests used in the evaluation of women for hirsutism and virilization are serum total or free testosterone and DHEA-S.[46,211] Elevation of DHEA-S concentration suggests an adrenal origin of androgens, whereas elevations in testosterone indicate an adrenal or ovarian source. Neoplastic disease is unlikely if the serum testosterone concentration is less than 200 ng/dL (6.9 nmol/L), the DHEA-S concentration is less than 700 µg/dL (19 µmol/L), or 17-KS concentrations are less than 30 mg/dL (1 mmol/L).[46,186,207] Regardless of the source of excess androgen production, the androstanediol glucuronide concentration is elevated in more than 90% of women with hirsutism because it is a marker of excessive DHT production in skin. Concentrations of SHBG can be decreased in hirsute women, so there has been some debate over whether total testosterone or bioavailable testosterone (free and weakly bound testosterone) is more clinically informative in diagnosing hirsutism. The reader is directed to a review by Wheeler that discusses many of these issues.[212]

Polycystic ovary syndrome is primarily a clinical diagnosis, and few laboratory tests are needed. Provided that other causes of oligoamenorrhea or amenorrhea have been ruled out (thyroid disease, hyperprolactinemia), given a history of androgen excess, the only condition that needs to be excluded is 21-hydroxylase–deficient nonclassic CAH; this can be done by measuring 17-hydroxyprogesterone (early morning; follicular phase). If the result is less than 200 ng/dL (6.1 nmol/L), nonclassic CAH can be excluded. Serum testosterone measurement is not necessary if clear hirsutism is present. Testosterone concentrations greater than 60 ng/dL (2 nmol/L) are consistent with PCOS.[191] FSH concentrations are often disproportionately normal or low. Patients with PCOS usually have E_2 concentrations greater than 40 pg/mL (147 pmol/L) and therefore experience withdrawal bleeding in response to a progestin challenge.

Morning plasma 17α-hydroxyprogesterone concentrations are measured to evaluate *nonclassic* or *late-onset 21-hydroxylase deficiency* (NCAH). A concentration less than 200 ng/dL (6.1 nmol/L) excludes this diagnosis, and a concentration greater than 1500 ng/dL (45 nmol/L) in nonpregnant women is confirmatory. When basal concentrations between 200 and 1500 ng/dL (6.1–45 nmol/L) are found, an ACTH stimulation test should be performed. NCAH typically has a 17α-hydroxyprogesterone concentration greater than 1500 ng/dL (45 nmol/L), and classic CAH has a response over 2000 ng/dL (60 nmol/L).[94,155,206,211] Patients with attenuated forms of CAH usually have normal concentrations of FSH and LH. About one-half have elevated testosterone and androstenedione concentrations.[73] Most of these patients also have increased concentrations of DHEA-S, and more than 90% have supranormal concentrations of androstanediol glucuronide.[21,213]

Other Factors. Hypothalamic dysfunction consists of those disorders that disrupt the frequency or amplitude of GnRH. Rarely is this due to a lesion or tumor. However, most commonly, disruption occurs in response to psychological stress, depression, severe weight loss, anorexia nervosa, or strenuous exercise.[104,172] A syndrome known as the *female athletic triad* has been described. This syndrome is prevalent in women who exercise vigorously, and it is associated with amenorrhea, disordered eating, and osteoporosis. Competitive long-distance runners, gymnasts, and professional ballet dancers appear to be at highest risk. Although the mechanism for the disturbance is unclear, symptoms and laboratory profiles are similar to those of other forms of hypothalamic amenorrhea. LH and FSH concentrations are normal or low, and E_2 concentrations are low. As a result of chronic low estrogen, bone mineral content is low and the incidence of stress fractures is increased.[104,171]

Several hormone-producing tumors of the ovary, pituitary gland, and adrenal glands occur in combination with amenorrhea.[46,90,215,216] This amenorrhea may be confused with pregnancy if the tumors produce hCG. Choriocarcinoma of the uterus or ovary may produce large amounts of hCG that cause hyperthyroidism because of the slight thyrotropic action of hCG. Granulosa–theca cell tumors are usually associated with estrogen secretion that results in amenorrhea and irregular menses and, rarely, excessive androgen with associated virilization.[46,90]

Many drugs produce amenorrhea (see Box 68.2), particularly phenothiazines and other psychotropic drugs such as haloperidol, pimozide, or clozapine.[172] Phenothiazine-induced amenorrhea is usually associated with hyperprolactinemia and galactorrhea. Drugs that affect the normal pathway of dopamine secretion will produce amenorrhea by decreasing the secretion of norepinephrine. Because norepinephrine is important in controlling the synthesis and secretion of GnRH, any alteration in its synthesis or secretion will result in menstrual abnormalities.[104,179] Older formulations of oral contraceptive pills utilized higher doses of estrogen that were thought to have suppressive effects on the HPO axis. This is no longer the case. Normal menses should resume shortly after the cessation of combined oral contraceptive pills.[104] If menses has not resumed after ceasing the oral contraceptive pill, evaluation is warranted. If other causes of amenorrhea are suspected, evaluation should not be delayed.

POINTS TO REMEMBER

- GnRH stimulates LH and FSH release, which control oocyte maturation and ovulation and increase estradiol and progesterone production.
- Estradiol is transported in blood tightly bound to SHBG and loosely bound to albumin, while progesterone is bound to corticosteroid binding globulin.
- Estradiol and progesterone both inhibit and stimulate LH and FSH release, with the type of regulation dependent on the stage of the menstrual cycle and the serum steroid hormone concentration.
- PCOS is defined by hyperandrogenism and oligo/anovulation and remains a diagnosis of exclusion based primarily on clinical evaluation.
- Pituitary secretion of hCG is often seen in postmenopausal women, and the pituitary origin can be confirmed by the presence of concurrent elevated serum serum FSH.

INFERTILITY

Infertility is defined as the inability to conceive after 1 year of unprotected intercourse.[46,217,218] It has been estimated that 93% of healthy couples practicing unprotected intercourse should expect to conceive within 1 year.[219] A specific cause of infertility is identified in approximately 80% of couples: one-third are due to female factors alone, one-third to male factors alone, and one-third to a combination of problems.

Primary infertility refers to couples or patients who have had no previous successful pregnancies. Secondary infertility encompasses patients who have previously conceived but are currently unable to conceive. These types of infertility generally share common causes.

Infertility problems often arise as a result of hormonal dysfunction of the hypothalamic-pituitary-gonadal axis. Measurements of peptide and steroid hormones in the serum are therefore essential aspects of the evaluation of infertility. This section focuses on hormonal and biochemical aspects of evaluating infertility.

Male Infertility

A list of the most common male infertility factors is given in Box 68.4. One algorithm for the evaluation of male infertility is shown in Fig. 68.11. Initial evaluation of male infertility should include a detailed history and physical examination. The physical examination should pay particular attention to (1) the external genitalia—for evidence of proper androgenization; (2) hair pattern—degree of virilization; (3) breast abnormalities—gynecomastia and or discharge; and (4) neurologic findings—sense of smell and visual impairments. The history must include (1) reproductive history, including living children and any pregnancies that resulted in miscarriage; (2) prescribed medications; (3) recreational and performance-enhancing drug and alcohol use; (4) systemic illness; and (5) potential toxin exposure. Sexual history should include sexual technique, frequency of intercourse, and use of any lubricants. Issues of potency must be distinguished from those of

BOX 68.4 Male Infertility Factors

Endocrine Disorders

Hypothalamic dysfunction (Kallmann syndrome)
Pituitary failure (tumor, radiation, surgery)
Hyperprolactinemia (drug, tumor)
Androgen insensitivity syndrome (AIS)
Exogenous androgens
Thyroid disorders
Adrenal hyperplasia
Testicular failure

Anatomic

Congenital absence of vas deferens
Obstructed vas deferens
Congenital abnormalities of ejaculatory system
Varicocele
Retrograde ejaculation

Abnormal Spermatogenesis

Unexplained azoospermia
Chromosomal abnormalities
Mumps orchitis
Cryptorchidism
Chemical or radiation exposure

Abnormal Motility

Absent cilia (Kartagener syndrome)
Antibody formation

Psychosocial

Unexplained impotence
Decreased libido

Modified from Morell V. Basic infertility assessment. *Primary Care* 1997;24:195–204.

AT A GLANCE

Evaluating Male Infertility

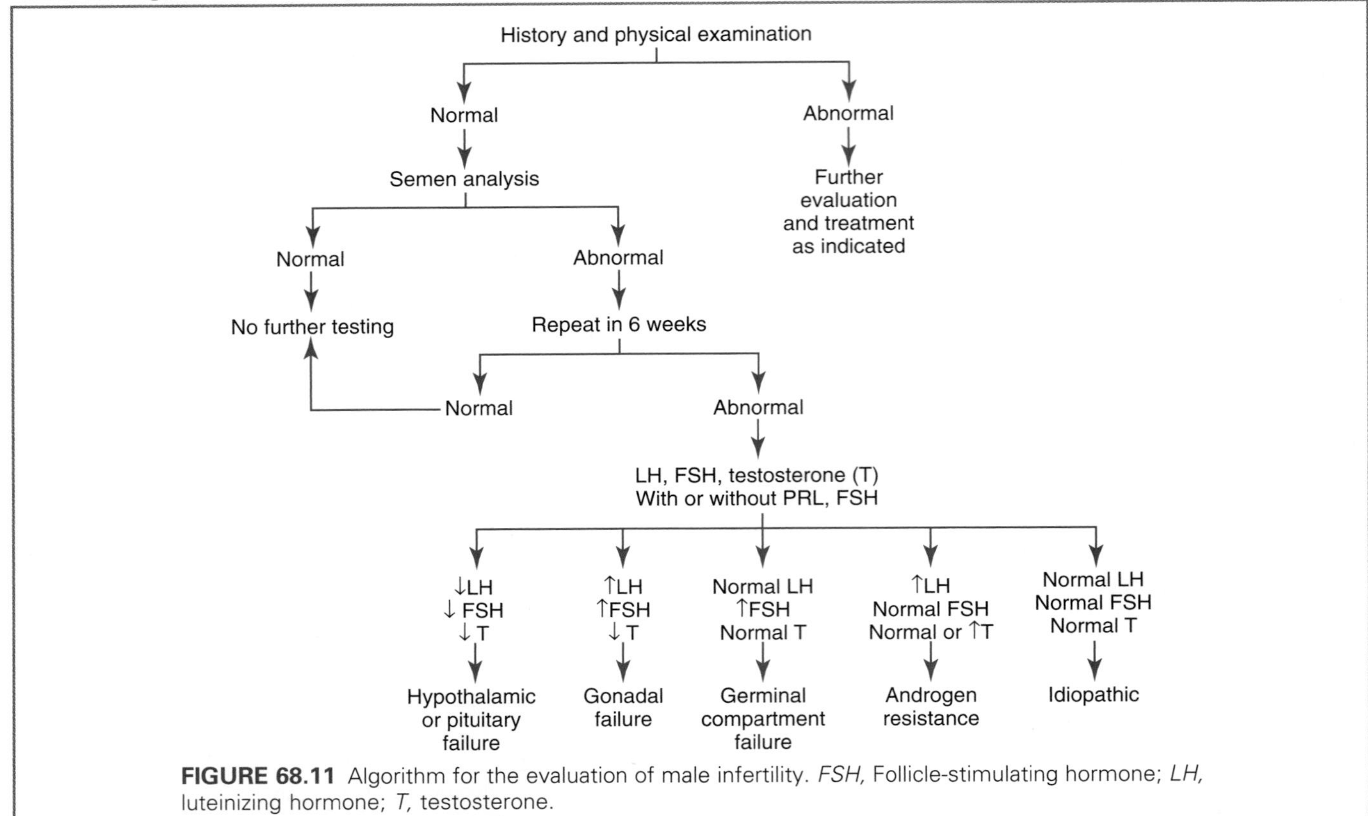

FIGURE 68.11 Algorithm for the evaluation of male infertility. *FSH,* Follicle-stimulating hormone; *LH,* luteinizing hormone; *T,* testosterone.

infertility or subfertility. All abnormalities in the history and physical examination should be pursued. Testosterone should be measured, especially when the patient history or physical examination suggests deficient development of secondary sex characteristics. Laboratory evaluation of male infertility should begin with evaluation of semen, which should be followed by evaluation of endocrine parameters.

Evaluation of Semen

Semen analysis measures ejaculate volume, pH, sperm count, motility, forward progression, and morphology. Semen should be analyzed within 1 hour after collection. Although semen analysis is not a test for infertility, it is considered the most important laboratory test in the evaluation of male fertility. Controversy exists as to what constitutes a "normal" semen profile. With the exception of the *azoospermic* male (defined as no sperm in the ejaculate), the lines between fertility and infertility are blurred and are intimately associated with the status of the female partner's reproductive function. However, clinical studies of infertile men and World Health Organization (WHO) guidelines have helped establish limits of adequacy (Table 68.3).[220,221] If semen analysis is normal, it is unlikely that other laboratory testing will be useful. If semen analysis is abnormal, it should be repeated in approximately 6 weeks. A new approach to semen analysis for investigation of infertility uses a monoclonal antibody to sperm protein SP-10. A version of the test is available to check the success of vasectomy.[222,223]

TABLE 68.3 Normal Seminal Fluid Values

Parameter	Value
Ejaculate volume	>1.5 mL (1.4–1.7)*
Sperm density	>15 million/mL (12–16)*
Total sperm count	>39 million/ejaculate (33–46)*
Motility	>32% progressive motility (31–34); >40% total (38–42)*
Morphology	>4.0% normal (3–4)*
pH	7.2–8.0*
Color	Gray-white-yellow
Liquefaction	Within 40 minutes
Fructose	>1200 μg/mL
Acid phosphatase	100–300 μg/mL
Citric acid	>3 mg/mL
Inositol	>1 mg/mL
Zinc	>75 μg/mL
Magnesium	>70 μg/mL
Prostaglandins (PGE_1 + PGE_2)	30–200 μg/mL
Glycerylphosphorylcholine	>650 μg/mL
Carnitine	>250 μg/mL
Glucosidase	>20 mU per ejaculate

*Values from World Health Organization. Cooper TG, et al. World Health Organization reference values for human semen characteristics. *Hum Reprod Update* 2010;3:231.

Evaluation of Obstruction

Obstruction of the male reproductive tract will result in male infertility, and analysis of specific semen parameters has proved a useful adjunct to physical examination in the evaluation of male reproductive tract obstruction. Testosterone produced after administration of hCG causes the seminal vesicles, epididymis, and prostate to increase the volume of ejaculate. An appropriate increase in serum testosterone without change in the ejaculate volume may indicate mechanical blockage. Absence of, or a decrease in, specific biochemical markers such as acid phosphatase and citric acid (from prostate), fructose, and prostaglandins (from seminal vesicles) can assist determination of the location of blockage.[224] Low seminal glucosidase concentrations in the presence of testes of normal size and consistency, normal semen volume, and normal serum FSH, have been used as an indication of obstruction (usually in the epididymis) or congenital bilateral absence of the vas deferens (a condition associated with mutations of the cystic fibrosis gene).[225]

Evaluation of Endocrine Parameters

If severe oligospermia or azoospermia is found, then measurement of serum testosterone, LH, and FSH concentrations is warranted, with or without measurement of prolactin and TSH. Hyperprolactinemia is a cause of secondary testicular dysfunction.[5] Prolactin excess likely causes hypogonadism by impairing GnRH release. It also leads to underandrogenization and erectile dysfunction (see earlier section "Erectile Dysfunction"). If hyperprolactinemia is found, it is imperative to check for hypothyroidism because elevated TRH concentrations can result in hyperprolactinemia. Pituitary adenomas and drugs such as anxiolytics, antihypertensives, serotonergics, and histamine H_2 receptor antagonists also increase serum prolactin.[226] Hyperthyroidism and hypothyroidism will alter spermatogenesis. Hyperthyroidism affects both pituitary and testicular function, with alterations in the secretion of releasing hormones and increased conversion of androgens to estrogens.

Patients with borderline or suppressed testosterone concentrations can be evaluated with an *hCG stimulation test*. With this test, an injection of 5000 IU hCG is administered intramuscularly following collection of a basal, early-morning testosterone sample. Serum testosterone is measured 72 hours later. Hypogonadal men show a depressed rise in testosterone concentration in response to this challenge. Doubling of testosterone concentration over baseline is consistent with normal Leydig cell function.[227] Failure to increase testosterone to greater than 150 ng/dL (5 nmol/L) indicates primary hypogonadism.[228] Alternatively, sperm counts may be evaluated before and after administration of clomiphene citrate or hCG. This represents more of a trial-and-error approach but is simpler to perform than a formal hCG stimulation test and is often preferred in clinical practice. Letrozole, an aromatase inhibitor, is also used to improve semen parameters is hypogonadal men.[229]

Testosterone is essential for normal sperm development (see Fig. 68.3). Therefore any disorder that results in hypogonadism (and thus low testosterone concentrations) results in infertility. Among the causes are hypogonadotropic and hypergonadotropic hypogonadism.

Hypergonadotropic Hypogonadism. Measurement of the concentration of FSH is indicated in men with sperm count lower than 5 to 10 million/mL. Elevated concentrations of FSH indicate Sertoli cell dysfunction and, in azoospermic men, primary germinal cell failure, Sertoli cell–only syndrome, or genetic conditions such as Klinefelter syndrome.[230] Radiotherapy and gonadotoxic chemotherapy can also lead to testicular failure with azoospermia. Elevated FSH (>120 IU/L) in the setting of decreased testosterone (<200 ng/dL, 7 nmol/L) and oligospermia indicate primary testicular failure.

Hypogonadotropic Hypogonadism. Decreased concentrations of testosterone (<200 ng/dL, 7 nmol/L) and decreased concentrations of FSH (<10 IU/L) are suggestive of hypogonadotropic hypogonadism. Administering GnRH may help to distinguish between gonadal insufficiencies caused by pituitary versus hypothalamic failure. Because the pituitary is sensitive to sex steroids for appropriate gonadotropin secretion, patients with long-standing hypogonadism should be given exogenous testosterone for 1 week before the GnRH stimulation test is administered. One approach to this test involves the intravenous injection of 100 μg of GnRH with measurement of FSH and LH concentrations at 0, 30, 60, 120, and 180 minutes after injection. Results of the GnRH test are classified as follows. An increase in serum gonadotropins of 10 IU/L or more over baseline is normal. If little to no increase in gonadotropins is seen, pituitary disease is likely. Patients with hypothalamic disease will demonstrate a delayed but significant increase of 7 IU/L or more within 180 minutes.[228] The most common cause of hypothalamic hypogonadism is *congenital idiopathic hypogonadotropic hypogonadism* (IHH) or its variant, Kallmann syndrome (see earlier section "Male Reproductive Abnormalities").[231] An adult-onset form of IHH has been recognized as a potentially treatable form of male infertility.[232] Molecular diagnosis using fluorescence in situ hybridization (FISH) analysis is now offered to families with X-linked Kallmann syndrome. This is the most common type of testing performed, but it will detect only major deletions in the *KAL* gene. Genome microarray analysis and prenatal diagnosis also are now available.

Mutations in the X chromosome gene, *DAX1*, also have been known to cause hypogonadotropic hypogonadism in association with congenital adrenal hypoplasia. This gene encodes an orphan nuclear hormone receptor that has a critical role in development of the hypothalamus, pituitary, adrenal, and gonads.[230] FISH analysis is also available for the diagnosis of *DAX1* mutations.

Y-Chromosome Microdeletions

Deletions in either of the azoospermia factor regions (*AZF1* and *AZF2*) on the long arm of the Y chromosome are associated with an inability to make sperm. In addition, genes such as *SRY* (sex-determining region Y) are on the short arm of chromosome Y. Deletion of these regions is associated with azoospermia or, less frequently, oligospermia. The incidence of Y microdeletions in idiopathic nonobstructive azoospermic men is 8% to 18%.[230] Testing for Y-chromosome microdeletions includes polymerase chain reaction (PCR) of specific regions of the Y chromosome to identify microdeletions. Tests should span *AZF1 (AZFa)* and *AZF2* (*AZFb* and *AZFc*) and other regions thought to encode putative spermatogenesis genes.[230] The utility of testing for Y-chromosome microdeletions is to provide additional information as to whether or not sperm might be retrieved on a testicular sperm extraction procedure.

Immunologic Parameters

Antibodies to sperm surface antigens have been explored as a cause of infertility. They are thought to impair fertility by decreasing motility, increasing agglutination, and impairing the ability of sperm to penetrate human ova.[233] However, this is controversial, and laboratory testing for antisperm antibodies is rarely performed.[234]

Female Infertility

Evaluating female infertility is more complex than evaluating infertility of the male. A list of the most common female infertility factors is given in Box 68.5. One algorithm for the evaluation of female infertility is shown in Fig. 68.12. This evaluation should be considered after 1 year of unprotected intercourse in women with regular menses younger than 35. If a woman is over the age of 35 or if the woman or her partner has a history of issues that would contribute to infertility, this workup should ensue sooner. Examples of issues that would prompt earlier workup include irregular menses, history of pelvic inflammatory disease or sexually transmitted infection, and history of exposure to gonadotoxic agents.

BOX 68.5 Female Infertility Factors

- Ovarian or Hormonal Factors
- Metabolic disease
  - Thyroid
  - Liver
  - Obesity
  - Androgen excess
  - Polycystic ovarian syndrome
- Hypergonadotropic hypogonadism
  - Menopause
  - Luteal phase deficiency
  - Gonadal dysgenesis
  - Primary ovarian insufficiency (autoimmune, cytotoxic, chemotherapy, radiation, tumor)
  - Resistant ovary syndrome
- Hypogonadotropic hypogonadism
  - Hyperprolactinemia (tumor, drugs)
  - Hypothalamic insufficiency (Kallmann syndrome)
  - Pituitary insufficiency (tumor, necrosis, thrombosis, stress, exercise, anorexia)
- Tubal Factors
  - Occlusion or scarring
  - Salpingitis isthmica nodosa
  - Infectious salpingitis
- Cervical Factors
  - Stenosis
  - Inflammation or infection
  - Abnormal mucous viscosity
- Uterine Factors
  - Leiomyomata
  - Congenital malformation
  - Adhesions
  - Endometritis or abnormal endometrium
- Psychosocial Factors
  - Decreased libido
  - Anorgasmia
- Iatrogenic
- Immunologic (Antisperm Antibodies)

Modified from Morell V. Basic infertility assessment. *Primary Care* 1997;24:195–204.

Initial Evaluation of Female Infertility

The initial evaluation of female infertility should include a detailed history and physical examination. The physical examination should include evaluation of (1) the external genitalia and hair pattern (for signs of androgen excess, including clitoromegaly, hirsutism, and virilization), (2) the pelvis (for masses, nodularity, or tenderness), (3) the breasts (for signs of galactorrhea), (4) neurologic findings (sense of smell and visual impairments), (5) the thyroid (for enlargement or nodules), and (6) body mass index. All abnormalities in the history and physical examination should be pursued. A thorough medical and surgical history is also necessary, including an assessment of the patient's gravidity and parity, coital frequency, duration of infertility, and prior workup and treatment for infertility. History of sexually transmitted infections, assessment of previous cervical cytologic and human papillomavirus (HPV) testing and treatment, and a menstrual history also should be obtained. Concentrations of TSH, testosterone, and prolactin should be measured if menstrual cycles are absent or irregular or if signs of galactorrhea or thyroid abnormalities are present. Ovulation reserve testing as discussed here should be considered in cases where diminished ovarian reserve is suspected.

Evaluation of Ovulation. In the menstruating woman, the next step would be to determine whether ovulation occurs. No current laboratory tests will confirm ovum release. However, measurement of the concentration of midluteal plasma progesterone does indicate that a corpus luteum was formed. Other methods, such as measurement of the LH surge (to predict ovulation) and basal body temperature (to detect a midcycle rise in progesterone), have been used to assess ovulation.

Progesterone Measurement. Measurement of the concentration of serum progesterone is the primary assay used for the evaluation of ovulation.[235,236] It is important to note that an increase in progesterone concentration indicates that a corpus luteum has been formed, but it does not confirm that the oocyte was actually released. Beginning immediately after ovulation, serum progesterone concentrations rise (see Fig. 68.9); they peak within 5 to 9 days during the midluteal phase (days 21 to 23).[236] If ovulation does not occur, the corpus luteum fails to form, and the expected cyclic rise in progesterone concentration is subnormal. If pregnancy occurs, hCG maintains the corpus luteum, and progesterone production continues to rise. Midluteal progesterone concentrations greater than 300 ng/dL (9.5 nmol/L) indicate that ovulation has taken place.[237]

Basal Body Temperature. Basal body temperature charts have long been accepted as simple, cost-effective indicators of ovulation. Ovulation is associated with a rapid rise in body temperature (by 0.2° to 0.5°F, or 0.1° to 0.3°C), which persists through the luteal phase. The rise in temperature is due to increased progesterone concentration. However, similar to progesterone, the rise in body temperature is evident only retrospectively and therefore does not predict imminent ovulation in a way helpful for timing intercourse.

Measurement of the Luteinizing Hormone Surge. Luteinizing hormone appears in the urine just after the serum LH

AT A GLANCE

Evaluating Female Infertility

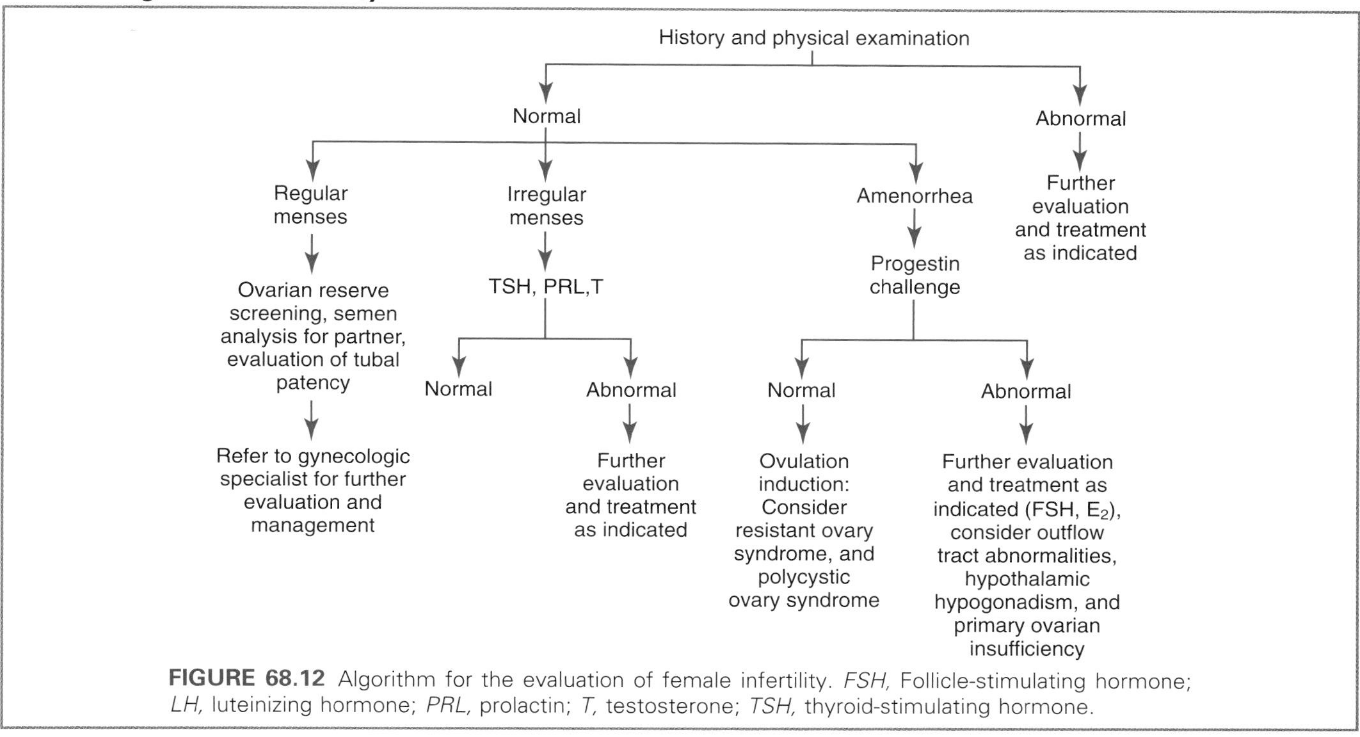

FIGURE 68.12 Algorithm for the evaluation of female infertility. *FSH,* Follicle-stimulating hormone; *LH,* luteinizing hormone; *PRL,* prolactin; *T,* testosterone; *TSH,* thyroid-stimulating hormone.

surge and 24 to 36 hours before ovulation (see Fig. 68.9). Measurement of LH does not confirm ovulation or provide insight into the cause of anovulation, but rather indicates when ovulation should occur and provides a guide with which to time intercourse. Methods for laboratory measurement of LH are given in Chapter 65.

Monoclonal technology has led to the use of *home LH kits* that not only provide accurate information as to the timing of ovulation but may reduce stress and costs associated with infertility programs because these tests are performed at home and are comparatively inexpensive.[238] Most home ovulation kits consist of a "dipstick" that uses a two-site, double monoclonal enzyme-linked immunoassay. Urine is applied to the test pad, and capillary action draws fluid across the pad. LH in the urine first is bound to an anti-LH antibody that is coupled to an enzyme conjugate, or colloidal gold. The LH-antibody complex then migrates to a region coated with a second anti-LH antibody. Once bound to this site, the substrate-enzyme reaction or colloidal gold complexes result in a color change that is proportional to the amount of LH present. A reference region is provided. A test result that matches or is darker in color than the reference region is considered a positive result, indicating that the LH surge is occurring. These tests effectively predict ovulation in 70% of women.[239] In one study of 26 normal women, home LH kits had a 92% positive predictive value for ovulation to occur within 48 hours of a positive urine LH screen.[240] The clinical utility of these devices is controversial, however,[241] and no studies have been performed to determine whether the use of home LH devices alters outcomes in women not being treated for infertility. A few studies have been published to look at outcomes in infertility patients, but the results are mixed when compared with serum LH testing or basal body temperature.[241] On the other hand, studies comparing urinary LH surge testing to ultrasound monitoring and human chorionic gonadotropin injections to monitor and trigger ovulation for intrauterine insemination have found no differences in chances of pregnancy between the two approaches, although the cost and time commitment to the latter option is clearly more involved.[242,243]

Evaluation of Endocrine Parameters

Disorders of hypothalamus, pituitary, and ovary are endocrine causes of infertility.

Hypergonadotropic Hypogonadism. Premature ovarian failure is indicated by repeatedly elevated basal FSH concentrations (>30 IU/L) or a single elevation of greater than 40 IU/L in a woman younger than 40 years. These patients are often hypoestrogenic (E_2 <20 pg/mL, 73 pmol/L)[236] and do not respond to a progestin challenge because their endometrium is atrophic (see earlier section on evaluation of secondary amenorrhea). A pelvic ultrasound will reveal a thin endometrium. Basal serum FSH has been used as an indicator of relative ovarian reserve. Fig. 68.13 shows the relationship between rising serum FSH and the reduced rate of successful pregnancy. A precipitous drop occurs at concentrations greater than 20 IU/L.

Assessing Ovarian Reserve. Women in their mid to late 30s and early 40s with infertility constitute the largest portion of the total infertility population. These women are also at increased risk for miscarriage. This reflects a diminished ovarian reserve as a result of follicular depletion and a decline in oocyte quality. As women age, serum FSH concentrations in the early follicular phase begin to increase. It has been

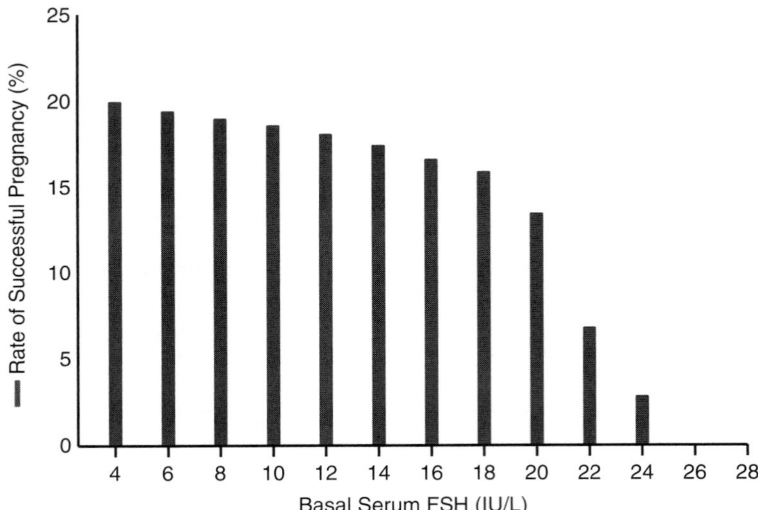

FIGURE 68.13 The relationship between increasing follicle-stimulating hormone (FSH) concentrations and decreased percentage of successful pregnancies. (Modified from Jones H, Toner JP. The infertile couple. *N Engl J Med* 1993;329:1710–5.)

suggested that this is due to a decline in the number of small follicles secreting inhibin B.

The concomitant measurement of follicular phase serum FSH and E_2 is a popular screening test for assessing ovarian reserve. In general, day 3 FSH concentrations greater than 20 to 25 IU/L are considered to be elevated and associated with poor reproductive outcome.[244] Concomitant measurement of serum E_2 concentration adds to the predictive power of an isolated FSH determination. Early follicular phase E_2 concentrations greater than 75 to 80 pg/mL (275–294 pmol/L) may be associated with poor response to ovarian stimulation and pregnancy outcome, although these concentrations may also be slightly elevated in women with PCOS.[245]

More recently anti-Müllerian hormone (AMH) (also known as Müllerian-inhibiting substance [MIS]) has emerged as a helpful indicator of ovarian reserve. AMH regulates follicle development and maturation as well as E_2 production.[246] AMH is produced by small, growing follicles but ceases to be produced during FSH-dependent follicular growth or in atretic follicles.[247] Serum AMH remains relatively constant throughout the menstrual cycle and decreases with age,[248,249] leading to its promotion as a marker of ovarian reserve and reduced reproductive capacity.[250-253] However, additional reports have demonstrated noticeable intraindividual variation in serum AMH.[254,255] This observation, coupled with the lack of standardization of AMH assays or clearly defined reference intervals,[199] concerns about sample stability,[256,257] and successful pregnancy in childhood lymphoma survivors with low serum AMH,[258] has led to concerns regarding the use of AMH to classify a patient's ovarian status.

Current literature suggests the most beneficial application of AMH measurement is not in AMH's ability to predict the chance of pregnancy but rather in predicting response to controlled ovarian stimulation used in assisted reproductive techniques.[259-262] Patients with elevated serum AMH concentrations are often "high responders" and are at risk of ovarian hyperstimulation syndrome (OHSS) if a standard ovarian stimulation protocol is used. As a result, these women may undergo a modified stimulation protocol to minimize the risk of OHSS. At the other end of the spectrum, women with low serum AMH concentrations are considered "low responders" and often require greater ovarian stimulation to ensure successful oocyte collection. Using AMH in conjunction with another screen of ovarian reserve (like ovarian antral follicle count [AFC] as measured by transvaginal ultrasound) can be quite helpful in optimizing the approach to ovarian stimulation for fertility treatment.

Inhibin B is produced by developing follicles, and concentrations peak during the follicular phase. Concentrations of inhibin B can be used in conjunction with serum FSH and E_2 to assess ovarian function. However, measurement of inhibin adds little to the more established use of serum FSH and E_2, AMH, and/or AFC. Measurement of inhibins, therefore, remains of research interest only.

Hypogonadotropic Hypogonadism. In hypogonadotropic hypogonadism, serum E_2 concentrations are less than 40 pg/mL (147 pmol/L); therefore there is no withdrawal bleeding with a progestin challenge because the endometrium is thin.[263] Decreased LH (<10 IU/L) and decreased FSH (<10 IU/L) are also present.[236] Hyperprolactinemia can cause hypogonadotropic hypogonadic infertility. The upper limit of normal plasma prolactin in an amenorrheic, hypoestrogenic, nonpregnant woman is 400 to 500 mIU/mL (20–25 ng/mL). If estrogen status is normal, maximum prolactin concentrations vary from 600 to 800 IU/L (30–40 ng/mL).[264] Thyroid-stimulating hormone should be measured to exclude hypothyroidism. Prolactin concentrations can be elevated in patients with PCOS and those taking medications such as antidepressants, cimetidine, and methyldopa, and in stressful conditions. Prolactin concentrations can be elevated if drawn later in the day or after a meal, so they should be drawn fasting, early in the day. In cases where hyperprolactinemia is noted, radiographic imaging of the pituitary is indicated to rule out pituitary adenoma or empty sella syndrome.

Ovulatory Factors. Ovulatory dysfunction is difficult to diagnose because it will manifest in the presence or absence of normal menses. Metabolic diseases of many types affect ovulatory function, including those that result in androgen excess. PCOS, which results in androgen excess, is the most common cause of anovulation and was discussed in detail earlier in the chapter. In women with hirsutism, CAH should be considered. 21-Hydroxylase deficiency or 3-β-hydroxysteroid deficiency may be present in up to 26% of cases.[265] Elevated follicular phase serum 17-hydroxyprogesterone concentrations require further evaluation for these conditions. In addition, it is possible for ovulatory dysfunction to be secondary to liver or thyroid disorders.

As with male infertility, hypogonadism (hypergonadotropic or hypogonadotropic) results in female infertility. Causes of hypergonadotropic hypogonadism include primary ovarian insufficiency (POI), gonadal dysgenesis, resistant ovary syndrome, menopause, and luteal phase deficiency. Causes of hypogonadotropic hypogonadism include pituitary or hypothalamic insufficiency and hyperprolactinemia. Many of these pathologic states have been discussed in the earlier section "Irregular Menses."

Historically, ovulation with inadequate luteinization and reduced progesterone secretion during the luteal phase was termed *luteal phase deficiency*. Currently, luteal phase deficiency is defined as a short luteal phase defined by less than 10 days between ovulation and menses or less than 13 days between the LH surge and menses.[46] Decreased progesterone production is presumed to be responsible, but this may follow insufficient follicular phase FSH secretion, abnormal LH surge, or other endocrine abnormalities.[266] While serum progesterone measurement or endometrial biopsy was used historically to diagnose luteal phase deficiency, it remains a clinical diagnosis defined by length of the luteal phase. It is often treated by using clomiphene citrate or aromatase inhibitors early in the follicular phase to improve follicular recruitment and subsequent luteal function, or with progesterone supplementation in the luteal phase. The clinical significance of luteal phase deficiency remains unclear.[267]

Postcoital Test. The postcoital test has been used historically to evaluate infertility; however, it has been shown to have limited utility.[268]

Immunologic Factors. Antisperm antibodies have been proposed to contribute to female infertility. However, this topic is controversial, and laboratory testing for antisperm antibodies is rarely performed.[234]

Assisted Reproduction

Couples with a multitude of infertility problems, including unidentified causes and persistent infertility despite standard treatments, may benefit from assisted reproductive techniques (ART). If no definable cause is identified, standard initial therapy consists of ovulation induction with intrauterine insemination for three cycles before progression to more aggressive techniques such as controlled ovarian hyperstimulation (COH) with inseminations or in vitro fertilization (IVF) with or without intracytoplasmic sperm injection (ICSI).[269] If very low sperm counts are present, it is often reasonable to proceed directly to IVF with ICSI (see below). Significant tubal pathology often warrants proceeding directly to IVF.

The laboratory plays an important role in the process of controlled ovarian hyperstimulation. The principle involves administration of gonadotropins to stimulate follicular growth, followed by hCG to stimulate follicular maturation and ovulation. Clinical, laboratory, and ultrasound monitoring of the treatment cycle is necessary to (1) identify the dose and length of therapy, (2) determine when or whether to administer hCG, and (3) obtain an adequate ovulatory response while avoiding hyperstimulation.[270]

Infertility treatments involve procedures that deliver a concentrated sperm sample directly to the uterus (intrauterine insemination) or assisted reproductive techniques. The latter are techniques that involve acquiring fertile ova using transvaginal ultrasound and assisting fertilization in the laboratory with conventional IVF or ICSI in the fallopian tubes using gamete intrafallopian transfer (GIFT) or zygote intrafallopian transfer (ZIFT).[271] IVF then requires embryo transfer back into the uterus. Very few GIFT or ZIFT procedures are performed today owing to the availability of improved embryo culture techniques. The latest successful techniques include direct ovum fertilization using direct micropipette ICSI of the sperm.[272] This procedure provides hope to even the azoospermic man for whom testicular aspiration may yield a few nonmotile sperm. ICSI is widely used today for non–male factor infertility cases as well, and it is employed in about 50% to 60% of IVF cycles.

Despite these advances, the 2012 Centers for Disease Control and Prevention (CDC) surveillance summary of ART reported that only 35.9% (35,780 out of 99,665) of all embryo transfers using fresh autologous oocytes performed in the United States resulted in a clinical pregnancy.[273] Multiple embryos are often transferred during a single ART cycle to improve the chance of pregnancy, which frequently results in multiple-gestation pregnancies. In 2012, 29% of ART cycles resulted in multiple-gestation pregnancy. With an understanding of the risks associated with multiple-gestation pregnancies[274] and the pressures to improve the success rate of ART, substantial research effort is focused on selecting embryos with the highest probability of successful implantation and healthy development, leading ultimately to a single live birth.[275] More emphasis is placed on single-embryo transfer.[276] Noninvasive approaches beyond morphology have been evaluated for embryo selection, including sampling of embryo culture medium to evaluate glucose consumption or other metabolic parameters, and embryo selection using time-lapse imaging, although neither of these has proven to be as good as preimplantation genetic screening (PGS) for identifying euploid embryos for transfer.[277-281] The drawback of PGS is that it is invasive, and it often requires freezing the embryos because many clinics do not have the facilities to perform the analysis of the cells in time for a fresh transfer. Thus PGS often requires additional time and cost commitment to an IVF cycle. Work on improving IVF outcomes has also focused on assessing endometrial receptivity to facilitate embryo transfer during the relatively brief window of the menstrual cycle when the endometrium is most likely to support blastocyst implantation.[282-286] Large clinical trials are required to definitively prove the clinical benefit of any of these techniques, but it is hoped that further optimization and eventual concurrent use of multiple techniques will improve the success rate of ART, while minimizing the occurrence of multiple-gestation pregnancies.

ANALYTICAL METHODS FOR REPRODUCTIVE HORMONES

A variety of methods are available for measuring sex steroids in body fluids. Currently, the most common method is

POINTS TO REMEMBER

Facts About Infertility

- A specific cause of infertility is identified in 80% of infertile couples.
- Infertility often arises as a result of hormonal dysfunction of the hypothalamic-pituitary-gonadal axis.
- Laboratory measurement of serum hormone concentrations is an integral part of the workup of both female and male infertility.

nonisotopic immunoassay. However, use of mass spectrometry to measure sex steroids is increasing. Some of the advantages and disadvantages are discussed in this chapter. Methods used for reproductive protein hormones are discussed in Chapters 65 and 69. Methods used for reproductive steroid hormones are discussed here.

Measurement of Sex Steroids by Mass Spectrometry

Although immunoassays are the predominant method for the detection and measurement of sex steroids (E_2, testosterone, progesterone, etc.), they are associated with considerable analytical problems. For example, automated testosterone immunoassays (nonisotopic) perform well in healthy adult males and estradiol immunoassays perform well in healthy premenopausal females but are unacceptable for use in children or adult patients with low hormone concentrations due to accuracy and imprecision problems at the low end of detectability. Studies by Wang and associates comparing testosterone measurement by the four most commonly used automated direct immunoassay platforms against an LC-MS/MS reference method indicate acceptable correlation only in the adult male range.[287] Immunoassay methods failed to accurately and precisely detect concentrations of testosterone below 100 ng/dL (3.47 nmol/L).[287] Because concentrations of testosterone in women, children, and hypogonadal men typically fall below 100 ng/dL (3.47 nmol/L), measurement by immunoassay is not recommended. In addition, there is a clinical demand for the measurement of low concentrations of E_2 (<25 pg/mL or <90 pmol/L)—for example, in the setting of breast cancer risk assessment among postmenopausal women or following response to aromatase inhibitor treatment.[288] Again, these demands are not met by current automated immunoassays and call for a more sensitive approach.[289]

Mass spectrometry–based methods have been described for several of the sex steroids, including testosterone, DHT, E_2, and progesterone.[290-294] In addition, methods are available to measure precursors and metabolites, including DHEA, DHEA-S, androstenedione, and androstenedione glucuronide.[295-297] Tandem mass spectrometry coupled with liquid chromatography (HPLC) offers several advantages over traditional immunoassays, including lower limits of detection, enhanced specificity, small sample size, decreased lot-to-lot variability, and the possibility of analyzing multiple steroids within the same sample. This ability to simultaneously measure a variety of analytes provides the opportunity for steroid profiling, which may enhance diagnostic capabilities. Because of these advantages, the Endocrine Society suggested using extraction and chromatography followed by MS or MS/MS as a potential gold standard for measurement of testosterone.[298] For a more thorough discussion of tandem mass spectrometry and steroid analysis, the reader is directed to Chapters 17 and 66 and a review by Soldin and Soldin.[299]

However, this technology has some disadvantages, including the requirement for highly trained personnel, high costs of equipment and maintenance, and lack of standardization. Because testosterone and estradiol assays are not standardized, observations from clinical studies that demonstrate increased disease risk at a given steroid hormone concentration cannot be transferred to other institutions that utilize a different assay method.[300] As a result, generalized cutoffs associated with disease risk cannot be defined, universally accepted reference intervals and clinical decision points cannot be established, and patient care guidelines either do not exist or cannot be applied. These differences in assay performance are attributed to differences in assay accuracy, specificity, imprecision, and calibration that are most pronounced in steroid hormone immunoassays, but mass spectrometric assays also require standardization.[301,302]

To address these issues, the Centers for Disease Control and Prevention (CDC) has developed the Hormone Standardization (HoSt) program.[303,304] In the initial phase, 40 samples with known hormone concentrations established using the CDC reference method are distributed to participating laboratories to facilitate assay calibration. In the second phase, participating laboratories are issued quarterly challenges to ensure the established calibration remains accurate. Following implementation of the HoSt program, mean bias between participating mass spectrometric testosterone methods and the CDC reference method decreased by 50% from 2007 to 2011.[303]

Methods for Determination of Total Testosterone in Blood

Circulating testosterone comprises three different forms or pools: a non-protein-bound or "free" form, a weakly bound form, and a tightly bound form. The weakly bound form is associated with albumin, and the tightly bound form is associated with sex hormone–binding globulin (SHBG), which is also known as testosterone/estradiol-binding globulin. The term *total testosterone* refers to serum measurements of free testosterone, albumin-bound testosterone, and SHBG-bound testosterone. Bioavailable testosterone includes circulating free testosterone and albumin-bound testosterone. Testosterone bound to SHBG is not biologically active, whereas the free form is available for target cells. Albumin-bound testosterone is also available to target tissues because testosterone can dissociate from the albumin carrier and rapidly diffuse into target cells.[12]

Methods

A 2014 College of American Pathologists (CAP) survey reports that 1560 out of 1592 (98%) participating laboratories measure the concentration of circulating testosterone (both protein-bound and non-protein-bound forms) using nonisotopic enzyme immunoassays. The remaining 32 laboratories utilize mass spectrometry.[305]

Direct (no extraction required) immunoassay methods have been developed for the determination of testosterone in serum or plasma.[306,307] In these methods, the steroid must be displaced from its binding proteins (albumin and SHBG), and results of the assay depend on the effectiveness of the displacement. Methods used to release testosterone from endogenous binding proteins include use of salicylates, surfactants, pH alterations, temperature changes, and competing steroids such as estrone or estradiol. Most of the direct immunologic methods use antisera generated against a C_{19} testosterone-protein conjugate. These assays have demonstrated variable precision agreement with mass spectrophotometry and established RIA methods.[308-310] However, most routine immunoassays are not sensitive enough to measure very low testosterone concentrations such as those found in women, children, or hypogonadal men. The Endocrine Society recommends use of a highly sensitive method such as a liquid chromatography/mass spectrometry/mass spectrometry (LC-MS/MS) method whenever low testosterone concentrations are suspected.[298]

Gas chromatography combined with mass spectrometry (GC-MS) remains the reference method for testosterone measurement, although LC-MS/MS reference methods are also in use.[311] Mass spectrometric reference methods are often used to assess the bias of routine immunoassay methods as discussed earlier.[308,312,313] Several other mass spectrometry–based methods have been described.[291,293]

Regardless of immunoassay type, almost all testosterone antisera show some degree of cross-reactivity with DHT (typically 3% to 5%) but show negligible cross-reactivity with other androgens. Assays that use antisera generated against the C-19 position provide maximum analytical specificity with respect to endogenous steroids. However, cross-reactions with 19-nonsteroids used in contraceptive preparations sometimes cause a problem. In most clinical situations, estimation of testosterone without prior separation of DHT is permitted because plasma concentrations of DHT are only 10% to 20% of those for testosterone. Moreover, testosterone and DHT are the two most important androgens in the systemic circulation; even when a method measures the concentrations of both, clinically useful information about the total androgen load is obtained. DHEA-S has been reported to cross-react in some testosterone assays.[314] If specific estimation of testosterone concentration is required, mass spectrometry is recommended.

Specimen Collection and Storage. Serum or heparinized plasma is used to measure total testosterone. Testosterone is subject to diurnal variation, reaching a peak concentration at between 0400 and 0800 hours. Therefore morning specimens are preferred. Serum/plasma samples are stable for up to 24 hours at room temperature, up to 1 week refrigerated, and up to 1 year frozen at −20°C.[315,316] DHEA supplementation should be avoided before testing.[317]

Reference Intervals. Example reference intervals for total testosterone in serum are listed in Table 68.4.[318,319]

Comments. Estimation of SHBG in serum is useful for interpreting blood concentrations of total testosterone and for calculating androgen index and bioavailable testosterone. Immunoassays for measurement of SHBG in the routine laboratory have been developed.[320] SHBG concentrations are increased by estradiol and decreased by testosterone[321] and therefore change with age.[322]

Methods for the Determination of Free and Bioavailable Testosterone in Blood

In cases where SHBG concentrations are altered, as in women, aging men, and illness, it has been argued that measurements of free or bioavailable testosterone more accurately reflect

TABLE 68.4 Reference Intervals for Total Testosterone in Serum

Testosterone (Method: LC/MS/MS)	ng/dL	nmol/L
Adults		
18–69 y, males	250–1100	8.7–38.2
females	2–45	0.07–1.6
70–89 y, males	90–890	3.1–30.9
70–94 y, females	2–40	0.07–1.4
1st-trimester pregnancy	20–135	0.7–4.7
2nd-trimester pregnancy	11–153	0.4–5.3
3rd-trimester pregnancy	11–146	0.4–5.1
Children		
Cord blood, males	17–61	0.6–2.1
females	16–44	0.6–1.5
1–10 d, males	≤187	≤6.5
females	≤24	≤0.8
1–3 mo, males	72–344	2.5–11.9
females	≤17	≤0.59
3–5 mo, males	≤201	≤7.0
females	≤12	≤0.4
5–7 mo, males	≤59	≤2.1
females	≤13	≤0.5
7–12 mo, males	≤16	≤0.6
females	≤11	≤0.4
1–5.9 y, males	≤5	≤0.2
females	≤8	≤0.3
6–7.9 y, males	≤25	≤0.9
females	≤20	≤0.7
8–10.9 y, males	≤42	≤1.5
females	≤35	≤1.2
11–11.9 y, males	≤260	≤9.0
females	≤40	≤1.4
12–13.9 y, males	≤420	≤14.6
females	≤40	≤1.4
14–17.9 y, males	≤1000	≤34.7
females	≤40	≤1.4
Tanner Stages		
I, males	≤5	≤0.2
females	≤8	≤0.3
II, males	≤167	≤5.8
females	≤24	≤0.8
III, males	21–719	0.7–25.0
females	≤28	≤1.0
IV, males	25–912	0.9–31.7
females	≤31	≤1.1
V, males	110–975	3.8–33.8
females	≤33	≤1.2

From Nakamoto JM, Mason PW, eds. The Quest Diagnostics manual: endocrinology, test selection and interpretation, 5th ed. Capistrano, Calif.: Quest Diagnostics/Nichols Institute, 2012. Prior to use, laboratories should verify the transferability of these reference intervals to their patient population following the methods described in Chapter 8.

TABLE 68.5 Reference Intervals for Free Testosterone in Serum

Free Testosterone (Method: Tracer Equilibrium Dialysis)	pg/mL	pmol/L	Free Fraction, % of Total
Men			
18–69 y	35.0–155.0	121–538	1.5–2.2
70–89 y	30.0–135.0	104–468	1.5–2.2
Women			
18–69 y	0.1–6.4	0.4–22.2	0.5–2.0
70–89 y	0.2–3.7	0.7–12.8	0.5–2.0
Pregnancy			
1st trimester	0.5–6.0	1.7–20.8	0.15–0.66
2nd trimester	0.2–3.1	0.7–10.8	0.10–0.34
3rd trimester	0.2–4.1	0.7–14.2	0.15–0.51
Children, Males			
5–9 y	≤5.3	≤18.4	0.44–1.78
10–13 y	0.7–52.0	2.4–180	0.53–3.33
14–17 y	18.0–111.0	62–385	1.05–2.91
Children, Females			
5–9 y	0.2–5.0	0.7–17.4	0.28–1.81
10–13 y	0.1–7.4	0.3–25.7	0.36–3.16
14–17 y	0.5–3.9	1.7–13.5	0.41–2.34

From Nakamoto JM, Mason PW, eds. The Quest Diagnostics manual: Endocrinology, test selection and interpretation, 5th ed. Capistrano, Calif.: Quest Diagnostics/Nichols Institute, 2012. Prior to use, laboratories should verify the transferability of these reference intervals to their patient population following the methods described in Chapter 8.

androgen status. Excellent reviews of various methods used to measure this fraction of testosterone are available.[212]

The three methods routinely used in clinical practice include:

1. Estimation of the free testosterone fraction by equilibrium dialysis or ultrafiltration
2. Estimation of combined free and weakly bound (bioavailable) testosterone fractions by selective precipitation of the tightly bound form
3. Calculation of free and weakly bound testosterone concentrations by mathematical modeling

Methods not recommended for use in clinical practice include:

1. Estimation of free hormone using a direct (analog tracer) radioimmunoassay
2. Calculation of the androgen index using indices that reflect the ratios of testosterone pools

Each approach is discussed in turn in the following sections. Example reference intervals for free testosterone and percent free testosterone in serum are listed in Table 68.5 and those for bioavailable testosterone in Table 68.6.[†]

[†]Laboratories should verify that these ranges are appropriate for use in their own settings.

TABLE 68.6 Reference Intervals for Bioavailable Testosterone in Serum

Bioavailable Testosterone (Method: Calculation)	ng/dL	nmol/L
Adults		
18–69 y, males	110–575	3.8–20.0
females	0.5–8.5	0.02–0.3
70–89 y, males	15–150	0.5–5.2
females	0.5–8.8	0.02–0.3
Children		
1–11.9 y, males	≤5.4	≤0.2
females	≤3.4	≤0.1
12–13.9 y, males	≤140	≤4.9
females	≤3.4	≤0.1
14–17.9 y, males	8.0–210	0.3–7.3
females	≤7.8	≤0.3

From Nakamoto JM, Mason PW, eds. The Quest Diagnostics manual: Endocrinology, test selection and interpretation, 5th ed. Capistrano, Calif.: Quest Diagnostics/Nichols Institute, 2012. Prior to use, laboratories should verify the transferability of these reference intervals to their patient population following the methods described in Chapter 8.

Equilibrium Dialysis/Ultrafiltration

Only a small fraction (1% to 2%) of unconjugated testosterone exists in the free state (non-protein-bound) in serum or plasma. None of the conventional assay methods, including RIA, is sufficiently sensitive to quantify free steroid directly in a protein-free ultrafiltrate of plasma. Instead, free steroid is estimated in plasma by adding a known amount of radiolabeled compound to the sample and allowing labeled and unlabeled compounds to reach equilibrium in their competition for the same binding sites on proteins. Bound and free radiolabeled fractions are then separated, and the ratio of free labeled to total labeled compound is determined. At equilibrium, this ratio is taken as a measure of the free testosterone fraction. An estimate of serum free testosterone can be calculated by multiplying the free testosterone fraction by the total testosterone concentration. A detailed procedure for the equilibrium dialysis method is included in the third edition of this textbook.[323]

Most of the problems with this procedure have involved tracer impurities and separation of bound and free labeled fractions. Several separation techniques have been used, including equilibrium dialysis, membrane ultrafiltration, and steady-state gel filtration. Deficiencies associated with these techniques include a requirement for a large sample volume, the need for complicated correction of sample volume changes that occur during the separation, and difficulties involved in collecting and measuring radioactivity in numerous fractions of each sample. Equilibrium dialysis has been used most often in the past, but serious errors often arise from the sample dilution required by this method.[324] Symmetric dialysis of undiluted samples is reported to be less susceptible to tracer contamination and dilution effects.[325] Ultrafiltration appears to overcome these problems and to obviate errors due to dilution.[326] Due to the labor-intensive nature of both equilibrium dialysis and ultrafiltration, these methods are used almost exclusively at reference laboratories.

Selective Precipitation

Selective precipitation of SHBG with ammonium sulfate is also used to measure bioavailable testosterone. With this technique, aliquots of serum or plasma are first incubated with radiolabeled testosterone. Testosterone bound to SHBG is then precipitated with 50% ammonium sulfate. The samples are centrifuged, and aliquots of the supernatant containing free and albumin-bound testosterone (also known as *non-SHBG-bound testosterone*) are radioactively counted. The percentage of radio label not bound to SHBG is subsequently multiplied by the total testosterone concentration to obtain the bioavailable testosterone.[212] Similar to equilibration dialysis and ultrafiltration methods, performance of selective precipitation is generally limited to reference laboratories.

Calculated Free Testosterone

Methods based on mathematical modeling use algorithms to derive non-SHBG-bound testosterone. These algorithms assume that when concentrations of total testosterone, SHBG, and albumin and the constants for binding of testosterone to SHBG and albumin are known, free testosterone and bioavailable testosterone can be calculated. These calculations are based on a proper estimation of the association constant for binding of testosterone to SHBG and albumin. The reader is directed to other references for further details on this method.[212,327,328] Because automated assays are available for total testosterone, SHBG, and albumin, calculation-based methods of measuring free testosterone are inexpensive and suitable for routine use in nonreference labs. Calculation-based methods also generate results that correlate well with equilibrium dialysis.[15,38] However, various association constants for SHBG have been reported, and conditions resulting in abnormal plasma protein concentrations, such as nephrotic syndrome, cirrhosis, and pregnancy, require adjustments in the assumption for albumin concentration.

Several different algorithms based on concentrations measured with a gold standard technique have been proposed.[329-331] Algorithms for calculating bioavailable testosterone are available free online (http://www.issam.ch/freetesto.htm); however, these sources do not always provide a reference for which algorithm is being used.

While calculated free testosterone algorithms are convenient and correlate well with equilibrium dialysis, it should be noted that no consensus has been reached about their use. De Ronde and colleagues compared five algorithms and concluded that they are not transferable to samples from other laboratories unless revalidation using laboratory-specific assays has been performed.[332] Likewise, Giton and colleagues reported that instead of using theoretical association constants, optimal paired association constants should be determined for each studied population.[333] Because this is impossible for the average clinician to do, these authors suggest using ammonium sulfate precipitation. Finally, Dechaud and colleagues reported an age-associated discrepancy between calculated and measured bioavailable testosterone, suggesting that a simplified law of mass action cannot predict variations in steroid distribution in serum.[334] These authors state that consensus is needed regarding the proper measurement of bioavailable testosterone for therapeutic decisions.

Direct (Analog Tracer) Radioimmunoassay

Several RIA procedures are commercially available for the direct estimation of free testosterone.[14,212,307,335,336] These assays use a labeled derivative (analog) of testosterone that, in theory, retains the ability to react with exogenous antitestosterone antibodies but is restricted from interacting with testosterone-binding proteins in the serum sample. In practice, development of an analog that does not interact with endogenous proteins has been difficult to achieve.

Advantages of RIA analog methods include a small sample requirement, relatively rapid results, a simple procedure, and the option to measure free testosterone without the need to measure total testosterone.[14,15,307,336] However, some have reported that direct RIAs are grossly inaccurate, underestimating free testosterone concentrations by manyfold.[14,15,337,338] For example, one study in females revealed that free testosterone concentrations obtained by two different analog assays were 15% to 35% and 25% to 30% of those obtained by ultrafiltration.[339] As a result, direct RIAs are not recommended by the Endocrine Society,[38] and they have largely been replaced by calculation methods based on total testosterone, SHBG, and albumin concentrations.[340]

Androgen Index

This index is a ratio of testosterone and SHBG multiplied by 100.[212] Although this is only an indicator of free testosterone, some have found it to be useful in the evaluation of hirsutism.[341] Other reports have indicated that the free androgen index is not a reliable parameter of free testosterone because of its variability as a function of SHBG concentration.[14,15,342] Use of the androgen index remains primarily of research interest.

Methods for the Determination of Testosterone Precursors and Metabolites in Blood

Several biosynthetic precursors and metabolites of testosterone are measured using specific immunoassays (directly or after sample extraction), chromatography, or LC-MS/MS.[291,295-297] Examples include DHT, 3α-androstanediol glucuronide, and androstenedione. Example reference intervals for these analytes in serum are listed in Table 68.7.

Methods for the Determination of Dehydroepiandrosterone and Its Sulfate

Measurements of DHEA or its sulfated conjugate, DHEA-S, in serum and plasma are important for investigations of adrenal androgen production, such as assessment of adrenal hyperplasia, adrenal tumors, adrenarche, delayed puberty, or hirsutism. DHEA-S in circulation originates primarily from the adrenal glands, although in men some may be derived from the testes; none is produced by the ovaries. DHEA is secreted almost entirely by the adrenal glands.

DHEA concentrations exhibit a circadian rhythm that reflects the secretion of ACTH; these concentrations vary during the menstrual cycle. DHEA-S concentrations, however, do not exhibit a circadian rhythm because of their longer circulating half-life.[175] Concentrations in serum are increased in cord blood and drop precipitously at birth. Concentrations in premature infants in general are much higher than those in full-term infants. Pregnancy and oral contraceptives induce a modest reduction, and glucocorticoids induce a marked decrease. Patients with polycystic ovary disease often have

TABLE 68.7 Reference Intervals for Dihydrotestosterone (DHT), 3α-Androstanediol Glucuronide, and Androstenedione in Serum

	ng/dL	nmol/L
Dihydrotestosterone (DHT) (Method: LC/MS/MS)		
Adult men	16–79	0.55–2.7
Adult women	5–46	0.17–1.6
3α-Androstanediol Glucuronide (Method: RIA)		
Men	260–1500	5.5–32
Women	60–300	1.3–6.4
Children		
Prepubertal	10–60	0.2–1.3
Tanner II–III		
Males	19–164	0.4–4.5
Females	33–244	0.7–5.2
Androstenedione (Method: LC/MS/MS)		
Men		
18–30 y	50–220	1.7–7.7
31–50 y	40–190	1.4–6.6
51–60 y	50–220	1.7–7.7
Women		
Follicular	35–250	1.2–8.7
Luteal	30–235	1.0–8.2
Postmenopausal	20–75	0.7–2.6
Children		
Premature infants (31–35 weeks)	≤480	≤16.8
Term infants	≤290	≤10.1
1–12 mo	6–78	0.2–2.7
1–4 y	5–51	0.2–1.8
5–9 y	6–115	0.2–4.0
10–13 y	12–221	0.4–7.7
14–17 y	22–225	0.8–7.9
Tanner II–III		
Males	17–82	0.6–2.9
Females	43–180	1.5–6.3
Tanner IV–V		
Males	57–150	2.0–5.2
Females	73–220	2.6–7.7

From Nakamoto JM, Mason PW, eds. The Quest Diagnostics manual: endocrinology, test selection and interpretation, 5th ed. Capistrano, Calif.: Quest Diagnostics/Nichols Institute, 2012. Prior to use, laboratories should verify the transferability of these reference intervals to their patient population following the methods described in Chapter 8.

elevated concentrations of DHEA-S, suggesting an adrenal androgen contribution to the defect in this disorder.[343] Concentrations of DHEA-S are also elevated in CAH and with adrenal cortical tumors (concentrations higher with adrenal carcinoma than with adrenal adenoma).[175] However, concentrations are not elevated in women with virilizing ovarian tumors. Glucocorticoid administration for several days suppresses concentrations in patients with adrenal hyperplasia. DHEA is commercially available in health food stores; therefore increased serum concentrations may be due to exogenous use.

Methods

According to a 2014 CAP survey, all participating laboratories used nonisotopic immunoassays for the measurement of DHEA-S.[305] Other methods include competitive protein-binding assays and GC-MS.[30,344,345] Immunoassays for DHEA-S demonstrate significant cross-reactivity with DHEA, androstenedione, and androsterone, yet the relative concentrations of these steroids have a minimal effect on assay performance.

Specimen Collection and Storage. Serum or plasma (preserved with ethylenediaminetetraacetic acid [EDTA]) is suitable for DHEA or DHEA-S immunoassays.[346-348] Early-morning collection, before 10:30 a.m., is preferred for DHEA.[346,347,349] DHEA-S specimens are stable for at least 1 day at room temperature. Refrigerated serum/plasma samples (4° to 8°C) are stable for up to 14 days, and those frozen at −20°C are stable for longer than 1 year.[315,316,350]

Reference Intervals. Example reference intervals for serum concentrations of DHEA-S and DHEA are listed in Table 68.8.[318,319,348]

Comments. Analysis of DHEA by immunoassay usually requires pretreatment of serum samples because the serum concentration of DHEA is 1000-fold lower than that of DHEA-S. Several extraction and chromatographic procedures have been suggested for this purpose. Celite is the preferred adsorbent, and dichloromethane and ethyl acetate are common choices for extraction solvents. Commercial RIA kits using solid-phase separation techniques and ^{125}I-labeled DHEA are widely available for convenient measurement of serum concentrations. A typical kit method will detect as little as 3 ng/dL (0.1 nmol/L) of DHEA.[346,347] Cross-reactivity of antisera with related steroids is relatively low, with some exceptions (androstanediol, about 6%; androstenedione, about 2%; and testosterone, about 1%). Between-extraction precision, expressed as a coefficient of variation, is less than ±12% at a DHEA concentration of 120 ng/dL (4.1 nmol/L).

Determination of 17-Ketosteroids in Urine

The 17-ketosteroids (KS) are metabolites of steroids that contain a keto group at C-17 and include androsterone, epiandrosterone, etiocholanolone, DHEA, 11-keto- and 11β-hydroxyandrosterone, and 11-keto- and 11β- hydroxyetiocholanolone. In men, approximately one-third of total urinary 17-KS represents metabolites of testosterone secreted by the testes, whereas most of the remaining two-thirds is derived from steroids produced by the adrenal glands. In women, who normally excrete smaller quantities than men, total 17-KS concentrations are derived almost exclusively from the adrenal glands. Thus the main purpose of measuring these steroid metabolites is to assess adrenal androgen production.

Measurement of DHEA-S in serum serves as a more convenient marker for adrenal androgen production than does urinary 17-KS excretion because 24-hour urine collection is not required and because many drugs interfere with the 17-KS assay.[351] For these reasons, many clinicians now prefer concentrations for plasma DHEA-S to those for urinary 17-KS.

Methods for the Detection of Anabolic Steroids

Detection of exogenous steroids used to improve athletic performance poses a challenge for the laboratory, given the

TABLE 68.8 Reference Intervals for Dehydroepiandrosterone Sulfate (DHEA-S) and Unconjugated Dehydroepiandrosterone (DHEA) in Serum

Dehydroepiandrosterone Sulfate (DHEA-S) (Method: Immunochemiluminometric Assay)	μg/dL	μmol/L
Men		
18–29 y	110–510	3.0–14.0
30–39 y	110–370	3.0–10.0
40–49 y	45–345	1.2–9.4
50–59 y	25–240	0.7–6.5
≥60 y	≤204	≤5.5
Women		
18–29 y	45–320	1.2–8.7
30–39 y	40–325	1.1–8.8
40–49 y	25–220	0.7–6.0
50–59 y	15–170	0.4–4.6
≥60 y	≤145	≤3.9
Children		
0–1 mo, male	≤316	≤8.6
female	15–261	0.4–7.1
1–6 mo, male	≤58	≤1.6
female	≤74	≤2.0
7–12 mo, male	≤26	≤0.7
female	≤26	≤0.7
1–3 y, male	≤15	≤0.4
female	≤22	≤0.6
4–6 y, male	≤27	≤0.7
female	≤34	≤0.9
7–9 y, male	≤91	≤2.5
female	≤92	≤2.5
10–13 y, male	≤138	≤3.7
female	≤148	≤4.0
14–16 y, male	38–340	1.0–9.2
female	37–307	1.0–8.3
Tanner stages		
I, male	≤89	≤2.4
female	≤46	≤1.2
II, male	≤81	≤2.2
female	15–113	0.4–3.1
III, male	22–126	0.6–3.4
female	42–162	1.1–4.4
IV, male	33–177	0.9–4.8
female	42–241	1.1–6.5
V, male	110–510	3.0–13.8
female	45–320	1.2–8.7

Dehydroepiandrosterone (DHEA) (Method: LC/MS/MS)	ng/dL	nmol/L
Men	61–1636	2.1–56.4
Women	102–1185	3.5–40.9
Children		
1–5 y	≤377	≤13.0
6–9 y	19–592	0.7–20.4
10–13 y	42–1067	1.4–36.8
14–17 y	137–1489	4.7–51.3

From Nakamoto JM, Mason PW, eds. The Quest Diagnostics manual: Endocrinology, test selection and interpretation, 5th ed. Capistrano, Calif.: Quest Diagnostics/Nichols Institute, 2012. Prior to use, laboratories should verify the transferability of these reference intervals to their patient population following the methods described in Chapter 8.

variety of exogenous anabolic steroids, which include both natural and synthetic testosterone analogs. Since the 1980s, GC-MS has been the method of choice to detect anabolic steroids.[352] The ratio of testosterone to epitestosterone (17 α-epimer) in urine has been used as a screening test for the detection of anabolic steroid abuse. A ratio of testosterone to epitestosterone greater than 6:1 suggests exogenous steroid use, and further testing should be performed for confirmation.[353,354] Others have suggested the ratio of testosterone to LH in the urine as an indication of testosterone doping. Detailed studies of these ratios are available.[355] Because hCG stimulates testosterone production by the testes, hCG has been placed on the World Anti-Doping Agency list of prohibited substances for male athletes. Measurement of intact hCG, free β subunit, and β-core fragment in the urine of male athletes is therefore an important consideration for antidoping laboratories.[356] For a more in-depth discussion of analytical considerations around drug monitoring in athletes, the reader is referred to the review by Bowers.[352]

Methods for the Determination of Estradiol in Blood

Both chromatography–mass spectrometry and immunoassay-based methods are used to measure estrogens in blood. GC-MS methods utilizing isotope dilution provide the most accurate and reliable measurement of E_2.[272,357-359] The main steps in these reference methods include solvent extraction, chromatographic fractionation, and chemical derivatization before analysis. Validation of immunoassay methods by this technique has become important in many external quality assurance programs.

Immunoassays consist of both indirect (extraction required) and direct (no extraction required) methods. The most common antigen used to prepare antibodies for E_2 assays is estradiol-6-(*O*-carboxymethyl) oxime conjugated to bovine serum albumin.[360] Cross-reactivity with other C-18 steroids is usually very minor because the 3- and 17-hydroxyl groups are left free. A 2014 CAP survey reported that all participating laboratories utilized direct enzyme immunoassays for routine measurement of E_2 concentrations.[305] Evaluation of estrogen concentrations in men, women taking aromatase inhibitors, postmenopausal women, and children requires the use of mass spectrometry–based methods described earlier.

To measure E_2 directly without extraction and chromatography, the steroid must be displaced from its binding proteins. The displacing agents used in commercial methods often are not disclosed, but in some systems, effective displacement is achieved by adding 8-anilino-1-naphthalene sulfonic acid

(ANS) or a large excess of a competing steroid such as dihydrotestosterone to the sample.[360]

Caution should be exercised when assaying samples from subjects who are receiving oral contraceptives or estrogen replacement therapy because cross-reacting steroids may cause elevated results. Most notably, cross-reactivity with estrone is as high as 10% for some assays, but much lower (<1%) for others. This is likely due to a difference in the specificity of the antibody used for E_2. Similar effects have been observed for metabolites conjugated at the 3 position, such as estrone-3-sulfate and estrone-3-glucuronide.[361,362]

Several immunoassays for E_2 have been developed and adapted for use on fully automated immunoassay systems.[363] All are heterogeneous assays (separation step needed), but most are direct assays and do not require preliminary extraction. Most procedures offer the convenience of solid-phase separation methods. For routine clinical applications, the greatest experience is with enzyme immunoassays. Most commercial enzyme immunoassays use horseradish peroxidase or alkaline phosphatase to label E_2 antigens; enzyme activity is determined using a variety of photometric,[362,364,365] fluorescent,[366-369] or chemiluminescent substrates.[370] A semiautomated "ultrasensitive" chemiluminescent immunoassay for E_2 has been described.[371] This method is advantageous because it is reportedly capable of accurately measuring low concentrations (<50 pmol/L) of E_2 observed in perimenopausal and postmenopausal women, healthy men, and children.

Taieb and colleagues compared detection limits and functional sensitivities of nine automated E_2 immunoassays.[372] They concluded that functional sensitivities, defined as the lowest concentration of analyte that can be measured with a run-to-run imprecision of 20%, were twofold to fourfold higher than detection limits of the tests. It is also important to note that none of the assays analyzed in this study had the functional sensitivity required for evaluation of serum E_2 measurements in men, menopausal women, and children.[373] Functional sensitivities ranged from 5.5 to 46 pg/mL (20–169 pmol/L). These assays have been optimized for clinical applications such as monitoring of ovarian stimulation for IVF, in which high E_2 concentrations are expected, but the values obtained depend on the method used.[374] The authors suggest that until E_2 assays are better standardized, reference intervals and cutoff points used as clinical decision criteria must be evaluated and modified, if necessary, for each assay.

Estradiol Assay Standardization

Specimen Collection and Storage. Serum and plasma (with EDTA or heparin as anticoagulant) have been used. Specimens should be centrifuged and separated within 24 hours. Serum/plasma specimens may be stored at room temperature for 1 day, refrigerated for 3 days, or frozen for up to 1 year.[315,316,35] Oral contraceptives have been known to alter E_2 concentrations.

Reference Intervals. Example reference intervals for serum concentrations of E_2 are listed in Table 68.9.

TABLE 68.9 Reference Intervals for Estradiol (E2) in Serum

Estradiol (Method: LC/MS/MS)	pg/mL	pmol/L
Men	≤29	≤106
Women		
Follicular	39–375	143–1377
Midcycle peak	94–762	345–2797
Luteal phase	48–440	176–1615
Postmenopausal	≤10	≤37
Children		
Prepubertal (1–9 y), males	≤4	≤15
females	≤16	≤59
10–11 y, males	≤12	≤44
females	≤65	≤239
12–14 y, males	≤24	≤88
females	≤142	≤521
15–17 y, males	≤31	≤114
females	≤283	≤1040

From Nakamoto JM, Mason PW, eds. The Quest Diagnostics manual: Endocrinology, test selection and interpretation, 5th ed. Capistrano, Calif.: Quest Diagnostics/Nichols Institute, 2012. Prior to use, laboratories should verify the transferability of these reference intervals to their patient population following the methods described in Chapter 8.

Methods for the Determination of Estriol in Blood

Except for purposes of fetal aneuploidy screening, measurement of E_3 has little clinical value because in nonpregnant women, E_3 is derived almost exclusively from E_2. A 2014 CAP survey reported that automated enzymatic immunoassay methods account for all unconjugated E_3 measurements.[305] Several of these assays have been validated for use in maternal serum screening.[375,376]

Specimen Collection and Storage

E_3 serum or plasma specimens are stable at room temperature for 24 hours; they can be refrigerated for 2 days and frozen at −20 °C for up to 1 year.[316]

Methods for the Determination of Estrone in Blood

Estrone determinations have limited clinical utility. Normally, blood estrone concentrations parallel E_2 concentrations throughout the menstrual cycle, but at slightly lower concentrations. For a specific analysis of estrone, the interested reader is directed to other references.[377,378]

Methods for the Determination of Progesterone in Blood

A 2014 CAP survey reported that enzyme immunoassays accounted for all progesterone assays used by survey participants.[305] Initial immunoassays for serum progesterone measurement used organic solvents to remove the steroid from endogenous binding proteins such as corticosteroid-binding globulin and albumin. Direct (nonextraction) measurement of progesterone in serum or plasma is considered the method of choice for routine applications. Various antigens have been used to prepare antisera for progesterone assays. Cross-reactivity is most prominent with 5α-pregnanediol ranging from 6% to 11%.

Several immunoassays are available on fully automated immunoassay systems.[379-382] All are heterogeneous assays that require separation of free and antibody-bound fractions. Enzymes appear to be the most widely used nonradioactive label. Alkaline phosphatase and horseradish peroxidase coupled to progesterone or antiprogesterone antibodies are particularly popular. An assortment of photometric,[362,383,384] fluorescent,[380,382,385] and luminescent[386,387] substrates are available for monitoring the enzyme activity of the antibody-bound fraction. Direct time-resolved fluoroimmunoassays for progesterone have been described.[388,389]

Although automated immunoassays are less labor intensive than RIAs and yield results in less time without the need for radioactivity, these assays do not have adequate functional sensitivity for the measurement of low progesterone concentrations in men, postmenopausal women, and children. Taieb and colleagues analyzed the detection limits and functional sensitivities of eight automated progesterone methods.[372] They reported that functional sensitivities (10–45 ng/dL or 0.32–1.43 nmol/L), defined as the lowest concentration of analyte that could be measured with a run-to-run imprecision of 20%, ranged from twofold to fourfold higher than the manufacturer-stated detection limit (6–15 ng/dL or 0.19–0.48 nmol/L). Automated progesterone assays have been optimized for use in in vitro fertilization protocols as a rapid, cost-effective way to evaluate ovarian stimulation and monitor ovulation.

Double-isotope derivative methods[390] and competitive protein-binding assays[391] have been applied to the measurement of serum progesterone, but these methods require extensive purification of the steroid and are labor intensive. GC procedures using flame ionization, electron capture, or nitrogen detection have been used to improve the accuracy of progesterone analysis.[344,391] However, these methods are time-consuming and often require solvent extraction, chromatography, and derivatization before the steroid is quantitated. GC-MS has been recommended as a reference method for progesterone determination. The GC-MS method of Thienpont and colleagues[292] uses heptafluorobutyric ester derivatives and 19-$^{2}H_3$-progesterone as internal standards.

Plasma concentrations of 17α-hydroxyprogesterone are measured to evaluate 21-hydroxylase deficiency. For specific methods regarding this analyte, the reader is referred to a review by Wallace.[123]

Specimen Collection and Storage

Serum or plasma (with heparin or EDTA as anticoagulant) is used and should be separated within 24 hours.[348] The patient need not be fasting, and no special handling procedures are necessary.[392,393] Serum/plasma specimens may be stored at room temperature for 24 hours and refrigerated at 4° to 8°C for up to 3 days or at −20°C for up to 1 year.[315,316,350]

Reference Intervals

Example reference intervals for serum concentrations of progesterone are listed in Table 68.10.[318,319]

Measurement of Salivary Sex Steroids

Measurement of steroid concentrations in saliva has the potential to serve as a noninvasive and convenient procedure for the assessment of "serum free" steroid concentrations. However, primarily because of rapid fluctuations in salivary concentration necessitating the collection of multiple samples, salivary testing for sex steroids is not commonplace. For further discussion of salivary steroid measurements, the reader is referred to a review by Wood.[394]

TABLE 68.10 Reference Intervals for Progesterone in Serum

Progesterone (Method: LC/MS/MS)	ng/mL	nmol/L
Men		
18–29 y	≤0.3	≤1.0
30–39 y	≤0.2	≤0.6
40–49 y	≤0.2	≤0.6
50–59 y	≤0.2	≤0.6
Women		
Follicular phase	≤2.7	≤8.6
Luteal phase	3.0–31.4	≤100
Postmenopausal	≤0.2	≤0.6
Children		
5–9 y, male	≤0.7	≤2.2
female	≤0.6	≤1.9
10–13 y, male	≤1.2	≤3.8
female	≤10.2	≤32.4
14–17 y, male	≤0.8	≤2.5
female	≤11.9	≤38

From Nakamoto JM, Mason PW, eds. The Quest Diagnostics manual: Endocrinology, test selection and interpretation, 5th ed. Capistrano, Calif.: Quest Diagnostics/Nichols Institute, 2012. Prior to use, laboratories should verify the transferability of these reference intervals to their patient population following the methods described in Chapter 8.

POINTS TO REMEMBER

- Measurement of total serum steroid hormone concentrations requires displacement of hormone from its binding proteins.
- Immunoassay remains the most common method of steroid hormone measurement, but mass spectrometry is becoming more widely used.
- Automated testosterone and estradiol immunoassays are acceptable for use in healthy adult men and women, respectively, but most lack sufficient accuracy and precision for use in children and adults with low steroid hormone concentrations.
- Mass spectrometry–based methods offer improved accuracy and a lower limit of detection but require highly trained personnel and increased equipment costs.
- Free testosterone is most accurately measured by equilibrium dialysis or ultrafiltration in a reference laboratory. Direct immunoassay measurement of free testosterone is not recommended.

SELECTED REFERENCES

For a full list of references for this chapter, please refer to ExpertConsult.com.

14. Morley JE, Patrick P, Perry HM 3rd. Evaluation of assays available to measure free testosterone. *Metabolism* 2002;**51**:554–9.

36. Layton JB, Li D, Meier CR, et al. Testosterone lab testing and initiation in the United Kingdom and the United States, 2000 to 2011. *J Clin Endocrinol Metab* 2014;**99**:835–42.

38. Bhasin S, Cunningham GR, Hayes FJ, et al. Testosterone therapy in men with androgen deficiency syndromes: an Endocrine Society clinical practice guideline. *J Clin Endocrinol Metab* 2010;**95**:2536–59.
44. Vigen R, O'Donnell CI, Baron AE, et al. Association of testosterone therapy with mortality, myocardial infarction, and stroke in men with low testosterone levels. *JAMA* 2013;**310**:1829–36.
46. Carr BR. Disorders of the ovary and female reproductive tract. In: Williams RH, Foster DW, Kronenberg HM, et al., editors. *Williams textbook of endocrinology*. 9th ed. Philadelphia: W.B. Saunders; 1998. p. 751–817.
48. Jaffe RB. Disorders of sexual development. In: Yen SSC, Jaffe RB, Barbieri RL, editors. *Reproductive endocrinology: Physiology, pathophysiology, and clinical management*. 4th ed. Philadelphia: W.B. Saunders Co; 1999. p. 363–87.
73. Yen SSC. The human menstrual cycle: neuroendocrine regulation. In: Yen SSC, Jaffe RB, Barbieri RL, editors. *Reproductive endocrinology: physiology, pathophysiology, and clinical management*. 4th ed. Philadelphia: W.B. Saunders Co; 1999. p. 191–217.
110. Santen RJ, Allred DC, Ardoin SP, et al. Postmenopausal hormone therapy: an Endocrine Society scientific statement. *J Clin Endocrinol Metab* 2010;**95**:s1–66.
116. Gronowski AM, Fantz CR, Parvin CA, et al. Use of serum FSH to identify perimenopausal women with pituitary HCG. *Clin Chem* 2008;**54**:652–6.
181. Practice Committee of American Society for Reproductive Medicine. Current evaluation of amenorrhea. *Fertil Steril* 2008;**90**:S219–25.
190. Legro RS, Arslanian SA, Ehrmann DA, et al. Diagnosis and treatment of polycystic ovary syndrome: an Endocrine Society clinical practice guideline. *J Clin Endocrinol Metab* 2013;**98**:4565–92.
199. Dewailly D, Andersen CY, Balen A, et al. The physiology and clinical utility of anti-Mullerian hormone in women. *Hum Reprod Update* 2014;**20**:370–85.
259. La Marca A, Giulini S, Tirelli A, et al. Anti-Mullerian hormone measurement on any day of the menstrual cycle strongly predicts ovarian response in assisted reproductive technology. *Hum Reprod* 2007;**22**:766–71.
261. Nelson SM. Biomarkers of ovarian response: current and future applications. *Fertil Steril* 2013;**99**:963–9.
274. Practice Committee of American Society for Reproductive M. Multiple gestation associated with infertility therapy: an American Society for Reproductive Medicine Practice Committee opinion. *Fertil Steril* 2012;**97**:825–34.
275. Montag M, Toth B, Strowitzki T. New approaches to embryo selection. *Reprod Biomed Online* 2013;**27**:539–46.
288. Demers LM. Testosterone and estradiol assays: current and future trends. *Steroids* 2008;**73**:1333–8.
298. Rosner W, Auchus RJ, Azziz R, et al. Position statement: utility, limitations, and pitfalls in measuring testosterone: an Endocrine Society position statement. *J Clin Endocrinol Metab* 2007;**92**:405–13.

69

Pregnancy and Its Disorders

*Melanie L. Yarbrough, Molly Stout, and Ann M. Gronowski**

ABSTRACT

Background

The clinical laboratory has an important role in monitoring pregnancy when an expectant mother is being treated. In contrast to most clinical situations in which a physician is caring for one patient, the physician must simultaneously care for both a mother and her fetus. The usual results for many clinical measurements no longer apply during pregnancy, further complicating the management of the patients.

Content

This chapter reviews the biology of pregnancy and discusses laboratory tests used to detect, evaluate, and monitor both normal and abnormal pregnancies. The physiologic changes associated with normal pregnancy are described along with a discussion on events surrounding conception and development of the fetus. Although most pregnancies progress without problems, complications can arise in the mother, placenta, or fetus. Diagnosis and management of maternal complications such as ectopic pregnancy, trophoblastic disease, preeclampsia, and liver disease as well as fetal complications including hemolytic disease of the newborn and vertically transmitted infections are highlighted. Laboratory testing is available to screen for and diagnose many fetal anomalies such as chromosomal abnormalities and neural tube defects. A detailed discussion of prenatal screening for fetal anomalies is provided. Lastly, this chapter will examine the chemistry, biochemistry, methods, and clinical significance of specific laboratory tests used in the management of pregnancy.

The clinical laboratory has an important role in monitoring pregnancy.[1] In contrast to most clinical situations, when treating an expectant mother, a physician must simultaneously care for more than one patient. The health of the mother and that of her fetus are intertwined, each affecting the other; thus pregnancy management must consider both. This chapter reviews the biology of pregnancy and discusses laboratory tests used to detect, evaluate, and monitor both normal and abnormal pregnancies.

HUMAN PREGNANCY

To appreciate the role of laboratory tests in pregnancy health care, it is necessary to understand fundamental topics, such as (1) the processes of conception, embryo development, and fetal growth; (2) the role of the placenta; (3) the importance and composition of amniotic fluid; (4) the maternal physiologic adaptations to pregnancy; and (5) the functional maturation of the fetus.

Conception and the Embryo and Fetus

Normal human pregnancy (ie, gestation) lasts approximately 40 weeks, as measured from the first day of the last normal menstrual period, a date commonly represented by the abbreviations LMP or LNMP. The anticipated date of birth of an infant is commonly referred to as the *expected date of confinement,* or EDC. During pregnancy, a woman undergoes dramatic physiologic and hormonal changes. When talking with patients, physicians customarily divide pregnancy into four time intervals. The first three time intervals are called *trimesters,* each of which is approximately 13 weeks. The last time interval, 37 to 42 weeks, is coined *term.* By convention, the first trimester, 0 to 13 weeks, begins on the first day of the last menses.

Ovulation occurs on approximately the 14th day of the regular menstrual cycle (see Chapter 68). If conception occurs, the ovum is fertilized, usually in the fallopian tube, and becomes a *zygote,* which is then carried down the tube into the uterus. The zygote divides, becoming a *morula.* After 50 to 60 cells are present, the morula develops a cavity, the primitive *yolk sac,* and thus becomes a *blastocyst,* which implants into the uterine wall about 5 days after fertilization. The cells on the exterior wall of the blastocyst, *trophoblasts,* synergistically invade the uterine endometrium and develop into chorionic villi, creating the placenta. Trophoblasts are subdivided into syncytiotrophoblasts and cytotrophoblasts, depending on location and cellular morphology.

At this stage, the product of conception is referred to as an *embryo.* A cavity called the *amnion* forms and enlarges with the accumulation of *amniotic fluid.* Nourished by the placenta and protected by the amniotic fluid, an embryo undergoes rapid cell division, differentiation, and growth. From combinations of three primary cell types, *ectoderm, mesoderm,* and *endoderm,* organs begin to form through a process called *organogenesis.* At 10 weeks, an embryo has developed most major structures and is now referred to as a *fetus.* At 13 weeks, the fetus weighs approximately 13 g and is approximately 8 cm long.

*The authors gratefully acknowledge the original contributions of George J. Knight, Edward Ashwood, David Grenache, and Geralyn Lambert-Messerlian, upon which portions of this chapter are based.

Rapid fetal growth occurs during the 13 to 26 weeks of the second trimester. By the end of the second trimester, the fetus weighs approximately 700 g and is 30 cm long. Although organogenesis is complete by the second trimester, fetal organ maturation continues through the rest of pregnancy. In the third trimester fetal growth and maturation continue, and toward the end of the third trimester there is a slight deceleration in the rate of fetal growth. By the end of the third trimester, the fetus weighs approximately 3200 g and is about 50 cm long. Term pregnancy is defined as 37 weeks or more. Recently, the definition of term pregnancy was subdivided into *early term* (37 0/7 to 38 6/7 weeks), *full term* (39 0/7 to 40 6/7 weeks), *and late term* (41 0/7 to 41 6/7 weeks). Term birth is defined as delivery at or beyond 37 weeks.[2] Normal labor, defined as rhythmic uterine contractions causing cervical dilation and eventually delivery of the fetus and placenta, normally occurs during this period.

Placenta

The placenta and the umbilical cord form the primary link between fetus and mother. The placenta grows throughout pregnancy and is normally delivered through the birth canal immediately after the birth of the infant.

Function

The placenta (1) keeps the maternal and fetal circulation systems separate, (2) nourishes the fetus, (3) eliminates fetal wastes, and (4) produces hormones vital to pregnancy. It is composed of large collections of fetal vessels called *villi.* These villi are finger-like projections that insert into blood-filled spaces called the intervillous spaces. Each intervillous space contains maternal blood that bathes the fetal villi and facilitates bidirectional exchange between mother and fetus. For substances to move from the maternal circulation to the fetal circulation, they must cross through the trophoblasts and several membranes. The transfer of any substance depends largely on the (1) concentration gradient between the maternal and fetal circulatory systems, (2) presence or absence of circulating binding proteins, (3) lipid solubility of the substance, and (4) presence of facilitated transport, such as ion pumps or receptor-mediated endocytosis (Box 69.1). The placenta is an effective barrier to the movement of large proteins and hydrophobic compounds bound to plasma proteins. Maternal immunoglobulin (Ig)G crosses the placenta via receptor-mediated endocytosis. Because of its long half-life, maternally produced IgG protects a newborn through passive immunity for the first 6 months of life. Antibody assays with low limits of detection may be positive in infants up to age 18 months because of the persistence of maternal antibodies.

Placental Hormones

The placenta produces several protein and steroid hormones (Fig. 69.1). The major protein hormones are human chorionic gonadotropin (hCG) and human placental lactogen (hPL). Steroid hormones including progesterone, estradiol, estriol, and estrone are synthesized in complex joint pathways involving maternal, placental, and fetal contributions. Generally, hormone production by the placenta increases in proportion to the increase in placental mass. Therefore, concentrations of hormones derived from the placenta, such as hPL, increase in maternal peripheral blood as the placenta increases in size. The hormone hCG, which peaks at the end of the first trimester, is an exception.

BOX 69.1 Normal Placental Transport

No Transport
Most proteins
Maternal IgM, IgA
Maternal and fetal erythrocytes

Limited Passive Transport
Unconjugated steroids
Steroid sulfates
Free fatty acids

Passive Transport
Molecules up to 5000 Da having lipid solubility
Oxygen
Carbon dioxide
Sodium and chloride
Urea
Ethanol

Active Transport Across Cell Membranes
Glucose
Many amino acids
Calcium

Receptor-Mediated Endocytosis
Maternal IgG
Low-density lipoprotein

Ig, Immunoglobulin.

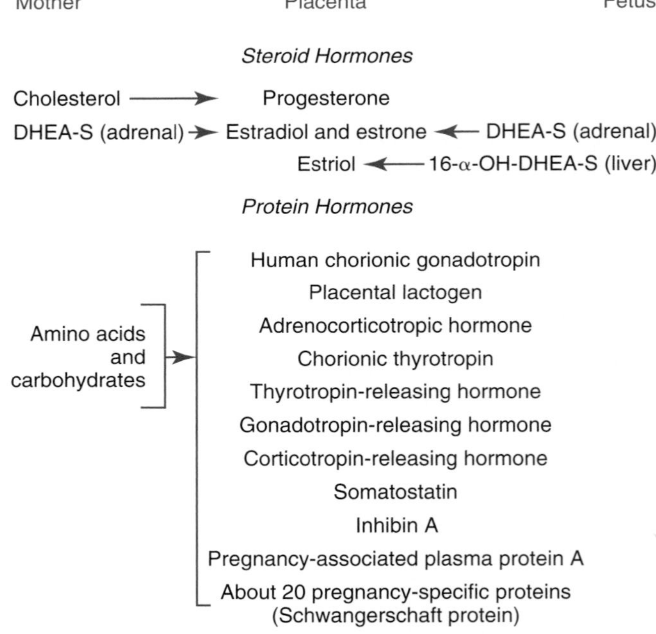

FIGURE 69.1 Schematic representation of steroid and protein hormone production by the placenta.

Chorionic Gonadotropin. One of the most important placental hormones is hCG. It stimulates the ovary to produce progesterone by maintaining the corpus luteum, which, in turn, prevents menstruation, thereby protecting the pregnancy. hCG is produced primarily by the syncytiotrophoblasts of the placenta. Hyperglycosylated hCG is believed to be produced by the more invasive extravillous cytotrophoblasts.[3] The chemistry, biochemistry, and methods for measuring hCG are discussed later in this chapter.

Placental Lactogen. PL, also known as human placental lactogen (hPL) and human chorionic somatomammotropin (hCS), is a single polypeptide chain of 191 amino acids having two intramolecular disulfide bridges and a molecular mass of 22,279 Da. The structure of hPL is exceptionally homologous (96%) with growth hormone (GH) and less so with prolactin (67%). Five genes on chromosome 17 compose a gene family that codes for both GH and hPL.[4] hPL production has been localized by immunofluorescence studies to the syncytiotrophoblastic cells of the placenta. The increase in maternal serum hPL concentration with advancing gestational age is directly correlated with the increasing mass of placental tissue and of functional syncytiotrophoblastic tissue.[5] The placental secretion near term is 1 to 2 g/day, the largest of any known human hormone.

hPL has many biologic activities, including (1) lactogenic, (2) metabolic, (3) somatotropic, (4) erythropoietic, and (5) aldosterone-stimulating effects. In addition, either directly or in synergism with prolactin, hPL has a significant role in preparing the mammary glands for lactation. The many metabolic activities of hPL closely resemble those of GH, including (1) inhibition of glucose uptake, (2) enhanced lipolysis leading to increased mobilization of free fatty acids, and (3) enhancement of nitrogen retention. Because glucose is the primary energy substrate for a fetus, it has been suggested that the glucose-sparing action of hPL may be a strategy to direct maternal metabolism toward greater use of fat for the mother's requirements, thereby sparing maternal glucose for fetal use. Rare normal pregnancies have been reported in which complete absence of hPL was noted. Although hPL was used in the past to evaluate fetal well-being, currently there is no clinical utility to hPL measurement.[6]

Placental Steroids. The placenta produces a wide variety of steroid hormones, including estrogen and progesterone, with large amounts of estrogens produced at term. The chemistry of these steroids is described in Chapter 68. Maternal cholesterol is the main precursor for placental progesterone production. Biosynthesis of estrogens by the placenta differs from that of the ovaries because the placenta has no 17α-hydroxylase. Thus each of the estrogens—estrone (E_1), estradiol (E_2), and estriol (E_3)—must be synthesized from C-19 intermediates that already have a hydroxyl group at position 17. In nonpregnant women, the ovaries secrete 100 to 600 µg/day of estradiol, of which about 10% is metabolized to estriol. During late pregnancy, the placenta produces 50 to 150 mg/day of estriol and 15 to 20 mg/day of estradiol and estrone. Secretion of estrogens and progesterone throughout pregnancy ensures (1) appropriate development of the endometrium, (2) uterine growth, (3) adequate uterine blood supply, and (4) preparation of the uterus for labor. Although measurement of estriol in the third trimester was used in the past to assess fetal well-being, most obstetricians now consider this practice obsolete.[7] Estriol measurements as a component in maternal serum screening for aneuploidy are useful in the second trimester of pregnancy for risk estimation for fetal trisomy 21 and 18 (see later discussion on maternal serum screening for fetal defects).

Amniotic Fluid

Throughout intrauterine life, the fetus lives within a fluid-filled compartment. The amniotic fluid provides a medium in which a fetus readily moves. It cushions a fetus against possible injury, helps maintain a constant temperature, and is inhaled and swallowed by the fetus during normal fetal lung development. This fluid is a dynamic medium whose volume and chemical composition are controlled within relatively narrow limits.

Volume and Dynamics

The volume of amniotic fluid increases progressively until 34 weeks' gestation, when it decreases slightly through the 40th week and then more sharply declines until the 42nd week.[8] The volume is 200 to 300 mL at 16 weeks, 400 to 1400 mL at 26 weeks, 300 to 2000 mL at 34 weeks, and 300 to 1400 mL at 40 weeks. The volume at any given moment is a function of several interrelated fluid fluxes. Direct measurements in primates and indirect measurements in humans have been used to derive a mathematical model of amniotic fluid volume.[9] At term, total fluid fluxes into and out of the amniotic cavity are large (≈60 mL/h) and result in complete exchange of the amniotic fluid volume twice per day. Gross unidirectional fluid volume shifts occur episodically: into the amniotic cavity by fetal urination and out of the cavity by fetal swallowing. These unidirectional shifts begin at the end of the first trimester and increase linearly until approximately 30 weeks. Fetal swallowing and urination then exponentially increase, peaking at term at about 1000 mL/day. Bidirectional water exchanges—so-called intramembranous fluxes—occur across the following surfaces: (1) placenta (mother-fetus), (2) umbilical vessels, through the substance of the umbilical cord (fetus–amniotic fluid), (3) fetal skin (fetus–amniotic fluid), and (4) fetal membranes (amniotic fluid–mother). These exchanges increase in a linear fashion throughout pregnancy. At term, they are approximately 400 mL/day. The fetal tracheobronchial tree is filled with amniotic fluid. Although lung fluid transport contributes a small volume, fetal inhalation is required for normal fetal lung development and is the mechanism of surfactant transport from the fetal lungs into the amniotic fluid.

Pathologic decreases and increases in amniotic fluid volume are encountered frequently in clinical practice. Intrauterine growth retardation and anomalies of the fetal urinary tract, such as bilateral renal agenesis or obstruction of the urethra, are associated with *oligohydramnios,* an abnormally low amniotic fluid volume. Increased fluid volume is known as *hydramnios* (also termed *polyhydramnios*). Conditions associated with hydramnios include (1) maternal diabetes mellitus, (2) severe Rh isoimmune disease, (3) fetal esophageal atresia, (4) multifetal pregnancy, (5) anencephaly, and (6) spina bifida.

Composition

Early in gestation, the composition of the amniotic fluid resembles a complex dialysate of the maternal serum. As a fetus grows, the amniotic fluid changes in several ways (Table 69.1). Most notably, the sodium concentration and osmolality decrease and concentrations of urea, creatinine, and uric acid increase.[10] The activities of many enzymes in amniotic fluid have been studied with respect to both gestational age and fetal status but have not been found to be clinically useful.

TABLE 69.1 Composition of Amniotic Fluid (Mean Values)

	GESTATIONAL AGE (WK)		
Component	**15**	**25**	**40**
Sodium, mmol/L	136	138	126
Potassium, mmol/L	3.9	4.0	4.3
Chloride, mmol/L	111	109	103
Bicarbonate, mmol/L	16	18	16
Urea nitrogen, mg/dL (mmol urea/L)	11 (3.9)	11 (3.9)	18 (6.4)
Creatinine, mg/dL (μmol/L)	0.8 (71)	0.9 (80)	2.2 (194)
Glucose, mg/dL (mmol/L)	47 (2.6)	39 (2.2)	32 (1.8)
Uric acid, mg/dL (mmol/L)	4.0 (0.24)	5.7 (0.34)	10.4 (0.61)
Total protein, g/dL (g/L)	0.5 (5)	0.8 (8)	0.3 (3)
Bilirubin, mg/dL (μmol/L)	0.13 (2.2)	0.14 (2.4)	0.04 (0.7)
Osmolality, mOsm/kg H_2O	272	272	255

From Benzie RJ, Doran TA, Harkins JL, Owen VM, Porter CJ. Composition of the amniotic fluid and maternal serum in pregnancy. *Am J Obstet Gynecol* 1974;119:798–810.

The major lipids of interest are the phospholipids (PL), whose type and concentrations reflect fetal lung maturity (discussed further later). Numerous steroid and protein hormones are also present in amniotic fluid.[11] The rare syndrome of congenital adrenal hyperplasia has been diagnosed antenatally by measuring 17-hydroxyprogesterone and pregnanetriol in the amniotic fluid near term.[12] Measurements of thyroid-stimulating hormone (TSH) and thyroxine in amniotic fluid may be useful in cases of fetal thyroid disease.[13] No other diagnostic uses for amniotic fluid hormone measurements are in common use. Prostaglandins (PGs) E_1, E_2, $F_{1\alpha}$, and $F_{2\alpha}$ all are found in low concentrations in amniotic fluid and increase gradually during pregnancy. PGE_2 and $PGF_{2\alpha}$ concentrations are very high during active labor.[14] Attempts to demonstrate an acute rise in PGE_2 or $PGF_{2\alpha}$ immediately before the onset of labor, at the initiation of parturition, have been unsuccessful.

Early in pregnancy, little or no particulate matter is found in the amniotic fluid. By 16 weeks' gestation, large numbers of cells are present, having been shed from the surfaces of the amnion, skin, and tracheobronchial tree. These cells have proved to be of great utility in antenatal diagnosis and are the cellular source for DNA used for karyotype analysis after amniocentesis. As pregnancy continues to progress, scalp hair and *lanugo* (fine hair on the body of the fetus) are shed into the fluid and contribute to its turbidity. Production of surfactant particles in the lung, termed *lamellar bodies,* greatly increases the haziness of the fluid. At term, amniotic fluid contains gross particles of *vernix caseosa,* the oily substance composed of sebum and desquamated epithelial cells covering the fetal skin.

Normal fetuses do not defecate during pregnancy. If severely stressed, a fetus may pass stool that is called *meconium.* This heterogeneous material contains many bile pigments and therefore stains the amniotic fluid green. Meconium-stained amniotic fluid is a sign of fetal stress.

POINTS TO REMEMBER

Placenta

- A major function of the placenta is production of several protein and steroid hormones.
- hCG is a protein hormone that maintains the corpus luteum on the ovary to produce progesterone, which protects the pregnancy by preventing menstruation. Later in pregnancy, progesterone is synthesized by the placenta.
- hPL is a protein hormone that regulates maternal and fetal metabolism to facilitate growth and development of the fetus.
- Major steroid hormones, including progesterone and estriol, are synthesized by the fetoplacental unit.

Amniotic Fluid

- Amniotic fluid provides a medium to cushion and protect the fetus.
- Early in gestation, the composition of the amniotic fluid resembles a complex dialysate of the maternal serum.
- Toward the end of the first trimester, the fetal kidneys begin to produce urine, which becomes the main component of amniotic fluid.
- Fetal cells shed in amniotic fluid are a source of DNA for karyotype analysis for suspected aneuploidy.
- Decreases and increases in amniotic fluid volume are indicative of potential pathophysiologic changes in pregnancy.

Maternal Adaptation

During pregnancy a woman undergoes dramatic physiologic and hormonal changes. The large quantities of estrogens, progesterone, PL, and corticosteroids produced during pregnancy affect various metabolic, physiologic, and endocrinologic systems. In addition, the woman experiences (1) an increase in resistance to angiotensin, (2) a predominance of lipid metabolism over glucose use, and (3) increased synthesis by the liver of thyroid- and steroid-binding proteins, fibrinogen, and other proteins characteristic of pregnancy. As a result of such changes, many of the laboratory reference intervals for nonpregnant patients are not appropriate for pregnant patients. Lockitch[15] has developed reference intervals for over 70 analytes in normal pregnancy. Her study group included a small sample size of 29 pregnant subjects tested from 16 weeks to term and also postpartum. Mean values for selected tests expressed as a percentage of control means are presented in Table 69.2. It should be noted that these reference intervals will vary depending on the testing method.

Hematologic Changes

The maternal blood volume increases during pregnancy by an average of 45%. The plasma volume increases more than the red blood cell mass; therefore, despite augmented erythropoiesis, the hemoglobin concentration, erythrocyte count, and hematocrit decrease during normal pregnancy, producing the so-called physiologic anemia of pregnancy. Hemoglobin concentrations at term average 12.6 g/dL(126 g/L), compared

TABLE 69.2 Mean Serum and Plasma Laboratory Values During Normal Pregnancies Expressed as a Percentage of the Nonpregnant Mean ($n = 29$)

	TIME OF GESTATION		
Analyte	**12 wk**	**32 wk**	**Term**
Sodium	97	98	97
Potassium	95	95	100
Bicarbonate	85	85	81
Chloride	98	100	99
Urea nitrogen	77	63	77
Creatinine	71	74	81
Fasting glucose	98	94	94
Bilirubin, unconjugated	56	67	78
Albumin	93	78	78
Protein	92	83	83
Uric acid	68	92	120
Calcium	98	94	97
Free ionized calcium	99	101	102
Parathyroid hormone, intact	—	—	140
1,25-Dihydroxyvitamin D	—	—	400
Phosphate	108	97	96
Magnesium	92	87	87
Alkaline phosphatase	90	203	347
Creatine kinase	87	86	135
α_1-Antitrypsin	129	174	191
Transferrin	105	160	170
Cholesterol	100	144	156
HDL-cholesterol	121	119	130
LDL-cholesterol	80	118	146
Fasting triglycerides	141	300	349
Iron	112	94	94
Iron-binding capacity	95	139	144
Transferrin saturation	136	68	64
Zinc protoporphyrin	107	109	144
Ferritin	81	33	59
Thyroxine	103	107	100
Triiodothyronine	100	121	121
Free thyroxine	98	72	74
Thyroxine-binding globulin	114	155	182
Thyroid-stimulating hormone	111	122	139
Cortisol	111	301	309
Aldosterone	—	—	1500
Prolactin	—	—	800
Hemoglobin	95	90	96
Hematocrit	94	91	97
Leukocyte count	144	167	240
Prothrombin time	99	97	97
Activated partial thromboplastin time	95	91	93
Platelet count	98	96	100
Fibrinogen	119	154	165

HDL, High-density lipoprotein; *LDL,* low-density lipoprotein.
Data from Lockitch G, editor. *Handbook of diagnostic biochemistry and hematology in normal pregnancy.* Boca Raton, FL: CRC Press, 1993.

with 13.3 g/dL (133 g/L) for the nonpregnant state. The leukocyte count varies considerably during pregnancy, from 4000 to 13,000/µL. During labor and puerperium (the interval immediately after delivery), leukocyte counts may be markedly increased.

The concentrations of several blood coagulation factors are increased during pregnancy. For example, plasma fibrinogen increases by approximately 65%, from 275 to 450 mg/dL (8.1 to 13.2 µmol/L); this increase contributes to the increase in sedimentation rate. Other clotting factors also increase, including factors VII, VIII, IX, and X. Prothrombin and factors V and XII do not change, whereas factors XI and XIII decrease slightly. Even though the platelet count remains unchanged in most women and the prothrombin time and activated partial thromboplastin time shorten slightly (see Table 69.2), pregnancy increases the risk of thromboembolism up to five times that of nonpregnant women.

Biochemical Changes

During pregnancy, electrolytes show little change, but an approximately 40% increase in cholesterol, PL, and free fatty acids is seen. Triglycerides increase by about 3-fold over the course of gestation. Plasma albumin is decreased to an average of 3.4 g/dL (34 g/L) in late pregnancy; plasma globulin concentrations increase slightly. Several of the plasma transport proteins, including thyroxine-binding globulin, cortisol-binding globulin, and sex hormone–binding globulin, increase markedly. Serum cholinesterase activity is reduced, whereas alkaline phosphatase activity in serum is tripled, mainly as the result of an increase in very heat-stable alkaline phosphatase of placental origin. In addition, creatine kinase can markedly increase upon delivery.

Renal Function

Pregnancy increases the glomerular filtration rate to about 170 mL/min/1.73m^2 by 20 weeks, and therefore increases the clearance of urea, creatinine, and uric acid. Concentrations of these three analytes are slightly decreased in serum for much of the pregnancy. As term approaches, the glomerular filtration rate begins to return to the nonpregnant rate. Urea and creatinine concentrations rise slightly during the last 4 weeks. During this time, tubular reabsorption of uric acid increases dramatically, which increases the serum uric acid compared with the nonpregnant state. Glucosuria up to 1000 mg/day (5.55 mmol/day) may be present due to the increased glomerular filtration rate, which presents more fluid to the tubules and therefore lowers the renal glucose threshold. Protein loss in the urine can increase to up to 300 mg/day.

Endocrine Changes

The action of progesterone prevents menses and thus allows pregnancy to continue. In early pregnancy, progesterone is produced by the corpus luteum of the maternal ovary in response to hCG. In later stages the placenta directly produces enough progesterone to maintain the pregnancy.

Throughout pregnancy, plasma parathyroid hormone is increased by approximately 40%, with almost no change in the plasma free ionized calcium fraction, thus suggesting a new set point for the secretion of parathyroid hormone. Calcitonin does not increase predictably during pregnancy, whereas 1,25-dihydroxyvitamin D is increased during pregnancy and promotes increased intestinal calcium absorption to support the calcium requirements for fetal skeletal development.

An increased estrogen concentration stimulates increased hepatic production of cortisol-binding globulin. The hepatic clearance of cortisol decreases. Thus, the absolute plasma concentrations of both total and free cortisol are several times higher during pregnancy. The diurnal rhythm of cortisol, higher in the morning and lower in the evening, is maintained. Increased plasma aldosterone and deoxycorticosterone concentrations are observed.

Increasing estrogen concentrations throughout pregnancy increase the secretion of prolactin up to tenfold. Conversely, high estrogen concentrations during pregnancy suppress the secretion of luteinizing hormone (LH) and follicle-stimulating hormone (FSH) below the detection limit. Baseline concentrations of other pituitary hormones such as TSH remain nearly unchanged (see Table 69.2), but the growth hormone (GH) response to provocative stimuli is blunted.

Although normal pregnancy is a euthyroid state, many changes occur in thyroid function. High concentrations of thyroxine-binding globulin raise the concentration of total thyroxine and triiodothyronine, but a slight decrease in free thyroxine concentration occurs during the second and third trimesters. A slight reciprocal increase in TSH was reported by Lockitch.[15] Thyroglobulin is significantly increased, especially in the third trimester.[16] Very few (<0.2% of) pregnant individuals develop hyperthyroidism, and hypothyroidism is very rare.[17] Postpartum thyroid dysfunction is common and is frequently unrecognized and misdiagnosed as routine postpartum symptoms of fatigue and weight changes. The fetal thyroid-pituitary axis functions independently from the mother's axis by the end of the first trimester. However, if the mother has preexisting Graves' disease (hyperthyroidism caused by autoantibodies that stimulate the thyroid), those antibodies can cross the placenta, causing hyperthyroidism in the fetus. If the mother has anti-TSH autoantibodies, the infant can develop transient hypothyroidism.[15]

Functional Development of the Fetus

Fetal organs mature during the third trimester but not at the same rate. This section reviews the lung, liver, kidneys, and blood maturation in the fetus.

Lungs and Pulmonary Surfactant

In normal air-breathing lungs, a substance called *pulmonary surfactant* coats the alveolar epithelium and responds to alveolar volume changes by reducing surface tension in the alveolar wall during expiration. Surfactant is needed because the surface tension is an inverse function of the radius of the airway. Thus small alveoli have a higher collapsing force than larger alveoli. Surfactant opposes the force and keeps the small alveoli from collapsing. Specialized alveolar cells called *type II granular pneumocytes* synthesize pulmonary surfactant and package it into laminated storage granules called *lamellar bodies.*[18,19] These storage granules are 1 to 5 μm in diameter and contain PL, cholesterol, and protein.[20] After exocytosis into the alveolar space, lamellar bodies unfold into a structure known as tubular myelin, which supplies the lipids necessary for regulation of surface tension in the lungs.[18] Pulmonary surfactant production starts as early as 20 weeks' gestation,[19] but adequate amounts do not accumulate until about 36 weeks. Exudation of pulmonary fluid (via the trachea) and fetal breathing movements transport lamellar bodies into the amniotic fluid.

The newborn lung contains 100 times more surfactant per cm^3 than the adult lung. Excessive surfactant is needed at birth as the newborn transitions from breathing water to breathing air. Surfactant overcomes the surface tension produced in water-filled alveoli that are admitting air for the first time.

Pulmonary surfactant is a complex mixture of lipids and proteins; less than 5% is composed of carbohydrates. The principal PLs present in surfactant are lecithin (phosphatidylcholine) and phosphatidylglycerol, while phosphatidylinositol and sphingomyelin are present in much lower abundance.[21] The synthesis of lecithin gradually increases from 28 weeks' gestation until birth, with the highest production occurring at week 36. Similarly, phosphatidylinositol first appears at 28 weeks' gestation, but reaches peak production at between 32 and 35 weeks. Phosphatidylglycerol is the last PL to be produced, appearing in surfactant at 36 weeks and continuing to rise until birth (see Chapter 34).[22] The protein fraction of lamellar bodies is approximately 4% and is composed of four surfactant-specific proteins, SP-A, SP-B, SP-C, and SP-D.[23,24]

Liver

Hematopoiesis occurs in the liver during the first two trimesters and is transferred to the fetal bone marrow during the third trimester. The liver is also responsible for production of specific proteins (such as albumin and clotting factors), metabolism and detoxification of many compounds, and secretion of substances such as bilirubin. A clinically useful protein produced by the liver is alpha-fetoprotein (AFP). Bilirubin secretion and detoxification mechanisms are immature until late in pregnancy and even in the first few months after birth. Thus premature infants often have high serum bilirubin concentrations and metabolize drugs poorly.

Kidneys

Toward the end of the first trimester, the fetal kidneys begin to produce urine, which becomes the main component of amniotic fluid. Early nephrons cannot produce concentrated urine, and pH regulation is also limited. Complete maturation occurs after birth. Although kidneys are not required for fetal survival, amniotic fluid is required for normal lung development. Without fluid to breathe, the fetal lungs fail to properly develop. Thus newborns without kidneys die of pulmonary failure.

Fetal Blood Development

Fetal blood is produced first by the embryonic yolk sac, then by the liver, and finally by the fetal bone marrow. The yolk sac produces three embryonic hemoglobins: Portland ($\zeta_{2\gamma2}$), Gower-1 ($\zeta_{2\varepsilon2}$), and Gower-2 ($\alpha_{2\varepsilon2}$). These normal embryonic hemoglobins are of little importance in clinical chemistry because they are present in fetal blood only in the first trimester.

With the switch of erythropoiesis to the fetal liver and spleen, fetal hemoglobin (HbF) production begins. HbF consists of two α- and two γ-chains ($\alpha_{2\gamma2}$). Small amounts of adult hemoglobin, HbA ($\alpha_{2\beta2}$), are also produced, but HbF predominates during the remainder of fetal life.

As the fetal bone marrow begins red cell production, HbA production increases. At birth, fetal blood contains 75% HbF and 25% HbA. HbF production rapidly diminishes during the first year of postnatal life. In normal adults, less than 1% of hemoglobin is HbF. The difference between fetal and adult hemoglobin is very significant because HbF has a higher affinity for oxygen than does HbA. Thus in the placenta, oxygen is released from the maternal HbA, diffuses into the chorionic villi, and preferentially binds to the fetal HbF. In addition, 2,3-diphosphoglycerate (2,3-DPG) does not bind HbF and therefore cannot decrease its affinity for oxygen.

MATERNAL AND FETAL HEALTH ASSESSMENT

For optimum health care during pregnancy a woman should consult her physician before conception.[25,26] Unfortunately, 49% of pregnancies in the United States are unintended; the percentage is higher for unmarried women.[27] Preconception evaluation should include a medical, reproductive, and family history; physical examination; and laboratory tests.

Laboratory Testing

The following laboratory tests are recommended as part of a preconception evaluation: (1) hematocrit, (2) blood type and Rh compatibility, (3) erythrocyte antibody screen, (4) Papanicolaou smear (or human papillomavirus test), (5) urinalysis, (6) rubella titer, (7) rapid plasma reagin test, (8) gonococcal and chlamydia DNA test, (9) cystic fibrosis carrier status,[28] (10) human immunodeficiency virus (HIV) antibody levels,[29] and (11) hepatitis B surface antigen levels.[30] Depending on demographic risks, genetic testing for disorders such as Tay-Sachs disease, thalassemia, and sickle cell disease should be offered.[31] A careful diet history is warranted. Folic acid supplementation should be recommended to reduce the risk of neural tube defects.[32] Women at high risk for diabetes mellitus should be screened for this disorder (see Chapter 57).

Many laboratory tests are useful for managing normal and abnormal pregnancies. Screening for fetal neural tube defects and aneuploidy should be offered to all pregnant patients. Depending on diabetes risk, glucose tolerance testing should be performed immediately or at 24 to 28 weeks (see Chapter 57 for details). Maternal observation and recording of fetal movements,[33] ultrasound examination (biophysical profile), and fetal heart rate patterns (non–stress test and contraction stress tests)[34] are the currently accepted methods for monitoring fetal well-being.

Diagnosis and Dating of Pregnancy

The most important aspects of pregnancy management are detection of pregnancy and establishing accurate estimates of gestational age. The most useful test for detecting pregnancy is the hCG test. Qualitative tests for hCG in blood or urine are used to screen for pregnancy. Urine hCG tests can detect pregnancy around the day of missed menses. False-positive or increased serum hCG test results have been obtained from qualitative and quantitative assays when human antimouse antibodies or heterophile antibodies are present (see Chapter 23).[35,36] If suspected, investigative experiments include testing a urine specimen for the presence of hCG, serially diluting the serum to confirm an appropriate dose response, testing the serum using a different hCG method, and retesting the serum after treatment with interfering antibody blocking agents.

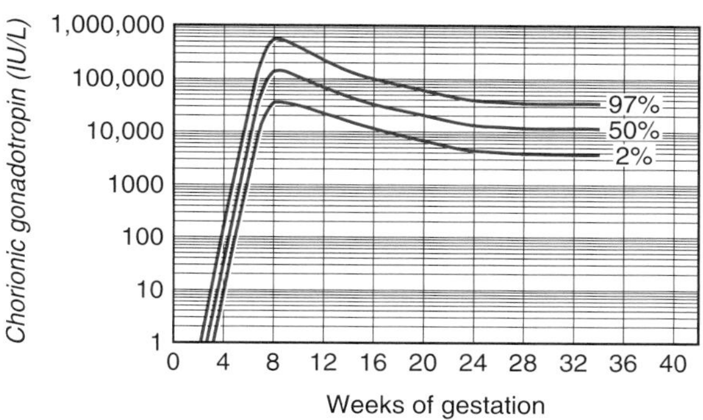

FIGURE 69.2 Concentration of chorionic gonadotropin (hCG) in maternal serum as a function of gestational age. Lines represent the 2nd, 50th, and 97th percentiles. The maternal serum values from 14 to 25 weeks are medians calculated from 24,229 pregnancies from testing performed at ARUP Laboratories, Inc., from January to October 1997. (From Ashwood ER. Evaluating health and maturation of the unborn: the role of the clinical laboratory. *Clin Chem* 1992;38:1523–9, with permission.)

Obstetricians measure the length of pregnancy in terms of *weeks,* not trimesters. To establish accurate dates, obstetricians rely predominantly on menstrual history and ultrasound measurements, although a physical exam, detection and quantification of hCG, and the presence of fetal heart tones may also be useful in certain circumstances. In the first 8 weeks of pregnancy, the hCG concentration in maternal serum rises geometrically (Fig. 69.2). Detectable amounts (>5 IU/L) are present in the serum 8 to 11 days after conception,[37] which is in the third week of pregnancy as measured from the LMP.[38] hCG usually becomes detectable in the urine 1 to 3 days later, although this interval is highly variable.[37] For women aged 13 to 40, serum hCG concentrations of 5 IU/L or greater are consistent with pregnancy. Higher values are infrequently seen in older, nonpregnant women and are thought to be caused by hCG secreted by the pituitary gland.[39] Concentrations in approximately half of pregnant women reach 25 IU/L on the first day of their missed period. The peak concentration occurs at about 8 to 10 weeks and is about 100,000 IU/L. Subsequently, hCG concentrations start to decline in serum and urine, and by the end of the second trimester, a 90% reduction from peak concentration has usually occurred. During the first several weeks of pregnancy, a hyperglycosylated variant of hCG is the predominant form of hCG produced.[3] This quickly switches to intact hCG. In the first trimester, maternal serum hCG is about 96% to 98% intact, 1% to 3% β-subunit, and up to 1% α-subunit. During the second trimester, subunit synthesis becomes unbalanced and the serum distribution shifts to 92% to 98% intact, 1% to 7% α-subunit, and up to 1% β-subunit.[40] Concentrations are approximately constant during the third trimester, with the predominant species being intact hCG. The presence of twins approximately doubles hCG concentrations.[41] In urine, hCG beta core fragment is the predominant form of hCG after approximately 5 weeks of pregnancy.[42]

COMPLICATIONS OF PREGNANCY

Although most pregnancies progress without problems, complications can arise in the mother, placenta, or fetus.

AT A GLANCE

Laboratory Evaluation of Maternal Health

First Prenatal Visit:
- Complete blood count (CBC)
- Rh(D) typing and antibody screen
- Pap smear
- Urinalysis
- Urine culture
- Rubella immunity
- Varicella immunity
- Hepatitis B screening
- HIV antibody test
- STI testing
  - Syphilis
  - Chlamydia

Women at Increased Risk May Also Receive Testing for the Following:
- Genetic testing for inherited disease
- Cystic fibrosis carrier testing
- Hemoglobinopathies
- Gonorrhea
- Tuberculosis
- Toxoplasma
- Hepatitis C

Additional Testing Later in Pregnancy:
- Detection of fetal anomalies
  - Maternal serum screening (first and second trimester)
  - Cell free fetal DNA screening (at 10 week's gestation or later)
- Oral glucose tolerance testing (between 24–28 weeks' gestation)
- Group B Strep cultures (between 35–37 weeks' gestation)

Abnormal Pregnancies

Conditions arising primarily in the mother include (1) ectopic pregnancy, (2) hyperemesis gravidarum, (3) preeclampsia, (4) HELLP syndrome (see later), (5) liver disease, and (6) hemolytic disease of the newborn. The clinician must distinguish abnormal changes in laboratory tests from normal physiologic changes induced by pregnancy (see Table 69.2).

Ectopic Pregnancy and Threatened Abortion

When a fertilized egg implants in a location other than the body of the uterus, the condition is called an *ectopic pregnancy.* Most abnormal implantations occur in the fallopian tube; they can also occur in the abdomen, although this is rare. Common symptoms of ectopic pregnancy include abdominal pain, vaginal bleeding, and adnexal mass. Tubal rupture from the expanding nondistensible fallopian tube can cause a life-threatening hemorrhage and is a common cause of maternal death from ectopic pregnancy. From 2006–2010 there were 16.0 pregnancy-related deaths per 100,000 live births in the United States; 3% were due to ectopic pregnancy.[43] Management of ectopic pregnancy can be surgical or medical (with methotrexate).[44,45] Early detection and proper management of ectopic pregnancy are the most effective means of preventing maternal morbidity and mortality.

Ultrasound examination is used to evaluate women with symptoms. When ultrasound is nondiagnostic, quantitative measurements of serum hCG are used to identify women with ectopic pregnancy or abnormal intrauterine pregnancy. These conditions frequently produce abnormal hCG concentrations and slow rates of increase[46] (see At a Glance: Evaluation of Ectopic Pregnancy).

An accurate gestational age is the best predictor of when an intrauterine pregnancy should be detected with transvaginal ultrasound. Failure to detect a gestational sac by sonography 24 days or longer after conception is presumptive evidence of an ectopic pregnancy or fetal demise.[47] An intrauterine pregnancy should be visible by ultrasonography at an hCG concentration of 1500 to 2000 IU/L, but this concentration has a clinical sensitivity of only 42% and a clinical specificity of 81% for the detection of ectopic pregnancy when no intrauterine gestational sac is visualized.[48]

When hCG concentrations are less than 1500 IU/L and ultrasonography is nondiagnostic, serial testing of hCG is used clinically. In normal intrauterine pregnancy, during the second through fifth weeks, the hCG doubles every 48 hours. After 5 weeks' gestation, the doubling time gradually lengthens to 2 to 3 days.[49] An increase in hCG of at least 53% over 48 hours is 99% specific for excluding an ectopic pregnancy,[50] but as many as 35% of ectopic gestations produce an increase greater than this.[51] hCG can be followed if rising appropriately until the discriminatory zone of 1500 to 2000 IU/L is reached, at which point ultrasonography can be repeated. If hCG does not increase appropriately, the differential diagnosis includes pregnancy failure and ectopic pregnancy, and repeat ultrasonographic examinations to rule out ectopic pregnancy should be undertaken.

The serum progesterone concentration is often low in mothers with an abnormal pregnancy.[52] For example, a serum progesterone level of less than 6 ng/mL (19.1 nmol/L) predicts an abnormal pregnancy outcome with 81% confidence for asymptomatic women within 8 weeks of their last menses,[53] but an average serum progesterone level in nonviable pregnancies was 10 ng/mL (31.8 nmol/L). For women with clinical symptoms of abnormal pregnancy, measurement of both hCG and progesterone is more predictive of abnormal pregnancy than a single hCG measurement. In a large outcome study, 97% of the patients with hCG of less than 3000 IU/L and progesterone of less than 12.6 ng/mL (40.1 nmol/L) had an abnormal pregnancy outcome, whereas those with hCG greater than 3000 IU/L or progesterone greater than 12.6 ng/mL (40.1 nmol/L) had a normal pregnancy.[54] McCord and associates[55] reported that in women at risk for ectopic pregnancy, a progesterone cutoff of 17.5 ng/mL (55.7 nmol/L) detected 92% of ectopic cases (clinical sensitivity), but had a very poor clinical specificity of about 14%. Investigators concluded that patients with progesterone levels greater than 17.5 ng/mL (55.7 nmol/L) needed no additional laboratory tests. A progesterone cutoff above 8 ng/mL (25.4 nmol/L) had a clinical sensitivity of 81% and a clinical specificity of 88%. In general, progesterone concentrations of 25 ng/mL (79.5 nmol/L) or more are associated with a viable intrauterine pregnancy.[56]

Preeclampsia and Eclampsia

Preeclampsia is a pregnancy condition characterized by hypertension and other end-organ involvement, including

AT A GLANCE

Evaluation of Ectopic Pregnancy

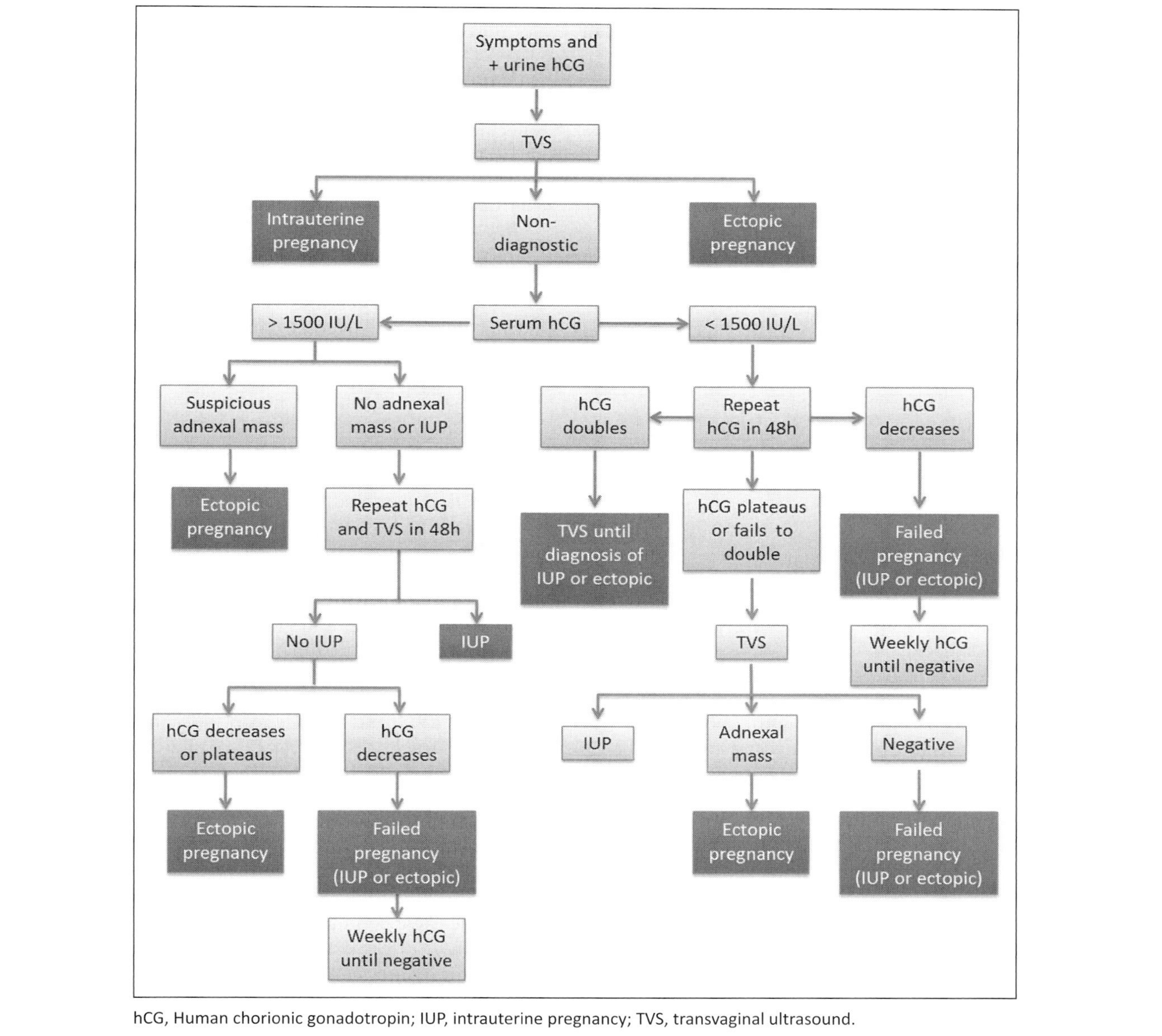

hCG, Human chorionic gonadotropin; IUP, intrauterine pregnancy; TVS, transvaginal ultrasound.

Modified from Gala RB. Ectopic pregnancy. In: *Williams gynecology*. New York: McGraw-Hill; 2008.

proteinuria, cerebral vasospasm, hematologic abnormalities such as hemolysis and thrombocytopenia, and transaminitis. It can occur any time after 20 weeks (although there are cases of preeclampsia occurring at less than 20 weeks in abnormal pregnancies such as molar pregnancies). It affects 3% to 5% of pregnancies and continues to be a major cause of maternal and perinatal mortality.[57,58] If the mother develops generalized seizures, the condition is called eclampsia.

The disorder manifests with placental ischemia and endothelial dysfunction that leads to intravascular deposition of fibrin with subsequent end-organ damage.[59] Most maternal deaths are due to central nervous system complications, but ischemic liver damage may also occur. The only cure for preeclampsia is delivery of the placenta.[60]

The cause of preeclampsia has not been elucidated,[60] but research suggests that increased circulating soluble fms-like tyrosine kinase 1 (sFlt-1) may have a role.[61] Although there are currently no effective preventive measures or treatments for preeclampsia, the ability to predict who will develop preeclampsia could allow for the development of preventive medicines. Therefore, many biomarkers have been examined in an attempt to predict the onset of preeclampsia. The most promising of these are angiogenic factors such as vascular endothelial growth factor, placental growth factor, sFlt-1, and soluble endoglin. Several studies have shown that aberrant expression of these angiogenic factors precedes the onset of preeclampsia.[61-64] A systematic review of 34 studies on these markers found significant differences in marker concentrations before 30 weeks' gestation between women who developed preeclampsia and women who remained healthy.[65] While these differences were statistically different, little difference was seen prior to 16 weeks' gestation and the poor sensitivity and specificity of individual factors suggested that these markers are not clinically useful for early prediction of preeclampsia. Ongoing research is investigating the possibility of combining biomarkers to increase their predictive capabilities.

AT A GLANCE

Diagnostic Criteria for Preeclampsia

Mild Preeclampsia	Severe Preeclampsia
Hypertension: Blood pressure ≥ 140/90 mm Hg (or mean arterial pressure of ≥105 mm Hg) **AND** Proteinuria: ≥300 mg of protein in 24-h urine collection or ≥1+ protein on urine dipstick **OR**	Systolic blood pressure of ≥160 mm Hg and/or diastolic blood pressure of ≥110 mm Hg on two occasions 6 h apart
In patients with hypertension in the absence of proteinuria, new onset of any of the following is diagnostic of preeclampsia:	Oliguria (<500 mL in 24 h)
Platelet count <100,000/µl	Cerebral or visual disturbances
Serum creatinine >1.1 mg/dL [97 µmol/L] or doubling of serum creatinine in the absence of other renal disease	Pulmonary edema or cyanosis
Liver transaminases elevated to twice the normal concentration	Epigastric or right upper–quadrant pain
Pulmonary edema	Impaired liver function
Cerebral or visual symptoms	Thrombocytopenia

Modified from Hypertension in pregnancy: report of the American College of Obstetricians and Gynecologists' Task Force on Hypertension in Pregnancy. *Obstet Gynecol* 2013;122:1122.

HELLP Syndrome

The HELLP syndrome (*h*emolysis, *e*levated *l*iver enzymes, and *l*ow platelet counts in association with *p*reeclampsia) is a life-threatening obstetric complication that occurs in 0.1% of pregnancies. Its most prominent features are thrombocytopenia and disseminated intravascular coagulation (see Chapter 71). Most cases occur between 27 and 36 weeks' gestation, but the syndrome also may occur postpartum. Women typically present with epigastric or right upper quadrant pain, malaise, nausea, vomiting, and headache.[67,68] Jaundice occurs in 5% of patients. Lactate dehydrogenase values may be very high, reflecting high levels of red blood cell hemolysis, and alanine aminotransferase (ALT) and aspartate aminotransferase (AST) are usually 2 to 10 times their upper reference limits. Treatment is delivery. Recurrence rates are 3% to 27%.

Liver Disease

Several liver disorders are unique to pregnancy.[69,70] These include (1) hyperemesis gravidarum, (2) cholestasis of pregnancy, and (3) fatty liver of pregnancy. These disorders must be distinguished from the normal physiologic changes of pregnancy (see Table 69.2). Significant changes normally seen in pregnancy include a dilutional decrease in serum albumin and an increase of alkaline phosphatase (from the placenta). Notably, total bilirubin, 5′-nucleotidase, gamma-glutamyl transpeptidase, ALT, and AST are unchanged in mothers with a normal pregnancy. Changes in these analytes reflect hepatobiliary disease. Also discussed in this section are (1) non–pregnancy-related liver disease in pregnancy, (2) differential diagnosis, and (3) effect of pregnancy on preexisting liver disease.

Hyperemesis Gravidarum. Hyperemesis gravidarum is characterized by nausea and vomiting and, in severe cases, dehydration and malnutrition. It typically occurs in the first trimester. When hyperemesis is severe enough to cause dehydration, abnormal liver enzyme values—usually less than four times the upper reference limit—are seen in approximately 50% of patients.[70] Mild hyperbilirubinemia may occur. However, significant liver disease does not occur, and liver biopsy results are normal. Low-birth-weight babies are common, especially for women who develop malnutrition.

During pregnancy, increased hCG concentrations are associated with suppressed thyroid-stimulating hormone (TSH) concentrations. hCG has thyrotropic effects and can bind TSH receptors and suppress TSH production. TSH is frequently suppressed in patients with highly increased concentrations of hCG that occur with hyperemesis gravidarum, gestational trophoblastic disease, and choriocarcinoma. Lockwood and colleagues demonstrated that at hCG concentrations of more than 400,000 IU/L, TSH is consistently suppressed (≤0.2 µIU/mL). Interestingly, most patients with hCG concentrations of more than 200,000 IU/L lack overt hyperthyroid symptoms.[71]

Cholestasis of Pregnancy. Pregnancy does not preclude the acquisition or aggravation of non—pregnancy-related liver disease. Thus, cholestasis during pregnancy may reflect the presence of (1) hepatotoxicity from drugs, (2) primary biliary cirrhosis, (3) Dubin-Johnson syndrome, or (4) cholelithiasis (see Chapter 61). Abdominal ultrasound, endoscopic retrograde cholangiography, or liver biopsy may be necessary to exclude these conditions.

The onset of cholestasis during pregnancy usually occurs in the third trimester and is manifested clinically by diffuse pruritus and, in 10% of patients, jaundice. The typical features of cholestasis, including pale stools and dark urine, are present and last until delivery. Women who experience cholestasis while taking oral contraceptives usually develop cholestasis of pregnancy. The serum bilirubin rarely exceeds 5 mg/dL (85.5 µmol/L). Alkaline phosphatase is typically two to four times the upper reference limit. Aminotransferase enzyme concentrations are mildly increased and may precede the increase of bile acids. The prothrombin time may be increased because of vitamin K malabsorption. Although many clinicians order serum bile acids in this setting,[72] this test is offered by only a few clinical laboratories, often requiring the diagnosis to be made on clinical symptoms. The condition is associated with an increased risk for preterm delivery and possibly fetal death, and has an increased risk for recurrence with subsequent pregnancies.[73]

Fatty Liver of Pregnancy. Fatty liver of pregnancy occurs in approximately 1 in 10,000 pregnancies and is characterized by accumulation of microvesicular fat in the hepatocytes.[74]

Many of the cases of this maternal disorder are caused by an inherited mitochondrial fatty acid oxidation disorder in the fetus, long-chain 3-hydroxyacyl-CoA dehydrogenase deficiency.[75] Mothers carrying fetuses with this disorder are 50 times more likely to develop fatty liver of pregnancy.[76] The disease typically occurs at week 37 and is manifested clinically by the rapid onset of malaise, nausea, vomiting, and abdominal pain. Mild increases in aminotransferase enzyme concentrations occur, with the AST increase typically greater than that of ALT but both typically less than six times the upper reference interval. Serum bilirubin is usually greater than 6 mg/dL (102.6 μmol/L). Life-threatening hypoglycemia may occur.[59] Hyperuricemia, presumably from tissue destruction and renal failure, is characteristic. Liver histology shows acute fatty infiltration with little necrosis or inflammation. The fat is microvesicular and pericentral in the cell, similar to what is seen in Reye syndrome. If untreated, fulminant hepatic failure with hepatic encephalopathy ensues. Treatment is immediate delivery, at which time rapid recovery usually occurs. The infant and maternal mortality rates are approximately 50% and 20%, respectively.

Differential Diagnosis. It is often difficult to distinguish the various liver diseases of pregnancy from each other and from naturally occurring liver diseases not unique to pregnancy. Acute fatty liver is suggested when nausea, vomiting, and abdominal pain are followed by jaundice, hypoglycemia, and encephalopathy that occurs in the presence of a small or normal-sized liver. The white blood cell count is usually increased above 15,000 cells/μL and ALT concentrations are typically four to six times the upper reference interval. Hypoalbuminemia, hyperuricemia, hypoglycemia, and DIC are typical. Hepatic ultrasound and computed tomography usually demonstrate fatty liver when present. In preeclampsia and the HELLP syndrome, the liver is usually enlarged, ALT concentrations are usually lower, bilirubin concentrations are mildly increased or normal, glucose is normal, and hypertension is present; in the absence of eclampsia, mentation is normal. Hyperuricemia is uncommon. Marked increases in aminotransferase enzyme concentrations suggest hepatic infarction or viral hepatitis (see below). Liver biopsy may be needed to differentiate non–pregnancy-related causes of liver disease, but should not be used to differentiate acute fatty liver from preeclampsia or HELLP syndrome because the treatment is the same for all of these conditions—delivery of the infant.[77]

Effect of Pregnancy on Preexisting Liver Disease. Conception and full-term parturition do not usually occur in women who have cirrhosis. However, liver disease is not a reason for termination. The hypervolemia associated with pregnancy may aggravate cirrhosis and predispose to bleeding from esophageal varices.[78]

Autoimmune chronic hepatitis is usually associated with amenorrhea, but pregnancy may occur after treatment to remission with corticosteroids.

Neonatal Thyroid Function

During the first trimester of pregnancy, the fetus is dependent on the mother for its supply of thyroid hormone. Low maternal thyroid hormone concentrations (overt or subclinical hypothyroidism) have been associated with adverse outcomes, such as preterm delivery,[79] fetal death, and a reduced IQ in children.[80,81] Women with untreated thyroid deficiency in pregnancy are also more likely to have permanent hypothyroidism after pregnancy (64%) than are euthyroid mothers.[80]

Later in pregnancy, the fetal thyroid–pituitary axis functions independently from the mother's axis in most cases. However, if the mother has preexisting Graves' disease (see Chapter 67), her IgG autoantibodies can cross the placenta and stimulate the fetal thyroid gland. Thus the fetus can develop hyperthyroidism. Measurement of TSH-receptor antibodies by thyrotropin-binding inhibitory immunoglobulin or thyroid-stimulating immunoglobulin assay is useful for assessing the risk of fetal or neonatal Graves' disease.

An association between an underactive thyroid gland during pregnancy and delayed neurodevelopment in the offspring is well known. In 1999, Haddow and colleagues suggested that even subclinical hypothyroidism could result in a lower IQ in the offspring of affected women.[80] For this reason, there has been discussion about routine screening of pregnant women for thyroid function. The American Association of Clinical Endocrinologists guidelines indicate that TSH screening should be routine before pregnancy or during the first trimester, and if the TSH is more than 10 mIU/L or if the TSH is 5 to 10 mIU/L and the patient has goiter or positive anti–thyroid peroxidase antibodies, then thyroid hormone replacement therapy should be initiated.[82] In contrast, the American Thyroid Association and the Endocrine Society only recommend screening pregnant women who are at high risk of overt hypothyroidism (eg, history of thyroid dysfunction, thyroid peroxidase antibodies positive, goiter).[83] If the TSH is more than 10 mIU/L, the guidelines suggest that thyroid hormone replacement therapy be initiated. The American College of Obstetricians and Gynecologists (ACOG) has recommended against screening all pregnant women for hypothyroidism, as there is lack of evidence that treatment of women with subclinical hypothyroidism will improve maternal or infant outcomes.[84] Regardless, when thyroid hormone is tested, the results should be interpreted using pregnancy-specific reference intervals.[85]

Hemolytic Disease of the Newborn

Hemolytic disease of the newborn (HDN) is a fetal hemolytic disorder caused by maternal antibodies directed against antigen on fetal erythrocytes. Commonly used synonyms for this disorder are *isoimmunization disease, Rh isoimmune disease, Rh disease,* or *D isoimmunization.* Any of a large number of erythrocyte surface antigens—Rh (CcDEe), A, B, Kell, Duffy, Kidd, and others—may be responsible for isoimmune hemolysis. When severe, the disorder is known as *erythroblastosis fetalis* and is life-threatening to the fetus and newborn. In the past, disease severity was assessed by measuring the amount of bilirubin in the amniotic fluid, and a description of methods for measurement of amniotic fluid bilirubin is available in previous editions of this textbook. This method is no longer widely practiced, however. Presently, the noninvasive ultrasonographic determination of middle fetal cerebral artery velocity has replaced amniotic fluid bilirubin measurements.[86,87]

Rh Blood Groups. Two genes, *RhD* and *RhCE,* encode for erythrocyte membrane proteins that are antigenic. Both are located on chromosome 1p about 30 kb apart. Approximately 15% of Caucasians, 5% of Africans, and less than 1% of Asians are RhD negative. The most prevalent RhD-negative allele is a deletion.[88] Exon 5 of *RhCE* has two common polymorphisms producing *E* or *e* antigen. Exon 2 of *RhCE* has two common polymorphisms producing *C* or *c* antigen.

Etiology. Maternal sensitization may occur in response to a blood transfusion or a pregnancy in which the mother is exposed to fetal red blood cells carrying the antigen that the mother lacks. Antibodies against RhD are the most common cause of HDN, although antibodies against other erythrocyte antigens can also cause disease.

The resulting maternal antibodies are actively transported across the placenta and into the fetus, where they cause destruction of the fetal erythrocytes. The severity of the resulting hemolysis is influenced by antibody specificity, titer, and transfer rate, as well as the functional maturity of the fetal spleen in which the sensitized erythrocytes are destroyed.

Destruction of the fetal erythrocytes, which is the central problem, produces several other problems. For example, fetal anemia imposes an extra burden on the fetal heart to provide an adequate oxygen supply to fetal tissues. Anemia stimulates the fetal marrow and extramedullary erythropoiesis in the liver and spleen to replace the destroyed erythrocytes. Extramedullary erythropoiesis destroys hepatocytes and leads to decreased production of serum albumin and decreased oncotic pressure in the intravascular space.

When severe, the composite outcome of these is high-output congestive heart failure and generalized fetal edema, a condition referred to as *hydrops fetalis,* which carries a very grave prognosis. Without therapeutic intervention via red blood cell transfusion into the umbilical cord, intrauterine demise soon follows.

If a fetus survives, the newborn will encounter a number of problems. While the fetus is in utero, the placenta and mother perform the functions of respiration and removal of bilirubinoid pigments resulting from hemolysis. Newborns must assume these functions for themselves in the presence of hydrops. The lungs are edematous, and pleural effusions and ascites physically restrict their ability to expand. The damaged liver is unable to conjugate and excrete bilirubin adequately. When bilirubin accumulates in the blood to excessive concentrations, it passes through the blood-brain barrier to deposit in the brain and destroy brain cells. This form of brain damage is termed *kernicterus.* Although kernicterus was not a concern in the hydropic fetus, it is a significant concern in these sick newborns. A severely erythroblastotic baby can be one of the most challenging cases in a neonatal intensive care unit.

Prophylaxis. An anti-RhD immune globulin, RhoGAM (Ortho Clinical Diagnostics, Raritan, New Jersey), has been used in the United States since 1968;[89] other similar products were introduced in 1971 and later. A 300-µg dose is administered intramuscularly to a mother potentially exposed to 15 mL or less of RhD-positive fetal erythrocytes following abortion, fetomaternal hemorrhage, amniocentesis, chorionic villus sampling (CVS), or delivery.[86] Use of anti-RhD immune globulin has been responsible for the dramatic reduction in the incidence of HDN. In addition to recognized fetomaternal hemorrhage, undetected transplacental fetomaternal bleeding during an apparently normal pregnancy can lead to antepartum sensitization. This would not be prevented by immediate postpartum administration of RhD immunoglobulin; therefore, antepartum administration at 28 weeks' gestation is recommended for RhD-negative women. Despite this immune prophylaxis, a small number of sensitized pregnancies continue to occur.

Clinical Management of Mothers Sensitized to RhD. To identify sensitized women, an alloantibody screen is performed at the first prenatal visit.[90] If an antibody to an erythrocyte antigen is identified, the titer is determined.[86] The critical anti-RhD titer, defined as the titer associated with risk for fetal hydrops, is usually 1:8 to 1:32, although studies of critical titer are quite disparate.[91] For all sensitized women, the paternal erythrocyte phenotype is determined. If the father is homozygous RhD-negative, then no follow-up studies are required. If he is D-positive, then zygosity is determined. Although this has historically been estimated from Rh antigen phenotypes (D, C/c, E/e) in conjunction with gene frequency tables based on race, DNA testing for RhD zygosity is more reliable. If the father is homozygous, then all of his offspring can be assumed to be RhD positive, negating the need for fetal RhD testing. Fetal RhD genotyping from cultured amniocytes is required if the father is heterozygous or is not available for testing. To guard against a false negative caused by a paternal RhD gene rearrangement (occurring in about 1.5% of Caucasians), the father can also be genotyped. A frequent occurrence in those of African ancestry is an RhD pseudogene; the patient is RhD-negative by serology, but RhD-positive on genotype. If the fetus is RhD-genotype–positive, the mother (who is RhD-negative serologically) should be tested for her RhD genotype. In the United States, as well as other parts of the world, fetal Rh genotyping using cell-free fetal DNA that circulates in maternal blood is now available (see Chapter 53).[92]

For sensitized mothers with an at-risk fetus, serial titers are performed on maternal serum every month until 24 weeks' gestation, and then every 2 weeks thereafter. If a critical titer of anti-D is detected, ultrasound Doppler measurements are used to determine the peak velocity of blood flow in the fetal middle cerebral artery. Higher velocity is a strong indicator of fetal anemia. Historically, amniocentesis was performed every 10 to 14 days to assess the bilirubin concentration in amniotic fluid. The procedure was originally called ΔOD_{450},[93] but the preferred clinical chemistry term is ΔA_{450}. Therapy for fetal anemia involves intrauterine percutaneous umbilical cord red blood cell transfusion. If fetal hydrops develops later in gestation (weeks 35 or beyond) or multiple transfusions have been required over the course of the pregnancy, delivery timing is decided balancing the risks of continued intrauterine development versus the risk for prematurity.

Trophoblastic Disease

Serum hCG determinations are very useful for monitoring patients with germ cell–derived neoplasms or other hCG-producing tumors, such as lung carcinoma. The use of hCG in these diseases is discussed in Chapter 31.

Vertically Transmitted Infections

Infections acquired during pregnancy and birth are significant contributors to fetal and neonatal morbidity and mortality rates. Testing is widely available to screen for many causes of perinatal and intrapartum infections. Timely recognition of infection is critical to initiate appropriate therapy to prevent transmission or limit congenital defects in the fetus or neonate.

TORCH Infections

TORCH infections refer to a group of infectious diseases that commonly cause in utero infections. The TORCH acronym typically includes the diseases (1) *t*oxoplasmosis, (2) *o*ther infections, (3) *r*ubella, (4) *c*ytomegalovirus, and (5) *h*erpes simplex virus. Historically, this term referred to pathogens that caused diseases with a similar presentation of rash and ocular findings.[94] However, the "other" category has expanded to include pathogens such as varicella zoster virus (VZV), syphilis, and parvovirus B19, with a wide variety of symptoms.

Screening for TORCH infections is useful for discriminating between recent or prior infection and for identifying women who lack immunity to a disease. Women who lack immunity are vaccinated or counseled on the use of infection-control practices to prevent infection during pregnancy.[95]

Toxoplasmosis. Toxoplasmosis is caused by the parasite *Toxoplasma gondii,* which is acquired orally via the consumption of undercooked meats or unpasteurized dairy products and through contact with cysts shed in cat feces. Prior infection in the mother usually results in lasting immunity and protection of the fetus. However, primary infection during pregnancy may result in congenital toxoplasmosis if transmission of parasites across the placenta occurs.[96] Most infants with congenital toxoplasmosis have asymptomatic or subclinical disease. If left untreated, infection can lead to vision loss, intellectual disability, deafness, and seizures in affected children.

Maternal serologic screening for toxoplasmosis is not routinely done in the United States, although screening programs are in place in other countries with a higher prevalence of disease. Maternal screening should be completed as part of the diagnostic workup if a pregnant woman experiences a mononucleosis-like illness but has a negative heterophile test[97] or if fetal abnormalities are detected by ultrasound.[98] The diagnosis of maternal infection is based on the detection of *Toxoplasma*-specific antibodies. A positive IgM result concurrent with a negative IgG finding may occur during early acute infection or may be a false positive. If IgG remains negative upon retesting after 2 weeks, the IgM is likely a false positive. The presence of *Toxoplasma*-specific IgM and IgG does not reliably predict recent infection, as IgM antibodies may remain detectable for up to 2 years after primary infection in a substantial portion of women.[99] Therefore, IgG avidity testing may be performed in a pregnant woman in the first 12 to 16 weeks of gestation. A high IgG avidity largely rules out an infection acquired during gestation; however, low IgG avidity does not necessarily indicate recent infection, as low avidity can persist for years in some women.[100,101]

Other Infections (Syphilis, Parvovirus Infection, Varicella Zoster Virus Infection). The "other" category in the TORCH acronym encompasses a host of vertically transmitted infections such as syphilis, parvovirus B19 infection, and VZV infection.

Syphilis. Congenital syphilis, caused by the bacteria *Treponema pallidum,* can result in stillbirth, hydrops fetalis, or prematurity. Because of the severe morbidity associated with the infection, routine syphilis screening is recommended for all pregnant women. The Centers for Disease Control and Prevention (CDC) recommends screening during the first prenatal visit, and rescreening in the third trimester is recommended in high-risk women, those who live in areas with a high syphilis prevalence, and those who were previously untested.[102]

Serologic testing methods for syphilis include treponemal-specific and nontreponemal tests. Treponemal tests include the *T. pallidum* particle agglutination (TP-PA) test and the fluorescent treponemal antibody absorption (FTA-Abs) test. These are confirmatory tests that detect antibodies against treponemal cellular components. Although they display excellent sensitivity and specificity, they are labor intensive and cannot be used to follow disease, because they remain positive even with treatment. Nontreponemal tests, including venereal disease research laboratory and rapid plasma reagin tests, detect antibodies to a cardiolipin-cholesterol-lecithin antigen produced in response to syphilis infection. Although these tests lack specificity, they are rapid and inexpensive and can be used to detect active infection and monitor effective treatment. Dilution of samples should be considered in patients with a high clinical suspicion for syphilis due to a potential hook effect with the rapid plasma reagin and venereal disease research laboratory tests.[103,104] In most settings, nontreponemal testing is used for initial screening and positive results are confirmed by treponemal-specific testing.[105] Because treponemal-specific testing using enzyme immunoassay (TP-EIA) can be automated and is often less expensive, some laboratories have initiated a reverse screening approach in which treponemal testing is followed up with a nontreponemal test.[106] However, because of the prevalence of syphilis in the United States, the use of a treponemal assay as a screening test yields a low positive predictive value.[107]

Parvovirus B19 Infection. Although 35% to 65% of pregnant women have antibodies to parvovirus B19,[108,109] an acute infection of a susceptible woman during pregnancy may lead to fetal loss or hydrops fetalis. Parvovirus B19 infects erythroid precursor cells in the fetus and causes fetal anemia and resulting hydrops. Although routine screening is not performed because clinical screening and treatment for fetal anemia is available, pregnant women who are exposed to or exhibit symptoms of parvovirus infection should undergo serologic testing for parvovirus B19-specific IgG and IgM to determine if they are susceptible to or have a current infection. If maternal diagnosis is inconclusive and clinical suspicion of fetal infection is high, detection of parvovirus B19 DNA by PCR in amniotic fluid can confirm the diagnosis of fetal infection.[110] After diagnosis of an acute infection, fetal surveillance for the development of fetal anemia (Doppler velocity of the middle cerebral artery) is undertaken. If anemia develops, the fetus can undergo treatment with intracordal red blood cell transfusion.

Varicella Zoster Virus Infection. VZV is a herpesvirus that causes distinct forms of disease. Primary infection results in a vesicular rash known as varicella (chickenpox). Later, reactivation of latent VZV causes herpes zoster (shingles). Primary infection acquired during early pregnancy may result in congenital varicella syndrome, which is characterized by skin lesions, eye disease, skeletal abnormalities, and neurologic defects.[111] Additionally, acute primary varicella is associated with a significant risk for maternal death because infections during pregnancy are associated with a higher risk for encephalitis and pneumonia than adult infections outside of pregnancy. Reactivation of latent infection in the mother is not associated with development of congenital varicella syndrome.

The incidence of varicella among adults declined in the United States after the introduction of the varicella vaccine in 1995.[112] The varicella immunity status of pregnant women should be established by verification of previous infection or vaccination by history or through serologic testing. Although the risk of transmission of primary VZV infection during pregnancy is small, the outcome is severe. If exposed to VZV, a seronegative woman should be given VZV immunoglobulin to decrease the risk of development of congenital varicella syndrome in the fetus.[111] If fetal infection is suspected, detection of VZV DNA by PCR of amniotic fluid and ultrasound evaluation for fetal abnormalities such as microcephaly or intrauterine growth restriction are useful in the assessment of congenital varicella syndrome in the fetus of an infected mother.[113]

Rubella. Rubella infection of adults or children causes symptoms including rash, headache, and fever that are usually mild or subclinical; however, maternal-to-fetal transmission of the virus can cause serious fetal defects, including miscarriage, stillbirth, and congenital rubella syndrome. Infants with congenital rubella syndrome frequently exhibit congenital heart defects, hearing impairment, and eye abnormalities.[114] These defects are mostly limited to maternal infections that are acquired before 16 weeks' gestation.[115] Congenital rubella syndrome is very rare in developed countries with established rubella vaccination programs.

In general, vaccination or previous infection is protective against intrauterine rubella infection. Therefore, serologic testing for rubella-specific IgG in pregnant women is recommended to assess rubella immunity status. If a woman is identified as nonimmune, the recommendation is for vaccination with measles, mumps, and rubella vaccine in the postpartum period. The CDC does not recommend testing for IgM, because of the high rate of false positives that occur as a result of the low prevalence of the infection in the United States.[116]

Cytomegalovirus Infection. Human cytomegalovirus (CMV) is a ubiquitous virus that is the most common cause of congenital viral infection. Approximately 40,000 infants are born with congenital CMV infection annually in the United States. The highest risk for maternal-to-fetal transmission of CMV occurs during primary infection. However, recurrent infection during pregnancy can also result in CMV transmission to a fetus.[117] The majority of congenital infections are asymptomatic, but around 10% of infants born to women with primary CMV infection have symptoms[118] that range from jaundice and petechial rash at birth to later complications such as hearing loss, vision impairment, and developmental delays in surviving infants.

Currently, no professional organization or governmental agency worldwide recommends prenatal CMV testing to establish the serologic status of pregnant women, because no effective vaccine and no useful treatment are available.[119] Serologic testing is routinely performed in some countries in Europe, however.[120] Additionally, maternal antibodies do not prevent reinfection or reactivation of CMV; thus, the potential for fetal transmission is still possible. Instead, women should be counseled on infection-control practices such as proper hand hygiene, because most CMV infections in pregnant women are acquired from contact with bodily fluids such as saliva and the urine of infected children.[95] This practice has been shown to reduce the CMV seroconversion rate in women during pregnancy.[121]

If primary maternal CMV infection is suspected, demonstration of seroconversion can confirm the diagnosis. However, such confirmation is only occasionally achieved due to the lack of routine antenatal screening for CMV. CMV-specific IgM is a highly sensitive but not specific marker of primary CMV infection, because CMV IgM can be present during primary infection, reinfection, or reactivation. Therefore, measurement of CMV IgG avidity has been used as a specific indicator of primary CMV infection. If measured before 16 weeks' gestation, high anti-CMV IgG avidity indicates that CMV infection likely occurred prior to conception.[122,123] The presence of low-avidity CMV-specific IgG in combination with CMV-specific IgM is highly suggestive of a recent primary CMV infection.[124] For more information on the diagnosis of and laboratory testing for CMV infection in children or adults, see Chapter 48.

Herpes Simplex Virus Infection. Herpes simplex virus (HSV) infection is widespread among women of childbearing age, and transmission of the virus to a neonate is a cause of major illness and even death. Infected infants may have localized infections of the mouth, eyes, or skin, and others have central nervous system disease or disseminated infection. The risk of transmission of genital HSV from an infected mother to her fetus is much higher when infection is acquired near the time of delivery.[125,126] Maternal genital HSV infection that is acquired earlier in pregnancy does not increase the rates of neonatal infection if HSV seroconversion has been completed before labor begins.[127] Diagnostic testing methods for HSV include viral culture, immunohistochemical staining, serologic testing, and nucleic acid testing (see Chapters 48 and 79).

Perinatal Infections

Besides TORCH infections, there are a number of infectious agents that can cause severe neonatal complications upon maternal-to-fetal transmission. These include (1) human immunodeficiency virus (HIV), (2) hepatitis B virus, (3) chlamydia and gonorrhea, and (4) group B *Streptococcus.*

Human Immunodeficiency Virus Infection. Human immunodeficiency virus (HIV) causes acquired immunodeficiency disease (AIDS). About half of the estimated 38 million people worldwide infected with HIV are women of childbearing age, with an overwhelming majority of those living in sub-Saharan Africa.[128] Most children living with HIV were infected by mother-to-child transmission during pregnancy or the perinatal period. Approximately 8700 babies are born to HIV-infected women each year in the United States,[129] and many of those women are unaware of their HIV status. Therefore, the CDC recommends that all pregnant women should be screened for HIV early in pregnancy, and retesting is recommended during the third trimester for women with a high risk of acquiring HIV infection.[130,131] In the United States, women should be screened using an opt-out approach, meaning a woman is notified that she will be tested for HIV as part of routine prenatal testing unless she declines. A review of HIV testing strategies across Europe found that 14 of 24 countries surveyed routinely offer universal screening for HIV using the opt-out approach.[132]

Third-generation screening tests for HIV consist of serologic testing for HIV IgM and IgG antibody detection. Fourth-generation assays also include virologic testing against the p24 antigen, which shortens the window period for detection of acute infection by several days.[133,134] Prenatal HIV screening has reduced perinatal HIV infection because women who test positive can be started on antiretroviral therapy and managed appropriately during delivery to reduce the risk of transmission.[135] For more information on laboratory testing methods available for the management of HIV-positive patients, see Chapters 48 and 79.

Viral Hepatitis. Viral hepatitis occurs with the same frequency in pregnancy as would be expected in a comparable age group.[136] Symptoms include malaise, nausea, vomiting, dark urine, and mild fever. The AST and ALT levels are virtually always greater than 10 times the upper reference interval and usually greater than 20 times the upper reference interval.

Women who acquire hepatitis B late in pregnancy or who are chronic carriers are more likely to transmit the disease to their babies. This is especially so if the mother is HBeAg positive (see Chapter 61). Possible outcomes in the infant include rare occurrences of fulminant hepatitis, mild hepatitis, and chronic hepatitis, which occur in up to 90% of HBeAg-positive women. All pregnant women should be screened for hepatitis B with HBsAg.[30] If positive, their babies should be immunized with hepatitis B immune globulin in addition to the hepatitis B vaccine. Vertical transmission of hepatitis C has been documented, and the overall risk of transmission is about 5%, with higher rates in some subgroups, such as women coinfected with HIV.[137] Because there is no available treatment for the newborn and because a significant proportion of infants with vertically acquired infection clear the infection, screening is recommended only for women with specific risk factors, such as HIV infection or intravenous drug use.

Chlamydial Infection and Gonorrhea. *Chlamydia trachomatis* and *Neisseria gonorrheae* are bacteria that are among the most commonly reported causes of sexually transmitted disease. Complications of chlamydial infection include ectopic pregnancy and infertility, and transmission of *Chlamydia* to a neonate via the birth canal of an infected woman can lead to conjunctivitis and pneumonia. Gonococcal infection of a pregnant woman is associated with premature rupture of membranes, preterm birth, and spontaneous abortion. Perinatal infection of a neonate most commonly causes conjunctivitis, though localized infection of other mucosal surfaces may arise. The CDC recommends that all pregnant women be screened for chlamydial infection during the initial prenatal visit, while screening for gonorrhea is recommended for pregnant women at risk for gonococcal infection or those living in a high prevalence area. Nucleic acid testing methods for detection of chlamydial infection and gonorrhea exhibit high analytical sensitivity and specificity and are described in detail in Chapter 48.

Group B Streptococcus. Group B streptococcus (GBS or *Streptococcus agalactiae*) is a gram-positive bacterium that is the most common cause of bacterial perinatal infections.[138] GBS colonizes the vagina and rectum of pregnant women, and vertical transmission occurs if GBS invades the amniotic fluid after the onset of labor or rupture of the membranes. Although colonized women are asymptomatic and GBS is considered a normal transient vaginal microbe, early-onset GBS infection in neonates is characterized by sepsis, pneumonia, or meningitis. Neonatal infection can be minimized by administration of antibiotics to colonized women during delivery.

The CDC recommends that all pregnant women be screened by rectovaginal culture for GBS colonization at 35 to 37 weeks' gestation. A rapid screening method is needed for women with no prenatal care or those who deliver before testing is completed. Current work is focused on molecular techniques such as DNA-based RT-PCR.[139] Although there are FDA-approved rapid tests available, they are not commonly used due to their cost and the need for continuous availability in the laboratory.[138] Details about GBS testing methods are described in Chapter 48.

Trichomonas *Infection.* Trichomoniasis is an infection of the urogenital tract caused by the protozoan *Trichomonas vaginalis.* The organism has been linked to an increased risk for preterm birth, premature rupture of membranes, and delivery of an infant with a decreased birth weight in infected women.[140] Rarely, vertical transmission can occur during delivery, leading to vaginitis, urinary tract infection, or respiratory distress. Screening for *Trichomonas* is not recommended as part of routine prenatal care in asymptomatic women.[102] However, because of possible adverse outcomes in pregnancy, pregnant women exhibiting symptoms of *Trichomonas* infection should be evaluated and treated appropriately.

Preterm Delivery

The leading cause of neonatal morbidity and mortality in the United States is preterm delivery, defined as delivery before 37 weeks' gestation; approximately 300,000 to 500,000 preterm births occur each year.[141] According to the World Health Organization (WHO), preterm birth rates are highest in North America and Africa, at 10.6% and 11.9%, respectively, while Europe has the lowest preterm birth rate at 6.2%.[142] Rupture of the fetal membranes prior to the onset of uterine contractions is known as premature rupture of membranes (PROM). When PROM occurs at less than 37 completed weeks' gestation, it is referred to as preterm PROM and is responsible for nearly one-third of preterm deliveries.[143]

Infants born before 37 weeks' gestation are usually of low birth weight (<2500 g) and are vulnerable to numerous complications, including (1) infection, (2) necrotizing enterocolitis, and (3) intraventricular hemorrhage, and often develop (4) *respiratory distress syndrome* (RDS). Some are of very low birth weight (<1500 g). According to the National Center for Health Statistics,[144] in 2012 8.0% of all U.S. liveborn infants were of low birth weight and 1.4% were of very low birth weight. Most of these infants will spend time in intensive care units at a cost of up to $3500 per day.

The cause of preterm labor is unknown, but it is likely that many factors are involved and several mechanisms have been supported by a considerable amount of clinical and experimental evidence. These include (1) pathologic distention of the uterus, (2) decidual hemorrhage, (3) activation of the maternal-fetal hypothalamic-pituitary-adrenal axis, and (4) intrauterine infection or inflammation.[145]

Premature Rupture of Membranes

Preterm PROM (PPROM) is a complication in 3% of pregnancies.[143] Risk factors for PPROM include (1) a history of PPROM, (2) genital tract infection, (3) antepartum bleeding, and (4) smoking. Most women who experience PPROM will deliver their infants within 1 week. Management of PPROM varies according to the gestational age of the fetus and the presence or absence of maternal or fetal infection. When PROM occurs at 34 to 36 weeks' gestation, the infant should be delivered, because this has been shown to reduce maternal and fetal infection rates compared with expectant management.[146] When it occurs prior to 34 weeks, expectant management with close fetal and maternal monitoring is undertaken, including in-patient hospitalization, antibiotic therapy, and corticosteroids to accelerate fetal lung development.[147]

The diagnosis of PROM is often difficult, and the commonly used tests to detect it lack clinical sensitivity and specificity.[148,149] These include (1) direct observation of fluid leaking from the cervix or pooling in the posterior fornix of the vagina, (2) ultrasound for the detection of oligohydramnios, (3) nitrazine (pH) and (4) fern tests, and (5) detection of placental alpha microglobulin-1 protein.

Fetal Lung Maturity

Respiratory distress syndrome (RDS), also called *hyaline membrane disease,* is the most common critical problem encountered in clinical management of preterm newborns. The worldwide incidence of RDS is 1% of live births and 10% to 15% of live preterm births (<37 weeks or <2500 g).[150] The risk of RDS is affected strongly by the gestational age at the time of birth, with a likelihood of less than 5% at 37 weeks, 20% at 34 weeks, and 60% at 29 weeks. In 2010, RDS was the eighth leading cause of death in infants in the United States.[151] Affected infants require supplemental oxygen and mechanical ventilation to remain properly oxygenated. The disorder is caused by a deficiency of *pulmonary surfactant.* In normal lungs, surfactant coats the alveolar epithelium and responds to alveolar volume changes by reducing the surface tension in the alveolar wall during expiration. When the quantity of surfactant is deficient, many of the alveoli collapse on expiration and thereby overinflate the remaining airways. The lungs become progressively noncompliant (stiff), and blood flowing through the capillary beds of collapsed alveoli fails to oxygenate. During the first few hours of life, affected infants develop tachypnea with or without cyanosis, nasal flaring, expiratory grunting, and intercostal retractions. The disease worsens during the next few days and is usually worse on the third or fourth day of life. Infants at risk for developing RDS are treated with intratracheal administration of exogenous surfactant immediately at birth.[152]

Very rarely, respiratory distress in a term newborn is caused by a mutation in the gene encoding for SP-B.[153] This condition, termed *congenital alveolar proteinosis,* is often fatal. A significant derangement in lamellar body production occurs in these cases. Study of the genetic variation suggests that there may be mild, nonfatal cases of this disorder.[154]

PRENATAL SCREENING FOR FETAL DEFECTS

Prenatal screening is the process of identifying pregnancies at sufficiently high risk of a serious birth defect, such as an open neural tube defect or Down syndrome. The risk for Down syndrome calculated using screening tests is more accurate than the use of maternal age alone, and the American College of Obstetricians and Gynecologists (ACOG) recommends that women of all ages be offered screening.[155] In Europe, the policies and recommendations for prenatal screening vary greatly by country. For example, in France all women must be offered prenatal screening by law and the costs of testing and

POINTS TO REMEMBER

Complications of Pregnancy

- When a fertilized egg implants in a location other than the body of the uterus, the condition is called an ectopic pregnancy.
- For women with clinical symptoms of abnormal pregnancy, measurement of both hCG and progesterone is more predictive of abnormal pregnancy than a single hCG measurement.
- Preeclampsia is characterized by hypertension, proteinuria, and, often, edema. Eclampsia is characterized by the development of seizures in conjunction with preeclampsia.
- TORCH (*t*oxoplasmosis, *o*ther infections, *r*ubella, *c*ytomegalovirus, and *h*erpes simplex virus) infections refer to a group of infectious diseases that commonly cause in utero infection.
- The diagnosis of PROM is often difficult, and the commonly used tests to detect it lack clinical sensitivity and specificity.
- Respiratory distress syndrome in a neonate is most commonly caused by a deficiency of pulmonary surfactant due to prematurity, which results in collapse of the alveoli.

Differential Diagnosis of Liver Disease

- Acute fatty liver is suggested in a patient with nausea and vomiting in the presence of jaundice, hypoglycemia, and encephalopathy with a small or normal-sized liver. ALT concentrations are typically 4 to 6 times the upper reference limit. Hepatic ultrasound and CT usually demonstrate fatty liver.
- Preeclampsia and the HELLP syndrome are characterized by an enlarged liver, lower ALT concentrations, mildly increased or normal bilirubin levels, normal glucose values, and hypertension.
- Marked increases in aminotransferase enzyme values suggest hepatic infarction or viral hepatitis.
- Liver biopsy may differentiate non–pregnancy-related causes of liver disease. Biopsy is not necessary to differentiate acute fatty liver from preeclampsia or HELLP syndrome because the treatment is the same for all of these conditions—delivery of the infant.

Hemolytic Disease of the Newborn

- HDN is a fetal hemolytic disorder caused by maternal antibodies directed against antigen on fetal erythrocytes.
- Maternal sensitization may occur in response to blood transfusion or exposure of the mother to fetal red blood cells carrying antigen that the mother lacks.
- To identify sensitized women, an alloantibody screen is performed. If an antibody to an erythrocyte antigen is identified, the titer is determined to monitor the risk for fetal hydrops.
- Fetal RhD genotyping may be required in a sensitized mother if the father is heterozygous or is not available for testing. The genotype is determined using cultured amniocytes or circulating cell-free fetal DNA.
- Noninvasive ultrasonographic determination of middle fetal cerebral artery velocity is useful to assess disease severity
- The use of anti-RhD immune globulin has dramatically reduced the incidence of HDN.

follow-up are reimbursed, while Ireland lacks a national policy for prenatal screening.[156] Screening rates vary and are high in some countries such as England (61%) and France (84%) but relatively low in others such as the Netherlands (26%).[157] The majority of countries in Europe focus on informing women of screening options to facilitate an informed decision and making the testing available if desired.[157]

In addition to prenatal screening tests for maternal serum analytes, detection of cell-free fetal DNA (cffDNA) in maternal blood holds promise for high-quality noninvasive screening or diagnosis of some fetal aneuploidies. Prenatal screening of cffDNA is highly sensitive and specific for Down syndrome in both high-risk and routine pregnancies.[158-160] However, cffDNA testing does not assess for the risk of neural tube defects and is not recommended for multiple gestations. Because of this and the lack of data on low-risk pregnancies, the ACOG recommends measurement of maternal serum analytes for routine prenatal screening.[161] A more detailed discussion of this technique and its applications can be found in Chapter 53.

Terminology and Method of Risk Calculation in Prenatal Screening

Calculation of risk in prenatal screening depends on the pregnant woman's prior risk and the pattern of test results.

Multiple of the Median

Understanding the published literature and clinical screening requires an understanding of the multiple of the median (MoM), the statistic used to normalize analyte values. The initial step in calculating a MoM is to develop a set of median values for each week (or day) of gestation, using the laboratory's own assay values measured on the population to be screened. Individual test results are then expressed as a MoM by dividing each individual test result by the median for the relevant gestational age. This convention was originally developed to take into account the large differences among centers in AFP assay values seen in the United Kingdom 1977 collaborative study.[162] The MoM is now universally used as a common factor for converting analyte values into an interpretative unit and serves as the starting point for calculating screening results for neural tube defects, Down syndrome, and trisomy 18.[163-165]

Calculating Individualized Patient-Specific Risks Using Multiple Biochemical Measurements

Measurements of each analyte are made on a serum sample, and the results in mass units are converted to MoM for the appropriate week of gestation. This MoM value is then adjusted for other variables, such as maternal weight and race (as described later in this chapter). Patient-specific Down syndrome risks are calculated using the adjusted MoM values along with the woman's maternal age at expected delivery by employing an algorithm that uses overlapping multivariate log Gaussian distributions.

The individualized risk (patient-specific risk) for any given condition is determined by multiplying the a priori risk for that condition by a likelihood ratio that is calculated using the woman's analyte measurements (ie, Patient risk = A priori risk × Likelihood ratio). This basic equation is used to calculate the patient-specific risk for neural tube defects, Down syndrome, trisomy 18, or any other condition in which the distributions of analytes for the unaffected and affected population have been determined. The a priori risk is obtained from large epidemiologic studies that ascertain the prevalence for the condition under consideration. For example, a woman's age is used to define her a priori risk for having a fetus with Down syndrome. Furthermore, because of spontaneous fetal losses during pregnancy, age-related risks are higher in the first trimester than at term. The likelihood ratio is determined by calculating the ratio of the heights of the affected and unaffected overlapping population distributions for any specified MoM value. When multiple tests are used, a single likelihood ratio is calculated using the overlapping distributions for each test but with the correlation between tests taken into account. This final calculated risk, rather than the analyte concentrations themselves, is the screening variable upon which clinical decisions are made and is typically reported as a ratio such as 1:100, 1:625, or 1: 10,000.

The test performance (detection and false-positive rates) achievable depends on many factors, including (1) the analyte combination chosen, (2) the risk cutoff chosen, (3) the method of dating used to establish gestational age, and (4) the maternal ages of the women being tested. Table 69.3 summarizes the impact of these factors and demonstrates how choices of second trimester test combination and risk cutoff affect detection and screen-positive rates.

Reporting Individual Results

The maternal serum screening report should contain the following information: (1) the concentrations and MoM values for measured analytes, (2) an interpretation as screen positive or screen negative, (3) the Down syndrome risk estimate (along with risks for other abnormalities such as trisomy 18), and (4) recommendations for possible further action. Physician-provided information should include (1) the specimen collection date, (2) identification as a first or second specimen, (3) the date of LMP or gestational age confirmed by ultrasound and maternal birth date (or age), (4) the relevant pregnancy history, (5) the number of fetuses (if known), (6) the maternal race, and (7) the presence or absence of preconceptional maternal diabetes requiring insulin therapy.

Prenatal Screening Tests

Maternal serum screening for neural tube defects began in the 1970s using second-trimester serum specimens. Since then, maternal serum screening has expanded to include partial detection of Down syndrome, trisomy 18, and Smith-Lemli-Opitz syndrome. However, because of the large number of pregnancies screened, and the interest in other fetal conditions and their possible association with abnormal maternal serum analyte concentrations, a wealth of associations between rarer conditions and screening results has been published. These findings are never diagnostic and are reported rarely by the screening laboratory. In certain circumstances, however, the healthcare provider may recommend pursuing a more extensive medical evaluation.

Neural Tube Defects

Neural tube defects are serious abnormalities that occur early in embryonic development. By 19 days after fertilization, the area that is to form the central nervous system (brain and

TABLE 69.3 Screening Performance According to Second-Trimester Risk Cutoff and Screening Test

Risk Cutoff															
Screening test (all	1 in 100			1 in 150			1 in 200			1 in 250			1 in 300		
include maternal age)	DR (%)	FPR (%)	OAPR	DR (%)	FPR (%)	OAPR	DR (%)	FPR (%)	OAPR	DR (%)	FPR (%)	OAPR	DR (%)	FPR (%)	OAPR
Integrated*	87	1.2	1:06	89	1.6	1:08	90	2.1	1:10	91	2.6	1:12	92	3	1:14
Serum Integrated*															
PAPP-A at 10 weeks†	82	1.8	1:10	85	2.6	1:14	87	3.3	1:17	88	4	1:20	89	4.6	1:23
PAPP-A at 11 weeks	79	2	1:11	82	2.9	1:16	85	3.8	1:20	86	4.6	1:23	87	5.3	1:27
Combined*	77	1.8	1:10	81	2.6	1:14	83	3.4	1:18	85	4.2	1:22	86	4.9	1:25
Quadruple	74	2.5	1:15	79	3.6	1:20	82	4.7	1:25	84	5.7	1:30	86	6.6	1:34

Free β-hCG, rather than total hCG, measured in tests that use second-trimester markers.

*All with first-trimester markers at 11 weeks except †.

DR, Detection rate; *FPR,* false-positive rate; *OAPR,* odds of being affected given a positive result.

Modified from Wald NJ, Rodeck C, Hackshaw AK, Rudnicka A. SURUSS in perspective. *Semin Perinatol* 2005;29:225–35.

spinal cord) has differentiated into a plate of cells. The flat plate then rolls up, and its edges fuse into a hollow neural tube that drops into the embryo to develop just underneath what will become the skin of the back. Neural tube formation is normally complete 4 weeks after fertilization. Failure of neural tube fusion leads to permanent developmental defects of the brain or spinal cord, or both. These defects include *anencephaly, meningomyelocele* (which is commonly called *spina bifida*), and *encephalocele*. Although there are many heterogeneous causes, about 90% fall into the classification of multifactorial inheritance.[166] Folic acid deficiency is clearly associated with increased frequency of neural tube closure defects.[167] The cause in these cases may be derangement of homocysteine metabolism caused by the folate deficiency.[168] Estimates attribute 70% or more of all neural tube defects to folate deficiency.[169] Since 1997, grain products in the United States and Canada have been fortified with 140 µg folic acid/100 g,[170] but the amount added is unlikely to be sufficient to reduce the birth prevalence by more than about 30%, the reduction that is commonly reported in observational trials.[171] Organizations such as the March of Dimes are conducting vigorous campaigns to educate women about the need for folic acid supplementation before becoming pregnant, as recommended by the CDC.[172] Most vitamin supplements contain 400 µg of folic acid, which is the recommended daily allowance.[173] Data published in 2009 suggest that vitamin B_{12} is also necessary.[174]

The birth prevalence of open neural tube defects varies with factors such as geographic location (higher in the eastern United States, lower in the West), race (lower in African-Americans), ethnicity (higher in Scotch-Irish), family history (higher with prior births of affected individuals),[175] and maternal weight (higher in obese women).[176,177] An average figure for the United States is 1 open neural tube defect per 1000 pregnancies (about 1 in 2000 for each individual defect). Almost all cases of anencephaly and about 95% of meningomyeloceles are open, with no overlying skin, and therefore are in direct communication with the amniotic fluid. Thus the fetal serum proteins normally present in amniotic fluid at low concentrations gain access in large quantities to the amniotic fluid. The increased amniotic fluid AFP concentration leads to increased amounts in the maternal circulation. Thus, only open neural tube defects are detected by maternal serum AFP screening.[162]

Prenatal Screening. In the early 1970s, Brock and colleagues demonstrated increased AFP concentrations in amniotic fluid of mothers carrying fetuses affected with an open neural tube defect (eg, anencephaly, open spina bifida).[178] Subsequently, it was shown that AFP concentrations were also increased in maternal serum (in the second trimester).[179] Concentrations in serum in affected and unaffected pregnancies overlapped considerably, however, indicating that maternal serum AFP would be useful only as an initial screening test to identify women at high risk for having an affected fetus (Fig. 69.3). These women would then need to be referred for diagnostic procedures (eg, high-resolution ultrasound and, if indicated, amniocentesis for measurement of AFP and acetylcholinesterase in amniotic fluid) to determine if the fetus had an open neural tube defect. A large collaborative study conducted in the United Kingdom in 1977 showed that maternal serum AFP screening for open neural tube defects in the second trimester of pregnancy was feasible, and the final report provided

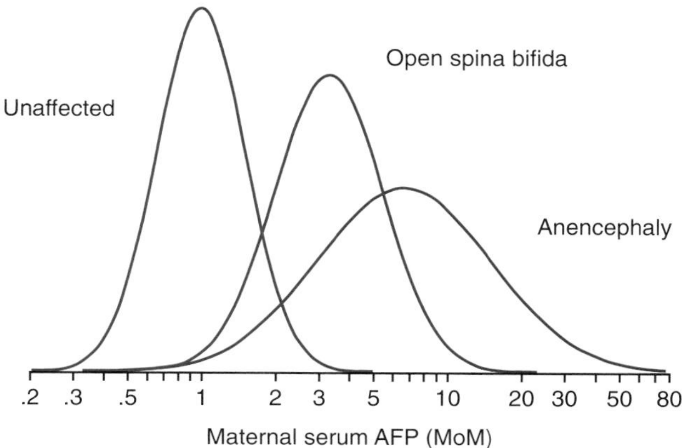

FIGURE 69.3 Distribution of maternal serum alpha-fetoprotein (AFP) measurements in unaffected pregnancies and in pregnancies affected with open spina bifida or anencephaly.

estimates of screening performance in terms of detection and false-positive rates.[162] A family history of neural tube defects in either parent increases the risk that the fetus is affected by 5-fold to 15-fold, but more than 90% of all infants with neural tube defects are born to unsuspecting parents who have no recognized risk factor for the disorder.[180,181] Maternal serum AFP testing thus provided a screening method that was available to all women to identify pregnancies at high risk or to estimate the numerical risk of having a fetus with an open neural tube defect.[164] In the 1980s, the use of maternal serum AFP to screen for open neural tube defects became a standard of care in the United States. The ACOG,[155] the American Society of Human Genetics,[182] and the American Academy of Pediatrics[183] have issued official statements supporting its use. Because of improvements in ultrasound technology, many countries such as England and Canada use fetal imaging techniques rather than maternal serum AFP measurement as a first-line test for structural fetal anomalies.[184]

Optimal screening occurs between 16 and 18 completed weeks' gestation, a time when the distributions of results for affected and unaffected pregnancies are maximally different, and when time for follow-up studies is adequate. Screening at 15 weeks is acceptable, but screening for open neural tube defects prior to 14 weeks is difficult to justify.[162,169] Although a patient-specific risk can be used when screening for open neural tube defects,[164] nearly all laboratories define a screen-positive result as AFP at or above a fixed MoM cutoff. The two most commonly used AFP MoM cutoffs in the United States are 2.0 and 2.5 MoM, yielding initial screen-positive rates of 3% to 5% and 1% to 3%, respectively. Observed rates are more likely to be at the lower end of the cited ranges if many pregnancies are dated by ultrasound. This improvement is a result of the finding that increased AFP values attributable to underestimated gestational age, fetal demise, and twin gestation will usually have been identified. The lower initial positive rate at 2.5 MoM is associated with a reduced detection rate for open spina bifida: 70% to 75% as compared with 80% to 85% at 2.0 MoM.[162,185] Nearly all cases of anencephaly are detected by maternal serum AFP screening.

Follow-Up Testing. Women who have a positive screening test result for open neural tube defects should be offered genetic counseling and further testing. A low-resolution ultrasound examination may verify the gestational age and identify other possible reasons for the increased AFP test results (eg, inaccurate gestational dating, recent fetal demise, twins). Patients who have an unexplained high maternal serum AFP result are offered high-resolution ultrasound or amniocentesis for measurement of amniotic fluid AFP and acetylcholinesterase (AChE), or both.

Compared with maternal serum, the distribution of amniotic fluid AFP concentrations in pregnancies affected with open neural tube defects is far more separated from unaffected pregnancies.[186] However, amniotic fluid AFP measurements are not by themselves diagnostic because of rare false-positive results. If the amniotic fluid is contaminated with even a small amount of fetal blood, as many as 2% to 3% of the results can be falsely positive.[186] All abnormal amniotic fluid AFP results must be confirmed by measurement of amniotic fluid AChE. The combination of amniotic fluid AFP and AChE is virtually diagnostic for an open neural tube defect.[186,187]

High-resolution ultrasound will almost always confirm a chemical diagnosis of a neural tube defect. Anencephaly is readily identifiable, and ultrasound diagnosis of open spina bifida is considerably enhanced by the presence of two cranial signs (known as the lemon and banana signs).[188,189] The lemon sign is a "pinched" skull in the frontal region resulting in a lemon shape compared with the normal egg shape. The banana sign is a reduction in the transverse diameter of the cerebellum, causing the two cerebellar hemispheres to assume a curved, "banana" shape. Ultrasound diagnosis of open neural tube defects is now so reliable that it is sometimes used for diagnosis in women with increased maternal serum AFP without waiting for amniotic fluid measurements.

Down Syndrome

Down syndrome is the most common serious disorder of the autosomal chromosomes in live-born infants, occurring in 1 in 700 live births. An extra copy of the long-arm region q22.1 to q22.3 of chromosome 21 results in a phenotype consisting of moderate to severe mental retardation, hypotonia, congenital heart defects, and flat facial profile. Chromosome 21 is the smallest chromosome, making up about 1.7% of the human genome. Most often an affected child has three copies of chromosome 21 (ie, trisomy 21), but 5% of cases are caused by translocations and 1% of cases are mosaics. The risk increases slowly up to age 30 and then steadily increases between ages 30 to 45 (Fig. 69.4) to a plateau.[190]

Prenatal Screening. In 1984, a major expansion of biochemical prenatal screening became possible when an association between second-trimester maternal serum AFP and fetal Down syndrome was reported.[191] Maternal serum AFP concentrations are about 25% lower in Down syndrome than in unaffected pregnancies. The association of AFP and Down syndrome was found to be independent of maternal age.[192] Before this discovery, the only available screening test for Down syndrome involved asking a woman her age. Women 35 years or older at the time of delivery would be offered amniocentesis and fetal karyotyping. Down syndrome screening using maternal age is based on the well-documented increase in risk for having a baby with Down syndrome as maternal age increases (see Fig. 69.4). The independence of maternal serum AFP measurements and maternal age established that it was possible to offer a screening method to younger women, in whom most cases of Down syndrome occur. Maternal serum AFP screening for Down syndrome also introduced the concept of using risk, rather than analyte concentration, as the screening variable for identifying high-risk women.[192] The effectiveness of maternal serum AFP screening in younger women was subsequently established.[193]

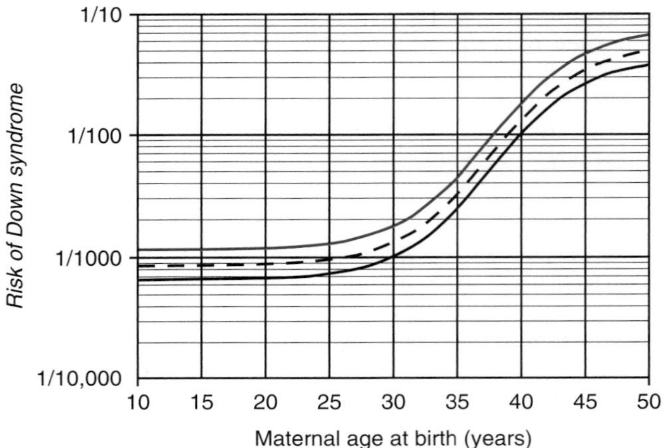

FIGURE 69.4 The relationship of maternal age and the risk of having a pregnancy affected with Down syndrome. *Red line,* first-trimester risk; *dashed line,* second-trimester risk; *solid black line,* term risk. The term risk is calculated from 1/(1+exp(7.33–4.211/(1+exp(–0.2815×(age–37.23–0.5))))). (Morris JK, Mutton DE, Alberman E. Revised estimates of the maternal age specific live birth prevalence of Down's syndrome. *J Med Screen* 2002;9:2–6.)

Unconjugated estriol (uE_3),[194] a product of the fetoplacental unit, is also about 25% lower in pregnancies with Down syndrome. In contrast, concentrations of hCG were found to be about twice as high.[195] In 1988, a method was proposed for combining maternal age with measurements of these three analytes (the triple test) into a single Down syndrome risk estimate.[165] A fourth analyte, inhibin A, was introduced as a clinical marker for Down syndrome screening in the late 1990s. Concentrations are two times higher in Down syndrome versus unaffected pregnancies.[196] The "quadruple test" provides approximately 80% detection at a 5% false-positive rate. Two large trials have confirmed its performance.[197,198] Table 69.4 shows general patterns of first- and second-trimester analytes associated with various disorders.[199,200]

Follow-Up Testing. Women who have a positive screening test result for increased risk of Down syndrome are usually referred for genetic counseling and further testing. A low-resolution ultrasound examination may be offered as a way to verify gestational age and to identify other possible reasons for the positive test result. One of the most common reasons for increased Down syndrome risk is overestimated gestational age. Up to one-third of women with positive second-trimester Down syndrome screening results who are dated by the last menstrual period are found to be too early in their pregnancies for reliable screening (<15 weeks) or reclassified as low risk after ultrasound revision of gestational age.[201] Women who are still at increased risk after the ultrasound examination should be offered amniocentesis to obtain fetal cells for karyotyping. Although some second-trimester ultrasound findings are associated with Down syndrome (eg, nuchal fold and shortened femur and humeral length), these findings are

TABLE 69.4 Conditions Associated With Various Maternal Serum Screening Result Patterns

	SECOND TRIMESTER				FIRST TRIMESTER		
Condition	**AFP**	**hCG**	**uE_3**	**InhA**	**PAPP-A**	**hCG**	**NT**
Amniocentesis	Normal to high	—	—	—	—	—	—
Anencephaly	Very high	—	Very low	—	—	—	—
Congenital nephrosis, duodenal atresia, encephalocele, esophageal atresia, gastroschisis, hydrocephalus, Meckel syndrome, omphalocele, sacrococcygeal teratoma	High	—	—	—	—	—	—
Cystic hygroma	High	—	—	—	—	—	Increased
Down syndrome	Low	High	Low	High	Low	High	Increased
Fetal blood contamination	High to very high	Unchanged	Unchanged	Unchanged	—	—	—
Molar pregnancy	Very low	Very high	Very low	Normal	—	—	—
Molar pregnancy (partial)	Low to normal	Very high	Low to normal	Normal	—	—	—
Myelomeningocele (open spina bifida)	High	—	—	—	—	—	—
Normal pregnancy	Low, normal, or high	Low, normal, or high	Low, normal, or high	Low, normal, or high	—	—	—
Overestimated gestational age	Low	High	Low	Normal	—	—	—
Preeclampsia	Normal to high	High	—	—	—	—	—
Pseudocyesis (imaginary pregnancy)	Undetectable	Undetectable	Undetectable	Undetectable	—	—	—
Smith-Lemli-Opitz syndrome	Low	Low	Very low	—	—	—	—
Spontaneous or impending pregnancy loss	Variable	Low or high	Low	Low or high	—	—	—
Steroid sulfatase deficiency (fetal)	Unchanged	Unchanged	Very low	Unchanged	—	—	—
Triploidy (paternal)	Variable	High	Low	High	Variable	Very high	—
Triploidy (maternal)	Variable	Low	Low	Low	Variable	Very low	—
Trisomy 13	Variable	Variable	Variable	Variable	Very low	Low	Increased
Trisomy 18	Low	Low	Very low	Normal	Very low	Very low	Increased
Turner syndrome without hydrops	Low	Low	Very low	Low	Variable	Variable	Increased
Turner syndrome with hydrops	Low	High	Very low	High	Variable	Variable	Increased
Twins and other multiple gestations	High	High	High	High	High	High	—
Underestimated gestational age	High	Low	High	Normal	—	—	—

AFP, α-Fetoprotein; *hCG*, human chorionic gonadotropin; *inhA*, inhibin A; *NT*, nuchal translucency; *PAPP-A*, pregnancy-associated plasma protein A; *uE_3*, unconjugated estriol.

not diagnostic.[202] The only way to diagnose Down syndrome is via fetal karyotype. However, the benefits of accurately diagnosing a chromosome abnormality in gestation must be weighed against the potential for harm with amniocentesis. Even amniocentesis performed by an experienced obstetrician using ultrasonography for guidance has a procedure-related rate of fetal loss of about 1 in 200 to 1 in 500.[203,204] Given that about 1 in 30 women with an initial screen-positive test result (high risk) will have a fetus with a chromosome abnormality, the offer of the invasive procedure is reasonable.

Women who have a screen positive result in the first trimester may be offered CVS to diagnose Down syndrome. This procedure is performed between the 10th and 12th weeks, carries a slightly higher risk of fetal loss than amniocentesis,[205] and is not available to patients in some geographic regions. Lastly, although most patients opt for screening tests before proceeding with invasive testing, diagnostic tests of amniocentesis and CVS are available to any woman regardless of her risk, should she choose to have them.

Trisomy 18

Trisomy 18 (Edwards syndrome) is caused by a nondisjunction event during meiosis that results in a fetus having an extra copy of chromosome 18. Although it occurs in only 1 in 8000 births, it is probably the most common chromosome defect at the time of conception. The dramatic change in prevalence is due to the very high fetal loss rate both before 8 weeks (>80%) and during the second and third trimesters (≈70%). Approximately 25% of affected fetuses have meningomyelocele (spina bifida) or omphalocele (abdominal wall defect). A high cesarean section rate has been reported for undiagnosed cases.[163] Following birth, half of the infants die within the first 5 days and 90% die within 100 days.[206]

Prenatal Screening. Prenatal screening studies have found that fetal trisomy 18 has a distinctive triple-marker pattern that is different from the Down syndrome pattern (see Table 69.4).[207] It is the least common of the three disorders considered for second-trimester maternal serum screening. It is also the one that is least compatible with life. For these reasons, a screening program exclusively devoted to the prenatal identification of trisomy 18 is unjustified. However, given that the serum analytes are already being measured to screen for Down syndrome and open neural tube defects, an additional interpretation of these analytes to quantify the risk of fetal trisomy 18 is warranted. Because the birth prevalence of trisomy 18 is one-tenth that of Down syndrome,[163] the percentage of women identified as screen positive must be correspondingly lower than that for Down syndrome.

In trisomy 18 pregnancies, the AFP (median = 0.65 MoM), uE_3 (0.43 MoM), and hCG concentrations (0.36 MoM) are low. A method for trisomy 18 risk calculation was published and is often included in prenatal screening programs.[163,208] The risk-based algorithm showed that at a second-trimester risk cutoff of 1:100, 60% of trisomy 18 pregnancies could be identified, with about 0.5% of women having an initial positive screen.[163]

Follow-Up Testing. In contrast to the screening protocols for open neural tube defects and Down syndrome, a dating ultrasound is not recommended as the first step after a finding of increased risk of trisomy 18. The second-trimester serum marker pattern is not consistent with incorrect gestational dating, and amniocentesis should be offered.[209,210] A high proportion of fetuses with trisomy 18 will have abnormal but nondiagnostic second-trimester ultrasound findings (eg, heart defects and clenched fists).[211] CVS may be offered to patients at high risk of trisomy 18 based on first-trimester screening results.

Smith-Lemli-Opitz Syndrome

Smith-Lemli-Opitz syndrome (SLOS) is caused by a defect in cholesterol synthesis. SLOS is inherited as an autosomal recessive mutation and occurs rarely, in about 1 of every 100,000 Caucasian pregnancies.[212] Children affected with SLOS have mental and growth deficiencies and other structural malformations of the skeleton, kidneys, genitals, lungs, and heart.[213]

Prenatal Screening. Second-trimester risk assessment for SLOS is possible using a multivariate Gaussian algorithm specific for this disorder. The marker pattern in affected pregnancies includes low AFP and hCG (median = 0.72 and 0.76 MoM, respectively), with very low uE_3 (0.21 MoM) concentrations (see Table 69.4).[214] Only pregnancies with a very high risk (1 in 50 or greater) are classified as screen positive for SLOS and recommended for diagnostic testing by amniocentesis. In this manner, 83% of SLOS cases can be identified at a 0.3% positive rate.[212] It is noteworthy that there is a high rate of fetal loss and other chromosomal (3.3%) or structural abnormalities (5.8%) among patients with false positive tests.

Follow-Up Testing. Patients at risk for SLOS should be offered genetic counseling to discuss the risks and benefits of diagnosis by amniocentesis. High amniotic fluid concentrations of the precursor 7-dehydrocholesterol are diagnostic of the disorder.[215]

Other Aneuploidies

Although chromosome disorders other than trisomies 21 and 18 are not part of routine screening, the marker patterns exhibited in maternal serum for some aneuploidies are similar. In particular, hydropic Turner syndrome and triploidy of paternal origin have serum marker patterns resembling that of Down syndrome pregnancy and are sometimes identified as high risk using this algorithm. Similarly, Turner syndrome without hydrops and triploidy of maternal origin are sometimes identified by the trisomy 18 risk algorithm. The pattern for trisomy 13 is variable (see Table 69.4).

Newer Screening Algorithms

Following extensive use of screening tests in the second trimester, new tests have been introduced that use serum collected in the first trimester.

First-Trimester Combined Test. For patients seeking early diagnosis, screening for Down syndrome in the first trimester (10 to 13 weeks' gestation) is available. First-trimester screening involves measurement of maternal serum pregnancy–associated plasma protein-A (PAPP-A) concentration, which is relatively low in Down syndrome pregnancy (median = 0.4 to 0.5 MoM between 10 and 13 weeks), and hCG (free beta subunit or total) concentration, which is relatively high in Down syndrome (median = 1.7 to 2.2 MoM).[216] In combination with maternal age, these two serum tests yield a detection rate of 60% at a 5% false-positive rate.[217] A third marker is used to improve first-trimester screening performance ultrasound measurements of nuchal translucency (NT), the subcutaneous space between the skin and cervical spine; this marker has been shown to be increased (2.0 MoM) in fetuses with Down syndrome.[218,219] Increased NT measurements are also a nonspecific finding for many fetal structural abnormalities,[220] and therefore are only useful as a screening test.[221] NT measurements alone detect 60% or more of the Down syndrome cases at a 5% screen positive rate, making NT the best single screening test described to date.[222]

However, neither ultrasound findings nor serum tests in the first trimester have sufficient predictive power to be used alone. In 2003 and 2005, two independent large multicenter trials demonstrated that a combination of NT and serum tests (the combined test) was comparable or slightly better than the second-trimester quadruple test for Down syndrome screening, detecting 85% of cases at a 5% false-positive rate. These trials were critical in proving the efficacy of first-trimester screening because they accounted for fetal losses between the first and second trimesters. The National Screening Committee of the United Kingdom National Health Service advocates the use of the combined test for Down syndrome prenatal screening.[223]

Reports have described trisomy 18 detection using first-trimester combined screening.[224] The pattern of markers in affected pregnancies consists of an increased NT measurement (median about 3.2 MoM), with reduced PAPP-A (0.18 MoM) and hCG (0.28 MoM) in the first trimester.[224] Estimates for the performance of first-trimester combined testing in the detection of trisomy 18 are varied, likely as the result of a high fetal loss rate and difficulties in complete ascertainment. The most optimistic estimates suggest that 90% to 100% of trisomy 18 cases can be detected with only 0.2% to 2.0% being called screen positive,[225,226] but a large multicenter study with the more comprehensive outcome tracking suggests that detection rates are closer to 80% for a 0.3% positive rate.[227]

Although first-trimester screening has obvious advantages, it also has limitations. First, unlike the second-trimester screening test, detection and false-positive rates are dependent on the gestational week of testing as shown in Table 69.5. The screening performance of PAPP-A and hCG measurements improves with advancing gestational age within the first trimester, while the performance of NT sonography decreases. Even so, these markers perform best when used simultaneously. Second, to be reliable, NT measurements must be performed at specialized referral centers that employ sonographers who have undergone rigorous training and participate in ongoing quality control programs. Routine office ultrasound is unsuitable for obtaining NT measurements. Therefore, access for women in some rural areas is limited. NT measurements are relatively expensive, as first-trimester ultrasound examinations are not routine, and third-party payers may be reluctant to reimburse these costs. The ACOG recommends that first-trimester screening be offered only with appropriately trained sonographers, a quality assurance program for NT, and access to diagnosis by CVS.[155] Last, routine screening for open neural tube defects using maternal serum AFP would still need to be performed, as such screening is not effective in the first trimester.[162,169]

TABLE 69.5 Expected Down Syndrome False-Positive Rates (FPRs) for a Detection Rate of 85% During the First Trimester

Test	WEEKS GESTATION			
Combinations*	11	12	13	11–13 Combined
NT	27	37	54	39
PAPP-A	43	51	60	51
Free hCGβ	56	50	42	50
Total hCG	72	61	45	60
NT, PAPP-A, and free hCGβ	5.3	6.1	7.6	6.3
NT, PAPP-A and total hCG	6.8	7.2	7.3	7.1

*Maternal age is used with each test combination.
hCG, Human chorionic gonadotropin; *NT,* nuchal translucency; *PAPP-A,* pregnancy-associated plasma protein A.
Modified from Palomaki GE, Lambert-Messerlian GM, Canick JA. A summary analysis of Down syndrome markers in the late first trimester. *Adv Clin Chem* 2007;43:177–210.

Combining First- and Second-Trimester Markers Into a Single Integrated Screening Test. The integrated test takes advantage of first- and second-trimester markers and avoids most of the limitations of stand-alone first-trimester screening.[228] With this approach, measurements of NT and PAPP-A are made in the first trimester but are not interpreted or acted upon until testing in the second trimester is complete. In the second trimester, a serum is drawn and a quadruple test performed. Results from all six tests (NT, PAPP-A, AFP, uE_3, hCG, and inhibin A) are then combined into a single risk estimate. This approach detects 85% of Down syndrome cases with only a 1% false-positive rate.[228] Studies involving more than 47,000 and 38,000 pregnancies at multiple centers obtained results consistent with this estimate.[229,230]

Given the low false-positive rate of the integrated test, fewer amniocenteses are needed and, hence, fewer fetal losses occur per Down syndrome case diagnosed. The integrated screen has been shown to be a cost-effective approach to Down syndrome screening, again on the basis of fewer costly diagnostic tests and affected liveborns.[231] Most of the cost in integrated screening comes from the NT ultrasound. Although NT alone is the best univariate screening marker, integrated screening can be offered effectively and at a lower cost by using a modified test based only on the serum markers (serum integrated). Maternal serum PAPP-A concentrations are measured at 10 to 13 weeks and combined with a second-trimester quad test for a five-marker screening panel. The serum integrated test gives an 85% detection of Down syndrome cases with about a 3% false-positive rate. A summary of detection and false-positive rates for second-trimester and integrated screening tests is illustrated in Fig. 69.5. The impact of different risk cutoffs and choice of screening test on test performance is shown in Table 69.3.

An alternative approach to integrated screening is the sequential integrated test, in which women at the very highest risk for Down syndrome pregnancy (1 in 25 or higher) at the first-trimester phase are alerted and recommended for diagnostic testing.[232,233] All remaining women (≈98%) proceed to second-trimester blood collection for a full integrated risk analysis. The advantages of this approach are that very high-risk women are afforded the opportunity for early diagnosis, and most patients have the safest and most effective screening strategy. The sequential integrated test offers an 85% detection rate with a 2% to 3% false-positive rate. This assumes that all patients have a first-trimester NT scan because a serum PAPP-A alone in the first trimester is not sufficient for calculation of interim risk. Contingent screening has been proposed whereby patients at very high and very low risk receive results in the first trimester, while those with an interim risk go on to have the second part of the full integrated screening test.[232,233] See the At a Glance box *Down Syndrome Screening Tests.*

Adjustments for Factors That Influence Analyte Measurements

Prenatal screening for both open neural tube defects and Down syndrome is optimized when each woman's analyte concentration is compared with those of other women (the

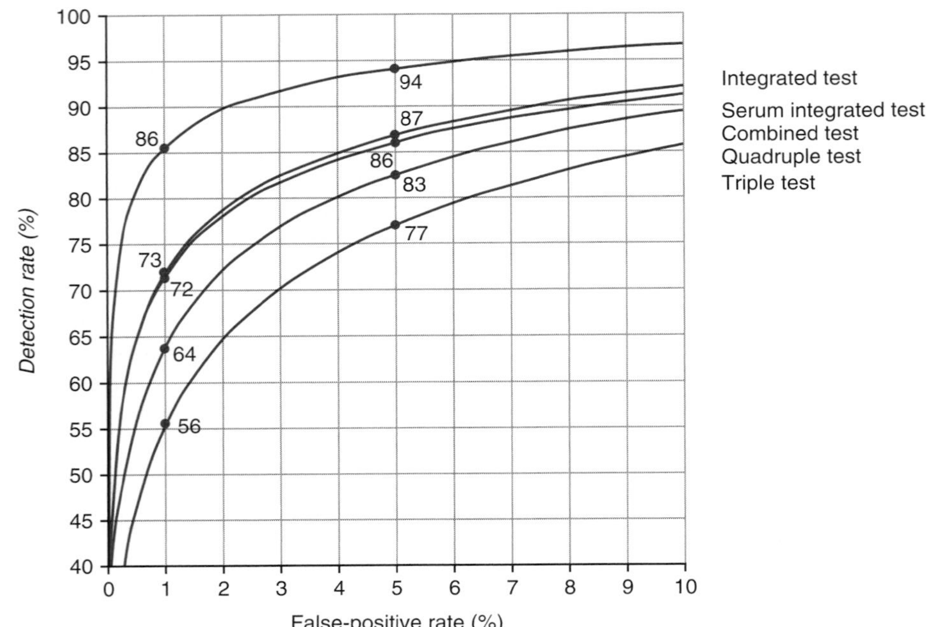

FIGURE 69.5 Receiver operating characteristic curves for tests used to screen for Down syndrome. (Reprinted with permission from Wald NJ, Rodeck C, Hackshaw AK, Rudnicka A. SURUSS in perspective. *Semin Perinatol* 2005;29:225–35.)

AT A GLANCE

Down Syndrome Screening Tests

Test Name	AFP	hCG	uE3	DIA	PAPP-A	NT	Trimester
Quadruple	✔	✔	✔	✔			2nd
Integrated					✔	✔	1st
	✔	✔	✔	✔			2nd
Serum integrated					✔		1st
	✔	✔	✔	✔			2nd
Sequential		✔			✔	✔	1st
	✔	✔	✔	✔			2nd

AFP, Alpha-fetoprotein; *DIA,* dimeric inhibin A; *hCG,* human chorionic gonadotropin; *NT,* nuchal translucency; *PAPP-A,* pregnancy-associated plasma A; *uE3,* unconjugated estriol.

reference group) who are "similar" to her in many respects.[234] In addition to gestational age, this "similarity" extends to other factors that have been shown to affect analyte concentrations, including (1) maternal weight, (2) race, (3) the presence of insulin-dependent diabetes (IDD), and (4) multiple pregnancy. Taking into account these factors increases the accuracy of the interpretation.

Maternal Weight

As maternal weight increases, the average concentration of analyte values decreases, likely because a fixed amount of analyte is diluted in an increased maternal blood volume. For example, heavier women have, on average, lower AFP values and are less likely than lighter-weight women to be screen positive for neural tube defects. Without taking maternal weight into account, screening is less effective in heavier women because their MoM values are inappropriately low. The importance of adjusting AFP MoM values for weight is reinforced by studies showing that heavier women have about a twofold to fourfold increased risk for open spina bifida.[176,177] No association between maternal weight and Down syndrome has been reported. The weight effect is also significant for hCG, inhibin A, and PAPP-A, but less so for uE_3. Maternal weight is taken into account for all serum markers by adjusting each woman's MoM values by a factor corresponding to the expected MoM value for women with her weight (Fig. 69.6). These factors are empirically derived from the screened population in a manner that is similar to deriving median analyte concentrations for each gestational age. Optimally, each laboratory should derive its own maternal weight adjustment factors for each analyte, because the average maternal weight may differ from that seen in other laboratories. These adjustment factors should be applied only over the maternal weight range in which they have been

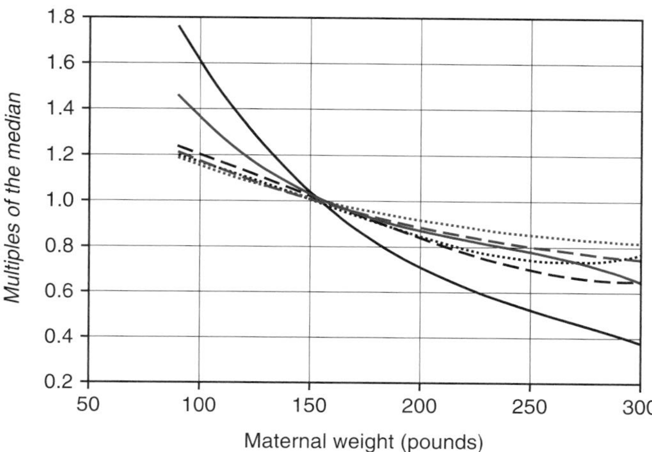

FIGURE 69.6 The relationship of AFP, uE_3, hCG, inhibin A, and PAPP-A (expressed as multiples of the median [MoM]) and maternal weight. The horizontal line at 1.0 MoM is the value found for a woman of average weight. *Red solid line*, AFP; *red dashed line*, inhA; *red dotted line*, uE_3; *black solid line*, PAPP-A; *black dashed line*, first-trimester hCG; *black dotted line*, second-trimester hCG.

shown to be appropriate. For example, if few or no data are available to derive adjustment factors for women weighing more than 300 pounds, then the laboratory should be careful in extrapolating factors to these women from data on women of lower weight. Laboratories should limit the range of adjustment using upper (and lower) truncation limits. If a woman's weight is outside these limits, adjustment should be applied as if the woman were at the respective limit. An effective model for all analytes is a linear reciprocal model. Maternal weights are stratified into weight groups and regressed against the reciprocal of maternal weight. This model and its application have been described in detail elsewhere.[234,235] Distributions of maternal weight vary within each racial group, with Asian women tending to have lower maternal weight than Caucasians, and African Americans weighing more. It is optimal to apply adjustment equations for each racial group to correct marker concentrations for weight.

Maternal Race

For second-trimester markers, African-American women have maternal serum AFP and hCG concentrations that are 10% to 15% higher than those found in Caucasian women.[234] Inhibin A concentrations are about 8% lower in African Americans,[236] and uE_3 concentrations are not different in these two populations. In the first trimester, serum PAPP-A (1.35 to 1.57 MoM) and hCG (1.11 to 1.21 MoM) concentrations are significantly increased in African-American women.[237-239] For other racial or ethnic groups, data are limited or small effects have been noted on marker concentrations; therefore, routine adjustments are not generally performed.

Adjustment for these differences can be accomplished in two ways. The first is to calculate a MoM value for African-American women using medians derived from the Caucasian population, and then to divide the resulting MoM by a factor corresponding to the ratio between values in the two populations (ie, 1.10 to 1.15). For example, if an African-American woman has a maternal serum AFP MoM of 1.60 calculated using median values from the Caucasian population, her adjusted MoM is 1.45 (1.60/1.10). The second approach is to calculate a separate set of medians using values measured on the African-American population.

Strong evidence suggests that the birth prevalence of open neural tube defects in African-American women is half or less than that in Caucasian women from the same geographic region.[240] Thus, at any given maternal serum AFP MoM, an African-American woman has half the risk of a Caucasian woman of having a pregnancy affected by an open neural tube defect. Limited information is available on the AFP concentrations in African-American women with an open neural tube defect, but what is published indicates that screening in this population should be equally effective. The prevalence of neural tube defects has declined since the practice of folic acid fortification was introduced, particularly in African-American women.[241] Data from California suggest that Hispanic women have the highest rates of neural tube defects (0.112%) as compared with Caucasians (0.096%) and Black or Asian women (0.075%).[242]

Insulin-Dependent Diabetes

Maternal serum AFP values in women who require insulin before pregnancy (type I) have been reported to be systematically lower by about 20% (0.88 MoM).[243] Women with type II diabetes, taking insulin or other oral agents, or on dietary restriction before pregnancy, also show reduced second-trimester maternal serum AFP concentrations.[244] However, controversy is ongoing regarding the need for adjustment of AFP concentrations in diabetic women when weight correction has been applied.[245] Some studies show that reduced AFP concentrations persist in diabetic women even after weight adjustment [244]; others suggest that reduced AFP concentrations can be completely explained by weight effects.[245] Debate also continues regarding whether the degree of glycemic control has an impact on maternal serum AFP concentrations in diabetic mothers.[246]

Second-trimester concentrations of uE_3 were also significantly reduced (0.95 MoM) in women with preexisting diabetes and may warrant adjustment. In contrast, alterations of second-trimester hCG and inhibin A concentrations are small, and whether or not they are taken into account will have little impact on the resulting Down syndrome risk. Similarly, first-trimester PAPP-A and hCG concentrations were not significantly altered in women with insulin-dependent diabetes (IDD).[247]

There is no compelling evidence to indicate that the rate of Down syndrome births in women with IDD is substantially different from that in the general population.[248] However, evidence suggests that the birth prevalence of open neural tube defects is higher by up to a factor of 5.[249] Thus at a given AFP MoM concentration, women with IDD are at a substantially higher risk of open neural tube defects than the general population. This can be taken into account by lowering the AFP MoM cutoff from, for example, 2.0 to 1.5. It is not possible to define the associated detection rate for diabetic mothers because no large series of maternal serum AFP measurements in IDD women with a fetus affected with an open neural tube defect have been published.

Twin Pregnancy

Maternal serum AFP concentrations in twin pregnancies are about twice the concentration found in singleton pregnancies (ie, ≈2.0 MoM).[234] Among singleton pregnancies with open spina bifida, the median serum AFP MoM is about 3.5.[162] Thus the expected maternal serum AFP in the average twin pregnancy affected with open spina bifida is thought to be around 4.5 MoM (1.0 MoM contributed by the unaffected fetus and 3.5 MoM from the fetus with open spina bifida). Screening performance in twin pregnancies therefore will not be as effective as in singleton pregnancies because the AFP distributions are less separated. Although most affected twin pregnancies are discordant for open neural tube defects, if both twins are affected (seen in about 5% of affected twin pregnancies), the screening performance can be expected to approach that in singleton pregnancies.

Calculation of Down syndrome risk requires that the distribution of analyte values for all tests in both unaffected and affected pregnancies be known. These distributions are well defined for AFP, uE_3, hCG, inhibin A, and PAPP-A in singleton pregnancies; thus reliable risks can be calculated. The distributions of these analytes are also available for a twin pregnancy unaffected by Down syndrome; the median MoMs in an unaffected twin pregnancy for AFP, uE_3, hCG, inhibin A, and PAPP-A are about 2.0, 1.7, 1.9, 2.0, and 1.8, respectively.[234,238,247] Fewer data are available for concentrations of these analytes in twin pregnancies affected with Down syndrome. A further complication is that in approximately one-third of pregnancies, both twins will be affected (monozygotic), and in two-thirds of pregnancies, only one twin will be affected (dizygotic). Screening will be less effective when only one twin is affected. Reports suggest that first-trimester serum marker concentrations differ in monozygotic and dizygotic twin pregnancies, with lower values in the former group.[250,251] Another difficulty is that the prevalence of Down syndrome is not well defined in twin pregnancies. Based on the rate of monozygotic and dizygotic twins, the prevalence of Down syndrome would be predicted to be 1.67 times higher in twin pregnancies. However, published data indicate that the prevalence of Down syndrome in twin pregnancies is actually similar to that found in singleton pregnancies.[252,253]

Given these limitations, calculation of only an approximate risk (sometimes called a *pseudorisk*) for twin pregnancy is possible.[254] This is accomplished by dividing the MoM value for each analyte by the corresponding median found in unaffected twin pregnancies. The twin pregnancy risk is then computed in the same way as for singleton pregnancies. If fetus-specific nuchal translucency measurements are available, adjusted serum marker results are used with *each* NT value to get a fetus-specific risk. The overall risk for the pregnancy is then calculated by adding the risk for each fetus in a dichorionic (presumed dizygotic) pregnancy, and averaging them for a monochorionic (presumed monozygotic) pregnancy. The resulting pseudorisk is compared with the same risk cutoff value used for women with singleton pregnancies to identify twin pregnancies as screen positive. This twin screening protocol will (1) correctly rank the pregnancies from highest to lowest risk and (2) yield a screen-positive rate similar to the rate found for singleton pregnancies at any given screening cutoff. The Down syndrome pseudorisk, however, may not be correct. Screen-positive women with twin pregnancies can be informed that their test results place them in a high-risk group but that their actual risk is uncertain. Performance of this screening and interpretation of risk for triplets and higher gestations is not recommended because of the limited data available. Typically for higher-order multiple gestations, nuchal translucency alone is performed. Additional factors that need to be considered when such screening is offered are the increased difficulty and fetal loss associated with multiple needle insertions necessary during amniocentesis, and loss of the unaffected twin should an affected twin be identified and selectively terminated.[255]

Pregnancies Achieved by Assisted Reproductive Technologies

Because women are choosing to become pregnant at more advanced chronologic ages, the use of assisted reproductive technologies, such as in vitro fertilization, for conception is increasing. Previous studies have shown that women who achieve pregnancy by IVF are about twice as likely to have a positive result after second-trimester Down syndrome screening than are women who achieve pregnancy spontaneously.[256] The increased rate is avoided with adjustment of certain MoM values. In particular, concentrations of uE_3 tend to be reduced (0.9 MoM), and hCG and inhibin A increased (1.1 to 1.2 MoM), in pregnancies achieved by IVF.[256,257] Correction of these MoMs restores an appropriate screen-positive rate. Pregnancies achieved by intrauterine insemination, with or without ovulation induction, show a similar trend in marker concentrations; however, this reproductive technology is less often reported to screening programs and therefore is difficult to take into account for risk analysis. In contrast, IVF pregnancies involving donation of oocytes have a unique marker pattern with relatively increased maternal serum AFP and inhibin A concentrations. Because these results provide opposing effects on risk, screen-positive rates are not increased and adjustment is not needed.[257]

The effects of assistive reproductive technologies on first-trimester screening markers are less pronounced. Although serum PAPP-A and hCG concentrations are slightly altered in IVF pregnancies (PAPP-A = 0.9 MoM; hCG = 1.1 MoM) relative to spontaneously achieved pregnancies, most studies show that these changes are not sufficient to lead to increased screen-positive rates.[257,258] Adjustment of first-trimester screening markers for ART pregnancies is less critical than adjustment of second-trimester markers, and, if done, would provide only a minimal improvement in screening performance. Expected and observed screen-positive rates in various assistive reproductive technologies pregnancies are shown in Table 69.6.[257]

Use of Epidemiologic Monitoring in Quality Control

In prenatal screening, the interpretative unit for each analyte is the MoM, which takes into account variables such as gestational age, maternal weight, race, and other factors. Expressing these results in MoMs allows the calculation of a patient-specific risk for Down syndrome. One of the most common causes of poor laboratory performance is the use of incorrect median values, either because those values are inappropriate for the method being used or because systematic shifts in assay values have occurred. Poor analytic performance also occurs when an assay is nonspecific or relatively inaccurate. Ensuring that median values (and, by extension, MoM values) are accurate is one of the most important responsibilities of the screening laboratory. The following discussions are adapted from an article by Knight and Palomaki[259] that discusses in detail the process of epidemiologic monitoring.

TABLE 69.6 Down Syndrome Screen Positive Rates (%) Observed (95% Confidence Intervals) and Expected for Assisted Reproductive Technologies

Type of Assisted Reproductive Technology	n	FIRST TRIMESTER		SECOND TRIMESTER	
		Observed	Expected	Observed	Expected
In vitro fertilization with ovulation induction	277	8.6 (5.3–11.9)	5.5	20.2 (15.4–25.0)	14.7
Intrauterine insemination with ovulation induction	323	3.4 (1.4–5.4)	4.2	21.2 (16.6–25.7)	11.9
Intrauterine insemination without ovulation induction	247	6.1 (3.1–9.1)	4.3	19.1 (14.1–24.0)	12.3
In vitro fertilization with ovulation induction and egg donation	59	3.4 (0.0–8.0)	2.5	12.3 (3.8–20.8)	7.4
In vitro fertilization with egg donation	56	1.8 (0.0–5.3)	1.0	7.4 (0.4–14.4)	3.9

Modified from Lambert-Messerlian G, Dugoff L, Vidaver J, Canick JA, Malone FD, Ball RH, et al. First- and second-trimester Down syndrome screening markers in pregnancies achieved through assisted reproductive technologies (ART): a FASTER trial study. *Prenat Diagn* 2006;26:672–8.

Definition of Epidemiologic Monitoring

A powerful method for evaluating and monitoring the appropriateness of medians is epidemiologic monitoring. This process involves gathering data from the screened population to calculate the detection (proportion of affected pregnancies with positive test results) and screen-positive (proportion of screened pregnancies with a positive test result) rates. These rates are then to be compared with expectations based on the maternal age distribution of the population studied. Obtaining a detection rate is difficult because complete ascertainment of all pregnancy outcomes is required, and it can take years before a sufficient number of affected pregnancies occur to allow reliable estimates. In practice, the screen-positive rate is used for epidemiologic monitoring because a reliable estimate can be calculated in a short time, and it is not necessary to have outcome information. For prenatal screening, the positive rate is defined as the proportion of women with test results falling at or above a specified AFP MoM (for open neural tube defect screening) or a specified risk cutoff value (Down syndrome screening). These rates are in fact similar to false-positive rates because few screen-positive individuals have true-positive results (ie, they do have an affected fetus). For this reason, the term *initial positive rate* (IPR) has been suggested, because it more accurately describes what is being calculated. The IPR can be used to assess whether medians are appropriate, because it will be shifted upward or downward if medians are incorrect for the population being screened. Further, once the IPR is shown to be within acceptable limits, continuous monitoring can help detect shifts in assay values.

Establishing Assay-Specific and Population-Specific Median Values

Another important responsibility of the prenatal screening laboratory is to establish assay-specific and population-specific median values for each analyte used in screening or to show that median values obtained from another source are appropriate. Relatively small errors in median values have a disproportionate impact on both the accuracy of the calculated risk and the number of women identified as screen positive. Values measured on the same patients and the same proficiency testing samples have been known to vary greatly among methods, depending on the analyte measured.[260] Median values therefore are not directly transferable between reagent sets from different methods. Median values sometimes differ among laboratories even when the same methodology is employed. This difference is caused by such factors as the reliability of gestational dating, race, and maternal weight; even apparently subtle differences in assay instrumentation; or changes in manufacturer lot numbers of reagents or calibrators.[261]

Median values must be routinely monitored and updated as necessary. Median values provided in package inserts are not acceptable for many of the reasons already given. It has been recommended that median values should be established using at least 100 values per week of gestation in the screening period. In practice, however, obtaining 100 serum samples for each gestational week is very difficult even for large laboratories. Given these constraints, the following strategies are recommended for obtaining reliable median values, categorized according to whether a laboratory is implementing a screening test for the first time or is updating an existing set of median values.

Two alternatives are available when a laboratory is establishing median values for the first time. The first and optimal method is to obtain measurements on 300 to 500 patient specimens using the assay selected for screening. Establishing that all of these samples come from unaffected singleton pregnancies is not necessary because the prevalence of conditions that produce abnormal values (eg, twins, fetal demise, open fetal defects) is small and will have minimal impact.[234] Data are used to derive median values for each completed week of gestation. Appropriate weighted regression analysis is then used to fit the observed data. The regression equation is used to predict "smoothed" medians for each week of gestation. Usually the median value is found at each completed week and is regressed against the average gestational age for that week. This technique helps reduce the effects of outliers. Weighting takes into account the reliability of these summary estimates and usually is based on the square root of the number of samples observed at each week.

Measurements of the concentrations of AFP, uE_3, and PAPP-A increase by a constant proportion—about 15% per week for AFP, 25% per week for uE_3 measurements, and 50% for PAPP-A. A log-linear model best fits this relationship (log of the measurements [y-axis] is regressed against gestational age [x-axis]). The regression model for hCG versus gestational age fits an exponential model similar to that used for radioactive decay. Measurements of inhibin A are relatively flat, but experience has shown that a cubic model fits the data, with a minimum found between 16 and 18 weeks' gestation.[262] Figs. 69.7 to 69.10 are graphical representations of the weighted regression equations and resulting smoothed medians for the

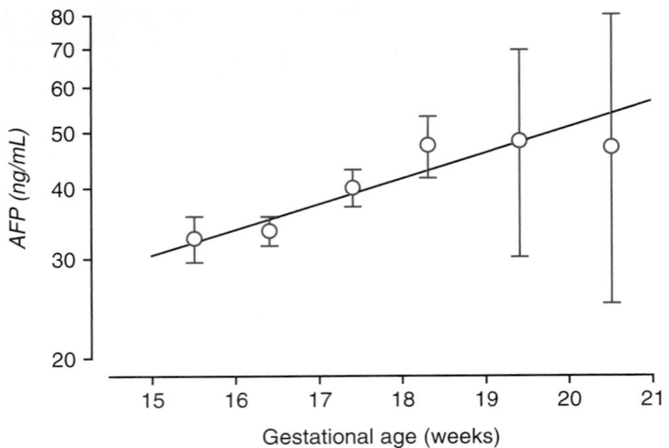

FIGURE 69.7 Computation of median values for maternal serum alpha-fetoprotein (AFP) in the second trimester. The observed average gestational age from Table 69.7 is plotted on the horizontal axis and the median of that week's AFP measurements on the vertical logarithmic axis. The thin vertical lines represent the 95% confidence intervals of the medians. The line represents the results of a linear regression analysis of log AFP versus age weighted by the square root of the number of samples. The equation of that line in completed weeks is median $AFP=10^{0.04465\times(weeks)+0.8334}$. The corresponding equation for day-specific medians is median $AFP=10^{0.006378\times(days)+0.8142}$.

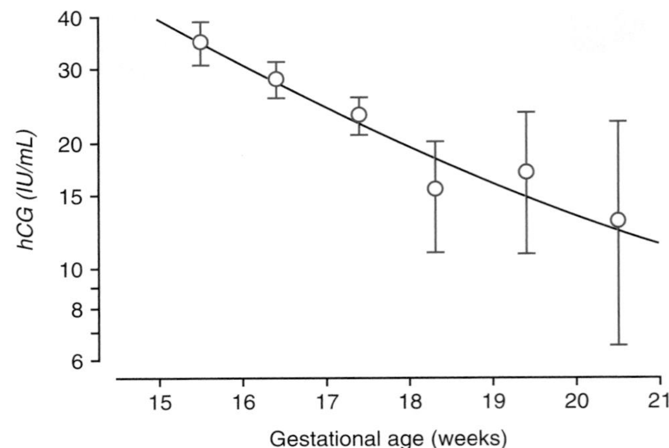

FIGURE 69.9 Computation of median values for maternal serum hCG in the second trimester. The observed average gestational age from Table 69.7 is plotted on the horizontal axis and the median of that week's hCG measurements on the vertical logarithmic axis. The thin vertical lines represent the 95% confidence intervals of the medians. The line represents the results of a nonlinear regression analysis weighted by the square root of the number of samples. The equation of that curve in completed weeks is hCG median = $39.69\times e^{-0.3001\times(weeks-14)}+5.93$. The corresponding equation for day-specific medians is hCG median = $45.14\times e^{-0.04287\times(days)}+5.93$.

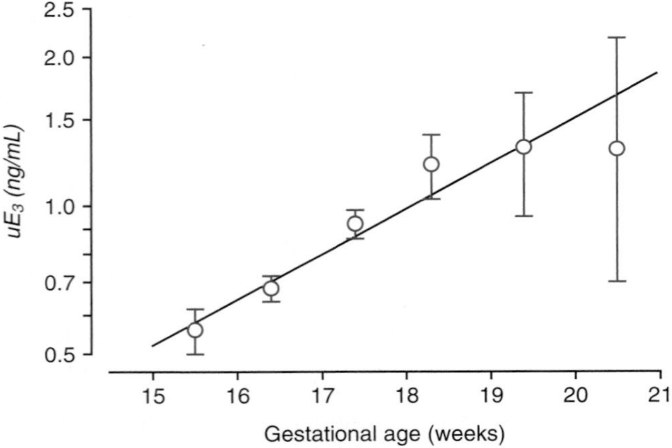

FIGURE 69.8 Computation of median values for maternal serum unconjugated estriol (uE_3) in the second trimester. The observed average gestational age from Table 69.7 is plotted on the horizontal axis and the median of that week's uE_3 measurements on the vertical logarithmic axis. The thin vertical lines represent the 95% confidence intervals of the medians. The line represents the results of a linear regression analysis of log uE_3 versus age weighted by the square root of the number of samples. The equation of that line in completed weeks is median $uE_3=10^{0.09165\times(weeks)-1.618}$. The corresponding equation for day-specific medians is median $uE_3=10^{0.01309\times(days)-1.657}$. SI unit (nmol/L) conversion factor: 3.47.

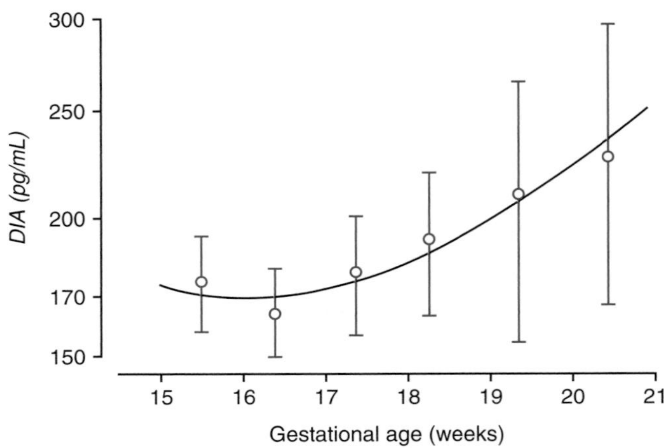

FIGURE 69.10 Computation of median values for maternal serum dimeric inhibin A (DIA) in the second trimester. The observed average gestational age from Table 69.7 is plotted on the horizontal axis and the median of that week's inhibin A measurements on the vertical logarithmic axis. The thin vertical lines represent the 95% confidence intervals of the medians. The line represents the results of a quadratic regression analysis weighted by the square root of the number of samples. The equation of that curve in completed weeks is inhibin A median $= 3.404\times weeks^2-106.7\times weeks+1005.7$. The corresponding equation for day-specific medians is inhibin A median $= 0.06947\times days^2-15.66\times days+1052$. SI unit (ng/mL) conversion factor: 1.

second-trimester markers (the legends contain the respective median regression equations). The data are provided in Table 69.7. Fig. 69.11 shows medians and weighted regression lines for first-trimester PAPP-A and total hCG.

Some laboratories use "day-specific" medians rather than weekly medians, where a different median value is used for each day of pregnancy. Although individual pregnancies cannot be reliably dated to within 1 day, a consistent day-by-day change in analyte concentrations is noted when data from a group of pregnant women is observed. Table 69.8 shows observed and regressed medians for uE_3 for a group of ultrasound-dated women in their 17th week of gestation. The observed median concentrations clearly increase during that week. The regressed median for 16 weeks, 0 days, is quite

TABLE 69.7 Observed and Regressed Median Values for Four Second-Trimester Down Syndrome Analytes

Week of Gestation	Mean GA	Number Studied	AFP (ng/mL)		uE_3 (ng/mL)		hCG (IU/mL)		InhA (pg/mL)	
			Obs	Reg	Obs	Reg	Obs	Reg	Obs	Reg
15	15.5	79	32.6	31.8	0.56	0.57	34.9	35.3	175	171
16	16.4	183	33.6	35.3	0.68	0.71	28.4	27.7	164	170
17	17.4	94	40.0	39.1	0.92	0.87	23.3	22.1	179	176
18	18.3	29	47.4	43.4	1.21	1.08	15.5	17.9	191	188
19	19.4	8	48.2	48.0	1.31	1.33	17.0	14.8	210	207
20	20.5	4	47.0	53.2	1.30	1.64	13.0	12.5	227	233
Average or total	16.7	397								

AFP, Alpha-fetoprotein; *GA*, gestational age; *hCG*, human chorionic gonadotropin; *InhA*, inhibin A; *Obs*, observed median; *Reg*, regressed median; *uE_3*, unconjugated estriol. SI conversion factors: AFP (μg/L) = 1; uE3 (nmol/L) = 3.47, InhA (ng/L) = 1.

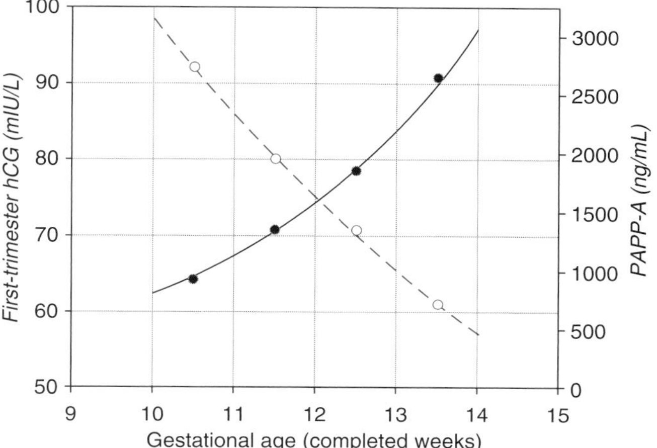

FIGURE 69.11 Typical median values for maternal serum pregnancy–associated plasma protein-A (PAPP-A) and total hCG in the first trimester. The observed average gestational age is plotted on the horizontal axis and the median of that week's PAPP-A or total hCG measurements on the vertical logarithmic axis. The PAPP-A median = $10^{(1.4633 + 0.144601 \times \text{weeks})}$. The total hCG median = $385.1 \times 0.98069^{\text{days}}$.

different from the median for 16 weeks, 6 days. If weekly medians were to have been used instead, all of these samples would have been interpreted against a single median of approximately 0.74 ng/mL (0.74 μg/L) (2.6 nmol/L).

An acceptable alternative for the generation of new median data is to identify an established laboratory that is willing to share its reliable median values. Then, 25 to 50 specimens are assayed at each laboratory. These specimens are selected so that their results span the analytic measurement range. The two sets of values are compared using linear regression analysis (after appropriate transformations) to establish the relationship between the two assays. The regression equation is applied to the reliable set of median values to derive a set of medians appropriate for the laboratory. These median values are used temporarily until values from 300 to 500 patients are available for the analysis provided earlier.

Laboratories must update existing median values in several situations. Significant differences in values on the same patient specimens are common when a new lot of the reagents or reagents from a different manufacturer are

TABLE 69.8 Observed and Regressed Day-Specific Medians for Unconjugated Estriol During the 17th Week of Gestation

Gestational Age (Week, Day)	Number of Observations	uE_3, ng/mL (nmol/L) Observed	Regressed
16,0	195	0.67 (2.3)	0.68 (2.4)
16,1	225	0.69 (2.4)	0.70 (2.4)
16,2	228	0.71 (2.5)	0.72 (2.5)
16,3	219	0.76 (2.6)	0.74 (2.6)
16,4	186	0.78 (2.7)	0.76 (2.6)
16,5	191	0.80 (2.8)	0.79 (2.7)
16,6	175	0.78 (2.7)	0.81 (2.8)

used. In this situation, the relationship between the new and old methods is established by regression analysis of values measured on the same patient specimens. If a periodic adjustment is required, the laboratory should carefully choose the characteristics of the population to be used (eg, race, method of dating, time period) and should verify that the assay has been providing consistent results over the time period of interest. This is done by routinely monitoring the median MoM over time (epidemiologic monitoring) as discussed in greater detail later in this chapter. Resulting data are then analyzed, as described previously.

Epidemiologic Monitoring of Open Neural Tube Defect Screening

In maternal serum AFP screening for open neural tube defects, the IPR is the proportion of women with values above the specified MoM cutoff value. For example, at a screening cutoff value of 2.5 MoM, IPRs should be 1% to 3%. When new medians are implemented, the IPR can be used to determine if the medians are appropriate by comparing the expected with the observed IPRs. If the IPR falls outside the expected range, it is possible that the medians are incorrect for the assay being used or for the population being screened. For example, if the IPR at a cutoff of 2.5 MoM is 5%, median values may be too low, resulting in too many high MoMs and too many women having screen-positive results.

Once the IPR is shown to be within an acceptable range, ongoing monitoring of this rate serves as a check on shifts in assay calibration caused by changes in (1) reagent lots, (2) reagent deterioration, (3) poor technical performance, and (4) other factors. Simultaneous monitoring of the IPR and the results of quality control (QC) samples can facilitate identification of shifts in assay values. If, for instance, the IPR at a 2.5 AFP MoM cutoff increases from 2% to 4%, and at the same time some or all of the values of QC samples shift significantly upward by 10% or more, the change is consistent with an upward shift in assay calibration. The IPR increases when the assay values increase because individual AFP values are interpreted by using medians generated from data gathered in the past. In the example given previously, it may be necessary to calculate new medians or adjust existing median values to take into account the assay shift.

It is difficult to provide an absolute rule as to how large a change in the IPR is sufficient to warrant recomputing medians. Factors other than the assay can affect the IPR. For example, a significant increase in the number of pregnancies dated by ultrasound will reduce the IPR because incorrectly dated pregnancies will be identified before the AFP test is done. However, consider that an upward shift in AFP values of just 10% can increase the IPR by more than 50% (eg, from 2% to 3%) with little gain in detection. In effect, more interventions (ultrasound examinations or amniocenteses, or both) will be required to detect each case of neural tube defect. Therefore, if a change in the IPR of 50% or more occurs simultaneously with an identifiable shift in assay values of 10% or more, medians need to be recalculated. Laboratories may wish to have stricter warning limits (eg, shifts of 25% or more in the IPR occurring simultaneously with a change of 7% or more in QC samples). When these rules are applied, enough values should be used to ensure that a reliable IPR can be calculated (generally 300 to 500 values will ensure reliability) and that observed changes are statistically significant. Further, the change should occur over several kit lots. Otherwise the laboratory may be tracking random error. The IPR can also be calculated using a moving window to improve reliability. For example, consider a laboratory that screens 300 women per month. In addition to calculating a monthly IPR, the lab could calculate a cumulative 3-month moving window by adding the current month's data and dropping data from the oldest month. The actual time period for both the individual and a cumulative moving window will be determined by how many samples are screened per unit of time by any given laboratory.

Epidemiologic Monitoring of Down Syndrome Screening

In screening for Down syndrome, the IPR is the proportion of women with a risk at or above the cutoff value. In contrast to neural tube defect screening, the IPR for Down syndrome screening is influenced by each of the analytes used in the risk calculation. Therefore, monitoring the IPR does not provide information on which assay(s) might be responsible when an inappropriate IPR is obtained. Consequently, it is necessary to individually monitor each assay separately. Individual monitoring of each assay can be accomplished according to the following rationale. When individual MoM values are calculated for each patient using gestational age–specific medians, MoM values can be analyzed collectively without regard for the gestational week. If the medians are appropriate, the resulting distribution of MoM values will have a grand median MoM of 1.00. The center of the distribution is typically expressed as the median, rather than as the mean, because MoM distributions are not Gaussian on the linear scale.

Initial application of the grand MoM is done to ensure that when medians are first implemented, they are appropriate for the assay and population being screened. This is accomplished by calculating the grand MoM using values from 300 to 500 individuals screened after the new set of medians is implemented. The grand MoM should be 1.00, within statistical limits. A convenient approach is to plot the grand MoM values on a graph, thus facilitating the detection of trends. IPR observations can be plotted on the same graph. If the IPR begins to trend in a positive or negative direction, the grand MoM for each assay can be examined to determine if one of the analytes is paralleling the IPR change. If a significant change in one of the assays has occurred, corrective action should be taken (eg, recalculating medians). For example, suppose the IPR shows a significant upward trend (eg, from 6% to 9%), and over the same time period the median MoM of the uE_3 assay significantly decreases (eg, from 1.03 to 0.91). Because low uE_3 values are associated with increased risk for fetal Down syndrome, it is possible that the change in the uE_3 assay is responsible for the increase in IPR. The next step would be to examine QC specimen values to determine whether a corresponding downward shift in values has occurred. If a shift has occurred, it is appropriate to recalculate and implement a new set of uE_3 medians using data collected after the time when the change in the uE_3 assay occurred (or to apply an adjustment factor to the old medians). A simultaneous change in two assays can complicate monitoring because the IPR might not change if the shift in one analyte value increases risk and the shift in the other analyte decreases risk. Simultaneous monitoring of the IPR and the median MoM for each analyte is recommended. IPRs should be calculated only when sufficient patient values are available (typically, 300 to 500 samples) to ensure a statistically reliable rate. Further, a single IPR or median MoM that deviates from expected should serve as only as a warning to examine QC data more closely.

Laboratories need to have an action limit in place to determine how much variability is to be allowed in the grand MoM, which is the median value of MoM values from all patients. To accomplish this, one should consider the impact on the Down syndrome detection rate and the IPR of a 10% downward shift in uE_3 values (grand MoM of 0.90). This is simulated by recalculating MoM values after assay values are artificially shifted down by 10%, followed by mathematical modeling of the detection rate and the associated IPR. Such an assay shift effectively changes the MoM for any given sample, because current assay values are interpreted using reference data collected in the past. When uE_3 values shift downward by 10%, the detection rate increases only slightly, from 59% to 62%. However, the IPR increases from 4.8% to 6.7%, a 40% increase. Thus, what might be viewed as a small shift in assay values has a large impact on the IPR, with little corresponding gain in cases detected. Relatively large changes in the IPR accompanying small shifts in assay values are one of the primary reasons for closely monitoring assays to ensure that the amniocentesis referral rate is maintained within reasonable limits. Given these facts, screening laboratories should consider important, as a minimum, a consistent deviation of 10% from 1.00 MoM (range 0.90 to 1.10). Laboratories may wish to consider setting up stricter warning limits, such as 7% (assuming this percentage is based on sufficient numbers of samples to yield statistically significant results). With this limit, median MoM values outside the range of 0.93 to 1.07 would be considered sufficiently deviant to warrant further investigation to determine whether a problem exists.

Although the IPR for laboratories screening for Down syndrome using multiple tests is generally about 5% in an unselected pregnancy population, it may be affected by various factors (other than incorrect medians), including the type of tests used, the screening cutoff value chosen, and the maternal age distribution of the screened population. For example, if screening applied primarily to older women, the IPR will be substantially higher because older women are collectively more likely to be screen-positive because of their higher age-specific risks. For example, if the triple test is being used to screen women of age 35 years and older at a term risk cutoff of 1:250, approximately 25% of women will be screen positive.[263] The method of gestational dating will also affect the IPR. Laboratories with a high percentage of pregnancies dated by the first day of the LMP will have a higher IPR than do laboratories where most gestational ages have been provided from ultrasound measurements because there is more variability in the accuracy of dating a population by LMP than by ultrasound.[201]

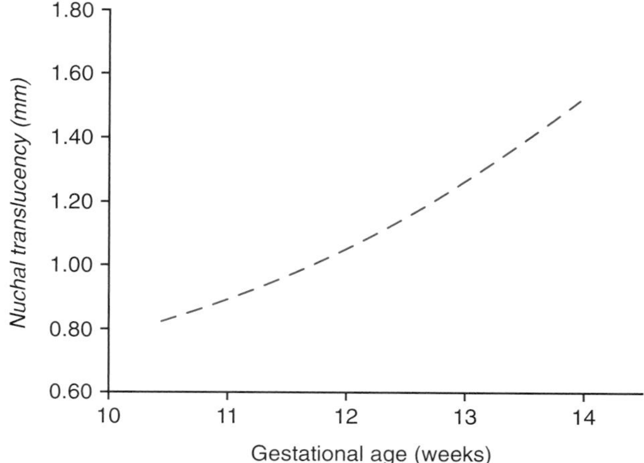

FIGURE 69.12 Typical medians for nuchal translucency during the first trimester.

Epidemiologic Monitoring of Nuchal Translucency Measurements

The introduction of the ultrasound measurement of nuchal translucency (NT) as part of the Down syndrome screening test has led to a new era in epidemiologic monitoring. Although serum screening analytes are under the day-to-day control of the laboratory, NT ultrasound is performed outside of the laboratory, at multiple locations, and by many individuals. This situation is comparable to trying to report uniform screening results with each patient's AFP measurement being run in a different lab using a different assay and reagent lot.

To bring uniformity to NT measurements, credentialing agencies have been established to train and certify sonographers. Examples of these agencies include the Fetal Medicine Foundation in the United Kingdom and the Nuchal Translucency Quality Review program, a subsidiary organization of the Society for Maternal-Fetal Medicine (SMFM). Certification involves didactic and hands-on training along with image review. NT should be used in screening by sonographers only after training has been provided and when quality assurance measures are in place.[155] Previous studies have clearly shown that without such training, the performance of NT as a marker for Down syndrome is erratic, with anywhere from 0% to 100% of cases detected prenatally.[217]

The laboratory has the responsibility of establishing NT median data for each sonographer and monitoring the performance over time. To determine a median equation, preliminary data should be submitted to the laboratory that include a series of paired NT and crown-rump length measurements. Regression analysis, as described earlier, provides an appropriate median equation. NT data should fit a log-linear regression and should increase by about 25% per gestational week (Fig. 69.12).[264] A single median equation may be used for all sonographers but is not likely to provide optimal interpretations for each individual sonographer. Even when all sonographers are trained using a single method, median NT results show marked variation.[265] A better approach is to generate an NT median equation for each sonographer or each group of sonographers for whom measurements are similar. Improved screening performance is observed when median data are made more specific.[266,267]

The task of monitoring NT performance over time is daunting given the variable relationship between sonography and laboratory staff at different institutions and the sheer numbers of sonographers who may be submitting data to one laboratory. A further complication is that a single sonographer may submit very few data points to a laboratory, and longtime intervals may be required before it is possible to conduct a meaningful review of results. Nevertheless, objective criteria upon which sonography data should be judged have been identified. As with serum markers, NT data, once normalized for gestational age, should center at a median of 1.0 MoM. The distribution of NT values in unaffected pregnancies generally has a standard deviation of the log MoM in the range of 0.1. The rate of increase with advancing gestational age between 10 and 13 weeks' gestation should be about 25% per week, as shown in Fig. 69.13.[268] Examination of NT data over time can be performed in-house or obtained externally through services provided to laboratories by the Nuchal Translucency Quality Review (NTQR) (www.ntqr.org) or the NT Monitor (www.ipmms.org) program. Regardless of method, ongoing quality assessment of NT data is essential for screening accuracy.[269]

External Proficiency Testing

All laboratories performing prenatal screening should participate in an external proficiency testing program that distributes unknown specimens reflecting the concentrations of analytes found in pregnancy. These programs will evaluate the laboratory's ability to convert analyte values into a MoM using the laboratory's own median equations, to make screening recommendations, to adjust for variables that influence analyte values, and to calculate patient-specific risks. In the United States, the College of American Pathologists (CAP) provides a second-trimester program (CAP Maternal Screening Survey FP) with approximately 200 enrolled laboratories. Five second-trimester serum and two

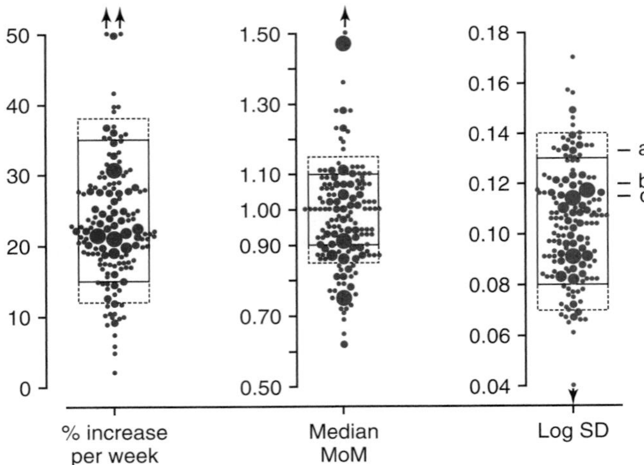

FIGURE 69.13 Summary of quality assessment parameters for 140 sonographers, showing the increase per week *(left column)*, the median NT MoM *(center column)*, and *the* logarithmic standard deviation *(right column)*. (Reprinted from Palomaki GE, Neveux LM, Donnenfeld A, et al. Quality assessment of routine nuchal translucency measurements: a North American laboratory perspective. *Genet Med* 2008;10:131–8.)

amniotic fluid proficiency samples are distributed three times each year. The CAP program has information on its website (www.cap.org) that assists participants with risk calculation verification depending on the parameter set used. New York State also has an external proficiency testing program that is required for laboratories serving New York State residents. Five serum and five amniotic fluid samples are distributed three times each year. A similar interlaboratory proficiency program for first-trimester screening markers is available through the Women and Infants Hospital of Rhode Island at www.ipmms.org. External proficiency programs for maternal serum screening are offered in other countries; guidelines for country-specific testing programs should be consulted for more information.

LABORATORY TESTS

In this section of the chapter, we review methods for measurement of (1) hCG, (2) AFP, (3) uE_3, (4) inhibin A, (5) PAPP-A, and (6) fetal lung maturity.

Chorionic Gonadotropin Testing

Measurement of hCG is used to (1) detect pregnancy and its abnormalities (eg, ectopic and molar pregnancies), (2) screen for Down syndrome and trisomy 18, and (3) monitor the course of a patient with a cancer that produces hCG. Because hCG has these diverse uses, many assays are used, including qualitative urine and serum devices and quantitative serum assays.

Chemistry

hCG is a glycoprotein containing a protein core with branched carbohydrate side chains that usually terminate with sialic acid. The hormone is a heterodimer composed of two nonidentical, non–covalently bound glycoprotein subunits, alpha (α) and beta (β) (see Chapter 36). When the hCG dimer is dissociated, the hormone activity is lost. However, a major part of the original activity is restored by equimolar recombination of the two subunits. The hCGα subunit contains 92 amino acids, 2 carbohydrate side chains, and 5 disulfide bridges. The molecular mass of the α subunit is estimated to be 14,900 Da, of which 10,200 is the protein component. hCGβ consists of 145 amino acids and has six carbohydrate side chains and six disulfide bridges. The molecular mass of the β subunit is estimated to be 23,000. Thus the heterodimer has a molecular weight of approximately 37,900 Da and has a higher carbohydrate proportion than any other human hormone.

The hCG carbohydrate composition changes as pregnancy progresses. In the first few weeks of pregnancy, more than 80% of immunoreactive hCG is a large molecular mass form (MW 41,000 to 42,000 Da), with additional monosaccharides in its carbohydrate chains, called *hyperglycosylated hCG* (hCG-H).[270] Serum concentrations of hCG-H decline rapidly after the fourth week, and the 37,900-Da molecular mass form predominates for the remainder of the pregnancy.[271] In addition to hCG and hCG-H, maternal serum includes numerous other hCG variants. To avoid confusion, the International Federation of Clinical Chemistry and Laboratory Medicine (IFCC) has recommended a specific nomenclature for the identification of intact hCG and its variants.[272] These include (1) nicked hCG (hCGn), (2) the free α subunit (hCGα), (3) the free β subunit (hCGβ), (4) the nicked free β subunit (hCGβn), and (5) the beta core fragment. hCGn is produced from enzymatic cleavage of peptide bonds in hCGβ at position 44–45 (and, after prolonged incubation, at position 51–52).[273] Nicking inactivates the hormone and may reduce the ability to bind some hCG antibodies. Other nicking sites are at β44–45, β47–48, and α70–71.[274] hCG beta core fragment is the terminal degradation product of hCGβ and represents the 73–amino acid core of hCGβ. It is composed of two pieces of the β-subunit, residues 6–40 and residues 55–92, held together by disulfide bridges.[275] hCG beta core fragment is detected only in urine and has a molecular mass of 13,000 Da.

Urine contains predominantly hCG beta core fragment and to a lesser degree unmodified hCG and hCGn. Clearance occurs both in the liver and through the kidneys and varies for the different hCG forms. Hepatic clearance[276] is approximately 2 $mL/min/m^2$, and renal clearance is approximately 0.4 $mL/min/m^2$. A study using highly specific immunoassays for hCG, hCGβ, and hCGα found that disappearance after term pregnancy was triphasic.[277] Rapid, medium, and slow half-lives were, respectively: hCG, 3.6, 18, and 53 hours; hCGβ, 1.0, 23, and 194 hours; and hCGα, 0.63, 6.0, and 22 hours.

Biochemistry

hCG is synthesized in the cytotrophoblast and syncytiotrophoblast cells of the placenta. Minute amounts are also made in the pituitary of men and nonpregnant women,[39,278,279] and, similar to many other pituitary hormones, it is secreted in a pulsatile fashion (see Chapter 36).[280] A single gene located on chromosome 6 encodes the α subunit of all four glycoprotein hormones (TSH, LH [luteinizing hormone], FSH, and hCG). Chromosome 19 contains a family of seven genes that encode the hCGβ subunit, though only three appear to be active.[281] Separate messenger RNAs are transcribed from the respective genes, and the α and β subunits are translated from each. The subunits spontaneously combine in the rough endoplasmic reticulum and are then continuously secreted into the maternal circulation.

Synthesis of hCGβ peaks at about 8 to 10 weeks' gestation, but production of the α subunit continues to increase and appears to be a function of the mass of the placenta. The production of hCGβ in the syncytiotrophoblasts may be under paracrine control of gonadotropin-releasing hormone (GnRH) produced in cytotrophoblasts. Studies suggest that the cytotrophoblasts produce inhibin, which stimulates hCG production.[282] The number of cytotrophoblasts peaks at about the same time the hCGβ production peaks. In the second trimester, more than 99% of hCG is the dimer form; only a small amount circulates as free hCGβ.[40]

Extensive homology exists between the peptide portions of hCGβ and LHβ subunits. Investigators have proposed that a single base pair deletion in the ancestral LHβ gene lengthened the subunit from 115 amino acids to 145 amino acids; 80% of the first 115 amino acids in both β subunits are identical, but 20 additional amino acid residues are unique in hCGβ.[283]

Physiology

hCG stimulates the corpus luteum in the ovary to make progesterone during the first weeks of pregnancy. The placenta makes inadequate amounts of progesterone during this time. No specific receptor for hCG is known; it binds to and activates the LH receptor in cells of the corpus luteum in the maternal ovary. Species other than primates and horses use LH for this function. Glycation of the α subunit has a dominant role[284] in signal transduction, an increase in intracellular cyclic adenosine monophosphate (cAMP). The cAMP increase in turn stimulates the production of progesterone, a steroid that prevents menses and thus facilitates pregnancy. hCG binds weakly to TSH receptors in the maternal thyroid, and extremely increased hCG concentrations have the potential to be thyrotropic. A study of 63 women with an hCG concentration greater than 400,000 IU/L revealed that TSH was suppressed and free thyroxine was increased in 100% and 80% of specimens, respectively. However, only four women had clinical signs and symptoms of hyperthyroidism.[71]

hCG-H is synthesized by the invasive cytotrophoblast cells and appears to have an autocrine function that modulates cytotrophoblast invasion of the myometrium in early pregnancy.[285]

hCG Assays

Of historical note, Vaitukaitis and colleagues took advantage of the uniqueness of hCGβ to produce the first specific assay for hCG, which used polyclonal antibodies raised against the β subunit.[286] Subsequently, highly specific monoclonal antibodies have been produced that recognize epitopes on the hCG dimer and hCGβ. The molecular epitope structure and the specificities of some of these antibodies have been described.[287]

Currently, bioassays, receptor assays, and agglutination inhibition assays are obsolete. The historical bioassays are interesting, however, because they exploit the physiologic effect of hCG.[288-292]

Qualitative hCG Tests. Numerous tests for the qualitative detection of hCG in urine or serum are available as over-the-counter (home) or point-of-care (POC) devices, and their use for the rapid identification of pregnancy is well established. Qualitative detection of hCG in urine is a test granted waived status under the Clinical Laboratory Improvement Amendments of 1988 (CLIA '88); therefore this is performed at home and at the POC. In contrast, the use of serum as a sample matrix is considered a moderately complex test, even when the test device itself is approved for use with urine or serum. The difference in test complexity status is due to the requirement that serum, rather than whole blood, should be analyzed, and that centrifugation of the specimen is necessary. As such, qualitative serum hCG tests are performed in laboratories, neither at home or in POC situations.

POC devices are single-use tests that utilize immunochromatography for the rapid qualitative detection of hCG when its concentration exceeds a detection threshold, which is frequently 25 IU/L. Cervinski and colleagues[293] evaluated the analytic lower limit of detection of 12 different brands of qualitative hCG tests (6 OTC and 6 POC devices) using urine specimens collected from 10 women in early pregnancy (within 10 days of expected menses). Detection limits varied from 6 to 100 IU/L for POC devices and from 0.5 to 25 IU/L for the OTC devices.[293] Considerable variation was noted across devices tested with a single specimen and within a device tested with different specimens; this was attributed to the heterogeneous mixture of hCG variants in pregnancy urine. The lower analytic limits of detection of the OTC devices was thought to be a function of the specimen volume used to perform those tests, which is approximately five times greater than volumes required for POC hCG tests.

First-morning specimens are preferred for qualitative urine pregnancy tests because they are concentrated and contain abundant hCG. Urine applied to the device is absorbed into a nitrocellulose bed. hCG is concentrated into a narrow band as the urine migrates. A dye- or latex bead–labeled anti-hCG antibody in the device binds to the migrating hCG and passes through a zone having solid-phase capture antibody to hCG. The appearance of a colored line indicates a positive test. An area of solid-phase antibody with specificity to the labeled anti-hCG antibody is located separate from the test band and controls for the addition of adequate specimen volume. False-positive results may occur because of the presence in serum of interfering substances such as interfering antibodies.[36] The test area of some devices may darken over time even in the absence of hCG; therefore delayed interpretation of the test band has been known to produce a false-positive result. False-negative results are more commonly encountered and occur if the hCG concentration is below the detection threshold (eg, a dilute urine), during early gestational age, or if hCG is extremely increased due to the high-dose hook effect. False-negative results have also been caused by increased concentrations of hCG beta core fragment because of its ability to bind one of the two anti-hCG reagent antibodies, thus preventing the binding of dimeric hCG.[294] Because hCG beta core fragment is a predominant hCG variant in urine after the fifth week of pregnancy, this hCG "hook effect" is an important consideration in healthcare settings where qualitative pregnancy tests are often performed beyond the first few weeks of pregnancy.

Exactly how soon after fertilization and implantation hCG becomes detectable in the urine varies considerably between women. Using a highly sensitive quantitative hCG test, Wilcox and colleagues[295] demonstrated that 90% of pregnancies were detectable on the day of the missed menses, while 100% were detectable 11 or more days later.

The simplicity and speed with which results are obtained make these tests valuable for pregnancy confirmation, but they may miss the diagnosis of a very early or abnormal pregnancy.

Quantitative hCG Tests. All commonly used hCG tests are high-performance immunometric assays designed to measure hCG over a wide range of concentrations. Upper limits of detection vary from 400 to 15,000 IU/L, and so specimen dilution is frequently required to obtain an absolute measurement. The lowest detectable concentration of these assays is from 1 to 2 IU/L.

The measurement of hCG is complicated by its molecular heterogeneity; considerable variation in measured hCG concentrations is observed between the different assays. One reason for this variation is the use of different antibody pairs in different hCG assays. Antibodies to hCG will recognize epitopes on the α subunit, the β subunit, or the αβ heterodimer,[287] and so analytic specificity is dependent upon the specific pair of antibodies utilized. Another source of variation is the reference material used to calibrate hCG assays. Most hCG assays are calibrated against the World Health Organization (WHO) Fourth (75/589) International Standard, which contains purified urinary hCG with an activity value of 9300 IU/mg determined by bioassay. However, these reference materials also contain substantial amounts of hCGn and hCGβ; this is problematic in that some hCG assays overrecognize or underrecognize these variants or may not detect them at all. A new preparation, the Fifth (07/364) International Standard, is now available that is highly purified from urine to remove the hCGn and hCGβ present in previous standards and is used by a minority of current assays. An evaluation of the use of hCG assays calibrated to the new standard for second-trimester Down syndrome screening found that hCG measurement using the new assay strongly correlated to the current method, although a proportional increase in hCG concentration using the new assay necessitated a calculation of new medians.[296]

Current hCG assays lack harmonization. This is due to the fact that various antibodies recognize the hCG variants differently. In addition, the secondary hCG standards that assay manufacturers provide to the end-user for assay calibration vary greatly in terms of purity. As a consequence, results from different hCG assays are not the same and cannot be directly compared.[297-299] In an effort to address some of these problems, the IFCC established the Working Group for the Standardization of hCG in 1994. This group prepared highly purified standards for 6 hCG variants and calibrated them in molar concentration.[272,274] These preparations are designated *reference reagents* (RR) and contain hCG (99/688), hCGn (99/642), hCGβ (99/650), hCGβn (99/692), hCGγcf, and hCGα (99/720).

Because of variation between hCG assays, median hCG values calculated for maternal serum screening are not transferable and should be considered method specific. hCG measurements in early pregnancy generally are expressed as international units per liter (IU/L). A typical hCG concentration at 16 weeks is approximately 30,000 IU/L, and many screening laboratories express hCG concentrations in international units per milliliter (eg, 30,000 IU/L is expressed as 30 IU/mL) (see Fig. 69.2). A simple alternative is to use kilo-international units per liter, consistent with the international system for SI units, in which concentrations are expressed per liter.

Immunoassays specific for free hCGβ are commercially available outside the United States (see http://www.perkinelmer.com/products/default.xhtml) and may be preferred for first-trimester screening.[300]

Specimen Collection and Handling. Serum is used for quantitative hCG assays and is obtained from fasting or nonfasting women by standard phlebotomy techniques. Blood specimens are collected into suitable tubes without anticoagulants, are allowed to clot at room temperature, and are centrifuged to obtain clear serum. hCG is stable in maternal serum and can be shipped at ambient temperature and stored at 4 to 8°C for 1 week.[301] If testing is to be delayed beyond 1 week, serum should be stored at −20°C or −70°C for long-term storage. As with most biologic materials, repeated freezing and thawing of the specimen should be avoided. Serum specimens showing gross hemolysis, gross lipemia, or turbidity should be avoided.

Specificity of hCG Assays

Modern hCG immunoassays should have little or no cross-reactivity with LH. Testing of serum samples with high physiologic LH concentrations has been used to ascertain that this hormone does not significantly influence the hCG results. Serum from postmenopausal women is a convenient source of specimens with high LH.

As discussed above, there is considerable variation between different hCG assays in regard to their detection of specific hCG variants. hCG assays are classified on the basis of their analytic specificity into those that detect only dimeric hCG, those that detect hCG and hCGβ, and those that detect hCG, hCGβ, and hCG beta core fragment.[297,299]

Clinical Significance of hCG Assays

Measurement of hCG assists in diagnosing and dating pregnancy, identifying ectopic pregnancies and other abnormalities, managing certain neoplasms, and predicting the risk of Down syndrome and trisomy 18. Each of these clinical uses was discussed earlier in this chapter or in Chapter 31. Typical values during pregnancy are shown in Fig. 69.2.

Alpha-Fetoprotein Testing

Measurement of AFP in maternal serum and amniotic fluid is used extensively throughout the United States and the United Kingdom for prenatal detection of some serious fetal anomalies. Use of AFP in nonpregnant patients for monitoring certain cancers is described in Chapter 31.

Chemistry

A fetal protein having α-electrophoretic motility was discovered in 1956 by Bergstrand and Czar.[302] Gitlin subsequently named this substance *α-fetoprotein*.[303,304] This glycoprotein has a molecular weight of approximately 70,000 Da. The gene, located within q11–22 on chromosome 4, is part of a family of genes that also codes for albumin and vitamin D–binding protein (also called *group-specific component* and *Gc globulin*).[305] The protein is composed of carbohydrate and a single polypeptide chain containing 591 amino acids. The complete amino acid sequence was reported in 1987.[306] The carbohydrate composition varies depending on the organ of synthesis, length of gestation, and source of the specimen (fetal serum vs. amniotic fluid).[307] Although determination of the carbohydrate content does not appear to be useful diagnostically in the setting of pregnancy, it may be useful in the diagnosis of hepatocellular carcinoma.[308] Heterogeneity has been demonstrated by electrophoresis and dissimilar binding to various lectins, such as concanavalin A.

Biochemistry

AFP is produced initially by the fetal yolk sac in small quantities and then by the fetal liver in larger quantities as the yolk sac degenerates. Trace amounts are also produced in the fetal gut and kidneys. Early in embryonic life, this protein has a high concentration in fetal serum, reaching about one-tenth the concentration of albumin. Maximal concentration in the fetal serum (≈3 million μg/L) is reached at about 9 weeks' gestation. The concentration then declines steadily to about 20,000 μg/L at term (Fig. 69.14).[304] The increase and decrease in concentration of AFP in the amniotic fluid roughly parallel those in the fetal serum, but the concentration is two to three orders of magnitude lower (≈15,000 μg/L at 16 weeks' gestation). The relationship with respect to maternal serum concentration is slightly more complicated because of several factors, including the (1) fetal-maternal transfer, (2) rapid growth of the fetus, (3) relatively constant size of the mother, (4) maternal clearance of the protein, and (5) variation of the volume of distribution in the mother with maternal weight. AFP is first detectable (≈5 μg/L) in maternal serum at about the 10th week of gestation. The concentration increases about 15% per week to a peak of approximately 180 μg/L at about 25 weeks. The concentration in maternal serum then subsequently declines slowly until term. A typical 16-week concentration is approximately 35 μg/L (see Fig. 69.7).[234] After birth, the maternal serum AFP rapidly decreases to less than 2 μg/L. In an infant, serum AFP declines exponentially to reach adult concentrations by the 10th month of life.[309]

The distribution of serum AFP concentrations in a population of pregnant mothers is Gaussian after logarithmic transformation.[162] Factors that affect the concentration of AFP in maternal serum include (1) gestational age, (2) maternal weight, (3) the presence of insulin-dependent maternal diabetes mellitus, (4) maternal race, (5) the number of fetuses present, (6) fetal renal disorders that cause proteinuria, and (7) fetal structural anomalies.

Amniotic fluid AFP has been measured as early as 8 weeks.[310] It rapidly decreases to a low point at 11 weeks, and then increases to reach a second maximum at 13 weeks. The concentration then falls in a log-linear fashion until 25 weeks, when the decline steepens. Several studies have shown that AChE used in combination with amniotic fluid AFP can aid in the detection of open neural tube defects from 13 to 25 weeks of pregnancy.[311]

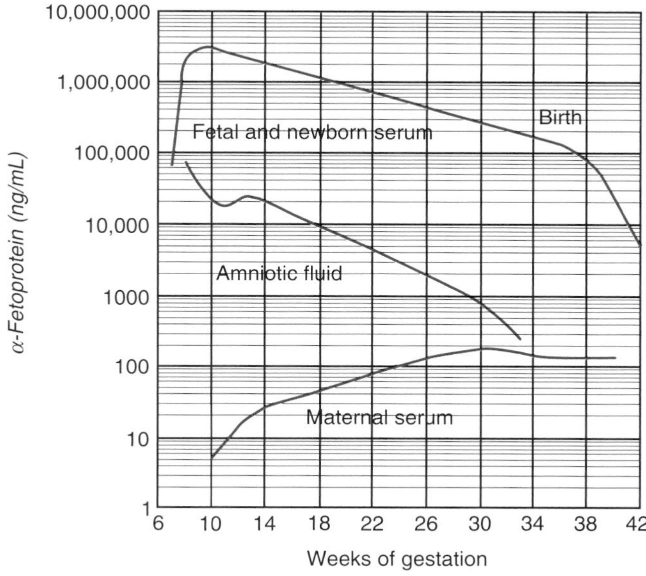

FIGURE 69.14 Concentrations of alpha-fetoprotein (AFP) in fetal and newborn serum, maternal serum, and amniotic fluid. Maternal serum values are medians calculated from 24,232 pregnancies, and amniotic fluid values are medians calculated from 1544 pregnancies from testing performed at ARUP Laboratories, Inc., from January to October 1997. SI unit conversion factor AFP (μg/L) = 1. (Fetal serum values are from Gitlin D. Normal biology of alpha-fetoprotein. *Ann N Y Acad Sci* 1975;259:7–16. Newborn serum values are from Wu JT, Roan Y, Knight JA. Serum AFP levels in normal infants: their clinical and physiological significance. In: Mizejewski G, Porter IH, editors. *Alpha-fetoprotein and congenital disorders.* Orlando, FL: Academic Press, 1985:111–21.)

Methods for Determining Alpha-Fetoprotein

Although AFP was traditionally measured by radioimmunoassay (RIA), newer methods use immunoenzymometric assay (IEMA) or chemiluminescent immunoassay (CIA) because of their (1) lower detection limits, (2) increased precision, (3) speed, (4) avoidance of radioactivity, and (5) ease of automation.[312] As indicated by the 2015 CAP survey FP, most laboratories in the United States measure AFP by using automated systems available from a number of vendors, and all of these systems perform satisfactorily.[260]

Calibration. Although two essentially equivalent international materials (WHO Reference Preparation for AFP [72–225] and British Standard [72–227]), both calibrated in international units, are available, most laboratories in the United States report AFP in nanograms per milliliter (ie, micrograms per liter). The relationship between nanograms and international units usually is given as 1.21 ng = 1 IU, but conversion factors may vary by manufacturer, perhaps reflecting differences in the carbohydrate content of respective calibrators.[313]

Specimen Collection and Handling

Serum specimens are obtained from nonfasting women through standard phlebotomy techniques. AFP is very stable in maternal serum and can be shipped at ambient temperature and stored at 4 to 8°C for 1 week or at −20°C for years.[301]

Clinical Significance of Alpha-Fetoprotein Testing

Maternal serum and amniotic fluid AFP are useful tests for detecting some serious fetal anomalies. Maternal serum AFP is increased in 85% to 95% of cases of fetal open neural tube defect[162] and is low in about 30% of cases of fetal Down syndrome.[191,192] Because maternal serum screening for fetal defects involves multiple tests, this subject was discussed earlier under Prenatal Screening. It is noteworthy that AFP is not required for healthy pregnancy. For example, a mutation of the AFP gene, which resulted in the complete absence of this protein in maternal serum or amniotic fluid, was not associated with fetal malformations or pregnancy complications.[314]

Measuring Amniotic Fluid Alpha-Fetoprotein

Amniotic fluid AFP is measured using the same immunoassays as for maternal serum AFP after a suitable dilution (usually 1:50 to 1:200). Results are expressed in nanograms per milliliter, micrograms per liter, or kilo IU per liter, and most laboratories use mass units. AFP in amniotic fluid is less stable than in serum; leaving samples at room temperature for prolonged periods, such as might occur during processing for chromosome analysis, results in degradation of amniotic fluid AFP. Refrigeration of amniotic fluid will compromise the chromosome analysis. Therefore, a portion of the collected fluid should be placed in the refrigerator as soon as possible after collection. Samples sent to reference laboratories should be shipped for next-day delivery at ambient temperature or on ice packs if the outside temperature is high. The presence of fetal blood in amniotic fluid samples has been known to increase AFP results, and laboratories should note the presence of blood in the report. In the event of an increased amniotic fluid AFP result (usually >2.0 or 2.5 MoM), the laboratory should test for the presence of fetal blood. Laboratories that measure amniotic fluid AFP need to establish medians for each week between 13 and 25 weeks' gestation. A method has been published that allows extrapolation to 13 weeks using data from 14 to 25 weeks.[315] Medians from the ARUP Laboratories (Salt Lake City, Utah) are shown graphically in Fig. 69.14.

Measuring Amniotic Fluid Acetylcholinesterase

AChE is an essential confirmatory test for samples with increased amniotic fluid AFP. Normal amniotic fluid contains a group of nonspecific cholinesterases referred to as pseudocholinesterase (PChE). Cerebrospinal fluid contains high concentrations of the neural enzyme AChE, and in cases of fetal open neural tube defects (and in about 80% of cases with defects of the abdominal wall), fluid leaks from the open lesion and allows AChE to enter the amniotic fluid.

The usual technique for identification of AChE is fractionation by polyacrylamide gel electrophoresis followed by incubation of the gel with the substrate acetylcholine and copper ions. AChE migrates more rapidly than PChE and appears as a distinct white precipitate band below the PChE band. To confirm that the second band is AChE, inhibition of the enzyme activity in the band by the specific AChE inhibitor 1,5-bis(4-allyldimethylammoniumphenyl)pentan-3-one dibromide (BW284C51) must be documented. Since no method is available commercially, laboratories have to develop their own assay systems using published methodology.[316,317] Enzyme immunoassay using a monoclonal antibody specific for neurally derived AChE has also been used.[318]

Unconjugated Estriol Testing

Measurement of unconjugated estriol (uE_3) is used in screening for Down syndrome. This steroid, rather than total estriol (unconjugated plus conjugated estriol), is the most specific of the estrogens for identifying a fetus with Down syndrome.

Chemistry

Estriol is an estrogen with hydroxyl groups at positions 3, 16, and 17 (see Chapter 68). Its systematic name is 1,3,5(10)-estriene-3,16-α,17-β-triol. Although present in nonpregnant patients in very low concentrations, during late pregnancy this estrogen predominates. Only a minor amount (≈10%) of the hormone circulates in plasma unconjugated,[319] and, because of its low solubility, this form is strongly bound to sex hormone–binding globulin. The majority exist as conjugates of glucuronate and sulfate (Fig. 69.15). Conjugation, which occurs in the maternal liver, makes the hormone more soluble and thus permits renal clearance.

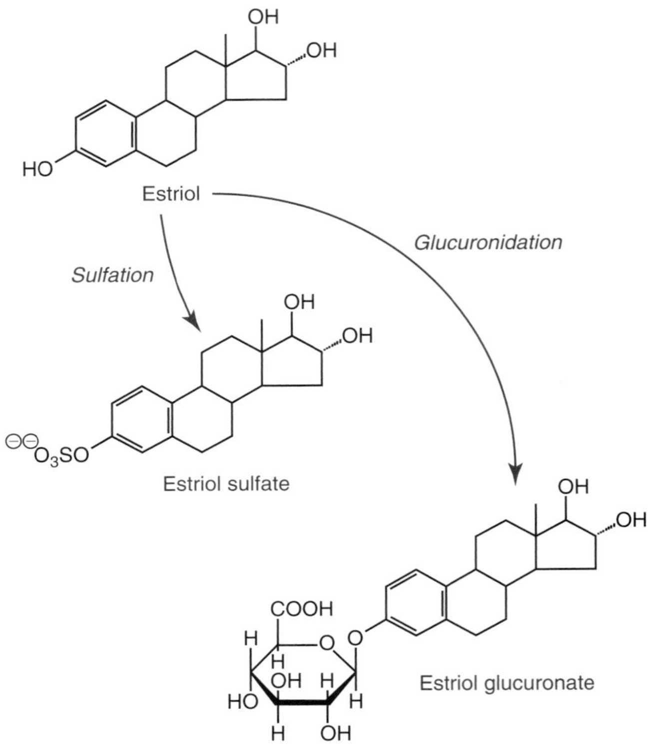

FIGURE 69.15 Forms of estriol present in maternal serum. Glucuronidation and sulfation can also occur at the other hydroxyl positions.

Biochemistry

Estriol is produced in very large amounts during the last trimester of pregnancy. The biosynthetic pathway requires three organs to be fully functioning: fetal adrenal, fetal liver, and placenta (Fig. 69.16). The fetal adrenal cortex possesses a unique zone for the production of steroids. The demand for estriol is so great that the size of the fetal adrenal is 10 to 20 times larger than the adult adrenal. The fetal cortex accounts for approximately 80% of the adrenal weight. The fetal adrenal avidly binds low-density lipoprotein to take in cholesterol, which is converted to two major steroid intermediates: pregnenolone sulfate and dehydroepiandrosterone sulfate (DHEA-S). These intermediates are secreted into the fetal circulation. The fetal liver, possessing 16α-hydroxylase, converts DHEA-S to 16α-hydroxy-DHEA-S, which is secreted back into the fetal circulation. Finally the placenta synthesizes estriol from 16α-hydroxy-DHEA-S. Approximately 90% of maternal serum estriol is derived from this fetal-placental pathway. A minor amount is made using precursors from the maternal ovary. The relationship of maternal serum uE_3 to gestational age in the second trimester is log-linear, increasing

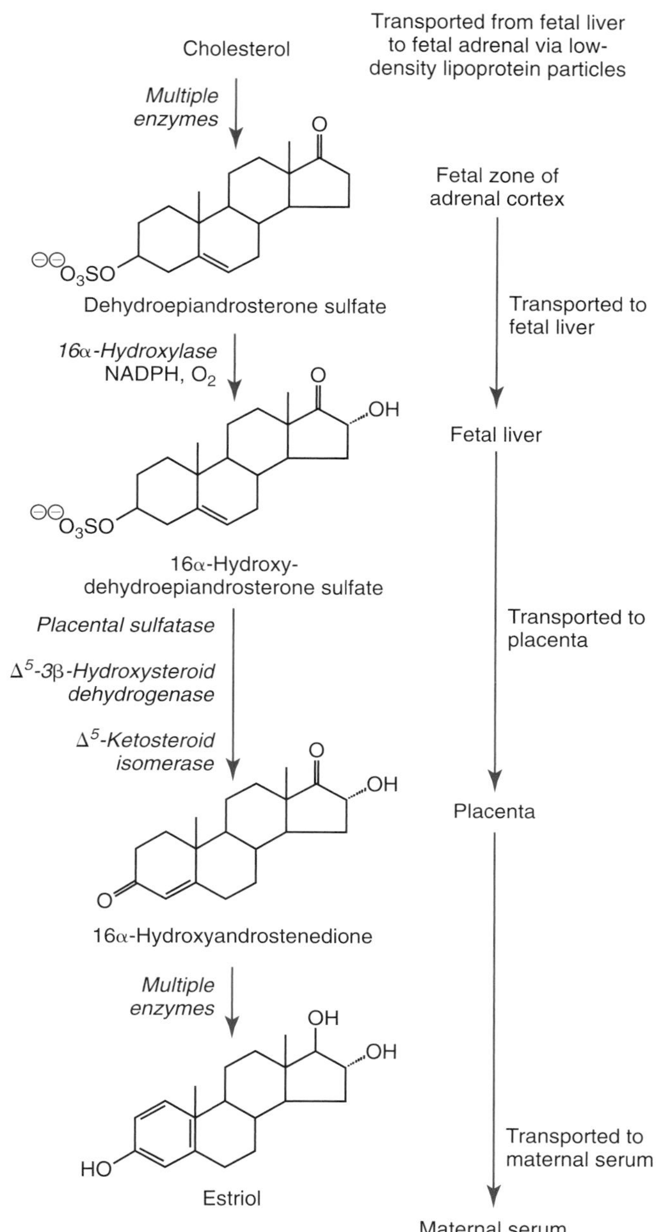

FIGURE 69.16 Biosynthetic pathway for estriol during pregnancy.

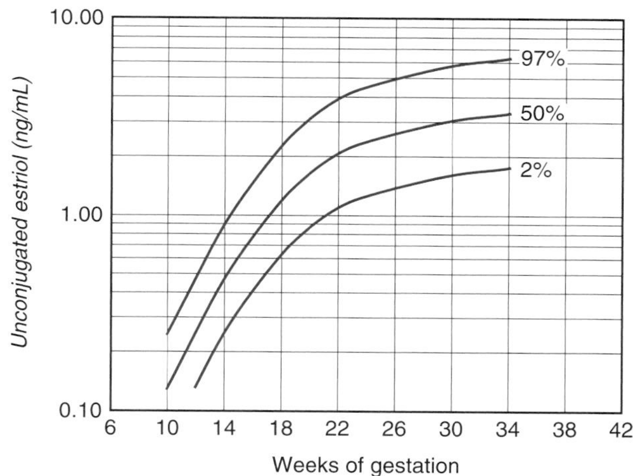

FIGURE 69.17 Concentration of unconjugated estriol (uE_3) in maternal serum as a function of gestational age. Lines represent the 2nd, 50th, and 97th percentiles. Maternal serum values from 14 to 25 weeks are medians calculated from 11,309 pregnancies from testing performed at ARUP Laboratories, Inc., from January to October 1997. SI unit conversion factor: uE3 (nmol/L) = 3.47.

at a rate of 20% to 25% per gestational week[234] (Fig. 69.17). Concentrations typical for the second trimester of pregnancy are 0.70 to 2.50 μg/L (2.43 to 8.68 nmol/L), depending on the assay used. Serum concentrations of estriol conjugates are fivefold to tenfold higher than serum concentrations of uE_3 during pregnancy.

Methods for Determining Unconjugated Estriol

The determination of uE_3 is made difficult by its low concentration. Until 2002, uE_3 was measured by ultrasensitive RIA methods. Subsequently, nonisotopic assays become available, usually as part of automated systems. The correlation between these methods and the RIA methods is fair (r^2 = 0.8), and most have not been clinically validated. A clinical outcome study using a nonisotopic method yielded Down syndrome screening performance equivalent to a previously validated RIA.[320] In addition, concentrations of estrone, estriol-3-sulfate, and estriol-3-glucuronide up to 1000 ng/mL cross-react less than 0.03% in current assays. Values obtained with various uE_3 assays vary widely as judged using the CAP proficiency testing Survey FP.[260] Conversion to MoM reduces the between-method differences, but uE_3 is still the most variable of the screening analytes.

Calibration. Assays for uE_3 are calibrated by the use of chemically pure estriol. Estriol values are reported in mass units (nanograms per milliliter or micrograms per liter) or SI units (nanomoles per liter). The equation for converting mass to SI units is 1 ng/ml = 3.47 nmol/L. Although pure uE_3 is available for calibrating uE_3 assays, commercial reagents yield values on clinical specimens that differ by factors of 2 to 3.[260]

Specimen Collection and Handling. Maternal serum specimens are obtained from nonfasting women by standard phlebotomy techniques. Of the four analytes currently used for screening, uE_3 is the least stable, and, consequently, requirements for collection, storage, and shipment are dictated by this analyte. The uE_3 concentration increases in blood at room temperature and at 4°C, because the conjugated forms are able to spontaneously deconjugate to form the parent hormone.[234] Therefore, collected blood should be allowed to clot, and serum should be removed promptly. If serum separator tubes are used, specimens should be centrifuged promptly after collection. Shipment of whole blood is not preferred. If whole blood is shipped through the mail, next-day delivery is essential. uE_3 is stable in serum for up to 7 days at 2 to 4°C (unpublished data, Foundation for Blood Research, Woman and Infant's Hospital, and ARUP Laboratories). The concentration of uE_3 increases when sera have been stored for longer than 4 days at room temperature.

Clinical Significance of Unconjugated Estriol Testing

Any disruption in the biosynthetic pathway will lead to very low maternal serum uE_3. Conditions that cause disruption include (1) fetal anencephaly, (2) placental sulfatase deficiency, (3) fetal death, (4) chromosome abnormalities, (5) molar pregnancy, and (6) Smith-Lemli-Opitz syndrome.[321,322] Placental sulfatase deficiency presents in the infant as X-linked ichthyosis. It is present in approximately 1 in every 2000 males. Because of the lack of uE_3, the mother often has a delayed onset of labor and the cesarean section rate is significantly higher in these mothers. SLOS is a serious, rare birth defect that is the result of an inborn error in cholesterol metabolism, 7-dehydrosterol-7-reductase deficiency. Down syndrome leads to a modest decrease in uE_3. Screening for Down syndrome is now the most common application of uE_3 measurements.[323]

Inhibin A Testing

Inhibins are members of the transforming growth factor-β (TGFβ) superfamily of proteins. As described in Chapter 68, inhibin is a negative feedback regulator of FSH secretion in both males and females. Inhibin A and B are proven bioactive forms. The placenta produces large quantities of inhibin A that completely suppress FSH.

Chemistry

Inhibins are proteins consisting of dimers of dissimilar subunits (α and β) linked by disulfide bridges. The β-subunit occurs in two closely related forms (β_A and β_B), leading to two types of dimeric inhibin (dimeric inhibin A, $\alpha\beta_A$ and dimeric inhibin B, $\alpha\beta_B$). The mature form of inhibin, which has a molecular mass of approximately 30,000 Da, is produced by cleavage of larger precursor forms. In follicular fluid and serum, mature inhibins, precursors of inhibins (particularly the processed form of the free α-subunit, pro-αC), and intermediate molecules of varying molecular weight are present.[324] Another group of related molecules, the activins, are dimers consisting of just the β-subunits.[325] Inhibin/activin β_C, β_D, and β_E subunits have also been identified, but are less well understood. Inhibin A is the only form within the inhibin/activin family of proteins that provides sufficient discrimination to be useful for use in Down syndrome screening.[326]

Biochemistry

Inhibins, and the closely related activins, are proteins that suppress or stimulate FSH secretion. In the reproductive system, inhibin and activin subunits are expressed in the placenta, as well as in the granulosa cells of the ovary and by the Sertoli cells of the testis. Inhibin A and inhibin B have distinctive serum profiles during the human menstrual cycle. Inhibin A rises from 10 to 20 ng/L in the follicular phase and peaks at ovulation (≈60 ng/L), before decreasing to basal amounts in the luteal phase. In postmenopausal women, the concentrations of both forms of inhibin are below 5 ng/L.[327] Men secrete inhibin B, but not inhibin A, from the testis into serum. Inhibin A is produced by the fetoplacental unit beginning in early pregnancy. Inhibin A concentrations exhibit a complex pattern during the course of pregnancy, rising to a peak at 8 to 10 weeks' gestation, declining to a minimum at 17 weeks of pregnancy, and then resuming to slowly increase at term (see Fig. 69.10). Unlike the other screening tests, average inhibin concentrations change relatively little from 15 to 20 weeks' gestation. A typical value at 17 weeks' gestation is 175 ng/L (175 pg /mL). Recently, inhibin/activin β_C and β_E subunits were localized in placental tissues, implying a potential role in pregnancy.[328,329]

Assay Methods for Inhibin A

Inhibin assays used for Down syndrome screening must measure only dimeric inhibin A and not the free α subunits and the precursors of higher molecular weight, which also circulate in blood. The original inhibin assays were enzyme-linked immunosorbent assay (ELISA) or RIAs and used antibodies directed against epitopes on the α-subunit that measured all forms of inhibin, including precursors. These assays are referred to as total inhibin or immunoreactive inhibin assays. Highly specific assays using monoclonal antibodies are available that measure only dimeric inhibin A. Specific inhibin A assays provide better screening performance than the nonspecific total inhibin assays.[326] An automated method for inhibin A measurement was released by Beckman Coulter in 2007 and has been shown to have acceptable analytic and clinical performance.[330] Typical values in the second trimester of pregnancy range from 50 to 400 pg/mL (50 to 400 ng/L), as shown in Fig. 69.10.

Specimen Collection and Handling. Serum specimens are obtained from nonfasting women by standard phlebotomy techniques. Inhibin A is stable in maternal serum and can be shipped at ambient temperature and stored at 4 to 8°C for 1 week.[301]

Clinical Significance of Inhibin A Testing

In addition to the usefulness of inhibin A as a predictor of Down syndrome risk discussed previously, inhibin A and B measurements have found additional applications as tumor markers for ovarian cancer and in the evaluation of male infertility.[326,331]

Pregnancy-Associated Plasma Protein A Testing

Pregnancy-associated plasma protein A is a unique serum marker for Down syndrome pregnancy in that concentrations are low in the first trimester (median = 0.34 MoM) but are normal in the second trimester (1.11 MoM).[229] PAPP-A concentrations in the maternal serum during the first trimester of pregnancy are associated with fetal and placental health and development.

Chemistry

The human PAPP-A gene is found on chromosome 9 and consists of 22 exons. It is translated into a 1626–amino acid product, of which 1546 amino acids compose the mature protein. Circulating PAPP-A is part of a larger molecular complex that includes two subunits of PAPP-A covalently bound to two subunits of pro major basic protein (pro MBP), forming a heterotetramer (Fig. 69.18).[332] The PAPP-A complex has a very high molecular weight of about 500 kDa.

Biochemistry

PAPP-A is a zinc-containing metalloproteinase glycoprotein. It is expressed at low concentrations in all tissues, but high amounts of PAPP-A protein and mRNA are localized in placental tissues throughout gestation. PAPP-A immunoreactivity is found in syncytiotrophoblast cells,[333] and the eosinophil major basic protein (pro-MBP) subunit is found in cytotrophoblast cells. Maternal serum PAPP-A concentrations increase as gestation proceeds to term. Concentrations of PAPP-A are critical to normal fetal growth because of its role as an insulin-like growth factor–binding protein (IGFBP)

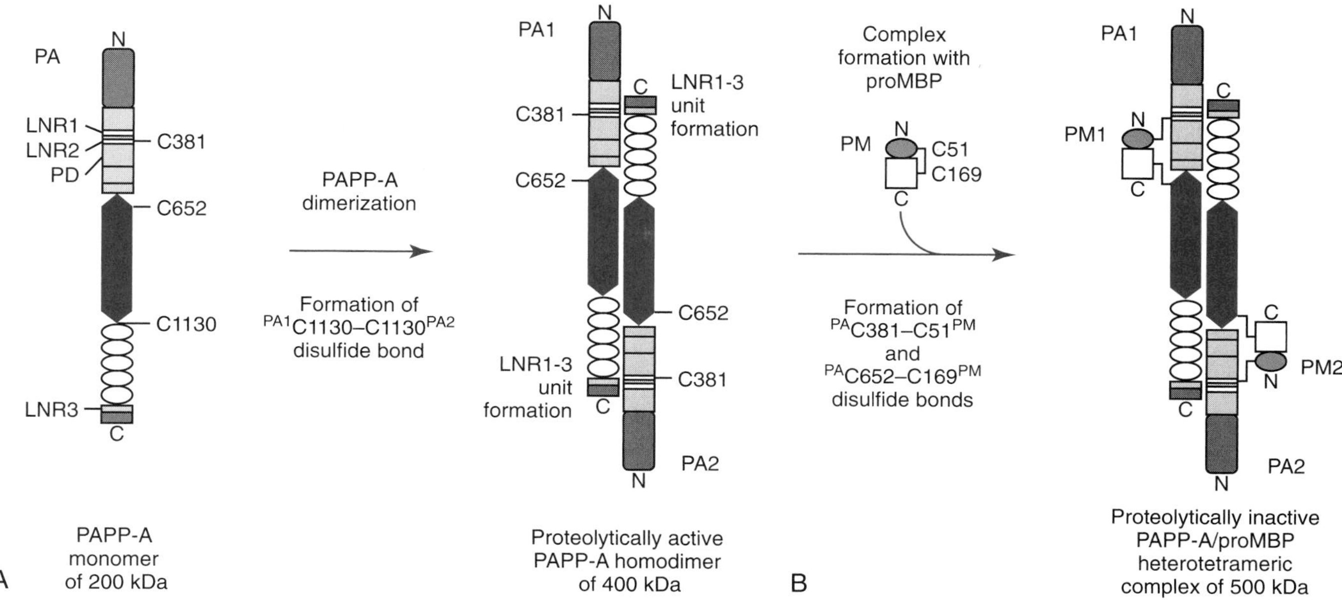

FIGURE 69.18 PAPP-A monomer, homodimer, and heterotetrameric complex. (Reprinted from Boldt HB, Conover CA. Pregnancy-associated plasma protein-A (PAPP-A): a local regulator of IGF bioavailability through cleavage of IGFBPs. *Growth Horm IGF Res* 2007;17:10–18.)

protease. PAPP-A regulates the action of insulin-like growth factor II (IGF-II) by cleaving its binding protein and thereby increasing bioavailable forms. PAPP-A predominantly cleaves IGFBP-4, a reaction that is dependent on the presence of IGF-II.[332]

Of note, the pro-MBP subunits are inactive precursor forms of MBP that are found in eosinophil crystalloid bodies and function in inflammatory responses.

Assay Methods for PAPP-A

PAPP-A was initially measured in pregnancy serum using antibody pairs in an ELISA format[334] and was later optimized for limit of detection[335] and detection of the PAPP-A: pro-MBP complex.[336] PAPP-A immunoassays are now commercially available in the United States on routine clinical chemistry platforms. There are significant between-method differences, and efforts to achieve standardization are currently under way.

Specimen Collection and Handling. Serum specimens are obtained from nonfasting women by standard phlebotomy techniques. A small increase in PAPP-A concentrations has been reported for collection in plastic versus glass tubes,[337] along with a significant decrease for heparin or EDTA plasma tubes versus serum.[338] EDTA chelates zinc and hence changes the protein configuration and heparin masks the antigenic sites. PAPP-A was stable with up to nine freeze-thaw cycles.[339] First-trimester serum PAPP-A concentrations are stable in serum at 4°C for 1 week or longer, depending on the assay used for testing.[301,340]

Clinical Significance of PAPP-A Testing

Low PAPP-A concentrations early in pregnancy have been associated with (1) Down syndrome, (2) a high rate of fetal loss, (3) poor fetal growth (intrauterine growth restriction [IUGR]), (4) premature delivery, (5) hypertension, and (6) preeclampsia.[341,342] Low PAPP-A concentrations have been reported in the second trimester of pregnancies with Cornelia de Lange syndrome, a serious developmental malformation syndrome of unknown origin.[343]

In addition to placental tissues, PAPP-A has been localized in tissues of the (1) colon, (2) kidney, (3) endometrium,[344] and (4) ovary, in (5) fibroblasts, and in (6) vascular smooth muscle cells and (7) osteoblasts.[332] Functional roles for PAPP-A in bone formation[345] and wound healing[346] have been described. Furthermore, ultrasensitive cardiac-specific measurements of PAPP-A have utility in the detection of acute coronary syndromes,[347] with higher concentrations indicative of a relatively poor prognosis.[348,349]

POINTS TO REMEMBER

Prenatal Screening

- Prenatal screening for detection of fetal anomalies should be offered to all women, regardless of age.
- Screening of maternal serum for AFP, hCG, uE_3, and inhibin A together with nuchal translucency measurement is useful to identify women with increased risk for having a fetus with anomalies such as a neural tube defect, Down syndrome, and trisomy 18.
- Down syndrome is associated with increased nuchal thickness and decreased concentrations of AFP and uE_3 and increased concentrations of hCG and inhibin-A in maternal serum.
- An increased risk for neural tube defects is associated with increased serum AFP.
- Trisomy 18 is associated with decreased concentrations of AFP, estriol, uE_3, and hCG.
- Cell-free fetal DNA in maternal blood can be used for high-quality noninvasive screening of fetal aneuploidies.

Fetal Fibronectin Testing

Determining the risk of preterm labor would help clinicians manage those at high risk more aggressively, thereby lowering the incidence of preterm delivery. In 1991, the fetal fibronectin (fFN) concentration in cervical and vaginal secretions was proposed as a test to aid in predicting preterm delivery.[350] While patients with a negative test result have only an approximately 1% chance of delivering in 1 week,[351] the positive predictive value of fFN is low. Several metaanalyses revealed that fFN is of limited utility in predicting preterm birth within 7 days of sample collection.[352-354]

Placental Alpha-Microglobulin-1 Testing

Placental alpha-microglobulin-1 (PAMG-1) is a placental glycoprotein first identified in 1977.[355] During pregnancy, PAMG-1 is secreted into the amniotic fluid, where it is present at a high concentration (2000 to 25,000 ng/mL) relative to that of maternal blood (5 to 25 ng/mL) or cervicovaginal fluid with intact membranes (0.05 to 2 ng/mL).[356] A test for PAMG-1 that exploits these large differences in concentrations has been developed for clinical use as an aid for the detection of premature rupture of membranes.

The commercially available test is a rapid immunochromatographic method that utilizes two monoclonal antibodies for the rapid detection of PAMG-1 in cervicovaginal fluid. The specimen is collected using a polyester swab that is placed into the vagina for 1 minute. The fluid obtained is eluted off the swab by rinsing it in a vial containing a buffer solution for 1 minute. A test strip is then placed into the buffer for 10 minutes. The test result is determined by visual inspection of a test and a control line on the lateral flow device. The analytic limit of detection of the test is 5 ng/mL.

Two studies have reported that this test is more sensitive and specific for the detection of PROM than clinical assessment or the nitrazine or ferning tests.[356,357] A study by Cousins and colleagues[357] included 203 women presenting with suspected PROM. The diagnosis of PROM was based on two positive results from a retrospective review of patient medical records and amniotic fluid, nitrazine testing, or fern testing. The clinical sensitivity of the test was 99% with a specificity of 100%.

In a prospective study of 184 women with suspected PROM, Lee and colleagues[356] evaluated this test against conventional clinical criteria. Women were diagnosed with PROM if amniotic fluid was observed leaking from the cervix or if any two of the following were true: (1) pooling of amniotic fluid was present in the posterior fornix, (2) a nitrazine test was positive, or (3) microscopic ferning was detected. The definitive diagnosis of PROM was made after delivery and was based on a review of the clinical record. The test was noted to be 99% sensitive and 88% specific compared with 87% and 100%, respectively, for the conventional assessment. Three false-positive results were unexplained, but it was speculated that they may have been caused by small leakages of amniotic fluid that were clinically unapparent. Compared with the nitrazine test alone, this test was significantly more sensitive (99% vs. 88%), with the same specificity (88%).

Contamination with large amounts of blood will cause a false-positive result. False-negative results may occur if the specimen is collected 12 or more hours after a rupture that is subsequently obstructed by the fetus or is resealed.

Tests for Evaluating Fetal Lung Maturity

Fetal lung maturity (FLM) tests help to assess the risk of a fetus to develop respiratory distress syndrome (RDS). The most common situation in which an FLM test is ordered is before repeat cesarean delivery when the age of gestation is uncertain. Another major indication is anticipated early delivery because of some medical or obstetric indication, such as (1) preterm labor, (2) premature rupture of the membranes, (3) worsening maternal hypertension, (4) severe renal disease, (5) intrauterine growth restriction, or (6) fetal distress. Results indicating immaturity of the fetal lungs might cause postponement of elective delivery or prompt active interventions to suppress preterm labor. Pharmacologic administration of corticosteroids is recommended for women between 24 and 34 weeks' gestation who are likely to deliver in the next week.[358] This therapy accelerates pulmonary maturation and prevents respiratory distress syndrome.

Numerous tests of amniotic fluid for FLM have been developed. All FLM tests exhibit high sensitivity for immaturity and an excellent predictive value of a mature result.[359] Despite performing well, the number of FLM tests performed each year in the United States has declined and several studies have demonstrated that FLM testing does not improve fetal morbidity or mortality.[360-362]

In 2008, the ACOG issued a revised practice bulletin concerning FLM.[141] This bulletin discourages FLM testing before 32 weeks of gestation or when delivery is mandated due to fetal or maternal indications and specifies that assessment of FLM is indicated prior to a scheduled delivery at less than 39 weeks of gestation, if it cannot be inferred from clinical history. However, the practice of scheduled deliveries at less than 39 weeks of gestation is now strongly discouraged by ACOG, unless delivery is justified by medical or obstetric complications.[363] Thus testing for FLM is becoming infrequent.

Standards of laboratory practice for FLM testing were published in 1997 and 2006 that make several recommendations regarding specimen collection, handling, centrifugation, and mixing that remain valid today.[1,364]

Collection and Handling of Amniotic Fluid for Fetal Lung Maturity Assessment

Fetal lung liquids contribute to amniotic fluid, resulting in an exchange of surfactants from the developing lungs to the amniotic fluid. Therefore, amniotic fluid is the required specimen for FLM testing, and it is obtained by transabdominal amniocentesis, usually during real-time sonographic visualization (see Chapter 4). In a multifetal pregnancy, there are usually separate sacs, each of which should be sampled. Vaginal pool specimens are rarely adequate for testing. Clinicians should seriously consider amniocentesis in patients with ruptured membranes.[1]

Fetal Lung Maturity Tests

Currently available methods for fetal lung maturity testing include (1) lamellar body count, (2) phosphatidylglycerol measurement, and the (3) lecithin/sphingomyelin ratio.

Lamellar Body Counts. The similarity in size between lamellar bodies (1 to 5 mm or 1.7 to 7.3 fL)[18] and platelets (2 to 4 mm or 5 to 7 fL) permits the use of automated hematologic cell counters to determine the lamellar body count (LBC).[365,366]

All clinical outcomes studies[365,367-379] have reported that LBC has high clinical sensitivity (95% to 100%) but low clinical specificity (≈70%) for the prediction of RDS. A metaanalysis[380] reported that at a fixed clinical sensitivity of 95%, the LBC specificity was 80%, whereas the L/S ratio specificity was 70%. Because LBC is a simple and rapid method that is reliably predictive of fetal lung maturity, this method has been suggested as a suitable replacement for the fluorescence polarization method that was widely used before its discontinuation.[381]

Determination of Lecithin/Sphingomyelin Ratio. The concentration of lecithin, a major surface-active component of lung surfactant, increases throughout the third trimester. Sphingomyelin, a minor component of pulmonary surfactant, is mainly derived from sources other than the lung and its concentration remains relatively constant. Thus, the sphingomyelin concentration is used as an internal standard for comparison with the rising lecithin concentration. The concentration of lecithin relative to sphingomyelin, the L/S ratio, tends to rise with increasing gestational age.[382]

Most laboratories use a commercially available method for L/S determination. However, because many techniques are available, laboratories should be very careful when establishing medical decision limits.[383-385] The L/S ratio is a labor-intensive test that has poor within- and between-lab precision; this may be why very few laboratories perform it.

About 1% of babies delivered within 24 hours of obtaining an L/S ratio of greater than 2.5 are expected to develop RDS. Thus, the L/S ratio has a high sensitivity for detecting lung immaturity. In contrast to the high degree of reliability of a prediction of maturity, only one-third of the babies predicted to be immature will in fact develop RDS. Test results are adversely affected by both the blood and the meconium.[386] Vaginal contamination of specimens obtained from a pool of fluid that has been present in the vagina for a relatively brief period does not affect either test.[387,388]

Measurement of Phosphatidylglycerol. Phosphatidylglycerol is present at relatively low concentrations exclusively in the lung. Measureable quantities of phosphatidylglycerol first appear in amniotic fluid several weeks after lecithin appears.[22] Therefore, phosphatidylglycerol is considered a late marker of FLM. Concentrations of phosphatidylglycerol were first measured by thin-layer chromatography in conjunction with lecithin and sphingomyelin in order to improve the poor specificity of the L/S ratio.[389] However, it soon became a stand-alone marker for FLM and its qualitative detection was made possible by the development of a rapid agglutination test that uses antiphosphatidylglycerol antibodies (AmnioStat-FLM-PG, Irvine Scientific, Santa Ana, California).[390]

Results for this test are reported as either negative (immature) or positive (mature). This nomenclature is opposite that used for other FLM tests, with positive meaning immature. RDS rarely develops in an infant when a positive phosphatidylglycerol result is obtained.

Several clinical outcome studies using AmnioStat have been reported.[390-395] Although positive phosphatidylglycerol results are about 99% predictive of maturity, negative results are highly unpredictive (RDS develops in about 25% of cases with a negative phosphatidylglycerol, depending on the population) and are therefore not useful clinically. Determination of phosphatidylglycerol is also useful for specimens contaminated with blood or meconium, as phosphatidylglycerol is not found in either substance.[391,396]

SELECTED REFERENCES

For a full list of references for this chapter, please refer to ExpertConsult.com.

7. Cunningham FG, MacDonald PC, Gant NF. *The placental hormones. Williams Obstetrics*. 18th ed. Norwalk, CN: Appleton & Lange; 1989. p. 67–85.
15. Lockitch GM, editor. *Handbook of diagnostic biochemistry and hematology in normal pregnancy*. Boca Raton, FL: CRC Press; 1993.
42. McChesney R, Wilcox AJ, O'Connor JF, et al. Intact HCG, free HCG beta subunit and HCG beta core fragment: longitudinal patterns in urine during early pregnancy. *Hum Reprod* 2005;**20**:928–35.
61. Levine RJ, Maynard SE, Qian C, et al. Circulating angiogenic factors and the risk of preeclampsia. *N Engl J Med* 2004;**350**: 672–83.
85. Lambert-Messerlian G, McClain M, Haddow JE, et al. First- and second-trimester thyroid hormone reference data in pregnant women: a FaSTER (First- and Second-Trimester Evaluation of Risk for aneuploidy) Research Consortium study. *Am J Obstet Gynecol* 2008;**199**: 62.e1–6.
87. Mari G, Deter RL, Carpenter RL, et al. Noninvasive diagnosis by Doppler ultrasonography of fetal anemia due to maternal red-cell alloimmunization. Collaborative Group for Doppler Assessment of the Blood Velocity in Anemic Fetuses. *N Engl J Med* 2000;**342**:9–14.
102. Workowski KA, Bolan GA, Centers for Disease Control and Prevention. Sexually transmitted diseases treatment guidelines, 2015. *MMWR Recomm Rep* 2015;**64**: 1–137.
107. Sena AC, White BL, Sparling PF. Novel *Treponema pallidum* serologic tests: a paradigm shift in syphilis screening for the 21st century. *Clin Infect Dis* 2010;**51**:700–8.
148. Palmer OM, Grenache DG, Gronowski AM. The NACB laboratory medicine practice guidelines for point-of-care reproductive testing. *Point of Care* 2007;**6**:265–72.
155. Practice Bulletin No. 163: Screening for fetal aneuploidy. *Obstet Gynecol* 2016;**127**:e123–37.
159. Norton ME, Jacobsson B, Swamy GK, et al. Cell-free DNA analysis for noninvasive examination of trisomy. *N Engl J Med* 2015;**372**:1589–97.
161. Committee Opinion No. 640: Cell-free DNA screening for fetal aneuploidy. *Obstet Gynecol* 2015;**126**:e31–7.
162. Wald NJ, Cuckle H, Brock JH, et al. Maternal serum-alpha-fetoprotein measurement in antenatal screening for anencephaly and spina bifida in early pregnancy. Report of U.K. collaborative study on alpha-fetoprotein in relation to neural-tube defects. *Lancet* 1977;**1**:1323–32.
198. Wald NJ, Huttly WJ, Hackshaw AK. Antenatal screening for Down's syndrome with the quadruple test. *Lancet* 2003;**361**:835–6.
201. Haddow JE, Palomaki GE, Knight GJ, et al. Prenatal screening for Down's syndrome with use of maternal serum markers. *N Engl J Med* 1992;**327**:588–93.
234. Haddow JE, Palomaki GE, Knight GJ, et al. *Variables which influence levels of AFP, uE3, and hCG and/or risk for*

Down syndrome. Foundation for Blood Research handbook, vol. II. Screening for Down syndrome. Scarborough, ME: Foundation for Blood Research; 1998. p. 1–48.

298. Gronowski AM, Grenache DG. Characterization of the hCG variants recognized by different hCG immunoassays: an important step toward standardization of hCG measurements. *Clin Chem* 2009;**55**:1447–9.

359. Yarbrough ML, Grenache DG, Gronowski AM. Fetal lung maturity testing: the end of an era. *Biomark Med* 2014;**8**:509–15.

70

Newborn Screening and Inborn Errors of Metabolism*

Marzia Pasquali and Nicola Longo

ABSTRACT

Background

Newborn screening can detect many metabolic disorders, allowing early initiation of treatment to prevent morbidity and mortality. The introduction of tandem mass spectrometry (MS/MS) has dramatically increased the number of conditions detectable at birth to include several inborn errors of amino acid metabolism, fatty acid oxidation, and organic acidemias.

Content

This chapter describes a range of metabolic disorders amenable to newborn screening. Amino acids and acylcarnitine are currently detected by MS/MS. The concentration of amino acids increases with inborn errors of amino acid metabolism (for example, phenylalanine in phenylketonuria). Acylcarnitine analysis can identify disorders of the intermediary metabolism of amino acids (organic acidemias) and disorders of the carnitine cycle and fatty acid oxidation. For each condition, the specific abnormal metabolite(s) is(are) indicated with the most appropriate way to confirm or exclude the diagnosis. In some cases, diagnostic metabolites disappear or are markedly reduced after the newborn period so DNA testing is indicated for diagnostic purposes. Early identification of metabolic disorders allows prompt therapeutic intervention and improves long-term outcome. Available therapies for metabolic disorders are also discussed in this chapter, together with the appropriate monitoring procedures.

Inborn errors of metabolism (IEM) affect the ability to convert nutrients or to use them for energy production. IEM typically present in the newborn period or in infancy. Some diseases, however, such as fatty acid oxidation defects or milder variants of classic metabolic disorders, may not be detected until adulthood. Despite the long asymptomatic period, their consequences can still be devastating and lead to death. Therefore identification and treatment of these diseases before irreversible damage occurs is critical. Clinical biochemical genetics is the discipline that deals with the diagnosis and treatment of patients with inborn errors of metabolism. In contrast to other, more common diseases, the treatment of IEM is lifelong and requires frequent monitoring. The biochemical diagnosis of IEM and treatment monitoring involve analysis of metabolites, enzymatic activity, and/or molecular structure. Because of technological advances (such as the introduction of tandem mass spectrometry [MS/MS] allowing the simultaneous detection of multiple analytes) and improved outcome of patients with IEM identified and treated early, many more IEM are now included in newborn screening programs than hitherto.

*The authors gratefully acknowledge the contributions by Drs. Piero Rinaldo, Si Houn Hahn, and Dietrich Matern to the previous edition on which portions of this chapter are based.

AT A GLANCE

IEMs

- Inborn errors of metabolism (IEMs) usually present in early infancy, although there are cases that can become symptomatic in late childhood or adulthood.
- Symptoms include vomiting, lethargy, seizures, and coma, leading to death. Symptoms may become evident only under environmental stress, such as fasting, infections, and exercise.
- The diagnosis requires specific biochemical genetics tests, such as amino acids analysis in plasma and urine, organic acids analysis in urine, measurement of carnitine and acylcarnitines in plasma, and enzyme assay. DNA testing confirms the diagnosis.
- Treatment is available and effective for most IEMs and consists of a special diet supplemented with vitamins/cofactors/drugs.
- The prognosis is good if treatment is initiated early, before symptoms occur.
- Newborn screening can identify many of these disorders presymptomatically.

INBORN ERRORS OF METABOLISM: CLINICAL PRESENTATION

Inborn errors of metabolism are due to impaired activity of enzymes, transporters, or cofactors and result in the

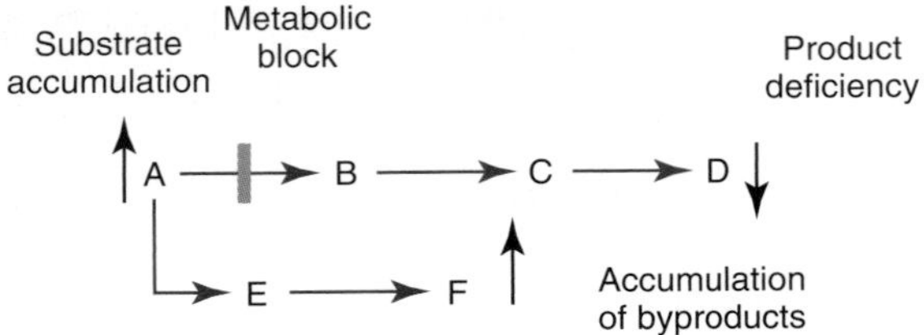

FIGURE 70.1 Schematic of metabolic pathway. The substrate A is converted by a series of reactions into product D. If one of the enzymes *(arrows)* is defective (metabolic block), the substrate of the reaction will accumulate (A in this case) and can enter alternative pathways of metabolism, leading to the formation of by-products (E and F in this case). At the same time, the concentration of the product of the reaction (D) will decrease.

accumulation of abnormal metabolites (substrates) proximal to the metabolic block or decreased formation or essential products. Fig. 70.1 shows a hypothetical metabolic pathway in which the substrate (A) needs to be converted into the product (D), with arrows representing individual enzymes. If an enzyme is defective (vertical rectangle), the concentration of substrate A will increase, and formation of product D will decrease. The substrate A can accumulate to very high concentrations, becoming substrate of enzymes not usually involved in its metabolism and producing abnormal by-products (E and F) through alternative pathways. The accumulation of specific metabolites and their by-products within organs and tissues and/or the lack of reaction products is the chemical basis of the pathology observed in different inborn errors of metabolism. At the same time, the measurement of some of these metabolites or their by-products is the basis of biochemical diagnostic testing for IEM and early detection by newborn screening programs.

Symptoms of inborn errors of metabolism usually appear early in infancy, although some conditions only become symptomatic in late childhood or adulthood. Signs and symptoms include failure to thrive, seizures, mental retardation, organs failure, and even death. Inborn errors of metabolism can be divided into three broad categories based on the effect of their metabolic derangement.[1]

1. Intoxication effect. The metabolites accumulating in the body produce a toxic effect on different organs. The patient may become acutely ill after a symptom-free period of time, usually 24 to 72 hours, and concomitantly with the ingestion of the substrates that cannot be adequately metabolized, such as proteins or sugars. Amino acidopathies (eg, phenylketonuria, maple syrup urine disease, homocystinuria), urea cycle defects (eg, citrullinemia, argininosuccinic aciduria, ornithine transcarbamylase deficiency), organic acidemias (eg, propionic acidemia, methylmalonic acidemia, glutaric acidemia type I), and disorders of sugar metabolism (galactosemia, hereditary fructose intolerance) belong to this group. Some of these disorders, such as phenylketonuria, affect primarily the brain, causing severe intellectual disability but without acute decompensation. In other disorders (eg, organic acidemias), symptoms appear shortly after protein intake (usually after the first few feedings) and include vomiting, lethargy, seizures, and coma, leading rapidly to death if not recognized and treated appropriately.
2. Energy deficiency. The symptoms in these disorders are due to impaired energy production. In some cases, patients may not be symptomatic for a long period of time, until energy requirements are increased due to involuntary fasting, illnesses, infection, or strenuous exercise. Disorders of fatty acid oxidation are classic examples of these disorders. They include medium-chain acyl-CoA dehydrogenase deficiency, very long-chain acyl-CoA dehydrogenase deficiency, carnitine uptake defect, and carnitine palmitoyl transferase deficiency I and II. The accumulation of fatty acids or other intermediates can also have an intoxication effect.[2] Other diseases in this group are glycogen storage disorders, in which hypoglycemia can occur in the presence or absence of any stress, mitochondrial disorders, and congenital lactic acidosis, in which the clinical course is progressive even in the absence of triggering conditions.[3]
3. Disorders of complex molecules. These result from defects in the synthesis or the catabolism of complex molecules. These disorders are progressive, independent of intercurrent events, and not related to food intake. The metabolism of complex molecules is altered in all lysosomal disorders, peroxisomal disorders, disorders of intracellular trafficking, and processing. For some of these disorders, a therapy is now available that is usually more effective if initiated before irreversible organ damage has occurred. For this reason, some of these conditions (eg, Pompe disease, mucopolysaccharidosis type 1) have been recommended for inclusion in newborn screening panels.

INBORN ERRORS OF METABOLISM: DIAGNOSIS

The clinical symptoms of metabolic disorders such as lethargy, failure to thrive, vomiting, and seizures overlap with those due to common conditions, such as sepsis or liver disease; however, routine laboratory tests in the symptomatic patient and a high index of suspicion can point in the right direction. For example, hyperammonemia without metabolic acidosis can suggest a defect of the urea cycle; hypoketotic hypoglycemia, usually with hyperammonemia, to various degrees leans toward a fatty acid oxidation impairment; and hyperammonemia with metabolic acidosis and ketosis is more suggestive of an organic acidemia (Table 70.1). The diagnosis of IEM requires specific tests that are usually performed in biochemical genetics laboratories. Amino acid analysis in plasma, urine (in few cases), and cerebrospinal fluid (in even fewer cases); organic acids analysis in urine; and carnitine and acylcarnitine profile in plasma represent the core group of tests necessary for the diagnosis of IEM. In contrast to most common chemistry tests, biochemical genetics tests are complex and require specialized personnel to perform them and interpret the results. Each profile should be interpreted in the context of clinical history, physical signs, and other laboratory studies by a board-certified doctoral scientist or physician with specialized training in metabolic disease and analytic testing. When the results are suggestive of a metabolic disorder, the interpretation should also include information about the disease and suggest additional tests to confirm the diagnosis when appropriate.

Some metabolic disorders can be treated by dietary modifications that usually consist of a lifelong dietary regimen in which the nutrient that cannot be metabolized properly is restricted, often with supplementation of vitamins and other nutrients, cofactors, and, in some cases, medications. Because

TABLE 70.1 Biochemical Findings in Disorders of Amino Acid, Fatty Acid, and Organic Acid Metabolism

	Organic Acidurias	Fatty Acid Oxidation Disorders	Urea Cycle Disorders	MSUD	NKHG
Neurological distress	I	I/ED	I	I	I
Metabolic acidosis	+++	–	+	+	–
Ketonuria (ketone bodies)	+++	–	–	+	–
Hyperammonemia	+	+	+++	–	–
Hypoglycemia (fasting)	+	+++	–	–	–
Lactic acidemia	++	+	–	–	–

ED, Energy deficiency; *I*, intoxication type of neurological distress (see text); *MSUD*, maple syrup urine disease; *NKHG*, nonketotic hyperglycinemia; +, possibly present; ++, frequently present; +++, typically present with high diagnostic significance; –, not typically present.

of the excellent outcome for many metabolic patients when the treatment is initiated before symptoms or any damage has occurred, a major focus of biochemical genetics has been on early identification of IEM in the newborn period through universal newborn screening.

PRENATAL DIAGNOSIS

Despite constant progress in medical treatment, several IEMs result in severe morbidity and, in some cases, mortality early in life. Most of these disorders are inherited as autosomal recessive traits (Table 70.2). Therefore the recurrence risk in subsequent pregnancies of the same couple is 25%. Genetic counseling of parents consists of a balanced assessment of (1) familial risk factors (parental consanguinity and ethnic origin); (2) risk of pregnancy loss as a consequence of the sampling procedure (0.5% to 1.0% by chorionic villus sampling [CVS], 0.5% by amniocentesis); (3) risk of maternal complications; (4) the clinical validity of the prenatal test; (5) the burden of the disease; and (6) the variable phenotypic expression of the disease, even within the same family.[4]

Methods used for prenatal diagnosis of IEM have different requirements in terms of timing, sample collection, and options for independent confirmation. CVS is typically performed at 10 to 13 weeks of gestational age, has a higher risk of fetal loss compared to classic amniocentesis, and may not provide accurate results owing to contamination with maternal tissue, which can make this approach unreliable, and confined placental mosaicism. On the other hand, certain enzymes, such as those of the glycine cleavage pathway defective in glycine encephalopathy, are only expressed in chorionic villi cells, rendering this procedure the only possibility when DNA testing is not possible.[5] Amniocentesis is performed later in pregnancy (14–20 weeks) and provides both amniocytes and amniotic fluid to be used for independent and complementary diagnostic methods. Reliance on separate tests based on independent methods performed by laboratories with adequate experience is strongly encouraged to avoid the occurrence of either incorrect or inconclusive results. In some IEM (eg, organic acidemias), amniotic fluid can be tested for the presence or absence of specific metabolites, in addition to providing amniocytes for enzyme assay and/or DNA analysis. The combination of at least two independent tests (eg, enzyme assay plus DNA analysis; metabolite analysis plus enzyme or DNA) should give more confidence in establishing a prenatal diagnosis. Before entertaining a prenatal diagnosis, one should make sure that the proband (individual first brought to medical attention in which the diagnosis was established) related to the index case has a diagnosis confirmed by traditional methods, including enzymology when appropriate. If DNA analysis is considered, the mutations of the index case should be known and should have been confirmed as causative of the disease. The major advantages of direct metabolite analysis in amniotic fluid are the independence from tissue expression and a rapid turnaround time. However, direct metabolites analysis in amniotic fluid has been reported only for a very limited number of diseases.

NEWBORN SCREENING

Newborn screening is a public health activity aimed at the early identification of conditions for which timely intervention can lead to the elimination or reduction of morbidity, mortality, and disabilities. It is an important and effective component of preventive medicine. Originally instituted in the 1960s for the early detection of phenylketonuria (PKU), the number of diseases screened for in the newborn period has dramatically increased with the introduction of MS/MS multiplex analysis of acylcarnitine and amino acid profiles (for further discussion on chromatographic separation and mass spectrometry, refer to Chapters 16 and 17, respectively).[6] For several IEMs, newborn screening is providing the opportunity to define their incidence, natural history, prospective screening experience, and effectiveness of treatment.[7] The complexity of the interpretation of MS/MS newborn screening results has prompted the development of algorithms for appropriate confirmatory testing and differential diagnosis of all detectable IEM (http://www.ncbi.nlm.nih.gov/books/NBK55827/).

Although the metabolic disorders identified by MS/MS represent the largest group of diseases identifiable by newborn screening, other IEM, endocrine, and hematological disorders (such as galactosemia, biotinidase deficiency, cystic fibrosis, congenital hypothyroidism, congenital adrenal hyperplasia, storage disorders, and hemoglobinopathies) are identifiable using more traditional screening methods (eg, enzyme assays, immunoassays, electrophoresis). The advances in therapeutic interventions for IEM are continuously expanding the role of newborn screening. Newborn screening does not identify all metabolic disorders, and some patients can be missed by newborn screening. Therefore a symptomatic patient, at any age, should be investigated despite normal newborn screening results.

TABLE 70.2 **Clinical and Laboratory Characteristics of Disorders of Amino Acid Metabolism**

Common Name	OMIM* No.	Inheritance	Enzyme/Transport Defect	Incidence (US)	Major Clinical Features	Major Biochemical Marker(s)
Disorders of Aromatic Amino Acid Metabolism						
Classical phenylketonuria (PKU)	261600	AR	Phenylalanine hydroxylase	1:23,000	Mental retardation, fair complexion, and pigmentation	Phenylalanine (B), phenylpyruvic (U), phenyllactic (U), 2-OH phenylacetic (U)
Defect of biopterin cofactor biosynthesis	233910	AR	GTP cyclohydrolase I	<1:100,000	Progressive mental retardation, seizures, muscle tone abnormalities, microcephaly, movement disorder	Phenylalanine (B), low neopterin and biopterin (U), low 5-HIAA and HVA (CSF)
Defect of biopterin cofactor biosynthesis	261640	AR	6-Pyruvoyltetrahydropterin synthase	<1:100,000	Progressive mental retardation, seizures, muscle tone abnormalities, microcephaly, movement disorder	Phenylalanine (B), high neopterin, low biopterin (U), low 5-HIAA, HVA (CSF)
Defect of biopterin cofactor regeneration	261630	AR	Dihydropterin reductase (DHPR)	<1:100,000	Progressive mental retardation, spasticity, dystonia, myoclonus, microcephaly, movement disorder	Phenylalanine (B), high biopterin (U), low 5-HIAA, HVA (CSF), low DHPR activity in DBS
Defect of biopterin cofactor regeneration	264070	AR	Pterin-4a-carbinolamine dehydratase	<1:100,000	Transient muscle tone abnormalities, long-term outcome usually benign	Phenylalanine (B), high neopterin, and primapterin (U)
Defect of biopterin cofactor regeneration (brain specific)	612716	AR	Sepiapterin reductase (SPR)	<1:100,000	Progressive mental retardation, dystonia, myoclonus, movement disorder	High 7,8-dihydropterin, low 5-HIAA, HVA (CSF) ADDED activity in DBS
Tyrosinemia type I	276700	AR	Fumarylacetoacetase	<1:100,000	Cirrhosis, hepatocellular carcinoma, rickets, renal Fanconi syndrome, neuropathic pain	Tyrosine (B), succinylacetone (U), 4-OH phenylpyruvic, 4-OH phenyllactic (U)
Tyrosinemia type II	276600	AR	Tyrosine aminotransferase	<1:100,000	Corneal ulcers, keratosis on palms and soles, photophobia, pain to extremities	Tyrosine (B), 4-OH phenylpyruvic, 4-OH phenyllactic (U)
Tyrosinemia type III	276710	AR	4-Hydroxyphenylpyruvate dioxygenase	<1:100,000	Developmental delay	Tyrosine (B), 4-OH phenylpyruvic, 4-OH phenyllactic (U)
Hawkinsinuria	140350	AD	4-Hydroxyphenylpyruvate dioxygenase	<1:100,000	Failure to thrive, hepatocellular dysfunction	2-Cystenyl-1,4-dihydrocyclohexenylacetate (U), 4-hydroxycyclohexylacetic acid (U)
Disorders of Branched-Chain Amino Acid Metabolism						
Maple syrup disease (MSUD IA, IB, II)	248600	AR	Branched-chain ketoacid dehydrogenase complex	1:200,000 (1:378 Mennonite)	Hypotonia, lethargy, seizures, coma, vomiting, ketosis, pancreatitis, brain edema	Branched-chain amino acids (B), allo isoleucine (B), branched-chain 2-ketoacids, and branched-chain 2-hydroxy acids (U)

E3 deficiency	246900	AR	Dihydrolipoyl dehydrogenase (E3)	<1:100,000	Failure to thrive, hypotonia, developmental delay, seizures, coma, lactic acidosis, hypoglycemia	Branched-chain amino acids (B), allo isoleucine (B), lactic and pyruvic acids (B,U), 2-ketoglutaric acid, branched-chain 2-ketoacids, and branched-chain 2-hydroxy acids (U)
Disorders of Sulfur Amino Acid Metabolism						
Hypermethioninemia	250850	AR	Methionine adenosyltransferase	<1:100,000	Fetid breath, demyelination	Methionine (B)
S-Adenosylhomocysteine hydrolase deficiency	180960	AR	S-Adenosylhomocysteine hydrolase	Unknown	Developmental delay, hypotonia, hepatocellular dysfunction, white matter atrophy, abnormal myelination	Methionine (B), total plasma homocysteine, mildly elevated (B), elevated S-adenosylhomocysteine, and S-adenosylmethionine (B)
Glycine-N-methyltransferase deficiency	606664	AR	Glycine N-methyltransferase	Unknown	Hepatomegaly	Methionine (B), S-adenosylmethionine (B)
Homocystinuria	236200	AR	Cystathionine beta-synthase	1:450,000	Mental retardation, ectopia lensis, skeletal anomalies	Free homocystine, total homocysteine, and methionine (B,U)
Sulfite oxidase deficiency	272300	AR	Sulfite oxidase	<1:100,000	Mental retardation, seizures, ectopia lensis, dysmorphic features, muscle tone abnormalities	S-sulfocysteine and taurine (B,U); low cystine (B,U)
Molybdenum cofactor deficiency	252150	AR	Sulfite oxidase, xanthine dehydrogenase, aldehyde oxidase	<1:100,000	Mental retardation, seizures, ectopia lensis, dysmorphic features, muscle tone abnormalities	S-sulfocysteine and taurine (B,U); low cystine (B,U); elevated hypoxanthine and xanthine (U); low uric acid (B)
Urea Cycle Disorders						
N-Acetylglutamate synthase deficiency	237310	AR	N-Acetylglutamate synthase	<1:1,000,000	Hyperammonemia, lethargy, hypothermia, apnea, brain edema, coma	Glutamine, alanine (B), low citrulline, and arginine (B)
CPS-I deficiency	237300	AR	Carbamoylphosphate I synthetase	<1:100,000	Hyperammonemia, lethargy, hypothermia, apnea, brain edema, coma	Glutamine, alanine (B), low citrulline, arginine (B)
OTC deficiency	311250	X-linked	Ornithine transcarbamylase	>1:50,000	Hyperammonemia, lethargy, hypothermia, apnea, brain edema, coma	Orotic (U), glutamine, alanine (B), low citrulline, arginine (B)
Citrullinemia	603470	AR	Argininosuccinate synthase	1:150,000	Hyperammonemia, lethargy, hypothermia, apnea, brain edema, coma	Citrulline (B), orotic (U)

Continued

TABLE 70.2 Clinical and Laboratory Characteristics of Disorders of Amino Acid Metabolism—cont'd

Common Name	OMIM* No.	Inheritance	Enzyme/Transport Defect	Incidence (US)	Major Clinical Features	Major Biochemical Marker(s)
Citrullinemia type II (citrin deficiency)	603471 (adult onset); 605814, neonatal onset)	AR	Aspartate/glutamate mitochondrial exchanger	<1:100,000	Cholestatic jaundice, hepatocellular dysfunction, episodic hyperammonemia, neurological/psychiatric symptoms	Citrulline, methionine, lysine (B), orotic (U), elevated galactose (B) in neonatal onset
Argininosuccinic acidemia	207900	AR	Argininosuccinate lyase	1:300,000	Hyperammonemia, lethargy, hypothermia, apnea, brain edema, coma, trichorrexis nodosa	Argininosuccinic (B,U), citrulline (B), low arginine (B)
Argininemia	207800	AR	Arginase	<1:100,000	Progressive spasticity, mental retardation	Arginine (B, CSF), orotic acid (U)
HHH syndrome	238970	AR	Mitochondrial ornithine transporter	<1:100,000	Mental retardation, seizures, pyramidal signs, compromised sense of vibration, episodic hyperammonemia	Ornithine (B,U), homocitrulline (U)
Miscellaneous Disorders of Amino Acid Metabolism						
Nonketotic hyperglycinemia	605899	AR	Glycine cleavage system (P, H, T, L proteins)	<1:100,000	Lethargy, seizures, myoclonic jerks, hypotonia, hiccups	Glycine (B,CSF,U), CSF Gly/Plasma Gly ratio >0.09
Gyrate atrophy of the choroid and retina	258870	AR	Ornithine aminotransferase	<1:100,000	Myopia, night blindness, progressive loss of peripheral vision	Ornithine (B)
Hyperprolinemia type I	239500	AR	Proline oxidase	<1:100,000	Clinically benign (most likely); renal disease, neurological manifestations (disputed)	Proline (B,U), hydroxyproline, glycine (U)
Hyperprolinemia type II	239510	AR	Delta 1-Pryrroline-5-carboxylate dehydrogenase	<1:100,000	Mental retardation, pyridoxine responsive seizures	Proline (B,U), Pyrroline 5-carboxylic (U)
Disorders of Amino Acid Membrane Transport						
Cystinuria	220100	AR	Absorption of cystine and dibasic amino acids in renal tubule and GI tract	>1:25,000	Nephrolithiasis	Cystine, lysine, ornithine, arginine (U)
Lysinuric protein intolerance (LPI)	222700	AR	Cationic amino acids transporter (SLC7A7)	<1:100,000	Failure to thrive, alveolar proteinosis, hepatosplenomegaly, pancreatitis, diarrhea, osteoporosis, hypotonia, postprandial hyperammonemia	Lysine, arginine, ornithine (U), orotic acid (U)
Hartnup disease	234500	AR	Neutral amino acids transporter 1 (SLC6A19)	>1:50,000	Ataxia, seizures, photodermatitis (pellagra-like)	Hyperexcretion of ALA, SER, THR, VAL, LEU, ILE, PHE, TYR, TRP, HIS, GLN, ASN (U)

**OMIM,* Online Mendelian inheritance in man (www.ncbi.nlm.nih.gov/entrez/query.fcgi?db=OMIM); *DBS,* dried blood spot; NBS, newborn screening; *5-HIAA,* 5-hydroxyindoleacetic acid; *HVA,* homovanillic acid.

POINTS TO REMEMBER

Inborn Errors of Metabolism

- Inborn errors of metabolism can present at any age but are more frequent in childhood.
- Unexplained metabolic acidosis, hyperammonemia, hypoglycemia, or abnormalities of liver function should prompt investigation for inborn errors of metabolism.
- Newborn screening identifies infants at risk for a metabolic disorder.
- MS/MS measures the concentration of amino acids and acylcarnitines and is becoming the preferred method in newborn screening programs.
- The diagnosis is confirmed biochemically by measuring plasma amino acids (by ion exchange chromatography or LC-MS/MS), urine organic acids (by gas chromatography/MS), and plasma acylcarnitine profile (by MS/MS).
- DNA testing or enzyme assay is necessary to definitively confirm the diagnosis of a metabolic disorder

EVALUATION OF SYMPTOMATIC PATIENTS

The most informative samples are those collected from patients during an acute metabolic decompensation. When possible, urine and blood should be collected at the same time. In several diseases, especially in fatty acid oxidation disorders, the diagnostic abnormalities may not be detectable when the patient has recovered from the acute episode. Urine and plasma or serum samples can be stored at −20°C until the need for specialized tests has been determined. Quantitative profiling of amino acids, carnitine, and acylcarnitines in plasma, and organic acids and acylglycines in urine are the biochemical investigations necessary to diagnose these disorders. Alternatively, a blood spot on filter paper may provide enough material for one or more of the investigations described in this chapter. In the case of death, collection of body fluids and tissue should be performed according to available protocols.[8,9]

POSTMORTEM SCREENING

Among IEM, fatty acid oxidation (FAO) disorders are those recognized more often after the diagnosis of an affected sibling or as a cause of sudden death.[10] Early reports attributed up to 5% of sudden death in children younger than 5 years of age to FAO,[11] and there is mounting evidence that some of these disorders can cause mortality in adults as well.[12] The postmortem evaluation of unexpected death, independently of age, especially when there is evidence of an acute illness or infection, should consider FAO as a cause. This can be accomplished by the analysis of acylcarnitines in blood and bile spots.[2] Reference intervals for acylcarnitines in postmortem blood and bile spots are listed in Table 70.3.

Blood and bile can be collected on filter paper identical to the cards used for newborn screening and shipped to the laboratory at room temperature once properly dried. In cases with a higher index of suspicion, an effort should be made to collect and freeze a specimen of liver[11] and collect a skin biopsy for establishing fibroblast culture that can be used, if needed, to confirm a diagnosis. Although fatty infiltration of the liver and/or other organs (eg, heart, muscle, and kidneys) is a common observation in FAO disorders, cardiac arrhythmia can occur with or without macroscopic steatosis, and a possible underlying FAO disorder should be considered in the evaluation of a case of sudden death, even in adults. In cases of sudden infant death, if parental permission to perform an autopsy is not granted, any leftover specimens or any unused portion of the blood spots collected for newborn screening, if still available, may be useful samples to obtain a diagnosis.

BIOCHEMICAL GENETICS TESTS: ANALYTICAL CONSIDERATIONS

In addition to the clinical presentation and routine laboratory tests, the diagnosis of patients with IEM relies on specific tests such as ion-exchange chromatography and liquid chromatography with tandem mass spectrometry (LC-MS/MS) for amino acids analysis, gas-chromatography-mass spectrometry (GC-MS) for organic acids analysis, tandem mass spectrometry (MS/MS) with (LC-MS/MS) or without liquid chromatographic separation for acylcarnitines profile, and LC-MS/MS or GC-MS for acylglycine profile. The combination of these tests, using different specimen types, is the key to the biochemical confirmation of metabolic disorders, whose diagnosis is then definitively confirmed using DNA testing or enzyme transport protein assays.

Analyses of plasma amino acids, urine organic acids, and plasma acylcarnitines are the mainstay for the diagnosis of most aminoacidopathies, organic acidemias, and disorders of FAO. To allow the early identification of asymptomatic patients by newborn screening, the diagnostic sensitivity and specificity of these methods need to be very high to detect even low concentrations of diagnostic metabolites. Furthermore, availability of age-appropriate reference intervals is necessary because the concentration of several metabolites (eg, acylcarnitines) changes rapidly with age.

Amino Acid Analysis

Several methods can be used for the analysis of amino acids in biological fluids (plasma, urine, CSF), and most involve chromatographic separation of the amino acids with precolumn (HPLC, GC methods) or postcolumn (ion exchange chromatography or IEC) derivatization, followed by detection by UV, fluorescence, or mass spectrometry.[13-18] IEC is the most frequently used method for amino acid analysis, although many laboratories are now using novel MS-MS–based methods. The challenges with amino acid analysis are the needs to cover a wide range of concentrations, have a very low detection limit, and have a high upper limit of linearity. In addition to these analytical requirements, isomers may need to be separated and quantified. With IEC, the sample (plasma, urine, or CSF) is deproteinized and injected onto an ion-exchange column (typically a Lithium column). The amino acids are separated based on their pKa by changing the pH and the ionic strength of the eluting buffers and the temperature of the column. Acidic amino acids are eluted first, followed by neutral and then basic amino acids. After their elution from the column, amino acids are mixed with ninhydrin at 135°C to form a colored adduct. The intensity of the color is proportional to the concentration of the amino acid. The absorbance is read at two different wavelengths: 570 nm (maximum absorbance for amino acids) and 440 nm

TABLE 70.3 Acylcarnitine Reference Intervals in Postmortem Blood and Bile Dried Spots

		BLOOD (*n* = 448)		BILE (*n* = 525)	
		Median (μmol/L)	**5th to 95th Percentile**	**Median (μmol/L)**	**5th to 95th Percentile**
Acetylcarnitine	C2	73.87	23.55–181.22	87.34	20.44–245.72
Acrylylcarnitine	C3:1	0.03	0.01–0.12	0.07	0.02–0.30
Propionylcarnitine	C3	2.95	0.55–8.01	2.07	0.36–8.10
Iso-/butyrylcarnitine	C4	4.24	0.79–14.49	1.81	0.50–5.75
Tiglylcarnitine	C5:1	0.07	0.02–0.21	0.13	0.03–0.53
Isovaleryl/2-CH_3 butyrylcarnitine	C5	0.65	0.18–1.73	0.85	0.19–2.90
3-OH butyrylcarnitine	C4-OH	1.97	0.35–6.25	0.65	0.12–2.26
Hexanoylcarnitine	C6	0.61	0.12–1.58	0.56	0.12–3.31
3-OH isovalerylcarnitine	C5-OH	0.28	0.10–0.74	0.22	0.06–0.67
Heptanoylcarnitine	C7	0.05	0.01–0.14	0.12	0.03–0.75
3-OH hexanoylcarnitine	C6-OH	0.14	0.03–0.45	0.16	0.03–0.59
Octenoylcarnitine	C8:1	0.16	0.03–0.48	2.56	0.18–36.01
Octanoylcarnitine	C8	0.35	0.19–1.02	0.63	0.19–6.46
Malonylcarnitine	C3-DC	0.12	0.03–0.32	0.22	0.04–0.96
Decadienoylcarnitine	C10:2	0.03	0.01–0.08	0.26	0.03–3.93
Decenoylcarnitine	C10:1	0.05	0.01–0.15	0.58	0.06–11.80
Decanoylcarnitine	C10	0.09	0.02–0.37	0.35	0.05–6.47
Methylmalonylcarnitine	C4-DC	0.29	0.09–0.81	0.30	0.06–0.92
3-OH decenoylcarnitine	C10:1-OH	0.05	0.02–0.14	0.18	0.04–1.97
Glutarylcarnitine (3-OH C10)	C5-DC	0.07	0.02–0.21	0.18	0.04–1.53
Dodecenoylcarnitine	C12:1	0.03	0.01–0.13	0.30	0.03–13.50
Dodecanoylcarnitine	C12	0.17	0.07–0.61	0.49	0.08–7.40
3-OH dodecenoylcarnitine	C12:1-OH	0.04	0.01–0.11	0.24	0.04–4.86
3-OH dodecanoylcarnitine	C12-OH	0.04	0.01–0.18	0.28	0.03–2.28
Tetradecadienoylcarnitine	C14:2	0.06	0.01–0.26	0.36	0.04–9.49
Tetradecenoylcarnitine	C14:1	0.07	0.02–0.30	0.30	0.03–12.49
Tetradecanoylcarnitine	C14	0.14	0.04–0.47	0.25	0.04–3.81
3-OH tetradecenoylcarnitine	C14:1-OH	0.04	0.01–0.10	0.15	0.03–2.60
3-OH tetradecanoylcarnitine	C14-OH	0.03	0.01–0.08	0.11	0.02–1.15
Hexadecenoylcarnitine	C16:1	0.07	0.02–0.28	0.15	0.03–2.73
Hexadecanoylcarnitine	C16	0.53	0.10–1.74	0.42	0.09–3.39
3-OH hexadecenoylcarnitine	C16:1-OH	0.06	0.02–0.24	0.24	0.04–1.45
3-OH hexadecanoylcarnitine	C16-OH	0.04	0.01–0.12	0.27	0.03–1.48
Octadecadienoylcarnitine	C18:2	0.18	0.03–0.55	0.22	0.03–2.93
Octadecenoylcarnitine	C18:1	0.53	0.11–1.69	0.38	0.07–3.75
Octadecanoylcarnitine	C18	0.43	0.12–1.34	0.36	0.06–2.13
3-OH octadecadienoylcarnitine	C18:2-OH	0.03	0.01–0.08	0.09	0.01–0.55
3-OH octadecenoylcarnitine	C18:1-OH	0.04	0.01–0.11	0.10	0.02–1.01
3-OH octadecanoylcarnitine	C18-OH	0.03	0.01–0.10	0.07	0.00–0.66

(maximum absorbance for imino acids, such as proline and hydroxyproline). The concentration of amino acids is calculated using an internal standard and external calibration. The identification of the individual amino acids relies on retention time, the ratio of the absorbance at the two wavelengths—440 and 570 nm—and, if uncertainty remains, by spiking the sample with a standard.

The use of LC-MS/MS–based methods for amino acids analysis is rapidly expanding. Although in some cases the preparation of the samples may take longer than IEC, the separation time required is much shorter. These methods have also increased analytical sensitivity and specificity and have allowed the identification of patients with milder forms of metabolic disorders in which the characteristic amino acid is present at a concentration not detectable by conventional IEC.[19] From the analytical point of view, it is important to have isotopically labeled internal standards for the amino acids quantified during the analysis to guarantee accurate results.

The specimen of choice is plasma collected under fasting conditions. In the case of infants and small children, the sample should be collected at least 2 hours after the last feed. Collection of serum should be avoided because of artifacts deriving from the clotting process. Blood should be collected with an anticoagulant (lithium or sodium heparin); plasma should be immediately separated and frozen until the time of analysis. Storage of samples at inappropriate temperature (eg, room temperature or refrigerated) can result in deamination of glutamine and binding of sulfur amino acids to protein. The pool of most amino acids in red blood cells is very similar to that in plasma; however, some amino acids are present at a higher concentrations in red blood cells (eg, aspartic acid, taurine, glutamic acid), and therefore hemolysis will result in an artificially increased concentration of those amino acids. In addition, red blood cells contain the enzyme arginase that converts arginine to ornithine and urea. Hemolysis may release this enzyme, resulting in decreased concentrations of arginine and increased ornithine. Results of plasma amino acids analysis are usually expressed in μmol/L.

Measurements of urine amino acids are useful only in the investigation of disorders of amino acids transport (eg, cystinuria, lysinuric protein intolerance, Hartnup disorder), prolidase deficiency, hypophosphatasia (with excess phosphoethanolamine), and sulfite oxidase deficiency. A random urine sample, without preservative, is usually sufficient. Specific reabsorption studies may require a timed (24-hour) urine collection. The sample should be collected without preservatives and kept refrigerated until the end of the collection. Urine samples, like plasma, should be frozen as soon as possible and kept frozen until analysis. Results are usually normalized for creatinine.[20]

Analysis of CSF amino acids is performed for very specific cases, such as in the diagnostic investigation of glycine encephalopathy (nonketotic hyperglycinemia), and in disorders of serine metabolism. CSF should be collected in such a way to avoid blood contamination, frozen immediately, and kept frozen until analysis. Results of CSF amino acid analysis are expressed in μmol/L. Amino acid results, regardless of specimen type, should be correlated with the clinical status, diet, and medications.

Urine Organic Acid Analysis by Gas Chromatography–Mass Spectrometry

The term *organic acids* includes metabolites of almost all pathways of intermediary metabolism, as well as exogenous compounds. Organic acids are analyzed by GC–MS; they are separated based on their volatility and solubility in the stationary nonpolar liquid phase of the capillary GC column. Prior to GC–MS analysis, organic acids must be extracted, usually with an organic solvent; derivatized by conversion (most frequently) to volatile trimethylsilyl (TMS) derivatives; and dissolved in organic solvents before analysis.[17,21,22] In organic acid analysis by GC–MS, the mass spectrometer is the detector. This allows the positive identification of organic acids not only by retention times but also by their characteristic fragmentation spectrum. A random urine specimen is routinely used for this analysis, but the most informative samples for the diagnosis of IEM are those collected during acute metabolic decompensation. Organic acid analysis of blood or CSF is usually not sufficiently informative to establish a diagnosis. The identification of the organic acids present in the sample relies on the use of a good reference library of spectral data, while the interpretation of organic acid profiles can be challenging because hundreds of compounds are present in a specimen. Recognition of abnormal patterns and possible interferences due to dietary or medications artifacts, knowledge about metabolic disorders and their presentation, and information about clinical status of the patients are among the key factors for correct interpretation of the results.

Plasma Acylcarnitine Profile

Acylcarnitines derive from conjugation of carnitine with acyl-CoAs. Carnitine (β-hydroxy-γ-trimethylammoniumbutyrate) is a water-soluble molecule essential in the transfer of long-chain fatty acids inside mitochondria for beta-oxidation. In addition to this, carnitine binds acyl residues accumulating in several organic acidemias and in FAO disorders to facilitate their excretion. In the presence of a metabolic block (organic acidemia or FAO disorder), specific acylcarnitines, derived from conjugation of carnitine with acyl-CoAs upstream of the metabolic block, accumulate, producing a pattern that is characteristic for each disease or group of diseases. For this reason, acylcarnitine analysis plays an essential role in the diagnosis of metabolic disorders. The analysis is usually performed by MS/MS with or without liquid chromatographic separation prior to MS/MS detection.[23,24] Plasma or serum is the biological fluid of choice, while whole blood spotted on filter paper is used for screening of newborns. The concentration of acylcarnitines in plasma differs from the concentration in whole blood, especially for long-chain acylcarnitines. This is probably due to binding of long-chain acylcarnitines to the membranes of blood cells, resulting in reduced long-chain species in plasma. The plasma for analysis of acylcarnitines should be separated immediately after collection and kept frozen until analysis. Hemolysis can result in increased long-chain acylcarnitines and mislead the diagnosis; therefore hemolyzed samples are unacceptable for acylcarnitine testing. Storage of the sample at room temperature or even refrigerated may result in hydrolysis and, consequently, reduced concentrations of acylcarnitines. Urine acylcarnitine analysis is performed only in the diagnostic workup of specific disorders, such as glutaric acidemia type I, and only if equivocal results are obtained with other tests. The quantification of acylcarnitines is usually performed using stable isotope dilution, keeping in mind that deuterated internal standards are not available for all the acylcarnitine species identified. Caution should be taken when comparing acylcarnitine results from different laboratories because the values may change, depending on the internal standards used.[25]

Reference Intervals

Age-appropriate reference intervals should be used in the interpretation of biochemical genetics tests. Reference intervals for urine organic acids, urine acylglycines, plasma, and urine acylcarnitines are listed in Tables 70.3 to 70.6. These reference intervals are derived from one laboratory and they may not be universally applicable. Laboratories should ideally develop their own reference intervals.

Enzyme Assay and DNA Testing

Several IEMs produce a characteristic pattern of metabolites that is not observed in other conditions, but for most, the diagnosis needs to be confirmed by a more specific method involving measurement of the activity of the putatively defective enzyme or transporter and/or DNA testing. This confirmation is critical because for many conditions, specific therapy, if available, needs to be continued for life or is very invasive (eg, for a bone marrow transplant). In addition, for some metabolic disorders there is genotype-phenotype correlation with specific mutations affecting the overall

TABLE 70.4 Reference Intervals of Selected Organic Acids and Acylglycines in Urine (mmol/mol Creatinine)

Age Groups	0–1 Month	1–6 Months	6 Months–5 Years	>5 Years
Acetylaspartic acid*	nd–13	nd–13	nd–13	nd–13
cis-Aconitic acid	5–31	10–97	10–97	3–44
Adipic acid	9–37	9–37	nd–15	nd–5
Azelaic acid	nd–1	nd–1	nd–1	nd–1
Butyrylglycine*	0.1–2	0.1–2	0.1–2	0.1–2
trans-Cinnamoylglycine*	0.1–8	0.1–8	0.1–8	0.1–8
Citric acid	nd–1045	104–268	0–656	87–639
Dodecanedioic acid*	nd–0.05	nd–0.05	nd–0.05	nd–0.05
Ethylmalonic acid*	0.4–17	0.4–17	0.4–17	0.4–17
Fumaric acid	10–45	4–45	1–27	2–4
Glutaric acid*	0.5–13	0.5–13	0.5–13	0.5–13
Glyceric acid*	nd–39	nd–184	nd–70	0–60
Glycolic acid*	nd–62	nd–104	3–121	nd–166
Glyoxylic acid*	nd–13	0–16	nd–7	nd–9
Hexadecanedioic acid*	nd–0.4	nd–0.4	nd–0.4	nd–0.4
Hexanoylglycine*	0.1–1.2	0.1–1.2	0.1–1.2	0.1–1.2
Homogentisic acid	nd–10	nd–10	nd–10	nd–10
Homovanillic acid*	nd–22	nd–22	nd–8	nd–7
3-Hydroxy butyric acid	nd–5	nd–5	nd–5	nd–10
2-Hydroxy glutaric acid	nd–15	nd–15	nd–15	nd–15
5-Hydroxy indoleacetic acid*	nd–12	nd–12	nd–12	nd–9
4-Hydroxy phenyllactic acid	nd–50	nd–10	nd–10	nd–10
4-Hydroxy phenylpyruvic acid	nd–20	nd–5	nd–5	nd–5
Isobutyrylglycine*	nd–9	0–9	0–9	0–9
Isocitric acid	0–368	0–67	0–77	16–99
Isovalerylglycine*	0.2–10	0.2–10	0.2–10	0.2–10
2-Ketoglutaric acid	22–567	63–552	36–103	41–82
Lactic acid	46–348	57–346	21–38	20–101
Malic acid	0–52	8–73	4–57	17–47
2-Methylbutyrylglycine*	0.2–5	0.2–5	0.2–5	0.2–5
Methylmalonic acid*	nd–3.6	nd–3.6	nd–3.6	nd–3.6
Methylsuccinic acid*	0–12	0–12	0–12	0–12
Octanoylglycine*	0.1–1.2	0.1–1.2	0.1–1.2	0.1–1.2
Orotic acid	1.4–5.3	1.0–3.2	0.5–3.3	0.4–1.2
Oxalic acid*	51–931	7–567	7–352	nd–187
3-Phenylpropionylglycine*	nd–0.6	nd–0.6	nd–0.6	nd–0.6
Pimelic acid	nd–1	nd–1	nd–1	nd–1
Pyroglutamic acid	nd–61	nd–61	nd–61	nd–61
Pyruvic acid	24–123	8–90	3–19	6–9
Sebacic acid	3–16	3–16	nd–8	nd–8
Suberic acid	4–20	4–20	nd–8	nd–8
Suberylglycine*	nd–5.4	nd–5.4	nd–5.4	nd–5.4
Succinic acid	35–547	34–156	16–118	29–87
Tetradecanedioic acid*	nd–0.40	nd–0.40	nd–0.40	nd–0.40
Uracil*	nd–32	nd–32	nd–21	nd–17
Uric acid*	359–2644	359–2644	185–1134	199–1034
Vanilylmandelic acid*	nd–15	nd–10	nd–7	nd–5

nd, Not detected.
*Measured using a stable isotope-labeled internal standard.
TIC detection limit: 0.1 mmol/mol creatinine.
SIM detection limit (with stable isotope labeled internal standard): 0.01 mmol/mol creatinine.

prognosis. For some diseases, such as phenylketonuria, the mutant enzyme is expressed only in the liver, and it is not practical and unacceptably invasive to obtain diagnostic confirmation by enzyme assay. DNA testing (by sequencing the whole gene) in this case can prove more useful. For several other conditions, the missing enzyme is expressed in blood cells or in fibroblasts that can be obtained by skin biopsy, a relatively noninvasive procedure. It must be noted that, with the decrease in the costs, DNA testing is becoming more and more popular to provide final diagnostic confirmation.

TABLE 70.5 Acylcarnitine Reference Intervals in Plasma

		0–7 DAYS (*n* =143)		8 D–7 YR (*n* = 2677)		>7 YR (*n* = 834)	
		Median (μmol/L)	5th–95th Percentile	Median (μmol/L)	5th–95th Percentile	Median (μmol/L)	5th–95th Percentile
Acetylcarnitine	C2	8.37	2.82–19.67	10.45	4.70–33.66	8.45	3.29–25.72
Acrylylcarnitine	C3:1	0.01	0.00–0.03	0.01	0.00–0.03	0.01	0.00–0.03
Propionylcarnitine	C3	0.34	0.07–1.85	0.49	0.17–1.27	0.45	0.17–1.49
Iso-/Butyrylcarnitine	C4	0.27	0.13–0.70	0.31	0.16–0.74	0.30	0.15–1.05
Tiglylcarnitine	C5:1	0.01	0.00–0.06	0.01	0.00–0.05	0.02	0.00–0.10
Isovaleryl/2-CH_3 butyrylcarnitine	C5	0.15	0.04–0.42	0.15	0.05–0.44	0.14	0.06–0.51
3-OH butyrylcarnitine	C4-OH	0.04	0.01–0.15	0.04	0.01–0.29	0.03	0.01–0.19
Hexanoylcarnitine	C6	0.05	0.01–0.49	0.06	0.02–0.20	0.05	0.02–0.21
3-OH isovalerylcarnitine	C5-OH	0.03	0.01–0.15	0.02	0.01–0.07	0.02	0.01–0.19
Heptanoylcarnitine	C7	0.01	0.00–0.05	0.01	0.00–0.04	0.01	0.00–0.06
3-OH hexanoylcarnitine	C6-OH	0.02	0.00–0.07	0.02	0.01–0.06	0.02	0.00–0.07
Octenoylcarnitine	C8:1	0.18	0.03–0.45	0.19	0.06–0.53	0.19	0.06–0.72
Octanoylcarnitine	C8	0.16	0.08–1.40	0.15	0.08–0.41	0.16	0.08–0.45
Malonylcarnitine	C3-DC	0.03	0.01–0.08	0.03	0.01–0.09	0.04	0.01–0.17
Decadienoylcarnitine	C10:2	0.03	0.01–0.07	0.02	0.01–0.07	0.02	0.01–0.11
Decenoylcarnitine	C10:1	0.09	0.03–0.41	0.12	0.04–0.37	0.14	0.03–0.46
Decanoylcarnitine	C10	0.10	0.02–0.51	0.13	0.04–0.44	0.14	0.03–0.58
Methylmalonylcarnitine	C4-DC	0.01	0.00–0.03	0.01	0.00–0.03	0.01	0.00–0.06
3-OH decenoylcarnitine	C10:1-OH	0.03	0.01–0.11	0.02	0.01–0.05	0.03	0.01–0.11
Glutarylcarnitine (3-OH C10)	C5-DC	0.02	0.00–0.11	0.02	0.00–0.06	0.02	0.00–0.12
Dodecenoylcarnitine	C12:1	0.04	0.01–0.29	0.05	0.01–0.19	0.06	0.01–0.21
Dodecanoylcarnitine	C12	0.07	0.02–0.33	0.07	0.03–0.18	0.06	0.02–0.18
3-OH dodecenoylcarnitine	C12:1-OH	0.02	0.00–0.07	0.01	0.00–0.05	0.02	0.00–0.08
3-OH dodecanoylcarnitine	C12-OH	0.02	0.00–0.08	0.01	0.00–0.03	0.01	0.00–0.04
Tetradecadienoylcarnitine	C14:2	0.03	0.01–0.12	0.03	0.01–0.12	0.03	0.01–0.12
Tetradecenoylcarnitine	C14:1	0.05	0.01–0.39	0.05	0.01–0.23	0.05	0.01–0.24
Tetradecanoylcarnitine	C14	0.04	0.01–0.23	0.03	0.01–0.10	0.02	0.01–0.12
3-OH tetradecenoylcarnitine	C14:1-OH	0.02	0.01–0.08	0.02	0.01–0.05	0.02	0.01–0.07
3-OH tetradecanoylcarnitine	C14-OH	0.01	0.00–0.06	0.01	0.00–0.03	0.01	0.00–0.04
Hexadecenoylcarnitine	C16:1	0.04	0.01–0.24	0.03	0.01–0.10	0.03	0.01–0.09
Hexadecanoylcarnitine	C16	0.17	0.05–0.67	0.10	0.04–0.23	0.09	0.04–0.21
3-OH hexadecenoylcarnitine	C16:1-OH	0.01	0.00–0.30	0.01	0.00–0.05	0.01	0.00–0.04
3-OH hexadecanoylcarnitine	C16-OH	0.01	0.00–0.08	0.01	0.00–0.03	0.01	0.00–0.03
Octadecadienoylcarnitine	C18:2	0.04	0.01–0.12	0.05	0.02–0.16	0.06	0.02–0.15
Octadecenoylcarnitine	C18:1	0.12	0.03–0.38	0.13	0.05–0.35	0.14	0.04–0.33
Octadecanoylcarnitine	C18	0.04	0.01–0.20	0.05	0.02–0.11	0.05	0.02–0.10
3-OH octadecadienoylcarnitine	C18:2-OH	0.01	0.00–0.04	0.01	0.00–0.02	0.01	0.00–0.02
3-OH octadecenoylcarnitine	C18:1-OH	0.01	0.00–0.04	0.01	0.00–0.03	0.01	0.00–0.03
3-OH octadecanoylcarnitine	C18-OH	0.01	0.00–0.03	0.01	0.00–0.02	0.01	0.00–0.02

The major limitation of DNA sequencing is that for certain conditions the same biochemical abnormality can be caused by deficiency of any of a number of genes (for example, in methylmalonic acidemia), or multiple genes might be required to encode all of the subunits of a single enzyme (such as in maple syrup urine disease). For this reason, gene panels now evaluate multiple genes at once, particularly by using next-generation sequencing. DNA sequencing may not identify all mutations causing a disease. It can miss single exon deletions and duplications, and it can identify new variations whose clinical significance is unclear because they have not been reported in other affected patients. In these cases, biochemical (including enzyme assay) and molecular investigations need to be performed together to confirm or exclude the diagnosis of a metabolic disorder.

DISORDERS OF AMINO ACID METABOLISM

The concentrations of individual amino acids in physiological fluids reflect a balance between their intake, their release from the catabolism of endogenous proteins, their filtration and reabsorption by the kidney, and their utilization by the body either to synthesize proteins or to produce energy. Changes in any of these processes can affect protein and amino acid metabolism with either accumulation or excessive losses of one or more amino acids.

Inborn errors of amino acid metabolism can present at any time in a person's life, but most become evident in infancy and early childhood. Affected patients may have failure to thrive, neurological symptoms, digestive problems, psychomotor retardation, and a wide spectrum of laboratory

TABLE 70.6 **Acylcarnitine Reference Intervals in Urine**

		0–7 DAYS (*n* = 20)		8 D–7 YR (*n* = 20)		>7 YR (*n* = 20)	
		Mean (mmol/mol Creatinine)	Range (mmol/mol Creatinine)	Mean (mmol/mol Creatinine)	Range (mmol/mol Creatinine)	Mean (mmol/mol Creatinine)	Range (mmol/mol Creatinine)
Acetylcarnitine	C2	1.13	0.19–2.92	4.30	0.07–16.46	0.35	0.04–1.26
Acrylylcarnitine	C3:1	0.02	0.00–0.06	0.01	0.00–0.04	0.00	0.00–0.00
Propionylcarnitine	C3	0.06	0.01–0.20	0.23	0.01–1.20	0.02	0.00–0.06
Iso-/Butyrylcarnitine	C4	0.14	0.02–0.36	0.79	0.02–2.74	0.10	0.01–0.29
Tiglylcarnitine	C5:1	0.05	0.01–0.14	0.10	0.00–0.34	0.01	0.00–0.03
Isovaleryl/2-CH_3 butyrylcarnitine	C5	0.09	0.00–0.25	0.39	0.00–1.53	0.03	0.00–0.07
3-OH butyrylcarnitine	C4-OH	0.03	0.01–0.06	0.09	0.00–0.26	0.01	0.00–0.03
Hexanoylcarnitine	C6	0.03	0.01–0.06	0.05	0.00–0.16	0.01	0.00–0.04
3-OH isovalerylcarnitine	C5-OH	0.09	0.00–0.19	0.17	0.01–0.52	0.02	0.01–0.05
Benzoylcarnitine	BZC	0.02	0.00–0.05	0.11	0.01–0.37	0.01	0.00–0.04
Heptanoylcarnitine	C7	0.02	0.00–0.06	0.04	0.00–0.15	0.00	0.00–0.01
3-OH hexanoylcarnitine	C6-OH	0.02	0.01–0.06	0.08	0.00–0.32	0.00	0.00–0.01
Octenoylcarnitine	C8:1	0.12	0.01–0.36	0.84	0.02–4.30	0.09	0.01–0.23
Octanoylcarnitine	C8	0.26	0.02–0.82	0.14	0.01–0.61	0.02	0.00–0.05
Malonylcarnitine	C3-DC	0.10	0.02–0.22	0.13	0.01–0.50	0.02	0.00–0.04
Decadienoylcarnitine	C10:2	0.04	0.00–0.09	0.17	0.01–0.48	0.03	0.01–0.08
Decenoylcarnitine	C10:1	0.05	0.01–0.13	0.24	0.01–0.65	0.03	0.01–0.07
Decanoylcarnitine	C10	0.03	0.01–0.08	0.04	0.00–0.21	0.01	0.00–0.02
Methylmalonylcarnitine	C4-DC	0.14	0.03–0.25	0.15	0.02–0.57	0.02	0.01–0.05
3-OH decenoylcarnitine	C10:1-OH	0.12	0.01–0.25	0.08	0.01–0.26	0.01	0.00–0.03
Glutarylcarnitine (3-OH C10)	C5-DC	0.14	0.03–0.31	0.13	0.01–0.37	0.03	0.01–0.06
Dodecenoylcarnitine	C12:1	0.01	0.00–0.03	0.03	0.00–0.07	0.00	0.00–0.01
Dodecanoylcarnitine	C12	0.05	0.01–0.10	0.05	0.00–0.19	0.01	0.00–0.02
Adipoylcarnitine	C6-DC	0.17	0.04–0.40	0.19	0.01–0.81	0.03	0.00–0.13
3-OH dodecenoylcarnitine	C12:1-OH	0.07	0.01–0.25	0.07	0.00–0.27	0.01	0.00–0.03
3-OH dodecanoylcarnitine	C12-OH	0.05	0.01–0.12	0.05	0.00–0.16	0.01	0.00–0.01
Tetradecadienoylcarnitine	C14:2	0.12	0.01–0.55	0.01	0.00–0.02	0.00	0.00–0.00
Tetradecenoylcarnitine	C14:1	0.05	0.00–0.24	0.05	0.00–0.21	0.01	0.00–0.01
Tetradecanoylcarnitine	C14	0.05	0.01–0.11	0.09	0.00–0.39	0.01	0.00–0.02
3-OH tetradecenoylcarnitine	C14:1-OH	0.04	0.01–0.10	0.04	0.00–0.14	0.01	0.00–0.01
3-OH tetradecanoylcarnitine	C14-OH	0.03	0.01–0.07	0.03	0.00–0.09	0.00	0.00–0.02
Hexadecenoylcarnitine	C16:1	0.01	0.00–0.03	0.01	0.00–0.04	0.00	0.00–0.00
Hexadecanoylcarnitine	C16	0.05	0.01–0.13	0.05	0.00–0.18	0.01	0.00–0.02
3-OH hexadecenoylcarnitine	C16:1-OH	0.32	0.00–2.06	0.01	0.00–0.02	0.00	0.00–0.00
3-OH hexadecanoylcarnitine	C16-OH	0.05	0.00–0.24	0.01	0.00–0.05	0.00	0.00–0.00
Octadecadienoylcarnitine	C18:2	0.08	0.00–0.37	0.01	0.00–0.02	0.00	0.00–0.00
Octadecenoylcarnitine	C18:1	0.01	0.00–0.03	0.01	0.00–0.02	0.00	0.00–0.00
Octadecanoylcarnitine	C18	0.01	0.00–0.02	0.01	0.00–0.05	0.00	0.00–0.00
3-OH octadecadienoylcarnitine	C18:2-OH	0.01	0.00–0.02	0.00	0.00–0.01	0.00	0.00–0.00
3-OH octadecenoylcarnitine	C18:1-OH	0.01	0.00–0.03	0.01	0.00–0.03	0.00	0.00–0.00
3-OH octadecanoylcarnitine	C18-OH	0.01	0.00–0.03	0.01	0.00–0.02	0.00	0.00–0.00

findings. If not diagnosed promptly and treated properly, these disorders can result in poor growth, mental retardation, and death.

Table 70.3 shows a summary of the most common disorders of amino acid metabolism and transport and their characteristics. Several of these disorders are discussed as examples in the following section.

Classic Phenylketonuria and Other Hyperphenylalaninemias

The hyperphenylalaninemias result from the impaired conversion of phenylalanine to tyrosine leading to increased concentration of phenylalanine in body fluids. They are caused by a primary deficiency of phenylalanine hydroxylase, the enzyme converting phenylalanine into tyrosine (Fig. 70.2), or, in rare cases (<2% of total cases in the United States), by a defect in the synthesis (Fig. 70.3) or recycling (Fig. 70.4) of the essential cofactor tetrahydrobiopterin. The combined incidence of these conditions is about 1 : 16,500 live births.[26] In phenylketonuria (PKU), there is accumulation of phenylalanine and other metabolites such as phenyllactate and phenylpyruvate (phenylketones). Increased phenylalanine interferes with neurotransmitter synthesis and uptake, leading to the clinical symptoms of PKU.[27]

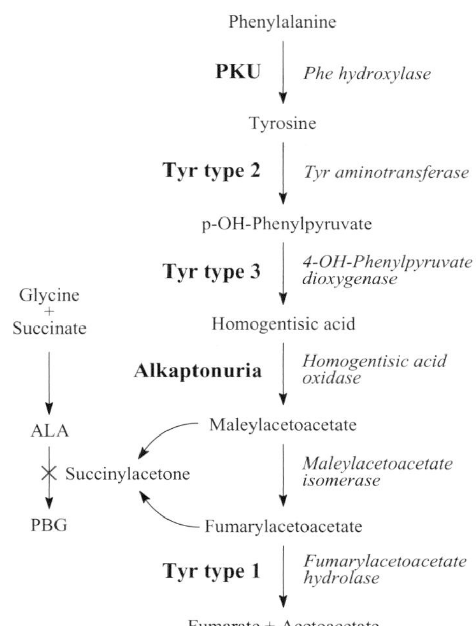

FIGURE 70.2 Metabolism of phenylalanine and tyrosine. Many different enzymes are required for the conversion of phenylalanine to fumarate and acetoacetate that can be subsequently oxidized to CO_2 and water. The disease caused by deficiency of any of these enzymes is indicated at the left of the arrows representing the function of the enzyme. In humans, there is no reported deficiency of maleylacetoacetate isomerase. *ALA,* Delta aminolevulinic acid; *PBG,* porphobilinogen; *PKU,* phenylketonuria; *Tyr,* Tyrosinemia.

Patients with PKU appear normal at birth, apart from an increased incidence of gastroesophageal reflux in those with very high phenylalanine concentrations. Delays in development, chronic eczema, and acquired microcephaly become evident after a few months of life. The abnormal brain development results in intellectual disability. This and all other problems can be prevented by a diet low in phenylalanine that needs to be initiated no later than 3 weeks of age for optimal outcome. For this reason, all infants in developed countries are screened shortly after birth for this condition. In utero, phenylalanine is removed from the child by the placenta. After birth, phenylalanine begins to accumulate as the child begins to feed and is exposed to proteins. Therefore, for optimal results, infants should be screened after at least 24 hours of life, when at least one feed has been given, to ensure an adequate rise in phenylalanine concentration. The diagnosis of PKU is confirmed by plasma amino acid analysis. In each infant, with even minimally increased serum phenylalanine, cofactor defects need to be excluded by measuring urine pterin profile and activity of dihydropteridine reductase (DHPR) in blood cells. Hyperphenylalaninemia due to phenylalanine hydroxylase deficiency is diagnosed biochemically when plasma phenylalanine concentrations are above the normal reference interval with a normal urine pterin profile and normal DHPR activity. Phenylalanine hydroxylase is expressed only in the liver, and confirmation of the diagnosis is performed by DNA sequencing of the phenylalanine hydroxylase (PAH) gene.

In patients with PKU due to phenylalanine hydroxylase deficiency, dietary treatment with a formula restricted in phenylalanine and supplemented with tyrosine should be started as soon as possible, and ideally before 3 weeks of age.[27] The phenylalanine-restricted diet needs to be continued for life. Phenylalanine concentrations are monitored periodically and should remain between 60 and 360 μmol/L (normal 30 and 80 μmol/L) to ensure adequate brain development.[28] If the concentration of phenylalanine is too low, the growth of the child can be compromised, and if it is too high, there can be impairment of executive functioning. High concentrations of phenylalanine in the first years of life lead to mental retardation. Phenylalanine at high concentrations is teratogenic and, depending on the concentration and period of exposure during pregnancy, can cause increased risk of spontaneous abortion, congenital heart defects, facial dysmorphism, microcephaly, and developmental delay (even in the absence of microcephaly) in the fetuses of women with PKU. Adverse pregnancy outcome in pregnant women with PKU can be minimized by maintaining phenylalanine concentrations less than 360 μmol/L.[29]

In approximately 2% of cases, hyperphenylalaninemia is due to a deficiency of biosynthesis (see Fig. 70.3) or recycling (see Fig. 70.4) of the cofactor tetrahydrobiopterin (BH_4). BH_4 is also a cofactor for tyrosine and tryptophan hydroxylases (see Fig. 70.4).[30] Infants with BH_4 deficiencies show signs of neurological involvement despite adequate dietary control of phenylalanine concentrations. The impairment of tyrosine and tryptophan hydroxylases reduces the synthesis of the neurotransmitters dopamine and serotonin, with severe neurological consequences. BH_4 is also a cofactor for nitric oxide synthase, which catalyzes the generation of nitric oxide from arginine, although the clinical consequences of this latter impairment are not known.

Five enzyme deficiencies leading to BH_4 deficiency have been reported (see Table 70.2). One of these, sepiapterin reductase deficiency, impairs BH_4 synthesis only in the brain because alternative pathways are available for its synthesis in the liver. As a result, patients with this latter condition have normal activity of phenylalanine hydroxylase in the liver and no hyperphenylalaninemia.[31] Among patients with BH_4 deficiencies and increased phenylalanine, 50% of cases are due to 6-pyruvoyltetrahydropterin synthase (6-PTPS) deficiency. These patients are clinically indistinguishable from those with classic PKU (due to phenylalanine hydroxylase deficiency) when identified through newborn screening but progressively deteriorate with loss of head control, truncal hypotonia with hypertonia of the extremities, drooling, swallowing difficulties, and myoclonic seizures between 2 and 6 months of age.[30] Treatment of these patients requires BH4, which usually normalizes the concentration of phenylalanine (except in some cases of DHPR deficiency), and neurotransmitter precursors (L-Dopa/carbidopa and 5-OH-tryptophan) and obviates the need for tyrosine and tryptophan hydroxylase to generate these substances.

Infants with benign hyperphenylalaninemia (phenylalanine <360 μmol/L) are occasionally identified by newborn screening because of a moderately increased blood concentration of phenylalanine. These patients have a partial deficiency of phenylalanine hydroxylase with residual enzyme activity up to 35% of normal. Although detected by neonatal screening, they remain healthy without dietary treatment. The possibility of an underlying cofactor deficiency should be ruled out. Phenylalanine, however, needs to be monitored

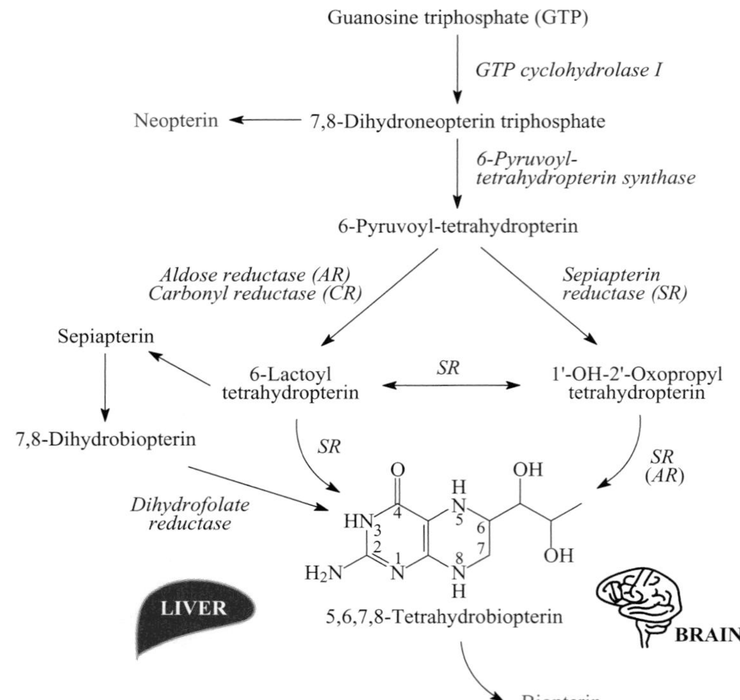

FIGURE 70.3 Biosynthesis of tetrahydrobiopterin (BH4). BH4 synthesis requires three different enzymes: GTP-cyclohydrolase 1, 6-pyruvoyltetrahydropterin synthase, and sepiapterin reductase. Some steps can be performed differently in the brain, which is strongly dependent on sepiapterin reductase, as compared to the liver that can perform the same reaction by the combined action of different enzymes. This leads to tetrahydrohydrobiopterin deficiency only in the brain in sepiapterin reductase deficiency without an increase in plasma phenylalanine because sufficient synthesis of the cofactor is retained in the liver. The origin of the commonly measured neopterin, biopterin, and sepiapterin is indicated. (Modified from Longo N. Disorders of biopterin metabolism. *J Inherit Metab Dis* 2009;32[3]:333–42.)

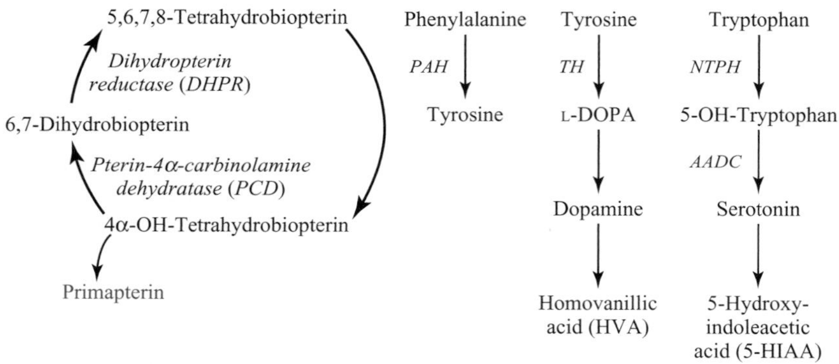

FIGURE 70.4 Regeneration of tetrahydrobiopterin. Tetrahydrobiopterin provides electrons for the hydroxylation of phenylalanine, tyrosine, and tryptophan by action of phenylalanine hydroxylase (PAH), tyrosine hydroxylase (TH), and neuronal tryptophan hydroxylase (NTPH), respectively. Reduction of 4 alpha-OH-tetrahydrobiopterin back to the active form requires the sequential action of pterin-4-alpha-carbinolamine dehydratase and dihydropteridine reductase. In the absence of pterin-4-alpha-carbinolamine dehydratase, the substrate is spontaneously converted to primapterin that can be detected in urine. (Modified from Longo N. Disorders of biopterin metabolism. *J Inherit Metab Dis* 2009;32[3]:333–42.)

periodically because, depending on the diet, its concentration can increase to a concentration requiring therapy.

Tyrosinemia Type 1

Hepatorenal tyrosinemia (tyrosinemia type 1, TYR1) is an autosomal recessive disease caused by deficiency of the enzyme fumarylacetoacetate hydrolase (see Fig. 70.2), expressed primarily in the liver and kidneys.[32] The incidence of TYR1 is approximately 1 in 100,000, with clustering of cases in the Lac-St. Jean region of Quebec (Canada). Patients with tyrosinemia type 1 can present before 6 months of age with severe liver involvement or after 6 months of age with chronic failure to thrive, mild hepatocellular dysfunction, renal involvement, and rickets due to renal Fanconi syndrome.[32] They can have extreme irritability due to peripheral neuropathy mimicking acute intermittent porphyria. This is caused by an accumulation of 5-aminolevulinic acid owing to inhibition of δ-aminolevulinic dehydratase by succinylacetone,[32] a toxic compound that accumulates in tyrosinemia type 1. Untreated patients can develop liver cirrhosis and are at very high risk for liver cancer.

Patients with TYR1 have increased concentrations of tyrosine in the plasma, but this elevation is not usually as marked as in patients with other forms of tyrosinemia, as is in tyrosinemia types 2 and 3, transient tyrosinemia of the newborn, prematurity, hepatocellular dysfunction of almost any cause (including those caused by gluconeogenesis disorders, galactosemia, fructosemia, peroxisomal disorders, mitochondrial DNA depletion syndrome), and as a result of diets very rich in protein. The biochemical diagnosis is based on the detection in the urine organic acids of succinylacetone (4,6-dioxaneheptanoic acid), the by-product of fumarylacetoacetic acid production, which is the intermediate immediately upstream of the enzyme defect.[32] TYR1 can be identified by newborn screening only when succinylacetone is used as primary marker because tyrosine is not usually increased in the newborn period in these patients.[33]

Therapy consists of a diet low in tyrosine and phenylalanine (the precursor of tyrosine) and NTBC [2-(2-nitro-4-trifluoromethylbenzoyl)-1,3-cyclohexanedione], an inhibitor of 4-hydroxyphenylpyruvate dioxygenase, the enzyme located upstream of fumarylacetoacetate hydrolase (see Fig. 70.2). NTBC prevents the synthesis of succinylacetone, which becomes undetectable in the urine almost immediately after initiation of treatment. Thereafter, periodical monitoring of blood or urine for succinylacetone is required. The adequacy of the diet is monitored by plasma amino acids. The measurement of α-fetoprotein is also used to monitor these patients because liver cancer is a complication of this condition. Liver transplantation is indicated in patients progressing to liver failure despite therapy or with liver cancer.[32]

Homocystinuria

Homocystinuria, characterized by increased concentration of the sulfur-containing amino acid homocystine in blood and urine, can be caused by at least seven genetically different disorders (Fig. 70.5). Methionine, homocysteine, and cysteine are linked by the methylation cycle and the trans-sulfuration pathway.[34] Conversion of methionine into homocysteine proceeds via the formation of S-adenosyl intermediates, including S-adenosylmethionine, the methyl group donor in several transmethylation reactions. Homocysteine is then condensed with serine by cystathionine β-synthase to form cystathionine. By the action of cystathionase, cysteine is generated and can participate in protein, glutathione, and taurine synthesis. Homocysteine can also be remethylated back to methionine by the action of methionine synthase, an enzyme that requires methylfolate and methylcobalamin as cofactors. Defects in any of these steps can result in homocystinuria. The most common form is classic homocystinuria, which is caused by reduced activity of cystathionine β-synthase. The worldwide incidence is approximately 1 : 300,000 live births,[35] with a very high incidence in Qatar (1 : 1,800).[36] Clinical manifestations are nonspecific at first and may include failure to thrive and

POINTS TO REMEMBER

Aromatic Amino Acid Metabolism

- Phenylketonuria is characterized by the accumulation of phenylalanine, which is toxic for the brain.
- Defects in the synthesis or recycling of tetrahydrobiopterin, an essential cofactor for phenylalanine hydroxylase, can also cause hyperphenylalaninemia.
- In tyrosinemia type 1, the accumulation of succinylacetone causes rickets (a consequence of succinylacetone-induced renal Fanconi syndrome), liver failure, and liver cancer.
- Therapy consists in diets restricted of the offending amino acid and, in the case of tyrosinemia, NTBC, which blocks production of succinylacetone.
- Therapy is monitored by measuring plasma amino acids in phenylketonuria and tyrosinemia type 1 and urine organic acids or succinylacetone in tyrosinemia type 1.

developmental delay. Patients can present in childhood or adolescence with (1) ophthalmological problems such as downward dislocation of the lens and myopia, (2) bone abnormalities with marfanoid habitus and pectus excavatum, (3) osteoporosis, (4) intellectual disability, and (5) psychiatric disturbances. Thromboembolic episodes can be seen even in children and are a major cause of morbidity and mortality.

The biochemical diagnosis is performed by plasma amino acid analysis, which shows increased plasma concentrations of methionine (especially in children) and the presence of the disulfide homocystine. Total plasma homocysteine (measured after reduction of all disulfide bonds and the release of homocysteine from proteins) is also markedly increased in this condition. It can be measured by immunoassay, HPLC, or MS-MS. Increased homocystine and total plasma homocysteine are also observed in (1) defects of homocysteine remethylation such as 5,10-methylene-tetrahydrofolate reductase deficiency, (2) methionine synthase *(cblG)*, (3) methionine synthase reductase *(cblE)* deficiency, (4) 5-methyl-tetrahydrofolate–homocysteine–methyltransferase deficiency, (5) vitamin B12 deficiency, and (6) in disorders of cobalamin metabolism (*cblC, cblD, cblF,* and *cblJ*). Patients with *cblC, cblF,* and *cblJ* and some patients with *cblD* defects have methylmalonic aciduria in addition to homocystinuria because the synthesis of adenosylcobalamin (the cofactor of methylmalonylCoA mutase) is impaired in addition to the synthesis of methylcobalamin (the cofactor of methionine synthase).[37] The clinical manifestations of homocysteine remethylation defects are prevalently neurological and include developmental delay, seizures, and ataxia, usually with acquired microcephaly.

Classic homocystinuria is detected in newborn screening by an increased plasma methionine concentration. Methionine can also be increased in liver disease, diets rich in protein, and other, rarer disorders of sulfur amino acid metabolism (S-adenosylhomocysteine hydrolase deficiency, glycine N-methyltransferase deficiency, methionine adenosyltransferase [MAT] deficiency). In these cases, homocystine is absent, and total plasma homocysteine is normal or only mildly increased. Defects in remethylation of homocysteine could potentially be identified by newborn screening by having very low concentrations of methionine. In these latter conditions, plasma amino acid analysis shows the presence

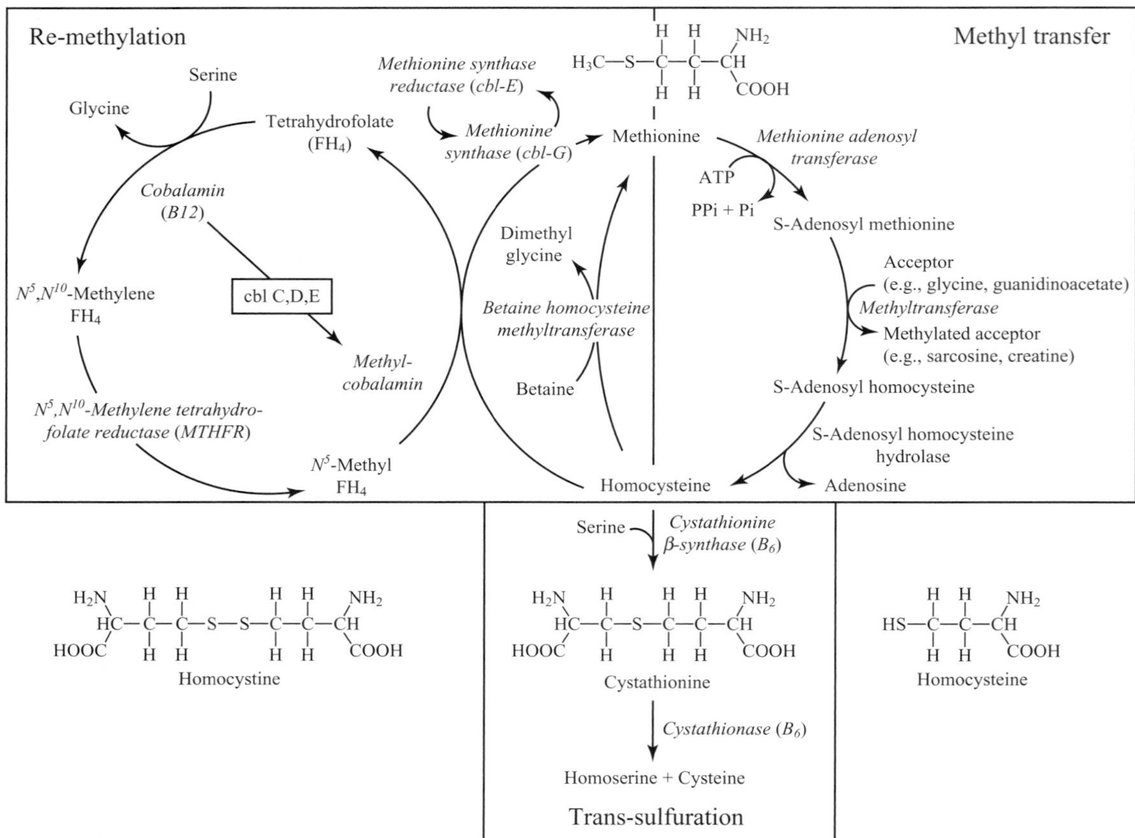

FIGURE 70.5 Sulfur amino acid metabolism. Methionine transfers a methyl group during its conversion to homocysteine. Defects in methyl transfer or in the subsequent metabolism of homocysteine by the pyridoxal phosphate (vitamin B_6)-dependent cystathionine beta-synthase increase plasma methionine concentrations. Homocysteine is transformed into methionine via remethylation. This occurs through methionine synthase, a reaction requiring methylcobalamin and folic acid. Deficiencies in these enzymes or lack of cofactors is associated with decreased or normal methionine concentrations. In an alternative pathway, homocysteine can be remethylated by betaine: homocysteine methyl transferase. The chemical structures of homocystine (detected by plasma amino acids) and homocysteine (detected by a separate test) are also shown.

of homocystine, but the concentration of methionine is low. Definitive confirmation of diagnosis requires DNA testing, now available through the analysis of panels containing all known genes capable of causing homocystinuria. Complementation studies in fibroblasts may still be helpful to define the basis of cases with negative mutation analysis.

Therapy for classic homocystinuria requires high doses of pyridoxine (the cofactor of cystathionine β-synthase), a special diet low in methionine, and administration of betaine that can donate the methyl group to homocysteine to generate methionine. Defects of vitamin B_{12} metabolism require high doses of intramuscular hydroxycobalamin and oral betaine.[34] Mild genetic variations in the methylenetetrahydrofolate reductase gene are frequent in the general population, and it is unclear whether therapy is necessary. Severe remethylation defects are treated with folinic acid, vitamin B_{12}, and betaine.[38]

Maple Syrup Urine Disease

Leucine, isoleucine, and valine are essential branched-chain amino acids. After transamination, they undergo decarboxylation by branched-chain α-ketoacid dehydrogenase, a complex enzyme that requires thiamin pyrophosphate as a cofactor.[39] This complex is composed of four subunits: $E_1\alpha$, $E_1\beta$, E_2, and E_3. The E_3 subunit is shared by two other dehydrogenases: pyruvate dehydrogenase and α-ketoglutarate dehydrogenase.[39] A defect of any component of the complex causes maple syrup urine disease (MSUD), an autosomal recessive disorder with an incidence of approximately 1:200,000 live births.[26] There are several forms of this disease, depending on the severity of the mutations: (1) the classic form, which is the most severe and is characterized by very high plasma concentrations of branched-chain amino acids; (2) forms responsive to pharmacological amounts of thiamine (thiamin-responsive MSUD);[40] (3) intermediate or intermittent forms triggered by high consumption of proteins or catabolic state (in which endogenous proteins released mostly by the muscle are degraded to produce energy); and (4) E3 deficiency, with combined deficiency of pyruvate and alpha-ketoglutarate dehydrogenase.[41]

Classic MSUD presents with poor feeding and vomiting during the first week of life, followed by lethargy and coma within a few days. This usually follows a normal birth and an uneventful first few days of life, during which branched-chain amino acids, especially leucine, increase to

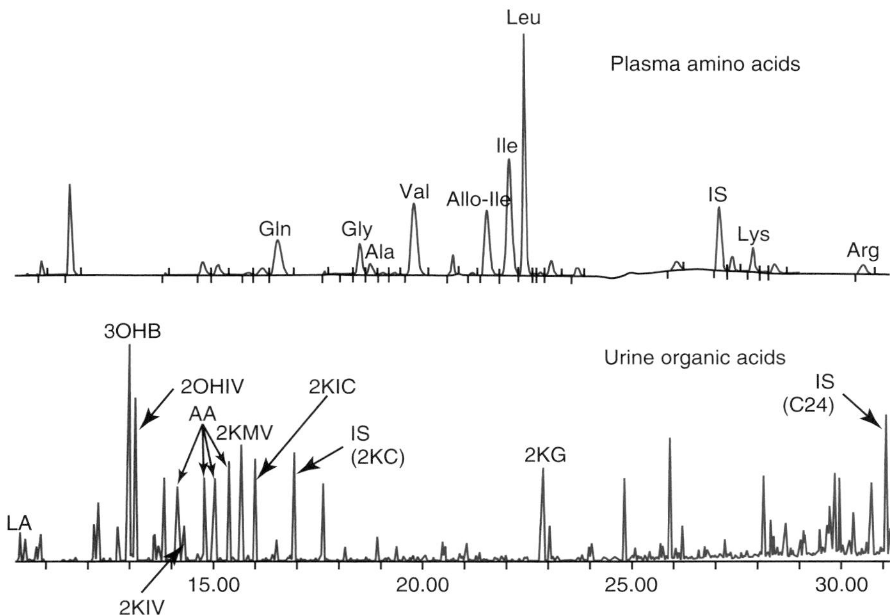

FIGURE 70.6 Plasma amino acids (by ion exchange chromatography) and urine organic acids (by gas chromatography/mass spectrometry) in maple syrup urine disease (branched-chain ketoacid dehydrogenase deficiency). *Top:* All 3 branched-chain amino acids (leucine, valine, and isoleucine) become increased in maple syrup urine disease. Alloisoleucine, an amino acid not normally present, is also present in this condition. *Bottom:* Urine organic acids show the presence of the characteristic metabolites 2-OH-isovaleric acid (2OHIV), 2-ketoisovaleric acid (2KIV), 2-ketomethylvaleric acid (2KMV), and 2-ketoisocaproic (2KIC). Lactic acid (LA) and ketones (3-OH-butyric acid [3OHB] and acetoacetate [AAA]) are also increased. 2-Ketocaproic acid (2KC) and tetracosane (C24) are used as internal standards (IS).

toxic concentrations. Leucine accumulates within the brain, causing cerebral edema, which is responsible for the progressive worsening of neurological symptoms. The results of routine laboratory analyses are mostly unremarkable except for the presence of ketonuria.

Some patients with significant residual enzyme activity can have recurrent episodes of vomiting or a neurological presentation (developmental delays, seizures) even after 1 year of age without any acute event. Other patients can also have intermittent episodes of acute decompensation with vomiting, ataxia, and lethargy progressing to coma. Once they recover, patients may return to a normal status with no obvious sequelae but may have persistent neurological deficits with seizures.[41]

MSUD should be suspected on the basis of the clinical presentation. The odor of maple syrup is not always present or appreciated in the newborn period and can be better appreciated by smelling the ear wax following otoscopic examination. The presence of ketones in the urine analysis can further suggest the diagnosis, as can the rapid urine test with 2,4-dinitrophenylhydrazine (DNPH), which forms a characteristic precipitate. Newborn screening can identify increased concentrations of leucine and isoleucine, with normal concentrations of other amino acids (such as phenylalanine) whose metabolism in not affected. Patients with milder forms of the disease can be missed by screening.[42] Initial biochemical confirmation is performed by plasma amino acid analysis, which shows a marked increase in leucine (usually the prominent amino acid), isoleucine, and valine, in addition to the pathognomonic presence of L-alloisoleucine (Fig. 70.6). Alloisoleucine is a stereoisomer derived through stepwise racemization and keto-enol tautomerization of (2*S*) 2-keto-3-methylvaleric acid to its (2*R*) enantiomer, followed by transamination.[43] The 2-keto-acids, the substrates immediately upstream of the enzyme block, are responsible for the positive DNPH test. Urine organic acid analysis shows the presence of the characteristic branched-chain ketoacids and increased excretion of 2-hydroxyisovaleric acid during episodes of decompensation (see Fig. 70.6).

Cornerstones of treatment are dietary products restricted in all three branched-chain amino acids, high-dose thiamin (in responsive cases), and valine and isoleucine supplements (these two amino acids become depleted with the degree of protein restriction required to lower leucine concentrations). Acute episodes are life-threatening and require aggressive treatment of brain edema (owing to intracellular leucine accumulation coupled to loss of sodium in urine) with intravenous mannitol, careful maintenance of sodium concentrations above 135 mmol/L with administration of 3% sodium chloride, administration of sufficient calories with intravenous glucose, and the use of lipids to block catabolism.[44] Dialysis is sometimes necessary to rapidly remove excess leucine.[45] Liver transplantation is curative for MSUD, and the explanted liver can be used to transplant other patients on the waiting list in domino because extrahepatic tissues have significant branched-chain ketoacid dehydrogenase activity.[46]

Urea Cycle Defects

The urea cycle disposes of the nitrogen groups of amino acids before their carbon skeleton is metabolized to gluconeogenic

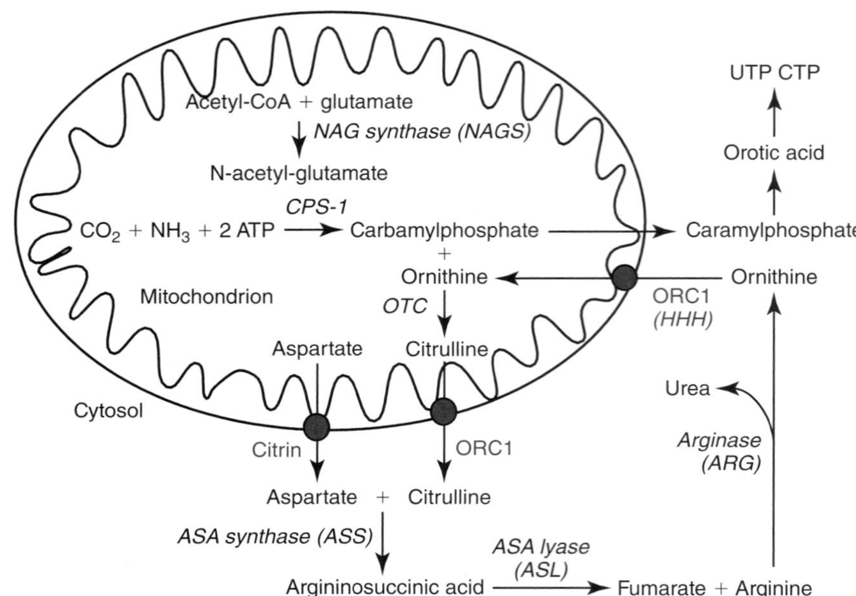

FIGURE 70.7 The urea cycle leads to the formation of urea starting from ammonia (NH_3). It requires many enzymes and mitochondrial transporters, any of which can be defective and impair the function of the urea cycle. *ASL,* Argininosuccinate lyase; *ASS,* argininosuccinate synthase; *ARG,* arginase; *citrin,* aspartate/glutamate exchanger; *CPS-1,* carbamyl phosphate synthase 1; *CTP,* cytidine triphosphate; *NAGS,* N-acetylglutamate synthase; *ORC1,* ornithine/citrulline mitochondrial transporter; *OTC,* ornithine transcarbamylase; *UTP,* uridine triphosphate.

POINTS TO REMEMBER

Sulfur and Branched-Chain Amino Acid Metabolism

- Classic homocystinuria is caused by deficiency of cystathionine β-synthase and results in the accumulation of homocysteine and methionine.
- Clinical manifestations of classic homocystinuria include dislocation of the lens and myopia, bone abnormalities with marfanoid habitus and pectus excavatum, osteoporosis, intellectual disability, psychiatric disturbances, and thromboembolic episodes.
- Defective remethylation of homocysteine to methionine can also cause homocystinuria, in this case with low plasma methionine concentrations.
- The clinical manifestations of homocysteine remethylation defects are prevalently neurological and include developmental delay, seizures, and ataxia.
- Maple syrup urine disease (MSUD) is caused by a block in the degradation of the branched-chain amino acids—isoleucine, leucine, and valine—with the corresponding ketoacids being responsible for the typical odor.
- Diagnosis relies on measurement of plasma amino acids and total plasma homocysteine (homocystinuria) or organic acids (MSUD).
- Clinical manifestations of MSUD include vomiting, lethargy progressing to coma, developmental delay, and ataxia.

(most amino acids) or ketogenic precursors (leucine and lysine), or both (isoleucine, phenylalanine, tyrosine, and tryptophan). The cycle requires the combined action of different enzymes and mitochondrial transporters (Fig. 70.7). Ornithine enters mitochondria through a specific transporter: the ornithine/citrulline exchanger (ORC1); there, it combines with carbamyl phosphate by the action of ornithine transcarbamylase (OTC). Synthesis of carbamyl phosphate requires the ammonia generated from the nitrogen group of amino acids, carbon dioxide, two molecules of ATP, and the action of carbamyl phosphate synthase 1 (CPS-1). The activity of this enzyme is dependent on an allosteric activator—N-acetyl glutamate—which is synthesized by N-acetylglutamate synthase (NAGS). The reaction between ornithine and carbamyl phosphate generates citrulline that exits mitochondria through the agency of (ORC1).[47] In the cytoplasm, citrulline combines with aspartate that is exported from mitochondria by the citrin transporter (aspartate/glutamate exchanger) through the action of argininosuccinate synthase (ASS). Argininosuccinate is cleaved by a lyase (ASL) into arginine and fumarate. Finally, arginase (ARG) generates urea and ornithine to restart the cycle. Deficiency of any of these enzymes or transporters can impair the function of the urea cycle and cause hyperammonemia. Newborn screening can identify increased plasma citrulline in citrullinemia type 1 (ASS deficiency) or 2 (citrin deficiency), and argininosuccinate in argininosuccinate lyase (ASL) deficiency. Increased plasma ornithine and homocitrulline should theoretically be the markers for hyperammonemia, hyperornithinemia, and homocitrullinuria syndrome (ORC1 deficiency/HHH syndrome), but it is unclear whether newborns with this condition show increases of these amino acids. Low citrulline with increased glutamine can be found in NAGS, CPS-1, and OTC deficiency, although appropriate cutoffs for citrulline or for other potentially useful markers, such as the ratio glutamate : citrulline, have not yet been established for the consistent identification of these conditions. OTC deficiency can be differentiated from the other two conditions by the increased urinary excretion of orotic acid that is formed from the carabamylphosphate that is unable to enter the urea cycle.

Patients with urea cycle defects may present at any age.[48] In the neonatal period, there is usually a brief interval between birth and the appearance of clinical manifestations, with the most severe cases presenting even before the results of newborn screening are available.[49] Hyperammonemia and the accumulation of glutamine in the brain lead to poor feeding, vomiting, lethargy, or irritability, progressing to coma and death. This is due to the toxic effects of ammonia and to the brain edema caused by glutamine and glutamate accumulation. Milder cases, in which the enzymatic block is not complete, present later in life, often triggered by excess protein intake or catabolic state secondary to fasting or infections. In infancy, the symptoms are similar to the neonatal period but less severe and more variable. Neurological abnormalities also include ataxia and irritability. These patients are often misdiagnosed as having gastrointestinal disorders, food allergies, behavioral problems, or nonspecific hepatitis. In children and adults, chronic neurological problems are characterized by learning difficulties, intellectual disability, behavioral problems, and recurrent vomiting, which occasionally deteriorates to acute decompensation with severe encephalopathy.[48] Arginase deficiency differs from the other urea cycle disorders because of the usually milder hyperammonemia and a clinical picture of spastic displegia, frequently misdiagnosed as cerebral palsy.[50]

The dominant laboratory findings in urea cycle defects are hyperammonemia and abnormalities of liver function, with variably increased transaminases and prolonged prothrombin (PT) and partial thromboplastin (PTT) times. Measurements of plasma amino acids, urine orotic acid, and, in some cases, urine amino acids are necessary for the diagnosis of these disorders. Other conditions that can cause hyperammonemia, such as organic acidemias and fatty acid oxidation defects, can be excluded by urine organic acid and plasma acylcarnitine profile. Increased plasma glutamine and alanine, seen when plasma amino acid analysis is performed, is a common finding in all urea cycle defects. Citrulline is the amino acid key to the diagnosis of the specific defects. Citrulline is low or undetectable in proximal defects of the urea cycle (NAGS, CPS-1, or OTC deficiency). Urine orotic acid is increased in OTC deficiency, but it is normal or low in NAGS and CPS-1 deficiency. A marked increase in plasma citrulline is found in argininosuccinic acid synthase deficiency, a condition commonly known as citrullinemia type 1. A twofold to fivefold increase of plasma citrulline in the presence of argininosuccinic acid is indicative of argininosuccinic acid lyase deficiency. A mild increase of plasma citrulline without argininosuccinic acid can also be seen in citrin deficiency (citrullinemia type 2) or, with other biochemical abnormalities and a severe clinical picture, in the neonatal variant of pyruvate carboxylase deficiency.

Acute hyperammonemia should be treated promptly as a medical emergency. Calories should be provided as intravenous glucose and lipids, using insulin if possible to reverse the catabolic state. A variety of conjugating agents (benzoate, phenylacetate, phenylbutyrate) are used to deplete the nitrogen pool through the excretion of their glycine and glutamine conjugates. Citrulline and/or arginine supplementation provide substrates of the urea cycle downstream of the specific block to allow protein synthesis to resume. If these therapies, along with the reversal of catabolism, fail to effectively reduce blood ammonia within hours, hemodialysis must be instituted. Long-term therapy consists of a diet low in proteins supplemented with citrulline (in OTC and CPS-1deficiency) or arginine (in ASS and ASL deficiency) and the oral administration of ammonia scavengers (eg, phenylbutyrate, benzoate, or glycerol phenylbutyrate).[48,49] NAGS deficiency responds to therapy with oral N-carbamylglutamate, a precursor of N-acetylglutamate.[51]

Glycine Encephalopathy (Nonketotic Hyperglycinemia)

Glycine is the simplest amino acid and can be metabolized by means of several pathways. The major catabolic pathway for glycine is through the glycine cleavage system, a four-peptide complex (proteins P, H, T, and L) attached to the inner mitochondrial membrane in liver, brain, kidney, and placenta.[5,52] One carbon is converted to carbon dioxide, and the other is transferred to tetrahydrofolate to form hydroxymethyltetrahydrofolate, which may either react with another mole of glycine to produce serine or form methyltetrahydrofolate, which serves as a methyl donor.[5,52,53]

Glycine encephalopathy or nonketotic hyperglycinemia (NKHG) is a severe condition caused by a defect in any of the P, T, or H proteins of the glycine cleavage system.[53] Patients with the classic form of the disease present within the first days of life with lethargy, poor sucking, severe hypotonia, hiccups, seizures, and apnea. Most of these patients die in the first few months of life or survive with profound developmental delays. Few patients have been described with transient NKHG, which disappears within the first 6 months of life. Atypical variants of NKHG have been diagnosed in patients with rather disparate manifestations, having in common in most cases seizures and delays of different degree of severity.[53]

Patients with glycine encephalopathy have no defined abnormalities on routine laboratory testing. Newborn screening is not reliable in identifying patients affected by the condition. The disease is characterized by increased plasma and CSF glycine concentrations with no other notable abnormalities (Fig. 70.8) and by unremarkable urine organic acid and plasma acylcarnitine profiles (performed to exclude ketotic hyperglycinemia, caused by organic acidemias such as propionic or methylmalonic acidemia). The concentration of glycine can vary in plasma from being mildly to markedly increased, but it is always high in the CSF (>30 μmol/L). The calculated CSF:plasma glycine concentration ratio (>0.08, reference interval: <0.04) is critical in the diagnosis of this condition,[5] but caution should be used in the interpretation of the ratio when the plasma and CSF specimens are not collected simultaneously (no more than 1 hour apart). Organic acidemias, such as propionic and methylmalonic acidemia, can present with increased plasma and CSF glycine, in the range observed in NKHG. In this case, analysis of urine organic acids should reveal the metabolites characteristic of the organic acidemia. Contamination of CSF with blood results in increased concentration of glycine; however, when it occurs, concentrations of other (unrelated) amino acids are also increased. Seizure medications, such as valproate, can inhibit the glycine cleavage system, resulting in increased plasma and CSF glycine. The diagnosis of NKHG is confirmed by enzyme assay or molecular analysis,[5] although some atypical, late-onset cases might have no identifiable mutations in the P, H, or T genes.[53]

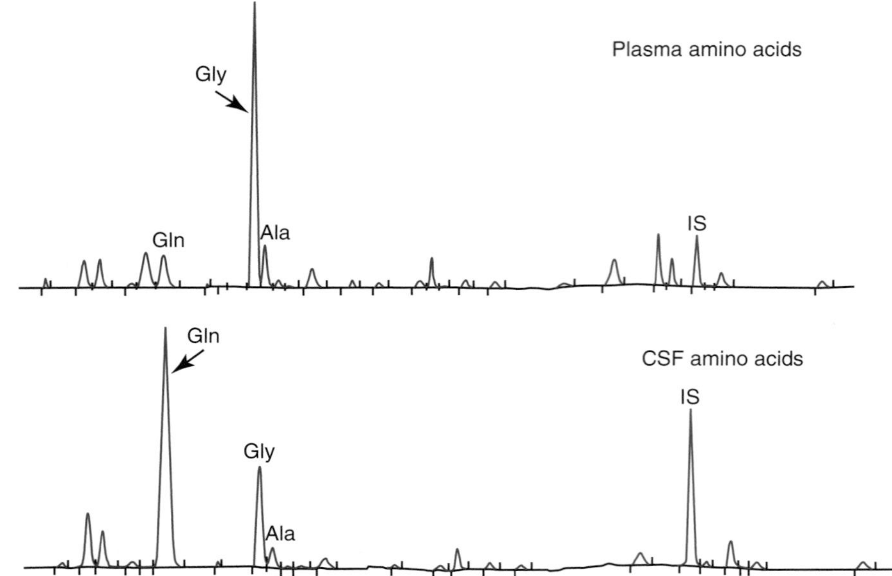

FIGURE 70.8 Plasma *(top)* and cerebrospinal fluid (CSF, *bottom*) amino acids (by ion exchange chromatography) in glycine encephalopathy. Glycine becomes the predominant amino acid in the plasma amino acids *(top)* and much higher than normal in the cerebrospinal fluid *(bottom)* compared to glutamine that physiologically is the predominant amino acid. *Ala,* Alanine; *Gln,* glutamine; *Gly,* glycine; *IS,* Internal Standard.

No effective treatment is known. Sodium benzoate binds glycine and decreases its concentration. It may be of help in milder forms of the disease. Treatment of seizures is indicated, although there is no treatment to prevent progression of the disease in severe cases.

POINTS TO REMEMBER

Urea Cycle Defects and Glycine Encephalopathy

- The nitrogen group of all amino acids is disposed through the urea cycle, whose blockage results in increased ammonia concentrations.
- Ornithine transcarbamylase deficiency is the most common urea cycle defect; it affects males more severely, being X-linked.
- Plasma amino acid analysis shows increased glutamine concentrations in all urea cycle defects, with concentrations of citrulline being the key to the diagnosis. Urine orotic acid excretion is also increased in most urea cycle defects, with the exception of GPS-1 and NAGS deficiency.
- Therapy consists of a low-protein diet and administration of phenylbutyrate, which can bind and reduce glutamine concentrations.
- In glycine encephalopathy, the accumulation of the neurotransmitter glycine damages the brain, causing seizures and delays.
- There is no effective therapy for severe forms of glycine encephalopathy.

ORGANIC ACIDEMIAS

Organic acidemias are IEM characterized by the accumulation of intermediates in the catabolic pathways of amino acids. These intermediates are water-soluble compounds containing one or more carboxyl groups (organic acids) and other functional groups (-keto, -hydroxy). They are either normal metabolites present in excessive amount or metabolites not normally present but derived from activation of alternative pathways in response to a specific metabolic block (see Fig. 70.1).

They have heterogeneous clinical presentations, with many of them causing the accumulation of organic compounds, resulting in metabolic acidosis (pH 6.85–7.30, [H^+] 50–141 nmol/L) with low bicarbonate (<5–15 mmol/L) and sometimes hyperammonemia. They differ from renal tubular acidosis because of a significant anion gap, represented by the organic anions not measured in routine chemistry panels. The biochemical diagnosis of organic acidemias is accomplished by urine organic acid analysis by GC-MS in addition to plasma amino acids and plasma acylcarnitine analysis. Table 70.7 summarizes the most common organic acidemias.

Disorders of Propionate Metabolism

Propionyl-CoA is an intermediate in the catabolism of isoleucine, valine, threonine, methionine, pyrimidines (uracil and thymine), and cholesterol and is the final product of the β-oxidation of odd-chain fatty acids. Propionyl-CoA is converted by a biotin-dependent carboxylase (propionyl-CoA carboxylase) to methylmalonyl-CoA, which is then converted to succinyl-CoA by an adenosylcobalamin-dependent mutase (methylmalonyl-CoA mutase) for oxidation in the tricarboxylic acid cycle.[54] Primary or secondary defects of these two enzymes (propionyl-CoA carboxylase and methylmalonyl-CoA mutase) were among the first organic acidurias to be discovered, and their natural history has been characterized perhaps better than any other inborn error of organic acid metabolism.[54]

Propionic acidemia (PA) and methylmalonic acidemia (MMA) are pan-ethnic disorders, but their combined incidence varies considerably, with estimates ranging from 1:2000 to 1:5000 (Saudi Arabia and Greenland)[55] to

TABLE 70.7 Clinical and Laboratory Characteristics of Disorders of Organic Acid Metabolism

Common Name	OMIM* No.	Inheritance	Enzyme/Transport Defect	Incidence (US)	Major Clinical Features	Major Biochemical Marker(s)
Disorders of Propionate Metabolism and Related Cofactors						
Propionic acidemia	232000, 232050	AR	Propionyl-CoA carboxylase (subunit alpha, beta)	1:240,000	Failure to thrive, developmental delay, hypotonia, neutropenia, lethargy progressing to coma, vomiting, hyperammonemia, metabolic acidosis	GLY (not in the neonatal period), propionylcarnitine (B), methylcitric acid, 3-OH propionic acid, propionylglycine, tiglylglycine (U)
Multiple carboxylase deficiency	253270	AR	Holocarboxylase synthase	1:2,000,000	Alopecia, perioral skin erosions, hearing loss, developmental delay, hypotonia, seizures, breathing problems, dehydration, ketoacidosis, lactic acidemia	Lactic acid, C5OH-carnitine, C3-carnitine (B), 3OH-isovaleric acid, 3-methylcrotonylglycine, 3OH-propionic acid, methylcitric acid, lactate, tiglylglycine (U)
Methylmalonic acidemia (mut^0 and mut^-)	251000	AR	Methylmalonyl-CoA mutase	1:160,000	Failure to thrive, anorexia, developmental delay, hypotonia, dehydration, ketoacidosis, vomiting, hyperammonemia	GLY, MMA, propionylcarnitine (B), MMA, methylcitric acid, 3OH-propionic acid (U)
Methylmalonic acidemia (cblA and cblB)	251100	AR	Mitochondrial cobalamin reductase	1:400,000	Failure to thrive, anorexia, developmental delay, hypotonia, dehydration, ketoacidosis	MMA, propionylcarnitine (B), MMA, methylcitric acid (U)
Methylmalonic acidemia (cblC): combined methylmalonic acidemia/ homocystinuria	277400	AR	Methionine synthase; methylmalonyl-CoA mutase	<1:100,000	Failure to thrive, developmental delay, hypotonia, megaloblastic anemia, hemolytic uremic syndrome, apnea, seizures, dehydration, ketoacidosis	MMA, tHcy, propionylcarnitine (B), MMA, methylcitric acid (U)
Methylmalonic acidemia (cblD): combined methylmalonic acidemia/ homocystinuria; Variant 1: Homocystinuria only; Variant 2: Methylmalonic acidemia only	277410	AR	Methionine synthase; methylmalonyl-CoA mutase	<1:100,000	Failure to thrive, developmental delay, hypotonia, megaloblastic anemia, hemolytic uremic syndrome, apnea, seizures, dehydration, ketoacidosis	MMA, tHcy, propionylcarnitine (B), MMA, methylcitric acid (U)
Methylmalonic acidemia (cblF)	277380	AR	Vitamin B12 lysosomal release	<1:100,000	Failure to thrive, developmental delay, hypotonia	MMA (B,U); tHCy (B,U)
Other Disorders of Branched-Chain Amino Acid Metabolism						
Isovaleric acidemia	243500	AR	Isovaleryl-CoA dehydrogenase	<1:100,000	Episodic vomiting, lethargy, coma, sweaty feet odor, dehydration, ketoacidosis	Isovalerylcarnitine (B), 3OH-isovaleric acid, isovalerylglycine (U)
3-Methylcrotonylglycinuria	210200	AR	3-Methylcrotonyl-CoA carboxylase	>1:60,000	Episodic vomiting, lethargy, coma, dehydration, ketoacidosis	C5OH-carnitine (B), 3OH-isovaleric acid, 3-methylcrotonylglycine (U)

Continued

TABLE 70.7 Clinical and Laboratory Characteristics of Disorders of Organic Acid Metabolism—cont'd

Common Name	OMIM* No.	Inheritance	Enzyme/Transport Defect	Incidence (US)	Major Clinical Features	Major Biochemical Marker(s)
3-Methylglutaconic aciduria	250950	AR	3-Methylglutaconyl-CoA hydratase	<1:100,000	Speech defect, mental retardation, hypertonia, spasticity, hypoglycemia, acidosis	C5OH-carnitine (B), 3OH-isovaleric acid, 3-methylglutaconic acid (U)
3-Hydroxy-3-methylglutaric aciduria	246450	AR	3-Hydroxy-3-methylglutaryl-CoA lyase	<1:100,000	Episodic vomiting, hypotonia, hypoglycemia, metabolic acidosis, hepatomegaly	C5OH-carnitine (B), 3OH-isovaleric acid, 3-methylglutaconic acid, 3-OH-3-methylglutaric acid (U)
2-Methylbutyrylglycinuria	600301	AR	2-Methylbutyryl-CoA dehydrogenase	<1:100,000 (1:500 Hmong)	Developmental delay, seizures, progressive muscle weakness, hypoglycemia, acidosis. Lack of symptoms also possible.	C5-carnitine (B), 2-methylbutyrylglycine (U)
2-Methyl-3-hydroxybutyric aciduria	300438	X-linked	2-Methyl-3-hydroxybutyryl-CoA dehydrogenase	<1:100,000	Progressive loss of mental and motor skills, acidosis	C5OH-carnitine, C5:1-carnitine (B), 2-methyl-3-OH-butyric acid, tiglylglycine (U)
Beta-ketothiolase deficiency	203750	AR	Beta-ketothiolase	<1:100,000	Episodic vomiting, lethargy, hypotonia, mental retardation, speech problems, ketoacidosis, seizures	C5OH-carnitine, C5:1-carnitine (B), 2-methyl-3-OH-butyric acid, 2-methylacetoacetic, tiglylglycine (U)
Isobutyrylglycinuria	611283	AR	Isobutyryl-CoA dehydrogenase	<1:100,000	Anemia, dilated cardiomyopathy	C4-carnitine (B), isobutyrylglycine (U)
3-Hydroxyisobutyric aciduria	Pending	AR	3-Hydroxyisobutyryl-CoA dehydrogenase or methylmalonic semialdehyde dehydrogenase	<1;100,000	Congenital anomalies, short stature, hypotonia, episodic ketoacidosis	3OH-isobutyric acid, 2-ethylhydracrylic acid (U)
Miscellaneous Disorders of Organic Acid Metabolism						
Alkaptonuria	203500	AR	Homogentisic dioxygenase	<1:100,000	Arthritis, ochronosis, heart valvulitis	Homogentisic acid (U)

Biotinidase deficiency	253260	AR	Biotinidase	>1:75,000	Alopecia, periorificial skin rash, conjunctivitis, developmental delay, hypotonia	Low biotinidase activity (B); 3OH-isovaleric acid and 3-methylcrotonylglycine (U) and C5OH-carnitine (B) may be elevated
4-OH butyric aciduria	271980	AR	Succinic semialdehyde dehydrogenase	<1:100,000	Developmental delay, ataxia, hypotonia, seizures, hyperkinetic behavior	4-OH butyric acid (U)
Canavan disease	271900	AR	N-aspartoacylase	<1:100,000 (1:5,000 Ashkenazi)	Hypotonia, developmental delay, macrocephaly, optic atrophy, seizures, progressive neurological degeneration	N-acetyl aspartic acid (U)
Ethylmalonic encephalopathy	602473	AR	Mitochondrial matrix protein (*ETHE1*)	<1:100,000	Hypotonia, spastic tetraparesis, petechiae, orthostatic acrocyanosis, diarrhea, lactic acidosis, developmental delay	C4-, C5-carnitines (B), EMA, lactic acid, isobutyrylglycine, 2-methylbutyrylglycine (U)
Glutaric acidemia type I	231670	AR	Glutaryl-CoA dehydrogenase	>1:75,000 (1:500 Amish)	Macrocephaly, hypotonia, abnormal movements, frontotemporal atrophy, basal ganglia lesions	C5DC-carnitine (B,U), glutaric acid, 3-OH glutaric acid (U)
Glyceroluria	307030	X-linked	Glycerol kinase	<1:100,000	Failure to thrive, episodic vomiting, developmental delay, bone fractures, acidosis, adrenal insufficiency	Pseudo-hypertriglyceridemia (B), glycerol (B, U)
Hyperoxaluria type I	259900	AR	Alanine:glyoxylate aminotransferase	<1:100,000	Urolithiasis, nephrocalcinosis, renal failure	Oxalic acid, glycolic acid (U)
Hyperoxaluria type II	260000	AR	D-Glyceric dehydrogenase	<1:100,000	Urolithiasis, hematuria, urinary tract infections, rarely nephrocalcinosis and renal failure	Oxalic acid, glyceric acid (U)
Malonic acidemia	248360	AR	Malonyl-CoA decarboxylase	<1:100,000	Short stature, cardiomyopathy, GI symptoms, hypotonia, developmental delay, hypoglycemia, acidosis	C3DC-carnitine (B), malonic acid, methylmalonic acid (U)
Pyroglutamic aciduria	266130	AR	Glutathione synthase	<1:100,000	Mental retardation, ataxia, spastic tetraparesis, seizures, acidosis, hemolytic anemia, neutropenia	Pyroglutamic (U)
Mevalonic aciduria	251170	AR	Mevalonate kinase	<1:100,000	Failure to thrive, developmental delay, ataxia, hypotonia, hepatosplenomegaly, skin rashes, diarrhea	Mevalonic acid, mevalonolactone (U)

**OMIM,* Online Mendelian inheritance in man (www.ncbi.nlm.nih.gov/entrez/query.fcgi?db=OMIM); *NBS,* newborn screening; *MMA,* methylmalonic acid; *EMA,* ethylmalonic acid; *RFLP,* restriction fragment length polymorphism; *NAA,* N-acetylaspartic acid.

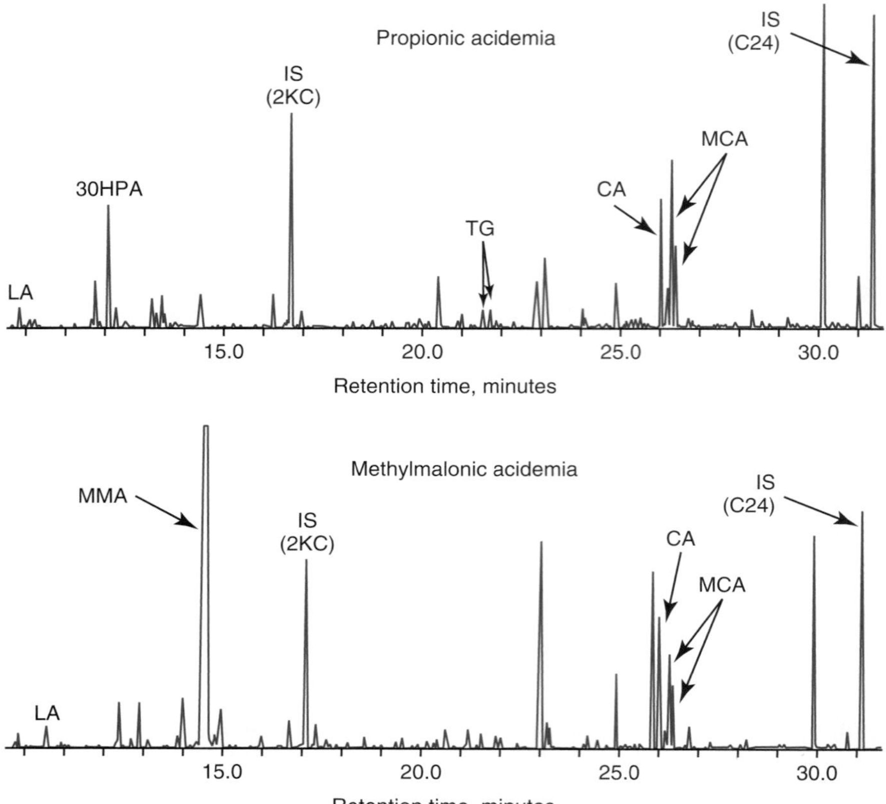

FIGURE 70.9 Urine organic acids (by gas chromatography/mass spectrometry) in propionic *(top)* and methylmalonic *(bottom)* acidemia. *Top:* Methylcitric acid (MCA) is the characteristic metabolite of propionic acidemia and is present in excess, even in milder forms of this condition. Other metabolites are 3-OH-propionic acid (3OHPA), tiglylglycine (TG), and propionylglycine (not seen in this chromatogram). Bottom: Methylmalonic acid (MMA) is markedly increased in patients with methylmalonic acidemia. Methylcitric acid can also be present in excess. *CA,* Citric acid; *LA,* lactic acid; *IS,* internal standard.

1 : 100,000 (see Table 70.7 for an incidence of each condition). Patients with PA and MMA typically are born at term with no pregnancy complications and present with an intoxication type of picture several hours to days after birth. Prominent manifestations include vomiting, hypotonia or hypertonia, lethargy, apnea, hypothermia, and rapid onset of coma. Routine laboratory investigations show severe metabolic acidosis and ketonuria (a finding of critical significance never to be overlooked in the newborn period); lactic acidemia and hyperammonemia are often present,[54] with the latter being extremely severe as in defects of the urea cycle. Similarly, there can be neutropenia and thromobocytopenia caused by bone marrow suppression. Complications of these disorders include cardiomyopathy (mostly in propionic acidemia), acute and chronic pancreatitis, and progressive renal failure (in MMA).[54] Patients who survive the initial event have developmental delay, hypotonia or hypertonia, and variable cognitive and neurological sequelae that are linked to the number and severity of acute episodes.

Both conditions, MMA and PA, are identified through newborn screening by the increased concentration of C3-carnitine. The use of second-tier tests (tests performed on the same blood spot used for the routine newborn screening) for the determination of methylmalonic acid and methylcitric acid, the characteristic metabolites of MMA and PA, respectively, are available and increase sensitivity and specificity of newborn screening.[56] Mildly increased C3 carnitine can also be seen in patients with vitamin B_{12} deficiency and sometimes with hyperbilirubinemia. Diagnosis is confirmed by urine organic acid analysis, which shows increased 2-methylcitric acid, together with other propionate metabolites, in PA, and markedly increased methylmalonic acid in MMA (Fig. 70.9). There are variant forms of PA, in which the presentation is neurological, without ketosis or acidosis. In these cases, the only abnormal metabolite detected by urine organic acid analysis is 2-methylcitric acid. Newborn screening should be able to identify even these mild variants. Plasma amino acid analysis can show hyperglycinemia, although patients with PA in the neonatal period may have normal glycine concentrations. Acylcarnitine analysis reveals increased propionylcarnitine in both PA and MMA, sometimes associated with carnitine deficiency. Treatment is based on the restriction of precursor amino acids (valine, methionine, isoleucine, threonine) and supplementation with carnitine and cofactors—biotin or hydroxycobalamin—as indicated.

Isovaleric Acidemia

Isovaleric acidemia (IVA) is a disorder of leucine catabolism caused by a deficiency of isovaleryl-CoA dehydrogenase.[57] The

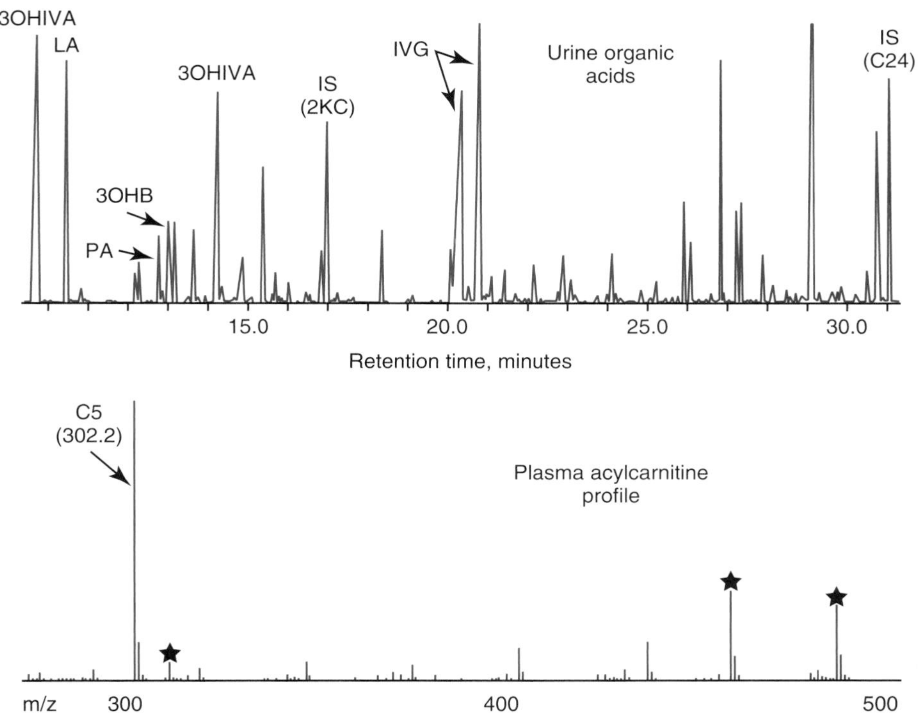

FIGURE 70.10 Urine organic acids (by gas chromatography/mass spectrometry) *(top)* and plasma acylcarnitine profile (by tandem mass spectrometry) *(bottom)* in isovaleric acidemia. Top: 3-OH-Isovaleric acid (3OHIVA) and isovalerylglycine (IVG) are the characteristic metabolites of isovaleric acidemia. In this sample, lactic acid (LA), pyruvic acid (PA), and 3-OH-butyric acid (3OHB) were also increased. *IS,* Internal standard. Bottom: C5 (Isovaleryl)-carnitine is markedly increased in patients with classic isovaleric acidemia. Internal standards are indicated with an asterisk.

clinical presentation can be with severe metabolic acidosis and hyperammonemia, leading to death shortly after birth. Milder variants present with vomiting and failure to thrive, evolving into acute presentation triggered by fever or other illnesses. One revealing feature of this IEM is the characteristic odor of "sweaty feet." Newborn screening by MS/MS reveals increased C5-carnitine (Fig. 70.10). The diagnosis is confirmed by urine organic acid analysis showing increased isovalerylglycine as the major by-product, followed by 3-hydroxyisovaleric acid (see Fig. 70.10). The marker for IVA in newborn screening is C5-carnitine; however, increased C5-carnitine can also reflect 2-methyl-butyryl-CoA dehydrogenase deficiency, an inherited disorder of isoleucine metabolism, characterized by variable excretion of 2-methylbutyrylglycine. In these patients, urine organic acid analysis may not detect 2-methylbutyrylglycine; therefore acylglycine analysis should also be performed in the investigation of an increased C5-carnitine concentration with normal urine organic acids. In several patients identified by newborn screening, the excretion of isovalerylglycine is only moderately increased, possibly due to a milder form of the disease.[57] Treatment with a low-protein diet, glycine (250 mg/kg/day), and carnitine (50–100 mg/kg/day) supplements allows for a good prognosis, but acute episodes of metabolic decompensation can be life-threatening at any age.

Glutaric Acidemia Type 1

Glutaric acidemia type 1 (GA-1) results from an inherited defect in glutaryl-CoA dehydrogenase, an enzyme involved in the degradation of lysine, hydroxylysine, and tryptophan. Affected individuals may have macrocephaly at birth or develop it in the first year of life.[58] They have mild hypotonia, and they can develop acute dystonia and spasticity caused by degeneration of the basal ganglia that is usually triggered by fever, infections, or dehydration. Brain imaging of affected individuals demonstrates frontotemporal atrophy and, after a crisis, the characteristic sequelae of acute striatal degeneration and shrinkage of the caudate nucleus and putamen.[59] Hypotonia followed by spasticity, abnormal movements, seizures, mild hypoglycemia, and metabolic acidosis have also been associated with acute events.

Diagnosis of this condition is confirmed by urine organic acid analysis, which shows massive excretion of glutaric and 3-hydroxyglutaric acids. This is associated with increased concentrations of glutarylcarnitine in plasma. Some patients, referred to as low excretors, show a more subtle biochemical phenotype with normal or mildly increased glutaric acid and mildly increased excretion of 3-hydroxyglutaric acid.[58] In these patients the concentration of plasma glutarylcarnitine can be normal, although they tend to have increased urinary excretion of glutarylcarnitine.[59] Infants with GA-1 have usually increased glutarylcarnitine identifiable by newborn screening, although some low excretors can be missed. Glutarylcarnitine can also be increased in patients with kidney failure but usually in association with other acylcarnitine species.

The treatment consists of a diet restricted in lysine and tryptophan with carnitine supplementation. Prompt treatment of infections or other illnesses and prevention of metabolic decompensation are also critical components of the treatment of this disease.

POINTS TO REMEMBER

Organic Acidemias

- Organic acidemias are disorders of the intermediary metabolism of amino acids.
- Propionic, methylmalonic, and isovaleric acidemia can present shortly after birth, with lethargy progressing to coma and death, associated with severe metabolic acidosis and hyperammonemia.
- Degeneration of the basal ganglia can occur in glutaric acidemia type 1, usually triggered by fever, infections, or dehydration.
- Diagnosis depends on the demonstration of characteristic metabolites on urine organic acid analysis and plasma acylcarnitine profile.
- Therapy consists of diets low in precursor amino acids and supplements of vitamins and carnitine.

DISORDERS OF THE CARNITINE CYCLE AND FATTY ACID OXIDATION

Carnitine (β-hydroxy-γ-trimethylammonium butyrate) plays an essential role in the transport of long-chain fatty acids inside mitochondria for β-oxidation. During periods of fasting or high energy demands, the main substrates for energy production in the liver, cardiac muscle, and skeletal muscle are fatty acids released from adipose tissue. The brain cannot utilize directly fatty acids because they cannot cross the blood–brain barrier; however, it can oxidize ketone bodies derived from β-oxidation of fatty acids in the liver (FAO).[60] If FAO is impaired, fatty acids will still be released by the adipose tissue during fasting or high energy demands but will accumulate in the liver, heart, or skeletal muscle. In the liver, impaired oxidation of fatty acids will result in steatosis and decreased production of ketones. Ketones are used by the heart, skeletal muscle, and brain as an energy source sparing glucose, while in the liver, the increased acetyl-CoA, derived from β-oxidation of fatty acids, stimulates gluconeogenesis, mostly from the carbon skeleton of amino acids released from skeletal muscle. The excessive utilization of glucose and lack of gluconeogenesis cause hypoglycemia that, in addition to decreased availability of ketones, decreases the energy supply for the brain, causing loss of consciousness, seizures, and coma. The accumulation of fats in the heart and skeletal muscle can cause cardiomyopathy and myopathy in addition to fatal arrhythmias.

Long-chain fatty acids, released from the adipose tissue, enter mitochondria for subsequent β-oxidation through the carnitine cycle (Fig. 70.11). This cycle requires enzymes and transporters that accumulate carnitine within the cell (OCTN2 carnitine transporter), conjugate it with long-chain fatty acids to form long-chain acylcarnitines (carnitine palmitoyl transferase 1, CPT1), transfer the acylcarnitines across the inner plasma membrane (carnitine-acylcarnitine translocase,

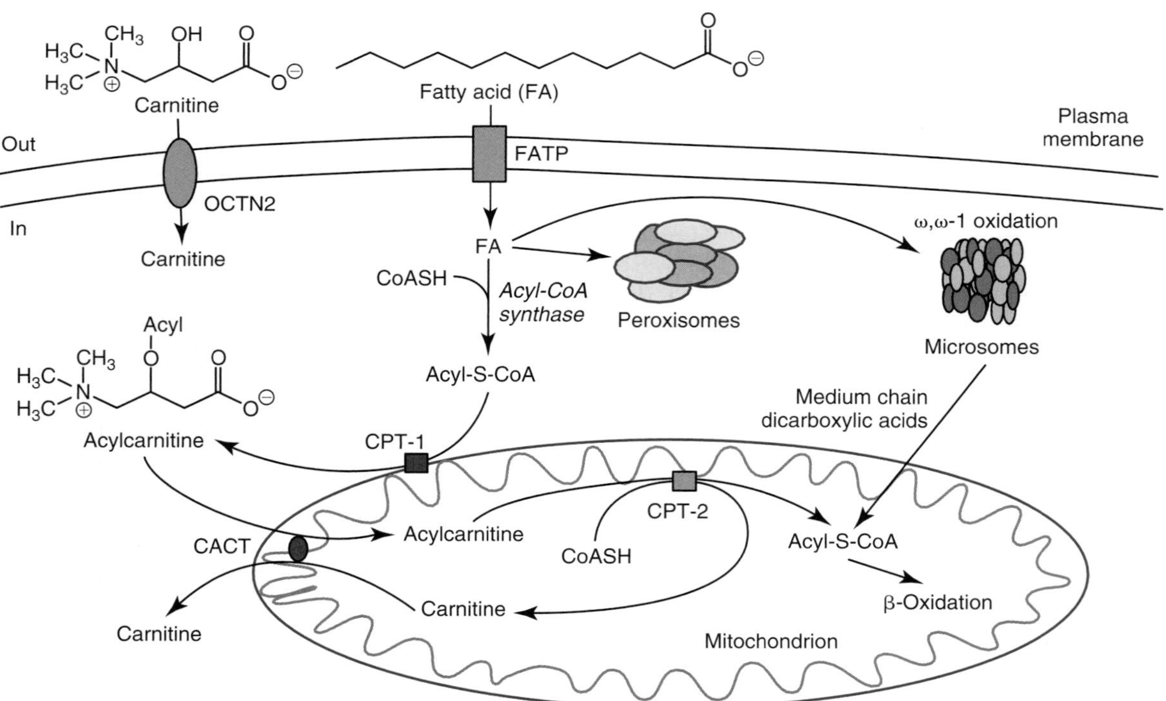

FIGURE 70.11 The carnitine cycle in fatty acid oxidation. The carnitine cycle is responsible for delivering long-chain fatty acid to the mitochondrial matrix for subsequent beta oxidation. *FATP,* Fatty acid transporter protein; *FA,* fatty acid; *CPT-1,* carnitine palmitoyl transferase-1; *CPT-2,* carnitine palmitoyl transferase-2; *CACT,* carnitine acyl carnitine translocase. (Modified from Longo N, Amat di San Filippo C, Pasquali M. Disorders of carnitine transport and the carnitine cycle. *Am J Med Genet C Semin Med Genet* 2006;142[2]:77–85.)

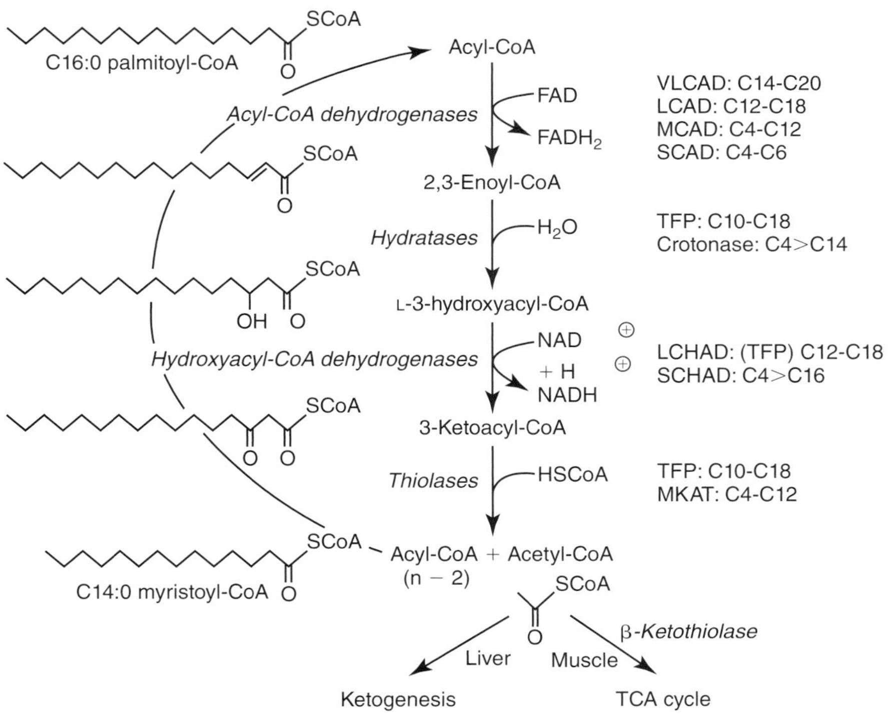

FIGURE 70.12 Beta oxidation of fatty acids. In the mitochondrial matrix, long-chain fatty acids undergo a series of steps to progressively shorten the fatty acids of two carbon units (acetyl-CoA) through a series of enzymatic reactions. Dehydrogenases with different carbon chain length specificity (very long-chain acyl CoA dehydrogenase (VLCAD), long-chain acyl CoA dehydrogenase (LCAD), medium-chain acyl CoA dehydrogenase (MCAD), and short-chain acyl CoA dehydrogenase (SCAD)—introduce a double bond between C2 and C3. A trifunctional protein (TFP) adds water and cleaves two carbon atoms from the long-chain fatty acid. This is done through the sequential action of a hydratase (enoyl-CoA hydratase), a β-hydroxyacyl-CoA dehydrogenase (long-chain-3-OH-acyl-CoA dehydrogenase [LCHAD]), and a thiolase (acyl-CoA acetyltransferase). The two carbon units generated can be completely oxidized in the muscle to CO_2 or generate ketone bodies in the liver that can be exported to provide energy to other organs.

CACT), and conjugate the fatty acids back to coenzyme A for subsequent beta oxidation (carnitine palmitoyl transferase 2, CPT2). Medium- and short-chain fatty acids can cross the mitochondrial membrane independently from the carnitine cycle. In the mitochondrial matrix, long-chain fatty acids undergo a series of enzymatic reactions to progressively shorten their chain of two carbon units (acetyl-CoA). Dehydrogenases with different carbon chain length specificity—from C18 to C4, very long-chain acyl CoA dehydrogenase (VLCAD), long-chain acyl CoA dehydrogenase (LCAD), medium-chain acyl CoA dehydrogenase (MCAD), short-chain acyl CoA dehydrogenase (SCAD)—introduce a double bond between C2 and C3 (Fig. 70.12). A trifunctional protein (TFP) adds water and cleaves two carbon atoms from the long-chain fatty acid. This is done through the sequential action of a hydratase (enoyl-CoA hydratase), a β-hydroxyacyl-CoA dehydrogenase (long-chain 3-OH-acyl-CoA dehydrogenase, LCHAD), and a thiolase (acyl-CoA acetyltransferase). The two-carbon units generated can be completely oxidized in the muscle to carbon dioxide or generate ketone bodies in the liver that can be exported to provide energy to other organs.

Deficiency in any of these steps will lead to impaired energy production—in most cases aggravated by fasting or catabolic state. The characteristics of disorders of the carnitine cycle and of FAO are summarized in Table 70.8 and are discussed in more detail below.

Carnitine Uptake Defect

Carnitine uptake defect (CUD), or primary carnitine deficiency, is an autosomal recessive disorder of the carnitine cycle affecting FAO. It is caused by a lack of functional organic cation transporter novel 2 (OCTN2). Primary carnitine deficiency has an incidence of about 1:40,000 newborns in the US population, but it has a much higher incidence in the Faroe Islands (1:720).[61] The lack of the plasma membrane carnitine transporter results in urinary carnitine wasting, low plasma carnitine concentrations (0–5 μmol/L, normal 25–50 μmol/L), and decreased intracellular carnitine accumulation. Patients with primary carnitine deficiency lose significant amounts (50% to 95%) of the filtered carnitine in urine, and their heterozygous parents lose two to three times the normal amount, explaining their mildly reduced plasma carnitine concentrations.[62] Patients can present with hepatic encephalopathy or cardiomyopathy triggered by fasting or infection. Routine laboratory studies can show hypoglycemia with minimal or no ketonuria, hyperammonemia with variably increased liver function tests, and, sometimes, increased plasma creatine kinase activity. Some

TABLE 70.8 **Clinical and Laboratory Characteristics of Fatty Acid Oxidation Disorders**

Common Name	OMIM* No.	Inheritance	Enzyme/Transport Defect	Incidence (US)	Major Clinical Features	Major Biochemical Marker(s)
Carnitine uptake defect	212140	AR	Carnitine transporter	1:40,000	Hypoglycemia, cardiomyopathy, fasting intolerance, hypoketotic hypoglycemia, sudden death	Low free carnitine (B), low long-chain acylcarnitines (B), decreased urinary carnitine reabsorption
CPT-I A deficiency (liver)	255120	AR	Carnitine palmitoyl transferase I	<1:100,000	Liver disease, hypotonia, renal tubular acidosis, fasting intolerance, hypoketotic hypoglycemia	High free carnitine (B), low long-chain acylcarnitines (B)
Translocase deficiency	212138	AR	Carnitine acylcarnitine translocase	<1:100,000	Cardiomyopathy, liver disease, fasting intolerance, hypoketotic hypoglycemia	C16/C18 acylcarnitines (B)
CPT-II deficiency	600649 608836 255110	AR	Carnitine palmitoyl transferase II	<1:100,000	Cardiomyopathy, liver disease, congenital anomalies. Adult-onset myopathy. Fasting/exercise/cold intolerance, myoglobinuria	C16/C18 acylcarnitines (B)
VLCAD deficiency	201475	AR	Very long-chain acyl-CoA dehydrogenase	>1:75,000	Spectrum from early-onset cardiomyopathy, coma, liver disease, fasting intolerance, hypoketotic hypoglycemia to adult-onset myopathy	C14:1-carnitine (B)
LCHAD deficiency	600890	AR	Long-chain 3-hydroxyacyl-CoA dehydrogenase	>1:75,000	Cardiomyopathy, liver disease, retinopathy, peripheral neuropathy, fasting intolerance, hypoketotic hypoglycemia, myoglobinuria. Maternal AFLP/HELLP syndrome	C16-OH/C18-OH acylcarnitines (B); C6-C14 3-OH dicarboxylic acids (U)
TFP deficiency	600890 143450	AR	Trifunctional protein	<1:100,000	Cardiomyopathy, liver disease, retinopathy, peripheral neuropathy, fasting intolerance, hypoketotic hypoglycemia, myoglobinuria. Maternal AFLP/HELLP syndrome	C16-OH/C18-OH acylcarnitines (B); C6-C14 3-OH dicarboxylic acids (U)
Glutaric acidemia type II	231680	AR	Electron transfer flavoprotein (ETF), ETF ubiquinone oxidoreductase	<1:100,000	Cardiomyopathy, liver disease, congenital anomalies. Adult-onset myopathy. Hypoketotic hypoglycemia, myoglobinuria	C4 to C18 acylcarnitines (B); C5-C10 dicarboxylic acid, ethylmalonic acid, C4-C8 acylglycines (U)
MCAD deficiency	201450	AR	Medium-chain acyl-CoA dehydrogenase	>1:15,000	Liver disease, fasting intolerance, hypoketotic hypoglycemia	C6, C8 and C10 acylcarnitines (B); suberic acid, hexanoylglycine, suberylglycine (U)
M/SCHAD deficiency	609975 231530		Medium/short-chain 3-hydroxyacyl-CoA dehydrogenase	<1:100,000	Liver disease, hyperinsulinemia, hypoglycemia	C4OH-carnitine (B), insulin (B)
SCAD deficiency	201470		Short-chain acyl-CoA dehydrogenase	>1:50,000	Mostly benign; developmental delay, hypotonia, seizures (may be observed)	C4-carnitine (B); ethylmalonic acid, methylsuccinic acid, butyrylglycine (U)

**OMIM,* Online Mendelian inheritance in man (www.ncbi.nlm.nih.gov/entrez/query.fcgi?db=OMIM); *NBS,* newborn screening; *AFLP,* acute fatty liver of pregnancy; *HELLP syndrome,* hemolysis, elevated liver enzymes, and low platelet count.

patients have been completely asymptomatic for all of their life and have been diagnosed following the birth of a child with low carnitine concentrations found on the newborn screening.[63] Some children who were diagnosed only because they had an affected sibling had only developmental delays. Newborn screening can identify reduced free carnitine in blood spots. Low carnitine concentrations in newborn blood spots can indicate a carnitine deficiency in the newborn or in the mother. Maternal carnitine deficiency can be due to carnitine uptake defect or can be secondary to an undiagnosed organic acidemia or FAO defect. Diagnosis of CUD is further suspected by finding extremely reduced concentration of free, total, and acylated carnitine (free carnitine <9 μmol/L, normal 25–50 μmol/L) with unremarkable urine organic acids. In symptomatic patients, urine organic acids may reveal a nonspecific dicarboxylic aciduria. Diagnosis is confirmed by demonstrating reduced carnitine transport (<10% of normal) in skin fibroblasts and/or DNA testing, although the latter can fail to identify some of the causative mutations. Therapy consists of lifelong carnitine (100–300 mg/kg per day) supplementation.

Carnitine Palmitoyl Transferase 1 Deficiency

Carnitine palmitoyl transferase 1 (CPT-1) conjugates fatty acids to carnitine, allowing their subsequent mitochondrial import (see Fig. 70.11). The three different isoforms of CPT-1 with tissue-specific expression encoded by different genes are liver-type (CPT-1A) encoded by a gene on 11q13, muscle-type (CPT-1B) encoded by a gene on 22q13, and brain-type (CPT-1C), whose gene maps to 19q13.[64] Only deficiency of the liver type, CPT-1A, has been demonstrated in humans. CPT-1 deficiency is usually triggered by fasting or viral illnesses. Affected children usually present between birth and 18 months of age with altered mental status and hepatomegaly. Routine laboratory evaluation indicates nonketotic hypoglycemia, mild hyperammonemia, increased liver function tests, and increased plasma free fatty acids. Newborn screening can identify increased concentration of free carnitine with low concentration of long-chain acylcarnitines (C16 and C18) and increased free carnitine/(C16+C18) ratio. This latter ratio allows discrimination of increased free carnitine due to carnitine supplements from CPT-1 deficiency.[65] Plasma carnitine concentrations are usually increased in classic cases but can be normal in milder cases. In these cases, DNA testing or assay of CPT-1 activity in fibroblasts is required to confirm or exclude the diagnosis. Therapy consists of avoidance of fasting, benefiting from nighttime feeds with uncooked cornstarch, and a low-fat diet rich in medium-chain triglycerides, which do not need the carnitine cycle for β-oxidation in liver mitochondria.

Carnitine-Acylcarnitine Translocase Deficiency

Carnitine-acylcarnitine translocase (CACT) operates a carnitine/acylcarnitine exchange across the inner mitochondrial membrane (see Fig. 70.11). CACT deficiency presents most often in the neonatal period with seizures, arrhythmia, and apnea. These episodes are frequently triggered by fasting or by the physiologic stress of birth. Patients with milder forms present in childhood with attacks triggered by fever, infections, and fasting as other FAO defects. Fasting hypoglycemia and seizures have been reported in these patients.

In neonatal cases and during acute attacks, routine laboratory testing reveals nonketotic hypoglycemia and hyperammonemia with increased creatine kinase activity and abnormal liver function tests. This disease is identified on newborn screening by increased C16- and C18:1- carnitine in blood spots, often in addition to low free carnitine. Diagnosis is confirmed by a plasma acylcarnitine profile, which shows a marked increase in long-chain acylcarnitines and decreased concentrations of free carnitine. This abnormal profile, however, is not distinguishable from that of neonatal CPT-2 deficiency, and direct assay of carnitine-acylcarnitine translocase in fibroblasts or DNA analysis is needed for diagnostic confirmation. Therapy consists of frequent feedings with a diet rich in carbohydrates; low in fat, most of which should be medium-chain triglycerides; and supplemented with carnitine. This therapy improves the acylcarnitine profile and prevents further attacks of hypoglycemia and arrhythmia.[66]

Carnitine Palmitoyl Transferase 2 Deficiency

Carnitine palmitoyl transferase 2 (CPT-2) deficiency presents most frequently in adolescents or young adults with muscle pain with or (in most cases) without myoglobinuria accompanied by increased serum creatine kinase activity precipitated by strenuous exercise, cold, fever, or prolonged fasting. Myoglobinuria can cause kidney failure and death. CPT-2 deficiency can also present in infancy and in the neonatal period.[64] The neonatal form, which is rapidly fatal, presents shortly after birth (from a few hours to 4 days) with respiratory distress, seizures, hepatomegaly, cardiomegaly, cardiac arrhythmia, and, in many cases, dysmorphic features, renal dysgenesis, and neuronal migration defects. The infantile variety usually presents between 6 and 24 months of age with recurrent attacks of hypoketotic hypoglycemia, causing loss of consciousness and seizures; liver failure; and transient hepatomegaly. Several children also have heart involvement with cardiomyopathy and arrhythmia. Episodes are triggered by infections, fever, and fasting.

Routine laboratory testing usually indicates hyperammonemia, metabolic acidosis, and hypoketotic hypoglycemia with increased creatine kinase. Newborn screening can reveal the same increase of long-chain acylcarnitines (C16, C18:1) seen in CACT deficiency, with carnitine deficiency being absent in patients with milder forms. Diagnosis is confirmed by a plasma acylcarnitine profile and by enzyme assay in fibroblasts and/or DNA analysis to differentiate from CACT deficiency. The late-onset CPT-2 deficiency responds to limitation of exercise, restriction of fat and long-chain fatty acids with increased dietary carbohydrates, and avoidance of fasting.

Very Long-Chain Acyl-CoA Dehydrogenase Deficiency

Very long-chain acyl-CoA dehydrogenase (VLCAD) catalyzes the first step of the fatty acid β-oxidation spiral (see Fig. 70.12). In the mid-1980s, patients with VLCAD deficiency were initially described as having long-chain acyl-CoA dehydrogenase (LCAD) deficiency.[67] However, affected patients were subsequently shown to have VLCAD deficiency.[68] The severity of the phenotype correlates with the genotype,[69] with earlier and more severe presentation observed in patients with the most severe deficiency. Patients with VLCAD deficiency can present in infancy with cardiomyopathy, cardiac

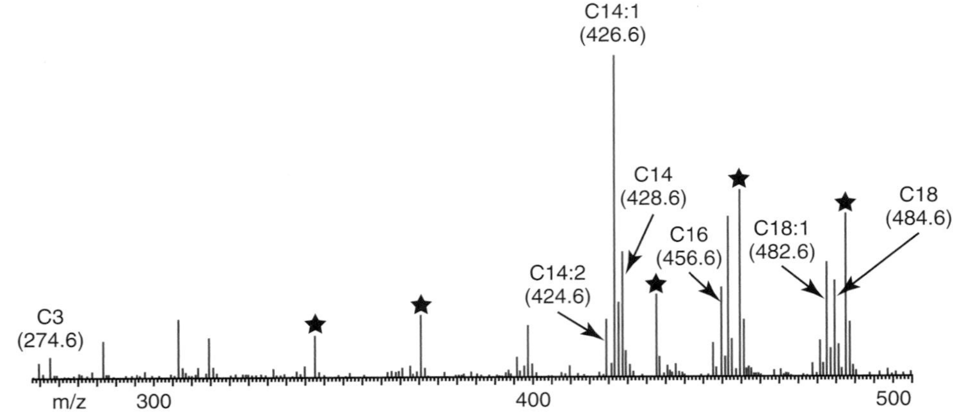

FIGURE 70.13 Plasma acylcarnitine profile (by tandem mass spectrometry) in VLCAD deficiency. C14:1-Carnitine is the diagnostic metabolite in VLCAD deficiency with elevation of other long-chain acylcarnitines (C14-, C16, C18-, C14:2-, and C18:1-carnitine). Internal standards are indicated with an asterisk.

arrest, hypoglycemia, and other hepatic symptoms. This form is rapidly fatal. Older children can present with hypoketotic hypoglycemia and hepatomegaly with or without cardiomyopathy. The milder form presents in adolescents or adults with muscle weakness and pain without cardiac and hepatic involvement.[70]

Routine laboratory testing during acute episodes reveals hypoketotic hypoglycemia and an increase in creatine kinase and transaminase activities. Increased concentration of C14:1-carnitine in the first newborn screen blood spot is often the only abnormality detected, and it may no longer be present in subsequent screens or diagnostic tests (plasma acylcarnitine profile). For this reason, in all infants with increased C14:1 carnitine on the newborn screening, the diagnosis of VLCAD deficiency needs to be confirmed or excluded by genetic analysis of the VLCAD gene and, in some cases, specific enzyme assay or FAO studies in vitro.[71] Therapy for this condition consists of avoidance of fasting, prompt treatment of infections, and a low-fat diet with medium-chain triglycerides providing most of the calories from lipids. Low-dose carnitine supplements (25 mg/kg per day) are sometimes given. Fig. 70.13 shows a characteristic plasma acylcarnitine profile of VLCAD deficiency.

Trifunctional Protein and Long-Chain 3-Hydroxy Acyl-CoA Dehydrogenase Deficiencies

The trifunctional protein (TFP) is a hetero-octamer containing four α- and four β-subunits encoded by two different genes.[72] The α-subunit harbors the activities of the second and third step of fatty acid β-oxidation, long-chain enoyl-CoA hydratase (LCEH), and long-chain 3-hydroxy acyl-CoA dehydrogenase (LCHAD). The β-subunit harbors long-chain 3-ketoacyl-CoA thiolase (LCKAT), which catalyzes the last step in β-oxidation of long-chain fatty acids. Mutations in either gene may cause complete TFP deficiency, and a prevalent mutation in the *HADHA* gene encoding the α-subunit (c.G1528C, p.E474Q) causes isolated LCHAD deficiency.[73] A genotype–phenotype correlation has also emerged for TFP deficiency, with residual enzyme activity being associated with a milder, later-onset phenotype. The three clinical phenotypes are a severe neonatal presentation with cardiomyopathy, Reye-like symptoms, and early death; a hepatic form with recurrent hypoketotic hypoglycemia; and a milder later-onset neuromyopathic phenotype with episodic myoglobinuria. Patients with LCHAD or TFP deficiencies may also develop pigmentary retinopathy and a peripheral neuropathy whose pathophysiology remains obscure. In addition, mothers of these patients can have significant complications with acute fatty liver of pregnancy or hemolysis, increased liver enzymes, and low platelets (HELLP) syndrome,[74] possibly due to the transplacental passage of 3-OH-fatty acids and related acylcarnitines.[75] This complication can occur in mothers independently of the fetal phenotype.[73]

Newborn screening can identify inceased C16:OH- and C18:1-OH-carnitines in blood spots of infants with LCHAD/TFP deficiency. A plasma acylcarnitine profile can identify the same abnormalities with the increase of additional long-chain acylcarnitines (Fig. 70.14). Urine organic acids collected at the time of an acute episode can show hypoketotic C6-C10 dicarboxylic aciduria and C6-C14 3-hydroxydicarboxylic aciduria with prominent unsaturated species. The urine organic acid profile rapidly normalizes with therapy and is normal in asymptomatic patients. Therapy for these conditions consists of avoidance of fasting, prompt treatment of infections, and a low-fat diet with medium-chain triglycerides providing most of the calories from lipids. Low-dose carnitine supplements (25 mg/kg per day) may be given.

Medium-Chain Acyl CoA Dehydrogenase Deficiency

Medium-chain acyl-CoA dehydrogenase deficiency (MCAD) is the most common disorder of FAO, with an estimated frequency of 1 : 17,000.[26,76,77] The symptoms of the disease are variable, from completely asymptomatic patients to hypoglycemia, lethargy, coma, and sudden death. Symptoms are usually triggered by fasting or illness. Although the majority of patients present in the first year of life, clinical symptoms can occur at any time, and as many as 20% of patients die before they are diagnosed.[78]

Patients with MCAD deficiency are identified by MS/MS newborn screening because of the characteristic acylcarnitine profile, with increased concentration of C6- (hexanoyl), C8- (octanoyl) and C10:1- (decenoyl) carnitine and increased C8/C2 and C8/C10 ratios (Fig. 70.15). Urine organic acid and urine

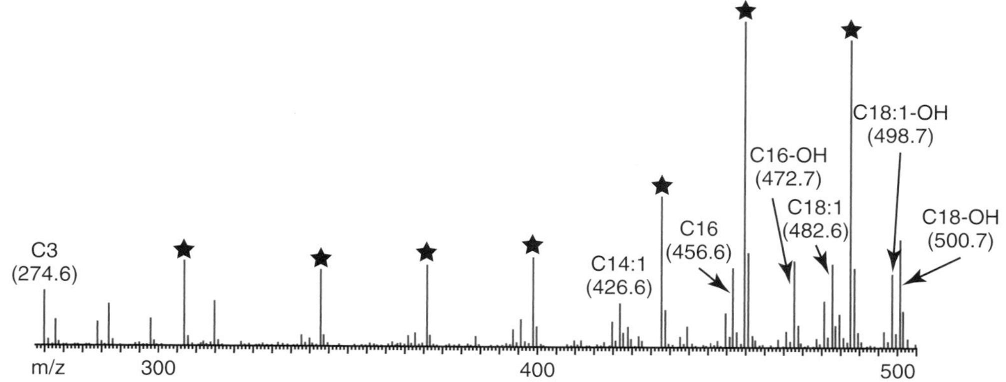

FIGURE 70.14 Plasma acylcarnitine profile (by tandem mass spectrometry) in TFP/LCHAD deficiency. 3-OH-Long-chain acylcarnitines (C16-OH-, C18-OH-, C18:1-OH-carnitine) become elevated in both TFP and LCHAD deficiency in addition to long-chain acylcarnitines. Internal standards are indicated with an *asterisk*.

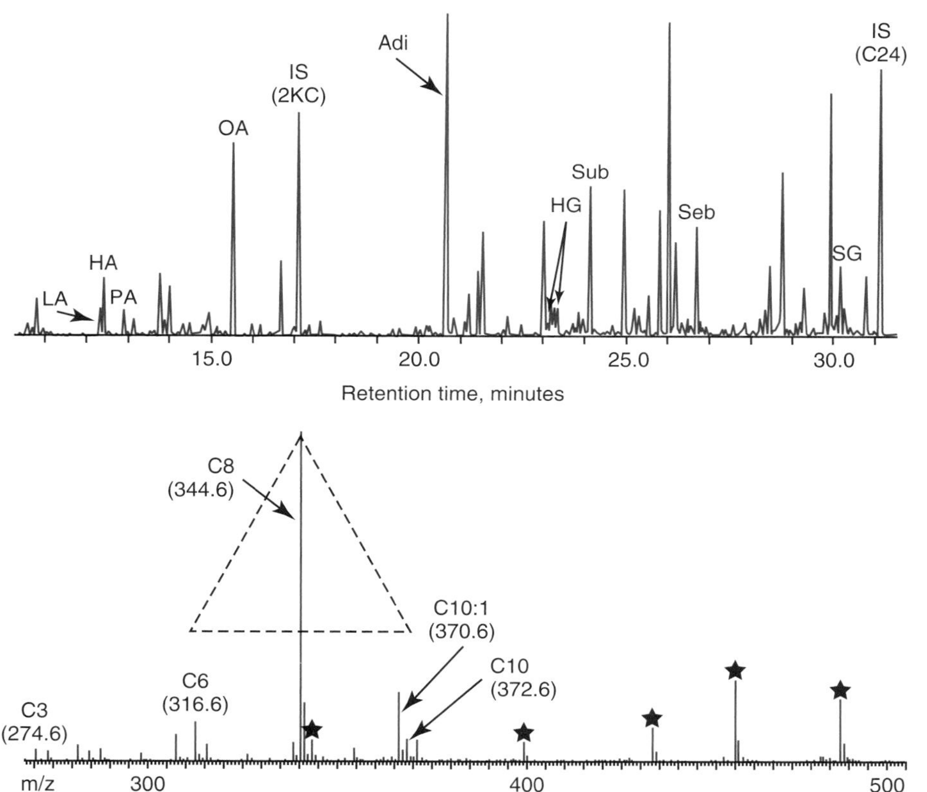

FIGURE 70.15 Urine organic acids (by gas chromatography/mass spectrometry) *(top, asterisk)* and plasma acylcarnitine profile (by tandem mass spectrometry) *(bottom)* in MCAD deficiency. Patients with MCAD deficiency can have dicarboxylic aciduria (increased excretion of adipic [Adi], suberic [Sub] and sebacic [Seb] acids, usually in a descending pattern, with adipic being the most increased) during episodes of decompensation or fasting. Hexanoic acid (HA) and octanoic acid (OA) can also be present during decompensation. Hexanoylglycine (HG) and suberylglycine (SG) are the diagnostic metabolites that usually remain present even when the patient is well compensated. Phenylpropionylglycine can appear in older patients as well. Urine acylglycine analysis is more effective than urine organic acid analysis for their quantification. *LA,* Lactic acid; *PA,* pyruvic acid; *IS,* internal standard. Bottom: The plasma acylcarnitine profile is characterized by increased C8-, C6-, and C10:1-carnitine, with the C8-carnitine peak at the vertex of a triangle over the other two increased species (indicated by the dotted lines). In carriers for this condition, C8-carnitine can be increased, but it is not usually the highest peak on visual inspection. Internal standards are indicated with an asterisk.

acylglycine analyses conducted during metabolic crisis show increased excretion of saturated and unsaturated dicarboxylic acids (adipic, suberic, sebacic), little or absent ketones, and increased excretion of hexanoylglycine and suberylglycine. Phenylpropionylglycine may be present, although it is usually in older patients. When patients are metabolically stable, the urinary concentration of these analytes is greatly reduced, although hexanoylglycine and suberylglycine remain detectable. The abnormal plasma acylcarnitine profile is almost always present. Follow-up of an abnormal newborn screening for MCAD deficiency should include analysis of urine organic acids, urine acylglycines, and plasma acylcarnitine profile. The diagnosis can be confirmed by DNA analysis. Among patients presenting with clinical symptoms, 98% carry at least one copy of the common mutation p.K304E, with 80% being homozygous for this mutation.[79] In newborns detected prospectively by newborn screening, the p.Y42H mutation has been found frequently in association with the common mutation p.K304E.[79] The p.Y42H mutation has not yet been reported in patients with clinical symptoms[79] and is associated with lower concentrations of diagnostic metabolites in blood and urine.[80]

The treatment consists of avoidance of fasting, low-fat diet, carnitine supplementation, and institution of an emergency plan in case of illness or other metabolic stress. Early diagnosis through newborn screening and early initiation of treatment lead to improved outcome.

Short-Chain Acyl-CoA Dehydrogenase Deficiency

Short-chain acyl-CoA dehydrogenase (SCAD) deficiency has been associated with a variety of clinical phenotypes, ranging from catastrophic illness in the neonatal period, hypotonia, developmental delay, seizures, myopathy, and others.[81,82] The lack of a consistent phenotype and the large number of infants identified with mild variants of this condition led to a reevaluation of this condition, with the conclusion that true SCAD deficiency lacks clinical significance.[81] In this condition, butyryl-CoA is subjected to alternative metabolism with carboxylation to ethylmalonic acid (EMA) mediated by propionyl-CoA carboxylase and conjugation with carnitine and glycine. The most useful biochemical markers of SCAD deficiency are therefore EMA and butyrylglycine in urine and butyrylcarnitine (C4) in plasma. These can be detected by newborn screening, although several programs in Europe no longer screen for this condition.[81] SCAD deficiency needs to be differentiated from ethylmalonic encephalopathy, a fatal mitochondrial disorder impairing the ability to remove sulfide[83,84] and multiple acyl-CoA dehydrogenase deficiency (in which ethylmalonic acid may accumulate). Urine organic acid, urine acylglycine, and plasma acylcarnitine profiles can differentiate among these conditions. In doubtful cases, DNA analysis can identify common and rare variants in the SCAD gene. There is no treatment required for SCAD deficiency.

Multiple Acyl-CoA Dehydrogenase Deficiency

Multiple Acyl CoA dehydrogenase (MAD) deficiency, also known as glutaric acidemia type 2 or glutaric aciduria type 2 (GA-2/MADD), is an autosomal recessive disorder of fatty acid, amino acid, and choline metabolism caused by mutations in the genes encoding the α- or β-subunit of electron transfer flavoprotein (ETF, genes *ETFA* and *ETFB*) or ETF ubiquinone oxidoreductase (ETFQO, gene *ETFDH*). The proteins encoded by these genes form a complex involved in electron transfer in the mitochondrial respiratory chain. MAD deficiency impairs electron transfer from many dehydrogenases (including SCAD, MCAD, VLCAD, glutarylCoA, and isovaleryl-CoA dehydrogenase), resulting in the accumulation of substrates of these enzymes.[85] Birth prevalence is estimated at 1:200,000. The neonatal-onset forms (severe MADD or S-MADD, types 1 and 2) are usually fatal and are characterized by nonketotic hypoglycemia, metabolic acidosis, multisystem involvement, accumulation of abnormal acylcarnitines in plasma, and excretion of large amounts of abnormal organic acid metabolites. Congenital anomalies (with cystic degeneration of the kidney, pachygyria, and other anomalies) are part of the type 1 S-MADD. The late-onset form (mild MADD, M-MADD, type 3) presents with symptoms ranging from hypoglycemic encephalopathy, sometimes combined with cardiomyopathy and childhood death, to fasting-induced episodes of lethargy, vomiting, hypoglycemia, metabolic acidosis, and hepatomegaly to exercise-induced myopathy. However, all three forms of GA-2/MADD can result in a severe outcome and premature death.

The diagnosis of GA-2/MADD can be suspected by NBS with MS/MS (increase of multiple acylcarnitines, usually with C10 and C12 being the highest peaks) and confirmed by urine organic acids (with the presence of hexanoylglycine, dicarboxylic aciduria, and the presence of 2-hydroxyglutaric acid; Fig. 70.16, top), plasma acylcarnitine profile (with an increase in multiple, though not necessarily all, acylcarnitines, including C4-[butyryl-/isobutyryl-], C5- [isovaleryl-], glutaryl- [C5-DC]-, decanoyl- [C10-], lauroyl- [C12-], and other long-chain acylcarnitines [C14- to C18-]) (Fig. 70.16, bottom). Enzyme assay in fibroblasts or DNA testing for the three genes *(ETFA, ETFB, ETFDH)* is necessary to exclude the diagnosis because the increase of acylcarnitine concentrations may be mild and detectable only during an acute metabolic crisis. Therapy consists of fasting avoidance; supplementation with coenzyme Q10, riboflavin, and carnitine; and the use of ketones.[85,86]

POINTS TO REMEMBER

Carnitine Cycle and Fatty Acid Oxidation Defects

- Most disorders of the carnitine cycle and fatty acid oxidation are triggered by fasting when fatty acids become the major source of energy production.
- These disorders present with hypoketotic hypoglycemia, cardiomyopathy, and sudden cardiac death.
- Diagnosis requires measurement of plasma acylcarnitines and, in some cases, DNA testing because biochemical abnormalities might disappear when the patient is well compensated.
- Therapy consists of fasting avoidance and supportive treatment with intravenous glucose if the patient is unable to eat. Medium-chain fatty acids and carnitine supplements are effective in some conditions.

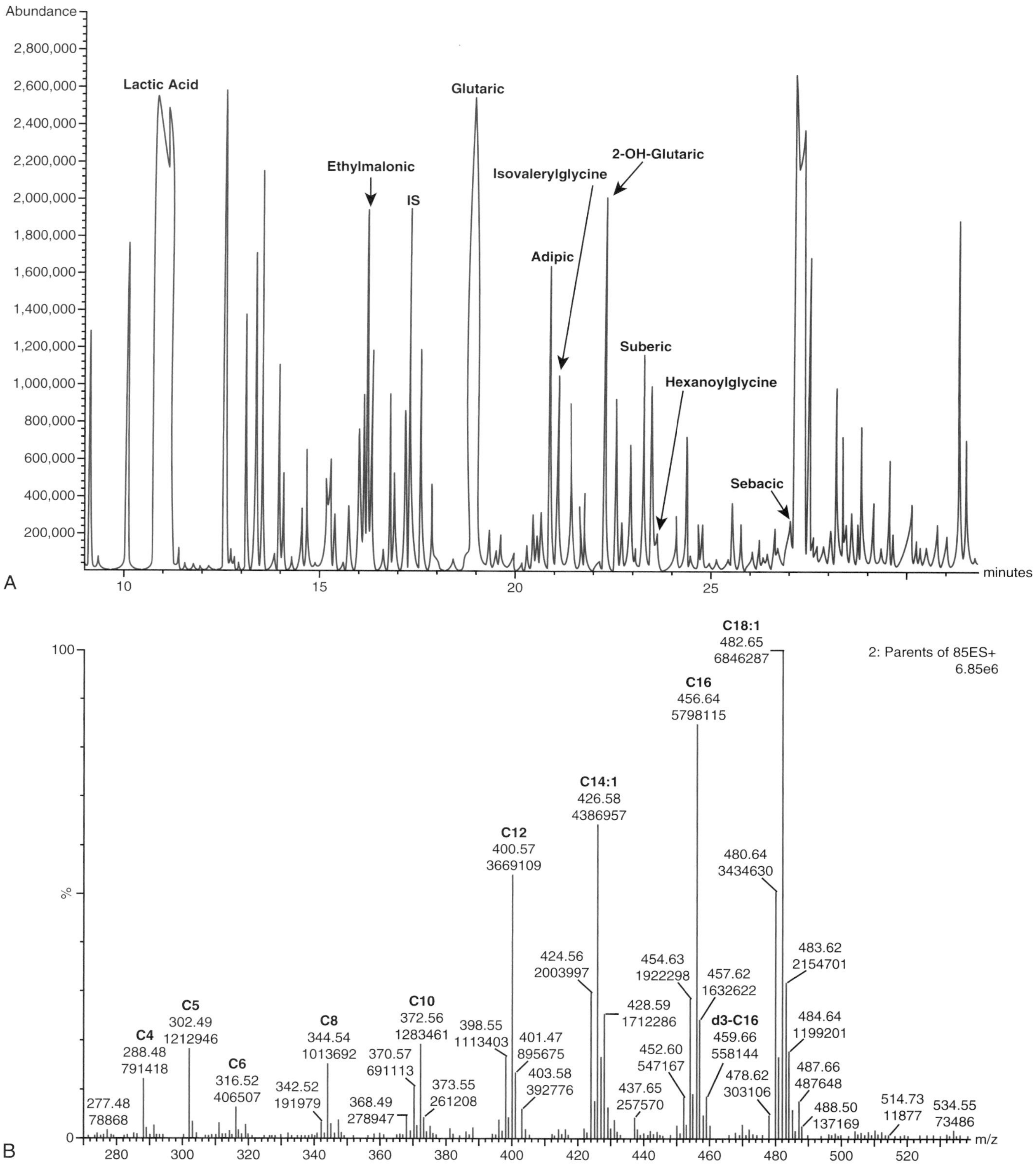

Abundance
2,800,000
2,600,000
2,400,000
2,200,000
2,000,000
1,800,000
1,600,000
1,400,000
1,200,000
1,000,000
800,000
600,000
400,000
200,000
Lactic Acid
Glutaric
Ethylmalonic
IS
Isovalerylglycine
2-OH-Glutaric
Adipic
Suberic
Hexanoylglycine
Sebacic
10
15
20
25
minutes
A

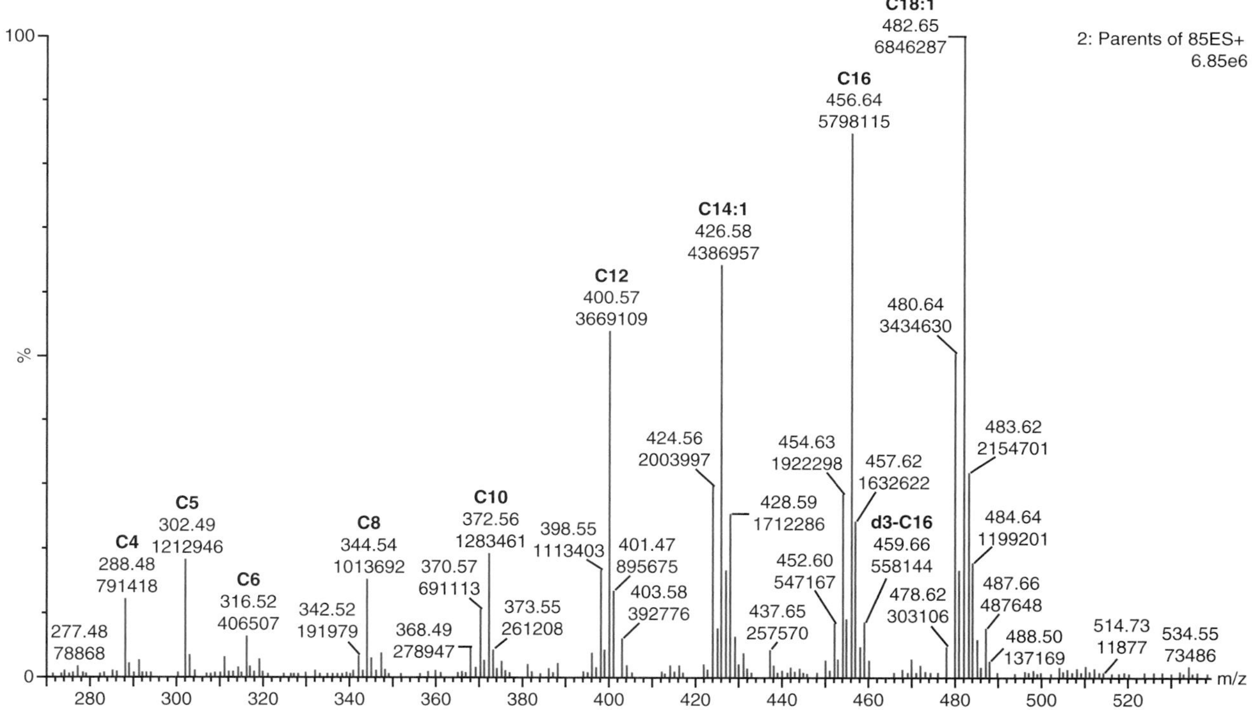

FIGURE 70.16 Urine organic acids (by gas chromatography/mass spectrometry) *(top)* and plasma acylcarnitine profile (by tandem mass spectrometry) *(bottom)* in MAD deficiency. A, In MAD deficiency, in addition to glutaric acid, other metabolites elevated are isovaleric, lactic and pyruvic, ethylmalonic, 2-OH-glutaric, and dicarboxylic acids, reflecting impairment of multiple dehydrogenases. *IS,* Internal standard. **B,** Acylcarnitine profile in a patient with GA-2/MAD deficiency at 2 days of age, symptomatic at diagnosis. Note marked elevation of C5-, C12-, and C14:1-carnitine.

SELECTED REFERENCES

For a full list of references for this chapter, please refer to ExpertConsult.com.

1. Saudubray JM, Sedel F, Walter JH. Clinical approach to treatable inborn metabolic diseases: an introduction. *J Inherit Metab Dis* 2006;**29**:261–74.
6. Chace DH, Kalas TA. A biochemical perspective on the use of tandem mass spectrometry for newborn screening and clinical testing. *Clin Biochem* 2005;**38**:296–309.
19. De Biase I, Liu A, Yuzyuk T, et al. Quantitative amino acid analysis by liquid chromatography-tandem mass spectrometry: implications for the diagnosis of argininosuccinic aciduria. *Clin Chim Acta* 2015;**442**:73–4.
20. Pasquali M, Longo N. Amino acids. In: Blau N, Duran M, Gibson KM, et al., editors. *Physician's guide to the diagnosis, treatment, and follow-up of inherited metabolic diseases, Vol.* Berlin: Springer-Verlag; 2014. p. 749–60.
26. Therrell BL Jr, Lloyd-Puryear MA, Camp KM, et al. Inborn errors of metabolism identified via newborn screening: ten-year incidence data and costs of nutritional interventions for research agenda planning. *Mol Genet Metab* 2014;**113**:14–26.
28. Camp KM, Parisi MA, Acosta PB, et al. Phenylketonuria scientific review conference: state of the science and future research needs. *Mol Genet Metab* 2014;**112**:87–122.
30. Longo N. Disorders of biopterin metabolism. *J Inherit Metab Dis* 2009;**32**:333–42.
32. Scott CR. The genetic tyrosinemias. *Am J Med Genet C Semin Med Genet* 2006;**142C**:121–6.
35. Shinawi M. Hyperhomocysteinemia and cobalamin disorders. *Mol Genet Metab* 2007;**90**:113–21.
44. Strauss KA, Puffenberger EG, Morton DH. Maple syrup urine disease. In: Pagon RA, Adam MP, Ardinger HH, et al., editors. *Genereviews(r), Vol.* Seattle (WA): 1993.
49. Nassogne MC, Heron B, Touati G, et al. Urea cycle defects: management and outcome. *J Inherit Metab Dis* 2005;**28**: 407–14.
54. Deodato F, Boenzi S, Santorelli FM, et al. Methylmalonic and propionic aciduria. *Am J Med Genet C Semin Med Genet* 2006;**142C**:104–12.
56. Matern D, Tortorelli S, Oglesbee D, et al. Reduction of the false-positive rate in newborn screening by implementation of ms/ms-based second-tier tests: the Mayo Clinic experience (2004-2007). *J Inherit Metab Dis* 2007;**30**:585–92.
57. Vockley J, Ensenauer R. Isovaleric acidemia: new aspects of genetic and phenotypic heterogeneity. *Am J Med Genet C Semin Med Genet* 2006;**142C**:95–103.
58. Hedlund GL, Longo N, Pasquali M. Glutaric acidemia type 1. *Am J Med Genet C Semin Med Genet* 2006;**142C**:86–94.
60. Longo N, Amat di San Filippo C, Pasquali M. Disorders of carnitine transport and the carnitine cycle. *Am J Med Genet C Semin Med Genet* 2006;**142C**:77–85.
63. Schimmenti LA, Crombez EA, Schwahn BC, et al. Expanded newborn screening identifies maternal primary carnitine deficiency. *Mol Genet Metab* 2007;**90**:441–5.
69. Andresen BS, Olpin S, Poorthuis BJ, et al. Clear correlation of genotype with disease phenotype in very-long-chain acyl-coa dehydrogenase deficiency. *Am J Hum Genet* 1999;**64**: 479–94.
79. Andresen BS, Dobrowolski SF, O'Reilly L, et al. Medium-chain acyl-coa dehydrogenase (mcad) mutations identified by ms/ms-based prospective screening of newborns differ from those observed in patients with clinical symptoms: identification and characterization of a new, prevalent mutation that results in mild mcad deficiency. *Am J Hum Genet* 2001;**68**: 1408–18.

SECTION VI

Hematology and Coagulation

Exam questions, case studies, and additional resources are available on ExpertConsult.com.
*Full versions of these chapters are available electronically on ExpertConsult.com.

71

Hemostasis

Russell A. Higgins, Steve Kitchen, and Dong Chen

ABSTRACT

Background

Hemostasis is a physiologic process involving coagulation proteins, platelets, and blood vessels that maintains blood in the fluid state under normal conditions but rapidly forms a blood clot at sites of injury. Pathophysiologic conditions of bleeding or thrombosis have necessitated the development of laboratory tests to diagnose and monitor these disorders.

Content

This chapter describes prothrombotic and antithrombotic contributions of platelets, plasma proteins, and blood vessels, setting the stage for a discussion of laboratory testing and pathologic disorders. Platelet and von Willebrand factor tests are discussed in the context of platelet disorders and von Willebrand disease. Unique preanalytical variables and end point detection methods for coagulation assays are described. Prothrombin time (PT), activated partial thromboplastin time (aPTT), thrombin time, and fibrinogen are used in the initial evaluation of hemorrhage, whereas mixing studies and measurement of specific coagulation factors narrow the diagnosis to inherited (eg, hemophilia A) or acquired disorders. D-Dimer testing is a marker of fibrinolysis used to assess disseminated intravascular coagulation or to exclude venous thromboembolism (VTE). Heritable thrombotic disorders may be investigated with protein C, protein S, antithrombin assays, factor V Leiden (FVL) mutation, and prothrombin *G20210A* mutation. Diagnosis of heparin-induced thrombocytopenia (HIT), antiphospholipid syndrome (APS), or thrombotic thrombocytopenic purpura requires clinicopathologic correlation and knowledge of specialized laboratory methods. aPTT is commonly used to monitor heparin therapy, but an increasing number of laboratories use heparin assays (anti-Xa methods). The international normalized ratio (INR) has been devised to monitor vitamin K antagonists, but newer direct oral anticoagulants pose new monitoring challenges.

72

Red Blood Cell Morphology and Indices With Clinical Chemistry Interface

Hooman H. Rashidi and Ralph Green

ABSTRACT

Background

A fundamental understanding of laboratory tests in hematology and associated peripheral blood smear findings are essential in analysis of certain chemistry test results. The overlap between hematology and chemistry is also an important aspect in most chemistry and hematology laboratories. Rigorous quality control to ensure precision and accuracy apply to both. Perturbations of blood chemistry may influence hematologic measurements, and hematologic abnormalities may affect analyte determinations in the clinical chemistry laboratories.

Content

This chapter describes the basic concepts and definitions in hematology, specifically looking at the most common peripheral blood smear red blood cell findings and the overlap of certain hematology and chemistry tests. Multiple substances and hematologic conditions can introduce spurious results in various aspects of laboratory medicine, especially within hematology and chemistry domains. Certain substances and conditions can lead to false increases or false decreases in various test results, and, if not corrected or noticed, they may lead or contribute to adverse patient outcomes. Being aware of such substances and conditions in patient management and in the scope of accurate laboratory test usage will ultimately enhance patient care and minimize adverse effects and unnecessary treatments.

73

Automated Hematology

Devon Chabot-Richards, Qian-Yun Zhang, and Tracy I. George

ABSTRACT

Background

The roots of automated hematology began with manual microscopy and laborious cell counting techniques. Using the Coulter principle and advances in laboratory methodology, automated hematology is now rapid and inexpensive, with the complete blood cell count (CBC) being one of the most commonly ordered tests in medicine.

Content

This chapter describes the principles of automated hematology, including how we measure red blood cells (RBCs), white blood cells (WBCs), and platelets from whole blood. Next, the laboratory parameters that are derived from the measurement of RBCs, WBCs, and platelets are discussed. These include standard laboratory measurements of the CBC that help describe anemia, such as the mean corpuscular volume, to newer measurements which quantitate immature granulocytes, immature platelets, and immature reticulocytes. The uses of recently introduced laboratory parameters in automated hematology are also described.

SECTION VII

Microbiology

Exam questions, case studies, and additional resources are available on ExpertConsult.com.
*Full versions of these chapters are available electronically on ExpertConsult.com.

74

Bacteriology

Christopher D. Doern and Betty A. Forbes

ABSTRACT

Background
The diagnosis of bacterial infection is one of the most important services provided by the clinical microbiology laboratory. The past decade has borne witness to a significant shift in the manner in which clinical microbiologists identify bacteria. With the widespread adoption of matrix-assisted laser desorption/ionization time-of-flight mass spectrometry (MALDI-TOF MS) and molecular methods such as 16S rDNA sequencing, clinical microbiologists are increasingly less reliant on traditional, growth-based, biochemical and metabolic methods.

Content
This chapter will describe bacteriology as it will likely be practiced going forward rather than reiterating how it has traditionally been practiced. As a means of introduction, the process of specimen submission to the clinical microbiology laboratory is overviewed. Identification of bacteria is then discussed in addition to the key principles in biochemical identification. Of note, organism categorization will be discussed in the context of modern diagnostic methods such as MALDI-TOF MS and sequence-based identification. In addition, this chapter will include a comprehensive discussion of bacterial infections with a focus on the laboratory methods required to diagnose them.

75

Antimicrobial Susceptibility Testing

Romney M. Humphries and April N. Abbott

ABSTRACT

Background

Antimicrobial susceptibility testing is one of the most important tasks of the clinical microbiology laboratory. Antimicrobial resistance is common, and early recognition of patients with resistant pathogens and appropriate optimization of their antimicrobial therapy significantly improves outcomes.

Content

This chapter reviews the key aspects of antimicrobial susceptibility testing of bacteria, mycobacteria, and yeast. In most circumstances, antimicrobial susceptibility testing (AST) is performed by evaluating the effect of antimicrobial agents on the growth of an organism, in culture. The relative effect (measured as either a zone of inhibition surrounding a disk containing the antimicrobial, or a minimum inhibitory concentration for dilution methods) is interpreted using clinical breakpoints set by international standards organizations. Standardization of AST is achieved through use of consistent inoculum concentrations, test media, and incubation conditions. The concepts of surrogate agent testing, detection of resistance mechanisms, use of commercial systems, and molecular methods for susceptibility testing are discussed. In some instances, additional testing is required to detect important resistance, including methicillin-resistant *Staphylococcus aureus* and vancomycin-resistant *Enterococcus.* β-lactam resistance in the *Enterobacteriaceae* is presented, along with key concepts for testing *Streptococcus pneumoniae,* β-hemolytic *Streptococcus* spp., *Neisseria gonorrhoeae, Pseudomonas aeruginosa, Acinetobacter baumannii,* and *Stenotrophomonas maltophilia.* Common antimicrobials used in clinical practice are also discussed.

76

Mycobacteriology

*Adam J. Caulfield, Rachael M. Liesman, Derrick J. Chen, and Nancy L. Wengenack**

ABSTRACT

Background

There are currently approximately 180 recognized species of mycobacteria. Although some species are strictly environmental organisms, several are significant human pathogens, including *Mycobacterium tuberculosis*. *M. tuberculosis* complex is responsible for nearly 1.4 million deaths each year, and nontuberculous mycobacteria, such as *M. avium* complex (MAC), are also responsible for significant morbidity and mortality.

Content

This chapter describes the laboratory methods used for the detection and identification of *Mycobacterium* species. Methods used for mycobacteria detection and identification are continually evolving to achieve more rapid, cost effective, and accurate results. Traditional microbiologic methods such as morphology and biochemical profiling have given way to molecular methods of detection and identification; however, acid-fast staining and culture for mycobacteria remain at the core of any diagnostic algorithm. After growth in culture, molecular technologies such as nucleic acid hybridization probes, matrix-assisted laser desorption/ionization time-of-flight mass spectrometry (MALDI-TOF MS), and DNA sequencing are used for definitive species identification. Nucleic acid amplification methods allow for culture-independent direct detection of the *M. tuberculosis* complex and MAC within respiratory specimens, as well as prediction of susceptibility to anti-infective therapy, which leads to more rapid diagnoses and appropriate patient care.

*This chapter is adapted in part with permission from Caulfield AJ, Wengenack NL. Diagnosis of active tuberculosis disease: from microscopy to molecular techniques. *J Clin Tuberc Other Mycobact Dis* 2016;4:33–43.

77

Mycology

*Ingibjörg Hilmarsdóttir, Audrey N. Schuetz, and Anna F. Lau**

ABSTRACT

Background

Ubiquitous in nature, fungi may be opportunistic organisms in compromised hosts or primary pathogens in immunocompetent individuals. Commensal fungi reside in the human body as normal flora and cause opportunistic infections. Diagnosis of fungal infections relies on assessment of several factors, including geographical exposure, underlying host condition, clinical manifestations, and diagnostic accuracy of laboratory tests such as culture, anatomic pathology tests, immunological assays, and molecular tests.

Content

A perspective on the importance of fungi in their natural environment is provided, and their differences in relation to other microorganisms are highlighted. Prevalent and emerging fungal infections are discussed, and a review of nomenclature changes in medical mycology is listed with the understanding of continued uncertainty regarding phylogenetic relationships between fungal taxa. Preanalytical, analytical, and postanalytical procedures for the laboratory diagnosis of fungal infections are reviewed, with emphasis on fungal morphology and issues that require close communication with the clinical team. Common histopathologic and cytologic features related to anatomic pathology are discussed. Given the suboptimal sensitivity, specificity, and relatively long turnaround time for culture-based detection and identification of fungi, a review of nonphenotypic methods such as mass spectrometry, immunological assays, and molecular tests is provided. Finally, the principal features of fungal infections are summarized, including patient populations affected, clinical manifestations, relevant diagnostic approaches and tests, and therapeutic issues related to antifungal resistance.

*We are grateful to Gabriel Lecso of the Service de Parasitologie-Mycologie, Hôpital Universitaire Pitié-Salpêtrière, Paris, France, for his collection of photographs that greatly enhanced the value of our chapter.

78

Parasitology

Esther Babady and Bobbi S. Pritt

ABSTRACT

Background
Parasites are an important cause of human morbidity and mortality worldwide. They include a diverse array of single-celled eukaryotic organisms (protozoa), multicellular worms (helminths), and arthropods that live in or on the human body and can cause mild to severe life-threatening disease. While many parasites primarily infect impoverished individuals in tropical and subtropical regions of the world, others cause infection in the world's temperate regions including those living in resource-rich, affluent countries. The study of parasitology has gained a renewed importance in recent decades due to the ease in which humans, animals, and food can move rapidly and widely across the globe and the increased number of individuals who are immunocompromised and at risk for severe disease.

Content
This chapter provides an overview of human parasitology and the general laboratory approaches for identifying important parasites in various specimens. Both conventional and state-of-the-art diagnostic methods are covered, including light microscopy, serology, antigen detection, and nucleic acid amplification. Particular attention is paid to testing in blood and stool, as these are the most common specimens received in the clinical laboratory for detection of parasites. The most important human parasites are discussed individually, with an emphasis on the fundamental clinical and biologic information needed for accurate diagnosis and management of infection. The categories of parasites covered include the blood and tissue protozoa, intestinal protozoa, intestinal helminths, tissue helminths, and medically important arthropods.

79

Virology

Blake W. Buchan and Neil W. Anderson

ABSTRACT

Background

Viral illness has a wide variety of clinical manifestations, ranging from focal to systemic, and affecting nearly every organ system. Infections may be asymptomatic, acute, or chronic in nature. The viruses causing these syndromes are diverse, but unrelated viruses may cause clinically indistinguishable disease. Combined, these factors drive the importance of rapid and accurate laboratory diagnosis to enable effective patient management.

Content

This chapter discusses the use of qualitative and quantitative nucleic acid amplification and detection methods to diagnose and monitor viral infections. It also provides alternative diagnostic methods for those syndromes not optimally diagnosed by molecular techniques. Specific topics covered in this chapter include viral infections of the respiratory tract, viral illness in immunocompromised populations, infections of the central nervous system, sexually transmitted viral illness, viral hepatitis, viral hemorrhagic fever, and diagnosis of vaccine-preventable viral infections. The epidemiology of the key organisms responsible for each of the clinical syndromes is highlighted, and the factors impacting laboratory diagnosis and interpretation of results are discussed. Examples include optimal specimen type, availability of standardized assays, utility of qualitative versus quantitative results, multiplexed detection strategies, and potential shortcomings of current diagnostic approaches.

SECTION VIII

Transfusion Medicine

Exam questions, case studies, and additional resources are available on ExpertConsult.com.
*Full versions of these chapters are available electronically on ExpertConsult.com.

80

Blood Groups, Pretransfusion Testing, and Red Blood Cell Transfusion

Karen Quillen

ABSTRACT

Background

Pretransfusion compatibility testing hinges on a solid understanding of the blood group antigens expressed on red blood cells. To optimize transfusion safety for the patient, clinical laboratories that provide pretransfusion testing also need a working familiarity with blood management concepts and subsets of challenging transfusion patients.

Content

This chapter outlines the salient historical facts and clinical significance of the major blood group systems, including the ABO, Rh D and CE, Kell, Kidd, Duffy, MN/Ss, I, Lewis, and P groups. Testing methods are described in detail, including ABO and Rh(D) determination, common ABO and D antigen variants that present in the transfusion service, different cross-matching methods, and the nuances of the direct antiglobulin test. Recent advances in molecular testing are outlined with specific examples of situations where such testing may be valuable. The issues of immunohematologic testing in the prenatal population are covered, including the management and prevention of Rh(D) isoimmunization. Patients with sickle cell disease and autoimmune hemolytic anemia are presented as examples of transfusion recipients who require special handling in pretransfusion testing. Concepts surrounding patient-centered blood management and evidence-based transfusion triggers are outlined.

81

Blood Components, Blood Donor Screening, and Transfusion Reactions

*John P Manis**

ABSTRACT

Transfusion of blood requires multiple steps including blood donation from healthy volunteers, manufacture and testing of blood components, and finally administration of the product to a patient. Nearly 15 million blood products are transfused annually in the United States, and all of these products are derived from healthy volunteer blood donors. Red cells, platelets, plasma, and cryoprecipitate are manufactured using relatively simple and widely available methods to supply the demand for blood. The safety of the blood supply is ensured using donor history questionnaires, laboratory testing, and quality measures to keep these biologic products derived from millions of donors therapeutically consistent. Transfusion of blood is a very safe procedure, though reactions can occur both in an acute (within 24 hours) or a delayed fashion. Transfusion reactions can range from mild allergic or febrile reactions to life-threatening acute hemolytic reactions. Understanding the process of obtaining, manufacturing, and transfusing blood is critical to interpret clinical outcomes of blood administration and to treat adverse events.

*The author would like to acknowledge Karen Quillen, MD, MPH, for her review of this chapter.

Reference Information for the Clinical Laboratory

*Khosrow Adeli, Ferruccio Ceriotti, and Michelle Nieuwesteeg**

ABSTRACT

Background
Accurate reference intervals established in healthy subjects are essential for appropriate interpretation of laboratory test results and to assist clinicians in diagnosis, monitoring, and treatment of disease. To facilitate interpretation of laboratory tests, reference intervals must be appropriately stratified based on key covariates, including age, gender, and ethnicity, which can alter "normal" analyte concentrations. When establishing or implementing reference intervals, it is important to consider the effect of these covariates as well as regional and methodologic variances. Notably, reference intervals are often method- and population-dependent; thus reference intervals and clinical decision limits may vary across laboratories. Reference intervals from one laboratory should not be adopted by another laboratory without first ensuring that the proper transference and verification have been completed.

Content
This chapter provides reference information for biochemical markers in serum, plasma, urine markers, and other body fluids, as well as for therapeutic drug monitoring and toxicology, hematologic parameters, and critical risk values. Where possible, method, age, and sex-specific partitions and values for both conventional and SI units are included. Reference publications are listed to support the values reported in this chapter. The reference information presented here has been updated using current studies where possible; however, some values were obtained from the previous edition. Most pediatric values were obtained from the Canadian Laboratory Initiative on Pediatric Reference Intervals (CALIPER) study.

OVERVIEW

Reference intervals are defined as "limiting values within which a specified percentage (usually 95%) of apparently healthy individuals' results would fall"—usually the 2.5th and 97.5th centiles of the test result distribution in the reference (healthy) population.

Reference limits and intervals provide valuable information to medical practitioners in their interpretation of quantitative laboratory test results, serving as health-associated benchmarks to which individual test results can be compared. Although the concept of reference intervals and their utility appears straightforward, the process of establishing accurate and reliable reference intervals is considerably complex and involved, requiring recruitment of a large number of healthy individuals. This is particularly challenging for pediatric populations. Each clinical laboratory is responsible for ensuring the validity of reference intervals issued with their test results. Accrediting and licensing organizations and regulatory bodies governing medical laboratory best practices require that individual laboratories establish or verify reference intervals for all quantitative test methods, the exception being for tests that employ clinical decision limits (eg, cholesterol, hemoglobin A_{1C}). It is important to note that values from apparently healthy and diseased populations may overlap significantly. Therefore reference intervals, although useful as a guide for clinicians, should not be used as absolute indicators of health and disease. Unfortunately, reference intervals are obtained with analytical procedures that produce results traceable only to the corresponding reference system and thus cannot be directly applied by any laboratory, because standardized methods, particularly for immunoassays, practically do not exist. Therefore the presented reference intervals are all, more or less, method-dependent. Moreover, it is not yet clear to what extent ethnicity and local environmental factors could influence the reference intervals for specific analytes. For these reasons the reference intervals presented in the following tables are for general informational purposes only. Each individual laboratory should generate its own set of reference intervals or validate published reference intervals based on the CLSI C28-A3 guidelines (CLSI document C28-A3. Wayne PAL Clinical and Laboratory Standards Institute 2008, p. 76).

Reference Information Tables and Figures

- **Table A.1.** Pediatric and Adult Reference Intervals for Biochemical Markers (Serum, Plasma, and Urine)
- **Figure A.1–A.10.** Dynamic changes in biochemical markers in children and adults (scatter graphs for 10 common chemistry and endocrine tests) shown in print version, all other graphs for remaining tests (121 graphs) can be found online at ExpertConsult.com.

*The chapter is based on that of WL Roberts, GA McMillan, CA Burtis, and DE Bruns, Reference Information for the Clinical Laboratory, from the fifth edition of this textbook.

TABLE A.1 Pediatric and Adult Reference Intervals for Biochemical Markers (Serum, Plasma, and Urine

Analyte	Specimen	Condition	REFERENCE INTERVALS Conventional Units	Conversion Factor	SI Units	Reference Publication
Acetaldehyde	WB (F^-/Ox)		mg/dL	22.7	µmol/L	
			<0.2		<4.5	1
		Occup exp	<0.5		<11.4	
		Toxic	1–2		22.7–45.4	
Acetylaspartic acid	U				mmol/mol creatinine	
					<14	1
α_1-Acid glycoprotein	S		mg/dL	0.01	g/L	
Pediatric values (0–19 y) based on Abbott Architect method		0–<6 mo	21–85		0.2–0.9	8
		6 mo–<5 y	48–201		0.5–2.0	
		5–<19 y	48–114		0.5–1.1	
		Adult (20–60 y)	50–120		0.5–1.2	
cis-Aconitic acid	U				mmol/mol creatinine	
		0–1 mo			5–31	1
		1–6 mo			10–97	
		6 mo–5 y			10–97	
		>5 y			3–44	
Adipic acid	U				mmol/mol creatinine	
		0–6 mo			9–37	1
		6 mo–5 y			<16	
		>5 y			<6	
Adipocarnitine	U				mmol/mol creatinine	
		0–7 d			0.04–0.40	1
		8 d–7 y			0.01–0.81	
		>7 y			0.00–0.13	
Adrenocorticotropic hormone (ACTH)	P, EDTA		pg/mL	0.22	pmol/L	
ACTH reference intervals may vary depending on immunoassay methods.		Cord	50–570		11–125	1
		Newborn	10–185		2.2–41	
		Adult (0800–0900)	<120		<26	
		Adult (24 h, supine)	<85		<19	
Alanine	P		mg/dL	112.2	µmol/L	
		Premature, 1 d	2.44–4.24		274–476	1
		Newborn, 1 d	2.10–3.65		236–410	
		1–3 mo	1.19–3.71		134–416	
		2–6 mo	1.58–3.68		177–413	
		9 mo–2 y	0.88–2.79		99–313	
		3–10 y	1.22–2.71		137–305	
		6–18 y	1.72–4.85		193–545	
		Adult	1.87–5.88		210–661	
	U, 24 h		mg/d	11.2	µmol/d	
		10 d–7 wk	4.1–9.3		46–104	
		3–12 y	9.1–39.2		102–439	
		Adult	7.9–48.3		88–541	

TABLE A.1 **Pediatric and Adult Reference Intervals for Biochemical Markers (Serum, Plasma, and Urine—cont'd**

Analyte	Specimen	Condition	REFERENCE INTERVALS Conventional Units	Conversion Factor	SI Units	Reference Publication
			μmol/g creatinine	0.113	μmol/mol creatinine	
		0–1 mo	554–2957		62.6–334.1	
		1–6 mo	613–2874		59.3–324.8	
		6 mo–1 y	428–2064		48.4–233.2	
		1–2 y	389–1497		44.0–169.2	
		2–3 y	255–1726		28.8–195.0	
Alanine aminotransferase	S		U/L	0.017	μkat/L	
With pyridoxal phosphate		0–<1 y	5–51		0.08–0.85	4
Values (0–<3 y) based on Abbott Architect method		1–<3 y	11–30		0.18–0.50	
Values (3–79 y) based on OCD Vitros method		3–5 y	15–33		0.26–0.56	
		6–8 y	16–37		0.27–0.63	9
		9–11 y	18–39		0.31–0.66	
		12–17 y, M	17–50		0.29–0.85	
		12–49 y, F	14–41		0.24–0.70	
		18–49 y, M	18–78		0.31–1.33	
		50–79 y, M	20–62		0.34–1.05	
		50–79 y, F	16–44		0.27–0.75	
Without pyridoxal phosphate	S	0–<1 y	5–33		0.08–0.56	4
		1–<13 y	9–25		0.15–0.43	
		13–19 y	8–22		0.14–0.37	
Albumin (BCG)	S		g/dL	10	g/L	
		3–5 y	3.9–5.0		39–50	9
		6–15 y	4.1–5.1		41–51	
		16–29 y, M	4.6–5.3		46–53	
		16–54 y, F	3.9–5.0		39–50	
		30–54 y, M	4.4–5.1		44–51	
		55–79 y	4.2–5.0		42–50	
	CSF, lumbar	See Table 82.2				1
		Adult				
		20–60 y	3.5–5.2		35–52	
		60–90 y	3.2–4.6		32–46	
		>90 y	2.9–4.5		29–45	
Values (3–79 y) based on OCD Vitros method	U		mg/L	1	mg/L	
		3–5 y	1.5–21.5		1.5–21.5	10
		6–8 y	1.5–37.8		1.5–37.8	
		9–19 y	1.5–169.6		1.5–169.6	
		20–29 y	1.5–74.6		1.5–74.6	
		30–39 y	1.5–36.8		1.5–36.8	
		40–79 y	1.5–47.2		1.5–47.2	
Albumin-creatinine ratio (NKDEP guidelines; see also Chapter 32)			mg/mmol		mg/g creatinine	
		M	<2.5		<22	
		F	<3.5		<30	
Aldolase	S		U/L	0.017	μkat/L	
		Child				1
		10–24 mo	10–40		0.17–0.68	
		25 mo–16 y	5–20		0.09–0.34	
		Adult	2.5–10.0		0.04–0.13	

Continued

TABLE A.1 Pediatric and Adult Reference Intervals for Biochemical Markers (Serum, Plasma, and Urine—cont'd

			REFERENCE INTERVALS			
Analyte	**Specimen**	**Condition**	**Conventional Units**	**Conversion Factor**	**SI Units**	**Reference Publication**
Aldosterone	S		ng/dL	0.0277	nmol/L	
		Cord blood	40–200		1.11–5.54	1
		Premature infants	19–141		0.53–3.91	
Full-term infants						
		3 d	7–184		0.19–5.10	
		1 wk	5–175		0.03–4.85	
		1–12 mo	5–90		0.14–2.49	
		1–2 y	7–54		0.19–1.50	
		2–10 y (supine)	3–35		0.08–0.97	
		2–10 y (upright)	5–80		0.14–2.22	
		10–15 y (supine)	2–22		0.06–0.61	
		10–15 y (upright)	4–48		0.11–1.33	
Adult						
		Supine	3–16		0.08–0.44	
		Upright	7–30		0.19–0.83	
	U, 24 hr		μg/d	nmol/d	μg/g creatinine	
		Newborns (1–3 d)	0.5–5	2.771–14	20–140	1
		Prepubertal children				
		4–10 y	1–8	3–22	4–22	
		Adults	3–19	8–51	1.5–20	
Aluminum	S, P		μg/L	0.0371	μmol/L	
			<5.51		<0.2	1
		Patients on hemodialysis	20–550		0.74–20.4	
		Al medication	<30		<1.11	
	U		5–30		0.19–1.11	
Ammonia nitrogen	P (Hep)		μg N/dL	0.714	μmol N/L	
		Newborn	90–150		64–107	1
		0–2 wk	79–129		56–92	
		>1 mo	29–70		21–50	
		Adult	15–45		11–32	
	U, 24 h		mg N/d	0.0714	mmol N/d	
		Infant	560–2900		40–207	1
		Adult	140–1500		10–107	
Amylase	S		U/L	0.017	μkat/L	
Values (0–<19 y) based on Abbott Architect method		0–14 d	3–10		0.05–0.17	4
		15 d–<13 wk	2–22		0.03–0.37	
		13 wk–<1 y	3–50		0.05–0.83	
		1–<19 y	25–101		0.42–1.68	
IFCC, 37°C		Adult	31–107		0.52–1.78	12
Androgen index, free (FAI)					%	
		0–<1 y, F			0.04–1.32	7
		1–<9 y, F			0.04–1.32	
		9–<14 y, F			0.12–2.63	
		14–19 y, F			0.59–6.50	
		0–<1 y, M			0.02–32.72	
		1–<9 y, M			0.03–0.60	
		9–<14 y, M			0.15–34.68	
		14–<19 y, M			3.58–83.30	
		Note: FAI should not be used in men if testosterone levels exceed SHBG binding capacity.				

TABLE A.1 **Pediatric and Adult Reference Intervals for Biochemical Markers (Serum, Plasma, and Urine—cont'd**

Analyte	Specimen	Condition	REFERENCE INTERVALS Conventional Units	Conversion Factor	SI Units	Reference Publication
3α-Androstanediol glucuronide	S	Levels may exceed SHBG binding capacity	ng/dL	0.0213	nmol/L	
		Child, prepubertal	10–60		0.2–1.3	1
		Adult, M	260–1500		5.5–32	
		Adult, F	60–300		1.3–6.4	
Androstenedione (LC-MS/MS)	S		ng/L			
		6–24 mo	25–150			29
		2–3 y	<110			
		4–5 y	23–170			
		6–7 y	10–290			
		7–9 y	30–300			
		10–11 y	70–390			
		12–13 y	100–640			
		14–15 y	180–940			
		16–17 y	300–1130			
		18–40 y	330–1340			
		40–67 y	280–890			
Vasopressin (Antidiuretic hormone [ADH])	P, EDTA	mOsm/kg	ng/L	0.926	pmol/L	
		270–280	<1.5		<1.4	1
		280–285	<2.5		<2.3	
		285–290	1–5		0.9–4.6	
		290–294	2–7		1.9–6.5	
		295–300	4–12		3.7–11.1	
Antimony	P (Hep)		µg/dL	82.1	nmol/L	
			0.014–0.090		1.15–7.39	1
	U		µg/L	8.21	nmol/L	
			<10		<82.1	
			mg/L		µmol/L	
		Toxic	>1		>8.21	
Antistreptolysin-O (ASO)	S		IU/mL	1	kIU/L	
Values (0–<19 y) based on Abbott Architect method		0–<6 mo	0–0		0–0	4
		6 mo–<1 y	0–30		0–30	
		1–<6 y	0–104		0–104	
		6–<19 y	0–331		0–331	
		Adult	<20–364		<20–364	24
α_1-Antitrypsin	S		mg/dL	0.01	g/L	
Values (0–<19 y) based on Abbott Architect method		0–<19 y	110–181		1.1–1.8	8
		Adult (20–60 y)	90–200		0.9–2.0	1
Apolipoprotein AI	S		mg/dL	0.01	g/L	
Values (0–<6 y) based on Abbott Architect method		0–14 d, F	71–97		0.7–1.0	4
		0–14 d, M	62–91		0.6–0.9	
		15 d–<1 y	53–175		0.5–1.8	
		1–<6 y	80–164		0.8–1.6	
Values (6–79 y) based on OCD Vitros method		6–15 y	100–180		1.0–1.8	10
		16–39 y, M	80–170		0.8–1.7	
		F	100–200		1.0–2.0	
		40–79 y M	120–200		1.2–2.0	
		F	110–230		1.1–2.3	

Continued

TABLE A.1 **Pediatric and Adult Reference Intervals for Biochemical Markers (Serum, Plasma, and Urine—cont'd**

Analyte	Specimen	Condition	REFERENCE INTERVALS			Reference Publication
			Conventional Units	Conversion Factor	SI Units	
Apolipoprotein B-100	S		mg/dL	0.01	g/L	
Values (0–<6 y) based on Abbott Architect method		0–14 d	9–67		0.1–0.7	4
		15 d–<1 y	19–123		0.2–1.2	
		1–<6 y	41–93		0.4–0.9	
Values (6–79 y) based on OCD Vitros method		6–13 y	50–100		0.5–1.0	10
		14–29 y	40–110		0.4–1.1	
		30–79 y	60–140		0.6–1.4	
Arginine	P		mg/dL	57.4	µmol/L	
		Premature, 1 d	0.17–1.57		10–90	1
		Newborn, 1 d	0.38–1.53		22–88	
		1–3 mo	0.38–1.30		22–74	
		2–6 mo	0.98–2.47		56–142	
		9 mo–2 y	0.19–1.13		11–65	
		3–10 y	0.40–1.50		23–86	
		6–18 y	0.77–2.26		44–130	
		Adult	0.37–2.40		21–138	
	U, 24 h		mg/d	5.74	µmol/d	
		10 d–7 wk	<1.2		<7	
		3–12 y	<5.1		<29	
		Adult	<50.2		<288	
			mg/g creatinine	0.65	mmol/mol creatinine	
		Adult	0–4		0–2.7	
Arsenic	WB (Hep)		µg/L	0.0113	µmol/L	
		Not exposed	2–23		0.03–0.31	1
		Chronic poisoning	100–500		1.33–6.65	
		Acute poisoning	600–9300		7.98–124	
		Not exposed	2–23		0.03–0.31	
Ascorbic acid (see vitamin C)						1
Asparagine	P		mg/dL	75.7	µmol/L	
		1–3 mo	0.08–0.44		6–33	1
		3 mo–6 y	0.95–1.90		72–144	
		6–18 y	0.42–0.82		32–62	
		Adult	0.40–0.91		30–69	
	U, 24 h		mg/d	7.57	µmol/d	
		Adult	4.5–13.2		34–100	
			mg/g creatinine	0.86	mmol/mol creatinine	
		Adult	2–10		1.8–8.6	
Aspartate aminotransferase	S		U/L	0.017	µkat/L	
With pyridoxal phosphate		0–14 d	23–186		0.38–3.10	4
Values (0–<3 y) based on Abbott Architect method		15 d–<1 y	23–83		0.38–1.38	
		1–<3 y	26–55		0.43–0.92	
Values (3–79 y) based on OCD Vitros method		3–5 y	28–52		0.48–0.88	9
		6–11 y, M	25–47		0.43–0.80	
		F	23–44		0.39–0.75	
		12–17 y, M	18–36		0.31–0.61	
		12–19 y, F	15–34		0.26–0.58	

TABLE A.1 Pediatric and Adult Reference Intervals for Biochemical Markers (Serum, Plasma, and Urine—cont'd

Analyte	Specimen	Condition	REFERENCE INTERVALS Conventional Units	Conversion Factor	SI Units	Reference Publication
		18–54 y, M	18–54		0.31–0.92	
		20–54 y, F	18–34		0.31–0.58	
		55–79 y	18–39		0.31–0.66	4
Without pyridoxal phosphate	S	0–14 d	32–162		0.54–2.75	
Values (0–<19 y) based on Abbott Architect method		15 d–<1 y	20–67		0.34–1.14	
		1–<7 y	21–44		0.36–0.75	
		7–<12 y	18–36		0.31–0.61	
		12–19 y, M	14–35		0.24–0.60	
		F	13–26		0.22–0.44	
Aspartic acid	P		mg/dL	75.1	µmol/L	
		Premature, 1 d	0–0.39		0–30	1
		Newborn, 1 d	<0.2 1		<16	
		1–3 mo	0–0.15		0–8	
		9 mo–2 y	<0.12		<9	
		19 mo–10 y	<0.27		<20	
		6–18 y	<0.19		<14	
		Adult	<0.32		<24	
	U, 24 h		mg/d	7.51	µmol/d	
		3–12 y	<5.1		<38	
		Adult	<26.2		<197	
			mg/g creatinine	0.85	mmol/mol creatinine	
		Adult	0–4		0.1–3.7	
Azelaic acid	U				mmol/mol creatinine	
					<1.1	1
Beryllium	U, 24 h		µg/L	0.111	µmol/L	
		Negative	None detected		None detected	1
		Toxic	>20		>2.22	
Bilirubin, direct (conjugated)	S		mg/dL	17.1	µmol/L	
Values (0–<19 y) based on Abbott Architect method		0–14 d	0.33–0.71		5.7–12.1	4
		15 d–<1 y	0.05–0.30		0.8–5.2	
		1–<9 y	0.05–0.20		0.8–3.4	
		9–<13 y	0.10–0.29		0.8–5.0	
		13–<19 y, F	0.10–0.39		1.7–6.7	
		13–<19 y, M	0.11–0.42		1.9–7.1	
Bilirubin, total	S		mg/dL	17.1	µmol/L	
Values (0–<3 y) based on Abbott Architect method		0–14 d	0.19–16.6		3.3–283.8	4
		15 d–<1 y	0.05–0.68		0.8–11.7	
		1–<3 y	0.05–0.40		0.8–6.8	
Values (3–79 y) based on OCD Vitros method						9
		3–5 y	0.1–0.5		1.0–8.8	
		6–15 y	0.1–0.9		1.0–15.6	
		16–48 y, M	0.2–1.1		3.0–18	
		F	0.1–0.9		1.0–16	
		49–79 y, M	0.1–1.2		2.0–19.9	
		F	0.1–1.0		1.0–16.6	
	U		Negative		Negative	1
	Amf	See Table 82.2				
Conjugated	S		0.0–0.2		0.0–3.4	

Continued

TABLE A.1 **Pediatric and Adult Reference Intervals for Biochemical Markers (Serum, Plasma, and Urine—cont'd**

Analyte	Specimen	Condition	REFERENCE INTERVALS Conventional Units	Conversion Factor	SI Units	Reference Publication
Biotin	WB	Healthy			0.5–2.20 nmol/L	1
		Deficiency			<0.5 nmol/L	
BNP (see Chapter 58)	U					1
Cadmium	WB (Hep)		µg/L	8.897	nmol/L	
		Nonsmokers	0.3–1.2		2.7–10.7	1
		Smokers	0.6–3.9		5.3–34.7	
	U, 24 h		µg/L		µmol/L	
		Toxic range	100–3000		0.9–26.7	
Calcitonin	S, P		pg/mL	1	ng/L	
		Men	<8.8		<8.8	1
		Women	<5.8		<5.8	
		Athyroidal	<0.5		<0.5	
Calcium, ionized (free)	S, P (Hep)		mg/dL	0.25	mmol/L	
		Adults	4.6–5.3		1.15–1.33	1
Calcium, total	S, P (Hep)		mg/dL	0.25	mmol/L	
Values (0–<3 y) based on Abbott Architect method		0–<1 y	8.5–11.0		2.13–2.74	4
		1–<3 y	9.2–10.5		2.29–2.63	
Values (3–79 y) based on OCD Vitros method		3–5 y	9.4–10.6		2.35–2.64	9
		6–15 y	9.3–10.5		2.33–2.62	
		16–19	9.2–10.4		2.3–2.60	
		20–39 y, M	9.1–10.4		2.28–2.60	
		20–39 y, F	9.0–10.1		2.24–2.53	
		40–79 y	9.0–10.2		2.24–2.56	
β-Carotene HPLC	S		µg/dL	0.0186	µmol/L	
			10–85		0.19–1.58	1
Cancer antigen 15–3	S		U/mL	1	kU/L	
			<30		<30	1
Cancer antigen 19–9	S		U/mL	1	kU/L	
			<37		<37	1
Cancer antigen 27.29	S		U/mL	1	kU/L	
			<37.7		<37.7	1
Cancer antigen 50	S		U/mL	1	kU/L	
			<14–20		<14–20	1
Cancer antigen 72–4	S		U/mL	1	kU/L	
			<6		<6	1
Cancer antigen 125	S		U/mL	1	kU/L	
			<35		<35	1
Cancer antigen 242	S		U/mL	1	kU/L	
			<20		<20	1
Cancer antigen 549	S		U/mL	1	kU/L	
			<11		<11	1
Carbon dioxide, partial pressure PCO_2	WB, arterial (Hep)		mm Hg	0.133	kPa	
		Newborn	27–40		3.59–5.32	1
		Infant	27–41		3.59–5.45	
		Adult, M	35–48		4.66–6.38	
		Adult, F	32–45		4.26–5.99	

TABLE A.1 **Pediatric and Adult Reference Intervals for Biochemical Markers (Serum, Plasma, and Urine—cont'd**

Analyte	Specimen	Condition	REFERENCE INTERVALS Conventional Units	Conversion Factor	SI Units	Reference Publication
Carbon dioxide, total (tCO_2)			mEq/L	1	mmol/L	
Values (0–<6 y) based on Abbott Architect method		0–14 d	5–20		5–20	4
		15 d–<1 y	10–24		10–24	
		1–<5 y	14–24		14–24	
		5–<6 y	17–26		17–26	
Values (6–79 y) based on OCD Vitros method		6–79 y	19–26		19–26	9
	WB					1
	Arterial		19–24		19–24	
	Venous		22–26		22–26	
Carbon monoxide	WB (EDTA)		%HbCO	0.01	HbCO Fraction	
		Nonsmokers	0.5–1.5		0.005–0.015	1
		Smokers				
		1–2 packs/d	4–5		0.04–0.05	
		>2 packs/d	8–9		0.08–0.09	
		Toxic	>20		>0.20	
		Lethal	>50		>0.5	
Carcinoembryonic antigen (CEA)	S		ng/mL	1	µg/L	
Values based on the Roche method		Nonsmokers	<3		<3	1
		Smokers	<5		<5	
Catecholamines						1
Epinephrine	P	Adults	pg/mL	5.46	pmol/L	
		Supine (30 min)	<50		<273	
		Sitting (15 min)	<60		<328	
		Standing (30 min)	<90		<491	
Norepinephrine	P	Adults	pg/mL	5.91	pmol/L	
		Supine (30 min)	110–410		650–2423	
		Sitting (15 min)	120–680		709–4019	
		Standing (30 min)	125–700		739–4137	
Dopamine	P	Adults	pg/mL	6.53	pmol/L	
		Supine (30 min)	<87		<475	
		Sitting (15 min)	<87		<475	
		Standing (30 min)	<87		<475	
Epinephrine *See Chapter 63, Table 63.1	U, 24 h					
Norepinephrine *See Chapter 63, Table 63.1	U, 24 h					
Dopamine *See Chapter 63, Table 63.1	U, 24 h					
Ceruloplasmin	P		mg/L	0.001	g/L	
		Cord (term)	50–330		0.05–0.33	
Pediatric values (0–19 y) based on Abbott Architect method		0–<2 mo	74–237		0.07–0.24	8
		2–<6 mo	135–330		0.13–0.33	
		6 mo–<1 y	137–389		0.14–0.39	
		1–<8 y	217–433		0.22–0.43	
		8–<14 y	205–402		0.21–0.40	
		14–<19 y, F	208–432		0.21–0.43	
		14–<19 y, M	170–348		0.17–0.35	

Continued

TABLE A.1 Pediatric and Adult Reference Intervals for Biochemical Markers (Serum, Plasma, and Urine—cont'd

Analyte	Specimen	Condition	REFERENCE INTERVALS Conventional Units	Conversion Factor	SI Units	Reference Publication
		Adult, M	220–400		0.22–0.40	1
		Adult, F with no contraceptive	250–600		0.25–0.60	
		Adult, F without contraceptives (estrogen)	270–660		0.27–0.66	
		Adult, pregnant F	300–1200		0.3–1.20	
			mg/dL	0.01	g/L	
		Adult (20–60 y)	20–60		0.2–0.6	
Chloride (Cl)	S, P		mEq/L	1	mmol/L	
Values (3–79 y) based on OCD Vitros method		3–5 y	100–107		100–107	9
		6–11 y	101–107		101–107	
		12–29 y, M	101–106		101–106	
		F	100–107		100–107	
		30–79 y	102–108		102–108	
	U, 24 h		mEq/d	1	mmol/d	1
		Infant	2–10		2–10	
		Child <6 y	15–40		15–40	
		6–10 y, M	36–110		36–110	
		F	18–74		18–74	
		10–14 y, M	64–176		64–176	
		F	36–173		36–173	
		Adult	110–250		110–250	
		>60 y	95–195		95–195	
	Sweat (iontophoresis)	See Table 82.2				
Cholesterol	S		mg/dL	0.0259	mmol/L	
Reference Limits						
Values (0–<3 y) based on Abbott Architect method		0–14 d F	46–125		1.19.24	4
		0–14 d M	42–109		1.09–2.82	
		15 d–<1 y	64–237		1.66–6.14	
		1–<3 y	112–208		2.90–5.39	
Values (3–79 y) based on OCD Vitros method		3–5 y	120–216		3.11–5.59	9
		6–15 y	116–205		3.00–5.31	
		16–19 y	100–182		2.59–4.71	
		20–29 y	116–228		3.00–5.91	
		30–39 y	147–266		3.81–6.89	
		40–79 y	139–274		3.60–7.10	
		Note: The more recent guidelines suggest that risk stratification should rely only on the 10-year atherosclerotic cardiovascular disease risk calculation (2013 ACC/AHA guideline on the treatment of blood cholesterol to reduce atherosclerotic cardiovascular risk in adults).				1
Clinical Decision Limits		Coronary heart disease risk Child				27
		Desirable	<170		<4.40	
		Borderline high	170–199		4.40–5.15	
		High	>200		>5.15	
		Coronary heart disease risk, Adult				1
		Desirable	<200		<5.18	
		Borderline high	200–239		5.18–6.19	
		High	>239		>6.19	
		Note: Cholesterol should not be used on its own for risk prediction.				

TABLE A.1 Pediatric and Adult Reference Intervals for Biochemical Markers (Serum, Plasma, and Urine—cont'd

			REFERENCE INTERVALS			
Analyte	**Specimen**	**Condition**	**Conventional Units**	**Conversion Factor**	**SI Units**	**Reference Publication**
Cholinesterase (37°C)	S		U/L	0.017	μkat/L	
		M	40–78		0.68–1.33	1
		F	33–76		0.56–1.29	
Cholinesterase activity with dibucaine inhibitor (ChEDi)	S		U/L	0.017	μkat/L	
		0–<1 mo	797–2478		13–41	8
Pediatric values (0–<19 y) based on Abbott Architect method		1 mo–<19 y	1523–3280		25–55	
Chorionic gonadotropin intact molecule	S		mIU/mL	1	IU/L	
		Male and nonpregnant female	<5.0		<5.0	1
		Female, pregnancy (wk of gestation)				
		4 wk	5–100		5–100	
		5 wk	200–3000		200–3000	
		6 wk	10,000–80,000		10,000–80,000	
		7–14 wk	90,000–500,000		90,000–500,000	
		15–26 wk	5000–80,000		5000–80,000	
			*Values based on the Second International Standard for hCG.			
		Trophoblastic disease	>100,000		>100,000	
	U		Negative		Negative	
			Half of pregnancies are detected on the first day of the missed menstrual period.		Half of pregnancies are detected on the first day of the missed menstrual period.	
Chromium			μg/L	19.23	nmol/L	
	WB (Hep)		0.7–28.0		14–538	1
	S		0.1–0.2		2–3	
			μg/d	19.23	nmol/d	
	U, 24 h		0.1–2.0		1.9–38.4	
			μg/L	19.23	nmol/L	
	RBC		20–36		384–692	
Chymotrypsin (37°C)	F		12 U/g stool	1	12 U/g stool	1
trans-Cinnamoylglycine	U				mmol/mol creatinine	
					0.1–8.0	1
Citric acid	U				mmol/mol creatinine	
		0–1 mo			<1046	1
		1–6 mo			104–268	
		6 mo–5 y			0–656	
		>5 y			87–639	

Continued

TABLE A.1 **Pediatric and Adult Reference Intervals for Biochemical Markers (Serum, Plasma, and Urine—cont'd**

Analyte	Specimen	Condition	REFERENCE INTERVALS Conventional Units	Conversion Factor	SI Units	Reference Publication
Cobalt			μg/L	16.97	nmol/L	
	S		0.11–0.45		1.9–7.6	1
	U		1–2		17.0–34.0	
			μg/kg		nmol/kg	
	RBC		16–46		272–781	
Complement C3	S		mg/dL	0.01	g/L	
Values (0–<19 y) based on Abbott Architect method		0–14 d	50–121		0.5–1.2	4
		15 d–<1 y	51–160		0.5–1.6	
		1–<19 y	83–152		0.8–1.5	
		Adult (20–60 y)	90–180		0.9–1.8	1
Complement C4	S		mg/dL	0.01	g/L	
Values (0–<19 y) based on Abbott Architect method		0–<1 y	7–30		0.1–0.3	4
		1–<19 y	13–37		0.1–0.4	
		Adult (20–60 y)	10–40		0.1–0.4	1
Copper	S		μg/dL	0.157	μmol/L	
		Birth-6 mo	20–70		3.1–10.9	1
		Deficiency	<30		<5	
		6 y	90–190		14.1–29.8	
		12 y	80–160		12.5–25.1	
		Adult, M	70–140		10.9–21.9	
		F	80–155		12.5–24.3	
		Deficiency	50		8	
		Pregnancy, at term	118–302		18.5–47.4	
		Blacks	Blacks 8–12% higher		Blacks 8–12% higher	
	U, 24 h		μg/dL	0.157	μmol/L	
		Adults	<60 μg/24 h		1.0 μmol/24 h	
		Wilson disease	>200 μg/24 h		>3 μmol/24 h	
Cortisol, free (see also Chapter 66)	S		μg/dL	27.6	nmol/L	
		0800 h	0.6–1.6		17–44	1
		1600 h	0.2–0.9		6–15	
	Sal	See Table 82.2				
	U, 24 h	Child	μg/d	2.76	nmol/d	
		1–10 y	2–27		6–74	
		2–11 y	1–21		3–58	
		11–20 y	5–55		14–152	
		12–16 y	2–38		6–105	
		Adult	μg/d	2.76	nmol/d	
		Extracted	20–90		55–248	
		Unextracted (HPLC)	<50		<138 nmol/d	See Chapter 66
Cortisol, total	S		μg/dL	27.6	nmol/L	
		Cord blood	5–17		138–469	1
Pediatric values (2 d–<19 y) based on Abbott Architect method		2–<15 d	1–12		13–340	2
		15 d–<1 y	1–17		14–458	
		1–<9 y	2–11		48–297	
		9–<14 y	2–13		60–349	
		14–<17 y	3–16		77–453	
		17–<19 y	4–18		97–506	
		Adult	μg/dL	27.6	nmol/L	1
		0800 h	3–21		83–580	
		0800 h	5–23		138–635	

TABLE A.1 Pediatric and Adult Reference Intervals for Biochemical Markers (Serum, Plasma, and Urine—cont'd

Analyte	Specimen	Condition	REFERENCE INTERVALS Conventional Units	Conversion Factor	SI Units	Reference Publication
		1600 h	3–16		83–441	
		2000 h	<50% of 0800 h values		<50% of 0800 h values	
Creatine kinase, myocardial bound (CKMB), mass* (see Chapter 58)						
C-reactive protein (CRP), high sensitivity	S		mg/L	1	mg/L	
Values (0–<3 y) based on Abbott Architect method		0–14 d	0.3–6.1		0.3–6.1	4
		15 d–<3 y	0.1–1.0		0.1–1.0	
Values (3–79 y) based on OCD Vitros method		3–5 y	0.1–2.4		0.1–2.4	10
		6–11 y	0.1–5.9		0.1–5.9	
		12–13 y	0.1–1.9		0.1–1.9	
		14–16 y	0.1–2.9		0.1–2.9	
		17–39 y, M	0.1–6.0		0.1–6.0	
		F	0.1–12.1		0.1–12.1	
		40–79 y	0.1–8.8		0.1–8.8	
		Males				
		American	0.3–8.6		0.3–8.6	1
		White American	0.2–12.3		0.2–12.3	
		African American	0.1–8.2		0.1–8.2	
		Mexican American	0.2–6.3		0.2–6.3	
		European	0.3–8.6		0.3–8.6	
		Japanese	<7.8		<7.8	
		Females				
		American	0.2–9.1		0.2–9.1	
		European	0.3–8.8		0.3–8.8	
Creatine kinase (CK)	S		U/L	0.017	μkat/L	
IFCC, 37°C		M	46–171		0.78–2.90	1
		F	34–145		0.58–2.47	
CK isoenzymes	S	Fraction 2 (MB)	<5.0 μg/L	1	<5.0 μg/L	1
		Relative index MB/total	<3.9%	0.01	<0.039 fractional activity	
Creatinine			mg/dL	88.4	μmol/L	
Enzymatic	S	0–14 d	0.32–0.92		28–81	4
Values (0–<3 y) based on Abbott Architect method		15 d–<2 y	0.10–0.36		9–32	
		2–<3 y	0.20–0.43		18–38	
Values (3–79 y) based on OCD Vitros method		3–5 y	0.31–0.51		28–45	9
		6–7 y	0.36–0.56		32–49	
		8–9 y	0.37–0.63		32–56	
		10–11 y	0.43–0.68		38–60	
		12–15 y, M	0.47–0.91		42–81	
		12–16 y, F	0.48–0.84		42–74	
		16–79 y, M	0.71–1.16		63–102	
		17–79 y, F	0.56–0.96		49–85	
	U		mg/dL	0.0884	mmol/L	

Continued

TABLE A.1 Pediatric and Adult Reference Intervals for Biochemical Markers (Serum, Plasma, and Urine—cont'd

Analyte	Specimen	Condition	REFERENCE INTERVALS Conventional Units	Conversion Factor	SI Units	Reference Publication
Values (3–79 y) based on OCD Vitros method		3–5 y	14.71–151.58		1–13	9
		6–11 y	13.57–195.70		1–17	
		12–13 y	21.49–214.93		2–19	
		14–29 y	19.23–305.43		2–27	
		30–79 y, M	14.71–294.12		1–26	
		F	12.44–229.64		1–20	
Jaffe			mg/dL	88.4	µmol/L	
	S	Cord	0.60–1.20		53–106	1
		0–14 d	0.42–1.05		37–93	4
		15 d–<1 y	0.31–0.53		28–47	
		1–<4 y	0.39–0.55		34–48	
		4–<7 y	0.44–0.65		39–57	
		7–<12 y	0.52–0.69		46–61	
		12–<15 y	0.57–0.80		50–71	
		15–<17 y, F	0.59–0.86		52–76	
		M	0.65–1.04		58–92	
		17–<19 y, F	0.60–0.88		53–78	
		M	0.69–1.10		61–97	
		18–60 y, M	0.90–1.30		80–115	1
		F	0.60–1.10		53–97	
		60–90 y, M	0.80–1.30		71–115	
		F	0.60–1.20		53–106	
		>90 y, M	1.00–1.70		88–150	
		F	0.60–1.30		53–115	
Jaffe, manual	U, 24 h		mg/kg/d	8.84	µmol/kg/d	
		Infant	8–20		71–177	1
		Child	8–22		71–194	
		Adolescent	8–30		71–265	
		Adult, M	14–26		124–230	
		F	11–20		97–177	
Creatinine clearance (see Glomerular filtration rate)						
C-Telopeptide	S		ng/L	1	ng/L	
		0–<1 y	210–4390		210–4390	8
Values (0–<19 y) based on Abbott Architect method		1–<6 y	350–4480		350–4480	
		6–<19 y	780–6790		780–6790	
		Men	<1009		<1009	1
		Premenopausal women	<574		<574	
	U, 24 h		mg/mol creatinine	1	mg/mol creatinine	
		Men	0–505		0–505	1
		Premenopausal women	0–476		0–476	
Cyanide	WB (Ox)		mg/L	38.5	µmol/L	
		Nonsmokers	<0.2		<7.7	1
		Smokers	<0.4		<15.4	
		Nitroprusside therapy	Up to 100 without toxicity		Up to 3850	
		Toxic	>1		38.5	

TABLE A.1 Pediatric and Adult Reference Intervals for Biochemical Markers (Serum, Plasma, and Urine—cont'd

			REFERENCE INTERVALS			
Analyte	**Specimen**	**Condition**	**Conventional Units**	**Conversion Factor**	**SI Units**	**Reference Publication**
Cystatin C	S		mg/L	1	mg/L	
Pediatric values (0–<19 y) based on Abbott Architect method		0–<1 mo	1.49–2.85		1.49–2.85	8
		1–<5 mo	1.01–1.92		1.01–1.92	
		5 mo–<1 y	0.75–1.53		0.75–1.53	
		1–<2 y, F	0.60–1.20		0.60–1.20	
		1–<2 y, M	0.77–1.85		0.77–1.85	
		2–<19 y	0.62–1.11		0.62–1.11	
		Adult, F	0.61–1.05		0.61–1.05	13
		M	0.71–1.21		0.71–1.21	
Cystine	S		mg/dL	83.3	μmol/L	
		Premature, 1 d	0.54–1.02		45–85	1
		Newborn, 1 d	0.43–1.01		36–84	
		1–3 mo	0.15–1.15		13–96	
		2–6 mo	0.64–0.97		53–81	
		3–10 y	0.54–0.92		45–77	
		6–18 y	0.43–0.70		36–58	
		Adult	0.40–1.40		33–117	
	U, 24 h		mg/d	8.33	μmol/d	
		10 d–7 wk	2.16–3.37		18–28	
		3–12 y	4.9–30.9		41–257	
		Adult	<38.1		<317	
			mg/g creatinine	0.94	mmol/mol creatinine	
		Adult	2–14		1.9–13.1	
Dehydroepiandrosterone, unconjugated	S		ng/dL	0.0347	nmol/L	
		Children				1
		6–9 y, M	13–187		0.45–6.49	
		6–9 y, F	18–189		0.62–6.55	
		10–11 y, M	31–205		1.07–7.11	
		10–11 y, F	112–224		3.88–7.77	
		12–14 y, M	83–258		2.88–8.95	
		12–14 y, F	98–360		3.40–12.5	
		Adult				
		M	180–1250		6.25–43.4	
		F	130–980		4.51–34.0	
Dehydroepiandrosterone sulfate	S		μg/dL	0.027	μmol/L	
Pediatric values (0–<19 y) based on Abbott Architect method		Children				8
		0–<2 mo	1110–>1565		30.1–>42.5	
		2–<6 mo	25–599		0.7–16.3	
		6 mo–<1 y	6–184		0.2–5.0	
		1–<6 y	3–117		0.1–3.2	
		6–<9 y	5–159		0.2–4.3	
		9–<13 y	35–281		0.9–7.6	
		13–<16 y	58–479		1.6–13.0	
		16–<19 y, F	152–595		4.1–16.1	
		16–<19 y, M	129–700		3.5–19.0	
		Pubertal levels,				
		Tanner stage				1
		1, M	5–265		0.1–7.2	
		1, F	5–125		0.1–3.4	
		2, M	15–380		0.4–10.3	
		2, F	15–150		0.4–4.0	

Continued

TABLE A.1 Pediatric and Adult Reference Intervals for Biochemical Markers (Serum, Plasma, and Urine—cont'd

			REFERENCE INTERVALS			
Analyte	**Specimen**	**Condition**	**Conventional Units**	**Conversion Factor**	**SI Units**	**Reference Publication**
		3, M	60–505		1.6–13.6	
		3, F	20–535		0.5–14.4	
		4, M	65–560		1.8–15.1	
		4, F	35–485		0.9–13.1	
		5, M	165–500		4.4–13.5	
		5, F	75–530		2.0–14.3	
		Adults				
		18–30 y, M	125–619		3.4–16.7	
		18–30 y, F	45–380		1.2–10.3	
		31–50 y, M	5–532		1.6–12.2	
		31–50 y, F	12–379		0.8–10.2	
		51–60 y, M	20–413		0.5–11.1	
		61–83 y, M	10–285		0.3–7.7	
		Postmenopausal F	30–260		0.8–7.0	
11-Deoxycortisol	S		ng/dL	0.0289	nmol/L	
		Cord blood	295–554		9–16	1
		Children and adults	20–158		0.6–4.6	
Deoxypyridinoline	U		µmol/mol creatinine	1	µmol/mol creatinine	
		Men	2.3–5.4		2.3–5.4	1
		Premenopausal women	3.0–7.4		3.0–7.4	
Dihydrotestosterone	S		ng/dL	0.0334	nmol/L	
		Child, prepubertal	<3		<0.10	1
		Adult, M	30–85		1.03–2.92	
		Adult, F	4–22		0.14–0.76	
Dodecanedioic acid	U				µmol/mol creatinine	
					<0.06	1
Dopamines	P, S		pg/mL		nmol/L	
L-Dopa (1-dodecenoylcarnitine)		Normotensive adults	1042–2366	0.0051	5.3–12.0	1
DOPAC (3,4-dihydroxyphenylacetic acid)			674–2636	0.0059	4.0–15.7	
DHPG (3,4-dihydroxyphenylglycol)			797–1208	0.0059	4.7–7.1	
DU-PAN-2			U/mL	1	kU/L	
			<401		<401	1
Estradiol	S		pg/mL	3.69	pmol/L	
Values (15 d–<19 y) based on Abbott Architect method		Child				
		15 d–<1 y	<25		<92	5
		1–<9 y, F	<10		<37	
		9–<11 y, F	<48		<176	
		11–<12 y, F	<94		<345	
		12–<14 y, F	11–172		39–631	
		14–19 y, F	<255		<936	
		1–<11 y, M	<13		<46	
		11–<13 y, M	<26		<95	
		13–<15 y, M	<28		<102	
		15–<19 y, M	<38		<141	
		Adults				1
		M	10–50		37–184	

TABLE A.1 Pediatric and Adult Reference Intervals for Biochemical Markers (Serum, Plasma, and Urine—cont'd

Analyte	Specimen	Condition	REFERENCE INTERVALS Conventional Units	Conversion Factor	SI Units	Reference Publication
		F				
		Early follicular phase	20–150		73–550	
		Late follicular phase	40–350		147–1285	
		Midcycle	150–750		550–2753	
		Luteal phase	30–450		110–1652	
		Postmenopausal	<21		<74	
Tanner (Values based on Abbott Architect method)		Pubertal levels				
		Tanner stage				
		1, M	<19		<68	5
		1, F	<20		<74	
		2, M	<18		<67	
		2, F	<26		<96	
		3, M	<21		<76	
		3, F	<86		<317	
		4, M	<35		<128	
		4, F	13–141		49–517	
		5, M	17–34		64–126	
		5, F	19–208		69–762	
Estriol, free (unconjugated, uE3)	S		ng/mL	3.47	nmol/L	
		Males and nonpregnant females	<2.0		<6.9	1
		Pregnancy, wk of gestation				
		16	0.30–1.05		1.04–3.64	
		18	0.63–2.30		2.19–7.98	
		34	5.3–18.3		18.4–63.5	
		35	5.2–26.4		18.0–91.6	
		36	8.2–28.1		28.4–97.5	
		37	8.0–30.1		27.8–104.0	
		38	8.6–38.0		29.8–131.9	
		39	7.2–34.3		25.0–119.0	
		40	9.6–28.9		33.3–100.3	
	Amf	See Table 82.2				
Estriol, total (E3)	S		ng/mL	3.47	nmol/L	
		Pregnancy, wk of gestation				1
		34	38–140		132–486	
		35	31–140		108–486	
		36	35–330		121–1145	
		37	45–260		156–902	
		38	48 -350		167–1215	
		39	59–570		205–1978	
		40	95–460		330–1596	
	U, 24 h		μg/d	3.47	nmol/d	
		M	1.0–11.0		3.5–38.2	
		F				
		Follicular phase	0–15.0		0–52.0	
		Ovulatory phase	13.0–54.0		45.1–187.4	
		Luteal phase	8.0–60.0		27.8–208.2	
		Postmenopausal	0–11.0		0–38.2	

Continued

TABLE A.1 Pediatric and Adult Reference Intervals for Biochemical Markers (Serum, Plasma, and Urine—cont'd

			REFERENCE INTERVALS			
Analyte	**Specimen**	**Condition**	**Conventional Units**	**Conversion Factor**	**SI Units**	**Reference Publication**
		Pregnancy				
		1st trimester	0–800		0–2776	
		2nd trimester	800–12,000		2776–41,640	
		3rd trimester	5000–50,000		17,350–173,500	
	Amf	See Table 82.2				
Estrone	S		pg/mL	3.69	pmol/L	
		M	15–65		55–240	1
		F				
		Early follicular phase	15–150		55–555	
		Late follicular phase	100–250		370–925	
		Luteal phase	15–200		55–740	
Ethanol	WB (Ox)		mg/dL	0.217	mmol/L	
		Impairment	50–100		11–22	1
		Depression of CNS	>100		>21.7	
		Fatalities reported	>400		>86.8	
Ethylmalonic acid	U				mmol/mol creatinine	
					0.4–17	1
Ferritin	S		ng/mL	1	μg/L	
Values (4 d–<3 y) based on Abbott Architect method		4–<15 d	99.6–717.0		99.6–717.0	2
		15 d–<6 mo	14.0–647.2		14.0–647.2	
		6 mo–<1 y	8.4–181.9		8.4–181.9	
		1–<3 y	5.3–99.9		5.3–99.9	
Values (3–79 y) based on the Siemens Immulite method		3–5 y	10.7–85.2		10.7–85.2	10
		6–16 y, M	16.2–106.7		16.2–106.7	
		6–24 y, F	9.6–81.9		9.6–81.9	
		17–37 y, M	39.3–439.4		39.3–439.4	
		25–49 y, F	6.5–147.1		6.5–147.1	
		38–79 y, M	45.8–714.8		45.8–714.8	
		50–79 y, F	6.0–362.6		6.0–362.6	
α-Fetoprotein (AFP)	S		mg/dL	0.01	g/L	
		Fetal, 1st trimester	200–400		2.0–4.0	1
		Cord blood	<5		<0.05	
Pediatric values based on Abbott Architect method			ng/mL	1	μg/L	
		0–<1 mo	>2000		>2000	3
		1–<3 mo	9.80–1359.0		9.80–1359.0	
		3–<6 mo	4.15–274.70		4.15–274.70	2
		6 mo–<1 y	2.66–148.21		2.66–148.21	
		1–<3 y	2.88–20.94		2.88–20.94	
		3–<19 y	0.89–4.48		0.89–4.48	
		Adult (85% of population)	<8.5		<8.5	1
		Adult (100% of population)	<15		<15	
	Maternal serum		ng/mL (median)	1	μg/L (median)	
		Wk of gestation				
		14th	25.6		25.6	
		15th	29.9		29.9	
		16th	34.8		34.8	
		17th	40.6		40.6	

TABLE A.1 Pediatric and Adult Reference Intervals for Biochemical Markers (Serum, Plasma, and Urine—cont'd

Analyte	Specimen	Condition	REFERENCE INTERVALS Conventional Units	Conversion Factor	SI Units	Reference Publication
		18th	47.3		47.3	
		19th	55.1		55.1	
		20th	64.3		64.3	
		21th	74.9		74.9	
		Tumor marker	ng/mL	1	μg/L	
		Early marker	10–20		10–20	
		Cancer	>1000		>1000	
	Amf	See Table 82.2				
Fluoride	S		mg/L	52.6	μmol/L	
			0.2–3.2		10.5–168	1
Folate			ng/mL	2.265	nmol/L	
Values (5 d–<6 y) based on Abbott Architect method	S	5 d–<1 y	>10.6		>23.9	2
		1–<3 y	>3.9		>8.7	
		3–<6 y	>11.9		>27.0	
Values (6–79 y) based on Siemens Immulite method		6–18 y	8.2–30.6		18.6–69.3	10
		19–79 y	9.5–39.0		21.5–88.4	
	Erythrocyte	3–5 y	294.7–883.4		703.1–2012.9	1
		6–79 y	228.2–998.7		541.4–2110.6	
		Note: Reference limits for erythrocytes depend on the level of supplementation in the country.				
	S Deficiency		<1.4		<3.2	
	Erythrocyte deficiency		<110		<252	
Follicle-stimulating hormone (FSH)	S		mIU/mL	1	IU/L	
Values (30 d–<19 y) based on Abbott Architect method		30 d–<1 y, F	0.4–10.4		0.4–10.4	5
		1–<9 y, F	0.4–5.5		0.4–5.5	
		9–<11 y, F	0.4–4.2		0.4–4.2	
		11–19 y, F	0.3–7.8		0.3–7.8	
		30 d–<1 y, M	0.1–2.4		0.1–2.4	
		1–<5 y, M	<0.9		<0.9	
		5–<10 y, M	<1.6		<1.6	
		10–<13 y, M	0.4–3.9		0.4–3.9	
		13–<19 y, M	0.8–5.1		0.8–5.1	
		Pubertal levels, Tanner stage				
		1, M	<1.5		<1.5	
		1, F	0.6–4.1		0.6–4.1	
		2, M	<3.0		<3.0	
		2, F	0.3–5.8		0.3–5.8	
		3, M	0.4–6.2		0.4–6.2	
		3, F	0.1–7.2		0.1–7.2	
		4, M	0.6–5.1		0.6–5.1	
		4, F	0.3–7.0		0.3–7.0	
		5, M	0.8–7.2		0.8–7.2	
		5, F	0.4–8.6		0.4–8.6	
		M (23–70 y)	1.4–15.4		1.4–15.4	1
		F				
		Follicular phase	1.4–9.9		1.4–9.9	
		Midcycle peak	0.2–17.2		0.2–17.2	
		Luteal phase	1.1–9.2		1.1–9.2	
		Postmenopausal	19.3–100.6		19.3–100.6	

Continued

TABLE A.1 Pediatric and Adult Reference Intervals for Biochemical Markers (Serum, Plasma, and Urine—cont'd

Analyte	Specimen	Condition	REFERENCE INTERVALS Conventional Units	Conversion Factor	SI Units	Reference Publication
Fructosamine	S	Child	5% below adult levels			1
		Adult	205–285 μmol/L		205–285 μmol/L	
Fumaric acid	U				mmol/mol creatinine	
		0–1 mo			10–45	1
		1–6 mo			4–45	
		6 mo–5 y			1–27	
		>5 y			2–4	
Glomerular filtration rate (endogenous) based on KDIGO	Categories		mL/ min/1.73 m^2	0.00963	mL/s/m^2	
	G1	Normal or high	≥90		≥0.87	26
	G2	Mildly decreased	60–89		0.58–0.86	
	G3a	Mildly to moderately decreased	45–59		0.43–0.57	
	G3b	Moderately to severely decreased	30–44		0.29–0.42	
	G4	Severely decreased	15–29		0.14–0.28	
	G5	Kidney failure	<15		<0.14	
Glucagon	P (Hep or EDTA)	Adult	ng/L		ng/L	
			70–180		70–180	1
	Amf	See Table 82.2				
Glucose	S, fasting		mg/dL	0.0555	mmol/L	
		Cord	45–96		2 .5–5.3	1
		Premature	20–60		1.1–3.3	
		Neonate	30–60		1.7–3.3	
		Newborn				
		1 d	40–60		2.2–3.3	
		>1 d	50–80		2.8–4.5	
		Child	60–100		3.3–5.6	
		Adult	74–100		4.1–5.6	
		>60 y	82–115		4.6–6.4	
		>90 y	75–121		4.2–6.7	
		Decision Limits				
		Normal glucose metabolism	≤100		≤5.55	
		Diabetes	≥126		≥7.00	
	CSF	See Table 82.2				
	U		1–15		0.1–0.8	
	U, 24 h		<0.5 g/d	5.55	<2.8 mmol/d	
Glucose-6-phosphate dehydrogenase (G-6-PD) in erythrocytes, WHO and ICSH	WB (ACD, EDTA, or Hep)		7.9–16.3 U/g Hb	64.5	510–1050 U/ mmol Hb	1
			230–470 U/ 10^{12} RBC	10^{-3}	0.23–0.47 nU/ RBC	
			2.69–5.53 U/ mL RBC	1	2.69–5.53 U/ mL RBC	
Glutamic acid	P		mg/dL	68	μmol/L	
		Premature, 1 d	0–1.98		0–135	1
		Newborn, 1 d	0.29–1.57		20–107	
		6 mo–3 y	0.28–1.47		19–100	

TABLE A.1 Pediatric and Adult Reference Intervals for Biochemical Markers (Serum, Plasma, and Urine—cont'd

Analyte	Specimen	Condition	REFERENCE INTERVALS Conventional Units	Conversion Factor	SI Units	Reference Publication
		3–10 y	0.34–3.68		23–250	
		6–18 y	0.10–0.96		7–65	
		Adult	0.21–2.82		14–192	
	U 24 h		mg/d	6.8	µmol/d	
		10 d–7 wk	0.3–1.5		2–10	
		Adult	<33.8		<230	
			mg/g creatinine	0.77	mmol/mol creatinine	
		Adult	2–6		1.5–4.7	
Glutamine	P		mg/dL	68.5	µmol/L	
		3 mo–6 y	6.93–10.89		475–746	1
		6–18 y	5.26–10.80		360–740	
		Adult	5.78–10.38		396–711	
	U, 24 h		mg/d	6.85	µmol/d	
		10 d–7 wk	12.4–25.8		85–177	
		3–12 y	20.4–113.7		140–779	
		Adult	43.8–151.8		300–1040	
			mg/g creatinine	0.77	mmol/mol creatinine	
		Adult	2–78		2–60	
γ-Glutamyltransferase	S		U/L	0.017	µkat/L	
Values (0–<3 y) based on Abbott Architect method		0–<14 d	23–219		0.38–3.65	4
		15 d–<1 y	8–127		0.13–2.12	
		1–<3 y	6–16		0.10–0.27	
Values (3–79 y) based on OCD Vitros method		3–5 y	11–20		0.19–0.34	9
		6–14 y, M	10–26		0.17–0.44	
		6–17 y, F	9–24		0.15–0.41	
		15–19 y, M	10–33		0.17–0.56	
		18–35 y, F	12–38		0.20–0.65	
		20–35 y, M	12–62		0.20–1.05	
		36–79 y, M	13–109		0.22–1.85	
		36–79 y, F	10–54		0.17–0.92	
Glutaric acid	U				mmol/mol creatinine	
					0.5–13	1
Glycated hemoglobin (HbA_{1c})	WB (EDTA, Hep or Ox)		%		mmol/mol (IFCC)	
Values (6–79 y) based on OCD Vitros method		6–39 y	4.9–6.1		30–43	10
		40–79 y	5.0–6.3		31–45	
		Cutoff for diagnosis	≥6.5 (NGSP)		≥48	30
Glyceric acid	U				mmol/mol creatinine	
		0–1 mo			<40	1
		1–6 mo			<185	
		6 mo–5 y			<71	
		>5y			<61	
Glycine	P		mg/dL	133.3	µmol/L	
		Premature 1 d	0–7.57		0–1010	1
		Newborn 1 d	1.68–3.86		224–514	
		1–3 mo	0.79–1.67		106–222	
		2–6 mo	1.31–2.22		175–296	
		9 mo–2 y	0.42–2.31		56–308	

Continued

TABLE A.1 Pediatric and Adult Reference Intervals for Biochemical Markers (Serum, Plasma, and Urine—cont'd

Analyte	Specimen	Condition	REFERENCE INTERVALS Conventional Units	Conversion Factor	SI Units	Reference Publication
		3–10 y	0.88–1.67		117–223	
		6–18 y	1.18–2.27		158–302	
		Adult	0.90–4.16		120–554	
	U, 24 h		mg/d	13.3	μmol/d	
		10 d–7 wk	14.6–9.2		194–787	
		3–12 y	12.4–106.8		165–1420	
		Adult	59.0–294.6		785–3918	
			mg/g creatinine	1.51	mmol/mol creatinine	
		Adult	12–108		18.2–163	
Glycolic acid	U				mmol/mol creatinine	
		0–1 mo			<63	1
		1–6 mo			<105	
		6 mo–5 y			2–121	
		>5 y			<167	
Glyoxylic acid	U				mmol/mol creatinine	
		0–1 mo			<14	1
		1–6 mo			<17	
		6 mo–5 y			<8	
		>5 y			<10	
Growth hormone	S		ng/mL	1	μg/L	
		Basal	2–5		2–5	1
		Insulin tolerance test	>10		>10	
		Arginine	>7.5		>7.5	
		L-Dopa	>7.5		>7.5	
Haptoglobin	S		mg/dL	0.01	g/L	
Values (0–<19 y) based on Abbott Architect method		0–14 d	0–10		0–0.1	4
		15 d–<1 y	7–221		0.1–2.2	
		1–<12 y	7–163		0.1–1.6	
		12–<19 y	7–179		0.1–1.8	
		Adult (20–60 y)	30–200		0.3–2.0	1
High-density lipoprotein cholesterol (HDL-C)	S		mg/dL	0.0259	mmol/L	
Reference Intervals						
Values (0–<3 y) based on Abbott Architect method		0–14 d	15–42		0.4–1.1	4
		15 d–<1 y	12–71		0.3–1.9	
		1–<3 y	32–63		0.8–1.6	
Values (3–79 y) based on OCD Vitros method		3–5 y	31–73		0.8–1.9	9
		6–14 y	35–81		0.9–2.1	
		15–79 y, M	31–70		0.8–1.8	
		F	35–89		0.9–2.3	
Clinical Decision Limits		Pediatric	mg/dL	0.0259	mmol/L	
		Acceptable	>45		>1.2	27
		Borderline	40–45		1.0–1.2	
		Low	<40		<1.0	
	ATP II classification					
		Low	<40		<1.0	1
		High	>59		>1.5	

TABLE A.1 Pediatric and Adult Reference Intervals for Biochemical Markers (Serum, Plasma, and Urine—cont'd

Analyte	Specimen	Condition	REFERENCE INTERVALS Conventional Units	Conversion Factor	SI Units	Reference Publication
Histidine	P		mg/dL	64.5	μmol/L	
		Premature, 1 d	0.16–1.40		10–90	1
		Newborn, 1 d	0.76–1.77		49–114	
		1–3 mo	0.66–1.30		43–83	
		2–6 mo	1.49–2.12		96–137	
		9 mo–2 y	0.37–1.74		24–112	
		3–10 y	0.37–1.32		24–85	
		6–18 y	0.99–1.64		64–106	
		Adult	0.50–1.66		32–107	
	U, 24 h		mg/d	6.45	μmol/d	
		10 d–7 wk	16.0–38.6		103–249	
		3–12 y	47.4–199.2		306–1285	
		Adult	72.9–440.8		470–2843	
			mg/g creatinine	0.73	mmol/mol creatinine	
		Adult	1–141		1–103	
Homocysteine, total	S, P		μmol/L	1	μmol/L	
		Folate-supplemented diet				1
		<15 y	<8		<8	
		15–65 y	<12		<12	
		>65 y	<16		<16	
		No folate supplementation				
		<15 y	<10		<10	
		15–65 y	<15		<15	
		>65 y	<20		<20	
Values (5 d–<6 y) based on Abbott Architect method		5 d–<1 y	2.9–10.0		2.9–10.0	2
		1–<6 y	2.8–7.6		2.8–7.6	
Values (6–79 y) based on OCD Vitros method		6–12 y	1.7–6.9		1.7–6.9	10
		13–25 y, M	3.6–10.6		3.6–10.6	
		13–39 y, F	2.9–9.5		2.9–9.5	
		26–79 y, M	5.2–14.1		5.2–14.1	
		40–79 y, F	3.7–10.9		3.7–10.9	
Homogentisic acid	U				mmol/mol creatinine	
					<11	1
Homovanillic acid (HVA)	U, 24 h		mg/d	5.49	μmol/d	
		3–6 y	1.4–4.3		8–24	1
		6–10 y	2.1–4.7		12–26	
		10–16 y	2.4–8.7		13–48	
		16–83 y	1.4–8.8		8–48	
	U	*See Chapter 63, Table 63.6				1
3-Hydroxybutyric acid	U				mmol/mol creatinine	
		0–5 y			<6	1
		>5 y			<11	

Continued

TABLE A.1 **Pediatric and Adult Reference Intervals for Biochemical Markers (Serum, Plasma, and Urine—cont'd**

Analyte	Specimen	Condition	REFERENCE INTERVALS Conventional Units	Conversion Factor	SI Units	Reference Publication
2-Hydroxyglutaric acid	U				mmol/mol creatinine	
					<16	1
5-Hydroxyindoleacetic acid		*See Chapter 63, Table 63.16				
4-Hydroxyphenyllactic acid	U				mmol/mol creatinine	
		0–1 mo			<51	1
		>1mo			<11	
4-Hydroxyphenylpyruvic acid	U				mmol/mol creatinine	
		0–1 mo			<21	1
		>1mo			<6	
17-Hydroxyprogesterone			ng/dL	0.03	nmol/L	
		Cord blood	900–5000		27.3–151.5	1
		Premature	26–568		0.8–17.0	
Values (4 d–<19 y) based on Abbott Architect method		4 d–<1 y	<130		<4.2	5
		1–<10 y	<35		<1.1	
		10–<15 y	13–90		0.4–2.7	
		15–<19 y, F	20–1030		0.6–32.6	
		15–<19 y, M	20–60		0.5–1.8	
Tanner values based on Abbott Architect method		Puberty-Tanner stage				
		1, M	<44		<1.4	
		1, F	<28		<0.9	
		2, M	<44		<1.4	
		2, F	13–41		0.4–1.3	
		3, M	<50		<1.6	
		3, F	16–47		0.5–1.5	
		4, M	<41		<1.3	
		4, F	19–72		0.6–2.3	
		5, M	13–50		0.4–1.6	
		5, F	<1028		<34.4	
		Adults				1
		M	27–199		0.8–6.0	
		F				
		Follicular phase	15–70		0.4–2.1	
		Luteal phase	35–290		1.0–8.7	
		Pregnancy	200–1200		6.0–36.0	
For LC-MSMS reference intervals please see: *Clin Chem* 2006;52:1559–1567		Post ACTH	<320		<9.6	
		Postmenopausal	<70		<2.1	
Hydroxyproline	P		mg/dL	76.3	μmol/L	
		Premature, 1 d	0–1.56		0–120	1
		6–18 y, M	<0.66		<50	
		6–18 y, F	<0.58		<44	
		Adult, M	<0.55		<42	
		Adult, F	<0.45		<34	
	U, 24 h		mg/d	7.63	μmol/d	
		Adult	<1.4		<11	
			mg/g creatinine	0.863	mmol/mol creatinine	
		Adult	19–36		16–31	

TABLE A.1 Pediatric and Adult Reference Intervals for Biochemical Markers (Serum, Plasma, and Urine—cont'd

			REFERENCE INTERVALS			
Analyte	**Specimen**	**Condition**	**Conventional Units**	**Conversion Factor**	**SI Units**	**Reference Publication**
Immunoglobulin A	S, P		mg/dL	0.01	g/L	
Values (0–<19 y) based on Abbott Architect method		0–<1 y	1–29		0.0–0.3	4
		1–<3 y	4–90		0.0–0.9	
		3–<6 y	26–147		0.3–1.5	
		6–<14 y	47–221		0.5–2.2	
		14–<19 y	53–287		0.5–2.9	
		Adult (20–60 y)	70–400		0.7–4.0	1
		Adult (>60 y)	90–4 10		0.9–4.1	
	Saliva	See Table 82.2				
	CSF	See Table 82.2				
Immunoglobulin D	S		IU/mL	1	kIU/L	
		Adult (20–60 y)	0–160		0–160	1
			ng/mL	1	µg/L	
			0–384		0–384	
Immunoglobulin E	S		kIU/L	2.4	µg/L	
Values (0–<19 y) based on Abbott Architect method		0–<7 y	<25–440		<60–1057	8
		7–<19 y	<25–450		<60–1079	
		Adult (20–60 y)	0–160		0–380	1
Immunoglobulin G	S		mg/dL	0.01	g/L	
Pediatric values (0–<19 y) based on Abbott Architect method		0–14 d	320–1407		3.2–14.1	4
		15 d–<1 y	108–702		1.1–7.0	
		1–<4 y	316–1148		3.2–11.5	
		4–<10 y	542–1358		5.4–13.6	
		10–<19 y	658–1534		6.6–15.3	
		Adult (20–60 y)	700–1600		7.0–16.0	1
		Adult (>60 y)	600–1560		6.0–15.6	
	CSF	See Table 82.2				
Immunoglobulin M	S		mg/dL	0.01	g/L	
Values (0–<19 y) based on Abbott Architect method		0–14 d	5–35		0.1–0.4	4
		15 d–13 wk	12–71		0.1–0.7	
		13 wk–<1 y	16–86		0.2–0.9	
		1–<19 y, F	48–186		0.5–1.9	
		1–<19 y, M	39–151		0.4–1.5	
		Adult (20–60 y)	40–230		0.4–2.3	1
		Adult (>60 y)	30–360		0.3–3.6	
	CSF	See Table 82.2				
Inhibin A	S		pg/mL	1	ng/L	
		M	1.0–3.6		1.0–3.6	1
		F (cycling; days of cycle)				
		Early follicular phase (−14 to −10 d)	5.5–28.2		5.5–28.2	
		Midfollicular phase (−9 to −4 d)	7.9–34.5		7.9–34.5	
		Late follicular phase (−3 to −1 d)	19.5–102.3		19.5–102 .3	
		Midcycle (d 0)	49.9–155.5		49.9–155.5	
		Early luteal (1–3 d)	35.9–132.7		35.9–132.7	
		Midluteal (4–11 d)	13.2–159.6		13.2–159.6	
		Late luteal (12–14 d)	7.3–89.9		7.3–89.9	
		IVF, peak levels	354–1690		354–1690	

Continued

TABLE A.1 Pediatric and Adult Reference Intervals for Biochemical Markers (Serum, Plasma, and Urine—cont'd

			REFERENCE INTERVALS			
Analyte	**Specimen**	**Condition**	**Conventional Units**	**Conversion Factor**	**SI Units**	**Reference Publication**
		PCOS, ovulatory	5.7–16.0		5.7–16.0	
		Postmenopausal	1.0–3.9		1.0–3.9	
Insulin	S		µIU/mL	6	pmol/L	
Values (0–<6 y) based on Abbott Architect method		0–<1 y	1.0–23.4		7–163	8
		1–<6 y	1.3–40.2		9–279	
Values (6–79 y) based on Siemens Immulite and ADVIA Centaur methods		6–10 y	0.4–13.0		3–93	10
		11–19 y	2.1–19.5		15–140	
		20–79 y	2.4–21.8		17–157	
Insulin-like growth factor-I	S		ng/mL	1	µg/L	
		1–2 y				1
		M	31–160		31–160	
		F	11–206		11–206	
		3–6 y				
		M	16–288		16–288	
		F	70–316		70–316	
		7–10 y				
		M	136–385		136–385	
		F	123–396		123–396	
		11–12 y				
		M	136–440		136–440	
		F	191–462		191–462	
		13–14 y				
		M	165–616		165–616	
		F	286–660		286–660	
		15–18 y				
		M	134–836		134–836	
		F	152–660		152–660	
		19–25 y				
		M	202–433		202–433	
		F	231–550		231–550	
		Adult (25–85 y)				
		M	135–449		135–449	
		F	135–449		135–449	
Insulin-like growth factor II	S		ng/mL	1	µg/L	
		Child				1
		Prepubertal	334–642		334–642	
		Pubertal	245–737		245–737	
		Adult	288–736		288–736	
		GH deficiency	51–299		51–299	
Iodine	U		µg/dL	0.079	µmol/L	
Values based on manual microplate analysis		3–5 y	5–83		0.39–6.58	9
		6–79 y	1–49		0.09–3.88	
Iron			µg/dL	1	µmol/L	
Values based on Abbott Architect method		0–<14 y	16–128		2.8–22.9	4
		14–<19 y, F	20–162		3.5–29.0	
		14–<19 y, M	31–168		5.5–30.0	
Isocitric acid	U				mmol/mol creatinine	
		0–1 mo			0–368	1
		1–6 mo			0–67	

TABLE A.1 Pediatric and Adult Reference Intervals for Biochemical Markers (Serum, Plasma, and Urine—cont'd

Analyte	Specimen	Condition	REFERENCE INTERVALS Conventional Units	Conversion Factor	SI Units	Reference Publication
		6 mo–5 y			0–77	
		>5 y			16–99	
Isoleucine	P		mg/dL	76.3	µmol/L	
		Premature, 1 d	0.26–0.78		20–60	1
		Newborn, 1 d	0.35–0.69		27–53	
		1–3 mo	0.59–0.95		45–73	
		2–6 mo	0.50–1.61		38–123	
		9 mo–2 y	0.34–1.23		26–94	
		3–10 y	0.37–1.10		28–84	
		6–18 y	0.50–1.24		38–95	
		Adult	0.48–1.28		37–98	
	U		mg/d	7.62	µmol/d	
		10 d-7 wk	Trace-0.4		Trace-3	
		3–12 y	2–7		15–53	
		Adult	5–24		38–183	
			mg/g creatinine	0.86	mmol/mol creatinine	
		Adult	1–5		0.8–4.4	1
L-Lactate	WB (Hep)		mg/dL	0.111	mmol/L	
		At bed rest				
		Venous	5–12		0.56–1.39	1
		Arterial	<22		<2.5	
			16–17		1.78–1.88	
	CSF	See Table 82.2				
	U, 24 h	Adult				
					mmol/mol creatinine	
		0–1 mo			46–348	
		1–6 mo			57–346	
		6 mo-5 y			21–38	
		>5 y			20–101	
	Gastric fluid	See Table 82.2				
Lactate dehydrogenase (LD)	S		U/L	0.017	µkat/L	
		24 mo–12 y	180–360		3.1–6.1	1
		12 y-60 y	125–220		2.1–3.7	
Lead	WB (Hep)		µg/dL	0.0483	µmol/L	
		Child	<25		<1.21	1
		Adult	<25		<1.21	
		Toxic	>99		>4.78	
	U, 24 h		µg/L		µmol/L	
			<80		<0.39	
Leucine	P		mg/dL	76.3	µmol/L	
		Premature, 1 d	0.26–1.58		20–120	1
		Newborn, 1 d	0.62–1.43		47–109	
		1–3 mo	10.58–2.14		44–164	
		9 mo–2 y	0.59–2.03		45–155	
		3–10 y	0.73–2.33		56–178	
		6–18 y	1.03–2.28		79–174	
		Adult	0.98–2.29		75–175	
	U, 24 h		mg/d	7.624	µmol/d	
		10 d–7 wk	0.9–2.0		7–15	
		3–12 y	3–11		23–84	

Continued

TABLE A.1 Pediatric and Adult Reference Intervals for Biochemical Markers (Serum, Plasma, and Urine—cont'd

Analyte	Specimen	Condition	REFERENCE INTERVALS Conventional Units	Conversion Factor	SI Units	Reference Publication
		Adult	2.6–8.1 mg/g creatinine	0.86	20–62 mmol/mol creatinine	
		Adult	0–8		0–6.8	
Lipase	S		U/L	0.017	µkat/L	
Values (0–<19 y) based on Abbott Architect method		0–<19 y	4–39		0.07–0.65	4
37°C		Adult	<38		<0.65	1
Low-density lipoprotein cholesterol (LDL-C) (measured)	S		mg/dL	0.0259	mmol/L	
Reference Intervals		6–24 y, F	46–143		1.2–3.7	9
Values (6–79 y) based on OCD Vitros method		25–49 y, M	62–189		1.6–4.9	
		F	50–178		1.3–4.6	
		50–79 y	73–189		1.9–4.9	
		Note: The more recent guidelines suggest that risk stratification should rely only on the 10-year atherosclerotic cardiovascular disease risk calculation (2013 ACC/AHA guideline on the treatment of blood cholesterol to reduce atherosclerotic cardiovascular risk in adults).				
Clinical Decision Limits			mg/dL	0.0259	mmol/L	
		Risk for coronary heart disease, Child				27
		Acceptable	<110		<2.8	
		Borderline	110–129		<3.3	
		High	>130		>3.4	
		Risk for coronary heart disease, Adults				1
		Optimal	<100		<2.59	
		Near/above optimal	100–129		2.59–3.34	
		Borderline high	130–159		3.37–4.12	
		High	160–189		4.15–4.90	
		Very high	>189		>4.90	
Lecithin-to-sphingomyelin ratio	Amf	See Table 82.2				1
Luteinizing hormone (LH)			mIU/mL	1	IU/L	
Values (4d–<19 y) based on Abbott Architect method		4 d–<3 mo F	<2.4		<2.4	5
		3 mo–<1 y F	<1.2		<1.2	
		1–<10 y, F	<0.3		<0.3	
		10–<13 y, F	<4.3		<4.3	
		13–<15 y, F	0.4–6.5		0.4–6.5	
		15–<17 y, F	<13.1		<13.1	
		17–<19 y, F	<8.4		<8.4	
Tanner values based on Abbott Architect method		Pubertal levels, Tanner stage				
		1, M	<1.2		<1.2	
		1, F	<0.1		<0.1	
		2, M	<1.2		<1.2	
		2, F	<2.3		<2.3	
		3, M	<2.3		<2.3	
		3, F	<7.4		<7.4	

TABLE A.1 Pediatric and Adult Reference Intervals for Biochemical Markers (Serum, Plasma, and Urine—cont'd

Analyte	Specimen	Condition	REFERENCE INTERVALS Conventional Units	Conversion Factor	SI Units	Reference Publication
		4, M	<4.9		<4.9	
		4, F	0.3–6.7		0.3–6.7	
		5, M	0.6–5.9		0.6–5.9	
		5, F	0.4–21.2		0.4–21.2	
		M (23–70 y)	1.2–7.8		1.2–7.8	1
		F				
		Follicular phase	1.7–15.0		1.7–15.0	
		Midcycle peak	21.9–56.6		21.9–56.6	
		Luteal phase	0.6–16.3		0.6–16.3	
		Postmenopausal	14.2–52.3		14.2–52.3	
Lysine	P		mg/dL	68.5	μmol/L	
		Premature, 1 d	1.01–4.53		70–310	1
		Newborn, 1 d	1.66–3.93		114–269	
		1–3 mo	0.54–2.46		37–169	
		9 mo–2 y	0.66–2.10		45–144	
		3–10 y	1.04–2.20		71–151	
		6–18 y	1.58–3.40		108–233	
		Adult	1.21–3.47		83–238	
	U, 24 h		mg/d	6.85	μmol/d	
		10 d–7 wk	5.7–10.9		39–75	
		3–12 y	9.3–93.7		64–642	
		Adult	3.1–153.0		21–1048	
			mg/g creatinine	0.77	mmol/mol creatinine	
		Adult	4–12		3.2–9.2	
α_2-Macroglobulin	S		mg/dL	0.01	g/L	
		Adult (20–60 y)	130–300		1.3–3.0	1
Magnesium AAS	S		mg/dL	0.4114	mmol/L	
		Newborn, 2–4 d	1.5–2.2		0.62–0.91	1
		5 mo–6 y	1.7–2.3		0.70–0.95	
		6–12 y	1.7–2.l		0.70–0.86	
		>12 y	1.6–2.6		0.66–1.07	
			mg/24 h	0.04114	mmol/24 h	
	U, 24 h		12–291		0.50–12.0	
Magnesium, free	S		mmol/L	1.0	mmol/L	
			0.45–0.60		0.45–0.60	1
Magnesium, total (enzymatic)	S		mg/dL	0.4114	mmol/L	
		0–14 d	1.99–3.94		0.82–1.62	4
		15 d–<1 y	1.97–3.09		0.81–1.27	
		1–<19 y	2.09–2.84		0.86–1.17	
Malic acid	U				mmol/mol creatinine	
		0–1 mo			0–52	1
		1–6 mo			8–73	
		6 mo–5 y			4–57	
		>5 y			17–47	
Manganese			μg/L	18.0	nmol/L	
	WB (Hep)		5–15		90–270	1
	S		0.5–1.3		9–24	

Continued

TABLE A.1 Pediatric and Adult Reference Intervals for Biochemical Markers (Serum, Plasma, and Urine—cont'd

Analyte	Specimen	Condition	REFERENCE INTERVALS Conventional Units	Conversion Factor	SI Units	Reference Publication
	U, collect in metal-free container		0.5–9.8		9.1–178	
		Toxic conc	>19		>342	
Mercury			µg/L	4.99	nmol/L	
	WB (EDTA)		0.6–59		3.0–294.4	1
	U, 24 h		<20		<99.8	
		Toxic conc	>150		>748.5	
		Lethal conc	>800		>3992	
Metanephrines (in serum, plasma)						1
Normetanephrine (free)	S, P	*See Chapter 63				1
Metanephrine (free)	S, P	*See Chapter 63				1
Normetanephrine (total)	S, P	*See Chapter 63				1
Metanephrine (total)	S, P	*See Chapter 63				1
Metanephrines (total in urine)						
Metanephrine	U, 24 h	*See Chapter 63, Table 63.10				1
Metanephrine	U	*See Chapter 63, Table 63.10				1
Normetanephrine	U, 24 h	*See Chapter 63, Table 63.10				1
Normetanephrine	U	*See Chapter 63, Table 63.10				1
Methanol		See Tables 82.3 and 82.5				
Methemoglobin (MetHb)	WB (EDTA, Hep or ACD)		g/dL	155	µmol/L	
			0.06–0.24		9.3–37.2	1
			% of total Hb		Mass fraction of total Hb	
			0.04–1.52		0.0004–0.0152	
Methionine			mg/dL	67.7	µmol/L	
	P	Premature, 1 d	0.38–0.66		25–45	1
		Newborn, 1 d	0.13–0.61		9–41	
		1–3 mo	0.05–0.57		3–39	
		2–6 mo	0.24–0.73		16–49	
		9 mo–2 y	0.04–0.43		3–29	
		3–10 y	0.16–0.24		11–16	
		6–18 y	0.24–0.55		16–37	
		Adult	0.09–0.60		6–40	
			mg/d	6.7	µmol/d	
		10 d–7 wk	0.1–1.9		0.7–13	
		3–12 y	3–14		20–95	
		Adult	<9.1		<63	
			mg/g creatinine	0.76	mmol/mol creatinine	
		Adult	0–9.5		0–7.2	
2-Methylbutyrylglycine	U				mmol/mol creatinine	
					0.2–5	1

TABLE A.1 Pediatric and Adult Reference Intervals for Biochemical Markers (Serum, Plasma, and Urine—cont'd

Analyte	Specimen	Condition	REFERENCE INTERVALS Conventional Units	Conversion Factor	SI Units	Reference Publication
Methylsuccinic acid	U				mmol/mol creatinine	
					0–12	1
β_2-Microglobulin	S		mg/dL	10	mg/L	
Values (0–<19 y) based on Abbott Architect method		0–<3 mo, F	0.19–0.58		1.9–5.8	1
		0–<3 mo, M	0.19–0.47		1.9–4.7	
		3 mo–<2 y	0.13–0.45		1.3–4.5	
		2–<19 y	0.12–0.23		1.2–2.3	
			mg/dL (mean)	10	mg/L (mean)	
		0–59 y	0.19		1.9	
		60–69 y	0.21		2.1	
		>70 y	0.24		2.4	
Molybdenum			μg/L		nmol/L	
	S		0.1–3.0	10.42	1.0–31.3	1
	U, 24 h		40–60 μg/d		416–625 nmol/d	
Niacin	U, 24 h		mg/d	7.3	μmol/d	
			2.4–6.4		17.5–46.7	1
Nickel			μg/L	17	nmol/L	
	S or P (Hep)		0.14–1.0		2.4–17.0	1
	WB		1.0–28.0		17–476	
			μg/d		nmol/d	
	U, 24 h		0.1–10		2–170	
N-telopeptide (BCE = bone collagen equivalents)	S		nmol BCE/L	1.0	nmol BCE/L	
		Men	5.4–24.2		5.4–24.2	1
		Premenopausal women	6.2–19.0		6.2–19.0	
			nmol BCE/ mmol creatinine	1.0	nmol BCE/ mmol creatinine	
		Men	3–63		3–63	
		Premenopausal women	5–65		5–65	
Nuclear matrix protein 22 (NMP-22)	S		U/mL	1.0	kU/L	
			<10		<10	1
Orotic acid					mmol/mol creatinine	
	U	0–1 mo			1.4–5.3	1
		1–6 mo			1.0–3.2	
		6 mo–5 y			0.5–3.3	
		>5 y			0.4–1.2	
Osteocalcin	S		ng/mL	1.0	μg/L	
		Adult, M	3.0–13.0		3.0–13.0	1
		Adult, F				
		Premenopausal	0.4–8.2		0.4–8.2	
		Postmenopausal	1.5–11.0		1.5–11.0	
Oxalic acid					mmol/mol creatinine	
	U	0–1 mo			51–931	1
		1–6 mo			7–567	

Continued

TABLE A.1 Pediatric and Adult Reference Intervals for Biochemical Markers (Serum, Plasma, and Urine—cont'd

Analyte	Specimen	Condition	REFERENCE INTERVALS Conventional Units	Conversion Factor	SI Units	Reference Publication
		6 mo–5 y			7–352	
		>5 y			<188	
2-Oxoglutaric acid	S				mmol/mol creatinine	
		0–1 mo			22–567	1
		1–6 mo			63–552	
		6 mo–5 y			36–103	
		>5 y			41–82	
Oxygen, partial pressure (PO_2)	Cord blood		mm Hg	0.133	kPa	
	Arterial		5.7–30.5		0.8–4.0	1
	Venous		17.4–41.0		2.3–5.5	
	WB, arterial	Birth	8–24		1.06–3.19	
		5–10 min	33–75		4.39–9.96	
		30 min	31–85		4.12–11.31	
		1 h	55–80		7.32–10.64	
		1 d	54–95		7.18–12.64	
		2 d–60 y	83–108		11.04–14.36	
		>60 y	>80		> 10.64	
		>70 y	>70		>9.31	
		>80 y	>60		>7.98	
		>90 y	>50		>6.65	
Oxygen, saturation (sO_2)	WB, arterial		Percent saturation	0.01	Fraction saturation	
		Newborn	40–90		0.40–0.90	1
		Thereafter	94–93		0.94–0.98	
Oxytocin	P, EDTA		μU/mL	1.0	mU/L	
		M	1.1–1.9		1.0–1.9	1
		F				
		Nonpregnant	1.0–1.8		1.0–1.8	
		Second stage of labor	3.2–5.3		3.2–5.3	
Pantothenic acid			μg/L	0.0046	μmol/L	
	WB		344–583		1.57–2.66	1
			mg/d	4.53	μmol/d	
	U, 24 h		1–15		5–68	
Parathyroid hormone, intact	S		pg/mL	0.106	pmol/L	
Values (6 d–<3 y) based on Abbott Architect method		6 d–<1 y	6–89		0.7–9.4	2
		1–<3 y	16–63		1.7–6.7	
Values (3–79 y) based on DiaSorin LIAISON method		3–5 y	7–29		0.7–3.1	10
		6–11 y	7–30		0.7–3.2	
		12–15 y	8–36		0.8–3.8	
		16–29 y	8–32		0.8–3.4	
		30–79 y	9–42		1.0–4.4	
Parathyroid hormone, (1–84)	S		pg/mL	1.0	ng/L	
			6–40		6–40	1
Parathyroid hormone-related peptide (PTHrP)	S		pmol/L	1.0	pmol/L	
			<1.4		<1.4	1

TABLE A.1 Pediatric and Adult Reference Intervals for Biochemical Markers (Serum, Plasma, and Urine—cont'd

Analyte	Specimen	Condition	REFERENCE INTERVALS Conventional Units	Conversion Factor	SI Units	Reference Publication
pH (37°C)	WB, arterial		pH	1.0	pH	
		Cord blood				1
		Arterial	7.18–7.38		7.18–7.38	
		Venous	7.25–7.45		7.25–7.45	
		Newborn				
		Premature, 48 h	7.35–7.50		7.35–7.50	
		Full term				
		Birth	7.11–7.36		7.11–7.36	
		5–10 min	7.09–7.30		7.09–7.30	
		30 min	7.21–7.38		7.21–7.38	
		1 h	7.26–7.49		7.26–7.49	
		1 d	7.29–7.45		7.29–7.45	
		Children, adults				
		Arterial	7.35–7.45		7.35–7.45	
		Venous	7.32–7.43		7.32–7.43	
		Adults				
		60–90 y	7.31–7.42		7.31–7.42	
		>90 y	7.26–7.43		7.26–7.43	
Phenylalanine			mg/dL	60.5	μmol/L	
	Dry blood spot		<2.1		<122	1
	P	Premature	2.0–7.5		121–454	
		Newborn	1.2–3.4		73–205	
		Phenylketonuric 2–3 d	>4.5		>272	
		Phenylketonuric untreated	15–30		907–1815	
		Adult	0.8–1.8			
			mg/d	6.05	μmol/d	
	U, 24 h	10 d DiaSorin LIAISON 7 wk	1.2–1.7		7–10	
		3–13 y	4.0–17.5		24–106	
		Adult	<16.5		<100	
			mg/g creatinine	0.68	mmol/mol creatinine	
		Adult	2–10		1.3–6.9	
3-Phenylpropionylglycine	U				mmol/mol creatinine	
					<0.7	1
Phosphate	S		mg/dL	0.323	mmol/L	
Values (0–<3 y) based on Abbott Architect method		0–14 d	5.6–10.5		1.80–3.40	4
		15 d–<1 y	4.8–8.4		1.54–2.72	
		1–<3 y	4.3–6.8		1.38–2.19	
Values (3–79 y) based on OCD Vitros method		3–5 y	4.4–6.0		1.41–1.94	9
		6–10 y	4.4–5.7		1.41–1.85	
		11–15 y, M	3.8–5.9		1.24–1.91	
		F	3.6–5.6		1.16–1.81	
		16–47 y	2.9–4.7		0.95–1.52	
		48–79 y, M	2.8–4.7		0.89–1.52	
		F	3.1–4.8		0.99–1.54	
	U, 24 h		g/d	32.3	mmol/d	
		Adults	0.4–1.3		12.9–42.0	

Continued

TABLE A.1 Pediatric and Adult Reference Intervals for Biochemical Markers (Serum, Plasma, and Urine—cont'd

Analyte	Specimen	Condition	REFERENCE INTERVALS Conventional Units	Conversion Factor	SI Units	Reference Publication
Phosphatase, acid tartrate resistant 37°C	S		U/L	0.017	μkat/L	
		Children	3.4–9.0		0.05–0.15	1
		Adult	1.5–4.5		0.03–0.08	
Phosphatase, alkaline IFCC, 37°C	S		U/L	0.017	μkat/L	
Values (0–<3 y) based on Abbott Architect method		0–14 d	90–273		1.50–4.55	4
		15 d–<1 y	134–518		2.23–8.63	
		1–<3 y	156–369		2.60–6.15	
Values (3–79 y) based on OCD Vitros method		3–5 y	144–327		2.45–5.56	9
		6–10 y	153–367		2.60–6.24	
		11–15 y, M	113–438		1.92–7.45	
		11–15 y, F	64–359		1.09–6.10	
		16–21 y, M	56–167		0.95–2.84	
		16–29 y, F	44–107		0.75–1.82	
		22–79 y, M	50–116		0.85–1.97	
		30–79 y, F	46–122		0.78–2.07	
Phosphatase, alkaline (bone specific, by immunoabsorption)	S		U/L	1.0	U/L	
		Men	15.0–41.3		15.0–41.3	1
		Premenopausal women	11.6–29.6		11.6–29.6	
Phosphatase, alkaline isoenzymes						1
Percentage of Total Activity	<1 y	1–15 y	Adult	Pregnant women	Postmenopausal women	
Biliary	3–6	2–5	1–3	1–3	0–12	
Liver	20–34	22–34	17–35	5–17	17–48	
Bone	20–30	21–30	13–19	8–14	8–21	
Placental	8–19	5–17	13–21	53–69	7–15	
Renal	1–3	0–1	0–2	3–6	0–2	
Intestinal	0–2	0–1	0–1	0–1	0–1	
Fraction Activity	<1 y	1–15 y	Adult	Pregnant women	Postmenopausal women	
Biliary	0.03–0.06	0.02–0.05	0.01–0.03	0.01–0.03	0.0–0.12	
Liver	0.20–0.34	0.22–0.34	0.17–0.35	0.05–0.17	0.17–0.48	
Bone	0.20–0.30	0.21–0.30	0.13–0.19	0.08–0.14	0.08–0.21	
Placental	0.08–0.19	0.05–0.17	0.13–0.21	0.53–0.69	0.07–0.15	
Renal	0.01–0.03	0.0–0.01	0.0–0.02	0.03–0.06	0.0–0.02	
Intestinal	0.0–0.02	0.0–0.01	0.0–0.01	0.0–0.01	0.0–0.01	
Pimelic acid	U				mmol/mol creatinine <1.1	1
Porphobilinogen	U, 24 h		mg/L <2.26	4.42	μmol/L <10	1

TABLE A.1 **Pediatric and Adult Reference Intervals for Biochemical Markers (Serum, Plasma, and Urine—cont'd**

Analyte	Specimen	Condition	REFERENCE INTERVALS Conventional Units	Conversion Factor	SI Units	Reference Publication
Porphyrins, total	U, 24h				nmol/L	
					20–320	1
	Feces				nmol/L g dry wt	
					10–200	
	Erythrocytes				µmol/L erythrocytes	
					0.4–1.7	
Potassium (K)			mEq/L	1.0	mmol/L	
	S	Premature cord	5.0–10.2		5.0–10.2	1
		Premature, 48 h	3.0–6.0		3.0–6.0	
		Newborn cord	5.6–12.0		5.6–12.0	
		Newborn	3.7–5.9		3.7–5.9	
		Infant	4.1–5.3		4.1–5.3	
Values (3–79 y) based on OCD Vitros method		3–5 y	3.9–4.6		3.9–4.6	9
		6–79 y	3.8–4.9		3.8–4.9	
			mEq/d	1.0	mmol/d	
	U, 24 h	6–10 y				
		M	17–54		17–54	1
		F	8–37		8–37	
		10–14 y				
		M	22–57		22–57	
		F	18–58		18–58	
		Adult	25–125		25–125	
Proinsulin	S		pmol/L	1.0	pmol/L	
			1.1–6.9		1.1–6.9	1
Prolactin	S		ng/mL	21.0	mIU/L	
		Cord blood	45–539		945–11319	1
Values (4 d–<19 y) based on Abbott Architect method		4–<30 d	13–213		273–4473	5
		30 d–<1 y	6–114		126–2394	
		1–<19 y	4–23		84–483	
		Puberty, Tanner stage				
		1, M	3–20		63–420	
		1, F	2–20		42–420	
		2, M	4–19		84–399	
		2, F	4–23		84–483	
		3, M	4–23		84–483	
		3, F	4–23		84–483	
		4, M	6–20		126–420	
		4, F	6–23		126–483	
		5, M	7–32		147–672	
		5, F	5–23		105–483	
		Adult				1
		M	3.0–14.7		63.0–308.7	
		F	3.8–23.0		79.8–483.0	
		Pregnancy, 3rd trimester	95–473		1995–9933	
Proline			mg/dL	86.9	µmol/L	
	P	Premature, 1 d	0.92–4.36		80–380	1
		Newborn, 1 d	1.23–3.18		107–277	
		1–3 mo	0.89–3.73		77–325	
		9 mo–2 y	0.59–2.13		51–185	
		3–10 y	0.78–1.70		68–148	
		6–18 y	0.67–3.72		58–324	

Continued

TABLE A.1 Pediatric and Adult Reference Intervals for Biochemical Markers (Serum, Plasma, and Urine—cont'd

Analyte	Specimen	Condition	REFERENCE INTERVALS Conventional Units	Conversion Factor	SI Units	Reference Publication
	U, 24 h	Adult	1.17–3.86		102–336	
			mg/d	8.69	μmol/d	
		10 d–7 wk	3.2–11.0		28–96	
		3–12 y	Trace		Trace	
		Adult	Trace		Trace	
			μmol/g creatinine	0.113	μmol/mol creatinine	
		0–1 mo	70–2300		7.91–259.9	
		1–6 mo	<600		<67.8	
		6 mo–1 y	<300		<33.9	
		1–2 y	<270		<30.5	
		2–3 y	<220		<24.9	
Propionylcarnitine					μmol/L	
	P	0–7 d			0.07–1.85	1
		8 d–7 y			0.17–1.27	
		>7 y			0.17–1.49	
	WB spots				0.55–8.01	
	Bile spots				0.36–8.10	
					mmol/mol creatinine	
	U	0–7 d			0.01–0.20	
		8 d–7 y			0.01–1.20	
		>7 y			0.00–0.06	
Prostate-specific antigen (PSA)	S		ng/mL	1.0	μg/L	
		M				1
		40–49 y	0–2.5		0–2.5	
		50–59 y	0–3.5		0–3.5	
		60–69 y	0–4.5		0–4.5	
		70–79 y	0–6.5		0–6.5	
Protein, total			g/dL	10	g/ L	
	Cord		4.8–8.0		48–80	1
	S	Premature	3.6–6.0		36–60	
Values (0–<3 y) based on Abbott Architect method		0–14 d	5.3–8.3		53–83	4
		15 d–<1 y	4.4–7.1		44–71	
		1–<3 y	6.1–7.5		61–75	
Values (3–79 y) based on OCD Vitros method		3–5 y	6.3–8.1		63–81	9
		6–19 y	6.8–8.2		68–82	
		20–29 y	6.5–8.3		65–83	
		30–79 y	6.5–7.8		65–78	
	U, 24 h		mg/dL	10	mg/L	1
		Adult	1–14		10–140	
		Excretion	mg/d	0.001	g/d	
		Adult	<100		<0.1	
		Pregnancy	<150		<0.15	
	CSF	See Table 82.2				
Pyroglutamic acid	U				mmol/mol creatinine	
					<62	1
Pyruvic acid			mg/dL	0.114	μmol/L	
	WB, arterial	Adult	0.2–0.7		0.02–0.08	1
	WB, venous	Adult	0.3–0.9		0.03–0.10	
	CSF	See Table 82.2				

TABLE A.1 **Pediatric and Adult Reference Intervals for Biochemical Markers (Serum, Plasma, and Urine—cont'd**

Analyte	Specimen	Condition	REFERENCE INTERVALS Conventional Units	Conversion Factor	SI Units	Reference Publication
	U, 24 h	Adult			<1.1 mmol/d	
					mmol/mol creatinine	
	U	0–1 mo			24–123	
		1–6 mo			8–90	
		6 mo–5 y			3–19	
		>5 y			6–9	
Retinol-binding protein (RBP)			mg/dL	10	mg/L	
	S	Birth	1.1–3.4		11–34	1
		6 mo	1.8–5.0		18–50	
		Adult	3.0–6.0		30–60	
Reverse triiodothyronine (rT_3)	S		ng/dL	0.0154	nmol/L	
		Cord (>37 wk)	130–300		2.00–4.62	1
		Children				
		1 d	83–194		1.28–2.99	
		2 d	107–209		1.65–3.22	
		3 d	102–166		1.57–2.56	
		1 mo–20 y	10–35		0.15–0.54	
		Adult	10–28		0.15–0.43	
		Maternal serum (15–40 wk)	11–33		0.17–0.51	
		Amniotic serum (17–22 wk)	163–599		2.51–9.22	
Rheumatoid factor (RF)	S		IU/mL	1	kIU/L	
Values (0–<19 y) based on Abbott Architect method		0–14 d	9.0–17.1		9.0–17.1	4
		15 d–<19 y	9.0–9.0		9.0–9.0	
		Adult	<7.5–14		<7.5–14	24
Riboflavin (vitamin B_2)			µg/dL	26.6	nmol/L	
	S		4–24		106–638	1
	Erythrocytes		10–50		266–1330	
			µg/g creatinine	0.3	µmol/mol creatinine	
	U		>80		>24	
			µg/d	2 .66	nmol/d	
	U, 24 h		>100		>266	
Sebacic acid	U	0–1 mo			mmol/mol creatinine	1
		1–6 mo			3–16	
		>6 mo			3–26	
					<9	
Selenium	S		µg/L	0.0127	µmol/L	
		Neonates	<8.0 (deficiency)		<0.10 (deficiency)	1
		<2 y	16–71		0.2–0.9	
		2–4 y	40–103		0.5–1.3	
		4–16 y	55–134		0.7–1.7	
		Adults	63–160		0.8–2.0	
	WB (Hep)		58–234		0.74–2.97	
	U, 24 h		7–160		0.09–2.03	
		Toxic conc	>400		>5.08	
Serotonin		*See Chapter 63, Table 63.15				11

Continued

TABLE A.1 Pediatric and Adult Reference Intervals for Biochemical Markers (Serum, Plasma, and Urine—cont'd

			REFERENCE INTERVALS			
Analyte	**Specimen**	**Condition**	**Conventional Units**	**Conversion Factor**	**SI Units**	**Reference Publication**
Sex hormone–binding globulin (SHBG)	S		nmol/L	1	nmol/L	
Values (4 d–<19 y) based on Abbott Architect method		4 d–<1 mo	14.4–120.2		14.4–120.2	5
		1 mo–<1 y	36.2–229.0		36.2–229.0	
		1–<8 y	41.8–188.7		41.8–188.7	
		8–<11 y	26.4–162.4		26.4–162.4	
		11–<13 y	14.9–107.8		14.9–107.8	
		13–<15 y	11.2–98.2		11.2–98.2	
		15–<17 y, F	9.8–84.1		9.8–84.1	
		17–<19 y, F	10.8–154.6		10.8–154.6	
Tanner values based on Abbott Architect method		Puberty, Tanner stage				
		1, M	23.4–156.8		23.4–156.8	
		1, F	21.1–210.1		21.1–210.1	
		2, M	27.5–133.4		27.5–133.4	
		2, F	29.6–140.7		29.6–140.7	
		3, M	17.4–160.1		17.4–160.1	
		3, F	23.7–101.7		23.7–101.7	
		4, M	12.2–79.4		12.2–79.4	
		4, F	12.1–125.6		12.1–125.6	
		5, M	7.7–49.4		7.7–49.4	
		5, F	15.3–92.5		15.3–92.5	
		Adult				25
		20 y	13.1–53.2		13.1–53.2	
		30 y	13.5–57.4		13.5–57.4	
		40 y	15.3–65.3		15.3–65.3	
		50 y	18.4–75.6		18.4–75.6	
		60 y	22.6–87.6		22.6–87.6	
		70 y	27.8–101.0		27.8–101.0	
		80 y	33.8–115.4		33.8–115.4	
Sodium (Na)			mEq/L	1.0	mmol/L	
		Premature cord	116–140		116–140	1
		Premature, 48 h	128–148		128–148	
		Newborn cord	126–166		126–166	
		Newborn	133–146		133–146	
		Infant	139–146		139–146	
Values (3–79 y) based on OCD Vitros method		3–5 y	135–142		135–142	9
		6–15 y	136–143		136–143	
		16–49 y, M	137–143		137–143	
		F	137–142		137–142	
		50–79 y	136–143		136–143	
	U, 24 h	6–10 y	mEq/d	1.0	mmol/d	1
		M	41–115		41–115	
		F	20–69		20–69	
		10–14 *y*				
		M	63–177		63–177	
		F	48–168		48–168	
		Adult				
		M	40–220		40–220	
		F	27–287		27–287	
Suberic acid	U				mmol/mol creatinine	
		0–6 mo			4–20	1
		>6 mo			<9	

TABLE A.1 Pediatric and Adult Reference Intervals for Biochemical Markers (Serum, Plasma, and Urine—cont'd

Analyte	Specimen	Condition	REFERENCE INTERVALS Conventional Units	Conversion Factor	SI Units	Reference Publication
Succinic acid	U				mmol/mol creatinine	
		0–1 mo			35–547	1
		1–6 mo			34–156	
		6 mo–5 y			16–118	
		> 5y			29–87	
Testosterone, bioavailable (Vermeulen equation)	S		ng/dL	0.0347	nmol/L	
Values (0–<19 y) based on Abbott Architect method		0–<1 y, F	0.29–6.05		0.01–0.21	7
		1–<9 y, F	0.29–6.05		0.01–0.21	
		9–<14 y, F	0.58–10.95		0.02–0.38	
		14–<19 y, F	3.75–23.05		0.13–0.80	
		0–<1 y, M	0–121.9		0.01–4.23	
		1–<9 y, M	0.29–2.88		0.01–0.10	
		9–<14 y, M	0.58–161.69		0.02–5.62	
		14–<19 y, M	12.1–346.69		0.42–12.03	
		Adult				
		M	66–417		2.29–14.5	1
		F	0.6–5.0		0.02–0.17	
Testosterone, free (Vermeulen Equation)	S		pg/mL	3.47	pmol/L	
		Cord, M	5–22		17.4–76.3	1
		Cord, F	4–19		13.9–55.5	
Values (0–<19 y) based on Abbott Architect method		0–<1 y, F	0.1–2.6		0.4–9.0	7
		1–<9 y, F	0.1–2.6		0.4–9.0	
		9–<14 y, F	0.3–4.7		1.0–16.3	
		14–<19 y, F	1.4–9.9		4.9–34.4	
		0–<1 y, M	0.03–57.2		0.1–198.6	
		1–<9 y, M	0.1–1.2		0.4–4.2	
		9–<14 y, M	0.4–72.2		1.4–250.7	
		14–<19 y, M	5.0–142.3		17.4–494.1	
		Adult				
		M	50–210		174–729	
		F	1.0–8.5		3.5–29.5	
Testosterone, total	S		ng/dL	0.0347	nmol/L	
		Cord, M	13–55		0.45–1.91	1
		Cord, F	5–45		0.17–1.56	
		Premature				
		M	37–198		1.28–6.87	
		F	5–22		0.17–0.76	
Values (4d–<19 y) based on Abbott Architect method		4 d–<9 y, F	1–62		0.0–2.15	5
		9–<13 y, F	<28		<0.98	
		13–<15 y, F	10–44		0.36–1.54	
		15–<19 y, F	14–49		0.49–1.70	
		4 d–<6 mo, M	9–299		0.3–10.37	
		6 mo–<9 y, M	<36		<1.24	
		9–<11 y, M	<23		<0.81	
		11–<14 y, M	<444		<15.42	
		14–<16 y, M	36–632		1.25–21.94	
		16–<19 y, M	148–794		5.13–27.55	

Continued

TABLE A.1 **Pediatric and Adult Reference Intervals for Biochemical Markers (Serum, Plasma, and Urine—cont'd**

Analyte	Specimen	Condition	REFERENCE INTERVALS Conventional Units	Conversion Factor	SI Units	Reference Publication
Tanner values based on Abbott Architect method		1, M	<18		<0.62	
		1, F	<19		<0.67	
		2, M	<25		<0.85	
		2, F	<20		<0.69	
		3, M	<543		<18.85	
		3, F	<42		<1.45	
		4, M	9–636		0.30–22.08	
		4, F	9–42		0.31–1.44	
		5, M	100–760		3.46–26.36	
		5, F	4–50		0.13–1.72	
		Adult				
		M	260–1000		9–34.72	1
		F	15–70		0.52–2.43	
Tetradecanedioic acid	U				mmol/mol creatinine	
					<0.5	1
Thallium			μg/L	4.89	nmol/L	
	WB (Hep)		<5		<24 .5	1
			mg/L		μmol/L	
		Toxic	0.1–8.0		0.5–390	
			μg/L	4.89	Nmol/L	
	U, 24 h		<2.0		<9.8	
			mg/L		μmol/L	
		Toxic	1.0–20.0		4.9–97.8	
Thiocyanate	S		mg/dL	172.4	μmol/L	
		Nonsmokers	<0.4		<69	1
		Smokers	<1.2		<207	
		Nitroprusside therapy	0.6–2.9		103–500	
		Toxic	>5		>862	
Threonine	P		mg/dL	84	μmol/L	
		Premature, 1 d	1.14–3.98		95–335	1
		Newborn, 1 d	1.36–3.99		114–335	
		1–3 mo	0.75–2.67		64–224	
		2–6 mo	2.27–4.33		191–364	
		3–10 y	0.50–1.13		42–95	
		6–18 y	0.88–2.40		74–202	
		Adult	0.94–2.30		79–193	
	U, 24 h		mg/d	8.40	μmol/d	
		10 d–7 wk	1.5–11.9		13–100	
		3–12 y	10.1–29.6		85–249	
		Adult	14.3–46.7		120–392	
			mg/g creatinine	0.95	mmol/mol creatinine	
		Adult	0–28		0–27	
Thyroglobulin (TG)	S		ng/mL	1.0	μg/L	
		Adult euthyroid	3–42		3–42	1
		Athyroidic patient	<5		<5	
Thyrotropin (thyroid-stimulating hormone) (TSH)			μIU/mL	1.0	mIU/L	
	S	Premature, 28–36 wk	0.7–27.0		0.7–27.0	1
		Cord blood (>37 wk)	2.3–13.2		2.3–13.2	

TABLE A.1 Pediatric and Adult Reference Intervals for Biochemical Markers (Serum, Plasma, and Urine—cont'd

Analyte	Specimen	Condition	REFERENCE INTERVALS Conventional Units	Conversion Factor	SI Units	Reference Publication
Values (4 d–<19 y) based on Abbott Architect method		4 d–<6 mo	0.7–4.8		0.7–4.8	2
		6 mo–<14 y	0.7–4.2			
		14–<19 y	0.5–3.4		0.5–3.4	
		Adults				1
		21–54 y	0.4–4.2		0.4–4.2	
		55–87 y	0.5–8.9		0.5–8.9	
		Pregnancy	µU/mL	1.0	mU/L	
		1st trimester	0.1–2.5		0.1–2.5	28
		2nd trimester	0.2–3.0		0.2–3.0	
		3rd trimester	0.3–3.0		0.3–3.0	
	WB (heel puncture)	Newborn screen	<20		<20	
Thyroxine-binding globulin (TBG)			mg/dL	10	mg/L	
	S	Cord	3.6–9.6		36–96	1
		Children				
		4 mo–1 y	3.1–5.6		31–56	
		1–5 y	2.9–5.4		29–54	
		5–10 y	2.5–5.0		25–50	
		10–15 y	2.1–4.6		21–46	
		Adult				
		M	1.2–2.5		12–25	
		F	1.4–3.0		14–30	
		F (oral contraceptive)	1.5–5.5		15–55	
Thyroxine (T_4), total			µg/dL	12.9	nmol/L	
Values (7 d–<19 y) based on Abbott Architect method	S	7 d–<1 y	5.9–13.7		76–176	2
		1–<9 y	6.2–10.3		79–133	
		9–<12 y	5.5–9.3		71–120	
		12–<14 y, F	5.1–8.3		65–107	
		12–<14 y, M	5.0–8.3		65–107	
		14–<19 y, F	5.5–13.0		70–167	
		Adults (15–60 y)				1
		M	4.6–10.5		59–135	
		F	5.5–11.0		65–138	
		>60 y	5.0–10.7		65–138	
		Newborn screen				
		1–5 d	>7.5		>97	
		6 d	>6.5		>84	
Thyroxine, free (FT_4)	S		ng/dL	12.9	pmol/L	
		Newborns (1–4 d)	2.2–5.3		28.4–68.4	1
Values (5 d–<19 y) based on Abbott Architect method		5–15 d	1.1–3.2		13.5–41.3	2
		15–<30 d	0.7–2.5		8.7–32.5	
		30 d–<1 y	0.9–1.7		11.4–21.9	
		1–<19 y	0.9–1.4		11.4–17.6	
		Adults (21–87 y)	0.8–2.7		10.3–34.7	1
		Pregnancy				
		1st trimester	0.7–2.0		9.0–25.7	
		2nd and 3rd trimesters	0.5–1.6		6.4–20.6	
Thyroxine, free index (FT_4I)	S		µg/dL	12 .9	nmol/L	
		Cord	6.0–13.2		77–170	1
		Infants				

Continued

TABLE A.1 Pediatric and Adult Reference Intervals for Biochemical Markers (Serum, Plasma, and Urine—cont'd

			REFERENCE INTERVALS			
Analyte	Specimen	Condition	Conventional Units	Conversion Factor	SI Units	Reference Publication
		1–3 d	9.9–17.5		128–226	
		1 wk	7.5–15.1		97–195	
		1–12 mo	5.0–13.0		65–168	
		Children				
		1–10 y	5.4–12.8		70–165	
		Pubertal child and adult	4.2–13.0		54–168	
Transferrin	S		mg/dL	0.01	g/L	
Values (0–<19 y) based on Abbott Architect method		0–<9 wk	104–224		1.0–2.2	4
		9 wk–<1 y	107–324		1.1–3.2	
		1–<19 y	220–337		2.2–3.4	
		20–60 y	200–360		2.0–3.6	1
		>60 y	160–340		1.6–3.4	
Transketolase, erythrocyte	Erythrocytes		U/g Hb	64.53	kU/mol Hb	
			0.75–1.30		48.4–83.9	1
Transthyretin (prealbumin)	S		mg/dL	10	mg/L	
Values (0–<19 y) based on Abbott Architect method		0–14 d	2–12		20–120	4
		15 d–<1 y	5–24		50–240	
		1–<5 y	12–23		120–230	
		5–<13 y	14–26		140–260	
		13–<16 y	18–31		180–310	
		16–<19 y, F	17–33		170–330	
		16–<19 y, M	20–35		200–350	
		Adult (20–60 y)	20–40		200–400	1
Triglycerides	S		mg/dL	0.0113	mmol/L	
Reference Intervals						
Values (0–<6 y) based on Abbott Architect method		0–14 d	82–259		0.9–2.9	4
		15 d–<1 y	53–258		0.6–2.9	
		1–<6 y	44–197		0.5–2.2	
Values (6–79 y) based on OCD Vitros method		6–29 y	35–186		0.4–2.1	9
		30–79 y M	44–301		0.5–3.4	
		F	35–212		0.4–2.4	
Clinical Decision Limits		Recommended cutoff points, Child	mg/dL	0.0113	mmol/L	27
		0–9 y				
		Acceptable	<75		<0.9	
		Borderline	75–99		0.9–1.1	
		High	>100		>1.1	
		10–19 y				
		Acceptable	<90		<1.0	
		Borderline	90–129		1.0–1.5	
		High	>130		>1.5	
		Recommended cutoff points, Adult	mg/dL	0.0113	mmol/L	1
		Normal	<150		<1.70	
		High	150–199		1.70–2.25	
		Hypertriglyceridemic	200–499		2.26–5.64	
		Very high	>499		>5.64	
Triiodothyronine (T_3), free			pg/dL	0.0154	pmol/L	
	S	Cord	15–391		0.2–6.0	1

TABLE A.1 Pediatric and Adult Reference Intervals for Biochemical Markers (Serum, Plasma, and Urine—cont'd

Analyte	Specimen	Condition	REFERENCE INTERVALS Conventional Units	Conversion Factor	SI Units	Reference Publication
Values (4 d–<19 y) based on Abbott Architect method		4 d–<1 y	234–487		3.6–7.5	2
		1–<12 y	279–442		4.3–6.8	
		12–<15 y, F	247–396		3.8–6.1	
		12–<15 y, M	286–435		4.4–6.7	
		15–<19 y, F	234–370		3.6–5.7	
		15–<19 y, M	227–383		3.5–5.9	
		Adult	210–440		3.2–6.8	1
		Pregnancy	200–380		3.1–5.9	
Triiodothyronine (T_3), total	S		ng/dL	0.0154	nmol/L	
		Cord (>37 wk)	5–141		0.08–2.17	1
Values (4 d–<19 y) based on Abbott Architect method		4 d–<1 y	85–234		1.33–3.60	2
		1–<12 y	113–189		1.74–2.91	
		12–<15 y	98–176		1.50–2.71	
		15–<17 y, F	92–142		1.42–2.18	
		15–<17 y, M	94–156		1.44–2.40	
		17–<19 y	90–168		1.38–2.58	
		Adults				1
		20–50 y	70–204		1.08–3.14	
		50–90 y	40–181		0.62–2.79	
		Pregnancy				
		1st trimester	81–190		1.25–2.93	
		2nd and 3rd trimesters	100–260		1.54–4.00	
Tryptophan			mg/dL	49	µmol/L	
	P	Premature, 1 d	0–1.23		0–60	1
		Newborn, 1 d	<1.37		<67	
		1–16 y	0.49–1.61		24–79	
		>16 y	0.41–1.94		20–95	
			mg/d	4.9	µmol/d	
	U, 24 h	Adult	5–39		25–191	
			mg/g		mmol/mol	
		Adult	<30		<16.5	
Tumor-associated trypsin inhibitor (TATI)			ng/mL	1.0	µg/L	
	S		3–21		3–21	1
	U		7–51		7–51	
Tyrosine	P		mg/dL	55.2	mmol/L	
		Premature, 1 d	0–5.79		0–320	1
		Newborn, 1 d	0.76–1.79		42–99	
		1–3 mo	0.54–2.42		30–134	
		2–6 mo	1.30–3.91		72–216	
		9 mo-2 y	0.20–2.21		1–122	
		3–10 y	0.56–1.29		31–71	
		6–18 y	0.78–1.59		43–88	
		Adult	0.40–1.58		22–87	
	U, 24 h		mg/d	5.52	µmol/d	
		10 d–7 wk	4.0–7.2		22–40	
		3–12 y	7.2–30.4		40–168	
		Adult	12.0–55.1		66–304	
			mg/g creatinine	0.62	mmol/mol creatinine	
		Adult	0–23		0–14.2	

Continued

TABLE A.1 Pediatric and Adult Reference Intervals for Biochemical Markers (Serum, Plasma, and Urine—cont'd

Analyte	Specimen	Condition	REFERENCE INTERVALS Conventional Units	Conversion Factor	SI Units	Reference Publication
Uracil	U				mmol/mol creatinine	1
		0–6 mo			<33	
		6 mo–5 y			<22	
		>5 y			<18	
Urea	S		mg/dL	0.357	mmol/L	
Values (0–<3 y) based on Abbott Architect method		0–<14 d	3–23		1.0–8.2	4
		15 d–<1 y	3–17		1.2–6.0	
		1–<3 y	9–22		3.2–7.9	
Values (3–79) based on OCD Vitros method		3–5 y	9–19		3.1–6.9	9
		6–7 y	8–21		2.8–7.5	
		8–19 y, M	8–20		2.9–7.0	
		20–39 y, M	9–22		3.3–7.9	
		40–59 y, M	10–24		3.5–8.6	
		8–59 y, F	8–19		2.7–6.7	
		60–79 y	10–26		3.6–9.2	
	U, 24 h		g/d	0.0357	mol/d	
			10–20		0.43–0.71	1
Uric acid	S		mg/dL	59.48	µmol/L	
Values (0–<3 y) based on Abbott Architect method		0–14 d	2.8–12.7		167–755	4
		15 d–<1 y	1.6–6.3		95–375	
		1–<3 y	1.8–4.9		107–291	
Values (3–79 y) based on OCD Vitros method		3–<5 y	2.0–4.9		117–291	9
		5–8 y	1.9–5.0		116–295	
		9–10 y	2.4–5.5		142–326	
		11–12 y	2.6–5.8		156–345	
		13–79 y, M	3.7–7.7		218–459	
		F	2.5–6.2		147–366	
Valine	P		mg/dL	85.5	µmol/L	
		Premature, 1 d	0.34–2.70		30–230	1
		Newborn, 1 d	0.94–2.88		80–246	
		1–3 mo	1.13–3.4 1		96–292	
		9 mo–2 y	0.67–3.07		57–262	
		3–10 y	1.50–3.31		128–283	
		6–18 y	1.83–3.37		156–288	
		Adult	1.65–3.71		141–317	
	U, 24 h		mg/d	8.55	µmol/d	
		10 d–7 wk	1.4–3.2		12–27	
		3–12 y	1.8–6.0		15–51	
		Adult	2.5–11.9		21–102	
Vanillylmandelic acid (VMA)	U, 24 h	*See Chapter 63, Table 63.6				1
Vitamin A	S		µg/dL	0.0349	µmol/L	
Values (0–<19 y) based on Abbott Architect method		0–<1 y	8–54		0.3–1.9	6
		1–<11 y	28–44		1.0–1.6	
		11–<16 y	25–55		0.9–1.9	
		16–<19 y	29–75		1.0–2.6	
		Adult	30–80		1.05–2.8	1
Vitamin B_1 (thiamine diphosphate)	WB		90–140 nmol/L	1	90–140 nmol/L	
	Erythrocytes		280–590 ng/g Hb	0.146	40.3–85.0 µmol/mol Hb	1

TABLE A.1 Pediatric and Adult Reference Intervals for Biochemical Markers (Serum, Plasma, and Urine—cont'd

Analyte	Specimen	Condition	REFERENCE INTERVALS Conventional Units	Conversion Factor	SI Units	Reference Publication
Vitamin B_2 (see riboflavin)						
Vitamin B_6	P (EDTA)		ng/mL	4.046	nmol/L	
			5–30		20–121	1
		Deficiency	<5		<20.2	
Vitamin B_{12}			ng/L	0.733	pmol/L	
Reference Intervals						2
Values (5 d–< 3 y) based on Abbott Architect method		5 d–<1 y	259–1576		191–1163	
		1–<3 y	283–1613		209–1190	
Values (3–79 y) based on Siemens Immulite method		3–5 y	310–988		229–729	10
		6–8 y	321–985		237–727	
		9–11 y	276–969		204–715	
		12–79 y	188–908		139–670	
Clinical Decision Limits						
		Acceptable (WHO)	>201		>147	1
		Deficiency (WHO)	<150		<110	
Vitamin C (ascorbic acid)	S		mg/dL	56.78	μmol/L	
			0.4–1.5		23–85	1
		Deficiency	<0.2		<11	
	Leukocyte		20–53 μg/10^8 leukocytes	0.057	1.14–3.01 fmol/10^8 leukocytes	
		Deficiency	<10 μg/108 leukocytes		<0.57 fmol/108 leukocytes	
Vitamin D 25(OH)D	S		ng/mL	2.5	nmol/L	
Values (5 d–<3 y) based on Abbott Architect method		5–<15 d	2–34		4–85	2
		15 d–<3 mo	6–41		15–101	
		3 mo–<1 y	7–47		17–118	
		1–<3 y	13–55		33–137	
Values (3–79 y) based on DiaSorin LIAISON method						10
	P	3–5 y	13–42		33–104	
		6–79 y	8–46		21–116	
		Deficiency	<20		<50	14
1,25(OH)2D			pg/mL	2.4	pmol/L	
			15–60		36–144	1
Vitamin E	S		mg/dL	23.2	μmol/L	
		Premature neonates	0.1–0.5		2.3–11.6	1
Values (0–<19 y) based on Abbott Architect method		0–<1 y	0.2–2.1		4.9–49.6	6
		1–<19 y	0.6–1.4		14.5–33.0	
		Adults	0.5–1.8		12–42	1
Vitamin E: Total cholesterol ratio		1–19 y			3.7–6.7	6
		1–19 y			8.5–44.5	
Vitamin K	S		ng/mL	2.22	nmol/L	
			0.13–1.19		0.29–2.64	1
Zinc	S		μg/dL	0.153	μmol/L	
			80–120		12–18	1
		Deficiency	<30		<5	
	U, 24 h		0.2–1.3 mg/ 24 h	15.3	3–21 μmol/ 24 h	

- **Table A.2.** Reference Intervals for Biochemical Markers in Other Body Fluids
- **Table A.3.** Reference Information for Toxicology and Therapeutic Drugs
- **Table A.4.** Pediatric and Adult Reference Intervals for Hematologic Markers
- **Table A.5.** Critical Values for Biochemical and Hematologic Markers

CHAPTER OUTLINE

Tables A.1 to A.5 include up-to-date reference interval information obtained from recent initiatives to establish adult and pediatric reference intervals for a wide range of biochemical and hematologic markers. As much as possible, data from recent a priori reference interval studies have been used to update each table and provide robust reference information obtained from large studies based on healthy populations. Where no new data were available, original reference intervals were adopted from the previous (fifth edition) tables.[1]

Table A.1 combines biochemical marker reference interval information for both children and adults. Most pediatric reference intervals listed in this chapter are based on recent data published by the Canadian Laboratory Initiative on Pediatric Reference Intervals (CALIPER), a national research project that has established age- and sex-specific reference intervals using data collected from thousands of healthy community children and adolescents.[2-8] The majority of CALIPER reference intervals were determined based on Abbott Architect assays, as indicated in the table. For specific hematology tests, chemistry, and special endocrine markers, both pediatric and adult reference values were obtained through the recent Canadian Health Measures Survey (CHMS) based on a study of approximately 12,000 children, adults, and elderly.[9-11] CHMS reference intervals were determined based on a number of platforms (Ortho Clinical Diagnostics, Raritan, New Jersey; Siemens New York, New York; other), as specified in the tables. Other reference intervals were adopted from reference tables in the fifth edition of this text[1] and other sources.[12-14]

Table A.2 lists reference intervals for routine tests performed on body fluids. Intervals were derived from the fifth edition of this text,[1] as well as from Zhang and associates.[15]

Table A.3 provides reference information for therapeutic drug monitoring, with toxicology tests shown in a separate table. Reference intervals were derived from the fifth edition of this text,[1] as well as from Hiemke and colleagues.[16]

Table A.4 depicts common hematologic markers based on the recent CHMS database.[11]

Text continued on p. 1816

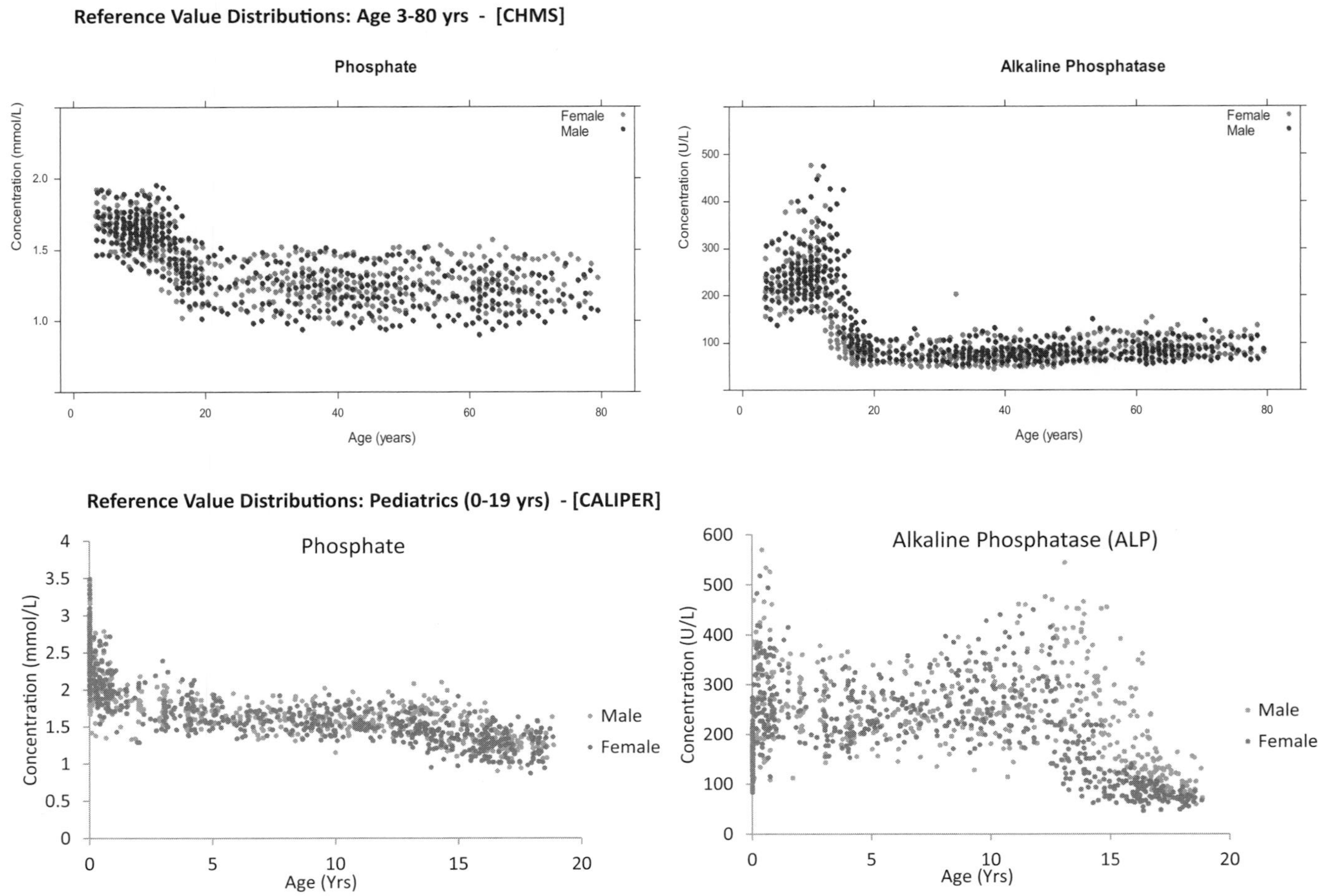

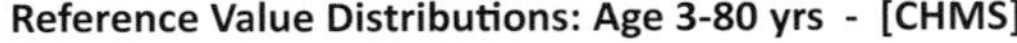

FIGURE A.1 Reference value distributions for phosphate (mmol/L) and alkaline phosphatase (ALP; U/L) based on data from the Canadian Health Measures Survey[10] *(top panel)* or the CALIPER cohort of healthy community children and adolescents[4] *(bottom panel)*.

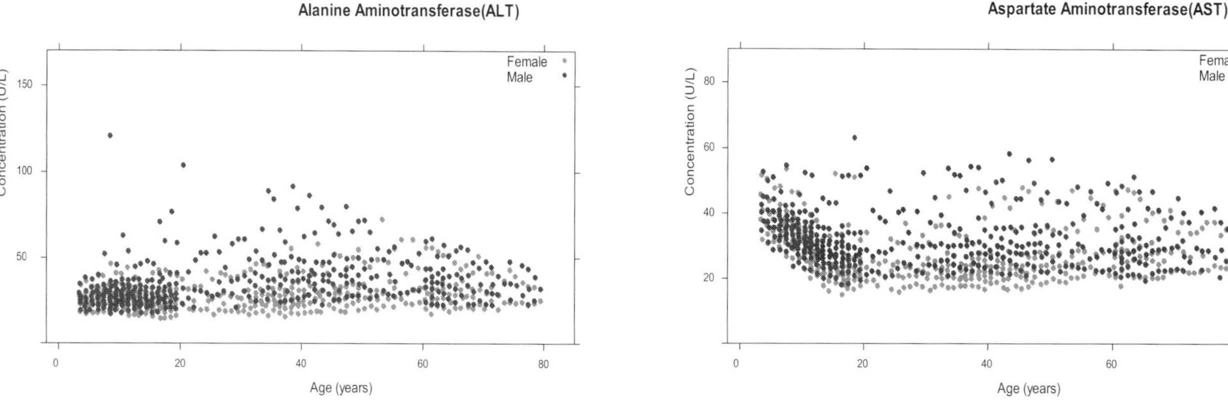

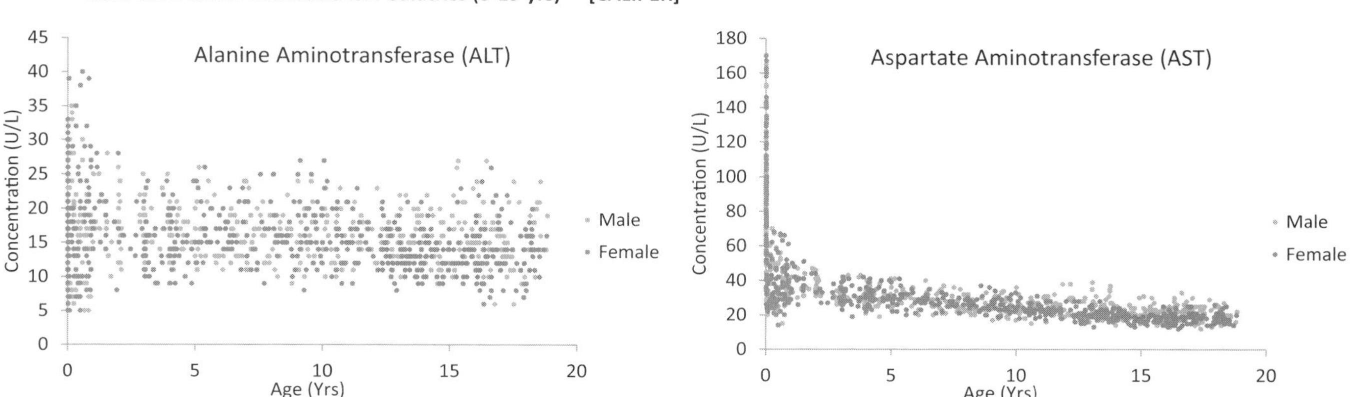

FIGURE A.2 Reference value distributions for alanine aminotransferase (*ALT;* U/L) and aspartate aminotransferase (*AST;* U/L) based on data from the Canadian Health Measures Survey[10] *(top panel)* or the CALIPER cohort of healthy community children and adolescents[4] *(bottom panel).*

Reference Value Distributions: Age 3-80 yrs - [CHMS]

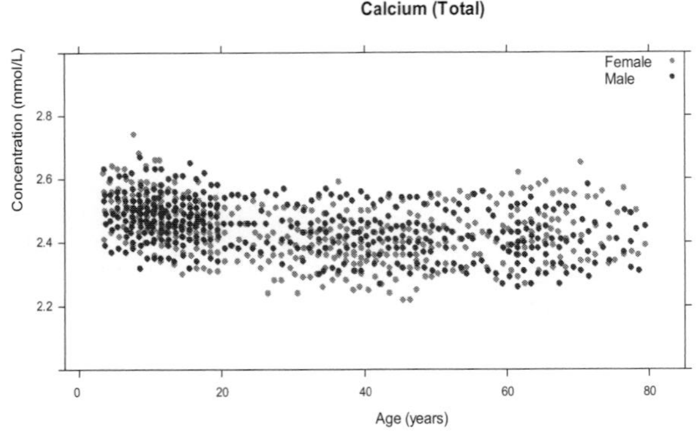

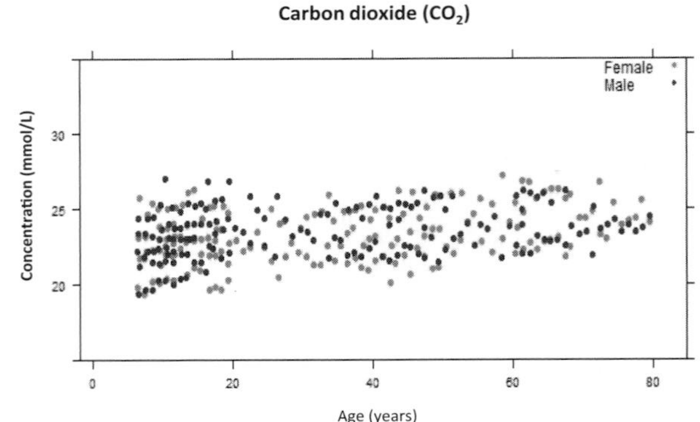

Reference Value Distributions: Pediatrics (0-19 yrs) - [CALIPER]

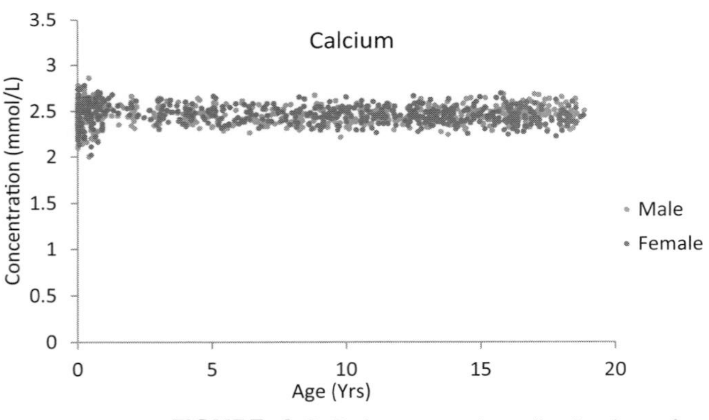

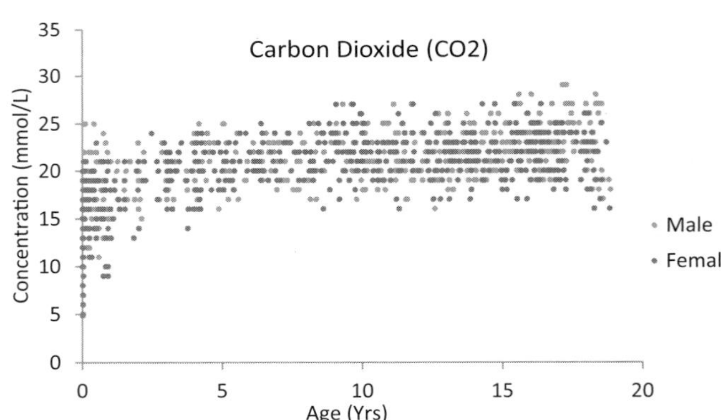

FIGURE A.3 Reference value distributions for calcium (total; mmol/L) and carbon dioxide (CO_2, mmol/L) based on data from the Canadian Health Measures Survey[10] *(top panel)* or the CALIPER cohort of healthy community children and adolescents[4] *(bottom panel)*.

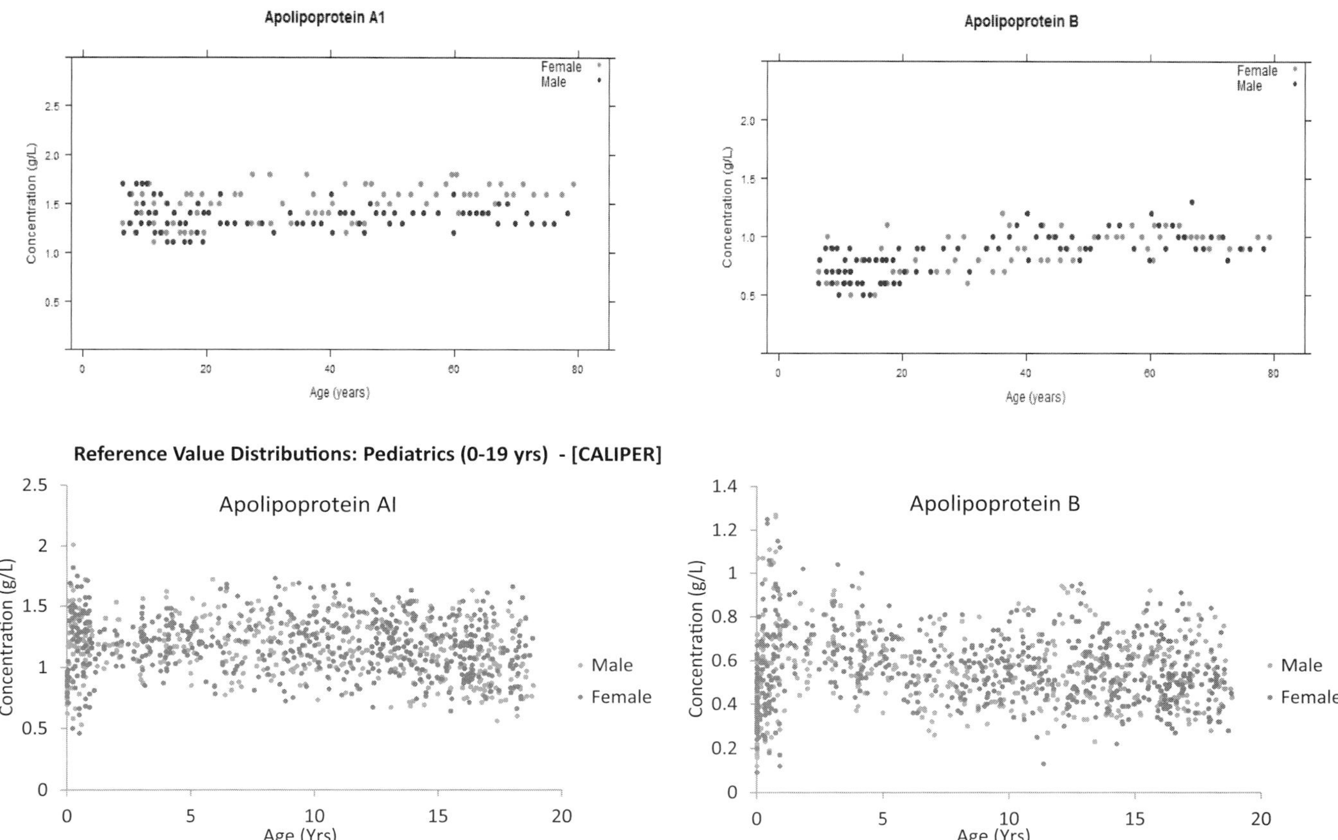

FIGURE A.4 Reference value distributions for apolipoproten A1 (g/L) and apolipoprotein B (g/L) based on data from the Canadian Health Measures Survey[11] *(top panel)* or the CALIPER cohort of healthy community children and adolescents[4] *(bottom panel).*

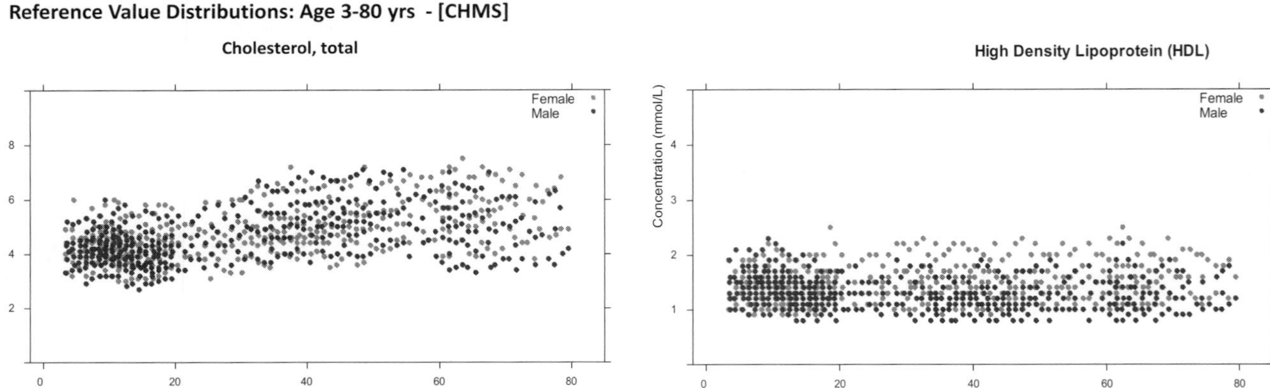

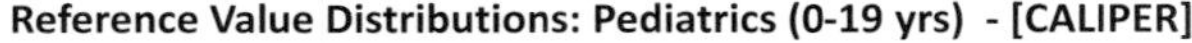

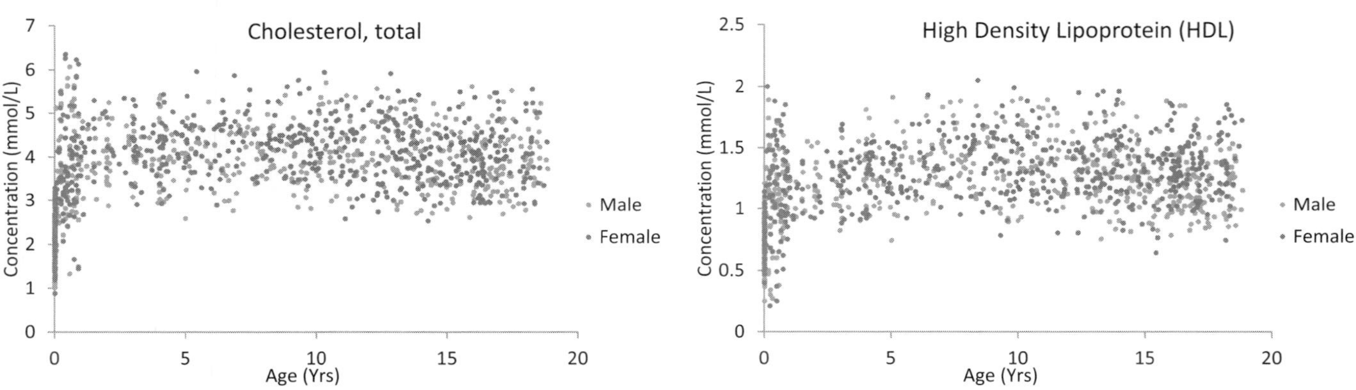

FIGURE A.5 Reference value distributions for cholesterol (total; mmol/L) and high-density lipoprotein (*HDL;* mmol/L) based on data from the Canadian Health Measures Survey[10] *(top panel)* or the CALIPER cohort of healthy community children and adolescents[4] *(bottom panel).*

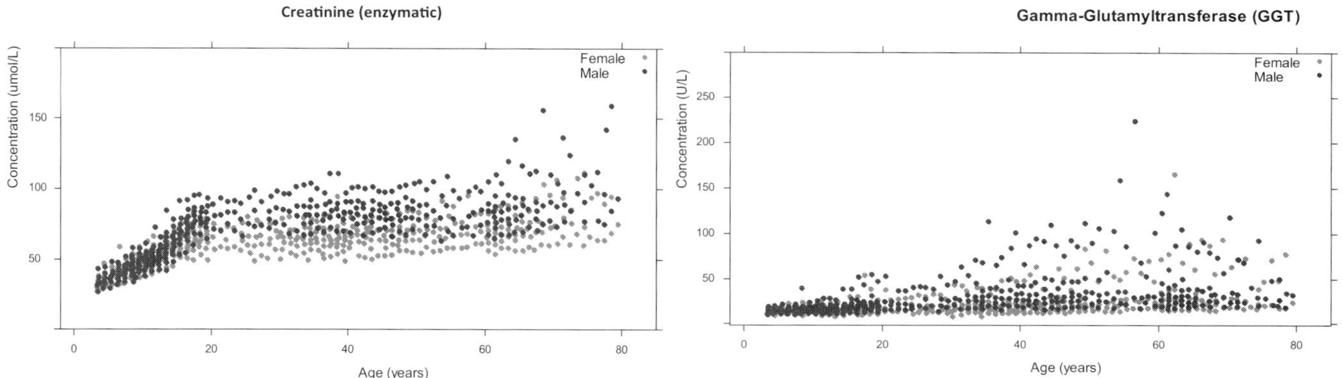

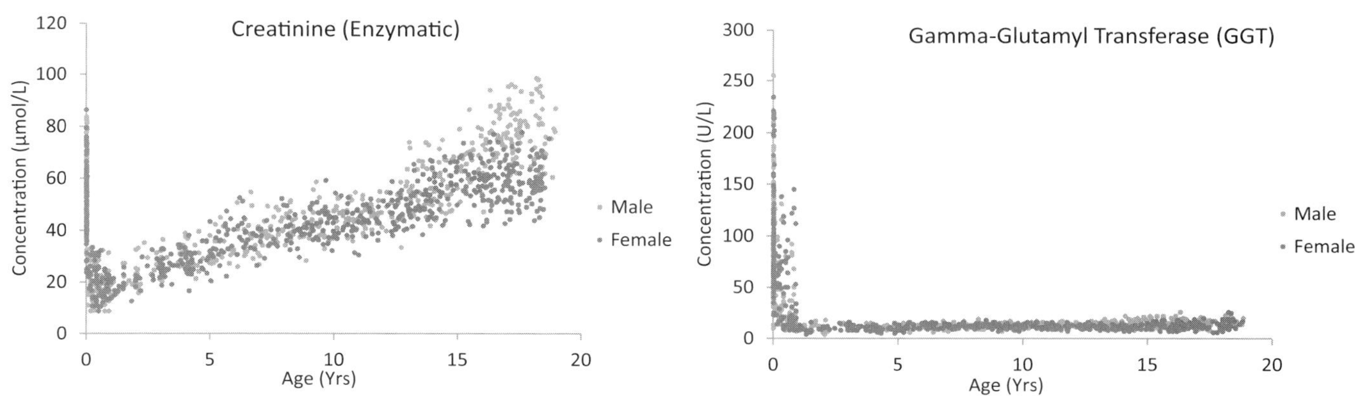

FIGURE A.6 Reference value distributions for creatinine (enzymatic; mmol/L) and γ-glutamyltransferase (*GGT;* U/L) based on data from the Canadian Health Measures Survey[10] *(top panel)* or the CALIPER cohort of healthy community children and adolescents[4] *(bottom panel).*

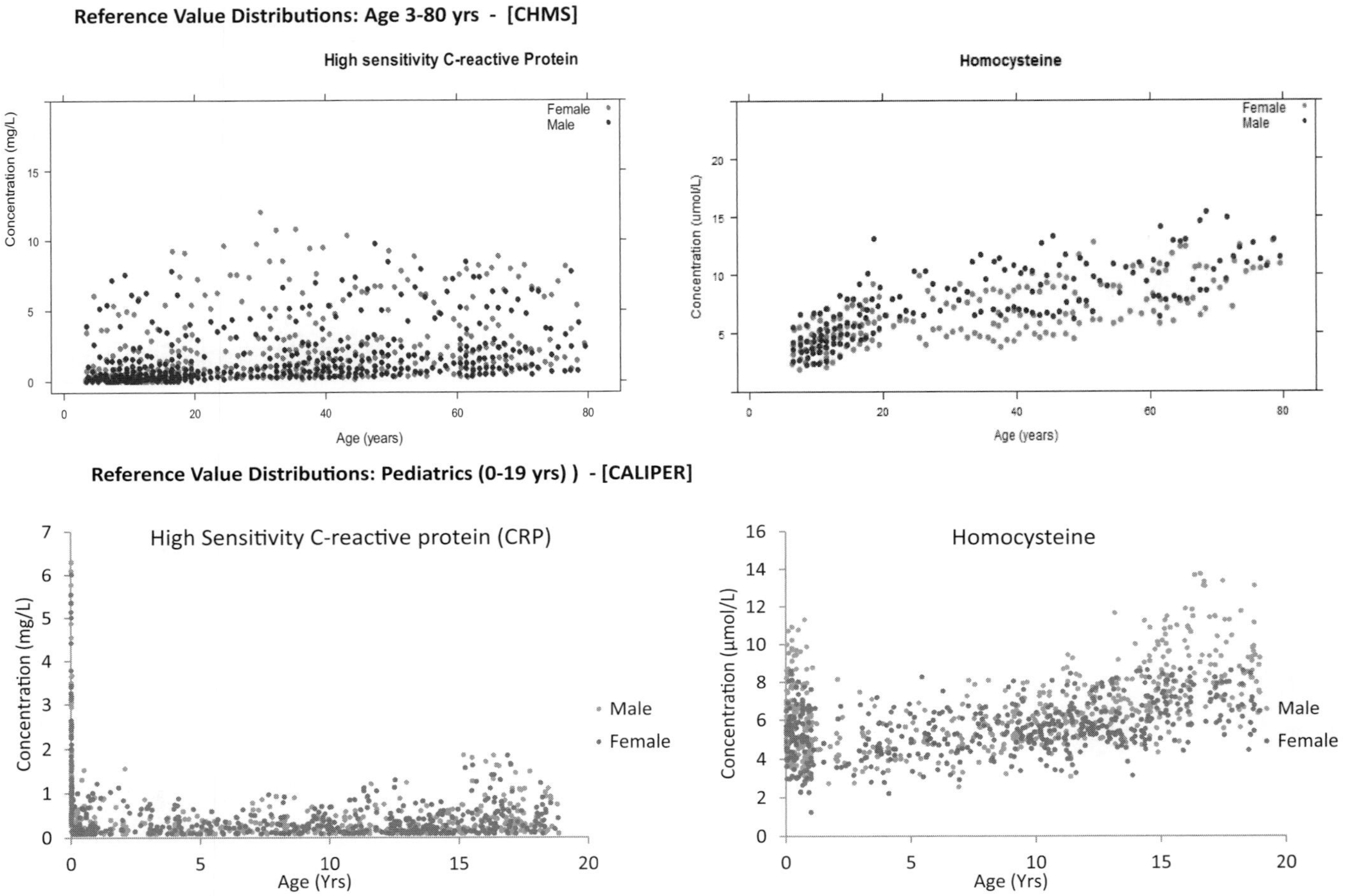

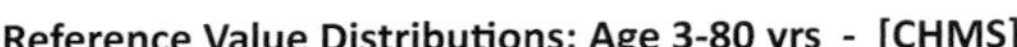

FIGURE A.7 Reference value distributions for high-sensitivity C-reactive protein (*CRP;* mg/L) and homocysteine (µmol/L) based on data from the Canadian Health Measures Survey[11] *(top panel)* or the CALIPER cohort of healthy community children and adolescents[2,4] *(bottom panel).*

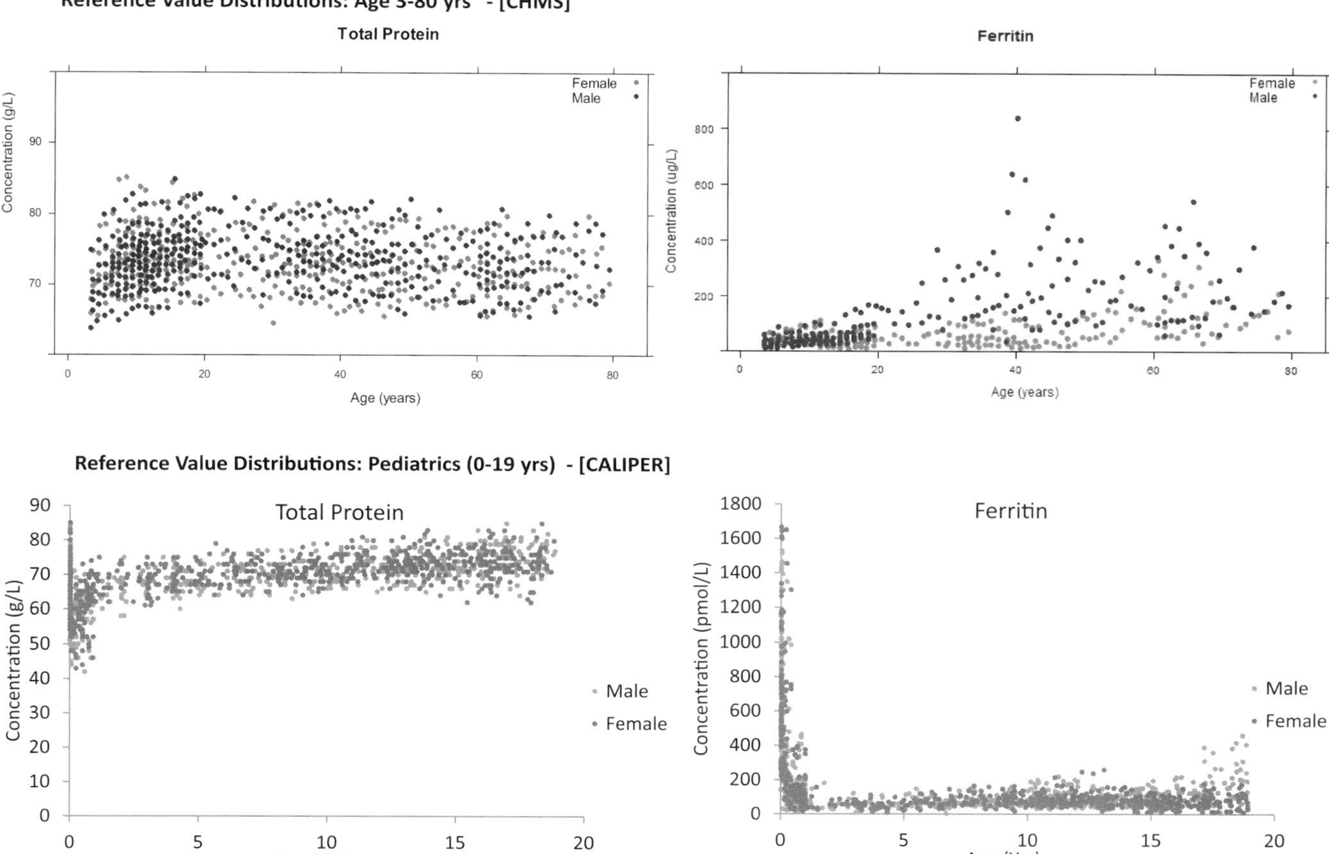

FIGURE A.8 Reference value distributions for total protein (g/L) and ferritin based on data from the Canadian Health Measures Survey[10,11] (*top panel;* μg/L) or the CALIPER cohort of healthy community children and adolescents[2,4] (*bottom panel;* pmol/L).

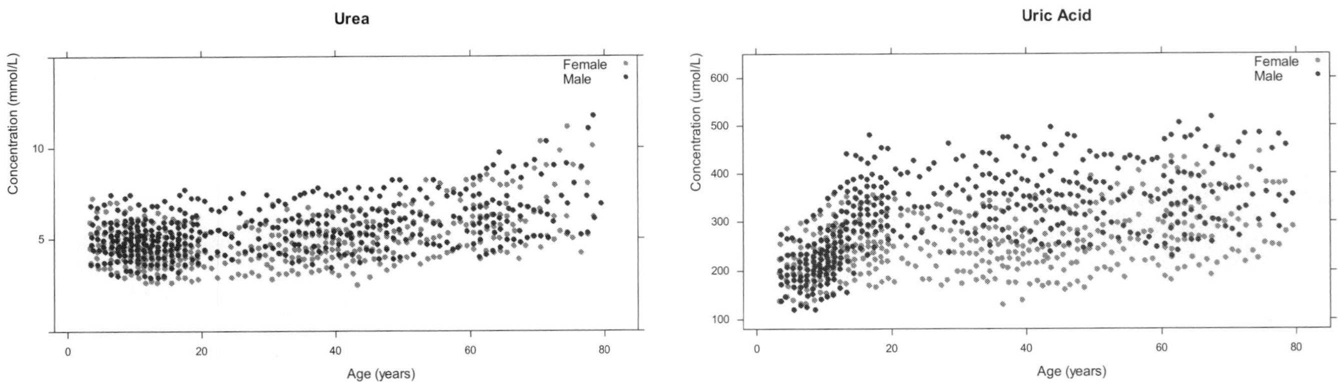

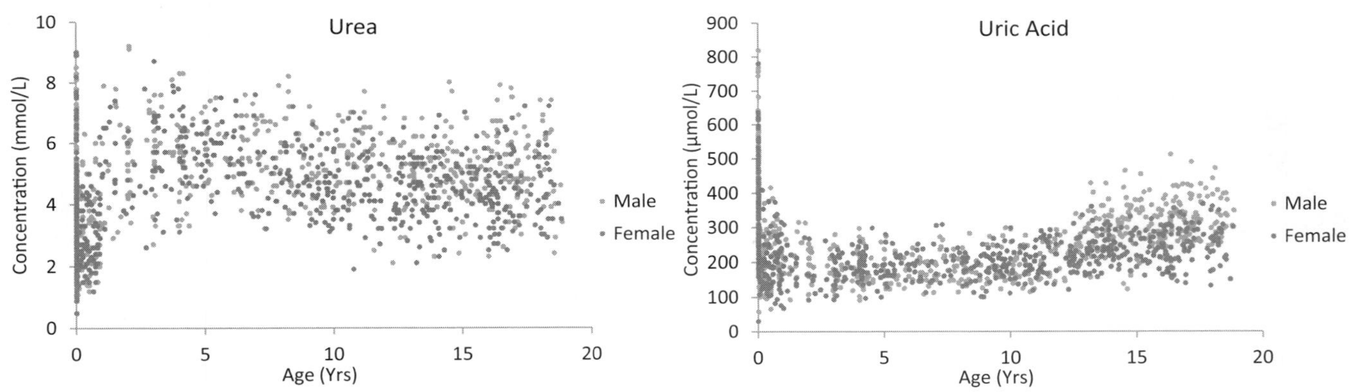

FIGURE A.9 Reference value distributions for urea (mmol/L) and uric acid (µmol/L) based on data from the Canadian Health Measures Survey[10] *(top panel)* or the CALIPER cohort of healthy community children and adolescents[4] *(bottom panel)*.

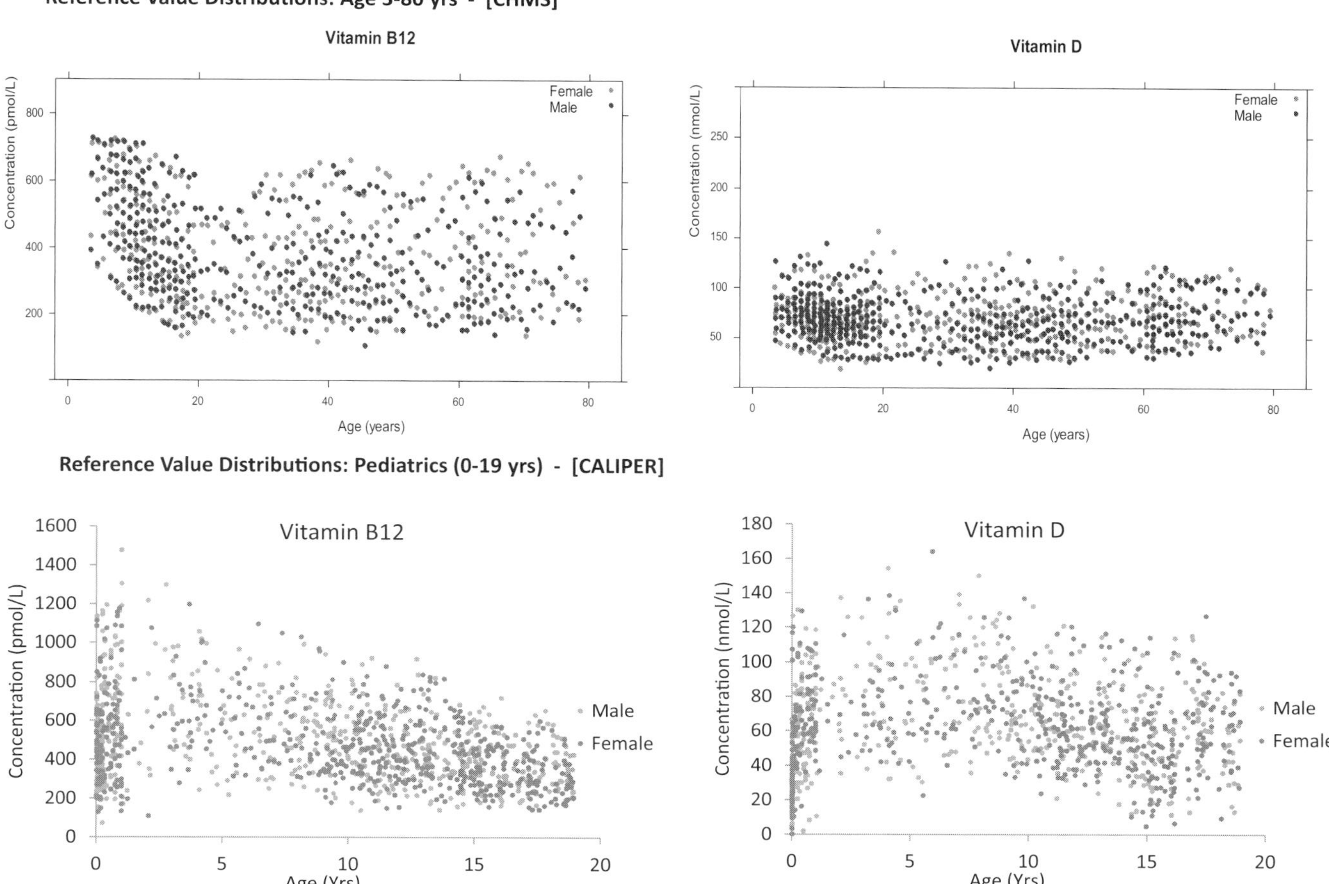

FIGURE A.10 Reference value distributions for vitamin B_{12} (pmol/L) and vitamin D (nmol/L) based on data from the Canadian Health Measures Survey[11] *(top panel)* or the CALIPER cohort of healthy community children and adolescents[2] *(bottom panel)*.

TABLE 82.2 Reference Intervals for Biochemical Markers in Other Body Fluids

			REFERENCE INTERVALS			
Analyte	**Specimen**	**Condition**	**Conventional Units**	**Conversion Factor**	**SI Units**	**Reference Publication**
α-Fetoprotein (AFP)	Amf	Weeks of Gestation	ng/mL	1	μg/L	1
		14	25.6		25.6	
		15	29.9		29.9	
		16	34.8		34.8	
		17	40.6		40.6	
		18	47.3		47.3	
		19	55.1		55.1	
		20	64.3		64.3	
		21	74.9		74.9	
Albumin	CSF, lumbar		mg/dL	10	mg/L	1
			17.7–25.1		177–251	
Bilirubin	Amf		mg/dL	17.1	μmol/L	1
		28 wk	<0.075		<1.28	
			$\Delta A_{450} < 0.048$			
		40 wk	<0.025		<0.43	
			$\Delta A_{450} < 0.02$			
Chloride	Sweat		mEq/L	1	mmol/L	1
	(iontophoresis)	Normal	5–35		5–35	
		Marginal	30–70		30–70	
		Cystic fibrosis	60–200		60–200	
Cortisol, free	Sal		ng/mL	2.76	nmol/L	
		0700 h	1.4–10.1		4–30	1
		2200 h	0.7–2.2		2–6	
Estriol, free (unconjugated uE_3)	Amf	Weeks of Gestation	ng/mL	3.47	nmol/L	1
		16–20	1.0–3.2		3.5–11	
		20–24	2 .1–7.8		7.3–27	
		24–28	2.1–7.8		7.3–27	
		28–32	4.0–13.6		14–47	
		32–36	3.6–15.5		12–54	
		36–38	4.6–18.0		16–62	
		38–40	5.4–19.8		19–69	
Estriol, total (E_3)	Amf	Weeks of Gestation	ng/mL	3.47	nmol/L	1
		21–32	5–50		17–174	
		33–35	90–240		312–833	
		36–41	150–213		521–739	
Glucagon	Amf		ng/L	1	ng/L	1
		Midgestation	23–63		23–63	
		Term	41–193		41–193	
Glucose	CSF		mg/dL	0.0555	mmol/L	1
		Infant, child	60–80		3.3–4.5	
		Adult	40–70		2.2–3.9	
Immunoglobulin A	CSF		mg/dL	10	mg/L	1
			0.0–0.6		0.0–6.0	
	Sal		<11		<0.11	
Immunoglobulin G	CSF		mg/dL	10	mg/L	1
			0–5.5		0–55	
Immunoglobulin M	CSF		mg/dL	10	mg/L	1
			0.0–1.3		0–13	
L-Lactate	CSF	Child	mg/d	0.0111	mmol/d	1
			496–1982		5.5–22	
		Adult	mg/dL	0.111	mmol/L	15
			9.1–18.8		1.01–2.09	
	Gastric fluid		Negative		Negative	1

TABLE 82.2 Reference Intervals for Biochemical Markers in Other Body Fluids—cont'd

Analyte	Specimen	Condition	REFERENCE INTERVALS Conventional Units	Conversion Factor	SI Units	Reference Publication
L/S Ratio	Amf	State of fetal maturity	Ratio	1	Ratio	1
		Immature	<1.5		<1.5	
		Transitional	1.6–2.4		1.6–2.4	
		Mature	>2.5		>2.5	
		Diabetic	>2.5		>2.5	
Protein, total	CSF		mg/dL	10	mg/L	1
		Premature	15–130		150–1300	
		Full-term newborn	40–120		400–1200	
		<1 mo	20 -80		200–800	
		>1 mo	15–40		150–400	
		Ventricular fluid	5–15		50–150	
		Cisternal fluid	15–25		150–250	
	Amf		g/dL	10	g/L	
		Early pregnancy	0.2–1.7		2.0–17.0	
		Late pregnancy	0.175–0.705		1.8–7.1	
Pyruvate	CSF		mg/dL	0.114	mmol/L	15
		Adult	0.3–1.3		0.03–0.15	
Serotonin	CSF		ng/mL	5.68	nmol/L	1
			1.0–2.1		5.7- 12.0	

Amf, Amniotic fluid; *CSF*, cerebrospinal fluid; *L/S*, lecithin-to-sphingomyelin ratio; *Sal*, saliva.

TABLE 82.3 Reference Information for Toxicology and Therapeutic Drugs

Drug	Specimen	Status	REFERENCE VALUES Conventional Units	Conversion Factor	SI Units	Reference Publication
Acetaminophen (Tylenol)	S or P		μg/mL	6.62	μmol/L	1
		Therap	10–30		66–199	
		Toxic				
		4 h after dose	>200		>1324	
		12 h after dose	>50		>331	
Amikacin (Amikin)	S or P		μg/mL	1.71	μmol/L	1
		Therap				
		Peak	25–35		43–60	
		Trough				
		Less severe infection	1–4		2–7	
		Severe infection	4–8		7–14	
		Toxic				
		Peak	>40		>68	
		Trough	>10		>17	
		Peak/MIC	>10		>17	
Aminocaproic acid (Amicar)	S or P		μg/mL	7.62	μmol/L	1
		Therap				
		Trough	100–400		762–3048	
Amiodarone (Cordarone)	S or P		μg/mL	1.47	μmol/L	1
		Therap	0.5–2.0		1–3	
		Toxic	>2.5		>4	

Continued

TABLE 82.3 Reference Information for Toxicology and Therapeutic Drugs—cont'd

Drug	Specimen	Status	REFERENCE VALUES Conventional Units	Conversion Factor	SI Units	Reference Publication
Amitriptyline (Elavil) + nortriptyline	S or P		ng/mL	3.61	nmol/L	1
		Therap	80–200		289–722	
		Toxic	>500 (sum)		>1805	
Amobarbital (Amytal)	S or P		µg/mL	4.42	µmol/L	1
		Therap	1–5		4–22	
		Toxic	>10		>44	
Amoxapine (Asendin) + 8-hydroxy amoxapine	S or P		ng/mL	3 .19	nmol/L	1
		Therap	200–600		638–1914	
		Toxic	>600		>1914	
Amphetamine (Adderall)	S or P		ng/mL	7.40	nmol/L	1
		Therap	20–30		148–222	
		Toxic	>200		>1480	
Bromide as bromine	S or P		µg/mL	0.0125	mmol/L	1
		Therap	750–1500		9–19	
		Toxic	>1250		>16	
Bupropion (Wellbutrin, Zyban)	S or P		ng/mL	3.62	nmol/L	1
		Therap	25–100		91–362	
		Toxic	>100		>362	
Caffeine	S or P		µg/mL	5.15	µmol/L	1
		Therap	8–20		41–103	
		Toxic	>20		>103	
Carbamazepine (Tegretol)	S or P		µg/mL	4.23	µmol/L	1
		Therap	4–12		17–51	
		Toxic	>15		>63	
Carbamazepine-10,11-epoxide (carbamazepine metabolite)	S or P		µg/mL	3.97	µmol/L	1
		Therap	0.4–4		2–16	
		Toxic	>8		>32	
Carbenicillin (Geopen)	S or P		µg/mL	2.64	µmol/L	1
		Therap	Dependent on MIC of specific organism			
		Toxic	>250 (neurotoxicity)		>660	
Chloral hydrate (Noctec) as trichloroethanol	S or P		µg/mL	6.69	µmol/L	1
		Therap	2–12		13–80	
		Toxic	>20		>134	
Chloramphenicol (Chloromycetin)	S or P		µg/mL	3.09	µmol/L	1
		Therap	10–25		31–77	
		Toxic	>25		>77	
		Gray baby syndrome	>40		>124	
Chlordiazepoxide (Librium) + nordiazepine	S or P		ng/mL	0.003	µmol/L	1
		Therap	700–1000		2–3	
		Toxic	>5000		>17	

TABLE 82.3 **Reference Information for Toxicology and Therapeutic Drugs—cont'd**

			REFERENCE VALUES			
Drug	**Specimen**	**Status**	**Conventional Units**	**Conversion Factor**	**SI Units**	**Reference Publication**
Chlorpromazine (Thorazine)	S or P		ng/mL	3.14	nmol/L	1
		Therap				
		Adult	30–300		94–942	
		Child	40–80		126–251	
		Toxic	>750		>2355	
Cimetidine (Tagamet)	S or P		μg/mL	3.96	μmol/L	1
		Therap				
		Trough	0.5–1.2		2–5	
		Toxic	>1.3		>5	
Ciprofloxacin (Cipro)	S or P		μg/mL	3.02	μmol/L	1
		Therap				
		Peak (oral dose)	0.5–1.5		2–5	
		Peak (IV dose)	<5.0		<15	
		Toxic	>5.0		>15	
		Gram positive				
		AUC/MIC	>30			
		Gram negative				
		AUC/MIC	>125			
Clomipramine (Anafranil) + norclomipramine	S or P		ng/mL	3.18	nmol/L	1
		Therap	175–450		556–1431	
		Toxic	>400 (sum)		>1272	
Clonazepam (Klonopin)	S or P		ng/mL	3.17	nmol/L	1
		Therap	20–70		63–222	
		Toxic	>80		>254	
Clonidine (Catapres)	S or P		ng/mL	4.35	nmol/L	1
		Therap	1.0–2.0		4–9	
Clorazepate (Tranxene) (see Nordiazepam)						
Clozapine (Clozaril)	S or P		ng/mL	3.06	nmol/L	1
		Therap	350–600		1071–1836	
		Toxic	>900		>2754	
Codeine	S or P		ng/mL	3.34	nmol/L	1
		Therap	10–100		33–334	
		Toxic	>1100		>3340	
Cyclosporin A (Sandimmune)	WB		ng/mL	0.83	nmol/L	1
		Therap				
		12 h after dose	50–350		42 -291	
		Toxic	>350		>291	
Delavirdine (Rescriptor)	S or P		μg/mL	1.80	μmol/L	1
		Therap				
		Trough	3–8		5–14	
		Peak	14–16		25–29	
		Toxic	>16		>29	
Desipramine (Norpramin)	S or P		ng/mL	3.75	nmol/L	1
		Therap	100–300		375–1126	
		Toxic	>400		>1502	
Diazepam (Valium) + nordiazepine	S or P		ng/mL	3.51	nmol/L	1
		Therap	100–1000		351–3512	
		Toxic	>5000		>17,559	

Continued

TABLE 82.3 Reference Information for Toxicology and Therapeutic Drugs—cont'd

			REFERENCE VALUES			
Drug	**Specimen**	**Status**	**Conventional Units**	**Conversion Factor**	**SI Units**	**Reference Publication**
Digitoxin	S or P		ng/mL	1.31	nmol/L	1
	≥8 h after dose	Therap	10–30		13–39	
		Toxic	>45		>59	
Digoxin (Lanoxin)	S or P		ng/mL	1.28	nmol/L	1
	≥12 h after dose	Therap	0.5–2.0		0.6–3.0	
		In heart failure	0.5–0.8		0.6–1.0	
		Toxic	>1.5		>2.0	
Disopyramide (Norpace)	S or P		µg/mL	2.95	µmol/L	1
		Therap	2.8–7.5		8–22	
		Toxic	>5		> 15	
Doxepin (Sinequan, Adapin) + nordoxepin	S or P		ng/mL	3.58	nmol/L	1
		Therap	50–150		179–537	
		Toxic	>500		>1790	
Efavirenz (Sustiva)	S or P		µg/mL	3.16	µmol/L	1
		Therap	1–4		3–13	
		Toxic	>4		>13	
Ephedrine (Ectasule)	S or P		µg/mL	6.05	µmol/L	1
		Therap	0.05–0.10		0.3–0.6	
		Toxic	>2		>12	
Ethanol	WB (Ox)		mg/dL	0.217	mmol/L	1
		Impairment	50–100		11–22	
		Depression of CNS	>100		>21.7	
		Fatalities reported	>400		>86.8	
Ethchlorvynol (Placidyl)	S or P		µg/mL	6.92	µmol/L	1
		Therap	2–8		14–55	
		Toxic	>20		>138	
Ethosuximide (Zarontin)	S or P		µg/mL	7.08	µmol/L	1
		Therap	40–100		283–708	
		Toxic	>150		>1062	
Everolimus (Zortress)	WB		ng/mL	1.04	nmol/L	1
		Therap	3–15		3–16	
		Toxic	>15		>16	
Felbamate (Felbatol)	S or P		µg/mL	4.2	µmol/L	1
		Therap	30–60		126–252	
		Toxic	>120		>504	
Fenoprofen (Nalfon)	S or P		µg/mL	4.12	µmol/L	1
		Therap	20–65		82–268	
Flecainide (Tambocor)	S or P		µg/mL	2.4 1	µmol/L	1
		Therap	0.2–1.0		0.5–2.0	
		Toxic	>1.0		>2.0	
5-Flucytosine (Ancobon)	S or P		µg/mL	7.75	µmol/L	1
		Peak	>25		>194	
		Toxic	>100		>775	
Fluoxetine (Prozac) + norfluoxetine	S or P		ng/mL	3.23	nmol/L	1
		Therap	120–300		388–969	
		Toxic	>1000		>3230	
Fluphenazine (Modecate)	S or P		ng/mL	2.29	nmol/L	1
		Therap	0.5–2		1–5	
		Toxic	>100		>229	

TABLE 82.3 Reference Information for Toxicology and Therapeutic Drugs—cont'd

Drug	Specimen	Status	REFERENCE VALUES Conventional Units	Conversion Factor	SI Units	Reference Publication
Flurazepam (Dalmane)	S or P		µg/mL	2.58	µmol/L	1
		Toxic	>0.2		>0.5	
Gabapentin (Neurontin)	S or P		µg/mL	5.84	µmol/L	1
		Therap	2–20		12–117	
		Toxic	>12		>70	
Gentamicin (Garamycin)	S or P		µg/mL	2.09	µmol/L	1
		Therap				
		Peak				
		Less severe infection	5–8		11–17	
		Severe infection	8–10		17–21	
		Trough				
		Less severe infection	<1		<2	
		Moderate infection	<2		<4	
		Severe infection	<4		<8	
		Toxic				
		Peak	>10		>21	
		Trough	>2		>4	
		Peak/MIC	>10		>21	
Glutethimide (Doriden)	S or P		µg/mL	4.60	µmol/L	1
		Therap	2–6		9–28	
		Toxic	>5		>23	
Haloperidol (Haldol)	S or P		ng/mL	2.66	nmol/L	1
		Therap	5–17		13–45	
		Toxic	>42		>112	
Hydromorphone (Dilaudid)	S or P		ng/mL	3.50	nmol/L	1
		Therap	1–3		4–11	
		Toxic	>100		>350	
Ibuprofen (Motrin)	S or P		µg/mL	4.85	µmol/L	1
		Therap	10–50		49–243	
		Toxic	>200		>970	
Imipramine (Tofranil) + desipramine	S or P		ng/mL	3.57	nmol/L	1
		Therap	150–300		536–1071	
		Toxic	>400 (sum)		>1428	
Indinavir (Crixivan)	S or P		µg/mL	1.41	µmol/L	1
		Therap				
		Trough	>0.1		>0.14	
		Peak	8–10		11–14	
		Toxic	>10		>14	
Isoniazid (Hyzyd, Nydrazid)	S or P		µg/mL	7.29	µmol/L	1
		Therap	1–7		7–15	
		Toxic	>20		>146	
Itraconazole (Sporanox) + hydroxyitraconazole	S or P		µg/mL	1.42	µmol/L	1
		Therap	>1.5		>2	

Continued

TABLE 82.3 Reference Information for Toxicology and Therapeutic Drugs—cont'd

Drug	Specimen	Status	REFERENCE VALUES Conventional Units	Conversion Factor	SI Units	Reference Publication
Kanamycin (Kantrex)	S or P		µg/mL	2.06	µmol/L	1
		Therap				
		Peak	25–35		52–72	
		Trough				
		Less severe infection	1–4		2–8	
		Severe infection	4–8		8–17	
		Toxic				
		Peak	>35		>72	
		Trough	>10		>21	
		Peak/MIC	>10		>21	
Lamivudine (Epivir, 3TC)	S or P		µg/mL	4.36	µmol/L	1
		Therap	>0.4		>2	
Lamotrigine (Lamictal)	S or P		µg/mL	3.91	µmol/L	1
		Therap	2.5–15		10–59	
Levetiracetam (Keppra)	S or P		µg/mL	5.88	µmol/L	1
		Therap	12–46		71–270	
Lidocaine (Xylocaine)	S or P		µg/mL	4.27	µmol/L	1
	≥45 min after bolus dose	Therap	1.5–5		6–12	
		Toxic	>6		>26	
Lithium (Eskalith)	S or P		mEq/L	1.0	mmol/L	1
		Therap	0.5–1.2		0.5–1	
		Toxic	>2		>2	
Lorazepam (Ativan)	S or P		ng/mL	3.11	nmol/L	1
		Therap	50–240		156–746	
Maprotiline (Ludiomil)	S or P		ng/mL	3.60	nmol/L	1
		Therap	125–200		450–720	
		Toxic	>300		>1080	
Meperidine (Demerol)	S or P		ng/mL	4.04	nmol/L	1
		Therap	70–500		283–2020	
		Toxic	>1000		>4004	
Mephobarbital (Mebaral)	S or P		µg/mL	4.06	µmol/L	1
		Therap	1–7		4–28	
		Toxic	>15		>61	
Meprobamate (Equanil)	S or P		µg/mL	4.58	µmol/L	1
		Therap	6–12		28–55	
		Toxic	>60		>275	
Methadone (Dolophine)	S or P		ng/mL	3.23	nmol/L	1
		Therap	100–400		320–1280	
		Toxic	>2000		>6460	
Methamphetamine (Desoxyn)	S or P		µg/mL	6.70	µmol/L	
		Therap	0.01–0.05		0.07–0.34	1
		Toxic	>0.5		>3	
Methanol			mg/L	0.0312	mmol/L	1
	WB (F/Ox)		<1.5		<0.05	
		Toxic	>200		>6.24	
	U	Occup exp	<50		<1.56	
			ppm		mmol/L	
	Breath		0.8		0.03	
		Occup exp	2.5		0.08	

TABLE 82.3 **Reference Information for Toxicology and Therapeutic Drugs—cont'd**

			REFERENCE VALUES			
Drug	**Specimen**	**Status**	**Conventional Units**	**Conversion Factor**	**SI Units**	**Reference Publication**
Methaqualone (Quaalude)	S or P		μg/mL	4.00	μmol/L	1
		Therap	2–3		8–12	
		Toxic	>10		>40	
Methotrexate (Trexall, Rheumatrex)	S or P		μg/mL	2.20	μmol/L	1
		Toxic				
		24 h after high-dose therapy	≥10		≥22	
		48 h after high-dose therapy	≥1		≥2	
		72 h after high-dose therapy	≥0.1		≥0.2	
Methsuximide (Celontin) as normethsuximide	S or P		μg/mL	5.29	μmol/L	1
		Therap	10–40		53–212	
		Toxic	>40		>212	
Methyldopa (Aldomet)	S or P		μg/mL	4 .73	μmol/L	1
		Therap	1–5		5–24	
		Toxic	>7		>33	
Methyprylon (Noludar)	S or P		μg/mL	5.46	μmol/L	1
		Therap	8–10		43–55	
		Toxic	>50		273	
Mexiletine (Mexitil)	S or P		μg/mL	5.58	μmol/L	1
		Therap	0.5–2		3–11	
		Toxic	>2.0		>11	
Morphine	S or P		ng/mL	3.50	nmol/L	1
		Therap	10–80		35–280	
		Toxic	>200		>700	
Mycophenolate mofetil (CellCept) as mycophenolic acid	S or P		μg/mL	3.12	μmol/L	1
		Therap	1.3–3.5		4–11	
		Toxic	>12		>38	
Nefazodone (Serzone)	S or P		ng/mL	2.13	nmol/L	1
		Therap	25–2500		53–5325	
		Toxic	>2500		>5325	
Nelfinavir (Viracept)	S or P		μg/mL	1.76	μmol/L	1
		Therap	>1		>2	
		Toxic	>6		>11	
Netilmicin (Netromycin)	S or P		μg/mL	2.10	μmol/L	1
		Therap				
		Peak				
		Less severe infection	5–8		10–17	
		Severe infection	8–10		17–21	
		Trough				
		Less severe infection	<1		<2	
		Moderate infection	<2		<4	
		Severe infection	<4		<8	
		Toxic				
		Peak	>10		>21	
		Trough	>2		>4	

Continued

TABLE 82.3 **Reference Information for Toxicology and Therapeutic Drugs—cont'd**

Drug	Specimen	Status	Conventional Units	Conversion Factor	SI Units	Reference Publication
			REFERENCE VALUES			
Nevirapine (Viramune)	S or P		µg/mL	3.76	µmol/L	1
		Therap	>3.5		<13.2	
		Toxic	>12		>45.1	
Nordiazepine, active metabolite of several benzodiazepines	S or P		ng/mL	3.76	nmol/L	1
		Therap	100–500		376–1880	
		Toxic	>500		>1880	
Nortriptyline (Aventyl)	S or P		ng/mL	3.80	nmol/L	1
		Therap	70–170		266–646	
		Toxic	>500		>1900	
Olanzapine (Zyprexa)	S or P		ng/mL	3.20	nmol/L	1
		Therap	20–80		64–256	
		Toxic	>1000		>3200	
Oxazepam (Serax)	S or P		µg/mL	3.49	µmol/L	1
		Therap	0.2–1.4		0.7–5	
Oxcarbazepine (Trileptal) as monohydroxy oxcarbazepine (MHD)	S or P		µg/mL	3.97	µmol/L	1
	S or P	Therap	3–35		12–139	
		Toxic	>40		>159	
Oxycodone (Percodan)	S or P		ng/mL	3.17	nmol/L	1
		Therap	10–100		32–317	
		Toxic	>200		>634	
Paraldehyde (Paral)	S or P		µg/mL	7.57	µmol/L	1
		Therap				
		Sedation	10–100		76–757	
		Anesthesia	>200		>1514	
		Toxic	>200		>1514	
		Lethal	>500		>3785	
Paroxetine (Paxil)	S or P		ng/mL	3.04	nmol/L	1
		Therap	70–120		231–365	
Pentazocine (Talwin)	S or P		µg/mL	3.50	µmol/L	1
		Therap	0.05–0.2		0.2–0.7	
		Toxic	>1.0		>4	
Pentobarbital (Nembutal)	S or P		µg/mL	4.42	µmol/L	1
		Therap				
		Hypnotic	1–5		4–22	
		Therap coma	20–50		88–221	
		Toxic	>10		>44	
Perphenazine (Apo-Perphenazine)	S or P		µg/mL	2.48	µmol/L	1
		Therap	0.6–2.4		2–6	
		Toxic	>12		>30	
Phenacetin	S or P		µg/mL	5.58	µmol/L	1
		Therap	1–30		6–167	
		Toxic	50–250		279–1395	
Phenobarbital (Luminal)	S or P		µg/mL	4.31	µmol/L	1
		Therap	10–40		43–173	
		Toxic				
		Slowness, ataxia, nystagmus	35–80		151–345	
		Coma, with reflexes	65–117		280–504	
		Coma, without reflexes	>100		>431	

TABLE 82.3 Reference Information for Toxicology and Therapeutic Drugs—cont'd

Drug	Specimen	Status	REFERENCE VALUES Conventional Units	Conversion Factor	SI Units	Reference Publication
Phensuximide (Milontin) + norphensuximide	S or P		μg/mL	5.29	μmol/L	1
		Therap	40–60		212–317	
Phenylbutazone (Butazolidin)	S or P		μg/mL	3.24	μmol/L	1
		Therap	50–100		162–324	
		Toxic	>100		>324	
Phenytoin (Dilantin)	S or P		μg/mL	3.96	μmol/L	1
		Therap	10–20		40–79	
		Free	1.0–2.0		4–8	
		Toxic	>20		>79	
Posaconazole (Noxafil)	S or P		μg/mL	1.43	μmol/L	1
		Therap	>1.25		>2	
Primidone (Mysoline) + phenobarbital	S or P		μg/mL	4.58	μmol/L	1
		Therap	5–10		23–46	
		Toxic	>15		>69	
Procainamide (Pronestyl) + *N*-acetylprocainamide (NAPA)	S or P		μg/mL	4.25	μmol/L	1
		Therap	4–10		17–42	
			12–18 (NAPA)	3.61	43–65	
		Toxic	>12		>51	
			>40 (NAPA)		>144	
Propafenone (Rythmol)	S or P		μg/mL	2.93	μmol/L	1
		Therap	0.5–2.0		1.5–6	
		Toxic	>2		>6	
Propoxyphene (Darvon)	S or P		μg/mL	2.95	μmol/L	1
		Therap	0.1–0.4		0.3–1.0	
		Toxic	>0.5		>2	
Propranolol (Inderal)	S or P		ng/mL	3.86	nmol/L	1
		Therap	20–100		77–386	
Protriptyline (Vivactil)	S or P		ng/mL	3.80	nmol/L	1
		Therap	70–260		266–988	
		Toxic	>500		>1900	
Quetiapine (Seroquel)	S or P		ng/mL	0.00261	μmol/L	16
		Therap	100–500		0.26–1.3	
		Toxic	>1000		>2.6	
Quinidine (BioQuin)	S or P		μg/mL	3.08	μmol/L	1
		Therap	2–5		6–14	
		Toxic	>6		>19	
Risperidone + 9-hydroxyrisperidone (Risperdal)	S or P		ng/mL	2.44	nmol/L	1
		Therap	20–60		49–146	
Ritonavir (Norvir)	S or P		μg/mL	1.39	μmol/L	1
		Therap	>2		>3	
		Toxic	>22		>31	
Salicylates as salicylic acid or with chronic ingestion	S or P		μg/mL	0.00727	mmol/L	1
		Therap				
		Analgesia, antipyresis	<100		<0.7	
		Antiinflammatory	150–300		1–2	
		Toxic	>100		>0.7	
		Lethal, 24+ h after a dose	>500		>4	

Continued

TABLE 82.3 Reference Information for Toxicology and Therapeutic Drugs—cont'd

Drug	Specimen	Status	Conventional Units (Reference Values)	Conversion Factor (Reference Values)	SI Units (Reference Values)	Reference Publication
Saquinavir (Fortovase, Invirase)	S or P		μg/mL	1.49	μmol/L	1
		Therap	>0.25		>0.4	
		Toxic	>6.0		>9	
Secobarbital (Seconal)	S or P		μg/mL	4.2	μmol/L	1
		Therap	1–2		4.2–8.4	
		Toxic	>5		>21.0	
Sertraline (Zoloft)	S or P		ng/mL	3.27	nmol/L	1
		Therap	10–50		33–164	
		Toxic	>300		>981	
Sirolimus (Rapamune, Rapamycin)	WB		ng/mL	1.10	nmol/L	1
		Therap	4–20		4–22	
		Toxic	>20		>22	
Sotalol (Betapace, Sorine)	S or P		μg/mL	3.67	μmol/L	1
		Therap	1–3		4–11	
Streptomycin	S or P		μg/ml	1.72	μmol/L	1
		Therap				
		Trough	<5		<9	
		Peak	20–30		34–52	
		Peak/MIC	>10		>17.2	
		Toxic	>50		>86	
Sulfonamides as sulfanilamide	S or P		mg/mL	5.81	mmol/L	1
		Therap	5–15		29–87	
		Toxic	>20		>116	
Tacrolimus (FK 506, Prodraf)	WB		ng/mL	1.24	nmol/L	1
		Therap	3–20		4–25	
		Toxic	>20		>25	
Teicoplanin (Targocid)	S or P		μg/mL	0.53	μmol/L	1
		Peak	>10		>5	
Theophylline (Uniphyl)	S or P		μg/mL	5.55	μmol/L	1
		Therap				
		Bronchodilator	8–20		44–111	
		Premature apnea	6–13		33–72	
		Toxic	>20		>111	
Thiopental (Pentothal)	S or P		μg/mL	4.13	μmol/L	1
		Hypnotic	1–5		4–21	
		Coma	30–100		124–413	
		Anesthesia	7–130		29–536	
		Toxic	>10		>41	
Thioridazine (Mellaril)	S or P		μg/mL	2.7	μmol/L	1
		Therap	0.2–2.0		0.5–5	
		Toxic	>10		>27	
Tiagabine (Gabitril)	S or P		ng/mL	2.66	nmol/L	1
		Therap	20–200		53–532	
		Toxic	>520		>1383	

TABLE 82.3 **Reference Information for Toxicology and Therapeutic Drugs—cont'd**

			REFERENCE VALUES			
Drug	**Specimen**	**Status**	**Conventional Units**	**Conversion Factor**	**SI Units**	**Reference Publication**
Tobramycin (Nebcin)	S or P		μg/mL	2.14	μmol/L	1
		Therap				
		Peak				
		Less severe infection	5–8		11–17	
		Severe infection	8–10		17–21	
		Trough				
		Less severe infection	<1		<2	
		Moderate infection	<2		<4	
		Severe infection	<4		<9	
		Toxic				
		Peak	>10		>21	
		Trough	>2		>4	
		Peak/MIC	>10		>21	
Tocainide (Tonocard)	S or P		μg/mL	5.20	μmol/L	1
		Therap	6–15		31–78	
		Toxic	>15		>78	
Tolbutamide (Orinase)	S or P		μg/mL	3.70	μmol/L	1
		Therap	90–240		333–888	
		Toxic	>640		>2368	
Topiramate (Topamax)	S or P		μg/mL	2.95	μmol/L	1
		Therap	5–20		15–59	
		Toxic	>12		>36	
Trazodone (Desyrel)	S or P		ng/mL	2.68	nmol/L	1
		Therap	650–1500		1748–4020	
		Toxic	>4000		>10,720	
Trimipramine (Surmontil)	S or P		ng/mL	3.40	nmol/L	1
		Therap	150–350		510–1190	
		Toxic	>500		>1700	
Valproic acid (Depakene)	S or P		μg/mL	6.93	μmol/L	1
		Therap	50–100		346–693	
		Toxic	>100		>693	
Vancomycin (Vancocin)	S or P		μg/mL	0.69	μmol/L	1
		Therap				
		Peak	20–40		14–28	
		Trough	>10		>7	
		Toxic	>80		>55	
Venlafaxine (Effexor) + desmethylvenlafaxine	S or P		ng/mL	3.61	nmol/L	1
		Therap	195–400		704–1444	
		Toxic	>1000 (sum)		>3610	
Vigabatrin (Sabril)	S or P		μg/mL	7.74	μmol/L	1
		Therap	0.8–36		6–279	
Voriconazole (Vfend)	S or P		μg/mL	2.86	μmol/L	
		Therap	1–6		3–17	
		Toxic	>6		>17	

Continued

TABLE 82.3 Reference Information for Toxicology and Therapeutic Drugs—cont'd

			REFERENCE VALUES			
Drug	**Specimen**	**Status**	**Conventional Units**	**Conversion Factor**	**SI Units**	**Reference Publication**
Warfarin (Coumadin)	S or P		μg/mL	3.24	μmol/L	1
		Therap	1–10		3–32	
		Toxic	>10		>32	
Zidovudine (AZT, Retrovir)	S or P		μg/mL	3.74	μmol/L	1
		Therap	>0.2		>0.8	
Zonisamide (Zonegran)	S or P		μg/mL	4.71	μmol/L	1
		Therap	10–40		47–188	

AUC, Area under the curve; *CNS,* central nervous system; *F,* fluoride ion; *MIC,* minimum inhibitory concentration; *Occup exp,* occupational exposure; *Ox,* oxalate; *P,* plasma; *S,* serum; *Therap,* therapeutic; *U,* urine; *WB,* whole blood.

TABLE 82.4 Pediatric and Adult Reference Intervals for Hematologic Markers Based on the Canadian Health Measures Survey

		REFERENCE INTERVALS				
Analyte	**Age**	**Conventional Units**	**Conversion Factor**	**SI Units**	**Instrument/Method**	**Reference Publication**
Basophils		$10^3/\mu L$	1	$10^9/L$	**Coulter DxH300C, HmX**	11
	3–5 y	0.0–0.1		0.0–0.1	Volume, scatter, conductivity measurements	
	6–79 y	0.0–0.9		0.0–0.9		
Eosinophils		$10^3/\mu L$	1	$10^9/L$	**Coulter DxH300C, HmX**	11
	3–5 y	0.0–0.5		0.0–0.5	Volume, scatter, conductivity measurements	
	6–11 y	0.0–0.5		0.0–0.5		
	12–79 y	0.1–0.2		0.1–0.2		
Fibrinogen		mg/dL	0.01	g/L	**Sysmex CA-500 SERIES analyzer**	11
	12–13 y	180–350		1.8–3.5	Clauss method,	
	14–39 y, M	210–370		2.1–3.7	Photooptical clot detection (turbidity measurement)	
	14–39 y, F	200–420		2.0–4.2		
	40–79 y	200–420		2.0–4.2		
Hematocrit		%	0.01	L/L	**Coulter DxH300C, HmX**	11
	3–5 y	34–42		0.34–0.42	Calculation using RBC and MCV	
	6–7 y	34–42		0.34–0.42		
	8–11 y	35–43		0.35–0.43		
	12–15 y, M	38–47		0.38–0.47		
	16–79 y, M	40–50		0.40–0.50		
	12–79 y, F	35–43		0.35–0.43		
Hemoglobin		g/dL	10	g/L	**Coulter DxH300C, HmX**	11
	3–5 y	11.4–14.3		113.5–143.1	Absorbance measurement using cyanmethemoglobin	
	6–8 y	11.5–14.3		114.7–143.0		
	9–10 y	11.8–14.7		118.4–146.9		
	11–14 y, M	12.4–15.7		124.2–156.5		
	15–19 y, M	13.3–16.9		132.5–169.0		
	20–79 y, M	13.6–16.9		136–168.9		
	11–79 y, F	11.9–14.8		119.3–148.4		
Lymphocytes		$10^3/\mu L$	1	$10^9/L$	**Coulter DxH300C, HmX**	11
	3–5 y	1.6–5.3		1.6–5.3	Volume, scatter, conductivity measurements	
	6–11 y	1.4–3.9		1.4–3.9		
	12–79 y	1.0–3.2		1.0–3.2		
Mean corpuscular hemoglobin		Pg	1	pg	**Coulter DxH300C**	11
	3–5 y	26.1–30.7		26.1–30.7	Calculation using hemoglobin and RBC	
	6–15 y	26.3–31.7		26.3–31.7		
	16–79 y	27.6–33.3		27.6–33.3		

TABLE 82.4 **Pediatric and Adult Reference Intervals for Hematologic Markers Based on the Canadian Health Measures Survey—cont'd**

Analyte	Age	REFERENCE INTERVALS Conventional Units	Conversion Factor	SI Units	Instrument/Method	Reference Publication
Mean corpuscular hemoglobin concentration		g/dL	10	g/L	**Coulter DxH300C**	11
	3–5 y	32.4–34.9		324–348.8	Calculation using hemoglobin and RBC	
	6–79 y	32.5–35.2		324.5–352.3		
Mean corpuscular volume		fL	1	fL	**Coulter DxH300C**	11
	3–5 y	77.2–89.5		77.2–89.5	Conductivity measurements	
	6–11 y	77.891.1		77.891.1		
	12–14 y	79.9–93.0		79.9–93.0		
	15–79 y	82.5–98.0		82.5–98.0		
Mean platelet volume		fL	1	fL	**Coulter DxH300C**	11
	3–5 y	6.4–9.5		6.4–9.5	Volume, scatter, conductivity measurements	
	6–11 y	6.6–9.8		6.6–9.8		
	12–79 y	7.0–10.3		7.0–10.3		
Monocytes		$10^3/\mu L$	1	$10^9/L$	**Coulter DxH300C, HmX**	11
	3–5 y	0.3–0.9		0.3–0.9	Volume, scatter, conductivity measurements	
	6–44 y	0.2–0.8		0.2–0.8		
	45–79 y, M	0.3–0.9		0.3–0.9		
	45–79 y, F	0.2–0.8		0.2–0.8		
Neutrophils		$10^3/\mu L$	1	$10^9/L$	**Coulter DxH300C, HmX**	11
	3–5 y	1.6–7.8		1.6–7.8	Volume, scatter, conductivity measurements	
	6–16 y, M	1.4–6.1		1.4–6.1		
	6–14 y, F	1.5–6.5		1.5–6.5		
	15–50 y, F	2.0–7.4		2.0–7.4		
	17–50 y, M	1.8–7.2		1.8–7.2		
	51 - 79 y	2.0–6.4		2.0–6.4		
Platelet count		$10^3/\mu L$	1	$10^9/L$	**Coulter DxH300C**	11
	3–5 y	187.4–444.6		187.4–444.6	Volume, scatter, conductivity measurements	
	6–9 y	186.7–400.4		186.7–400.4		
	10–13 y	176.9–381.3		176.9–381.3		
	14–26 y, M	138.7–319.6		138.7–319.6		
	F	158.1–361.6		158.1–361.6		
	27–50 y, M	152.6–322.4		152.6–322.4		
	F	141.7–362.1		141.7–362.1		
	60–79 y	142.6–347.7		142.6–347.7		
Red blood cell count		$10^6/\mu L$	1	$10^{12}/L$	**Coulter DxH300C**	11
	3–5 y	4.0–5.1		4.0–5.1	Volume, scatter, conductivity measurements	
	6–10 y	4.1–5.2		4.1–5.2		
	11–14 y	4.2–5.3		4.2–5.3		
	15–49 y, M	4.3–5.7		4.3–5.7		
	50–79 y, M	4.2–5.5		4.2–5.5		
	15–79 y, F	3.8–5.0		3.8–5.0		
Red cell distribution width		%	1	%	**Coulter DxH300C**	11
	3–5 y	11.3–13.4		11.3–13.4	Volume, scatter, conductivity measurements	
	6–80 y	11.4–13.5		11.4–13.5		
White blood cell count		$10^3/\mu l$	1	$10^9/L$	**Coulter DxH300C**	11
	3–5 y	4.4–12.9		4.4–12.9	Volume, scatter, conductivity measurements	
	6–79 y	3.8–10.4		3.8–10.4		

TABLE 82.5 Critical Values (Risk Thresholds) for Biochemical and Hematologic Markers

	REFERENCE INTERVALS				
	Conventional Units		SI Units		
Parameter	Lower Limit	Upper Limit	Lower Limit	Upper Limit	Reference Publication
Albumin (children)	g/dL 1.7	6.8	g/L 17	68	1
Aminotransferases	U/L —	1000	µkat/L —	16.7	17
Ammonia	µg/dL —	187	µmol/L —	110	1, 17, 18
Anion gap			mmol/L —	20	17
Bilirubin (newborn)	mg/dL —	15	mmol/L —	257	1, 17
Calcium (total)	mg/dL 6.6	14	mmol/L 1.65	3.5	17, 18, 19
Calcium (children)	mg/dL 6.5	12.7	mmo/L 1.63	3.18	1
Calcium (free)	mg/dL 3.1	6.3	mmol/L 0.78	1.6	1, 17, 18, 19
Carbon dioxide, total			mmol/L 10	40	1
Chloride (adult)			mmol/L 80	120	1
Creatinine (adult)	mg/dL —	5	mmol/L —	442	1
Creatinine (children)	mg/dL —	3.8	µmol/L —	336	1
Creatine kinase	U/L —	1000	µkat/L —	16.7	17
Glucose	mg/dL 40	500	mmol/L 2.22	27.8	18
Glucose (children)	mg/dL 46	445	mmol/L 2.56	24.72	1
Glucose (newborn)	mg/dL 30	325	mmol/L 1.67	18.06	1,17
Glucose, CSF (adult)	mg/dL 40	200	mmol/L 2.22	11.11	1
Glucose, CSF (children)	mg/dL 31	—	mmol/L 1.72	—	1
Lactate CSF	mg/dL —	30.6	mmol/L —	3.4	1
Lactate plasma	mg/dL —	45	mmol/L —	5	17
Lactate plasma (children)	mg/dL —	36.9	mmol/L —	4.1	1
Lactate dehydrogenase	U/L —	1000	µkat/L —	16.7	17
Lipase	U/L —	700	µkat/L —	11.7	17
Magnesium	mg/dL 1	4.9	mmol/L 0.41	2	1, 17
Osmolality			mOsm/kg 240	330	17

TABLE 82.5 **Critical Values (Risk Thresholds) for Biochemical and Hematologic Markers—cont'd**

	REFERENCE INTERVALS				
	Conventional Units		SI Units		
Parameter	**Lower Limit**	**Upper Limit**	**Lower Limit**	**Upper Limit**	**Reference Publication**
Osmolar gap			mOsm/Kg		
			—	10	17
Phosphate	mg/dL		mmol/L		
	1	9	0.32	2.9	1, 17
Potassium			mmol/L		
			2.8	6.2	1, 17
Potassium (newborn)			mmol/L		
			2.8	7.8	1
Protein (children)	g/dL		g/L		
	3.4	9.5	34	95	1
Protein, CSF (children)	mg/dL		mg/L		
	—	188	—	1880	1
Sodium			mmol/L		
			120	160	1, 17, 18, 19
T_4 (free)	ng/dL		pmol/L		
	—	3.5	—	4.5	17
Urea nitrogen	mg/dL		mmol/L		
	—	100	—	35.6	17
Urea	mg/dL		mmol/L		
	—	214	—	35.6	17
Urea nitrogen (children)	mg/dL		mmol/L		
	—	55	—	19.6	1
Uric acid	mg/dL		mmol/L		
	—	13	—	0.767	1, 17
Uric acid (children)	mg/dL		—		
	—	12	—	0.708	1
pH	7.2	7.6	7.2	7.6	1, 17
PCO_2	mm Hg		kPa		
	20	70	2.7	9.45	1
PO_2	mm Hg		kPa		
	40	—	5.3	—	1
PO_2 children	mm Hg		kPa		
	45	125	6.0	16.7	1
PO_2 newborn	mm Hg		kPa		
	35	90	4.7	12.0	1
Hematocrit (adult)	%		L/L		
	20	60	0.20	0.60	1
Hematocrit (newborn)	%		L/L		
	33	71	0.33	0.71	1
Hemoglobin (adult)	g/dL		g/L		
	7.0	20	70	200	1
Hemoglobin (newborn)	g/dL		g/L		
	10.0	22	100	2204	1
Leukocytes (adult)	10^3/mL		10^9/L		
	2	30	2	30	1
Leukocytes (children)	10^3/mL		10^9/L		
	2	43	2	43	1
Neutrophil count	10^3/mL		10^9/L		
	0.5	—	0.5	—	18
Platelet count	10^3/mL		10^9/L		
	20	1000	20	1000	17

Continued

TABLE 82.5 **Critical Values (Risk Thresholds) for Biochemical and Hematologic Markers—cont'd**

	REFERENCE INTERVALS				
	Conventional Units		SI Units		
Parameter	**Lower Limit**	**Upper Limit**	**Lower Limit**	**Upper Limit**	**Reference Publication**
Blasts	Any seen (first report only)				1
Drepanocytes	Presence of sickle cells or aplastic cells				1
Prothrombin time (INR)	—	5			18, 20
aPTT	Second		Second		
	—	100	—	100	20
Antithrombin	%				
	28	—	—		20
Fibrinogen	mg/dL		g/L		
	80	—	0.8	—	1
Digoxin	ng/mL		nmol/L		
	—	2.2	—	2.8	19
Digitoxin	mg/L		nmol/L		
	—	40	—	52	17
Ethanol	g/L		mmol/L		
CSF	—	3.5	—	66	17
CSF	Cells/μL				
WBC (0–1 y)	—	>30			1
WBC (1–4 y)	—	>20			
WBC (5–17 y)	—	>10			
WBC (>17 y)	—	>5			
Malignant cells, blasts, or microorganisms	Any Applies to other sterile body fluids				1

aPTT, Activated partial thromboplastin time; *CSF,* cerebrospinal fluid; *INR,* international normalized ratio; T_4, thyroxine; *WBC,* white blood cell.

Table A.5, in addition to reference intervals, provides a table of critical risk intervals. Notification of critical results to clinical staff is an important postanalytical process in all acute-care clinical laboratories. Data from a number of sources (references 1 and 17-20; CLSI, guideline GP47; Wayne PA: CLSI; 2015:100) has been used to generate a table of recommended intervals to assist laboratories when establishing and updating their critical risk result management policy.

Finally, biological variation is an important factor to consider when interpreting laboratory test results in a clinical setting. Biological variation represents the physiologic changes that occur within and between individuals for a specific analyte. Biological variation is important to consider for establishing the usual amounts of fluctuation for a given analyte when monitoring or following a patient, and for establishing quality specifications. Biological variation data have not been included in this chapter, but further information on biological variation in adults can be found from a number of sources.[21,22] Within-day pediatric biological variation information has also been recently published.[23] Chapter 7 provides detailed information about biological variation.

REFERENCES

1. Roberts WL, McMillan GA. Reference information for the clinical laboratory. In: Burtis DA, Burns DE, editors. *Tietz Textbook of Clinical Chemistry and Molecular Diagnostics.* 5th ed. St. Louis: Elsevier; 2013. p. 2131–88.
2. Bailey D, Colantonio D, Kyriakopoulou L, et al. Marked biological variance in endocrine and biochemical markers in childhood: establishment of pediatric reference intervals using healthy community children from the CALIPER cohort. *Clin Chem* 2013;**59**:1393–405.
3. Bevilacqua V, Chan MK, Chen Y, et al. Pediatric population reference value distributions for cancer biomarkers and covariate-stratified reference intervals in the CALIPER cohort. *Clin Chem* 2014;**60**:1532–42.
4. Colantonio DA, Kyriakopoulou L, Chan MK, et al. Closing the gaps in pediatric laboratory reference intervals: a CALIPER database of 40 biochemical markers in a healthy and multiethnic population of children. *Clin Chem* 2012;**58**:854–68.
5. Konforte D, Shea JL, Kyriakopoulou L, et al. Complex biological pattern of fertility hormones in children and adolescents: a study of healthy children from the CALIPER

cohort and establishment of pediatric reference intervals. *Clin Chem* 2013;**59**:1215–27.
6. Raizman JE, Cohen AH, Teodoro-Morrison T, et al. Pediatric reference value distributions for vitamins A and E in the CALIPER cohort and establishment of age-stratified reference intervals. *Clin Biochem* 2014;**47**:812–15.
7. Raizman JE, Quinn F, Armbruster DA, et al. Pediatric reference intervals for calculated free testosterone, bioavailable testosterone and free androgen index in the CALIPER cohort. *Clin Chem Lab Med* 2015;**53**:e239–43.
8. Kelly J, Raizman JE, Bevilacqua V, et al. Complex reference value distribution and partitioned reference intervals across the pediatric age for 14 special chemistry and endocrine markers in the CALIPER cohort of healthy community children and adolescents. *Clin Chim Acta* 2015;**450**: 169–202.
9. Adeli K, Higgins V, Nieuwesteeg M, et al. Biochemical marker reference values for pediatric, adult and geriatric age groups: establishment of robust pediatric and adult reference intervals based on the Canadian Health Measures Survey. *Clin Chem* 2015;**61**:1049–62.
10. Adeli K, Higgins V, Nieuwesteeg M, et al. Complex reference value distributions for endocrine and special chemistry biomarkers across pediatric, adult and geriatric age: establishment of robust pediatric and adult reference intervals based on the Canadian Health Measures Survey. *Clin Chem* 2015;**61**:1063–74.
11. Adeli K, Raizman JE, Chen Y, et al. Complex biological profile of hematological markers across pediatric, adult, and geriatric ages: establishment of robust pediatric and adult reference intervals based on the Canadian Health Measures Survey. *Clin Chem* 2015;**61**:1075–86.
12. Schumann G, Aoki R, Ferrero CA, et al. IFCC primary reference procedures for the measurement of catalytic activity concentrations of enzymes at 37 degrees C. *Clin Chem Lab Med* 2006;**44**:1146–55.
13. Ichihara K, Ceriotti F, Kazuo M, et al. The Asian project for collaborative derivation of reference intervals: (2) results of non-standardized analytes and transference of reference intervals to the participating laboratories on the basis of cross-comparison of test results. *Clin Chem Lab Med* 2013;**51**:1443–57.
14. Holick MF. Vitamin D deficiency. *N Engl J Med* 2007;**357**: 266–81.
15. Zhang WM, Natowicz MR. Cerebrospinal fluid lactate and pyruvate concentrations and their ratio. *Clin Biochem* 2013;**46**:694–7.
16. Hiemke C, Baumann P, Bergemann N, et al. AGNP Consensus guidelines for therapeutic drug monitoring in psychiatry: update 2011. *Pharmacopsychiatry* 2011;**44**:195–235.
17. Thomas L. Critical limits of laboratory results for urgent clinician notification. *eJIFCC* 2003;**14**(1):<www.ifcc.org/ifccfiles/docs/140103200303.pdf>.
18. Hashim IA, Cuthbert JA, Critical Values Working Group. Establishing, harmonizing and analyzing critical values in a large academic health center. *Clin Chem Lab Med* 2014;**52**:1129–35.
19. Piva E, Pelloso M, Penello L, et al. Laboratory critical values: automated notification supports effective clinical decision making. *Clin Biochem* 2014;**47**:1163–8.
20. Pai M, Moffat KA, Plumhoff E, et al. Critical values in the coagulation laboratory: results of a survey of the North American Specialized Coagulation Laboratory Association. *Am J Clin Pathol* 2011;**136**:836–41.
21. Westgard J Desirable biological variation database specifications. <https://www.westgard.com/biodatabase1.htm>.
22. Westgard J <https://www.westgard.com>.
23. Bailey D, Bevilacqua V, Colantonio DA, et al. Pediatric within-day biological variation and quality specificaions for 38 biochemical markers in the CALIPER cohort. *Clin Chem* 2014;**60**:518–29.
24. Fuentes-Arderiu X, Ferré-Masferrer M, Gonzàlez-Alba JM, et al. Multicentric reference values for some quantities measured with Tina-Quant® reagents systems and RD/Hitachi analysers. *Scand J Clin Lab Invest* 2001;**61**:273–6.
25. Bjerner J, Biernat D, Fosså SD, et al. Reference intervals for serum testosterone, SHBG, LH and FSH in males from the NORIP project. *Scand J Clin Lab Invest* 2009;**69**: 873–9.
26. KDIGO Clinical practice guideline for the evaluation and management of chronic kidney disease. *Kidney Int Suppl* 2013;**3**(1):<http://www.kdigo.org/clinical_practice_guidelines/pdf/CKD/KDIGO_2012_CKD_GL.pdf>.
27. National Heart, Lung and Blood Institute. Integrated guidelines for cardiovascular health and risk reduction in children and adolescents. <http://www.nhlbi.nih.gov/health-pro/guidelines/current/cardiovascular-health-pediatric-guidelines>.
28. Stagnaro-Green A, Abalovich M, Alexander E, et al. Guidelines of the American Thyroid Association for the diagnosis and management of thyroid disease during pregnancy and postpartum. *Thyroid* 2011;**21**:1081–125.
29. Kushnir MM, Blamires T, Rockwood AL, et al. Liquid chromatography: tandem mass spectrometry assay for androstenedione, dehydroepiandrosterone, and testosterone with pediatric and adult reference intervals. *Clin Chem* 2010;**56**:1138–47.
30. World Health Organization. *Use of glycated hemoglobin A1c in the diagnosis of diabetes mellitis*. WHO; 2011. p. 1–25.

ABBREVIATIONS

ACC: American College of Cardiology
ACD: Anticoagulant Citrate Dextrose
AHA: American Heart Association
Amf: Amniotic fluid
ATP III: Adult Treatment Panel III
AUC: Area under the curve
CNS: Central nervous system
CSF: Cerebrospinal fluid
EDTA: Ethylenediaminetetraacetic acid
F: Female, fluoride ion
Hb: Hemoglobin
HbCO: Carboxyhemoglobin
hCG: Human chorionic gonadotropin
Hep: Heparin
HPLC: High-performance liquid chromatography
ICSH: International Council for Standardization in Haematology
IVF: In vitro fertilization
KDIGO: Kidney Disease Improving Global Outcomes
LC-MS/MS: Liquid chromatography with dual mass spectrometry

L/S: Lecithin-to-sphingomyelin ratio
M: Male
NGSP: National Glycohemoglobin Standardization Program
NKDEP: National Kidney Disease Educational Program
Occup exp: Occupational exposure
Ox: Oxalate
P: Plasma
PCOS: Polycystic ovary syndrome
RBC: Red blood cells
S: Serum
Sal: Saliva
SHBG: Sex hormone–binding hormone
U: Urine
WB: Whole blood
WHO: World Health Organization

INDEX

Page numbers followed by *f* indicate figures, *t* indicate tables, and *b* indicate boxes.

D

E

M

N

O

P

U